DRUG INFORMATION HANDBOOK for ONCOLOGY

An Extensive Guide to Combination Chemotherapy Regimens

American Pharmacists Association®
Improving medication use. Advancing patient care.

APhA

Lexicomp is the official drug reference for the American Pharmacists Association.

14th Edition

SENIOR EDITOR

Diedra L. Bragalone,
PharmD, MBA, BCOP, BCPS

Lexicomp®

DRUG
INFORMATION
HANDBOOK
for ONCOLOGY

An Extensive Guide to Combination
Chemotherapy Regimens

American Pharmacists Association

NEW EDITION

SENIOR EDITOR

Dedra L. Snodgrass,
Pharm, MBA, BCOP, BCPS

DRUG INFORMATION HANDBOOK for ONCOLOGY

A Complete Guide to Combination Chemotherapy Regimens

Diedra L. Bragalone, PharmD, MBA, BCOP, BCPS
Pharmacotherapy Specialist
Wolters Kluwer

Lexicomp®

APhA

NOTICE

This data is intended to serve the user as a handy reference and not as a complete drug information resource. It does not include information on every therapeutic agent available. The publication covers more than 300 commonly used drugs and is specifically designed to present important aspects of drug data in a more concise format than is typically found in medical literature or product material supplied by manufacturers.

The nature of drug information is that it is constantly evolving because of ongoing research and clinical experience and is often subject to interpretation. While great care has been taken to ensure the accuracy of the information and recommendations presented, the reader is advised that the authors, editors, reviewers, contributors, and publishers cannot be responsible for the continued currency of the information or for any errors, omissions, or the application of this information, or for any consequences arising therefrom. Therefore, the author(s) and/or the publisher shall have no liability to any person or entity with regard to claims, loss, or damage caused, or alleged to be caused, directly or indirectly, by the use of information contained herein. Because of the dynamic nature of drug information, readers are advised that decisions regarding drug therapy must be based on the independent judgment of the clinician, changing information about a drug (eg, as reflected in the literature and manufacturer's most current product information), and changing medical practices. Therefore, this data is designed to be used in conjunction with other necessary information and is not designed to be solely relied upon by any user. The user of this data hereby and forever releases the authors and publishers of this data from any and all liability of any kind that might arise out of the use of this data. The editors are not responsible for any inaccuracy of quotation or for any false or misleading implication that may arise due to the text or formulas as used or due to the quotation of revisions no longer official.

Certain contributors have written for this book in their private capacities. No official support or endorsement by any federal or state agency or pharmaceutical company is intended or inferred.

The publishers have made every effort to trace any third party copyright holders, if any, for borrowed material. If they have inadvertently overlooked any, they will be pleased to make the necessary arrangements at the first opportunity.

If you have any suggestions or questions regarding any information presented in this data, please contact our drug information pharmacists at (855) 633-0577. Book revisions are available at our website at http://www.wolterskluwercdi.com/clinical-notices/revisions/.

This manual was produced using LIMS — A complete publishing service of Wolters Kluwer Clinical Drug Information, Inc.

Lexicomp®

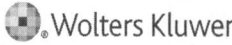 Wolters Kluwer

ISBN 978-1-59195-351-7

TABLE OF CONTENTS

ONCOLOGY EDITORIAL ADVISORY PANEL

ONCOLOGY OFF-LABEL REVIEW PANEL MEMBERS

Diedra L. Bragalone, PharmD, MBA, BCOP, BCPS
Pharmacotherapy Specialist
Wolters Kluwer

Stephanie S. Minich, PharmD, BCOP
Pharmacotherapy Specialist
Wolters Kluwer

Corey A. Carter, MD
Chief of Thoracic Oncology
John P. Murtha Cancer Center, Walter Reed National Military Medical Center

Mark T. Holdsworth, PharmD
Associate Professor of Pharmacy & Pediatrics and Pharmacy Practice Area Head
College of Pharmacy, The University of New Mexico

Polly E. Kintzel, PharmD, BCPS, BCOP
Clinical Pharmacy Specialist − Oncology
Spectrum Health

Omer N. Koc, MD
Staff Physician
Hematology and Medical Oncology Department, Cleveland Clinic

Nicholas A. Link, PharmD, BCOP
Clinical Specialist, Oncology
Hillcrest Hospital

Heidi Trinkman, PharmD
Pediatric Hematology/Oncology Clinical Pharmacy Specialist
Cook Children's Medical Center

DRUG INTERACTIONS EDITORIAL ADVISORY PANEL

EDITORIAL ADVISORY PANEL

Susan Cornell, PharmD, CDE, FAPhA, FAADE
Associate Professor
Department of Pharmacy Practice
Assistant Director of Experimental Education
Midwestern University, Chicago College of Pharmacy

Marilyn Cortell, RDH, MS, FAADH
Associate Professor
New York City College of Technology, City University of New York

Harold L. Crossley, DDS, MS, PhD
Professor Emeritus
Baltimore College of Dental Surgery, University of Maryland Baltimore

Melanie W. Cucchi, BS, PharmD, RPh
Clinical Manager
Wolters Kluwer

Laura Cummings, PharmD, BCPS
Pharmacotherapy Specialist
Wolters Kluwer

William J. Dana, PharmD, FASHP
Pharmacy Quality Assurance
Harris County Hospital District

Lacey Davis, PharmD, BCPS
Clinical Pharmacist – Hospice, Palliative Care, and Post-Acute Care
Aultman Hospital

Beth Deen, PharmD, BDNSP
Senior Pediatric Clinical Pharmacy Specialist
Cook Children's Medical Center

Jodi Dreiling, PharmD, BCPS
Pharmacotherapy Specialist in Critical Care
Akron General Medical Center

Kim S. Dufner, PharmD
Clinical Manager
Wolters Kluwer

Teri Dunsworth, PharmD, FCCP, BCPS
Pharmacotherapy Specialist
Wolters Kluwer

Michael S. Edwards, PharmD, MBA, BCOP
Chief, Oncology Pharmacy and *Director, Oncology Pharmacy Residency Program*
Walter Reed Army Medical Center

Vicki L. Ellingrod, PharmD, BCPP
Head, Clinical Pharmacogenomics Laboratory and *Associate Professor*
Department of Psychiatry, Colleges of Pharmacy and Medicine, University of Michigan

Kelley K. Engle, BSPharm
Pharmacotherapy Contributor
Stow, Ohio

Christopher Ensor, PharmD, BCPS (AQ-CV)
Clinical Pharmacy Specialist, Thoracic Transplantation
University of Pittsburgh Medical Center

Erin Fabian, PharmD, RPh, BCPS
Pharmacotherapy Specialist
Wolters Kluwer

Elizabeth A. Farrington, PharmD, FCCP, FCCM, FPPAG, BCPS
Pharmacist III - Pediatrics
New Hanover Regional Medical Center

Margaret A. Fitzgerald, MS, APRN, BC, NP-C, FAANP
President
Fitzgerald Health Education Associates, Inc.
Family Nurse Practitioner
Greater Lawrence Family Health Center

Carole W. Fuseck, MSN, RN, ACCNS-AG, VA-BC
Clinical Nurse Specialist, Critical Care
Louis Stokes Cleveland Department of Veteran Affairs Medical Center

Jason C. Gallagher, PharmD, BCPS
Clinical Pharmacy Specialist, Infectious Diseases and *Clinical Associate Professor*
Temple University Hospital

Michael A. Kahn, DDS
Professor and Chairman
Department of Oral and Maxillofacial Pathology, Tufts University School of Dental Medicine

Julie J. Kelsey, PharmD
Clinical Specialist
Women's Health and Family Medicine, Department of Pharmacy Services, University of Virginia Health System

Patrick J. Kiel, PharmD, BCPS, BCOP
Clinical Pharmacy Specialist
Hematology and Stem Cell Transplant, Indiana University Simon Cancer Center

Polly E. Kintzel, PharmD, BCPS, BCOP
Clinical Pharmacy Specialist – Oncology
Spectrum Health

Michael Klepser, PharmD, FCCP
Professor of Pharmacy
Department of Pharmacy Practice, Ferris State University

Sandra Knowles, RPh, BScPhm
Drug Policy Research Specialist
Li Ka Shing Institute, St. Michael's Hospital

Omer N. Koc, MD
Staff Physician
Hematology and Medical Oncology Department, Cleveland Clinic

Jill M. Kolesar, PharmD, FCCP, BCPS
Associate Professor
School of Pharmacy, University of Wisconsin Paul P. Carbone Comprehensive Cancer Center

Susannah E. Koontz, PharmD, BCOP
Principal and Consultant
Pediatric Hematology/Oncology and Stem Cell Transplantation/Cellular Therapy, Koontz Oncology Consulting, LLC

Donna M. Kraus, PharmD, FAPhA, FPPAG, FCCP
Associate Professor of Pharmacy Practice and *Pediatric Clinical Pharmacist*
Departments of Pharmacy Practice and Pediatrics, University of Illinois

Daniel L. Krinsky, RPh, MS
Manager, MTM Services
Giant Eagle Pharmacy
Assistant Professor
Department of Pharmacy Practice, Northeast Ohio Medical University (NEOMED)

Tim T.Y. Lau, PharmD, ACPR, FCSHP
Pharmacotherapeutic Specialist in Infectious Diseases
Pharmaceutical Sciences, Vancouver General Hospital

Lisiane Leal
Pharmacotherapy Contributor
Porto Alegre, Brazil

Mandy C. Leonard, PharmD, BCPS
Assistant Professor
Cleveland Clinic Lerner College of Medicine of Case Western University
Assistant Director, Drug Information Services
Cleveland Clinic

Jonathan Leung, PharmD, BCPS, BCPP
Neuropsychiatric Clinical Pharmacist
Mayo Clinic

John J. Lewin III, PharmD, BCPS
Clinical Specialist, Neurosciences Critical Care
The Johns Hopkins Hospital

Jeffrey D. Lewis, PharmD, MACM
Associate Dean and Associate Professor of Pharmacy Practice
Cedarville University School of Pharmacy

John Lindsley, PharmD, BCPS
Cardiology Clinical Pharmacy Specialist
The Johns Hopkins Hospital

10

Kevin M. Mulieri, BS, PharmD
Pediatric Hematology/Oncology
Clinical Specialist
Penn State Milton S. Hershey
Medical Center
Instructor of Pharmacology
Penn State College of Medicine

Naoto Nakagawa, PharmD, PhD
Chief Pharmacist
Drug Information Center, Japan

Lynne Nakashima, PharmD
Professional Practice Leader,
Clinical Professor
B.C. Cancer Agency, Vancouver
Centre, University of BC

Carrie Nemerovski, PharmD, BCPS
Pharmacotherapy Specialist
Wolters Kluwer

Elizabeth A. Neuner, PharmD, BCPS
Infectious Diseases Clinical Specialist
Cleveland Clinic

Kimberly Novack, PharmD, BCPS
Clinical Pharmacy Specialist, Cystic
Fibrosis and *Pharmacy Clinical*
Coordinator
Nationwide Children's Hospital

Carlene N. Oliverio, PharmD, BCPS
Clinical Content Specialist
Wolters Kluwer

Neeta O'Mara, PharmD, BCPS
Clinical Pharmacist
Dialysis Clinic

Tom Palma, MS, RPh
Medical Science Pharmacist
Wolters Kluwer

Susie H. Park, PharmD, BCPP
Assistant Professor of Clinical
Pharmacy
University of Southern Califormia

Nicole Passerrello, PharmD, BCPS
Pharmacotherapy Specialist
Wolters Kluwer

Gayle Pearson, BSPharm, MSA
Drug Information Pharmacist
Peter Lougheed Centre, Alberta Health
Services

Rebecca Pettit, PharmD, MBA, BCPS
Pediatric Pulmonary Clinical Pharmacy
Specialist
Riley Hospital for Children, Indiana
University Health, Department of
Pharmacy

Jennifer L. Placencia, PharmD
Neonatal Clinical Pharmacy Specialist
Texas Children's Hospital

Amy L. Potts, PharmD, BCPS
Assistant Director
Department of Pharmacy
PGY1 & *PGY2 Residency Program*
Director
Monroe Carell Jr. Children's Hospital at
Vanderbilt

Sally Rafie, PharmD, BCPS
Medical Safety Pharmacist
UC San Diego Health System

Esta Razavi, PharmD
Clinical Editor
Wolters Kluwer

James Reissig, PharmD
Assistant Director, Clinical Services
Akron General Medical Center

A.J. (Fred) Remillard, PharmD
Assistant Dean, Research and
Graduate Affairs
College of Pharmacy and Nutrition,
University of Saskatchewan

Elizabeth Rich, RN, BSN, BA
Registered Nurse – Medical Intensive
Care Unit
Cleveland Clinic

P. David Rogers, PharmD, PhD, FCCP
Director, Clinical and Translational
Therapeutics
University of Tennessee College of
Pharmacy

Amy Rybarczyk, PharmD, BCPS
Pharmacotherapy Specialist, Internal
Medicine
Akron General Medical Center

Elizabeth A. Tomsik, PharmD, BCPS
Senior Director
Content, Wolters Kluwer

David M. Weinstein, PhD, RPh
Senior Director, Clinical Content
Wolters Kluwer

Leslye Trachte, PharmD
Pharmacotherapy Contributor
Lawton, Oklahoma

Sarah White, PharmD, BCPS
Pharmacotherapy Contributor
Medford, Oregon

Dana Travis, RPh
Pharmacotherapy Specialist
Wolters Kluwer

Greg Wiggers, PharmD, PhD
Pharmacotherapy Specialist
Wolters Kluwer

Heidi Trinkman, PharmD
Pediatric Hematology/Oncology
Clinical Pharmacy Specialist
Cook Children's Medical Center

Sherri J. Willard Argyres, MA, PharmD
Medical Science Pharmacist
Wolters Kluwer

Jennifer Trofe-Clark, PharmD
Clinical Transplant Pharmacist
Hospital of The University of Pennsylvania

John C. Williamson, PharmD, BCPS
Pharmacy Clinical Coordinator,
Infectious Diseases
Wake Forest Baptist Health

Amy Van Orman, PharmD, BCPS
Pharmacotherapy Specialist
Wolters Kluwer

Nathan Wirick, PharmD, BCPS
Clinical Specialist in Infectious
Diseases and Antibiotic Management
Hillcrest Hospital

Carlos Vidotti
Pharmacotherapy Contributor
Brasilia DF, Brazil

Wende Wood, RPh, BSPharm, BCPP
Pharmacotherapy Contributor
Toronto, Ontario, Canada

Geoffrey Wall, RPh, PharmD, FCCP, BCPS, CGP
Professor of Clinical Sciences and
Associate Professor of Pharmacy
Practice
Drake University

Richard L. Wynn, BSPharm, PhD
Professor of Pharmacology
Baltimore College of Dental Surgery,
University of Maryland

Kristin Watson, PharmD, BCPS
Assistant Professor, Cardiology and
Clinical Pharmacist, Cardiology
Service
Heart Failure Clinic, University of
Maryland Medical Center

Jessica Zatroch, DDS
Private Practice Dentist
Willoughby Hills, OH

PREFACE

The *Drug Information Handbook for Oncology* was designed to meet the needs of all oncology professionals involved in prescribing, preparing, and administering therapy. Presented in a concise and uniform format, this book contains monographs with information pertaining to both antineoplastic agents and ancillary or supportive care medications. This handbook serves as a portable quick reference while providing comprehensive oncology-related drug information. Organized like a dictionary for ease-of-use, a drug monograph can be quickly located by generic name.

The Chemotherapy Regimen section provides a comprehensive presentation of cancer chemotherapy regimens. The regimens are listed alphabetically by regimen name (acronym). An index lists regimens by indication. In addition, a special Combination Chemotherapy Regimen field in each drug monograph will link you to the applicable regimens.

A special topics section addresses issues regarding Cancer Treatment-Related Complications (eg, chemotherapy-induced peripheral neuropathy, mucositis and stomatitis, management of chemotherapy-induced nausea and vomiting, common toxicity criteria, prevention and management of infections); Cancer-Related Topics (eg, chemotherapy and cancer treatment during pregnancy, chemotherapy and obesity, principles of anticancer therapy, venous thromboembolism in the cancer patient); and Safe Handling of Hazardous Drugs.

The appendix section includes information related to conversions, renal function, comparative drug charts, and laboratory reference values for adults. A pharmacologic category index provides a practical approach to categorizing drugs by their respective therapeutic classification.

We know you will find this handbook to be a valuable source of information and we welcome comments or suggestions to further improve future editions.

USE OF THE DRUG INFORMATION HANDBOOK FOR ONCOLOGY

The *Drug Information Handbook for Oncology* is divided into six sections.

The first section is a compilation of introductory text pertinent to the use of this book.

The drug information section of the handbook, in which all drugs are listed alphabetically, details information pertinent to each drug. Extensive cross-referencing is provided by US brand names, Canadian brand names, and index terms.

The Chemotherapy Regimen section provides a comprehensive presentation of cancer chemotherapy regimens. The regimens are listed alphabetically by regimen name (acronym). An index at the beginning of this section lists regimens by indications. In addition, a special Combination Chemotherapy Regimen field in each drug monograph will link you to the applicable regimens.

The Special Topics section contains important cancer-related issues (ie, chemotherapy and cancer treatment during pregnancy, chemotherapy and obesity, principles of anticancer therapy, and safe handling of hazardous drugs). These issues are discussed in detail.

The fifth section is an appendix section.

The last section of this handbook is an index listing drugs in their unique pharmacologic category.

Alphabetical Listing of Drugs

Drug information is presented in a consistent format and provides the following:

Generic Name	US adopted name
Pronunciation Guide	Phonetic pronunciation
Related Information	Cross-reference to other pertinent drug information found elsewhere in this handbook
Brand Names: US	Trade names (manufacturer-specific) found in the United States. The symbol [DSC] appears after trade names that have been recently discontinued.
Brand Names: Canada	Trade names found in Canada
Index Terms	Other names or accepted abbreviations of the generic drug. May also include common brand names no longer available; this field is used to create cross-references to monographs.
Pharmacologic Category	Unique systematic classification of medications

◀ Use | Information pertaining to FDA- or Canadian-approved indications for the drug

Labeled Contraindications | Information pertaining to inappropriate use of the drug as dictated by approved labeling

Pregnancy Risk Factor | Five categories established by the FDA to indicate the potential of a systemically absorbed drug for causing risk to fetus

Pregnancy Considerations | A summary of human and/or animal information pertinent to or associated with the use of the drug as it relates to clinical effects on the fetus, newborn, or pregnant woman

Breast-feeding Considerations | Information pertinent to or associated with the human use of the drug as it relates to clinical effects on the nursing infant or postpartum woman

Warnings/Precautions | Precautionary considerations, hazardous conditions related to use of the drug, and disease states or patient populations in which the drug should be cautiously used. Boxed warnings, when present, are clearly identified and are adapted from the FDA approved labeling. Consult the product labeling for the exact black box warning through the manufacturer's or the FDA website.

Adverse Reactions | Side effects grouped by percentage of incidence (if known) and/or body system

Drug Interactions

Metabolism/Transport Effects | If a drug has demonstrated involvement with cytochrome P450 enzymes, or other metabolism or transport proteins, this field will identify the drug as an inhibitor, inducer, or substrate of the specific enzyme(s) (eg, CYP1A2 or UGT1A1). CYP450 isoenzymes are identified as substrates (minor or major), inhibitors (weak, moderate, or strong), and inducers (weak or strong).

Avoid Concomitant Use | Designates drug combinations which should not be used concomitantly, due to an unacceptable risk:benefit assessment. Frequently, the concurrent use of the agents is explicitly prohibited or contraindicated by the product labeling.

Increased Effect/Toxicity | Drug combinations that result in a increased or toxic therapeutic effect between the drug listed in the monograph and other drugs or drug classes

Decreased Effect | Drug combinations that result in a decreased therapeutic effect between the drug listed in the monograph and other drugs or drug classes

Food Interactions | Possible important interactions between the drug listed in the monograph and food, alcohol, or other beverages

Storage/Stability	Information regarding storage and stability of commercially available products and products that have been reconstituted, diluted, or otherwise prepared. Provides the time and conditions for which a solution or mixture will maintain potency.
Preparation for Administration	Provides information regarding the preparation of drug products prior to administration, including dilution, reconstitution, etc.
Mechanism of Action	How the drug works in the body to elicit a response
Pharmacodynamics/ Kinetics	The magnitude of a drug's effect depends on the drug concentration at the site of action. The pharmacodynamics are expressed in terms of onset of action and duration of action. Pharmacokinetics are expressed in terms of absorption, distribution, protein binding, metabolism, bioavailability, half-life, time to peak serum concentration, and elimination.
Dosing	The amount of drug to be typically given or taken during therapy; may include the following:
Adult	The recommended amount of drug to be given to adult patients
Adult & Geriatric	This combined field is only used to indicate that no specific adjustments for elderly patients were identified. However, other issues should be considered (eg, renal or hepatic impairment).
Geriatric	A suggested amount of drug to be given to elderly patients; may include adjustments from adult dosing (lack of information in the monograph may imply that the drug is not used in the elderly patient or no specific adjustments could be identified)
Pediatric	Suggested amount of drug to be given to neonates, infants, and children. The following age group definitions are utilized to characterize age-related dosing unless otherwise specified in the monograph: Neonate (0 to 28 days of age), infant (>28 days to 1 year of age), children (1 to 12 years of age), and adolescent (13 to 18 years of age).
Renal Impairment	Suggested dosage adjustments based on compromised renal function; may include dosing instructions for patients on dialysis
Hepatic Impairment	Suggested dosage adjustments based on compromised liver function
Obesity	Dosing adjustment or dosing considerations for the obese adult patient. Obesity is defined as a BMI $\geq$30 kg/m^2 (based on the World Health Organization [WHO]).
Adjustment for Toxicity	Suggested dosage adjustments in the event specific toxicities related to therapy are noted, such as hematologic toxicities related to cancer chemotherapy

17

◀ Combination Regimens — List of combination chemotherapy regimens in which the drug is a component

Usual Infusion Concentrations — Information describing the usual concentrations of drugs for continuous infusion administration in the pediatric and adult populations as appropriate. Concentrations are derived from the literature, manufacturer's recommendation, or organizational recommendations (eg, the Institute for Safe Medication Practices [ISMP]) and are universally established. Institution-specific standard concentrations may differ from those listed.

Administration — Information regarding the recommended final concentrations, rates of administration for parenteral drugs, or other guidelines or relevant information to properly administer medications

Vesicant/Extravasation Risk — Indicates whether the drug is considered to be a vesicant and likely to cause significant morbidity if the infusion infiltrates soft tissues

Emetic Potential — Likelihood that the drug will cause nausea or vomiting

Extemporaneous Preparations — Directions for preparing liquid formulations from solid drug products. May include stability information and references.

Monitoring Parameters — Laboratory tests and patient physical parameters that should be monitored for safety and efficacy of drug therapy

Test Interactions — Listing of assay interferences when relevant; (B) = Blood; (S) = Serum; (U) = Urine

Dietary Considerations — Specific dietary modifications and/or restrictions (eg, information about sodium content)

Additional Information — Pertinent information about specific brands

Product Availability — Provides availability information on products that have been approved by the FDA, but not yet available for use. Estimates for when a product may be available are included, when this information is known. May also provide any unique or critical drug availability issues.

Prescribing and Access Restrictions — Provides information on any special requirements regarding the prescribing, obtaining, or dispensing of drugs, including access restrictions pertaining to drugs with REMS elements and those drugs with access restrictions that are not REMS-related

Medication Guide Available — Identifies drugs that have an FDA-approved Medication Guide

Dosage Forms Considerations — More specific Information regarding product concentrations, ingredients, package sizes, amount of doses per container, and other important details pertaining to various formulations of medications

Dosage Forms	Information with regard to form, strength, and availability of the drug in the United States. **Note:** Additional formulation information (eg, excipients, preservatives) is included when available. Please consult product labeling for further information.
Dosage Forms: Canada	Information with regard to form, strength, and availability of products that are uniquely available in Canada but currently are not available in the United States
Controlled Substance	Contains controlled substance schedule information as assigned by the United States Drug Enforcement Administration (DEA) or Canadian Controlled Substance Act (CDSA). CDSA information is only provided for drugs available in Canada and not available in the US

Chemotherapy Regimens

The Chemotherapy Regimen section provides a comprehensive presentation of cancer chemotherapy regimens. The regimens are listed alphabetically by regimen name (acronym). An index lists regimens by indications. In addition, a special Combination Chemotherapy Regimen field in each drug monograph will guide you to the applicable regimens.

Special Topics

Important cancer-related issues (ie, preventing and managing infections, mucositis and stomatitis, chemotherapy and cancer treatment during pregnancy, chemotherapy and obesity, principles of anticancer therapy, chronic pain management [cancer], hospice [end of life] care, palliative care medicine [cancer], hematopoietic stem cell transplantation, safe handling of hazardous drugs, venous thromboembolism in the cancer patient) are discussed in detail.

Appendix

The appendix offers a compilation of tables, guidelines, nomograms, algorithms, and conversion information which can often be helpful when considering patient care.

Pharmacologic Category Index

This index provides a useful listing of drugs by their pharmacologic classification.

PREGNANCY CATEGORIES

Pregnancy Categories (sometimes referred to as pregnancy risk factors) are a letter system presented under the *Teratogenic Effects* subsection of the product labeling. The system was initiated in 1979. The categories were required to be part of the package insert for prescription drugs that are systemically absorbed. The Food and Drug Administration (FDA) has updated prescribing labeling requirements and as of June 2015, the pregnancy categories will no longer be part of new product labeling. Prescription products which currently have a pregnancy category letter will be phasing this out of their product information.

The categories are defined as follows:

A   Adequate and well-controlled studies in pregnant women have not shown that the drug increases the risk of fetal abnormalities.

B   Animal reproduction studies show no evidence of impaired fertility or harm to the fetus; however, no adequate and well-controlled studies have been conducted in pregnant women.
or
Animal reproduction studies have shown adverse events; however, studies in pregnant women have not shown that the drug increases the risk of abnormalities.

C   Animal reproduction studies have shown an adverse effect on the fetus. There are no adequate and well-controlled studies in humans and the benefits from the use of the drug in pregnant women may be acceptable, despite its potential risks.
or
Animal reproduction studies have not been conducted.

D   Based on human data, the drug can cause fetal harm when administered to pregnant women, but the potential benefits from the use of the drug may be acceptable, despite its potential risks.

X   Studies in animals or humans have demonstrated fetal abnormalities (or there is positive evidence of fetal risk based on reports and/or marketing experience) and the risk of using the drug in pregnant women clearly outweighs any possible benefit (for example, safer drugs or other forms of therapy are available).

In 2008, the Food and Drug Administration (FDA) proposed new labeling requirements which would eliminate the use of the pregnancy category system and replace it with scientific data and other information specific to the use of the drug in pregnant women. These proposed changes were suggested because the current category system may be misleading. For instance, some practitioners may believe that risk increases from category A to B to C to D to X, which is not the intent. In addition, practitioners may not be aware that some medications are categorized based on animal data, while others are based on human data. The new labeling requirements will contain pregnancy and lactation subsections, each describing a risk summary, clinical considerations, and section for specific data.

For full descriptions of the final rule, refer to the following website: http://www.fda.gov/Drugs/DevelopmentApprovalProcess/DevelopmentResources/Labeling/ucm093307.htm

REDUCING ONCOLOGY MEDICATION ERRORS

Medication errors occurring in patients receiving treatment and supportive care for cancer remain a serious problem. Risk factors are numerous and include the multiple numbers and cycles of medication, the various routes of administration, the various locations of administration (which can progress from inpatient to ambulatory care to home administration), and the fact that patients from the very young to the elderly are frequently administered these agents. Many of the antineoplastic agents have a narrow therapeutic index and can produce unexpected toxicities with the slightest alteration in dosage. Subtherapeutic dosing may also be detrimental, producing less toxicity, but possibly resulting in decreased efficacy and affecting patient outcomes.

The incidence of medication errors in oncology patients noted in the published literature range from 3% to 4% in adult and pediatric inpatient and ambulatory settings, and from 10% to 20% for patients receiving oral antineoplastic therapy at home. Although the numbers appear small in some settings and many of the published medication errors are caught before reaching the patient ("near misses"), the impact can be disastrous. Published literature indicates that antineoplastic agents rank second only to central nervous system medications in causing fatal medication errors.

Medication errors involving chemotherapy and supportive care have been documented in all stages of the drug therapy process, from prescribing to compounding, dispensing, and administration, including patient self-medication at home. Various risk factors for medication errors have been identified at each stage. Accordingly, institutions and health care organizations have developed and continue to refine various standards, consensus documents, policies/procedures, and other safeguards to minimize the safety risk. Examples are noted in the following paragraphs.

Anticancer therapy should be based on standard regimens and modalities selected according to the patient's diagnosis and ability to tolerate treatment. Investigational therapy must be administered by way of an institutional review board-approved clinical trial or single patient Investigational New Drug (IND) license (compassionate use).

Facilities providing chemotherapy should establish and ensure that members of the oncology team have appropriate education, training, demonstrated competency, credentialing, and continuing education to care for patients receiving antineoplastic therapy. Staff must also be educated on safe handling of hazardous agents. Additionally, and fundamental to most safety strategies, is the standardization of the prescribing and documentation process through established guidelines, policies, and procedures which should be followed by all health care professionals involved. The use of collaboratively developed preprinted order forms or predefined computer generated order sets for approved protocols or treatment plans is one method to facilitate standardization. Examples of standardizing of the ordering processes, medication nomenclature, dosing, and other elements are noted below.

MEDICATION PRESCRIBING AND VERIFICATION

- Do not permit or accept verbal orders for chemotherapy, except for withholding or discontinuation of treatment.

- While there are certain situations in which treatment is urgent, do not permit or accept "STAT" orders for chemotherapy.

- Use redundant checks and verifications (by a second individual) at different points of the chemotherapy medication use process, (eg, prescribing, preparation, dispensing, administration).

- Individuals verifying orders that contain calculations should independently perform their own calculations, rather than checking another's mathematical work.

MEDICATION ORDER

Elements of information that should be included on a medication order for chemotherapy include the following:

- The patient's full name and at least one other unique identifier, such as medical record number or date of birth

- Date and time that the order was written or generated

- Date(s) and time(s) that that specific treatments are to be administered

- Treatment cycle and day number

- Patient-specific dosing poarameters, such as height, weight (including dosing weight), and body surface area

- Pertinent and current patient-specific laboratory values

- Medication(s) listed by generic name(s)

- Calculated doses for administration; schedule, and duration of administration

- Route of administration; rate of administration

- Patient's medication, food, and device allergies and sensitivities

- Name and credentials of prescriber

- Contact information for prescriber

- Protocol number or publication citation supporting ordered regimen

MEDICATION NAMES

Chemotherapy agents are highly susceptible to sound-alike/look-alike confusion (eg, fluorouracil/flucytosine/fluocinonide, leucovorin/Leukine/Alkeran/Leukeran) so particular precaution should be heeded to ensure correct drug identified by those interpreting the order.

- Use full generic names including descriptive terms, (eg, liposomal). Brand names should be reserved for products when they assist in further identifying the correct product (eg, combination product or liposomal vs nonliposomal formulation).

- Use full study name and/or protocol number with investigational antineoplastic treatments.

- Avoid abbreviated medication names, (eg, CTX, HN$_2$, MTX, VCR, or generalized generic terms [eg, "platinum" which can create confusion between CISplatin, CARBOplatin, and oxaliplatin]).

- Avoid investigational names for medications **with FDA approval** (eg, VP-16, FK-506, CBDCA).

- Utilize TALLman lettering (eg, DAUNOrubicin/DOXOrubicin, VinBLAStine/VinCRIStine).

- Omit the use of numbers within a medication name (eg, fluorouracil is correct, 5-fluorouracil is **incorrect**; mercaptopurine is correct, 6-mercaptopurine is **incorrect**).

- Avoid abbreviated names or acronyms for multidrug regimens, (eg, MOPP, ICE, ProMACE).

- Avoid or minimize look-alike drug product containers in the procurement process.

MEDICATION DOSE AND DURATION

- Include variables used for dosage calculations on the chemotherapy orders to allow for necessary double-checks, (eg, height [centimeters], weight [kilograms], BSA, laboratory test results or creatinine clearance). It is recommended that organizations standardize equations used for BSA and creatinine clearance calculations and situations when dosing should be based on actual or ideal body weight.

- Use guideline-based and/or manufacturer's recommendations for adjustment of dose based on body size. As an example, use of actual body weight for dose calculation in obese patients receiving treatment with curative intent is recommended. In comparison, the manufacturer of ixabepilone recommends capping the calculated dose amount at 88 mg for patients who are larger than 2.2 m^2 (40 mg/m^2/dose).

- Use guideline-based and/or manufacturer's recommendations for adjustment of dose based on organ function. As an example, for carboplatin dose calculation using the Calvert formula, the Food and Drug Administration recommends capping the calculated creatinine clearance (representing glomerular filtration rate) at a value of 125 mL/minute.

- Provide supporting references and/or rationale when doses vary from a standard regimen or are prescribed as flat doses to allow for necessary double-checks.

- Provide complete dosing information including calculated dose with reduction noted with rationale, total volume and solution to administer dose (if applicable), route of administration, rate or number of hours or days that dose is to be administered, which specific days dose is to be administered and total dose per treatment course, cycle or cumulative lifetime (if applicable). In some situations, clearly defining when to initiate therapy (Day 0 or Day 1) may be necessary for clarity.

Example: Patient = 1.8 m^2
Drug "X" 50 mg/m^2/day IV push for 3 days = 90 mg IV push on Days 3, 4, and 5
(Total Dose Drug "X" per cycle = 150 mg/m^2 = 270 mg)

* Always use a leading zero for numbers less than 1 (0.5 mg is correct and .5 mg is **incorrect**) and never use a trailing zero for whole numbers (2 mg is correct and 2.0 mg is **incorrect**).

* For doses that are greater than 1,000 dosing units, use properly placed commas to prevent 10-fold errors (100,000 units is correct and 100000 units is **incorrect**).

* Avoid dangerous, error-prone abbreviations (eg, regardless of letter-case: U, IU, QD, QOD, µg, cc, @, MS, MS04, MgS04). Regarding the example above, the terminology "IV push" is commonly used and accepted. However, consider using the complete term "intravenous push," and stating the rate of infusion for the "push" dose to minimize confusion.

* Establish regimen-specific appropriate monitoring (eg, laboratory tests) and follow-up intervals.

* Establish dosing and administration constraints including maximum single doses, maximum doses within specified time limits and acceptable routes and rates of administration.

* Consider verification of lifetime dosing limits for certain agents, including DOXOrubicin, DAUNOrubicin, EPIrubicin, IDArubicin, and bleomycin.

VINCA ALKALOID ADMINISTRATION

The vinca alkaloids vinblastine, vincristine, vincristine liposomal, and vinorelbine are for intravenous administration only. Inadvertent intrathecal administration of a vinca alkaloid can cause serious neurologic toxicity and is usually fatal. The Institute for Safe Medication Practices (ISMP) recommends admixture of vinca alkaloids in a minibag with volume of compatible fluid that is too large for intrathecal administration (adult patients, 50 mL; pediatric patients, 25 mL) in order to prevent inadvertent intrathecal administration.

INTRATHECAL CHEMOTHERAPY

* During the admixture process, intrathecal agents should not be prepared during the preparation of any other agents.

* After preparation, keep in an isolated location or container clearly marked with a label identifying as "intrathecal" use only.

* Delivery to the patient should only be with other medications intended for administration into the central nervous system.

ORAL CHEMOTHERAPY

Medication errors involving oral chemotherapy in both adult and pediatric patients are being increasingly reported and like other routes of administration, the origin of the error ranges from prescribing to dispensing to patient self-administration. Oral chemotherapy should go through the same double-check system in which parenteral chemotherapy is processed.

The following recommendations should be adhered to for oral chemotherapy (Goldspiel 2015):

- Drug doses and schedules should be described as the amount to be taken per dose (not as a total daily dose divided).

- Medication orders, instructions, and patient instructions should be clearly documented in the treatment plan and the number of doses to be administered should be clearly identified.

- Doses with solid dosage forms should specify if and how doses are to be rounded to the nearest tablet/capsule size.

- Only the quantity necessary to cover the administration period until the next clinical evaluation should be ordered.

- If appropriate, instructions on how the medication should be administered with regard to food should be provided; information on foods interacting with the medication should be provided.

- Oral chemotherapy medications ordered should be provided with parenteral chemotherapy orders to allow for appropriate medication screening/review.

- Oral chemotherapy medications ordered should be included on the patient's home medication list to allow for appropriate medication screening/review.

- Oral chemotherapy medications ordered should be communicated to the pharmacist to allow for appropriate medication screening/review.

- Patient instructions should be provided, along with instructions on what to do for missed doses.

- Patients should be provided with detailed instructions regarding anticipated adverse effects and which adverse events require contacting the health care professional.

- Safe handling, storage, and disposal instructions should be provided.

- Necessary supportive care recommendations and ancillary medications should be provided.

- Discourage refills on oral chemotherapy (if feasible).

- Patients should be educated as appropriate on access and cost of the intended oral chemotherapy.

Patient noncompliance with the prescribed dose regimen is a concern for institutional, outpatient, and retail practices. A major risk factor for these errors is the multiple dosage strengths for many agents, which must be combined to provide the prescribed dose. The prescriber, the pharmacist, and the patient should be cautious and very clear in the process of prescribing, dispensing, and administering the desired dose. Increased emphasis on patient counseling and additional techniques, such as pill counts, may decrease error risk and increase adherence.

Written or electronic patient education material should be provided before or at the time that oral chemotherapy is prescribed. Patient education should include the purpose for the medication; instructions for medication administration; common or potentially serious side effects; storage, safe handling, and disposal; potential drug-drug and drug-food interactions; a plan for missed doses; and access and cost information. Documentation of patient understanding should occur.

THE ROLE OF TECHNOLOGY

Computerized provider order entry (CPOE) and bar-code technology have been adopted by some institutions and practices in an effort to improve safety and efficiency and enhance communication between health care providers. Both technology tools have been shown to be useful, but certainly do not replace the need for continued surveillance and safety checks in all stages of the chemotherapy order process. For example, CPOE has been shown to decrease prescribing errors, but has little or no impact on dispensing and administration mistakes.

THE ROLE OF THE CANCER PATIENT

The patient remains the one constant in every health practitioner encounter, and could provide vigilance and support in identifying and preventing errors in his/her therapy. The majority of cancer patients are knowledgeable about their disease and their treatments, and can serve as a valuable resource in error prevention. Institutions should foster an environment which encourages patient participation. Informed consent for chemotherapy must be obtained prior to chemotherapy administration. A policy to assess adherence or oral chemotherapy should be developed.

Provide patient education, including information on:

- Medication(s), schedule, and planned duration
- Management of missed doses
- Possible short- and long-term adverse effects, including possible risks to future fertility (if applicable)
- Symptoms that should trigger notification of health care provider (and who to notify)
- Proper handling and storage of oral medications and proper disposal of unused medications

Medication errors are inevitable in all health care scenarios, including oncology. When such events occur, the issues of appropriate disclosure and follow-up are first priorities. The published literature has provided some insight to disclosure and to the support required by the patient and the health care team in such events. References addressing this issue are among the list at the end of the chapter.

ON-GOING INSTITUTIONAL REVIEW TO INCREASE ONCOLOGY MEDICATION SAFETY

Institutions and oncology practices should constantly review the chemotherapy order process and look for opportunities to promote a culture of safety:

- Consistent education to the health care team on all aspects of chemotherapy management

- Re-engineer processes if needed, as per the following examples:

    - Centralize the pharmaceutical chemotherapy compound process

    - Observe work flow: Minimize nursing interruptions during the administration of oncology medications, which has been shown to affect the incidence and severity of errors with high-risk medications

    - Restrict certain high-risk medications from specific hospital or clinic locations, such as keeping vinca alkaloids away from certain procedure areas to minimize risk of wrong route administration

    - Special packaging and warning labels for high-alert medications

    - Computer pop-up alerts

- Document, review, and discuss all oncology medication errors, including the "near misses"; not for punitive measures, but as teaching tools to improve the oncology medication process.

- Enhance communication among all health care team members (ie, utilize or improve the medication reconciliation process).

SELECTED READINGS

Aboumatar HJ, Winner L, Davis R, et al. Applying lean sigma solutions to mistake-proof the chemotherapy preparation process. *Jt Comm J Qual Patient Saf.* 2010;36(2):79-86.

Bartel SB. Safe practices and financial considerations in using oral chemotherapeutic agents. *Am J Health Syst Pharm.* 2007;64(9 Suppl 5):S8-S14.

Bonnabry P, Cingria L, Ackermann M, Sadeghipour F, Bigler L, Mach N. Use of a prospective risk analysis method to improve the safety of the cancer chemotherapy process. *Int J Qual Health Care.* 2006;18(1):9-16.

Brunetti L, Santell JP, Hicks RW. The impact of abbreviations on patient safety. *Jt Comm J Qual Patient Saf.* 2007;33(9):576-583.

Cooke DL, Dunscombe PB, Lee RC. Using a survey of incident reporting and learning practices to improve organisational learning at a cancer care centre. *Qual Saf Health Care.* 2007;16 (5):342-348.

Crossno CL, Cartwright JA, Hargrove FR. Using CPOE to improve communication, safety, and policy compliance when ordering pediatric chemotherapy. *Hosp Pharm.* 2007;42(4):368–373.

DuBeshter B, Griggs J, Angel C, et al. Chemotherapy dose limits set by users of a computer order entry system. *Hosp Pharm.* 2006;41(2):136-142.

Goldspiel B, Hoffman JM, Griffith NL, et al. ASHP guidelines on preventing medication errors with chemotherapy and biotherapy. *Am J Health Syst Pharm.* 2015;72(6):e6-e35.

Griggs JJ, Mangu PB, Anderson H, et al. Appropriate chemotherapy dosing for obese adult patients with cancer: American Society of Clinical Oncology clinical practice guideline. *J Clin Oncol.* 2012;30(13):1553-1561.

Harris TJ, Northfelt DW. Chemotherapy error: practical approaches to increasing patient safety. *J Patient Safety.* 2005;1(4):215-219.

Institute for Safe Medication Practices. 2014-2015 targeted medication safety best practices for hospitals. Available at http://www.ismp.org/tools/bestpractices/TMSBP-for-Hospitals.pdf. Accessed October 14, 2014.

Kozakiewicz JM, Benis LJ, Fisher SM, Marseglia JB. Safe chemotherapy administration: using failure mode and effects analysis in computerized prescriber order entry. *Am J Health Syst Pharm.* 2005;62(17):1813-1816.

Markert A, Thierry V, Kleber M, Behrens M, Engelhardt M. Chemotherapy safety and severe adverse events in cancer patients: strategies to efficiently avoid chemotherapy errors in in- and outpatient treatment. *Int J Cancer.* 2009;124(3):722-728.

Neuss MN, Polovich M, McNiff K, et al. 2013 updated American Society of Clinical Oncology/ Oncology Nursing Society chemotherapy administration safety standards including standards for the safe administration and management of oral chemotherapy. *J Oncol Pract.* 2013;9(2 Suppl):5s-13s.

Poon EG, Keohane CA, Yoon CS, et al. Effect of bar-code technology on the safety of medication administration. *N Engl J Med.* 2010;362(18):1698-1707.

Rinke ML, Shore AD, Morlock L, Hicks RW, Miller MR. Characteristics of pediatric chemotherapy medication errors in a national error reporting database. *Cancer.* 2007;110(1):186-195.

Schwappach DL, Hochreutener MA, Wernli M. Oncology nurses' perceptions about involving patients in the prevention of chemotherapy administration errors. *Oncol Nurs Forum.* 2010;37(2):E84-E91.

Schwappach DL, Wernli M. Chemotherapy patients' perceptions of drug administration safety. *J Clin Oncol.* 2010;28(17):2896-2901.

Schwappach DL, Wernli M. Medication errors in chemotherapy: incidence, types and involvement of patients in prevention. A review of the literature. *Eur J Cancer Care (Engl).* 2010;19(3):285-292.

To err is human: building a safer health system. Kohn LT, Corrigan JM, Donaldson MS, eds. Washington, D.C.: National Academy Press; 2000.

Trbovich P, Prakash V, Stewart J, Trip K, Savage P. Interruptions during the delivery of high-risk medications. *J Nurs Adm.* 2010;40(5):211-218.

Walsh KE, Dodd KS, Seetharaman K, et al. Medication errors among adults and children with cancer in the outpatient setting. *J Clin Oncol.* 2009;27(6):891-896.

Weingart SN, Price J, Duncombe D, et al. Patient-reported safety and quality of care in outpatient oncology. *Jt Comm J Qual Patient Saf.* 2007;33(2):83-94.

Weingart SN, Simchowitz B, Eng TK, et al. The You CAN campaign: teamwork training for patients and families in ambulatory oncology. *Jt Comm J Qual Patient Saf.* 2009;35(2):63-71.

Weingart SN, Toro J, Spencer J, et al. Medication errors involving oral chemotherapy. *Cancer.* 2010;116(10):2455-2464.

Westbrook JI, Woods A, Rob MI, Dunsmuir WT, Day RO. Association of interruptions with an increased risk and severity of medication administration errors. *Arch Intern Med.* 2010;170(8):683-690.

ALPHABETICAL LISTING OF DRUGS

- ◆ **Abbott-43818** *see* Leuprolide *on page 1030*
- ◆ **Abbott-Olanzapine ODT (Can)** *see* OLANZapine *on page 1242*
- ◆ **ABCD** *see* Amphotericin B Cholesteryl Sulfate Complex *on page 95*
- ◆ **Abelcet** *see* Amphotericin B (Lipid Complex) *on page 99*
- ◆ **ABI-007** *see* PACLitaxel (Protein Bound) *on page 1292*
- ◆ **Abiraterone** *see* Abiraterone Acetate *on page 30*

Abiraterone Acetate (a bir A ter one AS e tate)

Related Information
Palliative Care Medicine (Cancer) *on page 2252*
Brand Names: US Zytiga
Brand Names: Canada Zytiga
Index Terms Abiraterone; CB7630
Pharmacologic Category Antiandrogen; Antineoplastic Agent, Antiandrogen
Use Prostate cancer: Treatment of metastatic, castration-resistant prostate cancer (in combination with prednisone)
Labeled Contraindications Women who are or may become pregnant

Canadian labeling: Additional contraindication (not in U.S. labeling): Hypersensitivity to abiraterone acetate or any component of the formulation or container

Pregnancy Considerations Adverse effects were observed in animal reproduction studies at doses resulting in less systemic exposure than in humans. Adverse effects were also observed in the reproductive system of animals during toxicology and pharmacology studies. Based on the mechanism of action, abiraterone may cause fetal harm or fetal loss if administered during pregnancy. Abiraterone is not indicated for use in women and is specifically contraindicated in women who are or may become pregnant. It is not known if abiraterone is excreted in semen, therefore, men should use a condom and another method of birth control during treatment and for 1 week following therapy if having intercourse with a woman of reproductive age. Women who are or may become pregnant should wear gloves if contact with tablets may occur.

Breast-Feeding Considerations Not indicated for use in women

Warnings/Precautions Hazardous agent - use appropriate precautions for handling and disposal (NIOSH 2014 [group 1]). Significant increases in liver enzymes have been reported (higher likelihood in patients with baseline elevations), generally occurring in the first 3 months of treatment. May require dosage reduction, treatment interruption, and/ or discontinuation. ALT, AST, and bilirubin should be monitored prior to treatment, every 2 weeks for 3 months and monthly thereafter; patients with hepatic impairment, elevations in liver function tests, or experiencing hepatotoxicity require more frequent monitoring (see Dosage Adjustment for Hepatic Impairment and Monitoring Parameters). Evaluate liver function promptly with signs or symptoms of hepatotoxicity. The safety of retreatment after significant elevations (ALT or AST >20 times the upper limit of normal [ULN] and/or total bilirubin >10 times ULN) has not been evaluated. Do not use in patients with preexisting severe hepatic impairment (Child-Pugh class C); dosage reduction is recommended in patients with baseline moderate impairment. Canadian labeling (not in U.S. labeling) also recommends avoiding use in patients with preexisting moderate hepatic impairment.

Concurrent infection, stress, or interruption of daily corticosteroids is associated with reports of adrenocortical insufficiency. Monitor closely for signs and symptoms of adrenocorticoid insufficiency, which could be masked by adverse events associated with mineralocorticoid excess. Diagnostic testing for adrenal insufficiency may be clinically indicated. Increased corticosteroid doses may be required before, during, and after stress. May cause increased mineralocorticoid levels, which may result in hypertension, hypokalemia and fluid retention (including grades 3 and 4 events). Concomitant administration with corticosteroids reduces the incidence and severity of these adverse events. Control hypertension and correct hypokalemia prior to and during treatment. Use with caution in patients with cardiovascular disease (particularly heart failure, recent MI, or ventricular arrhythmia); patients with left ventricular ejection fraction (LVEF) <50% or NYHA class III or IV heart failure were excluded from clinical trials. Monitor at least monthly for hypertension, hypokalemia, and fluid retention.

Abiraterone must be administered on an empty stomach (administer at least 1 hour before and 2 hours after any food); abiraterone AUC (exposure) may be increased up to 10-fold if administered with a meal. Potentially significant drug-drug interactions may exist, requiring dose or frequency adjustment, additional monitoring, and/or selection of alternative therapy.

Adverse Reactions Note: Adverse reactions reported for use in combination with prednisone.

>10%:

Cardiovascular: Edema (25% to 27%; grades 3/4: ≤2%; includes anasarca, peripheral edema, pitting edema), hypertension (9% to 22%; grades 3/4: 1% to 4%)

Central nervous system: Fatigue (39%), insomnia (14%)

Dermatologic: Bruise (13%)

Endocrine & metabolic: Hypertriglyceridemia (63%), hyperglycemia (57%), hypernatremia (33%), hypokalemia (17% to 28%; grades 3/4: 3% to 5%), hypophosphatemia (24%; grades 3/4: 7%), hot flash (19% to 22%)

Gastrointestinal: Constipation (23%), diarrhea (18% to 22%), dyspepsia (6% to 11%)

Genitourinary: Urinary tract infection (12%)

Hematologic & oncologic: Lymphocytopenia (38%; grades 3/4: 9%)

Hepatic: Increased serum ALT (11% to 42%; grades 3/4: 1% to 6%), increased serum AST (37%; grades 3/4: 3%)

Neuromuscular & skeletal: Joint swelling (30%, includes arthralgia, arthritis, joint discomfort, joint stiffness), myalgia (26%; includes muscle rigidity, muscle spasm, musculoskeletal discomfort, musculoskeletal pain)

Respiratory: Cough (11% to 17%), upper respiratory infection (5% to 13%), dyspnea (12%), nasopharyngitis (11%)

1% to 10%:

Cardiovascular: Cardiac arrhythmia (7%; includes atrial fibrillation, atrial tachycardia, bradycardia, cardiac conduction disturbance, complete atrioventricular block, supraventricular tachycardia, tachycardia), chest pain (4%, includes angina pectoris, chest discomfort, unstable angina pectoris), cardiac failure (2%; includes cardiogenic shock, cardiomegaly, cardiomyopathy, congestive heart failure, left ventricular dysfunction, reduced ejection fraction)

Central nervous system: Falling (6%)

Dermatologic: Skin rash (8%)

◀

Genitourinary: Hematuria (10%), groin pain (7%), urinary frequency (7%), nocturia (6%)

Hepatic: Increased serum bilirubin (7%; grades 3/4: <1%)

Neuromuscular & skeletal: Bone fracture (6%)

Miscellaneous: Fever (9%)

<1%, postmarketing, and/or case reports: Adrenocortical insufficiency, myopathy (includes rhabdomyolysis), noninfectious pneumonitis

Drug Interactions

Metabolism/Transport Effects Substrate of CYP3A4 (major); **Note:** Assignment of Major/Minor substrate status based on clinically relevant drug interaction potential; **Inhibits** CYP1A2 (weak), CYP2C19 (moderate), CYP2C8 (weak), CYP2C9 (moderate), CYP2D6 (moderate), P-glycoprotein, SLCO1B1

Avoid Concomitant Use

Avoid concomitant use of Abiraterone Acetate with any of the following: Amodiaquine; Bosutinib; CYP3A4 Inducers (Strong); Indium 111 Capromab Pendetide; PAZOPanib; Silodosin; Thioridazine; Topotecan; VinCRIStine (Liposomal)

Increased Effect/Toxicity

Abiraterone Acetate may increase the levels/effects of: Afatinib; Amodiaquine; Bosentan; Bosutinib; Brentuximab Vedotin; Cannabis; Cilostazol; Citalopram; Colchicine; CYP1A2 Substrates; CYP2C19 Substrates; CYP2C8 Substrates; CYP2C9 Substrates; CYP2D6 Substrates; Dabigatran Etexilate; DOXOrubicin (Conventional); Dronabinol; Edoxaban; Eliglustat; Everolimus; Fesoterodine; Ledipasvir; Metoprolol; Naloxegol; Nebivolol; PAZOPanib; P-glycoprotein/ABCB1 Substrates; Prucalopride; Ranolazine; Rifaximin; Silodosin; Tetrahydrocannabinol; Thioridazine; TiZANidine; Topotecan; VinCRIStine (Liposomal)

The levels/effects of Abiraterone Acetate may be increased by: Osimertinib; Propafenone

Decreased Effect

Abiraterone Acetate may decrease the levels/effects of: Choline C 11; Clopidogrel; Codeine; Indium 111 Capromab Pendetide; Tamoxifen; TraMADol

The levels/effects of Abiraterone Acetate may be decreased by: Bosentan; CYP3A4 Inducers (Moderate); CYP3A4 Inducers (Strong); Dabrafenib; Deferasirox; Osimertinib; Siltuximab; Spironolactone; St Johns Wort; Tocilizumab

Food Interactions Taking abiraterone with food will increase systemic exposure (up to 10-fold). Management: Do not administer with food. Abiraterone must be taken on an empty stomach, at least 1 hour before and 2 hours after food.

Storage/Stability Store at 20°C to 25°C (68°F to 77°F); excursions are permitted between 15°C and 30°C (59°F and 86°F).

Mechanism of Action Selectively and irreversibly inhibits CYP17 (17 alpha-hydroxylase/C17,20-lyase), an enzyme required for androgen biosynthesis which is expressed in testicular, adrenal, and prostatic tumor tissues. Inhibits the formation of the testosterone precursors dehydroepiandrosterone (DHEA) and androstenedione.

Pharmacodynamics/Kinetics

Distribution: V_{dss}: 19,669 ± 13,358 L

Protein binding: >99%; to albumin and alpha$_1$-acid glycoprotein

Metabolism: Abiraterone acetate is hydrolyzed to the active metabolite abiraterone; further metabolized to inactive metabolites abiraterone sulphate and N-oxide abiraterone sulphate via CYP3A4 and SULT2A1

Bioavailability: Systemic exposure is increased by food

Half-life elimination: 14.4 to 16.5 hours (Acharya 2012)

Time to peak: 2 hours (Acharya 2012)

Excretion: Feces (~88%); urine (~5%)

Dosing

Adult & Geriatric Prostate cancer, metastatic, castration-resistant: Oral: 1000 mg once daily (in combination with prednisone 5 mg twice daily)

Dosage adjustment for concomitant strong CYP3A4 inducers: Avoid concomitant strong CYP3A4 inducers; if a strong CYP3A4 inducer must be administered concurrently, increase the abiraterone frequency to twice daily (eg, from 1000 mg once daily to 1000 mg twice daily). Upon discontinuation of the strong CYP3A4 inducer, reduce abiraterone back to the prior dose and frequency.

Renal Impairment No dosage adjustment necessary.

Hepatic Impairment

Hepatic impairment *prior to* treatment initiation:

Mild (Child-Pugh class A): No dosage adjustment necessary.

Moderate (Child-Pugh class B):

U.S. labeling: 250 mg once daily. Permanently discontinue if ALT and/or AST >5 times the upper limit of normal (ULN) or total bilirubin >3 times ULN during treatment.

Canadian labeling: Use is not recommended.

Severe (Child-Pugh class C): Do not use.

Hepatotoxicity *during* treatment:

U.S. labeling:

ALT and/or AST >5 times ULN or total bilirubin >3 times ULN: Withhold treatment until liver function tests return to baseline or ALT and AST ≤2.5 times ULN and total bilirubin ≤1.5 times ULN, then reinitiate at 750 mg once daily.

Recurrent hepatotoxicity on 750 mg/day: Withhold treatment until liver function tests return to baseline or ALT and AST ≤2.5 times ULN and total bilirubin ≤1.5 times ULN, then reinitiate at 500 mg once daily.

Recurrent hepatotoxicity on 500 mg once daily: Discontinue treatment

Canadian labeling:

ALT or AST >5 times ULN or total bilirubin >3 times ULN:

Withhold treatment until liver function tests normalize, then (when hepatic function returns to baseline) reinitiate at 500 mg once daily

Recurrent hepatotoxicity on 500 mg once daily: Discontinue treatment

ALT >20 times ULN (any time during treatment): Discontinue permanently.

Adjustment for Toxicity Hepatotoxicity: Refer to Dosing: Hepatic Impairment.

Combination Regimens

Prostate cancer: Abiraterone-Prednisone (Prostate) on page 1820

Administration Administer abiraterone orally on an empty stomach, at least 1 hour before and 2 hours after food. **Note:** The prescribing information describes when to give food with respect to abiraterone; no food should be consumed for at least 2 hours before or for at least 1 hour after the abiraterone dose. Swallow tablets whole with water. Do not crush or chew.

◀ Hazardous agent; use appropriate precautions for handling and disposal (NIOSH 2014 [group 1]). Women who are or may become pregnant should wear gloves if handling the tablets.

Monitoring Parameters ALT, AST, and bilirubin prior to treatment, every 2 weeks for 3 months and monthly thereafter; if baseline moderate hepatic impairment (Child-Pugh class B), monitor ALT, AST, and bilirubin prior to treatment, weekly for the first month, every 2 weeks for 2 months then monthly thereafter. If hepatotoxicity develops during treatment (and only after therapy is interrupted and liver function tests have returned to safe levels), monitor ALT, AST, and bilirubin every 2 weeks for 3 months and monthly thereafter. Monitoring of testosterone levels is not necessary. Serum potassium (prior to treatment and at least monthly).

Monitor for signs and symptoms of adrenocorticoid insufficiency; if clinically indicated, consider appropriate diagnostics to confirm adrenal insufficiency. Monitor blood pressure and for fluid retention (prior to treatment and at least monthly).

Dosage Forms Excipient information presented when available (limited, particularly for generics); consult specific product labeling.
Tablet, Oral:
Zytiga: 250 mg

- ◆ **ABLC** see Amphotericin B (Lipid Complex) on page 99
- ◆ **Abraxane** see PACLitaxel (Protein Bound) on page 1292
- ◆ **Abraxane for Injectable Suspension (Can)** see PACLitaxel (Protein Bound) on page 1292
- ◆ **Absorica** see ISOtretinoin on page 973
- ◆ **Abstral** see FentaNYL on page 692
- ◆ **ABX-EGF** see Panitumumab on page 1316
- ◆ **Accel-Olanzapine (Can)** see OLANZapine on page 1242
- ◆ **Accutane** see ISOtretinoin on page 973
- ◆ **Acetoxymethylprogesterone** see MedroxyPROGESTERone on page 1074
- ◆ **ACH-Anastrozole (Can)** see Anastrozole on page 112
- ◆ **ACH-Bicalutamide (Can)** see Bicalutamide on page 207
- ◆ **ACH-Letrozole (Can)** see Letrozole on page 1019
- ◆ **Ach-Mycophenolate (Can)** see Mycophenolate on page 1177
- ◆ **ACH-Temozolomide (Can)** see Temozolomide on page 1608
- ◆ **Aciclovir** see Acyclovir (Systemic) on page 35
- ◆ **Aciclovir** see Acyclovir (Topical) on page 42
- ◆ **Aclasta (Can)** see Zoledronic Acid on page 1790
- ◆ **4-(9-Acridinylamino) Methanesulfon-m-Anisidide** see Amsacrine on page 105
- ◆ **Acridinyl Anisidide** see Amsacrine on page 105
- ◆ **ACT-D** see DACTINomycin on page 431
- ◆ **ACT-Anastrozole (Can)** see Anastrozole on page 112
- ◆ **ACT Bicalutamide (Can)** see Bicalutamide on page 207
- ◆ **ACT Ciprofloxacin (Can)** see Ciprofloxacin (Systemic) on page 327
- ◆ **ACT Fluconazole (Can)** see Fluconazole on page 725

- **ACT-Imatinib (Can)** *see* Imatinib *on page 882*
- **Actinomycin** *see* DACTINomycin *on page 431*
- **Actinomycin D** *see* DACTINomycin *on page 431*
- **Actinomycin CI** *see* DACTINomycin *on page 431*
- **Actiq** *see* FentaNYL *on page 692*
- **Activase** *see* Alteplase *on page 78*
- **Activase rt-PA (Can)** *see* Alteplase *on page 78*
- **Activated Factor XIII** *see* Factor XIII Concentrate (Human) *on page 688*
- **Active-Tramadol** *see* TraMADol *on page 1672*
- **ACT Levofloxacin (Can)** *see* Levofloxacin (Systemic) *on page 1038*
- **ACT Nabilone (Can)** *see* Nabilone *on page 1187*
- **ACT Olanzapine (Can)** *see* OLANZapine *on page 1242*
- **ACT Olanzapine ODT (Can)** *see* OLANZapine *on page 1242*
- **ACT Ondansetron (Can)** *see* Ondansetron *on page 1253*
- **ACT Oxycodone CR (Can)** *see* OxyCODONE *on page 1277*
- **ACT Raloxifene (Can)** *see* Raloxifene *on page 1451*
- **ACT Temozolomide (Can)** *see* Temozolomide *on page 1608*
- **ACV** *see* Acyclovir (Systemic) *on page 35*
- **ACV** *see* Acyclovir (Topical) *on page 42*
- **Acycloguanosine** *see* Acyclovir (Systemic) *on page 35*
- **Acycloguanosine** *see* Acyclovir (Topical) *on page 42*

Acyclovir (Systemic) (ay SYE kloe veer)

Brand Names: US Zovirax
Brand Names: Canada Acyclovir Sodium for Injection; Acyclovir Sodium Injection; Apo-Acyclovir; Mylan-Acyclovir; ratio-Acyclovir; Teva-Acyclovir; Zovirax
Index Terms Aciclovir; ACV; Acycloguanosine; Zovirax
Pharmacologic Category Antiviral Agent
Use

Oral:

Herpes zoster (shingles): Acute treatment of herpes zoster (shingles).
Herpes simplex virus (HSV), genital: Treatment of initial episodes and the management of recurrent episodes of genital herpes.
Varicella (chickenpox): Treatment of varicella (chickenpox).

Injection:

Herpes simplex virus (HSV), mucocutaneous infection in immunocompromised patients: Treatment of initial and recurrent mucosal and cutaneous herpes simplex (HSV-1 and HSV-2) in immunocompromised patients.
Herpes simplex virus (HSV), genital infection (severe): Treatment of severe initial clinical episodes of genital herpes in immunocompetent patients.
Herpes simplex encephalitis: Treatment of herpes simplex encephalitis.
Herpes simplex virus (HSV), neonatal: Treatment of neonatal herpes infections.
Herpes zoster (shingles) in immunocompromised patients: Treatment of herpes zoster (shingles) in immunocompromised patients.

Pregnancy Risk Factor B

◀ **Dosing**

Adult & Geriatric

Herpes simplex virus (HSV), genital infection:

Immunocompetent:

IV: Initial episode, severe: 5 mg/kg/dose every 8 hours for 5 to 7 days **or** 5 to 10 mg/kg/dose every 8 hours for 2 to 7 days, follow with oral therapy to complete at least 10 days of therapy (CDC 2010)

Oral:

Initial episode: 200 mg 5 times daily while awake for 10 days **or** 400 mg 3 times daily for 7 to 10 days (CDC 2010)

Recurrence:

Manufacturer's labeling: **Note:** begin at earliest signs of disease: 200 mg 5 times daily while awake for 5 days

Alternate recommendation: 400 mg 3 times daily for 5 days **or** 800 mg twice daily for 5 days **or** 800 mg 3 times daily for 2 days (CDC 2010)

Chronic suppression: 400 mg twice daily or 200 mg 3 to 5 times daily, for up to 12 months followed by re-evaluation

HIV-infected patients (off-label use) (HHS [OI adult 2015]):

Initial or recurrent episodes: 400 mg 3 times daily for 5 to 14 days

Chronic suppressive therapy: 400 mg twice daily; continue indefinitely regardless of CD4 count in patients with severe recurrences of genital herpes or in patients who want to minimize frequency of recurrences

HSV encephalitis: IV: Independent of HIV status:

Manufacturer's labeling: 10 mg/kg/dose every 8 hours for 10 days

Alternate recommendation: 10 mg/kg/dose every 8 hours for 14 to 21 days (*Red Book* [AAP 2012])

HSV, mucocutaneous treatment:

Immunocompromised:

IV:

Manufacturer's labeling: 5 mg/kg/dose every 8 hours for 7 days

Alternate recommendations: 5 to 10 mg/kg/dose every 8 hours for 7 days (Leflore 2000)

Oral (off-label use): 400 mg 5 times daily for 7 days (Leflore 2000)

HIV-infected patients: (off-label use)

IV: 5 mg/kg/dose every 8 hours; may switch to oral after lesions begin to heal (HHS [OI adult 2015])

Oral: After initial IV therapy, may switch to 400 mg 3 times daily; continue until lesions are completely healed (HHS [OI adult 2015])

HSV, orolabial (cold sores) (off-label use): Oral:

Immunocompetent:

Treatment: (episodic/recurrent): 200 to 400 mg 5 times daily for 5 days (Cernik 2008; Leflore 2000; Spruance 1990).

Chronic suppression: 400 mg 2 times daily (has been clinically evaluated for up to 1 year) (Cernik 2008; Rooney 1993)

HIV-infected patients: Treatment: 400 mg 3 times daily for 5 to 10 days (HHS [OI adult 2015])

Herpes zoster (shingles), treatment:

Manufacturer's labeling:

IV: Immunocompromised: 10 mg/kg/dose every 8 hours for 7 days

Oral: Immunocompetent: 800 mg 5 times daily for 7 to 10 day

Alternate recommendations: HIV-infected patients (HHS [OI adult 2015]):

IV: *Extensive cutaneous lesions or visceral involvement:* 10 to 15 mg/kg/dose every 8 hours until clinical improvement; switch to oral famciclovir or valacyclovir (preferred) or acyclovir (alternative) to complete a 10 to 14 day course when formation of new lesions has ceased and signs/symptoms of visceral infection are improving

Oral (off-label use): *Acute localized infection (as an alternative to valacyclovir or famciclovir):* 800 mg 5 times daily for 7 to 10 days; consider longer duration if lesions resolve slowly

Prevention of early HSV reactivation in seropositive hematopoietic stem cell transplant (HSCT) recipients (off-label use): Note: Start at the beginning of conditioning therapy and continue until engraftment or until mucositis resolves (~30 days) (Tomblyn 2009)

Oral: 400 to 800 mg twice daily

IV: 250 mg/m^2 every 12 hours

Prevention of late HSV reactivation in seropositive HSCT recipients (off-label use): Oral: 800 mg twice daily; continue therapy for 1 year after HSCT (Tomblyn 2009).

Prevention of HSV reactivation in seropositive patients undergoing acute myeloid leukemia induction or reinduction (off-label use): Oral: 400 mg twice daily; continue during active therapy and throughout periods of neutropenia (Bergmann 1995; Freifeld 2011)

Prevention of VZV reactivation in HSCT recipients (off-label use): Oral: 800 mg twice daily; continue therapy for 1 year after HSCT (Tomblyn 2009).

Prophylaxis of CMV in low-risk allogeneic HSCT (off-label use; alternate therapy): Note: Begin at engraftment and continue to day 100; requires close monitoring for CMV reactivation (due to weak activity); not for use in patients at high risk for CMV disease (Tomblyn 2009)

Oral: 800 mg 4 times daily

IV: 500 mg/m^2 every 8 hours

Varicella (chickenpox), treatment: Begin treatment within the first 24 hours of rash onset:

Oral:

Immunocompetent (>40 kg): 800 mg 4 times daily for 5 days

HIV-infected patients (off-label use): *Uncomplicated cases (as an alternative to valacyclovir or famciclovir):* 800 mg 5 times daily for 5 to 7 days (HHS [OI adult 2015])

IV: HIV- infected patients (off-label use): Severe or complicated cases: 10 to 15 mg/kg/dose every 8 hours for 7 to 10 days; may switch to oral famciclovir or valacyclovir (preferred) or acyclovir (alternative) after defervescence if no evidence of visceral involvement (HHS [OI adult 2015])

Varicella-zoster virus acute retinal necrosis (ARN) in HIV-infected patients (off-label use): IV: 10 to 15 mg/kg/dose every 8 hours for 10 to 14 days, followed by valacyclovir for 6 weeks plus intravitreal ganciclovir twice weekly for 1 to 2 doses (HHS [OI adult 2015])

Pediatric

Herpes simplex virus (HSV), genital infection:

IV: Children ≥12 years and Adolescents: Immunocompetent: Initial episode, severe: 5 mg/kg/dose every 8 hours for 5 to 7 days **or** 5 to 10 mg/kg/dose every 8 hours for 2 to 7 days, follow with oral therapy to complete at least 10 days of therapy (CDC 2010)

Oral:

Infants and Children <12 years: Immunocompetent (off-label use):

Initial episode: 40 to 80 mg/kg/day divided into 3 to 4 doses for 5-10 days (maximum: 1,000 mg daily) (*Red Book* [AAP 2012])

Chronic suppression: 40 to 80 mg/kg/day in 3 divided doses for ≤12 months; (maximum: 1,000 mg daily) (*Red Book* [AAP 2009])

Children ≥12 years and Adolescents: Immunocompetent (off-label use):

Initial episode: 200 mg every 4 hours while awake (5 times daily) **or** 400 mg 3 times daily for 7 to 10 days; treatment can be extended beyond 10 days if healing is not complete (CDC 2010; *Red Book* [AAP 2012])

Chronic suppression: 800 mg daily in 2 divided doses for ≤12 continuous months (*Red Book* [AAP 2012])

Children: HIV-exposed/-positive (off-label use):

Children <45 kg:

Initial episode: 60 mg/kg/day divided into 3 doses daily for 5 to 14 days (maximum: 1,200 mg daily) (CDC 2009)

Chronic suppression: 20 mg/kg/dose twice daily (maximum dose: 400 mg) (CDC 2009)

Children ≥45 kg:

Initial episode: 400 mg twice daily for 5 to 14 days (CDC 2009)

Chronic suppression: 20 mg/kg/dose twice daily (maximum dose: 400 mg) (CDC 2009)

Children <12 years: Recurrent infection: Non-HIV-exposed/-positive: Oral: 20 to 25 mg/kg/dose twice daily; maximum dose: 400 mg (Bradley 2011)

Children ≥12 years: Recurrent infection: Non-HIV-exposed/-positive: 200 mg every 4 hours while awake (5 times daily) for 5 days **or** 800 mg twice daily for 5 days **or** 800 mg 3 times daily for 2 days (CDC 2010; *Red Book* [AAP 2012])

Adolescents: HIV-positive patients: (off-label use): Refer to adult dosing.

HSV encephalitis: IV:

Infants and Children 3 months to <12 years:

Immunocompetent:

Manufacturer's labeling: 20 mg/kg/dose every 8 hours for 10 days. **Note:** Doses ≥20 mg/kg may be associated with a higher incidence of nephrotoxicity (*Red Book* [AAP 2012])

Alternate recommendation: 10 to 15 mg/kg/dose every 8 hours for 14 to 21 days (*Red Book* [AAP 2012])

HIV-exposed/-positive: 10 mg/kg/dose every 8 hours for 21 days; do not discontinue therapy until a repeat HSV DNA PCR assay of the cerebrospinal fluid is negative (CDC 2009)

Children ≥12 years and Adolescents: Independent of HIV status:

Manufacturer's labeling: 10 mg/kg/dose every 8 hours for 10 days

Alternate recommendation: 10 mg/kg/dose every 8 hours for 14 to 21 days (*Red Book* [AAP 2012])

HSV gingivostomatitis (off-label use): HIV-exposed/-positive:

Mild, symptomatic: Oral: Infants and Children: 20 mg/kg/dose 3 times daily for 5 to 10 days (maximum dose: 400 mg) (CDC 2009)

Moderate to severe, symptomatic: IV: Infants and Children: 5 to 10 mg/kg/dose every 8 hours; **Note:** switch to oral therapy once lesions begin to regress (CDC 2009)

HSV, mucocutaneous treatment:
Immunocompromised:
IV:
Infants, Children, and Adolescents: 10 mg/kg/dose every 8 hours for 7 to 14 days (*Red Book* [AAP 2012])
Oral (off-label use):
Children ≥2 years and Adolescents: 1,000 mg daily in 3 to 5 divided doses for 7 to 14 days; some suggest the maximum daily dose should not exceed 80 mg/kg/day (*Red Book* [AAP 2009]; Red Book [AAP 2012])
HIV-infected patients (off-label use): Adolescents: IV, Oral: Refer to adult dosing.
Suppression, chronic (cutaneous, ocular) episodes: Immunocompromised:
Oral:
Infants and Children (HIV-exposed/-positive): 20 mg/kg/dose twice daily for 5 to 14 days; maximum dose: 400 mg (CDC 2009)
Children and Adolescents ≥12 years (independent of HIV status): 400 mg twice daily for up to 12 months (*Red Book* [AAP 2012])

HSV, neonatal: IV: Infants: Birth to 3 months: Treatment:
Manufacturer's labeling: 10 mg/kg/dose every 8 hours for 10 days
Alternate recommendations: 20 mg/kg/dose every 8 hours for 14 days (skin and mucous membrane disease) to 21 days (CNS disease) (CDC 2010; Kimberlin 2013; *Red Book* [AAP 2012])

HSV, orolabial (cold sores) (off-label use): Oral:
Immunocompetent: Chronic suppression: Children: 30 mg/kg/day in 3 divided doses for up to 12 months (maximum: 1,000 mg/day). **Note:** Re-evaluate after 12 months (*Red Book* [AAP 2012])
HIV-infected patients: Treatment: Adolescents: Refer to adult dosing.

Herpes zoster (shingles), treatment:
IV:
Immunocompetent (off-label use):
Infants: 10 mg/kg/dose every 8 hours for 7 to 10 days (*Red Book* [AAP 2012])
Children ≥1 year and Adolescents: 500 mg/m^2/dose every 8 hours for 7 to 10 days; some experts recommend 10 mg/kg/dose every 8 hours (*Red Book* [AAP 2012])
Immunocompromised:
Children <12 years: (off-label dose): 10 mg/kg/dose every 8 hours for 7 to 10 days (*Red Book* [AAP 2012])
Children ≥12 years and Adolescents: Manufacturer's labeling: Refer to adult dosing.
HIV-infected patients: Adolescents (off-label dose): *Extensive cutaneous lesions or visceral involvement:* Refer to adult dosing.
Oral:
Immunocompetent:
Manufacturer's labeling: Children ≥2 years and Adolescents: Refer to adult dosing.

◀

Alternate recommendations: Children ≥12 years and Adolescents: 800 mg 5 times daily for 5 to 7 days (*Red Book* [AAP 2012])

Immunocompromised: HIV-infected patients (off-label use): *Acute localized infection (as an alternative to valacyclovir or famciclovir):* Adolescents: Refer to adult dosing.

Prevention of HSV reactivation in HIV-exposed/-positive patients (off-label use): Oral: Children: 20 mg/kg/dose twice daily (maximum: 400 mg per dose) (CDC 2009)

Prevention of early HSV reactivation in seropositive hematopoietic stem cell transplant (HSCT) recipients (off-label use): Note: Start at the beginning of conditioning therapy and continue until engraftment or until mucositis resolves (~30 days) (Tomblyn 2009):
Oral:
Infants, Children, and Adolescents <40 kg (alternate therapy): 60 to 90 mg/kg/day in 2 to 3 divided doses
Children and Adolescents ≥40 kg: 400 to 800 mg twice daily
IV:
Infants, Children, and Adolescents <40 kg: 250 mg/m^2 every 8 hours or 125 mg/m^2 every 6 hours (maximum daily dose: 80 mg/kg/day)
Children and Adolescents ≥40 kg: 250 mg/m^2 every 12 hours

Prevention of late HSV reactivation in seropositive HSCT recipients (off-label use): Note: Continue therapy for 1 year after HSCT (Tomblyn 2009).
Infants, Children, and Adolescents <40 kg: Oral: 60 to 90 mg/kg/day in 2 to 3 divided doses (maximum dose: 800 mg twice daily)
Children and Adolescents ≥40 kg: Oral: 800 mg twice daily

Prevention of VZV reactivation in HSCT recipients (off-label use): Note: Continue therapy for 1 year after HSCT (Tomblyn 2009)
Infants, Children, and Adolescents <40 kg: Oral: 60 to 80 mg/kg/day in 2 to 3 divided doses
Children and Adolescents ≥40 kg: Oral: 800 mg twice daily

Prophylaxis of CMV in low-risk allogeneic HSCT (off-label use; alternate therapy): Note: Begin at engraftment and continue to day 100; requires close monitoring for CMV reactivation (due to weak activity); not for use in patients at high risk for CMV disease (Tomblyn 2009)
Oral:
Infants, Children, and Adolescents <40 kg: 600 mg/m^2 4 times daily
Children and Adolescents ≥40 kg: 800 mg 4 times daily
IV: Infants, Children, and Adolescents: 500 mg/m^2 every 8 hours

Varicella (chickenpox), treatment: Begin treatment within the first 24 hours of rash onset:
Oral:
Immunocompetent:
Children ≥2 years and ≤40 kg: 20 mg/kg/dose (maximum: 800 mg per dose) 4 times daily for 5 days
Children >40 kg: Refer to adult dosing.
HIV-infected patients (off-label use):
Infants and Children: Mild, uncomplicated disease and no or moderate immune suppression: 20 mg/kg/dose (maximum dose: 800 mg) 4 times daily for 7 to 10 days or until no new lesions for 48 hours (CDC 2009)

Adolescents: Uncomplicated cases (as an alternative to valacyclovir or famciclovir): Refer to adult dosing.

IV:

Immunocompetent (off-label use): Children ≥2 years: 10 mg/kg/dose or 500 mg/m^2/dose every 8 hours for 7 to 10 days (CDC 2009; *Red Book* [AAP 2012])

Immunocompromised (off-label use):

Infants (off-label dose): 10 mg/kg/dose every 8 hours for 7 to 10 days (*Red Book* [AAP 2012])

Children and Adolescents (off-label dose): 500 mg/m^2/dose every 8 hours for 7 to 10 days; some experts recommend 10 mg/kg/dose every 8 hours (*Red Book* [AAP 2012])

HIV-exposed/-positive (off-label use):

Infants: 10 mg/kg/dose every 8 hours for 7 to 10 days or until no new lesions for 48 hours (CDC 2009)

Children ≥1 year: 10 mg/kg/dose or 500 mg/m^2/dose every 8 hours for 7 to 10 days or until no new lesions for 48 hours (CDC 2009)

Adolescents: Refer to adult dosing.

Varicella-zoster virus acute retinal necrosis in HIV-exposed/-positive patients (off-label use): IV:

Infants and Children: 10 to 15 mg/kg/dose every 8 hours for 10 to 14 days, followed by oral acyclovir or valacyclovir for 4 to 6 weeks (CDC 2009)

Adolescents: Refer to adult dosing.

Renal Impairment

Oral:

CrCl 10-25 mL/minute/1.73 m^2: Normal dosing regimen 800 mg 5 times daily: Administer 800 mg every 8 hours

CrCl <10 mL/minute/1.73 m^2:

Normal dosing regimen 200 mg 5 times daily or 400 mg every 12 hours: Administer 200 mg every 12 hours

Normal dosing regimen 800 mg 5 times daily: Administer 800 mg every 12 hours

Intermittent hemodialysis (IHD): Dialyzable (60% reduction following a 6-hour session):

Normal dosing regimen 200 mg 5 times daily or 400 mg every 12 hours: Administer 200 mg every 12 hours; administer after hemodialysis on dialysis days

Normal dosing regimen 800 mg 5 times daily: Administer 800 mg every 12 hours; administer after hemodialysis on dialysis days

IV:

CrCl 25-50 mL/minute/1.73 m^2: Administer recommended dose every 12 hours

CrCl 10-25 mL/minute/1.73 m^2: Administer recommended dose every 24 hours

CrCl <10 mL/minute/1.73 m^2: Administer 50% of recommended dose every 24 hours

Intermittent hemodialysis (IHD) (administer after hemodialysis on dialysis days): Dialyzable (60% reduction following a 6-hour session): 2.5-5 mg/kg every 24 hours (Heintz 2009). **Note:** Dosing dependent on the assumption of 3 times weekly, complete IHD sessions.

Peritoneal dialysis (PD): Administer 50% of normal dose once daily; no supplemental dose needed (Aronoff 2007)

◀

Continuous renal replacement therapy (CRRT) (Heintz 2009; Trotman 2005): Drug clearance is highly dependent on the method of renal replacement, filter type, and flow rate. Appropriate dosing requires close monitoring of pharmacologic response, signs of adverse reactions due to drug accumulation, as well as drug concentrations in relation to target trough (if appropriate). The following are general recommendations only (based on dialysate flow/ultrafiltration rates of 1-2 L/hour and minimal residual renal function) and should not supersede clinical judgment:

CVVH: 5-10 mg/kg every 24 hours

CVVHD/CVVHDF: 5-10 mg/kg every 12-24 hours

Note: The higher end of dosage range (eg, 10 mg/kg every 12 hours for CVVHDF) is recommended for viral meningoencephalitis and varicella-zoster virus infections.

Hepatic Impairment Oral, IV: There are no dosage adjustments provided in the manufacturer's labeling; use caution in patients with severe impairment.

Obesity Obese patients should be dosed using ideal body weight.

Additional Information Complete prescribing information should be consulted for additional detail.

Dosage Forms Excipient information presented when available (limited, particularly for generics); consult specific product labeling.

Capsule, Oral:

Zovirax: 200 mg [contains fd&c blue #2 (indigotine), parabens]

Generic: 200 mg

Solution, Intravenous, as sodium [strength expressed as base]:

Generic: 50 mg/mL (10 mL, 20 mL)

Solution Reconstituted, Intravenous, as sodium [strength expressed as base]:

Generic: 500 mg (1 ea); 1000 mg (1 ea)

Suspension, Oral:

Zovirax: 200 mg/5 mL (473 mL) [contains methylparaben, propylparaben; banana flavor]

Generic: 200 mg/5 mL (473 mL)

Tablet, Oral:

Zovirax: 400 mg

Zovirax: 800 mg [contains fd&c blue #2 (indigotine)]

Generic: 400 mg, 800 mg

Acyclovir (Topical) (ay SYE kloe veer)

Brand Names: US Sitavig; Zovirax

Brand Names: Canada Zovirax

Index Terms Aciclovir; ACV; Acycloguanosine

Pharmacologic Category Antiviral Agent, Topical

Use Herpes virus:

Buccal tablet: Treatment of recurrent herpes labialis (cold sores) in immunocompetent adults.

Cream: Treatment of recurrent herpes labialis (cold sores) in immunocompetent children ≥12 years of age, adolescents, and adults.

Ointment: Management of initial genital herpes and in limited non-life-threatening mucocutaneous herpes simplex virus infections in immunocompromised patients.

Pregnancy Risk Factor B

Dosing
Adult & Geriatric
Genital HSV: Topical ointment: Initial episode: 1/2" ribbon of ointment for a 4" square surface area every 3 hours (6 times daily) for 7 days

Herpes labialis (cold sores):
Topical cream: Apply 5 times daily for 4 days
Buccal tablet: Apply one 50 mg tablet as a single dose to the upper gum region (canine fossa).

Mucocutaneous HSV (non-life-threatening, immunocompromised): Topical ointment: 1/2" ribbon of ointment for a 4" square surface area every 3 hours (6 times daily) for 7 days

Pediatric Herpes labialis (cold sores): Children ≥12 years and Adolescents: Topical cream: Refer to adult dosing.

Renal Impairment There are no dosage adjustments provided in the manufacturer's labeling. However, dosage adjustment is unlikely due to low systemic absorption.

Hepatic Impairment There are no dosage adjustments provided in the manufacturer's labeling. However, dosage adjustment is unlikely due to low systemic absorption.

Additional Information Complete prescribing information should be consulted for additional detail.

Dosage Forms Excipient information presented when available (limited, particularly for generics); consult specific product labeling. [DSC] = Discontinued product

Cream, External:
Zovirax: 5% (2 g [DSC], 5 g) [contains cetostearyl alcohol, propylene glycol]
Ointment, External:
Zovirax: 5% (30 g)
Generic: 5% (5 g, 15 g, 30 g)
Tablet, Buccal:
Sitavig: 50 mg [contains milk protein concentrate]

◆ **Acyclovir Sodium for Injection (Can)** *see* Acyclovir (Systemic) *on page 35*

◆ **Acyclovir Sodium Injection (Can)** *see* Acyclovir (Systemic) *on page 35*

◆ **AD32** *see* Valrubicin *on page 1717*

◆ **Adcetris** *see* Brentuximab Vedotin *on page 237*

◆ **Ado Trastuzumab** *see* Ado-Trastuzumab Emtansine *on page 43*

Ado-Trastuzumab Emtansine (a do tras TU zoo mab em TAN seen)
Related Information
Common Toxicity Criteria *on page 2122*
Safe Handling of Hazardous Drugs *on page 2292*

Brand Names: US Kadcyla
Brand Names: Canada Kadcyla
Index Terms Ado Trastuzumab; Adotrastuzumab; T-DM1; Trastuzumab Emtansine; Trastuzumab-DM1; Trastuzumab-MCC-DM1
Pharmacologic Category Antineoplastic Agent, Anti-HER2; Antineoplastic Agent, Antibody Drug Conjugate; Antineoplastic Agent, Antimicrotubular; Antineoplastic Agent, Monoclonal Antibody

Use Breast cancer, metastatic: Treatment (single-agent) of HER2-positive, metastatic breast cancer in patients who previously received trastuzumab and a taxane, separately or in combination, and have either received prior therapy for metastatic disease or developed disease recurrence during or within 6 months of completing adjuvant therapy.

Labeled Contraindications

US labeling: There are no contraindications in the manufacturer's labeling.

Canadian labeling: Hypersensitivity to trastuzumab emtansine or any component of the formulation.

Pregnancy Considerations Animal reproduction studies have not been conducted. **[US Boxed Warning]: Exposure to ado-trastuzumab emtansine may cause embryo-fetal death or birth defects. Effective contraception must be used in women of reproductive potential.** Oligohydramnios, pulmonary hypoplasia, skeletal malformations and neonatal death were observed following trastuzumab exposure during pregnancy (trastuzumab is the antibody component of ado-trastuzumab emtansine). The DM1 component of the ado-trastuzumab emtansine formulation is toxic to rapidly dividing cells and is also expected to cause fetal harm. Pregnancy status should be verified prior to therapy. Effective contraception is recommended during therapy and for 7 months after the last dose for women of childbearing potential.

If ado-trastuzumab emtansine exposure occurs during pregnancy or within 7 months prior to conception, healthcare providers should report the exposure to the Genentech Adverse Event Line (888-835-2555). Women exposed to ado-trastuzumab emtansine during pregnancy or within 7 months prior to conception are encouraged to enroll in MotHER Pregnancy Registry (1-800-690-6720).

European Society for Medical Oncology (ESMO) guidelines for cancer during pregnancy recommend delaying treatment with HER-2 targeted agents until after delivery in pregnant patients with HER-2 positive disease (Peccatori 2013).

Breast-Feeding Considerations It is not known if ado-trastuzumab emtansine is excreted into breast milk. Endogenous immunoglobulins are found in breast milk. Due to the potential for serious adverse reactions in the nursing infant, the decision to discontinue ado-trastuzumab emtansine or discontinue breast-feeding during treatment should take in account the wash-out period for the trastuzumab component and the benefits of treatment to the mother. Canadian labeling recommends avoiding breast-feeding for 7 months after completion of therapy.

Warnings/Precautions Hazardous agent - use appropriate precautions for handling and disposal (NIOSH 2014 [group 1]).

[US Boxed Warning]: May result in left ventricular ejection fraction (LVEF) reductions. Evaluate left ventricular function (in all patients) prior to and at least every 3 months during treatment; withhold for clinically significant left ventricular function decreases. Treatment interruption or dosage reductions are required inpatients who develop decreased LVEF. Use has not been studied in patients with LVEF <50% at baseline, with a history of symptomatic CHF, serious arrhythmia, or recent history (within 6 months) of MI or unstable angina.

[US Boxed Warning]: Serious hepatotoxicity, including liver failure and death, has been reported. Monitor transaminases and bilirubin at baseline and prior to each dose. Increases (transaminases or total bilirubin)

may require dose reductions or discontinuation. Hepatotoxicity is typically manifested by asymptomatic and transient increases in transaminases, although fatal cases of drug induced liver injury and hepatic encephalopathy have occurred; may be confounded by comorbidities or concomitant hepatotoxic medications. Use has not been studied in patients with baseline serum transaminases >2.5 times ULN or bilirubin >1.5 times ULN, or in patients with active hepatitis B or C virus. Cases of nodular regenerative hyperplasia (NRH), a rare liver disorder characterized by widespread benign transformation of hepatic parenchyma into small regenerative nodules, have been observed (by biopsy). NRH may develop into noncirrhotic portal hypertension. Consider NRH in patients with clinical symptoms of portal hypertension and/or cirrhosis-like pattern seen on liver CT scan, although without associated transaminase elevations or other manifestations of cirrhosis. Diagnosis of NRH is confirmed by histopathology; permanently discontinue if histopathology confirms NRH.

[US Boxed Warning]: Exposure to ado-trastuzumab emtansine may cause embryo-fetal death or birth defects. Effective contraception must be used in women of reproductive potential. Pregnancy status should be verified prior to therapy; effective contraception is recommended during therapy and for 7 months after the last dose for women of childbearing potential.

Infusion reactions (flushing, chills, fever, bronchospasm, dyspnea, wheezing, hypotension, and/or tachycardia) have been reported. After termination of infusion, these reactions generally resolved within several hours to a day. Medications for the treatment of reactions should be available for immediate use. Monitor closely for infusion reactions, especially during initial infusion. If reaction occurs, decrease infusion rate; for severe infusion reactions, interrupt infusion; permanently discontinue for life-threatening reactions. Serious allergic/anaphylactic reaction was observed (rare). Use is not recommended in patients who had trastuzumab permanently discontinued due to infusion reaction or hypersensitivity (has not been evaluated).

Thrombocytopenia may occur (nadir achieved: by day 8; generally resolves to ≤ grade 1 by the next scheduled dose); the incidence of thrombocytopenia may be higher in patients of Asian ancestry; monitor platelet count at baseline and prior to each dose; may require treatment interruption or dose reduction. Monitor closely if at bleeding risk due to thrombocytopenia and/or concomitant anticoagulant use. Has not been studied in patients with platelets <100,000/mm³ at treatment initiation. Neutropenia and anemia have also occurred. Hemorrhagic events, including central nervous system, respiratory, and gastrointestinal hemorrhage, have been observed; some hemorrhages were fatal. Some events occurred in patients who were receiving anticoagulation or antiplatelet therapy, or in patients with thrombocytopenia, although bleeding also occurred in patients without additional risk factors. Use caution when administering with antiplatelet agents or anticoagulants; consider additional monitoring when indicated. Local reactions (erythema, irritation, pain, swelling, or tenderness) secondary to extravasation have been noted; these were generally mild and typically occurred within 24 hours of infusion; monitor infusion site during infusion for possible infiltration. Sensory peripheral neuropathy has been reported, usually grade 1, although grade 3 peripheral neuropathy was also described; monitor for signs and symptoms of neuropathy; may require treatment interruption and/or dose reduction. Interstitial lung disease (ILD), including pneumonitis has been reported; some cases resulted in acute ▶

respiratory distress syndrome and/or fatalities; permanently discontinue with diagnosis of ILD or pneumonitis. Signs and symptoms of pneumonitis include dyspnea, cough, fatigue, and pulmonary infiltrates; may or may not occur in correlation with infusion reaction. Patients with dyspnea at rest (due to advance malignancy complications or comorbidity) may be at increased risk for pulmonary toxicity.

[US Boxed Warning]: Ado-trastuzumab emtansine and conventional trastuzumab are NOT interchangeable. Do not substitute. In Canada, the generic name for Kadcyla is trastuzumab emtansine (ie, lacks Ado- prefix) and may be confused with conventional trastuzumab. Verify product label prior to reconstitution and administration to prevent medication errors. Potentially significant drug-drug or drug-food interactions may exist, requiring dose or frequency adjustment, additional monitoring, and/or selection of alternative therapy. Establish HER2 overexpression or gene amplification status prior to treatment; has only been studied in patients with evidence of HER2 overexpression, either as 3+ IHC (Dako Herceptest™) or FISH amplification ratio ≥2 (Dako *HER2* FISH pharmDx™ test); there is only limited data on patients with breast cancer positive by FISH and 0 or 1+ by IHC.

Adverse Reactions

>10%:

Central nervous system: Fatigue (36%), headache (28%), peripheral neuropathy (21%; grades 3/4: 2%), insomnia (12%)

Dermatologic: Skin rash (12%)

Endocrine & metabolic: Decreased serum potassium (33%; grade 3: 3%)

Gastrointestinal: Nausea (40%), constipation (27%), diarrhea (24%), abdominal pain (19%), vomiting (19%), xerostomia (17%), stomatitis (14%)

Hematologic & oncologic: Decreased platelet count (83% [nadir by day 8]; grade 3: 14%; grade 4: 3%), decreased hemoglobin (60%; grade 3: 4%; grade 4: 1%), decreased neutrophils (39%; grade 3: 3%; grade 4: <1%), hemorrhage (32%; grades 3/4: 2%), thrombocytopenia (31%; grades 3/4: 15%; Asians grades 3/4: 45%), anemia (14%; grades 3/4: 4%)

Hepatic: Increased serum AST (98%; grades 3/4: <8%), increased serum ALT (82%; grades 3/4: <6%), increased serum transaminases (29%), increased serum bilirubin (17%)

Neuromuscular & skeletal: Musculoskeletal pain (36%), arthralgia (19%), weakness (18%), myalgia (14%)

Respiratory: Epistaxis (23%), cough (18%), dyspnea (12%)

Miscellaneous: Fever (19%)

1% to 10%:

Cardiovascular: Peripheral edema (7%), hypertension (5%; grades 3/4: 1%), left ventricular dysfunction (2%; grades 3/4: <1%)

Central nervous system: Dizziness (10%), chills (8%)

Dermatologic: Pruritus (6%)

Endocrine & metabolic: Hypokalemia (10%; grades 3/4: 3%)

Gastrointestinal: Dyspepsia (9%), dysgeusia (8%)

Genitourinary: Urinary tract infection (9%)

Hematologic & oncologic: Neutropenia (7%; grades 3/4: 2%)

Hepatic: Increased serum alkaline phosphatase (5%)

Hypersensitivity: Hypersensitivity (2%)

Immunologic: Antibody development (5%)

Ophthalmic: Blurred vision (5%), conjunctivitis (4%), dry eye syndrome (4%), increased lacrimation (3%)

Respiratory: Pneumonitis (≤1%)

Miscellaneous: Infusion related reaction (1%)

<1%: Anaphylactoid reaction, hepatic encephalopathy, hepatotoxicity, nodular regenerative hyperplasia, portal hypertension

Drug Interactions

Metabolism/Transport Effects Substrate of CYP3A4 (major); **Note:** Assignment of Major/Minor substrate status based on clinically relevant drug interaction potential

Avoid Concomitant Use

Avoid concomitant use of Ado-Trastuzumab Emtansine with any of the following: BCG (Intravesical); Belimumab; CloZAPine; Conivaptan; CYP3A4 Inhibitors (Strong); Dipyrone; Fusidic Acid (Systemic); Idelalisib; Natalizumab; Pimecrolimus; Tacrolimus (Topical); Tofacitinib; Vaccines (Live)

Increased Effect/Toxicity

Ado-Trastuzumab Emtansine may increase the levels/effects of: Belimumab; CloZAPine; Fingolimod; Leflunomide; Natalizumab; Tofacitinib; Vaccines (Live)

The levels/effects of Ado-Trastuzumab Emtansine may be increased by: Aprepitant; Conivaptan; CYP3A4 Inhibitors (Moderate); CYP3A4 Inhibitors (Strong); Dasatinib; Denosumab; Dipyrone; Fosaprepitant; Fusidic Acid (Systemic); Idelalisib; Ivacaftor; Luliconazole; Mifepristone; Netupitant; Osimertinib; Palbociclib; Pimecrolimus; Roflumilast; Simeprevir; Stiripentol; Tacrolimus (Topical); Trastuzumab

Decreased Effect

Ado-Trastuzumab Emtansine may decrease the levels/effects of: BCG (Intravesical); Coccidioides immitis Skin Test; Sipuleucel-T; Vaccines (Inactivated); Vaccines (Live)

The levels/effects of Ado-Trastuzumab Emtansine may be decreased by: Echinacea; Osimertinib

Storage/Stability Store intact vials at 2°C to 8°C (36°F to 46°F). Do not freeze or shake intact vials, reconstituted solution, or solutions diluted for infusion. Reconstituted vials do not contain preservative and should be used immediately, although may be stored for up to 24 hours at 2°C to 8°C (36°F to 46°F). Solutions diluted for infusion should be used immediately, although may be stored at 2°C to 8°C (36°F to 46°F) for up to 24 hours prior to use. This storage time is additional to that allowed for the reconstituted vials.

Preparation for Administration Hazardous agent; use appropriate precautions for handling and disposal (NIOSH 2014 [group 1]). Check vial labels to assure appropriate product is being reconstituted (ado-trastuzumab emtansine and conventional trastuzumab are different products and are **NOT** interchangeable).

Slowly inject sterile water for injection into the vial (5 mL for 100 mg vial or 8 mL for 160 mg vial) to a reconstituted concentration of 20 mg/mL. Gently swirl vial until completely dissolved. Reconstituted solution will be clear or slightly opalescent (there should be no visible particles) and colorless to pale brown. Dilute for infusion by adding to 250 mL sodium chloride 0.9%; gently invert bag to mix (do not shake).

Mechanism of Action Ado-trastuzumab emtansine is a HER2-antibody drug conjugate which incorporates the HER2 targeted actions of trastuzumab with the microtubule inhibitor DM1 (a maytansine derivative). The conjugate, which is linked via a stable thioether linker, allows for selective delivery into HER2 overexpressing cells, resulting in cell cycle arrest and apoptosis.

◀ **Pharmacodynamics/Kinetics**
Distribution: V_d: 3.13 L
Protein binding: DM1: 93%
Metabolism: DM1 undergoes hepatic metabolism via CYP3A4/5
Half-life elimination: ~4 days
Time to peak: Near the end of the infusion

Dosing

Adult & Geriatric Note: Do not substitute ado-trastuzumab emtansine (US) or trastuzumab emtansine (Canada) for or with conventional trastuzumab; products are different and are **NOT** interchangeable.

Breast cancer, metastatic, HER2+: IV: 3.6 mg/kg every 3 weeks until disease progression or unacceptable toxicity; Maximum dose: 3.6 mg/kg
Missed or delayed doses: If a planned dose is missed or delayed, administer as soon as possible (at the dose and rate most recently tolerated), do not wait until the next planned cycle. Then adjust schedule to maintain a 3-week interval between doses.

Renal Impairment
CrCl ≥30 mL/minute: No dosage adjustment necessary.
CrCl <30 mL/minute: There are no dosage adjustments provided in the manufacturer's labeling (has not been studied).

Hepatic Impairment
Hepatic impairment prior to treatment initiation: There are no dosage adjustments provided in the manufacturer's labeling (has not been studied).
Hepatotoxicity during treatment: Refer to Adjustment for Toxicity.

Adjustment for Toxicity Note: After a dose reduction is implemented, do not re-escalate dose.
Infusion-related reaction: Slow infusion rate or interrupt infusion. Permanently discontinue if life-threatening infusion reactions occur.
Dose levels for dosage reductions and/or discontinuation:
Starting dose: 3.6 mg/kg
First dose reduction: Reduce dose to 3 mg/kg
Second dose reduction: Reduce dose to 2.4 mg/kg
Further reductions necessary: Discontinue treatment.
Hematologic toxicity:
Grade 3 thrombocytopenia (platelets 25,000/mm^3 to <50,000/mm^3): Withhold treatment until platelet count recovers to ≤ grade 1 (platelets ≥75,000/mm^3), then resume treatment at the same dose level.
Grade 4 thrombocytopenia (platelets <25,000/mm^3): Withhold treatment until platelet count recovers to ≤ grade 1 (platelets ≥75,000/mm^3), then resume treatment with one dose level reduction.
Cardiotoxicity:
LVEF >45%: Continue treatment.
LVEF 40% to ≤45% and decrease is <10% points from baseline: Continue treatment and repeat LVEF assessment within 3 weeks.
LVEF 40% to ≤45% and decrease is ≥10% points from baseline: Withhold treatment and repeat LVEF assessment within 3 weeks; if repeat LVEF has not recovered to within 10% points from baseline, discontinue treatment.
LVEF <40%: Withhold treatment and repeat LVEF assessment within 3 weeks; if repeat LVEF is confirmed <40%, discontinue treatment.
HF (symptomatic): Discontinue treatment.

Hepatotoxicity:
Grade 2 ALT, AST elevations (>2.5 to ≤5 times ULN): Continue at same dose level.
Grade 3 ALT, AST elevations (>5 to ≤20 times ULN): Withhold until ALT, AST recover to ≤ grade 2, then resume with one dose level reduction.
Grade 4 ALT, AST elevations (>20 times ULN): Permanently discontinue treatment.
Grade 2 hyperbilirubinemia (>1.5 to ≤3 times ULN): Withhold until bilirubin recovers to ≤ grade 1 (≤1.5 times ULN), then resume at the same dose level.
Grade 3 hyperbilirubinemia (>3 to ≤10 times ULN): Withhold until bilirubin recovers to ≤ grade 1, then resume with one dose level reduction.
Grade 4 hyperbilirubinemia (>10 times ULN): Permanently discontinue treatment.
Concomitant ALT, AST >3 times ULN and total bilirubin >2 times ULN: Permanently discontinue treatment.
Nodular regenerative hyperplasia: Permanently discontinue treatment.
Peripheral neuropathy, grade 3 or 4: Temporarily discontinue until resolves to ≤ grade 2.
Pulmonary toxicity: Interstitial lung disease or pneumonitis: Permanently discontinue.
Combination Regimens
Breast cancer: Ado-Trastuzumab Emtansine (Breast) on page 1826
Administration Check label to ensure appropriate product is being administered (ado-trastuzumab emtansine [US] or trastuzumab emtansine [Canada] and conventional trastuzumab are different products and are **NOT** interchangeable).

Infuse over 90 minutes (first infusion) or over 30 minutes (subsequent infusions if prior infusions were well tolerated) through a 0.2 or 0.22 micron inline nonprotein adsorptive polyethersulfone filter. Do not administer IV push or bolus. Do not administer with other medications.

Closely monitor infusion site during administration. Monitor patient during infusion for signs of infusion-related reactions (eg, fever, chills); monitor for at least 90 minutes following initial infusion and (if tolerated) for at least 30 minutes following subsequent infusions.

Hazardous agent; use appropriate precautions for handling and disposal (NIOSH 2014 [group 1]).
Emetic Potential Low (10% to 30%)
Monitoring Parameters Platelet count (at baseline and prior to each dose), transaminases and bilirubin (at baseline and prior to each dose); verify pregnancy status prior to treatment initiation; HER2 expression status. Evaluate left ventricular function (prior to and at least every 3 months during treatment; for LVEF <40% or 40% to 45% with ≥10% absolute decrease below baseline value, reassess within 3 weeks). Monitor infusion site during infusion for possible infiltration; monitor for infusion reactions (during infusion and for 90 minutes after initial infusion and for 30 minutes after subsequent infusions); signs and symptoms of bleeding, neuropathy, and/or pulmonary toxicity
Dosage Forms Excipient information presented when available (limited, particularly for generics); consult specific product labeling.
Solution Reconstituted, Intravenous [preservative free]:
Kadcyla: 100 mg (1 ea); 160 mg (1 ea) [contains mouse protein (murine) (hamster)]

- ◆ **ADR (error-prone abbreviation)** *see* DOXOrubicin (Conventional) *on page 553*
- ◆ **AdreView™** *see* Iobenguane I 123 *on page 940*
- ◆ **Adria** *see* DOXOrubicin (Conventional) *on page 553*
- ◆ **Adriamycin** *see* DOXOrubicin (Conventional) *on page 553*
- ◆ **Adriamycin PFS (Can)** *see* DOXOrubicin (Conventional) *on page 553*
- ◆ **Adrucil** *see* Fluorouracil (Systemic) *on page 740*
- ◆ **Advagraf (Can)** *see* Tacrolimus (Systemic) *on page 1576*
- ◆ **Advate** *see* Antihemophilic Factor (Recombinant) *on page 119*
- ◆ **Adynovate** *see* Antihemophilic Factor (Recombinant [Pegylated]) *on page 123*

Afatinib (a FA ti nib)

Related Information

Common Toxicity Criteria *on page 2122*

Management of EGFR Inhibitor Toxicities: Dermatologic, Ocular, and Gastro-intestinal *on page 2179*

Safe Handling of Hazardous Drugs *on page 2292*

Brand Names: US Gilotrif

Brand Names: Canada Giotrif

Index Terms Afatinib Dimaleate; BIBW 2992

Pharmacologic Category Antineoplastic Agent, Epidermal Growth Factor Receptor (EGFR) Inhibitor; Antineoplastic Agent, Tyrosine Kinase Inhibitor

Use

Non-small cell lung cancer, metastatic: First-line treatment of metastatic non-small cell lung cancer (NSCLC) in patients whose tumors have epidermal growth factor receptor (EGFR) exon 19 deletions or exon 21 (L858R) substitution mutations as detected by an approved test.

Limitations of use: Safety and efficacy have not been established in patients whose tumors express EGFR mutations other than exon 19 deletion or exon 21 (L858R) substitution.

Labeled Contraindications

U.S. labeling: There are no contraindications listed in the manufacturer's labeling.

Canadian labeling: Hypersensitivity to afatinib or any component of the formulation.

Pregnancy Considerations Adverse events were observed in animal reproduction studies. Based on its mechanism of action, afatinib is expected to cause fetal harm if used during pregnancy. Women of reproductive potential should use highly-effective contraception during therapy and for at least 2 weeks after treatment has been discontinued.

Breast-Feeding Considerations It is not known if afatinib is excreted into breast milk. Due to the potential for serious adverse reactions in the nursing infant, the U.S. manufacturer's labeling recommends a decision be made whether to discontinue nursing or to discontinue the drug, taking into account the importance of treatment to the mother. The Canadian labeling recommends avoiding breast-feeding during therapy and for at least 2 weeks after treatment has been discontinued.

Warnings/Precautions Hazardous agent – use appropriate precautions for handling and disposal (meets NIOSH 2014 criteria). Cutaneous reactions (eg, acneiform rash, erythema, and rash) are common; grade 3 reactions (characterized by bullous, blistering, and exfoliating lesions) and palmar-plantar erythrodysesthesia syndrome were also seen in clinical trials. May require therapy interruption and dosage reduction; discontinue if life-threatening cutaneous lesions occur. Patients should be cautioned to avoid sun exposure and/or utilize adequate sun protection. Paronychia requiring dose reduction and discontinuation of therapy has been observed. In clinical trials, diarrhea and stomatitis frequently occurred in patients treated with afatinib; diarrhea was observed in the majority of patients and typically appeared within the first 6 weeks of therapy. Dehydration and renal impairment may occur as a consequence of diarrhea; monitor closely. Patients may require antidiarrheal therapy (eg, loperamide); initiate at the onset of diarrhea and continue until free of loose bowel movements for 12 hours. May necessitate therapy interruption and dosage reduction. The Canadian labeling recommends avoiding use in patients with GI disorders associated with diarrhea (eg, Crohn disease, malabsorption).

Decreases from baseline in left ventricular ejection fraction (LVEF) were noted in some patients receiving afatinib. Patients with abnormal LVEF or a significant cardiac history were excluded from clinical trials; use with caution in patients with cardiac risk factors and/or decreased LVEF. Keratitis was reported rarely in clinical trials; monitor for signs/symptoms of keratitis (eg, acute or worsening eye inflammation, blurred vision, eye pain, lacrimation, light sensitivity, red eye). Interrupt therapy in patients with suspected keratitis and consider discontinuation if diagnosis of ulcerative keratitis is confirmed (permanently discontinue for persistent ulcerative keratitis). Use with caution in patients with a history of keratitis, severe dry eye, ulcerative keratitis, or who wear contact lens (risk factor for keratitis and ulceration). Interstitial lung disease (ILD) or ILD-like reactions occurred in a small percentage of patients treated with afatinib (some fatal). ILD incidence appeared to be higher in Asian as compared to non-Asian patients. Monitor closely for signs/symptoms of ILD (eg, acute respiratory distress syndrome, allergic alveolitis, lung infiltration, pneumonitis). Interrupt therapy for suspected ILD; discontinue therapy with confirmed diagnosis.

Hepatic function test abnormalities (some fatal) were observed in clinical trials. Monitor liver function tests periodically; may require therapy interruption and dosage reduction. Discontinue if severe hepatic impairment occurs during therapy. Closely monitor patients with moderate-to-severe renal impairment, may require dosage adjustments if not tolerated. The Canadian labeling does not recommend use in severe hepatic or severe renal impairment. Potentially significant drug-drug interactions may exist, requiring dose or frequency adjustment, additional monitoring, and/or selection of alternative therapy. Safety and efficacy have not been established in patients with non-small cell lung cancer whose tumors express EGFR mutations other than exon 19 deletion or exon 21 (L858R) substitution. Increased mortality has been observed in a clinical trial evaluating afatinib in combination with vinorelbine for HER2-positive metastatic breast cancer (not an approved use). This combination was also associated with a higher incidence of adverse events (eg, diarrhea, rash), as well as fatalities due to infection and cancer progression. Afatinib should not be used in combination with vinorelbine for the treatment of HER2-positive metastatic breast cancer. Contains lactose;

Canadian labeling recommends avoiding use in patients with hereditary conditions of galactose intolerance, Lapp lactase deficiency, or glucose-galactose malabsorption.

Adverse Reactions

>10%:

Dermatologic: Acneiform eruption (90%; grade 3: 16%), paronychia (58%; grade 3: 11%), xeroderma (31%), pruritus (21%), cheilitis (12%)

Endocrine & metabolic: Weight loss (17%; grade 3: 1%), hypokalemia (11%; grades 3/4: 4%)

Gastrointestinal: Diarrhea (96%; grade 3: 15%), stomatitis (71%; grade 3: 9%), decreased appetite (29%; grade 3: 4%), vomiting (23%)

Genitourinary: Cystitis (13%; grade 3: 1%)

Hepatic: Increased serum ALT (11%; grades 3/4: 2%), increased serum AST (8%; grades 3/4: 2%)

Ophthalmic: Conjunctivitis (11%)

Respiratory: Epistaxis (17%), rhinorrhea (11%)

Miscellaneous: Fever (12%)

1% to 10%:

Central nervous system: Fatigue (<2%)

Dermatologic: Palmar-plantar erythrodysesthesia (7%)

Ophthalmic: Keratitis (2%; grade 3: <1%)

Renal: Renal insufficiency (6%; grade 3: >1%)

Respiratory: Pneumonitis (>1%; Asian descent: 2%)

<1%, postmarketing, and/or case reports: Pancreatitis, pneumonia, sepsis

Drug Interactions

Metabolism/Transport Effects Substrate of BCRP, P-glycoprotein; **Inhibits** BCRP, P-glycoprotein

Avoid Concomitant Use There are no known interactions where it is recommended to avoid concomitant use.

Increased Effect/Toxicity

Afatinib may increase the levels/effects of: Porfimer; Verteporfin

The levels/effects of Afatinib may be increased by: Lumacaftor; P-glycoprotein/ABCB1 Inhibitors

Decreased Effect

The levels/effects of Afatinib may be decreased by: Lumacaftor; P-glycoprotein/ABCB1 Inducers

Food Interactions Administration with a high-fat meal decreases C_{max} by 50% and AUC by 39% as compared to the fasted state. Management: Take at least 1 hour before or 2 hours (U.S. labeling) or 3 hours (Canadian labeling) after a meal.

Storage/Stability Store at 25°C (77°F); excursions are permitted between 15°C and 30°C (59°F and 86°F). Dispense in original bottle; protect from high humidity and light.

Mechanism of Action Highly selective blocker of the ErbB family, including EGFR (ErbB1), HER2 (ErbB2), and HER4 (ErbB4); covalently and irreversibly binds to the intracellular tyrosine kinase domain, resulting in tumor growth inhibition and tumor regression

Pharmacodynamics/Kinetics

Absorption: Decreased with high-fat meals

Protein binding: ~95%

Metabolism: Covalently adducted to proteins and nucleophilic small molecules (minimal enzymatic metabolism) (Wind, 2013)

Bioavailability: Tablets: 92% (as compared to an oral solution)
Half-life elimination: 37 hours
Time to peak: 2 to 5 hours
Excretion: Feces (85%); urine (4%); primarily as unchanged drug

Dosing

Adult & Geriatric Non-small cell lung cancer (NSCLC), metastatic, with EGFR exon 19 deletions or exon 21 (L858R) substitution mutations:
Oral: 40 mg once daily until disease progression or unacceptable toxicity
Missed doses:
  U.S. labeling: Do not take a missed dose within 12 hours of next dose
  Canadian labeling: Do not take a missed dose within 8 hours of next dose

Dosage adjustment for concomitant therapy:
U.S. labeling:
  P-gp inhibitors: If concomitant therapy is not tolerated, reduce afatinib daily dose by 10 mg. Upon discontinuation of the P-gp inhibitor, resume previous dose as tolerated.
  P-gp inducers: Increase afatinib daily dose by 10 mg if on chronic concomitant therapy with a P-gp inducer. Resume previous dose 2 to 3 days after discontinuation of P-gp inducer.
Canadian labeling: Avoid concurrent use with strong P-gp inhibitors or inducers. If concurrent use with a P-gp inhibitor is necessary, administer simultaneously with or after afatinib; monitor closely for adverse effects. The manufacturer labeling does not provide specific recommendations when concurrent use of a P-gp inducer is necessary.

Renal Impairment

Preexisting mild impairment (CrCl ≥60 mL/minute): No dosage adjustment is necessary.

Preexisting moderate-to-severe impairment (CrCl <60 mL/minute): There are no dosage adjustments provided in the manufacturer's labeling (has not been studied in patients with severe impairment [CrCl <30 mL/minute]); closely monitor and adjust dose if necessary. The Canadian labeling recommends avoiding use if CrCl <30 mL/minute.

Renal toxicity during treatment: If ≥ grade 2 renal toxicity occurs, withhold therapy. Upon improvement to baseline or ≤ grade 1, resume therapy at 10 mg per day less than previous dose.

Hepatic Impairment

Preexisting mild-to-moderate impairment (Child-Pugh class A or B): No dosage adjustment is necessary.

Preexisting severe impairment (Child-Pugh class C):
U.S. labeling: There are no dosage adjustments provided in the manufacturer's labeling (has not been studied); closely monitor and adjust dose if necessary.
Canadian labeling: Avoid use.

Hepatotoxicity during treatment: Withhold therapy for ≥ grade 3 hepatic dysfunction. Upon improvement to baseline or ≤ grade 1, resume therapy at 10 mg per day less than previous dose. Permanently discontinue for severe afatinib-induced hepatic impairment.

Adjustment for Toxicity Note: Permanently discontinue for intolerability or severe reaction occurring at a dose of 20 mg daily. The Canadian labeling recommends permanently discontinuing therapy for toxicities that do not resolve to ≤ grade 1 within 14 days of therapy interruption.

Cardiovascular: Permanently discontinue for symptomatic left ventricular dysfunction.

Dermatologic: Withhold therapy for prolonged (>7 days) or intolerable grade 2 or higher cutaneous reactions. Upon improvement to baseline or ≤ grade 1, resume therapy at 10 mg per day less than previous dose. Discontinue permanently for life-threatening bullous, blistering, or exfoliative skin lesions.

Gastrointestinal:

Diarrhea: Greater than or equal to grade 2 diarrhea that persists for ≥2 consecutive days despite antidiarrheal therapy: Interrupt therapy until resolution to ≤ grade 1, then resume at 10 mg per day less than previous dose.

Nausea/vomiting: Canadian labeling (not in U.S. labeling): Intolerable grade 2 or persistent (≥7 days) nausea/vomiting despite antiemetic therapy: Interrupt therapy until resolution to ≤ grade 1, then resume at 10 mg per day less than previous dose.

Ocular: Interrupt therapy for suspected keratitis; consider discontinuation if diagnosis of ulcerative keratitis is confirmed. Permanently discontinue for persistent ulcerative keratitis.

Pulmonary: Interrupt therapy for suspected interstitial lung disease (ILD); permanently discontinue if diagnosis is confirmed.

Other toxicity:

Greater than or equal to grade 3 adverse reactions: Withhold therapy for ≥ grade 3 adverse reactions. Upon improvement to baseline or ≤ grade 1, resume therapy at 10 mg per day less than previous dose.

Other poorly tolerated grade 2 adverse reactions persisting ≥7 days: Canadian labeling (not in U.S. labeling): Interrupt therapy until resolution to ≤ grade 1, then resume at 10 mg per day less than previous dose.

Combination Regimens

Lung cancer (non-small cell): Afatinib (NSCLC Regimen) on page 1827

Administration

U.S. labeling: Administer orally at least 1 hour before or 2 hours after a meal. Do not take a missed dose within 12 hours of the next dose. Hazardous agent; use appropriate precautions for handling and disposal (meets NIOSH 2014 criteria).

Canadian labeling: Administer orally at least 1 hour before or 3 hours after a meal. Do not take a missed dose within 8 hours of the next dose. Swallow whole with water.

Emetic Potential Minimal (<10%)

Monitoring Parameters EGFR mutation status; liver and renal function (periodically); monitor for skin toxicity, diarrhea, signs/symptoms of dehydration; monitor for signs/symptoms of interstitial lung disease (eg, acute respiratory distress syndrome, allergic alveolitis, lung infiltration, pneumonitis) and keratitis (eg, acute or worsening eye inflammation, blurred vision, eye pain, lacrimation, light sensitivity, red eye). Consider left ventricular ejection fraction assessment prior to and during therapy in patients with cardiac risk factors or conditions that may impair left ventricular function.

Dietary Considerations Take at least 1 hour before or 2 hours (U.S. labeling) or 3 hours (Canadian labeling) after a meal.

Dosage Forms Excipient information presented when available (limited, particularly for generics); consult specific product labeling.

Tablet, Oral:

Gilotrif: 20 mg

Gilotrif: 30 mg, 40 mg [contains fd&c blue #2 (indigotine)]

Dosage Forms: Canada Excipient information presented when available (limited, particularly for generics); consult specific product labeling.
Tablet, Oral:
  Giotrif: 20 mg, 30 mg, 40 mg

- **Afatinib Dimaleate** *see* Afatinib *on page 50*
- **Afinitor** *see* Everolimus *on page 656*
- **Afinitor Disperz** *see* Everolimus *on page 656*
- **Aflibercept I.V.** *see* Ziv-Aflibercept (Systemic) *on page 1785*
- **AG-013736** *see* Axitinib *on page 155*
- **Agrylin** *see* Anagrelide *on page 109*
- **AHF** *see* Antihemophilic Factor (Recombinant [Porcine Sequence]) *on page 123*
- **AHF (Human)** *see* Antihemophilic Factor (Human) *on page 117*
- **AHF (Recombinant)** *see* Antihemophilic Factor (Recombinant) *on page 119*
- **AHF (Recombinant [Pegylated])** *see* Antihemophilic Factor (Recombinant [Pegylated]) *on page 123*
- **AHF (Recombinant)** *see* Antihemophilic Factor (Recombinant [Porcine Sequence]) *on page 123*
- **A-hydroCort** *see* Hydrocortisone (Systemic) *on page 824*
- **A-Hydrocort** *see* Hydrocortisone (Systemic) *on page 824*
- **AJ-PIP/TAZ (Can)** *see* Piperacillin and Tazobactam *on page 1388*
- **Akynzeo** *see* Netupitant and Palonosetron *on page 1195*
- **ALA** *see* Aminolevulinic Acid *on page 94*
- **5-ALA** *see* Aminolevulinic Acid *on page 94*
- **Albumin-Bound Paclitaxel** *see* PACLitaxel (Protein Bound) *on page 1292*
- **Albumin-Stabilized Nanoparticle Paclitaxel** *see* PACLitaxel (Protein Bound) *on page 1292*
- **Aldara** *see* Imiquimod *on page 897*
- **Aldara P (Can)** *see* Imiquimod *on page 897*

Aldesleukin (al des LOO kin)

Related Information
  Management of Chemotherapy-Induced Nausea and Vomiting in Adults *on page 2142*
  Prevention of Chemotherapy-Induced Nausea and Vomiting in Children *on page 2203*
  Principles of Anticancer Therapy *on page 2261*
Brand Names: US Proleukin
Brand Names: Canada Proleukin
Index Terms IL-2; Interleukin 2; Interleukin-2; Lymphocyte Mitogenic Factor; Recombinant Human Interleukin-2; T-Cell Growth Factor; TCGF; Thymocyte Stimulating Factor
Pharmacologic Category Antineoplastic Agent, Biological Response Modulator; Antineoplastic Agent, Miscellaneous
Use
  Melanoma, metastatic: Treatment of metastatic melanoma
  Renal cell cancer, metastatic: Treatment of metastatic renal cell cancer

Limitations of use: Careful patient selection is necessary. Assess performance status (PS); patients with a more favorable PS (Eastern Cooperative Oncology Group [ECOG] PS 0) at treatment initiation respond better to aldesleukin (higher response rate and lower toxicity). Experience in patients with ECOG PS >1 is limited.

Labeled Contraindications Hypersensitivity to aldesleukin or any component of the formulation; patients with abnormal thallium stress or pulmonary function tests; patients who have had an organ allograft. **Re-treatment is contraindicated** in patients who have experienced sustained ventricular tachycardia (≥5 beats), uncontrolled or unresponsive cardiac arrhythmias, chest pain with ECG changes consistent with angina or MI, cardiac tamponade, intubation >72 hours, renal failure requiring dialysis for >72 hours, coma or toxic psychosis lasting >48 hours, repetitive or refractory seizures, bowel ischemia/perforation, or GI bleeding requiring surgery.

Pregnancy Considerations Adverse events were observed in animal reproduction studies. Use during pregnancy only if benefits to the mother outweigh potential risk to the fetus. Effective contraception is recommended for fertile males and/or females using this medication.

Breast-Feeding Considerations It is not known if aldesleukin is excreted in breast milk. Due to the potential for serious adverse reactions in the breast-feeding infant, a decision should be made to discontinue breast-feeding or to discontinue the drug, taking into account the importance of treatment to the mother.

Warnings/Precautions [U.S. Boxed Warning]: Aldesleukin therapy has been associated with capillary leak syndrome (CLS), characterized by vascular tone loss and extravasation of plasma proteins and fluid into extravascular space. CLS results in hypotension and reduced organ perfusion, which may be severe and can result in death. Cardiac arrhythmia, angina, myocardial infarction, respiratory insufficiency (requiring intubation), gastrointestinal bleeding or infarction, renal insufficiency, edema and mental status changes are also associated with CLS. CLS onset is immediately after treatment initiation. Monitor fluid status and organ perfusion status carefully; consider fluids and/or pressor agents to maintain organ perfusion. **[U.S. Boxed Warning]: Therapy should be restricted to patients with normal cardiac and pulmonary functions as defined by thallium stress and formal pulmonary function testing. Extreme caution should be used in patients with a history of prior cardiac or pulmonary disease** and in patients who are fluid-restricted or where edema may be poorly tolerated. Withhold treatment for signs of organ hypoperfusion, including altered mental status, reduced urine output, systolic BP <90 mm Hg or cardiac arrhythmia. Once blood pressure is normalized, may consider diuretics for excessive weight gain/edema. Recovery from CLS generally begins soon after treatment cessation. Perform a thorough clinical evaluation prior to treatment initiation; exclude patients with significant cardiac, pulmonary, renal, hepatic, or central nervous system impairment from treatment. Patients with a more favorable performance status prior to treatment initiation are more likely to respond to aldesleukin treatment, with a higher response rate and generally lower toxicity.

[U.S. Boxed Warning]: Should be administered under the supervision of an experienced cancer chemotherapy physician in a facility with cardiopulmonary or intensive specialists and intensive care facilities available. Adverse effects are frequent and sometimes fatal. May exacerbate preexisting or initial presentation of autoimmune diseases and inflammatory disorders;

exacerbation and/or new onset have been reported with aldesleukin and interferon alfa combination therapy. Thyroid disease (hypothyroidism, biphasic thyroiditis, and thyrotoxicosis) may occur; the onset of hypothyroidism is usually 4 to 17 weeks after treatment initiation; may be reversible upon treatment discontinuation (Hamnvik, 2011). Patients should be evaluated and treated for CNS metastases and have a negative scan prior to treatment; new neurologic symptoms and lesions have been reported in patients without preexisting evidence of CNS metastases (symptoms generally improve upon discontinuation, however, cases with permanent damage have been reported). Mental status changes (irritability, confusion, depression) can occur and may indicate bacteremia, sepsis, hypoperfusion, CNS malignancy, or CNS toxicity. May cause seizure; use with caution in patients with seizure disorder. Ethanol use may increase CNS adverse effects.

[U.S. Boxed Warning]: Impaired neutrophil function is associated with treatment; patients are at risk for disseminated infection (including sepsis and bacterial endocarditis), and central line-related gram-positive infections. Treat preexisting bacterial infection appropriately prior to treatment initiation. Antibiotic prophylaxis that has been associated with a reduced incidence of staphylococcal infections in aldesleukin studies includes the use of oxacillin, nafcillin, ciprofloxacin, or vancomycin. Monitor for signs of infection or sepsis during treatment.

[U.S. Boxed Warning]: Withhold treatment for patients developing moderate-to-severe lethargy or somnolence; continued treatment may result in coma. Standard prophylactic supportive care during high-dose aldesleukin treatment includes acetaminophen to relieve constitutional symptoms and an H_2 antagonist to reduce the risk of GI ulceration and/or bleeding. May impair renal or hepatic function; patients must have a serum creatinine ≤1.5 mg/dL prior to treatment. Concomitant nephrotoxic or hepatotoxic agents may increase the risk of renal or hepatic toxicity. Potentially significant drug-drug interactions may exist, requiring dose or frequency adjustment, additional monitoring, and/or selection of alternative therapy. Enhancement of cellular immune function may increase the risk of allograft rejection in transplant patients. An acute array of symptoms resembling aldesleukin adverse reactions (fever, chills, nausea, rash, pruritus, diarrhea, hypotension, edema, and oliguria) were observed within 1 to 4 hours after iodinated contrast media administration, usually when given within 4 weeks after aldesleukin treatment, although has been reported several months after aldesleukin treatment. The incidence of dyspnea and severe urogenital toxicities is potentially increased in elderly patients. Aldesleukin doses >12 to 15 million units/m^2 are associated with a moderate emetic potential; antiemetics are recommended to prevent nausea and vomiting (Dupuis, 2011).

Adverse Reactions

>10%:

Cardiovascular: Hypotension (71%; grade 4: 3%), peripheral edema (28%), tachycardia (23%), edema (15%), vasodilation (13%), supraventricular tachycardia (12%; grade 4: 1%), cardiovascular disorder (11%; includes blood pressure changes, HF and ECG changes)

Central nervous system: Chills (52%), confusion (34%; grade 4: 1%), fever (29%; grade 4: 1%), malaise (27%), somnolence (22%), anxiety (12%), pain (12%), dizziness (11%)

Dermatologic: Rash (42%), pruritus (24%), exfoliative dermatitis (18%)

◄

Endocrine & metabolic: Acidosis (12%; grade 4: 1%), hypomagnesemia (12%), hypocalcemia (11%)

Gastrointestinal: Diarrhea (67%; grade 4: 2%), vomiting (19% to 50%; grade 4: 1%), nausea (19% to 35%), stomatitis (22%), anorexia (20%), weight gain (16%), abdominal pain (11%)

Hematologic: Thrombocytopenia (37%; grade 4: 1%), anemia (29%), leukopenia (16%)

Hepatic: Hyperbilirubinemia (40%; grade 4: 2%), AST increased (23%; grade 4: 1%)

Neuromuscular & skeletal: Weakness (23%)

Renal: Oliguria (63%; grade 4: 6%), creatinine increased (33%; grade 4: 1%)

Respiratory: Dyspnea (43%; grade 4: 1%), lung disorder (24%; includes pulmonary congestion, rales, and rhonchi), cough (11%), respiratory disorder (11%; includes acute respiratory distress syndrome, infiltrates and pulmonary changes)

Miscellaneous: Antibody formation (66% to 74%), infection (13%; grade 4: 1%)

1% to 10%:

Cardiovascular: Arrhythmia (10%), cardiac arrest (grade 4: 1%), MI (grade 4: 1%), ventricular tachycardia (grade 4: 1%)

Central nervous system: Coma (grade 4: 2%), stupor (grade 4: 1%), psychosis (grade 4: 1%)

Gastrointestinal: Abdomen enlarged (10%)

Hematologic: Coagulation disorder (grade 4: 1%; includes intravascular coagulopathy)

Hepatic: Alkaline phosphatase increased (10%)

Renal: Anuria (grade 4: 5%), acute renal failure (grade 4: 1%)

Respiratory: Rhinitis (10%), apnea (grade 4: 1%)

Miscellaneous: Sepsis (grade 4: 1%)

<1%, postmarketing, and/or case reports: Agitation, allergic interstitial nephritis, anaphylaxis, angioedema, asthma, atrial arrhythmia, AV block, blindness (transient or permanent), bowel infarction/necrosis/perforation, bradycardia, bullous pemphigoid, BUN increased, capillary leak syndrome, cardiomyopathy, cellulitis, cerebral edema, cerebral lesions, cerebral vasculitis, cholecystitis, colitis, crescentic IgA glomerulonephritis, Crohn's disease exacerbation, delirium, depression (severe; leading to suicide), diabetes mellitus, duodenal ulcer, encephalopathy, endocarditis, eosinophilia, extrapyramidal syndrome, gastritis, hematemesis, hemoptysis, hemorrhage (including cerebral, gastrointestinal, retroperitoneal, subarachnoid, subdural), hepatic failure, hepatitis, hepatosplenomegaly, hypertension, hyperuricemia, hyper-/hypoventilation, hypothermia, hyperthyroidism, hypoxia, inflammatory arthritis, injection site necrosis, insomnia, intestinal obstruction, intestinal perforation, leukocytosis, lymphocytopenia, malignant hyperthermia, meningitis, mydriasis, myocardial ischemia, myocarditis, myopathy, myositis, neuralgia, neuritis, neuropathy, neutropenia, NPN increased, oculobulbar myasthenia gravis, optic neuritis, organ perfusion decreased, pancreatitis, paranoia, pericardial effusion, pericarditis, peripheral gangrene, phlebitis, pneumonia, pneumothorax, pulmonary edema, pulmonary embolus, respiratory acidosis, respiratory arrest, respiratory failure, rhabdomyolysis, scleroderma, seizure, shock, Stevens-Johnson syndrome, stroke, syncope, thrombosis, thyroiditis, tracheoesophageal fistula, transient ischemic attack, tubular necrosis, urticaria, ventricular extrasystoles

Drug Interactions
Metabolism/Transport Effects None known.
Avoid Concomitant Use
Avoid concomitant use of Aldesleukin with any of the following: BCG (Intravesical); CloZAPine; Corticosteroids; Dipyrone
Increased Effect/Toxicity
Aldesleukin may increase the levels/effects of: CloZAPine; DULoxetine; Hypotensive Agents; Iodinated Contrast Agents; Levodopa; RisperiDONE

The levels/effects of Aldesleukin may be increased by: ARIPiprazole; ARIPiprazole Lauroxil; Barbiturates; Dipyrone; Interferons (Alfa); Nicorandil
Decreased Effect
Aldesleukin may decrease the levels/effects of: BCG (Intravesical)

The levels/effects of Aldesleukin may be decreased by: Corticosteroids

Storage/Stability Store intact vials under refrigeration at 2°C to 8°C (36°F to 46°F). Protect from light. Plastic (polyvinyl chloride) bags result in more consistent drug delivery and are recommended. According to the manufacturer, reconstituted vials and solutions diluted for infusion are stable for 48 hours at room temperature or refrigerated although refrigeration is preferred because they do not contain preservatives. Do not freeze.

Preparation for Administration Reconstitute vials with 1.2 mL SWFI (preservative free) to a concentration of 18 million units (1.1 mg)/1 mL (sterile water should be injected towards the side of the vial). Gently swirl; do not shake. Further dilute with 50 mL of D5W. Smaller volumes of D5W should be used for doses ≤1.5 mg; avoid concentrations <30 mcg/mL and >70 mcg/mL (an increased variability in drug delivery has been seen). Plastic (polyvinyl chloride) bags result in more consistent drug delivery and are recommended. Filtration may result in loss of bioactivity. Addition of 0.1% albumin has been used to increase stability and decrease the extent of sorption if low final concentrations cannot be avoided.

Avoid bacteriostatic water for injection and NS for reconstitution or dilution; increased aggregation may occur.

Mechanism of Action Aldesleukin is a human recombinant interleukin-2 product which promotes proliferation, differentiation, and recruitment of T and B cells, natural killer (NK) cells, and thymocytes; causes cytolytic activity in a subset of lymphocytes and subsequent interactions between the immune system and malignant cells; can stimulate lymphokine-activated killer (LAK) cells and tumor-infiltrating lymphocytes (TIL) cells.

Pharmacodynamics/Kinetics
Absorption: Oral: Not absorbed

Distribution: Primarily into plasma, lymphocytes, lungs, liver, kidney, and spleen; V_d: 6.3 to 7.9 L (Whittington 1993)

Metabolism: Renal (metabolized to amino acids in the cells lining the proximal convoluted tubules of the kidney)

Half-life elimination: IV:
  Children: Distribution: 14 ± 6 minutes; Elimination: 51 ± 11 minutes
  Adults: Distribution: 13 minutes; Terminal: 85 minutes

Excretion: Urine (primarily as metabolites)

Dosing
Adult & Geriatric Consider premedication with an antipyretic to reduce fever, an H_2 antagonist for prophylaxis of gastrointestinal irritation/bleeding, antiemetics, and antidiarrheals; continue for 12 hours after the last aldesleukin

dose. Antibiotic prophylaxis is recommended to reduce the incidence of infection. Aldesleukin doses >12 to 15 million units/m^2 are associated with a moderate emetic potential; antiemetics are recommended to prevent nausea and vomiting.

Renal cell carcinoma, metastatic: IV: 600,000 units/kg every 8 hours for a maximum of 14 doses; repeat after 9 days for a total of 28 doses per course; re-treat if tumor shrinkage observed (and if no contraindications) at least 7 weeks after hospital discharge date

or

Off-label dosing: 720,000 units/kg every 8 hours for up to 12 doses; repeat with a second cycle 10 to 15 days later (Klapper, 2008)

Melanoma, metastatic: IV:

Single-agent use: 600,000 units/kg every 8 hours for a maximum of 14 doses; repeat after 9 days for a total of 28 doses per course; re-treat if tumor shrinkage observed (and if no contraindications) at least 7 weeks after hospital discharge date

or

Off-label dosing: 720,000 units/kg every 8 hours for 12 to 15 doses; repeat with a second cycle ~14 days after the first dose of the initial cycle (Smith, 2008)

Combination biochemotherapy (off-label use): 9 million units/m^2/day continuous infusion over 24 hours for 4 days every 3 weeks for up to 4 cycles (Atkins, 2008) **or** 9 million units/m^2/day continuous infusion over 24 hours days 5 to 8, 17 to 20, and 26 to 29 every 42 days for up to 5 cycles (Eton, 2002) **or** 9 million units/m^2/day continuous infusion over 24 hours for 4 days every 3 weeks for 6 cycles (Legha, 1998)

Pediatric Consider premedication with an antipyretic to reduce fever, an H$_2$ antagonist for prophylaxis of gastrointestinal irritation/bleeding, antiemetics, and antidiarrheals; continue for 12 hours after the last aldesleukin dose. Antibiotic prophylaxis is recommended to reduce the incidence of infection. Aldesleukin doses >12 to 15 million units/m^2 are associated with a moderate emetic potential; antiemetics are recommended to prevent nausea and vomiting (Dupuis, 2011).

Neuroblastoma (off-label use): IV: 3 million units/m^2/day continuous infusion over 24 hours daily for 4 days during week 1 and 4.5 million units/m^2/day continuous infusion over 24 hours daily for 4 days during week 2 of cycles 2 and 4 (regimen also includes isotretinoin, dinutuximab, and sargramostim) (Yu, 2010).

Renal Impairment Adults:

Renal impairment prior to treatment initiation:

Serum creatinine ≤1.5 mg/dL: There are no dosage adjustments provided in the manufacturer's labeling.

Serum creatinine >1.5 mg/dL: Do not initiate treatment.

Renal toxicity during treatment:

Serum creatinine >4.5 mg/dL (or ≥4 mg/dL with severe volume overload, acidosis, or hyperkalemia): Withhold dose; may resume when <4 mg/dL and fluid/electrolyte status is stable.

Persistent oliguria or urine output <10 mL/hour for 16 to 24 hours with rising serum creatinine: Withhold dose; may resume when urine output >10 mL/hour with serum creatinine decrease of >1.5 mg/dL or normalization.

Hemodialysis: Re-treatment is contraindicated in patients with renal failure requiring dialysis for >72 hours.

Hepatic Impairment Adults:

Hepatic impairment prior to treatment initiation: There are no dosage adjustments provided in the manufacturer's labeling.

Hepatotoxicity during treatment: Signs of hepatic failure (encephalopathy, increasing ascites, liver pain, hypoglycemia): Withhold dose and discontinue treatment for balance of cycle; may initiate a new course if indicated only after at least 7 weeks past resolution of all signs of hepatic failure (including hospital discharge).

Adjustment for Toxicity Withhold or interrupt a dose for toxicity; do not reduce the dose.

Cardiovascular toxicity:

Atrial fibrillation, supraventricular tachycardia, or bradycardia that is persistent, recurrent, or requires treatment: Withhold dose; may resume when asymptomatic with full recovery to normal sinus rhythm.

Systolic BP <90 mm Hg (with increasing pressor requirements): Withhold dose; may resume treatment when systolic BP ≥90 mm Hg and stable or pressor requirements improve.

Any ECG change consistent with MI, ischemia or myocarditis (with or without chest pain), or suspected cardiac ischemia: Withhold dose; may resume when asymptomatic, MI/myocarditis have been ruled out, suspicion of angina is low, or there is no evidence of ventricular hypokinesia.

CNS toxicity: Mental status change, including moderate confusion or agitation: Withhold dose; may resume when resolved completely.

Dermatologic toxicity: Bullous dermatitis or marked worsening of preexisting skin condition: Withhold dose; may treat with antihistamines or topical products (do not use topical steroids); may resume with resolution of all signs of bullous dermatitis.

Gastrointestinal: Stool guaiac repeatedly >3-4+: Withhold dose; may resume with negative stool guaiac.

Infection: Sepsis syndrome, clinically unstable: Withhold dose; may resume when sepsis syndrome has resolved, patient is clinically stable, and infection is under treatment.

Respiratory toxicity: Oxygen saturation <90%: Withhold dose; may resume when >90%.

Re-treatment with aldesleukin is contraindicated with the following toxicities: Sustained ventricular tachycardia (≥5 beats), uncontrolled or unresponsive cardiac arrhythmias, chest pain with ECG changes consistent with angina or MI, cardiac tamponade, intubation >72 hours, renal failure requiring dialysis for >72 hours, coma or toxic psychosis lasting >48 hours, repetitive or refractory seizures, bowel ischemia/perforation, or GI bleeding requiring surgery

Combination Regimens

Melanoma: CVD-Interleukin-Interferon (Melanoma) on page 1926

Renal cell cancer: Interleukin 2-Interferon Alfa-2 (RCC) on page 2018

Administration Aldesleukin doses >12 to 15 million units/m^2 are associated with a moderate emetic potential; antiemetics are recommended to prevent nausea and vomiting (Dupuis, 2011).

◀ Administer as IV infusion over 15 minutes (do not administer with an inline filter). Allow solution to reach room temperature prior to administration. Flush before and after with D5W, particularly if maintenance IV line contains sodium chloride. Some off-label uses/doses are infused as a continuous infusion (Legha, 1998; Yu, 2010). Has also been administered by SubQ injection (off-label route).

Emetic Potential Children and Adults:
>12 million units/m^2: Moderate (30% to 90%)
≤12 million units/m^2: Low (10% to 30%)

Monitoring Parameters

Baseline and periodic: CBC with differential and platelets, blood chemistries including electrolytes, renal and hepatic function tests, and chest x-ray; pulmonary function tests and arterial blood gases (baseline), thallium stress test (prior to treatment). Monitor thyroid function tests (TSH at baseline then every 2-3 months during aldesleukin treatment [Hamnvik, 2011]).

Monitoring during therapy should include daily (hourly if hypotensive) vital signs (temperature, pulse, blood pressure, and respiration rate), weight and fluid intake and output; in a patient with a decreased blood pressure, especially systolic BP <90 mm Hg, cardiac monitoring for rhythm should be conducted. If an abnormal complex or rhythm is seen, an ECG should be performed; vital signs in these hypotension patients should be taken hourly and central venous pressure (CVP) checked; monitor for change in mental status, and for signs of infection.

Additional Information 18 x 10^6 units = 1.1 mg protein

Dosage Forms Excipient information presented when available (limited, particularly for generics); consult specific product labeling.

Solution Reconstituted, Intravenous [preservative free]:
Proleukin: 22,000,000 units (1 ea)

Alemtuzumab (ay lem TU zoo mab)

Related Information

Chemotherapy and Obesity *on page 2220*
Common Toxicity Criteria *on page 2122*
Management of Chemotherapy-Induced Nausea and Vomiting in Adults *on page 2142*
Prevention and Management of Infections *on page 2196*
Prevention of Chemotherapy-Induced Nausea and Vomiting in Children *on page 2203*
Principles of Anticancer Therapy *on page 2261*

Brand Names: US Campath; Lemtrada

Brand Names: Canada Lemtrada; MabCampath

Index Terms Anti-CD52 Monoclonal Antibody; Campath; Campath-1H; Humanized IgG1 Anti-CD52 Monoclonal Antibody; MoAb CD52; Monoclonal Antibody Campath-1H; Monoclonal Antibody CD52

Pharmacologic Category Antineoplastic Agent, Anti-CD52; Antineoplastic Agent, Monoclonal Antibody; Monoclonal Antibody

Use

B-cell chronic lymphocytic leukemia: Campath or MabCampath [Canadian product]: Treatment (as a single agent) of B-cell chronic lymphocytic leukemia (B-CLL)

Multiple sclerosis, relapsing: Lemtrada: Treatment of patients with relapsing forms of multiple sclerosis (MS), generally who have had an inadequate response to 2 or more medications indicated for the treatment of MS.

Labeled Contraindications

U.S. labeling: There are no contraindications listed in the manufacturer's Campath labeling. Lemtrada is contraindicated in patients infected with HIV (due to prolonged reduction in CD4+ lymphocytes).

Canadian labeling:

Lemtrada: Hypersensitivity to alemtuzumab or any component of the formulation; HIV infection; active or latent tuberculosis; severe active infections; active malignancies; concurrent antineoplastic or immunosuppressive therapy; history of progressive multifocal leukoencephalopathy (PML)

MabCampath: Known type 1 hypersensitivity or anaphylactic reactions to alemtuzumab or any component of the formulation; active infections; underlying immunodeficiency (eg, seropositive for HIV); active secondary malignancies; current or history of progressive multifocal leukoencephalopathy (PML)

Pregnancy Considerations Adverse events were observed in animal reproduction studies. Human IgG is known to cross the placental barrier; therefore, alemtuzumab may also cross the barrier and cause fetal B- and T-lymphocyte depletion. Use during pregnancy only if the benefit to the mother outweighs the potential risk to the fetus. Effective contraception is recommended during and for at least 6 months (Campath) or 4 months (Lemtrada) after treatment for women of childbearing potential and men of reproductive potential.

Breast-Feeding Considerations Human IgG is excreted in breast milk; therefore, alemtuzumab may also be excreted in milk. Due to the potential for serious adverse reactions in the nursing infant, the decision to discontinue alemtuzumab or to discontinue breast-feeding should take into account the importance of treatment to the mother and the half-life of alemtuzumab. The Canadian labeling recommends discontinuing nursing during treatment and for at least 3 months (MabCampath) or 4 months (Lemtrada) after completing treatment course.

Warnings/Precautions [U.S. Boxed Warning (Lemtrada)]: Alemtuzumab causes serious, sometimes fatal, autoimmune conditions, such as immune thrombocytopenia and antiglomerular basement membrane disease, in patients receiving alemtuzumab for the treatment of multiple sclerosis (MS). Monitor complete blood counts with differential, serum creatinine levels, and urinalysis with urine cell counts at periodic intervals for 48 months after the last dose of alemtuzumab. Monitor for symptoms of immune thrombocytopenia (easy bruising, petechiae, spontaneous mucocutaneous bleeding, heavy menstrual bleeding) in patients receiving alemtuzumab for MS. Monitor for nephropathy symptoms (eg, elevated serum creatinine, hematuria, proteinuria). Alveolar hemorrhage manifesting as hemoptysis may be present in antiglomerular basement membrane disease. Glomerular nephropathies require urgent evaluation; may lead to renal failure if not treated. Prompt intervention is necessary for autoimmune cytopenias. Idiopathic thrombocytopenic purpura, thyroid disorders, autoimmune hemolytic anemia, autoimmune pancytopenia, undifferentiated connective tissue disorders, acquired hemophilia A, rheumatoid arthritis, vitiligo, retinal pigment epitheliopathy have been reported in patients receiving alemtuzumab for MS. Guillain-Barre syndrome and chronic inflammatory demyelinating polyradiculoneuropathy have been reported in patients receiving alemtuzumab for other uses. Alemtuzumab may increase the risk for other autoimmune conditions.

◀

Autoimmune thyroid disorders occurred in over one-third of patients receiving alemtuzumab for MS. In a trial evaluating alemtuzumab versus interferon beta-1a in patients with MS, thyroid dysfunction occurred more frequently in patients taking alemtuzumab (34% versus 6.5%) (Daniels, 2014). The incidence of the first episode of thyroid dysfunction increased annually the first 3 years (year 1: 4.6%; year 2: 13.3%; year 3: 16.1%) then gradually decreased thereafter. Among patients with alemtuzumab-related thyroid dysfunction, Graves' hyperthyroidism occurred most commonly (23%), followed by hypothyroidism and subacute thyroiditis (7% and 4%, respectively). Thyroid dysfunction (thyroiditis, Graves' disease) has also been reported with alemtuzumab use for the treatment of other conditions. For B-CLL treatment, TSH monitoring is recommended; monitor TSH at baseline and every 2 to 3 months during alemtuzumab treatment (Hamnvik, 2011). For MS, monitor TSH at baseline and every 3 months until 48 months after last infusion or longer or at any time during therapy if clinically indicated.

[U.S. Boxed Warning]: Serious and potentially fatal infusion-related reactions may occur; monitor for infusion reaction; carefully monitor during infusion; withhold treatment for serious or grade 3 or 4 infusion reactions. For B-cell chronic lymphocytic leukemia (B-CLL), gradual escalation to the recommended maintenance dose is required at initiation and with treatment interruptions (for ≥7 days) to minimize infusion-related reactions. For multiple sclerosis, must be administered in a setting with appropriate equipment and personnel to manage anaphylaxis or serious infusion reaction; monitor for 2 hours after each infusion; inform patients that serious infusion reactions may also occur after the 2-hour monitoring period. Infusion reactions have been reported more than 24 hours after infusion. In patients treated for B-CLL, infusion reaction symptoms may include acute respiratory distress syndrome, anaphylactic shock, angioedema, bronchospasm, cardiac arrest, cardiac arrhythmias, chills, dyspnea, fever, hypotension, myocardial infarction, pulmonary infiltrates, rash, rigors, syncope, or urticaria. The incidence of infusion reaction is highest during the first week of B-CLL treatment. Premedicate with acetaminophen and an oral antihistamine. Medications for the treatment of reactions should be available for immediate use. Use caution and carefully monitor blood pressure in patients with ischemic heart disease and patients on antihypertensive therapy. For B-CLL, reinitiate with gradual dose escalation if treatment is withheld ≥7 days. Similar infusion reactions have been observed with use in the treatment of multiple sclerosis; premedication with corticosteroids for initial 3 days of each treatment course is recommended. Antihistamines and/or antipyretics may also be considered. Consider additional monitoring in patients with existing cardiovascular or respiratory compromise (the Canadian labeling recommends obtaining an ECG prior to each treatment course). Observe for infusion-related reactions; advise patients to monitor for signs/symptoms of infusion reaction, particularly during the 24 hours following infusion.

[U.S. Boxed Warning (Campath)]: Serious and fatal cytopenias (including pancytopenia, bone marrow hypoplasia, autoimmune hemolytic anemia, and autoimmune idiopathic thrombocytopenia) have occurred. Single doses >30 mg or cumulative weekly doses >90 mg are associated with an increased incidence of pancytopenia. Severe prolonged myelosuppression, hemolytic anemia, pure red cell aplasia, bone marrow aplasia, and bone marrow hypoplasia have also been reported with use at the normal dose for the treatment of B-CLL. Discontinue for serious hematologic or other serious toxicity (except lymphopenia) until the event resolves. Permanently discontinue if autoimmune anemia or autoimmune thrombocytopenia occurs. Patients receiving blood products should only receive irradiated blood products due to the potential for transfusion-associated GVHD during lymphopenia.

[U.S. Boxed Warning (Campath)]: Serious and potentially fatal infections (bacterial, viral, fungal, and protozoan) have been reported. Administer prophylactic medications against PCP pneumonia and herpes viral infections during treatment and for at least 2 months following last dose or until CD4+ counts are ≥200 cells/mm^3 (whichever is later). Severe and prolonged lymphopenia may occur; CD4+ counts usually return to ≥200 cells/mm^3 within 2 to 6 months; however, CD4+ and CD8+ lymphocyte counts may not return to baseline levels for more than 1 year. Withhold treatment during serious infections; may be reinitiated upon resolution of infection. Monitor for CMV infection (during and for at least 2 months after completion of therapy); initiate appropriate antiviral treatment and withhold alemtuzumab for CMV infection or confirmed CMV viremia (withhold alemtuzumab during CMV antiviral treatment). For patients being treated for MS, initiate antiviral prophylaxis (for herpetic viral infections) beginning on the first day of treatment and continue for at least 2 months or until CD4+ lymphocyte count is ≥200/mm^3. In clinical trials for MS, infections seen more commonly in alemtuzumab-treated patients included nasopharyngitis, urinary tract infection, upper respiratory tract infection, sinusitis, herpetic infections, influenza, and bronchitis; serious cases of appendicitis, gastroenteritis, pneumonia, herpes zoster, and tooth infection also occurred. Consider delaying treatment in patients with active infection until infection is controlled. Patients should be screened for human papilloma virus (HPV) and tuberculosis as clinically necessary. Progressive multifocal leukoencephalopathy (PML) been reported with use (rarely); withhold therapy immediately for signs/symptoms suggestive of PML. According to the Canadian labeling, alemtuzumab is contraindicated in patients with a history of PML.

[U.S. Boxed Warning (Lemtrada)]: Alemtuzumab may cause an increased risk of malignancies, including thyroid cancer, melanoma, and lymphoproliferative disorders, Perform baseline and yearly skin exams. Other malignant neoplasm (breast cancer or basal cell carcinoma) has been observed (rarely) in patients receiving treatment for MS. Use of Lemtrada in patients with active malignancies is contraindicated; use caution if initiating treatment in patients with preexisting malignancy (Canadian labeling).

Pneumonitis (hypersensitivity or fibrosis) has been reported. Monitor for symptoms (dyspnea, cough, wheezing, hemoptysis, chest pain/tightness). Alemtuzumab is associated with a moderate emetic potential in the oncology setting; antiemetics may be recommended to prevent nausea and vomiting (Basch, 2011; Roila, 2010). Potentially significant drug-drug interactions may exist, requiring dose or frequency adjustment, additional monitoring, and/or selection of alternative therapy. If considering Lemtrada treatment for use in a patient who has previously received Campath/MabCampath, consider the additive and long-lasting immune system effects. Patients should not be immunized with live, viral vaccines during or recently after treatment. The ability to respond to any vaccine following therapy is unknown. Testing for antibodies to varicella zoster virus (VZV) is recommended prior to initiation of Lemtrada if history of chickenpox or VZV vaccination status is unknown. When using for the treatment of multiple sclerosis, complete necessary immunizations at least 6 weeks prior to initiating alemtuzumab. Determine if patient has a history varicella or vaccination for VZV; if not, test for VZV antibodies and consider vaccinations for antibody-negative patients; postpone alemtuzumab treatment for 6 weeks following VZV vaccination.

Alemtuzumab is not recommended for use in MS patients with inactive disease or who are stable on other treatment. Patients should commit to at least 48 months of follow-up after the last infusion. Alemtuzumab has not been studied in MS patients infected with HBV or HCV; consider screening patients at increased risk of infection prior to initiating treatment. Use with caution in HBV or HCV carriers; patients may be at risk for viral reactivation. **[U.S. Boxed Warning (Lemtrada)]: Due to the risk of autoimmunity, infusion reactions, and malignancies, alemtuzumab is available only through restricted distribution under a Risk Evaluation Mitigation Strategy (REMS) Program when used for the treatment of MS. Contact 1-855-676-6326 to enroll in the Lemtrada REMS program.** Prescribers and pharmacies must be certified with the REMS program, and patients and healthcare facilities must be enrolled and comply with ongoing monitoring.

Adverse Reactions Adverse reactions listed below are reflective of both the U.S. and Canadian product information.

>10%:

Central nervous system: Headache (44% to 52%), fatigue (8% to 21%), insomnia (11% to 17%), paresthesia (10% to 12%)

Dermatologic: Skin rash (43% to 53%), urticaria (15% to 17%), pruritus (13% to 17%)

Endocrine & metabolic: Thyroid disease (13% to 34%)

Gastrointestinal: Nausea (16% to 22%), diarrhea (12%), oral candidiasis (3% to 12%)

Genitourinary: Urinary tract infection (18% to 19%), vulvovaginal candidiasis (3% to 12%)

Hematologic & oncologic: Lymphocytopenia (6% to 100%)

Immunologic: Antibody development (8% to 85%; no effect on drug efficacy; anti-alemtuzumab: 2%)

Infection: Infection (71%), herpes virus infection (16%), fungal infection (12% to 13%)

Local: Infusion related reaction (92%)

Neuromuscular & skeletal: Arthralgia (12% to 13%), limb pain (13%), back pain (12%)

Respiratory: Nasopharyngitis (24% to 25%), upper respiratory tract infection (15% to 16%), oropharyngeal pain (11%), sinusitis (11%)

Miscellaneous: Fever (26% to 30%)

1% to 10%:

Cardiovascular: Flushing (10%), chest discomfort (7% to 8%), tachycardia (6% to 8%), peripheral edema (5%), palpitations (4%), bradycardia (3%), hypotension (3%), chest pain (2%), cold extremities (1%)

Central nervous system: Chills (9% to 10%), dizziness (10%), anxiety (7%), pain (5% to 7%), vertigo (4%), equilibrium disturbance (3%), hyperthermia (3%), increased body temperature (3%), drowsiness (2%), facial hypoesthesia (2%), hypertonia (2%)

Dermatologic: Skin rash (generalized; 7% to 8%), erythema (6%), acne vulgaris (3%), allergic dermatitis (3%), alopecia (3%), erythematous rash (3%), hyperhidrosis (3%), pruritic rash (3%), papular rash (2%), pruritus (generalized; 2%), skin blister (1%), xeroderma (1%)

Endocrine & metabolic: Hypothyroidism (5%), hypermenorrhea (4%), hyperthyroidism (4%), chronic lymphocytic thyroiditis (2%), Graves' disease (2%), thyroid stimulating hormone suppression (2%), goiter (1%)

Gastrointestinal: Vomiting (10%), abdominal pain (5% to 10%), oral herpes (9%), dyspepsia (6% to 9%), dysgeusia (8%), gastroenteritis (4%), upper abdominal pain (4%), abdominal distention (2%), oral mucosa ulcer (1%)

Genitourinary: Occult blood in urine (4% to 8%), uterine hemorrhage (5%), hematuria (3%), cystitis (2%), fungal vaginosis (2%), increase in urinary protein (2%), irregular menses (2%), proteinuria (2%), abnormal urinalysis (1%), herpes genitalis (1%), vaginal hemorrhage (1%)

Hematologic & oncologic: Bruise (10%), decreased CD-4 cell count (5% to 6%), decreased CD-8 cell counts (5% to 6%), decreased absolute lymphocyte count (4% to 5%), decreased T cell lymphocytes (4%), reduction of B-cells (4%), abnormal white blood cell differential (lymphocyte percentage decreased: 3%; lymphocyte percentage increased: 2%), immune thrombocytopenia (2%), nonthrombocytopenic purpura (2%), hematoma (1%), petechia (1%)

Hypersensitivity: Cytokine release syndrome (2%)

Infection: Influenza (8%), herpes zoster (4%), bacterial infection (3%), herpes simplex infection (2%), human papilloma virus infection (2%)

Local: Catheter pain (1%)

Neuromuscular & skeletal: Myalgia (6% to 7%), myasthenia (7%), muscle spasm (6%), weakness (5% to 6%), neck pain (5%), joint sprain (2%), joint swelling (2%), musculoskeletal chest pain (2%)

Ophthalmic: Blurred vision (5%), conjunctivitis (2%), Graves' ophthalmopathy (1%)

Otic: Otalgia (3%), otic infection (3%)

Respiratory: Cough (9%), dyspnea (8% to 9%), bronchitis (7%), epistaxis (5%), pharyngitis (4%), rhinitis (4%), sinus congestion (3%), nasal congestion (2%), wheezing (2%), bronchospasm (1%)

<1%, postmarketing, and/or case reports: Abnormal gait, abnormal hepatic function tests, acquired blood coagulation disorder, agitation, allodynia, altered blood pressure, amenorrhea, anaphylactic shock, anaphylaxis, anemia, angina pectoris, angioedema, anti-GBM disease, antithyroid antibody positive, aphthous stomatitis, aplastic anemia, asthma, ataxia, atrial fibrillation, autoimmune hemolytic anemia, autoimmune thrombocytopenia, bacterial vaginosis, bacteriuria, bacteriuria (asymptomatic), burning sensation, candidiasis, cardiac failure, cardiomyopathy, casts in urine, catheter-site erythema, catheter-site reaction (rash), cellulitis, cervical dysplasia, cervicitis, choking sensation, chronic inflammatory demyelinating polyradiculoneuropathy, connective tissue disease (undifferentiated), constipation, constriction of the pharynx, crystalluria, cutaneous papilloma, decreased appetite, decreased free T4, decreased hematocrit, decreased hemoglobin, decreased monocytes, decreased neutrophils, decreased T3 level, dehydration, depression, desquamation, diaphoresis, disturbance in attention, dry eye syndrome, dysesthesia, dysmenorrhea, dysphagia, dyssomnia, dysuria, ecchymoses, eczema, edema, eosinopenia, eosinophilia, Epstein-Barr-associated lymphoproliferative disorder, Epstein-Barr infection, esophageal candidiasis, esophagitis, eye pain, eyelid edema, facial edema, facial pain, facial swelling, feeling of heaviness, flatulence, fungal skin infection, furuncle, gastritis, gastroesophageal reflux disease, gastrointestinal disease, gingival hemorrhage, gingival pain, gingivitis, glossalgia, glycosuria, graft versus host disease (transfusion associated), Guillain-Barre syndrome, hematochezia, hemiparesis, hemolytic anemia, hemophilia A (acquired [anti-Factor VIII

antibodies]), hemoptysis, hiccups, hyperemia, hyperesthesia, hypersensitivity reaction, hypopigmentation, increased blood pressure, increased free T4, increased heart rate, increased monocytes, increased serum alkaline phosphatase, increased serum ALT, increased serum AST, increased serum bilirubin, increased T3 level, infusion site reaction, iron deficiency anemia, irritability, joint stiffness, labyrinthitis, laryngitis, leukocytosis, leukocyturia, limb pain, local alterations in temperature sensations, lower respiratory tract infection, lymphoproliferative disorder, macular eruption, maculopapular rash, major hemorrhage, malignant lymphoma, malignant melanoma, malignant neoplasm of thyroid, membranous glomerulonephritis, memory impairment, meningitis due to listeria monocytogenes, meningitis (herpes), menstrual disease, microcytic anemia, migraine, mucosal inflammation, multiple sclerosis, muscle spasticity, musculoskeletal pain, natural killer cell count increased, neutropenia, night sweats, noncardiac chest pain, onychomycosis, optic neuropathy, oropharyngeal blistering, ostealgia, ovarian cyst, pain at injection site, painful respiration, pallor, pancytopenia, papule, periorbital edema, peripheral neuropathy, pharyngeal erythema, photophobia, pityriasis rosea, pleurisy, pneumonia, pneumonitis, pollakiuria, positive direct Coombs test, postherpetic neuralgia, presyncope, progressive multifocal leukoencephalopathy, protozoal infection, prurigo, pruritus of ear, psychomotor agitation, pyelonephritis, reactivation of disease, reduced ejection fraction, respiratory congestion (upper), respiratory tract infection, restless leg syndrome, restlessness, retinal pigment changes (epitheliopathy), rheumatoid arthritis, rhinorrhea, seasonal allergy, sensation of cold, sensory disturbance, serum sickness, skin hyperpigmentation, skin infection, skin irritation, skin lesion, stiffness, streptococcal pharyngitis, subacute thyroiditis, suicidal ideation, suicidal tendencies, syncope, tachypnea, throat irritation, thrombocytopenia, thyroiditis, tinea, tinea pedis, tinea versicolor, tinnitus, tongue discoloration, tonsillitis, tooth abscess, tooth infection, toothache, tracheobronchitis, tuberculosis, tumor lysis syndrome, type 1 diabetes mellitus, upper airway symptoms (cough syndrome), urethritis, urinary incontinence, urinary urgency, urine abnormality, vaginal infection, varicella, viral infection, viral respiratory tract infection, visual disturbance, vitiligo, voice disorder, weight gain, weight loss, xerostomia

Drug Interactions

Metabolism/Transport Effects None known.

Avoid Concomitant Use

Avoid concomitant use of Alemtuzumab with any of the following: BCG (Intravesical); Belimumab; CloZAPine; Dipyrone; Natalizumab; Pimecrolimus; Tacrolimus (Topical); Tofacitinib; Vaccines (Live)

Increased Effect/Toxicity

Alemtuzumab may increase the levels/effects of: Belimumab; CloZAPine; Fingolimod; Leflunomide; Natalizumab; Tofacitinib; Vaccines (Live)

The levels/effects of Alemtuzumab may be increased by: Denosumab; Dipyrone; Pimecrolimus; Roflumilast; Tacrolimus (Topical); Trastuzumab

Decreased Effect

Alemtuzumab may decrease the levels/effects of: BCG (Intravesical); Coccidioides immitis Skin Test; Sipuleucel-T; Vaccines (Inactivated); Vaccines (Live)

The levels/effects of Alemtuzumab may be decreased by: Echinacea

Storage/Stability

Campath: Prior to dilution, store intact (30 mg/1 mL) vials at 2°C to 8°C (36°F to 46°F); do not freeze (if accidentally frozen, thaw in refrigerator prior to administration). Do not shake; protect from light. Following dilution, store at room temperature or refrigerate; protect from light; use within 8 hours. Discard unused portion in the vial.

Lemtrada: Prior to dilution, store intact vials at 2°C to 8°C (36°F to 46°F). Do not freeze. Do not shake; protect from light. Following dilution, store at room temperature or refrigerate; use within 8 hours.

MabCampath [Canadian product]: Prior to dilution, store vials at 2°C to 8°C (36°F to 46°F). Do not freeze (discard vial if frozen). Do not shake. Protect from light. Following dilution, store at room temperature or refrigerate; use within 8 hours.

Preparation for Administration

Campath, MabCampath [Canadian product]: Dilute for infusion in 100 mL NS or D5W. Compatible in polyvinylchloride (PVC) bags. Gently invert the bag to mix the solution. Do not shake prior to use.

Lemtrada: Withdraw 12 mg (1.2 mL) from vial and add to 100 mL bag of NS or D5W. Gently invert the bag to mix the solution.

Mechanism of Action Binds to CD52, a nonmodulating antigen present on the surface of B and T lymphocytes, a majority of monocytes, macrophages, NK cells, and a subpopulation of granulocytes. After binding to CD52$^+$ cells, an antibody-dependent lysis of malignant cells occurs. In multiple sclerosis, alemtuzumab immunomodulatory effects may include alteration in the number, proportions, and properties of some lymphocyte subsets following treatment.

Pharmacodynamics/Kinetics

Distribution: V_d: IV: Campath: 0.18 L/kg (range: 0.1 to 0.4 L/kg); Lemtrada: 14.1 L

Metabolism: Campath: Clearance decreases with repeated dosing (due to loss of CD52 receptors in periphery), resulting in a sevenfold increase in AUC after 12 weeks of therapy.

Half-life elimination: IV: Campath: 11 hours (following first 30 mg dose; range: 2 to 32 hours); 6 days (following the last 30 mg dose; range: 1 to 14 days); Lemtrada: ~2 weeks

Dosing

Adult & Geriatric

B-cell chronic lymphocytic leukemia (B-CLL): Campath: IV: Gradually escalate to a maintenance of 30 mg per dose 3 times weekly on alternate days for a total duration of therapy of up to 12 weeks (Hillmen, 2007; Keating, 2002)

Note: Dose escalation is required; usually accomplished in 3 to 7 days. Single doses >30 mg or cumulative doses >90 mg/week increase the incidence of pancytopenia. Pretreatment (with acetaminophen 500 to 1,000 mg and diphenhydramine 50 mg) is recommended prior to the first dose, with dose escalations, and as clinically indicated; IV glucocorticoids may be used for severe infusion-related reactions. Administer antiviral prophylaxis (for herpetic viral infections) and *Pneumocystis jiroveci* pneumonia (PCP) prophylaxis; continue for at least 2 months after completion of alemtuzumab and until CD4+ lymphocyte count is ≥200/mm^3. Reinitiate with gradual dose escalation if treatment is withheld ≥7 days. Alemtuzumab is associated with a moderate emetic potential in the oncology setting; antiemetics may be recommended to prevent nausea and vomiting (Basch, 2011; Roila, 2010).

Dose escalation: Initial: 3 mg daily beginning on day 1; if tolerated (infusion reaction ≤ grade 2), increase to 10 mg daily; if tolerated (infusion reaction ≤ grade 2), may increase to maintenance of 30 mg per dose 3 times weekly if required.

B-CLL (off-label route): SubQ: Initial: 3 mg on day 1; if tolerated 10 mg on day 3; if tolerated increase to 30 mg on day 5; maintenance: 30 mg per dose 3 times weekly for a maximum of 18 weeks (Lundin, 2002) **or** 3 mg on day 1; if tolerated 10 mg on day 2; if tolerated 30 mg on day 3, followed by 30 mg per dose 3 times weekly for 4 to 12 weeks (Stilgenbauer, 2009)

Multiple sclerosis, relapsing: Lemtrada: IV: 12 mg daily for 5 consecutive days (total 60 mg), followed 12 months later by 12 mg daily for 3 consecutive days (total 36 mg); total duration of therapy: 24 months.

Note: Premedicate with corticosteroids (methylprednisolone 1,000 mg or equivalent) immediately prior to alemtuzumab for the first 3 days of each treatment course. Antihistamines and/or antipyretics may also be considered. Administer antiviral prophylaxis (for herpetic viral infections) beginning on the first day of treatment and continue for at least 2 months after completion of alemtuzumab and until CD4+ lymphocyte count is ≥200/mm^3. In some clinical trials patients received an additional 12 mg daily for 3 consecutive days 12 months later (total duration of 36 months) (CAMMS223, 2008; Coles, 2012).

Autoimmune cytopenias, CLL-induced, refractory (off-label use): IV, SubQ: Gradually escalate to a maintenance of 10 to 30 mg per dose 3 times weekly for 4 to 12 weeks (Karlsson, 2007; Osterborg, 2009)

Graft versus host disease (GVHD), acute, steroid refractory, treatment (off-label use): IV: 10 mg daily for 5 consecutive days, then 10 mg weekly on days 8, 15, and 22 if CR not achieved (Martinez, 2009) **or** 10 mg weekly until symptom resolution (Schnitzler, 2009)

Renal transplant, induction (off-label use): IV: 30 mg as a single dose at the time of transplant (Hanaway, 2011)

Stem cell transplant (allogeneic) conditioning regimen (off-label use): IV: 20 mg daily for 5 days (in combination with fludarabine and melphalan) beginning 8 days prior to transplant (Mead, 2010) **or** beginning 7 days prior to transplant (Van Besien, 2009)

T-cell prolymphocytic leukemia (T-PLL; off-label use): IV: Initial test dose 3 mg or 10 mg, followed by dose escalation to 30 mg per dose 3 times weekly as tolerated until maximum response (Dearden, 2001) **or** Initial dose: 3 mg day 1, if tolerated increase to 10 mg day 2, if tolerated increase to 30 mg on day 3 (days 1, 2, and 3 are consecutive days), followed by 30 mg per dose every Monday, Wednesday, Friday for a total of 4 to 12 weeks (Keating, 2002)

Renal Impairment There are no dosage adjustments provided in the manufacturer's labeling (has not been studied).

Hepatic Impairment There are no dosage adjustments provided in the manufacturer's labeling (has not been studied).

Obesity *American Society for Blood and Marrow Transplantation (ASBMT) practice guideline committee position statement on chemotherapy dosing in obesity:* Utilize a flat dose based on the regimen selected for hematopoietic stem cell transplant conditioning in adults (Bubalo, 2014).

Adjustment for Toxicity
Dosage adjustment for nonhematologic toxicity:
Treatment of B-CLL: Campath:
Note: If treatment is withheld ≥7 days, reinitiate at 3 mg with re-escalation to 10 mg and then 30 mg.
Grade 3 or 4 infusion reaction: Withhold infusion
Serious infection or other serious adverse reaction: Withhold alemtuzumab until resolution
Autoimmune anemia or autoimmune thrombocytopenia: Discontinue alemtuzumab
Treatment of MS: Lemtrada: Serious infusion reaction: Consider immediate discontinuation

Dosage adjustment for hematologic toxicity (severe neutropenia or thrombocytopenia, not autoimmune): Treatment of B-CLL: Campath:
Note: If treatment is withheld ≥7 days, reinitiate at 3 mg with re-escalation to 10 mg and then 30 mg.
ANC <250/mm^3 and/or platelet count ≤25,000/mm^3:
First occurrence: Withhold treatment; resume at 30 mg per dose when ANC ≥500/mm^3 and platelet count ≥50,000/mm^3
Second occurrence: Withhold treatment; resume at 10 mg per dose when ANC ≥500/mm^3 and platelet count ≥50,000/mm^3
Third occurrence: Discontinue alemtuzumab.
Patients with a baseline ANC ≤250/mm^3 and/or a baseline platelet count ≤25,000/mm^3 at initiation of therapy: If ANC and/or platelet counts decrease to ≤50% of the baseline value:
First occurrence: Withhold treatment; resume at 30 mg per dose upon return to baseline values
Second occurrence: Withhold treatment; resume at 10 mg per dose upon return to baseline values
Third occurrence: Discontinue alemtuzumab.

Administration
Campath or MabCampath [Canadian product]: Administer by IV infusion over 2 hours. Premedicate with diphenhydramine 50 mg and acetaminophen 500 to 1000 mg 30 minutes before each infusion. IV glucocorticoids have been effective in decreasing severe infusion-related events. Start anti-infective prophylaxis. Other drugs should not be added to or simultaneously infused through the same IV line. Do not give IV push or bolus. Compatible in polyvinylchloride (PVC) or polyethylene lined administration sets or low protein binding filters.
Campath: SubQ (off-label route): SubQ administration has been studied (Lundin, 2002; Stilgenbauer, 2009); an increased rate of injection site reactions has been observed, with only rare incidences of chills or infusion-like reactions typically observed with IV infusion. A longer dose escalation time (1 to 2 weeks) may be needed due to injection site reactions (Lundin, 2002). Premedicate with diphenhydramine 50 mg and acetaminophen 500 to 1000 mg 30 minutes before dose. The subQ route should **NOT** be used for the treatment of T-PLL (Deardon, 2011).
Alemtuzumab is associated with a moderate emetic potential in the oncology setting; antiemetics may be recommended to prevent nausea and vomiting (Basch, 2011; Roila, 2010).
Lemtrada: Administer by IV infusion over 4 hours (beginning within 8 hours after dilution); do not administer by IV push or IV bolus. Do not infuse other medications through the same IV line. Premedicate with corticosteroids

(methylprednisolone 1,000 mg or equivalent) for first 3 days of each treatment course. Administer in a setting with personnel and equipment appropriate to manage infusion reactions. Monitor vital signs prior to and periodically during the infusion. Infusion reactions should be managed symptomatically; consider discontinuing immediately for severe infusion reaction. Observe for at least 2 hours after each infusion, longer if clinically indicated.

Emetic Potential
Children: Minimal (<10%)
Adults: Moderate (30% to 90%)

Monitoring Parameters Campath: CBC with differential and platelets (weekly, more frequent if worsening); signs and symptoms of infection; CD4+ lymphocyte counts (after treatment until recovery); CMV antigen (routinely during and for 2 months after treatment); consider TSH at baseline and then every 2 to 3 months during alemtuzumab treatment (Hamnvik, 2011). Monitor closely for infusion reactions (including hypotension, rigors, fever, shortness of breath, bronchospasm, chills, and/or rash); vital signs (prior to and during infusion); carefully monitor BP especially in patients with ischemic heart disease or on antihypertensive medications;

Lemtrada: CBC with differential prior to initiation then monthly until 48 months after last infusion; serum creatinine prior to initiation then monthly until 48 months after last infusion or at any time during therapy if clinically indicated; urinalysis with urine cell counts (prior to initiation then monthly); signs/symptoms of infection; TSH at baseline and every 3 months until 48 months after last infusion or longer or at any time during therapy if clinically indicated; observe for at least 2 hours after each infusion, longer if clinically indicated; ECG prior to each treatment course; annual HPV screening; signs/symptoms of PML; baseline and annual skin exams (for melanoma).

Test Interactions May interfere with diagnostic serum tests that utilize antibodies.

Prescribing and Access Restrictions As of September 4, 2012, alemtuzumab (Campath) is no longer commercially available in the United States (or Europe); a restricted distribution program will allow access (free of charge) for appropriate patients. Information on necessary documentation and requirements is available at Campath Distribution Program (1-877-422-6728) or Genzyme Medical Information (1-800-745-4447, option 2).

Medication Guide Available Yes

Dosage Forms Excipient information presented when available (limited, particularly for generics); consult specific product labeling.
Solution, Intravenous [preservative free]:
  Campath: 30 mg/mL (1 mL) [contains edetate disodium dihydrate, mouse protein (murine) (hamster), polysorbate 80]
  Lemtrada: 12 mg/1.2 mL (1.2 mL) [contains edetate disodium dihydrate, mouse protein (murine) (hamster), polysorbate 80]

Dosage Forms: Canada Excipient information presented when available (limited, particularly for generics); consult specific product labeling.
Injection, solution [preservative free]:
  MabCampath: 30 mg/mL (1 mL) [contains edetate disodium, polysorbate 80]
Injection, solution [preservative free]:
  Lemtrada: 10 mg/mL (1.2 mL) [contains edetate disodium, polysorbate 80]

◆ **Alimta** see PEMEtrexed on page 1368

Alitretinoin (Topical) (a li TRET i noyn)

Brand Names: US Panretin

Pharmacologic Category Antineoplastic Agent, Retinoic Acid Derivative

Use Topical treatment of cutaneous lesions in AIDS-related Kaposi's sarcoma. Not indicated when systemic therapy is necessary (eg, >10 new lesions in previous month, symptomatic visceral involvement, symptomatic pulmonary Kaposi's sarcoma, symptomatic lymphedema)

Pregnancy Risk Factor D

Dosing

Adult Kaposi's sarcoma: Topical: Initial: Apply gel twice daily to cutaneous lesions; may gradually increase application frequency to 3-4 times daily based on lesion tolerance. Response may be observed within 2 weeks of initiation, but typically a longer period is required (some patients have required >14 weeks). Continue therapy for as long as patients derives benefit (in clinical trials, therapy lasted up to 96 weeks).

Renal Impairment No dosage adjustment provided in manufacturer's labeling; however, systemic absorption is not extensive making the need for a dose adjustment appear unlikely.

Hepatic Impairment No dosage adjustment provided in manufacturer's labeling; however, systemic absorption is not extensive making the need for a dose adjustment appear unlikely.

Adjustment for Toxicity Reduce application frequency for application site toxicity; for severe reactions, temporarily discontinue therapy until symptoms resolve.

Additional Information Complete prescribing information should be consulted for additional detail.

Dosage Forms Excipient information presented when available (limited, particularly for generics); consult specific product labeling.

Gel, External:

Panretin: 0.1% (60 g)

◆ **Alkeran** *see* Melphalan *on page 1080*

◆ **Alloprin (Can)** *see* Allopurinol *on page 73*

Allopurinol (al oh PURE i nole)

Related Information

Mucositis and Stomatitis *on page 2186*

Brand Names: US Aloprim; Zyloprim

Brand Names: Canada Alloprin; Apo-Allopurinol; JAMP-Allopurinol; Mar-Allopurinol; Novo-Purol; Zyloprim

Index Terms Allopurinol Sodium

Pharmacologic Category Antigout Agent; Xanthine Oxidase Inhibitor

Use

Oral:

Calcium oxalate calculi: Management of recurrent calcium oxalate calculi (with uric acid excretion >800 mg/day in men and >750 mg/day in women)

Gout: Management of primary or secondary gout (acute attack, tophi, joint destruction, uric acid lithiasis, and/or nephropathy)

Lesch-Nyhan syndrome: *Canadian labeling:* Additional use (not in U.S. labeling): Management of hyperuricemia associated with Lesch-Nyhan syndrome

◀ **Malignancies:** Management of hyperuricemia associated with cancer treatment for leukemia, lymphoma, or solid tumor malignancies

IV: **Malignancies:** Management of hyperuricemia associated with cancer treatment for leukemia, lymphoma, or solid tumor malignancies

Labeled Contraindications

Severe hypersensitivity reaction to allopurinol or any component of the formulation

Canadian labeling: Additional contraindications (not in U.S. labeling): Nursing mothers and children (except those with hyperuricemia secondary to malignancy or Lesch-Nyhan syndrome)

Pregnancy Considerations Adverse events were observed in some animal reproduction studies. Allopurinol crosses the placenta (Torrance, 2009). An increased risk of adverse fetal events has not been observed (limited data) (Hoeltzenbein, 2013).

Breast-Feeding Considerations Allopurinol and its metabolite are excreted into breast milk; the metabolite was also detected in the serum of the nursing infant (Kamilli, 1993). The U.S. manufacturer recommends caution be used when administering allopurinol to nursing women. The Canadian labeling contraindicates use in nursing women except those with hyperuricemia secondary to malignancy.

Warnings/Precautions Do not use to treat asymptomatic hyperuricemia. Has been associated with a number of hypersensitivity reactions, including severe reactions (vasculitis and Stevens-Johnson syndrome); discontinue at first sign of rash. Consider HLA-B*5801 testing in patients at a higher risk for allopurinol hypersensitivity syndrome (eg, Koreans with stage 3 or worse CKD and Han Chinese and Thai descent regardless of renal function) prior to initiation of therapy (ACR guidelines [Khanna, 2012]). Reversible hepatotoxicity has been reported; use with caution in patients with preexisting hepatic impairment. Bone marrow suppression has been reported; use caution with other drugs causing myelosuppression. Caution in renal impairment, dosage adjustments needed. Full effect on serum uric acid levels in chronic gout may take several weeks to become evident; gradual titration is recommended. Potentially significant drug-drug interactions may exist, requiring dose or frequency adjustment, additional monitoring, and/or selection of alternative therapy.

Adverse Reactions

Most commonly reported:

Dermatologic: Skin rash

Endocrine & metabolic: Gout (acute)

Gastrointestinal: Diarrhea, nausea

Hepatic: Increased liver enzymes, increased serum alkaline phosphatase

<1%, postmarketing, and/or case reports: Abdominal pain, ageusia, agranulocytosis, alopecia, angioedema, aplastic anemia, arthralgia, bronchospasm, cataract, cholestatic jaundice, drowsiness, dysgeusia, dyspepsia, ecchymoses, eczematoid dermatitis, eosinophilia, epistaxis, exfoliative dermatitis, fever, gastritis, gynecomastia, headache, hepatic necrosis, hepatitis, hepatomegaly, hepatotoxicity (idiosyncratic) (Chalasani, 2014), hyperbilirubinemia, hypersensitivity reaction, leukocytosis, leukopenia, lichen planus, macular retinitis, myopathy, necrotizing angiitis, nephritis, neuritis, neuropathy, onycholysis, pancreatitis, paresthesia, pruritus, purpura, renal failure, skin granuloma (annulare), Stevens-Johnson syndrome, thrombocytopenia, toxic epidermal necrolysis, toxic pustuloderma, uremia, vasculitis, vesicobullous dermatitis, vomiting

Drug Interactions

Metabolism/Transport Effects None known.

Avoid Concomitant Use

Avoid concomitant use of Allopurinol with any of the following: Didanosine; Pegloticase; Tegafur

Increased Effect/Toxicity

Allopurinol may increase the levels/effects of: Amoxicillin; Ampicillin; Aza-THIOprine; Bendamustine; CarBAMazepine; ChlorproPAMIDE; Cyclophos-phamide; Didanosine; Doxofylline; Mercaptopurine; Pegloticase; Theophylline Derivatives; Vitamin K Antagonists

The levels/effects of Allopurinol may be increased by: ACE Inhibitors; Loop Diuretics; Thiazide Diuretics

Decreased Effect

Allopurinol may decrease the levels/effects of: Tegafur

The levels/effects of Allopurinol may be decreased by: Antacids

Storage/Stability

Powder for injection: Store at controlled room temperature of 20°C to 25°C (68°F to 77°F). Following preparation, intravenous solutions should be stored at 20°C to 25°C (68°F to 77°F). Do not refrigerate reconstituted and/or diluted product. Must be administered within 10 hours of solution preparation.

Tablet: Store at controlled room temperature of 20°C to 25°C (68°F to 77°F). Protect from moisture and light.

Preparation for Administration Reconstitute powder for injection with SWFI. Further dilution with NS or D_5W (50 to 100 mL) to ≤6 mg/mL is recommended.

Mechanism of Action Allopurinol inhibits xanthine oxidase, the enzyme responsible for the conversion of hypoxanthine to xanthine to uric acid. Allopurinol is metabolized to oxypurinol which is also an inhibitor of xanthine oxidase; allopurinol acts on purine catabolism, reducing the production of uric acid without disrupting the biosynthesis of vital purines.

Pharmacodynamics/Kinetics

Onset of action: Gout: 2 to 3 days, peak effect: 1 to 2 weeks; Hyperuricemia associated with chemotherapy: Maximum effect: 27 hours (Coiffier, 2008)

Absorption: Oral: ~80% to 90% from GI tract; Rectal: Poor and erratic

Distribution: V_d: ~1.6 L/kg; V_{ss}: 0.84 to 0.87 L/kg; enters breast milk

Protein binding: <1%

Metabolism: ~75% to active metabolites, chiefly oxypurinol

Bioavailability: 49% to 53%

Half-life elimination:

Normal renal function: Parent drug: 1 to 3 hours; Oxypurinol: 18 to 30 hours

End-stage renal disease: Prolonged

Time to peak, plasma: Oral: Allopurinol: 1.54 hours; Oxipurinol: 4.5 hours

Excretion: Urine (76% as oxypurinol, 12% as unchanged drug); feces (20%)

Allopurinol and oxypurinol are dialyzable

Dosing

Adult & Geriatric Note: Oral doses >300 mg should be given in divided doses.

◀ **Gout (chronic):** Oral:

Manufacturer's labeling: Initial: 100 mg once daily; increase at weekly intervals in increments of 100 mg/day as needed to achieve desired serum uric acid level. Usual dosage range: 200 to 300 mg/day in mild gout; 400 to 600 mg/day in moderate to severe tophaceous gout. Maximum daily dose: 800 mg/day.

Alternative dosing (off-label): Initial: 100 mg daily, increasing the dose gradually in increments of 100 mg/day every 2 to 5 weeks as needed to achieve desired serum uric acid level of ≤6 mg/dL (ACR guidelines [Khanna, 2012]; EULAR guidelines [Zhang, 2006]; McGill, 2010). Some patients may require therapy targeted at a serum uric acid level <5 mg/dL to control symptoms. Allopurinol may be initiated during an acute gout attack so long as antiinflammatory therapy has been initiated as well (ACR guidelines [Khanna, 2012]).

Management of hyperuricemia associated with chemotherapy and/or radiation therapy:

Oral:

U.S. labeling: 600 to 800 mg daily in divided doses

Canadian labeling: 600 to 800 mg daily in 2 to 3 divided doses for 2 to 3 days prior to chemotherapy/radiation therapy then adjust dose per serum uric acid level; for ongoing management, 300 to 400 mg daily is usually sufficient to control serum uric levels.

Alternative dosing (off-label; intermediate risk for tumor lysis syndrome): Intermediate risk for tumor lysis syndrome: 10 mg/kg daily divided every 8 hours (maximum dose: 800 mg daily) **or** 50 to 100 mg/m^2 every 8 hours (maximum dose: 300 mg/m^2 daily), begin 1 to 2 days before initiation of induction chemotherapy; may continue for 3 to 7 days after chemotherapy (Coiffier, 2008)

IV: **Note:** Intravenous daily dose can be given as a single infusion or in equally divided doses at 6-, 8-, or 12-hour intervals.

Manufacturer's labeling: 200 to 400 mg/m^2 daily (maximum: 600 mg daily) beginning 1 to 2 days before chemotherapy

Alternative dosing (off-label; intermediate risk for tumor lysis syndrome): 200 to 400 mg/m^2 daily (maximum dose: 600 mg daily) in 1 to 3 divided doses beginning 1 to 2 days before the start of induction chemotherapy; may continue for 3 to 7 days after chemotherapy (Coiffier, 2008)

Recurrent calcium oxalate stones: Oral: 200 to 300 mg daily in single or divided doses; may adjust dose as needed to control hyperuricosuria

Pediatric

Management of hyperuricemia associated with chemotherapy and/or radiation therapy:

Oral: **Note:** Oral doses >300 mg should be given in divided doses.

U.S. labeling:

Children <6 years: 150 mg daily

Children 6 to 10 years: 300 mg daily

Children >10 years: Refer to adult dosing.

Canadian labeling:

Children 6 to 10 years: 10 mg/kg daily (do not exceed adult dosing); adjust dose as necessary after 48 hours

Alternative dosing (off-label; intermediate risk for tumor lysis syndrome): Intermediate risk for tumor lysis syndrome: 10 mg/kg daily divided every 8 hours (maximum dose: 800 mg daily) **or** 50 to 100 mg/m^2 every 8 hours (maximum dose: 300 mg/m^2 daily), begin 12 to 24 hours (children) or 1 to 2 days (adults) before initiation of induction chemotherapy; may continue for 3 to 7 days after chemotherapy (Coiffier, 2008)

IV: **Note:** Intravenous daily dose can be given as a single infusion or in equally divided doses at 6-, 8-, or 12-hour intervals.

Manufacturer's labeling: Starting dose: 200 mg/m^2 daily beginning 1 to 2 days before chemotherapy

Alternative dosing (off-label; intermediate risk for tumor lysis syndrome) 200 to 400 mg/m^2 daily (maximum dose: 600 mg daily) in 1 to 3 divided doses beginning 1 to 2 days before the start of induction chemotherapy; may continue for 3 to 7 days after chemotherapy (Coiffier, 2008)

Management of hyperuricemia associated with Lesch-Nyhan syndrome: *Canadian labeling (not in U.S. labeling):* Children 6 to 10 years: Oral: 10 mg/kg daily in 1 to 3 divided doses; adjust dose as necessary after 48 hours

Renal Impairment

Manufacturer's labeling: Oral, IV: Lower doses are required in renal impairment due to potential for accumulation of allopurinol and metabolites.

CrCl 10 to 20 mL/minute: 200 mg daily

CrCl 3 to 10 mL/minute: ≤100 mg daily

CrCl <3 mL/minute: ≤100 mg/dose at extended intervals

Alternative dosing (off-label):

Management of hyperuricemia associated with chemotherapy: Dosage reduction of 50% is recommended in renal impairment (Coiffier, 2008)

Gout: Oral:

Initiate therapy with 50 to 100 mg daily, and gradually increase to a maintenance dose to achieve a serum uric acid level of ≤6 mg/dL (with close monitoring of serum uric acid levels and for hypersensitivity) (Dalbeth, 2007).

or

In patients with stage 4 CKD or worse, initiate therapy at 50 mg/day, increasing the dose every 2 to 5 weeks to achieve desired uric acid levels of ≤6 mg/dL; doses >300 mg/day are permitted so long as they are accompanied by appropriate patient education and monitoring for toxicity (eg, pruritus, rash, elevated hepatic transaminases). Some patients may require therapy targeted at a serum uric acid level <5 mg/dL to control symptoms (ACR guidelines; Khanna, 2012)

Hemodialysis: Initial: 100 mg alternate days given postdialysis, increase cautiously to 300 mg based on response. If dialysis is on a daily basis, an additional 50% of the dose may be required postdialysis (Dalbeth, 2007)

Hepatic Impairment There are no dosage adjustments provided in the U.S. manufacturer's labeling. The Canadian labeling suggests that a dose reduction is necessary but does not provide specific dosing recommendations.

Administration

Oral: Administer after meals with plenty of fluid.

IV: The rate of infusion depends on the volume of the infusion; infuse maximum single daily doses (600 mg/day) over ≥30 minutes. Whenever possible, therapy should be initiated at 24 to 48 hours before the start of chemotherapy known to cause tumor lysis (including adrenocorticosteroids). IV daily dose can be administered as a single infusion or in equally divided doses at 6-, 8-, or 12-hour interval.

Extemporaneous Preparations A 20 mg/mL oral suspension may be made with tablets and either a 1:1 mixture of Ora-Sweet® and Ora-Plus® or a 1:1 mixture of Ora-Sweet® SF and Ora-Plus® or a 1:4 mixture of cherry syrup concentrate and simple syrup, NF. Crush eight 300 mg tablets in a mortar and reduce to a fine powder. Add small portions of chosen vehicle and mix to a uniform paste; mix while adding the vehicle in incremental proportions to **almost** 120 mL; transfer to a calibrated bottle, rinse mortar with vehicle, and add quantity of vehicle sufficient to make 120 mL. Label "shake well". Stable for 60 days refrigerated or at room temperature (Allen, 1996; Nahata, 2004).

Allen LV Jr and Erickson MA 3rd, "Stability of Acetazolamide, Allopurinol, Azathioprine, Clonazepam, and Flucytosine in Extemporaneously Compounded Oral Liquids," *Am J Health Syst Pharm*, 1996, 53(16):1944-9.

Nahata MC, Pai VB, and Hipple TF, *Pediatric Drug Formulations*, 5th ed, Cincinnati, OH: Harvey Whitney Books Co, 2004.

Monitoring Parameters CBC, serum uric acid levels every 2 to 5 weeks during dose titration until desired level is achieved; every 6 months thereafter (ACR guidelines [Khanna, 2012]), I & O, hepatic and renal function, especially at start of therapy; signs and symptoms of hypersensitivity

Dietary Considerations Fluid intake should be administered to yield neutral or slightly alkaline urine and an output of ~2 L (in adults).

Dosage Forms Excipient information presented when available (limited, particularly for generics); consult specific product labeling. [DSC] = Discontinued product

Solution Reconstituted, Intravenous, as sodium [strength expressed as base, preservative free]:
  Aloprim: 500 mg (1 ea)
  Generic: 500 mg (1 ea [DSC])
Tablet, Oral:
  Zyloprim: 100 mg, 300 mg [scored]
  Generic: 100 mg, 300 mg

Dosage Forms: Canada Note: Refer also to Dosage Forms.
Excipient information presented when available (limited, particularly for generics); consult specific product labeling.
Tablet, Oral, as sodium:
  Zyloprim: 200 mg [scored]

Alteplase (AL te plase)

Brand Names: US Activase; Cathflo Activase

Brand Names: Canada Activase rt-PA; Cathflo Activase

Index Terms Alteplase, Recombinant; Alteplase, Tissue Plasminogen Activator, Recombinant; tPA

Pharmacologic Category Thrombolytic Agent
Use
Activase:
Acute ischemic stroke: Treatment of acute ischemic stroke (AIS)
Pulmonary embolism: Management of acute massive pulmonary embolism (PE)
ST-elevation myocardial infarction: Management of ST-elevation myocardial infarction (STEMI) for the lysis of thrombi in coronary arteries.
Limitations of use: The risk of stroke may outweigh the benefit produced by thrombolytic therapy in patients whose acute myocardial infarction (MI) puts them at low risk for death or heart failure.
Recommended criteria for treatment:
STEMI (ACCF/AHA [O'Gara 2013]): Ischemic symptoms within 12 hours of treatment or evidence of ongoing ischemia 12 to 24 hours after symptom onset with a large area of myocardium at risk or hemodynamic instability.
STEMI ECG definition: New ST-segment elevation at the J point in at least 2 contiguous leads of ≥2 mm (0.2 mV) in men or ≥1.5 mm (0.15 mV) in women in leads V_2-V_3 and/or ≥1 mm (0.1 mV) in other contiguous precordial leads or limb leads. New or presumably new left bundle branch block (LBBB) may interfere with ST-elevation analysis and should not be considered diagnostic in isolation.
At non-PCI-capable hospitals, the ACCF/AHA recommends thrombolytic therapy administration when the anticipated first medical contact (FMC)-to-device time at a PCI-capable hospital is >120 minutes due to unavoidable delays.
AIS: Onset of stroke symptoms within 3 hours of treatment
Acute PE: Age ≤75 years: Documented massive PE (defined as acute PE with sustained hypotension [SBP <90 mm Hg for ≤15 minutes or requiring inotropic support], persistent profound bradycardia [HR <40 bpm with signs or symptoms of shock], or pulselessness); alteplase may be considered for submassive PE with clinical evidence of adverse prognosis (eg, new hemodynamic instability, worsening respiratory insufficiency, severe right ventricular (RV) dysfunction, or major myocardial necrosis) and low risk of bleeding complications. **Note:** Not recommended for patients with low-risk PE (eg, normotensive, no RV dysfunction, normal biomarkers) or submassive acute PE with minor RV dysfunction, minor myocardial necrosis, and no clinical worsening (AHA [Jaff 2011]).
Cathflo Activase: Restoration of function to central venous access device
Pregnancy Risk Factor C
Dosing
Adult & Geriatric
Acute ischemic stroke: Activase: IV: Within 3 hours of the onset of symptom onset (labeled use) **or** within 3 to 4.5 hours of symptom onset (off-label use; Hacke 2008; Jauch 2013): **Note:** Perform noncontrast-enhanced CT or MRI prior to administration. Initiation of anticoagulants (eg, heparin) or antiplatelet agents (eg, aspirin) within 24 hours after starting alteplase is not recommended; however, initiation of aspirin within 24 to 48 hours after stroke onset is recommended (Jauch 2013). Initiation of SubQ heparin (≤10,000 units) or equivalent doses of low molecular weight heparin for prevention of DVT during the first 24 hours of the 3 to 4.5 hour window trial did not increase incidence of intracerebral hemorrhage (Hacke 2008).
Recommended total dose: 0.9 mg/kg (maximum total dose: 90 mg)

◄

Patients ≤100 kg: Load with 0.09 mg/kg (10% of 0.9 mg/kg dose) as an IV bolus over 1 minute, followed by 0.81 mg/kg (90% of 0.9 mg/kg dose) as a continuous infusion over 60 minutes.

Patients >100 kg: Load with 9 mg (10% of 90 mg) as an IV bolus over 1 minute, followed by 81 mg (90% of 90 mg) as a continuous infusion over 60 minutes.

Central venous catheter clearance: Cathflo Activase (1 mg/mL): Intra-catheter:

Patients <30 kg: 110% of the internal lumen volume of the catheter, not to exceed 2 mg/2 mL; retain in catheter for 0.5 to 2 hours; may instill a second dose if catheter remains occluded

Patients ≥30 kg: 2 mg/2 mL; retain in catheter for 0.5 to 2 hours; may instill a second dose if catheter remains occluded

Pulmonary embolism (PE) (acute massive): Activase: IV: 100 mg over 2 hours; may be administered as a 10 mg bolus followed by 90 mg over 2 hours as was done in patients with submassive PE (Konstantinides 2002). Institute or resume parenteral anticoagulation near the end of or immediately following the alteplase infusion when the partial thromboplastin time or thrombin time returns to twice normal or less. **Note:** Use in submassive PE is off-label.

ST-elevation myocardial infarction (STEMI): Activase: IV: **Note:** Manufacturer's labeling recommends 3-hour infusion regimen; however, accelerated regimen preferred by the ACCF/AHA (O'Gara 2013).

Accelerated regimen (weight-based):

Patients >67 kg: Total dose: 100 mg over 1.5 hours; administered as a 15 mg IV bolus over 1 to 2 minutes followed by infusions of 50 mg over 30 minutes, then 35 mg over 1 hour. Maximum total dose: 100 mg

Patients ≤67 kg: Infuse 15 mg IV bolus over 1 to 2 minutes followed by infusions of 0.75 mg/kg (not to exceed 50 mg) over 30 minutes then 0.5 mg/kg (not to exceed 35 mg) over 1 hour. Maximum total dose: 100 mg

Note: Thrombolytic should be administered within 30 minutes of hospital arrival. Generally, there is only a small trend for benefit of therapy after a delay of 12 to 24 hours from symptom onset, but thrombolysis may be considered for selected patients with ongoing ischemic pain and extensive ST elevation; however, primary PCI is preferred in these patients. Administer concurrent aspirin, clopidogrel, and anticoagulant therapy (ie, unfractionated heparin, enoxaparin, or fondaparinux) with alteplase (O'Gara 2013).

Acute peripheral arterial occlusion (off-label use): Intra-arterial:

Weight-based regimen: 0.001 to 0.02 mg/kg/hour (maximum dose: 2 mg/hour) (Semba 2000)

or

Fixed-dose regimen: 0.12 to 2 mg/hour (Semba 2000)

Note: The ACC/AHA guidelines state that thrombolysis is an effective and beneficial therapy for those with acute limb ischemia (Rutherford categories I and IIa) of <14 days duration (Hirsch 2006). The optimal dosage and concentration has not been established; a number of intra-arterial delivery techniques are employed with continuous infusion being the most common (Ouriel 2004). The Advisory Panel to the Society for Cardiovascular and Interventional Radiology on Thrombolytic Therapy recommends dosing of ≤2 mg/hour and concomitant administration of subtherapeutic heparin (aPTT 1.25 to 1.5 times baseline) (Semba 2000). Duration of alteplase infusion dependent upon size and location of the thrombus; typically between 6 to 48 hours (Disini 2008).

Frostbite (off-label use): Note: For use in patients with deep frostbite injury with potential significant morbidity (eg, extending proximally to the proximal interphalangeal joints of digits), without contraindications to the use of alteplase, who present within 24 hours of injury. Use of alteplase in the field is not recommended; administer treatment in a facility capable of intensive-care monitoring (WMS [McIntosh 2014]). Additional data may be necessary to further define the role of alteplase in the treatment of frostbite. Intra-arterial: 2 to 4 mg bolus followed by a continuous intra-arterial infusion of 0.5 to 1 mg/hour (total dose if bilateral extremity involvement) via femoral or brachial artery; administer with continuous infusion heparin via an intra-arterial catheter. Discontinue alteplase if fibrinogen levels decrease to <150 mg/dL, if reperfusion is complete (as evidenced by angiography), or after a period of 48 hours whether or not reperfusion is achieved (Bruen 2007; Ibrahim 2015).

Parapneumonic effusions and empyema (off-label use): Intrapleural: 10 mg (diluted in 30 mL of normal saline) administered twice daily for a total of 3 days; each alteplase dose was followed >2 hours later by an intrapleural dornase alfa dose (with a 1-hour dwell time for each drug) (Rahman 2011). Some clinicians suggest consideration of fibrinolytic use in patients in whom treatment with at least 24 hours of chest tube drainage has failed and who are poor surgical candidates (Hamblin 2010). Dosing for this indication has not been established. Alteplase monotherapy dosing regimens have varied (range: 10 to 100 mg) and produced conflicting results in small trials and case series. These regimens have also included variations in chest tube sizes, number of doses, patient positions (still vs rotation), and clamping durations (Thommi 2007; Thommi 2012).

Prosthetic valve thrombosis, right-sided (any size thrombus) or left-sided (thrombus area <0.8 cm^2, recent onset [<14 days] of NYHA class I to II symptoms), or left-sided (thrombus area ≥0.8 cm^2) when contraindications to surgery exist (off-label use) (ACCP [Guyatt 2012]; AHA/ACC [Nishimura 2014]; Alpert 2003; Roudaut 2003): IV:

High-dose regimen: Load with 10 mg, followed by 90 mg over 90 to 180 minutes (without heparin during infusion)

Low-dose regimen (preferred for very small adults): Load with 20 mg, followed by 10 mg/hour for 3 hours (without heparin during infusion)

Note: After successful administration of alteplase, heparin infusion should be introduced until warfarin achieves therapeutic INR (aortic: 3.0 to 4.0; mitral: 3.5 to 4.5) (Bonow 2008). The 2012 ACCP guidelines for antithrombotic therapy make no recommendation regarding INR range after prosthetic valve thrombosis.

Pulmonary embolism (PE) (submassive) (off-label use): Activase: IV: 100 mg over 2 hours; administered as a 10 mg bolus followed by 90 mg over 2 hours (Konstantinides 2002). Institute or resume parenteral anticoagulation near the end of or immediately following the alteplase infusion when the partial thromboplastin time or thrombin time returns to twice normal or less. **Note:** Not recommended for submassive PE with minor RV dysfunction, minor myocardial necrosis, and no clinical worsening or low-risk PE (ie, normotensive, no RV dysfunction, normal biomarkers) (AHA [Jaff 2011]).

◄ **Pediatric**

Central venous catheter clearance: Intracatheter:

Patients <30 kg: 110% of the internal lumen volume of the catheter, not to exceed 2 mg/2 mL; retain in catheter for 0.5 to 2 hours; may instill a second dose if catheter remains occluded

Patients ≥30 kg: 2 mg/2 mL; retain in catheter for 0.5 to 2 hours; may instill a second dose if catheter remains occluded

Parapneumonic effusions and empyema (off-label use): Infants >3 months, Children, and Adolescents: Intrapleural: 4 mg (diluted in 40 mL of normal saline), with the first dose administered at time of chest tube placement (with a 1-hour dwell time); repeat every 24 hours for a total of 3 doses; or 0.1 mg/kg (maximum: 3 mg) (diluted in 10 to 30 mL of normal saline), with the first dose administered after pigtail catheter (chest tube) placement (45- to 60-minute dwell time) and repeat doses administered every 8 hours for 3 days (total of 9 doses) (Bradley 2011; Hawkins 2004; St Peter 2009). Dosing for this indication has not been established. Several intrapleural dosage regimens have been evaluated and have included variations in chest tube sizes, number of doses, patient positions (still vs rotation), and clamping durations.

Renal Impairment There are no dosage adjustments provided in the manufacturer's labeling. Plasma clearance is rapid and mediated primarily by the liver; therefore, degree of renal impairment is unlikely to influence elimination of alteplase. Hemostatic defects due to severe renal disease may increase the risk for bleeding.

Hepatic Impairment There are no dosage adjustments provided in the manufacturer's labeling. Plasma clearance is rapid and mediated primarily by the liver. Significant hepatic impairment and hemostatic defects due to severe hepatic disease may increase the risk for bleeding.

Additional Information Complete prescribing information should be consulted for additional detail.

Dosage Forms Excipient information presented when available (limited, particularly for generics); consult specific product labeling.

Solution Reconstituted, Injection:

Cathflo Activase: 2 mg (1 ea)

Solution Reconstituted, Intravenous:

Activase: 50 mg (1 ea); 100 mg (1 ea)

◆ **Alteplase, Recombinant** *see* Alteplase *on page 78*

◆ **Alteplase, Tissue Plasminogen Activator, Recombinant** *see* Alteplase *on page 78*

◆ **Alti-MPA (Can)** *see* MedroxyPROGESTERone *on page 1074*

Altretamine (al TRET a meen)

Related Information

Management of Chemotherapy-Induced Nausea and Vomiting in Adults *on page 2142*

Prevention of Chemotherapy-Induced Nausea and Vomiting in Children *on page 2203*

Safe Handling of Hazardous Drugs *on page 2292*

Brand Names: US Hexalen

Brand Names: Canada Hexalen

Index Terms Hexamethylmelamine; HMM; HXM

Pharmacologic Category Antineoplastic Agent, Alkylating Agent

Use Palliative treatment of persistent or recurrent ovarian cancer

Labeled Contraindications Hypersensitivity to altretamine or any component of the formulation; preexisting severe bone marrow suppression or severe neurologic toxicity

Pregnancy Considerations Teratogenic effects were noted in animal studies. There are no adequate and well-controlled studies in pregnant women. May cause fetal harm if administered during pregnancy. Women of childbearing potential should avoid becoming pregnant while on therapy.

Breast-Feeding Considerations Due to the potential for toxicity in the nursing infant, breast-feeding is not recommended.

Warnings/Precautions Hazardous agent - use appropriate precautions for handling and disposal (NIOSH 2014 [group 1]). **[U.S. Boxed Warning]: Peripheral blood counts and neurologic examinations should be done routinely before each cycle and during treatment.** Dose-related bone marrow suppression is common; use with caution in patients previously treated with other myelosuppressive agents. Peripheral neuropathy and neurotoxicity (ataxia, dizziness, vertigo, mood disorders, and disorders of consciousness) have been reported; usually occur in patients receiving continuous high-dose daily treatment and is generally reversible upon discontinuation. Altretamine is associated with a high emetic potential; antiemetics are recommended to prevent nausea and vomiting (Dupuis, 2011; Roila, 2010). Has been administered safely to patients with preexisting neuropathy (due to cisplatin); close monitoring is required. Concurrent use of altretamine and MAO inhibitors may cause severe orthostatic hypotension. **[U.S. Boxed Warning]: Should be administered under the supervision of an experienced cancer chemotherapy physician.**

Adverse Reactions

>10%:

Gastrointestinal: Nausea/vomiting (33%; severe 1%)

Hematologic: Anemia (33%), leukopenia (5% to 15%; grade 4: <1%)

Neuromuscular & skeletal: Peripheral sensory neuropathy (31%; mild: 9%; moderate-to-severe: 9%)

1% to 10%:

Central nervous system: Fatigue, seizure

Gastrointestinal: Anorexia

Hematologic: Thrombocytopenia

Hepatic: Alkaline phosphatase increased

Renal: BUN increased, serum creatinine increased

<1%, postmarketing, and/or case reports: Alopecia, ataxia, depression, dizziness, hepatotoxicity, mood disorders, neurotoxicity, pruritus, rash, vertigo

Drug Interactions

Metabolism/Transport Effects None known.

Avoid Concomitant Use

Avoid concomitant use of Altretamine with any of the following: BCG (Intravesical); CloZAPine; Dipyrone; Natalizumab; Pimecrolimus; Tacrolimus (Topical); Tofacitinib; Vaccines (Live)

Increased Effect/Toxicity

Altretamine may increase the levels/effects of: CloZAPine; Fingolimod; Leflunomide; MAO Inhibitors; Natalizumab; Tofacitinib; Tricyclic Antidepressants; Vaccines (Live)

The levels/effects of Altretamine may be increased by: Denosumab; Dipyrone; Pimecrolimus; Roflumilast; Tacrolimus (Topical); Trastuzumab

Decreased Effect

Altretamine may decrease the levels/effects of: BCG (Intravesical); Coccidioides immitis Skin Test; Sipuleucel-T; Vaccines (Inactivated); Vaccines (Live)

The levels/effects of Altretamine may be decreased by: Echinacea; Multivitamins/Fluoride (with ADE); Multivitamins/Minerals (with ADEK, Folate, Iron); Multivitamins/Minerals (with AE, No Iron); Pyridoxine

Storage/Stability Store at 25°C (77°F); excursions permitted to 15°C to 30°C (59°F to 86°F).

Mechanism of Action Altretamine structurally resembles alkylating agents, although has demonstrated activity in tumors resistant to classic alkylating agents. Cytotoxic effect not fully characterized, however it is theorized that metabolically activated oxidative N-demethylation intermediates bind to and damage DNA.

Pharmacodynamics/Kinetics

Absorption: Well absorbed

Distribution: Distributed into tissues high in lipid content and into tumor tissue

Metabolism: Hepatic; rapid and extensive oxidative N-demethylation to active metabolites (pentamethylmelamine and tetramethylmelamine)

Half-life elimination: ~7 hours (range: 2-10 hours)

Time to peak, plasma: 0.5-3 hours

Excretion: Urine (90%, <1% as unchanged drug)

Dosing

Adult & Geriatric Note: Altretamine is associated with a high emetic potential; antiemetics are recommended to prevent nausea and vomiting (Roila, 2010)

Ovarian cancer, persistent or recurrent: Oral: 260 mg/m^2/day in 4 divided doses for 14 or 21 days of a 28-day cycle

Renal Impairment No dosage adjustment provided in manufacturer's labeling (has not been studied).

Hepatic Impairment No dosage adjustment provided in manufacturer's labeling (has not been studied).

Obesity *ASCO Guidelines for appropriate chemotherapy dosing in obese adults with cancer:* Utilize patient's actual body weight (full weight) for calculation of body surface area- or weight-based dosing, particularly when the intent of therapy is curative; manage regimen-related toxicities in the same manner as for nonobese patients; if a dose reduction is utilized due to toxicity, consider resumption of full weight-based dosing with subsequent cycles, especially if cause of toxicity (eg, hepatic or renal impairment) is resolved (Griggs, 2012).

Adjustment for Toxicity Temporarily withhold for 14 days or longer, and resume dose at 200 mg/m^2/day for any of the following:

Platelet count <75,000/mm^3

White blood cell count <2000/mm^3 or granulocyte count <1000/mm^3

Progressive neurotoxicity

Gastrointestinal intolerance not responsive to antiemetic regimens

Discontinue if neurotoxicity does not stabilize at 200 mg/m^2/day.

Administration Altretamine is associated with a high emetic potential; antiemetics are recommended to prevent nausea and vomiting (Dupuis, 2011; Roila, 2010)

Administer total daily dose orally as 4 divided doses after meals and at bedtime.

Hazardous agent; use appropriate precautions for handling and disposal (NIOSH 2014 [group 1]).

Emetic Potential Children and Adults: High (>90%)

Monitoring Parameters CBC with differential (before each cycle and regularly during treatment), neurologic examination (before each cycle and regularly during treatment)

Dietary Considerations Should be taken after meals (and at bedtime).

Dosage Forms Excipient information presented when available (limited, particularly for generics); consult specific product labeling.

Capsule, Oral:

Hexalen: 50 mg

◆ **AmBisome** see Amphotericin B (Liposomal) *on page 102*

◆ **AMD3100** see Plerixafor *on page 1392*

◆ **A-Methapred** see MethylPREDNISolone *on page 1125*

◆ **Amethopterin** see Methotrexate *on page 1104*

◆ **AMG 073** see Cinacalcet *on page 324*

◆ **AMG-162** see Denosumab *on page 499*

◆ **AMG 531** see RomiPLOStim *on page 1498*

◆ **Amicar** see Aminocaproic Acid *on page 91*

Amifostine (am i FOS teen)

Related Information

Chemotherapy-Induced Peripheral Neuropathy *on page 2116*

Management of Chemotherapy-Induced Nausea and Vomiting in Adults *on page 2142*

Prevention of Chemotherapy-Induced Nausea and Vomiting in Children *on page 2203*

Brand Names: US Ethyol

Brand Names: Canada Ethyol

Index Terms Ethiofos; Gammaphos; WR-2721; YM-08310

Pharmacologic Category Antidote; Chemoprotective Agent

Use Reduce the incidence of moderate-to-severe xerostomia in patients undergoing postoperative radiation treatment for head and neck cancer, where the radiation port includes a substantial portion of the parotid glands; reduce the cumulative renal toxicity associated with repeated administration of cisplatin

Labeled Contraindications Hypersensitivity to aminothiol compounds or any component of the formulation

Pregnancy Considerations Adverse events have been observed in animal reproduction studies.

Breast-Feeding Considerations It is not known if amifostine is excreted in breast milk. Due to the potential for adverse reactions in the nursing infant, the manufacturer recommends that breast-feeding should be discontinued during treatment.

◀ **Warnings/Precautions** Patients who are hypotensive or dehydrated should not receive amifostine. Interrupt antihypertensive therapy for 24 hours before treatment; patients who cannot safely stop their antihypertensives 24 hours before, should not receive amifostine. Adequately hydrated prior to treatment and keep in a supine position during infusion. Monitor blood pressure every 5 minutes during the infusion. If hypotension requiring interruption of therapy occurs, patients should be placed in the Trendelenburg position and given an infusion of normal saline using a separate IV line; subsequent infusions may require a dose reduction. Infusions >15 minutes are associated with a higher incidence of adverse effects. Use caution in patients with cardiovascular and cerebrovascular disease and any other patients in whom the adverse effects of hypotension may have serious adverse events.

Serious cutaneous reactions, including erythema multiforme, Stevens-Johnson syndrome, toxic epidermal necrolysis, toxoderma and exfoliative dermatitis have been reported with amifostine. May be delayed, developing up to weeks after treatment initiation. Cutaneous reactions have been reported more frequently when used as a radioprotectant. Discontinue treatment for severe/serious cutaneous reaction, or with fever. Withhold treatment and obtain dermatologic consultation for rash involving lips or mucosa (of unknown etiology outside of radiation port) and for bullous, edematous or erythematous lesions on hands, feet, or trunk; reinitiate only after careful evaluation.

Amifostine doses >300 mg/m² are associated with a moderate emetic potential (Dupuis, 2011). It is recommended that antiemetic medication, including dexamethasone 20 mg IV and a serotonin 5-HT$_3$ receptor antagonist be administered prior to and in conjunction with amifostine. Rare hypersensitivity reactions, including anaphylaxis and allergic reaction, have been reported; discontinue if allergic reaction occurs; do not rechallenge. Medications for the treatment of hypersensitivity reactions should be available.

Reports of clinically-relevant hypocalcemia are rare, but serum calcium levels should be monitored in patients at risk of hypocalcemia, such as those with nephrotic syndrome; may require calcium supplementation. Should not be used (in patients receiving chemotherapy for malignancies other than ovarian cancer) where chemotherapy is expected to provide significant survival benefit or in patients receiving definitive radiotherapy, unless within the context of a clinical trial.

Adverse Reactions

>10%:

Cardiovascular: Hypotension (15% to 61%; grades 3/4: 3% to 8%; dose dependent)

Gastrointestinal: Nausea/vomiting (53% to 96%; grades 3/4: 8% to 30%; dose dependent)

1% to 10%: Endocrine & metabolic: Hypocalcemia (clinically significant: 1%)

<1%, postmarketing, and/or case reports: Apnea, anaphylactoid reactions, anaphylaxis, arrhythmia, atrial fibrillation, atrial flutter, back pain, bradycardia, cardiac arrest, chest pain, chest tightness, chills, cutaneous eruptions, dizziness, erythema multiforme, exfoliative dermatitis, extrasystoles, dyspnea, fever, flushing, hiccups, hypersensitivity reactions (fever, rash, hypoxia, dyspnea, laryngeal edema), hypertension (transient), hypoxia, malaise, MI, myocardial ischemia, pruritus, rash (mild), renal failure, respiratory arrest, rigors, seizure, sneezing, somnolence, Stevens-Johnson syndrome, supraventricular tachycardia, syncope, tachycardia, toxic epidermal necrolysis, toxoderma, urticaria

Drug Interactions

Metabolism/Transport Effects None known.

Avoid Concomitant Use There are no known interactions where it is recommended to avoid concomitant use.

Increased Effect/Toxicity

The levels/effects of Amifostine may be increased by: Antihypertensives

Decreased Effect There are no known significant interactions involving a decrease in effect.

Storage/Stability Store intact vials of lyophilized powder at room temperature of 20°C to 25°C (68°F to 77°F). Reconstituted solutions (500 mg/10 mL) and solutions for infusion are chemically stable for up to 5 hours at room temperature (25°C) or up to 24 hours under refrigeration (2°C to 8°C).

Preparation for Administration For IV infusion, reconstitute intact vials with 9.7 mL 0.9% sodium chloride injection and dilute in 0.9% sodium chloride to a final concentration of 5-40 mg/mL. For SubQ administration, reconstitute with 2.5 mL NS or SWFI.

Mechanism of Action Prodrug that is dephosphorylated by alkaline phosphatase in tissues to a pharmacologically-active free thiol metabolite. The free thiol is available to bind to, and detoxify, reactive metabolites of cisplatin; and can also act as a scavenger of free radicals that may be generated (by cisplatin or radiation therapy) in tissues.

Pharmacodynamics/Kinetics

Distribution: V_d: 3.5 L; unmetabolized prodrug is largely confined to the intravascular compartment; active metabolite is distributed into normal tissues with high concentrations in bone marrow, GI mucosa, skin, liver, and salivary glands

Protein binding: 4%

Metabolism: Hepatic dephosphorylation to two metabolites (active-free thiol and disulfide)

Half-life elimination: 9.3 minutes (Fouladi, 2001); Adults: ~8 to 9 minutes

Excretion: Urine (as metabolites)

Clearance, plasma: 2.17 L/minute

Dosing

Adult & Geriatric Note: Amifostine doses >300 mg/m^2 are associated with a moderate emetic potential. Antiemetic medication, including dexamethasone 20 mg IV and a serotonin 5-HT$_3$ receptor antagonist, is recommended prior to and in conjunction with amifostine.

Cisplatin-induced renal toxicity, reduction: IV: 910 mg/m^2 once daily over 15 minutes 30 minutes prior to cytotoxic therapy

For 910 mg/m^2 doses, the manufacturer suggests the following blood pressure-based adjustment schedule:

The infusion of amifostine should be interrupted if the systolic blood pressure decreases significantly from baseline, as defined below:

Decrease of 20 mm Hg if baseline systolic blood pressure <100

Decrease of 25 mm Hg if baseline systolic blood pressure 100-119

Decrease of 30 mm Hg if baseline systolic blood pressure 120-139

Decrease of 40 mm Hg if baseline systolic blood pressure 140-179

Decrease of 50 mm Hg if baseline systolic blood pressure ≥180

If blood pressure returns to normal within 5 minutes (assisted by fluid administration and postural management) and the patient is asymptomatic, the infusion may be restarted so that the full dose of amifostine may be administered. If the full dose of amifostine cannot be administered, the dose of amifostine for subsequent cycles should be 740 mg/m^2.

◀ **Xerostomia from head and neck cancer, reduction:**
   IV: 200 mg/m^2 over 3 minutes once daily 15-30 minutes prior to radiation therapy **or**
   SubQ (off-label route): 500 mg once daily prior to radiation therapy
   Prevention of radiation proctitis in rectal cancer (off-label use): IV: 340 mg/m^2 once daily prior to radiation therapy (Keefe, 2007; Peterson, 2008)

Renal Impairment No dosage adjustment provided in manufacturer's labeling.

Hepatic Impairment No dosage adjustment provided in manufacturer's labeling.

Administration Amifostine doses >300 mg/m^2 are associated with a moderate emetic potential; antiemetics are recommended to prevent nausea/vomiting (Dupuis, 2011)

IV: Administer over 3 minutes (prior to radiation therapy) or 15 minutes (prior to cisplatin); administration as a longer infusion is associated with a higher incidence of side effects. Patients should be kept in supine position during infusion. **Note:** SubQ administration (off-label) has been used.

Emetic Potential Children and Adults:
>300 mg/m^2: Moderate (30% to 90%)
≤300 mg/m^2: Low (10% to 30%)

Monitoring Parameters Blood pressure should be monitored every 5 minutes during the infusion and after administration if clinically indicated; serum calcium levels (in patients at risk for hypocalcemia). Evaluate for cutaneous reactions prior to each dose.

Additional Information Oncology Comment: The American Society of Clinical Oncology (ASCO) guidelines for the use of protectants for chemotherapy and radiation (Hensley, 2008) recommend the use of amifostine for prevention of nephrotoxicity due to cisplatin-based chemotherapy and to decrease the incidence of acute and delayed radiation therapy-induced xerostomia. The ASCO guidelines do not recommend the use of amifostine to reduce the incidence of neutropenia or thrombocytopenia associated with chemotherapy or radiation therapy, neurotoxicity or ototoxicity associated with platinum-based chemotherapy, radiation therapy-induced mucositis associated with head and neck cancer, or esophagitis due to chemotherapy in patients with non-small cell lung cancer. Additionally, the guidelines do not support the use of amifostine in patients with head and neck cancer receiving concurrent platinum-based chemotherapy.

Dosage Forms Excipient information presented when available (limited, particularly for generics); consult specific product labeling.
Solution Reconstituted, Intravenous:
  Ethyol: 500 mg (1 ea)
  Generic: 500 mg (1 ea)
Solution Reconstituted, Intravenous [preservative free]:
  Generic: 500 mg (1 ea)

Amikacin (am i KAY sin)

Brand Names: Canada Amikacin Sulfate Injection, USP; Amikin
Index Terms Amikacin Sulfate
Pharmacologic Category Antibiotic, Aminoglycoside

Use Treatment of serious infections (bone infections, respiratory tract infections, endocarditis, and septicemia) due to organisms resistant to gentamicin and tobramycin, including *Pseudomonas*, *Proteus*, *Serratia*, and other gram-negative bacilli; documented infection of mycobacterial organisms susceptible to amikacin

Pregnancy Risk Factor D

Dosing

Adult & Geriatric Individualization is critical because of the low therapeutic index

In underweight and nonobese patients, use of total body weight (TBW) instead of ideal body weight for determining the initial mg/kg/dose is widely accepted (Nicolau, 1995). Ideal body weight (IBW) also may be used to determine doses for patients who are neither underweight nor obese (Gilbert 2009).

Initial and periodic peak and trough plasma drug levels should be determined, particularly in critically-ill patients with serious infections or in disease states known to significantly alter aminoglycoside pharmacokinetics (eg, cystic fibrosis, burns, or major surgery). Manufacturer recommends a maximum daily dose of 15 mg/kg/day (or 1.5 g/day in heavier patients). Higher doses may be warranted based on therapeutic drug monitoring or susceptibility information.

Usual dosage range:

IM, IV: 5-7.5 mg/kg/dose every 8 hours; **Note:** Some clinicians suggest a daily dose of 15-20 mg/kg for all patients with normal renal function. This dose is at least as efficacious with similar, if not less, toxicity than conventional dosing.

Intrathecal/intraventricular (off-label route): Meningitis (susceptible gram-negative organisms): 5-50 mg/day

Indication-specific dosing:

Endophthalmitis, bacterial (off-label use): Intravitreal: 0.4 mg/0.1 mL NS in combination with vancomycin

Hospital-acquired pneumonia (HAP): IV: 20 mg/kg/day with antipseudomonal beta-lactam or carbapenem (American Thoracic Society/ATS guidelines)

Meningitis (susceptible gram-negative organisms):

IV: 5 mg/kg every 8 hours (administered with another bactericidal drug)

Intrathecal/intraventricular (off-label route): Usual dose: 30 mg/day (IDSA 2004); Range: 5-50 mg/day (with concurrent systemic antimicrobial therapy) (Gilbert, 1986; Guardado 2008; IDSA 2004; Kasiakou 2005)

***Mycobacterium avium* complex (MAC) (off-label use):** IV: Adjunct therapy (with macrolide, rifamycin, and ethambutol): 8-25 mg/kg 2-3 times weekly for first 2-3 months for severe disease (maximum single dose for age >50 years: 500 mg) (Griffith 2007)

Mycobacterium fortuitum, M. chelonae,* or *M. abscessus: IV: 10-15 mg/kg daily for at least 2 weeks with high dose cefoxitin

Pediatric Usual dosage range: Infants and Children: IM, IV: 5-7.5 mg/kg/dose every 8 hours

Note: Individualization is critical because of the low therapeutic index

Use of ideal body weight (IBW) for determining the mg/kg/dose appears to be more accurate than dosing on the basis of total body weight (TBW)

◀ Initial and periodic peak and trough plasma drug levels should be determined, particularly in critically-ill patients with serious infections or in disease states known to significantly alter aminoglycoside pharmacokinetics (eg, cystic fibrosis, burns, or major surgery). Manufacturer recommends a maximum daily dose of 15 mg/kg/day (or 1.5 g/day in heavier patients). Higher doses may be warranted based on therapeutic drug monitoring or susceptibility information.

Renal Impairment

Some patients may require larger or more frequent doses if serum levels document the need (ie, cystic fibrosis or febrile granulocytopenic patients).

CrCl ≥60 mL/minute: Administer every 8 hours

CrCl 40-60 mL/minute: Administer every 12 hours

CrCl 20-40 mL/minute: Administer every 24 hours

CrCl <20 mL/minute: Loading dose, then monitor levels

Intermittent hemodialysis (IHD) (administer after hemodialysis on dialysis days): Dialyzable (20%; variable; dependent on filter, duration, and type of HD): 5-7.5 mg/kg every 48-72 hours. Follow levels. Redose when pre-HD concentration <10 mg/L; redose when post-HD concentration <6-8 mg/L (Heintz 2009). **Note:** Dosing dependent on the assumption of 3 times/week, complete IHD sessions.

Peritoneal dialysis (PD): Dose as CrCl <20 mL/minute: Follow levels.

Continuous renal replacement therapy (CRRT) (Heintz 2009; Trotman 2005): Drug clearance is highly dependent on the method of renal replacement, filter type, and flow rate. Appropriate dosing requires close monitoring of pharmacologic response, signs of adverse reactions due to drug accumulation, as well as drug concentrations in relation to target trough (if appropriate). The following are general recommendations only (based on dialysate flow/ultrafiltration rates of 1-2 L/hour and minimal residual renal function) and should not supersede clinical judgment:

CVVH/CVVHD/CVVHDF: Loading dose of 10 mg/kg followed by maintenance dose of 7.5 mg/kg every 24-48 hours

Note: For severe gram-negative rod infections, target peak concentration of 15-30 mg/L; redose when concentration <10 mg/L (Heintz 2009).

Hepatic Impairment No dosage adjustment provided in manufacturer's labeling.

Obesity In moderate obesity (TBW/IBW ≥1.25) or greater, (eg, morbid obesity [TBW/IBW >2]), initial dosage requirement may be estimated using a dosing weight of IBW + 0.4 (TBW - IBW) (Traynor, 1995).

Additional Information Complete prescribing information should be consulted for additional detail.

Dosage Forms Excipient information presented when available (limited, particularly for generics); consult specific product labeling.

Solution, Injection, as sulfate:

Generic: 500 mg/2 mL (2 mL); 1 g/4 mL (4 mL)

Solution, Injection, as sulfate [preservative free]:

Generic: 1 g/4 mL (4 mL)

◆ **Amikacin Sulfate** see Amikacin on page 88

◆ **Amikacin Sulfate Injection, USP (Can)** see Amikacin on page 88

◆ **Amikin (Can)** see Amikacin on page 88

◆ **2-Amino-6-Mercaptopurine** see Thioguanine on page 1637

◆ **2-Amino-6-Methoxypurine Arabinoside** see Nelarabine on page 1191

Aminocaproic Acid (a mee noe ka PROE ik AS id)

Brand Names: US Amicar

Index Terms EACA; Epsilon Aminocaproic Acid

Pharmacologic Category Antifibrinolytic Agent; Antihemophilic Agent; Hemostatic Agent; Lysine Analog

Use To enhance hemostasis when fibrinolysis contributes to bleeding (causes may include cardiac surgery, hematologic disorders, neoplastic disorders, abruptio placentae, hepatic cirrhosis, and urinary fibrinolysis)

Labeled Contraindications Disseminated intravascular coagulation (without heparin); evidence of an active intravascular clotting process

Pregnancy Considerations Animal reproduction studies have not been conducted.

Breast-Feeding Considerations It is not known if aminocaproic acid is excreted in breast milk. The manufacturer recommends that caution be exercised when administering aminocaproic acid to nursing women

Warnings/Precautions Avoid rapid IV administration (may induce hypotension, bradycardia, or arrhythmia); rapid injection of undiluted solution is not recommended. Use with caution in patients with renal disease; aminocaproic acid may accumulate in patients with decreased renal function. Intrarenal obstruction may occur secondary to glomerular capillary thrombosis or clots in the renal pelvis and ureters. Do not use in hematuria of upper urinary tract origin unless possible benefits outweigh risks. Do not administer without a definite diagnosis of laboratory findings indicative of hyperfibrinolysis. Inhibition of fibrinolysis may promote clotting or thrombosis; more likely due to the presence of DIC. Skeletal muscle weakness ranging from mild myalgias and fatigue to severe myopathy with rhabdomyolysis and acute renal failure has been reported with prolonged use. Monitor CPK; discontinue treatment with a rise in CPK. Do not administer with factor IX complex concentrates or anti-inhibitor coagulant complexes; may increase risk for thrombosis.

Benzyl alcohol and derivatives: Some dosage forms may contain benzyl alcohol; large amounts of benzyl alcohol (≥99 mg/kg/day) have been associated with a potentially fatal toxicity ("gasping syndrome") in neonates; the "gasping syndrome" consists of metabolic acidosis, respiratory distress, gasping respirations, CNS dysfunction (including convulsions, intracranial hemorrhage), hypotension and cardiovascular collapse (AAP ["Inactive" 1997]; CDC, 1982); some data suggests that benzoate displaces bilirubin from protein binding sites (Ahlfors, 2001); avoid or use dosage forms containing benzyl alcohol with caution in neonates. See manufacturer's labeling.

Adverse Reactions Frequency not defined.

Cardiovascular: Arrhythmia, bradycardia, edema, hypotension, intracranial hypertension, peripheral ischemia, syncope, thrombosis

Central nervous system: Confusion, delirium, dizziness, fatigue, hallucinations, headache, malaise, seizure, stroke

Dermatologic: Rash, pruritus

Gastrointestinal: Abdominal pain, anorexia, cramps, diarrhea, GI irritation, nausea, vomiting

Genitourinary: Dry ejaculation

Hematologic: Agranulocytosis, bleeding time increased, leukopenia, thrombocytopenia

Local: Injection site necrosis, injection site pain, injection site reactions

Neuromuscular & skeletal: CPK increased, myalgia, myositis, myopathy, rhabdomyolysis (rare), weakness

◀ Ophthalmic: Vision decreased, watery eyes

Otic: Tinnitus

Renal: BUN increased, intrarenal obstruction (glomerular capillary thrombosis), myoglobinuria (rare), renal failure (rare)

Respiratory: Dyspnea, nasal congestion, pulmonary embolism

Miscellaneous: Allergic reaction, anaphylactoid reaction, anaphylaxis

Postmarketing and/or case reports: Hepatic lesion, hyperkalemia, myocardial lesion

Drug Interactions

Metabolism/Transport Effects None known.

Avoid Concomitant Use

Avoid concomitant use of Aminocaproic Acid with any of the following: Anti-inhibitor Coagulant Complex (Human); Factor IX (Human); Factor IX (Recombinant); Factor IX Complex (Human) [(Factors II, IX, X)]

Increased Effect/Toxicity

Aminocaproic Acid may increase the levels/effects of: Anti-inhibitor Coagulant Complex (Human); Factor IX (Human); Factor IX (Recombinant); Factor IX Complex (Human) [(Factors II, IX, X)]; Fibrinogen Concentrate (Human)

The levels/effects of Aminocaproic Acid may be increased by: Fibrinogen Concentrate (Human); Tretinoin (Systemic)

Decreased Effect There are no known significant interactions involving a decrease in effect.

Storage/Stability Store intact vials, tablets, and syrup at 15°C to 30°C (59°F to 86°F). Do not freeze injection or syrup. Solutions diluted for IV use in D$_5$W or NS to concentrations of 10-100 mg/mL are stable at 4°C (39°F) and 23°C (73°F) for 7 days (Zhang, 1997).

Preparation for Administration Dilute IV solution in D$_5$W, 0.9% sodium chloride, or Ringer's injection.

Mechanism of Action Binds competitively to plasminogen; blocking the binding of plasminogen to fibrin and the subsequent conversion to plasmin, resulting in inhibition of fibrin degradation (fibrinolysis).

Pharmacodynamics/Kinetics

Onset of action: ~1 to 72 hours

Distribution: Widely through intravascular and extravascular compartments; V$_d$: Oral: 23 L; IV: 30 L

Metabolism: Minimally hepatic

Bioavailability: Oral: 100%

Half-life elimination: 1 to 2 hours

Time to peak: Oral: 1.2 ± 0.45 hours

Excretion: Urine (65% as unchanged drug, 11% as metabolite)

Dosing

Adult & Geriatric

Acute bleeding: Oral, IV: Loading dose: 4-5 g during the first hour, followed by 1 g/hour for 8 hours (or 1.25 g/hour using oral solution) or until bleeding controlled (maximum daily dose: 30 g)

Control of bleeding with severe thrombocytopenia (off-label use) (Bartholomew, 1989; Gardner, 1980):

Initial: IV: 100 mg/kg (maximum dose: 5 g) over 30-60 minutes

Maintenance: Oral, IV: 1-4 g every 4-8 hours or 1 g/hour (maximum daily dose: 24 g)

Control of oral bleeding in congenital and acquired coagulation disorder (off-label use): Oral: 50-60 mg/kg every 4 hours (Mannucci, 1998)

Prevention of dental procedure bleeding in patients on oral anticoagulant therapy (off-label use): Oral rinse: Hold 4 g/10 mL in mouth for 2 minutes then spit out. Repeat every 6 hours for 2 days after procedure (Souto, 1996). Concentration and frequency may vary by institution and product availability.

Prevention of perioperative bleeding associated with cardiac surgery (off-label use): IV: Loading dose of 75-150 mg/kg (typically 5-10 g), followed by 10-15 mg/kg/hour (typically 1 g/hour); may add 2-2.5 g/L of cardiopulmonary bypass circuit priming solution (Gravlee, 2008)

or

Loading dose of 10 g followed by 2 g/hour during surgery; no medication added to the bypass circuit (Fergusson, 2008)

or

10 g over 20-30 minutes prior to skin incision, followed by 10 g after heparin administration then 10 g at discontinuation of cardiopulmonary bypass (Vander Salm, 1996)

Traumatic hyphema (off-label use): Oral: 50 mg/kg/dose every 4 hours (maximum daily dose: 30 g) for 5 days (Brandt, 2001; Crouch, 1999)

Pediatric

Prevention of perioperative bleeding associated with cardiac surgery (off-label use): IV: 100 mg/kg given over 20-30 minutes after induction and prior to incision, 100 mg/kg during cardiopulmonary bypass, and 100 mg/kg after heparin reversal over 3 hours (Chauhan, 2004)

Prevention of bleeding associated with extracorporeal membrane oxygenation (ECMO) (off-label use): IV: 100 mg/kg prior to or immediately after cannulation, followed by 25-30 mg/kg/hour for up to 72 hours (Downard, 2003; Horwitz, 1998; Wilson, 1993)

Prevention of perioperative bleeding associated with spinal surgery (eg, idiopathic scoliosis) (off-label use): Children and Adolescents: IV: 100 mg/kg given over 15-20 minutes after induction, followed by 10 mg/kg/hour for the remainder of the surgery; discontinue at time of wound closure (Florentino-Pineda, 2001; Florentino-Pineda, 2004)

Traumatic hyphema (off-label use): Oral: Refer to adult dosing.

Renal Impairment May accumulate in patients with decreased renal function. When used during cardiopulmonary bypass in anephric patients, a normal or slightly reduced loading dose and a continuous infusion rate of 5 mg/kg/hour has been recommended (Gravlee, 2008).

Hepatic Impairment No dosage adjustment provided in the manufacturer's labeling.

Usual Infusion Concentrations: Adult IV infusion: 5000 mg in 250 mL (concentration: 20 mg/mL) of D_5W, NS, or Ringer's injection

Administration Rapid IV injection (IVP) of undiluted solution is not recommended due to possible hypotension, bradycardia, and arrhythmia.

IV: May administer loading dose over 15-60 minutes depending on indication; a continuous infusion may be necessary.

Monitoring Parameters Fibrinogen, fibrin split products, creatine phosphokinase (with long-term therapy), BUN, creatinine

Dosage Forms Excipient information presented when available (limited, particularly for generics); consult specific product labeling. [DSC] = Discontinued product

Solution, Intravenous:

Generic: 250 mg/mL (20 mL)

Solution, Oral:
Amicar: 25% (236.5 mL) [contains edetate disodium, methylparaben, propyl-paraben, saccharin sodium; raspberry flavor]
Syrup, Oral:
Amicar: 25% (473 mL) [raspberry flavor]
Generic: 25% (237 mL [DSC], 473 mL [DSC])
Tablet, Oral:
Amicar: 500 mg, 1000 mg [scored]
Generic: 500 mg [DSC], 1000 mg [DSC]

Aminolevulinic Acid (a MEE noh lev yoo lin ik AS id)

Brand Names: US Levulan Kerastick
Brand Names: Canada Levulan Kerastick
Index Terms 5-ALA; 5-Aminolevulinic Acid; ALA; Amino Levulinic Acid; Amino-levulinic Acid HCl; Aminolevulinic Acid Hydrochloride
Pharmacologic Category Photosensitizing Agent, Topical; Topical Skin Product
Use Actinic keratoses: Treatment of minimally to moderately thick actinic keratoses of the face or scalp; to be used in conjunction with blue light illumination
Pregnancy Risk Factor C
Dosing
Adult & Geriatric
Note: Should only be applied by qualified medical personnel (not intended for application by patients).
Actinic keratoses: Topical: Apply to actinic keratoses (**not** perilesional skin) followed 14 to 18 hours later by blue light illumination. Application/treatment may be repeated at a treatment site (once) after 8 weeks.
Renal Impairment There are no dosage adjustments provided in the manufacturer's labeling.
Hepatic Impairment There are no dosage adjustments provided in the manufacturer's labeling.
Additional Information Complete prescribing information should be consulted for additional detail.
Dosage Forms Excipient information presented when available (limited, particularly for generics); consult specific product labeling.
Solution Reconstituted, External, as hydrochloride:
Levulan Kerastick: 20% (1 ea) [contains alcohol, usp, isopropyl alcohol, laureth, polyethylene glycol]

◆ **Amino Levulinic Acid** see Aminolevulinic Acid on page 94

◆ **5-Aminolevulinic Acid** see Aminolevulinic Acid on page 94

◆ **Aminolevulinic Acid HCl** see Aminolevulinic Acid on page 94

◆ **Aminolevulinic Acid Hydrochloride** see Aminolevulinic Acid on page 94

◆ **AMJ 9701** see Palifermin on page 1304

◆ **AMN107** see Nilotinib on page 1198

◆ **Amnesteem** see ISOtretinoin on page 973

◆ **Amphadase** see Hyaluronidase on page 820

◆ **Amphotec** see Amphotericin B Cholesteryl Sulfate Complex on page 95

◆ **Amphotec® (Can)** see Amphotericin B Cholesteryl Sulfate Complex on page 95

Amphotericin B Cholesteryl Sulfate Complex
(am foe TER i sin bee kole LES te ril SUL fate KOM plecks)
Brand Names: US Amphotec
Brand Names: Canada Amphotec®
Index Terms ABCD; Amphotericin B Colloidal Dispersion
Pharmacologic Category Antifungal Agent, Parenteral
Use Treatment of invasive aspergillosis in patients who have failed amphotericin B deoxycholate treatment, or who have renal impairment or experience unacceptable toxicity which precludes treatment with amphotericin B deoxycholate in effective doses.
Pregnancy Risk Factor B
Dosing
Adult & Geriatric Aspergillosis (invasive), treatment: *Usual dosage range:* 3-4 mg/kg/day. **Note:** 6 mg/kg/day has been used for treatment of life-threatening invasive aspergillosis in immunocompromised patients (Bowden, 2002).
Premedication: For patients who experience chills, fever, hypotension, nausea, or other nonanaphylactic infusion-related immediate reactions, premedicate with the following drugs 30-60 minutes prior to drug administration: A nonsteroidal with or without diphenhydramine **or** acetaminophen with diphenhydramine **or** hydrocortisone 50-100 mg with or without a nonsteroidal and diphenhydramine (Paterson, 2008).
Test dose: For patients receiving their first dose in a new treatment course, a small amount (10 mL of the final preparation, containing between 1.6-8.3 mg) infused over 15-30 minutes is recommended. The patient should then be observed for an additional 30 minutes.
Pediatric Refer to adult dosing.
Renal Impairment
Mild to moderate impairment: No dosage adjustment provided in manufacturer's labeling. However, no pharmacokinetic changes were noted in patients with mild-to-moderate impairment.
Severe impairment: No dosage adjustment provided in manufacturer's labeling (has not been studied).
Hepatic Impairment No dosage adjustment provided in manufacturer's labeling (has not been studied).
Additional Information Complete prescribing information should be consulted for additional detail.
Dosage Forms Excipient information presented when available (limited, particularly for generics); consult specific product labeling.
Suspension Reconstituted, Intravenous:
Amphotec: 50 mg (1 ea); 100 mg (1 ea) [contains edetate disodium, hydrochloric acid, lactose, sodium cholesteryl sulfate, tromethamine]

♦ **Amphotericin B Colloidal Dispersion** *see* Amphotericin B Cholesteryl Sulfate Complex *on page 95*

Amphotericin B (Conventional)
(am foe TER i sin bee con VEN sha nal)
Brand Names: Canada Fungizone
Index Terms Amphotericin B Deoxycholate; Amphotericin B Desoxycholate; Conventional Amphotericin B
Pharmacologic Category Antifungal Agent, Parenteral

◀ **Use**

Life-threatening fungal infections: Treatment of patients with progressive, potentially life-threatening fungal infections: Aspergillosis, cryptococcosis (torulosis), North American blastomycosis, systemic candidiasis, coccidioidomycosis, histoplasmosis, zygomycosis (including mucormycosis due to susceptible species of the genera *Absidia, Mucor,* and *Rhizopus*), and infections due to related susceptible species of *Conidiobolus, Basidiobolus,* and sporotrichosis.

Leishmaniasis: May be useful in the treatment of American mucocutaneous leishmaniasis, but it is not the drug of choice as primary therapy.

Pregnancy Risk Factor B

Dosing

Adult & Geriatric Note: Premedication: For patients who experience infusion-related immediate reactions, premedicate with the following drugs 30 to 60 minutes prior to drug administration: NSAID and/or diphenhydramine **or** acetaminophen with diphenhydramine **or** hydrocortisone. If the patient experiences rigors during the infusion, meperidine may be administered.

Test dose: IV: 1 mg infused over 20 to 30 minutes. Many clinicians believe a test dose is unnecessary.

Susceptible fungal infections: IV: Adults: 0.3 to 1.5 mg/kg/day; 1 to 1.5 mg/kg over 4 to 6 hours every other day may be given once therapy is established; aspergillosis, rhinocerebral mucormycosis, often require 1 to 1.5 mg/kg/day; do not exceed 1.5 mg/kg/day

Aspergillosis, disseminated: IV: 0.6 to 0.7 mg/kg/day for 3 to 6 months

Aspergillosis (invasive) in HIV-infected patients (off-label use): IV: 1 mg/kg once daily until infection resolution and CD4 count >200 cells/mm^3 (HHS [OI adult 2015])

Bone marrow transplantation (prophylaxis): IV: Low-dose amphotericin B 0.1 to 0.25 mg/kg/day has been administered after bone marrow transplantation to reduce the risk of invasive fungal disease.

Candidemia (neutropenic or non-neutropenic): IV: 0.5 to 1 mg/kg/day until 14 days after first negative blood culture and resolution of signs and symptoms (Pappas 2009)

Candidiasis, chronic, disseminated: IV: 0.5 to 0.7 mg/kg/day for 3 to 6 months and resolution of radiologic lesions (Pappas 2009)

Coccidioidomycosis in HIV-infected patients with severe, non-meningeal infection (ie, diffuse pulmonary or severely ill with extrathoracic disseminated disease) (off-label use): IV: 0.7 to 1 mg/kg/day until clinical improvement, then initiate triazole therapy (eg, fluconazole or itraconazole) (HHS [OI adult 2015])

Dematiaceous fungi: IV: 0.7 mg/kg/day in combination with an azole

Endocarditis: IV: 0.6 to 1 mg/kg/day (with or without flucytosine) for 6 weeks after valve replacement; **Note:** If isolates susceptible and/or clearance demonstrated, guidelines recommend step-down to fluconazole; also for long-term suppression therapy if valve replacement is not possible (Pappas 2009)

Endophthalmitis, fungal (off-label use):

Intravitreal: 5 to 12.5 mcg (with or without concomitant systemic therapy) (Brod 1990)

IV: 0.7 to 1 mg/kg/day (with flucytosine) for at least 4 to 6 weeks (Pappas 2009)

Esophageal candidiasis: IV: 0.3 to 0.7 mg/kg/day for 14 to 21 days after clinical improvement (Pappas 2009)

Histoplasmosis: Chronic, severe pulmonary or disseminated: IV: 0.5 to 1 mg/kg/day for 7 days, then 0.8 mg/kg every other day (or 3 times/week) until total dose of 10 to 15 mg/kg; may continue itraconazole as suppressive therapy (lifelong for immunocompromised patients)

Meningitis:

Candidal: IV: 0.7 to 1 mg/kg/day (with or without flucytosine) for at least 4 weeks; **Note:** Liposomal amphotericin favored by IDSA guidelines based on decreased risk of nephrotoxicity and potentially better CNS penetration (Pappas 2009)

Cryptococcal or Coccidioides: Intrathecal: Initial: 0.01 to 0.05 mg as single daily dose; may increase daily in increments of 0.025 to 0.1 mg as tolerated (maximum: 1.5 mg/day; most patients will tolerate a maximum dose of ~0.5 mg/treatment). Once titration to a maximum tolerated dose is achieved, that dose is administered daily. Once CSF improvement noted, may decrease frequency on a weekly basis (eg, 5 times/week, then 3 times/week, then 2 times/week, then once weekly, then once every other week, then once every 2 weeks, etc) until administration occurs once every 6 weeks. Typically, concurrent oral azole therapy is maintained (Stevens 2001). **Note:** IDSA notes that the use of intrathecal amphotericin for cryptococcal meningitis is generally discouraged and rarely necessary (Perfect 2010).

Histoplasma: IV: 0.5 to 1 mg/kg/day for 7 days, then 0.8 mg/kg every other day (or 3 times/week) for 3 months total duration; follow with fluconazole suppressive therapy for up to 12 months

Meningoencephalitis, cryptococcal (Perfect 2010): IV:

HIV positive: Induction: 0.7 to 1 mg/kg/day (plus flucytosine 100 mg/kg/day) for 2 weeks, then change to oral fluconazole for at least 8 weeks; alternatively, amphotericin (0.7 to 1 mg/kg/day) may be continued uninterrupted for 4 to 6 weeks; maintenance: amphotericin 1 mg/kg/week for ≥1 year may be considered, but inferior to use of azoles

HIV negative: Induction: 0.7 to 1 mg/kg/day (plus flucytosine 100 mg/kg/day) for 2 weeks (low-risk patients), ≥4 weeks (non-low-risk, but without neurologic complication, immunosuppression, underlying disease, and negative CSF culture at 2 weeks), >6 weeks (neurologic complication or patients intolerant of flucytosine) Follow with azole consolidation/maintenance treatment.

Oropharyngeal candidiasis: IV: 0.3 mg/kg/day for 7 to 14 days (Pappas 2009)

Osteoarticular candidiasis: IV: 0.5 to 1 mg/kg/day for several weeks, followed by fluconazole for 6 to 12 months (osteomyelitis) or 6 weeks (septic arthritis) (Pappas 2009)

Penicillium marneffei: IV: 0.6 mg/kg/day for 2 weeks

Pneumonia: Cryptococcal (mild-to-moderate): IV:

HIV positive: 0.5 to 1 mg/kg/day

HIV negative: 0.5 to 0.7 mg/kg/day (plus flucytosine) for 2 weeks

Sporotrichosis: Pulmonary, meningeal, osteoarticular or disseminated: IV: Total dose of 1 to 2 g, then change to oral itraconazole or fluconazole for suppressive therapy

Urinary tract candidiasis (IDSA [Pappas 2009]):

Fungus balls: IV: 0.5 to 0.7 mg/kg/day with or without flucytosine 25 mg/kg 4 times daily

Pyelonephritis: IV: 0.5 to 0.7 mg/kg/day with or without flucytosine 25 mg/kg 4 times daily for 2 weeks

Symptomatic cystitis: IV: 0.3 to 0.6 mg/kg/day for 1 to 7 days

◄

Bladder irrigation in patients with C. krusei or fluconazole-resistant C. glabrata: Irrigate with 50 mcg/mL solution instilled periodically or continuously for 5 to 7 days or until cultures are clear. **Note:** Recommended for use in conjunction with other treatment modalities (Fisher 2011).

Pediatric Note: Premedication: For patients who experience infusion-related immediate reactions, premedicate with the following drugs 30 to 60 minutes prior to drug administration: NSAID and/or diphenhydramine **or** acetaminophen with diphenhydramine **or** hydrocortisone. If the patient experiences rigors during the infusion, meperidine may be administered.

Test dose: IV: Infants and Children: 0.1 mg/kg/dose to a maximum of 1 mg; infuse over 30 to 60 minutes. Many clinicians believe a test dose is unnecessary.

Susceptible fungal infections: IV: Infants and Children: Maintenance dose: 0.25 to 1 mg/kg/day given once daily; infuse over 2 to 6 hours. Once therapy has been established, amphotericin B can be administered on an every-other-day basis at 1 to 1.5 mg/kg/dose; cumulative dose: 1.5 to 2 g over 6 to 10 weeks

Note: Duration of therapy varies with nature of infection: Usual duration is 4 to 12 weeks or cumulative dose of 1 to 4 g.

Indication-specific dosing:

Infants and Children:

Aspergillosis (HIV-exposed/-positive): IV: 1 to 1.5 mg/kg/day once daily (CDC 2009)

Candidiasis (HIV-exposed/-positive):

Invasive: IV: 0.5 to 1.5 mg/kg/day once daily (CDC 2009)

Esophageal: IV: 0.3 to 0.5 mg/kg/day once daily (CDC 2009)

Oropharyngeal, refractory: IV: 0.3 to 0.5 mg/kg/day (CDC 2009)

Coccidioidomycosis (HIV-exposed/-positive): IV: 0.5 to 1 mg/kg/day (CDC 2009)

Cryptococcus, CNS disease (HIV-exposed/-positive): IV: 0.7 to 1 mg/kg/day plus flucytosine; **Note:** Minimum 2 week induction followed by consolidation and chronic suppressive therapy; may increase amphotericin dose to 1.5 mg/kg/day if flucytosine is not tolerated.

Cryptococcus, disseminated (non-CNS disease) or severe pulmonary disease (HIV-exposed/-positive): IV: 0.7 to 1 mg/kg/day once daily with or without flucytosine

Histoplasma, CNS or severe disseminated: IV: 1 mg/kg/day once daily (CDC 2009)

Adolescents:

Aspergillosis (invasive) in HIV-infected patients (off-label use): IV: Refer to adult dosing.

Coccidioidomycosis in HIV-infected patients with severe, non-meningeal infection (ie, diffuse pulmonary or severely ill with extrathoracic disseminated disease) (off-label use): IV: Refer to adult dosing.

Renal Impairment

If renal dysfunction is due to the drug, the daily total can be decreased by 50% or the dose can be given every other day. IV therapy may take several months.

Renal replacement therapy: Poorly dialyzed; no supplemental dose or dosage adjustment necessary, including patients on intermittent hemodialysis or CRRT.

Peritoneal dialysis (PD): Administration in dialysate: 1 to 2 mg/L of peritoneal dialysis fluid either with or without low-dose IV amphotericin B (a total dose of 2 to 10 mg/kg given over 7 to 14 days). Precipitate may form in ionic dialysate solutions.

Hepatic Impairment No dosage adjustment provided in manufacturer's labeling.

Additional Information Complete prescribing information should be consulted for additional detail.

Dosage Forms Excipient information presented when available (limited, particularly for generics); consult specific product labeling.

Solution Reconstituted, Injection, as desoxycholate:

Generic: 50 mg (1 ea)

◆ **Amphotericin B Deoxycholate** *see* Amphotericin B (Conventional)
on page 95

◆ **Amphotericin B Desoxycholate** *see* Amphotericin B (Conventional)
on page 95

Amphotericin B (Lipid Complex)
(am foe TER i sin bee LIP id KOM pleks)

Brand Names: US Abelcet

Brand Names: Canada Abelcet

Index Terms ABLC

Pharmacologic Category Antifungal Agent, Parenteral

Use Treatment of invasive fungal infection in patients who are refractory to or intolerant of conventional amphotericin B (amphotericin B deoxycholate) therapy

Pregnancy Risk Factor B

Dosing

Adult & Geriatric Note: Premedication: For patients who experience infusion-related immediate reactions, premedicate with the following drugs 30 to 60 minutes prior to drug administration: A nonsteroidal anti-inflammatory agent ± diphenhydramine **or** acetaminophen with diphenhydramine **or** hydrocortisone. If the patient experiences rigors during the infusion, meperidine may be administered.

Usual dose: IV: 5 mg/kg once daily

Manufacturer's labeling: Invasive fungal infections (when patients are intolerant or refractory to conventional amphotericin B): IV: 5 mg/kg/day

Indication-specific dosing:

Aspergillosis, invasive (alternative to preferred therapy): IV: 5 mg/kg/day; duration of treatment depends on site of infection, extent of disease and level of immunosuppression (Walsh 2008)

Aspergillosis (invasive) in HIV-infected patients (alternative to preferred therapy) (off-label use): 5 mg/kg/day; treat until infection appears to be resolved and CD4 count >200 cells/mm^3 (HHS [OI adult 2015])

Blastomycosis, moderately severe to severe (off-label dose): IV: 3 to 5 mg/kg/day for 1 to 2 weeks or until improvement, followed by oral itraconazole (Chapman 2008)

◄ **Candidiasis (off-label dose):** IV:
Chronic disseminated candidiasis, pericarditis or myocarditis due to Candida, suppurative thrombophlebitis: 3 to 5 mg/kg/day. **Note:** In chronic disseminated candidiasis, transition to fluconazole after several weeks in stable patients is preferred (Pappas 2009)
CNS candidiasis: 3 to 5 mg/kg/day (with or without flucytosine) for several weeks, followed by fluconazole (Pappas 2009)
Endocarditis due to Candida, infected pacemaker, ICD, or VAD: 3 to 5 mg/kg/day (with or without flucytosine); continue to treat for 4 to 6 weeks after device removal unless device cannot be removed then chronic suppression with fluconazole is recommended (Pappas 2009)

Coccidioidomycosis, progressive, disseminated (alternative to preferred therapy) (off-label dose): IV: 2 to 5 mg/kg/day (Galgiani 2005)

Coccidioidomycosis in HIV-infected patients with severe, nonmeningeal infection (ie, diffuse pulmonary or severely ill with extrathoracic disseminated disease) (off-label use): 4 to 6 mg/kg/day until clinical improvement, then switch to fluconazole or itraconazole (HHS [OI adult 2015])

Cryptococcosis: IV:
Cryptococcal meningitis in HIV-infected patients (alternative to preferred therapy) (off-label use): Induction therapy: 5 mg/kg/day with flucytosine for at least 2 weeks, followed by fluconazole for consolidation therapy (HHS [OI adult 2015]; Perfect 2010). **Note:** If flucytosine is not given due to intolerance, duration of amphotericin B lipid complex therapy should be 4 to 6 weeks (Perfect 2010).
Cryptococcal meningoencephalitis in HIV-negative patients and nontransplant patients (as an alternative to conventional amphotericin B): Induction therapy: 5 mg/kg/day (with flucytosine if possible) for ≥4 weeks followed by oral fluconazole. **Note:** If flucytosine is not given or treatment is interrupted, consider prolonging induction therapy for an additional 2 weeks (Perfect 2010).
Cryptococcal meningoencephalitis in transplant recipients: Induction therapy: 5 mg/kg/day (with flucytosine) for at least 2 weeks, followed by oral fluconazole **Note:** If flucytosine is not given, duration of amphotericin B lipid complex therapy should be 4 to 6 weeks (Perfect 2010).
Nonmeningeal cryptococcosis: Induction therapy: 5 mg/kg/day (with flucytosine if possible) for ≥4 weeks may be used for severe pulmonary cryptococcosis or for cryptococcemia with evidence of high fungal burden, followed by oral fluconazole. **Note:** If flucytosine is not given or treatment is interrupted, consider prolonging induction therapy for an additional 2 weeks (Perfect 2010).

Histoplasmosis: IV:
Acute pulmonary (moderately severe to severe): 5 mg/kg/day for 1 to 2 weeks, followed by oral itraconazole (Wheat 2007)
Moderate to severe disseminated disease in HIV-infected patients (alternative to preferred therapy) (off-label use): 3 mg/kg/day for at least 2 weeks, followed by itraconazole maintenance therapy (HHS [OI adult 2015])
Progressive disseminated (alternative to preferred therapy): 5 mg/kg/day for 1 to 2 weeks, followed by oral itraconazole (Wheat 2007)

Leishmaniasis (visceral) in HIV-infected patients (off-label use; HHS [OI adult 2015]):
Chronic maintenance therapy (for patients with a CD4 count <200 cells/mm^3: 3 mg/kg every 21 days (HHS [OI adult 2015])

Sporotrichosis (off-label dose): IV:

Meningeal: 5 mg/kg/day for 4 to 6 weeks, followed by oral itraconazole (Kauffman 2007)

Pulmonary, osteoarticular, and disseminated: 3 to 5 mg/kg/day, followed by oral itraconazole after a favorable response is seen with amphotericin initial therapy (Kauffman 2007)

Pediatric Note: Premedication: For patients who experience infusion-related immediate reactions, premedicate with the following drugs 30 to 60 minutes prior to drug administration: A nonsteroidal anti-inflammatory agent ± diphenhydramine **or** acetaminophen with diphenhydramine **or** hydrocortisone. If the patient experiences rigors during the infusion, meperidine may be administered.

Usual dose: 5 mg/kg once daily

Manufacturer's labeling: Invasive fungal infections (when patients are intolerant or refractory to conventional amphotericin B): Children: IV: 5 mg/kg/day

Indication-specific dosing:

Aspergillosis (HIV-positive patients) (alternative to preferred therapy): Infants and Children: IV: 5 mg/kg/day for ≥12 weeks (CDC [pediatric 2009])

Adolescents: Refer to adult dosing.

Candidiasis, invasive (HIV-positive patients) (alternative to preferred therapy): Infants and Children: IV: 5 mg/kg/day; treatment duration based on clinical response, treat until 2 to 3 weeks after last positive blood culture (CDC [pediatric 2009])

Coccidioidomycosis in HIV-infected patients with severe, nonmeningeal infection (ie, diffuse pulmonary or severely ill with extrathoracic disseminated disease) (off-label use): Adolescents: Refer to adult dosing.

Cryptococcosis:

Cryptococcus neoformans, disseminated disease (non-CNS disease) (HIV-positive patients): Infants and Children: IV: 5 mg/kg/day (with or without flucytosine); treatment duration of non-CNS disease varies by clinical response and site/severity of infection (CDC [pediatric 2009])

Cryptococcal meningitis in HIV-infected patients (as an alternative to preferred therapy) (off-label use): Adolescents: Refer to adult dosing.

Histoplasmosis in HIV-infected patients with moderate to severe disseminated disease (alternative to preferred therapy): Adolescents: Refer to adult dosing.

Leishmaniasis (visceral), chronic maintenance therapy in HIV-infected patients (off-label use): Adolescents: Refer to adult dosing.

Renal Impairment

Manufacturer's labeling: No dosage adjustment provided in manufacturer's labeling (has not been studied).

Alternate recommendations (Aronoff 2007):

Intermittent hemodialysis: Not hemodialyzable; no supplemental dosage necessary.

Peritoneal dialysis: No supplemental dosage necessary.

Continuous renal replacement therapy (CRRT): No supplemental dosage necessary.

Hepatic Impairment No dosage adjustment provided in manufacturer's labeling (has not been studied).

◀ **Additional Information** Complete prescribing information should be consulted for additional detail.

Dosage Forms Excipient information presented when available (limited, particularly for generics); consult specific product labeling.

Suspension, Intravenous:

Abelcet: 5 mg/mL (20 mL)

Amphotericin B (Liposomal) (am foe TER i sin bee lye po SO mal)

Brand Names: US AmBisome

Brand Names: Canada AmBisome

Index Terms Amphotericin B Liposome; L-AmB; Liposomal Amphotericin; Liposomal Amphotericin B

Pharmacologic Category Antifungal Agent, Parenteral

Use

Cryptococcal meningitis in HIV-infected patients: Treatment of cryptococcal meningitis in HIV-infected patients.

Fungal infections, empiric therapy: Empiric treatment in febrile neutropenic patients with presumed fungal infection.

Fungal infections, systemic therapy: Treatment of systemic infections caused by *Aspergillus* sp, *Candida* sp, and/or *Cryptococcus* sp in patients refractory to conventional amphotericin B deoxycholate therapy or when renal impairment or unacceptable toxicity precludes the use of the deoxycholate formulation.

Leishmaniasis (visceral): Treatment of visceral leishmaniasis.

Pregnancy Risk Factor B

Dosing

Adult & Geriatric

Usual dosage range: IV: 3 to 6 mg/kg/day; **Note:** Higher doses (7.5 to 15 mg/kg/day) have been used clinically in special cases (CDC 2013; Kauffman 2012; Walsh 2001)

Note: Premedication: For patients who experience nonanaphylactic immediate infusion-related reactions, premedicate with the following drugs 30 to 60 minutes prior to drug administration: A nonsteroidal anti-inflammatory agent ± diphenhydramine; **or** acetaminophen with diphenhydramine; **or** hydrocortisone. If the patient experiences rigors during the infusion, meperidine may be administered.

Indication-specific dosing: IV:

Aspergillus **(systemic infection):** 3 to 5 mg/kg/day

Aspergillosis (invasive) in HIV-infected patients (alternative to preferred therapy) (off-label use): 5 mg/kg/day until infection resolution and CD4 count >200 cells/mm^3 (HHS [OI adult 2015])

Candidiasis:

Empiric therapy: 3 to 5 mg/kg/day (Pappas 2009)

Endocarditis: 3 to 5 mg/kg/day (with or without flucytosine) for 6 weeks after valve replacement; Note: If isolates susceptible and/or clearance demonstrated, guidelines recommend step-down to fluconazole; also for long-term suppression therapy if valve replacement is not possible (Pappas 2009)

General invasive disease: 3 to 5 mg/kg/day with oral flucytosine (off-label combination; Pappas 2009)

Meningitis: 3 to 5 mg/kg/day with or without oral flucytosine (off-label combination; Pappas 2009)

Osteoarticular: 3 to 5 mg/kg/day for several weeks, followed by fluconazole for 6 to 12 months (osteomyelitis) or 6 weeks (septic arthritis) (Pappas 2009)

Systemic infection: Manufacturer's labeling: 3 to 5 mg/kg/day

Coccidioidomycosis in HIV-infected patients with severe, non-meningeal infection (ie, diffuse pulmonary or severely ill with extrathoracic, disseminated disease) (off-label use): 4 to 6 mg/kg/day until clinical improvement, then initiate triazole therapy (eg, fluconazole or itraconazole) (HHS [OI adult 2015])

Cryptococcus **(systemic infection):** 3 to 5 mg/kg/day

Cryptococcal meningitis in HIV-infected patients:

Manufacturer's labeling: 6 mg/kg/day

Alternate recommendations: 3 to 4 mg/kg/day in combination with oral flucytosine (HHS [OI adult 2015])

Fungal sinusitis: Limited data in immunocompromised patients have shown efficacy with 3 to 10 mg/kg/day (Barron 2005; Pagano 2004; Rokicka 2006). **Note:** An azole antifungal is recommended if causative organism is *Aspergillus* spp or *Pseudallescheria boydii* (*Scedosporium* sp).

Histoplasmosis in HIV-infected patients (off-label use; HHS [OI adult 2015]):

Moderately severe to severe disseminated disease: Induction therapy: 3 mg/kg/day for at least 2 weeks, followed by oral itraconazole for maintenance therapy

Histoplasma meningitis: Induction therapy: 5 mg/kg/day for 4 to 6 weeks, followed by oral itraconazole for maintenance therapy

Leishmaniasis (cutaneous) in HIV-infected patients (off-label use): 2 to 4 mg/kg/day for 10 days or an interrupted schedule (eg, 4 mg/kg on days 1 through 5, and then on days 10, 17, 24, 31, 38). Total dose administered should be 20 to 60 mg/kg (HHS [OI adult 2015])

Leishmaniasis (visceral):

Immunocompetent: 3 mg/kg/day on days 1 through 5, and 3 mg/kg/day on days 14 and 21; a repeat course may be given in patients who do not achieve parasitic clearance

Immunocompromised: 4 mg/kg/day on days 1 through 5, and 4 mg/kg/day on days 10, 17, 24, 31, and 38

Leishmaniasis (visceral) in HIV-infected patients (off-label use; HHS [OI adult 2015]):

Treatment: 2 to 4 mg/kg/day **or** an interrupted schedule (eg, 4 mg/kg on days 1 through 5, and then on days 10, 17, 24, 31, and 38). Total dose administered: 20 to 60 mg/kg

Chronic maintenance therapy (for patients with a CD4 count <200 cells/mm^3): 4 mg/kg every 2 to 4 weeks

Meningitis (secondary to contaminated [eg, Exserohilum rostratum] steroid products), severe or in patients not improving with voriconazole monotherapy (off-label use) (CDC 2013; Kauffman 2012): IV: 5 to 6 mg/kg/day in combination with voriconazole for ≥3 months; a higher dose (7.5 mg/kg/day) may be considered in patients who are not improving. **Note:** Consult an infectious disease specialist and current CDC guidelines for specific treatment recommendations.

Osteoarticular infection (secondary to contaminated [eg, *Exserohilum rostratum*] steroid products), severe or in patients with clinical instability (off-label use) (CDC 2013; Kauffman 2012): IV: 5 mg/kg/day in combination with voriconazole for ≥3 months. **Note:** Consult an infectious disease specialist and current CDC guidelines for specific treatment recommendations.

***Penicillium marneffei* infection in HIV-infected patients (off-label use):** 3 to 5 mg/kg/day for 2 weeks, followed by oral itraconazole for 10 weeks, followed by chronic maintenance therapy (HHS [OI adult 2015])

Pediatric

Usual dosage range: Infants, Children, and Adolescents: IV: 3 to 6 mg/kg/day

Note: Premedication: For patients who experience nonanaphylactic immediate infusion-related reactions, premedicate with the following drugs 30 to 60 minutes prior to drug administration: A nonsteroidal anti-inflammatory agent ± diphenhydramine; **or** acetaminophen with diphenhydramine; **or** hydrocortisone. If the patient experiences rigors during the infusion, meperidine may be administered.

Indication-specific dosing:

Infants, Children, and Adolescents: IV:

Empiric therapy: 3 mg/kg/day

Cryptococcal meningitis in HIV-exposed/infected patients:

Infants and Children: 6 mg/kg/dose once daily; may coadminister with flucytosine (HHS [OI pediatric 2013]; off-label combination)

Adolescents: Refer to adult dosing.

Systemic fungal infections *(Aspergillus, Candida, Cryptococcus)*; non-HIV-exposed/-infected: 3 to 5 mg/kg/day

Systemic fungal infections (HIV-exposed/-infected [HHS (OI pediatric 2013; OI adult 2015)]; off-label use):

Infants and Children:

Candidiasis, invasive: 5 mg/kg/dose once daily

Coccidioidomycosis (severe illness with respiratory compromise due to diffuse pulmonary or disseminated non-meningitic disease): 5 mg/kg/dose once daily until clinical improvement, then initiate triazole therapy (eg, fluconazole or itraconazole); dosage may be increased to 10 mg/kg/dose once daily for life-threatening infection.

Cryptococcus, disseminated (non-CNS): 3 to 5 mg/kg/dose once daily (may consider addition of oral flucytosine)

Histoplasmosis:

CNS infection: 5 mg/kg/dose once daily

Disseminated: 3 to 5 mg/kg/day once daily

Adolescents: Refer to adult dosing.

Leishmaniasis (cutaneous) in HIV-infected patients (off-label use): Adolescents: Refer to adult dosing.

Leishmaniasis (visceral):

Immunocompetent: 3 mg/kg/day on days 1 to 5, and 3 mg/kg/day on days 14 and 21; a repeat course may be given in patients who do not achieve parasitic clearance

Immunocompromised: 4 mg/kg/day on days 1 to 5, and 4 mg/kg/day on days 10, 17, 24, 31, and 38

Leishmaniasis (visceral) in HIV-infected patients (off-label use): Adolescents: Refer to adult dosing.

***Penicillium marneffei* infection in HIV-infected patients (off-label use):** Adolescents: Refer to adult dosing.

Renal Impairment

There are no dosage adjustments provided in the manufacturer's labeling; has been successfully administered to patients with preexisting renal impairment.

End-stage renal disease (ESRD) on intermittent hemodialysis (IHD) (administer after hemodialysis on dialysis days): Poorly dialyzed; no dosage adjustment necessary (Heintz 2009)

CVVH/CVVHD/CVVHDF: No dosage adjustment necessary (Heintz 2009)

Hepatic Impairment

There are no dosage adjustments provided in the manufacturer's labeling (has not been studied).

Additional Information Complete prescribing information should be consulted for additional detail.

Dosage Forms Excipient information presented when available (limited, particularly for generics); consult specific product labeling.

Suspension Reconstituted, Intravenous:

AmBisome: 50 mg (1 ea) [contains cholesterol, distearoyl phosphatidylglycerol, hydrogenated soy phosphatidylcholine, sodium succinate hexahydrate, sucrose, tocopherol, dl-alpha]

◆ **Amphotericin B Liposome** see Amphotericin B (Liposomal) on page 102

◆ **AMSA** see Amsacrine on page 105

◆ **Amsacrin** see Amsacrine on page 105

Amsacrine (AM sah kreen)

Related Information

Management of Drug Extravasations on page 2159

Safe Handling of Hazardous Drugs on page 2292

Brand Names: Canada AMSA PD

Index Terms 4-(9-Acridinylamino) Methanesulfon-m-Anisidide; Acridinyl Anisidide; AMSA; Amsacrin; m-AMSA

Pharmacologic Category Antineoplastic Agent, Miscellaneous

Use Note: Not approved in the US.

Acute leukemia: Remission induction in refractory acute leukemia in adults

Labeled Contraindications Hypersensitivity to amsacrine, acridine derivatives (eg, acriflavine), or any component of the formulation; preexisting drug-induced or radiation therapy-induced bone marrow suppression

Pregnancy Considerations Animal reproduction studies have not been conducted. Women of childbearing potential should avoid becoming pregnant while receiving treatment.

Breast-Feeding Considerations It is not known if amsacrine is excreted in breast milk. Breast-feeding should be discontinued prior to treatment.

Warnings/Precautions Hazardous agent - use appropriate precautions for handling and disposal (NIOSH 2014 [group 1]).

Amsacrine is a potent bone marrow suppressant; effects may be prolonged and may require supportive therapy. Monitor CBC with differential during induction therapy. Leukopenia is generally transient. The WBC nadir usually occurs at 11 to 13 days after treatment; recovery usually occurs by days 17 to 25. Anemia and thrombocytopenia may also occur. Monitor for infection (due to neutropenia) and bleeding (due to thrombocytopenia). Hematologic toxicity may require dose reduction, therapy interruption or treatment delay. Doses higher than recommended may result in severe and prolonged marrow suppression.

◀ Arrhythmia, heart failure, bradycardia, and tachycardia have been reported. Risk factors for arrhythmia may include hypokalemia and a history of anthracycline therapy. Correct fluid and electrolyte imbalance prior to treatment initiation. Serum potassium should be >4 mEq/L prior to administration (Arlin, 1988). The risk for arrhythmia is decreased by ensuring normal potassium levels. Monitor ECG during and after infusion.

Vesicant; ensure proper needle or catheter placement prior to and during infusion. Avoid extravasation. Extravasation may result in severe irritation or necrosis. Tumor lysis syndrome may occur; adequate hydration and prophylactic uric acid reduction should be considered prior to or during treatment; monitor closely.

Use with caution in patients with significant hepatic impairment (bilirubin >2 mg/dL); toxicity may be increased. Hepatic metabolism and biliary excretion are major routes of elimination. Dosage reductions may be recommended. Evaluate hepatic function prior to and during treatment. Use with caution in patients with significant renal impairment (BUN >20 mg/dL; serum creatinine >1.2 mg/dL); toxicity may be increased. Dosage reductions may be recommended. Evaluate renal function prior to and during treatment. Potentially significant drug-drug interactions may exist, requiring dose or frequency adjustment, additional monitoring, and/or selection of alternative therapy. Avoid vaccination with live virus vaccines during treatment. Amsacrine contains N,N-dimethylacetamide, which is incompatible with many closed system transfer devices (CSTDs); the plastic components of CSTDs may dissolve and result in subsequent leakage and potential infusion of dissolved plastic into the patient (ISMP [Smetzer 2015]). The manufacturer reports a low risk of microbial contamination and infection exists with use of AMSA PD injection (50 mg/mL); risk may be further minimized with the use of Sartorius sterile filters (Minisart SRP [PTFE] 0.2 micrometer, 15 mm; provided by the manufacturer) prior to transferring AMSA PD to the diluent. Monitor for signs/symptoms of infection during therapy (Health Canada 2014).

Adverse Reactions

>10%:

Gastrointestinal: Nausea (>10%), vomiting (>10%), stomatitis (>10%), diarrhea (>10%), perirectal abscess (>10%), abdominal pain (>10%)

Hematologic: Myelosuppression, leukopenia (nadir: 11-13 days; recovery: days 17-25)

Frequency not defined:

Cardiovascular: Atrial tachyarrhythmia, atrial tachycardia, atrial fibrillation, bradycardia, cardiomyopathy (rare), cardiopulmonary arrest, CHF (rare); ECG changes (QT prolongation, nonspecific ST segment or T wave changes); ejection fraction decreased, hypotension, sinus tachycardia, tachycardia, ventricular arrhythmia, ventricular extrasystoles, ventricular fibrillation, ventricular tachyarrhythmia

Central nervous system: Confusion, dizziness, emotional lability, fever, headache, hypoesthesia, lethargy, seizure

Dermatologic: Alopecia, cutaneous inflammatory reaction, dermatologic reaction, purpura, rash (purpuric or maculopapular), urticaria

Gastrointestinal: Anorexia, dysphagia, gingivitis, gum hemorrhage, hematemesis, weight changes

Genitourinary: Orange-red discoloration of the urine

Hematologic: Anemia, granulocytopenia, hemorrhage, pancytopenia, thrombocytopenia

Hepatic: Alkaline phosphatase increased, AST increased, bilirubin increased, hepatic insufficiency, hepatitis, hepatotoxicity, jaundice, progressive liver failure

Local: Injection site inflammation, phlebitis

Neuromuscular & skeletal: Musculoskeletal pain, paresthesia, weakness

Renal: BUN increased, creatinine increased, hematuria, proteinuria, renal failure

Respiratory: Dyspnea

Miscellaneous: Allergic reaction, infection

Drug Interactions

Metabolism/Transport Effects None known.

Avoid Concomitant Use

Avoid concomitant use of Amsacrine with any of the following: BCG (Intravesical); CloZAPine; Dipyrone; Natalizumab; Pimecrolimus; Tacrolimus (Topical); Tofacitinib; Vaccines (Live)

Increased Effect/Toxicity

Amsacrine may increase the levels/effects of: CloZAPine; Fingolimod; Leflunomide; Natalizumab; Tofacitinib; Vaccines (Live)

The levels/effects of Amsacrine may be increased by: Denosumab; Dipyrone; Pimecrolimus; Roflumilast; Tacrolimus (Topical); Trastuzumab

Decreased Effect

Amsacrine may decrease the levels/effects of: BCG (Intravesical); Coccidioides immitis Skin Test; Sipuleucel-T; Vaccines (Inactivated); Vaccines (Live)

The levels/effects of Amsacrine may be decreased by: Echinacea

Storage/Stability Store intact ampuls and diluent vials at controlled room temperature of 15°C to 25°C (59°F to 77°F). Concentrated amsacrine should not be stored in plastic syringes for >15 minutes. Reconstituted vials may be stored at room temperature for up to 24 hours, under ambient light conditions. Solutions diluted for administration are stable for up to 7 days in glass or Abbott plastic containers, however, the manufacturer recommends use within 24 hours when stored at room temperature and 72 hours if refrigerated.

Preparation for Administration Note: A low risk of microbial contamination exists with use of AMSA PD injection (50 mg/mL); risk may be further minimized with the use of Sartorius sterile filters (Minisart SRP [PTFE] 0.2 micrometer, 15 mm; provided by the manufacturer) prior to transferring AMSA PD to the diluent (Health Canada 2014).

Hazardous agent; use appropriate precautions for handling and disposal (NIOSH 2014 [group 1]). Reconstitute by adding 1.5 mL amsacrine to diluent vial (containing 13.5 mL L-lactic acid), resulting in a 5 mg/mL reconstituted solution. Glass syringes should be used, however if using plastic syringes, do not allow concentrated amsacrine to remain in plastic syringe for >15 minutes. Further dilute appropriate dose in 500 mL D_5W (the solution may be mixed in plastic bags when diluted for infusion). Amsacrine contains N,N-dimethylacetamide, which is incompatible with many closed system transfer devices (CSTDs); the plastic components of CSTDs may dissolve and result in subsequent leakage and potential infusion of dissolved plastic into the patient (ISMP [Smetzer 2015]).

◀ **Mechanism of Action** Amsacrine has been shown to inhibit DNA synthesis by binding to, and intercalating with, DNA; inhibits topoisomerase II activity.

Pharmacodynamics/Kinetics

Protein binding: 85% to 95% (Hall, 1983)

Metabolism: Hepatic

Half-life elimination: Terminal: Mean 7.4 hours; range: 6 to 10 hours (Hall, 1983)

Excretion: Bile (primarily); urine (35%; 20% as unchanged drug)

Dosing

Adult & Geriatric

Acute leukemia: IV:

Induction: 75 to 125 mg/m^2/day for 5 days every 3 to 4 weeks (125 mg/m^2/day is preferred; two courses may be necessary to achieve induction; increase dose by 20% in second and subsequent cycles if marrow hypoplasia not achieved and in absence of significant toxicity in previous course.)

Maintenance: Once remission has been achieved, maintenance dose should be ~50% of induction dose, administered every 4 to 8 weeks, depending on blood cell counts and marrow recovery

Acute myeloid leukemia (off-label dosing): IV: 120 mg/m^2 over 60 minutes on days 3, 5, and 7 of induction cycle 2 (in combination with cytarabine) (Löwenberg, 2011) **or** 120 mg/m^2 over 60 minutes on days 4, 5, and 6 of induction cycle 2 (in combination with cytarabine ± G-CSF) (Löwenberg, 2003)

Renal Impairment

BUN >20 mg/dL and/or serum creatinine >1.2 mg/dL: Dosage reduction is recommended; however there are no specific adjustments provided in the manufacturer's labeling. The following adjustments have been reported: Hall, 1983:

Serum creatinine 1.2 to 1.8 mg/dL: No dosage adjustment necessary.

Serum creatinine 2 to 3 mg/dL, oliguric patients: Reduce dose by 30% to 40%; may increase subsequent dose based on toxicity.

Hepatic Impairment Bilirubin >2 mg/dL: Dosage reduction is recommended; however, there are no specific adjustments provided in the manufacturer's labeling. The following adjustments have been reported:

Hall, 1983: Bilirubin >2 mg/dL: Reduce dose by 30% to 40%; may increase subsequent dose based on toxicity.

Koren, 1992: Severe hepatic dysfunction: Reduce dose by at least 50%

Adjustment for Toxicity Consider decreasing dose by 20% if life-threatening infection or hemorrhage occurred in previous cycle; delay second and subsequent cycles until recovery from myelosuppression or evidence of leukemic infiltrate is evident.

Administration IV: Infuse over 60 to 90 minutes.

Amsacrine contains N,N-dimethylacetamide, which is incompatible with many closed system transfer devices (CSTDs); the plastic components of CSTDs may dissolve and result in subsequent leakage and potential infusion of dissolved plastic into the patient (ISMP [Smetzer 2015]).

Vesicant; ensure proper needle or catheter placement prior to and during infusion; avoid extravasation.

Extravasation management: If extravasation occurs, stop infusion immediately and disconnect (leave cannula/needle in place); gently aspirate extravasated solution (do **NOT** flush the line); remove needle/cannula; elevate extremity.

Hazardous agent; use appropriate precautions for handling and disposal (NIOSH 2014 [group 1]).

Vesicant/Extravasation Risk Vesicant

Monitoring Parameters CBC with differential, bone marrow studies, electrolytes (serum potassium), hepatic function, renal function; ECG (during and after infusion); monitor for infection, bleeding, monitor fluid status, signs/symptoms of tumor lysis syndrome; monitor infusion site during infusion.

Product Availability Not available in the US

Dosage Forms: Canada Excipient information presented when available (limited, particularly for generics); consult specific product labeling.
Injection, solution [preservative free]:
  AMSA PD: 50 mg/mL (1.5 mL) [supplied with L-lactic acid 0.0353 M 13.5 mL]

♦ **AMSA PD (Can)** see Amsacrine on page 105

Anagrelide (an AG gre lide)

Brand Names: US Agrylin

Brand Names: Canada Agrylin; Dom-Anagrelide; Mylan-Anagrelide; PMS-Anagrelide; Sandoz-Anagrelide

Index Terms Anagrelide Hydrochloride; BL4162A

Pharmacologic Category Antiplatelet Agent; Phosphodiesterase-3 Enzyme Inhibitor

Use Thrombocythemia: Treatment of thrombocythemia associated with myeloproliferative disorders to reduce the risk of thrombosis and reduce associated symptoms (including thrombohemorrhagic events)

Labeled Contraindications There are no contraindications listed in the manufacturer's labeling.

Pregnancy Considerations Adverse events were observed in some animal reproduction studies. Data regarding use of anagrelide during pregnancy is limited. The manufacturer recommends effective contraception in women of childbearing potential.

Breast-Feeding Considerations It is not known if anagrelide is excreted in breast milk. Due to the potential for serious adverse reactions in the nursing infant, a decision should be made whether to discontinue nursing or to discontinue the drug, taking into account the importance of treatment to the mother.

Warnings/Precautions Major hemorrhagic events have occurred when used concomitantly with aspirin. Monitor closely for bleeding, particularly when used concurrently with other agents known to increase bleeding risk (eg, anticoagulants, NSAIDs, antiplatelet agents, other phosphodiesterase 3 (PDE3) inhibitors, and selective serotonin reuptake inhibitors). Ventricular tachycardia and torsades de pointes have been reported. As with other PDE3 inhibitors, anagrelide may cause vasodilation, tachycardia, palpitations and heart failure. PDE3 inhibitors are associated with decreased survival (compared to placebo) in patients with class III or IV heart failure. Dose-related increases in heart rate and mean QTc interval have been observed in a clinical trial. The maximum change in mean heart rate was ~8 beats per minute (bpm) at a dose of 0.5 mg and ~29 bpm with a 2.5 mg dose. The maximum mean change in QTc I (individual subject correlation) from placebo was 7 ms and 13 ms with doses of 0.5 mg and 2.5 mg, respectively. Use is not recommended in patients with hypokalemia, congenital long QT syndrome, a known history of acquired QTc prolongation, or when using concomitant therapy which may prolong the QTc interval. Hypotension accompanied by dizziness may occur, particularly with higher doses. Use with caution in patients with cardiovascular disease (eg, heart failure, bradyarrhythmias, electrolyte abnormalities); consider periodic ECGs; benefits should outweigh risks. Pretreatment cardiovascular evaluation (including ECG) and careful monitoring during treatment is recommended. Interstitial lung disease (including allergic alveolitis, eosinophilic pneumonia, and interstitial pneumonitis) has been associated with use; onset is from 1 week to several years, usually presenting with progressive dyspnea with lung infiltrations; symptoms usually improve after discontinuation. Use caution in patients with mild to moderate hepatic dysfunction; dosage reduction and careful monitoring are required for moderate hepatic impairment; use has not been studied in patients with severe impairment. Hepatic impairment increases anagrelide exposure and may increase the risk of QTc prolongation. Monitor liver function prior to and during treatment. Renal abnormalities (including renal failure) have been observed with anagrelide use; may be associated with preexisting renal impairment, although dosage adjustment due to renal insufficiency was not required; monitor closely in patients with renal insufficiency. Potentially significant drug-drug interactions may exist, requiring dose or frequency adjustment, additional monitoring, and/or selection of alternative therapy.

Adverse Reactions Frequency not always defined; reactions similar in adult and pediatric patients unless otherwise noted.

Cardiovascular: Palpitations (26%), edema (21%), peripheral edema (9%), chest pain (8%), tachycardia (8%), angina pectoris (1% to <5%), cardiac arrhythmia (1% to <5%), cardiac failure (1% to <5%), hypertension (1% to <5%), orthostatic hypotension (1% to <5%), syncope (1% to <5%), vasodilatation (1% to <5%), atrial fibrillation, cardiomegaly, cardiomyopathy, cerebrovascular accident, complete atrioventricular block, decreased diastolic pressure (pediatric patients), increased heart rate (pediatric patients), myocardial infarction, pericardial effusion, systolic hypotension (pediatric patients)

Central nervous system: Headache (44%), dizziness (15%), pain (15%), malaise (6%), paresthesia (6%), amnesia (1% to <5%), chills (1% to <5%), confusion (1% to <5%), depression (1% to <5%), drowsiness (1% to <5%), insomnia (1% to <5%), migraine (1% to <5%), nervousness (1% to <5%), fatigue (pediatric patients)

Dermatologic: Skin rash (8%), pruritus (6%), alopecia (1% to <5%)

Gastrointestinal: Diarrhea (26%), nausea (17%), abdominal pain (16%), flatulence (10%), vomiting (10%), anorexia (8%), dyspepsia (5%), constipation (1% to <5%), gastritis (1% to <5%), gastrointestinal hemorrhage (1% to <5%), pancreatitis

Hematologic & oncologic: Anemia (1% to <5%), bruise (1% to <5%), hemorrhage (1% to <5%), thrombocytopenia (1% to <5%)

Hepatic: Increased liver enzymes (1% to <5%)

Neuromuscular & skeletal: Weakness (23%), back pain (6%), arthralgia (1% to <5%), myalgia (1% to <5%), muscle cramps (pediatric patients)

Ophthalmic: Diplopia (1% to <5%), visual field defect (1% to <5%)

Otic: Tinnitus (1% to <5%)

Renal: Hematuria (1% to <5%), renal failure (1%)

Respiratory: Dyspnea (12%), cough (6%), epistaxis (1% to <5%), flu-like symptoms (1% to <5%), pneumonia (1% to <5%), pleural effusion, pulmonary hypertension, pulmonary fibrosis, pulmonary infiltrates

Miscellaneous: Fever (9%)

<1%, postmarketing, and/or case reports: Eosinophilic pneumonitis, hepato-toxicity, hypersensitivity pneumonitis, increased serum ALT (>3 x ULN), increased serum AST (>3 x ULN), interstitial nephritis, interstitial pneumonitis, leukocytosis, prolonged Q-T interval on ECG, skin photosensitivity (pediatric patients), torsades de pointes, ventricular tachycardia

Drug Interactions

Metabolism/Transport Effects None known.

Avoid Concomitant Use

Avoid concomitant use of Anagrelide with any of the following: Highest Risk QTc-Prolonging Agents; Ivabradine; Mifepristone; Moderate Risk QTc-Prolonging Agents; Urokinase

Increased Effect/Toxicity

Anagrelide may increase the levels/effects of: Agents with Antiplatelet Properties; Anticoagulants; Apixaban; Cilostazol; Collagenase (Systemic); Dabigatran Etexilate; Deoxycholic Acid; Highest Risk QTc-Prolonging Agents; Ibritumomab; Obinutuzumab; Riociguat; Rivaroxaban; Salicylates; Thrombolytic Agents; Tositumomab and Iodine I 131 Tositumomab; Urokinase

The levels/effects of Anagrelide may be increased by: Glucosamine; Herbs (Anticoagulant/Antiplatelet Properties); Ibrutinib; Ivabradine; Limaprost; MAO Inhibitors; Mifepristone; Moderate Risk QTc-Prolonging Agents; Multivitamins/Fluoride (with ADE); Multivitamins/Minerals (with ADEK, Folate, Iron); Multivitamins/Minerals (with AE, No Iron); Omega-3 Fatty Acids; Pentosan Polysulfate Sodium; Pentoxifylline; Prostacyclin Analogues; QTc-Prolonging Agents (Indeterminate Risk and Risk Modifying); Tipranavir; Vitamin E; Vitamin E (Oral)

Decreased Effect There are no known significant interactions involving a decrease in effect.

Storage/Stability Store at 25°C (77°F); excursions permitted to 15°C to 30°C (59°F to 86°F). Protect from light.

Mechanism of Action Anagrelide appears to inhibit cyclic nucleotide phosphodiesterase and the release of arachidonic acid from phospholipase, possibly by inhibiting phospholipase A_2. It also causes a dose-related reduction in platelet production, which results from decreased megakaryocyte hypermaturation (disrupts the postmitotic phase of maturation).

Pharmacodynamics/Kinetics Note: In pediatric patients 7-14 years; data has shown a decreased maximum serum concentration (48%) and AUC (55%) compared to adults when normalized to dose and bodyweight.

Onset of action: Initial: Within 7 to 14 days; complete response (platelets ≤600,000/mm^3): 4 to 12 weeks

Duration: 6 to 24 hours; upon discontinuation, platelet count begins to rise within 4 days

Metabolism: Hepatic, partially via CYP1A2; to two major metabolites, RL603 and 3-hydroxy anagrelide

Bioavailability: Food has no clinically significant effect

Half-life elimination: Anagrelide: 1.5 hours, similar data reported in pediatric patients 7-14 years; 3-hydroxy anagrelide: 2.5 hours

◄ Time to peak, serum: 1 hour, similar data reported in pediatric patients 7-14 years

Excretion: Urine (<1% as unchanged drug)

Dosing

Adult & Geriatric

Thrombocythemia: Oral: Initial: 0.5 mg 4 times daily or 1 mg twice daily (most patients will experience adequate response at dose ranges of 1.5 to 3 mg per day)

Note: Maintain initial dose for ≥1 week, then adjust to the lowest effective dose to reduce and maintain platelet count <600,000/mm^3 ideally to the normal range; the dose must not be increased by >0.5 mg per day in any 1 week; maximum single dose: 2.5 mg; maximum daily dose: 10 mg

Thrombocythemia, essential (off-label dosing): Oral: Initial: 0.5 mg twice daily for 1 week, then adjust dose to maintain platelet counts at normal (≤450,000/mm^3) or near normal (450,000/mm^3 to 600,000/mm^3) levels (Gisslinger, 2013).

Pediatric Thrombocythemia: Oral: Initial: 0.5 mg once daily (range: 0.5 mg 1 to 4 times daily)

Note: Maintain initial dose for ≥1 week, then adjust to the lowest effective dose to reduce and maintain platelet count <600,000/mm^3 ideally to the normal range; the dose must not be increased by >0.5 mg per day in any 1 week; maximum single dose: 2.5 mg; maximum daily dose: 10 mg

Renal Impairment No dosage adjustment necessary; monitor closely.

Hepatic Impairment

Moderate impairment (Child-Pugh score 7 to 9): Initial: 0.5 mg once daily; maintain for at least 1 week with careful monitoring of cardiovascular status; the dose must not be increased by >0.5 mg per day in any 1 week.

Severe impairment (Child-Pugh score ≥10): Avoid use.

Administration May be administered without regard to food.

Monitoring Parameters Platelet count (every 2 days during the first week of treatment and at least weekly until the maintenance dose is reached; continue to monitor after cessation of treatment); CBC with differential (monitor closely during first 2 weeks of treatment), liver function (ALT and AST; baseline and during treatment), BUN, and serum creatinine (monitor closely during first weeks of treatment); serum electrolytes; blood pressure; heart rate; cardiovascular exam, including ECG (pretreatment; monitor during therapy); signs/symptoms of interstitial lung disease; monitor for thrombosis or bleeding

Dosage Forms Excipient information presented when available (limited, particularly for generics); consult specific product labeling.

Capsule, Oral:

Agrylin: 0.5 mg

Generic: 0.5 mg, 1 mg

♦ **Anagrelide Hydrochloride** see Anagrelide on page 109

♦ **Anandron (Can)** see Nilutamide on page 1205

Anastrozole (an AS troe zole)

Brand Names: US Arimidex

Brand Names: Canada ACH-Anastrozole; ACT-Anastrozole; Apo-Anastrozole; Arimidex; Auro-Anastrozole; Bio-Anastrozole; JAMP-Anastrozole; Mar-Anastrozole; Med-Anastrozole; Mint-Anastrozole; Mylan-Anastrozole; Nat-Anastrozole; PMS-Anastrozole; RAN-Anastrozole; Riva-Anastrozole; Sandoz-Anastrozole; Taro-Anastrozole; Teva-Anastrozole; Zinda-Anastrozole

Index Terms ICI-D1033; ZD1033

Pharmacologic Category Antineoplastic Agent, Aromatase Inhibitor

Use Breast cancer:

First-line treatment of locally-advanced or metastatic breast cancer (hormone receptor-positive or unknown) in postmenopausal women

Adjuvant treatment of early hormone receptor-positive breast cancer in postmenopausal women

Treatment of advanced breast cancer in postmenopausal women with disease progression following tamoxifen therapy

Labeled Contraindications Hypersensitivity to anastrozole or any component of the formulation; use in women who are or may become pregnant

Canadian labeling: Additional contraindications (not in U.S. labeling): Lactating women

Pregnancy Considerations Adverse events were observed in animal reproduction studies. Anastrozole is contraindicated in women who are or may become pregnant (may cause fetal harm if administered during pregnancy). Use in premenopausal women with breast cancer does not provide any clinical benefit.

Breast-Feeding Considerations It is not known if anastrozole is excreted in breast milk. Due to the potential for serious adverse reactions in the nursing infant, a decision should be made whether to discontinue nursing or to discontinue the drug, taking into account the importance of treatment to the mother. The Canadian labeling contraindicates use in lactating women.

Warnings/Precautions Hazardous agent - use appropriate precautions for handling and disposal (NIOSH 2014 [group 1]). Use is contraindicated in women who are or may become pregnant. Anastrozole offers no clinical benefit in premenopausal women with breast cancer. Patients with preexisting ischemic cardiac disease have an increased risk for ischemic cardiovascular events.

Due to decreased circulating estrogen levels, anastrozole is associated with a reduction in bone mineral density (BMD); decreases (from baseline) in total hip and lumbar spine BMD have been reported. Patients with preexisting osteopenia are at higher risk for developing osteoporosis (Eastell, 2008). When initiating anastrozole treatment, follow available guidelines for bone mineral density management in postmenopausal women with similar fracture risk; concurrent use of bisphosphonates may be useful in patients at risk for fractures.

Elevated total cholesterol levels (contributed to by LDL cholesterol increases) have been reported in patients receiving anastrozole; use with caution in patients with hyperlipidemias; cholesterol levels should be monitored/managed in accordance with current guidelines for patients with LDL elevations. Plasma concentrations in patients with stable hepatic cirrhosis were within the range of concentrations seen in normal subjects across all clinical trials; use has not been studied in patients with severe hepatic impairment.

Adverse Reactions

>10%:

Cardiovascular: Vasodilatation (25% to 36%), ischemic heart disease (4%; 17% in patients with preexisting ischemic heart disease), hypertension (2% to 13%), angina pectoris (2%; 12% in patients with preexisting ischemic heart disease), edema (7% to 11%)

Central nervous system: Fatigue (19%), mood disorder (19%), headache (9% to 18%), pain (11% to 17%), depression (2% to 13%)

Dermatologic: Skin rash (6% to 11%)

◀ Endocrine & metabolic: Hot flash (12% to 36%)

Gastrointestinal: Gastrointestinal distress (29% to 34%), nausea (11% to 20%), vomiting (8% to 13%)

Neuromuscular & skeletal: Weakness (13% to 19%), arthritis (17%), arthralgia (2% to 15%), back pain (10% to 12%), ostealgia (6% to 12%), osteoporosis (11%)

Respiratory: Pharyngitis (6% to 14%), dyspnea (8% to 11%), increased cough (7% to 11%)

1% to 10%:

Cardiovascular: Peripheral edema (5% to 10%), chest pain (5% to 7%), venous thrombosis (2% to 4%; including pulmonary embolism, thrombophlebitis, retinal vein thrombosis), myocardial infarction (1%)

Central nervous system: Insomnia (2% to 10%), dizziness (5% to 8%), paresthesia (5% to 7%), anxiety (2% to 6%), confusion (2% to 5%), drowsiness (2% to 5%), malaise (2% to 5%), nervousness (2% to 5%), carpal tunnel syndrome (3%), hypertonia (3%), cerebrovascular insufficiency (2%), lethargy (1%)

Dermatologic: Alopecia (2% to 5%), pruritus (2% to 5%), diaphoresis (1% to 5%)

Endocrine & metabolic: Hypercholesterolemia (9%), increased serum cholesterol (9%), weight gain (2% to 9%), increased gamma-glutamyl transferase (2% to 5%), weight loss (2% to 5%)

Gastrointestinal: Constipation (7% to 9%), diarrhea (7% to 9%), abdominal pain (6% to 9%), anorexia (5% to 8%), dyspepsia (7%), gastrointestinal disease (7%), xerostomia (4% to 6%)

Genitourinary: Mastalgia (2% to 8%), urinary tract infection (2% to 8%), pelvic pain (5% to 7%), vulvovaginitis (6%), vaginal dryness (1% to 5%), vaginal hemorrhage (1% to 5%), vaginal discharge (4%), vaginitis (4%), leukorrhea (2% to 3%)

Hematologic & oncologic: Lymphedema (10%), breast neoplasm (5%), neoplasm (5%), anemia (2% to 5%), leukopenia (2% to 5%), tumor flare (3%)

Hepatic: Increased serum alkaline phosphatase (2% to 5%), increased serum ALT (2% to 5%), increased serum AST (2% to 5%)

Infection: Infection (2% to 9%)

Neuromuscular & skeletal: Bone fracture (1% to 10%), arthrosis (7%), myalgia (2% to 6%), neck pain (2% to 5%), pathological fracture (2% to 5%)

Ophthalmic: Cataract (6%)

Respiratory: Flu-like symptoms (2% to 7%), sinusitis (2% to 6%), bronchitis (2% to 5%), rhinitis (2% to 5%)

Miscellaneous: Accidental injury (2% to 10%), cyst (5%), fever (2% to 5%)

<1%, postmarketing, and/or case reports: Anaphylaxis, angioedema, cerebral infarction, cerebral ischemia, decreased bone mineral density, dermal ulcer, endometrial carcinoma, erythema multiforme, hepatitis, hepatomegaly, hypercalcemia, hypersensitivity angiitis (including anaphylactoid purpura [IgA vasculitis]), increased serum bilirubin, jaundice, joint stiffness, pulmonary embolism, retinal thrombosis, skin blister, skin lesion, Stevens-Johnson syndrome, tenosynovitis (stenosing), urticaria

Drug Interactions

Metabolism/Transport Effects Inhibits CYP1A2 (weak), CYP2C8 (weak), CYP2C9 (weak)

Avoid Concomitant Use

Avoid concomitant use of Anastrozole with any of the following: Amodiaquine; Estrogen Derivatives

Increased Effect/Toxicity
Anastrozole may increase the levels/effects of: Amodiaquine; Methadone; TiZANidine

Decreased Effect
The levels/effects of Anastrozole may be decreased by: Estrogen Derivatives; Tamoxifen

Storage/Stability Store at 20°C to 25°C (68°F to 77°F).

Mechanism of Action Potent and selective nonsteroidal aromatase inhibitor. By inhibiting aromatase, the conversion of androstenedione to estrone, and testosterone to estradiol, is prevented, thereby decreasing tumor mass or delaying progression in patients with tumors responsive to hormones. Anastrozole causes an 85% decrease in estrone sulfate levels.

Pharmacodynamics/Kinetics
Onset of estradiol reduction: 70% reduction after 24 hours; 80% after 2 weeks of therapy

Duration of estradiol reduction: 6 days

Absorption: Well absorbed; extent of absorption not affected by food

Protein binding, plasma: 40%

Metabolism: Extensively hepatic (~85%) via N-dealkylation, hydroxylation, and glucuronidation; primary metabolite (triazole) inactive

Half-life elimination: ~50 hours

Time to peak, plasma: ~2 hours without food; 5 hours with food

Excretion: Feces; urine (urinary excretion accounts for ~10% of total elimination, mostly as metabolites)

Dosing
Adult & Geriatric

Breast cancer, advanced: Postmenopausal females: Oral: 1 mg once daily; continue until tumor progression

Breast cancer, early (adjuvant treatment): Postmenopausal females: Oral: 1 mg once daily. **Note:** The American Society of Clinical Oncology (ASCO) guidelines for Adjuvant Endocrine Therapy of Hormone-Receptor Positive Breast Cancer (Focused Update) recommend a maximum duration of 5 years of aromatase inhibitor (AI) therapy for postmenopausal women; AIs may be combined with tamoxifen for a total duration of up to 10 years of endocrine therapy. Refer to the guidelines for specific recommendations based on menopausal status and tolerability (Burstein, 2014).

Breast cancer, risk reduction (off-label use): Postmenopausal females ≥40 years: Oral: 1 mg once daily for 5 years (Cuzick, 2014)

Renal Impairment No dosage adjustment necessary.

Hepatic Impairment
Mild to moderate impairment or stable hepatic cirrhosis: No dosage adjustment necessary.

Severe hepatic impairment: There are no dosage adjustments provided in the manufacturer's labeling (has not been studied).

Administration May be administered with or without food. Hazardous agent; use appropriate precautions for handling and disposal (NIOSH 2014 [group 1]).

Monitoring Parameters
Bone mineral density; total cholesterol and LDL

Breast cancer risk reduction (off-label use): Bone mineral density at baseline, mammograms, and clinical breast exam at baseline and at least every 2 years (Cuzick, 2014)

Dosage Forms Excipient information presented when available (limited, particularly for generics); consult specific product labeling.
Tablet, Oral:
  Arimidex: 1 mg
  Generic: 1 mg

◆ **Ancobon** see Flucytosine on page 731

◆ **Androcur® (Can)** see Cyproterone on page 402

◆ **Androcur® Depot (Can)** see Cyproterone on page 402

◆ **Androxy** see Fluoxymesterone on page 750

Anidulafungin (ay nid yoo la FUN jin)

Brand Names: US Eraxis
Brand Names: Canada Eraxis
Index Terms LY303366
Pharmacologic Category Antifungal Agent, Parenteral; Echinocandin
Use Treatment of candidemia and other forms of Candida infections (including those of intra-abdominal, peritoneal, and esophageal locus)
Pregnancy Risk Factor B
Dosing
  Adult & Geriatric
  Aspergillosis (invasive) in HIV-infected patients: IV: 200 mg on day 1, then 100 mg once daily until infection resolution and CD4 count >200 cells/mm^3 (HHS [OI adult 2015])
  Candidemia, intra-abdominal or peritoneal candidiasis: IV: Initial dose: 200 mg on day 1; subsequent dosing: 100 mg daily; treatment should continue until 14 days after last positive culture
  Esophageal candidiasis: IV: Initial dose: 100 mg on day 1; subsequent dosing: 50 mg daily; treatment should continue for a minimum of 14 days and for at least 7 days after symptom resolution
  Pediatric Aspergillosis (invasive) in HIV-infected patients (off-label use): Adolescents: IV: Refer to adult dosing.
  Renal Impairment No dosage adjustment necessary, including dialysis patients.
  Hepatic Impairment No dosage adjustment necessary.
  Additional Information Complete prescribing information should be consulted for additional detail.
  Dosage Forms Excipient information presented when available (limited, particularly for generics); consult specific product labeling.
  Solution Reconstituted, Intravenous [preservative free]:
    Eraxis: 50 mg (1 ea); 100 mg (1 ea) [contains polysorbate 80]

◆ **Anti-D Immunoglobulin** see Rh$_o$(D) Immune Globulin on page 1471

◆ **131 I Anti-B1 Antibody** see Tositumomab and Iodine I 131 Tositumomab on page 1663

◆ **131 I-Anti-B1 Monoclonal Antibody** see Tositumomab and Iodine I 131 Tositumomab on page 1663

◆ **Antibody-Drug Conjugate SGN-35** see Brentuximab Vedotin on page 237

◆ **Anti-CD20 Monoclonal Antibody** see RiTUXimab on page 1482

◆ **Anti-CD20-Murine Monoclonal Antibody I-131** see Tositumomab and Iodine I 131 Tositumomab on page 1663

◆ **Anti-CD30 ADC SGN-35** *see* Brentuximab Vedotin *on page* 237

◆ **Anti-CD30 Antibody-Drug Conjugate SGN-35** *see* Brentuximab Vedotin *on page* 237

◆ **Anti-CD52 Monoclonal Antibody** *see* Alemtuzumab *on page* 62

◆ **anti-c-erB-2** *see* Trastuzumab *on page* 1685

◆ **anti-ERB-2** *see* Trastuzumab *on page* 1685

Antihemophilic Factor (Human)

(an tee hee moe FIL ik FAK tor HYU man)

Brand Names: US Hemofil M; Koate-DVI; Monoclate-P

Brand Names: Canada Hemofil M

Index Terms AHF (Human); Factor VIII (Human); Kaote DVI

Pharmacologic Category Antihemophilic Agent; Blood Product Derivative

Use

Hemophilia A: Prevention and treatment of hemorrhagic episodes in patients with hemophilia A (classic hemophilia); perioperative management of hemophilia A.

Note: Can be of significant therapeutic value in patients with acquired factor VIII inhibitors not exceeding 10 Bethesda units/mL

Limitations of use: Not effective in controlling bleeding in patients with von Willebrand disease and therefore is not indicated for this use.

Pregnancy Risk Factor C

Dosing

Adult & Geriatric Hemophilia: IV: Individualize dosage based on coagulation studies performed prior to treatment and at regular intervals during treatment. In general, administration of factor VIII 1 unit/kg will increase circulating factor VIII levels by ~2 units/dL. **Refer to product information for specific manufacturer recommended dosing.** Alternatively, the World Federation of Hemophilia (WFH) has recommended general dosing for factor VIII products.

Dosage based on desired factor VIII increase (%):

To calculate dosage needed based on desired factor VIII increase (%):

Body weight (kg) x 0.5 units/kg x desired factor VIII increase (%) = units factor VIII required

For example:

50 kg x 0.5 units/kg x 30 (% increase) = 750 units factor VIII

Dosage based on expected factor VIII increase (%):

It is also possible to calculate the **expected** % factor VIII increase:

(# units administered x 2%/units/kg) divided by body weight (kg) = expected % factor VIII increase

For example:

(1400 units x 2%/units/kg) divided by 70 kg = 40%

◀ World Federation of Hemophilia (WFH) treatment recommendations when no significant resource constraint exists (WFH [Srivastava 2013]):

2013 World Federation of Hemophilia
Treatment Recommendations
(When No Significant Resource Constraint Exists)

Site of Hemorrhage/ Clinical Situation	Desired Factor VIII Level to Maintain	Duration
Joint	40 to 60 units/dL	1 to 2 days, may be longer if response is inadequate
Superficial muscle/no neurovascular compromise	40 to 60 units/dL	2 to 3 days, sometimes longer if response is inadequate
Iliopsoas and deep muscle with neurovascular injury, or substantial blood loss	Initial: 80 to 100 units/dL	Initial: 1 to 2 days
	Maintenance: 30 to 60 units/dL	Maintenance: 3 to 5 days, sometimes longer as secondary prophylaxis during physiotherapy
CNS/Head	Initial: 80 to 100 units/dL	Initial: 1 to 7 days
	Maintenance: 50 units/dL	Maintenance: 8 to 21 days
Throat and neck	Initial: 80 to 100 units/dL	Initial: 1 to 7 days
	Maintenance: 50 units/dL	Maintenance: 8 to 14 days
Gastrointestinal	Initial: 80 to 100 units/dL	Initial: 7 to 14 days
	Maintenance: 50 units/dL	Maintenance: Not specified
Renal	50 units/dL	3 to 5 days
Deep laceration	50 units/dL	5 to 7 days
Surgery (major)	Preop: 80 to 100 units/dL	
	Postop: 60 to 80 units/dL	Postop: 1 to 3 days
	Postop: 40 to 60 units/dL	Postop: 4 to 6 days
	Postop: 30 to 50 units/dL	Postop: 7 to 14 days
Surgery (minor)	Preop: 50 to 80 units/dL	
	Postop: 30 to 80 units/dL	Postop: 1 to 5 days depending on procedure type

Note: Factor VIII level may either be expressed as units/dL or as %. Dosing frequency most commonly corresponds to the half-life of factor VIII but should be determined based on an assessment of factor VIII levels before the next dose.

Continuous infusion (for patients who require prolonged periods of treatment [eg, intracranial hemorrhage or surgery] to avoid peaks and troughs associated with intermittent infusions) (Batorova 2002; Batorova 2012; Poon 2012; Rickard 1995; WFH [Srivastava 2013]): Following initial bolus to achieve the desired factor VIII level, initiate 2 to 4 units/kg/hour; adjust dose based on frequent factor assays and calculation of factor VIII clearance at steady-state using the following equations:

Factor VIII clearance (mL/kg/hour) = (current infusion rate in units/kg/hour) divided by (plasma level in units/mL)

New infusion rate (units/kg/hour) = (factor VIII clearance in mL/kg/hour) x (desired plasma level in units/mL)

Pediatric Refer to adult dosing.

Renal Impairment There are no dosage adjustments provided in the manufacturer's labeling.

Hepatic Impairment There are no dosage adjustments provided in the manufacturer's labeling.

Additional Information Complete prescribing information should be consulted for additional detail.

Dosage Forms Considerations

Strengths expressed with approximate values. Consult individual vial labels for exact potency within each vial.

Hemofil M packaged contents may contain natural rubber latex.

Dosage Forms Excipient information presented when available (limited, particularly for generics); consult specific product labeling. [DSC] = Discontinued product

Kit, Intravenous:

Monoclate-P: ~250 units, ~500 units, ~1000 units, ~1500 units [contains mouse protein (murine) (hamster)]

Solution Reconstituted, Intravenous:

Koate-DVI: ~500 units (1 ea) [contains albumin human, polyethylene glycol, polysorbate 80]

Solution Reconstituted, Intravenous [preservative free]:

Hemofil M: ~250 units (1 ea) [contains albumin human, mouse protein (murine) (hamster), polyethylene glycol]

Hemofil M: ~250 units (1 ea) [contains mouse protein (murine) (hamster), polyethylene glycol]

Hemofil M: ~500 units (1 ea) [contains albumin human, mouse protein (murine) (hamster), polyethylene glycol]

Hemofil M: ~500 units (1 ea) [contains mouse protein (murine) (hamster), polyethylene glycol]

Hemofil M: ~1000 units (1 ea); ~1700 units (1 ea) [contains albumin human, mouse protein (murine) (hamster), polyethylene glycol]

Koate-DVI: ~250 units (1 ea); ~500 units (1 ea [DSC]); ~1000 units (1 ea) [contains albumin human, polyethylene glycol, polysorbate 80]

Antihemophilic Factor (Recombinant)

(an tee hee moe FIL ik FAK tor ree KOM be nant)

Brand Names: US Advate; Eloctate; Helixate FS; Kogenate FS; Kogenate FS Bio-Set; Novoeight; Nuwiq; Recombinate; Xyntha; Xyntha Solofuse

Brand Names: Canada Advate; Helixate FS; Kogenate FS; Xyntha; Xyntha Solofuse

Index Terms AHF (Recombinant); Efraloctocog Alfa; Factor VIII (Recombinant); Moroctocog Alfa; Nuwiq; Octacog Alfa; rAHF

Pharmacologic Category Antihemophilic Agent

Use Hemophilia A:

Control and prevention of bleeding episodes: For the prevention and control of bleeding episodes in adults and children with hemophilia A.

Perioperative management: For surgical prophylaxis in adults and children with hemophilia A.

Routine prophylaxis to prevent or reduce the frequency of bleeding (Advate, Eloctate, Helixate FS, Kogenate FS, Novoeight, Nuwiq, Xyntha [Canadian labeling; not in US labeling]): For routine prophylactic treatment to prevent or reduce the frequency of bleeding episodes in adults and children with hemophilia A.

Routine prophylaxis to prevent bleeding episodes and joint damage (Helixate FS, Kogenate FS): For routine prophylactic treatment to reduce the frequency of bleeding episodes and the risk of joint damage in children without preexisting joint damage.

Pregnancy Risk Factor C

◀ **Dosing**

Adult & Geriatric Hemophilia A: IV: Individualize dosage based on coagulation studies performed prior to treatment and at regular intervals during treatment. In general, administration of factor VIII 1 unit/kg will increase circulating factor VIII levels by ~2 units/dL. **Refer to product information for specific manufacturer recommended dosing.** Alternatively, the World Federation of Hemophilia (WFH) has recommended general dosing for factor VIII products.

Dosage based on desired factor VIII increase (%):
To calculate dosage needed based on desired factor VIII increase (%):
[Body weight (kg) x desired factor VIII increase (%)] divided by 2 (%/units/kg) = units factor VIII required
For example:
50 kg x 30 (% increase) divided by 2 = 750 units factor VIII
Dosage based on expected factor VIII increase (%):
It is also possible to calculate the **expected** % factor VIII increase:
[# units administered x 2 (%/units/kg)] divided by body weight (kg) = expected % factor VIII increase
For example:
[1,400 units x 2] divided by 70 kg = 40%
World Federation of Hemophilia (WFH) treatment recommendations when no significant resource constraint exists (WFH [Srivastava 2013]):

2013 World Federation of Hemophilia Treatment Recommendations (When No Significant Resource Constraint Exists)

Site of Hemorrhage/ Clinical Situation	Desired Factor VIII Level to Maintain	Duration
Joint	40 to 60 units/dL	1 to 2 days, may be longer if response is inadequate
Superficial muscle/no neurovascular compromise	40 to 60 units/dL	2 to 3 days, sometimes longer if response is inadequate
Iliopsoas and deep muscle with neurovascular injury, or substantial blood loss	*Initial:* 80 to 100 units/dL	*Initial:* 1 to 2 days
	Maintenance: 30 to 60 units/dL	*Maintenance:* 3 to 5 days, sometimes longer as secondary prophylaxis during physiotherapy
CNS/Head	*Initial:* 80 to 100 units/dL	*Initial:* 1 to 7 days
	Maintenance: 50 units/dL	*Maintenance:* 8 to 21 days
Throat and neck	*Initial:* 80 to 100 units/dL	*Initial:* 1 to 7 days
	Maintenance: 50 units/dL	*Maintenance:* 8 to 14 days
Gastrointestinal	*Initial:* 80 to 100 units/dL	*Initial:* 7 to 14 days
	Maintenance: 50 units/dL	*Maintenance:* Not specified
Renal	50 units/dL	3 to 5 days
Deep laceration	50 units/dL	5 to 7 days

(continued)

2013 World Federation of Hemophilia Treatment Recommendations (When No Significant Resource Constraint Exists) *(continued)*

Site of Hemorrhage/ Clinical Situation	Desired Factor VIII Level to Maintain	Duration
Surgery (major)	*Preop:* 80 to 100 units/dL	
	Postop: 60 to 80 units/dL	*Postop:* 1 to 3 days
	Postop: 40 to 60 units/dL	*Postop:* 4 to 6 days
	Postop: 30 to 50 units/dL	*Postop:* 7 to 14 days
Surgery (minor)	*Preop:* 50 to 80 units/dL	
	Postop: 30 to 80 units/dL	*Postop:* 1 to 5 days depending on procedure type

Note: Factor VIII level may either be expressed as units/dL or as %. Dosing frequency most commonly corresponds to the half-life of factor VIII but should be determined based on an assessment of factor VIII levels before the next dose.

Continuous infusion (for patients who require prolonged periods of treatment [eg, intracranial hemorrhage or surgery] to avoid peaks and troughs associated with intermittent infusions) (Batorova 2002; Batorova 2012; Poon 2012; Rickard 1995; WFH [Srivastava 2013]): Following initial bolus to achieve the desired factor VIII level, initiate 2 to 4 units/kg/hour; adjust dose based on frequent factor assays and calculation of factor VIII clearance at steady-state using the following equations:

Factor VIII clearance (mL/kg/hour) = (current infusion rate in units/kg/hour) divided by (plasma level in units/mL)

New infusion rate (units/kg/hour) = (factor VIII clearance in mL/kg/hour) x (desired plasma level in units/mL)

Routine prophylaxis to prevent or reduce the frequency of bleeding episodes: IV:

Advate: 20 to 40 units/kg every other day (3 to 4 times weekly). Alternatively, an every-third-day dosing regimen may be used to target factor VIII trough levels of ≥1%.

Eloctate: 50 units/kg every 4 days; may adjust within the range of 25 to 65 units/kg at 3- to 5-day intervals based on patient response.

Helixate FS: 25 units/kg 3 times weekly

Kogenate FS: 25 units/kg 3 times weekly

Novoeight: 20 to 50 units/kg 3 times weekly **or** 20 to 40 units/kg every other day

Nuwiq: 30 to 40 units/kg every other day

Xyntha (Canadian labeling; not in US labeling): Treatment experienced patients: 25 to 35 units/kg 3 times weekly

Pediatric Hemophilia A: Children and Adolescents: IV: Refer to adult dosing.
Note: Children <6 years may require higher doses and/or more frequent administration.

Routine prophylaxis to prevent bleeding episodes:

Advate: Refer to adult dosing.

Eloctate: 50 units/kg every 4 days; may adjust within the range of 25 to 65 units/kg at 3- to 5-day intervals based on patient response. More frequent or higher doses up to 80 units/kg may be required in children <6 years.

Helixate FS: Children: 25 units/kg every other day

◀ Novoeight:
  Children: 25 to 60 units per kg 3 times weekly **or** 25 to 50 units/kg every other day
  Adolescents: Refer to adult dosing
  Xyntha (Canadian labeling; not in US labeling): Adolescents (treatment experienced): Refer to adult dosing.
  Routine prophylaxis to prevent bleeding episodes and joint damage (without preexisting joint damage) (Helixate FS, Kogenate FS): 25 units/kg every other day

Renal Impairment There are no dosage adjustments provided in the manufacturer's labeling.

Hepatic Impairment There are no dosage adjustments provided in the manufacturer's labeling.

Additional Information Complete prescribing information should be consulted for additional detail.

Product Availability Nuwiq: FDA approved September 2015; availability anticipated in early 2016.

Dosage Forms Considerations Strengths expressed with approximate values. Consult individual vial labels for exact potency within each vial.

Dosage Forms Excipient information presented when available (limited, particularly for generics); consult specific product labeling.

Kit, Intravenous:
  Kogenate FS: 250 units, 500 units, 1000 units [contains mouse protein (murine) (hamster)]
  Nuwiq: 250 units
Kit, Intravenous [preservative free]:
  Helixate FS: 250 units, 500 units, 1000 units, 2000 units, 3000 units [contains polysorbate 80]
  Kogenate FS: 2000 units, 3000 units [contains mouse protein (murine) (hamster)]
  Kogenate FS Bio-Set: 250 units, 500 units, 1000 units, 2000 units, 3000 units
  Nuwiq: 500 units, 1000 units, 2000 units
  Xyntha: 250 units, 500 units, 1000 units, 2000 units [albumin free; contains mouse protein (murine) (hamster), polysorbate 80]
  Xyntha Solofuse: 250 units, 500 units, 1000 units, 2000 units, 3000 units [albumin free; contains mouse protein (murine) (hamster), polysorbate 80]
Solution Reconstituted, Intravenous [preservative free]:
  Advate: 250 units (1 ea); 500 units (1 ea); 1000 units (1 ea); 1500 units (1 ea); 2000 units (1 ea); 3000 units (1 ea); 4000 units (1 ea) [albumin free; contains polysorbate 80]
  Eloctate: 250 units (1 ea); 500 units (1 ea); 750 units (1 ea); 1000 units (1 ea); 1500 units (1 ea); 2000 units (1 ea); 3000 units (1 ea)
  Novoeight: 250 units (1 ea); 500 units (1 ea); 1000 units (1 ea); 1500 units (1 ea); 2000 units (1 ea); 3000 units (1 ea) [contains mouse protein (murine) (hamster), polysorbate 80]
  Nuwiq: 250 units (1 ea); 500 units (1 ea); 1000 units (1 ea); 2000 units (1 ea)
  Recombinate: 220-400 units (1 ea); 401-800 units (1 ea); 801-1240 units (1 ea); 1241-1800 units (1 ea); 1801-2400 units (1 ea) [contains albumin human, polyethylene glycol, polysorbate 80]

Antihemophilic Factor (Recombinant [Pegylated])
(an tee hee moe FIL ik FAK tor ree KOM be nant PEG i late ed)

Index Terms Adynovate; AHF (Recombinant [Pegylated]); Factor VIII (Recombinant [Pegylated])

Pharmacologic Category Antihemophilic Agent

Use Hemophilia A:

Treatment and control of bleeding episodes: For the on-demand treatment and control of bleeding episodes in adults and children 12 years and older with hemophilia A.

Routine prophylaxis to reduce the frequency of bleeding: For routine prophylaxis to reduce the frequency of bleeding episodes in adults and children 12 years and older with hemophilia A.

Limitations of use: Not indicated for the treatment of von Willebrand disease

Additional Information Complete prescribing information should be consulted for additional detail.

Product Availability Adynovate: FDA approved November 2015; anticipated availability is currently undetermined

Antihemophilic Factor (Recombinant [Porcine Sequence]) (an tee hee moe FIL ik FAK tor ree KOM be nant POR sine SEE kwens)

Brand Names: US Obizur

Index Terms AHF; AHF (Recombinant); Factor VIII; Factor VIII (Recombinant); pFVIII; rAHF; rpFVIII

Pharmacologic Category Antihemophilic Agent

Use

Acquired hemophilia A: Treatment of bleeding episodes in adults with acquired hemophilia A

Limitations of use: Not indicated for the treatment of congenital hemophilia A or von Willebrand disease; safety and efficacy of has not been established in patients with baseline anti- porcine factor VIII inhibitor titer >20 BU.

Pregnancy Risk Factor C

Dosing

Adult & Geriatric

Acquired hemophilia A: IV: **Note:** Dose, dosing frequency, and duration based on location and severity of bleeding, target factor VIII levels, and clinical condition of the patient. Plasma levels of factor VIII should not exceed 200% of normal or 200 units/dL.

Minor to moderate hemorrhage: 200 units/kg initially to achieve factor VIII plasma level 50% to 100% of normal; titrate subsequent doses to maintain recommended factor VIII trough levels and individual clinical response; dose every 4 to 12 hours (frequency may be adjusted based on clinical response/factor VIII levels).

Major hemorrhage: 200 units/kg initially to achieve factor VIII plasma level 100% to 200% (for acute bleed) or 50% to 100% (after acute bleed is controlled, if required) of normal; titrate subsequent doses to maintain recommended factor VIII trough levels and individual clinical response; dose every 4 to 12 hours (frequency may be adjusted based on clinical response/factor VIII levels).

Renal Impairment There are no dosage adjustments provided in the manufacturer's labeling.

Hepatic Impairment There are no dosage adjustments provided in the manufacturer's labeling.

◄ **Additional Information** Complete prescribing information should be consulted for additional detail.

Product Availability Obizur: Health Canada approved October 2015; anticipated availability is currently unknown.

Dosage Forms Excipient information presented when available (limited, particularly for generics); consult specific product labeling.
Solution Reconstituted, Intravenous:
  Obizur: 500 units (1 ea) [contains mouse protein (murine) (hamster), polysorbate 80]

♦ **Anti-PD-1 human monoclonal antibody MDX-1106** see Nivolumab on page 1209

♦ **Anti-PD-1 Monoclonal Antibody MK-3475** see Pembrolizumab on page 1362

Antithrombin (an tee THROM bin)

Brand Names: US ATryn; Thrombate III
Brand Names: Canada Antithrombin III NF; Thrombate III®
Index Terms Antithrombin Alfa; Antithrombin III; AT; AT-III; hpAT; rhAT; rhATIII
Pharmacologic Category Anticoagulant; Blood Product Derivative
Use
Treatment of antithrombin deficiency: Thrombate III: Antithrombin III (human) is indicated for the treatment of patients with hereditary antithrombin (AT) deficiency in connection with surgical or obstetrical procedures or when they suffer from thromboembolism.

Prevention of thromboembolic events: ATryn: Recombinant antithrombin is indicated for the prevention of perioperative and peripartum thromboembolic events in patients with hereditary antithrombin deficiency.
Limitations of use: ATryn is not indicated for treatment of thromboembolic events in patients with hereditary antithrombin deficiency.

Pregnancy Risk Factor B (Thrombate III); C (ATryn)
Dosing
Adult & Geriatric Antithrombin deficiency: IV:
ATryn: Prophylaxis of thrombosis during perioperative and peripartum procedures:
Dosing is individualized based on pretherapy antithrombin (AT) activity levels. Therapy should begin before delivery or ~24 hours prior to surgery to obtain target AT activity levels. Dosing should be targeted to keep levels between 80% to 120% of normal. Loading dose should be given as a 15-minute infusion, followed by maintenance dose as a continuous infusion. Doses may be calculated based on the following formulas:
Surgical patients (nonpregnant):
Loading dose: [(100 - baseline AT activity level) **divided** by 2.3] x body weight (kg) = units of antithrombin required
Maintenance infusion: [(100 - baseline AT activity level) **divided** by 10.2] x body weight (kg) = units of antithrombin required/hour
Pregnant patients: **Note:** Pregnant women undergoing surgical procedures (other than a Cesarean section) should also be dosed according to the formula below.
Loading dose: [(100 - baseline AT activity level) **divided** by 1.3] x body weight (kg) = units of antithrombin required
Maintenance infusion: [(100 - baseline AT activity level) **divided** by 5.4] x body weight (kg) = units of antithrombin required/hour

Dosing adjustments: Adjustments should be made based on AT activity levels to maintain levels between 80% to 120% of normal. Surgery or delivery may rapidly decrease AT levels; check AT level just after surgery or delivery. The first AT level should be obtained 2 hours after initiation and adjusted as follows:

AT activity level <80%: Increase dose by 30%; recheck AT level 2 hours after adjustment. Alternatively, an additional bolus dose (using loading dose formula) may be needed to rapidly restore AT levels. Calculate the additional bolus/loading dose using the last available AT activity result. After additional loading/bolus dose given, resume maintenance infusion at the same rate prior to bolus administration.

AT activity level 80% to 120%: No dosage adjustment needed; recheck AT level in 6 hours

AT activity level >120%: Decrease dose by 30%; recheck AT level 2 hours after adjustment

Thrombate III: Prophylaxis of thrombosis during surgical or obstetrical procedures or treatment of thromboembolism:

Initial loading dose: Dosing is individualized based on pretherapy antithrombin (AT) levels. The initial dose should raise AT levels to 120% and may be calculated based on the following formula:

[(desired AT level % - baseline AT level %) x body weight (kg)] **divided** by 1.4 = units of antithrombin required

For example, if a 70 kg adult patient had a baseline AT level of 57%, the initial dose would be

[(120% - 57%) x 70] divided by 1.4 = 3150 units

Maintenance dose: In general, subsequent dosing should be targeted to keep levels between 80% to 120% which may be achieved by administering 60% of the initial loading dose every 24 hours. Adjustments may be made by adjusting dose or interval. Maintain level within normal range for 2-8 days depending on type of procedure/situation.

Renal Impairment There are no dosage adjustments provided in the manufacturer's labeling.

Hepatic Impairment There are no dosage adjustments provided in the manufacturer's labeling.

Additional Information Complete prescribing information should be consulted for additional detail.

Dosage Forms Excipient information presented when available (limited, particularly for generics); consult specific product labeling.

Solution Reconstituted, Intravenous:

Thrombate III: 500 units (1 ea); 1000 units (1 ea)

ATryn: 1750 units (1 ea)

◆ **Antithrombin III** see Antithrombin on page 124

◆ **Antithrombin III NF (Can)** see Antithrombin on page 124

◆ **Antithrombin Alfa** see Antithrombin on page 124

Antithymocyte Globulin (Equine)

(an te THY moe site GLOB yu lin, E kwine)

Related Information

Chemotherapy and Obesity *on page 2220*
Hematopoietic Stem Cell Transplantation *on page 2272*

Brand Names: US Atgam

Brand Names: Canada Atgam

Index Terms Antithymocyte Immunoglobulin; ATG; Horse Antihuman Thymocyte Gamma Globulin; Lymphocyte Immune Globulin

Pharmacologic Category Immune Globulin; Immunosuppressant Agent; Polyclonal Antibody

Use

Aplastic anemia: Treatment of moderate-to-severe aplastic anemia in patients not considered suitable candidates for bone marrow transplantation

Limitations of use: The usefulness of antithymocyte globulin (equine) has not be demonstrated in patients with aplastic anemia who are suitable candidates for transplantation, or in aplastic anemia secondary to neoplastic disease, storage disease, myelofibrosis, Fanconi syndrome, or in patients with known prior treatment with myelotoxic agents or radiation therapy

Renal transplantation: Management of allograft rejection in renal transplantation, either in combination with conventional treatments for the management of acute rejection, or as an adjunct treatment in the prevention of rejection

Labeled Contraindications History of severe systemic reaction (eg, anaphylactic reaction) to prior administration of antithymocyte globulin or other equine gamma globulins

Pregnancy Considerations Adverse events were observed in some animal reproduction studies. Women exposed to Atgam during pregnancy may be enrolled in the National Transplantation Pregnancy Registry (877-955-6877).

Breast-Feeding Considerations It is not known if antithymocyte globulin (equine) is excreted into breast milk. Due to the potential for serious adverse reactions in the nursing infant, the manufacturer recommends a decision be made whether to discontinue nursing or to discontinue the drug, taking into account the importance of treatment to the mother.

Warnings/Precautions [U.S. Boxed Warning]: Should only be used by physicians experienced in immunosuppressive therapy in the management of renal transplantation or aplastic anemia. Adequate laboratory and supportive medical resources must be readily available in the facility for patient management. Hypersensitivity and anaphylactic reactions may occur; discontinue for symptoms of anaphylaxis; immediate treatment (including epinephrine 1:1000) should be available. Systemic reaction (rash, dyspnea, hypotension, tachycardia, or anaphylaxis) precludes further administration of antithymocyte globulin (equine; ATG). Respiratory distress, hypotension, or pain (chest, flank, or back) may indicate an anaphylactoid/anaphylactic reaction. Serious immune-mediated reactions have been reported (rare), including anaphylaxis, infusion reactions, and serum sickness. Skin testing is recommended prior to administration of the initial ATG dose. A positive skin test is suggestive of an increased risk for systemic allergic reactions with an infusion, although anaphylaxis may occur in patients who display negative skin tests. If ATG treatment is deemed appropriate following a positive skin test, the first infusion should be administered in a controlled environment with intensive life support immediately available.

Discontinue if severe and unremitting thrombocytopenia and/or leukopenia occur in solid organ transplant patients. Clinically significant hemolysis has been reported (rarely); severe and unremitting hemolysis may require treatment discontinuation; chest, flank or back pain may indicate hemolysis. Abnormal hepatic function tests have been observed in patients with aplastic anemia and other hematologic disorders receiving ATG. ATG is an immunosuppressant; monitor closely for signs of infection. An increased incidence of cytomegalovirus (CMV) infection has been reported in studies. Administer via central line due to chemical phlebitis that may occur with a peripheral vein. Dose must be administered over at least 4 hours. Patient may need to be pretreated with an antipyretic, antihistamine, and/or corticosteroid. Intradermal skin testing is recommended prior to first-dose administration. Product of equine and human plasma; may have a risk of transmitting disease, including a theoretical risk of Creutzfeldt-Jakob disease (CJD). Product potency and activity may vary from lot to lot. Potentially significant drug-drug interactions may exist, requiring dose or frequency adjustment, additional monitoring, and/or selection of alternative therapy. Live viral vaccines may not replicate and antibody response may be reduced if administered during ATG treatment. Patients should not be immunized with attenuated live viral vaccines for 6 months after treatment.

Adverse Reactions

>10%:
Central nervous system: Chills, fever, headache
Dermatologic: Pruritus, rash, urticaria, wheal/flare
Hematologic: Leukopenia, thrombocytopenia
Neuromuscular & skeletal: Arthralgia

1% to 10%:
Cardiovascular: Bradycardia, cardiac irregularity, chest pain, edema, heart failure, hyper-/hypotension, myocarditis
Central nervous system: Agitation, encephalitis, lethargy, lightheadedness, listlessness, seizure, viral encephalopathy
Gastrointestinal: Diarrhea, nausea, stomatitis, vomiting
Hepatic: Hepatosplenomegaly, liver function tests abnormal
Local: Injection site reactions (pain, redness, swelling), phlebitis, thrombophlebitis, burning soles/palms
Neuromuscular & skeletal: Aches, back pain, joint stiffness, myalgia
Ocular: Periorbital edema
Renal: Proteinuria, renal function tests abnormal
Respiratory: Dyspnea, pleural effusion, respiratory distress
Miscellaneous: Anaphylactic reaction, diaphoresis, lymphadenopathy, night sweats, serum sickness, viral infection

<1%, postmarketing, and/or case reports: Abdominal pain, acute renal failure, anaphylactoid reaction, anemia, aplasia, apnea, confusion, cough, deep vein thrombosis, disorientation, dizziness, eosinophilia, epigastric pain, epistaxis, erythema, faintness, flank pain, GI bleeding, GI perforation, granulocytopenia, hemolysis, hemolytic anemia, herpes simplex reactivation, hiccups, hyperglycemia, iliac vein obstruction, infection, involuntary movement, kidney enlarged/ruptured, laryngospasm, malaise, neutropenia, pancytopenia, paresthesia, pulmonary edema, renal artery thrombosis, rigidity, sore mouth/throat, tachycardia, toxic epidermal necrosis, tremor, vasculitis, viral hepatitis, weakness, wound dehiscence

Drug Interactions

Metabolism/Transport Effects None known.

◀ **Avoid Concomitant Use**

Avoid concomitant use of Antithymocyte Globulin (Equine) with any of the following: BCG (Intravesical); Natalizumab; Pimecrolimus; Tacrolimus (Topical); Tofacitinib; Vaccines (Live)

Increased Effect/Toxicity

Antithymocyte Globulin (Equine) may increase the levels/effects of: Fingolimod; Leflunomide; Natalizumab; Tofacitinib; Vaccines (Live)

The levels/effects of Antithymocyte Globulin (Equine) may be increased by: Denosumab; Pimecrolimus; Roflumilast; Tacrolimus (Topical); Trastuzumab

Decreased Effect

Antithymocyte Globulin (Equine) may decrease the levels/effects of: BCG (Intravesical); Coccidioides immitis Skin Test; Sipuleucel-T; Vaccines (Inactivated); Vaccines (Live)

The levels/effects of Antithymocyte Globulin (Equine) may be decreased by: Echinacea

Storage/Stability Refrigerate ampules at 2°C to 8°C (36°F to 46°F). Do not freeze. Do not shake. Solutions diluted for infusion are stable for 24 hours (including infusion time) under refrigeration. Allow infusion solution to reach room temperature prior to administration.

Preparation for Administration Dilute into inverted bottle of sterile vehicle to ensure that undiluted lymphocyte immune globulin does not contact air. Gently rotate or swirl to mix; do not shake (to avoid excessive foaming and/or denaturation of the protein). Final concentration should not exceed 4 mg/mL. May be diluted in NS, $D_5^1/4$NS, or $D_5^1/2$NS **(do not use D_5W; low salt concentrations may result in precipitation)**. Inspect for particulate matter or discoloration prior to administration (solution may be transparent to slightly opalescent, colorless to faintly pink or brown, and may develop a slight granular or flaky deposit during storage).

Mechanism of Action Immunosuppressant involved in the elimination of antigen-reactive T lymphocytes (killer cells) in peripheral blood or alteration in the function of T-lymphocytes, which are involved in humoral immunity and partly in cell-mediated immunity; induces complete or partial hematologic response in aplastic anemia

Pharmacodynamics/Kinetics

Distribution: Poor into lymphoid tissues; binds to circulating lymphocytes, granulocytes, platelets, bone marrow cells

Half-life elimination: 5.7 ± 3 days

Excretion: Urine (~1%)

Dosing

Adult & Geriatric Note: Test dose: A skin test is recommended prior to administration of the initial dose. Test initially with an epicutaneous prick of undiluted antithymocyte globulin (ATG); if no wheal in 10 minutes, then use 0.02 mL intradermally of a 1:1000 dilution of ATG in normal saline along with a separate saline control of 0.02 mL; observe in 10 minutes. A positive skin reaction consists of a wheal with the initial prick test (undiluted) or ≥3 mm in diameter larger than the saline control with the diluted intradermal test. Alternatively, a 0.1 mL test dose (5 mg/mL concentration) may be administered intradermally along with a separate saline control; erythema larger than 5 mm in diameter (compared to the control) is considered a positive test (Molldrem, 2002). A positive skin test is suggestive of an increased risk for systemic allergic reactions with an infusion, although anaphylaxis may occur in patients who display negative skin tests. If ATG treatment is deemed appropriate following a positive skin test, the first infusion should be administered in a controlled environment with intensive life support immediately available. A systemic reaction precludes further administration of the drug.

Note: Consider premedication with an antihistamine, corticosteroids, and/or an antipyretic.

Aplastic anemia protocol: IV: 10 to 20 mg/kg/day for 8 to 14 days, then if needed, may administer every other day for 7 more doses for a total of 21 doses in 28 days **or**
Off-label dosing: 40 mg/kg/day for 4 days in combination with cyclosporine (Rosenfeld, 1995; Scheinberg, 2011)

Renal transplantation rejection, prophylaxis: IV: 15 mg/kg/day for 14 days, then give every other day for 7 more doses for a total of 21 doses in 28 days; the initial dose should be administered within 24 hours before or after transplantation (range: 10 to 30 mg/kg/day)

Renal transplantation rejection, treatment: IV: 10 to 15 mg/kg/day for 14 days, then if needed, may administer every other day for 7 more doses for a total of 21 doses in 28 days (range: 10 to 30 mg/kg/day)

Acute graft-versus-host disease (GVHD) treatment (off-label use): IV: 30 mg/kg/dose every other day for 6 doses (MacMillan, 2007) **or** 15 mg/kg/dose twice daily for 10 doses (MacMillan, 2002)

Myelodysplastic syndromes, refractory, lower-risk disease (off-label use): IV: 40 mg/kg/dose once daily for 4 days; an intradermal test dose was administered prior to treatment (Molldrem, 2002)

Pediatric Note: See adult dosing for notes on intradermal skin testing and premedication.

Aplastic anemia protocol: IV: 10 to 20 mg/kg/day for 8 to 14 days; then if needed, may administer every other day for 7 more doses for a total of 21 doses in 28 days **or**
Off-label dosing (in combination with cyclosporine):
Children >10 kg and Adolescents: 40 mg/kg/day for 4 days (Rosenfeld, 1995)
Children >2 years and Adolescents: 40 mg/kg/day for 4 days (Scheinberg, 2011)

Renal transplantation: IV:
Rejection prophylaxis: 15 mg/kg/day for 14 days, then give every other day for 7 more doses for a total of 21 doses in 28 days; the initial dose should be administered within 24 hours before or after transplantation (range: 5 to 25 mg/kg/day)
Rejection treatment: 10 to 15 mg/kg/day for 14 days, then if needed, may administer every other day for 7 more doses for a total of 21 doses in 28 days (range: 5 to 25 mg/kg/day)

Acute GVHD treatment (off-label use): IV: 30 mg/kg/dose every other day for 6 doses (MacMillan, 2007) **or** 15 mg/kg/dose twice daily for 10 doses (MacMillan, 2002)

Renal Impairment There are no dosage adjustments provided in the manufacturer's labeling.

Hepatic Impairment There are no dosage adjustments provided in the manufacturer's labeling.

Obesity *American Society for Blood and Marrow Transplantation (ASBMT) practice guideline committee position statement on chemotherapy dosing in obesity:* Utilize actual body weight (full weight) to calculate mg/kg dosing for hematopoietic stem cell transplant conditioning regimens (Bubalo, 2014).

◀ **Adjustment for Toxicity**
  Anaphylaxis: Discontinue infusion immediately; administer epinephrine. May
    require corticosteroids, respiration assistance, and/or other resuscitative
    measures. Do not resume infusion.
  Hemolysis (severe and unremitting): May require discontinuation of
    treatment.
  Leukopenia (severe and unremitting) in renal transplant patients: Discontinue
    treatment.
  Thrombocytopenia (severe and unremitting) in renal transplant patients:
    Discontinue treatment.
Administration Infuse over at least 4 hours through a 0.2 to 1 micron inline
  filter. Allow solution to reach room temperature prior to infusion. Infusion must
  be completed with 24 hours of preparation. May cause vein irritation (chemical
  phlebitis) if administered peripherally; high flow veins are preferred to reduce
  phlebitis (infuse into vascular shunt, arterial venous fistula, or high-flow central
  vein).

  Monitor closely throughout the infusion for allergic reactions. Appropriate
  resuscitative equipment should be nearby during administration. May require
  premedication with an antipyretic, antihistamine, and/or a corticosteroid to
  prevent reactions. Discontinue infusion for anaphylaxis or respiratory distress.
  Administer epinephrine, corticosteroids, antihistamines, and/or antipyretics as
  indicated to manage reactions.

  Due to possible infusion-related reactions, it may be preferable to avoid
  initiating treatment late in the day or on weekends; consider withholding
  beta-blockers prior to administration to avoid suppressing compensatory
  responses to anaphylaxis (Scheinberg, 2012).
Monitoring Parameters CBC with differential and platelet count, monitor vital
  signs during administration; monitor for infusion reactions
Dosage Forms Excipient information presented when available (limited,
  particularly for generics); consult specific product labeling.
  Injectable, Intravenous:
    Atgam: 50 mg/mL (5 mL) [thimerosal free]

Antithymocyte Globulin (Rabbit)
(an te THY moe site GLOB yu lin RAB bit)
Related Information
  Chemotherapy and Obesity *on page 2220*
  Hematopoietic Stem Cell Transplantation *on page 2272*
Brand Names: US Thymoglobulin
Brand Names: Canada Thymoglobulin
Index Terms Antithymocyte Immunoglobulin; rATG
Pharmacologic Category Immune Globulin; Immunosuppressant Agent;
  Polyclonal Antibody
Use Renal transplant rejection: Treatment of acute rejection of renal trans-
  plant; used in conjunction with concomitant immunosuppression
Labeled Contraindications Hypersensitivity to antithymocyte globulin, rabbit
  proteins, or any component of the formulation; acute or chronic infection
Pregnancy Considerations Animal reproduction studies have not been
  conducted. Women exposed to thymoglobulin during pregnancy may be
  enrolled in the National Transplantation Pregnancy Registry (877-955-6877).

Breast-Feeding Considerations This product has not been evaluated in nursing women; the manufacturer recommends that breast-feeding be discontinued if therapy is needed.

Warnings/Precautions [U.S. Boxed Warning]: Should only be used by physicians experienced in immunosuppressive therapy for the treatment of renal transplant patients. Medical surveillance is required during the infusion. Initial dose must be administered over at least 6 hours into a high flow vein; patient may need pretreatment with an antipyretic, antihistamine, and/or corticosteroid. Hypersensitivity and fatal anaphylactic reactions can occur; immediate treatment (including epinephrine 1:1000) should be available. An increased incidence of lymphoma, post-transplant lymphoproliferative disease (PTLD), other malignancies, or severe infections may develop following concomitant use of immunosuppressants and prolonged use or overdose of antithymocyte globulin. Appropriate antiviral, antibacterial, antiprotozoal, and/or antifungal prophylaxis is recommended. Reversible neutropenia or thrombocytopenia may result from the development of cross-reactive antibodies.

Release of cytokines by activated monocytes and lymphocytes may cause fatal cytokine release syndrome (CRS) during administration of antithymocyte globulin. Rapid infusion rates of have been associated with CRS in case reports. Symptoms range from a mild, self-limiting "flu-like reaction" to severe, life-threatening reactions. Severe or life-threatening symptoms include hypotension, acute respiratory distress syndrome, pulmonary edema, myocardial infarction, and tachycardia. Patients should not be immunized with attenuated live viral vaccines during or shortly after treatment; safety of immunization following therapy has not been studied. Potentially significant drug-drug interactions may exist, requiring dose or frequency adjustment, additional monitoring, and/or selection of alternative therapy.

Adverse Reactions

>10%:

Cardiovascular: Hypertension, peripheral edema, tachycardia

Central nervous system: Chills, fever, headache, pain, malaise

Endocrine & metabolic: Hyperkalemia

Gastrointestinal: Abdominal pain, diarrhea, nausea

Genitourinary: Urinary tract infection

Hematologic: Leukopenia, thrombocytopenia

Neuromuscular & skeletal: Weakness

Respiratory: Dyspnea

Miscellaneous: Antirabbit antibody development, cytomegalovirus infection, sepsis, systemic infection

1% to 10%:

Central nervous system: Dizziness

Gastrointestinal: Gastritis, gastrointestinal moniliasis

Miscellaneous: Herpes simplex infection, oral moniliasis

Postmarketing and/or case reports: Anaphylaxis, cytokine release syndrome, PTLD, neutropenia, serum sickness (delayed)

Drug Interactions

Metabolism/Transport Effects None known.

Avoid Concomitant Use

Avoid concomitant use of Antithymocyte Globulin (Rabbit) with any of the following: BCG (Intravesical); Natalizumab; Pimecrolimus; Tacrolimus (Topical); Tofacitinib; Vaccines (Live)

Increased Effect/Toxicity

Antithymocyte Globulin (Rabbit) may increase the levels/effects of: Fingolimod; Leflunomide; Natalizumab; Tofacitinib; Vaccines (Live)

The levels/effects of Antithymocyte Globulin (Rabbit) may be increased by: Denosumab; Pimecrolimus; Roflumilast; Tacrolimus (Topical); Trastuzumab

Decreased Effect

Antithymocyte Globulin (Rabbit) may decrease the levels/effects of: BCG (Intravesical); Coccidioides immitis Skin Test; Sipuleucel-T; Vaccines (Inactivated); Vaccines (Live)

The levels/effects of Antithymocyte Globulin (Rabbit) may be decreased by: Echinacea

Storage/Stability Store powder under refrigeration at 2°C to 8°C (36°F to 46°F); do not freeze. Protect from light. Reconstituted product is stable for up to 24 hours at room temperature; however, since it contains no preservatives, it should be used immediately following reconstitution.

Preparation for Administration Allow vials to reach room temperature, then reconstitute each vial with SWFI 5 mL. Rotate vial gently until dissolved. Prior to administration, further dilute one vial in 50 mL saline or dextrose (total volume is usually 50-500 mL depending on total number of vials needed per dose). Mix by gently inverting infusion bag once or twice.

Mechanism of Action Polyclonal antibody which appears to cause immunosuppression by acting on T-cell surface antigens and depleting CD4 lymphocytes

Pharmacodynamics/Kinetics

Onset of action (T-cell depletion): Within 1 day

Duration: Lymphopenia may persist ≥1 year

Half-life elimination, plasma: 2 to 3 days

Dosing

Adult & Geriatric Treatment of acute renal transplant rejection: IV: 1.5 mg/kg/day for 7 to 14 days

Pediatric Refer to adult dosing.

Obesity *American Society for Blood and Marrow Transplantation (ASBMT) practice guideline committee position statement on chemotherapy dosing in obesity:* Utilize actual body weight (full weight) to calculate mg/kg dosing for hematopoietic stem cell transplant conditioning regimens (Bubalo, 2014).

Adjustment for Toxicity

WBC count 2,000 to 3,000 cells/mm^3 or platelet count 50,000 to 75,000 cells/mm^3: Reduce dose by 50%.

WBC count <2,000 cells/mm^3 or platelet count <50,000 cells/mm^3: Consider discontinuing treatment.

Administration The first dose should be infused over at least 6 hours through a high-flow vein. Subsequent doses should be administered over at least 4 hours. Administer through an in-line 0.22 micron filter. Premedication with corticosteroids, acetaminophen, and/or an antihistamine may reduce infusion-related reactions.

Monitoring Parameters Lymphocyte profile, CBC with differential and platelet count; vital signs during administration; signs and symptoms of infection

Test Interactions Potential interference with rabbit antibody-based immunoassays

Dosage Forms Excipient information presented when available (limited, particularly for generics); consult specific product labeling.
Solution Reconstituted, Intravenous:
  Thymoglobulin: 25 mg (1 ea) [contains glycine, mannitol, sodium chloride]

◆ **Antithymocyte Immunoglobulin** *see* Antithymocyte Globulin (Equine) *on page 126*

◆ **Antithymocyte Immunoglobulin** *see* Antithymocyte Globulin (Rabbit) *on page 130*

◆ **Anti-VEGF Monoclonal Antibody** *see* Bevacizumab *on page 191*

◆ **Anti-VEGF rhuMAb** *see* Bevacizumab *on page 191*

◆ **Anzemet** *see* Dolasetron *on page 548*

◆ **AP24534** *see* PONATinib *on page 1403*

◆ **APC8015** *see* Sipuleucel-T *on page 1528*

◆ **APO-066** *see* Deferiprone *on page 486*

◆ **Apo-Acyclovir (Can)** *see* Acyclovir (Systemic) *on page 35*

◆ **Apo-Allopurinol (Can)** *see* Allopurinol *on page 73*

◆ **Apo-Anastrozole (Can)** *see* Anastrozole *on page 112*

◆ **Apo-Benzydamine (Can)** *see* Benzydamine *on page 190*

◆ **Apo-Bicalutamide (Can)** *see* Bicalutamide *on page 207*

◆ **Apo-Ciproflox (Can)** *see* Ciprofloxacin (Systemic) *on page 327*

◆ **Apo-Cyclosporine (Can)** *see* CycloSPORINE (Systemic) *on page 385*

◆ **Apo-Desmopressin (Can)** *see* Desmopressin *on page 505*

◆ **Apo-Dexamethasone (Can)** *see* Dexamethasone (Systemic) *on page 513*

◆ **Apo-Famciclovir® (Can)** *see* Famciclovir *on page 689*

◆ **Apo-Fentanyl Matrix (Can)** *see* FentaNYL *on page 692*

◆ **Apo-Fluconazole (Can)** *see* Fluconazole *on page 725*

◆ **Apo-Flutamide (Can)** *see* Flutamide *on page 751*

◆ **Apo-Haloperidol (Can)** *see* Haloperidol *on page 807*

◆ **Apo-Hydromorphone (Can)** *see* HYDROmorphone *on page 830*

◆ **Apo-Hydroxyurea (Can)** *see* Hydroxyurea *on page 839*

◆ **Apo-Imatinib (Can)** *see* Imatinib *on page 882*

◆ **Apo-Imiquimod (Can)** *see* Imiquimod *on page 897*

◆ **Apo-Ketoconazole (Can)** *see* Ketoconazole (Systemic) *on page 991*

◆ **Apo-Letrozole (Can)** *see* Letrozole *on page 1019*

◆ **APO-Levofloxacin (Can)** *see* Levofloxacin (Systemic) *on page 1038*

◆ **Apo-Linezolid (Can)** *see* Linezolid *on page 1049*

◆ **Apo-Lorazepam (Can)** *see* LORazepam *on page 1058*

◆ **Apo-Medroxy (Can)** *see* MedroxyPROGESTERone *on page 1074*

◆ **Apo-Methotrexate (Can)** *see* Methotrexate *on page 1104*

◆ **Apo-Metoclop (Can)** *see* Metoclopramide *on page 1134*

◆ **Apo-Mycophenolate (Can)** *see* Mycophenolate *on page 1177*

◆ **Apo-Oflox (Can)** *see* Ofloxacin (Systemic) *on page 1240*

◆ **Apo-Olanzapine (Can)** *see* OLANZapine *on page 1242*

Aprepitant (ap RE pi tant)

Related Information

Management of Chemotherapy-Induced Nausea and Vomiting in Adults *on page* 2142

Palliative Care Medicine (Cancer) *on page* 2252

Prevention of Chemotherapy-Induced Nausea and Vomiting in Children *on page* 2203

Brand Names: US Emend

Brand Names: Canada Emend

Index Terms L 754030; MK 869

Pharmacologic Category Antiemetic; Substance P/Neurokinin 1 Receptor Antagonist

Use

Chemotherapy-induced nausea and vomiting: Prevention of acute and delayed nausea and vomiting associated with moderately- and highly-emetogenic chemotherapy (in combination with other antiemetics) in patients ≥12 years and patients <12 years who weigh at least 30 kg.

Postoperative nausea and vomiting: Prevention of postoperative nausea and vomiting (PONV) in adults.

Limitations of use: Aprepitant has not been studied for the management of existing nausea and vomiting. Chronic, continuous administration is not recommended (chronic use may alter aprepitant's drug interaction profile).

Labeled Contraindications Hypersensitivity to aprepitant or any component of the formulation; concurrent use with pimozide

Pregnancy Considerations Adverse events were not observed in animal reproduction studies. Efficacy of hormonal contraceptive may be reduced during and for 28 days following the last aprepitant dose; alternative or additional methods of contraception should be used both during treatment with fosaprepitant or aprepitant and for at least 1 month following the last fosaprepitant/aprepitant dose.

Breast-Feeding Considerations It is not known if aprepitant is excreted in breast milk. According to the manufacturer, the decision to breast-feed during therapy should take into account the risk of exposure to the infant and the benefits of treatment to the mother.

Warnings/Precautions Potentially significant drug-drug interactions may exist, requiring dose or frequency adjustment, additional monitoring, and/or selection of alternative therapy. Use caution with severe hepatic impairment (Child-Pugh class C); has not been studied. Due to a risk of significantly increased pimozide plasma concentrations and potential for QT prolongation, concurrent use with pimozide is contraindicated. Other CYP3A4-mediated drug interactions may occur. In patients receiving concurrent warfarin, a clinically significant decrease in INR or prothrombin time (PT) may occur; monitor INR/PT for 2 weeks (particularly at 7 to 10 days) following aprepitant administration. Hypersensitivity reactions, including anaphylactic reactions have been reported. Pediatric patients should be at least 30 kg and be able to swallow capsules whole. Not approved for prevention of postoperative nausea and vomiting in children.

Adverse Reactions Adverse reactions may be reported in combination with other antiemetic agents. As reported for highly emetogenic cancer chemotherapy or moderately emetogenic cancer chemotherapy, unless otherwise noted as reported for postoperative nausea and vomiting (PONV).

>10%:

Central nervous system: Fatigue (adults: 13%; children & adolescents: 5%)

Hematologic & oncologic: Neutropenia (children & adolescents: 13%; adults: <3%)

0.5% to 10%:

Cardiovascular: Hypotension (PONV: 6%), bradycardia (PONV: <3%), flushing (<3%), palpitations (<3%), peripheral edema (<3%), syncope (PONV: <3%)

Central nervous system: Headache (children & adolescents: 9%), dizziness (<3% to 5%), anxiety (<3%), hypoesthesia (PONV: <3%), hypothermia (PONV: <3%), malaise (<3%), peripheral neuropathy (<3%)

Dermatologic: Alopecia (<3%), hyperhidrosis (<3%), skin rash (<3%), urticaria (<3%)

Endocrine & metabolic: Dehydration (≤3%), decreased serum albumin (PONV: <3%), decreased serum potassium (PONV: <3%), decreased serum sodium (<3%), hot flash (<3), hypokalemia (<3%), hypovolemia (PONV: <3%), increased serum glucose (PONV: <3%), weight loss (<3%)

Gastrointestinal: Constipation (PONV: 9%), diarrhea (6% to 9%), dyspepsia (≤7%), abdominal pain (≤6%), hiccups (4% to 5%), decreased appetite (<3% to 5%), dysgeusia (<3%), eructation (<3%), flatulence (<3%), gastritis (<3%), gastroesophageal reflux disease (<3%), nausea (<3%), vomiting (<3%), xerostomia (<3%)

Genitourinary: Proteinuria (<3%)

Hematologic & oncologic: Decreased hemoglobin (children & adolescents: 5%), decreased white blood cell count (≤4%), anemia (<3%), febrile neutropenia (<3%), hematoma (PONV: <3%), thrombocytopenia (<3%)

Hepatic: Increased serum ALT (3%), increased serum alkaline phosphatase (<3%), increased serum AST (<3%), increased serum bilirubin (PONV: <3%)

Infection: Candidiasis (<3%), postoperative infection (PONV: <3%)

Neuromuscular & skeletal: Weakness (≤7%), musculoskeletal pain (<3%)

Renal: Increased blood urea nitrogen (<3%)

Respiratory: Cough (<3% to 5%), dyspnea (<3%), hypoxia (PONV: <3%), oropharyngeal pain (<3%), pharyngitis (<3%), respiratory depression (PONV: <3%)

Miscellaneous: Wound dehiscence (PONV: <3%)

<0.5%, postmarketing, and/or case reports: Anaphylaxis, angioedema, hypersensitivity reaction, pruritus, Stevens-Johnson syndrome, toxic epidermal necrolysis

Drug Interactions

Metabolism/Transport Effects Substrate of CYP1A2 (minor), CYP2C19 (minor), CYP3A4 (major); **Note:** Assignment of Major/Minor substrate status based on clinically relevant drug interaction potential; **Inhibits** CYP2C19 (weak), CYP2C9 (weak), CYP3A4 (moderate); **Induces** CYP2C9 (strong)

Avoid Concomitant Use

Avoid concomitant use of Aprepitant with any of the following: Bosutinib; Cisapride; Cobimetinib; Conivaptan; CYP3A4 Inducers (Strong); CYP3A4 Inhibitors (Moderate); CYP3A4 Inhibitors (Strong); Domperidone; Flibanserin; Fusidic Acid (Systemic); Ibrutinib; Idelalisib; Ivabradine; Lomitapide; Naloxegol; Olaparib; Pimozide; Simeprevir; Tolvaptan; Trabectedin; Ulipristal

Increased Effect/Toxicity

Aprepitant may increase the levels/effects of: Apixaban; ARIPiprazole; Avanafil; Bosentan; Bosutinib; Brexpiprazole; Bromocriptine; Budesonide (Systemic); Budesonide (Systemic, Oral Inhalation); Budesonide (Topical); Cannabis; Cilostazol; Cisapride; Cobimetinib; Colchicine; Corticosteroids (Systemic); CYP3A4 Substrates; Dapoxetine; Dofetilide; Domperidone; DOXOrubicin (Conventional); Dronabinol; Eletriptan; Eliglustat; Eplerenone; Everolimus; FentaNYL; Flibanserin; Halofantrine; Hydrocodone; Ibrutinib; Ifosfamide; Ivabradine; Ivacaftor; Lomitapide; Lurasidone; Naloxegol; NiMODipine; Olaparib; OxyCODONE; Pimecrolimus; Pimozide; Propafenone; Ranolazine; Salmeterol; Saxagliptin; Simeprevir; Sirolimus; Sonidegib; Suvorexant; Tetrahydrocannabinol; Tolvaptan; Trabectedin; Ulipristal; Vilazodone; Vindesine; Zopiclone; Zuclopenthixol

The levels/effects of Aprepitant may be increased by: Conivaptan; CYP3A4 Inhibitors (Moderate); CYP3A4 Inhibitors (Strong); Dasatinib; Fosaprepitant; Fusidic Acid (Systemic); Idelalisib; Luliconazole; Osimertinib; Palbociclib; Stiripentol

Decreased Effect

Aprepitant may decrease the levels/effects of: Contraceptives (Estrogens); Contraceptives (Progestins); CYP2C9 Substrates; Diclofenac (Systemic); PARoxetine; TOLBUTamide; Warfarin

The levels/effects of Aprepitant may be decreased by: Bosentan; CYP3A4 Inducers (Moderate); CYP3A4 Inducers (Strong); Dabrafenib; Deferasirox; Osimertinib; PARoxetine; Siltuximab; St Johns Wort; Tocilizumab

Food Interactions Aprepitant serum concentration may be increased when taken with grapefruit juice. Management: Avoid concurrent use.

Storage/Stability Store at room temperature of 20°C to 25°C (68°F to 77°F).

Mechanism of Action Prevents acute and delayed vomiting by inhibiting the substance P/neurokinin 1 (NK_1) receptor; augments the antiemetic activity of 5-HT_3 receptor antagonists and corticosteroids to inhibit acute and delayed phases of chemotherapy-induced emesis.

Pharmacodynamics/Kinetics

Distribution: V_d: ~70 L; crosses the blood-brain barrier

Protein binding: >95%

Metabolism: Extensively hepatic via CYP3A4 (major); CYP1A2 and CYP2C19 (minor); forms 7 metabolites (weakly active)

Bioavailability: ~60% to 65%

Half-life elimination: Terminal: ~9 to 13 hours

Time to peak, plasma: Adult: ~3 hours; Pediatric: ~4 hours

Excretion: Primarily via metabolism

Dosing

Adult & Geriatric

Prevention of chemotherapy-induced nausea/vomiting:

Manufacturer's labeling:

Prevention of nausea/vomiting associated with highly-emetogenic chemotherapy: Oral: 125 mg 1 hour prior to chemotherapy on day 1, followed by 80 mg once daily on days 2 and 3 (in combination with a 5-HT$_3$ antagonist antiemetic on day 1 and dexamethasone on days 1 to 4)

Prevention of nausea/vomiting associated with moderately-emetogenic chemotherapy: Oral: 125 mg 1 hour prior to chemotherapy on day 1, followed by 80 mg once daily on days 2 and 3 (in combination with a 5-HT$_3$ antagonist antiemetic and dexamethasone on day 1)

Guideline recommendations:

Prevention of nausea/vomiting associated with highly-emetogenic chemotherapy (including anthracycline and cyclophosphamide [AC] regimens): Oral:

American Society of Clinical Oncology (ASCO; Basch, 2011): 125 mg prior to chemotherapy on day 1, followed by 80 mg once daily on days 2 and 3 (in combination with a 5-HT$_3$ antagonist antiemetic on day 1 and dexamethasone on days 1 to 4 or days 1 to 3)

Multinational Association of Supportive Care in Cancer (MASCC) and European Society of Medical Oncology (ESMO) (Roila, 2010): 125 mg prior to chemotherapy on day 1, followed by 80 mg once daily on days 2 and 3 (in combination with a 5-HT$_3$ antagonist antiemetic on day 1 and dexamethasone on days 1 to 4 **or** day 1 only [AC regimen])

Prevention of postoperative nausea/vomiting (PONV): Oral: 40 mg within 3 hours prior to anesthesia induction

Pediatric

Manufacturer's labeling:

Prevention of nausea/vomiting associated with highly-emetogenic chemotherapy: Children <12 years and ≥30 kg, Children ≥12 years, and Adolescents: Oral: 125 mg 1 hour prior to chemotherapy on day 1, followed by 80 mg once daily on days 2 and 3 (in combination with a 5-HT$_3$ antagonist antiemetic on day 1 and dexamethasone on days 1 to 4 [reduce dexamethasone dose to 50% of recommended dose])

Prevention of nausea/vomiting associated with moderately-emetogenic chemotherapy: Children <12 years and ≥30 kg, Children ≥12 years, and Adolescents: Oral: 125 mg 1 hour prior to chemotherapy on day 1, followed by 80 mg once daily on days 2 and 3 (in combination with a 5-HT$_3$ antagonist antiemetic and dexamethasone on day 1 [reduce dexamethasone dose to 50% of recommended dose])

Pediatric guideline recommendations: **Prevention of nausea/vomiting associated with highly-emetogenic chemotherapy:** *Pediatric Oncology Group of Ontario (POGO):* Children ≥12 years and Adolescents: Oral: 125 mg prior to chemotherapy on day 1, followed by 80 mg once daily on days 2 and 3 (Dupuis, 2013). The antiemetic regimen also includes a 5-HT$_3$ antagonist and dexamethasone.

Renal Impairment
No dosage adjustment necessary.
ESRD undergoing dialysis: No dosage adjustment necessary.
Hepatic Impairment
Mild-to-moderate impairment (Child-Pugh class A or B): No dosage adjustment necessary.
Severe impairment (Child-Pugh class C): Use with caution; no data available; may require additional monitoring for adverse reactions.

Administration
Swallow capsule whole (according to the manufacturer).
Prevention of chemotherapy-induced nausea/vomiting: Administer with or without food. First dose should be given 1 hour prior to chemotherapy; subsequent doses should be given 1 hour prior to chemotherapy or in the morning (if no chemotherapy is administered).
Prevention of postoperative nausea/vomiting: Administer within 3 hours prior to induction; follow health care provider instructions about food/drink restrictions prior to surgery.

Extemporaneous Preparations A 20 mg/mL oral aprepitant suspension may be prepared with capsules and a 1:1 combination of Ora-Sweet and Ora-Plus (or Ora-Blend). Empty the contents of four 125 mg capsules into a mortar and reduce to a fine powder (process will take 10-15 minutes). Add small portions of vehicle and mix to a uniform paste. Add sufficient vehicle to form a liquid; transfer to a graduated cylinder, rinse mortar with vehicle, and add quantity of vehicle sufficient to make 25 mL. Label "shake well" and "refrigerate". Stable for 90 days refrigerated.

Dupuis LL, Lingertat-Walsh K, and Walker SE, "Stability of an Extemporaneous Oral Liquid Aprepitant Formulation," *Support Care Cancer*, 2009, 17(6):701-6.

Monitoring Parameters In patients receiving concurrent warfarin, monitor INR/PT for 2 weeks (particularly at 7 to 10 days) following aprepitant administration; signs/symptoms of hypersensitivity reaction.

Dosage Forms Excipient information presented when available (limited, particularly for generics); consult specific product labeling.
Capsule, Oral:
Emend: 40 mg, 80 mg, 125 mg, 80 mg & 125 mg

Arsenic Trioxide (AR se nik tri OKS id)

Related Information

Common Toxicity Criteria *on page 2122*

Management of Chemotherapy-Induced Nausea and Vomiting in Adults *on page 2142*

Management of Drug Extravasations *on page 2159*

Prevention of Chemotherapy-Induced Nausea and Vomiting in Children *on page 2203*

Safe Handling of Hazardous Drugs *on page 2292*

Brand Names: US Trisenox

Brand Names: Canada Trisenox

Index Terms Arsenic (III) Oxide; As_2O_3; ATO

Pharmacologic Category Antineoplastic Agent, Miscellaneous

Use Acute promyelocytic leukemia: Remission induction and consolidation in patients with acute promyelocytic leukemia (APL) who are refractory to, or have relapsed from, retinoid and anthracycline chemotherapy, and whose APL is characterized by the presence of the t(15;17) translocation or PML/RAR-alpha gene expression

Labeled Contraindications

Hypersensitivity to arsenic or any component of the formulation

Canadian labeling: Additional contraindications (not in US labeling): Pregnancy; breast-feeding

Pregnancy Considerations Adverse events have been observed in animal reproduction studies. Arsenic crosses the human placenta. In studies of women exposed to high levels of arsenic from drinking water, cord blood levels were similar to maternal serum levels. Dimethylarsinic acid (DMA) was the form of arsenic found in the fetus. An increased risk of low birth weight and still births were observed in women who ingested high levels of dietary arsenic. Women of childbearing potential should avoid pregnancy; effective contraception should be used during and after therapy. The Canadian labeling contraindicates use in pregnant women. It also recommends that women of childbearing potential avoid pregnancy, and male patients wear condoms during intercourse with women who are pregnant or of childbearing potential during therapy and for 3 months following therapy discontinuation.

Breast-Feeding Considerations Arsenic is naturally found in breast milk; concentrations range from 0.2 to 6 mcg/kg. In studies of women exposed to high levels of arsenic from drinking water, breast milk concentrations were low (~3.1 mcg/kg) and did not correlate with maternal serum levels. The possible effect of maternal arsenic trioxide therapy on breast milk concentrations is not known. Due to the potential for serious adverse reactions in a nursing infant, the manufacturer recommends discontinuing breast-feeding during therapy. The Canadian labeling contraindicates use in nursing women and recommends avoiding nursing during treatment and for 3 months after therapy discontinuation.

Warnings/Precautions Hazardous agent - use appropriate precautions for handling and disposal (NIOSH 2014 [group 1]). **[US Boxed Warnings]: May prolong the QT interval and lead to torsade de pointes or complete AV block, which may be fatal. Risk factors for torsade de pointes include extent of prolongation, HF, a history of torsade de pointes, preexisting QT interval prolongation, patients taking medications known to prolong the QT interval or potassium-wasting diuretics, and conditions which cause hypokalemia or hypomagnesemia. If possible, discontinue all** ▶

◄ medications known to prolong the QT interval. **[US Boxed Warning]: A baseline 12-lead ECG, serum electrolytes (potassium, calcium, magnesium), and creatinine should be obtained prior to treatment.** QT prolongation was observed 1 to 5 weeks after infusion, and returned to baseline by 8 weeks after infusion. Monitor ECG at baseline and then weekly; more frequently if clinically indicated. If baseline QTc >500 msec, correct prior to treatment. If QTc >500 msec during treatment, reassess, correct contributing factors, and consider temporarily withholding treatment. If syncope or irregular heartbeat develop during therapy, hospitalize patient for monitoring; assess electrolytes and do not reinitiate until QTc <460 msec, electrolyte abnormalities are corrected and syncope/irregular heartbeat has resolved.

[US Boxed Warning]: May cause APL differentiation syndrome (formerly called retinoic-acid-APL [RA-APL] syndrome), which is characterized by dyspnea, fever, weight gain, pulmonary infiltrates, and pleural or pericardial effusions, with or without leukocytosis. May be fatal. High-dose steroids (dexamethasone 10 mg IV twice daily for at least 3 days or until signs/symptoms subside; initiate immediately if APL differentiation syndrome is suspected) have been used for treatment; in general, most patients may continue arsenic trioxide during treatment of APL differentiation syndrome. May lead to the development of hyperleukocytosis (leukocytes ≥10,000/mm^3); did not correlate with baseline WBC counts and generally was not as high during consolidation as observed during induction treatment. Use with caution in patients with hepatic impairment; in patients with severe hepatic impairment, monitor closely for toxicity. Use with caution in patients with severe renal impairment (dose reduction may be warranted); systemic exposure to metabolites may be higher; has not been studied in dialysis patients. Monitor electrolytes, CBC with differential, and coagulation parameters at least twice a week during induction and weekly during consolidation; more frequently if clinically indicated. Arsenic trioxide is associated with a moderate emetic potential; antiemetics are recommended to prevent nausea and vomiting (Dupuis 2011). Potentially significant interactions may exist, requiring dose or frequency adjustment, additional monitoring, and/or selection of alternative therapy.

Adverse Reactions

>10%:

Cardiovascular: Tachycardia (55%), edema (40%), QT interval >500 msec (40%), chest pain (25%; grades 3/4: 5%), hypotension (25%; grades 3/4: 5%)

Central nervous system: Fatigue (63%), fever (63%), headache (60%), insomnia (43%), anxiety (30%), dizziness (23%), depression (20%), pain (15%)

Dermatologic: Dermatitis (43%), pruritus (33%), bruising (20%), dry skin (15%), erythema (13%)

Endocrine & metabolic: Hypokalemia (50%; grades 3/4: 13%), hyperglycemia (45%; grades 3/4: 13%), hypomagnesemia (45%; grades 3/4: 13%), hyperkalemia (18%; grades 3/4: 5%)

Gastrointestinal: Nausea (75%), abdominal pain (58%), vomiting (58%), diarrhea (53%), sore throat (35%), constipation (28%), anorexia (23%), appetite decreased (15%), weight gain (13%)

Genitourinary: Vaginal hemorrhage (13%)

Hematologic: Leukocytosis (50%; grades 3/4: 3%), APL differentiation syndrome (23%; grades 3/4: 8%), anemia (20%; grades 3/4: 5%), thrombocytopenia (18%; grades 3/4: 13%), febrile neutropenia (13%; grades 3/4: 8%)

Hepatic: ALT increased (20%; grades 3/4: 5%), AST increased (13%; grades 3/4: 3%)

Local: Injection site: Pain (20%), erythema (13%)

Neuromuscular & skeletal: Rigors (38%), arthralgia (33%), paresthesia (33%), myalgia (25%), bone pain (23%), back pain (18%), limb pain (13%), neck pain (13%), tremor (13%)

Respiratory: Cough (65%), dyspnea (53%; grades 3/4: 10%), epistaxis (25%), hypoxia (23%), pleural effusion (20%), sinusitis (20%), postnasal drip (13%), upper respiratory tract infection (13%), wheezing (13%)

Miscellaneous: Herpes simplex (13%), diaphoresis (13%)

1% to 10%:

Cardiovascular: Hypertension (10%), flushing (10%), pallor (10%), palpitation (10%), facial edema (8%), abnormal ECG (not QT prolongation) (8%), atrial dysrhythmia (5%), torsade de pointes (3%)

Central nervous system: Seizure (8%; grades 3/4: 5%), somnolence (8%), agitation (5%), coma (5%), confusion (5%)

Dermatologic: Hyperpigmentation (8%), petechia (8%), skin lesions (8%), urticaria (8%), local exfoliation (5%)

Endocrine & metabolic: Hypocalcemia (10%), hypoglycemia (8%), intermenstrual bleeding (8%), acidosis (5%)

Gastrointestinal: Dyspepsia (10%), loose stools (10%), abdominal distension (8%), abdominal tenderness (8%), caecitis (children: 8%), fecal incontinence (8%), gastrointestinal hemorrhage (8%), hemorrhagic diarrhea (8%), oral blistering (8%), weight loss (8%), xerostomia (8%), oral candidiasis (5%)

Genitourinary: Incontinence (5%)

Hematologic: Neutropenia (10%; grades 3/4: 10%), DIC (8%), hemorrhage (8%)

Local: Injection site edema (10%)

Neuromuscular & skeletal: Weakness (10%)

Ocular: Blurred vision (10%), eye irritation (10%), dry eye (8%), eyelid edema (5%), painful red eye (5%)

Otic: Earache (8%), tinnitus (5%)

Renal: Renal failure (8%; grades 3/4: 3%), renal impairment (8%), oliguria (5%)

Respiratory: Breath sounds decreased (10%), crepitations (10%), rales (10%), hemoptysis (8%), pulmonary edema (children: 8%), rhonchi (8%), tachypnea (8%), nasopharyngitis (5%)

Miscellaneous: Bacterial infection (8%), herpes zoster (8%), lymphadenopathy (8%), night sweats (8%), hypersensitivity (5%), sepsis (5%; grades 3/4: 5%)

<1%, postmarketing, and/or case reports: Acute respiratory distress syndrome, AV block, capillary leak syndrome, CHF, dysphagia, enuresis, heart block, hypoalbuminemia, hyponatremia, hypophosphatemia, lipase increased, mitochondrial myopathy, mucosal inflammation, neuralgia, oropharyngeal pain, pancytopenia, peripheral neuropathy, pneumonitis, pulmonary infiltrate, respiratory distress, stomatitis, ventricular extrasystoles, ventricular tachycardia

Drug Interactions

Metabolism/Transport Effects None known.

Avoid Concomitant Use

Avoid concomitant use of Arsenic Trioxide with any of the following: BCG (Intravesical); CloZAPine; Dipyrone; Highest Risk QTc-Prolonging Agents; Ivabradine; Mifepristone; Moderate Risk QTc-Prolonging Agents

◀ **Increased Effect/Toxicity**
Arsenic Trioxide may increase the levels/effects of: CloZAPine; Highest Risk QTc-Prolonging Agents

The levels/effects of Arsenic Trioxide may be increased by: Dipyrone; Ivabradine; Mifepristone; Moderate Risk QTc-Prolonging Agents; QTc-Prolonging Agents (Indeterminate Risk and Risk Modifying)

Decreased Effect
Arsenic Trioxide may decrease the levels/effects of: Antidiabetic Agents; BCG (Intravesical)

Storage/Stability Store at 25°C (77°F); excursions permitted to 15°C to 30°C (59°F to 86°F); do not freeze. Following dilution, solution for infusion is stable for 24 hours at room temperature or 48 hours when refrigerated.

Preparation for Administration Hazardous agent; use appropriate precautions for handling and disposal (NIOSH 2014 [group 1]). Dilute with 100 to 250 mL D_5W or 0.9% NaCl. Discard unused portion of ampule.

Mechanism of Action Induces apoptosis in APL cells via morphological changes and DNA fragmentation; also damages or degrades the fusion protein promyelocytic leukemia (PML)-retinoic acid receptor (RAR) alpha

Pharmacodynamics/Kinetics
Distribution: V_{dss}: Arsenious acid (As^{III}): 562 L; widely distributed throughout body tissues; dependent on body weight and increases as body weight increases; orally administered arsenic trioxide distributes into the CNS

Metabolism: Arsenic trioxide is immediately hydrolyzed to the active form, arsenious acid (As^{III}) which is methylated (hepatically) to the less active pentavalent metabolites, monomethylarsonic acid (MMA^V) and dimethylarsinic acid (DMA^V) by methyltransferases; As^{III} is also oxidized to the minor metabolite, arsenic acid (As^V)

Half-life elimination: As^{III}: 10 to 14 hours; MMA^V: ~32 hours; DMA^V: ~72 hours

Time to peak: As^{III}: At the end of infusion (2 hours); MMA^V and DMA^V; ~10 to 24 hours

Excretion: Urine (MMA^V, DMA^V, and 15% of a dose as unchanged As^{III})

Dosing
Adult *Note:* Arsenic trioxide is associated with a moderate emetic potential; antiemetics are recommended to prevent nausea and vomiting.

Acute promyelocytic leukemia (APL), relapsed or refractory: IV:
Induction: 0.15 mg/kg once daily until bone marrow remission; maximum: 60 doses for induction

Consolidation: 0.15 mg/kg once daily starting 3 to 6 weeks after completion of induction therapy; maximum: 25 doses over a period of up to 5 weeks for consolidation

APL, newly diagnosed (off-label use): IV:
Low/intermediate risk (Lo-Coco 2013):
Induction: 0.15 mg/kg/day; administer daily until bone marrow remission (in combination with tretinoin)

Consolidation: 0.15 mg/kg/day; administer 5 days/week for 4 weeks every 8 weeks for a total of 4 cycles (in combination with tretinoin)

High-risk:
Consolidation therapy after remission induction with tretinoin, daunorubicin and cytarabine (Powell 2010): Two consolidation courses (2 weeks apart): 0.15 mg/kg/day 5 days/week for 5 weeks

In combination with tretinoin in patients unable to tolerate anthracycline-based therapy (Estey 2006; Ravandi 2009):

Induction (beginning 10 days after initiation of tretinoin): 0.15 mg/kg/day until bone marrow remission; maximum: 75 doses for induction

Consolidation: 0.15 mg/kg/day Monday through Friday for 4 weeks every 8 weeks for 4 cycles (weeks 1 to 4, 9 to 12, 17 to 20, and 25 to 28)

APML 4 protocol (Iland 2012):

Induction: 0.15 mg/kg/day over 2 hours on days 9 to 36 (in combination with tretinoin and age-adjusted idarubicin)

Consolidation (2 cycles): 0.15 mg/kg/day on days 1 to 28 of consolidation cycle 1 (in combination with tretinoin); 0.15 mg/kg/day on days 1 to 5, 8 to 12, 15 to 19, 22 to 26, and 29 to 33 of consolidation cycle 2 (in combination with tretinoin)

Pediatric Note: Arsenic trioxide is associated with a moderate emetic potential; antiemetics are recommended to prevent nausea and vomiting (Dupuis 2011).

Acute promyelocytic leukemia (APL), relapsed or refractory: Children ≥4 years (US labeling) or ≥5 years (Canadian labeling): IV: Refer to adult dosing. **Note:** The Canadian labeling recommends dosing obese pediatric patients based on ideal body weight.

APL, newly diagnosed (off-label use): IV:

Induction, consolidation, and maintenance (Mathews 2006):

Induction: 0.15 mg/kg/day (maximum dose: 10 mg); administer daily until bone marrow remission; maximum: 60 doses for induction

Consolidation: 0.15 mg/kg/day (maximum dose: 10 mg) for 4 weeks, starting 4 weeks after completion of induction therapy

Maintenance: 0.15 mg/kg/dose (maximum dose: 10 mg) administered 10 days per month for 6 months, starting 4 weeks after completion of consolidation therapy

Children >1 year and Adolescents (APML 4 protocol; Iland 2012):

Induction: 0.15 mg/kg/day over 2 hours on days 9 to 36 (in combination with tretinoin and idarubicin)

Consolidation (2 cycles): 0.15 mg/kg/day on days 1 to 28 of consolidation cycle 1 (in combination with tretinoin); 0.15 mg/kg/day on days 1 to 5, 8 to 12, 15 to 19, 22 to 26, and 29 to 33 of consolidation cycle 2 (in combination with tretinoin)

Renal Impairment

Mild-to-moderate impairment (CrCl ≥30 mL/minute): There are no dosage adjustments provided in the manufacturer's labeling.

Severe renal impairment (CrCl <30 mL/minute): Use with caution (systemic exposure to metabolites may be higher); may require dosage reduction; monitor closely for toxicity.

Dialysis patients: There are no dosage adjustments provided in the manufacturer's labeling (has not been studied).

Hepatic Impairment There are no dosage adjustments provided in the manufacturer's labeling; use with caution. Patients with severe impairment (Child-Pugh class C) should be monitored closely for toxicity.

Adjustment for Toxicity Consider delaying infusion if a severe non-hematologic reaction occurs (eg, neurologic or dermatologic toxicity) until the toxicity has improved to ≤ grade 1.

◀ **Combination Regimens**
Leukemia, acute promyelocytic:
Tretinoin-Arsenic Trioxide (APL) on page 2095
Tretinoin-Daunorubicin-Cytarabine Induction, Consolidation, Maintenance (APL) on page 2097

Administration Arsenic trioxide is associated with a moderate emetic potential; antiemetics are recommended to prevent nausea and vomiting (Dupuis 2011). For relapsed/refractory APL, administer as an IV infusion over 1 to 2 hours. For newly diagnosed APL (off-label use), infusion rate may vary; refer to specific protocol. If acute vasomotor reactions occur, the infusion duration may be extended to up to 4 hours. Does not require administration via a central venous catheter.

Hazardous agent; use appropriate precautions for handling and disposal (NIOSH 2014 [group 1]).

Vesicant/Extravasation Risk May be an irritant

Emetic Potential Children and Adults: Moderate (30% to 90%)

Monitoring Parameters Monitor electrolytes (potassium, calcium, and magnesium), CBC with differential, serum creatinine, hepatic function, blood glucose, and coagulation parameters at baseline then at least twice weekly during induction and at least weekly during consolidation; more frequent monitoring may be necessary in unstable patients; baseline then weekly 12-lead ECG; signs/symptoms of APL differentiation syndrome (unexplained fever, dyspnea and/or weight gain, abnormal chest auscultatory findings or radiographic abnormalities)

Dosage Forms Excipient information presented when available (limited, particularly for generics); consult specific product labeling.
Solution, Intravenous:
Trisenox: 10 mg/10 mL (10 mL)

◆ **Artificial Saliva** see Saliva Substitute on page 1511
◆ **Arzerra** see Ofatumumab on page 1235
◆ **As₂O₃** see Arsenic Trioxide on page 139
◆ **AsmalPred [DSC]** see PrednisoLONE (Systemic) on page 1421
◆ **AsmalPred Plus [DSC]** see PrednisoLONE (Systemic) on page 1421
◆ **ASNase** see Asparaginase (E. coli) on page 144
◆ **Asparaginase** see Asparaginase (E. coli) on page 144

Asparaginase (*E. coli*) (a SPEAR a ji nase e ko lye)
Related Information
Common Toxicity Criteria on page 2122
Management of Chemotherapy-Induced Nausea and Vomiting in Adults on page 2142
Prevention of Chemotherapy-Induced Nausea and Vomiting in Children on page 2203

Brand Names: US Elspar [DSC]
Brand Names: Canada Kidrolase

Index Terms *E. coli* Asparaginase; ASNase; Asparaginase; Elspar; L-ASP; L-asparaginase (*E. coli*)

Pharmacologic Category Antineoplastic Agent, Enzyme; Antineoplastic Agent, Miscellaneous

Use Acute lymphoblastic leukemia: Treatment of acute lymphoblastic leukemia (ALL) (in combination with other chemotherapy)

Labeled Contraindications Known hypersensitivity to asparaginase (*E. coli*-derived) or any component of the formulation; hepatic insufficiency, pancreatitis, pregnancy, breast-feeding, recent yellow fever vaccination, concurrent administration with phenytoin

Pregnancy Considerations Use is contraindicated.

Warnings/Precautions [Canadian Boxed Warning]: Allergic reactions may occur during therapy, particularly in patients with known hypersensitivity to other forms of L-asparaginase. Observe for reactions following administration; reactions generally occur 30 to 60 minutes following administration (although may also occur beyond that time). Immediate treatment for hypersensitivity reactions should be available during administration. Discontinue if serious allergic reaction occurs. Prior exposure to asparaginase is a risk factor for allergic reactions; IV administration (compared to IM or SubQ administration) and younger age also may be associated with hypersensitivity reactions (Stock 2011; Woo 2000). Patients who have an allergic reaction to *E. coli* asparaginase may also react to asparaginase (*Erwinia*) or to pegaspargase.

[Canadian Boxed Warning]: Should be administered under the supervision of an experienced cancer chemotherapy physician in a setting where full resuscitative facilities are immediately available.

[Canadian Boxed Warning]: Adverse effects on liver function may be observed including exacerbation of preexisting liver impairment (due to prior therapy or underlying disease). Physicians should carefully consider therapeutic benefits versus toxicity risks. Altered liver function tests (eg, increased AST, ALT, alkaline phosphatase, bilirubin, and decreased serum albumin, plasma fibrinogen) may occur; fulminant hepatic failure has also occurred. Fatty liver may be observed on biopsy. Use with caution and monitor liver function tests at least weekly during therapy; discontinue therapy for any significant changes. May induce excessive ammonia production; monitor for signs of metabolic encephalopathy (confusion, stupor, coma).

Serious thrombosis, including sagittal sinus thrombosis may occur; discontinue with serious thrombotic events. Anticoagulation prophylaxis during therapy may be considered in some patients (Farge 2013). The risk for thrombosis may be higher in adult patients (Stock 2011). Increased prothrombin time, partial thromboplastin time and hypofibrinogenemia may occur; cerebrovascular thrombosis and hemorrhage have been reported; monitor coagulation parameters at baseline and periodically during and after therapy; use cautiously in patients with an underlying coagulopathy. Replacement therapy should be instituted if fibrinogen <1g/L or ATIII <60%; if ineffective, treatment should preferably be suspended and resumed only when the laboratory parameters have normalized.

May cause hyperglycemia/glucose intolerance (possibly irreversible). Cases of diabetic ketoacidosis have been observed; monitor blood glucose as clinically necessary. May cause serious and possibly fulminant or fatal pancreatitis; promptly evaluate patients with abdominal pain. May consider continuing ▶

145

therapy for asymptomatic chemical pancreatitis (amylase or lipase >3 times ULN) or only radiologic abnormalities; monitor closely for rising amylase and/or lipase levels (Stock 2011). Discontinue permanently for clinical pancreatitis (eg, vomiting, severe abdominal pain) with amylase/lipase elevation >3 times ULN for >3 days and/or development of a pancreatic pseudocyst. Avoid alcohol use (Stock 2011).

Posterior reversible encephalopathy syndrome (PRES) has been observed in patients treated with asparaginase (in combination with other chemotherapy agents). Monitor for signs/symptoms of PRES (eg, altered mental status, headache, hypertension, seizures, visual disturbances); interrupt therapy for suspected PRES. Control blood pressure and closely monitor for seizure activity. Appropriate measures must be taken to prevent tumor lysis syndrome and subsequent hyperuricemia and uric acid nephropathy; monitor, consider antihyperuricemic therapy, hydration and urinary alkalization.

Do not interchange E. coli asparaginase for Erwinia asparaginase or pegaspargase; ensure the proper formulation, route of administration, and dose prior to administration. The E. coli and the Erwinia strains of asparaginase differ slightly in their gene sequencing, and have slight differences in their enzyme characteristics. Both are highly specific for asparagine and have <10% activity for the D-isomer.

Adverse Reactions Frequency not defined.

Cardiovascular: Cerebrovascular accident (hemorrhagic stroke and thrombotic stroke [Morgan 2011]), thrombosis (including cerebral thrombosis)

Central nervous system: Central nervous system disease (adults; includes delusion, disorientation, mild depression, Parkinsonian-like syndrome, personality disorder, seizure), cerebral hemorrhage, cerebrovascular hemorrhage (Morgan 2011)

Endocrine & metabolic: Amenorrhea, decreased glucose tolerance, hyperammonemia (with clinical signs of metabolic encephalopathy [eg, impaired consciousness with coma, confusion, and stupor]), hypercholesterolemia, hyperglycemia, hypertriglyceridemia, hypoalbuminemia, hypocholesterolemia, increased uric acid, weight loss

Gastrointestinal: Abdominal pain (infrequent), acute pancreatitis (may be fatal), cholestatic injury, diarrhea (infrequent), intestinal perforation (rare), nausea (frequent, but rarely severe; may be secondary to increased blood urea nitrogen and increased uric acid), vomiting (frequent, but rarely severe; may be secondary to increased blood urea nitrogen and increased uric acid)

Genitourinary: Azoospermia

Hematologic: Antithrombin III deficiency, blood coagulation disorder (change in hemostatic function), bone marrow depression, decreased clotting factors (factors VII, VIII, IX, and X), decreased plasminogen, hypofibrinogenemia, prolonged partial thromboplastin time, prolonged prothrombin time

Hepatic: Hepatic injury, hepatotoxicity (usually mild and regressive, but may be fatal rarely), hyperbilirubinemia, increased serum alkaline phosphatase, increased serum ALT, increased serum AST (mild), jaundice, liver steatosis

Hypersensitivity: Allergic reactions (includes anaphylactic shock, anaphylaxis, bronchospasm, edema, hypotension, laryngeal edema, skin rash, urticaria; onset usually within 1 hour of administration and risk increasing with increasing number of exposures)

Immunologic: Increased serum globulins (beta and gamma)

Infection: Septicemia (during bone marrow depression)

Renal: Increased blood urea nitrogen, renal failure

Respiratory: Respiratory distress (with retrosternal pressure)
Miscellaneous: Fever

Drug Interactions

Metabolism/Transport Effects None known.

Avoid Concomitant Use There are no known interactions where it is recommended to avoid concomitant use.

Increased Effect/Toxicity

Asparaginase (E. coli) may increase the levels/effects of: Dexamethasone (Systemic)

Decreased Effect There are no known significant interactions involving a decrease in effect.

Storage/Stability Intact vials of powder should be refrigerated at 2°C to 8°C (36°F to 48°F). Reconstituted solution should be used immediately after preparation, although is stable for 3 hours at room temperature or 72 hours refrigerated.

Preparation for Administration Reconstitute each vial with 4 mL sterile water for injection; rotate gently, do not shake. For IM administration, the US manufacturer recommended reconstitution of the lyophilized powder with 2 mL NS to a concentration of 5000 units/mL; however, some institutions reconstitute with 1 mL NS for IM use, resulting in a concentration of 10,000 units/mL. Shake well, but not too vigorously. A 5 micron filter may be used to remove fiber-like particles in the solution (do not use a 0.2 micron filter; has been associated with loss of potency).

Standard IM dilution: 5,000 units/mL (10,000 units/mL has been used by some institutions)

Standard IV dilution: Dilute in 50 to 250 mL NS or D_5W

Mechanism of Action In leukemic cells, asparaginase hydrolyzes L-asparagine to ammonia and L-aspartic acid, leading to depletion of asparagine. Leukemia cells, especially lymphoblasts, require exogenous asparagine; normal cells can synthesize asparagine. Asparagine depletion in leukemic cells leads to inhibition of protein synthesis and apoptosis. Asparaginase is cycle-specific for the G_1 phase.

Pharmacodynamics/Kinetics

Distribution: IV: Slightly higher than plasma volume; <1% CSF penetration
Metabolism: Systemically degraded
Half-life elimination: IM: 34 to 49 hours; IV: 8 to 30 hours
Time to peak, plasma: IM: 14 to 24 hours

Dosing

Adult & Geriatric Note: Dose, frequency, number of doses, and start date may vary by protocol and treatment phase.

Acute lymphoblastic leukemia (ALL; Canadian labeling): IM, IV:

Daily administration: 200 to 1,000 units/kg/day for 28 consecutive days; continue induction therapy for an additional 14 days if not in remission or begin maintenance therapy if in remission

Intermittent administration: 400 units/kg on Monday and Wednesday and 600 units/kg on Friday; repeat for 4 weeks; continue induction therapy for an additional 2 weeks if not in remission or begin maintenance therapy if in remission

Hyper-CVAD regimen (off-label dosing): IV 20,000 units weekly for 4 doses (starting on day 2) during either months 7 and 19 or months 7 and 11 of intensification phase (Thomas 2010)

◄   *Larson regimen (off-label dosing):* SubQ: 6000 units/m²/dose on days 5, 8, 11, 15, 18, and 22 (induction phase) and on days 15, 18, 22, and 25 (early intensification phase) (Larson, 1995)

    Linker regimen (off-label dosing): IM:

      Remission induction: 6000 units/m²/dose on days 17-28; if bone marrow on day 28 is positive for residual leukemia: 6000 units/m²/dose on days 29-35 (Linker, 1991)

      Consolidation (Treatment A; cycles 1, 3, 5, and 7): 12,000 units/m²/dose on days 2, 4, 7, 9, 11, and 14 (Linker, 1991)

Lymphoblastic lymphoma (off-label use): Hyper-CVAD regimen: IV: 20,000 units weekly for 4 doses (starting on day 2) for 2 cycles (months 7 and 11) during maintenance phase (Thomas 2004)

Pediatric Note: Dose, frequency, number of doses, and start date may vary by protocol and treatment phase.

Acute lymphoblastic leukemia (ALL): Children and Adolescents: Refer to adult dosing.

    CCG 1922 protocol (off-label dosing): IM: 6,000 units/m²/dose 3 times weekly for 9 doses beginning either on day 2, 3, or 4 (induction phase) and 6,000 units/m²/dose on Monday, Wednesday, and Friday for 6 doses beginning day 3 (delayed intensification phase) (Bostrom 2004)

    DFCI-ALL Consortium protocol 00-01 (off-label dosing): IM: 25,000 units/m² for 1 dose (induction phase) and 25,000 units/m²/dose weekly for 30 weeks (intensification phase) (Vrooman 2013)

    DFCI-ALL Consortium protocol 95-01 (off-label dosing): IM: 25,000 units/m² for 1 dose on day 4 (induction phase) and 25,000 units/m²/dose weekly for 20 weeks (intensification phase) (Moghrabi 2007)

    Hyper-CVAD regimen (off-label dosing): Adolescents ≥13 years: Refer to adult dosing.

Lymphoblastic lymphoma (off-label use): Adolescents >15 years: Refer to adult dosing.

Renal Impairment There are no dosage adjustments provided in the manufacturer's labeling.

Hepatic Impairment Use is contraindicated in patients with hepatic insufficiency. The following adjustments have been recommended for hepatotoxicity during treatment (Stock 2011):

ALT/AST >3 to 5 times ULN: Continue therapy.

ALT/AST >5 to 20 times ULN: Delay next dose until transaminases <3 times ULN.

ALT/AST >20 times ULN: Discontinue therapy if takes longer than 1 week for transaminases to return to <3 times ULN.

Direct bilirubin <3 mg/dL: Continue therapy.

Direct bilirubin 3.1 to 5 mg/dL: Hold asparaginase and resume when direct bilirubin <2 mg/dL; consider switching to alternate asparaginase product.

Direct bilirubin >5 mg/dL: Discontinue asparaginase; do not substitute other asparaginase products; do not make up for missed doses.

Adjustment for Toxicity

Allergic reaction/hypersensitivity: Discontinue for severe reactions.

Neurotoxicity (posterior reversible encephalopathy syndrome; PRES): Interrupt therapy for suspected PRES; control blood pressure and closely monitor for seizure activity.

Pancreatitis: Discontinue permanently (per manufacturer).

Thrombotic event: Discontinue for serious reactions.

The following adjustments have also been recommended (Stock 2011):

Hyperammonemia-related fatigue: Continue therapy for grade 2 toxicity. If grade 3 toxicity occurs, reduce dose by 25%; resume full dose when toxicity ≤ grade 2 (make up for missed doses). If grade 4 toxicity occurs, reduce dose by 50%; resume full dose when toxicity ≤ grade 2 (make up for missed doses).

Hyperglycemia: Continue therapy for uncomplicated hyperglycemia. If hyperglycemia requires insulin therapy, hold asparaginase (and any concomitant corticosteroids) until blood glucose controlled; resume dosing at prior dose level. For life-threatening hyperglycemia or toxicity requiring urgent intervention, hold asparaginase (and corticosteroids) until blood glucose is controlled with insulin; resume asparaginase and do not make up for missed doses.

Hypersensitivity reactions: May continue dosing for urticaria without bronchospasm, hypotension, edema, or need for parenteral intervention. If wheezing or other symptomatic bronchospasm with or without urticaria, angioedema, hypotension, and/or life-threatening hypersensitivity reactions occur, discontinue asparaginase.

Hypertriglyceridemia: If serum triglyceride level <1,000 mg/dL, continue asparaginase but monitor closely for pancreatitis. If triglyceride level >1,000 mg/dL, hold asparaginase and monitor; resume therapy at prior dose level after triglyceride level returns to baseline.

Pancreatitis:

Asymptomatic amylase or lipase >3 times ULN (chemical pancreatitis) or radiologic abnormalities only: Continue asparaginase and monitor levels closely.

Symptomatic amylase or lipase >3 times ULN: Hold asparaginase until enzyme levels stabilize or are declining.

Symptomatic pancreatitis or clinical pancreatitis (abdominal pain with amylase or lipase >3 times ULN for >3 days and/or development of pancreatic pseudocyst): Permanently discontinue asparaginase.

Thrombosis and bleeding, CNS:

Thrombosis: Continue therapy for abnormal laboratory findings without a clinical correlate. If grade 3 toxicity occurs, discontinue therapy; if CNS signs/symptoms are fully resolved and further asparaginase doses are required, may resume therapy at a lower dose and/or longer intervals between doses. Discontinue therapy for grade 4 toxicity.

Hemorrhage: Discontinue therapy; do not withhold therapy for abnormal laboratory findings without a clinical correlate. If grade 3 toxicity occurs, discontinue therapy; if CNS signs/symptoms are fully resolved and further asparaginase doses are required, may resume therapy at a lower dose and/or longer intervals between doses. Discontinue therapy for grade 4 toxicity.

Thrombosis and bleeding, non-CNS:

Thrombosis: Continue therapy for abnormal laboratory findings without a clinical correlate. If grade 3 or 4 toxicity occurs, withhold therapy until acute toxicity and clinical signs resolve and anticoagulant therapy is stable or completed. Do not withhold therapy for abnormal laboratory findings without clinical correlate.

◄   Hemorrhage: If grade 2 bleeding in conjunction with hypofibrinogenemia occurs, withhold therapy until bleeding ≤ grade 1. Do not withhold therapy for abnormal laboratory findings without clinical correlate. For grade 3 or 4 bleeding, withhold therapy until bleeding ≤ grade 1 and until acute toxicity and clinical signs resolve and coagulant replacement therapy is stable or completed.

Combination Regimens

Leukemia, acute lymphocytic:
CALGB 8811 Regimen (ALL) on page 1853
CALGB 9111 Regimen (ALL) on page 1854
Hyper-CVAD (Leukemia, Acute Lymphocytic) on page 2006
Linker Protocol (ALL) on page 2030
PVA (POG 8602) on page 2069
PVDA on page 2071

Administration May be administered IM (preferred for intermittent administration) or IV; has been administered SubQ (off-label route; Larson, 1995) in specific protocols. May administer corticosteroids 1 to 2 days prior to initiating reinduction therapy (to prevent hypersensitivity reaction). Observe patients for 1 hour after administration; have epinephrine, diphenhydramine, and hydrocortisone at the bedside. A physician should be readily accessible.

IM: Doses should be given as a deep intramuscular injection into a large muscle; volumes >2 mL should be divided and administered in 2 separate sites.

IV: Infuse over at least 30 minutes through the side arm of a NS or D_5W infusion.

Emetic Potential Children and Adults: Minimal (<10%)

Monitoring Parameters CBC with differential, amylase, lipase, triglycerides, liver function prior to and weekly during therapy, coagulation parameters (baseline and prior to each injection), blood glucose, uric acid. Monitor for allergic reaction; monitor for onset of abdominal pain and mental status changes. Monitor vital signs during administration.

Product Availability US product, Elspar, was discontinued more than 1 year ago.

Dosage Forms Excipient information presented when available (limited, particularly for generics); consult specific product labeling. [DSC] = Discontinued product

Solution Reconstituted, Injection:
Elspar: 10,000 units (1 ea [DSC])

Dosage Forms: Canada Excipient information presented when available (limited, particularly for generics); consult specific product labeling. [DSC] = Discontinued product

Solution Reconstituted, Injection:
Kidrolase: 10,000 units (1 ea)

Asparaginase (*Erwinia*) (a SPEAR a ji nase er WIN i ah)

Related Information

Common Toxicity Criteria on page 2122

Management of Chemotherapy-Induced Nausea and Vomiting in Adults on page 2142

Prevention of Chemotherapy-Induced Nausea and Vomiting in Children on page 2203

Brand Names: US Erwinaze

Brand Names: Canada Erwinase

Index Terms *Erwinia chrysanthemi*; Asparaginase *Erwinia chrysanthemi*; L-asparaginase (*Erwinia*)

Pharmacologic Category Antineoplastic Agent, Enzyme; Antineoplastic Agent, Miscellaneous

Use Acute lymphoblastic leukemia: Treatment (in combination with other chemotherapy) of acute lymphoblastic leukemia (ALL) in patients with hypersensitivity to *E. coli*-derived asparaginase

Labeled Contraindications

History of serious hypersensitivity reactions, including anaphylaxis to asparaginase (*Erwinia*) or any component of the formulation; history of serious pancreatitis, serious thrombosis, or serious hemorrhagic event with prior asparaginase treatment

Canadian labeling: Additional contraindications (not in the U.S. labeling): Women who are or may become pregnant

Pregnancy Considerations Adverse events were observed in animal reproduction studies.

Breast-Feeding Considerations It is not known if asparaginase *Erwinia chrysanthemi* is excreted in breast milk. Due to the potential for serious adverse reactions in the nursing infant, the manufacturer recommends a decision be made to discontinue nursing or to discontinue the drug, taking into account the importance of treatment to the mother.

Warnings/Precautions Serious hypersensitivity reactions (grade 3 and 4), including anaphylaxis, have occurred in 5% of patients in clinical trials. Immediate treatment for hypersensitivity reactions should be available during treatment; discontinue for serious hypersensitivity reactions (and administer appropriate treatment).

Pancreatitis has been reported in 5% of patients in clinical trials; promptly evaluate with symptoms suggestive of pancreatitis. For mild pancreatitis, withhold treatment until signs and symptoms subside and amylase levels return to normal; may resume after resolution. Discontinue for severe or hemorrhagic pancreatitis characterized by abdominal pain >72 hours and amylase ≥2 x ULN. Further use is contraindicated if severe pancreatitis is diagnosed.

Serious thrombotic events, including sagittal sinus thrombosis and pulmonary embolism, have been reported with asparaginase formulations. Decreases in fibrinogen, protein C activity, protein S activity, and antithrombin III have been noted following a 2-week treatment course administered intramuscularly. Discontinue for hemorrhagic or thrombotic events; may resume treatment after resolution (contraindicated with history of serious thrombosis or hemorrhagic event with prior asparaginase treatment).

In clinical trials, 4% of patients experienced glucose intolerance; may be irreversible; monitor glucose levels (baseline and periodic) during treatment; may require insulin administration.

Do not interchange *Erwinia* asparaginase for *E. coli* asparaginase or pegaspargase; ensure the proper formulation, route of administration, and dose prior to administration.

Adverse Reactions Frequency of adverse reactions is for both IM and IV routes unless specified.

>10%: Hypersensitivity: Hypersensitivity reaction (14% [IV: ≤37%]; grades 3/4: 4%; includes anaphylaxis, urticaria)

◄ 1% to 10%:

    Cardiovascular: Thrombosis (2% [IV: ≤7%]; grades 3/4: ≤1%; includes pulmonary embolism and cerebrovascular accident)

    Endocrine & metabolic: Hyperglycemia (4% [IV: ≤17%]; grades 3/4: 4%), abnormal transaminase (4%), decreased glucose tolerance (4%)

    Gastrointestinal: Nausea (3% [IV: ≤20%]), vomiting (3% [IV: ≤17%]), pancreatitis (4%; grades 3/4: <1%), abdominal pain (1%), diarrhea (1%), mucositis (1%)

    Local: Injection site reaction (3%)

    Miscellaneous: Fever (4%)

<1%, postmarketing, and/or case reports: Acute renal failure, anorexia, azotemia, bone marrow depression (rare), changes in serum lipids, chills, decreased serum albumin, decreased serum cholesterol, disseminated intravascular coagulation, headache, hemorrhage, hepatomegaly, hyperammonemia, hyperbilirubinemia, irritability, malabsorption syndrome, proteinuria, seizure, transient ischemic attacks, weight loss

Drug Interactions

Metabolism/Transport Effects None known.

Avoid Concomitant Use There are no known interactions where it is recommended to avoid concomitant use.

Increased Effect/Toxicity

Asparaginase (Erwinia) may increase the levels/effects of: Dexamethasone (Systemic)

Decreased Effect There are no known significant interactions involving a decrease in effect.

Storage/Stability Store intact vials refrigerated at 2°C to 8°C (36°F to 46°F). Protect from light. Within 15 minutes of reconstitution, withdraw appropriate volume for dose into a polypropylene syringe. Do not freeze or refrigerate reconstituted solution; discard if not administered within 4 hours.

Preparation for Administration Reconstitute each vial with 1 mL of preservative free sodium chloride 0.9% (NS) to obtain a concentration of 10,000 units/mL, or with 2 mL preservative free NS to obtain a concentration of 5,000 units/mL. Gently direct the NS down the wall of the vial (do not inject forcefully into or onto the powder). Dissolve by gently swirling or mixing; do not shake or invert the vial. Resulting reconstituted solution should be clear and colorless and free of visible particles or protein aggregates. Within 15 minutes of reconstitution, withdraw appropriate volume for dose into a polypropylene syringe. If administering intravenously, slowly inject the appropriate volume of reconstituted solution into a NS 100 mL infusion bag; do not shake or squeeze the bag. Administer within 4 hours of reconstitution.

Mechanism of Action Asparaginase catalyzes the deamidation of asparagine to aspartic acid and ammonia, reducing circulating levels of asparagine. Leukemia cells lack asparagine synthetase and are unable to synthesize asparagine. Asparaginase reduces the exogenous asparagine source for the leukemic cells, resulting in cytotoxicity specific to leukemic cells.

Pharmacodynamics/Kinetics Half-life elimination: IM: ~16 hours (Asselin, 1993; Avramis, 2005); IV: ~7.5 hours

Dosing

    Adult Note: If administering IV, consider monitoring nadir serum asparaginase activity (NSAA) levels; if desired levels are not achieved, change to IM administration.

Acute lymphoblastic leukemia (ALL): IM, IV:
As a substitute for pegaspargase: 25,000 units/m^2 3 times weekly (Mon, Wed, Fri) for 6 doses for each planned pegaspargase dose
As a substitute for asparaginase (E. coli): 25,000 units/m^2 for each scheduled asparaginase (*E. coli*) dose

ALL induction: *Canadian labeling (not in the U.S. labeling):* SubQ: 10,000 units/m^2 days 1, 3, and 5 of week 4 and day 1 of week 5 (in combination with prednisolone, vincristine, mercaptopurine, and methotrexate) **or** 10,000 units/m^2 3 times weekly (starting week 4) for 4 weeks (in combination with prednisolone, vincristine, and daunorubicin)

Pediatric Note: If administering IV, consider monitoring nadir serum asparaginase activity (NSAA) levels; if desired levels are not achieved, change to IM administration.

Acute lymphoblastic leukemia (ALL): Children ≥1 year and Adolescents: IM, IV: Refer to adult dosing.

ALL induction: *Canadian labeling (not in the U.S. labeling):*
Children <14 years: IM: 6,000 units/m^2 3 times weekly for 9 doses beginning day 4 of week 1 (in combination with vincristine, prednisone, methotrexate, and daunorubicin)
Children >14 years: SubQ: Refer to adult dosing.

Renal Impairment There are no dosage adjustments provided in the manufacturer's labeling.

Hepatic Impairment There are no dosage adjustments provided in the manufacturer's labeling; however, the following adjustments have been recommended for other asparaginase products for hepatotoxicity during treatment (Stock 2011):
ALT/AST >3 to 5 times ULN: Continue therapy
ALT/AST >5 to 20 times ULN: Delay next dose until transaminases <3 times ULN
ALT/AST >20 times ULN: Discontinue therapy if takes longer than 1 week for transaminases to return to <3 times ULN.
Direct bilirubin <3 mg/dL: Continue therapy
Direct bilirubin 3.1 to 5 mg/dL: Hold asparaginase and resume when direct bilirubin <2 mg/dL; consider switching to alternate asparaginase product.
Direct bilirubin >5 mg/dL: Discontinue asparaginase; do not substitute other asparaginase products; do not make up for missed doses.

Adjustment for Toxicity
Hemorrhagic or thrombotic event: Discontinue treatment; may resume treatment upon symptom resolution.
Pancreatitis:
Mild pancreatitis: Withhold treatment until signs and symptoms subside and amylase levels return to normal; may resume after resolution.
Severe or hemorrhagic pancreatitis (abdominal pain >72 hours and amylase ≥2 x ULN): Discontinue treatment; further use is contraindicated.
Serious hypersensitivity reaction: Discontinue treatment.

The following adjustments have also been recommended for asparaginase products (Stock 2011):
Hyperammonemia-related fatigue: Continue therapy for grade 2 toxicity. If grade 3 toxicity occurs, reduce dose by 25%; resume full dose when toxicity ≤ grade 2 (make up for missed doses). If grade 4 toxicity occurs, reduce dose by 50%; resume full dose when toxicity ≤ grade 2 (make up for missed doses).

◄ **Hyperglycemia:** Continue therapy for uncomplicated hyperglycemia. If hyperglycemia requires insulin therapy, hold asparaginase (and any concomitant corticosteroids) until blood glucose controlled; resume dosing at prior dose level. For life-threatening hyperglycemia or toxicity requiring urgent intervention, hold asparaginase (and corticosteroids) until blood glucose is controlled with insulin; resume asparaginase and do not make up for missed doses.

Hypersensitivity reactions: May continue dosing for urticaria without bronchospasm, hypotension, edema, or need for parenteral intervention. If wheezing or other symptomatic bronchospasm with or without urticaria, angioedema, hypotension, and/or life-threatening hypersensitivity reactions occur, discontinue asparaginase.

Hypertriglyceridemia: If serum triglyceride level <1000 mg/dL, continue asparaginase but monitor closely for pancreatitis. If triglyceride level >1,000 mg/dL, hold asparaginase and monitor; resume therapy at prior dose level after triglyceride level returns to baseline.

Pancreatitis:

Asymptomatic amylase or lipase >3 times ULN (chemical pancreatitis) or radiologic abnormalities only: Continue asparaginase and monitor levels closely.

Symptomatic amylase or lipase >3 times ULN: Hold asparaginase until enzyme levels stabilize or are declining.

Symptomatic pancreatitis or clinical pancreatitis (abdominal pain with amylase or lipase >3 times ULN for >3 days and/or development of pancreatic pseudocyst): Permanently discontinue asparaginase.

Thrombosis and bleeding, CNS:

Thrombosis: Continue therapy for abnormal laboratory findings without a clinical correlate. If grade 3 toxicity occurs, discontinue therapy; if CNS signs/symptoms are fully resolved and further asparaginase doses are required, may resume therapy at a lower dose and/or longer intervals between doses. Discontinue therapy for grade 4 toxicity.

Hemorrhage: Discontinue therapy; do not withhold therapy for abnormal laboratory findings without a clinical correlate. If grade 3 toxicity occurs, discontinue therapy; if CNS signs/symptoms are fully resolved and further asparaginase doses are required, may resume therapy at a lower dose and/or longer intervals between doses. Discontinue therapy for grade 4 toxicity.

Thrombosis and bleeding, non-CNS:

Thrombosis: Continue therapy for abnormal laboratory findings without a clinical correlate. If grade 3 or 4 toxicity occurs, withhold therapy until acute toxicity and clinical signs resolve and anticoagulant therapy is stable or completed. Do not withhold therapy for abnormal laboratory findings without clinical correlate.

Hemorrhage: If grade 2 bleeding in conjunction with hypofibrinogenemia occurs, withhold therapy until bleeding ≤ grade 1. Do not withhold therapy for abnormal laboratory findings without clinical correlate. For grade 3 or 4 bleeding, withhold therapy until bleeding ≤ grade 1 and until acute toxicity and clinical signs resolve and coagulant replacement therapy is stable or completed.

Administration

IM: The volume of each single injection site should be limited to 2 mL; use multiple injections for volumes >2 mL.

IV: Infuse over 1 hour; do not infuse other medications through the same IV line.

Canadian labeling (additional administration route not in the U.S. labeling): May also be administered SubQ (IM and SubQ are preferred).

Emetic Potential Children and Adults: Minimal (<10%)

Monitoring Parameters CBC with differential, amylase, lipase, triglycerides, liver enzymes, blood glucose (baseline and periodically during treatment), coagulation parameters; for IV administration, consider monitoring nadir serum asparaginase activity (NSAA) levels. Monitor for symptoms of hypersensitivity, symptoms of pancreatitis, thrombosis, or hemorrhage.

Prescribing and Access Restrictions Erwinaze is distributed through Accredo Health Group, Inc. (1-877-900-9223).

Dosage Forms Excipient information presented when available (limited, particularly for generics); consult specific product labeling.

Solution Reconstituted, Intramuscular:

Erwinaze: 10,000 units (1 ea)

Axitinib (ax I ti nib)

Related Information

Management of Chemotherapy-Induced Nausea and Vomiting in Adults *on page 2142*

Safe Handling of Hazardous Drugs *on page 2292*

Brand Names: US Inlyta

Brand Names: Canada Inlyta

Index Terms AG-013736

◀ **Pharmacologic Category** Antineoplastic Agent, Tyrosine Kinase Inhibitor; Antineoplastic Agent, Vascular Endothelial Growth Factor (VEGF) Inhibitor

Use Renal cell carcinoma, advanced: Treatment of advanced renal cell carcinoma after failure of one prior systemic therapy.

Labeled Contraindications There are no contraindications listed within the manufacturer's labeling.

Pregnancy Considerations Teratogenic, embryotoxic, and fetotoxic events were observed in animal reproduction studies when administered in doses less than the normal human dose. Based on its mechanism of action and because axitinib inhibits angiogenesis (a critical component of fetal development), adverse effects on pregnancy would be expected. Women of childbearing potential should be advised to avoid pregnancy during therapy.

Breast-Feeding Considerations It is not known if axitinib is excreted in breast milk. Due to the potential for serious adverse reactions in the nursing infant, the manufacturer recommends a decision be made whether to discontinue nursing or to discontinue the drug, taking into account the importance of treatment to the mother.

Warnings/Precautions Hazardous agent - use appropriate precautions for handling and disposal (meets NIOSH 2014 criteria). May cause hypertension; the median onset is within the first month, and has been observed as early as 4 days after treatment initiation. Hypertensive crisis has been reported. Blood pressure should be well-controlled prior to treatment initiation. Monitor blood pressure and treat with standard antihypertensive therapy. Persistent hypertension (despite antihypertensive therapy) may require dose reduction; discontinue if severe and persistent despite concomitant antihypertensives (or dose reduction), or with evidence of hypertensive crisis. Monitor for hypotension if on antihypertensive therapy and axitinib is withheld or discontinued. Cardiac failure, including fatal events, has been observed rarely. Monitor for signs/symptoms of cardiac failure throughout therapy; management may require permanent therapy discontinuation.

Gastrointestinal perforation and fistulas (including a fatality) have been reported. Monitor for signs/symptoms throughout treatment. Has not been studied in patients with recent active gastrointestinal bleeding; use is not recommended.

Arterial thrombotic events (cerebrovascular accident, MI, retinal artery occlusion, and transient ischemic attack), with fatalities, have been reported. Venous thrombotic events, including pulmonary embolism, deep vein thrombosis, retinal vein occlusion and retinal vein thrombosis, have been observed (with some fatalities). Use with caution in patients with a history of or risks for arterial or venous thrombotic events; has not been studied in patients within 12 months of an arterial thrombotic event or within 6 months of a venous thrombotic event. Hemorrhagic events (cerebral hemorrhage, gastrointestinal hemorrhage, hematuria, hemoptysis, and melena) have been reported (with some fatalities). Temporarily interrupt treatment with any hemorrhage requiring medical intervention.

Cases of reversible posterior leukoencephalopathy syndrome (RPLS) have been reported. Symptoms of RPLS include confusion, headache, hypertension (mild-to-severe), lethargy, seizure, blindness and/or other vision, or neurologic disturbances; interrupt treatment and manage hypertension. MRI is recommended to confirm RPLS diagnosis. Discontinue axitinib if RPLS is confirmed. The safety of reinitiating axitinib in patients previously experiencing RPLS is unknown.

Hypothyroidism occurs commonly with tyrosine kinase inhibitors, including axitinib. Hyperthyroidism has also been reported. Monitor thyroid function at baseline and periodically throughout therapy. Thyroid disorders should be treated according to standard practice to achieve/maintain euthyroid state. Proteinuria is associated with use. Monitor for proteinuria at baseline and periodically throughout therapy. If moderate or severe proteinuria occurs, reduce dose or temporarily withhold treatment. Although the effect on wound healing has not been studied with axitinib, vascular endothelial growth factor (VEGF) receptor inhibitors are associated with impaired wound healing. Discontinue treatment at least 24 hours prior to scheduled surgery; treatment reinitiation should be guided by clinical judgment and wound assessment. Has not been studied in patients with evidence of untreated brain metastases; use is not recommended. Systemic exposure to axitinib is increased in patients with moderate hepatic impairment; dose reductions are recommended. Has not been studied in patients with severe hepatic impairment. Increases in ALT have been observed during treatment; monitor liver function tests. Potentially significant drug-drug interactions may exist, requiring dose or frequency adjustment, additional monitoring, and/or selection of alternative therapy.

Adverse Reactions

>10%:

Cardiovascular: Hypertension (40%; grades 3/4: 16%)

Central nervous system: Fatigue (39%), dysphonia (31%), headache (14%)

Dermatologic: Palmar-plantar erythrodysesthesia syndrome (27%; grades 3/4: 5%), rash (13%; grades 3/4: <1%)

Endocrine & metabolic: Bicarbonate decreased (44%), hypocalcemia (39%), hyperglycemia (28%), hypothyroidism (19%; grades 3/4: <1%), hypernatremia (17%), hyperkalemia (15%), hypoalbuminemia (15%), hyponatremia (13%), hypophosphatemia (13%), hypoglycemia (11%)

Gastrointestinal: Diarrhea (55%; grades 3/4: 11%), appetite decreased (34%), nausea (32%; grades 3/4: 3%), lipase increased (3% to 27%), amylase increased (25%), weight loss (25%), vomiting (24%; grades 3/4: 3%), constipation (20%), mucosal inflammation (15%), stomatitis (15%), abdominal pain (8% to 14%), taste alteration (11%)

Hematologic: Anemia (4% to 35%; grades 3/4: <1%), lymphopenia (33%; grades 3/4: 3%), hemorrhage (16%; grades 3/4 1%), thrombocytopenia (15%; grades 3/4: <1%), leukopenia (11%)

Hepatic: Alkaline phosphatase increased (30%), ALT increased (22%; grades 3/4: <1%), AST increased (20%; grades 3/4: <1%)

Neuromuscular & skeletal: Weakness (21%), arthralgia (15%), limb pain (13%)

Renal: Creatinine increased (55%), proteinuria (11%; grade 3: 3%)

Respiratory: Cough (15%), dyspnea (15%)

1% to 10%:

Cardiovascular: Venous thrombotic events (grades 3/4: 3%), arterial thrombotic events (2%; grade 3/4: 1%), deep vein thrombosis (1%), transient ischemic attack (1%)

Central nervous system: Dizziness (9%)

Dermatologic: Dry skin (10%), pruritus (7%), alopecia (4%), erythema (2%)

Endocrine & metabolic: Dehydration (6%), hyperthyroidism (1%)

Gastrointestinal: Dyspepsia (10%), hemorrhoids (4%), rectal hemorrhage (2%), fistula (1%), gastrointestinal perforation (≤1%)

Hematologic: Hemoglobin increased (9%), polycythemia (1%)

Neuromuscular & skeletal: Myalgia (7%)

Ocular: Retinal vein occlusion/thrombosis (1%)

Otic: Tinnitus (3%)

Renal: Hematuria (3%)

Respiratory: Epistaxis (6%), hemoptysis (2%), pulmonary embolism (2%)

<1%, postmarketing, and/or case reports: Cerebral bleeding, cerebrovascular accident, fever, hypertensive crisis, heart failure, neutropenia, reversible posterior leukoencephalopathy syndrome (RPLS)

Drug Interactions

Metabolism/Transport Effects Substrate of CYP1A2 (minor), CYP2C19 (minor), CYP3A4 (major), UGT1A1; **Note:** Assignment of Major/Minor substrate status based on clinically relevant drug interaction potential

Avoid Concomitant Use

Avoid concomitant use of Axitinib with any of the following: Conivaptan; CYP3A4 Inducers (Moderate); CYP3A4 Inducers (Strong); CYP3A4 Inhibitors (Strong); Fusidic Acid (Systemic); Grapefruit Juice; Idelalisib; St Johns Wort

Increased Effect/Toxicity

Axitinib may increase the levels/effects of: Bisphosphonate Derivatives

The levels/effects of Axitinib may be increased by: Aprepitant; Conivaptan; CYP3A4 Inhibitors (Moderate); CYP3A4 Inhibitors (Strong); Dasatinib; Fosaprepitant; Fusidic Acid (Systemic); Grapefruit Juice; Idelalisib; Ivacaftor; Luliconazole; Mifepristone; Netupitant; Osimertinib; Palbociclib; Simeprevir; Stiripentol

Decreased Effect

The levels/effects of Axitinib may be decreased by: CYP3A4 Inducers (Moderate); CYP3A4 Inducers (Strong); Deferasirox; Osimertinib; Siltuximab; St Johns Wort; Tocilizumab

Food Interactions Axitinib serum concentrations may be increased when taken with grapefruit or grapefruit juice. Management: Avoid concurrent use.

Storage/Stability Store at 20°C to 25°C (68°F to 77°F); excursions permitted to 15°C to 30°C (59°F to 86°F).

Mechanism of Action Axitinib is a selective second generation tyrosine kinase inhibitor which blocks angiogenesis and tumor growth by inhibiting vascular endothelial growth factor receptors (VEGFR-1, VEGFR-2, and VEGFR-3).

Pharmacodynamics/Kinetics

Absorption: Rapid (Rugo, 2005)

Distribution: V_d: 160 L

Protein binding: >99%; to albumin (primarily) and to alpha$_1$ acid glycoprotein (AAG)

Metabolism: Hepatic; primarily via CYP3A4/5 and to a lesser extend via CYP1A2, CYP2C19 and UGT1A1

Bioavailability: 58%

Half-life elimination: 2.5 to 6 hours

Time to peak: 2.5 to 4 hours

Excretion: Feces (~41%; 12% as unchanged drug); urine (~23%; as metabolites)

Dosing

Adult Renal cell cancer, advanced: Oral: Initial: 5 mg twice daily (approximately every 12 hours)

Dose increases: If dose is tolerated (no adverse events above grade 2, blood pressure is normal and no antihypertensive use) for at least 2 consecutive weeks, may increase the dose to 7 mg twice daily, and then further increase (using the same tolerance criteria) to 10 mg twice daily.

Dose decreases: For adverse events, reduce dose from 5 mg twice daily to 3 mg twice daily; further reduce to 2 mg twice daily if adverse events persist.

Dosage adjustment for strong CYP3A4 inhibitors: Avoid concomitant administration with strong CYP3A4 inhibitors (eg, clarithromycin, itraconazole, ketoconazole, nefazodone, protease inhibitors, telithromycin, voriconazole, grapefruit juice); if concomitant administration with a strong CYP3A4 inhibitor cannot be avoided, ~50% dosage reduction is recommended; adjust dose based on individual tolerance and safety. When the strong CYP3A4 inhibitor is discontinued, resume previous axitinib dose after 3-5 half-lives of the inhibitor have passed.

Geriatric Refer to adult dosing. No adjustment necessary.

Renal Impairment

Mild to severe renal impairment (CrCl 15 to <89 mL/minute): No initial dosage adjustment necessary.

End-stage renal disease (ESRD) There are no dosage adjustments provided in the manufacturer's labeling; use with caution.

Hepatic Impairment

Mild impairment (Child-Pugh class A): No starting dosage adjustment necessary.

Moderate impairment (Child-Pugh class B): Reduce starting dose by ~50%; increase or decrease based on individual tolerance.

Severe impairment (Child-Pugh class C): There are no dosage adjustments provided in the manufacturer's labeling (has not been studied).

Adjustment for Toxicity

Adverse events: May require temporary interruption, dose decreases (reduce dose from 5 mg twice daily to 3 mg twice daily; further reduce to 2 mg twice daily) or discontinuation

Cardiac failure: May require permanent discontinuation

Hypertension: Treat with standard antihypertensive therapy.

Persistent hypertension: May require dose reduction

Severe, persistent (despite antihypertensives and dose reduction), or evidence of hypertensive crisis: Discontinue treatment

Hemorrhage: Any bleeding requiring medical intervention: Temporarily interrupt treatment.

Proteinuria (moderate-to-severe): Reduce dose or temporarily interrupt treatment.

Combination Regimens

Renal cell cancer: Axitinib (RCC Regimen) on page 1828

Administration Oral: Swallow tablet whole with a glass of water. May be taken with or without food. If a dose is missed or vomited, do not make up; resume dosing with the next scheduled dose. A suspension may be prepared for nasogastric administration (refer to Extemporaneous Preparations information).

Hazardous agent; use appropriate precautions for handling and disposal (meets NIOSH 2014 criteria).

Emetic Potential Minimal (<10%)

Extemporaneous Preparations Hazardous agent – use appropriate precautions for handling and disposal (meets NIOSH 2014 criteria). For patients unable to swallow tablets whole, a suspension may be prepared for nasogastric tube administration (for doses of 2 to 10 mg). Place a 20 mL tightly capped amber syringe in a small drinking glass, with the open end of the syringe pointing up. Place the appropriate axitinib dose in the open syringe barrel; add 15 mL of USP grade water (do not use tap water or bottled water) to the syringe. Allow at least 10 minutes to dissolve the tablets; avoid direct light. Place the plunger of the syringe into the barrel, invert the syringe so the tip is pointing upward and remove the cap. Expel excess air; replace the cap until ready for use (keep syringe tip facing up). Prior to administration, gently invert the syringe several times to ensure a uniform suspension. Flush the nasogastric feeding tube with 15 mL of USP grade water before administration. After administering the dose, draw up 10 mL of USP grade water (into the same syringe which contained the dose) and flush the feeding tube; repeat this step 5 additional times to ensure the entire dose has been administered. Lastly, flush the feeding tube with a separate syringe containing 15 mL of USP grade water. Administer within 15 minutes of preparation.

Borst DL, Arruda LS, MacLean E, Pithavala YK, Morgado JE. Common questions regarding clinical use of axitinib in advanced renal cell carcinoma. Am J Health Syst Pharm. 2014;71 (13):1092-1096.

Monitoring Parameters Hepatic function (ALT, AST, and bilirubin; baseline and periodic), thyroid function (baseline and periodic), urinalysis (for proteinuria; baseline and periodically); blood pressure, signs/symptoms of RPLS, gastrointestinal bleeding/perforation/fistula, signs/symptoms cardiac failure

Thyroid function testing recommendations (Hamnvik, 2011):
Preexisting levothyroxine therapy: Obtain baseline TSH levels, then monitor every 4 weeks until levels and levothyroxine dose are stable, then monitor every 2 months
Without preexisting thyroid hormone replacement: TSH at baseline, then monthly for 4 months, then every 2-3 months

Dietary Considerations May be taken without regard to food. Avoid grapefruit and grapefruit juice.

Prescribing and Access Restrictions Available from select specialty pharmacies. Further information may be obtained at 877-744-5675 or www.inlytahcp.com.

Dosage Forms Excipient information presented when available (limited, particularly for generics); consult specific product labeling.
Tablet, Oral:
Inlyta: 1 mg, 5 mg

◆ **AY-25650** see Triptorelin on page 1703

◆ **5-Aza-2'-deoxycytidine** see Decitabine on page 474

AzaCITIDine (ay za SYE ti deen)

Related Information

Management of Chemotherapy-Induced Nausea and Vomiting in Adults *on page 2142*

Prevention of Chemotherapy-Induced Nausea and Vomiting in Children *on page 2203*

Safe Handling of Hazardous Drugs *on page 2292*

Brand Names: US Vidaza

Brand Names: Canada Vidaza

Index Terms 5-Azacytidine; 5-AZC; AZA-CR; Azacytidine; Ladakamycin

Pharmacologic Category Antineoplastic Agent, Antimetabolite; Antineoplastic Agent, DNA Methylation Inhibitor

Use

US labeling:

Myelodysplastic syndromes: Treatment of myelodysplastic syndromes (MDS) in patients with the following French-American-British (FAB) classification subtypes: Refractory anemia or refractory anemia with ringed sideroblasts (if accompanied by neutropenia or thrombocytopenia or requiring transfusions), refractory anemia with excess blasts, refractory anemia with excess blasts in transformation, and chronic myelomonocytic leukemia.

Canadian labeling:

Acute myeloid leukemia: Treatment of acute myeloid leukemia (AML) with 20% to 30% blasts and myelodysplasia-related features (previously referred to as multilineage dysplasia), according to World Health Organization (WHO) classification.

Myelodysplastic syndromes: Treatment of Intermediate-2 and high-risk myelodysplastic syndromes (MDS) (according to International Prognostic Scoring System) in adults who are not eligible for hematopoietic stem cell transplantation.

Labeled Contraindications Hypersensitivity to azacitidine, mannitol, or any component of the formulation; advanced malignant hepatic tumors

Pregnancy Considerations Adverse events were observed in animal reproduction studies. Women of childbearing potential should be advised to avoid pregnancy during treatment. In addition, males should be advised to avoid fathering a child while on azacitidine therapy. The Canadian labeling recommends women of childbearing potential use effective contraception during and up to 3 months after therapy and males to avoid fathering a child during therapy and for 6 months after the last dose.

Breast-Feeding Considerations It is not known if azacitidine is excreted in breast milk. Due to the potential for serious adverse reactions in the nursing infant, a decision should be made to discontinue the drug or to discontinue breast-feeding, taking into account the importance of treatment to the mother.

Warnings/Precautions Hazardous agent; use appropriate precautions for handling and disposal (NIOSH 2014 [group 1]). May cause hepatotoxicity in patients with preexisting hepatic impairment. Progressive hepatic coma leading to death has been reported in patients with extensive tumor burden due to metastatic disease, especially those with a baseline albumin <30 g/L. Patients with hepatic impairment were excluded from clinical studies for myelodysplastic syndrome (MDS). Use is contraindicated in patients with advanced malignant hepatic tumors. Renal toxicities, including serum creatinine elevations, renal tubular acidosis (serum bicarbonate decrease to <20 mEq/L associated with alkaline urine and serum potassium <3 mEq/L), and renal

◀ failure (some fatal), have been reported with intravenous azacitidine when used in combination with other chemotherapy agents. Withhold or reduce the dose with unexplained decreases in serum bicarbonate <20 mEq/L or if elevations in BUN or serum creatinine occur. Patients with renal impairment may be at increased risk for renal toxicity. Severe renal impairment did not have a major effect on azacitidine exposure after multiple subcutaneous administrations and no dosage adjustment is necessary for the first cycle, however, monitor closely for toxicity (azacitidine and metabolites are excreted renally).

Neutropenia, thrombocytopenia, and anemia are common; may cause therapy delays and/or dosage reductions; monitor blood counts prior to each cycle (at a minimum), and more frequently if clinically indicated. Azacitidine is associated with a moderate emetic potential (Basch 2011; Dupuis 2011; Roila 2010); antiemetics are recommended to prevent nausea and vomiting. Injection site reactions commonly occurred with subcutaneous administration. Potentially significant drug-drug interactions may exist, requiring dose or frequency adjustment, additional monitoring, and/or selection of alternative therapy.

Some dosage forms may contain polysorbate 80 (also known as Tweens). Hypersensitivity reactions, usually a delayed reaction, have been reported following exposure to pharmaceutical products containing polysorbate 80 in certain individuals (Isaksson 2002; Lucente 2000; Shelley 1995). Thrombocytopenia, ascites, pulmonary deterioration, and renal and hepatic failure have been reported in premature neonates after receiving parenteral products containing polysorbate 80 (Alade 1986; CDC 1984). See manufacturer's labeling.

Adverse Reactions

>10%:

Cardiovascular: Peripheral edema (7% to 19%), chest pain (16%)

Central nervous system: Fatigue (13% to 36%), rigors (26%), headache (22%), dizziness (19%), anxiety (5% to 13%), depression (12%), insomnia (9% to 11%), malaise (11%), pain (11%)

Dermatologic: Erythema (7% to 17%), pallor (16%), skin lesion (15%), skin rash (10% to 14%), pruritus (12%), diaphoresis (11%)

Endocrine & metabolic: Weight loss (≤16%), pitting edema (15%), hypokalemia (6% to 13%)

Gastrointestinal: Nausea (48% to 71%), vomiting (27% to 54%), constipation (34% to 50%), diarrhea (36%), anorexia (13% to 21%), abdominal pain (11% to 16%), abdominal tenderness (12%)

Hematologic & oncologic: Thrombocytopenia (66% to 70%; grades 3/4: 58%), anemia (51% to 70%; grades 3/4: 14%), neutropenia (32% to 66%; grades 3/4: 61%), leukopenia (18% to 48%; grades 3/4: 15%), bruise (19% to 31%), petechia (11% to 24%), febrile neutropenia (14% to 16%; grades 3/4: 13%), bone marrow depression (nadir: days 10 to 17; recovery: days 28 to 31)

Local: Injection site reactions (14% to 29%): Erythema (35% to 43%; more common with IV administration), pain (19% to 23%; more common with IV administration), bruising (5% to 14%)

Neuromuscular & skeletal: Weakness (29%), arthralgia (22%), limb pain (20%), back pain (19%), myalgia (16%)

Respiratory: Cough (11% to 30%), dyspnea (5% to 29%), pharyngitis (20%), epistaxis (16%), nasopharyngitis (15%), upper respiratory infection (9% to 13%), pneumonia (11%), rales (9% to 11%)

Miscellaneous: Fever (30% to 52%)

5% to 10%:

Cardiovascular: Heart murmur (10%), hypertension (≤9%), tachycardia (9%), hypotension (7%), syncope (6%), chest wall pain (5%)

Central nervous system: Lethargy (7% to 8%), hypoesthesia (5%), post-operative pain (5%)

Dermatologic: Night sweats (9%), cellulitis (8%), rash at injection site (6%), urticaria (6%), skin nodules (5%), xeroderma (5%)

Gastrointestinal: Gingival hemorrhage (10%), stomatitis (8%), dyspepsia (6% to 7%), hemorrhoids (7%), abdominal distention (6%), loose stools (6%), dysphagia (5%), tongue ulcer (5%)

Genitourinary: Urinary tract infection (8% to 9%), dysuria (8%), hematuria (≤6%)

Hematologic & oncologic: Lymphadenopathy (10%), hematoma (9%), oral mucosal petechiae (8%), postprocedural hemorrhage (6%), oral hemorrhage (5%)

Hypersensitivity: Transfusion reaction (7%)

Infection: Herpes simplex infection (9%)

Local: Itching at injection site (7%), hematoma at injection site (6%), injection site granuloma (5%), induration at injection site (5%), skin discoloration at injection site (5%), swelling at injection site (5%)

Neuromuscular & skeletal: Muscle cramps (6%)

Respiratory: Rhinorrhea (10%), wheezing (9%), abnormal breath sounds (8%), nasal congestion (6%), pharyngolaryngeal pain (6%), pleural effusion (6%), post nasal drip (6%), rhinitis (6%), rhonchi (6%), atelectasis (5%), sinusitis (5%)

Miscellaneous: Lymphadenopathy (10%), herpes simplex (9%), night sweats (9%), transfusion reaction (7%), mouth hemorrhage (5%)

<5%, postmarketing, and/or case reports: Abscess (limb, perirectal), aggravated bone pain, agranulocytosis, anaphylactic shock, atrial fibrillation, azotemia, bacterial infection, blastomycosis, bone marrow failure, cardiac failure, cardiorespiratory arrest, catheter site hemorrhage, cellulitis, cerebral hemorrhage, cholecystectomy, cholecystitis, congestive cardiomyopathy, decreased serum bicarbonate, dehydration, diverticulitis, fibrosis (interstitial and alveolar), gastrointestinal hemorrhage, glycosuria, hemophthalmos, hemoptysis, hepatic coma, hypersensitivity reaction, hypophosphatemia, increased serum creatinine, injection site infection, interstitial pulmonary disease, intracranial hemorrhage, leukemia cutis, melena, neutropenic sepsis, orthostatic hypotension, pancytopenia, pneumonitis, polyuria, pulmonary infiltrates, pyoderma gangrenosum, renal failure, renal tubular acidosis, respiratory distress, seizure, sepsis, sepsis syndrome, septic shock, splenomegaly, Sweet's syndrome, tissue necrosis at injection site, toxoplasmosis, tumor lysis syndrome

Drug Interactions

Metabolism/Transport Effects None known.

Avoid Concomitant Use

Avoid concomitant use of AzaCITIDine with any of the following: BCG (Intravesical); CloZAPine; Dipyrone; Natalizumab; Pimecrolimus; Tacrolimus (Topical); Tofacitinib; Vaccines (Live)

◀ **Increased Effect/Toxicity**

AzaCITIDine may increase the levels/effects of: CloZAPine; Fingolimod; Leflunomide; Natalizumab; Tofacitinib; Vaccines (Live)

The levels/effects of AzaCITIDine may be increased by: Denosumab; Dipyrone; Pimecrolimus; Roflumilast; Tacrolimus (Topical); Trastuzumab

Decreased Effect

AzaCITIDine may decrease the levels/effects of: BCG (Intravesical); Coccidioides immitis Skin Test; Sipuleucel-T; Vaccines (Inactivated); Vaccines (Live)

The levels/effects of AzaCITIDine may be decreased by: Echinacea

Storage/Stability Prior to reconstitution, store intact vials at room temperature of 25°C (77°F); excursions permitted to 15°C to 30°C (59°F to 86°F).
US labeling:

IV solution: **Solutions for IV administration have very limited stability and must be prepared immediately prior to each dose.** Administration must be completed within 1 hour of (vial) reconstitution.

SubQ suspension: Following reconstitution, suspension may be stored at room temperature for up to 1 hour prior to immediate administration (administer within 1 hour of reconstitution). If administration is delayed, refrigerate reconstituted suspension immediately (either in vial or syringe); may be stored for up to 8 hours (if reconstituted with room temperature SWFI) or up to 22 hours (if reconstituted with refrigerated SWFI). After removal from refrigerator, may be allowed up to 30 minutes to reach room temperature prior to immediate administration.

Canadian labeling:

SubQ suspension: Following reconstitution, suspension may be stored at room temperature for up to 45 minutes prior to immediate administration; discard if not administered within 45 minutes. Alternatively, may reconstitute prior to administration and store suspension in refrigerator at 2°C to 8°C (36°F to 46°F) for up to 8 hours. After removal from refrigerator, may be allowed up to 30 minutes to reach room temperature prior to immediate administration.

Preparation for Administration Hazardous agent; use appropriate precautions for handling and disposal (NIOSH 2014 [group 1]). If reconstituted solution comes in contact with skin, wash immediately and thoroughly with soap and water; if comes in contact with mucous membranes, flush thoroughly with water.

IV: Reconstitute vial with 10 mL SWFI to form a 10 mg/mL solution; vigorously shake or roll vial until solution is dissolved and clear. Mix in 50 to 100 mL of NS or lactated Ringer's injection for infusion.

SubQ: Slowly add 4 mL SWFI to each vial, resulting in a concentration of 25 mg/mL. Vigorously shake or roll vial until a suspension is formed (suspension will be cloudy). The manufacturer recommends dividing doses >4 mL equally into 2 syringes. Do not filter after reconstitution (may remove active drug). Resuspend contents of syringe by vigorously rolling between palms immediately prior to administration.

Discard unused portion (does not contain preservatives); do not save unused portions for later administration.

Mechanism of Action Antineoplastic effects may be a result of azacitidine's ability to promote hypomethylation of DNA, restoring normal gene differentiation and proliferation. Azacitidine also exerts direct toxicity to abnormal hematopoietic cells in the bone marrow.

Pharmacodynamics/Kinetics
Absorption: SubQ: Rapid and complete
Distribution: V_d: IV: 76 ± 26 L; does not cross blood-brain barrier
Metabolism: Hepatic; hydrolysis to several metabolites
Bioavailability: SubQ: ~89%
Half-life elimination: IV, SubQ: ~4 hours
Time to peak, plasma: SubQ: 30 minutes
Excretion: Urine (50% to 85%); feces (<1%)

Dosing
Adult Note: Azacitidine is associated with a moderate emetic potential (Basch 2011; Roila 2010); antiemetics are recommended to prevent nausea and vomiting.

Myelodysplastic syndromes (MDS):
US labeling: IV, SubQ: Initial cycle: 75 mg/m²/day for 7 days. Subsequent cycles: 75 mg/m²/day for 7 days every 4 weeks; dose may be increased to 100 mg/m²/day if no benefit is observed after 2 cycles and no toxicity other than nausea and vomiting have occurred. Patients should be treated for a minimum of 4 to 6 cycles; treatment may be continued as long as patient continues to benefit.

Canadian labeling: SubQ: Initial cycle: 75 mg/m²/day for 7 days. Subsequent cycles: If no toxicity observed with initial treatment continue 75 mg/m²/day for 7 days every 4 weeks; dose reductions and/or therapy interruption may be required for hematologic or renal toxicity. Patients should be treated for a minimum of 6 cycles and then as long as patient continues to benefit or until disease progression.

Note: Alternate (off-label) schedules (which have produced hematologic response) have been used for convenience in community oncology centers (Lyons 2009): SubQ:
75 mg/m²/day for 5 days (Mon-Fri), 2 days rest (Sat, Sun), then 75 mg/m²/day for 2 days (Mon, Tues); repeat cycle every 28 days **or**
50 mg/m²/day for 5 days (Mon-Fri), 2 days rest (Sat, Sun), then 50 mg/m²/day for 5 days (Mon-Fri); repeat cycle every 28 days **or**
75 mg/m²/day for 5 days (Mon-Fri), repeat cycle every 28 days

Acute myeloid leukemia (AML): Canadian labeling (off-label use in US): SubQ: 75 mg/m²/day for 7 days every 4 weeks for at least 6 cycles; treatment may be continued as long as patient continues to benefit or until disease progression or unacceptable toxicity (Fenaux 2010). Dose reductions and/or therapy interruption may be required for hematologic or renal toxicity.

Dosage adjustment based on serum electrolytes: If serum bicarbonate falls to <20 mEq/L (unexplained decrease): Reduce dose by 50% for next treatment course.

Geriatric Refer to adult dosing. Due to the potential for decreased renal function in the elderly, select dose carefully and closely monitor renal function.

Renal Impairment
Renal impairment at *baseline:*
Mild to moderate impairment (CrCl ≥30 mL/minute): No dosage adjustment necessary (Douvali 2012).
Severe impairment (CrCl <30 mL/minute): No dosage adjustment necessary for cycle 1; due to renal excretion of azacitidine and metabolites, monitor closely for toxicity.

Renal toxicity *during* treatment:

US labeling: Unexplained increases in BUN or serum creatinine: Delay next cycle until values reach baseline or normal, then reduce dose by 50% for next treatment course.

Canadian labeling: Unexplained increases in serum creatinine or BUN ≥2 fold above baseline and above the upper limit of normal (ULN): Delay next cycle until values reach baseline or normal, then reduce dose by 50% for next treatment course.

Hepatic Impairment No dosage adjustment provided in the manufacturer's labeling (has not been studied). Use is contraindicated in patients with advanced malignant hepatic tumors.

Adjustment for Toxicity

US labeling: Hematologic toxicity: MDS:

For baseline WBC ≥3 x 10^9/L, ANC ≥1.5 x 10^9/L, and platelets ≥75 x 10^9/L:

Nadir count: ANC <0.5 x 10^9/L or platelets <25 x 10^9/L: Administer 50% of dose during next treatment course

Nadir count: ANC 0.5 to 1.5 x 10^9/L or platelets 25-50 x 10^9/L: Administer 67% of dose during next treatment course

Nadir count: ANC >1.5 x 10^9/L or platelets >50 x 10^9/L: Administer 100% of dose during next treatment course

For baseline WBC <3 x 10^9/L, ANC <1.5 x 10^9/L, or platelets <75 x 10^9/L: Adjust dose as follows based on nadir counts and bone marrow biopsy cellularity at the time of nadir, unless clear improvement in differentiation at the time of the next cycle:

WBC or platelet nadir decreased 50% to 75% from baseline and bone marrow biopsy cellularity at time of nadir 30% to 60%: Administer 100% of dose during next treatment course

WBC or platelet nadir decreased 50% to 75% from baseline and bone marrow biopsy cellularity at time of nadir 15% to 30%: Administer 50% of dose during next treatment course

WBC or platelet nadir decreased 50% to 75% from baseline and bone marrow biopsy cellularity at time of nadir <15%: Administer 33% of dose during next treatment course

WBC or platelet nadir decreased >75% from baseline and bone marrow biopsy cellularity at time of nadir 30% to 60%: Administer 75% of dose during next treatment course

WBC or platelet nadir decreased >75% from baseline and bone marrow biopsy cellularity at time of nadir 15% to 30%: Administer 50% of dose during next treatment course

WBC or platelet nadir decreased >75% from baseline and bone marrow biopsy cellularity at time of nadir <15%: Administer 33% of dose during next treatment course

Note: If a nadir defined above occurs, administer the next treatment course 28 days after the start of the preceding course as long as WBC and platelet counts are >25% above the nadir and rising. If a >25% increase above the nadir is not seen by day 28, reassess counts every 7 days. If a 25% increase is not seen by day 42, administer 50% of the scheduled dose.

Canadian labeling: AML, MDS:

For baseline WBC ≥3 x 10^9/L, ANC ≥1.5 x 10^9/L, and platelets ≥75 x 10^9/L prior to first treatment:

Nadir count: ANC ≤1 x 10^9/L or platelets ≤50 x 10^9/L: If hematologic toxicity is observed, delay treatment

Nadir count: ANC ≤1 x 10^9/L or platelets ≤50 x 10^9/L: Delay treatment until ANC and platelets have recovered (to at least the nadir plus half the difference between nadir and baseline); if recovery achieved within 14 days, no dosage adjustment is necessary; if recovery not achieved within 14 days administer 50% of dose during next treatment course

Nadir count: ANC >1 x 10^9/L or platelets >50 x 10^9/L: If recovery not achieved within 14 days administer 100% of dose during next treatment course

For baseline WBC <3 x 10^9/L, ANC <1.5 x 10^9/L, or platelets <75 x 10^9/L prior to first treatment:

WBC or ANC or platelets decreased <50%, or decreased >50% but with improvement in any cell line differentiation: No delay or dose adjustment is necessary during next treatment course.

WBC or ANC or platelets decreased >50% with no improvement in cell line differentiation: Delay treatment until platelet count and ANC recovery. If recovery occurs within 14 days no dosage adjustment is necessary in the next treatment course. If recovery is not achieved within 14 days determine bone marrow cellularity. If bone marrow cellularity is >50% no dosage adjustment is necessary during next treatment course. If bone marrow cellularity is ≤50% delay treatment until recovery and reduce dose during next treatment course as follows:

Bone marrow cellularity 15 to 50%: Administer 50% of dose if recovery achieved >21 days or administer 100% of dose if recovery achieved >14 to ≤21 days

Bone marrow cellularity <15%: Administer 33% of dose if recovery achieved >21 days or administer 100% of dose if recovery achieved >14 to ≤21 days

Note: Resume 28 day treatment cycles following dose modifications.

Missed doses: Missed doses should be added to the end of the current dosing cycle; do not administer at time of next dose (ie, double dose).

Combination Regimens

Leukemia, acute myeloid: Azacitidine (AML Regimen) on page 1828
Myelodysplastic syndrome: Azacitidine (MDS Regimen) on page 1828

Administration Azacitidine is associated with a moderate emetic potential (Basch 2011; Dupuis 2011; Roila 2010); antiemetics are recommended to prevent nausea and vomiting.

SubQ: The manufacturer recommends equally dividing volumes >4 mL into 2 syringes and injecting into 2 separate sites; however, policies for maximum SubQ administration volume may vary by institution; interpatient variations may also apply. Rotate sites for each injection (thigh, abdomen, or upper arm). Administer subsequent injections at least 1 inch from previous injection sites; do not inject into tender, bruised, red, or hard areas. Allow refrigerated suspensions to come to room temperature (up to 30 minutes) prior to administration. Resuspend by inverting the syringe 2 to 3 times and then rolling the syringe between the palms for 30 seconds.

IV: Infuse over 10 to 40 minutes; infusion must be completed within 1 hour of (vial) reconstitution.

Hazardous agent; use appropriate precautions for handling and disposal (NIOSH 2014 [group 1]). If azacitidine suspension comes in contact with the skin, immediately wash with soap and water. If it comes into contact with mucous membranes, flush thoroughly with water.

Emetic Potential Children and Adults: Moderate (30% to 90%)

◄ **Monitoring Parameters** Monitor liver function tests, electrolytes CBC with differential and platelets, renal function (BUN and serum creatinine) at baseline, prior to each cycle, and more frequently if indicated. Also monitor for nausea/vomiting and for injection site reactions.

Dosage Forms Excipient information presented when available (limited, particularly for generics); consult specific product labeling.

Suspension Reconstituted, Injection:

Generic: 100 mg (1 ea)

Suspension Reconstituted, Injection [preservative free]:

Vidaza: 100 mg (1 ea)

Generic: 100 mg (1 ea)

Aztreonam (Systemic) (AZ tree oh nam)

Brand Names: US Azactam; Azactam in Dextrose

Index Terms Azthreonam

Pharmacologic Category Antibiotic, Miscellaneous

Use Treatment of patients with urinary tract infections, lower respiratory tract infections, septicemia, skin/skin structure infections, intra-abdominal infections, and gynecological infections caused by susceptible gram-negative bacilli

Pregnancy Risk Factor B

Dosing

Adult & Geriatric

Urinary tract infection: IM, IV: 500 mg to 1 g every 8 to 12 hours

Moderately severe systemic infections: 1 g IV or IM or 2 g IV every 8 to 12 hours. **Note:** IV route preferred for septicemia, intra-abdominal abscess, or peritonitis; higher doses (8 to 12 g daily) may be needed for patients with cystic fibrosis (Zobell, 2013) or other infections (Solomkin, 2010).

Severe systemic or life-threatening infections (eg, *Pseudomonas aeruginosa*): IV: 2 g every 6 to 8 hours; maximum: 8 g daily. **Note:** Higher doses (8 to 12 g daily) may be needed for patients with cystic fibrosis (Zobell, 2013) or other infections (Solomkin, 2010).

Surgical (perioperative) prophylaxis (off-label use): IV: 2 g within 60 minutes prior to surgery. Doses may be repeated in 4 hours if procedure is lengthy or if there is excessive blood loss (Bratzler, 2013).

Pediatric

Mild-to-moderate infections: Infants ≥9 months, Children, and Adolescents: IV: 30 mg/kg/dose every 8 hours; maximum: 120 mg/kg/day (8 g daily)

Moderate-to-severe infections: Infants ≥9 months, Children, and Adolescents: IV: 30 mg/kg/dose every 6 to 8 hours; maximum: 120 mg/kg/day (8 g daily)

Cystic fibrosis: Infants ≥9 months, Children, and Adolescents: IV: 50 mg/kg/dose every 6 to 8 hours (ie, up to 200 mg/kg/day); maximum: 8 g daily. **Note:** Higher doses (8 to 12 g daily) may be needed for patients with cystic fibrosis (Zobell, 2013).

Surgical (perioperative) prophylaxis (off-label use): Children ≥1 year and Adolescents: IV: 30 mg/kg within 60 minutes prior to surgery (maximum: 2,000 mg per dose). Doses may be repeated in 4 hours if procedure is lengthy or if there is excessive blood loss (Bratzler, 2013).

Renal Impairment

IM, IV: Adults: Following initial dose, maintenance doses should be given as follows:

CrCl 10 to 30 mL/minute: 50% of usual dose at the usual interval

CrCl <10 mL/minute: 25% of usual dosage at the usual interval

Intermittent hemodialysis (IHD): Dialyzable (20% to 50%): Loading dose of 500 mg, 1 g, or 2 g, followed by 25% of initial dose at usual interval; for serious/life-threatening infections, administer 12.5% of initial dose after each hemodialysis session (given in addition to the maintenance doses). Alternatively, may administer 500 mg every 12 hours (Heintz, 2009). **Note:** Dosing dependent on the assumption of 3 times/week, complete IHD sessions.

Peritoneal dialysis (PD): Administer as for CrCl <10 mL/minute (Aronoff, 2007)

Continuous renal replacement therapy (CRRT) (Heintz, 2009; Trotman, 2005): Drug clearance is highly dependent on the method of renal replacement, filter type, and flow rate. Appropriate dosing requires close monitoring of pharmacologic response, signs of adverse reactions due to drug accumulation, as well as drug concentrations in relation to target trough (if appropriate). The following are general recommendations only (based on dialysate flow/ultrafiltration rates of 1 to 2 L/hour and minimal residual renal function) and should not supersede clinical judgment:

CVVH: Loading dose of 2 g followed by 1 to 2 g every 12 hours

CVVHD/CVVHDF: Loading dose of 2 g followed by either 1 g every 8 hours **or** 2 g every 12 hours (Heintz, 2009)

Hepatic Impairment No dosage adjustment provided in manufacturer's labeling. Use with caution (minor hepatic elimination occurs).

Additional Information Complete prescribing information should be consulted for additional detail.

Dosage Forms Excipient information presented when available (limited, particularly for generics); consult specific product labeling.

Solution, Intravenous:

Azactam in Dextrose: 1 g (50 mL); 2 g (50 mL) [sodium free]

Solution Reconstituted, Injection:

Azactam: 1 g (1 ea); 2 g (1 ea) [sodium free]

Generic: 1 g (1 ea); 2 g (1 ea)

Aztreonam (Oral Inhalation) (AZ tree oh nam)

Brand Names: US Cayston

Brand Names: Canada Cayston
Index Terms Azthreonam
Pharmacologic Category Antibiotic, Miscellaneous
Use Improve respiratory symptoms in cystic fibrosis (CF) patients with *Pseudomonas aeruginosa*
Pregnancy Risk Factor B
Dosing
  Adult Cystic fibrosis: Inhalation (nebulizer): 75 mg 3 times daily (at least 4 hours apart) for 28 days; do not repeat for 28 days after completion
  Pediatric
    Cystic fibrosis: Children ≥7 years and Adolescents: Inhalation (nebulizer): 75 mg 3 times daily (at least 4 hours apart) for 28 days; do not repeat for 28 days after completion
  Renal Impairment Dosage adjustment not required for mild, moderate, or severe renal impairment.
  Hepatic Impairment There are no dosage adjustments provided in the manufacturer's labeling.
Additional Information Complete prescribing information should be consulted for additional detail.
Prescribing and Access Restrictions Cayston (aztreonam inhalation solution) is only available through a select group of specialty pharmacies and cannot be obtained through a retail pharmacy. Because Cayston may only be used with the Altera Nebulizer System, it can only be obtained from the following specialty pharmacies; IV Solutions/Maxor; Foundation Care; Pharmaceutical Specialties Inc; TLCRx/ ModernHEALTH; and Walgreens Specialty Pharmacy. This network of specialty pharmacies ensures proper access to both the drug and device. To obtain the medication and proper nebulizer, contact the Cayston Access Program at 1-877-7CAYSTON (1-877-722-9786) or at www.cayston.com.
Dosage Forms Excipient information presented when available (limited, particularly for generics); consult specific product labeling.
  Solution Reconstituted, Inhalation [preservative free]:
    Cayston: 75 mg (84 mL) [arginine free]

◆ **B1939** *see* EriBULin *on page* 624
◆ **Bacillus Calmette-Guérin (BCG) Live** *see* BCG (Intravesical) *on page* 174
◆ **Bactrim** *see* Sulfamethoxazole and Trimethoprim *on page* 1560
◆ **Bactrim DS** *see* Sulfamethoxazole and Trimethoprim *on page* 1560
◆ **BAL8557** *see* Isavuconazonium Sulfate *on page* 972

Basiliximab (ba si LIK si mab)

Related Information
  Hematopoietic Stem Cell Transplantation *on page* 2272
Brand Names: US Simulect
Brand Names: Canada Simulect
Pharmacologic Category Immunosuppressant Agent; Monoclonal Antibody
Use Renal transplant rejection: Prophylaxis of acute organ rejection in renal transplantation in combination with cyclosporine (modified) and corticosteroids
Labeled Contraindications Known hypersensitivity to basiliximab or any component of the formulation

Pregnancy Considerations Adverse effects were not observed in animal reproduction studies. IL-2 receptors play an important role in the development of the immune system. Women of childbearing potential should use effective contraceptive measures before beginning treatment, during, and for 4 months after completion of basiliximab treatment. The National Transplantation Pregnancy Registry (NTPR, Temple University) is a registry for pregnant women taking immunosuppressants following any solid organ transplant. The NTPR encourages reporting of all immunosuppressant exposures during pregnancy in transplant recipients at 877-955-6877.

Breast-Feeding Considerations It is not known if basiliximab is excreted in human milk. Because many immunoglobulins are secreted in milk and the potential for serious adverse reactions exists, a decision should be made to discontinue nursing or discontinue the drug, taking into account the importance of the drug to the mother. The Canadian labeling recommends women avoid nursing for 4 months following the last dose.

Warnings/Precautions To be used as a component of an immunosuppressive regimen which includes cyclosporine and corticosteroids. The incidence of lymphoproliferative disorders and/or opportunistic infections may be increased by immunosuppressive therapy. Severe hypersensitivity reactions, occurring within 24 hours, have been reported. Reactions, including anaphylaxis, have occurred both with the initial exposure and/or following re-exposure after several months. Use caution during re-exposure to a subsequent course of therapy in a patient who has previously received basiliximab; patients in whom concomitant immunosuppression was prematurely discontinued due to abandoned transplantation or early graft loss are at increased risk for developing a severe hypersensitivity reaction upon re-exposure. Discontinue permanently if a severe reaction occurs. Medications for the treatment of hypersensitivity reactions should be available for immediate use. Treatment may result in the development of human antimurine antibodies (HAMA); however, limited evidence suggesting the use of muromonab-CD3 or other murine products is not precluded. **[U.S. Boxed Warning]: Should be administered under the supervision of a physician experienced in immunosuppression therapy and organ transplant management.** In renal transplant patients receiving basiliximab plus prednisone, cyclosporine, and mycophenolate, new-onset diabetes, glucose intolerance, and impaired fasting glucose were observed at rates significantly higher than observed in patients receiving prednisone, cyclosporine, and mycophenolate without basiliximab (Aasebo, 2010). Potentially significant drug-drug interactions may exist, requiring dose or frequency adjustment, additional monitoring, and/or selection of alternative therapy.

Adverse Reactions Administration of basiliximab did not appear to increase the incidence or severity of adverse effects in clinical trials. Adverse events were reported in 96% of both the placebo and basiliximab groups.

>10%:

  Cardiovascular: Hypertension, peripheral edema

  Central nervous system: Fever, headache, insomnia, pain

  Dermatologic: Acne, wound complications

  Endocrine & metabolic: Hypercholesterolemia, hyperglycemia, hyper-/hypo-kalemia, hyperuricemia, hypophosphatemia

  Gastrointestinal: Abdominal pain, constipation, diarrhea, dyspepsia, nausea, vomiting

  Genitourinary: Urinary tract infection

  Hematologic: Anemia

  Neuromuscular & skeletal: Tremor

Respiratory: Dyspnea, infection (upper respiratory)

Miscellaneous: Viral infection

3% to 10%:

Cardiovascular: Abnormal heart sounds, angina, arrhythmia, atrial fibrillation, chest pain, generalized edema, heart failure, hypotension, tachycardia

Central nervous system: Agitation, anxiety, depression, dizziness, fatigue, hypoesthesia, malaise

Dermatologic: Cyst, hypertrichosis, pruritus, rash, skin disorder, skin ulceration

Endocrine & metabolic: Acidosis, dehydration, diabetes mellitus, fluid overload, glucocorticoids increased, hyper-/hypocalcemia, hyperlipemia, hypertriglyceridemia, hypoglycemia, hypomagnesemia, hyponatremia, hypoproteinemia

Gastrointestinal: Abdomen enlarged, esophagitis, flatulence, gastroenteritis, GI hemorrhage, gingival hyperplasia, melena, moniliasis, stomatitis (including ulcerative), weight gain

Genitourinary: Bladder disorder, dysuria, genital edema (male), impotence, ureteral disorder, urinary frequency, urinary retention

Hematologic: Hematoma, hemorrhage, leukopenia, polycythemia, purpura, thrombocytopenia, thrombosis

Neuromuscular & skeletal: Arthralgia, arthropathy, back pain, cramps, fracture, hernia, leg pain, myalgia, neuropathy, paresthesia, rigors, weakness

Ocular: Abnormal vision, cataract, conjunctivitis

Renal: Albuminuria, hematuria, nonprotein nitrogen increased, oliguria, renal function abnormal, renal tubular necrosis

Respiratory: Bronchitis, bronchospasm, cough, pharyngitis, pneumonia, pulmonary edema, rhinitis, sinusitis

Miscellaneous: Accidental trauma, cytomegalovirus (CMV) infection, herpes infection (simplex and zoster), infection, sepsis

Postmarketing and/or case reports: Anaphylaxis, capillary leak syndrome, cytokine release syndrome, diabetes (new onset), fasting glucose impaired, glucose intolerance, hypersensitivity reaction (including heart failure, hypotension, tachycardia, bronchospasm, dyspnea, pulmonary edema, respiratory failure, sneezing, pruritus, rash, urticaria), lymphoproliferative disease

Drug Interactions

Metabolism/Transport Effects None known.

Avoid Concomitant Use

Avoid concomitant use of Basiliximab with any of the following: BCG (Intravesical); Belimumab; Natalizumab; Pimecrolimus; Tacrolimus (Topical); Tofacitinib; Vaccines (Live)

Increased Effect/Toxicity

Basiliximab may increase the levels/effects of: Belimumab; Fingolimod; Leflunomide; Natalizumab; Tofacitinib; Vaccines (Live)

The levels/effects of Basiliximab may be increased by: Denosumab; Pimecrolimus; Roflumilast; Tacrolimus (Topical); Trastuzumab

Decreased Effect

Basiliximab may decrease the levels/effects of: BCG (Intravesical); Coccidioides immitis Skin Test; Sipuleucel-T; Vaccines (Inactivated); Vaccines (Live)

The levels/effects of Basiliximab may be decreased by: Echinacea

Storage/Stability Store intact vials refrigerated at 2°C to 8°C (36°F to 46°F). Should be used immediately after reconstitution; however, if not used immediately, reconstituted solution may be stored at 2°C to 8°C for up to 24 hours or at room temperature for up to 4 hours. Discard the reconstituted solution if not used within 24 hours.

Preparation for Administration Reconstitute with preservative-free sterile water for injection (reconstitute 10 mg vial with 2.5 mL, 20 mg vial with 5 mL). Shake gently to dissolve. May further dilute reconstituted solution with 25 mL (10 mg) or 50 mL (20 mg) 0.9% sodium chloride or dextrose 5% in water. When mixing the solution, gently invert the bag to avoid foaming. Do not shake solutions diluted for infusion.

Mechanism of Action Chimeric (murine/human) immunosuppressant monoclonal antibody which blocks the alpha-chain of the interleukin-2 (IL-2) receptor complex; this receptor is expressed on activated T lymphocytes and is a critical pathway for activating cell-mediated allograft rejection

Pharmacodynamics/Kinetics

Duration: Mean: 36 days (determined by IL-2R alpha saturation)

Distribution: Mean: V_d: Children 1 to 11 years: 4.8 ± 2.1 L; Adolescents 12 to 16 years: 7.8 ± 5.1 L; Adults: 8.6 ± 4.1 L

Half-life elimination: Children 1 to 11 years: 9.5 days; Adolescents 12 to 16 years: 9.1 days; Adults: Mean: 7.2 days

Dosing

Adult & Geriatric Note: Patients previously administered basiliximab should only be re-exposed to a subsequent course of therapy with extreme caution.

Acute renal transplant rejection prophylaxis: IV: 20 mg within 2 hours prior to transplant surgery, followed by a second 20 mg dose 4 days after transplantation. The second dose should be withheld if complications occur (including severe hypersensitivity reactions or graft loss).

Acute cardiac transplant rejection prophylaxis (off-label use): IV: 20 mg on the day of transplant, followed by a second dose 4 days after transplantation (Mehra, 2005); usually given within the first hour postoperatively

Acute liver transplant rejection prophylaxis (off-label use): IV: 20 mg within 6 hours of organ reperfusion, followed by a second 20 mg dose 4 days after transplantation (Neuhaus, 2002)

Treatment of refractory acute GVHD (off-label use): IV: 20 mg on days 1 and 4; may repeat for recurrent acute GVHD (Schmidt-Hieber, 2005). Additional data may be necessary to further define the role of basiliximab in this condition.

Pediatric Note: Patients previously administered basiliximab should only be re-exposed to a subsequent course of therapy with extreme caution.

Acute renal transplant rejection prophylaxis: IV: **Note:** Use in pediatric patients is not approved in the Canadian labeling (limited pharmacokinetic data available).

Children <35 kg: 10 mg within 2 hours prior to transplant surgery, followed by a second 10 mg dose 4 days after transplantation; the second dose should be withheld if complications occur (including severe hypersensitivity reactions or graft loss)

Children ≥35 kg: Refer to adult dosing

Renal Impairment There are no dosage adjustments provided in the manufacturer's labeling.

Hepatic Impairment There are no dosage adjustments provided in the manufacturer's labeling.

◄ **Administration** For intravenous administration only. Infuse as a bolus or IV infusion over 20-30 minutes. (Bolus dosing is associated with nausea, vomiting, and local pain at the injection site.) Administer only after assurance that patient will receive renal graft and immunosuppression. For the treatment of acute GVHD (off-label use), the dose was diluted in 250 mL NS and administered over 30 minutes (Schmidt-Hieber, 2005).

Monitoring Parameters Signs and symptoms of acute rejection; hypersensitivity, infection

Dosage Forms Excipient information presented when available (limited, particularly for generics); consult specific product labeling.

Solution Reconstituted, Intravenous [preservative free]:

Simulect: 10 mg (1 ea); 20 mg (1 ea)

♦ **BAY 43-9006** *see* SORAfenib *on page 1547*

♦ **BAY 73-4506** *see* Regorafenib *on page 1466*

♦ **BAY88-8223** *see* Radium Ra 223 Dichloride *on page 1448*

♦ **Baycadron [DSC]** *see* Dexamethasone (Systemic) *on page 513*

BCG (Intravesical) (bee see jee)

Related Information

Safe Handling of Hazardous Drugs *on page 2292*

Brand Names: US TheraCys; Tice BCG

Brand Names: Canada ImmuCyst; Oncotice

Index Terms Bacillus Calmette-Guérin (BCG) Live; BCG, Live

Pharmacologic Category Antineoplastic Agent, Biological Response Modulator

Use

Bladder cancer: Treatment and prophylaxis of carcinoma in situ of the urinary bladder; prophylaxis of primary or recurrent superficial or minimally invasive (stage Ta and/or T1) papillary tumors following transurethral resection

Limitations of use: BCG (intravesical) is not recommended for stage Ta low-grade papillary tumors unless judged to be at high risk for recurrence. BCG (intravesical) is not recommended for immunization against tuberculosis.

Labeled Contraindications Known hypersensitivity to any component of BCG (intravesical), after a previous administration of BCG (intravesical), or after a previous administration of a medicinal product containing the same substances; hypersensitivity to latex (TheraCys); immunosuppressed patients or persons with congenital or acquired immune deficiencies (eg, HIV infection, leukemia, lymphoma, cancer therapy, immunosuppressive therapy such as corticosteroids); active tuberculosis; concurrent febrile illness, urinary tract infection, or gross hematuria; current symptoms or previous history of a systemic BCG reaction; recent (TheraCys: <14 days; TICE BCG: <7 to 14 days) biopsy, transurethral resection (TUR), or traumatic catheterization

Pregnancy Considerations Animal reproduction studies have not been conducted. BCG (intravesical) is not recommended for use in pregnant women. Women of childbearing potential should be advised to avoid pregnancy while on BCG (intravesical) therapy.

Breast-Feeding Considerations It is not known if BCG (intravesical) is excreted in breast milk. Due to the potential for serious adverse reactions in the nursing infant, a decision should be made to discontinue breast-feeding or avoid use of BCG (intravesical), taking into account the importance of BCG (intravesical) to the mother.

Warnings/Precautions Hazardous agent - Use appropriate precautions for handling and disposal (NIOSH 2014 [group 1]).

[US Boxed Warning]: Contains live, attenuated mycobacteria. Use appropriate precautions for handling and disposal. BCG is a biohazard; proper preparation technique, handling, and disposal of all equipment in contact with BCG as a biohazard material is recommended. BCG infections have been reported in healthcare workers due to accidental exposure (needlestick, skin laceration); nosocomial infections have been reported in patients (including immunosuppressed patients) receiving parenteral medications prepared in areas where BCG was prepared. To avoid cross contamination, do not prepare parenteral medications in an area where BCG has been prepared. Determine PPD status prior to use. Prior to intravesical instillation, patients with a positive PPD test should be further assessed for signs and/or symptoms of active or latent tuberculosis.

[US Boxed Warning]: May cause disseminated (including fatal) infections following intravesical administration. Instillation to actively bleeding mucosa may promote systemic BCG infection or sepsis; postpone treatment for at least 1 to 2 weeks (depending on product) following TUR, biopsy, traumatic catheterization (may resume original schedule after 14 days), or gross hematuria. Do not use in patients with concurrent infections. Use caution in patients with aneurysms and prosthetic devices; ectopic BCG infection may occur at these sites. If signs and symptoms of a systemic BCG infection occur, permanently discontinue BCG treatment and begin therapy with 2 or more antimycobacterial agents while conducting a diagnostic evaluation. Infection from BCG (intravesical) is not sensitive to pyrazinamide. Do not use prophylactic antimycobacterial therapy to prevent local adverse events during treatment (there is no data to support use and may alter efficacy). If a bacterial urinary tract infection occurs, withhold therapy until complete resolution.

A systemic granulomatous illness occurring following exposure to BCG is referred to as a systemic BCG reaction when any of the following are present without another detectable etiology: Fever ≥39.5°C for ≥12 hours or ≥38.5°C for ≥48 hours; pneumonitis; hepatitis; organ dysfunction outside of the GU tract with granulomatous inflammation; clinical signs of sepsis. A systemic BCG reaction is more likely to occur with intravesical administration <14 days after a biopsy, transurethral resection (TUR), or traumatic catheterization. Fatalities have been reported with systemic BCG reactions.

Intravesical instillations should be postponed during antibiotic therapy; antibiotics may reduce the efficacy of therapy. BCG (intravesical) may cause symptoms of bladder irritability which usually begin 4 to 6 hours after instillation and may last 24 to 72 hours; symptoms may increase in severity following each instillation. Intravesical instillation may be associated with increased risk of severe local reactions in the presence of small bladder capacity; use with caution. Packaging may contain natural latex rubber. BCG (intravesical) is not a vaccine for the prevention of cancer. Information is not available for interchanging products used for intravesical administration. Potentially significant drug-drug interactions may exist, requiring dose or frequency adjustment, additional monitoring, and/or selection of alternative therapy.

◄ **Adverse Reactions** Adverse events should be reported to MEDWATCH (800-FDA-1088 or www.fda.gov/medwatch) or the manufacturer.

>10%:

Central nervous system: Malaise (≤40%), chills (9% to 34%), pain (≤17%)

Gastrointestinal: Nausea (≤16%), vomiting (≤16%), anorexia (≤11%)

Genitourinary: Dysuria (52% to 60%), irritable bladder (50% to 60%), urinary frequency (40% to ≤50%), urinary urgency (6% to ≤50%), hematuria (26% to 39%; grade ≥33% to 7%), cystitis (6% to 30%), urinary tract infection (2% to 18%; grade ≥3: ≤1%)

Hematologic & oncologic: Anemia (≤21%)

Respiratory: Flu-like symptoms (24% to 33%; grade ≥3: ≤9%)

Miscellaneous: Fever (17% to 38%; grade ≥3: ≤8%)

1% to 10%:

Central nervous system: Fatigue (≤7%), dizziness (≤2%), headache (≤2%)

Dermatologic: Diaphoresis (3%), skin rash (≤3%)

Endocrine & metabolic: Weight loss (≤2%)

Gastrointestinal: Diarrhea (≤6%), abdominal pain (2% to 3%), hepatic granuloma (≤1%)

Genitourinary: Genital pain (10%), nephrotoxicity (10%), hemorrhagic cystitis (9%), bladder spasm (≤8%), bladder pain (≤6%), urinary incontinence (2% to 6%), nocturia (5%), bladder contraction (≤5%), urine deposits (2%), epididymitis (≤1%), orchitis (≤1%), prostatitis (≤1%), pyuria (≤1%), urethritis (≤1%), urinary tract obstruction (≤1%)

Hematologic & oncologic: Leukopenia (≤5%), blood coagulation disorder (≤1%); thrombocytopenia (≤1%)

Hepatic: Hepatitis (≤1%)

Hypersensitivity: Hypersensitivity (2%)

Infection: Sepsis (3%; BCG sepsis: ≤1%), genital abscess (≤2%), genital inflammation (≤2%)

Neuromuscular & skeletal: Arthritis (≤7%), arthralgia (≤7%), myalgia (≤7%), muscle cramps (≤4%), rigors (3%)

Respiratory: Pulmonary infection (3%), pneumonitis (≤1%)

<1%, postmarketing, and/or case reports: Adverse drug effect (systemic BCG reaction; may include fever ≥39.5°C (≥103.1°F) for ≥12 hours; fever ≥38.5°C (≥101.3°F) for ≥48 hours; pneumonitis; hepatitis; other organ dysfunction outside of the GU tract with granulomatous inflammation on biopsy; or the classical signs of sepsis, including circulatory collapse, acute respiratory distress, and DIC), conjunctivitis, constipation, erythema nodosum, flank pain, granulomatous choreoretinitis, increased blood urea nitrogen, increased serum creatinine, infection, interstitial pulmonary disease, iritis, keratitis, *Mycobacterium bovis* (includes infection of bone, bone marrow, kidney, lung, liver, lymph nodes, prostate), nephritis (includes glomerulonephritis, interstitial nephritis, renal tubulo-interstitial nephritis), pneumonia, pyelonephritis, Reiter's syndrome, renal abscess, renal failure, urinary retention (includes bladder tamponade and increased post-void residual urine volume), uveitis

Drug Interactions

Metabolism/Transport Effects None known.

Avoid Concomitant Use

Avoid concomitant use of BCG (Intravesical) with any of the following: Antibiotics; Hexaminolevulinate; Immunosuppressants; Myelosuppressive Agents

Increased Effect/Toxicity There are no known significant interactions involving an increase in effect.

Decreased Effect

BCG (Intravesical) may decrease the levels/effects of: Hexaminolevulinate

The levels/effects of BCG (Intravesical) may be decreased by: Antibiotics; Immunosuppressants; Myelosuppressive Agents

Storage/Stability Store intact vials at 2°C to 8°C (36°F to 46°F). Protect from light. After reconstitution, store TheraCys at 2°C to 25°C (35°F to 77°F) and store TICE BCG at 2°C to 8°C (36°F to 46°F). Use within 2 hours of mixing.

Preparation for Administration Hazardous agent; use appropriate precautions for handling and disposal (NIOSH 2014 [group 1]). Prepare using aseptic technique. Do not prepare parenteral medications in an area where BCG has been prepared. Do not filter.

TheraCys: Reconstitute with 3 mL of sterile preservative free saline and shake gently to create a fine, even suspension (avoid foaming). Withdraw contents (~3 mL) and further dilute with sterile preservative free saline to a final volume of 50 mL.

TICE BCG: Reconstitute with 1 mL sterile preservative free saline using a 3 mL syringe. Add to vial and swirl gently to form a homogenous suspension (forceful agitation may cause clumping). Dispense into a catheter tip syringe containing 49 mL of sterile preservative free saline. Mix by gently rotating the syringe. May also order reconstitution accessories from manufacturer.

Mechanism of Action BCG (intravesical) is an attenuated strain of bacillus Calmette-Guérin (*Mycobacterium bovis*) used as a biological response modifier. BCG, when used intravesicularly for treatment of bladder carcinoma *in situ*, is thought to cause a local, chronic inflammatory response involving macrophage and leukocyte infiltration of the bladder. BCG (intravesical) is active immunotherapy which stimulates the host's immune mechanism to reject the tumor.

Dosing

Adult & Geriatric

Bladder cancer: Intravesicular:

TheraCys: Induction: One dose (81 mg or one vial) instilled into bladder (retain for up to 2 hours) once weekly for 6 weeks beginning at least 14 days after biopsy or transurethral resection, followed by maintenance therapy of 81 mg (one vial) at 3, 6, 12, 18, and 24 months after initial dose.

TICE BCG: Induction: One dose (~50 mg or one vial) instilled into the bladder (retain for 2 hours) once weekly for 6 weeks beginning 7 to 14 days after biopsy (may repeat cycle 1 time if tumor remission not achieved), followed by maintenance therapy of ~50 mg (one vial) approximately once a month for at least 6 to 12 months.

Renal Impairment There are no dosage adjustments provided in the manufacturer's labeling.

Hepatic Impairment There are no dosage adjustments provided in the manufacturer's labeling.

Administration For intravesicular (bladder instillation) administration only; **do not administer IV, SubQ, IM, or intradermally**.

Intravesicular: Patients should not drink fluids for 4 hours prior to instillation. Empty or drain bladder. Instill BCG (intravesical) by gravity; retain for as long as possible, up to 2 hours. Patient should lie prone for at least 15 minutes, then rotate positions (lie on right side, left side, abdomen, and back) every 15 minutes to maximize bladder surface exposure (TICE BCG); for TheraCys, ▶

patient may be in an upright position after the first 15 minutes. Following bladder instillation, patients should be instructed to void in a seated position in order to avoid the splashing of urine; burning may occur with the first void following therapy. Prior to flushing, disinfect the urine for 15 minutes with an equal amount of household bleach (this should be done for the first 6 hours after therapy). After administration, patients should drink plenty of water in order to flush the bladder.

Hazardous agent; use appropriate precautions for handling and disposal (NIOSH 2014 [group 1]).

Monitoring Parameters

PPD test prior to treatment

Intravesical treatment: Signs and symptoms of toxicity/infection following every treatment. Signs that antituberculous therapy may be needed: Flu-like symptoms ≥72 hours, fever ≥101.3°F, systemic symptoms which worsen with each treatment, persistently abnormal liver function tests, prostatitis, epididymitis or orchitis of >2 to 3 day duration

Dosage Forms Excipient information presented when available (limited, particularly for generics); consult specific product labeling.

Suspension Reconstituted, Intravesical:

Tice BCG: 50 mg (1 ea)

Suspension Reconstituted, Intravesical [preservative free]:

TheraCys: 81 mg (1 ea) [contains monosodium glutamate (sodium glutamate)]

♦ **BCG, Live** see BCG (Intravesical) on page 174

♦ **BCNU** see Carmustine on page 284

♦ **Bebulin** see Factor IX Complex (Human) [(Factors II, IX, X)] on page 677

♦ **Bebulin VH** see Factor IX Complex (Human) [(Factors II, IX, X)] on page 677

♦ **Becenum** see Carmustine on page 284

♦ **Beleodaq** see Belinostat on page 178

Belinostat (be LIN oh stat)

Related Information

Safe Handling of Hazardous Drugs on page 2292

Brand Names: US Beleodaq

Index Terms PXD101

Pharmacologic Category Antineoplastic Agent, Histone Deacetylase (HDAC) Inhibitor

Use Peripheral T-cell lymphoma: Treatment of relapsed or refractory peripheral T-cell lymphoma (PTCL)

Labeled Contraindications There are no contraindications listed in the manufacturer's labeling.

Pregnancy Considerations Animal reproduction studies have not been conducted. Belinostat is a genotoxic drug that targets dividing cells; embryofetal toxicity is expected if exposure occurs during pregnancy. Based on animal data, belinostat may also impair male fertility. Women of reproductive potential should avoid pregnancy during treatment with belinostat.

Breast-Feeding Considerations It is not known if belinostat is excreted in breast milk. Due to the potential for serious adverse reactions in the nursing infant, the manufacturer recommends that a decision be made whether to discontinue nursing or to discontinue the drug, taking into account the importance of treatment to the mother.

Warnings/Precautions Hazardous agent – Use appropriate precautions for handling and disposal (meets NIOSH 2014 criteria).

May cause thrombocytopenia, leukopenia (neutropenia and lymphopenia), and/or anemia. Monitor blood counts at baseline and weekly during treatment. May require dosage reduction, treatment delay, or discontinuation. Serious infections (occasionally fatal), including pneumonia and sepsis, have occurred with treatment. Do not administer in patients with an active infection. Heavily pretreated patients (history of extensive or intensive prior chemotherapy) may be at higher risk for life-threatening infections.

May cause liver function test abnormalities and fatal hepatotoxicity. Monitor liver function tests at baseline and prior to each cycle. May require dosage reduction, treatment delay, or permanent discontinuation (based on the severity of the hepatotoxicity). Belinostat is metabolized hepatically and increased exposure is expected to occur in patients with hepatic impairment. Patients with moderate to severe hepatic impairment (total bilirubin >1.5 times ULN) were excluded from clinical studies. Tumor lysis syndrome (TLS) has been observed; closely monitor patients with advanced disease and/or high tumor burden. If TLS occurs, initiate appropriate treatment. Nausea, vomiting, and diarrhea occur with belinostat; may require management with antiemetic and antidiarrheal medications. In a phase 1 study, nausea/vomiting generally occurred at the end of the infusion each day (rarely persisting beyond day 5 each cycle) and was managed with standard antiemetics (Steele, 2011).

Belinostat is primarily metabolized by UGT1A1; the initial dose should be reduced in patients known to be homozygous for UGT1A1*28 allele. Potentially significant drug-drug interactions may exist, requiring dose or frequency adjustment, additional monitoring, and/or selection of alternative therapy.

Adverse Reactions
>10%:
  Cardiovascular: Peripheral edema (20%), prolonged Q-T interval on ECG (11%; grades 3/4: 4%)
  Central nervous system: Fatigue (37%; grades 3/4: 5%), chills (16%; grades 3/4: 1%), headache (15%)
  Dermatologic: Skin rash (20%; grades 3/4: 1%), pruritus (16%; grades 3/4: 3%)
  Endocrine & metabolic: Increased lactate dehydrogenase (16%; grades 3/4: 2%), hypokalemia (12%; grades 3/4: 4%)
  Gastrointestinal: Nausea (42%; grades 3/4: 1%), vomiting (29%; grades 3/4: 1%), constipation (23%; grades 3/4: 1%), diarrhea (23%; grades 3/4: 2%), decreased appetite (15%; grades 3/4: 2%), abdominal pain (11%; grades 3/4: 1%)
  Hematologic & oncologic: Anemia (32%; grades 3/4: 11%), thrombocytopenia (16%; grades 3/4: 7%)
  Local: Pain at injection site (14%)
  Respiratory: Dyspnea (22%; grades 3/4: 6%), cough (19%)
  Miscellaneous: Fever (35%; grades 3/4: 2%)
1% to 10%:
  Cardiovascular: Hypotension (10%; grades 3/4: 3%), phlebitis (10%; grades 3/4: 1%)
  Central nervous system: Dizziness (10%)
  Infection: Infection (>2%)

Renal: Increased serum creatinine (>2%)

Respiratory: Pneumonia (>2%)

Miscellaneous: Multi-organ failure (>2%)

<1%, postmarketing, and/or case reports: Abnormal hepatic function tests, febrile neutropenia, hepatic failure, hepatotoxicity, leukopenia, sepsis, tumor lysis syndrome, ventricular fibrillation

Drug Interactions

Metabolism/Transport Effects Substrate of CYP2A6 (minor), CYP2C9 (minor), CYP3A4 (minor), P-glycoprotein, UGT1A1; **Note:** Assignment of Major/Minor substrate status based on clinically relevant drug interaction potential; **Inhibits** CYP2C8 (weak), CYP2C9 (weak)

Avoid Concomitant Use

Avoid concomitant use of Belinostat with any of the following: Amodiaquine; Atazanavir; BCG (Intravesical); CloZAPine; Dipyrone

Increased Effect/Toxicity

Belinostat may increase the levels/effects of: Amodiaquine; CloZAPine

The levels/effects of Belinostat may be increased by: Atazanavir; Dipyrone

Decreased Effect

Belinostat may decrease the levels/effects of: BCG (Intravesical)

Storage/Stability Store intact vials at 20°C to 25°C (68°F to 77°F); excursions are permitted between 15°C and 30°C (59°F and 86°F). Retain in original package until use. The reconstituted solution may be stored for 12 hours at 15°C to 25°C (59°F to 77°F). Solutions diluted for infusion may be stored for up to 36 hours (including infusion time) at 15°C to 25°C (59°F to 77°F).

Preparation for Administration Hazardous agent; use appropriate precautions for handling and disposal (meets NIOSH 2014 criteria). Reconstitute each 500 mg vial with SWFI 9 mL to a concentration of 50 mg/mL. Swirl vial contents until there are no visible particles in the reconstituted solution. Further dilute the appropriate dose in NS 250 mL; do not use if cloudy or precipitate is present.

Mechanism of Action Histone deacetylase (HDAC) inhibitor which catalyzes acetyl group removal from protein lysine residues (of histone and some nonhistone proteins). Inhibition of histone deacetylase results in accumulation of acetyl groups, leading to cell cycle arrest and apoptosis. Belinostat has preferential cytotoxicity toward tumor cells versus normal cells.

Pharmacodynamics/Kinetics

Distribution: ~114 L/m^2 (Steele, 2011); mean volume of distribution approaches total body water

Protein binding: 93% to 96%

Metabolism: Hepatic; predominantly via UGT1A1, also by CYP2A6, CYP2C9, and CYP3A4 to the amide and acid metabolites

Half-life elimination: 1.1 hours

Time to peak: At end of infusion (Steele, 2011)

Excretion: Urine (~40%, predominantly as metabolites; <2% as unchanged drug)

Dosing

Adult & Geriatric Note: ANC should be ≥1000/mm^3 and platelets should be ≥50,000/mm^3 prior to each cycle

Peripheral T-cell lymphoma, relapsed or refractory: IV: 1000 mg/m^2 daily on days 1 to 5 every 21 days until disease progression or unacceptable toxicity (O'Connor, 2013)

Dosage adjustment for patients with reduced UGT1A1 activity: Reduce initial dose to 750 mg/m² for patients known to be homozygous for UGT1A1*28 allele.

Renal Impairment

CrCl >39 mL/minute: Exposure is not altered (dosage adjustment is not likely necessary).

CrCl ≤39 mL/minute: There are no dosage adjustments provided in the manufacturer's labeling (data is insufficient to recommend a dose).

Hepatic Impairment

Mild hepatic impairment: There are no dosage adjustments provided in the manufacturer's labeling (exposure is expected to be increased in hepatic impairment).

Moderate to severe hepatic impairment (total bilirubin >1.5 times ULN): There are no dosage adjustments provided in the manufacturer's labeling (data is insufficient to recommend a dose).

Obesity *ASCO Guidelines for appropriate chemotherapy dosing in obese adults with cancer:* Utilize patient's actual body weight (full weight) for calculation of body surface area- or weight-based dosing, particularly when the intent of therapy is curative; manage regimen-related toxicities in the same manner as for nonobese patients; if a dose reduction is utilized due to toxicity, consider resumption of full weight-based dosing with subsequent cycles, especially if cause of toxicity (eg, hepatic or renal impairment) is resolved (Griggs, 2012).

Adjustment for Toxicity

Hematologic toxicity: ANC should be ≥1000/mm³ and platelets should be ≥50,000/mm³ prior to each cycle and prior to resuming treatment following a delay due to toxicity. Resume subsequent treatment according to the following parameters:

Platelets ≥25,000/mm³ and nadir ANC ≥500/mm³: No dosage adjustment necessary (continue treatment without modification).

Nadir ANC <500/mm³ and any platelet count: Reduce dose by 25% (to 750 mg/m²).

Platelets <25,000/mm³ and any nadir ANC: Reduce dose by 25% (to 750 mg/m²).

Recurrent nadir ANC <500/mm³ and/or recurrent nadir platelets <25,000/mm³ following 2 dosage reductions: Discontinue treatment.

Nonhematologic toxicity: Nonhematologic toxicities should be grade 2 or lower prior to retreatment. Resume subsequent treatment according to the following parameters:

Any grade 3 or 4 toxicity (except nausea, vomiting, or diarrhea): Reduce dose by 25% (to 750 mg/m²).

Recurrent grade 3 or 4 toxicity following 2 dosage reductions: Discontinue treatment.

Grade 3 or 4 nausea, vomiting, or diarrhea: Manage with supportive care; reduce the dose only if duration is >7 days with supportive management.

Administration IV: Infuse over 30 minutes using a 0.22-micron inline filter; if infusion site pain or other symptoms associated with infusion occur, may increase infusion time to 45 minutes.

Hazardous agent; use appropriate precautions for handling and disposal (meets NIOSH 2014 criteria).

Emetic Potential Low (10% to 30%)

Monitoring Parameters Monitor CBC with platelets and differential at baseline and weekly; serum chemistries (including renal and hepatic functions tests) at baseline and before each cycle; monitor for signs/symptoms of gastrointestinal toxicity (eg, nausea, vomiting, diarrhea), tumor lysis syndrome, and infection.

Dosage Forms Excipient information presented when available (limited, particularly for generics); consult specific product labeling.

Solution Reconstituted, Intravenous:

Beleodaq: 500 mg (1 ea)

Bendamustine (ben da MUS teen)

Related Information

Common Toxicity Criteria *on page 2122*

Management of Chemotherapy-Induced Nausea and Vomiting in Adults *on page 2142*

Management of Drug Extravasations *on page 2159*

Prevention of Chemotherapy-Induced Nausea and Vomiting in Children *on page 2203*

Safe Handling of Hazardous Drugs *on page 2292*

Brand Names: US Treanda

Brand Names: Canada Treanda

Index Terms Bendamustine Hydrochloride; Cytostasan; SDX-105

Pharmacologic Category Antineoplastic Agent, Alkylating Agent; Antineoplastic Agent, Alkylating Agent (Nitrogen Mustard)

Use

Chronic lymphocytic leukemia: Treatment of chronic lymphocytic leukemia (CLL)

Non-Hodgkin lymphoma: Treatment of indolent B-cell non-Hodgkin lymphoma (NHL) which has progressed during or within 6 months of rituximab treatment or a rituximab-containing regimen

Labeled Contraindications Hypersensitivity (eg, anaphylactic or anaphylactoid reactions) to bendamustine or any component of the formulation

Pregnancy Considerations Adverse events were observed in animal reproduction studies. May cause fetal harm if administered during pregnancy. For women and men of reproductive potential, the US labeling recommends effective contraception during and for 3 months after treatment. The Canadian labeling recommends effective contraception beginning 2 weeks prior to treatment and for ≥1 month after treatment.

Breast-Feeding Considerations It is not known if bendamustine is excreted in breast milk. Due to the potential for serious adverse reactions in the nursing infant, the decision to discontinue bendamustine or discontinue breast-feeding should take into account the benefits of treatment to the mother.

Warnings/Precautions Hazardous agent - use appropriate precautions for handling and disposal (NIOSH 2014 [group 1]). Myelosuppression (neutropenia, thrombocytopenia, and anemia) is a common toxicity; may require therapy delay and/or dose reduction; monitor blood counts frequently (nadirs typically occurred in the third week of treatment). Complications due to febrile neutropenia and severe thrombocytopenia have been reported (some fatal). ANC should recover to ≥1000/mm^3 and platelets to ≥75,000/mm^3 prior to cycle initiation. Pneumonia, sepsis, and septic shock have been reported; fatalities due to infection have occurred; patients with myelosuppression are more susceptible to infection; monitor closely.

Infusion reactions, including chills, fever, pruritus, and rash are common; rarely, anaphylactic and anaphylactoid reactions have occurred, particularly with the second or subsequent cycle(s). Patients who experienced grade 3 or higher allergic reactions should not be rechallenged. Consider premedication with antihistamines, antipyretics, and corticosteroids for patients with a history of grade 1 or 2 infusion reaction. Discontinue for severe allergic reaction or grade 4 infusion reaction; consider discontinuation with grade 3 infusion reaction. Rash, toxic skin reactions and bullous exanthema have been reported with monotherapy and in combination with other antineoplastics; may be progressive or worsen with continued treatment; discontinue bendamustine treatment for severe or progressive skin reaction; monitor closely; withhold or discontinue bendamustine treatment for severe or progressive skin reaction. The risk for severe skin toxicity is increased with concurrent use of allopurinol and other medications known to cause skin toxicity; Stevens-Johnson syndrome (SJS) and toxic epidermal necrolysis (TEN) have been reported. TEN has also been reported when used in combination with rituximab. Bendamustine is an irritant with vesicant-like properties; ensure proper needle or catheter placement prior to and during infusion; avoid extravasation; erythema, marked swelling, and pain have been reported with extravasation. Bendamustine is associated with a moderate emetic potential (Basch 2011; Dupuis 2011; Roila 2010); antiemetics are recommended to prevent nausea and vomiting.

Tumor lysis syndrome (usually occurring in the first treatment cycle) may occur as a consequence of antineoplastic treatment, including treatment with bendamustine. May lead to life-threatening acute renal failure; vigorous hydration and prophylactic measures (eg, antihyperuricemic therapy) should be instituted prior to treatment in high-risk patients; monitor closely. **Note:** Allopurinol may increase the risk for bendamustine skin toxicity. May cause hypokalemia; monitor potassium closely during therapy, particularly in patients with cardiac disease.

Per manufacturer's labeling, use with caution in patients with mild hepatic impairment. However, a pharmacokinetic study showed only slight differences in bendamustine AUC and C_{max} in patients with mild hepatic impairment (defined in the study as total bilirubin 1 to 1.5 times ULN or AST greater than ULN), as compared to patients with normal hepatic function (Owen 2010). Use is not recommended in patients with moderate (AST or ALT 2.5 to 10 times ULN and total bilirubin 1.5 to 3 times ULN) or severe (total bilirubin >3 times ULN) hepatic impairment.

Use with caution in patients with mild-to-moderate renal impairment. The U.S. and Canadian product labels do not recommend use in patients with CrCl <40 mL/minute. A pharmacokinetic study illustrated only slight differences in bendamustine AUC and C_{max} in patients with mild (CrCl >50 to ≤80 mL/minute) and moderate (CrCl >30 to ≤50 mL/minute) renal dysfunction, compared to patients with normal renal function (Owen 2010). A retrospective safety study found no significant difference in lab toxicities between CLL patients with renal impairment (CrCl <40 mL/minute) compared to those without renal impairment, although an increase in grades 3/4 thrombocytopenia and grades 3/4 BUN increases were detected in patients with renal impairment (Nordstrom 2012); monitor blood counts and renal function. **Note:** UK labeling (Levact prescribing information, October 2010) recommends no dosage adjustment for patients with CrCl >10 mL/minute. Secondary malignancies (including myelodysplastic syndrome, myeloproliferative disorders, acute myeloid leukemia and bronchial cancer) and premalignant diseases have been reported in patients who have received bendamustine. Potentially significant drug-drug interactions may exist, requiring dose or frequency adjustment, additional monitoring, and/or selection of alternative therapy.

Two formulations of bendamustine are available: A liquid solution formulation (45 mg/0.5 mL and 180 mg/2 mL) and the powder for reconstitution (5 mg/mL after reconstitution). Concentrations, storage, and compatibility differ between formulations. Use caution when selecting bendamustine formulation for preparation and administration. Bendamustine solution (45 mg/0.5 mL and 180 mg/ 2 mL) contains N,N-dimethylacetamide, which is incompatible with closed-system transfer devices (CSTDs), adapters, and syringes containing polycarbonate or acrylonitrile-butadiene-styrene (ABS). When used to prepare or transfer the concentrated bendamustine solution into the infusion bag, the plastic components of these devices may dissolve, resulting in subsequent leakage and potential infusion of dissolved plastic into the patient (ISMP [Smetzer 2015]). Do not use the liquid solution formulation if CSTDs, adapters, and syringes containing polycarbonate or ABS are used **prior** to dilution in the infusion bag; according to the bendamustine manufacturer, after dilution into the infusion bag, devices containing polycarbonate or ABS (including infusion sets) may be used.

Adverse Reactions

>10%:

Cardiovascular: Peripheral edema (NHL 13%; grades 3/4: <1%)

Central nervous system: Fatigue (NHL 57% [grades 3/4: 11%]; CLL 9%), headache (21%), dizziness (14%), chills (6% to 14%), insomnia (13%)

Dermatologic: Skin rash (8% to 16%; grades 3/4: ≤3%)

Endocrine & metabolic: Weight loss (NHL 18% [grades 3/4: 2%]; CLL 7%); dehydration (14%)

Gastrointestinal: Nausea (NHL 75% [grades 3/4: 4%]; CLL 20% [grades 3/4: <1%]), vomiting (NHL 40% [grades 3/4: 3%]; CLL 16% [grades 3/4: <1%]), diarrhea (NHL 37% [grades 3/4: 3%]; CLL 9% [grades 3/4: 1%]), constipation (NHL 29%; grades 3/4: <1%), anorexia (NHL 23%; grades 3/4: 2%), stomatitis (NHL 15%; grades 3/4: <1%), decreased appetite (NHL 13%; grades 3/4: <1%), abdominal pain (NHL 5% to 13%; grades 3/4: 1%), dyspepsia (11%)

Hematologic & oncologic: Lymphocytopenia (NHL 99% [grades 3/4: 94%]; CLL 68% [grades 3/4: 47%]), bone marrow depression (grades 3/4: 98%; nadir: In week 3), leukopenia (NHL 94% [grades 3/4: 56%]; CLL 61% [grades 3/4: 28%]), decreased hemoglobin (88% to 89%; grades 3/4: 11% to 13%), decreased neutrophils (NHL 86% [grades 3/4: 60%]; CLL 75% [grades 3/4: 43%]), thrombocytopenia (77% to 86%; grades 3/4: NHL 25%; CLL 11%)

Hepatic: Increased serum bilirubin (34%; grades 3/4: 3%)

Neuromuscular & skeletal: Back pain (14%), weakness (8% to 11%)

Respiratory: Cough (NHL 22%; CLL 4%), dyspnea (16%)

Miscellaneous: Fever (NHL 34%; CLL 24%)

1% to 10%:

Cardiovascular: Tachycardia (7%), chest pain (6%), hypotension (6%), exacerbation of hypertension (≤3%)

Central nervous system: Anxiety (8%), depression (6%), pain (6%)

Dermatologic: Pruritus (5% to 6%), hyperhidrosis (5%), night sweats (5%), xeroderma (5%)

Endocrine & metabolic: Hypokalemia (9%), hyperuricemia (7%; grades 3/4: 2%), hyperglycemia (grades 3/4: 3%), hypocalcemia (grades 3/4: 2%), hyponatremia (grades 3/4: 2%)

Gastrointestinal: Gastroesophageal reflux disease (10%), xerostomia (9%), dysgeusia (7%), oral candidiasis (6%), abdominal distention (5%)

Genitourinary: Urinary tract infection (10%)

Hematologic & oncologic: Febrile neutropenia (6%)

Hepatic: Increased serum ALT (grades 3/4: 3%), increased serum AST (grades 3/4: 1%)

Hypersensitivity: Hypersensitivity (5%; grades 3/4: 1%)

Infection: Herpes zoster (10%), infection (6%; grades 3/4: 2%), herpes simplex infection (3%)

Local: Infusion site reaction (6%), catheter pain (5%)

Neuromuscular & skeletal: Arthralgia (6%), limb pain (5%), ostealgia (5%)

Renal: Increased serum creatinine (grades 3/4: 2%)

Respiratory: Upper respiratory tract infection (10%), sinusitis (9%), pharyngolaryngeal pain (8%), pneumonia (8%), nasopharyngitis (6% to 7%), nasal congestion (5%), wheezing (5%)

<1%, postmarketing, and/or case reports: Acute renal failure, alopecia, anaphylaxis, bronchogenic carcinoma, bullous rash, cardiac failure, dermatitis, dermatological reaction (toxic), drowsiness, erythema, exacerbation of hepatitis B, hemolysis, infusion related reaction, malaise, mucositis, myelodysplastic syndrome, myeloid leukemia (acute), myeloproliferative disease, pneumonitis, pulmonary fibrosis, sepsis, septic shock, skin necrosis, Stevens-Johnson syndrome, toxic epidermal necrolysis, tumor lysis syndrome

Drug Interactions

Metabolism/Transport Effects Substrate of BCRP, CYP1A2 (minor), P-glycoprotein; **Note:** Assignment of Major/Minor substrate status based on clinically relevant drug interaction potential

Avoid Concomitant Use

Avoid concomitant use of Bendamustine with any of the following: BCG (Intravesical); CloZAPine; Dipyrone

Increased Effect/Toxicity

Bendamustine may increase the levels/effects of: CloZAPine

The levels/effects of Bendamustine may be increased by: Allopurinol; CYP1A2 Inhibitors (Strong); Dipyrone

Decreased Effect

Bendamustine may decrease the levels/effects of: BCG (Intravesical)

The levels/effects of Bendamustine may be decreased by: CYP1A2 Inducers (Strong)

Storage/Stability

Powder for solution: Prior to reconstitution, store intact vials up to 25°C (77°F); excursions are permitted up to 30°C (86°F). Protect from light. The solution in the vial (reconstituted with SWFI) is stable for 30 minutes (transfer to 500 mL infusion bag within that 30 minutes). The solution diluted in 500 mL for infusion is stable for 24 hours refrigerated (2°C to 8°C ([36°F to 46°F]) or 3 hours at room temperature (15°C to 30°C [59°F to 86°F]) and room light. Infusion must be completed within these time frames.

◀ Solution: Store intact vials between 2°C to 8°C (36°F to 46°F); protect from light. Solutions diluted for infusion are stable for up to 24 hours when stored at 2°C to 8°C (36°F to 46°F) or for up to 2 hours when stored at 15°C to 30°C (59°F to 86°F) and room light. Infusion must be completed within these time frames.

Preparation for Administration Hazardous agent; use appropriate precautions for handling and disposal (NIOSH 2014 [group 1]).

Two formulations of bendamustine are available: a liquid solution formulation (45 mg/0.5 mL and 180 mg/2 mL) and the powder for reconstitution (5 mg/mL after reconstitution). Concentrations, storage, and compatibility differ between formulations. Use caution when selecting bendamustine formulation for preparation and administration. Do not mix or combine the two formulations.

Powder for solution (for reconstitution): Reconstitute 25 mg vial with 5 mL and 100 mg vial with 20 mL of sterile water for injection to a concentration of 5 mg/mL; powder usually dissolves within 5 minutes (do not use if particulates are visible). Within 30 minutes of reconstitution, dilute appropriate dose for infusion in 500 mL NS (or $D_{2.5}\frac{1}{2}$NS) to a final concentration of 0.2 to 0.6 mg/mL; mix thoroughly. Closed-system transfer devices (CSTDs) or adaptors containing polycarbonate or acrylonitrile-butadiene-styrene (ABS) are safe to use with the lyophilized powder formulation.

Solution: Prior to administration, dilute appropriate dose (using polypropylene syringes with a metal needle and polypropylene hub) in 500 mL NS (or $D_{2.5}\frac{1}{2}$NS) to a final concentration of 0.2 to 0.7 mg/mL; resulting solution should be colorless to yellow. Bendamustine contains N,N-dimethylacetamide, which is incompatible with CSTDs, adapters, and syringes containing polycarbonate or ABS. When used to prepare or transfer the concentrated bendamustine solution into the infusion bag, the plastic components of these devices may dissolve, resulting in subsequent leakage and potential infusion of dissolved plastic into the patient (ISMP [Smetzer 2015]). If using a syringe to withdraw and transfer bendamustine solution from the vial into the infusion bag, only use polypropylene syringes (translucent in appearance) with a metal needle and polypropylene hub. **After** dilution into the infusion bag, devices containing polycarbonate or ABS (including infusion sets) may be used.

Mechanism of Action Bendamustine is an alkylating agent (nitrogen mustard derivative) with a benzimidazole ring (purine analog) which demonstrates only partial cross-resistance (*in vitro*) with other alkylating agents. It leads to cell death via single and double strand DNA cross-linking. Bendamustine is active against quiescent and dividing cells. The primary cytotoxic activity is due to bendamustine (as compared to metabolites).

Pharmacodynamics/Kinetics

Distribution: V_{ss}: ~20 to 25 L

Protein binding: 94% to 96%

Metabolism: Hepatic (extensive), via CYP1A2 to active (minor) metabolites gamma-hydroxy bendamustine (M3) and N-desmethyl-bendamustine (M4); also via hydrolysis to low cytotoxic metabolites, monohydroxy bendamustine (HP1) and dihydroxy bendamustine (HP2)

Half-life elimination: Bendamustine: ~40 minutes; M3: ~3 hours; M4: ~30 minutes

Time to peak, serum: At end of infusion

Excretion: Feces (~25%); urine (~50%; ~3% as active parent drug)

Dosing

Adult & Geriatric Note: Bendamustine is associated with a moderate emetic potential (Basch 2011; Roila 2010); antiemetics are recommended to prevent nausea and vomiting.

Chronic lymphocytic leukemia (CLL): IV: 100 mg/m^2 over 30 minutes on days 1 and 2 of a 28-day treatment cycle (as a single agent) for up to 6 cycles (Knauf 2009; Knauf 2012)

CLL, first-line treatment (off-label dosing): IV: 90 mg/m^2 on days 1 and 2 of a 28-day treatment cycle (in combination with rituximab) for up to 6 cycles (Fischer 2012)

CLL, relapsed/refractory (off-label dosing): IV: 70 mg/m^2 on days 1 and 2 of a 28-day treatment cycle (in combination with rituximab) for up to 6 cycles (Fischer 2011)

Non-Hodgkin lymphomas: IV:

Lymphoma, indolent B-cell, refractory: 120 mg/m^2 over 60 minutes on days 1 and 2 of a 21-day treatment cycle (as a single agent) for up to 8 cycles (Kahl 2010)

Lymphoma, indolent B-cell, follicular, or mantle cell, first-line (off-label use): 90 mg/m^2 over 30 to 60 minutes on days 1 and 2 of a 28-day treatment cycle (in combination with rituximab) for up to 6 cycles (Rummel, 2013) **or** 90 mg/m^2 over 30 minutes on days 1 and 2 of a 28-day treatment cycle (in combination with rituximab) for 6 to 8 cycles (Flinn, 2014)

Lymphoma, follicular, relapsed or refractory (off-label use): 90 mg/m^2 over 60 minutes on days 1 and 2 of a 35-day treatment cycle (in combination with bortezomib and rituximab) for 5 cycles (Fowler 2011)

Lymphoma, mantle cell, relapsed or refractory (off-label use): 90 mg/m^2 over 30 minutes on days 2 and 3 of a 28-day treatment cycle (in combination with rituximab) for up to 4 cycles (Rummel 2005)

Hodgkin lymphoma, relapsed or refractory (off-label use): IV: 120 mg/m^2 over 30 minutes on days 1 and 2 of a 28-day treatment cycle for up to 6 cycles (Moskowitz 2013)

Multiple myeloma, salvage therapy (off-label use): IV: 90 to 100 mg/m^2 on days 1 and 2 of a 28-day treatment cycle for at least 2 cycles (Knop, 2005) **or** 75 mg/m^2 on days 1 and 2 of a 28-day treatment cycle (in combination with lenalidomide and dexamethasone) for up to 8 cycles (Lentzsch, 2012)

Waldenström macroglobulinemia, refractory (off-label use): IV: 90 mg/m^2 on days 1 and 2 of a 28-day treatment cycle (in combination with rituximab) for 6 cycles (Treon 2011) **or** 90 mg/m^2 over 30 minutes on days 2 and 3 of a 28-day treatment cycle (in combination with rituximab) for 4 cycles (Rummel 2005)

Renal Impairment

CrCl <40 mL/minute: Use is not recommended in the U.S. and Canadian manufacturers' labeling.

Study data suggest minor changes in systemic exposure may occur with mild-to-moderate renal impairment. Based on a pharmacokinetic study (patients receiving 120 mg/m^2 for 2 days every 21 days), only slight differences in bendamustine AUC and C_{max} were demonstrated in patients with mild (CrCl >50 to ≤80 mL/minute) and moderate (CrCl >30 to ≤50 mL/minute) renal dysfunction, compared to patients with normal renal function (Owen 2010). A retrospective study of bendamustine in CLL and NHL patients with renal impairment (CrCl <40 mL/minute) compared to those without (CrCl ≥60 mL/minute) found no significant difference in lab toxicities in CLL patients with renal impairment compared to those without renal impairment, although an increase in grades 3/4 thrombocytopenia was noted in NHL patients and grades 3/4 BUN increases were higher when combining data for CLL and NHL (Nordstrom 2012).

Note: UK manufacturer's labeling (Levact [prescribing information], October 2010) recommends no dosage adjustment for patients with CrCl >10 mL/minute.

Hepatic Impairment

Mild impairment: Per U.S. and Canadian manufacturers' labeling, use with caution. However, a pharmacokinetic study showed only slight differences in bendamustine AUC and C_{max} in patients with mild hepatic impairment (defined in the study as total bilirubin 1-1.5 times ULN or AST greater than ULN), compared to patients with normal hepatic function (Owen 2010).

Moderate impairment (AST or ALT 2.5-10 times ULN and total bilirubin 1.5-3 times ULN): Use is not recommended.

Severe impairment (total bilirubin >3 times ULN): Use is not recommended.

Obesity *American Society of Clinical Oncology (ASCO) Guidelines for appropriate chemotherapy dosing in obese adults with cancer:* Utilize patient's actual body weight (full weight) for calculation of body surface area- or weight-based dosing, particularly when the intent of therapy is curative; manage regimen-related toxicities in the same manner as for nonobese patients; if a dose reduction is utilized due to toxicity, consider resumption of full weight-based dosing with subsequent cycles, especially if cause of toxicity (eg, hepatic or renal impairment) is resolved (Griggs 2012).

Adjustment for Toxicity

Infusion reactions:

Grade 1 or 2: Consider premedication with antihistamines, antipyretics, and corticosteroids in subsequent cycles

Grade 3: Consider discontinuing treatment

Grade 4: Discontinue treatment

Skin reaction, severe or progressive: Withhold or discontinue treatment

Treatment delay:

Hematologic toxicity ≥ grade 4: Delay treatment until resolves (ANC ≥1000/mm^3, platelets ≥75,000/mm^3)

Nonhematologic toxicity ≥ grade 2 (clinically significant): Delay treatment until resolves to ≤ grade 1

Dose modification CLL:

Hematologic toxicity ≥ grade 3: Reduce dose to 50 mg/m^2 on days 1 and 2 of each treatment cycle. For recurrent hematologic toxicity (≥ grade 3), further reduce dose to 25 mg/m^2 on days 1 and 2 of the treatment cycle. May cautiously re-escalate dose in subsequent cycles.

Nonhematologic toxicity ≥ grade 3 (clinically significant): Reduce dose to 50 mg/m^2 on days 1 and 2 of the treatment cycle with discretion. May cautiously re-escalate dose in subsequent cycles.

Dose modification in NHL:

Hematologic toxicity grade 4: Reduce dose to 90 mg/m^2 on days 1 and 2 of each treatment cycle. For recurrent hematologic toxicity (grade 4), further reduce dose to 60 mg/m^2 on days 1 and 2 of each treatment cycle.

Nonhematologic toxicity ≥ grade 3: Reduce dose to 90 mg/m^2 on days 1 and 2 of the treatment cycle with discretion. For recurrent toxicity ≥ grade 3, further reduce dose to 60 mg/m^2 on days 1 and 2 of each treatment cycle.

Combination Regimens

Leukemia, chronic lymphocytic:

Lymphoma, non-Hodgkin (Follicular):

Multiple myeloma:

Administration Infuse over 30 minutes for the treatment of CLL and over 60 minutes for NHL; administration times for off-label uses/doses vary by protocol. Bendamustine solution (45 mg/0.5 mL and 180 mg/2 mL) contains N, N-dimethylacetamide, which is incompatible with closed-system transfer devices (CSTDs), adapters, and syringes containing polycarbonate or acrylonitrile-butadiene-styrene (ABS). After dilution of bendamustine solution into the infusion bag, devices containing polycarbonate or ABS (including infusion sets) may be used.

Consider premedication with antihistamines, antipyretics, and corticosteroids for patients with a previous grade 1 or 2 infusion reaction to bendamustine. Bendamustine is associated with a moderate emetic potential (Basch 2011; Dupuis 2011; Roila 2010); antiemetics are recommended to prevent nausea and vomiting.

Irritant with vesicant-like properties; ensure proper needle or catheter placement prior to and during infusion. Avoid extravasation; monitor IV site for redness, swelling, or pain.

Extravasation management: If extravasation occurs, stop infusion immediately and disconnect (leave cannula/needle in place); gently aspirate extravasated solution (do **NOT** flush the line); remove needle/cannula; elevate extremity. Apply dry cold compresses for 20 minutes 4 times daily (Perez Fildago 2012). May be managed with sodium thiosulfate in the same manner as mechlorethamine extravasation (Schulmeister 2011).

Sodium thiosulfate 1/6 M solution (instructions for mechlorethamine): Inject subcutaneously into extravasation area using 2 mL for each mg of drug suspected to have extravasated (Perez Fidalgo 2012; Polovich 2009).

Hazardous agent; use appropriate precautions for handling and disposal (NIOSH 2014 [group 1]).

Vesicant/Extravasation Risk Irritant with vesicant-like properties; there are case reports of erythema, swelling, and pain from extravasation

Emetic Potential Children and Adults: Moderate (30% to 90%)

◀ **Monitoring Parameters** CBC with differential and platelets (monitored weekly [initially] in clinical trials); serum creatinine; ALT, AST, and total bilirubin; monitor potassium and uric acid levels in patients at risk for tumor lysis syndrome; monitor for infusion reactions anaphylaxis, infection, and dermatologic toxicity; monitor IV site during and after infusion.

Canadian labeling also recommends periodic monitoring of blood pressure, serum glucose, and ECG (in patients with cardiac disease particularly if concomitant electrolyte disturbances).

Dosage Forms Excipient information presented when available (limited, particularly for generics); consult specific product labeling.
Solution, Intravenous:
    Treanda: 45 mg/0.5 mL (0.5 mL); 180 mg/2 mL (2 mL) [contains propylene glycol]
Solution Reconstituted, Intravenous:
    Treanda: 25 mg (1 ea); 100 mg (1 ea)

◆ **Bendamustine Hydrochloride** see Bendamustine on page 182
◆ **BeneFIX** see Factor IX (Recombinant) on page 684
◆ **BeneFix (Can)** see Factor IX (Recombinant) on page 684
◆ **Benzmethyzin** see Procarbazine on page 1436

Benzydamine (ben ZID a meen)

Brand Names: Canada Apo-Benzydamine; Dom-Benzydamine; Novo-Benzydamine; Pharixia; Tantum
Index Terms Benzydamine HCl; Benzydamine Hydrochloride; Benzydamine Mouthwash; Difflam
Pharmacologic Category Anti-inflammatory, Locally Applied; Local Anesthetic, Oral
Use Note: Not approved in the US
  Mucositis: Symptomatic relief of oropharyngeal mucositis due to radiation therapy
  Pharyngitis (acute): Relief of acute sore throat pain
Dosing
  Adult & Geriatric
    Mucositis: Oral rinse: 15 mL (undiluted solution) as a gargle or rinse 3 or 4 times daily (depending on mucositis severity); contact with inflamed mucosa should be maintained for at least 30 seconds, followed by expulsion from the mouth. Begin the day before radiation therapy, continue during radiation therapy, and after until satisfactory improvement occurs.
    Pharyngitis (acute): Oral rinse: Gargle with 15 mL (undiluted solution) every 1½ to 3 hours until symptoms resolve. Patient should expel solution from mouth following use; solution should not be swallowed.
  Pediatric
    Mucositis: Children ≥6 years and Adolescents: Oral rinse: Refer to adult dosing.
    Pharyngitis (acute): Children ≥6 years and Adolescents: Oral rinse: Refer to adult dosing.
  Renal Impairment There are no dosage adjustments provided in the manufacturer's labeling; use with caution (some absorption may occur and elimination is renal).
  Hepatic Impairment There are no dosage adjustments provided in the manufacturer's labeling.

Additional Information Complete prescribing information should be consulted for additional detail.

Product Availability Not available in the US

Dosage Forms: Canada Excipient information presented when available (limited, particularly for generics); consult specific product labeling.
Oral rinse: 0.15% (100 mL, 250 mL)

♦ **Benzydamine HCl** *see* Benzydamine *on page 190*

♦ **Benzydamine Hydrochloride** *see* Benzydamine *on page 190*

♦ **Benzydamine Mouthwash** *see* Benzydamine *on page 190*

Bevacizumab (be vuh SIZ uh mab)

Related Information
Chemotherapy-Induced Peripheral Neuropathy *on page 2116*
Common Toxicity Criteria *on page 2122*
Management of Chemotherapy-Induced Nausea and Vomiting in Adults *on page 2142*
Prevention of Chemotherapy-Induced Nausea and Vomiting in Children *on page 2203*
Principles of Anticancer Therapy *on page 2261*

Brand Names: US Avastin

Brand Names: Canada Avastin

Index Terms Anti-VEGF Monoclonal Antibody; Anti-VEGF rhuMAb; rhuMAb-VEGF

Pharmacologic Category Antineoplastic Agent, Monoclonal Antibody; Antineoplastic Agent, Vascular Endothelial Growth Factor (VEGF) Inhibitor; Vascular Endothelial Growth Factor (VEGF) Inhibitor

Use

Cervical cancer, persistent/recurrent/metastatic: Treatment of persistent, recurrent, or metastatic cervical cancer (in combination with paclitaxel and either cisplatin or topotecan). **Note:** Not an approved use in Canada.

Colorectal cancer, metastatic: First- or second-line treatment of metastatic colorectal cancer (CRC) (in combination with fluorouracil-based chemotherapy); second-line treatment of metastatic CRC (in combination with fluoropyrimidine-irinotecan- or fluoropyrimidine-oxaliplatin-based chemotherapy) after progression on a first-line treatment containing bevacizumab.
Limitations of use: Not indicated for the adjuvant treatment of colon cancer.

Glioblastoma: Treatment of progressive glioblastoma (as a single agent).
Limitations of use: Effectiveness is based on improvement in objective response rate.

Non-small cell lung cancer, nonsquamous: First-line treatment of unresectable, locally advanced, recurrent or metastatic nonsquamous non-small cell lung cancer (NSCLC) (in combination with carboplatin and paclitaxel).

Ovarian (epithelial), fallopian tube, or primary peritoneal cancer (platinum-resistant recurrent): Treatment of platinum-resistant recurrent epithelial ovarian, fallopian tube, or primary peritoneal cancer (in combination with paclitaxel, doxorubicin [liposomal], or topotecan) in patients who received no more than 2 prior chemotherapy regimens. According to the Canadian labeling, patients should not have received prior VEGF-targeted therapy (including bevacizumab).

◀ **Ovarian (epithelial), fallopian tube, or primary peritoneal cancer (platinum-sensitive recurrent):** Canadian labeling: Treatment of first recurrence platinum-sensitive epithelial ovarian, fallopian tube, or primary peritoneal cancer (in combination with carboplatin and gemcitabine). Patients should not have received prior VEGF-targeted therapy (including bevacizumab).

Renal cell carcinoma, metastatic: Treatment of metastatic renal cell carcinoma (RCC) (in combination with interferon alfa). **Note:** Not an approved use in Canada.

Labeled Contraindications There are no contraindications listed in the manufacturer's labeling.

Canadian labeling: Hypersensitivity to bevacizumab, any component of the formulation, Chinese hamster ovary cell products or other recombinant human or humanized antibodies; untreated CNS metastases

Pregnancy Considerations Based on its mechanism of action, bevacizumab would be expected to cause fetal harm if administered to a pregnant woman. Information from postmarketing reports following exposure in pregnancy is limited. Adequate contraception during therapy and for ≥6 months following the last dose is recommended due to the long half-life of bevacizumab. Bevacizumab treatment may also increase the risk of ovarian failure and impair fertility; long term effects on fertility are not known.

Breast-Feeding Considerations It is not known if bevacizumab is excreted in breast milk. Immunoglobulins are excreted in breast milk, and it is assumed that bevacizumab may appear in breast milk. Because of the potential for serious adverse reactions in the nursing infant, breast-feeding is not recommended. The half-life of bevacizumab is up to 50 days (average 20 days), and this should be considered when decisions are made concerning breast-feeding resumption.

Note: Canadian labeling recommends to discontinue breast-feeding during treatment and to avoid breast-feeding a minimum of 6 months following discontinuation of treatment.

Warnings/Precautions [US Boxed Warning]: Gastrointestinal (GI) perforation (sometimes fatal) has occurred in 0.3 to 3.2% of clinical study patients receiving bevacizumab; discontinue (permanently) if GI perforation occurs. All cervical cancer patients with GI perforation had a history of prior pelvic radiation. GI perforation was observed in patients with platinum-resistant ovarian cancer, although patients with evidence of recto-sigmoid involvement (by pelvic exam), bowel involvement (on CT scan), or clinical symptoms of bowel obstruction were excluded from the study; avoid bevacizumab use in these ovarian cancer patient populations. Most cases occur within 50 days of treatment initiation; monitor patients for signs/symptoms (eg, fever, abdominal pain with constipation and/or nausea/vomiting). GI fistula (including enterocutaneous, esophageal, duodenal, and rectal fistulas), and intra-abdominal abscess have been reported in patients receiving bevacizumab for colorectal cancer, ovarian cancer, and other cancers (not related to treatment duration). Non-GI fistula formation (including tracheoesophageal, bronchopleural, biliary, vaginal, vesical, renal, bladder, and female tract fistulas) has been observed (rarely fatal), most commonly within the first 6 months of treatment. Gastrointestinal-vaginal fistulas have been reported in cervical cancer patients, all of whom had received prior pelvic radiation; patients may also have bowel obstructions requiring surgical intervention and diverting ostomies. Permanently discontinue in patients who develop internal organ fistulas, tracheoesophageal (TE) fistula, or any grade 4 fistula. **[US Boxed Warning]: The incidence of wound healing and surgical**

complications, including serious and fatal events, is increased in patients who have received bevacizumab; discontinue with wound dehiscence. Although the appropriate interval between withholding bevacizumab and elective surgery has not been defined, bevacizumab should be discontinued at least 28 days prior to surgery and should not be reinitiated for at least 28 days after surgery and until wound is fully healed. In a retrospective review of central venous access device placements, a greater risk of wound dehiscence was observed when port placement and bevacizumab administration were separated by <14 days (Erinjeri 2011).

[US Boxed Warning]: Severe or fatal hemorrhage, including hemoptysis, gastrointestinal bleeding, central nervous system hemorrhage, epistaxis, and vaginal bleeding have been reported (up to 5 times more frequently if receiving bevacizumab). Avoid use in patients with serious hemorrhage or recent hemoptysis (≥2.5 mL blood). Serious or fatal pulmonary hemorrhage has been reported in patients receiving bevacizumab (primarily in patients with non–small cell lung cancer with squamous cell histology [not an FDA-approved indication]). Intracranial hemorrhage, including cases of grade 3 or 4 hemorrhage, has occurred in patients with previously treated glioblastoma. Treatment discontinuation is recommended in all patients with intracranial or other serious hemorrhage. Use with caution in patients with CNS metastases; once case of CNS hemorrhage was observed in an ongoing study of NSCLC patients with CNS metastases. Use in patients with untreated CNS metastases is contraindicated in the Canadian labeling. Use with caution in patients at risk for thrombocytopenia.

Bevacizumab is associated with an increased risk for arterial thromboembolic events (ATE), including cerebral infarction, stroke, MI, TIA, angina, and other ATEs, when used in combination with chemotherapy. History of ATE, diabetes, or ≥65 years of age may present an even greater risk. Although patients with cancer are already at risk for venous thromboembolism (VTE), a meta-analysis of 15 controlled trials has demonstrated an increased risk for VTE in patients who received bevacizumab (Nalluri 2008). Cervical cancer patients receiving bevacizumab plus chemotherapy may be at increased risk of grade 3 or higher VTE compared to those patients who received chemotherapy alone. Permanently discontinue therapy in patients with severe ATE or life-threatening (grade 4) VTE, including pulmonary embolism; the safety of treatment reinitiation after ATE has not been studied.

Use with caution in patients with cardiovascular disease. Among approved and nonapproved uses evaluated thus far, the incidence of heart failure (HF) and/or left ventricular dysfunction (including LVEF decline), is higher in patients receiving bevacizumab plus chemotherapy when compared to chemotherapy alone. Bevacizumab may potentiate the cardiotoxic effects of anthracyclines. HF is more common with prior anthracycline exposure and/or left chest wall irradiation. The safety of therapy resumption or continuation in patients with cardiac dysfunction has not been studied. In studies of patients with metastatic breast cancer (an off-label use), the incidence of grades 3 or 4 HF was increased in patients receiving bevacizumab plus paclitaxel, compared to the control arm. Patients with metastatic breast cancer who had received prior anthracycline therapy had a higher rate of HF compared to those receiving paclitaxel alone (3.8% vs 0.6% respectively). A meta-analysis of 5 studies which enrolled patients with metastatic breast cancer who received bevacizumab suggested an association with an increased risk of heart failure; all trials included in the analysis enrolled patients who either received prior or were receiving concurrent anthracycline therapy (Choueiri 2011).

Bevacizumab may cause and/or worsen hypertension; the incidence of severe hypertension in increased with bevacizumab. Use caution in patients with preexisting hypertension and monitor BP closely (every 2 to 3 weeks during treatment; regularly after discontinuation if bevacizumab-induced hypertension occurs or worsens). Permanent discontinuation is recommended in patients who experience a hypertensive crisis or hypertensive encephalopathy. Temporarily discontinue in patients who develop uncontrolled hypertension. An increase in diastolic and systolic blood pressures were noted in a retrospective review of patients with renal insufficiency (CrCl ≤60 mL/minute) who received bevacizumab for renal cell cancer (Gupta 2011). Cases of posterior reversible encephalopathy syndrome (PRES) have been reported. Symptoms (which include headache, seizure, confusion, lethargy, blindness and/or other vision, or neurologic disturbances) may occur from 16 hours to 1 year after treatment initiation. Resolution of symptoms usually occurs within days after discontinuation; however, neurologic sequelae may remain. PRES may be associated with hypertension; discontinue bevacizumab and begin management of hypertension, if present. The safety of treatment reinitiation after PRES is not known.

Infusion reactions (eg, hypertension, hypertensive crisis, wheezing, oxygen desaturation, hypersensitivity [including anaphylactic/anaphylactoid reactions], chest pain, rigors, headache, diaphoresis) may occur with the first infusion (uncommon); interrupt therapy in patients experiencing severe infusion reactions and administer appropriate therapy; there are no data to address routine premedication use or reinstitution of therapy in patients who experience severe infusion reactions. Cases of necrotizing fasciitis, including fatalities, have been reported (rarely); usually secondary to wound healing complications, GI perforation or fistula formation. Discontinue in patients who develop necrotizing fasciitis. Proteinuria and/or nephrotic syndrome have been associated with bevacizumab; risk may be increased in patients with a history of hypertension; thrombotic microangiopathy has been associated with bevacizumab-induced proteinuria. Withhold treatment for ≥2 g proteinuria/24 hours and resume when proteinuria is <2 g/24 hours; discontinue in patients with nephrotic syndrome. Elderly patients (≥65 years of age) are at higher risk for adverse events, including thromboembolic events and proteinuria; serious adverse events occurring more frequently in the elderly also include weakness, deep thrombophlebitis, sepsis, hyper-/hypotension, MI, CHF, diarrhea, constipation, anorexia, leukopenia, anemia, dehydration, hypokalemia, and hyponatremia. Potentially significant drug-drug interactions may exist, requiring dose or frequency adjustment, additional monitoring, and/or selection of alternative therapy. Microangiopathic hemolytic anemia (MAHA) has been reported when bevacizumab has been used in combination with sunitinib. Concurrent therapy with sunitinib and bevacizumab is also associated with dose-limiting hypertension in patients with metastatic renal cell cancer. The incidence of hand-foot syndrome is increased in patients treated with bevacizumab plus sorafenib in comparison to those treated with sorafenib monotherapy. When used in combination with myelosuppressive chemotherapy, increased rates of severe or febrile neutropenia and neutropenic infection were reported. Bevacizumab, in combination with chemotherapy (or biologic therapy), is associated with an increased risk of treatment-related mortality; a higher risk of fatal adverse events was identified in a meta-analysis of 16 trials in which bevacizumab was used for the treatment of various cancers (breast cancer, colorectal cancer, non-small cell lung cancer, pancreatic cancer, prostate cancer, and renal cell cancer) and compared to chemotherapy alone (Ranpura 2011). When bevacizumab is used in combination with myelosuppressive chemotherapy, increased rates of severe or febrile neutropenia and neutropenic infection have been reported. In premenopausal women receiving bevacizumab in combination with mFOLFOX (fluorouracil/oxaliplatin based chemotherapy) the incidence of ovarian failure (amenorrhea ≥3 months) was higher (34%) compared to women who received mFOLFOX alone (2%); ovarian function recovered in some patients after treatment was discontinued; premenopausal women should be informed of the potential risk of ovarian failure. Serious eye infections and vision loss due to endophthalmitis have been reported from intravitreal administration (off-label use/route).

Adverse Reactions Percentages reported as monotherapy and as part of combination chemotherapy regimens. Some studies only reported hematologic toxicities grades ≥4 and nonhematologic toxicities grades ≥3.

>10%:

Cardiovascular: Hypertension (12% to 34%; grades 3/4: 5% to 18%), venous thromboembolism (secondary: 21%; with oral anticoagulants), peripheral edema (15%), hypotension (7% to 15%), venous thromboembolism (8% to 14%; grades 3/4: 5% to 15%), arterial thrombosis (6%; grades 3/4: 3%)

Central nervous system: Fatigue (33% to 80%; grades 3/4: 4% to 19%), pain (8% to 62%; grades 3/4: 8%), headache (22% to 37%; grades 3/4: 3% to 4%), dizziness (19% to 26%), taste disorder (14% to 21%), peripheral sensory neuropathy (17% to 18%), anxiety (17%)

Dermatologic: Alopecia (6% to 32%), palmar-plantar erythrodysesthesia (11%), exfoliative dermatitis (>10%), xeroderma (>10%)

Endocrine & metabolic: Ovarian failure (34%), hyperglycemia (26%), hypomagnesemia (24%), weight loss (15% to 21%), hyponatremia (19%; grades 3/4: 4%), hypoalbuminemia (16%)

Gastrointestinal: Abdominal pain (50% to 61%; grades 3/4: 8%), vomiting (47% to 52%; grades 3/4: 11%), anorexia (35% to 43%), constipation (40%; grades 3/4: 4%), decreased appetite (34%), diarrhea (21%; grades 3/4: 1% to 34%), stomatitis (15% to 32%), gastrointestinal hemorrhage (19% to 24%), dyspepsia (17% to 24%), nausea (grades 3/4: 12%)

Genitourinary: Proteinuria (4% to 36%; grades >2%: grades 3/4: ≤7%; median onset: 5.6 months; median time to resolution: 6.1 months), urinary tract infection (22%; grades 3/4: -8%), pelvic pain (14%; grades 3/4: 6%)

Hematologic & oncologic: Hemorrhage (40%; grades 3/4: ≤7%), leukopenia (grades 3/4: 37%), pulmonary hemorrhage (4% to 31%), neutropenia (12%; grades ≥3: 8% to 27%, grade 4: 27%), lymphocytopenia (12%; grades 3/4: 6%)

Infection: Infection (55%; serious: 7% to 14%; pneumonia, catheter infection, or wound infection)

Neuromuscular & skeletal: Myalgia (19%), back pain (12%; grades 3/4: 6%)

Renal: Increased serum creatinine (16%)

Respiratory: Upper respiratory tract infection (40% to 47%), epistaxis (17% to 35%), dyspnea (25% to 26%), rhinitis (3% to >10%)

Miscellaneous: Postoperative wound complication (including dehiscence, 1% to 15%)

◀ 1% to 10%:

Cardiovascular: Thrombosis (8% to 10%), deep vein thrombosis (6% to 9%; grades 3/4: 9%), syncope (grades 3/4: 3%), intra-abdominal thrombosis (venous, grades 3/4: 3%), left ventricular dysfunction (grades 3/4: 1%), pulmonary embolism (1%)

Central nervous system: Voice disorder (5% to 9%)

Dermatologic: Dermal ulcer (6%), cellulitis (grades 3/4: 3%), acne vulgaris (1%)

Endocrine & metabolic: Dehydration (grades 3/4: 4% to 10%), hypokalemia (grades 3/4: 7%)

Gastrointestinal: Xerostomia (4% to 7%), rectal pain (6%), colitis (1% to 6%), intestinal obstruction (grades 3/4: 4%), gingival hemorrhage (minor, 2% to 4%), gastrointestinal perforation (≤3%), gastroesophageal reflux disease (2%), gastrointestinal fistula (≤2%), gingivitis (2%), oral mucosa ulcer (2%), gastritis (1%), gingival pain (1%)

Genitourinary: Vaginal hemorrhage (4%)

Hematologic & oncologic: Febrile neutropenia (5%), neutropenic infection (grades 3/4: 5%), thrombocytopenia (5%), hemorrhage (CNS; 5%; grades 3/4: 1%)

Infection: Abscess (tooth, 2%)

Neuromuscular & skeletal: Weakness (grades 3/4: 10%), dysarthria (8%)

Ophthalmic: Blurred vision (2%)

Otic: Tinnitus (2%), deafness (1%)

Respiratory: Pneumonitis (grades 3/4: 5%)

Miscellaneous: Fistula (gastrointestinal-vaginal; 8%), fistula (anal; 6%; grades 3/4: 4%), infusion related reaction (<3%), fistula (≤2%)

<1%, postmarketing, and/or case reports: Anaphylaxis, anastomotic ulcer, angina pectoris, antibody development (anti-bevacizumab and neutralizing), bladder fistula, bronchopleural fistula, cerebral infarction, conjunctival hemorrhage, endophthalmitis (infectious and sterile), eye discomfort, eye pain, fistula of bile duct, fulminant necrotizing fasciitis, gallbladder perforation, gastrointestinal ulcer, hemolytic anemia (microangiopathic; when used in combination with sunitinib), hemoptysis, hemorrhagic stroke, hypersensitivity, hypertensive crisis, hypertensive encephalopathy, increased intraocular pressure, inflammation of anterior segment of eye (toxic anterior segment syndrome) (Sato 2010), intestinal necrosis, intraocular inflammation (iritis, vitritis), mesenteric thrombosis, myocardial infarction, nasal septum perforation, nephrotic syndrome, ocular hyperemia, osteonecrosis of the jaw, pancytopenia, permanent vision loss, polyserositis, pulmonary hypertension, rectal fistula, renal failure, renal fistula, renal thrombotic microangiopathy, retinal detachment, retinal hemorrhage, reversible posterior leukoencephalopathy syndrome, sepsis, tracheoesophageal fistula, transient ischemic attacks, vaginal fistula, visual disturbance, vitreous hemorrhage, vitreous opacity

Drug Interactions

Metabolism/Transport Effects None known.

Avoid Concomitant Use

Avoid concomitant use of Bevacizumab with any of the following: BCG (Intravesical); Belimumab; CloZAPine; Dipyrone; SUNItinib

Increased Effect/Toxicity

Bevacizumab may increase the levels/effects of: Antineoplastic Agents (Anthracycline, Systemic); Belimumab; Bisphosphonate Derivatives; CloZAPine; SORAfenib; SUNItinib

The levels/effects of Bevacizumab may be increased by: Dipyrone; SUNItinib

Decreased Effect

Bevacizumab may decrease the levels/effects of: BCG (Intravesical)

Storage/Stability Store intact vials at 2°C to 8°C (36°F to 46°F) in original carton; do not freeze. Protect from light; do not shake. Diluted solutions are stable for up to 8 hours under refrigeration. Discard unused portion of vial.

Preparation for Administration Dilute in 100 mL NS prior to infusion (the manufacturer recommends a total volume of 100 mL). Do not mix with dextrose-containing solutions.

Mechanism of Action Bevacizumab is a recombinant, humanized monoclonal antibody which binds to, and neutralizes, vascular endothelial growth factor (VEGF), preventing its association with endothelial receptors, Flt-1 and KDR. VEGF binding initiates angiogenesis (endothelial proliferation and the formation of new blood vessels). The inhibition of microvascular growth is believed to retard the growth of all tissues (including metastatic tissue).

Pharmacodynamics/Kinetics

Distribution: V_d: 46 mL/kg

Half-life elimination:

IV:

Pediatric patients (age: 1 to 21 years): Median: 11.8 days (range: 4.4 to 14.6 days) (Glade Bender 2008)

Adults: ~20 days (range: 11 to 50 days)

Intravitreal: ~5 to 10 days (Bakri 2007; Krohne 2008)

Dosing

Adult & Geriatric

Cervical cancer, persistent/recurrent/metastatic: IV: 15 mg/kg every 3 weeks (in combination with paclitaxel and either cisplatin or topotecan) until disease progression or unacceptable toxicity (Tewari 2014)

Colorectal cancer, metastatic, in combination with fluorouracil-based chemotherapy: IV: 5 mg/kg every 2 weeks (in combination with bolus-IFL) **or** 10 mg/kg every 2 weeks (in combination with FOLFOX4)

Canadian labeling: 5 mg/kg every 2 weeks (in combination with fluorouracil-based chemotherapy)

Colorectal cancer, metastatic, following first-line therapy containing bevacizumab: IV: 5 mg/kg every 2 weeks **or** 7.5 mg/kg every 3 weeks (in combination with fluoropyrimidine-irinotecan or fluoropyrimidine-oxaliplatin based regimen)

Glioblastoma: IV: 10 mg/kg every 2 weeks as monotherapy **or** (off-label dosing) 10 mg/kg every 2 weeks (in combination with irinotecan) (Vredenburgh 2007)

Non-small cell lung cancer (nonsquamous cell histology): IV: 15 mg/kg every 3 weeks (in combination with carboplatin and paclitaxel) for 6 cycles followed by maintenance treatment (off-label use) of bevacizumab 15 mg/kg every 3 weeks as monotherapy until disease progression or unacceptable toxicity (Sandler 2006)

◀ **Ovarian (epithelial), fallopian tube, or primary peritoneal cancer (platinum-resistant recurrent):** IV: 10 mg/kg every 2 weeks (in combination with weekly paclitaxel, every 4 week doxorubicin [liposomal], or days 1, 8, and 15 topotecan) **or** 15 mg/kg every 3 weeks (in combination with every 3 week topotecan) (Pujade-Lauraine 2014)

Ovarian (epithelial), fallopian tube, or primary peritoneal cancer (platinum-sensitive recurrent): Canadian labeling: IV: 15 mg/kg every 3 weeks (in combination with carboplatin and gemcitabine) for 6 to 10 cycles then continue with bevacizumab (monotherapy) until disease progression or unacceptable toxicity (Aghajanian 2012).

Renal cell cancer, metastatic: IV: 10 mg/kg every 2 weeks (in combination with interferon alfa) **or** (off-label dosing) 10 mg/kg every 2 weeks as monotherapy (Yang 2003)

Age-related macular degeneration (off-label use/route): Intravitreal: 1.25 mg (0.05 mL) monthly for 3 months, then may be given scheduled (monthly) or as needed based on monthly ophthalmologic assessment (Chakravarthy 2013; Martin 2012)

Breast cancer, metastatic (off-label use): IV: 10 mg/kg every 2 weeks (in combination with paclitaxel) (Miller 2007)

Endometrial cancer, recurrent or persistent (off-label use): IV: 15 mg/kg every 3 weeks (as monotherapy) until disease progression or unacceptable toxicity (Aghajanian 2011)

Soft tissue sarcoma, angiosarcoma, metastatic or locally advanced (off-label use): IV: 15 mg/kg every 3 weeks until disease progression or unacceptable toxicity (Agulnik 2013). Additional data may be necessary to further define the role of bevacizumab in this condition.

Renal Impairment There are no dosage adjustments provided in the manufacturer's labeling.

Hepatic Impairment There are no dosage adjustments provided in the manufacturer's labeling.

Adjustment for Toxicity IV administration (systemic): There are no recommended dosage reductions. Temporary suspension is recommended for severe infusion reactions, at least 4 weeks prior to (and after) elective surgery, in moderate-to-severe proteinuria (in most studies, treatment was withheld for ≥2 g proteinuria/24 hours), or in patients with severe hypertension which is not controlled with medical management. Permanent discontinuation is recommended (by the manufacturer) in patients who develop wound dehiscence and wound healing complications requiring intervention, necrotizing fasciitis, fistula (gastrointestinal and nongastrointestinal), gastrointestinal perforation, intra-abdominal abscess, hypertensive crisis, hypertensive encephalopathy, serious bleeding/hemorrhage, severe arterial thromboembolic event, life-threatening (grade 4) venous thromboembolic events (including pulmonary embolism), nephrotic syndrome, or PRES.

Combination Regimens

Colorectal cancer:
Bevacizumab-Fluorouracil-Leucovorin (Colorectal) on page 1841
Bevacizumab + FOLFIRI (Colorectal) on page 1842
Bevacizumab FOLFOX (Colorectal) on page 1842
Bevacizumab + XELOX (Colorectal) on page 1846
Endometrial cancer: Bevacizumab (Endometrial Regimen) on page 1841
Lung cancer (non-small cell):
Bevacizumab-Carboplatin-Paclitaxel (NSCLC) on page 1839
Bevacizumab-Carboplatin-Pemetrexed (NSCLC) on page 1839
Bevacizumab-Cisplatin-Gemcitabine (NSCLC) on page 1840
Ovarian cancer:
Bevacizumab-Carboplatin-Gemcitabine (Ovarian) on page 1839
Bevacizumab-Doxorubicin (Liposomal) (Ovarian) on page 1841
Bevacizumab-Paclitaxel (Ovarian) on page 1845
Bevacizumab-Topotecan Daily (Ovarian) on page 1845
Bevacizumab-Topotecan Weekly (Ovarian) on page 1846
Renal cell cancer:
Bevacizumab-Interferon Alfa (RCC) on page 1844
Bevacizumab (RCC Regimen) on page 1845
Soft tissue sarcoma (angiosarcoma): Bevacizumab (Angiosarcoma Regimen) on page 1838

Administration

IV: Infuse the initial dose over 90 minutes. The second infusion may be shortened to 60 minutes if the initial infusion is well tolerated. The third and subsequent infusions may be shortened to 30 minutes if the 60-minute infusion is well tolerated. Monitor closely during the infusion for signs/symptoms of an infusion reaction. After tolerance at the 90-, 60-, and 30-minute infusion rates has been established, some institutions use an off-label 10-minute infusion rate (0.5 mg/kg/minute) for bevacizumab dosed at 5 mg/kg (Reidy 2007). In a study evaluating the safety of the 0.5 mg/kg/minute infusion rate, proteinuria and hypertension incidences were not increased with the shorter infusion time (Shah 2013). Do not administer IV push. Do not administer with dextrose solutions. Temporarily withhold bevacizumab for 4 weeks prior to elective surgery and for at least 4 weeks (and until the surgical incision is fully healed) after surgery.

Intravitreal injection (off-label use/route): Adequate local anesthesia and a topical broad-spectrum antimicrobial agent should be administered prior to the procedure.

Emetic Potential Children and Adults: Minimal <10%

Monitoring Parameters
Monitor closely during the infusion for signs/symptoms of an infusion reaction. Monitor CBC with differential; signs/symptoms of gastrointestinal perforation, fistula, or abscess (including abdominal pain, constipation, vomiting, and fever); signs/symptoms of bleeding, including hemoptysis, gastrointestinal, and/or CNS bleeding, and/or epistaxis. Monitor blood pressure every 2 to 3 weeks; more frequently if hypertension develops during therapy. Continue to monitor blood pressure after discontinuing due to bevacizumab-induced hypertension. Monitor for proteinuria/nephrotic syndrome with urine dipstick; collect 24-hour urine in patients with ≥2+ reading. Monitor for signs/symptoms of thromboembolism (arterial and venous).

AMD (off-label use): Monitor intraocular pressure and retinal artery perfusion

◄ **Dosage Forms** Excipient information presented when available (limited, particularly for generics); consult specific product labeling.
Solution, Intravenous [preservative free]:
Avastin: 100 mg/4 mL (4 mL); 400 mg/16 mL (16 mL)

Bexarotene (Systemic) (beks AIR oh teen)

Related Information
Common Toxicity Criteria *on page 2122*
Management of Chemotherapy-Induced Nausea and Vomiting in Adults *on page 2142*
Prevention of Chemotherapy-Induced Nausea and Vomiting in Children *on page 2203*
Safe Handling of Hazardous Drugs *on page 2292*

Brand Names: US Targretin
Index Terms 3-methyl TTNEB
Pharmacologic Category Antineoplastic Agent, Retinoic Acid Derivative
Use Cutaneous T-cell lymphoma, refractory: Treatment of cutaneous manifestations of cutaneous T-cell lymphoma in patients who are refractory to at least one prior systemic therapy

Labeled Contraindications
Known hypersensitivity to bexarotene or any component of the formulation; pregnancy
Documentation of allergenic cross-reactivity for retinoids is limited. However, because of similarities in chemical structure and/or pharmacologic actions, the possibility of cross-sensitivity cannot be ruled out with certainty.

Pregnancy Considerations [U.S. Boxed Warning]: Bexarotene is a retinoid, a drug class associated with birth defects in humans; do not administer during pregnancy. Bexarotene caused birth defects when administered orally to pregnant rats. It must not be given to a pregnant woman or a woman who intends to become pregnant. If a woman becomes pregnant while taking the drug, it must be stopped immediately and appropriate counseling be given. In women of childbearing potential, therapy should be started on the second or third day of a normal menstrual period. Either abstinence or 2 forms of reliable contraception (one should be nonhormonal) must be used for at least 1 month before initiating therapy, during therapy, and for 1 month following discontinuation of bexarotene. A negative pregnancy test (sensitivity of at least 50 milliunits/mL) within 1 week prior to beginning therapy, and monthly thereafter is required for women of childbearing potential. A maximum 1 month supply is recommended so that pregnancy tests may be evaluated. Male patients must use a condom during any sexual contact with women of childbearing age during therapy, and for at least 1 month following discontinuation of bexarotene.

Breast-Feeding Considerations It is not known if bexarotene is excreted into breast milk. Due to the potential for serious adverse reactions in a nursing infant, breast-feeding is not recommended by the manufacturer.

Warnings/Precautions Hazardous agent - use appropriate precautions for handling and disposal (NIOSH 2014 [group 1]). **[U.S. Boxed Warning]: Bexarotene is a retinoid, a drug class associated with birth defects in humans; do not administer during pregnancy. Bexarotene caused birth defects when administered orally to pregnant rats.** Pregnancy test needed within 1 week before initiation and every month thereafter. Effective contraception must be in place 1 month before initiation, during therapy, and for at least 1 month after discontinuation. Male patients with sexual partners who are pregnant, possibly pregnant, or who could become pregnant, must use condoms during sexual intercourse during treatment and for at least 1 month after last dose.

Bexarotene induces significant lipid abnormalities in a majority of patients (elevated triglycerides and total cholesterol, and decreased high-density lipoprotein [HDL]) and usually occur within 2 to 4 weeks; effects are reversible on discontinuation or generally mitigated by dose reduction and/or antilipemic therapy. Monitor fasting lipid panel; may require dose reduction, treatment interruption, and/or concomitant antilipemic therapy. Fasting triglycerides should be normal (or normalized with appropriate therapy) prior to initiation; triglycerides should be maintained <400 mg/dL. In studies, HMG-CoA reductase inhibitors were used to manage lipids; gemfibrozil is not recommended due to potential for drug interactions. Pancreatitis associated with hypertriglyceridemia has been reported. Interrupt treatment and evaluate if pancreatitis is suspected. Cutaneous T-cell lymphoma patients with risk factors for pancreatitis (eg, prior pancreatitis, uncontrolled hyperlipidemia, excessive ethanol consumption, uncontrolled diabetes, biliary tract disease, concomitant medications causing hyperlipidemia or concomitant medications associated with pancreatic toxicity) may be at increased risk for bexarotene-associated pancreatitis. Dose-related elevations in ALT, AST, and bilirubin have been reported; cases of cholestasis and liver failure (fatal) have occurred. Monitor for liver function test abnormalities and temporarily withhold or discontinue if ALT, AST, or bilirubin are >3 times the upper limit of normal (ULN). Liver function test elevations resolved within 1 month in most patients following dose reduction or discontinuation. Bexarotene rapidly suppresses thyroid-stimulating hormone (TSH) levels by directly inhibiting TSH secretion and also affects thyroid hormone metabolism (Hamnvik, 2011). Reductions in total thyroxine (T_4) and thyroid-stimulating hormone (TSH) are reversible. Hypothyroidism commonly occur. Monitor thyroid functions tests, including free T_4 levels at baseline and during treatment Thyroid supplementation is usually required; patients already receiving thyroid hormone therapy may require increased thyroid hormone doses to achieve therapeutic levels (Hamnvik, 2011). Grade 1 to 3 leukopenia has occurred (predominantly as neutropenia); the incidence is higher with doses >300 mg/m²/day. The onset of leukopenia was generally 4 to 8 weeks. Grade 3 and 4 neutropenia have occurred. Leukopenia and neutropenia typically resolved within 30 days after discontinuation or dose reduction. Monitor complete blood cell count (CBC) with differential at baseline and periodically during treatment. Leukopenia and neutropenia were rarely associated with severe conditions or serious adverse events. Any new visual abnormalities experienced by the patient should be evaluated by an ophthalmologist (cataracts may develop or worsen, especially in the geriatric population).

Retinoids are associated with photosensitivity; phototoxicity (sunburn, sunlight sensitivity) has occurred with bexarotene when patients were exposed to direct sunlight; advise patients to minimize exposure to sunlight and artificial ultraviolet light during treatment. Use with extreme caution in patients with hepatic impairment; bexarotene undergoes extensive hepatic elimination. Due to the potential for additive toxicities, patients should be advised to limit additional vitamin A intake (in studies, additional vitamin A was limited to ≤15,000 units/day). Use caution with diabetic patients; may enhance the actions of insulin, sulfonylureas or thiazolidinediones, resulting in hypoglycemia in patients receiving these agents (hypoglycemia has not been observed with bexarotene monotherapy). Monitor blood glucose as necessary. Potentially significant drug-drug interactions may exist, requiring dose or frequency adjustment, additional monitoring, and/or selection of alternative therapy.

Adverse Reactions

>10%:

Cardiovascular: Peripheral edema (11% to 13%)

Central nervous system: Headache (30% to 42%), fever (5% to 17%), chills (10% to 13%), insomnia (5% to 11%)

Dermatologic: Rash (17% to 23%), exfoliative dermatitis (10% to 28%), dry skin (9% to 11%), alopecia (4% to 11%)

Endocrine & metabolic: Hyperlipidemia (79%), hypercholesteremia (32% to 62%), hypothyroidism (29% to 53%)

Gastrointestinal: Diarrhea (7% to 42%), anorexia (2% to 23%), nausea (8% to 16%), vomiting (4% to 13%), abdominal pain (4% to 11%)

Hematologic: Leukopenia (17% to 47%), anemia (6% to 25%), hypochromic anemia (4% to 13%)

Hepatic: LDH increased (7% to 13%)

Neuromuscular & skeletal: Weakness (20% to 45%), back pain (2% to 11%)

Miscellaneous: Infection (13% to 23%; bacterial: 1% to 13%), flu-like syndrome (4% to 13%)

<10%:

Cardiovascular: Angina pectoris, cerebrovascular accident, chest pain, heart failure (right), hypertension, syncope, tachycardia

Central nervous system: Agitation, ataxia, confusion, depression, dizziness, hyperesthesia, subdural hematoma

Dermatologic: Acne, cellulitis, cheilitis, maculopapular rash, photosensitivity, pustular rash, serous drainage, skin nodule, skin rash, skin sensitivity, sunburn, vesicular bullous rash

Endocrine & metabolic: Breast pain, hypoproteinemia, hyperglycemia

Gastrointestinal: Amylase increased, colitis, constipation, dyspepsia, flatulence, gastroenteritis, gingivitis, melena, pancreatitis, weight loss/gain, xerostomia

Genitourinary: Dysuria, hematuria, urinary incontinence, urinary tract infection, urinary urgency

Hematologic: Coagulopathy, eosinophilia, hemorrhage, lymphocytosis, thrombocythemia, thrombocytopenia

Hepatic: ALT increased, AST increased, bilirubin increased, hepatic failure

Neuromuscular & skeletal: Arthralgia, arthrosis, bone pain, myalgia, myasthenia, neuropathy

Ocular: Blepharitis, cataracts (new and worsening), conjunctivitis, corneal lesion, dry eyes, keratitis, visual field defects

Otic: Ear pain, otitis externa

Renal: Albuminuria, creatinine increased, renal function abnormal

Respiratory: Bronchitis, cough, dyspnea, hemoptysis, hypoxia, pharyngitis, pleural effusion, pneumonia, pulmonary edema, rhinitis

Miscellaneous: Monilia, sepsis

Drug Interactions

Metabolism/Transport Effects Substrate of CYP3A4 (minor); **Note:** Assignment of Major/Minor substrate status based on clinically relevant drug interaction potential; **Induces** CYP3A4 (moderate)

Avoid Concomitant Use

Avoid concomitant use of Bexarotene (Systemic) with any of the following: Antihepaciviral Combination Products; Axitinib; BCG (Intravesical); Bedaquiline; Bosutinib; CloZAPine; Cobimetinib; Dipyrone; Flibanserin; Gemfibrozil; Multivitamins/Fluoride (with ADE); Multivitamins/Minerals (with ADEK, Folate, Iron); Multivitamins/Minerals (with AE, No Iron); Nisoldipine; Olaparib; Palbociclib; Ranolazine; Simeprevir; Sonidegib; Tetracycline Derivatives; Vitamin A

Increased Effect/Toxicity

Bexarotene (Systemic) may increase the levels/effects of: Clarithromycin; CloZAPine; Ifosfamide; Porfimer; Verteporfin

The levels/effects of Bexarotene (Systemic) may be increased by: CARBOplatin; Dipyrone; Gemfibrozil; Multivitamins/Fluoride (with ADE); Multivitamins/Minerals (with ADEK, Folate, Iron); Multivitamins/Minerals (with AE, No Iron); PACLitaxel (Conventional); Tetracycline Derivatives; Vitamin A

Decreased Effect

Bexarotene (Systemic) may decrease the levels/effects of: Antihepaciviral Combination Products; ARIPiprazole; AtorvaSTATin; Axitinib; BCG (Intravesical); Bedaquiline; Bosutinib; Clarithromycin; Cobimetinib; Contraceptives (Estrogens); Contraceptives (Progestins); CYP3A4 Substrates; Daclatasvir; FentaNYL; Flibanserin; Hydrocodone; Ibrutinib; Ifosfamide; NiMODipine; Nisoldipine; Olaparib; PACLitaxel (Conventional); Palbociclib; Ranolazine; Rolapitant; Saxagliptin; Simeprevir; Sonidegib; Tamoxifen

Food Interactions Bioavailability is increased when administered with a fat-containing meal. Management: Administer with food.

Storage/Stability Store at 2°C to 25°C (36°F to 77°F). Protect from light. Avoid humidity and high temperatures after opening bottle.

Mechanism of Action Selectively binds to and activates retinoid X receptors (RXRs). Once activated, RXRs function as transcription factors to regulate the expression of genes which control cellular differentiation and proliferation. Bexarotene inhibits the growth *in vitro* of some tumor cell lines of hematopoietic and squamous cell origin and induces tumor regression *in vivo* in some animal models.

Pharmacodynamics/Kinetics

Absorption: Improved 48% by a fat-containing meal

Protein binding: >99% to plasma proteins

Metabolism: Hepatic via CYP3A4 isoenzyme to four metabolites; further metabolized by glucuronidation

Half-life elimination: ~7 hours

Time to peak: ~2 hours

Excretion: Feces (primarily); urine (minimal, <1%)

Dosing

Adult & Geriatric

Cutaneous T-cell lymphoma, refractory: Oral: Initial: 300 mg/m^2 once daily taken as a single daily dose; if well tolerated, but no tumor response after 8 weeks, may increase to 400 mg/m^2 once daily; continue as long as clinical benefit is demonstrated (bexarotene was administered in studies for up to 97 weeks).

Mycosis fungoides/Sezary syndrome, refractory/resistant (off-label dose): Oral: 75 to 150 mg daily in combination with PUVA; maximum dose: 300 mg daily (Rupoli, 2010; Singh, 2004)

◄ **Renal Impairment** There are no dosage adjustments provided in the manufacturer's labeling (has not been studied); however, although renal elimination is a minor excretion pathway, renal insufficiency may result in significant protein binding changes and alter pharmacokinetics of bexarotene.

Hepatic Impairment There are no dosage adjustments provided in the manufacturer's labeling (has not been studied); however, hepatic impairment would be expected to result in decreased clearance of bexarotene due to the extensive hepatic contribution to elimination.

Obesity *ASCO Guidelines for appropriate chemotherapy dosing in obese adults with cancer:* Utilize patient's actual body weight (full weight) for calculation of body surface area- or weight-based dosing, particularly when the intent of therapy is curative; manage regimen-related toxicities in the same manner as for nonobese patients; if a dose reduction is utilized due to toxicity, consider resumption of full weight-based dosing with subsequent cycles, especially if cause of toxicity (eg, hepatic or renal impairment) is resolved (Griggs, 2012).

Adjustment for Toxicity If necessitated by toxicity, may decrease dose from 300 mg/m²/day to 200 mg/m²/day, then to 100 mg/m²/day, or temporarily hold. Upon recovery, may titrate dose upward with careful monitoring.

Hepatotoxicity: If AST, ALT, or bilirubin >3 times ULN, consider withholding or discontinuing therapy.

Hypertriglyceridemia: Consider dose reduction, treatment interruption, and or antilipemic therapy.

Leukopenia and neutropenia: Leukopenia and neutropenia resolved after dose reduction or discontinuation.

Combination Regimens

Lymphoma, non-Hodgkin (CTCL): Bexarotene (NHL-CTCL Regimen) on page 1847

Administration Administer with a meal. Hazardous agent; use appropriate precautions for handling and disposal (NIOSH 2014 [group 1]). Avoid contact with broken or leaking capsules; if contact occurs, wash immediately with soap and water. If it is necessary to manipulate the capsules (eg, to prepare an oral suspension), it is recommended to double glove, wear a protective gown, and prepare in a controlled device (NIOSH, 2014).

Emetic Potential Children and Adults: Low (10% to 30%)

Extemporaneous Preparations Hazardous agent: Use appropriate precautions for handling and disposal (NIOSH 2014 [group 1]). When manipulating capsules, NIOSH recommends double gloving, a protective gown, and preparation in a controlled device; if not prepared in a controlled device, respiratory and eye protection as well as ventilated engineering controls are recommended (NIOSH, 2014).

A 1 mg/mL oral suspension may be prepared with capsules. Cut one 75 mg capsule in half, rinse the interior contents of the capsule, and suspend with 75 mL sterile water. Administer immediately after preparation. To ensure administration of full dose, rinse empty glass with half a glass of water and administer residue.

Targretin data on file, Eisai Inc.

Monitoring Parameters If female, pregnancy test within 1 week before initiation then monthly while on bexarotene; fasting lipid panel (before initiation, then weekly until lipid response established [usually 2 to 4 weeks] and then at 8-week intervals thereafter); liver function tests (baseline, then at 1, 2, and 4 weeks after initiation, then at 8-week intervals thereafter if stable); monitor thyroid function tests (including free T_4) at baseline and weekly for the first 5 to 7 weeks, then every 1 to 2 months (Hamnvik, 2011); CBC with differential (baseline and periodic); blood glucose (in diabetic patients); ophthalmic exam (if visual abnormalities occur)

Test Interactions Treatment with bexarotene may interfere with CA125 assay values in patients with ovarian cancer (per manufacturer's labeling).

Dietary Considerations Avoid grapefruit juice.

Dosage Forms Excipient information presented when available (limited, particularly for generics); consult specific product labeling.

Capsule, Oral:
Targretin: 75 mg
Generic: 75 mg

Bexarotene (Topical) (beks AIR oh teen)

Related Information
Safe Handling of Hazardous Drugs *on page 2292*

Brand Names: US Targretin

Pharmacologic Category Antineoplastic Agent, Retinoic Acid Derivative

Use Cutaneous T-cell lymphoma: Topical treatment of cutaneous lesions in patients with refractory or persistent cutaneous T-cell lymphoma (stage 1A and 1B) or who have not tolerated other therapies

Labeled Contraindications
Known hypersensitivity to bexarotene or any component of the formulation; pregnancy

Documentation of allergenic cross-reactivity for drugs in this class is limited. However, because of similarities in chemical structure and/or pharmacologic actions, the possibility of cross-sensitivity cannot be ruled out with certainty.

Pregnancy Considerations Bexarotene is a retinoid, a drug class associated with birth defects in humans; do not administer during pregnancy. Bexarotene caused birth defects when administered orally to pregnant rats. It must not be given to a pregnant woman or a woman who intends to become pregnant. If a woman becomes pregnant while using the gel, it must be stopped immediately and appropriate counseling be given. In women of childbearing potential, therapy should be started on the second or third day of a normal menstrual period. Either abstinence or two forms of reliable contraception (one should be nonhormonal) must be used for at least 1 month before initiating therapy, during therapy, and for 1 month following discontinuation of bexarotene. A negative pregnancy test (sensitivity of at least 50 milliunits/mL) within 1 week prior to beginning therapy, and monthly thereafter is required for women of childbearing potential. Males patients must use a condom during any sexual contact with women of childbearing age during therapy, and for 1 month following discontinuation of bexarotene

Breast-Feeding Considerations It is not known if bexarotene is excreted into breast milk. Due to the potential for serious adverse reactions in a nursing infant, a decision should be made to discontinue bexarotene gel or to discontinue breast-feeding during therapy, taking into account the importance of treatment to the mother.

Warnings/Precautions Hazardous agent - use appropriate precautions for handling and disposal (NIOSH 2014 [group 1]). **Bexarotene is a retinoid, a drug class associated with birth defects in humans; do not administer during pregnancy.** Pregnancy test needed 1 week before initiation and every month thereafter. Effective contraception must be in place 1 month before initiation, during therapy, and for at least 1 month after discontinuation. Male ▶

patients with sexual partners who are pregnant, possibly pregnant, or who could become pregnant, must use condoms during sexual intercourse during treatment and for 1 month after last dose. May induce lipid abnormalities; reversible on discontinuation. Use with caution in patients with known hypersensitivity to other retinoids. Retinoids may cause photosensitization; minimize sunlight and artificial UV light exposure during treatment. Due to the potential for additive toxicities, patients should be advised to limit additional vitamin A intake to <15,000 units/day. Patients should avoid insect repellents containing N,N-diethyl-meta-toluamide (DEET) while using topical bexarotene (animal studies demonstrated increased DEET toxicity). Potentially significant drug-drug interactions may exist, requiring dose or frequency adjustment, additional monitoring, and/or selection of alternative therapy.

Adverse Reactions

Cardiovascular: Edema (10%)

Central nervous system: Headache (14%), weakness (6%), pain (30%)

Dermatologic: Rash (14% to 72%), pruritus (6% to 40%), contact dermatitis (14%), exfoliative dermatitis (6%)

Endocrine & metabolic: Hyperlipidemia (10%)

Hematologic: Leukopenia (6%), lymphadenopathy (6%)

Neuromuscular & skeletal: Paresthesia (6%)

Respiratory: Cough (6%), pharyngitis (6%)

Miscellaneous: Diaphoresis (6%), infection (18%)

Drug Interactions

Metabolism/Transport Effects Substrate of CYP3A4 (minor); **Note:** Assignment of Major/Minor substrate status based on clinically relevant drug interaction potential

Avoid Concomitant Use There are no known interactions where it is recommended to avoid concomitant use.

Increased Effect/Toxicity

Bexarotene (Topical) may increase the levels/effects of: Porfimer; Verteporfin

The levels/effects of Bexarotene (Topical) may be increased by: Multivitamins/Fluoride (with ADE); Multivitamins/Minerals (with ADEK, Folate, Iron); Multivitamins/Minerals (with AE, No Iron); Vitamin A

Decreased Effect There are no known significant interactions involving a decrease in effect.

Storage/Stability Store at 25°C (77°F); excursions are permitted between 15°C and 30°C (59°F and 86°F). Avoid exposure to high temperatures and humidity after the tube is opened. Protect from light. Keep away from open flame.

Mechanism of Action Binds to and activates retinoid X receptor subtypes. Once activated, these receptors function as transcription factors that regulate the expression of genes which control cellular differentiation and proliferation.

Pharmacodynamics/Kinetics

Onset: Response may be seen at 4 weeks, although longer application may be required for response (range: up to 56 weeks).

Absorption: Systemically absorbed following topical application (1% gel: generally less than 5 ng/mL and did not exceed 55 ng/mL)

Protein binding: >99% to plasma proteins

Dosing

Adult & Geriatric

Cutaneous T-cell lymphoma: Topical: Apply to lesions once every other day for first week, then increase on a weekly basis to once daily, 2 times daily, 3 times daily, and finally 4 times daily, according to individual lesion tolerance. Continue as long as deriving benefit. Response is usually observed with application at 2 to 4 times daily. May decrease frequency if local toxicity occurs; for severe irritation, temporarily withhold for a few days until symptoms subside.

Renal Impairment There are no dosage adjustments provided in the manufacturer's labeling (has not been studied); however, although renal elimination is a minor excretion pathway, renal insufficiency may result in significant protein binding changes and altered pharmacokinetics of bexarotene.

Hepatic Impairment There are no dosage adjustments provided in the manufacturer's labeling (has not been studied); however, hepatic impairment would be expected to result in decreased clearance of bexarotene due to the extensive hepatic contribution to elimination.

Administration Using a clean, dry finger, apply a sufficient amount to cover lesion with a generous coating. Allow gel to dry before covering with clothing. Avoid application to normal skin; do not apply near mucosal surfaces. Use of occlusive dressings is not recommended. If applying after bathing/showering, wait 20 minutes prior to application. Avoid bathing/showering/swimming for at least 3 hours following application (if possible). Following application, wipe excess gel from finger with a disposable tissue and wash hands with soap and water. Hazardous agent; use appropriate precautions for handling and disposal (NIOSH 2014 [group 1]).

Monitoring Parameters If female, pregnancy test 1 week before initiation then monthly while on bexarotene

Dosage Forms Excipient information presented when available (limited, particularly for generics); consult specific product labeling.

Gel, External:

Targretin: 1% (60 g) [contains alcohol, usp]

♦ **Bexxar [DSC]** *see* Tositumomab and Iodine I 131 Tositumomab *on page 1663*

♦ **Bexxar (Can)** *see* Tositumomab and Iodine I 131 Tositumomab *on page 1663*

♦ **BIBW 2992** *see* Afatinib *on page 50*

Bicalutamide (bye ka LOO ta mide)

Related Information

Safe Handling of Hazardous Drugs *on page 2292*

Brand Names: US Casodex

Brand Names: Canada ACH-Bicalutamide; ACT Bicalutamide; Apo-Bicalutamide; Casodex; Dom-Bicalutamide; JAMP-Bicalutamide; Mylan-Bicalutamide; PHL-Bicalutamide; PMS-Bicalutamide; PRO-Bicalutamide; RAN-Bicalutamide; Sandoz-Bicalutamide; Teva-Bicalutamide

Index Terms CDX; ICI-176334

Pharmacologic Category Antineoplastic Agent, Antiandrogen

◄ **Use**

Prostate cancer, metastatic: Treatment of stage D_2 metastatic prostate cancer (in combination with an LHRH agonist)

Limitation of use: Bicalutamide 150 mg daily is not approved for use alone or with other treatments

Labeled Contraindications

Hypersensitivity to bicalutamide or any component of the formulation; use in women, especially women who are or may become pregnant

Canadian labeling: Additional contraindications (not in U.S. labeling): Patients with localized prostate cancer undergoing watchful waiting; children

Pregnancy Considerations Adverse events were observed in animal reproduction studies. Bicalutamide use is contraindicated in women. Androgen receptor inhibition during pregnancy may affect fetal development.

Breast-Feeding Considerations Bicalutamide is not indicated for use in women.

Warnings/Precautions Hazardous agent - use appropriate precautions for handling and disposal (NIOSH 2014 [group 1]). Rare cases of death or hospitalization due to hepatitis have been reported postmarketing. Use with caution in moderate-to-severe hepatic dysfunction. Hepatotoxicity generally occurs within the first 3 to 4 months of use; patients should be monitored for signs and symptoms of liver dysfunction. Bicalutamide should be discontinued if patients have jaundice or ALT is >2 times the upper limit of normal. Androgen-deprivation therapy may increase the risk for cardiovascular disease (Levine, 2010). Androgen deprivation therapy may cause prolongation of the QT/QTc interval (Garnick, 2004); evaluate risk versus benefit in patients with congenital long QT syndrome, heart failure, frequent electrolyte abnormalities, and in patients taking medication known to prolong the QT interval. Correct electrolytes prior to initiation and consider periodic electrolyte and ECG monitoring.

Anemia may occur with testosterone suppression; monitor CBC periodically as indicated. Interstitial lung disease has been reported rarely (including fatalities) although mostly at dosages greater than what is recommended; promptly evaluate any worsening of respiratory symptoms (eg, dyspnea, cough and fever). Prolonged use of antiandrogen therapy is associated with decreased bone mineral density and an increased risk of osteoporosis and fracture (Smith, 2003); alcohol abuse, familial history of osteoporosis, and/or chronic use of drugs capable of decreasing bone mass (eg, corticosteroids) may increase risk. Evaluate risk carefully before initiating therapy.

May cause gynecomastia, breast pain, or lead to spermatogenesis inhibition. When used in combination with LHRH agonists, a loss of glycemic control and decrease in glucose tolerance has been reported in patients with diabetes; monitor. May cause gynecomastia or breast pain (at higher, off-label doses), or lead to spermatogenesis inhibition. Potentially significant drug-drug interactions may exist, requiring dose or frequency adjustment, additional monitoring, and/or selection of alternative therapy. Discontinue use immediately if disease worsens; decreased prostate specific antigen (PSA) levels and/or clinical improvement may be observed in some patients when antiandrogen therapy is held due to worsening of disease. The Canadian labeling recommends monitoring patients for 6 to 8 weeks after interrupting therapy to observe for withdrawal response.

Adverse Reactions Adverse reaction percentages reported as part of combination regimen with an LHRH analogue unless otherwise noted.

>10%:
  Cardiovascular: Peripheral edema (13%)
  Central nervous system: Pain (35%)
  Endocrine & metabolic: Hot flash (53%), gynecomastia (9%; monotherapy [150 mg]: 38% to 73% [McLeod 2006])
  Gastrointestinal: Constipation (22%), nausea (15%), diarrhea (12%), abdominal pain (11%)
  Genitourinary: Mastalgia (6%; monotherapy [150 mg]: 39% to 85% [McLeod 2006]), pelvic pain (21%), hematuria (12%), nocturia (12%)
  Hematologic & oncologic: Anemia (11%)
  Infection: Infection (18%)
  Neuromuscular & skeletal: Back pain (25%), weakness (22%)
  Respiratory: Dyspnea (13%)
≥2% to 10%:
  Cardiovascular: Chest pain (8%), hypertension (8%), angina pectoris (2% to <5%), cardiac arrest (2% to <5%), cardiac failure (2% to <5%), coronary artery disease (2% to <5%), edema (2% to <5%), myocardial infarction (2% to <5%), syncope (2% to <5%)
  Central nervous system: Dizziness (10%), paresthesia (8%), headache (7%), insomnia (7%), myasthenia (7%), anxiety (5%), chills (2% to <5%), confusion (2% to <5%), drowsiness (2% to <5%), hypertonia (2% to <5%), nervousness (2% to <5%), neuropathy (2% to <5%), depression (4%)
  Dermatologic: Skin rash (9%), diaphoresis (6%), alopecia (2% to <5%), pruritus (2% to <5%), xeroderma (2% to <5%)
  Endocrine & metabolic: Weight loss (7%), hyperglycemia (6%), weight gain (5%), decreased libido (2% to <5%), dehydration (2% to <5%), gout (2% to <5%), hypercholesterolemia (2% to <5%)
  Gastrointestinal: Dyspepsia (7%), anorexia (6%), flatulence (6%), vomiting (6%), dysphagia (2% to <5%), hernia (2% to <5%), melena (2% to <5%), periodontal abscess (2% to <5%), xerostomia (2% to <5%)
  Genitourinary: Urinary tract infection (9%), impotence (7%), difficulty in micturition (5%), urinary retention (5%), dysuria (2% to <5%), urinary urgency (2% to <5%), urinary incontinence (4%)
  Hematologic & oncologic: Gastrointestinal carcinoma (2% to <5%), rectal hemorrhage (2% to <5%), skin carcinoma (2% to <5%)
  Hepatic: Increased liver enzymes (7%), increased serum alkaline phosphatase (5%)
  Infection: Herpes zoster (2% to <5%), sepsis (2% to <5%)
  Neuromuscular & skeletal: Ostealgia (9%), arthritis (5%), leg cramps (2% to <5%), myalgia (2% to <5%), neck pain (2% to <5%), pathological fracture (4%)
  Ophthalmic: Cataract (2% to <5%)
  Renal: Polyuria (6%), hydronephrosis (2% to <5%), increased blood urea nitrogen (2% to <5%), increased serum creatinine (2% to <5%)
  Respiratory: Cough (8%), pharyngitis (8%), flu-like symptoms (7%), bronchitis (6%), asthma (2% to <5%), epistaxis (2% to <5%), sinusitis (2% to <5%), pneumonia (4%), rhinitis (4%)
  Miscellaneous: Cyst (2% to <5%), fever (2% to <5%)

◀ <1%, postmarketing, and/or case reports: Decreased glucose tolerance, decreased hemoglobin, decreased white blood cell count, hepatic failure, hepatitis, hepatotoxicity, hypersensitivity (including angioedema and urticaria), increased serum ALT, increased serum AST, increased serum bilirubin, interstitial pneumonitis, interstitial pulmonary disease (most often at doses >50 mg), pulmonary fibrosis, skin photosensitivity

Drug Interactions

Metabolism/Transport Effects Inhibits CYP3A4 (weak)

Avoid Concomitant Use

Avoid concomitant use of Bicalutamide with any of the following: Astemizole; Cisapride; Indium 111 Capromab Pendetide; Pimozide; Terfenadine

Increased Effect/Toxicity

Bicalutamide may increase the levels/effects of: ARIPiprazole; Astemizole; Cisapride; Dofetilide; Flibanserin; Hydrocodone; Lomitapide; NiMODipine; Pimozide; Porfimer; Terfenadine; Verteporfin; Vitamin K Antagonists

Decreased Effect

Bicalutamide may decrease the levels/effects of: Choline C 11; Indium 111 Capromab Pendetide

Storage/Stability Store at room temperature of 20°C to 25°C (68°F to 77°F).

Mechanism of Action Androgen receptor inhibitor; pure nonsteroidal antiandrogen that binds to androgen receptors; specifically a competitive inhibitor for the binding of dihydrotestosterone and testosterone; prevents testosterone stimulation of cell growth in prostate cancer

Pharmacodynamics/Kinetics

Absorption: Well absorbed; unaffected by food

Protein binding: 96%

Metabolism: Extensively hepatic; glucuronidation and oxidation of the R (active) enantiomer to inactive metabolites; the S enantiomer is inactive

Half-life elimination:

　Active enantiomer: ~6 days

　Active enantiomer (in patients with severe liver disease): ~10 days

　R-isomer (in patients with severe liver disease): Increased ~76%

Time to peak, plasma: Active enantiomer: ~31 hours

Excretion: Urine and feces

Dosing

Adult & Geriatric

Prostate cancer, metastatic: Oral: 50 mg once daily (in combination with an LHRH analogue)

Prostate cancer, locally-advanced, high recurrence risk (off-label use): Oral: 150 mg once daily (as monotherapy) (McLeod, 2006). Additional trials may be necessary to further define the role of bicalutamide in this condition.

Renal Impairment No dosage adjustment necessary.

Hepatic Impairment

Hepatic impairment at treatment initiation: Mild, moderate, or severe impairment: No dosage adjustment is necessary. Use with caution in patients with moderate-to-severe impairment; clearance may be delayed in severe impairment (based on a limited number of patients).

Hepatic impairment during treatment: ALT >2 times ULN or jaundice develops: Discontinue immediately.

Administration Dose should be taken at the same time each day, either in the morning or in the evening. May be administered with or without food. Treatment for metastatic cancer should be started concomitantly with an LHRH analogue.

Hazardous agent; use appropriate precautions for handling and disposal (NIOSH 2014 [group 1]).

Monitoring Parameters Periodically monitor CBC, ECG, echocardiograms, serum testosterone, luteinizing hormone, and prostate specific antigen (PSA). Liver function tests should be obtained at baseline and repeated regularly during the first 4 months of treatment, and periodically thereafter; monitor for signs and symptoms of liver dysfunction (discontinue if jaundice is noted or ALT is >2 times the upper limit of normal). Monitor blood glucose in patients with diabetes. If initiating bicalutamide in patients who are on warfarin, closely monitor prothrombin time.

Dosage Forms Excipient information presented when available (limited, particularly for generics); consult specific product labeling.
Tablet, Oral:
Casodex: 50 mg
Generic: 50 mg

Bleomycin (blee oh MYE sin)

Related Information
Brand Names: Canada Blenoxane; Bleomycin Injection, USP
Index Terms Blenoxane; Bleo; Bleomycin Sulfate; BLM
Pharmacologic Category Antineoplastic Agent, Antibiotic

◀ **Use**

   Head and neck cancers: Treatment of squamous cell carcinomas of the head and neck

   Hodgkin lymphoma: Treatment of Hodgkin lymphoma

   Malignant pleural effusion: Sclerosing agent for malignant pleural effusion

   Testicular cancer: Treatment of testicular cancer

Labeled Contraindications Hypersensitivity to bleomycin or any component of the formulation

Pregnancy Considerations Adverse effects were observed in animal reproduction studies. According to the manufacturer, women of childbearing potential should avoid becoming pregnant during bleomycin treatment. The European Society for Medical Oncology has published guidelines for diagnosis, treatment, and follow-up of cancer during pregnancy; the guidelines recommend referral to a facility with expertise in cancer during pregnancy and encourage a multidisciplinary team (obstetrician, neonatologist, oncology team). In general, if chemotherapy is indicated, it should be avoided in the first trimester and there should be a 3-week time period between the last chemotherapy dose and anticipated delivery, and chemotherapy should not be administered beyond week 33 of gestation (Peccatori 2013). When multiagent therapy is needed to treat Hodgkin lymphoma during pregnancy, bleomcyin (as a component of the ABVD [doxorubicin, bleomycin, vinblastine, and dacarbazine] regimen) may be used, starting with the second trimetster (Follows 2014; Peccatori 2013).

Breast-Feeding Considerations It is not known if bleomycin is excreted in breast milk. Due to the potential for serious adverse reactions in the nursing infant, breast-feeding is not recommended by the manufacturer.

Warnings/Precautions Hazardous agent - use appropriate precautions for handling and disposal (NIOSH 2014 [group 1]). **[U.S. Boxed Warning]: Occurrence of pulmonary fibrosis (commonly presenting as pneumonitis; occasionally progressing to pulmonary fibrosis) is the most severe toxicity. Risk is higher in elderly patients or patients receiving >400 units total lifetime dose;** other possible risk factors include smoking and patients with prior radiation therapy or receiving concurrent oxygen (especially high inspired oxygen doses). A review of patients receiving bleomycin for the treatment of germ cell tumors suggests risk for pulmonary toxicity is increased in patients >40 years of age, with glomerular filtration rate <80 mL/minute, advanced disease, and cumulative doses >300 units (O'Sullivan, 2003). Pulmonary toxicity may include bronchiolitis obliterans and organizing pneumonia (BOOP), eosinophilic hypersensitivity, and interstitial pneumonitis, progressing to pulmonary fibrosis (Sleijfer, 2001); pulmonary toxicity may be due to a lack of the enzyme which inactivates bleomycin (bleomycin hydrolase) in the lungs (Morgan, 2011; Sleijfer, 2001). If pulmonary changes occur, withhold treatment and investigate if drug-related. In children, a younger age at treatment, cumulative dose ≥400 units/m^2 (combined with chest irradiation), and renal impairment are associated with a higher incidence of pulmonary toxicity (Huang, 2011).

A severe idiosyncratic reaction consisting of hypotension, mental confusion, fever, chills, and wheezing (similar to anaphylaxis) has been reported in 1% of lymphoma patients treated with bleomycin. Since these reactions usually occur after the first or second dose, careful monitoring is essential after these doses. Use caution when administering O_2 during surgery to patients who have received bleomycin; the risk of bleomycin-related pulmonary toxicity is increased. Use caution with renal impairment (CrCl <50 mL/minute), may require dose adjustment. May cause renal or hepatic toxicity. **[U.S. Boxed Warning]: Should be administered under the supervision of an experienced cancer chemotherapy physician.** Potentially significant drug-drug interactions may exist, requiring dose or frequency adjustment, additional monitoring, and/or selection of alternative therapy. Some products available internationally may have vial strength and dosing expressed as international units or milligrams (instead of units or USP units); refer to prescribing information for specific dosing information.

Adverse Reactions

>10%:

Dermatologic: Pain at the tumor site, phlebitis. About 50% of patients develop erythema, rash, striae, induration, hyperkeratosis, vesiculation, and peeling of the skin, particularly on the palmar and plantar surfaces of the hands and feet. Hyperpigmentation (50%), alopecia, nailbed changes may also occur. These effects appear dose related and reversible with discontinuation.

Gastrointestinal: Stomatitis and mucositis (30%), anorexia, weight loss

Respiratory: Tachypnea, rales, acute or chronic interstitial pneumonitis, and pulmonary fibrosis (5% to 10%); hypoxia and death (1%). Symptoms include cough, dyspnea, and bilateral pulmonary infiltrates. The pathogenesis is not certain, but may be due to damage of pulmonary, vascular, or connective tissue. Response to steroid therapy is variable and somewhat controversial.

Miscellaneous: Acute febrile reactions (25% to 50%)

1% to 10%:

Dermatologic: Skin thickening, diffuse scleroderma, onycholysis, pruritus

Miscellaneous: Anaphylactoid-like reactions (characterized by hypotension, confusion, fever, chills, and wheezing; onset may be immediate or delayed for several hours); idiosyncratic reactions (1% in lymphoma patients)

<1%, postmarketing, and/or case reports: Angioedema, cerebrovascular accident, cerebral arteritis, chest pain, coronary artery disease, flagellate hyperpigmentation, hepatotoxicity, malaise, MI, myelosuppression (rare), myocardial ischemia, nausea, pericarditis, Raynaud's phenomenon, renal toxicity, scleroderma-like skin changes, Stevens-Johnson syndrome, thrombotic microangiopathy, toxic epidermal necrolysis, vomiting

Drug Interactions

Metabolism/Transport Effects None known.

Avoid Concomitant Use

Avoid concomitant use of Bleomycin with any of the following: BCG (Intravesical); Brentuximab Vedotin; Natalizumab; Pimecrolimus; Tacrolimus (Topical); Tofacitinib; Vaccines (Live)

Increased Effect/Toxicity

Bleomycin may increase the levels/effects of: Fingolimod; Leflunomide; Natalizumab; Tofacitinib; Vaccines (Live)

The levels/effects of Bleomycin may be increased by: Brentuximab Vedotin; Denosumab; Filgrastim; Gemcitabine; Pimecrolimus; Roflumilast; Sargramostim; Tacrolimus (Topical); Trastuzumab

Decreased Effect

Bleomycin may decrease the levels/effects of: BCG (Intravesical); Coccidioides immitis Skin Test; Phenytoin; Sipuleucel-T; Vaccines (Inactivated); Vaccines (Live)

The levels/effects of Bleomycin may be decreased by: Echinacea

◀ **Storage/Stability** Refrigerate intact vials of powder. Intact vials are stable for up to 4 weeks at room temperature. Solutions reconstituted in NS are stable for up to 28 days refrigerated and 14 days at room temperature; however, the manufacturer recommends stability of 24 hours in NS at room temperature.

Preparation for Administration Hazardous agent; use appropriate precautions for handling and disposal (NIOSH 2014 [group 1]). For IV use, reconstitute 15-unit vial with 5 mL with NS and the 30-unit vial with 10 mL NS; for IM or SubQ use, reconstitute 15-unit vial with 1-5 mL of SWFI, BWFI, or NS and the 30-unit vial with 2-10 mL of SWFI, BWFI, or NS. For intrapleural use, mix in 50-100 mL of NS.

Mechanism of Action Inhibits synthesis of DNA; binds to DNA leading to single- and double-strand breaks; also inhibits (to a lesser degree) RNA and protein synthesis

Pharmacodynamics/Kinetics

Absorption: IM and intrapleural administration: 30% to 50% of IV serum concentrations; intraperitoneal and SubQ routes produce serum concentrations equal to those of IV

Distribution: V_d: 22 L/m²; highest concentrations in skin, kidney, lung, heart tissues; lowest in testes and GI tract; does not cross blood-brain barrier

Protein binding: 1%

Metabolism: Via several tissues including hepatic, GI tract, skin, pulmonary, renal, and serum

Half-life elimination: Biphasic (renal function dependent):

Children: 2.1 to 3.5 hours

Adults:

Normal renal function: Initial: 1.3 hours; Terminal: 9 hours

End-stage renal disease: Initial: 2 hours; Terminal: 30 hours

Time to peak, serum: IM: Within 30 minutes

Excretion: Urine (50% to 70% as active drug)

Dosing

Adult Note: The risk for pulmonary toxicity increases with age >70 years and cumulative lifetime dose of >400 units. **International considerations:** Dosages below expressed as USP units; 1 USP unit = 1 mg (by potency) = 1,000 international units (Stefanou, 2001).

Test dose for lymphoma patients: IM, IV, SubQ: Because of the possibility of an anaphylactoid reaction, the manufacturer recommends administering 1 to 2 units of bleomycin before the first 1 to 2 doses; monitor vital signs every 15 minutes; wait a minimum of 1 hour before administering remainder of dose; if no acute reaction occurs, then the regular dosage schedule may be followed. **Note:** Test doses may not be predictive of a reaction (Lam, 2005) and/or may produce false-negative results.

Hodgkin lymphoma (off-label dosing): IV:

ABVD: 10 units/m² days 1 and 15 of a 28-day treatment cycle (in combination with doxorubicin, vinblastine, and dacarbazine) (Straus, 2004)

BEACOPP: 10 units/m² day 8 of a 21-day treatment cycle (in combination with etoposide, doxorubicin, cyclophosphamide, vincristine, procarbazine, and prednisone) (Dann, 2007; Diehl, 2003)

Stanford V: 5 units/m²/dose in weeks 2, 4, 6, 8, 10 and 12 (in combination with mechlorethamine, vinblastine, vincristine, doxorubicin, etoposide, and prednisone) (Horning, 2002; Horning, 2000)

Testicular cancer (off-label dosing): IV: BEP: 30 units/dose days 1, 8, and 15 of a 21-day treatment cycle for 4 cycles (in combination with etoposide and cisplatin) (Culine, 2008; Nichols, 1998)

Ovarian germ cell cancer (off-label use): IV: 30 units/dose days 1, 8, and 15 of a 21-day treatment cycle for 3 cycles (Williams, 1994) **or** 15 units/m² day 1 of a 21-day treatment cycle for 4 cycles (Cushing, 2004); in combination with etoposide and cisplatin

Malignant pleural effusion: Intrapleural: 60 units as a single instillation; mix in 50 to 100 mL of NS

Geriatric Refer to adult dosing. The incidence of pulmonary toxicity is higher in patients >70 years of age.

Pediatric Note: The risk for pulmonary toxicity increases with age >70 years and cumulative lifetime dose of >400 units. **International considerations:** Dosages below expressed as USP units; 1 USP unit = 1 mg (by potency) = 1,000 international units (Stefanou, 2001).

Test dose for lymphoma patients: IM, IV, SubQ: Because of the possibility of an anaphylactoid reaction, the manufacturer recommends administering 1 to 2 units of bleomycin before the first 1 to 2 doses; monitor vital signs every 15 minutes; wait a minimum of 1 hour before administering remainder of dose; if no acute reaction occurs, then the regular dosage schedule may be followed. **Note:** Test doses may not be predictive of a reaction (Lam, 2005) and/or may produce false-negative results.

Hodgkin lymphoma (off-label dosing): IV: ABVD: IV: 10 units/m² days 1 and 15 of a 28-day treatment cycle (in combination with doxorubicin, vinblastine, and dacarbazine) (Hutchinson, 1998)

Renal Impairment

The U.S. labeling recommends the following adjustments (creatinine clearance should be estimated using the Cockcroft-Gault formula):

CrCl >50 mL/minute: No dosage adjustment necessary.
CrCl 40-50 mL/minute: Administer 70% of normal dose
CrCl 30-40 mL/minute: Administer 60% of normal dose
CrCl 20-30 mL/minute: Administer 55% of normal dose
CrCl 10-20 mL/minute: Administer 45% of normal dose
CrCl 5-10 mL/minute: Administer 40% of normal dose

The Canadian labeling recommends the following adjustment: CrCl ≤40 mL/minute: Reduce dose by 40% to 75%.

The following adjustments have also been recommended:

Aronoff, 2007: Adults: Continuous renal replacement therapy (CRRT): Administer 75% of dose

Kintzel, 1995: Adults:
CrCl 46-60 mL/minute: Administer 70% of dose
CrCl 31-45 mL/minute: Administer 60% of dose
CrCl <30 mL/minute: Consider use of alternative drug

Hepatic Impairment There are no dosage adjustments provided in the manufacturer's labeling (has not been studied); however, adjustment for hepatic impairment is not necessary (King, 2001).

Obesity *ASCO Guidelines for appropriate chemotherapy dosing in obese adults with cancer:* Fixed doses (dosing which is independent of body weight or BSA), are used in some protocols (eg, testicular cancer); due to toxicity concerns, the same fixed dose should also be considered for obese patients (Griggs, 2012).

◀ **Adjustment for Toxicity**
Pulmonary changes: Discontinue until determined not to be drug-related.
Pulmonary diffusion capacity for carbon monoxide (DL_{CO}) <30% to 35% of
baseline: Discontinue treatment.

Combination Regimens

Lymphoma, Hodgkin:
ABVD Early Stage (Hodgkin) on page 1820
ABVD (Hodgkin) on page 1821
BEACOPP-14 (Hodgkin) on page 1829
BEACOPP Escalated (Hodgkin) on page 1830
BEACOPP Escalated Plus Standard (Hodgkin) on page 1830
BEACOPP Standard (Hodgkin) on page 1832
C-MOPP/ABV Hybrid (Hodgkin) on page 1919
MOPP/ABVD (Hodgkin) on page 2039
MOPP/ABV Hybrid (Hodgkin) on page 2040
Stanford V (Hodgkin) on page 2085
Ovarian cancer: BEP (Ovarian) on page 1837
Testicular cancer: BEP (Testicular) on page 1838

Administration

IV doses should be administered slowly over 10 minutes (according to the
manufacturer's labeling).
IM or SubQ: May cause pain at injection site
Intrapleural: 60 units in 50 to 100 mL NS; use of topical anesthetics or opioid
analgesia is usually not necessary

Hazardous agent; use appropriate precautions for handling and disposal
(NIOSH 2014 [group 1]).

Vesicant/Extravasation Risk May be an irritant

Emetic Potential Children and Adults: Minimal (<10%)

Monitoring Parameters Pulmonary function tests, including total lung volume, forced vital capacity, diffusion capacity for carbon monoxide; vital
capacity, total lung capacity and pulmonary capillary blood volume may be
better indicators of changes induced by bleomycin (Sleifjer, 2001); chest x-ray,
renal function, liver function, temperature initially; check body weight at regular
intervals

Additional Information One unit of bleomycin equivalent to 1 mg of activity;
in the U.S. dosing is no longer expressed using milligrams (Perry, 2012).

International considerations: One USP unit of bleomycin = 1 mg (by potency) =
1000 international units (Stefanou, 2001)

Dosage Forms Excipient information presented when available (limited,
particularly for generics); consult specific product labeling.
Solution Reconstituted, Injection:
Generic: 15 units (1 ea); 30 units (1 ea)
Solution Reconstituted, Injection [preservative free]:
Generic: 15 units (1 ea); 30 units (1 ea)

◆ **Bleomycin Injection, USP (Can)** see Bleomycin on page 211
◆ **Bleomycin Sulfate** see Bleomycin on page 211

Blinatumomab (blin a TOOM oh mab)

Related Information
Common Toxicity Criteria *on page 2122*
Principles of Anticancer Therapy *on page 2261*

Brand Names: US Blincyto

Index Terms MT103

Pharmacologic Category Antineoplastic Agent, Anti-CD19/CD3; Antineoplastic Agent, Monoclonal Antibody

Use Acute lymphoblastic leukemia: Treatment of Philadelphia chromosome-negative (Ph-) relapsed or refractory B-cell precursor acute lymphoblastic leukemia (ALL)

Labeled Contraindications Known hypersensitivity to blinatumomab or any component of the formulation

Pregnancy Considerations Animal reproductions studies have not been conducted.

Breast-Feeding Considerations It is not known if blinatumomab is excreted in breast milk. Due to the potential for serious adverse reactions in the nursing infant, the manufacturer recommends a decision be made to discontinue nursing or to discontinue the drug, taking into account the importance of treatment to the mother.

Warnings/Precautions [U.S. Boxed Warning]: Cytokine release syndrome (CRS), which may be life-threatening or fatal, has occurred. Interrupt or discontinue therapy as recommended. Infusion reactions have also occurred, and may be difficult to distinguish from CRS. CRS symptoms may include pyrexia, headache, nausea, weakness, hypotension, increased transaminases, and elevated total bilirubin. In some patients, disseminated intravascular coagulation (DIC), capillary leak syndrome (CLS), and hemophagocytic lymphohistiocytosis/macrophage activation syndrome (HLH/MAS) have been reported in the setting of CRS. Monitor closely for signs/symptoms of these conditions; may require therapy interruption or discontinuation. CRS which was life-threatening or fatal occurred rarely. **[U.S. Boxed Warning]: Neurological toxicities, which may be severe, life-threatening, or fatal, have occurred. Interrupt or discontinue therapy as recommended.** Neurotoxicity has occurred in approximately half of patients in clinical trials. The median time to onset was 7 days. Grade 3 or higher neurotoxicity (eg, encephalopathy, convulsions, speech disorders, disturbances in consciousness, confusion and disorientation, and coordination and balance disorders) has also been observed. Patients are at risk for loss of consciousness due to neurologic events while taking blinatumomab; advise patients to avoid driving, participating in hazardous occupations, or operating heavy or dangerous machinery during treatment. Monitor patients for signs/symptoms of neurotoxicity; may require therapy interruption or discontinuation. The majority of symptoms resolved after interrupting therapy. Leukoencephalopathy (as seen on MRI) has been reported, particularly in those patients who received prior treatment with cranial irradiation and antileukemia chemotherapy (eg, high dose methotrexate or intrathecal cytarabine).

Neutropenia and neutropenic fever, including life-threatening episodes, have been reported. Monitor blood counts throughout therapy; may require therapy interruption if prolonged neutropenia occurs. Anemia and thrombocytopenia may also occur. Serious infections such as sepsis, pneumonia, bacteremia, opportunistic infections, and catheter-related infections have been reported in approximately one-fourth of patients in clinical trials (may be life-threatening or ▶

217

fatal). Consider prophylactic antibiotics if appropriate, and monitor closely for signs/symptoms of infection. Treat promptly if infection occurs. Transient increases in liver enzymes (associated both with and without CRS) may occur during therapy. The median time to enzyme elevation was 15 days; grade 3 or higher elevations were observed in a small percentage of patients. Monitor ALT, AST, GGT, and total bilirubin at baseline and during treatment. Interrupt therapy if transaminases are >5 times ULN or if bilirubin is >3 times ULN. Life-threatening or fatal tumor lysis syndrome (TLS) has been observed. Administer measures to prevent TLS (eg, pretreatment nontoxic cytoreduction, and hydration during treatment). Monitor for signs/symptoms of TLS (eg, acute renal failure, hyperkalemia, hypocalcemia, hyperuricemia, and/or hyperphosphatemia); may require treatment interruption or discontinuation. Elderly patients experienced an increased rate of neurotoxicity (including cognitive disorder), encephalopathy, confusion, and serious infections as compared to patients less than 65 years. Preparation and administration errors have occurred. Do not flush infusion line, particularly when changing infusion bags or at completion of infusion; may result in overdose and complications. IV bag volume will be more than the volume administered to the patient (240 mL) to account for IV line priming and to ensure that the full dose is administered. Follow preparation and administration instructions carefully. Refer to manufacturer labeling for further information.

Adverse Reactions

>10%:

Cardiovascular: Peripheral edema (25%; ≥ grade 3: <1%), chest pain (11%; ≥ grade 3: 1%), hypotension (11%; ≥ grade 3: 2%)

Central nervous system: Neurotoxicity (50%; ≥ grade 3: 15%; incidence increased in older adults), headache (36%; ≥ grade 3: 3%), fatigue (17%; ≥ grade 3: 1%), chills (15%), insomnia (15%), dizziness (14%; ≥ grade 3: <1%)

Dermatologic: Skin rash (21%; ≥ grade 3: 2%)

Endocrine & metabolic: Hypokalemia (23%; ≥ grade 3: 6%), hypomagnesemia (12%), hyperglycemia (11%; ≥ grade 3: 7%), weight gain (11%)

Gastrointestinal: Nausea (25%), constipation (20%; ≥ grade 3: <1%), diarrhea (20%; ≥ grade 3: 1%), abdominal pain (15%; ≥ grade 3: 2%), vomiting (13%)

Hematologic & oncologic: Febrile neutropenia (25%; ≥ grade 3: 23%), anemia (18%; ≥ grade 3: 13%), neutropenia (16%; ≥ grade 3: 15%), thrombocytopenia (11%; ≥ grade 3: 8%)

Hepatic: Increased serum ALT (12%; ≥ grade 3: 6%), increased serum AST (11%; ≥ grade 3: 4%)

Hypersensitivity: Cytokine release syndrome (including cytokine storms) (11%; ≥ grade 3: 1%)

Infection: Infection (44%; ≥ grade 3: 25%), bacterial infection (19%; ≥ grade 3: 12%), fungal infection (15%; ≥ grade 3: 7%), viral infection (13%; ≥ grade 3: 4%)

Neuromuscular & skeletal: Tremor (20%; ≥ grade 3: 1%), back pain (14%; ≥ grade 3: 2%), limb pain (12%; ≥ grade 3: 1%), ostealgia (11%; ≥ grade 3: 3%)

Respiratory: Cough (19%), dyspnea (15%; ≥ grade 3: 5%)

Miscellaneous: Fever (62%; ≥ grade 3: 7%)

1% to 10%:

Cardiovascular: Hypertension (8%; ≥ grade 3: 5%), tachycardia (8%), edema (5%)

Central nervous system: Confusion (7%), brain disease (5%), paresthesia (5%), aphasia (4%), disorientation (3%), convulsions (2%), memory impairment (2%), cognitive dysfunction (1%), loss of consciousness

Endocrine & metabolic: Hypophosphatemia (6%; ≥ grade 3: 5%), increased gamma-glutamyl transferase (6%), hypoalbuminemia (4%)

Gastrointestinal: Decreased appetite (10%; ≥ grade 3: 3%)

Hematologic & oncologic: Decreased serum immunoglobulins (9%), leukopenia (9%; ≥ grade 3: 8%), tumor lysis syndrome (4%), leukocytosis (2%), lymphocytopenia (1%)

Hepatic: Increased serum bilirubin (8%), increased liver enzymes (1%)

Hypersensitivity: Cytokine storm (1%), hypersensitivity (1%)

Infection: Sepsis (7%; ≥ grade 3: 6%)

Neuromuscular & skeletal: Arthralgia (10%; ≥ grade 3: 2%)

Respiratory: Pneumonia (9%; ≥ grade 3: 8%)

<1%, postmarketing, and/or case reports: Bronchospasm, capillary leak syndrome, leukoencephalopathy, speech disturbance

Drug Interactions

Metabolism/Transport Effects None known.

Avoid Concomitant Use

Avoid concomitant use of Blinatumomab with any of the following: BCG (Intravesical); CloZAPine; Dipyrone; Natalizumab; Pimecrolimus; Tacrolimus (Topical); Tofacitinib; Vaccines (Live)

Increased Effect/Toxicity

Blinatumomab may increase the levels/effects of: CloZAPine; Fingolimod; Leflunomide; Natalizumab; Tofacitinib; Vaccines (Live)

The levels/effects of Blinatumomab may be increased by: Denosumab; Dipyrone; Pimecrolimus; Roflumilast; Tacrolimus (Topical); Trastuzumab

Decreased Effect

Blinatumomab may decrease the levels/effects of: BCG (Intravesical); Coccidioides immitis Skin Test; Sipuleucel-T; Vaccines (Inactivated); Vaccines (Live)

The levels/effects of Blinatumomab may be decreased by: Echinacea

Storage/Stability Store intact vials (drug and solution stabilizer) in the original package at 2°C to 8°C (36°F to 46°F); protect from light. Do not freeze. Intact vials of both drug and stabilizer may be stored for up to 8 hours at room temperature. Reconstituted solution is stable for up to 4 hours at 23°C to 27°C (73°F to 81°F) or up to 24 hours at 2°C to 8°C (36°F to 46°F). Solutions diluted for infusion are stable for up to 48 hours at 23°C to 27°C (73°F to 81°F) or up to 8 days at 2°C to 8°C (36°F to 46°F). Infusion should be completed within these time frames; if IV bag of solution for infusion is not administered within the time frames and temperatures indicated, discard; do not refrigerate again.

Preparation for Administration All doses should be prepared in a prefilled 250 mL NS bag. Prefilled 250 mL NS bags typically contain overfill to a volume of 265 to 275 mL and dose calculations are based on a starting volume of 265 to 275 mL (if necessary, adjust the bag volume to achieve a starting volume between 265 and 275 mL). Final bag volume will be more than the volume administered to the patient (240 mL) to account for IV line priming and to ensure that the full dose is administered. Use only polyolefin, PVC non-diethylhexylphthalate (non-DEHP), or ethyl vinyl acetate (EVA) infusion bags or pump cassettes. IV solution stabilizer provided is used to coat the prefilled NS bag prior to addition of reconstituted blinatumomab. Therefore, the IV solution stabilizer is added to the NS bag; do NOT use IV solution stabilizer for reconstitution of blinatumomab. Preparation and administration errors have occurred; follow preparation instructions carefully. Refer to manufacturer labeling for further information.

9 mcg daily dose infused over 24 hours at a rate of 10 mL/hour: Transfer **5.5 mL** of IV solution stabilizer to the prefilled 250 mL NS bag using a 10 mL syringe; gently mix to avoid foaming. Reconstitute **one** vial of lyophilized powder with 3 mL of preservative-free SWFI; direct stream toward the side of the vial and gently swirl to avoid excess foaming. Do not shake; final reconstituted concentration is 12.5 **mcg**/mL. Reconstituted solution should be clear to slightly opalescent, colorless to slightly yellow; do not use if cloudy or if precipitation occurs. Transfer **0.83 mL** of reconstituted solution into the prefilled NS bag; gently mix. Remove air from the IV bag; prime IV line with the prepared infusion solution only (do not prime with NS). If not used immediately, store at 2°C to 8°C (36°F to 46°F) for up to 8 days (infusion must be completed within this time frame).

9 mcg daily dose infused over 48 hours at a rate of 5 mL/hour: Transfer 5.5 **mL** of IV solution stabilizer to the prefilled 250 mL NS bag using a 10 mL syringe; gently mix to avoid foaming. Reconstitute **one** vial of lyophilized powder with 3 mL of preservative-free SWFI; direct stream toward the side of the vial and gently swirl to avoid excess foaming. Do not shake; final reconstituted concentration is 12.5 **mcg**/mL. Reconstituted solution should be clear to slightly opalescent, colorless to slightly yellow; do not use if cloudy or if precipitation occurs. Transfer **1.7 mL** of reconstituted solution into the prefilled NS bag; gently mix. Remove air from the IV bag; prime IV line with the prepared infusion solution only (do not prime with NS). If not used immediately, store at 2°C to 8°C (36°F to 46°F) for up to 8 days (infusion must be completed within this time frame).

28 mcg daily dose infused over 24 hours at a rate of 10 mL/hour: Transfer **5.6 mL** of IV solution stabilizer to the prefilled 250 mL NS bag using a 10 mL syringe; gently mix to avoid foaming. Reconstitute **one** vial of lyophilized powder with 3 mL of preservative-free SWFI; direct stream toward the side of the vial and gently swirl to avoid excess foaming. Do not shake; final reconstituted concentration is 12.5 **mcg**/mL. Reconstituted solution should be clear to slightly opalescent, colorless to slightly yellow; do not use if cloudy or if precipitation occurs. Transfer **2.6 mL** of reconstituted solution into the prefilled NS bag; gently mix. Remove air from the IV bag; prime IV line with the prepared infusion solution only (do not prime with NS). If not used immediately, store at 2°C to 8°C (36°F to 46°F) for up to 8 days (infusion must be completed within this time frame).

28 mcg daily dose infused over 48 hours at a rate of 5 mL/hour: Transfer **5.6 mL** of IV solution stabilizer to the prefilled 250 mL NS bag using a 10 mL syringe; gently mix to avoid foaming. Use 2 vials of lyophilized powder; reconstitute each vial with 3 mL of preservative-free SWFI; direct stream toward the side of the vial and gently swirl to avoid excess foaming. Do not shake; final reconstituted concentration in each vial is 12.5 mcg/mL. Reconstituted solution should be clear to slightly opalescent, colorless to slightly yellow; do not use if cloudy or if precipitation occurs. Transfer **5.2 mL** (2.7 mL from one vial and the remaining 2.5 mL from the second vial) of reconstituted solution into the prefilled NS bag; gently mix. Remove air from the IV bag; prime IV line with the prepared infusion solution only (do not prime with NS). If not used immediately, store at 2°C to 8°C (36°F to 46°F) for up to 8 days (infusion must be completed within this time frame).

Mechanism of Action Blinatumomab is a bispecific CD19-directed CD3 T-cell engager which binds to CD19 expressed on B-cells and CD3 expressed on T-cells. It activates endogenous T cells by connecting CD3 in the T-cell receptor complex with CD19 on B-cells (malignant and benign), thus forming a cytolytic synapse between a cytotoxic T-cell and the cancer target B-cell (Topp, 2014). Blinatumomab mediates the production of cytolytic proteins, release of inflammatory cytokines, and proliferation of T cells, which result in lysis of CD19-positive cells.

Pharmacodynamics/Kinetics

Distribution: 4.52 L

Half-life elimination: 2.11 hours

Excretion: Urine (negligible amounts)

Dosing

Adult & Geriatric Note: Hospitalization is recommended for the first 9 days of cycle 1, and the first 2 days of cycle 2. Consider hospitalization or close observation by a healthcare professional (or hospitalization) is recommended for initiation of all subsequent cycles or for therapy reinitiation (eg, treatment is interrupted for 4 or more hours). Do **not** flush infusion line, particularly when changing infusion bags or at completion of infusion; may result in overdose and complications. Premedicate with dexamethasone 20 mg IV one hour prior to the first dose of each cycle, prior to a step dose (eg, Cycle 1 day 8), or when restarting therapy after an interruption of ≥4 hours.

Acute lymphoblastic leukemia (B-cell precursor), Philadelphia chromosome-negative, relapsed/refractory: Adults ≥45 kg: IV: Each treatment cycle consists of 4 weeks of continuous infusion followed by a 2-week treatment-free interval (allow at least 2 weeks treatment-free between cycles). Therapy involves 2 induction cycles followed by 3 additional cycles for consolidation (total of up to 5 cycles).

Cycle 1: 9 **mcg** daily administered as a continuous infusion on days 1 to 7, followed by 28 **mcg** daily as a continuous infusion on days 8 to 28 of a 6-week treatment cycle

Cycles 2 through 5: 28 **mcg** daily administered as a continuous infusion on days 1 to 28 of a 6-week treatment cycle

Renal Impairment

CrCl ≥30 mL/minute: No dosage adjustment necessary.

CrCl <30 mL/minute: There are no dosage adjustments provided in the manufacturer's labeling (has not been studied).

Hemodialysis: There are no dosage adjustments provided in the manufacturer's labeling (has not been studied).

Hepatic Impairment

There are no dosage adjustments provided in the manufacturer's labeling (has not been studied).

Hepatotoxicity during treatment: Interrupt therapy if transaminases are >5 times ULN or if bilirubin is >3 times ULN.

Adjustment for Toxicity If the interruption after an adverse event is no longer than 7 days, continue the same cycle to a total of 28 days of infusion inclusive of days before and after the interruption in that cycle. If an interruption due to an adverse event is longer than 7 days, start a new cycle.

◀

Cytokine release syndrome (CRS):
Grade 3: Interrupt therapy until resolved, then resume dosing at 9 **mcg** daily. Increase dose to 28 **mcg** daily after 7 days if toxicity does not recur.
Grade 4: Discontinue permanently

Neurologic toxicity:
Grade 3: Interrupt therapy for at least 3 days and until toxicity is ≤ grade 1 (mild), then resume dosing at 9 **mcg** daily. Increase dose to 28 **mcg** daily after 7 days if toxicity does not recur. If toxicity occurred at the 9 **mcg** daily dose, or if it takes more than 7 days to resolve, discontinue permanently.
Grade 4: Discontinue permanently
Seizure: Discontinue permanently if more than 1 seizure occurs.

Other clinically relevant toxicity:
Grade 3: Interrupt therapy until toxicity is ≤ grade 1 (mild), then resume dosing at 9 mcg daily. Increase dose to 28 mcg daily after 7 days if toxicity does not recur. If toxicity takes more than 14 days to resolve, discontinue permanently.
Grade 4: Discontinue permanently

Administration IV: Administer 240 mL as a continuous IV infusion at a constant flow rate of 10 mL/hour for 24 hours or 5 mL/hour for 48 hours (depending on dose, duration, and/or concentration) through a dedicated lumen. Use a programmable, lockable, non-elastomeric infusion pump with an alarm; IV tubing should include a sterile, nonpyrogenic, low protein-binding, 0.2 micron in-line filter. Only use polyolefin, PVC non-di-ethylhexylphthalate (non-DEHP), or ethyl vinyl acetate (EVA) infusion bags, pump cassettes and IV tubing. IV tubing should be primed with prepared infusion solution, not NS. Premedicate with dexamethasone 20 mg IV one hour prior to the first dose of each cycle, prior to a step dose (such as cycle 1 day 8), or when restarting therapy after an interruption of ≥4 hours.

Do not flush infusion line, particularly when changing infusion bags or at completion of infusion; may result in excess dosage and complications. Do not infuse other medications through the same line.

Emetic Potential Low (10% to 30%)

Monitoring Parameters CBC with differential, liver function tests (ALT, AST, GGT, and total bilirubin) at baseline and throughout therapy; signs/symptoms of cytokine release syndrome, neurotoxicity, infection, and tumor lysis syndrome

Medication Guide Available Yes

Dosage Forms Excipient information presented when available (limited, particularly for generics); consult specific product labeling.
Solution Reconstituted, Intravenous [preservative free]:
Blincyto: 35 mcg (1 ea) [contains polysorbate 80]

Bortezomib (bore TEZ oh mib)

Related Information

Chemotherapy-Induced Peripheral Neuropathy *on page 2116*

Common Toxicity Criteria *on page 2122*

Hematopoietic Stem Cell Transplantation *on page 2272*

Hypercalcemia of Malignancy *on page 2241*

Management of Chemotherapy-Induced Nausea and Vomiting in Adults *on page 2142*

Management of Drug Extravasations *on page 2159*

Prevention and Management of Infections *on page 2196*

Prevention of Chemotherapy-Induced Nausea and Vomiting in Children *on page 2203*

Principles of Anticancer Therapy *on page 2261*

Safe Handling of Hazardous Drugs *on page 2292*

Brand Names: US Velcade

Brand Names: Canada Bortezomib For Injection; Velcade

Index Terms LDP-341; MLN341; PS-341

Pharmacologic Category Antineoplastic Agent; Proteasome Inhibitor

Use

Mantle cell lymphoma: Treatment of mantle cell lymphoma

Multiple myeloma: Treatment of multiple myeloma

Labeled Contraindications Hypersensitivity (excluding local reactions) to bortezomib, boron, mannitol, or any component of the formulation; administration via the intrathecal route

Pregnancy Considerations Adverse effects (fetal loss and decreased fetal weight) were observed in animal reproduction studies at doses less than the equivalent human dose (based on BSA). Women of reproductive potential should avoid becoming pregnant and should use effective contraception during treatment. The Canadian labeling recommends that females and males of reproductive potential use effective contraception during treatment and for 3 months following treatment.

Breast-Feeding Considerations It is not known if bortezomib is excreted in breast milk. Due to the potential for serious adverse reactions in the nursing infant, the decision to discontinue bortezomib or to discontinue breast-feeding should take into account the benefits of treatment to the mother.

Warnings/Precautions Hazardous agent - use appropriate precautions for handling and disposal (NIOSH 2014 [group 1]). May cause or worsen peripheral neuropathy (usually sensory but may be mixed sensorimotor); risk may be increased with previous use of neurotoxic agents or preexisting peripheral neuropathy (patients with preexisting neuropathy should use only after risk versus benefit assessment); monitor for signs and symptoms; adjustment of dose and/or schedule may be required. The incidence of grades 2 and 3 peripheral neuropathy may be lower with SubQ route (compared to IV); consider SubQ administration in patients with preexisting or at high risk for peripheral neuropathy; the majority of patients with ≥ grade 2 peripheral neuropathy have improvement in or resolution of symptoms with dose adjustments or discontinuation; in a study of elderly patients receiving a weekly bortezomib schedule with combination chemotherapy, the incidence of peripheral neuropathy was significantly reduced without an effect on outcome (Boccadoro, 2010; Palumbo, 2009). May cause hypotension (including postural and orthostatic); use caution with dehydration, history of syncope, or medications associated with hypotension (may require adjustment of antihypertensive medication, hydration, and mineralocorticoids and/or sympa-thomimetics). Has been associated with the development or exacerbation of heart failure (HF) and decreased left ventricular ejection fraction (LVEF); monitor closely in patients with risk factors for HF or existing heart disease, although HF and decreased LVEF have been observed in patients without risk factors. Has also been associated with isolated reports of QTc prolongation.

Pulmonary disorders (some fatal) including pneumonitis, interstitial pneumo-nia, lung infiltrates, and acute respiratory distress syndrome (ARDS) have been reported. Pulmonary hypertension (without left heart failure or significant pulmonary disease has been reported rarely). Promptly evaluate with new or worsening cardiopulmonary symptoms; therapy interruption may be required. Tumor lysis syndrome has been reported; risk is increased in patients with high tumor burden prior to treatment. Posterior reversible leukoencephalopathy syndrome (PRES, formerly RPLS) has been reported (rarely). Symptoms of PRES include confusion, headache, hypertension, lethargy, seizure, blindness and/or other vision, or neurologic disturbances; discontinue bortezomib if PRES occurs. MRI is recommended to confirm PRES diagnosis. The safety of reinitiating bortezomib in patients previously experiencing PRES is unknown. Progressive multifocal leukoencephalopathy (PML) has been rarely observed; monitor closely and evaluate promptly. Herpes (zoster and simplex) reactivation has been reported with bortezomib; consider antiviral prophylaxis during therapy. Hematologic toxicity, including grade 3 and 4 neutropenia and severe thrombocytopenia, may occur (nadirs generally occur following the last dose of a cycle and recover prior to the next cycle); risk is increased in patients with pretreatment platelet counts <75,000/μL; frequent monitoring is required throughout treatment; may require dosage or schedule adjustments; withhold treatment for platelets <30,000/μL. Management with platelet transfusions and supportive care may be necessary. Hemorrhage (gastrointestinal and intra-cerebral) due to low platelet count has been observed. Acute liver failure has been reported (rarely) in patients receiving multiple concomitant medications and with serious underlying conditions. Hepatitis, transaminase increases, and hyperbilirubinemia have also been reported; interrupt therapy to assess reversibility. Use caution in patients with hepatic dysfunction; reduced initial doses are recommended for moderate and severe hepatic impairment (expo-sure is increased); closely monitor for toxicities. Hyper- and hypoglycemia may occur in diabetic patients receiving oral hypoglycemics; may require adjust-ment of diabetes medications. Nausea, vomiting, diarrhea or constipation may occur; may require antiemetics or antidiarrheals; ileus may occur; administer fluid and electrolytes to prevent dehydration (monitor closely); interrupt therapy for severe symptoms.

Potentially significant drug-drug/drug-food interactions may exist, requiring dose or frequency adjustment, additional monitoring, and/or selection of alternative therapy. Coadministration of strong CYP3A4 inhibitors may increase bortezomib exposure; monitor for toxicity and consider dose reduction if concurrent therapy cannot be avoided. Efficacy may be reduced when administered with strong CYP3A4 inducers; concomitant use is not recom-mended.

For IV or SubQ administration only. Intrathecal administration is contra-indicated; inadvertent intrathecal administration has resulted in death. Borte-zomib should **NOT** be prepared during the preparation of any intrathecal medications. After preparation, keep bortezomib in a location **away** from the separate storage location recommended for intrathecal medications.

Bortezomib should **NOT** be delivered to the patient at the same time with any medications intended for central nervous system administration. The reconstituted concentrations for IV and SubQ administration are different; use caution when calculating the volume for each route and dose. The manufacturer provides stickers to facilitate identification of the route for reconstituted vials.

Adverse Reactions Incidences reported are associated with monotherapy. Additional adverse reactions reported with mono- or combination therapy; frequency not defined.

Cardiovascular: Hypotension (8% to 9%; grades 3/4: ≤2%), cardiac disease (treatment emergent; 8%), acute pulmonary edema (≤1%), cardiac failure (≤1%), cardiogenic shock (≤1%), pulmonary edema (≤1%), aggravated atrial fibrillation, angina pectoris, atrial flutter, atrioventricular block, bradycardia, cerebrovascular accident, deep vein thrombosis, edema, embolism (peripheral), facial edema, hemorrhagic stroke, hypertension, ischemic heart disease, myocardial infarction, pericardial effusion, pericarditis, peripheral edema, phlebitis, portal vein thrombosis, pulmonary embolism, septic shock, sinoatrial arrest, subdural hematoma, torsades de pointes, transient ischemic attacks, ventricular tachycardia

Central nervous system: Peripheral neuropathy (IV 35% to 54%; SubQ 37%; grade ≥2: 24% to 39%; grade ≥3: SubQ 5% to 6%; IV 7% to 15%; grade 4: <1%), fatigue (7% to 52%), neuralgia (23%), headache (10% to 19%), paresthesia (7% to 19%), dizziness (10% to 18%; excludes vertigo), agitation, anxiety, ataxia, brain disease, cerebral hemorrhage, chills, coma, confusion, cranial nerve palsy, dysarthria, dysautonomia, dysesthesia, insomnia, malaise, mental status changes, motor dysfunction, paralysis, psychosis, seizure, spinal cord compression, suicidal ideation, vertigo

Dermatologic: Skin rash (12% to 23%), pruritus, urticaria

Endocrine & metabolic: Dehydration (2%), amyloid heart disease, hyperglycemia (diabetic patients), hyperkalemia, hypernatremia, hyperuricemia, hypocalcemia, hypoglycemia (diabetic patients), hypokalemia, hyponatremia, weight loss

Gastrointestinal: Diarrhea (19% to 52%), nausea (14% to 52%), constipation (24% to 34%), vomiting (9% to 29%), anorexia (14% to 21%), abdominal pain (11%), decreased appetite (11%), cholestasis, duodenitis (hemorrhagic), dysphagia, fecal impaction, gastritis (hemorrhagic), gastroenteritis, gastroesophageal reflux disease, hematemesis, intestinal obstruction, intestinal perforation, melena, oral candidiasis, pancreatitis, paralytic ileus, peritonitis, stomatitis

Genitourinary: Bladder spasm, hematuria, hemorrhagic cystitis, urinary incontinence, urinary retention, urinary tract infection

Hematologic & oncologic: Thrombocytopenia (16% to 52%; grade 3: 5% to 24%; grade 4: 3% to 7%; nadir: Day 11; recovery: By day 21), neutropenia (5% to 27%; grade 3: 8% to 18%; grade 4: 2% to 4%; nadir: Day 11; recovery: By day 21), anemia (12% to 23%; grade 3: 4% to 6%; grade 4: <1%). leukopenia (18% to 20%; grade 3: 5%; grade 4: ≤1%), hemorrhage (≥ grade 3: 2%), disseminated intravascular coagulation, febrile neutropenia, lymphocytopenia, oral mucosal petechiae

Hepatic: Ascites, hepatic failure, hepatic hemorrhage, hepatitis, hyperbilirubinemia

Hypersensitivity: Anaphylaxis, angioedema, hypersensitivity, hypersensitivity angiitis

Infection: Herpes zoster (reactivation; 6% to 11%), herpes simplex infection (1% to 3%), herpes zoster (1% to 2%), aspergillosis, bacteremia, listeriosis, toxoplasmosis

Local: Injection site reaction (mostly redness; SubQ 6%), irritation at injection site (IV 5%), catheter infection

Neuromuscular & skeletal: Weakness (7% to 16%), arthralgia, back pain, bone fracture, limb pain, myalgia, ostealgia

Ophthalmic: Blurred vision, conjunctival infection, conjunctival irritation, diplopia

Otic: Auditory impairment

Renal: Bilateral hydronephrosis, nephrolithiasis, proliferative glomerulonephritis, renal failure

Respiratory: Dyspnea (11%), pneumonia (1% to 3%), adult respiratory distress syndrome, aspiration pneumonia, atelectasis, bronchitis, chronic obstructive pulmonary disease (exacerbation), cough, epistaxis, hemoptysis, hypoxia, laryngeal edema, nasopharyngitis, pleural effusion, pneumonitis, pulmonary hypertension, pulmonary infiltrates (including diffuse), respiratory tract infection, sinusitis

Miscellaneous: Fever (8% to 23%)

<1%, postmarketing, and/or case reports: Acute ischemic stroke, amyloidosis, blindness, cardiac arrest, cardiac tamponade, cardiorespiratory arrest, deafness (bilateral), decreased left ventricular ejection fraction, dysgeusia, dyspepsia, herpes meningoencephalitis, increased gamma-glutamyl transferase, increased serum alkaline phosphatase, increased serum transaminases, interstitial pneumonitis, ischemic colitis, ocular herpes simplex, optic neuritis, progressive multifocal leukoencephalopathy, prolonged QT interval on ECG, respiratory failure, respiratory insufficiency, reversible posterior leukoencephalopathy syndrome, sepsis, SIADH, Stevens-Johnson syndrome, subarachnoid hemorrhage, Sweet syndrome, syncope, tachycardia, toxic epidermal necrolysis, tumor lysis syndrome

Drug Interactions

Metabolism/Transport Effects Substrate of CYP1A2 (minor), CYP2C19 (major), CYP2C9 (minor), CYP2D6 (minor), CYP3A4 (major); **Note:** Assignment of Major/Minor substrate status based on clinically relevant drug interaction potential; **Inhibits** CYP1A2 (weak), CYP2C19 (moderate), CYP2C9 (weak), CYP2D6 (weak)

Avoid Concomitant Use

Avoid concomitant use of Bortezomib with any of the following: BCG (Intravesical); CloZAPine; CYP3A4 Inducers (Strong); Dipyrone; Green Tea; St Johns Wort

Increased Effect/Toxicity

Bortezomib may increase the levels/effects of: ARIPiprazole; Cilostazol; Citalopram; CloZAPine; CYP2C19 Substrates; Highest Risk QTc-Prolonging Agents; Moderate Risk QTc-Prolonging Agents; TiZANidine

The levels/effects of Bortezomib may be increased by: CYP3A4 Inhibitors (Strong); Dipyrone; Mifepristone; Osimertinib

Decreased Effect

Bortezomib may decrease the levels/effects of: BCG (Intravesical); Clopidogrel

The levels/effects of Bortezomib may be decreased by: Ascorbic Acid; Bosentan; CYP2C19 Inducers (Strong); CYP3A4 Inducers (Moderate); CYP3A4 Inducers (Strong); Dabrafenib; Deferasirox; Green Tea;

Multivitamins/Fluoride (with ADE); Multivitamins/Minerals (with ADEK, Folate, Iron); Multivitamins/Minerals (with AE, No Iron); Osimertinib; Siltuximab; St Johns Wort; Tocilizumab

Storage/Stability Prior to reconstitution, store intact vials at 25°C (77°F); excursions are permitted between 15°C and 30°C (59°F and 86°F). Once reconstituted, the manufacturer recommends use within 8 hours of reconstitution. However, stability studies have demonstrated solutions of 1 mg/mL (vial or syringe) may be stored at room temperature for up to 3 days, or under refrigeration for up to 5 days (Andre, 2005); or refrigerated in the original vial for up to 15 days (Vanderloo, 2010). Protect from light. After preparation, keep bortezomib in a location away from the separate storage location recommended for intrathecal medications.

Preparation for Administration Note: The reconstituted concentrations for IV and SubQ administration are different; the manufacturer provides stickers to facilitate identification of the route for reconstituted vials. The amount contained in each vial may exceed the prescribed dose; use care with dosage and volume calculations.

Hazardous agent; use appropriate precautions for handling and disposal (NIOSH 2014 [group 1]). Reconstitute only with normal saline (NS). Reconstituted solutions should be clear and colorless.

IV: Reconstitute each 3.5 mg vial with 3.5 mL NS to a concentration of 1 mg/mL.

SubQ: Reconstitute each 3.5 mg vial with 1.4 mL NS to a concentration of 2.5 mg/mL (Moreau, 2011). If injection site reaction occurs, the more dilute 1 mg/mL concentration may be used SubQ.

Mechanism of Action Bortezomib inhibits proteasomes, enzyme complexes which regulate protein homeostasis within the cell. Specifically, it reversibly inhibits chymotrypsin-like activity at the 26S proteasome, leading to activation of signaling cascades, cell-cycle arrest, and apoptosis.

Pharmacodynamics/Kinetics

Distribution: 498 to 1884 L/m^2; distributes widely to peripheral tissues

Protein binding: ~83%

Metabolism: Hepatic primarily via CYP2C19 and 3A4 and to a lesser extent CYP1A2; forms metabolites (inactive) via deboronization followed by hydroxylation

Half-life elimination: Single dose: IV: 9 to 15 hours; Multiple dosing: 1 mg/m^2: 40 to 193 hours; 1.3 mg/m^2: 76 to 108 hours

Dosing

Adult & Geriatric Note: Consecutive doses should be separated by at least 72 hours.

Multiple myeloma (first-line therapy; in combination with melphalan and prednisone): IV, SubQ: 1.3 mg/m^2 days 1, 4, 8, 11, 22, 25, 29, and 32 of a 42-day treatment cycle for 4 cycles, followed by 1.3 mg/m^2 days 1, 8, 22, and 29 of a 42-day treatment cycle for 5 cycles.

Retreatment may be considered for multiple myeloma patients who had previously responded to bortezomib (either as monotherapy or in combination) and who have relapsed at least 6 months after completing prior bortezomib therapy; initiate at the last tolerated dose.

Transplant-eligible patients (first-line therapy; in combination with other chemotherapy agents) (Canadian labeling): IV: 1.3 mg/m^2 days 1, 4, 8, and 11 followed by a rest period of up to 20 days (equals one treatment cycle); administer 3 to 6 cycles.

◄ *Alternative first-line therapy (off-label dosing):*

CyBorD regimen: IV: 1.5 mg/m^2 days 1, 8, 15, and 22 of a 28-day treatment cycle for 4 cycles (may continue beyond 4 cycles) in combination with cyclophosphamide and dexamethasone (Khan, 2012)

PAD regimen: IV: Induction: 1.3 mg/m^2 days 1, 4, 8, and 11 of a 28-day treatment cycle for 3 cycles (in combination with doxorubicin and dexamethasone), followed by conditioning/stem cell transplantation, and then maintenance bortezomib 1.3 mg/m^2 once every 2 weeks for 2 years (Sonneveld, 2012)

VRd regimen: IV: 1.3 mg/m^2 days 1, 4, 8, and 11 of a 21-day treatment cycle for 8 cycles (in combination with lenalidomide and dexamethasone) (Kumar, 2012; Richardson, 2010)

Patients ≥65 years: IV: 1.3 mg/m^2 days 1, 8, 15, and 22 of a 35-day treatment cycle, in combination with **either** melphalan and prednisone or melphalan, prednisone, and thalidomide (Boccadoro, 2010; Bringhen, 2010; Palumbo, 2009)

Multiple myeloma (relapsed): IV, SubQ: 1.3 mg/m^2 twice weekly for 2 weeks on days 1, 4, 8, and 11 of a 21-day treatment cycle. Therapy extending beyond 8 cycles may be administered by the standard schedule or may be given once weekly for 4 weeks (days 1, 8, 15, and 22), followed by a 13-day rest (days 23 through 35).

Retreatment may be considered for multiple myeloma patients who had previously responded to bortezomib (either as monotherapy or in combination) and who have relapsed at least 6 months after completing prior bortezomib therapy; initiate at the last tolerated dose. Administer twice weekly for 2 weeks on days 1, 4, 8, and 11 of a 21-day treatment cycle (either as a single-agent or in combination with dexamethasone) for a maximum of 8 cycles.

Alternative relapsed therapy (off-label dosing): IV: 1.3 mg/m^2 days 1, 4, 8, and 11 of a 21-day treatment cycle for at least 8 cycles or until disease progression or unacceptable toxicity (in combination with liposomal doxorubicin) (Orlowski, 2007)

Mantle cell lymphoma (first-line therapy; in combination with rituximab, cyclophosphamide, doxorubicin, and prednisone [VcR-CAP]): IV: 1.3 mg/m^2 days 1, 4, 8, 11 of a 21-day treatment cycle for 6 cycles. If response first documented at cycle 6, treatment for an additional 2 cycles is recommended.

Mantle cell lymphoma (relapsed): IV, SubQ: 1.3 mg/m^2 twice weekly for 2 weeks on days 1, 4, 8, and 11 of a 21-day treatment cycle. Therapy extending beyond 8 cycles may be administered by the standard schedule or may be given once weekly for 4 weeks (days 1, 8, 15, and 22), followed by a 13-day rest (days 23 through 35).

Cutaneous or peripheral T-cell lymphoma, relapsed/refractory (off-label use): IV: 1.3 mg/m^2 twice weekly for 2 weeks on days 1, 4, 8, and 11 of a 21-day treatment cycle (Zinzani, 2007); additional data may be necessary to further define the role of bortezomib in this condition.

Follicular lymphoma, relapsed/refractory (off-label use): IV: 1.3 mg/m^2 days 1, 4, 8, and 11 of a 28-day treatment cycle, in combination with bendamustine and rituximab for 6 cycles (Friedberg, 2011) **or** 1.6 mg/m^2 days 1, 8, 15, and 22 of a 35-day treatment cycle, in combination with bendamustine and rituximab for 5 cycles (Fowler, 2011)

Systemic light-chain amyloidosis (off-label use): IV: 1.3 mg/m^2 days 1, 4, 8, and 11 of a 21-day treatment cycle (with or without dexamethasone) (Kastritis, 2010)

Waldenström's macroglobulinemia, relapsed/refractory (off-label use):
IV: 1.3 mg/m² days 1, 4, 8, and 11 of a 21-day treatment cycle (Chen, 2007) **or** 1.3 mg/m² days 1, 4, 8, and 11 of a 21-day treatment cycle (in combination with dexamethasone and rituximab) (Treon, 2009) **or** 1.6 mg/m² days 1, 8, and 15 of a 28-day treatment cycle (in combination with rituximab) (Ghobrial, 2010)

Renal Impairment No dosage adjustment is necessary. Dialysis may reduce bortezomib concentrations; administer postdialysis (Leal, 2011).

Hepatic Impairment

Mild impairment (bilirubin ≤1 times ULN and AST >ULN or bilirubin >1 to 1.5 times ULN): No initial dose adjustment is necessary (LoRusso, 2012).

Moderate (bilirubin >1.5 to 3 times ULN) and severe impairment (bilirubin >3 times ULN): Reduce initial dose to 0.7 mg/m² in the first cycle; based on patient tolerance, may consider dose escalation to 1 mg/m² (LoRusso, 2012) or further dose reduction to 0.5 mg/m² in subsequent cycles

Obesity *ASCO Guidelines for appropriate chemotherapy dosing in obese adults with cancer:* Utilize patient's actual body weight (full weight) for calculation of body surface area- or weight-based dosing, particularly when the intent of therapy is curative; manage regimen-related toxicities in the same manner as for nonobese patients; if a dose reduction is utilized due to toxicity, consider resumption of full weight-based dosing with subsequent cycles, especially if cause of toxicity (eg, hepatic or renal impairment) is resolved (Griggs, 2012).

Adjustment for Toxicity

Myeloma (first-line therapy):

Platelets should be ≥70,000/mm³, ANC should be ≥1000/mm³, and nonhematologic toxicities should resolve to grade 1 or baseline prior to therapy initiation.

Platelets ≤30,000/mm³ or ANC ≤750/mm³ on bortezomib day(s) (except day 1): Withhold bortezomib; if several bortezomib doses in consecutive cycles are withheld, reduce dose 1 level (1.3 mg/m²/dose reduced to 1 mg/m²/dose; 1 mg/m²/dose reduced to 0.7 mg/m²/dose)

Grade ≥3 nonhematological toxicity (other than neuropathy): Withhold bortezomib until toxicity resolves to grade 1 or baseline. May reinitiate bortezomib at 1 dose level reduction (1.3 mg/m²/dose reduced to 1 mg/m²/dose; 1 mg/m²/dose reduced to 0.7 mg/m²/dose).

Neuropathic pain and/or peripheral sensory or motor neuropathy: See "Neuropathic pain and/or peripheral sensory or motor neuropathy" toxicity adjustment guidelines below.

Mantle cell lymphoma (first-line therapy):

Platelets should be ≥100,000/mm³, ANC should be ≥1,500/mm³, hemoglobin should be ≥8 g/dL, and nonhematologic toxicities should resolve to grade 1 or baseline prior to each cycle (cycle 2 and beyond).

Platelets <25,000/mm³ or ≥ grade 3 neutropenia on bortezomib day(s) (except day 1): Withhold bortezomib for up to 2 weeks until platelets are ≥25,000/mm³ and/or ANC ≥750/mm³, then reduce dose 1 level (1.3 mg/m²/dose reduced to 1 mg/m²/dose; 1 mg/m²/dose reduced to 0.7 mg/m²/dose). If hematologic toxicity does not resolve after withholding therapy, discontinue bortezomib.

Grade ≥3 nonhematological toxicity (other than neuropathy): Withhold bortezomib until toxicity resolves to ≤ grade 2. May reinitiate bortezomib at 1 dose level reduction (1.3 mg/m²/dose reduced to 1 mg/m²/dose; 1 mg/m²/dose reduced to 0.7 mg/m²/dose).

Neuropathic pain and/or peripheral sensory or motor neuropathy: See "Neuropathic pain and/or peripheral sensory or motor neuropathy" toxicity adjustment guidelines below.

Relapsed multiple myeloma and mantle cell lymphoma:

Grade 3 nonhematological (excluding neuropathy) or grade 4 hematological toxicity: Withhold until toxicity resolved; may reinitiate with a 25% dose reduction (1.3 mg/m^2/dose reduced to 1 mg/m^2/dose; 1 mg/m^2/dose reduced to 0.7 mg/m^2/dose)

Neuropathic pain and/or peripheral sensory, motor, or autonomic neuropathy:

Note: Consider subQ administration in patients with preexisting or at high risk for peripheral neuropathy.

Grade 1 (asymptomatic; deep tendon reflex loss or paresthesia) without pain or loss of function: No action needed

Grade 1 with pain or grade 2 (moderate symptoms; limiting instrumental activities of daily living): Reduce dose to 1 mg/m^2

Grade 2 with pain or grade 3 (severe symptoms; limiting self-care activities of daily living): Withhold until toxicity resolved, may reinitiate at 0.7 mg/m^2 once weekly

Grade 4 (life-threatening consequences with urgent intervention indicated) and/or severe autonomic neuropathy: Discontinue therapy.

Combination Regimens

Amyloidosis: Bortezomib-Dexamethasone (Amyloidosis) on page 1848

Lymphoma, non-Hodgkin (Follicular): Bendamustine-Bortezomib-Rituximab (NHL-Follicular) on page 1833

Lymphoma, non-Hodgkin (Mantle Cell): VcR-CAP (NHL-Mantle Cell) on page 2106

Multiple myeloma:

Bortezomib-Dexamethasone (Multiple Myeloma) on page 1848

Bortezomib-Doxorubicin-Dexamethasone (Multiple Myeloma) on page 1849

Bortezomib-Doxorubicin (Liposomal) on page 1849

Bortezomib-Doxorubicin (Liposomal)-Dexamethasone on page 1850

Bortezomib-Melphalan-Prednisone-Thalidomide on page 1850

Cyclophosphamide-Bortezomib-Dexamethasone (Multiple Myeloma) on page 1927

Lenalidomide-Bortezomib-Dexamethasone (Multiple Myeloma) on page 2026

Melphalan-Prednisone-Bortezomib (Multiple Myeloma) on page 2033

Panobinostat-Bortezomib-Dexamethasone (Multiple Myeloma) on page 2059

Waldenstrom Macroglobulinemia:

Bortezomib-Dexamethasone-Rituximab (Waldenstrom Macroglobulinemia) on page 1848

Bortezomib-Rituximab (Waldenstrom Macroglobulinemia) on page 1850

Bortezomib (Waldenstrom Macroglobulinemia) on page 1851

Administration Note: The reconstituted concentrations for IV and SubQ administration are different; use caution when calculating the volume for each route and dose. Consider SubQ administration in patients with preexisting or at high risk for peripheral neuropathy.

IV: Administer via rapid IV push (3-5 seconds). When administering in combination with rituximab for first-line therapy of mantle cell lymphoma, administer bortezomib prior to rituximab.

SubQ: Subcutaneous administration of bortezomib 1.3 mg/m^2 days 1, 4, 8, and 11 of a 21-day treatment cycle has been studied in a limited number of patients with relapsed multiple myeloma; doses were administered subcutaneously (concentration of 2.5 mg/mL) into the thigh or abdomen, rotating the injection site with each dose; injections at the same site within a single cycle were avoided (Moreau, 2010; Moreau, 2011). Response rates were similar to IV administration; decreased incidence of grade 3 or higher adverse events were observed with SubQ administration. Administer at least 1 inch from an old site and never administer to tender, bruised, erythematous, or indurated sites. If injection site reaction occurs, the more dilute 1 mg/mL concentration may be used SubQ (or IV administration of 1 mg/mL concentration may be considered).

For IV or SubQ administration only; fatalities have been reported with inadvertent intrathecal administration. Bortezomib should **NOT** be delivered to the patient at the same time with any medications intended for central nervous system administration.

Hazardous agent; use appropriate precautions for handling and disposal (NIOSH 2014 [group 1]).

Vesicant/Extravasation Risk May be an irritant; extravasation has not been associated with tissue damage

Emetic Potential
Children: Minimal (<10%)
Adults: Low (10% to 30%)

Monitoring Parameters CBC with differential and platelets (monitor frequently throughout therapy); liver function tests (in patients with existing hepatic impairment); signs/symptoms of peripheral neuropathy, dehydration, hypotension, PRES, or PML; renal function, baseline chest x-ray and then periodic pulmonary function testing (with new or worsening pulmonary symptoms)

Dietary Considerations Green tea and green tea extracts may diminish the therapeutic effect of bortezomib and should be avoided (Golden, 2009). Avoid grapefruit juice. Avoid additional, nondietary sources of ascorbic acid supplements, including multivitamins containing ascorbic acid (may diminish bortezomib activity) during treatment, especially 12 hours before and after bortezomib treatment (Perrone, 2009).

Dosage Forms Excipient information presented when available (limited, particularly for generics); consult specific product labeling.
Solution Reconstituted, Injection:
Velcade: 3.5 mg (1 ea)

♦ **Bortezomib For Injection (Can)** see Bortezomib on page 223
♦ **Bosulif** see Bosutinib on page 231

Bosutinib (boe SUE ti nib)
Related Information
Common Toxicity Criteria on page 2122
Management of Chemotherapy-Induced Nausea and Vomiting in Adults on page 2142
Principles of Anticancer Therapy on page 2261
Safe Handling of Hazardous Drugs on page 2292
Brand Names: US Bosulif
Brand Names: Canada Bosulif

Index Terms Bosutinib Monohydrate; SKI-606

Pharmacologic Category Antineoplastic Agent, BCR-ABL Tyrosine Kinase Inhibitor; Antineoplastic Agent, Tyrosine Kinase Inhibitor

Use Chronic myelogenous leukemia (CML):

US labeling: Treatment of chronic, accelerated, or blast phase Philadelphia chromosome-positive (Ph+) CML in patients resistant or intolerant to prior therapy

Canadian labeling: Treatment of chronic, accelerated or blast phase Philadelphia chromosome-positive (Ph+) CML in patients resistant or intolerant to prior therapy and for whom subsequent treatment with imatinib, nilotinib, and dasatinib is not appropriate

Labeled Contraindications

Hypersensitivity to bosutinib or any component of the formulation

Canadian labeling: Additional contraindications (not in US labeling): History of long QT syndrome or with persistent QT interval >480 milliseconds; uncorrected hypokalemia or hypomagnesemia; hepatic impairment

Pregnancy Considerations Adverse events were observed in animal reproduction studies. Based on the mechanism of action, bosutinib may cause fetal harm if administered in pregnancy. Females of reproductive potential should use effective contraception during bosutinib treatment and for at least 30 days after completion of treatment. The Canadian labeling suggests that semen from male patients (including those who have undergone successful vasectomy) receiving bosutinib may pose a risk to a developing fetus and recommends that male patients use effective contraception while receiving treatment, during any treatment interruptions, and for at least 4 weeks after discontinuation of treatment.

Breast-Feeding Considerations It is not known if bosutinib is excreted in breast milk. Due to the potential for serious adverse reactions in the nursing infant, the decision to discontinue bosutinib or discontinue breast-feeding should take into account the benefits of treatment to the mother.

Warnings/Precautions Hazardous agent - use appropriate precautions for handling and disposal (meets NIOSH 2014 criteria).

Diarrhea, nausea, vomiting, and abdominal pain may occur. Monitor; may require treatment interruption, dose reduction, or discontinuation. For patients experiencing diarrhea (all grades), the median time to onset was 2 days; median duration (per event) was 1 day; manage diarrhea with antidiarrheals and/or fluid replacement. Nausea and vomiting may be managed with antiemetics and fluid replacement. Acute pancreatitis has been reported; use caution in patients with a prior history of pancreatitis. The Canadian labeling recommends interruption of therapy in patients with elevated amylase/lipase accompanied by abdominal symptoms and evaluation to rule out pancreatitis.

Bleeding events (eg, GI, ophthalmic, pericardial, cerebral, vaginal) have been reported. Anemia, neutropenia, and thrombocytopenia may also occur. May require treatment interruption, dose reduction, or discontinuation. Monitor blood counts weekly during first month, then monthly thereafter (or as clinically indicated). Fluid retention, manifesting as pericardial effusion, pleural effusion, pulmonary edema and/or peripheral edema may occur; may be severe. Monitor for fluid retention (eg, weight gain) and manage appropriately; may require treatment interruption, dose reduction, or discontinuation. QTcF >500 milliseconds was observed rarely (≤0.8%) in clinical trials (Abbas 2012; Cortes 2012); patients with significant or uncontrolled cardiovascular disease (including prolonged QT interval at baseline) were not studied. The Canadian labeling recommends obtaining an ECG (baseline and as clinically indicated there-after), correction of preexisting hypokalemia and/or hypomagnesemia and periodic monitoring of serum potassium and magnesium.

Bosutinib exposure is increased in patients with hepatic impairment; dose reduction is recommended (Canadian labeling contraindicates use in patients with hepatic impairment at baseline). Hepatotoxicity has been reported during treatment; dose reductions may be necessary. Monitor liver function. ALT and AST elevations may occur, usually with an onset in the first 3 months of treatment (median onset was ~30 to 33 days; median duration was 21 days). One case of drug-induced liver injury has been reported; full recovery occurred after discontinuation. Bosutinib exposure is increased in patients with moderate or severe renal impairment. Declines in glomerular filtration rates throughout bosutinib treatment have been observed in clinical studies; monitor renal function at baseline and during therapy, particularly in patients with preexisting impairment or other risk factors for renal dysfunction. Consider dosage adjustment in patients with renal dysfunction at baseline or with treatment emergent impairment. Bone fracture and mineral abnormalities (eg, hypophosphatemia) has been reported (Bosulif Canadian product monograph 2014); monitor patients with severe osteoporosis or endocrine disease (eg, hyperparathyroidism) for mineral abnormalities and/or changes in bone density.

Potentially significant drug-drug interactions may exist, requiring dose or frequency adjustment, additional monitoring, and/or selection of alternative therapy. Proton pump inhibitors (PPIs) may decrease bosutinib effects; consider using short acting antacids or H_2 antagonists instead of PPIs; separate administration of antacids or H_2 antagonists from bosutinib by at least 2 hours.

Adverse Reactions

>10%:

Cardiovascular: Edema (14%; grades 3/4: <1%)

Central nervous system: Fatigue (20% to 26%), headache (18% to 20%), dizziness (10% to 13%)

Dermatologic: Skin rash (34% to 35%), pruritus (8% to 11%)

Endocrine & metabolic: Hypophosphatemia (50% [Gambacorti–Passerini 2014]; grades 3/4: 7%), hypokalemia (18%; grades 3/4: 2% [Gambacorti-Passerini 2014])

Gastrointestinal: Diarrhea (76% to 84%; grades 3/4: 5% to 9%), nausea (46% to 47%; grades 3/4: 1% to 2%), vomiting (37% to 42%; grades 3/4: 3% to 4%), abdominal pain (29% to 40%; grades 3/4: 1% to 5%), increase serum lipase (15% to 38%; grades 3/4: 3% to 9% [Cortes 2012, Gambacorti–Passerini 2014]), decreased appetite (13% to 14%)

Hematologic & oncologic: Thrombocytopenia (40% to 42%; grades 3/4: 26% to 37%), anemia (23% to 37%; grades 3/4: 9% to 26%), neutropenia (16% to 19%; grades 3/4: 11% to 18%)

Hepatic: Increased serum ALT (10% to 20%; grades 3/4: 5% to 7%), increased serum AST (11% to 16%; grades 3/4: 3% to 4%)

Neuromuscular & skeletal: Arthralgia (13% to 14%), back pain (7% to 12%), weakness (10% to 11%)

Respiratory: Cough (20% to 21%), dyspnea (10% to 19%), respiratory tract infection (10% to 12%), nasopharyngitis (5% to 12%)

Miscellaneous: Fever (22% to 36%)

1% to 10%:

Cardiovascular: Pericardial effusion (grades 3/4: <1%), chest pain, prolonged Q-T interval on ECG

Central nervous system: Pain

Dermatologic: Acne vulgaris, urticaria

Endocrine & metabolic: Dehydration, hyperkalemia

Gastrointestinal: Dysgeusia, gastritis

Hematologic & oncologic: Febrile neutropenia

Hepatic: Hepatic insufficiency, hepatotoxicity, increased serum bilirubin

Hypersensitivity: Hypersensitivity reaction

Infection: Influenza

Neuromuscular & skeletal: Increased creatine phosphokinase, myalgia

Otic: Tinnitus

Renal: Increased serum creatinine, renal failure

Respiratory: Bronchitis, pleural effusion, pneumonia

<1%, postmarketing, and/or case reports: Anaphylactic shock, erythema multiforme, exfoliative dermatitis, fixed drug eruption, gastrointestinal hemorrhage, hepatic injury, pancreatitis, pericarditis, pulmonary edema, pulmonary hypertension, respiratory failure

Drug Interactions

Metabolism/Transport Effects Substrate of CYP3A4 (major); **Note:** Assignment of Major/Minor substrate status based on clinically relevant drug interaction potential; **Inhibits** P-glycoprotein

Avoid Concomitant Use

Avoid concomitant use of Bosutinib with any of the following: BCG (Intravesical); Bitter Orange; CloZAPine; Conivaptan; CYP3A4 Inducers (Moderate); CYP3A4 Inducers (Strong); CYP3A4 Inhibitors (Moderate); CYP3A4 Inhibitors (Strong); Dipyrone; Fusidic Acid (Systemic); Idelalisib; P-glycoprotein/ABCB1 Inhibitors; Pomegranate; St Johns Wort; Star Fruit

Increased Effect/Toxicity

Bosutinib may increase the levels/effects of: CloZAPine; Highest Risk QTc-Prolonging Agents; Moderate Risk QTc-Prolonging Agents

The levels/effects of Bosutinib may be increased by: Bitter Orange; Conivaptan; CYP3A4 Inhibitors (Moderate); CYP3A4 Inhibitors (Strong); Dasatinib; Dipyrone; Fosaprepitant; Fusidic Acid (Systemic); Idelalisib; Luliconazole; Osimertinib; Palbociclib; P-glycoprotein/ABCB1 Inhibitors; Pomegranate; Star Fruit; Stiripentol

Decreased Effect

Bosutinib may decrease the levels/effects of: BCG (Intravesical)

The levels/effects of Bosutinib may be decreased by: Antacids; CYP3A4 Inducers (Moderate); CYP3A4 Inducers (Strong); Deferasirox; H2-Antagonists; Osimertinib; Proton Pump Inhibitors; Siltuximab; St Johns Wort; Tocilizumab

Food Interactions Grapefruit juice may increase bosutinib plasma concentration. Management: Avoid grapefruit juice during bosutinib therapy. Additionally the Canadian labeling recommends avoiding products containing Seville oranges, pomegranate and star fruit during therapy; may increase bosutinib plasma concentrations.

Storage/Stability Store at 20°C to 25°C (68°F to 77°F); excursions permitted to 15°C to 30°C (59°F to 86°F).

Mechanism of Action BCR-ABL tyrosine kinase inhibitor (TKI); inhibits BCR-ABL kinase that promotes CML. Also inhibits SRC family (including SRC, LYN, and HCK). Bosutinib has minimal activity against c-KIT and platelet-derived growth factor receptor (PDGFR), which are nonspecific targets associated with toxicity in other TKIs (Cortes 2012). Bosutinib has activity in 16 of 18 imatinib-resistant BCR-ABL mutations, with the exceptions of the T315I and V299L mutants (Cortes 2011).

Pharmacodynamics/Kinetics

Onset:

Median time to complete hematologic response (in responders): 2 weeks (Cortes 2011)

Median time to major cytogenetic response (in responders): 12.3 weeks (Cortes 2011)

Median time to first complete cytogenic response: 12.9 weeks (Cortes 2012)

Absorption: Slow (Abbas 2012)

Distribution: V_d: 6,080 ± 1,230 L

Protein binding: 94% to plasma proteins

Metabolism: Hepatic via CYP3A4, primarily to inactive metabolites oxydechlorinated (M2) bosutinib and N-desmethylated (M5) bosutinib, also to bosutinib N-oxide (M6)

Half-life elimination: 22 to 27 hours (Cortes 2011)

Time to peak: 4 to 6 hours

Excretion: Feces (~91%); urine (3%)

Dosing

Adult & Geriatric Philadelphia chromosome-positive chronic myelogenous leukemia (Ph+CML): Oral: 500 mg once daily; continue until disease progression or unacceptable toxicity. **Note:** If complete hematologic response is not achieved by week 8 or complete cytogenetic response is not achieved by week 12, in the absence of grade 3 or higher adverse reactions, consider increasing the dose from 500 mg once daily to 600 mg once daily.

Missed doses: If a dose is missed beyond 12 hours, skip the dose and resume the usual dose the following day

Renal Impairment

Preexisting impairment:

Mild impairment (CrCl >50 to 80 mL/minute): There are no dosage adjustments provided in manufacturer's labeling, however, based on the pharmacokinetics, the need for dosage adjustment is not likely.

Moderate impairment (CrCl 30 to 50 mL/minute): Initial: 400 mg once daily.

Severe impairment (CrCl <30 mL/minute): Reduce dose to 300 mg once daily (this dose is predicted to result in an AUC similar to that of patients with normal renal function, however, there is no efficacy data for this dose in CML patients with renal impairment).

Renal toxicity during treatment: If unable to tolerate initial dose, reduce dose per adjustment recommendations for toxicity (withhold treatment until resolved, then consider resuming at 400 mg once daily; if clinically appropriate, may re-escalate dose to 500 mg once daily).

Hemodialysis: There are no dosage adjustments provided in the manufacturer's labeling (has not been studied).

Hepatic Impairment

Preexisting impairment (mild, moderate, or severe):

US labeling: Child-Pugh class A, B, or C: Reduce initial dose to 200 mg once daily (this dose is predicted to result in an AUC similar to that of patients with normal hepatic function, however, there is no efficacy data for this dose in CML patients with hepatic impairment).

Canadian labeling: Use is contraindicated in hepatic impairment.

Hepatotoxicity during treatment:

ALT or AST >5 times ULN: Withhold treatment until recovery to ≤2.5 times ULN and resume at 400 mg once daily thereafter. If recovery to ≤2.5 times ULN takes >4 weeks: Discontinue bosutinib.

ALT or AST ≥3 times ULN in conjunction with bilirubin elevation >2 times ULN and alkaline phosphatase <2 times ULN: Discontinue bosutinib.

Adjustment for Toxicity

Hematologic toxicity: ANC <1000/mm^3 or platelets <50,000/mm^3: Withhold treatment until ANC ≥1000/mm^3 **and** platelets ≥50,000/mm^3; if recovery occurs within 2 weeks, resume treatment at the same dose. If ANC and platelets remain low for >2 weeks, upon recovery, resume treatment with the dose reduced by 100 mg. If cytopenia recurs, withhold until recovery and resume treatment with the dose reduced by an additional 100 mg. Doses <300 mg daily have not been evaluated.

Nonhematologic toxicity:

Diarrhea: Grade 3 or 4 (≥7 stools/day increase over baseline): Withhold treatment until recovery to ≤ grade 1; may resume at 400 mg once daily.

Other clinically significant nonhematologic toxicity, moderate or severe: Withhold treatment until resolved, then consider resuming at 400 mg once daily; may re-escalate dose to 500 mg once daily if clinically appropriate.

Combination Regimens

Leukemia, chronic myelogenous: Bosutinib (CML Regimen) on page 1851

Administration Oral: Administer with food. Swallow tablet whole; do not crush or break. Hazardous agent; use appropriate precautions for handling and disposal (meets NIOSH 2014 criteria).

Emetic Potential Minimal (<10%)

Monitoring Parameters CBC with differential and platelets (weekly during first month, then monthly thereafter, or as clinically indicated); hepatic enzymes (monthly for first 3 months or as clinically indicated; monitor more frequently with transaminase elevations); renal function (at baseline and throughout therapy); diarrhea episodes; fluid/edema status (eg, weight gain)

Canadian labeling: Additional recommendations (not in US labeling): ECG (baseline then as clinically indicated); serum electrolytes and lipase/amylase (baseline, frequently during treatment, and as clinically indicated); bone density (patients with severe osteoporosis or endocrine disease)

Dietary Considerations Take with food.

Dosage Forms Excipient information presented when available (limited, particularly for generics); consult specific product labeling.

Tablet, Oral:

Bosulif: 100 mg, 500 mg

◆ **Bosutinib Monohydrate** *see* Bosutinib *on page 231*

◆ **BRAF(V600E) Kinase Inhibitor RO5185426** *see* Vemurafenib *on page 1734*

◆ **Brentuximab** *see* Brentuximab Vedotin *on page 237*

Brentuximab Vedotin (bren TUX i mab ve DOE tin)

Related Information

Management of Chemotherapy-Induced Nausea and Vomiting in Adults *on page 2142*

Principles of Anticancer Therapy *on page 2261*

Safe Handling of Hazardous Drugs *on page 2292*

Brand Names: US Adcetris

Brand Names: Canada Adcetris

Index Terms Anti-CD30 ADC SGN-35; Anti-CD30 Antibody-Drug Conjugate SGN-35; Antibody-Drug Conjugate SGN-35; Brentuximab; SGN-35

Pharmacologic Category Antineoplastic Agent, Anti-CD30; Antineoplastic Agent, Antibody Drug Conjugate; Antineoplastic Agent, Monoclonal Antibody

Use

Anaplastic large cell lymphoma (systemic): Treatment of systemic anaplastic large cell lymphoma after failure of at least 1 prior multiagent chemotherapy regimen

Hodgkin lymphoma: Treatment of classical Hodgkin lymphoma after failure of at least 2 prior multiagent chemotherapy regimens (in patients who are not autologous hematopoietic stem cell transplant candidates) or after failure of autologous hematopoietic stem cell transplant

Hodgkin lymphoma (post-autologous hematopoietic stem cell transplantation): Treatment (maintenance therapy) of classical Hodgkin lymphoma in patients at high risk of relapse or progression as post–autologous hematopoietic stem cell transplant consolidation

Labeled Contraindications

US labeling: Concurrent use with bleomycin

Canadian labeling: Hypersensitivity to brentuximab or any component of the formulation; concurrent use with bleomycin; patients who have or have history of progressive multifocal leukoencephalopathy

Pregnancy Considerations Adverse events were observed in animal reproduction studies. Based on the mechanism of action, may cause fetal harm if administered to a pregnant woman.

Breast-Feeding Considerations It is not known if brentuximab vedotin is excreted in breast milk. Due to the potential for serious adverse reactions in the nursing infant, the manufacturer recommends a decision be made to discontinue nursing or to discontinue the drug, taking into account the importance of treatment to the mother.

Warnings/Precautions Hazardous agent - use appropriate precautions for handling and disposal (NIOSH 2014 [group 1]).

[US Boxed Warning]: Cases of progressive multifocal leukoencephalopathy (PML) and death due to JC virus infection have been reported. Immunosuppression due to prior chemotherapy treatments or underlying disease may also contribute to PML development. New-onset signs/symptoms of central nervous system abnormalities (eg, changes in mood, memory, cognition, motor incoordination and/or weakness, speech and/or visual disturbances) should receive prompt evaluation with neurology consultation, brain MRI, and lumbar puncture or brain biopsy. The time to initial symptom onset varies from treatment initiation, with some cases occurring within 3 months of initial drug exposure. Withhold treatment with new-onset symptoms suggestive of PML; discontinue if diagnosis of PML is confirmed.

Peripheral neuropathy is common and is generally cumulative; usually sensory neuropathy, although motor neuropathy has also been observed; neuropathy completely resolved in nearly half of patients; almost one-third had partial improvement. Monitor for symptoms of neuropathy (hypoesthesia, hyperesthesia, paresthesia, discomfort, burning sensation, neuropathic pain, or weakness); dose interruption, reduction or discontinuation may be recommended for new or worsening neuropathy.

Grade 3 or 4 neutropenia, thrombocytopenia, and anemia may occur; neutropenia may be severe and/or prolonged (≥1 week); neutropenic fever also has been reported; monitor blood counts prior to each dose and consider more frequent monitoring for patients with Grade 3 or 4 neutropenia; may require growth factor support, dose interruption, reduction or discontinuation. Serious infections, including opportunistic infections (eg, pneumonia, bacteremia, sepsis/septic shock) have been reported (some fatal); monitor for signs or symptoms of bacterial, fungal, or viral infections. Infusion reactions, including anaphylaxis have been reported; monitor during infusion. For anaphylaxis, immediately and permanently discontinue and administer appropriate medical intervention. For infusion-related reaction, interrupt infusion and administer appropriate medical intervention; premedicate for subsequent infusions (with acetaminophen, an antihistamine, and/or a corticosteroid).

Noninfectious pulmonary toxicity (eg, pneumonitis, interstitial lung disease, acute respiratory distress syndrome), some fatal, has been reported in patients receiving brentuximab vedotin. Monitor for signs/symptoms of pulmonary toxicity (eg, cough, dyspnea). Withhold treatment and perform prompt diagnostic evaluation and management for new or worsening pulmonary symptoms. Due to the risk for pulmonary injury, concurrent use with bleomycin is contraindicated. In a study comparing brentuximab combined with ABVD (doxorubicin, bleomycin, vinblastine, and dacarbazine) to brentuximab combined with AVD (doxorubicin, vinblastine, and dacarbazine), the occurrence of pulmonary toxicity was higher in the brentuximab/ABVD group. Pulmonary symptoms/toxicities reported with brentuximab in combination with ABVD consisted of cough, dyspnea, and interstitial infiltration/inflammation; most patients responded to corticosteroids. Potentially significant drug-drug interactions may exist, requiring dose or frequency adjustment, additional monitoring, and/or selection of alternative therapy.

Serious hepatotoxicity, including fatalities, has occurred; cases were consistent with hepatocellular injury, with elevations of transaminases and/or bilirubin. Some have occurred after the initial dose or after rechallenge. The risk for hepatotoxicity may be increased with preexisting liver disease, elevated baseline liver enzymes, and concurrent medications. Monitor liver enzymes and bilirubin. Treatment delay, dose reduction or discontinuation may be required for new, worsening, or recurrent hepatotoxicity. Avoid use in patients with moderate to severe hepatic impairment (Child-Pugh classes B and C). The frequency of grade 3/4 toxicities (and deaths) was increased in patients with moderate or severe impairment (compared to patients with normal hepatic function). A component of brentuximab vedotin, the microtubule-disrupting agent monomethylauristatin E (MMAE) is excreted hepatically. MMAE exposure is increased ~2.2-fold in patients with hepatic impairment.

Avoid use in patients with severe renal impairment (CrCl <30 mL/minute). The frequency of grade 3/4 toxicities (and deaths) was increased in patients with severe impairment (compared to patients with normal renal function). A component of brentuximab vedotin, the microtubule-disrupting agent MMAE is excreted renally; MMAE exposure is increased in patients with severe impairment. Stevens-Johnson syndrome (SJS) and toxic epidermal necrolysis (TEN) have been reported (some fatal). Discontinue (and begin appropriate management) if SJS or TEN occur. Tumor lysis syndrome (TLS) may occur; risk of TLS is higher in patients with a high tumor burden or with rapid tumor proliferation; monitor closely.

Adverse Reactions

>10%:

Cardiovascular: Peripheral edema (4% to 16%)

Central nervous system: Peripheral sensory neuropathy (52% to 53%; grade 3: 8% to 10%), fatigue (41% to 49%), pain (7% to 28%), headache (16% to 19%), insomnia (14% to 16%), dizziness (11% to 16%), peripheral motor neuropathy (7% to 16%; grade 3: 3% to 4%), chills (12% to 13%), anxiety (7% to 11%)

Dermatologic: Skin rash (27% to 31%), pruritus (17% to 19%), alopecia (13% to 14%), night sweats (9% to 12%)

Endocrine & metabolic: Weight loss (6% to 12%)

Gastrointestinal: Nausea (38% to 42%), diarrhea (29% to 36%), abdominal pain (9% to 25%), vomiting (17% to 22%), constipation (16% to 19%), decreased appetite (11% to 16%)

Hematologic & oncologic: Neutropenia (54% to 55%; grade 3: 12% to 15%; grade 4: 6% to 9%), anemia (33% to 52%; grade 3: 2% to 8%; grade 4: ≤2%), thrombocytopenia (16% to 28%; grade 3: 5% to 7%; grade 4: 2% to 5%), lymphadenopathy (10% to 11%)

Immunologic: Antibody development (antibrentuximab; transient: 30%; persistent: 7%)

Neuromuscular & skeletal: Arthralgia (9% to 19%), myalgia (16% to 17%), back pain (10% to 14%)

Respiratory: Upper respiratory tract infection (12% to 47%), cough (17% to 25%), dyspnea (13% to 19%), oropharyngeal pain (9% to 11%)

Miscellaneous: Fever (29% to 38%), infusion related reaction (grades 1/2: 12%)

1% to 10%:

Cardiovascular: Septic shock (3%), supraventricular cardiac arrhythmia (3%), pulmonary embolism (2%)

Dermatologic: Xeroderma (4% to 10%)

Genitourinary: Urinary tract infection (3%)

Neuromuscular & skeletal: Muscle spasm (9% to 10%), limb pain (3% to 10%)

Renal: Pyelonephritis (2%)

Respiratory: Pneumonitis (2%), pneumothorax (2%)

<1%, postmarketing, and/or case reports: Anaphylaxis, febrile neutropenia, hepatotoxicity, hyperglycemia, infection (including pneumonia, bacteremia, sepsis), JC virus infection, pancreatitis, progressive multifocal leukoencephalopathy, pulmonary toxicity, Stevens-Johnson syndrome, toxic epidermal necrolysis, tumor lysis syndrome

Drug Interactions

Metabolism/Transport Effects Substrate of CYP3A4 (minor), P-glycoprotein; **Note:** Assignment of Major/Minor substrate status based on clinically relevant drug interaction potential

◄ **Avoid Concomitant Use**

Avoid concomitant use of Brentuximab Vedotin with any of the following: BCG (Intravesical); Belimumab; Bleomycin; Natalizumab; Pimecrolimus; Tacrolimus (Topical); Tofacitinib; Vaccines (Live)

Increased Effect/Toxicity

Brentuximab Vedotin may increase the levels/effects of: Belimumab; Bleomycin; Fingolimod; Leflunomide; Natalizumab; Tofacitinib; Vaccines (Live)

The levels/effects of Brentuximab Vedotin may be increased by: CYP3A4 Inhibitors (Strong); Denosumab; Lumacaftor; P-glycoprotein/ABCB1 Inhibitors; Pimecrolimus; Ranolazine; Roflumilast; Tacrolimus (Topical); Trastuzumab

Decreased Effect

Brentuximab Vedotin may decrease the levels/effects of: BCG (Intravesical); Coccidioides immitis Skin Test; Sipuleucel-T; Vaccines (Inactivated); Vaccines (Live)

The levels/effects of Brentuximab Vedotin may be decreased by: CYP3A4 Inducers (Strong); Echinacea; Lumacaftor; P-glycoprotein/ABCB1 Inducers

Storage/Stability Store intact vials refrigerated at 2°C to 8°C (36°F to 46°F) in the original carton. Protect from light. Reconstituted solution should be diluted immediately; however, may be stored refrigerated for up to 24 hours; do not freeze. Solutions diluted for infusion should be used immediately after preparation; however, may be stored for 24 hours refrigerated (do not freeze); use within 24 hours of initial reconstitution.

Preparation for Administration Hazardous agent: Use appropriate precautions for handling and disposal (NIOSH 2014 [group 1]). Reconstitute each 50 mg vial with 10.5 mL sterile water for injection (SWFI), resulting in a concentration of 5 mg/mL. Direct SWFI toward the vial wall; do not direct toward the cake or powder. Swirl gently to dissolve, do not shake. Reconstituted solution should be clear to slightly opalescent without visible particles. Further dilute in at least 100 mL of either NS, D_5W, or lactated Ringer's to a final concentration of 0.4 to 1.8 mg/mL; gently invert bag to mix. Do not mix with other medications. Use within 24 hours of initial reconstitution.

Mechanism of Action Brentuximab vedotin is an antibody drug conjugate (ADC) directed at CD30 consisting of 3 components: 1) a CD30-specific chimeric IgG1 antibody cAC10; 2) a microtubule-disrupting agent, monomethylauristatin E (MMAE); and 3) a protease cleavable dipeptide linker (which covalently conjugates MMAE to cAC10). The conjugate binds to cells which express CD30, and forms a complex which is internalized within the cell and releases MMAE. MMAE binds to the tubules and disrupts the cellular microtubule network, inducing cell cycle arrest (G2/M phase) and apoptosis.

Pharmacodynamics/Kinetics

Distribution: V_{dss}: ADC: 6 to 10 L

Metabolism: MMAE: Minimal, primarily via oxidation by CYP3A4/5

Half-life elimination: Terminal: ADC: ~4 to 6 days

Time to peak: ADC: At end of infusion; MMAE: ~1 to 3 days

Excretion: MMAE: Feces (~72%, primarily unchanged); urine

Dosing

Adult & Geriatric

Hodgkin lymphoma, refractory: IV: 1.8 mg/kg (maximum dose: 180 mg) every 3 weeks, continue until disease progression or unacceptable toxicities

Hodgkin lymphoma, maintenance therapy after autologous hemato-poietic stem cell transplantation (HSCT): IV: 1.8 mg/kg (maximum dose: 180 mg) every 3 weeks, continue until a maximum of 16 cycles, disease progression, or unacceptable toxicity. Begin therapy within 4 to 6 weeks post HSCT or upon recovery from HSCT.

Systemic anaplastic large cell lymphoma (sALCL), refractory: IV: 1.8 mg/kg (maximum dose: 180 mg) every 3 weeks, continue until disease progression or unacceptable toxicities

Renal Impairment
CrCl ≥30 mL/minute: Initial: No dosage adjustment necessary.
CrCl <30 mL/minute: Initial: Avoid use.

Hepatic Impairment
Mild impairment (Child-Pugh class A): Initial: 1.2 mg/kg (maximum dose: 120 mg) every 3 weeks.
Moderate to severe impairment (Child-Pugh class B or C): Avoid use.

Adjustment for Toxicity
Hematologic toxicity:
Grade 3 or 4 neutropenia: Withhold treatment until resolves to baseline or ≤ grade 2, consider growth factor support in subsequent cycles.
Recurrent grade 4 neutropenia (despite the use of growth factor support): Consider reducing the dose to 1.2 mg/kg or discontinuing treatment
Grade 3 or 4 thrombocytopenia (Canadian labeling): Monitor closely; dose delays or platelet transfusions may be considered.

Nonhematologic toxicities:
Anaphylaxis: Discontinue immediately and permanently
Infusion reaction: Interrupt infusion and administer appropriate medical intervention. Premedicate subsequent infusions with acetaminophen, an antihistamine, and/or a corticosteroid.
Peripheral neuropathy, new or worsening grade 2 or 3: Withhold treatment until improves or returns to grade 1 or baseline; then resume with dose reduced to 1.2 mg/kg
Peripheral neuropathy, grade 4: Discontinue treatment
Progressive multifocal leukoencephalopathy (PML): Withhold treatment with new-onset symptoms suggestive of PML; discontinue if PML diagnosis confirmed
Pulmonary toxicity: Withhold treatment with new-onset or worsening pulmonary symptoms during evaluation and until symptomatic improvement
Stevens-Johnson syndrome or toxic epidermal necrolysis: Discontinue and administer appropriate medical intervention

Combination Regimens
Lymphoma, Hodgkin: Brentuximab (Hodgkin Regimen) on page 1851

Administration Infuse over 30 minutes. Do not administer as IV push or bolus; do not mix or infuse with other medications. Hazardous agent; use appropriate precautions for handling and disposal (NIOSH 2014 [group 1]).

Emetic Potential Low (10% to 30%)

Monitoring Parameters CBC with differential prior to each dose (more frequently if clinically indicated); liver and renal function tests. Monitor for infusion reaction, tumor lysis syndrome, signs/symptoms of progressive multi-focal leukoencephalopathy (PML), and for signs of neuropathy (hypoesthesia, hyperesthesia, paresthesia, discomfort, burning sensation, or neuropathic pain or weakness), dermatologic toxicity, pulmonary toxicity, or infection.

Dosage Forms Excipient information presented when available (limited, particularly for generics); consult specific product labeling.
Solution Reconstituted, Intravenous [preservative free]:
  Adcetris: 50 mg (1 ea) [contains polysorbate 80]

◆ **BRL 43694** see Granisetron on page 801
◆ **BTK inhibitor PCI-32765** see Ibrutinib on page 856
◆ **Buscopan (Can)** see Scopolamine (Systemic) on page 1520
◆ **Bussulfam** see Busulfan on page 242

Busulfan (byoo SUL fan)
Related Information
Chemotherapy and Obesity on page 2220
Fertility and Cancer Therapy on page 2137
Hematopoietic Stem Cell Transplantation on page 2272
Management of Chemotherapy-Induced Nausea and Vomiting in Adults on page 2142
Management of Drug Extravasations on page 2159
Prevention of Chemotherapy-Induced Nausea and Vomiting in Children on page 2203
Safe Handling of Hazardous Drugs on page 2292
Brand Names: US Busulfex; Myleran
Brand Names: Canada Busulfex; Myleran
Index Terms Bussulfam; Busulfanum; Busulphan
Pharmacologic Category Antineoplastic Agent, Alkylating Agent
Use
Chronic myeloid leukemia (CML):
  Injection: Conditioning regimen prior to allogeneic hematopoietic progenitor cell transplantation for CML (in combination with cyclophosphamide)
  Tablets: Palliative treatment of CML
Labeled Contraindications Hypersensitivity to busulfan or any component of the formulation; oral busulfan is contraindicated in patients without a definitive diagnosis of CML
Pregnancy Considerations Adverse events were observed in animal reproduction studies. May cause fetal harm if administered during pregnancy. The solvent in IV busulfan, DMA, is also associated with teratogenic effects and may impair fertility. Women and men of childbearing potential should use effective contraception to avoid pregnancy during and after busulfan treatment.
Breast-Feeding Considerations It is not known if busulfan is excreted in breast milk. According to the manufacturer, the decision to discontinue breast-feeding during therapy or to discontinue busulfan should take into account the benefits of treatment to the mother; breast-feeding should be discontinued during IV busulfan treatment.
Warnings/Precautions Hazardous agent - use appropriate precautions for handling and disposal (NIOSH 2014 [group 1]). **[US Boxed Warning]: Severe and prolonged bone marrow suppression commonly occurs; reduce dose or discontinue oral busulfan for unusual suppression; may require bone marrow biopsy. Hematopoietic progenitor cell transplantation is required to prevent potentially fatal complications from prolonged myelosuppression due to IV busulfan.** May result in severe neutropenia, thrombocytopenia, anemia, bone marrow failure, and/or severe pancytopenia; pancytopenia may be prolonged (1 month up to 2 years) and may be

reversible. When used for transplantation, monitor CBC with differential daily during treatment and until engraftment. The onset of neutropenia is a median of 4 days post-transplant; recovery is within a median of 13 days following allogeneic transplant (with prophylactic G-CSF use in most patients). Thrombocytopenia occurred at a median of 5 to 6 days. Use with caution in patients with compromised bone marrow reserve (due to prior treatment or radiation therapy). Monitor closely for signs of infection (due to neutropenia) or bleeding (due to thrombocytopenia). May require antibiotic therapy and platelet and red blood cell support.

Seizures have been reported with IV busulfan and with high-dose oral busulfan. When using as a conditioning regimen for transplant, initiate prophylactic anticonvulsant therapy (eg, phenytoin, levetiracetam, benzodiazepines, or valproic acid) prior to treatment. Use with caution in patients predisposed to seizures, with a history of seizures, head trauma, or with other medications associated with inducing seizures. Phenytoin increases busulfan clearance by ≥15%; busulfan kinetics and dosing recommendations for high-dose HSCT conditioning were studied with concomitant phenytoin. If alternate anticonvulsants are used, busulfan clearance may be decreased and dosing should be monitored accordingly.

Bronchopulmonary dysplasia with pulmonary fibrosis ("busulfan lung") is associated with chronic busulfan use; onset is delayed with symptoms occurring at an average of 4 years (range: 4 months to 10 years) after treatment; may be fatal. Symptoms generally include a slow onset of cough, dyspnea, and fever (low-grade), although acute symptomatic onset may also occur. Diminished diffusion capacity and decreased pulmonary compliance have been noted with pulmonary function testing. Differential diagnosis should rule out opportunistic pulmonary infection or leukemic pulmonary infiltrates; may require lung biopsy. Discontinue busulfan if toxicity develops. Pulmonary toxicity may be additive if administered with other cytotoxic agents also associated with pulmonary toxicity. Cardiac tamponade as been reported in children with thalassemia treated with high-dose oral busulfan in combination with cyclophosphamide. Abdominal pain and vomiting preceded tamponade in most children. Monitor for signs/symptoms and evaluate/treat promptly if cardiac tamponade is suspected. Busulfan has been causally related to the development of secondary malignancies (tumors and acute leukemias); chromosomal alterations may also occur. Chronic low-dose busulfan has been associated with ovarian failure (including failure to achieve puberty). Busulfan is associated with a moderate emetic potential (depending on dose and/or administration route); antiemetics may be recommended to prevent nausea and vomiting (Dupuis 2011).

High busulfan area under the concentration versus time curve (AUC) values (>1500 micromolar•minute) are associated with increased risk of hepatic sinusoidal obstruction syndrome (SOS; formerly called veno-occlusive disease [VOD]) due to conditioning for allogenic HSCT; patients with a history of radiation therapy, prior chemotherapy (≥3 cycles), or prior stem cell transplantation are at increased risk; monitor liver function tests (serum transaminases, alkaline phosphatase, and bilirubin) daily until 28 days posttransplant to detect hepatotoxicity (which may preclude hepatic SOS). Oral busulfan doses above 16 mg/kg (based on IBW) and concurrent use with alkylating agents may also increase the risk for hepatic SOS. The solvent in IV busulfan, dimethylacetamide (DMA), may impair fertility. N,N-dimethylacetamide is incompatible with many closed-system transfer devices (CSTDs) used for preparing injectable antineoplastics (ISMP [Smetzer 2015]). DMA may also be associated with hepatotoxicity, hallucinations, somnolence, lethargy, and confusion. **[US Boxed Warning]: According to the manufacturer, oral busulfan should not be used until CML diagnosis has been established. The responsible health care provider should be experienced in assessing response to chemotherapy.** Cellular dysplasia in many organs has been observed (in addition to lung dysplasia); giant hyperchromatic nuclei have been noted in adrenal glands, liver, lymph nodes, pancreas, thyroid, and bone marrow. May obscure routine diagnostic cytologic exams (eg, cervical smear). Potentially significant drug-drug interactions may exist, requiring dose or frequency adjustment, additional monitoring, and/or selection of alternative therapy.

Adverse Reactions

IV:

>10%:

Cardiovascular: Tachycardia (44%), hypertension (36%; grades 3/4: 7%), edema (28% to 79%), thrombosis (33%), chest pain (26%), vasodilation (25%), hypotension (11%; grades 3/4: 3%)

Central nervous system: Insomnia (84%), fever (80%), anxiety (72% to 75%), headache (69%), chills (46%), pain (44%), dizziness (30%), depression (23%), confusion (11%)

Dermatologic: Rash (57%), pruritus (28%), alopecia (17%)

Endocrine & metabolic: Hypomagnesemia (77%), hyperglycemia (66% to 67%; grades 3/4: 15%), hypokalemia (64%), hypocalcemia (49%), hypophosphatemia (17%)

Gastrointestinal: Vomiting (43% to 100%), nausea (83% to 98%), mucositis/stomatitis (79% to 97%; grades 3/4: 26%), anorexia (85%), diarrhea (84%; grades 3/4: 5%), abdominal pain (72%), dyspepsia (44%), constipation (38%), xerostomia (26%), rectal disorder (25%), abdominal fullness (23%)

Hematologic: Myelosuppression (≤100%), neutropenia (100%; onset: 4 days; median recovery: 13 days [with G-CSF support]), thrombocytopenia (98%; median onset: 5-6 days), lymphopenia (children: 79%), anemia (69%)

Hepatic: Hyperbilirubinemia (49%; grades 3/4: 30%), ALT increased (31%; grades 3/4: 7%), hepatic sinusoidal obstruction syndrome (SOS; venoocclusive disease) (adults: 8% to 12%; children: 21%), alkaline phosphatase increased (15%), jaundice (12%)

Local: Injection site inflammation (25%), injection site pain (15%)

Neuromuscular & skeletal: Weakness (51%), back pain (23%), myalgia (16%), arthralgia (13%)

Renal: Creatinine increased (21%), oliguria (15%)

Respiratory: Rhinitis (44%), lung disorder (34%), cough (28%), epistaxis (25%), dyspnea (25%), pneumonia (children: 21%), hiccup (18%), pharyngitis (18%)

Miscellaneous: Infection (51%; includes severe bacterial, viral [CMV], and fungal infections), allergic reaction (26%)

1% to 10%:

Cardiovascular: Arrhythmia (5%), cardiomegaly (5%), atrial fibrillation (2%), ECG abnormal (2%), heart block (2%), heart failure (grade 3/4: 2%), pericardial effusion (2%), tamponade (children with thalassemia: 2%), ventricular extrasystoles (2%), hypervolemia

Central nervous system: Lethargy (7%), hallucination (5%), agitation (2%), delirium (2%), encephalopathy (2%), seizure (2%), somnolence (2%), cerebral hemorrhage (1%)

Dermatologic: Vesicular rash (10%), vesiculobullous rash (10%), skin discoloration (8%), maculopapular rash (8%), acne (7%), exfoliative dermatitis (5%), erythema nodosum (2%)
Endocrine & metabolic: Hyponatremia (2%)
Gastrointestinal: Ileus (8%), weight gain (8%), esophagitis (grade 3: 2%), hematemesis (2%), pancreatitis (2%)
Hematologic: Prothrombin time increased (2%)
Hepatic: Hepatomegaly (6%)
Renal: Hematuria (8%), dysuria (7%), hemorrhagic cystitis (grade 3/4: 7%), BUN increased (3%; grades 3/4: 2%)
Respiratory: Asthma (8%), alveolar hemorrhage (5%), hyperventilation (5%), hemoptysis (3%), pleural effusion (3%), sinusitis (3%), atelectasis (2%), hypoxia (2%)

Oral: Frequency not defined:
Dermatologic: Hyperpigmentation of skin (5% to 10%), rash
Endocrine & metabolic: Amenorrhea, ovarian suppression
Gastrointestinal: Xerostomia
Hematologic: Myelosuppression (anemia, leukopenia, thrombocytopenia)

IV and/or Oral: Infrequent, postmarketing, and/or case reports: Acute leukemias, adrenal insufficiency, alopecia (permanent), aplastic anemia (may be irreversible), azoospermia, bronchopulmonary dysplasia, capillary leak syndrome, cataracts (rare), cheilosis, cholestatic jaundice, corneal thinning, dry skin, endocardial fibrosis, erythema multiforme, esophageal varices, gynecomastia, hepatic dysfunction, hepatocellular atrophy, hyperuricemia, hyperuricosuria, interstitial pulmonary fibrosis, malignant tumors, myasthenia gravis, neutropenic fever, ocular (lens) changes, ovarian failure, pancytopenia, porphyria cutanea tarda, pulmonary fibrosis, radiation myelopathy, radiation recall (skin rash), sepsis, sterility, testicular atrophy, thrombotic microangiopathy (TMA), tumor lysis syndrome, urticaria
Drug Interactions
Metabolism/Transport Effects None known.
Avoid Concomitant Use
Avoid concomitant use of Busulfan with any of the following: BCG (Intravesical); CloZAPine; Dipyrone; Natalizumab; Pimecrolimus; Tacrolimus (Topical); Tofacitinib; Vaccines (Live)
Increased Effect/Toxicity
Busulfan may increase the levels/effects of: CloZAPine; Fingolimod; Ifosfamide; Leflunomide; Natalizumab; Tofacitinib; Vaccines (Live)

The levels/effects of Busulfan may be increased by: Acetaminophen; Antifungal Agents (Azole Derivatives, Systemic); Denosumab; Dipyrone; MetroNIDAZOLE (Systemic); Pimecrolimus; Propacetamol; Roflumilast; Tacrolimus (Topical); Trastuzumab
Decreased Effect
Busulfan may decrease the levels/effects of: BCG (Intravesical); Coccidioides immitis Skin Test; Sipuleucel-T; Vaccines (Inactivated); Vaccines (Live)

The levels/effects of Busulfan may be decreased by: Echinacea; Fosphenytoin; Phenytoin

◄ **Storage/Stability**

Injection: Store intact vials under refrigeration at 2°C to 8°C (36°F to 46°F). Solutions diluted in sodium chloride (NS) injection or dextrose 5% in water (D₅W) for infusion are stable for up to 8 hours at room temperature (25°C (77°F)); the infusion must also be completed within that 8-hour timeframe. Dilution of busulfan injection in NS is stable for up to 12 hours refrigerated (2°C to 8°C); the infusion must be completed within that 12-hour timeframe. Tablet: Store at 25°C (77°F); excursions permitted to 15°C to 30°C (59°F to 86°F).

Preparation for Administration Hazardous agent; use appropriate precautions for handling and disposal (NIOSH 2014 [group 1]). Injection: Dilute in NS or D₅W. The dilution volume should be 10 times the volume of busulfan injection, ensuring that the final concentration of busulfan is 0.5 mg/mL. Always add busulfan to the diluent, and not the diluent to the busulfan. Mix with several inversions. Do not use polycarbonate syringes or filters for preparation or administration. Busulfan for injection contains N,N-dimethylacetamide, which is incompatible with many closed-system transfer devices (CSTDs); the plastic components of CSTDs may dissolve and result in subsequent leakage and potential infusion of dissolved plastic into the patient (ISMP [Smetzer 2015]).

Mechanism of Action Busulfan is an alkylating agent which reacts with the N-7 position of guanosine and interferes with DNA replication and transcription of RNA. Busulfan has a more marked effect on myeloid cells than on lymphoid cells and is also very toxic to hematopoietic stem cells. Busulfan exhibits little immunosuppressive activity. Interferes with the normal function of DNA by alkylation and cross-linking the strands of DNA.

Pharmacodynamics/Kinetics

Absorption: Rapid and complete

Distribution: V_d: Pediatric (IV): ~0.64 L/kg; crosses blood brain barrier and distributes into CSF with levels equal to plasma

Protein binding: ~32% to plasma proteins and 47% to red blood cells

Metabolism: Extensively hepatic (may increase with multiple doses); glutathione conjugation followed by oxidation

Bioavailability: Oral: Children ≥13 years and adults: 80% ± 20%; Children 1.5 to 6 years: 68% ± 31%

Half-life elimination: 2 to 3 hours

Time to peak, serum: Oral: ~1 hour; IV: Within 5 minutes

Excretion: Urine (25% to 60% predominantly as metabolites; <2% as unchanged drug)

Dosing

Adult Note: Premedicate with prophylactic anticonvulsant therapy (eg, phenytoin, levetiracetam, benzodiazepines, or valproic acid) beginning 12 hours prior to high-dose busulfan treatment and continuing for 24 hours after the last busulfan dose. Busulfan is associated with a moderate emetic potential (depending on dose and/or administration route); antiemetics may be recommended to prevent nausea and vomiting (Dupuis 2011). Antiemetics are recommended when used for transplantation.

Chronic myelogenous leukemia (CML), palliation (manufacturer's labeling): *Oral:*

Remission induction: 60 mcg/kg/day or 1.8 mg/m²/day; usual range: 4 to 8 mg/day; titrate dose (or withhold) to maintain leukocyte counts ≥15,000/mm³ (doses >4 mg/day should be reserved for patients with the most compelling symptoms)

Maintenance: When leukocyte count ≥50,000/mm³: Resume induction dose **or** (if remission <3 months) 1 to 3 mg/day (to control hematologic status and prevent relapse)

Hematopoietic stem cell (HSCT) conditioning regimen:

IV: 0.8 mg/kg/dose (ideal or actual body weight, whichever is lower) every 6 hours for 4 days (a total of 16 doses) beginning 7 days prior to transplant (followed by cyclophosphamide).

Obesity: For obese or severely-obese patients, use of an adjusted body weight [IBW + 0.25 x (actual − IBW)] is recommended (by the manufacturer).

Reduced intensity conditioning regimen (off-label dosing): 0.8 mg/kg/day for 4 days starting 5 days prior to transplant (in combinations with fludarabine) (Ho 2009)

Oral (off-label use): 1 mg/kg/dose every 6 hours for 16 doses (in combination with cyclophosphamide) (Socié 2001) **or** 1 mg/kg/dose every 6 hours for 16 doses beginning 9 days prior to transplant (in combination with cyclophosphamide) (Cassileth 1993) **or** 0.44 mg/kg/dose every 6 hours for 16 doses (in combination with cyclophosphamide) (Anderson 1996) **or** 1 mg/kg/dose every 6 hours for 16 doses beginning 6 days prior to transplant (in combination with melphalan) (Fermand 2005)

Essential thrombocythemia (off-label use): Oral: 2 to 4 mg daily (Fabris 2009; Tefferi 2011)

Polycythemia vera, refractory (off-label use): Oral: 2 to 4 mg daily (Tefferi 2011)

Geriatric Oral (refer to individual protocols): Start with lowest recommended doses for adults.

Pediatric Note: Premedicate with prophylactic anticonvulsant therapy (eg, phenytoin, levetiracetam, benzodiazepines, or valproic acid) beginning 12 hours prior to high-dose busulfan treatment and continuing for 24 hours after the last busulfan dose. Busulfan is associated with a moderate emetic potential (depending on dose and/or administration route); antiemetics may be recommended to prevent nausea and vomiting (Dupuis 2011). Antiemetics are recommended when used for transplantation.

Chronic myelogenous leukemia (CML), palliation (manufacturer's labeling): Oral:

Remission induction: 60 mcg/kg/day or 1.8 mg/m²/day; titrate dose (or withhold) to maintain leukocyte counts ≥15,000/mm³ (doses >4 mg/day should be reserved for patients with the most compelling symptoms)

Maintenance: When leukocyte count ≥50,000/mm³: Resume induction dose **or** (if remission <3 months) 1 to 3 mg/day (to control hematologic status and prevent relapse)

Hematopoietic stem cell transplant (HSCT) conditioning regimens:

IV:

≤12 kg: 1.1 mg/kg/dose (actual body weight) every 6 hours for 16 doses (over 4 days) (followed by cyclophosphamide)

>12 kg: 0.8 mg/kg/dose (actual body weight) every 6 hours for 16 doses (over 4 days) (followed by cyclophosphamide)

Adjust dose to desired AUC (900 to 1,350 micromolar•minute) at the completion of dose 1 using the following formula:

Adjusted dose (mg) = Actual dose (mg) x [target AUC (micromolar•minute) / actual AUC (micromolar•minute)]

◀ Reduced intensity conditioning regimen (off-label dosing): 0.8 mg/kg/dose for 1 dose 7 to 10 days prior to transplant, followed by ~0.8 mg/kg/dose (busulfan kinetics calculated after initial dose) every 6 hours for 7 doses beginning 3 to 6 days prior to transplant (in combination with fludarabine and antithymocyte globulin) (Pulsipher 2009)

Oral (off-label use): 1 mg/kg/dose every 6 hours for 16 doses beginning 9 days prior to transplant (in combination with cyclophosphamide) (Cassileth 1998)

Renal Impairment

IV: There are no dosage adjustments provided in the manufacturer's labeling (has not been studied).

Oral: There are no dosage adjustments provided in the manufacturer's labeling (elimination appears to be independent of renal function); however, it has been suggested that adjustment is not necessary (Aronoff 2007).

Hepatic Impairment

IV: There are no dosage adjustments provided in the manufacturer's labeling (has not been studied).

Oral: There are no dosage adjustments provided in the manufacturer's labeling.

Obesity *American Society for Blood and Marrow Transplantation (ASBMT) practice guideline committee position statement on chemotherapy dosing in obesity (Bubalo 2014):*

Busulfan (oral): **Note:** For doses over 12 mg/kg, utilize pharmacokinetically targeted dosage (as appropriate for disease state). When busulfan and cyclophosphamide are used in combination for HSCT conditioning, the maximum tolerated busulfan dose is 4 mg/kg/day for 4 days. The maximum tolerated busulfan dose has not been determined when used in combination with other agents.

Body surface area (BSA) dosing: Adults and pediatrics: Utilize actual body weight (ABW) to calculate BSA

Weight based dosing (mg/kg): Adults: Utilize ABW25 for obese and non-obese patients; Pediatric: Utilize actual body weight (ABW)

ABW25: Adjusted wt (kg) = Ideal body weight (kg) + 0.25 [actual wt (kg) - ideal body weight (kg)]

Administration Busulfan is associated with a moderate emetic potential (depending on dose and/or administration route); antiemetics may be recommended to prevent nausea and vomiting (Dupuis 2011). Antiemetics are recommended when used for transplantation.

Intravenous busulfan should be infused over 2 hours via central line. Use an administration set with a minimal residual priming volume (2 to 5 mL for adults and 1 to 3 mL for pediatrics). Flush line before and after each infusion with 5 mL D_5W or NS. Do not use polycarbonate syringes or filters for preparation or administration. Busulfan injection contains N,N-dimethylacetamide, which is incompatible with many closed-system transfer devices (CSTDs); the plastic components of CSTDs may dissolve and result in subsequent leakage and potential infusion of dissolved plastic into the patient (ISMP [Smetzer 2015]).

HSCT only: To facilitate ingestion of high oral doses, may insert multiple tablets into gelatin capsules.

Hazardous agent; use appropriate precautions for handling and disposal (NIOSH 2014 [group 1]). Avoid exposure to crushed or broken tablets; if it is necessary to manipulate the tablets (eg, to prepare an oral solution), it is recommended to double glove, wear a protective gown, and prepare in a controlled device (NIOSH 2014).

Vesicant/Extravasation Risk May be an irritant

Emetic Potential

Children:
IV: Moderate (30% to 90%)
Oral: Minimal (<10%) to Low (10% to 30%)
Adults:
IV: Moderate (30% to 90%)
Oral ≥4 mg/day: Moderate (30% to 90%)
Oral <4 mg/day: Minimal (<10%)

Extemporaneous Preparations Hazardous agent: Use appropriate precautions for handling and disposal (NIOSH 2014 [group 1]). When manipulating tablets, NIOSH recommends double gloving, a protective gown, and preparation in a controlled device; if not prepared in a controlled device, respiratory and eye protection as well as ventilated engineering controls are recommended (NIOSH 2014).

A 2 mg/mL oral suspension can be prepared in a vertical flow hood with tablets and simple syrup. Crush one-hundred-twenty 2 mg tablets in a mortar and reduce to a fine powder. Add small portions of simple syrup and mix to a uniform paste; mix while adding the simple syrup in incremental proportions to **almost** 120 mL; transfer to a graduated cylinder, rinse mortar and pestle with simple syrup, and add quantity of vehicle sufficient to make 120 mL. Transfer contents of the graduated cylinder into an amber prescription bottle. Label "shake well", "refrigerate", and "caution chemotherapy". Stable for 30 days.
Allen LV, "Busulfan Oral Suspension," *US Pharm*, 1990, 15:94-5.

Monitoring Parameters

CBC with differential and platelet count (weekly for palliative treatment; daily until engraftment for HSCT); liver function tests (evaluate transaminases, alkaline phosphatase, and bilirubin daily for at least 28 days post transplant) and signs/symptoms of sinusoidal obstruction syndrome. Monitor for signs/symptoms of cardiac tamponade.

If conducting therapeutic drug monitoring for AUC calculations in HSCT, monitor blood samples at appropriate collections times (record collection times). Do not collect blood sample during busulfan infusion; collect blood sample from a different port than that used for infusion. Blood samples should be placed on wet ice immediately after collection and should be centrifuged (at 4°C [39.2°F]) within 1 hour. The plasma, harvested into appropriate cryovial storage tubes, should be frozen immediately at −20°C (−4°F). All plasma samples should be sent frozen (on dry ice) to the assay laboratory for the determination of plasma busulfan concentrations.

Dosage Forms Excipient information presented when available (limited, particularly for generics); consult specific product labeling.

Solution, Intravenous:
Busulfex: 6 mg/mL (10 mL)
Tablet, Oral:
Myleran: 2 mg

◆ **Busulfanum** see Busulfan on page 242

◆ **Busulfex** see Busulfan on page 242

♦ **Busulphan** *see* Busulfan *on page 242*

♦ **C2B8 Monoclonal Antibody** *see* RiTUXimab *on page 1482*

♦ **2C4 Antibody** *see* Pertuzumab *on page 1380*

♦ **C225** *see* Cetuximab *on page 311*

Cabazitaxel (ca baz i TAKS el)

Related Information

Common Toxicity Criteria *on page 2122*

Management of Chemotherapy-Induced Nausea and Vomiting in Adults *on page 2142*

Safe Handling of Hazardous Drugs *on page 2292*

Brand Names: US Jevtana

Brand Names: Canada Jevtana

Index Terms RPR-116258A; XRP6258

Pharmacologic Category Antineoplastic Agent, Antimicrotubular; Antineoplastic Agent, Taxane Derivative

Use Prostate cancer, metastatic: Treatment of hormone-refractory metastatic prostate cancer (in combination with prednisone) in patients previously treated with a docetaxel-containing regimen

Labeled Contraindications Severe hypersensitivity to cabazitaxel or any component of the formulation, or to other medications formulated with polysorbate 80; neutrophil count ≤1,500/mm^3; severe hepatic impairment (total bilirubin >3 times ULN)

Canadian labeling: Additional contraindications (not in US labeling): Hepatic impairment (bilirubin ≥ULN or AST and/or ALT ≥1.5 times ULN); concomitant vaccination with yellow fever vaccine

Pregnancy Considerations Adverse events have been observed in animal reproduction studies. Cabazitaxel is not indicated for use in women. May cause fetal harm if administered during pregnancy. Pregnant women should avoid exposure to cabazitaxel.

Breast-Feeding Considerations It is not known if cabazitaxel is excreted in breast milk. Cabazitaxel is not indicated for use in women. Due to the potential for serious adverse reactions in the nursing infant, the manufacturer recommends a decision be made to discontinue nursing or to discontinue the drug, taking into account the importance of treatment to the mother.

Warnings/Precautions Hazardous agent - use appropriate precautions for handling and disposal (NIOSH 2014 [group 1]). **[US Boxed Warning]: Severe hypersensitivity reactions, including generalized rash, erythema, hypotension, and bronchospasm may occur; immediate discontinuation is required if hypersensitivity is severe; administer appropriate supportive medications. Premedicate with an IV antihistamine, corticosteroid and H$_2$ antagonist prior to infusion. Use in patients with history of severe hypersensitivity to cabazitaxel or other medications formulated with polysorbate 80 is contraindicated.** Observe closely during infusion, especially during the first and second infusions; reaction may occur within minutes. Do not rechallenge after severe hypersensitivity reactions.

[US Boxed Warning]: Deaths due to neutropenia have been reported. Cabazitaxel is contraindicated in patients with neutrophil count ≤1,500/mm^3; monitor blood counts frequently. Neutropenia, anemia, thrombocytopenia, and/or pancytopenia may occur with use; grade 3 and 4 neutropenia was observed in over 80% of patients treated with cabazitaxel in a clinical trial. Dose reductions are recommended following neutropenic fever or prolonged neutropenia. Administration of WBC growth factors may reduce the risk of complications due to neutropenia; consider primary WBC growth factor prophylaxis in high-risk patients (eg, >65 years of age, poor performance status, history of neutropenic fever, extensive prior radiation, poor nutrition status, or other serious comorbidities); secondary prophylaxis and therapeutic WBC growth factors should be considered in all patients with increased risk for neutropenic complications. Use cautiously in patients with hemoglobin <10 g/dL. Monitor complete blood counts weekly during cycle 1 and prior to subsequent treatment cycles, or as clinically indicated. Patients ≥65 years of age are more likely to experience certain adverse reactions, including grade 3 and 4 neutropenia and neutropenic fever. Fatigue, asthenia, pyrexia, dizziness, urinary tract infection, and dehydration also occurred more frequently in elderly patients compared to younger patients. Death due to causes other than disease progression (within 30 days of the last cabazitaxel dose) was higher in elderly patients versus younger patients.

Use is contraindicated in patients with severe hepatic impairment (total bilirubin >3 times ULN). Dose reduction is necessary in patients with mild impairment (total bilirubin >1 to ≤1.5 times ULN or AST >1.5 times ULN) and moderate impairment (total bilirubin >1.5 to ≤3 times ULN); use with caution and monitor closely. Due to extensive hepatic metabolism, cabazitaxel exposure is increased in patients with hepatic impairment. Renal failure (including rare fatalities) has been reported from clinical trials; generally associated with dehydration, sepsis, or obstructive uropathy; use with caution in patients with severe renal impairment (CrCl <30 mL/minute) and end-stage renal disease. Nausea, vomiting, and diarrhea may occur. Diarrhea may be severe and may result in dehydration and electrolyte imbalance; fatalities have been reported. Per the manufacturer, antiemetic prophylaxis is recommended. Antidiarrheal medication and fluid and electrolyte replacement may be necessary. Diarrhea ≥ grade 3 may require treatment delay and or dosage reduction. Gastro-intestinal hemorrhage and perforation, enterocolitis, neutropenic enterocolitis, and ileus (some fatal) have also been observed. Use with caution in patients at risk of developing gastrointestinal complications (eg, elderly patients, those with neutropenia or a prior history of pelvic radiation, adhesions, GI ulceration or bleeding, concomitant use of steroids, NSAIDs, antiplatelet or anticoagulant medications). Evaluate promptly if symptoms such as abdominal pain and tenderness, fever, persistent constipation, and diarrhea (with or without neu-tropenia) occur. May require treatment interruption and/or therapy discontinu-ation.

Failure to properly reconstitute the concentrated vial of cabazitaxel with the correct amount of diluent may lead to higher dosage being administered and increased risk of toxicity. Follow manufacturer instructions carefully. Potentially significant drug-drug interactions may exist, requiring dose or frequency adjustment, additional monitoring, and/or selection of alternative therapy.

Some dosage forms may contain polysorbate 80 (also known as Tweens). Hypersensitivity reactions, usually a delayed reaction, have been reported following exposure to pharmaceutical products containing polysorbate 80 in certain individuals (Isaksson 2002; Lucente 2000; Shelley 1995). Thrombocy-topenia, ascites, pulmonary deterioration, and renal and hepatic failure have been reported in premature neonates after receiving parenteral products containing polysorbate 80 (Alade 1986; CDC 1984). See manufacturer's labeling.

◀ **Adverse Reactions Note:** Adverse reactions reported for combination therapy with prednisone.

>10%:

Central nervous system: Fatigue (37%), fever (12%)

Gastrointestinal: Diarrhea (47%; grades 3/4: 6%), nausea (34%), vomiting (22%), constipation (20%), abdominal pain (17%), anorexia (16%), taste alteration (11%)

Hematologic: Anemia (98%; grades 3/4: 11%), leukopenia (96%; grades 3/4: 69%), neutropenia (94%; grades 3/4: 82%; nadir: 12 days [range: 4-17 days]), thrombocytopenia (48%; grades 3/4: 4%)

Neuromuscular & skeletal: Weakness (20%), back pain (16%), peripheral neuropathy (13%; grades 3/4: <1%), arthralgia (11%)

Renal: Hematuria (17%)

Respiratory: Dyspnea (12%), cough (11%)

1% to 10%:

Cardiovascular: Peripheral edema (9%), arrhythmia (5%), hypotension (5%)

Central nervous system: Dizziness (8%), headache (8%), pain (5%)

Dermatologic: Alopecia (10%)

Endocrine & metabolic: Dehydration (5%)

Gastrointestinal: Dyspepsia (10%), weight loss (9%), mucosal inflammation (6%)

Genitourinary: Urinary tract infection (8%), dysuria (7%)

Hematologic: Neutropenic fever (grades 3/4: 7%)

Hepatic: ALT increased (grades 3/4: ≤1%), AST increased (grades 3/4: ≤1%), bilirubin increased (grades 3/4: ≤1%)

Neuromuscular & skeletal: Muscle spasm (7%)

<1%, postmarketing, and/or case reports: Colitis, electrolyte imbalance, enterocolitis, gastritis, gastrointestinal hemorrhage, gastrointestinal perforation, hypersensitivity (eg, rash, erythema, hypotension, bronchospasm), intestinal obstruction, neutropenic enterocolitis, renal failure, sepsis, septic shock

Drug Interactions

Metabolism/Transport Effects Substrate of CYP2C8 (minor), CYP3A4 (major); **Note:** Assignment of Major/Minor substrate status based on clinically relevant drug interaction potential

Avoid Concomitant Use

Avoid concomitant use of Cabazitaxel with any of the following: BCG (Intravesical); CloZAPine; Conivaptan; Dipyrone; Fusidic Acid (Systemic); Idelalisib; Natalizumab; Pimecrolimus; Tacrolimus (Topical); Tofacitinib; Vaccines (Live)

Increased Effect/Toxicity

Cabazitaxel may increase the levels/effects of: Antineoplastic Agents (Anthracycline, Systemic); CloZAPine; DOXOrubicin (Conventional); Fingolimod; Leflunomide; Natalizumab; Tofacitinib; Vaccines (Live)

The levels/effects of Cabazitaxel may be increased by: Aprepitant; Conivaptan; CYP3A4 Inhibitors (Moderate); CYP3A4 Inhibitors (Strong); Dasatinib; Denosumab; Dipyrone; Fosaprepitant; Fusidic Acid (Systemic); Idelalisib; Ivacaftor; Luliconazole; Mifepristone; Netupitant; Osimertinib; Palbociclib; Pimecrolimus; Platinum Derivatives; Roflumilast; Simeprevir; Stiripentol; Tacrolimus (Topical); Trastuzumab

Decreased Effect

Cabazitaxel may decrease the levels/effects of: BCG (Intravesical); Coccidioides immitis Skin Test; Sipuleucel-T; Vaccines (Inactivated); Vaccines (Live)

The levels/effects of Cabazitaxel may be decreased by: Bosentan; CYP3A4 Inducers (Moderate); CYP3A4 Inducers (Strong); Dabrafenib; Deferasirox; Echinacea; Enzalutamide; Mitotane; Osimertinib; Siltuximab; St Johns Wort; Tocilizumab

Food Interactions Grapefruit juice may increase the levels/effects of cabazitaxel. Management: Avoid grapefruit juice.

Storage/Stability Store intact vials at 25°C (77°F); excursions permitted between 15°C and 30°C (59°F and 86°F). Do not refrigerate. Do not prepare or administer in PVC-containing infusion containers or polyurethane infusion sets. The US labeling indicates the initial reconstituted solution (at 10 mg/mL) is stable for 30 minutes in the vial and that solutions for infusion are stable for up to 8 hours at room temperature (includes the 1 hour infusion) or 24 hours refrigerated (includes the 1 hour infusion). The Canadian labeling indicates the initial reconstituted solution (at 10 mg/mL) is stable for 1 hour in the vial and that solutions for infusion are stable for up to 8 hours at room temperature (includes the 1 hour infusion) or 48 hours refrigerated (includes the 1 hour infusion).

Preparation for Administration Hazardous agent; use appropriate precautions for handling and disposal (NIOSH 2014 [group 1]). Do not prepare or administer in PVC-containing infusion containers or polyurethane infusion sets. Cabazitaxel and diluent vials contain overfill. **Preparation requires 2 steps.** Slowly inject the **entire contents** of the provided diluent vial into the cabazitaxel 60 mg/1.5 mL vial, directing the diluent down the vial wall. Mix gently by inverting the vial for at least 45 seconds; do not shake. Allow vial to sit so that foam dissipates and solution appears homogeneous. This results in an intermediate reconstituted concentration of 10 mg/mL. The US labeling recommends to further dilute within 30 minutes into a 250 mL D_5W or NS non-PVC infusion container to final concentration of 0.1 to 0.26 mg/mL (total doses >65 mg will require a larger infusion volume; final concentration should not exceed 0.26 mg/mL). The Canadian labeling recommends further dilution of the reconstituted vial occur within 60 minutes. Gently invert container to mix. Do not use infusion solutions if crystals or precipitate appear; discard if this occurs. Infusion should be completed within 8 hours if stored at room temperature. For infusion solutions stored under refrigeration, the US labeling recommends that the infusion be completed within 24 hours. The Canadian labeling recommends that the infusion be completed within 48 hours.

Mechanism of Action Cabazitaxel is a taxane derivative which is a microtubule inhibitor; it binds to tubulin promoting assembly into microtubules and inhibiting disassembly which stabilizes microtubules. This inhibits microtubule depolymerization and cell division, arresting the cell cycle and inhibiting tumor proliferation. Unlike other taxanes, cabazitaxel has a poor affinity for multidrug resistance (MDR) proteins, therefore conferring activity in resistant tumors.

Pharmacodynamics/Kinetics

Distribution: V_{dss}: 4,864 L; has greater CNS penetration than other taxanes

Protein binding: 89% to 92%; primarily to serum albumin and lipoproteins

Metabolism: Extensively hepatic; primarily via CYP3A4 and 3A5; also via CYP2C8 (minor)

Half-life elimination: Terminal: 95 hours

Excretion: Feces (76% as metabolites); Urine (~4%)

◀ **Dosing**

Adult Note: Premedicate at least 30 minutes prior to each dose of cabazitaxel with an antihistamine (eg, diphenhydramine IV 25 mg or equivalent), a corticosteroid (eg, dexamethasone 8 mg IV or equivalent), and an H_2 antagonist (eg, ranitidine 50 mg IV or equivalent). Per the manufacturer, antiemetic prophylaxis (oral or IV) is also recommended.

Prostate cancer, metastatic: IV: 25 mg/m^2 once every 3 weeks (in combination with prednisone)

Dosage adjustment for concomitant use with strong CYP3A inhibitors: Concomitant use with strong CYP3A inhibitors (eg, ketoconazole, itraconazole, clarithromycin, protease inhibitors, nefazodone, telithromycin, voriconazole) may increase cabazitaxel plasma concentrations; avoid concurrent use. If concomitant use cannot be avoided, consider reducing cabazitaxel dose by 25%.

Renal Impairment

Mild to moderate renal impairment (CrCl ≥30 mL/minute): No dosage adjustment necessary.

Severe renal impairment (CrCl <30 mL/minute) or end-stage renal disease: Use with caution; monitor closely.

Hepatic Impairment

US labeling:

Mild impairment (total bilirubin >1 to ≤1.5 times ULN or AST ≥1.5 times ULN): Reduce dose to 20 mg/m^2.

Moderate impairment (total bilirubin >1.5 to ≤3 times ULN with any AST): Reduce dose to 15 mg/m^2 (based on tolerability; efficacy of this dose is not known).

Severe impairment (total bilirubin >3 times ULN): Use is contraindicated.

Canadian labeling: Hepatic impairment (bilirubin ≥1 times ULN or AST and/or ALT ≥1.5 times ULN): Use is contraindicated.

Obesity ASCO Guidelines for appropriate chemotherapy dosing in obese adults with cancer: Utilize patient's actual body weight (full weight) for calculation of body surface area- or weight-based dosing, particularly when the intent of therapy is curative; manage regimen-related toxicities in the same manner as for nonobese patients; if a dose reduction is utilized due to toxicity, consider resumption of full weight-based dosing with subsequent cycles, especially if cause of toxicity (eg, hepatic or renal impairment) is resolved (Griggs 2012).

Adjustment for Toxicity

Hematologic toxicity:

Neutropenia ≥ grade 3 for >1 week despite WBC growth factors: Delay treatment until ANC >1,500/mm^3 and then reduce dose to 20 mg/m^2 with continued WBC growth factor secondary prophylaxis.

Neutropenic fever or neutropenic infection: Delay treatment until improvement/resolution and ANC >1,500/mm^3 and then reduce dose to 20 mg/m^2 with continued WBC growth factor secondary prophylaxis.

Persistent hematologic toxicity (despite dosage reduction): Discontinue treatment.

Nonhematologic toxicity:

Severe hypersensitivity: Discontinue immediately.

Diarrhea ≥ grade 3 or persistent despite appropriate medication, fluids, and electrolyte replacement: Delay treatment until improves or resolves and then reduce dose to 20 mg/m^2.

Persistent diarrhea (despite dosage reduction): Discontinue treatment.

Peripheral neuropathy (grade 2): Delay treatment until improves or resolves and then reduce dose to 20 mg/m^2

Persistent peripheral neuropathy (despite dosage reduction) or ≥ grade 3 peripheral neuropathy: Discontinue treatment

Combination Regimens

Prostate cancer: Cabazitaxel-Prednisone (Prostate) on page 1852

Administration IV: Infuse over 1 hour using a 0.22-micron inline filter. Do not use polyurethane-containing infusion sets for administration. Allow to reach room temperature prior to infusion. Premedicate with an antihistamine, a corticosteroid, and an H$_2$ antagonist at least 30 minutes prior to infusion. Observe closely during infusion (for hypersensitivity). Per the manufacturer, antiemetic prophylaxis (oral or IV) is also recommended.

Hazardous agent; use appropriate precautions for handling and disposal (NIOSH 2014 [group 1]).

Emetic Potential Low (10% to 30%)

Monitoring Parameters CBC with differential and platelets (weekly during first cycle, then prior to each treatment cycle and as clinically indicated); hepatic/renal function. Monitor for hypersensitivity reactions (especially during the first and second infusions). Monitor for signs/symptoms of gastrointestinal disorders (eg, nausea, vomiting, diarrhea, gastrointestinal hemorrhage and perforation, ileus, colitis, abdominal pain/tenderness)

Dietary Considerations Avoid grapefruit juice.

Dosage Forms Excipient information presented when available (limited, particularly for generics); consult specific product labeling.

Solution, Intravenous:

Jevtana: 60 mg/1.5 mL (1.5 mL) [contains alcohol, usp, polysorbate 80]

Cabozantinib (ka boe ZAN ti nib)

Related Information

Common Toxicity Criteria on page 2122

Management of Chemotherapy-Induced Nausea and Vomiting in Adults on page 2142

Principles of Anticancer Therapy on page 2261

Safe Handling of Hazardous Drugs on page 2292

Brand Names: US Cometriq

Index Terms BMS-907351; Cabozantinib s-Malate; XL184

Pharmacologic Category Antineoplastic Agent, Tyrosine Kinase Inhibitor; Antineoplastic Agent, Vascular Endothelial Growth Factor (VEGF) Inhibitor

Use Thyroid cancer, medullary: Treatment of progressive, metastatic medullary thyroid cancer (MTC)

Labeled Contraindications There are no contraindications listed in the manufacturer's labeling.

Pregnancy Considerations Based on its mechanism of action, adverse effects on pregnancy would be expected. In animal reproduction studies, teratogenic effects (fetal loss, malformations, and skeletal/visceral variations) were observed with doses below the recommended human dose. Patients (male and female) should use effective contraception during therapy and for up to 4 months after therapy completion.

Breast-Feeding Considerations It is not known if cabozantinib is excreted into breast milk. According to the manufacturer, the decision to discontinue cabozantinib or to discontinue breast-feeding should take into account the benefits of treatment to the mother.

Warnings/Precautions Hazardous agent - use appropriate precautions for handling and disposal (meets NIOSH 2014 criteria). Palmar-plantar erythrodysesthesia syndrome (PPES) was commonly observed in clinical trials; severe PPES (≥ grade 3) also occurred frequently. May require dosage reduction and/or discontinuation. Cabozantinib inhibits vascular endothelial growth factor receptors 1, 2, and 3; wound complications have been reported with therapy. Hold treatment at least 28 days prior to scheduled surgery; resume based on judgment of adequate wound healing post surgery. Withhold treatment in patients with dehiscence or other wound healing complications requiring intervention. **[US Boxed Warning]: Serious and occasionally fatal hemorrhage (including hemoptysis and gastrointestinal) has occurred with therapy. Monitor for signs/symptoms of bleeding and do not administer to patients with severe hemorrhage** or a recent history of hemorrhage or hemoptysis.

Stage 1 or 2 hypertension was observed in more than half of cabozantinib-treated patients and occurred more frequently than in placebo-treated patients. Monitor blood pressure prior to therapy initiation and frequently thereafter; withhold for hypertension that is uncontrolled with appropriate medical management. May require cabozantinib dosage reduction and/or therapy discontinuation. An increased incidence of thrombotic events was seen in cabozantinib-treated patients versus placebo; discontinue therapy in patients who develop an acute myocardial infarction or other clinically significant arterial thromboembolic event. Proteinuria occurred in a small number of patients receiving cabozantinib as compared to placebo; nephrotic syndrome was also reported (rare). Monitor urine protein regularly and discontinue therapy if nephrotic syndrome develops.

[US Boxed Warning]: Serious gastrointestinal (GI) perforations and fistulas have been reported; discontinue for GI perforation or fistulation formation. GI fistula may be fatal. Tracheal/esophageal fistulas were also noted; some cases were fatal. Monitor for signs/symptoms of perforations and fistulas; if observed, discontinue therapy. Reversible posterior leukoencephalopathy syndrome (RPLS), also referred to as posterior reversible leukoencephalopathy syndrome (PRES), occurred rarely in clinical studies. Monitor for signs/symptoms of RPLS (seizures, headache, visual disturbances, confusion or altered mental function); if diagnosis confirmed, discontinue therapy.

Osteonecrosis of the jaw occurred rarely; oral examinations should be performed prior to and periodically throughout therapy. Patients should maintain proper oral hygiene practices; if possible, withhold therapy for at least 28 days prior to scheduled invasive dental procedures. Safety and efficacy of cabozantinib have not been established in patients with serum bilirubin ≥1.5 times ULN. Use is not recommended in moderate or severe hepatic impairment; pharmacokinetics have not been studied and there are limited data in patients with serum bilirubin >1.5 times ULN. Avoid the use of concomitant strong CYP3A4 inducers and/or strong CYP3A4 inhibitors. Dosage adjustments are required if concurrent therapy is unavoidable.

Adverse Reactions

>10%:

Cardiovascular: Hypertension (33%; grades 3/4: 8%)

Central nervous system: Fatigue (41%), dysphonia (20%), headache (18%), dizziness (14%)

Dermatologic: Palmar-plantar erythrodysesthesia (50%; grades 3/4: 13%), hair color changes (34%), dry skin (19%), rash (19%), alopecia (16%), erythema (11%)

Endocrine & metabolic: Hypocalcemia (52%), hypophosphatemia (28%), hypomagnesemia (19%), hypokalemia (18%)

Gastrointestinal: Diarrhea (63%), stomatitis (51%), weight loss (48%), appetite decreased (46%), nausea (43%), oral pain (36%), abnormal taste (34%), abdominal pain (27%), constipation (27%), vomiting (24%), dysphagia (13%), dyspepsia (11%)

Hematologic: Lymphopenia (53%; grades 3/4: 16%), neutropenia (35%; grades 3/4: 3%), thrombocytopenia (35%)

Hepatic: ALT increased (86%), AST increased (86%), alkaline phosphatase increased (52%), hyperbilirubinemia (25%)

Neuromuscular & skeletal: Weakness (21%), arthralgia (14%), muscle spasms (12%)

1% to 10%:

Cardiovascular: Venous thromboembolism (6%), arterial thromboembolism (2%)

Central nervous system: Anxiety (9%)

Dermatologic: Hyperkeratosis (7%)

Endocrine & metabolic: Hyponatremia (10%), dehydration (7%)

Gastrointestinal: Hemorrhoids (9%), gastrointestinal perforation (3%), gastrointestinal fistula (1%)

Hematologic: Hemorrhage (≥ grade 3: 3%)

Neuromuscular & skeletal: Musculoskeletal chest pain (9%), paresthesia (7%), peripheral neuropathy (5%), osteonecrosis of the jaw (1%)

Renal: Proteinuria (2%)

Miscellaneous: Nongastrointestinal fistula (4%)

<1%: Reversible posterior leukoencephalopathy syndrome (RPLS), wound healing impaired

Drug Interactions

Metabolism/Transport Effects Substrate of CYP2C9 (minor), CYP3A4 (major); **Note:** Assignment of Major/Minor substrate status based on clinically relevant drug interaction potential; **Inhibits** P-glycoprotein

Avoid Concomitant Use

Avoid concomitant use of Cabozantinib with any of the following: Conivaptan; CYP3A4 Inducers (Strong); CYP3A4 Inhibitors (Strong); Dexamethasone (Systemic); Fusidic Acid (Systemic); Grapefruit Juice; Idelalisib; St Johns Wort

Increased Effect/Toxicity

Cabozantinib may increase the levels/effects of: Bisphosphonate Derivatives

The levels/effects of Cabozantinib may be increased by: Aprepitant; Conivaptan; CYP3A4 Inhibitors (Moderate); CYP3A4 Inhibitors (Strong); Dasatinib; Fosaprepitant; Fusidic Acid (Systemic); Grapefruit Juice; Idelalisib; Ivacaftor; Luliconazole; Mifepristone; Netupitant; Osimertinib; Palbociclib; Simeprevir; Stiripentol

Decreased Effect

The levels/effects of Cabozantinib may be decreased by: Bosentan; CYP3A4 Inducers (Moderate); CYP3A4 Inducers (Strong); Dabrafenib; Deferasirox; Dexamethasone (Systemic); Osimertinib; Siltuximab; St Johns Wort; Tocilizumab

◀ **Food Interactions** A high-fat meal increased C_{max} and AUC by 41% and 57%, respectively compared to the fasted state. Cabozantinib serum concentrations may be increased when taken with grapefruit or grapefruit juice. Management: Must be taken on an empty stomach, at least 1 hour before and 2 hours after food. Avoid concurrent use with grapefruit or grapefruit juice.

Storage/Stability Store at 20°C to 25°C (68°F to 77°F); excursions permitted from 15°C to 30°C (59°F to 86°F).

Mechanism of Action Cabozantinib is a potent inhibitor of proinvasive receptor tyrosine kinases (RTKs), including AXL, FLT-3, KIT, MET, RET, TIE-2, TRKB, and VEGFR-1, -2, and -3; induces apoptosis of cancer cells and suppresses tumor growth, metastasis, and angiogenesis (Yakes, 2011).

Pharmacodynamics/Kinetics

Distribution: V_d: ~349 L

Protein binding: ≥99.7% to plasma proteins

Metabolism: Hepatic via CYP3A4

Half-life elimination: ~55 hours

Time to peak: 2 to 5 hours

Excretion: Feces (54%); urine (27%)

Dosing

Adult Medullary thyroid cancer, metastatic: Oral: 140 mg once daily until disease progression or unacceptable toxicity occurs; do not exceed 180 mg daily

Missed doses: Do not take a missed dose within 12 hours of the next dose.

Renal cell cancer, clear cell, advanced (off-label use; second-line therapy): Oral: 60 mg once daily, continue as long as benefiting clinically or until unacceptable toxicity occurs (Choueiri 2015)

Dosage adjustment for concomitant CYP3A4 inhibitors/inducers:

Strong CYP3A4 inhibitors: Avoid concomitant use; if concomitant use is required, **reduce** the daily dose of cabozantinib by 40 mg (ie, from 140 mg to 100 mg daily or from 100 mg to 60 mg daily). If the strong inhibitor is discontinued, allow ~2-3 days to elapse prior to adjusting the cabozantinib dose upwards to the dose used prior to the initiation of the strong inhibitor.

Strong CYP3A4 inducers: Avoid concomitant use; if concomitant use is required, **increase** the daily dose by 40 mg (ie, from 140 mg to 180 mg daily or from 100 mg to 140 mg daily). If the strong inducer is discontinued, allow ~2-3 days to elapse prior to reducing the cabozantinib dose to the dose used prior to the initiation of the strong inducer.

Renal Impairment

Mild-to-moderate impairment (CrCl ≥30 mL/minute): No dosage adjustment necessary.

Severe impairment (CrCl <30 mL/minute): There are no dosage adjustments provided in the manufacturer's labeling (has not been studied).

Hepatic Impairment

Mild impairment: There are no dosage adjustments provided in the manufacturer's labeling (limited data available in patients with total bilirubin >1.5 times ULN).

Moderate or severe impairment: Use is not recommended (has not been studied).

Adjustment for Toxicity

Hematologic: Withhold therapy for grade 4 hematologic adverse reactions. Upon return to baseline or improvement to grade 1, reduce the dose to 100 mg daily. If previously receiving 100 mg daily, resume therapy at 60 mg daily. If previously receiving 60 mg daily, resume at 60 mg daily if tolerated; otherwise, discontinue therapy.

Other toxicity: Grade 3 or higher nonhematologic toxicity or intolerable grade 2 toxicity: Upon return to baseline or improvement to grade 1, reduce the dose to 100 mg daily. If previously receiving 100 mg daily, resume therapy at 60 mg daily. If previously receiving 60 mg daily, resume at 60 mg daily if tolerated; otherwise, discontinue therapy.

Permanently discontinue for:

Malignant hypertension, hypertensive crisis, persistent uncontrolled hypertension despite optimal therapy

Nephrotic syndrome

Reversible posterior leukoencephalopathy syndrome (RPLS)

Serious arterial thromboembolic event (eg, MI or cerebral infarction)

Severe hemorrhage

Visceral perforation or fistula formation

Administration Administer orally on an empty stomach (1 hour before or 2 hours after eating). Swallow whole; do not open capsules. Hazardous agent; use appropriate precautions for handling and disposal (meets NIOSH 2014 criteria).

Emetic Potential Minimal (<10%)

Monitoring Parameters Renal function, liver function, CBC with differential and platelets, serum electrolytes; blood pressure (prior to initiation and regularly during therapy); monitor for perforations, fistulas, signs/symptoms of bleeding, palmar-plantar erythrodysesthesia syndrome (PPES), reversible posterior leukoencephalopathy syndrome (RPLS), proteinuria (regularly during therapy), osteonecrosis of the jaw (perform oral examination prior to initiation and periodically during therapy), wound healing complications, diarrhea, stomatitis

Dietary Considerations Avoid grapefruit and grapefruit juice throughout therapy.

Prescribing and Access Restrictions Distribution of Cometriq is limited to Diplomat Specialty Pharmacy (855-253-3273).

Dosage Forms Excipient information presented when available (limited, particularly for generics); consult specific product labeling.

Capsule, oral [each package contains four blister cards; each card contains the following]:

Cometriq: 60 mg daily-dose: 20 mg (21s)

Cometriq: 100 mg daily-dose: 80 mg (7s) and 20 mg (7s)

Cometriq: 140 mg daily-dose: 80 mg (7s) and 20 mg (21s)

◆ **Cabozantinib s-Malate** see Cabozantinib on page 255

◆ **Caelyx (Can)** see DOXOrubicin (Liposomal) on page 565

◆ **CAFdA** see Clofarabine on page 350

◆ **CAL-101** see Idelalisib on page 867

◆ **Calcimar (Can)** see Calcitonin on page 259

Calcitonin (kal si TOE nin)

Brand Names: US Fortical; Miacalcin

◀ **Brand Names: Canada** Calcimar
Index Terms Calcitonin (Salmon); Salcatonin
Pharmacologic Category Antidote; Hormone
Use
Injection:
  Hypercalcemia: Adjunctive therapy for hypercalcemia
  Paget disease: Treatment of symptomatic Paget disease of bone (osteitis deformans) in patients who are nonresponsive or intolerant to alternative therapy
  Postmenopausal osteoporosis: Treatment of osteoporosis in women more than 5 years postmenopause
Intranasal:
  Postmenopausal osteoporosis: Treatment of postmenopausal osteoporosis in women more than 5 years postmenopause
Pregnancy Risk Factor C
Dosing
  Adult & Geriatric
    Paget's disease, symptomatic *(Miacalcin):* IM, SubQ: 100 units daily. **Note:** Due to the risk of malignancy associated with prolonged calcitonin use, the Canadian labeling recommends limiting therapy in most patients to ≤3 months; under exceptional circumstances (eg, impending pathologic fracture), therapy may be extended to ≤6 months
    Hypercalcemia *(Miacalcin):* Initial: IM, SubQ: 4 units/kg every 12 hours; after 1 to 2 days, may increase up to 8 units/kg every 12 hours; if the response remains unsatisfactory after 2 more days, may further increase up to a maximum of 8 units/kg every 6 hours
    Postmenopausal osteoporosis:
      Miacalcin: IM, SubQ: 100 units daily
      Fortical, Miacalcin: Intranasal: 200 units (1 spray) in one nostril once daily
  Renal Impairment There are no dosage adjustments provided in the manufacturer's labeling.
  Hepatic Impairment There are no dosage adjustments provided in the manufacturer's labeling.
Additional Information Complete prescribing information should be consulted for additional detail.
Dosage Forms Excipient information presented when available (limited, particularly for generics); consult specific product labeling.
Solution, Injection:
  Miacalcin: 200 units/mL (2 mL) [contains phenol]
Solution, Nasal:
  Fortical: 200 units/actuation (3.7 mL)
  Miacalcin: 200 units/actuation (3.7 mL)
  Generic: 200 units/actuation (3.7 mL)
Dosage Forms: Canada Refer to Dosage Forms. Intranasal solution is not available in Canada.

- **Camptosar** *see* Irinotecan (Conventional) *on page 949*
- **Camptothecin-11** *see* Irinotecan (Conventional) *on page 949*
- **Cancidas** *see* Caspofungin *on page 291*
- **CanesOral (Can)** *see* Fluconazole *on page 725*
- **CAPE** *see* Capecitabine *on page 261*

Capecitabine (ka pe SITE a been)

Related Information

Chemotherapy and Obesity *on page 2220*

Common Toxicity Criteria *on page 2122*

Management of Chemotherapy-Induced Nausea and Vomiting in Adults *on page 2142*

Management of EGFR Inhibitor Toxicities: Dermatologic, Ocular, and Gastrointestinal *on page 2179*

Mucositis and Stomatitis *on page 2186*

Prevention of Chemotherapy-Induced Nausea and Vomiting in Children *on page 2203*

Safe Handling of Hazardous Drugs *on page 2292*

Brand Names: US Xeloda

Brand Names: Canada Teva-Capecitabine; Xeloda

Index Terms CAPE

Pharmacologic Category Antineoplastic Agent, Antimetabolite; Antineoplastic Agent, Antimetabolite (Pyrimidine Analog)

Use

Breast cancer, metastatic:

Monotherapy: Treatment of metastatic breast cancer resistant to both paclitaxel and an anthracycline-containing regimen or resistant to paclitaxel in patients for whom further anthracycline therapy is not indicated

Combination therapy: Treatment of metastatic breast cancer (in combination with docetaxel) after failure of a prior anthracycline-containing regimen

Colorectal cancer: First-line treatment of metastatic colorectal cancer when treatment with a fluoropyrimidine alone is preferred; adjuvant therapy of Dukes' C colon cancer after complete resection of the primary tumor when fluoropyrimidine therapy alone is preferred

Labeled Contraindications Known hypersensitivity to capecitabine, fluorouracil, or any component of the formulation; severe renal impairment (CrCl <30 mL/minute)

Pregnancy Considerations Adverse effects were observed in animal reproduction studies. Fetal harm may occur if administered during pregnancy. Women of childbearing potential should use effective contraceptives to avoid pregnancy during treatment.

Breast-Feeding Considerations It is not known if capecitabine is excreted in breast milk. Due to the potential for serious adverse reactions in the nursing infant, the decision to discontinue capecitabine or to discontinue breast-feeding should take into account the importance of treatment to the mother.

Warnings/Precautions Hazardous agent - use appropriate precautions for handling and disposal (NIOSH 2014 [group 1]). Bone marrow suppression may occur, hematologic toxicity is more common when used in combination therapy; use with caution; dosage adjustments may be required. Product labeling recommends that patients with baseline platelets <100,000/mm³ and/or neutrophils <1,500/mm³ not receive capecitabine therapy and also to ▶

withhold for grade 3 or 4 hematologic toxicity during treatment. Patients with certain homozygous or heterozygous mutations of the dihydropyrimidine dehydrogenase (DPD) enzyme are at increased risk for acute early-onset (potentially severe, life-threatening, or fatal) toxicity due to total or near total absence of DPD activity. Toxicity may include mucositis/stomatitis, diarrhea, neutropenia, and neurotoxicity. Patients with partial DPD activity are also at risk for severe, life-threatening, or fatal toxicity. May require therapy interruption or permanent discontinuation, depending on the onset, duration, and severity of toxicity observed. No capecitabine dose has been shown to be safe in patients with complete DPD deficiency; data is insufficient to recommend a dose in patients with partial DPD activity.

Capecitabine may cause diarrhea (may be severe); median time to first occurrence of grade 2 to 4 diarrhea was 34 days; median duration of grades 3 or 4 diarrhea was 5 days. Withhold treatment for grades 2 to 4 diarrhea; subsequent doses should be reduced after grade 3 or 4 diarrhea or recurrence of grade 2 diarrhea. Antidiarrheal therapy (eg, loperamide) is recommended. Necrotizing enterocolitis (typhlitis) has been reported. Dehydration may occur rapidly in patients with diarrhea, nausea, vomiting, anorexia, and/or weakness; adequately hydrate prior to treatment initiation. Elderly patients may be a higher risk for dehydration. **Note:** Canadian labeling recommends treatment interruption for dehydration requiring IV hydration lasting <24 hours and dosage reduction if IV hydration required for ≥24 hours; correct precipitating factors and ensure rehydration prior to resuming therapy.

Hand-and-foot syndrome is characterized by numbness, dysesthesia/paresthesia, tingling, painless or painful swelling, erythema, desquamation, blistering, and severe pain; median onset is 79 days (range: 11 to 360 days). If grade 2 or 3 hand-and-foot syndrome occurs, interrupt administration of capecitabine until decreases to grade 1. Following grade 3 hand-and-foot syndrome, decrease subsequent doses of capecitabine. Stevens-Johnson syndrome and toxic epidermal necrolysis (TEN) have been reported (some fatal); permanently discontinue capecitabine if a severe dermatologic or mucocutaneous reaction occurs. In patients with colorectal cancer, treatment with capecitabine immediately following 6 weeks of fluorouracil/leucovorin (FU/LV) therapy has been associated with an increased incidence of grade ≥3 toxicity, when compared to patients receiving the reverse sequence, capecitabine (two 3-week courses) followed by FU/LV (Hennig, 2008).

Grade 3 and 4 hyperbilirubinemia have been observed in patients with and without hepatic metastases at baseline (median onset: 64 days). Transaminase and alkaline phosphatase elevations have also been reported. If capecitabine-related grade 3 or 4 hyperbilirubinemia occurs, Interrupt treatment until bilirubin ≤3 times ULN. Use with caution in patients with mild to moderate hepatic impairment due to liver metastases; effect of severe hepatic impairment has not been studied. Dehydration may occur, resulting in acute renal failure (may be fatal); concomitant use with nephrotoxic agents and baseline renal dysfunction may increase the risk. Use with caution in patients with mild to moderate renal impairment; reduce dose with moderate impairment (exposure to capecitabine and metabolites is increased) and carefully monitor and reduce subsequent dose (with any grade 2 or higher adverse effect) with mild to moderate impairment; use is contraindicated in severe impairment. Use with caution in patients ≥60 years of age, the incidence of treatment-related adverse events may be higher.

Cardiotoxicity has been observed with capecitabine, including myocardial infarction, ischemia, angina, dysrhythmias, cardiac arrest, cardiac failure, sudden death, ECG changes, and cardiomyopathy; may be more common in patients with a history of coronary artery disease. **[US Boxed Warning]: Capecitabine may increase the anticoagulant effects of warfarin; bleeding events, including death, have occurred with concomitant use. Clinically significant increases in prothrombin time (PT) and INR have occurred within several days to months after capecitabine initiation (in patients previously stabilized on anticoagulants), and may continue up to 1 month after capecitabine discontinuation; may occur in patients with or without liver metastases. Monitor PT and INR frequently and adjust anticoagulation dosing accordingly. An increased risk of coagulopathy is correlated with a cancer diagnosis and age >60 years.** Other potentially significant drug-drug interactions may exist, requiring dose or frequency adjustment, additional monitoring, and/or selection of alternative therapy.

An investigational uridine prodrug, uridine triacetate (formerly called vistonuridine), has been studied in a limited number of cases of fluoropyrimidine overdose. Of 17 patients receiving uridine triacetate beginning within 8 to 96 hours after fluorouracil overdose, all patients fully recovered (von Borstel, 2009). Updated data has described a total of 28 patients treated with uridine triacetate for fluorouracil overdose (including overdoses related to continuous infusions delivering fluorouracil at rates faster than prescribed), all of whom recovered fully (Bamat, 2010). An additional case report describes accidental capecitabine ingestion by a 22 month old child; uridine triacetate was initiated approximately 7 hours after exposure. The patient received uridine triacetate every 6 hours for a total of 20 doses through nasogastric tube administration; he was asymptomatic throughout his course and was discharged with normal laboratory values (Kanie, 2011). Refer to Uridine Triacetate monograph.

Adverse Reactions Frequency listed derived from monotherapy trials. Incidence reported for all indications and usage, unless otherwise noted. Frequency not always defined.

>10%:

Cardiovascular: Edema (≤15%)

Central nervous system: Fatigue (≤42%), paresthesia (stage IV breast cancer: 21%; grades 3/4: 1%), pain (≤12%)

Dermatologic: Palmar-plantar erythrodysesthesia (54% to 60%; grades ≥3: 11% to 17%), dermatitis (27% to 37%, grades ≥3: 1%)

Gastrointestinal: Diarrhea (47% to 57%, grades 3/4: 2% to 13%), nausea (34% to 43%; stage IV breast cancer: 53%), vomiting (metastatic colorectal cancer, stage IV breast cancer: 27% to 37%; Dukes' C colon cancer: 15%), abdominal pain (metastatic colorectal cancer: 35%; stage IV breast cancer: 20%; Dukes' C colon cancer: 14%), decreased appetite (26%), stomatitis (22% to 25%), anorexia (stage IV breast cancer: 23%; Dukes' C colon cancer: 9%), constipation (9% to 15%)

Hematologic & oncologic: Lymphocytopenia (stage IV breast cancer: 94%; stage IV breast cancer, grades 3/4: 15% to 44%), anemia (72% to 80%, grades 3/4: ≤3%), neutropenia (≤26%, grades 3/4: ≤3%), thrombocytopenia (stage IV breast cancer: 24%; all: grades 3/4: 1% to 3%)

Hepatic: Hyperbilirubinemia (Metastatic colorectal cancer: 48%; stage IV breast cancer: 22%; all: grades 3/4: 2% to 23%)

Neuromuscular & skeletal: Weakness (≤42%)

Ophthalmic: Eye irritation (13% to 15%)

Miscellaneous: Fever (7% to 18%)

1% to 10%:
Cardiovascular: Venous thrombosis (8%), chest pain (≤6%), atrial fibrillation (<5%), bradycardia (<5%), collapse (<5%), extrasystoles (<5%), pericardial effusion (<5%), ventricular premature contractions (<5%), angina pectoris, cardiac arrest, cardiac arrhythmia, cardiac failure, cardiomyopathy, ECG changes, ischemic heart disease, myocardial infarction

Central nervous system: Lethargy (10%), peripheral sensory neuropathy (10%), headache (5% to 10%), insomnia (≤8%), dizziness (6% to 8%), ataxia (<5%), depression (≤5%), mood changes (5%), abnormal gait (<5%), brain disease (<5%), dysarthria (<5%), dysphasia (<5%), equilibrium disturbance (<5%), irritability (<5%), myasthenia (<5%), sedation (<5%), vertigo (<5%)

Dermatologic: Nail disease (≤7%), skin discoloration (7%), skin rash (7%), alopecia (6%), erythema (6%), dermal ulcer (<5%), pruritus (<5%)

Endocrine & metabolic: Dehydration (7%), hot flash (<5%), hypokalemia (<5%), hypomagnesemia (<5%), increased thirst (<5%), weight gain (<5%), decreased serum calcium (Dukes' C colon cancer: grades 3/4: 2%), increased serum calcium (Dukes' C colon cancer: grades 3/4: 1%)

Gastrointestinal: Gastrointestinal motility disorder (10%), GI inflammation (upper: 8%), oral discomfort (grades 3/4: 10%), dyspepsia (6% to 8%), upper abdominal pain (7%), intestinal obstruction (≤6%), dysgeusia (6%), gastrointestinal hemorrhage (6%), abdominal distention (<5%), dysphagia (<5%), rectal pain (<5%), toxic dilation of intestine (<5%), increased serum alanine aminotransferase (Dukes' C colon cancer: grades 3/4: 2%), sore throat (2%), necrotizing enterocolitis

Hematologic & oncologic: Hemorrhage (<5%), lymphedema (<5%), granulocytopenia (Dukes' C colon cancer: grades 3/4: 3%), immune thrombocytopenia (1%)

Hepatic: Abnormal hepatic function tests (<5%)

Hypersensitivity: Drug-induced hypersensitivity (<5%)

Infection: Viral infection (metastatic colorectal cancer: 5%)

Neuromuscular & skeletal: Back pain (10%), myalgia (≤9%), arthralgia (8%), limb pain (stage IV breast cancer: 6%), tremor (<5%)

Ophthalmic: Visual disturbance (metastatic colorectal cancer: 5%), conjunctivitis (≤5%), keratoconjunctivitis (<5%)

Respiratory: Cough (≤7%), chest mass (<5%), dyspnea (<5%), flu-like symptoms (<5%), hemoptysis (<5%), hoarseness (<5%), pharyngeal disease (metastatic colorectal cancer: 5%), epistaxis (≤3%), laryngitis (1%)

<1%, postmarketing, and/or case reports (limited to important or life-threatening): Acute renal failure, arthritis, ascites, asthma, blood coagulation disorder, bone marrow depression, bronchitis, bronchopneumonia, bronchospasm, cachexia, cerebrovascular accident, cholestatic hepatitis, confusion, cutaneous lupus erythematosus, diaphoresis, ecchymoses, esophagitis, fibrosis, flu-like symptoms, fungal infection, gastric ulcer, gastroenteritis, gastrointestinal perforation, hepatic failure, hepatic fibrosis, hepatitis, hypersensitivity, hypertension, hypertriglyceridemia, hypotension, jaundice, keratitis, lacrimal stenosis, leukoencephalopathy, leukopenia, loss of consciousness, myocarditis, nocturia, ostealgia, pancytopenia, phlebitis (venous), photophobia, pneumonia, pulmonary embolism, radiation recall phenomenon, renal insufficiency, respiratory distress, sepsis, Stevens-Johnson syndrome, syncope, tachycardia, toxic epidermal necrolysis

Drug Interactions

Metabolism/Transport Effects Inhibits CYP2C9 (strong)

Avoid Concomitant Use

Avoid concomitant use of Capecitabine with any of the following: BCG (Intravesical); CloZAPine; Dipyrone; Gimeracil; Natalizumab; Pimecrolimus; Tacrolimus (Topical); Tofacitinib; Vaccines (Live)

Increased Effect/Toxicity

Capecitabine may increase the levels/effects of: Bosentan; Carvedilol; CloZAPine; CYP2C9 Substrates; Diclofenac (Systemic); Dronabinol; Fingolimod; Fosphenytoin; Lacosamide; Leflunomide; Natalizumab; Ospemifene; Parecoxib; Phenytoin; Ramelteon; Tetrahydrocannabinol; Tofacitinib; Vaccines (Live); Vitamin K Antagonists

The levels/effects of Capecitabine may be increased by: Cannabis; Cimetidine; Denosumab; Dipyrone; Gimeracil; Leucovorin Calcium-Levoleucovorin; MetroNIDAZOLE (Systemic); Pimecrolimus; Roflumilast; Tacrolimus (Topical); Trastuzumab

Decreased Effect

Capecitabine may decrease the levels/effects of: BCG (Intravesical); Coccidioides immitis Skin Test; Sipuleucel-T; Vaccines (Inactivated); Vaccines (Live)

The levels/effects of Capecitabine may be decreased by: Echinacea

Food Interactions Food reduced the rate and extent of absorption of capecitabine. Management: Administer within 30 minutes after a meal.

Storage/Stability Store at room temperature of 25°C (77°F); excursions permitted between 15°C and 30°C (59°F and 86°F). Keep bottle tightly closed.

Mechanism of Action Capecitabine is a prodrug of fluorouracil. It undergoes hydrolysis in the liver and tissues to form fluorouracil which is the active moiety. Fluorouracil is a fluorinated pyrimidine antimetabolite that inhibits thymidylate synthetase, blocking the methylation of deoxyuridylic acid to thymidylic acid, interfering with DNA, and to a lesser degree, RNA synthesis. Fluorouracil appears to be phase specific for the G_1 and S phases of the cell cycle.

Pharmacodynamics/Kinetics

Absorption: Rapid and extensive (rate and extent reduced by food)

Protein binding: <60%; ~35% to albumin

Metabolism:

Hepatic: Inactive metabolites: 5'-deoxy-5-fluorocytidine, 5'-deoxy-5-fluorouridine

Tissue: Enzymatically metabolized to fluorouracil, which is then metabolized to active metabolites, 5-fluoroxyuridine monophosphate (F-UMP) and 5-5-fluoro-2'-deoxyuridine-5'-O-monophosphate (F-dUMP)

Half-life elimination: ~0.75 hour

Time to peak: 1.5 hours; Fluorouracil: 2 hours

Excretion: Urine (96%, 57% as α-fluoro-β-alanine; <3% as unchanged drug); feces (<3%)

◀ **Dosing**
Adult

Breast cancer, metastatic: Oral: 1,250 mg/m^2 twice daily for 2 weeks, every 21 days (as either monotherapy or in combination with docetaxel)

Breast cancer, metastatic (off-label dosing): Oral: 1,000 mg/m^2 twice daily (in combination with ixabepilone) on days 1 to 14 of a 3-week cycle until disease progression or unacceptable toxicity (Thomas, 2007)

Breast cancer, metastatic, HER2+ (off-label dosing): Oral: 1,000 mg/m^2 twice daily (in combination with lapatinib) on days 1 to 14 of a 3-week cycle until disease progression or unacceptable toxicity (Geyer, 2006) or 1,250 mg/m^2 twice daily (in combination with trastuzumab) on days 1 to 14 of a 3-week cycle (Bartsch, 2007)

Breast cancer, metastatic, HER2+ with brain metastases, first-line therapy (off-label dosing): Oral: 1,000 mg/m^2 twice daily (in combination with lapatinib) on days 1 to 14 of a 3-week cycle until disease progression or unacceptable toxicity (Bachelot, 2012)

Colorectal cancer, metastatic: Oral: 1,250 mg/m^2 twice daily for 2 weeks, every 21 days. **Note:** Capecitabine toxicities, particularly hand-foot syndrome, may be higher in North American populations; therapy initiation at doses of 1,000 mg/m^2 twice daily (for 2 weeks every 21 days) may be considered (Haller, 2008).

Colorectal cancer (off-label dosing): Oral: 1,000 mg/m^2 twice daily (in combination with oxaliplatin) on days 1 to 14 of a 3-week cycle for 8 or 16 cycles (Cassidy, 2008; Haller, 2011; Schmoll, 2007)

Dukes' C colon cancer, adjuvant therapy: Oral: 1,250 mg/m^2 twice daily for 2 weeks, every 21 days, for a recommended total duration of 24 weeks (8 cycles of 2 weeks of drug administration and 1 week rest period).

Esophageal and gastric cancers (off-label uses): Oral:

Preoperative or definitive chemoradiation: 800 mg/m^2 twice daily (in combination with cisplatin and radiation) on days 1 to 5 weekly for 5 weeks (Lee, 2007) **or** 625 mg/m^2 twice daily (in combination with oxaliplatin and radiation) on days 1 to 5 weekly for 5 weeks (Javle, 2009)

Postoperative chemoradiation: 625 to 825 mg/m^2 twice daily during radiation therapy (Lee, 2006)

Locally advanced or metastatic (chemoradiation not indicated): 1,000 to 1,250 mg/m^2 twice daily (monotherapy or in combination with cisplatin with or without trastuzumab) on days 1 to 14 of a 3-week cycle (Bang, 2010; Hong, 2004; Kang, 2009) **or** 625 mg/m^2 twice daily (in combination with epirubicin and cisplatin or oxaliplatin) on days 1 to 21 of a 3-week cycle for up to 8 cycles (Cunningham, 2008; Sumpter, 2005)

Hepatobiliary cancers, advanced (off-label use): Oral: 650 mg/m^2 twice daily (in combination with gemcitabine) on days 1 to 14 of a 3-week cycle (Knox, 2005) **or** 1,000 mg/m^2 twice daily (in combination with oxaliplatin) on days 1 to 14 of a 3-week cycle (Nehls, 2008) **or** 1,250 mg/m^2 twice daily (in combination with cisplatin) on days 1 to 14 of a 3-week cycle (Kim, 2003); all regimens continued until disease progression or unacceptable toxicity

Neuroendocrine (pancreatic/islet cell) tumors, metastatic or unresectable (off label use): Oral: 750 mg/m^2 twice daily (in combination with temozolomide) on days 1 to 14 of a 4-week cycle (Strosberg, 2011)

Ovarian, fallopian tube, or peritoneal cancer, platinum-refractory (off label use): Oral: 1,000 mg/m^2 twice daily on days 1 to 14 of a 3-week cycle until disease progression or unacceptable toxicity (Wolf, 2006)

Pancreatic cancer, metastatic (off-label use): Oral: 1,250 mg/m^2 twice daily on days 1 to 14 of a 3-week cycle (Cartwright, 2002) **or** 830 mg/m^2 twice daily (in combination with gemcitabine) on days 1 to 21 of a 4-week cycle until disease progression or unacceptable toxicity (Cunningham, 2009)

Unknown primary cancer (off-label use): Oral: 1,000 mg/m^2 twice daily (in combination with oxaliplatin) on days 1 to 14 of a 3-week cycle for up to 6 cycles or until disease progression (Hainsworth, 2010) **or** 800 mg/m^2 twice daily (in combination with carboplatin and gemcitabine) on days 1 to 14 of a 3-week cycle for up to 8 cycles or until disease progression or unacceptable toxicity (Schneider, 2007)

Geriatric The elderly may be more sensitive to the toxic effects of fluorouracil. Insufficient data are available to provide dosage modifications.

Renal Impairment Note: Renal function may be estimated using the Cockcroft-Gault formula for dosage adjustment purposes.

Renal impairment at treatment initiation:

CrCl ≥51 mL/minute: Initial: No dosage adjustment necessary.

CrCl 30 to 50 mL/minute: Initial: Administer 75% of usual dose (Cassidy, 2002; Poole, 2002; Xeloda prescribing information, 2015)

CrCl <30 mL/minute: Use is contraindicated (Poole, 2002; Xeloda prescribing information, 2015)

Renal toxicity during treatment: Refer to Dosage Adjustment for Toxicity.

Hepatic Impairment

Hepatic impairment at treatment initiation:

Mild to moderate impairment: No starting dose adjustment necessary (Ecklund, 2005; Superfin, 2007); however, carefully monitor patients.

Severe hepatic impairment: There are no dosage adjustments provided in the manufacturer's labeling (has not been studied).

Hepatotoxicity during treatment: Hyperbilirubinemia, grade 3 or 4: Interrupt treatment until bilirubin ≤3 times ULN; refer to Dosage Adjustment for Toxicity for dosage recommendations.

Obesity *ASCO Guidelines for appropriate chemotherapy dosing in obese adults with cancer:* Utilize patient's actual body weight (full weight) for calculation of body surface area- or weight-based dosing, particularly when the intent of therapy is curative; manage regimen-related toxicities in the same manner as for nonobese patients; if a dose reduction is utilized due to toxicity, consider resumption of full weight-based dosing with subsequent cycles, especially if cause of toxicity (eg, hepatic or renal impairment) is resolved (Griggs, 2012).

Adjustment for Toxicity

See table on next page (**Note:** Capecitabine dosing recommendations apply to both monotherapy and when used in combination therapy with docetaxel).

Monitor carefully for toxicity and adjust dose as necessary. Doses reduced for toxicity should not be increased at a later time. For combination therapy, also refer to docetaxel product labeling for docetaxel dose modifications. If treatment delay is required for either capecitabine or docetaxel, withhold both agents until appropriate to resume combination treatment.

Recommended Capecitabine Dose Modifications

Toxicity Grades	During a Course of Therapy	Dose Adjustment for Next Cycle (% of starting dose)
Grade 1	Maintain dose level	Maintain dose level
Grade 2		
1st appearance	Interrupt until resolved to grade 0 to 1	100%
2nd appearance	Interrupt until resolved to grade 0 to 1	75%
3rd appearance	Interrupt until resolved to grade 0 to 1	50%
4th appearance	Discontinue treatment permanently	
Grade 3		
1st appearance	Interrupt until resolved to grade 0 to 1	75%
2nd appearance	Interrupt until resolved to grade 0 to 1	50%
3rd appearance	Discontinue treatment permanently	
Grade 4 1st appearance	Discontinue permanently **or** If in the patient's best interest to continue, interrupt until resolved to grade 0 to 1	50%

Dosage adjustments for hematologic toxicity in combination therapy with ixabepilone:

Neutrophils <500/mm^3 for ≥7 days or neutropenic fever: Hold for concurrent diarrhea or stomatitis until neutrophils recover to >1000/mm^3, then continue at same dose

Platelets <25,000/mm^3 (or <50,000/mm^3 with bleeding): Hold for concurrent diarrhea or stomatitis until platelets recover to >50,000/mm^3, then continue at same dose

Combination Regimens

Biliary adenocarcinoma: Gemcitabine-Capecitabine (Biliary Cancer) on page 1990

Breast cancer:
Capecitabine (Breast Regimen) on page 1856
Capecitabine-Docetaxel (Breast) on page 1856
Capecitabine-Ixabepilone (Breast) on page 1858
Capecitabine + Lapatinib (Breast) on page 1858
Capecitabine-Trastuzumab (Breast) on page 1859

Colorectal cancer:
Bevacizumab + XELOX (Colorectal) on page 1846
XELOX (Colorectal) on page 2111

Esophageal cancer:
Cisplatin-Capecitabine (Esophageal Cancer) on page 1889
Epirubicin-Cisplatin-Capecitabine (Gastric/Esophageal) on page 1956
Epirubicin-Oxaliplatin-Capecitabine (Gastric/Esophageal) on page 1957
Irinotecan-Capecitabine (Esophageal Cancer) on page 2019

Gastric cancer:
Capecitabine-Docetaxel (Gastric Cancer) on page 1857
Capecitabine-Oxaliplatin (Gastric) on page 1859
Cisplatin-Capecitabine (Gastric Cancer) on page 1889
Epirubicin-Cisplatin-Capecitabine (Gastric/Esophageal) on page 1956
Epirubicin-Oxaliplatin-Capecitabine (Gastric/Esophageal) on page 1957
Irinotecan-Capecitabine (Gastric Cancer) on page 2020
Trastuzumab-Cisplatin-Capecitabine (Gastric Cancer) on page 2093
Gastrointestinal cancer: CAPOX (Biliary Cancer) on page 1860
Pancreatic cancer:
Capecitabine-Gemcitabine (Pancreatic) on page 1858
CAPOX (Pancreatic) on page 1861
GTX (Pancreatic) on page 2001

Administration Usually administered in 2 divided doses taken 12 hours apart. Doses should be taken with water within 30 minutes after a meal. Swallow tablets whole; do not cut or crush.

Hazardous agent; use appropriate precautions for handling and disposal (NIOSH 2014 [group 1]). If it is necessary to manipulate the tablets (eg, to prepare an oral solution), it is recommended to double glove, wear a protective gown, and prepare in a controlled device (NIOSH, 2014).

Emetic Potential Children and Adults: Low (10% to 30%)

Extemporaneous Preparations Hazardous agent: Use appropriate precautions for handling and disposal (NIOSH 2014 [group 1]). When manipulating tablets, NIOSH recommends double gloving, a protective gown, and preparation in a controlled device; if not prepared in a controlled device, respiratory and eye protection as well as ventilated engineering controls are recommended (NIOSH, 2014).

A 10 mg/mL oral solution may be made with tablets. Crush four 500 mg tablets in a mortar and reduce to a fine powder; add to 200 mL water. Capecitabine tablets are water soluble (data on file from Roche). Administer immediately after preparation, 30 minutes after a meal.

Judson IR, Beale PJ, Trigo JM, et al, "A Human Capecitabine Excretion Balance and Pharmacokinetic Study After Administration of a Single Oral Dose of ^{14}C-Labelled Drug," *Invest New Drugs*, 1999, 17(1):49-56.

Monitoring Parameters Renal function should be estimated at baseline to determine initial dose. During therapy, CBC with differential, hepatic function, and renal function should be monitored. Monitor INR closely if receiving concomitant warfarin. Monitor for diarrhea, dehydration, hand-foot syndrome, Stevens-Johnson syndrome, toxic epidermal necrolysis, stomatitis, and cardiotoxicity.

Dosage Forms Excipient information presented when available (limited, particularly for generics); consult specific product labeling.
Tablet, Oral:
Xeloda: 150 mg, 500 mg
Generic: 150 mg, 500 mg

◆ **Caphosol®** see Saliva Substitute *on page 1511*

◆ **Caprelsa** see Vandetanib *on page 1728*

◆ **Carac** see Fluorouracil (Topical) *on page 747*

CARBOplatin (KAR boe pla tin)

Related Information

Chemotherapy and Obesity *on page 2220*

Chemotherapy-Induced Peripheral Neuropathy *on page 2116*

Hematopoietic Stem Cell Transplantation *on page 2272*

Management of Chemotherapy-Induced Nausea and Vomiting in Adults *on page 2142*

Management of Drug Extravasations *on page 2159*

Prevention of Chemotherapy-Induced Nausea and Vomiting in Children *on page 2203*

Safe Handling of Hazardous Drugs *on page 2292*

Brand Names: Canada Carboplatin Injection; Carboplatin Injection BP

Index Terms CBDCA; Paraplatin

Pharmacologic Category Antineoplastic Agent, Alkylating Agent; Antineoplastic Agent, Platinum Analog

Use Ovarian cancer: Initial treatment of advanced ovarian cancer in combination with other established chemotherapy agents; palliative treatment of recurrent ovarian cancer after prior chemotherapy, including cisplatin-based treatment

Labeled Contraindications History of severe allergic reaction to carboplatin, cisplatin, other platinum-containing formulations, mannitol, or any component of the formulation; should not be used in patients with severe bone marrow depression or significant bleeding

Pregnancy Considerations Embryotoxicity and teratogenicity have been observed in animal reproduction studies. May cause fetal harm if administered during pregnancy. Women of childbearing potential should avoid becoming pregnant during treatment.

Breast-Feeding Considerations It is not known if carboplatin is excreted in breast milk. Due to the potential for toxicity in nursing infants, breast-feeding is not recommended.

Warnings/Precautions Hazardous agent - use appropriate precautions for handling and disposal (NIOSH 2014 [group 1]). High doses have resulted in severe abnormalities of liver function tests. **[US Boxed Warning]: Bone marrow suppression, which may be severe, is dose related; may result in infection (due to neutropenia) or bleeding (due to thrombocytopenia); anemia may require blood transfusion;** reduce dosage in patients with bone marrow suppression; cycles should be delayed until WBC and platelet counts have recovered. Patients who have received prior myelosuppressive therapy and patients with renal dysfunction are at increased risk for bone marrow suppression. Anemia is cumulative.

When calculating the carboplatin dose using the Calvert formula and an estimated glomerular filtration rate (GFR), the laboratory method used to measure serum creatinine may impact dosing. Compared to other methods, standardized isotope dilution mass spectrometry (IDMS) may underestimate serum creatinine values in patients with low creatinine values (eg, ≤0.7 mg/dL) and may overestimate GFR in patients with normal renal function. This may result in higher calculated carboplatin doses and increased toxicities. If using IDMS, the Food and Drug Administration (FDA) recommends that clinicians consider capping estimated GFR at a maximum of 125 mL/minute to avoid potential toxicity.

[US Boxed Warning]: Anaphylactic-like reactions have been reported with carboplatin; may occur within minutes of administration. Epinephrine, corticosteroids and antihistamines have been used to treat symptoms. The risk of allergic reactions (including anaphylaxis) is increased in patients previously exposed to platinum therapy. Skin testing and desensitization protocols have been reported (Confina-Cohen, 2005; Lee, 2004; Markman, 2003). When administered as sequential infusions, taxane derivatives (docetaxel, paclitaxel) should be administered before the platinum derivatives (carboplatin, cisplatin) to limit myelosuppression and to enhance efficacy. Ototoxicity may occur when administered concomitantly with aminoglycosides. Clinically significant hearing loss has been reported to occur in pediatric patients when carboplatin was administered at higher than recommended doses in combination with other ototoxic agents (eg, aminoglycosides). In a study of children receiving carboplatin for the treatment of retinoblastoma, those <6 months of age at treatment initiation were more likely to experience ototoxicity; long-term audiology monitoring is recommended (Qaddoumi, 2012). Loss of vision (usually reversible within weeks of discontinuing) has been reported with higher than recommended doses.

Use caution in elderly patients; may cause or exacerbate syndrome of inappropriate antidiuretic hormone secretion or hyponatremia; monitor sodium closely with initiation or dosage adjustments in older adults (Beers Criteria). Peripheral neuropathy occurs infrequently, the incidence of peripheral neuropathy is increased in patients >65 years of age and those who have previously received cisplatin treatment. Patients >65 years of age are more likely to develop severe thrombocytopenia.

Limited potential for nephrotoxicity unless administered concomitantly with aminoglycosides. **[US Boxed Warning]: Vomiting may occur.** Carboplatin is associated with a moderate emetic potential in adult patients and a high emetic potential in pediatric patients; antiemetics are recommended to prevent nausea and vomiting (Basch, 2011; Dupuis, 2011; Roila, 2010). May be severe in patients who have received prior emetogenic therapy. **[US Boxed Warning]: Should be administered under the supervision of an experienced cancer chemotherapy physician.**

Adverse Reactions Percentages reported with single-agent therapy.

>10%:

Central nervous system: Pain (23%)

Endocrine & metabolic: Hyponatremia (29% to 47%), hypomagnesemia (29% to 43%), hypocalcemia (22% to 31%), hypokalemia (20% to 28%)

Gastrointestinal: Vomiting (65% to 81%), abdominal pain (17%), nausea (without vomiting: 10% to 15%)

Hematologic & oncologic: Bone marrow depression (dose related and dose limiting; nadir at ~21 days with single-agent therapy), anemia (71% to 90%; grades 3/4: 21%), leukopenia (85%; grades 3/4: 15% to 26%), neutropenia (67%; grades 3/4: 16% to 21%), thrombocytopenia (62%; grades 3/4: 25% to 35%)

Hepatic: Increased serum alkaline phosphatase (24% to 37%), increased serum AST (15% to 19%)

Hypersensitivity: Hypersensitivity (2% to 16%)

Neuromuscular & skeletal: Weakness (11%)

Renal: Decreased creatinine clearance (27%), increased blood urea nitrogen (14% to 22%)

◀ 1% to 10%:
   Central nervous system: Peripheral neuropathy (4% to 6%), neurotoxicity (5%)
   Dermatologic: Alopecia (2% to 3%)
   Gastrointestinal: Constipation (6%), diarrhea (6%), dysgeusia (1%), mucositis (≤1%), stomatitis (≤1%)
   Hematologic & oncologic: Bleeding complications (5%), hemorrhage (5%)
   Hepatic: Increased serum bilirubin (5%)
   Infection: Infection (5%)
   Ophthalmic: Visual disturbance (1%)
   Otic: Ototoxicity (1%)
   Renal: Increased serum creatinine (6% to 10%)
<1%, postmarketing, and/or case reports (Limited to important or life-threatening): Anaphylaxis, anorexia, bronchospasm, cardiac failure, cerebrovascular accident, dehydration, embolism, erythema, febrile neutropenia, hemolytic anemia (acute), hemolytic-uremic syndrome, hypertension, hypotension, injection site reaction (pain, redness, swelling), limb ischemia (acute), malaise, metastases, pruritus, skin rash, tissue necrosis (associated with extravasation), urticaria, vision loss

Drug Interactions
Metabolism/Transport Effects None known.
Avoid Concomitant Use
   Avoid concomitant use of CARBOplatin with any of the following: BCG (Intravesical); CloZAPine; Dipyrone; Natalizumab; Pimecrolimus; SORAfenib; Tacrolimus (Topical); Tofacitinib; Vaccines (Live)
Increased Effect/Toxicity
   CARBOplatin may increase the levels/effects of: Bexarotene (Systemic); CloZAPine; Fingolimod; Leflunomide; Natalizumab; Taxane Derivatives; Tofacitinib; Topotecan; Vaccines (Live)

   The levels/effects of CARBOplatin may be increased by: Aminoglycosides; Denosumab; Dipyrone; Pimecrolimus; Roflumilast; SORAfenib; Tacrolimus (Topical); Trastuzumab
Decreased Effect
   CARBOplatin may decrease the levels/effects of: BCG (Intravesical); Coccidioides immitis Skin Test; Fosphenytoin-Phenytoin; Sipuleucel-T; Vaccines (Inactivated); Vaccines (Live)

   The levels/effects of CARBOplatin may be decreased by: Echinacea
Storage/Stability Store intact vials at room temperature at 25°C (77°F); excursions permitted to 15°C to 30°C (59°F to 86°F). Protect from light. Further dilution to a concentration as low as 0.5 mg/mL is stable at room temperature (25°C) for 8 hours in NS or D$_5$W. Stability has also been demonstrated for dilutions in D$_5$W in PVC bags at room temperature for 9 days (Benaji, 1994); however, the manufacturer recommends use within 8 hours due to lack of preservative. Multidose vials are stable for up to 14 days after opening when stored at 25°C (77°F) following multiple needle entries.
Preparation for Administration Hazardous agent; use appropriate precautions for handling and disposal (NIOSH 2014 [group 1]).
   Solution for injection: Manufacturer's labeling states solution can be further diluted to concentrations as low as 0.5 mg/mL in NS or D$_5$W; however, most clinicians generally dilute dose in either 100 mL or 250 mL of NS or D$_5$W. Concentrations used for desensitization vary based on protocol.

Needles or IV administration sets that contain aluminum should not be used in the preparation or administration of carboplatin; aluminum can react with carboplatin resulting in precipitate formation and loss of potency.

Mechanism of Action Carboplatin is a platinum compound alkylating agent which covalently binds to DNA; interferes with the function of DNA by producing interstrand DNA cross-links

Pharmacodynamics/Kinetics

Distribution: V_d: 16 L (based on a dose of 300 to 500 mg/m^2); into liver, kidney, skin, and tumor tissue

Protein binding: Carboplatin: 0%; Platinum (from carboplatin): Irreversibly binds to plasma proteins

Metabolism: Minimally hepatic to aquated and hydroxylated compounds

Half-life elimination: CrCl >60 mL/minute: Carboplatin: 2.6 to 5.9 hours (based on a dose of 300 to 500 mg/m^2); Platinum (from carboplatin): ≥5 days

Excretion: Urine (~70% as carboplatin within 24 hours; 3% to 5% as platinum within 1 to 4 days)

Dosing

Adult Note: Doses for adults are commonly calculated by the target AUC using the Calvert formula, where **Total dose (mg) = Target AUC x (GFR + 25)**. If estimating glomerular filtration rate (GFR) instead of a measured GFR, the Food and Drug Administration (FDA) recommends that clinicians consider capping estimated GFR at a maximum of 125 mL/minute to avoid potential toxicity. Carboplatin is associated with a moderate emetic potential in adult patients; antiemetics are recommended to prevent nausea and vomiting (Basch, 2011; Roila, 2010).

Ovarian cancer, advanced: *Manufacturer's labeling:* IV: 360 mg/m^2 every 4 weeks (as a single agent) **or** 300 mg/m^2 every 4 weeks (in combination with cyclophosphamide) **or** Target AUC 4 to 6 (single agent; in previously-treated patients)

Off-label dosing for advanced ovarian cancer: IV: Target AUC 5 to 7.5 every 3 weeks (in combination with paclitaxel) (Ozols, 2003; Parmar, 2003) **or** Target AUC 5 every 3 weeks (in combination with docetaxel) (Vasey, 2004)

Bladder cancer (off-label use): IV: Target AUC 5 every 3 weeks (in combination with gemcitabine) (Bamias, 2006) **or** Target AUC 6 every 3 weeks (in combination with paclitaxel) (Vaughn, 2002)

Breast cancer, metastatic (off-label use): IV: Target AUC 6 every 3 weeks (in combination with trastuzumab and paclitaxel) (Robert, 2006) **or** Target AUC 6 every 3 weeks (in combination with trastuzumab and docetaxel) (Pegram, 2004; Valero, 2011)

Cervical cancer, recurrent or metastatic (off-label use): IV: Target AUC 5 every 3 weeks (in combination with paclitaxel) (Pectasides, 2009) **or** Target AUC 5 to 6 every 4 weeks (in combination with paclitaxel) (Tinker, 2005) **or** 400 mg/m^2 every 28 days (as a single agent) (Weiss, 1990)

Endometrial cancer (off-label use): IV: Target AUC 5 every 3 weeks (in combination with paclitaxel) (Pectasides, 2008) **or** Target AUC 2 on days 1, 8, and 15 every 28 days (in combination with paclitaxel) (Secord, 2007)

Esophageal cancer (off-label use): IV: Target AUC 2 on days 1, 8, 15, 22, and 29 for 1 cycle (in combination with paclitaxel) (van Meerten, 2006) **or** Target AUC 5 every 3 weeks (in combination with paclitaxel) (El-Rayes, 2004)

Head and neck cancer (off-label use): IV: Target AUC 5 every 3 weeks (in combination with cetuximab) (Chan, 2005) **or** Target AUC 5 every 3 weeks (in combination with cetuximab and fluorouracil) (Vermorken, 2008) **or** 300 mg/m^2 every 4 weeks (in combination with fluorouracil) (Forastiere, 1992) **or** Target AUC 6 every 3 weeks (in combination with paclitaxel) (Clark, 2001)

Hodgkin lymphoma, relapsed or refractory (off-label use): IV: Target AUC 5 (maximum dose: 800 mg) for 2 cycles (in combination with ifosfamide and etoposide) (Moskowitz, 2001)

Malignant pleural mesothelioma (off-label use): IV: Target AUC 5 every 3 weeks (in combination with pemetrexed) (Castagneto, 2008; Ceresoli, 2006)

Melanoma, advanced or metastatic (off-label use): IV: Target AUC 2 days on 1, 8, and 15 every 4 weeks (in combination with paclitaxel) (Rao, 2006)

Non-Hodgkin lymphomas, relapsed or refractory (off-label use): IV: Target AUC 5 (maximum dose: 800 mg) per cycle for 3 cycles (in combination with rituximab, ifosfamide and etoposide) (Kewalramani, 2004)

Non-small cell lung cancer (off-label use): IV: Target AUC 6 every 3 to 4 weeks (in combination with paclitaxel) (Ramalingam, 2008; Schiller, 2002; Strauss, 2008) **or** Target AUC 6 every 3 weeks (in combination with bevacizumab and paclitaxel) (Sandler, 2006) **or** Target AUC 5 every 3 weeks (in combination with pemetrexed) (Gronberg, 2009) **or** in combination with radiation therapy and paclitaxel (Belani, 2005):

Target AUC 6 every 3 weeks for 2 cycles **or**

Target AUC 6 every 3 weeks for 2 cycles; then target AUC 2 weekly for 7 weeks **or**

Target AUC 2 every week for 7 weeks; then target AUC 6 every 3 weeks for 2 cycles

Sarcomas: Ewing sarcoma, osteosarcoma (off-label uses): IV: 400 mg/m^2/day for 2 days every 21 days (in combination with ifosfamide and etoposide) (van Winkle, 2005)

Small cell lung cancer (off-label use): IV: Target AUC 6 every 3 weeks (in combination with etoposide) (Skarlos, 2001) **or** Target AUC 5 every 3 weeks (in combination with irinotecan) (Hermes, 2008) **or** Target AUC 5 every 28 days (in combination with irinotecan) (Schmittel, 2006)

Testicular cancer (off-label use): IV: Target AUC 7 as a one-time dose (Oliver, 2011) **or** 700 mg/m^2/day for 3 days beginning 5 days prior to peripheral stem cell infusion (in combination with etoposide) for 2 cycles (Einhorn, 2007)

Thymic malignancies (off-label use): IV: Target AUC 5 every 3 weeks (in combination with paclitaxel) (Lemma, 2008)

Unknown primary adenocarcinoma (off-label use): IV: Target AUC 6 every 3 weeks (in combination with paclitaxel) (Briasoulis, 2000) **or** Target AUC 6 every 3 weeks (in combination with docetaxel) (Greco, 2000) **or** Target AUC 6 every 3 weeks (in combination with paclitaxel and etoposide) (Hainsworth, 2006) **or** Target AUC 5 every 3 weeks (in combination with paclitaxel and gemcitabine) (Greco, 2002)

Geriatric The Calvert formula should be used to calculate dosing for elderly patients. Refer to adult dosing.

Pediatric Carboplatin is associated with a high emetic potential in pediatric patients; antiemetics are recommended to prevent nausea and vomiting (Dupuis, 2011).

Central nervous system tumors (off-label use):

Glioma: IV: 175 mg/m^2 weekly for 4 weeks every 6 weeks, with a 2-week recovery period between courses (in combination with vincristine) (Packer, 1997)

Neuroblastoma, localized and unresectable: IV: Children ≥10 kg: 200 mg/m^2/day days 1, 2, and 3 every 21 days for 2 cycles (in combination with etoposide for 2 cycles then followed by cyclophosphamide, doxorubicin and vincristine) (Rubie, 1998) **or** Children <1 year: 6.6 mg/kg/day days 1, 2, and 3 (in combination with etoposide for 2 cycles, then followed by cyclophosphamide, doxorubicin, and vincristine) (Rubie, 2001)

Sarcomas: Ewing sarcoma, osteosarcoma (off-label uses): IV: 400 mg/m^2/day for 2 days every 21 days (in combination with ifosfamide and etoposide) (van Winkle, 2005)

Renal Impairment Note: Dose determination with Calvert formula uses GFR and, therefore, inherently adjusts for renal dysfunction.

The manufacturer's labeling recommends the following dosage adjustments for single-agent therapy: Adults:

Baseline CrCl 41 to 59 mL/minute: Initiate at 250 mg/m^2 and adjust subsequent doses based on bone marrow toxicity

Baseline CrCl 16 to 40 mL/minute: Initiate at 200 mg/m^2 and adjust subsequent doses based on bone marrow toxicity

Baseline CrCl ≤15 mL/minute: There are no dosage adjustments provided in the manufacturer's labeling.

The following dosage adjustments have also been recommended:

Aronoff, 2007:

Adults (**Note:** For dosing based on **mg/m^2**):

GFR >50 mL/minute: No dosage adjustment is necessary

GFR 10 to 50 mL/minute: Administer 50% of the dose

GFR <10 mL/minute: Administer 25% of the dose

Hemodialysis: Administer 50% of dose

Continuous ambulatory peritoneal dialysis (CAPD): Administer 25% of dose

Continuous renal replacement therapy (CRRT): 200 mg/m^2

Children:

GFR <50 mL/minute: Use Calvert formula incorporating patient's GFR

Hemodialysis, peritoneal dialysis, continuous renal replacement therapy (CRRT): Use Calvert formula incorporating patient's GFR

Janus, 2010: Hemodialysis: Carboplatin dose (mg) = Target AUC x 25; administer on a nondialysis day, hemodialysis should occur between 12-24 hours after carboplatin dose

Hepatic Impairment There are no dosage adjustments provided in the manufacturer's labeling; however, carboplatin undergoes minimal hepatic metabolism therefore dosage adjustment may not be needed.

Obesity

American Society of Clinical Oncology (ASCO) Guidelines for appropriate chemotherapy dosing in obese adults with cancer: Dosing based on GFR should be considered in obese patients; GFR should not exceed 125 mL/minute (Griggs, 2012).

American Society for Blood and Marrow Transplantation (ASBMT) practice guideline committee position statement on chemotherapy dosing in obesity: Utilize actual body weight (full weight) for calculation of body surface area (when applicable) in carboplatin dosing for hematopoietic stem cell transplant conditioning regimens in adults. Based on the literature, there is no consensus for carboplatin dosing based on AUC in transplant conditioning regimens or dosing adjustments during transplant for obese patients (Bubalo, 2014).

Adjustment for Toxicity Platelets <50,000 cells/mm^3 or ANC <500 cells/mm^3: Administer 75% of dose

Combination Regimens

Bladder cancer: Carboplatin-Gemcitabine (Bladder) on page 1867

Bone sarcoma (Ewing sarcoma): Ifosfamide-Carboplatin-Etoposide (Ewing Sarcoma) on page 2014

Bone sarcoma (osteosarcoma): Ifosfamide-Carboplatin-Etoposide (Osteosarcoma) on page 2015

Breast cancer:
  Carboplatin (Breast Regimen) on page 1861
  Carboplatin-Docetaxel-Trastuzumab (Breast) on page 1862
  Carboplatin-Paclitaxel-Trastuzumab (Breast) on page 1872

Cervical cancer: Carboplatin-Paclitaxel (Cervical Cancer) on page 1868

Endometrial cancer: Carboplatin-Paclitaxel (Endometrial) on page 1869

Esophageal cancer: Paclitaxel-Carboplatin (Esophageal Cancer) on page 2050

Head and neck cancer:
  Carboplatin-Cetuximab (Head and Neck Cancer) on page 1861
  Cetuximab-Carboplatin-Fluorouracil (Head and Neck Cancer) on page 1880
  Fluorouracil-Carboplatin (Head and Neck Cancer) on page 1977

Lung cancer (non-small cell):
  Bevacizumab-Carboplatin-Paclitaxel (NSCLC) on page 1839
  Bevacizumab-Carboplatin-Pemetrexed (NSCLC) on page 1839
  Carboplatin-Gemcitabine (NSCLC) on page 1867
  Carboplatin-Paclitaxel (NSCLC) on page 1870
  Carboplatin-Paclitaxel (Protein Bound) (NSCLC) on page 1872
  Carboplatin-Pemetrexed (NSCLC) on page 1874
  EC (NSCLC) on page 1953

Lung cancer (small cell):
  Carboplatin-Etoposide (Small Cell Lung Cancer) on page 1865
  Carboplatin-Irinotecan (Small Cell Lung Cancer) on page 1868

Lymphoma, Hodgkin:
  Gemcitabine-Dexamethasone-Carboplatin (Hodgkin) on page 1991
  ICE (Hodgkin) on page 2013

Lymphoma, non-Hodgkin: ICE (Lymphoma, non-Hodgkin) on page 2013

Lymphoma, non-Hodgkin (DLBCL):
  R-ICE (NHL-DLBCL) on page 2076
  Rituximab-Gemcitabine-Dexamethasone-Carboplatin (NHL-DLBCL) on page 2081

Malignant pleural mesothelioma: Carboplatin-Pemetrexed (Mesothelioma) on page 1874

Neuroblastoma: CE-CAdO (Neuroblastoma) on page 1877

Ovarian cancer:
  Bevacizumab-Carboplatin-Gemcitabine (Ovarian) on page 1839
  Carboplatin-Docetaxel (Ovarian) on page 1862
  Carboplatin-Doxorubicin (Liposomal) (Ovarian) on page 1864
  Carboplatin-Etoposide (Ovarian Germ Cell Tumor) on page 1864
  Carboplatin-Gemcitabine (Ovarian) on page 1868
  Carboplatin-Paclitaxel (Ovarian) on page 1871

Retinoblastoma:
  Carboplatin-Etoposide (Retinoblastoma) on page 1865
  Carboplatin-Etoposide-Vincristine (Retinoblastoma) on page 1866
  Carboplatin-Vincristine (Retinoblastoma) on page 1875
Testicular cancer: Carboplatin (Testicular Regimen) on page 1874
Thymoma/Thymic carcinoma: Carboplatin-Paclitaxel (Thymoma/Thymic) on page 1872
Unknown primary, adenocarcinoma:
  Carboplatin-Docetaxel (Unknown Primary, Adenocarcinoma) on page 1863
  Carboplatin-Etoposide-Paclitaxel (Unknown Primary, Adenocarcinoma) on page 1864
  Carboplatin-Paclitaxel (Unknown Primary, Adenocarcinoma) on page 1873
Unknown primary, squamous cell: Carboplatin-Docetaxel (Unknown Primary, Squamous Cell) on page 1863

Administration Carboplatin is associated with a moderate emetic potential in adult patients and a high emetic potential in pediatric patients; antiemetics are recommended to prevent nausea and vomiting (Basch, 2011; Dupuis, 2011; Roila, 2010).

Infuse over at least 15 minutes; usually infused over 15 to 60 minutes, although some protocols may require infusions up to 24 hours. When administered as a part of a combination chemotherapy regimen, sequence of administration may vary by regimen; refer to specific protocol for sequence recommendation.

Needles or IV administration sets that contain aluminum should not be used in the preparation or administration of carboplatin; aluminum can react with carboplatin resulting in precipitate formation and loss of potency.

Hazardous agent; use appropriate precautions for handling and disposal (NIOSH 2014 [group 1]).

Vesicant/Extravasation Risk May be an irritant

Emetic Potential Children: High (>90%)
  Adults: Moderate (30% to 90%)

Monitoring Parameters CBC (with differential and platelet count), serum electrolytes, serum creatinine and BUN, creatinine clearance, liver function tests; audiology evaluations (children <6 months of age)

Dosage Forms Excipient information presented when available (limited, particularly for generics); consult specific product labeling.
Solution, Intravenous:
  Generic: 50 mg/5 mL (5 mL); 150 mg/15 mL (15 mL); 450 mg/45 mL (45 mL); 600 mg/60 mL (60 mL)
Solution, Intravenous [preservative free]:
  Generic: 50 mg/5 mL (5 mL); 150 mg/15 mL (15 mL); 450 mg/45 mL (45 mL); 600 mg/60 mL (60 mL)
Solution Reconstituted, Intravenous:
  Generic: 150 mg (1 ea)

◆ **Carboplatin Injection (Can)** see CARBOplatin on page 270
◆ **Carboplatin Injection BP (Can)** see CARBOplatin on page 270
◆ **Carboxypeptidase-G2** see Glucarpidase on page 793
◆ **Cardiolite** see Technetium Tc 99m Sestamibi on page 1602

Carfilzomib (kar FILZ oh mib)

Related Information

Common Toxicity Criteria *on page 2122*

Management of Chemotherapy-Induced Nausea and Vomiting in Adults *on page 2142*

Safe Handling of Hazardous Drugs *on page 2292*

Brand Names: US Kyprolis

Index Terms CFZ; PR-171

Pharmacologic Category Antineoplastic Agent; Proteasome Inhibitor

Use Multiple myeloma, relapsed/refractory: Treatment (monotherapy) of multiple myeloma in patients who have received at least 2 prior therapies (including bortezomib and an immunomodulatory agent) and have demonstrated disease progression on or within 60 days of completion of the last therapy; treatment of multiple myeloma (in combination with lenalidomide and dexamethasone) in patients who have received 1 to 3 prior therapies.

Labeled Contraindications There are no contraindications listed in the manufacturer's labeling.

Pregnancy Considerations Adverse events were observed in animal reproduction studies. Based on the mechanism of action, adverse fetal events would be expected to occur with use in pregnant women. Females of reproductive potential are advised to avoid pregnancy during therapy; effective contraception should be used during treatment and for at least 2 weeks following therapy completion.

Breast-Feeding Considerations It is not known if carfilzomib is excreted in breast milk. Due to the potential for serious adverse reactions in the breast-feeding infant, the manufacturer recommends against breast-feeding while on carfilzomib; a decision should be made to discontinue breast-feeding or to discontinue the drug, taking into account the importance of treatment to the mother and the health benefits of breast-feeding. The appropriate timing to restart breast-feeding after treatment discontinuation should be determined with the health care provider.

Warnings/Precautions Hazardous agent - use appropriate precautions for handling and disposal (meets NIOSH 2014 criteria). Thrombocytopenia (including grade 4) was observed in patients receiving carfilzomib, with platelet nadirs occurring between day 8 and day 15 of each 28-day treatment cycle, and recovery to baseline by the start of the next cycle. Monitor platelets closely and adjust dose or withhold therapy if necessary. Anemia, lymphopenia, leukopenia, and neutropenia were also observed. Death caused by cardiac arrest has occurred within 24 hours of drug administration. Carfilzomib has been associated with new-onset or worsening of heart failure (HF), pulmonary edema, decreased left ventricular ejection fraction (LVEF), restrictive cardiomyopathy, myocardial ischemia, and myocardial infarction (including fatalities). Cardiac events typically were observed early in therapy (<5 cycles). Patients 75 years of age or older have an increased risk of heart failure. Monitor closely for cardiac complications and for volume overload (due to pretreatment hydration), particularly in patients at risk for heart failure; withhold carfilzomib therapy for grade 3 or 4 cardiac events until recovery. Patients with New York Heart Association Class III and IV heart failure, recent myocardial infarction (within 3 to 6 months), and conduction abnormalities not managed by medication were excluded from clinical trials and may be at increased risk for cardiac complications. Hypertension has occurred with use; hypertensive crisis and hypertensive emergency have also been reported (some events were fatal). Monitor blood pressure throughout therapy; if hypertension cannot be adequately controlled, interrupt carfilzomib therapy and evaluate; assess risks versus benefits when determining to restart treatment.

Acute respiratory distress syndrome (ARDS), acute respiratory failure, and acute diffuse-infiltrative pulmonary disease (eg, pneumonitis and interstitial lung disease) have occurred in a small number of patients (some events were fatal); discontinue therapy if any of these drug-induced pulmonary toxicities occur. Pulmonary arterial hypertension (PAH) was observed (including grade 3 or higher events) in studies; perform cardiac imaging or other testing as appropriate, and withhold carfilzomib until PAH is resolved or returns to baseline. Dyspnea (including grade 3 or higher events) has been reported; monitor closely. Withhold carfilzomib until pulmonary symptom resolution or return to baseline. Renal toxicity (eg, renal impairment, acute renal failure, renal failure) has been reported with carfilzomib. Acute renal failure was observed more frequently in patients receiving carfilzomib monotherapy for advanced relapsed/refractory multiple myeloma; renal failure risk is greater when patients have a baseline reduced creatinine clearance. Monitor renal function closely; may require therapy interruption or dose reduction.

Thrombocytopenic thrombotic purpura/hemolytic uremic syndrome (TTP/HUS) has been reported (some fatal); monitor for signs/symptoms. Interrupt therapy if TTP/HUS diagnosis is suspected and manage appropriately (eg, plasma exchange as clinically necessary). If TTP/HUS diagnosis is excluded, may consider reinitiating therapy; the safety of restarting carfilzomib after a TTP/HUS diagnosis is not known. Posterior reversible encephalopathy syndrome (PRES) has been reported rarely with use; symptoms include seizure, headache, lethargy, confusion, blindness, altered consciousness, hypertension, and other visual/neurological disturbances. Discontinue therapy if PRES diagnosis is suspected; the safety of reinitiating therapy after PRES diagnosis is not known. Venous thromboembolism (eg, deep vein thrombosis and pulmonary embolism) has been observed, particularly when used as part of combination therapy with lenalidomide and dexamethasone. Thromboprophylaxis is recommended when appropriate, based on patients' underlying risk factors, treatment regimen, and clinical status.

Infusion reactions such as chills, fever, arthralgia, myalgia, shortness of breath, hypotension, facial flushing, facial edema, vomiting, weakness, syncope, chest tightness, or angina may occur immediately following or within 24 hours of carfilzomib infusion (may be life-threatening). To lessen the incidence and intensity of infusion reactions, administer dexamethasone prior to drug administration. Tumor lysis syndrome (TLS), including fatalities has been observed. TLS risk is increased in multiple myeloma patients with a high tumor burden. Adequately hydrate patients prior to carfilzomib therapy and monitor closely for signs and symptoms of TLS; consider use of antihyperuricemic agents. If TLS occurs, interrupt treatment until resolved.

Hepatic failure, including fatal cases, has been reported rarely (<1%). Increased transaminases and hyperbilirubinemia have also been observed. Interrupt carfilzomib therapy in patients with grade 3 or higher hepatic toxicity until resolved or recovered to baseline (may require dose reduction if appropriate to reinitiate); monitor liver enzymes regularly.

Potentially significant interactions may exist, requiring dose or frequency adjustment, additional monitoring, and/or selection of alternative therapy. Consult drug interactions database for more detailed information. Vials contain the excipient cyclodextrin (sulfobutyl ether beta-cyclodextrin), which may accumulate in patients with renal insufficiency, although the clinical significance of this finding is uncertain (Luke 2010).

Adverse Reactions

>10%:

Cardiovascular: Peripheral edema (24%), hypertension (14%), chest wall pain (11%)

Central nervous system: Fatigue (56%), fever (30%), headache (28%), insomnia (18%), chills (16%), dizziness (13%), hypoesthesia (12%), pain (12%)

Endocrine & metabolic: Hypokalemia (14%), hypomagnesemia (14%), hyperglycemia (12%), hypercalcemia (11%), hypophosphatemia (11%)

Gastrointestinal: Nausea (45%), diarrhea (33%), vomiting (22%), constipation (21%), anorexia (12%)

Hematologic: Anemia (47%; grade 3: 21%; grade 4: 1%), thrombocytopenia (36%; grade 3: 13%; grade 4: 10%), lymphopenia (24%; grade 3: 16%; grade 4: 2%), neutropenia (21%; grade 3: 10%; grade 4: 1%), leukopenia (14%; grade 3: 5%; grade 4:<1%)

Hepatic: AST increased (13%; grade 3: 3%; grade 4: <1%)

Neuromuscular & skeletal: Back pain (20%), arthralgia (16%), muscle spasms (14%), peripheral neuropathy (14%; grade 3: 1%), weakness (14%), limb pain (13%)

Renal: Creatinine increased (24%; grade 3: 3%; grade 4: <1%)

Respiratory: Dyspnea (35%; grade 3: 5%; grade 4: <1%), upper respiratory tract infection (28%), cough (26%), pneumonia (13%; grade 3: 10%; grade 4: <1%)

1% to 10%:

Cardiovascular: Cardiac failure (7%; includes CHF, pulmonary edema, ejection fraction decrease)

Endocrine & metabolic: Hyponatremia (10%)

Renal: Renal failure (9%)

Respiratory: Pulmonary arterial hypertension (2%)

Miscellaneous: Herpes zoster reactivation (2%)

<1%, postmarketing, and/or case reports: Bilirubin increased, hepatic failure, infusion reaction, intracranial hemorrhage, multiorgan failure, myocardial ischemia, neutropenic fever, sepsis, tumor lysis syndrome

Drug Interactions

Metabolism/Transport Effects Substrate of P-glycoprotein; **Inhibits** P-glycoprotein

Avoid Concomitant Use

Avoid concomitant use of Carfilzomib with any of the following: BCG (Intravesical); CloZAPine; Dipyrone

Increased Effect/Toxicity

Carfilzomib may increase the levels/effects of: CloZAPine

The levels/effects of Carfilzomib may be increased by: Dipyrone; Lumacaftor; P-glycoprotein/ABCB1 Inhibitors; Ranolazine

Decreased Effect

Carfilzomib may decrease the levels/effects of: BCG (Intravesical)

The levels/effects of Carfilzomib may be decreased by: Lumacaftor; P-glycoprotein/ABCB1 Inducers

Storage/Stability Store intact vials refrigerated at 2°C to 8°C (36°F to 46°F). Store in original carton until use to protect from light. Reconstituted drug (in the vial or in a syringe) and preparations diluted for infusion are stable for 4 hours at room temperature or for 24 hours refrigerated at 2°C to 8°C (36°F to 46°F).

Preparation for Administration Hazardous agent; use appropriate precautions for handling and disposal (meets NIOSH 2014 criteria). Reconstitute with 29 mL sterile water for injection to a concentration of 2 mg/mL (directing solution onto the inside wall of the vial to avoid foaming). Gently invert and/or swirl vial slowly for ~1 minute to mix; do not shake. If foaming results, allow solution to sit for 2 to 5 minutes until foaming resolves. Reconstituted solution should be clear and colorless. May further dilute dose in 50 mL D_5W. The amount contained in each vial may exceed the prescribed dose; use care with dosage and volume calculations. Discard unused portion of the vial.

Mechanism of Action Carfilzomib inhibits proteasomes, which are responsible for intracellular protein homeostasis. Specifically, it is a potent, selective, and irreversible inhibitor of chymotrypsin-like activity of the 20S proteasome, leading to cell cycle arrest and apoptosis.

Pharmacodynamics/Kinetics

Distribution: V_{dss}: 28 L; penetrates all tissues extensively except the brain (Kortuem 2013)

Protein binding: 97%

Metabolism: Rapid and extensive; peptidase cleavage and epoxide hydrolysis; minimal metabolism through cytochrome P450-mediated mechanisms

Half-life elimination: Doses ≥15 mg/m^2: <1 hour on day 1 of cycle 1

Excretion: Urine (25%, primarily as metabolites)

Dosing

Adult & Geriatric Note: Hydrate with oral fluids (30 mL/kg) at least 48 hours prior to initiating cycle 1, as well as with 250 to 500 mL normal saline (or other appropriate IV fluid) before dosing (recommended) and after (if needed) administration during cycle 1 (continue oral and/or IV hydration in subsequent cycles if necessary); monitor for evidence of volume overload and adjust hydration based on individual needs. Premedicate with dexamethasone (4 mg orally or IV, or the recommended dexamethasone dose when used in combination therapy) 30 minutes to 4 hours prior to all doses in cycle 1, and as needed with future cycles to reduce the incidence and severity of infusion reaction. Consider antiviral prophylaxis for patients with a history of herpes zoster infection. Thromboprophylaxis is recommended when administering in combination with lenalidomide and dexamethasone.

Multiple myeloma, relapsed/refractory (single-agent): IV: **Note:** Patients with a body surface area (BSA) >2.2 m^2 should be dosed based upon a maximum BSA of 2.2 m^2. Dose adjustments for weight changes of ≤20% are not necessary, per manufacturer labeling. Continue until disease progression or unacceptable toxicity.

Cycle 1: 20 mg/m^2 on days 1 and 2; if tolerated, increase dose to 27 mg/m^2 on days 8, 9, 15, and 16 of a 28-day treatment cycle

Cycles 2 to 12: 27 mg/m^2 days 1, 2, 8, 9, 15, and 16 of a 28-day treatment cycle

Cycle 13 and beyond: 27 mg/m^2 on days 1, 2, 15, and 16 of a 28-day treatment cycle

Multiple myeloma, relapsed/refractory (combination therapy [with lena-lidomide and dexamethasone]) (Stewart 2015): IV:

Cycle 1: 20 mg/m^2 on days 1 and 2 followed by 27 mg/m^2 on days 8, 9, 15, and 16.

Cycles 2 to 12: 27 mg/m^2 on days 1, 2, 8, 9, 15, and 16.

Cycles 13 to 18: 27 mg/m^2 on days 1, 2, 15, and 16; lenalidomide and dexamethasone may be continued (until disease progression or unaccept-able toxicity)

Renal Impairment

Preexisting renal impairment: There are no dosage adjustments provided in the manufacturer's labeling; however, results from a phase 2 study in patients with renal impairment indicate that the pharmacokinetics and safety of carfilzomib were unchanged in this patient population; no dosage adjustment is necessary in patients with baseline dysfunction, including patients on hemodialysis (Badros 2013). **Note:** Dialysis clearance of carfilzomib has not been studied; per manufacturer labeling, administer postdialysis.

Renal toxicity during treatment: Serum creatinine ≥2 times baseline, CrCl <15 mL/minute or CrCl decreases to ≤50% of baseline, or patient requires dialysis: Withhold dose and monitor renal function. If renal toxicity is due to carfilzomib, resume dosing when renal function has improved to within 25% of baseline; resume with a reduced dose by 1 dose level (from 27 mg/m^2 to 20 mg/m^2 or from 20 mg/m^2 to 15 mg/m^2). If toxicity is not due to carfilzomib, restart at the discretion of the prescriber.

Hepatic Impairment Preexisting hepatic impairment: There are no dosage adjustments provided in the manufacturer's labeling (has not been studied; patients with ALT or AST ≥3 times ULN and bilirubin ≥2 times ULN were excluded from clinical trials).

Hepatotoxicity during treatment: Grade 3 or 4 elevation of bilirubin, trans-aminases, or other liver abnormalities: Withhold dose until resolved or at baseline. After resolution, if appropriate to reinitiate, consider restarting at a reduced dose level (from 27 mg/m^2 to 20 mg/m^2 or from 20 mg/m^2 to 15 mg/m^2) with frequent monitoring of hepatic function.

Obesity *ASCO Guidelines for appropriate chemotherapy dosing in obese adults with cancer:* In general, utilize patient's actual body weight (full weight) for calculation of body surface area- or weight-based dosing, particularly when the intent of therapy is curative; manage regimen-related toxicities in the same manner as for nonobese patients; if a dose reduction is utilized due to toxicity, consider resumption of full weight-based dosing with subsequent cycles, especially if cause of toxicity (eg, hepatic or renal impairment) is resolved (Griggs 2012). **Note:** According to the manufacturer, patients with a body surface area (BSA) >2.2 m^2 should be dosed based upon a maximum BSA of 2.2 m^2; dose adjustments for weight changes of ≤20% are not necessary.

Adjustment for Toxicity

Hematologic toxicity:

ANC <500/mm^3: Withhold dose; continue at same dose level if ANC recovers to ≥500/mm^3. For subsequent ANC levels <500/mm^3, withhold dose and consider reducing dose by one dose level (from 27 mg/m^2 to 20 mg/m^2 or from 20 mg/m^2 to 15 mg/m^2) if ANC ≥500/mm^3 when restarting.

Platelets: <10,000/mm^3 or evidence of bleeding with thrombocytopenia: Withhold dose; continue at same dose level if platelets recover to ≥10,000/mm^3 and bleeding is controlled. For subsequent platelet levels <10,000/mm^3, withhold dose and consider reducing dose by one dose level (from 27 mg/m^2 to 20 mg/m^2 or from 20 mg/m^2 to 15 mg/m^2) if platelets ≥10,000/mm^3 when restarting.

Nonhematologic toxicity:

Cardiac: Grade 3 or 4, new-onset or worsening of heart failure, decreased left ventricular function, or myocardial ischemia: Withhold dose until resolved or at baseline. After resolution, if appropriate to reinitiate, consider restarting at a reduced dose level (from 27 mg/m^2 to 20 mg/m^2 or from 20 mg/m^2 to 15 mg/m^2).

Hypertension, severe or life-threatening: If hypertension cannot be adequately controlled, withhold dose and evaluate. After resolution, if appropriate to reinitiate (if risk versus benefit ratio is acceptable), consider restarting at a reduced dose level (from 27 mg/m^2 to 20 mg/m^2 or from 20 mg/m^2 to 15 mg/m^2).

Pulmonary toxicity

Acute respiratory distress syndrome, acute respiratory failure, and acute diffuse infiltrative pulmonary disease (drug-induced): Discontinue therapy.

Pulmonary hypertension: Withhold dose until resolved or at baseline. After resolution, if appropriate to reinitiate after severe or life-threatening pulmonary hypertension (if risk versus benefit ratio is acceptable), consider restarting at a reduced dose level (from 27 mg/m^2 to 20 mg/m^2 or from 20 mg/m^2 to 15 mg/m^2).

Grade 3 or 4 dyspnea: Withhold dose until resolved or at baseline. After resolution, if appropriate to reinitiate (if risk versus benefit ratio is acceptable), consider restarting (at next scheduled treatment) at a reduced dose level (from 27 mg/m^2 to 20 mg/m^2 or from 20 mg/m^2 to 15 mg/m^2).

Tumor lysis syndrome: Interrupt treatment until resolved.

Other grade 3 or 4 nonhematologic toxicities: Withhold dose until resolved or at baseline. After resolution, consider restarting (at next scheduled treatment) at a reduced dose level (from 27 mg/m^2 to 20 mg/m^2 or from 20 mg/m^2 to 15 mg/m^2).

Combination Regimens

Multiple myeloma:

Carfilzomib, Lenalidomide, Dexamethasone (Multiple Myeloma) on page 1875

Carfilzomib (Multiple Myeloma Regimen) on page 1876

Administration IV: Administer over 10 minutes. Do not administer as an IV bolus. Hydrate with oral fluids (30 mL/kg) at least 48 hours prior to initiating cycle 1, as well as with 250 to 500 mL NS (or other appropriate IV fluid) prior to (recommended) and after (if needed) each dose in cycle 1; continue oral and/or IV hydration in subsequent cycles (if necessary). Flush line before and after carfilzomib with NS or D$_5$W. Do not administer with other medications. Premedicate with dexamethasone (4 mg orally or IV, or the recommended dexamethasone dose when used in combination therapy) 30 minutes to 4 hours prior to all doses in cycle 1, and as needed with future cycles to reduce the incidence and severity of infusion reaction. Hazardous agent; use appropriate precautions for handling and disposal (meets NIOSH 2014 criteria).

Emetic Potential Low (10% to 30%)

Monitoring Parameters CBC with differential and platelets (monitor frequently throughout therapy); renal function, pulmonary function (with new or worsening pulmonary symptoms), liver function tests, blood pressure. Signs/symptoms of infusion-related reactions, congestive heart failure, tumor lysis syndrome, peripheral neuropathy, posterior reversible encephalopathy syndrome, thrombocytopenic thrombotic purpura/hemolytic uremic syndrome, and venous thromboembolic events. Monitor for evidence of volume overload due to pre- and posthydration.

Dosage Forms Excipient information presented when available (limited, particularly for generics); consult specific product labeling.

Solution Reconstituted, Intravenous:

Kyprolis: 60 mg (1 ea)

♦ **Carimune NF** see Immune Globulin on page 903

Carmustine (kar MUS teen)

Related Information

Chemotherapy and Obesity on page 2220

Hematopoietic Stem Cell Transplantation on page 2272

Management of Chemotherapy-Induced Nausea and Vomiting in Adults on page 2142

Management of Drug Extravasations on page 2159

Prevention of Chemotherapy-Induced Nausea and Vomiting in Children on page 2203

Safe Handling of Hazardous Drugs on page 2292

Brand Names: US BiCNU; Gliadel Wafer

Brand Names: Canada BiCNU; Gliadel Wafer

Index Terms BCNU; Becenum; bis(chloroethyl) nitrosourea; bis-chloronitrosourea; Carmustine Polymer Wafer; Carmustine Sustained-Release Implant Wafer; Carmustinum; WR-139021

Pharmacologic Category Antineoplastic Agent, Alkylating Agent; Antineoplastic Agent, Alkylating Agent (Nitrosourea)

Use

Brain tumors:

Injection: Palliative treatment of brain tumors including glioblastoma, brainstem glioma, medulloblastoma, astrocytoma, ependymoma, and metastatic brain tumors

Wafer (implant): Treatment of newly-diagnosed high-grade malignant glioma (as an adjunct to surgery and radiation); treatment of recurrent glioblastoma multiforme (as adjunct to surgery)

Hodgkin lymphoma, relapsed/refractory: Injection: Palliative treatment (secondary) of Hodgkin lymphoma (in combination with other antineoplastics) that has relapsed with or was refractory to primary therapy

Multiple myeloma: Injection: Palliative treatment of multiple myeloma (in combination with prednisone)

Non-Hodgkin lymphomas, relapsed/refractory: Injection: Palliative treatment (secondary) of non-Hodgkin lymphoma (in combination with other antineoplastics) that has relapsed with or was refractory to primary therapy

Labeled Contraindications

IV: Hypersensitivity to carmustine or any component of the formulation

Implant: There are no contraindications listed in the manufacturer's labeling.

Pregnancy Considerations Adverse events have been observed in animal reproduction studies. Carmustine may cause fetal harm if administered to a pregnant woman. Women of childbearing potential should use effective contraception to avoid becoming pregnant while on treatment. May impair fertility. Advise males of potential risk of infertility and to seek fertility/family planning counseling prior to receiving carmustine wafer implants.

Breast-Feeding Considerations It is not known if carmustine is excreted in breast milk. Due to the potential for serious adverse reactions in the nursing infant, the manufacturer recommends breast-feeding be discontinued during treatment.

Warnings/Precautions Hazardous agent - use appropriate precautions for handling and disposal (NIOSH 2014 [group 1]).

Injection:

[US Boxed Warning]: Bone marrow suppression, primarily thrombocytopenia (which may lead to bleeding) and leukopenia (which may lead to infection), is the most common and severe toxicity. Hematologic toxicity is generally delayed; monitor blood counts for at least 6 weeks following treatment. The manufacturer suggests not administering more frequently than every 6 weeks for approved doses/uses. Myelosuppression is cumulative; consider nadir blood counts from prior dose for dosage adjustment. Patients must have platelet counts >100,000/mm^3 and leukocytes >4,000/mm^3 for a repeat dose. Myelosuppression generally occurs 4 to 6 weeks after administration; thrombocytopenia occurs at ~4 weeks and persists for 1 to 2 weeks; leukopenia occurs at 5 to 6 weeks and persists for 1 to 2 weeks. Anemia may occur (less common and less severe than leukopenia or thrombocytopenia). Long-term use is associated with the development of secondary malignancies (acute leukemias and bone marrow dysplasias).

[US Boxed Warnings]: Dose-related pulmonary toxicity may occur; patients receiving cumulative doses >1,400 mg/m^2 are at higher risk. Delayed onset of pulmonary fibrosis may occur years after treatment (may be fatal), particularly in children. Pulmonary toxicity has occurred in children up to 17 years after treatment; this occurred in ages 1 to 16 for the treatment of intracranial tumors; cumulative doses ranged from 770 to 1,800 mg/m^2 (in combination with cranial radiotherapy). Pulmonary toxicity is characterized by pulmonary infiltrates and/or fibrosis and has been reported from 9 days to 43 months after nitrosourea treatment (including carmustine). Although pulmonary toxicity generally occurs in patients who have received prolonged treatment, pulmonary fibrosis has been reported with cumulative doses <1,400 mg/m^2. In addition to high cumulative doses, other risk factors for pulmonary toxicity include history of lung disease and baseline predicted forced vital capacity (FVC) or carbon monoxide diffusing capacity (DL$_{CO}$) <70%. Baseline and periodic pulmonary function tests are recommended. For high-dose treatment (transplant; off-label dose), acute lung injury may occur ~1 to 3 months post transplant; advise patients to contact their transplant physician for dyspnea, cough, or fever; interstitial pneumonia may be managed with a course of corticosteroids. Children are at higher risk of delayed pulmonary toxicity with IV carmustine.

Reversible increases in transaminases, bilirubin, and alkaline phosphatase have been reported (rare). Monitor liver function tests periodically during treatment. Renal failure, progressive azotemia, and decreased kidney size have been reported in patients who have received large cumulative doses or

◀ prolonged treatment. Renal toxicity has also been reported in patients who have received lower cumulative doses. Monitor renal function tests periodically during treatment.

Carmustine is associated with a moderate to high emetic potential (dose-related); antiemetics are recommended to prevent nausea and vomiting (Basch, 2011; Dupuis, 2011). Injection site burning and local tissue reactions, including swelling, pain, erythema, and necrosis have been reported. Monitor infusion site closely for infiltration or injection site reactions. Off-label administration (intraarterial intracarotid route) has been associated with ocular toxicity. Consider initiating IV treatment at the lower end of the dose range in elderly patients. The diluent for IV carmustine contains ethanol.

Wafer implant:
Seizures occurred in patients who received carmustine wafer implants, including new or worsening seizures and treatment-emergent seizures. Just over half of treatment-emergent seizures occurred within 5 days of surgery; the median onset of first new or worsened post-operative seizure was 4 days. Optimal anti-seizure therapy should be initiated prior to surgery. Monitor for seizures. Brain edema has been reported in patients with newly diagnosed glioma, including one report of intracranial mass effect unresponsive to corticosteroids which led to brain herniation. Monitor closely for intracranial hypertension related to brain edema, inflammation, or necrosis of brain tissue surrounding resection. Re-operation to remove wafers (or remnants) may be necessary for refractory cases. Cases of meningitis have occurred in patients with recurrent glioma receiving wafer implants. Two cases were bacterial (one patient required removal of implants 4 days after implantation and the other developed meningitis following reoperation for recurrent tumor). Another case was determined to be chemical meningitis and resolved with corticosteroids. Monitor postoperatively for signs/symptoms of meningitis and CNS infection.

Monitor closely for known craniotomy-related complications (seizure, intracranial infection, abnormal wound healing, brain edema). Wafer migration may occur; avoid communication between the resection cavity and the ventricular system to prevent wafer migration; communications larger than the wafer should be closed prior to implantation; wafer migration into the ventricular system may cause obstructive hydrocephalus. Monitor for signs/symptoms of obstructive hydrocephalus.

Impaired neurosurgical wound healing, including would dehiscence, delayed healing, and subdural, subgleal or wound effusions may occur with carmustine wafer implant treatment; cerebrospinal fluid leaks have also been reported. Monitor post-operatively for impaired neurosurgical wound healing.

[US Boxed Warning]: Should be administered under the supervision of an experienced cancer chemotherapy physician. Potentially significant drug-drug interactions may exist, requiring dose or frequency adjustment, additional monitoring, and/or selection of alternative therapy.

Adverse Reactions
IV: Frequency not defined:
Cardiovascular: Cardiac arrhythmia (with high doses), chest pain, flushing (with rapid infusion), hypotension, tachycardia
Central nervous system: Dizziness, headache
Dermatologic: Burning sensation of skin (after skin contact), hyperpigmentation (after skin contact)

Gastrointestinal: Nausea (common; dose related), vomiting (common; dose related)

Hematologic & oncologic: Leukopenia (common; onset: 5 to 6 weeks; recovery: After 1 to 2 weeks), thrombocytopenia (common: onset: ~4 weeks; recovery: After 1 to 2 weeks), anemia, febrile neutropenia, malignant neoplasm (secondary; acute leukemia, bone marrow dysplasias)

Hepatic: Increased serum alkaline phosphatase, increased serum bilirubin, increased serum transaminases

Hypersensitivity: Hypersensitivity reaction

Infection: Infection (with high doses)

Local: Burning sensation at injection site, erythema at injection site, pain at injection site, swelling at injection site, tissue necrosis at injection site, venous thrombosis at injection site (rare)

Ophthalmic: Neuroretinitis, suffusion of the conjunctiva (with rapid infusion)

Renal: Azotemia (progressive; with long-term therapy), nephron atrophy (with long-term therapy), nephrotoxicity, renal failure (with long-term therapy)

Respiratory: Interstitial pneumonitis (with high doses), lung hypoplasia, pulmonary fibrosis (occurring up to 17 years after treatment), pulmonary infiltrates

Wafer:

>10%:

Central nervous system: Seizure (37%; new or worsening: 20%), cerebral edema (4% to 23%), depression (16%)

Dermatologic: Skin rash (5% to 12%)

Gastrointestinal: Nausea (22%), vomiting (21%), constipation (19%)

Genitourinary: Urinary tract infection (21%)

Neuromuscular & skeletal: Weakness (22%)

Miscellaneous: Wound healing impairment (14% to 16%), fever (12%)

1% to 10%:

Cardiovascular: Chest pain (5%)

Central nervous system: Intracranial hypertension (9%), cerebral hemorrhage (6%), meningitis (4%)

Gastrointestinal: Abdominal pain (8%)

Infection: Abscess (local 6%)

Neuromuscular & skeletal: Back pain (7%)

<1%, postmarketing, and/or case reports: Sepsis

Drug Interactions

Metabolism/Transport Effects None known.

Avoid Concomitant Use

Avoid concomitant use of Carmustine with any of the following: BCG (Intravesical); CloZAPine; Dipyrone; Natalizumab; Pimecrolimus; Tacrolimus (Topical); Tofacitinib; Vaccines (Live)

Increased Effect/Toxicity

Carmustine may increase the levels/effects of: CloZAPine; Fingolimod; Leflunomide; Natalizumab; Tofacitinib; Vaccines (Live)

The levels/effects of Carmustine may be increased by: Cimetidine; Denosumab; Dipyrone; Melphalan; Pimecrolimus; Roflumilast; Tacrolimus (Topical); Trastuzumab

◄ **Decreased Effect**

Carmustine may decrease the levels/effects of: BCG (Intravesical); Coccidioides immitis Skin Test; Sipuleucel-T; Vaccines (Inactivated); Vaccines (Live)

The levels/effects of Carmustine may be decreased by: Echinacea

Storage/Stability

Injection: Store intact vials and provided diluent under refrigeration at 2°C to 8°C (36°F to 46°F). Carmustine has a low melting point (30.5°C to 32°C [86.9°F to 89.6°F]); exposure to temperature at or above the melting point will cause the drug to liquefy and appear as an oil film on the vials. If drug liquefies, discard the vials as this is a sign of decomposition.

Reconstituted solutions are stable for 24 hours refrigerated (2°C to 8°C) and protected from light. Examine reconstituted vials for crystal formation prior to use. If crystals are observed, they may be redissolved by warming the vial to room temperature with agitation.

Solutions diluted to a concentration of 0.2 mg/mL in D_5W are stable for 8 hours at room temperature (25°C) in glass and protected from light. Although the manufacturer recommends only glass containers be used, stability of a 1 mg/mL solution in D_5W has also been demonstrated for up to 6 hours (with a 6% to 7% loss of potency) in polyolefin containers (Trissel, 2006).

Wafer: Store at or below -20°C (-4°F). Unopened outer foil pouches may be kept at room temperature for up to 6 hours at a time for up to 3 cycles within a 30-day period.

Preparation for Administration Hazardous agent; use appropriate precautions for handling and disposal (NIOSH 2014 [group 1]).

Injection: Reconstitute initially with 3 mL of supplied diluent (dehydrated alcohol injection, USP); then further dilute with SWFI (27 mL), this provides a concentration of 3.3 mg/mL in ethanol 10%; protect from light; further dilute for infusion with D_5W using a non-PVC container (eg, glass or polyolefin).

Implant: Each wafer is packaged within 2 nested aluminum foil pouches; the inner pouch is sterile and is designed to maintain sterility and protect from moisture; the outer wrap is not sterile. Deliver to the operating room in the unopened outer aluminum foil pouch. Do not open until the wafers are ready to be implanted. Follow manufacturer's instructions for opening the pouch, being careful not to apply pressure to the wafer.

Mechanism of Action Interferes with the normal function of DNA and RNA by alkylation and cross-linking the strands of DNA and RNA, and by possible protein modification; may also inhibit enzyme processes by carbamylation of amino acids in protein

Pharmacodynamics/Kinetics

Distribution: IV: 3.3 L/kg; readily crosses blood-brain barrier producing CSF levels >50% of blood plasma levels; highly lipid soluble

Metabolism: Rapidly hepatic; forms active metabolites

Half-life elimination: IV: Biphasic: Initial: 1.4 minutes; Secondary: 22 minutes (active metabolites: Plasma half-life of 67 minutes)

Excretion: IV: Urine (~60% to 70%) within 96 hours; lungs (~10% as CO_2)

Dosing

Adult & Geriatric Note: Carmustine (IV) is associated with a moderate to high emetic potential (dose-related); antiemetics are recommended to prevent nausea and vomiting (Basch, 2011; Dupuis, 2011).

Brain tumors, Hodgkin lymphoma, multiple myeloma, non-Hodgkin lymphoma (per manufacturer labeling): IV: 150 to 200 mg/m^2 every 6 weeks or 75 to 100 mg/m^2/day for 2 days every 6 weeks

Glioblastoma multiforme (recurrent), glioma (malignant, newly-diagnosed high-grade): Implantation (wafer): 8 wafers (7.7 mg each) implanted intracranially into in the resection cavity (total dose 61.6 mg); should the size and shape not accommodate 8 wafers, the maximum number of wafers feasible (up to 8) should be placed

Indication-specific dosing:

Brain tumor, primary (off-label doses): IV:

80 mg/m^2/day for 3 days every 8 weeks for 6 cycles (Brandes, 2004)

200 mg/m^2 every 8 weeks [maximum cumulative dose: 1500 mg/m^2] (Selker, 2002)

Hodgkin lymphoma, relapsed or refractory (off-label dose): IV: Mini-BEAM regimen: 60 mg/m^2 day 1 every 4 to 6 weeks (in combination with etoposide, cytarabine, and melphalan) (Colwill, 1995; Martin, 2001)

Multiple myeloma, relapsed, refractory (off-label dose): IV: VBMCP regimen: 20 mg/m^2 day 1 every 35 days (in combination with vincristine, melphalan, cyclophosphamide, and prednisone) (Kyle, 2006; Oken, 1997)

Mycosis fungoides, early stage (off-label use; Zackheim, 2003): Topical:

Ointment (10 mg/100 grams petrolatum): Apply (with gloves) once daily to affected areas

Solution (0.2% solution in alcohol; dilute 5 mL in 60 mL water): Apply (with gloves) once daily to affected areas

Stem cell or bone marrow transplant, autologous (off-label use): IV:

BEAM regimen: 300 mg/m^2 6 days prior to transplant (in combination with etoposide, cytarabine, and melphalan) (Chopra, 1993; Linch, 2010)

CBV regimen: 600 mg/m^2 3 days prior to transplant (in combination with cyclophosphamide and etoposide) (Reece, 1991)

Renal Impairment

IV: There are no dosage adjustments provided in the manufacturer's labeling. The following dosage adjustments have been reported (Kintzel, 1995):

CrCl 46 to 60 mL/minute: Administer 80% of dose

CrCl 31 to 45 mL/minute: Administer 75% of dose

CrCl ≤30 mL/minute: Consider use of alternative drug.

Wafer implant: There are no dosage adjustments provided in the manufacturer's labeling.

Hepatic Impairment

IV: Dosage adjustment may be necessary; however, no specific guidelines are available.

Wafer implant: There are no dosage adjustments provided in the manufacturer's labeling.

Obesity

*American Society of Clinical Oncology (ASCO) Guidelines for appropriate chemotherapy dosing in obese adults with cancer (**Note: Excludes HSCT dosing**):* Utilize patient's actual body weight (full weight) for calculation of body surface area- or weight-based dosing, particularly when the intent of therapy is curative; manage regimen-related toxicities in the same manner as for nonobese patients; if a dose reduction is utilized due to toxicity, consider resumption of full weight-based dosing with subsequent cycles, especially if cause of toxicity (eg, hepatic or renal impairment) is resolved (Griggs, 2012).

American Society for Blood and Marrow Transplantation (ASBMT) practice guideline committee position statement on chemotherapy dosing in obesity: Utilize actual body weight (full weight) for calculation of body surface area in carmustine dosing for hematopoietic stem cell transplant conditioning regimens in adult patients weighing ≤120% of their ideal body weight (IBW). In patients weighing >120% IBW, utilize adjusted body weight 25% (ABW25) to calculate BSA (Bubalo, 2014).

ABW25: Adjusted wt (kg) = Ideal body weight (kg) + 0.25 [actual wt (kg) - ideal body weight (kg)]

Adjustment for Toxicity Hematologic toxicity: Based on nadir counts with previous dose (manufacturer's labeling). IV:

If leukocytes ≥3,000/mm^3 and platelets ≥75,000/mm^3: Administer 100% of dose

If leukocytes 2,000 to 2,999/mm^3 or platelets 25,000 to 74,999/mm^3: Administer 70% of dose

If leukocytes <2,000/mm^3 or platelets <25,000/mm^3: Administer 50% of dose

Combination Regimens

Lymphoma, Hodgkin:

Dexa-BEAM (Hodgkin) on page 1937

mini-BEAM (Hodgkin) on page 2037

Multiple myeloma: VBMCP (Multiple Myeloma) on page 2105

Administration

Carmustine (IV) is associated with a moderate to high emetic potential (dose-related); antiemetics are recommended to prevent nausea and vomiting (Basch, 2011; Dupuis, 2011).

Injection: Irritant (alcohol-based diluent). Significant absorption to PVC containers; should be prepared in either glass or polyolefin containers. Infuse over at least 2 hours (infusions <2 hours may lead to injection site pain or burning); infuse through a free-flowing saline or dextrose infusion, or administer through a central catheter to alleviate venous pain/irritation.

High-dose carmustine (transplant dose; off-label use): Infuse over a least 2 hours to avoid excessive flushing, agitation, and hypotension; was infused over 1 hour in some trials (Chopra, 1993). **High-dose carmustine may be fatal if not followed by stem cell rescue.** Monitor vital signs frequently during infusion; patients should be supine during infusion and may require the Trendelenburg position, fluid support, and vasopressor support.

Implant: Double glove before handling; outer gloves should be discarded as chemotherapy waste after handling wafers. Any wafer or remnant that is removed upon repeat surgery should be discarded as chemotherapy waste. The outer surface of the external foil pouch is not sterile. Open pouch gently; avoid pressure on the wafers to prevent breakage. Wafers that are broken in half may be used, however, wafers broken into more than 2 pieces should be discarded in a biohazard container. Slight overlapping of wafers during placement is acceptable. Oxidized regenerated cellulose (Surgicel) may be placed over the wafer to secure; irrigate cavity prior to closure.

Topical (off-label use): Apply solution with brush or gauze pads; ointment and solution should be applied while wearing gloves to involved areas only; avoid contact with eyes or mouth (Zackheim, 2003).

Hazardous agent; use appropriate precautions for handling and disposal (NIOSH 2014 [group 1]).

Vesicant/Extravasation Risk Irritant; infiltration may result in local pain, erythema, swelling, burning and skin necrosis; the alcohol-based diluent may be an irritant, especially with high doses.

Emetic Potential
Children and Adults:
>250 mg/m^2: High (>90%)
≤250 mg/m^2: Moderate (30% to 90%)

Monitoring Parameters
Injection: CBC with differential and platelet count (weekly for at least 6 weeks after a dose), pulmonary function tests (FVC, DL$_{CO}$; at baseline and frequently during treatment), liver function (periodically), renal function tests (periodically); monitor blood pressure and vital signs during administration, monitor infusion site for possible infiltration

Wafer: Monitor postoperatively for seizures, impaired neurosurgical wound healing, and signs/symptoms of meningitis, CNS infection, and obstructive hydrocephalus; monitor closely for intracranial hypertension related to brain edema, inflammation, or necrosis of brain tissue surrounding resection.

Dosage Forms Excipient information presented when available (limited, particularly for generics); consult specific product labeling.
Solution Reconstituted, Intravenous:
BiCNU: 100 mg (1 ea) [contains alcohol, usp]
Wafer, Implant:
Gliadel Wafer: 7.7 mg (8 ea) [contains polifeprosan 20]

♦ **Carmustine Polymer Wafer** see Carmustine on page 284

♦ **Carmustine Sustained-Release Implant Wafer** see Carmustine on page 284

♦ **Carmustinum** see Carmustine on page 284

♦ **Casodex** see Bicalutamide on page 207

Caspofungin (kas poe FUN jin)

Brand Names: US Cancidas
Brand Names: Canada Cancidas
Index Terms Caspofungin Acetate
Pharmacologic Category Antifungal Agent, Parenteral; Echinocandin
Use Treatment of invasive *Aspergillus* infections in patients who are refractory or intolerant of other therapies; treatment of candidemia and other *Candida* infections (intra-abdominal abscesses, peritonitis, pleural space); treatment of esophageal candidiasis; empirical treatment for presumed fungal infections in febrile neutropenic patients
Pregnancy Risk Factor C
Dosing
Adult & Geriatric Note: Duration of caspofungin treatment should be determined by patient status and clinical response.
Aspergillosis (invasive): IV: Initial dose: 70 mg on day 1; subsequent dosing: 50 mg once daily. Duration of therapy should be a minimum of 6 to 12 weeks or throughout period of immunosuppression and until lesions have resolved (Walsh 2008). Salvage treatment with 70 mg once daily (off-label dosing) has been reported (Maertens 2006).
Aspergillosis (invasive) in HIV-infected patients (off-label use): Adolescents and Adults: IV: Initial dose: 70 mg on day 1; subsequent dosing: 50 mg once daily. Continue until infection resolution and CD4 count >200 cells/mm^3 (HHS [OI adult 2015]).

◀ **Candidemia:** IV: Initial dose: 70 mg on day 1; subsequent dosing: 50 mg once daily; generally continue for at least 14 days after the last positive culture or longer if neutropenia warrants. Higher doses (150 mg once daily infused over ~2 hours) compared to the standard adult dosing regimen (50 mg once daily) have not demonstrated additional benefit or toxicity in patients with invasive candidiasis (Betts 2009).

Esophageal candidiasis: IV: 50 mg once daily; continue for 7 to 14 days after symptom resolution. **Note:** The majority of patients studied for this indication also had oropharyngeal involvement.

Esophageal candidiasis in HIV-infected patients (off-label use): Adolescents and Adults: IV: 50 mg once daily; continue for 14 to 21 days (HHS [OI adult 2015]).

Empiric therapy: IV: Initial dose: 70 mg on day 1; subsequent dosing: 50 mg once daily; continue until resolution of neutropenia; if fungal infection confirmed, continue for a minimum of 14 days (continue for at least 7 days after resolution of both neutropenia and clinical symptoms); if clinical response inadequate, may increase up to 70 mg once daily if tolerated, but increased efficacy not demonstrated.

Dosage adjustment with concomitant use of an enzyme inducer:
Patients receiving rifampin: 70 mg caspofungin once daily
Patients receiving carbamazepine, dexamethasone, efavirenz, nevirapine, or phenytoin (and possibly other enzyme inducers): May require an increased dose of caspofungin 70 mg once daily.

Pediatric

Aspergillosis (invasive), candidemia, esophageal candidiasis, empiric therapy: Infants ≥3 months, Children, and Adolescents ≤17 years: IV: Initial dose: 70 mg/m^2 on day 1, subsequent dosing: 50 mg/m^2 once daily, if clinical response inadequate, may increase to 70 mg/m^2 once daily if tolerated, but increased efficacy not demonstrated (maximum dose, loading or maintenance: 70 mg). Duration of caspofungin treatment should be determined by patient status and clinical response; refer to adult dosing for indication-specific recommended durations.

Aspergillosis (invasive) in HIV-infected patients (off-label use): Adolescents: IV: Refer to adult dosing.

Esophageal candidiasis in HIV-infected patients (off-label use): Adolescents: IV: Refer to adult dosing.

Dosage adjustment with concomitant use of an enzyme inducer:
Patients receiving carbamazepine, dexamethasone, efavirenz, nevirapine, phenytoin, or rifampin (and possibly other enzyme inducers): Consider 70 mg/m^2 once daily (maximum: 70 mg daily)

Renal Impairment No dosage adjustment necessary.
End-stage renal disease (ESRD) requiring hemodialysis: Poorly dialyzed; no supplemental dose or dosage adjustment necessary, including patients on intermittent hemodialysis (IHD), peritoneal dialysis, or continuous renal replacement therapy (eg, CVVHD).

Hepatic Impairment

Adults:
Mild insufficiency (Child-Pugh class A): No dosage adjustment necessary.
Moderate insufficiency (Child-Pugh class B): 70 mg on day 1 (where recommended), followed by 35 mg once daily
Severe insufficiency (Child-Pugh class C): No dosage adjustment provided in manufacturer's labeling (has not been studied).

Children: Mild-to-severe insufficiency (Child-Pugh classes A, B, or C): No dosage adjustment provided in manufacturer's labeling (has not been studied).

Additional Information Complete prescribing information should be consulted for additional detail.

Dosage Forms Excipient information presented when available (limited, particularly for generics); consult specific product labeling.

Solution Reconstituted, Intravenous, as acetate:

Cancidas: 50 mg (1 ea); 70 mg (1 ea)

♦ **Caspofungin Acetate** see Caspofungin on page 291

♦ **Cathflo Activase** see Alteplase on page 78

♦ **Catridecacog** see Factor XIII A-Subunit (Recombinant) on page 687

♦ **Cayston** see Aztreonam (Oral Inhalation) on page 169

♦ **CB-1348** see Chlorambucil on page 317

♦ **CB7630** see Abiraterone Acetate on page 30

♦ **CBDCA** see CARBOplatin on page 270

♦ **CC-4047** see Pomalidomide on page 1396

♦ **CC-5013** see Lenalidomide on page 1003

♦ **CCI-779** see Temsirolimus on page 1616

♦ **CCNU** see Lomustine on page 1054

♦ **2-CdA** see Cladribine on page 344

♦ **CDDP** see CISplatin on page 334

♦ **CDX** see Bicalutamide on page 207

♦ **CeeNU** see Lomustine on page 1054

♦ **CeeNU [DSC]** see Lomustine on page 1054

Cefepime (SEF e pim)

Brand Names: US Maxipime

Brand Names: Canada Maxipime

Index Terms Cefepime Hydrochloride

Pharmacologic Category Antibiotic, Cephalosporin (Fourth Generation)

Use

Febrile neutropenia: Treatment (empiric monotherapy) of febrile neutropenic patients.

Intra-abdominal infections: Treatment of complicated intra-abdominal infections, in combination with metronidazole, caused by *Escherichia coli*, viridans group streptococci, *Pseudomonas aeruginosa*, *Klebsiella pneumoniae*, *Enterobacter* species, or *Bacteroides fragilis*.

Pneumonia (moderate to severe): Treatment of moderate to severe pneumonia caused by *Streptococcus pneumoniae*, including cases associated with concurrent bacteremia, *P. aeruginosa*, *K. pneumoniae*, or *Enterobacter* species.

Skin and skin structure infections: Treatment of moderate to severe uncomplicated skin and skin structure infections caused by *Staphylococcus aureus* (methicillin-susceptible isolates only) or *Streptococcus pyogenes*.

◄ **Urinary tract infections (including pyelonephritis):** Treatment of complicated and uncomplicated urinary tract infections (UTIs), including pyelonephritis, caused by *E. coli* or *K. pneumoniae*, when the infection is severe, or caused by *E. coli*, *K. pneumoniae*, or *Proteus mirabilis*, when the infection is mild to moderate, including cases associated with concurrent bacteremia with these microorganisms.

Pregnancy Risk Factor B

Dosing

Adult & Geriatric

Febrile neutropenia, monotherapy: IV: 2 g every 8 hours for 7 days or until the neutropenia resolves

Intra-abdominal infections, complicated, severe (in combination with metronidazole): IV: **Note:** 2010 IDSA guidelines recommend a duration of 4 to 7 days (provided source controlled). Not recommended for hospital-acquired intra-abdominal infections (IAI) associated with multidrug-resistant gram negative organisms or in mild-to-moderate community-acquired IAIs due to risk of toxicity and the development of resistant organisms (Solomkin, [IDSA] 2010).

Due to *P. aeruginosa*: 2 g every 8 hours for 7 to 10 days

Not due to *P. aeruginosa*: 2 g every 8 to 12 hours for 7 to 10 days

Pneumonia: IV: **Note:** Duration of therapy may vary considerably for healthcare associated pneumonia (7 to 21 days). In absence of *Pseudomonas*, and if appropriate empiric treatment used and patient responsive, it may be clinically appropriate to reduce duration of therapy to 7 to 10 days (American Thoracic Society Guidelines, 2005).

Due to *P. aeruginosa*: 1 to 2 g every 8 hours for 10 days; **Note:** Longer courses (eg, 14 to 21 days) may be required (American Thoracic Society Guidelines, 2005).

Not due to *P. aeruginosa*: 1 to 2 g every 8 to 12 hours for 10 days

Skin and skin structure infection, uncomplicated: IV: 2 g every 12 hours for 10 days

Urinary tract infections, complicated and uncomplicated:

Mild-to-moderate: IM, IV: 0.5 to 1 g every 12 hours for 7 to 10 days

Severe: IV: 2 g every 12 hours for 10 days

Brain abscess, postneurosurgical prevention (off-label use): IV: 2 g every 8 hours with vancomycin (Tunkel, 2004)

Prosthetic joint infection, *Enterobacter spp.* or *Pseudomonas aeruginosa* (off-label use): IV: 2 g every 12 hours for 4 to 6 weeks; **Note:** When treating *P. aeruginosa*, consider addition of an aminoglycoside (Osmon, 2013)

Pediatric

Infants ≥2 months, Children, and Adolescents ≤16 years (≤40 kg):

Febrile neutropenia: IV: 50 mg/kg/dose every 8 hours for 7 days or until neutropenia resolves (maximum: 2 g/dose)

Pneumonia: IV:

Due to *P. aeruginosa*: 50 mg/kg/dose every 8 hours for 10 days (maximum: 2 g/dose)

Not due to *P. aeruginosa*: 50 mg/kg/dose every 12 hours for 10 days (maximum: 2 g/dose)

Skin and skin structure infections (uncomplicated): IV: 50 mg/kg/dose every 12 hours for 10 days (maximum: 2 g/dose)

Urinary tract infections, complicated and uncomplicated: IV, IM: 50 mg/kg/dose every 12 hours for 7 to 10 days (maximum: 1 g/dose); **Note:** IM may be considered for mild-to-moderate infection only.

Intra-abdominal infection, complicated (off-label use): IV: **Note:** IDSA 2010 guidelines recommend duration of 4 to 7 days (provided source controlled): 50 mg/kg/dose every 12 hours in combination with metronidazole (Solomkin [IDSA], 2010)

Children >40 kg and Adolescents >16 years:

Febrile neutropenia, monotherapy: IV: 2 g every 8 hours for 7 days or until the neutropenia resolves

Intra-abdominal infections, complicated, severe (in combination with metronidazole): IV: **Note:** IDSA 2010 guidelines recommend duration of 4 to 7 days (provided source controlled) (Solomkin, [IDSA] 2010).

Due to *P. aeruginosa*: 2 g every 8 hours for 7 to 10 days

Not due to *P. aeruginosa*: 2 g every 8 to 12 hours for 7 to 10 days

Pneumonia: IV:

Due to *P. aeruginosa*: 1 to 2 g every 8 hours for 10 days

Not due to *P. aeruginosa*: 1 to 2 g every 8 to 12 hours for 10 days

Skin and skin structure infections, uncomplicated: IV: 2 g every 12 hours for 10 days

Urinary tract infections, complicated and uncomplicated:

Mild-to-moderate: IM, IV: 0.5 to 1 g every 12 hours for 7 to 10 days

Severe: IV: 2 g every 12 hours for 10 days

Renal Impairment

Adults: Recommended maintenance schedule based on creatinine clearance (may be estimated using the Cockcroft-Gault formula), compared to normal dosing schedule: See table.

Cefepime Hydrochloride

Creatinine Clearance (mL/minute)	Recommended Maintenance Schedule			
>60 (normal recommended dosing schedule)	500 mg every 12 hours	1 g every 12 hours	2 g every 12 hours	2 g every 8 hours
30-60	500 mg every 24 hours	1 g every 24 hours	2 g every 24 hours	2 g every 12 hours
11-29	500 mg every 24 hours	500 mg every 24 hours	1 g every 24 hours	2 g every 24 hours
<11	250 mg every 24 hours	250 mg every 24 hours	500 mg every 24 hours	1 g every 24 hours

Intermittent hemodialysis (IHD) (administer after hemodialysis on dialysis days): IV: Initial: 1 g (single dose) on day 1. Maintenance: 0.5-1 g every 24 hours **or** 1-2 g every 48-72 hours (Heintz, 2009) **or** 2 g 3 times weekly after dialysis (Perez, 2012). **Note:** Dosing dependent on the assumption of 3 times weekly, complete IHD sessions.

Peritoneal dialysis (PD): Removed to a lesser extent than hemodialysis; administer normal recommended dose every 48 hours

◄ Continuous renal replacement therapy (CRRT) (Heintz, 2009; Trotman, 2005): Drug clearance is highly dependent on the method of renal replacement, filter type, and flow rate. Appropriate dosing requires close monitoring of pharmacologic response, signs of adverse reactions due to drug accumulation, as well as drug concentrations in relation to target trough (if appropriate). The following are general recommendations only (based on dialysate flow/ultrafiltration rates of 1-2 L/hour and minimal residual renal function) and should not supersede clinical judgment:

CVVH: Loading dose of 2 g followed by 1-2 g every 12 hours

CVVHD/CVVHDF: Loading dose of 2 g followed by either 1 g every 8 hours or 2 g every 12 hours. **Note:** Dosage of 1 g every 8 hours results in similar steady-state concentrations as 2 g every 12 hours and is more cost effective (Heintz, 2009).

Note: Consider higher dosage of 4 g/day if treating *Pseudomonas* or life-threatening infections in order to maximize time above MIC (Trotman, 2005). Dosage of 2 g every 8 hours may be needed for gram-negative rods with MIC ≥4 mg/L (Heintz, 2009).

Children: No dosage adjustment provided in the manufacturer's labeling; however, similar dosage adjustments to adults would be anticipated based on comparable pharmacokinetics between children and adults.

Hepatic Impairment No dosage adjustment necessary.

Additional Information Complete prescribing information should be consulted for additional detail.

Dosage Forms Excipient information presented when available (limited, particularly for generics); consult specific product labeling.

Solution, Intravenous, as hydrochloride:
Generic: 1 g/50 mL (50 mL); 2% (100 mL)
Solution Reconstituted, Injection, as hydrochloride:
Maxipime: 1 g (1 ea); 2 g (1 ea)
Generic: 1 g (1 ea); 2 g (1 ea)
Solution Reconstituted, Intravenous, as hydrochloride:
Maxipime: 1 g (1 ea); 2 g (1 ea)
Generic: 1 g/50 mL (1 ea); 2 g/50 mL (1 ea)

◆ **Cefepime Hydrochloride** see Cefepime on page 293

CefTAZidime (SEF tay zi deem)

Brand Names: US Fortaz; Fortaz in D5W; Tazicef
Brand Names: Canada Ceftazidime For Injection; Fortaz
Index Terms Tazidime
Pharmacologic Category Antibiotic, Cephalosporin (Third Generation)
Use

Bacterial septicemia: Treatment of septicemia caused by *Pseudomonas aeruginosa*, *Klebsiella* spp., *Haemophilus influenzae*, *Escherichia coli*, *Serratia* spp., *Streptococcus pneumoniae*, and *Staphylococcus aureus* (methicillin-susceptible strains).

Bone and joint infections: Treatment of bone and joint infections caused by *Pseudomonas aeruginosa*, *Klebsiella* spp., *Enterobacter* spp., and *Staphylococcus aureus* (methicillin-susceptible strains).

CNS infections: Treatment of meningitis caused by *Haemophilus influenzae* and *Neisseria meningitidis*. Ceftazidime has also been used successfully in cases of meningitis due to *Pseudomonas aeruginosa* and *Streptococcus pneumoniae*.

Empiric therapy in the immunocompromised patient: Empiric treatment of infections in immunocompromised patients.

Gynecologic infections: Treatment of endometritis, pelvic cellulitis, and other infections of the female genital tract caused by *Escherichia coli.*

Intra-abdominal infections: Treatment of peritonitis caused by *Escherichia coli, Klebsiella* spp., and *Staphylococcus aureus* (methicillin-susceptible strains) and polymicrobial intra-abdominal infections caused by aerobic and anaerobic organisms and some *Bacteroides* spp. (many strains of *Bacteroides fragilis* are resistant).

Lower respiratory tract infections: Treatment of lower respiratory tract infections, including pneumonia, caused by *Pseudomonas aeruginosa* and other *Pseudomonas* spp.; *Haemophilus influenzae*, including ampicillin-resistant strains; *Klebsiella* spp.; *Enterobacter* spp.; *Proteus mirabilis*; *Escherichia coli*; *Serratia* spp.; *Citrobacter* spp.; *Streptococcus pneumoniae*; and *Staphylococcus aureus* (methicillin-susceptible strains).

Skin and skin-structure infections: Treatment of skin and skin-structure infections caused by *Pseudomonas aeruginosa*; *Klebsiella* spp.; *Escherichia coli*; *Proteus* spp.; including *Proteus mirabilis* and indole-positive *Proteus*; *Enterobacter* spp.; *Serratia* spp.; *Staphylococcus aureus* (methicillin-susceptible strains); and *Streptococcus pyogenes* (group A beta-hemolytic streptococci).

Urinary tract infections (UTI): Treatment of complicated and uncomplicated UTIs caused by *Pseudomonas aeruginosa*; *Enterobacter* spp.; *Proteus* spp., including *Proteus mirabilis* and indole-positive *Proteus*; *Klebsiella* spp.; and *Escherichia coli.*

Pregnancy Risk Factor B

Dosing

Adult & Geriatric

Bacterial arthritis (gram negative bacilli): IV: 1-2 g every 8 hours

Cystic fibrosis: IV:

Manufacturer's labeling: 90 to 150 mg/kg/day every 8 hours (maximum: 6 g daily)

Alternative recommendations: Intermittent IV infusion: 200 to 400 mg/kg/day divided every 6 to 8 hours (maximum: 8 to 12 g daily); **or** by continuous IV infusion: 100 to 200 mg/kg/day (maximum: 12 g daily) (Zobell, 2013)

Empiric therapy in immunocompromised patients: IV: 2 g every 8 hours

Endophthalmitis, bacterial (off-label use): Intravitreal: 2 to 2.25 mg/0.1 mL NS in combination with vancomycin (Jackson, 2003; Roth, 1997)

Intra-abdominal infection, severe (in combination with metronidazole): IV: 2 g every 8 hours for 4 to 7 days (provided source controlled). Not recommended for hospital-acquired intra-abdominal infections (IAI) associated with multidrug-resistant gram negative organisms or in mild-to-moderate community-acquired IAIs due to risk of toxicity and the development of resistant organisms (Solomkin, 2010).

Melioidosis (off-label use): IV: Note: Switching to meropenem therapy is indicated if patient condition worsens (eg, organ failure, new infection focus development, repeat blood cultures remained positive). Oral eradication therapy is recommended after the intensive (acute) phase treatment is complete (Lipsitz, 2012).

Severe, acute phase: 50 mg/kg/dose every 8 hours (maximum dose: 2 g) or 2 g for one dose, followed by 6 g daily by continuous infusion for ≥10 days with or without TMP/SMX (Lipsitz, 2012).

Peritonitis (CAPD) (off-label route; Li, 2010): Intraperitoneal:

Intermittent: 1 to 1.5 g every 24 hours per exchange in the long dwell (≥6 hours)

Continuous (per liter exchange): Loading dose: 500 mg; maintenance dose: 125 mg. **Note:** If patient has residual renal function (eg, >100 mL/day urine output), empirically increase each dose by 25%.

Pneumonia:

Uncomplicated: IM, IV: 500 mg to 1 g every 8 hours

Hospital-acquired pneumonia (off-label dose): IV: 2 g every 8 hours (ATS/IDSA, 2005)

Prosthetic joint infection, *Pseudomonas aeruginosa* (alternative to cefepime or meropenem): IV: 2 g every 8 hours for 4 to 6 weeks (consider addition of an aminoglycoside) (Osmon, 2013)

Skin and soft tissue infections: IV, IM: 500 mg to 1 g every 8 hours

Severe infections, including meningitis, CNS infection, osteomyelitis, gynecological: IV: 2 g every 8 hours

Urinary tract infections: IV, IM:

Uncomplicated: 250 mg every 12 hours

Complicated: 500 mg every 8 to 12 hours

Pediatric

Susceptible infections: IV:

Children 1 month to 12 years: 30 to 50 mg/kg/dose every 8 hours; maximum dose: 6 g/day (higher doses reserved for immunocompromised patients, cystic fibrosis, or meningitis)

Children ≥12 years: Refer to adult dosing.

Indication-specific dosing:

Cystic fibrosis: Infants, Children, and Adolescents: IV:

Manufacturer's labeling: 150 mg/kg/day divided every 8 hours (maximum: 6 g daily)

Alternative recommendations: 200 to 300 mg/kg/day divided every 8 hours (maximum: 6 g daily) (*Red Book* [AAP], 2012)

Melioidosis (off-label use): IV: **Note:** Switching to meropenem therapy is indicated if patient condition worsens (eg, organ failure, new infection focus development, repeat blood cultures remained positive). Oral eradication therapy is recommended after the intensive (acute) phase treatment is complete (Lipsitz, 2012).

Severe, acute phase: Infants >3 months, Children, and Adolescents: 50 mg/kg/dose every 8 hours (maximum dose: 2 g) or 2 g for one dose, followed by 6 g daily by continuous infusion for ≥10 days with or without TMP/SMX (Lipsitz, 2012). **Note:** Depending on infection severity, the dose for patients ≥3 months can be ≤40 mg/kg (maximum dose: 2 g) (Lipsitz, 2012).

Renal Impairment Note: If the dose recommended in the dosing section is lower than that recommended for patients with renal insufficiency as outlined below, the lower dose should be used. In severe infections, when the usual dose would be ceftazidime 6 g/day in patients without renal impairment, consider increasing the doses below by 50% or increase the dosing frequency. Further dosage adjustments should be determined by infection severity, susceptibility and patient response to therapy.

CrCl 31 to 50 mL/minute: 1 g every 12 hours

CrCl 16 to 30 mL/minute: 1 g every 24 hours

CrCl 6 to 15 mL/minute: 500 mg every 24 hours

CrCl <5 mL/minute: 500 mg every 48 hours

Intermittent hemodialysis (IHD) (administer after hemodialysis on dialysis days): Dialyzable (50% to 100%): 500 mg to 1 g every 24 hours **or** 1 to 2 g every 48 to 72 hours (Heintz, 2009). **Note:** Dosing dependent on the assumption of 3 times per week, complete IHD sessions.

Peritoneal dialysis (PD): IV:
Intermittent: Loading dose of 1 g, followed by 500 mg every 24 hours
Continuous: Loading dose of 1 g, followed by 500 mg every 24 hours. **Note:** an additional 125 mg per liter of exchange fluid may be added to the dialysate if clinically warranted.

Continuous renal replacement therapy (CRRT) (Heintz, 2009; Trotman, 2005): Drug clearance is highly dependent on the method of renal replacement, filter type, and flow rate. Appropriate dosing requires close monitoring of pharmacologic response, signs of adverse reactions due to drug accumulation, as well as drug concentrations in relation to target trough (if appropriate). The following are general recommendations only (based on dialysate flow/ultrafiltration rates of 1 to 2 L/hour and minimal residual renal function) and should not supersede clinical judgment:

CVVH: Loading dose of 2 g followed by 1 to 2 g every 12 hours
CVVHD/CVVHDF: Loading dose of 2 g followed by either 1 g every 8 hours **or** 2 g every 12 hours. **Note:** Dosage of 1 g every 8 hours results in similar steady-state concentrations as 2 g every 12 hours and is more cost effective. Dosage of 2 g every 8 hours may be needed for gram-negative rods with MIC ≥4 mg/L (Heintz, 2009).

Note: For patients receiving CVVHDF, some recommend giving a loading dose of 2 g followed by 3 g over 24 hours as a continuous IV infusion to maintain concentrations ≥4 times the MIC for susceptible pathogens (Heintz, 2009).

Hepatic Impairment No dosage adjustment necessary.

Additional Information Complete prescribing information should be consulted for additional detail.

Dosage Forms Excipient information presented when available (limited, particularly for generics); consult specific product labeling. [DSC] = Discontinued product

Solution, Intravenous, as sodium [strength expressed as base]:
Fortaz in D5W: 1 g (50 mL); 2 g (50 mL)
Tazicef: 1 g/50 mL (50 mL)

Solution Reconstituted, Injection:
Fortaz: 500 mg (1 ea); 1 g (1 ea); 2 g (1 ea); 6 g (1 ea)
Tazicef: 1 g (1 ea); 2 g (1 ea); 6 g (1 ea)
Generic: 500 mg (1 ea [DSC]); 1 g (1 ea); 2 g (1 ea); 6 g (1 ea); 100 g (1 ea)

Solution Reconstituted, Injection [preservative free]:
Generic: 1 g (1 ea); 2 g (1 ea); 6 g (1 ea)

Solution Reconstituted, Intravenous:
Fortaz: 1 g (1 ea); 2 g (1 ea)
Tazicef: 1 g (1 ea); 2 g (1 ea)
Generic: 1 g/50 mL (1 ea); 2 g/50 mL (1 ea)

◆ **Ceftazidime For Injection (Can)** see CefTAZidime on page 296

CefTRIAXone (sef trye AKS one)

Brand Names: US Rocephin

Brand Names: Canada Ceftriaxone for Injection; Ceftriaxone for Injection USP; Ceftriaxone Sodium for Injection; Ceftriaxone Sodium for Injection BP

Index Terms Ceftriaxone Sodium

◄ **Pharmacologic Category** Antibiotic, Cephalosporin (Third Generation)
Use
  Bacterial infections:
    Treatment: Treatment of lower respiratory tract infections, acute bacterial otitis media, skin and skin structure infections, bone and joint infections, intra-abdominal and urinary tract infections, pelvic inflammatory disease (PID), uncomplicated gonorrhea, bacterial septicemia, and meningitis
    Prophylaxis: Used in surgical (perioperative) prophylaxis
Pregnancy Risk Factor B
Dosing
  Adult & Geriatric
    Dosage range: IM, IV: Usual dose: 1 to 2 g every 12 to 24 hours, depending on the type and severity of infection
    Acute bacterial rhinosinusitis, severe infection requiring hospitalization (off-label use): IV: 1 to 2 g every 12 to 24 hours for 5 to 7 days (Chow 2012)
    Arthritis, septic (off-label use): IV: 1 to 2 g once daily (Coiffier 2014; Dalla Vestra 2008; Harwood 2008; Raad 2004). Additional data may be necessary to further define the role of ceftriaxone in this condition.
    Bacterial enteric infections in HIV-infected patients (empiric treatment) (off-label use): Adolescents: IV: 1 g every 24 hours (HHS [OI adult 2015])
    Bite wounds (animal) (off-label use): IV: 1 g every 12 hours in combination with clindamycin or metronidazole for anaerobic coverage
    Brain abscess (off-label use):
      Empiric: IV: 2 g every 12 hours with metronidazole (Brouwer 2014; Louvois 2000). Additional data may be necessary to further define the role of ceftriaxone in this condition.
      Enterobacteriaceae or *Haemophilus spp.:* IV: 2 g every 12 hours; **Note:** Often isolated in mixed infection, combination therapy may be needed (Brouwer 2014).
    Chancroid (off-label use): IM: 250 mg as single dose (CDC 2010)
    Cholecystitis, mild-to-moderate: IV: 1 to 2 g every 12 to 24 hours for 4 to 7 days (provided source controlled) (Solomkin 2010)
    Gonococcal infections:
      Uncomplicated cervicitis, pharyngitis, proctitis, urethritis, vulvovaginitis (off-label dose): IM: 250 mg in a single dose with oral azithromycin (preferred) or oral doxycycline (alternative) (CDC 2012)
      Conjunctivitis (off-label use): IM: 1 g in a single dose (CDC 2010)
      Disseminated (off-label use): IM, IV: 1 g once daily for 24 to 48 hours may switch to cefixime (after improvement noted) to complete a total of 7 days of therapy (CDC 2010)
      Endocarditis (off-label use): IV: 1 to 2 g every 12 hours for at least 28 days (CDC 2010)
      Epididymitis, acute (off-label use): IM: 250 mg in a single dose with doxycycline (CDC 2010)
      Meningitis: IV: 1 to 2 g every 12 hours for 10 to 14 days (CDC 2010)
    Infective endocarditis (off-label use): IM, IV:
      Native valve: 2 g once daily for 2 to 4 weeks; **Note:** If using 2-week regimen or for relatively penicillin-resistant streptococcus, concurrent gentamicin is recommended; for HACEK organisms, duration of therapy is 4 weeks (Baddour 2005).
      Prosthetic valve: 2 g once daily for 6 weeks (with or without gentamicin [dependent on penicillin MIC]); for HACEK organisms, duration of therapy is 4 weeks (Baddour 2005).

Enterococcus faecalis (resistant to penicillin, aminoglycoside, and vanco-mycin), native or prosthetic valve: 2 g twice daily for ≥8 weeks adminis-tered concurrently with ampicillin (Baddour 2005)

Prophylaxis: 1 g 30 to 60 minutes before procedure (Wilson 2007). Intra-muscular injections should be avoided in patients who are receiving anticoagulant therapy. In these circumstances, orally administered regi-mens should be given whenever possible. Intravenously administered antibiotics should be used for patients who are unable to tolerate or absorb oral medications.

Note: American Heart Association (AHA) guidelines now recommend prophylaxis only in patients undergoing invasive procedures and in whom underlying cardiac conditions may predispose to a higher risk of adverse outcomes should infection occur. As of April 2007, routine prophylaxis for GI/GU procedures is no longer recommended by the AHA.

Intra-abdominal infection, complicated, community-acquired, mild-to-moderate (in combination with metronidazole): IV: 1 to 2 g every 12 to 24 hours for 4 to 7 days (provided source controlled) (Solomkin 2010)

Lyme neuroborreliosis (off-label use): IV: 2 g once daily for 14 days (Halperin 2007)

Meningitis (empiric treatment): IV: 2 g every 12 hours for 7 to 14 days (longer courses may be necessary for selected organisms)

Meningococcal disease, invasive, high-risk patient contacts (chemo-prophylaxis) (off-label use): IM: 250 mg in a single dose (CDC 2005; Red Book [AAP 2012])

Pelvic inflammatory disease: IM: 250 mg in a single dose plus doxycycline (with or without metronidazole) (CDC 2010)

Prophylaxis against sexually-transmitted diseases following sexual assault: IM: 250 mg as a single dose (in combination with azithromycin and metronidazole) (CDC 2010)

Prosthetic joint infection: IV:

Staphylococci, oxacillin-susceptible: 1 to 2 g every 24 hours for 2 to 6 weeks (in combination with rifampin) followed by oral antibiotic treatment and suppressive regimens (Osmon 2013)

Streptococci, beta-hemolytic: 2 g every 24 hours for 4 to 6 weeks (Osmon 2013)

Pyelonephritis (acute, uncomplicated): Females: IV: 1 to 2 g once daily (Stamm 1993). Many physicians administer a single parenteral dose before initiating oral therapy (Warren 1999).

Septic/toxic shock (off-label use): IV: 2 g once daily; with clindamycin for toxic shock

Skin and soft tissue necrotizing infection (off-label use) (IDSA [Stevens 2014]): Note: Continue until further debridement is not necessary, patient has clinically improved, and patient is afebrile for 48 to 72 hours.

Due to *Aeromonas hydrophilia:* IV: 1 to 2 g once daily in combination with doxycycline

Due to *Vibrio vulnificus:* IV: 1 g once daily in combination with doxycycline

Surgical (perioperative) prophylaxis: IV: 1 g 30 minutes to 2 hours before surgery

Manufacturer's labeling: 1 g 30 minutes to 2 hours before surgery

Alternate dosing: 1 to 2 g within 60 minutes prior to surgery (Bratzler 2013)

Alternate dosing for colorectal procedures: 2 g within 60 minutes prior to surgery with concomitant metronidazole (Bratzler 2013)

Cholecystectomy: 1 to 2 g every 12 to 24 hours, discontinue within 24 hours unless infection outside gallbladder suspected (Solomkin 2010)

◀ **Surgical site infections (intestinal or genitourinary tract surgery, surgery of axilla, or perineum) (off-label use):** IV: 1 g every 24 hours, in combination with metronidazole (IDSA [Stevens 2014])

Syphilis (off-label use): IM, IV: 1 g once daily for 10 to 14 days; **Note:** Alternative treatment for early syphilis, optimal dose, and duration have not been defined (CDC 2010).

Typhoid fever (off-label use): IV: 2 g every 12 to 24 hours for 10 to 14 days; **Note:** Usually reserved for fluoroquinolone resistant disease (WHO 2003).

Whipple disease (off-label use): IV: Initial: 2 g once daily for 10 to 14 days, then oral therapy (sulfamethoxazole and trimethoprim preferred) (Feurle 2010; Feurle 2013)

Pediatric

Dosage range: Infants, Children, and Adolescents: Usual dose: IM, IV:

Mild-to-moderate infections: 50 to 75 mg/kg/day in 1 to 2 divided doses every 12 to 24 hours (maximum: 2,000 mg daily); continue until at least 2 days after signs and symptoms of infection have resolved

Serious infections: 80-100 mg/kg/day in 1 to 2 divided doses (maximum: 4,000 mg daily)

Acute bacterial rhinosinusitis, severe infection requiring hospitalization (off-label use): IV: 50 mg/kg/day divided every 12 hours for 10 to 14 days (Chow 2012)

Bacterial enteric infections in HIV-infected patients (empiric treatment) (off-label use): Adolescents: IV: Refer to adult dosing.

Community-acquired pneumonia (CAP) (IDSA/PIDS [Bradley 2011]) (off-label use): Infants >3 months and Children: IV: 50 to 100 mg/kg/day once daily or divided every 12 hours (maximum: 2,000 mg daily). **Note:** May consider addition of vancomycin or clindamycin to empiric therapy if community-acquired MRSA suspected. Use the higher end of the range for penicillin-resistant *S. pneumoniae*; in children ≥5 years, a macrolide antibiotic should be added if atypical pneumonia cannot be ruled out; preferred in patients not fully immunized for *H. influenzae* type b and *S. pneumoniae*, or significant local resistance to penicillin in invasive pneumococcal strains.

Epididymitis, acute (off-label use): Children >8 years (and ≥45 kg) and Adolescents: IM: 250 mg in a single dose with a concomitant doxycycline regimen (CDC 2010; Red Book [AAP 2012])

Epiglottis (off-label use): IV: 100 mg/kg/day as a single dose on day 1, then 50 mg/kg as a single dose on day 2 (Sawyer 1994) or 75 mg/kg once daily for 10 to 14 days (Low 2003). Additional data may be necessary to further define the role of ceftriaxone in this condition.

Gonococcal infections:

Arthritis (CDC 2010): IM, IV:

≤45 kg: 50 mg/kg/dose once daily (maximum: 1,000 mg) for 7 days

>45 kg: 50 mg/kg/dose once daily (maximum: 2,000 mg) for 7 days

Bacteremia (CDC 2010): IM, IV:

≤45 kg: 50 mg/kg/dose once daily (maximum: 1,000 mg) for 7 days

>45 kg: 50 mg/kg/dose once daily (maximum: 2,000 mg) for 7 days

Conjunctivitis (off-label use): IM, IV:

<45 kg: 50 mg/kg in a single dose (maximum: 1,000 mg) (Red Book [AAP 2012])

≥45 kg: Refer to adult dosing.

Disseminated (off-label use): IM, IV:

Infants: 25 to 50 mg/kg/dose once daily for 7 days (10 to 14 days for meningitis) (CDC 2010); **Note:** Use contraindicated in hyperbilirubinemic neonates.

Children <45 kg: 25 to 50 mg/kg dose once daily (maximum: 1,000 mg) for 7 days (CDC 2010)

Children >45 kg: Refer to adult dosing.

Endocarditis (off-label use):

≤45 kg: IM, IV: 50 mg/kg/day divided every 12 hours (maximum: 2,000 mg daily) for at least 28 days (Red Book [AAP 2012])

>45 kg: IV: Refer to adult dosing.

Meningitis: IV:

≤45 kg: 50 mg/kg/day divided every 12 hours (maximum: 2,000 mg daily); usual duration of treatment is 10 to 14 days (Red Book [AAP 2012])

>45 kg: Refer to adult dosing.

Prophylaxis (due to maternal gonococcal infection): IM, IV: 25 to 50 mg/kg as a single dose (maximum: 125 mg) (CDC 2010)

Uncomplicated cervicitis, pharyngitis, proctitis, urethritis, vulvovaginitis (off-label use) (CDC 2010):

≤45 kg: IM: 125 mg as a single dose (with or without azithromycin or erythromycin) (Red Book [AAP 2012])

>45 kg: Refer to adult dosing.

Infective endocarditis (off-label use): IM, IV:

Native valve: 100 mg/kg once daily (maximum: 2,000 mg daily) for 2 to 4 weeks; **Note:** If using 2-week regimen or for relatively penicillin-resistant streptococcus, concurrent gentamicin is recommended; for HACEK organisms, duration of therapy is 4 weeks (Baddour 2005)

Prosthetic valve: 100 mg/kg once daily (maximum: 2,000 mg daily) for 6 weeks (with or without gentamicin [dependent on penicillin MIC]); for HACEK organisms, duration of therapy is 4 weeks (Baddour 2005)

Enterococcus faecalis (resistant to penicillin, aminoglycoside, and vancomycin), native or prosthetic valve: 100 mg/kg/day divided every 12 hours for ≥8 weeks administered concurrently with ampicillin (Baddour 2005)

Prophylaxis: 50 mg/kg 30 to 60 minutes before procedure; maximum dose: 1,000 mg (Red Book [AAP 2012]; Wilson 2007). Intramuscular injections should be avoided in patients who are receiving anticoagulant therapy. In these circumstances, orally administered regimens should be given whenever possible. Intravenously administered antibiotics should be used for patients who are unable to tolerate or absorb oral medications.

Note: American Heart Association (AHA) guidelines now recommend prophylaxis only in patients undergoing invasive procedures and in whom underlying cardiac conditions may predispose to a higher risk of adverse outcomes should infection occur. As of April 2007, routine prophylaxis for GI/GU procedures is no longer recommended by the AHA.

Lyme disease (off-label use): IM, IV:

Atrioventricular heart block or carditis: 50 to 75 mg/kg once daily (maximum: 2,000 mg) for 2 to 3 weeks (Red Book [AAP 2012])

Encephalitis or other late neurologic disease: 50 to 75 mg/kg once daily (maximum: 2,000 mg) for 2 to 4 weeks (Red Book [AAP 2012])

Neuroborreliosis: 50 to 75 mg/kg once daily (maximum: 2,000 mg) for 14 days (Halperin 2007)

Meningitis: 50 to 75 mg/kg once daily (maximum: 2,000 mg) for 2 weeks (Red Book [AAP 2012])

Persistent or recurrent arthritis: 50 to 75 mg/kg once daily (maximum: 2,000 mg) for 2 to 4 weeks (Red Book [AAP 2012])

Meningitis (empiric treatment): IM, IV: Loading dose of 100 mg/kg (maximum: 4,000 mg), followed by:

Manufacturer's labeling: 100 mg/kg/day divided every 12 to 24 hours (maximum: 4,000 mg daily); usual duration of treatment is 7 to 14 days

Alternate dosing: 80 to 100 mg/kg/day divided every 12 to 24 hours (maximum: 4,000 mg daily) (Tunkel 2004)

Meningococcal disease, invasive, high-risk patient contacts (chemoprophylaxis) (off-label use):

Children and Adolescents <15 years: IM: 125 mg in a single dose (CDC 2005; Red Book [AAP 2012]).

Adolescents ≥15 years: Refer to adult dosing.

Otitis media: IM:

Acute: 50 mg/kg in a single dose (maximum: 1,000 mg)

Persistent or relapsing (off-label dose): 50 mg/kg once daily for 3 days (AAP 2014; Lieberthal 2013)

Pneumonia: IV: 50 to 75 mg/kg once daily

Prophylaxis against sexually-transmitted diseases following sexual assault (off-label use):

≤45 kg: IM: 125 mg in a single dose (in combination with azithromycin and metronidazole) (CDC 2010)

>45 kg: Refer to adult dosing.

Shigella dysentery type 1 (off-label dose): IM: 50 to 100 mg/kg/day for 2 to 5 days (WHO 2005)

Skin/skin structure infections: IM, IV: 50 to 75 mg/kg/day in 1 to 2 divided doses (maximum: 2,000 mg daily)

Surgical (perioperative) prophylaxis (off-label dose): Children ≥1 year: IV: 50 to 75 mg/kg within 60 minutes prior to surgery (maximum: 2,000 mg) (Bratzler 2013)

Typhoid fever (off-label use): IV: 80 mg/kg once daily for 14 days (Stephens 2002)

Renal Impairment There are no dosage adjustments provided in the manufacturer's labeling; however, in patients with concurrent renal and hepatic impairment, maximum daily dose should not exceed 2 g.

ESRD requiring dialysis: Poorly dialyzed; no supplemental dose or dosage adjustment necessary, including patients on intermittent hemodialysis, peritoneal dialysis, or continuous renal replacement therapy (eg, CVVHD) (Aronoff 2007).

Hepatic Impairment There are no dosage adjustments provided in the manufacturer's labeling; however, in patients with concurrent renal and hepatic impairment, maximum daily dose should not exceed 2 g.

Additional Information Complete prescribing information should be consulted for additional detail.

Dosage Forms Excipient information presented when available (limited, particularly for generics); consult specific product labeling.

Solution, Intravenous:

Generic: 20 mg/mL (50 mL); 40 mg/mL (50 mL)

Solution Reconstituted, Injection:

Rocephin: 500 mg (1 ea); 1 g (1 ea)

Generic: 250 mg (1 ea); 500 mg (1 ea); 1 g (1 ea); 2 g (1 ea); 100 g (1 ea)

Solution Reconstituted, Intravenous:

Generic: 1 g (1 ea); 2 g (1 ea); 10 g (1 ea)

- ◆ **Ceftriaxone for Injection (Can)** *see* CefTRIAXone *on page* 299
- ◆ **Ceftriaxone for Injection USP (Can)** *see* CefTRIAXone *on page* 299
- ◆ **Ceftriaxone Sodium** *see* CefTRIAXone *on page* 299
- ◆ **Ceftriaxone Sodium for Injection (Can)** *see* CefTRIAXone *on page* 299
- ◆ **Ceftriaxone Sodium for Injection BP (Can)** *see* CefTRIAXone *on page* 299
- ◆ **CellCept** *see* Mycophenolate *on page* 1177
- ◆ **CellCept Intravenous** *see* Mycophenolate *on page* 1177
- ◆ **CellCept I.V. (Can)** *see* Mycophenolate *on page* 1177

Ceritinib (se RI ti nib)

Related Information
Safe Handling of Hazardous Drugs *on page* 2292

Brand Names: US Zykadia

Brand Names: Canada Zykadia

Index Terms LDK378

Pharmacologic Category Antineoplastic Agent, Anaplastic Lymphoma Kinase Inhibitor; Antineoplastic Agent, Tyrosine Kinase Inhibitor

Use
US labeling: **Non-small cell lung cancer, metastatic:** Treatment of patients with anaplastic lymphoma kinase (ALK)-positive metastatic non-small cell lung cancer (NSCLC) who have progressed on or are intolerant to crizotinib.

Canadian labeling: **Non-small cell lung cancer, locally advanced or metastatic:** Treatment of patients with ALK-positive locally advanced (not amenable to curative therapy) or metastatic NSCLC who have progressed on or are intolerant to crizotinib.

Labeled Contraindications
There are no contraindications listed in the manufacturer's US labeling.

Canadian labeling: Hypersensitivity to ceritinib or any component of the formulation; congenital long QT syndrome or persistent Fridericia-corrected electrocardiogram interval (QTcF) of >500 msec.

Pregnancy Considerations Adverse events were observed in animal reproduction studies. Based on its mechanism of action, ceritinib may cause fetal harm if administered to a pregnant woman. Women of reproductive potential should use effective contraception during and for at least 2 weeks following therapy discontinuation. The Canadian labeling recommends women and men of reproductive potential use effective contraception during and for up to 3 months following therapy discontinuation.

Breast-Feeding Considerations It is not known if ceritinib is excreted in breast milk. Due to the potential for serious adverse reactions in the nursing infant, breast-feeding is not recommended by the manufacturer.

Warnings/Precautions Hazardous agent – use appropriate precautions for handling and disposal (meets NIOSH 2014 criteria). Symptomatic bradycardia may occur; heart rate <50 beats/minute has occurred. If possible, avoid concurrent use with other agents known to cause bradycardia (eg, beta blockers, nondihydropyridine calcium channel blockers, clonidine, digoxin). Monitor heart rate and blood pressure regularly. If symptomatic bradycardia (not life-threatening) occurs, withhold treatment until recovery to asymptomatic bradycardia or to a heart rate of ≥60 beats/minute, evaluate concurrent medications, and adjust ceritinib dose. Permanently discontinue for life-threatening bradycardia due to ceritinib; if life-threatening bradycardia occurs and concurrent medications associated with bradycardia can be discontinued or ▶

dose adjusted, restart ceritinib at a reduced dose (with frequent monitoring). QTc interval prolongation has occurred in clinical studies, and may be concentration-dependent. QT prolongation may lead to an increased risk for ventricular tachyarrhythmias (eg, torsades de pointes) or sudden death. Correct electrolyte abnormalities prior to initiating therapy. Periodically monitor ECG and electrolytes in patients with heart failure, bradyarrhythmias, electrolyte abnormalities, or who are taking medications known to prolong the QTc interval. May require treatment interruption, dosage reduction, or discontinuation. Avoid use in patients with congenital long QTc syndrome. The Canadian labeling contraindicates use in patients with congenital long QTc syndrome or persistent QTcF of >500 msec. Permanently discontinue in patients who develop QTc interval prolongation in combination with torsades de pointes or polymorphic ventricular tachycardia or signs/symptoms of serious arrhythmia.

Diarrhea, nausea, vomiting, or abdominal pain occurred in the majority of patients in clinical trials; over one-third of patients required dose reductions due to severe or persistent gastrointestinal toxicity. Manage symptoms medically with appropriate therapy (eg, antidiarrheals, antiemetics, fluid replacement) as indicated. May require therapy interruption and dosage reduction. Ceritinib is associated with a moderate emetic potential; antiemetics may be needed to prevent nausea and vomiting. If vomiting occurs, do not administer an additional dose; continue with the next scheduled dose. Hepatotoxicity has been observed in patients treated with ceritinib in clinical trials, including ALT levels >5 times ULN in over one-quarter of patients. Concurrent ALT elevations >3 times ULN with total bilirubin >2 times ULN (with normal alkaline phosphatase) occurred rarely. Monitor liver function tests (eg, ALT, AST, total bilirubin) monthly and as clinically necessary, more frequently in patients who develop transaminase abnormalities. May require therapy interruption, dosage reduction, and/or discontinuation. Use with caution in patients with hepatic impairment (has not been studied in patients with moderate or severe impairment). Ceritinib is metabolized and eliminated hepatically; systemic exposure and toxicities may be increased in patients with hepatic dysfunction. Although rare, pancreatitis (with fatality) has been reported. Grade 3 to 4 lipase and amylase elevations occurred in clinical trials. Monitor lipase and amylase prior to treatment and periodically during treatment as clinically necessary. May require treatment interruption and dose reduction.

Hyperglycemia, including grade 3 and 4 toxicity, has been observed in ceritinib-treated patients. The risk of grade 3 or 4 hyperglycemia increases significantly in diabetic patients or those with glucose intolerance; risk is also increased in patients receiving corticosteroids. Monitor fasting blood glucose levels at baseline and as clinically necessary, particularly in patients with diabetes. May require initiation or optimization of antihyperglycemic therapy. Temporarily interrupt therapy for hyperglycemia until adequately controlled; reduce dose upon recovery. If adequate glycemic control is not possible with medical management, permanently discontinue ceritinib. Severe and life-threatening interstitial lung disease (ILD)/pneumonitis (some fatal) may occur. Monitor for signs/symptoms of pulmonary toxicity; permanently discontinue in patients diagnosed with treatment-related ILD/pneumonitis. Potentially significant interactions may exist, requiring dose or frequency adjustment, additional monitoring, and/or selection of alternative therapy. In vitro studies indicate that ceritinib solubility and bioavailability may be decreased at higher pH; concurrent use with proton pump inhibitors, H$_2$-receptor antagonists, or antacids has not been evaluated.

Adverse Reactions

>10%:
Central nervous system: Fatigue (52%), neuropathy (17%; including paresthesia, muscular weakness, gait disturbance, peripheral neuropathy, hypoesthesia, peripheral sensory neuropathy, dysesthesia, neuralgia, peripheral motor neuropathy, hypotonia, polyneuropathy)

Dermatologic: Skin rash (16%; including maculopapular rash, acneiform dermatitis)

Endocrine & metabolic: Increased serum glucose (49%; grades 3/4: 13%), decreased serum phosphate (36%)

Gastrointestinal: Diarrhea (86%; grades 3/4: 6%), nausea (80%; grades 3/4: 4%), vomiting (60%; grades 3/4: 4%), abdominal pain (54%), decreased appetite (34%), constipation (29%), increased serum lipase (28%), disease of esophagus (16%; including dyspepsia, gastroesophageal reflux disease, dysphagia)

Hematologic & oncologic: Decreased hemoglobin (84%)

Hepatic: Increased serum ALT (80%; grades 3/4: 27%), increased serum AST (75%; grades 3/4: 13%), increased serum bilirubin (15%; grades 3/4: 1%)

Renal: Increased serum creatinine (58%)

1% to 10%:
Cardiovascular: Prolonged Q-T interval on ECG (4%; >60 msec increase from baseline: 3%; >500 msec: <1%), bradycardia (3%), sinus bradycardia (1%)

Ophthalmic: Visual disturbance (9%; including vision impairment, blurred vision, photopsia, accommodation disorder, presbyopia, reduced visual acuity)

Respiratory: Interstitial pulmonary disease (4%; grades 3/4: 3%)

Drug Interactions

Metabolism/Transport Effects Substrate of CYP3A4 (major), P-glycoprotein; **Note:** Assignment of Major/Minor substrate status based on clinically relevant drug interaction potential; **Inhibits** CYP2C9 (moderate), CYP3A4 (strong)

Avoid Concomitant Use

Avoid concomitant use of Ceritinib with any of the following: Ado-Trastuzumab Emtansine; Alfuzosin; Aprepitant; Astemizole; Avanafil; Axitinib; Barnidipine; Bosutinib; Bradycardia-Causing Agents; Bromocriptine; Cabozantinib; Cobimetinib; Conivaptan; Crizotinib; CYP3A4 Inducers (Strong); CYP3A4 Inhibitors (Strong); Dabrafenib; Dapoxetine; Domperidone; Dronedarone; Eletriptan; Eplerenone; Everolimus; Flibanserin; Fusidic Acid (Systemic); Grapefruit Juice; Halofantrine; Highest Risk QTc-Prolonging Agents; Ibrutinib; Idelalisib; Irinotecan Products; Isavuconazonium Sulfate; Ivabradine; Lapatinib; Lercanidipine; Lomitapide; Lovastatin; Lurasidone; Macitentan; Mifepristone; Naloxegol; Nilotinib; NiMODipine; Nisoldipine; Olaparib; Osimertinib; Palbociclib; Pimozide; Ranolazine; Red Yeast Rice; Regorafenib; Salmeterol; Silodosin; Simeprevir; Simvastatin; Sonidegib; St Johns Wort; Suvorexant; Tamsulosin; Terfenadine; Ticagrelor; Tolvaptan; Toremifene; Trabectedin; Ulipristal; Vemurafenib; VinCRIStine (Liposomal); Vorapaxar

Increased Effect/Toxicity

Ceritinib may increase the levels/effects of: Ado-Trastuzumab Emtansine; Alfuzosin; Almotriptan; Alosetron; Apixaban; Aprepitant; ARIPiprazole; ARIPiprazole Lauroxil; Astemizole; Avanafil; Axitinib; Barnidipine; Bedaquiline; Bortezomib; Bosentan; Bosutinib; Brentuximab Vedotin; Brexpiprazole;

Brinzolamide; Bromocriptine; Budesonide (Nasal); Budesonide (Oral Inhalation); Budesonide (Systemic); Budesonide (Systemic, Oral Inhalation); Budesonide (Topical); Cabazitaxel; Cabozantinib; Cannabis; Cariprazine; Cilostazol; Cobimetinib; Colchicine; Conivaptan; Crizotinib; CYP2C9 Substrates; CYP3A4 Substrates; Dabrafenib; Daclatasvir; Dapoxetine; Dasatinib; Dienogest; Domperidone; DOXOrubicin (Conventional); Dronabinol; Dronedarone; Drospirenone; Dutasteride; Eletriptan; Eplerenone; Erlotinib; Estazolam; Etizolam; Everolimus; FentaNYL; Fesoterodine; Flibanserin; Fluticasone (Nasal); Fluticasone (Oral Inhalation); Gefitinib; Halofantrine; Highest Risk QTc-Prolonging Agents; Hydrocodone; Ibrutinib; Imatinib; Imidafenacin; Irinotecan Products; Isavuconazonium Sulfate; Ivabradine; Ivacaftor; Ixabepilone; Lacosamide; Lapatinib; Lercanidipine; Levobupivacaine; Levomilnacipran; Lomitapide; Lovastatin; Lurasidone; Macitentan; Maraviroc; MedroxyPROGESTERone; MethylPREDNISolone; Moderate Risk QTc-Prolonging Agents; Naloxegol; Nilotinib; NiMODipine; Nisoldipine; Olaparib; Osimertinib; Ospemifene; Oxybutynin; OxyCODONE; Palbociclib; Panobinostat; Parecoxib; Paricalcitol; PAZOPanib; Pimecrolimus; Pimozide; PONATinib; Pranlukast; PrednisoLONE (Systemic); PredniSONE; Ramelteon; Ranolazine; Red Yeast Rice; Regorafenib; Repaglinide; Retapamulin; Rilpivirine; RomiDEPsin; Ruxolitinib; Salmeterol; Saxagliptin; Sildenafil; Silodosin; Simeprevir; Simvastatin; Sonidegib; SORAfenib; Suvorexant; Tacrolimus (Systemic); Tadalafil; Tamsulosin; Tasimelteon; Terfenadine; Tetrahydrocannabinol; Ticagrelor; Tofacitinib; Tolterodine; Tolvaptan; Toremifene; Trabectedin; TraMADol; Ulipristal; Vardenafil; Vemurafenib; Vilazodone; VinCRIStine (Liposomal); Vindesine; Vorapaxar; Zopiclone

The levels/effects of Ceritinib may be increased by: Bradycardia-Causing Agents; Bretylium; Conivaptan; Corticosteroids; CYP3A4 Inhibitors (Moderate); CYP3A4 Inhibitors (Strong); Fusidic Acid (Systemic); Grapefruit Juice; Idelalisib; Ivabradine; Luliconazole; Mifepristone; Netupitant; P-glycoprotein/ABCB1 Inhibitors; QTc-Prolonging Agents (Indeterminate Risk and Risk Modifying); Stiripentol

Decreased Effect

Ceritinib may decrease the levels/effects of: Antidiabetic Agents; Ifosfamide; Prasugrel; Ticagrelor

The levels/effects of Ceritinib may be decreased by: Bosentan; CYP3A4 Inducers (Moderate); CYP3A4 Inducers (Strong); Deferasirox; P-glycoprotein/ABCB1 Inducers; Siltuximab; St Johns Wort; Tocilizumab

Food Interactions

A high-fat meal increases AUC and C_{max} by 73% and 41%, respectively and a low-fat meal increases AUC and C_{max} by 58% and 43%, respectively; systemic exposure when administered with a meal may exceed that of a typical dose, and may result in increased toxicity. Management: Administer on an empty stomach, at least 2 hours before or after a meal.

Grapefruit and grapefruit juice may inhibit the metabolism of ceritinib and increase its systemic exposure. Management: Avoid grapefruit juice during therapy.

Storage/Stability Store at 25°C (77°F); excursions are permitted between 15°C and 30°C (59°F and 86°F).

Mechanism of Action Potent inhibitor of anaplastic lymphoma kinase (ALK), a tyrosine kinase involved in the pathogenesis of non-small cell lung cancer. ALK gene abnormalities due to mutations or translocations may result in expression of oncogenic fusion proteins (eg, ALK fusion protein) which alter signaling and expression and result in increased cellular proliferation and survival in tumors which express these fusion proteins. ALK inhibition reduces proliferation of cells expressing the genetic alteration. Ceritinib also inhibits insulin-like growth factor 1 receptor (IGF-1R), insulin receptor (InsR), and ROS1. Ceritinib has demonstrated activity in crizotinib-resistant tumors in NSCLC xenograft models.

Pharmacodynamics/Kinetics

Absorption: AUC and C_{max} increased 73% and 41%, respectively, when administered with a high-fat meal, and 58% and 43%, respectively when taken with a low-fat meal (when compared to fasting)

Distribution: 4,230 L (following a single dose), with a small preferential distribution to red blood cells versus plasma

Protein binding: 97% to human plasma proteins

Metabolism: Primarily hepatic via CYP3A

Half-life elimination: 41 hours

Time to peak: ~4 to 6 hours

Excretion: Feces (~92% with 68% as unchanged drug); urine (~1%)

Dosing

Adult & Geriatric Note: Ceritinib is associated with a moderate emetic potential; antiemetics may be needed to prevent nausea and vomiting.

Non-small cell lung cancer (ALK-positive), metastatic: Oral: 750 mg once daily; continue until disease progression or unacceptable toxicity.

Missed doses: If a dose is missed, take the missed dose unless the next dose is due within 12 hours. If vomiting occurs, do not administer an additional dose, patients should continue with the next scheduled dose.

Dosage adjustment for concomitant therapy:

Strong CYP3A4 inhibitors:

US labeling: Avoid concomitant use of strong CYP3A inhibitors; if concurrent administration cannot be avoided, reduce ceritinib dose by approximately one-third (rounded to the nearest multiple of the 150 mg strength). After discontinuation of the strong CYP3A inhibitor, resume ceritinib therapy at the dose used prior to initiation of the CYP3A4 inhibitor.

Canadian labeling: Avoid concomitant use of strong CYP3A inhibitors.

Strong CYP3A4 inducers: Avoid concurrent use of strong CYP3A inducers (eg, carbamazepine, phenytoin, rifampin, and St John's wort) during treatment with ceritinib.

Renal Impairment

CrCl ≥30 to 90 mL/minute: No dosage adjustment is necessary.

CrCl <30 mL/minute: There are no dosage adjustments provided in the manufacturer's labeling (has not been studied).

Hepatic Impairment

Preexisting mild impairment (total bilirubin ≤ULN and AST >ULN **or** total bilirubin >1 to 1.5 times ULN and any AST): No dosage adjustment is necessary.

Preexisting moderate or severe impairment: There are no dosage adjustments provided in the manufacturer's labeling (has not been studied). Ceritinib is primarily metabolized and eliminated hepatically; exposure is likely increased in patients with hepatic impairment.

Hepatotoxicity during treatment:

ALT or AST >5 times ULN with total bilirubin ≤2 times ULN (US labeling) or ≤1.5 times ULN (Canadian labeling): Interrupt therapy until recovery to baseline or ALT/AST ≤3 times ULN, then resume with a 150 mg dose reduction.

ALT or AST >3 times ULN with total bilirubin >2 times ULN (US labeling) or >1.5 times ULN (Canadian labeling) in the absence of cholestasis or hemolysis: Permanently discontinue therapy.

Adjustment for Toxicity Note: Over half of patients initiating treatment required at least 1 dose reduction; the median time to the first dose reduction was 7 weeks. Discontinue if patients are unable to tolerate 300 mg daily.

Cardiac:

Bradycardia (heart rate <50 beats per minute [US labeling] or <60 beats per minute [Canadian labeling]):

US labeling: Symptomatic bradycardia (not life-threatening): Interrupt therapy and evaluate concomitant medications known to cause brady-cardia. Upon recovery to asymptomatic bradycardia or to a heart rate ≥60 beats per minute, adjust the dose.

Canadian labeling: Interrupt therapy and evaluate for concomitant medication known to cause bradycardia. Upon recovery to asymptomatic bradycardia or to a heart rate ≥60 beats per minute:

If concomitant medication is identified and discontinued or its dose adjusted, reinitiate ceritinib at its previous dose.

If no concomitant medication is identified or if it is identified but not discontinued or not dose-adjusted, reinitiate ceritinib with a 150 mg dose reduction.

Symptomatic bradycardia (life-threatening or requiring intervention) in patients taking concomitant medications known to cause bradycardia/hypotension:

US labeling: Interrupt therapy until recovery to asymptomatic bradycardia or to a heart rate ≥60 beats per minute. If the concomitant medication can be adjusted or discontinued, resume ceritinib therapy with the dose reduced by 150 mg.

Canadian labeling: Interrupt therapy until recovery to asymptomatic bradycardia or to a heart rate ≥60 beats per minute. If concomitant medication can be discontinued or its dose adjusted, resume ceritinib with the dose reduced by 300 mg; monitor frequently; permanently discontinue ceritinib for recurrence.

Symptomatic bradycardia (life-threatening) in patients not taking concomitant medications known to cause bradycardia/hypotension: Permanently discontinue therapy.

QTc prolongation:

QTc interval >500 msec on at least 2 separate ECGs: Interrupt therapy until QTc interval is <481 msec or recovers to baseline if baseline QTc is ≥481 msec, then resume therapy with a 150 mg dose reduction.

QTc prolongation in combination with torsades de pointes, polymorphic ventricular tachycardia, or signs/symptoms of serious arrhythmia: Permanently discontinue therapy.

Gastrointestinal:

Severe or intolerable nausea, vomiting, or diarrhea (despite appropriate management): Interrupt therapy until improved, then resume treatment with a 150 mg dose reduction.

Lipase or amylase elevation >2 times ULN: Interrupt therapy and monitor serum lipase and amylase; upon recovery to <1.5 times ULN, resume treatment with a 150 mg dose reduction.

Metabolic: Persistent hyperglycemia >250 mg/dL (despite optimal antihyperglycemic therapy): Interrupt therapy until hyperglycemia is adequately controlled, then resume therapy with a 150 mg dose reduction. If hyperglycemia cannot be controlled, discontinue ceritinib permanently.

Pulmonary: Treatment-related interstitial lung disease/pneumonitis (any grade): Permanently discontinue therapy.

Combination Regimens

Lung cancer (non-small cell): Ceritinib (NSCLC Regimen) on page 1879

Administration

Ceritinib is associated with a moderate emetic potential; antiemetics may be needed to prevent nausea and vomiting.

Administer orally on an empty stomach (at least 2 hours before or 2 hours after a meal). Hazardous agent; use appropriate precautions for handling and disposal (meets NIOSH 2014 criteria).

The Canadian labeling recommends that the capsule not be crushed or chewed.

Emetic Potential Moderate (30% to 90%).

Monitoring Parameters ALK positivity; CBC, renal function, liver function, fasting blood glucose (baseline and as clinically necessary), lipase and amylase (baseline and periodically as clinically necessary); electrolytes (baseline and periodically thereafter); cardiac monitoring (heart rate and QTc interval); blood pressure; signs/symptoms of gastrointestinal and pulmonary toxicity; signs/symptoms of pancreatitis.

Dietary Considerations Avoid grapefruit and grapefruit juice.

Dosage Forms Excipient information presented when available (limited, particularly for generics); consult specific product labeling.

Capsule, Oral:

Zykadia: 150 mg [contains fd&c blue #2 (indigotine)]

◆ **Cerubidine** see DAUNOrubicin (Conventional) on page 463

◆ **Cervarix** see Papillomavirus (Types 16, 18) Vaccine (Human, Recombinant) on page 1332

◆ **Cesamet** see Nabilone on page 1187

Cetuximab (se TUK see mab)

Related Information

Common Toxicity Criteria on page 2122

Management of Chemotherapy-Induced Nausea and Vomiting in Adults on page 2142

Management of EGFR Inhibitor Toxicities: Dermatologic, Ocular, and Gastrointestinal on page 2179

Prevention of Chemotherapy-Induced Nausea and Vomiting in Children on page 2203

Principles of Anticancer Therapy on page 2261

Brand Names: US Erbitux

Brand Names: Canada Erbitux

Index Terms C225; IMC-C225; MOAB C225

Pharmacologic Category Antineoplastic Agent, Epidermal Growth Factor Receptor (EGFR) Inhibitor; Antineoplastic Agent, Monoclonal Antibody

◄ **Use**

Colorectal cancer, metastatic: Treatment of *KRAS* wild-type (without mutation), epidermal growth factor receptor (EGFR)-expressing metastatic colorectal cancer as determined by approved tests (in combination with FOLFIRI [irinotecan, fluorouracil, and leucovorin] as first-line treatment, in combination with irinotecan [in patients refractory to irinotecan-based chemotherapy], or as a single agent in patients who have failed irinotecan- and oxaliplatin-based chemotherapy or who are intolerant to irinotecan).

Limitation of use: Cetuximab is not indicated for the treatment of *RAS*-mutant colorectal cancer or when results of the *RAS* mutation tests are unknown.

Head and neck cancer, squamous cell: Treatment of squamous cell cancer of the head and neck (as a single agent for recurrent or metastatic disease after platinum-based chemotherapy failure; in combination with radiation therapy as initial treatment of locally or regionally advanced disease; in combination with platinum and fluorouracil-based chemotherapy as first-line treatment of locoregional or metastatic disease).

Labeled Contraindications

There are no contraindications listed in the manufacturer's US labeling.

Canadian labeling: Known severe hypersensitivity to cetuximab or any component of the formulation

Pregnancy Considerations Adverse events were observed in animal reproduction studies. Human IgG is known to cross the placenta. Because cetuximab inhibits epidermal growth factor (EGF), a component of fetal development, adverse effects on pregnancy would be expected. The manufacturer recommends that males and females use effective contraception during therapy and for 6 months following the last dose of cetuximab.

Breast-Feeding Considerations It is not known if cetuximab is excreted in breast milk. IgG antibodies can be detected in breast milk. Due to the potential for serious adverse reactions in the nursing infant, the manufacturer recommends that the decision to discontinue cetuximab or discontinue breast-feeding should take into account the benefits of treatment to the mother. If breast-feeding is interrupted for cetuximab treatment, based on the half-life, breast-feeding should not be resumed for at least 60 days following the last cetuximab dose.

Warnings/Precautions [US Boxed Warning]: In clinical trials, serious infusion reactions have been reported in approximately 3% of patients; fatal outcome has been reported rarely (less than 1 in 1,000); interrupt infusion promptly and permanently discontinue for serious infusion reactions. Reactions have included airway obstruction (bronchospasm, stridor, hoarseness), hypotension, loss of consciousness, shock, myocardial infarction (MI), and/or cardiac arrest. Premedicate with an intravenous (IV) H_1 antagonist 30 to 60 minutes prior to the first dose; premedication for subsequent doses is based on clinical judgment and with consideration of prior reaction to the initial infusion. The use of nebulized albuterol-based premedication to prevent infusion reaction has been reported (Tra, 2008). Approximately 90% of reactions occur with the first infusion despite the use of prophylactic antihistamines. Immediate treatment for anaphylactic/anaphylactoid reactions should be available during administration. The manufacturer recommends monitoring patients for at least 1 hour following completion of infusion, or longer if a reaction occurs. Mild to moderate infusion reactions are managed by slowing the infusion rate (by 50%) and administering antihistamines. Patients with preexisting IgE antibody against cetuximab (specific for galactose-α-1,3-galactose) are reported to have a higher incidence of severe hypersensitivity reaction. Severe hypersensitivity reaction has been reported more frequently in patients living in the middle south area of the United States, including North Carolina and Tennessee (Chung, 2008; O'Neil, 2007).

[US Boxed Warning]: In patients with squamous cell head and neck cancer, cardiopulmonary arrest and/or sudden death has occurred in 2% of patients receiving radiation therapy in combination with cetuximab and in 3% of patients receiving combination chemotherapy (platinum and fluorouracil-based) with cetuximab. Closely monitor serum electrolytes (magnesium, potassium, calcium) during and after cetuximab treatment (monitor for at least 8 weeks after treatment). Use with caution in patients with history of coronary artery disease, heart failure, and arrhythmias; fatalities have been reported. Interstitial lung disease has been reported; use with caution in patients with preexisting lung disease; interrupt treatment for acute onset or worsening of pulmonary symptoms; permanently discontinue with confirmed interstitial lung disease.

Acneiform rash has been reported in 76% to 88% of patients (severe in 1% to 17%), usually developing within the first 2 weeks of therapy; may require dose modification; generally resolved after discontinuation in most patients, although persisted beyond 28 days in some patients. Acneiform rash should be treated with topical and/or oral antibiotics; topical corticosteroids are not recommended. In colorectal cancer, the presence of acneiform rash correlates with treatment response and prolonged survival (Cunningham, 2004). Life-threatening and fatal bullous mucocutaneous disease (with blisters, erosions, and skin sloughing) has been observed with cetuximab; etiology is not determined; may be due to EGFR inhibition or to idiosyncratic immune-related effects (eg, Stevens-Johnson syndrome, toxic epidermal necrolysis). Other dermatologic toxicities, including dry skin, fissures, hypertrichosis, paronychial inflammation, and skin infections, have been reported; related ocular toxicities (blepharitis, conjunctivitis, keratitis, ulcerative keratitis with decreased visual acuity) may also occur. Monitor closely for dermatologic toxicities and potential infectious sequelae. Sunlight may exacerbate skin reactions (limit sun exposure).

Hypomagnesemia is common (may be severe); the onset of electrolyte disturbance may occur within days to months after initiation of treatment; monitor magnesium, calcium, and potassium during treatment and for at least 8 weeks after completion; may require electrolyte replacement. Non-neutralizing anti-cetuximab antibodies were detected in 5% of evaluable patients. In a study of radiation therapy **and** cisplatin with or without cetuximab in patients with squamous cell head and neck cancer, an increase in the incidence of adverse reactions (eg, grade 3/4 mucositis, radiation recall, acneiform rash, electrolyte abnormalities, cardiac events including ischemia) was noted in patients receiving cetuximab, including fatal reactions; there was no improvement in the primary end point of progression-free survival.

In patients with colorectal cancer, cetuximab is only indicated for EGFR-expressing metastatic colorectal cancer without *RAS* (*KRAS* or *NRAS*) mutations. Determine *RAS* mutation status prior to treatment (with an approved test). Patients with a codon 12 and 13 (exon 2), codon 59 and 61 (exon 3), and codon 117 and 146 (exon 4) *RAS* mutation are unlikely to benefit from EGFR inhibitor therapy (while experiencing toxicities) and should not receive cetuximab treatment; cetuximab is not effective for colorectal cancer with RAS mutations. Cetuximab is also reported to be ineffective in patients with *BRAF*

V600E mutation (Di Nicolantonio, 2008). The American Society of Clinical Oncology (ASCO) provisional clinical opinion (Allegra 2009) recommends genotyping tumor tissue for KRAS mutation in all patients with metastatic colorectal cancer (genotyping may be done on archived specimens). In trials for colorectal cancer, evidence of EGFR expression was required, although the response rate did not correlate with either the percentage of cells positive for EGFR or the intensity of expression. EGFR expression has been detected in nearly all patients with head and neck cancer; therefore laboratory evidence of EGFR expression is not necessary for head and neck cancers.

Adverse Reactions

>10%:

Central nervous system: Fatigue (91%), malaise (≤73%), pain (59%), peripheral sensory neuropathy (45%; grades 3/4: 1%), headache (19% to 38%), insomnia (27%), confusion (18%), chills (≤16%), rigors (≤16%), anxiety (14%), depression (14%)

Dermatologic: Desquamation (95%), acneiform eruption (15% to 88%; grades 3/4: 1% to 18%), radiodermatitis (86%), xeroderma (14% to 57%), pruritus (14% to 47%), skin rash (28% to 44%), changes in nails (31%), acne vulgaris (14% to 22%), paronychia (20%), palmar-plantar erythrodysesthesia (19%), skin fissure (19%), alopecia (12%)

Endocrine & metabolic: Weight loss (15% to 84%), hypomagnesemia (6% to 55%), dehydration (13% to 25%), hypocalcemia (12%), hypokalemia (12%)

Gastrointestinal: Diarrhea (19% to 72%), nausea (49% to 64%), abdominal pain (59%), constipation (53%), vomiting (40%), stomatitis (31% to 32%), anorexia (25% to 30%), dyspepsia (14% to 16%), xerostomia (12%)

Hematologic & oncologic: Neutropenia (49%; grades 3/4: 31%), leukopenia (grades 3/4: 17%)

Hepatic: Increased serum alanine aminotransferase (43%), increased serum aspartate aminotransferase (38%), increased serum alkaline phosphatase (33%)

Infection: Infection (13% to 44%), infection without neutropenia (38%)

Local: Application site reaction (18%)

Neuromuscular & skeletal: Weakness (≤73%), ostealgia (15%), arthralgia (14%)

Ophthalmic: Conjunctivitis (10% to 18%)

Respiratory: Dyspnea (49%), cough (30%), pharyngitis (26%)

Miscellaneous: Fever (22% to 29%), infusion related reaction (10% to 18%; grades 3/4: 2% to 5%)

1% to 10%:

Cardiovascular: Cardiorespiratory arrest (2% to 3%), ischemic heart disease (2%)

Dermatologic: Hypertrichosis

Gastrointestinal: Dysgeusia (10%)

Immunologic: Antibody development (5%)

Infection: Sepsis (1% to 4%)

Renal: Renal failure (1%: colorectal cancer patients; frequency not defined in other populations)

<1%, postmarketing, and/or case reports: Abscess, aseptic meningitis, blepharitis, bronchospasm, bullous pemphigoid, cardiac arrhythmia, cellulitis, cheilitis, corneal ulcer, electrolyte disturbance, hoarseness, hypotension, interstitial pulmonary disease, keratitis, loss of consciousness, mucosal inflammation, myocardial infarction, pulmonary embolism, shock, skin infection, Stevens-Johnson syndrome, stridor, toxic epidermal necrolysis

Drug Interactions

Metabolism/Transport Effects None known.

Avoid Concomitant Use There are no known interactions where it is recommended to avoid concomitant use.

Increased Effect/Toxicity There are no known significant interactions involving an increase in effect.

Decreased Effect There are no known significant interactions involving a decrease in effect.

Storage/Stability Store intact vials refrigerated at 2°C to 8°C (36°F to 46°F); do not freeze. Preparations in infusion containers are stable for up to 12 hours refrigerated at 2°C to 8°C (36°F to 46°F) and up to 8 hours at room temperature of 20°C to 25°C (68°F to 77°F).

Preparation for Administration Reconstitution is not required. Appropriate dose should be added to empty sterile container (may contain a small amount of visible white, amorphous cetuximab particles); do not shake or dilute. Discard unused portion of the vial; discard any remaining solution in infusion container after 8 hours at room temperature or after 12 hours refrigerated.

Mechanism of Action Recombinant human/mouse chimeric monoclonal antibody which binds specifically to the epidermal growth factor receptor (EGFR, HER1, c-ErbB-1) and competitively inhibits the binding of epidermal growth factor (EGF) and other ligands. Binding to the EGFR blocks phosphorylation and activation of receptor-associated kinases, resulting in inhibition of cell growth, induction of apoptosis, and decreased matrix metalloproteinase and vascular endothelial growth factor production. EGFR signal transduction results in *RAS* wild-type activation; cells with *RAS* mutations appear to be unaffected by EGFR inhibition.

Pharmacodynamics/Kinetics

Distribution: V_d: ~2 to 3 L/m^2

Half-life elimination: ~112 hours (range: 63 to 230 hours)

Dosing

Adult & Geriatric Note: Premedicate with an H_1 antagonist (eg, diphenhydramine) IV 30 to 60 minutes prior to the first dose; premedication for subsequent doses is based on clinical judgment.

Colorectal cancer, metastatic, KRAS wild-type (without mutation): IV:
Initial loading dose: 400 mg/m^2 infused over 120 minutes
Maintenance dose: 250 mg/m^2 infused over 60 minutes weekly until disease progression or unacceptable toxicity
Note: If given in combination with FOLFIRI (irinotecan, fluorouracil, and leucovorin), complete cetuximab infusion 1 hour prior to FOLFIRI.

Head and neck cancer (squamous cell): IV:
Initial loading dose: 400 mg/m^2 infused over 120 minutes
Maintenance dose: 250 mg/m^2 infused over 60 minutes weekly
Note: If given in combination with radiation therapy, administer loading dose 1 week prior to initiation of radiation course; weekly maintenance dose should be completed 1 hour prior to radiation for the duration of radiation therapy (6 to 7 weeks). If given in combination with chemotherapy, administer loading dose on the day of initiation of platinum and fluorouracil-based chemotherapy, cetuximab infusion should be completed 1 hour prior to initiation of chemotherapy; weekly maintenance dose should be completed 1 hour prior to chemotherapy; continue until disease progression or unacceptable toxicity. Monotherapy weekly doses should be continued until disease progression or unacceptable toxicity

◄ **Colorectal cancer, advanced, biweekly administration (off-label dosing):** IV: 500 mg/m² every 2 weeks (initial dose infused over 120 minutes, subsequent doses infused over 60 minutes) in combination with irinotecan (Pfeiffer 2008)

Non-small cell lung cancer (NSCLC), EGFR-expressing, advanced (off-label use): IV: Initial loading dose: 400 mg/m², followed by maintenance dose: 250 mg/m² weekly in combination with cisplatin and vinorelbine for up to 6 cycles, then as monotherapy until disease progression or unacceptable toxicity (Pirker 2009; Pirker 2012)

Squamous cell skin cancer, unresectable (off-label use): IV: Initial loading dose: 400 mg/m², followed by maintenance dose: 250 mg/m² weekly until disease progression (Maubec 2011)

Renal Impairment There are no dosage adjustments provided in the manufacturer's labeling.

Hepatic Impairment There are no dosage adjustments provided in the manufacturer's labeling.

Adjustment for Toxicity

Infusion reactions, grade 1 or 2 and nonserious grade 3: Reduce the infusion rate by 50% and continue to use prophylactic antihistamines

Infusion reactions, severe: Immediately and permanently discontinue treatment

Pulmonary toxicity:

Acute onset or worsening pulmonary symptoms: Hold treatment

Interstitial lung disease: Permanently discontinue

Skin toxicity, mild to moderate: No dosage modification required

Acneiform rash, severe (grade 3 or 4):

First occurrence: Delay cetuximab infusion 1 to 2 weeks

If improvement, continue at 250 mg/m²

If no improvement, discontinue therapy

Second occurrence: Delay cetuximab infusion 1 to 2 weeks

If improvement, continue at reduced dose of 200 mg/m²

If no improvement, discontinue therapy

Third occurrence: Delay cetuximab infusion 1 to 2 weeks

If improvement, continue at reduced dose of 150 mg/m²

If no improvement, discontinue therapy

Fourth occurrence: Discontinue therapy

Combination Regimens

Colorectal cancer:

Cetuximab Biweekly (Colorectal Regimen) on page 1879

Cetuximab (Biweekly)-Irinotecan (Colorectal) on page 1879

Cetuximab (Colorectal Regimen) on page 1882

Cetuximab + FOLFIRI (Colorectal) on page 1882

Cetuximab-Irinotecan (Colorectal) on page 1883

Head and neck cancer:

Carboplatin-Cetuximab (Head and Neck Cancer) on page 1861

Cetuximab-Carboplatin-Fluorouracil (Head and Neck Cancer) on page 1880

Cetuximab-Cisplatin-Fluorouracil (Head and Neck Cancer) on page 1880

Cisplatin-Cetuximab (Head and Neck Cancer) on page 1889

Paclitaxel-Cetuximab on page 2050

Lung cancer, non-small cell: Cetuximab-Cisplatin-Vinorelbine (NSCLC) on page 1881

Squamous cell carcinoma: Cetuximab (Squamous Cell Regimen) on page 1884

Administration Administer via IV infusion; loading dose over 2 hours, weekly maintenance dose over 1 hour. Do not administer as IV push or bolus. Do not shake or dilute. Administer via infusion pump or syringe pump. Following the infusion, an observation period (1 hour) is recommended; longer observation time (following an infusion reaction) may be required. Premedication with an H_1 antagonist prior to the initial dose is recommended. The maximum infusion rate is 10 mg/minute. Administer through a low protein-binding 0.22 micrometer in-line filter.

For biweekly administration (off-label frequency and dose), the initial dose was infused over 120 minutes and subsequent doses infused over 60 minutes (Pfeiffer 2007; Pfeiffer 2008).

Emetic Potential Children and Adults: Minimal (<10%)

Monitoring Parameters Vital signs during infusion and observe for at least 1 hour postinfusion. Patients developing dermatologic toxicities should be monitored for the development of complications. Periodic monitoring of serum magnesium, calcium, and potassium are recommended to continue over an interval consistent with the half-life (8 weeks); monitor closely (during and after treatment) for cetuximab plus radiation therapy. *KRAS* genotyping of tumor tissue in patients with colorectal cancer

Dosage Forms Excipient information presented when available (limited, particularly for generics); consult specific product labeling.

Solution, Intravenous [preservative free]:

Erbitux: 100 mg/50 mL (50 mL); 200 mg/100 mL (100 mL) [contains galactose-alpha-1,3-galactose]

♦ **CFZ** see Carfilzomib on page 278

♦ **CGP-42446** see Zoledronic Acid on page 1790

♦ **CGP-57148B** see Imatinib on page 882

♦ **CGS-20267** see Letrozole on page 1019

♦ **CGX-625** see Omacetaxine on page 1248

♦ **ch14.18** see Dinutuximab on page 530

♦ **Chloditan** see Mitotane on page 1155

♦ **Chlodithane** see Mitotane on page 1155

Chlorambucil (klor AM byoo sil)

Related Information

Fertility and Cancer Therapy on page 2137

Management of Chemotherapy-Induced Nausea and Vomiting in Adults on page 2142

Prevention of Chemotherapy-Induced Nausea and Vomiting in Children on page 2203

Safe Handling of Hazardous Drugs on page 2292

Brand Names: US Leukeran

Brand Names: Canada Leukeran®

Index Terms CB-1348; Chlorambucilum; Chloraminophene; Chlorbutinum; WR-139013

Pharmacologic Category Antineoplastic Agent, Alkylating Agent; Antineoplastic Agent, Alkylating Agent (Nitrogen Mustard)

Use

Chronic lymphocytic leukemia (CLL): Management of CLL

Lymphomas: Management of Hodgkin lymphoma and non-Hodgkin lymphomas (NHL)

Canadian labeling: Additional uses (not in U.S. labeling): Management of Waldenström's macroglobulinemia

Labeled Contraindications Hypersensitivity to chlorambucil or any component of the formulation; hypersensitivity to other alkylating agents (may have cross-hypersensitivity); prior (demonstrated) resistance to chlorambucil

Canadian labeling: Additional contraindications (not in U.S. labeling): Use within 4 weeks of a full course of radiation or chemotherapy

Pregnancy Considerations Animal reproduction studies have demonstrated teratogenicity. Chlorambucil crosses the human placenta. Following exposure during the first trimester, case reports have noted adverse renal effects (unilateral agenesis). Women of childbearing potential should avoid becoming pregnant while receiving treatment. **[U.S. Boxed Warning]: Affects human fertility; probably mutagenic and teratogenic as well**; chromosomal damage has been documented. Reversible and irreversible sterility (when administered to prepubertal and pubertal males), azoospermia (in adult males) and amenorrhea (in females) have been observed. Fibrosis, vasculitis and depletion of primordial follicles have been noted on autopsy of the ovaries.

Breast-Feeding Considerations It is not known if chlorambucil is excreted in breast milk. Due to the potential for serious adverse reactions in the nursing infant, the decision to discontinue chlorambucil or to discontinue breast-feeding should take into account the benefits of treatment to the mother.

Warnings/Precautions Hazardous agent - use appropriate precautions for handling and disposal (NIOSH 2014 [group 1]). Seizures have been observed; use with caution in patients with seizure disorder or head trauma; history of nephrotic syndrome and high pulse doses are at higher risk of seizures. **[U.S. Boxed Warning]: May cause severe bone marrow suppression;** neutropenia may be severe. Reduce initial dosage if patient has received myelosuppressive or radiation therapy within the previous 4 weeks, or has a depressed baseline leukocyte or platelet count. Irreversible bone marrow damage may occur with total doses approaching 6.5 mg/kg. Progressive lymphopenia may develop (recovery is generally rapid after discontinuation). Avoid administration of live vaccines to immunocompromised patients. Rare instances of severe skin reactions (eg, erythema multiforme, Stevens-Johnson syndrome, toxic epidermal necrolysis) have been reported; discontinue promptly if skin reaction occurs.

Chlorambucil is primarily metabolized in the liver. Dosage reductions should be considered in patients with hepatic impairment. **[U.S. Boxed Warning]: Affects human fertility; carcinogenic in humans and probably mutagenic and teratogenic as well;** chromosomal damage has been documented. Reversible and irreversible sterility (when administered to prepubertal and pubertal males), azoospermia (in adult males) and amenorrhea (in females) have been observed. **[U.S. Boxed Warning]: Carcinogenic;** acute myelocytic leukemia and secondary malignancies may be associated with chronic therapy. Duration of treatment and higher cumulative doses are associated with a higher risk for development of leukemia. Potentially significant drug-drug interactions may exist, requiring dose or frequency adjustment, additional monitoring, and/or selection of alternative therapy.

Adverse Reactions Frequency not always defined.

Central nervous system: Agitation (rare), ataxia (rare), confusion (rare), drug fever, fever, focal/generalized seizure (rare), hallucinations (rare)

Dermatologic: Angioneurotic edema, erythema multiforme (rare), rash, skin hypersensitivity, Stevens-Johnson syndrome (rare), toxic epidermal necrolysis (rare), urticaria

Endocrine & metabolic: Amenorrhea, infertility, SIADH (rare)

Gastrointestinal: Diarrhea (infrequent), nausea (infrequent), oral ulceration (infrequent), vomiting (infrequent)

Genitourinary: Azoospermia, cystitis (sterile)

Hematologic: Neutropenia (onset: 3 weeks; recovery: 10 days after last dose), bone marrow failure (irreversible), bone marrow suppression, anemia, leukemia (secondary), leukopenia, lymphopenia, pancytopenia, thrombocytopenia

Hepatic: Hepatotoxicity, jaundice

Neuromuscular & skeletal: Flaccid paresis (rare), muscular twitching (rare), myoclonia (rare), peripheral neuropathy, tremor (rare)

Respiratory: Interstitial pneumonia, pulmonary fibrosis

Miscellaneous: Allergic reactions, malignancies (secondary)

Drug Interactions

Metabolism/Transport Effects None known.

Avoid Concomitant Use

Avoid concomitant use of Chlorambucil with any of the following: BCG (Intravesical); CloZAPine; Dipyrone; Natalizumab; Pimecrolimus; Tacrolimus (Topical); Tofacitinib; Vaccines (Live)

Increased Effect/Toxicity

Chlorambucil may increase the levels/effects of: CloZAPine; Fingolimod; Leflunomide; Natalizumab; Tofacitinib; Vaccines (Live)

The levels/effects of Chlorambucil may be increased by: Denosumab; Dipyrone; Pimecrolimus; Roflumilast; Tacrolimus (Topical); Trastuzumab

Decreased Effect

Chlorambucil may decrease the levels/effects of: BCG (Intravesical); Coccidioides immitis Skin Test; Sipuleucel-T; Vaccines (Inactivated); Vaccines (Live)

The levels/effects of Chlorambucil may be decreased by: Echinacea

Food Interactions Absorption is decreased when administered with food. Management: Administer preferably on an empty stomach.

Storage/Stability Store in refrigerator at 2°C to 8°C (36°F to 46°F).

Mechanism of Action Alkylating agent; interferes with DNA replication and RNA transcription by alkylation and cross-linking the strands of DNA

Pharmacodynamics/Kinetics

Absorption: Rapid and complete (>70%); reduced with food

Distribution: V_d: ~0.3 L/kg

Protein binding: ~99%; primarily to albumin

Metabolism: Hepatic (extensively); primarily to active metabolite, phenylacetic acid mustard

Half-life elimination: ~1.5 hours; Phenylacetic acid mustard: ~1.8 hours

Time to peak, plasma: Within 1 hour; Phenylacetic acid mustard: 1.2-2.6 hours

Excretion: Urine (~20% to 60%, primarily as inactive metabolites, <1% as unchanged drug or phenylacetic acid mustard)

◀ **Dosing**

Adult Note: With bone marrow lymphocytic infiltration involvement (in CLL, Hodgkin lymphoma, or NHL), the maximum dose is 0.1 mg/kg/day. While short treatment courses are preferred, if maintenance therapy is required, the maximum dose is 0.1 mg/kg/day.

Chronic lymphocytic leukemia (CLL): Oral:

U.S. labeling: 0.1 mg/kg/day for 3-6 weeks **or** 0.4 mg/kg pulsed doses administered intermittently, biweekly, or monthly (increased by 0.1 mg/kg/dose until response/toxicity observed)

Canadian labeling: Initial: 0.15 mg/kg/day until WBC is 10,000/mm^3; interrupt treatment for 4 weeks, then may resume at 0.1 mg/kg/day until response (generally ~2 years)/toxicity observed

Off-label dosing for CLL: 0.4 mg/kg day 1 every 2 weeks; if tolerated may increase by 0.1 mg/kg with each treatment course to a maximum dose of 0.8 mg/kg and maximum of 24 cycles (Eichhorst, 2009) **or** 30 mg/m^2 day 1 every 2 weeks (in combination with prednisone) (Raphael, 1991) **or** 40 mg/m^2 day 1 every 4 weeks until disease progression or complete remission or response plateau for up to a maximum of 12 cycles (Rai, 2000)

Hodgkin lymphoma: Oral:

U.S. labeling: 0.2 mg/kg/day for 3-6 weeks

Canadian labeling: 0.2 mg/kg/day for 4-8 weeks

Non-Hodgkin lymphomas (NHL): Oral:

U.S. labeling: 0.1 mg/kg/day for 3-6 weeks

Canadian labeling: Initial: 0.1-0.2 mg/kg/day for 4-8 weeks; for maintenance treatment, reduce dose or administer intermittently

Waldenström's macroglobulinemia (U.S. off-label use): Oral: 0.1 mg/kg/day (continuously) for at least 6 months **or** 0.3 mg/kg/day for 7 days every 6 weeks for at least 6 months (Kyle, 2000)

Geriatric Refer to adult dosing. Begin at the lower end of dosing range(s)

Pediatric Nephrotic syndrome, steroid sensitive (off-label use): Oral: 0.2 mg/kg once daily for ~8 weeks (Hodson, 2010)

Renal Impairment No dosage adjustment provided in manufacturer's labeling; however, renal elimination of unchanged chlorambucil and active metabolite (phenylacetic acid mustard) is minimal and renal impairment is not likely to affect elimination. The following adjustments have been recommended: Adults:

Aronoff, 2007:

CrCl >50 mL/minute: No adjustment necessary.

CrCl 10-50 mL/minute: Administer 75% of dose.

CrCl <10 mL/minute: Administer 50% of dose.

Peritoneal dialysis (PD): Administer 50% of dose.

Kintzel, 1995: Based on the pharmacokinetics, dosage adjustment is not indicated

Hepatic Impairment Chlorambucil undergoes extensive hepatic metabolism. Although dosage reduction should be considered in patients with hepatic impairment, no dosage adjustment is provided in the manufacturer's labeling (data is insufficient).

Obesity *ASCO Guidelines for appropriate chemotherapy dosing in obese adults with cancer:* Utilize patient's actual body weight (full weight) for calculation of body surface area- or weight-based dosing, particularly when the intent of therapy is curative; manage regimen-related toxicities in the same manner as for nonobese patients; if a dose reduction is utilized due to

toxicity, consider resumption of full weight-based dosing with subsequent cycles, especially if cause of toxicity (eg, hepatic or renal impairment) is resolved (Griggs, 2012). **Note:** The manufacturer recommends the maximum dose should not exceed 0.1 mg/kg/day if maintenance therapy is required and with bone marrow infiltration.

Adjustment for Toxicity
Skin reactions: Discontinue treatment
Hematologic:
WBC or platelets below normal: Reduce dose.
Severely depressed WBC or platelet counts: Discontinue.
Persistently low neutrophil or platelet counts or peripheral lymphocytosis: May be suggestive of bone marrow infiltration; if infiltration confirmed, do not exceed 0.1 mg/kg/day.
Concurrent or within 4 weeks (before or after) of chemotherapy/radiotherapy: Initiate treatment cautiously; reduce dose; monitor closely.

Combination Regimens
Leukemia, chronic lymphocytic:
Chlorambucil (CLL Regimen) on page 1884
Chlorambucil-Obinutuzumab (CLL) on page 1884
Chlorambucil-Ofatumumab (CLL) on page 1885
Chlorambucil-Prednisone (CLL) on page 1885
Lymphoma, Hodgkin: ChIVPP (Hodgkin) on page 1886

Administration May be administered as a single daily dose; preferably on an empty stomach.

Hazardous agent; use appropriate precautions for handling and disposal (NIOSH 2014 [group 1]).

Emetic Potential Children and Adults: Minimal (<10%)

Extemporaneous Preparations Hazardous agent: Use appropriate precautions for handling and disposal (NIOSH 2014 [group 1]).

A 2 mg/mL oral suspension may be prepared with tablets. Crush sixty 2 mg tablets in a mortar and reduce to a fine powder. Add small portions of methylcellulose 1% and mix to a uniform paste (total methylcellulose: 30 mL); mix while adding simple syrup in incremental proportions to **almost** 60 mL; transfer to a graduated cylinder, rinse mortar and pestle with simple syrup, and add quantity of vehicle sufficient to make 60 mL. Transfer contents of graduated cylinder to an amber prescription bottle. Label "shake well", "refrigerate", and "protect from light". Stable for 7 days refrigerated.

Dressman JB and Poust RI, "Stability of Allopurinol and of Five Antineoplastics in Suspension," *Am J Hosp Pharm*, 1983, 40(4):616-8.

Nahata MC, Pai VB, and Hipple TF, *Pediatric Drug Formulations*, 5th ed, Cincinnati, OH: Harvey Whitney Books Co, 2004.

Monitoring Parameters Liver function tests, CBC with differential (weekly, with WBC monitored twice weekly during the first 3-6 weeks of treatment)

Dosage Forms Excipient information presented when available (limited, particularly for generics); consult specific product labeling.
Tablet, Oral:
Leukeran: 2 mg

◆ **Chlorambucilum** see Chlorambucil on page 317
◆ **Chloraminophene** see Chlorambucil on page 317
◆ **Chlorbutinum** see Chlorambucil on page 317
◆ **Chlorethazine** see Mechlorethamine (Systemic) on page 1067

♦ **Chlorethazine Mustard** *see* Mechlorethamine (Systemic) *on page 1067*

♦ **Chlormeprazine** *see* Prochlorperazine *on page 1441*

♦ **2-Chlorodeoxyadenosine** *see* Cladribine *on page 344*

ChlorproMAZINE (klor PROE ma zeen)

Brand Names: Canada Chlorpromazine Hydrochloride Inj; Teva-Chlorpromazine

Index Terms Chlorpromazine Hydrochloride; CPZ; Thorazine

Pharmacologic Category Antimanic Agent; First Generation (Typical) Antipsychotic

Use

Behavioral problems: Treatment of severe behavioral problems in children 1 to 12 years of age marked by combativeness and/or explosive hyperexcitable behavior (out of proportion to immediate provocations).

Bipolar disorder: Treatment of manic episodes associated with bipolar disorder.

Hiccups: Treatment of intractable hiccups.

Hyperactivity: Short-term treatment of hyperactive children who show excessive motor activity with accompanying conduct disorders consisting of some or all of the following symptoms: impulsivity, difficulty sustaining attention, aggressiveness, mood lability, and poor frustration tolerance.

Nausea/Vomiting: Management of nausea and vomiting.

Porphyria, acute intermittent: Treatment of acute intermittent porphyria.

Schizophrenia/Psychotic disorders: Treatment of schizophrenia and psychotic disorders.

Surgery: Management of restlessness and apprehension prior to surgery.

Tetanus: Adjunctive therapy in the treatment of tetanus.

Dosing

Adult & Geriatric

Bipolar disorder/psychotic disorders/schizophrenia:

Oral: Range: 30 to 800 mg daily in 2 to 4 divided doses, initiate at lower doses and titrate as needed; usual dose: 200 to 800 mg daily; some patients may require 1 to 2 g daily, however, therapeutic gain is limited at doses >1 g daily

IM: Initial: 25 mg, may repeat (25 to 50 mg) in 1 to 4 hours, gradually increase to a maximum of 400 mg/dose every 4 to 6 hours until patient is controlled; usual dose: 200 to 800 mg daily

Intractable hiccups:

Oral, IM: 25 to 50 mg 3 to 4 times/day

IV (refractory to oral or IM treatment): 25 to 50 mg via slow IV infusion

Nausea and vomiting:

Oral: 10 to 25 mg every 4 to 6 hours as needed

IM: 25 to 50 mg every 3 to 4 hours as needed

IV (during surgery): 2 mg per fractional injection at 2 minute intervals using a 1 mg/mL solution; do not exceed 25 mg

Porphyria, acute intermittent:

Oral: 25 to 50 mg 3 to 4 times daily; usually may be discontinued after several weeks although maintenance therapy may be necessary

IM: 25 mg 3 or 4 times daily (until patient can tolerate oral administration)

Presurgical apprehension:

Oral: 25 to 50 mg 2 to 3 hours prior to surgery

IM: 12.5 to 25 mg 1 to 2 hours prior to surgery

Tetanus: IM, IV: 25 to 50 mg 3 or 4 times daily; titrate to response

Pediatric

Behavior problems; severe: Note: Begin with low doses and gradually titrate as needed to lowest effective dose; route of administration should be determined by severity of symptoms.

Infants ≥6 months, Children, and Adolescents weighing ≤45.5 kg:

Oral: Initial: 0.55 mg/kg/dose every 4 to 6 hours as needed; may titrate as required; in severe cases, higher doses may be required (50 to 100 mg daily); in older children, higher daily doses (200 mg daily or higher) may be necessary; maximum daily dose: 500 mg/**day**; daily doses >500 mg have not been shown to further improve behavior in pediatric patients with severe mental impairment

IM, IV (off-label): Initial: 0.55 mg/kg/dose every 6-8 hours as needed; may titrate as required in severe cases (Kliegman, 2007)

Maximum recommended daily doses:

Children <5 years or weighing <22.7 kg: 40 mg/**day**

Children ≥5 years and Adolescents or weighing 22.7 to 45.5 kg: 75 mg/**day**

Adolescents weighing >45.5 kg:

Oral: Range: 30 to 800 mg daily in 2 to 4 divided doses, initiate at lower doses and titrate as needed; usual dose is 200 mg daily

IM, IV (off-label): 25 mg initially, may repeat (25 to 50 mg) in 1 to 4 hours, gradually increase to a maximum of 400 mg/dose every 4 to 6 hours until patient controlled; usual dose 200 to 800 mg daily (Kliegman, 2007)

Nausea and vomiting, treatment (non-CINV):

Infants ≥6 months, Children, and Adolescents weighing ≤45.5 kg: Oral, IM, IV: 0.55 mg/kg/dose every 6 to 8 hours as needed; in severe cases, higher doses may be needed; usual maximum daily dose: IM, IV:

Children <5 years or weighing <22.7 kg: 40 mg/**day**

Children ≥5 years and Adolescents or weighing 22.7 to 45.5 kg: 75 mg/**day**

Adolescents weighing >45.5 kg:

Oral: 10 to 25 mg every 4 to 6 hours as needed

IM, IV: Initial: 25 mg; if tolerated (no hypotension), then may give 25 to 50 mg every 4 to 6 hours as needed

Prevention of chemotherapy-associated nausea and vomiting (Pediatric Oncology Group of Ontario [POGO] dosing recommendation): Highly or moderately emetogenic chemotherapy (patients who cannot receive corticosteroids): Infants ≥6 months, Children, and Adolescents: IV: 0.5 mg/kg/dose every 6 hours (in combination with ondansetron or granisetron); if not controlled, may increase up to 1 mg/kg/dose; monitor for sedation, maximum dose: 50 mg (Dupuis, 2013)

Presurgical apprehension: Infants ≥6 months, Children, and Adolescents:

Oral: 0.55 mg/kg 2 to 3 hours prior to surgery; maximum dose 50 mg

IM: 0.55 mg/kg/dose 1 to 2 hours prior to surgery; maximum dose 25 mg

Tetanus:

Infants ≥6 months, Children, and Adolescents weighing ≤45.5 kg: IM, IV: 0.55 mg/kg/dose every 6 to 8 hours; in severe cases higher doses may be needed

Usual maximum daily dose:

Children <5 years or weighing <22.7 kg: 40 mg/**day**

Children ≥5 years and Adolescents or weighing 22.7 to 45.5 kg: 75 mg/**day**

Adolescents weighing ≥45.5 kg: IM, IV: 25 to 50 mg every 6 to 8 hours; begin with low dose titrate to response

Renal Impairment There are no dosage adjustments provided in the manufacturer's labeling; use with caution. Not dialyzable (0% to 5%)

Hepatic Impairment There are no dosage adjustments provided in the manufacturer's labeling; use with caution.

Additional Information Complete prescribing information should be consulted for additional detail.

Dosage Forms Excipient information presented when available (limited, particularly for generics); consult specific product labeling.

Solution, Injection, as hydrochloride:
  Generic: 25 mg/mL (1 mL); 50 mg/2 mL (2 mL)
Tablet, Oral, as hydrochloride:
  Generic: 10 mg, 25 mg, 50 mg, 100 mg, 200 mg

- ◆ **Chlorpromazine Hydrochloride** *see* ChlorproMAZINE *on page* 322
- ◆ **Chlorpromazine Hydrochloride Inj (Can)** *see* ChlorproMAZINE *on page* 322
- ◆ **Ciclosporin** *see* CycloSPORINE (Systemic) *on page* 385
- ◆ **Cilastatin and Imipenem** *see* Imipenem and Cilastatin *on page* 893

Cinacalcet (sin a KAL cet)

Brand Names: US Sensipar

Brand Names: Canada Sensipar

Index Terms AMG 073; Cinacalcet Hydrochloride

Pharmacologic Category Calcimimetic

Use

Hyperparathyroidism, primary: Treatment of severe hypercalcemia in adult patients with primary hyperparathyroidism for whom parathyroidectomy would be indicated on the basis of serum calcium levels, but who are unable to undergo parathyroidectomy

Hyperparathyroidism, secondary: Treatment of secondary hyperparathyroidism in adult patients with chronic kidney disease (CKD) on dialysis.

Limitation of use: Not indicated for use in patients with CKD who are not on dialysis (due to the increased risk of hypocalcemia)

Parathyroid carcinoma: Treatment of hypercalcemia in adult patients with parathyroid carcinoma

Labeled Contraindications

Serum calcium lower than the lower limit of normal range

Canadian labeling: Additional contraindications (not in U.S. labeling): Hypersensitivity to any component of the formulation

Pregnancy Considerations Adverse events have been observed in animal reproduction studies. Women who become pregnant during cinacalcet treatment are encouraged to enroll in Amgen's Pregnancy Surveillance Program (1-800-772-6436).

Breast-Feeding Considerations It is not known if cinacalcet is excreted in breast milk. Due to the potential for clinically significant adverse reactions in the nursing infant, the manufacturer recommends a decision be made whether to discontinue nursing or the drug, taking into account the importance of treatment to the mother. Women who choose to continue nursing during cinacalcet treatment are encouraged to enroll in Amgen's Lactation Surveillance Program (1-800-772-6436).

Warnings/Precautions Life-threatening and fatal events associated with hypocalcemia have occurred. Use is contraindicated if the serum calcium is less than the lower limit of the normal range. Monitor serum calcium and for symptoms of hypocalcemia (eg, muscle cramps, myalgia, paresthesia, seizure, tetany); may require treatment interruption, dose reduction, or initiation (or dose increases) of calcium-based phosphate binder and/or vitamin D to raise serum calcium depending on calcium levels or symptoms of hypocalcemia. Use with caution in patients with a seizure disorder (seizure threshold is lowered by significant serum calcium reductions); monitor calcium levels closely. Adynamic bone disease may develop if intact parathyroid hormone (iPTH) levels are suppressed <100 pg/mL; reduce dose or discontinue use of cinacalcet and/or vitamin D if iPTH levels decrease below 150 pg/mL.

Use caution in patients with moderate-to-severe hepatic impairment (Child-Pugh classes B and C); monitor serum calcium, serum phosphorus and iPTH closely. In the U.S., the long-term safety and efficacy of cinacalcet has not been evaluated in chronic kidney disease (CKD) patients with hyperparathyroidism not requiring dialysis. Not indicated for CKD patients not receiving dialysis. Although possibly related to lower baseline calcium levels, clinical studies have shown an increased incidence of hypocalcemia (<8.4 mg/dL) in patients not requiring dialysis. Cases of idiosyncratic hypotension, worsening of heart failure, and/or arrhythmia have been reported in patients with impaired cardiovascular function; may correlate with decreased serum calcium. QT prolongation and ventricular arrhythmia secondary to hypocalcemia have also been reported. Potentially significant interactions may exist, requiring dose or frequency adjustment, additional monitoring, and/or selection of alternative therapy.

Adverse Reactions

>10%:

Cardiovascular: Hypotension (12%)

Central nervous system: Paresthesia (14% to 29%), headache (≤21%), fatigue (12% to 21%), depression (10% to 18%)

Endocrine & metabolic: Hypocalcemia (<8.4 mg/dL: 6% to 75%; <7.5 mg/dL: 29% to 33%), dehydration (≤24%), hypercalcemia (12% to 21%), hypoparathyroidism (intact parathyroid hormone <100 pg/mL: ≤11%)

Gastrointestinal: Nausea (30% to 66%), vomiting (26% to 52%), diarrhea (21%), anorexia (6% to 21%), constipation (5% to 18%), abdominal pain (11%)

Hematologic & oncologic: Anemia (6% to 17%)

Neuromuscular & skeletal: Bone fracture (12% to 21%), muscle spasm (11% to 18%), arthralgia (6% to 17%), weakness (5% to 17%), myalgia (15%), back pain (12%), limb pain (10% to 12%)

Respiratory: Dyspnea (13%), cough (12%), upper respiratory tract infection (8% to 12%)

1% to 10%:

Cardiovascular: Hypertension (7%)

Central nervous system: Dizziness (7% to 10%), noncardiac chest pain (6%), seizure (≤3%)

Endocrine & metabolic: Hyperkalemia (8%)

Gastrointestinal: Upper abdominal pain (8%), dyspepsia (7%), decreased appetite (6%)

Hypersensitivity: Hypersensitivity reaction (9%)

Infection: Localized infection (dialysis access site; 5%)

Postmarketing and/or case reports: Adynamic bone disease, angioedema, cardiac arrhythmia, cardiac failure, hypotension (idiosyncratic), prolonged Q-T interval on ECG (secondary to hypocalcemia), skin rash, urticaria, ventricular arrhythmia (secondary to hypocalcemia)

Drug Interactions

Metabolism/Transport Effects Substrate of CYP1A2 (minor), CYP2D6 (minor), CYP3A4 (major); **Note:** Assignment of Major/Minor substrate status based on clinically relevant drug interaction potential; **Inhibits** CYP2D6 (strong)

Avoid Concomitant Use

Avoid concomitant use of Cinacalcet with any of the following: Conivaptan; Fusidic Acid (Systemic); Idelalisib; Mequitazine; Pimozide; Tamoxifen; Thioridazine

Increased Effect/Toxicity

Cinacalcet may increase the levels/effects of: ARIPiprazole; ARIPiprazole Lauroxil; AtoMOXetine; Brexpiprazole; CYP2D6 Substrates; Dapoxetine; DOXOrubicin (Conventional); DULoxetine; Eliglustat; Fesoterodine; Iloperidone; Mequitazine; Metoprolol; Nebivolol; Pimozide; Propafenone; Tamsulosin; Tetrabenazine; Thioridazine; TraMADol; Tricyclic Antidepressants; Vortioxetine

The levels/effects of Cinacalcet may be increased by: Aprepitant; Conivaptan; CYP3A4 Inhibitors (Moderate); CYP3A4 Inhibitors (Strong); Dasatinib; Fosaprepitant; Fusidic Acid (Systemic); Idelalisib; Ivacaftor; Luliconazole; Mifepristone; Netupitant; Osimertinib; Palbociclib; Simeprevir; Stiripentol

Decreased Effect

Cinacalcet may decrease the levels/effects of: Codeine; Hydrocodone; Iloperidone; Tacrolimus (Systemic); Tamoxifen; TraMADol

The levels/effects of Cinacalcet may be decreased by: Osimertinib

Food Interactions Food increases bioavailability. Management: Administer with food or shortly after a meal.

Storage/Stability Store at 25°C (77°F); excursions permitted to 15°C to 30°C (59°F to 86°F).

Mechanism of Action Increases the sensitivity of the calcium-sensing receptor on the parathyroid gland thereby, concomitantly lowering parathyroid hormone (PTH), serum calcium, and serum phosphorus levels, preventing progressive bone disease and adverse events associated with mineral metabolism disorders.

Pharmacodynamics/Kinetics

Distribution: V_d: ~1,000 L

Protein binding: ~93% to 97%

Metabolism: Hepatic (extensive) via CYP3A4, 2D6, 1A2; forms inactive metabolites

Half-life elimination: Terminal: 30 to 40 hours; moderate hepatic impairment: 65 hours; severe hepatic impairment: 84 hours

Time to peak, plasma: ~2 to 6 hours; increased with food.

Excretion: Urine ~80% (as metabolites); feces ~15%

Dosing

Adult & Geriatric Note: Do not titrate dose more frequently than every 2 to 4 weeks. May be used alone or in combination with vitamin D and/or phosphate binders. Dosage adjustment may be required in patients on concurrent CYP3A4 inhibitors.

Hyperparathyroidism, primary: Oral: Initial: 30 mg twice daily; increase dose incrementally (to 60 mg twice daily, 90 mg twice daily, and 90 mg 3 or 4 times daily) as necessary to normalize serum calcium levels.

Hyperparathyroidism, secondary: Oral: Initial: 30 mg once daily; increase dose incrementally (to 60 mg once daily, 90 mg once daily, 120 mg once daily, and 180 mg once daily) as necessary to maintain intact parathyroid hormone (iPTH) level between 150 to 300 pg/mL.

Parathyroid carcinoma: Oral: Initial: 30 mg twice daily; increase dose incrementally (to 60 mg twice daily, 90 mg twice daily, and 90 mg 3 to 4 times daily) as necessary to normalize serum calcium levels.

Renal Impairment No dosage adjustment necessary.

Hepatic Impairment

Mild impairment (Child-Pugh class A): No dosage adjustment necessary.

Moderate to severe impairment (Child-Pugh class B or C); may have an increased exposure to cinacalcet and increased half-life. Dosage adjustments may be necessary based on serum calcium, serum phosphorus, and/or iPTH.

Adjustment for Toxicity Dosage adjustment for hypocalcemia:

If serum calcium >7.5 mg/dL but <8.4 mg/dL **or** if hypocalcemia symptoms occur: Use calcium-containing phosphate binders and/or vitamin D to raise calcium levels.

If serum calcium <7.5 mg/dL **or** if hypocalcemia symptoms persist and the dose of vitamin D cannot be increased: Withhold cinacalcet until serum calcium ≥8 mg/dL and/or symptoms of hypocalcemia resolve. Reinitiate cinacalcet at the next lowest dose.

If iPTH <150 pg/mL: Reduce dose or discontinue cinacalcet and/or vitamin D.

Administration Administer with food or shortly after a meal. Do not break or divide tablet; should be taken whole.

Monitoring Parameters

Monitor for signs/symptoms of hypocalcemia. Monitor serum calcium and iPTH concentrations closely in patients on concurrent CYP3A4 inhibitors, with hepatic impairment or with seizure disorders.

Hyperparathyroidism, secondary: Serum calcium and phosphorus levels prior to initiation and within a week of initiation and frequently during dose titration; iPTH should be measured 1 to 4 weeks after initiation or dosage adjustment (wait at least 12 hours after dose before drawing iPTH levels). After the maintenance dose is established, obtain serum calcium levels monthly.

Parathyroid carcinoma and hyperparathyroidism, primary: Serum calcium levels prior to initiation and within a week of initiation or dosage adjustment; once maintenance dose is established, obtain serum calcium every 2 months.

Dosage Forms Excipient information presented when available (limited, particularly for generics); consult specific product labeling.

Tablet, Oral:

Sensipar: 30 mg, 60 mg, 90 mg

◆ **Cinacalcet Hydrochloride** *see* Cinacalcet *on page 324*

◆ **Cipro** *see* Ciprofloxacin (Systemic) *on page 327*

◆ **Cipro XL (Can)** *see* Ciprofloxacin (Systemic) *on page 327*

Ciprofloxacin (Systemic) (sip roe FLOKS a sin)

Brand Names: US Cipro; Cipro in D5W; Cipro XR

◄ **Brand Names: Canada** ACT Ciprofloxacin; Apo-Ciproflox; Auro-Ciprofloxacin; Cipro; Cipro XL; Ciprofloxacin Injection; Ciprofloxacin Injection USP; Ciprofloxacin Intravenous Infusion; Ciprofloxacin Intravenous Infusion BP; Dom-Ciprofloxacin; JAMP-Ciprofloxacin; Mar-Ciprofloxacin; Mint-Ciproflox; Mint-Ciprofloxacin; Mylan-Ciprofloxacin; PHL-Ciprofloxacin; PMS-Ciprofloxacin; PMS-Ciprofloxacin XL; PRO-Ciprofloxacin; RAN-Ciprofloxacin; ratio-Ciprofloxacin; Riva-Ciprofloxacin; Sandoz-Ciprofloxacin; Septa-Ciprofloxacin; Taro-Ciprofloxacin; Teva-Ciprofloxacin

Index Terms Ciprofloxacin Hydrochloride; Proquin XR

Pharmacologic Category Antibiotic, Fluoroquinolone

Use

Children: Complicated urinary tract infections and pyelonephritis due to *E. coli*. **Note:** Although effective, ciprofloxacin is not the drug of first choice in children.

Children and Adults: To reduce incidence or progression of disease following exposure to aerolized *Bacillus anthracis*; prophylaxis and treatment of plague, including pneumonic and septicemic plague, due to *Yersinia pestis*.

Adults: Treatment of the following infections when caused by susceptible bacteria: Urinary tract infections; acute uncomplicated cystitis in females; chronic bacterial prostatitis; lower respiratory tract infections (including acute exacerbations of chronic bronchitis); acute sinusitis; skin and skin structure infections; bone and joint infections; complicated intra-abdominal infections (in combination with metronidazole); infectious diarrhea; typhoid fever due to *Salmonella typhi* (eradication of chronic typhoid carrier state has not been proven); uncomplicated cervical and urethra gonorrhea (due to *N. gonorrhoeae*); nosocomial pneumonia; empirical therapy for febrile neutropenic patients (in combination with piperacillin)

Note: As of April 2007, the CDC no longer recommends the use of fluoroquinolones for the treatment of gonococcal disease.

Pregnancy Risk Factor C

Dosing

Adult Note: Extended release tablets and immediate release formulations are not interchangeable. Unless otherwise specified, oral dosing reflects the use of immediate release formulations.

Anthrax:

Inhalational (postexposure prophylaxis):
Oral: 500 mg every 12 hours for 60 days
IV: 400 mg every 12 hours for 60 days

Cutaneous (treatment, CDC guidelines): Oral: Immediate release formulation: 500 mg every 12 hours for 60 days. **Note:** In the presence of systemic involvement, extensive edema, lesions on head/neck, refer to IV dosing for treatment of inhalational/gastrointestinal/oropharyngeal anthrax.

Inhalational/gastrointestinal/oropharyngeal (treatment, CDC guidelines): IV: 400 mg every 12 hours. **Note:** Initial treatment should include two or more agents predicted to be effective (per CDC recommendations). Continue combined therapy for 60 days.

Bacterial enteric infections in HIV-infected patients (empiric treatment) (off-label use; HHS [OI adult 2015]):
Oral: 500 to 750 mg every 12 hours
IV: 400 mg every 12 hours

Bite wounds (animal, human) (off-label use) (IDSA [Stevens 2014]):
Note: Recommended as an alternative therapy for human bite wound in patients hypersensitive to beta-lactams.
Oral: 500 to 750 mg twice daily; in combination with metronidazole
IV: 400 mg every 12 hours; in combination with metronidazole

Bone/joint infections:
Oral: 500 to 750 mg twice daily for 4 to 8 weeks
IV:
Mild/moderate: 400 mg every 12 hours for 4 to 8 weeks
Severe/complicated: 400 mg every 8 hours for 4 to 8 weeks

Chancroid (off-label use): Oral: 500 mg twice daily for 3 days (CDC 2010)

Cystitis, acute uncomplicated:
Oral, immediate release: 250 mg every 12 hours for 3 days
Oral, extended release (Cipro XR): 500 mg every 24 hours for 3 days

Endocarditis due to HACEK organisms (off-label use) (Baddour 2005):
Note: Not first-line option; use only if intolerant of beta-lactam therapy:
Oral: 500 mg every 12 hours for 4 weeks (native valve) or 6 weeks (prosthetic valve)
IV: 400 mg every 12 hours for 4 weeks (native valve) or 6 weeks (prosthetic valve)

Epididymitis, chlamydial (off-label use): Oral: 500 mg single dose (Canadian STI Guidelines 2008)

Febrile neutropenia: IV: 400 mg every 8 hours for 7 to 14 days (combination therapy with piperacillin generally recommended)

Gonococcal infections:
Urethral/cervical gonococcal infections: Oral: 250 to 500 mg as a single dose (CDC recommends concomitant doxycycline or azithromycin due to possible coinfection with *Chlamydia*); **Note:** As of April 2007, the CDC no longer recommends the use of fluoroquinolones for the treatment of uncomplicated gonococcal disease.

Granuloma inguinale (donovanosis) (off-label use): Oral: 750 mg twice daily for at least 3 weeks (and until lesions have healed) (CDC 2010)

Infectious diarrhea: Oral:
Salmonella: 500 mg twice daily for 5 to 7 days
Shigella (including Shigella dysentery type 1) (off-label regimen): 500 mg twice daily for 3 days (IDSA 2001)
Traveler's diarrhea (off-label regimen): Mild: 750 mg as a single dose (CDC 2012; de la Cabada Bauch 2011); Severe: 500 mg twice daily for 3 days (IDSA 2001)
Vibrio cholerae (off-label regimen): 1 g as a single (CDC 2011)

Infectious diarrhea due to *Salmonella, Shigella, or Campylobacter* in HIV-infected patients (off-label use; HHS [OI adult 2015]): Note: Patients with bacteremia due to *Campylobacter* should receive additional therapy with an aminoglycoside
Oral: 500 to 750 mg every 12 hours
IV: 400 mg every 12 hours)
Duration of therapy: Oral, IV:
Salmonella: Without bacteremia: 7 to 14 days (CD4 count ≥200 cells/mm^3) or 2 to 6 weeks (CD4 count <200 cells/mm^3); With bacteremia: 14 days or longer based on clinical condition (CD4 count ≥200 cells/mm^3) or 2 to 6 weeks (CD4 count <200 cells/mm^3)
Shigella or *Campylobacter:* Gastroenteritis: 7 to 10 days; Bacteremia: ≥14 days; Recurrent infections: *Campylobacter:* 2 to 6 weeks; *Shigella:* ≤6 weeks

Intra-abdominal, complicated, community-acquired (in combination with metronidazole): Note: Avoid using in settings where *E. coli* susceptibility to fluoroquinolones is <90%:

Oral: 500 mg every 12 hours for 7 to 14 days

IV: 400 mg every 12 hours for 7 to 14 days; **Note:** 2010 IDSA guidelines recommend treatment duration of 4 to 7 days (provided source controlled)

Lower respiratory tract:

Oral: 500 to 750 mg twice daily for 7 to 14 days

IV: 400 mg every 8 to 12 hours for 7 to 14 days

Meningococcal meningitis prophylaxis (off-label use): Oral: 500 mg as a single dose (CDC 2005)

Nosocomial pneumonia: IV: 400 mg every 8 hours for 10 to 14 days

Periodontitis (off-label use): Oral: 500 mg every 12 hours for 8 to 10 days (Rams 1992)

Plague:

Manufacturer's labeling:

Oral: 500 to 750 mg every 12 hours for 14 days

IV: 400 mg every 8 to 12 hours for 14 days

Alternate dosing:

Contained casualty management: IV: 400 mg twice daily for 10 days. Can switch to oral administration when clinically indicated (Bossi 2004; CDC [plague] 2012; Inglesby 2000).

Mass casualty management: Oral: 500 mg twice daily for 10 days (Inglesby 2000)

Mass casualty postexposure prophylaxis: Oral: 500 mg twice daily for 7 days (Bossi 2004; CDC [plague] 2012; Inglesby 2000).

Prostatitis (chronic, bacterial):

Oral: 500 mg every 12 hours for 28 days

IV: 400 mg every 12 hours for 28 days

Sinusitis (acute):

Oral: 500 mg every 12 hours for 10 days

IV: 400 mg every 12 hours for 10 days

Skin/skin structure infections:

Oral: 500 to 750 mg twice daily for 7 to 14 days

IV: Mild to moderate: 400 mg every 12 hours for 7 to 14 days; Severe/complicated: 400 mg every 8 hours for 7 to 14 days

Skin and soft tissue necrotizing infection due to *Aeromonas hydrophila* (off-label use): IV: 400 mg every 12 hours; in combination with doxycycline. Continue treatment until further debridement is not necessary, patient has clinically improved, and patient is afebrile for 48 to 72 hours (IDSA [Stevens 2014]).

Spontaneous bacterial peritonitis (prevention) (off-label use): Oral: Long-term prophylaxis: 500 mg once daily (preferred) (Terg 2008). Weekly dosing of 750 mg orally for long-term prophylaxis has been studied, but concerns regarding quinolone bacterial resistance limit use (AASLD [Runyon 2012]; Roulachon 1995). American Association for the Study of Liver Diseases (AASLD) guidelines note that intermittent dosing (ie, 5 days/week, weekly) of antibiotics, although shown to be effective in SBP prevention, may be inferior to daily dosing due to development of bacterial resistance. Daily dosing regimens are preferred (AASLD [Runyon 2012]).

Surgical (preoperative) prophylaxis (off-label use): IV: 400 mg within 120 minutes prior to surgical incision (Bratzler 2013)

Surgical site infection (intestinal or GU tract, perineum, or axilla) (off-label use) (IDSA [Stevens 2014]):
Oral: 750 mg every 12 hours, in combination with metronidazole
IV: 400 mg every 12 hours, in combination with metronidazole

Tularemia (off-label use):
Contained casualty management: IV: 400 mg twice daily for 10 days. Can switch to oral administration when clinically indicated (Dennis 2001).
Mass casualty management or postexposure prophylaxis: Oral: 500 or 750 mg twice daily for 14 days. At least 14 days of therapy is recommended in oral regimens (Bossi [tularemia] 2004; Dennis 2001; Stevens 2014).

Typhoid fever: Oral: 500 mg every 12 hours for 10 days

Urinary tract infection:
Oral, immediate release: 250 to 500 mg every 12 hours for 7 to 14 days
IV: 200 to 400 mg every 8 to 12 hours for 7 to 14 days

Urinary tract infection, complicated (including pyelonephritis): Oral, extended release (Cipro XR): 1000 mg every 24 hours for 7 to 14 days

Geriatric Refer to adult dosing. Adjust dose carefully based on renal function.

Pediatric Note: Extended release tablets and immediate release formulations are not interchangeable. Unless otherwise specified, oral dosing reflects the use of immediate release formulations.

Anthrax:
Inhalational (postexposure prophylaxis):
Oral: 15 mg/kg/dose every 12 hours for 60 days; maximum: 500 mg/dose
IV: 10 mg/kg/dose every 12 hours for 60 days; do **not** exceed 400 mg/dose (800 mg/day)
Cutaneous (treatment, CDC guidelines): Oral: 10 to 15 mg/kg every 12 hours for 60 days (maximum: 1000 mg/day); amoxicillin 80 mg/kg/day divided every 8 hours is an option for completion of treatment after clinical improvement. **Note:** In the presence of systemic involvement, extensive edema, lesions on head/neck, refer to IV dosing for treatment of inhalational/gastrointestinal/oropharyngeal anthrax.
Inhalational/gastrointestinal/oropharyngeal (treatment, CDC guidelines): IV: Initial: 10 to 15 mg/kg every 12 hours for 60 days (maximum: 500 mg/dose); switch to oral therapy when clinically appropriate; refer to adult dosing for notes on combined therapy and duration

Bacterial enteric infections in HIV-infected patients (empiric treatment) (off-label use): Adolescents: Refer to adult dosing

Community-acquired pneumonia (CAP) (IDSA/PIDS 2011): *H. influenzae,* moderate-to-severe infection (alternative to ampicillin, ceftriaxone, or cefotaxime): Infants >3 months and Children: IV: 30 mg/kg/day divided every 12 hours

Cystic fibrosis (off-label use): Children 5 to 17 years:
Oral: 40 mg/kg/day divided every 12 hours administered following 1 week of IV therapy has been reported in a clinical trial; total duration of therapy: 10 to 21 days (Rubio 1997)
IV: 30 mg/kg/day divided every 8 hours for 1 week, followed by oral therapy, has been reported in a clinical trial (Rubio 1997)

Infectious diarrhea due to *Salmonella*, *Shigella*, or *Campylobacter* in HIV-infected patients (off-label dose): Adolescents: Refer to adult dosing.

Shigella dysentery type 1 (off-label use): Oral: 30 mg/kg/day in 2 divided doses for 3 days (WHO 2005)

Plague:

Manufacturer's labeling: Infants, Children, and Adolescents:

Oral: 15 mg/kg/dose every 8 to 12 hours for 10 to 21 days; maximum: 500 mg/dose

IV: 10 mg/kg/dose every 8 to 12 hours for 10 to 21 days; maximum: 400 mg/dose

Alternate dosing: Children and Adolescents:

Contained casualty management: IV: 15 mg/kg twice daily for 10 days (maximum: 1000 mg/day). Can switch to oral administration when clinically indicated (CDC [plague] 2014; Inglesby 2000).

Mass casualty management: Oral: 20 mg/kg twice daily for 10 days (maximum: 1000 mg/day) (Inglesby 2000)

Mass casualty postexposure prophylaxis: Oral: 20 mg/kg twice daily for 7 days (maximum: 1000 mg/day) (CDC [plague] 2014; Inglesby 2000)

Surgical (preoperative) prophylaxis (off-label use): Children ≥1 year: IV: 10 mg/kg within 120 minutes prior to surgical incision (maximum: 400 mg/dose) (Bratzler 2013)

Urinary tract infection (complicated) or pyelonephritis: Children 1 to 17 years:

Oral: 20 to 40 mg/kg/day in 2 divided doses (every 12 hours) for 10 to 21 days; maximum: 1,500 mg/day. **Note:** 30 to 40 mg/kg/day reserved for severe infections (*Red Book* 2012).

IV: 6 to 10 mg/kg every 8 hours for 10 to 21 days (maximum: 400 mg/dose)

Renal Impairment Adults:

Manufacturer's labeling:

Oral, immediate release:

CrCl >50 mL/minute: No dosage adjustment necessary.

CrCl 30 to 50 mL/minute: 250 to 500 mg every 12 hours

CrCl 5 to 29 mL/minute: 250 to 500 mg every 18 hours

ESRD on intermittent hemodialysis (IHD)/peritoneal dialysis (PD) (administer after dialysis on dialysis days): 250 to 500 mg every 24 hours

Oral, extended release:

CrCl ≥30 mL/minute: No dosage adjustment necessary.

CrCl <30 mL/minute: 500 mg every 24 hours

ESRD on intermittent hemodialysis (IHD)/peritoneal dialysis (PD) (administer after dialysis on dialysis days): 500 mg every 24 hours

IV:

CrCl ≥30 mL/minute: No dosage adjustment necessary.

CrCl 5 to 29 mL/minute: 200 to 400 mg every 18 to 24 hours

Alternate recommendations: Oral (immediate release), IV:

CrCl >50 mL/minute: No dosage adjustment necessary (Aronoff 2007).

CrCl 10 to 50 mL/minute: Administer 50% to 75% of usual dose every 12 hours (Aronoff 2007).

CrCl <10 mL/minute: Administer 50% of usual dose every 12 hours (Aronoff 2007).

Intermittent hemodialysis (IHD) (administer after hemodialysis on dialysis days): Minimally dialyzable (<10%): Oral: 250 to 500 mg every 24 hours **or** IV: 200 to 400 mg every 24 hours (Heintz 2009). **Note:** Dosing dependent on the assumption of 3 times weekly, complete IHD sessions.

Continuous renal replacement therapy (CRRT) (Heintz 2009; Trotman 2005): Drug clearance is highly dependent on the method of renal replacement, filter type, and flow rate. Appropriate dosing requires close monitoring of pharmacologic response, signs of adverse reactions due to drug accumulation, as well as drug concentrations in relation to target trough (if appropriate). The following are general recommendations only (based on dialysate flow/ultrafiltration rates of 1 to 2 L/hour and minimal residual renal function) and should not supersede clinical judgment:

CVVH/CVVHD/CVVHDF: IV: 200 to 400 mg every 12 to 24 hours

Hepatic Impairment There are no dosage adjustments provided in manufacturer's labeling. Use with caution in severe impairment.

Additional Information Complete prescribing information should be consulted for additional detail.

Medication Guide Available Yes

Dosage Forms Excipient information presented when available (limited, particularly for generics); consult specific product labeling.

Solution, Intravenous:
Cipro in D5W: 200 mg/100 mL (100 mL) [latex free]
Generic: 200 mg/100 mL (100 mL); 400 mg/200 mL (200 mL); 200 mg/20 mL (20 mL); 400 mg/40 mL (40 mL)

Solution, Intravenous [preservative free]:
Cipro in D5W: 200 mg/100 mL (100 mL); 400 mg/200 mL (200 mL) [latex free]
Generic: 200 mg/100 mL (100 mL); 400 mg/200 mL (200 mL); 200 mg/20 mL (20 mL); 400 mg/40 mL (40 mL)

Suspension Reconstituted, Oral:
Cipro: 250 mg/5 mL (100 mL); 500 mg/5 mL (100 mL) [strawberry flavor]
Generic: 250 mg/5 mL (100 mL); 500 mg/5 mL (100 mL)

Tablet, Oral, as hydrochloride [strength expressed as base]:
Cipro: 250 mg, 500 mg
Generic: 100 mg, 250 mg, 500 mg, 750 mg

Tablet Extended Release 24 Hour, Oral, as base and hydrochloride [strength expressed as base]:
Cipro XR: 500 mg, 1000 mg
Generic: 500 mg, 1000 mg

◆ **Ciprofloxacin Hydrochloride** see Ciprofloxacin (Systemic) on page 327

◆ **Ciprofloxacin Injection (Can)** see Ciprofloxacin (Systemic) on page 327

◆ **Ciprofloxacin Injection USP (Can)** see Ciprofloxacin (Systemic) on page 327

◆ **Ciprofloxacin Intravenous Infusion (Can)** see Ciprofloxacin (Systemic) on page 327

◆ **Ciprofloxacin Intravenous Infusion BP (Can)** see Ciprofloxacin (Systemic) on page 327

◆ **Cipro in D5W** see Ciprofloxacin (Systemic) on page 327

◆ **Cipro XR** see Ciprofloxacin (Systemic) on page 327

◆ **cis-DDP** see CISplatin on page 334

◆ **cis-Diamminedichloroplatinum** see CISplatin on page 334

CISplatin (SIS pla tin)

Related Information

Chemotherapy and Obesity *on page 2220*

Chemotherapy-Induced Peripheral Neuropathy *on page 2116*

Fertility and Cancer Therapy *on page 2137*

Hematopoietic Stem Cell Transplantation *on page 2272*

Management of Chemotherapy-Induced Nausea and Vomiting in Adults *on page 2142*

Management of Drug Extravasations *on page 2159*

Prevention of Chemotherapy-Induced Nausea and Vomiting in Children *on page 2203*

Safe Handling of Hazardous Drugs *on page 2292*

Brand Names: Canada Cisplatin Injection; Cisplatin Injection BP; Cisplatin Injection, Mylan STD

Index Terms CDDP; cis-DDP; cis-Diamminedichloroplatinum; cis-platinum; DDP; Platinol; Platinol-AQ

Pharmacologic Category Antineoplastic Agent, Alkylating Agent; Antineoplastic Agent, Platinum Analog

Use

Bladder cancer, advanced: Treatment (as a single agent) of advanced bladder cancer (transitional cell) in patients who are no longer candidates for local therapy including surgery and/or radiation therapy

Ovarian cancer, metastatic: Treatment of metastatic ovarian cancer (in combination with other chemotherapy agents) in patients who have previously received appropriate surgery and/or radiation therapy, or as a single agent for refractory tumors in patients who have not previously received cisplatin

Testicular cancer, metastatic: Treatment of metastatic testicular cancer (in combination with other chemotherapy agents) in patients who have previously received appropriate surgery and/or radiation therapy

Labeled Contraindications History of allergic reactions to cisplatin, other platinum-containing compounds, or any component of the formulation; preexisting renal impairment; myelosuppressed patients; hearing impairment

Pregnancy Considerations Adverse effects have been observed in animal reproduction studies. Women of childbearing potential should be advised to avoid pregnancy during treatment. May case fetal harm if administered during pregnancy.

Breast-Feeding Considerations Cisplatin is excreted in breast milk. Breast-feeding is not recommended by the manufacturer.

Warnings/Precautions Hazardous agent - use appropriate precautions for handling and disposal (NIOSH 2014 [group 1]). **[US Boxed Warning]: Doses >100 mg/m²/cycle (once every 3 to 4 weeks) are rare; verify with the prescriber. Exercise caution to avoid inadvertent overdose due to potential sound-alike/look-alike confusion between CISplatin and CARBOplatin or prescribing practices that fail to differentiate daily doses from the total dose per cycle.** At the approved dose, cisplatin should not be administered more frequently than once every 3 to 4 weeks. Patients should receive adequate hydration, with or without diuretics, prior to and for 24 hours after cisplatin administration. **[US Boxed Warning]: Cumulative renal toxicity associated with cisplatin is severe.** Monitor serum creatinine, blood urea nitrogen, creatinine clearance, and serum electrolytes (calcium, magnesium, potassium, and sodium) closely. According to the manufacturer's labeling, use is contraindicated in patients with preexisting renal impairment and renal function must return to normal prior to administering subsequent cycles; some literature recommends reduced doses with renal impairment. Nephrotoxicity may be potentiated by aminoglycosides.

Use caution in the elderly; may cause or exacerbate syndrome of inappropriate antidiuretic hormone secretion or hyponatremia; monitor sodium closely with initiation or dosage adjustments in older adults (Beers Criteria). Elderly patients may be more susceptible to nephrotoxicity and peripheral neuropathy; select dose cautiously and monitor closely.

[US Boxed Warning]: Dose-related toxicities include myelosuppression, nausea, and vomiting. Cisplatin is associated with a high emetic potential; antiemetics are recommended to prevent nausea and vomiting (Basch, 2011; Dupuis, 2011; Roila, 2010). Nausea and vomiting are dose-related and may be immediate and/or delayed. Diarrhea may also occur. **[US Boxed Warning]: Ototoxicity, which may be more pronounced in children, is manifested by tinnitus and/or loss of high frequency hearing and occasionally, deafness; may be significant.** Ototoxicity is cumulative and may be severe. Audiometric testing should be performed at baseline and prior to each dose. Certain genetic variations in the thiopurine S-methyltransferase (TPMT) gene may be associated with an increased risk of ototoxicity in children administered conventional cisplatin doses (Pussegoda, 2013). Controversy may exist regarding the role of TPMT variants in cisplatin ototoxicity (Ratain, 2013; Yang, 2013); the association has not been consistent across populations and studies. Children without the TPMT gene variants may still be at risk for ototoxicity. Cumulative dose, prior or concurrent exposure to other ototoxic agents (eg, aminoglycosides, carboplatin), prior cranial radiation, younger age, and type of cancer may also increase the risk for ototoxicity in children (Knight, 2005; Landier, 2014). Pediatric patients should receive audiometric testing at baseline, prior to each dose, and for several years after discontinuing therapy. An international grading scale (SIOP Boston scale) has been developed to assess ototoxicity in children (Brock, 2012). Severe (and possibly irreversible) neuropathies (including stocking-glove paresthesias, areflexia, and loss of proprioception/vibratory sensation) may occur with higher than recommended doses or more frequent administration; may require therapy discontinuation. Seizures, loss of motor function, loss of taste, leukoencephalopathy, and posterior reversible leukoencephalopathy syndrome (PRES [formerly RPLS]) have also been described. Serum electrolytes, particularly magnesium and potassium, should be monitored and replaced as needed during and after cisplatin therapy.

[US Boxed Warning]: Anaphylactic-like reactions have been reported; may include facial edema, bronchoconstriction, tachycardia, and hypotension and may occur within minutes of administration; symptoms may be managed with epinephrine, corticosteroids, and/or antihistamines. Hyperuricemia has been reported with cisplatin use, and is more pronounced with doses >50 mg/m^2; consider antihyperuricemic therapy to reduce uric acid levels. Local infusion site reactions may occur; monitor infusion site during administration; avoid extravasation. Secondary malignancies have been reported with cisplatin in combination with other chemotherapy agents. Potentially significant drug-drug interactions may exist, requiring dose or frequency adjustment, additional monitoring, and/or selection of alternative therapy. **[US Boxed Warning]: Should be administered under the supervision of an experienced cancer chemotherapy physician. Adequate diagnostic and**

◀ **treatment facilities and appropriate management of potential complications should be readily available.** Cisplatin is a vesicant at higher concentrations, and an irritant at lower concentrations; ensure proper needle or catheter placement prior to and during infusion; avoid extravasation. Local infusion site reactions may occur; monitor infusion site during administration.

Adverse Reactions

>10%:

Central nervous system: Neurotoxicity (peripheral neuropathy is dose and duration dependent)

Gastrointestinal: Nausea and vomiting (76% to 100%)

Genitourinary: Nephrotoxicity (28% to 36%; acute renal failure and chronic renal insufficiency)

Hematologic & oncologic: Anemia (≤40%), leukopenia (25% to 30%; nadir: Day 18 to 23; recovery: By day 39; dose related), thrombocytopenia (25% to 30%; nadir: Day 18 to 23; recovery: By day 39; dose related)

Hepatic: Increased liver enzymes

Otic: Ototoxicity (children 40% to 60%; adults 10% to 31%; as tinnitus, high frequency hearing loss)

1% to 10%: Local: Local irritation

<1%, postmarketing, and/or case reports: Alopecia (mild), ageusia, anaphylaxis, aortic thrombosis (Fernandes 2011), autonomic neuropathy, bradycardia (Schlumbrecht 2015), bronchoconstriction, cardiac arrhythmia, cardiac failure, cerebral arteritis, cerebrovascular accident, dehydration, diarrhea, extravasation, heart block, hemolytic anemia (acute), hemolytic-uremic syndrome, hiccups, hypercholesterolemia, hyperuricemia, hypocalcemia, hypokalemia, hypomagnesemia, hyponatremia, hypophosphatemia, hypotension, increased serum amylase, ischemic heart disease, leukoencephalopathy, Lhermitte's sign, myocardial infarction, neutropenic enterocolitis (Furonaka 2005), optic neuritis, pancreatitis (Trivedi 2005), papilledema, peripheral ischemia (acute), phlebitis (Tokuda 2014), reversible posterior leukoencephalopathy syndrome, seizure, SIADH, skin rash, tachycardia, tetany, thrombotic thrombocytopenic purpura, vision color changes, vision loss

Drug Interactions

Metabolism/Transport Effects None known.

Avoid Concomitant Use

Avoid concomitant use of CISplatin with any of the following: BCG (Intravesical); CloZAPine; Dipyrone; Natalizumab; Pimecrolimus; Tacrolimus (Topical); Tofacitinib; Vaccines (Live)

Increased Effect/Toxicity

CISplatin may increase the levels/effects of: Aminoglycosides; CloZAPine; Fingolimod; Leflunomide; Natalizumab; Taxane Derivatives; Tofacitinib; Topotecan; Vaccines (Live); Vinorelbine

The levels/effects of CISplatin may be increased by: Denosumab; Dipyrone; Loop Diuretics; Pimecrolimus; Roflumilast; Tacrolimus (Topical); Trastuzumab

Decreased Effect

CISplatin may decrease the levels/effects of: BCG (Intravesical); Coccidioides immitis Skin Test; Fosphenytoin-Phenytoin; Sipuleucel-T; Vaccines (Inactivated); Vaccines (Live)

The levels/effects of CISplatin may be decreased by: Alpha-Lipoic Acid; Echinacea

Storage/Stability Store intact vials at 15°C to 25°C (59°F to 77°F). Protect from light. Do not refrigerate solution (precipitate may form). Further dilution **stability is dependent on the chloride ion concentration** and should be mixed in solutions of NS (at least 0.3% NaCl). According to the manufacturer, after initial entry into the vial, solution is stable for 28 days protected from light or for at least 7 days under fluorescent room light at room temperature.

Further dilutions in NS, D_5/0.45% NaCl or D_5/NS to a concentration of 0.05 to 2 mg/mL are stable for 72 hours at 4°C to 25°C.

Preparation for Administration Hazardous agent; use appropriate precautions for handling and disposal (NIOSH 2014 [group 1]). Must be diluted prior to infusion; dilute in NS, D_5/0.45% NaCl or D_5/NS to a concentration of 0.05 to 2 mg/mL. The infusion solution should have a final sodium chloride concentration ≥0.2%. Do **NOT** dilute in D_5W. Needles or IV administration sets that contain aluminum should not be used in the preparation or administration; aluminum can react with cisplatin resulting in precipitate formation and loss of potency.

Mechanism of Action Inhibits DNA synthesis by the formation of DNA cross-links; denatures the double helix; covalently binds to DNA bases and disrupts DNA function; may also bind to proteins; the *cis*-isomer is 14 times more cytotoxic than the *trans*-isomer; both forms cross-link DNA but cis-platinum is less easily recognized by cell enzymes and, therefore, not repaired. Cisplatin can also bind two adjacent guanines on the same strand of DNA producing intrastrand cross-linking and breakage.

Pharmacodynamics/Kinetics

Distribution: IV: Rapidly into tissue; high concentrations in kidneys, liver, ovaries, uterus, and lungs

Protein binding: >90% (O'Dwyer 2000)

Metabolism: Nonenzymatic; inactivated (in both cell and bloodstream) by sulfhydryl groups; covalently binds to glutathione and thiosulfate

Half-life elimination: Initial: 14 to 49 minutes; Beta: 0.7 to 4.6 hours; Gamma: 24 to 127 hours (O'Dwyer 2000)

Excretion: Urine (>90%); feces (minimal)

Dosing

Adult VERIFY ANY CISPLATIN DOSE EXCEEDING 100 mg/m² PER COURSE. Pretreatment hydration with 1 to 2 L of IV fluid is recommended. Cisplatin is associated with a high emetic potential; antiemetics are recommended to prevent nausea and vomiting (Basch 2011; Roila 2010).

Bladder cancer, advanced: IV: 50 to 70 mg/m² every 3 to 4 weeks; heavily pretreated patients: 50 mg/m² every 4 weeks

Ovarian cancer, metastatic: IV:

Single agent: 100 mg/m² every 4 weeks

Combination therapy: 75 to 100 mg/m² every 4 weeks or (off-label dosing) 75 mg/m² every 3 weeks (Ozols 2003)

Intraperitoneal (off-label route): 100 mg/m² on day 2 of a 21-day treatment cycle (in combination with IV and intraperitoneal paclitaxel) for 6 cycles (Armstrong 2006)

Testicular cancer, metastatic: IV: 20 mg/m²/day for 5 days repeated every 3 weeks (in combination with bleomycin and etoposide) (Cushing 2004; Saxman 1998)

CISPLATIN

Testicular germ cell tumor, malignant (off-label dosing): IV: 25 mg/m^2 on days 2 to 5 every 3 weeks (in combination with paclitaxel and ifosfamide) for 4 cycles (Kondagunta 2005) **or** 20 mg/m^2 on days 1 to 5 every 3 weeks (in combination with bleomycin and etoposide) for 4 cycles (Nichols 1998) **or** 20 mg/m^2 on days 1 to 5 every 3 weeks (in combination with etoposide and ifosfamide) for 4 cycles (Nichols 1998)

Breast cancer, triple-negative (off-label use): IV: Neoadjuvant therapy (single agent): 75 mg/m^2 on day 1 every 3 weeks for 4 cycles (Silver 2010). Additional data may be necessary to further define the role of cisplatin in this setting.

Cervical cancer (off-label use): IV: 75 mg/m^2 on day 1 every 3 weeks (in combination with fluorouracil and radiation) for 3 cycles (Morris 1999) **or** 70 mg/m^2 on day 1 every 3 weeks for 4 cycles (in combination with fluorouracil; cycles 1 and 2 given concurrently with radiation) (Peters 2000) **or** 50 mg/m^2 on day 1 every 4 weeks (in combination with radiation and fluorouracil) for 2 cycles (Whitney 1999)

Endometrial carcinoma, recurrent, metastatic, or high-risk (off-label use): IV: 50 mg/m^2 on day 1 every 3 weeks (in combination with doxorubicin ± paclitaxel) for 7 cycles or until disease progression or unacceptable toxicity (Fleming 2004)

Esophageal and gastric cancers (off-label uses): IV:

CF regimen: 100 mg/m^2 over 30 minutes on days 1 and 29 (preoperative chemoradiation; in combination with fluorouracil) (Tepper 2008)

ECF, ECX regimens: 60 mg/m^2 on day 1 every 21 days for up to 8 cycles in combination with epirubicin (E) and either fluorouracil (F) or capecitabine (X) (Cunningham 2008) **or**

ECF regimen: 60 mg/m^2 on day 1 every 21 days for 3 preoperative and 3 postoperative cycles in combination with epirubicin and fluorouracil (Cunningham 2006)

TCF or DCF regimen: 75 mg/m^2 on day 1 every 3 weeks (in combination with docetaxel and fluorouracil) until disease progression or unacceptable toxicity (Ajani 2007; Van Cutsem 2006)

Head and neck cancer (off-label use): IV:

Locally-advanced disease: 100 mg/m^2 every 3 weeks for 3 doses (with concurrent radiation) (Bernier 2004; Cooper 2004) **or** 75 mg/m^2 every 3 weeks (in combination with docetaxel and fluorouracil) for 4 cycles or until disease progression or unacceptable toxicity (if no disease progression after 4 cycles, chemotherapy was followed by radiation) (Vermorken 2007) **or** 100 mg/m^2 every 3 weeks (in combination with docetaxel and fluorouracil) for 3 cycles or until disease progression or unacceptable toxicity (chemotherapy was followed by chemoradiation) (Posner 2007)

Metastatic disease: 100 mg/m^2 every 3 weeks (in combination with fluorouracil and cetuximab) until disease progression or unacceptable toxicity or a maximum of 6 cycles (Vermorken 2008)

Hodgkin lymphoma, relapsed/refractory (off-label use): IV:

DHAP regimen: 100 mg/m^2 continuous infusion over 24 hours on day 1 for 2 cycles; median duration between cycle 1 and 2 was 16 days (in combination with dexamethasone and cytarabine) (Josting 2002)

ESHAP regimen: 25 mg/m^2/day on days 1 to 4 (in combination with etoposide, methylprednisolone, and cytarabine) every 3 to 4 weeks for 3 or 6 cycles (Aparicio 1999)

Malignant pleural mesothelioma (off-label use): IV: 75 mg/m^2 on day 1 of each 21-day cycle (in combination with pemetrexed) (Vogelzang 2003) **or** 100 mg/m^2 on day 1 of a 28-day cycle (in combination with gemcitabine)

(Nowak 2002) **or** 80 mg/m^2 on day 1 of a 21-day cycle (in combination with gemcitabine) (van Haarst 2002)

Multiple myeloma (off-label use): IV: VDT-PACE regimen: 10 mg/m^2/day administered as a continuous infusion on days 1 to 4 of each cycle; repeat every 4 to 6 weeks (in combination with bortezomib, dexamethasone, thalidomide, doxorubicin, cyclophosphamide, and etoposide) (Lee 2003; Pineda-Roman 2008)

Non-Hodgkin lymphoma, relapsed/refractory: IV:

DHAP regimen: 100 mg/m^2 continuous infusion over 24 hours on day 1 every 3 to 4 weeks for 6 to 10 cycles (in combination with dexamethasone and cytarabine) (Velasquez 1988)

ESHAP regimen: 25 mg/m^2/day continuous infusion over 24 hours on days 1 to 4 every 3 to 4 weeks for 6 to 8 cycles (in combination with etoposide, methylprednisolone, and cytarabine) (Velasquez 1994)

Non-small cell lung cancer (NSCLC; off-label use): IV: **Note:** There are multiple cisplatin-containing regimens for the treatment of NSCLC. Listed below are several commonly used regimens:

100 mg/m^2 on day 1 every 4 weeks (in combination with etoposide) for 3 to 4 cycles; (Arriagada 2007), or

100 mg/m^2 on day 1 every 4 weeks (in combination with vinorelbine) (Kelly 2001; Wozniak 1998), or

100 mg/m^2 on day 1 every 4 weeks (in combination with gemcitabine) (Comella 2000), or

80 mg/m^2 on day 1 every 3 weeks (in combination with gemcitabine) (Ohe 2007), or

75 mg/m^2 on day 1 every 3 weeks (in combination with pemetrexed) for up to 6 cycles or until disease progression or unacceptable toxicity (Scagliotti 2008)

Osteosarcoma (off-label use; combination chemotherapy): Adults <30 years: IV: 60 mg/m^2/day for 2 days on weeks 2, 7, 25, and 28 (neoadjuvant) or weeks 5, 10, 25, and 28 (adjuvant) in combination with methotrexate, leucovorin, doxorubicin, cyclophosphamide, bleomycin, and dactinomycin (Goorin 2003)

Penile cancer, metastatic (off-label use): IV: 25 mg/m^2 over 2 hours on days 1, 2, and 3 every 3 to 4 weeks (in combination with paclitaxel and ifosfamide) for 4 cycles (Pagliaro 2010)

Small cell lung cancer (SCLC; off-label use): IV:

Limited-stage disease: 60 mg/m^2 on day 1 every 3 weeks for 4 cycles (in combination with etoposide and concurrent radiation) (Turrisi 1999)

Extensive-stage disease: 80 mg/m^2 on day 1 every 3 weeks (in combination with etoposide) for 4 cycles (Lara 2009) or a maximum of 8 cycles (Ihde 1994) **or** 60 mg/m^2 on day 1 every 4 weeks for 4 cycles (in combination with irinotecan) (Lara 2009)

Geriatric Refer to adult dosing. Select dose cautiously and monitor closely in the elderly; may be more susceptible to nephrotoxicity and peripheral neuropathy.

Pediatric VERIFY ANY CISPLATIN DOSE EXCEEDING 100 mg/m^2 PER COURSE. Pretreatment hydration is recommended. Cisplatin is associated with a high emetic potential; antiemetics are recommended to prevent nausea and vomiting (Dupuis 2011).

Germ cell tumors (off-label use; combination chemotherapy): IV: 20 mg/m^2/day on days 1 to 5 or 100 mg/m^2 on day 1 of a 21-day treatment cycle (Pinkerton 1986)

◀ **Hepatoblastoma (off-label use; combination chemotherapy):** IV: 80 mg/m^2 continuous infusion over 24 hours on day 1 of a 21-day treatment cycle (Pritchard 2000)

Medulloblastoma (off-label use; combination chemotherapy): IV: 75 mg/m^2 on either day 0 or day 1 of each chemotherapy cycle (Packer 2006)

Neuroblastoma, high-risk (off-label use; combination chemotherapy): IV: 50 mg/m^2/day on days 0 to 3 of a 21-day cycle (cycles 3 and 5) (Naranjo 2011) **or** 50 mg/m^2/day on days 1 to 4 (cycles 3, 5, and 7) (Kushner 1994)

Osteosarcoma (off-label use; combination chemotherapy): IV: 60 mg/m^2/day for 2 days on weeks 2, 7, 25, and 28 (neoadjuvant) or weeks 5, 10, 25, and 28 (adjuvant) in combination with methotrexate, leucovorin, doxorubicin, cyclophosphamide, bleomycin, and dactinomycin (Goorin 2003)

Renal Impairment Note: The manufacturer(s) recommend that repeat courses of cisplatin should not be given until serum creatinine is <1.5 mg/dL and/or BUN is <25 mg/dL and use is contraindicated in preexisting renal impairment. The following adjustments have been recommended.

Aronoff 2007:

CrCl 10 to 50 mL/minute: Administer 75% of dose

CrCl <10 mL/minute: Administer 50% of dose

Hemodialysis: Partially cleared by hemodialysis

Administer 50% of dose posthemodialysis

Continuous ambulatory peritoneal dialysis (CAPD): Administer 50% of dose

Continuous renal replacement therapy (CRRT): Administer 75% of dose

Janus 2010: Hemodialysis: Reduce initial dose by 50%; administer post hemodialysis or on nondialysis days.

Kintzel 1995:

CrCl 46 to 60 mL/minute: Administer 75% of dose

CrCl 31 to 45 mL/minute: Administer 50% of dose

CrCl <30 mL/minute: Consider use of alternative drug

Hepatic Impairment There are no dosage adjustments provided in the manufacturer's labeling. However, cisplatin undergoes nonenzymatic metabolism and predominantly renal elimination; therefore, dosage adjustment is likely not necessary.

Obesity *ASCO Guidelines for appropriate chemotherapy dosing in obese adults with cancer:* Utilize patient's actual body weight (full weight) for calculation of body surface area- or weight-based dosing, particularly when the intent of therapy is curative; manage regimen-related toxicities in the same manner as for nonobese patients; if a dose reduction is utilized due to toxicity, consider resumption of full weight-based dosing with subsequent cycles, especially if cause of toxicity (eg, hepatic or renal impairment) is resolved (Griggs 2012).

Combination Regimens

Biliary adenocarcinoma: Gemcitabine-Cisplatin (Biliary Cancer) on page 1991

Bladder cancer:

Cisplatin-Docetaxel-Gemcitabine (Bladder) on page 1891

Cisplatin-Fluorouracil (Bladder Cancer) on page 1896

Cisplatin-Gemcitabine (Bladder) on page 1903

CMV (Bladder) on page 1920

Dose Dense MVAC (Bladder Cancer) on page 1948

MVAC (Bladder) on page 2042

PCG (Bladder) on page 2060

Administration Cisplatin is associated with a high emetic potential; antiemetics are recommended to prevent nausea and vomiting (Basch 2011; Dupuis 2011; Roila 2010). Pretreatment hydration with 1 to 2 L of fluid is recommended prior to cisplatin administration; adequate post hydration and urinary output (>100 mL/hour) should be maintained for 24 hours after administration.

IV: Infuse over 6 to 8 hours (according to the manufacturer's labeling); has also been infused (off-label rates) over 30 minutes to 3 hours, at a rate of 1 mg/minute, or as a continuous infusion; infusion rate varies by protocol (refer to specific protocol for infusion details). Do not administer as a rapid IV injection. Also refer to specific protocol for information regarding recommended concomitant hydration and diuretics.

Intraperitoneal (off-label route): Solution was prepared in warmed saline and infused as rapidly as possible through an implantable intraperitoneal catheter (Armstrong 2006).

Needles or IV administration sets that contain aluminum should not be used in the preparation or administration; aluminum may react with cisplatin resulting in precipitate formation and loss of potency.

Vesicant (at higher concentrations); ensure proper needle or catheter placement prior to and during infusion; avoid extravasation.

Extravasation management: If extravasation occurs, stop infusion immediately and disconnect (leave cannula/needle in place); gently aspirate extravasated solution (do **NOT** flush the line); initiate sodium thiosulfate antidote; elevate extremity.

Sodium thiosulfate 1/6 M solution: Inject 2 mL into existing IV line for each 100 mg of cisplatin extravasated; then consider also injecting 1 mL as 0.1 mL subcutaneous injections (clockwise) around the area of extravasation, may repeat subcutaneous injections several times over the next 3 to 4 hours (Ener 2004).

Dimethyl sulfoxide (DMSO) may also be considered an option: Apply to a region covering twice the affected area every 8 hours for 7 days; begin within 10 minutes of extravasation; do not cover with a dressing (Perez Fidalgo 2012).

Hazardous agent; use appropriate precautions for handling and disposal (NIOSH 2014 [group 1]).

Vesicant/Extravasation Risk Vesicant (>0.4 mg/mL); Irritant (≤0.4 mg/mL)

Emetic Potential Children and Adults: High (>90%)

Monitoring Parameters Renal function (serum creatinine, BUN, CrCl [baseline and before each cycle]); electrolytes (particularly calcium, magnesium, potassium, and sodium [baseline and before each cycle]); CBC with differential and platelet count (weekly); liver function tests (periodic); urine output, urinalysis; audiography (baseline and prior to each subsequent dose, and following treatment in children), neurologic exam (with high dose); monitor infusion site during infusion

Dietary Considerations Some products may contain sodium.

Dosage Forms Excipient information presented when available (limited, particularly for generics); consult specific product labeling.

Solution, Intravenous:

Generic: 50 mg/50 mL (50 mL); 100 mg/100 mL (100 mL)

Solution, Intravenous [preservative free]:

Generic: 50 mg/50 mL (50 mL); 100 mg/100 mL (100 mL); 200 mg/200 mL (200 mL)

- ◆ **Cisplatin Injection (Can)** *see* CISplatin *on page* 334
- ◆ **Cisplatin Injection BP (Can)** *see* CISplatin *on page* 334
- ◆ **Cisplatin Injection, Mylan STD (Can)** *see* CISplatin *on page* 334
- ◆ **cis-platinum** *see* CISplatin *on page* 334
- ◆ *Cis*-**Retinoic Acid** *see* ISOtretinoin *on page* 973
- ◆ **13-*cis*-Retinoic Acid** *see* ISOtretinoin *on page* 973
- ◆ **CIS-SULFUR COLLOID** *see* Technetium Tc 99m Sulfur Colloid *on page* 1602
- ◆ **13-*cis*-Vitamin A Acid** *see* ISOtretinoin *on page* 973
- ◆ **Citrovorum Factor** *see* Leucovorin Calcium *on page* 1023
- ◆ **CL-118,532** *see* Triptorelin *on page* 1703
- ◆ **CL-184116** *see* Porfimer *on page* 1409
- ◆ **CL-232315** *see* MitoXANtrone *on page* 1159

Cladribine (KLA dri been)

Related Information

Common Toxicity Criteria *on page* 2122
Management of Chemotherapy-Induced Nausea and Vomiting in Adults *on page* 2142
Management of Drug Extravasations *on page* 2159
Prevention of Chemotherapy-Induced Nausea and Vomiting in Children *on page* 2203
Safe Handling of Hazardous Drugs *on page* 2292

Brand Names: US Leustatin [DSC]
Brand Names: Canada Cladribine Injection
Index Terms 2-CdA; 2-Chlorodeoxyadenosine; Leustatin
Pharmacologic Category Antineoplastic Agent, Antimetabolite; Antineoplastic Agent, Antimetabolite (Purine Analog)
Use Treatment of active hairy cell leukemia
Labeled Contraindications Hypersensitivity to cladribine or any component of the formulation
Pregnancy Considerations Teratogenic effects and fetal mortality were observed in animal reproduction studies. May cause fetal harm if administered during pregnancy. Women of reproductive potential should use highly effective contraception during treatment.
Breast-Feeding Considerations Due to the potential for serious adverse reactions in the nursing infant, the decision to discontinue cladribine or to discontinue breast-feeding should take into account the importance of treatment to the mother.
Warnings/Precautions Hazardous agent - use appropriate precautions for handling and disposal (NIOSH 2014 [group 1]). **[U.S. Boxed Warning]: Dose-dependent, reversible myelosuppression (neutropenia, anemia, and thrombocytopenia) is common and generally reversible;** use with caution in patients with preexisting hematologic or immunologic abnormalities; monitor blood counts, especially during the first 4-8 weeks after treatment. **[U.S. Boxed Warning]: Serious, dose-related neurologic toxicity (including irreversible paraparesis and quadriparesis) has been reported with continuous infusions of higher doses (4-9 times the FDA-approved dose); may also occur at approved doses (rare).** Neurotoxicity may be delayed and may present as progressive, irreversible weakness; diagnostics with electromyography and nerve conduction studies were consistent with demyelinating

disease. **[U.S. Boxed Warning]: Acute nephrotoxicity (eg, acidosis, anuria, increased serum creatinine), possibly requiring dialysis, has been reported with high doses (4-9 times the FDA-approved dose), particularly when administered with other nephrotoxic agents.** Use with caution in patients with renal or hepatic impairment. Fever (>100°F) may occur, with or without neutropenia, observed more commonly in the first month of treatment. Infections (bacterial, viral, and fungal) were reported more commonly in the first month after treatment (generally mild or moderate in severity, although serious infections including sepsis have been reported); the incidence is reduced in the second month; due to neutropenia and T-cell depletion, risk versus benefit of treatment should be evaluated in patients with active infections. Administration of live vaccines is not recommended during treatment with cladribine (may increase the risk of infection due to immunosuppression). Use caution in patients with high tumor burden; tumor lysis syndrome may occur (rare). **[U.S. Boxed Warning]: Should be administered under the supervision of an experienced cancer chemotherapy physician.**

Benzyl alcohol and derivatives: Weekly (7-day) infusion preparation recommends further dilution with bacteriostatic normal saline which contains benzyl alcohol; large amounts of benzyl alcohol (≥99 mg/kg/day) have been associated with a potentially fatal toxicity ("gasping syndrome") in neonates; the "gasping syndrome" consists of metabolic acidosis, respiratory distress, gasping respirations, CNS dysfunction (including convulsions, intracranial hemorrhage), hypotension, and cardiovascular collapse (AAP ["Inactive" 1997]; CDC, 1982); some data suggests that benzoate displaces bilirubin from protein binding sites (Ahlfors, 2001); avoid or use dosage forms containing benzyl alcohol with caution in neonates. See manufacturer's labeling.

Adverse Reactions
>10%:
Central nervous system: Fever (33% to 69%; ≥100°F: 67%; ≥104°F: 11%), fatigue (11% to 45%), headache (7% to 22%)
Dermatologic: Rash (10% to 27%)
Gastrointestinal: Nausea (22% to 28%), appetite decreased (8% to 17%), vomiting (9% to 13%)
Hematologic: Neutropenia (grade 4: 70%; recovery: by week 5); anemia (1% to 37%; recovery: by week 8); myelosuppression (34%; prolonged), neutropenic fever (8% to 47%; severe: 32%), thrombocytopenia (grade 4: 12%; recovery: by day 12)
Local: Injection site reactions (9% to 19%)
Respiratory: Abnormal breath sounds (4% to 11%)
Miscellaneous: Infection (month 1: 28% [serious: 6%]; month 2: 6%)
1% to 10%:
Cardiovascular: Edema (2% to 6%), tachycardia (2% to 6%), thrombosis (2%)
Central nervous system: Chills (2% to 9%), dizziness (6% to 9%), insomnia (3% to 7%), malaise (5% to 7%), pain (6%), anxiety (1%)
Dermatologic: Purpura (10%), petechiae (2% to 8%), pruritus (2% to 6%), erythema (6%), hyperhidrosis (3%), bruising (1% to 2%)
Gastrointestinal: Diarrhea (7% to 10%), constipation (4% to 9%), abdominal pain (4% to 6%), flatulence (1%)
Local: Phlebitis (2%)
Neuromuscular & skeletal: Weakness (6% to 9%), myalgia (6% to 7%), arthralgia (3% to 5%), muscle weakness (1%)
Respiratory: Cough (7% to 10%), abnormal chest sounds (9%), dyspnea (5% to 7%), epistaxis (5%), rales (1%)

◀ Miscellaneous: Diaphoresis (9%)

<1%, postmarketing, and/or case reports: Aplastic anemia, bacteremia, bilirubin increased, CD4 lymphocytopenia (nadir: 4-6 months), cellulitis, consciousness decreased, confusion, conjunctivitis, hemolytic anemia, hypereosinophilia, hypersensitivity, myelodysplastic syndrome, opportunistic infections (cytomegalovirus, fungal infections, herpes virus infections, listeriosis, *Pneumocystis jirovecii*), pancytopenia (prolonged), paraparesis, pneumonia, polyneuropathy (with high doses), progressive multifocal leukoencephalopathy (PML), pulmonary interstitial infiltrates, quadriparesis (reported at high doses), renal dysfunction (with high doses), renal failure, septic shock, Stevens-Johnson syndrome, stroke, toxic epidermal necrolysis, transaminases increased, tuberculosis reactivation, tumor lysis syndrome, urticaria

Drug Interactions

Metabolism/Transport Effects None known.

Avoid Concomitant Use

Avoid concomitant use of Cladribine with any of the following: BCG (Intravesical); CloZAPine; Dipyrone; Natalizumab; Pimecrolimus; Tacrolimus (Topical); Tofacitinib; Vaccines (Live)

Increased Effect/Toxicity

Cladribine may increase the levels/effects of: CloZAPine; Fingolimod; Leflunomide; Natalizumab; Tofacitinib; Vaccines (Live)

The levels/effects of Cladribine may be increased by: Denosumab; Dipyrone; Pimecrolimus; Roflumilast; Tacrolimus (Topical); Trastuzumab

Decreased Effect

Cladribine may decrease the levels/effects of: BCG (Intravesical); Coccidioides immitis Skin Test; Sipuleucel-T; Vaccines (Inactivated); Vaccines (Live)

The levels/effects of Cladribine may be decreased by: Echinacea

Storage/Stability

Store intact vials refrigerated at 2°C to 8°C (36°F to 46°F). Protect from light. A precipitate may develop at low temperatures and may be resolubilized at room temperature or by shaking the solution vigorously. Inadvertent freezing does not affect the solution; if freezing occurs prior to dilution, allow to thaw naturally prior to reconstitution; do not heat or microwave; do not refreeze.

24-hour continuous infusion: Dilutions for infusion should be used promptly; if not used promptly, the 24-hour infusion may be stored refrigerated for up to 8 hours prior to administration.

7-day continuous infusion: Dilutions for infusion should be used promptly; if not used promptly, the 7-day infusion may be stored refrigerated for up to 8 hours prior to administration. Reconstituted solution is stable for 7 days (when diluted in bacteriostatic NS) in a CADD® medication cassette reservoir. For patients weighing >85 kg, the effectiveness of the preservative in the bacteriostatic diluent may be reduced (due to dilution).

Preparation for Administration Hazardous agent; use appropriate precautions for handling and disposal (NIOSH 2014 [group 1]).

A precipitate may develop at low temperatures and may be resolubilized at room temperature or by shaking the solution vigorously. Inadvertent freezing does not affect the solution; if freezing occurs prior to dilution, allow to thaw naturally; do not heat or microwave; do not refreeze.

To prepare a 24-hour continuous infusion: Dilute in 500 mL NS. The manufacturer recommends filtering with a 0.22 micron hydrophilic syringe filter prior to adding to infusion bag.

To prepare a 7-day continuous infusion: Dilute to a total volume of 100 mL in a CADD medication cassette reservoir using bacteriostatic NS. Filter diluent and cladribine with a 0.22 micron hydrophilic filter prior to adding to cassette/reservoir.

Mechanism of Action A purine nucleoside analogue; prodrug which is activated via phosphorylation by deoxycytidine kinase to a 5'-triphosphate derivative (2-CdAMP). This active form incorporates into DNA to result in the breakage of DNA strand and shutdown of DNA synthesis and repair. This also results in a depletion of nicotinamide adenine dinucleotide and adenosine triphosphate (ATP). Cladribine is cell-cycle nonspecific.

Pharmacodynamics/Kinetics

Distribution: V_d: ~9 L/kg; penetrates CSF (CSF concentrations are ~25% of plasma concentrations)

Protein binding: ~20%

Half-life elimination: After a 2-hour infusion (with normal renal function): 5.4 hours

Excretion: Urine (18%)

Dosing

Adult & Geriatric Details concerning dosing in combination regimens should also be consulted.

Hairy cell leukemia: IV: 0.09 mg/kg/day continuous infusion for 7 days for 1 cycle **or** (off-label dosing) 0.1 mg/kg/day continuous infusion for 7 days for 1 cycle (Goodman, 2003; Saven, 1998)

Acute myeloid leukemia, induction (off-label use): IV: CLAG or CLAG-M regimen: 5 mg/m²/day over 2 hours for 5 days; a second induction may be administered if needed (Robak, 2000; Wierzbowska, 2008; Wrzesień-Kuś, 2003)

Chronic lymphocytic leukemia (off-label use): IV: 0.1 mg/kg/day continuous infusion for 7 days every 4-5 weeks (Saven, 1995) **or** 0.14 mg/kg/day over 2 hours for 5 days every 28 days for 3-6 cycles (Byrd, 2003)

Mantle cell lymphoma (off-label use): IV: 5 mg/m²/day over 2 hours for 5 days every 4 weeks for 2-6 cycles (Inwards, 2008; Rummel, 1999) **or** 5 mg/m²/day over 2 hours for 5 days every 4 weeks for 2-6 cycles (in combination with rituximab) (Inwards, 2008)

Waldenström's macroglobulinemia (off-label use):

IV: 0.1 mg/kg/day continuous infusion for 7 days every 4 weeks for 2 cycles (Dimopoulos, 1994)

SubQ: 0.1 mg/kg/day for 5 consecutive days every month for 4 cycles (in combination with rituximab) (Laszlo, 2010)

Pediatric

Acute myeloid leukemia (off-label use): IV: 8.9 mg/m²/day continuous infusion for 5 days for 1 or 2 courses (Krance, 2001) **or** 9 mg/m²/day over 30 minutes for 5 days for 1 course (in combination with cytarabine) (Crews, 2002; Rubnitz, 2009)

Langerhans cell histiocytosis, refractory (off-label use): IV: 5 mg/m²/day over 2 hours for 5 days every 21 days for up to 6 cycles (Weitzman, 2009)

◀ **Renal Impairment** No dosage adjustment provided in the manufacturer's labeling (due to inadequate data); use with caution. The following adjustments have been used (Aronoff, 2007):

Adults:

CrCl 10-50 mL/minute: Administer 75% of dose

CrCl <10 mL/minute: Administer 50% of dose

Continuous ambulatory peritoneal dialysis (CAPD): Administer 50% of dose

Children:

CrCl 10-50 mL/minute: Administer 50% of dose

CrCl <10 mL/minute: Administer 30% of dose

Hemodialysis: Administer 30% of dose

Continuous renal replacement therapy (CRRT): Administer 50% of dose

Hepatic Impairment No dosage adjustment provided in the manufacturer's labeling (due to inadequate data); use with caution.

Obesity ASCO Guidelines for appropriate chemotherapy dosing in obese adults with cancer: Utilize patient's actual body weight (full weight) for calculation of body surface area- or weight-based dosing, particularly when the intent of therapy is curative; manage regimen-related toxicities in the same manner as for nonobese patients; if a dose reduction is utilized due to toxicity, consider resumption of full weight-based dosing with subsequent cycles, especially if cause of toxicity (eg, hepatic or renal impairment) is resolved (Griggs, 2012).

Combination Regimens

Leukemia, acute myeloid:

CLAG (AML Induction) on page 1916

CLAG-M (AML Induction) on page 1917

Lymphoma, non-Hodgkin (Mantle Cell): Cladribine-Rituximab (NHL-Mantle Cell) on page 1916

Waldenstrom Macroglobulinemia: Cladribine-Rituximab (Waldenstrom Macroglobulinemia) on page 1916

Administration

IV: Administer as a continuous infusion. May also be administered over 30 minutes or over 2 hours (off-label administration rates) depending on indication and/or protocol.

SubQ (off-label route): May also be administered SubQ (Laszlo, 2010)

Hazardous agent; use appropriate precautions for handling and disposal (NIOSH 2014 [group 1]).

Vesicant/Extravasation Risk May be an irritant.

Emetic Potential Children and Adults: Minimal (<10%)

Monitoring Parameters CBC with differential (particularly during the first 4-8 weeks post-treatment), renal and hepatic function; bone marrow biopsy (after CBC has normalized, to confirm treatment response); monitor for fever; monitor for signs/symptoms of neurotoxicity

Dosage Forms Excipient information presented when available (limited, particularly for generics); consult specific product labeling. [DSC] = Discontinued product

Solution, Intravenous:

Leustatin: 1 mg/mL (10 mL [DSC])

Generic: 1 mg/mL (10 mL [DSC])

Solution, Intravenous [preservative free]:

Generic: 1 mg/mL (10 mL)

◆ **Cladribine Injection (Can)** see Cladribine on page 344

Clodronate (KLOE droh nate)

Brand Names: Canada Bonefos; Clasteon

Index Terms Clodronate Disodium

Pharmacologic Category Bisphosphonate Derivative

Use Note: Not approved in the US

Hypercalcemia of malignancy: Management of hypercalcemia of malignancy

Osteolytic bone metastases: Management of osteolysis due to bone metastases of malignancy

Dosing

Adult & Geriatric

Hypercalcemia of malignancy:

IV:

Clasteon

Single infusion: 1,500 mg as a single dose

Multiple infusions: 300 mg once daily; treatment duration should not exceed 10 days

Bonefos: Multiple infusions: 300 mg once daily; treatment duration should not exceed 7 days

Oral: Recommended daily maintenance dose following calcium normalization with IV therapy:

Clasteon: Range: 1,600 mg (4 capsules) to 2,400 mg (6 capsules) given in a single dose or in 2 divided doses; maximum recommended daily dose: 3,200 mg (8 capsules).

Bonefos: Range: 1,600 mg (4 capsules) to 2,400 mg (6 capsules) given in a single dose or in 2 divided doses; maximum recommended daily dose: 3,200 mg (8 capsules).

Osteolytic bone metastases:

IV:

Clasteon:

Single infusion: 1,500 mg as a single dose

Multiple infusions: 300 mg once daily; treatment duration should not exceed 10 days

Bonefos: Multiple infusions: 300 mg once daily; treatment duration should not exceed 7 days

Oral:

Clasteon: Recommended daily maintenance dose following IV therapy: Range: 1,600 mg (4 capsules) to 2,400 mg (6 capsules) given in a single dose or in 2 divided doses; maximum recommended daily dose: 3,200 mg (8 capsules).

Bonefos: Initial: 1,600 mg/day; may be increased to a maximum of 3,200 mg/day

Note: Retreatment: Limited data suggest that patients who develop hypercalcemia following discontinuation of therapy or during oral therapy may be retreated with Bonefos or Clasteon at a higher oral dosage (up to 3,200 mg/day) or by IV infusion with Clasteon (1,500 mg as single dose or 300 mg once daily) or Bonefos (300 mg once daily).

◀ **Renal Impairment**
Clasteon:
Serum creatinine (S_{cr}) >5 mg/dL: Use is contraindicated.
S_{cr} ≥2.5 to 5 mg/dL: There are no specific dosage adjustments provided in manufacturer's labeling; however, the manufacturer recommends considering a dose reduction or withholding therapy.
Bonefos: **Note:** S_{cr} >5 mg/dL: Use is contraindicated.
IV:
CrCl: 50 to 80 mL/minute: Administer 75% to 100% of normal dose.
CrCl: 12 to 49 mL/minute: Administer 50% to 75% of normal dose.
CrCl: <12 mL/minute: Administer 50% of normal dose.
Oral: **Note:** Daily doses >1,600 mg should not be used continuously.
CrCl: >50 mL/minute: No dosage adjustment necessary.
CrCl: 30 to 50 mL/minute: Administer 75% of normal dose.
CrCl: <30 mL/minute: Administer 50% of normal dose.
Hepatic Impairment There are no dosage adjustments provided in the manufacturer's labeling; however, elimination is predominantly renal.
Additional Information Complete prescribing information should be consulted for additional detail.
Product Availability Not available in the US
Dosage Forms: Canada Excipient information presented when available (limited, particularly for generics); consult specific product labeling.
Capsule, oral:
Bonefos, Clasteon: 400 mg
Injection, solution:
Bonefos: 60 mg/mL (5 mL)
Clasteon: 30 mg/mL (10 mL)

◆ **Clodronate Disodium** see Clodronate on page 349

Clofarabine (klo FARE a been)
Related Information
Chemotherapy and Obesity on page 2220
Common Toxicity Criteria on page 2122
Management of Chemotherapy-Induced Nausea and Vomiting in Adults on page 2142
Prevention and Management of Infections on page 2196
Prevention of Chemotherapy-Induced Nausea and Vomiting in Children on page 2203
Safe Handling of Hazardous Drugs on page 2292
Brand Names: US Clolar
Brand Names: Canada Clolar
Index Terms CAFdA; Clofarex
Pharmacologic Category Antineoplastic Agent, Antimetabolite; Antineoplastic Agent, Antimetabolite (Purine Analog)
Use Acute lymphoblastic leukemia: Treatment of relapsed or refractory acute lymphoblastic leukemia (ALL) in patients 1 to 21 years of age (after at least 2 prior regimens)
Labeled Contraindications There are no contraindications listed in the manufacturer's U.S. labeling.

Canadian labeling: Hypersensitivity to clofarabine or any component of the formulation; symptomatic CNS involvement; history of serious heart, liver, kidney, or pancreas disease; severe hepatic impairment (AST and/or ALT >5 x ULN, and/or bilirubin >3 x ULN); severe renal impairment (CrCl <30 mL/minute)

Pregnancy Considerations Adverse events were observed in animal reproduction studies. May cause fetal harm if administered to a pregnant woman. Women of childbearing potential should be advised to use effective contraception and avoid becoming pregnant during therapy.

Breast-Feeding Considerations It is not known if clofarabine is excreted in breast milk. Due to the potential for serious adverse reactions in the nursing infant, breast-feeding should be avoided during clofarabine treatment.

Warnings/Precautions Hazardous agent - use appropriate precautions for handling and disposal (NIOSH 2014 [group 1]). Cytokine release syndrome (eg, tachypnea, tachycardia, hypotension, pulmonary edema) may develop into capillary leak syndrome, systemic inflammatory response syndrome (SIRS), and organ dysfunction; discontinue with signs/symptoms of SIRS or capillary leak syndrome (rapid onset respiratory distress, hypotension, pleural/pericardial effusion, and multiorgan failure) and consider supportive treatment with diuretics, corticosteroids, and/or albumin. Prophylactic corticosteroids may prevent or diminish the signs/symptoms of cytokine release. May require dosage reduction. Monitor blood pressure during 5 days of treatment; discontinue if hypotension develops. Monitor if on concurrent medications known to affect blood pressure. Dose-dependent, reversible myelosuppression (neutropenia, thrombocytopenia, and anemia) is common; may be severe and prolonged. Monitor blood counts and platelets. May be at increased risk for infection due to neutropenia; opportunistic infection or sepsis (may be severe or fatal) is increased due to prolonged neutropenia and immunocompromised state; monitor for signs and symptoms of infection and treat promptly if infection develops. May require therapy discontinuation. Serious and fatal hemorrhages (including cerebral, gastrointestinal, and pulmonary hemorrhage) have occurred, usually associated with thrombocytopenia. Monitor and manage coagulation parameters.

Serious and fatal cases of Stevens-Johnson syndrome (SJS) and toxic epidermal necrolysis (TEN) have been reported. Discontinue clofarabine for exfoliative or bullous rash, or if SJS or TEN are suspected. Clofarabine is associated with a moderate emetic potential; antiemetics are recommended to prevent nausea and vomiting (Basch, 2011; Dupuis, 2011; Roila, 2010). Serious and fatal enterocolitis (including neutropenic colitis, cecitis, and *C. difficile* colitis) has been reported, usually occurring within 30 days of treatment, and when used in combination with other chemotherapy. May lead to complication including necrosis, perforation, hemorrhage or sepsis. Monitor for signs/symptoms of enterocolitis and manage promptly.

Has not been studied in patients with hepatic impairment; use with caution (per manufacturer's labeling). Canadian labeling contraindicates use in severe impairment or in patients with a history of serious hepatic disease. Transaminases and bilirubin may be increased during treatment; transaminase elevations generally occur within 10 days of administration and persist for ≤15 days. In some cases, hepatotoxicity was severe and fatal. The risk for hepatotoxicity, including hepatic sinusoidal obstruction syndrome (SOS; formerly called veno-occlusive disease), is increased in patients who have previously undergone a hematopoietic stem cell transplant. Monitor liver function closely; may require therapy interruption or discontinuation; discontinue if SOS is suspected. Elevated creatinine, acute renal failure, and hematuria were observed in clinical studies. Monitor renal function closely; may require dosage reduction or therapy discontinuation. A pharmacokinetic study demonstrated that systemic exposure increases as creatinine clearance decreases (CrCl <60 mL/minute) (Bonate, 2011). Dosage reduction required for moderate renal impairment (CrCl 30-60 mL/minute); use with caution in patients with CrCl <30 mL/minute (has not been studied). Canadian labeling contraindicates use in severe impairment or in patients with a history of serious kidney disease. Minimize the use of drugs known to cause renal toxicity during the 5-day treatment period; avoid concomitant hepatotoxic medications. Tumor lysis syndrome/hyperuricemia may occur as a consequence of leukemia treatment, including treatment with clofarabine, usually occurring in the first treatment cycle. May lead to life-threatening acute renal failure; adequate hydration and prophylactic antihyperuricemic therapy throughout treatment will reduce the risk/effects of tumor lysis syndrome; monitor closely. Potentially significant drug-drug interactions may exist, requiring dose or frequency adjustment, additional monitoring, and/or selection of alternative therapy.

Adverse Reactions

>10%:

Cardiovascular: Tachycardia (35%), hypotension (29%; grade 3: 11%; grade 4: 8%), flushing (19%), hypertension (13%), edema (12%)

Central nervous system: Headache (43%), chills (34%), fatigue (34%), anxiety (21%), pain (15%)

Dermatologic: Pruritus (43%), skin rash (38%), palmar-plantar erythrodysesthesia (16%), erythema (11%)

Gastrointestinal: Vomiting (78%; grades 3/4: 9%), nausea (73%; grades 3/4: 15%), diarrhea (56%), abdominal pain (8% to 35%), anorexia (30%), gingival bleeding (17%), mucosal inflammation (16%), oral candidiasis (11%)

Genitourinary: Hematuria (13%)

Hematologic & oncologic: Leukopenia (grades 3/4: 88%), anemia (83%; grades 3/4: 75%), lymphocytopenia (grades 3/4: 82%), thrombocytopenia (81%; grades 3/4: 80%), neutropenia (grades 3/4: 10% to 64%), febrile neutropenia (55%; grades 3/4: 54%), petechia (26%)

Hepatic: Increased serum ALT (81%; grades 3/4: 43% to 44%), increased serum AST (74%; grades 3/4: 36%), increased bilirubin (45%; grades 3/4: 13%)

Infection: Infection (83%; includes bacterial, fungal, and viral), sepsis (including septic shock; 17%),

Local: Catheter infection (12%)

Neuromuscular & skeletal: Limb pain (30%), myalgia (14%)

Renal: Creatinine increased (50%; grades 3/4: 8%)

Respiratory: Epistaxis (27%), dyspnea (13%), pleural effusion (12%)

Miscellaneous: Fever (39%)

1% to 10%:

Cardiovascular: Pericardial effusion (8%), capillary leak syndrome (4%), hepatic veno-occlusive disease (2%)

Central nervous system: Drowsiness (10%), irritability (10%), lethargy (10%), agitation (5%), mental status changes (1% to 4%)

Dermatologic: Cellulitis (8%), pruritic rash (8%)

Gastrointestinal: Rectal pain (8%), pseudomembranous colitis (7%), stomatitis (7%), pancreatitis (1% to 4%), typhlitis (1% to 4%)

Hematologic & oncologic: Tumor lysis syndrome (grade 3: 6%), oral mucosal petechiae (5%)

Hepatic: Jaundice (8%), hyperbilirubinemia (1% to 4%; grade 4: 2%)

Hypersensitivity: Hypersensitivity (1% to 4%)

Infection: Herpes simplex infection (10%), bacteremia (9%), candidiasis (7%), herpes zoster (7%), staphylococcal bacteremia (6%), staphylococcal sepsis (5%), sepsis syndrome (2%)

Neuromuscular & skeletal: Back pain (10%), ostealgia (10%), weakness (10%), arthralgia (9%)

Respiratory: Pneumonia (10%), respiratory distress (10%), tachypnea (9%), upper respiratory tract infection (5%), pulmonary edema (1% to 4%)

<1%, postmarketing, and/or case reports: Bone marrow failure, confusion, enterocolitis (occurs more frequently within 30 days of treatment and with combination chemotherapy), exfoliative dermatitis, gastrointestinal hemorrhage, hallucination (Jeha, 2006), hepatomegaly (Jeha, 2006), hypokalemia (Jeha, 2006), hyponatremia, hypophosphatemia, increased right ventricular pressure (Jeha, 2006), left ventricular systolic dysfunction (Jeha, 2006), major hemorrhage (including cerebral and pulmonary; majority of cases associated with thrombocytopenia), pancytopenia, Stevens-Johnson syndrome, syncope, toxic epidermal necrolysis

Drug Interactions

Metabolism/Transport Effects None known.

Avoid Concomitant Use

Avoid concomitant use of Clofarabine with any of the following: BCG (Intravesical); CloZAPine; Dipyrone; Natalizumab; Pimecrolimus; Tacrolimus (Topical); Tofacitinib; Vaccines (Live)

Increased Effect/Toxicity

Clofarabine may increase the levels/effects of: CloZAPine; Fingolimod; Leflunomide; Natalizumab; Tofacitinib; Vaccines (Live)

The levels/effects of Clofarabine may be increased by: Denosumab; Dipyrone; Pimecrolimus; Roflumilast; Tacrolimus (Topical); Trastuzumab

Decreased Effect

Clofarabine may decrease the levels/effects of: BCG (Intravesical); Coccidioides immitis Skin Test; Sipuleucel-T; Vaccines (Inactivated); Vaccines (Live)

The levels/effects of Clofarabine may be decreased by: Echinacea

Storage/Stability Store intact vials at room temperature of 25°C (77°F); excursions permitted to 15°C to 30°C (59°F to 86°F). Solutions diluted for infusion in D$_5$W or NS may be stored for 24 hours at room temperature.

Preparation for Administration Hazardous agent; use appropriate precautions for handling and disposal (NIOSH 2014 [group 1]). Clofarabine should be diluted with NS or D$_5$W to a final concentration of 0.15 to 0.4 mg/mL. Manufacturer recommends the product be filtered through a 0.2 micron filter prior to dilution.

Mechanism of Action Clofarabine, a purine (deoxyadenosine) nucleoside analog, is metabolized to clofarabine 5'-triphosphate. Clofarabine 5'-triphosphate decreases cell replication and repair as well as causing cell death. To decrease cell replication and repair, clofarabine 5'-triphosphate competes with deoxyadenosine triphosphate for the enzymes ribonucleotide reductase and DNA polymerase. Cell replication is decreased when clofarabine 5'-triphosphate inhibits ribonucleotide reductase from reacting with deoxyadenosine triphosphate to produce deoxynucleotide triphosphate which is needed for ▶

DNA synthesis. Cell replication is also decreased when clofarabine 5'-triphosphate competes with DNA polymerase for incorporation into the DNA chain; when done during the repair process, cell repair is affected. To cause cell death, clofarabine 5'-triphosphate alters the mitochondrial membrane by releasing proteins, an inducing factor and cytochrome C.

Pharmacodynamics/Kinetics

Distribution: V_d: Children: 172 L/m^2 or 5.8 L/kg (Bonate, 2011); Elderly: 268 L/kg (Bonate, 2011)

Protein binding: 47%, primarily to albumin

Metabolism: Intracellulary by deoxycytidine kinase and mono- and diphosphokinases to active metabolite clofarabine 5'-triphosphate; limited hepatic metabolism (0.2%)

Half-life elimination: Children: ~5 hours; Children and Adults: 7 hours (Bonate, 2011)

Excretion: Urine (49% to 60%, as unchanged drug)

Dosing

Adult Note: Consider prophylactic corticosteroids (hydrocortisone 100 mg/m^2 on days 1 to 3) to prevent signs/symptoms of capillary leak syndrome or systemic inflammatory response syndrome (SIRS), and hydration and antihyperuricemic therapy (to reduce the risk of tumor lysis syndrome/hyperuricemia). Calculate body surface area (BSA) prior to each cycle, utilizing actual body weight. Clofarabine is associated with a moderate emetic potential; antiemetics are recommended to prevent nausea and vomiting (Basch, 2011; Roila, 2010).

Acute lymphoblastic leukemia (ALL) relapsed or refractory: Adults ≤21 years: IV: 52 mg/m^2/day days 1 through 5; repeat every 2 to 6 weeks; subsequent cycles should begin no sooner than 14 days from day 1 of the previous cycle (subsequent cycles may be administered when ANC ≥750/mm^3)

Acute lymphoblastic leukemia, relapsed/refractory (ALL; off-label population): IV:

Induction: 40 mg/m^2 once daily for 5 days; may repeat induction cycle once in 3 to 6 weeks if needed (depending on marrow response and recovery) (Kantarjian, 2003)

Consolidation: 30 mg/m^2 once daily for 5 days (or last tolerated induction dose, whichever is lower); repeat every 4 weeks for up to a maximum of 6 consolidation cycles (Kantarjian, 2003)

Acute myeloid leukemia (AML), refractory (off-label use): Adults <70 years: IV:

Induction: 25 mg/m^2/day for 5 days (in combination with cytarabine and filgrastim) may repeat one time after 21 days if needed (Becker, 2011)

Consolidation: 20 mg/m^2/day for 5 days (in combination with cytarabine and filgrastim) for 1 or 2 cycles (Becker, 2011)

Pediatric Note: Consider prophylactic corticosteroids (hydrocortisone 100 mg/m^2 on days 1 to 3) to prevent signs/symptoms of capillary leak syndrome or systemic inflammatory response syndrome (SIRS), and hydration and antihyperuricemic therapy (to reduce the risk of tumor lysis syndrome/hyperuricemia). Calculate body surface area (BSA) prior to each cycle, utilizing actual body weight. Clofarabine is associated with a moderate emetic potential; antiemetics are recommended to prevent nausea and vomiting (Dupuis, 2011).

Acute lymphoblastic leukemia (ALL), relapsed or refractory: Children ≥1 year and Adolescents: IV: 52 mg/m^2/day days 1 through 5; repeat every 2 to 6 weeks; subsequent cycles should begin no sooner than 14 days from day 1 of the previous cycle (subsequent cycles may be administered when ANC ≥750/mm^3)

Langerhans cell histiocytosis, refractory (off-label use): Children 1 to 18 years: IV: 25 mg/m^2/day days 1 through 5; repeat every 28 days for 2 to 8 cycles (Simko, 2014). Additional data may be necessary to further define the role of clofarabine in this condition.

Renal Impairment Clofarabine undergoes renal elimination and exposure is increased as creatinine clearance decreases (Bonate, 2011).

Renal impairment at baseline:

U.S. labeling:

CrCl 30-60 mL/minute: Reduce dose by 50%

CrCl <30 mL/minute: There are no dosage adjustments provided in the manufacturer's labeling; use with caution (has not been studied).

Canadian labeling:

CrCl ≥30 mL/minute: There are no dosage adjustments provided in the manufacturer's labeling; use with caution (has not been studied).

CrCl <30 mL/minute: Use is contraindicated.

Renal toxicity during treatment: Grade 3 or higher increase in serum creatinine: Discontinue clofarabine; may reinitiate with a 25% dose reduction after patient is stable and organ function recovers to baseline

Hepatic Impairment

Hepatic impairment at baseline: There are no dosage adjustments provided in the manufacturer's labeling; use with caution (has not been studied). Canadian labeling contraindicates use in severe impairment.

Hepatotoxicity during treatment: Grade 3 or higher increase in bilirubin: Discontinue clofarabine; may reinitiate with a 25% dose reduction after patient is stable and organ function recovers to baseline.

Obesity *American Society for Blood and Marrow Transplantation (ASBMT) practice guideline committee position statement on chemotherapy dosing in obesity:* Utilize actual body weight (full weight) for calculation of body surface area in clofarabine dosing for hematopoietic stem cell transplant conditioning regimens in pediatrics and adults (Bubalo, 2014).

Adjustment for Toxicity

Hematologic toxicity: ANC <500/mm^3 lasting ≥4 weeks: Reduce dose by 25% for next cycle

Nonhematologic toxicity:

Clinically significant infection: Withhold treatment until infection is under control, then restart at full dose

Grade 3 toxicity excluding infection, nausea and vomiting, and transient elevations in transaminases and bilirubin: Withhold treatment; may reinitiate with a 25% dose reduction with resolution or return to baseline

Grade ≥3 increase in creatinine or bilirubin: Discontinue; may reinitiate with 25% dosage reduction when creatinine or bilirubin return to baseline and patient is stable; administer antihyperuricemic therapy for elevated uric acid.

Grade 4 toxicity (noninfectious): Discontinue treatment.

Capillary leak or systemic inflammatory response syndrome (SIRS) early signs/symptoms (eg, hypotension, tachycardia, tachypnea, pulmonary edema): Discontinue clofarabine; institute supportive measures. May

◀ consider reinitiating with a 25% dose reduction after patient is stable and organ function recovers to baseline.

Dermatologic toxicity: Exfoliative or bullous rash, or suspected Stevens-Johnson syndrome or toxic epidermal necrolysis: Discontinue clofarabine.

Hypotension (during the 5 days of infusion): Discontinue clofarabine. If hypotension is transient and resolves (without pharmacologic intervention), may reinitiate with 25% dosage reduction (Canadian labeling).

Combination Regimens

Leukemia, acute lymphocytic: Clofarabine (ALL Regimen) on page 1917
Leukemia, acute myeloid: Clofarabine-Cytarabine (AML) on page 1917

Administration

Clofarabine is associated with a moderate emetic potential; antiemetics are recommended to prevent nausea and vomiting (Basch, 2011; Dupuis, 2011; Roila, 2010).

IV infusion: Infuse over 2 hours for relapsed/refractory ALL. May be infused over 1 hour for some off-label protocols (Becker, 2011; Kantarjian, 2003). Continuous IV fluids are encouraged to decrease adverse events and tumor lysis effects. Hypotension may be a sign of capillary leak syndrome or systemic inflammatory response syndrome (SIRS). Discontinue if the patient becomes hypotensive during administration; may consider therapy reinitiation with a 25% dose reduction after return to baseline. Do not administer any other medications through the same intravenous line.

Hazardous agent; use appropriate precautions for handling and disposal (NIOSH 2014 [group 1]).

Emetic Potential Children and Adults: Moderate (30% to 90%)

Monitoring Parameters CBC with differential and platelets (daily during treatment, then 1 to 2 times weekly or as necessary); liver and kidney function (during 5 days of clofarabine administration); coagulation parameters, blood pressure, cardiac function, and respiratory status during infusion; signs and symptoms of tumor lysis syndrome, infection, hepatic sinusoidal obstruction syndrome, enterocolitis, and cytokine release syndrome (tachypnea, tachycardia, hypotension, pulmonary edema); hydration status

Dosage Forms Excipient information presented when available (limited, particularly for generics); consult specific product labeling.

Solution, Intravenous [preservative free]:
Clolar: 1 mg/mL (20 mL)

◆ **Clofarex** *see* Clofarabine *on page* 350
◆ **Clolar** *see* Clofarabine *on page* 350

Clotrimazole (Oral) (kloe TRIM a zole)

Index Terms Mycelex

Pharmacologic Category Antifungal Agent, Imidazole Derivative; Antifungal Agent, Oral Nonabsorbed

Use

Oropharyngeal candidiasis (treatment): Local treatment of oropharyngeal candidiasis.

Oropharyngeal candidiasis (prophylaxis): To reduce the incidence of oropharyngeal candidiasis in immunocompromised patients undergoing chemotherapy, radiotherapy, or steroid therapy utilized in the treatment of leukemia, solid tumors, or renal transplantation.

Pregnancy Risk Factor C

Dosing
Adult & Geriatric
Oropharyngeal candidiasis (prophylaxis): Oral: 10 mg dissolved slowly 3 times daily for the duration of chemotherapy or until steroids are reduced to maintenance levels.

Oropharyngeal candidiasis (treatment): Oral: 10 mg dissolved slowly 5 times daily for 14 consecutive days. Note: When used for initial treatment in patients with HIV-1, duration of therapy is 7 to 14 days (DHHS [adult] 2014; DHHS [pediatric] 2013).

Pediatric Oropharyngeal candidiasis (treatment): Children ≥3 years and Adolescents: Refer to adult dosing.

Renal Impairment There are no dosage adjustments provided in the manufacturer's labeling.

Hepatic Impairment There are no dosage adjustments provided in the manufacturer's labeling.

Additional Information Complete prescribing information should be consulted for additional detail.

Dosage Forms Excipient information presented when available (limited, particularly for generics); consult specific product labeling.
Lozenge, Mouth/Throat:
Generic: 10 mg (70 ea, 140 ea)
Troche, Mouth/Throat:
Generic: 10 mg

- **CMA-676** see Gemtuzumab Ozogamicin on page 786
- **C-Met/Hepatocyte Growth Factor Receptor Tyrosine Kinase Inhibitor PF-02341066** see Crizotinib on page 366
- **C-Met/HGFR Tyrosine Kinase Inhibitor PF-02341066** see Crizotinib on page 366
- **CMV Hyperimmune Globulin** see Cytomegalovirus Immune Globulin (Intravenous-Human) on page 419
- **CMV-IGIV** see Cytomegalovirus Immune Globulin (Intravenous-Human) on page 419
- **CNTO 328** see Siltuximab on page 1525
- **Coagulation Factor I** see Fibrinogen Concentrate (Human) on page 711
- **Coagulation Factor VIIa** see Factor VIIa (Recombinant) on page 676

Cobimetinib (koe bi ME ti nib)
Related Information
Safe Handling of Hazardous Drugs on page 2292
Brand Names: US Cotellic
Index Terms Cobimetinib Fumarate; Cotellic; GDC-0973; XL518
Pharmacologic Category Antineoplastic Agent, MEK Inhibitor
Use
Melanoma, unresectable or metastatic: Treatment of unresectable or metastatic melanoma in patients with a BRAF V600E or V600K mutation (in combination with vemurafenib)

Limitations of use: Not indicated for treatment of patients with wild-type BRAF melanoma

Labeled Contraindications There are no contraindications listed in the manufacturer's labeling.

◀ **Pregnancy Considerations** Adverse events were observed in animal reproduction studies. Based on the mechanism of action, cobimetinib would be expected to cause fetal harm. Women of reproductive potential should use effective contraception during therapy and for 2 weeks after the final dose.

Breast-Feeding Considerations It is not known if cobimetinib is excreted in breast milk. The manufacturer does not recommend breast-feeding during therapy or for 2 weeks after the final dose.

Warnings/Precautions Hazardous agent – Use appropriate precautions for handling and disposal (meets NIOSH 2014 criteria).

New primary cutaneous malignancies may occur. Malignancies included cutaneous squamous cell carcinoma (cuSCC) or keratoacanthoma (KA), basal cell carcinoma (BCC), and second primary melanoma. The median time to detection of first cuSCC or KA was 4 months (range: 2 to 11 months); the median time to first detection of BCC was 4 months (range: 1 to 13 months). Dermatologic exams should be performed prior to initiation, every 2 months during treatment, and for 6 months following discontinuation of cobimetinib/vemurafenib combination therapy. Suspicious lesions should be managed with excision and dermatopathologic evaluation. Dosage adjustment is not recommended for new cutaneous malignancies. Vemurafenib may be associated with the development of noncutaneous malignancy; monitor for signs/symptoms of noncutaneous malignancy during combination treatment.

Hemorrhage, including major symptomatic bleeding in a critical area/organ, may occur with cobimetinib. Grade 3 to 4 bleeding has occurred. Cerebral hemorrhage, gastrointestinal bleeding, reproductive system hemorrhage, and hematuria have been reported. May require treatment interruption, dose reduction, and/or discontinuation. Symptomatic or asymptomatic declines in left ventricular ejection fraction (LVEF) may occur with cobimetinib. Safety has not been established in patients with baseline LVEF below the institutional lower limit of normal (LLN) or below 50%. Assess LVEF (by echocardiogram or MUGA scan) prior to therapy initiation, 1 month after initiation, and every 3 months thereafter until cobimetinib is discontinued. May require treatment interruption, dose reduction and/or discontinuation. Also assess LVEF at ~2 weeks, 4 weeks, 10 weeks, 16 weeks, and then as clinically indicated after a dose reduction or treatment interruption. The median time to first onset of LVEF decline was 4 months (range: 23 days to 13 months). Decreased LVEF resolved to >LLN or within 10% of baseline at nearly two-thirds of patients with a median time to resolution of 3 months (range: 4 days to 12 months).

Severe rash and other skin reactions (including grades 3 and 4) may occur; some events required hospitalization. The median time to onset of grade 3 and 4 rash events was 11 days (range: 3 days to ~3 months); most patients with grades 3 and 4 rash experienced complete resolution at a median time of 21 days (range: 4 days to 17 months). May require treatment interruption, dose reduction and/or discontinuation. Photosensitivity was reported in nearly one-half of patients (may be severe). The median time to first onset of photosensitivity was 2 months (range: 1 day to 14 months); the median duration was 3 months (range: 2 days to 14 months). Photosensitivity resolved in nearly two-thirds of patients. Advise patients to avoid sun exposure, wear protective clothing, and use a broad-spectrum UVA/UVB sunscreen and lip balm (SPF 30 or higher) when outdoors. Photosensitivity may require treatment interruption, dose reduction, and/or discontinuation. Ocular toxicities may occur, including serous retinopathy (fluid accumulation under retina layers). Chorioretinopathy and retinal detachment have been reported; retinal vein occlusion has also been reported (case report). The time to first onset of serous retinopathy ranged between 2 days to 9 months with a duration of 1 day to 15 months. Perform ophthalmic examinations regularly during treatment, and with reports of new or worsening visual disturbances. If serous retinopathy is diagnosed, interrupt treatment until visual symptoms improve; may require treatment interruption, dose reduction, and/or discontinuation.

Hepatotoxicity (including grades 3 or 4 transaminase, total bilirubin, or alkaline phosphatase elevations) may occur with cobimetinib. Monitor liver function test at baseline and monthly during treatment, or as clinically necessary. Grade 3 and 4 elevations may require treatment interruption, dose reduction, and/or discontinuation. Rhabdomyolysis and creatine phosphokinase (CPK) elevations may occur with cobimetinib. The median time to first occurrence of grade 3 or 4 CPK elevations was 16 days (range: 12 days to 11 months), with a median time to resolution of 15 days (range: 9 days to 11 months). Obtain baseline serum CPK and creatinine levels at baseline, periodically during treatment and as clinically indicated. If CPK is elevated, evaluate for signs/symptoms of rhabdomyolysis or other etiology. Depending on severity, may require treatment interruption, dose reduction, and/or discontinuation.

Prior to initiating therapy, confirm BRAF V600K or V600E mutation status with an approved test; approved for use in patients with BRAF V600K and BRAF V600E mutations. Not indicated for use in patients with wild-type BRAF melanoma. Potentially significant drug-drug interactions may exist, requiring dose or frequency adjustment, additional monitoring, and/or selection of alternative therapy.

Adverse Reactions

Percentages reported as part of combination chemotherapy regimens.

>10%:

Cardiovascular: Decreased left ventricular ejection fraction (grades 2/3: 26%), hypertension (15%)

Dermatologic: Skin photosensitivity (46% to 47%, grades 3/4: 4%; includes solar dermatitis and sunburn), acneiform eruption (16%, grades 3/4: 2%)

Endocrine & metabolic: Hypophosphatemia (68%), increased gamma-glutamyl transferase (65%; grades 3/4: 21%), hypoalbuminemia (42%), hyponatremia (38%), hyperkalemia (26%), hypokalemia (25%), hypocalcemia (24%)

Gastrointestinal: Diarrhea (60%), nausea (41%), vomiting (24%), stomatitis (14%; includes aphthous stomatitis, mucositis, and oral mucosa ulcer)

Hematologic & oncologic: Lymphocytopenia (73%, grades 3/4: 10%), anemia (69%; grades 3/4: 3%), thrombocytopenia (18%), hemorrhage (13%, grades 3/4: 1%; includes bruise, ecchymoses, epistaxis, gingival hemorrhage, hematemesis, hematochezia, hemoptysis, hemorrhoidal bleeding, hypermenorrhea, melena, menometrorrhagia, nail bed bleeding, pulmonary hemorrhage, purpura, rectal hemorrhage, rupture of ovarian cyst, subarachnoid hemorrhage, subgaleal hematoma, traumatic hematoma, uterine hemorrhage, and vaginal hemorrhage)

Hepatic: Increased serum AST (73%, grades 3/4: 7% to 8%), increased serum alkaline phosphatase (71%, grades 3/4: 7%), increased serum ALT (68%, grades 3/4: 11%)

Neuromuscular & Skeletal: Increased creatine phosphokinase (79%, grades 3/4: 12% to 14%)

◄ Ophthalmic: Visual impairment (15%, grades 3/4: <1%; includes blurred vision, decreased visual acuity), chorioretinopathy (13%, grades 3/4: <1%), retinal detachment (12%, grades 3/4: 2%; includes detachment of macular retinal pigment epithelium and retinal pigment epithelium detachment)

Renal: Increased serum creatinine (100%; grades 3/4: 3%)

Miscellaneous: Fever (28%)

1% to 10%:

Central nervous system: Chills (10%)

Dermatologic: Skin rash (grades 3/4: 16%; grade 4: 2%; rash resulting in hospitalization: 3%)

Gastrointestinal: Gastrointestinal hemorrhage (4%)

Genitourinary: Genitourinary tract hemorrhage (2%), hematuria (2%)

Hematologic & oncologic: Keratoacanthoma (≤6%), squamous cell carcinoma of skin (≤6%), basal cell carcinoma (5%)

Hepatic: Abnormal bilirubin levels (grades 3/4: 2%)

<1%, postmarketing, and/or case reports: Cerebral hemorrhage, malignant melanoma (second primary), malignant neoplasm (noncutaneous)

Drug Interactions

Metabolism/Transport Effects Substrate of CYP3A4 (major), P-glycoprotein; **Note:** Assignment of Major/Minor substrate status based on clinically relevant drug interaction potential

Avoid Concomitant Use

Avoid concomitant use of Cobimetinib with any of the following: Conivaptan; CYP3A4 Inducers (Moderate); CYP3A4 Inducers (Strong); CYP3A4 Inhibitors (Moderate); CYP3A4 Inhibitors (Strong); Fusidic Acid (Systemic); Idelalisib

Increased Effect/Toxicity

Cobimetinib may increase the levels/effects of: Porfimer; Verteporfin

The levels/effects of Cobimetinib may be increased by: Conivaptan; CYP3A4 Inhibitors (Moderate); CYP3A4 Inhibitors (Strong); Dasatinib; Fosaprepitant; Fusidic Acid (Systemic); Idelalisib; Ivacaftor; Luliconazole; Osimertinib; Palbociclib; Simeprevir; Stiripentol

Decreased Effect

The levels/effects of Cobimetinib may be decreased by: CYP3A4 Inducers (Moderate); CYP3A4 Inducers (Strong); Deferasirox; Osimertinib; Siltuximab; Tocilizumab

Storage/Stability Store below 30°C (86°F).

Mechanism of Action Cobimetinib is a potent and selective inhibitor of the mitogen-activated extracellular kinase (MEK) pathway (Larkin 2014); it reversibly inhibits MEK1 and MEK2, which are upstream regulators of the extracellular signal-related kinase (ERK) pathway. The ERK pathway promotes cellular proliferation. MEK1 and MEK2 are part of the BRAF pathway, which is activated by BRAF V600E and K mutations. Vemurafenib targets a different kinase in the RAS/RAF/MEK/ERK pathway; when cobimetinib and vemurafenib are used in combination, increased apoptosis and reduced tumor growth occurs.

Pharmacodynamics/Kinetics

Distribution: 806 L

Protein binding: 95%; to plasma proteins

Metabolism: Hepatic: via CYP3A4 oxidation and UGT2B7 glucuronidation

Bioavailability, absolute: 46%

Half-life elimination, mean: 44 hours (range: 23 to 70 hours)

Time to peak, median: 2.4 hours (range: 1 to 24 hours)

Excretion: Feces (76%; ~7 as unchanged drug); Urine (~18%; ~2% as unchanged drug)

Dosing

Adult & Geriatric

Melanoma, unresectable or metastatic (with BRAF V600E or V600K mutations): Oral: 60 mg once daily days 1 to 21 of each 28-day treatment cycle (in combination with vemurafenib); continue until disease progression or unacceptable toxicity (Larkin 2014).

Missed doses: If a dose is missed or if vomiting occurs after a dose is taken, resume with the next scheduled dose (do not take an additional dose).

Dosage adjustment for concurrent CYP3A4 inhibitors: Avoid concurrent use of strong or moderate CYP3A4 inhibitors with cobimetinib. If concurrent short-term use (≤14 days) of a moderate CYP3A4 inhibitor cannot be avoided, reduce the cobimetinib dose from 60 mg to 20 mg; after the moderate CYP3A4 inhibitor is discontinued, resume the previous dose of 60 mg. If the current dose is 40 or 20 mg daily, alternatives to the strong or moderate CYP3A4 inhibitor should be used.

Renal Impairment

CrCl 30 to 89 mL/minute: No dosage adjustment is necessary.

CrCl <30 mL/minute: There is no dosage adjustment provided in the manufacturer's labeling (has not been established).

Hepatic Impairment

Hepatic impairment prior to treatment:

Mild impairment (total bilirubin ≤ULN and AST >ULN **or** total bilirubin >ULN to ≤1.5 times ULN and any AST): No dosage adjustment is necessary.

Moderate to severe impairment: There is no dosage adjustment provided in the manufacturer's labeling (has not been studied); however, exposure may be increased.

Hepatotoxicity during treatment:

First occurrence of grade 4 lab abnormality (ALT, AST, or alkaline phosphatase >20 times ULN or total bilirubin >10 times ULN) or hepatotoxicity: Withhold cobimetinib for up to 4 weeks; if improves to grades 0 or 1, resume at the next lower dose level. Permanently discontinue if not improved to grade 0 or 1 within 4 weeks.

Recurrent grade 4 lab abnormality or hepatotoxicity: Permanently discontinue.

Adjustment for Toxicity

Recommended cobimetinib dose reductions for toxicity (vemurafenib may also require dosage adjustment):

First dose reduction: 40 mg once daily

Second dose reduction: 20 mg once daily

Subsequent modification (if unable to tolerate 20 mg once daily): Permanently discontinue

Cardiotoxicity:

Asymptomatic cardiomyopathy (absolute decrease in LVEF >10% [from baseline] and less than the institutional lower limit of normal [LLN]): Withhold cobimetinib for 2 weeks and repeat LVEF. If LVEF ≥ LLN **and** absolute decrease from baseline is ≤10%, resume at the next lower dose level. Permanently discontinue if LVEF < LLN **or** absolute decrease from baseline is >10%.

Symptomatic cardiomyopathy (symptomatic LVEF decrease from baseline): Withhold cobimetinib for up to 4 weeks and repeat LVEF. If symptoms resolve **and** LVEF ≥ LLN **and** absolute decrease from baseline is ≤10%, resume at the next lower dose level. Permanently discontinue if symptoms persist **or** LVEF < LLN **or** absolute decrease from baseline is >10%.

CPK elevation or rhabdomyolysis:

Grade 4 CPK elevation (>10 times ULN) or any CPK elevation with myalgia: Withhold cobimetinib for up to 4 weeks; if improves to grade 3 or lower, resume at the next lower dose level. Permanently discontinue if not improved within 4 weeks.

Dermatologic toxicity:

Grade 2 (intolerable) or grade 3 or 4: Withhold or reduce dose.

New primary cutaneous or noncutaneous malignancies: No cobimetinib dosage modification is necessary.

Hemorrhage:

Grade 3: Withhold cobimetinib for up to 4 weeks; if improves to grades 0 or 1, resume at the next lower dose level. Permanently discontinue if not improved within 4 weeks.

Grade 4: Permanently discontinue.

Ocular:

Serous retinopathy: Withhold cobimetinib for up to 4 weeks; if signs/ symptoms improve, resume at the next lower dose level. Permanently discontinue if not improved or symptoms recur within 4 weeks at the lower dose.

Retinal vein occlusion: Permanently discontinue.

Photosensitivity:

Grade 2 (intolerable), grade 3 or 4: Withhold cobimetinib for up to 4 weeks; if improves to grades 0 or 1, resume at the next lower dose level. Permanently discontinue if not improved within 4 weeks.

Other toxicities:

Grade 2 (intolerable), or any grade 3: Withhold cobimetinib for up to 4 weeks; if improves to grades 0 or 1, resume at the next lower dose level. Permanently discontinue if not improved within 4 weeks.

Grade 4, first occurrence: Withhold cobimetinib until adverse reaction improves to grade 0 or 1 and then resume at the next lower dose level or permanently discontinue.

Grade 4, recurrent: Permanently discontinue.

Administration Oral: May be administered with or without food.

Hazardous agent; use appropriate precautions for handling and disposal (meets NIOSH 2014 criteria). NIOSH recommends single gloving for administration of intact tablets (NIOSH 2014).

Monitoring Parameters

BRAF V600K or V600E mutation status (prior to treatment); liver function tests (baseline and monthly during treatment, more frequently if clinically indicated); creatine phosphokinase and serum creatinine (baseline and periodically during treatment, more frequently if clinically indicated). Assess left ventricular ejection fraction (LVEF) by echocardiogram or MUGA scan prior to therapy initiation, 1 month after initiation, and every 3 months thereafter until cobimetinib is discontinued; also assess LVEF at ~2 weeks, 4 weeks, 10 weeks, 16 weeks, and then as clinically indicated after a dose reduction or treatment interruption.

Dermatologic exams (baseline, every 2 months during treatment, and for 6 months following discontinuation); ophthalmic examinations (regularly during treatment and with reports of new or worsening visual disturbances); monitor for signs/symptoms of dermatologic toxicity, hemorrhage, noncutaneous malignancy, photosensitivity, and rhabdomyolysis.

Prescribing and Access Restrictions Available through specialty pharmacies. Further information may be obtained from the manufacturer, Genentech, at 1-888-249-4918, or at http://www.cotellic.com.

Dosage Forms Excipient information presented when available (limited, particularly for generics); consult specific product labeling.

Tablet, Oral:

Cotellic: 20 mg

◆ **Cobimetinib Fumarate** *see* Cobimetinib *on page 357*

Codeine (KOE deen)

Brand Names: Canada Codeine Contin; PMS-Codeine; ratio-Codeine

Index Terms Codeine Phosphate; Codeine Sulfate; Methylmorphine

Pharmacologic Category Analgesic, Opioid; Antitussive

Use

Pain: Management of mild-to-moderately-severe pain

Cough: *Canadian labeling:* Additional use (not in US labeling): Relief of exhausting, nonproductive cough which does not respond to nonopioid antitussives

Pregnancy Risk Factor C

Dosing

Adult

Cough: Oral:

Canadian labeling:

Immediate release tablet: 15 mg to 30 mg every 6 to 8 hours as needed (maximum: 120 mg/day).

Oral solution: 5 mL (25 mg) every 6 to 8 hours as needed.

Alternative recommendation (off-label use in US): Reported doses vary; range: 7.5 to 120 mg/day as a single dose or in divided doses (Bolser 2006; Smith 2010); **Note:** The American College of Chest Physicians does not recommend the routine use of codeine as an antitussive in patients with upper respiratory infections (Bolser 2006).

Pain management (analgesic): Oral: **Note:** These are guidelines and do not represent the maximum doses that may be required in all patients. Doses should be titrated to pain relief/prevention.

Immediate release (tablet, oral solution): Initial: 15 to 60 mg every 4 hours as needed; maximum total daily dose: 360 mg/day; patients with prior opioid exposure may require higher initial doses. **Note:** The American Pain Society recommends an initial dose of 30 to 60 mg for adults with moderate pain (American Pain Society 2008).

Controlled release: Codeine Contin [Canadian product]: **Note:** Titrate at intervals of ≥48 hours until adequate analgesia has been achieved. Daily doses >600 mg/day should not be used; patients requiring higher doses should be switched to an opioid approved for use in severe pain. In patients who receive both Codeine Contin and an immediate release or combination codeine product for breakthrough pain, the rescue dose of immediate release codeine product should be ≤12.5% of the total daily Codeine Contin dose.

Opioid-naive patients: Initial: 50 mg every 12 hours

◄

Conversion from immediate release codeine preparations: Immediate release codeine preparations contain ~75% codeine base. Therefore, patients who are switching from immediate release codeine preparations may be transferred to a ~25% lower total daily dose of Codeine Contin, equally divided into 2 daily doses every 12 hours.

*Conversion from a combination codeine product (eg, codeine with acet-aminophen **or** aspirin):* See table:

Number of 30 mg Codeine Combination Tablets Daily	Initial Dose of Codeine Contin	Maintenance Dose of Codeine Contin
≤6	50 mg every 12 h	100 mg every 12 h
7-9	100 mg every 12 h	150 mg every 12 h
10-12	150 mg every 12 h	200 mg every 12 h
>12	200 mg every 12 h	200-300 every 12 h (maximum: 300 mg every 12 h)

Conversion from another opioid analgesic: Using the patient's current opioid dose, calculate an equivalent daily dose of immediate release codeine. A ~25% lower dose of Codeine Contin should then be initiated, equally divided into 2 daily doses.

Discontinuation of therapy: **Note:** Gradual dose reduction is recommended if clinically appropriate. Initially reduce the total daily dose by 50% and administer equally divided into 2 daily doses for 2 days followed by a 25% reduction every 2 days thereafter.

Geriatric Refer to adult dosing. Use with caution and consider initiation at the low end of the dosing range; reduced initial dosages may be necessary.

Pediatric

Cough: *Canadian labeling:* Children ≥12 years and Adolescents: Oral: Refer to adult dosing.

Pain management (analgesic): Oral: **Note:** These are guidelines and do not represent the maximum doses that may be required in all patients. Doses should be titrated to pain relief/prevention.)

Canadian labeling: Children ≥12 years and Adolescents:

Immediate release (tablet, oral solution): Refer to adult dosing.

Controlled release: Use is not recommended (has not been studied)

Alternative recommendations (off-label use in US): Immediate release (tablet, oral solution): Initial: 0.5 to 1 mg/kg/dose every 4 hours as needed; maximum: 60 mg/dose (American Pain Society 2008)

Renal Impairment

US labeling: There are no specific dosage adjustments provided in the manufacturers labeling; however, clearance may be reduced; active metabolites may accumulate. Initiate at lower doses or longer dosing intervals followed by careful titration.

Canadian labeling:

Immediate release (tablet, oral solution):

CrCl >50 mL/minute: No dosage adjustment necessary.

CrCl 10 to 50 mL/minute: Administer 75% of dose and titrate carefully as needed.

CrCl <10 mL/minute: Administer 50% of dose and titrate carefully as needed.

Controlled release: There are no dosage adjustments provided in the manufacturer labeling; however, a reduced dosage is recommended

Alternate recommendations: The following guidelines have been used by some clinicians (Aronoff 2007):
CrCl 10 to 50 mL/minute: Administer 75% of dose
CrCl <10 mL/minute: Administer 50% of dose

Hepatic Impairment There are no dosage adjustments provided in the manufacturer's labeling (has not been studied); however, initial lower doses or longer dosing intervals followed by careful titration are recommended.

Additional Information Complete prescribing information should be consulted for additional detail.

Medication Guide Available Yes

Dosage Forms Excipient information presented when available (limited, particularly for generics); consult specific product labeling. [DSC] = Discontinued product
Solution, Oral, as sulfate:
Generic: 30 mg/5 mL (500 mL [DSC])
Tablet, Oral, as sulfate:
Generic: 15 mg, 30 mg, 60 mg

Dosage Forms: Canada Excipient information presented when available (limited, particularly for generics); consult specific product labeling.
Solution, Oral, as phosphate: 25 mg/5 mL
Tablet, Controlled Release:
Codeine Contin: 50 mg, 100 mg, 150 mg, 200 mg

Controlled Substance C-II

◆ **Codeine Contin (Can)** *see* Codeine *on page 363*
◆ **Codeine Phosphate** *see* Codeine *on page 363*
◆ **Codeine Sulfate** *see* Codeine *on page 363*
◆ **CO Exemestane (Can)** *see* Exemestane *on page 672*
◆ **CO Famciclovir (Can)** *see* Famciclovir *on page 689*
◆ **Co-Fentanyl (Can)** *see* FentaNYL *on page 692*
◆ **CO Fluconazole (Can)** *see* Fluconazole *on page 725*
◆ **Cometriq** *see* Cabozantinib *on page 255*
◆ **Compazine** *see* Prochlorperazine *on page 1441*
◆ **Compound F** *see* Hydrocortisone (Systemic) *on page 824*
◆ **Compro** *see* Prochlorperazine *on page 1441*
◆ **CO Mycophenolate (Can)** *see* Mycophenolate *on page 1177*
◆ **Conventional Amphotericin B** *see* Amphotericin B (Conventional) *on page 95*
◆ **Conventional Cytarabine** *see* Cytarabine (Conventional) *on page 403*
◆ **Conventional Daunomycin** *see* DAUNOrubicin (Conventional) *on page 463*
◆ **Conventional Doxorubicin** *see* DOXOrubicin (Conventional) *on page 553*
◆ **Conventional Irinotecan** *see* Irinotecan (Conventional) *on page 949*
◆ **Conventional Paclitaxel** *see* PACLitaxel (Conventional) *on page 1284*
◆ **Conventional Trastuzumab** *see* Trastuzumab *on page 1685*
◆ **Conventional Vincristine** *see* VinCRIStine *on page 1746*
◆ **ConZip** *see* TraMADol *on page 1672*
◆ **Corifact** *see* Factor XIII Concentrate (Human) *on page 688*
◆ **Cortef** *see* Hydrocortisone (Systemic) *on page 824*

- **Cortisol** *see* Hydrocortisone (Systemic) *on page 824*
- **Cosmegen** *see* DACTINomycin *on page 431*
- **Cotellic** *see* Cobimetinib *on page 357*
- **Cotellic** *see* Cobimetinib *on page 357*
- **Co-Trimoxazole** *see* Sulfamethoxazole and Trimethoprim *on page 1560*
- **CO Valacyclovir (Can)** *see* ValACYclovir *on page 1712*
- **Co-Vidarabine** *see* Pentostatin *on page 1375*
- **CP358774** *see* Erlotinib *on page 628*
- **CPDG2** *see* Glucarpidase *on page 793*
- **CPG2** *see* Glucarpidase *on page 793*
- **CPM** *see* Cyclophosphamide *on page 372*
- **CPT-11** *see* Irinotecan (Conventional) *on page 949*
- **CPZ** *see* ChlorproMAZINE *on page 322*
- **13-CRA** *see* ISOtretinoin *on page 973*
- **CRA-032765** *see* Ibrutinib *on page 856*
- **Cresemba** *see* Isavuconazonium Sulfate *on page 972*

Crizotinib (kriz OH ti nib)

Related Information

Common Toxicity Criteria *on page 2122*

Management of Chemotherapy-Induced Nausea and Vomiting in Adults *on page 2142*

Principles of Anticancer Therapy *on page 2261*

Safe Handling of Hazardous Drugs *on page 2292*

Brand Names: US Xalkori

Brand Names: Canada Xalkori

Index Terms C-Met/Hepatocyte Growth Factor Receptor Tyrosine Kinase Inhibitor PF-02341066; C-Met/HGFR Tyrosine Kinase Inhibitor PF-02341066; MET Tyrosine Kinase Inhibitor PF-02341066; PF-02341066

Pharmacologic Category Antineoplastic Agent, Anaplastic Lymphoma Kinase Inhibitor; Antineoplastic Agent, Tyrosine Kinase Inhibitor

Use Non-small cell lung cancer, metastatic: Treatment of patients with metastatic non-small cell lung cancer (NSCLC) whose tumors are anaplastic lymphoma kinase (ALK)-positive (as detected by an approved test)

Labeled Contraindications

U.S. labeling: There are no contraindications listed in the manufacturer's labeling.

Canadian labeling: Hypersensitivity to crizotinib or any component of the formulation; congenital long QT syndrome or with persistent Fridericia-corrected QT interval (QTcF) ≥500 msec

Pregnancy Considerations Adverse events have been observed in animal reproduction studies. Based on the mechanism of action, crizotinib may cause fetal harm if administered during pregnancy. Women of childbearing potential should use adequate contraception during treatment and for at least 45 days after the last crizotinib dose; men of reproductive potential should use adequate contraception methods during and for at least 90 days after treatment. The Canadian labeling recommends adequate contraception during treatment and for at least 90 days after the last dose for both males and females.

Breast-Feeding Considerations It is not known if crizotinib is excreted in breast milk. Due to the potential for serious adverse reactions in the nursing infant, the manufacturer recommends against breast-feeding during treatment and for 45 days after the final dose.

Warnings/Precautions Hazardous agent - use appropriate precautions for handling and disposal (NIOSH 2014 [group 1]). Approved for use only in patients with metastatic non-small cell lung cancer (NSCLC) who test positive for the abnormal anaplastic lymphoma kinase (ALK) gene. The Vysis ALK break-apart FISH probe kit is approved to test for the gene abnormality.

Fatalities due to crizotinib-induced hepatotoxicity have occurred. Grade 3 or 4 ALT increases (usually asymptomatic and reversible) have been observed in clinical trials. May require dosage interruption and/or reduction; permanent discontinuation was necessary in some cases; elevations in ALT or AST >5 x ULN were observed; concurrent ALT or AST elevations ≥3 x ULN and total bilirubin elevations ≥2 x ULN (without alkaline phosphatase elevations) occurred rarely. Transaminase elevation onset generally was within 2 months of treatment initiation. Monitor liver function tests, including ALT and total bilirubin every 2 weeks during the first 2 months of therapy, then monthly and as clinically necessary. Use with caution in patients with hepatic impairment (has not been studied); crizotinib is extensively metabolized in the liver and liver impairment is likely to increase crizotinib levels.

Severe, life-threatening, and potentially fatal interstitial lung disease (ILD)/ pneumonitis has been associated with crizotinib. Onset was generally within 3 months of treatment initiation. Monitor for pulmonary symptoms which may indicate ILD/pneumonitis; exclude other potential causes (eg, disease progression, infection, other pulmonary disease, or radiation therapy). Permanently discontinue if treatment-related ILD/pneumonitis is confirmed.

Symptomatic bradycardia may occur; heart rate <50 beats/minute has occurred. If possible, avoid concurrent use with other agents known to cause bradycardia (eg, beta blockers, nondihydropyridine calcium channel blockers, clonidine, digoxin). Monitor heart rate and blood pressure regularly. If symptomatic bradycardia (not life-threatening) occurs, withhold treatment until recovery to asymptomatic bradycardia or to a heart rate of ≥60 beats/minute, evaluate concurrent medications, and potentially reduce crizotinib dose. Permanently discontinue for life-threatening bradycardia due to crizotinib; if life-threatening bradycardia occurs and concurrent medications associated with bradycardia can be discontinued or dose adjusted, restart crizotinib at a reduced dose (with frequent monitoring). QTc prolongation has been observed; consider periodic monitoring of ECG and electrolytes in patients with heart failure, bradyarrhythmias, electrolyte abnormalities, or who are taking medications known to prolong the QT interval. May require treatment interruption, dosage reduction, or discontinuation. Avoid use in patients with congenital long QT syndrome. Canadian labeling contraindicates use in patients with congenital long QT syndrome or persistent QTcF ≥500 msec.

Ocular toxicities (eg, blurred vision, diplopia, photophobia, photopsia, visual acuity decreased, visual brightness, visual field defect, visual impairment, and/ or vitreous floaters) commonly occur. Onset is generally within 1 week of treatment initiation. Grade 4 visual field defect with vision loss had been reported (rare); optic atrophy and optic nerve disorder have been reported as potential causes of vision loss. Discontinue with new onset of severe visual loss (best corrected vision less than 20/200 in one or both eyes). Obtain ophthalmic evaluation (including best corrected visual acuity, retinal photographs, visual fields, optical coherence tomography, and other evaluations as appropriate). The risks of re-starting crizotinib after severe vision loss have not been evaluated; the decision to resume therapy should consider the potential benefits of treatment. Reduce initial dose in patients with severe renal impairment not requiring dialysis. Potentially significant drug-drug and drug-food interactions may exist, requiring dose or frequency adjustment, additional monitoring, and/or selection of alternative therapy. Avoid concomitant use with strong CYP3A4 inhibitors and inducers and with CYP3A4 substrates. Crizotinib is associated with a moderate emetic potential; antiemetics may be needed to prevent nausea and vomiting.

Adverse Reactions Frequency not always defined.

Cardiovascular: Edema (31% to 49%), bradycardia (5% to 15%; grades 3/4: 1%), pulmonary embolism (6%), prolonged Q-T interval on ECG (5% to 6%; grades 3/4: 2% to 3%), syncope (1% to 3%), cardiac arrhythmia, septic shock

Central nervous system: Fatigue (27% to 29%), neuropathy (19% to 25%; includes dysesthesia, gait disturbance, hypoesthesia, muscular weakness, neuralgia, peripheral neuropathy, parasthesia, peripheral sensory neuropathy, polyneuropathy, burning sensation in skin), headache (22%), dizziness (18% to 22%)

Dermatologic: Skin rash (9% to 11%)

Endocrine & metabolic: Hypophosphatemia (28% to 32%), hypokalemia (18%), weight loss (10%), weight gain (8%), diabetic ketoacidosis (≤2%)

Gastrointestinal: Diarrhea (60% to 61%), nausea (55% to 56%), vomiting (46% to 47%), constipation (42% to 43%), decreased appetite (30%), abdominal pain (26%), dysgeusia (26%), dyspepsia (8% to 14%), dysphagia (10%)

Hematologic & oncologic: Neutropenia (49% to 52%; grades 3/4: 11% to 12%), lymphocytopenia (48% to 51%; grades 3/4: 7% to 9%)

Hepatic: Increased serum ALT (76% to 79%; grades 3/4: 11% to 17%), increased serum AST (61% to 66%; grades 3/4: 6% to 9%), hepatic failure (1%)

Infection: Sepsis (≤5%)

Neuromuscular & skeletal: Limb pain (16%), muscle spasm (8%)

Ophthalmic: Visual disturbance (60% to 71%; grades 3/4: <1%; grade 4: <1%; onset: <2 weeks; includes blurred vision, diplopia, photophobia, photopsia, visual acuity decreased, visual brightness, visual field defect, visual impairment, vitreous floaters)

Renal: Renal cyst (3% to 5%)

Respiratory: Upper respiratory tract infection (26% to 32%), adult respiratory distress syndrome (≤5%), interstitial pulmonary disease (≤5%; grades 3/4: 1%; includes acute respiratory distress syndrome, pneumonitis), pneumonia (≤5%), respiratory failure (≤5%), dyspnea (2%)

Miscellaneous: Fever (19%)

<1%, postmarketing, and/or case reports: Hepatotoxicity

Drug Interactions

Metabolism/Transport Effects Substrate of CYP3A4 (major), P-glycoprotein; **Note:** Assignment of Major/Minor substrate status based on clinically relevant drug interaction potential; **Inhibits** CYP2B6 (moderate), CYP3A4 (moderate), OCT1, OCT2, P-glycoprotein

Avoid Concomitant Use

Avoid concomitant use of Crizotinib with any of the following: Alfentanil; Aprepitant; Bosutinib; Ceritinib; Cobimetinib; Conivaptan; CycloSPORINE (Systemic); CYP3A4 Inducers (Strong); CYP3A4 Inhibitors (Strong); Dihydroergotamine; Domperidone; Ergotamine; FentaNYL; Flibanserin; Fusidic Acid (Systemic); Grapefruit Juice; Highest Risk QTc-Prolonging Agents; Ibrutinib; Idelalisib; Ivabradine; Lomitapide; Mifepristone; Naloxegol; Olaparib; PAZOPanib; Pimozide; QuiNIDine; Silodosin; Simeprevir; Sirolimus; St Johns Wort; Tacrolimus (Systemic); Tolvaptan; Topotecan; Trabectedin; Ulipristal; VinCRIStine (Liposomal)

Increased Effect/Toxicity

Crizotinib may increase the levels/effects of: Afatinib; Alfentanil; Apixaban; Aprepitant; ARIPiprazole; Avanafil; Bosentan; Bosutinib; Bradycardia-Causing Agents; Brentuximab Vedotin; Brexpiprazole; Bromocriptine; Budesonide (Systemic); Budesonide (Systemic, Oral Inhalation); Budesonide (Topical); BuPROPion; Cannabis; Ceritinib; Cilostazol; Cobimetinib; Colchicine; CycloSPORINE (Systemic); CYP2B6 Substrates; CYP3A4 Substrates; Dabigatran Etexilate; Dapoxetine; Dihydroergotamine; Domperidone; DOXOrubicin (Conventional); Dronabinol; Edoxaban; Eletriptan; Eplerenone; Ergotamine; Everolimus; FentaNYL; Flibanserin; Highest Risk QTc-Prolonging Agents; Hydrocodone; Ibrutinib; Imatinib; Ivabradine; Ivacaftor; Lacosamide; Ledipasvir; Lomitapide; Lurasidone; Moderate Risk QTc-Prolonging Agents; Naloxegol; NiMODipine; Nintedanib; Olaparib; OxyCODONE; PAZOPanib; P-glycoprotein/ABCB1 Substrates; Pimecrolimus; Pimozide; Prucalopride; QuiNIDine; Ranolazine; Rifaximin; Rivaroxaban; Salmeterol; Saxagliptin; Silodosin; Simeprevir; Sirolimus; Sonidegib; Suvorexant; Tacrolimus (Systemic); Tetrahydrocannabinol; Tolvaptan; Topotecan; Trabectedin; Ulipristal; Vilazodone; VinCRIStine (Liposomal); Vindesine; Zopiclone

The levels/effects of Crizotinib may be increased by: Bretylium; Conivaptan; CYP3A4 Inhibitors (Moderate); CYP3A4 Inhibitors (Strong); Dasatinib; Fosaprepitant; Fusidic Acid (Systemic); Grapefruit Juice; Idelalisib; Ivabradine; Luliconazole; Mifepristone; Netupitant; Palbociclib; P-glycoprotein/ABCB1 Inhibitors; QTc-Prolonging Agents (Indeterminate Risk and Risk Modifying); Ruxolitinib; Stiripentol; Tofacitinib

Decreased Effect

Crizotinib may decrease the levels/effects of: Ifosfamide

The levels/effects of Crizotinib may be decreased by: Bosentan; CYP3A4 Inducers (Moderate); CYP3A4 Inducers (Strong); Dabrafenib; Deferasirox; P-glycoprotein/ABCB1 Inducers; Siltuximab; St Johns Wort; Tocilizumab

Food Interactions Grapefruit juice may increase serum crizotinib levels. Management: Avoid grapefruit and grapefruit juice.

Storage/Stability Store between 20°C and 25°C (68°F and 77°F); excursions are permitted between 15°C and 30°C (59°F and 86°F).

Mechanism of Action Tyrosine kinase receptor inhibitor, which inhibits anaplastic lymphoma kinase (ALK), Hepatocyte Growth Factor Receptor (HGFR, c-MET), and Recepteur d'Origine Nantais (RON). ALK gene abnormalities due to mutations or translocations may result in expression of oncogenic fusion proteins (eg, ALK fusion protein) which alter signaling and expression and result in increased cellular proliferation and survival in tumors which express these fusion proteins. Approximately 2% to 7% of patients with NSCLC have the abnormal echinoderm microtubule-associated protein-like 4, or EML4-ALK gene (which has a higher prevalence in never smokers or light smokers and in

◀ patients with adenocarcinoma). Crizotinib selectively inhibits ALK tyrosine kinase, which reduces proliferation of cells expressing the genetic alteration.

Pharmacodynamics/Kinetics

Distribution: V_{ss}: 1772 L

Protein binding: 91%

Metabolism: Hepatic, via CYP3A4/5

Bioavailability: 43% (range: 32% to 66%); bioavailability is reduced 14% with a high-fat meal

Half-life elimination: Terminal: 42 hours

Time to peak: 4 to 6 hours

Excretion: Feces (63%; 53% as unchanged drug); urine (22%; 2% as unchanged drug)

Dosing

Adult & Geriatric Note: Crizotinib is associated with a moderate emetic potential; antiemetics may be needed to prevent nausea and vomiting.

Non-small cell lung cancer (NSCLC), metastatic (ALK-positive): Oral: 250 mg twice daily, continue treatment until disease progression or unacceptable toxicity

Missed doses: If a dose is missed, take as soon as remembered unless it is <6 hours prior to the next scheduled dose (skip the dose if <6 hours before the next dose); do not take 2 doses at the same time to make up for a missed dose. If vomiting occurs after dose, administer the next dose at the regularly scheduled time.

Renal Impairment

Mild to moderate impairment (CrCl 30-89 mL/minute): No dosage adjustment necessary.

Severe impairment (CrCl <30 mL/minute) not requiring dialysis: Initial: 250 mg once daily.

Hepatic Impairment

Hepatotoxicity **prior to** treatment: No dosage adjustment provided in manufacturer's labeling (has not been studied); crizotinib undergoes extensive hepatic metabolism and systemic exposure may be increased with impairment; use with caution.

Hepatotoxicity **during** treatment:

Grade 3 or 4 ALT or AST elevation (ALT or AST >5 x ULN) with ≤ grade 1 total bilirubin elevation (total bilirubin ≤1.5 x ULN): Withhold treatment until recovery to baseline or ≤ grade 1 (<3 x ULN), then resume at a reduced dose (200 mg twice daily).

Recurrent grade 3 or 4 ALT or AST elevation with ≤ grade 1 total bilirubin elevation: Withhold treatment until recovery to baseline or ≤ grade 1, then resume at the next lower reduced dose (250 mg once daily).

Recurrent grade 3 or 4 ALT or AST elevation on 250 mg once daily: Permanently discontinue.

Grade 2, 3, or 4 ALT or AST elevation (ALT or AST >3 x ULN) with concurrent grade 2, 3, or 4 total bilirubin elevation (>1.5 x ULN) in the absence of cholestasis or hemolysis: Permanently discontinue.

Adjustment for Toxicity Note: If dose reduction is necessary, reduce dose to 200 mg orally twice daily; if necessary, further reduce to 250 mg once daily. If unable to tolerate 250 mg once daily, permanently discontinue therapy.

Hematologic toxicity (except lymphopenia, unless lymphopenia is associated with clinical events such as opportunistic infection):

Grade 3 toxicity (WBC 1,000 to 2,000/mm^3, ANC 500 to 1,000/mm^3, platelets 25,000 to 50,000/mm^3), grade 3 anemia: Withhold treatment until recovery to ≤ grade 2, then resume at the same dose and schedule.

Grade 4 toxicity (WBC <1,000/mm^3, ANC <500/mm^3, platelets <25,000/mm^3), grade 4 anemia: Withhold treatment until recovery to ≤ grade 2, then resume at 200 mg twice daily.

Recurrent grade 4 toxicity on 200 mg twice daily: Withhold treatment until recovery to ≤ grade 2, then resume at 250 mg once daily.

Recurrent grade 4 toxicity on 250 mg once daily: Permanently discontinue.

Nonhematologic toxicities:

Cardiovascular toxicities:

QTc prolongation:

Grade 3 QTc prolongation (QTc >500 msec without life-threatening signs or symptoms) on at least 2 separate ECGs: Withhold treatment until recovery to baseline or to ≤ grade 1 (QTc ≤480 msec), then resume at 200 mg twice daily.

Recurrent grade 3 QTc prolongation at 200 mg twice daily: Withhold treatment until recovery to baseline or to ≤ grade 1, then resume at 250 mg once daily.

Recurrent grade 3 QTc prolongation at 250 mg once daily: Permanently discontinue.

Grade 4 QTc prolongation (QTc >500 msec or ≥60 msec change from baseline with life-threatening symptoms): Permanently discontinue.

Bradycardia:

Grade 2 bradycardia (symptomatic with medical intervention indicated) or grade 3 bradycardia (severe/medically significant with intervention indicated): Withhold until recovery to asymptomatic bradycardia or to a heart rate of ≥60 beats/minute and evaluate concomitant medications. If contributing concomitant medication is identified and discontinued (or dose adjusted), then resume crizotinib at the previous dose. If no contributing concomitant medication is identified (or cannot be discontinued or dose adjusted), resume crizotinib at a reduced dose.

Grade 4 bradycardia (life-threatening with urgent intervention indicated): Withhold until recovery to asymptomatic bradycardia or to a heart rate of ≥60 beats/minute and evaluate concomitant medications. If contributing concomitant medication is identified and discontinued (or dose adjusted), then resume crizotinib at 250 mg once daily with frequent monitoring. If no contributing concomitant medication is identified, permanently discontinue crizotinib. Permanently discontinue for recurrence.

Hepatotoxicity: Refer to Dosage Adjustment in Hepatic Impairment.

Ocular toxicity: Visual loss (grade 4 visual disorder) or new onset of severe visual loss (best corrected vision less than 20/200 in one or both eyes): Discontinue during evaluation of severe vision loss.

Pulmonary toxicity: Interstitial lung disease (ILD)/pneumonitis (any grade; not attributable to disease progression, infection, other pulmonary disease or radiation therapy): Permanently discontinue.

Combination Regimens

Lung cancer (non-small cell): Crizotinib (NSCLC Regimen) on page 1926

◄ **Administration**

Crizotinib is associated with a moderate emetic potential; antiemetics may be needed to prevent nausea and vomiting.

Swallow capsules whole (do not crush, dissolve, or open capsules). Administer with or without food. If vomiting occurs after dose, administer the next dose at the regularly scheduled time.

Hazardous agent; use appropriate precautions for handling and disposal (NIOSH 2014 [group 1]).

Emetic Potential Moderate (30% to 90%)

Monitoring Parameters ALK positivity; CBC with differential monthly and as clinically appropriate (monitor more frequently if grades 3 or 4 abnormalities observed or with fever or infection), liver function tests every 2 weeks for the first 2 months, then monthly and as clinically appropriate (monitor more frequently if grades 2, 3, or 4 abnormalities observed); renal function (baseline and periodic). Monitor pulmonary symptoms (for interstitial lung disease [ILD]/pneumonitis). Monitor heart rate and blood pressure; consider monitoring ECG and electrolytes in patients with heart failure, bradycardia, bradyarrhythmias, electrolyte abnormalities, or who are taking medications known to prolong the QT interval. Obtain ophthalmic evaluation (including best corrected visual acuity, retinal photographs, visual fields, optical coherence tomography, and other evaluations as appropriate) if severe visual loss occurs.

Dietary Considerations Avoid grapefruit and grapefruit juice.

Prescribing and Access Restrictions Available through specialty pharmacies. Further information may be obtained from the manufacturer, Pfizer, at 1-877-744-5675, or at http://www.pfizerpro.com

Dosage Forms Excipient information presented when available (limited, particularly for generics); consult specific product labeling.

Capsule, Oral:

Xalkori: 200 mg, 250 mg

◆ **CsA** see CycloSPORINE (Systemic) on page 385

◆ **CTX** see Cyclophosphamide on page 372

◆ **CyA** see CycloSPORINE (Systemic) on page 385

Cyclophosphamide (sye kloe FOS fa mide)

Related Information

Chemotherapy and Cancer Treatment During Pregnancy on page 2214

Chemotherapy and Obesity on page 2220

Fertility and Cancer Therapy on page 2137

Hematopoietic Stem Cell Transplantation on page 2272

Management of Chemotherapy-Induced Nausea and Vomiting in Adults on page 2142

Management of Drug Extravasations on page 2159

Mucositis and Stomatitis on page 2186

Prevention of Chemotherapy-Induced Nausea and Vomiting in Children on page 2203

Principles of Anticancer Therapy on page 2261

Safe Handling of Hazardous Drugs on page 2292

Brand Names: Canada Procytox

Index Terms CPM; CTX; CYT; Cytoxan; Neosar

Pharmacologic Category Antineoplastic Agent, Alkylating Agent; Antineoplastic Agent, Alkylating Agent (Nitrogen Mustard); Antirheumatic Miscellaneous; Immunosuppressant Agent

Use

Oncology uses: Treatment of acute lymphoblastic leukemia (ALL), acute myelocytic leukemia (AML), breast cancer, chronic lymphocytic leukemia (CLL), chronic myeloid leukemia (CML), Hodgkin lymphoma, mycosis fungoides, multiple myeloma, neuroblastoma, non-Hodgkin lymphomas (including Burkitt lymphoma), ovarian adenocarcinoma, and retinoblastoma

Limitations of use: Although potentially effective as a single-agent in susceptible malignancies, cyclophosphamide is more frequently used in combination with other chemotherapy drugs

Canadian labeling: Additional use (not in US labeling): Treatment of lung cancer

Nononcology uses: *US labeling:* Nephrotic syndrome: Treatment of minimal change nephrotic syndrome (biopsy proven) in children who are unresponsive or intolerant to corticosteroid therapy

Limitations of use: The safety and efficacy for the treatment of nephrotic syndrome in adults or in other renal diseases has not been established.

Labeled Contraindications

US labeling: Hypersensitivity to cyclophosphamide or any component of the formulation; urinary outflow obstruction

Canadian labeling: Hypersensitivity to cyclophosphamide or its metabolites, urinary outflow obstructions, severe myelosuppression, severe renal or hepatic impairment, active infection (especially varicella zoster), severe immunosuppression

Pregnancy Considerations Cyclophosphamide crosses the placenta and can be detected in amniotic fluid (D'Incalci 1982). Based on the mechanism of action, cyclophosphamide may cause fetal harm if administered during pregnancy. Adverse events (including ectrodactylia) were observed in human studies following exposure to cyclophosphamide. Women of childbearing potential should avoid pregnancy while receiving cyclophosphamide and for up to 1 year after completion of treatment. Males with female partners who are or may become pregnant should use a condom during and for at least 4 months after cyclophosphamide treatment. Cyclophosphamide may cause sterility in males and females (may be irreversible) and amenorrhea in females. When treatment is needed for lupus nephritis, cyclophosphamide should be avoided in women who are pregnant or those who wish to preserve their fertility (Hahn 2012). Chemotherapy, if indicated, may be administered to pregnant women with breast cancer as part of a combination chemotherapy regimen (common regimens administered during pregnancy include doxorubicin (or epirubicin), cyclophosphamide, and fluorouracil); chemotherapy should not be administered during the first trimester, after 35 weeks gestation, or within 3 weeks of planned delivery (Amant 2010; Loibl 2006).

Breast-Feeding Considerations Cyclophosphamide is excreted into breast milk. Leukopenia and thrombocytopenia were noted in an infant exposed to cyclophosphamide while nursing. The mother was treated with one course of cyclophosphamide 6 weeks prior to delivery then cyclophosphamide IV 6 mg/kg (300 mg) once daily for 3 days beginning 20 days postpartum. Complete blood counts were obtained in the breast-feeding infant on each day of therapy; WBC and platelets decreased by day 3 (Durodola 1979). Due to the potential for serious adverse effects in the nursing infant, a decision should be made to discontinue cyclophosphamide or to discontinue breast-feeding, taking into account the importance of treatment to the mother.

Warnings/Precautions Hazardous agent - use appropriate precautions for handling and disposal (NIOSH 2014 [group 1]).

Cyclophosphamide is associated with the development of hemorrhagic cystitis, pyelitis, ureteritis, and hematuria. Hemorrhagic cystitis may rarely be severe or fatal. Bladder fibrosis may also occur, either with or without cystitis. Urotoxicity is due to excretion of cyclophosphamide metabolites in the urine and appears to be dose- and treatment duration-dependent, although may occur with short-term use. Increased hydration and frequent voiding is recommended to help prevent cystitis; some protocols utilize mesna to protect against hemorrhagic cystitis. Monitor urinalysis for hematuria or other signs of urotoxicity. Severe or prolonged hemorrhagic cystitis may require medical or surgical treatment. While hematuria generally resolves within a few days after treatment is with-held, it may persist in some cases. Discontinue cyclophosphamide with severe hemorrhagic cystitis. Exclude or correct any urinary tract obstructions prior to treatment initiation (use is contraindicated with bladder outlet obstruction). Use with caution (if at all) in patients with active urinary tract infection. Use with caution in patients with renal impairment; dosage adjustment may be needed. Decreased renal excretion and increased serum levels (cyclophosphamide and metabolites) may occur in patients with severe renal impairment (CrCl 10 to 24 mL/minute); monitor for signs/symptoms of toxicity. Use is contraindicated in severe impairment in the Canadian labeling. Cyclophosphamide and metabolites are dialyzable; differences in amount dialyzed may occur due to dialysis system used. If dialysis is required, maintain a consistent interval between administration and dialysis.

Leukopenia, neutropenia, thrombocytopenia, and anemia may commonly occur; may be dose related. Bone marrow failure has been reported. Bone marrow failure and severe immunosuppression may lead to serious (and fatal) infections, including sepsis and septic shock, or may reactive latent infections. Antimicrobial prophylaxis may be considered in appropriate patients. Initiate antibiotics for neutropenic fever; antifungal and antiviral medications may also be necessary. Monitor blood counts during treatment. Avoid use if neutrophils are ≤1,500/mm^3 and platelets are <50,000/mm^3. Consider growth factors (primary or secondary prophylaxis) in patients at increased risk for complications due to neutropenia. Platelet and neutrophil nadirs are usually at weeks 1 and 2 of treatment and recovery is expected after ~20 days. Severe myelo-suppression may be more prevalent in heavily pretreated patients or in patients receiving concomitant chemotherapy and/or radiation therapy. Monitor for infections; immunosuppression and serious infections may occur; serious infections may require dose reduction, or interruption or discontinuation of treatment.

Cardiotoxicity has been reported (some fatal), usually with high doses associated with transplant conditioning regimens, although may rarely occur with lower doses. Cardiac abnormalities do not appear to persist. Cardiotoxicities reported have included arrhythmias (supraventricular and ventricular [some with QT prolongation]), congestive heart failure, heart block, hemopericardium (secondary to hemorrhagic myocarditis and myocardial necrosis), myocarditis (including hemorrhagic), pericarditis, pericardial effusion including cardiac tamponade, and tachyarrhythmias. Cardiotoxicity is related to endothelial capillary damage; symptoms may be managed with diuretics, ACE inhibitors, beta-blockers, or inotropics (Floyd 2005). The risk for cardiotoxicity may be increased with higher doses, advanced age, and in patients with prior radiation to the cardiac region, and in patients who have received prior or concurrent cardiotoxic medication. Use with caution in patients with preexisting cardiovascular disease or those at risk for cardiotoxicity. For patients with cardiac risk factors or preexisting cardiac disease, monitor during treatment.

Pulmonary toxicities, including pneumonitis, pulmonary fibrosis, pulmonary veno-occlusive disease, and acute respiratory distress syndrome, have been reported. Monitor for signs/symptoms of pulmonary toxicity. Consider pulmonary function testing to assess the severity of pneumonitis (Morgan 2011). Cyclophosphamide-induced pneumonitis is rare and may present as early (within 1 to 6 months) or late onset (several months to years). Early onset may be reversible with discontinuation; late onset is associated with pleural thickening and may persist chronically (Malik 1996). In addition, late onset pneumonitis (>6 months after therapy initiation) may be associated with increased mortality.

Hepatic sinusoidal obstruction syndrome (SOS), formerly called veno-occlusive liver disease (VOD), has been reported in patients receiving chemotherapy regimens containing cyclophosphamide. A major risk factor for SOS is cytoreductive conditioning transplantation regimens with cyclophosphamide used in combination with total body irradiation or busulfan (or other agents). Other risk factors include preexisting hepatic dysfunction, prior radiation to the abdominal area, and low performance status. Children <3 years of age are reported to be at increased risk for hepatic SOS; monitor for signs or symptoms of hepatic SOS, including bilirubin >1.4 mg/dL, unexplained weight gain, ascites, hepatomegaly, or unexplained right upper quadrant pain (Arndt 2004). SOS has also been reported in patients receiving long-term lower doses for immunosuppressive indications. Use with caution in patients with hepatic impairment; dosage adjustment may be needed. Use is contraindicated in severe impairment in the Canadian labeling. The conversion between cyclophosphamide to the active metabolite may be reduced in patients with severe hepatic impairment, potentially reducing efficacy.

Nausea and vomiting commonly occur. Cyclophosphamide is associated with a moderate to high emetic potential (depending on dose, regimen, or administration route); antiemetics are recommended to prevent nausea and vomiting (Basch 2011; Dupuis 2011; Roila 2010). Stomatitis/mucositis may also occur. Anaphylactic reactions have been reported; cross-sensitivity with other alkylating agents may occur. Hyponatremia associated with increased total body water, acute water intoxication, and a syndrome resembling SIADH (syndrome of inappropriate secretion of antidiuretic hormone) has been reported; some have been fatal. May interfere with wound healing. May impair fertility; interferes with oogenesis and spermatogenesis. Effect on fertility is generally dependent on dose and duration of treatment and may be irreversible. The age at treatment initiation and cumulative dose were determined to be risk factors for ovarian failure in cyclophosphamide use for the treatment of systemic lupus erythematosus (SLE) (Mok 1998). Potentially significant drug-drug interactions may exist, requiring dose or frequency adjustment, additional monitoring, and/or selection of alternative therapy. Secondary malignancies (bladder cancer, myelodysplasia, acute leukemias, lymphomas, thyroid cancer, and sarcomas) have been reported with both single-agent and with combination chemotherapy regimens; onset may be delayed (up to several years after treatment). Bladder cancer usually occurs in patients previously experiencing hemorrhagic cystitis; risk may be reduced by preventing hemorrhagic cystitis.

◀ **Adverse Reactions** Frequency not defined.

Dermatologic: Alopecia (reversible; onset: 3-6 weeks after start of treatment)

Endocrine & metabolic: Amenorrhea, azoospermia, gonadal suppression, oligospermia, oogenesis impaired, sterility

Gastrointestinal: Abdominal pain, anorexia, diarrhea, mucositis, nausea/vomiting (dose-related), stomatitis

Genitourinary: Hemorrhagic cystitis

Hematologic: Anemia, leukopenia (dose-related; recovery: 7-10 days after cessation), myelosuppression, neutropenia, neutropenic fever, thrombocytopenia

Miscellaneous: Infection

Postmarketing and/or case reports: Acute respiratory distress syndrome, anaphylactic reactions, anaphylaxis, arrhythmias (with high-dose [HSCT] therapy), bladder/urinary fibrosis, blurred vision, cardiac tamponade (with high-dose [HSCT] therapy), cardiotoxicity, confusion, C-reactive protein increased, dizziness, dyspnea, ejection fraction decreased, erythema multiforme, gastrointestinal hemorrhage, hearing disorders, heart block, heart failure (with high-dose [HSCT] therapy), hematuria, hemopericardium, hemorrhagic colitis, hemorrhagic myocarditis (with high-dose [HSCT] therapy), hemorrhagic ureteritis, hepatic sinusoidal obstruction syndrome (SOS; formerly called veno-occlusive liver disease), hepatitis, hepatotoxicity, hypersensitivity reactions, hyperuricemia, hypokalemia, hyponatremia, interstitial pneumonitis, interstitial pulmonary fibrosis (with high doses), jaundice, latent infection reactivation, LDH increased, malaise, mesenteric ischemia (acute), methemoglobinemia (with high-dose [HSCT] therapy), multiorgan failure, myocardial necrosis (with high-dose [HSCT] therapy), neurotoxicity, neutrophilic eccrine hidradenitis, ovarian fibrosis, pancreatitis, pericarditis, pigmentation changes (skin/fingernails), pneumonia, pulmonary hypertension, pulmonary infiltrates, pulmonary veno-occlusive disease, pyelonephritis, radiation recall, rash, renal tubular necrosis, reversible posterior leukoencephalopathy syndrome (RPLS), rhabdomyolysis, secondary malignancy, septic shock, sepsis, SIADH, Stevens-Johnson syndrome, testicular atrophy, thrombocytopenia (immune mediated), thrombotic disorders (arterial and venous), toxic epidermal necrolysis, toxic megacolon, tumor lysis syndrome, weakness, wound healing impaired

Drug Interactions

Metabolism/Transport Effects Substrate of CYP2A6 (minor), CYP2B6 (major), CYP2C19 (minor), CYP2C9 (minor), CYP3A4 (minor); **Note:** Assignment of Major/Minor substrate status based on clinically relevant drug interaction potential; **Induces** CYP2B6 (weak/moderate), CYP2C9 (weak/moderate)

Avoid Concomitant Use

Avoid concomitant use of Cyclophosphamide with any of the following: BCG (Intravesical); Belimumab; CloZAPine; Dipyrone; Etanercept; Natalizumab; Pimecrolimus; Tacrolimus (Topical); Tofacitinib; Vaccines (Live)

Increased Effect/Toxicity

Cyclophosphamide may increase the levels/effects of: Amiodarone; Antineoplastic Agents (Anthracycline, Systemic); CloZAPine; CycloSPORINE (Systemic); Fingolimod; Leflunomide; Natalizumab; Sargramostim; Succinylcholine; Tofacitinib; Vaccines (Live)

The levels/effects of Cyclophosphamide may be increased by: Allopurinol; AzaTHIOprine; Belimumab; CYP2B6 Inhibitors (Moderate); Denosumab; Dipyrone; Etanercept; Filgrastim; Pentostatin; Pimecrolimus; Protease

Inhibitors; Quazepam; Roflumilast; Tacrolimus (Topical); Thiazide Diuretics; Trastuzumab

Decreased Effect

Cyclophosphamide may decrease the levels/effects of: BCG (Intravesical); Coccidioides immitis Skin Test; CycloSPORINE (Systemic); Sipuleucel-T; Vaccines (Inactivated); Vaccines (Live)

The levels/effects of Cyclophosphamide may be decreased by: CYP2B6 Inducers (Strong); Dabrafenib; Echinacea; Lumacaftor

Storage/Stability

Injection powder for reconstitution: Store intact vials of powder ≤25°C (77°F). Exposure to excessive temperatures during transport or storage may cause active ingredient to melt (vials with melting may have a clear to yellow viscous liquid which may appear as droplets); do not use vials with signs of melting. Solutions reconstituted in sterile water for injection should be further diluted immediately; do not inject SWFI reconstituted solution directly. Reconstituted solutions in normal saline (NS) are stable for 24 hours at room temperature and for 6 days refrigerated at 2°C to 8°C (36°F to 46°F). Solutions diluted for infusion in 1/2NS or NS are stable for 24 hours at room temperature and for 6 days refrigerated; solutions diluted in D5W or D5NS are stable for 24 hours at room temperature and for 36 hours refrigerated.

Capsules: Store at 20°C to 25°C (68°F to 77°F); excursions are permitted between 15°C and 30°C (59°F and 86°F).

Tablets: Store tablets at ≤25°C (77°F); brief excursions are permitted up to 30°C (86°F); protect from temperatures >30°C (86°F).

Preparation for Administration Hazardous agent; use appropriate precautions for handling and disposal (NIOSH 2014 [group 1]).

Injection powder for reconstitution: Reconstitute with 25 mL for a 500 mg vial, 50 mL for a 1000 mg vial, or 100 mL for a 2000 mg vial to a concentration of 20 mg/mL using NS only for direct IV push, or NS or SWFI for IV infusion; swirl gently to mix. For IV infusion, further dilute for infusion in D5W, 1/2NS, or D5NS, to a minimum concentration of 2 mg/mL.

Mechanism of Action Cyclophosphamide is an alkylating agent that prevents cell division by cross-linking DNA strands and decreasing DNA synthesis. It is a cell cycle phase nonspecific agent. Cyclophosphamide also possesses potent immunosuppressive activity. Cyclophosphamide is a prodrug that must be metabolized to active metabolites in the liver.

Pharmacodynamics/Kinetics

Absorption: Oral: Well absorbed

Distribution: V_d: 30 to 50 L (approximates total body water); crosses into CSF (not in high enough concentrations to treat meningeal leukemia)

Protein binding: ~20%; some metabolites are bound at >60%

Metabolism: Hepatic to active metabolites acrolein, 4-aldophosphamide, 4-hydroperoxycyclophosphamide, and nor-nitrogen mustard

Bioavailability: >75%

Half-life elimination: IV: 3 to 12 hours

Time to peak: Oral: ~1 hour; IV: Metabolites: 2 to 3 hours

Excretion: Urine (10 to 20% as unchanged drug); feces (4%)

Dosing

Adult Cyclophosphamide is associated with a moderate to high emetic potential (depending on dose, regimen, or administration route); antiemetics are recommended to prevent nausea and vomiting (Basch 2011; Roila 2010).

◄ ***US labeling:* Malignancy:**
IV: 40 to 50 mg/kg in divided doses over 2 to 5 days **or** 10 to 15 mg/kg every 7 to 10 days **or** 3 to 5 mg/kg twice weekly
Oral: 1 to 5 mg/kg/day (initial and maintenance dosing)

***Canadian labeling:* Malignancy:**
IV: Initial: 40 to 50 mg/kg (1500 to 1800 mg/m^2) administered as 10 to 20 mg/kg/day over 2 to 5 days; Maintenance: 10 to 15 mg/kg (350 to 550 mg/m^2) every 7 to 10 days **or** 3 to 5 mg/kg (110 to 185 mg/m^2) twice weekly
Oral: Initial 1 to 5 mg/kg/day (depending on tolerance); Maintenance: 1 to 5 mg/kg/day

Indication specific and/or off-label uses/dosing:

Acute lymphoblastic leukemia (off-label dosing): Multiple-agent regimens:

Hyper-CVAD regimen: IV: 300 mg/m^2 over 3 hours (with mesna) every 12 hours for 6 doses on days 1, 2, and 3 during odd-numbered cycles (cycles 1, 3, 5, 7) of an 8-cycle phase (Kantarjian 2004)

CALGB8811 regimen: IV:
Adults <60 years: Induction phase: 1200 mg/m^2 on day 1 of a 4-week cycle; Early intensification phase: 1000 mg/m^2 on day 1 of a 4-week cycle (repeat once); Late intensification phase: 1000 mg/m^2 on day 29 of an 8-week cycle (Larson 1995)
Adults ≥60 years: Induction phase: 800 mg/m^2 on day 1 of a 4-week cycle; Early intensification phase: 1000 mg/m^2 on day 1 of a 4-week cycle (repeat once); Late intensification phase: 1000 mg/m^2 on day 29 of an 8-week cycle (Larson 1995)

Breast cancer (off-label dosing):

AC regimen: IV: 600 mg/m^2 on day 1 every 21 days (in combination with doxorubicin) for 4 cycles (Fisher 1990)

CEF regimen: Oral: 75 mg/m^2/day days 1 to 14 every 28 days (in combination with epirubicin and fluorouracil) for 6 cycles (Levine 1998)

CMF regimen: Oral: 100 mg/m^2/day days 1 to 14 every 28 days (in combination with methotrexate and fluorouracil) for 6 cycles (Levine 1998) **or** IV: 600 mg/m^2 on day 1 every 21 days (in combination with methotrexate and fluorouracil); Goldhirsch 1998)

Chronic lymphocytic leukemia (off-label dosing): IV: R-FC regimen: 250 mg/m^2/day for 3 days every 28 days (in combination with rituximab and fludarabine) for 6 cycles (Robak 2010)

Ewing sarcoma (off-label use): IV: VAC/IE regimen: VAC: 1200 mg/m^2 (plus mesna) on day 1 of a 21-day treatment cycle (in combination with vincristine and doxorubicin [with dactinomycin when maximum doxorubicin dose reached]), alternates with IE (ifosfamide and etoposide) for a total of 17 cycles (Grier 2003)

Gestational trophoblastic tumors, high-risk (off-label use): IV: EMA/CO regimen: 600 mg/m^2 on day 8 of 2-week treatment cycle (in combination with etoposide, methotrexate, dactinomycin, and vincristine), continue for at least 2 treatment cycles after a normal hCG level (Escobar 2003; Lurain 2006)

Granulomatosis with polyangiitis (GPA; Wegener granulomatosis) (off-label use; in combination with glucocorticoids):

Low-dose: Oral: 1.5 to 2 mg/kg/day (Jayne 2003; Stone 2010) or 2 mg/kg/day until remission, followed by 1.5 mg/kg/day for 3 additional months (de Groot 2009; Harper 2012)

Pulse: IV: 15 mg/kg (maximum dose: 1200 mg) every 2 weeks for 3 doses, followed by maintenance pulses of either 15 mg/kg IV (maximum dose: 1200 mg) every 3 weeks or 2.5 to 5 mg/kg/day orally on days 1, 2, and 3 every 3 weeks for 3 months after remission achieved (de Groot 2009; Harper 2012)

Hodgkin lymphoma (off-label dosing): IV:

BEACOPP regimen: 650 mg/m^2 on day 1 every 3 weeks (in combination with bleomycin, etoposide, doxorubicin, vincristine, procarbazine, and prednisone) for 8 cycles (Diehl 2003)

BEACOPP escalated regimen: 1200 mg/m^2 on day 1 every 3 weeks (in combination with bleomycin, etoposide, doxorubicin, vincristine, procarbazine, and prednisone) for 8 cycles (Diehl 2003)

Multiple myeloma (off-label dosing): Oral: CyBorD regimen: 300 mg/m^2 on days 1, 8, 15, and 22 every 4 weeks (in combination with bortezomib and dexamethasone) for 4 cycles; may continue beyond 4 cycles (Khan 2012)

Non-Hodgkin lymphoma (off-label dosing): IV:

R-CHOP regimen: 750 mg/m^2 on day 1 every 3 weeks (in combination with rituximab, doxorubicin, vincristine, and prednisone) for 8 cycles (Coiffier 2002)

R-EPOCH (dose adjusted) regimen: 750 mg/m^2 on day 5 every 3 weeks (in combination with rituximab, etoposide, prednisone, vincristine, and doxorubicin) for 6 to 8 cycles (Garcia-Suarez 2007)

CODOX-M/IVAC (Burkitt lymphoma): Cycles 1 and 3 (CODOX-M): 800 mg/m^2 on day 1, followed by 200 mg/m^2 on days 2 to 5 (Magrath 1996) **or** 800 mg/m^2 on days 1 and 2 (Lacasce 2004), in combination with vincristine, doxorubicin, and methotrexate; CODOX-M alternates with IVAC (etoposide, ifosfamide, and cytarabine) for a total of 4 cycles

Lupus nephritis (off-label use): IV: 500 mg once every 2 weeks for 6 doses or 500 to 1000 mg/m^2 once every month for 6 doses (Hahn 2012) **or** 500 to 1000 mg/m^2 every month for 6 months, then every 3 months for a total of at least 2.5 years (Austin 1986; Gourley 1996)

Ovarian germ cell tumors (malignant; off-label use): IV: 150 mg/m^2 on days 1 to 5 every 28 days (in combination with dactinomycin and vincristine) for at least 10 cycles (Slayton 1985)

Small cell lung cancer (SCLC), refractory (off-label use): IV: 1000 mg/m^2 (maximum: 2000 mg) on day 1 every 3 weeks (in combination with doxorubicin and vincristine) until disease progression or unacceptable toxicity (von Pawel 1999)

Stem cell transplant conditioning (off-label use): IV:

Nonmyeloablative transplant (allogeneic): 750 mg/m^2/day for 3 days beginning 5 days prior to transplant (in combination with fludarabine) (Khouri 2008)

Myeloablative transplant:

100 mg/kg (based on IBW, unless actual weight <95% of IBW) as a single dose 2 days prior to transplant (in combination with total body irradiation and etoposide) (Thompson 2008)

50 mg/kg/day for 4 days beginning 5 days before transplant (with or without antithymocyte globulin [equine]) (Champlin 2007)

50 mg/kg/day for 4 days beginning 5 days prior to transplant (in combination with busulfan) (Cassileth 1993)

60 mg/kg/day for 2 days (in combination with busulfan and total body irradiation) (Anderson 1996)

1,800 mg/m^2/day for 4 days beginning 7 days prior to transplant (in combination with etoposide and carmustine) (Reece 1991)

◀ **Geriatric** Refer to adult dosing; adjust for renal clearance.

Pediatric Cyclophosphamide is associated with a moderate to high emetic potential (depending on dose, regimen, or administration route); antiemetics are recommended to prevent nausea and vomiting (Dupuis 2011).

US labeling:

Malignancy:

IV: 40 to 50 mg/kg in divided doses over 2 to 5 days **or** 10 to 15 mg/kg every 7 to 10 days **or** 3 to 5 mg/kg twice weekly

Oral: 1 to 5 mg/kg/day (initial and maintenance dosing)

Nephrotic syndrome, corticosteroid refractory or intolerant, or corticosteroid sparing: Oral: Initial: 2 mg/kg once daily for 8 to 12 weeks (maximum cumulative dose: 168 mg/kg); treatment beyond 90 days may increase the potential for sterility in males; treatment beyond 1 course is not recommended (Lombel 2013)

Canadian labeling: **Malignancy:**

IV: Initial: 2 to 8 mg/kg (60 to 250 mg/m^2) in divided doses for 6 or more days; Maintenance: 10 to 15 mg/kg every 7 to 10 days or 30 mg/kg every 3 to 4 weeks or when bone marrow function recovers

Oral: Initial: 2 to 8 mg/kg (60 to 250 mg/m^2) in divided doses for 6 or more days; Maintenance: 2 to 5 mg/kg (50 to 150 mg/m^2) twice weekly

Indication specific and/or off-label uses/dosing:

Ewing sarcoma (off-label use): IV: VAC/IE regimen: VAC: 1200 mg/m^2 (plus mesna) on day 1 of a 21-day treatment cycle (in combination with vincristine and doxorubicin [then dactinomycin when maximum doxorubicin dose reached]), alternates with IE (ifosfamide and etoposide) for a total of 17 cycles (Grier 2003)

Hodgkin lymphoma (off-label dosing): IV: BEACOPP escalated regimen: 1200 mg/m^2 on day 0 of a 21-day treatment cycle (in combination with bleomycin, etoposide, doxorubicin, vincristine, prednisone, and procarbazine) for 4 cycles (Kelly 2011)

Lupus nephritis (off-label use): IV: 500 to 1000 mg/m^2 every month for 6 months, then every 3 months for a total of 2.5 to 3 years (Austin 1986; Gourley 1996; Lehman 2000)

Ovarian germ cell tumors (malignant; off-label use): IV: 150 mg/m^2 on days 1 to 5 every 28 days (in combination with dactinomycin and vincristine) for at least 10 cycles (Slayton 1985)

Neuroblastoma (off-label dosing): IV: CE-CAdO regimen, courses 3 and 4: 300 mg/m^2 days 1 to 5 every 21 days for 2 cycles (Rubie 1998) **or** 10 mg/kg days 1 to 5 every 21 days for 2 cycles (Rubie 2001). **Note:** Decreased doses may be recommended for newborns or children <10 kg.

Stem cell transplant conditioning (off-label use): Myeloablative transplant: IV: 50 mg/kg/day for 4 days beginning 5 days before transplant (with or without antithymocyte globulin [equine]) (Champlin 2007)

Wilms tumor, relapsed (off-label use): Infants, Children, and Adolescents: IV (in combination with vincristine, doxorubicin, mesna, etoposide, filgrastim, and radiation therapy) (Green 2007):

Pediatrics ≤30 kg: 14.7 mg/kg days 1 to 5 of weeks 3, 9, 15, and 21 and 14.7 mg/kg days 1 to 3 of weeks 6, 12, 18, and 24

Pediatrics >30 kg: 440 mg/m^2 days 1 to 5 of weeks 3, 9, 15, and 21 and 440 mg/m^2 days 1 to 3 of weeks 6, 12, 18, and 24

Renal Impairment

US labeling: There are no dosage adjustments provided in the manufacturer's labeling (use with caution; elevated levels of metabolites may occur).

Canadian labeling:

Mild impairment: There are no dosage adjustments provided in the manufacturer's labeling

Moderate impairment: Dose reduction may be necessary; manufacturer's labeling does not provide specific dosing recommendations

Severe impairment: Use is contraindicated.

The following adjustments have also been recommended:

Aronoff 2007: Children and Adults:

CrCl ≥10 mL/minute: No dosage adjustment required.

CrCl <10 mL/minute: Administer 75% of normal dose.

Hemodialysis: Moderately dialyzable (20% to 50%); administer 50% of normal dose; administer after hemodialysis

Continuous ambulatory peritoneal dialysis (CAPD): Administer 75% of normal dose.

Continuous renal replacement therapy (CRRT): Administer 100% of normal dose.

Janus 2010: Hemodialysis: Administer 75% of normal dose; administer after hemodialysis

Hepatic Impairment
The conversion between cyclophosphamide to the active metabolite may be reduced in patients with severe hepatic impairment, potentially reducing efficacy.

US labeling: There are no dosage adjustments provided in the manufacturer's labeling.

Canadian labeling:

Mild-to-moderate impairment: There are no dosage adjustments provided in the manufacturer's labeling.

Severe impairment: Use is contraindicated.

The following adjustments have been recommended (Floyd 2006):

Serum bilirubin 3.1 to 5 mg/dL or transaminases >3 times ULN: Administer 75% of dose.

Serum bilirubin >5 mg/mL: Avoid use.

Obesity

*American Society of Clinical Oncology (ASCO) Guidelines for appropriate chemotherapy dosing in obese adults with cancer (**Note: Excludes HSCT dosing**): Utilize patient's actual body weight (full weight) for calculation of body surface area- or weight-based dosing, particularly when the intent of therapy is curative; manage regimen-related toxicities in the same manner as for nonobese patients; if a dose reduction is utilized due to toxicity, consider resumption of full weight-based dosing with subsequent cycles, especially if cause of toxicity (eg, hepatic or renal impairment) is resolved (Griggs 2012).*

American Society for Blood and Marrow Transplantation (ASBMT) practice guideline committee position statement on chemotherapy dosing in obesity (Bubalo 2014):

Cy200 (cyclophosphamide total dose of 200 mg/kg): Use the lesser of IBW or actual body weight (ABW).

Cy120 (cyclophosphamide total dose of 120 mg/kg): Use either IBW or ABW for patients ≤120% IBW (preferred method for adults of all body sizes); use ABW25 for patients >120% IBW (preferred for pediatric patients).

ABW25: Adjusted wt (kg) = Ideal body weight (kg) + 0.25 [actual wt (kg) - ideal body weight (kg)]

Adjustment for Toxicity

Hematologic toxicity: May require dose reduction or treatment interruption; Canadian labeling recommends reducing initial dose by 30% to 50% if bone marrow function compromised (due to prior radiation therapy, prior chemotherapy, or tumor infiltration)

Hemorrhagic cystitis, severe: Discontinue treatment.

Combination Regimens

Bone sarcoma (Ewing sarcoma):
Brain tumor:
Breast cancer:
Gestational trophoblastic tumor:
Leukemia, acute lymphocytic:
Leukemia, chronic lymphocytic:
Lung cancer (small cell):

◀ **Administration**

Cyclophosphamide is associated with a moderate to high emetic potential (depending on dose, regimen, or administration route); antiemetics are recommended to prevent nausea and vomiting (Basch 2011; Dupuis 2011; Roila 2010).

IV: Infusion rate may vary based on protocol (refer to specific protocol for infusion rate). Administer by direct IV injection (if reconstituted in NS), IVPB, or continuous IV infusion

Bladder toxicity: To minimize bladder toxicity, increase normal fluid intake during and for 1 to 2 days after cyclophosphamide dose. Most adult patients will require a fluid intake of at least 2 L/day. High-dose regimens should be accompanied by vigorous hydration with or without mesna therapy. Morning administration may be preferred to ensure adequate hydration throughout the day.

Hematopoietic stem cell transplant: Approaches to reduction of hemorrhagic cystitis include infusion of 0.9% NaCl 3 $L/m^2/24$ hours, infusion of 0.9% NaCl 3 $L/m^2/24$ hours with continuous 0.9% NaCl bladder irrigation 300 to 1000 mL/hour, and infusion of 0.9% NaCl 1.5 to 3 $L/m^2/24$ hours with intravenous mesna. Hydration should begin at least 4 hours before cyclophosphamide and continue at least 24 hours after completion of cyclophosphamide. The dose of daily mesna used may be 67% to 100% of the daily dose of cyclophosphamide. Mesna can be administered as a continuous 24-hour intravenous infusion or be given in divided doses every 4 hours. Mesna should begin at the start of treatment, and continue at least 24 hours following the last dose of cyclophosphamide.

Oral: Tablets are not scored and should not be cut, chewed, or crushed. Swallow capsules whole; do not open, crush, or chew. To minimize bladder toxicity, increase normal fluid intake. Morning administration may be preferred to ensure adequate hydration throughout the day; do not administer tablets/capsules at bedtime.

Hazardous agent; use appropriate precautions for handling and disposal (NIOSH 2014 [group 1]). Wear gloves when handling capsules/tablets and container. NIOSH recommends single gloving for administration of intact capsules or tablets (NIOSH 2014). Avoid exposure to broken capsules; if contact occurs, wash hands immediately and thoroughly.

Vesicant/Extravasation Risk May be an irritant

Emetic Potential

Children:

IV:

≥1,000 mg/m^2: High (>90%)

<1,000 mg/m^2: Moderate (30% to 90%)

Oral: Moderate (30% to 90%)

Adults:

IV:

≥1,500 mg/m^2: High (>90%)

<1,500 mg/m^2: Moderate (30% to 90%)

Oral: Moderate (30% to 90%)

Extemporaneous Preparations Hazardous agent: Use appropriate precautions for handling and disposal (NIOSH 2014 [group 1]). When compounding an oral solution or suspension, NIOSH recommends double gloving, a protective gown, and preparation in a controlled device; if not prepared in a controlled device, respiratory and eye protection as well as ventilated engineering controls are recommended (NIOSH 2014).

Liquid solutions for oral administration may be prepared by dissolving cyclo-phosphamide injection in Aromatic Elixir, N.F. Store refrigerated (in glass container) for up to 14 days.

Cyclophosphamide Prescribing Information, Baxter Healthcare Corporation, Deerfield, Il, May, 2013.

A 10 mg/mL oral suspension may be prepared by reconstituting one 2 g vial for injection with 100 mL of NaCl 0.9%, providing an initial concentration of 20 mg/mL. Mix this solution in a 1:1 ratio with either Simple Syrup, NF or Ora-Plus® to obtain a final concentration of 10 mg/mL. Label "shake well" and "refrigerate". Stable for 56 days refrigerated.

Kennedy R, Groepper D, Tagen M, et al, "Stability of Cyclophosphamide in Extemporaneous Oral Suspensions," *Ann Pharmacother,* 2010, 44(2):295-301.

Monitoring Parameters CBC with differential and platelets, BUN, UA, serum electrolytes, serum creatinine; monitor for signs/symptoms of hemorrhagic cystitis or other urinary/renal toxicity, pulmonary, cardiac, and/or hepatic toxicity

Additional Information In patients with CYP2B6 G516T variant allele, cyclophosphamide metabolism is markedly increased; metabolism is not influenced by CYP2C9 and CYP2C19 isotypes (Xie 2006).

Dosage Forms Excipient information presented when available (limited, particularly for generics); consult specific product labeling.

Capsule, Oral:
  Generic: 25 mg, 50 mg
Solution Reconstituted, Injection:
  Generic: 500 mg (1 ea); 1 g (1 ea); 2 g (1 ea)
Tablet, Oral:
  Generic: 25 mg, 50 mg

Dosage Forms: Canada Additional dosage forms available in Canada. Excipient information presented when available (limited, particularly for generics); consult specific product labeling.

Injection, powder for reconstitution: 200 mg

◆ **Cyclosporin A** see CycloSPORINE (Systemic) *on page 385*

CycloSPORINE (Systemic) (SYE kloe spor een)

Related Information

Hematopoietic Stem Cell Transplantation *on page 2272*
Safe Handling of Hazardous Drugs *on page 2292*

Brand Names: US Gengraf; Neoral; SandIMMUNE

Brand Names: Canada Apo-Cyclosporine; Neoral; Sandimmune I.V.; Sandoz-Cyclosporine

Index Terms Ciclosporin; CsA; CyA; Cyclosporin A

Pharmacologic Category Calcineurin Inhibitor; Immunosuppressant Agent

Use

Cyclosporine modified:

  Transplant rejection prophylaxis: Prophylaxis of organ rejection in kidney, liver, and heart transplants (has been used with azathioprine and/or corticosteroids)

  Rheumatoid arthritis: Treatment of severe, active rheumatoid arthritis (RA) not responsive to methotrexate alone

  Psoriasis: Treatment of severe, recalcitrant plaque psoriasis in nonimmunocompromised adults unresponsive to or unable to tolerate other systemic therapy

Cyclosporine non-modified: Transplant rejection (prophylaxis/treatment): Prophylaxis of organ rejection in kidney, liver, and heart transplants (has been used with azathioprine and/or corticosteroids; treatment of chronic organ rejection)

Canadian labeling: Additional uses (not in US labeling):

Cyclosporine modified: Nephrotic syndrome: Induction and maintenance of remission in steroid dependent/resistant nephrotic syndrome due to glomerular disease (eg, minimal change nephropathy, membranous glomerulonephritis, focal and segmental glomerulosclerosis); maintenance of steroid induced remission allowing for steroid dose reduction or withdrawal.

Cyclosporine modified/non-modified: Bone marrow transplantation: Prophylaxis of graft rejection following bone marrow transplantation; prophylaxis or treatment of graft-versus-host disease (GVHD)

Labeled Contraindications

Hypersensitivity to cyclosporine or any component of the formulation. IV cyclosporine is contraindicated in hypersensitivity to polyoxyethylated castor oil (Cremophor EL).

Rheumatoid arthritis and psoriasis patients with abnormal renal function, uncontrolled hypertension, or malignancies. Concomitant treatment with PUVA or UVB therapy, methotrexate, other immunosuppressive agents, coal tar, or radiation therapy are also contraindications for use in patients with psoriasis.

Canadian labeling: Additional contraindications (not in US labeling): Concurrent use with bosentan; rheumatoid arthritis and psoriasis patients with primary or secondary immunodeficiency excluding autoimmune disease, uncontrolled infection, or malignancy (excluding non-melanoma skin cancer).

Pregnancy Considerations Adverse events were not observed following the use of oral cyclosporine in animal reproduction studies (using doses that were not maternally toxic). In humans, cyclosporine crosses the placenta; maternal concentrations do not correlate with those found in the umbilical cord. Cyclosporine may be detected in the serum of newborns for several days after birth (Claris 1993). Based on clinical use, premature births and low birth weight were consistently observed in pregnant transplant patients (additional pregnancy complications also present). Formulations may contain alcohol; the alcohol content should be taken into consideration in pregnant women.

The pharmacokinetics of cyclosporine may be influenced by pregnancy (Grimer 2007). Cyclosporine may be used in pregnant renal, liver, or heart transplant patients (Cowan 2012; EBPG Expert Group on Renal Transplantation 2002; McGuire 2009; Parhar 2012). If therapy is needed for psoriasis, other agents are preferred; however, cyclosporine may be used as an alternative agent along with close clinical monitoring; use should be avoided during the first trimester if possible (Bae 2012). If treatment is needed for lupus nephritis, other agents are recommended to be used in pregnant women (Hahn 2012).

Following transplant, normal menstruation and fertility may be restored within months; however, appropriate contraception is recommended to prevent pregnancy until 1-2 years following the transplant to improve pregnancy outcomes (Cowan 2012; EBPG Expert Group on Renal Transplantation 2002; McGuire 2009; Parhar 2012).

A pregnancy registry has been established for pregnant women taking immunosuppressants following any solid organ transplant (National Transplantation Pregnancy Registry, Temple University, 877-955-6877).

A pregnancy registry has also been established for pregnant women taking Neoral for psoriasis or rheumatoid arthritis (Neoral Pregnancy Registry for Psoriasis and Rheumatoid Arthritis, Thomas Jefferson University, 888-522-5581).

Breast-Feeding Considerations Cyclosporine is excreted in breast milk. Concentrations of cyclosporine in milk vary widely and breast-feeding during therapy is generally not recommended (Bae 2012; Cowan 2012). Due to the potential for serious adverse in the breast-feeding infant, a decision should be made to discontinue cyclosporine or to discontinue breast-feeding, taking into account the importance of treatment to the mother. Formulations may contain alcohol which may be present in breast milk and could be absorbed orally by the breast-feeding infant.

Warnings/Precautions Hazardous agent - use appropriate precautions for handling and disposal (NIOSH 2014 [group 2]).

[US Boxed Warning]: Increased risk of lymphomas and other malignancies (including fatal outcomes), **particularly skin cancers;** risk is related to intensity/duration of therapy and the use of more than one immunosuppressive agent; all patients should avoid excessive sun/UV light exposure. **[US Boxed Warning]: May cause hypertension; risk is increased with increasing doses/duration.** Use caution when changing dosage forms.

[US Boxed Warning]: Renal impairment, including structural kidney damage has occurred (when used at high doses); risk is increased with increasing doses/duration; monitor renal function closely. Elevations in serum creatinine and BUN generally respond to dosage reductions. Use caution with other potentially nephrotoxic drugs (eg, acyclovir, aminoglycoside antibiotics, amphotericin B, ciprofloxacin); monitor renal function closely with concomitant use. If significant renal impairment occurs, reduce the dose of the coadministered medication or consider alternative treatment. Elevations in serum creatinine and BUN associated with nephrotoxicity generally respond to dosage reductions. In renal transplant patients with rapidly rising BUN and creatinine, carefully evaluate to differentiate between cyclosporine-associated nephrotoxicity and renal rejection episodes. In cases of severe rejection that fail to respond to pulse steroids and monoclonal antibodies, switching to an alternative immunosuppressant agent may be preferred to increasing cyclosporine to excessive blood concentrations.

[US Boxed Warning]: Increased risk of infection with use; serious and fatal infections have been reported. Bacterial, viral, fungal, and protozoal infections (including opportunistic infections) have occurred. Polyoma virus infections, such as the JC virus and BK virus, may result in serious and sometimes fatal outcomes. The JC virus is associated with progressive multifocal leukoencephalopathy (PML), and PML has been reported in patients receiving cyclosporine. PML may be fatal and presents with hemiparesis, apathy, confusion, cognitive deficiencies, and ataxia; consider neurologic consultation as indicated. The BK virus is associated with nephropathy, and polyoma virus-associated nephropathy (PVAN) has been reported in patients receiving cyclosporine. PVAN is associated with serious adverse effects including renal dysfunction and renal graft loss. If PML or PVAN occur in transplant patients, consider reducing immunosuppression therapy as well as the risk that reduced immunosuppression poses to grafts.

Hepatotoxicity (transaminase and bilirubin elevations) and liver injury, including cholestasis, jaundice, hepatitis, and liver failure, has been reported. These events were mainly in patients with confounding factors including infections, coadministration with other potentially hepatotoxic medications, underlying conditions, and significant comorbidities. Fatalities have also been reported rarely, primarily in transplant patients. Increased hepatic enzymes and bilirubin have occurred, usually in the first month and when used at high doses; improvement is usually seen with dosage reduction.

Should be used initially with corticosteroids in transplant patients. Significant hyperkalemia (with or without hyperchloremic metabolic acidosis) and hyperuricemia have occurred with therapy. Syndromes of microangiopathic hemolytic anemia and thrombocytopenia have occurred and may result in graft failure; it is accompanied by platelet consumption within the graft. Syndrome may occur without graft rejection. Although management of the syndrome is unclear, discontinuation or reduction of cyclosporine, in addition to streptokinase and heparin administration or plasmapheresis, has been associated with syndrome resolution. However, resolution seems to be dependent upon early detection of the syndrome via indium 111 labeled platelet scans.

May cause seizures, particularly if used with high-dose corticosteroids. Encephalopathy (including posterior reversible encephalopathy syndrome [PRES]) has also been reported; predisposing factors include hypertension, hypomagnesemia, hypocholesterolemia, high-dose corticosteroids, high cyclosporine serum concentration, and graft-versus-host disease (GVHD). Encephalopathy may be more common in patients with liver transplant compared to kidney transplant. Other neurotoxic events, such as optic disc edema (including papilloedema and potential visual impairment), have been rarely reported primarily in transplant patients.

[US Boxed Warning]: The modified/non-modified formulations are not bioequivalent; cyclosporine (modified) has increased bioavailability as compared to cyclosporine (non-modified) and the products cannot be used interchangeably without close monitoring. Cyclosporine (modified) refers to the oral solution and capsule dosage formulations of cyclosporine in an aqueous dispersion (previously referred to as "microemulsion"). Potentially significant drug-drug/drug-food interactions may exist, requiring dose or frequency adjustment, additional monitoring, and/or selection of alternative therapy. Gingival hyperplasia may occur; avoid concomitant nifedipine in patients who develop gingival hyperplasia (may increase frequency of hyperplasia). Monitor cyclosporine concentrations closely following the addition, modification, or deletion of other medication. Live, attenuated vaccines may be less effective; vaccination should be avoided. Make dose adjustments based on cyclosporine blood concentrations. **[US Boxed Warning]: Cyclosporine non-modified absorption is erratic; monitor blood concentrations closely. [US Boxed Warning]: Prescribing and dosage adjustment should only be under the direct supervision of an experienced physician. Adequate laboratory/medical resources and follow-up are necessary.** Anaphylaxis has been reported with IV use; reserve for patients who cannot take oral form. **[US Boxed Warning]: Risk of skin cancer may be increased in transplant patients.** Due to the increased risk for nephrotoxicity in renal transplantation, avoid using standard doses of cyclosporine in combination with everolimus; reduced cyclosporine doses are recommended; monitor cyclosporine concentrations closely. Cyclosporine and everolimus combination therapy may increase the risk for proteinuria. Cyclosporine combined with either everolimus or sirolimus may increase the risk for thrombotic micro-angiopathy/thrombotic thrombocytopenic purpura/hemolytic uremic syndrome (TMA/TTP/HUS). Cyclosporine has extensive hepatic metabolism and exposure is increased in patients with severe hepatic impairment; may require dose reduction.

Patients with psoriasis should avoid excessive sun exposure. **[US Boxed Warning]: Risk of skin cancer may be increased with a history of PUVA and possibly methotrexate or other immunosuppressants, UVB, coal tar, or radiation.**

Rheumatoid arthritis: If receiving other immunosuppressive agents, radiation or UV therapy, concurrent use of cyclosporine is not recommended.

Products may contain corn oil, ethanol (consider alcohol content in certain patient populations, including pregnant or breast-feeding women, patients with liver disease, seizure disorders, alcohol dependency, or pediatrics), or propylene glycol; injection also contains the vehicle Cremophor EL (polyoxyethylated castor oil), which has been associated with hypersensitivity (anaphylactic) reactions. Due to the risk for anaphylaxis, IV cyclosporine should be reserved for use in patients unable to take an oral formulation. Some dosage forms may contain propylene glycol; large amounts are potentially toxic and have been associated hyperosmolality, lactic acidosis, seizures, and respiratory depression; use caution (AAP 1997; Zar 2007).

Adverse Reactions Adverse reactions reported with systemic use, including rheumatoid arthritis, psoriasis, and transplantation (kidney, liver, and heart). Percentages noted include the highest frequency regardless of indication/dosage. Frequencies may vary for specific conditions or formulation.

>10%:
  Cardiovascular: Hypertension (8% to 53%), edema (5% to 14%)
  Central nervous system: Headache (2% to 25%), paresthesia (1% to 11%)
  Dermatologic: Hypertrichosis (5% to 19%)
  Endocrine & metabolic: Hirsutism (21% to 45%), increased serum triglycerides (15%), female genital tract disease (9% to 11%)
  Gastrointestinal: Nausea (2% to 23%), diarrhea (3% to 13%), gingival hyperplasia (2% to 16%), abdominal distress (<1% to 15%), dyspepsia (2% to 12%)
  Genitourinary: Urinary tract infection (kidney transplant: 21%)
  Infection: Increased susceptibility to infection (3% to 25%), viral infection (kidney transplant: 16%)
  Neuromuscular & skeletal: Tremor (7% to 55%), leg cramps (2% to 12%)
  Renal: Increased serum creatinine (16% to ≥50%), renal insufficiency (10% to 38%)
  Respiratory: Upper respiratory tract infection (1% to 14%)

Kidney, liver, and heart transplant only (≤2% unless otherwise noted):
  Cardiovascular: Chest pain (≤4%), flushing (<1% to 4%), glomerular capillary thrombosis, myocardial infarction
  Central nervous system: Convulsions (1% to 5%), anxiety, confusion, lethargy, tingling sensation
  Dermatologic: Skin infection (7%), acne vulgaris (1% to 6%), nail disease (brittle fingernails), hair breakage, night sweats, pruritus

Endocrine & metabolic: Gynecomastia (<1% to 4%), hyperglycemia, hypo-magnesemia, weight loss

Gastrointestinal: Vomiting (2% to 10%), anorexia, aphthous stomatitis, con-stipation, dysphagia, gastritis, hiccups, pancreatitis

Genitourinary: Hematuria

Hematologic & oncologic: Leukopenia (<1% to 6%), lymphoma (<1% to 6%), anemia, thrombocytopenia, upper gastrointestinal hemorrhage

Hepatic: Hepatotoxicity (<1% to 7%)

Infection: Localized fungal infection (8%), cytomegalovirus disease (5%), septicemia (5%), abscess (4%), fungal infection (systemic: 2%)

Neuromuscular & skeletal: Arthralgia, myalgia, weakness

Ophthalmic: Conjunctivitis, visual disturbance

Otic: Hearing loss, tinnitus

Respiratory: Sinusitis (<1% to 7%), pneumonia (6%)

Miscellaneous: Fever

Rheumatoid arthritis only (1% to <3% unless otherwise noted):

Cardiovascular: Chest pain (4%), cardiac arrhythmia (2%), abnormal heart sounds, cardiac failure, myocardial infarction, peripheral ischemia

Central nervous system: Dizziness (8%), pain (6%), insomnia (4%), depres-sion (3%), migraine (2% to 3%), anxiety, drowsiness, emotional lability, hypoesthesia, lack of concentration, malaise, neuropathy, nervousness, paranoia, vertigo

Dermatologic: Cellulitis, dermatological reaction, dermatitis, diaphoresis, dyschromia, eczema, enanthema, folliculitis, nail disease, pruritus, urticaria, xeroderma

Endocrine & metabolic: Menstrual disease (3%), decreased libido, diabetes mellitus, goiter, hot flash, hyperkalemia, hyperuricemia, hypoglycemia, increased libido, weight gain, weight loss

Gastrointestinal: Vomiting (9%), flatulence (5%), gingivitis (4%), constipation, dysgeusia, dysphagia, enlargement of salivary glands, eructation, esoph-agitis, gastric ulcer, gastritis, gastroenteritis, gingival hemorrhage, glossitis, peptic ulcer, tongue disease, xerostomia

Genitourinary: Leukorrhea (1%), breast fibroadenosis, hematuria, mastalgia, nocturia, urine abnormality, urinary incontinence, urinary urgency, uterine hemorrhage

Hematologic & oncologic: Purpura (3% to 4%), anemia, carcinoma, leukope-nia, lymphadenopathy

Hepatic: Hyperbilirubinemia

Infection: Abscess (including renal), bacterial infection, candidiasis, fungal infection, herpes simplex infection, herpes zoster, viral infection

Neuromuscular & skeletal: Arthralgia, bone fracture, dislocation, myalgia, stiffness, synovial cyst, tendon disease, weakness

Ophthalmic: Cataract, conjunctivitis, eye pain, visual disturbance

Otic: Tinnitus, deafness, vestibular disturbance

Renal: Abscess (renal), increased blood urea nitrogen, polyuria, pyeloneph-ritis

Respiratory: Cough (5%), dyspnea (5%), sinusitis (4%), abnormal breath sounds, bronchospasm, epistaxis, tonsillitis

Psoriasis only (1% to <3% unless otherwise noted):

Cardiovascular: Chest pain, flushing

Central nervous system: Psychiatric disturbance (4% to 5%), pain (3% to 4%), dizziness, insomnia, nervousness, vertigo

Dermatologic: Acne vulgaris, folliculitis, hyperkeratosis, pruritus, skin rash, xeroderma

Endocrine & metabolic: Hot flash

Gastrointestinal: Abdominal distention, constipation, gingival hemorrhage, increased appetite

Genitourinary: Urinary frequency

Hematologic & oncologic: Abnormal erythrocytes, altered platelet function, blood coagulation disorder, carcinoma, hemorrhagic diathesis

Hepatic: Hyperbilirubinemia

Neuromuscular & skeletal: Arthralgia (1% to 6%)

Ophthalmic: Visual disturbance

Respiratory: Flu-like symptoms (8% to 10%), bronchospasm (5%), cough (5%), dyspnea (5%), rhinitis (5%), respiratory tract infection

Miscellaneous: Fever

Postmarketing and/or case reports (any indication): Anaphylaxis/anaphylactoid reaction (possibly associated with Cremophor EL vehicle in injection formulation), brain disease, central nervous system toxicity, cholestasis, cholesterol increased, exacerbation of psoriasis (transformation to erythrodermic or pustular psoriasis), fatigue, gout, haemolytic uremic syndrome, hepatic insufficiency, hepatitis, hyperbilirubinemia, hyperkalemia, hyperlipidemia, hypertrichosis, hyperuricemia, hypomagnesemia, impaired consciousness, increased susceptibility to infection (including JC virus and BK virus), jaundice, leg pain (possibly a manifestation of Calcineurin-Inhibitor Induced Pain Syndrome), malignant lymphoma, migraine, myalgia, myopathy, myositis, papilledema, progressive multifocal leukoencephalopathy, pseudotumor cerebri, pulmonary edema (noncardiogenic), renal disease (polyoma virus-associated), reversible posterior leukoencephalopathy syndrome, rhabdomyolysis, thrombotic microangiopathy

Drug Interactions

Metabolism/Transport Effects Substrate of CYP3A4 (major), P-glycoprotein; **Note:** Assignment of Major/Minor substrate status based on clinically relevant drug interaction potential; **Inhibits** BSEP, CYP2C9 (weak), CYP3A4 (weak), P-glycoprotein, SLCO1B1

Avoid Concomitant Use

Avoid concomitant use of CycloSPORINE (Systemic) with any of the following: Aliskiren; AtorvaSTATin; BCG (Intravesical); Bosentan; Bosutinib; Cholic Acid; Conivaptan; Crizotinib; Dronedarone; Enzalutamide; Eplerenone; Foscarnet; Fusidic Acid (Systemic); Idelalisib; Lercanidipine; Lovastatin; Mifepristone; Natalizumab; PAZOPanib; Pimecrolimus; Pimozide; Pitavastatin; Potassium-Sparing Diuretics; Silodosin; Simeprevir; SimvaSTATin; Sitaxentan; Tacrolimus (Systemic); Tacrolimus (Topical); Tofacitinib; Topotecan; Vaccines (Live); VinCRIStine (Liposomal)

Increased Effect/Toxicity

CycloSPORINE (Systemic) may increase the levels/effects of: Afatinib; Aliskiren; Ambrisentan; ARIPiprazole; AtorvaSTATin; Boceprevir; Bosentan; Bosutinib; Brentuximab Vedotin; Calcium Channel Blockers (Dihydropyridine); Calcium Channel Blockers (Nondihydropyridine); Caspofungin; Cholic Acid; Colchicine; Dabigatran Etexilate; Dexamethasone (Systemic); Digoxin; Dofetilide; DOXOrubicin (Conventional); Dronedarone; Edoxaban; Eluxadoline; Etoposide; Etoposide Phosphate; Everolimus; Ezetimibe; Fibric Acid Derivatives; Fimasartan; Fingolimod; Flibanserin; Fluvastatin; Hydrocodone; Imipenem; Ledipasvir; Leflunomide; Lercanidipine; Lomitapide; Loop Diuretics; Lovastatin; Methotrexate; MethylPREDNISolone; Minoxidil (Systemic);

Minoxidil (Topical); MitoXANtrone; Naloxegol; Natalizumab; Neuromuscular-Blocking Agents; NiMODipine; Nonsteroidal Anti-Inflammatory Agents; PAZOPanib; P-glycoprotein/ABCB1 Substrates; Pimozide; Pitavastatin; Pravastatin; PredniSOLONE (Systemic); PredniSONE; Protease Inhibitors; Prucalopride; Ranolazine; Repaglinide; Rifaximin; Rosuvastatin; Silodosin; Simeprevir; Simvastatin; Sirolimus; Sitaxentan; Tacrolimus (Systemic); Tacrolimus (Topical); Ticagrelor; Tofacitinib; Topotecan; Vaccines (Live); VinCRIStine (Liposomal)

The levels/effects of CycloSPORINE (Systemic) may be increased by: AcetaZOLAMIDE; Aminoglycosides; Amiodarone; Amphotericin B; Androgens; Angiotensin II Receptor Blockers; Antifungal Agents (Azole Derivatives, Systemic); Aprepitant; Boceprevir; Bromocriptine; Calcium Channel Blockers (Nondihydropyridine); Carvedilol; Chloramphenicol; Conivaptan; Crizotinib; Cyclophosphamide; CYP3A4 Inhibitors (Moderate); CYP3A4 Inhibitors (Strong); Dasatinib; Denosumab; Dexamethasone (Systemic); Eplerenone; Ezetimibe; Fluconazole; Fosaprepitant; Foscarnet; Fusidic Acid (Systemic); GlyBURIDE; Grapefruit Juice; Idelalisib; Imatinib; Imipenem; Ivacaftor; Lercanidipine; Luliconazole; Macrolide Antibiotics; Melphalan; Methotrexate; MethylPREDNISolone; Metoclopramide; Metreleptin; Mifepristone; Netupitant; Nonsteroidal Anti-Inflammatory Agents; Norfloxacin; Ombitasvir, Paritaprevir, and Ritonavir; Ombitasvir, Paritaprevir, Ritonavir, and Dasabuvir; Omeprazole; Osimertinib; Palbociclib; P-glycoprotein/ABCB1 Inhibitors; Pimecrolimus; Potassium-Sparing Diuretics; Pravastatin; PredniSOLONE (Systemic); PredniSONE; Protease Inhibitors; Pyrazinamide; Quinupristin; Ranolazine; Ritonavir; Roflumilast; Simeprevir; Sirolimus; Stiripentol; Sulfonamide Derivatives; Tacrolimus (Systemic); Tacrolimus (Topical); Telaprevir; Temsirolimus; Trastuzumab

Decreased Effect

CycloSPORINE (Systemic) may decrease the levels/effects of: BCG (Intravesical); Coccidioides immitis Skin Test; GlyBURIDE; Mycophenolate; Sipuleucel-T; Vaccines (Inactivated); Vaccines (Live)

The levels/effects of CycloSPORINE (Systemic) may be decreased by: Adalimumab; Armodafinil; Ascorbic Acid; Barbiturates; Bosentan; CarBAMazepine; Colesevelam; Cyclophosphamide; CYP3A4 Inducers (Moderate); CYP3A4 Inducers (Strong); Dabrafenib; Deferasirox; Dexamethasone (Systemic); Echinacea; Efavirenz; Enzalutamide; Fibric Acid Derivatives; Fosphenytoin; Griseofulvin; Imipenem; MethylPREDNISolone; Metreleptin; Mitotane; Modafinil; Multivitamins/Fluoride (with ADE); Multivitamins/Minerals (with ADEK, Folate, Iron); Multivitamins/Minerals (with AE, No Iron); Nafcillin; Orlistat; Osimertinib; P-glycoprotein/ABCB1 Inducers; Phenytoin; PrednisoLONE (Systemic); PredniSONE; Rifamycin Derivatives; Sevelamer; Siltuximab; Somatostatin Analogs; St Johns Wort; Sulfinpyrazone; Sulfonamide Derivatives; Tocilizumab; Vitamin E; Vitamin E (Oral)

Food Interactions Grapefruit juice increases cyclosporine serum concentrations. Management: Avoid grapefruit juice.

Storage/Stability

Capsules (modified): Store in the original unit-dose container at 20°C to 25°C (68°F to 77°F).

Capsules (non-modified): Store at 25°C (77°F); excursions are permitted between 15°C and 30°C (59°F and 86°F). An odor may be detected upon opening the unit-dose container, which will dissipate shortly thereafter. This odor does not affect the quality of the product.

Injection: Store below 30°C (86°F) or at controlled room temperature (product dependent). Protect from light. Stability of injection of parenteral admixture at room temperature (25°C) is 6 hours in PVC; 12 to 24 hours in Excel, PAB containers, or glass. The manufacturer recommends discarding diluted infusion solutions after 24 hours.

Oral solution (modified): Store in the original container at 20°C to 25°C (68°F to 77°F). Do not store in the refrigerator. Once opened, use within 2 months. At temperatures below 20°C (68°F), the solution may gel; light flocculation or the formation of a light sediment also may occur. There is no impact on product performance or dosing using the syringe provided. Allow to warm to room temperature (25°C [77°F]) to reverse these changes.

Oral solution (non-modified): Store in the original container at temperatures below 30°C (86°F). Do not store in the refrigerator. Protect from freezing. Once opened, use within 2 months.

Preparation for Administration Hazardous agent - use appropriate precautions for handling and disposal (NIOSH 2014 [group 2]).

Injection: To minimize leaching of DEHP, non-PVC containers and sets should be used for preparation and administration.

Sandimmune injection: Injection should be further diluted (1 mL [50 mg] of concentrate in 20-100 mL of D_5W or NS) for administration by intravenous infusion.

Oral solution: Should be mixed in glass containers (not in plastic).

Mechanism of Action Inhibition of production and release of interleukin II and inhibits interleukin II-induced activation of resting T-lymphocytes.

Pharmacodynamics/Kinetics

Absorption: Oral:

Cyclosporine (non-modified): Erratic and incomplete; dependent on presence of food, bile acids, and GI motility; larger oral doses are needed in pediatrics due to shorter bowel length and limited intestinal absorption

Cyclosporine (modified): Erratic and incomplete; increased absorption, up to 30% when compared to cyclosporine (non-modified); less dependent on food, bile acids, or GI motility when compared to cyclosporine (non-modified)

Distribution: Widely in tissues and body fluids including the liver, pancreas, and lungs

V_{dss}: 4-6 L/kg in renal, liver, and marrow transplant recipients (slightly lower values in cardiac transplant patients; children <10 years have higher values); ESRD: 3.49 L/kg

Protein binding: 90% to 98% to lipoproteins

Metabolism: Extensively hepatic via CYP3A4; forms at least 25 metabolites; extensive first-pass effect following oral administration

Bioavailability: Oral:

Cyclosporine (non-modified): Dependent on patient population and transplant type (<10% in adult liver transplant patients and as high as 89% in renal transplant patients); bioavailability of Sandimmune capsules and oral solution are equivalent; bioavailability of oral solution is ~30% of the IV solution

Children: 28% (range: 17% to 42%); gut dysfunction common in BMT patients and oral bioavailability is further reduced

Cyclosporine (modified): Bioavailability of Neoral capsules and oral solution are equivalent:

Children: 43% (range: 30% to 68%)

Adults: 23% greater than with cyclosporine (non-modified) in renal transplant patients; 50% greater in liver transplant patients

◀ Half-life elimination: Oral: May be prolonged in patients with hepatic impairment and shorter in pediatric patients due to the higher metabolism rate

Cyclosporine (non-modified): Biphasic: Alpha: 1.4 hours; Terminal: 19 hours (range: 10-27 hours)

Cyclosporine (modified): Biphasic: Terminal: 8.4 hours (range: 5-18 hours)

Time to peak, serum: Oral:

Cyclosporine (non-modified): 2-6 hours; some patients have a second peak at 5-6 hours

Cyclosporine (modified): Renal transplant: 1.5-2 hours

Excretion: Primarily feces; urine (6%, 0.1% as unchanged drug and metabolites)

Dosing

Adult Neoral/Gengraf and Sandimmune are not bioequivalent and cannot be used interchangeably.

Psoriasis: Oral: Cyclosporine (modified): Initial dose: 2.5 mg/kg daily, divided twice daily

Titration:

US labeling: Increase by 0.5 mg/kg daily if insufficient response is seen after 4 weeks of treatment. Additional dosage increases may be made every 2 weeks if needed (maximum dose: 4 mg/kg daily)

Canadian labeling: Increase by 0.5 to 1 mg/kg daily if insufficient response is seen after 4 weeks of treatment. Additional dosage increases may be made every 4 weeks if needed (maximum dose: 5 mg/kg daily)

Discontinue if no benefit is seen by 6 weeks of therapy at the maximum dose. Once patients are adequately controlled, the dose should be decreased to the lowest effective dose. Doses lower than 2.5 mg/kg daily may be effective. The Canadian labeling recommends 6 attempting to wean patients off therapy if no relapse occurs within 6 months of achieving remission. Treatment longer than 1 year is not recommended.

Note: Increase the frequency of blood pressure monitoring after each alteration in dosage of cyclosporine. Cyclosporine dosage should be decreased by 25% to 50% in patients with no history of hypertension who develop sustained hypertension during therapy and, if hypertension persists, treatment with cyclosporine should be discontinued.

Rheumatoid arthritis: Oral: Cyclosporine (modified): Initial dose: 2.5 mg/kg daily, divided twice daily; salicylates, NSAIDs, and oral glucocorticoids may be continued (refer to Drug Interactions)

Titration:

US labeling: Dose may be increased by 0.5 to 0.75 mg/kg daily if insufficient response is seen after 8 weeks of treatment; additional dosage increases may be made again at 12 weeks (maximum dose: 4 mg/kg daily). Discontinue if no benefit is seen by 16 weeks of therapy.

Canadian labeling: If insufficient response to initial dose after 6 weeks, may increase dose gradually as tolerated (maximum dose: 5 mg/kg daily); maintenance therapy should be individualized to the lowest effective and tolerable dose; may take up to 12 weeks before full effect is achieved.

Note: Increase the frequency of blood pressure monitoring after each alteration in dosage of cyclosporine. Cyclosporine dosage should be decreased by 25% to 50% in patients with no history of hypertension who develop sustained hypertension during therapy and, if hypertension persists, treatment with cyclosporine should be discontinued.

Solid organ transplant (newly transplanted patients): Adjunct therapy with corticosteroids is recommended. Initial dose should be given 4 to 12 hours prior to transplant or may be given postoperatively; adjust initial dose to achieve desired plasma concentration.

Oral: Dose is dependent upon type of transplant and formulation:

Cyclosporine (modified):

Renal: 9 ± 3 mg/kg daily, in 2 divided doses

Liver: 8 ± 4 mg/kg daily, in 2 divided doses

Heart: 7 ± 3 mg/kg daily, in 2 divided doses

Cyclosporine (non-modified): Initial doses of 10 to 14 mg/kg daily have been used for renal transplants (the manufacturer's labeling includes dosing from initial clinical trials of 15 mg/kg daily [range: 14 to 18 mg/kg daily]; however, this higher dosing level is rarely used any longer). Continue initial dose daily for 1 to 2 weeks; taper by 5% per week to a maintenance dose of 5 to 10 mg/kg daily; some renal transplant patients may be dosed as low as 3 mg/kg daily

Note: When using the non-modified formulation, cyclosporine levels may increase in liver transplant patients when the T-tube is closed; dose may need decreased

IV: Cyclosporine (non-modified): Manufacturer's labeling: Initial dose: 5 to 6 mg/kg daily or one-third of the oral dose as a single dose, infused over 2 to 6 hours; use should be limited to patients unable to take capsules or oral solution; patients should be switched to an oral dosage form as soon as possible.

Note: Many transplant centers administer cyclosporine as "divided dose" infusions (in 2 to 3 doses daily) or as a continuous (24-hour) infusion; dosages range from 3 to 7.5 mg/kg daily. Specific institutional protocols should be consulted.

Note: Conversion to cyclosporine (modified) from cyclosporine (non-modified): Start with daily dose previously used and adjust to obtain preconversion cyclosporine trough concentration. Plasma concentrations should be monitored every 4 to 7 days and dose adjusted as necessary, until desired trough level is obtained. When transferring patients with previously poor absorption of cyclosporine (non-modified), monitor trough levels at least twice weekly (especially if initial dose exceeds 10 mg/kg daily); high plasma levels are likely to occur.

Acute graft versus host disease (GVHD), prevention (off-label use in the US): IV followed by oral:

Initial: IV: 3 mg/kg daily 1 day prior to transplant; may convert to oral therapy when tolerated; titrate dose to appropriate cyclosporine trough concentration (in combination with methotrexate); taper per protocol (refer to specific references for tapering and target trough details); discontinue 6 months post-transplant in the absence of acute GVHD (Ratanatharathorn 1998; Ruutu 2013; Storb 1986a; Storb 1986b)

or

Initial: IV: 5 mg/kg (continuous infusion over 20 hours) each day for 6 days (loading dose) starting 2 days prior to transplant, then 3 mg/kg over 20 hours each day for 11 days starting on post-transplant day 4, then 3.75 mg/kg over 20 hours each day for 21 days starting on day 15, then **oral** (in 2 divided daily doses): 10 mg/kg daily days 36 to 83, then 8 mg/kg daily days 84 to 97, then 6 mg/kg daily days 98 to 119, then 4 mg/kg daily days 120 to 180, then discontinue (in combination with methotrexate +/- corticosteroid) (Chao 1993; Chao 2000)

Bone marrow transplantation *(Canadian labeling):* **Note:** IV administration is preferred for initial therapy.

Oral: Cyclosporine (modified): Initial: 12.5 to 15 mg/kg daily in 2 divided doses beginning 1 day prior to transplant; Maintenance: ~12.5 mg/kg daily in 2 divided doses every 12 hours for at least 3 to 6 months (higher doses may be required in patients with gastrointestinal conditions which may decrease absorption); decrease dose gradually to zero by 1 year following transplant. Patients who develop GVHD after discontinuation of cyclosporine may be reinitiated on therapy with a loading dose of 10 to 12.5 mg/kg followed by the previously established maintenance dose. Patients with mild, chronic GVHD should be treated with lowest effective dose.

IV: Cyclosporine (non-modified): Initial: 3 to 5 mg/kg daily or one-third of the oral dose as a single dose (infused over 2 to 6 hours) beginning 1 day prior to transplant; Maintenance: May continue initial dose for up to 2 weeks; however, patients should be switched to an oral dosage form as soon as possible.

Focal segmental glomerulosclerosis (off-label use in the US): Oral: Initial: 3.5 to 5 mg/kg daily divided every 12 hours (in combination with oral prednisone) (Braun 2008; Cattran 1999)

Interstitial cystitis (bladder pain syndrome) (off-label use): Oral: Initial: 2 to 3 mg/kg/day in 2 divided doses (maximum of 300 mg daily). Once symptom relief is established, the dose can be tapered as tolerated (to as low as 1 mg/kg as a single daily dose) and in some cases can be stopped with continued benefit. Treatment duration was at least 6 months to more than 1 year in some patients (Forrest 2012; Sairanen 2004; Sairanen 2005; Sairanen 2008).

Nephrotic syndrome *(Canadian labeling):* Oral: Cyclosporine (modified):
Initial: 3.5 mg/kg daily in 2 divided doses every 12 hours; titrate for induction of remission and renal function. Adjunct therapy with low-dose oral corticosteroids is recommended for patients with an inadequate response to cyclosporine (particularly if steroid-resistant).

Maintenance: Dose is individualized based on proteinuria, serum creatinine, and tolerability but should be maintained at lowest effective dose; maximum dose: 5 mg/kg daily. Discontinue if no improvement is observed after 3 months.

Lupus nephritis (off-label use): Oral: Cyclosporine (modified): Initial: 4 mg/kg daily for 1 month (reduce dose if trough concentrations >200 ng/mL); reduce dose by 0.5 mg/kg every 2 weeks to a maintenance dose of 2.5 to 3 mg/kg daily (Moroni 2006)

Ulcerative colitis, severe (steroid-refractory) (off-label use):

IV: Cyclosporine (non-modified): 2 to 4 mg/kg daily, infused continuously over 24 hours. (Lichtiger 1994; Van Assche 2003). **Note:** Some studies suggest no therapeutic difference between low-dose (2 mg/kg) and high-dose (4 mg/kg) cyclosporine regimens (Van Assche 2003).

Oral: Cyclosporine (modified): 2.3 to 3 mg/kg every 12 hours (De Saussure 2005; Weber 2006)

Note: Patients responsive to IV therapy should be switched to oral therapy when possible.

Geriatric Refer to adult dosing. **Sandimmune and Neoral/Gengraf are not bioequivalent and cannot be used interchangeably.**

Pediatric

Bone marrow transplantation *(Canadian labeling)*: **Note:** IV administration is preferred for initial therapy.

Oral: Cyclosporine (modified): Initial: 12.5 to 15 mg/kg daily in 2 divided doses beginning 1 day prior to transplant; Maintenance: ~12.5 mg/kg daily in 2 divided doses every 12 hours for at least 3 to 6 months (higher doses may be required in patients with gastrointestinal conditions which may decrease absorption); decrease dose gradually to zero by 1 year following transplant. Patients who develop graft versus host disease (GVHD) after discontinuation of cyclosporine may be reinitiated on therapy with a loading dose of 10 to 12.5 mg/kg followed by the previously established maintenance dose. Patients with mild, chronic GVHD should be treated with lowest effective dose.

IV: Cyclosporine (non-modified): Initial: 3 to 5 mg/kg daily or one-third of the oral dose as a single dose (infused over 2 to 6 hours) beginning 1 day prior to transplant; Maintenance: may continue initial dose for up to 2 weeks; however, patients should be switched to an oral dosage form as soon as possible.

Nephrotic syndrome *(Canadian labeling)*: Oral: Cyclosporine (modified):

Initial: 4.2 mg/kg daily in 2 divided doses every 12 hours; titrate for induction of remission and renal function. Adjunct therapy with low-dose oral corticosteroids is recommended for patients with an inadequate response to cyclosporine (particularly if steroid-resistant).

Maintenance: Dose is individualized based on proteinuria, serum creatinine, and tolerability but should be maintained at lowest effective dose; maximum dose: 6 mg/kg daily. Discontinue if no improvement is observed after 3 months.

Solid organ transplant: Refer to adult dosing. Children may require, and are able to tolerate, larger doses than adults.

Renal Impairment

Nephrotic syndrome: *Canadian labeling:* Initial: 2.5 mg/kg daily

Serum creatinine levels >30% above pretreatment levels: Take another sample within 2 weeks; if the level remains >30% above pretreatment levels, decrease dosage of cyclosporine (modified) by 25% to 50%.

Psoriasis (severe):

Abnormal renal function prior to treatment: Use is contraindicated.

Abnormal renal function during treatment:

US labeling:

Serum creatinine levels ≥25% above pretreatment levels: Take another sample within 2 weeks; if the level remains ≥25% above pretreatment levels, decrease dosage of cyclosporine (modified) by 25% to 50%. If two dosage adjustments do not reverse the increase in serum creatinine levels, treatment should be discontinued.

Serum creatinine levels ≥50% above pretreatment levels: Decrease cyclosporine dosage by 25% to 50%. If two dosage adjustments do not reverse the increase in serum creatinine levels, treatment should be discontinued.

Canadian labeling: Serum creatinine levels >30% above pretreatment levels: Decrease dosage of cyclosporine (modified) by 25% to 50%. If dosage adjustment does not reverse the increase in serum creatinine levels within 30 days, discontinue treatment.

◀ **Rheumatoid arthritis:**
Abnormal renal function prior to treatment: Use is contraindicated.
Abnormal renal function during treatment: *Canadian labeling:*
Serum creatinine levels >30% above pretreatment levels: Take another sample within 2 weeks; if the level remains ≥30% above pretreatment levels, manufacturer labeling recommends reducing dose but does not provide specific dosing recommendation. If dosage adjustment does not reverse the increase in serum creatinine levels within 30 days, discontinue treatment.
Serum creatinine levels >50% above pretreatment levels: Reduce dose by 50%; if dosage adjustment does not reverse the increase in serum creatinine levels within 30 days, discontinue treatment.
Hemodialysis: Supplemental dose is not necessary.
Peritoneal dialysis: Supplemental dose is not necessary.

Hepatic Impairment
Mild-to-moderate impairment: There are no dosage adjustments provided in the manufacturer's labeling; monitor blood concentrations.
Severe impairment: There are no dosage adjustments provided in the manufacturer's labeling; however, metabolism is extensively hepatic (exposure is increased). Monitor blood concentrations; may require dose reduction.

Administration
Oral solution: Do not administer liquid from plastic or styrofoam cup. May dilute Neoral oral solution with orange juice or apple juice. May dilute Sandimmune oral solution with milk, chocolate milk, or orange juice. Avoid changing diluents frequently. Mix thoroughly and drink at once. Use syringe provided to measure dose. Mix in a glass container and rinse container with more diluent to ensure total dose is taken. Do not rinse syringe before or after use (may cause dose variation).
Administer this medication consistently with relation to time of day and meals.
Combination therapy with renal transplantation:
Everolimus: Administer cyclosporine at the same time as everolimus
Sirolimus: Administer cyclosporine 4 hours prior to sirolimus
IV: The manufacturer recommends that following dilution, intravenous admixture be administered over 2-6 hours. However, many transplant centers administer as divided doses (2-3 doses/day) or as a 24-hour continuous infusion. Discard solution after 24 hours. Anaphylaxis has been reported with IV use; reserve for patients who cannot take oral form. Patients should be under continuous observation for at least the first 30 minutes of the infusion, and should be monitored frequently thereafter. Maintain patent airway; other supportive measures and agents for treating anaphylaxis should be present when IV drug is given. To minimize leaching of DEHP, non-PVC sets should be used for administration.

Hazardous agent - use appropriate precautions for handling and disposal (NIOSH 2014 [group 2]).

Monitoring Parameters Monitor plasma concentrations periodically and following the addition, modification, or deletion of other medications. Monitor renal function (serum creatinine and BUN) after any cyclosporine dosage changes or addition, modification, or deletion of other medications. Monitor blood pressure after any cyclosporine dosage changes or addition, modification, or deletion of other medications. Monitor for hypersensitivity reactions (IV cyclosporine). Monitor for signs/symptoms of hepatotoxicity, secondary malignancy, infection.

Nephrotic syndrome (Canadian labeling): Baseline blood pressure (2 readings within 2 weeks), fasting serum creatinine (at least 3 levels within 2 weeks), creatinine clearance, urinalysis, CBC, liver function, serum uric acid, serum potassium, and malignancy screening (eg, skin, mouth, lymph nodes). Biweekly monitoring of blood pressure for initial 3 months and then monthly thereafter, frequent monitoring of renal function and periodic cyclosporine trough levels are recommended during therapy. Consider renal biopsy in patients with steroid-dependent minimal change neuropathy who have been maintained on therapy >1 year.

Transplant patients: Cyclosporine trough levels, serum electrolytes, renal function, hepatic function, blood pressure, lipid profile

Psoriasis therapy: Baseline blood pressure, serum creatinine (2 levels each), BUN, CBC, serum magnesium, potassium, uric acid, lipid profile. Biweekly monitoring of blood pressure, complete blood count, serum creatinine, and levels of BUN, uric acid, potassium, lipids, and magnesium during the first 3 months of treatment for psoriasis. Monthly monitoring is recommended after this initial period. (**Note:** The Canadian labeling recommends bimonthly monitoring of serum creatinine after the initial period if serum creatinine remains stable and cyclosporine dose is ≤2.5 mg/kg daily, and monthly monitoring for higher doses). Also evaluate any atypical skin lesions prior to therapy. Increase the frequency of blood pressure monitoring after each alteration in dosage of cyclosporine.

Rheumatoid arthritis: Baseline blood pressure, and serum creatinine (2 levels each); serum creatinine every 2 weeks for first 3 months, then monthly if patient is stable. Increase the frequency of blood pressure monitoring after each alteration in dosage of cyclosporine. Additional Canadian labeling recommendations include CBC, hepatic function, urinalysis, serum potassium and uric acid (baseline and periodic thereafter).

Test Interactions Specific whole blood assay for cyclosporine may be falsely elevated if sample is drawn from the same central venous line through which dose was administered (even if flush has been administered and/or dose was given hours before); cyclosporine metabolites cross-react with radioimmunoassay and fluorescence polarization immunoassay

Dietary Considerations Avoid grapefruit juice with oral cyclosporine use.

Dosage Forms Considerations

Cyclosporine (modified): Gengraf and Neoral

Cyclosporine (non-modified): SandIMMUNE

Cyclosporine injection contains polyoxyethylated castor oil (Cremophor EL)

Dosage Forms Excipient information presented when available (limited, particularly for generics); consult specific product labeling. [DSC] = Discontinued product

Capsule, Oral:

Gengraf: 25 mg, 100 mg [DSC] [contains cremophor el, fd&c blue #2 (indigotine)]

Gengraf: 100 mg [contains fd&c blue #2 (indigotine)]

Neoral: 25 mg, 100 mg [contains alcohol, usp]

SandIMMUNE: 25 mg, 100 mg

Generic: 25 mg, 50 mg, 100 mg

Solution, Intravenous:

SandIMMUNE: 50 mg/mL (5 mL) [contains alcohol, usp, cremophor el]

Generic: 50 mg/mL (5 mL)

◄

Solution, Oral:
  Gengraf: 100 mg/mL (50 mL) [contains propylene glycol]
  Neoral: 100 mg/mL (50 mL) [contains alcohol, usp]
  SandIMMUNE: 100 mg/mL (50 mL) [contains alcohol, usp]
  Generic: 100 mg/mL (50 mL)

Dosage Forms: Canada
Excipient information presented when available (limited, particularly for generics); consult specific product labeling.
Capsule, Oral:
  Neoral: 10 mg, 25 mg, 50 mg, 100 mg [contains alcohol]
Solution, Intravenous:
  SandIMMUNE IV: 50 mg/mL (1 mL, 5 mL) [contains alcohol, cremophor el]
Solution, Oral:
  Neoral: 100 mg/mL (50 mL) [contains alcohol, propylene glycol]

◆ **Cyklokapron** see Tranexamic Acid on page 1681

Cyproheptadine (si proe HEP ta deen)

Brand Names: Canada Euro-Cyproheptadine; PMS-Cyproheptadine

Index Terms Cyproheptadine Hydrochloride; Periactin

Pharmacologic Category Histamine H_1 Antagonist; Histamine H_1 Antagonist, First Generation; Piperidine Derivative

Use Perennial and seasonal allergic rhinitis and other allergic symptoms including urticaria

Labeled Contraindications Hypersensitivity to cyproheptadine or any component of the formulation; narrow-angle glaucoma; bladder neck obstruction; pyloroduodenal obstruction; symptomatic prostatic hyperplasia; stenosing peptic ulcer; concurrent use of MAO inhibitors; use in debilitated elderly patients; use in premature and term newborns due to potential association with SIDS; breast-feeding

Pregnancy Considerations Adverse events have been observed in some animal reproduction studies. Maternal antihistamine use has generally not resulted in an increased risk of birth defects; however, information specific to cyproheptadine is limited. Antihistamines are recommended for the treatment of rhinitis, urticaria, and pruritus with rash in pregnant women (although second generation antihistamines may be preferred). Antihistamines are not recommended for treatment of pruritus associated with intrahepatic cholestasis in pregnancy.

Breast-Feeding Considerations It is not known if cyproheptadine is excreted into breast milk. Premature infants and newborns have a higher risk of intolerance to antihistamines. Use while breast-feeding is contraindicated by the manufacturer. Antihistamines may decrease maternal serum prolactin concentrations when administered prior to the establishment of nursing.

Warnings/Precautions May cause CNS depression, which may impair physical or mental abilities; patients must be cautioned about performing tasks which require mental alertness (eg, operating machinery or driving). Effects may be potentiated when used with other sedative drugs or ethanol. Use with caution in patients with cardiovascular disease; increased intraocular pressure; respiratory disease; or thyroid dysfunction. In the elderly, avoid use of this potent anticholinergic agent due to increased risk of confusion, dry mouth, constipation, and other anticholinergic effects; clearance decreases in patients of advanced age (Beers Criteria). Antihistamines may cause excitation in young children.

Adverse Reactions Frequency not defined.

Cardiovascular: Extrasystoles, hypotension, palpitations, tachycardia

Central nervous system: Ataxia, chills, confusion, dizziness, drowsiness, euphoria, excitement, fatigue, hallucination, headache, hysteria, insomnia, irritability, nervousness, neuritis, paresthesia, restlessness, sedation, seizure, vertigo

Dermatologic: Diaphoresis, skin photosensitivity, skin rash, urticaria

Gastrointestinal: Abdominal pain, anorexia, cholestasis, constipation, diarrhea, increased appetite, nausea, vomiting, xerostomia

Genitourinary: Difficulty in micturition, urinary frequency, urinary retention

Hematologic & oncologic: Agranulocytosis, hemolytic anemia, leukopenia, thrombocytopenia

Hepatic: Hepatic failure, hepatitis, jaundice

Hypersensitivity: Anaphylactic shock, angioedema, hypersensitivity reaction

Neuromuscular & skeletal: Tremor

Ophthalmic: Blurred vision, diplopia

Otic: Labyrinthitis (acute), tinnitus

Respiratory: Nasal congestion, pharyngitis, thickening of bronchial secretions

Drug Interactions

Metabolism/Transport Effects None known.

Avoid Concomitant Use

Avoid concomitant use of Cyproheptadine with any of the following: Aclidinium; Azelastine (Nasal); Cimetropium; Eluxadoline; Glucagon; Glycopyrrolate; Ipratropium (Oral Inhalation); Levosulpiride; MAO Inhibitors; Orphenadrine; Paraldehyde; Potassium Chloride; Thalidomide; Tiotropium; Umeclidinium

Increased Effect/Toxicity

Cyproheptadine may increase the levels/effects of: AbobotulinumtoxinA; Alcohol (Ethyl); Analgesics (Opioid); Anticholinergic Agents; Azelastine (Nasal); Buprenorphine; Cimetropium; CNS Depressants; Eluxadoline; Glucagon; Glycopyrrolate; Hydrocodone; Methotrimeprazine; Metyrosine; Mirabegron; Mirtazapine; OnabotulinumtoxinA; Orphenadrine; Paraldehyde; Potassium Chloride; Pramipexole; Ramosetron; RimabotulinumtoxinB; ROPINIRole; Rotigotine; Suvorexant; Thalidomide; Thiazide Diuretics; Tiotropium; Topiramate; Zolpidem

The levels/effects of Cyproheptadine may be increased by: Aclidinium; Brimonidine (Topical); Cannabis; Doxylamine; Dronabinol; Droperidol; HydrOXYzine; Ipratropium (Oral Inhalation); Kava Kava; Magnesium Sulfate; MAO Inhibitors; Methotrimeprazine; Mianserin; Minocycline; Nabilone; Perampanel; Pramlintide; Rufinamide; Sodium Oxybate; Tapentadol; Tetrahydrocannabinol; Umeclidinium

Decreased Effect

Cyproheptadine may decrease the levels/effects of: Acetylcholinesterase Inhibitors; Benzylpenicilloyl Polylysine; Betahistine; Gastrointestinal Agents (Prokinetic); Hyaluronidase; Itopride; Levosulpiride; MAO Inhibitors; Secretin; Selective Serotonin Reuptake Inhibitors

The levels/effects of Cyproheptadine may be decreased by: Acetylcholinesterase Inhibitors; Amphetamines

Storage/Stability
Oral solution: Store at 15°C to 30°C (59°F to 86°F); protect from light.
Oral syrup: Store at 20°C to 25°C (68°F to 77°F); excursions permitted to 15°C to 30°C (59°F to 86°F); protect from light.
Oral tablets: Store at 20°C to 25°C (68°F to 77°F).

Mechanism of Action A potent antihistamine and serotonin antagonist, competes with histamine for H_1-receptor sites on effector cells in the gastrointestinal tract, blood vessels, and respiratory tract

Pharmacodynamics/Kinetics
Metabolism: Primarily by hepatic glucuronidation via UGT1A (Walker, 1996)
Half-life elimination: Metabolites: ~16 hours (Paton, 1985)
Time to peak, plasma: 6-9 hours (Paton, 1985)
Excretion: Urine (~40% primarily as metabolites); feces (2% to 20%)

Dosing
Adult
Allergic conditions: Oral: 4-20 mg daily divided every 8 hours (not to exceed 0.5 mg/kg/day); some patients may require up to 32 mg daily for adequate control of symptoms
Migraine headache prophylaxis (off-label use): Oral: 2 mg every 12 hours (with or without propranolol) (Holland, 2012; Rao, 2000)
Serotonin syndrome (off-label use): Oral: Initial: 12 mg followed by 2 mg every 2 hours or 4-8 mg every 6 hours as needed for symptom control (Boyer, 2005; Sun-Edelstein, 2008)
Spasticity associated with spinal cord damage (off-label use): Oral: Initial: 2-4 mg every 8 hours; maximum: 8 mg every 8 hours (Barbeau, 1982; Wainberg, 1990)
Geriatric Refer to adult dosing. Initiate therapy at the lower end of the dosage range.

Pediatric
Allergic conditions: Oral: 0.25 mg/kg/day or 8 mg/m^2/day in 2-3 divided doses **or**
Children 2-6 years: 2 mg every 8-12 hours (not to exceed 12 mg daily)
Children 7-14 years: 4 mg every 8-12 hours (not to exceed 16 mg daily)
Migraine headache prophylaxis (off-label use): Oral: 4 mg every 8-12 hours

Renal Impairment No dosage adjustment provided in manufacturer's labeling. However, elimination is diminished in renal insufficiency.
Hepatic Impairment No dosage adjustment provided in manufacturer's labeling.

Test Interactions Diagnostic antigen skin test results may be suppressed; false positive serum TCA screen

Dosage Forms Excipient information presented when available (limited, particularly for generics); consult specific product labeling.
Syrup, Oral, as hydrochloride:
Generic: 2 mg/5 mL (10 mL, 473 mL)
Tablet, Oral, as hydrochloride:
Generic: 4 mg

◆ **Cyproheptadine Hydrochloride** see Cyproheptadine on page 400

Cyproterone (sye PROE ter one)
Brand Names: Canada Androcur®; Androcur® Depot; Novo-Cyproterone
Index Terms Cyproterone Acetate; SH 714

Pharmacologic Category Antiandrogen; Antineoplastic Agent, Antiandrogen
Use Note: Not approved in the US
Palliative treatment of advanced prostate cancer
Dosing
Adult & Geriatric
Prostate cancer, advanced (palliative treatment): Males:
Oral: 200-300 mg daily in 2-3 divided doses (maximum: 300 mg daily); following orchiectomy, reduce dose to 100-200 mg daily
IM: 300 mg (3 mL) once weekly; reduce dose in orchiectomized patients to 300 mg every 2 weeks
Note: May interchange between oral and IM administration during chronic therapy; dosages should remain within usual ranges (oral: 100-300 mg daily; IM: 300 mg weekly or every 2 weeks).
Treatment of paraphilia/hypersexuality (off-label use; Guay, 2009; Reilly, 2000): Males (**Note:** Avoid use if active pituitary pathology, hepatic failure, or thromboembolic disease):
Oral: 50-600 mg daily
IM: 300-600 mg weekly or every other week
Renal Impairment Has not been studied in patients with renal impairment. Use with caution; 33% of cyproterone is excreted renally.
Hepatic Impairment Use is contraindicated with hepatic impairment or liver disease.
Additional Information Complete prescribing information should be consulted for additional detail.
Product Availability Not available in the US
Dosage Forms: Canada Excipient information presented when available (limited, particularly for generics); consult specific product labeling.
Injection, solution, as acetate: 100 mg/mL (3 mL)
Androcur® Depot: 100 mg/mL (3 mL) [contains benzyl benzoate and castor oil]
Tablet, as acetate: 50 mg
Androcur®: 50 mg

Cytarabine (Conventional) (sye TARE a been con VEN sha nal)
Related Information
Brand Names: Canada Cytarabine Injection; Cytosar
Index Terms Ara-C; Arabinosylcytosine; Conventional Cytarabine; Cytarabine; Cytarabine Hydrochloride; Cytosar-U; Cytosine Arabinosine Hydrochloride

◀ **Pharmacologic Category** Antineoplastic Agent, Antimetabolite; Antineoplastic Agent, Antimetabolite (Pyrimidine Analog)

Use

Acute myeloid leukemia: Remission induction (in combination with other chemotherapy medications) in acute myeloid leukemia (AML)

Acute lymphocytic leukemia: Treatment of acute lymphocytic leukemia (ALL)

Chronic myeloid leukemia: Treatment of chronic myeloid leukemia (CML; blast phase)

Meningeal leukemia: Prophylaxis and treatment of meningeal leukemia

Labeled Contraindications Hypersensitivity to cytarabine or any component of the formulation

Pregnancy Considerations Adverse effects were demonstrated in animal reproduction studies. Limb and ear defects have been noted in case reports of cytarabine exposure during the first trimester of pregnancy. The following have also been noted in the neonate: Pancytopenia, WBC depression, electrolyte abnormalities, prematurity, low birth weight, decreased hematocrit or platelets. Risk to the fetus is decreased if treatment can be avoided during the first trimester; however, women of childbearing potential should be advised of the potential risks.

Breast-Feeding Considerations It is not known if cytarabine is excreted in breast milk. Due to the potential for serious adverse reactions in the nursing infant, the decision to discontinue cytarabine or to discontinue breast-feeding should take into account the importance of treatment to the mother.

Warnings/Precautions Hazardous agent - use appropriate precautions for handling and disposal (NIOSH 2014 [group 1]). **[U.S. Boxed Warning]: Myelosuppression (leukopenia, thrombocytopenia and anemia) is the major toxicity of cytarabine.** Use with caution in patients with prior drug-induced bone marrow suppression. Monitor blood counts frequently; once blasts are no longer apparent in the peripheral blood, bone marrow should be monitored frequently. Monitor for signs of infection or neutropenic fever due to neutropenia or bleeding due to thrombocytopenia. **[U.S. Boxed Warning]: Toxicities (less serious) include nausea, vomiting, diarrhea, abdominal pain, oral ulcerations and hepatic dysfunction.** In adults, doses >1000 mg/m^2 are associated with a moderate emetic potential (Basch, 2011; Roila, 2010). In pediatrics, doses >200 mg/m^2 are associated with a moderate emetic potential and 3000 mg/m^2 is associated with a high emetic potential (Dupuis, 2011); antiemetics are recommended to prevent nausea and vomiting.

High-dose regimens are associated with CNS, gastrointestinal, ocular (reversible corneal toxicity and hemorrhagic conjunctivitis; prophylaxis with ophthalmic corticosteroid drops is recommended), pulmonary toxicities and cardiomyopathy. Neurotoxicity associated with high-dose treatment may present as acute cerebellar toxicity (with or without cerebral impairment), personality changes, or may be severe with seizure and/or coma; may be delayed, occurring up to 3 to 8 days after treatment has begun. Risk factors for neurotoxicity include cumulative cytarabine dose, prior CNS disease and renal impairment; high-dose therapy (>18 g/m^2 per cycle) and age >50 years also increase the risk for cerebellar toxicity (Herzig, 1987). Tumor lysis syndrome and subsequent hyperuricemia may occur; monitor, consider antihyperuricemic therapy and hydrate accordingly. Potentially significant drug-drug interactions may exist, requiring dose or frequency adjustment, additional monitoring, and/or selection of alternative therapy. There have been case reports of fatal cardiomyopathy when high dose cytarabine was used in combination with cyclophosphamide as a preparation regimen for transplantation.

Use with caution in patients with impaired renal and hepatic function; may be at higher risk for CNS toxicities; dosage adjustments may be necessary. Sudden respiratory distress, rapidly progressing to pulmonary edema and cardiomegaly has been reported with high dose cytarabine. May present as severe dyspnea with a rapid onset and refractory hypoxia with diffuse pulmonary infiltrates, leading to respiratory failure; may be fatal (Morgan, 2011). Cytarabine (ARA-C) syndrome is characterized by fever, myalgia, bone pain, chest pain (occasionally), maculopapular rash, conjunctivitis, and malaise; generally occurs 6 to 12 hours following administration; may be managed with corticosteroids. Anaphylaxis resulting in acute cardiopulmonary arrest has been reported (rare). There have been reports of acute pancreatitis in patients receiving continuous infusion cytarabine and in patients receiving cytarabine who were previously treated with L-asparaginase. **[U.S. Boxed Warning]: Should be administered under the supervision of an experienced cancer chemotherapy physician. Due to the potential toxicities, induction treatment with cytarabine should be in a facility with sufficient laboratory and supportive resources.** Some products may contain benzyl alcohol; do not use products containing benzyl alcohol or products reconstituted with bacteriostatic diluent intrathecally or for high-dose cytarabine regimens. Benzyl alcohol is associated with gasping syndrome in premature infants. Delayed progressive ascending paralysis has been reported in two children who received combination chemotherapy with IV and intrathecal cytarabine at conventional doses for the treatment of acute myeloid leukemia (was fatal in one patient). When used for intrathecal administration, should not be prepared during the preparation of any other agents; after preparation, store intrathecal medications in an isolated location or container clearly marked with a label identifying as "intrathecal" use only; delivery of intrathecal medications to the patient should only be with other medications also intended for administration into the central nervous system (Jacobson, 2009).

Adverse Reactions

Frequent:

Central nervous system: Fever

Dermatologic: Rash

Gastrointestinal: Anal inflammation, anal ulceration, anorexia, diarrhea, mucositis, nausea, vomiting

Hematologic: Myelosuppression, neutropenia (onset: 1 to 7 days; nadir [biphasic]: 7 to 9 days and at 15 to 24 days; recovery [biphasic]: 9 to 12 days and at 24 to 34 days), thrombocytopenia (onset: 5 days; nadir: 12 to 15 days; recovery 15 to 25 days), anemia, bleeding, leukopenia, megaloblastosis, reticulocytes decreased

Hepatic: Hepatic dysfunction, transaminases increased (acute)

Local: Thrombophlebitis

Less frequent:

Cardiovascular: Chest pain, pericarditis

Central nervous system: Dizziness, headache, neural toxicity, neuritis

Dermatologic: Alopecia, pruritus, skin freckling, skin ulceration, urticaria

Gastrointestinal: Abdominal pain, bowel necrosis, esophageal ulceration, esophagitis, pancreatitis, sore throat

Genitourinary: Urinary retention

Hepatic: Jaundice

Local: Injection site cellulitis
Ocular: Conjunctivitis
Renal: Renal dysfunction
Respiratory: Dyspnea
Miscellaneous: Allergic edema, anaphylaxis, sepsis

Infrequent and/or case reports: Acute respiratory distress syndrome, amylase increased, angina, aseptic meningitis, cardiopulmonary arrest (acute), cerebral dysfunction, cytarabine syndrome (bone pain, chest pain, conjunctivitis, fever, maculopapular rash, malaise, myalgia); exanthematous pustulosis, hepatic sinusoidal obstruction syndrome (SOS; veno-occlusive disease), hyperuricemia, injection site inflammation (SubQ injection), injection site pain (SubQ injection), interstitial pneumonitis, lipase increased, paralysis (intrathecal and IV combination therapy), reversible posterior leukoencephalopathy syndrome (RPLS), rhabdomyolysis, toxic megacolon

Adverse events associated with high-dose cytarabine (CNS, gastrointestinal, ocular, and pulmonary toxicities are more common with high-dose regimens):
Cardiovascular: Cardiomegaly, cardiomyopathy (in combination with cyclophosphamide)
Central nervous system: Cerebellar toxicity, coma, neurotoxicity (up to 55% in patients with renal impairment), personality change, somnolence
Dermatologic: Alopecia (complete), desquamation, rash (severe)
Gastrointestinal: Gastrointestinal ulcer, pancreatitis, peritonitis, pneumatosis cystoides intestinalis
Hepatic: Hyperbilirubinemia, liver abscess, liver damage, necrotizing colitis
Neuromuscular & skeletal: Peripheral neuropathy (motor and sensory)
Ocular: Corneal toxicity, hemorrhagic conjunctivitis
Respiratory: Pulmonary edema, syndrome of sudden respiratory distress
Miscellaneous: Sepsis

Adverse events associated with intrathecal cytarabine administration:
Central nervous system: Accessory nerve paralysis, fever, necrotizing leukoencephalopathy (with concurrent cranial irradiation, intrathecal methotrexate, and intrathecal hydrocortisone), neurotoxicity, paraplegia
Gastrointestinal: Dysphagia, nausea, vomiting
Ocular: Blindness (with concurrent systemic chemotherapy and cranial irradiation), diplopia
Respiratory: Cough, hoarseness
Miscellaneous: Aphonia

Drug Interactions
Metabolism/Transport Effects None known.
Avoid Concomitant Use
Avoid concomitant use of Cytarabine (Conventional) with any of the following: BCG (Intravesical); CloZAPine; Dipyrone; Natalizumab; Pimecrolimus; Tacrolimus (Topical); Tofacitinib; Vaccines (Live)

Increased Effect/Toxicity
Cytarabine (Conventional) may increase the levels/effects of: CloZAPine; Fingolimod; Leflunomide; Natalizumab; Tofacitinib; Vaccines (Live)

The levels/effects of Cytarabine (Conventional) may be increased by: Denosumab; Dipyrone; Pimecrolimus; Roflumilast; Tacrolimus (Topical); Trastuzumab

Decreased Effect

Cytarabine (Conventional) may decrease the levels/effects of: BCG (Intravesical); Coccidioides immitis Skin Test; Flucytosine; Sipuleucel-T; Vaccines (Inactivated); Vaccines (Live)

The levels/effects of Cytarabine (Conventional) may be decreased by: Echinacea

Storage/Stability Store intact vials of powder for reconstitution at 20°C to 25°C (68°F to 77°F); store intact vials of solution at 15°C to 30°C (59°F to 86°F).

IV:

Powder for reconstitution: Reconstituted solutions should be stored at room temperature and used within 48 hours.

For IV infusion: Solutions for IV infusion diluted in D$_5$W or NS are stable for 8 days at room temperature, although the manufacturer recommends administration as soon as possible after preparation.

Intrathecal: Administer as soon as possible after preparation. After preparation, store intrathecal medications in an isolated location or container clearly marked with a label identifying as "intrathecal" use only.

Preparation for Administration Hazardous agent; use appropriate precautions for handling and disposal (NIOSH 2014 [group 1]). **Note:** Solutions containing bacteriostatic agents may be used for SubQ and standard-dose (100 to 200 mg/m^2) IV cytarabine preparations, but should not be used for the preparation of either intrathecal doses or high-dose IV therapies.

IV:

Powder for reconstitution: Reconstitute with bacteriostatic water for injection (for standard-dose).

For IV infusion: Further dilute in 250 to 1000 mL 0.9% NaCl or D$_5$W.

Intrathecal: Powder for reconstitution: Reconstitute with preservative free sodium chloride 0.9%; may further dilute to preferred final volume (volume generally based on institution or practitioner preference; may be up to 12 mL) with Elliott's B solution, sodium chloride 0.9% or lactated Ringer's. Intrathecal medications should not be prepared during the preparation of any other agents.

Triple intrathecal therapy (TIT): Cytarabine 30 to 50 mg with hydrocortisone sodium succinate 15 to 25 mg and methotrexate 12 mg are reported to be compatible together in a syringe (Cheung, 1984) and cytarabine 18 to 36 mg with hydrocortisone 12 to 24 mg and methotrexate 6 to 12 mg, prepared to a final volume of 6 to 12 mL, is reported compatible as well (Lin, 2008).

Intrathecal preparations should be administered as soon as possible after preparation because intrathecal preparations are preservative free.

Mechanism of Action Inhibits DNA synthesis. Cytarabine gains entry into cells by a carrier process, and then must be converted to its active compound, aracytidine triphosphate. Cytarabine is a pyrimidine analog and is incorporated into DNA; however, the primary action is inhibition of DNA polymerase resulting in decreased DNA synthesis and repair. The degree of cytotoxicity correlates linearly with incorporation into DNA; therefore, incorporation into the DNA is responsible for drug activity and toxicity. Cytarabine is specific for the S phase of the cell cycle (blocks progression from the G$_1$ to the S phase).

Pharmacodynamics/Kinetics

Distribution: V$_d$: Total body water; widely and rapidly since it enters the cells readily; crosses blood-brain barrier with CSF levels of 40% to 50% of plasma level

◀ Metabolism: Primarily hepatic; metabolized by deoxycytidine kinase and other nucleotide kinases to aracytidine triphosphate (active); about 86% to 96% of dose is metabolized to inactive uracil arabinoside (ARA-U); intrathecal administration results in little conversion to ARA-U due to the low levels of deaminase in the cerebral spinal fluid

Half-life elimination: IV: Initial: 7 to 20 minutes; Terminal: 1 to 3 hours; Intrathecal: 2 to 6 hours

Time to peak, plasma: SubQ: 20 to 60 minutes

Excretion: Urine (~80%; 90% as metabolite ARA-U) within 24 hours

Dosing

Adult & Geriatric Note: Doses >1000 mg/m^2 are associated with a moderate emetic potential in adults (Basch, 2011; Roila, 2010); antiemetics are recommended to prevent nausea and vomiting.

Acute myeloid leukemia (AML) remission induction: IV: Standard-dose (manufacturer's labeling; in combination with other chemotherapy agents): 100 mg/m^2/day continuous infusion for 7 days **or** 200 mg/m^2/day continuous infusion (as 100 mg/m^2 over 12 hours every 12 hours) for 7 days

Indication-specific dosing:

AML induction: IV:

7 + 3 regimens (a second induction course may be administered if needed; refer to specific references): 100 mg/m^2/day continuous infusion for 7 days (in combination with daunorubicin **or** idarubicin **or** mitoxantrone) (Arlin, 1990; Dillman, 1991; Fernandez, 2009; Vogler, 1992; Wiernik, 1992) **or** (Adults <60 years) 200 mg/m^2/day continuous infusion for 7 days (in combination with daunorubicin) (Dillman, 1991)

Low intensity therapy (off-label dosing): Adults ≥65 years: SubQ: 20 mg/m^2/day for 14 days out of every 28-day cycle for at least 4 cycles (Fenaux, 2010) **or** 10 mg/m^2 every 12 hours for 21 days; if complete response not achieved, may repeat a second course after 15 days (Tilly, 1990)

AML consolidation (off-label use): IV:

5 + 2 regimens: 100 mg/m^2/day continuous infusion for 5 days (in combination with daunorubicin **or** idarubicin **or** mitoxantrone) (Arlin, 1990; Wiernik, 1992)

5 + 2 + 5 regimen: 100 mg/m^2/day continuous infusion for 5 days (in combination with daunorubicin **and** etoposide) (Bishop, 1996)

Single-agent: Adults ≤60 years: 3000 mg/m^2 over 3 hours every 12 hours on days 1, 3, and 5 (total of 6 doses); repeat every 28 to 35 days for 4 courses (Mayer, 1994)

AML salvage treatment (off-label use): IV:

CLAG regimen: 2000 mg/m^2/day over 4 hours for 5 days (in combination with cladribine and G-CSF); may repeat once if needed (Wrzesień-Kuś, 2003)

CLAG-M regimen: 2000 mg/m^2/day over 4 hours for 5 days (in combination with cladribine, G-CSF, and mitoxantrone); may repeat once if needed (Wierzbowska, 2008)

FLAG regimen: 2000 mg/m^2/day over 4 hours for 5 days (in combination with fludarabine and G-CSF); may repeat once if needed (Montillo, 1998)

GCLAC regimen: Adults 18 to 70 years (Becker, 2011):

Induction: 2,000 mg/m^2 over 2 hours once daily for 5 days (in combination with clofarabine and filgrastim; administer 4 hours after initiation of clofarabine); may repeat induction once if needed.

Consolidation: 1,000 mg/m^2 over 2 hours once daily for 5 days (in combination with clofarabine and filgrastim; administer 4 hours after initiation of clofarabine) for 1 or 2 cycles

HiDAC (high-dose cytarabine) ± an anthracycline: 3000 mg/m^2 over 1 hour every 12 hours for 6 days (total of 12 doses) (Herzig, 1985)

MEC regimen: 1,000 mg/m^2/day over 6 hours for 6 days (in combination with mitoxantrone and etoposide) (Amadori, 1991) **or**

Adults <60 years: 500 mg/m^2/day continuous infusion days 1, 2, and 3 and days 8, 9, and 10 (in combination with mitoxantrone and etoposide); may administer a second course if needed (Archimbaud, 1991; Archimbaud, 1995)

Acute promyelocytic leukemia (APL) induction (off-label dosing): IV: 200 mg/m^2/day continuous infusion for 7 days beginning on day 3 of treatment (in combination with tretinoin and daunorubicin) (Ades, 2006; Ades, 2008; Powell, 2010)

APL consolidation (off-label use): IV:

In combination with idarubicin and tretinoin: High-risk patients (WBC ≥10,000/mm^3) (Sanz, 2010): Adults ≤60 years:

First consolidation course: 1000 mg/m^2/day for 4 days

Third consolidation course: 150 mg/m^2 every 8 hours for 4 days

In combination with idarubicin, tretinoin, and thioguanine: High-risk patients (WBC >10,000/mm^3) (Lo Coco, 2010): Adults ≤61 years:

First consolidation course: 1000 mg/m^2/day for 4 days

Third consolidation course: 150 mg/m^2 every 8 hours for 5 days

In combination with daunorubicin (Ades, 2006; Ades, 2008):

First consolidation course: 200 mg/m^2/day for 7 days

Second consolidation course:

Age ≤60 years and low risk (WBC <10,000/mm^3): 1000 mg/m^2 every 12 hours for 4 days (8 doses)

Age <50 years and high risk (WBC ≥10,000/mm^3): 2000 mg/m^2 every 12 hours for 5 days (10 doses)

Age 50 to 60 years and high risk (WBC ≥10,000/mm^3): 1500 mg/m^2 every 12 hours for 5 days (10 doses) (Ades, 2008)

Age >60 years and high risk (WBC ≥10,000/mm^3): 1000 mg/m^2 every 12 hours for 4 days (8 doses)

Acute lymphocytic leukemia (ALL; off-label dosing):

Induction regimen, relapsed or refractory: IV: 3000 mg/m^2 over 3 hours daily for 5 days (in combination with idarubicin [day 3]) (Weiss, 2002)

Dose-intensive regimen: IV: 3000 mg/m^2 over 2 hours every 12 hours days 2 and 3 (4 doses/cycle) of even numbered cycles (in combination with methotrexate; alternates with Hyper-CVAD) (Kantarjian, 2000)

CALGB 8811 regimen (Larson, 1995): SubQ

Early intensification phase: 75 mg/m^2/dose days 1 to 4 and 8 to 11 (4-week cycle; repeat once)

Late intensification phase: 75 mg/m^2/dose days 29 to 32 and 36 to 39

Linker protocol: Adults <50 years: IV: 300 mg/m^2/day days 1, 4, 8, and 11 of even numbered consolidation cycles (in combination with teniposide) (Linker, 1991)

Chronic lymphocytic leukemia (CLL; off-label use): *OFAR regimen:* IV: 1000 mg/m^2/dose over 2 hours days 2 and 3 every 4 weeks for up to 6 cycles (in combination with oxaliplatin, fludarabine, and rituximab) (Tsimberidou, 2008)

◀ **Primary central nervous system (CNS) lymphoma (off-label use):** IV: 2000 mg/m^2 over 1 hour every 12 hours days 2 and 3 (total of 4 doses) every 3 weeks (in combination with methotrexate and followed by whole brain irradiation) for a total of 4 courses (Ferreri, 2009)

Hodgkin lymphoma, relapsed or refractory (off-label use): IV:

DHAP regimen: 2000 mg/m^2 over 3 hours every 12 hours day 2 (total of 2 doses/cycle) for 2 cycles (in combination with dexamethasone and cisplatin) (Josting, 2002)

ESHAP regimen: 2000 mg/m^2 day 5 (in combination with etoposide, methylprednisolone, and cisplatin) every 3 to 4 weeks for 3 or 6 cycles (Aparicio, 1999)

Mini-BEAM regimen: 100 mg/m^2 every 12 hours days 2 to 5 (total of 8 doses) every 4 to 6 weeks (in combination with carmustine, etoposide, and melphalan) (Colwill, 1995; Martin, 2001)

BEAM regimen (transplant preparative regimen): 200 mg/m^2 twice daily for 4 days beginning 5 days prior to transplant (in combination with carmustine, etoposide, and melphalan) (Chopra, 1993)

Non-Hodgkin lymphomas (off-label use): IV:

CALGB 9251 regimen: Cycles 2, 4, and 6: 150 mg/m^2/day continuous infusion days 4 and 5 (Lee, 2001; Rizzieri, 2004)

CODOX-M/IVAC regimen:

Adults ≤60 years: Cycles 2 and 4 (IVAC): 2000 mg/m^2 every 12 hours days 1 and 2 (total of 4 doses/cycle) (IVAC is combination with ifosfamide, mesna, and etoposide; IVAC alternates with CODOX-M) (Magrath, 1996)

Adults ≤65 years: Cycles 2 and 4 (IVAC): 2000 mg/m^2 over 3 hours every 12 hours days 1 and 2 (total of 4 doses/cycle) (IVAC is combination with ifosfamide, mesna, and etoposide; IVAC alternates with CODOX-M) (Mead, 2008)

Adults >65 years: Cycles 2 and 4 (IVAC): 1000 mg/m^2 over 3 hours every 12 hours days 1 and 2 (total of 4 doses/cycle) (IVAC is combination with ifosfamide, mesna, and etoposide; IVAC alternates with CODOX-M) (Mead, 2008)

DHAP regimen:

Adults ≤70 years: 2000 mg/m^2 over 3 hours every 12 hours day 2 (total of 2 doses/cycle) every 3 to 4 weeks for 6 to 10 cycles (in combination with dexamethasone and cisplatin) (Velasquez, 1988)

Adults >70 years: 1000 mg/m^2 over 3 hours every 12 hours day 2 (total of 2 doses/cycle) every 3 to 4 weeks for 6 to 10 cycles (in combination with dexamethasone and cisplatin) (Velasquez, 1988)

ESHAP regimen: 2000 mg/m^2 over 2 hours day 5 every 3 to 4 weeks for 6 to 8 cycles (in combination with etoposide, methylprednisolone, and cisplatin) (Velasquez, 1994)

BEAM regimen (transplant preparative regimen): 200 mg/m^2 twice daily for 3 days beginning 4 days prior to transplant (in combination with carmustine, etoposide, and melphalan) (Linch, 2010) **or** 100 mg/m^2 over 1 hour every 12 hours for 4 days beginning 5 days prior to transplant (in combination with carmustine, etoposide, and melphalan) (van Imhoff, 2005)

Meningeal leukemia: Intrathecal: **Note:** Optimal intrathecal chemotherapy dosing should be based on age rather than on body surface area (BSA); CSF volume correlates with age and not to BSA (Bleyer, 1983; Kerr, 2001).

Dosing provided in the manufacturer's labeling is BSA-based (usual dose 30 mg/m^2 every 4 days; range: 5 to 75 mg/m^2 once daily for 4 days or once every 4 days until CNS findings normalize, followed by 1 additional treatment).

Off-label uses or doses for intrathecal therapy: Intrathecal:

CNS prophylaxis (ALL): 100 mg weekly for 8 doses, then every 2 weeks for 8 doses, then monthly for 6 doses (high-risk patients) **or** 100 mg on day 7 or 8 with each chemotherapy cycle for 4 doses (low risk patients) **or** 16 doses (high-risk patients) (Cortes, 1995)

  or as part of intrathecal triple therapy (TIT): 40 mg days 0 and 14 during induction, days 1, 4, 8, and 11 during CNS therapy phase, every 18 weeks during intensification and maintenance phases (Storring, 2009)

CNS prophylaxis (APL, as part of TIT): 50 mg per dose; administer 1 dose prior to consolidation and 2 doses during each of 2 consolidation phases (total of 5 doses) (Ades, 2006; Ades, 2008)

CNS leukemia treatment (ALL, as part of TIT): 40 mg twice weekly until CSF cleared (Storring, 2009)

CNS lymphoma treatment: 50 mg twice a week for 4 weeks, then weekly for 4-8 weeks, then every other week for 4 weeks, then every 4 weeks for 4 doses (Glantz, 1999)

Leptomeningeal metastases treatment: 25 to 100 mg twice weekly for 4 weeks, then once weekly for 4 weeks, then a maintenance regimen of once a month (Chamberlain, 2010) **or** 40 to 60 mg per dose (DeAngelis, 2005)

Pediatric Note: Doses >200 mg/m^2 are associated with a moderate emetic potential and 3000 mg/m^2 is associated with a high emetic potential (Dupuis, 2011); antiemetics are recommended to prevent nausea and vomiting.

Acute myeloid leukemia (AML) remission induction: IV: Standard-dose (manufacturer's labeling labeling; in combination with other chemotherapy agents): 100 mg/m^2/day continuous infusion for 7 days **or** 200 mg/m^2/day continuous infusion (as 100 mg/m^2 over 12 hours every 12 hours) for 7 days

Indication-specific dosing:

AML induction: *7 + 3 regimen:* IV:

Children <3 years (off-label dosing): 3.3 mg/kg/day continuous infusion for 7 days; minimum of 2 courses (in combination with daunorubicin) (Woods, 1990)

Children ≥3 years: 100 mg/m^2/day continuous infusion for 7 days; minimum of 2 courses (in combination with daunorubicin) (Woods, 1990)

AML consolidation (off-label use): *5 + 2 + 5 regimen:* IV: Adolescents ≥15 years: 100 mg/m^2/day continuous infusion for 5 days for 2 consolidation courses (in combination with daunorubicin and etoposide) (Bishop, 1996)

AML salvage treatment (off-label use):

Clofarabine/Cytarabine regimen: Induction: IV: Children ≥1 year and Adolescents: 1,000 mg/m^2/day over 2 hours for 5 days (in combination with clofarabine; cytarabine is administered 4 hours after initiation of clofarabine) for up to 2 induction cycles (Cooper, 2014)

FLAG regimen: IV: Children ≥11 years: 2,000 mg/m^2/day over 4 hours for 5 days (in combination with fludarabine and G-CSF); may repeat once if needed (Montillo, 1998)

MEC regimen: IV:

Children ≥5 years: 1,000 mg/m^2/day over 6 hours for 6 days (in combination with etoposide and mitoxantrone) (Amadori, 1991)

Adolescents ≥15 years: 500 mg/m²/day continuous infusion days 1, 2, and 3 and days 8, 9, and 10 (in combination with mitoxantrone and etoposide); may administer a second course if needed (Archimbaud, 1991; Archimbaud, 1995)

Acute lymphocytic leukemia (ALL; off-label dosing): *POG 8602/PVA regimen, intensification phase:* IV: Children ≥1 year: 1,000 mg/m² continuous infusion over 24 hours day 1 (beginning 12 hours after start of methotrexate) every 3 weeks or every 12 weeks for 6 cycles (Land, 1994)

Non-Hodgkin lymphomas (off-label use):

CODOX-M/IVAC regimen: IV: Children ≥3 years: Cycles 2 and 4 (IVAC): 2,000 mg/m² every 12 hours days 1 and 2 (total of 4 doses/cycle) (IVAC is combination with ifosfamide, mesna and etoposide; IVAC alternates with CODOX-M) (Magrath, 1996)

High-dose cytarabine: IV: Children >1 year and Adolescents: 3,000 mg/m² over 3 hours every 12 hours on days 2 and 3 (secondary phase; total of 4 doses) in combination with methotrexate and intrathecal methotrexate/cytarabine (Bowman, 1996)

Meningeal leukemia: Intrathecal: **Note:** Optimal intrathecal chemotherapy dosing should be based on age rather than on body surface area (BSA); CSF volume correlates with age and not to BSA (Bleyer, 1983; Kerr, 2001). Dosing provided in the manufacturer's labeling is BSA-based (usual dose 30 mg/m² every 4 days; range: 5 to 75 mg/m² once daily for 4 days or once every 4 days until CNS findings normalize, followed by 1 additional treatment).

Age-based intrathecal dosing (off-label; Woods, 1990): Intrathecal:

CNS prophylaxis:

<1 year: 20 mg per dose

1 to 1.99 years: 30 mg per dose

2 to 2.99 years: 50 mg per dose

≥3 years: 70 mg per dose

ALL CNS prophylaxis, age-specific doses from literature:

Administer on day 0 of induction therapy (Gaynon, 1993):

1 to <2 years: 30 mg per dose

2 to <3 years: 50 mg per dose

≥3 years: 70 mg per dose

Administer as part of triple intrathecal therapy (TIT) on days 1 and 15 of induction therapy; days 1, 15, 50, and 64 (standard risk patients) or days 1, 15, 29, and 43 (high-risk patients) during consolidation therapy; day 1 of reinduction therapy, and during maintenance therapy (very high-risk patients receive on days 1, 22, 45, and 59 of induction, days 8, 22, 36, and 50 of consolidation therapy, days 8 and 38 of reinduction therapy, and during maintenance) (Lin, 2007):

<1 year: 18 mg per dose

1 to 2 years: 24 mg per dose

2 to 3 years: 30 mg per dose

≥3 years: 36 mg per dose

Administer on day 0 of induction therapy, then as part of TIT on days 7, 14, and 21 during consolidation therapy; as part of TIT on days 0, 28, and 35 for 2 cycles of delayed intensification therapy, and then maintenance treatment as part of TIT on day 0 every 12 weeks for 38 months (boys) or 26 months (girls) from initial induction treatment (Matloub, 2006):

1 to <2 years: 16 mg per dose

2 to <3 years: 20 mg per dose

≥3 years: 24 to 30 mg per dose

Administer on day 15 of induction therapy, days 1 and 15 of reinduction phase; and day 1 of cycle 2 of maintenance 1A phase (Pieters, 2007):
<1 year: 15 mg per dose
≥1 year: 20 mg per dose

Treatment, CNS leukemia (ALL): Intrathecal: Administer as part of TIT weekly until CSF remission, then every 4 weeks throughout continuation treatment (Lin, 2007):
<1 year: 18 mg per dose
1 to 2 years: 24 mg per dose
2 to 3 years: 30 mg per dose
≥3 years: 36 mg per dose

Renal Impairment There are no dosage adjustments provided in the manufacturer's labeling; however, the following adjustments have been recommended:

Aronoff, 2007 (cytarabine 100 to 200 mg/m^2): Children and Adults: No adjustment necessary

Kintzel, 1995 (high-dose cytarabine 1 to 3 g/m^2):
CrCl 46 to 60 mL/minute: Administer 60% of dose
CrCl 31 to 45 mL/minute: Administer 50% of dose
CrCl <30 mL/minute: Consider use of alternative drug

Smith, 1997 (high-dose cytarabine; ≥2 g/m^2/dose):
Serum creatinine 1.5 to 1.9 mg/dL or increase (from baseline) of 0.5 to 1.2 mg/dL: Reduce dose to 1 g/m^2/dose
Serum creatinine ≥2 mg/dL or increase (from baseline) of >1.2 mg/dL: Reduce dose to 0.1 g/m^2/day as a continuous infusion

Hemodialysis: In 4 hour dialysis sessions (with high flow polysulfone membrane) 6 hours after cytarabine 1 g/m^2 over 2 hours, 63% of the metabolite ARA-U was extracted from plasma (based on a single adult case report) (Radeski, 2011)

Hepatic Impairment Dose may need to be adjusted in patients with liver failure since cytarabine is partially detoxified in the liver. There are no dosage adjustments provided in the manufacturer's labeling; however, the following adjustments have been recommended:

Floyd, 2006: Transaminases (any elevation): Administer 50% of dose; may increase subsequent doses in the absence of toxicities

Koren, 1992 (dose level not specified): Bilirubin >2 mg/dL: Administer 50% of dose; may increase subsequent doses in the absence of toxicities

Obesity

American Society of Clinical Oncology (ASCO) Guidelines for appropriate chemotherapy dosing in obese adults with cancer: Utilize patient's actual body weight (full weight) for calculation of body surface area- or weight-based dosing, particularly when the intent of therapy is curative; manage regimen-related toxicities in the same manner as for nonobese patients; if a dose reduction is utilized due to toxicity, consider resumption of full weight-based dosing with subsequent cycles, especially if cause of toxicity (eg, hepatic or renal impairment) is resolved (Griggs, 2012).

American Society for Blood and Marrow Transplantation (ASBMT) practice guideline committee position statement on chemotherapy dosing in obesity: Utilize actual body weight (full weight) for calculation of body surface area in cytarabine dosing for hematopoietic stem cell transplant conditioning regimens in pediatrics and adults (Bubalo, 2014).

◄ **Combination Regimens**

Lymphoma, non-Hodgkin (DLBCL):
DHAP (NHL-DLBCL) on page 1938
R-DHAP (NHL-DLBCL) on page 2073
Lymphoma, non-Hodgkin (Mantle cell): Rituximab-Hyper-CVAD (NHL-Mantle Cell) on page 2082

Administration

IV: Infuse standard dose therapy for AML (100 to 200 mg/m^2/day) as a continuous infusion. Infuse high-dose therapy (off-label) over 1 to 3 hours (usually). Other rates have been used, refer to specific reference.

In adults, doses >1000 mg/m^2 are associated with a moderate emetic potential (Basch, 2011; Roila, 2010). In pediatrics, doses >200 mg/m^2 are associated with a moderate emetic potential and 3000 mg/m^2 is associated with a high emetic potential (Dupuis, 2011); antiemetics are recommended to prevent nausea and vomiting.

Intrathecal: Intrathecal doses should be administered as soon as possible after preparation.

May also be administered SubQ.

Hazardous agent; use appropriate precautions for handling and disposal (NIOSH 2014 [group 1]).

Emetic Potential

Children:
3000 mg/m^2: High (>90%)
>200 mg/m^2 to <3000 mg/m^2: Moderate (30% to 90%)
≤200 mg/m^2: Low (10% to 30%)
Adults:
>1000 mg/m^2: Moderate (30% to 90%)
≤1000 mg/m^2: Low (10% to 30%)

Monitoring Parameters Liver function tests, CBC with differential and platelet count, serum creatinine, BUN, serum uric acid

Dosage Forms Excipient information presented when available (limited, particularly for generics); consult specific product labeling.
Solution, Injection:
Generic: 20 mg/mL (25 mL); 100 mg/mL (20 mL)
Solution, Injection [preservative free]:
Generic: 20 mg/mL (5 mL, 50 mL); 100 mg/mL (20 mL)
Solution Reconstituted, Injection:
Generic: 100 mg (1 ea); 500 mg (1 ea); 1 g (1 ea)

Cytarabine (Liposomal) (sye TARE a been lye po SO mal)

Related Information

Common Toxicity Criteria on page 2122
Management of Chemotherapy-Induced Nausea and Vomiting in Adults on page 2142
Safe Handling of Hazardous Drugs on page 2292

Brand Names: US DepoCyt

Brand Names: Canada DepoCyt

Index Terms Cytarabine Lipid Complex; Cytarabine Liposome; DepoFoam-Encapsulated Cytarabine; DTC 101; Liposomal Cytarabine

Pharmacologic Category Antineoplastic Agent, Antimetabolite; Antineoplastic Agent, Antimetabolite (Pyrimidine Analog)

Use Lymphomatous meningitis: Intrathecal treatment of lymphomatous meningitis

◀ **Labeled Contraindications** Hypersensitivity to cytarabine or any component of the formulation; active meningeal infection

Pregnancy Considerations Adverse effects were observed in animal reproductive studies with conventional cytarabine. Conventional cytarabine has been associated with fetal malformations when given as a component of systemic combination chemotherapy during the first trimester. Systemic exposure following intrathecal administration of cytarabine liposomal is negligible; however, women of childbearing potential should avoid becoming pregnant during treatment.

Breast-Feeding Considerations It is not known if cytarabine (liposomal) is excreted in breast milk; the systemic exposure following intrathecal administration of cytarabine (liposomal) is negligible. Due to the potential for serious adverse reactions in the nursing infant, a decision should be made to discontinue cytarabine (liposomal) or to discontinue breast-feeding, taking into account the importance of treatment to the mother.

Warnings/Precautions Hazardous agent - use appropriate precautions for handling and disposal (NIOSH 2014 [group 1]). **[US Boxed Warning]: Chemical arachnoiditis (nausea, vomiting, headache, fever) occurs commonly; may be fatal if untreated. Dexamethasone should be administered concomitantly with cytarabine (liposomal) to diminish chemical arachnoid symptoms;** the incidence and severity of chemical arachnoiditis is reduced with dexamethasone. If chemical arachnoiditis is suspected, exclude other possible inflammatory, infectious, or neoplastic conditions. Toxic effects may be related to a single dose or to cumulative administration and usually occur within 5 days, although may occur at any time during treatment. Monitor continuously for development of neurotoxicity; dose reduction or discontinuation may be necessary. Hydrocephalus has been reported and may be precipitated by chemical arachnoiditis.

May cause neurotoxicity (including myelopathy), which may lead to permanent neurologic deficit (rare). The risk for neurotoxicity is increased when administered with other antineoplastic agents or with cranial/spinal irradiation. CSF flow blockage may lead to increased free cytarabine concentrations in the CSF and increases the risk for neurotoxicity; consider assessing CSF flow prior to administration. Persistent (extreme) somnolence, hemiplegia, visual disturbances (including blindness; may be total and permanent), deafness, cranial nerve palsies have been reported. Signs/symptoms of peripheral neuropathy (eg, pain, numbness, paresthesia, weakness, impaired bowel/bladder control) have also been reported. Combined neurologic features (cauda equina syndrome) have been reported in some cases. If neurotoxicity develops, reduce subsequent doses or discontinue treatment. Headache, nausea, and fever are early signs of neurotoxicity. Transient elevations in CSF protein and CSF white blood cell counts have been observed following administration.

For intrathecal use only. Intrathecal medications should not be prepared during the preparation of any other agents. After preparation, store intrathecal medications in an isolated location or container clearly marked with a label identifying as "intrathecal" use only. Delivery of intrathecal medications to the patient should only be with other medications intended for administration into the central nervous system (Jacobson, 2009).

Adverse Reactions
>10%:
Cardiovascular: Peripheral edema (11%)

416

Central nervous system: Chemical arachnoiditis (without dexamethasone premedication: 100%; with dexamethasone premedication: 33% to 42%; grade 4: 19% to 30%; onset: ≤5 days); headache (56%), confusion (33%), fever (32%), fatigue (25%), seizure (20% to 22%), dizziness (18%), lethargy (16%), insomnia (14%), memory impairment (14%), pain (14%)

Endocrine & metabolic: Dehydration (13%)

Gastrointestinal: Nausea (46%), vomiting (44%), constipation (25%), diarrhea (12%), appetite decreased (11%)

Genitourinary: Urinary tract infection (14%)

Hematologic: Anemia (12%), thrombocytopenia (3% to 11%)

Neuromuscular & skeletal: Weakness (40%), back pain (24%), abnormal gait (23%), limb pain (15%), neck pain (14%), arthralgia (11%), neck stiffness (11%)

Ocular: Blurred vision (11%)

1% to 10%:

Cardiovascular: Tachycardia (9%), hypotension (8%), hypertension (6%), syncope (3%), edema (2%)

Central nervous system: Agitation (10%), hypoesthesia (10%), depression (8%), anxiety (7%), sensory neuropathy (3%)

Dermatologic: Pruritus (2%)

Endocrine & metabolic: Hypokalemia (7%), hyponatremia (7%), hyperglycemia (6%)

Gastrointestinal: Abdominal pain (9%), dysphagia (8%), anorexia (5%), hemorrhoids (3%), mucosal inflammation (3%)

Genitourinary: Incontinence (7%), urinary retention (5%)

Hematologic: Neutropenia (10%), contusion (2%)

Neuromuscular & skeletal: Muscle weakness (10%), tremor (9%), peripheral neuropathy (3% to 4%), abnormal reflexes (3%)

Otic: Hypoacusis (6%)

Respiratory: Dyspnea (10%), cough (7%), pneumonia (6%)

Miscellaneous: Diaphoresis (2%)

<1%, postmarketing, and/or case reports: Anaphylaxis, bladder control impaired, blindness, bowel control impaired, cauda equine syndrome, cranial nerve palsies, CSF protein increased, CSF WBC increased, deafness, encephalopathy, hemiplegia, hydrocephalus, infectious meningitis, intracranial pressure increased, myelopathy, neurologic deficit, numbness, papilledema, somnolence, visual disturbance

Drug Interactions

Metabolism/Transport Effects None known.

Avoid Concomitant Use

Avoid concomitant use of Cytarabine (Liposomal) with any of the following: BCG (Intravesical); Tofacitinib

Increased Effect/Toxicity

Cytarabine (Liposomal) may increase the levels/effects of: Fingolimod; Tofacitinib

Decreased Effect

Cytarabine (Liposomal) may decrease the levels/effects of: BCG (Intravesical)

Storage/Stability

Store intact vial at 2°C to 8°C (36°F to 46°F); protect from freezing. Avoid aggressive agitation. Withdraw from the vial immediately prior to administration; solutions should be used within 4 hours of withdrawal from the vial.

After preparation, store intrathecal medications in an isolated location or container clearly marked with a label identifying as "intrathecal" use only (Jacobson, 2009).

Preparation for Administration Hazardous agent; use appropriate precautions for handling and disposal (NIOSH 2014 [group 1]). Gloves should be worn during preparation and administration. Allow vial to warm to room temperature. Particles may settle in diluent over time, and may be resuspended with gentle agitation or inversion immediately prior to withdrawing from the vial. Do not agitate aggressively. Withdraw from the vial immediately prior to administration. No further reconstitution or dilution is required. Do not mix with any other medications. Intrathecal medications should not be prepared during the preparation of any other agents (Jacobson, 2009).

Mechanism of Action Cytarabine liposomal is a sustained-release formulation of the active ingredient cytarabine, an antimetabolite which acts through inhibition of DNA synthesis and is cell cycle-specific for the S phase of cell division. Cytarabine is converted intracellularly to its active metabolite cytarabine-5'-triphosphate (ara-CTP). Ara-CTP also appears to be incorporated into DNA and RNA; however, the primary action is inhibition of DNA polymerase, resulting in decreased DNA synthesis and repair. The liposomal formulation allows for gradual release, resulting in prolonged exposure.

Pharmacodynamics/Kinetics

Absorption: Systemic exposure following intrathecal administration is negligible since transfer rate from CSF to plasma is slow

Half-life elimination, CSF: 6 to 82 hours

Time to peak, CSF: Intrathecal: <1 hour

Dosing

Adult & Geriatric Note: Initiate dexamethasone 4 mg twice daily (oral or IV) for 5 days, beginning on the day of cytarabine liposomal administration.

Lymphomatous meningitis: Intrathecal:

Induction: 50 mg every 14 days for a total of 2 doses (weeks 1 and 3)

Consolidation: 50 mg every 14 days for 3 doses (weeks 5, 7, and 9), followed by an additional dose at week 13

Maintenance: 50 mg every 28 days for 4 doses (weeks 17, 21, 25, and 29)

Renal Impairment There are no dosage adjustments provided in the manufacturer's labeling (has not been studied).

Hepatic Impairment There are no dosage adjustments provided in the manufacturer's labeling (has not been studied).

Adjustment for Toxicity If drug-related neurotoxicity develops, reduce dose to 25 mg. If toxicity persists, discontinue treatment.

Administration For intrathecal use only. Dose should be removed from vial immediately before administration (must be administered within 4 hours of removal from the vial). An in-line filter should **NOT** be used. Administer directly into the CSF via an intraventricular reservoir or by direct injection into the lumbar sac. Injection should be made slowly (over 1 to 5 minutes). Patients should lie flat for 1 hour after lumbar puncture. After administration, observe for immediate toxic reactions.

Hazardous agent; use appropriate precautions for handling and disposal (NIOSH 2014 [group 1]). Gloves should be worn during preparation and administration. If contact with skin occurs, immediately wash with soap and water; if contact with mucous membranes occurs, flush thoroughly with water.

Monitoring Parameters Monitor closely for signs of an immediate reaction; chemical arachnoiditis; neurotoxicity

Dosage Forms Excipient information presented when available (limited, particularly for generics); consult specific product labeling.

Suspension, Intrathecal:

DepoCyt: 50 mg/5 mL (5 mL) [contains cholesterol, dioleoylphosphatidylcholine (dopc), dipalmitoylphosphatidylglycerol (dppg), triolein]

♦ **Cytarabine Hydrochloride** see Cytarabine (Conventional) on page 403

♦ **Cytarabine Injection (Can)** see Cytarabine (Conventional) on page 403

♦ **Cytarabine Lipid Complex** see Cytarabine (Liposomal) on page 415

♦ **Cytarabine Liposome** see Cytarabine (Liposomal) on page 415

♦ **CytoGam®** see Cytomegalovirus Immune Globulin (Intravenous-Human) on page 419

Cytomegalovirus Immune Globulin (Intravenous-Human) (sye toe meg a low VYE rus i MYUN GLOB yoo lin in tra VEE nus HYU man)

Brand Names: US CytoGam®

Brand Names: Canada CytoGam®

Index Terms CMV Hyperimmune Globulin; CMV-IGIV

Pharmacologic Category Blood Product Derivative; Immune Globulin

Use Prophylaxis of cytomegalovirus (CMV) disease associated with kidney, lung, liver, pancreas, and heart transplants; concomitant use with ganciclovir should be considered in organ transplants (other than kidney) from CMV seropositive donors to CMV seronegative recipients

Pregnancy Risk Factor C

Dosing

Adult & Geriatric

Prophylaxis of CMV disease in kidney transplant: IV:

Initial dose (within 72 hours of transplant): 150 mg/kg/dose

2-, 4-, 6-, and 8 weeks after transplant: 100 mg/kg/dose

12- and 16 weeks after transplant: 50 mg/kg/dose

Prophylaxis of CMV disease in liver, lung, pancreas, or heart transplant: IV:

Initial dose (within 72 hours of transplant): 150 mg/kg/dose

2-, 4-, 6-, and 8 weeks after transplant: 150 mg/kg/dose

12- and 16 weeks after transplant: 100 mg/kg/dose

Treatment of severe CMV pneumonitis in hematopoietic stem cell transplant (off-label use; in combination with ganciclovir): IV: 400 mg/kg on days 1, 2, and 7, followed by 200 mg/kg on day 14; if still symptomatic, may administer an additional 200 mg/kg on day 21 (Reed, 1988) **or** 150 mg/kg twice weekly (Alexander, 2010)

Pediatric Prophylaxis of CMV disease in kidney, liver, lung, pancreas, or heart transplant: Children and Adolescents: IV: Refer to adult dosing.

Renal Impairment No dosage adjustment provided in manufacturer's labeling; use with caution. Infuse at minimum rate possible.

Hepatic Impairment No dosage adjustment provided in manufacturer's labeling.

Additional Information Complete prescribing information should be consulted for additional detail.

Dosage Forms Excipient information presented when available (limited, particularly for generics); consult specific product labeling.

Injection, solution [preservative free]:

CytoGam®: 50 mg (± 10 mg)/mL (50 mL) [contains sodium 20-30 mEq/L, human albumin, and sucrose 50 mg/mL]

Dabrafenib (da BRAF e nib)

Brand Names: US Tafinlar

Brand Names: Canada Tafinlar

Index Terms GSK2118436

Pharmacologic Category Antineoplastic Agent, BRAF Kinase Inhibitor

Use Melanoma:

US labeling: Treatment of unresectable or metastatic melanoma in patients with a BRAF V600E mutation (single agent therapy) or in patients with BRAF V600E or BRAF V600K mutations (in combination with trametinib); confirm BRAF V600E or BRAF V600K mutation status with an approved test prior to treatment.

Canadian labeling: Treatment of unresectable or metastatic melanoma in patients with a BRAF V600 mutation (as detected by a validated test) as single agent therapy or in combination with trametinib.

Limitations of use: Not indicated for treatment of patients with wild-type BRAF melanoma.

Labeled Contraindications

There are no contraindications listed in the manufacturer's US labeling.

Canadian labeling: Hypersensitivity to dabrafenib or any component of the formulation.

Pregnancy Considerations Adverse effects were observed in animal reproduction studies. Based on its mechanism of action, dabrafenib would be expected to cause fetal harm if administered to a pregnant woman. Females of reproductive potential should use a highly effective nonhormonal contraceptive during therapy and for at least 2 weeks [US labeling] or at least 4 weeks [Canadian labeling] (for single-agent therapy) or 4 months (for combination therapy with trametinib) after treatment is complete; hormonal contraceptives may not be effective. Spermatogenesis may be impaired in males (observed in animal studies); family planning and fertility counseling should be considered prior to therapy.

Breast-Feeding Considerations It is not known if dabrafenib is excreted into breast milk. Due to the potential for serious adverse reactions in the nursing infant, the manufacturer recommends a decision be made whether to discontinue nursing or to discontinue the drug, taking into account the importance of treatment to the mother.

Warnings/Precautions Hazardous agent – use appropriate precautions for handling and disposal (meets NIOSH 2014 criteria). Serious adverse reactions (retinal vein occlusion, interstitial lung disease) that occur with single-agent trametinib may also occur when dabrafenib is administered in combination with trametinib. Cardiomyopathy may be observed when concomitantly with trametinib. The median time to onset of cardiomyopathy was ~3 months (range: 27 to 253 days) when used in combination with trametinib. Assess LVEF (by echocardiogram or MUGA scan) prior to combination therapy initiation, at 1 month, and then at 2- to 3-month intervals while on combination therapy. Cardiac dysfunction may require dabrafenib treatment interruption (see Trametinib monograph for dosage modifications). Cardiomyopathy resolved following therapy adjustments and/or interruption. QTcF prolongation >60 msec above baseline or to >500 msec was reported, both as a single agent or when used in combination with trametinib. Hemorrhage, including symptomatic bleeding in a critical area/organ, may occur when dabrafenib is used in combination with trametinib. Major bleeding events (some fatal) included intracranial or gastrointestinal hemorrhage. May require treatment interruption and dosage reduction; permanently discontinue dabrafenib (and trametinib) for all grade 4 hemorrhagic events and any grade 3 event that does not improve with therapy interruption. Venous thromboembolism events (some fatal) may occur when dabrafenib is used in combination with trametinib. DVT and PE occurred at an increased incidence with combination therapy. Patients should seek immediate medical attention with symptoms of DVT or PE (shortness of breath, chest pain, arm/leg swelling). Dabrafenib therapy may be continued for uncomplicated DVT or PE; permanently discontinue dabrafenib (and trametinib) for life-threatening PE.

Serious febrile reactions and fever (any severity) complicated by hypotension, rigors or chills, dehydration, or renal failure were observed during dabrafenib single-agent therapy and when used in combination with trametinib. The median time to initial fever (single-agent therapy) was 11 days (range: 1 to 202 days); median duration was 3 days (range: 1 to 129 days). In patients treated with combination therapy, the median time to onset of fever was 30 days and duration was 6 days. Interrupt dabrafenib therapy for fever ≥38.5°C (101.3°F) or for any other serious febrile reaction complicated by hypotension, rigors/chills, dehydration, or renal failure; evaluate promptly for signs/symptoms of infection. Dosage reduction (or discontinuation) may be required; when resuming therapy after a febrile reaction, may require prophylactic administration of antipyretics. Hyperglycemia may occur while on therapy (either as a single agent or in combination with trametinib); may require initiation of insulin or oral hypoglycemic agent therapy (or an increased dose if already taking). Monitor serum glucose as clinically necessary, particularly in patients with preexisting diabetes or hyperglycemia. Instruct patients to report symptoms of severe hyperglycemia (eg, polydipsia, polyuria).

Serious dermatologic toxicity (eg, rash, dermatitis, acneiform rash, palmar-plantar erythrodysesthesia syndrome, erythema) may occur when used in combination with trametinib (known complication of single-agent trametinib therapy); some patients required hospitalization for severe toxicity or for secondary skin infections. The median time to onset and resolution of skin toxicity for combination therapy was 37 days (range: 1 to 225 days) and 33 days (range: 3 to 421 days), respectively. Monitor for dermatologic toxicity and signs/symptoms of secondary infections. Treatment interruption, dose reduction, and/or therapy discontinuation may be necessary. Cutaneous squamous cell carcinoma and keratoacanthoma (cuSCC) and melanoma were observed during single agent dabrafenib therapy at an increased incidence compared with control therapy in clinical trials. The median time to the first occurrence of cuSCC was 9 weeks (range: 1 to 53 weeks); approximately one-third of patients who developed cuSCC had more than one occurrence (with continued treatment). The median time between diagnosis of the first and second lesions was 6 weeks. When used in combination with trametinib, cuSCC occurred less frequently than with single-agent dabrafenib therapy; time to diagnosis ranged from 136 to 197 days after the initiation of combination treatment. Basal cell carcinoma (BCC) occurs more frequently with combination versus single-agent therapy; the incidence of BCC is 9% for combination therapy versus 2% for single-agent dabrafenib. The time to BCC diagnosis ranged from 28 to 249 days for patients receiving combination therapy. Dermatologic evaluations should be performed prior to initiating therapy, every 2 months during therapy, and for up to 6 months post discontinuation. There are case reports of noncutaneous malignancies, including pancreatic cancer (KRAS mutation-positive), colorectal cancer (recurrent NRAS mutation-positive), hand and neck cancer, and glioblastoma, with combination therapy; monitor for signs/symptoms of noncutaneous malignancies. Dabrafenib should be permanently discontinued if RAS mutation-positive noncutaneous malignancies develop (no trametinib dosage reduction is required).

Retinal pigment epithelial detachments (RPED) were seen in clinical trials when used in combination with trametinib (known complication of trametinib single-agent therapy). Detachments were typically bilateral and multifocal and occurred in the macular area of the retina. Promptly refer patients for ophthalmological evaluations if loss of vision or other visual disturbances occur; dabrafenib dosage modification is not necessary for RPED (trametinib therapy modification may be required). In clinical trials, ophthalmic exams (including retinal evaluation) were performed prior to and regularly during treatment with combination therapy. Uveitis and iritis have been reported with dabrafenib single-agent therapy and when used in combination with trametinib; manage symptomatically with ophthalmic steroid and mydriatic drops. May require dabrafenib treatment interruption (does not require alteration in trametinib therapy). Monitor for signs/symptoms of uveitis (eg, eye pain, photophobia, vision changes).

Potentially significant drug-drug interactions may exist, requiring dose or frequency adjustment, additional monitoring, and/or selection of alternative therapy. Drugs affecting gastric pH (eg, proton pump inhibitors, H2-receptor antagonists, antacids) may alter dabrafenib solubility, resulting in decreased bioavailability. Clinical trials have not been performed to evaluate concomitant administration and its effect on dabrafenib efficacy. Patients with glucose-6-phosphate dehydrogenase (G6PD) deficiency may be at risk for hemolytic anemia when administered dabrafenib; use with caution and closely observe for signs/symptoms of hemolytic anemia. Not indicated for treatment of patients with wild-type BRAF melanoma. Exposing wild-type cells to BRAF inhibitors such as dabrafenib may result in paradoxical activation of MAP-kinase signaling and increased cell proliferation. Prior to initiating therapy, confirm BRAF V600E or BRAF V600K mutations (US labeling) or BRAF V600 mutations (Canadian labeling) status with an approved test. Data regarding single-agent use in patients with BRAF V600K mutation is limited; compared to BRAF V600E mutation, lower response rates have been observed with BRAF

V600K mutation. Data regarding other less common BRAF V600 mutations is lacking.

Adverse Reactions

Monotherapy:

>10%:

Cardiovascular: Peripheral edema (17%)

Central nervous system: Fatigue (40%), headache (28% to 32%), chills (17%)

Dermatologic: Dermatological reaction (68%), skin rash (17% to 53%), hyperkeratosis (37%), alopecia (22%), palmar-plantar erythrodysesthesia (20%), pruritus (13%)

Endocrine & metabolic: Hyperglycemia (49% to 50%; grades 3/4: 2% to 6%), hypophosphatemia (37% to 40%), increased gamma-glutamyl transferase (38%), hyponatremia (8% to 36%), hypoalbuminemia (23%), hypokalemia (23%), hyperkalemia (15%)

Gastrointestinal: Diarrhea (28%), abdominal pain (21%), nausea (21%), decreased appetite (19%), vomiting (15%), constipation (11%)

Hematologic & oncologic: Lymphocytopenia (40%; grades 3/4: 6%), anemia (28%), papilloma (27%), leukopenia (21%), malignant neoplasm of skin (keratoacanthoma and squamous cell carcinoma; 7% to 19%; grades 3/4: 4%)

Hepatic: Increased serum alkaline phosphatase (19% to 26%), increased serum AST (15%), increased serum ALT (11%)

Neuromuscular & skeletal: Arthralgia (27% to 34%), myalgia (11% to 23%), limb pain (19%), back pain (11% to 12%)

Respiratory: Cough (12% to 21%)

Miscellaneous: Fever (26% to 28%; grades 3/4: ≤4%)

1% to 10%:

Cardiovascular: Prolonged Q-T interval on ECG (>60 msec from baseline: 2%; >500 msec: 2%)

Central nervous system: Dizziness (9%), insomnia (8%)

Dermatologic: Actinic keratosis (9%), night sweats (6%), xeroderma (6%), acneiform eruption (4%), erythema (2%)

Endocrine & metabolic: Hypocalcemia (9%), hypomagnesemia (6%), hypercalcemia (4%), dehydration (2%)

Gastrointestinal: Pancreatitis (<10%), xerostomia (6%)

Genitourinary: Urinary tract infection (9%)

Hematologic & oncologic: Neutropenia (9%; grades 3/4: 2%), thrombocytopenia (8%), basal cell carcinoma (2%), hemorrhage (2%), malignant melanoma (2%)

Hypersensitivity: Hypersensitivity (bullous rash, <10%)

Neuromuscular & skeletal: Muscle spasm (4%)

Ophthalmic: Uveitis (including iritis, 1%)

Renal: Interstitial nephritis (<10%), increased serum creatinine (9%)

Respiratory: Nasopharyngitis (10%)

Miscellaneous: Febrile reaction (2%)

Combination therapy with trametanib:

>10%:

Cardiovascular: Peripheral edema (28% to 31%), prolonged Q-T interval on ECG (>60 msec from baseline: 13%; >500 msec: 4%)

Central nervous system: Chills (50% to 58%), fatigue (53% to 57%), headache (29% to 37%), insomnia (11% to 18%), dizziness (13% to 16%)

Dermatologic: Dermatological reaction (65%; 3% required hospitalization), skin rash (43% to 45%), night sweats (15% to 24%), xeroderma (9% to 18%), acneiform eruption (11% to 16%), actinic keratosis (7% to 15%), erythema (6% to 15%), pruritus (11%)

Endocrine & metabolic: Hyperglycemia (58% to 67%; grades 3/4: 5% to 6%), increased gamma-glutamyl transferase (54% to 56%), hyponatremia (48% to 55%), hypoalbuminemia (43% to 53%), hypophosphatemia (41% to 47%), hypokalemia (15% to 29%), hyperkalemia (18% to 22%), hypocalcemia (13% to 20%), hypercalcemia (15% to 19%), hypomagnesemia (2% to 18%), dehydration (6% to 11%)

Gastrointestinal: Nausea (44% to 46%), vomiting (40% to 43%), diarrhea (26% to 36%), abdominal pain (24% to 33%), decreased appetite (22% to 30%), constipation (17% to 22%), xerostomia (11%)

Genitourinary: Urinary tract infection (6% to 13%)

Hematologic & oncologic: Leukopenia (46% to 62%; grades 3/4: 4% to 5%), lymphocytopenia (55% to 59%; grades 3/4: 19% to 22%), anemia (46% to 55%; grades 3/4: 4% to 7%), neutropenia (37% to 55%; grades 3/4: 2% to 13%), thrombocytopenia (31%; grades 3/4: 2% to 4%), hemorrhage (11% to 16%; major hemorrhage [intracranial or gastric]: 5%)

Hepatic: Increased serum alkaline phosphatase (60% to 67%), increased serum AST (54% to 60%), increased serum ALT (35% to 42%), hyperbilirubinemia (7% to 15%)

Neuromuscular & skeletal: Arthralgia (27% to 44%), myalgia (22% to 24%), back pain (11% to 18%), limb pain (11% to 16%), muscle spasm (2% to 16%)

Renal: Increased serum creatinine (20% to 24%)

Respiratory: Cough (11% to 29%), oropharyngeal pain (7% to 13%)

Miscellaneous: Fever (57% to 71%; grades 3/4: 5% to 9%), febrile reaction (25%)

1% to 10%:

Cardiovascular: Hypertension (<10%), cardiomyopathy (≤9%), venous thromboembolism (deep vein thrombosis or pulmonary embolism; 7%)

Dermatologic: Cellulitis (<10%), folliculitis (<10%), hyperhidrosis (<10%), hyperkeratosis (<10%), palmar-plantar erythrodysesthesia (<10%), paronychia (<10%), pustular rash (<10%), secondary skin infection (3%)

Endocrine & metabolic: Hyperglycemia (grade 3: 5% to 6%)

Gastrointestinal: Pancreatitis (<10%), stomatitis (<10%)

Hematologic & oncologic: Cutaneous papilloma (<10%), basal cell carcinoma (9%), malignant neoplasm of skin (keratoacanthoma and squamous cell carcinoma; 7%)

Neuromuscular & skeletal: Weakness (<10%)

Ophthalmic: Blindness (transient; <10%), blurred vision (<10%), retinal detachment (pigment epithelium; 1%), uveitis (1%)

Renal: Renal failure (2% to 7%)

<1%: Glioblastoma, malignant neoplasm of colon and rectum (recurrent NRAS mutation-positive), malignant neoplasm of head and neck, pancreatic adenocarcinoma (KRAS mutation-positive)

Drug Interactions

Metabolism/Transport Effects Substrate of BCRP, CYP2C8 (major), CYP3A4 (major), P-glycoprotein; **Note:** Assignment of Major/Minor substrate status based on clinically relevant drug interaction potential; **Inhibits** BCRP, SLCO1B1; **Induces** CYP2B6 (weak/moderate), CYP2C19 (weak/moderate), CYP2C8 (weak/moderate), CYP2C9 (weak/moderate), CYP3A4 (moderate)

Avoid Concomitant Use
Avoid concomitant use of Dabrafenib with any of the following: Axitinib; Bedaquiline; Bosutinib; Cobimetinib; Conivaptan; CYP2C8 Inducers (Strong); CYP2C8 Inhibitors (Strong); CYP3A4 Inducers (Strong); CYP3A4 Inhibitors (Strong); Flibanserin; Fusidic Acid (Systemic); Idelalisib; Nisoldipine; Olaparib; Palbociclib; PAZOPanib; Ranolazine; Simeprevir; Sonidegib

Increased Effect/Toxicity
Dabrafenib may increase the levels/effects of: Highest Risk QTc-Prolonging Agents; Moderate Risk QTc-Prolonging Agents; PAZOPanib; Topotecan

The levels/effects of Dabrafenib may be increased by: Conivaptan; CYP2C8 Inhibitors (Moderate); CYP2C8 Inhibitors (Strong); CYP3A4 Inhibitors (Moderate); CYP3A4 Inhibitors (Strong); Deferasirox; Fusidic Acid (Systemic); Idelalisib; Luliconazole; Mifepristone; Osimertinib; Trametinib

Decreased Effect
Dabrafenib may decrease the levels/effects of: Antidiabetic Agents; ARIPiprazole; Axitinib; Bedaquiline; Bosutinib; Cobimetinib; Contraceptives (Estrogens); Contraceptives (Progestins); CYP2B6 Substrates; CYP2C19 Substrates; CYP2C8 Substrates; CYP2C9 Substrates; CYP3A4 Substrates; Daclatasvir; FentaNYL; Flibanserin; Ibrutinib; Nisoldipine; Olaparib; Palbociclib; Proton Pump Inhibitors; Ranolazine; Saxagliptin; Simeprevir; Sonidegib

The levels/effects of Dabrafenib may be decreased by: Antacids; CYP2C8 Inducers (Strong); CYP3A4 Inducers (Strong); H2-Antagonists; Osimertinib; Proton Pump Inhibitors; St Johns Wort

Food Interactions Administration with a high-fat meal decreased C_{max} and AUC by 51% and 31%, respectively, and delayed median T_{max} by ~4 hours. Management: Administer 1 hour before or 2 hours after a meal.

Storage/Stability Store at 25°C (77°F); excursions permitted to 15°C to 30°C (59°F to 86°F).

Mechanism of Action Selectively inhibits some mutated forms of the protein kinase B-raf (BRAF). BRAF V600 mutations result in constitutive activation of the BRAF pathway; through BRAF inhibition, dabrafenib inhibits tumor cell growth. The combination of dabrafenib and trametinib allows for greater inhibition of the MAPK pathway, resulting in BRAF V600 melanoma cell death (Flaherty, 2012).

Pharmacodynamics/Kinetics
Absorption: Decreased with a high-fat meal

Distribution: 70.3 L

Protein binding: 99.7% to plasma proteins

Metabolism: Hepatic via CYP2C8 and CYP3A4 to hydroxy-dabrafenib (active) which is further metabolized via CYP3A4 oxidation to desmethyl-dabrafenib (active)

Bioavailability: 95%

Half-life elimination: Parent drug: 8 hours; Hydroxy-dabrafenib (active metabolite): 10 hours; Desmethyl-dabrafenib (active metabolite): 21-22 hours

Time to peak: 2 hours; delayed with a high-fat meal

Excretion: Feces (71%); urine (23%; metabolites only)

Dosing
Adult & Geriatric
US labeling:
Melanoma, metastatic or unresectable (with BRAF V600E mutation): Oral: 150 mg twice daily (approximately every 12 hours) until disease progression or unacceptable toxicity (single-agent therapy)

Melanoma, metastatic or unresectable (with BRAF V600E or BRAF V600K mutation): Oral: 150 mg twice daily (approximately every 12 hours) until disease progression or unacceptable toxicity (in combination with trametinib)

Canadian labeling: **Melanoma, metastatic or unresectable (with BRAF V600 mutation):** Oral: 150 mg twice daily (approximately every 12 hours) until disease progression or unacceptable toxicity (single-agent therapy or in combination with trametinib)

Missed doses: A missed dose may be administered up to 6 hours prior to the next dose; do not administer if <6 hours until the next dose.

Renal Impairment

Mild to moderate impairment (GFR ≥30 mL/minute/1.73 m^2): No dosage adjustment necessary.

Severe impairment (GFR <30 mL/minute/1.73 m^2): There are no dosage adjustments provided in the manufacturer's labeling (has not been studied)

Hepatic Impairment

Mild impairment: No dosage adjustment necessary.

Moderate to severe impairment: There are no dosage adjustments provided in the manufacturer's labeling (has not been studied); however, metabolism is primarily hepatic and exposure may be increased in patients with moderate to severe impairment.

Adjustment for Toxicity

Recommended dabrafenib dose reductions for toxicity:

First dose reduction: 100 mg twice daily

Second dose reduction: 75 mg twice daily

Third dose reduction: 50 mg twice daily

Subsequent modifications (if unable to tolerate 50 mg twice daily): Permanently discontinue.

Note: If using combination therapy, refer to Trametinib monograph for recommended trametinib dose reductions.

Cardiac:

Asymptomatic, 10% or greater absolute decrease in LVEF from baseline and LVEF is below institutional lower limits of normal (LLN) from pretreatment value: No dabrafenib dosage modification is necessary.

>20% absolute decrease in LVEF from baseline and LVEF is below institutional LLN: Interrupt dabrafenib therapy; if improved, may resume at the same dose.

Symptomatic heart failure: Interrupt dabrafenib therapy; if improved, may resume at the same dose.

Dermatologic:

Intolerable grade 2 skin toxicity or grade 3 or 4 skin toxicity: Interrupt dabrafenib therapy for up to 3 weeks. If toxicity improves within 3 weeks, resume at a lower dose level. If toxicity does not improve within 3 weeks following therapy interruption, permanently discontinue dabrafenib.

New primary cutaneous malignancy: No dabrafenib dosage modification is necessary.

Fever:

Fever of 38.5°C to 40°C (101.3°F to 104°F): Interrupt dabrafenib therapy until temperature normalizes. Resume at the same or lower dose level.

Fever >40°C (104°F) and/or fever complicated by rigors, hypotension, dehydration, or renal failure: Interrupt dabrafenib therapy until temperature normalizes. Resume at a lower dose level or permanently discontinue.

Hemorrhage:

Grade 3 hemorrhage: Interrupt dabrafenib therapy. If hemorrhage improves, resume at a lower dose level. If hemorrhage does not improve following therapy interruption, permanently discontinue dabrafenib.

Grade 4 hemorrhage: Permanently discontinue dabrafenib.

Ocular:

Uveitis and iritis: Interrupt dabrafenib therapy for up to 6 weeks. If improves to ≤ grade 1 within 6 weeks following therapy interruption, resume at the same dose. If does not improve, permanently discontinue dabrafenib.

Grade 2 or 3 retinal pigment epithelial detachments (RPED): No dabrafenib dosage modification is necessary.

Retinal vein occlusion: No dabrafenib dosage modification is necessary.

Pulmonary: Interstitial lung disease or pneumonitis: No dabrafenib dosage modification is necessary.

Venous thromboembolism:

Uncomplicated DVT or PE: No dabrafenib dosage modification is necessary.

Life-threatening PE: Permanently discontinue dabrafenib.

Other toxicity:

Intolerable grade 2 or any grade 3 toxicity: Interrupt dabrafenib therapy until resolution to ≤ grade 1; resume at a lower dose level. If toxicity does not improve following therapy interruption, permanently discontinue dabrafenib.

Grade 4 toxicity (first occurrence): Interrupt dabrafenib therapy until resolution to ≤ grade 1; consider resuming at a lower dose level or permanently discontinue.

Grade 4 toxicity (recurrent after dosage reduction): Permanently discontinue dabrafenib.

New primary noncutaneous malignancy (RAS mutation-positive): Permanently discontinue dabrafenib.

Combination Regimens

Melanoma:

Dabrafenib (Melanoma Regimen) on page 1934

Dabrafenib-Trametinib (Melanoma) on page 1934

Administration Administer orally at least 1 hour before or 2 hours after a meal; doses should be ~12 hours apart. Do not open, crush, or break capsules. A missed dose may be administered up to 6 hours prior to the next dose. When administered in combination with trametinib, take the once-daily dose of trametinib at the same time each day with either the morning or evening dose of dabrafenib.

Hazardous agent; use appropriate precautions for handling and disposal (meets NIOSH 2014 criteria).

Emetic Potential Minimal (<10%)

Monitoring Parameters BRAFV600 mutation status; serum glucose (particularly in patients with preexisting diabetes mellitus or hyperglycemia); electrolytes; renal function; dermatologic evaluations prior to initiation, every 2 months during therapy, and for up to 6 months following discontinuation to assess for new cutaneous malignancies; monitor for febrile drug reactions and signs/symptoms of infections; signs/symptoms of uveitis (eg, eye pain, photophobia, vision changes), monitor for signs/symptoms of hemolytic anemia.

For patients receiving combination therapy with trametinib: Hepatic function (Canadian labeling recommends approximately every 4 weeks for 6 months after initiation then periodically as clinically indicated); CBC (baseline and periodically during therapy); assess LVEF (by echocardiogram or MUGA scan) at baseline, 1 month after therapy initiation, and then at 2- to 3-month intervals; monitor for signs/symptoms of hemorrhage, venous thromboembolism, interstitial lung disease, and RPED, or retinal vein occlusion.

Dietary Considerations Administer at least 1 hour before or 2 hours after a meal.

Medication Guide Available Yes

Dosage Forms Excipient information presented when available (limited, particularly for generics); consult specific product labeling.

Capsule, Oral:

Tafinlar: 50 mg, 75 mg

Dacarbazine (da KAR ba zeen)

Related Information

Management of Chemotherapy-Induced Nausea and Vomiting in Adults *on page 2142*

Prevention of Chemotherapy-Induced Nausea and Vomiting in Children *on page 2203*

Safe Handling of Hazardous Drugs *on page 2292*

Brand Names: Canada Dacarbazine for Injection

Index Terms DIC; Dimethyl Triazeno Imidazole Carboxamide; DTIC; DTIC-Dome; Imidazole Carboxamide; Imidazole Carboxamide Dimethyltriazene; WR-139007

Pharmacologic Category Antineoplastic Agent, Alkylating Agent (Triazene)

Use Treatment of malignant melanoma, Hodgkin lymphoma

Labeled Contraindications Hypersensitivity to dacarbazine or any component of the formulation

Pregnancy Considerations [U.S. Boxed Warning]: This agent is carcinogenic and/or teratogenic when used in animals; adverse effects have been observed in animal studies. There are no adequate and well-controlled trials in pregnant women; use in pregnancy only if the potential benefit outweighs the potential risk to the fetus.

Breast-Feeding Considerations Due to the potential for serious adverse reactions in the nursing infant, breast-feeding is not recommended.

Warnings/Precautions Hazardous agent - use appropriate precautions for handling and disposal (NIOSH 2014 [group 1]). **[U.S. Boxed Warnings]: Bone marrow suppression is a common toxicity;** leukopenia and thrombocytopenia may be severe; may result in treatment delays or discontinuation; monitor closely. **Hepatotoxicity with hepatocellular necrosis and hepatic vein thrombosis has been reported (rare),** usually with combination chemotherapy, but may occur with dacarbazine alone. The half-life is increased in patients with renal and/or hepatic impairment; use caution, monitor for toxicity and consider dosage reduction. Anaphylaxis may occur following dacarbazine administration. Extravasation may result in tissue damage and severe pain. **[U.S. Boxed Warnings]: May be carcinogenic and/or teratogenic. Should be administered under the supervision of an experienced cancer chemotherapy physician.** Carefully evaluate the potential benefits of therapy against the risk for toxicity. Dacarbazine is associated with a high emetic potential; antiemetics are recommended to prevent nausea and vomiting (Basch, 2011; Dupuis, 2011; Roila, 2010).

Adverse Reactions Frequency not always defined.
Dermatologic: Alopecia
Gastrointestinal: Nausea and vomiting (>90%), anorexia
Hematologic: Myelosuppression (onset: 5-7 days; nadir: 7-10 days; recovery: 21-28 days), leukopenia, thrombocytopenia
Local: Pain on infusion
Infrequent, postmarketing, and/or case reports: Anaphylactic reactions, anemia, diarrhea, eosinophilia, erythema, facial flushing, facial paresthesia, flu-like syndrome (fever, myalgia, malaise), hepatic necrosis, hepatic vein occlusion, liver enzymes increased (transient), paresthesia, photosensitivity, rash, renal functions test abnormalities, taste alteration, urticaria

Drug Interactions

Metabolism/Transport Effects Substrate of CYP1A2 (major), CYP2E1 (major); **Note:** Assignment of Major/Minor substrate status based on clinically relevant drug interaction potential

Avoid Concomitant Use
Avoid concomitant use of Dacarbazine with any of the following: BCG (Intravesical); CloZAPine; Dipyrone; Natalizumab; Pimecrolimus; Tacrolimus (Topical); Tofacitinib; Vaccines (Live)

Increased Effect/Toxicity
Dacarbazine may increase the levels/effects of: CloZAPine; Fingolimod; Leflunomide; Natalizumab; Tofacitinib; Vaccines (Live)

The levels/effects of Dacarbazine may be increased by: Abiraterone Acetate; CYP1A2 Inhibitors (Moderate); CYP1A2 Inhibitors (Strong); CYP2E1 Inhibitors (Moderate); CYP2E1 Inhibitors (Strong); Deferasirox; Denosumab; Dipyrone; MAO Inhibitors; Peginterferon Alfa-2b; Pimecrolimus; Roflumilast; Tacrolimus (Topical); Trastuzumab; Vemurafenib

Decreased Effect
Dacarbazine may decrease the levels/effects of: BCG (Intravesical); Coccidioides immitis Skin Test; Sipuleucel-T; Vaccines (Inactivated); Vaccines (Live)

The levels/effects of Dacarbazine may be decreased by: Cannabis; CYP1A2 Inducers (Strong); Cyproterone; Echinacea; Osimertinib; SORAfenib; Teriflunomide

Storage/Stability Store intact vials under refrigeration (2°C to 8°C). Protect from light. The following stability information has also been reported: Intact vials are stable for 3 months at room temperature (Cohen, 2007). Reconstituted solution is stable for 24 hours at room temperature (20°C) and 96 hours under refrigeration (4°C) when protected from light, although the manufacturer recommends use within 72 hours if refrigerated and 8 hours at room temperature. Solutions for infusion (in D_5W or NS) are stable for 24 hours at room temperature if protected from light. Decomposed drug turns pink.

Preparation for Administration Hazardous agent; use appropriate precautions for handling and disposal (NIOSH 2014 [group 1]). The manufacturer recommends reconstituting 100 mg and 200 mg vials with 9.9 mL and 19.7 mL SWFI, respectively, to a concentration of 10 mg/mL; some institutions use different standard dilutions (eg, 20 mg/mL).

Standard IV dilution: Dilute in 250-1000 mL D_5W or NS.

◀ **Mechanism of Action** Alkylating agent which is converted to the active alkylating metabolite MTIC [(methyl-triazene-1-yl)-imidazole-4-carboxamide] via the cytochrome P450 system. The cytotoxic effects of MTIC are manifested through alkylation (methylation) of DNA at the O^6, N^7 guanine positions which lead to DNA double strand breaks and apoptosis. Non-cell cycle specific.

Pharmacodynamics/Kinetics

Distribution: V_d: 0.6 L/kg, exceeding total body water; suggesting binding to some tissue (probably liver)

Protein binding: ~5%

Metabolism: Extensively hepatic to the active metabolite MTIC [(methyl-triazene-1-yl)-imidazole-4-carboxamide]

Half-life elimination: Biphasic: Initial: 20-40 minutes, Terminal: 5 hours; Patients with renal and hepatic dysfunction: Initial: 55 minutes, Terminal: 7.2 hours

Excretion: Urine (~40% as unchanged drug)

Dosing

Adult & Geriatric Note: Dacarbazine is associated with a high emetic potential; antiemetics are recommended to prevent nausea and vomiting (Basch, 2011; Roila, 2010).

Hodgkin lymphoma (combination chemotherapy): IV: 375 mg/m²/dose days 1 and 15 every 4 weeks (ABVD regimen)

Metastatic melanoma: IV: 250 mg/m²/dose days 1-5 every 3 weeks

Metastatic melanoma (off-label dosing; in combination with cisplatin and vinblastine): IV:. 800 mg/m² on day 1 every 3 weeks (Atkins, 2008; Eton, 2002)

Soft tissue sarcoma (off-label use; MAID regimen): IV: 250 mg/m²/day continuous infusion for 4 days every 3 weeks (total of 1000 mg/m²/cycle) (Antman, 1993; Antman, 1998)

Pediatric Note: Dacarbazine is associated with a high emetic potential; antiemetics are recommended to prevent nausea and vomiting (Dupuis, 2011).

Hodgkin lymphoma (combination chemotherapy): IV: 375 mg/m²/dose days 1 and 15 every 4 weeks (ABVD regimen; Hutchinson, 1998)

Renal Impairment The FDA-approved labeling does not contain dosage adjustment guidelines. The following guidelines have been used by some clinicians (Kintzel, 1995):

CrCl 46-60 mL/minute: Administer 80% of dose

CrCl 31-45 mL/minute: Administer 75% of dose

CrCl <30 mL/minute: Administer 70% of dose

Hepatic Impairment The FDA-approved labeling does not contain adjustment guidelines. May cause hepatotoxicity; monitor closely for signs of toxicity.

Obesity *ASCO Guidelines for appropriate chemotherapy dosing in obese adults with cancer:* Utilize patient's actual body weight (full weight) for calculation of body surface area- or weight-based dosing, particularly when the intent of therapy is curative; manage regimen-related toxicities in the same manner as for nonobese patients; if a dose reduction is utilized due to toxicity, consider resumption of full weight-based dosing with subsequent cycles, especially if cause of toxicity (eg, hepatic or renal impairment) is resolved (Griggs, 2012).

Combination Regimens

Lymphoma, Hodgkin:

ABVD Early Stage (Hodgkin) on page 1820
ABVD (Hodgkin) on page 1821

MOPP/ABVD (Hodgkin) on page 2039
Melanoma:
Cisplatin-Vinblastine-Dacarbazine (Melanoma) on page 1912
CVD-Interleukin-Interferon (Melanoma) on page 1926
Soft tissue sarcoma:
AD (Soft Tissue Sarcoma) on page 1826
MAID (Soft Tissue Sarcoma) on page 2031

Administration Dacarbazine is associated with a high emetic potential; antiemetics are recommended to prevent nausea and vomiting (Basch, 2011; Dupuis, 2011; Roila, 2010).

Infuse over 30 to 60 minutes; rapid infusion may cause severe venous irritation. May also be administered as a continuous infusion (off-label administration rate) depending on the protocol.

Extravasation management: Local pain, burning sensation, and irritation at the injection site may be relieved by local application of hot packs. If extravasation occurs, apply cold packs. Protect exposed tissue from light following extravasation.

Hazardous agent; use appropriate precautions for handling and disposal (NIOSH 2014 [group 1]).

Vesicant/Extravasation Risk May be an irritant

Emetic Potential Children and Adults: High (>90%)

Monitoring Parameters CBC with differential, liver function

Dosage Forms Excipient information presented when available (limited, particularly for generics); consult specific product labeling.
Solution Reconstituted, Intravenous:
  Generic: 100 mg (1 ea); 200 mg (1 ea)
Solution Reconstituted, Intravenous [preservative free]:
  Generic: 200 mg (1 ea)

♦ **Dacarbazine for Injection (Can)** see Dacarbazine on page 428

♦ **Dacogen** see Decitabine on page 474

♦ **DACT** see DACTINomycin on page 431

DACTINomycin (dak ti noe MYE sin)

Related Information

Management of Chemotherapy-Induced Nausea and Vomiting in Adults on page 2142
Management of Drug Extravasations on page 2159
Safe Handling of Hazardous Drugs on page 2292

Brand Names: US Cosmegen

Brand Names: Canada Cosmegen

Index Terms ACT-D; Actinomycin; Actinomycin Cl; Actinomycin D; DACT

Pharmacologic Category Antineoplastic Agent, Antibiotic

Use Treatment of Wilms' tumor, childhood rhabdomyosarcoma, Ewing's sarcoma, metastatic testicular tumors (nonseminomatous), gestational trophoblastic neoplasm; regional perfusion (palliative or adjunctive) of locally recurrent or locoregional solid tumors (sarcomas, carcinomas and adenocarcinomas)

Labeled Contraindications Hypersensitivity to dactinomycin or any component of the formulation; patients with concurrent or recent chickenpox or herpes zoster

◀ **Pregnancy Considerations [U.S. Boxed Warning]: Avoid exposure during pregnancy.** Adverse effects have been observed in animal reproduction studies. Women of childbearing potential are advised not to become pregnant. When used for gestational trophoblastic neoplasm, unfavorable outcomes have been reported when subsequent pregnancies occur within 6 months of treatment. It is recommended to use effective contraception for 6 months to 1 year after therapy (Matsui 2004; Seckl 2013)

Breast-Feeding Considerations It is not known if dactinomycin is excreted in human breast milk. According to the manufacturer labeling, due to the potential for serious adverse reactions in the nursing infant, the decision to discontinue dactinomycin or to discontinue breast-feeding during therapy should take into account the benefits of treatment to the mother.

Warnings/Precautions [U.S. Boxed Warning]: Hazardous agent - use appropriate precautions for handling and disposal (NIOSH 2014 [group 1]). If accidental exposure occurs, immediately irrigate copiously for at least 15 minutes with water, saline, or balanced ophthalmic irrigation solution (eye exposure) and at least 15 minutes with water (skin exposure); prompt ophthalmic or medical consultation is also recommended. Contaminated clothing should be destroyed and shoes thoroughly cleaned prior to reuse.

Vesicant; ensure proper needle or catheter placement prior to and during infusion; avoid extravasation. **[U.S. Boxed Warning]: Extremely corrosive to soft tissues; if extravasation occurs during IV use, severe damage to soft tissues will occur; has led to contracture of the arm (rare). Avoid inhalation of vapors or contact with skin, mucous membrane, or eyes; avoid exposure during pregnancy.** Recommended for IV administration only. The manufacturer recommends intermittent ice (15 minutes 4 times/day) for suspected extravasation.

May cause hepatic sinusoidal obstruction syndrome (SOS; formerly called veno-occlusive liver disease); use with caution in hepatobiliary dysfunction. Monitor for signs or symptoms of hepatic SOS, including bilirubin >1.4 mg/dL, unexplained weight gain, ascites, hepatomegaly, or unexplained right upper quadrant pain (Arndt, 2004). The risk of fatal SOS is increased in children <4 years of age.

Dactinomycin potentiates the effects of radiation therapy; use with caution in patients who have received radiation therapy; reduce dosages in patients who are receiving dactinomycin and radiation therapy simultaneously; combination with radiation therapy may result in increased toxicity (eg, GI toxicity, myelosuppression, severe oropharyngeal mucositis). Avoid dactinomycin use within 2 months of radiation treatment for right-sided Wilms' tumor, may increase the risk of hepatotoxicity.

Dactinomycin is associated with a high emetic potential; antiemetics are recommended to prevent nausea and vomiting (Basch, 2011; Dupuis, 2011). Toxic effects may be delayed in onset (2-4 days following a course of treatment) and may require 1-2 weeks to reach maximum severity. Discontinue treatment with severe myelosuppression, diarrhea, or stomatitis. Long-term observation of cancer survivors is recommended due to the increased risk of second primary tumors following treatment with radiation and antineoplastic agents. Regional perfusion therapy may result in local limb edema, soft tissue damage, and possible venous thrombosis; leakage of dactinomycin into systemic circulation may result in hematologic toxicity, infection, impaired wound healing, and mucositis. Dosage is usually expressed in **MICRO**grams and should be calculated on the basis of body surface area (BSA) in obese or edematous adult patients (to relate dose to lean body mass). Avoid administration of live vaccines during dactinomycin treatment. Avoid use in infants <6 months of age (toxic effects may occur more frequently). May be associated with an increased risk of myelosuppression in the elderly; use with caution. **[U.S. Boxed Warning]: Should be administered under the supervision of an experienced cancer chemotherapy physician.** Potentially significant drug-drug interactions may exist, requiring dose or frequency adjustment, additional monitoring, and/or selection of alternative therapy.

Adverse Reactions Frequency not defined.

Central nervous system: Fatigue, fever, lethargy, malaise

Dermatologic: Acne, alopecia (reversible), cheilitis, erythema multiforme, increased pigmentation, sloughing, or erythema of previously irradiated skin; skin eruptions, Stevens-Johnson syndrome, toxic epidermal necrolysis

Endocrine & metabolic: Growth retardation, hyperuricemia, hypocalcemia

Gastrointestinal: Abdominal pain, anorexia, diarrhea, dysphagia, esophagitis, GI ulceration, mucositis, nausea, pharyngitis, proctitis, stomatitis, vomiting

Hematologic: Agranulocytosis, anemia, aplastic anemia, febrile neutropenia, leukopenia, myelosuppression (onset: 7 days, nadir: 14-21 days, recovery: 21-28 days), neutropenia, pancytopenia, reticulocytopenia, thrombocytopenia, thrombocytopenia (immune mediated)

Hepatic: Ascites, bilirubin increased, hepatic failure, hepatitis, hepatomegaly, hepatopathy thrombocytopenia syndrome, hepatotoxicity, liver function test abnormality, hepatic sinusoidal obstruction syndrome (SOS; veno-occlusive liver disease)

Local: Erythema, edema, epidermolysis, pain, tissue necrosis, and ulceration (following extravasation)

Neuromuscular & skeletal: Myalgia

Renal: Renal function abnormality

Respiratory: Pneumonitis

Miscellaneous: Anaphylactoid reaction, infection, sepsis (including neutropenic sepsis)

Drug Interactions

Metabolism/Transport Effects None known.

Avoid Concomitant Use

Avoid concomitant use of DACTINomycin with any of the following: BCG (Intravesical); CloZAPine; Dipyrone; Natalizumab; Pimecrolimus; Tacrolimus (Topical); Tofacitinib; Vaccines (Live)

Increased Effect/Toxicity

DACTINomycin may increase the levels/effects of: CloZAPine; Fingolimod; Leflunomide; Natalizumab; Tofacitinib; Vaccines (Live)

The levels/effects of DACTINomycin may be increased by: Denosumab; Dipyrone; Pimecrolimus; Roflumilast; Tacrolimus (Topical); Trastuzumab

Decreased Effect

DACTINomycin may decrease the levels/effects of: BCG (Intravesical); Coccidioides immitis Skin Test; Sipuleucel-T; Vaccines (Inactivated); Vaccines (Live)

The levels/effects of DACTINomycin may be decreased by: Echinacea

◄ **Storage/Stability** Store at controlled room temperature of 20°C to 25°C (68°F to 77°F). Protect from light and humidity. According to the manufacturer's labeling, recommended final concentrations (≥10 mcg/mL) are stable for 10 hours at room temperature but should be administered within 4 hours due to the lack of preservative.

Preparation for Administration Hazardous agent; use appropriate precautions for handling and disposal (NIOSH 2014 [group 1]). Reconstitute initially with 1.1 mL of preservative-free SWFI to yield a concentration of 500 mcg/mL (diluent containing preservatives will cause precipitation). May further dilute in D_5W or NS in glass or polyvinyl chloride (PVC) containers to a recommended concentration of ≥10 mcg/mL; final concentrations <10 mcg/mL are not recommended. Cellulose ester membrane filters may partially remove dactinomycin from solution and should not be used during preparation or administration.

Mechanism of Action Binds to the guanine portion of DNA intercalating between guanine and cytosine base pairs inhibiting DNA and RNA synthesis and protein synthesis

Pharmacodynamics/Kinetics

Distribution: Children: Extensive extravascular distribution (59-714 L) (Veal, 2005); does not penetrate blood-brain barrier

Metabolism: Minimal

Half-life elimination: ~36 hours; Children: Range: 14-43 hours (Veal, 2005)

Excretion: ~30% in urine and feces within 1week

Dosing

Adult Note: Medication orders for dactinomycin are commonly written in MICROgrams (eg, 150 mcg) although many regimens list the dose in MILLIgrams (eg, mg/kg or mg/m²). The dose intensity per 2-week cycle should not exceed 15 mcg/kg/day for 5 days or 400-600 mcg/m²/day for 5 days. The manufacturer recommends calculation of the dosage for obese or edematous adult patients on the basis of body surface area in an effort to relate dosage to lean body mass. Dactinomycin is associated with a high emetic potential; antiemetics are recommended to prevent nausea and vomiting (Basch, 2011).

Testicular cancer, metastatic: IV: 1000 mcg/m² on day 1 (in combination with cyclophosphamide, bleomycin, cisplatin, and vinblastine)

Gestational trophoblastic neoplasm: IV: 12 mcg/kg/day for 5 days (as a single agent) **or** 500 mcg/dose on days 1 and 2 (in combination with etoposide, methotrexate, leucovorin, vincristine, cyclophosphamide, and cisplatin) **or** (off-label dosing for low-risk disease) 1.25 mg/m2 every 2 weeks as a single agent (Osborne, 2011)

Wilms tumor, Ewing's sarcoma, rhabdomyosarcoma: IV: 15 mcg/kg/day for 5 days (in various combination regimens and schedules)

Regional perfusion (dosages and techniques may vary by institution; obese patients and patients with prior chemotherapy or radiation therapy may require lower doses): Lower extremity or pelvis: 50 mcg/kg; Upper extremity: 35 mcg/kg

Osteosarcoma (off-label use): IV: 600 mcg/m² on days 1, 2, and 3 of weeks 15, 31, 34, 39, and 42 (as part of a combination chemotherapy regimen) (Goorin, 2003)

Ovarian (germ cell) tumor (off-label use): IV: 500 mcg daily for 5 days every 4 weeks (in combination with vincristine and cyclophosphamide) (Gershenson, 1985) **or** 300 mcg/m²/day for 5 days every 4 weeks (in combination with vincristine and cyclophosphamide) (Slayton, 1985)

Geriatric Refer to adult dosing. Elderly patients are at increased risk of myelosuppression; dosing should begin at the low end of the dosing range.

Pediatric Note: Medication orders for dactinomycin are commonly written in MICROgrams (eg, 150 mcg) although many regimens list the dose in MILLIgrams (eg, mg/kg or mg/m^2). The dose intensity per 2-week cycle should not exceed 15 mcg/kg/day for 5 days or 400-600 mcg/m^2/day for 5 days. Dactinomycin is associated with a high emetic potential; antiemetics are recommended to prevent nausea and vomiting (Dupuis, 2011).

Wilms tumor, rhabdomyosarcoma, Ewing's sarcoma: Children >6 months: IV: 15 mcg/kg/day for 5 days (in various combination regimens and schedules)

Off-label dosing:

Rhabdomyosarcoma: IV:

VAC regimen:

Children <1 year: 25 mcg/kg every 3 weeks, weeks 0 to 45 (in combination with vincristine and cyclophosphamide, and mesna); dose omission required following radiation therapy (Raney, 2011)

Children ≥1 year: 45 mcg/kg (maximum dose: 2500 mcg) every 3 weeks, weeks 0 to 45 (in combination with vincristine and cyclophosphamide, and mesna); dose omission required following radiation therapy (Raney, 2011)

Wilms tumor: IV:

DD-4A regimen: 45 mcg/kg on day 1 every 6 weeks for 54 weeks (in combination with doxorubicin and vincristine) (Green, 1998)

EE-4A regimen: 45 mcg/kg on day 1 every 3 weeks for 18 weeks (in combination with vincristine) (Green, 1998)

VAD regimen:

Children <1 year: 750 mcg/m^2 every 6 weeks for 1 year (stage III disease) (in combination with vincristine and doxorubicin) (Pritchard, 1995)

Children ≥1 year: 1500 mcg/m^2 every 6 weeks for 1 year (stage III disease) (in combination with vincristine and doxorubicin) (Pritchard, 1995)

Osteosarcoma (off-label use): IV: 600 mcg/m^2 on days 1, 2, and 3 of weeks 15, 31, 34, 39, and 42 (as part of a combination chemotherapy regimen) (Goorin, 2003)

Renal Impairment There are no dosage adjustments provided in the manufacturer's labeling; however, based on the amount of urinary excretion, dosage adjustments may not be necessary.

Hepatic Impairment

U.S. labeling: There are no dosage adjustments provided in manufacturer's labeling.

Canadian labeling:

Mild impairment: There are no dosage adjustments provided.

Moderate-severe impairment: Dose reduction may be considered; 33% to 50% dose reductions for patients with hyperbilirubinemia have been recommended by some clinicians.

Off-label dosing: Any transaminase increase: Reduce dose by 50%; may increase by monitoring toxicities (Floyd, 2006).

Obesity *ASCO Guidelines for appropriate chemotherapy dosing in obese adults with cancer:* Utilize patient's actual body weight (full weight) for calculation of body surface area- or weight-based dosing, particularly when the intent of therapy is curative; manage regimen-related toxicities in the same manner as for nonobese patients; if a dose reduction is utilized due to

toxicity, consider resumption of full weight-based dosing with subsequent cycles, especially if cause of toxicity (eg, hepatic or renal impairment) is resolved (Griggs, 2012).

Combination Regimens

Bone sarcoma (Ewing sarcoma): VAC Alternating With IE (Ewing Sarcoma) on page 2102

Gestational trophoblastic tumor:
  EMA/CO (Gestational Trophoblastic Tumor) on page 1954
  EMA/EP (Gestational Trophoblastic Tumor) on page 1954
  EMA (Gestational Trophoblastic Tumor) on page 1955
  MAC (Gestational Trophoblastic Tumor) on page 2031

Ovarian cancer: VAC (Ovarian) on page 2102

Soft tissue sarcoma (rhabdomyosarcoma):
  VAC Pulse on page 2103
  VAC (Rhabdomyosarcoma) on page 2103

Wilms' tumor:
  DD-4A (Wilms' Tumor) on page 1936
  EE-4A (Wilms' Tumor) on page 1953
  VAD (Wilms' Tumor) on page 2104

Administration Dactinomycin is associated with a high emetic potential; antiemetics are recommended to prevent nausea and vomiting (Basch, 2011; Dupuis, 2011).

IV: Administer by slow IV push or infuse over 10-15 minutes. Do not filter with cellulose ester membrane filters. Do not administer IM or SubQ.

Vesicant; ensure proper needle or catheter placement prior to and during infusion; avoid extravasation.

Extravasation management: If extravasation occurs, stop infusion immediately and disconnect (leave cannula/needle in place); gently aspirate extravasated solution (do **NOT** flush the line); remove needle/cannula; elevate extremity. Apply dry cold compresses for 20 minutes 4 times a day for 1-2 days (Perez Fildago, 2012).

Hazardous agent; use appropriate precautions for handling and disposal (NIOSH 2014 [group 1]).

Vesicant/Extravasation Risk Vesicant

Emetic Potential Children and Adults: High (>90%)

Monitoring Parameters CBC with differential and platelet count, liver function tests, and renal function tests; monitor for signs/symptoms of hepatic SOS, including unexplained weight gain, ascites, hepatomegaly, or unexplained right upper quadrant pain (Arndt, 2004)

Test Interactions May interfere with bioassays of antibacterial drug levels

Dosage Forms Excipient information presented when available (limited, particularly for generics); consult specific product labeling. [DSC] = Discontinued product

Solution Reconstituted, Intravenous:
  Cosmegen: 0.5 mg (1 ea)
Solution Reconstituted, Intravenous [preservative free]:
  Generic: 0.5 mg (1 ea [DSC])

Dalteparin (dal TE pa rin)

Related Information

Venous Thromboembolism in the Cancer Patient *on page* 2267

Brand Names: US Fragmin

Brand Names: Canada Fragmin

Index Terms Dalteparin Sodium

Pharmacologic Category Anticoagulant; Anticoagulant, Low Molecular Weight Heparin

Use Prevention of deep vein thrombosis (DVT) which may lead to pulmonary embolism, in patients requiring abdominal surgery who are at risk for thromboembolism complications (eg, patients >40 years of age, obesity, patients with malignancy, history of DVT or pulmonary embolism, and surgical procedures requiring general anesthesia and lasting >30 minutes); prevention of DVT in patients undergoing hip-replacement surgery; patients immobile during an acute illness; prevention of ischemic complications in patients with unstable angina or non-Q-wave myocardial infarction on concurrent aspirin therapy; in patients with cancer, extended treatment (6 months) of acute symptomatic venous thromboembolism (DVT and/or PE) to reduce the recurrence of venous thromboembolism

Canadian labeling: Additional use (off-label use in U.S.): Treatment of acute DVT; prevention of venous thromboembolism (VTE) in patients at risk of VTE undergoing general surgery; anticoagulant in extracorporeal circuit during hemodialysis and hemofiltration

Labeled Contraindications Hypersensitivity to dalteparin (eg, pruritus, rash, anaphylactic reactions) or any component of the formulation; history of heparin-induced thrombocytopenia (HIT) or HIT with thrombosis; hypersensitivity to heparin or pork products; active major bleeding; patients with unstable angina, non-Q-wave MI, or prolonged venous thromboembolism prophylaxis undergoing epidural/neuraxial anesthesia

Note: Use of dalteparin in patients with current HIT or HIT with thrombosis is **not** recommended and considered contraindicated due to high cross-reactivity to heparin-platelet factor-4 antibody (Guyatt [ACCP], 2012; Warkentin, 1999).

Canadian labeling: Additional contraindications (not in U.S. labeling): Septic endocarditis, major blood clotting disorders; acute gastroduodenal ulcer; cerebral hemorrhage; severe uncontrolled hypertension; diabetic or hemorrhagic retinopathy; other diseases that increase risk of hemorrhage; injuries to and operations on the CNS, eyes, and ears

Pregnancy Considerations Adverse effects were not observed in animal reproduction studies. Low molecular weight heparin (LMWH) does not cross the placenta; increased risks of fetal bleeding or teratogenic effects have not been reported (Bates, 2012).

LMWH is recommended over unfractionated heparin for the treatment of acute venous thromboembolism (VTE) in pregnant women. LMWH is also recommended over unfractionated heparin for VTE prophylaxis in pregnant women with certain risk factors. LMWH should be discontinued at least 24 hours prior to induction of labor or a planned cesarean delivery. For women undergoing cesarean section and who have additional risk factors for developing VTE, the prophylactic use of LMWH may be considered. For women who require long-term anticoagulation with warfarin and who are considering pregnancy, LMWH substitution should be done prior to conception when possible. When choosing therapy, fetal outcomes (ie, pregnancy loss, malformations), maternal out-comes (ie, VTE, hemorrhage), burden of therapy, and maternal preference should be considered (Guyatt, 2012). LMWH may also be used in women with mechanical heart valves (consult current guidelines for details) (Bates, 2012; Nishimura, 2014).

Multiple-dose vials contain benzyl alcohol (avoid in pregnant women due to association with gasping syndrome in premature infants); use of preservative-free formulation is recommended.

Breast-Feeding Considerations In lactating women receiving prophylactic doses of dalteparin, small amounts of anti-xa activity was noted in breast milk. The milk/plasma ratio was <0.025 to 0.224. Oral absorption of low molecular weight heparin is extremely low, and is therefore unlikely to cause adverse events in a nursing infant. Use of LMWH may be continued in breast-feeding women (Guyatt, 2012).

Warnings/Precautions [U.S. Boxed Warning]: Spinal or epidural hema-tomas, including subsequent paralysis, may occur with recent or antici-pated neuraxial anesthesia (epidural or spinal) or spinal puncture in patients anticoagulated with LMWH or heparinoids. Consider risk versus benefit prior to spinal procedures; risk is increased by the use of concomitant agents which may alter hemostasis, the use of indwelling epidural catheters for analgesia, a history of spinal deformity or spinal surgery, as well as traumatic or repeated epidural or spinal punctures. Optimal timing between neuraxial procedures and dalteparin administra-tion is not known. Delay placement or removal of catheter for at least 12 hours after administration of 2,500 units once daily, at least 15 hours after the administration of 5,000 units once daily, and at least 24 hours after the administration of higher doses (200 units/kg once daily, 120 units/kg twice daily) and consider doubling these times in patients with creatinine clearance <30 mL/minute; risk of neuraxial hematoma may still exist since antifactor Xa levels are still detectable at these time points. Upon removal of catheter, consider delaying next dose of dalteparin for at least 4 hours. Patient should be observed closely for bleeding, signs and symptoms of neurological impair-ment, bowel and/or bladder dysfunction if therapy is administered during or immediately following diagnostic lumbar puncture, epidural anesthesia, or spinal anesthesia. If neurological compromise is noted, urgent treatment is necessary. If spinal hematoma is suspected, diagnose and treat immediately; spinal cord decompression may be considered although it may not prevent or reverse neurological sequelae. Use of dalteparin is contraindicated in patients undergoing epidural/neuraxial anesthesia. Patient should be observed closely for bleeding if dalteparin is administered during or immediately following diagnostic lumbar puncture, epidural anesthesia, or spinal anesthesia.

Use with caution in patients with preexisting thrombocytopenia, recent child-birth, subacute bacterial endocarditis, peptic ulcer disease, pericarditis or pericardial effusion, liver or renal function impairment, recent lumbar puncture, vasculitis, concurrent use of aspirin (increased bleeding risk), previous hyper-sensitivity to heparin, heparin-associated thrombocytopenia. Monitor platelet count closely. Cases of dalteparin-induced thrombocytopenia and thrombosis (similar to heparin-induced thrombocytopenia [HIT]), some complicated by organ infarction, limb ischemia, or death, have been observed. In patients with a history of HIT or HIT with thrombosis, dalteparin is contraindicated. Consider discontinuation of therapy in any patient developing significant thrombocyto-penia (eg, <100,000/mm^3) and/or thrombosis related to initiation of dalteparin especially when associated with a positive *in vitro* test for antiplatelet antibodies. Use caution in patients with congenital or drug-induced thrombocytopenia or platelet defects.

Monitor patient closely for signs or symptoms of bleeding. Certain patients are at increased risk of bleeding. Risk factors include bacterial endocarditis; congenital or acquired bleeding disorders; active ulcerative or angiodysplastic GI diseases; severe uncontrolled hypertension; hemorrhagic stroke; or use shortly after brain, spinal, or ophthalmology surgery; in patients treated concomitantly with platelet inhibitors; recent GI bleeding; thrombocytopenia or platelet defects; hypertensive or diabetic retinopathy; or in patients undergoing invasive procedures. Protamine may be considered as a partial reversal agent in overdose situations (consult Protamine monograph for dosing recommendations).

Use with caution in patients with severe renal impairment or severe hepatic impairment; accumulation may occur with repeated dosing increasing the risk for bleeding. Heparin can cause hyperkalemia by affecting aldosterone. Similar reactions could occur with dalteparin. Monitor for hyperkalemia. Do **not** administer intramuscularly. Not to be used interchangeably (unit for unit) with heparin or any other low molecular weight heparins.

Benzyl alcohol and derivatives: Some dosage forms may contain benzyl alcohol and should not be used in pregnant women. In neonates, large amounts of benzyl alcohol (≥99 mg/kg/day) have been associated with a potentially fatal toxicity ("gasping syndrome"); the "gasping syndrome" consists of metabolic acidosis, respiratory distress, gasping respirations, CNS dysfunction (including convulsions, intracranial hemorrhage), hypotension, and cardiovascular collapse (AAP ["Inactive" 1997]; CDC, 1982); some data suggests that benzoate displaces bilirubin from protein binding sites (Ahlfors, 2001); avoid or use dosage forms containing benzyl alcohol with caution in neonates. See manufacturer's labeling.

There is no consensus for adjusting/correcting the weight-based dosage of LMWH for patients who are morbidly obese (BMI ≥40 kg/m^2). The American College of Chest Physicians Practice Guidelines suggest consulting with a pharmacist regarding dosing in bariatric surgery patients and other obese patients who may require higher doses of LMWH (Gould, 2012).

Adverse Reactions Note: As with all anticoagulants, bleeding is the major adverse effect of dalteparin. Hemorrhage may occur at virtually any site. Risk is dependent on multiple variables.

>10%: Hematologic & oncologic: Hemorrhage (3% to 14%), thrombocytopenia (including heparin-induced thrombocytopenia, <1%; cancer clinical trials: ~11%)

1% to 10%:

Hematologic & oncologic: Major hemorrhage (≤6%), wound hematoma (3%)

Hepatic: Increased serum ALT (>3 x ULN: 4% to 10%), increased serum AST (>3 x ULN: 5% to 9%)

Local: Pain at injection site (≤12%), hematoma at injection site (≤7%)

<1% (Limited to important or life-threatening): Alopecia, anaphylactoid reaction, gastrointestinal hemorrhage, hemoptysis, hypersensitivity reaction (fever, pruritus, rash, injections site reaction, bullous eruption), postoperative wound bleeding, skin necrosis, subdural hematoma, thrombosis (associated with heparin-induced thrombocytopenia). Spinal or epidural hematomas can occur following neuraxial anesthesia or spinal puncture, resulting in paralysis.

◀ **Drug Interactions**

Metabolism/Transport Effects None known.

Avoid Concomitant Use

Avoid concomitant use of Dalteparin with any of the following: Apixaban; Dabigatran Etexilate; Edoxaban; Hemin; Omacetaxine; Rivaroxaban; Urokinase; Vorapaxar

Increased Effect/Toxicity

Dalteparin may increase the levels/effects of: ACE Inhibitors; Aliskiren; Angiotensin II Receptor Blockers; Anticoagulants; Canagliflozin; Collagenase (Systemic); Deferasirox; Deoxycholic Acid; Eplerenone; Ibritumomab; Nintedanib; Obinutuzumab; Omacetaxine; Palifermin; Potassium Salts; Potassium-Sparing Diuretics; Rivaroxaban; Tositumomab and Iodine I 131 Tositumomab

The levels/effects of Dalteparin may be increased by: 5-ASA Derivatives; Agents with Antiplatelet Properties; Apixaban; Dabigatran Etexilate; Dasatinib; Edoxaban; Hemin; Herbs (Anticoagulant/Antiplatelet Properties); Ibrutinib; Limaprost; Nonsteroidal Anti-Inflammatory Agents; Omega-3 Fatty Acids; Pentosan Polysulfate Sodium; Pentoxifylline; Prostacyclin Analogues; Salicylates; Sugammadex; Thrombolytic Agents; Tibolone; Tipranavir; Urokinase; Vitamin E; Vitamin E (Oral); Vorapaxar

Decreased Effect

Dalteparin may decrease the levels/effects of: Factor X (Human)

The levels/effects of Dalteparin may be decreased by: Estrogen Derivatives; Progestins

Storage/Stability Store at 20°C to 25°C (68°F to 77°F). Multidose vials may be stored for up to 2 weeks at room temperature after entering.

Preparation for Administration Canadian labeling: If necessary, may dilute in isotonic sodium chloride or dextrose solutions to a concentration of 20 units/ mL. Use within 24 hours of mixing.

Mechanism of Action Low molecular weight heparin analog with a molecular weight of 4000-6000 daltons; the commercial product contains 3% to 15% heparin with a molecular weight <3000 daltons, 65% to 78% with a molecular weight of 3000-8000 daltons and 14% to 26% with a molecular weight >8000 daltons; while dalteparin has been shown to inhibit both factor Xa and factor IIa (thrombin), the antithrombotic effect of dalteparin is characterized by a higher ratio of antifactor Xa to antifactor IIa activity (ratio = 4)

Pharmacodynamics/Kinetics

Onset of action: Anti-Xa activity: Within 1-2 hours

Duration: >12 hours

Distribution: V_d: 40-60 mL/kg

Protein binding: Low affinity for plasma proteins (Howard, 1997)

Bioavailability: SubQ: 81% to 93%

Half-life elimination (route dependent): Anti-Xa activity: 2-5 hours; prolonged in chronic renal insufficiency: 3.7-7.7 hours (following a single 5000 unit dose)

Time to peak, serum: Anti-Xa activity: ~4 hours

Excretion: Primarily renal (Howard, 1997)

Dosing

Adult & Geriatric Note: Each 2500 units of anti-Xa activity is equal to 16 mg of dalteparin.

Anticoagulant for hemodialysis and hemofiltration: IV: Canadian labeling (not in U.S. labeling):

Chronic renal failure with no other bleeding risks:

Hemodialysis/filtration ≤4 hours: IV bolus: 5,000 units

Hemodialysis/filtration >4 hours: IV bolus: 30-40 units/kg, followed by an infusion of 10-15 units/kg/hour (typically produces plasma concentrations of 0.5-1 units anti-Xa/mL)

Acute renal failure and high bleeding risk: IV bolus: 5-10 units/kg, followed by an infusion of 4-5 units/kg/hour (typically produces plasma concentrations of 0.2-0.4 units anti-Xa/mL)

DVT prophylaxis: Note: In morbidly obese patients (BMI ≥40 kg/m^2), increasing the prophylactic dose by 30% may be appropriate (Nutescu, 2009):

Abdominal surgery:

Low-to-moderate DVT risk: SubQ: 2500 units 1-2 hours prior to surgery, then once daily for 5-10 days postoperatively

High DVT risk: SubQ: 5000 units the evening prior to surgery and then once daily for 5-10 days postoperatively. Alternatively in patients with malignancy: 2500 units 1-2 hours prior to surgery, 2500 units 12 hours later, then 5000 units once daily for 5-10 days postoperatively.

General surgery with risk factors for VTE: Canadian labeling (not in U.S. labeling): 2500 units 1-2 hours preoperatively followed by 2500-5000 units every morning (may administer 2500 units no sooner than 4 hours after surgery and 8 hours after previous dose provided hemostasis has been achieved) or if other risk factors are present (eg, malignancy, heart failure), then may administer 5000 units the evening prior to surgery followed by 5000 units every evening postoperatively; continue treatment until patient is mobilized (approximately ≥5-7 days)

Total hip replacement surgery: SubQ: **Note:** Three treatment options are currently available. Dose is given for 5-10 days, although up to 14 days of treatment have been tolerated in clinical trials. The American College of Chest Physicians (ACCP) recommends a minimum duration of at least 10-14 days; extended duration of up to 35 days is suggested (Guyatt, 2012).

Postoperative regimen:

Initial: 2500 units 4-8 hours after surgery (or later if hemostasis not achieved). The ACCP recommends initiation ≥12 hours after surgery if postoperative regimen chosen (Guyatt, 2012).

Maintenance: 5000 units once daily; allow at least 6 hours to elapse after initial postsurgical dose (adjust administration time accordingly)

Preoperative regimen (starting day of surgery):

Initial: 2500 units within 2 hours **before** surgery. The ACCP recommends initiation ≥12 hours before surgery if preoperative regimen chosen (Guyatt, 2012). At 4-8 hours **after** surgery (or later if hemostasis not achieved), administer 2500 units.

Maintenance: 5000 units once daily; allow at least 6 hours to elapse after initial postsurgical dose (adjust administration time accordingly)

Preoperative regimen (starting evening prior to surgery):

Initial: 5000 units 10-14 hours **before** surgery. The ACCP recommends initiation ≥12 hours before surgery if preoperative regimen chosen (Guyatt, 2012). At 4-8 hours **after** surgery (or later if hemostasis not achieved), administer 5000 units.

Maintenance: 5000 units once daily, allowing 24 hours between doses

Immobility during acute illness: 5000 units once daily

◄ **Unstable angina or non-Q-wave myocardial infarction:** SubQ: 120 units/kg body weight (maximum dose: 10,000 units) every 12 hours for up to 5-8 days with concurrent aspirin therapy. Discontinue dalteparin once patient is clinically stable.

Obesity: Use actual body weight to calculate dose; dose capping at 10,000 units recommended (Nutescu, 2009).

Venous thromboembolism, extended treatment in cancer patients: SubQ:

Initial (month 1): 200 units/kg (maximum dose: 18,000 units) once daily for 30 days

Maintenance (months 2-6): ~150 units/kg (maximum dose: 18,000 units) once daily. If platelet count between $50,000\text{-}100,000/mm^3$, reduce dose by 2,500 units until platelet count recovers to $\geq100,000/mm^3$. If platelet count $<50,000/mm^3$, discontinue dalteparin until platelet count recover to $>50,000/mm^3$.

Obesity: Use actual body weight to calculate dose; dose capping is not recommended (Nutescu, 2009). However, the manufacturer recommends a maximum dose of 18,000 units per day for the treatment of VTE in cancer patients.

DVT (with or without PE) treatment in noncancer patients (off-label use in U.S.): SubQ: 200 units/kg once daily (Feissinger, 1996; Jaff, 2011; Wells, 2005) **or** 100 units/kg twice daily (Jaff, 2011). Use of once daily administration is suggested (Guyatt, 2012).

Canadian labeling: SubQ: 200 units/kg once daily (maximum dose: 18,000 units/day) **or** alternatively, may adapt dose as follows (SubQ):

46-56 kg: 10,000 units once daily

57-68 kg: 12,500 units once daily

69-82 kg: 15,000 units once daily

≥83 kg: 18,000 units once daily

Note: If increased bleeding risk, may give 100 units/kg SubQ twice daily. Concomitant treatment with a vitamin-K antagonist is usually initiated immediately.

Obesity: Use actual body weight to calculate dose; dose capping is not recommended (Nutescu, 2009). One study demonstrated similar anti-Xa levels after 3 days of therapy in obese patients (>40% above IBW; range: 82-190 kg) compared to those ≤20% above IBW or between 20% to 40% above IBW (Wilson, 2001).

Pregnant women (off-label use): 200 units/kg/dose once daily or 100 units/kg/dose every 12 hours. Discontinue ≥24 hours prior to the induction of labor or cesarean section. Dalteparin therapy may be substituted with heparin near term. Continue anticoagulation therapy for ≥6 weeks postpartum (minimum duration of therapy: 3 months). LMWH or heparin therapy is preferred over warfarin during pregnancy (Bates, 2012).

Mechanical heart valve (aortic or mitral position) to bridge anticoagulation (off-label use): 100 units/kg/dose every 12 hours (ACCP [Douketis, 2012]). **Note:** If used in pregnant patients, target anti-Xa level of 0.8 to 1.2 units/mL, 4 to 6 hours postdose (AHA/ACC [Nishimura, 2014]).

Prevention of recurrent venous thromboembolism in pregnancy (off-label use): SubQ: 5000 units once daily. Therapy should continue for 6 weeks postpartum in high-risk women (Bates, 2012).

Renal Impairment Half-life is increased in patients with chronic renal failure, use with caution, accumulation can be expected; specific dosage adjustments have not been recommended. Accumulation was not observed in critically ill patients with severe renal insufficiency (CrCl <30 mL/minute) receiving prophylactic doses (5000 units) for a median of 7 days (Douketis, 2008). In cancer patients, receiving treatment for venous thromboembolism, if CrCl <30 mL/minute, manufacturer recommends monitoring anti-Xa levels to determine appropriate dose.

Hepatic Impairment No dosage adjustment provided in manufacturer's labeling; use with caution.

Obesity Refer to indication-specific dosing for obesity-related information (may not be available for all indications).

Administration

For deep SubQ injection; may be injected in a U-shape to the area surrounding the navel, the upper outer side of the thigh, or the upper outer quadrangle of the buttock. Use thumb and forefinger to lift a fold of skin when injecting dalteparin to the navel area or thigh. Insert needle at a 45- to 90-degree angle. The entire length of needle should be inserted. Do not expel air bubble from fixed-dose syringe prior to injection. Air bubble (and extra solution, if applicable) may be expelled from graduated syringes. In order to minimize bruising, do not rub injection site.

To convert from IV unfractionated heparin (UFH) infusion to SubQ dalteparin (Nutescu, 2007): Calculate specific dose for dalteparin based on indication, discontinue UFH and begin dalteparin within 1 hour

To convert from SubQ dalteparin to IV UFH infusion (Nutescu, 2007): Discontinue dalteparin; calculate specific dose for IV UFH infusion based on indication; omit heparin bolus/loading dose

Converting from SubQ dalteparin dosed every 12 hours: Start IV UFH infusion 10-11 hours after last dose of dalteparin

Converting from SubQ dalteparin dosed every 24 hours: Start IV UFH infusion 22-23 hours after last dose of dalteparin

IV (Canadian labeling; not an approved route in U.S. labeling): Administer as bolus IV injection or as continuous infusion. Recommended concentration for infusion: 20 units/mL.

Monitoring Parameters Periodic CBC including platelet count; stool occult blood tests; monitoring of PT and PTT is not necessary. Once patient has received 3-4 doses, anti-Xa levels, drawn 4-6 hours after dalteparin administration, may be used to monitor effect in patients with severe renal dysfunction or if abnormal coagulation parameters or bleeding should occur. For patients >190 kg, if anti-Xa monitoring is available, adjusting dose based on anti-Xa levels is recommended; if anti-Xa monitoring is unavailable, reduce dose if bleeding occurs (Nutescu, 2009).

Dosage Forms Excipient information presented when available (limited, particularly for generics); consult specific product labeling. [DSC] = Discontinued product

Solution, Subcutaneous:
Fragmin: 25,000 units/mL (3.8 mL [DSC]); 95,000 units/3.8 mL (3.8 mL) [contains benzyl alcohol]
Solution, Subcutaneous [preservative free]:
Fragmin: 10,000 units/mL (1 mL); 2500 units/0.2 mL (0.2 mL); 5000 units/0.2 mL (0.2 mL); 7500 units/0.3 mL (0.3 mL); 12,500 units/0.5 mL (0.5 mL); 15,000 units/0.6 mL (0.6 mL); 18,000 units/0.72 mL (0.72 mL)

♦ **Dalteparin Sodium** *see* Dalteparin *on page 437*

Daratumumab (dar a TOOM ue mab)

Brand Names: US Darzalex

Index Terms JNJ-54767414

Pharmacologic Category Antineoplastic Agent, Anti-CD38; Antineoplastic Agent, Monoclonal Antibody

Use Multiple myeloma, relapsed/refractory: Treatment of multiple myeloma in patients who have received at least 3 prior lines of therapy including a proteasome inhibitor (PI) and an immunomodulatory agent or who are double-refractory to a PI and an immunomodulatory agent.

Labeled Contraindications There are no contraindications listed in the manufacturer's labeling.

Pregnancy Considerations Animal reproduction studies have not been conducted. Daratumumab is a monoclonal antibody; monoclonal antibodies are known to cross the placenta. Based on the mechanism of action, daratumumab may cause myeloid or lymphoid cell depletion and decreased bone density in the fetus. Females of reproduction potential should use effective contraception during therapy and for 3 months after treatment is complete. The administration of live vaccines should be deferred for neonates and infants exposed to daratumumab in utero until a hematology evaluation can be completed.

Breast-Feeding Considerations It is not known if daratumumab is excreted into breast milk. Daratumumab is a monoclonal antibody; monoclonal antibodies can be detected in breast milk and are not expected to enter the neonatal or infant circulation in substantial amounts. According to the manufacturer, the decision to breast-feed during therapy should take into account the risk of exposure to the infant and the benefits of treatment to the mother.

Warnings/Precautions Severe infusion reactions may occur (including bronchospasm, hypoxia, dyspnea, and hypertension), mostly during the first infusion. Other signs and symptoms include cough, wheezing, larynx and throat tightness/irritation, laryngeal edema, pulmonary edema, nasal congestion, and allergic rhinitis. Less commonly reported symptoms include hypotension, headache, rash urticarial, pruritus, nausea, vomiting, and chills. Infusion reactions were reported in approximately 50% of patients in clinical trials. Reactions may also be seen during subsequent infusions, and generally occur either during the infusion or within 4 hours of completion (median onset was 1.5 hours [range: up to ~9 hours]); some reactions occurred up to 48 hours after the infusion. Premedication with antihistamines, antipyretics, and corticosteroids is required; interrupt infusion for any reaction and manage as appropriate. Reduce the infusion rate for grade 1, 2, or 3 reaction; permanently discontinue therapy for grade 4 infusion reaction. Administer in a facility with immediate access to resuscitative measures (eg, glucocorticoids, epinephrine, bronchodilators, and/or oxygen). Administer oral corticosteroids on the first and second day after infusion to reduce the risk of delayed infusion reactions. Consider short- and long-acting bronchodilators and inhaled corticosteroids for patients with obstructive pulmonary disorders; monitor closely.

Lymphopenia, neutropenia, thrombocytopenia, and anemia (including grade 3 and 4 toxicity) were commonly reported as treatment emergent adverse reactions in clinical trials. Monitor complete blood counts as clinically necessary. Daratumumab (a human IgG kappa monoclonal antibody) may be detected on serum protein electrophoresis and immunofixation assays which monitor for endogenous M-protein. Interference with these assays by daratumumab may affect the determination of complete response and disease progression in some patients with IgG kappa myeloma protein. Through binding to CD38 on red blood cells, daratumumab use may result in a positive indirect antiglobulin test (Coombs test). Daratumumab-mediated Coombs test positivity may persist for up to 6 months after the last infusion. In addition, daratumumab (bound to red blood cells) masks antibody detection to minor antigens in the patient's serum; ABO and Rh blood type determination are not affected. Notify blood transfusion centers and blood banks that a patient has received daratumumab, and type and screen patients prior to therapy initiation.

Adverse Reactions

Cardiovascular: Hypertension (10%)

Central nervous system: Fatigue (39%), headache (12%), chills (10%)

Gastrointestinal: Nausea (27%), diarrhea (16%), constipation (15%), decreased appetite (15%), vomiting (14%)

Hematologic & oncologic: Lymphocytopenia (72%; grade: 3: 30%; grade 4: 10%), neutropenia (60%; grade 3: 17%; grade 4: 3%), thrombocytopenia (48%; grade 3: 10%; grade 4: 8%), anemia (45%; grade 3: 19%)

Infection: Herpes zoster (3%)

Local: Infusion site reaction (first infusion: 46% to 48%; grade 3: 3%; second infusion: 5%; subsequent infusions: 4%)

Neuromuscular & skeletal: Back pain (23%), arthralgia (17%), leg pain (15%), musculoskeletal chest pain (12%)

Respiratory: Cough (21%), upper respiratory (20%), nasal congestion (17%), dyspnea (15%), nasopharyngitis (15%), pneumonia (6% to 11%)

Miscellaneous: Fever (3% to 21%), physical health deterioration (3%)

Drug Interactions

Metabolism/Transport Effects None known.

Storage/Stability Store intact vials at 2°C to 8°C (36°F to 46°F). Do not freeze or shake; protect from light. Solutions diluted for infusion may be stored for up to 24 hours at 2°C to 8°C (36°F to 46°F) if protected from light; do not freeze. Use immediately after coming to room temperature; infusion should be completed within 15 hours. Discard any unused portion of the solution.

Preparation for Administration Determine the appropriate dose and volume of daratumumab required (based on patient's actual body weight); daratumumab should be colorless to pale yellow (do not use if opaque particles, discoloration, or other foreign particles are observed). Remove the volume of 0.9% sodium chloride injection from the infusion bag that is equal to the required volume of the daratumumab dose. Add the appropriate daratumumab volume to a 1,000 mL (first infusion) or 500 mL (subsequent infusions) 0.9% sodium chloride bag; gently invert to mix (do not shake). Infusion bags/containers must be made of polyvinylchloride (PVC), polypropylene (PP), polyethylene (PE) or polyolefin blend (PP+PE). If the diluted solution is refrigerated prior to use, allow to come to room temperature before administration. After dilution, may develop very small translucent to white proteinaceous particles; do not use if discolored or if visibly opaque or foreign particles are observed.

Mechanism of Action Daratumumab is an IgG1κ human monoclonal antibody directed against CD38. CD38 is a cell surface glycoprotein which is highly expressed on myeloma cells, yet is expressed at low levels on normal lymphoid and myeloid cells (Lokhorst 2015). By binding to CD38, daratumumab inhibits the growth of CD38 expressing tumor cells by inducing apoptosis directly through Fc mediated cross linking as well as by immune-mediated tumor cell lysis through complement dependent cytotoxicity, antibody dependent cell mediated cytotoxicity, and antibody dependent cellular phagocytosis.

◀ **Pharmacodynamics/Kinetics**
Distribution: Central: 4.7 ± 1.3 L
Half-life elimination: 18 ± 9 days

Dosing

Adult & Geriatric Note: Premedicate approximately 1 hour prior to infusion with an IV corticosteroid, an oral antipyretic, and an oral or IV antihistamine. Post-infusion, administer an oral corticosteroid on the first and second day after each infusion to reduce the risk of delayed infusion reactions. To prevent herpes zoster reactivation, initiate antiviral prophylaxis within 1 week of starting daratumumab and continue for 3 months following completion of treatment. Per the manufacturer, daratumumab dosing should be based on actual body weight.

Multiple myeloma, relapsed/refractory: Adults: IV:
Weeks 1 to 8: 16 mg/kg once weekly
Weeks 9 to 24: 16 mg/kg once every 2 weeks
Weeks 25 and beyond: 16 mg/kg once every 4 weeks until disease progression
Missed dose: If a dose is missed, administer as soon as possible and adjust the schedule accordingly (maintain the treatment interval).

Premedications:
Corticosteroid: IV: Methylprednisolone 100 mg or equivalent intermediate- or long-acting corticosteroid; following the second infusion, the dose may be decreased (eg, methylprednisolone 60 mg or equivalent) **plus**
Antipyretic: Oral: Acetaminophen 650 to 1000 mg **plus**
Antihistamine: IV or Oral: Diphenhydramine 25 to 50 mg or equivalent

Post-infusion medication: Administer an oral corticosteroid (eg, methyl-prednisolone 20 mg or equivalent) on the first and second day after all infusions. In patients with a history of obstructive pulmonary disorder, consider short and long-acting bronchodilators and inhaled corticosteroids post-infusion. If no major infusion reactions occur during the first 4 infusions, these additional inhaled post-infusion medications may be discontinued.

Renal Impairment Preexisting impairment: No dosage adjustment is necessary.

Hepatic Impairment

Mild impairment (total bilirubin 1 to 1.5 times ULN or AST >ULN): No dosage adjustment necessary.

Moderate to severe impairment (total bilirubin >1.5 times ULN and any AST): There are no dosage adjustments provided in the manufacturer's labeling (has not been studied).

Adjustment for Toxicity

Infusion reactions: Immediately interrupt infusion for reaction of any severity. Manage symptoms as clinically appropriate.

Grade 1 or 2 (mild to moderate) infusion reaction: Once symptoms resolve, resume the infusion at no more than 50% of the rate at which the reaction occurred. If no further reactions are observed, may escalate the infusion rate as appropriate (see Administration).

Grade 3 (severe) infusion reaction: If symptoms improve to grade 2 or lower, consider resuming the infusion at no more than 50% of the rate at which the reaction occurred. If no further reactions are observed, may escalate the infusion rate as appropriate (see Administration). If a grade 3 reaction recurs, repeat the steps above. Permanently discontinue if a grade 3 infusion reaction occurs for the third time.

Grade 4 (life-threatening) infusion reaction: Permanently discontinue.

Administration For IV infusion only. Do not administer IV push or as a bolus. Premedicate with an IV corticosteroid, acetaminophen, and an IV or oral antihistamine (see Dosing) approximately 60 minutes prior to administration. Infuse in an environment equipped to monitor for and manage infusion reactions. Administer with an infusion set fitted with a flow regulator and with an inline, sterile, non-pyrogenic, low protein-binding polyethersulfone filter (0.22 or 0.2 micrometer). Polyurethane, polybutadiene, polyvinylchloride, polypropylene, or polyethylene administration sets are required. Do not exceed infusion rates below. Do not mix with or infuse with other medications. Begin infusion immediately after infusion bag reaches room temperature (if refrigerated). Infusion should be completed within 15 hours. Interrupt infusion for any severity of infusion reaction; if the reaction resolves or improves to ≤ grade 2, may resume infusion (see Dosage Adjustment for Toxicity). If infusion cannot be completed, do not save unused portion for reuse. Post-infusion, administer an oral corticosteroid on the first and second day after all infusions to reduce the risk of delayed infusion reactions. In patients with a history of obstructive pulmonary disorder, consider short and long-acting bronchodilators and inhaled corticosteroids post-infusion.

Infusion rate:

First infusion (1,000 mL volume): Infuse at 50 mL/hour for the first hour. If no infusion reactions occur, may increase the rate by 50 mL/hour every hour (maximum rate: 200 mL/hour).

Second infusion (500 mL volume): Infuse at 50 mL/hour for the first hour. Escalate the rate only if there were no grade 1 or greater infusion reactions during the first 3 hours of the first infusion. If no infusion reactions occur, may increase the rate by 50 mL/hour every hour (maximum rate: 200 mL/hour).

Subsequent infusions (500 mL volume): Escalate the rate only if there were no grade 1 or greater infusion reactions during a final infusion rate of ≥100 mL/hour in the first 2 infusions. Infuse at 100 mL/hour for the first hour. If no infusion reactions occur, may increase the rate by 50 mL/hour every hour (maximum rate: 200 mL/hour).

Monitoring Parameters Complete blood cell counts as clinically necessary; type and screen (blood type) prior to initiating therapy; signs/symptoms of infusion reactions.

Test Interactions Daratumumab binds to CD38 on red blood cells and results in a positive indirect antiglobulin test (Coombs test), which may persist for up to 6 months after the last infusion. Daratumumab may also mask antibody detection to minor antigens in the patient's serum. Mitigation methods include treating reagent red blood cells with dithiothreitol (DTT) to disrupt daratumumab binding or genotyping. As the Kell blood group system is also sensitive to DTT, K-negative units should be supplied after ruling out or identifying alloantibodies using DTT-treated red blood cells.

Daratumumab may be detected on both serum protein electrophoresis and immunofixation assays used for multiple myeloma endogenous M-protein monitoring, and may affect the determination of complete response and disease progression of some patients with IgG kappa myeloma protein. In patients with persistent very good partial response, consider other methods to evaluate the depth of treatment response.

◀ **Dosage Forms** Excipient information presented when available (limited, particularly for generics); consult specific product labeling.
Solution, Intravenous [preservative free]:
Darzalex: 100 mg/5 mL (5 mL); 400 mg/20 mL (20 mL) [contains mouse protein (murine) (hamster)]

Darbepoetin Alfa (dar be POE e tin AL fa)

Related Information
Palliative Care Medicine (Cancer) *on page 2252*

Brand Names: US Aranesp (Albumin Free)

Brand Names: Canada Aranesp

Index Terms Darbepoetin Alfa Polysorbate; Erythropoiesis-Stimulating Agent (ESA); Erythropoiesis-Stimulating Protein; NESP; Novel Erythropoiesis-Stimulating Protein

Pharmacologic Category Colony Stimulating Factor; Erythropoiesis-Stimulating Agent (ESA); Hematopoietic Agent

Use

Anemia: Treatment of anemia due to concurrent myelosuppressive chemotherapy in patients with cancer (nonmyeloid malignancies) receiving chemotherapy (palliative intent) for a planned minimum of 2 additional months of chemotherapy; treatment of anemia due to chronic kidney disease (including patients on dialysis and not on dialysis)

Limitations of use: In clinical trials, darbepoetin alfa has not demonstrated improved quality of life, fatigue, or well-being. Darbepoetin alfa is **not** indicated for use under the following conditions:
- Cancer patients receiving hormonal therapy, therapeutic biologic products, or radiation therapy unless also receiving concurrent myelosuppressive chemotherapy
- Cancer patients receiving myelosuppressive chemotherapy when the expected outcome is curative
- As a substitute for red blood cell (RBC) transfusion in patients requiring immediate correction of anemia

Labeled Contraindications Serious allergic reaction to darbepoetin alfa or any component of the formulation; uncontrolled hypertension; pure red cell aplasia (PRCA) that begins after treatment with darbepoetin alfa or other erythropoietin protein drugs

Pregnancy Considerations Adverse events were observed in animal reproduction studies. Women who become pregnant during treatment with darbepoetin alfa are encouraged to enroll in Amgen's Pregnancy Surveillance Program (800-772-6436).

Breast-Feeding Considerations It is not known if darbepoetin alfa is excreted in breast milk. The manufacturer recommends that caution be exercised when administering darbepoetin alfa to nursing women.

Warnings/Precautions [US Boxed Warning]: Erythropoiesis-stimulating agents (ESAs) increased the risk of serious cardiovascular events, myocardial infarction, stroke, venous thromboembolism, vascular access thrombosis, and/or tumor progression in clinical studies when administered to target hemoglobin levels >11 g/dL (and provide no additional benefit); a rapid rise in hemoglobin (>1 g/dL over 2 weeks) may also contribute to these risks. **[US Boxed Warning]: A shortened overall survival and/or increased risk of tumor progression or recurrence has been reported in studies with breast, cervical, head and neck, lymphoid, and**

non–small cell lung cancer patients. It is of note that in these studies, patients received ESAs to a target hemoglobin of ≥12 g/dL; although risk has not been excluded when dosed to achieve a target hemoglobin of <12 g/dL. **[US Boxed Warnings]: To decrease these risks, and risk of cardio- and thrombovascular events, use ESAs in cancer patients only for the treatment of anemia related to concurrent myelosuppressive chemotherapy and use the lowest dose needed to avoid red blood cell transfusions. Discontinue ESA following completion of the chemotherapy course. ESAs are <u>not</u> indicated for patients receiving myelosuppressive therapy when the anticipated outcome is curative.** A dosage modification is appropriate if hemoglobin levels rise >1 g/dL per 2-week time period during treatment (Rizzo 2010). Use of ESAs has been associated with an increased risk of venous thromboembolism (VTE) without a reduction in transfusions in patients >65 years of age with cancer (Hershman 2009). Improved anemia symptoms, quality of life, fatigue, or well-being have not been demonstrated in controlled clinical trials. **[US Boxed Warning]: Because of the risks of decreased survival and increased risk of tumor growth or progression, health care providers and hospitals must enroll and comply with the ESA APPRISE (Assisting Providers and Cancer Patients with Risk Information for the Safe use of ESAs) Oncology Program to prescribe or dispense ESAs to cancer patients.** Prescribers and patients will have to provide written documentation of discussed risks prior to each course.

[US Boxed Warning]: An increased risk of death, serious cardiovascular events, and stroke was reported in patients with chronic kidney disease (CKD) administered ESAs to target hemoglobin levels ≥11 g/dL; use the lowest dose sufficient to reduce the need for RBC transfusions. An optimal target hemoglobin level, dose or dosing strategy to reduce these risks has not been identified in clinical trials. Hemoglobin rising >1 g/dL in a 2-week period may contribute to the risk (dosage reduction recommended). The American College of Physicians recommends against the use of ESAs in patients with mild to moderate anemia and heart failure or coronary heart disease (ACP [Qaseem 2013]). The American College of Cardiology Foundation/American Heart Association (ACCF/AHA) 2013 Heart Failure Guidelines do not provide a clear recommendation on the use of ESAs in anemic heart failure patients. The effects of ESAs on quality of life measures, morbidity, and mortality are potentially modest and still unclear. The authors declined to provide an official recommendation regarding the use of ESAs pending the completion of ongoing randomized trials (ACCF/AHA [Yancy 2013]).

CKD patients who exhibit an inadequate hemoglobin response to ESA therapy may be at a higher risk for cardiovascular events and mortality compared to other patients. ESA therapy may reduce dialysis efficacy (due to increase in red blood cells and decrease in plasma volume); adjustments in dialysis parameters may be needed. Patients treated with epoetin may require increased heparinization during dialysis to prevent clotting of the extracorporeal circuit. CKD patients not requiring dialysis may have a better response to darbepoetin alfa and may require lower doses. Increased mortality was observed in patients undergoing coronary artery bypass surgery who received epoetin; these deaths were associated with thrombotic events. An increased risk of deep vein thrombosis (DVT) has been observed in patients treated with epoetin undergoing surgical orthopedic procedures. Darbepoetin alfa is **not** approved for reduction in allogeneic red blood cell transfusions in patients scheduled for surgical procedures. The risk for seizures is increased with darbepoetin alfa use in patients with CKD; use with caution in patients with a history of seizures. Monitor closely for neurologic symptoms during the first several months of therapy. Use with caution in patients with hypertension; hypertensive encephalopathy has been reported. Use is contraindicated in patients with uncontrolled hypertension. If hypertension is difficult to control, reduce or hold darbepoetin alfa. Due to the delayed onset of erythropoiesis, darbepoetin alfa is **not** recommended for acute correction of severe anemia or as a substitute for emergency transfusion.

Prior to treatment, correct or exclude deficiencies of iron, vitamin B_{12}, and/or folate, as well as other factors that may impair erythropoiesis (inflammatory conditions, infections, bleeding). Prior to and during therapy, iron stores must be evaluated. Supplemental iron is recommended if serum ferritin <100 mcg/L or serum transferrin saturation <20%; most patients with CKD will require iron supplementation. Poor response should prompt evaluation of these potential factors, as well as possible malignant processes and hematologic disease (thalassemia, refractory anemia, myelodysplastic disorder), occult blood loss, hemolysis, osteitis fibrosa cystic, and/or bone marrow fibrosis. Severe anemia and pure red cell aplasia (PRCA) with associated neutralizing antibodies to erythropoietin has been reported, predominantly in patients with CKD receiving SubQ darbepoetin alfa (the intravenous (IV) route is preferred for hemodialysis patients). Cases have also been reported in patients with hepatitis C who were receiving ESAs, interferon, and ribavirin. Patients with a sudden loss of response to darbepoetin alfa (with severe anemia and a low reticulocyte count) should be evaluated for PRCA with associated neutralizing antibodies to erythropoietin; discontinue treatment (permanently) in patients with PRCA secondary to neutralizing antibodies to erythropoietin. Antibodies may cross-react; do not switch to another ESA in patients who develop antibody-mediated anemia.

The American Society of Clinical Oncology (ASCO) and American Society of Hematology (ASH) 2010 updates to the clinical practice guidelines for the use of ESAs in patients with cancer indicate that ESAs are appropriate when used according to the parameters identified within the Food and Drug Administration (FDA)-approved labeling for epoetin and darbepoetin alfa (Rizzo 2010). ESAs are an option for chemotherapy-associated anemia when the hemoglobin has fallen to <10 g/dL to decrease the need for RBC transfusions. ESAs should only be used in conjunction with concurrent chemotherapy. Although the FDA label now limits ESA use to the palliative setting, the ASCO/ASH guidelines suggest using clinical judgment in weighing risks versus benefits as formal outcomes studies of ESA use defined by intent of chemotherapy treatment have not been conducted.

Potentially serious allergic reactions have been reported (rarely), including anaphylactic reactions, angioedema, bronchospasm, rash, and urticaria. Discontinue immediately (and permanently) in patients who experience serious allergic/anaphylactic reactions. Some products may contain latex. Some dosage forms may contain polysorbate 80 (also known as Tweens). Hypersensitivity reactions, usually a delayed reaction, have been reported following exposure to pharmaceutical products containing polysorbate 80 in certain individuals (Isaksson 2002; Lucente 2000; Shelley 1995). Thrombocytopenia, ascites, pulmonary deterioration, and renal and hepatic failure have been reported in premature neonates after receiving parenteral products containing polysorbate 80 (Alade 1986; CDC 1984). See manufacturer's labeling.

Adverse Reactions
>10%:
Cardiovascular: Hypertension (31%), peripheral edema (17%), edema (6% to 13%)

Gastrointestinal: Abdominal pain (10% to 13%)

Respiratory: Dyspnea (17%), cough (12%)

1% to 10%:
Cardiovascular: Angina pectoris, hypotension, myocardial infarction, pulmonary embolism, thromboembolism, thrombosis of vascular graft (arteriovenous), vascular injury (vascular access complications)

Central nervous system: Cerebrovascular disease

Dermatologic: Erythema, skin rash

Endocrine & metabolic: Hypervolemia

<1%, postmarketing, and/or case reports: Anaphylaxis, anemia (associated with neutralizing antibodies; severe; with or without other cytopenias), angioedema, bronchospasm, cerebrovascular accident, hypersensitivity reaction, hypertensive encephalopathy, pure red cell aplasia, seizure, tumor growth (progression/recurrence; cancer patients), urticaria

Drug Interactions
Metabolism/Transport Effects None known.

Avoid Concomitant Use There are no known interactions where it is recommended to avoid concomitant use.

Increased Effect/Toxicity

Darbepoetin Alfa may increase the levels/effects of: Lenalidomide; Thalidomide

The levels/effects of Darbepoetin Alfa may be increased by: Nandrolone

Decreased Effect There are no known significant interactions involving a decrease in effect.

Storage/Stability Store at 2°C to 8°C (36°F to 46°F); do not freeze. Do not shake. Protect from light. Store in original carton until use. The following stability information has also been reported: May be stored at room temperature for up to 7 days (Cohen 2007).

Mechanism of Action Induces erythropoiesis by stimulating the division and differentiation of committed erythroid progenitor cells; induces the release of reticulocytes from the bone marrow into the bloodstream, where they mature to erythrocytes. There is a dose-response relationship with this effect. This results in an increase in reticulocyte counts followed by a rise in hematocrit and hemoglobin levels. When administered SubQ or IV, darbepoetin alfa's half-life is ~3 times that of epoetin alfa concentrations.

Pharmacodynamics/Kinetics
Onset of action: Increased hemoglobin levels not generally observed until 2 to 6 weeks after initiating treatment

Absorption: SubQ: Slow

Distribution: V_d: 0.06 L/kg

Bioavailability: CKD: SubQ: Adults: ~37% (range: 30% to 50%); Children: 54% (range: 32% to 70%)

Half-life elimination:
CKD: Adults:
IV: 21 hours
SubQ: Nondialysis patients: 70 hours (range: 35 to 139 hours); Dialysis patients: 46 hours (range: 12 to 89 hours)
Cancer: Adults: SubQ: 74 hours (range: 24 to 144 hours); Children: 49 hours

◀ **Note:** Darbepoetin alfa half-life is approximately 3-fold longer than epoetin alfa following IV administration

Time to peak: SubQ:

CKD: Adults: 48 hours (range: 12 to 72 hours; independent of dialysis); Children: 36 hours (range: 10 to 58 hours)

Cancer: Adults: 71 to 90 hours (range: 28 to 123 hours); Children: 71 hours (range: 21 to 143 hours)

Dosing

Adult & Geriatric Note: Evaluate iron status in all patients before and during treatment and maintain iron repletion.

Anemia associated with chronic kidney disease (CKD): Individualize dosing and use the lowest dose necessary to reduce the need for red blood cell (RBC) transfusions.

*Chronic kidney disease patients **ON dialysis*** (IV route is preferred for hemodialysis patients; initiate treatment when hemoglobin is <10 g/dL; reduce dose or interrupt treatment if hemoglobin approaches or exceeds 11 g/dL): IV, SubQ: Initial: 0.45 mcg/kg once weekly **or** 0.75 mcg/kg once every 2 weeks **or** conversion from epoetin alfa: Epoetin alfa doses of <1,500 to ≥90,000 units per week may be converted to darbepoetin alfa doses ranging from 6.25 to 200 mcg per week (see adult column in conversion table below).

*Chronic kidney disease patients **NOT on dialysis*** (consider initiating treatment when hemoglobin is <10 g/dL; use only if rate of hemoglobin decline would likely result in RBC transfusion and desire is to reduce risk of alloimmunization or other RBC transfusion-related risks; reduce dose or interrupt treatment if hemoglobin exceeds 10 g/dL): IV, SubQ: Initial: 0.45 mcg/kg once every 4 weeks

Dosage adjustments for chronic kidney disease patients (either on dialysis or not on dialysis): Do not increase dose more frequently than every 4 weeks (dose decreases may occur more frequently).

If hemoglobin increases >1 g/dL in any 2-week period: Decrease dose by ≥25%

If hemoglobin does not increase by >1 g/dL after 4 weeks: Increase dose by 25%

Inadequate or lack of response: If adequate response is not achieved over 12 weeks, further increases are unlikely to be of benefit and may increase the risk for adverse events; use the minimum effective dose that will maintain a hemoglobin level sufficient to avoid RBC transfusions **and** evaluate patient for other causes of anemia; discontinue treatment if responsiveness does not improve

Anemia due to chemotherapy in cancer patients: Initiate treatment only if hemoglobin <10 g/dL and anticipated duration of myelosuppressive chemotherapy is at least 2 additional months. Titrate dosage to use the minimum effective dose that will maintain a hemoglobin level sufficient to avoid RBC transfusions. Discontinue darbepoetin alfa following completion of chemotherapy.

SubQ: Initial: 2.25 mcg/kg once weekly **or** 500 mcg once every 3 weeks until completion of chemotherapy

Dosage adjustments:

Increase dose: If hemoglobin does not increase by 1 g/dL **and** remains below 10 g/dL after initial 6 weeks (for patients receiving weekly therapy only), increase dose to 4.5 mcg/kg once weekly (no dosage adjustment if using every-3-week dosing).

Reduce dose by 40% if hemoglobin increases >1 g/dL in any 2-week period **or** hemoglobin reaches a level sufficient to avoid RBC transfusion. Withhold dose if hemoglobin exceeds a level needed to avoid RBC transfusion. Resume treatment with a 40% dose reduction when hemoglobin approaches a level where transfusions may be required.

Discontinue: On completion of chemotherapy or if after 8 weeks of therapy there is no hemoglobin response or RBC transfusions still required

Symptomatic anemia associated with MDS (off-label use): SubQ: 150 to 300 mcg once weekly (Giraldo 2006; Stasi 2005) **or** 500 mcg once every 2 to 3 weeks (Gabrilove 2008)

Conversion from epoetin alfa to darbepoetin alfa in CKD (on dialysis): See table

Conversion From Epoetin Alfa to Darbepoetin Alfa in Chronic Kidney Disease (Estimated Initial Dose)

Previous Dosage of Epoetin Alfa (units/week)	Children Darbepoetin Alfa Dosage (mcg/week)	Adults Darbepoetin Alfa Dosage (mcg/week)
<1,500	Not established	6.25
1,500 to 2,499	6.25	6.25
2,500 to 4,999	10	12.5
5,000 to 10,999	20	25
11,000 to 17,999	40	40
18,000 to 33,999	60	60
34,000 to 89,999	100	100
≥90,000	200	200

Note: In patients receiving epoetin alfa 2 to 3 times per week, darbepoetin alfa is administered once weekly. In patients receiving epoetin alfa once weekly, darbepoetin alfa is administered once every 2 weeks. The darbepoetin alfa dose to be administered every 2 weeks is derived by adding together 2 weekly epoetin alfa doses and then converting to the appropriate darbepoetin alfa dose. Titrate dose to hemoglobin response thereafter. The dose conversion in this table does not accurately estimate the once-monthly dose in chronic kidney disease (CKD) patients not on dialysis.

Pediatric Note: Evaluate iron status in all patients before and during treatment and maintain iron repletion.

Anemia associated with chronic kidney disease (CKD): Individualize dosing and use the lowest dose necessary to reduce the need for red blood cell (RBC) transfusions.

Chronic kidney disease patients ON dialysis (IV route is preferred for hemodialysis patients; initiate treatment when hemoglobin is <10 g/dL; reduce dose or interrupt treatment if hemoglobin approaches or exceeds 12 g/dL): IV, SubQ: Initial: 0.45 mcg/kg once weekly or conversion from epoetin alfa: Initial dose: Epoetin alfa doses of 1,500 to ≥90,000 units per week may be converted to darbepoetin alfa doses ranging from 6.25 to 200 mcg per week (see conversion table in adult dosing).

Chronic kidney disease patients **NOT on dialysis** (consider initiating treatment when hemoglobin is <10 g/dL; use only if rate of hemoglobin decline would likely result in RBC transfusion and desire is to reduce risk of alloimmunization or other RBC transfusion-related risks; reduce dose or interrupt treatment if hemoglobin exceeds 12 g/dL): IV, SubQ: Initial: 0.45 mcg/kg once weekly or 0.75 mcg/kg once every 2 weeks

Dosage adjustments for chronic kidney disease patients: Do not increase dose more frequently than every 4 weeks (dose decreases may occur more frequently).

If hemoglobin increases >1 g/dL in any 2-week period: Decrease dose by ≥25%

If hemoglobin does not increase by >1 g/dL after 4 weeks: Increase dose by 25%

Inadequate or lack of response: If adequate response is not achieved over 12 weeks, further increases are unlikely to be of benefit and may increase the risk for adverse events; use the minimum effective dose that will maintain a hemoglobin level sufficient to avoid RBC transfusions **and** evaluate patient for other causes of anemia; discontinue treatment if responsiveness does not improve

Renal Impairment No dosage adjustment necessary.

Hepatic Impairment There are no dosage adjustments provided in the manufacturer's labeling.

Administration May be administered by SubQ or IV injection. The IV route is recommended in hemodialysis patients. Do not shake; vigorous shaking may denature darbepoetin alfa, rendering it biologically inactive. Do not dilute or administer in conjunction with other drug solutions. Discard any unused portion of the vial; do not pool unused portions.

Monitoring Parameters Hemoglobin (at least once per week until maintenance dose established and after dosage changes; monitor less frequently once hemoglobin is stabilized); CKD patients should be also be monitored at least monthly following hemoglobin stability); iron stores (transferrin saturation and ferritin) prior to and during therapy; serum chemistry (CKD patients); blood pressure; fluid balance (CKD patients); seizures (CKD patients following initiation for first few months, includes new-onset or change in seizure frequency or premonitory symptoms)

Cancer patients: Examinations recommended by the ASCO/ASH guidelines (Rizzo 2010) prior to treatment include peripheral blood smear (in some situations a bone marrow exam may be necessary), assessment for iron, folate, or vitamin B_{12} deficiency, reticulocyte count, renal function status, and occult blood loss; during ESA treatment, assess baseline and periodic iron, total iron-binding capacity, and transferrin saturation or ferritin levels.

Dietary Considerations Supplemental iron intake may be required in patients with low iron stores.

Prescribing and Access Restrictions As a requirement of the REMS program, access to this medication is restricted. Healthcare providers and hospitals must be enrolled in the ESA APPRISE (Assisting Providers and Cancer Patients with Risk Information for the Safe use of ESAs) Oncology Program (866-284-8089; http://www.esa-apprise.com) to prescribe or dispense ESAs (ie, darbepoetin alfa, epoetin alfa) to patients with cancer.

Medication Guide Available Yes

Dosage Forms Excipient information presented when available (limited, particularly for generics); consult specific product labeling.

Solution, Injection [preservative free]:

Aranesp (Albumin Free): 25 mcg/mL (1 mL); 40 mcg/mL (1 mL); 25 mcg/0.42 mL (0.42 mL); 60 mcg/mL (1 mL); 40 mcg/0.4 mL (0.4 mL); 100 mcg/mL (1 mL); 60 mcg/0.3 mL (0.3 mL); 100 mcg/0.5 mL (0.5 mL); 150 mcg/0.75 mL (0.75 mL); 200 mcg/mL (1 mL); 300 mcg/mL (1 mL); 200 mcg/0.4 mL (0.4 mL); 300 mcg/0.6 mL (0.6 mL) [albumin free; contains polysorbate 80]

Aranesp (Albumin Free): 10 mcg/0.4 mL (0.4 mL) [contains mouse protein (murine) (hamster), polysorbate 80]

Aranesp (Albumin Free): 150 mcg/0.3 mL (0.3 mL) [contains polysorbate 80]

Solution Prefilled Syringe, Injection [preservative free]:

Aranesp (Albumin Free): 25 mcg/0.42 mL (0.42 mL); 40 mcg/0.4 mL (0.4 mL) [albumin free; contains polysorbate 80]

Aranesp (Albumin Free): 150 mcg/0.3 mL (0.3 mL); 500 mcg/mL (1 mL) [contains polysorbate 80]

◆ **Darbepoetin Alfa Polysorbate** *see* Darbepoetin Alfa *on page 448*

◆ **Darzalex** *see* Daratumumab *on page 444*

Dasatinib (da SA ti nib)

Related Information

Common Toxicity Criteria *on page 2122*

Management of Chemotherapy-Induced Nausea and Vomiting in Adults *on page 2142*

Prevention of Chemotherapy-Induced Nausea and Vomiting in Children *on page 2203*

Principles of Anticancer Therapy *on page 2261*

Safe Handling of Hazardous Drugs *on page 2292*

Brand Names: US Sprycel

Brand Names: Canada Sprycel

Index Terms BMS-354825

Pharmacologic Category Antineoplastic Agent, BCR-ABL Tyrosine Kinase Inhibitor; Antineoplastic Agent, Tyrosine Kinase Inhibitor

Use

Acute lymphoblastic leukemia: Treatment of Philadelphia chromosome-positive (Ph+) acute lymphoblastic leukemia (ALL) with resistance or intolerance to prior therapy.

Chronic myeloid leukemia: Treatment of newly diagnosed Ph+ chronic myeloid leukemia (CML) in chronic phase; treatment of chronic, accelerated, or myeloid or lymphoid blast phase Ph+ CML with resistance or intolerance to prior therapy, including imatinib.

Labeled Contraindications

US labeling: There are no contraindications listed in the manufacturer's labeling.

Canadian labeling: Hypersensitivity to dasatinib or any other component of the formulation; breast-feeding

Pregnancy Considerations Dasatinib crosses the placenta, with fetal plasma and amniotic concentrations comparable to maternal concentrations. Adverse effects, including hydrops fetalis and fetal leukopenia and thrombocytopenia have been reported following maternal exposure to dasatinib. Women of reproductive potential should use effective contraception during and for 30 days after the final dose to avoid becoming pregnant. Pregnant women are advised to avoid contact with crushed or broken tablets.

Breast-Feeding Considerations It is not known if dasatinib is excreted in breast milk. According to the manufacturer, due to the potential for serious adverse reactions in the nursing infant, breast-feeding is not recommended during treatment and for 2 weeks following the final dose.

Warnings/Precautions Hazardous agent - use appropriate precautions for handling and disposal (NIOSH 2014 [group 1]). Severe dose-related bone marrow suppression (thrombocytopenia, neutropenia, anemia) is associated with treatment (usually reversible); dosage adjustment and/or temporary interruption may be required for severe myelosuppression; the incidence of myelosuppression is higher in patients with advanced chronic myeloid leukemia (CML) and Ph+ acute lymphoblastic leukemia (ALL). Monitor blood counts every 2 weeks for 12 weeks and then every 3 months thereafter or as clinically indicated (for chronic phase CML) or weekly for the first 2 months, then monthly thereafter or as clinically necessary (for accelerated or blast phase CML or for ALL). Fatal intracranial and GI hemorrhage have been reported in association with dasatinib use. Severe hemorrhage (including CNS, GI) may occur due to thrombocytopenia; in addition to thrombocytopenia, dasatinib may also cause platelet dysfunction. Concomitant medications that inhibit platelet function or anticoagulants may increase the risk of bleeding. Potentially significant drug-drug interactions may exist, requiring dose or frequency adjustment, additional monitoring, and/or selection of alternative therapy. Use caution with patients taking anticoagulants or medications interfering with platelet function; not studied in clinical trials. Avoid concomitant use with CYP3A4 inducers and inhibitors; if concomitant use cannot be avoided, consider dasatinib dosage adjustments. Elevated gastric pH may reduce dasatinib bioavailability; avoid concomitant use with proton pump inhibitors and H_2 blockers. If needed, may consider antacid administration at least 2 hours before or 2 hours after the dasatinib dose.

Cardiomyopathy, diastolic dysfunction, heart failure (congestive), left ventricular dysfunction, and MI have been reported; monitor for signs and symptoms of cardiac dysfunction. Dasatinib may cause fluid retention, including pleural and pericardial effusions, pulmonary hypertension, and generalized or superficial edema. A prompt chest x-ray (or other appropriate diagnostic imaging) is recommended for symptoms suggestive of effusion (new or worsening dyspnea on exertion or at rest, pleuritic chest pain, or dry cough). Fluid retention may be managed with supportive care (diuretics or corticosteroids); thoracentesis and oxygen therapy may be necessary for severe fluid retention; consider dose reduction or treatment interruption. Utilizing once-daily dosing is associated with a decreased frequency of fluid retention. The risk for pleural effusion is increased in patients with hypertension, prior cardiac history and a twice a day administration schedule; interrupt treatment for grade ≥2 effusion; may consider reinitiating at a reduced dose after resolution (Quintás-Cardama, 2007). Use caution in patients where fluid accumulation may be poorly tolerated, such as in cardiovascular disease (HF or hypertension) and pulmonary disease. Patients 65 years of age and older are more likely to experience toxicity (compared with younger patients). Dasatinib may increase the risk for pulmonary arterial hypertension (PAH). PAH may occur at any time after starting treatment, including after >12 months of therapy. Evaluate for underlying cardiopulmonary disease prior to therapy initiation and during therapy; evaluate and rule out alternative etiologies in patients with symptoms suggestive of PAH (eg, dyspnea, fatigue, hypoxia, fluid retention) and interrupt therapy if symptoms are severe. Discontinue permanently with confirmed PAH diagnosis (may be reversible upon discontinuation).

May prolong QT interval; there are reports of patients with QTcF >500 msec. Use caution in patients at risk for QT prolongation, including patients with long QT syndrome, patients taking antiarrhythmic medications or other medications that lead to QT prolongation or potassium-wasting diuretics, patients with cumulative high-dose anthracycline therapy, and conditions which cause hypokalemia or hypomagnesemia. Correct hypokalemia and hypomagnesemia prior to and during dasatinib therapy. Cases of severe mucocutaneous dermatologic reactions (including Stevens-Johnson syndrome and erythema multiforme) have been reported with dasatinib. Discontinue dasatinib if severe mucocutaneous reaction occurs and other etiologies have been ruled out. Use caution with hepatic impairment due to extensive hepatic metabolism. Tumor lysis syndrome (TLS) has been reported in patients with resistance to imatinib therapy, usually in patients with advanced phase disease. Risk for TLS is higher in patients with advanced stage disease and/or a high tumor burden; monitor patients at risk more frequently. Maintain adequate hydration and correct uric acid levels prior to treatment; monitor electrolyte levels.

Adverse Reactions

≥10%:

Cardiovascular: Facial edema, peripheral edema

Central nervous system: Headache (12% to 33%), fatigue (8% to 26%), pain (11%)

Dermatologic: Skin rash (11% to 21%; includes drug eruption, erythema, erythema multiforme, erythematous rash, erythrosis, exfoliative rash, follicular rash, heat rash, macular rash, maculopapular rash, milia, papular rash, pruritic rash, pustular rash, skin exfoliation, skin irritation, urticaria vesiculosa, vesicular rash), pruritus (12%)

Endocrine & metabolic: Fluid retention (19% to 48%; grades 3/4: 1% to 8%; cardiac-related: 9%)

Gastrointestinal: Diarrhea (17% to 31%), nausea (8% to 24%), vomiting (5% to 16%), abdominal pain (7% to 12%)

Hematologic & oncologic: Thrombocytopenia (grades 3/4: 22% to 85%), neutropenia (grades 3/4: 29% to 79%), anemia (grades 3/4: 13% to 74%), hemorrhage (8% to 26%; grades 3/4: 1% to 9%), febrile neutropenia (4% to 12%; grades 3/4: 4% to 12%)

Infection: Infection (9% to 14%; includes bacterial, fungal, viral)

Local: Localized edema (3% to 22%; grades 3/4: ≤1%; superficial)

Neuromuscular & skeletal: Musculoskeletal pain (<22%), myalgia (7% to 13%), arthralgia (≤13%)

Respiratory: Pleural effusion (5% to 28%; grades 3/4: ≤7%), dyspnea (3% to 24%)

Miscellaneous: Fever (6% to 18%)

1% to <10%:

Cardiovascular: Cardiac conduction disturbance (7%), ischemic heart disease (4%), cardiac disease (≤4%; includes cardiac failure, cardiomyopathy, diastolic dysfunction, ejection fraction decreased, left ventricular dysfunction, ventricular failure), edema (≤4%; generalized), pericardial effusion (≤4%; grades 3/4: ≤1%), prolonged Q-T interval on ECG (≤1%), cardiac arrhythmia, chest pain, flushing, hypertension, palpitations, tachycardia

Central nervous system: Chills, depression, dizziness, drowsiness, insomnia, myasthenia, neuropathy, peripheral neuropathy

Dermatologic: Acne vulgaris, alopecia, dermatitis, eczema, hyperhidrosis, urticaria, xeroderma

Endocrine & metabolic: Hyperuricemia, weight gain, weight loss

Gastrointestinal: Constipation (10%), gastrointestinal hemorrhage (2% to 9%; grades 3/4: 1% to 7%), abdominal distention, change in appetite, colitis (including neutropenic colitis), dysgeusia, dyspepsia, enterocolitis, gastritis, mucositis, stomatitis

Hematologic & oncologic: CNS hemorrhage (≤3%; grades 3/4: ≤3%), bruise

Hepatic: Increased serum bilirubin (grades 3/4: ≤6%), increased serum ALT (grades 3/4: ≤5%), increased serum AST (grades 3/4: ≤4%), ascites (≤1%)

Infection: Herpes virus infection, sepsis

Neuromuscular & skeletal: Muscle spasm (5%), stiffness, weakness

Ophthalmic: Blurred vision, decreased visual acuity, dry eye syndrome, visual disturbance

Otic: Tinnitus

Renal: Increased serum creatinine (grades 3/4: ≤8%)

Respiratory: Pulmonary hypertension (≤5%; grades 3/4: ≤1%), pulmonary edema (≤4%; grades 3/4: ≤3%), cough, pneumonia (bacterial, viral, or fungal), pneumonitis, pulmonary infiltrates, upper respiratory tract infection

Miscellaneous: Soft tissue injury (oral)

<1%, postmarketing, and/or case reports: Abnormal gait, abnormal platelet aggregation, abnormal T waves on ECG, acute coronary syndrome, acute pancreatitis, acute respiratory distress, amnesia, anal fissure, angina pectoris, anxiety, arthritis, asthma, ataxia, atrial fibrillation, atrial flutter, bronchospasm, bullous skin disease, cardiac arrest, cardiomegaly, cerebrovascular accident, cholecystitis, cholestasis, confusion, conjunctivitis, convulsions, coronary artery disease, cor pulmonale, cranial nerve palsy (facial), decreased libido, deep vein thrombosis, dehydration, dementia, dermal ulcer, diabetes mellitus, dyschromia, dysphagia, embolism, emotional lability, epistaxis, equilibrium disturbance, erythema nodosum, esophagitis, fibrosis (dermal), fistula (anal), gastroesophageal reflux disease, gastrointestinal disease (protein wasting), gingival hemorrhage, gynecomastia, hearing loss, hematoma, hematuria, hemoptysis, hemorrhage (ocular), hepatitis, hypercholesterolemia, hypersensitivity, hypersensitivity angiitis, hyperthyroidism, hypoalbuminemia, hypotension, hypothyroidism, increased creatine phosphokinase, increased gamma-glutamyl transferase, increased lacrimation, increased pulmonary artery pressure, increased troponin, inflammation (panniculitis), interstitial pulmonary disease, intestinal obstruction, livedo reticularis, lymphadenopathy, lymphocytopenia, malaise, menstrual disease, myocardial infarction, myocarditis, nail disease, optic neuritis, osteonecrosis, ototoxicity (hemorrhage), palmar-plantar erythrodysesthesia, pancreatitis, pericarditis, petechia, photophobia, pleuropericarditis, prolongation P-R interval on ECG, proteinuria, pulmonary embolism, pure red cell aplasia, renal failure, renal insufficiency, rhabdomyolysis, skin photosensitivity, Stevens-Johnson syndrome, Sweet's syndrome, syncope, tendonitis, thrombophlebitis, thrombosis, thyroiditis, transient ischemic attacks, tremor, tumor lysis syndrome, upper gastrointestinal tract ulcer, urinary frequency, uterine hemorrhage, vaginal hemorrhage, ventricular arrhythmia, ventricular tachycardia, vertigo, voice disorder

Drug Interactions

Metabolism/Transport Effects Substrate of CYP3A4 (major); **Note:** Assignment of Major/Minor substrate status based on clinically relevant drug interaction potential; **Inhibits** CYP3A4 (weak)

Avoid Concomitant Use

Avoid concomitant use of Dasatinib with any of the following: BCG (Intravesical); CloZAPine; Conivaptan; Dipyrone; Fusidic Acid (Systemic); H2-Antagonists; Idelalisib; Natalizumab; Pimecrolimus; Pimozide; Proton Pump Inhibitors; St Johns Wort; Tacrolimus (Topical); Tofacitinib; Vaccines (Live)

Increased Effect/Toxicity

Dasatinib may increase the levels/effects of: Acetaminophen; Agents with Antiplatelet Properties; Anticoagulants; ARIPiprazole; CloZAPine; CYP3A4 Substrates; Fingolimod; Flibanserin; Highest Risk QTc-Prolonging Agents; Hydrocodone; Leflunomide; Lomitapide; Moderate Risk QTc-Prolonging Agents; Natalizumab; NiMODipine; Pimozide; Propacetamol; Tofacitinib; Vaccines (Live)

The levels/effects of Dasatinib may be increased by: Acetaminophen; Aprepitant; Conivaptan; CYP3A4 Inhibitors (Moderate); CYP3A4 Inhibitors (Strong); Denosumab; Dipyrone; Fosaprepitant; Fusidic Acid (Systemic); Idelalisib; Ivacaftor; Luliconazole; Mifepristone; Netupitant; Osimertinib; Palbociclib; Pimecrolimus; Roflumilast; Simeprevir; Stiripentol; Tacrolimus (Topical); Trastuzumab; Voriconazole

Decreased Effect

Dasatinib may decrease the levels/effects of: BCG (Intravesical); Coccidioides immitis Skin Test; Sipuleucel-T; Vaccines (Inactivated); Vaccines (Live)

The levels/effects of Dasatinib may be decreased by: Antacids; Bosentan; CYP3A4 Inducers (Moderate); CYP3A4 Inducers (Strong); Dabrafenib; Deferasirox; Dexamethasone (Systemic); Echinacea; Enzalutamide; H2-Antagonists; Mitotane; Osimertinib; Proton Pump Inhibitors; Siltuximab; St Johns Wort; Tocilizumab

Food Interactions Dasatinib serum concentrations may be increased when taken with grapefruit or grapefruit juice. Management: Avoid concurrent use.

Storage/Stability Store at 20°C to 25°C (68°F to 77°F); excursions permitted to 15°C to 30°C (59°F to 86°F).

Mechanism of Action BCR-ABL tyrosine kinase inhibitor; targets most imatinib-resistant BCR-ABL mutations (except the T315I and F317V mutants) by distinctly binding to active and inactive ABL-kinase. Kinase inhibition halts proliferation of leukemia cells. Also inhibits SRC family (including SRC, LKC, YES, FYN); c-KIT, EPHA2 and platelet derived growth factor receptor (PDGFRβ)

Pharmacodynamics/Kinetics

Distribution: 2505 L

Protein binding: Dasatinib: 96%; metabolite (active): 93%

Metabolism: Hepatic (extensive); metabolized by CYP3A4 (primarily), flavin-containing mono-oxygenase-3 (FOM-3) and uridine diphosphate-glucuronosyltransferase (UGT) to an active metabolite and other inactive metabolites (the active metabolite plays only a minor role in the pharmacology of dasatinib)

Half-life elimination: Terminal: 3 to 5 hours

Time to peak, plasma: 0.5 to 6 hours

Excretion: Feces (~85%, 19% as unchanged drug); urine (~4%, 0.1% as unchanged drug)

◄ **Dosing**

Adult & Geriatric Note: The effect of discontinuation on long-term disease outcome after achieving cytogenetic response (including complete cytogenetic response) or major molecular response is not known.

Chronic myelogenous leukemia (CML), Philadelphia chromosome-positive (Ph+), newly diagnosed in chronic phase: Oral: 100 mg once daily until disease progression or unacceptable toxicity. In clinical studies, a dose escalation to 140 mg once daily was allowed in patients not achieving hematologic or cytogenetic response at recommended initial dosage.

CML, Ph+, resistant or intolerant: Oral:

Chronic phase: 100 mg once daily until disease progression or unacceptable toxicity. In clinical studies, a dose escalation to 140 mg once daily was allowed in patients not achieving hematologic or cytogenetic response at recommended initial dosage.

Accelerated or blast phase: 140 mg once daily until disease progression or unacceptable toxicity. In clinical studies, a dose escalation to 180 mg once daily was allowed in patients not achieving hematologic or cytogenetic response at recommended initial dosage.

Acute lymphoblastic leukemia (ALL), Ph+: Oral: 140 mg once daily until disease progression or unacceptable toxicity. In clinical studies, a dose escalation to 180 mg once daily was allowed in patients not achieving hematologic or cytogenetic response at recommended initial dosage.

Gastrointestinal stromal tumors (GIST; off-label use): Oral: 70 mg twice daily (Montemurro, 2012; Trent, 2011).

Missed doses: If a dose is missed, take the next regularly scheduled dose; 2 doses should not be taken at the same time.

Dosage adjustment for concomitant CYP3A4 inhibitors: Avoid concomitant administration with strong CYP3A4 inhibitors (eg, clarithromycin, itraconazole, ketoconazole, nefazodone, protease inhibitors, telithromycin, voriconazole, grapefruit juice); if concomitant administration with a strong CYP3A4 inhibitor cannot be avoided, consider reducing dasatinib from 100 mg once daily to 20 mg once daily **or** from 140 mg once daily to 40 mg once daily, with careful monitoring. If reduced dose is not tolerated, the strong CYP3A4 inhibitor must be discontinued or dasatinib therapy temporarily held until concomitant inhibitor use has ceased. When a strong CYP3A4 inhibitor is discontinued, allow a washout period (~1 week) prior to adjusting dasatinib dose upward.

Dosage adjustment for concomitant CYP3A4 inducers: Avoid concomitant administration with strong CYP3A4 inducers (eg, carbamazepine, dexamethasone, phenobarbital, phenytoin, rifabutin, rifampin, St John's wort); if concomitant administration with a strong CYP3A4 inducer cannot be avoided, consider increasing the dasatinib dose with careful monitoring.

Renal Impairment There are no dosage adjustments provided in the manufacturer's labeling. However, <4% of dasatinib and metabolites are renally excreted.

Hepatic Impairment No initial dosage adjustment is necessary; use with caution. Transaminase or bilirubin elevations during treatment may be managed with treatment interruption or dose reduction.

Adjustment for Toxicity

Hematologic toxicity: Note: Growth factor support may be considered in patients with resistant myelosuppression.

Chronic phase CML (100 mg daily starting dose): For ANC <500/mm^3 or platelets <50,000/mm^3, withhold treatment until ANC ≥1000/mm^3 and platelets ≥50,000/mm^3; then resume treatment at the original starting dose if recovery occurs in ≤7 days. If platelets <25,000/mm^3 or recurrence of ANC <500/mm^3 for >7 days, withhold treatment until ANC ≥1000/mm^3 and platelets ≥50,000/mm^3; then resume treatment at 80 mg once daily (second episode). For third episode, further reduce dose to 50 mg once daily (for newly diagnosed patients) or discontinue (for patients resistant or intolerant to prior therapy)

Accelerated or blast phase CML and Ph+ ALL (140 mg once daily starting dose): For ANC <500/mm^3 or platelets <10,000/mm^3, if cytopenia unrelated to leukemia, withhold treatment until ANC ≥1000/mm^3 and platelets ≥20,000/mm^3; then resume treatment at the original starting dose. If cytopenia recurs, withhold treatment until ANC ≥1000/mm^3 and platelets ≥20,000/mm^3; then resume treatment at 100 mg once daily (second episode) or 80 mg once daily (third episode). For cytopenias related to leukemia (confirm with marrow aspirate or biopsy), consider dose escalation to 180 mg once daily.

Nonhematologic toxicity: Withhold treatment until toxicity improvement or resolution; if appropriate, resume treatment at a reduced dose based on the event severity and recurrence.

Dermatologic toxicities: Manage rash with antihistamines or topical or systemic steroids (Khoury, 2009), or treatment interruption, dose reduction, or discontinuation. Discontinue if dasatinib-related severe mucocutaneous reaction occurs.

Fluid retention: Manage with diuretics, short courses of corticosteroids, and/or supportive care. Severe pleural effusions may require thoracentesis and oxygen therapy; consider dose reduction or treatment interruption. For grade 3 pleural effusion, withhold treatment until resolves to grade 1 or lower and consider corticosteroids (eg, prednisone 20 to 40 mg/day for 3 to 4 days), diuretics, thoracentesis and/or pleurodesis; may resume dasatinib at a decreased dose when effusion resolves (Khoury, 2009).

Pulmonary arterial hypertension: Discontinue with confirmed pulmonary arterial hypertension.

Combination Regimens

Leukemia, acute lymphocytic: Dasatinib (ALL Regimen) on page 1934
Leukemia, chronic myelogenous: Dasatinib (CML Regimen) on page 1935
Soft tissue sarcoma (gastrointestinal stromal tumor [GIST]): Dasatinib (GIST Regimen) on page 1935

Administration Administer once daily (morning or evening). May be taken without regard to food. Swallow whole; do not break, crush, or chew tablets. Take with a meal if GI upset occurs (Khoury, 2009).

Hazardous agent; use appropriate precautions for handling and disposal (NIOSH 2014 [group 1]). Avoid exposure to crushed tablets. Although crushing of the tablets is not recommended, if it is necessary to manipulate the tablets (eg, to prepare an oral suspension), it is recommended to double glove, wear a protective gown, and prepare in a controlled device (NIOSH 2014).

Emetic Potential Children and Adults: Minimal (<10%)

Extemporaneous Preparations Hazardous agent: Use appropriate precautions for handling and disposal (NIOSH 2014 [group 1]). When manipulating tablets, NIOSH recommends double gloving, a protective gown, and preparation in a controlled device; if not prepared in a controlled device, respiratory and eye protection as well as ventilated engineering controls are recommended (NIOSH 2014).

An oral suspension may be prepared by dissolving dasatinib tablet(s) for one dose in 30 mL chilled orange or apple juice (without preservatives). After 5 minutes, swirl the contents for 3 seconds and repeat the process every 5 minutes for a total of 20 minutes following addition of tablet(s). Minimize time between end of 20 minutes and administration since suspension will taste more bitter if allowed to stand longer. Swirl contents of container one last time, then administer immediately. To ensure the full dose is administered, rinse container with 15 mL juice and administer residue. May be administered orally (or by nasogastric tube). Discard any unused portion after 60 minutes.
Sprycel data on file, Bristol-Myers Squibb

Monitoring Parameters CBC with differential every 2 weeks for 12 weeks and then every 3 months thereafter or as clinically indicated (for chronic phase chronic myeloid leukemia [CML]) **or** weekly for 2 months, then monthly or as clinically necessary (for accelerated or blast phase CML or for acute lymphoblastic leukemia [ALL]); bone marrow biopsy; liver function tests, electrolytes including calcium, phosphorus, magnesium; monitor for fluid retention; monitor for signs/symptoms of cardiac dysfunction; ECG monitoring if at risk for QTc prolongation; chest x-ray is recommended for symptoms suggestive of pleural effusion (eg, cough, dyspnea); signs/symptoms of tumor lysis syndrome and dermatologic reactions.

Thyroid function testing recommendations (Hamnvik, 2011):
Preexisting levothyroxine therapy: Obtain baseline TSH levels, then monitor every 4 weeks until levels and levothyroxine dose are stable, then monitor every 2 months
Without preexisting thyroid hormone replacement: TSH at baseline, then monthly for 4 months, then every 2 to 3 months

Dietary Considerations Avoid grapefruit juice.

Dosage Forms Excipient information presented when available (limited, particularly for generics); consult specific product labeling.
Tablet, Oral:
Sprycel: 20 mg, 50 mg, 70 mg, 80 mg, 100 mg, 140 mg

◆ **Daunomycin** see DAUNOrubicin (Conventional) on page 463

◆ **DAUNOrubicin Citrate** see DAUNOrubicin (Liposomal) on page 470

◆ **DAUNOrubicin Citrate (Liposomal)** see DAUNOrubicin (Liposomal) on page 470

◆ **DAUNOrubicin Citrate Liposome** see DAUNOrubicin (Liposomal) on page 470

DAUNOrubicin (Conventional) (daw noe ROO bi sin con VEN sha nal)

Related Information

Chemotherapy and Cancer Treatment During Pregnancy *on page 2214*

Chemotherapy and Obesity *on page 2220*

Management of Chemotherapy-Induced Nausea and Vomiting in Adults *on page 2142*

Management of Drug Extravasations *on page 2159*

Prevention of Chemotherapy-Induced Nausea and Vomiting in Children *on page 2203*

Principles of Anticancer Therapy *on page 2261*

Safe Handling of Hazardous Drugs *on page 2292*

Brand Names: Canada Cerubidine; Daunorubicin Hydrochloride for Injection

Index Terms Cerubidine; Conventional Daunomycin; Daunomycin; DAUNOrubicin Hydrochloride; Rubidomycin Hydrochloride

Pharmacologic Category Antineoplastic Agent, Anthracycline; Antineoplastic Agent, Topoisomerase II Inhibitor

Use

Acute lymphocytic leukemia: Treatment (remission induction) of acute lymphocytic leukemia (ALL) in children and adults (in combination with other chemotherapy)

Acute myeloid leukemia: Treatment (remission induction) of acute myeloid leukemia (AML) in adults (in combination with other chemotherapy)

Labeled Contraindications Hypersensitivity to daunorubicin or any component of the formulation

Pregnancy Considerations Adverse events have been observed in animal reproduction studies. Daunorubicin crosses the placenta. Women of reproductive potential should avoid pregnancy.

Breast-Feeding Considerations It is not known if daunorubicin is excreted into breast milk. Due to the potential for serious adverse reactions in the nursing infant, the manufacturer recommends a decision be made whether to discontinue nursing or to discontinue the drug, taking into account the importance of treatment to the mother.

Warnings/Precautions Hazardous agent - use appropriate precautions for handling and disposal (NIOSH 2014 [group 1]). **[U.S. Boxed Warning]: Potent vesicant; if extravasation occurs, severe local tissue damage leading to ulceration and necrosis, and pain may occur. For IV administration only. NOT for IM or SubQ administration. Administer through a rapidly flowing IV line.** Ensure proper needle or catheter placement prior to and during infusion. Avoid extravasation. **[U.S. Boxed Warning]: Severe bone marrow suppression may occur when used at therapeutic doses; may lead to infection or hemorrhage.** Use with caution in patients with drug-induced bone marrow suppression (preexisting), unless the therapy benefit outweighs the toxicity risk. Monitor blood counts at baseline and frequently during therapy.

[U.S. Boxed Warning]: May cause cumulative, dose-related myocardial toxicity; may lead to heart failure. May occur either during treatment or may be delayed (months to years after cessations of treatment). The incidence of irreversible myocardial toxicity increases as the total cumulative (lifetime) dosages approach 550 mg/m^2 in adults, 400 mg/m^2 in adults receiving chest radiation, 300 mg/m^2 in children >2 years of age, or 10 mg/kg in children <2 years of age. Total cumulative dose should take into account prior treatment with other anthracyclines or anthracenediones, previous or concomitant treatment with cardiotoxic agents or irradiation of chest. Although the risk increases with cumulative dose, irreversible cardiotoxicity may occur at any dose level. Patients with preexisting heart disease, hypertension, concurrent administration of other antineoplastic agents, prior or concurrent chest irradiation, advanced age; and infants and children are at increased risk. Monitor left ventricular (LV) function (baseline and periodic) with ECHO or MUGA scan; monitor ECG. Cardiotoxicity may occur more frequently in elderly patients. Use with caution in patients with impaired renal function and/or poor marrow reserve due to advanced age; dosage adjustment may be necessary. Infants and children are at increased risk for developing delayed cardiotoxicity; long-term periodic cardiac function monitoring is recommended.

[U.S. Boxed Warning]: Dosage reductions are recommended in patients with renal or hepatic impairment; significant impairment may result in increased toxicities. May cause tumor lysis syndrome and hyperuricemia. Urinary alkalinization and prophylaxis with an antihyperuricemic agent may be necessary. Monitor electrolytes, renal function, and hydration status. Use with caution in patients who have received radiation therapy; reduce dosage in patients who are receiving radiation therapy simultaneously. Secondary leukemias may occur when used with combination chemotherapy or radiation therapy. **[U.S. Boxed Warning]: Should be administered under the supervision of an experienced cancer chemotherapy physician.** Use caution when selecting product for preparation and dispensing; indications, dosages, and adverse event profiles differ between conventional daunorubicin hydrochloride solution and daunorubicin liposomal. Potentially significant drug-drug interactions may exist, requiring dose or frequency adjustment, additional monitoring, and/or selection of alternative therapy.

Adverse Reactions

>10%:

Cardiovascular: Transient ECG abnormalities (supraventricular tachycardia, S-T wave changes, atrial or ventricular extrasystoles); generally asymptomatic and self-limiting. CHF, dose related, may be delayed for 7-8 years after treatment.

Dermatologic: Alopecia (reversible), radiation recall

Gastrointestinal: Mild nausea or vomiting, stomatitis

Genitourinary: Discoloration of urine (red)

Hematologic: Myelosuppression (onset: 7 days; nadir: 10-14 days; recovery: 21-28 days), primarily leukopenia; thrombocytopenia and anemia

1% to 10%:

Dermatologic: Skin "flare" at injection site; discoloration of saliva, sweat, or tears

Endocrine & metabolic: Hyperuricemia

Gastrointestinal: Abdominal pain, GI ulceration, diarrhea

<1%, postmarketing, and/or case reports: Anaphylactoid reaction, arrhythmia, bilirubin increased, cardiomyopathy, hepatitis, infertility; local (cellulitis, pain, thrombophlebitis at injection site); MI, myocarditis, nail banding, neutropenic typhlitis, onycholysis, pericarditis, pigmentation of nailbeds, secondary leukemia, skin rash, sterility, systemic hypersensitivity (including urticaria, pruritus, angioedema, dysphagia, dyspnea); transaminases increased

Drug Interactions

Metabolism/Transport Effects Substrate of P-glycoprotein

Avoid Concomitant Use

Avoid concomitant use of DAUNOrubicin (Conventional) with any of the following: BCG (Intravesical); CloZAPine; Dipyrone; Natalizumab; Pimecrolimus; Tacrolimus (Topical); Tofacitinib; Vaccines (Live)

Increased Effect/Toxicity

DAUNOrubicin (Conventional) may increase the levels/effects of: CloZAPine; Fingolimod; Leflunomide; Natalizumab; Tofacitinib; Vaccines (Live)

The levels/effects of DAUNOrubicin (Conventional) may be increased by: Bevacizumab; Cyclophosphamide; Denosumab; Dipyrone; Lumacaftor; P-glycoprotein/ABCB1 Inhibitors; Pimecrolimus; Ranolazine; Roflumilast; Tacrolimus (Topical); Taxane Derivatives; Trastuzumab

Decreased Effect

DAUNOrubicin (Conventional) may decrease the levels/effects of: BCG (Intravesical); Cardiac Glycosides; Coccidioides immitis Skin Test; Sipuleucel-T; Vaccines (Inactivated); Vaccines (Live)

The levels/effects of DAUNOrubicin (Conventional) may be decreased by: Cardiac Glycosides; Echinacea; Lumacaftor; P-glycoprotein/ABCB1 Inducers

Storage/Stability

Solution: Store intact vials at 2°C to 8°C (36°F to 46°F). Protect from light. Retain in carton until time of use. Solution prepared for infusion may be stored at 20°C to 25°C (68°F to 77°F) for up to 24 hours. Discard unused portion.

Lyophilized powder [Canadian product]: Store intact vials of powder at 15°C to 30°C (59°F to 86°F). Protect from light. Retain in carton until time of use. Reconstituted daunorubicin is stable for 24 hours at room temperature or 48 hours when refrigerated at 2°C to 8°C (36°F to 46°F). Protect reconstituted solution from light.

Preparation for Administration Hazardous agent; use appropriate precautions for handling and disposal (NIOSH 2014 [group 1]). Dilute vials of powder for injection [Canadian product] with 4 mL SWFI for a final concentration of 5 mg/mL. May further dilute solution or reconstituted daunorubicin solution in D_5W or NS for infusion.

Mechanism of Action Inhibits DNA and RNA synthesis by intercalation between DNA base pairs and by steric obstruction. Daunomycin intercalates at points of local uncoiling of the double helix. Although the exact mechanism is unclear, it appears that direct binding to DNA (intercalation) and inhibition of DNA repair (topoisomerase II inhibition) result in blockade of DNA and RNA synthesis and fragmentation of DNA.

Pharmacodynamics/Kinetics

Distribution: Distributes widely into tissues, particularly the liver, kidneys, lung, spleen, and heart; does not distribute into the CNS

Metabolism: Primarily hepatic to daunorubicinol (active), then to inactive aglycones, conjugated sulfates, and glucuronides

Half-life elimination: Initial: 45 minutes; Terminal: 18.5 hours; Daunorubicinol plasma half-life: ~27 hours

Excretion: Feces (40%); urine (~25% as unchanged drug and metabolites)

Dosing

Adult & Geriatric Daunorubicin is associated with a moderate emetic potential; antiemetics are recommended to prevent nausea and vomiting (Basch, 2011; Roila, 2010).

◄ *Manufacturer's labeling:* **Note:** Cumulative doses above 550 mg/m^2 in adults without risk factors for cardiotoxicity and above 400 mg/m^2 in adults receiving chest irradiation are associated with an increased risk of cardiomyopathy.

Acute lymphocytic leukemia (ALL):
IV: 45 mg/m^2 on days 1, 2, and 3 (in combination with vincristine, prednisone, and asparaginase)

Acute myeloid leukemia (AML):
Adults <60 years: Induction: IV: 45 mg/m^2 on days 1, 2, and 3 of the first course of induction therapy; subsequent courses: 45 mg/m^2 on days 1 and 2 (in combination with cytarabine)
Adults ≥60 years: Induction: IV: 30 mg/m^2 on days 1, 2, and 3 of the first course of induction therapy; subsequent courses: 30 mg/m^2 on days 1 and 2 (in combination with cytarabine)

Indication-specific dosing (off-label dosing):
ALL:
CALGB 8811 regimen: IV: 45 mg/m^2 (in patients <60 years) or 30 mg/m^2 (in patients ≥60 years) on days 1, 2, and 3 of induction (Course I; 4 week cycle), in combination with cyclophosphamide, prednisone, vincristine, and asparaginase (Larson, 1995)
CCG 1961: Adults ≤21 years: IV: Induction: 25 mg/m^2 once weekly for 4 weeks (in combination with vincristine, prednisone, and asparaginase) (Nachman, 2009)
GRAALL-2003: Adults ≤60 years: IV:
Induction: 50 mg/m^2 on days 1, 2, and 3 **and** 30 mg/m^2 on days 15 and 16 (in combination with prednisone, vincristine, asparaginase, cyclophosphamide, and G-CSF support) (Huguet, 2009)
Late intensification: 30 mg/m^2 on days 1, 2, and 3 (in combination with prednisone, vincristine, asparaginase, cyclophosphamide, and G-CSF support) (Huguet, 2009)
MRC UKALLXII/ECOG E2993: Adults <60 years: IV: Induction (Phase I): 60 mg/m^2 on days 1, 8, 15, and 22 (in combination with vincristine, asparaginase, and prednisone) (Rowe, 2005)
PETHEMA ALL-96: Adults ≤30 years: IV:
Induction: 30 mg/m^2 on days 1, 8, 15, and 22 (in combination with vincristine, prednisone, asparaginase, and cyclophosphamide) (Ribera, 2008)
Consolidation-2/Reinduction: 30 mg/m^2 on days 1, 2, 8, and 9 (in combination with vincristine, dexamethasone, asparaginase, and cyclophosphamide) (Ribera, 2008)
Protocol 8707: Adults ≤60 years: IV: Induction and Consolidation 2A cycles: 60 mg/m^2 on days 1, 2, and 3 (in combination with vincristine, prednisone, and asparaginase). An additional 60 mg/m^2 daunorubicin dose may be administered on day 15 of induction if bone marrow biopsy on day 14 shows residual disease (Linker, 2002)

AML: Induction:
CCG 2891: Adults <21 years: IV: 20 mg/m^2/day continuous infusion on days 0 to 4 and 10 to 14 (in combination with dexamethasone, cytarabine, thioguanine, and etoposide) (Woods, 1996)
Adults <60 years: IV: 90 mg/m^2 on days 1, 2, and 3 (in combination with cytarabine). If residual disease was observed on day 12 to day 14 bone marrow biopsy, 45 mg/m^2 for 3 days was administered (in combination with cytarabine) (Fernandez, 2009).

Adults <60 years: IV: 60 mg/m² on days 1, 2, and 3 (in combination with cytarabine and cladribine); may repeat if partial remission occurs (Holowiecki, 2012).

Adults ≥60 years: IV: 45 or 90 mg/m² on days 1, 2, and 3 (in combination with cytarabine); the escalated 90 mg/m² dose was associated with increased remission rates and overall survival in the subgroup of patients 60 to 65 years of age as compared to patients >65 years (Lowenberg, 2009)

Acute promyelocytic leukemia (APL):

Induction: Adults: IV: 50 mg/m² on days 3, 4, 5, and 6 (in combination with ATRA and cytarabine) (Powell, 2010) **or** 60 mg/m² on days 1, 2, and 3 (in combination with ATRA and cytarabine) (Ades, 2008)

Consolidation: Adults: IV: 50 mg/m² on days 1, 2, and 3 for 2 cycles (in combination with ATRA; arsenic trioxide was administered for 2 cycles prior to daunorubicin and ATRA) (Powell, 2010) **or** 60 mg/m² on days 1, 2, and 3 during cycle 1 of consolidation (in combination with cytarabine), followed by 45 mg/m² on days 1, 2, and 3 during cycle 2 of consolidation (in combination with cytarabine) (Ades, 2008)

Pediatric Daunorubicin is associated with a moderate emetic potential; antiemetics are recommended to prevent nausea and vomiting (Dupuis, 2011).

Manufacturer's labeling: **Note:** Cumulative doses above 300 mg/m² in children >2 years or 10 mg/kg in children <2 years of age are associated with an increased risk of cardiomyopathy.

Acute lymphocytic leukemia (ALL):

Children <2 years or BSA <0.5 m²: Remission induction: IV: 1 mg/kg/dose on day 1 every week for up to 4 to 6 cycles (in combination with vincristine and prednisone)

Children ≥2 years and BSA ≥0.5 m²: Remission induction: IV: 25 mg/m² on day 1 every week for up to 4 to 6 cycles (in combination with vincristine and prednisone)

Indication-specific dosing (off-label dosing):

ALL:

CCG 1961: Children ≥10 years and Adolescents: IV: Induction: 25 mg/m² once weekly for 4 weeks (in combination with vincristine, prednisone, and asparaginase) (Nachman, 2009)

GRAALL-2003: Adolescents ≥15 years: IV:

Induction: 50 mg/m² on days 1, 2, and 3 **and** 30 mg/m² on days 15 and 16 (in combination with prednisone, vincristine, asparaginase, cyclophosphamide, and G-CSF support) (Huguet, 2009)

Late intensification: 30 mg/m² on days 1, 2, and 3 (in combination with prednisone, vincristine, asparaginase, cyclophosphamide, and G-CSF support) (Huguet, 2009)

MRC UKALLXII/ECOG E2993: Adolescents ≥15 years: IV: Induction (Phase I): 60 mg/m² on days 1, 8, 15, and 22 (in combination with vincristine, asparaginase, and prednisone) (Rowe, 2005)

PETHEMA ALL-96: Adolescents ≥15 years: IV:

Induction: 30 mg/m² on days 1, 8, 15, and 22 (in combination with vincristine, prednisone, asparaginase, and cyclophosphamide) (Ribera, 2008)

Consolidation-2/Reinduction: 30 mg/m² on days 1, 2, 8, and 9 (in combination with vincristine, dexamethasone, asparaginase, and cyclophosphamide) (Ribera, 2008)

Acute myeloid leukemia (AML): Induction:

CCG 2891:

Children <3 years: IV: 0.67 mg/kg/day continuous infusion on days 0 to 4 and 10 to 14 (in combination with dexamethasone, cytarabine, thioguanine, and etoposide) (Woods, 1996)

Children ≥3 years and Adolescents: IV: 20 mg/m^2/day continuous infusion on days 0 to 4 and 10 to 14 (in combination with dexamethasone, cytarabine, thioguanine, and etoposide) (Woods, 1996)

MRC AML 10/12: Children ≤14 years: IV: 50 mg/m^2 on days 1, 3, and 5 for 2 cycles (in combination with cytarabine and etoposide) (Gibson, 2005)

Renal Impairment The manufacturer's labeling recommends the following adjustment: S_{cr} >3 mg/dL: Administer 50% of normal dose

The following adjustments have also been recommended (Aronoff, 2007):

Adults: No dosage adjustment necessary.

Children:

CrCl <30 mL/minute: Administer 50% of dose

Hemodialysis/continuous ambulatory peritoneal dialysis (CAPD): Administer 50% of dose

Hepatic Impairment The manufacturer's labeling recommends the following adjustments:

Serum bilirubin 1.2 to 3 mg/dL: Administer 75% of dose

Serum bilirubin >3 mg/dL: Administer 50% of dose

The following adjustments have also been recommended (Floyd, 2006):

Serum bilirubin 1.2 to 3 mg/dL: Administer 75% of dose

Serum bilirubin 3.1 to 5 mg/dL: Administer 50% of dose

Serum bilirubin >5 mg/dL: Avoid use

Combination Regimens

Leukemia, acute lymphocytic:

CALGB 8811 Regimen (ALL) on page 1853

CALGB 9111 Regimen (ALL) on page 1854

DVP on page 1952

Linker Protocol (ALL) on page 2030

PVDA on page 2071

Leukemia, acute myeloid:

5 + 2 (Cytarabine-Daunorubicin) (AML Induction) on page 1816

5 + 2 (Cytarabine-Daunorubicin) (AML Postremission) on page 1816

5 + 2 + 5 (Cytarabine-Daunorubicin-Etoposide) (AML Consolidation) on page 1817

7 + 3 (Cytarabine-Daunorubicin) (AML Induction) on page 1817

7 + 3 + 7 (Cytarabine-Daunorubicin-Etoposide) (AML Induction) on page 1819

Cytarabine (High Dose)-Daunorubicin (AML Induction) on page 1931

Cytarabine (High Dose)-Daunorubicin-Etoposide (AML Induction) on page 1932

Leukemia, acute promyelocytic:

Tretinoin-Daunorubicin (APL) on page 2096

Tretinoin-Daunorubicin-Cytarabine Induction, Consolidation, Maintenance (APL) on page 2097

Administration Daunorubicin is associated with a moderate emetic potential; antiemetics are recommended to prevent nausea and vomiting (Basch, 2011; Dupuis, 2011; Roila, 2010).

For IV administration only. Do not administer IM or SubQ. Administer as slow IV push over 1 to 5 minutes into the tubing of a rapidly infusing IV solution of D_5W or NS or may dilute further and infuse over 15 to 30 minutes.

Vesicant; ensure proper needle or catheter placement prior to and during infusion; avoid extravasation.

Extravasation management: If extravasation occurs, stop infusion immediately and disconnect (leave cannula/needle in place); gently aspirate extravasated solution (do **NOT** flush the line); remove needle/cannula; elevate extremity. Initiate antidote (dexrazoxane or dimethyl sulfate [DMSO]). Apply dry cold compresses for 20 minutes 4 times daily for 1 to 2 days (Perez Fidalgo, 2012); withhold cooling beginning 15 minutes before dexrazoxane infusion; continue withholding cooling until 15 minutes after infusion is completed. Topical DMSO should not be administered in combination with dexrazoxane; may lessen dexrazoxane efficacy.

> *Dexrazoxane:* Adults: 1000 mg/m^2 (maximum dose: 2000 mg) IV (administer in a large vein remote from site of extravasation) over 1 to 2 hours days 1 and 2, then 500 mg/m^2 (maximum dose: 1000 mg) IV over 1-2 hours day 3; begin within 6 hours of extravasation. Day 2 and day 3 doses should be administered at approximately the same time (± 3 hours) as the dose on day 1 (Mouridsen, 2007; Perez Fidalgo, 2012). **Note:** Reduce dexrazoxane dose by 50% in patients with moderate to severe renal impairment (CrCl <40 mL/minute).

> *DMSO:* Children and Adults: Apply topically to a region covering twice the affected area every 8 hours for 7 days; begin within 10 minutes of extravasation; do not cover with a dressing (Perez Fidalgo, 2012).

Hazardous agent; use appropriate precautions for handling and disposal (NIOSH 2014 [group 1]).

Vesicant/Extravasation Risk Vesicant

Emetic Potential Children and Adults: Moderate (30% to 90%)

Monitoring Parameters CBC with differential and platelet count, liver function test, ECG, left ventricular ejection function (echocardiography [ECHO] or multigated radionuclide angiography [MUGA] scan), renal function test, signs/symptoms of extravasation

Dosage Forms Excipient information presented when available (limited, particularly for generics); consult specific product labeling.
Injectable, Intravenous:
  Generic: 5 mg/mL (4 mL)
Injectable, Intravenous [preservative free]:
  Generic: 5 mg/mL (4 mL, 10 mL)

◆ **DAUNOrubicin Hydrochloride** *see* DAUNOrubicin (Conventional) *on page 463*

◆ **Daunorubicin Hydrochloride for Injection (Can)** *see* DAUNOrubicin (Conventional) *on page 463*

DAUNOrubicin (Liposomal) (daw noe ROO bi sin lye po SO mal)

Related Information

Common Toxicity Criteria *on page 2122*

Management of Chemotherapy-Induced Nausea and Vomiting in Adults *on page 2142*

Management of Drug Extravasations *on page 2159*

Safe Handling of Hazardous Drugs *on page 2292*

Brand Names: US DaunoXome

Index Terms DAUNOrubicin Citrate; DAUNOrubicin Citrate (Liposomal); DAU-NOrubicin Citrate Liposome; Liposomal DAUNOrubicin

Pharmacologic Category Antineoplastic Agent, Anthracycline; Antineoplastic Agent, Topoisomerase II Inhibitor

Use

Kaposi sarcoma: First-line treatment of advanced HIV-associated Kaposi sarcoma

Limitation of use: Daunorubicin (liposomal) is not recommended in HIV-related Kaposi sarcoma which is less than advanced.

Labeled Contraindications

Hypersensitivity to daunorubicin (liposomal) or any component of the formulation

Documentation of allergenic cross-reactivity for drugs in this class is limited. However, because of similarities in chemical structure and/or pharmacologic actions, the possibility of cross-sensitivity cannot be ruled out with certainty.

Pregnancy Considerations Adverse events were observed in animal reproduction studies. May cause fetal harm if administered during pregnancy. Women of childbearing potential should avoid becoming pregnant while receiving treatment.

Breast-Feeding Considerations Based on information from daunorubicin (conventional), it is not known if daunorubicin (liposomal) is excreted into breast milk. Daunorubicin (liposomal) is indicated for advanced HIV-associated Kaposi sarcoma. In the United States, where formula is accessible, affordable, safe, and sustainable, and the risk of infant mortality due to diarrhea and respiratory infections is low, complete avoidance of breast-feeding by HIV-infected women is recommended to decrease potential transmission of HIV (DHHS [perinatal], 2012).

Warnings/Precautions Hazardous agent - use appropriate precautions for handling and disposal (NIOSH 2014 [group 1]). **[US Boxed Warning]: Due to the potential for cardiac toxicity and heart failure, monitor cardiac function regularly, especially in patients with previous therapy with anthracyclines, thoracic radiation, or who have preexisting cardiac disease.** Cardiomyopathy is usually associated with a decrease left in ventricular ejection fraction (LVEF). Although the risk increases with cumulative dose, irreversible cardiotoxicity may occur with anthracycline treatment at any dose level. Patients who have received prior anthracycline therapy (DOXOrubicin >300 mg/m^2 or equivalent), with preexisting heart disease, hypertension, concurrent administration of other antineoplastic agents, prior or concurrent chest irradiation, and advanced age are at increased risk. Evaluate LVEF prior to treatment and periodically during treatment (at cumulative doses of daunorubicin liposomal 320 mg/m^2 and every 160 mg/m^2 thereafter or every 160 mg/m^2 in patients at higher risk).

[US Boxed Warning]: May cause bone marrow suppression, particularly neutropenia (may be severe). Monitor blood counts. Monitor closely for infections (including opportunistic infections). **[US Boxed Warning]: Reduce dosage in patients with hepatic impairment.** Use caution with renal impairment; may require dose adjustment. **[US Boxed Warning]: The lipid component is associated with infusion-related reactions (back pain, flushing, chest tightness) usually within the first 5 minutes of infusion and subsides with interruption of the infusion, and generally does not recur if the infusion is resumed at a lower rate.** Monitor for infusion reactions; interrupt infusion if reaction occurs, and resume at reduced infusion rate.

Although not reported with daunorubicin (liposomal), daunorubicin (conventional) is associated with local tissue necrosis if extravasated. Potentially significant drug-drug interactions may exist, requiring dose or frequency adjustment, additional monitoring, and/or selection of alternative therapy. **[US Boxed Warning]: Should be administered under the supervision of an experienced cancer chemotherapy physician.**

Adverse Reactions Frequency not always defined.

Cardiovascular: Edema (11%), chest pain (10%), angina pectoris (≤5%), atrial fibrillation (≤5%), cardiac arrest (≤5%), cardiac tamponade (≤5%), hypertension (≤5%), myocardial infarction (≤5%), palpitations (≤5%), pericardial effusion (≤5%), pulmonary hypertension (≤5%), sinus tachycardia (≤5%), supraventricular tachycardia (≤5%), syncope (≤5%), tachycardia (≤5%), ventricular premature contractions (≤5%), decreased left ventricular ejection fraction (3%; reduction of 20% to 25%), cardiomyopathy (cumulative, dose-related; total dose above 300 mg/m^2)

Central nervous system: Fatigue (49%), headache (25%), rigors (19%), neuropathy (13%), depression (10%), malaise (10%), dizziness (8%), insomnia (6%), abnormality in thinking (≤5%), amnesia (≤5%), anxiety (≤5%), ataxia (≤5%), confusion (≤5%), drowsiness (≤5%), emotional lability (≤5%), hallucination (≤5%), hypertonia (≤5%), meningitis (≤5%), seizure (≤5%)

Dermatologic: Diaphoresis (14%), alopecia (8%), pruritus (7%), folliculitis (≤5%), seborrhea (≤5%), xeroderma (≤5%)

Endocrine & metabolic: Dehydration (≤5%), hot flash (≤5%), increased thirst (≤5%)

Gastrointestinal: Nausea (54%), diarrhea (38%), abdominal pain (23%), anorexia (23%), vomiting (23%), stomatitis (10%), constipation (7%), tenesmus (5%), dental caries (≤5%), dysgeusia (≤5%), dysphagia (≤5%), gastritis (≤5%), gastrointestinal hemorrhage (≤5%), gingival hemorrhage (≤5%), hemorrhoids (≤5%), hiccups (≤5%), increased appetite (≤5%), melena (≤5%), xerostomia (≤5%)

Genitourinary: Dysuria (≤5%), nocturia (≤5%)

Hematologic & oncologic: Neutropenia (<1,000 cells/mm^3: 36%; grade 4: 15%), lymphadenopathy (≤5%), splenomegaly (≤5%), bone marrow depression (especially granulocytes; platelets and erythrocytes less effected), severe granulocytopenia (may be associated with fever and result in infection)

Hepatic: Hepatomegaly (≤5%)

Hypersensitivity: Hypersensitivity reaction (24%)

Infection: Opportunistic infection (40%; median time to first infection/illness: 214 days)

Local: inflammation at injection site (≤5%)

Neuromuscular & skeletal: Back pain (16%), arthralgia (7%), myalgia (7%), abnormal gait (≤5%), hyperkinesia (≤5%), tremor (≤5%)

Ophthalmic: Visual disturbance (5%), conjunctivitis (≤5%), eye pain (≤5%)

Otic: Deafness (≤5%), otalgia (≤5%), tinnitus (≤5%)

Renal: Polyuria (≤5%)

Respiratory: Cough (28%), dyspnea (26%), rhinitis (12%), sinusitis (8%), flu-like symptoms (5%), hemoptysis (≤5%), increased bronchial secretions (≤5%), pulmonary infiltrates (≤5%)

Miscellaneous: Fever (47%), infusion-related reaction (14%; includes back pain, flushing, chest tightness)

Drug Interactions

Metabolism/Transport Effects Substrate of P-glycoprotein

Avoid Concomitant Use

Avoid concomitant use of DAUNOrubicin (Liposomal) with any of the following: BCG (Intravesical); CloZAPine; Dipyrone; Natalizumab; Pimecrolimus; Tacrolimus (Topical); Tofacitinib; Vaccines (Live)

Increased Effect/Toxicity

DAUNOrubicin (Liposomal) may increase the levels/effects of: CloZAPine; Fingolimod; Leflunomide; Natalizumab; Tofacitinib; Vaccines (Live)

The levels/effects of DAUNOrubicin (Liposomal) may be increased by: Bevacizumab; Cyclophosphamide; Denosumab; Dipyrone; Lumacaftor; P-glycoprotein/ABCB1 Inhibitors; Pimecrolimus; Ranolazine; Roflumilast; Tacrolimus (Topical); Taxane Derivatives; Trastuzumab

Decreased Effect

DAUNOrubicin (Liposomal) may decrease the levels/effects of: BCG (Intravesical); Cardiac Glycosides; Coccidioides immitis Skin Test; Sipuleucel-T; Vaccines (Inactivated); Vaccines (Live)

The levels/effects of DAUNOrubicin (Liposomal) may be decreased by: Cardiac Glycosides; Echinacea; Lumacaftor; P-glycoprotein/ABCB1 Inducers

Storage/Stability Store intact vials at 2°C to 8°C (36°F to 46°F); do not freeze. Protect from light. Diluted daunorubicin liposomal for infusion may be refrigerated at 2°C to 8°C (36°F to 46°F) for a maximum of 6 hours (if not used immediately).

Preparation for Administration Hazardous agent; use appropriate precautions for handling and disposal (NIOSH 2014 [group 1]). The only fluid that may be mixed with daunorubicin (liposomal) is D_5W. Dilute with an equivalent volume of D_5W to a 1:1 solution (to a concentration of 1 mg daunorubicin liposomal/mL). Must **not** be mixed with saline, bacteriostatic agents (such as benzyl alcohol), or any other solution. Do not mix with other medications.

Mechanism of Action Liposomal preparation of daunorubicin; liposomes have been shown to penetrate solid tumors more effectively, possibly because of their small size and longer circulation time. Once in tissues, daunorubicin is released (over time). Daunorubicin inhibits DNA and RNA synthesis by intercalation between DNA base pairs and by steric obstruction; and intercalates at points of local uncoiling of the double helix. Although the exact mechanism is unclear, it appears that direct binding to DNA (intercalation) and inhibition of DNA repair (topoisomerase II inhibition) result in blockade of DNA and RNA synthesis and fragmentation of DNA.

Pharmacodynamics/Kinetics

Distribution: V_d: ~5 to 8 L

Metabolism: Daunorubicinol (major active metabolite) is detected at low levels in plasma

Half-life elimination: Distribution: 4.4 hours

Excretion: Primarily feces; some urine

Dosing

Adult & Geriatric Note: DAUNOrubicin (liposomal) is different from the conventional DAUNOrubicin formulation; do **NOT** substitute (indications and doses are different).

Kaposi sarcoma: IV: 40 mg/m^2 once every 2 weeks; continue until disease progression.

Renal Impairment Serum creatinine >3 mg/dL: Administer 50% of normal dose.

Hepatic Impairment

Bilirubin 1.2 to 3 mg/dL: Administer 75% of normal dose.

Bilirubin >3 mg/dL: Administer 50% of normal dose.

Obesity *ASCO Guidelines for appropriate chemotherapy dosing in obese adults with cancer:* Utilize patient's actual body weight (full weight) for calculation of body surface area- or weight-based dosing, particularly when the intent of therapy is curative; manage regimen-related toxicities in the same manner as for nonobese patients; if a dose reduction is utilized due to toxicity, consider resumption of full weight-based dosing with subsequent cycles, especially if cause of toxicity (eg, hepatic or renal impairment) is resolved (Griggs 2012).

Adjustment for Toxicity

ANC <750/mm^3: Withhold treatment.

Infusion reactions (back pain, flushing, chest tightness): Temporarily interrupt infusion; may resume at a slower rate.

Combination Regimens

Leukemia, acute lymphocytic: Hyper-CVAD (Leukemia, Acute Lymphocytic) on page 2006

Administration Infuse over 1 hour; do not mix with other drugs. Do NOT administer with an in-line filter. Avoid extravasation.

Hazardous agent; use appropriate precautions for handling and disposal (NIOSH 2014 [group 1]).

Vesicant/Extravasation Risk May be an irritant

Emetic Potential Low (10% to 30%).

Monitoring Parameters CBC with differential and platelets (prior to each dose), liver function tests, renal function tests; evaluate cardiac function (baseline left ventricular ejection fraction [LVEF] prior to treatment initiation; repeat LVEF at total cumulative doses of 320 mg/m^2, and every 160 mg/m^2 thereafter; patients with preexisting cardiac disease, history of prior chest irradiation, or history of prior anthracycline treatment should have baseline LVEF and every 160 mg/m^2 thereafter); signs and symptoms of infection or disease progression; monitor closely for infusion reactions

Dosage Forms Considerations Daunorubicin (liposomal) injection contains sucrose 2,125 mg/25 mL

Dosage Forms Excipient information presented when available (limited, particularly for generics); consult specific product labeling.

Injectable, Intravenous [preservative free]:

DaunoXome: 2 mg/mL (25 mL) [pyrogen free]

◆ **DaunoXome** see DAUNOrubicin (Liposomal) on page 470

◆ **DAVA** see Vindesine on page 1760

◆ **dCF** see Pentostatin on page 1375

◆ **DDAVP** see Desmopressin on page 505

◆ **DDAVP Melt (Can)** *see* Desmopressin *on page 505*

◆ **DDAVP Rhinal Tube (Can)** *see* Desmopressin *on page 505*

◆ **DDAVP Rhinyle (Can)** *see* Desmopressin *on page 505*

◆ **DDP** *see* CISplatin *on page 334*

◆ **Deacetyl Vinblastine Carboxamide** *see* Vindesine *on page 1760*

◆ **1-Deamino-8-D-Arginine Vasopressin** *see* Desmopressin *on page 505*

◆ **Decadron** *see* Dexamethasone (Systemic) *on page 513*

◆ **Decapeptyl (Can)** *see* Triptorelin *on page 1703*

Decitabine (de SYE ta been)

Related Information

Common Toxicity Criteria *on page 2122*

Management of Chemotherapy-Induced Nausea and Vomiting in Adults *on page 2142*

Prevention of Chemotherapy-Induced Nausea and Vomiting in Children *on page 2203*

Safe Handling of Hazardous Drugs *on page 2292*

Brand Names: US Dacogen

Index Terms 5-Aza-2'-deoxycytidine; 5-Aza-dCyd; Deoxyazacytidine; Dezocitidine

Pharmacologic Category Antineoplastic Agent, Antimetabolite; Antineoplastic Agent, DNA Methylation Inhibitor

Use Myelodysplastic syndromes: Treatment of myelodysplastic syndromes (MDS), including previously treated and untreated, de novo and secondary MDS of all French-American-British (FAB) subtypes (refractory anemia, refractory anemia with ringed sideroblasts, refractory anemia with excess blasts, refractory anemia with excess blasts in transformation, and chronic myelomonocytic leukemia) and intermediate-1, intermediate-2, and high-risk International Prognostic Scoring System (IPSS) groups

Labeled Contraindications There are no contraindications listed in the manufacturer's labeling.

Pregnancy Considerations Adverse events were observed in animal reproduction studies. Based on the mechanism of action, decitabine may cause fetal harm if administered during pregnancy. Women of childbearing potential should be advised to use effective contraception to avoid pregnancy during treatment and for 1 month after treatment. In addition, males should be advised to avoid fathering a child while on decitabine therapy and for 2 months after treatment.

Breast-Feeding Considerations Because of the potential for serious adverse reactions in the nursing infant, a decision should be made to discontinue breast-feeding or the drug, taking into account the importance of treatment to the mother.

Warnings/Precautions Hazardous agent - use appropriate precautions for handling and disposal (NIOSH 2014 [group 1]). Neutropenia and thrombocytopenia commonly occur; anemia and neutropenic fever have also been reported. Myelosuppression and worsening neutropenia are more common in first two treatment cycles and may not correlate with progression of underlying MDS. Hematologic toxicity may require dosage adjustment (after the first cycle), growth factor support, and/or antimicrobial agents. Monitor for infection. Potentially significant drug-drug interactions may exist, requiring dose or frequency adjustment, additional monitoring, and/or selection of alternative therapy.

Adverse Reactions

>10%:

Cardiovascular: Peripheral edema (25% to 27%), pallor (23%), edema (5% to 18%), cardiac murmur (16%), hypotension (6% to 11%)

Central nervous system: Fever (6% to 53%), fatigue (46%), headache (23% to 28%), insomnia (14% to 28%), dizziness (18% to 21%), chills (16%), pain (5% to 13%), confusion (8% to 12%), lethargy (12%), anxiety (9% to 11%), hypoesthesia (11%)

Dermatologic: Petechiae (12% to 39%), bruising (9% to 22%), rash (11% to 19%), erythema (5% to 14%), cellulitis (9% to 12%), lesions (5% to 11%), pruritus (9% to 11%)

Endocrine & metabolic: Hyperglycemia (6% to 33%), hypoalbuminemia (7% to 24%), hypomagnesemia (5% to 24%), hypokalemia (12% to 22%), hyperkalemia (13%), hyponatremia (19%)

Gastrointestinal: Nausea (40% to 42%), constipation (30% to 35%), diarrhea (28% to 34%), vomiting (16% to 25%), anorexia/appetite decreased (8% to 23%), abdominal pain (5% to 14%), oral mucosal petechiae (13%), stomatitis (11% to 12%), dyspepsia (10% to 12%)

Hematologic: Neutropenia (38% to 90%; grades 3/4: 37% to 87%; recovery 28-50 days), thrombocytopenia (27% to 89%; grades 3/4: 24% to 85%), anemia (31% to 82%; grades 3/4: 22%), febrile neutropenia (20% to 29%; grades 3/4: 23%), leukopenia (6% to 28%; grades 3/4: 22%), lymphadenopathy (12%)

Hepatic: Hyperbilirubinemia (6% to 14%), alkaline phosphatase increased (11%)

Local: Tenderness (11%)

Neuromuscular & skeletal: Rigors (22%), arthralgia (17% to 20%), limb pain (18% to 19%), back pain (17% to 18%), weakness (15%)

Respiratory: Cough (27% to 40%), dyspnea (29%), pneumonia (20% to 22%), pharyngitis (16%), lung crackles (14%), epistaxis (13%)

5% to 10%:

Cardiovascular: Tachycardia (8%), chest pain/discomfort (6% to 7%), facial edema (6%), hypertension (6%), heart failure (5%)

Central nervous system: Depression (9%), malaise (5%)

Dermatologic: Alopecia (8%), dry skin (8%), urticaria (6%)

Endocrine & metabolic: Hyperuricemia (10%), LDH increased (8%), bicarbonate increased (6%), dehydration (6% to 8%), hypochloremia (6%), bicarbonate decreased (5%), hypoproteinemia (5%)

Gastrointestinal: Mucosal inflammation (9%), weight loss (9%), gingival bleeding (8%), hemorrhoids (8%), loose stools (7%), tongue ulceration (7%), dysphagia (5% to 6%), oral candidiasis (6%), toothache (6%), abdominal distension (5%), gastroesophageal reflux (5%), glossodynia (5%), lip ulceration (5%), oral pain (5%), tooth abscess (5%)

Genitourinary: Urinary tract infection (7%), dysuria (6%), polyuria (5%)

Hematologic: Bacteremia (5% to 8%), hematoma (5%), pancytopenia (5%), thrombocythemia (5%)

Hepatic: Ascites (10%), AST increased (10%), hypobilirubinemia (5%)

Local: Catheter infection (8%), catheter site erythema (5%), catheter site pain (5%), injection site swelling (5%)

Neuromuscular & skeletal: Myalgia (5% to 9%), falling (8%), chest wall pain (7%), muscle spasm (7%), bone pain (6%), musculoskeletal pain/discomfort (5% to 6%), crepitation (5%)

Ocular: Blurred vision (6%)

Otic: Ear pain (6%)

Respiratory: Breath sounds abnormal (5% to 10%), hypoxia (10%), upper respiratory tract infection (10%), pharyngolaryngeal pain (8%), rales (8%), pulmonary edema (6%), sinusitis (5% to 6%), pleural effusion (5%), post-nasal drip (5%), sinus congestion (5%)

Miscellaneous: Candidal infection (10%), staphylococcal infection (7%), transfusion reaction (7%), night sweats (5%)

<5%, postmarketing, and/or case reports: Anaphylactic reaction, atrial fibrillation, bronchopulmonary aspergillosis, cardiomyopathy, cardiorespiratory arrest/failure, catheter site hemorrhage, cholecystitis, fungal infection, gastrointestinal hemorrhage, gingival pain, hemoptysis, hypersensitivity, intracranial hemorrhage, mental status change, MI, mycobacterium avium complex infection, peridiverticular abscess, pseudomonal lung infection, pulmonary embolism, pulmonary infiltrates, pulmonary mass, renal failure, respiratory arrest, sepsis, splenomegaly, supraventricular tachycardia, Sweet's syndrome (acute febrile neutrophilic dermatosis), urethral hemorrhage

Drug Interactions

Metabolism/Transport Effects None known.

Avoid Concomitant Use

Avoid concomitant use of Decitabine with any of the following: BCG (Intravesical); CloZAPine; Dipyrone

Increased Effect/Toxicity

Decitabine may increase the levels/effects of: CloZAPine

The levels/effects of Decitabine may be increased by: Dipyrone

Decreased Effect

Decitabine may decrease the levels/effects of: BCG (Intravesical)

Storage/Stability Store intact vials at 25°C (77°F); excursions permitted to 15°C to 30°C (59°F to 86°F). Solutions diluted for infusion may be stored for up to 4 hours prior to infusion refrigerated at 2°C to 8°C (36°F to 46°F) **if** prepared with cold infusion fluids. Infusion should begin within 15 minutes of preparation if room temperature infusion solutions are utilized.

Preparation for Administration Hazardous agent; use appropriate precautions for handling and disposal (NIOSH 2014 [group 1]). Vials should be reconstituted with 10 mL SWFI to a concentration of 5 mg/mL. Immediately further dilute with NS, D_5W, or lactated Ringer's to a final concentration of 0.1 to 1 mg/mL. Use appropriate precautions for handling and disposal. Solutions not administered within 15 minutes of preparation should be prepared with cold (2°C to 8°C [36°F to 46°F]) infusion solutions.

Mechanism of Action After phosphorylation, decitabine is incorporated into DNA and inhibits DNA methyltransferase causing hypomethylation and subsequent cell death (within the S-phase of the cell cycle).

Pharmacodynamics/Kinetics

Distribution: ~63 to 89 L/m^2 (Cashen 2008)

Metabolism: Possibly via deamination by cytidine deaminase

Half-life elimination: ~30 to 35 minutes

Dosing

Adult & Geriatric

Myelodysplastic syndromes (MDS): IV:

15 mg/m^2 over 3 hours every 8 hours (45 mg/m^2/day) for 3 days (135 mg/m^2/cycle) every 6 weeks; treatment is recommended for at least 4 cycles and may continue until the patient no longer benefits.

Adjustment for prolonged hematologic toxicity (ANC <1,000/mm^3 and platelets <50,000/mm^3):

>6 weeks but <8 weeks: Delay dose for up to 2 weeks and temporarily reduce dose to 11 mg/m^2 every 8 hours (33 mg/m^2/day) for 3 days (99 mg/m^2/cycle)

>8 weeks but <10 weeks: Assess for disease progression; if no disease progression, delay dose for up to 2 weeks and reduce dose to 11 mg/m^2 every 8 hours (33 mg/m^2/day) for 3 days (99 mg/m^2/cycle); maintain or increase dose with subsequent cycles if clinically indicated

or

20 mg/m^2 over 1 hour daily for 5 days every 28 days (delay subsequent treatment cycles until hematologic recovery [ANC ≥1,000/mm^3 and platelets ≥50,000/mm^3]); treatment is recommended for at least 4 cycles and may continue until the patient no longer benefits.

Acute myeloid leukemia (AML) (off-label use): Adults ≥60 years: IV: 20 mg/m^2 over 1 hour daily for 5 days every 28 days until relapse, disease progression, or unacceptable toxicity (Cashen 2010; Kantarjian 2012)

Renal Impairment

Preexisting impairment: There are no dosage adjustments provided in the manufacturer's labeling (has not been studied); use with caution.

Renal toxicity during treatment: Serum creatinine ≥2 mg/dL: Temporarily hold treatment until resolution.

Hepatic Impairment

Preexisting impairment: There are no dosage adjustments provided in the manufacturer's labeling (has not been studied); use with caution.

Hepatotoxicity during treatment: ALT and/or bilirubin ≥2 times ULN: Temporarily hold treatment until resolution.

Adjustment for Toxicity

Hematologic toxicity (ANC <1,000/mm^3 and platelets <50,000/mm^3): Delay and/or reduce dose; refer to adult dosing for recommendations specific to each MDS dosing regimen

Nonhematologic toxicity: Temporarily hold treatment until resolution for any of the following toxicities:

Serum creatinine ≥2 mg/dL

ALT, bilirubin ≥2 times ULN

Active or uncontrolled infection

Combination Regimens

Leukemia, acute myeloid: Decitabine (AML Regimen) on page 1936

Myelodysplastic syndrome: Decitabine (MDS Regimen) on page 1936

Administration Infuse over 1 to 3 hours. For the treatment of myelodysplastic syndromes, administer by IV infusion over 3 hours (15 mg/m^2 dose) or over 1 hour (20 mg/m^2 dose). For the treatment of acute myeloid leukemia (off-label use), administer by IV infusion over 1 hour (Cashen 2010; Kantarjian 2012). Premedication with antiemetics is recommended according to the manufacturer.

◄ Hazardous agent; use appropriate precautions for handling and disposal (NIOSH 2014 [group 1]).

Emetic Potential Children and Adults: Minimal (<10%)

Monitoring Parameters CBC with differential and platelets (with each cycle and more frequently if needed); liver enzymes (prior to treatment initiation and periodically); serum creatinine (prior to treatment initiation and periodically)

Dosage Forms Excipient information presented when available (limited, particularly for generics); consult specific product labeling.

Solution Reconstituted, Intravenous:
Dacogen: 50 mg (1 ea)
Generic: 50 mg (1 ea)

Deferasirox (de FER a sir ox)

Brand Names: US Exjade; Jadenu
Brand Names: Canada Exjade
Index Terms ICL670
Pharmacologic Category Chelating Agent
Use

Chronic iron overload due to transfusions: Treatment of chronic iron overload caused by blood transfusions (transfusional hemosiderosis) in patients 2 years and older.

Chronic iron overload in nontransfusion-dependent thalassemia syndromes: Treatment of chronic iron overload in patients 10 years and older with nontransfusion-dependent thalassemia syndromes and with a liver iron concentration (LIC) of at least 5 mg of iron per gram of liver dry weight (mg Fe/g dw) and a serum ferritin greater than 300 mcg/L (US labeling) or serum ferritin consistently above 800 mcg/L (Canadian labeling).

Limitations of use: Safety and efficacy of deferasirox in combination with other iron chelation therapies have not been established. Controlled studies of deferasirox in myelodysplastic syndromes and chronic iron overload due to transfusions have not been conducted.

Labeled Contraindications

Known hypersensitivity to deferasirox or any component of the formulation; CrCl <40 mL/minute or serum creatinine >2 times the age-appropriate ULN; poor performance status; high-risk myelodysplastic syndromes; advanced malignancies; platelet counts <50,000/mm^3

Canadian labeling: Additional contraindications (not in US labeling): MDS patients with <1 year life expectancy; CrCl <60 mL/minute

Pregnancy Considerations Adverse events were observed in animal reproduction studies. Information related to the use of deferasirox in pregnant women is limited (Vini 2011).

Breast-Feeding Considerations It is not known if deferasirox is excreted in breast milk. Due to the potential for serious adverse reactions in the nursing infant, the manufacturer recommends a decision be made to discontinue breast-feeding or to discontinue the drug, taking into account the importance of treatment to the mother.

Warnings/Precautions [US Boxed Warning]: Acute renal failure (including fatalities and cases requiring dialysis) may occur; observed more frequently in patients with comorbid conditions and advanced hematologic malignancies. Obtain serum creatinine and calculate creatinine clearance in duplicate at baseline prior to initiation, and monitor at least monthly thereafter; in patients with underlying renal dysfunction or at risk for acute renal failure, monitor creatinine weekly during the first

month then at least monthly thereafter. Dose reduction, interruption, or discontinuation should be considered for serum creatinine elevations. Monitor serum creatinine and/or CrCl more frequently if creatinine levels are increasing. Use with caution in renal impairment; dosage modification or treatment discontinuation may be required; reductions in initial dose are recommended for patients with CrCl 40 to 60 mL/minute; use is contraindicated in patients with CrCl <40 mL/minute (US labeling) or <60 mL/minute (Canadian labeling) or serum creatinine >2 times age-appropriate ULN. May cause proteinuria; monitor monthly. Renal tubular damage, including Fanconi syndrome, has also been reported, primarily in pediatric/adolescent patients with beta-thalassemia and serum ferritin levels <1,500 mcg/L.

[US Boxed Warning]: Hepatic injury and failure (including fatalities) may occur. Monitor transaminases and bilirubin at baseline, every 2 weeks for 1 month, then at least monthly thereafter. Hepatitis and elevated transaminases have also been reported. Hepatotoxicity is more common in patients >55 years of age and in patients with significant comorbidities (eg, cirrhosis, multiorgan failure). Reduce dose or temporarily interrupt treatment for severe or persistent increases in transaminases/bilirubin. [US Boxed Warning]: Avoid use in patients with severe (Child-Pugh class C) hepatic impairment; a dose reduction is required in patients with moderate (Child-Pugh class B) hepatic impairment. Monitor patients with mild (Child-Pugh class A) or moderate (Child-Pugh class B) impairment closely for efficacy and for adverse reactions requiring dosage reduction.

[US Boxed Warning]: Gastrointestinal (GI) hemorrhage (including fatalities) may occur; observed more frequently in elderly patients with advanced hematologic malignancies and/or low platelet counts; discontinue treatment for suspected GI hemorrhage or ulceration. Other GI effects including irritation and ulceration (sometimes complicated with GI perforation, including fatalities) have been reported. Use caution with concurrent medications that may increase risk of adverse GI effects (eg, NSAIDs, corticosteroids, anticoagulants, oral bisphosphonates). Monitor patients closely for signs/symptoms of GI ulceration/bleeding.

May cause skin rash (dose-related), including erythema multiforme; mild to moderate rashes may resolve without treatment interruption; for severe rash, interrupt and consider restarting at a lower dose with dose escalation and oral steroids; discontinue if erythema multiforme is suspected. Severe skin reactions, including Stevens-Johnson syndrome (SJS) and erythema multiforme, have also been reported; if suspected, discontinue immediately and evaluate. Do not reintroduce therapy. Hypersensitivity reactions, including severe reactions (anaphylaxis and angioedema) have been reported, onset is usually within the first month of treatment; discontinue if severe. Auditory (decreased hearing and high-frequency hearing loss) or ocular disturbances (lens opacities, cataracts, intraocular pressure elevation, and retinal disorders) have been reported (rare); monitor and consider dose reduction or treatment interruption. Bone marrow suppression (including agranulocytosis, neutropenia, thrombocytopenia, and worsening anemia) has been reported, risk may be increased in patients with preexisting hematologic disorders; monitor blood counts regularly; interrupt treatment in patients who develop cytopenias; may reinitiate once cause of cytopenia has been determined; use contraindicated if platelet count <50,000/mm^3. Potentially significant drug-drug interactions may exist, requiring dose or frequency adjustment, additional monitoring, and/or selection of alternative therapy. For transfusion-related iron overload, treatment should be initiated with evidence of chronic iron overload (ie, transfusion of ≥100 mL/kg of packed RBCs [eg, ≥20 units for a 40 kg individual] and serum ferritin consistently >1,000 mcg/L). For non-transfusion-dependent iron overload, initiate with liver iron concentration ≥5 mg Fe/g dry liver weight and serum ferritin >300 mcg/L. Prior to use, consider risk versus anticipated benefit with respect to individual patient's life expectancy and prognosis. Use with caution in elderly patients due to the higher incidence of toxicity (eg, hepatotoxicity) and fatal events during use. Overchelation of iron may increase development of toxicity; consider temporary interruption of treatment in transfusional iron overload when serum ferritin <500 mcg/L; in non-transfusion-dependent thalassemia when serum ferritin <300 mcg/L or hepatic iron concentration <3 mg Fe/g dry weight. May contain lactose; Canadian product labeling recommends avoiding use in patients with galactose intolerance, Lapp lactase deficiency, or glucose-galactose malabsorption syndromes. Deferasirox has a low affinity for binding with zinc and copper, may cause variable decreases in the serum concentration of these trace minerals.

Adverse Reactions Frequency not always defined.

>10%:

Central nervous system: Headache (Phatak 2010, Vichinsky 2007)

Dermatologic: Skin rash (dose related; 2% to 11%)

Gastrointestinal: Abdominal pain (dose related; 21% to 28%), nausea (dose related; 2% to 23%), vomiting (dose related; 10% to 21%), diarrhea (dose related; 5% to 20%)

Genitourinary: Proteinuria (19%)

Infection: Viral infection (Vichinsky 2007)

Renal: Increased serum creatinine (dose related; 2% to 38%)

Respiratory: Cough (Vichinsky 2007), nasopharyngitis (Vichinsky 2007)

1% to 10%:

Central nervous system: Fatigue (≤1%)

Hepatic: Increased serum ALT (2% to 8%)

Neuromuscular & skeletal: Arthralgia (Vichinsky 2007), back pain (Vichinsky 2007)

Respiratory: Pharyngolaryngeal pain (≤1%), respiratory tract infection (Vichinsky 2007), pharyngitis (Vichinsky 2007)

<1%, postmarketing, and/or case reports: Abnormal hepatic function tests, acute renal failure, agranulocytosis, alopecia, anaphylaxis, anemia (worsening), angioedema, anxiety, cataract, cholelithiasis, constipation (Vichinsky 2007), cytopenia, dizziness, drug fever, duodenal ulcer, dyschromia, edema, erythema multiforme, esophagitis, Fanconi's syndrome, fever, gastric ulcer, gastritis, gastrointestinal hemorrhage, gastrointestinal perforation, glycosuria, hearing loss (including high frequency), hematuria, hepatic failure, hepatic insufficiency, hepatitis, hyperactivity, hypersensitivity angiitis, hypersensitivity reaction, hypocalcemia, IgA vasculitis, increased intraocular pressure, increased serum bilirubin (Vichinsky 2007), insomnia, interstitial nephritis, maculopathy, neutropenia, nontuberculous mycobacterial infection, optic neuritis, pancreatitis (associated with gallstones), purpura, renal tubular disease, renal tubular necrosis, retinopathy, sleep disorder, Stevens-Johnson syndrome, thrombocytopenia, visual disturbance, urticaria

Drug Interactions

Metabolism/Transport Effects Substrate of UGT1A1; **Inhibits** CYP1A2 (moderate), CYP2C8 (moderate); **Induces** CYP3A4 (weak)

Avoid Concomitant Use
Avoid concomitant use of Deferasirox with any of the following: Aluminum Hydroxide; Amodiaquine; Theophylline; TiZANidine

Increased Effect/Toxicity
Deferasirox may increase the levels/effects of: Agomelatine; Amodiaquine; CYP1A2 Substrates; CYP2C8 Substrates; Pirfenidone; Repaglinide; Theophylline; TiZANidine

The levels/effects of Deferasirox may be increased by: Anticoagulants; Bisphosphonate Derivatives; Corticosteroids; Corticosteroids (Systemic); Nonsteroidal Anti-Inflammatory Agents

Decreased Effect
Deferasirox may decrease the levels/effects of: ARIPiprazole; CYP3A4 Substrates; Hydrocodone; NiMODipine; Saxagliptin

The levels/effects of Deferasirox may be decreased by: Aluminum Hydroxide; Bile Acid Sequestrants; Fosphenytoin; PHENobarbital; Phenytoin; Rifampin; Ritonavir

Food Interactions
Tablets for oral suspension: Bioavailability is increased variably when taken with food. Management: Take on an empty stomach at the same time each day at least 30 minutes before food. Maintain adequate hydration, unless instructed to restrict fluid intake.

Tablets: Bioavailability decreased slightly (not clinically meaningful) after a low-fat meal and increased after a high-fat meal. Management: Take on an empty stomach or with a light meal (containing ~250 calories and <7% fat content).

Storage/Stability Store at 25°C (77°F); excursions permitted to 15°C and 30°C (59°F and 86°F). Protect from moisture.

Mechanism of Action Selectively binds iron, forming a complex that is excreted primarily through the feces.

Pharmacodynamics/Kinetics
Distribution: Adults: 14.4 ± 2.7L

Protein binding: ~99% to serum albumin

Metabolism: Hepatic via glucuronidation by UGT1A1(primarily) and UGT1A3; minor oxidation by CYP450; undergoes enterohepatic recirculation

Bioavailability: Tablets for oral suspension: 70%; Tablets: 36% greater than tablets for oral suspension

Half-life elimination: 8 to 16 hours

Time to peak, plasma: Tablets and tablets for oral suspension: ~1.5 to 4 hours

Excretion: Feces (84%); urine (8%)

Dosing
Adult & Geriatric Note: Calculate dose to the nearest whole tablet size.

Conversion from Exjade to Jadenu: The dose for Jadenu should be ~30% lower (rounded to the nearest whole tablet).

Chronic iron overload due to transfusions: Oral: **Note:** Treatment should only be initiated with evidence of chronic iron overload (ie, transfusion of ≥100 mL/kg of packed red blood cells [eg, ≥20 units for a 40 kg individual] and serum ferritin consistently >1,000 mcg/L).

US labeling:

Exjade:

Initial: 20 mg/kg once daily

Maintenance: **Note:** Consider interrupting therapy for serum ferritin <500 mcg/L (risk of toxicity may be increased). Adjust dose every 3 to 6 months based on serum ferritin trends; adjust by 5 or 10 mg/kg/day;

titrate to individual response and treatment goals. In patients not adequately controlled with 30 mg/kg/day, doses up to 40 mg/kg/day may be considered for serum ferritin levels persistently >2,500 mcg/L and not decreasing over time (doses above 40 mg/kg/day are not recommended).

Jadenu:

Initial: 14 mg/kg once daily

Maintenance: **Note:** Consider interrupting therapy for serum ferritin <500 mcg/L (risk of toxicity may be increased). Adjust dose every 3 to 6 months based on serum ferritin trends; adjust by 3.5 or 7 mg/kg/day; titrate to individual response and treatment goals. In patients not adequately controlled with 21 mg/kg/day, doses up to 28 mg/kg/day may be considered for serum ferritin levels persistently >2,500 mcg/L and not decreasing over time (doses above 28 mg/kg/day are not recommended).

Canadian labeling: Dosing based on treatment goal and patient's individual transfusion rate:

Exjade:

Treatment goal: Maintenance of acceptable body iron levels:

Initial: 10 mg/kg once daily if transfused packed red blood cells (pRBCs) <7 mL/kg/month (approximately <2 units per month for an adult)

Initial: 20 mg/kg once daily if transfused pRBCs ≥7 mL/kg/month (approximately >2 units per month for an adult)

Treatment goal: Iron overload reduction:

Initial: 20 mg/kg once daily if transfused pRBCs <14 mL/kg/month (approximately <4 units per month for an adult)

Initial: 30 mg/kg once daily if transfused pRBCs ≥14 mL/kg/month (approximately >4 units per month for an adult)

Maintenance: **Note:** Consider interrupting therapy for serum ferritin <500 mcg/L (risk of toxicity may be increased).

Adjust dose every 3 to 6 months based on serum ferritin trends; adjust by 5 or 10 mg/kg/day; titrate to individual response and treatment goals. In patients with beta-thalassemia not adequately controlled with 30 mg/kg/day, doses up to 40 mg/kg/day may be considered. Do not exceed 30 mg/kg/day in non-beta-thalessemic patients.

Chronic iron overload in non-transfusion-dependent thalassemia syndromes: Oral:

US labeling: **Note:** Treatment should only be initiated with evidence of chronic iron overload (hepatic iron concentration ≥5 mg Fe/g dry weight and serum ferritin >300 mcg/L).

Exjade:

Initial: 10 mg/kg once daily. Consider increasing to 20 mg/kg once daily after 4 weeks if baseline hepatic iron concentration is >15 mg Fe/g dry weight.

Maintenance: Monitor serum ferritin monthly; if serum ferritin is <300 mcg/L, interrupt therapy and obtain hepatic iron concentration. Monitor hepatic iron concentration every 6 months; interrupt therapy if hepatic iron concentration <3 mg Fe/g dry weight. After 6 months of therapy, consider dose adjustment to a maximum of 20 mg/kg/day if hepatic iron concentration >7 mg Fe/g dry weight. Reduce dose to ≤10 mg/kg when hepatic iron concentration is 3 to 7 mg Fe/g dry weight. Do not exceed

20 mg/kg/day. After interruption, resume treatment when hepatic iron concentration >5 mg Fe/g dry weight.

Jadenu:

Initial: 7 mg/kg once daily. Consider increasing to 14 mg/kg once daily after 4 weeks if baseline hepatic iron concentration is >15 mg Fe/g dry weight.

Maintenance: Monitor serum ferritin monthly; if serum ferritin is <300 mcg/L, interrupt therapy and obtain hepatic iron concentration. Monitor hepatic iron concentration every 6 months; interrupt therapy if hepatic iron concentration <3 mg Fe/g dry weight. After 6 months of therapy, consider dose adjustment to a maximum of 14 mg/kg/day if hepatic iron concentration >7 mg Fe/g dry weight. Reduce dose to ≤7 mg/kg when hepatic iron concentration is 3 to 7 mg Fe/g dry weight. Do not exceed 14 mg/kg/day. After interruption, resume treatment when hepatic iron concentration >5 mg Fe/g dry weight.

Canadian labeling: **Note:** Treatment should only be initiated with evidence of chronic iron overload (hepatic iron concentration ≥5 mg Fe/g dry weight and serum ferritin consistently >800 mcg/L).

Exjade:

Initial: 10 mg/kg/day

Maintenance: Do not exceed 10 mg/kg/day in patients whose hepatic iron concentration was not evaluated and if serum ferritin ≤2,000 mcg/L. Monitor serum ferritin monthly; consider dose adjustment by 5 or 10 mg/kg/day every 3 to 6 months if hepatic iron concentration ≥7 mg Fe/g dry weight or serum transferrin levels consistently >2,000 mcg/L. Patients receiving >10 mg/kg should have their dose reduced to ≤10 mg/kg when hepatic iron concentration <7 mg Fe/g dry weight or serum ferritin <2,000 mcg/L. Interrupt therapy when hepatic iron concentration <3 mg Fe/g dry weight or serum ferritin <300 mcg/L. Doses above 20 mg/kg/day are not recommended.

Dosage adjustment with concomitant bile acid sequestrants (eg, cholestyramine, colesevelam, colestipol) or potent UGT inducers (eg, rifampin, phenytoin, phenobarbital, ritonavir): Avoid concomitant use; if coadministration necessary, consider increasing the initial dose of deferasirox dose by 50%; monitor serum ferritin and clinical response.

Pediatric Note: Calculate dose to the nearest whole tablet size. When calculating dose, consider changes in weight over time.

Chronic iron overload due to transfusions: Children ≥2 years and Adolescents: Refer to adult dosing.

Chronic iron overload in non-transfusion-dependent thalassemia syndromes: Children ≥10 years and Adolescents: Refer to adult dosing.

Conversion from Exjade to Jadenu: The dose for Jadenu should be ~30% lower (rounded to the nearest whole tablet).

Renal Impairment Creatinine clearance should be estimated using the Cockcroft-Gault formula.

Renal impairment at treatment initiation:

CrCl >60 mL/minute: No dosage adjustment necessary.

CrCl 40 to 60 mL/minute:

US labeling: Reduce initial dose by 50%.

Canadian labeling: Use is contraindicated

CrCl <40 mL/minute or serum creatinine >2 times age-appropriate ULN: Use is contraindicated.

◀ **Renal toxicity during treatment:**
US labeling:
Transfusional iron overload:
Adolescents ≥16 years and Adults: For increase in serum creatinine ≥33% above the average baseline, repeat within 1 week; if still elevated by ≥33%: Reduce daily dose by 10 mg/kg (for Exjade) **or** 7 mg/kg (for Jadenu)

Children ≥2 years to Adolescents 15 years: For increase in serum creatinine >33% above the average baseline level and above the age-appropriate ULN: Reduce daily dose by 10 mg/kg (for Exjade) **or** 7 mg/kg (for Jadenu)

All patients: CrCl <40 mL/minute or serum creatinine >2 times age-appropriate ULN: Discontinue treatment.

Non-transfusion-dependent thalassemia syndromes:
Adolescents ≥16 years and Adults: For increase in serum creatinine ≥33% above the average baseline, repeat within 1 week; if still elevated by ≥33%:

Exjade: Interrupt therapy if the dose is 5 mg/kg; reduce dose by 50% if the dose is 10 or 20 mg/kg

Jadenu: Interrupt therapy if the dose is 3.5 mg/kg; reduce dose by 50% if the dose is 7 or 14 mg/kg

Children ≥10 years to Adolescents 15 years: For increase in serum creatinine >33% above the average baseline level and above the age-appropriate ULN: Reduce daily dose by 5 mg/kg (for Exjade) **or** 3.5 mg/kg (for Jadenu)

All patients: CrCl <40 mL/minute or serum creatinine >2 times age-appropriate ULN: Discontinue treatment.

Canadian labeling:
Adolescents ≥16 years and Adults: For increase in serum creatinine >33% above the average pretreatment level for 2 consecutive weekly levels, reduce daily dose by 10 mg/kg.

Children ≥2 years and Adolescents <16 years: For increase in serum creatinine above the age-appropriate ULN for 2 consecutive levels, reduce daily dose by 10 mg/kg.

All patients: Progressive increase serum creatinine beyond ULN: Withhold treatment.

Hepatic Impairment
Hepatic impairment at treatment initiation:
Mild impairment (Child-Pugh class A): No dosage adjustment necessary; monitor closely for efficacy and for adverse reactions requiring dosage reduction.

Moderate impairment (Child-Pugh class B): Initial: Reduce dose by 50%; monitor closely for efficacy and for adverse reactions requiring dosage reduction.

Severe impairment (Child-Pugh class C): Avoid use.

Hepatic toxicity during treatment: Severe or persistent increases in transaminases/bilirubin: Reduce dose or temporarily interrupt treatment.

Adjustment for Toxicity
Bone marrow suppression: Interrupt treatment; may reinitiate once cause of cytopenia has been determined; use contraindicated if platelet count <50,000/mm^3

Dermatologic toxicity:
Rash (severe): Interrupt treatment; may reintroduce at a lower dose (with future dose escalation) and short-term oral corticosteroids.
Severe skin reaction (Stevens-Johnson syndrome, erythema multiforme): Discontinue and evaluate.
Gastrointestinal: Discontinue treatment for suspected GI ulceration or hemorrhage.
Hearing loss or visual disturbance: Consider dose reduction or treatment interruption.

Administration Oral:

Tablets (Jadenu): Swallow with water or other liquids at the same time each day. Take on an empty stomach or with a light meal (contains less than 7% fat content and ~250 calories). For patients who have difficulty swallowing whole tablets, may crush tablets and mix with soft foods (eg, yogurt, applesauce); consume entire mixture immediately after preparation (do not store for future use). Commercial crushers with serrated surfaces should be avoided for crushing a single 90 mg tablet.

Tablets for suspension (Exjade): Administer tablets by making an oral suspension; **do not chew or swallow tablets whole.** Completely disperse tablets in water, orange juice, or apple juice (use 3.5 ounces for total doses <1 g; 7 ounces for doses ≥1 g); stir to form a fine suspension and drink entire contents. Rinse remaining residue with more fluid; drink. Avoid dispersion of tablets in milk (due to slowed dissolution) or carbonated drinks (due to foaming) (Séchaud, 2008). Administer at same time each day on an empty stomach, at least 30 minutes before food. Do not take simultaneously with aluminum-containing antacids.

Do not take simultaneously with aluminum-containing antacids.

Monitoring Parameters Serum ferritin (baseline, monthly thereafter), iron levels (baseline), CBC with differential, serum creatinine and creatinine clearance (2 baseline assessments then monthly thereafter; in patients who are at increased risk of complications [eg, preexisting renal conditions, elderly, comorbid conditions, or receiving other potentially nephrotoxic medications]: weekly for the first month then at least monthly thereafter); hepatic iron concentration (non-transfusion-dependent thalassemia; baseline, every 6 months); urine protein (monthly); monitor serum creatinine and/or creatinine clearance more frequently if creatinine levels are increasing; serum transaminases (ALT/AST) and bilirubin (baseline, every 2 weeks for the first month, then monthly); baseline and annual auditory and ophthalmic examination (including slit lamp examinations and dilated fundoscopy); performance status (in patients with hematologic malignancies); signs/symptoms of GI ulcers or hemorrhage; cumulative number of RBC units received

Canadian labeling also recommends monitoring growth and body weight every 12 months in pediatric patients.

Dietary Considerations

Tablets for oral suspension: Bioavailability increased variably when taken with food; take on empty stomach 30 minutes before a meal.

Tablets: Bioavailability decreased slightly (not clinically meaningful) after a low-fat meal and increased after a high fat meal; take on an empty stomach or with a light meal (containing ~250 calories and <7% fat content).

Prescribing and Access Restrictions Deferasirox (Exjade) is only available through a restricted distribution program called EPASS Complete Care. Prescribers must enroll patients in this program in order to obtain the medication. For patient enrollment, contact 1-888-90-EPASS (1-888-903-7277).

◄ **Dosage Forms** Excipient information presented when available (limited, particularly for generics); consult specific product labeling.
Tablet, Oral:
  Jadenu: 90 mg, 180 mg, 360 mg
Tablet Soluble, Oral:
  Exjade: 125 mg, 250 mg, 500 mg

Deferiprone (de FER i prone)

Related Information
Safe Handling of Hazardous Drugs *on page 2292*

Brand Names: US Ferriprox

Index Terms APO-066

Pharmacologic Category Chelating Agent

Use
Transfusional iron overload: Treatment of transfusional iron overload due to thalassemia syndromes with inadequate response to other chelation therapy.
Limitation of use: Safety and effectiveness have not been established for the treatment of transfusional iron overload in patients with other chronic anemias.

Labeled Contraindications Hypersensitivity to deferiprone or any component of the formulation

Pregnancy Considerations Adverse effects have been observed in animal reproduction studies. Although there is limited data in humans, deferiprone may cause fetal harm if administered during pregnancy. During treatment with deferiprone in women of reproductive potential, pregnancy should be avoided.

Breast-Feeding Considerations It is not known if deferiprone is excreted in breast milk. Due to the potential for serious adverse reactions in the nursing infant, the manufacturer recommends a decision be made whether to discontinue nursing or to discontinue the drug, taking into account the importance of treatment to the mother.

Warnings/Precautions Hazardous agent - use appropriate precautions for handling and disposal (NIOSH 2014 [group 2]).

[US Boxed Warning]: May cause agranulocytosis, which may lead to serious infections (some fatal). Neutropenia may precede agranulocytosis; monitor absolute neutrophil count (ANC) prior to treatment initiation and weekly during therapy. If infection develops, interrupt treatment and monitor ANC more frequently. Patients should promptly report any symptoms which may indicate infection. Interrupt treatment if neutropenia (ANC <1,500/mm^3) develops; withhold other medications which may also be associated with neutropenia; monitor CBC, corrected WBC, ANC, and platelets daily until ANC recovery. If ANC <500/mm^3, consider hospitalization (and other clinically appropriate management); do not resume or rechallenge unless the potential benefits outweigh potential risks. Neutropenia and agranulocytosis were generally reversible upon discontinuation. Avoid concurrent use with other agents associated with neutropenia (or agranulocytosis).

ALT elevations in have been observed; monitor ALT and consider treatment interruption for persistent elevations. Lower plasma zinc concentrations have been observed; monitor zinc levels and supplement if necessary.

Adverse Reactions
>10%:
  Gastrointestinal: Nausea (13%)
  Genitourinary: Chromaturia (15%)

1% to 10%:

Central nervous system: Headache (3%)

Gastrointestinal: Abdominal pain/discomfort (10%), vomiting (10%), appetite increased (4%), diarrhea (3%), dyspepsia (2%), weight gain (2%), appetite decreased (1%)

Hematologic: Neutropenia (6% to 7%), agranulocytosis (2%)

Hepatic: ALT increased (8%), AST increased (1%)

Neuromuscular and skeletal: Arthralgia (10%), back pain (2%), limb pain (2%), arthropathy (1%)

<1%, postmarketing, and/or case reports: Acute respiratory distress syndrome, anaphylactic shock, atrial fibrillation, bilirubin increased, bruxism, cardiac failure, cerebellar syndrome, cerebral hemorrhage, chills, chondropathy, CPK increased, cryptococcal cutaneous infection, dehydration, depression, diplopia, enterocolitis, enteroviral encephalitis, epistaxis, fever, furuncle, gait disturbance, gastric ulcer, glycosuria, hemoglobinuria, hemoptysis, Henoch-Schönlein purpura (IgA vasculitis), hepatitis (infectious), hepatomegaly, hyperhydrosis, hyper-/hypotension, hypersensitivity, hypospadias, intracranial pressure increased, jaundice, metabolic acidosis, multiorgan failure, myositis, obsessive compulsive disorder, pancreatitis, pancytopenia, papilledema, parotid gland enlargement, periorbital edema, peripheral edema, pharyngitis, photosensitivity, pneumonia, pruritus, psychomotor skills impaired, pulmonary embolism, pustular rash, pyramidal tract syndrome, rash, rectal hemorrhage, retinal toxicity, seizure, sepsis, somnolence, subcutaneous abscess, thrombocytosis, torsade de pointes, trismus, urticaria, zinc levels decreased

Drug Interactions

Metabolism/Transport Effects Substrate of UGT1A6, UGT1A9, UGT2B15, UGT2B7

Avoid Concomitant Use There are no known interactions where it is recommended to avoid concomitant use.

Increased Effect/Toxicity

The levels/effects of Deferiprone may be increased by: UGT1A6 Inhibitors

Decreased Effect

The levels/effects of Deferiprone may be decreased by: Antacids; Calcium Salts; Iron Salts; Magnesium Salts; Multivitamins/Minerals (with ADEK, Folate, Iron); Multivitamins/Minerals (with AE, No Iron); Zinc Salts

Storage/Stability Store at 20°C to 25°C (68°F to 77°F); excursions permitted to 15°C to 30°C (59°F to 86°F).

Mechanism of Action Iron-chelating agent with affinity for ferric ion (iron III); binds to ferric ion and forms a 3:1 (deferiprone:iron) complex which is excreted in the urine. Has a lower affinity for other metals such as copper, aluminum, and zinc.

Pharmacodynamics/Kinetics

Absorption: Rapid

Distribution: 1.6 L/kg (in thalassemia patients)

Protein binding: <10%

Metabolism: Primarily by UGT 1A6; major metabolite (3-O-glucuronide) lacks iron-binding capacity

Half life elimination: 1.9 hours

Time to peak: ~1-2 hours

Excretion: Urine (75% to 90%; primarily as metabolite)

Dosing

Adult Note: Round dose to the nearest 250 mg (or 1/2 tablet). If serum ferritin falls consistently below 500 mcg/L, consider temporary treatment interruption.

Transfusional iron overload: Oral: Initial: 25 mg/kg 3 times/day (75 mg/kg/ day); individualize dose based on response and therapeutic goal; maximum dose: 33 mg/kg 3 times/day (99 mg/kg/day)

Geriatric Refer to adult dosing. Begin at the low end of dosing range.

Renal Impairment There are no dosage adjustments provided in the manufacturer's labeling (has not been studied).

Hepatic Impairment There are no dosage adjustments provided in the manufacturer's labeling (has not been studied).

Adjustment for Toxicity

ANC <1,500/mm^3: Interrupt treatment; do not rechallenge unless the potential benefit outweighs the risk

ANC 1,500/mm^3 and >500/mm^3: Interrupt treatment immediately and monitor until recovery; do not rechallenge unless the potential benefit outweighs the risk.

ANC <500/mm^3: In addition to treatment interruption, consider hospitalization (and other clinically-appropriate management); do not resume unless the potential benefits outweigh potential risks

Infection: Interrupt treatment; monitor ANC more frequently

Administration Administer in the morning, at mid day and in the evening. Administration with food may decrease nausea. Allow at least a 4-hour interval with foods containing polyvalent cations (iron, aluminum, zinc).

Hazardous agent - use appropriate precautions for handling and disposal (NIOSH 2014 [group 2]).

Monitoring Parameters Serum ferritin (every 2-3 months); ANC (at baseline and weekly during treatment); if ANC <1,500/mm^3, monitor CBC, WBC (corrected for nucleated RBCs), ANC, and platelets daily until ANC recovery; ALT (monthly); zinc levels; signs or symptoms of infection

Dietary Considerations May be taken with food to decrease nausea. Allow at least a 4-hour interval with foods containing iron, aluminum, and zinc.

Medication Guide Available Yes

Dosage Forms Excipient information presented when available (limited, particularly for generics); consult specific product labeling.

Tablet, Oral:

Ferriprox: 500 mg [scored]

Deferoxamine (de fer OKS a meen)

Brand Names: US Desferal

Brand Names: Canada Deferoxamine Mesylate for Injection; Desferal; PMS-Deferoxamine

Index Terms Deferoxamine Mesylate; Desferrioxamine; DFM

Pharmacologic Category Antidote; Chelating Agent

Use Adjunct in the treatment of acute iron intoxication; treatment of chronic iron overload secondary to multiple transfusions

Canadian labeling (off-label use in the U.S.): Diagnosis of aluminum overload; treatment of chronic aluminum overload in patients with end-stage renal failure undergoing maintenance dialysis

Labeled Contraindications Hypersensitivity to deferoxamine or any component of the formulation; patients with severe renal disease or anuria
Note: Canadian labeling does not include severe renal disease or anuria as contraindications.

Pregnancy Considerations Adverse events have been observed in animal reproduction studies. Toxic amounts of iron or deferoxamine have not been noted to cross the placenta; however, the metabolic effects of a maternal overdose may adversely affect the fetus. In case of acute iron toxicity, treatment during pregnancy should not be withheld (Chang 2011).

Breast-Feeding Considerations It is not known if deferoxamine is excreted in breast milk. The manufacturer recommends that caution be exercised when administering to nursing women.

Warnings/Precautions Flushing of the skin, hypotension, urticaria, and shock are associated with rapid IV infusion; administer IM, by slow subcutaneous or slow IV infusion only. Auditory disturbances (tinnitus and high frequency hearing loss) have been reported following prolonged administration, at high doses, or in patients with low ferritin levels; generally reversible with early detection and immediate discontinuation. Elderly patients are at increased risk for hearing loss. Audiology exams are recommended with long-term treatment. Ocular disturbances (blurred vision, cataracts, corneal opacities, decreased visual acuity, impaired peripheral, color, and night vision, optic neuritis, retinal pigment abnormalities, scotoma, visual loss/defect) have been reported following prolonged administration, at high doses, or in patients with low ferritin levels; generally reversible with early detection and immediate discontinuation. Elderly patients are at increased risk for ocular disorders. Periodic ophthalmic exams are recommended with long-term treatment.

Deferoxamine has been associated with acute respiratory distress syndrome following excessively high-dose IV treatment of acute iron intoxication or thalassemia (has been reported in children and adults). High deferoxamine doses and concurrent low ferritin levels are also associated with growth retardation. Growth velocity may partially resume to pretreatment velocity rates after deferoxamine dose reduction. Patients with iron overload are at increased susceptibility to infection with *Yersinia enterocolitica* and *Yersinia pseudotuberculosis*; treatment with deferoxamine may enhance this risk; if infection develops, discontinue therapy until resolved. Rare and serious cases of mucormycosis have been reported with use; withhold treatment with signs and symptoms of mucormycosis.

Increases in serum creatinine, acute renal failure and renal tubular disorders have been reported; monitor for changes in renal function. When iron is chelated with deferoxamine, the chelate is excreted renally. Deferoxamine is readily dialyzable. Treatment with deferoxamine in patients with aluminum toxicity may cause hypocalcemia and aggravate hyperparathyroidism. Deferoxamine may cause neurological symptoms (including seizure) in patients with aluminum-related encephalopathy receiving dialysis and may precipitate dialysis dementia onset.

Deferoxamine is **not** indicated for the treatment of primary hemochromatosis (treatment of choice is phlebotomy). Patients should be informed that urine may have a reddish color. Combination treatment with ascorbic acid (>500 mg/day in adults) and deferoxamine may impair cardiac function (rare), reversible upon discontinuation of ascorbic acid. If combination treatment is warranted, initiate ascorbic acid only after one month of regular deferoxamine treatment, do not exceed ascorbic acid dose of 200 mg/day for adults (in ▶

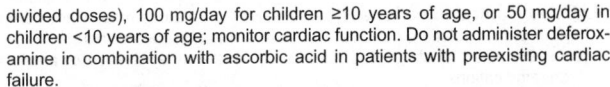

divided doses), 100 mg/day for children ≥10 years of age, or 50 mg/day in children <10 years of age; monitor cardiac function. Do not administer deferoxamine in combination with ascorbic acid in patients with preexisting cardiac failure.

Adverse Reactions Frequency not defined.

Cardiovascular: Flushing, hypotension, shock, tachycardia

Central nervous system: Brain disease (aluminum toxicity/dialysis-related), dizziness, headache, neuropathy (peripheral, sensory, motor, or mixed), paresthesia, seizure

Dermatologic: Skin rash, urticaria

Endocrine & metabolic: Growth suppression (children), hyperparathyroidism (aggravated), hypocalcemia

Gastrointestinal: Abdominal distress, abdominal pain, diarrhea, nausea, vomiting

Genitourinary: Dysuria, urine discoloration (reddish color)

Hematologic & oncologic: Dysplasia (metaphyseal; children <3 years; dose related), leukopenia, thrombocytopenia

Hepatic: Hepatic insufficiency, increased serum transaminases

Hypersensitivity: Anaphylaxis (with or without shock), angioedema, hypersensitivity

Infection: Infection (*Yersinia*, mucormycosis)

Local: Injection site reaction (burning, crust, edema, erythema, eschar, induration, infiltration, irritation, pain, pruritus, swelling, vesicles, wheal formation)

Neuromuscular & skeletal: Arthralgia, muscle spasm, myalgia

Ophthalmic: Blurred vision, cataract, chromatopsia, corneal opacity, decreased peripheral vision, decreased visual acuity, nocturnal amblyopia, optic neuritis, retinal pigment changes, scotoma, vision loss, visual field defect

Otic: Hearing loss, tinnitus

Renal: Acute renal failure, increased serum creatinine, renal tubular disease

Respiratory: Acute respiratory distress (dyspnea, cyanosis, and/or interstitial infiltrates), asthma

Miscellaneous: Fever

Drug Interactions

Metabolism/Transport Effects None known.

Avoid Concomitant Use There are no known interactions where it is recommended to avoid concomitant use.

Increased Effect/Toxicity

Deferoxamine may increase the levels/effects of: Prochlorperazine

The levels/effects of Deferoxamine may be increased by: Ascorbic Acid; Multivitamins/Fluoride (with ADE); Multivitamins/Minerals (with ADEK, Folate, Iron); Multivitamins/Minerals (with AE, No Iron)

Decreased Effect There are no known significant interactions involving a decrease in effect.

Storage/Stability Prior to reconstitution, store at ≤25°C (≤77°F). Following reconstitution, may be stored at room temperature for 24 hours, although the manufacturer recommends use begin within 3 hours of reconstitution. Do not refrigerate reconstituted solution. When stored at 30°C in polypropylene infusion pump syringes, deferoxamine 250 mg/mL in sterile water for injection retained 95% of initial concentration for 14 days (Stiles, 1996).

Preparation for Administration

IM: Reconstitute with sterile water for injection (500 mg vial with 2 mL SWFI; 2000 mg vial with 8 mL SWFI) to a final concentration of 213 mg/mL

IV: Reconstitute with sterile water for injection (500 mg vial with 5 mL SWFI; 2000 mg vial with 20 mL SWFI) to a final concentration of 95 mg/mL; further dilute for infusion in sodium chloride 0.9%, sodium chloride 0.45%, D_5W, or LR.

SubQ: Reconstitute with sterile water for injection (500 mg vial with 5 mL SWFI; 2000 mg vial with 20 mL SWFI) to a final concentration of 95 mg/mL

Mechanism of Action Complexes with trivalent ions (ferric ions) to form ferrioxamine, which is removed by the kidneys, slows accumulation of hepatic iron and retards or eliminates progression of hepatic fibrosis. Also known to inhibit DNA synthesis *in vitro*.

Pharmacodynamics/Kinetics

Absorption: IM, SubQ: Well absorbed

Distribution: Distributed throughout body fluids

Protein binding: <10%

Metabolism: Plasma enzymes; binds with iron to form ferrioxamine (iron complex)

Half-life elimination: 14 hours (plasma half-life: 20 to 30 minutes)

Excretion: Primarily urine (as unchanged drug and ferrioxamine); feces (via bile)

Dosing

Adult

Acute iron toxicity: Note: The IV route is used when severe toxicity is evidenced by cardiovascular collapse or systemic symptoms (coma, shock, metabolic acidosis, or gastrointestinal bleeding) or potentially severe intoxications (peak serum iron level >500 mcg/dL) (Perrone, 2011). When severe symptoms are not present, the IM route may be used (per the manufacturer).

IM, IV: Initial: 1,000 mg, may be followed by 500 mg every 4 hours for 2 doses; subsequent doses of 500 mg have been administered every 4 to 12 hours based on clinical response (maximum recommended dose: 6,000 mg/day [per manufacturer])

Canadian labeling:

IM: Initial: 90 mg/kg/dose (maximum/dose: 2,000 mg) followed by 45 mg/kg every 4 to 12 hours as needed (maximum: 6000 mg/24 hours)

IV: 15 mg/kg/hour up to a maximum of 80 mg/kg/dose or maximum of 6,000 mg/24 hours

Chronic iron overload:

IM: 500 to 1,000 mg/day (maximum: 1000 mg/day)

IV: 40 to 50 mg/kg/day (maximum: 60 mg/kg/day) over 8 to 12 hours for 5 to 7 days per week

SubQ: 1,000 to 2,000 mg/day or 20 to 40 mg/kg/day over 8 to 24 hours

Off-label dosing: IV, SubQ: 25 to 50 mg/kg over 8 to 10 hours 5 to 7 days per week (Brittenham, 2011)

Canadian labeling: IV, SubQ: 1,000 to 4,000 mg/day (20 to 60 mg/kg/day) over ~12 hours (may further increase iron excretion with infusion at the same dose over 24 hours). SubQ infusions are administered 4 to 7 days per week based on the degree of iron overload.

Diagnosis of aluminum-induced toxicity with CKD (off-label use; K/DOQI guidelines, 2003): IV: Test dose: 5 mg/kg during the last hour of dialysis if serum aluminum levels are 60 to 200 mcg/L, or clinical signs/symptoms of toxicity, or aluminum exposure prior to parathyroid surgery. Measure aluminum just prior to deferoxamine; remeasure 2 days later (test is positive if serum aluminum is ≥50 mcg/L). Do not use if aluminum serum levels are >200 mcg/L.

Canadian labeling: **Note:** Measure serum aluminum levels prior to and after administration of deferoxamine. IV: Test dose: 5 mg/kg/dose (infusion rate not to exceed 15 mg/kg/hour) following hemodialysis (preferred) or during the last hour of dialysis if serum aluminum levels are >60 mcg/L in association with serum ferritin levels >100 mcg/L; continuous rise in serum aluminum over the next 24 to 48 hours suggests overload. Remeasure serum aluminum levels prior to next hemodialysis, test is considered positive if serum aluminum levels increase >150 mcg/L above baseline.

Treatment of aluminum toxicity with CKD (off-label use; K/DOQI guidelines, 2003): IV:

Administer after diagnostic deferoxamine test dose. **Note:** The risk for deferoxamine-associated neurotoxicity is increased if aluminum serum levels are >200 mcg/L; withhold deferoxamine and administer intensive dialysis until <200 mcg/L.

Aluminum rise ≥300 mcg/L: 5 mg/kg once a week 5 hours before dialysis for 4 months

Aluminum rise <300 mcg/L: 5 mg/kg once a week during the last hour of dialysis for 2 months

Canadian labeling: Treatment should be considered for symptomatic patients with serum aluminum levels >60 mcg/L and a positive deferoxamine test dose.

Hemodialysis: IV: 5 mg/kg/dose (infusion rate not to exceed 15 mg/kg/hour) once weekly for 3 months following hemodialysis (preferred) or during the last hour of dialysis administered. Withhold treatment for 1 month then perform deferoxamine test. Further treatment is not recommended if 2 consecutive tests (performed 1 month apart) yield an increase in serum aluminum levels <75 mcg/L.

Continuous ambulatory or cyclic peritoneal dialysis: Intraperitoneal (preferred), IM, SubQ infusion (slow), or IV infusion (slow): 5 mg/kg/dose once weekly prior to final daily exchange

Geriatric Refer to adult dosing. May initiate at the lower end of the dosing range.

Pediatric

Acute iron toxicity: Children and Adolescents: **Note:** The IV route is used when severe toxicity is evidenced by cardiovascular collapse or systemic symptoms (coma, shock, metabolic acidosis, or gastrointestinal bleeding) or potentially severe intoxications (peak serum iron level >500 mcg/dL) (Perrone, 2011). When severe symptoms are not present, the IM route may be used (per the manufacturer).

IM: 90 mg/kg/dose every 8 hours (maximum: 6,000 mg/24 hours)

IV: 15 mg/kg/hour (maximum: 6,000 mg/24 hours)

Canadian labeling:

IM: Initial: 90 mg/kg/dose (maximum/dose: 1,000 mg) followed by 45 mg/kg every 4 to 12 hours as needed (maximum: 6,000 mg/24 hours)

IV: 15 mg/kg/hour up to a maximum of 80 mg/kg/dose or maximum of 6,000 mg/24 hours

Chronic iron overload: Children ≥3 years and Adolescents:

IV: 20 to 40 mg/kg/day over 8 to 12 hours for 5 to 7 days per week; dose should not exceed 40 mg/kg/day until growth has ceased

SubQ: 20 to 40 mg/kg/day over 8 to 12 hours (maximum: 1,000 to 2,000 mg/day)

Off-label dosing: IV, SubQ: 25 to 30 mg/kg over 8 to 10 hours 5 to 7 days per week (Brittenham, 2011)

Diagnosis of aluminum induced toxicity with CKD (off-label use; K/DOQI guidelines, 2003): Children and Adolescents: IV: Test dose: 5 mg/kg during the last hour of dialysis if serum aluminum levels are 60 to 200 mcg/L, or clinical signs/symptoms of toxicity, or aluminum exposure prior to para-thyroid surgery. Measure aluminum just prior to deferoxamine; remeasure 2 days later (test is positive if serum aluminum is ≥50 mcg/L). Do not use if aluminum serum levels are >200 mcg/L.

Treatment of aluminum toxicity with CKD (off-label use; K/DOQI guidelines, 2003): Children and Adolescents: IV: Administer after diagnostic deferoxamine test dose. **Note:** The risk for deferoxamine-associated neuro-toxicity is increased if aluminum serum levels are >200 mcg/L; withhold deferoxamine and administer intensive dialysis until <200 mcg/L.

Aluminum rise ≥300 mcg/L: 5 mg/kg once a week 5 hours before dialysis for 4 months

Aluminum rise <300 mcg/L: 5 mg/kg once a week during the last hour of dialysis for 2 months

Renal Impairment Severe renal disease or anuria: Use is contraindicated in the manufacturer's U.S. labeling.

The following adjustments have been used by some clinicians (Aronoff, 2007): Adults:

CrCl >50 mL/minute: No adjustment required

CrCl 10 to 50 mL/minute, CRRT: Administer 25% to 50% of normal dose

CrCl<10 mL/minute, hemodialysis, peritoneal dialysis: Avoid use

Hepatic Impairment There are no dosage adjustments provided in the manufacturer's labeling (has not been studied).

Administration

IV: Urticaria, flushing of the skin, hypotension, and shock have occurred following rapid IV administration; limiting infusion rate to 15 mg/kg/hour may help avoid infusion-related adverse effects.

Acute iron toxicity: The manufacturer states that the IM route is preferred; however, the IV route is generally preferred in patients with severe toxicity (ie, patients in shock). For the first 1,000 mg, infuse at 15 mg/kg/hour. Subsequent doses may be given over 4 to 12 hours at a rate not to exceed 125 mg/hour.

Chronic iron overload: Administer over 8 to 12 hours for 5 to 7 days per week; rate not to exceed 15 mg/kg/hour. In patients with poor compliance, defer-oxamine may be administered on the same day of blood transfusion, either prior to or following transfusion; do not administer concurrently with trans-fusion. Longer infusion times (24 hours) and IV administration may be required in patients with severe cardiac iron deposition (Brittenham, 2011).

Diagnosis or treatment of aluminum-induced toxicity with CKD: Administer dose over 1 hour, during the last hour of dialysis (K/DOQI guidelines, 2003).

SubQ: When administered for chronic iron overload, administration over 8 to 12 hours using a portable infusion pump is generally recommended; how-ever, longer infusion times (24 hours) may also be used. Topical anesthetic or glucocorticoid creams may be used for induration or erythema (Britten-ham, 2011).

IM: IM administration may be used for patients with acute iron toxicity that do not exhibit severe symptoms (per the manufacturer); may also be used in the treatment of chronic iron toxicity.

Monitoring Parameters Serum iron, ferritin, total iron-binding capacity, CBC with differential, renal function tests (serum creatinine), liver function tests, serum chemistries; ophthalmologic exam (visual acuity tests, fundoscopy, slit-lamp exam) and audiometry with long-term treatment; growth and body weight in children (every 3 months)

Dialysis patients: Serum aluminum (yearly; every 3 months in patients on aluminum-containing medications)

Aluminum-induced bone disease: Serum aluminum 2 days following test dose; test is considered positive if serum aluminum increases ≥50 mcg/L

Test Interactions TIBC may be falsely elevated with high serum iron concentrations or deferoxamine therapy. Imaging results may be distorted due to rapid urinary excretion of deferoxamine-bound gallium-67; discontinue deferoxamine 48 hours prior to scintigraphy.

Dietary Considerations Vitamin C supplements may need to be limited. The manufacturer recommends a maximum ascorbic acid dose of 200 mg/day in adults (given in divided doses), 100 mg/day in children ≥10 years of age, or 50 mg/day in children <10 years of age. Avoid concurrent use with ascorbic acid in patients with heart failure.

Dosage Forms Excipient information presented when available (limited, particularly for generics); consult specific product labeling. [DSC] = Discontinued product

Solution Reconstituted, Injection, as mesylate:
Desferal: 500 mg (1 ea); 2 g (1 ea [DSC])
Generic: 500 mg (1 ea); 2 g (1 ea)

◆ **Deferoxamine Mesylate** *see* Deferoxamine *on page* 488
◆ **Deferoxamine Mesylate for Injection (Can)** *see* Deferoxamine *on page* 488

Defibrotide (DE fib ro tide)

Index Terms DF; Prociclide

Pharmacologic Category Antiplatelet Agent; Thrombolytic Agent

Warnings/Precautions Predominant exclusion criteria from studies were clinically significant bleeding, >1 pressor agent to maintain blood pressure, neurotoxicity, intubated patients, grade B to D graft versus host disease (GVHD); grade B skin GVHD was allowed (Richardson, 2010; Richardson, 2011). Patients were excluded from studies if on prior or concurrent systemic tissue plasminogen activator use, concomitant anticoagulants (except when used for central line management or dialysis; patients on prior heparin were eligible if heparin was discontinued ≥12 hours prior to enrollment); or concomitant treatment with antithrombin III, other antithrombotics, ursodiol (unless for confirmed bile sludging), or nonsteroidal anti-inflammatory agents (Richardson, 2010). Defibrotide is derived from porcine tissue.

Adverse Reactions Frequency not defined.

Cardiovascular: Hypotension

Central nervous system: CNS hemorrhage, fever

Endocrine: Hot flashes

Gastrointestinal: Abdominal pain, cramping, diarrhea, diarrhea (hemorrhagic), gastrointestinal bleeding, hematemesis, mouth hemorrhage, nausea, vomiting

Hematologic: Hemorrhage/bleeding

Local: Thrombophlebitis

Renal: Hematuria, renal failure
Respiratory: Diffuse alveolar hemorrhage, epistaxis, pulmonary hemorrhage
Miscellaneous: Allergic reaction

Preparation for Administration Defibrotide was mixed in D_5W to a maximum concentration of 4 mg/mL (Richardson, 2010).

Mechanism of Action Defibrotide binds to and protects vascular hepatic endothelial cells (especially small vessels) by enhancing fibrinolysis and suppressing coagulation. Effects are local, with no significant effect on systemic coagulation. Has antithrombotic, anti-inflammatory, antiplatelet, and anti-ischemic properties.

Pharmacodynamics/Kinetics

Distribution: V_d: 0.04-0.05 L/kg (Palmer, 1993)
Excretion: Urine and feces (Palmer, 1993)

Dosing

Adult

Prevention of hepatic sinusoidal obstruction syndrome (SOS) in HSCT (off-label use): IV: 5 mg/kg twice daily for 21 days post-transplant (Dignan, 2007)

Treatment of hepatic SOS in HSCT (off-label use; begin treatment as soon as possible after SOS is suspected): IV: 6.25 mg/kg every 6 hours for at least 21 days (Richardson, 2009; Richardson, 2011)

Geriatric Refer to adult dosing.

Pediatric

Prevention of hepatic sinusoidal obstruction syndrome (SOS) in hematopoietic stem cell transplant (HSCT; off-label use): IV: 6.25 mg/kg every 6 hours beginning the same day as the conditioning regimen and continued for at least 14 and up to 30 days post-transplant (Corbacioglu, 2012)

Treatment of hepatic SOS in HSCT (off-label use; begin treatment as soon as possible after SOS is suspected): IV: Refer to adult dosing.

Administration IV: Infuse over 2 hours (Corbacioglu, 2012; Dignan, 2007; Richardson, 2002)

Monitoring Parameters Monitor for signs and symptoms of hepatic SOS; monitor for bleeding

Prescribing and Access Restrictions Defibrotide is an investigational agent available for the treatment of hepatic SOS through an Expanded Access Treatment IND Protocol (protocol 2006-05). Information on access is available at http://www.gentium.com/products/defibrotide/access-to-defibrotide.aspx.

Degarelix (deg a REL ix)

Related Information

Safe Handling of Hazardous Drugs on page 2292

Brand Names: US Firmagon

Brand Names: Canada Firmagon

Index Terms Degarelix Acetate; FE200486

Pharmacologic Category Antineoplastic Agent, Gonadotropin-Releasing Hormone Antagonist; Gonadotropin Releasing Hormone Antagonist

Use Prostate cancer, advanced: Treatment of advanced prostate cancer

Labeled Contraindications

Known hypersensitivity to degarelix or any component of the formulation; women who are or may become pregnant.

Documentation of allergenic cross-reactivity for drugs in this class is limited. However, because of similarities in chemical structure and/or pharmacologic actions, the possibility of cross-sensitivity can not be ruled out with certainty.

Pregnancy Considerations Adverse events were observed in animal reproduction studies. Use is contraindicated in women who are or may become pregnant.

Breast-Feeding Considerations It is not known if degarelix is excreted in breast milk. This product is not indicated for use in women.

Warnings/Precautions Hazardous agent - use appropriate precautions for handling and disposal (NIOSH 2014 [group 1]). Hypersensitivity reactions (including anaphylaxis, urticaria, and angioedema) have been reported. Discontinue for serious hypersensitivity reaction (immediately if dose not fully injected); manage hypersensitivity as clinically indicated. Do not rechallenge after serious hypersensitivity reaction.

Androgen deprivation therapy may prolong the QT interval; use with caution in patients with congenital long QT syndrome, a known history of QT prolongation or other risk factors for QT prolongation (eg, concomitant use of medications known to prolong QT interval, heart failure, and/or electrolyte abnormalities). Consider periodic electrolyte and ECG monitoring. Androgen-deprivation therapy may increase the risk for cardiovascular disease (Levine 2010) and decreased bone mineral density. Androgen deprivation therapy may be associated with an increased risk for insulin resistance and diabetes (Keating 2006).

Degarelix exposure is decreased in patients with hepatic impairment, dosage adjustment is not recommended in patients with mild-to-moderate hepatic impairment, although testosterone levels should be monitored. Has not been studied in patients with severe hepatic impairment; use with caution. Data for use in patients with moderate-to-severe renal impairment (CrCl <50 mL/minute) is limited; use with caution. Potentially significant drug-drug interactions may exist, requiring dose or frequency adjustment, additional monitoring, and/or selection of alternative therapy.

Adverse Reactions
>10%:

Central nervous system: Fatigue (3% to ≥10%)

Endocrine & metabolic: Hot flash (26%), increased gamma-glutamyl transferase (≥10%), weight loss (≥10%), weight gain (9% to ≥10%)

Hepatic: Increased serum transaminases (47%)

Local: Injection site reactions (35%, grade 3: ≤2%; pain at injection site [28%], erythema at injection site [17%], swelling at injection site [6%], induration at injection site [4%], injection site nodule [3%], injection site infection [including abscess, 1%])

Miscellaneous: Fever (1% to ≥10%)

1% to 10%:

Cardiovascular: Hypertension (6%)

Central nervous system: Chills (5%), dizziness (1% to 5%), headache (1% to 5%), insomnia (1% to 5%)

Dermatologic: Diaphoresis

Endocrine & metabolic: Hypercholesterolemia (3%), gynecomastia

Gastrointestinal: Constipation (5%), nausea (1% to 5%), diarrhea

Genitourinary: Urinary tract infection (5%), erectile dysfunction, testicular atrophy

Hepatic: Increased serum ALT (10%; grade 3: <1%), increased serum AST (5%; grade 3: <1%)

Immunologic: Antibody development (antidegarelix: 10%)

Neuromuscular & skeletal: Back pain (6%), arthralgia (5%), weakness (1% to 5%)

Miscellaneous: Night sweats (1% to 5%)

<1%, postmarketing, and/or case reports: Bone metastases (worsening), cerebrovascular accident, depression, hypersensitivity reaction (including anaphylaxis, urticaria, and angioedema), itching at injection site, local soreness/soreness at injection site, malignant lymphoma, mental status changes, myocardial infarction, osteoarthritis, prolonged Q-T interval on ECG, squamous cell carcinoma, unstable angina pectoris

Drug Interactions

Metabolism/Transport Effects None known.

Avoid Concomitant Use

Avoid concomitant use of Degarelix with any of the following: Indium 111 Capromab Pendetide

Increased Effect/Toxicity

Degarelix may increase the levels/effects of: Highest Risk QTc-Prolonging Agents; Moderate Risk QTc-Prolonging Agents

The levels/effects of Degarelix may be increased by: Mifepristone

Decreased Effect

Degarelix may decrease the levels/effects of: Indium 111 Capromab Pendetide

Storage/Stability Store at 25°C (77°F); excursions permitted to 15°C to 30°C (59°F to 86°F). Use within 1 hour of reconstitution. Do not shake the vials.

Preparation for Administration Hazardous agent; use appropriate precautions for handling and disposal (NIOSH 2014 [group 1]); wear gloves for preparation and administration. Reconstitute with provided prefilled syringe containing preservative free sterile water for injection (reconstitute each 120 mg vial with 3 mL; reconstitute the 80 mg vial with 4.2 mL). Swirl gently; do not shake (to prevent foaming). Dissolution usually takes a few minutes, although may take up to 15 minutes. May tilt the vial slightly if the powder adheres to the side of the vial. To withdraw for administration, turn the vial completely upside down and pull down on the plunger to withdraw all of the reconstituted solution from the vial to the syringe; expel all air bubbles. Administer within 1 hour of reconstitution. Use of concentrations other than those described in the manufacturer's labeling is not recommended.

Mechanism of Action Gonadotropin-releasing hormone (GnRH) antagonist which reversibly binds to GnRH receptors in the anterior pituitary gland, blocking the receptor and decreasing secretion of luteinizing hormone (LH) and follicle stimulation hormone (FSH), resulting in rapid androgen deprivation by decreasing testosterone production, thereby decreasing testosterone levels. Testosterone levels do not exhibit an initial surge, or flare, as is typical with GnRH agonists (Crawford 2011).

Pharmacodynamics/Kinetics

Onset of action: Rapid; ~96% of patients had testosterone levels ≤50 ng/dL within 3 days (Klotz 2008)

Distribution: V_d: >1000 L

Protein binding: ~90%

Metabolism: Hepatobiliary, via peptide hydrolysis

Bioavailability: Biphasic release: Rapid release initially, then slow release from depot formed after subcutaneous injection administration (Tornoe 2007). Bioavailability is decreased in patients with mild-to-moderate hepatic impairment.

Half-life elimination: Loading dose: SubQ: ~53 days

Time to peak, plasma: Loading dose: SubQ: Within 2 days

Excretion: Feces (~70% to 80%, primarily as peptide fragments); urine (~20% to 30%)

Dosing

Adult & Geriatric Prostate cancer, advanced: SubQ:

Loading dose: 240 mg administered as two 120 mg (3 mL) injections

Maintenance dose: 80 mg administered as one 4 mL injection every 28 days (beginning 28 days after initial loading dose)

Renal Impairment

CrCl 50 to 80 mL/minute: No dosage adjustment necessary.

CrCl <50 mL/minute: There are no dosage adjustments provided in the manufacturer's labeling; use with caution.

Hepatic Impairment

Mild-to-moderate hepatic impairment: No dosage adjustment necessary; monitor serum testosterone levels.

Severe hepatic impairment: There are no dosage adjustments provided in the manufacturer's labeling (has not been studied); use with caution.

Combination Regimens

Prostate cancer: Degarelix (Prostate Regimen) on page 1937

Administration Administer (deep) SubQ in the abdominal area by pinching skin and elevating SubQ tissue; insert needle at a 45 degree angle. Slowly inject over 30 seconds. For SubQ administration only; do not inject into a vein or into muscle. Avoid pressure exposed areas (eg, waistband, belt, or near ribs). Rotate injection site. Inject loading dose as two 3 mL injections (40 mg/mL) in different sites; maintenance dose should be administered as a single 4 mL injection (20 mg/mL); begin maintenance dose 28 days after initial loading dose.

Hazardous agent; use appropriate precautions for handling and disposal (NIOSH 2014 [group 1]).

Monitoring Parameters Prostate-specific antigen (PSA) periodically, serum testosterone levels (if PSA increases; in patients with hepatic impairment: monitor testosterone levels monthly until achieve castration levels, then consider monitoring every other month), liver function tests (at baseline); consider periodic monitoring of serum electrolytes (calcium, magnesium, potassium, sodium); bone mineral density; consider periodic ECG monitoring.

Screen for diabetes and cardiovascular risk (blood pressure, lipid profile, serum glucose) prior to initiating treatment and 3 to 6 months after initiation (Levine 2010).

Test Interactions Suppression of pituitary-gonadal function may affect diagnostic tests of pituitary gonadotropic and gonadal functions.

Dosage Forms Excipient information presented when available (limited, particularly for generics); consult specific product labeling.

Solution Reconstituted, Subcutaneous, as acetate:

Firmagon: 80 mg (1 ea); 120 mg (1 ea)

◆ **Degarelix Acetate** see Degarelix on page 495

◆ **Delta-9-tetrahydro-cannabinol** see Dronabinol on page 577

◆ **Delta-9 THC** *see* Dronabinol *on page 577*

◆ **Deltacortisone** *see* PredniSONE *on page 1426*

◆ **Deltadehydrocortisone** *see* PredniSONE *on page 1426*

◆ **Deltasone** *see* PredniSONE *on page 1426*

◆ **Demerol** *see* Meperidine *on page 1086*

◆ **4-Demethoxydaunorubicin** *see* IDArubicin *on page 862*

Denosumab (den OH sue mab)

Related Information
Hypercalcemia of Malignancy *on page 2241*

Brand Names: US Prolia; Xgeva

Brand Names: Canada Prolia; Xgeva

Index Terms AMG-162

Pharmacologic Category Bone-Modifying Agent; Monoclonal Antibody

Use

Hypercalcemia of malignancy (Xgeva): Treatment of hypercalcemia of malignancy refractory to bisphosphonate therapy

Osteoporosis/bone loss (Prolia): Treatment of osteoporosis in postmenopausal women at high risk of fracture; treatment of osteoporosis (to increase bone mass) in men at high risk of fracture; treatment of bone loss in men receiving androgen-deprivation therapy (ADT) for nonmetastatic prostate cancer; treatment of bone loss in women receiving aromatase inhibitor (AI) therapy for breast cancer

Tumors (Xgeva): Prevention of skeletal-related events (eg, fracture, spinal cord compression, bone pain requiring surgery/radiation therapy) in patients with bone metastases from solid tumors; treatment of giant cell tumor of the bone in adults and skeletally mature adolescents that is unresectable or where surgical resection is likely to result in severe morbidity

Limitation of use: Denosumab is NOT indicated for prevention of skeletal-related events in patients with multiple myeloma

Labeled Contraindications Hypersensitivity to denosumab or any component of the formulation; preexisting hypocalcemia; pregnancy (Prolia only)

Pregnancy Considerations Use of Prolia is contraindicated in pregnant women. Adverse events were observed in animal reproduction studies. Specifically, increased fetal loss, stillbirths, postnatal mortality, absent lymph nodes, abnormal bone growth, and decreased neonatal growth was observed in cynomolgus monkeys exposed to denosumab throughout pregnancy. Denosumab was measurable in the offspring at one month of age. Fetal exposure to monoclonal antibodies is expected to increase as pregnancy progresses. Women of reproductive potential should be advised to use effective contraception during denosumab treatment and for at least 5 months following the last dose. Studies of denosumab when used for osteoporosis/bone loss in men demonstrated that it is unlikely that a female partner or fetus would be exposed during unprotected sex to pharmacologically relevant denosumab concentrations via seminal fluid; however, exposure from seminal fluid of men receiving denosumab for other indications and higher doses is unknown and therefore their pregnant partners should be counseled regarding this potential risk.

Women exposed to denosumab during pregnancy should contact the Amgen Pregnancy Surveillance Program (800-772-6436).

Breast-Feeding Considerations It is not known if denosumab is excreted in breast milk. According to the manufacturer, the decision to discontinue denosumab or discontinue breast-feeding should take into account the benefits of treatment to the mother. In some animal studies, mammary gland development was impaired following exposure to denosumab during pregnancy, resulting in impaired lactation postpartum.

Warnings/Precautions Clinically significant hypersensitivity (including anaphylaxis) has been reported. May include throat tightness, facial edema, upper airway edema, lip swelling, dyspnea, pruritus, rash, urticaria, and hypotension. If anaphylaxis or clinically significant hypersensitivity occurs, initiate appropriate management and permanently discontinue. Denosumab may cause or exacerbate hypocalcemia; severe symptomatic cases (including fatalities) have been reported. An increased risk has been observed with increasing renal dysfunction, most commonly severe dysfunction (creatinine clearance <30 mL/minute and/or on dialysis), and with inadequate/no calcium supplementation. Monitor calcium levels; correct preexisting hypocalcemia prior to therapy. Monitor levels more frequently when denosumab is administered with other drugs that can also lower calcium levels. Use caution in patients with a history of hypoparathyroidism, thyroid surgery, parathyroid surgery, malabsorption syndromes, excision of small intestine, severe renal impairment/dialysis, or other conditions which would predispose the patient to hypocalcemia; monitor calcium, phosphorus, and magnesium closely during therapy (the manufacturer recommends monitoring within 14 days of injection [Prolia] or during the first weeks of therapy initiation [Xgeva]). Hypocalcemia lasting weeks to months (and requiring frequent monitoring) has been reported in postmarketing analyses. Administer calcium, vitamin D, and magnesium as necessary. Patients with severe renal impairment (CrCl <30 mL/minute) or those on dialysis may also develop marked elevations of serum parathyroid hormone (PTH). Incidence of infections may be increased, including serious skin infections, abdominal, urinary, ear, or periodontal infections. Endocarditis has also been reported following use. Patients should be advised to contact their healthcare provider if signs or symptoms of severe infection or cellulitis develop. Use with caution in patients with impaired immune systems or using concomitant immunosuppressive therapy; may be at increased risk for serious infections. Evaluate the need for continued treatment with serious infection.

Atypical femur fractures have been reported in patients receiving denosumab. The fractures may occur anywhere along the femoral shaft (may be bilateral) and commonly occur with minimal to no trauma to the area. Some patients experience prodromal pain weeks or months before the fracture occurs. Because these fractures also occur in osteoporosis patients not treated with denosumab, it is unclear if denosumab therapy is the cause for the fractures; concomitant glucocorticoids may contribute to fracture risk. Advise patients to report new/unusual hip, thigh, or groin pain; and if so, evaluate for atypical/incomplete fracture. Contralateral limb should be assessed if atypical fracture occurs. Consider interrupting therapy in patients who develop an atypical femoral fracture. Osteonecrosis of the jaw (ONJ) has been reported in patients receiving denosumab. ONJ may manifest as jaw pain, osteomyelitis, osteitis, bone erosion, tooth/periodontal infection, toothache, gingival ulceration/erosion. Risk factors include invasive dental procedures (eg, tooth extraction, dental implants, boney surgery); a diagnosis of cancer, concomitant chemotherapy, corticosteroids, immunosuppressive therapy, or angiogenesis inhibitors, poor oral hygiene, ill-fitting dentures; and comorbid disorders (anemia, coagulopathy, diabetes, infection, gingival infections, and other preexisting dental disease). Concomitant use with other medications associated with this condition may increase the risk of developing ONJ. In studies of patients with osseous metastasis, a longer duration of denosumab exposure was associated with a higher incidence of ONJ. Patients should maintain good oral hygiene during treatment. A dental exam and preventive dentistry is recommended prior to therapy initiation. The benefit:risk must be assessed by the treating physician and/or dentist/surgeon prior to any invasive dental procedure; avoid invasive procedures in patients with bone metastases receiving therapy for prevention of skeletal-related events. Patients developing ONJ while on denosumab therapy should receive care by a dentist or oral surgeon; extensive dental surgery to treat ONJ may exacerbate ONJ; evaluate individually and consider interrupting or discontinuing therapy if extensive dental surgery is necessary. Severe and occasionally incapacitating bone, joint, and/or muscle pain has been reported (time to onset of symptoms has varied from one day to several months after initiating therapy). Consider discontinuing use if severe symptoms develop.

Postmenopausal osteoporosis: For use in women at high risk for fracture which is defined as a history of osteoporotic fracture or multiple risk factors for fracture. May also be used in women who failed or did not tolerate other therapies.

Bone metastases: Denosumab is not indicated for the prevention of skeletal-related events in patients with multiple myeloma. In trials of with multiple myeloma patients, denosumab was noninferior to zoledronic acid in delaying time to first skeletal-related event and mortality was increased in a subset of the denosumab-treated group.

Breast cancer: The American Society of Clinical Oncology (ASCO) updated guidelines on the role of bone-modifying agents (BMAs) in the prevention and treatment of skeletal-related events for metastatic breast cancer patients (Van Poznak 2011). The guidelines recommend initiating a BMA (denosumab, pamidronate, zoledronic acid) in patients with metastatic breast cancer to the bone. There is currently no literature indicating the superiority of one particular BMA. Optimal duration is not defined; however, the guidelines recommend continuing therapy until substantial decline in patient's performance status. The ASCO guidelines are in alignment with package insert guidelines for dosing, renal dose adjustments, infusion times, prevention and management of osteonecrosis of the jaw, and monitoring of laboratory parameter recommendations. BMAs are not the first-line therapy for pain. BMAs are to be used as adjunctive therapy for cancer-related bone pain associated with bone metastasis, demonstrating a modest pain control benefit. BMAs should be used in conjunction with agents such as NSAIDs, opioid and nonopioid analgesics, corticosteroids, radiation/surgery, and interventional procedures.

Denosumab therapy results in significant suppression of bone turnover; the long term effects of treatment are not known but may contribute to adverse outcomes such as ONJ, atypical fractures, or delayed fracture healing; monitor. Use with caution in patients with renal impairment (CrCl <30 mL/minute) or patients on dialysis; risk of hypocalcemia is increased. Dose adjustment is not needed when administered at 60 mg every 6 months (Prolia); once-monthly dosing has not been evaluated in patients with renal impairment (Xgeva). Dermatitis, eczema, and rash (which are not necessarily specific to the injection site) have been reported; consider discontinuing if severe symptoms occur. Packaging may contain natural latex rubber. May impair bone growth in children with open growth plates or inhibit eruption of dentition. In pediatrics, indicated only for the treatment of giant cell tumor of the bone in adolescents who are skeletally mature. Do not administer Prolia and Xgeva to the same patient for different indications. Denosumab is intended for subcutaneous route only and should not be administered intravenously, intramuscularly, or intradermally.

Adverse Reactions A postmarketing safety program for Prolia is available to collect information on adverse events; more information is available at http://www.proliasafety.com. To report adverse events for either Prolia or Xgeva, prescribers may also call Amgen at 800-772-6436 or FDA at 800-332-1088.

Percentages noted with Prolia (60 mg every 6 months) unless specified as Xgeva (120 mg every 4 weeks):

>10%:

Cardiovascular: Hypertension (11%, Lewiecki 2007)

Central nervous system: Fatigue (Xgeva: ≤45%), headache (Xgeva: 13% to 24%), peripheral edema (5%; Xgeva: 24%)

Dermatologic: Dermatitis (4% to 11%), eczema (4% to 11%), skin rash (3% to 11%)

Endocrine & metabolic: Hypophosphatemia (Xgeva: 32%; grade 3: 10% to 15%), hypocalcemia (2%; Xgeva: 3% to 18%; grade 3: 3%)

Gastrointestinal: Nausea (Xgeva: 31%), decreased appetite (Xgeva: 24%), vomiting (Xgeva: 24%), constipation (Xgeva: 21%), diarrhea (Xgeva: 20%)

Hematologic & oncologic: Anemia (Xgeva: 21%)

Infection: Influenza (11%, Lewiecki 2007)

Neuromuscular & skeletal: Weakness (Xgeva: ≤45%), arthralgia (7% to 14%), limb pain (10% to 12%), back pain (8% to 12%)

Respiratory: Dyspnea (Xgeva: 21% to 27%), cough (Xgeva: 15%)

1% to 10%:

Cardiovascular: Angina pectoris (3%)

Central nervous system: Sciatica (5%)

Endocrine & metabolic: Hypercholesterolemia (7%)

Gastrointestinal: Flatulence (2%)

Hematologic & oncologic: Malignant neoplasm (new; 3% to 5%)

Infection: Serious infection (4%)

Neuromuscular & skeletal: Musculoskeletal pain (6%), ostealgia (4%), myalgia (3%), osteonecrosis (jaw; ≤2%; Xgeva ≤2%)

Ophthalmic: Cataract (≤5%)

Respiratory: Nasopharyngitis (7%), upper respiratory tract infection (5%)

<1%, postmarketing, and/or case reports: Anaphylaxis (both formulations), antibody development (both formulations), endocarditis, erythema, facial swelling, femur fracture (both formulations; diaphyseal, subtrochanteric), hypersensitivity (both formulations), hypotension, pancreatitis, severe hypocalcemia (symptomatic; both formulations), urticaria

Drug Interactions

Metabolism/Transport Effects None known.

Avoid Concomitant Use

Avoid concomitant use of Denosumab with any of the following: Belimumab

Increased Effect/Toxicity

Denosumab may increase the levels/effects of: Belimumab; Immunosuppressants

Decreased Effect There are no known significant interactions involving a decrease in effect.

Storage/Stability Store in original carton under refrigeration at 2°C to 8°C (36°F to 46°F). Do not freeze. Prior to use, bring to room temperature of 25°C (77°F) in original container (usually takes 15 to 30 minutes); do not use any other methods for warming. Use within 14 days once at room temperature. Protect from direct heat and light; do not expose to temperatures >25°C (77°F). Avoid vigorous shaking.

Mechanism of Action Denosumab is a monoclonal antibody with affinity for nuclear factor-kappa ligand (RANKL). Osteoblasts secrete RANKL; RANKL activates osteoclast precursors and subsequent osteolysis which promotes release of bone-derived growth factors, such as insulin-like growth factor-1 (IGF1) and transforming growth factor-beta (TGF-beta), and increases serum calcium levels. Denosumab binds to RANKL, blocks the interaction between RANKL and RANK (a receptor located on osteoclast surfaces), and prevents osteoclast formation, leading to decreased bone resorption and increased bone mass in osteoporosis. In solid tumors with bony metastases, RANKL inhibition decreases osteoclastic activity leading to decreased skeletal related events and tumor-induced bone destruction. In giant cell tumors of the bone (which express RANK and RANKL), denosumab inhibits tumor growth by preventing RANKL from activating its receptor (RANK) on the osteoclast surface, osteoclast precursors, and osteoclast-like giant cells.

Pharmacodynamics/Kinetics

Onset of action: Decreases markers of bone resorption by ~85% within 3 days; maximal reductions observed within 1 month

Hypercalcemia of malignancy: Time to response (median): 9 days; Time to complete response (median): 23 days (Hu 2014)

Duration: Markers of bone resorption return to baseline within 12 months of discontinuing therapy

Hypercalcemia of malignancy: Duration of response (median): 104 days; Duration of complete response (median): 34 days (Hu 2014)

Bioavailability: SubQ: 62%

Half-life elimination: ~25 to 28 days

Time to peak, serum: 10 days (range: 3 to 21 days)

Dosing

Adult & Geriatric Note: Administer calcium and vitamin D as necessary to prevent or treat hypocalcemia

Hypercalcemia of malignancy (Xgeva): SubQ: 120 mg every 4 weeks; during the first month, give an additional 120 mg on days 8 and 15 (Hu 2014)

Prevention of skeletal-related events in bone metastases from solid tumors (Xgeva): SubQ: 120 mg every 4 weeks (Fizazi 2011; Henry 2011; Stopeck 2010)

Treatment of androgen deprivation-induced bone loss in men with prostate cancer (Prolia): SubQ: 60 mg as a single dose, once every 6 months (Smith 2009)

Treatment of aromatase inhibitor-induced bone loss in women with breast cancer (Prolia): SubQ: 60 mg as a single dose, once every 6 months (Ellis 2008)

Treatment of giant cell tumor of the bone (Xgeva): SubQ: 120 mg once every 4 weeks; during the first month, give an additional 120 mg on days 8 and 15 (Blay 2011; Thomas 2010)

Treatment of osteoporosis in men or postmenopausal women (Prolia): SubQ: 60 mg as a single dose, once every 6 months

◄ **Pediatric Note:** Administer calcium and vitamin D as necessary to prevent or treat hypocalcemia

Treatment of giant cell tumor of the bone (Xgeva): Adolescents (skeletally mature) 13 to 17 years: SubQ: 120 mg once every 4 weeks; during the first month, give an additional 120 mg on days 8 and 15

Renal Impairment Monitor patients with severe impairment (CrCl <30 mL/minute or on dialysis) due to increased risk of hypocalcemia.

Prolia: No dosage adjustment is necessary.

Xgeva: There are no dosage adjustments provided in the manufacturer's labeling. However, in studies of patients with varying degrees of renal impairment, the degree of renal impairment had no effect on denosumab pharmacokinetics or pharmacodynamics.

Hepatic Impairment There are no dosage adjustments provided in the manufacturer's labeling (has not been studied).

Administration SubQ: Denosumab is intended for subcutaneous route only and should not be administered intravenously, intramuscularly, or intradermally. Prior to administration, bring to room temperature in original container (allow to stand ~15 to 30 minutes); do not warm by any other method. Solution may contain trace amounts of translucent to white protein particles; do not use if cloudy, discolored (normal solution should be clear and colorless to pale yellow), or contains excessive particles or foreign matter. Avoid vigorous shaking. Administer via SubQ injection in the upper arm, upper thigh, or abdomen.

Prolia: If a dose is missed, administer as soon as possible, then continue dosing every 6 months from the date of the last injection.

Monitoring Parameters Recommend monitoring of serum creatinine, serum calcium, phosphorus and magnesium (especially within the first 14 days of therapy [Prolia] or during the first weeks of therapy initiation [Xgeva]), signs and symptoms of hypocalcemia, especially in patients predisposed to hypocalcemia (severe renal impairment, thyroid/parathyroid surgery, malabsorption syndromes, hypoparathyroidism); infection, or dermatologic reactions; routine oral exam (prior to treatment); dental exam if risk factors for ONJ; monitor for sings/symptoms of hypersensitivity

Osteoporosis: Bone mineral density (BMD) should be re-evaluated every 2 years (or more frequently) after initiating therapy (NOF 2014); annual measurements of height and weight, assessment of chronic back pain; serum calcium and 25(OH)D; may consider monitoring biochemical markers of bone turnover

Dietary Considerations Ensure adequate calcium and vitamin D intake to prevent or treat hypocalcemia. Calcium 1000 mg/day and vitamin D ≥400 units/day is recommended in product labeling (Prolia). If dietary intake is inadequate, dietary supplementation is recommended. Women and men should consume:

Calcium: 1000 mg/day (men 50 to 70 years) **or** 1200 mg/day (women ≥51 years and men ≥71 years) (IOM 2011; NOF 2014)

Vitamin D: 800 to 1000 units/day (men and women ≥50 years) (NOF 2014). Recommended Dietary Allowance (RDA): 600 units/day (men and women ≤70 years) **or** 800 units/day (men and women ≥71 years) (IOM 2011).

Medication Guide Available Yes

Dosage Forms Excipient information presented when available (limited, particularly for generics); consult specific product labeling.
Solution, Subcutaneous [preservative free]:
Prolia: 60 mg/mL (1 mL) [contains mouse protein (murine) (hamster)]
Xgeva: 120 mg/1.7 mL (1.7 mL)

Desmopressin (des moe PRES in)

Brand Names: US DDAVP; DDAVP Rhinal Tube; Stimate
Brand Names: Canada Apo-Desmopressin; DDAVP; DDAVP Melt; DDAVP Rhinyle; Nocdurna; Octostim; PMS-Desmopressin; Teva-Desmopressin
Index Terms 1-Deamino-8-D-Arginine Vasopressin; Desmopressin Acetate
Pharmacologic Category Antihemophilic Agent; Hemostatic Agent; Hormone, Posterior Pituitary; Vasopressin Analog, Synthetic
Use

Injection:

Diabetes insipidus: Antidiuretic replacement therapy in the management of central (cranial) diabetes insipidus; management of the temporary polyuria and polydipsia following head trauma or surgery in the pituitary region.
Limitations of use: Desmopressin is ineffective for the treatment of nephrogenic diabetes insipidus.

Hemophilia A: For use in patients with hemophilia A with factor VIII coagulant activity levels >5% to maintain hemostasis during surgical procedures and postoperatively when administered 30 minutes prior to the scheduled procedure and to also stop bleeding due to spontaneous or trauma-induced injuries, such as hemarthroses, intramuscular hematomas, or mucosal bleeding.
Limitations of use: Not indicated for the treatment of hemophilia A with factor VIII coagulant activity levels ≤5%, for the treatment of hemophilia B, or in patients who have factor VIII antibodies. In certain clinical situations, it may be justified to try desmopressin with careful monitoring in patients with factor VIII levels between 2% and 5%.

Von Willebrand disease (type 1): For use in patients with mild to moderate classic von Willebrand disease (type 1) with factor VIII coagulant activity levels >5% to maintain hemostasis during surgical procedures and

◀ postoperatively when administered 30 minutes prior to the scheduled procedure and to stop bleeding due to spontaneous or trauma-induced injuries, such as hemarthroses, intramuscular hematomas, or mucosal bleeding.

Limitations of use: Patients with von Willebrand disease who are least likely to respond are those with severe homozygous von Willebrand disease with factor VIII coagulant activity and factor VIII von Willebrand factor antigen levels <1%; other patients may respond (variable) depending on the type of molecular defect they have. Check bleeding time and factor VIII coagulant activity, ristocetin cofactor activity, and von Willebrand factor antigen during administration of desmopressin to ensure that adequate levels are being achieved. Not indicated for the treatment of severe classic von Willebrand disease (type I) or when there is evidence of an abnormal molecular form of factor VIII antigen.

Intranasal:

Diabetes insipidus (DDAVP Rhinal tube): Antidiuretic replacement therapy in the management of central (cranial) diabetes insipidus; management of the temporary polyuria and polydipsia following head trauma or surgery in the pituitary region.

Limitation of use: Desmopressin is ineffective for the treatment of nephrogenic diabetes insipidus.

Hemophilia A (Stimate): For use in patients with hemophilia A with factor VIII coagulant activity levels >5% and to stop bleeding due to spontaneous or trauma-induced injuries, such as hemarthroses, intramuscular hematomas, or mucosal bleeding.

Limitations of use: Not indicated for the treatment of hemophilia A with factor VIII coagulant activity levels ≤5%, for the treatment of hemophilia B, or in patients who have factor VIII antibodies.

von Willebrand disease (type 1) (Stimate): For use in patients with mild to moderate classic von Willebrand disease (type 1) with factor VIII coagulant activity levels >5% and to stop bleeding due to spontaneous or trauma-induced injuries, such as hemarthroses, intramuscular hematomas, mucosal bleeding, or menorrhagia.

Limitations of use: Not indicated for the treatment of severe classic von Willebrand disease (type 1) or when there is evidence of an abnormal molecular form of factor VIII antigen.

Tablets:

Diabetes insipidus: Antidiuretic replacement therapy in the management of central diabetes insipidus; management of the temporary polyuria and polydipsia following head trauma or surgery in the pituitary region.

Limitation of use: Desmopressin is ineffective for the treatment of nephrogenic diabetes insipidus.

Primary nocturnal enuresis: Management of primary nocturnal enuresis, either alone or as an adjunct to behavioral conditioning or other non-pharmacologic intervention.

Labeled Contraindications Known hypersensitivity to desmopressin acetate or any component of the formulations; hyponatremia or a history of hyponatremia; moderate-to-severe renal impairment (CrCl <50 mL/minute). There are no contraindications listed in the Stimate prescribing information.

Canadian labeling: Additional contraindications (not in US labeling): Type 2B or platelet-type (pseudo) von Willebrand's disease (injection, intranasal, oral, sublingual); known hyponatremia, habitual or psychogenic polydipsia, cardiac insufficiency or other conditions requiring diuretic therapy (intranasal, sublingual); nephrosis, severe hepatic dysfunction (sublingual); primary nocturnal enuresis (intranasal)

Pregnancy Considerations Adverse events were not observed in animal reproduction studies. Anecdotal reports suggest congenital anomalies and low birth weight. However, causal relationship has not been established. Desmopressin has been used safely throughout pregnancy for the treatment of diabetes insipidus (Brewster, 2005; Schrier, 2010). The use of desmopressin is limited for the treatment of von Willebrand disease in pregnant women (NHLBI, 2007).

Breast-Feeding Considerations It is not known if desmopressin is excreted in breast milk. The manufacturer recommends that caution be exercised when administering desmopressin to nursing women.

Warnings/Precautions Severe allergic reactions have been reported with desmopressin; anaphylactic reactions have only occurred rarely with IV and intranasal administration. Desmopressin use may rarely lead to hyponatremia with associated signs and symptoms (eg, nausea/vomiting, headache, depressed reflexes, disorientation, irritability, muscle weakness/spasms/cramps) and extreme decreases in plasma osmolality, resulting in seizures, coma, respiratory arrest, and death. Risk factors for hyponatremia with desmopressin use include cystic fibrosis, renal dysfunction, heart failure, young age, advanced age, inappropriate high fluid intake, a higher than recommended dose, and concomitant use of medications known to either increase thirst or cause syndrome of inappropriate ADH secretion (SIADH). Fluid restriction during use is recommended. Monitor for signs/symptoms of hyponatremia Fluid intake should be adjusted downward in the elderly and in very young patients to decrease the possibility of water intoxication and hyponatremia. Use with caution in patients with habitual or psychogenic polydipsia. Patients consuming excessive amounts of water are at greater risk of hyponatremia. Use in these patients is contraindicated in Canadian labeling. Patients should be instructed to restrict fluid intake from 1 hour before to 8 hours after taking desmopressin tablets.

Acute cerebrovascular thrombosis and acute myocardial infarction have occurred (rare) with desmopressin injection; use with caution in patients predisposed to thrombus formation. Patients with type 2B von Willebrand disease requiring hemostasis should not be treated with desmopressin since may result in platelet aggregation, thrombocytopenia, and possibly thrombosis. Injection and intranasal desmopressin may cause a slight increase or transient decrease in blood pressure, and a compensatory increase in heart rate. Use with caution in patients with coronary artery insufficiency and/or hypertensive cardiovascular disease.

When using desmopressin for primary nocturnal enuresis, treatment should be interrupted if the patient experiences an acute illness (eg, fever, recurrent vomiting or diarrhea), vigorous exercise, or any condition associated with an increase in water consumption to prevent hyponatremia.

Consider alternative route of administration if changes in the nasal mucosa due to intranasal use (scarring, edema) occur leading to unreliable absorption. Some patients may demonstrate a change in response after long-term therapy (>6 months) characterized as decreased response or a shorter duration of response. Consider alternative route of administration (IV or intranasal) with inadequate therapeutic response at maximum recommended oral doses.

◄ **Adverse Reactions** Frequency may not be defined (may be dose or route related).

Cardiovascular: Decreased blood pressure (IV), increased blood pressure (IV), flushing (facial)

Central nervous system: Headache (2% to 5%), dizziness (intranasal; ≤3%), chills (intranasal; 2%), nostril pain (intranasal; ≤2%)

Dermatologic: Skin rash

Endocrine & metabolic: Hyponatremia, water intoxication

Gastrointestinal: Abdominal pain (intranasal; 2%) gastrointestinal disease (intranasal; ≤2%), nausea (intranasal; ≤2%), abdominal cramps, sore throat

Hepatic: Increased serum transaminases (transient; associated primarily with tablets)

Local: Burning sensation at injection site, erythema at injection site, swelling at injection site

Neuromuscular & Skeletal: Weakness (intranasal; ≤2%)

Ophthalmic: Abnormal lacrimation (intranasal; ≤2%), conjunctivitis (intranasal; ≤2%), ocular edema (intranasal; ≤2%)

Respiratory: Rhinitis (intranasal; 3% to 8%), epistaxis (intranasal; ≤3%), cough, nasal congestion, upper respiratory tract infection

<1%, postmarketing, and/or case reports: Abnormality in thinking, agitation, anaphylaxis (rare), balanitis, cerebral thrombosis (IV; acute), chest pain, coma, diarrhea, drowsiness, dyspepsia, edema, eye pruritus, hypersensitivity reaction (rare), insomnia, localized warm feeling, myocardial infarction (IV), pain, palpitations, photophobia, seizure, tachycardia, vomiting, vulvar pain

Drug Interactions

Metabolism/Transport Effects None known.

Avoid Concomitant Use

Avoid concomitant use of Desmopressin with any of the following: Tolvaptan

Increased Effect/Toxicity

Desmopressin may increase the levels/effects of: Lithium

The levels/effects of Desmopressin may be increased by: Analgesics (Opioid); CarBAMazepine; ChlorproMAZINE; LamoTRIgine; Nonsteroidal Anti-Inflammatory Agents; Selective Serotonin Reuptake Inhibitors; Tricyclic Antidepressants

Decreased Effect

The levels/effects of Desmopressin may be decreased by: Demeclocycline; Lithium; Tolvaptan

Storage/Stability

DDAVP:

Nasal spray: Store at controlled room temperature of 20°C to 25°C (68°F to 77°F). Keep nasal spray in upright position.

Rhinal Tube solution: Store refrigerated at 2°C to 8°C (36°F to 46°F). May store at controlled room temperature of 20°C to 25°C (68°F to 77°F) for up to 3 weeks.

Solution for injection: Store refrigerated at 2°C to 8°C (36°F to 46°F).

Tablet: Store at controlled room temperature of 20°C to 25°C (68°F to 77°F). Avoid excessive heat. Protect from light.

DDAVP Melt (CAN; not available in US): Store at 15°C to 25°C (59°F to 77°F) in original container. Protect from moisture.

Stimate nasal spray: Store at room temperature not to exceed 25°C (77°F). Discard 6 months after opening bottle. Store bottle in upright position.

Preparation for Administration

DDAVP injection: Hemophilia A and von Willebrand disease (type 1): Dilute solution for injection in 10 or 50 mL NS for IV infusion (10 mL for children ≤10 kg; 50 mL for adults and children >10 kg).

Stimate nasal spray: Press pump down 4 times to prime prior to initial use.

Mechanism of Action Synthetic analogue of the antidiuretic hormone arginine vasopressin. In a dose dependent manner, desmopressin increases cyclic adenosine monophosphate (cAMP) in renal tubular cells which increases water permeability resulting in decreased urine volume and increased urine osmolality; increases plasma levels of von Willebrand factor, factor VIII, and t-PA contributing to a shortened activated partial thromboplastin time (aPTT) and bleeding time.

Pharmacodynamics/Kinetics

Onset of action:

Intranasal: Antidiuretic: 15 to 30 minutes; Increased factor VIII and von Willebrand factor (vWF) activity (dose related): 30 minutes

Peak effect: Antidiuretic: 1 hour; Increased factor VIII and vWF activity: 1.5 hours

IV infusion: Increased factor VIII and vWF activity: 30 minutes (dose related)

Peak effect: 1.5 to 2 hours

Oral tablet: Antidiuretic: ~1 hour

Peak effect: 4 to 7 hours

Duration: Intranasal, Injection, Oral tablet: ~6 to 14 hours

Absorption: Sublingual: Rapid

Bioavailability: Intranasal: ~3.5%; Oral tablet: 5% compared to intranasal, 0.16% compared to IV

Half-life elimination: 2 to 4 hours; Renal impairment: 9 hours

Excretion: Urine (primarily)

Dosing

Adult & Geriatric

Diabetes insipidus: Note: Fluid restriction should be observed. Dosing should be individualized to response.

IV, SubQ: U.S. labeling: 2 to 4 mcg daily (0.5 to 1 mL) in 2 divided doses or one-tenth (1/10) of the maintenance intranasal dose. Fluid restriction should be observed.

IM, IV, SubQ: Canadian labeling: 1 to 4 mcg (0.25 to 1 mL) once daily or one-tenth (1/10) of the maintenance intranasal dose. Fluid restriction should be observed.

Intranasal (100 mcg/mL nasal solution): Usual dose range: 10 to 40 mcg daily (0.1 to 0.4 mL) as a single dose or divided 2 to 3 times daily; adjust morning and evening doses separately for an adequate diurnal rhythm of water turnover. Most adults require 10 mcg (0.1 mL) twice daily. **Note:** The nasal spray pump can only deliver doses of 10 mcg (0.1 mL) or multiples of 10 mcg (0.1 mL); if doses other than this are needed, the rhinal tube delivery system is preferred. Fluid restriction should be observed.

Oral:

US labeling: Initial: 0.05 mg twice daily; total daily dose should be increased or decreased as needed to obtain adequate antidiuresis (range: 0.1 to 1.2 mg divided 2 to 3 times daily). Fluid restriction should be observed.

◀ Canadian labeling: Initial: 0.1 mg 3 times daily; total daily dose should be increased or decreased as needed to obtain adequate antidiuresis (range: 0.3 to 1.2 mg divided 3 times daily). Fluid restriction should be observed.

Sublingual formulation [Canadian product]: Initial: 60 mcg 3 times daily; total daily dose should be increased or decreased as needed to obtain adequate antidiuresis. Usual maintenance: 120 to 720 mcg equally divided 2 or 3 times daily. Fluid restriction should be observed.

Nocturnal enuresis: *Oral:* Initial: 0.2 mg at bedtime; dose may be titrated up to 0.6 mg to achieve desired response.

Hemophilia A and von Willebrand disease (type 1):

IV: 0.3 mcg/kg by slow infusion; may repeat dose if needed (based on clinical response and laboratory results); if used preoperatively, administer 30 minutes before procedure

Canadian labeling (not in US labeling): Maximum IV dose: 20 mcg

Intranasal (using high concentration spray [1.5 mg/mL] [eg, Stimate]): <50 kg: 150 mcg (1 spray in a single nostril); ≥50 kg: 300 mcg (1 spray each nostril); repeat use is determined by the patient's clinical condition and laboratory work. If using preoperatively, administer 2 hours before surgery.

Uremic bleeding associated with acute or chronic renal failure (off-label use): IV: 0.4 mcg/kg over 10 minutes (Watson, 1984)

Prevention of surgical bleeding in patients with uremia (off-label use): IV: 0.3 mcg/kg over 30 minutes (Mannucci, 1983)

Pediatric

Diabetes insipidus: Note: Fluid restriction should be observed in these patients; younger patients more susceptible to plasma osmolality shifts and possible hyponatremia. Dosing should be individualized to response.

Parenteral:

US labeling: Children ≥12 years and Adolescents: IV, SubQ: Refer to adult dosing.

Alternative recommendations (off-label): Infants and Children <12 years: IV, SubQ: No definitive dosing available. Adult dosing should **not** be used in this age group; adverse events such as hyponatremia-induced seizures may occur. Dose should be reduced. Some have suggested an initial dosage range of 0.1 to 1 mcg daily in 1 or 2 divided doses (Cheetham, 2002). Initiate at low dose and increase as necessary. Closely monitor serum sodium levels and urine output; fluid restriction is recommended.

Canadian labeling: IM, IV, SubQ: Children and Adolescents: 0.4 mcg (0.1 mL) once daily or one-tenth ($^1/_{10}$) of the maintenance intranasal dose. Fluid restriction should be observed.

Intranasal (using 100 mcg/mL nasal solution [eg, DDAVP]):

Infants ≥3 months and Children ≤12 years: Usual dose range: 5 to 30 mcg daily (0.05 to 0.3 mL daily) as a single dose or divided 2 times daily; adjust morning and evening doses separately for an adequate diurnal rhythm of water turnover. **Note:** The nasal spray pump can only deliver doses of 10 mcg (0.1 mL) or multiples of 10 mcg (0.1 mL); if doses other than this are needed, the rhinal tube delivery system is preferred. Fluid restriction should be observed.

Adolescents: Refer to adult dosing.

Oral:

US labeling: Children ≥4 years and Adolescents: Refer to adult dosing.

Canadian labeling:

Children: Initial: 0.1 mg 3 times daily; total daily dose should be increased or decreased as needed to obtain adequate antidiuresis (range: 0.3 to 1.2 mg divided 3 times daily). Divide daily doses so that the evening dose is 2 times higher than the morning or afternoon dose to ensure adequate antidiuresis during the night. Fluid restriction should be observed.

Adolescents: Refer to adult dosing.

Sublingual formulation [Canadian product]:

Children: Initial: 60 mcg 3 times daily; total daily dose should be increased or decreased as needed to obtain adequate antidiuresis. Usual maintenance: 120 to 720 mcg equally divided 2 to 3 times daily; divide daily doses so that the evening dose is 2 times higher than the morning or afternoon dose to ensure adequate antidiuresis during the night. Fluid restriction should be observed.

Adolescents: Refer to adult dosing.

Hemophilia A and von Willebrand disease (type 1):

IV: Infants ≥3 months, Children, and Adolescents: Refer to adult dosing.

Note: Adverse events such as hyponatremia-induced seizures have been reported especially in young children using this dosing regimen (Das, 2005; Molnar, 2005; Smith, 1989; Thumfart, 2005; Weinstein, 1989). Fluid restriction and careful monitoring of serum sodium levels and urine output are necessary.

Intranasal (using high concentration spray [1.5 mg/mL] [eg, Stimate]): Infants ≥11 months, Children, and Adolescents: Refer to adult dosing.

Nocturnal enuresis:

Oral:

Children ≥6 years and Adolescents (US labeling) or Children ≥5 years and Adolescents (Canadian labeling): Initial: 0.2 mg at bedtime. Dose may be titrated up to 0.6 mg to achieve desired response. Fluid intake should be limited 1 hour prior to dose until the next morning, or at least 8 hours after administration.

Sublingual [Canadian product]: Children ≥5 years and Adolescents: Initial: 120 mcg administered 1 hour before bedtime; dose may be titrated up to a maximum of 360 mcg to achieve desired response. Fluid intake should be limited 1 hour prior to dose until the next morning, or at least 8 hours after administration.

Renal Impairment CrCl <50 mL/minute: Use is contraindicated according to the manufacturers (except 1.5 mg/mL nasal spray); however, has been used in acute and chronic renal failure patients experiencing uremic bleeding or for prevention of surgical bleeding (off-label uses) (Mannucci, 1983; Watson, 1984).

Hepatic Impairment There are no dosage adjustments provided in the manufacturer's labeling.

Administration

IM (Canadian labeling; not in US labeling), IV push, SubQ injection: Central diabetes insipidus: Withdraw dose from ampul into appropriate syringe size (eg, insulin syringe). Further dilution is not required. Administer as direct injection.

◀ IV infusion:

Hemophilia A, von Willebrand disease (type 1), and prevention of surgical bleeding in patients with uremia (off-label) (Mannucci, 1983): Infuse over 15 to 30 minutes

Acute uremic bleeding (off-label) (Watson, 1984a): May infuse over 10 minutes

Intranasal: Ensure that nasal passages are intact, clean, and free of obstruction prior to administration.

DDAVP: Nasal pump spray: Delivers 0.1 mL (10 mcg); for doses <10 mcg or for other doses which are not multiples, use rhinal tube. DDAVP Nasal spray delivers fifty 10 mcg doses. For 10 mcg dose, administer in one nostril. Any solution remaining after 50 doses should be discarded. Pump must be primed prior to first use.

DDAVP Rhinal tube: Insert top of dropper into tube (arrow marked end) in downward position. Squeeze dropper until solution reaches desired calibration mark. Disconnect dropper. Grasp the tube ¾ inch from the end and insert tube into nostril until the fingertips reach the nostril. Place opposite end of tube into the mouth (holding breath). Tilt head back and blow with a strong, short puff into the nostril (for very young patients, an adult should blow solution into the child's nose). Reseal dropper after use.

Oral:

Diabetes insipidus: Fluid restriction should be observed.

Primary nocturnal enuresis: Minimize fluid intake beginning 1 hour prior to administration and continue until the morning (for at least 8 hours).

May administer with or without food. Food may reduce/delay absorption although does not affect antidiuretic activity (Rittig, 1998).

Monitoring Parameters Blood pressure and pulse should be monitored during IV infusion

Note: For all indications, fluid intake, urine volume, and signs and symptoms of hyponatremia should be closely monitored especially in high-risk patient subgroups (eg, young children, elderly, patients with heart failure).

Diabetes insipidus: Urine specific gravity, plasma and urine osmolality, serum electrolytes

Hemophilia A: Factor VIII coagulant activity, factor VIII ristocetin cofactor activity, and factor VIII antigen levels, aPTT

von Willebrand disease: Factor VIII coagulant activity, factor VIII ristocetin cofactor activity, and factor VIII von Willebrand antigen levels, bleeding time

Nocturnal enuresis: Serum electrolytes if used for >7 days

Additional Information 10 mcg of desmopressin acetate is equivalent to 40 units

Dosage Forms Considerations

DDAVP and Minirin 5 mL bottles contain 50 sprays.

Stimate 2.5 mL bottles contain 25 sprays.

Dosage Forms

Excipient information presented when available (limited, particularly for generics); consult specific product labeling. [DSC] = Discontinued product

Solution, Injection, as acetate:

DDAVP: 4 mcg/mL (1 mL)

DDAVP: 4 mcg/mL (10 mL) [contains chlorobutanol (chlorobutol)]

Generic: 4 mcg/mL (1 mL, 10 mL)

Solution, Nasal, as acetate:

DDAVP: 0.01% (5 mL) [contains benzalkonium chloride]

DDAVP Rhinal Tube: 0.01% (2.5 mL) [contains chlorobutanol (chlorobutol)]

Stimate: 1.5 mg/mL (2.5 mL) [contains benzalkonium chloride]
Generic: 0.01% (2.5 mL, 5 mL)
Tablet, Oral, as acetate:
DDAVP: 0.1 mg
DDAVP: 0.1 mg [DSC], 0.2 mg [scored]
Generic: 0.1 mg, 0.2 mg

Dosage Forms: Canada Excipient information presented when available (limited, particularly for generics); consult specific product labeling.
Tablet, Sublingual, as acetate:
DDAVP® Melt: 60 mcg, 120 mcg, 240 mcg

♦ **Desmopressin Acetate** *see* Desmopressin *on page 505*

♦ **Detryptoreline** *see* Triptorelin *on page 1703*

Dexamethasone (Systemic) (deks a METH a sone)

Related Information

Corticosteroids Systemic Equivalencies *on page 2334*
Management of Chemotherapy-Induced Nausea and Vomiting in Adults *on page 2142*
Palliative Care Medicine (Cancer) *on page 2252*
Prevention and Management of Infections *on page 2196*

Brand Names: US Baycadron [DSC]; Dexamethasone Intensol; DexPak 10 Day; DexPak 13 Day; DexPak 6 Day; DoubleDex

Brand Names: Canada Apo-Dexamethasone; Dexasone; Dom-Dexamethasone; PHL-Dexamethasone; PMS-Dexamethasone; PRO-Dexamethasone; ratio-Dexamethasone

Index Terms Decadron; Dexamethasone Sodium Phosphate

Pharmacologic Category Anti-inflammatory Agent; Antiemetic; Corticosteroid, Systemic

Use Primarily as an anti-inflammatory or immunosuppressant agent in the treatment of a variety of diseases including those of allergic, dermatologic, gastrointestinal, endocrine, hematologic, inflammatory, neoplastic, nervous system, ophthalmic, renal, respiratory, rheumatic, and autoimmune origin; management of cerebral edema, chronic swelling, as a diagnostic agent, diagnosis of Cushing syndrome, antiemetic

Labeled Contraindications Hypersensitivity to dexamethasone or any component of the formulation, including sulfites; systemic fungal infections, cerebral malaria

Pregnancy Considerations Adverse events have been observed with corticosteroids in animal reproduction studies. Betamethasone crosses the placenta (Brownfoot 2013); and is partially metabolized by placental enzymes to an inactive metabolite (Murphy 2007). Some studies have shown an association between first trimester systemic corticosteroid use and oral clefts (Park-Wyllie 2000; Pradat 2003). Systemic corticosteroids may have an effect on fetal growth (decreased birth weight); however, information is conflicting (Lunghi 2010). Hypoadrenalism may occur in newborns following maternal use of corticosteroids during pregnancy; monitor.

Because antenatal corticosteroid administration may reduce the incidence of intraventricular hemorrhage, necrotizing enterocolitis, neonatal mortality, and respiratory distress syndrome, the injection is often used in patients with preterm premature rupture of membranes (membrane rupture between 24 0/7 weeks and 34 0/7 weeks of gestation) who are at risk of preterm ▶

delivery (ACOG 2013). When systemic corticosteroids are needed in pregnancy, it is generally recommended to use the lowest effective dose for the shortest duration of time, avoiding high doses during the first trimester (Leachman 2006; Lunghi 2010; Makol 2011; Østensen 2009).

Women exposed to dexamethasone during pregnancy for the treatment of an autoimmune disease may contact the OTIS Autoimmune Diseases Study at 877-311-8972.

Breast-Feeding Considerations Corticosteroids are excreted in human milk; information specific to dexamethasone has not been located. The manufacturer notes that when used systemically, maternal use of corticosteroids have the potential to cause adverse events in a nursing infant (eg, growth suppression, interfere with endogenous corticosteroid production. Due to the potential for serious adverse reactions in the nursing infant, the manufacturer recommends a decision be made whether to discontinue nursing or to discontinue the drug, taking into account the importance of treatment to the mother. If there is concern about exposure to the infant, some guidelines recommend waiting 4 hours after the maternal dose of an oral systemic corticosteroid before breast-feeding in order to decrease potential exposure to the nursing infant (based on a study using prednisolone) (Bae 2011; Leachman 2006; Makol 2011; Ost 1985).

Warnings/Precautions Corticosteroids are not approved for epidural injection. Serious neurologic events (eg, spinal cord infarction, paraplegia, quadriplegia, cortical blindness, stroke), some resulting in death, have been reported with epidural injection of corticosteroids, with and without use of fluoroscopy. Intra-articular injection may produce systemic as well as local effects. Appropriate examination of any joint fluid present is necessary to exclude a septic process. Avoid injection into an infected site. Do not inject into unstable joints. Patients should not overuse joints in which symptomatic benefit has been obtained as long as the inflammatory process remains active. Frequent intra-articular injection may result in damage to joint tissues.

Use with caution in patients with thyroid disease, hepatic impairment, renal impairment, cardiovascular disease, diabetes, glaucoma, cataracts, myasthenia gravis, osteoporosis, seizures, or GI diseases (diverticulitis, intestinal anastomoses, peptic ulcer, ulcerative colitis) due to perforation risk. Avoid ethanol may enhance gastric mucosal irritation. Use caution following acute MI (corticosteroids have been associated with myocardial rupture). Because of the risk of adverse effects, systemic corticosteroids should be used cautiously in the elderly in the smallest possible effective dose for the shortest duration. May affect growth velocity; growth should be routinely monitored in pediatric patients. Withdraw therapy with gradual tapering of dose.

May cause hypercorticism or suppression of hypothalamic-pituitary-adrenal (HPA) axis, particularly in younger children or in patients receiving high doses for prolonged periods. HPA axis suppression may lead to adrenal crisis. Withdrawal and discontinuation of a corticosteroid should be done slowly and carefully. Particular care is required when patients are transferred from systemic corticosteroids to inhaled products due to possible adrenal insufficiency or withdrawal from steroids, including an increase in allergic symptoms. Adult patients receiving >20 mg per day of prednisone (or equivalent) may be most susceptible. Fatalities have occurred due to adrenal insufficiency in asthmatic patients during and after transfer from systemic corticosteroids to aerosol steroids; aerosol steroids do not provide the systemic steroid needed to treat patients having trauma, surgery, or infections. Dexamethasone does not provide adequate mineralocorticoid activity in adrenal insufficiency (may be employed as a single dose while cortisol assays are performed). The lowest possible dose should be used during treatment; discontinuation and/or dose reductions should be gradual. Rare cases of anaphylactoid reactions have been observed in patients receiving corticosteroids. Patients may require higher doses when subject to stress (ie, trauma, surgery, severe infection).

Acute myopathy has been reported with high dose corticosteroids, usually in patients with neuromuscular transmission disorders; may involve ocular and/or respiratory muscles; monitor creatine kinase; recovery may be delayed. Perineal burning, tingling, pain and pruritus have been reported with IV administration. May occur more commonly in females, with higher doses, and with rapid administration. Symptom onset is sudden and usually resolves in <1 minute (Allan 1986; Neff 2002; Perron 2003; Singh 2011). Corticosteroid use may cause psychiatric disturbances, including depression, euphoria, insomnia, mood swings, and personality changes. Preexisting psychiatric conditions may be exacerbated by corticosteroid use. Prolonged use of corticosteroids may increase the incidence of secondary infection, mask acute infection (including fungal infections), prolong or exacerbate viral infections, or limit response to vaccines. Exposure to chickenpox or measles should be avoided; corticosteroids should not be used to treat ocular herpes simplex. Corticosteroids should not be used for cerebral malaria, fungal infections, or viral hepatitis. Close observation is required in patients with latent tuberculosis and/or TB reactivity; restrict use in active TB (only fulminating or disseminated TB in conjunction with antituberculosis treatment). Amebiasis should be ruled out in any patient with recent travel to tropic climates or unexplained diarrhea prior to initiation of corticosteroids.

Prolonged treatment with corticosteroids has been associated with the development of Kaposi sarcoma (case reports); if noted, discontinuation of therapy should be considered. High-dose corticosteroids should not be used to manage acute head injury. Some products may contain sodium sulfite, a sulfite that may cause allergic-type reactions including anaphylaxis and life-threatening or less severe asthmatic episodes in susceptible patients. Potentially significant drug-drug interactions may exist, requiring dose or frequency adjustment, additional monitoring, and/or selection of alternative therapy. Some dosage forms may contain propylene glycol; large amounts are potentially toxic and have been associated hyperosmolality, lactic acidosis, seizures, and respiratory depression; use caution (AAP ["Inactive" 1997]; Zar 2007).

Benzyl alcohol and derivatives: Some dosage forms may contain sodium benzoate/benzoic acid; benzoic acid (benzoate) is a metabolite of benzyl alcohol; large amounts of benzyl alcohol (≥99 mg/kg/day) have been associated with a potentially fatal toxicity ("gasping syndrome") in neonates; the "gasping syndrome" consists of metabolic acidosis, respiratory distress, gasping respirations, CNS dysfunction (including convulsions, intracranial hemorrhage), hypotension, and cardiovascular collapse (AAP ["Inactive" 1997]; CDC 1982); some data suggests that benzoate displaces bilirubin from protein binding sites (Ahlfors 2001); avoid or use dosage forms containing benzyl alcohol derivative with caution in neonates. See manufacturer's labeling.

Adverse Reactions Frequency not defined.

Cardiovascular: Arrhythmia, bradycardia, cardiac arrest, cardiomyopathy, CHF, circulatory collapse, edema, hypertension, myocardial rupture (post-MI), syncope, thromboembolism, vasculitis

Central nervous system: Depression, emotional instability, euphoria, headache, intracranial pressure increased, insomnia, malaise, mood swings, neuritis, personality changes, pseudotumor cerebri (usually following discontinuation), psychic disorders, seizure, vertigo

Dermatologic: Acne, allergic dermatitis, alopecia, angioedema, bruising, dry skin, erythema, fragile skin, hirsutism, hyper-/hypopigmentation, hypertrichosis, perianal pruritus (following IV injection), petechiae, rash, skin atrophy, skin test reaction impaired, striae, urticaria, wound healing impaired

Endocrine & metabolic: Adrenal suppression, carbohydrate tolerance decreased, Cushing's syndrome, diabetes mellitus, glucose intolerance decreased, growth suppression (children), hyperglycemia, hypokalemic alkalosis, menstrual irregularities, negative nitrogen balance, pituitary-adrenal axis suppression, protein catabolism, sodium retention

Gastrointestinal: Abdominal distention, appetite increased, gastrointestinal hemorrhage, gastrointestinal perforation, nausea, pancreatitis, peptic ulcer, ulcerative esophagitis, weight gain

Genitourinary: Altered (increased or decreased) spermatogenesis

Hepatic: Hepatomegaly, transaminases increased

Local: Postinjection flare (intra-articular use), thrombophlebitis

Neuromuscular & skeletal: Arthropathy, aseptic necrosis (femoral and humoral heads), fractures, muscle mass loss, myopathy (particularly in conjunction with neuromuscular disease or neuromuscular-blocking agents), neuropathy, osteoporosis, parasthesia, tendon rupture, vertebral compression fractures, weakness

Ocular: Cataracts, exophthalmos, glaucoma, intraocular pressure increased

Renal: Glucosuria

Respiratory: Pulmonary edema

Miscellaneous: Abnormal fat deposition, anaphylactoid reaction, anaphylaxis, avascular necrosis, diaphoresis, hiccups, hypersensitivity, impaired wound healing, infections, Kaposi's sarcoma, moon face, secondary malignancy

Drug Interactions

Metabolism/Transport Effects Substrate of CYP3A4 (major), P-glycoprotein; **Note:** Assignment of Major/Minor substrate status based on clinically relevant drug interaction potential; **Inhibits** P-glycoprotein; **Induces** CYP2A6 (weak/moderate), CYP2B6 (weak/moderate), CYP2C9 (weak/moderate), CYP3A4 (moderate), P-glycoprotein, UGT1A1

Avoid Concomitant Use

Avoid concomitant use of Dexamethasone (Systemic) with any of the following: Aldesleukin; Antihepaciviral Combination Products; Axitinib; BCG (Intravesical); Bedaquiline; Bosutinib; Cabozantinib; Cobimetinib; Conivaptan; Flibanserin; Fusidic Acid (Systemic); Idelalisib; Indium 111 Capromab Pendetide; Lapatinib; Mifepristone; Natalizumab; Nilotinib; Nisoldipine; Olaparib; Palbociclib; Pimecrolimus; Ranolazine; Rilpivirine; RomiDEPsin; Simeprevir; Sonidegib; Tacrolimus (Topical); Ticagrelor; Tofacitinib; VinCRIStine (Liposomal)

Increased Effect/Toxicity

Dexamethasone (Systemic) may increase the levels/effects of: Acetylcholinesterase Inhibitors; Amphotericin B; Androgens; Clarithromycin; CycloSPORINE (Systemic); Deferasirox; Fingolimod; Fosphenytoin; Ifosfamide; Leflunomide; Lenalidomide; Loop Diuretics; Natalizumab; Nicorandil; NSAID (COX-2 Inhibitor); NSAID (Nonselective); Phenytoin; Quinolone Antibiotics; Thalidomide; Thiazide Diuretics; Tofacitinib; Vaccines (Live); Warfarin

The levels/effects of Dexamethasone (Systemic) may be increased by: Aprepitant; Asparaginase (E. coli); Asparaginase (Erwinia); Conivaptan; CycloSPORINE (Systemic); CYP3A4 Inhibitors (Moderate); CYP3A4 Inhibitors (Strong); Denosumab; Estrogen Derivatives; Fosamprenavir; Fosaprepitant; Fusidic Acid (Systemic); Idelalisib; Indacaterol; Ivacaftor; Luliconazole; Mifepristone; Netupitant; Neuromuscular-Blocking Agents (Nondepolarizing); Osimertinib; P-glycoprotein/ABCB1 Inhibitors; Pimecrolimus; Roflumilast; Salicylates; Stiripentol; Tacrolimus (Topical); Telaprevir; Trastuzumab

Decreased Effect

Dexamethasone (Systemic) may decrease the levels/effects of: Aldesleukin; Antidiabetic Agents; Antihepaciviral Combination Products; ARIPiprazole; Axitinib; BCG (Intravesical); Bedaquiline; Bosutinib; Cabozantinib; Calcitriol (Systemic); Caspofungin; Clarithromycin; Cobicistat; Cobimetinib; Coccidioides immitis Skin Test; Corticorelin; CycloSPORINE (Systemic); CYP3A4 Substrates; Daclatasvir; Dasatinib; Elvitegravir; FentaNYL; Flibanserin; Fosamprenavir; Fosphenytoin; Hyaluronidase; Hydrocodone; Ibrutinib; Ifosfamide; Imatinib; Indium 111 Capromab Pendetide; Isoniazid; Ixabepilone; Lapatinib; Nilotinib; NiMODipine; Nisoldipine; Olaparib; Palbociclib; Phenytoin; Ranolazine; Rilpivirine; Rolapitant; RomiDEPsin; Salicylates; Saxagliptin; Simeprevir; Sipuleucel-T; Sonidegib; SUNitinib; Telaprevir; Ticagrelor; Triazolam; Urea Cycle Disorder Agents; Vaccines (Inactivated); Vaccines (Live); VinCRIStine (Liposomal)

The levels/effects of Dexamethasone (Systemic) may be decreased by: Antacids; Bile Acid Sequestrants; Bosentan; CYP3A4 Inducers (Moderate); CYP3A4 Inducers (Strong); Dabrafenib; Deferasirox; Echinacea; Enzalutamide; Fosphenytoin; Mifepristone; Mitotane; Osimertinib; P-glycoprotein/ABCB1 Inducers; Phenytoin; Siltuximab; St Johns Wort; Tocilizumab

Storage/Stability

Elixir: Store at 15°C to 30°C (59°F to 86°F); avoid freezing.

Injection: Store intact vials at 20°C to 25°C (68°F to 77°F); excursions permitted to 15°C to 30°C (59°F to 86°F). Protect from light, heat, and freezing. Diluted solutions should be used within 24 hours.

Oral concentrated solution (Intensol): Store at 20°C to 25°C (68°F to 77°F); do not freeze; do not use if precipitate is present; dispense only in original bottle and only with manufacturer-supplied calibrated dropper; discard open bottle after 90 days.

Oral solution: Store at 20°C to 25°C (68°F to 77°F).

Tablets: Store at 20°C to 25°C (68°F to 77°F); protect from moisture.

Preparation for Administration

Oral: Oral administration of dexamethasone for croup may be prepared using a parenteral dexamethasone formulation and mixing it with an oral flavored syrup (Bjornson 2004).

IV: May be given undiluted or further diluted in NS or D_5W. Use preservative-free product when used in neonates, especially premature infants.

Mechanism of Action A long acting corticosteroid with minimal sodium-retaining potential. Decreases inflammation by suppression of neutrophil migration, decreased production of inflammatory mediators, and reversal of increased capillary permeability; suppresses normal immune response. Dexamethasone's mechanism of antiemetic activity is unknown.

Pharmacodynamics/Kinetics

Onset of action: IV: Prompt

Absorption: Oral: 61% to 86%

Metabolism: Hepatic

Half-life elimination: Oral: ~4 hours (Czock 2005); IV: ~1 to 5 hours (Hochhaus 2001; Miyabo 1991; Rohdewald 1987; Toth 1999)

Time to peak, serum: Oral: 1 to 2 hours (Czock 2005); IM: ~30 to 120 minutes (Egerman 1997; Hochhaus 2001); IV: 5 to 10 minutes (free dexamethasone) (Miyabo 1991; Rohdewald 1987)

Excretion: Urine (~10%) (Duggan 1975; Miyabo 1991)

Dosing

Adult

Anti-inflammatory:

Oral, IM, IV: 0.75 to 9 mg/day in divided doses every 6 to 12 hours

Intra-articular, intralesional, or soft tissue: 0.4 to 6 mg/day

Extubation or airway edema: Oral, IM, IV: 0.5 to 2 mg/kg/day in divided doses every 6 hours beginning 24 hours prior to extubation and continuing for 4 to 6 doses afterwards

Cerebral edema: IV: 10 mg stat, 4 mg IM/IV (should be given as sodium phosphate) every 6 hours until response is maximized, then switch to oral regimen, then taper off if appropriate; dosage may be reduced after 2 to 4 days and gradually discontinued over 5 to 7 days

Dexamethasone suppression test (depression/suicide indicator) (off-label use): Oral: 1 mg at 11 PM, draw blood at 8 AM the following day for plasma cortisol determination

Cushing syndrome, diagnostic: Oral: 1 mg at 11 PM, draw blood at 8 AM; greater accuracy for Cushing's syndrome may be achieved by the following: Dexamethasone 0.5 mg by mouth every 6 hours for 48 hours (with 24-hour urine collection for 17-hydroxycorticosteroid excretion)

Differentiation of Cushing syndrome due to ACTH excess from Cushing due to other causes: Oral: Dexamethasone 2 mg every 6 hours for 48 hours (with 24-hour urine collection for 17-hydroxycorticosteroid excretion)

Multiple sclerosis (acute exacerbation): Oral: 30 mg/day for 1 week, followed by 4 to 12 mg/day for 1 month

Treatment of shock:

Addisonian crisis/shock (eg, adrenal insufficiency/responsive to steroid therapy): IV: 4 to 10 mg as a single dose, which may be repeated if necessary

Unresponsive shock (eg, unresponsive to steroid therapy): IV: 1 to 6 mg/kg as a single IV dose or up to 40 mg initially followed by repeat doses every 2 to 6 hours while shock persists

Physiological replacement: Oral, IM, IV (should be given as sodium phosphate): 0.03 to 0.15 mg/kg/day **or** 0.6 to 0.75 mg/m^2/day in divided doses every 6 to 12 hours

Acute mountain sickness (AMS)/high altitude cerebral edema (HACE) (off-label use):

Prevention: Oral: 2 mg every 6 hours **or** 4 mg every 12 hours starting on the day of ascent; may be discontinued after staying at the same elevation for 2 to 3 days or if descent is initiated; do not exceed a 10 day duration (Luks 2010). **Note:** In situations of rapid ascent to altitudes >3500 meters (such as rescue or military operations), 4 mg every 6 hours may be considered (Luks 2010).

Treatment: Oral, IM, IV:

AMS: 4 mg every 6 hours (Luks 2010)

HACE: Initial: 8 mg as a single dose; Maintenance: 4 mg every 6 hours until symptoms resolve (Luks 2010)

Antenatal fetal maturation (off-label use): IM: In women with preterm premature rupture of membranes (membrane rupture between 24 0/7 weeks and 34 0/7 weeks of gestation), a single course of corticosteroids is recommended if there is a risk of preterm delivery (ACOG 2013). Although the optimal corticosteroid and dose have not been determined, dexamethasone 6 mg every 12 hours for a total of 4 doses has been used in most studies (Brownfoot 2013).

Chemotherapy-associated nausea and vomiting, prevention (off-label use):

High emetic potential chemotherapy: Oral, IV: 12 mg on day 1 prior to chemotherapy (in combination with aprepitant or fosaprepitant and a $5HT_3$ antagonist on day 1) followed by 8 mg on days 2 to 3 or days 2 to 4 (with aprepitant on days 2 and 3 if aprepitant used on day 1) (Basch 2011; Roila 2010) **or** (if aprepitant/fosaprepitant not used): 20 mg day 1 (in combination with a $5HT_3$ antagonist on day 1) followed by 8 mg twice daily for 3 to 4 days (MASCC 2013)

Moderate emetic potential chemotherapy: Oral, IV: 8 mg on day 1 prior to chemotherapy (in combination with a $5HT_3$ antagonist on day 1) and 8 mg on days 2 and 3 (Basch 2011; Roila 2010)

Low emetic potential chemotherapy: Oral, IV: 8 mg prior to chemotherapy (Basch 2011; Roila 2010)

Multiple myeloma (off-label use): Oral: 40 mg once daily on days 1 to 4, 9 to 12, and 17 to 20 (as induction therapy) in combination with bortezomib and doxorubicin for 3 cycles (Sonneveld 2012) **or** 40 mg once weekly on days 1, 8, 15, and 22 every 28 days (in combination with lenalidomide) until disease progression (Rajkumar 2010) or 40 mg once weekly on days 1, 8, 15, and 22 every 28 days (in combination with pomalidomide) until disease progression or unacceptable toxicity (San Miguel 2013). **Note:** Multiple dexamethasone-containing regimens are available for the treatment of multiple myeloma. Refer to appropriate literature/guidelines for additional details.

Geriatric Refer to adult dosing. Use cautiously in the elderly in the smallest possible dose.

Pediatric

Anti-inflammatory and/or immunosuppressant: Oral, IM, IV: 0.08 to 0.3 mg/kg/day **or** 2.5 to 10 mg/m^2/day in divided doses every 6 to 12 hours

Extubation or airway edema: Oral, IM, IV: 0.5 to 2 mg/kg/day in divided doses every 6 hours beginning 24 hours prior to extubation and continuing for 4 to 6 doses afterwards

Cerebral edema: IV: Loading dose: 1 to 2 mg/kg/dose as a single dose; maintenance: 1 to 1.5 mg/kg/day (maximum: 16 mg/day) in divided doses every 4 to 6 hours, taper off over 1 to 6 weeks

Croup (laryngotracheobronchitis): Oral, IM, IV: 0.6 mg/kg once; usual maximum dose: 16 mg (doses as high as 20 mg have been used) (Bjornson 2004; Hegenbarth 2008; Rittichier 2000); a single oral dose of 0.15 mg/kg has been shown effective in children with mild to moderate croup (Russell 2004; Sparrow 2006)

Bacterial meningitis: Infants and Children >6 weeks: IV: 0.15 mg/kg/dose every 6 hours for the first 2 to 4 days of antibiotic treatment; start dexamethasone 10 to 20 minutes before or with the first dose of antibiotic

Physiologic replacement: Oral, IM, IV: 0.03 to 0.15 mg/kg/day or 0.6 to 0.75 mg/m^2/day in divided doses every 6 to 12 hours

◄ **Acute mountain sickness (AMS)/high altitude cerebral edema (HACE) (off-label use):** Oral, IM, IV: 0.15 mg/kg/dose every 6 hours; consider using for high altitude pulmonary edema because of associated HACE with this condition (Luks 2010; Pollard 2001)

Chemotherapy-associated nausea and vomiting, prevention (off-label use): Pediatric Oncology Group of Ontario guideline recommendations (Dupuis, 2013): Infants, Children, and Adolescents:

High emetic potential chemotherapy: Oral, IV: 6 mg/m^2/dose every 6 hours (in combination with a 5HT$_3$ antagonist and aprepitant [if no interaction with aprepitant and if ≥12 years]); reduce dexamethasone dose by 50% if administered concomitantly with aprepitant

Moderate emetic potential chemotherapy: Oral, IV:

BSA ≤0.6 m^2: 2 mg every 12 hours (in combination with a 5HT$_3$ antagonist)

BSA >0.6 m^2: 4 mg every 12 hours (in combination with a 5HT$_3$ antagonist)

Renal Impairment There are no dosage adjustments provided in the manufacturer's labeling; use with caution. Hemodialysis or peritoneal dialysis: Supplemental dose is not necessary.

Hepatic Impairment There are no dosage adjustments provided in the manufacturer's labeling.

Combination Regimens

Multiple myeloma:

Administration

Oral: Administer with meals to decrease GI upset.

IV: May administer the 4 mg/mL or 10 mg/mL concentration undiluted over ≤1 minute (Gahart 2015). Rapid administration may be associated with perineal irritation (especially with higher doses); consider further dilution and administration by IV intermittent infusion over 5 to 15 minutes (Allan 1986; Neff 2002; Perron 2003; Singh 2011).

IM: Administer the 4 mg/mL or 10 mg/mL concentration deep IM.

Intra-articular: Administer into affected joint using the 4 mg/mL concentration only.

Intralesional injection: Administer into affected area using the 4 mg/mL concentration only.

Soft tissue injection: Administer into affected tissue using the 4 mg/mL concentration only.

Monitoring Parameters Hemoglobin, occult blood loss, serum potassium, glucose, growth in children

Test Interactions May suppress the wheal and flare reactions to skin test antigens

Dietary Considerations May be taken with meals to decrease GI upset. May need diet with increased potassium, pyridoxine, vitamin C, vitamin D, folate, calcium, and phosphorus.

Additional Information Effects of inhaled/intranasal steroids on growth have been observed in the absence of laboratory evidence of HPA axis suppression, suggesting that growth velocity is a more sensitive indicator of systemic corticosteroid exposure in pediatric patients than some commonly used tests of HPA axis function. The long-term effects of this reduction in growth velocity associated with orally-inhaled and intranasal corticosteroids, including the impact on final adult height, are unknown. The potential for "catch up" growth following discontinuation of treatment with inhaled corticosteroids has not been adequately studied.

◄ **Withdrawal/tapering of therapy:** Corticosteroid tapering following short-term use is limited primarily by the need to control the underlying disease state; tapering may be accomplished over a period of days. Following longer-term use, tapering over weeks to months may be necessary to avoid signs and symptoms of adrenal insufficiency and to allow recovery of the HPA axis. Testing of HPA axis responsiveness may be of value in selected patients. Subtle deficits in HPA response may persist for months after discontinuation of therapy, and may require supplemental dosing during periods of acute illness or surgical stress.

Dosage Forms Excipient information presented when available (limited, particularly for generics); consult specific product labeling. [DSC] = Discontinued product

Concentrate, Oral:
 Dexamethasone Intensol: 1 mg/mL (30 mL) [contains alcohol, usp; unflavored flavor]

Elixir, Oral:
 Baycadron: 0.5 mg/5 mL (237 mL [DSC]) [contains alcohol, usp, benzoic acid, fd&c red #40, propylene glycol; raspberry flavor]
 Generic: 0.5 mg/5 mL (237 mL)

Kit, Injection, as sodium phosphate:
 DoubleDex: 10 mg/mL

Solution, Oral:
 Generic: 0.5 mg/5 mL (240 mL, 500 mL)

Solution, Injection, as sodium phosphate:
 Generic: 4 mg/mL (1 mL, 5 mL, 30 mL); 20 mg/5 mL (5 mL); 120 mg/30 mL (30 mL); 10 mg/mL (1 mL, 10 mL [DSC]); 100 mg/10 mL (10 mL)

Solution, Injection, as sodium phosphate [preservative free]:
 Generic: 4 mg/mL (1 mL); 10 mg/mL (1 mL)

Tablet, Oral:
 DexPak 10 Day: 1.5 mg [scored; contains fd&c red #40 aluminum lake]
 DexPak 13 Day: 1.5 mg [scored; contains fd&c red #40 aluminum lake]
 DexPak 6 Day: 1.5 mg [scored; contains fd&c red #40 aluminum lake]
 Generic: 0.5 mg, 0.75 mg, 1 mg, 1.5 mg, 2 mg, 4 mg, 6 mg

Dexrazoxane (deks ray ZOKS ane)

Related Information

Management of Chemotherapy-Induced Nausea and Vomiting in Adults *on page 2142*

Management of Drug Extravasations *on page 2159*

Prevention of Chemotherapy-Induced Nausea and Vomiting in Children *on page 2203*

Safe Handling of Hazardous Drugs *on page 2292*

Brand Names: US Totect; Zinecard

Brand Names: Canada Zinecard

Index Terms ICRF-187

Pharmacologic Category Antidote; Antidote, Extravasation; Chemoprotective Agent

Use

Prevention of cardiomyopathy associated with doxorubicin (Zinecard, generic products): To reduce the incidence and severity of cardiomyopathy associated with doxorubicin administration in women with metastatic breast cancer who have received a cumulative doxorubicin dose of 300 mg/m^2 and will benefit from continuing doxorubicin therapy to maintain tumor control. Not recommended for use with initial doxorubicin therapy.

Extravasation of anthracyclines (Totect): Treatment of extravasation resulting from intravenous anthracycline chemotherapy.

Labeled Contraindications

Zinecard:

US labeling: Use with chemotherapy regimens that do not contain an anthracycline

Canadian labeling: Hypersensitivity to dexrazoxane or any component of the formulation; use with chemotherapy regimens that do not contain an anthracycline; use as a chemotherapeutic agent

Totect: There are no contraindications listed in the manufacturer's labeling.

Pregnancy Considerations Adverse events were observed in animal reproduction studies using doses less than the equivalent human dose (based on BSA). May cause fetal harm if administered during pregnancy. Women of childbearing potential should use highly effective contraception to prevent pregnancy during treatment.

Breast-Feeding Considerations It is not known if dexrazoxane is excreted in breast milk. Due to the potential for serious adverse reactions in the nursing infant, a decision should be made to discontinue nursing or to discontinue dexrazoxane, taking into account the importance of treatment to the mother.

Warnings/Precautions Hazardous agent - use appropriate precautions for handling and disposal (NIOSH 2014 [group 2]).

Dexrazoxane may cause mild myelosuppression (leukopenia, neutropenia, and thrombocytopenia); myelosuppression may be additive with concurrently administered chemotherapeutic agents. Does not eliminate the potential for anthracycline-induced cardiac toxicity; carefully monitor cardiac function (LVEF) before and periodically during treatment. Potentially significant drug-drug interactions may exist, requiring dose or frequency adjustment, additional monitoring, and/or selection of alternative therapy. May interfere with the antitumor effect of chemotherapy when given concurrently with fluorouracil, doxorubicin and cyclophosphamide (FAC). Acute myeloid leukemia (AML) and myelodysplastic syndrome (MDS) have been reported in pediatric patients and some adult patients receiving dexrazoxane in combination with chemotherapy.

◀ When used for the prevention of cardiomyopathy, doxorubicin should be administered within 30 minutes after the completion of the dexrazoxane infusion (do not administer doxorubicin before dexrazoxane). Dosage adjustment required for moderate or severe renal insufficiency (clearance is reduced). Due to dosage adjustments for doxorubicin in hepatic impairment, a proportional dose reduction in dexrazoxane is recommended to maintain the dosage ratio of 10:1. Do not use DMSO in patients receiving dexrazoxane for anthracycline extravasation; may diminish dexrazoxane efficacy. For IV administration; not for local infiltration into extravasation site.

Adverse Reactions Note: Most adverse reactions are thought to be attributed to chemotherapy, except for increased myelosuppression, pain at injection site, and phlebitis.

Prevention of doxorubicin cardiomyopathy (reactions listed are those which were greater in the dexrazoxane arm in a comparison of chemotherapy plus dexrazoxane vs chemotherapy alone):
Cardiovascular: Phlebitis (6%)
Central nervous system: Fatigue (61%), neurotoxicity (17%)
Dermatologic: Erythema (5%)
Hematologic & oncologic: Bone marrow depression, granulocytopenia, leukopenia, thrombocytopenia
Infection: Infection (23%), sepsis (17%)
Local: Pain at injection site pain (12%)
Miscellaneous: Fever (34%)
Postmarketing, and/or case reports: Metastases (including acute myeloid leukemia, myelodysplastic syndrome)

Anthracycline extravasation:
Cardiovascular: Peripheral edema (10%), localized phlebitis (6%)
Central nervous system: Fatigue (13%), dizziness (11%), depression (8%), headache (6%), insomnia (5%)
Dermatologic: Alopecia (14%)
Endocrine & metabolic: Hypercalcemia (7%), hyponatremia (6%), increased lactate dehydrogenase (5%)
Gastrointestinal: Nausea (43%), vomiting (19%), diarrhea (11%), abdominal pain (6%), constipation (6%), anorexia (5%)
Hematologic & oncologic: Decreased white blood cell count (73%; grade 3: 25%; grade 4: 20%), decreased neutrophils (61%; grade 3: 22%; grade 4: 24%), decreased hemoglobin (43%; grade 3: 3%), anemia (6%), febrile neutropenia (3%), neutropenia (3%), leukopenia, thrombocytopenia
Hepatic: Increased serum AST (28%), increased serum ALT (22%), increased serum bilirubin (11%), increased serum alkaline phosphatase (4%)
Infection: Postoperative infection (16%)
Local: Pain at injection site (16%)
Renal: Increased serum creatinine (14%)
Respiratory: Dyspnea (8%), pneumonia (6%), cough (5%)
Miscellaneous: Fever (21%)

Drug Interactions
Metabolism/Transport Effects None known.
Avoid Concomitant Use
Avoid concomitant use of Dexrazoxane with any of the following: BCG (Intravesical); CloZAPine; Dimethyl Sulfoxide; Dipyrone

Increased Effect/Toxicity

Dexrazoxane may increase the levels/effects of: CloZAPine

The levels/effects of Dexrazoxane may be increased by: Dipyrone

Decreased Effect

Dexrazoxane may decrease the levels/effects of: BCG (Intravesical); DOX-Orubicin (Conventional)

The levels/effects of Dexrazoxane may be decreased by: Dimethyl Sulfoxide

Storage/Stability Note: Preparation and storage are product specific; refer to individual product labeling for further details. Discard unused solutions.

Totect: Store intact vials at 25°C (77°F); excursions permitted to 15°C to 30°C (59°F to 86°F). Protect from light. When reconstituted with the supplied diluent to a final concentration of 10 mg/mL the reconstituted solution is stable for 2 hours. Solutions for infusion are stable for 4 hours when stored at <25°C (77°F).

Zinecard: Store intact vials at 25°C (77°F); excursions permitted to 15°C to 30°C (59°F to 86°F). When reconstituted with sterile water for injection, the reconstituted solution is stable for 30 minutes at room temperature or 3 hours refrigerated at 2°C to 8°C (36°F to 46°F). Solutions diluted for infusion are stable for 1 hour when stored at room temperature or 4 hours refrigerated.

Dexrazoxane generic formulation (Mylan): Store intact vials at 20°C to 25°C (68°F to 77°F). Reconstituted solutions and solutions diluted for infusion are stable for 6 hours when stored at room temperature or refrigerated at 2°C to 8°C (36°F to 46°F).

Additional stability information: When studied as a 24-hour continuous infusion for the prevention of cardiomyopathy, solutions prepared with sodium lactate diluent and diluted to a final concentration of 0.1 or 0.5 mg/mL in D_5W were found to retain ≥90% of their initial concentration when stored at room temperature (ambient light conditions) for ≤24 hours (Tetef, 2001).

Preparation for Administration Hazardous agent; use appropriate precautions for handling and disposal (NIOSH 2014 [group 2]).

Note: Preparation and storage are product specific; refer to individual product labeling for further details. Discard unused solutions. Do not mix in the same container with other medications.

Totect: Reconstitute 500 mg vial with 50 mL of the supplied diluent (0.167 Molar sodium lactate injection) to a final concentration of 10 mg/mL. Prior to infusion, further dilute reconstituted dexrazoxane solution in NS 1000 mL.

Zinecard: Reconstitute vial with sterile water for injection to a concentration of dexrazoxane 10 mg/mL. Prior to infusion, further dilute reconstituted dexrazoxane solution in lactated Ringer's injection to a final concentration of 1.3-3 mg/mL.

Dexrazoxane generic formulation (Mylan): Reconstitute with the supplied diluent (0.167 Molar sodium lactate injection) to a final concentration of 10 mg/mL. Prior to infusion, further dilute reconstituted dexrazoxane solution with D_5W or NS to a final concentration of 1.3 to 5 mg/mL.

Mechanism of Action Derivative of ethylenediaminetetraacetic acid (EDTA); a potent intracellular chelating agent. As a cardioprotectant, dexrazoxane appears to be converted intracellularly to a ring-opened chelating agent that interferes with iron-mediated oxygen free radical generation thought to be responsible, in part, for anthracycline-induced cardiomyopathy. In the management of anthracycline extravasation, dexrazoxane may act by reversibly inhibiting topoisomerase II, protecting tissue from anthracycline cytotoxicity, thereby decreasing tissue damage.

◀ **Pharmacodynamics/Kinetics**
Distribution: V_d: 22 to 25 L/m^2
Protein binding: None
Half-life elimination: 2.1 to 2.5 hours
Excretion: Urine (42%)

Dosing

Adult & Geriatric

Prevention of doxorubicin cardiomyopathy: IV: A 10:1 ratio of dexrazoxane:doxorubicin (dexrazoxane 500 mg/m^2:doxorubicin 50 mg/m^2). **Note:** Cardiac monitoring should continue during dexrazoxane therapy; doxorubicin/dexrazoxane should be discontinued in patients who develop a decline in LVEF or clinical CHF.

Treatment of anthracycline extravasation: IV: 1000 mg/m^2 on days 1 and 2 (maximum dose: 2000 mg), followed by 500 mg/m^2 on day 3 (maximum dose: 1000 mg); begin treatment as soon as possible, within 6 hours of extravasation

Pediatric Prevention of doxorubicin cardiomyopathy associated with acute lymphoblastic leukemia treatment (high-risk patients; off-label use): IV: A 10:1 ratio of dexrazoxane:doxorubicin (eg, dexrazoxane 300 mg/m^2:doxorubicin 30 mg/m^2) was used in patients with high-risk acute lymphoblastic leukemia; dexrazoxane is administered immediately prior to the doxorubicin dose (Lipshultz, 2010; Moghrabi, 2007; Silverman, 2010)

Renal Impairment Note: Renal function may be estimated using the Cockcroft-Gault formula.
Mild (CrCl ≥40 mL/minute) impairment: No dosage adjustment necessary.
Moderate-to-severe (CrCl <40 mL/minute) impairment:
  Prevention of cardiomyopathy: Reduce dose by 50%, using a 5:1 dexrazoxane:doxorubicin ratio (dexrazoxane 250 mg/m^2:doxorubicin 50 mg/m^2)
  Anthracycline extravasation: Reduce dose by 50%

Hepatic Impairment

Prevention of cardiomyopathy: Since doxorubicin dosage is reduced in hyperbilirubinemia, a proportional reduction in dexrazoxane dosage is recommended (maintain a 10:1 ratio of dexrazoxane:doxorubicin)

Anthracycline extravasation: There are no dosage adjustments provided in the manufacturer's labeling (has not been studied).

Administration

Prevention of doxorubicin cardiomyopathy: Administer doxorubicin within 30 minutes after completion of the dexrazoxane infusion (do not administer doxorubicin before dexrazoxane).

Zinecard: Administer by rapid drip infusion over 15 minutes; do **not** administer by IV push

Dexrazoxane generic formulation (Mylan): Administer by slow IV push or rapid drip infusion

Treatment of anthracycline extravasation: Stop vesicant infusion immediately and disconnect IV line (leave needle/cannula in place); gently aspirate extravasated solution from the IV line (do **NOT** flush the line); remove needle/cannula; elevate extremity. Administer dexrazoxane IV over 1-2 hours; begin infusion as soon as possible, within 6 hours of extravasation. Day 2 and 3 doses should be administered at approximately the same time (±3 hours) as the dose on day 1. Infusion solution should be at room temperature prior to administration. Infuse in a large vein in an area remote from the extravasation. For IV administration only; not for local infiltration into extravasation.

Apply dry cold compresses for 20 minutes 4 times daily for 1-2 days (Pérez Fidalgo, 2012); withhold cooling beginning 15 minutes before dexrazoxane infusion; continue withholding cooling until 15 minutes after infusion is completed. Do not use DMSO in combination with dexrazoxane; may lessen efficacy.

Hazardous agent - use appropriate precautions for handling and disposal (NIOSH 2014 [group 2]).

Emetic Potential Children and Adults: Minimal (<10%)

Monitoring Parameters CBC with differential (frequent); liver function; serum creatinine; cardiac function (repeat monitoring at 400 mg/m^2, 500 mg/m^2, and with every 50 mg/m^2 of doxorubicin thereafter); monitor site of extravasation

Dosage Forms Excipient information presented when available (limited, particularly for generics); consult specific product labeling.

Solution Reconstituted, Intravenous:

Totect: 500 mg (1 ea) [pyrogen free]

Zinecard: 250 mg (1 ea); 500 mg (1 ea) [pyrogen free]

Generic: 250 mg (1 ea); 500 mg (1 ea)

◆ **Dezocitidine** *see* Decitabine *on page 474*

◆ **DF** *see* Defibrotide *on page 494*

◆ **dFdC** *see* Gemcitabine *on page 776*

◆ **dFdCyd** *see* Gemcitabine *on page 776*

◆ **DFM** *see* Deferoxamine *on page 488*

◆ **DHAD** *see* MitoXANtrone *on page 1159*

◆ **DHAQ** *see* MitoXANtrone *on page 1159*

◆ **DHPG Sodium** *see* Ganciclovir (Systemic) *on page 768*

◆ **Diaminocyclohexane Oxalatoplatinum** *see* Oxaliplatin *on page 1269*

◆ **DIC** *see* Dacarbazine *on page 428*

◆ **Difflam** *see* Benzydamine *on page 190*

◆ **Diflucan** *see* Fluconazole *on page 725*

◆ **Diflucan injection (Can)** *see* Fluconazole *on page 725*

◆ **Diflucan One (Can)** *see* Fluconazole *on page 725*

◆ **Diflucan PWS (Can)** *see* Fluconazole *on page 725*

◆ **Difluorodeoxycytidine Hydrochlorothiazide** *see* Gemcitabine *on page 776*

◆ **Dihematoporphyrin Ether** *see* Porfimer *on page 1409*

◆ **Dihydrohydroxycodeinone** *see* OxyCODONE *on page 1277*

◆ **Dihydromorphinone** *see* HYDROmorphone *on page 830*

◆ **Dihydroxyanthracenedione** *see* MitoXANtrone *on page 1159*

◆ **Dihydroxyanthracenedione Dihydrochloride** *see* MitoXANtrone *on page 1159*

◆ **Dihydroxydeoxynorvinkaleukoblastine** *see* Vinorelbine *on page 1764*

◆ **Dilaudid** *see* HYDROmorphone *on page 830*

◆ **Dilaudid-HP** *see* HYDROmorphone *on page 830*

Dimethyl Sulfoxide (dye meth il sul FOKS ide)

Related Information
Management of Drug Extravasations *on page 2159*

Brand Names: US Rimso-50

Brand Names: Canada Dimethyl Sulfoxide Irrigation, USP; Kemsol; Rimso-50

Index Terms Dimethylsulfoxide; DMSO

Pharmacologic Category Antidote, Extravasation; Urinary Tract Product

Use
Interstitial cystitis: Symptomatic relief of interstitial cystitis.

Limitation of use: There is no clinical evidence of effectiveness of dimethyl sulfoxide in the treatment of bacterial urinary tract infections.

Labeled Contraindications There are no contraindications listed in the manufacturer's labeling.

Pregnancy Considerations Adverse events have been observed in some animal reproduction studies.

Breast-Feeding Considerations It is not known if dimethyl sulfoxide is excreted in breast milk. The manufacturer recommends that caution be exercised when administering dimethyl sulfoxide to nursing women.

Warnings/Precautions For bladder instillation or topical administration for extravasation management (off-label use) only; not for IV or IM administration. Do not use in patients receiving dexrazoxane for anthracycline extravasation (Mourdisen, 2007); dimethyl sulfoxide (DMSO) may diminish dexrazoxane efficacy. Hypersensitivity reactions with intravesical administration have been reported rarely; hypersensitivity has also occurred with topical administration. If anaphylactoid symptoms occur, manage appropriately. Use with caution in patients with urinary tract malignancy; may be harmful due to vasodilatory effects. Lens changes and opacities have been observed in animal studies; full eye exams (including slit lamp) are recommended prior to use and periodically during treatment. A garlic-like taste may occur, beginning a few minutes after instillation and lasting for several hours. Garlic odor on the breath and skin may also occur and persist for up to 3 days. Bladder discomfort may occur; generally diminishes with repeated administration.

Adverse Reactions Frequency not defined.

Dermatologic: Body odor (garlic; duration: Up to 72 hours)

Gastrointestinal: Halitosis/unpleasant taste (garlic; onset: Within a few minutes after instillation; duration: Up to 72 hours)

Genitourinary: Bladder pain, cystitis (transient)

Local: Localized erythema (topical application; Perez Fidalgo, 2012)

Hypersensitivity: Hypersensitivity

Postmarketing and/or case reports: Contact dermatitis, cystitis (eosinophilic), pigment deposits on lens

Drug Interactions
Metabolism/Transport Effects Inhibits CYP2C19 (weak), CYP2C9 (weak)

Avoid Concomitant Use

Avoid concomitant use of Dimethyl Sulfoxide with any of the following: Dexrazoxane

Increased Effect/Toxicity

Dimethyl Sulfoxide may increase the levels/effects of: Sulindac

Decreased Effect

Dimethyl Sulfoxide may decrease the levels/effects of: Dexrazoxane

Storage/Stability Store at 20°C to 25°C (68°F to 77°F). Protect from strong light.

Mechanism of Action For management of cystitis, dimethyl sulfoxide (DMSO) has anti-inflammatory, analgesic, mast cell inhibition, and muscle relaxing effects (Chancellor, 2004). DMSO also has free-radical scavenger properties, which increases removal of vesicant drugs from tissues to minimize tissue damage in extravasation management (Perez Fidalgo, 2012).

Pharmacodynamics/Kinetics

Absorption: Topical: Absorbed

Distribution: Topical: Generally distributed into tissues and body fluid

Excretion: Urine and feces; some elimination via skin and lungs

Dosing

Adult & Geriatric

Interstitial cystitis: Bladder instillation: Instill 50 mL directly into bladder and retain for 15 minutes; repeat every 2 weeks until symptoms are relieved, then increase intervals between treatments **or** 50 mL directly into bladder and retain for 15 to 20 minutes every 1 to 2 weeks for 4 to 8 treatments (Chancellor, 2004)

Extravasation management (anthracyclines, mitomycin, or mitoxantrone; off-label use): Topical DMSO: Apply to a region covering twice the affected area every 8 hours for 7 days; begin within 10 minutes of extravasation; do not cover with a dressing (Perez Fidalgo, 2012)

Pediatric Extravasation management (anthracyclines, mitomycin, or mitoxantrone; off-label use): Children and Adolescents: Refer to adult dosing.

Administration

Intravesical: Instill directly into the bladder via catheter or syringe. To reduce bladder spasm, apply an analgesic lubricant (eg, lidocaine jelly) to urethra prior to catheter insertion; oral analgesics or belladonna and opium suppositories prior to administration may be of benefit. **Not for IV or IM use.**

Extravasation management (off-label use): Stop vesicant infusion immediately and disconnect IV line (leave needle/cannula in place); gently aspirate extravasated solution from the IV line (do **NOT** flush the line); remove needle/cannula; elevate extremity. Apply DMSO topically (within 10 minutes of extravasation) to extravasation site, covering an area twice the size of extravasation; allow to air dry; do not cover with a dressing (Perez Fidalgo, 2012). **Not for IV or IM use.**

Monitoring Parameters CBC, chemistry panel, liver and renal function tests about every 6 months; eye examinations and slit lamp examinations (baseline and periodically during treatment). For extravasation management, monitor and document extravasation site.

Dosage Forms Excipient information presented when available (limited, particularly for generics); consult specific product labeling.

Solution, Intravesical:

Rimso-50: 50% (50 mL)

◆ **Dimethylsulfoxide** see Dimethyl Sulfoxide on page 528

◆ **Dimethyl Sulfoxide Irrigation, USP (Can)** see Dimethyl Sulfoxide on page 528

◆ **Dimethyl Triazeno Imidazole Carboxamide** see Dacarbazine on page 428

Dinutuximab (din ue TUX i mab)

Related Information

Chemotherapy-Induced Peripheral Neuropathy *on page* 2116

Common Toxicity Criteria *on page* 2122

Principles of Anticancer Therapy *on page* 2261

Brand Names: US Unituxin

Index Terms ch14.18; MOAB Ch14.18

Pharmacologic Category Antineoplastic Agent, Anti-GD2; Antineoplastic Agent, Monoclonal Antibody

Use Neuroblastoma: Treatment of high-risk neuroblastoma (in combination with granulocyte-macrophage colony-stimulating factor [GM-CSF; sargramostim], interleukin-2 [IL-2; aldesleukin] and 13-cis-retinoic acid [RA; isotretinoin]) in pediatric patients who achieve at least a partial response to prior first-line multiagent, multimodality therapy.

Labeled Contraindications History of anaphylaxis to dinutuximab

Pregnancy Considerations Reproduction studies have not been completed with dinutuximab. Monoclonal antibodies cross the placenta, the largest amount during the third trimester of pregnancy. Based on the mechanism of action, dinutuximab may cause fetal harm. Women of reproductive potential should use effective contraception during therapy and for 2 months after the last dose.

Breast-Feeding Considerations It is not known if dinutuximab is excreted in breast milk. IgG molecules are excreted in breast milk. Due to the potential for serious adverse reactions in the nursing infant, breast-feeding is not recommended by the manufacturer.

Warnings/Precautions [US Boxed Warning]: Serious and potentially life-threatening infusion reactions occurred in approximately one-fourth of patients treated with dinutuximab. Administer required prehydration and premedication, including antihistamines, prior to each dinutuximab infusion. Monitor patients closely for signs and symptoms of an infusion reaction during and for at least 4 hours following completion of each dinutuximab infusion. Immediately interrupt dinutuximab for severe infusion reactions and permanently discontinue dinutuximab for anaphylaxis. Infusion reactions typically occurred during infusion or within 24 hours of completion and may include facial and upper airway edema, dyspnea, bronchospasm, stridor, urticaria, and hypotension. Infusion reactions may require blood pressure support, bronchodilator therapy, corticosteroids, infusion rate interruption and/or reduction, or permanent therapy discontinuation. Infusion should be in a facility with cardiopulmonary medication/equipment available. Severe capillary leak syndrome was reported in close to one-fourth of patients receiving dinutuximab. Immediately interrupt infusion if capillary leak syndrome develops; infusion rate reduction and/or therapy discontinuation may be necessary. Initiate appropriate management in patients with symptomatic or severe capillary leak syndrome. Severe hypotension occurred more frequently in patients receiving dinutuximab. Intravenous hydration is required prior to each infusion; closely monitor blood pressure during infusion. May require therapy interruption or discontinuation; initiate appropriate medical management in patients with a systolic blood pressure (SBP) less than lower limit of normal for age, or SBP that is decreased by more than 15% compared to baseline. Electrolyte abnormalities (such as hyponatremia, hypokalemia, and hypocalcemia) were reported in at least one-fourth of patients who received dinutuximab, including grade 3 or 4 events. In a study of a related anti-GD2 antibody, syndrome of inappropriate antidiuretic hormone secretion (SIADH) resulting in severe hyponatremia was reported. Monitor electrolytes closely during therapy.

[US Boxed Warning]: Dinutuximab causes severe neuropathic pain in the majority of patients. Administer intravenous opioids prior to, during, and for 2 hours following completion of the dinutuximab infusion. In clinical studies of patients with high-risk neuroblastoma, grade 3 peripheral sensory neuropathy occurred in 2% to 9% of patients. In clinical studies of dinutuximab and related GD2-binding antibodies, severe motor neuropathy was observed in adults. Resolution of motor neuropathy was not documented in all cases. Permanently discontinue dinutuximab for severe unresponsive pain, severe sensory neuropathy, or moderate to severe peripheral motor neuropathy. In patients who experienced peripheral sensory neuropathy of any grade, the median duration was 9 days (range: 3 to 163 days). Most patients experienced pain; severe pain was observed in over 50% of patients treated with dinutuximab; pain may occur despite analgesic/ opioid therapy. Pain typically occurred during infusion and included abdominal, generalized, extremity, or back pain, neuralgia, musculoskeletal chest pain, and arthralgia. Premedication with analgesics, including opioids, is required prior to each dose, during the infusion, and for 2 hours following the infusion. Severe pain may require reduction of the infusion rate or therapy discontinuation.

Severe (grade 3 or 4) anemia, neutropenia, thrombocytopenia, and neutropenic fever were observed in dinutuximab-treated patients. Monitor complete blood counts closely during treatment. Severe (grade 3 or 4) bacteremia was reported more frequently in dinutuximab-treated patients, and required intravenous antibiotics or other urgent interventions. Sepsis was also observed in patients receiving dinutuximab. Monitor closely for signs/symptoms of systemic infection; may require therapy interruption until resolution of infection. Hemolytic uremic syndrome (without documented infection) resulted in renal insufficiency, electrolyte abnormalities, anemia, and hypertension in a small number of patients. Atypical hemolytic uremic syndrome recurred in one patient upon rechallenge. Permanently discontinue if hemolytic uremic syndrome develops; manage supportively. Neurological ocular toxicity such as blurred vision, photophobia, mydriasis, fixed or unequal pupils, optic nerve disorder, and papilledema were reported in clinical trials. In patients who experienced complete resolution of ocular toxicity, the median duration of toxicity was 4 days (range: 0 to 221 days). May require therapy interruption, dosage reduction, or treatment discontinuation. Potentially significant interactions may exist, requiring dose or frequency adjustment, additional monitoring, and/or selection of alternative therapy.

Adverse Reactions Frequency not always defined.

>10%:

Cardiovascular: Hypotension (60%; grades 3/4: 16%), capillary leak syndrome (40%; grades ≥3: 6% to 23%), tachycardia (19%), edema (17%), hypertension (14%)

Central nervous system: Pain (85%; grades 3/4: 51%), peripheral neuropathy (13%; grades 3/4: 6%)

Dermatologic: Urticaria (37%; grades 3/4: 13%)

Endocrine & metabolic: Hyponatremia (58%; grades 3/4: 23%), hypokalemia (43%), hypoalbuminemia (33%), hypocalcemia (27%), hypophosphatemia (20%), hyperglycemia (18%), hypertriglyceridemia (16%), hypomagnesemia (12%)

Gastrointestinal: Increased serum alanine aminotransferase (56%), vomiting (46%), diarrhea (43%), increased serum aspartate aminotransferase (28%), decreased appetite (15%)

Genitourinary: Proteinuria (16%)

Hematologic & oncologic: Thrombocytopenia (66%; grades 3/4: 39%), lymphocytopenia (62%; grades 3/4: 51%), anemia (51%; grades 3/4: 34%), neutropenia (39%; grades 3/4: 34%), hemorrhage (17%; grades 3/4: 6%), febrile neutropenia (grades 3/4: 4%)

Infection: Sepsis (18%; grade 3/4: 16%), infection (device related, 16%; grade 3/4: 16%), bacteremia (grades 3/4: 13%)

Renal: Increased serum creatinine (15%)

Respiratory: Hypoxia (24%)

Miscellaneous: Fever (72%; grades 3/4: 40%), infusion related reaction (60%)

1% to 10%

Central nervous system: Peripheral sensory neuropathy (9%; grade 3: 1%), peripheral motor neuropathy (grade 3: 1%)

Endocrine & metabolic: Weight gain (10%), electrolyte disturbance

Gastrointestinal: Nausea (10%)

Hematologic & oncologic: Hemolytic-uremic syndrome (2%)

Hypersensitivity: Severe infusion related reaction

Ophthalmic: Blurred vision (2%), blepharoptosis, optic nerve damage, papilledema, photophobia

Renal: Renal insufficiency

<1%, postmarketing, and/or case reports: Diplopia, fixation of pupils, mydriasis

Drug Interactions

Metabolism/Transport Effects None known.

Avoid Concomitant Use

Avoid concomitant use of Dinutuximab with any of the following: BCG (Intravesical); Belimumab; CloZAPine; Dipyrone; Natalizumab; Pimecrolimus; Tacrolimus (Topical); Tofacitinib; Vaccines (Live)

Increased Effect/Toxicity

Dinutuximab may increase the levels/effects of: Belimumab; CloZAPine; DULoxetine; Fingolimod; Hypotensive Agents; Leflunomide; Levodopa; Natalizumab; RisperiDONE; Tofacitinib; Vaccines (Live)

The levels/effects of Dinutuximab may be increased by: ARIPiprazole; ARIPiprazole Lauroxil; Barbiturates; Denosumab; Dipyrone; Nicorandil; Pimecrolimus; Roflumilast; Tacrolimus (Topical); Trastuzumab

Decreased Effect

Dinutuximab may decrease the levels/effects of: BCG (Intravesical); Coccidioides immitis Skin Test; Sipuleucel-T; Vaccines (Inactivated); Vaccines (Live)

The levels/effects of Dinutuximab may be decreased by: Echinacea

Storage/Stability Store intact vials at 2°C to 8°C (36°F to 46°F); do not freeze. Do not shake. Keep the vial in the outer carton to protect from light. Solutions diluted for infusion should be stored at 2°C to 8°C (36°F to 46°F). Initiate infusion within 4 hours of preparation. Discard diluted solution 24 hours after preparation.

Preparation for Administration Must be diluted prior to infusion. Withdraw the required dinutuximab volume and inject into a 100 mL bag of NS. Mix by gentle inversion; do not shake. Discard unused vial contents. Initiate infusion within 4 hours of preparation. Do not use if cloudy, discolored (pronounced), or contains particulates.

Mechanism of Action Dinutuximab binds to the disialoganglioside GD2, which is highly expressed in neuroblastoma, most melanomas, and other tumors, as well as on normal tissues such as neurons, skin melanocytes, and peripheral sensory nerve fibers (Yu, 2010). By binding to CD2, dinutuximab induces cell lysis (of GD2-expressing cells) through antibody-dependent cell-mediated cytotoxicity (ADCC) and complement-dependent cytotoxicity (CDC).

Pharmacodynamics/Kinetics

Distribution: Pediatric: 5.4 L

Half-life elimination, terminal: 10 days

Dosing

Pediatric

Neuroblastoma, high-risk: IV: 17.5 mg/m^2/day for 4 consecutive days for a maximum of 5 cycles (in combination with GM-CSF [sargramostim], IL-2 [aldesleukin] and 13-cis-retinoic acid [isotretinoin]). Infuse on days 4, 5, 6, and 7 during cycles 1, 3, and 5 (cycles 1, 3, and 5 are 24 days in duration); infuse on days 8, 9, 10, and 11 during cycles 2 and 4 (cycles 2 and 4 are 32 days in duration).

Premedications:

Analgesics: Administer morphine 50 mcg/kg IV immediately prior to dinutuximab infusion initiation; continue as a morphine drip at an infusion rate of 20 to 50 mcg/kg/hour during and for 2 hours following completion of infusion. May administer additional doses of 25 to 50 mcg/kg IV as needed up to once every 2 hours followed by an increase in the drip rate in clinically stable patients. Consider conversion to fentanyl or hydromorphone if morphine is not tolerated; if pain is inadequately controlled with opioids, consider adjunct therapy with gabapentin or lidocaine.

Antihistamine: Administer an antihistamine (eg, diphenhydramine 0.5 to 1 mg/kg/dose; maximum dose 50 mg) IV over 10 to 15 minutes starting 20 minutes prior to dinutuximab infusion and every 4 to 6 hours as tolerated during the infusion.

Antipyretics: Administer acetaminophen (10 to 15 mg/kg/dose; maximum dose 650 mg) 20 minutes prior to each infusion and every 4 to 6 hours as needed for fever and pain. May administer ibuprofen (5 to 10 mg/kg/dose) every 6 hours as needed for control of persistent fever or pain.

IV hydration: Administer NS 10 mL/kg IV over 1 hour just prior to each dinutuximab infusion.

Renal Impairment There are no dosage adjustments provided in the manufacturer's labeling (has not been studied).

Hepatic Impairment There are no dosage adjustments provided in the manufacturer's labeling (has not been studied).

Adjustment for Toxicity

Anaphylaxis, grade 3 or 4: Permanently discontinue therapy.

Capillary leak syndrome:

Moderate to severe, but not life-threatening: Immediately interrupt infusion; upon resolution, resume infusion at 50% of the previous rate.

◄

Life-threatening: Discontinue infusion for the current cycle; in subsequent cycles, infuse at 50% of the previous rate. If life-threatening capillary leak syndrome recurs, permanently discontinue therapy.

Hemolytic uremic syndrome: Permanently discontinue therapy and administer supportive management.

Hyponatremia, grade 4 (despite appropriate fluid management): Permanently discontinue therapy.

Hypotension (symptomatic hypotension, systolic blood pressure [SBP] less than lower limit of normal for age, or SBP decreased by more than 15% compared to baseline): Interrupt infusion; upon resolution, resume infusion at 50% of the previous rate. If blood pressure remains stable for ≥2 hours, increase infusion rate as tolerated up to a maximum rate of 1.75 mg/m²/hour.

Infection (systemic)/sepsis, severe: Discontinue therapy until infection resolves; may resume therapy with subsequent cycles.

Infusion-related reaction:

Mild to moderate reaction (eg, transient rash, fever, rigors, and localized urticaria that respond promptly to symptomatic treatment): Reduce infusion rate by 50%; monitor closely. Upon resolution, gradually increase infusion rate up to a maximum of 1.75 mg/m²/hour.

Severe or prolonged reaction (eg, mild bronchospasm without other symptoms, angioedema that does not affect the airway): Immediately interrupt infusion; if symptoms resolve rapidly, resume infusion at 50% of the previous rate and monitor closely. If reaction recurs, discontinue therapy until the following day. If symptoms resolve and further treatment is warranted, premedicate with IV hydrocortisone 1 mg/kg (maximum 50 mg) and infuse at a rate of 0.875 mg/m²/hour in an intensive care unit. If reaction recurs again, permanently discontinue therapy.

Life-threatening reaction: Permanently discontinue therapy and administer supportive management.

Neuropathy:

Grade 4 sensory neuropathy or grade 3 sensory neuropathy that interferes with daily activities for more than 2 weeks: Permanently discontinue therapy.

Grade 2 peripheral motor neuropathy: Permanently discontinue therapy.

Ocular neurological disorders (eg, blurred vision, photophobia, mydriasis, fixed or unequal pupils, optic nerve disorder, eyelid ptosis, and/or papilledema): Discontinue infusion until symptom resolution; upon resolution, reduce **dose** by 50%. If reaction recurs, or if reaction is accompanied by visual impairment (eg, subtotal or total vision loss), permanently discontinue therapy.

Pain, severe (grade 3): Decrease the infusion rate to 0.875 mg/m²/hour. If pain is not adequately controlled despite rate reduction and use of maximum supportive measures, permanently discontinue therapy.

Serum sickness, grade 3 or 4: Permanently discontinue therapy.

Administration Administer as an IV infusion only; **do not administer as an IV push or bolus.** Administer NS 10 mL/kg IV over 1 hour just prior to each dinutuximab infusion. Premedicate with analgesics, an antihistamine, and an antipyretic prior to administration (see Dosing). Infuse in an environment equipped to monitor for and manage infusion reactions. Interrupt infusion for toxicity (see Dosing Adjustment for Toxicity).

Initiate infusion at a rate of 0.875 mg/m^2/hour for 30 minutes. Increase infusion rate gradually as tolerated to a maximum rate of 1.75 mg/m^2/hour to infuse over 10 to 20 hours each day. Monitor patients closely for signs and symptoms of an infusion reaction during and for at least 4 hours following completion of each dinutuximab infusion.

Monitoring Parameters CBC with differential, serum electrolytes, renal function, blood pressure; monitor for signs/symptoms of infusion reactions (during and for at least 4 hours after infusion), pain, peripheral neuropathy, capillary leak syndrome, infection/sepsis, hemolytic uremic syndrome, and ocular toxicity

Dosage Forms Excipient information presented when available (limited, particularly for generics); consult specific product labeling.

Solution, Intravenous [preservative free]:

Unituxin: 17.5 mg/5 mL (5 mL) [contains mouse protein (murine) (hamster)]

◆ **Disodium Thiosulfate Pentahydrate** see Sodium Thiosulfate on page 1540

◆ **5071-1DL(6)** see Megestrol on page 1076

◆ **4-DMDR** see IDArubicin on page 862

◆ **DMSO** see Dimethyl Sulfoxide on page 528

◆ **Docefrez** see DOCEtaxel on page 535

DOCEtaxel (doe se TAKS el)

Related Information

Chemotherapy and Cancer Treatment During Pregnancy on page 2214

Chemotherapy and Obesity on page 2220

Common Toxicity Criteria on page 2122

Management of Chemotherapy-Induced Nausea and Vomiting in Adults on page 2142

Management of Drug Extravasations on page 2159

Mucositis and Stomatitis on page 2186

Prevention of Chemotherapy-Induced Nausea and Vomiting in Children on page 2203

Safe Handling of Hazardous Drugs on page 2292

Brand Names: US Docefrez; Taxotere

Brand Names: Canada Docetaxel for Injection; Taxotere

Index Terms RP-6976

Pharmacologic Category Antineoplastic Agent, Antimicrotubular; Antineoplastic Agent, Taxane Derivative

Use

US labeling:

Docefrez:

Breast cancer: Treatment of breast cancer (locally advanced/metastatic) after prior chemotherapy failure

Non-small cell lung cancer: Treatment of locally advanced or metastatic non-small cell lung cancer (NSCLC)

Prostate cancer: Treatment of hormone-refractory metastatic prostate cancer

Taxotere:

Breast cancer: Treatment of breast cancer (locally advanced/metastatic) after prior chemotherapy failure, or adjuvant treatment of operable node-positive

Gastric cancer: Treatment of advanced gastric adenocarcinoma

◀ **Head and neck cancer:** Treatment of locally advanced squamous cell head and neck cancer

NSCLC: Treatment of locally advanced or metastatic NSCLC

Prostate cancer: Treatment of hormone refractory, metastatic prostate cancer

Canadian labeling:

Breast cancer: Treatment of breast cancer (locally advanced/metastatic or adjuvant treatment of operable node-positive)

Head and neck cancer: Treatment of recurrent and/or metastatic squamous cell head and neck cancer

NSCLC: Treatment of locally advanced or metastatic NSCLC

Ovarian cancer: Treatment of metastatic ovarian cancer following failure of first-line or subsequent chemotherapy

Prostate cancer: Treatment of hormone refractory, metastatic prostate cancer

Labeled Contraindications

Severe hypersensitivity to docetaxel or any component of the formulation; severe hypersensitivity to other medications containing polysorbate 80; neutrophil count <1500/mm^3

Canadian labeling: Additional contraindications (not in U.S. labeling): Severe hepatic impairment; pregnancy; breast-feeding

Pregnancy Considerations Adverse events have been observed in animal reproduction studies. An *ex vivo* human placenta perfusion model illustrated that docetaxel crossed the placenta at term. Placental transfer was low and affected by the presence of albumin; higher albumin concentrations resulted in lower docetaxel placental transfer (Berveiller, 2012). Some pharmacokinetic properties of docetaxel may be altered in pregnant women (van Hasselt, 2014). Women of childbearing potential should avoid becoming pregnant during therapy. A pregnancy registry is available for all cancers diagnosed during pregnancy at Cooper Health (877-635-4499).

Breast-Feeding Considerations It is not known if docetaxel is excreted into breast milk. Due to the potential for serious adverse reactions in nursing the infant, the US labeling recommends a decision be made to discontinue breast-feeding or the drug, taking into account the importance of treatment to the mother. The Canadian labeling contraindicates use in breast-feeding women.

Warnings/Precautions Hazardous agent - use appropriate precautions for handling and disposal (NIOSH 2014 [group 1]). **[US Boxed Warning]: Avoid use in patients with bilirubin exceeding upper limit of normal (ULN) or AST and/or ALT >1.5 times ULN in conjunction with alkaline phosphatase >2.5 times ULN; patients with isolated transaminase elevations >1.5 times ULN also had a higher rate of neutropenic fever, although no increased incidence of toxic death.** Patients with abnormal liver function are also at increased risk of other treatment-related adverse events, including grade 4 neutropenia, infections, and severe thrombocytopenia, stomatitis, skin toxicity or toxic death; obtain liver function tests prior to each treatment cycle. Canadian labeling contraindicates use in severe hepatic impairment. Canadian labeling contraindicates use in severe hepatic impairment. **[US Boxed Warnings]: Severe hypersensitivity reactions, characterized by generalized rash/erythema, hypotension, bronchospasms, or anaphylaxis may occur (may be fatal; has occurred in patients receiving corticosteroid premedication); minor reactions including flushing or localized skin reactions may also occur; do not administer to patients with a history of severe hypersensitivity to docetaxel or polysorbate 80 (component of**

formulation). Severe fluid retention, characterized by pleural effusion (requiring immediate drainage, ascites, peripheral edema (poorly tolerated), dyspnea at rest, cardiac tamponade, generalized edema, and weight gain, has been reported. Fluid retention may begin as lower extremity peripheral edema and become generalized with a median weight gain of 2 kg. In patients with breast cancer, the median cumulative dose to onset of moderate or severe fluid retention was 819 mg/m^2; fluid retention resolves in a median of 16 weeks after discontinuation. Observe for hypersensitivity, especially with the first two infusions. Discontinue for severe reactions; do not rechallenge if severe. Patients should be premedicated with a corticosteroid (starting one day prior to administration) to reduce the incidence and severity of hypersensitivity reactions and fluid retention; severity is reduced with dexamethasone premedication starting one day prior to docetaxel administration. Premedication with oral corticosteroids is recommended to decrease the incidence and severity of fluid retention and severity of hypersensitivity reactions. The manufacturer recommends dexamethasone 16 mg/day (8 mg twice daily) orally for 3 days, starting the day before docetaxel administration; for prostate cancer, when prednisone is part of the antineoplastic regimen, dexamethasone 8 mg orally is administered at 12 hours, 3 hours, and 1 hour prior to docetaxel.

[US Boxed Warning]: Patients with abnormal liver function, those receiving higher doses, and patients with non-small cell lung cancer and a history of prior treatment with platinum derivatives who receive single-agent docetaxel at a dose of 100 mg/m^2 are at higher risk for treatment-related mortality.

Neutropenia is the dose-limiting toxicity. Patients with increased liver function tests experienced more episodes of neutropenia with a greater number of severe infections. **[US Boxed Warning]: Patients with an absolute neutrophil count <1,500/mm^3 should not receive docetaxel.** Platelets should recover to >100,000/mm^3 prior to treatment. Monitor blood counts and liver function tests frequently; dose reduction or therapy discontinuation may be necessary.

Cutaneous reactions including erythema (with edema) and desquamation have been reported; may require dose reduction. Cystoid macular edema (CME) has been reported; if vision impairment occurs, a prompt comprehensive ophthalmic exam is recommended. If CME is diagnosed, initiate appropriate CME management and discontinue docetaxel (consider non-taxane treatments). In a study of patients receiving docetaxel for the adjuvant treatment of breast cancer, a majority of patients experienced tearing, which occurred in patients with and without lacrimal duct obstruction at baseline; onset was generally after cycle 1, but subsided in most patients within 4 months after therapy completion (Chan, 2013). Dosage adjustment is recommended with severe neurosensory symptoms (paresthesia, dysesthesia, pain); persistent symptoms may require discontinuation; reversal of symptoms may be delayed after discontinuation. Some docetaxel formulations contain alcohol (content varies by formulation), which may affect the central nervous system and cause symptoms of alcohol intoxication. Consider alcohol content and use with caution in patients for whom alcohol intake should be avoided or minimized. Patients should avoid driving or operating machinery immediately after the infusion. Treatment-related acute myeloid leukemia or myelodysplasia occurred in patients receiving docetaxel in combination with anthracyclines and/or cyclophosphamide. Fatigue and weakness (may be severe) have been

◀ reported; symptoms may last a few days up to several weeks; in patients with progressive disease, weakness may be associated with a decrease in performance status. Potentially significant drug-drug interactions may exist, requiring dose or frequency adjustment, additional monitoring, and/or selection of alternative therapy. Docetaxel is an irritant with vesicant-like properties; ensure proper needle or catheter placement prior to and during infusion; avoid extravasation.

Some dosage forms may contain polysorbate 80 (also known as Tweens). Hypersensitivity reactions, usually a delayed reaction, have been reported following exposure to pharmaceutical products containing polysorbate 80 in certain individuals (Isaksson, 2002; Lucente 2000; Shelley, 1995). Thrombocytopenia, ascites, pulmonary deterioration, and renal and hepatic failure have been reported in premature neonates after receiving parenteral products containing polysorbate 80 (Alade, 1986; CDC, 1984). See manufacturer's labeling.

Adverse Reactions Percentages reported for docetaxel monotherapy; frequency may vary depending on diagnosis, dose, liver function, prior treatment, and premedication. The incidence of adverse events was usually higher in patients with elevated liver function tests.

>10%:
  Central nervous system: Central nervous system toxicity (20% to 58%; severe: 6%; including neuropathy)
  Dermatologic: Alopecia (56% to 76%), dermatological reaction (20% to 48%; severe: ≤5%), nail disease (11% to 41%)
  Endocrine & metabolic: Fluid retention (13% to 60%; severe: 7% to 9%; dose dependent)
  Gastrointestinal: Stomatitis (19% to 53%; severe 1% to 8%), diarrhea (23% to 43%; severe: 5% to 6%), nausea (34% to 42%), vomiting (22% to 23%)
  Hematologic & oncologic: Neutropenia (84% to 99%; grade 4: 75% to 86%; nadir [median]: 7 days, duration [severe neutropenia]: 7 days; dose dependent), leukopenia (84% to 99%; grade 4: 32% to 44%), anemia (65% to 97%; dose dependent; grades 3/4: 8% to 9%), thrombocytopenia (8% to 14%; grade 4: 1%; dose dependent), febrile neutropenia (5% to 14%; dose dependent)
  Hepatic: Increased serum transaminases (4% to 19%)
  Hypersensitivity: Hypersensitivity (1% to 21%; with premedication 15%)
  Infection: Infection (1% to 34%; dose dependent)
  Neuromuscular & skeletal: Weakness (53% to 66%; severe 13% to 18%), myalgia (3% to 23%), neuromuscular reaction (16%)
  Respiratory: Pulmonary reaction (41%)
  Miscellaneous: Fever (31% to 35%)
1% to 10%:
  Cardiovascular: Decreased left ventricular ejection fraction (8% to 10%), hypotension (3%)
  Central nervous system: Peripheral motor neuropathy (4%; severe; mainly distal extremity weakness)
  Gastrointestinal: Dysgeusia (6%)
  Hepatic: Increased serum bilirubin (9%), increased serum alkaline phosphatase (4% to 7%)
  Local: Infusion site reactions (4%, including hyperpigmentation, inflammation, redness, dryness, phlebitis, extravasation, swelling of the vein)
  Neuromuscular and skeletal: Arthralgia (3% to 9%)

Ophthalmic: Epiphora (associated with canalicular stenosis [≤77% with weekly administration; ≤1% with every 3-week administration])

<1%, postmarketing, and/or case reports: Abdominal pain, acute myelocytic leukemia, acute respiratory distress, anaphylactic shock, anorexia, ascites, atrial fibrillation, atrial flutter, atrioventricular block, bradycardia, bronchospasm, cardiac arrhythmia, cardiac failure, cardiac tamponade, chest pain, chest tightness, colitis, confusion, conjunctivitis, constipation, cystoid macular edema, deep vein thrombosis, dehydration, disease of the lacrimal apparatus (duct obstruction), disseminated intravascular coagulation, drug fever, duodenal ulcer, dyspnea, ECG abnormality, erythema multiforme, esophagitis, gastrointestinal hemorrhage, gastrointestinal obstruction, gastrointestinal perforation, hearing loss, hemorrhagic diathesis, hepatitis, hypertension, hyponatremia, intestinal obstruction, interstitial pulmonary disease, ischemic colitis, ischemic heart disease, lacrimation, loss of consciousness (transient), lymphedema (peripheral), multiorgan failure, myelodysplastic syndrome, myocardial infarction, neutropenic enterocolitis, ototoxicity, pain, palmarplantar erythrodysesthesia, pericardial effusion, pleural effusion, pneumonia, pneumonitis, pruritus, pulmonary edema, pulmonary embolism, pulmonary fibrosis, radiation pneumonitis, radiation recall phenomenon, renal failure, renal insufficiency, respiratory failure, skin changes (scleroderma-like), seizure, sepsis, sinus tachycardia, Stevens-Johnson syndrome, subacute cutaneous lupus erythematosus, syncope, toxic epidermal necrolysis, tachycardia, thrombophlebitis, unstable angina pectoris, visual disturbance (transient)

Drug Interactions

Metabolism/Transport Effects Substrate of CYP3A4 (major), P-glycoprotein; **Note:** Assignment of Major/Minor substrate status based on clinically relevant drug interaction potential

Avoid Concomitant Use

Avoid concomitant use of DOCEtaxel with any of the following: BCG (Intravesical); CloZAPine; Conivaptan; Dipyrone; Fusidic Acid (Systemic); Idelalisib; Natalizumab; Pimecrolimus; Tacrolimus (Topical); Tofacitinib; Vaccines (Live)

Increased Effect/Toxicity

DOCEtaxel may increase the levels/effects of: Antineoplastic Agents (Anthracycline, Systemic); CloZAPine; Fingolimod; Leflunomide; Natalizumab; Tofacitinib; Vaccines (Live)

The levels/effects of DOCEtaxel may be increased by: Antifungal Agents (Azole Derivatives, Systemic); Conivaptan; CYP3A4 Inhibitors (Moderate); CYP3A4 Inhibitors (Strong); Dasatinib; Denosumab; Dipyrone; Dronedarone; Fusidic Acid (Systemic); Idelalisib; Ivacaftor; Luliconazole; Mifepristone; Netupitant; Osimertinib; Palbociclib; P-glycoprotein/ABCB1 Inhibitors; Pimecrolimus; Platinum Derivatives; Ranolazine; Roflumilast; Simeprevir; SORAfenib; Stiripentol; Tacrolimus (Topical); Trastuzumab

Decreased Effect

DOCEtaxel may decrease the levels/effects of: BCG (Intravesical); Coccidioides immitis Skin Test; Sipuleucel-T; Vaccines (Inactivated); Vaccines (Live)

The levels/effects of DOCEtaxel may be decreased by: Bosentan; CYP3A4 Inducers (Moderate); CYP3A4 Inducers (Strong); Dabrafenib; Deferasirox; Echinacea; Enzalutamide; Mitotane; Osimertinib; P-glycoprotein/ABCB1 Inducers; Siltuximab; St Johns Wort; Tocilizumab

◀ **Storage/Stability** Storage and stability may vary by manufacturer, refer to specific prescribing information.

Docetaxel 10 mg/mL: Store intact vials between 2°C to 25°C (36°F to 77°F) (actual recommendations may vary by generic manufacturer; consult manufacturer's labeling). Protect from bright light. Freezing does not adversely affect the product. Multi-use vials (80 mg/8 mL and 160 mg/16 mL) are stable for up to 28 days after first entry when stored between 2°C to 8°C (36°F to 46°F) and protected from light. Solutions diluted for infusion should be used within 4 hours of preparation, including infusion time.

Docetaxel 20 mg/mL concentrate:

Taxotere: Store intact vials between 2°C to 25°C (36°F to 77°F). Protect from bright light. Freezing does not adversely affect the product. Solutions diluted for infusion in non-PVC containers should be used within 6 hours of preparation, including infusion time, when stored between 2°C to 25°C (36°F to 77°F) or within 48 hours when stored between 2°C to 8°C (36°F to 46°F).

Generic formulations: Store intact vials at 25°C (77°F); excursions permitted between 15°C to 30°C (59°F to 86°F). Protect from light. Solutions diluted for infusion should be used within 4 hours of preparation, including infusion time.

Docetaxel lyophilized powder (Docefrez): Store intact vials between 2°C to 8°C (36°F to 46°F). Protect from light. Allow vials (and provided diluent) to stand at room temperature for 5 minutes prior to reconstitution. After reconstitution, may be stored refrigerated or at room temperature for up to 8 hours. Solutions diluted for infusion should be used within 6 hours of preparation, including infusion time. According to the manufacturer, physical and chemical in-use stability of the infusion solution (prepared as recommended) has been demonstrated in non-PVC bags up to 48 hours when stored between 2°C and 8°C (36°F and 46°F).

Two-vial formulation *(generic; concentrate plus diluent formulation):* Reconstituted solutions of the two-vial formulation are stable in the vial for 8 hours at room temperature or under refrigeration. Solutions diluted for infusion in polyolefin containers should be used within 4 hours of preparation, including infusion time.

Preparation for Administration Hazardous agent; use appropriate precautions for handling and disposal (NIOSH 2014 [group 1]).

Preparation instructions may vary by manufacturer, refer to specific prescribing information. **Note:** Some formulations contain overfill.

Note: Multiple concentrations: Docetaxel is available as a one-vial formulation at concentrations of 10 mg/mL (generic formulation) and 20 mg/mL (concentrate; Taxotere, and as a lyophilized powder (Docefrez) which is reconstituted (with provided diluent) to 20 mg/0.8 mL (20 mg vial) or 24 mg/mL (80 mg vial). Admixture errors have occurred due to the availability of various concentrations. Docetaxel was previously available as a two-vial formulation which included two vials (a concentrated docetaxel vial and a diluent vial), resulting in a reconstituted concentration of 10 mg/mL; the two-vial formulation has been discontinued by the Taxotere manufacturer (available generically).

One-vial formulations: Further dilute for infusion in 250 to 500 mL of NS or D₅W in a non-DEHP container (eg, glass, polypropylene, polyolefin) to a final concentration of 0.3 to 0.74 mg/mL. Gently rotate and invert manually to mix thoroughly; avoid shaking or vigorous agitation.

Taxotere: Use **only** a 21 gauge needle to withdraw docetaxel from the vial (larger bore needles, such as 18 gauge or 19 gauge needles, may cause stopper coring and rubber precipitates). If intact vials were stored refrigerated, allow to stand at room temperature for 5 minutes prior to dilution. Inspect vials prior to dilution; solution is supersaturated and may crystalize over time; do not use if crystalized.

Lyophilized powder: Dilute with the provided diluent (contains ethanol in polysorbate 80); add 1 mL to each 20 mg vial (resulting concentration is 20 mg/0.8 mL) and 4 mL to each 80 mg vial (resulting concentration is 24 mg/mL). Shake well to dissolve completely. Reconstituted solution is supersaturated and could crystallize over time; if crystals appear, discard the solution (should no longer be used). If air bubbles are present, allow to stand for a few minutes while air bubbles dissipate. Further dilute in 250 mL of NS or D_5W in a non-DEHP container (eg, glass, polypropylene, polyolefin) to a final concentration of 0.3 to 0.74 mg/mL (for doses >200 mg, use a larger volume of NS or D_5W, not to exceed a final concentration of 0.74 mg/mL). Mix thoroughly by manual agitation.

Two-vial formulation *(generic; concentrate plus diluent formulation):* Vials should be diluted with 13% (w/w) polyethylene glycol 400/water (provided with the drug) to a final concentration of 10 mg/mL. Do not shake. Further dilute for infusion in 250 to 500 mL of NS or D_5W in a non-DEHP container (eg, glass, polypropylene, polyolefin) to a final concentration of 0.3 to 0.74 mg/mL. Gently rotate to mix thoroughly. Do not use the two-vial formulation with the one-vial formulation for the same admixture product.

Mechanism of Action Docetaxel promotes the assembly of microtubules from tubulin dimers, and inhibits the depolymerization of tubulin which stabilizes microtubules in the cell. This results in inhibition of DNA, RNA, and protein synthesis. Most activity occurs during the M phase of the cell cycle.

Pharmacodynamics/Kinetics Exhibits linear pharmacokinetics at the recommended dosage range

Distribution: Extensive extravascular distribution and/or tissue binding; V_{dss}: 113 L (mean steady state)

Protein binding: ~94% to 97%, primarily to alpha$_1$-acid glycoprotein, albumin, and lipoproteins

Metabolism: Hepatic; oxidation via CYP3A4 to metabolites

Half-life elimination: Terminal: ~11 hours

Excretion: Feces (~75%, <8% as unchanged drug); urine (~6%)

Dosing

Adult & Geriatric Note: Premedicate with corticosteroids for 3 days, beginning one day prior to docetaxel administration, to reduce the severity of hypersensitivity reactions and fluid retention. Patients being treated for prostate cancer with concurrent prednisone should be premedicated with oral dexamethasone at 12 hours, 3 hours, and 1 hour prior to docetaxel administration.

US labeling:

Breast cancer: IV infusion:

Locally advanced or metastatic: 60 to 100 mg/m^2 every 3 weeks (as a single agent)

Operable, node-positive (adjuvant treatment): TAC regimen: 75 mg/m^2 every 3 weeks for 6 courses (in combination with doxorubicin and cyclophosphamide) (Mackey, 2013; Martin, 2005)

◄ *Adjuvant treatment (off-label dosing):* 75 mg/m² every 21 days (in combination with cyclophosphamide) for 4 cycles (Jones, 2006) **or** 75 mg/m² every 21 days (in combination with carboplatin and trastuzumab) for 6 cycles (Slamon, 2011)

Neoadjuvant treatment (off-label dosing): 75 mg/m² (cycle 1; if tolerated, may increase to 100 mg/m² in subsequent cycles) every 21 days for a total of 4 cycles (in combination with trastuzumab and pertuzumab) (Gianni, 2012)

Metastatic treatment (off-label dosing):

Every-3-week administration: 75 mg/m² (cycle 1; may increase to 100 mg/m² in subsequent cycles) every 21 days for at least 6 cycles (in combination with trastuzumab and pertuzumab) (Baselga, 2012; Swain, 2013) **or** 100 mg/m² every 21 days (in combination with trastuzumab) for at least 6 cycles (Marty, 2005) **or** 75 mg/m² every 21 days (in combination with capecitabine) until disease progression or unacceptable toxicity (O'Shaughnessy, 2002) **or** 60 mg/m², 75 mg/m², or 100 mg/m² every 21 days for at least 6 cycles until disease progression, unacceptable toxicity, or discontinuation (Harvey, 2006)

Weekly administration: 40 mg/m²/dose once a week (as a single agent) for 6 weeks followed by a 2-week rest, repeat until disease progression or unacceptable toxicity (Burstein, 2000) **or** 35 mg/m²/dose once weekly for 3 weeks, followed by a 1-week rest, may increase to 40 mg/m² once weekly for 3 weeks followed by a 1-week rest with cycle 2 (Rivera, 2008) **or** 35 mg/m²/dose once weekly (in combination with trastuzumab) for 3 weeks followed by a 1-week rest; repeat until disease progression or unacceptable toxicity (Esteva, 2002)

Non-small cell lung cancer: IV infusion: 75 mg/m² every 3 weeks (as a single agent or in combination with cisplatin)

Prostate cancer: IV infusion: 75 mg/m² every 3 weeks (in combination with prednisone)

Gastric adenocarcinoma: IV infusion: 75 mg/m² every 3 weeks (in combination with cisplatin and fluorouracil)

Sequential chemotherapy and chemoradiation (off-label dosing): Induction: 75 mg/m² on days 1 and 22 (in combination with cisplatin) for 2 cycles, followed by chemoradiation: 20 mg/m² weekly for 5 weeks (in combination with cisplatin and radiation) (Ruhstaller, 2009)

Locally advanced or metastatic disease (off-label dosing): 50 mg/m² on day 1 every 2 weeks (in combination with fluorouracil, leucovorin, and oxaliplatin) until disease progression or unacceptable toxicity up to a maximum of 8 cycles (Al-Batran, 2008)

Head and neck cancer: IV infusion: 75 mg/m² every 3 weeks (in combination with cisplatin and fluorouracil) for 3 or 4 cycles, followed by radiation therapy

Canadian labeling:

Breast cancer: IV infusion:

Locally advanced or metastatic: 75 mg/m² (as combination therapy) **or** 100 mg/m² (as a single agent) every 3 weeks

Operable, node-positive (adjuvant treatment): 75 mg/m² every 3 weeks for 6 courses (in combination with doxorubicin and cyclophosphamide)

Non-small cell lung cancer (locally advanced or metastatic), ovarian cancer (metastatic), head and neck cancer (recurrent and/or metastatic): IV infusion: 75 mg/m² (as combination therapy) **or** 100 mg/m² (as a single agent) every 3 weeks

Prostate cancer (hormone-refractory, metastatic): IV infusion: 75 mg/m^2 every 3 weeks (in combination with prednisone or prednisolone)

Off-label uses:

Bladder cancer, metastatic (off-label use): IV infusion: 100 mg/m^2 every 3 weeks (as a single agent) (McCaffrey, 1997) **or** 35 mg/m^2 on days 1 and 8 of a 21-day cycle (in combination with gemcitabine and cisplatin) for at least 6 cycles or until disease progression or unacceptable toxicity (Pectasides, 2002)

Esophageal cancer (off-label use): IV infusion:

Sequential chemotherapy and chemoradiation: Induction: 75 mg/m^2 on days 1 and 22 (in combination with cisplatin) for 2 cycles, followed by chemoradiation: 20 mg/m^2 weekly for 5 weeks (in combination with cisplatin and radiation) (Ruhstaller, 2009)

Definitive chemoradiation: 60 mg/m^2 on days 1 and 22 (in combination with cisplatin and radiation) for 1 cycle (Li, 2010)

Locally advanced or metastatic disease: 75 mg/m^2 on day 1 every 3 weeks (in combination with cisplatin and fluorouracil) (Ajani, 2007; Van Cutsem, 2006) **or** 50 mg/m^2 on day 1 every 2 weeks (in combination with fluorouracil, leucovorin, and oxaliplatin) until disease progression or unacceptable toxicity up to a maximum of 8 cycles (Al-Batran, 2008) **or** 35 mg/m^2 on days 1, 8, 15, 29, 36, 43, 50, and 57 (in combination with cisplatin, fluorouracil, and radiotherapy; neoadjuvant setting) (Pasini, 2013)

Ewing sarcoma, osteosarcoma (recurrent or progressive; off-label uses): 100 mg/m^2 on day 8 of a 21-day cycle (in combination with gemcitabine) (Navid, 2008)

Ovarian cancer (off-label use in US): IV infusion: 60 mg/m^2 every 3 weeks (in combination with carboplatin) for up to 6 cycles (Markman, 2001) **or** 75 mg/m^2 every 3 weeks (in combination with carboplatin) for 6 cycles (Vasey, 2004) **or** 35 mg/m^2 (maximum dose: 70 mg) weekly for 3 weeks followed by a 1-week rest (in combination with carboplatin) (Kushner, 2007)

Small cell lung cancer, relapsed (off-label use): IV infusion: 100 mg/m^2 every 3 weeks (Smyth, 1994)

Soft tissue sarcoma (off-label use): IV infusion: 100 mg/m^2 on day 8 of a 3-week treatment cycle (in combination with gemcitabine and filgrastim or pegfilgrastim) (Leu, 2004; Maki, 2007)

Unknown-primary, adenocarcinoma (off-label use): IV infusion: 65 mg/m^2 every 3 weeks (in combination with carboplatin) (Greco, 2000) **or** 75 mg/m^2 on day 8 of a 3-week treatment cycle (in combination with gemcitabine) for up to 6 cycles (Pouessel, 2004) **or** 60 mg/m^2 on day 1 of a 3-week treatment cycle (in combination with cisplatin) (Mukai, 2010)

Dosing adjustment for concomitant CYP3A4 inhibitors: Avoid the concomitant use of strong CYP3A4 inhibitors with docetaxel. If concomitant use of a strong CYP3A4 inhibitor cannot be avoided, consider reducing the docetaxel dose by 50% (based on limited pharmacokinetic data).

Pediatric Note: Premedicate with corticosteroids for 3 days, beginning one day prior to docetaxel administration, to reduce the severity of hypersensitivity reactions and fluid retention.

Ewing sarcoma, osteosarcoma (recurrent or progressive; off-label uses): Children ≥8 years and Adolescents: IV infusion: 100 mg/m^2 on day 8 of a 21-day cycle (in combination with gemcitabine) (Navid, 2008)

Renal Impairment Renal excretion is minimal (~6%), therefore, the need for dosage adjustments for renal dysfunction is unlikely (Janus, 2010; Li, 2007).

◀ Not removed by hemodialysis, may be administered before or after hemodialysis (Janus, 2010).

Hepatic Impairment

US labeling:

Total bilirubin greater than the ULN, or AST and/or ALT >1.5 times ULN concomitant with alkaline phosphatase >2.5 times ULN: Use is not recommended.

Hepatic impairment dosing adjustment specific for gastric or head and neck cancer:

AST/ALT >2.5 to ≤5 times ULN and alkaline phosphatase ≤2.5 times ULN: Administer 80% of dose

AST/ALT >1.5 to ≤5 times ULN and alkaline phosphatase >2.5 to ≤5 times ULN: Administer 80% of dose

AST/ALT >5 times ULN and /or alkaline phosphatase >5 times ULN: Discontinue docetaxel

Canadian labeling:

Serum bilirubin >ULN **or** AST and/or ALT >1.5 times ULN associated with alkaline phosphatase >2.5 times ULN: Avoid use.

Severe hepatic impairment: Use is contraindicated.

The following adjustments have also been used (Floyd, 2006):

Transaminases 1.6 to 6 times ULN: Administer 75% of dose.

Transaminases >6 times ULN: Use clinical judgment.

Obesity *ASCO Guidelines for appropriate chemotherapy dosing in obese adults with cancer:* Utilize patient's actual body weight (full weight) for calculation of body surface area- or weight-based dosing, particularly when the intent of therapy is curative; manage regimen-related toxicities in the same manner as for nonobese patients; if a dose reduction is utilized due to toxicity, consider resumption of full weight-based dosing with subsequent cycles, especially if cause of toxicity (eg, hepatic or renal impairment) is resolved (Griggs, 2012).

Adjustment for Toxicity

US labeling:

Note: Toxicity includes febrile neutropenia, neutrophils <500/mm^3 for >1 week, severe or cumulative cutaneous reactions; in non–small cell lung cancer, this may also include platelet nadir <25,000/mm^3 and other grade 3/4 nonhematologic toxicities.

Breast cancer (single agent): Patients dosed initially at 100 mg/m^2; reduce dose to 75 mg/m^2; **Note:** If the patient continues to experience these adverse reactions, the dosage should be reduced to 55 mg/m^2 or therapy should be discontinued; discontinue for peripheral neuropathy ≥ grade 3. Patients initiated at 60 mg/m^2 who do not develop toxicity may tolerate higher doses.

Breast cancer, adjuvant treatment (combination chemotherapy): TAC regimen should be administered when neutrophils are ≥1500/mm^3. Patients experiencing febrile neutropenia should receive G-CSF in all subsequent cycles. Patients with persistent febrile neutropenia (while on G-CSF), patients experiencing severe/cumulative cutaneous reactions, moderate neurosensory effects (signs/symptoms) or grade 3 or 4 stomatitis should receive a reduced dose (60 mg/m^2) of docetaxel. Discontinue therapy with persistent toxicities after dosage reduction.

Non-small cell lung cancer:

Monotherapy: Patients dosed initially at 75 mg/m^2 should have dose held until toxicity is resolved, then resume at 55 mg/m^2; discontinue for peripheral neuropathy ≥ grade 3.

Combination therapy (with cisplatin): Patients dosed initially at 75 mg/m^2 should have the docetaxel dosage reduced to 65 mg/m^2 in subsequent cycles; if further adjustment is required, dosage may be reduced to 50 mg/m^2.

Prostate cancer: Reduce dose to 60 mg/m^2; discontinue therapy if toxicities persist at lower dose.

Gastric cancer, head and neck cancer: Note: Cisplatin may require dose reductions/therapy delays for peripheral neuropathy, ototoxicity, and/or nephrotoxicity. Patients experiencing febrile neutropenia, documented infection with neutropenia or neutropenia >7 days should receive G-CSF in all subsequent cycles. For neutropenic complications despite G-CSF use, further reduce dose to 60 mg/m^2. Dosing with neutropenic complications in subsequent cycles should be further reduced to 45 mg/m^2. Patients who experience grade 4 thrombocytopenia should receive a dose reduction from 75 mg/m^2 to 60 mg/m^2. Discontinue therapy for persistent toxicities.

Gastrointestinal toxicity for docetaxel in combination with cisplatin and fluorouracil for treatment of gastric cancer or head and neck cancer:

Diarrhea, grade 3:

First episode: Reduce fluorouracil dose by 20%

Second episode: Reduce docetaxel dose by 20%

Diarrhea, grade 4:

First episode: Reduce fluorouracil and docetaxel doses by 20%

Second episode: Discontinue treatment

Stomatitis, grade 3:

First episode: Reduce fluorouracil dose by 20%

Second episode: Discontinue fluorouracil for all subsequent cycles

Third episode: Reduce docetaxel dose by 20%

Stomatitis, grade 4:

First episode: Discontinue fluorouracil for all subsequent cycles

Second episode: Reduce docetaxel dose by 20%

Canadian labeling: **Note:** Toxicity includes febrile neutropenia, neutrophils ≤500/mm^3 for >1 week, severe or cumulative cutaneous reactions, or severe neurosensory symptoms.

Patients initially dosed at 100 mg/m^2: Reduce dose to 75 mg/m^2; Patients initially dosed at 75 mg/m^2: Reduce dose to 60 mg/m^2. Discontinue therapy for persistent toxicities after dosage reduction.

Breast cancer, adjuvant treatment (combination chemotherapy): Patients experiencing febrile neutropenia should receive G-CSF in all subsequent cycles. Patients with persistent febrile neutropenia (while on G-CSF), patients experiencing severe/cumulative cutaneous reactions, severe neurosensory symptoms, or grade 3 or 4 stomatitis should have their dose reduced to 60 mg/m^2. Discontinue therapy with persistent toxicities after dosage reduction.

◀ **Concomitant use with capecitabine (treatment of metastatic breast cancer):**

Grade 2 toxicities:

First episode: Interrupt therapy until resolution to < grade 2, then resume docetaxel and capecitabine at previous dose; consider prophylactic measures if appropriate and/or possible

Second episode of same toxicity: Interrupt therapy until resolution to < grade 2, then resume docetaxel at 55 mg/m^2; reduce capecitabine dose to 75% of original dose

Further episodes of same toxicity: Discontinue docetaxel; interrupt capecitabine until resolution to < grade 2, then resume at 50% of original dose (third episode) or discontinue therapy altogether (fourth episode)

Grade 3 toxicities:

First episode: Occurring at time treatment is due: Interrupt docetaxel until resolution to < grade 2 (maximum delay ≤2 weeks), then resume docetaxel at 55 mg/m^2; reduce capecitabine dose to 75% of original dose (consider prophylactic measure if appropriate); if no resolution to < grade 2 within 2 weeks, discontinue docetaxel but may resume capecitabine at 75% of original dose after resolution to < grade 2. Occurring between cycles and resolves to < grade 2 by time of next treatment: Administer docetaxel at 55 mg/m^2 and reduce capecitabine dose to 75% of original dose; consider prophylactic measures if appropriate and/or possible.

Further episodes of same toxicity: Discontinue docetaxel; interrupt capecitabine until resolution to < grade 2, then resume capecitabine at 50% of original dose (second episode) or discontinue therapy altogether (third episode)

Grade 4 toxicities: First episode: Discontinue docetaxel and capecitabine therapy or if deemed clinically necessary, capecitabine may be continued at 50% of original dose

Combination Regimens

Bladder cancer:

Bone sarcoma (Ewing sarcoma):

Bone sarcoma (osteosarcoma):

Breast cancer:

Cervical cancer:

Esophageal cancer:
  Docetaxel-Cisplatin-Fluorouracil (Gastric/Esophageal Cancer) on page 1940
  Docetaxel-Oxaliplatin-Leucovorin-Fluorouracil (Esophageal Cancer) on page 1946
Gastric cancer:
  Capecitabine-Docetaxel (Gastric Cancer) on page 1857
  Docetaxel-Cisplatin-Fluorouracil (Gastric/Esophageal Cancer) on page 1940
Head and neck cancer: Docetaxel-Cisplatin-Fluorouracil (Head and Neck Cancer) on page 1941
Lung cancer (non-small cell):
  Cisplatin-Docetaxel (NSCLC) on page 1891
  Docetaxel-Gemcitabine (NSCLC) on page 1943
  Docetaxel (NSCLC Regimen) on page 1945
  Docetaxel-Ramucirumab (NSCLC) on page 1946
Lung cancer (small cell): Docetaxel (Small Cell Lung Cancer Regimen) on page 1947
Ovarian cancer:
  Carboplatin-Docetaxel (Ovarian) on page 1862
  Docetaxel (Ovarian Regimen) on page 1945
Pancreatic cancer: GTX (Pancreatic) on page 2001
Prostate cancer: Docetaxel-Prednisone (Prostate) on page 1946
Soft tissue sarcoma: Docetaxel-Gemcitabine (Soft Tissue Sarcoma) on page 1943
Unknown primary, adenocarcinoma:
  Carboplatin-Docetaxel (Unknown Primary, Adenocarcinoma) on page 1863
  Cisplatin-Docetaxel (Unknown Primary, Adenocarcinoma) on page 1891
  Docetaxel-Gemcitabine (Unknown Primary, Adenocarcinoma) on page 1944
Unknown primary, squamous cell:
  Carboplatin-Docetaxel (Unknown Primary, Squamous Cell) on page 1863
  Cisplatin-Docetaxel-Fluorouracil (Unknown Primary, Squamous Cell) on page 1890
  Cisplatin-Docetaxel (Unknown Primary, Squamous Cell) on page 1892
Uterine sarcoma: Docetaxel-Gemcitabine (Uterine Leiomyosarcoma) on page 1944

Administration Administer IV infusion over 1-hour through nonsorbing polyethylene lined (non-DEHP) tubing; in-line filter is not necessary (the use of a filter during administration is not recommended by the manufacturer). Infusion should be completed within 4 hours of final preparation. **Note:** Premedication with corticosteroids for 3 days, beginning the day before docetaxel administration, is recommended to reduce the incidence and severity of hypersensitivity reactions and fluid retention. Some docetaxel formulations contain alcohol (content varies by formulation); use with caution in patients for whom alcohol intake should be avoided or minimized.

Irritant with vesicant-like properties; avoid extravasation. Assure proper needle or catheter position prior to administration.

Extravasation management: If extravasation occurs, stop infusion immediately and disconnect (leave cannula/needle in place); gently aspirate extravasated solution (do **NOT** flush the line); remove needle/cannula; elevate extremity. Information conflicts regarding the use of warm or cold compresses (Perez Fidalgo, 2012; Polovich, 2009).

Hazardous agent; use appropriate precautions for handling and disposal (NIOSH 2014 [group 1]).

◀ **Vesicant/Extravasation Risk** Irritant with vesicant-like properties

Emetic Potential Children and Adults: Low (10% to 30%)

Monitoring Parameters CBC with differential, liver function tests, bilirubin, alkaline phosphatase, renal function; monitor for hypersensitivity reactions, neurosensory symptoms, gastrointestinal toxicity (eg, diarrhea, stomatitis), cutaneous reactions, visual impairment, fluid retention, epiphora, and canalicular stenosis

Dosage Forms Excipient information presented when available (limited, particularly for generics); consult specific product labeling. [DSC] = Discontinued product

Concentrate, Intravenous:
  Taxotere: 20 mg/mL (1 mL); 80 mg/4 mL (4 mL); 20 mg/0.5 mL (0.5 mL [DSC]) [contains alcohol, usp, polysorbate 80]
  Generic: 20 mg/mL (1 mL); 80 mg/4 mL (4 mL); 160 mg/8 mL (8 mL); 20 mg/0.5 mL (0.5 mL); 80 mg/2 mL (2 mL)
Concentrate, Intravenous [preservative free]:
  Generic: 20 mg/mL (1 mL); 80 mg/4 mL (4 mL); 140 mg/7 mL (7 mL); 160 mg/8 mL (8 mL)
Solution, Intravenous:
  Generic: 20 mg/2 mL (2 mL); 80 mg/8 mL (8 mL); 160 mg/16 mL (16 mL); 200 mg/20 mL (20 mL)
Solution Reconstituted, Intravenous:
  Docefrez: 20 mg (1 ea); 80 mg (1 ea) [contains alcohol, usp, polysorbate 80]

◆ **Docetaxel for Injection (Can)** see DOCEtaxel *on page 535*

Dolasetron (dol A se tron)

Related Information
Management of Chemotherapy-Induced Nausea and Vomiting in Adults *on page 2142*

Brand Names: US Anzemet

Brand Names: Canada Anzemet

Index Terms Dolasetron Mesylate; MDL 73,147EF

Pharmacologic Category Antiemetic; Selective 5-HT$_3$ Receptor Antagonist

Use

U.S. labeling:
  Injection: Prevention and treatment of postoperative nausea and vomiting in adults and children ≥2 years
  Oral: Prevention of nausea and vomiting associated with moderately emetogenic cancer chemotherapy (initial and repeat courses) in adults and children ≥2 years
Canadian labeling: Oral: Prevention of nausea and vomiting associated with emetogenic cancer chemotherapy (initial and repeat courses)

Labeled Contraindications

U.S. labeling:
  Injection: Hypersensitivity to dolasetron or any component of the formulation; intravenous administration is contraindicated when used for prevention of chemotherapy-associated nausea and vomiting
  Tablet: Hypersensitivity to dolasetron or any component of the formulation
Canadian labeling: Hypersensitivity to dolasetron or any component of the formulation; use in children and adolescents <18 years of age; use for the prevention or treatment of postoperative nausea and vomiting; concomitant use with apomorphine

Pregnancy Considerations Adverse events have not been observed in animal reproduction studies.

Breast-Feeding Considerations It is not known if dolasetron is excreted in breast milk. The manufacturer recommends that caution be exercised when administering dolasetron to nursing women.

Warnings/Precautions Dolasetron is associated with a number of dose-dependent increases in ECG intervals (eg, PR, QRS duration, QT/QTc, JT), usually occurring 1-2 hours after IV administration and usually lasting 6-8 hours; however, may last ≥24 hours and rarely lead to heart block or arrhythmia. Clinically relevant QT-interval prolongation may occur resulting in torsade de pointes, when used in conjunction with other agents that prolong the QT interval (eg, Class I and III antiarrhythmics). Avoid use in patients at greater risk for QT prolongation (eg, patients with congenital long QT syndrome, medications known to prolong QT interval, electrolyte abnormalities, and cumulative high-dose anthracycline therapy) and/or ventricular arrhythmia. Correct potassium or magnesium abnormalities prior to initiating therapy. IV formulations of 5-HT$_3$ antagonists have more association with ECG interval changes, compared to oral formulations. Reduction in heart rate may also occur with the 5-HT$_3$ antagonists. Use with caution in children and adolescents who have or may develop QTc prolongation; rare cases of supraventricular and ventricular arrhythmias, cardiac arrest, and MI have been reported in this population. ECG monitoring is recommended in patients with renal impairment and in the elderly.

Serotonin syndrome has been reported with 5-HT$_3$ receptor antagonists, predominantly when used in combination with other serotonergic agents (eg, SSRIs, SNRIs, MAOIs, mirtazapine, fentanyl, lithium, tramadol, and/or methylene blue). Some of the cases have been fatal. The majority of serotonin syndrome reports due to 5-HT$_3$ receptor antagonist have occurred in a post-anesthesia setting or in an infusion center. Serotonin syndrome has also been reported following overdose of another 5-HT$_3$ receptor antagonist. Monitor patients for signs of serotonin syndrome, including mental status changes (eg, agitation, hallucinations, delirium, coma); autonomic instability (eg, tachycardia, labile blood pressure, diaphoresis, dizziness, flushing, hyperthermia); neuromuscular changes (eg, tremor, rigidity, myoclonus, hyperreflexia, incoordination); gastrointestinal symptoms (eg, nausea, vomiting, diarrhea); and/or seizures. If serotonin syndrome occurs, discontinue 5-HT$_3$ receptor antagonist treatment and begin supportive management.

Use with caution in patients allergic to other 5-HT$_3$ receptor antagonists; cross-reactivity has been reported with other 5-HT$_3$ receptor antagonists. **For chemotherapy-associated nausea and vomiting, should be used on a scheduled basis, not on an "as needed" (PRN) basis,** since data support the use of this drug only in the prevention of nausea and vomiting (due to antineoplastic therapy) and not in the rescue of nausea and vomiting. Not intended for treatment of nausea and vomiting or for chronic continuous therapy. If the prophylaxis dolasetron dose for postoperative nausea and vomiting has failed, a repeat dose should not be administered as rescue or treatment for postoperative nausea and vomiting. Potentially significant drug-drug interactions may exist, requiring dose or frequency adjustment, additional monitoring, and/or selection of alternative therapy.

Some dosage forms may contain polysorbate 80 (also known as Tweens). Hypersensitivity reactions, usually a delayed reaction, have been reported following exposure to pharmaceutical products containing polysorbate 80 in certain individuals (Isaksson, 2002; Lucente 2000; Shelley, 1995). Thrombocytopenia, ascites, pulmonary deterioration, and renal and hepatic failure have been reported in premature neonates after receiving parenteral products containing polysorbate 80 (Alade, 1986; CDC, 1984). See manufacturer's labeling.

Adverse Reactions Adverse events may vary according to indication and route of administration.

>10%: Central nervous system: Headache (oral: 18% to 23%; IV: 9%)

1% to 10%:

Cardiovascular: Bradycardia (4% to 5%; may be severe after IV administration), tachycardia (≤3%), edema (<2%), facial edema (<2%), flushing (<2%), hypotension (<2%; may be severe after IV administration), orthostatic hypotension (<2%), peripheral edema (<2%), peripheral ischemia (<2%), phlebitis (<2%), sinus arrhythmia (<2%), thrombophlebitis (<2%)

Central nervous system: Fatigue (oral: 3% to 6%), dizziness (1% to 6%), pain (≤3%), abnormal dreams (<2%), agitation (<2%), anxiety (<2%), ataxia (<2%), chills (≤2%), confusion (<2%), depersonalization (<2%), paresthesia (<2%), shivering (≤2%), sleep disorder (<2%), twitching (<2%), vertigo (<2%)

Dermatologic: Diaphoresis (<2%), skin rash (<2%), urticaria (<2%)

Endocrine & metabolic: Increased gamma-glutamyl transferase (<2%)

Gastrointestinal: Diarrhea (oral: 2% to 5%), dyspepsia (≤3%), abdominal pain (<2%), anorexia (<2%), constipation (<2%), dysgeusia (<2%), pancreatitis (<2%)

Genitourinary: Dysuria (<2%), hematuria (<2%)

Hematologic and oncologic: Anemia (<2%), hematoma (<2%), prolonged prothrombin time (<2%), prolonged partial thromboplastin time (<2%), purpura (<2%), thrombocytopenia (<2%)

Hepatic: Hyperbilirubinemia (<2%), increased serum alkaline phosphatase (<2%)

Hypersensitivity: Anaphylaxis (<2%)

Local: Burning sensation at injection site (IV: <2%), pain at injection site (IV: <2%)

Neuromuscular & skeletal: Arthralgia (<2%), myalgia (<2%), tremor (<2%)

Ophthalmic: Photophobia (<2%), visual disturbance (<2%)

Otic: Tinnitus (<2%)

Renal: Acute renal failure (<2%), polyuria (<2%)

Respiratory: Bronchospasm (<2%), dyspnea (<2%), epistaxis (<2%)

<1%, postmarketing, and/or case reports: Abnormal T waves on ECG, appearance of U waves on ECG, atrial fibrillation, atrial flutter, atrioventricular block, bundle branch block (left and right), cardiac arrest, chest pain, extrasystoles (APCs or VPCs), increased serum ALT (transient), increased serum AST (transient), ischemic heart disease, nodal arrhythmia, palpitations, prolongation P-R interval on ECG (dose dependent), prolonged Q-T interval on ECG, serotonin syndrome, slow R wave progression, ST segment changes on ECG, syncope (may be severe after IV administration), torsades de pointes, ventricular arrhythmia, ventricular fibrillation cardiac arrest (IV), ventricular tachycardia (IV), wide complex tachycardia (IV), widened QRS complex on ECG (dose-dependent)

Drug Interactions

Metabolism/Transport Effects Substrate of CYP2C9 (minor), CYP3A4 (minor); **Note:** Assignment of Major/Minor substrate status based on clinically relevant drug interaction potential; **Inhibits** CYP2D6 (weak)

Avoid Concomitant Use

Avoid concomitant use of Dolasetron with any of the following: Apomorphine; Highest Risk QTc-Prolonging Agents; Ivabradine; Mequitazine; Mifepristone

Increased Effect/Toxicity

Dolasetron may increase the levels/effects of: Apomorphine; ARIPiprazole; Highest Risk QTc-Prolonging Agents; Mequitazine; Moderate Risk QTc-Prolonging Agents; Panobinostat; Serotonin Modulators

The levels/effects of Dolasetron may be increased by: Ivabradine; Mifepristone; QTc-Prolonging Agents (Indeterminate Risk and Risk Modifying)

Decreased Effect

Dolasetron may decrease the levels/effects of: Tapentadol; TraMADol

Food Interactions Food does not affect the bioavailability of oral doses.

Storage/Stability

Injection: Store intact vials at 20°C to 25°C (68°F to 77°F); excursions are permitted to 15°C to 30°C (59°F to 86°F). Protect from light. Solutions diluted for infusion are stable under normal lighting conditions at room temperature for 24 hours or under refrigeration for 48 hours.

Tablets: Store at 20°C to 25°C (68°F to 77°F). Protect from light.

Preparation for Administration May be administered undiluted, or diluted in 50 mL of a compatible solution (ie, 0.9% NS, D_5W, $D_5^{1/2}NS$, D_5LR, LR, and 10% mannitol injection).

Mechanism of Action Selective serotonin receptor (5-HT$_3$) antagonist, blocking serotonin both peripherally (primary site of action) and centrally at the chemoreceptor trigger zone

Pharmacodynamics/Kinetics

Absorption: Oral: Rapid and complete

Distribution: Hydrodolasetron: 5.8 L/kg

Protein binding: Hydrodolasetron: 69% to 77% (50% bound to alpha$_1$-acid glycoprotein)

Metabolism: Hepatic; rapid reduction by carbonyl reductase to hydrodolasetron (active metabolite); further metabolized by CYP2D6, CYP3A, and flavin monooxygenase

Bioavailability: Oral: ~75% (not affected by food)

Half-life elimination: Dolasetron: ≤10 minutes; hydrodolasetron: Adults: 6-8 hours; Children: 4-6 hours; Severe renal impairment: 11 hours; Severe hepatic impairment: 11 hours

Time to peak, plasma: Hydrodolasetron: IV: 0.6 hours; Oral: ~1 hour

Excretion: Urine ~67% (53% to 61% of the total dose as active metabolite hydrodolasetron); feces ~33%

Dosing

Adult & Geriatric Note: Use of intravenous dolasetron is contraindicated for the prevention of chemotherapy induced nausea and vomiting. In Canada, use of dolasetron is also contraindicated in the prevention and treatment of postoperative nausea and vomiting in adults.

U.S. labeling:

Prevention of chemotherapy-associated nausea and vomiting (including initial and repeat courses): Oral: 100 mg within 1 hour before chemotherapy

◄ **Postoperative nausea and vomiting:**
Prevention: IV: 12.5 mg ~15 minutes before cessation of anesthesia (do not exceed the recommended dose)
Treatment: IV: 12.5 mg as soon as nausea or vomiting present (do not exceed the recommended dose)

Canadian labeling: **Prevention of chemotherapy-associated nausea and vomiting (including initial and repeat courses):** Adults: Oral: 100 mg within 1 hour before chemotherapy

Pediatric Note: In Canada, use of dolasetron is contraindicated in children and adolescents <18 years of age.

Prevention of chemotherapy-associated nausea and vomiting (including initial and repeat courses): Children 2-16 years: Oral: 1.8 mg/kg within 1 hour before chemotherapy; maximum: 100 mg/dose

Postoperative nausea and vomiting: Children 2-16 years:
Prevention:
Oral: 1.2 mg/kg within 2 hours before surgery; maximum: 100 mg/dose
IV: 0.35 mg/kg ~15 minutes before cessation of anesthesia; maximum: 12.5 mg/dose
Treatment:
IV: 0.35 mg/kg as soon as nausea or vomiting present; maximum: 12.5 mg/dose

Renal Impairment No dosage adjustment necessary; however, ECG monitoring is recommended in patients with renal impairment.

Hepatic Impairment No dosage adjustment necessary.

Administration

IV injection may be given either undiluted as an IV push over 30 seconds or diluted in 50 mL of compatible fluid and infused over 15 minutes. Flush line before and after dolasetron administration.

Oral: When unable to administer in tablet form, dolasetron injection may be diluted in apple or apple-grape juice and taken orally; this dilution is stable for 2 hours at room temperature (Anzemet prescribing information, 2013).

Extemporaneous Preparations Dolasetron injection may be diluted in apple or apple-grape juice and taken orally; this dilution is stable for 2 hours at room temperature (Anzemet prescribing information, 2013).

A 10 mg/mL oral suspension may be prepared with tablets and either a 1:1 mixture of Ora-Plus and Ora-Sweet SF or a 1:1 mixture of strawberry syrup and Ora-Plus. Crush twelve 50 mg tablets in a mortar and reduce to a fine powder. Slowly add chosen vehicle to **almost** 60 mL; transfer to a calibrated bottle, rinse mortar with vehicle, and add quantity of vehicle sufficient to make 60 mL. Label "shake well" and "refrigerate". Stable for 90 days refrigerated.

Anzemet® prescribing information, sanofi-aventis U.S. LLC, Bridgewater, NJ, 2013.

Johnson CE, Wagner DS, and Bussard WE, "Stability of Dolasetron in Two Oral Liquid Vehicles," *Am J Health Syst Pharm*, 2003, 60(21):2242-4.

Monitoring Parameters ECG (in patients with cardiovascular disease, elderly, renally impaired, those at risk of developing hypokalemia and/or hypomagnesemia); potassium, magnesium

Additional Information Efficacy of dolasetron, for chemotherapy treatment, is enhanced with concomitant administration of dexamethasone 20 mg (increases complete response by 10% to 20%). Oral administration of the intravenous solution is equivalent to tablets.

Dosage Forms Excipient information presented when available (limited, particularly for generics); consult specific product labeling.
Solution, Intravenous, as mesylate:
 Anzemet: 20 mg/mL (0.625 mL, 5 mL, 25 mL)
Tablet, Oral, as mesylate:
 Anzemet: 50 mg, 100 mg

◆ **Dolasetron Mesylate** see Dolasetron on page 548
◆ **Dolophine** see Methadone on page 1099
◆ **Doloral (Can)** see Morphine (Systemic) on page 1167
◆ **Dom-Anagrelide (Can)** see Anagrelide on page 109
◆ **Dom-Benzydamine (Can)** see Benzydamine on page 190
◆ **Dom-Bicalutamide (Can)** see Bicalutamide on page 207
◆ **Dom-Ciprofloxacin (Can)** see Ciprofloxacin (Systemic) on page 327
◆ **Dom-Dexamethasone (Can)** see Dexamethasone (Systemic) on page 513
◆ **Dom-Fluconazole (Can)** see Fluconazole on page 725
◆ **Dom-Lorazepam (Can)** see LORazepam on page 1058
◆ **Dom-Medroxyprogesterone (Can)** see MedroxyPROGESTERone on page 1074
◆ **Dom-Ondansetron (Can)** see Ondansetron on page 1253
◆ **DOM-Valacyclovir (Can)** see ValACYclovir on page 1712
◆ **DoubleDex** see Dexamethasone (Systemic) on page 513
◆ **Doxil** see DOXOrubicin (Liposomal) on page 565

DOXOrubicin (Conventional) (doks oh ROO bi sin con VEN sha nal)
Related Information
 Chemotherapy and Cancer Treatment During Pregnancy on page 2214
 Chemotherapy and Obesity on page 2220
 Management of Chemotherapy-Induced Nausea and Vomiting in Adults on page 2142
 Management of Drug Extravasations on page 2159
 Prevention of Chemotherapy-Induced Nausea and Vomiting in Children on page 2203
 Principles of Anticancer Therapy on page 2261
 Safe Handling of Hazardous Drugs on page 2292
Brand Names: US Adriamycin
Brand Names: Canada Adriamycin PFS; Doxorubicin Hydrochloride For Injection, USP; Doxorubicin Hydrochloride Injection
Index Terms ADR (error-prone abbreviation); Adria; Conventional Doxorubicin; Doxorubicin HCl; Doxorubicin Hydrochloride; Hydroxydaunomycin Hydrochloride; Hydroxyldaunorubicin Hydrochloride
Pharmacologic Category Antineoplastic Agent, Anthracycline; Antineoplastic Agent, Topoisomerase II Inhibitor
Use
 Breast cancer: Treatment component of adjuvant therapy in women with evidence of axillary lymph node involvement following resection of primary breast cancer

◄ **Metastatic cancers or disseminated neoplastic conditions:** Treatment of acute lymphoblastic leukemia, acute myeloid leukemia, Wilms tumor, neuroblastoma, soft tissue and bone sarcomas, breast cancer, ovarian cancer, transitional cell bladder carcinoma, thyroid carcinoma, gastric carcinoma, Hodgkin lymphoma, non-Hodgkin lymphoma, and bronchogenic carcinoma in which the small cell histologic type is the most responsive compared with other cell types

Labeled Contraindications Hypersensitivity (including anaphylaxis) to doxorubicin, any component of the formulation, or to other anthracyclines or anthracenediones; recent MI (within past 4 to 6 weeks), severe myocardial insufficiency, severe arrhythmia; previous therapy with high cumulative doses of doxorubicin, daunorubicin, idarubicin, or other anthracycline and anthracenediones; severe persistent drug-induced myelosuppression or baseline neutrophil count <1500/mm^3; severe hepatic impairment (Child-Pugh class C or bilirubin >5 mg/dL)

Pregnancy Considerations Adverse events have been observed in animal reproduction studies. Based on the mechanism of action, doxorubicin may cause fetal harm if administered during pregnancy (according to the manufacturer's labeling). Advise patients (females of reproductive potential and males with female partners of reproductive potential) to use effective non-hormonal contraception during and for 6 months following therapy. Limited information is available from a retrospective study of women who received doxorubicin (in combination with cyclophosphamide) during the second or third (prior to week 35) trimester for the treatment of pregnancy-associated breast cancer (Ring, 2005). Some pharmacokinetic properties of doxorubicin may be altered in pregnant women (van Hasselt, 2014). The European Society for Medical Oncology (ESMO) has published guidelines for diagnosis, treatment, and follow-up of cancer during pregnancy (Peccatori 2013); the guidelines recommend referral to a facility with expertise in cancer during pregnancy and encourage a multidisciplinary team (obstetrician, neonatologist, oncology team). If chemotherapy is indicated, it should **not** be administered in the first trimester, but may begin in the second trimester. There should be a 3-week time period between the last chemotherapy dose and anticipated delivery, and chemotherapy should not be administered beyond week 33 of gestation.

A pregnancy registry is available for all cancers diagnosed during pregnancy at Cooper Health (877-635-4499).

Breast-Feeding Considerations Doxorubicin and its metabolites are excreted in breast milk. Due to the potential for serious adverse reactions in the nursing infant, the manufacturer recommends a decision be made whether to discontinue nursing or to discontinue the drug, taking into account the importance of treatment to the mother.

Warnings/Precautions Hazardous agent - use appropriate precautions for handling and disposal (NIOSH 2014 [group 1]). **[U.S. Boxed Warning]: May cause cumulative, dose-related, myocardial toxicity (early or delayed, including acute left ventricular failure and HF). The risk of cardiomyopathy increases with cumulative exposure and with concomitant cardiotoxic therapy; the incidence of irreversible myocardial toxicity increases as the total cumulative (lifetime) dosages approach 300 to 500 mg/m^2. Assess left ventricular ejection fraction (LVEF) with either an echocardiogram or MUGA scan before, during, and after therapy; increase the frequency of assessments as the cumulative dose exceeds 300 mg/m^2.** Cardiotoxicity is dose-limiting. Delayed cardiotoxicity may occur late in treatment or within months to years after completion of therapy, and is typically manifested by LVEF reduction and/or heart failure (may be life threatening). Subacute effects such as pericarditis and myocarditis may also occur. Early toxicity may consist of tachyarrhythmias, including sinus tachycardia, premature ventricular contractions, and ventricular tachycardia, as well as bradycardia. Electrocardiographic changes including ST-T wave changes, atrioventricular and bundle-branch block have also been reported. These effects are not necessarily predictive of subsequent delayed cardiotoxicity. Total cumulative dose should take into account prior treatment with other anthracyclines or anthracenediones, previous or concomitant treatment with other cardiotoxic agents or irradiation of chest. Although the risk increases with cumulative dose, irreversible cardiotoxicity may occur at any dose level. Patients with active or dominant cardiovascular disease, concurrent administration of cardiotoxic drugs, prior therapy with other anthracyclines or anthracenediones, prior or concurrent chest irradiation, advanced age, and infants and children are at increased risk. Alternative administration schedules (weekly or continuous infusions) have are associated with less cardiotoxicity.

[U.S. Boxed Warning]: Vesicant; if extravasation occurs, severe local tissue damage leading to tissue injury, blistering, ulceration, and necrosis may occur. Discontinue infusion immediately and apply ice to the affected area. For IV administration only. Do not administer IM or SubQ. Ensure proper needle or catheter placement prior to and during infusion. Avoid extravasation.

[U.S. Boxed Warning]: May cause severe myelosuppression, which may result in serious infection, septic shock, transfusion requirements, hospitalization, and death. Myelosuppression may be dose-limiting and primarily manifests as leukopenia and neutropenia; anemia and thrombocytopenia may also occur. The nadir typically occurs 10 to 14 days after administration with cell count recovery around day 21. Monitor blood counts at baseline and regularly during therapy.

[U.S. Boxed Warning]: Secondary acute myelogenous leukemia (AML) and myelodysplastic syndrome (MDS) have been reported following treatment. AML and MDS typically occur within one to three years of treatment; risk factors for development of secondary AML or MDS include treatment with anthracyclines in combination with DNA-damaging antineoplastics (eg, alkylating agents) and/or radiation therapy, heavily pretreated patients, and escalated anthracycline doses. May cause tumor lysis syndrome and hyperuricemia (in patients with rapidly growing tumors). Urinary alkalinization and prophylaxis with an antihyperuricemic agent may be necessary. Monitor electrolytes, renal function, and hydration status. **[U.S. Boxed Warning]: Dosage modification is recommended in patients with impaired hepatic function;** toxicities may be increased in patients with hepatic impairment. Use is contraindicated in patients with severe impairment (Child-Pugh class C or bilirubin >5 mg/dL). Monitor hepatic function tests (eg, transaminases, alkaline phosphatase, and bilirubin) closely. Use with caution in patients who have received radiation therapy; radiation recall may occur. May increase radiation-induced toxicity to the myocardium, mucosa, skin, and liver. Doxorubicin is associated with a moderate or high emetic potential (depending on dose or regimen); antiemetics are recommended to prevent nausea and vomiting (Basch, 2011; Dupuis, 2011; Roila, 2010). Potentially significant drug-drug interactions may exist, requiring dose or frequency adjustment, additional monitoring, and/or selection of alternative therapy.

In men, doxorubicin may damage spermatozoa and testicular tissue, resulting in possible genetic fetal abnormalities; may also result in oligospermia, azoospermia, and permanent loss of fertility (sperm counts have been reported to return to normal levels in some men, occurring several years after the end of therapy). In females of reproductive potential, doxorubicin may cause infertility and result in amenorrhea; premature menopause can occur. Children are at increased risk for developing delayed cardiotoxicity; long-term cardiac function monitoring is recommended. Doxorubicin may contribute to prepubertal growth failure in children; may also contribute to gonadal impairment (usually temporary). Radiation recall pneumonitis has been reported in children receiving concomitant dactinomycin and doxorubicin. **[U.S. Boxed Warning]: Should be administered under the supervision of an experienced cancer chemotherapy physician.** Use caution when selecting product for preparation and dispensing; indications, dosages and adverse event profiles differ between conventional doxorubicin hydrochloride solution and doxorubicin liposomal. Both formulations are the same concentration. As a result, serious errors have occurred.

Adverse Reactions Frequency not defined.

Cardiovascular:

Acute cardiotoxicity: Atrioventricular block, bradycardia, bundle branch block, ECG abnormalities, extrasystoles (atrial or ventricular), sinus tachycardia, ST-T wave changes, supraventricular tachycardia, tachyarrhythmia, ventricular tachycardia

Delayed cardiotoxicity: LVEF decreased, CHF (manifestations include ascites, cardiomegaly, dyspnea, edema, gallop rhythm, hepatomegaly, oliguria, pleural effusion, pulmonary edema, tachycardia); myocarditis, pericarditis

Central nervous system: Malaise

Dermatologic: Alopecia, itching, photosensitivity, radiation recall, rash; discoloration of saliva, sweat, or tears

Endocrine & metabolic: Amenorrhea, dehydration, infertility (may be temporary), hyperuricemia

Gastrointestinal: Abdominal pain, anorexia, colon necrosis, diarrhea, GI ulceration, mucositis, nausea, vomiting

Genitourinary: Discoloration of urine

Hematologic: Leukopenia/neutropenia (75%; nadir: 10-14 days; recovery: by day 21); thrombocytopenia and anemia

Local: Skin "flare" at injection site, urticaria

Neuromuscular & skeletal: Weakness

Postmarketing and/or case reports: Anaphylaxis, azoospermia, bilirubin increased, chills, coma (when in combination with cisplatin or vincristine), conjunctivitis, fever, gonadal impairment (children), growth failure (prepubertal), hepatitis, hyperpigmentation (nail, skin & oral mucosa), infection, keratitis, lacrimation, myelodysplastic syndrome, neutropenic fever, neutropenic typhlitis, oligospermia, onycholysis, peripheral neurotoxicity (with intra-arterial doxorubicin), phlebosclerosis, radiation recall pneumonitis (children), secondary acute myelogenous leukemia, seizure (when in combination with cisplatin or vincristine), sepsis, shock, Stevens-Johnson syndrome, systemic hypersensitivity (including urticaria, pruritus, angioedema, dysphagia, and dyspnea), toxic epidermal necrolysis, transaminases increased, urticaria

Drug Interactions

Metabolism/Transport Effects **Substrate** of CYP2D6 (major), CYP3A4 (major), P-glycoprotein; **Note:** Assignment of Major/Minor substrate status based on clinically relevant drug interaction potential; **Inhibits** CYP2B6 (moderate), CYP2D6 (weak); **Induces** P-glycoprotein

Avoid Concomitant Use

Avoid concomitant use of DOXOrubicin (Conventional) with any of the following: BCG (Intravesical); CloZAPine; Conivaptan; Dipyrone; Fusidic Acid (Systemic); Idelalisib; Natalizumab; Pimecrolimus; Tacrolimus (Topical); Tofacitinib; Vaccines (Live)

Increased Effect/Toxicity

DOXOrubicin (Conventional) may increase the levels/effects of: ARIPiprazole; CloZAPine; CYP2B6 Substrates; Fingolimod; Leflunomide; Mercaptopurine; Natalizumab; Tofacitinib; Vaccines (Live); Zidovudine

The levels/effects of DOXOrubicin (Conventional) may be increased by: Abiraterone Acetate; Bevacizumab; Conivaptan; Cyclophosphamide; CycloSPORINE (Systemic); CYP2D6 Inhibitors (Moderate); CYP2D6 Inhibitors (Strong); CYP3A4 Inhibitors (Moderate); CYP3A4 Inhibitors (Strong); Dasatinib; Denosumab; Dipyrone; Fosaprepitant; Fusidic Acid (Systemic); Idelalisib; Luliconazole; Mifepristone; Osimertinib; Palbociclib; Panobinostat; Peginterferon Alfa-2b; P-glycoprotein/ABCB1 Inhibitors; Pimecrolimus; Roflumilast; SORAfenib; Stiripentol; Tacrolimus (Topical); Taxane Derivatives; Trastuzumab

Decreased Effect

DOXOrubicin (Conventional) may decrease the levels/effects of: BCG (Intravesical); Cardiac Glycosides; Coccidioides immitis Skin Test; Sipuleucel-T; Stavudine; Vaccines (Inactivated); Vaccines (Live); Zidovudine

The levels/effects of DOXOrubicin (Conventional) may be decreased by: Bosentan; Cardiac Glycosides; CYP3A4 Inducers (Moderate); CYP3A4 Inducers (Strong); Dabrafenib; Deferasirox; Dexrazoxane; Echinacea; Enzalutamide; Mitotane; Osimertinib; Peginterferon Alfa-2b; P-glycoprotein/ABCB1 Inducers; Siltuximab; St Johns Wort; Tocilizumab

Storage/Stability

Lyophilized powder: Store powder at 20°C to 25°C (68°F to 77°F). Protect from light. Retain in carton until time of use. Discard unused portion from single-dose vials. Reconstituted doxorubicin is stable for 7 days at room temperature under normal room lighting and for 15 days when refrigerated at 2°C to 8°C (36°F to 46°F). Protect reconstituted solution from light.

Solution: Store refrigerated at 2°C to 8°C (36°F to 46°F). Protect from light. Retain in carton until time of use. Discard unused portion. Storage of vials of solution under refrigeration may result in formation of a gelled product; if gelling occurs, place vials at room temperature for 2 to 4 hours to return the product to a slightly viscous, mobile solution.

Preparation for Administration Hazardous agent; use appropriate precautions for handling and disposal (NIOSH 2014 [group 1]). Reconstitute lyophilized powder with NS (using 5 mL for the 10 mg vial; 10 mL for the 20 mg vial; or 25 mL for the 50 mg vial) to a final concentration of 2 mg/mL; gently shake until contents are dissolved. May further dilute doxorubicin solution or reconstituted doxorubicin solution in 50 to 1000 mL D_5W or NS for infusion. Unstable in solutions with a pH <3 or >7.

Mechanism of Action Inhibition of DNA and RNA synthesis by intercalation between DNA base pairs by inhibition of topoisomerase II and by steric obstruction. Doxorubicin intercalates at points of local uncoiling of the double helix. Although the exact mechanism is unclear, it appears that direct binding to DNA (intercalation) and inhibition of DNA repair (topoisomerase II inhibition) result in blockade of DNA and RNA synthesis and fragmentation of DNA. Doxorubicin is also a powerful iron chelator; the iron-doxorubicin complex can bind DNA and cell membranes and produce free radicals that immediately cleave the DNA and cell membranes.

Pharmacodynamics/Kinetics

Distribution: V_d: 809 to 1214 L/m^2; does not cross the blood-brain barrier

Protein binding, plasma: ~75%

Metabolism: Primarily hepatic to doxorubicinol (active), then to inactive aglycones, conjugated sulfates, and glucuronides

Half-life elimination:

Distribution: ~5 minutes

Terminal: 20 to 48 hours

Male: 54 hours; Female: 35 hours

Excretion: Feces (~40% as unchanged drug); urine (5% to 12% as unchanged drug and metabolites)

Dosing

Adult & Geriatric Doxorubicin is associated with a moderate to high emetic potential (depending on dose or regimen); antiemetics are recommended to prevent nausea and vomiting (Basch, 2011; Roila, 2010).

Manufacturer's labeling: **Note:** Lower dosages should be considered for patients with inadequate marrow reserve (due to advanced age, prior treatment, or neoplastic marrow infiltration). Cumulative doses above 550 mg/m^2 are associated with an increased risk of cardiomyopathy.

Breast cancer: IV: 60 mg/m^2 on day 1 of a 21-day cycle (in combination with cyclophosphamide) for 4 cycles

Metastatic solid tumors, leukemia, or lymphoma: IV:

Single-agent therapy: 60 to 75 mg/m^2 every 21 days

Combination therapy: 40 to 75 mg/m^2 every 21 to 28 days

Indication-specific dosing (off-label dosing):

Acute lymphoblastic leukemia: IV:

Hyper-CVAD regimen: 50 mg/m^2 on day 4 of Courses 1, 3, 5, and 7 (in combination with cyclophosphamide, vincristine, and dexamethasone); alternating cycles with high-dose methotrexate and cytarabine (Kantarjian, 2004)

CALGB 8811 regimen: 30 mg/m^2 on days 1, 8 and 15 of late intensification (Course IV; 8-week cycle); in combination with vincristine, dexamethasone, cyclophosphamide, thioguanine, and cytarabine (Larson, 1995)

Bladder cancer, transitional cell: IV: *Dose-dense MVAC regimen:* 30 mg/m^2 on day 2 every 14 days (in combination with methotrexate, vinblastine, and cisplatin) (Sternberg, 2001)

Breast cancer: IV:

CAF regimen: 30 mg/m^2 on days 1 and 8 every 28 days for 6 cycles (in combination with cyclophosphamide and fluorouracil) (Bull, 1978)

FAC regimen: 50 mg/m^2 on day 1 (or administered as a 72-hour continuous infusion) every 21 days for 6 cycles (in combination with fluorouracil and cyclophosphamide) (Assikis, 2003)

TAC regimen: 50 mg/m^2 on day 1 every 21 days for 6 cycles (in combination with docetaxel and cyclophosphamide) (Martin, 2005)

Ewing sarcoma: IV:

VAC/IE regimen: Adults ≤30 years: 75 mg/m^2 on day 1 every 21 days for 5 cycles (in combination with vincristine and cyclophosphamide; after 5 cycles, dactinomycin replaced doxorubicin), alternating cycles with ifosfamide and etoposide for a total of 17 cycles (Grier, 2003)

VAIA regimen: Adults <35 years: 30 mg/m^2/day on days 1 and 2 every 21 days (doxorubicin alternates with dactinomycin; in combination with vincristine and ifosfamide) (Paulussen, 2008)

VIDE regimen: 20 mg/m^2/day over 4 hours on days 1 to 3 every 21 days for 6 cycles (in combination with vincristine, ifosfamide, and etoposide) (Juergens, 2006)

Hodgkin lymphoma: IV:

ABVD regimen: 25 mg/m^2 on days 1 and 15 every 28 days (in combination with bleomycin, vinblastine, and dacarbazine) for 2 to 4 cycles (Bonadonna, 2004; Engert, 2010)

BEACOPP and escalated BEACOPP regimens: 25 mg/m^2 (BEACOPP) or 35 mg/m^2 (escalated BEACOPP) on day 1 every 21 days (in combination with bleomycin, etoposide, cyclophosphamide, vincristine, procarbazine, and prednisone) (Engert, 2009)

Stanford V regimen: 25 mg/m^2 on weeks 1, 3, 5, 7, 9, and 11 of a 12-week cycle (in combination with mechlorethamine, vinblastine, vincristine, bleomycin, etoposide, and prednisone) (Horning, 2002)

Non-Hodgkin lymphoma: IV:

CHOP or RCHOP regimen: 50 mg/m^2 on day 1 every 21 days (in combination with cyclophosphamide, vincristine, and prednisone +/- rituximab) (Coiffier, 2010; McKelvey, 1976)

Hyper-CVAD + rituximab regimen: 50 mg/m^2 administered as a continuous infusion over 24 hours on day 4 of Courses 1, 3, 5, and 7 (21-day treatment cycles; in combination with cyclophosphamide, vincristine, dexamethasone, and rituximab); alternating cycles with high-dose methotrexate and cytarabine (Thomas, 2006)

Dose-adjusted EPOCH or REPOCH regimen: 10 mg/m^2/day administered as a continuous infusion on days 1 to 4 every 21 days (in combination with etoposide, vincristine, cyclophosphamide, and prednisone +/- rituximab) (Garcia-Suarez, 2007; Wilson, 2002)

Nordic regimen (Maxi-CHOP): 75 mg/m^2 on day 1 every 21 days (in combination with cyclophosphamide, vincristine, prednisone, and rituximab), alternating cycles with high-dose cytarabine (Geisler, 2008)

Osteosarcoma: IV:

Cisplatin/doxorubicin regimen: Adults ≤40 years: 25 mg/m^2 (bolus infusion) on days 1 to 3 every 21 days (in combination with cisplatin) (Bramwell, 1992)

High-dose methotrexate/cisplatin/doxorubicin/ifosfamide regimen: Adults <40 years:

Preoperative: 75 mg/m^2 administered as a continuous infusion over 24 hours on day 3 of weeks 1 and 7 (in combination with methotrexate, cisplatin, and ifosfamide) (Bacci, 2003)

Postoperative: 90 mg/m^2 administered as a continuous infusion over 24 hours on weeks 13, 22, and 31 (in combination with methotrexate, cisplatin, and ifosfamide) (Bacci, 2003)

High-dose methotrexate/cisplatin/doxorubicin regimen: Adults <40 years: Preoperative: 60 mg/m^2 over 8 hours on days 9 and 36 (in combination with methotrexate and cisplatin) (Bacci, 2000)

Postoperative: 45 mg/m^2/day over 4 hours for 2 consecutive days (in combination with methotrexate, cisplatin +/- ifosfamide, +/- etoposide; refer to protocol for criteria, frequency, and other specific information) (Bacci, 2000)

Small cell lung cancer, recurrent: IV: *CAV regimen:* 45 mg/m^2 (maximum dose: 100 mg) on day 1 every 21 days (in combination with cyclophosphamide and vincristine) until disease progression or unacceptable toxicity or for at least 4 or 6 cycles past maximum response (von Pawel, 1999)

Soft tissue sarcoma: IV:

Nonspecific histologies:

AD regimen: 60 mg/m^2 on day 1 every 21 days (either as a bolus infusion or administered continuously over 96 hours; in combination with dacarbazine) (Zalupski, 1991)

AIM regimen: 30 mg/m^2 on days 1 and 2 every 21 days (in combination with ifosfamide and mesna) (Edmonson, 1993)

MAID regimen: 20 mg/m^2/day as a continuous infusion on days 1 to 3 every 21 days (in combination with ifosfamide, mesna, and dacarbazine) (Elias, 1989)

Single-agent regimen: 75 mg/m^2 on day 1 every 21 days until disease progression or unacceptable toxicity (Santoro, 1995)

Rhabdomyosarcoma:

VAC/IE regimen: Adults <21 years: 37.5 mg/m^2 on days 1 and 2 (administered over 18 hours each day) every 6 weeks (in combination with vincristine and cyclophosphamide), alternating cycles with ifosfamide and etoposide (Arndt, 1998)

VAI regimen (based on a limited number of patients): Adults: 25 mg/m^2/day on days 1 to 3 every 21 days (in combination with vincristine and ifosfamide) (Ogilvie, 2010)

Off-label uses:

Endometrial carcinoma, advanced: IV: 60 mg/m^2 on day 1 every 21 days for 8 cycles; maximum cumulative dose: 420 mg/m^2 (in combination with cisplatin) (Randall, 2006)

Multiple myeloma: IV:

PAD regimen: Induction: 9 mg/m^2/day on days 1 to 4 for 3 cycles (in combination with bortezomib and dexamethasone) (Sonneveld, 2012)

VDT-PACE regimen: 10 mg/m^2/day administered as a continuous infusion on days 1 to 4 of each cycle (in combination with bortezomib, dexamethasone, thalidomide, cisplatin, cyclophosphamide, and etoposide) (Lee, 2003; Pineda-Roman, 2008)

Thymomas and thymic malignancies: IV:

CAP regimen: 50 mg/m^2 on day 1 every 21 days for up to 8 cycles (in combination with cisplatin and cyclophosphamide) (Loehrer, 1994)

ADOC regimen: 40 mg/m^2 on day 1 every 21 days (in combination with cisplatin, vincristine, and cyclophosphamide) (Fornasiero, 1991)

Uterine sarcoma: IV: 60 mg/m^2 on day 1 every 21 days; maximum cumulative dose: 480 mg/m^2 (Omura, 1983) **or** 50 mg/m^2 (over 15 minutes) on day 1 every 21 days; maximum cumulative dose: 450 mg/m^2 (in combination with ifosfamide/mesna) (Sutton, 1996)

Waldenstrom macroglobulinemia: IV: *R-CHOP regimen:* 50 mg/m^2 on day 1 every 21 days for 4 to 8 cycles (in combination with cyclophospha-mide, vincristine, prednisone, and rituximab) (Buske, 2009)

Pediatric Doxorubicin is associated with a moderate to high emetic potential (depending on dose or regimen); antiemetics are recommended to prevent nausea and vomiting (Dupuis, 2011).

Manufacturer's labeling: **Note:** Lower dosages should be considered for patients with inadequate marrow reserve (due to advanced age, prior treatment, or neoplastic marrow infiltration). Cumulative doses above 550 mg/m^2 are associated with an increased risk of cardiomyopathy.

Metastatic solid tumors, leukemia, or lymphoma: Children and Adoles-cents: IV:

Single-agent therapy: 60 to 75 mg/m^2 every 21 days

Combination therapy: 40 to 75 mg/m^2 every 21 to 28 days

Indication-specific dosing (off-label dosing):

Acute lymphoblastic leukemia: IV:

DFCI Consortium Protocol 00-01: Children ≥1 year and Adolescents:

Induction: 30 mg/m^2/dose on days 0 and 1 of a 4-week cycle (Vroo-man, 2013)

CNS therapy: High-risk patients: 30 mg/m^2 on day 1 of a 3-week cycle (with dexrazoxane) (Vrooman, 2013)

Intensification: High-risk patients: 30 mg/m^2 on day 1 of every 3-week cycle (with dexrazoxane; cumulative doxorubicin dose: 300 mg/m^2) (Vrooman, 2013)

Ewing sarcoma: Children and Adolescents: IV:

VAC/IE regimen: 75 mg/m^2 on day 1 every 21 days for 5 cycles (in combination with vincristine and cyclophosphamide; after 5 cycles, dactinomycin replaced doxorubicin), alternating cycles with ifosfamide and etoposide for a total of 17 cycles (Grier, 2003)

VAIA regimen: 30 mg/m^2/day on days 1 and 2 every 21 days (doxorubicin alternates with dactinomycin; in combination with vincristine and ifosfa-mide) for 14 cycles (Paulussen, 2008)

VIDE regimen: 20 mg/m^2/day over 4 hours on days 1 to 3 every 21 days for 6 cycles (in combination with vincristine, ifosfamide, and etoposide) (Juergens, 2006)

Osteosarcoma: Children and Adolescents: IV:

Cisplatin/doxorubicin regimen: 25 mg/m^2 (bolus infusion) on days 1 to 3 every 21 days (in combination with cisplatin) (Bramwell, 1992)

High-dose methotrexate/cisplatin/doxorubicin/ifosfamide regimen:

Preoperative: 75 mg/m^2 administered as a continuous infusion over 24 hours on day 3 of weeks 1 and 7 (in combination with methotrexate, cisplatin, and ifosfamide) (Bacci, 2003)

Postoperative: 90 mg/m^2 administered as a continuous infusion over 24 hours on weeks 13, 22, and 31 (in combination with methotrexate, cisplatin, and ifosfamide) (Bacci, 2003)

High-dose methotrexate/cisplatin/doxorubicin regimen:

Preoperative: 60 mg/m^2 over 8 hours on days 9 and 36 (in combination with methotrexate and cisplatin) (Bacci, 2000)

Postoperative: 45 mg/m^2/day over 4 hours for 2 consecutive days (in combination with methotrexate, cisplatin +/- ifosfamide, +/- etoposide; refer to protocol for criteria, frequency, and other specific information) (Bacci, 2000)

◀ **Rhabdomyosarcoma:** Children and Adolescents: IV:

VAC/IE regimen: 37.5 mg/m^2 on days 1 and 2 (administered over 18 hours each day) every 6 weeks (in combination with vincristine and cyclophosphamide), alternating cycles with ifosfamide and etoposide (Arndt, 1998)

Renal Impairment

Mild, moderate, or severe impairment: No dosage adjustment provided in the manufacturers' labeling; however, adjustments are likely not necessary given limited renal excretion.

The following adjustments have also been recommended (Aronoff, 2007):

CrCl <50 mL/minute: No dosage adjustment necessary.

Hemodialysis: Supplemental dose is not necessary.

Hepatic Impairment

The manufacturers' labeling recommends the following adjustments:

Serum bilirubin 1.2 to 3 mg/dL: Administer 50% of dose.

Serum bilirubin 3.1 to 5 mg/dL: Administer 25% of dose.

Severe hepatic impairment (Child-Pugh class C or bilirubin >5 mg/dL): Use is contraindicated.

The following adjustments have also been recommended (Floyd, 2006):

Transaminases 2 to 3 times ULN: Administer 75% of dose.

Transaminases >3 times ULN: Administer 50% of dose.

Obesity *ASCO Guidelines for appropriate chemotherapy dosing in obese adults with cancer:* Utilize patient's actual body weight (full weight) for calculation of body surface area- or weight-based dosing, particularly when the intent of therapy is curative; manage regimen-related toxicities in the same manner as for nonobese patients; if a dose reduction is utilized due to toxicity, consider resumption of full weight-based dosing with subsequent cycles, especially if cause of toxicity (eg, hepatic or renal impairment) is resolved (Griggs, 2012).

Adjustment for Toxicity Cardiotoxicity: Discontinue in patients who develop signs/symptoms of cardiomyopathy.

Combination Regimens

Bladder cancer:

Dose Dense MVAC (Bladder Cancer) on page 1948

MVAC (Bladder) on page 2042

Bone sarcoma (Ewing sarcoma): VAC Alternating With IE (Ewing Sarcoma) on page 2102

Breast cancer:

AC (Breast) on page 1822

AC (Dose-Dense) followed by Paclitaxel (Dose-Dense) (Breast) on page 1822

AC (Dose-Dense) followed by Paclitaxel (Dose-Dense)-Trastuzumab (Breast) on page 1823

AC (Dose-Dense) followed by Paclitaxel Weekly (Breast) on page 1824

AC followed by Docetaxel Every 3 Weeks (Breast) on page 1824

AC followed by Paclitaxel-Trastuzumab (Breast) on page 1825

AC followed by Paclitaxel Weekly (Breast) on page 1825

CAF IV (Breast) on page 1852

CAF Oral (Breast) on page 1852

Doxorubicin (Breast Regimen) on page 1949

TAC (Breast) on page 2086

◀ Soft tissue sarcoma:

Wilms' tumor:

Administration Doxorubicin is associated with a moderate to high emetic potential (depending on dose or regimen); antiemetics are recommended to prevent nausea and vomiting (Basch, 2011; Dupuis, 2011; Roila, 2010).

Administer IV push over at least 3 to 10 minutes or by continuous infusion (infusion via central venous line recommended). Do not administer IM or SubQ. Rate of administration varies by protocol, refer to individual protocol for details. Protect from light until completion of infusion. Avoid contact with alkaline solutions. Monitor for local erythematous streaking along vein and/or facial flushing (may indicate rapid infusion rate); decrease the rate if occurs.

Vesicant; ensure proper needle or catheter placement prior to and during infusion; avoid extravasation.

Extravasation management: If extravasation occurs, stop infusion immediately and disconnect (leave cannula/needle in place); gently aspirate extravasated solution (do **NOT** flush the line); remove needle/cannula; elevate extremity. Initiate antidote (dexrazoxane or dimethyl sulfate [DMSO]). Apply dry cold compresses for 20 minutes 4 times daily for 1 to 2 days (Perez Fidalgo, 2012); withhold cooling beginning 15 minutes before dexrazoxane infusion; continue withholding cooling until 15 minutes after infusion is completed. Topical DMSO should not be administered in combination with dexrazoxane; may lessen dexrazoxane efficacy.

> *Dexrazoxane:* Adults: 1000 mg/m^2 (maximum dose: 2000 mg) IV (administer in a large vein remote from site of extravasation) over 1 to 2 hours days 1 and 2, then 500 mg/m^2 (maximum dose: 1000 mg) IV over 1 to 2 hours day 3; begin within 6 hours of extravasation. Day 2 and day 3 doses should be administered at approximately the same time (± 3 hours) as the dose on day 1 (Mouridsen, 2007; Perez Fidalgo, 2012). **Note:** Reduce dexrazoxane dose by 50% in patients with moderate to severe renal impairment (CrCl <40 mL/minute).

> *DMSO:* Children and Adults: Apply topically to a region covering twice the affected area every 8 hours for 7 days; begin within 10 minutes of extravasation; do not cover with a dressing (Perez Fidalgo, 2012).

Hazardous agent; use appropriate precautions for handling and disposal (NIOSH 2014 [group 1]).

Vesicant/Extravasation Risk Vesicant; see Management of Drug Extravasations on page 2159.

Emetic Potential

Children: Moderate (30% to 90%)

Adults:

≥60 mg/m^2 or when used in combination with cyclophosphamide: High (>90%)

<60 mg/m^2: Moderate (30% to 90%)

Monitoring Parameters CBC with differential and platelet count; liver function tests (bilirubin, ALT/AST, alkaline phosphatase); serum uric acid, calcium, potassium, phosphate and creatinine; hydration status; cardiac function (baseline, periodic, and followup): ECG, left ventricular ejection fraction (echocardiography [ECHO] or multigated radionuclide angiography [MUGA]); monitor infusion site

Dosage Forms Excipient information presented when available (limited, particularly for generics); consult specific product labeling. [DSC] = Discontinued product

Solution, Intravenous, as hydrochloride:
  Adriamycin: 2 mg/mL (5 mL, 10 mL, 25 mL, 100 mL)
  Generic: 2 mg/mL (5 mL, 10 mL, 25 mL, 100 mL)
Solution, Intravenous, as hydrochloride [preservative free]:
  Generic: 2 mg/mL (5 mL, 10 mL, 25 mL, 100 mL)
Solution Reconstituted, Intravenous, as hydrochloride:
  Adriamycin: 10 mg (1 ea); 20 mg (1 ea); 50 mg (1 ea)
  Generic: 10 mg (1 ea [DSC]); 50 mg (1 ea)
Solution Reconstituted, Intravenous, as hydrochloride [preservative free]:
  Generic: 10 mg (1 ea); 50 mg (1 ea [DSC])

DOXOrubicin (Liposomal) (doks oh ROO bi sin lye po SO mal)

Related Information

Common Toxicity Criteria *on page 2122*
Management of Chemotherapy-Induced Nausea and Vomiting in Adults *on page 2142*
Management of Drug Extravasations *on page 2159*
Prevention of Chemotherapy-Induced Nausea and Vomiting in Children *on page 2203*
Safe Handling of Hazardous Drugs *on page 2292*

Brand Names: US Doxil; Lipodox; Lipodox 50
Brand Names: Canada Caelyx; Myocet
Index Terms DOXOrubicin Hydrochloride (Liposomal); DOXOrubicin Hydrochloride Encapsulated Liposomes (Myocet); DOXOrubicin Hydrochloride Liposome; DOXOrubicin Hydrochloride Liposomes (Myocet); Lipodox; Liposomal DOXOrubicin; Pegylated DOXOrubicin Liposomal; Pegylated Liposomal DOXOrubicin; Pegylated Liposomal DOXOrubicin Hydrochloride (Doxil, Caelyx)
Pharmacologic Category Antineoplastic Agent, Anthracycline; Antineoplastic Agent, Topoisomerase II Inhibitor

Use

US labeling:

AIDS-related Kaposi sarcoma: Treatment of AIDS-related Kaposi sarcoma (after failure of or intolerance to prior systemic therapy)
Multiple myeloma: Treatment of multiple myeloma (in combination with bortezomib) in patients who are bortezomib- naïve and have received at least 1 prior therapy
Ovarian cancer, advanced: Treatment of progressive or recurrent ovarian cancer (after platinum-based treatment)

Canadian labeling: Treatment of metastatic breast cancer (as monotherapy [Caelyx] or in combination with cyclophosphamide [Myocet]); advanced ovarian cancer (after failure of first-line treatment [Caelyx]); AIDS-related Kaposi sarcoma (after failure of or intolerance to prior systemic therapy [Caelyx])

◄ **Labeled Contraindications**

Severe hypersensitivity (including anaphylaxis) to doxorubicin liposomal, conventional doxorubicin, or any component of the formulation

Canadian labeling (Caelyx): Additional contraindications (not in US labeling): Breast-feeding

Pregnancy Considerations Adverse events were observed in animal reproduction studies. May cause fetal harm if administered during pregnancy. Women and men of reproductive potential should use effective contraception during therapy and for 6 months after treatment. Doxorubicin liposomal may damage spermatozoa and testicular tissue in males and may result in oligospermia, azoospermia, and permanent loss of fertility. May cause amenorrhea, infertility, and premature menopause in females.

Breast-Feeding Considerations It is not known if doxorubicin liposomal is excreted in breast milk. Due to the potential for serious adverse reactions in the nursing infant, breast-feeding should be discontinued during treatment.

Warnings/Precautions Hazardous agent - use appropriate precautions for handling and disposal (NIOSH 2014 [group 1]).

[US Boxed Warning]: Doxorubicin liposomal may cause myocardial damage (including congestive heart failure) as the total cumulative dose of doxorubicin approaches 550 mg/m². In a clinical study of 250 patients with advanced cancer who were treated with doxorubicin liposomal, the risk of cardiotoxicity was 11% when the cumulative anthracycline dose was between 450 to 550 mg/m². Prior use of other anthracyclines or anthracenediones should be included in calculations of total cumulative dosage. The risk of cardiomyopathy may be increased at lower cumulative doses in patients with prior mediastinal irradiation. Myocardial damage may manifest as acute left ventricular failure; cardiotoxicity is defined as a >20% decrease in resting left ventricular ejection fraction (LVEF) from baseline (if LVEF remained in the normal range) or a >10% decrease from baseline (where LVEF was less than the institutional lower limit of normal). Some patients developed signs/symptoms of heart failure without documented evidence of cardiotoxicity. The risk of cardiomyopathy with doxorubicin is generally proportional to the cumulative exposure, although the relationship between cumulative doxorubicin liposomal dose and the risk of cardiotoxicity is not known. For Myocet [Canadian product], cardiotoxicity may occur as the cumulative (lifetime) dose approaches 750 mg/m². Anthracycline-induced cardiotoxicity may be delayed (after discontinuation of anthracycline treatment). Assess left ventricular function with echocardiogram or MUGA prior to and during treatment to detect acute changes; monitor after treatment to detect delayed cardiotoxicity. Use in patients with a history of cardiovascular disease only if potential benefits outweigh cardiovascular risk.

[US Boxed Warning]: Acute infusion-related reactions consisting of, but not limited to, flushing, shortness of breath, facial swelling, headache, chills, back pain, tightness in the chest or throat, and/or hypotension occurred in 11% of patients with solid tumors treated with doxorubicin liposomal. Serious, life-threatening and fatal infusion reactions have been reported. Infusion reactions have also included chest pain, pruritus, rash, cyanosis, syncope, tachycardia, bronchospasm, asthma, and apnea. Most reactions occurred during the first infusion. Some reactions have resulted in dose interruption. Medication and equipment to manage infusion reactions should be immediately available during infusion. Initiate infusion at a rate of 1 mg/minute, with the rate increased (to complete infusion over 60 minutes) as tolerated. If an infusion reaction occurs, temporarily interrupt infusion until resolved and resume at a reduced rate. Discontinue for serious or life-threatening infusion reactions.

Neutropenia, anemia, and thrombocytopenia may occur. Monitor blood counts. Treatment delay, dosage modification, or discontinuation may be required. Hematologic toxicity may occur at a higher frequency and severity with combination chemotherapy. Palmar-plantar erythrodysesthesia (hand-foot syndrome) has been reported in patients receiving doxorubicin liposomal; it is usually seen after 2 to 3 treatment cycles, although may also occur earlier; dosage modification may be required; in severe or debilitating cases, treatment discontinuation may be required. Pharmacokinetics in patients with hepatic impairment has not been adequately studied. Doxorubicin is predominantly eliminated hepatically; reduce doxorubicin liposomal dose in patients with serum bilirubin ≥1.2 mg/dL.

Cases of secondary oral cancers (primarily squamous cell carcinoma) have been reported with long-term (>1 year) doxorubicin liposomal exposure; these secondary oral malignancies have occurred during treatment and up to 6 years after treatment. The development of oral ulceration or discomfort should be monitored and further evaluated in patients with past or present use of doxorubicin liposomal. Tissue distribution of the liposomal doxorubicin compared to free doxorubicin may play a role in the development of oral secondary malignancies associated with long-term use.

Liposomal vs conventional formulation dosing: Liposomal formulations of doxorubicin should **NOT** be substituted for conventional doxorubicin hydrochloride on a mg-per-mg basis. Potentially significant drug-drug interactions may exist, requiring dose or frequency adjustment, additional monitoring, and/or selection of alternative therapy. Use of Caelyx [Canadian product] in splenectomized patients with AIDS-related Kaposi sarcoma is not recommended (has not been studied).

Adverse Reactions Frequency not always defined.

>10%:

  Cardiovascular: Cardiomyopathy (dose related: 11%; Kaposi sarcoma: <1%), cardiotoxicity (11%), chest tightness (11%), flushing (11%), hypotension (1% to 11%)

  Central nervous system: Fatigue (>20%), headache (≤11%)

  Dermatologic: Palmar-plantar erythrodysesthesia (ovarian cancer: ≤51%; grades 3/4: 24%), skin rash (grades 3/4: 29%, Kaposi sarcoma: 1% to 5%), alopecia (9% to 19%), facial swelling (11%)

  Gastrointestinal: Nausea (ovarian cancer: 46%; Kaposi sarcoma: 17% to 18%; grades 3/4: 5%), stomatitis (grades 3/4: 41%, Kaposi sarcoma: 5% to 8%), vomiting (grades 3/4: 33%; Kaposi sarcoma: 8%), constipation (>20%), diarrhea (grades 3/4: 21%; Kaposi sarcoma: 3% to 8%), anorexia (20%; Kaposi sarcoma: 1% to 5%), mucous membrane disease (14%; grades 3/4: 4%), dyspepsia 12%; grades 3/4: <1%)

  Hematologic & oncologic: Thrombocytopenia (dose related, Kaposi sarcoma: 1% to 61%), neutropenia (dose related: 4% to 49%), leukopenia (37%), anemia (16% to 58%; dose related <1% to 5%)

  Neuromuscular & skeletal: Weakness (grades 3/4: 40%; Kaposi sarcoma: 7% to 10%), back pain (grades 3/4: 11% to 12%; Kaposi sarcoma: 1% to 5%)

  Respiratory: Pharyngitis (16%; Kaposi sarcoma <1%), dyspnea (1% to 15%)

  Miscellaneous: Fever (21%; Kaposi sarcoma: 8% to 9%; grades 3/4: <1%), infusion related reaction (7% to 11%)

DOXORUBICIN (LIPOSOMAL)

1% to 10%:

Cardiovascular: Cardiac arrest (≤10%), chest pain (Kaposi sarcoma: 1% to 5%), deep thrombophlebitis (ovarian cancer: 1% to 10%), tachycardia (1% to 10%), vasodilation (ovarian cancer: 1% to 10%)

Central nervous system: Depression (ovarian cancer: 1% to 10%), dizziness (1% to 10%), drowsiness (1% to 10%), chills (Kaposi sarcoma: 1% to 5%)

Dermatologic: Acne vulgaris (ovarian cancer: 1% to 10%), ecchymoses (ovarian cancer: 1% to 10%), exfoliative dermatitis (ovarian cancer: 1% to 10%), fungal dermatitis (ovarian cancer: 1% to 10%), furunculosis (ovarian cancer: 1% to 10%), herpes simplex dermatitis (1% to 10%), pruritus (1% to 10%), skin discoloration (ovarian cancer: 1% to 10%), vesiculobullous dermatitis (ovarian cancer: 1% to 10%), xeroderma (ovarian cancer: 1% to 10%), maculopapular rash (≤10%)

Endocrine & metabolic: Hypercalcemia (ovarian cancer: 1% to 10%), hypokalemia (ovarian cancer: 1% to 10%), hyponatremia (ovarian cancer: 1% to 10%), weight loss (1% to 10%), dehydration (≤10%), hyperglycemia (1% to 5%)

Gastrointestinal: Dysphagia (1% to 10%), esophagitis (ovarian cancer: 1% to 10%), intestinal obstruction (ovarian cancer: 1% to 10%), oral candidiasis (1% to 10%), oral mucosa ulcer (1% to 10%), dysgeusia (1% to ≤10%), abdomen enlarged (ovarian cancer 1% to 5%), glossitis (1% to 5%), increased serum alanine aminotransferase (Kaposi sarcoma 1% to 5%), cachexia

Genitourinary: Hematuria (ovarian cancer: 1% to 10%), hemorrhagic cystitis, urinary tract infection (ovarian cancer: 1% to 10%), vulvovaginal candidiasis (ovarian cancer 1% to 10%)

Hematologic & oncologic: Rectal hemorrhage (ovarian cancer: 1% to 10%), hemolysis (1% to 5%), prolonged prothrombin time (1% to 5%), bone marrow depression (Kaposi sarcoma), progression of cancer (Kaposi sarcoma)

Hepatic: Hyperbilirubinemia (1% to 10%), increased serum alkaline phosphatase (Kaposi sarcoma 1% to 8%)

Hypersensitivity: Hypersensitivity reaction (Kaposi sarcoma 1% to 5%)

Infection: Infection (1% to 12%), herpes zoster (≤10%), paresthesia (5%), myalgia (ovarian cancer: 1% to 5%), neuropathy (ovarian cancer 1% to 5%), toxoplasmosis (Kaposi sarcoma)

Ocular: Dry eye syndrome (ovarian cancer: 1% to 10%), conjunctivitis (≤10%), retinitis (Kaposi sarcoma 1% to 5%) optic neuritis (Kaposi sarcoma)

Respiratory: Epistaxis (ovarian cancer: 1% to 10%), pneumonia (1% to 10%), rhinitis (ovarian cancer: 1% to 10%), sinusitis (ovarian cancer: 1% to 10%), increased cough (≤10%), cough (Kaposi sarcoma)

<1%, postmarketing, and/or case reports (Limited to important or life-threatening): Abnormal vision, abscess, acute brain syndrome, albuminuria, alkaline phosphatase increased anaphylactic reaction, anxiety, arthralgia, asthma, balanitis, blindness, bone pain, bronchitis, bundle branch block (Kaposi sarcoma), BUN increased, candidiasis (Kaposi sarcoma), cardiomegaly, cardiomyopathy, cellulitis, CHF, colitis, confusion, congestive heart failure (Kaposi sarcoma), creatinine increased, cryptococcosis, cryptococcosis (Kaposi sarcoma), diabetes mellitus, dysuria,edema, emotional lability, erythema multiforme, erythema nodosum, eosinophilia, fecal impaction, flatulence, flu-like syndrome, gastritis, hemorrhage, hepatic failure, hepatitis (Kaposi sarcoma), hepatosplenomegaly, hyperkalemia, hyperlipidemia, hypernatremia, hyperuricemia, hyperventilation, hypoglycemia, hypomagnesemia, hypophosphatemia, hypoproteinemia, hypothermia, injection site

568

hemorrhage, injection site pain, insomnia, jaundice, ketosis, lactic dehydro-genase increased, lymphadenopathy, lymphangitis, migraine, myositis, muscle spasm, optic neuritis, pain, pallor, palpitations (Kaposi sarcoma), pancreatitis, pericardial effusion, petechia, pneumothorax, peripheral edema, pleural effusion, pulmonary embolism, radiation injury, sclerosing cholangitis, seizure, secondary acute myelocytic leukemia, sepsis (Kaposi sarcoma), skin necrosis, skin ulcer, syncope, squamous cell carcinoma, Stevens-Johnson syndrome, tenesmus, thrombophlebitis (Kaposi sarcoma), thromboplastin decreased, thrombosis (Kaposi sarcoma), tinnitus, toxic epidermal necroly-sis, urticaria, vertigo (Kaposi sarcoma), ventricular arrhythmia (Kaposi sarcoma)

Drug Interactions

Metabolism/Transport Effects Substrate of CYP2D6 (major), CYP3A4 (major); **Note:** Assignment of Major/Minor substrate status based on clinically relevant drug interaction potential; **Inhibits** CYP2B6 (moderate)

Avoid Concomitant Use

Avoid concomitant use of DOXOrubicin (Liposomal) with any of the following: BCG (Intravesical); CloZAPine; Conivaptan; Dipyrone; Fusidic Acid (Sys-temic); Idelalisib; Natalizumab; Pimecrolimus; Tacrolimus (Topical); Tofaciti-nib; Vaccines (Live)

Increased Effect/Toxicity

DOXOrubicin (Liposomal) may increase the levels/effects of: CloZAPine; CYP2B6 Substrates; Fingolimod; Leflunomide; Natalizumab; Tofacitinib; Vac-cines (Live); Zidovudine

The levels/effects of DOXOrubicin (Liposomal) may be increased by: Abir-aterone Acetate; Aprepitant; Bevacizumab; Conivaptan; Cyclophosphamide; CYP2D6 Inhibitors (Moderate); CYP2D6 Inhibitors (Strong); CYP3A4 Inhib-itors (Moderate); CYP3A4 Inhibitors (Strong); Dasatinib; Denosumab; Dipyr-one; Fosaprepitant; Fusidic Acid (Systemic); Idelalisib; Ivacaftor; Luliconazole; Mifepristone; Netupitant; Osimertinib; Palbociclib; Panobino-stat; Peginterferon Alfa-2b; Pimecrolimus; Roflumilast; Simeprevir; Stiripen-tol; Tacrolimus (Topical); Taxane Derivatives; Trastuzumab

Decreased Effect

DOXOrubicin (Liposomal) may decrease the levels/effects of: BCG (Intra-vesical); Cardiac Glycosides; Coccidioides immitis Skin Test; Sipuleucel-T; Stavudine; Vaccines (Inactivated); Vaccines (Live); Zidovudine

The levels/effects of DOXOrubicin (Liposomal) may be decreased by: Bosentan; Cardiac Glycosides; CYP3A4 Inducers (Moderate); CYP3A4 Inducers (Strong); Dabrafenib; Deferasirox; Echinacea; Enzalutamide; Mito-tane; Osimertinib; Peginterferon Alfa-2b; Siltuximab; St Johns Wort; Tocili-zumab

Storage/Stability Store intact vials refrigerated at 2°C to 8°C (36°F to 46°F); avoid freezing.

Doxil, Caelyx: Solutions diluted for infusion should be refrigerated at 2°C to 8°C (36°F to 46°F); administer within 24 hours.

Myocet: Refer to product labeling for detailed reconstitution and preparation information. Following reconstitution, may be stored up to 8 hours at room temperature or up to 72 hours refrigerated at 2°C to 8°C (36°F to 46°F); do not freeze.

◀ **Preparation for Administration** Hazardous agent; use appropriate precautions for handling and disposal (NIOSH 2014 [group 1]).

Doxil, Caelyx: Dilute doses ≤90 in D_5W 250 mL prior to administration. Dilute doses >90 mg in D_5W 500 mL. Solution is not clear, but has a red, translucent appearance due to the liposomal dispersion. Dilute only in D_5W; do not use bacteriostatic agents; do not mix with other medications.

Myocet: Refer to product labeling for detailed reconstitution and preparation information.

Mechanism of Action Doxorubicin inhibits DNA and RNA synthesis by intercalating between DNA base pairs causing steric obstruction and inhibits topoisomerase-II at the point of DNA cleavage. Doxorubicin is also a powerful iron chelator. The iron-doxorubicin complex can bind DNA and cell membranes, producing free hydroxyl (OH) radicals that cleave DNA and cell membranes. Active throughout entire cell cycle. Doxorubicin liposomal is a pegylated formulation which protects the liposomes, and thereby increases blood circulation time.

Pharmacodynamics/Kinetics

Distribution: V_{dss}: ~2.7 to 2.8 L/m^2; largely confined to vascular fluid

Protein binding, plasma: Unknown; nonliposomal (conventional) doxorubicin: ~70%

Half-life elimination: Terminal: Distribution: ~4.7 to 5.2 hours, Elimination: ~52 to 55 hours

Metabolism: Hepatic and in plasma to doxorubicinol and the sulfate and glucuronide conjugates of 4-demethyl,7-deoxyaglycones

Dosing

Adult & Geriatric Liposomal formulations of doxorubicin should NOT be substituted for conventional doxorubicin hydrochloride on a mg-per-mg basis.

US labeling:

AIDS-related Kaposi sarcoma: IV: 20 mg/m^2 once every 21 days until disease progression or unacceptable toxicity

Multiple myeloma: IV: 30 mg/m^2 on day 4 every 21 days (in combination with bortezomib) for 8 cycles or until disease progression or unacceptable toxicity (Orlowski 2007)

Multiple myeloma, newly diagnosed (off-label dosing): IV: 40 mg/m^2 on day 1 every 4 weeks (in combination with vincristine and dexamethasone) for at least 4 cycles (Rifkin, 2006).

Ovarian cancer, advanced: IV: 50 mg/m^2 once every 28 days until disease progression or unacceptable toxicity

Ovarian cancer, advanced, recurrent (off- label dosing): IV: 40 mg/m^2 once every 28 days (as a single agent) until disease progression or unacceptable toxicity (Ferrandina, 2008; Rose, 2001) or 30 mg/m^2 once every 28 days (in combination with carboplatin) for at least 6 cycles (Pujade-Lauraine, 2010) or 40 mg/m^2 once every 28 days (in combination with bevacizumab) until disease progression or unacceptable toxicity (Pujade-Lauraine, 2014).

Canadian labeling:

AIDS-related Kaposi sarcoma (Caelyx): IV: 20 mg/m^2 once every 2 to 3 weeks; continue as long as responding and tolerating

Breast cancer, metastatic: IV:

Caelyx: 50 mg/m^2 once every 4 weeks until disease progression or unacceptable toxicity

Myocet: 60 to 75 mg/m^2 once every 3 weeks (in combination with cyclophosphamide)

Ovarian cancer, advanced (Caelyx): IV: 50 mg/m^2 once every 4 weeks until disease progression or unacceptable toxicity

Off-label uses/doses:

Breast cancer, metastatic (off-label use in US): IV: 50 mg/m^2 every 4 weeks (Keller, 2004)

Cutaneous T-cell lymphomas (off-label use): IV: 20 mg/m^2 days 1 and 15 every 4 weeks for 6 cycles (Dummer, 2012) **or** 20 mg/m^2 every 4 weeks (Wollina, 2003)

Hodgkin lymphoma, salvage treatment (off-label use): IV: GVD regimen: 10 mg/m^2 (post-transplant patients) or 15 mg/m^2 (transplant-naive patients) days 1 and 8 every 3 weeks (in combination with gemcitabine and vinorelbine) for 2 to 6 cycles (Bartlett, 2007)

Soft tissue sarcoma, advanced (off-label use): IV: 50 mg/m^2 every 4 weeks for 6 cycles (Judson, 2001)

Uterine sarcoma, advanced or recurrent (off-label use): IV: 50 mg/m^2 every 4 weeks until disease progression or unacceptable toxicity (Sutton, 2005)

Renal Impairment There are no dosage adjustments provided in the manufacturer's labeling (has not been studied).

Hepatic Impairment

US labeling: There are no dosage adjustments provided in the manufacturer's labeling. However, doxorubicin is predominantly hepatically eliminated and reduced doxorubicin liposomal doses are recommended in patients with serum bilirubin ≥1.2 mg/dL.

Canadian labeling:

Caelyx: AIDS-related Kaposi sarcoma:

Bilirubin 1.2 to 3 mg/dL: Administer 50% of normal dose

Bilirubin >3 mg/dL: Administer 25% of normal dose

Caelyx: Breast cancer and ovarian cancer:

Bilirubin 1.2 to 3 mg/dL: Initial dose: Administer 75% of normal dose; if tolerated and no change in bilirubin/hepatic enzymes, may increase to full dose with cycle 2

Bilirubin >3 mg/dL: Initial dose: Administer 50% of normal dose; if tolerated and no change in bilirubin/hepatic enzymes, may increase dose to 75% of normal dose for cycle 2; if cycle 2 dose tolerated, may increase to full dose for subsequent cycles.

Myocet: Breast cancer:

Bilirubin 1.2 to 3 mg/dL: Administer 50% of normal dose

Bilirubin >3 mg/dL: Administer 25% of normal dose

◀ **Obesity** *ASCO Guidelines for appropriate chemotherapy dosing in obese adults with cancer:* Utilize patient's actual body weight (full weight) for calculation of body surface area- or weight-based dosing, particularly when the intent of therapy is curative; manage regimen-related toxicities in the same manner as for nonobese patients; if a dose reduction is utilized due to toxicity, consider resumption of full weight-based dosing with subsequent cycles, especially if cause of toxicity (eg, hepatic or renal impairment) is resolved (Griggs, 2012).

Adjustment for Toxicity

US labeling: **Note:** Once a dosage reduction due to toxicity has been implemented, the dose should not be increased at a later time.

Recommended Dose Modification Guidelines

Toxicity Grade	Dose Adjustment
HAND-FOOT SYNDROME (HFS)	
1 (Mild erythema, swelling, or desquamation not interfering with daily activities)	No prior Grade 3 or 4 HFS toxicity: No dosage adjustment is necessary. Prior Grade 3 or 4 HFS toxicity: Delay dose up to 2 weeks and decrease dose by 25%.
2 (Erythema, desquamation, or swelling interfering with, but not precluding, normal physical activities; small blisters or ulcerations <2 cm in diameter)	Delay dosing up to 2 weeks or until resolved to Grade 0 or 1. If after 2 weeks there is no resolution, discontinue liposomal doxorubicin. If resolved to Grade 0 or 1 within 2 weeks and no prior Grade 3 or 4 HFS, continue treatment at previous dose. If a prior Grade 3 or 4 HFS has occurred, decrease dose by 25%.
3 (Blistering, ulceration, or swelling interfering with walking or normal daily activities; cannot wear regular clothing)	Delay dosing up to 2 weeks or until resolved to Grade 0 or 1, then decrease dose by 25%. If no resolution after 2 weeks, discontinue liposomal doxorubicin.
4 (Diffuse or local process causing infectious complications, or a bedridden state or hospitalization)	Delay dosing up to 2 weeks or until resolved to Grade 0 or 1, then decrease dose by 25%. If no resolution after 2 weeks, discontinue liposomal doxorubicin.
STOMATITIS	
1 (Painless ulcers, erythema, or mild soreness)	No prior Grade 3 or 4 toxicity: No dosage adjustment is necessary. Prior Grade 3 or 4 toxicity: Delay dose up to 2 weeks and decrease dose by 25%.
2 (Painful erythema, edema, or ulcers, but can eat)	Delay dosing up to 2 weeks or until resolved to Grade 0 or 1. If after 2 weeks there is no resolution, discontinue liposomal doxorubicin. If resolved to Grade 0 or 1 within 2 weeks and no prior Grade 3 or 4 stomatitis, continue treatment at previous dose. If prior Grade 3 or 4 stomatitis, decrease dose by 25%.
3 (Painful erythema, edema, or ulcers, and cannot eat)	Delay dosing up to 2 weeks or until resolved to Grade 0 or 1. Decrease dose by 25% and return to original dosing interval. If after 2 weeks there is no resolution, discontinue liposomal doxorubicin.
4 (Requires parenteral or enteral support)	Delay dosing up to 2 weeks or until resolved to Grade 0 or 1. Decrease dose by 25% and return to original dosing interval. If after 2 weeks there is no resolution, discontinue liposomal doxorubicin.

See table: "Hematologic Toxicity"

Hematologic Toxicity (see below for multiple myeloma)

Grade	ANC	Platelets	Modification
1	1,500 to 1,900/mm^3	75,000 to 150,000/mm^3	No dosage adjustment is necessary.
2	1,000 to <1,500/mm^3	50,000 to <75,000/mm^3	Delay until ANC ≥1,500/mm^3 and platelets ≥75,000/mm^3; resume treatment at previous dose.
3	500 to 999/mm^3	25,000 to <50,000/mm^3	Delay until ANC ≥1,500/mm^3 and platelets ≥75,000/mm^3; resume treatment at previous dose.
4	<500/mm^3	<25,000/mm^3	Delay until ANC ≥1,500/mm^3 and platelets ≥75,000/mm^3; resume at 25% dose reduction or continue at previous dose with granulocyte growth factor support.

Doxorubicin Liposomal Dosing Adjustment for Toxicity in Treatment with Bortezomib (for Multiple Myeloma) (see Bortezomib monograph for bortezomib dosage reduction with toxicity guidelines):

Fever ≥38°C and ANC <1,000/mm^3: If prior to doxorubicin liposomal treatment (day 4), do not administer (withhold); if after doxorubicin liposomal administered, reduce dose by 25% in next cycle.

ANC <500/mm^3, platelets <25,000/mm^3, hemoglobin <8 g/dL: If prior to doxorubicin liposomal treatment (day 4); do not administer (withhold); if after doxorubicin liposomal administered and if bortezomib dose reduction occurred for hematologic toxicity, reduce dose by 25% in next cycle

Grade 3 or 4 nonhematologic toxicity: Delay dose until resolved to grade <2 and then reduce dose by 25%

Neuropathic pain or peripheral neuropathy: No dose reductions needed for doxorubicin liposomal, refer to Bortezomib monograph for bortezomib dosing adjustment.

Canadian labeling:
Caelyx: Nonhematologic toxicity: Breast cancer, ovarian cancer:

Caelyx: Recommended Dose Modification Guidelines

Toxicity Grade	Week After Prior Caelyx Dose (Breast Cancer or Ovarian Cancer)	
	Weeks 4 and 5	Week 6
HAND-FOOT SYNDROME (HFS)		
1 (Mild erythema, swelling, or desquamation not interfering with daily activities)	Redose unless patient has experienced previous Grade 3 or 4 HFS toxicity. If so, wait an additional week	Decrease dose by 25%; return to 4-week interval
2 (Erythema, desquamation, or swelling interfering with, but not precluding, normal physical activities; small blisters or ulcerations <2 cm in diameter)	Wait an additional week	Decrease dose by 25%; return to 4-week interval
3 (Blistering, ulceration, or swelling interfering with walking or normal daily activities; cannot wear regular clothing)	Wait an additional week	Discontinue therapy

(continued)

Caelyx: Recommended Dose Modification Guidelines *(continued)*

Toxicity Grade	Week After Prior Caelyx Dose (Breast Cancer or Ovarian Cancer)	
	Weeks 4 and 5	Week 6
4 (Diffuse or local process causing infectious complications, or a bedridden state or hospitalization)	Wait an additional week	Discontinue therapy
STOMATITIS		
1 (Painless ulcers, erythema, or mild soreness)	Redose unless patient has experienced previous Grade 3 or 4 stomatitis. If so, wait an additional week.	Decrease dose by 25%; return to 4-week interval or if warranted, discontinue therapy
2 (Painful erythema, edema, or ulcers, but can eat)	Wait an additional week	Decrease dose by 25%; return to 4-week interval or if warranted, discontinue therapy
3 (Painful erythema, edema, or ulcers, and cannot eat)	Wait an additional week	Discontinue therapy
4 (Requires parenteral or enteral support)	Wait an additional week	Discontinue therapy

Caelyx: Hematologic toxicity: Breast cancer, ovarian cancer: Refer to US dosage adjustment for hematologic toxicity section.

Caelyx: Nonhematologic toxicity: AIDS-related Kaposi sarcoma:

Caelyx: Recommended Dose Modification Guidelines: Hand-Foot Syndrome (HFS) (AIDS-related Kaposi Sarcoma)

Toxicity Grade	Weeks Since Last Caelyx Dose (AIDS-related Kaposi Sarcoma)	
	3 Weeks	4 Weeks
HAND-FOOT SYNDROME (HFS)		
1 (Mild erythema, swelling, or desquamation not interfering with daily activities)	Redose unless patient has experienced previous Grade 3 or 4 skin toxicity. If so, wait an additional week	Decrease dose by 25%; return to 3-week interval
2 (Erythema, desquamation, or swelling interfering with, but not precluding, normal physical activities; small blisters or ulcerations <2 cm in diameter)	Wait an additional week	Decrease dose by 50%; return to 3-week interval
3 (Blistering, ulceration, or swelling interfering with walking or normal daily activities; cannot wear regular clothing)	Wait an additional week	Discontinue therapy
4 (Diffuse or local process causing infectious complications, or a bedridden state or hospitalization)	Wait an additional week	Discontinue therapy

Caelyx: Recommended Dose Modification Guidelines: Stomatitis (AIDS-related Kaposi Sarcoma)

STOMATITIS Toxicity grade:	Caelyx Dosage Adjustment (AIDS-related Kaposi Sarcoma)
1 (Painless ulcers, erythema, or mild soreness)	No dosage adjustment
2 (Painful erythema, edema, or ulcers, but can eat)	Wait 1 week and if symptoms improve, redose at 100% dose
3 (Painful erythema, edema, or ulcers, and cannot eat)	Wait 1 week and if symptoms improve, redose with a 25% dose reduction
4 (Requires parenteral or enteral support)	Wait 1 week and if symptoms improve, redose with a 50% dose reduction

Caelyx: Hematologic toxicity: AIDS-related Kaposi sarcoma:

Caelyx: Hematologic Toxicity (AIDS-related Kaposi Sarcoma)

Grade	ANC	Platelets	Modification
1	1,500 to 1,900/mm^3	75,000 to 150,000/mm^3	None
2	1,000 to <1,500/mm^3	50,000 to <75,000/mm^3	None
3	500 to 999/mm^3	25,000 to <50,000/mm^3	Wait until ANC ≥1,000/mm^3 and/or platelets ≥50,000/mm^3; redose with a 25% dose reduction.
4	<500/mm^3	<25,000/mm^3	Wait until ANC ≥1,000/mm^3 and/or platelets ≥50,000/mm^3; redose with a 50% dose reduction.

Myocet: Hematologic or gastrointestinal toxicity: Dosage reduction: If initial dose was 75 mg/m^2, reduce dose to 60 mg/m^2; if initial dose was 60 mg/m^2, reduce dose to 50 mg/m^2. If toxicity persists with subsequent cycles, consider reducing dose further (from 60 mg/m^2 to 50 mg/m^2 or from 50 mg/m^2 to 40 mg/m^2).

Neutropenia: If grade 4 neutropenia (ANC <500/mm^3) without fever lasting ≥7 days or grade 4 neutropenia of any duration with concurrent fever (≥38.5°C) occurs, consider reducing dose with subsequent cycles. **Note:** Prior to dose reductions, prophylactic cytokine therapy may be considered.

Thrombocytopenia or anemia: If grade 4 thrombocytopenia or anemia occurs, hold therapy until recovery to ≤ grade 2. Reduce dose with subsequent cycles or consider discontinuing treatment.

Gastrointestinal toxicity or mucositis: Grade 3 mucositis persisting ≥3 days, or grade 4 mucositis of any duration, or grade 3 or 4 gastrointestinal toxicity not responsive to interventions and/or prophylaxis: Consider dose reduction with subsequent cycles.

Combination Regimens

Breast cancer: Doxorubicin (Liposomal) (Breast Regimen) on page 1950
Lymphoma, Hodgkin: GVD (Hodgkin) on page 2002

◄ Multiple myeloma:

Ovarian cancer:

Administration Monitor for infusion reaction. For IV infusion only; do not administer IV push.

Doxil, Caelyx: Administer IVPB over 60 minutes; the manufacturer recommends infusing the first dose at initial rate of 1 mg/minute to minimize risk of infusion reactions; if no infusion-related reactions are observed, then increase the infusion rate for completion over 1 hour. Do **NOT** administer undiluted. Do **NOT** mix with in-line filters. Do not mix with other medications. Monitor for local erythematous streaking along vein and/or facial flushing (may indicate rapid infusion rate).

For multiple myeloma, administer doxorubicin liposomal after bortezomib on day 4 of each cycle.

Myocet: Infuse over 1 hour.

Irritant (Perez Fidalgo, 2012); monitor infusion site; avoid extravasation. Assure proper needle or catheter position prior to administration.

Extravasation management: If extravasation, infiltration, or burning/stinging sensation occurs, stop infusion immediately and disconnect (leave cannula/needle in place); gently aspirate extravasated solution (do **NOT** flush the line); remove needle/cannula; elevate extremity (Perez Fidalgo, 2012; Polovich, 2009). Do not apply pressure to the site. Apply ice to the site for 15 minutes 4 times a day for 3 days.

Hazardous agent; use appropriate precautions for handling and disposal (NIOSH 2014 [group 1]). If contact with skin/mucosa occurs, wash immediately with soap and water.

Vesicant/Extravasation Risk Irritant

Emetic Potential Children and Adults: Low (10% to 30%)

Monitoring Parameters CBC with differential and platelet count, liver function tests (ALT/AST, bilirubin, alkaline phosphatase); monitor infusion site, monitor for infusion reactions, hand-foot syndrome, stomatitis, and oral ulceration/discomfort suggestive of secondary oral malignancy

Cardiac function (left ventricular ejection fraction [LVEF]; baseline and periodic); echocardiography, or MUGA scan may be used.

Dosage Forms Excipient information presented when available (limited, particularly for generics); consult specific product labeling.

Injectable, Intravenous, as hydrochloride:

Doxil: 2 mg/mL (10 mL, 25 mL)

Lipodox: 2 mg/mL (10 mL)

Lipodox 50: 2 mg/mL (25 mL)

Generic: 2 mg/mL (10 mL, 25 mL)

Dosage Forms: Canada Excipient information presented when available (limited, particularly for generics); consult specific product labeling.
Injection, solution, as hydrochloride, pegylated:
  Caelyx: 2 mg/mL (10 mL, 25 mL)
Injection, encapsulated liposomes:
  Myocet: 3-vial kit (doxorubicin HCl for injection 50 mg/vial, liposomes for injection, and buffer for injection)

◆ **Doxorubicin HCl** see DOXOrubicin (Conventional) on page 553

◆ **Doxorubicin Hydrochloride** see DOXOrubicin (Conventional) on page 553

◆ **DOXOrubicin Hydrochloride Encapsulated Liposomes (Myocet)** see DOXOrubicin (Liposomal) on page 565

◆ **Doxorubicin Hydrochloride For Injection, USP (Can)** see DOXOrubicin (Conventional) on page 553

◆ **Doxorubicin Hydrochloride Injection (Can)** see DOXOrubicin (Conventional) on page 553

◆ **DOXOrubicin Hydrochloride (Liposomal)** see DOXOrubicin (Liposomal) on page 565

◆ **DOXOrubicin Hydrochloride Liposome** see DOXOrubicin (Liposomal) on page 565

◆ **DOXOrubicin Hydrochloride Liposomes (Myocet)** see DOXOrubicin (Liposomal) on page 565

Dronabinol (droe NAB i nol)

Related Information
Management of Chemotherapy-Induced Nausea and Vomiting in Adults on page 2142

Brand Names: US Marinol

Index Terms Delta-9 THC; Delta-9-tetrahydro-cannabinol; Tetrahydrocannabinol; THC

Pharmacologic Category Antiemetic; Appetite Stimulant

Use
Appetite stimulation in AIDS patients: Treatment of anorexia associated with weight loss in patients with AIDS.

Chemotherapy-induced nausea and vomiting: Treatment of nausea and vomiting associated with cancer chemotherapy in patients who have failed to respond adequately to conventional antiemetic treatments.

Labeled Contraindications Hypersensitivity to dronabinol, cannabinoids, sesame oil, or any component of the formulation.

Pregnancy Considerations Adverse events have been observed in animal reproduction studies.

Breast-Feeding Considerations Dronabinol is excreted in breast milk. Breast-feeding is not recommended by the manufacturer.

Warnings/Precautions Use with caution in patients with seizure disorders and in the elderly. May cause occasional hypotension, possible hypertension, syncope, or tachycardia; use with caution in patients with cardiac disorders. May cause CNS depression, which may impair physical or mental abilities; patients must be cautioned about performing tasks that require mental alertness (eg, operating machinery, driving).

◄ Administration with phenothiazines (eg, prochlorperazine) for the management of chemotherapy-induced nausea and vomiting may result in improved efficacy (compared to either drug alone) without additional toxicity. Use with caution in patients with a history of substance abuse, including alcohol abuse or dependence; potential for drug dependency exists. Tolerance, psychological and physical dependence may occur with prolonged use. May cause withdrawal symptoms upon abrupt discontinuation. Use with caution in patients with mania, depression, or schizophrenia; careful psychiatric monitoring is recommended.

Adverse Reactions Frequency not always specified.

>1%:

Cardiovascular: Palpitations, tachycardia, vasodilation/facial flushing

Central nervous system: Euphoria (8% to 24%, dose related), abnormal thinking (3% to 10%), dizziness (3% to 10%), paranoia (3% to 10%), somnolence (3% to 10%), amnesia, anxiety, ataxia, confusion, depersonalization, hallucination

Gastrointestinal: Abdominal pain (3% to 10%), nausea (3% to 10%), vomiting (3% to 10%)

Neuromuscular & skeletal: Weakness

<1%, postmarketing, and/or case reports: Conjunctivitis, depression, diarrhea, fatigue, fecal incontinence, flushing, hypotension, myalgia, nightmares, seizure, speech difficulties, tinnitus, vision difficulties

Drug Interactions

Metabolism/Transport Effects Substrate of CYP2C9 (minor), CYP3A4 (minor); **Note:** Assignment of Major/Minor substrate status based on clinically relevant drug interaction potential

Avoid Concomitant Use There are no known interactions where it is recommended to avoid concomitant use.

Increased Effect/Toxicity

Dronabinol may increase the levels/effects of: Alcohol (Ethyl); CNS Depressants; Sympathomimetics

The levels/effects of Dronabinol may be increased by: Anticholinergic Agents; Cocaine; CYP2C9 Inhibitors (Moderate); CYP2C9 Inhibitors (Strong); CYP3A4 Inhibitors (Moderate); CYP3A4 Inhibitors (Strong); MAO Inhibitors; Ritonavir

Decreased Effect

The levels/effects of Dronabinol may be decreased by: CYP3A4 Inducers (Strong)

Storage/Stability Store in a cool environment between 8°C and 15°C (46°F and 59°F) or refrigerated; protect from freezing.

Mechanism of Action Dronabinol (synthetic delta-9-tetrahydrocannabinol [delta-9-THC]), an active cannabinoid and natural occurring component of *Cannabis sativa L.* (marijuana), activates cannabinoid receptors CB_1 and CB_2. Activation of the CB_1 receptor produces marijuana-like effects on psyche and circulation, whereas activation of the CB_2 receptor does not. Dronabinol has approximately equal affinity for the CB_1 and CB_2 receptors; however, efficacy is less at CB_2 receptors. Activation of the cannabinoid system with dronabinol causes psychological effects that can be divided into 4 groups: affective (euphoria and easy laughter); sensory (increased perception of external stimuli and of the person's own body); somatic (feeling of the body floating or sinking in the bed); and cognitive (distortion of time perception, memory lapses, difficulty in concentration). Most effects (eg, analgesia, appetite enhancement, muscle relaxation, hormonal actions) are mediated by central cannabinoid receptors (CB_1), their distribution reflecting many of the medicinal benefits and adverse effects (Grotenhermen 2003).

Pharmacodynamics/Kinetics

Onset of action: ~0.5 to 1 hour

Peak effect: 2 to 4 hours

Duration: 4 to 6 hours (psychoactive effects); ≥24 hours (appetite stimulation)

Absorption: Oral: 90% to 95%; 10% to 20% of dose gets into systemic circulation

Distribution: V_d: ~10 L/kg; dronabinol is highly lipophilic

Protein binding: ~97%

Metabolism: Extensive first-pass hepatic primarily via microsomal hydroxylation to metabolites, some of which are active; 11-hydroxy-delta-9-tetrahydrocannabinol (11-OH-THC) is the major active metabolite

Half-life elimination: Dronabinol: 25 to 36 hours (terminal)

Time to peak, serum: 0.5 to 4 hours

Excretion: Feces (50%, 5% as unchanged drug); urine (10% to 15%)

Dosing

Adult & Geriatric Note: Use caution when increasing the dose of dronabinol because of the increased frequency of dose-related adverse reactions at higher dosages.

Appetite stimulation in AIDS patients: Oral: Initial: 2.5 mg twice daily (before lunch and dinner); for patients unable to tolerate this dosage, may reduce to 2.5 mg once daily (in the evening or at bedtime). May increase dose gradually based on response and tolerability (maximum: 20 mg per day [in divided doses]).

Chemotherapy-induced nausea and vomiting (manufacturer's labeling): Oral: 5 mg/m² administered 1 to 3 hours before chemotherapy, then give 5 mg/m²/dose every 2 to 4 hours after chemotherapy for a total of 4 to 6 doses/day; increase doses in increments of 2.5 mg/m² based on response and tolerability (maximum: 15 mg/m²/dose). **Note:** Initiate with the lowest recommended dose and titrate to response; most patients respond to 5 mg 3 to 4 times daily; based on initial results, the dose may be escalated during a chemotherapy cycle or with subsequent cycles.

Chemotherapy-induced nausea and vomiting, refractory (off-label dosing): Oral: 2.5 to 10 mg 3 or 4 times daily (Lohr 2008)

Pediatric

Chemotherapy-induced nausea and vomiting: Oral: Refer to adult dosing. Use caution when increasing the dose because of the increased frequency of dose-related adverse reactions at higher dosages.

Renal Impairment There are no dosage adjustments provided in the manufacturer's labeling.

Hepatic Impairment There are no dosage adjustments provided in the manufacturer's labeling.

Administration Oral: For appetite stimulation, administer twice-daily doses before lunch and dinner; administer single doses in the evening or at bedtime.

Monitoring Parameters CNS effects, heart rate, blood pressure, behavioral profile

Dietary Considerations Capsules contain sesame oil.

579

◀ **Dosage Forms** Excipient information presented when available (limited, particularly for generics); consult specific product labeling.
Capsule, Oral:
Marinol: 2.5 mg, 5 mg, 10 mg [contains sesame oil]
Generic: 2.5 mg, 5 mg, 10 mg
Controlled Substance C-III

♦ **Droxia** see Hydroxyurea on page 839
♦ **DTC 101** see Cytarabine (Liposomal) on page 415
♦ **DTIC** see Dacarbazine on page 428
♦ **DTIC-Dome** see Dacarbazine on page 428
♦ **D-Trp(6)-LHRH** see Triptorelin on page 1703
♦ **Duragesic** see FentaNYL on page 692
♦ **Duragesic MAT (Can)** see FentaNYL on page 692
♦ **Duramorph** see Morphine (Systemic) on page 1167
♦ **Durela (Can)** see TraMADol on page 1672
♦ **DVA** see Vindesine on page 1760
♦ **E7080** see Lenvatinib on page 1014
♦ **E7389** see EriBULin on page 624
♦ **EACA** see Aminocaproic Acid on page 91
♦ **E. coli Asparaginase** see Asparaginase (E. coli) on page 144
♦ **Econopred** see PrednisoLONE (Ophthalmic) on page 1424
♦ **Ecteinascidin** see Trabectedin on page 1665
♦ **Ecteinascidin 743** see Trabectedin on page 1665

Eculizumab (e kue LIZ oo mab)

Brand Names: US Soliris
Brand Names: Canada Soliris
Index Terms h5G1.1; Monoclonal Antibody 5G1.1; Monoclonal Antibody Anti-C5
Pharmacologic Category Monoclonal Antibody; Monoclonal Antibody, Complement Inhibitor
Use
Atypical hemolytic uremic syndrome: Treatment of atypical hemolytic uremic syndrome (aHUS) to inhibit complement-mediated thrombotic microangiopathy.
Limitation of use: Eculizumab is not indicated for the treatment of patients with Shiga toxin Escherichia coli-related hemolytic uremic syndrome.
Paroxysmal nocturnal hemoglobinuria: Treatment of paroxysmal nocturnal hemoglobinuria (PNH) to reduce hemolysis.
Labeled Contraindications Unresolved serious Neisseria meningitidis infection; patients not currently vaccinated against Neisseria meningitidis (unless risks of treatment delay outweigh risk of developing a meningococcal infection)
Pregnancy Considerations Adverse events were observed in animal reproduction studies. Eculizumab crosses the placenta and can be detected in cord blood. Pregnant women with PNH and their fetuses have high rates of morbidity and mortality during pregnancy and the postpartum period. Treatment of PNH with eculizumab has been shown to increase fetal survival and decrease

maternal complications (Kelly 2015). Use of eculizumab for the treatment of a HUS in pregnancy has also been described (Ardissino 2013).

Breast-Feeding Considerations Excretion of eculizumab into breast milk was not noted in breast milk samples from 10 women. In a separate case report, eculizumab was detected in the initial breast milk sample of a woman, but not subsequent samples (Kelly 2015). The manufacturer recommends that caution be used if administered to nursing women.

Warnings/Precautions [US Boxed Warning]: Meningococcal *(Neisseria meningitides)* **infections have occurred in patients receiving eculizumab; may be fatal or life-threatening if not detected and treated promptly. Monitor closely for early signs of meningococcal infection; evaluate and treat promptly if suspected. Follow current meningococcal immunization recommendations for patients with complement deficiencies. Vaccinate with meningococcal vaccine at least 2 weeks prior to initiation of treatment (unless the risks of delaying eculizumab outweigh the risk of developing meningococcal infection);** revaccinate according to current guidelines. Polyvalent meningococcal vaccines are recommended. If urgent treatment is necessary in an unvaccinated patient, administer meningococcal vaccine as soon as possible. Although the risk/benefits of prophylactic meningococcal antibiotic therapy have not been determined, prophylactic antibiotics were administered in clinical studies until at least 2 weeks after vaccination. Meningococcal infections developed in some patients despite vaccination. Discontinue eculizumab during the treatment of serious meningococcal infections. In addition to meningitis, the risk of other infections, especially encapsulated bacteria (eg, *Streptococcus pneumoniae, H. influenzae*) is increased with eculizumab treatment (because eculizumab blocks terminal complement activation). Aspergillus infections have occurred in immunocompromised and neutropenic patients. Children should receive vaccination for prevention of *S. pneumoniae, H. influenzae* according to current ACIP guidelines. Use caution in patients with concurrent systemic infection. Patients should be up to date with all immunizations before initiating therapy. **[US Boxed Warning]: Access is restricted through a REMS program. Prescribers must be enrolled in the program; enrollment and additional information is available at 1-888-765-4747.** Counsel patients on the risk of meningococcal infection; ensure patients are vaccinated and provide educational materials.

Infusion reactions, including anaphylaxis or hypersensitivity, may occur; interrupt infusion for severe reaction (eg, cardiovascular instability, respiratory compromise). Continue monitoring for 1 hour after completion of infusion. Patients with PNH who discontinue treatment may be at increased risk for serious hemolysis; monitor closely for at least 8 weeks after treatment discontinuation. When used for aHUS, monitor for at least 12 weeks after treatment discontinuation for signs/symptoms of thrombotic microangiopathy (TMA) complications (angina, dyspnea, mental status changes, seizure, or thrombosis; occurrence of two or repeated measurement of any one of the following: Serum creatinine elevation (≥25% from baseline or nadir), serum LDH elevation (≥25% from baseline or nadir), thrombocytopenia (platelet decrease by ≥25% compared to baseline or peak). If TMA complications occur after stopping eculizumab, consider reinitiation of treatment, plasmapheresis, plasma exchange, fresh frozen plasma infusion, and/or appropriate organ-specific measures. In clinical trials, anticoagulant therapy was continued in patients who were receiving these agents (due to history of or risk for thromboembolism) prior to initiation of eculizumab. Potentially significant drug-drug interactions may exist, requiring dose or frequency adjustment, additional monitoring, and/or selection of alternative therapy. The effect of anticoagulant therapy withdrawal is unknown; treatment with eculizumab should not alter anticoagulation management

Adverse Reactions Frequency reported for adolescent and adult patients ≥13 years unless otherwise noted.

>10%:

Cardiovascular: Hypertension (aHUS: 17% to 59%; infants, children, and adolescents 5 months through 17 years: 18%), peripheral edema (20% to 29%), tachycardia (aHUS: children 21%), hypotension (12% to 20%)

Central nervous system: Headache (37% to 50%; serious: 2%; infants, children, and adolescents 5 months through 17 years: 18%), insomnia (10% to 24%), fatigue (7% to 20%)

Dermatologic: Skin rash (infants ≥5 months, children, adolescents, and adults 12% to 18%), pruritus (6% to 15%)

Endocrine & metabolic: Hypokalemia (10% to 18%)

Gastrointestinal: Diarrhea (32% to 47%; infants, children, and adolescents 2 months through 17 years: 32%), vomiting (15% to 47%; infants, children, and adolescents 2 months through 17 years: 21% to 27%), nausea (12% to 40%), abdominal pain (15% to 30%), gastroenteritis (5% to 18%), dyspepsia (infants, children, and adolescents 5 months through 17 years: 14%)

Genitourinary: Urinary tract infection (15% to 35%; infants, children, and adolescents 5 months through 17 years: 18%), uropathy (infants, children, and adolescents 5 months through 17 years: 18%), proteinuria (5% to 12%)

Hematologic & oncologic: Anemia (17% to 35%; serious: 2%), neoplasm (6% to 30%), leukopenia (16% to 24%)

Local: Catheter infection (infants, children, and adolescents 5 months through 17 years: 14%)

Neuromuscular & skeletal: Weakness (15% to 20%), back pain (5% to 19%), arthralgia (6% to 17%), muscle spasm (infants, children, and adolescents 5 months through 17 years: 14%), limb pain (7% to 11%)

Ophthalmic: Eye disease (10% to 29%; infants, children, and adolescents 5 months through 17 years: 14%)

Renal: Renal insufficiency (15% to 29%)

Respiratory: Nasopharyngitis (18% to 55%; infants, children, and adolescents 5 months through 17 years: 27%), upper respiratory tract infection (infants ≥2 months, children, adolescents, and adults 5% to 40%), cough (infants ≥5 months, children, adolescents, and adults 12% to 36%), nasal congestion (aHUS: children 21%), rhinitis (infants, children, and adolescents 5 months through 17 years: 18%), bronchitis (10% to 18%), oropharyngeal pain (infants, children, and adolescents 5 months through 17 years: 14%)

Miscellaneous: Fever (infants, children, and adolescents 2 months through 17 years: 47% to 50%; adults 17% to 25%)

1% to 10%:

Gastrointestinal: Constipation (7%)

Immunologic: Antibody development (2% to 3%; neutralizing: 1%)

Infection: Herpes virus infection (7%), viral infection (serious: 2%), meningococcal infection (≤1%)

Neuromuscular & skeletal: Myalgia (7%)

Respiratory: Respiratory tract infection (7%), sinusitis (7%), flu-like symptoms (5%)

<1%, postmarketing, and/or case reports: Abdominal distention, anxiety, aspergillosis, cholangitis, dizziness, dysgeusia, endometritis, hematoma (mild), infusion related reaction, pyelonephritis

Drug Interactions

Metabolism/Transport Effects None known.

Avoid Concomitant Use

Avoid concomitant use of Eculizumab with any of the following: BCG (Intravesical); Belimumab; Natalizumab; Pimecrolimus; Tacrolimus (Topical); Tofacitinib; Vaccines (Live)

Increased Effect/Toxicity

Eculizumab may increase the levels/effects of: Belimumab; Fingolimod; Leflunomide; Natalizumab; Tofacitinib; Vaccines (Live)

The levels/effects of Eculizumab may be increased by: Denosumab; Pimecrolimus; Roflumilast; Tacrolimus (Topical); Trastuzumab

Decreased Effect

Eculizumab may decrease the levels/effects of: BCG (Intravesical); Coccidioides immitis Skin Test; Sipuleucel-T; Vaccines (Inactivated); Vaccines (Live)

The levels/effects of Eculizumab may be decreased by: Echinacea

Storage/Stability Prior to dilution, store intact vials at 2°C to 8°C (36°F to 46°F); do not freeze. Protect from light; do not shake. Following dilution, store at room temperature or refrigerate; protect from light; use within 24 hours. If refrigerated, allow admixture to reach room temperature prior to administration (do not use a heat source or warming).

Preparation for Administration Add eculizumab to an infusion bag and dilute with an equal volume of D_5W, sodium chloride 0.9%, sodium chloride 0.45%, or Ringer's injection to a final concentration of 5 mg/mL (eg, 300 mg to a total volume of 60 mL, 600 mg in a total volume of 120 mL, 900 mg in a total volume of 180 mL, or 1200 mg to a total volume of 240 mL). Gently invert bag to mix thoroughly; do not shake.

Mechanism of Action Terminal complement-mediated intravascular hemolysis is a key clinical feature of paroxysmal nocturnal hemoglobinuria (PNH); blocking the formation of membrane attack complex (MAC) results in stabilization of hemoglobin and a reduction in the need for RBC transfusions. Impairment of complement activity regulation leads to uncontrolled complement activation in atypical hemolytic uremic syndrome (aHUS). Eculizumab is a humanized monoclonal IgG antibody that binds to complement protein C5, preventing cleavage into C5a and C5b. Blocking the formation of C5b inhibits the subsequent formation of terminal complex C5b-9 or MAC.

Pharmacodynamics/Kinetics

Onset of action: PNH: Reduced hemolysis: ≤1 week

Distribution: PNH: 7.7 L; aHUS: 6.14 L

Half-life elimination: PNH: ~11 days (range: ~8-15 days); aHUS: ~12 days (during plasma exchange the half-life is reduced to 1.26 hours)

Dosing

Adult & Geriatric Note: Patients must receive meningococcal vaccine at least 2 weeks prior to treatment initiation; revaccinate according to current guidelines. Treatment should be administered at the recommended time interval although administration may be varied by ±2 days.

Atypical hemolytic uremic syndrome (aHUS): IV: Induction: 900 mg weekly for 4 doses; Maintenance: 1200 mg at week 5, then 1200 mg every 2 weeks

Supplemental dosing for patients receiving plasmapheresis or plasma exchange: If most recent dose was ≥600 mg, administer 600 mg within 60 minutes after each plasmapheresis or plasma exchange

Supplemental dosing for patients receiving fresh frozen plasma infusion: If most recent dose was ≥300 mg, administer 300 mg within 60 minutes prior to each infusion of fresh frozen plasma

Paroxysmal nocturnal hemoglobinuria (PNH): IV: 600 mg weekly for 4 doses, followed by 900 mg 1 week later; then 900 mg every 2 weeks

Pediatric Note: Patients must receive meningococcal vaccine at least 2 weeks prior to treatment initiation; revaccinate according to current guidelines. Treatment should be administered at the recommended time interval although administration may be varied by ±2 days.

Atypical hemolytic uremic syndrome (aHUS): IV:

Children 5 kg to <10 kg: Induction: 300 mg weekly for 1 dose; Maintenance: 300 mg at week 2, then 300 mg every 3 weeks

Children 10 kg to <20 kg: Induction: 600 mg weekly for 1 dose; Maintenance: 300 mg at week 2, then 300 mg every 2 weeks

Children 20 kg to <30 kg: Induction: 600 mg weekly for 2 doses; Maintenance: 600 mg at week 3, then 600 mg every 2 weeks

Children 30 kg to <40 kg: Induction: 600 mg weekly for 2 doses; Maintenance: 900 mg at week 3, then 900 mg every 2 weeks

Children ≥40 kg: Induction: 900 mg weekly for 4 doses; Maintenance: 1200 mg at week 5, then 1200 mg every 2 weeks

Supplemental dosing for patients receiving plasmapheresis or plasma exchange:

If most recent dose was 300 mg, administer 300 mg within 60 minutes after each plasmapheresis or plasma exchange

If most recent dose was ≥600 mg, administer 600 mg within 60 minutes after each plasmapheresis or plasma exchange

Supplemental dosing for patients receiving fresh frozen plasma infusion: If most recent dose was ≥300 mg, administer 300 mg within 60 minutes prior to each infusion of fresh frozen plasma

Renal Impairment There are no dosage adjustments provided in the manufacturer's labeling (has not been studied).

Hepatic Impairment There are no dosage adjustments provided in the manufacturer's labeling (has not been studied).

Administration IV: Allow to reach room temperature prior to administration. Infuse over 35 minutes in adults and over 1 to 4 hours in pediatric patients; do not administer as an IV push or bolus. Decrease infusion rate or discontinue for infusion reactions; do not exceed a maximum 2-hour duration of infusion in adults. Monitor for at least 1 hour following completion of infusion (for signs/symptoms of infusion reaction).

Monitoring Parameters CBC with differential, lactic dehydrogenase (LDH), serum creatinine, AST, urinalysis; early signs/symptoms of meningococcal infection; signs and symptoms of infusion reaction (during infusion and for 1 hour after infusion complete).

After discontinuation:

aHUS: Signs/symptoms of thrombotic microangiopathy (TMA) complications (monitor for at least 12 weeks after treatment discontinuation), including angina, dyspnea, mental status changes, seizure, or thrombosis; occurrence of two or repeated measurement of any one of the following: Serum creatinine elevation (≥25% from baseline or nadir), serum LDH elevation (≥25% from baseline or nadir), thrombocytopenia (platelet decrease by ≥25% compared to baseline or peak).

PNH: Signs and symptoms of intravascular hemolysis (monitor for at least 8 weeks after discontinuation), including anemia, fatigue, pain, dark urine, dyspnea, or thrombosis.

Prescribing and Access Restrictions Patients and providers must enroll with Soliris OneSource (1-888-765-4747) program prior to treatment initiation.

Medication Guide Available Yes

Dosage Forms Excipient information presented when available (limited, particularly for generics); consult specific product labeling.

Solution, Intravenous [preservative free]:

Soliris: 10 mg/mL (30 mL)

- ◆ **Efraloctocog Alfa** see Antihemophilic Factor (Recombinant) on page 119
- ◆ **Efudex** see Fluorouracil (Topical) on page 747
- ◆ **Eldisine** see Vindesine on page 1760
- ◆ **Eligard** see Leuprolide on page 1030
- ◆ **Elitek** see Rasburicase on page 1462
- ◆ **Ellence** see EPIrubicin on page 608
- ◆ **Eloctate** see Antihemophilic Factor (Recombinant) on page 119

Elotuzumab (el oh TOOZ ue mab)

Index Terms Empliciti; HuLuc63

Pharmacologic Category Antineoplastic Agent, Monoclonal Antibody; Antineoplastic Agent, SLAMF7 Monoclonal Antibody

Use Multiple myeloma: Treatment of multiple myeloma (in combination with lenalidomide and dexamethasone) in patients who have received 1 to 3 prior therapies

Labeled Contraindications There are no contraindications listed in the manufacturer's labeling.

Product Availability Empliciti: FDA approved November 2015; anticipated availability is December 2015

- ◆ **Eloxatin** see Oxaliplatin on page 1269
- ◆ **Elspar** see Asparaginase (E. coli) on page 144
- ◆ **Elspar [DSC]** see Asparaginase (E. coli) on page 144

Eltrombopag (el TROM boe pag)

Brand Names: US Promacta

Brand Names: Canada Revolade

Index Terms Eltrombopag Olamine; Revolade; SB-497115; SB-497115-GR

Pharmacologic Category Colony Stimulating Factor; Hematopoietic Agent; Thrombopoietic Agent

Use

Aplastic anemia, severe: Treatment of severe aplastic anemia in patients who have had an insufficient response to immunosuppressive therapy.

Chronic hepatitis C infection-associated thrombocytopenia: Treatment of thrombocytopenia in patients with chronic hepatitis C (CHC) to allow the initiation and maintenance of interferon-based therapy.

◄ **Chronic immune (idiopathic) thrombocytopenia:** Treatment of thrombocytopenia in adult and pediatric patients ≥1 year of age (US labeling) or adult patients (Canadian labeling) with chronic immune (idiopathic) thrombocytopenia (ITP) who have had insufficient response to corticosteroids, immune globulin, or splenectomy.

Limitations of use: For ITP, use eltrombopag only if the degree of thrombocytopenia and clinical condition increase the risk for bleeding. For chronic hepatitis C (CHC), use eltrombopag only if the degree of thrombocytopenia prevents initiation of or limits the ability to maintain interferon-based therapy. For CHC, safety and efficacy have not been established when used in combination with direct-acting antiviral agents without interferon for treatment of CHC infection.

Labeled Contraindications

US labeling: There are no contraindications listed in the manufacturer's labeling.

Canadian labeling: Hypersensitivity to eltrombopag or any component of the formulation; severe hepatic impairment (Child-Pugh class C)

Pregnancy Considerations Adverse effects were observed in animal reproduction studies. A Promacta pregnancy registry has been established to monitor outcomes of women exposed to eltrombopag during pregnancy (1-888-825-5249).

Breast-Feeding Considerations It is not known if eltrombopag is excreted in breast milk. Due to the potential for serious adverse effects in the nursing infant, a decision should be made to discontinue therapy or to discontinue breast-feeding, taking into account the importance of treatment to the mother.

Warnings/Precautions Liver enzyme elevations may occur; obtain ALT, AST, and bilirubin prior to treatment initiation, every 2 weeks during adjustment phase, then monthly (after stable dose established); obtain fractionation for elevated bilirubin levels. Repeat abnormal liver function tests within 3 to 5 days; if confirmed abnormal, monitor weekly until resolves, stabilizes, or returns to baseline. Discontinue treatment for ALT levels ≥3 times the upper limit of normal (ULN) in patients with normal hepatic function, or ≥3 times baseline in those with preexisting transaminase elevations and which are progressive, or persistent (≥4 weeks), or accompanied by increased direct bilirubin, or accompanied by clinical signs of liver injury or evidence of hepatic decompensation. Hepatotoxicity may reoccur with re-treatment after therapy interruption; however, if the benefit of treatment outweighs the hepatotoxicity risk, initiate carefully, and monitor liver function tests weekly during the dose adjustment phase; permanently discontinue if liver abnormalities persist, worsen, or recur with rechallenge. Use with caution in patients with preexisting hepatic impairment (clearance may be reduced); dosage reductions are recommended in patients with ITP (except children 1 to 5 years) and severe aplastic anemia who have hepatic dysfunction (no initial dose reductions are necessary in patients with chronic hepatitis C-related thrombocytopenia); monitor closely. The Canadian labeling contraindicates use in patients with severe impairment.

[US Boxed Warning]: May increase risk of hepatic decompensation when used in combination with interferon and ribavirin in patients with chronic hepatitis C. In clinical trials, patients with low albumin (<3.5 g/dL) or a Model for End-Stage Liver Disease (MELD) score ≥10 at baseline had an increased risk of hepatic decompensation; closely monitor these patients during therapy. If antiviral therapy is discontinued for hepatic decompensation according to interferon/ribavirin recommendations, eltrombopag should also be discontinued. Indirect hyperbilirubinemia is commonly observed with eltrombopag when used in combination with peginterferon and ribavirin. In addition, ascites, encephalopathy, and thrombotic events were reported more frequently than placebo in chronic hepatitis C trials.

May increase the risk for bone marrow reticulin formation or progression (Canadian labeling). Monitor peripheral blood smear for cellular morphologic abnormalities; analyze CBC monthly; discontinue treatment with onset of new or worsening abnormalities (eg, teardrop and nucleated RBC, immature WBC) or cytopenias and consider bone marrow biopsy (with staining for fibrosis).

Thromboembolism may occur with excessive increases in platelet levels. Use with caution in patients with known risk factors for thromboembolism (eg, Factor V Leiden, ATIII deficiency, antiphospholipid syndrome, chronic liver disease). Thrombotic events, primarily involving the portal venous system, were more commonly seen in eltrombopag-treated chronic hepatitis C patients with thrombocytopenia (when compared to placebo). Thrombotic events (including portal venous thrombosis) were also reported in a study of non-ITP thrombocytopenic patients with chronic liver disease undergoing elective invasive procedures receiving eltrombopag 75 mg once daily. Symptoms of portal vein thrombosis include abdominal pain, nausea, vomiting, and diarrhea. The risk for portal venous thrombosis is increased in thrombocytopenic patients with chronic liver disease receiving 75 mg once daily for 2 weeks as preparation for invasive procedures. Stimulation of cell surface thrombopoietin (TPO) receptors may increase the risk for hematologic malignancies (Canadian labeling).

Cataract formation or worsening was observed in clinical trials. Monitor regularly for signs and symptoms of cataracts; obtain ophthalmic exam at baseline and during therapy. Use with caution in patients at risk for cataracts (eg, advanced age, long-term glucocorticoid use). Potentially significant drug-drug interactions may exist, requiring dose or frequency adjustment, additional monitoring, and/or selection of alternative therapy. Take eltrombopag at least 2 hours before and 4 hours after antacids, minerals (eg, iron, calcium, aluminum, magnesium, selenium, zinc), or foods high in calcium; may reduce eltrombopag levels. Patients of East-Asian ethnicity (eg, Chinese, Japanese, Korean, Taiwanese) may have greater drug exposure (compared to non-East Asians); therapy should be initiated with lower starting doses in ITP and severe aplastic anemia patients. Use with caution in renal impairment (any degree) and monitor closely; initial dosage adjustment is not necessary.

Do not use to normalize platelet counts. *ITP:* Indicated only when the degree of thrombocytopenia and clinical conditions increase the risk for bleeding in patients with chronic immune ITP; use the lowest dose necessary to achieve and maintain platelet count ≥50,000/mm³. Discontinue if platelet count does not respond to a level to avoid clinically important bleeding after 4 weeks at the maximum recommended dose. *Chronic hepatitis C-associated thrombocytopenia:* Use only when thrombocytopenia prevents the initiation and maintenance of interferon-based therapy; discontinue if antiviral therapy is discontinued. Safety and efficacy have not been established when combined with direct acting antiviral medications approved for chronic hepatitis C genotype 1 infection therapy. *Severe aplastic anemia:* Use the lowest dose to achieve and maintain hematologic response. Discontinue if no hematologic response has occurred after 16 weeks of therapy, excessive platelet count

◄ responses or important liver test abnormalities. Consider discontinuation if new cytogenetic abnormalities are observed.

Adverse Reactions Adverse reactions and incidences reported are associated with adults unless otherwise indicated.

>10%:

Central nervous system: Fatigue (ITP: 4%; chronic hepatitis C: 28%; aplastic anemia: 28%), headache (ITP: 10%; chronic hepatitis C: 21%; aplastic anemia 21%), insomnia (chronic hepatitis C: 16%), chills (chronic hepatitis C: 14%), dizziness (aplastic anemia: 14%)

Dermatologic: Pruritus (chronic hepatitis C: 15%), ecchymosis (aplastic anemia: 12%)

Gastrointestinal: Nausea (ITP: 4% to 9%; chronic hepatitis C: 19%; aplastic anemia 33%), diarrhea (aplastic anemia: 21%; chronic hepatitis C: 19%; ITP: 9%; children: 9%), appetite decreased (chronic hepatitis C: 18%), abdominal pain (aplastic anemia 12%; children: 8%)

Hematologic & oncologic: Anemia (chronic hepatitis C: 40%), febrile neutropenia (aplastic anemia: 14%)

Hepatic: Hyperbilirubinemia (total bilirubin ≥1.5 x ULN: 76%; ITP and chronic hepatitis C: 6% to 8%), increased serum transaminases (aplastic anemia: 12%), abnormal hepatic function (ITP: 11%), increased serum ALT (children: 6%; ITP: 5% to 6%), increased serum AST (ITP: 4%; children: 4%)

Neuromuscular & skeletal: Limb pain (aplastic anemia: 19%), weakness (chronic hepatitis C: 16%), arthralgia (aplastic anemia: 12%), muscle spasm (aplastic anemia: 12%), myalgia (ITP and chronic hepatitis C: 5% to 12%)

Respiratory: Cough (aplastic anemia: 23%; chronic hepatitis C: 15%; children: 9%), flu-like syndrome (chronic hepatitis C: 18%), upper respiratory infection (children: 17%; ITP: 7%), dyspnea (aplastic anemia: 14%), oropharyngeal pain (aplastic anemia: 14%; children: 8%; ITP: 4%), nasopharyngitis (children: 12%), rhinorrhea (aplastic anemia: 12%, children: 4%)

Miscellaneous: Fever (chronic hepatitis C: 30%; aplastic anemia: 14%; children: 9%)

1% to 10%:

Cardiovascular: Peripheral edema (chronic hepatitis C: 10%), thrombosis (chronic hepatitis C: 3%)

Dermatologic: Alopecia (ITP: 2%; chronic hepatitis C: 10%), skin rash (children: 5%; ITP: 3%)

Gastrointestinal: Toothache (children: 6%), vomiting (ITP: 6%), xerostomia (ITP: 2%)

Genitourinary: Urinary tract infection (ITP: 5%)

Hematologic & oncologic: Thrombocytopenia (chronic hepatitis C: 3%)

Hepatic: Alkaline phosphatase increased (ITP: 2%)

Infection: Influenza (ITP: 3%)

Neuromuscular & skeletal: Back pain (ITP: 3%), paresthesia (ITP: 3%), musculoskeletal pain (ITP: 2%)

Ophthalmic: Cataract (ITP and chronic hepatitis C: 4% to 8%)

Respiratory: Rhinitis (children: 9%), pharyngitis (ITP: 4%)

<1%, postmarketing, and/or case reports: Abdominal distension, constipation, decreased visual acuity, deep vein thrombosis, desquamation, drowsiness, dry eye syndrome, dysesthesia, dysgeusia, dyspepsia, eye pain, facial swelling, fecal discoloration, foreign body sensation, glossalgia, hemorrhage, hemorrhoids, hot flash, hyperhidrosis, hypoesthesia, hypokalemia, increased hemoglobin, increased lacrimation, increased serum albumin, increased serum creatinine, increased serum total protein, lesion (hepatic), local

inflammation (wound), malaise, malignant neoplasm (rectosigmoid), night sweats, oral herpes, oropharyngeal blistering, ostealgia, portal vein thrombosis, pulmonary embolism, pulmonary infarct, retinal hemorrhage, retinal pigment changes, sinus tachycardia, sleep disorder, superficial thrombophlebitis, tachycardia, thromboembolic complications, thrombotic microangiopathy (with acute renal failure), upper abdominal pain, urticaria, vertigo

Drug Interactions

Metabolism/Transport Effects Substrate of BCRP, CYP1A2 (minor), CYP2C8 (minor), UGT1A1, UGT1A3; **Note:** Assignment of Major/Minor substrate status based on clinically relevant drug interaction potential; **Inhibits** BCRP, SLCO1B1, UGT1A1, UGT1A3, UGT1A4, UGT1A6, UGT1A9, UGT2B15, UGT2B7

Avoid Concomitant Use

Avoid concomitant use of Eltrombopag with any of the following: Irinotecan Products; PAZOPanib

Increased Effect/Toxicity

Eltrombopag may increase the levels/effects of: BCRP/ABCG2 Substrates; Deferiprone; Eluxadoline; Irinotecan Products; OATP1B1/SLCO1B1 Substrates; PAZOPanib; Rosuvastatin; Topotecan

Decreased Effect

The levels/effects of Eltrombopag may be decreased by: Aluminum Hydroxide; Calcium Salts; Iron Salts; Magnesium Salts; Multivitamins/Minerals (with ADEK, Folate, Iron); Multivitamins/Minerals (with AE, No Iron); Selenium; Sucralfate; Zinc Salts

Food Interactions Food, especially dairy products, may decrease the absorption of eltrombopag. Management: Take on an empty stomach at least 1 hour before or 2 hours after a meal. Separate intake from antacids, foods high in calcium, or minerals (eg, iron, calcium, aluminum, magnesium, selenium, zinc) by at least 4 hours.

Storage/Stability

Oral suspension: Store at 20°C to 25°C (68°F to 77°F); excursions permitted to 15°C to 30°C (59°F to 86°F). Once reconstituted (if not used immediately), the suspension may be stored for a maximum of 30 minutes between 20°C and 25°C (68°F to 77°F); excursions permitted to 15°C to 30°C (59°F to 86°F). Discard the mixture if not used within 30 minutes.

Tablets: Store at 20°C to 25°C (68°F to 77°F); excursions are permitted between 15°C and 30°C (59°F and 86°F). If present, do not remove desiccant. Dispense in original bottle.

Preparation for Administration The oral suspension must be reconstituted with cool or cold water only (do not use hot water). Fill the provided oral syringe with 20 mL of drinking water and empty into the mixing bottle. Add the appropriate eltrombopag dose to the mixing bottle; gently and slowly shake the bottle for at least 20 seconds to mix. If not used immediately, suspension may be stored for up to 30 minutes at room temperature; discard any solution if not used within 30 minutes. Following administration, discard suspension remaining in bottle in trash (do not dispose of in drain); clean supplies by removing plunger from oral syringe, rinse bottle, lid, syringe, and plunger under running water and air-dry (bottle may stain, this is normal); wash hands with soap and water. If powder or suspension spills during preparation or administration, consider wearing disposable gloves during spill clean-up to avoid staining skin.

Mechanism of Action Thrombopoietin (TPO) nonpeptide agonist which increases platelet counts by binding to and activating the human TPO receptor. ▶

◄ Activates intracellular signal transduction pathways to increase proliferation and differentiation of marrow progenitor cells. Does not induce platelet aggregation or activation.

Pharmacodynamics/Kinetics

Onset of action: Platelet count increase: Within 1 to 2 weeks

Peak platelet count increase: 14 to 16 days

Duration: Platelets return to baseline: 1 to 2 weeks after last dose

Protein binding: >99%

Metabolism: Extensive hepatic metabolism; via CYP 1A2, 2C8 oxidation and UGT 1A1, 1A3 glucuronidation

Bioavailability: ~52%; in adults, plasma AUC was increased by 22% with the oral suspension versus tablets

Half-life elimination: ~21 to 32 hours in healthy individuals; ~26 to 35 hours in patients with ITP

Time to peak, plasma: 2 to 6 hours

Excretion: Feces (~59%, 20% as unchanged drug, 21% glutathione-related conjugates); urine (31%, 20% glucuronide of the phenylpyrazole moiety)

Dosing

Adult & Geriatric Note: Do not use eltrombopag to normalize platelet counts.

Chronic immune (idiopathic) thrombocytopenia (ITP): Oral: **Note:** Use the lowest dose to achieve and maintain platelet count ≥50,000/mm^3 as needed to reduce the risk of bleeding. Discontinue if platelet count does not respond to a level that avoids clinically important bleeding after 4 weeks at the maximum daily dose of 75 mg.

Initial: 50 mg once daily (25 mg once daily for patients of East-Asian ethnicity [eg, Chinese, Japanese, Korean, Taiwanese]); dose should be titrated based on platelet response. Maximum dose: 75 mg once daily.

Dosage adjustment based on platelet response (US labeling):

Platelet count <50,000/mm^3 (≥2 weeks after treatment initiation or a dose increase): Increase daily dose by 25 mg (if taking 12.5 mg once daily, increase dose to 25 mg once daily prior to increasing the dose amount by 25 mg daily); maximum: 75 mg once daily

Platelet count ≥200,000/mm^3 and ≤400,000/mm^3 (at any time): Reduce daily dose by 25 mg (if taking 25 mg once daily, decrease dose to 12.5 mg once daily); reassess in 2 weeks

Platelet count >400,000/mm^3: Withhold dose; assess platelet count twice weekly; when platelet count <150,000/mm^3, resume with the daily dose reduced by 25 mg (if taking 25 mg once daily, resume with 12.5 mg once daily)

Platelet count >400,000/mm^3 after 2 weeks at the lowest dose: Discontinue treatment

Dosage adjustment based on platelet response (Canadian labeling):

Platelet count <50,000/mm^3 (≥2 weeks after treatment initiation or a dose increase): Increase daily dose by 25 mg; maximum: 75 mg once daily

Platelet count ≥200,000/mm^3 and ≤300,000/mm^3 (at any time): Reduce daily dose by 25 mg; reassess in 2 weeks

Platelet count >300,000/mm^3: Withhold dose; assess platelet count twice weekly; when platelet count <150,000/mm^3, resume with the daily dose reduced by 25 mg

Platelet count >300,000/mm^3 after 2 weeks at the lowest dose: Discontinue treatment

Chronic hepatitis C-associated thrombocytopenia: Oral: **Note:** Use the lowest dose to achieve the target platelet count necessary to initiate antiviral therapy (peginterferon and ribavirin) or to avoid dose reductions of peginterferon during antiviral therapy. Discontinue when antiviral therapy is stopped.

Initial: 25 mg once daily; dose should be titrated based on platelet response. Maximum dose: 100 mg once daily

Dosage adjustment based on platelet response (US labeling):

Platelet count <50,000/mm^3 (after at least 2 weeks): Increase daily dose by 25 mg every 2 weeks; maximum dose: 100 mg once daily

Platelet count ≥200,000/mm^3 and ≤400,000/mm^3 (at any time): Reduce daily dose by 25 mg; reassess in 2 weeks

Platelet count >400,000/mm^3: Withhold dose; assess platelet count twice weekly; when platelet count <150,000/mm^3, resume with the daily dose reduced by 25 mg (if taking 25 mg once daily, resume with 12.5 mg once daily)

Platelet count >400,000/mm^3 after 2 weeks at the lowest dose: Discontinue treatment

Dosage adjustment based on platelet response (Canadian labeling):

Platelet count <50,000/mm^3 (after at least 2 weeks): Increase daily dose by 25 mg every 2 weeks; maximum dose: 100 mg once daily

Platelet count ≥150,000/mm^3 and ≤200,000/mm^3: Reduce daily dose by 25 mg; reassess in 2 weeks

Platelet count >200,000/mm^3: Withhold dose; assess platelet count twice weekly; when platelet count <150,000/mm^3, resume with the daily dose reduced by 25 mg (if taking 25 mg once daily, consider resuming with 25 mg every other day)

Platelet count >200,000/mm^3 after 2 weeks at the lowest dose: Discontinue treatment

Severe aplastic anemia: Oral: **Note:** Use the lowest dose to achieve and maintain hematologic response. Hematologic response may take up to 16 weeks and requires dose titration. Discontinue therapy if hematologic response is not achieved after 16 weeks of treatment, for excessive platelet responses or for liver function abnormalities. Consider discontinuing if new cytogenetic abnormalities are observed.

Initial: 50 mg once daily (25 mg once daily for patients of East-Asian ethnicity); dose should be titrated based on platelet response. Maximum dose: 150 mg once daily.

Dosage adjustment based on platelet response (US labeling):

Platelet count <50,000/mm^3 (≥2 weeks after treatment initiation or a dose increase): Increase daily dose by 50 mg (if taking 25 mg once daily, increase dose to 50 mg once daily prior to increasing the dose amount by 50 mg daily); maximum: 150 mg once daily

Platelet count ≥200,000/mm^3 and ≤400,000/mm^3 (at any time): Reduce daily dose by 50 mg; reassess in 2 weeks

Platelet count >400,000/mm^3: Withhold dose for 1 week; when platelet count <150,000/mm^3, resume with the daily dose reduced by 50 mg

Platelet count >400,000/mm^3 after 2 weeks at the lowest dose: Discontinue treatment

Dosage adjustment based on platelet response (Canadian labeling):

Platelet count <50,000/mm^3 (≥2 weeks after treatment initiation or a dose increase): Increase daily dose by 50 mg (if taking 25 mg once daily, increase dose to 50 mg once daily prior to increasing the dose amount by 50 mg daily); maximum: 150 mg once daily

Platelet count ≥200,000/mm^3 and ≤300,000/mm^3 (at any time): Reduce daily dose by 50 mg (if taking 50 mg once daily, reduce daily dose by 25 mg); reassess in 2 weeks

Platelet count >300,000/mm^3: Withhold dose for at least 1 week; when platelet count <150,000/mm^3, resume with the daily dose reduced by 50 mg

Platelet count >300,000/mm^3 after 2 weeks at the lowest dose: Discontinue treatment

For patients who achieve tri-lineage response, including transfusion independence, lasting 8 weeks, may reduce the dose by 50%. If counts remain stable after 8 weeks at the reduced dose, discontinue and monitor blood counts. If platelets counts drop to <30,000/mm^3, hemoglobin to <9 g/dL, or ANC to <500/mm^3, may reinitiate at the prior effective dose.

Pediatric Note: Do not use eltrombopag to normalize platelet counts.

Chronic immune (idiopathic) thrombocytopenia (ITP): Note: Use the lowest dose to achieve and maintain platelet count ≥50,000/mm^3 as needed to reduce the risk of bleeding. Discontinue if platelet count does not respond to a level that avoids clinically important bleeding after 4 weeks at the maximum daily dose of 75 mg.

Children 1 to 5 years: Oral: Initial: 25 mg once daily; dose should be titrated based on platelet response (no dosage adjustment required for patients of East Asian ancestry). Maximum dose: 75 mg once daily.

Children ≥6 years and Adolescents: Oral: Refer to adult dosing

Renal Impairment

US labeling: No dosage adjustment is necessary.

Canadian labeling:

Mild to moderate impairment (CrCl ≥30 mL/minute): No dosage adjustment is necessary. Use with caution and monitor closely.

Severe impairment (CrCl <30 mL/minute): Use is generally not recommended.

Hepatic Impairment

Adjustment for hepatic impairment prior to initiating treatment:

Chronic ITP: **Note:** In patients with ITP and hepatic impairment, wait 3 weeks (instead of 2 weeks) after therapy initiation or subsequent dosage changes prior to increasing dose.

US labeling:

Mild, moderate, or severe impairment (Child-Pugh classes A, B, or C): Initial: 25 mg once daily

Patients of East-Asian ethnicity with hepatic impairment (Child-Pugh classes A, B, or C): Initial: Consider 12.5 mg once daily

Canadian labeling:

Mild or moderate impairment (Child-Pugh classes A or B): Initial: 25 mg once daily

Severe impairment (Child-Pugh class C): Use is contraindicated

Chronic hepatitis C-associated thrombocytopenia:

US labeling: Initial: No dosage adjustment is necessary

Canadian labeling:

Mild or moderate impairment (Child-Pugh classes A or B): Initial: No dosage adjustment is necessary

Severe impairment (Child-Pugh class C): Use is contraindicated

Severe aplastic anemia:

US labeling: Mild, moderate, or severe impairment (Child-Pugh classes A, B, or C): Initial: 25 mg once daily

Canadian labeling:

Mild or moderate impairment (Child-Pugh classes A or B): Initial: 25 mg once daily

Severe impairment (Child-Pugh class C): Use is contraindicated

Adjustment for hepatic impairment during treatment:

ALT levels ≥3 times the upper limit of normal (ULN) in patients with normal hepatic function or ≥3 times baseline in those with preexisting transaminase elevations **and** which are progressive, persistent (≥4 weeks), accompanied by increased direct bilirubin, or accompanied by clinical signs of liver injury or evidence of hepatic decompensation: Discontinue treatment. Hepatotoxicity may recur with re-treatment after therapy interruption, but if determined to be clinically beneficial, may cautiously resume treatment; monitor ALT weekly during dosage titration; permanently discontinue if liver function test elevations persist, worsen, or recur.

Administration Administer on an empty stomach, 1 hour before or 2 hours after a meal. Swallow tablets whole; do not crush and mix with food or liquids. Prepare the suspension with cool or cold water only (do not use hot water); discard any suspension not administered within 30 minutes after reconstitution. If powder or suspension spills during preparation or administration, consider wearing disposable gloves during spill clean-up to avoid staining skin. Do not administer concurrently with antacids, foods high in calcium, or minerals (eg, iron, calcium, aluminum, magnesium, selenium, zinc); administer eltrombopag at least 2 hours before and 4 hours after. Do not administer more than one dose within 24 hours.

Monitoring Parameters

Thrombocytopenia due to CHC and chronic ITP: Liver function tests, including ALT, AST, and bilirubin (baseline, every 2 weeks during dosage titration, then monthly; evaluate abnormal liver function tests within 3 to 5 days; monitor weekly until abnormalities resolve, stabilize, or return to baseline or if re-treating [not recommended] after therapy interruption for hepatotoxicity); bilirubin fractionation (for elevated bilirubin); CBC with differential and platelet count (weekly at initiation and during dosage titration, then monthly when stable; after cessation, monitor weekly for ≥4 weeks; when switching between the oral suspension and tablet, monitor platelet counts weekly for 2 weeks, then monthly when stable); peripheral blood smear (baseline and monthly when stable), bone marrow biopsy with staining for fibrosis (if peripheral blood smear reveals abnormality); ophthalmic exam (baseline and during treatment)

Severe aplastic anemia: CBC with differential and platelets (regularly throughout therapy), liver function tests (regularly throughout therapy); ophthalmic exam (baseline and during treatment)

Dietary Considerations Food, especially dairy products, may decrease the absorption of eltrombopag; allow at least 4 hours between dosing of eltrombopag and polyvalent cation intake (eg, dairy products, calcium-rich foods, multivitamins with minerals).

Product Availability Promacta oral suspension: FDA approved August 2015; anticipated availability is currently unknown.

Medication Guide Available Yes

◄ **Dosage Forms** Excipient information presented when available (limited, particularly for generics); consult specific product labeling.
Tablet, Oral:
Promacta: 12.5 mg
Promacta: 25 mg [contains fd&c yellow #6 aluminum lake]
Promacta: 50 mg [contains fd&c blue #2 aluminum lake]
Promacta: 75 mg
Dosage Forms: Canada Excipient information presented when available (limited, particularly for generics); consult specific product labeling.
Tablet, Oral:
Revolade: 25 mg, 50 mg, 75 mg

◆ **Eltrombopag Olamine** see Eltrombopag on page 585
◆ **Emcyt** see Estramustine on page 636
◆ **Emend** see Aprepitant on page 134
◆ **Emend** see Fosaprepitant on page 759
◆ **Emend® IV (Can)** see Fosaprepitant on page 759
◆ **EMLA** see Lidocaine and Prilocaine on page 1046
◆ **Empliciti** see Elotuzumab on page 585
◆ **EnovaRX-Tramadol** see TraMADol on page 1672

Enoxaparin (ee noks a PA rin)
Related Information
Venous Thromboembolism in the Cancer Patient on page 2267
Brand Names: US Lovenox
Brand Names: Canada Lovenox; Lovenox HP; Lovenox With Preservative
Index Terms Enoxaparin Sodium
Pharmacologic Category Anticoagulant; Anticoagulant, Low Molecular Weight Heparin
Use
Acute coronary syndromes: Unstable angina (UA), non-ST-elevation (NSTEMI), and ST-elevation myocardial infarction (STEMI)
DVT prophylaxis: Following hip or knee replacement surgery, abdominal surgery, or in medical patients with severely-restricted mobility during acute illness who are at risk for thromboembolic complications. **Note:** Patients at risk of thromboembolic complications who undergo abdominal surgery include those with one or more of the following risk factors: >40 years of age, obesity, general anesthesia lasting >30 minutes, malignancy, history of deep vein thrombosis or pulmonary embolism
DVT treatment (acute): Inpatient treatment (patients with or without pulmonary embolism) and outpatient treatment (patients without pulmonary embolism)
Labeled Contraindications
Hypersensitivity to enoxaparin, heparin, pork products, or any component of the formulation (including benzyl alcohol in multiple-dose vials); thrombocytopenia associated with a positive in vitro test for antiplatelet antibodies in the presence of enoxaparin; active major bleeding
Canadian labeling: Additional contraindications (not in U.S. labeling): Use of multiple-dose vials in newborns or premature neonates; history of confirmed or suspected immunologically-mediated heparin-induced thrombocytopenia; acute or subacute bacterial endocarditis; major blood clotting disorders;

active gastric or duodenal ulcer; hemorrhagic cerebrovascular accident (except if there are systemic emboli); severe uncontrolled hypertension; diabetic or hemorrhagic retinopathy; other conditions or diseases involving an increased risk of hemorrhage; injuries to and operations on the brain, spinal cord, eyes, and ears; spinal/epidural anesthesia when repeated dosing of enoxaparin (1 mg/kg every 12 hours or 1.5 mg/kg daily) is required, due to increased risk of bleeding.

Note: Use of enoxaparin in patients with current heparin-induced thrombocytopenia (HIT) or HIT with thrombosis is **not** recommended and considered contraindicated due to high cross-reactivity to heparin-platelet factor-4 antibody (Guyatt [ACCP], 2012; Warkentin, 1999).

Pregnancy Considerations Adverse events were not observed in animal reproduction studies. Low molecular weight heparin (LMWH) does not cross the placenta; increased risks of fetal bleeding or teratogenic effects have not been reported (Bates, 2012).

LMWH is recommended over unfractionated heparin for the treatment of acute venous thromboembolism (VTE) in pregnant women. LMWH is also recommended over unfractionated heparin for VTE prophylaxis in pregnant women with certain risk factors (eg, homozygous factor V Leiden, antiphospholipid antibody syndrome with ≥3 previous pregnancy losses). Prophylaxis is not routinely recommended for women undergoing assisted reproduction therapy; however, LMWH therapy is recommended for women who develop severe ovarian hyperstimulation syndrome. LMWH should be discontinued at least 24 hours prior to induction of labor or a planned cesarean delivery. For women undergoing cesarean section and who have additional risk factors for developing VTE, the prophylactic use of LMWH may be considered (Bates, 2012).

LMWH may also be used in women with mechanical heart valves (consult current guidelines for details) (Bates, 2012; Nishimura, 2014). Women who require long-term anticoagulation with warfarin and who are considering pregnancy, LMWH substitution should be done prior to conception when possible. When choosing therapy, fetal outcomes (ie, pregnancy loss, malformations), maternal outcomes (ie, VTE, hemorrhage), burden of therapy, and maternal preference should be considered (Bates, 2012). Monitoring antifactor Xa levels is recommended (Bates, 2012; Nishimura, 2014).

Multiple-dose vials contain benzyl alcohol (avoid in pregnant women due to association with gasping syndrome in premature infants); use of preservative-free formulations is recommended.

Breast-Feeding Considerations Small amounts of LMWH have been detected in breast milk; however, because it has a low oral bioavailability, it is unlikely to cause adverse events in a nursing infant. Enoxaparin product labeling does not recommend use in nursing women; however, antithrombotic guidelines state that use of LMWH may be continued in breast-feeding women (Guyatt, 2012).

Warnings/Precautions [U.S. Boxed Warning]: Spinal or epidural hematomas, including subsequent long-term or permanent paralysis, may occur with recent or anticipated neuraxial anesthesia (epidural or spinal anesthesia) or spinal puncture in patients anticoagulated with LMWH or heparinoids. Consider risk versus benefit prior to spinal procedures; risk is increased by the use of concomitant agents which may alter hemostasis, the use of indwelling epidural catheters, a history of spinal deformity or spinal surgery, as well as a history of traumatic or repeated

◄ **epidural or spinal punctures. Optimal timing between neuraxial proce-dures and enoxaparin administration is not known.** Delay placement or removal of catheter for at least 12 hours after administration of low-dose enoxaparin (eg, 30 to 60 mg/day) and at least 24 hours after high-dose enoxaparin (eg, 0.75 to 1 mg/kg twice daily or 1.5 mg/kg once daily) and consider doubling these times in patients with creatinine clearance <30 mL/minute; risk of neuraxial hematoma may still exist since antifactor Xa levels are still detectable at these time points. Patients receiving twice daily high-dose enoxaparin should have the second dose withheld to allow a longer time period prior to catheter placement or removal. Upon removal of catheter, consider withholding enoxaparin for at least 4 hours. **Patient should be observed closely for bleeding and signs and symptoms of neurological impairment if therapy is administered during or immediately following diagnostic lumbar puncture, epidural anesthesia, or spinal anesthesia. If neuro-logical compromise is noted, urgent treatment is necessary.** If spinal hematoma is suspected, diagnose and treat immediately; spinal cord decom-pression may be considered although it may not prevent or reverse neuro-logical sequelae.

Do not administer intramuscularly. Discontinue use 12 to 24 hours prior to CABG and dose with unfractionated heparin per institutional practice (ACCF/AHA [Anderson, 2013]). Not recommended for thromboprophylaxis in patients with prosthetic heart valves (especially pregnant women). Not to be used interchangeably (unit for unit) with heparin or any other low molecular weight heparins. Monitor patient closely for signs or symptoms of bleeding. Certain patients are at increased risk of bleeding. Risk factors include bacterial endocarditis; congenital or acquired bleeding disorders; active ulcerative or angiodysplastic GI diseases; severe uncontrolled hypertension; hemorrhagic stroke; use shortly after brain, spinal, or ophthalmic surgery; patients treated concomitantly with platelet inhibitors; recent GI bleeding or ulceration; renal dysfunction and hemorrhage; thrombocytopenia or platelet defects or history of heparin-induced thrombocytopenia; severe liver disease; hypertensive or diabetic retinopathy; or in patients undergoing invasive procedures. Protamine may be considered as a partial reversal agent in overdose situations (consult Protamine monograph for dosing recommendations). To minimize risk of bleeding following PCI, achieve hemostasis at the puncture site after PCI. If a closure device is used, sheath can be removed immediately. If manual compression is used, remove sheath 6 hours after the last IV/SubQ dose of enoxaparin. Do not administer further doses until 6 to 8 hours after sheath removal; observe for signs of bleeding/hematoma formation. Cases of enox-aparin-induced thrombocytopenia and thrombosis (similar to heparin-induced thrombocytopenia [HIT]), some complicated by organ infarction, limb ischemia, or death, have been observed. Use with extreme caution or avoid in patients with history of HIT, especially if administered within 100 days of HIT episode (Warkentin, 2001); monitor platelet count closely. Use is contraindicated in patients with thrombocytopenia associated with a positive *in vitro* test for antiplatelet antibodies in the presence of enoxaparin. Discontinue therapy and consider alternative treatment if platelets are <100,000/mm^3 and/or thrombosis develops. Use caution in patients with congenital or drug-induced thrombocytopenia or platelet defects. Risk of bleeding may be increased in women <45 kg and in men <57 kg. Use caution in patients with renal failure; dosage adjustment needed if CrCl <30 mL/minute. Use with caution in the elderly (delayed elimination may occur); dosage alteration/adjustment may be required (eg, omission of IV bolus in acute STEMI in patients ≥75 years of age). Monitor for hyperkalemia; can cause hyperkalemia possibly by suppress-ing aldosterone production.

Benzyl alcohol and derivatives: Some dosage forms may contain benzyl alcohol and should not be used in pregnant women. In neonates, large amounts of benzyl alcohol (≥99 mg/kg/day) have been associated with a potentially fatal toxicity ("gasping syndrome"); the "gasping syndrome" consists of metabolic acidosis, respiratory distress, gasping respirations, CNS dysfunction (including convulsions, intracranial hemorrhage), hypotension, and cardiovascular collapse (AAP ["Inactive" 1997]; CDC, 1982); some data suggests that benzoate displaces bilirubin from protein binding sites (Ahlfors, 2001); avoid or use dosage forms containing benzyl alcohol with caution in neonates. See manufacturer's labeling.

Safety and efficacy of prophylactic dosing of enoxaparin has not been established in patients who are obese (>30 kg/m^2) nor is there a consensus regarding dosage adjustments. The American College of Chest Physicians Practice Guidelines suggest consulting with a pharmacist regarding dosing in bariatric surgery patients and other obese patients who may require higher doses of LMWH (ACCP [Gould, 2012]).

Adverse Reactions As with all anticoagulants, bleeding is the major adverse effect of enoxaparin. Hemorrhage may occur at virtually any site. Risk is dependent on multiple variables. At the recommended doses, single injections of enoxaparin do not significantly influence platelet aggregation or affect global clotting time (ie, PT or aPTT).

1% to 10%:
Central nervous system: Confusion (2%), pain
Gastrointestinal: Nausea (3%), diarrhea (2%)
Hematologic & oncologic: Major hemorrhage (<1% to 4%; includes cases of intracranial, retroperitoneal, or intraocular hemorrhage; incidence varies with indication/population), thrombocytopenia (moderate 1%; severe 0.1%), anemia (<2%), bruise
Hepatic: Increased serum ALT (6%), increased serum AST (6%)
Local: Hematoma at injection site (9%), irritation at injection site, bruising at injection site, erythema at injection site, pain at injection site
Renal: Hematuria (≤2%)
Miscellaneous: Fever (5% to 8%)
<1%, postmarketing, and/or case reports: Alopecia, anaphylaxis, anaphylactoid reaction, eczematous rash (plaques), eosinophilia, epidural hematoma (spinal; after neuroaxial anesthesia or spinal puncture; risk may be increased with indwelling epidural catheter or concomitant use of other drugs affecting hemostasis), headache, hepatic injury (hepatocellular and cholestatic), hyperkalemia, hyperlipidemia (very rare), hypersensitivity angiitis, hypersensitivity reaction, hypertriglyceridemia, intracranial hemorrhage (up to 0.8%), osteoporosis (following long-term therapy), pruritic erythematous rash (patches), pruritus, purpura, retroperitoneal hemorrhage, severe anemia (hemorrhagic), shock, skin necrosis, thrombocythemia, thrombocytopenia, thrombosis (prosthetic value [in pregnant females] or associated with enoxaparin-induced thrombocytopenia; can cause limb ischemia or organ infarction), urticaria, vesicobullous rash

◀ **Drug Interactions**

Metabolism/Transport Effects None known.

Avoid Concomitant Use

Avoid concomitant use of Enoxaparin with any of the following: Apixaban; Dabigatran Etexilate; Edoxaban; Hemin; Omacetaxine; Rivaroxaban; Urokinase; Vorapaxar

Increased Effect/Toxicity

Enoxaparin may increase the levels/effects of: ACE Inhibitors; Aliskiren; Angiotensin II Receptor Blockers; Anticoagulants; Canagliflozin; Collagenase (Systemic); Deferasirox; Deoxycholic Acid; Eplerenone; Ibritumomab; Nintedanib; Obinutuzumab; Omacetaxine; Palifermin; Potassium Salts; Potassium-Sparing Diuretics; Rivaroxaban; Tositumomab and Iodine I 131 Tositumomab

The levels/effects of Enoxaparin may be increased by: 5-ASA Derivatives; Agents with Antiplatelet Properties; Apixaban; Dabigatran Etexilate; Dasatinib; Edoxaban; Hemin; Herbs (Anticoagulant/Antiplatelet Properties); Ibrutinib; Limaprost; Nonsteroidal Anti-Inflammatory Agents; Omega-3 Fatty Acids; Pentosan Polysulfate Sodium; Pentoxifylline; Prostacyclin Analogues; Salicylates; Sugammadex; Thrombolytic Agents; Tibolone; Tipranavir; Urokinase; Vitamin E; Vitamin E (Oral); Vorapaxar

Decreased Effect

Enoxaparin may decrease the levels/effects of: Factor X (Human)

The levels/effects of Enoxaparin may be decreased by: Estrogen Derivatives; Progestins

Storage/Stability Store at 25°C (77°F); excursions permitted to 15°C to 30°C (59°F to 86°F); do not freeze. Do not store multiple-dose vials for >28 days after first use.

Mechanism of Action Standard heparin consists of components with molecular weights ranging from 4000 to 30,000 daltons with a mean of 16,000 daltons. Heparin acts as an anticoagulant by enhancing the inhibition rate of clotting proteases by antithrombin III impairing normal hemostasis and inhibition of factor Xa. Low molecular weight heparins have a small effect on the activated partial thromboplastin time and strongly inhibit factor Xa. Enoxaparin is derived from porcine heparin that undergoes benzylation followed by alkaline depolymerization. The average molecular weight of enoxaparin is 4500 daltons which is distributed as (≤20%) 2000 daltons (≥68%) 2000 to 8000 daltons, and (≤15%) >8000 daltons. Enoxaparin has a higher ratio of antifactor Xa to antifactor IIa activity than unfractionated heparin.

Pharmacodynamics/Kinetics

Onset of action: Peak effect: SubQ: Antifactor Xa and antithrombin (antifactor IIa): 3 to 5 hours

Duration: 40 mg dose: Antifactor Xa activity: ~12 hours

Distribution: 4.3 L (based on antifactor Xa activity)

Protein binding: Does not bind to heparin binding proteins

Metabolism: Hepatic, to lower molecular weight fragments (little activity)

Half-life elimination, plasma: 2 to 4 times longer than standard heparin, independent of dose; based on anti-Xa activity: 4.5 to 7 hours

Excretion: Urine (40% of dose; 10% as active fragments)

Dosing

Adult Note: One mg of enoxaparin is equal to 100 units of anti-Xa activity (World Health Organization First International Low Molecular Weight Heparin Reference Standard). Weight-based doses (eg, 1 mg/kg) are commonly rounded to the nearest 10 mg; also see institution-specific rounding protocols if available. Most available prefilled syringes are graduated in 10 mg increments.

DVT prophylaxis: SubQ:

Obesity: **Note:** In morbidly-obese patients (BMI ≥40 kg/m^2), increasing the prophylactic dose by 30% may be appropriate for some indications (Nutescu, 2009). For bariatric surgery, dose increases may be >30% based on clinical trial data.

Abdominal surgery: 40 mg once daily, with initial dose given 2 hours prior to surgery; continue until risk of DVT has diminished (usually 7 to 10 days).

Hip replacement surgery:

Twice-daily dosing: 30 mg every 12 hours, with initial dose within 12 to 24 hours after surgery, and every 12 hours for at least 10 days or until risk of DVT has diminished or the patient is adequately anticoagulated on warfarin. The American College of Chest Physicians recommends initiation ≥12 hours preoperatively **or** ≥12 hours postoperatively; extended duration of up to 35 days suggested (Guyatt, 2012).

Once-daily dosing: 40 mg once daily, with initial dose within 9 to 15 hours before surgery, and daily for at least 10 days (or up to 35 days postoperatively) or until risk of DVT has diminished or the patient is adequately anticoagulated on warfarin. The American College of Chest Physicians recommends initiation ≥12 hours preoperatively **or** ≥12 hours postoperatively; extended duration of up to 35 days suggested (Guyatt, 2012).

Knee replacement surgery: 30 mg every 12 hours, with initial dose within 12 to 24 hours after surgery, and every 12 hours for at least 10 days or until risk of DVT has diminished or the patient is adequately anticoagulated on warfarin. The American College of Chest Physicians recommends initiation ≥12 hours preoperatively **or** ≥12 hours postoperatively; extended duration of up to 35 days suggested (Guyatt, 2012).

Medical patients with severely-restricted mobility during acute illness: 40 mg once daily; continue until risk of DVT has diminished (usually 6 to 11 days).

Bariatric surgery (off-label use): Roux-en-Y gastric bypass: Appropriate dosing strategies have not been clearly defined (Borkgren-Okonek, 2008; Scholten, 2002):

BMI ≤50 kg/m^2: 40 mg every 12 hours

BMI >50 kg/m^2: 60 mg every 12 hours

◀

> **Note:** The 2013 AACE/TOS/ASMBS bariatric surgery guidelines recommend, along with early ambulation, both sequential compression devices and subcutaneous LMWH or unfractionated heparin administered within 24 hours after surgery with consideration of extended prophylaxis for those who are at high risk for VTE (eg, history of DVT) (AACE/TOS/ASMBS [Mechanick, 2013]).

Prevention of recurrent venous thromboembolism in pregnancy (off-label use): 40 mg once daily. Therapy should continue for 6 weeks postpartum in high-risk women (Bates, 2012).

DVT treatment (acute): SubQ: **Note:** Start warfarin on the first or second treatment day and continue enoxaparin until INR is ≥2 for at least 24 hours (usually 5 to 7 days) (Guyatt, 2012).

Inpatient treatment (with or without pulmonary embolism): 1 mg/kg/dose every 12 hours or 1.5 mg/kg once daily.

Outpatient treatment (without pulmonary embolism): 1 mg/kg/dose every 12 hours.

Obesity: Use actual body weight to calculate dose; dose capping not recommended; use of twice daily dosing preferred (Nutescu, 2009)

Pregnant women (off-label use): 1 mg/kg/dose every 12 hours. Discontinue ≥24 hours prior to the induction of labor or cesarean section. Enoxaparin therapy may be substituted with heparin near term. Continue anticoagulation therapy for ≥6 weeks postpartum (minimum duration of therapy: 3 months). LMWH or heparin therapy is preferred over warfarin during pregnancy (Bates, 2012).

Percutaneous coronary intervention (PCI), adjunctive therapy (off-label dosing) (ACCF/AHA/SCAI [Levine, 2011]): IV:

If patient undergoing PCI has been treated with multiple doses of enoxaparin and PCI occurs within 8 hours after the last SubQ enoxaparin dose: No additional enoxaparin is needed.

If PCI occurs 8 to 12 hours after the last SubQ enoxaparin dose or the patient received only 1 therapeutic SubQ dose (eg, 1 mg/kg): Administer a single IV dose of 0.3 mg/kg.

If PCI occurs >12 hours after the last SubQ dose: May use an established anticoagulation regimen (eg, full-dose unfractionated heparin or bivalirudin).

If patient has not received prior anticoagulant therapy: 0.5 to 0.75 mg/kg IV bolus dose

ST-elevation MI (STEMI):

Patients <75 years of age: Initial: 30 mg IV single bolus plus 1 mg/kg (maximum: 100 mg for the first 2 doses only) SubQ every 12 hours. The first SubQ dose should be administered with the IV bolus. Maintenance: After first 2 doses, administer 1 mg/kg SubQ every 12 hours.

Patients ≥75 years of age: Initial: SubQ: 0.75 mg/kg every 12 hours (**Note:** No IV bolus is administered in this population); a maximum dose of 75 mg is recommended for the first 2 doses. Maintenance: After first 2 doses, administer 0.75 mg/kg SubQ every 12 hours

Obesity: Use weight-based dosing; a maximum dose of 100 mg is recommended for the first 2 doses (Nutescu, 2009)

Additional notes on STEMI treatment: Therapy may be continued for up to 8 days or until revascularization. Unless contraindicated, all patients should receive aspirin (indefinitely) and clopidogrel (ACCF/AHA [O'Gara, 2013]). In patients with STEMI receiving thrombolytics, initiate enoxaparin dosing between 15 minutes before and 30 minutes after fibrinolytic therapy.

Mechanical heart valve (aortic or mitral position) to bridge anticoagulation (off-label use): SubQ: 1 mg/kg every 12 hours (ACCP [Douketis, 2012]). **Note:** If used in pregnant patients, target anti-Xa level of 0.8 to 1.2 units/mL, 4 to 6 hours postdose (AHA/ACC [Nishimura, 2014]).

Unstable angina or non-ST-elevation MI (NSTEMI): SubQ: 1 mg/kg every 12 hours in conjunction with oral aspirin therapy; continue for the duration of hospitalization (a minimum of at least 2 days) or up to 8 days (ACCF/AHA [Anderson, 2013])

Obesity: Use actual body weight to calculate dose; dose capping not recommended (Nutescu, 2009)

Conversion:

Conversion from IV unfractionated heparin (UFH) infusion to SubQ enoxaparin (Nutescu, 2007): Calculate specific dose for enoxaparin based on indication, discontinue UFH and begin enoxaparin within 1 hour.

Conversion from SubQ enoxaparin to IV UFH infusion (Nutescu, 2007): Discontinue enoxaparin, calculate specific dose for IV UFH infusion based on indication, omit heparin bolus/loading dose:

Converting from SubQ enoxaparin dosed every 12 hours: Start IV UFH infusion 10 to 11 hours after last dose of enoxaparin

Converting from SubQ enoxaparin dosed every 24 hours: Start IV UFH infusion 22 to 23 hours after last dose of enoxaparin

Geriatric SubQ: Refer to adult dosing. Increased incidence of bleeding with doses of 1.5 mg/kg/day or 1 mg/kg every 12 hours; injection-associated bleeding and serious adverse reactions are also increased in the elderly. Careful attention should be paid to elderly patients, particularly those <45 kg. **Note:** Dosage alteration/adjustment may be required.

Pediatric Note: One mg of enoxaparin is equal to 100 units of anti-Xa activity (World Health Organization First International Low Molecular Weight Heparin Reference Standard).

Thromboembolism (off-label use; Monagle, 2012): SubQ:

Infants <2 months: Initial:

Prophylaxis: 0.75 mg/kg every 12 hours

Treatment: 1.5 mg/kg every 12 hours

Infants >2 months and Children ≤18 years: Initial:

Prophylaxis: 0.5 mg/kg every 12 hours

Treatment: 1 mg/kg every 12 hours

◀ Maintenance: See **Dosage Titration** table:

Enoxaparin Pediatric Dosage Titration[1]

Anti-Xa Result	Dose Titration	Time to Repeat Anti-Xa Measurement
<0.35 units/mL	Increase dose by 25%	4 h after next dose
0.35-0.49 units/mL	Increase dose by 10%	4 h after next dose
0.5-1 unit/mL	Keep same dosage	Next day, then 1 wk later, then monthly (4 h after dose)
1.1-1.5 units/mL	Decrease dose by 20%	Before next dose
1.6-2 units/mL	Hold dose for 3 h and decrease dose by 30%	Before next dose, then 4 h after next dose
>2 units/mL	Hold all doses until anti-Xa is 0.5 units/mL, then decrease dose by 40%	Before next dose and every 12 h until anti-Xa <0.5 units/mL

[1]Nomogram to be used for treatment dosing.

Modified from Duplaga BA, et al, "Dosing and Monitoring of Low-Molecular-Weight Heparins in Special Populations," *Pharmacotherapy*, 2001, 21(2):218-34.

Renal Impairment

CrCl ≥30 mL/minute: No specific adjustment recommended (per manufacturer); monitor closely for bleeding.

CrCl <30 mL/minute:

DVT prophylaxis in abdominal surgery, hip replacement, knee replacement, or in medical patients during acute illness: SubQ: 30 mg once daily. **Note:** The Canadian labeling recommends 20 to 30 mg once daily (based on risk/benefit assessment) for prophylaxis in abdominal or colorectal surgery or in medical patients during acute illness.

DVT treatment (inpatient or outpatient treatment in conjunction with warfarin): SubQ: 1 mg/kg once daily

STEMI:

<75 years: Initial: IV: 30 mg as a single dose with the first dose of the SubQ maintenance regimen administered at the same time as the IV bolus; Maintenance: SubQ: 1 mg/kg once daily. **Note:** Canadian labeling recommends a maximum dose of 100 mg for the first SubQ dose.

≥75 years of age: Omit IV bolus; Maintenance: SubQ: 1 mg/kg once daily. **Note:** Canadian labeling recommends a maximum dose of 100 mg for the first SubQ dose.

Unstable angina, NSTEMI: SubQ: 1 mg/kg once daily

Dialysis: Enoxaparin has not been FDA approved for use in dialysis patients. Its elimination is primarily via the renal route. Serious bleeding complications have been reported with use in patients who are dialysis dependent or have severe renal failure. LMWH administration at fixed doses without monitoring has greater unpredictable anticoagulant effects in patients with chronic kidney disease. If used, dosages should be reduced and anti-Xa levels frequently monitored, as accumulation may occur with repeated doses. Many clinicians would not use enoxaparin in this population especially without timely anti-Xa levels.

Hemodialysis: Supplemental dose is not necessary.

Peritoneal dialysis: Significant drug removal is unlikely based on physiochemical characteristics.

Hepatic Impairment There are no dosage adjustments provided in the manufacturer's labeling (has not been studied); use with caution.

Obesity Refer to indication-specific dosing for obesity-related information (may not be available for all indications).

Administration Note: Enoxaparin is available in 100 mg/mL and 150 mg/mL concentrations.

SubQ: Administer by deep SubQ injection alternating between the left or right anterolateral and left or right posterolateral abdominal wall. Do not mix with other infusions or injections. In order to minimize bruising, do not rub injection site. To avoid loss of drug from the 30 mg and 40 mg prefilled syringes, do not expel the air bubble from the syringe prior to injection.

IV: STEMI and PCI only: The U.S. labeling recommends using the multiple-dose vial to prepare IV doses. The Canadian labeling recommends either the multiple-dose vial or a prefilled syringe. Do not mix or coadminister with other medications; may be administered with NS or D$_5$W. Flush IV access site with a sufficient amount of NS or D$_5$W prior to and following IV bolus administration. When used prior to percutaneous coronary intervention or as part of treatment for ST-elevation myocardial infarction (STEMI), a single dose may be administered IV except when the patient is ≥75 years of age and is experiencing STEMI then only administer by SubQ injection.

Monitoring Parameters Platelets, occult blood, anti-Xa levels, serum creatinine; monitoring of PT and/or aPTT is not necessary. Routine monitoring of anti-Xa levels is not required, but has been utilized in patients with obesity and/or renal insufficiency. Monitoring anti-Xa levels is recommended in pregnant women receiving therapeutic doses of enoxaparin or when receiving enoxaparin for the prevention of thromboembolism with mechanical heart valves (Guyatt, 2012). For patients >190 kg, if anti-Xa monitoring is available, adjusting dose based on anti-Xa levels is recommended; if anti-Xa monitoring is unavailable, reduce dose if bleeding occurs (Nutescu, 2009). Monitor obese patients closely for signs/symptoms of thromboembolism.

Dosage Forms Excipient information presented when available (limited, particularly for generics); consult specific product labeling.

Solution, Injection, as sodium:
Lovenox: 300 mg/3 mL (3 mL) [contains benzyl alcohol, pork (porcine) protein]
Generic: 300 mg/3 mL (3 mL)
Solution, Subcutaneous, as sodium [preservative free]:
Lovenox: 30 mg/0.3 mL (0.3 mL); 40 mg/0.4 mL (0.4 mL); 60 mg/0.6 mL (0.6 mL); 80 mg/0.8 mL (0.8 mL); 100 mg/mL (1 mL); 120 mg/0.8 mL (0.8 mL); 150 mg/mL (1 mL) [contains pork (porcine) protein]
Generic: 30 mg/0.3 mL (0.3 mL); 40 mg/0.4 mL (0.4 mL); 60 mg/0.6 mL (0.6 mL); 80 mg/0.8 mL (0.8 mL); 100 mg/mL (1 mL); 120 mg/0.8 mL (0.8 mL); 150 mg/mL (1 mL)

◆ **Enoxaparin Sodium** see Enoxaparin on page 594
◆ **Entertainer's Secret® [OTC]** see Saliva Substitute on page 1511
◆ **Envarsus XR** see Tacrolimus (Systemic) on page 1576

Enzalutamide (en za LOO ta mide)

Related Information

Safe Handling of Hazardous Drugs on page 2292

Brand Names: US Xtandi

Brand Names: Canada Xtandi

▶

ENZALUTAMIDE

Index Terms MDV3100
Pharmacologic Category Antineoplastic Agent, Antiandrogen
Use Prostate cancer, metastatic: Treatment of metastatic, castration-resistant prostate cancer
Labeled Contraindications
Women who are or may become pregnant
Canadian labeling: Additional contraindications (not in US labeling): Hypersensitivity to enzalutamide or any component of the formulation; women who are lactating
Pregnancy Considerations Adverse effects were observed in animal reproduction studies. Enzalutamide is an androgen receptor inhibitor and would be expected to cause fetal harm based on its mechanism of action. Enzalutamide is not indicated for use in women and is specifically contraindicated for use in women who are or may become pregnant. Men using this medication should use a condom if having intercourse with a pregnant woman. A condom plus another effective method of birth control is recommended during therapy and for 3 months after treatment for men using this medication and who are having intercourse with a woman of reproductive potential.
Breast-Feeding Considerations Enzalutamide is not indicated for use in women.
Warnings/Precautions Hazardous agent - use appropriate precautions for handling and disposal (meets NIOSH 2014 criteria). Seizures were observed in clinical trials (onset: ~1 to 20 months after treatment initiation). Therapy was permanently discontinued and patients were not rechallenged; seizures resolved upon therapy cessation. Patients with predisposing factors for seizure were excluded from the trials; factors include seizure history, underlying brain injury with loss of consciousness, transient ischemic attack within the past 12 months, cerebral vascular accident, brain metastases, brain arteriovenous malformation, or (in one study) the use of concomitant medications which may lower the seizure threshold. Enzalutamide should be used with caution in patients with a history of seizure disorders or other predisposing factors. Discontinue permanently if seizures develop during treatment. Posterior reversible encephalopathy syndrome (PRES) has been reported in patients receiving enzalutamide. PRES is a neurological disorder which may present with rapidly evolving symptoms (headache, seizure, lethargy, confusion, blindness, and other visual/neurologic disturbances) with or without associated hypertension. PRES diagnosis may be confirmed with magnetic resonance imaging (MRI). Discontinue enzalutamide in patients who develop PRES.

Enzalutamide may cause hypospermatogenesis and may impair male fertility. Androgen-deprivation therapy may increase the risk of cardiovascular disease (Levine, 2010). An increase in systolic and diastolic blood pressures has been observed (Scher, 2012); may worsen preexisting hypertension.

Potentially significant drug-drug interactions may exist, requiring dose or frequency adjustment, additional monitoring, and/or selection of alternative therapy. May contain sorbitol; Canadian product labeling recommends avoiding use in patients with fructose intolerance.
Adverse Reactions
>10%:
Cardiovascular: Peripheral edema (12% to 15%), hypertension (6% to 14%)
Central nervous system: Fatigue (≤51%), falling (5% to 13%), headache (11% to 12%), dizziness (10% to 11%)
Endocrine & metabolic: Hot flash (18% to 20%), weight loss (12%)

Gastrointestinal: Constipation (23%), diarrhea (17% to 22%), decreased appetite (19%)

Hematologic & oncologic: Neutropenia (15%; grades 3/4: 1%)

Neuromuscular & skeletal: Weakness (≤51%), back pain (26% to 29%), arthralgia (21%), musculoskeletal pain (15%)

Respiratory: Upper respiratory tract infection (11% to 16%), dyspnea (11%)

1% to 10%:

Central nervous system: Myasthenia (10%), insomnia (8% to 9%), anxiety (7%), paresthesia (7%), cauda equina syndrome (≤7%), spinal cord compression (≤7%), altered mental status (4% to 6%), hypoesthesia (4%), hallucination (2%), restless leg syndrome (2%)

Dermatologic: Pruritus (4%), xeroderma (4%)

Endocrine & metabolic: Gynecomastia (3%)

Gastrointestinal: Dysgeusia (8%)

Genitourinary: Hematuria (7% to 9%), pollakiuria (5%)

Hematologic & oncologic: Thrombocytopenia (6%)

Hepatic: Increased serum bilirubin (3%)

Infection: Infection (≤6%; including sepsis)

Neuromuscular & skeletal: Bone fracture (4% to 9%), stiffness (3%)

Respiratory: Lower respiratory tract infection (8% to 9%), epistaxis (3%)

<1%: Reversible posterior leukoencephalopathy syndrome, seizure

Drug Interactions

Metabolism/Transport Effects Substrate of CYP2C8 (major), CYP3A4 (major); **Note:** Assignment of Major/Minor substrate status based on clinically relevant drug interaction potential; **Inhibits** BCRP, MRP2, P-glycoprotein; **Induces** CYP2C19 (weak/moderate), CYP2C9 (weak/moderate), CYP3A4 (strong)

Avoid Concomitant Use

Avoid concomitant use of Enzalutamide with any of the following: Abiraterone Acetate; Alfentanil; Antihepaciviral Combination Products; Apixaban; Apremilast; Aprepitant; Artemether; Axitinib; Bedaquiline; Boceprevir; Bortezomib; Bosutinib; Cabozantinib; Cariprazine; Ceritinib; CloZAPine; Cobimetinib; Crizotinib; CycloSPORINE (Systemic); CYP2C8 Inducers (Strong); CYP2C8 Inhibitors (Strong); CYP3A4 Inducers (Strong); Dabrafenib; Daclatasvir; Dienogest; Dihydroergotamine; Dronedarone; Eliglustat; Ergotamine; Everolimus; FentaNYL; Flibanserin; Fosphenytoin-Phenytoin; Ibrutinib; Idelalisib; Indium 111 Capromab Pendetide; Irinotecan Products; Isavuconazonium Sulfate; Itraconazole; Ivabradine; Ivacaftor; Lapatinib; Lumefantrine; Lurasidone; Macitentan; Mifepristone; Naloxegol; Netupitant; NIFEdipine; Nilotinib; NiMODipine; Nisoldipine; Olaparib; Osimertinib; Palbociclib; Panobinostat; PAZOPanib; Perampanel; Pimozide; PONATinib; Praziquantel; QuiNIDine; Ranolazine; Regorafenib; Rivaroxaban; Roflumilast; RomiDEPsin; Simeprevir; Sirolimus; Sonidegib; SORAfenib; St Johns Wort; Suvorexant; Tacrolimus (Systemic); Tasimelteon; Telaprevir; Ticagrelor; Tofacitinib; Tolvaptan; Toremifene; Trabectedin; Ulipristal; Vandetanib; Vemurafenib; VinCRIStine (Liposomal); Vorapaxar; Warfarin

Increased Effect/Toxicity

Enzalutamide may increase the levels/effects of: Clarithromycin; Ifosfamide

The levels/effects of Enzalutamide may be increased by: Clarithromycin; CYP2C8 Inhibitors (Moderate); CYP2C8 Inhibitors (Strong); CYP3A4 Inhibitors (Strong); Deferasirox

▶

◄ **Decreased Effect**

Enzalutamide may decrease the levels/effects of: Abiraterone Acetate; Alfentanil; Antihepaciviral Combination Products; Apixaban; Apremilast; Aprepitant; ARIPiprazole; ARIPiprazole Lauroxil; Artemether; Axitinib; Bedaquiline; Boceprevir; Bortezomib; Bosutinib; Brentuximab Vedotin; Brexpiprazole; Cabozantinib; Cannabidiol; Cannabis; Cariprazine; Ceritinib; Choline C 11; Clarithromycin; CloZAPine; Cobimetinib; Corticosteroids (Systemic); Crizotinib; CycloSPORINE (Systemic); CYP2C19 Substrates; CYP2C9 Substrates; CYP3A4 Substrates; Dabrafenib; Daclatasvir; Dasatinib; Dexamethasone (Systemic); Dienogest; Dihydroergotamine; DOXOrubicin (Conventional); Dronabinol; Dronedarone; Eliglustat; Ergotamine; Erlotinib; Etoposide; Etoposide Phosphate; Everolimus; Exemestane; FentaNYL; Flibanserin; Fosphenytoin-Phenytoin; Gefitinib; GuanFACINE; Hydrocortisone (Systemic); Ibrutinib; Idelalisib; Ifosfamide; Imatinib; Indium 111 Capromab Pendetide; Irinotecan Products; Isavuconazonium Sulfate; Itraconazole; Ivabradine; Ivacaftor; Ixabepilone; Lapatinib; Linagliptin; Lumefantrine; Lurasidone; Macitentan; Maraviroc; MethylPREDNISolone; Mifepristone; Naloxegol; Netupitant; NIFEdipine; Nilotinib; NiMODipine; Nisoldipine; Olaparib; Osimertinib; Palbociclib; Panobinostat; PAZOPanib; Perampanel; Pimozide; PONATinib; Praziquantel; PrednisoLONE (Systemic); PredniSONE; Propafenone; QUEtiapine; QuiNIDine; Ranolazine; Regorafenib; Rivaroxaban; Roflumilast; Rolapitant; RomiDEPsin; Saxagliptin; Simeprevir; Sirolimus; Sonidegib; SORAfenib; SUNItinib; Suvorexant; Tacrolimus (Systemic); Tadalafil; Tasimelteon; Telaprevir; Tetrahydrocannabinol; Ticagrelor; Tofacitinib; Tolvaptan; Toremifene; Trabectedin; Ulipristal; Vandetanib; Vemurafenib; Vilazodone; VinCRIStine (Liposomal); Vorapaxar; Vortioxetine; Warfarin; Zaleplon; Zuclopenthixol

The levels/effects of Enzalutamide may be decreased by: Bosentan; CYP2C8 Inducers (Strong); CYP3A4 Inducers (Moderate); CYP3A4 Inducers (Strong); Deferasirox; Siltuximab; St Johns Wort; Tocilizumab

Storage/Stability Store at 20°C to 25°C (68°F to 77°F); excursions permitted to 15°C to 30°C (59°F to 86°F). Protect from moisture; keep bottle tightly closed.

Mechanism of Action Enzalutamide is a pure androgen receptor signaling inhibitor; unlike other antiandrogen therapies, it has no known agonistic properties. It inhibits androgen receptor nuclear translocation, DNA binding, and coactivator mobilization, leading to cellular apoptosis and decreased prostate tumor volume.

Pharmacodynamics/Kinetics

Absorption: Rapid

Distribution: 110 L

Protein binding: Parent drug: 97% to 98% to primarily albumin; active metabolite: 95% to plasma proteins

Metabolism: Primarily hepatic via CYP2C8 (responsible for formation of active metabolite N-desmethyl enzalutamide) and CYP3A4

Half-life elimination: Parent drug: 5.8 days (range: 2.8 to 10.2 days); N-desmethyl enzalutamide: 7.8 to 8.6 days

Time to peak: 1 hour (range: 0.5 to 3 hours)

Excretion: Urine (71%); feces (14%); primarily as inactive metabolite

Dosing

Adult & Geriatric

Prostate cancer, metastatic, castration-resistant: Oral: 160 mg once daily

Dosage adjustment for concomitant strong CYP2C8 inhibitors: Avoid concomitant use if possible. If coadministration is necessary, reduce enzalutamide dose to 80 mg once daily. If the strong CYP2C8 inhibitor is discontinued, adjust the enzalutamide dose back up to the dose used prior to the initiation of the strong CYP2C8 inhibitor.

Dosage adjustment for concomitant strong CYP3A4 inducers: Avoid concomitant use if possible. If coadministration is necessary, increase the enzalutamide dose to 240 mg once daily. If the strong CYP3A4 inducer is discontinued, adjust the enzalutamide dose back to the dose used prior to the initiation of the strong CYP3A4 inducer.

Renal Impairment

Preexisting mild-to-moderate impairment (CrCl 30-89 mL/minute): No initial dosage adjustment necessary.

Preexisting severe impairment (CrCl <30 mL/minute), including end-stage renal disease: There are no dosage adjustments provided in the manufacturer's labeling (has not been studied).

Hepatic Impairment Preexisting mild, moderate, or severe impairment (Child-Pugh class A, B, or C): No dosage adjustment necessary. Canadian labeling recommends to avoid use in severe impairment.

Adjustment for Toxicity If ≥ grade 3 toxicity or intolerable side effects occur, withhold treatment for 1 week or until symptom(s) improve to ≤ grade 2, then resume at same dose, or reduce dose to 120 mg or 80 mg once daily, if necessary.

Seizures: Permanently discontinue treatment.

Combination Regimens

Prostate Cancer: Enzalutamide (Prostate Regimen) on page 1955

Administration May be administered with or without food; take at the same time each day. Swallow capsules whole; do not chew, dissolve, or open the capsules. Hazardous agent; use appropriate precautions for handling and disposal (meets NIOSH 2014 criteria).

Monitoring Parameters Monitor for signs/symptoms of seizure, loss of consciousness, dizziness, and hallucinations; CBC with differential and liver function tests (baseline and periodic); additional INR monitoring (if on warfarin); blood pressure (baseline and periodic), signs/symptoms of posterior reversible encephalopathy syndrome

Dosage Forms Excipient information presented when available (limited, particularly for generics); consult specific product labeling.

Capsule, Oral:

Xtandi: 40 mg

♦ **EPEG** see Etoposide on page 641

♦ **Epidoxorubicin** see EPIrubicin on page 608

♦ **Epipodophyllotoxin** see Etoposide on page 641

♦ **Epipodophyllotoxin** see Etoposide Phosphate on page 651

EPIrubicin (ep i ROO bi sin)

Related Information

Chemotherapy and Cancer Treatment During Pregnancy *on page 2214*

Management of Chemotherapy-Induced Nausea and Vomiting in Adults *on page 2142*

Management of Drug Extravasations *on page 2159*

Prevention of Chemotherapy-Induced Nausea and Vomiting in Children *on page 2203*

Safe Handling of Hazardous Drugs *on page 2292*

Brand Names: US Ellence

Brand Names: Canada Ellence; Epirubicin for Injection; Epirubicin Hydrochloride Injection; Pharmorubicin

Index Terms Epidoxorubicin; Epirubicin Hydrochloride; Pidorubicin; Pidorubicin Hydrochloride

Pharmacologic Category Antineoplastic Agent, Anthracycline; Antineoplastic Agent, Topoisomerase II Inhibitor

Use Breast cancer, adjuvant treatment: Adjuvant therapy component for primary breast cancer in patients with evidence of axillary node involvement following tumor resection

Labeled Contraindications Hypersensitivity to epirubicin, other anthracyclines, anthracenediones, or any component of the formulation; cardiomyopathy and/or heart failure; recent myocardial infarction, severe arrhythmias; previous treatment with anthracyclines up to the maximum cumulative dose

Pregnancy Considerations Adverse events were observed in animal reproduction studies. Women of childbearing potential should be advised to use effective contraception and avoid becoming pregnant during treatment. Men undergoing treatment should use effective contraception. Epirubicin may cause irreversible amenorrhea in premenopausal women.

Limited information is available from a retrospective study of women who received epirubicin (in combination with cyclophosphamide or weekly as a single-agent) during the second or third (prior to week 35) trimester for the treatment of pregnancy-associated breast cancer (Ring 2005) and from a study of women who received epirubicin (weekly as a single-agent) at gestational weeks 16 through 30 for the treatment of pregnancy-associated breast cancer (Peccatori 2009). Some pharmacokinetic properties of epirubicin may be altered in pregnant women (van Hasselt 2014). The European Society for Medical Oncology (ESMO) has published guidelines for diagnosis, treatment, and follow-up of cancer during pregnancy (Peccatori 2013); the guidelines recommend referral to a facility with expertise in cancer during pregnancy and encourage a multidisciplinary team (obstetrician, neonatologist, oncology team). If chemotherapy is indicated, it should not be administered in the first trimester, but may begin in the second trimester. There should be a 3-week time period between the last chemotherapy dose and anticipated delivery, and chemotherapy should not be administered beyond week 33 of gestation.

A pregnancy registry is available for all cancers diagnosed during pregnancy at Cooper Health (877-635-4499).

Breast-Feeding Considerations Excretion in human breast milk is unknown; however, other anthracyclines are excreted. Due to the potential for serious adverse reactions in the nursing infant, the manufacturer recommends a decision be made to discontinue nursing or to discontinue the drug, taking into account the importance of treatment to the mother.

Warnings/Precautions Hazardous agent - use appropriate precautions for handling and disposal (NIOSH 2014 [group 1]).

[US Boxed Warning]: Myocardial toxicity, including fatal heart failure (HF) may occur, particularly in patients who have received prior anthracyclines (or anthracenediones), prior or concomitant radiotherapy to the mediastinal/pericardial area, who have preexisting cardiac disease (active or dormant), or with concomitant cardiotoxic medications. Cardiotoxicity may be concurrent or delayed (months to years after treatment). The risk of HF is ~0.9% at a cumulative dose of 550 mg/m^2, ~1.6% at a cumulative dose of 700 mg/m^2, and ~3.3% at a cumulative dose of 900 mg/m^2. Cardiotoxicity may also occur at lower cumulative doses or without risk factors. The risk of delayed cardiotoxicity increases more steeply with cumulative doses >900 mg/m^2 and this dose should be exceeded only with extreme caution. The maximum cumulative dose used in adjuvant studies was 720 mg/m^2. Cardiotoxicity is dose-limiting. Early toxicity may consist of tachyarrhythmias, including sinus tachycardia, premature ventricular contractions, and ventricular tachycardia, as well as bradycardia. Electrocardiographic changes including ST-T wave changes, atrioventricular and bundle-branch block have also been reported. These effects are not necessarily predictive of subsequent delayed cardiotoxicity. Delayed toxicity is typically caused by cardiomyopathy which presents as decreased left ventricular ejection fraction (LVEF) and/or signs/symptoms of HF (eg, tachycardia, dyspnea, pulmonary edema, edema, hepatomegaly, ascites, pleural effusion, gallop rhythm). Total cumulative dose should take into account prior treatment with other anthracyclines or anthracenediones, previous or concomitant treatment with other cardiotoxic agents or irradiation of chest. Although the risk increases with cumulative dose, irreversible cardiotoxicity may occur at any dose level. Patients with active or dormant cardiovascular disease, concurrent administration of cardiotoxic drugs, prior therapy with other anthracyclines or anthracenediones, prior or concurrent chest irradiation, advanced age, and infants and children are at increased risk. Children are at increased risk for developing delayed cardiotoxicity. Regular monitoring of LVEF and discontinuation at the first sign of impairment is recommended especially in patients with cardiac risk factors or impaired cardiac function. Discontinue treatment with signs of decreased LVEF. The half-life of other cardiotoxic agents (eg, trastuzumab) must be considered in sequential therapy.

[US Boxed Warning]: May cause severe myelosuppression, including leukopenia, thrombocytopenia, and anemia. Myelosuppression is the dose-limiting toxicity. Obtain baseline and periodic blood counts. Patients should recover from myelosuppression due to prior chemotherapy treatment before beginning treatments. Severe neutropenia and severe infections may require supportive care. Thrombophlebitis and thromboembolic phenomena (including pulmonary embolism) have occurred.

[US Boxed Warning]: Dosage reduction is recommended in patients with mild-to-moderate hepatic impairment. Use is not recommended in severe hepatic impairment; predominantly hepatically eliminated; impaired hepatic function may lead to increased exposure and toxicity and in patients with serum creatinine >5 mg/dL (has not been studied in patients on dialysis). Monitor hepatic and renal function at baseline and during treatment. May cause tumor lysis syndrome (TLS), although generally does not occur in patients with breast cancer; if TLS risk is suspected, consider ▶

◀ monitoring serum uric acid, potassium, calcium, phosphate, and serum creatinine after initial administration; hydration and antihyperuricemic prophylaxis may minimize potential TLS complications. Radiation recall (inflammatory) has been reported; epirubicin may have radiosensitizing activity. **[US Boxed Warning]: Treatment with anthracyclines (including epirubicin) may increase the risk of secondary acute myeloid leukemia (AML). AML is more common when given in combination with other antineoplastic agents, in patients who have received multiple courses of previous chemotherapy, or with escalated anthracycline doses. In breast cancer patients, the risk for treatment-related AML or myelodysplastic syndrome (MDS) was estimated at 0.27% at 3 years, 0.46% at 5 years, and 0.55% at 8 years after treatment.** The latency period for secondary leukemias may be short (1 to 3 years).

[US Boxed Warning]: For IV administration only. Vesicant; if extravasation occurs, severe local tissue damage and necrosis may occur; not for IM or SubQ use. Injection in to a small vein or repeated administration in the same vein may result in venous sclerosis. Ensure proper needle or catheter placement prior to and during infusion. Avoid extravasation. If perivenous infiltration occurs, immediately discontinue infusion and restart in another vein. Women ≥70 years of age should be closely monitored for toxicity. Children may be at increased risk for developing acute and delayed cardiotoxicity; long-term periodic cardiac function monitoring is recommended. **[US Boxed Warning]: Should be administered under the supervision of an experienced cancer chemotherapy physician.** Epirubicin is associated with a moderate to high emetic potential (depending on dose or regimen); antiemetics are recommended to prevent nausea and vomiting (Basch 2011; Dupuis 2011; Roila 2010). Patients should recover from acute toxicities (stomatitis, myelosuppression, infections) prior to initiating treatment. Assess baseline labs (blood counts, bilirubin, ALT, AST, serum creatinine) and cardiac function (with LVEF). Prophylactic antibiotics should be administered with the CDF-120 regimen. Patients should not be immunized with live viral vaccines during or shortly after treatment. Inactivated vaccines may be administered (response may be diminished). Potentially significant interactions may exist, requiring dose or frequency adjustment, additional monitoring, and/or selection of alternative therapy.

Adverse Reactions Percentages reported as part of combination chemotherapy regimens.

>10%:

Central nervous system: Lethargy (1% to 46%)

Dermatologic: Alopecia (70% to 96%)

Endocrine & metabolic: Amenorrhea (69% to 72%), hot flashes (5% to 39%)

Gastrointestinal: Nausea/vomiting (83% to 92%; grades 3/4: 22% to 25%), mucositis (9% to 59%; grades 3/4: ≤9%), diarrhea (7% to 25%)

Hematologic: Leukopenia (50% to 80%; grades 3/4: 2% to 59%), neutropenia (54% to 80%; grades 3/4: 11% to 67%; nadir: 10-14 days; recovery: by day 21), anemia (13% to 72%; grades 3/4: ≤6%), thrombocytopenia (5% to 49%; grades 3/4: ≤5%)

Local: Injection site reactions (3% to 20%; grades 3/4: <1%)

Ocular: Conjunctivitis (1% to 15%)

Miscellaneous: Infection (15% to 22%; grades 3/4: ≤2%)

1% to 10%:
  Cardiovascular: LVEF decreased (asymptomatic; delayed: 1% to 2%), HF (0.4% to 1.5%)
  Central nervous system: Fever (1% to 5%)
  Dermatologic: Rash (1% to 9%), skin changes (1% to 5%)
  Gastrointestinal: Anorexia (2% to 3%)
  Hematologic: Neutropenic fever (grades 3/4: ≤6%)
<1%, postmarketing, case reports, and/or frequency not defined: Abdominal pain, acute lymphoid leukemia (ALL), acute myelogenous leukemia (AML), anaphylaxis, arrhythmia, arterial embolism, ascites, atrioventricular block, bradycardia, bundle-branch block, cardiomyopathy, chills, dehydration, dyspnea, ECG abnormalities, erythema, esophagitis, flushing, GI burning sensation, GI erosions/ulcerations, GI pain, GI bleeding, hepatomegaly, hyperpigmentation (oral mucosa, nails, skin), hypersensitivity, hyperuricemia, myelodysplastic syndrome, myocarditis, neutropenic typhlitis, phlebitis, photosensitivity, pneumonia, premature menopause, premature ventricular contractions, pulmonary edema, pulmonary embolism, radiation recall, sepsis, shock, sinus tachycardia, stomatitis, ST-T wave changes (nonspecific), tachyarrhythmias, thromboembolism, thrombophlebitis, toxic megacolon, transaminases increased, urine discoloration (red), urticaria, ventricular tachycardia

Drug Interactions

Metabolism/Transport Effects None known.

Avoid Concomitant Use

Avoid concomitant use of EPIrubicin with any of the following: BCG (Intravesical); Cimetidine; CloZAPine; Dipyrone; Natalizumab; Pimecrolimus; Tacrolimus (Topical); Tofacitinib; Vaccines (Live)

Increased Effect/Toxicity

EPIrubicin may increase the levels/effects of: CloZAPine; Fingolimod; Leflunomide; Natalizumab; Tofacitinib; Vaccines (Live)

The levels/effects of EPIrubicin may be increased by: Bevacizumab; Cimetidine; Cyclophosphamide; Denosumab; Dipyrone; Pimecrolimus; Roflumilast; Tacrolimus (Topical); Taxane Derivatives; Trastuzumab

Decreased Effect

EPIrubicin may decrease the levels/effects of: BCG (Intravesical); Cardiac Glycosides; Coccidioides immitis Skin Test; Sipuleucel-T; Vaccines (Inactivated); Vaccines (Live)

The levels/effects of EPIrubicin may be decreased by: Cardiac Glycosides; Echinacea

Storage/Stability Protect from light.

Solution: Store intact vials at 2°C to 8°C (36°F to 46°F); do not freeze. Protect from light. Product may "gel" at refrigerated temperatures; will return to slightly viscous solution after 2 to 4 hours at room temperature (15°C to 25°C). Discard unused solution from single dose vials within 24 hours of entry.

Lyophilized powder: Store at room temperature of 25°C (77°F); excursions permitted to 15°C to 30°C (59°F to 86°F). Reconstituted solutions are stable for 24 hours when stored at 2°C to 8°C (36°F to 46°F) or at room temperature. ▶

◄ **Preparation for Administration** Hazardous agent; use appropriate precautions for handling and disposal (NIOSH 2014 [group 1]). Reconstitute lyophilized powder with sterile water for injection (25 mL for the 50 mg vial) to a final concentration of 2 mg/mL. Shake vigorously; may take several minutes for dissolution. May be further diluted with sterile water for injection.

Mechanism of Action Epirubicin is an anthracycline antineoplastic agent; known to inhibit DNA and RNA synthesis by steric obstruction after intercalating between DNA base pairs; active throughout entire cell cycle. Intercalation triggers DNA cleavage by topoisomerase II, resulting in cytocidal activity. Also inhibits DNA helicase, and generates cytotoxic free radicals.

Pharmacodynamics/Kinetics

Distribution: V_{dss}: 21 to 27 L/kg

Protein binding: ~77% to albumin

Metabolism: Extensively via hepatic and extrahepatic (including RBCs) routes

Half-life elimination: Triphasic; Mean terminal: 33 hours

Excretion: Feces (34% to 35%); urine (20% to 27%)

Dosing

Adult Note: Patients receiving 120 mg/m^2/cycle as part of combination therapy (CEF-120 regimen) should also receive prophylactic antibiotic therapy with sulfamethoxazole/trimethoprim or a fluoroquinolone. Lower starting doses may be necessary for heavily pretreated patients, patients with preexisting myelosuppression, or with bone marrow involvement. If clinically reasonable, delay epirubicin therapy until other cardiotoxic agents with long half-lives (eg, trastuzumab) have been cleared. The recommended lifetime maximum dose is 900 mg/m^2. Epirubicin is associated with a moderate to high emetic potential (depending on dose or regimen); antiemetics are recommended to prevent nausea and vomiting (Basch 2011; Dupuis 2011; Roila 2010).

Breast cancer, adjuvant treatment: IV: Usual dose: 100-120 mg/m^2 per 3- or 4-week treatment cycle as follows:

60 mg/m^2 on days 1 and 8 every 28 days for 6 cycles in combination with cyclophosphamide and fluorouracil (CEF-120 regimen; Levine 2005) **or**

100 mg/m^2 on day 1 every 21 days for 6 cycles in combination with cyclophosphamide and fluorouracil (FEC-100 regimen; Bonneterre 2005) **or**

Breast cancer (off-label regimens): IV:

EC regimen: 100 mg/m^2 on day 1 every 21 days for 8 cycles in combination with cyclophosphamide (Piccart 2001) **or**

EP or EC regimen: 75 mg/m^2 on day 1 every 21 days for up to 6 cycles in combination with either paclitaxel or cyclophosphamide (Langley 2005) **or**

FEC regimen ± paclitaxel: 90 mg/m^2 on day 1 every 21 days for 6 cycles in combination with fluorouracil and cyclophosphamide or for 4 cycles in combination with fluorouracil and cyclophosphamide followed by paclitaxel (Martin 2008) **or**

FEC regimen followed by pertuzumab + trastuzumab + docetaxel: 100 mg/m^2 on day 1 every 21 days for 3 cycles in combination with fluorouracil and cyclophosphamide, followed by 3 cycles of pertuzumab, trastuzumab, and docetaxel (Schneeweiss 2013) **or**

CEF regimen: 50 mg/m^2 on days 1 and 8 every 21 or 28 days for 6 to 9 cycles in combination with cyclophosphamide and fluorouracil (Ackland 2001)

Esophageal cancer (off-label use): IV:

ECF, ECX, EOF, and EOX regimens: 50 mg/m^2 on day 1 every 21 days for up to 8 cycles in combination with cisplatin (C), oxaliplatin (O), fluorouracil (F), and/or capecitabine (X) (Cunningham 2008) **or**

ECF regimen: 50 mg/m^2 on day 1 every 21 days for 3 preoperative and 3 postoperative cycles in combination with cisplatin and fluorouracil (Cunningham 2006)

Gastric cancer (off-label use): IV:

ECF, ECX, EOF, and EOX regimens: 50 mg/m^2 on day 1 every 21 days for up to 8 cycles in combination with cisplatin (C), oxaliplatin (O), fluorouracil (F), and/or capecitabine (X) (Cunningham 2008; Waters 1999) **or**

ECF regimen: 50 mg/m^2 on day 1 every 21 days for 3 preoperative and 3 postoperative cycles in combination with cisplatin and fluorouracil (Cunningham 2006)

Osteosarcoma (off-label use): IV: 90 mg/m^2 on day 1 every 21 days for 3 cycles before surgery and 90 mg/m^2 on day 1 every 28 days for 3 cycles after surgery (in combination with cisplatin, ifosfamide and mesna) (Basaran 2007)

Soft tissue sarcoma (off-label use): IV: 25 mg/m^2 on days 1, 2, and 3 every 28 days for 4 cycles (in combination with ifosfamide and mesna) (Petrioli 2002) **or** 60 mg/m^2 on days 1 and 2 every 21 days for 5 cycles (in combination with ifosfamide, mesna, and filgrastim) (Frustaci 2001)

Dosage adjustment for toxicity (breast cancer; labeled dosing):

Note: Heavily-treated patients, patients with preexisting bone marrow depression or neoplastic bone marrow infiltration: Lower starting doses (75 to 90 mg/m^2) should be considered.

Delay day 1 dose of subsequent cycles until platelets are ≥100,000/mm^3, ANC ≥1500/mm^3, and nonhematologic toxicities have recovered to ≤ grade 1

Reduce day 1 dose in subsequent cycles to 75% of previous day 1 dose if patient experiences nadir platelet counts <50,000/mm^3, ANC <250/mm^3, neutropenic fever, or grade 3/4 nonhematologic toxicity during the previous cycle

For CEF-120 regimen, reduce day 8 dose to 75% of day 1 dose if platelet counts are 75,000 to 100,000/mm^3 and ANC is 1000 to 1499/mm^3; omit day 8 dose if platelets are <75,000/mm^3, ANC <1000/mm^3, or grade 3/4 nonhematologic toxicity

Geriatric Plasma clearance of epirubicin in elderly female patients was noted to be reduced by 35%. Although no initial dosage reduction is specifically recommended, particular care should be exercised in monitoring toxicity and adjusting subsequent dosage in elderly patients (particularly females >70 years of age).

Renal Impairment The manufacturer's labeling recommends lower doses (dose not specified) in patients with severe renal impairment (serum creatinine >5 mg/dL). Other sources (Aronoff 2007) suggest no dosage adjustment is needed for CrCl <50 mL/minute.

Hepatic Impairment The manufacturer's labeling recommends the following adjustments (based on clinical trial information):

Bilirubin 1.2 to 3 mg/dL or AST 2 to 4 times the upper limit of normal: Administer 50% of recommended starting dose

Bilirubin >3 mg/dL or AST >4 times the upper limit of normal: Administer 25% of recommended starting dose

Severe hepatic impairment: Use is not recommended (has not been studied).

Obesity *ASCO Guidelines for appropriate chemotherapy dosing in obese adults with cancer:* Utilize patient's actual body weight (full weight) for calculation of body surface area- or weight-based dosing, particularly when the intent of therapy is curative; manage regimen-related toxicities in the same manner as for nonobese patients; if a dose reduction is utilized due to toxicity, consider resumption of full weight-based dosing with subsequent cycles, especially if cause of toxicity (eg, hepatic or renal impairment) is resolved (Griggs 2012).

Combination Regimens

Bone sarcoma (osteosarcoma): Ifosfamide-Cisplatin-Epirubicin (Osteosarcoma) on page 2015

Breast cancer:

Cyclophosphamide-Epirubicin (Breast) on page 1929

Docetaxel-Trastuzumab followed by FEC (Breast) on page 1947

Epirubicin (Breast Regimen) on page 1955

FEC followed by Docetaxel Every 3 Weeks (Breast) on page 1966

FEC followed by Paclitaxel Weekly (Breast) on page 1967

FEC IV (Breast) on page 1967

FEC Oral (Breast) on page 1968

Esophageal cancer:

Epirubicin-Cisplatin-Capecitabine (Gastric/Esophageal) on page 1956

Epirubicin-Cisplatin-Fluorouracil (Gastric/Esophageal) on page 1956

Epirubicin-Oxaliplatin-Capecitabine (Gastric/Esophageal) on page 1957

Epirubicin-Oxaliplatin-Fluorouracil (Gastric/Esophageal) on page 1958

Gastric cancer:

Epirubicin-Cisplatin-Capecitabine (Gastric/Esophageal) on page 1956

Epirubicin-Cisplatin-Fluorouracil (Gastric/Esophageal) on page 1956

Epirubicin-Oxaliplatin-Capecitabine (Gastric/Esophageal) on page 1957

Epirubicin-Oxaliplatin-Fluorouracil (Gastric/Esophageal) on page 1958

Soft tissue sarcoma: Epirubicin-Ifosfamide (Soft Tissue Sarcoma) on page 1957

Administration Epirubicin is associated with a moderate to high emetic potential (depending on dose or regimen); antiemetics are recommended to prevent nausea and vomiting (Basch 2011; Dupuis 2011; Roila 2010).

IV: Infuse over 15 to 20 minutes or slow IV push; if lower doses due to dose reduction are administered, may reduce infusion time proportionally. Do not infuse over <3 minutes. Infuse into a free-flowing IV solution (NS or D_5W). Avoid the use of veins over joints or in extremities with compromised venous or lymphatic drainage.

Vesicant; ensure proper needle or catheter placement prior to and during infusion; avoid extravasation.

Extravasation management: If extravasation occurs, stop infusion immediately and disconnect (leave cannula/needle in place); gently aspirate extravasated solution (do **NOT** flush the line); remove needle/cannula; elevate extremity. Initiate antidote (dexrazoxane or dimethyl sulfate [DMSO]). Apply dry cold compresses for 20 minutes 4 times daily for 1 to 2 days (Perez Fidalgo 2012); withhold cooling beginning 15 minutes before dexrazoxane infusion; continue withholding cooling until 15 minutes after infusion is completed. Topical DMSO should not be administered in combination with dexrazoxane; may lessen dexrazoxane efficacy.

Dexrazoxane: Adults: 1,000 mg/m² (maximum dose: 2,000 mg) IV (administer in a large vein remote from site of extravasation) over 1 to 2 hours days 1 and 2, then 500 mg/m² (maximum dose: 1,000 mg) IV over 1 to 2 hours day 3; begin within 6 hours of extravasation. Day 2 and day 3 doses should be administered at approximately the same time (±3 hours) as the dose on day 1 (Mouridsen 2007; Perez Fidalgo 2012). **Note:** Reduce dexrazoxane dose by 50% in patients with moderate to severe renal impairment (CrCl <40 mL/minute).

DMSO: Children and Adults: Apply topically to a region covering twice the affected area every 8 hours for 7 days; begin within 10 minutes of extravasation; do not cover with a dressing (Perez Fidalgo 2012).

Hazardous agent; use appropriate precautions for handling and disposal (NIOSH 2014 [group 1]).

Vesicant/Extravasation Risk Vesicant

Emetic Potential
Children: Moderate (30% to 90%)
Adults:
>90 mg/m² or when used in combination with cyclophosphamide: High (>90%)
≤90 mg/m²: Moderate (30% to 90%)

Monitoring Parameters Baseline and repeated measurements of CBC with differential, liver function tests, serum creatinine, electrolytes, ECG, and LVEF. The method used for assessment of LVEF (echocardiogram or MUGA) should be consistent during routine monitoring. Monitor injection site during infusion for possible extravasation or local reactions.

Dosage Forms Excipient information presented when available (limited, particularly for generics); consult specific product labeling. [DSC] = Discontinued product
Solution, Intravenous, as hydrochloride [preservative free]:
Ellence: 50 mg/25 mL (25 mL); 200 mg/100 mL (100 mL)
Generic: 50 mg/25 mL (25 mL); 200 mg/100 mL (100 mL)
Solution Reconstituted, Intravenous, as hydrochloride:
Generic: 50 mg (1 ea); 200 mg (1 ea [DSC])

♦ **Epirubicin for Injection (Can)** *see* EPIrubicin *on page 608*

♦ **Epirubicin Hydrochloride** *see* EPIrubicin *on page 608*

♦ **Epirubicin Hydrochloride Injection (Can)** *see* EPIrubicin *on page 608*

♦ **Episil** *see* Mucosal Coating Agent *on page 1175*

♦ **EPO** *see* Epoetin Alfa *on page 615*

Epoetin Alfa (e POE e tin AL fa)

Related Information
Palliative Care Medicine (Cancer) *on page 2252*
Brand Names: US Epogen; Procrit
Brand Names: Canada Eprex
Index Terms rHuEPO; rHuEPO-α; EPO; Epoetin Alfa, Recombinant; Erythropoiesis-Stimulating Agent (ESA); Erythropoietin
Pharmacologic Category Colony Stimulating Factor; Erythropoiesis-Stimulating Agent (ESA); Hematopoietic Agent

◀ **Use**

Anemia: Treatment of anemia due to concurrent myelosuppressive chemo-therapy in patients with cancer (nonmyeloid malignancies) receiving chemo-therapy (palliative intent) for a planned minimum of 2 additional months of chemotherapy; treatment of anemia due to chronic kidney disease (including patients on dialysis and not on dialysis) to decrease the need for RBC transfusion; treatment of anemia associated with HIV (zidovudine) therapy when endogenous erythropoietin levels ≤500 mUnits/mL; reduction of allo-geneic RBC transfusion for elective, noncardiac, nonvascular surgery when perioperative hemoglobin is >10 to ≤13 g/dL and there is a high risk for blood loss

Limitations of use: Epoetin alfa has not been shown to improve quality of life, fatigue, or patient well-being. Epoetin alfa is **not** indicated for use under the following conditions:
- Cancer patients receiving hormonal therapy, therapeutic biologic products, or radiation therapy unless also receiving concurrent myelosuppressive chemotherapy
- Cancer patients receiving myelosuppressive chemotherapy when the expected outcome is curative
- Surgery patients who are willing to donate autologous blood
- Surgery patients undergoing cardiac or vascular surgery
- As a substitute for RBC transfusion in patients requiring immediate correction of anemia

Labeled Contraindications Serious allergic reactions to epoetin alfa or any component of the formulation; uncontrolled hypertension; pure red cell aplasia (PRCA) that begins after treatment with epoetin alfa or other epoetin protein drugs; multidose vials contain benzyl alcohol and are contraindicated in neonates, infants, pregnant women, and nursing women

Pregnancy Considerations Adverse events were observed in animal repro-duction studies. In vitro studies suggest that recombinant erythropoietin does not cross the human placenta (Reisenberger 1997). Polyhydramnios and intrauterine growth retardation have been reported with use in women with chronic kidney disease (adverse effects also associated with maternal dis-ease). Hypospadias and pectus excavatum have been reported with first trimester exposure (case report).

Recombinant erythropoietin alfa has been evaluated as adjunctive treatment for severe pregnancy associated iron deficiency anemia (Breymann 2001; Krafft 2009) and has been used in pregnant women with iron-deficiency anemia associated with chronic kidney disease (CKD) (Furaz-Czerpak 2012; Josephson 2007).

Amenorrheic premenopausal women should be cautioned that menstruation may resume following treatment with recombinant erythropoietin (Furaz-Czer-pak 2012). Multidose formulations containing benzyl alcohol are contraindi-cated for use in pregnant women; if treatment during pregnancy is needed, single dose preparations should be used.

Women who become pregnant during treatment with epoetin alfa are encour-aged to enroll in Amgen's Pregnancy Surveillance Program (1-800-772-6436).

Breast-Feeding Considerations Endogenous erythropoietin is found in breast milk (Semba 2002). It is not known if recombinant erythropoietin alfa is excreted into breast milk. The manufacturer recommends caution be used if the single dose vial preparation is administered to nursing women; use of the multiple dose vials containing benzyl alcohol is contraindicated in breast-feeding women. When administered enterally to neonates (mixed with human milk or infant formula), recombinant erythropoietin did not significantly increase serum EPO concentrations. If passage via breast milk does occur, risk to a nursing infant appears low (Juul 2003).

Warnings/Precautions [US Boxed Warning]: Erythropoiesis-stimulating agents (ESAs) increased the risk of serious cardiovascular events, myocardial infarction, stroke, venous thromboembolism, vascular access thrombosis, mortality, and/or tumor progression in clinical studies when administered to target hemoglobin levels >11 g/dL (and provide no additional benefit); a rapid rise in hemoglobin (>1 g/dL over 2 weeks) may also contribute to these risks. **[US Boxed Warning]: A shortened overall survival and/or increased risk of tumor progression or recurrence has been reported in studies with breast, cervical, head and neck, lymphoid, and non-small cell lung cancer patients.** It is of note that in these studies, patients received ESAs to a target hemoglobin of ≥12 g/dL; although risk has not been excluded when dosed to achieve a target hemoglobin of <12 g/dL. **[US Boxed Warnings]: To decrease these risks, and risk of cardio- and thrombovascular events, use the lowest dose needed to avoid red blood cell transfusions. Use ESAs in cancer patients only for the treatment of anemia related to concurrent myelosuppressive chemotherapy; discontinue ESA following completion of the chemotherapy course. ESAs are not indicated for patients receiving myelosuppressive therapy when the anticipated outcome is curative.** A dosage modification is appropriate if hemoglobin levels rise >1 g/dL per 2-week time period during treatment (Rizzo 2010). Use of ESAs has been associated with an increased risk of venous thromboembolism (VTE) without a reduction in transfusions in patients with cancer (Hershman 2009). Improved anemia symptoms, quality of life, fatigue, or well-being have not been demonstrated in controlled clinical trials. **[US Boxed Warning]: Because of the risks of decreased survival and increased risk of tumor growth or progression, health care providers and hospitals must enroll and comply with the ESA APPRISE (Assisting Providers and Cancer Patients with Risk Information for the Safe use of ESAs) Oncology Program to prescribe or dispense ESAs to cancer patients.** Prescribers and patients will have to provide written documentation of discussed risks prior to each new course.

[US Boxed Warning]: An increased risk of death, serious cardiovascular events, and stroke was reported in chronic kidney disease (CKD) patients administered ESAs to target hemoglobin levels ≥11 g/dL; use the lowest dose sufficient to reduce the need for RBC transfusions. An optimal target hemoglobin level, dose or dosing strategy to reduce these risks has not been identified in clinical trials. Hemoglobin rising >1 g/dL in a 2-week period may contribute to the risk (dosage reduction recommended). The American College of Physicians recommends against the use of ESAs in patients with mild to moderate anemia and heart failure or coronary heart disease (ACP [Qaseem 2013]). The ACCF/AHA 2013 Heart Failure Guidelines do not provide a clear recommendation on the use of erythropoiesis-stimulating agents (ESA) in anemic heart failure patients. The effects of ESAs on quality of life measures, morbidity, and mortality are potentially modest and still unclear. Additionally, the safety of epoetin alfa has not been well studied in this population. The authors declined to provide an official recommendation regarding the use of ESAs pending the completion of ongoing randomized trials (ACCF/AHA [Yancy 2013]).

Chronic kidney disease patients who exhibit an inadequate hemoglobin response to ESA therapy may be at a higher risk for cardiovascular events and mortality compared to other patients. ESA therapy may reduce dialysis efficacy (due to increase in red blood cells and decrease in plasma volume); adjustments in dialysis parameters may be needed. Patients treated with epoetin may require increased heparinization during dialysis to prevent clotting of the extracorporeal circuit. **[US Boxed Warning]: DVT prophylaxis is recommended in perisurgery patients due to the risk of DVT.** Increased mortality was also observed in patients undergoing coronary artery bypass surgery who received epoetin alfa; these deaths were associated with thrombotic events. Epoetin alfa is **not** approved for reduction of red blood cell transfusion in patients undergoing cardiac or vascular surgery and is **not** indicated for surgical patients willing to donate autologous blood.

Use with caution in patients with hypertension (contraindicated in uncontrolled hypertension) or with a history of seizures; hypertensive encephalopathy and seizures have been reported. If hypertension is difficult to control, reduce or hold epoetin alfa. An excessive rate of rise of hemoglobin is associated with hypertension or exacerbation of hypertension; decrease the epoetin alfa dose if the hemoglobin increase exceeds 1 g/dL in any 2-week period. Blood pressure should be controlled prior to start of therapy and monitored closely throughout treatment. The risk for seizures is increased with epoetin alfa use in patients with CKD; monitor closely for neurologic symptoms during the first several months of therapy. Due to the delayed onset of erythropoiesis, epoetin alfa is **not** recommended for acute correction of severe anemia or as a substitute for emergency transfusion.

Prior to treatment, correct or exclude deficiencies of iron, vitamin B_{12}, and/or folate, as well as other factors which may impair erythropoiesis (inflammatory conditions, infections, bleeding). Prior to and periodically during therapy, iron stores must be evaluated. Supplemental iron is recommended if serum ferritin <100 mcg/L or serum transferrin saturation <20%; most patients with chronic kidney disease will require iron supplementation. Poor response should prompt evaluation of these potential factors, as well as possible malignant processes and hematologic disease (thalassemia, refractory anemia, myelodysplastic disorder), occult blood loss, hemolysis, ostetis fibrosa cystic, and/or bone marrow fibrosis. Severe anemia and pure red cell aplasia (PRCA) with associated neutralizing antibodies to erythropoietin has been reported, predominantly in patients with CKD receiving SubQ epoetin alfa (the IV route is preferred for hemodialysis patients). Cases have also been reported in patients with hepatitis C who were receiving ESAs, interferon, and ribavirin. Patients with a sudden loss of response to epoetin alfa (with severe anemia and a low reticulocyte count) should be evaluated for PRCA with associated neutralizing antibodies to erythropoietin; discontinue treatment (permanently) in patients with PRCA secondary to neutralizing antibodies to epoetin alfa. Antibodies may cross-react; do not switch to another ESA in patients who develop antibody-mediated anemia.

The American Society of Clinical Oncology (ASCO) and American Society of Hematology (ASH) 2010 updates to the clinical practice guidelines for the use of ESAs in patients with cancer indicate that ESAs are appropriate when used according to the parameters identified within the FDA-approved labeling for epoetin and darbepoetin afla (Rizzo 2010). ESAs are an option for chemotherapy associated anemia when the hemoglobin has fallen to <10 g/dL to decrease the need for RBC transfusions. ESAs should only be used in conjunction with concurrent chemotherapy. Although the FDA label now limits ESA use to the palliative setting, the ASCO/ASH guidelines suggest using clinical judgment in weighing risks versus benefits as formal outcomes studies of ESA use defined by intent of chemotherapy treatment have not been conducted.

Potentially serious allergic reactions have been reported (rarely), including anaphylactic reactions, angioedema, bronchospasm, rash, and urticaria. Discontinue immediately (and permanently) in patients who experience serious allergic/anaphylactic reactions.

Some dosage forms may contain polysorbate 80 (also known as Tweens). Hypersensitivity reactions, usually a delayed reaction, have been reported following exposure to pharmaceutical products containing polysorbate 80 in certain individuals (Isaksson 2002; Lucente 2000; Shelley 1995). Thrombocytopenia, ascites, pulmonary deterioration, and renal and hepatic failure have been reported in premature neonates after receiving parenteral products containing polysorbate 80 (Alade 1986; CDC 1984). See manufacturer's labeling.

Some products may contain albumin.

Benzyl alcohol and derivatives: Some dosage forms may contain benzyl alcohol; large amounts of benzyl alcohol (≥99 mg/kg/day) have been associated with a potentially fatal toxicity ("gasping syndrome") in neonates; the "gasping syndrome" consists of metabolic acidosis, respiratory distress, gasping respirations, CNS dysfunction (including convulsions, intracranial hemorrhage), hypotension and cardiovascular collapse (AAP ["Inactive" 1997]; CDC 1982); some data suggests that benzoate displaces bilirubin from protein binding sites (Ahlfors 2001); avoid or use dosage forms containing benzyl alcohol with caution in neonates. See manufacturer's labeling.

Adverse Reactions

>10%:
  Cardiovascular: Hypertension (3% to 28%)
  Central nervous system: Fever (10% to 42%), headache (5% to 18%)
  Dermatologic: Pruritus (12% to 21%), rash (2% to 19%)
  Gastrointestinal: Nausea (35% to 56%), vomiting (12% to 28%)
  Local: Injection site reaction (7% to 13%)
  Neuromuscular & skeletal: Arthralgia (10% to 16%)
  Respiratory: Cough (4% to 26%)
1% to 10%:
  Cardiovascular: Deep vein thrombosis, edema, thrombosis
  Central nervous system: Chills, depression, dizziness, insomnia
  Dermatologic: Urticaria
  Endocrine & metabolic: Hyperglycemia, hypokalemia
  Gastrointestinal: Dysphagia, stomatitis, weight loss
  Hematologic: Leukopenia
  Local: Clotted vascular access
  Neuromuscular & skeletal: Bone pain, muscle spasm, myalgia
  Respiratory: Pulmonary embolism, respiratory congestion, upper respiratory infection

◄ <1%, postmarketing, and/or case reports: Allergic reaction, anaphylactic reaction, angioedema, bronchospasm, erythema, hypersensitivity reactions, hypertensive encephalopathy, MI, microvascular thrombosis, neutralizing antibodies, porphyria, pure red cell aplasia (PRCA), renal vein thrombosis, retinal artery thrombosis, seizure, stroke, tachycardia, temporal vein thrombosis, thrombophlebitis, TIA, tumor progression

Drug Interactions

Metabolism/Transport Effects None known.

Avoid Concomitant Use There are no known interactions where it is recommended to avoid concomitant use.

Increased Effect/Toxicity

Epoetin Alfa may increase the levels/effects of: Lenalidomide; Thalidomide

The levels/effects of Epoetin Alfa may be increased by: Nandrolone

Decreased Effect There are no known significant interactions involving a decrease in effect.

Storage/Stability Vials should be stored at 2°C to 8°C (36°F to 46°F); **Do not freeze. Do not shake.** Protect from light.

Single-dose 1 mL vial contains no preservative: Use one dose per vial. Do not re-enter vial; discard unused portions.

Single-dose vials (except 40,000 units/mL vial) are stable for 2 weeks at room temperature (Cohen 2007). Single-dose 40,000 units/mL vial is stable for 1 week at room temperature.

Multidose 1 mL or 2 mL vial contains preservative. Store at 2°C to 8°C after initial entry and between doses. Discard 21 days after initial entry.

Multidose vials (with preservative) are stable for 1 week at room temperature (Cohen 2007).

Prefilled syringes containing the 20,000 units/mL formulation with preservative are stable for 6 weeks refrigerated (2°C to 8°C) (Naughton 2003).

Dilutions of 1:10 and 1:20 (1 part epoetin alfa:19 parts sodium chloride) are stable for 18 hours at room temperature (Ohls 1996).

Prior to SubQ administration, preservative free solutions may be mixed with bacteriostatic NS containing benzyl alcohol 0.9% in a 1:1 ratio (Corbo 1992).

Dilutions of 1:10 in $D_{10}W$ with human albumin 0.05% or 0.1% are stable for 24 hours.

Preparation for Administration Prior to SubQ administration, preservative free solutions may be mixed with bacteriostatic NS containing benzyl alcohol 0.9% in a 1:1 ratio.

Mechanism of Action Induces erythropoiesis by stimulating the division and differentiation of committed erythroid progenitor cells; induces the release of reticulocytes from the bone marrow into the bloodstream, where they mature to erythrocytes. There is a dose response relationship with this effect. This results in an increase in reticulocyte counts followed by a rise in hematocrit and hemoglobin levels.

Pharmacodynamics/Kinetics

Onset of action: Several days

Peak effect: Hemoglobin level: 2 to 6 weeks

Distribution: V_d: 9 L; rapid in the plasma compartment; concentrated in liver, kidneys, and bone marrow

Metabolism: Some degradation does occur

Bioavailability: SubQ: ~21% to 31%; intraperitoneal epoetin alfa: 3% (Macdougall 1989)

Half-life elimination: Cancer: SubQ: 16 to 67 hours; Chronic kidney disease: IV: 4 to 13 hours

Time to peak, serum: Chronic kidney disease: SubQ: 5 to 24 hours

Excretion: Feces (majority); urine (small amounts, 10% unchanged in normal volunteers)

Dosing

Adult & Geriatric Note: Evaluate iron status in all patients before and during treatment and maintain iron repletion.

Anemia associated with chronic kidney disease (CKD): Individualize dosing and use the lowest dose necessary to reduce the need for RBC transfusions.

Chronic kidney disease patients ON dialysis (IV route is preferred for hemodialysis patients; initiate treatment when hemoglobin is <10 g/dL; reduce dose or interrupt treatment if hemoglobin approaches or exceeds 11 g/dL): IV, SubQ: Initial dose: 50 to 100 units/kg 3 times a week

Chronic kidney disease patients NOT on dialysis (consider initiating treatment when hemoglobin is <10 g/dL; use only if rate of hemoglobin decline would likely result in RBC transfusion and desire is to reduce risk of alloimmunization and/or other RBC transfusion-related risks; reduce dose or interrupt treatment if hemoglobin exceeds 10 g/dL): IV, SubQ: Initial dose: 50 to 100 units/kg 3 times a week

Dosage adjustments for chronic kidney disease patients (either on dialysis or not on dialysis): Do not increase dose more frequently than every 4 weeks (dose decreases may occur more frequently); avoid frequent dosage adjustments.

If hemoglobin does not increase by >1 g/dL after 4 weeks: Increase dose by 25%

If hemoglobin increases >1 g/dL in any 2-week period: Reduce dose by ≥25%

Inadequate or lack of response over a 12-week escalation period: Further increases are unlikely to improve response and may increase risks; use the minimum effective dose that will maintain a hemoglobin level sufficient to avoid RBC transfusions and evaluate patient for other causes of anemia. Discontinue therapy if responsiveness does not improve.

Anemia due to chemotherapy in cancer patients: Initiate treatment only if hemoglobin <10 g/dL and anticipated duration of myelosuppressive chemotherapy is at least 2 additional months. Titrate dosage to use the minimum effective dose that will maintain a hemoglobin level sufficient to avoid red blood cell transfusions. Discontinue erythropoietin following completion of chemotherapy. SubQ: Initial dose: 150 units/kg 3 times a week or 40,000 units once weekly until completion of chemotherapy

Dosage adjustments:

If hemoglobin does not increase by ≥1 g/dL **and** remains below 10 g/dL after initial 4 weeks: Increase to 300 units/kg 3 times a week or 60,000 units weekly; discontinue after 8 weeks of treatment if RBC transfusions are still required or there is no hemoglobin response

If hemoglobin exceeds a level needed to avoid red blood cell transfusion: Withhold dose; resume treatment with a 25% dose reduction when hemoglobin approaches a level where transfusions may be required.

If hemoglobin increases >1 g/dL in any 2-week period **or** hemoglobin reaches a level sufficient to avoid red blood cell transfusion: Reduce dose by 25%.

Anemia due to zidovudine in HIV-infected patients: Titrate dosage to use the minimum effective dose that will maintain a hemoglobin level sufficient to avoid red blood cell transfusions. Hemoglobin levels should not exceed 12 g/dL.

Serum erythropoietin levels ≤500 mUnits/mL and zidovudine doses ≤4200 mg/week): IV, SubQ: Initial: 100 units/kg 3 times a week; if hemoglobin does not increase after 8 weeks, increase dose by ~50 to 100 units/kg at 4 to 8 week intervals until hemoglobin reaches a level sufficient to avoid RBC transfusion; maximum dose: 300 units/kg. Withhold dose if hemoglobin exceeds 12 g/dL, may resume treatment with a 25% dose reduction once hemoglobin <11 g/dL. Discontinue if hemoglobin increase is not achieved with 300 units/kg for 8 weeks.

Surgery patients (perioperative hemoglobin should be >10 g/dL and ≤13 g/dL; DVT prophylactic anticoagulation is recommended): SubQ: Initial dose:

300 units/kg/day for 15 days total, beginning 10 days before surgery, on the day of surgery, and for 4 days after surgery **or**

600 units/kg once weekly for 4 doses, given 21-, 14-, and 7 days before surgery, and on the day of surgery

Symptomatic anemia associated with myelodysplastic syndrome (off-label use): SubQ: 150 to 300 units/kg once daily (Greenburg 2009) or 450 to 1000 units/kg/week in divided doses, 3 to 7 times a week (Hellström-Lindberg 1995) or 60,000 units once weekly (Park 2008)

Pediatric Note: Evaluate iron status in all patients before and during treatment and maintain iron repletion.

Anemia associated with chronic kidney disease (CKD): Individualize dosing and use the lowest dose necessary to reduce the need for RBC transfusions.

Chronic kidney disease patients **ON dialysis** (IV route is preferred for hemodialysis patients; initiate treatment when hemoglobin is <10 g/dL; reduce dose or interrupt treatment if hemoglobin approaches or exceeds 11 g/dL):

Pediatrics 1 month to 16 years: IV, SubQ: Initial dose: 50 units/kg 3 times a week

Dosage adjustments for chronic kidney disease patients: Do not increase dose more frequently than every 4 weeks (dose decreases may occur more frequently); avoid frequent dosage adjustments

If hemoglobin does not increase by >1 g/dL after 4 weeks: Increase dose by 25%

If hemoglobin increases >1 g/dL in any 2-week period: Reduce dose by ≥25%

Inadequate or lack of response over a 12-week escalation period: Further increases are unlikely to improve response and may increase risks; use the minimum effective dose that will maintain a hemoglobin level sufficient to avoid RBC transfusions and evaluate patient for other causes of anemia. Discontinue therapy if responsiveness does not improve.

Anemia due to chemotherapy in cancer patients: Initiate treatment only if hemoglobin <10 g/dL and anticipated duration of myelosuppressive chemotherapy is at least 2 additional months. Titrate dosage to use the minimum effective dose that will maintain a hemoglobin level sufficient to avoid red blood cell transfusions. Discontinue erythropoietin following completion of chemotherapy.

Children ≥5 years and Adolescents: IV: Initial dose: 600 units/kg once weekly until completion of chemotherapy.

Dosage adjustments:

If hemoglobin does not increase by ≥1 g/dL **and** remains <10 g/dL after initial 4 weeks: Increase to 900 units/kg (maximum dose: 60,000 units); discontinue after 8 weeks of treatment if RBC transfusions are still required or there is no hemoglobin response.

If hemoglobin exceeds a level needed to avoid red blood cell transfusion: Withhold dose; resume treatment with a 25% dose reduction when hemoglobin approaches a level where transfusions may be required.

If hemoglobin increases >1 g/dL in any 2-week period **or** hemoglobin reaches a level sufficient to avoid red blood cell transfusion: Reduce dose by 25%.

Anemia due to zidovudine in HIV-infected patients: Titrate dosage to use the minimum effective dose that will maintain a hemoglobin level sufficient to avoid red blood cell transfusions. Hemoglobin levels should not exceed 12 g/dL. Children 8 months to 17 years (based on limited data): IV, SubQ: Reported dosing range: 50 to 400 units/kg 2 to 3 times a week

Renal Impairment No dosage adjustment necessary.

Hepatic Impairment There are no dosage adjustments provided in the manufacturer's labeling.

Administration Do not shake.

SubQ is the preferred route of administration **except** in patients with CKD on hemodialysis.; usually administered undiluted, although may use a 1:1 dilution with bacteriostatic NS.

Patients with CKD on hemodialysis: IV route preferred; it may be administered into the venous line at the end of the dialysis procedure

Monitoring Parameters Transferrin saturation and serum ferritin (prior to and during treatment); hemoglobin (weekly after initiation and following dose adjustments until stable and sufficient to minimize need for RBC transfusion, CKD patients should be also be monitored at least monthly following hemoglobin stability); blood pressure; seizures (CKD patients following initiation for first few months, includes new-onset or change in seizure frequency or premonitory symptoms)

Cancer patients: Examinations recommended by the ASCO/ASH guidelines (Rizzo 2010) prior to treatment include: peripheral blood smear (in some situations a bone marrow exam may be necessary), assessment for iron, folate, or vitamin B_{12} deficiency, reticulocyte count, renal function status, and occult blood loss; during ESA treatment, assess baseline and periodic iron, total iron-binding capacity, and transferrin saturation or ferritin levels.

Prescribing and Access Restrictions As a requirement of the REMS program, access to this medication is restricted. Healthcare providers and hospitals must be enrolled in the ESA APPRISE (Assisting Providers and Cancer Patients with Risk Information for the Safe use of ESAs) Oncology Program (866-284-8089; http://www.esa-apprise.com) to prescribe or dispense ESAs (ie, epoetin alfa, darbepoetin alfa) to patients with cancer. ▶

Medication Guide Available Yes

Dosage Forms Excipient information presented when available (limited, particularly for generics); consult specific product labeling.

Solution, Injection:

Epogen: 10,000 units/mL (2 mL); 20,000 units/mL (1 mL) [contains benzyl alcohol]

Procrit: 10,000 units/mL (2 mL); 20,000 units/mL (1 mL) [contains benzyl alcohol]

Solution, Injection [preservative free]:

Epogen: 2000 units/mL (1 mL); 3000 units/mL (1 mL); 4000 units/mL (1 mL); 10,000 units/mL (1 mL)

Procrit: 2000 units/mL (1 mL); 3000 units/mL (1 mL); 4000 units/mL (1 mL); 10,000 units/mL (1 mL); 40,000 units/mL (1 mL)

Dosage Forms: Canada Excipient information presented when available (limited, particularly for generics); consult specific product labeling.

Injection, solution [preservative free]:

Eprex: 1000 units/0.5 mL (0.5 mL), 2000 units/0.5 mL (0.5 mL), 3000 units/0.3 mL (0.3 mL), 4000 units/0.4 mL (0.4 mL), 5000 units/0.5 mL (0.5 mL), 6000 units/0.6 mL (0.6 mL), 8000 units/0.8 mL (0.8 mL), 10,000 units/mL (1 mL), 20,000 units/0.5 mL (0.5 mL), 30,000 units/0.75 mL (0.75 mL), 40,000 units/mL (1 mL) [contains polysorbate 80; prefilled syringe, free of human serum albumin]

EriBULin (er i BUE lin)

Related Information

Common Toxicity Criteria on page 2122

Management of Chemotherapy-Induced Nausea and Vomiting in Adults on page 2142

Safe Handling of Hazardous Drugs on page 2292

Brand Names: US Halaven

Brand Names: Canada Halaven

Index Terms B1939; E7389; ER-086526; Eribulin Mesylate; Halichondrin B Analog

Pharmacologic Category Antineoplastic Agent, Antimicrotubular

Use Breast cancer, metastatic: Treatment of metastatic breast cancer in patients who have received at least 2 prior chemotherapy regimens for the treatment of metastatic disease (prior treatment should have included an anthracycline and a taxane in either the adjuvant or metastatic setting)

Labeled Contraindications There are no contraindications listed in the manufacturer's labeling.

Canadian labeling (not in U.S. labeling): Hypersensitivity to eribulin mesylate, halichondrin B, or its chemical derivatives.

Pregnancy Considerations Adverse effects were observed in animal reproduction studies. Based on its mechanism of action, eribulin would be expected to cause fetal harm if administered during pregnancy. Women of childbearing potential should use effective contraception to avoid pregnancy during eribulin treatment; the Canadian labeling recommends continuing effective contraception for at least 3 months after treatment.

Breast-Feeding Considerations It is not known if eribulin is excreted in breast milk. Due to the potential for serious adverse reactions in the nursing infant, a decision should be made to discontinue eribulin or to discontinue breast-feeding, taking into account the importance of treatment to the mother.

Warnings/Precautions Hazardous agent - use appropriate precautions for handling and disposal (NIOSH 2014 [group 1]). Hematologic toxicity, including severe neutropenia, has occurred; may require treatment delay and dosage reduction. A higher incidence of grade 4 neutropenia and neutropenic fever occurred in patients with ALT or AST >3 x ULN or bilirubin >1.5 x ULN. Monitor complete blood counts prior to each dose; more frequently if severe cytopenias develop. Patients with baseline neutrophils <1,500/mm^3 were not included in clinical studies.

Peripheral neuropathy commonly occurs and is the most frequent toxicity leading to discontinuation. Peripheral neuropathy may be prolonged (>1 year in 5% of patients); may require treatment delay. Monitor for signs of peripheral motor or sensory neuropathy. Some patients may have preexisting neuropathy because of prior chemotherapy; monitor closely for worsening.

QT prolongation was observed on day 8 of eribulin therapy (in an uncontrolled study); monitor ECG in patients with heart failure, bradyarrhythmia, with concomitant medication known to prolong the QT interval, or with electrolyte imbalance; correct hypokalemia and hypomagnesemia prior to treatment; monitor electrolytes periodically during treatment. Avoid use in patients with congenital long QT syndrome.

Dosage reduction required in patients with mild to moderate (Child-Pugh class A or B) hepatic impairment; use has not been studied in patients with severe hepatic impairment; transaminase or bilirubin elevations are associated with a higher incidence of grade 4 neutropenia and neutropenic fever. Dosage reduction required in patients with moderate or severe renal impairment (CrCl 15 to 49 mL/minute). Potentially significant drug-drug interactions may exist, requiring dose or frequency adjustment, additional monitoring, and/or selection of alternative therapy. Some products available internationally may have vial strength and dosing expressed as the base (instead of as the salt); refer to prescribing information for specific dosing information.

Adverse Reactions

>10%:

Central nervous system: Fatigue (≤54%), peripheral neuropathy (35%; grades 3/4: ≤8%), headache (19%)

Dermatologic: Alopecia (45%)

Endocrine & metabolic: Weight loss (21%)

Gastrointestinal: Nausea (35%), constipation (25%), anorexia (20%), diarrhea (18%), vomiting (18%)

Hematologic & oncologic: Neutropenia (82%; grades 3: 28%; grade 4: 29%; nadir: 13 days; recovery: 8 days), anemia (58%; grades 3/4: 2%)

Hepatic: Increased serum ALT (18%)

Neuromuscular & skeletal: Weakness (≤54%), arthralgia (≤22%), myalgia (≤22%), back pain (16%), ostealgia (12%), limb pain (11%)

Respiratory: Dyspnea (16%), cough (14%)

Miscellaneous: Fever (21%)

1% to 10%:

Cardiovascular: Peripheral edema (≥5% to <10%)

Central nervous system: Depression (≥5% to <10%), dizziness (≥5% to <10%), insomnia (≥5% to <10%), myasthenia (≥5% to <10%)

Dermatologic: Skin rash (≥5% to <10%)

Endocrine & metabolic: Hypokalemia (≥5% to <10%)

Gastrointestinal: Mucosal inflammation (9%), abdominal pain (≥5% to <10%), dysgeusia (≥5% to <10%), dyspepsia (≥5% to <10%), stomatitis (≥5% to <10%), xerostomia (≥5% to <10%)

Genitourinary: Urinary tract infection (10%)

Hematologic & oncologic: Febrile neutropenia (5%), thrombocytopenia (grades 3/4: 1%)

Neuromuscular & skeletal: Muscle spasm (≥5% to <10%)

Ophthalmic: Increased lacrimation (≥5% to <10%)

Respiratory: Upper respiratory tract infection (≥5% to <10%)

<1%, postmarketing, and/or case reports: Dehydration, drug-induced hypersensitivity, hepatotoxicity, hypomagnesemia, interstitial pulmonary disease, lymphocytopenia, neutropenic sepsis, pancreatitis, pneumonia, prolonged Q-T interval on ECG, sepsis

Drug Interactions

Metabolism/Transport Effects Substrate of CYP3A4 (minor); **Note:** Assignment of Major/Minor substrate status based on clinically relevant drug interaction potential

Avoid Concomitant Use

Avoid concomitant use of EriBULin with any of the following: BCG (Intravesical); CloZAPine; Dipyrone

Increased Effect/Toxicity

EriBULin may increase the levels/effects of: CloZAPine; Highest Risk QTc-Prolonging Agents; Moderate Risk QTc-Prolonging Agents

The levels/effects of EriBULin may be increased by: Dipyrone; Mifepristone

Decreased Effect

EriBULin may decrease the levels/effects of: BCG (Intravesical)

Storage/Stability Store intact vials at 25°C (77°F); excursions permitted between 15°C and 30°C (59°F and 86°F); do not freeze. Store in original carton. Undiluted solutions in a syringe and solutions diluted in normal saline for infusion are stable for up to 4 hours at room temperature or up to 24 hours refrigerated at 4°C (40°F).

Preparation for Administration Hazardous agent; use appropriate precautions for handling and disposal (NIOSH 2014 [group 1]). No dilution required. May prepare by drawing into a syringe for administration or may dilute in 100 mL normal saline. Discard unused portion of vial.

Mechanism of Action Eribulin is a non-taxane microtubule inhibitor which is a halichondrin B analog. It inhibits the growth phase of the microtubule by inhibiting formation of mitotic spindles causing mitotic blockage and arresting the cell cycle at the G_2/M phase; suppresses microtubule polymerization yet does not affect depolymerization.

Pharmacodynamics/Kinetics

Distribution: V_d: 43 to 114 L/m²

Protein binding: 49% to 65%

Metabolism: Negligible

Half-life, elimination: ~40 hours

Excretion: Feces (82%, predominantly as unchanged drug); urine (9%, primarily as unchanged drug)

Dosing

Adult & Geriatric Note: *International Considerations:* Some products available internationally may have vial strength and dosing expressed as the base (instead of as the salt). Refer to prescribing information for specific dosing information.

Breast cancer, metastatic: IV: Eribulin mesylate: 1.4 mg/m²/dose on days 1 and 8 of a 21-day treatment cycle

Renal Impairment Note: *International Considerations:* Some products available internationally may have vial strength and dosing expressed as the base (instead of as the salt). Refer to prescribing information for specific dosing information.

Mild impairment (CrCl ≥50 mL/minute): No dosage adjustment required.

Moderate impairment (CrCl 30 to 49 mL/minute): Reduce to eribulin mesylate 1.1 mg/m²/dose.

Severe impairment (CrCl 15 to 29 mL/minute): Reduce to eribulin mesylate 1.1 mg/m²/dose.

ESRD (*Canadian labeling*): Use is not recommended.

Hepatic Impairment Note: *International Considerations:* Some products available internationally may have vial strength and dosing expressed as the base (instead of as the salt). Refer to prescribing information for specific dosing information.

Mild hepatic impairment (Child-Pugh class A): Reduce to eribulin mesylate 1.1 mg/m²/dose.

Moderate hepatic impairment (Child-Pugh class B): Reduce to eribulin mesylate 0.7 mg/m²/dose.

Severe hepatic impairment (Child-Pugh class C): There are no dosage adjustments provided in the manufacturer's U.S. labeling (has not been studied); use is not recommended in the Canadian labeling.

Obesity *ASCO Guidelines for appropriate chemotherapy dosing in obese adults with cancer:* Utilize patient's actual body weight (full weight) for calculation of body surface area- or weight-based dosing, particularly when the intent of therapy is curative; manage regimen-related toxicities in the same manner as for nonobese patients; if a dose reduction is utilized due to toxicity, consider resumption of full weight-based dosing with subsequent cycles, especially if cause of toxicity (eg, hepatic or renal impairment) is resolved (Griggs, 2012).

Adjustment for Toxicity Note: *International Considerations:* Some products available internationally may have vial strength and dosing expressed as the base (instead of as the salt). Refer to prescribing information for specific dosing information.

◀ ANC <1,000/mm³ or platelets <75,000/mm³ or grade 3 or 4 nonhematologic toxicity on day 1 or 8: Withhold dose; may delay day 8 dose up to 1 week. If toxicity resolves to ≤ grade 2 by day 15 administer a reduced dose and wait at least 2 weeks before beginning the next cycle. Omit dose if not resolved to ≤ grade 2 by day 15. Do not re-escalate dose after reduction.

Permanently reduce dose from eribulin mesylate 1.4 mg/m² to 1.1 mg/m² for the following:

ANC <500/mm³ for >7 days

ANC <1000/mm³ with fever or infection

Platelets <25,000/mm³

Platelets <50,000/mm³ requiring transfusion

Nonhematologic toxicity of grade 3 or 4

Dose omission or delay due to toxicity on day 8 of prior cycle

Permanently reduce dose from eribulin mesylate 1.1 mg/m² to 0.7 mg/m² for occurrence of any of the above events; discontinue treatment if the above toxicities occur at the 0.7 mg/m² dose level.

Combination Regimens

Breast cancer: Eribulin (Breast Regimen) on page 1962

Administration IV: Infuse over 2 to 5 minutes. May be administered undiluted or diluted. Do not administer other medications through the same IV line, or through a line containing dextrose.

Hazardous agent; use appropriate precautions for handling and disposal (NIOSH 2014 [group 1]).

Emetic Potential Low (10% to 30%)

Monitoring Parameters CBC with differential prior to each dose; renal and liver function tests; serum electrolytes, including potassium and magnesium. Assess for peripheral neuropathy prior to each dose. Monitor ECG in patients with heart failure, bradyarrhythmia, with concomitant medication known to prolong the QT interval, and electrolyte abnormalities (eg, hypokalemia, hypomagnesemia).

Additional Information *International considerations:* Eribulin mesylate 1.4 mg is equivalent to eribulin (base) 1.23 mg.

Dosage Forms Excipient information presented when available (limited, particularly for generics); consult specific product labeling.

Solution, Intravenous, as mesylate:

Halaven: 1 mg/2 mL (2 mL) [contains alcohol, usp]

◆ **Eribulin Mesylate** *see* EriBULin *on page* 624

◆ **Erismodegib** *see* Sonidegib *on page* 1543

◆ **Erivedge** *see* Vismodegib *on page* 1771

Erlotinib (er LOE tye nib)

Related Information

Management of Chemotherapy-Induced Nausea and Vomiting in Adults *on page* 2142

Management of EGFR Inhibitor Toxicities: Dermatologic, Ocular, and Gastro-intestinal *on page* 2179

Prevention of Chemotherapy-Induced Nausea and Vomiting in Children *on page* 2203

Principles of Anticancer Therapy *on page* 2261

Safe Handling of Hazardous Drugs *on page* 2292

Brand Names: US Tarceva

Brand Names: Canada Tarceva

Index Terms CP358774; Erlotinib Hydrochloride; OSI-774

Pharmacologic Category Antineoplastic Agent, Epidermal Growth Factor Receptor (EGFR) Inhibitor; Antineoplastic Agent, Tyrosine Kinase Inhibitor

Use

Non-small cell lung cancer (NSCLC): First-line treatment of metastatic non-small cell lung cancer (NSCLC) in tumors with epidermal growth factor receptor (EGFR) exon 19 deletions or exon 21 (L858R) substitution mutations as detected by an approved test; treatment of locally advanced or metastatic NSCLC after failure of at least 1 prior chemotherapy regimen; maintenance treatment of locally advanced or metastatic NSCLC which has not progressed after 4 cycles of first-line platinum-based chemotherapy

Limitations of use: Use in combination with platinum-based chemotherapy is not recommended. First-line treatment in patients with metastatic NSCLC with EGFR mutations other than exon 19 deletion or exon 21 (L858R) substitution has not been evaluated.

Pancreatic cancer (not an approved use in Canada): First-line treatment of locally advanced, unresectable, or metastatic pancreatic cancer (in combination with gemcitabine)

Labeled Contraindications

There are no contraindications listed in the manufacturer's U.S. labeling.

Canadian labeling: Hypersensitivity to erlotinib or any component of the formulation

Pregnancy Considerations Adverse events were observed in animal reproduction studies. Based on the mechanism of action, may cause fetal harm if administered in pregnancy. Females of reproductive potential should be advised to avoid pregnancy; highly effective contraception is recommended during treatment and for at least 2 weeks after treatment has been completed.

Breast-Feeding Considerations It is not known if erlotinib is excreted in breast milk. Due to the potential for serious adverse reactions in the nursing infant, the decision to discontinue breast-feeding or discontinue erlotinib should take into account the benefits of treatment to the mother.

Warnings/Precautions Hazardous agent - use appropriate precautions for handling and disposal (NIOSH 2014 [group 1]). Rare, sometimes fatal, interstitial lung disease (ILD) has occurred; symptoms include acute respiratory distress syndrome, interstitial pneumonia, obliterative bronchiolitis, pneumonitis (including radiation and hypersensitivity), pulmonary fibrosis, and pulmonary infiltrates. The onset of symptoms has been within 5 days to more than 9 months after treatment initiation (median: 39 days). Interrupt treatment for unexplained new or worsening pulmonary symptoms (dyspnea, cough, and fever); permanently discontinue for confirmed ILD.

Hepatic failure and hepatorenal syndrome have been reported, particularly in patients with baseline hepatic impairment (although have also been observed in patients with normal hepatic function). Monitor liver function (transaminases, bilirubin, and alkaline phosphatase); patients with any hepatic impairment (total bilirubin >ULN; Child-Pugh class A, B, or C) should be closely monitored, including those with hepatic disease due to tumor burden. Dosage reduction, interruption, or discontinuation may be recommended for changes in hepatic function. Use with extreme caution in patients with total bilirubin >3 times ULN. Interrupt therapy if total bilirubin is >3 times ULN or transaminases are >5 times ULN in patients without preexisting hepatic impairment. In patients with baseline hepatic dysfunction or biliary obstruction, interrupt therapy if bilirubin doubles or transaminases triple from baseline values. Increased monitoring of liver function is required in patients with preexisting hepatic impairment or biliary obstruction. Acute renal failure, renal insufficiency, and hepatorenal syndrome have been reported, either secondary to hepatic impairment at baseline or due to severe dehydration; use with caution in patients with or at risk for renal impairment. Monitor closely for dehydration; monitor renal function and electrolytes in patients at risk for dehydration. If severe renal impairment develops, interrupt therapy until toxicity resolves. Gastrointestinal perforation has been reported with use; risk for perforation is increased with concurrent anti-angiogenic agents, corticosteroids, NSAIDs, and/or taxane based-therapy, and patients with history of peptic ulcers or diverticular disease; permanently discontinue in patients who develop perforation.

Bullous, blistering, or exfoliating skin conditions, some suggestive of Stevens-Johnson or toxic epidermal necrolysis (TEN) have been reported. An acne-like rash commonly appears on the face, back, and upper chest. Generalized or severe acneiform, erythematous or maculopapular rash may occur. Skin rash may correlate with treatment response and prolonged survival (Saif, 2008); management of skin rashes that are not serious should include alcohol-free lotions, topical antibiotics, or topical corticosteroids, or if necessary, oral antibiotics and systemic corticosteroids; avoid sunlight. Reduce dose or temporarily interrupt treatment for severe skin reactions; discontinue treatment for bullous, blistering or exfoliative skin toxicity. Corneal perforation and ulceration have been reported with use; decreased tear production, abnormal eyelash growth, keratoconjunctivitis sicca, or keratitis have also been reported and are known risk factors for corneal ulceration/perforation. Interrupt or discontinue treatment in patients presenting with eye pain or other acute or worsening ocular symptoms. Consider a baseline ophthalmologic exam and reassess for ocular toxicities at 4 to 8 weeks after treatment initiation (Renouf, 2012).

MI, CVA, and microangiopathic hemolytic anemia with thrombocytopenia have been reported (rarely) with erlotinib in combination with gemcitabine. Elevated INR and bleeding events (including fatal hemorrhage) have been reported; monitor prothrombin time and INR closely. Erlotinib levels may be lower in patients who smoke; advise patients to stop smoking. Smokers treated with 300 mg/day exhibited steady-state erlotinib levels comparable to former- and never-smokers receiving 150 mg/day (Hughes, 2009). Potentially significant drug-drug interactions may exist, requiring dose or frequency adjustment, additional monitoring, and/or selection of alternative therapy. Avoid concomitant use with proton pump inhibitors. If taken with an H_2-receptor antagonist (eg, ranitidine), administer erlotinib 10 hours after the H_2-receptor antagonist dose and at least 2 hours prior to the next H_2-receptor dose. If an antacid is necessary, separate dosing by several hours. In patients with NSCLC, EGFR mutations, specifically exon 19 deletions and exon 21 mutation (L858R), are associated with better response to erlotinib (Riely, 2006); erlotinib treatment is not recommended in patients with *K-ras* mutations; they are not likely to benefit from erlotinib treatment (Eberhard, 2005; Miller, 2008). Concurrent erlotinib plus platinum-based chemotherapy is not recommended for first line treatment of locally advanced or metastatic NSCLC due to a lack of clinical benefit. The cobas EGFR mutation test has been approved to detect EGFR mutation for first-line NSCLC treatment. Product may contain lactose; avoid use in patients with Lapp lactase deficiency, glucose-galactose malabsorption, or glucose intolerance.

Adverse Reactions
Adverse reactions reported with monotherapy:
>10%:
  Cardiovascular: Chest pain (≤18%)
  Central nervous system: Fatigue (9% to 52%)
  Dermatologic: Skin rash (49% to 85%; grade 3: 5% to 13%; grade 4: <1%;
    median onset: 8 days), xeroderma (4% to 21%), pruritus (7% to 16%),
    paronychia (4% to 16%), alopecia (14% to 15%), acne vulgaris (6% to 12%)
  Gastrointestinal: Diarrhea (20% to 62%; grade 3: 2% to 6%; grade 4: <1%;
    median onset: 12 days), anorexia (9% to 52%), nausea (23% to 33%),
    decreased appetite (≤28%), vomiting (13% to 23%), mucositis (≤18%),
    stomatitis (11% to 17%), abdominal pain (3% to 11%), constipation (≤8%)
  Genitourinary: Urinary tract infection (≤4%)
  Hematologic & oncologic: Anemia (≤11%; grade 4: 1%)
  Infection: Increased susceptibility to infection (4% to 24%)
  Miscellaneous: Fever (≤11%)
  Neuromuscular & skeletal: Weakness (≤53%), back pain (19%), arthralgia
    (≤13%), musculoskeletal pain (11%)
  Ophthalmic: Conjunctivitis (12% to 18%), keratoconjunctivitis sicca (12%)
  Respiratory: Cough (33% to 48%), dyspnea (41% to 45%; grades 3/4: 8%
    to 28%)
1% to 10%:
  Cardiovascular: Peripheral edema (≤5%)
  Central nervous system: Pain (≤9%), headache (≤7%), anxiety (≤5%),
    dizziness (≤4%), insomnia (≤4%), neurotoxicity (≤4%), paresthesia (≤4%),
    voice disorder (≤4%)
  Dermatologic: Folliculitis (≤8%), nail disease (≤7%), exfoliative dermatitis
    (5%), hypertrichosis (5%), skin fissure (5%), acneiform eruption (4% to
    5%), erythema (≤5%), dermatitis (4%), erythematous rash (≤4%), palmar-
    plantar erythrodysesthesia (≤4%), bullous dermatitis
  Endocrine & metabolic: Weight loss (4% to 5%)
  Gastrointestinal: Dyspepsia (≤5%), xerostomia (≤3%), taste disorder (≤1%)
  Hematologic & oncologic: Lymphocytopenia (≤4%; grade 3: 1%), leukopenia
    (≤3%), thrombocytopenia (≤1%)
  Hepatic: Hyperbilirubinemia (7%; grade 3: ≤1%), increased serum ALT (grade
    2: 2% to 4%; grade 3: 1% to 3%), increased gamma-glutamyl transferase
    (≤4%), hepatic failure (≤1%)
  Neuromuscular & skeletal: Muscle spasm (≤4%), musculoskeletal chest pain
    (≤4%), ostealgia (≤4%)
  Otic: Tinnitus (≤1%)
  Renal: Increased serum creatinine (≤1%), renal failure (≤1%),
  Respiratory: Nasopharyngitis (≤7%), epistaxis (≤4%), pulmonary embolism
    (≤4%), respiratory tract infection (≤4%), pneumonitis (3%), pulmonary
    fibrosis (3%)
<1%: Interstitial pulmonary disease

Adverse reactions reported with combination (erlotinib plus gemcitabine) therapy:
>10%:
  Cardiovascular: Edema (37%), thrombosis (grades 3/4: 11%)
  Central nervous system: Fatigue (73% to 79%), depression (19%), dizziness
    (15%), headache (15%), anxiety (13%)
  Dermatologic: Skin rash (70%), alopecia (14%)

Gastrointestinal: Nausea (60%), anorexia (52%), diarrhea (48%), abdominal pain (46%), vomiting (42%), weight loss (39%), stomatitis (22%), dyspepsia (17%), flatulence (13%)

Hepatic: Increased serum ALT (grade 2: 31%, grade 3: 13%, grade 4: <1%), increased serum AST (grade 2: 24%, grade 3: 10%, grade 4 <1%), hyper-bilirubinemia (grade 2: 17%, grade 3: 10%, grade 4: <1%)

Infection: Increased susceptibility to infection (39%)

Miscellaneous: Fever (36%)

Neuromuscular & skeletal: Ostealgia (25%), myalgia (21%), neuropathy (13%), rigors (12%)

Respiratory: Dyspnea (24%), cough (16%)

1% to 10%:

Cardiovascular: Cardiac arrhythmia (<5%), syncope (<5%), deep vein thrombosis (4%), cerebrovascular accident (3%; including cerebral hemorrhage), myocardial infarction (2%)

Gastrointestinal: Intestinal obstruction (<5%), pancreatitis (<5%)

Hematologic & oncologic: Hemolytic anemia (<5%), microangiopathic hemolytic anemia with thrombocytopenia (1%)

Renal: Renal insufficiency (<5%), renal failure (1%)

Respiratory: Interstitial pulmonary disease (<3%)

<1%: Bullous dermatitis, exfoliative dermatitis, hepatic failure

Mono- or combination therapy: <1%, postmarketing, and/or case reports: Acute peptic ulcer with hemorrhage, bronchiolitis, corneal perforation, corneal ulcer, decreased lacrimation, episcleritis, gastritis, gastrointestinal hemorrhage, gastrointestinal perforation, hearing loss, hematemesis, hematochezia, hepatorenal syndrome, hepatotoxicity, hirsutism, hyperpigmentation, hypokalemia, increased eyelash thickness, increased growth in number of eyelashes, keratitis, melena, misdirected growth of eyelashes, myopathy (in combination with statin therapy), ocular inflammation, peptic ulcer, rhabdomyolysis (in combination with statin therapy), skin photosensitivity, skin rash (acneiform; sparing prior radiation field), Stevens-Johnson syndrome, toxic epidermal necrolysis, tympanic membrane perforation, uveitis

Drug Interactions

Metabolism/Transport Effects Substrate of CYP1A2 (minor), CYP3A4 (major); **Note:** Assignment of Major/Minor substrate status based on clinically relevant drug interaction potential; **Inhibits** UGT1A1

Avoid Concomitant Use

Avoid concomitant use of Erlotinib with any of the following: Conivaptan; Fusidic Acid (Systemic); Idelalisib; Irinotecan Products; Proton Pump Inhibitors

Increased Effect/Toxicity

Erlotinib may increase the levels/effects of: Irinotecan Products; Warfarin

The levels/effects of Erlotinib may be increased by: Aprepitant; Ciprofloxacin (Systemic); Conivaptan; CYP3A4 Inhibitors (Moderate); CYP3A4 Inhibitors (Strong); Dasatinib; FluvoxaMINE; Fosaprepitant; Fusidic Acid (Systemic); Grapefruit Juice; Idelalisib; Ivacaftor; Luliconazole; Mifepristone; Netupitant; Osimertinib; Palbociclib; Simeprevir; Stiripentol

Decreased Effect

The levels/effects of Erlotinib may be decreased by: Antacids; Bosentan; CYP3A4 Inducers (Moderate); CYP3A4 Inducers (Strong); Dabrafenib; Deferasirox; Enzalutamide; H2-Antagonists; Mitotane; Osimertinib; Proton Pump Inhibitors; Siltuximab; St Johns Wort; Tocilizumab

Food Interactions Erlotinib bioavailability is increased with food. Grapefruit or grapefruit juice may decrease metabolism and increase erlotinib plasma concentrations. Management: Take on an empty stomach at least 1 hour before or 2 hours after the ingestion of food. Avoid grapefruit and grapefruit juice. Maintain adequate nutrition and hydration, unless instructed to restrict fluid intake.

Storage/Stability Store at 25°C (77°F); excursions are permitted between 15°C and 30°C (59°F and 86°F).

Mechanism of Action Reversibly inhibits overall epidermal growth factor receptor (HER1/EGFR) - tyrosine kinase activity. Intracellular phosphorylation is inhibited which prevents further downstream signaling, resulting in cell death. Erlotinib has higher binding affinity for EGFR exon 19 deletion or exon 21 L858R mutations than for the wild type receptor.

Pharmacodynamics/Kinetics

Absorption: Oral: 60% on an empty stomach; almost 100% on a full stomach

Distribution: 232 L

Protein binding: ~93% to albumin and alpha$_1$-acid glycoprotein

Metabolism: Hepatic, via CYP3A4 (major), CYP1A1 (minor), CYP1A2 (minor), and CYP1C (minor)

Bioavailability: Almost 100% when given with food; 60% without food

Half-life elimination: 36 hours

Time to peak, plasma: 4 hours

Excretion: Primarily as metabolites: Feces (83%; 1% as unchanged drug); urine (8%; <1% as unchanged drug)

Dosing

Adult & Geriatric

Non-small cell lung cancer (NSCLC), metastatic, first-line therapy in patients with EGFR exon 19 deletions or exon 21 (L858R) substitution mutations: Oral: 150 mg once daily until disease progression or unacceptable toxicity (Rosell, 2012; Zhou, 2011).

NSCLC, refractory: Oral: 150 mg once daily until disease progression or unacceptable toxicity (Shepherd, 2005)

NSCLC, maintenance therapy: Oral: 150 mg once daily until disease progression or unacceptable toxicity (Capuzzo, 2010)

Pancreatic cancer: Oral: 100 mg once daily until disease progression or unacceptable toxicity (in combination with gemcitabine) (Moore, 2007)

Dosage adjustment for concomitant CYP3A4 inhibitors/inducers:

CYP3A4 inhibitors: Avoid concurrent use if possible; consider dose reductions for severe adverse reactions if erlotinib is administered concomitantly with strong CYP3A4 inhibitors (eg, azole antifungals, clarithromycin, erythromycin, nefazodone, protease inhibitors, telithromycin, grapefruit, or grapefruit juice). Dose reduction (if required) should be done in decrements of 50 mg (after toxicity has resolved to baseline or ≤ grade 1).

Concomitant CYP3A4 and CYP1A2 inhibitor (eg, ciprofloxacin): Avoid concurrent use if possible; consider dose reductions in decrements of 50 mg if severe adverse reactions occur (after toxicity has resolved to baseline or ≤ grade 1).

CYP3A4 inducers: Alternatives to the enzyme-inducing agent should be utilized first. Concomitant administration with CYP3A4 inducers (eg, carbamazepine, phenobarbital, phenytoin, rifamycins, and St John's wort) may require increased erlotinib doses (increase as tolerated at 2-week intervals in 50 mg increments to a maximum of 450 mg); doses >150 mg daily should be considered with rifampin (the maximum erlotinib dose studied in combination with rifampin was 450 mg). Immediately reduce erlotinib dose to recommended starting dose when CYP3A4 inducer is discontinued.

Dosage adjustment for concomitant smoking: Increase dose at 2-week intervals in 50 mg increments to a maximum dose of 300 mg (with careful monitoring) in patients who continue to smoke; immediately reduce erlotinib dose to recommended starting dose upon smoking cessation.

Renal Impairment

Renal impairment at treatment initiation: There are no dosage adjustments provided in the manufacturer's labeling (has not been studied), although <9% of a single dose is excreted in the urine.

Renal toxicity during treatment: Withhold treatment for grades 3/4 renal toxicity (consider discontinuing) and for risk of renal failure due to dehydration; may resume after euvolemia re-established (at previous dose). If treatment withheld due to toxicity and therapy is resumed, reinitiate with a 50 mg dose reduction after toxicity has resolved to baseline or ≤ grade 1.

Hepatic Impairment

Hepatic impairment at treatment initiation:

U.S. labeling:

Total bilirubin > ULN or Child-Pugh classes A, B, and C: There are no dosage adjustments provided in the manufacturer's labeling; use with caution and monitor closely during treatment.

Total bilirubin >3 times ULN: Use extreme caution.

Canadian labeling:

Moderate impairment: There are no dosage adjustments provided in the manufacturer's labeling; however, a reduced dose should be considered.

Severe impairment (including total bilirubin >3 times ULN and/or transaminases >5 times ULN): Use is not recommended.

The following adjustments have also been studied: A reduced starting dose (75 mg once daily) has been recommended in patients with hepatic dysfunction (AST ≥3 times ULN or direct bilirubin 1-7 mg/dL), with individualized dosage escalation if tolerated (Miller, 2007); another study determined that pharmacokinetic and safety profiles were similar between patients with normal hepatic function and moderate hepatic impairment (O'Bryant, 2012).

Hepatotoxicity during treatment: U.S. labeling:

Patients with normal hepatic function at baseline: If total bilirubin >3 times ULN and/or transaminases >5 times ULN during use: Interrupt therapy (consider discontinuing); if treatment is resumed, reinitiate with a 50 mg dose reduction after bilirubin and transaminases return to baseline; discontinue treatment if there is no significant improvement or resolution within 3 weeks.

Patients with baseline hepatic impairment or biliary obstruction: If bilirubin doubles or transaminases triple over baseline during use: Interrupt therapy (consider discontinuing); if treatment is resumed, reinitiate with a 50 mg dose reduction after bilirubin and transaminases return to baseline; discontinue treatment if there is no significant improvement or resolution of hepatotoxicity within 3 weeks.

Adjustment for Toxicity

Dermatologic toxicity:

Bullous, blistering, or exfoliative skin toxicity (severe): Discontinue treatment.

Severe rash (unresponsive to medical management): Withhold treatment; may reinitiate with a 50 mg dose reduction after toxicity has resolved to baseline or ≤ grade 1.

Gastrointestinal toxicity:

Diarrhea: Manage with loperamide; in severe diarrhea (unresponsive to loperamide) or dehydration due to diarrhea, withhold treatment; may reinitiate with a 50 mg dose reduction after toxicity has resolved to baseline or ≤ grade 1.

Gastrointestinal perforation: Discontinue treatment.

Ocular toxicities:

Acute or worsening ocular toxicities (eg, eye pain): Interrupt and consider discontinuing treatment. If therapy is resumed, reinitiate with a 50 mg dose reduction after toxicity has resolved to baseline or ≤ grade 1.

Corneal perforation or severe ulceration: Discontinue treatment.

Keratitis (grade 3 or 4 or grade 2 persisting >2 weeks): Withhold treatment; may reinitiate with a 50 mg dose reduction after toxicity has resolved to baseline or ≤ grade 1.

Pulmonary symptoms: Acute onset (or worsening) of pulmonary symptoms (eg, dyspnea, cough, fever): Interrupt treatment and evaluate for drug-induced interstitial lung disease; discontinue permanently with development of interstitial lung disease

Combination Regimens

Lung cancer (non-small cell): Erlotinib (NSCLC Regimen) on page 1962

Pancreatic cancer: Erlotinib-Gemcitabine (Pancreatic) on page 1962

Administration The manufacturer recommends administration on an empty stomach (at least 1 hour before or 2 hours after the ingestion of food). Avoid concomitant use with proton pump inhibitors. If taken with an H_2-receptor antagonist (eg, ranitidine), administer erlotinib 10 hours after the H_2-receptor antagonist dose and at least 2 hours prior to the next H_2- receptor dose. If an antacid is necessary, separate dosing by several hours.

For patients unable to swallow whole, tablets may be dissolved in 100 mL water and administered orally or via feeding tube (silicone-based); to ensure full dose is received, rinse container with 40 mL water, administer residue and repeat rinse (data on file, Genentech [contact product manufacturer to obtain current information]; Siu, 2007; Soulieres, 2004).

Hazardous agent; use appropriate precautions for handling and disposal (NIOSH 2014 [group 1]).

Emetic Potential Children and Adults: Minimal (<10%)

Extemporaneous Preparations Hazardous agent; use appropriate precautions for handling and disposal (NIOSH 2014 [group 1]).

A suspension for oral or feeding tube (silicone-based) administration may be prepared by dissolving tablets needed for dose in 100 mL water. To ensure full dose is received, rinse container with 40 mL water, administer residue and repeat rinse. Administer immediately after preparation; stability of solution is unknown (Data on file from Genentech [contact product manufacturer to obtain current information]).

Siu LL, Soulieres D, Chen EX, et al, "Phase I/II Trial of Erlotinib and Cisplatin in Patients With Recurrent or Metastatic Squamous Cell Carcinoma of the Head and Neck: A Princess Margaret Hospital Phase II Consortium and National Cancer Institute of Canada Clinical Trials Group Study," *J Clin Oncol*, 2007, 25(16):2178-83.

Soulieres D, Senzer NN, Vokes EE, et al, "Multicenter Phase II Study of Erlotinib, an Oral Epidermal Growth Factor Receptor Tyrosine Kinase Inhibitor, in Patients With Recurrent or Metastatic Squamous Cell Cancer of the Head and Neck," *J Clin Oncol*, 2004, 22(1):77-85.

Monitoring Parameters Periodic liver function tests (transaminases, bilirubin, and alkaline phosphatase); monitor more frequently with worsening liver function; periodic renal function tests and serum electrolytes (in patients at risk for dehydration); hydration status; signs/symptoms of pulmonary toxicity; prothrombin time and INR (in patients on concomitant warfarin therapy); consider a baseline ophthalmologic exam and reassess for ocular toxicities at 4 to 8 weeks after treatment initiation (Renouf, 2012); EGFR mutation status in patients with NSCLC adenocarcinoma (Keedy, 2011); the cobas EGFR mutation test has been approved to detect EGFR mutation for first-line NSCLC treatment

Dietary Considerations Take this medicine on an empty stomach, 1 hour before or 2 hours after a meal. Avoid grapefruit juice.

Additional Information In patients with NSCLC, some factors which correlate positively with response to EGFR-tyrosine kinase inhibitor (TKI) therapy include patients who have never smoked, EGFR mutation, and patients of Asian origin. EGFR mutations, specifically exon 19 deletions and exon 21 mutation (L858R) correlate with response to tyrosine kinase inhibitors (Riely, 2006). *K-ras* mutations correlated with poorer outcome with EGFR-TKI therapy in patients with NSCLC (Cooley, 2008; Jackman, 2008; Masarelli, 2007; Shepherd, 2005).

Dosage Forms Excipient information presented when available (limited, particularly for generics); consult specific product labeling.
Tablet, Oral:
  Tarceva: 25 mg [contains fd&c yellow #6 (sunset yellow)]
  Tarceva: 100 mg, 150 mg

♦ **Erlotinib Hydrochloride** *see* Erlotinib *on page* 628

♦ **Erwinase (Can)** *see* Asparaginase (*Erwinia*) *on page* 150

♦ **Erwinaze** *see* Asparaginase (*Erwinia*) *on page* 150

♦ *Erwinia chrysanthemi* *see* Asparaginase (*Erwinia*) *on page* 150

♦ **Erythropoiesis-Stimulating Agent (ESA)** *see* Darbepoetin Alfa *on page* 448

♦ **Erythropoiesis-Stimulating Agent (ESA)** *see* Epoetin Alfa *on page* 615

♦ **Erythropoiesis-Stimulating Protein** *see* Darbepoetin Alfa *on page* 448

♦ **Erythropoietin** *see* Epoetin Alfa *on page* 615

Estramustine (es tra MUS teen)

Related Information
  Management of Chemotherapy-Induced Nausea and Vomiting in Adults *on page* 2142

Brand Names: US Emcyt

Brand Names: Canada Emcyt

Index Terms Estramustine Phosphate; Estramustine Phosphate Sodium

Pharmacologic Category Antineoplastic Agent, Alkylating Agent; Antineoplastic Agent, Antimicrotubular; Antineoplastic Agent, Hormone (Estrogen/Nitrogen Mustard)

Use

Prostate cancer: Treatment (palliative) of progressive or metastatic prostate cancer

Limitation of use: A clinical practice guideline from the American Society of Clinical Oncology (ASCO) and Cancer Care Ontario recommends that estramustine not be offered to men with metastatic castration-resistant prostate cancer due to a lack of benefit in survival or quality of life (Basch, 2014).

Labeled Contraindications Hypersensitivity to estramustine, estradiol, nitrogen mustard, or any component of the formulation; active thrombophlebitis or thromboembolic disorders (except where tumor mass is the cause of thromboembolic disorder and the benefit may outweigh the risk)

Canadian labeling: Additional contraindications (not in the U.S. labeling): Severe hepatic or cardiac disease

Pregnancy Considerations Estramustine is not indicated for use in women. Some men who were impotent on estrogen therapy have regained potency while taking estramustine; effective contraception should be used for male patients with partners of childbearing potential.

Breast-Feeding Considerations Estramustine is not indicated for use in women.

Warnings/Precautions Hazardous agent - use appropriate precautions for handling and disposal (NIOSH 2014 [group 1]). Glucose tolerance may be decreased; use with caution in patients with diabetes. Hypertension (monitor blood pressure periodically), peripheral edema (new-onset or exacerbation), or congestive heart disease may occur; use with caution in patients where fluid accumulation may be poorly tolerated, including cardiovascular disease (HF or hypertension), migraine, seizure disorder or renal dysfunction. Estrogen treatment for prostate cancer is associated with an increased risk of thrombosis and MI; (including fatalities); use caution with history of thrombophlebitis, thrombosis, or thromboembolic disease or history of cerebrovascular or coronary artery disease. Liver enzyme and bilirubin abnormalities may occur; monitor during and for 2 months after treatment. Use with caution in patients with hepatic impairment (may be metabolized poorly) or with metabolic bone diseases. Allergic reactions and angioedema, including airway involvement, have been reported with use. Patients with prostate cancer and osteoblastic metastases are at risk for hypocalcemia; monitor calcium. Estrogenic effects may decrease testosterone levels; may cause gynecomastia and/or impotence. Potentially significant drug-drug/drug-food interactions may exist, requiring dose or frequency adjustment, additional monitoring, and/or selection of alternative therapy. Avoid vaccination with live vaccines during treatment (risk of infection may be increased due to immunosuppression). Although the response to vaccines may be diminished, inactivated vaccines may be administered during treatment. Estramustine is associated with a moderate emetic potential; antiemetics are recommended to prevent nausea and vomiting. A clinical practice guideline from the American Society of Clinical Oncology (ASCO) and Cancer Care Ontario recommends that estramustine not be offered to men with metastatic castration-resistant prostate cancer due to a lack of benefit in survival or quality of life (Basch, 2014).

Adverse Reactions

>10%:

Cardiovascular: Edema (20%)

Endocrine & metabolic: Gynecomastia (75%), breast tenderness (71%), libido decreased

Gastrointestinal: Nausea (16%), diarrhea (13%), gastrointestinal upset (12%)

Hepatic: LDH increased (2% to 33%), AST increased (2% to 33%)

Respiratory: Dyspnea (12%)

1% to 10%:

Cardiovascular: CHF (3%), MI (3%), cerebrovascular accident (2%), chest pain (1%), flushing (1%)

Central nervous system: Lethargy (4%), insomnia (3%), emotional lability (2%), anxiety (1%), headache (1%)

Dermatologic: Bruising (3%), dry skin (2%), pruritus (2%), hair thinning (1%), rash (1%), skin peeling (1%)

Gastrointestinal: Anorexia (4%), flatulence (2%), burning throat (1%), gastrointestinal bleeding (1%), thirst (1%), vomiting (1%)

Hematologic: Leukopenia (4%), thrombocytopenia (1%)

Hepatic: Bilirubin increased (1% to 2%)

Local: Thrombophlebitis (3%)

Neuromuscular & skeletal: Leg cramps (9%)

Ocular: Tearing (1%)

Respiratory: Pulmonary embolism (2%), upper respiratory discharge (1%), hoarseness (1%)

<1%, postmarketing, and/or case reports: Allergic reactions, anemia, angina, angioedema, cerebrovascular ischemia, confusion, coronary ischemia, depression, glucose tolerance decreased, hyper-/hypocalcemia, hypertension, impotence, muscle weakness, venous thrombosis

Drug Interactions

Metabolism/Transport Effects None known.

Avoid Concomitant Use

Avoid concomitant use of Estramustine with any of the following: BCG (Intravesical); Natalizumab; Pimecrolimus; Tacrolimus (Topical); Tofacitinib; Vaccines (Live)

Increased Effect/Toxicity

Estramustine may increase the levels/effects of: Fingolimod; Leflunomide; Natalizumab; Tofacitinib; Vaccines (Live)

The levels/effects of Estramustine may be increased by: Clodronate; Denosumab; Pimecrolimus; Roflumilast; Tacrolimus (Topical); Trastuzumab

Decreased Effect

Estramustine may decrease the levels/effects of: BCG (Intravesical); Coccidioides immitis Skin Test; Sipuleucel-T; Vaccines (Inactivated); Vaccines (Live)

The levels/effects of Estramustine may be decreased by: Calcium Salts; Echinacea

Food Interactions Estramustine serum levels may be decreased if taken with milk or other dairy products, calcium supplements, and vitamins containing calcium. Management: Take on an empty stomach at least 1 hour before or 2 hours after eating.

Storage/Stability Store refrigerated at 2°C to 8°C (36°F to 46°F).

Mechanism of Action Estradiol and nornitrogen mustard carbamate-linked combination which has antiandrogen effects (due to estradiol) and antimicrotubule effects (due to nornitrogen mustard); causes a marked decrease in plasma testosterone and an increase in estrogen levels.

Pharmacodynamics/Kinetics

Absorption: Incomplete (Bergenheim, 1998)

Metabolism: Initially dephosphorylated in the GI tract, then hepatically oxidated and hydrolyzed to estramustine, estromustine (oxidized isomer of estramustine), estrone, and estradiol.

Bioavailability: Oral: 44% to 75% (Bergenheim, 1998)

Half-life elimination: Estromustine: 13.6 hours (range: 9-23 hours); Estrone: 16.5 hours (Bergenheim, 1998)

Time to peak: 2-3 hours (Bergenheim, 1998)

Excretion: Feces (primarily); urine (trace amounts) (Bergenheim, 1998)

Dosing

Adult & Geriatric Note: Estramustine is associated with a moderate emetic potential; antiemetics are recommended to prevent nausea and vomiting.

Prostate cancer, progressive or metastatic: Males: Oral: 14 mg/kg/day (range: 10-16 mg/kg/day) in 3 or 4 divided doses

Renal Impairment There are no dosage adjustments provided in the manufacturer's labeling; use with caution.

Hepatic Impairment There are no dosage adjustments provided in the manufacturer's labeling; use with caution (may be poorly metabolized).

Obesity *ASCO Guidelines for appropriate chemotherapy dosing in obese adults with cancer:* Utilize patient's actual body weight (full weight) for calculation of body surface area- or weight-based dosing, particularly when the intent of therapy is curative; manage regimen-related toxicities in the same manner as for nonobese patients; if a dose reduction is utilized due to toxicity, consider resumption of full weight-based dosing with subsequent cycles, especially if cause of toxicity (eg, hepatic or renal impairment) is resolved (Griggs, 2012).

Administration Estramustine is associated with a moderate emetic potential; antiemetics are recommended to prevent nausea and vomiting.

Administer on an empty stomach, at least 1 hour before or 2 hours after eating. Administer with water; do not administer with milk, milk-based products, or calcium products.

Hazardous agent; use appropriate precautions for handling and disposal (NIOSH 2014 [group 1]).

Emetic Potential Moderate (30% to 90%)

Monitoring Parameters Serum calcium, liver function tests (during and for 2 months following treatment); blood pressure

Dietary Considerations Should be taken at least 1 hour before or 2 hours after eating. Milk products and calcium-rich foods or supplements may impair the oral absorption of estramustine phosphate sodium.

Dosage Forms Excipient information presented when available (limited, particularly for generics); consult specific product labeling.

Capsule, Oral, as phosphate sodium:

Emcyt: 140 mg

♦ **Estramustine Phosphate** *see* Estramustine *on page 636*

♦ **Estramustine Phosphate Sodium** *see* Estramustine *on page 636*

♦ **ET-743** *see* Trabectedin *on page 1665*

Ethiodized Oil (eth EYE oh dyezd oyl)

Pharmacologic Category Diagnostic Agent, Radiologic Examination of GI Tract

Use

Hysterosalpingography: For hysterosalpingography in adults

Lymphography: For lymphography in adult and pediatric patients

Selective hepatic intra-arterial injection: For imaging tumors in adults with known hepatocellular carcinoma (HCC)

Pregnancy Risk Factor C

Dosing

Adult Use the smallest possible dose based on anatomical area to be visualized; dose varies with procedure. Refer to prescribing information for detailed dosing and administration information.

Hysterosalpingography: Inject in 2 mL increments into the endometrial cavity until tubal patency is observed; discontinue use if excessive discomfort develops. Reimage after 24 hours to determine if ethiodized oil has entered the peritoneal cavity.

Lymphography: Note: Inject into lymphatic vessel under radiological monitoring. Interrupt injection if patient experiences pain; discontinue injection if lymphatic blockage is present (to minimize entry into the venous circulation via lymphovenous channels) and/or as soon as ethiodized oil is radiographically evident in the thoracic duct (to minimize entry into the subclavian vein and pulmonary embolization). Obtain immediate postinjection images; reimage at 24 to 48 hours to evaluate nodal architecture.

Unilateral lymphography of upper extremities: 2 to 4 mL

Unilateral lymphography of lower extremities: 6 to 8 mL

Penile lymphography: 2 to 3 mL

Cervical lymphography: 1 to 2 mL

Selective hepatic intra-arterial injection: Note: Dose depends on tumor size, local blood flow in liver and tumor: Dosage range: 1.5 to 15 mL administered slowly under continuous radiologic monitoring; discontinue administration when stagnation or reflux is evident. Limit dose to the quantity required for adequate visualization; maximum total dose: 20 mL

Pediatric Use the smallest possible dose based on anatomical area to be visualized; dose varies with procedure. Refer to prescribing information for detailed dosing and administration information.

Lymphography: 1 to 6 mL according to area to be visualized; Maximum dose: 0.25 mL/kg.

Note: Inject into lymphatic vessel under radiological monitoring. Interrupt injection if patient experiences pain; discontinue injection if lymphatic blockage is present (to minimize entry into the venous circulation via lymphovenous channels) and/or as soon as ethiodized oil is radiographically evident in the thoracic duct (to minimize entry into the subclavian vein and pulmonary embolization). Obtain immediate postinjection images; reimage at 24 to 48 hours to evaluate nodal architecture.

Renal Impairment There are no dosage adjustments provided in the manufacturer's labeling.

Hepatic Impairment There are no dosage adjustments provided in the manufacturer's labeling.

Additional Information Complete prescribing information should be consulted for additional detail.

Dosage Forms Excipient information presented when available (limited, particularly for generics); consult specific product labeling.
Injection: Iodine 37% (10 mL)

◆ **Ethiofos** *see* Amifostine *on page 85*

◆ **Ethoxynaphthamido Penicillin Sodium** *see* Nafcillin *on page 1189*

◆ **Ethyol** *see* Amifostine *on page 85*

◆ **ETOP** *see* Etoposide Phosphate *on page 651*

◆ **Etopophos** *see* Etoposide Phosphate *on page 651*

Etoposide (e toe POE side)

Related Information

Chemotherapy and Obesity *on page 2220*
Hematopoietic Stem Cell Transplantation *on page 2272*
Management of Chemotherapy-Induced Nausea and Vomiting in Adults *on page 2142*
Management of Drug Extravasations *on page 2159*
Palliative Care Medicine (Cancer) *on page 2252*
Prevention of Chemotherapy-Induced Nausea and Vomiting in Children *on page 2203*
Safe Handling of Hazardous Drugs *on page 2292*

Brand Names: US Toposar

Brand Names: Canada Etoposide Injection; Etoposide Injection USP; Vepesid

Index Terms EPEG; Epipodophyllotoxin; VePesid; VP-16; VP-16-213; VP16

Pharmacologic Category Antineoplastic Agent, Podophyllotoxin Derivative; Antineoplastic Agent, Topoisomerase II Inhibitor

Use

Small cell lung cancer (oral and IV): Treatment (first-line) of small cell lung cancer (SCLC)

Testicular cancer (IV): Treatment of refractory testicular tumors (injectable formulation)

Canadian labeling: Treatment of small cell lung cancer (SCLC; first- and second-line); treatment of non-small cell lung cancer (NSCLC); treatment of non-Hodgkin lymphomas (first-line); treatment of testicular cancer (first-line [injectable formulation] and refractory)

Labeled Contraindications Hypersensitivity to etoposide or any component of the formulation

Canadian labeling: Additional contraindications (not in U.S. labeling): Severe leukopenia or thrombocytopenia; severe hepatic impairment; severe renal impairment

Pregnancy Considerations Adverse events were observed in animal reproduction studies. Fetal growth restriction and newborn myelosuppression have been observed following maternal use of regimens containing etoposide during pregnancy (NTP 2013; Peccatori 2013). The European Society for Medical Oncology has published guidelines for diagnosis, treatment, and follow-up of cancer during pregnancy. The guidelines recommend referral to a facility with expertise in cancer during pregnancy and encourage a multidisciplinary team (obstetrician, neonatologist, oncology team). In general, if chemotherapy is indicated, it should be avoided during in the first trimester, there should be a 3-week time period between the last chemotherapy dose and anticipated ▶

delivery, and chemotherapy should not be administered beyond week 33 of gestation. Guidelines for the treatment of SCLC are not provided (Peccatori 2013).

In women of reproductive potential, product labeling for etoposide phosphate notes that it may cause amenorrhea, infertility, or premature menopause; effective contraception should be used during therapy and for ≥6 months after the last dose. In males, azoospermia, oligospermia, or permanent loss of fertility may occur. In addition, spermatozoa and testicular tissue may be damaged. Males with female partners of reproductive potential should use condoms during therapy and for ≥4 months after the last dose.

Breast-Feeding Considerations Etoposide is excreted in breast milk. Based on data from one case report, concentrations are below the limit of detection 24 hours after the last dose (Azuno 1995). Due to the potential for serious adverse reactions in the nursing infant, the manufacturer recommends a decision be made whether to discontinue nursing or to discontinue the drug, taking into account the importance of treatment to the mother.

Warnings/Precautions Hazardous agent - use appropriate precautions for handling and disposal (NIOSH 2014 [group 1]). **[U.S. Boxed Warning]: Severe dose-limiting and dose-related myelosuppression with resulting infection or bleeding may occur.** Treatment should be withheld for platelets <50,000/mm^3 or absolute neutrophil count (ANC) <500/mm^3. May cause anaphylactic-like reactions manifested by chills, fever, tachycardia, bronchospasm, dyspnea, and hypotension. In addition, facial/tongue swelling, coughing, chest tightness, cyanosis, laryngospasm, diaphoresis, hypertension, back pain, loss of consciousness, and flushing have also been reported less commonly. Incidence is primarily associated with intravenous administration (up to 2%) compared to oral administration (<1%). Infusion should be interrupted and medications for the treatment of anaphylaxis should be available for immediate use. High drug concentration and rate of infusion, as well as presence of benzyl alcohol in the etoposide intravenous formulation have been suggested as contributing factors to the development of hypersensitivity reactions. Etoposide intravenous formulations may contain benzyl alcohol, while etoposide phosphate (the water soluble prodrug of etoposide) intravenous formulation does not contain benzyl alcohol. Case reports have suggested that etoposide phosphate has been used successfully in patients with previous hypersensitivity reactions to etoposide (Collier, 2008; Siderov, 2002). The use of concentrations higher than recommended were associated with higher rates of anaphylactic-like reactions in children.

Secondary acute leukemias have been reported with etoposide, either as monotherapy or in combination with other chemotherapy agents. Must be diluted; do not give IV push, infuse over at least 30 to 60 minutes; hypotension is associated with rapid infusion. If hypotension occurs, interrupt infusion and administer IV hydration and supportive care; decrease infusion upon reinitiation. Etoposide is an irritant; tissue irritation and inflammation have occurred following extravasation. Do not administer IM or SubQ. Dosage should be adjusted in patients with hepatic or renal impairment (Canadian labeling contraindicates use in severe hepatic and/or renal impairment). Use with caution in patients with low serum albumin; may increase risk for toxicities. Use with caution in elderly patients; may be more likely to develop severe myelosuppression and/or GI effects (eg, nausea/vomiting). **[U.S. Boxed Warning]: Should be administered under the supervision of an experienced cancer chemotherapy physician.**

Oral etoposide is associated with a low (adults) or moderate (children) emetic potential; antiemetics may be recommended to prevent nausea and vomiting (Dupuis, 2011; Roila, 2010). Potentially significant drug-drug interactions may exist, requiring dose or frequency adjustment, additional monitoring, and/or selection of alternative therapy.

Benzyl alcohol and derivatives: Some dosage forms may contain benzyl alcohol; large amounts of benzyl alcohol (≥99 mg/kg/day) have been associated with a potentially fatal toxicity ("gasping syndrome") in neonates; the "gasping syndrome" consists of metabolic acidosis, respiratory distress, gasping respirations, CNS dysfunction (including convulsions, intracranial hemorrhage), hypotension, and cardiovascular collapse (AAP ["Inactive" 1997]; CDC, 1982); some data suggests that benzoate displaces bilirubin from protein binding sites (Ahlfors, 2001); avoid or use dosage forms containing benzyl alcohol with caution in neonates. See manufacturer's labeling.

Injectable formulation contains alcohol (~33% v/v); may contribute to adverse reactions, especially with higher etoposide doses.

Polysorbate 80: Some dosage forms may contain polysorbate 80 (also known as Tweens). Hypersensitivity reactions, usually a delayed reaction, have been reported following exposure to pharmaceutical products containing polysorbate 80 in certain individuals (Isaksson, 2002; Lucente 2000; Shelley, 1995). Thrombocytopenia, ascites, pulmonary deterioration, and renal and hepatic failure have been reported in premature neonates after receiving parenteral products containing polysorbate 80 (Alade, 1986; CDC, 1984). See manufacturer's labeling.

Adverse Reactions Note: The following may occur with higher doses used in stem cell transplantation: Alopecia, ethanol intoxication, hepatitis, hypotension (infusion-related), metabolic acidosis, mucositis, nausea and vomiting (severe), secondary malignancy, skin lesions (resembling Stevens-Johnson syndrome).

>10%:
  Dermatologic: Alopecia (8% to 66%)
  Gastrointestinal: Nausea/vomiting (31% to 43%), anorexia (10% to 13%), diarrhea (1% to 13%)
  Hematologic: Leukopenia (60% to 91%; grade 4: 3% to 17%; nadir: 7-14 days; recovery: By day 20), thrombocytopenia (22% to 41%; grades 3/4: 1% to 20%; nadir: 9-16 days; recovery: By day 20), anemia (≤33%)

1% to 10%:
  Cardiovascular: Hypotension (1% to 2%; due to rapid infusion)
  Gastrointestinal: Stomatitis (1% to 6%), abdominal pain (up to 2%)
  Hepatic: Hepatic toxicity (up to 3%)
  Neuromuscular & skeletal: Peripheral neuropathy (1% to 2%)
  Miscellaneous: Anaphylactic-like reaction (IV infusion 1% to 2%; oral capsules <1%; including chills, fever, tachycardia, bronchospasm, dyspnea)

<1%, postmarketing, and/or case reports: Amenorrhea, back pain, blindness (transient/cortical), constipation, cough, cyanosis, diaphoresis, dysphagia, erythema, esophagitis, extravasation (induration/necrosis), facial swelling, fatigue, fever, hyperpigmentation, hypersensitivity, hypersensitivity-associated apnea, interstitial pneumonitis, laryngospasm, maculopapular rash, malaise, metabolic acidosis, MI, mucositis, myocardial ischemia, optic neuritis, ovarian failure, perivasculitis, pruritus, pulmonary fibrosis, radiation-recall dermatitis, rash, reversible posterior leukoencephalopathy syndrome ▶

◀ (RPLS), seizure, somnolence, Stevens-Johnson syndrome, tongue swelling, toxic epidermal necrolysis, toxic megacolon, urticaria, vasospasm, weakness

Drug Interactions

Metabolism/Transport Effects Substrate of CYP1A2 (minor), CYP2E1 (minor), CYP3A4 (major), P-glycoprotein; **Note:** Assignment of Major/Minor substrate status based on clinically relevant drug interaction potential; **Inhibits** CYP2C9 (weak)

Avoid Concomitant Use

Avoid concomitant use of Etoposide with any of the following: BCG (Intravesical); CloZAPine; Conivaptan; Dipyrone; Fusidic Acid (Systemic); Idelalisib; Natalizumab; Pimecrolimus; Tacrolimus (Topical); Tofacitinib; Vaccines (Live)

Increased Effect/Toxicity

Etoposide may increase the levels/effects of: CloZAPine; Fingolimod; Leflunomide; Natalizumab; Tofacitinib; Vaccines (Live); Vitamin K Antagonists

The levels/effects of Etoposide may be increased by: Aprepitant; Atovaquone; Conivaptan; CycloSPORINE (Systemic); CYP3A4 Inhibitors (Moderate); CYP3A4 Inhibitors (Strong); Dasatinib; Denosumab; Dipyrone; Fosaprepitant; Fusidic Acid (Systemic); Idelalisib; Ivacaftor; Luliconazole; Mifepristone; Netupitant; Osimertinib; Palbociclib; P-glycoprotein/ABCB1 Inhibitors; Pimecrolimus; Ranolazine; Roflumilast; Simeprevir; Stiripentol; Tacrolimus (Topical); Trastuzumab

Decreased Effect

Etoposide may decrease the levels/effects of: BCG (Intravesical); Coccidioides immitis Skin Test; Sipuleucel-T; Vaccines (Inactivated); Vaccines (Live)

The levels/effects of Etoposide may be decreased by: Bosentan; CYP3A4 Inducers (Moderate); CYP3A4 Inducers (Strong); Dabrafenib; Deferasirox; Enzalutamide; Mitotane; Osimertinib; P-glycoprotein/ABCB1 Inducers; Siltuximab; St Johns Wort; Tocilizumab

Storage/Stability

Capsules: Store oral capsules at 2°C to 8°C (36°F to 46°F); do not freeze. Dispense in a light-resistant container.

Injection: Store intact vials of injection at 20°C to 25°C (68°F to 77°F; do not freeze. According to the manufacturer's labeling, stability for solutions diluted for infusion in D_5W or NS (in glass or plastic containers) varies based on concentration; 0.2 mg/mL solutions are stable for 96 hours at room temperature and 0.4 mg/mL solutions are stable for 24 hours at room temperature (precipitation may occur at concentrations above 0.4 mg/mL).

Etoposide injection contains polysorbate 80 which may cause leaching of diethylhexyl phthalate (DEHP), a plasticizer contained in polyvinyl chloride (PVC) bags and tubing. Higher concentrations and longer storage time after preparation in PVC bags may increase DEHP leaching. Preparation in glass or polyolefin containers will minimize patient exposure to DEHP. When undiluted etoposide injection is stored in acrylic or ABS (acrylonitrile, butadiene and styrene) plastic containers, the containers may crack and leak.

Preparation for Administration Hazardous agent; use appropriate precautions for handling and disposal (NIOSH 2014 [group 1]). Etoposide should be diluted to a concentration of 0.2 to 0.4 mg/mL in D_5W or NS for administration. Diluted solutions have concentration-dependent stability: More concentrated solutions have shorter stability times. Precipitation may occur with concentrations >0.4 mg/mL.

Mechanism of Action Etoposide has been shown to delay transit of cells through the S phase and arrest cells in late S or early G_2 phase. The drug may inhibit mitochondrial transport at the NADH dehydrogenase level or inhibit uptake of nucleosides into HeLa cells. It is a topoisomerase II inhibitor and appears to cause DNA strand breaks. Etoposide does not inhibit microtubular assembly.

Pharmacodynamics/Kinetics

Absorption: Oral: Significant inter- and intrapatient variation

Distribution: Average V_d: 7 to 17 L/m²; poor penetration across the blood-brain barrier; CSF concentrations <5% of plasma concentrations

Protein binding: 94% to 98%

Metabolism: Hepatic, via CYP3A4 and 3A5, to various metabolites; in addition, conversion of etoposide to the O-demethylated metabolites (catechol and quinine) via prostaglandin synthases or myeloperoxidase occurs, as well as glutathione and glucuronide conjugation via GSTT1/GSTP1 and UGT1A1 (Yang, 2009)

Bioavailability: Oral: ~50% (range: 25% to 75%)

Half-life elimination: Terminal: IV: 4 to 11 hours; Children: Normal renal/hepatic function: 6 to 8 hours

Excretion:

Children: IV: Urine (~55% as unchanged drug) in 24 hours

Adults: IV: Urine (56%; 45% as unchanged drug) within 120 hours; feces (44%) within 120 hours

Dosing

Adult & Geriatric

U.S. labeling:

Small cell lung cancer (combination chemotherapy):

IV: 35 mg/m²/day for 4 days, up to 50 mg/m²/day for 5 days every 3 to 4 weeks

Oral: Due to poor bioavailability, oral doses should be twice the IV dose (and rounded to the nearest 50 mg)

Testicular cancer (combination chemotherapy): IV: 50 to 100 mg/m²/day for days 1 to 5 **or** 100 mg/m²/day on days 1, 3, and 5 repeated every 3 to 4 weeks

Canadian labeling: **Non-Hodgkin lymphoma (in combination with other agents), non-small cell lung cancer (alone or in combination), small cell lung cancer (first-line in combination; second-line alone or in combination), testicular cancer (in combination; oral therapy for refractory disease):**

IV: 50 to 100 mg/m²/day for 5 days

Oral: 100 to 200 mg/m²/day for 5 days; administer daily doses >200 mg in 2 divided doses.

Adult off-label uses and/or dosing:

Hematopoietic stem cell transplant conditioning regimen, lymphoid malignancies: IV: 60 mg/kg over 4 hours as a single dose 3 or 4 days prior to transplantation (Horning, 1994; Snyder, 1993; Weaver, 1994)

Non-small cell lung cancer: IV: 100 mg/m² days 1, 2, and 3 every 3 weeks for 4 cycles or every 4 weeks for 3 to 4 cycles (in combination with cisplatin) (Arriagada, 2004) **or** 50 mg/m² days 1 to 5 and days 29 to 33 (in combination with cisplatin and radiation therapy) (Albain, 2009)

Ovarian cancer, refractory: Oral: 50 mg/m² once daily for 21 days every 4 weeks until disease progression or unacceptable toxicity (Rose, 1998)

◄

Small cell lung cancer, limited stage (combination chemotherapy): IV: 120 mg/m^2/day on days 1, 2, and 3 every 3 weeks for 4 courses (Turrisi, 1999) **or** 100 mg/m^2/day on days 1, 2, and 3 for induction therapy, followed by consolidation chemotherapy (Saito, 2006) **or** 100 mg/m^2/day on days 1, 2, and 3 every 3 weeks up to a maximum of 6 cycles (Skarlos, 2001) **or** 100 mg/m^2/day IV on day 1, followed by 200 mg/m^2/day **orally** on days 2 through 4 every 3 weeks for a maximum of 5 courses (Sundstrom, 2002)

Small cell lung cancer, extensive stage (combination chemotherapy): 100 mg/m^2/day IV on days 1, 2, and 3 every 3 weeks for 4 cycles (Lara, 2009) **or** 100 mg/m^2/day IV on day 1, followed by 200 mg/m^2/day **orally** on days 2 through 4 every 3 weeks for a maximum of 5 courses (Sundstrom, 2002) **or** IV: 80 mg/m^2/day on days 1, 2, and 3 every 3 weeks up to 8 cycles (Ihede, 1994)

Testicular cancer (combination chemotherapy):

Nonseminoma: IV: 100 mg/m^2/day on days 1 through 5 every 21 days for 3 to 4 courses (Saxman, 1998)

Nonseminoma, metastatic (high-dose regimens): IV: 750 mg/m^2/day administered 5, 4, and 3 days before peripheral blood stem cell infusion, repeat for a second cycle after recovery of granulocyte and platelet counts (Einhorn, 2007) **or** 400 mg/m^2/day (beginning on cycle 3) on days 1, 2, and 3, with peripheral blood stem cell support, administered at 14- to 21-day intervals for 3 cycles (Kondagunta, 2007)

Thymoma, locally advanced or metastatic: IV: 120 mg/m^2 days 1, 2, and 3 every 3 weeks (in combination with cisplatin) for up to 8 cycles (Giaccone, 1996)

Unknown primary adenocarcinoma: Oral: 50 mg once daily on days 1, 3, 5, 7, and 9 alternating with 100 mg once daily on days 2, 4, 6, 8, and 10 every 3 weeks (in combination with paclitaxel and carboplatin) (Greco, 2000; Hainsworth, 2006)

Pediatric Note: Oral etoposide is associated with a moderate emetic potential; antiemetics may be recommended to prevent nausea and vomiting (Dupuis, 2011).

Acute myeloid leukemia (AML) induction (off-label use; combination chemotherapy) (Woods, 1996): IV:

<3 years: 3.3 mg/kg/day continuous infusion for 4 days

≥3 years: 100 mg/m^2/day continuous infusion for 4 days

Central nervous system tumors (off-label use; combination chemotherapy): IV:

<3 years: 6.5 mg/kg/dose days 3 and 4 of each 28-day "B" treatment cycle (Duffner, 1993)

≥3 years: 100 mg/m^2/day on days 1, 2, and 3 of a 3-week treatment cycle (Taylor, 2003)

≥6 years: 150 mg/m^2/day on days 3 and 4 of a 3-week treatment course (Kovnar, 1990)

Hematopoietic stem cell transplantation conditioning regimen: IV: 60 mg/kg/dose over 4 hours as a single dose 3 or 4 days prior to transplantation (Horning, 1994; Snyder, 1993)

Hodgkin lymphoma (off-label use): IV: 200 mg/m^2/day on days 1, 2, and 3 every 3 weeks (Kelly, 2002)

Neuroblastoma (off-label use): IV:

Induction: 100 mg/m^2/day on days 1 to 5 of each cycle (Kaneko, 2002)

Hematopoietic stem cell transplantation conditioning regimen: 200 mg/m^2/day for 4 days beginning 8 or 9 days prior to transplantation (Kaneko, 2002)

Sarcoma, refractory (off-label use): IV: 100 mg/m^2/day on days 1 to 5 of cycle; repeat cycle every 21 days (Van Winkle, 2005)

Renal Impairment Oral, IV:

The manufacturer's U.S. labeling recommends the following adjustments:

CrCl >50 mL/minute: No adjustment required.

CrCl 15 to 50 mL/minute: Administer 75% of dose

CrCl <15 mL minute: Data not available; consider further dose reductions

The following adjustments have also been recommended:

Aronoff, 2007:

Adults:

CrCl 10 to 50 mL/minute: Administer 75% of dose.

CrCl <10 mL minute: Administer 50% of dose.

Hemodialysis: Administer 50% of dose; supplemental posthemodialysis dose is not necessary.

Peritoneal dialysis: Administer 50% of dose; supplemental dose is not necessary.

Continuous renal replacement therapy (CRRT): Administer 75% of dose.

Children:

CrCl 10 to 50 mL/minute/1.73 m^2: Administer 75% of dose.

CrCl <10 mL minute/1.73 m^2: Administer 50% of dose.

Hemodialysis: Administer 50% of dose.

Peritoneal dialysis: Administer 50% of dose.

Continuous renal replacement therapy (CRRT): Administer 75% of dose and reduce for hyperbilirubinemia.

Janus, 2010: Hemodialysis: Reduce dose by 50%; not removed by hemodialysis so may be administered before or after dialysis

Kintzel, 1995:

CrCl 46 to 60 mL/minute: Administer 85% of dose

CrCl 31 to 45 mL/minute: Administer 80% of dose

CrCl ≤30 mL/minute: Administer 75% of dose

Hepatic Impairment

Manufacturer's U.S. labeling: There are no dosage adjustments provided in the manufacturer's labeling.

Canadian labeling:

Mild-to-moderate impairment: There are no dosage adjustments provided in the manufacturer's labeling.

Severe impairment: Use is contraindicated.

The following adjustments have also been recommended:

Donelli, 1998: Liver dysfunction may reduce the metabolism and increase the toxicity of etoposide. Normal doses of IV etoposide should be given to patients with liver dysfunction (dose reductions may result in subtherapeutic concentrations); however, use caution with concomitant liver dysfunction (severe) and renal dysfunction as the decreased metabolic clearance cannot be compensated by increased renal clearance.

Floyd, 2006: Bilirubin 1.5 to 3 mg/dL or AST >3 times ULN: Administer 50% of dose

King, 2001; Koren, 1992: Bilirubin 1.5 to 3 mg/dL or AST >180 units/L: Administer 50% of dose

Obesity

*American Society of Clinical Oncology (ASCO) Guidelines for appropriate chemotherapy dosing in obese adults with cancer (**Note:** Excludes HSCT dosing):* Utilize patient's actual body weight (full weight) for calculation of body surface area- or weight-based dosing, particularly when the intent of therapy is curative; manage regimen-related toxicities in the same manner as for nonobese patients; if a dose reduction is utilized due to toxicity, consider resumption of full weight-based dosing with subsequent cycles, especially if cause of toxicity (eg, hepatic or renal impairment) is resolved (Griggs, 2012).

American Society for Blood and Marrow Transplantation (ASBMT) practice guideline committee position statement on chemotherapy dosing in obesity: Utilize actual body weight (full weight) for calculation of body surface area (BSA) for BSA-based dosing and utilize adjusted body weight 25% (ABW25) for mg/kg dosing for hematopoietic stem cell transplant conditioning regimens in adults (Bubalo, 2014).

ABW25: Adjusted wt (kg) = Ideal body weight (kg) + 0.25 [actual wt (kg) - ideal body weight (kg)]

Adjustment for Toxicity Oral, IV:

Infusion (hypersensitivity) reactions: Interrupt infusion.

ANC <500/mm³ or platelets <50,000/mm³: Withhold treatment until recovery.

Severe adverse reactions (nonhematologic): Reduce dose or discontinue treatment.

WBC 2000-3000/mm³ or platelets 75,000-100,000/mm³: Canadian labeling (not in U.S. labeling): Reduce dose by 50%

Combination Regimens

Bone sarcoma (Ewing sarcoma):
Ifosfamide-Carboplatin-Etoposide (Ewing Sarcoma) on page 2014
Ifosfamide-Etoposide (Ewing Sarcoma) on page 2016
VAC Alternating With IE (Ewing Sarcoma) on page 2102
Bone sarcoma (osteosarcoma): Ifosfamide-Carboplatin-Etoposide (Osteosarcoma) on page 2015
Brain tumors:
CDDP/VP-16 on page 1877
COPE on page 1926
Gestational trophoblastic tumor:
EMA/CO (Gestational Trophoblastic Tumor) on page 1954
EMA/EP (Gestational Trophoblastic Tumor) on page 1954
EMA (Gestational Trophoblastic Tumor) on page 1955
Leukemia, acute lymphocytic: Hyper-CVAD (Leukemia, Acute Lymphocytic) on page 2006
Leukemia, acute myeloid:
5 + 2 + 5 (Cytarabine-Daunorubicin-Etoposide) (AML Consolidation) on page 1817
7 + 3 + 7 (Cytarabine-Daunorubicin-Etoposide) (AML Induction) on page 1819
Cytarabine (High Dose)-Daunorubicin-Etoposide (AML Induction) on page 1932
MEC-G (AML Induction) on page 2032
Mitoxantrone-Etoposide (AML Induction) on page 2037
Mitoxantrone-Etoposide-Cytarabine (AML) on page 2038
Lung cancer (non-small cell):
Cisplatin-Etoposide (NSCLC) on page 1894
EC (NSCLC) on page 1953

Administration

Oral etoposide is associated with a low (adults) or moderate (children) emetic potential; antiemetics may be recommended to prevent nausea and vomiting (Dupuis, 2011; Roila, 2010).

Oral: Doses ≤200 mg/day as a single once daily dose; doses >200 mg should be given in 2 divided doses. If necessary, the injection may be used for oral administration (see Extemporaneous Preparations). Canadian labeling recommends administering capsule on an empty stomach.

IV: Administer standard doses over at least 30 to 60 minutes to minimize the risk of hypotension. Higher (off-label) doses used in transplantation may be infused over longer time periods depending on the protocol. Etoposide injection contains polysorbate 80 which may cause leaching of diethylhexyl phthalate (DEHP), a plasticizer contained in polyvinyl chloride (PVC) tubing. Administration through non-PVC (low sorbing) tubing will minimize patient exposure to DEHP. Etoposide is an irritant; tissue irritation and inflammation have occurred following extravasation; avoid extravasation.

Concentrations >0.4 mg/mL are very unstable and may precipitate within a few minutes. For large doses, where dilution to ≤0.4 mg/mL is not feasible, consideration should be given to slow infusion of the undiluted drug through a running normal saline, dextrose or saline/dextrose infusion; or use of etoposide phosphate. Due to the risk for precipitation, an inline filter may be used; etoposide solutions of 0.1 to 0.4 mg/mL may be filtered through a 0.22 micron filter without damage to the filter; etoposide solutions of 0.2 mg/mL may be filtered through a 0.22 micron filter without significant loss of drug.

Hazardous agent; use appropriate precautions for handling and disposal (NIOSH 2014 [group 1]).

Vesicant/Extravasation Risk May be an irritant

Emetic Potential

Children:
Oral: Moderate (30% to 90%)
IV: Low (10% to 30%)
Adults:
Oral: Low (10% to 30%)
IV: Low (10% to 30%)

Extemporaneous Preparations Hazardous agent: Use appropriate precautions for handling and disposal (NIOSH 2014 [group 1]).

Etoposide 10 mg/mL oral solution: Dilute etoposide for injection 1:1 with normal saline to a concentration of 10 mg/mL. This solution is stable in plastic oral syringes for 22 days at room temperature. Prior to oral administration, further mix with fruit juice (orange, apple, or lemon; **NOT** grapefruit juice) to a concentration of <0.4 mg/mL; once mixed with fruit juice, use within 3 hours.
McLeod HL and Relling MV, "Stability of Etoposide Solution for Oral Use," *Am J Hosp Pharm*, 1992, 49(11):2784-5.

Monitoring Parameters CBC with differential; liver function (bilirubin, ALT, AST), albumin, renal function tests; vital signs (blood pressure); signs of an infusion reaction

Dosage Forms Excipient information presented when available (limited, particularly for generics); consult specific product labeling.
Capsule, Oral:
Generic: 50 mg

Solution, Intravenous:
  Toposar: 100 mg/5 mL (5 mL); 500 mg/25 mL (25 mL); 1 g/50 mL (50 mL)
    [contains alcohol, usp, polyethylene glycol 300, polysorbate 80]
  Generic: 100 mg/5 mL (5 mL); 500 mg/25 mL (25 mL); 1 g/50 mL (50 mL)

Etoposide Phosphate (e toe POE side FOS fate)

Related Information

Common Toxicity Criteria *on page 2122*

Management of Drug Extravasations *on page 2159*

Safe Handling of Hazardous Drugs *on page 2292*

Brand Names: US Etopophos

Index Terms Epipodophyllotoxin; ETOP

Pharmacologic Category Antineoplastic Agent, Podophyllotoxin Derivative; Antineoplastic Agent, Topoisomerase II Inhibitor

Use

Small cell lung cancer: First-line treatment of small cell lung cancer (in combination with other chemotherapy agents)

Testicular cancer, refractory: Treatment of refractory testicular tumors (in combination with other chemotherapy agents) in patients who have already received appropriate therapy with surgery, chemotherapy, and radiation

Labeled Contraindications Hypersensitivity to etoposide, etoposide phosphate, or any component of the formulation

Pregnancy Considerations Adverse events were observed in animal reproduction studies. Fetal growth restriction and newborn myelosuppression have been observed following maternal use of regimens containing etoposide during pregnancy (NTP 2013; Peccatori 2013). The European Society for Medical Oncology has published guidelines for diagnosis, treatment, and follow-up of cancer during pregnancy. The guidelines recommend referral to a facility with expertise in cancer during pregnancy and encourage a multidisciplinary team (obstetrician, neonatologist, oncology team). In general, if chemotherapy is indicated, it should be avoided during in the first trimester, there should be a 3-week time period between the last chemotherapy dose and anticipated delivery, and chemotherapy should not be administered beyond week 33 of gestation. Guidelines for the treatment of SCLC are not provided (Peccatori 2013).

In women of reproductive potential, etoposide phosphate may cause amenorrhea, infertility, or premature menopause; effective contraception should be used during therapy and for ≥6 months after the last dose. In males, azoospermia, oligospermia, or permanent loss of fertility may occur. In addition, spermatozoa and testicular tissue may be damaged. Males with female partners of reproductive potential should use condoms during therapy and for ≥4 months after the last dose.

Breast-Feeding Considerations Etoposide is excreted in breast milk (Azuno 1995). Due to the potential for serious adverse reactions in the nursing infant, the manufacturer recommends a decision be made whether to discontinue nursing or to discontinue the drug, taking into account the importance of treatment to the mother.

Warnings/Precautions Hazardous agent - use appropriate precautions for handling and disposal (NIOSH 2014 [group 1]). **[US Boxed Warning]: Severe myelosuppression with resulting infection or bleeding may occur.** Myelosuppression is dose-limiting; fatalities due to myelosuppression have been reported following etoposide administration. Hematologic toxicity may occur ▶

◀ both during or after therapy; the leukocyte nadir occurs at days 15 to 22; ANC nadir occurs at days 12 to 19, and the platelet nadir occurs at days 10 to 15. Marrow recovery usually occurs by day 21, although may be delayed. Treatment should be withheld for platelets <50,000/mm^3 or absolute neutrophil count (ANC) <500/mm^3. Monitor blood counts prior to therapy initiation and before each cycle of etoposide phosphate. May cause anaphylactic-like reactions manifested by chills, fever, tachycardia, bronchospasm, dyspnea, and hypotension. In addition, facial/tongue swelling, coughing, throat tightness, cyanosis, laryngospasm, diaphoresis, back pain, hypertension, flushing, apnea and loss of consciousness have also been reported less commonly. Anaphylactic-type reactions have occurred with the first infusion. Infusion should be interrupted and medications for the treatment of anaphylaxis should be available for immediate use. Underlying mechanisms behind the development of hypersensitivity reactions is unknown, but have been attributed to high drug concentration and rate of infusion. Another possible mechanism may be due to the differences between available etoposide intravenous formulations. Etoposide intravenous formulation contains polysorbate 80 and benzyl alcohol, while etoposide phosphate (the water soluble prodrug of etoposide) intravenous formulation does not contain either vehicle. Case reports have suggested that etoposide phosphate has been used successfully in patients with previous hypersensitivity reactions to etoposide (Collier 2008; Siderov 2002).

Secondary acute leukemias have been reported with etoposide, either as monotherapy or in combination with other chemotherapy agents. Dosage should be adjusted in patients with hepatic or renal impairment. Use with caution in patients with low serum albumin; may increase risk for toxicities. Doses of etoposide phosphate >175 mg/m^2 have not been evaluated. Each 100 mg vial of etoposide phosphate is equivalent to 100 mg of etoposide. Equivalent doses should be used when converting from etoposide to etoposide phosphate. Use caution in elderly patients (may be more likely to develop severe myelosuppression and/or GI effects. Etoposide phosphate may result in infertility in male and female patients. In addition, spermatozoa and testicular tissue damage may occur in males; amenorrhea and premature menopause may also occur in women. Males with female partners of childbearing potential should use condoms during therapy and for at least 4 months after the last dose; females of childbearing potential should use effective contraception during therapy and for 6 months after the last dose. Administer by slow IV infusion; hypotension has been reported with etoposide phosphate administration, generally associated with rapid IV infusion. Injection site reactions may occur; monitor infusion site closely. Potentially significant drug-drug interactions may exist, requiring dose or frequency adjustment, additional monitoring, and/or selection of alternative therapy. **[US Boxed Warning]: Should be administered under the supervision of an experienced cancer chemotherapy physician.**

Adverse Reactions Note: Also see adverse reactions for **etoposide;** etoposide phosphate is converted to etoposide, adverse reactions experienced with etoposide would also be expected with etoposide phosphate.

>10%:
  Central nervous system: Chills/fever (24%)
  Dermatologic: Alopecia (33% to 44%)
  Gastrointestinal: Nausea/vomiting (37%), anorexia (16%), mucositis (11%)

Hematologic: Leukopenia (91%; grade 4: 17%; nadir: day 15-22; recovery: usually by day 21), neutropenia (88%; grade 4: 37%; nadir: day 12-19; recovery: usually by day 21), anemia (72%; grades 3/4: 19%), thrombocytopenia (23%; grade 4: 9%; nadir: day 10-15; recovery: usually by day 21)

Neuromuscular & skeletal: Weakness/malaise (39%)

1% to 10%:

Cardiovascular: Hypotension (1% to 5%), hypertension (3%), facial flushing (2%)

Central nervous system: Dizziness (5%)

Dermatologic: Skin rash (3%)

Gastrointestinal: Constipation (8%), abdominal pain (7%), diarrhea (6%), taste perversion (6%)

Local: Extravasation/phlebitis (5%; including swelling, pain, cellulitis, necrosis, and/or skin necrosis at site of infiltration)

Miscellaneous: Anaphylactic-type reactions (3%; including chills, diaphoresis, fever, rigor, tachycardia, bronchospasm, dyspnea, pruritus)

<1%, postmarketing, and/or case reports: Acute leukemia (with/without pre-leukemia phase), anaphylactic-like reactions, back pain, blindness (transient, cortical), cough, cyanosis, diaphoresis, dysphagia, erythema, facial swelling, hepatic toxicity, hyperpigmentation, hypersensitivity-associated apnea, infection, interstitial pneumonitis, laryngospasm, maculopapular rash, neutropenic fever, optic neuritis, perivasculitis, pulmonary fibrosis, radiation recall dermatitis, seizure, Stevens-Johnson syndrome, tongue swelling, toxic epidermal necrolysis, urticaria

Drug Interactions

Metabolism/Transport Effects Substrate of CYP1A2 (minor), CYP2E1 (minor), CYP3A4 (major), P-glycoprotein; **Note:** Assignment of Major/Minor substrate status based on clinically relevant drug interaction potential; **Inhibits** CYP2C9 (weak)

Avoid Concomitant Use

Avoid concomitant use of Etoposide Phosphate with any of the following: BCG (Intravesical); CloZAPine; Conivaptan; Dipyrone; Fusidic Acid (Systemic); Idelalisib; Natalizumab; Pimecrolimus; Tacrolimus (Topical); Tofacitinib; Vaccines (Live)

Increased Effect/Toxicity

Etoposide Phosphate may increase the levels/effects of: CloZAPine; Fingolimod; Leflunomide; Natalizumab; Tofacitinib; Vaccines (Live); Vitamin K Antagonists

The levels/effects of Etoposide Phosphate may be increased by: Aprepitant; Conivaptan; CycloSPORINE (Systemic); CYP3A4 Inhibitors (Moderate); CYP3A4 Inhibitors (Strong); Dasatinib; Denosumab; Dipyrone; Fosaprepitant; Fusidic Acid (Systemic); Idelalisib; Ivacaftor; Luliconazole; Mifepristone; Netupitant; Osimertinib; Palbociclib; P-glycoprotein/ABCB1 Inhibitors; Pimecrolimus; Ranolazine; Roflumilast; Simeprevir; Stiripentol; Tacrolimus (Topical); Trastuzumab

Decreased Effect

Etoposide Phosphate may decrease the levels/effects of: BCG (Intravesical); Coccidioides immitis Skin Test; Sipuleucel-T; Vaccines (Inactivated); Vaccines (Live)

The levels/effects of Etoposide Phosphate may be decreased by: Bosentan; CYP3A4 Inducers (Moderate); CYP3A4 Inducers (Strong); Dabrafenib; Deferasirox; Enzalutamide; Mitotane; Osimertinib; P-glycoprotein/ABCB1 Inducers; Siltuximab; St Johns Wort; Tocilizumab

Storage/Stability Store intact vials under refrigeration at 2°C to 8°C (36°F to 46°F). Protect from light. Reconstituted solution is stable refrigerated at 2°C to 8°C (36°F to 46°F) for 7 days. At room temperature of 20°C to 25°C (68°F to 77°F), reconstituted solutions are stable for 24 hours when reconstituted with SWFI, D_5W, or NS, or for 48 hours when reconstituted with bacteriostatic water for injection with benzyl alcohol or bacteriostatic sodium chloride for injection with benzyl alcohol. Further diluted solutions for infusion are stable at room temperature 20°C to 25°C (68°F to 77°F) or under refrigeration 2°C to 8°C (36°F to 46°F) for up to 24 hours.

Preparation for Administration Hazardous agent; use appropriate precautions for handling and disposal (NIOSH 2014 [group 1]). Reconstitute vials with 5 mL or 10 mL SWFI, D_5W, NS, bacteriostatic water for injection with benzyl alcohol, or bacteriostatic sodium chloride for injection with benzyl alcohol to a concentration of 20 mg/mL or 10 mg/mL etoposide equivalent. These solutions may be administered without further dilution or may be diluted in D5W or NS to a concentration as low as 0.1 mg/mL.

Mechanism of Action Etoposide phosphate is converted *in vivo* to the active moiety, etoposide, by dephosphorylation. Etoposide inhibits mitotic activity; inhibits cells from entering prophase; inhibits DNA synthesis. Initially thought to be mitotic inhibitors similar to podophyllotoxin, but actually have no effect on microtubule assembly. However, have been shown to induce DNA strand breakage and inhibition of topoisomerase II (an enzyme which breaks and repairs DNA); etoposide acts in late S or early G2 phases.

Pharmacodynamics/Kinetics

Distribution: Average V_d: 7 to 17 L/m^2; poor penetration across blood-brain barrier; concentrations in CSF being <10% that of plasma

Protein binding: 97%

Metabolism:

Etoposide phosphate: Rapidly and completely converted to etoposide in plasma

Etoposide: Hepatic, via CYP3A4 and 3A5 to various metabolites; in addition, conversion of etoposide to the O-demethylated metabolites (catechol and quinine) via prostaglandin synthases or myeloperoxidase occurs, as well as glutathione and glucuronide conjugation via GSTT1/GSTP1 and UGT1A1 (Yang 2009)

Half-life elimination: Terminal: 4 to 11 hours; Children: Normal renal/hepatic function: 6 to 8 hours

Excretion: Urine (56%; 45% as etoposide) within 120 hours; feces (44%) within 120 hours

Children: Urine (~55% as etoposide) in 24 hours

Dosing

Adult & Geriatric Note: Etoposide phosphate is a prodrug of etoposide; equivalent doses should be used when converting from etoposide to etoposide phosphate. Each 100 mg vial of etoposide phosphate is equivalent to 100 mg of etoposide.

Small cell lung cancer (in combination with other approved chemotherapeutic drugs): IV: Etoposide 35 mg/m^2/day for 4 days up to 50 mg/m^2/day for 5 days. Courses are repeated at 3- to 4-week intervals after adequate recovery from toxicity.

Testicular cancer, refractory (in combination with other approved chemotherapeutic agents): IV: Etoposide 50 to 100 mg/m²/day on days 1 to 5 to 100 mg/m²/day on days 1, 3, and 5. Courses are repeated at 3- to 4-week intervals after adequate recovery from toxicity.

Indication-specific off-label dosing: Refer to Etoposide monograph.

Renal Impairment

CrCl >50 mL/minute: No dosage adjustment necessary.

CrCl 15 to 50 mL/minute: Administer 75% of dose.

CrCl <15 mL minute: Data are not available; consider further dose reductions.

Etoposide phosphate is rapidly and completely converted to etoposide in plasma, please refer to Etoposide monograph for additional renal dosing adjustments (for etoposide).

Hepatic Impairment There are no dosage adjustments provided in the manufacturer's labeling. Etoposide phosphate is rapidly and completely converted to etoposide in plasma; please refer to Etoposide monograph for etoposide hepatic dosing adjustments.

Obesity *ASCO Guidelines for appropriate chemotherapy dosing in obese adults with cancer (**Note:** Excludes HSCT dosing):* Utilize patient's actual body weight (full weight) for calculation of body surface area- or weight-based dosing, particularly when the intent of therapy is curative; manage regimen-related toxicities in the same manner as for nonobese patients; if a dose reduction is utilized due to toxicity, consider resumption of full weight-based dosing with subsequent cycles, especially if cause of toxicity (eg, hepatic or renal impairment) is resolved (Griggs 2012).

Adjustment for Toxicity

Hematologic (ANC <500/mm³ and/or platelets <50,000/mm³): Interrupt treatment until blood counts have sufficiently recovered.

Severe adverse reactions: Reduce dose, interrupt treatment, or discontinue.

Combination Regimens

Retinoblastoma: Carboplatin-Etoposide-Vincristine (Retinoblastoma) on page 1866

Administration Infuse by slow IV infusion over 5 to 210 minutes; risk of hypotension may increase with rate of infusion. Do not administer as a bolus injection.

Hazardous agent; use appropriate precautions for handling and disposal (NIOSH 2014 [group 1]).

Vesicant/Extravasation Risk May be an irritant

Emetic Potential Low (10% to 30%)

Monitoring Parameters CBC with differential and platelets (prior to initial treatment and each cycle), bilirubin, AST/ALT, renal function, vital signs (blood pressure)

Dosage Forms Excipient information presented when available (limited, particularly for generics); consult specific product labeling.

Solution Reconstituted, Intravenous [strength expressed as base]:

Etopophos: 100 mg (1 ea)

◆ **Etoposide Injection (Can)** *see* Etoposide *on page 641*

◆ **Etoposide Injection USP (Can)** *see* Etoposide *on page 641*

◆ **Euflex (Can)** *see* Flutamide *on page 751*

◆ **Eulexin** *see* Flutamide *on page 751*

◆ ***Euphorbia peplus* Derivative** *see* Ingenol Mebutate *on page 928*

◆ **Euro-Cyproheptadine (Can)** *see* Cyproheptadine *on page 400*

Everolimus (e ver OH li mus)

Related Information

Common Toxicity Criteria *on page 2122*

Management of Chemotherapy-Induced Nausea and Vomiting in Adults *on page 2142*

Prevention of Chemotherapy-Induced Nausea and Vomiting in Children *on page 2203*

Principles of Anticancer Therapy *on page 2261*

Safe Handling of Hazardous Drugs *on page 2292*

Brand Names: US Afinitor; Afinitor Disperz; Zortress

Brand Names: Canada Afinitor

Index Terms RAD001

Pharmacologic Category Antineoplastic Agent, mTOR Kinase Inhibitor; Immunosuppressant Agent; mTOR Kinase Inhibitor

Use

Breast cancer, advanced (Afinitor only): Treatment of advanced hormone receptor-positive, HER2-negative breast cancer in postmenopausal women (in combination with exemestane and after letrozole or anastrozole failure)

Pancreatic neuroendocrine tumors (Afinitor only): Treatment of locally advanced, metastatic or unresectable progressive pancreatic neuroendocrine tumors (PNET)

Limitations of use: Not indicated for the treatment of functional carcinoid tumors.

Renal angiomyolipoma with tuberous sclerosis complex (Afinitor only): Treatment of renal angiomyolipoma with tuberous sclerosis complex (TSC) not requiring immediate surgery

Renal cell carcinoma, advanced (Afinitor only): Treatment of advanced renal cell cancer (RCC) after sunitinib or sorafenib failure

Subependymal giant cell astrocytoma (Afinitor or Afinitor Disperz only): Treatment of subependymal giant cell astrocytoma (SEGA) associated with TSC which requires intervention, but cannot be curatively resected

Liver transplantation (Zortress only): Prophylaxis of organ rejection in liver transplantation (in combination with corticosteroids and reduced doses of tacrolimus)

Renal transplantation (Zortress only): Prophylaxis of organ rejection in renal transplant patients at low to moderate immunologic risk (in combination with basiliximab induction and concurrent with corticosteroids and reduced doses of cyclosporine)

Labeled Contraindications Hypersensitivity to everolimus, sirolimus, other rapamycin derivatives, or any component of the formulation.

Pregnancy Considerations Adverse events were observed in animal reproduction studies with exposures lower than expected with human doses. Based on the mechanism of action, may cause fetal harm if administered during pregnancy. Women of reproductive potential should be advised to avoid pregnancy and use highly effective birth control during treatment and for up to 8 weeks after everolimus discontinuation.

The National Transplantation Pregnancy Registry (NTPR) (Temple University) is a registry for pregnant women taking immunosuppressants following any solid organ transplant. The NTPR encourages reporting of all immunosuppressant exposures during pregnancy in transplant recipients at 877-955-6877.

Breast-Feeding Considerations It is not known if everolimus is excreted in breast milk. Due to the potential for serious adverse reactions in the nursing infant, breast-feeding should be avoided.

Warnings/Precautions Hazardous agent - use appropriate precautions for handling and disposal (NIOSH 2014 [group 1]).

To avoid potential contact with everolimus, caregivers should wear gloves when preparing suspension from tablets for oral suspension. Noninfectious pneumonitis, interstitial lung disease (ILD), and/or noninfectious fibrosis have been observed with mTOR inhibitors including everolimus; some cases were fatal. Symptoms include dyspnea, cough, hypoxia and/or pleural effusion; promptly evaluate worsening respiratory symptoms. Cases of ILD have been reported with pulmonary hypertension (including pulmonary arterial hypertension) as a secondary event. Consider opportunistic infections such as *Pneumocystis jiroveci* pneumonia (PCP) when evaluating clinical symptoms. May require treatment interruption followed by dose reduction (pneumonitis has developed even with reduced doses) and/or corticosteroid therapy; discontinue for grade 4 pneumonitis. Consider discontinuation for recurrence of grade 3 toxicity after dosage reduction. In patients who require steroid therapy for symptom management, consider PCP prophylaxis. Imaging may overestimate the incidence of clinical pneumonitis. **[US Boxed Warning]: Everolimus has immunosuppressant properties which may result in infection;** the risk of developing bacterial (including mycobacterial), viral, fungal and protozoal infections and for local, opportunistic (including polyomavirus infection), and/or systemic infections is increased; may lead to sepsis, respiratory failure, hepatic failure, or fatality. Polyomavirus infection in transplant patients may be serious and/or fatal. Polyoma virus-associated nephropathy (due to BK virus), which may result in serious cases of deteriorating renal function and renal graft loss, has been observed with use. JC virus-associated progressive multiple leukoencephalopathy (PML) may also be associated with everolimus use in transplantation. Reduced immunosuppression (taking into account the risks of rejection) should be considered with evidence of polyoma virus infection or PML. Reactivation of hepatitis B has been observed in patients receiving everolimus. Resolve preexisting invasive fungal infections prior to treatment initiation. Cases (some fatal) of *Pneumocystis jiroveci* pneumonia (PCP) have been reported with everolimus use. Consider PCP prophylaxis in patients receiving concomitant corticosteroid or other immunosuppressant therapy. In addition, transplant recipient patients should receive prophylactic therapy for PCP and for cytomegalovirus (CMV). Monitor for signs and symptoms of infection during treatment. Discontinue if invasive systemic fungal infection is diagnosed (and manage with appropriate antifungal therapy).

[US Boxed Warning]: Immunosuppressant use may result in the development of malignancy, including lymphoma and skin cancer. The risk is associated with treatment intensity and the duration of therapy. To minimize the risk for skin cancer, limit exposure to sunlight and ultraviolet light; wear protective clothing and use effective sunscreen.

[US Boxed Warning]: Due to the increased risk for nephrotoxicity in renal transplantation, avoid standard doses of cyclosporine in combination with everolimus; reduced cyclosporine doses are recommended when everolimus is used in combination with cyclosporine. Therapeutic monitoring of cyclosporine and everolimus concentrations is recommended. Monitor for proteinuria; the risk of proteinuria is increased when everolimus is used in combination with cyclosporine, and with higher serum everolimus concentrations. Everolimus and cyclosporine combination therapy may increase the risk for thrombotic microangiopathy/thrombotic thrombocytopenic purpura/hemolytic uremic syndrome (TMA/TTP/HUS); monitor blood counts. In liver transplantation, the tacrolimus dose and target range should be reduced to minimize the risk of nephrotoxicity. Eliminating calcineurin inhibitors from the immunosuppressive regimen may result in acute rejection. Elevations in serum creatinine (generally mild), renal failure, and proteinuria have been also observed with everolimus use; monitor renal function (BUN, creatinine, and/or urinary protein). Risk of nephrotoxicity may be increased when administered with calcineurin inhibitors (eg, cyclosporine, tacrolimus); dosage adjustment of calcineurin inhibitor is necessary. An increased incidence of rash, infection and dose interruptions have been reported in patients with renal insufficiency (CrCl ≤60 mL/minute) who received mTOR inhibitors for the treatment of renal cell cancer (Gupta, 2011); serum creatinine elevations and proteinuria have been reported. Monitor renal function (BUN, serum creatinine, urinary protein) at baseline and periodically, especially if risk factors for further impairment exist; pharmacokinetic studies have not been conducted; dosage adjustments are not required based on renal impairment. **[US Boxed Warning]: An increased risk of renal arterial and venous thrombosis has been reported with use in renal transplantation, generally within the first 30 days after transplant; may result in graft loss.** MTOR inhibitors are associated with an increase in hepatic artery thrombosis, most cases have been reported within 30 days after transplant and usually proceeded to graft loss or death; do not use everolimus prior to 30 days post liver transplant.

Potentially significant drug-drug/drug-food interactions may exist, requiring dose or frequency adjustment, additional monitoring, and/or selection of alternative therapy. In transplant patients, avoid the use of certain HMG-CoA reductase inhibitors (eg, simvastatin, lovastatin); may increase the risk for rhabdomyolysis due to the potential interaction with cyclosporine (which may be given in combination with everolimus for transplantation).

Use is associated with mouth ulcers, mucositis and stomatitis; manage with topical therapy; avoid the use of alcohol-, hydrogen peroxide-, iodine-, or thyme-based mouthwashes (due to the high potential for drug interactions, avoid the use of systemic antifungals unless fungal infection has been diagnosed). Everolimus is associated with the development of angioedema; concomitant use with other agents known to cause angioedema (eg, ACE inhibitors) may increase the risk. Everolimus use may delay wound healing and increase the occurrence of wound-related complications (eg, wound dehiscence, infection, incisional hernia, lymphocele, seroma); may require surgical intervention; use with caution in the peri-surgical period. Generalized edema, including peripheral edema and lymphedema, and local fluid accumulation (eg, pericardial effusion, pleural effusion, ascites) may also occur.

Everolimus exposure is increased in patients with hepatic impairment. For patients with breast cancer, PNET, RCC, or renal angiomyolipoma with mild and moderate hepatic impairment, reduced doses are recommended; in patients with severe hepatic impairment, use is recommended (at reduced doses) if the potential benefit outweighs risks. Reduced doses are recommended in transplant patients with hepatic impairment; pharmacokinetic information does not exist for renal transplant patients with severe impairment (Child-Pugh class B or C); monitor whole blood trough levels closely for patients with SEGA, reduced doses may be needed for mild and moderate hepatic impairment (based on therapeutic drug monitoring), and are recommended in severe hepatic impairment; monitor whole blood trough levels. The Canadian labeling recommends against the use of everolimus in patients <18 years of age with SEGA and hepatic impairment.

[US Boxed Warning]: Increased mortality (usually associated with infections) within the first 3 months after transplant was noted in a study of patients with *de novo* heart transplant receiving immunosuppressive regimens containing everolimus (with or without induction therapy). Use in heart transplantation is not recommended. Hyperglycemia, hyperlipidemia, and hypertriglyceridemia have been reported. Higher serum everolimus concentrations are associated with an increased risk for hyperlipidemia. Use has not been studied in patients with baseline cholesterol >350 mg/dL. Monitor fasting glucose and lipid profile prior to treatment initiation and periodically thereafter; monitor more frequently in patients with concomitant medications affecting glucose. Manage with appropriate medical therapy (if possible, optimize glucose control and lipids prior to treatment initiation). Antihyperlipidemic therapy may not normalize levels. May alter insulin and/or oral hypoglycemic therapy requirements in patients with diabetes; the risk for new onset diabetes is increased with everolimus use after transplantation. Decreases in hemoglobin, neutrophils, platelets, and lymphocytes have been reported; monitor blood counts at baseline and periodically. Increases in serum glucose are common; may alter insulin and/or oral hypoglycemic therapy requirements in patients with diabetes; the risk for new-onset diabetes is increased with everolimus use after transplantation. Patients should not be immunized with live viral vaccines during or shortly after treatment and should avoid close contact with recently vaccinated (live vaccine) individuals; consider the timing of routine immunizations prior to the start of therapy in pediatric patients treated for SEGA. In pediatric patients treated for SEGA, complete recommended series of live virus childhood vaccinations prior to treatment (if immediate everolimus treatment is not indicated); an accelerated vaccination schedule may be appropriate. Continue treatment with everolimus for renal cell cancer as long as clinical benefit is demonstrated or until occurrence of unacceptable toxicity. Safety and efficacy have not been established for the use of everolimus in the treatment of carcinoid tumors.

Tablets (Afinitor, Zortress) and tablets for oral suspension (Afinitor Disperz) are not interchangeable; Afinitor Disperz is only indicated in conjunction with therapeutic monitoring for the treatment of SEGA. Do not combine formulations to achieve total desired dose. May cause infertility; in females, menstrual irregularities, secondary amenorrhea, and increases in luteinizing hormone and follicle-stimulating hormone have occurred; azoospermia and oligospermia have been observed in males. Avoid use in patients with hereditary galactose intolerance, Lapp lactase deficiency, or glucose-galactose malabsorption; may result in diarrhea and malabsorption. The safety and efficacy of everolimus in renal transplantation patients with high-immunologic risk or in solid organ transplant other than renal or liver have not been established. **[US Boxed Warning]: In transplantation, everolimus should only be used by** ▶

◄ **physicians experienced in immunosuppressive therapy and management of transplant patients. Adequate laboratory and supportive medical
resources must be readily available.** For indications requiring whole blood
trough concentrations to determine dosage adjustments, a consistent method
should be used; concentration values from different assay methods may not be
interchangeable.

Adverse Reactions

Transplantation:

Frequency not always defined. Reactions occur in kidney and liver transplantation unless otherwise specified.

>10%:

Cardiovascular: Peripheral edema (kidney transplant: 45%; liver transplant:
18%), hypertension (kidney transplant: 30%; liver transplant: 17%)

Central nervous system: Headache (18% to 19%), insomnia (kidney transplant: 17%), procedural pain (kidney transplant: 15%)

Endocrine & metabolic: Diabetes mellitus (new onset: liver transplant: 32%;
kidney transplant: 9%), hypercholesterolemia (15% to 24%), hyperkalemia
(renal transplant: 18%), hypomagnesemia (kidney transplant: 14%), hypophosphatemia (kidney transplant: 13%), hyperglycemia (kidney transplant:
12%), hypokalemia (kidney transplant: 12%)

Gastrointestinal: Constipation (kidney transplant: 38%), nausea (kidney
transplant: 29%; liver transplant: 14%), diarrhea (19%), vomiting (kidney
transplant: 15%), abdominal pain (13%; upper abdominal pain, kidney
transplant: 2%)

Genitourinary: Urinary tract infection (kidney transplant: 22%), hematuria
(kidney transplant: 12%), dysuria (kidney transplant: 11%)

Hematologic & oncologic: Anemia (kidney transplant: 26%), leukopenia (3%
to 12%)

Infection: Infection (kidney transplant: 62%; liver transplant: 50%), viral
infection (liver transplant: 17%; kidney transplant: 10%), bacterial infection
(liver transplant: 16%), hepatitis C (liver transplant: 11%)

Local: Incisional pain (kidney transplant: 16%)

Neuromuscular & skeletal: Limb pain (kidney transplant: 12%), back pain
(kidney transplant: 11%)

Renal: Increased serum creatinine (kidney transplant: 18%)

Respiratory: Upper respiratory tract infection (kidney transplant: 16%)

Miscellaneous: Postoperative wound complication (kidney transplant: 35%;
liver transplant: 11%; includes incisional hernia, lymphocele, seroma,
wound dehiscence), fever (13% to 19%)

1% to 10%:

Cardiovascular: Hypertensive crisis (1%), angina pectoris, atrial fibrillation,
cardiac failure, chest discomfort, chest pain, deep vein thrombosis, edema,
hypotension, palpitations, pulmonary embolism, renal artery thrombosis,
syncope, tachycardia, venous thromboembolism

Central nervous system: Fatigue (9%), agitation, anxiety, chills, depression,
dizziness, drowsiness, hallucination, hemiparesis, hypoesthesia, lethargy,
malaise, migraine, myasthenia, neuralgia, pain, paresthesia

Dermatologic: Acneiform eruption, acne vulgaris, alopecia, cellulitis, diaphoresis, folliculitis, hypertrichosis, night sweats, onychomycosis, pruritus, skin
rash, tinea pedis

Endocrine & metabolic: Acidosis, amenorrhea, cushingoid appearance, cyanocobalamin deficiency, dehydration, fluid retention, gout, hirsutism, hypercalcemia, hyperparathyroidism, hypertriglyceridemia, hyperuricemia, hypocalcemia, hypoglycemia, hyponatremia, iron deficiency, ovarian cyst

Gastrointestinal: Stomatitis (kidney transplant: 8%), dyspepsia (kidney transplant: 4%), abdominal distention, anorexia, decreased appetite, dysphagia, epigastric distress, flatulence, gastroenteritis, gastroesophageal reflux disease, gingival hyperplasia, hematemesis, hemorrhoids, intestinal obstruction, oral candidiasis, oral herpes, oral mucosa ulcer, peritoneal effusion, peritonitis

Genitourinary: Erectile dysfunction (kidney transplant: 5%), bladder spasm, perinephric abscess, perinephric hematoma, pollakiuria, proteinuria, pyuria, scrotal edema, urethritis, urinary retention, urinary urgency

Hematologic & oncologic: Neoplasm (3% to 4%), leukocytosis, lymphadenopathy, lymphorrhea, neutropenia, pancytopenia, thrombocythemia, thrombocytopenia

Hepatic: Abnormal hepatic function tests (liver transplant: 7%), ascites (liver transplant: 4%), hepatitis (noninfections), increased liver enzymes, increased serum alkaline phosphatase, increased serum bilirubin

Hypersensitivity: Angioedema (<1%)

Infection: BK virus (kidney transplant: 1%), bacteremia, candidiasis, herpes virus infection, influenza, sepsis, wound infection

Neuromuscular & skeletal: Tremor (8% to 9%), arthralgia, joint swelling, muscle spasm, musculoskeletal pain, myalgia, osteomyelitis, osteonecrosis, osteoporosis, spondylitis, weakness

Ophthalmic: Blurred vision, cataract, conjunctivitis

Renal: Hydronephrosis, increased blood urea nitrogen, interstitial nephritis, polyuria, pyelonephritis, renal failure (acute), renal insufficiency, renal tubular necrosis

Respiratory: Cough (kidney transplant: 7%), atelectasis, bronchitis, dyspnea, epistaxis, lower respiratory tract infection, nasal congestion, nasopharyngitis, oropharyngeal pain, pleural effusion, pneumonia, pulmonary edema, rhinorrhea, sinus congestion, sinusitis, wheezing

Antineoplastic:

Antineoplastic indications include advanced hormone receptor-positive, HER2-negative breast cancer (advanced HR + BC), pancreatic neuroendocrine tumors (PNET), renal cell carcinoma (RCC), renal angiomyolipoma and tuberous sclerosis complex (TSC), and subependymal giant cell astrocytoma (SEGA)

>10%:

Cardiovascular: Edema (PNET: ≤39%), peripheral edema (PNET: ≤39%; advanced HR + BC, RCC, TSC: 13% to 25%), hypertension (PNET, RCC: 4% to 13%)

Central nervous system: Malaise (PNET: ≤45%), fatigue (advanced HR + BC, PNET, RCC: 31% to ≤45%; SEGA: 14%), headache (PNET: ≤30%; advanced HR + BC, RCC: 19% to 21%), migraine (PNET: ≤30%), behavioral problems (SEGA: 21%; includes abnormal behavior, aggressive behavior, agitation, anxiety, obsessive compulsive symptoms, panic attack), insomnia (advanced HR + BC, PNET, RCC, SEGA: 6% to 14%), dizziness (PNET, RCC: 7% to 12%)

◄ Dermatologic: Skin rash (PNET: 59%; advanced HR + BC: 39%; RCC, SEGA: 21% to 29%; may include allergic dermatitis, macular eruption, maculopapular rash, papular rash, urticaria), cellulitis (SEGA: 29%), acne vulgaris (TSC: 22%; SEGA: 10%), nail disease (PNET: 22%; RCC: 5%), pruritus (advanced HR + BC, PNET, RCC: 13% to 21%), xeroderma (PNET, RCC: 13%)

Endocrine & metabolic: Hypercholesterolemia (TSC, SEGA: 81% to 85%), decreased serum bicarbonate (PNET: 56%), hypertriglyceridemia (TSC: 52%; SEGA: 27%), hypophosphatemia (TSC: 49%; SEGA: 9%), decreased serum calcium (PNET: 37%), decreased serum albumin (advanced HR + BC: 33%; PNET: 13%), hyperglycemia (SEGA: 25%; advanced HR + BC: 14%), amenorrhea (TSC, SEGA: 15% to 17%)

Gastrointestinal: Stomatitis (advanced HR + BC, PNET, SEGA, TSC: 62% to 78%; grades 3/4: ≤9%; RCC: 44%, grades 3/4: ≤4%), diarrhea (PNET: 50%; advanced HR + BC, RCC: 30% to 33%; TSC, SEGA: 14% to 17%; may include bowel urgency, colitis, enteritis, enterocolitis, steatorrhea), abdominal pain (PNET: 36%; RCC: 9%), decreased appetite (advanced HR + BC, PNET: 30%; TSC: 6%), nausea (advanced HR + BC, RCC: 26% to 29%; SEGA: 8%), vomiting (15% to 29%), weight loss (advanced HR + BC, PNET: 25% to 28%; RCC: 9%), anorexia (RCC: 25%), dysgeusia (advanced HR + BC, PNET: 19% to 22%; RCC: 10%; TSC: 5%), mucositis (RCC: 19%; grades 3/4: ≤1%), constipation (advanced HR + BC, PNET, SEGA: 10% to 14%), xerostomia (advanced HR + BC, PNET, RCC: 8% to 11%)

Genitourinary: Urinary tract infection (PNET: 16%; advanced HR + BC, RCC: 5% to 10%), irregular menses (TSC, PNET: 10% to 11%)

Hematologic & oncologic: Increase in fasting plasma glucose (PNET: 75%, grades 3/4: 17%; TSC: 14%), prolonged partial thromboplastin time (SEGA: 72%), anemia (TSC: 61%; SEGA: 41%), lymphocytopenia (advanced HR + BC, PNET, RCC: 45% to 54%; advanced HR + BC, RCC grade 3: 11% to 16%, RCC grade 4: 2%; PNET grades 3/4: 16%; TSC: 20%, grade 3: 1%), thrombocytopenia (advanced HR + BC, PNET: 45% to 54%; advanced HR + BC grade 3: 3%, PNET grades 3/4: 3%; RCC, TSC: 19% to 23%, RCC grade 3: 1%), neutropenia (SEGA: 46%, grade 3: 9%; advanced HR + BC, PNET: 30% to 31%, PNET grades 3/4: 4%, advanced HR + BC grade 3: 2%; RCC 14%, grade 4: <1%), leukopenia (TSC: 37%)

Hepatic: Increased serum alkaline phosphatase (PNET: 74%; TSC: 32%, grade 3: 1%), increased serum AST (advanced HR + BC: 69%; PNET: 56%; RCC, TSC, SEGA: 23% to 33%; advanced HR + BC, RCC, TSC grade 3: ≤4%; advanced HR + BC, RCC grade 4: <1%), increased serum ALT (advanced HR + BC, PNET: 48% to 51%, advanced HR + BC grade 4: <1%; RCC, TSC, SEGA: 18% to 21%; RCC, TSC grade 3: 1%)

Infection: Infection (advanced HR + BC: 50%; RCC: 37%; advanced HR + BC, RCC grade 3: 4% to 7%; advanced HR + BC, RCC grade 4: 1% to 3%)

Neuromuscular & skeletal: Weakness (RCC: 33%; advanced HR + BC: 13%), arthralgia (advanced HR + BC, PNET, TSC: 13% to 20%), back pain (advanced HR + BC, PNET: 14% to 15%), limb pain (PNET, RCC, SEGA: 8% to 14%)

Renal: Increased serum creatinine (RCC: 50%; advanced HR + BC, PNET: 19% to 24%, advanced HR + BC, RCC grade 3: 1% to 2%, PNET grades 3/4: 2%)

Respiratory: Respiratory tract infection (SEGA: 31%, grade 3: 1%, grade 4: 1%; includes viral respiratory tract infection), cough (advanced HR + BC, PNET, RCC, TSC: 20% to 30%; includes productive cough), nasopharyngitis (PNET: ≤25%; advanced HR + BC, RCC: 6% to 10%), rhinitis (PNET: ≤25%), upper respiratory tract infection (PNET: ≤25%; TSC: 11%; advanced HR + BC: 5%), dyspnea (advanced HR + BC, PNET, RCC: 20% to 24%; includes dyspnea on exertion), epistaxis (advanced HR + BC, PNET, RCC: 17% to 22%; TSC, SEGA: 5% to 9%), pneumonitis (advanced HR + BC, PNET, RCC: 14% to 19%; TSC, SEGA: 1%; advanced HR + BC, PNET, RCC grade 3: 3% to 4%; advanced HR + BC, PNET grade 4: <1%; may include interstitial pulmonary disease, pulmonary alveolar hemorrhage, pulmonary alveolitis, pulmonary fibrosis, pulmonary infiltrates, pulmonary toxicity, restrictive pulmonary disease), oropharyngeal pain (PNET: 11%)

Miscellaneous: Fever (advanced HR + BC, PNET, RCC, SEGA: 15% to 31%)

1% to 10%:

Cardiovascular: Chest pain (RCC: 5%), tachycardia (RCC: 3%), cardiac failure (RCC: 1%), deep vein thrombosis (RCC: <1%)

Central nervous system: Depression (TSC: 5%), paresthesia (RCC: 5%), chills (RCC: 4%)

Dermatologic: Alopecia (advanced HR + BC: 10%), palmar-plantar erythrodysesthesia (RCC: 5%), erythema (RCC: 4%), onychoclasis (RCC: 4%), skin lesion (RCC: 4%), acneiform eruption (RCC: 3%)

Endocrine & metabolic: Diabetes mellitus (PNET: 10%; RCC: exacerbation of diabetes mellitus: 2%, new onset: <1%), hypermenorrhea (TSC, SEGA: 6% to 10%), menstrual disease (TSC, SEGA: 6% to 10%), increased luteinizing hormone (TSC, SEGA: 1% to 4%), increased follicle-stimulating hormone (TSC: 3%), ovarian cyst (TSC: 3%)

Gastrointestinal: Gastroenteritis (SEGA: 10%; includes viral gastroenteritis, gastrointestinal infection), hemorrhoids (RCC: 5%), dysphagia (RCC: 4%)

Genitourinary: Vaginal hemorrhage (TSC: 8%), dysmenorrhea (SEGA: 6%), uterine hemorrhage (SEGA: 6%), cystitis (advanced HR + BC: 3%)

Hematologic & oncologic: Hemorrhage (RCC: 3%)

Hepatic: Increased serum bilirubin (RCC: 3%; grade 3: <1%, grade 4: <1%)

Hypersensitivity: Hypersensitivity (TSC, SEGA: 3%; includes anaphylaxis, chest pain, dyspnea, flushing), angioedema (RCC, TSC: ≤1%)

Infection: Candidiasis (advanced HR + BC, RCC: <1%), hepatitis C (advanced HR + BC: <1%), sepsis (advanced HR + BC, RCC: <1%)

Neuromuscular & skeletal: Muscle spasm (PNET: 10%), jaw pain (RCC: 3%)

Ophthalmic: Eyelid edema (RCC: 4%), conjunctivitis (RCC: 2%)

Otic: Otitis media (TSC: 6%)

Renal: Renal failure (RCC: 3%)

Respiratory: Streptococcal pharyngitis (SEGA: 10%), pleural effusion (RCC: 7%), pneumonia (advanced HR + BC, RCC, SEGA: 4% to 6%), bronchitis (advanced HR + BC, RCC: 4%), pharyngolaryngeal pain (RCC: 4%), rhinorrhea (RCC: 3%), sinusitis (advanced HR + BC, RCC: 3%)

Miscellaneous: Postoperative wound complication (RC: <1%; wound healing impairment)

<1%, postmarketing, and/or case reports: Ageusia, arterial thrombosis, aspergillosis, azoospermia, cardiac arrest, cholecystitis, cholelithiasis, complex regional pain syndrome, contact dermatitis, decreased plasma testosterone, eczema, excoriation, gastritis, hemolytic uremic syndrome, hypersensitivity angiitis, male infertility, nephrotoxicity, noninfectious pneumonitis, oligospermia, pancreatitis (including acute pancreatitis), pericardial effusion, pharyngitis, pityriasis rosea, pneumonia due to *Pneumocystis jiroveci*, polyoma virus

infection, progressive multifocal leukoencephalopathy, reactivation of HBV, respiratory distress, seizure, thrombosis of vascular graft (kidney), thrombotic thrombocytopenic purpura

Drug Interactions

Metabolism/Transport Effects Substrate of CYP3A4 (major), P-glycoprotein; **Note:** Assignment of Major/Minor substrate status based on clinically relevant drug interaction potential

Avoid Concomitant Use

Avoid concomitant use of Everolimus with any of the following: BCG (Intravesical); CloZAPine; Conivaptan; CYP3A4 Inducers (Strong); CYP3A4 Inhibitors (Strong); Dipyrone; Fusidic Acid (Systemic); Grapefruit Juice; Idelalisib; Natalizumab; Pimecrolimus; St Johns Wort; Tacrolimus (Topical); Tofacitinib; Vaccines (Live); Voriconazole

Increased Effect/Toxicity

Everolimus may increase the levels/effects of: ACE Inhibitors; CloZAPine; Fingolimod; Leflunomide; Natalizumab; Tofacitinib; Vaccines (Live)

The levels/effects of Everolimus may be increased by: Conivaptan; Cyclo-SPORINE (Systemic); CYP3A4 Inhibitors (Moderate); CYP3A4 Inhibitors (Strong); Dasatinib; Denosumab; Dipyrone; Fosaprepitant; Fusidic Acid (Systemic); Grapefruit Juice; Idelalisib; Luliconazole; Mifepristone; Osimertinib; Palbociclib; P-glycoprotein/ABCB1 Inhibitors; Pimecrolimus; Roflumilast; Stiripentol; Tacrolimus (Topical); Trastuzumab; Voriconazole

Decreased Effect

Everolimus may decrease the levels/effects of: Antidiabetic Agents; BCG (Intravesical); Coccidioides immitis Skin Test; Sipuleucel-T; Vaccines (Inactivated); Vaccines (Live)

The levels/effects of Everolimus may be decreased by: Bosentan; CYP3A4 Inducers (Moderate); CYP3A4 Inducers (Strong); Dabrafenib; Deferasirox; Echinacea; Efavirenz; Osimertinib; P-glycoprotein/ABCB1 Inducers; Siltuximab; St Johns Wort; Tocilizumab

Food Interactions Grapefruit juice may increase levels of everolimus. Absorption with food may be variable. Management: Avoid grapefruit juice. Take with or without food, but be consistent with regard to food.

Storage/Stability Tablets and tablets for suspension: Store at room temperature of 25°C (77°F); excursions permitted to 15°C to 30°C (59°F to 86°F). Protect from light; protect from moisture.

Mechanism of Action Everolimus is a macrolide immunosuppressant and a mechanistic target of rapamycin (mTOR) inhibitor which has antiproliferative and antiangiogenic properties, and also reduces lipoma volume in patients with angiomyolipoma. Reduces protein synthesis and cell proliferation by binding to the FK binding protein-12 (FKBP-12), an intracellular protein, to form a complex that inhibits activation of mTOR (mechanistic target of rapamycin) serine-threonine kinase activity. Also reduces angiogenesis by inhibiting vascular endothelial growth factor (VEGF) and hypoxia-inducible factor (HIF-1) expression. Angiomyolipomas may occur due to unregulated mTOR activity in TSC-associated renal angiomyolipoma (Budde, 2012); everolimus reduces lipoma volume (Bissler, 2012).

Pharmacodynamics/Kinetics

Absorption: Rapid, but moderate

Protein binding: ~74%

Metabolism: Extensively metabolized in the liver via CYP3A4; forms 6 weak metabolites

Bioavailability:

Tablets: ~30%; systemic exposure reduced by 22% with a high-fat meal and by 32% with a light-fat meal

Tablets for suspension: AUC equivalent to tablets although peak concentrations are 20% to 36% lower; steady state concentrations are similar; systemic exposure reduced by 12% with a high-fat meal and by 30% with a low-fat meal

Half-life elimination: ~30 hours

Time to peak, plasma: 1 to 2 hours

Excretion: Feces (80%, based on solid organ transplant studies); Urine (~5%, based on solid organ transplant studies)

Dosing

Adult & Geriatric Note: Tablets (Afinitor, Zortress) and tablets for oral suspension (Afinitor Disperz) are not interchangeable; Afinitor Disperz is only indicated for the treatment of subependymal giant cell astrocytoma (SEGA), in conjunction with therapeutic monitoring. Do not combine formulations to achieve total desired dose.

Breast cancer, advanced, hormone receptor-positive, HER2-negative: Oral: 10 mg once daily (in combination with exemestane), continue treatment until disease progression or unacceptable toxicity

Pancreatic neuroendocrine tumors (PNET), advanced: Oral: 10 mg once daily, continue treatment until disease progression or unacceptable toxicity

Renal angiomyolipoma: Oral: 10 mg once daily, continue treatment until disease progression or unacceptable toxicity

Renal cell cancer, advanced (RCC): Oral: 10 mg once daily, continue treatment until disease progression or unacceptable toxicity

Liver transplantation, rejection prophylaxis (begin at least 30 days post-transplant): Oral: Initial: 1 mg twice daily; adjust maintenance dose if needed at a 4- to 5-day interval (from prior dose adjustment) based on serum concentrations, tolerability, and response; goal serum concentration is between 3 and 8 ng/mL (based on an LC/MS/MS assay method). If trough is <3 ng/mL, double total daily dose (using available tablet strengths); if trough >8 ng/mL on 2 consecutive measures, decrease dose by 0.25 mg twice daily. Administer in combination with tacrolimus (reduced dose required) and corticosteroids

Renal transplantation, rejection prophylaxis: Oral: Initial: 0.75 mg twice daily; adjust maintenance dose if needed at a 4- to 5-day interval (from prior dose adjustment) based on serum concentrations, tolerability, and response; goal serum concentration is between 3 and 8 ng/mL (based on an LC/MS/MS assay method). If trough is <3 ng/mL, double total daily dose (using available tablet strengths); if trough >8 ng/mL on 2 consecutive measures, decrease dose by 0.25 mg twice daily. Administer in combination with basiliximab induction and concurrently with cyclosporine (dose adjustment required) and corticosteroids

Subependymal giant cell astrocytoma (SEGA; dosing based on body surface area [BSA]): Oral: **Note:** Continue until disease progression or unacceptable toxicity.

Initial dose: 4.5 mg/m^2 once daily; round to nearest tablet (tablet or tablet for oral suspension) size.

If trough <5 ng/mL: Increase dose by 2.5 mg daily (tablets) or 2 mg daily (tablets for oral suspension).

◄ If trough >15 ng/mL: Reduce dose by 2.5 mg daily (tablets) or 2 mg daily (tablets for oral suspension). If dose reduction necessary in patients receiving the lowest strength available, administer every other day.

Therapeutic drug monitoring: Assess trough concentration ~2 weeks after initiation or with dosage modifications, initiation or changes to concurrent CYP3A4/P-glycoprotein (P-gp) inhibitor/inducer therapy, changes in hepatic impairment, or when changing dosage forms between tablets and tablets for oral suspension; adjust maintenance dose if needed at 2-week intervals to achieve and maintain trough concentrations between 5 and 15 ng/mL; once stable dose is attained and if BSA is stable throughout treatment, monitor trough concentrations every 6 to 12 months (monitor every 3 to 6 months if BSA is changing).

Carcinoid tumors, advanced (off-label use): Oral: 10 mg once daily (in combination with octreotide LAR) until disease progression or toxicity (Pavel, 2010)

Waldenström macroglobulinemia, relapsed or refractory (off-label use): Oral: 10 mg once daily until disease progression or toxicity (Ghobrial, 2010)

Dosage adjustment for concomitant CYP3A4 inhibitors/inducers and/or P-gp inhibitors:

Breast cancer, PNET, RCC, renal angiomyolipoma:

CYP3A4/P-gp inducers: Strong inducers: Avoid coadministration with strong CYP3A4/P-gp inducers (eg, carbamazepine, phenobarbital, phenytoin, rifabutin, rifampin, rifapentine, St John's wort); if concomitant use cannot be avoided, consider doubling the everolimus dose, using increments of 5 mg or less, with careful monitoring (Canadian labeling recommends a maximum daily dose of 20 mg in patients with renal angiomyolipoma). If the strong CYP3A4/P-gp enzyme inducer is discontinued, consider allowing 3 to 5 days to elapse prior to reducing the everolimus to the dose used prior to initiation of the CYP3A4/P-gp inducer.

CYP3A4/P-gp inhibitors:

Strong inhibitors: Avoid concomitant administration with strong CYP3A4/P-gp inhibitors (eg, atazanavir, clarithromycin, indinavir, itraconazole, ketoconazole, nefazodone, nelfinavir, ritonavir, saquinavir, telithromycin, voriconazole).

Moderate CYP3A4/P-gp inhibitors (eg, amprenavir, aprepitant, diltiazem, erythromycin, fluconazole, fosamprenavir, verapamil):

US labeling: Reduce everolimus dose to 2.5 mg once daily; may consider increasing from 2.5 mg to 5 mg once daily based on patient tolerance. When the moderate inhibitor is discontinued, allow ~2 to 3 days to elapse prior to adjusting the everolimus upward to the recommended starting dose or to the dose used prior to initiation of the moderate inhibitor.

Canadian labeling: Reduce everolimus dose by 50%; further reductions may be necessary for adverse reactions. If dose reduction is required for patients receiving the lowest available strength, consider alternate-day dosing. When the moderate inhibitor is discontinued, allow at least 3 days or 4 elimination half-lives to elapse prior to adjusting the everolimus to the dose used prior to initiation of the moderate inhibitor.

Renal transplantation: Dosage adjustments may be necessary based on everolimus serum concentrations

SEGA:

CYP3A4/P-gp inducers: Strong inducers:

US labeling: Avoid concomitant administration with strong CYP3A4/P-gp inducers (eg, carbamazepine, phenobarbital, phenytoin, rifabutin, rifampin, rifapentine, St John's wort); if concomitant use cannot be avoided, an initial starting everolimus dose of 9 mg/m^2 once daily is recommended, or, double the everolimus dose and assess tolerability; assess trough concentration after ~2 weeks; adjust dose as necessary based on therapeutic drug monitoring to maintain target trough concentrations of 5 to 15 ng/mL. If the strong CYP3A4 enzyme inducer is discontinued, reduce the everolimus dose by ~50% or to the dose used prior to initiation of the CYP3A4/P-gp inducer; reassess trough concentration after ~2 weeks.

Canadian labeling: Avoid concomitant administration with strong CYP3A4 inducers (eg, carbamazepine, oxcarbazepine, phenobarbital, phenytoin, rifampin, rifabutin, rifapentine, St John's wort); if concomitant use cannot be avoided and everolimus level <5 ng/mL, may increase daily dose by 2.5 mg every 2 weeks (tablets) or 2 mg every 2 weeks (tablets for oral suspension) until target everolimus trough concentration is 5 to 15 ng/mL. If the strong CYP3A4/P-gp inducer is discontinued, reduce everolimus to the dose used prior to initiation of the CYP3A4/P-gp inducer. Assess trough concentrations ~2 weeks after any change in dose or after any initiation or change in CYP3A4/P-gp inducer therapy.

CYP3A4/P-gp inhibitors:

Strong inhibitors: Avoid concomitant administration with strong CYP3A4/P-gp inhibitors (eg, atazanavir, clarithromycin, indinavir, itraconazole, ketoconazole, nefazodone, nelfinavir, ritonavir, saquinavir, telithromycin, voriconazole).

Moderate CYP3A4/P-gp inhibitors (eg, amprenavir, aprepitant, diltiazem, erythromycin, fluconazole, fosamprenavir, verapamil):

US labeling:

Currently taking a moderate CYP3A4/P-gp inhibitor and starting everolimus: 2.5 mg/m^2 once daily.

Currently taking everolimus and starting a moderate CYP3A4/P-gp inhibitor: Reduce everolimus dose by ~50%; if dose reduction is required for patients receiving the lowest strength available, administer every other day.

Discontinuing a moderate CYP3A4/P-gp inhibitor after concomitant use with everolimus: Discontinue moderate inhibitor and allow 2 to 3 days to elapse prior to resuming the everolimus dose used prior to initiation of the moderate inhibitor.

Therapeutic drug monitoring: Assess trough concentration ~2 weeks after everolimus initiation or dosage modifications, or initiation or changes to concurrent CYP3A4/P-gp inhibitor therapy; adjust maintenance dose if needed at 2-week intervals to achieve and maintain trough concentrations between 5 and 15 ng/mL.

Canadian labeling: Reduce everolimus dose by ~50% (if dose reduction is required for patients receiving the lowest strength available, consider alternate-day dosing). If the moderate inhibitor is discontinued, the everolimus dose should be returned to the dose used prior to initiation of the inhibitor.

◄

Therapeutic drug monitoring: Assess trough concentration ~2 weeks after everolimus initiation or dosage modifications, or initiation or changes to concurrent CYP3A4/P-gp inhibitor therapy. Maintain trough concentrations between 5 and 15 ng/mL; may increase dose within the target range to achieve higher concentrations as tolerated.

Pediatric Note: Tablets (Afinitor, Zortress) and tablets for oral suspension (Afinitor Disperz) are not interchangeable. Do not combine formulations to achieve total desired dose.

Subependymal giant cell astrocytoma (SEGA): Children ≥1 year: Refer to adult dosing.

Renal Impairment No dosage adjustment is necessary.

Hepatic Impairment

Mild impairment (Child-Pugh class A):

Breast cancer, PNET, RCC, renal angiomyolipoma: Reduce dose to 7.5 mg once daily; if not tolerated, may further reduce to 5 mg once daily.

Liver or renal transplantation: Reduce initial dose by ~33%; individualize subsequent dosing based on therapeutic drug monitoring (target trough concentration: 3 to 8 ng/mL).

SEGA:

U.S. labeling: Adjustment to initial dose may not be necessary; subsequent dosing is based on therapeutic drug monitoring (monitor ~2 weeks after initiation, dosage modifications, or after any change in hepatic status; target trough concentration: 5 to 15 ng/mL).

Canadian labeling: Initial:

Patients ≥18 years of age: 75% of usual dose based on calculated BSA (rounded to the nearest strength). Assess trough concentrations ~2 weeks after initiation, dosage modifications, or after any change in hepatic status. Target trough concentration: 5 to 15 ng/mL; may increase dose within the target range to achieve higher concentrations as tolerated.

Patients <18 years of age: Use is not recommended.

Moderate impairment (Child-Pugh class B):

Breast cancer, PNET, RCC, renal angiomyolipoma: Reduce dose to 5 mg once daily; if not tolerated, may further reduce to 2.5 mg once daily.

Liver or renal transplantation: Reduce initial dose by ~50%; individualize subsequent dosing based on therapeutic drug monitoring (target trough concentration: 3 to 8 ng/mL).

SEGA:

US labeling: Adjustment to initial dose may not be necessary; subsequent dosing is based on therapeutic drug monitoring (monitor ~2 weeks after initiation, dosage modifications, or after any change in hepatic status; target trough concentration: 5 to 15 ng/mL).

Canadian labeling: Initial:

Patients ≥18 years of age: 50% of usual dose based on calculated BSA (rounded to the nearest strength). Assess trough concentrations ~2 weeks after initiation, dosage modifications, or after any change in hepatic status. Target trough concentration: 5 to 15 ng/mL; may increase dose within the target range to achieve higher concentrations as tolerated.

Patients <18 years of age: Use is not recommended.

Severe impairment (Child-Pugh class C):

Breast cancer, PNET, RCC, renal angiomyolipoma: If potential benefit outweighs risks, a maximum dose of 2.5 mg once daily may be used.

Liver or renal transplantation: Reduce initial dose by ~50%; individualize subsequent dosing based on therapeutic drug monitoring (target trough concentration: 3 to 8 ng/mL).

SEGA:

US labeling: Reduce initial dose to 2.5 mg/m^2 once daily (or current dose by ~50%); subsequent dosing is based on therapeutic drug monitoring (monitor ~2 weeks after initiation, dosage modifications, or after any change in hepatic status; target trough concentration: 5 to 15 ng/mL).

Canadian labeling: Use is not recommended.

Adjustment for Toxicity

Breast cancer (adjustments apply to everolimus), PNET, RCC, renal angiomyolipoma, SEGA: Toxicities may require temporary dose interruption (with or without a subsequent dose reduction) or discontinuation; reduce everolimus dose by ~50% if dosage adjustment is necessary:

Noninfectious pneumonitis:

Grade 1 (asymptomatic radiological changes suggestive of pneumonitis): No dosage adjustment is necessary; monitor appropriately.

Grade 2 (symptomatic but not interfering with activities of daily living [ADL]): Consider interrupting treatment, rule out infection, and consider corticosteroids until symptoms improve to ≤ grade 1; reinitiate at a lower dose. Discontinue if recovery does not occur within 4 weeks.

Grade 3 (symptomatic, interferes with ADL; oxygen indicated): Interrupt treatment until symptoms improve to ≤ grade 1; rule out infection and consider corticosteroid treatment; may reinitiate at a lower dose. If grade 3 toxicity recurs, consider discontinuing.

Grade 4 (life-threatening; ventilatory support indicated): Discontinue treatment; rule out infection; consider corticosteroid treatment.

Stomatitis (avoid the use of products containing alcohol, hydrogen peroxide, iodine, or thyme derivatives):

Grade 1 (minimal symptoms, normal diet): No dosage adjustment is necessary; manage with mouth wash (nonalcoholic or isotonic salt water) several times a day

Grade 2 (symptomatic but can eat and swallow modified diet): Interrupt treatment until symptoms improve to ≤ grade 1; reinitiate at same dose; if stomatitis recurs at grade 2, interrupt treatment until symptoms improve to ≤ grade 1 and then reinitiate at a lower dose. Also manage with topical (oral) analgesics (eg, benzocaine, butyl aminobenzoate, tetracaine, menthol, or phenol) ± topical (oral) corticosteroids (eg, triamcinolone).

Grade 3 (symptomatic and unable to orally aliment or hydrate adequately): Interrupt treatment until symptoms improve to ≤ grade 1; then reinitiate at a lower dose. Also manage with topical (oral) analgesics (eg, benzocaine, butyl aminobenzoate, tetracaine, menthol, or phenol) ± topical (oral) corticosteroids (eg, triamcinolone).

Grade 4 (life-threatening symptoms): Discontinue treatment; initiate appropriate medical intervention.

Metabolic toxicity (eg, hyperglycemia, dyslipidemia):

Grade 1: No dosage adjustment is necessary; initiate appropriate medical intervention and monitor.

Grade 2: No dosage adjustment is necessary; manage with appropriate medical intervention and monitor.

Grade 3: Temporarily interrupt treatment; reinitiate at a lower dose; manage with appropriate medical intervention and monitor.

◀

Grade 4: Discontinue treatment; manage with appropriate medical intervention.

Nonhematologic toxicities (excluding pneumonitis, stomatitis, or metabolic toxicity):

Grade 1: If toxicity is tolerable, no dosage adjustment is necessary; initiate appropriate medical intervention and monitor.

Grade 2: If toxicity is tolerable, no dosage adjustment is necessary; initiate appropriate medical intervention and monitor. If toxicity becomes intolerable, temporarily interrupt treatment until improvement to ≤ grade 1 and reinitiate at the same dose; if toxicity recurs at grade 2, temporarily interrupt treatment until improvement to ≤ grade 1 and then reinitiate at a lower dose.

Grade 3: Temporarily interrupt treatment until improvement to ≤ grade 1; initiate appropriate medical intervention and monitor. May reinitiate at a lower dose; if toxicity recurs at grade 3, consider discontinuing.

Grade 4 (life-threatening symptoms): Discontinue treatment; initiate appropriate medical intervention.

Liver or renal transplantation:

Evidence of polyoma virus infection or PML: Consider reduced immunosuppression (taking into account the allograft risks associated with decreased immunosuppression)

Pneumonitis (grade 4 symptoms) or invasive systemic fungal infection: Discontinue

SEGA: *Severe/intolerable adverse reactions:* Temporarily interrupt or permanently discontinue treatment; if dose reduction is required upon reinitiation, reduce dose by ~50%; if dose reduction is required for patients receiving the lowest available strength, consider alternate-day dosing.

Combination Regimens

Breast cancer: Everolimus-Exemestane (Breast) on page 1965

Renal cell cancer: Everolimus (RCC Regimen) on page 1965

Waldenstrom Macroglobulinemia: Everolimus (Waldenstrom Macroglobulinemia) on page 1966

Administration May be taken with or without food; to reduce variability, take consistently with regard to food. Afinitor missed doses may be taken up to 6 hours after regularly scheduled time; if >6 hours, resume at next regularly scheduled time.

Tablets: Swallow whole with a glass of water. Do not break, chew, or crush (do not administer tablets that are crushed or broken). Avoid contact with or exposure to crushed or broken tablets.

Tablets for oral suspension: Administer as a suspension only. Administer immediately after preparation; discard if not administered within 60 minutes after preparation. Prepare suspension in water only. Do not break or crush tablets.

Preparation in an oral syringe: Place dose into 10 mL oral syringe (maximum: 10 mg/syringe; use an additional syringe for doses >10 mg). Draw ~5 mL of water and ~4 mL of air into oral syringe; allow to sit (tip up) in a container until tablets are in suspension (3 minutes). Gently invert syringe 5 times immediately prior to administration; administer contents, then add ~5 mL water and ~4 mL of air to same syringe, swirl to suspend remaining particles and administer entire contents.

Preparation in a small glass: Place dose into a small glass (≤100 mL) containing ~25 mL water (maximum: 10 mg/glass; use and additional glass for doses >10 mg); allow to sit until tablets are in suspension (3 minutes).

Stir gently with spoon immediately prior to administration; administer contents, then add ~25 mL water to same glass, swirl with same spoon to suspend remaining particles and administer entire contents.

Breast cancer, pancreatic neuroendocrine tumors, renal cell cancer, renal angiolipoma, SEGA: Administer at the same time each day.

Liver transplantation: Administer consistently ~12 hours apart; administer at the same time as tacrolimus.

Renal transplantation: Administer consistently ~12 hours apart; administer at the same time as cyclosporine.

Hazardous agent; use appropriate precautions for handling and disposal (NIOSH 2014 [group 1]). To avoid potential contact with everolimus, caregivers should wear gloves when preparing suspension from tablets for oral suspension. NIOSH recommends single gloving for administration of intact tablets (NIOSH 2014). Avoid exposure to crushed tablets. When it is necessary to manipulate the tablets (eg, to prepare an oral liquid or suspension), it is recommended to double glove, wear a protective gown, and prepare in a controlled device (NIOSH 2014).

Emetic Potential Children and Adults: Low (10% to 30%)

Extemporaneous Preparations Hazardous agent: Use appropriate precautions for handling and disposal (NIOSH 2014 [group 1]). When compounding an oral liquid or suspension, NIOSH recommends double gloving, a protective gown, and preparation in a controlled device; if not prepared in a controlled device, respiratory and eye protection as well as ventilated engineering controls are recommended (NIOSH 2014).

Tablets: An oral liquid may be prepared using tablets. Disperse tablet in ~30 mL (1 oz) of water; gently stir. Administer and rinse container with additional 30 mL (1 oz) water and administer to ensure entire dose is administered. Administer immediately after preparation.

Afinitor (everolimus) [prescribing information]. East Hanover, NJ: Novartis Pharmaceuticals Corporation; July 2012.

Tablets for oral suspension: Administer as a suspension only. Administer immediately after preparation; discard if not administered within 60 minutes after preparation. Prepare suspension in water only. Do not break or crush tablets.

Preparation in an oral syringe: Place dose into 10 mL oral syringe (maximum 10 mg/syringe; use an additional syringe for doses >10 mg). Draw ~5 mL of water and ~4 mL of air into oral syringe; allow to sit (tip up) in a container until tablets are in suspension (3 minutes). Gently invert syringe 5 times immediately prior to administration; administer contents, then add ~5 mL water and ~4 mL of air to same syringe, swirl to suspend remaining particles and administer entire contents.

Preparation in a small glass: Place dose into a small glass (≤100 mL) containing ~25 mL water (maximum 10 mg/glass; use an additional glass for doses >10 mg); allow to sit until tablets are in suspension (3 minutes). Stir gently with spoon immediately prior to administration; administer contents, then add ~25 mL water to same glass, swirl with same spoon to suspend remaining particles and administer entire contents.

Administer immediately after preparation; discard if not administered within 60 minutes after preparation.

Afinitor and Afinitor Disperz (everolimus) [prescribing information]. East Hanover, NJ: Novartis Pharmaceuticals Corporation; August 2012.

Monitoring Parameters CBC with differential (baseline and periodic), liver function; serum creatinine, urinary protein, and BUN (baseline and periodic); fasting serum glucose and lipid profile (baseline and periodic); monitor for signs and symptoms of infection, noninfectious pneumonitis, or malignancy

For liver or renal transplantation, monitor everolimus whole blood trough concentrations (based on an LC/MS/MS assay method), especially in patients with hepatic impairment, with concomitant CYP3A4 inhibitors and inducers, and when cyclosporine formulations or doses are changed; dosage adjustments should be made on trough concentrations obtained 4 to 5 days after a previous dosage adjustment; monitor cyclosporine concentrations; monitor for proteinuria

For SEGA, monitor everolimus whole blood trough concentrations ~2 weeks after treatment initiation or with dosage modifications, initiation or changes to concurrent CYP3A4/P-glycoprotein (P-gp) inhibitor/inducer therapy, changes in hepatic function and when changing dosage forms between Afinitor tablets and Afinitor Disperz. Maintain trough concentrations between 5 and 15 ng/mL; once stable dose is attained and if BSA is stable throughout treatment, monitor trough concentrations every 6 to 12 months (monitor every 3 to 6 months if BSA is changing).

Dietary Considerations Avoid grapefruit juice.

Medication Guide Available Yes

Dosage Forms Excipient information presented when available (limited, particularly for generics); consult specific product labeling.

Tablet, Oral:
Afinitor: 2.5 mg, 5 mg, 7.5 mg, 10 mg
Zortress: 0.25 mg, 0.5 mg, 0.75 mg
Tablet Soluble, Oral:
Afinitor Disperz: 2 mg, 3 mg, 5 mg

- ◆ **Evista** see Raloxifene on page 1451
- ◆ **Exalgo** see HYDROmorphone on page 830

Exemestane (ex e MES tane)

Related Information
Safe Handling of Hazardous Drugs on page 2292

Brand Names: US Aromasin

Brand Names: Canada Aromasin; CO Exemestane

Pharmacologic Category Antineoplastic Agent, Aromatase Inhibitor

Use Breast cancer: Treatment of advanced breast cancer in postmenopausal women whose disease has progressed following tamoxifen therapy; adjuvant treatment of postmenopausal women with estrogen receptor-positive early breast cancer following 2-3 years of tamoxifen (for a total of 5 consecutive years of adjuvant therapy).

Labeled Contraindications Known hypersensitivity to exemestane or any component of the formulation; women who are or may become pregnant; premenopausal women

Pregnancy Considerations Adverse events were observed in animal reproduction studies. Exemestane is not indicated for use in premenopausal women and use during pregnancy is contraindicated. Based on the mechanism of action, exemestane is expected to cause fetal harm if administered to a pregnant woman.

Breast-Feeding Considerations Exemestane is indicated for use only in postmenopausal women. Due to the potential for serious adverse reactions in the nursing infant, the manufacturer recommends a decision be made whether to discontinue nursing or to discontinue the drug, taking into account the importance of treatment to the mother.

Warnings/Precautions Hazardous agent - use appropriate precautions for handling and disposal (NIOSH 2014 [group 1]). Due to decreased circulating estrogen levels, exemestane is associated with a reduction in bone mineral density over time; decreases (from baseline) in lumbar spine and femoral neck density have been observed; assess bone mineral density at baseline in patients with, or at risk for osteoporosis; monitor exemestane therapy and initiate osteoporosis treatment if indicated. Due to high prevalence of vitamin D deficiency in women with breast cancer, assess 25-hydroxy vitamin D levels at baseline and supplement accordingly. Grade 3 or 4 lymphopenia has been observed with exemestane, although most patients had preexisting lower grade lymphopenia; some patients improved or recovered while continuing exemestane; lymphopenia did not result in a significant increase in viral infections, and no opportunistic infections were observed. Elevations of AST, ALT, alkaline phosphatase, and gamma glutamyl transferase >5 times ULN have been observed (rarely) in patients with advanced breast cancer; may be attributable to underlying liver and/or bone metastases. In patients with early breast cancer, elevations of bilirubin, alkaline phosphatase, and serum creatinine were more common with exemestane treatment than with tamoxifen or placebo. Potentially significant drug-drug interactions may exist, requiring dose or frequency adjustment, additional monitoring, and/or selection of alternative therapy. Not to be given with estrogen-containing agents. Dose adjustment recommended with concomitant strong CYP3A4 inducers.

Adverse Reactions

>10%:

Cardiovascular: Hypertension (5% to 15%)

Central nervous system: Fatigue (8% to 22%), insomnia (11% to 14%), pain (13%), headache (7% to 13%), depression (6% to 13%)

Dermatological: Hyperhidrosis (4% to 18%), alopecia (15%)

Endocrine & metabolic: Hot flashes (13% to 33%)

Gastrointestinal: Nausea (9% to 18%), abdominal pain (6% to 11%)

Hepatic: Alkaline phosphatase increased (14% to 15%)

Neuromuscular & skeletal: Arthralgia (15% to 29%)

1% to 10%:

Cardiovascular: Edema (6% to 7%); cardiac ischemic events (2%: MI, angina, myocardial ischemia); chest pain

Central nervous system: Dizziness (8% to 10%), anxiety (4% to 10%), fever (5%), confusion, hypoesthesia

Dermatologic: Dermatitis (8%), itching, rash

Endocrine & metabolic: Weight gain (8%)

Gastrointestinal: Diarrhea (4% to 10%), vomiting (7%), anorexia (6%), constipation (5%), appetite increased (3%), dyspepsia

Genitourinary: Urinary tract infection (2% to 5%)

Hepatic: Bilirubin increased (5% to 7%)

Neuromuscular & skeletal: Back pain (9%), limb pain (9%), myalgia (6%), osteoarthritis (6%), weakness (6%), osteoporosis (5%), pathological fracture (4%), paresthesia (3%), carpal tunnel syndrome (2%), cramps (2%)

Ocular: Visual disturbances (5%)

Renal: Creatinine increased (6%)

Respiratory: Dyspnea (10%), cough (6%), bronchitis, pharyngitis, rhinitis, sinusitis, upper respiratory infection

Miscellaneous: Flu-like syndrome (6%), lymphedema, infection

<1%, postmarketing, and/or case reports: Acute generalized exanthematous pustulosis, cardiac failure, cholestatic hepatitis, endometrial hyperplasia, gastric ulcer, GGT increased, hepatitis, hypersensitivity, neuropathy, osteo-chondrosis, pruritus, thromboembolism, transaminases increased, trigger finger, urticaria, uterine polyps

A dose-dependent decrease in sex hormone-binding globulin has been observed with daily doses of ≥2.5 mg. Serum luteinizing hormone and follicle-stimulating hormone levels have increased with this medicine.

Drug Interactions

Metabolism/Transport Effects Substrate of CYP3A4 (major); **Note:** Assignment of Major/Minor substrate status based on clinically relevant drug interaction potential; **Induces** CYP3A4 (weak)

Avoid Concomitant Use

Avoid concomitant use of Exemestane with any of the following: Estrogen Derivatives

Increased Effect/Toxicity

Exemestane may increase the levels/effects of: Methadone

The levels/effects of Exemestane may be increased by: Osimertinib

Decreased Effect

Exemestane may decrease the levels/effects of: ARIPiprazole; Hydrocodone; NiMODipine; Saxagliptin

The levels/effects of Exemestane may be decreased by: Bosentan; CYP3A4 Inducers (Moderate); CYP3A4 Inducers (Strong); Dabrafenib; Deferasirox; Enzalutamide; Estrogen Derivatives; Mitotane; Osimertinib; Siltuximab; St Johns Wort; Tocilizumab

Food Interactions Plasma levels increased by 40% when exemestane was taken with a fatty meal. Management: Administer after a meal.

Storage/Stability Store at 25°C (77°F); excursions permitted to 15°C to 30°C (59°F to 86°F).

Mechanism of Action Exemestane is an irreversible, steroidal aromatase inactivator. It is structurally related to androstenedione, and is converted to an intermediate that irreversibly blocks the active site of the aromatase enzyme, leading to inactivation ("suicide inhibition") and thus preventing conversion of androgens to estrogens in peripheral tissues. Significantly lowers circulating estrogens in postmenopausal breast cancers where growth is estrogen-dependent.

Pharmacodynamics/Kinetics

Absorption: Rapid and moderate (~42%) following oral administration; AUC and C_{max} increased by 59% and 39%, respectively, following a high-fat breakfast (compared to fasted state)

Distribution: Extensive into tissues

Protein binding: 90%, primarily to albumin and α_1-acid glycoprotein

Metabolism: Extensively hepatic; oxidation (CYP3A4) of methylene group, reduction of 17-keto group with formation of many secondary metabolites; metabolites are inactive

Half-life elimination: ~24 hours

Time to peak: Women with breast cancer: 1.2 hours

Excretion: Urine (<1% as unchanged drug, 39% to 45% as metabolites); feces (36% to 48%)

Dosing

Adult & Geriatric

Breast cancer, advanced: Postmenopausal females: Oral: 25 mg once daily; continue until tumor progression

Breast cancer, early (adjuvant treatment): Postmenopausal females: Oral: 25 mg once daily (following 2 to 3 years of tamoxifen therapy) for a total duration of 5 years of endocrine therapy (in the absence of recurrence or contralateral breast cancer). **Note:** The American Society of Clinical Oncology (ASCO) guidelines for Adjuvant Endocrine Therapy of Hormone Receptor-Positive Breast Cancer (Focused Update) recommend a maximum duration of 5 years of aromatase inhibitor (AI) therapy for postmenopausal women; AIs may be combined with tamoxifen for a total duration of up to 10 years of endocrine therapy. Refer to the guidelines for specific recommendations based on menopausal status and tolerability (Burstein 2014).

Breast cancer, early (first-line adjuvant treatment; off-label use): Postmenopausal females: Oral: 25 mg once daily for 5 years (Burstein 2010; van de Velde 2011). **Note:** ASCO guidelines for Adjuvant Endocrine Therapy of Hormone Receptor-Positive Breast Cancer (Focused Update) recommend a maximum duration of 5 years of aromatase inhibitor (AI) therapy for postmenopausal women; AIs may be combined with tamoxifen for a total duration of up to 10 years of endocrine therapy. Refer to the guidelines for specific recommendations based on menopausal status and tolerability (Burstein 2014).

Breast cancer, risk reduction (off-label use): Postmenopausal females ≥35 years: Oral: 25 mg once daily for 5 years (Goss 2011; Visvanathan 2013)

Dosage adjustment with strong CYP3A4 inducers: U.S. labeling: 50 mg once daily when used with potent inducers (eg, rifampin, phenytoin)

Renal Impairment No adjustment necessary (although the safety of chronic doses in patients with moderate-to-severe renal impairment has not been studied, dosage adjustment does not appear necessary).

Hepatic Impairment No adjustment necessary (although the safety of chronic doses in patients with moderate-to-severe hepatic impairment has not been studied, dosage adjustment does not appear necessary).

Combination Regimens

Breast cancer: Everolimus-Exemestane (Breast) on page 1965

Administration Administer after a meal. Hazardous agent; use appropriate precautions for handling and disposal (NIOSH 2014 [group 1]).

Monitoring Parameters 25-hydroxy vitamin D levels (at baseline); bone mineral density

Dietary Considerations Patients on aromatase inhibitor therapy should receive vitamin D and calcium supplements.

Dosage Forms Excipient information presented when available (limited, particularly for generics); consult specific product labeling.

Tablet, Oral:

Aromasin: 25 mg

Generic: 25 mg

◆ **Exjade** see Deferasirox on page 478

◆ **Extended Release Epidural Morphine** *see* Morphine (Liposomal) *on page 1173*

Factor VIIa (Recombinant) <small>(FAK ter SEV en aye ree KOM be nant)</small>

Brand Names: US NovoSeven RT

Brand Names: Canada Niastase; Niastase RT

Index Terms Coagulation Factor VIIa; Eptacog Alfa (Activated); rFVIIa

Pharmacologic Category Antihemophilic Agent

Use Bleeding episodes and perioperative management: Treatment of bleeding episodes and perioperative management in adults and children with hemophilia A or B with inhibitors, congenital factor VII (FVII) deficiency, and Glanzmann's thrombasthenia with refractoriness to platelet transfusions, with or without antibodies to platelets; treatment of bleeding episodes and perioperative management in adults with acquired hemophilia.

Pregnancy Risk Factor C

Dosing

Adult & Geriatric IV:

Hemophilia A or B with inhibitors:

Bleeding episodes: 90 mcg/kg every 2 hours until hemostasis is achieved or until the treatment is judged ineffective. Doses between 35 and 90 mcg/kg have been used successfully in clinical trials. The dose, interval, and duration of therapy may be adjusted based upon the severity of bleeding and the degree of hemostasis achieved. For patients experiencing severe bleeds, dosing should be continued at 3- to 6-hour intervals after hemostasis has been achieved and the duration of dosing should be minimized.

Perioperative management: 90 mcg/kg immediately before surgery (additional bolus doses may be administered for major surgery if required); repeat at 2-hour intervals for the duration of surgery. For minor surgery, continue 90 mcg/kg every 2 hours for 48 hours, then every 2 to 6 hours until healed. For major surgery, continue 90 mcg/kg every 2 hours for 5 days, then every 4 hours until healed.

Congenital factor VII deficiency:

Bleeding episodes: 15 to 30 mcg/kg every 4 to 6 hours until hemostasis is achieved. Doses as low as 10 mcg/kg have been effective.

Perioperative management: 15 to 30 mcg/kg immediately before surgery; repeat every 4 to 6 hours for the duration of surgery and until hemostasis achieved. Doses as low as 10 mcg/kg have been effective.

Acquired hemophilia:

Bleeding episodes: 70 to 90 mcg/kg every 2 to 3 hours until hemostasis is achieved.

Perioperative management: 70 to 90 mcg/kg immediately before surgery; repeat every 2 to 3 hours for the duration of surgery and until hemostasis achieved.

Glanzmann's thrombasthenia:

Bleeding episodes (refractory to platelet transfusions): 90 mcg/kg every 2 to 6 hours until hemostasis is achieved.

Perioperative management: 90 mcg/kg immediately before surgery; repeat at 2-hour intervals for the duration of surgery. Continue 90 mcg/kg every 2 to 6 hours to prevent postoperative bleeding. **Note:** Higher average infused doses (median: 100 mcg/kg) were noted for surgical patients who had clinical refractoriness with or without platelet-specific antibodies compared to those with neither.

Intracerebral hemorrhage (ICH) (warfarin-related) (off-label use; Freeman, 2004; Ilyas, 2008): 10 to 100 mcg/kg (see **"Note"** below) administered concurrently with IV vitamin K (to correct the nonfactor VII coagulation factors).

Note: Lower doses (10 to 20 mcg/kg) are generally preferred given the higher risk of thromboembolic complications with higher doses; response is highly variable; monitor INR frequently after administration since rebound increases in INR occur quickly given the short half-life of rFVIIa; duration of INR correction is dose dependent. Routine use as a sole agent is not recommended for warfarin-related ICH (Morgenstern, 2010).

Treatment of refractory bleeding after cardiac surgery in nonhemophiliac patients: Dosing not established; doses in the range of 35 to 70 mcg/kg have been recommended based on low-quality evidence (case series, observational studies) (Chapman, 2011; Ferraris, 2011; Karkouti, 2007); in patients with a left ventricular assist device, lower doses (ie, 10 to 20 mcg/kg) may be preferred to reduce thromboembolic events (Bruckner, 2009).

Pediatric

Congenital factor VII deficiency: Children and Adolescents: Refer to adult dosing.

Glanzmann's thrombasthenia: Children and Adolescents: Refer to adult dosing.

Hemophilia A or B with inhibitors: Children and Adolescents: Refer to adult dosing.

Renal Impairment There are no dosage adjustments provided the in manufacturer's labeling.

Hepatic Impairment There are no dosage adjustments provided in the manufacturer's labeling; use with caution.

Additional Information Complete prescribing information should be consulted for additional detail.

Dosage Forms Excipient information presented when available (limited, particularly for generics); consult specific product labeling.

Solution Reconstituted, Intravenous [preservative free]:

NovoSeven RT: 1 mg (1 ea); 2 mg (1 ea); 5 mg (1 ea); 8 mg (1 ea) [contains polysorbate 80]

- ◆ **Factor VIII** see Antihemophilic Factor (Recombinant [Porcine Sequence]) on page 123
- ◆ **Factor VIII (Human)** see Antihemophilic Factor (Human) on page 117
- ◆ **Factor VIII (Recombinant)** see Antihemophilic Factor (Recombinant) on page 119
- ◆ **Factor VIII (Recombinant [Pegylated])** see Antihemophilic Factor (Recombinant [Pegylated]) on page 123
- ◆ **Factor VIII (Recombinant)** see Antihemophilic Factor (Recombinant [Porcine Sequence]) on page 123

Factor IX Complex (Human) [(Factors II, IX, X)]
(FAK ter nyne KOM pleks HYU man FAKter too nyne ten)

Brand Names: US Bebulin; Bebulin VH; Profilnine; Profilnine SD

Index Terms 3 Factor PCC; 3-Factor PCC; PCC (Caution: Confusion-prone synonym); Prothrombin Complex Concentrate (Caution: Confusion-prone synonym); Three-Factor PCC

Pharmacologic Category Antihemophilic Agent; Blood Product Derivative; Prothrombin Complex Concentrate (PCC)

Use

Factor IX deficiency (hemophilia B [Christmas disease]): Prevention and control of bleeding in patients with factor IX deficiency (hemophilia B or Christmas disease)

Limitations of use: Not indicated for the treatment of other factor deficiencies (eg, factor II, VII, VIII, X), treatment of hemophilia A patients with inhibitors to factor VIII, or treatment of bleeding caused by low levels of liver-dependent coagulation factors.

Pregnancy Risk Factor C

Dosing

Adult & Geriatric Note: Factor IX complex (Human) [Factors II, IX, X] (Bebulin, Profilnine) contains low or nontherapeutic levels of factor VII component and should not be confused with Prothrombin Complex Concentrate (Human) [(Factors II, VII, IX, X), Protein C, Protein S] (Kcentra, Octaplex) which contains therapeutic levels of factor VII.

Control or prevention of bleeding in patients with factor IX deficiency (hemophilia B [Christmas disease]): Dosage is expressed in units of factor IX activity and must be individualized based on severity of factor IX deficiency, extent and location of bleeding, and clinical status of patient. Close laboratory monitoring of the factor IX level is required to determine proper dosage, particularly with severe hemorrhage and major surgery. Larger doses than those derived from the formula below may be required, especially if treatment is delayed. When multiple doses are required, administer at 24-hour intervals unless otherwise specified.

Formula for units required to raise blood level %:

Bebulin: In general, factor IX 1 unit/kg will increase the plasma factor IX level by 0.8%

Number of Factor IX units required = body weight (kg) x desired factor IX increase (as % of normal) x 1.2 units/kg

Profilnine: In general, factor IX 1 unit/kg will increase the plasma factor IX level by 1%:

Number of factor IX units required = bodyweight (kg) x desired factor IX increase (as % of normal) x 1 unit/kg

For example, to increase factor IX level to 25% of normal in a 70 kg patient: Number of factor IX units needed = 70 kg x 25 x 1 unit/kg = 1,750 units

As a general rule, the level of factor IX required for treatment of different conditions is listed below:

Hemorrhage: IV:

Minor bleeding (early hemarthrosis, minor epistaxis, gingival bleeding, mild hematuria):

Bebulin: Raise factor IX level to 20% of normal (typical initial dose: 25 to 35 units/kg); average duration of treatment is 1 day. A single dose is usually sufficient or a second dose may be given after 24 hours.

Profilnine: Raise factor IX level to 20% to 30% of normal (initial dose: 20 to 30 units/kg) every 16 to 24 hours for 1 to 2 days for minor hemorrhage or until hemorrhage stops and healing has been achieved.

Moderate bleeding (severe joint bleeding, early hematoma, major open bleeding, minor trauma, minor hemoptysis, hematemesis, melena, major hematuria):

Bebulin: Raise factor IX level to 40% of normal (typical initial dose: 50 to 65 units/kg); average duration of treatment is 2 days or until adequate wound healing.

Profilnine: Raise factor IX level to 20% to 30% of normal (initial dose: 20 to 30 units/kg) every 16 to 24 hours for 2 to 7 days for moderate hemorrhage or until hemorrhage stops and healing has been achieved.

Major bleeding (severe hematoma, major trauma, severe hemoptysis, hematemesis, melena):

Bebulin: Raise factor IX level to ≥60% of normal (typical initial dose: 75 to 90 units/kg); average duration of treatment is 2 to 3 days or until adequate wound healing.

Profilnine: Raise factor IX level to 30% to 50% of normal (initial dose: 30 to 50 units/kg) every 16 to 24 hours; following this treatment period, maintain factor IX levels at 20% of normal (maintenance dose: 20 units/kg) for 3 to 10 days or until healing has been achieved.

Surgical procedures: IV:

Dental surgery:

Bebulin: Raise factor IX level to 40% to 60% of normal on day of surgery (typical dose: 50 to 75 units/kg). One infusion, administered 1 hour prior to surgery, is generally sufficient for the extraction of one tooth; for the extraction of multiple teeth, replacement therapy may be required for up to 1 week (See dosing guidelines for *Minor Surgery*).

Profilnine: Raise factor IX level to 50% of normal immediately prior to procedure; maintain factor IX levels at 30% to 50% of normal (maintenance dose: 30 to 50 units/kg) every 16 to 24 hours for 7 to 10 days following surgery or until healing has been achieved.

Minor surgery:

Bebulin: Raise factor IX level to 40% to 60% of normal on day of surgery (typical initial dose: 50 to 75 units/kg). Decrease factor IX level from 40% to 60% of normal to 20% to 40% of normal during initial postoperative period (1 to 2 weeks or until adequate wound healing) [typical dose: 26 to 65 units/kg]. The preoperative dose should be given 1 hour prior to surgery. The average dosing interval may be every 12 hours initially, then every 24 hours later in the postoperative period.

Profilnine: Raise factor IX level to 30% to 50% of normal (initial dose: 30 to 50 units/kg) prior to surgery (**Note:** Surgery type not specified by the manufacturer); maintain factor IX levels at 30% to 50% of normal (maintenance dose: 30 to 50 units/kg) every 16 to 24 hours for 7 to 10 days following surgery or until healing is achieved.

Major surgery:

Bebulin: Raise factor IX level to ≥60% of normal on day of surgery (typical initial dose: 75 to 90 units/kg). Decrease factor IX level from ≥60% of normal to 20% to 60% of normal during initial postoperative period (1 to 2 weeks) [typical dose: 25 to 75 units/kg]; further decrease to maintain a factor IX level of 20% of normal during late postoperative period (≥3 weeks) and continuing until adequate wound healing is achieved [typical dose: 25 to 35 units/kg]. The preoperative dose should be given 1 hour prior to surgery. The average dosing interval may be every 12 hours initially, then every 24 hours later in the postoperative period.

Profilnine: Raise Factor IX level to 30% to 50% of normal (initial dose: 30 to 50 units/kg) prior to surgery (**Note:** Surgery type not specified by the manufacturer); maintain factor IX levels at 30% to 50% of normal (maintenance dose: 30 to 50 units/kg) every 16 to 24 hours for 7 to 10 days following surgery or until healing is achieved.

Warfarin associated hemorrhage (off-label use): IV: **Note:** Products contain low or nontherapeutic levels of factor VII component; therefore, additional fresh frozen plasma (FFP) or factor VIIa may be considered (Masotti 2011). When immediate INR reversal is required, concomitant use of 1 to 2 units of FFP should be considered to ensure acute INR reversal (Baker 2004; Holland 2009). Coadminister vitamin K (phytonadione) 5 to 10 mg by slow IV infusion (ACCP [Guyatt 2012]); vitamin K may be repeated every 12 hours if INR is persistently elevated. Dosing has not been established; the following regimens have been used with some success.

The following 2 methods have been suggested, but are not product specific:

Adjusted-dose regimen, weight based (Liumbruno 2009):

INR <2: 20 units/kg

INR 2 to 4: 30 units/kg

INR >4: 50 units/kg

Note: If after administration, INR remains >1.5 consider repeating dose appropriate for INR.

May also determine dose based on presenting INR and estimated functional prothrombin complex (PC) expressed as percentage of normal plasma levels (see table; Masotti 2011):

Units needed to be infused = (**target** % of functional PC to be reached - **current** estimated % of functional PC) x kg of body weight

Example:

Patient (weight: 70 kg) presents with INR of 4.5 which corresponds to an **estimated % functional PC** of 10% (see table). Target INR of 1.4 corresponds to an **estimated target % functional PC** of 40%.

Units needed to be infused = (40 - 10) x 70 kg = 2,100 units

Conversion of the INR to Estimated Functional Prothrombin Complex (PC)

INR Value	Estimated Functional PC
≥5	5%
4 to 4.9	10%
2.6 to 3.2	15%
2.2 to 2.5	20%
1.9 to 2.1	25%
1.7 to 1.8	30%
1.4 to 1.6	40%
1 to 1.3	100%

Warfarin associated intracranial hemorrhage (off-label use): IV: **Note:** Products contain low or nontherapeutic levels of factor VII component; therefore, additional FFP or factor VIIa may be considered (Masotti 2011).

When immediate INR reversal is required, concomitant use of 1 to 2 units of FFP should be considered to ensure acute INR reversal (Baker 2004; Chong 2010; Holland 2009). Coadminister vitamin K (phytonadione) 5 to 10 mg by slow IV infusion (ACCP [Guyatt 2012]); vitamin K may be repeated every 12 hours if INR is persistently elevated. Dosing has not been established; the following regimens have been used with some success.

Fixed-dose regimen, weight based (Frontera 2014): 50 units/kg irrespective of INR; if after administration INR is not corrected to <1.4, FFP may be administered. **Note:** Bebulin used during study.

Adjusted-dose regimen, weight based (Chong 2010):

INR <5: 30 units/kg

INR >5 (emergent): 50 units/kg

Note: Profilnine used during study. If after administration INR remains >1.2, consider repeating dose and administering more FFP until INR <1.2

Pediatric Control or prevention of bleeding in patients with factor IX deficiency (hemophilia B [Christmas disease]) (off-label use): IV: Refer to adult dosing.

Renal Impairment There are no dosage adjustments provided in the manufacturer's labeling.

Hepatic Impairment There are no dosage adjustments provided in the manufacturer's labeling; monitor factor IX levels. Use with caution due to the risk of thromboembolic complications.

Additional Information Complete prescribing information should be consulted for additional detail.

Dosage Forms Considerations

Strengths expressed as an approximate value. Consult individual vial labels for exact potency within each vial.

Bebulin VH packaged contents may contain natural rubber latex.

Dosage Forms Excipient information presented when available (limited, particularly for generics); consult specific product labeling.

Solution Reconstituted, Intravenous:

Bebulin: 200-1200 units (1 ea)

Bebulin VH: 200-1200 units (1 ea)

Profilnine: 500 units (1 ea); 1000 units (1 ea); 1500 units (1 ea) [contains polysorbate 80]

Profilnine SD: 500 units (1 ea); 1000 units (1 ea); 1500 units (1 ea) [contains polysorbate 80]

◆ **Factor IX Concentrate** see Factor IX (Human) *on page 681*

◆ **Factor IX Concentrate** see Factor IX (Recombinant) *on page 684*

Factor IX (Human) (FAK ter nyne HYU man)

Brand Names: US AlphaNine SD; Mononine

Brand Names: Canada Immunine VH

Index Terms Factor IX Concentrate

Pharmacologic Category Antihemophilic Agent; Blood Product Derivative

Use Prevention and control of bleeding in patients with hemophilia B (congenital factor IX deficiency or Christmas disease)

◄ **NOTE:** Contains **nondetectable levels of factors II, VII, and X.** Therefore, **NOT INDICATED** for replacement therapy of any other clotting factor besides factor IX or for reversal of anticoagulation due to either vitamin K antagonists or other anticoagulants (eg, dabigatran), for hemophilia A patients with factor VIII inhibitors, or for patients in a hemorrhagic state caused by reduced production of liver-dependent coagulation factors (eg, hepatitis, cirrhosis).

Pregnancy Risk Factor C
Dosing

Adult & Geriatric NOTE: Contains **nondetectable levels of factors II, VII, and X.** Therefore, **NOT INDICATED** for replacement therapy of any other clotting factor besides factor IX or for reversal of anticoagulation due to either vitamin K antagonists or other anticoagulants (eg, dabigatran), for hemophilia A patients with factor VIII inhibitors, or for patients in a hemorrhagic state caused by reduced production of liver-dependent coagulation factors (eg, hepatitis, cirrhosis).

Control or prevention of bleeding in patients with factor IX deficiency (hemophilia B or Christmas disease): IV: *AlphaNine SD, Mononine:* Dosage is expressed in units of factor IX activity; dosing must be individualized based on severity of factor IX deficiency, extent and location of bleeding, and clinical status of patient. Refer to product information for specific manufacturer recommended dosing. Alternatively, the World Federation of Hemophilia (WFH) has recommended general dosing for factor IX products.

Formula to determine units required to obtain desired factor IX level:
Note: If patient has severe hemophilia (ie, baseline factor IX level is or presumed to be <1%), then may just use "desired factor IX level" instead of "desired factor IX level increase".

Number of factor IX units required = patient weight (in kg) x desired factor IX level increase (as % or units/dL) x 1 unit/kg

For example, to attain an 80% level in a 70 kg patient who has a baseline level of 20%: Number of factor IX units needed = 70 kg x 60% x 1 unit/kg = 4200 units

Alternative dosing (off-label): Note: The following recommendations may vary from those found within prescribing information or practitioner preference.

Prophylaxis: 15 to 30 units/kg/dose twice weekly (Utrecht protocol; WFH [Srivastava 2013]) **or** 25 to 40 units/kg/dose twice weekly (Malmö protocol; WFH [Srivastava 2013]) **or** 40 to 100 units/kg/dose 2 to 3 times weekly (National Hemophilia Foundation, MASAC recommendation, 2007); optimum regimen has yet to be defined.

Treatment:

2013 World Federation of Hemophilia Treatment Recommendations (When No Significant Resource Constraint Exists):

Site of Hemorrhage/Clinical Situation	Desired Factor IX Level to Maintain	Duration
Joint	40 to 60 units/dL	1 to 2 days, may be longer if response is inadequate
Superficial muscle/no neurovascular compromise	40 to 60 units/dL	2 to 3 days, sometimes longer if response is inadequate
Iliopsoas and deep muscle with neurovascular injury, or substantial blood loss	*Initial:* 60 to 80 units/dL *Maintenance:* 30 to 60 units/dL	*Initial:* 1 to 2 days *Maintenance:* 3 to 5 days, sometimes longer as secondary prophylaxis during physiotherapy
CNS/head	*Initial:* 60 to 80 units/dL *Maintenance:* 30 units/dL	*Initial:* 1 to 7 days *Maintenance:* 8 to 21 days
Throat and neck	*Initial:* 60 to 80 units/dL *Maintenance:* 30 units/dL	*Initial:* 1 to 7 days *Maintenance:* 8 to 14 days
Gastrointestinal	*Initial:* 60 to 80 units/dL *Maintenance:* 30 units/dL	*Initial:* 7 to 14 days *Maintenance:* Not specified
Renal	40 units/dL	3 to 5 days
Deep laceration	40 units/dL	5 to 7 days
Surgery (major)	*Preop:* 60 to 80 units/dL	
	Postop: 40 to 60 units/dL 30 to 50 units/dL 20 to 40 units/dL	*Postop:* 1 to 3 days 4 to 6 days 7 to 14 days
Surgery (minor)	*Preop:* 50 to 80 units/dL	
	Postop: 30 to 80 units/dL	*Postop:* 1 to 5 days depending on procedure type

Note: Factor IX level may either be expressed as units/dL or as %. Dosing frequency most commonly corresponds to the half-life of factor IX but should be determined based on an assessment of factor IX levels before the next dose.

Continuous infusion (for patients who require prolonged periods of treatment [eg, intracranial hemorrhage or surgery] to avoid peaks and troughs associated with intermittent infusions) (Batorova, 2002; Poon, 2012; Rickard, 1995; WFH [Srivastava 2013]): Following initial bolus to achieve the desired factor IX level: Initiate 4 to 6 units/kg/hour; adjust dose based on frequent factor assays and calculation of factor IX clearance at steady-state using the following equations:

Factor IX clearance (mL/kg/hour) = (current infusion rate in units/kg/hour) divided by (plasma level in units/mL)

New infusion rate (units/kg/hour) = (factor IX clearance in mL/kg/hour) x (desired plasma level in units/mL)

Pediatric NOTE: Contains **nondetectable levels of factors II, VII, and X**. Therefore, **NOT INDICATED** for replacement therapy of any other clotting factor besides factor IX or for reversal of anticoagulation due to either vitamin K antagonists or other anticoagulants (eg, dabigatran), for hemophilia A patients with factor VIII inhibitors, or for patients in a hemorrhagic state caused by reduced production of liver-dependent coagulation factors (eg, hepatitis, cirrhosis).

◀

Control or prevention of bleeding in patients with factor IX deficiency (hemophilia B or Christmas disease): Infants, Children, and Adolescents: IV: *AlphaNine SD, Mononine:* Dosage is expressed in units of factor IX activity; dosing must be individualized based on severity of factor IX deficiency, extent and location of bleeding, and clinical status of patient. Refer to product information for specific manufacturer recommended dosing. Alternatively, the World Federation of Hemophilia (WFH) has recommended general dosing for factor IX products.

Formula to determine units required to obtain desired factor IX level:

Note: If patient has severe hemophilia (ie, baseline factor IX level is or presumed to be <1%), then may just use "desired factor IX level" instead of "desired factor IX level increase".

Number of factor IX units required = patient weight (in kg) x desired factor IX level increase (as % or units/dL) x 1 unit/kg

For example, to attain an 80% level in a 70 kg patient who has a baseline level of 20%: Number of factor IX units needed = 70 kg x 60% x 1 unit/kg = 4200 units

Alternative recommendations (off-label): Infants, Children, and Adolescents:

Prophylaxis, primary: Refer to adult dosing.

Treatment: Refer to adult dosing.

Additional Information Complete prescribing information should be consulted for additional detail.

Dosage Forms Considerations

Strengths expressed with approximate values. Consult individual vial labels for exact potency within each vial.

Dosage Forms Excipient information presented when available (limited, particularly for generics); consult specific product labeling.

Solution Reconstituted, Intravenous [preservative free]:

AlphaNine SD: 500 units (1 ea); 1000 units (1 ea); 1500 units (1 ea) [contains polysorbate 80]

Mononine: 250 units (1 ea); 500 units (1 ea); 1000 units (1 ea) [contains polysorbate 80]

Factor IX (Recombinant) (FAK ter nyne ree KOM be nant)

Brand Names: US Alprolix; BeneFIX; Ixinity; Rixubis

Brand Names: Canada BeneFix

Index Terms Factor IX Concentrate

Pharmacologic Category Antihemophilic Agent

Use Factor IX deficiency: Prevention and control of bleeding in patients with factor IX deficiency (hemophilia B [Christmas disease]); perioperative management in patients with hemophilia B; routine prophylaxis to prevent or reduce the frequency of bleeding episodes in patients with hemophilia B (Alprolix and Rixubis).

NOTE: Contains **only factor IX**. Therefore, **NOT INDICATED** for replacement therapy of any other clotting factor besides factor IX or for reversal of anticoagulation due to either vitamin K antagonists or other anticoagulants (eg, dabigatran), for hemophilia A patients with factor VIII inhibitors, or for patients in a hemorrhagic state caused by reduced production of liver-dependent coagulation factors (eg, hepatitis, cirrhosis).

Pregnancy Risk Factor C

Dosing

Adult & Geriatric NOTE: Contains **only factor IX**. Therefore, **NOT INDICATED** for replacement therapy of any other clotting factor besides factor IX or for reversal of anticoagulation due to either vitamin K antagonists or other anticoagulants (eg, dabigatran), for hemophilia A patients with factor VIII inhibitors, or for patients in a hemorrhagic state caused by reduced production of liver-dependent coagulation factors (eg, hepatitis, cirrhosis).

Control or prevention of bleeding in patients with factor IX deficiency (hemophilia B or Christmas disease): IV: Dosage is expressed in units of factor IX activity; dosing must be individualized based on severity of factor IX deficiency, extent and location of bleeding, clinical status of patient, and recovery of factor IX. As compared to Benefix, Ixinity, and Rixubis, Alprolix displays a longer half-life. Therefore, Alprolix dosing and frequency may differ. **Refer to product information for specific manufacturer recommended dosing.** Alternatively, the World Federation of Hemophilia (WFH) has recommended general dosing for factor IX products.

Formula for units required to raise blood level %: Note: If patient has severe hemophilia (ie, baseline factor IX level is or presumed to be <1%), then may just use "desired factor IX level" instead of "desired factor IX level *increase*". On average, the observed recovery for BeneFix is 0.8 units/dL per units/kg in adults.

Number of factor IX units required = patient weight (in kg) x desired factor IX level increase (as % or units/dL) x reciprocal of observed recovery (as units/kg per units/dL)

Alternative dosing (off-label): Note: The following recommendations may vary from those found within prescribing information or practitioner preference.

Prophylaxis: 15 to 30 units/kg/dose twice weekly (Utrecht protocol; WFH [Srivastava 2013]) **or** 25 to 40 units/kg/dose twice weekly (Malmö protocol; WFH [Srivastava 2013]) **or** 40 to 100 units/kg/dose 2 to 3 times weekly (National Hemophilia Foundation, MASAC recommendation, 2007); optimum regimen has yet to be defined.

Treatment:

2013 World Federation of Hemophilia Treatment Recommendations (When No Significant Resource Constraint Exists):

Site of Hemorrhage/Clinical Situation	Desired Factor IX Level to Maintain	Duration
Joint	40-60 units/dL	1-2 days, may be longer if response is inadequate
Superficial muscle/no neurovascular compromise	40-60 units/dL	2-3 days, sometimes longer if response is inadequate
Iliopsoas and deep muscle with neurovascular injury, or substantial blood loss	*Initial:* 60-80 units/dL *Maintenance:* 30-60 units/dL	*Initial:* 1-2 days *Maintenance:* 3-5 days, sometimes longer as secondary prophylaxis during physiotherapy
CNS/head	*Initial:* 60-80 units/dL *Maintenance:* 30 units/dL	*Initial:* 1-7 days *Maintenance:* 8-21 days
Throat and neck	*Initial:* 60-80 units/dL *Maintenance:* 30 units/dL	*Initial:* 1-7 days *Maintenance:* 8-14 days

(continued)

FACTOR IX (RECOMBINANT)

2013 World Federation of Hemophilia Treatment Recommendations (When No Significant Resource Constraint Exists): *(continued)*

Site of Hemorrhage/Clinical Situation	Desired Factor IX Level to Maintain	Duration
Gastrointestinal	*Initial:* 60-80 units/dL *Maintenance:* 30 units/dL	*Initial:* 7-14 days *Maintenance:* Not specified
Renal	40 units/dL	3-5 days
Deep laceration	40 units/dL	5-7 days
Surgery (major)	*Preop:* 60-80 units/dL	
	Postop: 40-60 units/dL 30-50 units/dL 20-40 units/dL	*Postop:* 1-3 days 4-6 days 7-14 days
Surgery (minor)	*Preop:* 50-80 units/dL	
	Postop: 30-80 units/dL	*Postop:* 1-5 days depending on procedure type

Note: Factor IX level may either be expressed as units/dL or as %. Dosing frequency most commonly corresponds to the half-life of factor IX but should be determined based on an assessment of factor IX levels before the next dose.

Continuous infusion (For patients who require prolonged periods of treatment [eg, intracranial hemorrhage or surgery] to avoid peaks and troughs associated with intermittent infusions) (Batorova, 2002; Poon, 2012; Rickard, 1995; WFH [Srivastava 2013]): **Note:** Evidence supporting the use of continuous infusion is primarily with BeneFix (Chowdary, 2001): Following initial bolus to achieve the desired factor IX level, initiate 4 to 6 units/kg/hour; adjust dose based on frequent factor assays and calculation of factor IX clearance at steady-state using the following equations:

Factor IX clearance (mL/kg/hour) = (current infusion rate in units/kg/hour)/ (plasma level in units/mL)

New infusion rate (units/kg/hour) = (factor IX clearance in mL/kg/hour) x (desired plasma level in units/mL)

Routine prophylaxis to prevent bleeding episodes in patients with factor IX deficiency (hemophilia B or Christmas disease): IV:

Alprolix: 50 units/kg once weekly or 100 units/kg once every 10 days; adjust dose based on individual response

Rixubis: 40 to 60 units/kg twice weekly; may titrate dose depending upon age, bleeding pattern, and physical activity

Pediatric NOTE: Contains **only factor IX.** Therefore, **NOT INDICATED** for replacement therapy of any other clotting factor besides factor IX or for reversal of anticoagulation due to either vitamin K antagonists or other anticoagulants (eg, dabigatran), for hemophilia A patients with factor VIII inhibitors, or for patients in a hemorrhagic state caused by reduced production of liver-dependent coagulation factors (eg, hepatitis, cirrhosis).

Control or prevention of bleeding in patients with factor IX deficiency (hemophilia B or Christmas disease): IV: Dosage is expressed in units of factor IX activity; dosing must be individualized based on severity of factor IX deficiency, extent and location of bleeding, clinical status of patient, and recovery of factor IX. As compared to Benefix, Ixinity, and Rixubis, Alprolix displays a longer half-life. Therefore, Alprolix dosing and frequency may differ. **Refer to product information for specific manufacturer recommended dosing.** Alternatively, the World Federation of Hemophilia (WFH) has recommended general dosing for factor IX products.

Formula for units required to raise blood level %: **Note:** If patient has severe hemophilia (ie, baseline factor IX level is or presumed to be <1%), then may just use "desired factor IX level" instead of "desired factor IX level *increase*". On average, the observed recovery for BeneFix is 0.7 units/dL per units/kg in children <15 years of age.

Infants, Children, and Adolescents: IV: Number of factor IX units required = patient weight (in kg) x desired factor IX level increase (as % or units/dL) x reciprocal of observed recovery (as units/kg per units/dL)

Alternative recommendations (off label): Infants, Children, and Adolescents:

Prophylaxis: Refer to adult dosing.

Treatment: Refer to adult dosing.

Routine prophylaxis to prevent bleeding episodes in patients with factor IX deficiency (hemophilia B or Christmas disease): IV:

Alprolix: 50 units/kg once weekly or 100 units/kg once every 10 days; adjust dose based on individual response

Rixubis:

Children <12 years: 60 to 80 units/kg twice weekly; may titrate dose depending upon age, bleeding pattern, and physical activity.

Children ≥12 years and Adolescents: 40 to 60 units/kg twice weekly; may titrate dose depending upon age, bleeding pattern, and physical activity.

Renal Impairment There are no dosage adjustments provided in the manufacturer's labeling; monitor factor IX levels.

Hepatic Impairment There are no dosage adjustments provided in the manufacturer's labeling; monitor factor IX levels. Use with caution due to the risk of thromboembolic complications.

Additional Information Complete prescribing information should be consulted for additional detail.

Dosage Forms Considerations Strengths expressed with approximate values. Consult individual vial labels for exact potency within each vial.

Dosage Forms Excipient information presented when available (limited, particularly for generics); consult specific product labeling.

Solution Reconstituted, Intravenous [preservative free]:

Alprolix: 500 units (1 ea); 1000 units (1 ea); 2000 units (1 ea); 3000 units (1 ea)

BeneFIX: 250 units (1 ea); 500 units (1 ea); 1000 units (1 ea); 2000 units (1 ea) [contains polysorbate 80]

Ixinity: 500 units (1 ea); 1000 units (1 ea); 1500 units (1 ea) [contains mouse protein (murine) (hamster), polysorbate 80]

Rixubis: 250 units (1 ea); 500 units (1 ea); 1000 units (1 ea); 2000 units (1 ea); 3000 units (1 ea) [contains polysorbate 80]

◆ **3 Factor PCC** *see* Factor IX Complex (Human) [(Factors II, IX, X)] *on page 677*

◆ **Factor 13** *see* Factor XIII Concentrate (Human) *on page 688*

Factor XIII A-Subunit (Recombinant)
(FAK ter THIR teen aye SUB yoo nit ree KOM be nant)

Brand Names: US Tretten

Brand Names: Canada Tretten

Index Terms Catridecacog; Recombinant Factor XIII A-Subunit; rFXIII

Pharmacologic Category Antihemophilic Agent

◄ **Use Factor XIII A-subunit deficiency:** Routine prophylaxis of bleeding in patients with congenital factor XIII A-subunit deficiency

Pregnancy Risk Factor C

Dosing

Adult & Geriatric Factor XIII A-subunit deficiency: IV: 35 units/kg once monthly to achieve a target trough level of factor XIII activity ≥10% using a validated assay; consider dose adjustment if adequate coverage is not achieved (higher doses may not increase the levels of tetrameric factor XIII).

Note: Treatment should be initiated under the supervision of a healthcare provider experienced in the treatment of rare bleeding disorders.

Pediatric Infants, Children, and Adolescents: Refer to adult dosing.

Renal Impairment No dosage adjustment provided in manufacturer's labeling.

Hepatic Impairment No dosage adjustment provided in manufacturer's labeling.

Additional Information Complete prescribing information should be consulted for additional detail.

Dosage Forms Excipient information presented when available (limited, particularly for generics); consult specific product labeling.

Solution Reconstituted, Intravenous:

Tretten: 2000-3125 units (1 ea)

Factor XIII Concentrate (Human)

(FAK ter THIR teen KON cen trate HYU man)

Brand Names: US Corifact

Brand Names: Canada Corifact

Index Terms Activated Factor XIII; Corifact; Factor 13; FXIII

Pharmacologic Category Antihemophilic Agent; Blood Product Derivative

Use Prophylaxis against bleeding episodes and management of perioperative surgical bleeding in patients with congenital factor XIII deficiency

Pregnancy Risk Factor C

Dosing

Adult & Geriatric Congenital factor XIII deficiency: IV:

Prophylaxis:

Initial: 40 units/kg

Maintenance: Dose adjustment should be based on factor XIII activity trough levels (target level of 5% to 20% using Berichrom activity assay) and clinical response; repeat every 28 days

One trough level of <5%: Increase dosage by 5 units/kg

Trough level of 5% to 20%: No dosage change

Two trough levels of >20%: Decrease dosage by 5 units/kg

One trough level of >25%: Decrease dosage by 5 units/kg

Perioperative management of surgical bleeding: Individualize dosing based on factor XIII activity level, type of surgery, and clinical response; monitor factor XIII activity levels during and after surgery:

If time since last prophylactic dose ≤7 days: Additional dose may not be needed.

If time since last prophylactic dose 8 to 21 days: Additional partial or full dose may be necessary based on factor XIII activity level

If time since last prophylactic dose 21 to 28 days: Administer full prophylactic dose

Pediatric Infants, Children, and Adolescents: Refer to adult dosing.

Renal Impairment There are no dosage adjustments provided in the manufacturer's labeling.

Hepatic Impairment There are no dosage adjustments provided in the manufacturer's labeling.

Additional Information Complete prescribing information should be consulted for additional detail.

Dosage Forms Excipient information presented when available (limited, particularly for generics); consult specific product labeling.

Kit, Intravenous [preservative free]:

Corifact: 1000-1600 units

Dosage Forms: Canada Note: Refer also to dosage forms.

Excipient information presented when available (limited, particularly for generics); consult specific product labeling.

Solution Reconstituted, Intravenous [preservative free]

Corifact: 200-320 units

Famciclovir (fam SYE kloe veer)

Brand Names: US Famvir

Brand Names: Canada Apo-Famciclovir®; Ava-Famciclovir; CO Famciclovir; Famvir®; PMS-Famciclovir; Sandoz-Famciclovir

Pharmacologic Category Antiviral Agent

Use Treatment of acute herpes zoster (shingles) in immunocompetent patients; treatment and suppression of recurrent episodes of genital herpes in immunocompetent patients; treatment of herpes labialis (cold sores) in immunocompetent patients; treatment of recurrent orolabial/genital (mucocutaneous) herpes simplex in HIV-infected patients

Pregnancy Risk Factor B

Dosing

Adult & Geriatric

Genital herpes simplex virus (HSV) infection: Oral: **Note:** Initiate therapy as soon as possible after diagnosis and within 72 hours of rash onset

Immunocompetent patients:

Initial episode: 250 mg 3 times/day for 7 to 10 days (CDC, 2010)

Recurrence: 1,000 mg twice daily for 1 day (**Note:** Initiate therapy as soon as possible and within 6 hours of symptoms/lesions onset)

Alternatively, the following regimens are also recommended: 125 mg twice daily for 5 days or 500 mg as a single dose, followed by 250 mg twice daily for 2 days (CDC, 2010). **Note:** Canadian labeling recommends 125 mg twice daily for 5 days.

Suppressive therapy: 250 mg twice daily for up to 1 year; **Note:** Duration not established, but efficacy/safety have been demonstrated for 1 year (CDC, 2010)

HIV-infected patients:

Manufacturer's labeling: Recurrent episodes: 500 mg twice daily for 7 days

Alternate dosing:

Initial or recurrent episodes: 500 mg twice daily for 5 to 14 days (HHS [OI adult 2015])

Chronic suppressive therapy (off-label use): 500 mg twice daily; continue indefinitely regardless of CD4 count in patients with severe recurrences of genital herpes or in patients who want to minimize frequency of recurrences (HHS [OI adult 2015])

◀

Herpes labialis/orolabial (cold sores): Oral: **Note:** Initiate therapy as soon as possible after diagnosis and within 72 hours of rash onset

Immunocompetent patients:

Recurrent episodes: 1,500 mg as a single dose; initiate therapy at first sign or symptom such as tingling, burning, or itching (initiated within 1 hour in clinical studies)

HIV patients:

Manufacturer's labeling: Recurrent episodes: 500 mg twice daily for 7 days

Alternate dosing: Treatment: 500 mg twice daily for 5 to 10 days (HHS [OI adult 2015])

Herpes zoster (shingles): Oral: **Note:** Initiate therapy as soon as possible after diagnosis and within 72 hours of rash onset

Immunocompetent patients: 500 mg every 8 hours for 7 days

HIV-infected patients (off-label use): 500 mg 3 times daily for 7 to 10 days; consider longer duration if lesions heal slowly (HHS [OI adult 2015])

Varicella infection (chickenpox) in HIV-infected patients (uncomplicated cases) (off-label use): Oral: 500 mg 3 times daily for 5 to 7 days (HHS [OI adult 2015])

Pediatric

Genital herpes simplex virus (HSV) in HIV-infected patients: Adolescents (off-label population): Oral:

Initial or recurrent episodes: 500 mg twice daily for 5 to 14 days (HHS [OI adult 2015])

Chronic suppressive therapy (off-label use): 500 mg twice daily; continue indefinitely regardless of CD4 count in patients with severe recurrences of genital herpes or in patients who want to minimize frequency of recurrences (HHS [OI adult 2015])

Herpes labialis/orolabial (cold sores) in HIV-infected patients: Adolescents (off-label population): Oral: Treatment: 500 mg twice daily for 5 to 10 days (HHS [OI adult 2015])

Herpes zoster (shingles) in HIV-infected patients (off-label use): Adolescents: Oral: 500 mg 3 times daily for 7 to 10 days; consider longer duration if lesions heal slowly (HHS [OI adult 2015])

Varicella infection (chickenpox) in HIV-infected patients (uncomplicated cases) (off-label use): Adolescents: Oral: 500 mg 3 times daily for 5 to 7 days (HHS [OI adult 2015])

Renal Impairment

Dosing adjustment in renal impairment:

Herpes zoster:

CrCl ≥60 mL/minute: No dosage adjustment necessary

CrCl 40-59 mL/minute: Administer 500 mg every 12 hours

CrCl 20-39 mL/minute: Administer 500 mg every 24 hours

CrCl <20 mL/minute: Administer 250 mg every 24 hours

Hemodialysis: Administer 250 mg after each dialysis session.

Recurrent genital herpes: Treatment:

U.S. labeling (single-day regimen):

CrCl ≥60 mL/minute: No dosage adjustment necessary

CrCl 40-59 mL/minute: Administer 500 mg every 12 hours for 1 day

CrCl 20-39 mL/minute: Administer 500 mg as a single dose

CrCl <20 mL/minute: Administer 250 mg as a single dose

Hemodialysis: Administer 250 mg as a single dose after a dialysis session.

Canadian labeling:
CrCl >20 mL/minute/1.73 m^2: No dosage adjustment necessary
CrCl <20 mL/minute/1.73 m^2: Administer 125 mg every 24 hours
Hemodialysis: Administer 125 mg after each dialysis session.

Recurrent genital herpes: Suppression:
CrCl ≥40 mL/minute: No dosage adjustment necessary
CrCl 20-39 mL/minute: Administer 125 mg every 12 hours
CrCl <20 mL/minute: Administer 125 mg every 24 hours
Hemodialysis: Administer 125 mg after each dialysis session.

Recurrent herpes labialis: Treatment (single-dose regimen):
CrCl ≥60 mL/minute: No dosage adjustment necessary
CrCl 40-59 mL/minute: Administer 750 mg as a single dose
CrCl 20-39 mL/minute: Administer 500 mg as a single dose
CrCl <20 mL/minute: Administer 250 mg as a single dose
Hemodialysis: Administer 250 mg as a single dose after a dialysis session.

Recurrent orolabial/genital (mucocutaneous) herpes in HIV-infected patients:
CrCl ≥40 mL/minute: No dosage adjustment necessary
CrCl 20-39 mL/minute: Administer 500 mg every 24 hours
CrCl <20 mL/minute: Administer 250 mg every 24 hours
Hemodialysis: Administer 250 mg after each dialysis session.

Hepatic Impairment
Mild-to-moderate impairment: No dosage adjustment is necessary
Severe impairment: No dosage adjustment provided in manufacturer's labeling; has not been studied. However, a 44% decrease in the C_{max} of penciclovir (active metabolite) was noted in patients with mild-to-moderate impairment; impaired conversion of famciclovir to penciclovir may affect efficacy.

Additional Information Complete prescribing information should be consulted for additional detail.

Dosage Forms Excipient information presented when available (limited, particularly for generics); consult specific product labeling.
Tablet, Oral:
Famvir: 125 mg, 250 mg, 500 mg
Generic: 125 mg, 250 mg, 500 mg

FentaNYL (FEN ta nil)

Brand Names: US Abstral; Actiq; Duragesic; Fentora; Ionsys; Lazanda; Onsolis [DSC]; Subsys

Brand Names: Canada Abstral; Apo-Fentanyl Matrix; Co-Fentanyl; Duragesic MAT; Fentanyl Citrate Injection, USP; Fentora; Mylan-Fentanyl Matrix Patch; PMS-Fentanyl MTX; RAN-Fentanyl Matrix Patch; Sandoz Fentanyl Patch; Teva-Fentanyl

Index Terms Fentanyl Citrate; Fentanyl Hydrochloride; Fentanyl Patch; Ionsys; OTFC (Oral Transmucosal Fentanyl Citrate)

Pharmacologic Category Analgesic, Opioid; Anilidopiperidine Opioid; General Anesthetic

Use

Injection:

Pain management: Relief of pain, preoperative medication.

Surgery: Adjunct to general or regional anesthesia.

Transdermal device (eg, Ionsys): **Postoperative pain, acute:** Short-term management of acute postoperative pain in adult patients requiring opioid analgesia in the hospital.

Limitations of use: Only for use in patients who are alert enough and have adequate cognitive ability to understand the directions for use. Not for home use. Transdermal device is for use only in patients in the hospital. Discontinue treatment with the device before patients leave the hospital. The device is for use after patients have been titrated to an acceptable level of analgesia using alternate opioid analgesics.

Transdermal patch (eg, Duragesic): **Chronic pain:** Management of pain in opioid-tolerant patients, severe enough to require daily, around-the-clock, long-term opioid treatment and for which alternative treatment options are inadequate.

Limitations of use: Because of the risks of addiction, abuse, and misuse with opioids, even at recommended doses, and because of the greater risks of overdose and death with extended-release opioid formulations, reserve fentanyl transdermal patch for use in patients for whom alternative treatment options (eg, nonopioid analgesics, immediate-release opioids) are ineffective, not tolerated, or would be otherwise inadequate to provide sufficient management of pain.

Transmucosal lozenge (eg, Actiq), buccal tablet (Fentora), buccal film (Onsolis), nasal spray (Lazanda), sublingual tablet (Abstral), sublingual spray (Subsys): **Cancer pain:** Management of breakthrough cancer pain in opioid-tolerant patients who are already receiving and who are tolerant to around-the-clock opioid therapy for their underlying persistent cancer pain.

Note: "Opioid-tolerant" patients are defined as patients who are taking at least:

Oral morphine 60 mg/day, **or**

Transdermal fentanyl 25 mcg/hour, **or**

Oral oxycodone 30 mg/day, **or**

Oral hydromorphone 8 mg/day, **or**

Oral oxymorphone 25 mg/day, **or**

Equianalgesic dose of another opioid for at least 1 week

Pregnancy Risk Factor C

Dosing

Adult Note: Ranges listed may not represent the maximum doses that may be required in some patients. Doses and dosage intervals should be titrated to pain relief/prevention. Monitor vital signs routinely. Single IM doses have duration of 1-2 hours, single IV doses last 0.5 to 1 hour.

Surgery:

Premedication: IM, slow IV: 50 to 100 mcg administered 30 to 60 minutes prior to surgery **or** slow IV: 25 to 50 mcg given shortly before induction (Barash, 2009)

Adjunct to general anesthesia: Slow IV:

Low dose: 1 to 2 mcg/**kg** depending on the indication (Miller, 2010); additional maintenance doses are generally not needed.

Moderate dose (fentanyl plus a sedative/hypnotic): Initial: 2 to 4 mcg/**kg**; Maintenance (bolus or infusion): 25 to 50 mcg every 15 to 30 minutes or 0.5 to 2 mcg/kg/**hour**. Discontinuing fentanyl infusion 30 to 60 minutes prior to the end of surgery will usually allow adequate ventilation upon emergence from anesthesia.

High dose (opioid anesthesia): 4 to 20 mcg/**kg** bolus then 2 to 10 mcg/kg/**hour** (Miller, 2010); **Note:** High-dose fentanyl (ie, 20 to 50 mcg/kg) is rarely used, but is still described in the manufacturer's label. The concept of fast-tracking and early intubation following cardiac surgery has essentially replaced high-dose fentanyl anesthesia.

Adjunct to regional anesthesia: 50 to 100 mcg IM or slow IV over 1 to 2 minutes. **Note:** An IV should be in place with regional anesthesia so the IM route is rarely used but still maintained as an option in the manufacturer's labeling.

Postoperative recovery: IM, slow IV: 50 to 100 mcg every 1 to 2 hours as needed.

Postoperative pain: Epidural (Canadian labeling; not in U.S. labeling): Initial: 100 mcg (diluted in 8 mL of preservative free NS to final concentration of 10 mcg/mL); may repeat with additional 100 mcg boluses on demand or alternatively may administer by continuous infusion at a rate of 1 mcg/kg/hour.

Pain management:

Postoperative pain, acute: Transdermal device (Ionsys): Apply one device to chest or upper outer arm only. Only the patient may activate the device (40 mcg dose of fentanyl per activation; maximum 6 doses per hour). Only one device may be applied at a time for up to 24 hours or 80 doses, whichever comes first. May be used for a maximum of 72 hours, with each subsequent device applied to a different skin site. If inadequate analgesia is achieved with one device, either provide additional supplemental analgesic medication or replace with an alternate analgesic medication. Refer to manufacturer's labeling for activation instructions.

Note: For hospital use only by patients under medical supervision and direction and only after patients have been titrated to an acceptable level of analgesia using another opioid analgesic.

Severe pain:

Intermittent dosing: IM, IV (off-label dose): Slow IV: 25 to 35 mcg (based on ~70 kg patient) **or** 0.35 to 0.5 mcg/kg every 30 to 60 minutes as needed (SCCM [Barr, 2013]). **Note:** After the first dose, if severe pain persists and adverse effects are minimal at the time of expected peak effect (eg, ~5 minutes after IV administration), may repeat dose (APS, 2008). In addition, since the duration of activity with IV administration is

◀ 30 to 60 minutes, more frequent administration may be necessary when administered by this route.

Patient-controlled analgesia (PCA) (off-label use; American Pain Society, 2008; Miller, 2010): Opioid-naive: IV:

Usual concentration: 10 mcg/mL

Demand dose: Usual: 10 to 20 mcg

Lockout interval: 4 to 10 minutes

Usual basal rate: ≤50 mcg/hour. **Note:** Continuous basal infusions are not recommended for initial programming and should rarely be used; consider limiting infusion rate to 10 mcg/hour if used (Grass, 2005).

Critically-ill patients (off-label dose): Slow IV: 25 to 35 mcg (based on ~70 kg patient) **or** 0.35 to 0.5 mcg/kg every 30 to 60 minutes as needed (SCCM [Barr, 2013]). **Note:** More frequent dosing may be needed (eg, mechanically-ventilated patients).

Continuous infusion: 50 to 700 mcg/hour (based on ~70 kg patient) **or** 0.7 to 10 mcg/kg/**hour** (SCCM [Barr, 2013]).

Alternative continuous infusion dosing: 1 to 2 mcg/kg bolus followed by an initial rate of 1 to 2 mcg/**kg**/hour (Peng, 1999) **or** 25 to 100 mcg bolus followed by an initial rate of 25 to 200 mcg/**hour** (Liu, 2003). **Note:** When pain is not controlled, may administer an additional small bolus dose (eg, 25 to 50 mcg) prior to increasing the infusion rate (Loper 1990; Peng, 1999; Salomaki, 1991).

Intrathecal (off-label use; American Pain Society, 2008): **Must be preservative-free.** Doses must be adjusted for age, injection site, and patient's medical condition and degree of opioid tolerance.

Single dose: 5 to 25 mcg; may provide adequate relief for up to 6 hours

Continuous infusion: Not recommended in acute pain management due to risk of excessive accumulation. For chronic cancer pain, infusion of very small doses may be practical (American Pain Society, 2008).

Epidural (off-label use; American Pain Society, 2008): **Must be preservative-free.** Doses must be adjusted for age, injection site, and patient's medical condition and degree of opioid tolerance

Single dose: 25 to 100 mcg; may provide adequate relief for up to 8 hours

Continuous infusion: 25 to 100 mcg/hour (fentanyl alone). When combined with a local anesthetic (eg, bupivacaine or ropivacaine), fentanyl requirement are less (Manion, 2011).

Breakthrough cancer pain: Transmucosal: For patients who are tolerant to and currently receiving opioid therapy for persistent cancer pain; dosing should be individually titrated to provide adequate analgesia with minimal side effects. Dose titration should be done if patient requires more than 1 dose/breakthrough pain episode for several consecutive episodes. Patients experiencing >4 breakthrough pain episodes per day should have the dose of their long-term opioid re-evaluated. **Patients must remain on around-the-clock opioids during use.**

Lozenge (Actiq): **Note:** Do **not** convert patients from any other fentanyl product to Actiq on a mcg-per-mcg basis. Patients previously using another fentanyl product should be initiated at a dose of 200 mcg; individually titrate to provide adequate analgesia while minimizing adverse effects.

Initial dose: 200 mcg (consumed over 15 minutes) for all patients; if after 30 minutes from the start of the lozenge (ie, 15 minutes following the completion of the lozenge), the pain is unrelieved, a second 200 mcg dose may be given over 15 minutes. A maximum of 1 additional dose can be given per pain episode; **must wait at least 4 hours before treating**

another episode. To limit the number of units in the home during titration, only prescribe an initial titration supply of six 200 mcg lozenges.

Dose titration: From the initial dose, closely follow patients and modify the dose until patient reaches a dose providing adequate analgesia using a single dosage unit per breakthrough cancer pain episode. If signs/symptoms of excessive opioid effects (eg, respiratory depression) occur, immediately remove the dosage unit from the patient's mouth, dispose of properly, and reduce subsequent doses. If adequate relief is not achieved 15 minutes after completion of the first dose (ie, 30 minutes after the start of the lozenge), only 1 additional lozenge of the same strength may be given for that episode; **must wait at least 4 hours before treating another episode.**

Maintenance dose: Once titrated to an effective dose, patients should generally use a single dosage unit per breakthrough pain episode. During any pain episode, if adequate relief is not achieved 15 minutes after completion of the first dose (ie, 30 minutes after the start of the lozenge), only 1 additional lozenge of the same strength may be given over 15 minutes for that episode; **must wait at least 4 hours before treating another episode**. Consumption should be limited to ≤4 units per day (once an effective breakthrough dose is found). If adequate analgesia is **not** provided after treating several episodes of breakthrough pain using the same dose, increase dose to next highest lozenge strength (initially dispense no more than 6 units of the new strength). Consider increasing the around-the-clock opioid therapy in patients experiencing >4 breakthrough pain episodes per day. If signs/symptoms of excessive opioid effects (eg, respiratory depression) occur, immediately remove the dosage unit from the patient's mouth, dispose of properly, and reduce subsequent doses.

Buccal film (Onsolis): **Note:** Do **not** convert patients from any other fentanyl product to Onsolis on a mcg-per-mcg basis. Patients previously using another fentanyl product should be initiated at a dose of 200 mcg; individually titrate to provide adequate analgesia while minimizing adverse effects.

Initial dose: 200 mcg for all patients; if after 30 minutes pain is unrelieved, the patient may use an alternative rescue medication as directed by their health care provider. Do **not** redose with Onsolis within an episode; buccal film should only be used once per breakthrough cancer pain episode. **Must wait at least 2 hours before treating another episode with buccal film.**

Dose titration: If titration required, increase dose in 200 mcg increments once per episode using multiples of the 200 mcg film (for doses up to 800 mcg); do not redose within a single episode of breakthrough pain and separate single doses by ≥2 hours. During titration, do not exceed 4 simultaneous applications of the 200 mcg films (800 mcg) (when using multiple films, do not place on top of each other; film may be placed on both sides of mouth); if >800 mcg required, treat next episode with one 1200 mcg film (maximum dose: 1200 mcg). Once maintenance dose is determined, all other unused films should be disposed of and that strength (using a single film) should be used. During any pain episode, if adequate relief is not achieved after 30 minutes following buccal film application, a rescue medication (as determined by health care provider) may be used.

Maintenance dose: Determined dose applied as a single film once per episode and separated by ≥2 hours (dose range: 200 to 1200 mcg); limit to 4 applications per day. Consider increasing the around-the-clock opioid therapy in patients experiencing >4 breakthrough pain episodes per day.

Buccal tablet (Fentora): **Note:** Do **not** convert patients from any other fentanyl product to Fentora on a mcg-per-mcg basis. Patients previously using another fentanyl product should be initiated at a dose of 100 mcg; individually titrate to provide adequate analgesia while minimizing adverse effects. For patients previously using the transmucosal lozenge (Actiq), the initial dose should be selected using the conversions listed; see *Conversion from lozenge (Actiq) to buccal tablet (Fentora)*.

Initial dose: 100 mcg for all patients unless patient already using Actiq; see *Conversion from lozenge (Actiq) to buccal tablet (Fentora)*; if after 30 minutes pain is unrelieved, the U.S. labeling suggests that a second 100 mcg dose may be administered (maximum of 2 doses per breakthrough pain episode). The Canadian labeling recommends only a single dose per breakthrough pain episode; patients experiencing breakthrough pain after administration may take an alternative analgesic as rescue medication after 30 minutes. **Must wait at least 4 hours before treating another episode with Fentora buccal tablet.**

Dose titration: If titration required, 100 mcg dose may be increased to 200 mcg using two 100 mcg tablets (one on each side of mouth) with the next breakthrough pain episode. If 200 mcg dose is not successful, patient can use four 100 mcg tablets (two on each side of mouth) with the next breakthrough pain episode. If titration requires >400 mcg per dose, titrate using 200 mcg tablets; do not use more than 4 tablets simultaneously (maximum single dose: 800 mcg). During any pain episode, if adequate relief is not achieved after 30 minutes following buccal tablet application, a second dose of same strength per breakthrough pain episode may be used. The Canadian labeling recommends only a single dose per breakthrough pain episode; patients experiencing breakthrough pain after administration may take an alternative analgesic as rescue medication after 30 minutes. **Must wait at least 4 hours before treating another episode with Fentora buccal tablet.**

Maintenance dose: Following titration, the effective maintenance dose using 1 tablet of the appropriate strength should be administered once per episode; if after 30 minutes pain is unrelieved, may administer a second dose of the same strength; The Canadian labeling recommends only a single dose per breakthrough pain episode; patients experiencing breakthrough pain after administration may take an alternative analgesic as rescue medication after 30 minutes. **Must wait ≥4 hours before treating another episode with Fentora buccal tablet.** Limit to 4 applications per day. Consider increasing the around-the-clock opioid therapy in patients experiencing >4 breakthrough pain episodes per day. Once an effective maintenance dose has been established, the buccal tablet may be administered sublingually (alternate route). To prevent confusion, patient should only have one strength available at a time. Once maintenance dose is determined, all other unused tablets should be disposed of and that strength (using a single tablet) should be used. Using more than four buccal tablets at a time has not been studied.

Conversion from lozenge (Actiq) to buccal tablet (Fentora):

Lozenge dose 200 to 400 mcg: Initial buccal tablet dose is 100 mcg; may titrate using multiples of 100 mcg

Lozenge dose 600 to 800 mcg: Initial buccal tablet dose is 200 mcg; may titrate using multiples of 200 mcg

Lozenge dose 1200 to 1600 mcg: Initial buccal tablet dose is 400 mcg (using two 200 mcg tablets); may titrate using multiples of 200 mcg

Nasal spray (Lazanda): **Note:** Do **not** convert patients from any other fentanyl product to Lazanda on a mcg-per-mcg basis. Patients previously using another fentanyl product should be initiated at a dose of 100 mcg; individually titrate to provide adequate analgesia while minimizing adverse effects.

Initial dose: 100 mcg (one 100 mcg spray in one nostril) for all patients; if after 30 minutes pain is unrelieved, an alternative rescue medication may be used as directed by their health care provider. **Must wait at least 2 hours before treating another episode with Lazanda nasal spray.** However, for the next pain episode, increase to a higher dose using the recommended dose titration steps.

Dose titration: If titration required, increase to a higher dose for the next pain episode using these titration steps **(Note: Must wait at least 2 hours before treating another episode with Lazanda nasal spray)**: If no relief with 100 mcg dose, increase to 200 mcg dose per episode (one 100 mcg spray in each nostril); if no relief with 200 mcg dose, increase to 400 mcg per episode (one 400 mcg spray in one nostril or two 100 mg sprays in each nostril); if no relief with 400 mcg dose, increase to 800 mcg dose per episode (one 400 mcg spray in each nostril). **Note:** Single doses >800 mcg have not been evaluated. There are no data supporting the use of a combination of dose strengths.

Maintenance dose: Once maintenance dose for breakthrough pain episode has been determined, use that dose for subsequent episodes. For pain that is not relieved after 30 minutes of Lazanda administration or if a separate breakthrough pain episode occurs within the 2 hour window before the next Lazanda dose is permitted, a rescue medication may be used. Limit Lazanda use to ≤4 episodes of breakthrough pain per day. If patient is experiencing >4 breakthrough pain episodes per day, consider increasing the around-the-clock, long-acting opioid therapy; if long-acting opioid therapy dose is altered, re-evaluate and retitrate Lazanda dose as needed. If response to maintenance dose changes (increase in adverse reactions or alterations in pain relief), dose readjustment may be necessary.

Sublingual spray (Subsys): **Note:** Do **not** convert patients from any other fentanyl product to Subsys on a mcg-per-mcg basis. Patients previously using another fentanyl product should be initiated at a dose of 100 mcg; individually titrate to provide adequate analgesia while minimizing adverse effects. For patients previously using the transmucosal lozenge (Actiq), the initial dose should be selected using the conversions listed; see *Conversion from lozenge (Actiq) to sublingual spray (Subsys)*.

Initial dose: 100 mcg for all patients unless patient already using Actiq; see *Conversion from lozenge (Actiq) to sublingual spray (Subsys)*. If pain is unrelieved, 1 additional 100 mcg dose may be given 30 minutes after administration of the first dose. A maximum of 2 doses can be given per breakthrough pain episode. **Must wait at least 4 hours before treating another episode with sublingual spray.**

◄ Dose titration: If titration required, titrate to a dose that provides adequate analgesia (with tolerable side effects) using the following titration steps: If no relief with 100 mcg dose, increase to 200 mcg dose (using one 200 mcg unit); if no relief with 200 mcg dose, increase to 400 mcg dose (using one 400 mcg unit); if no relief with 400 mcg dose, increase to 600 mcg dose (using one 600 mcg unit); if no relief with 600 mcg dose, increase to 800 mcg dose (using one 800 mcg unit); if no relief with 800 mcg dose, increase to 1200 mcg dose (using two 600 mcg units); if no relief with 1200 mcg dose, increase to 1600 mcg dose (using two 800 mcg units). During dose titration, if breakthrough pain unrelieved 30 minutes after Subsys administration, 1 additional dose using the same strength may be administered (maximum: 2 doses per breakthrough pain episode); **patient must wait 4 hours before treating another breakthrough pain episode with sublingual spray.**

Maintenance dose: Once maintenance dose for breakthrough pain episode has been determined, use that dose for subsequent episodes. If occasional episodes of unrelieved breakthrough pain occur following 30 minutes of Subsys administration, 1 additional dose using the same strength may be administered (maximum: 2 doses per breakthrough pain episode); **patient must wait 4 hours before treating another breakthrough pain episode with Subsys.** Once maintenance dose is determined, limit Subsys use to ≤4 episodes of breakthrough pain per day. If response to maintenance dose changes (increase in adverse reactions or alterations in pain relief), dose readjustment may be necessary. If patient is experiencing >4 breakthrough pain episodes per day, consider increasing the around-the-clock, long-acting opioid therapy.

Conversion from lozenge (Actiq) to sublingual spray (Subsys):

Lozenge dose 200 to 400 mcg: Initial sublingual spray dose is 100 mcg; may titrate using multiples of 100 mcg

Lozenge dose 600 to 800 mcg: Initial sublingual spray dose is 200 mcg; may titrate using multiples of 200 mcg

Lozenge dose 1,200 to 1,600 mcg: Initial sublingual spray dose is 400 mcg; may titrate using multiples of 400 mcg

Sublingual tablet (Abstral): **Note:** Do **not** convert patients from any other fentanyl product to Abstral on a mcg-per-mcg basis. Patients previously using another fentanyl product should be initiated at a dose of 100 mcg (except Actiq); individually titrate to provide adequate analgesia while minimizing adverse effects.

Initial dose:

U.S. labeling: 100 mcg for all patients; if pain is unrelieved, a second 100 mcg dose may be given 30 minutes after administration of the first dose. A maximum of 2 doses can be given per breakthrough pain episode. **Must wait at least 2 hours before treating another episode with sublingual tablet.**

Canadian labeling: 100 mcg for all patients; if pain is unrelieved 30 minutes after administration of Abstral, an alternative rescue medication (other than Abstral) may be given. Administer only 1 dose of Abstral per breakthrough pain episode. **Must wait at least 2 hours before treating another episode with sublingual tablet.**

Dose titration: If titration required, increase in 100 mcg increments (up to 400 mcg) over consecutive breakthrough episodes. If titration requires >400 mcg per dose, increase in increments of 200 mcg, starting with 600 mcg dose and titrating up to 800 mcg. During titration, patients may use multiples of 100 mcg and/or 200 mcg tablets for any single dose; do not exceed 4 tablets at one time; safety and efficacy of doses >800 mcg have not been evaluated. During dose titration, if breakthrough pain unrelieved 30 minutes after sublingual tablet administration, the U.S. labeling suggests that 1 additional dose using the same strength may be administered (maximum: 2 doses per breakthrough pain episode); the Canadian labeling recommends use of an alternative rescue medication and limits use of Abstral to 1 dose per breakthrough pain episode. **Patient must wait 2 hours before treating another breakthrough pain episode with sublingual tablet.**

Maintenance dose: Once maintenance dose for breakthrough pain episode has been determined, use only 1 tablet in the appropriate strength per episode; if pain is unrelieved with maintenance dose:

U.S. labeling: A second dose may be given after 30 minutes; maximum of 2 doses/episode of breakthrough pain; separate treatment of subsequent episodes by ≥2 hours; limit treatment to ≤4 breakthrough episodes per day.

Canadian labeling: Administer alternative rescue medication after 30 minutes; maximum of 1 Abstral dose/episode of breakthrough pain; separate treatment of subsequent episodes by ≥2 hours; limit treatment to ≤4 breakthrough episodes per day.

Consider increasing the around-the-clock long-acting opioid therapy in patients experiencing >4 breakthrough pain episodes per day; if long-acting opioid therapy dose altered, re-evaluate and retitrate Abstral dose as needed.

Conversion from lozenge (Actiq) to sublingual tablet (Abstral):

Lozenge dose 200 mcg: Initial sublingual tablet dose is 100 mcg; may titrate using multiples of 100 mcg

Lozenge dose 400 to 1,200 mcg: Initial sublingual tablet dose is 200 mcg; may titrate using multiples of 200 mcg

Lozenge dose 1,600 mcg: Initial sublingual tablet dose is 400 mcg; may titrate using multiples of 400 mcg

Chronic pain management (opioid-tolerant patients only): Transdermal patch: Discontinue or taper all other around-the-clock or extended release opioids when initiating therapy with fentanyl transdermal patch.

Initial: To convert patients from oral or parenteral opioids to transdermal patch, a 24-hour analgesic requirement should be calculated (based on prior opioid use). Using the tables, the appropriate initial dose can be determined. The initial fentanyl dosage may be approximated from the 24-hour morphine dosage equivalent and titrated to minimize adverse effects and provide analgesia. Substantial interpatient variability exists in relative potency. Therefore, it is safer to underestimate a patient's daily fentanyl requirement and provide breakthrough pain relief with rescue medication (eg, immediate release opioid) than to overestimate requirements. With the initial application, the absorption of transdermal fentanyl requires several hours to reach plateau; therefore transdermal fentanyl is inappropriate for management of acute pain. Change patch every 72 hours.

Conversion from continuous infusion of fentanyl: In patients who have adequate pain relief with a fentanyl infusion, fentanyl may be converted to transdermal dosing at a rate equivalent to the intravenous rate. A two-step taper of the infusion to be completed over 12 hours has been recommended (Kornick, 2001) after the patch is applied. The infusion is decreased to 50% of the original rate six hours after the application of the first patch, and subsequently discontinued twelve hours after application. ▶

Titration: Short-acting agents may be required until analgesic efficacy is established and/or as supplements for "breakthrough" pain. The amount of supplemental doses should be closely monitored. Appropriate dosage increases may be based on daily supplemental dosage using the ratio of 45 mg/24 hours of oral morphine to a 12.5 mcg/hour increase in fentanyl dosage (U.S. labeling) or using the ratio of 45 to 59 mg/24 hours of oral morphine to a 12 mcg/hour increase in fentanyl dosage (Canadian labeling).

Frequency of adjustment: The dosage should not be titrated more frequently than every 3 days after the initial dose or every 6 days thereafter. Titrate dose based on the daily dose of supplemental opioids required by the patient on the second or third day of the initial application. **Note:** Upon discontinuation, ~17 hours are required for a 50% decrease in fentanyl levels.

Frequency of application: The majority of patients may be controlled on every 72-hour administration; however, a small number of adult patients require every 48-hour administration.

Discontinuation: When discontinuing transdermal fentanyl and not converting to another opioid, use a gradual downward titration, such as decreasing the dose by 50% every 6 days, to reduce the possibility of withdrawal symptoms.

Dose conversion guidelines for transdermal fentanyl (see following tables).

Note: U.S. and Canadian dose conversion guidelines differ; consult appropriate table. The conversion factors in these tables are only to be used for the conversion from current opioid therapy to Duragesic. Conversion factors in this table cannot be used to convert from Duragesic to another opioid (doing so may lead to fatal overdose due to overestimation of the new opioid). These are not tables of equianalgesic doses.

U.S. Labeling: Dose Conversion Guidelines: Recommended Initial Duragesic Dose Based Upon Daily Oral Morphine Dose[1,2]

Oral 24-Hour Morphine (mg/day)	Duragesic Dose[3] (mcg/h)
60 to 134	25
135 to 224	50
225 to 314	75
315 to 404	100
405 to 494	125
495 to 584	150
585 to 674	175
675 to 764	200
765 to 854	225
855 to 944	250
945 to 1034	275
1035 to 1124	300

[1]The table should NOT be used to convert from transdermal fentanyl (Duragesic) to other opioid analgesics. Rather, following removal of the patch, titrate the dose of the new opioid until adequate analgesia is achieved.

[2]Recommendations are based on U.S. product labeling for Duragesic.

[3]Pediatric patients initiating therapy on a 25 mcg/hour Duragesic system should be opioid-tolerant and receiving at least 60 mg oral morphine equivalents per day.

U.S. Labeling: Dose Conversion Guidelines[1,2]

Current Analgesic	Daily Dosage (mg/day)			
Morphine (IM/IV)	10 to 22	23 to 37	38 to 52	53 to 67
Oxycodone (oral)	30 to 67	67.5 to 112	112.5 to 157	157.5 to 202
Codeine (oral)	150 to 447	-	-	-
Hydromorphone (oral)	8 to 17	17.1 to 28	28.1 to 39	39.1 to 51
Hydromorphone (IV)	1.5 to 3.4	3.5 to 5.6	5.7 to 7.9	8 to 10
Meperidine (IM)	75 to 165	166 to 278	279 to 390	391 to 503
Methadone (oral)	20 to 44	45 to 74	75 to 104	105 to 134
Fentanyl transdermal recommended dose (mcg/h)	25 mcg/h	50 mcg/h	75 mcg/h	100 mcg/h

[1]The table should NOT be used to convert from transdermal fentanyl (Duragesic) to other opioid analgesics. Rather, following removal of the patch, titrate the dose of the new opioid until adequate analgesia is achieved.

[2]Recommendations are based on U.S. product labeling for Duragesic.

Transdermal patch (Duragesic MAT [Canadian product]): Adults:

Canadian Labeling: Dose Conversion Guidelines (Adults): Recommended Initial Duragesic MAT Dose Based Upon Daily Oral Morphine Dose[1,2]

Oral 24-Hour Morphine (Current Dose in mg/day)	Duragesic MAT Dose (Initial Dose in mcg/h)
45 to 59	12
60 to 134	25
135 to 179	37
180 to 224	50
225 to 269	62
270 to 314	75
315 to 359	87
360 to 404	100
405 to 494	125
495 to 584	150
585 to 674	175
675 to 764	200
765 to 854	225
855 to 944	250
945 to 1034	275
1035 to 1124	300

[1]The table should NOT be used to convert from transdermal fentanyl (Duragesic MAT) to other opioid analgesics. Rather, following removal of the patch, titrate the dose of the new opioid until adequate analgesia is achieved.

[2]Recommendations are based on Canadian product labeling for Duragesic MAT.

Note: The 12 mcg/hour dose included in this table is to be used for incremental dose adjustment and is generally not recommended for initial dosing, except for patients in whom lower starting doses are deemed clinically appropriate.

Canadian Labeling: Dosing Conversion Guidelines (Adults)[1,2]

Current Analgesic	Daily Dosage (mg/day)						
Morphine[3] (IM/IV)	20 to 44	45 to 60	61 to 75	76 to 90	n/a[4]	n/a[4]	n/a[4]
Oxycodone (oral)	30 to 66	67 to 90	91 to 112	113 to 134	135 to 157	158 to 179	180 to 202
Codeine (oral)	150 to 447	448 to 597	598 to 747	748 to 897	898 to 1047	1048 to 1197	1198 to 1347
Hydromorphone (oral)	8 to 16	17 to 22	23 to 28	29 to 33	34 to 39	40 to 45	46 to 51
Hydromorphone (IV)	4 to 8.4	8.5 to 11.4	11.5 to 14.4	14.5 to 16.5	16.6 to 19.5	19.6 to 22.5	22.6 to 25.5
Fentanyl transdermal recommended dose (mcg/h)	25 mcg/h	37 mcg/h	50 mcg/h	62 mcg/h	75 mcg/h	87 mcg/h	100 mcg/h

[1]The table should NOT be used to convert from transdermal fentanyl (Duragesic MAT) to other opioid analgesics. Rather, following removal of the patch, titrate the dose of the new opioid until adequate analgesia is achieved.

[2]Recommendations are based on Canadian product labeling for Duragesic MAT.

[3]Morphine dose conversion based upon I.M to oral dose ratio of 1:3.

[4]Insufficient data available to provide specific dosing recommendations. Use caution; adjust dose conservatively.

Geriatric Elderly have been found to be twice as sensitive as younger patients to the effects of fentanyl. A wide range of doses may be used. When choosing a dose, take into consideration the following patient factors: age, weight, physical status, underlying disease states, other drugs used, type of anesthesia used, and the surgical procedure to be performed.

Transmucosal lozenge (eg, Actiq): In clinical trials, patients who were >65 years of age were titrated to a mean dose that was 200 mcg less than that of younger patients.

Pediatric Note: Ranges listed may not represent the maximum doses that may be required in some patients. Doses and dosage intervals should be titrated to pain relief/prevention. Monitor vital signs routinely. Single IM doses have duration of 1 to 2 hours, single IV doses last 0.5 to 1 hour.

Surgery adjunct to anesthesia (induction and maintenance): Children ≥2 years and Adolescents: IV: 2 to 3 mcg/**kg**/dose every 1 to 2 hours as needed

Breakthrough cancer pain: Adolescents ≥16 years: Transmucosal lozenge (Actiq): Refer to adult dosing.

Chronic pain management: Children ≥2 years and Adolescents (opioid-tolerant patients): Transdermal patch (U.S. labeling): Refer to adult dosing. **Note:** Canadian labeling does not approve of use in patients <18 years.

Pain management (off-label use): *Patient-controlled analgesia (PCA) (off-label use; American Pain Society, 2008):* Children <50 kg: IV: **Note:** Opioid-naive:

Usual concentration: 10 to 50 mcg/mL (varies by patient weight and institution)

Demand dose: 0.5 to 1 mcg/kg/dose

Lockout interval: 6 to 8 minutes

Usual basal rate (optional): ≤0.5 mcg/kg/**hour**. **Note:** Due to safety concerns, continuous basal infusions are not recommended for initial programming and should rarely be used (Grass, 2005).

Renal Impairment

Injection: No dosage adjustment provided in manufacturer's labeling; use with caution.

Transdermal (device): There are no dosage adjustments provided in the manufacturer's labeling (has not been studied); fentanyl pharmacokinetics may be altered in renal disease.

Transdermal (patch): Degree of impairment (ie, CrCl) not defined in manufacturer's labeling.

US labeling:

Mild-to-moderate impairment: Initial: Reduce dose by 50%.

Severe impairment: Use not recommended.

Canadian labeling: There are no specific dosage adjustments provided in the manufacturer's labeling; monitor closely for toxicity and reduce dose if necessary.

Transmucosal (buccal film/tablet, sublingual spray/tablet, lozenge) and nasal spray: Although fentanyl pharmacokinetics may be altered in renal disease, fentanyl can be used successfully in the management of breakthrough cancer pain. Doses should be titrated to reach clinical effect with careful monitoring of patients with severe renal disease.

Hepatic Impairment

Injection: No dosage adjustment provided in manufacturer's labeling; use with caution.

Transdermal (device): There are no dosage adjustments provided in the manufacturer's labeling (has not been studied); fentanyl pharmacokinetics may be altered in hepatic disease.

Transdermal (patch):

US labeling:

Mild-to-moderate impairment: Initial: Reduce dose by 50%.

Severe impairment: Use not recommended.

Canadian labeling: There are no specific dosage adjustments provided in the manufacturer's labeling; monitor closely for toxicity and reduce dose if necessary.

Transmucosal (buccal film/tablet, sublingual spray/tablet, lozenge) and nasal spray: Although fentanyl pharmacokinetics may be altered in hepatic disease, fentanyl can be used successfully in the management of breakthrough cancer pain. Doses should be titrated to reach clinical effect with careful monitoring of patients with severe hepatic disease.

◀ **Additional Information** Complete prescribing information should be consulted for additional detail.

Product Availability

Ionsys (iontophoretic transdermal system): FDA approved May 2015; availability anticipated in the third quarter of 2015. Information pertaining to this product within the monograph is pending revision. Consult prescribing information for additional information.

Onsolis: Reformulated product FDA approved August 2015; availability anticipated in 2016. Consult prescribing information for additional information.

Prescribing and Access Restrictions As a requirement of the REMS program, access is restricted.

Transmucosal immediate-release fentanyl products (eg, sublingual tablets and spray, oral lozenges, buccal tablets and soluble film, nasal spray) are only available through the Transmucosal Immediate-Release Fentanyl (TIRF) REMS ACCESS program. Enrollment in the program is required for outpatients, prescribers for outpatient use, pharmacies (inpatient and outpatient), and distributors. Enrollment is not required for inpatient administration (eg, hospitals, hospices, long-term care facilities), inpatients, and prescribers who prescribe to inpatients. Further information is available at 1-866-822-1483 or at www.TIRFREMSaccess.com

Note: Effective December, 2011, individual REMs programs for TIRF products were combined into a single access program (TIRF REMS Access). Prescribers and pharmacies that were enrolled in at least one individual REMS program for these products will automatically be transitioned to the single access program.

Medication Guide Available Yes

Dosage Forms Excipient information presented when available (limited, particularly for generics); consult specific product labeling. [DSC] = Discontinued product

Film, for buccal application, as citrate [strength expressed as base]:

Onsolis: 200 mcg (30s); 400 mcg (30s); 600 mcg (30s); 800 mcg (30s); 1200 mcg (30s) [DSC]

Injection, solution, as citrate [strength expressed as base, preservative free]:

Generic: 0.05 mg/mL (2 mL, 5 mL, 10 mL, 20 mL, 50 mL)

Liquid, sublingual, as base [spray]:

Subsys: 100 mcg (30s); 200 mcg (30s); 400 mcg (30s); 600 mcg (30s); 800 mcg (30s) [contains dehydrated ethanol 63.6%, propylene glycol]

Lozenge, oral, as citrate [strength expressed as base, transmucosal]:

Actiq: 200 mcg (30s); 400 mcg (30s); 600 mcg (30s); 800 mcg (30s); 1200 mcg (30s); 1600 mcg (30s) [contains sugar 2 g/lozenge; berry flavor]

Generic: 200 mcg (30s); 400 mcg (30s); 600 mcg (30s); 800 mcg (30s); 1200 mcg (30s); 1600 mcg (30s)

Patch, transdermal, as base:

Duragesic: 12 [delivers 12.5 mcg/hr] (5s) [contains ethanol 0.1 mL/10 cm^2; 5 cm^2]

Duragesic: 25 [delivers 25 mcg/hr] (5s) [contains ethanol 0.1 mL/10 cm^2; 10 cm^2]

Duragesic: 50 [delivers 50 mcg/hr] (5s) [contains ethanol 0.1 mL/10 cm^2; 20 cm^2]

Duragesic: 75 [delivers 75 mcg/hr] (5s) [contains ethanol 0.1 mL/10 cm^2; 30 cm^2]

Duragesic: 100 [delivers 100 mcg/hr] (5s) [contains ethanol 0.1 mL/10 cm²; 40 cm²]

Ionsys: 40 mcg/actuation (6s) [iontophoretic transdermal system]

Generic: 12 [delivers 12.5 mcg/hr] (5s); 25 [delivers 25 mcg/hr] (5s); 50 [delivers 50 mcg/hr] (5s); 75 [delivers 75 mcg/hr] (5s); 87.5 [delivers 87.5 mcg/hr] (5s); 100 [delivers 100 mcg/hr] (5s)

Powder, for prescription compounding, as citrate: USP: 100% (1 g)

Solution, intranasal, as citrate [strength expressed as base, spray]:
Lazanda: 100 mcg/spray (5 mL); 400 mcg/spray (5 mL) [delivers 8 metered sprays]

Tablet, for buccal application, as citrate [strength expressed as base]:
Fentora: 100 mcg (28s); 200 mcg (28s); 400 mcg (28s); 600 mcg (28s); 800 mcg (28s)

Tablet, sublingual, as citrate [strength expressed as base]:
Abstral: 100 mcg (12s, 32s); 200 mcg (12s, 32s); 300 mcg (12s, 32s); 400 mcg (12s, 32s); 600 mcg (32s); 800 mcg (32s)

Dosage Forms: Canada Excipient information presented when available (limited, particularly for generics); consult specific product labeling.

Patch, transdermal, as base: 12 mcg/hr (5s); 25 mcg/hr (5s); 50 mcg/hr (5s); 75 mcg/hr (5s); 100 mcg/hr (5s)

Duragesic MAT: 12 mcg/hr (5s)
Duragesic MAT: 25 mcg/hr (5s)
Duragesic MAT: 50 mcg/hr (5s)
Duragesic MAT: 75 mcg/hr (5s)
Duragesic MAT: 100 mcg/hr (5s)

Controlled Substance C-II

◆ **Fentanyl Citrate** see FentaNYL on page 692

◆ **Fentanyl Citrate Injection, USP (Can)** see FentaNYL on page 692

◆ **Fentanyl Hydrochloride** see FentaNYL on page 692

◆ **Fentanyl Patch** see FentaNYL on page 692

◆ **Fentora** see FentaNYL on page 692

◆ **Feraheme** see Ferumoxytol on page 708

Ferric Gluconate (FER ik GLOO koe nate)

Brand Names: US Ferrlecit; Nulecit [DSC]

Brand Names: Canada Ferrlecit

Index Terms Sodium Ferric Gluconate; Sodium Ferric Gluconate Complex

Pharmacologic Category Iron Salt

Use Iron deficiency anemia: Treatment of iron-deficiency anemia in patients undergoing hemodialysis in conjunction with erythropoietin therapy

Labeled Contraindications Known hypersensitivity to ferric gluconate or any component of the formulation

Pregnancy Considerations Adverse events were not observed in animal reproduction studies. It is recommended that pregnant women meet the dietary requirements of iron with diet and/or supplements in order to prevent adverse events associated with iron deficiency anemia in pregnancy. Treatment of iron deficiency anemia in pregnant women is the same as in nonpregnant women and in most cases, oral iron preparations may be used. Except in severe cases of maternal anemia, the fetus achieves normal iron stores regardless of maternal concentrations.

◀ **Breast-Feeding Considerations** Iron is normally found in breast milk. Breast milk or iron fortified formulas generally provide enough iron to meet the recommended dietary requirements of infants. The amount of iron in breast milk is generally not influenced by maternal iron status.

Warnings/Precautions Serious hypersensitivity reactions, including anaphylactic-type reactions, have occurred (may be life-threatening). Monitor during administration and for ≥30 minutes after administration and until clinically stable after infusion. Avoid rapid administration. Equipment for resuscitation and trained personnel experienced in handling medical emergencies should always be immediately available. Clinically significant hypotension may occur; usually resolves within 1-2 hours. May augment hemodialysis-induced hypotension. Use with caution in elderly patients. Use only in patients with documented iron deficiency; caution with hemoglobinopathies or other refractory anemias.

Benzyl alcohol and derivatives: Some dosage forms may contain benzyl alcohol; large amounts of benzyl alcohol (≥99 mg/kg/day) have been associated with a potentially fatal toxicity ("gasping syndrome") in neonates; the "gasping syndrome" consists of metabolic acidosis, respiratory distress, gasping respirations, CNS dysfunction (including convulsions, intracranial hemorrhage), hypotension and cardiovascular collapse (AAP ["Inactive" 1997]; CDC, 1982); some data suggests that benzoate displaces bilirubin from protein binding sites (Ahlfors, 2001); avoid or use dosage forms containing benzyl alcohol with caution in neonates. See manufacturer's labeling.

Adverse Reactions Percentages reported in adults unless otherwise noted:
>10%:
  Cardiovascular: Hypotension (children 35%; adults 29%), hypertension (children 23%; adults 13%), tachycardia (children 17%; adults 5%)
  Central nervous system: Headache (children 24%; adults 7%), dizziness (13%)
  Gastrointestinal: Vomiting (adults ≤35%; children 11%), nausea (adults ≤35%; children 9%), diarrhea (adults ≤35%; children 8%)
  Hematologic: Erythrocytes abnormal (11% [changes in morphology, color, or number])
  Local: Injection site reaction (33%)
  Neuromuscular & skeletal: Cramps (25%)
  Respiratory: Dyspnea (11%)
1% to 10%:
  Cardiovascular: Chest pain (10%), syncope (6%), edema (5%), angina pectoris, bradycardia, hypervolemia, MI, peripheral edema, vasodilation
  Central nervous system: Pain (10%), fever (children 9%; adults 5%), fatigue (6%), agitation, chills, consciousness decreased, lightheadedness, malaise, rigors, somnolence
  Dermatologic: Pruritus (6%), rash
  Endocrine & metabolic: Hyperkalemia (6%), hypoglycemia, hypokalemia
  Gastrointestinal: Abdominal pain (children 9%; adults 6%), anorexia, dyspepsia, eructation, flatulence, GI disorder, melena, rectal disorder
  Genitourinary: Menorrhagia, UTI
  Hematologic: Thrombosis (children 6%), anemia, leukocytosis, lymphadenopathy
  Neuromuscular & skeletal: Leg cramps (10%), weakness (7%), paresthesias (6%), arm pain, arthralgia, back pain, leg edema, myalgia
  Ocular: Arcus senilis, conjunctivitis, diplopia, puffy eyelids, redness of eyes, rolling of eyes, watery eyes

Otic: Deafness

Respiratory: Pharyngitis (children 9%), cough (6%), rhinitis (children 6%), upper respiratory infections (6%), pneumonia, pulmonary edema

Miscellaneous: Abscess, carcinoma, diaphoresis, flu-like symptoms, infection, sepsis

Postmarketing and/or case reports: Allergic reaction, anaphylactic reactions, convulsion, dry mouth, dysgeusia, facial flushing, hemorrhage, hypertonia, hypoesthesia, loss of consciousness, nervousness, pallor, phlebitis, shock, skin discoloration

Drug Interactions

Metabolism/Transport Effects None known.

Avoid Concomitant Use

Avoid concomitant use of Ferric Gluconate with any of the following: Dimercaprol

Increased Effect/Toxicity

The levels/effects of Ferric Gluconate may be increased by: ACE Inhibitors; Dimercaprol

Decreased Effect There are no known significant interactions involving a decrease in effect.

Storage/Stability Store at 20°C to 25°C (68°F to 77°F); excursions permitted to 15°C to 30°C (59°F to 86°F). Do not freeze. Use immediately after dilution.

Preparation for Administration For IV infusion, dilute ferric gluconate in 0.9% sodium chloride (children: 25 mL NS, adults: 100 mL NS).

Mechanism of Action Supplies a source to elemental iron necessary to the function of hemoglobin, myoglobin and specific enzyme systems; allows transport of oxygen via hemoglobin

Pharmacodynamics/Kinetics Half-life elimination: Bound iron: 1 hour

Dosing

Adult & Geriatric

Iron-deficiency anemia, hemodialysis patients: IV: 125 mg elemental iron per dialysis session. Most patients will require a cumulative dose of 1 g elemental iron over approximately 8 sequential dialysis treatments to achieve a favorable response.

Note: A test dose of 2 mL diluted in NS 50 mL administered over 60 minutes was previously recommended (not in current manufacturer labeling). Doses >125 mg are associated with increased adverse events.

Chemotherapy-associated anemia (off-label use): IV infusion: 125 mg once every week for 6 doses (Pedrazzoli, 2008) or for 8 doses (Henry, 2007)

Pediatric Iron-deficiency anemia, hemodialysis patients: Children ≥6 years: IV: 1.5 mg/kg of elemental iron (maximum: 125 mg/dose) per dialysis session. Doses >1.5 mg/kg are associated with increased adverse events.

Renal Impairment No dosage adjustment necessary. The ferric gluconate iron complex is not dialyzable.

Hepatic Impairment No dosage adjustment necessary.

Administration IV

Children: Administer diluted in 25 mL NS over 1 hour.

Adults: Administer diluted in 100 mL NS over 1 hour or administer undiluted, slowly at a rate of up to 12.5 mg/minute.

Monitoring Parameters Hemoglobin and hematocrit, serum ferritin, iron saturation; vital signs; signs and symptoms of hypersensitivity (monitor for ≥30 minutes following the end of administration and until clinically stable)

NKF K/DOQI guidelines recommend that iron status should be monitored monthly during initiation through the percent transferrin saturation (TSAT) and serum ferritin.

Chemotherapy-associated anemia (off-label use): Iron, total iron-binding capacity, transferrin saturation, or ferritin levels at baseline and periodically (Rizzo, 2011).

Test Interactions Serum or transferrin bound iron levels may be falsely elevated if assessed within 24 hours of ferric gluconate administration. Serum ferritin levels may be falsely elevated for 5 days after ferric gluconate administration.

Dosage Forms Considerations Strength of ferric gluconate injection is expressed as elemental iron.

Dosage Forms Excipient information presented when available (limited, particularly for generics); consult specific product labeling. [DSC] = Discontinued product

Solution, Intravenous:
Ferrlecit: 12.5 mg/mL (5 mL) [contains benzyl alcohol, sucrose]
Nulecit: 12.5 mg/mL (5 mL [DSC]) [contains benzyl alcohol, sucrose]
Generic: 12.5 mg/mL (5 mL)

◆ **Ferriprox** *see Deferiprone on page 486*
◆ **Ferrlecit** *see Ferric Gluconate on page 705*

Ferumoxytol (fer ue MOX i tol)

Brand Names: US Feraheme
Brand Names: Canada Feraheme
Pharmacologic Category Iron Salt
Use Iron-deficiency anemia in chronic kidney disease: Treatment of iron-deficiency anemia in adults with chronic kidney disease

Labeled Contraindications
Hypersensitivity to ferumoxytol, other IV iron products, or any component of the formulation
Canadian labeling: Additional contraindications (not in US labeling): Any known history of drug allergy, evidence of iron overload; anemia not caused by iron deficiency

Pregnancy Considerations Adverse events were observed in animal reproduction studies. The Canadian labeling recommends avoiding use in women of childbearing potential not using adequate contraception.

Breast-Feeding Considerations It is not known if ferumoxytol is excreted into breast milk. Due to the potential for serious adverse reactions in the nursing infant, the manufacturer recommends a decision be made whether to discontinue nursing or to discontinue the drug, taking into account the importance of treatment to the mother.

Warnings/Precautions [US Boxed Warning]: Serious hypersensitivity reactions, including anaphylactic-type reactions (some fatal), may occur, presenting with cardiac/cardiorespiratory arrest, clinically significant hypotension, syncope, or unresponsiveness even in patients who previously tolerated ferumoxytol. Equipment for resuscitation and trained personnel experienced in handling emergencies should be immediately available during use. Monitor patients for signs/symptoms of hypersensitivity reactions, including blood pressure and pulse during and ≥30 minutes (until clinically stable) following administration. Other

hypersensitivity reactions have also occurred (pruritus, rash, urticaria, wheezing). Patients with multiple drug allergies may have greater risk of anaphylaxis; elderly patients with multiple or serious comorbidities who develop hypersensitivity and/or hypotension after ferumoxytol may be at greater risk for serious adverse events.

Do not administer in the presence of tissue iron overload; periodic monitoring of hemoglobin, serum ferritin, serum iron, and transferrin saturation is recommended. Serum iron and transferrin-bound iron may be overestimated in laboratory assays if level is drawn during the first 24 hours following administration. Administration may alter magnetic resonance (MR) imaging; conduct anticipated MRI studies prior to use. MR imaging alterations may persist for ≤3 months following use, with peak alterations anticipated in the first 2 days following administration. If MR imaging is required within 3 months after administration, use T1- or proton density-weighted MR pulse sequences to decrease effect on imagining. Do not use T2-weighted sequence MR imaging prior to 4 weeks following ferumoxytol administration. Ferumoxytol does not interfere with X-ray, computed tomography (CT), positron emission tomography (PET), single photon emission computed tomography (SPECT), ultrasound or nuclear medicine imaging. Potentially significant drug-drug interactions may exist, requiring dose or frequency adjustment, additional monitoring, and/or selection of alternative therapy.

Adverse Reactions
1% to 10%:
Cardiovascular: Hypotension (≤3%), edema (2%), peripheral edema (2%), chest pain (1%), hypertension (1%)
Central nervous system: Dizziness (3%), headache (2%), fever (1%)
Dermatologic: Pruritus (1%), rash (1%)
Gastrointestinal: Diarrhea (4%), nausea (3%), constipation (2%), vomiting (2%), abdominal pain (1%)
Neuromuscular & skeletal: Back pain (1%), muscle spasms (1%)
Respiratory: Cough (1%), dyspnea (1%)
Miscellaneous: Hypersensitivity reactions (≤4%; serious reactions: <1%)
<1%, postmarketing, and/or case reports: Anaphylactic/anaphylactoid reactions, angioedema, cardiac/cardiorespiratory arrest, cardiac rhythm abnormalities, congestive heart failure, cyanosis, fatigue, hypotension (clinically significant); infusion site reactions (including bruising, burning, erythema, irritation, pain, swelling, warmth); ischemic myocardial events, loss of consciousness, pulse absent, syncope, tachycardia, unresponsiveness, urticaria, wheezing

Drug Interactions
Metabolism/Transport Effects None known.
Avoid Concomitant Use
Avoid concomitant use of Ferumoxytol with any of the following: Dimercaprol
Increased Effect/Toxicity
The levels/effects of Ferumoxytol may be increased by: Dimercaprol
Decreased Effect There are no known significant interactions involving a decrease in effect.
Storage/Stability Store intact vials at 20°C to 25°C (68°F to 77°F); excursions are permitted between 15°C and 30°C (59°F and 86°F). Solutions diluted in NS or D_5W at concentrations of 2 to 8 mg/mL elemental iron should be used immediately, but may be stored at 23°C to 27°C (73°F to 81°F) for up to 4 hours.

◀ **Preparation for Administration** Must be diluted prior to administration. To prepare for intravenous infusion, dilute in 50 to 200 mL of NS or D_5W.

Mechanism of Action Superparamagnetic iron oxide coated with a low molecular weight semisynthetic carbohydrate; iron-carbohydrate complex enters the reticuloendothelial system macrophages of the liver, spleen, and bone marrow where the iron is released from the complex. The released iron is either transported into storage pools or is transported via plasma transferrin for incorporation into hemoglobin.

Pharmacodynamics/Kinetics

Distribution: V_d: 3.16 L

Metabolism: Iron released from iron-carbohydrate complex after uptake in the reticuloendothelial system macrophages of the liver, spleen, and bone marrow

Half-life elimination: ~15 hours

Dialysis: Ferumoxytol is not removed by hemodialysis

Dosing

Adult & Geriatric Doses expressed in mg of **elemental** iron. **Note:** Test dose: Product labeling does not indicate need for a test dose.

Iron-deficiency anemia in chronic kidney disease: IV:

US labeling: 510 mg as an IV infusion, followed by a second 510 mg IV infusion 3 to 8 days after initial dose. Assess response at least 30 days following the second dose. The recommended dose may be readministered in patients with persistent or recurrent iron-deficiency anemia.

Canadian labeling:

Baseline hemoglobin >10 to 12 g/dL:

Body weight ≤50 kg: 510 mg as an IV infusion.

Body weight >50 kg: 510 mg as an IV infusion, followed by a second 510 mg IV infusion 2 to 8 days after initial dose.

Baseline hemoglobin ≤10 g/dL (regardless of weight): 510 mg as an IV infusion, followed by a second 510 mg IV infusion 2 to 8 days after initial dose.

Renal Impairment No dosage adjustment necessary.

Hemodialysis: Not removed by hemodialysis; however, administer dose after at least 1 hour of hemodialysis has been completed and once blood pressure has stabilized.

Hepatic Impairment There are no dosage adjustments provided in the manufacturer's labeling.

Administration

IV: Administer diluted as a slow IV infusion over at least 15 minutes. Patient should be in a reclined or semi-reclined position during the infusion; monitor for signs of hypersensitivity (including blood pressure and pulse) for at least 30 minutes after infusion. **Note:** Serious hypersensitivity reactions have been observed with rapid IV injection (<1 minute) (Macdougall, 2014; Vadhan-Raj, 2014). Wait ≥30 minutes between administration of ferumoxytol and other agents that may cause serious hypersensitivity reactions and/or hypotension (eg, chemotherapy, monoclonal antibodies).

Hemodialysis patients: Administer dose after at least 1 hour of hemodialysis has been completed and once blood pressure has stabilized.

Monitoring Parameters Hemoglobin, serum ferritin, serum iron, transferrin saturation (at least 1 month following second injection and periodically); signs/symptoms of hypersensitivity reactions, blood pressure, pulse (during and ≥30 minutes following administration)

Test Interactions May interfere with MR imaging; alterations may persist for ≤3 months following use, with peak alterations anticipated in the first 2 days following administration. If MR imaging is required within 3 months after administration, use T1- or proton density-weighted MR pulse sequences to decrease effect on imaging. Do not use T2-weighted sequence MR imaging prior to 4 weeks following administration.

Serum iron and transferrin-bound iron may be overestimated in laboratory assays if level is drawn during the first 24 hours following administration (due to contribution of iron in ferumoxytol).

Dosage Forms Considerations Strength of ferumoxytol is expressed as elemental iron

Dosage Forms Excipient information presented when available (limited, particularly for generics); consult specific product labeling.

Solution, Intravenous [preservative free]:

Feraheme: 510 mg/17 mL (17 mL)

Fibrinogen Concentrate (Human)
(fi BRIN o gin KON suhn trate HYU man)

Brand Names: US RiaSTAP

Index Terms Coagulation Factor I

Pharmacologic Category Blood Product Derivative

Use Congenital fibrinogen deficiency: Treatment of acute bleeding episodes in patients with congenital fibrinogen deficiency, including afibrinogenemia and hypofibrinogenemia.

Pregnancy Risk Factor C

Dosing

Adult & Geriatric Congenital fibrinogen deficiency: IV: **Note:** Adjust dose based on laboratory values and condition of patient. Maintain a target fibrinogen level of 100 mg/dL until hemostasis is achieved.

When baseline fibrinogen level is known:

Dose (mg/kg) = [Target level (mg/dL) - measured level (mg/dL)] **divided by** 1.7 (mg/dL per mg/kg body weight)

When baseline fibrinogen level is not known: 70 mg/kg

Pediatric Congenital fibrinogen deficiency: IV: Refer to adult dosing.

Renal Impairment There are no dosage adjustments provided in the manufacturer's labeling.

Hepatic Impairment There are no dosage adjustments provided in the manufacturer's labeling.

Additional Information Complete prescribing information should be consulted for additional detail.

Dosage Forms Excipient information presented when available (limited, particularly for generics); consult specific product labeling. [DSC] = Discontinued product

Injection, powder for reconstitution:

RiaSTAP: 900-1300 mg [contains albumin (human); exact potency labeled on vial]

Filgrastim (fil GRA stim)

Related Information

Hematopoietic Stem Cell Transplantation *on page* 2272

Brand Names: US Granix; Neupogen; Zarxio

Brand Names: Canada Neupogen

◀ **Index Terms** Filgrastim-Sndz; G-CSF; Granulocyte Colony Stimulating Factor; Tbo-Filgrastim; Tevagrastim

Pharmacologic Category Colony Stimulating Factor; Hematopoietic Agent

Use

Myelosuppressive chemotherapy recipients with nonmyeloid malignancies:

Neupogen, Zarxio: To decrease the incidence of infection (neutropenic fever) in patients with nonmyeloid malignancies receiving myelosuppressive chemotherapy associated with a significant incidence of severe neutropenia with fever.

Granix: To decrease the duration of severe neutropenia in patients with nonmyeloid malignancies receiving myelosuppressive chemotherapy associated with a clinically significant incidence of neutropenic fever.

Acute myeloid leukemia (AML) patients following induction or consolidation chemotherapy (Neupogen, Zarxio): To reduce the time to neutrophil recovery and the duration of fever following induction or consolidation chemotherapy in adults with AML.

Bone marrow transplantation (Neupogen, Zarxio): To reduce the duration of neutropenia and neutropenia-related events (eg, neutropenic fever) in patients with nonmyeloid malignancies receiving myeloablative chemotherapy followed by marrow transplantation.

Hematopoietic radiation injury syndrome, acute (Neupogen): To increase survival in patients acutely exposed to myelosuppressive doses of radiation.

Peripheral blood progenitor cell collection and therapy (Neupogen, Zarxio): Mobilization of autologous hematopoietic progenitor cells into the peripheral blood for apheresis collection.

Severe chronic neutropenia (Neupogen, Zarxio): Long-term administration to reduce the incidence and duration of neutropenic complications (eg, fever, infections, oropharyngeal ulcers) in symptomatic patients with congenital, cyclic, or idiopathic neutropenia.

Labeled Contraindications

Neupogen, Zarxio: History of serious allergic reactions to human granulocyte colony-stimulating factors, such as filgrastim or pegfilgrastim, or any component of the formulation

Granix: There are no contraindications listed in the manufacturer's labeling

Pregnancy Considerations Adverse events have been observed in animal reproduction studies. Filgrastim has been shown to cross the placenta in humans.

Women who become pregnant during Neupogen treatment are encouraged to enroll in the manufacturer's Pregnancy Surveillance Program (1-800-772-6436).

Breast-Feeding Considerations It is not known if filgrastim, filgrastim-sndz, or tbo-filgrastim is excreted in breast milk. The manufacturers recommend that caution be exercised when administering filgrastim products to breast-feeding women.

Women who are nursing during Neupogen treatment are encouraged to enroll in the manufacturer's Lactation Surveillance program (1-800-772-6436).

Warnings/Precautions Serious allergic reactions (including anaphylaxis) have been reported, usually with the initial exposure; may be managed symptomatically with administration of antihistamines, steroids, bronchodilators, and/or epinephrine. Allergic reactions may recur within days after the initial allergy management has been stopped. Do not administer filgrastim products to patients who experienced serious allergic reaction to filgrastim or pegfilgrastim. Permanently discontinue filgrastim products in patients with serious allergic reactions. Rare cases of splenic rupture have been reported (may be fatal); in patients with upper abdominal pain, left upper quadrant pain, or shoulder tip pain, withhold treatment and evaluate for enlarged spleen or splenic rupture. Moderate or severe cutaneous vasculitis has been reported, generally occurring in patients with severe chronic neutropenia on chronic therapy. Withhold treatment if cutaneous vasculitis occurs; may be restarted with a dose reduction once symptoms resolve and the absolute neutrophil count (ANC) has decreased. Capillary leak syndrome (CLS), characterized by hypotension, hypoalbuminemia, edema, and hemoconcentration, may occur in patients receiving human granulocyte colony-stimulating factors (G-CSF). CLS episode may vary in frequency and severity. If CLS develops, monitor closely and manage symptomatically (may require intensive care). CLS may be life-threatening if treatment is delayed.

White blood cell counts of $\geq 100,000/mm^3$ have been reported with filgrastim doses >5 mcg/kg/day. When filgrastim products are used as an adjunct to myelosuppressive chemotherapy, discontinue when ANC exceeds $10,000/mm^3$ after the ANC nadir has occurred (to avoid potential excessive leukocytosis). Doses that increase the ANC beyond $10,000/mm^3$ may not result in additional clinical benefit. Monitor complete blood cell count (CBC) twice weekly during therapy. In patients receiving myelosuppressive chemotherapy, filgrastim discontinuation generally resulted in a 50% decrease in circulating neutrophils within 1 to 2 days, and a return to pretreatment levels in 1 to 7 days. When used for peripheral blood progenitor cell collection, discontinue filgrastim products if leukocytes >$100,000/mm^3$. Thrombocytopenia has also been reported with filgrastim products; monitor platelet counts. Filgrastim products should not be routinely used in the treatment of established neutropenic fever. Colony-stimulating factors may be considered in cancer patients with febrile neutropenia who are at high risk for infection-associated complications or who have prognostic factors indicative of a poor clinical outcome (eg, prolonged and severe neutropenia, age >65 years, hypotension, pneumonia, sepsis syndrome, presence of invasive fungal infection, uncontrolled primary disease, hospitalization at the time of fever development) (Freifeld, 2011; Smith, 2006). Colony-stimulating factors (CSF) should not be routinely used for patients with neutropenia who are afebrile. Dose-dense regimens that require colony-stimulating factors should only be used within the context of a clinical trial or if supported by convincing evidence (Smith, 2015). Recommendations for the Use of WBC Growth Factors Clinical Practice Guideline Update recommend that prophylactic CSF be used in patients ≥65 years with diffuse aggressive lymphoma treated with curative chemotherapy (eg, rituximab, cyclophosphamide, doxorubicin, vincristine, prednisone), especially if patients have comorbid conditions (Smith, 2015). CSF use in pediatric patients is typically directed by clinical pediatric protocols. The American Society of Clinical Oncology (ASCO) Recommendations for the Use of WBC Growth Factors Clinical Practice Guideline Update states that CSFs may be reasonable as primary prophylaxis in pediatric patients when chemotherapy regimens with a high likelihood of febrile neutropenia are employed. Likewise, secondary CSF prophylaxis should be limited to high-risk patients. In pediatric cancers in which dose-intense chemotherapy (with a survival benefit) is used, CSFs should be given to facilitate chemotherapy administration. CSFs should not be used in the pediatric population for nonrelapsed acute lymphoblastic or myeloid leukemia when no infection is present (Smith, 2015). Do not use filgrastim products in the period 24 hours before to 24 hours after administration of cytotoxic chemotherapy because of the potential sensitivity of rapidly dividing myeloid cells to cytotoxic chemotherapy. Transient increase in neutrophil count is seen 1 to 2 days after filgrastim initiation; however, for sustained neutrophil response, continue until post-nadir ANC reaches 10,000/mm^3. Avoid simultaneous use of filgrastim products with chemotherapy and radiation therapy. Avoid concurrent radiation therapy with filgrastim; safety and efficacy have not been established with patients receiving radiation therapy. The G-CSF receptor through which filgrastim products act has been found on tumor cell lines. May potentially act as a growth factor for any tumor type (including myeloid malignancies and myelodysplasia). When used for stem cell mobilization, may release tumor cells from marrow, which could be collected in leukapheresis product; potential effect of tumor cell reinfusion is unknown.

May precipitate severe sickle cell crises, sometimes resulting in fatalities, in patients with sickle cell disorders (sickle cell trait or sickle cell disease); carefully evaluate potential risks and benefits. Discontinue in patients undergoing sickle cell crisis. Establish diagnosis of severe chronic neutropenia (SCN) prior to initiation; use prior to appropriate diagnosis of SCN may impair or delay proper evaluation and treatment for neutropenia due to conditions other than SCN. Based on findings of azotemia, hematuria (micro- and macroscopic), proteinuria, and renal biopsy, glomerulonephritis has occurred in patients receiving filgrastim. Glomerulonephritis usually resolved after filgrastim dose reduction or discontinuation. If glomerulonephritis is suspected, evaluate for cause; if likely due to filgrastim, consider dose reduction or treatment interruption. Myelodysplastic syndrome (MDS) and acute myeloid leukemia (AML) have been reported to occur in the natural history of congenital neutropenia (without cytokine therapy). Cytogenetic abnormalities and transformation to MDS and AML have been observed with filgrastim when used to manage SCN, although the risk for MDS and AML appears to be in patients with congenital neutropenia. Abnormal cytogenetics and MDS are associated with the development of AML. The effects of continuing filgrastim products in patients who have developed abnormal cytogenetics or MDS are unknown; consider risk versus benefits of continuing treatment. Acute respiratory distress syndrome (ARDS) has been reported. Evaluate patients who develop fever and lung infiltrates or respiratory distress for ARDS; discontinue in patients with ARDS. Reports of alveolar hemorrhage, manifested as pulmonary infiltrates and hemoptysis (requiring hospitalization), have occurred in healthy donors undergoing PBPC mobilization (off-label for use in healthy donors); hemoptysis resolved upon discontinuation. Increased bone marrow hematopoietic activity due to CSF use has been associated with transient bone-imaging changes; interpret results accordingly.

The packaging of some dosage forms may contain latex.

Some products available internationally may have vial strength and dosing expressed as units (instead of as micrograms). Refer to prescribing information for specific strength and dosing information.

Some dosage forms may contain polysorbate 80 (also known as Tweens). Hypersensitivity reactions, usually a delayed reaction, have been reported following exposure to pharmaceutical products containing polysorbate 80 in certain individuals (Isaksson, 2002; Lucente 2000; Shelley, 1995). Thrombocytopenia, ascites, pulmonary deterioration, and renal and hepatic failure have been reported in premature neonates after receiving parenteral products containing polysorbate 80 (Alade, 1986; CDC, 1984). See manufacturer's labeling.

Adverse Reactions

>10%:

Cardiovascular: Chest pain (5% to 13%)

Central nervous system: Fatigue (20%), dizziness (14%), pain (12%)

Dermatologic: Skin rash (2% to 14%)

Endocrine & metabolic: Increased lactate dehydrogenase (6% to ≤58%; reversible mild to moderate elevations), increased uric acid (≤58%; reversible mild to moderate elevations)

Gastrointestinal: Nausea (10% to 43%)

Hematologic & oncologic: Thrombocytopenia (5% to 38%), splenomegaly (≥5%; severe chronic neutropenia: 30%), petechia (17%)

Hepatic: Increased serum alkaline phosphatase (6% to 11%)

Neuromuscular & skeletal: Ostealgia (5% to 33%; dose and cycle related), back pain (2% to 15%)

Respiratory: Epistaxis (2% to 15%), cough (14%), dyspnea (13%)

Miscellaneous: Fever (12% to 48%; dose and cycle related)

1% to 10%:

Cardiovascular: Peripheral edema (≥5%), hypertension (≥4%), cardiac arrhythmia (≤3%), myocardial infarction (≤3%)

Central nervous system: Headache (7% to 10%), hypoesthesia (≥5%), insomnia (≥5%), malaise (≥5%), mouth pain (≥5%)

Dermatologic: Alopecia (≥5%), erythema (≥2%), maculopapular rash (≥2%)

Gastrointestinal: Vomiting (5% to 7%), constipation (≥2%), diarrhea (≥2%)

Genitourinary: Decreased appetite (≥5%), urinary tract infection (≥5%)

Hematologic & oncologic: Anemia (≥5%), leukocytosis (≤2%)

Hypersensitivity: Transfusion reaction (2% to 10%), hypersensitivity reaction (≥5%)

Immunologic: Antibody development (3%; no evidence of neutralizing response)

Infection: Sepsis (≥5%)

Neuromuscular & skeletal: Arthralgia (5% to 9%), limb pain (2% to 7%), muscle spasm (≥5%), musculoskeletal pain (≥5%) weakness (≥5%)

Respiratory: Bronchitis (≥5%), upper respiratory tract infection (≥5%)

<1%, postmarketing, and/or case reports: Anaphylaxis, capillary leak syndrome, cerebral hemorrhage, decreased bone mineral density, decreased hemoglobin, euthymia nodosum, exacerbation of psoriasis, facial edema, glomerulonephritis, hematuria, hemoptysis, hepatomegaly, hypersensitivity angiitis, hypotension, injection site reaction, osteoporosis, proteinuria, pulmonary alveolar hemorrhage, pulmonary infiltrates, renal insufficiency, respiratory distress syndrome, severe sickle cell crisis, splenic rupture, Sweet syndrome, tachycardia, urticaria, wheezing

Drug Interactions

Metabolism/Transport Effects None known.

Avoid Concomitant Use There are no known interactions where it is recommended to avoid concomitant use.

Increased Effect/Toxicity

Filgrastim may increase the levels/effects of: Bleomycin; Cyclophosphamide; Topotecan

Decreased Effect There are no known significant interactions involving a decrease in effect.

◄ **Storage/Stability**

Neupogen: Store at 2°C to 8°C (36°F to 46°F). Store in the original carton. Protect from light. Protect from direct sunlight. Avoid freezing; if frozen, thaw in the refrigerator before administration. Discard if frozen more than once. Do not shake. Transport via a pneumatic tube has not been studied. Prior to injection, allow to reach room temperature for up to 30 minutes and a maximum of 24 hours. Discard any vial or prefilled syringe left at room temperature for more than 24 hours. Solutions diluted for infusion may be stored at room temperature for up to 24 hours (infusion must be completed within 24 hours of preparation).

Extended storage information may be available for undiluted filgrastim; contact product manufacturer to obtain current recommendations. Sterility has been assessed and maintained for up to 7 days when prepared under strict aseptic conditions (Jacobson, 1996; Singh, 1994). The manufacturer recommends using within 24 hours due to the potential for bacterial contamination.

Granix: Store prefilled syringes at 2°C to 8°C (36°F to 46°F). Protect from light. Do not shake. May be removed from 2°C to 8°C (36°F to 46°F) storage for a single period of up to 5 days between 23°C to 27°C (73°F to 81°F). If not used within 5 days, the product may be returned to 2°C to 8°C (36°F to 46°F) up to the expiration date. Exposure to -1°C to -5°C (23°F to 30°F) for up to 72 hours and temperatures as low as -15°C to -25°C (5°F to -13°F) for up to 24 hours do not adversely affect stability. Discard unused product.

Zarxio: Store at 2°C to 8°C (36°F to 46°F). Store in the original carton. Protect from light. Avoid freezing; if frozen, thaw in the refrigerator before administration. Discard if frozen more than once. Do not shake. Transport via a pneumatic tube has not been studied. Prior to injection, allow to reach room temperature for up to 30 minutes and a maximum of 24 hours. Discard any prefilled syringe left at room temperature for more than 24 hours. Solutions diluted for infusion may be stored at room temperature for up to 24 hours (infusion must be completed within 24 hours of preparation).

Preparation for Administration Visually inspect prior to use; discard if discolored or if particulates are present.

Neupogen: **Do not dilute with saline at any time; product may precipitate.** Filgrastim (vial only; do not use prefilled syringe for IV preparation) may be diluted with D_5W to a concentration of 5 to 15 mcg/mL for IV infusion administration (minimum concentration: 5 mcg/mL). Concentrations of 5 to 15 mcg/mL require addition of albumin (final albumin concentration of 2 mg/mL) to prevent adsorption to plastics. Dilution to <5 mcg/mL is not recommended. Do not shake. May be prepared in glass bottles, polyvinyl chloride (PVC) or polyolefin bags, and polypropylene syringes. Discard unused portion of vial.

Granix: Remove needle shield and expel extra volume if needed (depending on dose). Prefilled syringe is single use; discard unused portion.

Zarxio: **Do not dilute with saline at any time; product may precipitate.** Filgrastim-sndz may be diluted with D_5W to a concentration of 5 to 15 mcg/mL for IV infusion administration. Concentrations of 5 to 15 mcg/mL require addition of albumin (final albumin concentration of 2 mg/mL) to prevent adsorption to plastics. Do not shake. May be prepared in glass, PVC, polyolefin, and polypropylene. Discard unused portion of syringe.

Mechanism of Action Filgrastim and tbo-filgrastim are granulocyte colony stimulating factors (G-CSF) produced by recombinant DNA technology. G-CSFs stimulate the production, maturation, and activation of neutrophils to increase both their migration and cytotoxicity.

Pharmacodynamics/Kinetics

Onset of action:

Filgrastim: 1 to 2 days

Tbo-filgrastim: Time to maximum ANC: 3 to 5 days

Duration:

Filgrastim: Neutrophil counts generally return to baseline within 4 days

Tbo-filgrastim: ANC returned to baseline by 21 days after completion of chemotherapy

Distribution: V_d: 150 mL/kg; Continuous infusion: No evidence of drug accumulation over a 11- to 20-day period

Metabolism: Systemically degraded

Bioavailability: Filgrastim: SubQ: 60% to 70%; Tbo-filgrastim: SubQ: 33%

Half-life elimination: Filgrastim: ~3.5 hours; Tbo-filgrastim: 3 to 4 hours

Time to peak, serum: SubQ: Filgrastim: 2 to 8 hours; Tbo-filgrastim: 4 to 6 hours

Dosing

Adult & Geriatric Note: Do not administer in the period 24 hours before to 24 hours after cytotoxic chemotherapy. May round the dose to the nearest vial size for convenience and cost minimization (Ozer, 2000). **International considerations:** Dosages below expressed as micrograms; 1 mcg = 100,000 units (Hoglund, 1998).

Myelosuppressive chemotherapy recipients with nonmyeloid malignancies (Neupogen, Zarxio): SubQ, IV: 5 mcg/kg/day; doses may be increased by 5 mcg/kg (for each chemotherapy cycle) according to the duration and severity of the neutropenia; continue for up to 14 days until the absolute neutrophil count (ANC) reaches 10,000/mm³. Discontinue if the ANC surpasses 10,000/mm³ after the expected chemotherapy-induced neutrophil nadir.

Myelosuppressive chemotherapy recipients with nonmyeloid malignancies (Granix): SubQ: 5 mcg/kg/day; continue until anticipated nadir has passed and neutrophil count has recovered to normal range.

Acute myeloid leukemia (AML) following induction or consolidation chemotherapy (Neupogen, Zarxio): SubQ, IV: 5 mcg/kg/day; doses may be increased by 5 mcg/kg (for each chemotherapy cycle) according to the duration and severity of the neutropenia; continue for up to 14 days until the ANC reaches 10,000/mm³. Discontinue if the ANC surpasses 10,000/mm³ after the expected chemotherapy-induced neutrophil nadir.

Bone marrow transplantation (Neupogen, Zarxio): IV infusion: 10 mcg/kg/day (administer ≥24 hours after chemotherapy and ≥24 hours after bone marrow infusion); adjust the dose according to the duration and severity of neutropenia; recommended steps based on neutrophil response:

When ANC >1,000/mm³ for 3 consecutive days: Reduce dose to 5 mcg/kg/day

If ANC remains >1,000/mm³ for 3 more consecutive days: Discontinue

If ANC decreases to <1,000/mm³: Resume at 5 mcg/kg/day.

If ANC decreases to <1,000/mm³ during the 5 mcg/kg/day dose: Increase dose to 10 mcg/kg/day and follow the above steps.

◀ **Hematopoietic radiation injury syndrome, acute (Neupogen):** SubQ: 10 mcg/kg once daily; begin as soon as possible after suspected or confirmed radiation doses >2 gray (Gy) and continue filgrastim until ANC remains >1,000/mm^3 for 3 consecutive CBCs or ANC exceeds 10,000/mm^3 after the radiation-induced nadir. ASCO guidelines recommend initiating within 24 hours of exposure of a dose ≥2 Gy and/or significant decrease in absolute lymphocyte count, or for anticipated neutropenia <500/mm^3 for ≥7 days (Smith, 2015).

Peripheral blood progenitor cell collection and therapy (Neupogen, Zarxio): SubQ: 10 mcg/kg daily, usually for 6 to 7 days (with apheresis occurring on days 5, 6, and 7). Begin at least 4 days before the first apheresis and continue until the last apheresis; discontinue for WBC >100,000/mm^3

Severe chronic neutropenia (Neupogen, Zarxio): SubQ:
Congenital: Initial: 6 mcg/kg/day in 2 divided doses; adjust the dose based on ANC and clinical response; mean dose: 6 mcg/kg/day
Idiopathic: Initial: 5 mcg/kg once daily; adjust the dose based on ANC and clinical response; mean dose: 1.2 mcg/kg/day
Cyclic: Initial: 5 mcg/kg once daily; adjust the dose based on ANC and clinical response; mean dose: 2.1 mcg/kg/day

Anemia in myelodysplastic syndrome (off-label use; in combination with epoetin): SubQ: 300 mcg weekly in 2 to 3 divided doses (Malcovati, 2013) **or** 1 mcg/kg once daily (Greenberg, 2009) **or** 75 mcg, 150 mcg, or 300 mcg per dose 3 times weekly (Hellstrom-Lindberg, 2003)

Hematopoietic stem cell mobilization in autologous transplantation in patients with non-Hodgkin lymphoma or multiple myeloma (in combination with plerixafor; off-label combination): SubQ: 10 mcg/kg once daily; begin 4 days before initiation of plerixafor; continue G-CSF on each day prior to apheresis for up to 8 days (DiPersio, 2009a; DiPersio, 2009b)

Hepatitis C treatment-associated neutropenia (off-label use): SubQ: 150 mcg once weekly to 300 mcg 3 times weekly; titrate to maintain ANC between 750 and 10,000/mm^3 (Younossi, 2008)

Pediatric Note: Do not administer in the period 24 hours before to 24 hours after cytotoxic chemotherapy. **International considerations:** Dosages below expressed as micrograms; 1 mcg = 100,000 units (Hoglund, 1998).

Myelosuppressive chemotherapy recipients with nonmyeloid malignancies (Neupogen, Zarxio): SubQ, IV: 5 mcg/kg/day; doses may be increased by 5 mcg/kg (for each chemotherapy cycle) according to the duration and severity of the neutropenia; continue for up to 14 days until the absolute neutrophil count (ANC) reaches 10,000/mm^3. Discontinue if the ANC surpasses 10,000/mm^3 after the expected chemotherapy-induced neutrophil nadir.

Bone marrow transplantation (Neupogen, Zarxio): IV infusion: 10 mcg/kg/ day (administer ≥24 hours after chemotherapy and ≥24 hours after bone marrow infusion); adjust the dose according to the duration and severity of neutropenia; recommended steps based on neutrophil response:
When ANC >1,000/mm^3 for 3 consecutive days: Reduce dose to 5 mcg/ kg/day
If ANC remains >1,000/mm^3 for 3 more consecutive days: Discontinue
If ANC decreases to <1,000/mm^3: Resume at 5 mcg/kg/day
If ANC decreases to <1,000/mm^3 during the 5 mcg/kg/day dose, increase dose to 10 mcg/kg/day and follow the above steps

Hematopoietic radiation injury syndrome, acute (Neupogen): SubQ: 10 mcg/kg once daily; begin as soon as possible after suspected or confirmed radiation doses >2 gray (Gy) and continue filgrastim until ANC remains >1,000/mm^3 for 3 consecutive CBCs or ANC exceeds 10,000/mm^3 after the radiation-induced nadir. ASCO guidelines recommend initiating within 24 hours of exposure of a dose ≥2 Gy and/or significant decrease in absolute lymphocyte count, or for anticipated neutropenia <500/mm^3 for ≥7 days (Smith, 2015).

Peripheral blood progenitor cell collection and therapy (Neupogen, Zarxio): SubQ: 10 mcg/kg daily, usually for 6 to 7 days (with apheresis occurring on days 5, 6, and 7). Begin at least 4 days before the first apheresis and continue until the last apheresis; discontinue for WBC >100,000/mm^3

Severe chronic neutropenia (Neupogen, Zarxio): Infants ≥1 month, Children, and Adolescents: SubQ:

Congenital: Initial: 6 mcg/kg/day in 2 divided doses; adjust the dose based on ANC and clinical response; mean dose: 6 mcg/kg/day

Idiopathic: Initial: 5 mcg/kg once daily; adjust the dose based on ANC and clinical response; mean dose: 1.2 mcg/kg/day

Cyclic: Initial: 5 mcg/kg once daily; adjust the dose based on ANC and clinical response; mean dose: 2.1 mcg/kg/day

Renal Impairment

Renal impairment at treatment initiation:

Neupogen, Zarxio: No dosage adjustment necessary.

Granix:

Mild impairment: No dosage adjustment necessary.

Moderate to severe impairment: There are no dosage adjustments provided in the manufacturer's labeling (has not been studied).

Renal toxicity during treatment: Glomerulonephritis due to filgrastim: Consider dose reduction or treatment interruption.

Hepatic Impairment

Neupogen, Zarxio: No dosage adjustment necessary.

Granix: There are no dosage adjustments provided in the manufacturer's labeling (has not been studied).

Combination Regimens

Bladder cancer:

Cisplatin-Docetaxel-Gemcitabine (Bladder) on page 1891

Dose Dense MVAC (Bladder Cancer) on page 1948

MVAC (Bladder) on page 2042

Bone sarcoma (Ewing sarcoma):

Docetaxel-Gemcitabine (Ewing Sarcoma) on page 1942

Cyclophosphamide-Topotecan (Ewing Sarcoma) on page 1930

Ifosfamide-Carboplatin-Etoposide (Ewing Sarcoma) on page 2014

Bone sarcoma (osteosarcoma):

Docetaxel-Gemcitabine (Osteosarcoma) on page 1943

Ifosfamide-Carboplatin-Etoposide (Osteosarcoma) on page 2015

Breast cancer:

AC (Dose-Dense) followed by Paclitaxel (Dose-Dense) (Breast) on page 1822

AC (Dose-Dense) followed by Paclitaxel Weekly (Breast) on page 1824

Endometrial cancer: Cisplatin-Doxorubin-Paclitaxel (Endometrial) on page 1893

Esophageal cancer: Paclitaxel-Cisplatin (Esophageal Cancer) on page 2050 ▶

◄

Administration Do not administer earlier than 24 hours after or in the 24 hours prior to cytotoxic chemotherapy.

IV (Neupogen, Zarxio): May be administered IV as a short infusion over 15 to 30 minutes (chemotherapy-induced neutropenia) or by continuous infusion (chemotherapy-induced neutropenia) or as an infusion of no longer than 24 hours (bone marrow transplantation).

SubQ: May be administered SubQ (chemotherapy-induced neutropenia, peripheral blood progenitor cell collection, severe chronic neutropenia, hematopoietic radiation injury syndrome). Administer into the outer upper arm, abdomen (except within 2 inches of navel), front middle thigh, or the upper outer buttocks area. Rotate injection site; do not inject into areas that are tender, red, bruised, hardened, or scarred, or sites with stretch marks.

Some patients (or caregivers) may be appropriate candidates for subQ self-administration with proper training; patients/caregivers should follow the manufacturer instructions for preparation and administration. Granix is available in prefilled syringes with and without a needle guard; the prefilled syringe without a safety needle guard is intended for patient/caregiver self-administration.

Monitoring Parameters

Chemotherapy-induced neutropenia: complete blood cell count (CBC) with differential and platelets prior to chemotherapy and twice weekly during growth factor treatment.

Bone marrow transplantation: CBC with differential and platelets frequently.

Hematopoietic radiation injury syndrome (acute): CBC at baseline (do not delay filgrastim for baseline CBC) and approximately every 3 days until ANC remains >1,000/mm^3 for 3 consecutive CBCs. Estimate absorbed radiation dose (radiation exposure) based on information from public health authorities, biodosimetry (if available), or clinical findings (eg, onset of vomiting or lymphocyte depletion kinetics).

Peripheral progenitor cell collection: Neutrophil counts after 4 days of filgrastim treatment.

Severe chronic neutropenia: CBC with differential and platelets twice weekly during the first month of therapy and for 2 weeks following dose adjustments; once clinically stable, monthly for 1 year and quarterly thereafter. Monitor bone marrow and karyotype prior to treatment; and monitor marrow and cytogenetics annually throughout treatment.

Test Interactions May interfere with bone imaging studies; increased hematopoietic activity of the bone marrow may appear as transient positive bone imaging changes

Dietary Considerations Some products may contain sodium.

Dosage Forms Considerations

Prefilled syringes: Granix, Neupogen: 300 mcg/0.5 mL (0.5 mL); 480 mcg/0.8 mL (0.8 mL)

Vials: Neupogen: 300 mcg/mL (1 mL); 480 mcg/1.6 mL (1.6 mL)

Dosage Forms Excipient information presented when available (limited, particularly for generics); consult specific product labeling.

Solution, Injection:

Neupogen: 300 mcg/mL (1 mL); 480 mcg/1.6 mL (1.6 mL) [contains polysorbate 80]

Solution, Injection [preservative free]:

Neupogen: 300 mcg/0.5 mL (0.5 mL); 480 mcg/0.8 mL (0.8 mL) [contains polysorbate 80]

Solution Prefilled Syringe, Injection [preservative free]:

Zarxio: 300 mcg/0.5 mL (0.5 mL); 480 mcg/0.8 mL (0.8 mL) [contains polysorbate 80]

◀ Solution Prefilled Syringe, Subcutaneous [preservative free]:
  Granix: 300 mcg/0.5 mL (0.5 mL); 480 mcg/0.8 mL (0.8 mL) [contains polysorbate 80]

◆ **Filgrastim-Sndz** *see* Filgrastim *on page 711*

◆ **Firmagon** *see* Degarelix *on page 495*

◆ **First-Vancomycin 25** *see* Vancomycin *on page 1720*

◆ **First-Vancomycin 50** *see* Vancomycin *on page 1720*

◆ **FK228** *see* RomiDEPsin *on page 1494*

◆ **FK506** *see* Tacrolimus (Systemic) *on page 1576*

◆ **Flagyl** *see* MetroNIDAZOLE (Systemic) *on page 1142*

◆ **Flagyl** *see* MetroNIDAZOLE (Systemic) *on page 1142*

◆ **Flagyl ER** *see* MetroNIDAZOLE (Systemic) *on page 1142*

◆ **Flebogamma [DSC]** *see* Immune Globulin *on page 903*

◆ **Flebogamma DIF** *see* Immune Globulin *on page 903*

◆ **Flo-Pred** *see* PrednisoLONE (Systemic) *on page 1421*

◆ **Floxuridin** *see* Floxuridine *on page 722*

Floxuridine (floks YOOR i deen)

Related Information
Management of Chemotherapy-Induced Nausea and Vomiting in Adults *on page 2142*
Safe Handling of Hazardous Drugs *on page 2292*

Brand Names: Canada FUDR®

Index Terms 5-FUDR; FdUrD; Floxuridin; Fluorodeoxyuridine; FUDR

Pharmacologic Category Antineoplastic Agent, Antimetabolite; Antineoplastic Agent, Antimetabolite (Pyrimidine Analog)

Use Colorectal cancer, hepatic metastases: Palliative management of hepatic metastases of colorectal cancer (administered by continuous regional intra-arterial infusion) in select patients considered incurable by surgical resection or other means.

Labeled Contraindications Poor nutritional states; depressed bone marrow function; potentially serious infections

Pregnancy Considerations Teratogenic effects have been observed in animal reproduction studies. Medications that inhibit DNA synthesis are known to be teratogenic in humans. Women of childbearing potential should avoid pregnancy.

Breast-Feeding Considerations It is not known if floxuridine is excreted in human milk; the manufacturer recommends against breast-feeding during floxuridine treatment.

Warnings/Precautions Hazardous agent - use appropriate precautions for handling and disposal (NIOSH 2014 [group 1]). Use with extreme caution in patients with renal or hepatic impairment. Bleeding may occur; discontinue if hemorrhage (from any site) occurs. May cause severe hematologic toxicity (anemia, leukopenia, and thrombocytopenia). Discontinue if white blood count <3500/mm^3 (or is falling rapidly) or if platelet count <100,000/mm^3. May cause gastrointestinal toxicity. Discontinue at the first sign of stomatitis or esophagopharyngitis; discontinue for intractable vomiting, diarrhea, or gastrointestinal ulceration/bleeding. Myocardial ischemia has been reported; discontinue if occurs. Toxicities may occur; monitor closely. Severe toxicities are more likely to occur in high risk patients, patients with prior pelvic irradiation, or in those who have received prior alkylating agents.

[U.S. Boxed Warning]: Should be administered under the supervision of a physician experienced in cancer chemotherapy and in intra-arterial treatment. [U.S. Boxed Warning]: Due to the risk for severe toxic reactions, the manufacturer recommends that patients be hospitalized for initiation of the first treatment course. Not intended for use as an adjuvant to surgery or in patients with known disease extending beyond an area of single-artery infusion. Potentially significant drug-drug interactions may exist, requiring dose or frequency adjustment, additional monitoring, and/or selection of alternative therapy.

Adverse Reactions

>10%:

Gastrointestinal: Diarrhea (may be dose limiting), stomatitis

Hematologic & oncologic: Anemia, bone marrow depression (nadir: 7-10 days; may be dose limiting), leukopenia, thrombocytopenia

1% to 10%:

Dermatologic: Alopecia, dermatitis, localized erythema, skin hyperpigmentation, skin photosensitivity

Gastrointestinal: Anorexia, biliary sclerosis, cholecystitis

Hepatic: Jaundice

<1%, postmarketing, and/or case reports: Abdominal cramps, abdominal pain, BSP abnormality, change in prothrombin time, decreased erythrocyte sedimentation rate, decreased serum total protein, duodenal ulcer, duodenitis, enteritis, fever, gastritis, gastroenteritis, gastrointestinal hemorrhage, gastrointestinal ulcer, glossitis, hemorrhage, hepatic abscess, increased erythrocyte sedimentation rate, increased lactate dehydrogenase, increased serum alkaline phosphatase, increased serum bilirubin, increased serum total protein, increased serum transaminases, infusion related reaction (arterial aneurysm; arterial ischemia; arterial thrombosis; embolism; fibromyositis; thrombophlebitis; hepatic necrosis; abscesses; infection at catheter site; bleeding at catheter site; catheter blocked, displaced, or leaking), ischemic heart disease, lethargy, malaise, nausea, pharyngitis, skin rash, vomiting, weakness

Drug Interactions

Metabolism/Transport Effects Inhibits CYP2C9 (strong)

Avoid Concomitant Use

Avoid concomitant use of Floxuridine with any of the following: BCG (Intravesical); CloZAPine; Dipyrone; Gimeracil; Natalizumab; Pimecrolimus; Tacrolimus (Topical); Tofacitinib; Vaccines (Live)

Increased Effect/Toxicity

Floxuridine may increase the levels/effects of: Bosentan; Carvedilol; CloZAPine; CYP2C9 Substrates; Diclofenac (Systemic); Dronabinol; Fingolimod; Fosphenytoin; Lacosamide; Leflunomide; Natalizumab; Ospemifene; Parecoxib; Phenytoin; Ramelteon; Tetrahydrocannabinol; Tofacitinib; Vaccines (Live)

The levels/effects of Floxuridine may be increased by: Cannabis; Cimetidine; Denosumab; Dipyrone; Gimeracil; Pimecrolimus; Roflumilast; Tacrolimus (Topical); Trastuzumab

◄ **Decreased Effect**

Floxuridine may decrease the levels/effects of: BCG (Intravesical); Coccidioides immitis Skin Test; Sipuleucel-T; Vaccines (Inactivated); Vaccines (Live)

The levels/effects of Floxuridine may be decreased by: Echinacea

Storage/Stability Store intact vials at 20°C to 25°C (68°F to 77°F). Reconstituted vials are stable for up to 2 weeks under refrigeration at 2°C to 8°C (36°F to 46°F).

Preparation for Administration Hazardous agent; use appropriate precautions for handling and disposal (NIOSH 2014 [group 1]). Reconstitute with 5 mL SWFI for a final concentration of 100 mg/mL. Further dilute in D_5W or NS to a volume appropriate for intra-arterial administration.

Mechanism of Action Floxuridine is catabolized to fluorouracil after intra-arterial administration, resulting in activity similar to fluorouracil; inhibits thymidylate synthetase and disrupts DNA and RNA synthesis.

Pharmacodynamics/Kinetics

Metabolism: Hepatic; Active metabolites: Floxuridine monophosphate (FUDR-MP) and fluorouracil; Inactive metabolites: Urea, CO_2, α-fluoro-β-alanine, α-fluoro-β-guanidopropionic acid, α-fluoro-β-ureidopropionic acid, and dihydrofluorouracil

Excretion: Urine (as fluorouracil, urea, α-fluoro-β-alanine, α-fluoro-β-guanidopropionic acid, α-fluoro-β-ureidopropionic acid, and dihydrofluorouracil; Respiratory (as exhaled gases [CO_2])

Dosing

Adult Colorectal cancer, hepatic metastases: Intra-arterial: 0.1-0.6 mg/kg/day as a continuous infusion; continue until intolerable toxicity

Renal Impairment No dosage adjustment provided in the manufacturer's labeling; use with extreme caution.

Hepatic Impairment No dosage adjustment provided in the manufacturer's labeling; use with extreme caution. The following adjustments have been recommended (Floyd, 2006):

Serum bilirubin 1.2 times ULN or alkaline phosphatase 1.2 times ULN: Administer 80% of dose

Serum bilirubin 1.5 times ULN; transaminases 3 times baseline or alkaline phosphatase 1.5 times ULN: Administer 50% of dose

Serum bilirubin 2 times ULN; transaminases >3 times baseline or alkaline phosphatase 2 times ULN: No recommendation is available

Obesity *ASCO Guidelines for appropriate chemotherapy dosing in obese adults with cancer:* Utilize patient's actual body weight (full weight) for calculation of body surface area- or weight-based dosing, particularly when the intent of therapy is curative; manage regimen-related toxicities in the same manner as for nonobese patients; if a dose reduction is utilized due to toxicity, consider resumption of full weight-based dosing with subsequent cycles, especially if cause of toxicity (eg, hepatic or renal impairment) is resolved (Griggs, 2012).

Adjustment for Toxicity

Hematologic: Discontinue if white blood count <3500/mm^3 (or is falling rapidly) or if platelet count <100,000/mm^3.

Nonhematologic toxicity: Discontinue for myocardial ischemia, stomatitis/esophagopharyngitis, vomiting (intractable), diarrhea, gastrointestinal ulceration/bleeding, hemorrhage (from any site).

Administration Administer as a continuous intra-arterial infusion using an infusion pump.

Hazardous agent; use appropriate precautions for handling and disposal (NIOSH 2014 [group 1]).

Emetic Potential Low (10% to 30%)

Monitoring Parameters CBC with differential and platelet count; liver function; signs/symptoms of stomatitis/esophagopharyngitis, gastrointestinal ulceration/bleeding, hemorrhage, vomiting, and diarrhea

Dosage Forms Excipient information presented when available (limited, particularly for generics); consult specific product labeling.
Solution Reconstituted, Injection:
Generic: 0.5 g (1 ea)

◆ **Flucinom** see Flutamide on page 751

Fluconazole (floo KOE na zole)

Brand Names: US Diflucan

Brand Names: Canada ACT Fluconazole; Apo-Fluconazole; CanesOral; CO Fluconazole; Diflucan; Diflucan injection; Diflucan One; Diflucan PWS; Dom-Fluconazole; Fluconazole Injection; Fluconazole Injection SDZ; Fluconazole Omega; Monicure; Mylan-Fluconazole; Novo-Fluconazole; PHL-Fluconazole; PMS-Fluconazole; PRO-Fluconazole; Riva-Fluconazole; Taro-Fluconazole

Index Terms Diflucan

Pharmacologic Category Antifungal Agent, Oral; Antifungal Agent, Parenteral

Use Treatment of candidiasis (esophageal, oropharyngeal, peritoneal, urinary tract, vaginal); systemic candida infections (eg, candidemia, disseminated candidiasis, and pneumonia); cryptococcal meningitis; antifungal prophylaxis in allogeneic bone marrow transplant recipients

Pregnancy Risk Factor C (single dose for vaginal candidiasis)/D (all other indications)

Dosing

Adult & Geriatric The daily dose of fluconazole is the same for both oral and IV administration

Usual dosage range: Oral, IV: 150 mg once **or** Loading dose: 200 to 800 mg; maintenance: 200 to 800 mg once daily; duration and dosage depend on location and severity of infection

Indication-specific dosing:

Blastomycosis (off-label use): Oral: *CNS disease:* Consolidation: 800 mg daily for ≥12 months and until resolution of CSF abnormalities (Chapman 2008)

Candidiasis: Oral, IV:

Candidemia (neutropenic and non-neutropenic): Loading dose: 800 mg (12 mg/kg) on day 1, then 400 mg daily (6 mg/kg/day) for 14 days after first negative blood culture and resolution of signs/symptoms. **Note:** Not recommended for patients with recent azole exposure, critical illness, or if *C. krusei* or *C. glabrata* are suspected (Pappas 2009).

Chronic, disseminated: 400 mg daily (6 mg/kg/day) until calcification or lesion resolution (Pappas 2009)

CNS candidiasis (alternative therapy): 400 to 800 mg daily (6 to 12 mg/kg/day) until CSF/radiological abnormalities resolved. **Note:** Recommended as alternative therapy in patients intolerant of amphotericin B (Pappas 2009).

Endocarditis, prosthetic valve (off-label use): 400 to 800 mg daily (6 to 12 mg/kg/day) for 6 weeks after valve replacement (as step-down in stable, culture-negative patients); long-term suppression in absence of valve replacement: 400 to 800 mg daily (Pappas 2009)

Endophthalmitis (off-label use): 400 to 800 mg daily (6 to 12 mg/kg/day) for 4 to 6 weeks until examination indicates resolution (Pappas 2009)

Esophageal:
Manufacturer's labeling: Loading dose: 200 mg on day 1, then maintenance dose of 100 to 400 mg daily for 21 days and for at least 2 weeks following resolution of symptoms

Alternative dosing: 200 to 400 mg daily for 14 to 21 days; suppressive therapy of 100 to 200 mg 3 times weekly may be used for recurrent infections (Pappas 2009)

Intertrigo (off-label use): 50 mg daily or 150 mg once weekly (Coldiron 1991; Nozickova 1998; Stengel 1994)

Oropharyngeal:
Manufacturer's labeling: Loading dose: 200 mg on day 1; maintenance dose 100 mg daily for ≥2 weeks. **Note:** Therapy with 100 mg daily is associated with resistance development (Rex 1995).

Alternative dosing: 100 to 200 mg daily for 7 to 14 days for uncomplicated, moderate-to-severe disease; chronic therapy of 100 mg 3 times weekly is recommended in immunocompromised patients with history of oropharyngeal candidiasis (OPC) (Pappas 2009)

Osteoarticular: 400 mg daily for 6 to 12 months (osteomyelitis) or 6 weeks (septic arthritis) (Pappas 2009)

Pacemaker (or ICD, VAD) infection (off-label use): 400 to 800 mg daily (6 to 12 mg/kg/day) for 4 to 6 weeks after device removal (as step-down in stable, culture-negative patients); long-term suppression when VAD cannot be removed: 400 to 800 mg daily (Pappas 2009)

Pericarditis or myocarditis: 400 to 800 mg daily for several months (Pappas 2009)

Peritonitis: 50 to 200 mg daily. **Note:** Some clinicians do not recommend using <200 mg daily (Chen 2004).

Prophylaxis:
Bone marrow transplant: 400 mg once daily. Patients anticipated to have severe granulocytopenia should start therapy several days prior to the anticipated onset of neutropenia and continue for 7 days after the neutrophil count is >1000 mm^3.

High-risk ICU patients in units with high incidence of invasive candidiasis: 400 mg once daily (Pappas 2009)

Neutropenic patients: 400 mg once daily for duration of neutropenia (Pappas 2009)

Peritoneal dialysis associated infection (concurrently treated with antibiotics), prevention of secondary fungal infection: 200 mg every 48 hours (Restrepo 2010)

Solid organ transplant: 200 to 400 mg once daily for at least 7 to 14 days (Pappas 2009)

Surgical (perioperative) prophylaxis in high-risk patients undergoing liver, pancreas, kidney, or pancreas-kidney transplantation (off-label use): IV: 400 mg given in the perioperative period and continued in the post-operative period for ≤28 days. Time of initiation and duration varies with transplant type and operative protocol (Bratzler 2013).

Thrombophlebitis, suppurative (off-label use): 400 to 800 mg daily (6 to 12 mg/kg/day) and as step-down in stable patients for ≥2 weeks (Pappas 2009)

Urinary tract:

Cystitis:

Manufacturer's labeling: UTI: 50 to 200 mg once daily

Asymptomatic, patient undergoing urologic procedure: 200 to 400 mg once daily several days before and after the procedure (Pappas 2009)

Symptomatic: 200 mg once daily for 2 weeks (Pappas 2009)

Fungus balls: 200 to 400 mg once daily (Pappas 2009)

Pyelonephritis: 200 to 400 mg once daily for 2 weeks (Pappas 2009)

Vaginal:

Uncomplicated: Manufacturer's labeling: 150 mg as a single oral dose

Complicated: 150 mg every 72 hours for 3 doses (Pappas 2009)

Recurrent: 150 mg once daily for 10 to 14 days, followed by 150 mg once weekly for 6 months (Pappas 2009), **or** fluconazole (oral) 100 mg, 150 mg, or 200 mg every third day for a total of 3 doses (day 1, 4, and 7), then 100 mg, 150 mg, or 200 mg dose weekly for 6 months (CDC 2010)

Coccidioidomycosis, treatment (off-label use):

HIV-infected (HHS [OI adult 2015]):

Meningeal infections (consultation with specialist is advised): IV, Oral: 400 to 800 mg once daily; patients who complete initial therapy should be considered for lifelong suppressive therapy using fluconazole 400 mg once daily if CD4 counts remain <250 cells/mm^3.

Mild infections (eg, focal pneumonia): Oral: 400 mg once daily; patients who complete initial therapy should be considered for lifelong suppressive therapy using fluconazole 400 mg once daily if CD4 counts remain <250 cells/mm^3.

Non-HIV infected (off-label use): Oral, IV:

Disseminated, extrapulmonary: 400 mg once daily (some experts use 2000 mg daily [Galgiani 2005])

Meningitis: 400 mg once daily (some experts use initial doses of 800 to 1000 mg daily), lifelong duration (Galgiani 2005)

Pneumonia, acute, uncomplicated: 200 to 400 mg daily for 3 to 6 months (Catanzaro 1995; Galgiani 2000)

Pneumonia, chronic progressive, fibrocavitary: 200 to 400 mg daily for 12 months (Catanzaro 1995; Galgiani 2000)

Pneumonia, diffuse: Consolidation after amphotericin B induction: 400 mg daily for 12 months (lifelong in chronically immunosuppressed) (Galgiani 2005)

Coccidioidomycosis, prophylaxis (off-label use): Oral:

HIV-infected patients (HHS [OI adult 2015]):

Primary prophylaxis in patients with a new positive IgM or IgG serologic test who live in disease-endemic areas and have CD4 counts <250 cells/mm^3: 400 mg once daily

Chronic suppressive therapy (secondary prophylaxis): 400 mg once daily ▶

◄

Solid organ transplant (off-label use): **Note:** Prophylaxis regimens in this setting have not been established; the following regimen has been proposed for transplant recipients who maintain residence in a *Coccidioides* spp endemic area.

Previous history >12 months prior to transplant: 200 mg once daily for 6 to 12 months (Vikram 2009; Vucicevic 2011)

Previous history ≤12 months prior to transplant: 400 mg once daily, lifelong treatment (Vikram 2009; Vucicevic 2011)

Positive serology before or at transplant: 400 mg once daily, lifelong treatment; if serology is negative at 12 months, consider a dose reduction to 200 mg daily (Vikram 2009; Vucicevic 2011)

No history (at risk for *de novo* post-transplant disease): some clinicians treat with 200 mg daily for 6 to 12 months (Vucicevic 2011)

Cryptococcosis:

Meningitis:

Manufacturer's labeling: Oral, IV: 400 mg for 1 dose, then 200 to 400 mg once daily for 10 to 12 weeks following negative CSF culture

Alternate dosing: HIV-infected:

Induction (alternative to preferred therapy): Oral, IV: 800 to 1,200 mg once daily with concomitant flucytosine for 6 weeks (Perfect 2010) **or** 400 to 800 mg once daily with concomitant flucytosine for at least 2 weeks (HHS [OI adult 2015]) **or** 1,200 mg once daily as monotherapy for at least 2 weeks (HHS [OI adult 2015])

Consolidation (preferred therapy): Oral, IV: 400 mg once daily for at least 8 weeks (HHS [OI adult 2015])

Maintenance (suppression) (preferred therapy): Oral: 200 mg once daily for at least 12 months; maintenance therapy may be stopped if the following criteria are fulfilled: induction, consolidation, and at least 12 months of maintenance therapy has been completed, patient remains asymptomatic from cryptococcal infection, and CD4 count ≥100 cells/mm^3 for ≥3 months and HIV RNA suppressed in response to effective ART (HHS [OI adult 2015])

Pulmonary (immunocompetent) (off-label use): 400 mg once daily for 6 to 12 months (Perfect 2010)

Pediatric The daily dose of fluconazole is the same for oral and IV administration

Usual dosage range: Oral, IV: Loading dose: 6 to 12 mg/kg/dose; maintenance: 3 to 12 mg/kg/dose once daily; duration and dosage depend on location and severity of infection

Indication-specific dosing:

Candidiasis: Oral, IV:

Esophageal:

Manufacturer's recommendation: Loading dose: 6 mg/kg/dose; maintenance: 3-12 mg/kg/dose once daily for 21 days and for at least 2 weeks following resolution of symptoms (maximum: 600 mg/day)

HIV-exposed/-infected: Loading dose: 6 mg/kg/dose once on day 1; maintenance: 3 to 6 mg/kg/dose once daily for 4 to 21 days (maximum: 400 mg/day) (CDC 2009)

Relapse suppression (HIV-exposed/-infected): 3 to 6 mg/kg/dose once daily (maximum: 200 mg/day) (CDC 2009)

Invasive disease (alternative therapy): 5 to 6 mg/kg/dose every 12 hours for ≥28 days (maximum: 600 mg/day) (CDC 2009)

Oropharyngeal:
> Manufacturer's recommendation: Loading dose: 6 mg/kg/dose; maintenance: 3 mg/kg/dose once daily for ≥2 weeks (maximum: 600 mg/day)
> HIV-exposed/-infected: 3 to 6 mg/kg/dose once daily for 7 to 14 days (maximum: 400 mg/day) (CDC 2009)

Surgical (perioperative) prophylaxis in high-risk patients undergoing liver, pancreas, kidney, or pancreas-kidney transplantation (off-label use): IV: 6 mg/kg given in the perioperative period and continued in the postoperative period for ≤28 days (maximum dose 400 mg). Time of initiation and duration varies with transplant type and operative protocol (Bratzler 2013).

Coccidioidomycosis: Oral, IV:

Children: *Meningeal infection, or in a stable patient with diffuse pulmonary or disseminated disease* (HIV-exposed/-infected):
> Treatment: 5 to 6 mg/kg/dose twice daily (maximum daily dose: 800 mg/**day**) (CDC 2009) followed by chronic suppressive therapy (see below)
> Relapse suppression: 6 mg/kg/dose once daily (maximum daily dose: 400 mg/**day**) (CDC 2009)

Adolescents: Treatment, primary prophylaxis, or chronic suppressive therapy (secondary prophylaxis): Refer to adult dosing.

Cryptococcosis: Oral, IV:

Meningitis: Manufacturer's labeling: 12 mg/kg/dose for 1 dose, then 6 to 12 mg/kg/day for 10-12 weeks following negative CSF culture

HIV-exposed/-infected:
> *CNS disease (alternative therapy in patients intolerant of amphotericin B):*
> Children:
>> Induction: 12 mg/kg/dose for 1 dose, then 6 to 12 mg/kg/day (maximum: 800 mg/day) for ≥2 weeks (in combination with flucytosine) (CDC 2009)
>> Consolidation: 10 to 12 mg/kg/day for 8 weeks (Perfect 2010) **or** 12 mg/kg/dose for 1 dose, then 6 to 12 mg/kg/day (maximum: 800 mg/day) for 8 weeks (CDC 2009)
>> Maintenance (suppression): 6 mg/kg/day (maximum: 200 mg/day) (CDC 2009; Perfect 2010)
> Adolescents: Refer to adult dosing.

> *Non-CNS disease, disseminated (including severe pulmonary disease) (alternative therapy; off-label use):* Induction: 12 mg/kg/dose for 1 dose, then 6 to 12 mg/kg/day (maximum: 600 mg/day) (CDC 2009)

> *Non-CNS disease, localized (including isolated pulmonary disease) (off-label use):* 12 mg/kg/dose for 1 dose, then 6 to 12 mg/kg/day (maximum: 600 mg/day). **Note:** Duration depends upon infection site and severity (CDC 2009). For patients with pulmonary disease (not delineated by severity), the IDSA recommends a duration of 6 to 12 months (Perfect 2010).

Primary antifungal prophylaxis in pediatric oncology patients (guideline recommendations; Science 2014): Oral, IV:

Allogeneic hematopoietic stem cell transplant (HSCT): Infants ≥1 month, Children, and Adolescents <19 years: 6 to 12 mg/kg/day (maximum: 400 mg/day), begin at the start of conditioning; continue until engraftment

Allogeneic HSCT with grades 2 to 4 acute graft-versus-host-disease (GVHD) or chronic extensive GVHD: Begin with GVHD diagnosis, continue until GVHD resolves:
> Infants ≥1 month and Children <13 years: 6 to 12 mg/kg/day (maximum: 400 mg/day)

◄ Adolescents ≥13 years (where posaconazole is contraindicated): 6 to 12 mg/kg/day (maximum: 400 mg/day)

Autologous HSCT with neutropenia anticipated >7 days: Infants ≥1 month, Children, and Adolescents <19 years: 6 to 12 mg/kg/day (maximum: 400 mg/day), begin at the start of conditioning; continue until engraftment

Acute myeloid leukemia (AML) or myelodysplastic syndromes (MDS): Infants ≥1 month, Children, and Adolescents <19 years: 6 to 12 mg/kg/day (maximum: 400 mg/day) during chemotherapy associated neutropenia; alternative antifungals may be suggested for children ≥13 years in centers with a high local incidence of mold infections or if fluconazole is not available

Renal Impairment

Manufacturer's labeling: **Note:** Renal function estimated using the Cockcroft-Gault formula

No adjustment for vaginal candidiasis single-dose therapy

For multiple dosing in adults, administer loading dose of 50 to 400 mg, then adjust daily doses as follows (dosage reduction in children should parallel adult recommendations):

CrCl >50 mL/minute: No dosage adjustment necessary

CrCl ≤50 mL/minute (no dialysis): Reduce dose by 50%

End-stage renal disease on intermittent hemodialysis (IHD):

Manufacturer's labeling: 100% of daily dose (according to indication) after each dialysis session; on non-dialysis days, patient should receive a reduced dose according to their CrCl.

Alternate recommendations: Doses of 200 to 400 mg every 48 to 72 hours **or** 100 to 200 mg every 24 hours have been recommended. **Note:** Dosing dependent on the assumption of 3 times/week, complete IHD sessions (Heintz 2009).

Continuous renal replacement therapy (CRRT) (Heintz 2009; Trotman 2005): Drug clearance is highly dependent on the method of renal replacement, filter type, and flow rate. Appropriate dosing requires close monitoring of pharmacologic response, signs of adverse reactions due to drug accumulation, as well as drug concentrations in relation to target trough (if appropriate). The following are general recommendations only (based on dialysate flow/ultrafiltration rates of 1 to 2 L/hour and minimal residual renal function) and should not supersede clinical judgment:

CVVH: Loading dose of 400 to 800 mg followed by 200 to 400 mg every 24 hours

CVVHD/CVVHDF: Loading dose of 400 to 800 mg followed by 400 to 800 mg every 24 hours (CVVHD or CVVHDF) **or** 800 mg every 24 hours (CVVHDF)

Note: Higher maintenance doses of 400 mg every 24 hours (CVVH), 800 mg every 24 hours (CVVHD), and 500 to 600 mg every 12 hours (CVVHDF) may be considered when treating resistant organisms and/or when employing combined ultrafiltration and dialysis flow rates of ≥2 L/hour for CVVHD/CVVHDF (Heintz 2009; Trotman 2005).

Hepatic Impairment There are no dosage adjustments provided in the manufacturer's labeling; use with caution.

Additional Information Complete prescribing information should be consulted for additional detail.

Dosage Forms Excipient information presented when available (limited, particularly for generics); consult specific product labeling.

Solution, Intravenous:

Generic: 100 mg (50 mL); 200 mg (100 mL); 400 mg (200 mL)

Solution, Intravenous [preservative free]:
  Generic: 200 mg (100 mL); 400 mg (200 mL)
Suspension Reconstituted, Oral:
  Diflucan: 10 mg/mL (35 mL); 40 mg/mL (35 mL) [orange flavor]
  Generic: 10 mg/mL (35 mL); 40 mg/mL (35 mL)
Tablet, Oral:
  Diflucan: 50 mg, 100 mg, 150 mg, 200 mg
  Generic: 50 mg, 100 mg, 150 mg, 200 mg

◆ **Fluconazole Injection (Can)** see Fluconazole on page 725

◆ **Fluconazole Injection SDZ (Can)** see Fluconazole on page 725

◆ **Fluconazole Omega (Can)** see Fluconazole on page 725

Flucytosine (floo SYE toe seen)

Brand Names: US Ancobon
Index Terms 5-FC; 5-Fluorocytosine; 5-Flurocytosine
Pharmacologic Category Antifungal Agent, Oral
Use Adjunctive treatment of systemic fungal infections (eg, septicemia, endocarditis, UTI, meningitis, or pulmonary) caused by susceptible strains of *Candida* or *Cryptococcus*
Pregnancy Risk Factor C
Dosing
  Adult & Geriatric Usual dosage ranges: Oral: 50 to 150 mg/kg/day in divided doses every 6 hours
  Cryptococcocal meningitis, treatment: Oral:
    Non-HIV-infected: Induction: 25 mg/kg/dose (with amphotericin B) every 6 hours for at least 4 weeks; if clinical improvement, may discontinue both amphotericin and flucytosine and follow with an extended course of fluconazole (Perfect 2010).
    HIV-infected: Oral: Induction: 25 mg/kg/dose (with an amphotericin B formulation [liposomal amphotericin B is preferred]) every 6 hours for at least 2 weeks (HHS [OI adult 2015]).
  Endocarditis (off-label use): Oral: 100 mg/kg daily in 3 or 4 divided doses (with amphotericin B) for at least 4 to 6 weeks after valve replacement (Gould 2012; Pappas 2009)
  Pediatric
  Cryptococcocal meningitis, treatment:
    Non-HIV-infected: Children (off-label population): Oral: Induction: 25 mg/kg/dose (with amphotericin B) every 6 hours for at least 4 weeks; if clinical improvement, may discontinue both amphotericin and flucytosine and follow with an extended course of fluconazole (Perfect 2010).
    HIV-infected: Adolescents (off-label population): Refer to adult dosing.
  Renal Impairment No dosage adjustment provided in manufacturer's labeling (**Note:** Manufacturer recommends dose reduction); however, the following adjustments have been recommended:
    Adults (based upon dosing of 25 mg/kg every 6 hours):
      CrCl >40 mL/minute: No dosage adjustment recommended (Perfect 2010)
      CrCl 20 to 40 mL/minute: 50% of standard dose every 6 hours (Perfect 2010)
      CrCl 10 to 20 mL/minute: 25% of standard dose every 6 hours (Perfect 2010)

◀

ESRD on intermittent hemodialysis (IHD): 25 to 50 mg/kg every 48 to 72 hours; administer dose after hemodialysis (Drew 1999; HHS [OI adult 2015])

Adults and Adolescents (HIV-infected patients) (based upon dosing of 25 mg/kg every 6 hours) (HHS [OI adult 2015]):

CrCl >40 mL/minute: No dosage adjustment recommended

CrCl 20 to 40 mL/minute: 25 mg/kg every 12 hours

CrCl 10 to ≤20 mL/minute: 25 mg/kg every 24 hours

CrCl <10 mL/minute: 25 mg/kg every 48 hours

ESRD on intermittent hemodialysis (IHD): 25 to 50 mg/kg every 48 to 72 hours; administer dose after hemodialysis

Infants, Children, and non-HIV positive Adolescents (based upon dosing of 100 to 150 mg/kg/day divided every 6 hours) (Aronoff 2007): **Note:** Flucytosine should be avoided in children with severe renal impairment (DHHS [pediatric] 2013):

CrCl 30 to 50 mL/minute: 25 to 37.5 mg/kg every 8 hours

CrCl 10 to 29 mL/minute: 25 to 37.5 mg/kg every 12 hours

CrCl <10 mL/minute: 25 to 37.5 mg/kg every 24 hours

Hemodialysis: 25 to 37.5 mg/kg every 24 hours

Peritoneal dialysis: 25 to 37.5 mg/kg every 24 hours

Continuous renal replacement therapy: 25 to 37.5 mg/kg every 8 hours (monitor serum concentrations)

Hepatic Impairment No dosage adjustment provided in manufacturer's labeling; use with caution.

Additional Information Complete prescribing information should be consulted for additional detail.

Dosage Forms Excipient information presented when available (limited, particularly for generics); consult specific product labeling.

Capsule, Oral:

Ancobon: 250 mg, 500 mg

Generic: 250 mg, 500 mg

◆ **Fludara** see Fludarabine on page 732

Fludarabine (floo DARE a been)

Related Information

Chemotherapy and Obesity on page 2220

Hematopoietic Stem Cell Transplantation on page 2272

Management of Chemotherapy-Induced Nausea and Vomiting in Adults on page 2142

Prevention and Management of Infections on page 2196

Prevention of Chemotherapy-Induced Nausea and Vomiting in Children on page 2203

Safe Handling of Hazardous Drugs on page 2292

Brand Names: US Fludara

Brand Names: Canada Fludara; Fludarabine Phosphate for Injection; Fludarabine Phosphate for Injection, USP; Fludarabine Phosphate Injection, PPC STD.

Index Terms 2F-ara-AMP; Fludarabine Phosphate

Pharmacologic Category Antineoplastic Agent, Antimetabolite; Antineoplastic Agent, Antimetabolite (Purine Analog)

Use

Chronic lymphocytic leukemia: Treatment of progressive or refractory B-cell chronic lymphocytic leukemia (CLL)

Canadian labeling: Second-line treatment of chronic lymphocytic leukemia (CLL); second-line treatment of low-grade, refractory non-Hodgkin lymphoma (NHL)

Labeled Contraindications Hypersensitivity of fludarabine or any component of the formulation

Canadian labeling: Additional contraindications (not in US labeling): Severe renal impairment (CrCl <30 mL/minute); decompensated hemolytic anemia; concurrent use with pentostatin

Pregnancy Considerations Adverse events were observed in animal reproduction studies. Based on the mechanism of action, fludarabine may cause fetal harm if administered during pregnancy. Effective contraception is recommended during and for 6 months after treatment for women and men with female partners of reproductive potential.

Breast-Feeding Considerations It is not known if fludarabine is excreted in breast milk. Due to the potential for serious adverse reactions in the nursing infant, a decision should be made to discontinue breast-feeding or to discontinue fludarabine, taking into account the importance of treatment to the mother.

Warnings/Precautions Hazardous agent - use appropriate precautions for handling and disposal (NIOSH 2014 [group 1]). Use with caution in patients with renal insufficiency (clearance of the primary metabolite 2-fluoro-ara-A is reduced); dosage reductions are recommended (monitor closely for excessive toxicity); use of the IV formulation is not recommended if CrCl <30 mL/minute. Canadian labeling contraindicates use of oral and IV formulations if CrCl <30 mL/minute. Use with caution in patients with preexisting hematological disorders (particularly granulocytopenia) or preexisting central nervous system disorder (epilepsy), spasticity, or peripheral neuropathy. **[US Boxed Warning]: Higher than recommended doses are associated with severe neurologic toxicity (delayed blindness, coma, death); similar neurotoxicity (agitation, coma, confusion and seizure) has been reported with standard CLL doses.** Neurotoxicity symptoms due to high doses appear from 21 to 60 days following the last fludarabine dose, although neurotoxicity has been reported as early as 7 days and up to 225 days. Possible neurotoxic effects of chronic administration are unknown. Caution patients about performing tasks which require mental alertness (eg, operating machinery or driving).

[US Boxed Warning]: Life-threatening (and sometimes fatal) autoimmune effects, including hemolytic anemia, autoimmune thrombocytopenia/ thrombocytopenic purpura (ITP), Evans syndrome, and acquired hemophilia have occurred; monitor closely for hemolysis; discontinue fludarabine if hemolysis occurs; the hemolytic effects usually recur with fludarabine rechallenge. **[US Boxed Warning]: Severe bone marrow suppression (anemia, thrombocytopenia, and neutropenia) may occur;** may be cumulative. Severe myelosuppression (trilineage bone marrow hypoplasia/aplasia) has been reported (rare) with a duration of significant cytopenias ranging from 2 months to 1 year. First-line combination therapy is associated with prolonged cytopenias, with anemia lasting up to 7 months, neutropenia up to 9 months, and thrombocytopenia up to 10 months; increased age is predictive for prolonged cytopenias (Gill, 2010).

◀ Use with caution in patients with documented infection, fever, immunodeficiency, or with a history of opportunistic infection; prophylactic anti-infectives should be considered for patients with an increased risk for developing opportunistic infections. Progressive multifocal leukoencephalopathy (PML) due to JC virus (usually fatal) has been reported with use; usually in patients who had received prior and/or other concurrent chemotherapy; onset ranges from a few weeks to 1 year; evaluate any neurological change promptly. Avoid vaccination with live vaccines during and after fludarabine treatment. May cause tumor lysis syndrome; risk is increased in patients with large tumor burden prior to treatment. Patients receiving blood products should only receive irradiated blood products due to the potential for transfusion related GVHD. Potentially significant drug-drug interactions may exist, requiring dose or frequency adjustment, additional monitoring, and/or selection of alternative therapy. **[US Boxed Warnings]: Do not use in combination with pentostatin; may lead to severe, even fatal pulmonary toxicity. Should be administered under the supervision of an experienced cancer chemotherapy physician.**

Adverse Reactions

>10%:

Cardiovascular: Edema (8% to 19%)

Central nervous system: Fever (60% to 69%), fatigue (10% to 38%), pain (20% to 22%), chills (11% to 19%)

Dermatologic: Rash (15%)

Gastrointestinal: Nausea/vomiting (31% to 36%), anorexia (7% to 34%), diarrhea (13% to 15%), gastrointestinal bleeding (3% to 13%)

Genitourinary: Urinary tract infection (2% to 15%)

Hematologic: Myelosuppression (nadir: 10-14 days; recovery: 5-7 weeks; dose-limiting toxicity), anemia (60%), neutropenia (grade 4: 59%; nadir: ~13 days), thrombocytopenia (55%; nadir: ~16 days)

Neuromuscular & skeletal: Weakness (9% to 65%), myalgia (4% to 16%), paresthesia (4% to 12%)

Ocular: Visual disturbance (3% to 15%)

Respiratory: Cough (10% to 44%), pneumonia (16% to 22%), dyspnea (9% to 22%), upper respiratory infection (2% to 16%)

Miscellaneous: Infection (33% to 44%), diaphoresis (1% to 13%)

1% to 10%:

Cardiovascular: Angina (≤6%), arrhythmia (≤3%), cerebrovascular accident (≤3%), heart failure (≤3%), MI (≤3%), supraventricular tachycardia (≤3%), deep vein thrombosis (1% to 3%), phlebitis (1% to 3%), aneurysm (≤1%), transient ischemic attack (≤1%)

Central nervous system: Malaise (6% to 8%), headache (≤3%), sleep disorder (1% to 3%), cerebellar syndrome (≤1%), depression (≤1%), mentation impaired (≤1%)

Dermatologic: Alopecia (≤3%), pruritus (1% to 3%), seborrhea (≤1%)

Endocrine & metabolic: Hyperglycemia (1% to 6%), dehydration (≤1%)

Gastrointestinal: Stomatitis (≤9%), esophagitis (≤3%), constipation (1% to 3%), mucositis (≤2%), dysphagia (≤1%)

Genitourinary: Dysuria (3% to 4%), hesitancy (≤3%)

Hematologic: Hemorrhage (≤1%)

Hepatic: Cholelithiasis (≤3%), liver function tests abnormal (1% to 3%), liver failure (≤1%)

Neuromuscular & skeletal: Osteoporosis (≤2%), arthralgia (≤1%)

Otic: Hearing loss (2% to 6%)

Renal: Hematuria (2% to 3%), renal failure (≤1%), renal function test abnormal (≤1%), proteinuria (≤1%)

Respiratory: Pharyngitis (≤9%), allergic pneumonitis (≤6%), hemoptysis (1% to 6%), sinusitis (≤5%), bronchitis (≤1%), epistaxis (≤1%), hypoxia (≤1%)

Miscellaneous: Anaphylaxis (≤1%), tumor lysis syndrome (≤1%)

<1%, postmarketing, and/or case reports: Acute respiratory distress syndrome, agitation, blindness, bone marrow fibrosis, cerebral hemorrhage, coma, confusion, Epstein-Barr virus (EBV) associated lymphoproliferation, EBV reactivation, erythema multiforme, Evans syndrome, flank pain, hemolytic anemia (autoimmune), hemophilia (acquired), hemorrhagic cystitis, hepatic enzymes increased, herpes zoster reactivation, hyperkalemia, hyperphosphatemia, hyperuricemia, hypocalcemia, interstitial pulmonary infiltrate, metabolic acidosis, myelodysplastic syndrome/acute myeloid leukemia (usually associated with prior or concurrent treatment with other anticancer agents), opportunistic infection, optic neuritis, optic neuropathy, pancreatic enzymes abnormal, pancytopenia, pemphigus, pericardial effusion, peripheral neuropathy, pneumonitis, progressive multifocal leukoencephalopathy (PML), pulmonary fibrosis, pulmonary hemorrhage, respiratory distress, respiratory failure, Richter's syndrome, seizure, skin cancer (new onset or exacerbation), Stevens-Johnson syndrome, thrombocytopenia (autoimmune), thrombocytopenic purpura (autoimmune), toxic epidermal necrolysis, trilineage bone marrow aplasia, trilineage bone marrow hypoplasia, urate crystalluria, wrist drop

Also observed: Neurologic syndrome characterized by cortical blindness, coma, and paralysis [36% at doses >96 mg/m^2 for 5-7 days; <0.2% at doses <125 mg/m^2/cycle (onset of neurologic symptoms may be delayed for 3-4 weeks)]

Drug Interactions

Metabolism/Transport Effects None known.

Avoid Concomitant Use

Avoid concomitant use of Fluadarabine with any of the following: BCG (Intravesical); CloZAPine; Dipyrone; Natalizumab; Pentostatin; Pimecrolimus; Tacrolimus (Topical); Tofacitinib; Vaccines (Live)

Increased Effect/Toxicity

Fludarabine may increase the levels/effects of: CloZAPine; Fingolimod; Leflunomide; Natalizumab; Pentostatin; Tofacitinib; Vaccines (Live)

The levels/effects of Fludarabine may be increased by: Denosumab; Dipyrone; Pentostatin; Pimecrolimus; Roflumilast; Tacrolimus (Topical); Trastuzumab

Decreased Effect

Fludarabine may decrease the levels/effects of: BCG (Intravesical); Coccidioides immitis Skin Test; Sipuleucel-T; Vaccines (Inactivated); Vaccines (Live)

The levels/effects of Fludarabine may be decreased by: Echinacea; Imatinib

Storage/Stability

IV: Store intact vials under refrigeration or at room temperature, as specified according to each manufacturer's labeling. Reconstituted solution or vials of the solution for injection that have been punctured (in use) should be used within 8 hours.

Tablet [Canadian product]: Store at 15°C to 30°C (59°F to 86°F); should be kept within packaging until use.

◄ **Preparation for Administration** Hazardous agent; use appropriate precautions for handling and disposal (NIOSH 2014 [group 1]).

Lyophilized vials: Reconstitute with 2 mL SWFI; further dilute in 100 to 125 mL D_5W or NS.

Solution for injection: Dilute in 100 to 125 mL D_5W or NS.

Mechanism of Action Fludarabine inhibits DNA synthesis by inhibition of DNA polymerase and ribonucleotide reductase; also inhibits DNA primase and DNA ligase I

Pharmacodynamics/Kinetics

Distribution: V_d: 38 to 96 L/m^2; widely with extensive tissue binding

Protein binding: 2-fluoro-ara-A: ~19% to 29%

Metabolism: IV: Fludarabine phosphate is rapidly dephosphorylated in the plasma to 2-fluoro-ara-A (active metabolite), which subsequently enters tumor cells and is phosphorylated by deoxycytidine kinase to the active triphosphate derivative (2-fluoro-ara-ATP)

Bioavailability: Oral: 2-fluoro-ara-A: 50% to 65%

Half-life elimination: 2-fluoro-ara-A: ~20 hours

Time to peak, plasma: Oral: 1 to 2 hours

Excretion: Urine (60%, 23% as 2-fluoro-ara-A) within 24 hours

Dosing

Adult & Geriatric

Chronic lymphocytic leukemia (CLL), progressive or refractory:

IV: 25 mg/m^2/day for 5 days every 28 days

Oral (Canadian labeling; not available in U.S.): 40 mg/m^2 once daily for 5 days every 28 days

CLL combination regimens (off-label dosing): IV:

FC: 30 mg/m^2/day for 3 days every 28 days for 6 cycles (in combination with cyclophosphamide) (Eichhorst, 2006) **or** 20 mg/m^2/day for 5 days every 28 days for 6 cycles (in combination with cyclophosphamide) (Flinn, 2007)

FCR: 25 mg/m^2/day for 3 days every 28 days for 6 cycles (in combination with cyclophosphamide and rituximab) (Keating, 2005; Robak, 2010; Wierda, 2005)

FR: 25 mg/m^2/day for 5 days every 28 days for 6 cycles (in combination with rituximab) (Byrd, 2003)

OFAR: 30 mg/m^2/day for 2 days every 28 days for 6 cycles (in combination with oxaliplatin, cytarabine, and rituximab) (Tsimberidou, 2008)

Acute myeloid leukemia (AML), high-risk patients (off-label use): IV: 30 mg/m^2/day for 5 days induction therapy, followed by post remission therapy of 30 mg/m^2/day for 4 days every other cycle (in combination with cytarabine with or without filgrastim) (Borthakur, 2008)

AML, refractory (off-label use): IV: 30 mg/m^2/day for 5 days (in combination with cytarabine and filgrastim), may repeat once for partial remission (Montillo, 1998) **or** 30 mg/m^2/day for 5 days for 1 or 2 cycles (in combination with cytarabine, idarubicin, and filgrastim) (Virchis, 2004)

Non-Hodgkin lymphomas: IV:

Canadian labeling: 25 mg/m^2 for 5 days every 28 days; dosage adjustment may be necessary for hematologic or nonhematologic toxicity.

Follicular lymphoma (off-label use):

FCR: 25 mg/m^2/day for 3 days every 21 days for 4 cycles (in combination with cyclophosphamide and rituximab) (Sacchi, 2007)

FCMR: 25 mg/m^2/day for 3 days every 28 days for 4 cycles (in combination with cyclophosphamide, mitoxantrone, and rituximab) (Forstpointner, 2004; Forstpointner, 2006)

FND: 25 mg/m^2/day for 3 days every 28 days for up to 8 cycles (in combination with mitoxantrone and dexamethasone) (McLaughlin, 1996; Tsimberidou, 2002)

FNDR: 25 mg/m^2/day for 3 days every 28 days for up to 8 cycles (in combination with mitoxantrone, dexamethasone, and rituximab) (McLaughlin, 2000)

FR: 25 mg/m^2/day for 5 days every 28 days for 6 cycles (in combination with rituximab) (Czuczman, 2005)

Mantle cell lymphoma (off-label use):

FC: 20 mg/m^2/day for 4 to 5 days or 25 mg/m^2/day for 3-5 days (in combination with cyclophosphamide) (Cohen, 2001)

FCMR: 25 mg/m^2/day for 3 days every 28 days for 4 cycles (in combination with cyclophosphamide, mitoxantrone, and rituximab) (Forstpointner, 2004; Forstpointner, 2006)

Waldenstron macroglobulinemia (off-label use): IV: 25 mg/m^2/day for 5 days every 28 days (Foran, 1999) **or** 25 mg/m^2/day for 5 days every 28 days for 6 cycles (in combination with rituximab) (Treon, 2009)

Stem cell transplant (allogeneic) conditioning regimen, reduced-intensity, (off-label use): IV: 30 mg/m^2/dose for 6 doses beginning 10 days prior to transplant **or** 30 mg/m^2/dose for 5 days beginning 6 days prior to transplant (in combination with busulfan with or without antithymocyte globulin) (Schetelig, 2003)

Stem cell transplant (allogeneic) nonmyeloablative conditioning regimen (off-label use): IV: 30 mg/m^2/dose for 3 doses beginning 5 days prior to transplant (in combination with cyclophosphamide and rituximab) (Khouri, 2008) **or** 30 mg/m^2/dose for 3 doses beginning 4 days prior to transplant (in combination with total body irradiation) (Rezvani, 2008)

Pediatric

Acute myeloid leukemia (AML) (off-label use): IV: 10.5 mg/m^2 bolus infusion followed by a continuous infusion of 30.5 mg/m^2/day for 48 hours (Lange, 2008)

Acute lymphocytic leukemia (ALL) or AML, relapsed (off-label use): IV: 10.5 mg/m^2 bolus over 15 minutes followed by a continuous infusion of 30.5 mg/m^2/day for 48 hours (Avramis, 1998)

Stem cell transplant (allogeneic) conditioning regimen, reduced-intensity (off-label use): IV: 30 mg/m^2/dose for 6 doses beginning 7-10 days prior to transplant (in combination with busulfan and antithymocyte globulin) (Pulsipher, 2009)

Renal Impairment

U.S. labeling: Adults: CLL: IV:

CrCl 50-79 mL/minute: Decrease dose to 20 mg/m^2.

CrCl 30-49 mL/minute: Decrease dose to 15 mg/m^2.

CrCl <30 mL/minute: Avoid use.

Canadian labeling: CLL (Oral, IV), NHL (IV):

CrCl 30-70 mL/minute: Reduce dose by up to 50%.

CrCl <30 mL/minute: Use is contraindicated.

The following guidelines have been used by some clinicians: Aronoff, 2007: IV:

Adults:

CrCl 10-50 mL/minute: Administer 75% of dose.

CrCl <10 mL/minute: Administer 50% of dose.

Hemodialysis: Administer after dialysis

Continuous ambulatory peritoneal dialysis (CAPD): Administer 50% of dose.

Continuous renal replacement therapy (CRRT): Administer 75% of dose.

Children:

CrCl 30-50 mL/minute: Administer 80% of dose.

CrCl <30 mL/minute: Not recommended.

Hemodialysis: Administer 25% of dose

Continuous ambulatory peritoneal dialysis (CAPD): Not recommended.

Continuous renal replacement therapy (CRRT): Administer 80% of dose.

Hepatic Impairment There are no dosage adjustments provided in the manufacturer's labeling.

Obesity

American Society of Clinical Oncology (ASCO) Guidelines for appropriate chemotherapy dosing in obese adults with cancer (**Note:** *Excludes leukemias and HSCT dosing):* Utilize patient's actual body weight (full weight) for calculation of body surface area- or weight-based dosing, particularly when the intent of therapy is curative; manage regimen-related toxicities in the same manner as for nonobese patients; if a dose reduction is utilized due to toxicity, consider resumption of full weight-based dosing with subsequent cycles, especially if cause of toxicity (eg, hepatic or renal impairment) is resolved (Griggs, 2012).

American Society for Blood and Marrow Transplantation (ASBMT) practice guideline committee position statement on chemotherapy dosing in obesity: Utilize actual body weight (full weight) for calculation of body surface area in fludarabine dosing for hematopoietic stem cell transplant conditioning regimens in adults (Bubalo, 2014).

Adjustment for Toxicity

Hematologic or nonhematologic toxicity (other than neurotoxicity): Consider treatment delay or dosage reduction.

Hemolysis: Discontinue treatment.

Neurotoxicity: Consider treatment delay or discontinuation.

Combination Regimens

Leukemia, acute myeloid:

FLAG (AML Induction) on page 1968

FLAG-IDA (AML Induction) on page 1970

Leukemia, chronic lymphocytic:

Fludarabine-Cyclophosphamide (CLL) on page 1971

Fludarabine-Cyclophosphamide-Rituximab (CLL) on page 1973

Fludarabine-Rituximab (CLL) on page 1976

OFAR (CLL) on page 2045

Lymphoma, non-Hodgkin:

Fludarabine-Cyclophosphamide-Mitoxantrone-Rituximab on page 1972

Fludarabine-Mitoxantrone-Dexamethasone (NHL) on page 1975

Fludarabine-Mitoxantrone-Dexamethasone-Rituximab on page 1975

Lymphoma, non-Hodgkin (Follicular):

Fludarabine-Cyclophosphamide-Rituximab (NHL-Follicular) on page 1974

Fludarabine-Rituximab (NHL-Follicular) on page 1976

Lymphoma, non-Hodgkin (Mantle Cell): Fludarabine-Cyclophosphamide (NHL-Mantle Cell) on page 1973

Administration

IV: The manufacturer recommends administering over ~30 minutes. Continuous infusions and IV bolus over 15 minutes have been used for some off-label protocols (refer to individual studies for infusion rate details).

Oral: Tablet [Canadian product] may be administered with or without food; should be swallowed whole with water; do not chew, break, or crush.

Hazardous agent; use appropriate precautions for handling and disposal (NIOSH 2014 [group 1]).

Emetic Potential Children and Adults:

Oral: Low (10% to 30%)

IV: Minimal (<10%)

Monitoring Parameters CBC with differential, platelet count, AST, ALT, serum creatinine, serum albumin, uric acid; monitor for signs of infection and neurotoxicity

Dosage Forms Excipient information presented when available (limited, particularly for generics); consult specific product labeling. [DSC] = Discontinued product

Solution, Intravenous, as phosphate:

Generic: 50 mg/2 mL (2 mL)

Solution, Intravenous, as phosphate [preservative free]:

Generic: 50 mg/2 mL (2 mL [DSC])

Solution Reconstituted, Intravenous, as phosphate:

Fludara: 50 mg (1 ea)

Generic: 50 mg (1 ea)

Solution Reconstituted, Intravenous, as phosphate [preservative free]:

Generic: 50 mg (1 ea)

Dosage Forms: Canada Excipient information presented when available (limited, particularly for generics); consult specific product labeling.

Tablet, as phosphate:

Fludara: 10 mg

Fluorouracil (Systemic) (flure oh YOOR a sil)

Related Information

Chemotherapy and Cancer Treatment During Pregnancy *on page 2214*

Management of Chemotherapy-Induced Nausea and Vomiting in Adults *on page 2142*

Management of Drug Extravasations *on page 2159*

Management of EGFR Inhibitor Toxicities: Dermatologic, Ocular, and Gastrointestinal *on page 2179*

Mucositis and Stomatitis *on page 2186*

Prevention of Chemotherapy-Induced Nausea and Vomiting in Children *on page 2203*

Safe Handling of Hazardous Drugs *on page 2292*

Brand Names: US Adrucil

Brand Names: Canada Fluorouracil Injection

Index Terms 5-Fluorouracil; 5-Fluracil; 5-FU; Fluoro Uracil; Fluouracil; FU

Pharmacologic Category Antineoplastic Agent, Antimetabolite; Antineoplastic Agent, Antimetabolite (Pyrimidine Analog)

Use Treatment of breast cancer, colon cancer, rectal cancer, pancreatic cancer, and stomach (gastric) cancer

Labeled Contraindications Hypersensitivity to fluorouracil or any component of the formulation; poor nutritional states; depressed bone marrow function; potentially serious infections

Pregnancy Considerations Adverse effects (increased resorptions, embryo-lethality, and teratogenicity) have been observed in animal reproduction studies. Based on the mechanism of action, fluorouracil may cause fetal harm if administered during pregnancy (according to the manufacturer's labeling). The National Comprehensive Cancer Network (NCCN) breast cancer guidelines (v.3.2012) state that chemotherapy, if indicated, may be administered to pregnant women with breast cancer as part of a combination chemotherapy regimen (common regimens administered during pregnancy include doxorubicin, cyclophosphamide, and fluorouracil); chemotherapy should not be administered during the first trimester, after 35 weeks gestation, or within 3 weeks of planned delivery.

Breast-Feeding Considerations Based on the mechanism of action, the manufacturer's labeling recommends against breast-feeding if receiving fluorouracil.

Warnings/Precautions Hazardous agent - use appropriate precautions for handling and disposal (NIOSH 2014 [group 1]). Use with caution in patients with impaired kidney or liver function. Discontinue if intractable vomiting or diarrhea, precipitous falls in leukocyte or platelet counts, gastrointestinal ulcer or bleeding, stomatitis, or esophagopharyngitis, hemorrhage, or myocardial ischemia occurs. Use with caution in poor-risk patients who have had high-dose pelvic radiation or previous use of alkylating agents and in patients with widespread metastatic marrow involvement. Palmar-plantar erythrodysesthesia (hand-foot) syndrome has been associated with use (symptoms include a tingling sensation, which may progress to pain, and then to symmetrical swelling and erythema with tenderness; desquamation may occur; with treatment interruption, generally resolves over 5-7 days).

Continuous infusion: Serious errors have occurred when doses administered by continuous ambulatory infusion pumps have inadvertently been given over 1 to 4 hours instead of the intended extended continuous infusion duration.

Depending on protocol, infusion duration may range from 46 hours to 7 days for continuous infusions of fluorouracil. Ambulatory pumps utilized for continuous infusions should have safeguards to allow for detection of programming errors. If using an elastomeric device for ambulatory continuous infusion, carefully select and double check the flow rate on the device. Appropriate prescribing (in single daily doses [not course doses] with instructions to infuse over a specific time period), appropriate training/certification/education of staff involved with dispensing and administration processes, and independent double checks should be utilized throughout dispensing and administration procedures (ISMP [Smetzer 2015]).

An investigational uridine prodrug, uridine triacetate (formerly called vistonuridine), has been studied in a limited number of cases of fluorouracil overdose. Of 17 patients receiving uridine triacetate beginning within 8-96 hours after fluorouracil overdose, all patients fully recovered (von Borstel, 2009). Updated data has described a total of 28 patients treated with uridine triacetate for fluorouracil overdose (including overdoses related to continuous infusions delivering fluorouracil at rates faster than prescribed), all of whom recovered fully (Bamat, 2010). Refer to Uridine Triacetate monograph.

Administration to patients with a genetic deficiency of dihydropyrimidine dehydrogenase (DPD) has been associated with prolonged clearance and increased toxicity (diarrhea, neutropenia, and neurotoxicity) following administration; rechallenge has resulted in recurrent toxicity (despite dose reduction). **[U.S. Boxed Warning]: Should be administered under the supervision of an experienced cancer chemotherapy physician; the manufacturer's labeling recommends hospitalizing patients during the first treatment course due to the potential for severe toxicity.** Potentially significant drug-drug interactions may exist, requiring dose or frequency adjustment, additional monitoring, and/or selection of alternative therapy.

Adverse Reactions Toxicity depends on duration of treatment and/or rate of administration

Cardiovascular: Angina, arrhythmia, heart failure, MI, myocardial ischemia, vasospasm, ventricular ectopy

Central nervous system: Acute cerebellar syndrome, confusion, disorientation, euphoria, headache, nystagmus, stroke

Dermatologic: Alopecia, dermatitis, dry skin, fissuring, nail changes (nail loss), palmar-plantar erythrodysesthesia syndrome, pruritic maculopapular rash, photosensitivity, Stevens-Johnson syndrome, toxic epidermal necrolysis, vein pigmentation

Gastrointestinal: Anorexia, bleeding, diarrhea, esophagopharyngitis, mesenteric ischemia (acute), nausea, sloughing, stomatitis, ulceration, vomiting

Hematologic: Agranulocytosis, anemia, leukopenia (nadir: days 9-14; recovery by day 30), pancytopenia, thrombocytopenia

Local: Thrombophlebitis

Ocular: Lacrimation, lacrimal duct stenosis, photophobia, visual changes

Respiratory: Epistaxis

Miscellaneous: Anaphylaxis, generalized allergic reactions

Drug Interactions

Metabolism/Transport Effects Inhibits CYP2C9 (strong)

Avoid Concomitant Use

Avoid concomitant use of Fluorouracil (Systemic) with any of the following: BCG (Intravesical); CloZAPine; Dipyrone; Gimeracil; Natalizumab; Pimecrolimus; Tacrolimus (Topical); Tofacitinib; Vaccines (Live)

◀

Increased Effect/Toxicity

Fluorouracil (Systemic) may increase the levels/effects of: Bosentan; Carvedilol; CloZAPine; CYP2C9 Substrates; Diclofenac (Systemic); Dronabinol; Fingolimod; Fosphenytoin; Lacosamide; Leflunomide; Natalizumab; Ospemifene; Parecoxib; Phenytoin; Ramelteon; Tetrahydrocannabinol; Tofacitinib; Vaccines (Live); Vitamin K Antagonists

The levels/effects of Fluorouracil (Systemic) may be increased by: Cannabis; Cimetidine; Denosumab; Dipyrone; Gemcitabine; Gimeracil; Leucovorin Calcium-Levoleucovorin; MetroNIDAZOLE (Systemic); Pimecrolimus; Roflumilast; SORAfenib; Tacrolimus (Topical); Trastuzumab

Decreased Effect

Fluorouracil (Systemic) may decrease the levels/effects of: BCG (Intravesical); Coccidioides immitis Skin Test; Sipuleucel-T; Vaccines (Inactivated); Vaccines (Live)

The levels/effects of Fluorouracil (Systemic) may be decreased by: Echinacea; SORAfenib

Storage/Stability Store intact vials at room temperature. Do not refrigerate or freeze. Protect from light. Slight discoloration may occur during storage; does not usually denote decomposition. If exposed to cold, a precipitate may form; **gentle** heating to 60°C (140°F) will dissolve the precipitate without impairing the potency. According to the manufacturer, pharmacy bulk vials should be used within 4 hours of initial entry. Solutions for infusion should be used promptly. Fluorouracil 50 mg/mL in NS was stable in polypropylene infusion pump syringes for 7 days when stored at 30°C (86°F) (Stiles, 1996). Stability of fluorouracil 1 mg/mL or 10 mg/mL in NS or D_5W in PVC bags was demonstrated for up to 14 days at 4°C (39.2°F) and 21°C (69.8°F) (Martel, 1996). Stability of undiluted fluorouracil (50 mg/mL) in ethylene-vinyl acetate ambulatory pump reservoirs was demonstrated for 3 days at 4°C (39.2°F) (precipitate formed after 3 days) and for 14 days at 33°C (91.4°F) (Martel, 1996). Stability of undiluted fluorouracil (50 mg/mL) in PVC ambulatory pump reservoirs was demonstrated for 5 days at 4°C (39.2°F) (precipitate formed after 5 days) and for 14 days at 33°C (91.4°F) (Martel, 1996).

Preparation for Administration Hazardous agent; use appropriate precautions for handling and disposal (NIOSH 2014 [group 1]). May dispense in a syringe or dilute in 50-1000 mL NS or D_5W for infusion.

Mechanism of Action A pyrimidine analog antimetabolite that interferes with DNA and RNA synthesis; after activation, F-UMP (an active metabolite) is incorporated into RNA to replace uracil and inhibit cell growth; the active metabolite F-dUMP, inhibits thymidylate synthetase, depleting thymidine triphosphate (a necessary component of DNA synthesis).

Pharmacodynamics/Kinetics

Distribution: Penetrates extracellular fluid, CSF, and third space fluids (eg, pleural effusions and ascitic fluid), marrow, intestinal mucosa, liver and other tissues

Metabolism: Hepatic (90%); via a dehydrogenase enzyme; FU must be metabolized to active metabolites, 5-fluoroxyuridine monophosphate (F-UMP) and 5-5-fluoro-2'-deoxyuridine-5'-O-monophosphate (F-dUMP)

Half-life elimination: 16 minutes (range: 8-20 minutes); two metabolites, F-dUMP and F-UMP, have prolonged half-lives depending on the type of tissue

Excretion: Primarily metabolized in the liver; excreted in lung (as expired CO_2) and urine (7% to 20% as unchanged drug within 6 hours; also as metabolites within 9-10 hours)

Dosing

Adult & Geriatric Details concerning dosing in combination regimens should be consulted:

Breast cancer (off-label dosing): IV:

CEF regimen: 500 mg/m² on days 1 and 8 every 28 days (in combination with cyclophosphamide and epirubicin) for 6 cycles (Levine, 1998)

CMF regimen: 600 mg/m² on days 1 and 8 every 28 days (in combination with cyclophosphamide and methotrexate) for 6 cycles (Goldhirsch, 1998; Levine, 1998)

FAC regimen: 500 mg/m² on days 1 and 8 every 21-28 days (in combination with cyclophosphamide and doxorubicin) for 6 cycles (Assikis, 2003)

Colorectal cancer (off-label dosing): IV:

FLOX regimen: 500 mg/m² bolus on days 1, 8, 15, 22, 29, and 36 (1 hour after leucovorin) every 8 weeks (in combination with leucovorin and oxaliplatin) for 3 cycles (Kuebler, 2007)

FOLFOX6 and mFOLFOX6 regimen: 400 mg/m² bolus on day 1, followed by 1200 mg/m²/day continuous infusion for 2 days (over 46 hours) every 2 weeks (in combination with leucovorin and oxaliplatin) until disease progression or unacceptable toxicity (Cheeseman, 2002)

FOLFIRI regimen: 400 mg/m² bolus on day 1, followed by 1200 mg/m²/day continuous infusion for 2 days (over 46 hours) every 2 weeks (in combination with leucovorin and irinotecan) until disease progression or unacceptable toxicity; after 2 cycles, may increase continuous infusion fluorouracil dose to 1500 mg/m²/day (over 46 hours) (Andre, 1999)

Roswell Park regimen: 500 mg/m² (bolus) on days 1, 8, 15, 22, 29, and 36 (1 hour after leucovorin) every 8 weeks (in combination with leucovorin) for 4 cycles (Haller, 2005)

Gastric cancer (off-label dosing): IV:

CF regimen: 750-1000 mg/m²/day continuous infusion days 1-4 and 29-32 of a 35-day treatment cycle (preoperative chemoradiation; in combination with cisplatin) (Tepper, 2008; NCCN Gastric Cancer Guidelines v2.2012)

ECF regimen (resectable disease): 200 mg/m²/day continuous infusion days 1-21 every 3 weeks (in combination with epirubicin and cisplatin) for 6 cycles (3 cycles preoperatively and 3 cycles postoperatively) (Cunningham, 2006)

ECF or EOF regimen (advanced disease): 200 mg/m²/day continuous infusion days 1-21 every 3 weeks (in combination with epirubicin and either cisplatin or oxaliplatin) for a planned duration of 24 weeks (Sumpter, 2005)

TCF or DCF regimen: 750 mg/m²/day continuous infusion days 1-5 every 3 weeks or 1000 mg/m²/day continuous infusion days 1-5 every 4 weeks (in combination with docetaxel and cisplatin) until disease progression or unacceptable toxicity (Ajani, 2007; Van Cutsem, 2006; NCCN Gastric Cancer Guidelines v2.2012)

ToGA regimen (HER2-positive): 800 mg/m²/day continuous infusion days 1-5 every 3 weeks (in combination with cisplatin and trastuzumab) until disease progression or unacceptable toxicity (Bang, 2010)

Pancreatic cancer (off-label dosing): IV:

Chemoradiation therapy: 250 mg/m²/day continuous infusion for 3 weeks prior to and then throughout radiation therapy (Regine, 2008)

Fluorouracil-Leucovorin: 425 mg/m²/day (bolus) days 1-5 every 28 days (in combination with leucovorin) for 6 cycles (Neoptolemos, 2010)

◄   *FOLFIRINOX regimen:* 400 mg/m^2 bolus on day 1, followed by 1200 mg/m^2/day continuous infusion for 2 days (over 46 hours) every 14 days (in combination with leucovorin, irinotecan, and oxaliplatin) until disease progression or unacceptable toxicity for a recommended 12 cycles (Conroy, 2011)

Anal carcinoma (off-label use): IV: 1000 mg/m^2/day continuous infusion days 1-4 and days 29-32 (in combination with mitomycin and radiation therapy) (Ajani, 2008)

Bladder cancer (off-label use): IV: 500 mg/m^2/day continuous infusion days 1-5 and days 16-20 (in combination with mitomycin and radiation therapy) (James, 2012)

Cervical cancer (off-label use): IV: 1000 mg/m^2/day continuous infusion days 1-4 (in combination with cisplatin and radiation therapy) every 3 weeks for 3 cycles (Eifel, 2004)

Esophageal cancer (off-label use): IV:

CF regimen: 750-1000 mg/m^2/day continuous infusion days 1-4 and 29-32 of a 35-day treatment cycle (preoperative chemoradiation; in combination with cisplatin) (Tepper, 2008; NCCN Esophageal and Esophagogastric Junction Cancers Guidelines v2.2012)

ECF regimen (resectable disease): 200 mg/m^2/day continuous infusion days 1-21 every 3 weeks (in combination with epirubicin and cisplatin) for 6 cycles (3 cycles preoperatively and 3 cycles postoperatively) (Cunningham, 2006)

ECF or EOF regimen (advanced disease): 200 mg/m^2/day continuous infusion days 1-21 every 3 weeks (in combination with epirubicin and either cisplatin or oxaliplatin) for a planned duration of 24 weeks (Sumpter, 2005)

TCF or DCF regimen: 750 mg/m^2/day continuous infusion days 1-5 every 3 weeks or 1000 mg/m^2/day continuous infusion days 1-5 every 4 weeks (in combination with docetaxel and cisplatin) until disease progression or unacceptable toxicity (Ajani, 2007; Van Cutsem, 2006; NCCN Esophageal and Esophagogastric Junction Cancers Guidelines v2.2012)

Head and neck cancer, squamous cell (off-label use): IV:

Platinum-Fluorouracil regimen: 1000 mg/m^2/day continuous infusion days 1-4 every 3 weeks (in combination with cisplatin) for at least 6 cycles (Gibson, 2005) **or** 600 mg/m^2/day continuous infusion days 1-4, 22-25, and 43-46 (in combination with carboplatin and radiation) (Denis, 2004; Bourhis, 2012)

TPF regimen: 1000 mg/m^2/day continuous infusion days 1-4 every 3 weeks (in combination with docetaxel and cisplatin) for 3 cycles, and followed by chemoradiotherapy (Posner, 2007) **or** 750 mg/m^2/day continuous infusion days 1-5 every 3 weeks (in combination with docetaxel and cisplatin) for up to 4 cycles (Vermorken, 2007)

Platinum, 5-FU, and cetuximab regimen: 1000 mg/m^2/day continuous infusion days 1-4 every 3 weeks (in combination with either cisplatin or carboplatin and cetuximab) for a total of up to 6 cycles (Vermorken, 2008)

Hepatobiliary cancer (off-label use): IV: 600 mg/m^2 (bolus) on days 1, 8, and 15 every 4 weeks (in combination with gemcitabine and leucovorin) (Alberts, 2005)

Renal Impairment No dosage adjustment provided in the manufacturer's labeling; however, extreme caution should be used in patients with renal impairment. The following adjustments have been recommended:

CrCl <50 mL/minute and continuous renal replacement therapy (CRRT): No dosage adjustment necessary (Aronoff, 2007).

Hemodialysis:

Administer standard dose following hemodialysis on dialysis days (Janus, 2010).

Administer 50% of standard dose following hemodialysis (Aronoff, 2007).

Hepatic Impairment No dosage adjustment provided in the manufacturer's labeling; however, extreme caution should be used in patients with hepatic impairment. The following adjustments have been recommended:

Floyd, 2006: Bilirubin >5 mg/dL: Avoid use.

Koren, 1992: Hepatic impairment (degree not specified): Administer <50% of dose, then increase if toxicity does not occur.

Obesity *ASCO Guidelines for appropriate chemotherapy dosing in obese adults with cancer:* Utilize patient's actual body weight (full weight) for calculation of body surface area- or weight-based dosing, particularly when the intent of therapy is curative; manage regimen-related toxicities in the same manner as for nonobese patients; if a dose reduction is utilized due to toxicity, consider resumption of full weight-based dosing with subsequent cycles, especially if cause of toxicity (eg, hepatic or renal impairment) is resolved (Griggs, 2012).

Adjustment for Toxicity *According to the manufacturer, treatment should be discontinued for the following:* Stomatitis or esophagopharyngitis, leukopenia (WBC <3500/mm^3), rapidly falling white blood cell count, intractable vomiting, diarrhea, frequent bowel movements, watery stools, gastrointestinal ulcer or bleeding, thrombocytopenia (platelets <100,000/mm^3), hemorrhage

Combination Regimens

Anal cancer: Fluorouracil-Mitomycin (Anal Cancer) on page 1983
Breast cancer:
  CAF IV (Breast) on page 1852
  CAF Oral (Breast) on page 1852
  Cisplatin-Fluorouracil (Bladder Cancer) on page 1896
  CMF Oral (Breast) on page 1918
  Docetaxel-Trastuzumab followed by FEC (Breast) on page 1947
  FEC followed by Docetaxel Every 3 Weeks (Breast) on page 1966
  FEC followed by Paclitaxel Weekly (Breast) on page 1967
  FEC IV (Breast) on page 1967
  FEC Oral (Breast) on page 1968
Cervical cancer: Cisplatin-Fluorouracil (Cervical Cancer) on page 1897
Colorectal cancer:
  Bevacizumab-Fluorouracil-Leucovorin (Colorectal) on page 1841
  Bevacizumab + FOLFIRI (Colorectal) on page 1842
  Bevacizumab FOLFOX (Colorectal) on page 1842
  Cetuximab + FOLFIRI (Colorectal) on page 1882
  FLOX (Colorectal) on page 1970
  Fluorouracil-Leucovorin on page 1979
  Fluorouracil-Leucovorin-Irinotecan (Saltz Regimen) (Colorectal) on page 1981
  FOLFIRI (Colorectal) on page 1983
  FOLFOX1 (Colorectal) on page 1984
  FOLFOX2 (Colorectal) on page 1985

Administration IV: Administration rate varies by protocol; refer to specific reference for protocol. May be administered by IV push, IV bolus, or as a continuous infusion. Avoid extravasation (may be an irritant).

Hazardous agent; use appropriate precautions for handling and disposal (NIOSH 2014 [group 1]).

Vesicant/Extravasation Risk May be an irritant

Emetic Potential Children and Adults: Low (10% to 30%)

Monitoring Parameters CBC with differential and platelet count, renal function tests, liver function tests, signs of palmar-plantar erythrodysesthesia syndrome, stomatitis, diarrhea, hemorrhage, or gastrointestinal ulcers or bleeding

Dietary Considerations Increase dietary intake of thiamine.

Dosage Forms Excipient information presented when available (limited, particularly for generics); consult specific product labeling.
Solution, Intravenous:
Adrucil: 500 mg/10 mL (10 mL); 2.5 g/50 mL (50 mL); 5 g/100 mL (100 mL)
Generic: 500 mg/10 mL (10 mL); 1 g/20 mL (20 mL); 2.5 g/50 mL (50 mL); 5 g/100 mL (100 mL)

Fluorouracil (Topical) (flure oh YOOR a sil)

Related Information
Management of EGFR Inhibitor Toxicities: Dermatologic, Ocular, and Gastrointestinal *on page 2179*
Safe Handling of Hazardous Drugs *on page 2292*

Brand Names: US Carac; Efudex; Fluoroplex; Tolak

Brand Names: Canada Efudex; Fluoroplex

Index Terms 5-Fluorouracil; 5-FU; FU; Topical Fluorouracil

Pharmacologic Category Antineoplastic Agent, Antimetabolite; Antineoplastic Agent, Antimetabolite (Pyrimidine Analog); Topical Skin Product

Use
Actinic or solar keratosis: Management of multiple actinic or solar keratoses
Basal cell carcinoma (5%): Treatment of superficial basal cell carcinomas when conventional methods are impractical (eg, due to multiple lesions or difficult treatment sites)
Limitations of use: Establish diagnosis of superficial basal cell carcinoma prior to treatment (use has not been proven effective in other types of basal cell carcinomas); surgery is preferred with isolated, easily accessible basal cell carcinomas because success with such lesions is almost 100% and the success rate with fluorouracil cream and solution is ~93%.

Labeled Contraindications Hypersensitivity to fluorouracil or any component of the formulation; dihydropyrimidine dehydrogenase (DPD) enzyme deficiency; women who are or may become pregnant

Pregnancy Considerations Animal reproduction studies have not been conducted with topical fluorouracil, although teratogenic effects have been observed in animal studies with parenteral administration. Adverse effects have been reported following use of topical fluorouracil products in humans. Use is contraindicated during pregnancy. Women of reproductive potential should use effective contraception during and for one month after the final application of topical fluorouracil.

Breast-Feeding Considerations It is not known if fluorouracil (topical) is excreted in breast milk. Due to the potential for serious adverse reactions in the nursing infant, a decision should be made to discontinue nursing or to discontinue the drug, taking into account the importance of treatment to the mother.

Warnings/Precautions Hazardous agent - use appropriate precautions for handling and disposal (NIOSH 2014 [group 1]). Individuals lacking dihydropyrimidine dehydrogenase (DPD) enzyme activity may exhibit severe toxicity with topical fluorouracil. Life-threatening systemic toxicity has been reported with the topical use of fluorouracil 5% in a patient with DPD enzyme deficiency; signs/symptoms included bloody diarrhea, stomatitis, esophagus, stomach, and small bowel inflammation, severe abdominal pain, vomiting, chills, fever, erythematous skin rash, neutropenia, and thrombocytopenia. It is unknown if patients with profound DPD enzyme deficiency would develop systemic toxicity with lower concentrations of topical fluorouracil. Discontinue if signs of DPD deficiency develop.

When applied to a lesion, erythema followed by vesiculation, desquamation, erosion and reepithelialization occurs. Local reactions and alterations in skin appearance may persist for several weeks after discontinuation. Bruising, burning, crusting, dryness, edema, irritation, pain, pruritus, scaling scarring, soreness, stinging, and ulceration may commonly result from topical therapy. Increased absorption through ulcerated or inflamed skin is possible. May be associated with delayed-type hypersensitivity reactions, including allergic contact dermatitis. Severe pruritus or eczema (at the application site or at a distant site) may be indicative of hypersensitivity; patch testing may not be useful in the evaluation of these reactions; discontinue immediately for signs of hypersensitivity. Topical fluorouracil is associated with photosensitivity, including severe sunburn. Avoid prolonged exposure to sunlight or UV irradiation during treatment; reaction intensity may be increased.

Appropriate use: Avoid topical application to mucous membranes due to potential for local inflammation and ulceration; cases of miscarriage and a birth defect (ventricular septal defect) have been reported when fluorouracil was applied to mucous membrane areas during pregnancy. The use of occlusive dressings with topical preparations may increase the severity of inflammation in nearby skin areas (a porous gauze dressing may be applied for cosmetic reasons without increase in reaction). Avoid eyelids, eyes, and periocular area when applying (corneal and conjunctival disorders have occurred with topical fluorouracil). Wash hands well following application; if ocular exposure occurs, flush with large amounts of water.

Benzyl alcohol and derivatives: Some dosage forms may contain benzyl alcohol; large amounts of benzyl alcohol (≥ 99 mg/kg/day) have been associated with a potentially fatal toxicity ("gasping syndrome") in neonates; the "gasping syndrome" consists of metabolic acidosis, respiratory distress, gasping respirations, CNS dysfunction (including convulsions, intracranial hemorrhage), hypotension and cardiovascular collapse (AAP ["Inactive"], 1997; CDC, 1982); some data suggests that benzoate displaces bilirubin from protein binding sites (Ahlfors, 2001); avoid or use dosage forms containing benzyl alcohol with caution in neonates. See manufacturer's labeling. Some dosage forms contain peanut oil.

Adverse Reactions

>10%:

Dermatologic: Application site scaling ($\leq 95\%$), application site dryness (70% to $\leq 95\%$), application site crusting (87%), application site skin erosion (25% to 68%)

Local: Application site erythema (90% to 99%), application site reaction (92% to 97%), application site stinging ($\leq 87\%$), application site burning (60% to $\leq 87\%$), application site pruritus (85%), application site edema (14% to 69%), application site pain (31% to 61%)

1% to 10%:

Central nervous system: Headache (4%)

Dermatologic: Skin irritation (1% to 2%)

Infection: Common cold (5%)

Ophthalmic: Eye irritation (3% to 7%; burning, watering, sensitivity, stinging, itching)

Respiratory: Sinusitis (5%)

<1%, postmarketing, and/or case reports: Allergic contact dermatitis, alopecia, anxiety, bullous pemphigoid, burning sensation of skin, chronic lympocytic leukemia, conjunctival disease, conjunctivitis, corneal disease, eosinophilia, eye irritation, herpes simplex infection, hyperpigmentation, ichthyosis, inflammation, insomnia, irritability, lacrimation, leukocytosis, medicine-like taste, muscle tenderness, nasal discomfort, pain, pancytopenia, pruritus, scarring, skin blister, skin irritation, skin neoplasm (nonmelanoma), skin photosensitivity, skin rash, skin tenderness, stomatitis, suppuration, swelling, swelling of eye, telangiectasia, thrombocytopenia, toxic granulations, ulcer, urticaria

Drug Interactions

Metabolism/Transport Effects Inhibits CYP2C9 (weak)

Avoid Concomitant Use There are no known interactions where it is recommended to avoid concomitant use.

Increased Effect/Toxicity

Fluorouracil (Topical) may increase the levels/effects of: Fosphenytoin; Phenytoin; Vitamin K Antagonists

The levels/effects of Fluorouracil (Topical) may be increased by: Gemcitabine; Leucovorin Calcium-Levoleucovorin; SORAfenib

Decreased Effect

The levels/effects of Fluorouracil (Topical) may be decreased by: SORAfenib

Storage/Stability Store at controlled room temperature of 15°C to 30°C (59°F to 86°F). Do not freeze.

Mechanism of Action A pyrimidine antimetabolite that interferes with DNA synthesis by blocking the methylation of deoxyuridylic acid to thymidylic acid; blocks DNA synthesis to prevent cell proliferation of fast growing cells and cause cell death.

Pharmacodynamics/Kinetics

Absorption: ~6% of a topical dose is absorbed systemically (5% cream)

Time to Peak: ~1 hour following application (4% cream)

Dosing

Adult & Geriatric

Actinic or solar keratosis: Topical:

Cream (0.5%): Apply thin film to lesions once daily for up to 4 weeks, as tolerated

Cream (1%): Apply to lesions twice daily for 2 to 6 weeks

Cream (4%): Apply to lesions once daily for 4 weeks as tolerated

Cream (5%) or solution (2% and 5%): Apply to lesions twice daily for 2 to 4 weeks; complete healing may not be evident for 1 to 2 months following treatment

Superficial basal cell carcinoma: Topical: Cream (5%) or solution (5%): Apply to affected lesions twice daily for 3 to 6 weeks; treatment may be continued for up to 10 to 12 weeks

Renal Impairment There are no dosage adjustments provided in the manufacturer's labeling.

Hepatic Impairment There are no dosage adjustments provided in the manufacturer's labeling.

Administration Topical: Apply 10 minutes after washing, rinsing, and drying the affected area. Apply a sufficient amount to cover lesions, preferably using a nonmetal applicator or suitable glove.

Cream (4%): Apply after washing, rinsing, and drying the affected area. Apply a sufficient amount to cover lesions of the face, ears, and/or scalp with a thin film, using fingertips to gently massage uniformly into skin.

If applied with fingertip, wash hands immediately after application. Do not cover area with an occlusive dressing. Topical preparations are for external use only; not for ophthalmic, oral, mucous membrane, or intravaginal use.

Hazardous agent; use appropriate precautions for handling and disposal (NIOSH 2014 [group 1]).

Dosage Forms Excipient information presented when available (limited, particularly for generics); consult specific product labeling.

Cream, External:

Carac: 0.5% (30 g) [contains methylparaben, polysorbate 80, propylene glycol, propylparaben, trolamine (triethanolamine)]

Efudex: 5% (40 g)

Fluoroplex: 1% (30 g) [contains benzyl alcohol]

Tolak: 4% (40 g) [contains cetyl alcohol, methylparaben, peanut oil, propylparaben]

Generic: 0.5% (30 g); 5% (40 g)

Solution, External:

Generic: 2% (10 mL); 5% (10 mL)

◆ **Fluorouracil Injection (Can)** see Fluorouracil (Systemic) on page 740

◆ **Fluouracil** see Fluorouracil (Systemic) on page 740

Fluoxymesterone (floo oks i MES te rone)

Brand Names: US Androxy

Index Terms Androxy; Halotestin

Pharmacologic Category Androgen

Use Replacement therapy in the treatment of delayed male puberty; male hypogonadism (primary or hypogonadotropic); inoperable metastatic female breast cancer

Pregnancy Risk Factor X

Dosing

Adult & Geriatric

Hypogonadism (Males): Oral: 5-20 mg daily

Delayed puberty (Males): Oral: 2.5-20 mg daily for 4-6 months

Inoperable breast carcinoma (Females): Oral: 10-40 mg daily in divided doses for ≥3 months

Renal Impairment No dosage adjustment provided in manufacturer's labeling; use with caution.

Hepatic Impairment No dosage adjustment provided in manufacturer's labeling; use with caution.

Additional Information Complete prescribing information should be consulted for additional detail.

Dosage Forms Excipient information presented when available (limited, particularly for generics); consult specific product labeling.

Tablet, Oral:

Androxy: 10 mg [scored; contains fd&c blue #1 aluminum lake, fd&c yellow #10 aluminum lake, fd&c yellow #6 aluminum lake]

Controlled Substance C-III

◆ **5-Fluracil** see Fluorouracil (Systemic) on page 740

♦ **5-Flurocytosine** *see* Flucytosine *on page 731*

Flutamide (FLOO ta mide)

Related Information

Safe Handling of Hazardous Drugs *on page 2292*

Brand Names: Canada Apo-Flutamide; Euflex; PMS-Flutamide; Teva-Flutamide

Index Terms Eulexin; Flucinom; Flugerel; Niftolid; SCH 13521

Pharmacologic Category Antineoplastic Agent, Antiandrogen

Use Prostate cancer: Management of locally confined Stage B_2 to C and Stage D_2 metastatic prostate cancer (in combination with a luteinizing hormone-releasing hormone [LHRH] agonist). For Stage B_2 to C prostate cancer, flutamide treatment (and goserelin) should start 8 weeks prior to initiating radiation therapy and continue during radiation therapy. To achieve treatment benefit in Stage D_2 metastatic prostate cancer, initiate flutamide with the LHRH agonist and continue until disease progression.

Labeled Contraindications Hypersensitivity to flutamide or any component of the formulation; severe hepatic impairment (evaluate baseline hepatic enzymes prior to treatment).

Pregnancy Considerations Adverse events have been observed in animal reproduction studies. May cause fetal harm if administered in pregnancy. Flutamide is not indicated for use in women.

Breast-Feeding Considerations According to the manufacturer, this product is not indicated for use in women. Information related to use in nursing women has not been located.

Warnings/Precautions Hazardous agent - use appropriate precautions for handling and disposal (NIOSH 2014 [group 1]). **[U.S. Boxed Warning]: Hospitalization and death (rare) due to liver failure have been reported in patients taking flutamide. Elevated serum transaminase levels, jaundice, hepatic encephalopathy, and acute hepatic failure have been reported. Hepatotoxicity was reversible after discontinuation in some cases. In about 50% of the cases, the onset of hepatotoxicity was within the first 3 months of treatment. Monitor serum transaminase levels at baseline, monthly for 4 months, and periodically thereafter. Also obtain liver function tests at the first symptoms suggestive of liver dysfunction (nausea, vomiting, abdominal pain, fatigue, anorexia, "flu-like" symptoms, hyperbilirubinuria, jaundice, or right upper quadrant tenderness). Use is not recommended in patients with ALT values greater than 2 times ULN; discontinue use immediately in patients with jaundice or if ALT rises above 2 times ULN.** Use is contraindicated in patients with severe hepatic impairment. Androgen-deprivation therapy may increase the risk for cardiovascular disease (Levine, 2010). Not indicated for use in women and should not be used in women, particularly for nonserious or nonlife-threatening conditions.

Potentially significant drug-drug interactions may exist, requiring dose or frequency adjustment, additional monitoring, and/or selection of alternative therapy. Patients with glucose-6 phosphate dehydrogenase deficiency or hemoglobin M disease or smokers are at risk of toxicities associated with aniline exposure, including methemoglobinemia, hemolytic anemia, and cholestatic jaundice. Monitor methemoglobin levels. Gynecomastia may occur in patients receiving flutamide in combination with medical castration.

◀ **Adverse Reactions**
>10%:
Endocrine & metabolic: Hot flash (46% to 61%), galactorrhea (9% to 42%), decreased libido (36%), increased lactate dehydrogenase (transient; mild)
Gastrointestinal: Diarrhea (12% to 40%), vomiting (11% to 12%)
Genitourinary: Impotence (33%), cystitis (16%), breast tenderness
Hematologic & oncologic: Rectal hemorrhage (14%), tumor flare
Hepatic: Increased serum AST (transient; mild)
1% to 10%:
Cardiovascular: Edema (4%), hypertension (1%)
Central nervous system: Anxiety, confusion, depression, dizziness, drowsiness, headache, insomnia, nervousness
Dermatologic: Skin rash (3% to 8%), ecchymoses, pruritus
Endocrine & metabolic: Gynecomastia (9%)
Gastrointestinal: Nausea (9%), proctitis (8%), gastric distress (4% to 6%), anorexia (4%), constipation, dyspepsia, increased appetite
Genitourinary: Hematuria (7%)
Hematologic & oncologic: Anemia (6%), leukopenia (3%), thrombocytopenia (1%)
Infection: Herpes zoster
Neuromuscular & skeletal: Weakness (1%)
<1%, postmarketing, and case reports: Cholestatic jaundice, hemolytic anemia, hepatic encephalopathy, hepatic failure, hepatic necrosis, hepatitis, hypersensitivity pneumonitis, increased blood urea nitrogen, increased gamma-glutamyl transferase, increased serum ALT, increased serum bilirubin, increased serum creatinine, jaundice, macrocytic anemia, malignant neoplasm of breast (male), methemoglobinemia, myocardial infarction, oligospermia, pulmonary embolism, skin photosensitivity, sulfhemoglobinemia, thrombophlebitis, urine discoloration (amber, yellow-green)

Drug Interactions
Metabolism/Transport Effects Substrate of CYP1A2 (major), CYP3A4 (major); **Note:** Assignment of Major/Minor substrate status based on clinically relevant drug interaction potential; **Inhibits** CYP1A2 (weak)

Avoid Concomitant Use
Avoid concomitant use of Flutamide with any of the following: Conivaptan; Fusidic Acid (Systemic); Idelalisib; Indium 111 Capromab Pendetide

Increased Effect/Toxicity
Flutamide may increase the levels/effects of: Prilocaine; Sodium Nitrite; TiZANidine

The levels/effects of Flutamide may be increased by: Abiraterone Acetate; Aprepitant; Conivaptan; CYP1A2 Inhibitors (Moderate); CYP1A2 Inhibitors (Strong); CYP3A4 Inhibitors (Moderate); CYP3A4 Inhibitors (Strong); Dapsone (Topical); Dasatinib; Deferasirox; Fosaprepitant; Fusidic Acid (Systemic); Idelalisib; Ivacaftor; Luliconazole; Mifepristone; Netupitant; Nitric Oxide; Osimertinib; Palbociclib; Peginterferon Alfa-2b; Simeprevir; Stiripentol; Vemurafenib

Decreased Effect
Flutamide may decrease the levels/effects of: Choline C 11; Indium 111 Capromab Pendetide

The levels/effects of Flutamide may be decreased by: Bosentan; Cannabis; CYP1A2 Inducers (Strong); CYP3A4 Inducers (Moderate); CYP3A4 Inducers

(Strong); Cyproterone; Dabrafenib; Deferasirox; Enzalutamide; Mitotane; Osimertinib; Siltuximab; St Johns Wort; Teriflunomide; Tocilizumab

Storage/Stability Store at 25°C (77°F); excursions permitted to 15°C to 30°C (59°F to 86°F). Dispense with a child-resistant closure in a tight, light-resistant container.

Mechanism of Action Nonsteroidal antiandrogen that inhibits androgen uptake and/or inhibits binding of androgen in target tissues.

Pharmacodynamics/Kinetics

Absorption: Oral: Rapid and complete

Protein binding: Parent drug: 94% to 96%; 2-hydroxyflutamide: 92% to 94%

Metabolism: Extensively hepatic to ≥6 metabolites, primarily 2-hydroxyfluta-mide (active)

Half-life elimination: ~6 hours (2-hydroxyflutamide)

Time to peak: ~2 hours (2-hydroxyflutamide)

Excretion: Primarily urine (as metabolites); feces (~4%)

Dosing

Adult & Geriatric Prostate cancer, metastatic: Males: Oral: 250 mg 3 times daily (every 8 hours)

Renal Impairment No dosage adjustment is necessary in patients with chronic renal insufficiency.

Hepatic Impairment

Mild to moderate impairment: There are no dosage adjustments provided in the manufacturer's labeling.

Severe impairment: Use is contraindicated.

Administration May be administered with or without food. Administer orally in 3 divided doses (every 8 hours). Hazardous agent; use appropriate precautions for handling and disposal (NIOSH 2014 [group 1]).

Monitoring Parameters Serum transaminases (at baseline, monthly for 4 months, and periodically thereafter); monitor liver function tests at the first sign or symptom of liver dysfunction (eg, nausea, vomiting, abdominal pain, fatigue, anorexia, flu-like symptoms, hyperbilirubinuria, jaundice, or right upper quadrant tenderness); monitor prostate specific antigen (PSA)

Dosage Forms Excipient information presented when available (limited, particularly for generics); consult specific product labeling.

Capsule, Oral:

Generic: 125 mg

Dosage Forms: Canada Excipient information presented when available (limited, particularly for generics); consult specific product labeling.

Tablet, Oral: 250 mg

◆ **Folinate Calcium** see Leucovorin Calcium on page 1023

◆ **Folinic Acid (error prone synonym)** see Leucovorin Calcium on page 1023

◆ **Folotyn** see PRALAtrexate on page 1417

Fondaparinux (fon da PARE i nuks)

Related Information

Venous Thromboembolism in the Cancer Patient on page 2267

Brand Names: US Arixtra

Brand Names: Canada Arixtra

Index Terms Fondaparinux Sodium

Pharmacologic Category Anticoagulant; Anticoagulant, Factor Xa Inhibitor

◀ **Use**

Acute deep vein thrombosis: Treatment of acute deep vein thrombosis (DVT) in conjunction with warfarin.

Acute pulmonary embolism: Treatment of acute pulmonary embolism (PE) in conjunction with warfarin.

Deep vein thrombosis prophylaxis: Prophylaxis of DVT in patients undergoing surgery for hip replacement, knee replacement, hip fracture (including extended prophylaxis following hip fracture surgery), or abdominal surgery (in patients at risk for thromboembolic complications).

Canadian labeling: Additional uses; not approved in the US: Management of unstable angina or non-ST segment elevation myocardial infarction (UA/NSTEMI) for the prevention of death and subsequent MI; management of ST segment elevation MI (STEMI) for the prevention of death and myocardial reinfarction

Labeled Contraindications Serious hypersensitivity (eg, angioedema, anaphylactoid/anaphylactic reactions) to fondaparinux or any component of the formulation; severe renal impairment (CrCl <30 mL/minute); body weight <50 kg (prophylaxis); active major bleeding; bacterial endocarditis; thrombocytopenia associated with a positive *in vitro* test for antiplatelet antibody in the presence of fondaparinux

Pregnancy Considerations Adverse events have not been observed in animal reproduction studies. Based on case reports, small amounts of fondaparinux have been detected in the umbilical cord following multiple doses during pregnancy (Dempfle, 2004). Use of fondaparinux in pregnancy should be limited to those women who have severe allergic reactions to heparin, including heparin-induced thrombocytopenia, and who cannot receive danaparoid (Guyatt, 2012).

Breast-Feeding Considerations It is not known if fondaparinux is excreted in breast milk. The manufacturer recommends caution be used if administered to nursing women. The use of alternative anticoagulants is preferred (Guyatt, 2012). The Canadian labeling does not recommend use in breast-feeding women.

Warnings/Precautions [U.S. Boxed Warning]: Spinal or epidural hematomas, including subsequent long-term or permanent paralysis, may occur with recent or anticipated neuraxial anesthesia (epidural or spinal anesthesia) or spinal puncture in patients anticoagulated with LMWH, heparinoids, or fondaparinux. Consider risk versus benefit prior to spinal procedures; risk is increased by the use of concomitant agents which may alter hemostasis (such as NSAIDS, platelet inhibitors, or other anticoagulants), the use of indwelling epidural catheters, a history of spinal deformity or spinal surgery, as well as a history of traumatic or repeated epidural or spinal punctures. Patient should be observed closely for bleeding and signs and symptoms of neurological impairment (eg, midline back pain, sensory and motor deficits [numbness, tingling, weakness in lower limbs], bowel or bladder dysfunction) if therapy is administered during or immediately following diagnostic lumbar puncture, epidural anesthesia, or spinal anesthesia. **Optimal timing between administration of fondaparinux and neuraxial procedures is unknown.**

Monitor patient closely for signs or symptoms of bleeding. Certain patients are at increased risk of bleeding. Risk factors include bacterial endocarditis; congenital or acquired bleeding disorders; active ulcerative and angiodysplastic GI disease; uncontrolled arterial hypertension; hemorrhagic stroke;

recent intracranial hemorrhage; or use shortly after brain, spinal, or ophthalmology surgery; in patients treated concomitantly with platelet inhibitors; or thrombocytopenia or platelet defects; diabetic retinopathy; patients <50 kg. Risk of major bleeding may be increased if initial dose is administered earlier than recommended (initiation recommended at 6 to 8 hours following surgery). Do not administer with other agents that increase the risk of hemorrhage unless they are essential for the management of the underlying condition (eg, vitamin K antagonists for treatment of VTE). PT and aPTT are insensitive measures of fondaparinux activity. If unexpected changes in coagulation parameters or major bleeding occur, discontinue fondaparinux (elevated aPTT associated with bleeding events have been reported in postmarketing data).

Thrombocytopenia has occurred with administration, including very rare reports of thrombocytopenia with thrombosis similar to heparin-induced thrombocytopenia (HIT); however, has been used in patients with current or history of HIT due to a lack of an immune-mediated effect on platelets (ACCP [Guyatt, 2012]; Savi, 2005). Use is contraindicated in patients with thrombocytopenia associated with a positive in vitro test for antiplatelet antibodies in the presence of fondaparinux. Monitor patients closely and discontinue therapy if platelets fall to <100,000/mm^3 (US labeling) or <50,000/ mm^3 (Canadian labeling).

The administration of fondaparinux as the sole anticoagulant is **not recommended** during PCI due to an increased risk for guiding-catheter thrombosis. Use of an anticoagulant with antithrombin activity (eg, unfractionated heparin) is recommended as adjunctive therapy to PCI even if prior treatment with fondaparinux (must take into account whether GP IIb/IIIa antagonists have been administered) (ACCF/AHA [Anderson, 2013]; Levine, 2011). Use of fondaparinux during primary PCI is not recommended. In STEMI patients undergoing primary PCI for reperfusion, the use of fondaparinux prior to and during PCI is not recommended (Canadian labeling).

Use with caution in patients with hepatic impairment and in the elderly. Use with caution in patients with CrCl 30 to 50 mL/minute; contraindicated in patients with CrCl <30 mL/minute. Periodically monitor renal function; discontinue if severe renal dysfunction or labile function develops. Increased risk of bleeding in patients <50 kg; use with caution; dosage reduction recommended. Contraindicated in patients <50 kg when used for prophylactic therapy. Potentially significant interactions may exist, requiring dose or frequency adjustment, additional monitoring, and/or selection of alternative therapy.

For subcutaneous administration; not for IM administration. The needle guard may contain natural latex rubber. For STEMI patients (Canadian labeling; off-label use in United States) may administer initial dose IV. Do not use interchangeably (unit for unit) with low molecular weight heparins, heparin, or heparinoids. Discontinue use 24 hours prior to CABG and dose with unfractionated heparin per institutional practice (ACCF/AHA [Anderson, 2013]). Following discontinuation, the anticoagulant effects of fondaparinux may persist for 2 to 4 days and even longer in patients with renal impairment.

Adverse Reactions As with all anticoagulants, bleeding is the major adverse effect. Hemorrhage may occur at any site. Risk appears increased by a number of factors including renal dysfunction, age (>75 years), and weight (<50 kg).

>10%: Hematologic & oncologic: Anemia (2% to 20%)

1% to 10%:

Cardiovascular: Hypotension (≤4%)

Central nervous system: Insomnia (≤5%), dizziness (≤4%), confusion (1% to 3%)

Dermatologic: Increased wound secretion (≤5%), skin blister (≤3%)

Endocrine & metabolic: Hypokalemia (≤4%)

Hematologic & oncologic: Purpura (≤4%), thrombocytopenia (50,000 to 100,000/mm^3: 3%), hematoma (2% to 3%), minor hemorrhage (2% to 3%), major hemorrhage (1% to 3%; risk of major hemorrhage increased as high as 5% in patients receiving initial dose <6 hours following surgery), postoperative hemorrhage (≤2%)

Hepatic: Increased serum ALT (>3 × ULN: 1% to 3%), increased serum AST (>3 × ULN: <1% to ≤2%)

Infection: postoperative wound infection (abdominal surgery: 5%)

Respiratory: Epistaxis (VTE: 1%)

<1%, postmarketing, and/or case reports: Anaphylactoid reaction, anaphylaxis, angioedema, catheter site thrombosis (during PCI; without heparin), elevated aPTT associated with bleeding, epidural hematoma, hemorrhagic death, injection site reaction (bleeding at injection site, skin rash, pruritus), intracranial hemorrhage, reoperation due to bleeding, severe thrombocytopenia (<50,000/mm^3), spinal hematoma, thrombocytopenia (with thrombosis)

Drug Interactions

Metabolism/Transport Effects None known.

Avoid Concomitant Use

Avoid concomitant use of Fondaparinux with any of the following: Apixaban; Dabigatran Etexilate; Edoxaban; Hemin; Omacetaxine; Rivaroxaban; Urokinase; Vorapaxar

Increased Effect/Toxicity

Fondaparinux may increase the levels/effects of: Anticoagulants; Collagenase (Systemic); Deferasirox; Deoxycholic Acid; Ibritumomab; Nintedanib; Obinutuzumab; Omacetaxine; Rivaroxaban; Tositumomab and Iodine I 131 Tositumomab

The levels/effects of Fondaparinux may be increased by: Agents with Antiplatelet Properties; Apixaban; Dabigatran Etexilate; Dasatinib; Edoxaban; Hemin; Herbs (Anticoagulant/Antiplatelet Properties); Ibrutinib; Limaprost; Nonsteroidal Anti-Inflammatory Agents; Omega-3 Fatty Acids; Pentosan Polysulfate Sodium; Prostacyclin Analogues; Salicylates; Sugammadex; Thrombolytic Agents; Tibolone; Tipranavir; Urokinase; Vitamin E; Vitamin E (Oral); Vorapaxar

Decreased Effect

Fondaparinux may decrease the levels/effects of: Factor X (Human)

The levels/effects of Fondaparinux may be decreased by: Estrogen Derivatives; Progestins

Storage/Stability Store at 25°C (77°F); excursions permitted to 15°C to 30°C (59°F to 86°F).

Canadian labeling: Store <25°C (77°F); do not freeze. For IV infusion, use immediately once diluted in NS; can also be stored for up to 24 hours at 15°C to 30°C (59°F to 86°F).

Preparation for Administration Canadian labeling: For IV administration: May mix with 25 mL or 50 mL NS

Mechanism of Action Fondaparinux is a synthetic pentasaccharide that causes an antithrombin III-mediated selective inhibition of factor Xa. Neutralization of factor Xa interrupts the blood coagulation cascade and inhibits thrombin formation and thrombus development.

Pharmacodynamics/Kinetics

Absorption: SubQ: Rapid and complete

Distribution: V_d: 7 to 11 L; mainly in blood

Protein binding: ≥94% to antithrombin III

Bioavailability: SubQ: 100%

Half-life elimination: 17 to 21 hours; prolonged with renal impairment and in the elderly

Time to peak: SubQ: ~2 to 3 hours

Excretion: Urine (up to 77%, unchanged drug)

Dosing

Adult & Geriatric Note: PT and aPTT are insensitive measures of fondaparinux activity. If unexpected changes in coagulation parameters or major bleeding occur, discontinue fondaparinux.

DVT prophylaxis: SubQ: Adults ≥50 kg: 2.5 mg once daily. **Note:** Prophylactic use contraindicated in patients <50 kg. Initiate dose after hemostasis has been established, no earlier than 6 to 8 hours postoperatively.

DVT prophylaxis with history of HIT (off-label use): SubQ: 2.5 mg once daily (Blackmer, 2009; Harenberg, 2004; Parody, 2003)

Usual duration: 5 to 9 days (up to 10 days following abdominal surgery or up to 11 days following hip fracture, hip replacement, or knee replacement was administered in clinical trials). The American College of Chest Physicians recommends a minimum of 10 to 14 days for patients undergoing total hip arthroplasty, total knee arthroplasty, or hip fracture surgery; extended duration of up to 35 days suggested (Guyatt, 2012).

Acute DVT/PE treatment: SubQ: **Note:** Start warfarin on the first or second treatment day and continue fondaparinux until INR is ≥2 for at least 24 hours (usually 5 to 7 days) (Guyatt, 2012):

<50 kg: 5 mg once daily

50 to 100 kg: 7.5 mg once daily

>100 kg: 10 mg once daily

Usual duration: 5 to 9 days (administered up to 26 days in clinical trials)

Acute coronary syndrome (Canadian labeling; off-label use in United States):

UA/NSTEMI: SubQ: 2.5 mg once daily; initiate as soon as possible after presentation; treat for the duration of hospitalization, up to 8 days (ACCF/AHA [Anderson, 2013]; Yusuf 2006a)

STEMI: IV: 2.5 mg once; subsequent doses (starting the following day): SubQ: 2.5 mg once daily; treat for the duration of the hospitalization, up to 8 days, or until revascularization (ACCF/AHA [O'Gara, 2013]; Yusuf, 2006b)

Note: Discontinue fondaparinux 24 hours prior to coronary artery bypass graft (CABG) surgery; instead, administer unfractionated heparin per institutional practice (ACCF/AHA [Anderson, 2013]).

Acute symptomatic superficial vein thrombosis (≥5 cm in length) of the legs (off-label use): SubQ: 2.5 mg once daily for 45 days (Decousus, 2010; Guyatt, 2012)

◀ **Acute thrombosis (unrelated to HIT) in patients with a past history of HIT (off-label use; Guyatt, 2012; Warkentin, 2011):** SubQ:

<50 kg: 5 mg once daily

50 to 100 kg: 7.5 mg once daily

>100 kg: 10 mg once daily

Renal Impairment

CrCl >50 mL/minute: There are no dosage adjustments provided in the manufacturer's labeling. Total clearance is reduced ~25% compared to patients with normal renal function.

CrCl 30 to 50 mL/minute: Use caution; total clearance ~40% lower compared to patients with normal renal function. When used for thromboprophylaxis, the American College of Chest Physicians suggests a 50% reduction in dose or use of low-dose heparin instead of fondaparinux (Garcia, 2012).

CrCl <30 mL/minute: Use is contraindicated.

Hepatic Impairment

Mild-to-moderate impairment (Child-Pugh class A and B): No dosage adjustment necessary; monitor for signs of bleeding.

Severe impairment (Child-Pugh class A and B): There are no dosage adjustment provided in the manufacturer's labeling (has not been studied). Use with caution; monitor closely for signs of bleeding.

Administration For SubQ administration; do **not** administer IM. Alternate injection sites. Do not expel air bubble from syringe before injection. Administer according to recommended regimen; when used for DVT prophylaxis, early initiation (before 6 hours after orthopedic surgery) has been associated with increased bleeding. For STEMI patients (Canadian labeling; off-label use in United States) may administer initial dose as IV push or mix in NS and infuse over 1 to 2 minutes; flush tubing with NS after infusion to ensure complete administration for fondaparinux.

To convert from IV unfractionated heparin (UFH) infusion to SubQ fondaparinux (Nutescu, 2007): Calculate specific dose for fondaparinux based on indication, discontinue UFH, and begin fondaparinux within 1 hour

To convert from SubQ fondaparinux to IV UFH infusion (Nutescu, 2007): Discontinue fondaparinux; calculate specific dose for IV UFH infusion based on indication; omit heparin bolus/loading dose

For subQ fondaparinux dosed every 24 hours: Start IV UFH infusion 22 to 23 hours after last dose of fondaparinux

Monitoring Parameters Periodically monitor CBC, platelet count, serum creatinine, and occult blood testing of stools. Anti-Xa activity of fondaparinux can be measured by the assay if fondaparinux is used as the calibrator.

Test Interactions International standards of heparin or LMWH are not the appropriate calibrators for antifactor Xa activity of fondaparinux.

Dosage Forms Excipient information presented when available (limited, particularly for generics); consult specific product labeling.

Solution, Subcutaneous, as sodium:

Generic: 2.5 mg/0.5 mL (0.5 mL); 5 mg/0.4 mL (0.4 mL); 7.5 mg/0.6 mL (0.6 mL); 10 mg/0.8 mL (0.8 mL)

Solution, Subcutaneous, as sodium [preservative free]:

Arixtra: 2.5 mg/0.5 mL (0.5 mL); 5 mg/0.4 mL (0.4 mL); 7.5 mg/0.6 mL (0.6 mL); 10 mg/0.8 mL (0.8 mL)

Generic: 2.5 mg/0.5 mL (0.5 mL); 5 mg/0.4 mL (0.4 mL); 7.5 mg/0.6 mL (0.6 mL); 10 mg/0.8 mL (0.8 mL)

◆ **Fondaparinux Sodium** *see* Fondaparinux *on page 753*

- ◆ **5-Formyl Tetrahydrofolate** *see* Leucovorin Calcium *on page 1023*
- ◆ **Fortaz** *see* CefTAZidime *on page 296*
- ◆ **Fortaz in D5W** *see* CefTAZidime *on page 296*
- ◆ **Fortical** *see* Calcitonin *on page 259*

Fosaprepitant (fos a PRE pi tant)

Related Information

Management of Chemotherapy-Induced Nausea and Vomiting in Adults *on page 2142*

Brand Names: US Emend

Brand Names: Canada Emend® IV

Index Terms Aprepitant Injection; Fosaprepitant Dimeglumine; L-758,298; MK 0517

Pharmacologic Category Antiemetic; Substance P/Neurokinin 1 Receptor Antagonist

Use Prevention of acute and delayed nausea and vomiting associated with moderately- and highly-emetogenic chemotherapy (in combination with other antiemetics)

Labeled Contraindications Hypersensitivity to fosaprepitant, aprepitant, polysorbate 80, or any component of the formulation; concurrent use with pimozide or cisapride

Canadian labeling: Additional contraindications (not in U.S. labeling): Concurrent use with astemizole or terfenadine

Pregnancy Considerations Adverse events were not observed in animal reproduction studies for aprepitant. Efficacy of hormonal contraceptive may be reduced; alternative or additional methods of contraception should be used both during treatment with fosaprepitant or aprepitant and for at least 1 month following the last fosaprepitant/aprepitant dose.

Breast-Feeding Considerations It is not known if fosaprepitant is excreted in breast milk. Due to the potential for serious adverse reactions in the nursing infant, the manufacturer recommends a decision be made whether to discontinue nursing or to discontinue the drug, taking into account the importance of treatment to the mother.

Warnings/Precautions Fosaprepitant is rapidly converted to aprepitant, which has a high potential for drug interactions. Potentially significant drug-drug interactions may exist, requiring dose or frequency adjustment, additional monitoring, and/or selection of alternative therapy. Immediate hypersensitivity has been reported (rarely) with fosaprepitant; stop infusion with hypersensitivity symptoms (dyspnea, erythema, flushing, or anaphylaxis); do not reinitiate. Some dosage forms may contain polysorbate 80 (also known as Tweens). Hypersensitivity reactions, usually a delayed reaction, have been reported following exposure to pharmaceutical products containing polysorbate 80 in certain individuals (Isaksson, 2002; Lucente 2000; Shelley, 1995). Thrombocytopenia, ascites, pulmonary deterioration, and renal and hepatic failure have been reported in premature neonates after receiving parenteral products containing polysorbate 80 (Alade, 1986; CDC, 1984). See manufacturer's labeling. Use caution with hepatic impairment; has not been studied in patients with severe hepatic impairment (Child-Pugh class C). Not studied for treatment of existing nausea and vomiting. Chronic continuous administration of fosaprepitant is not recommended.

◄ **Adverse Reactions** Adverse reactions reported with aprepitant and fosaprepitant (as part of a combination chemotherapy regimen) occurring at a higher frequency than standard antiemetic therapy:

1% to 10%:

Central nervous system: Fatigue (1% to 3%), headache (2%)

Gastrointestinal: Anorexia (2%), constipation (2%), dyspepsia (2%), diarrhea (1%), eructation (1%)

Hepatic: ALT increased (1% to 3%), AST increased (1%)

Local: Injection site reactions (3%; includes erythema, induration, pain, pruritus, or thrombophlebitis)

Neuromuscular & skeletal: Weakness (3%)

Miscellaneous: Hiccups (5%)

<1%, postmarketing, and/or case reports: Abdominal distention, abdominal pain, acid reflux, acne, alkaline phosphatase increased, anaphylactic reaction, anemia, angioedema, anxiety, bradycardia, candidiasis, cardiovascular disorder, chest discomfort, chills, cognitive disorder, conjunctivitis, cough, disorientation, dizziness, dream abnormality, duodenal ulcer (perforating), dysarthria, dyspnea, dysuria, edema, epigastric distress, erythema, euphoria, feces hard, flatulence, flushing, gait disturbance, gastroesophageal reflux disease, hematuria (microscopic), hot flush, hyperglycemia, hyperhidrosis, hypersensitivity reaction, hypertension, hypoesthesia, hyponatremia, insomnia, lethargy, malaise, miosis, muscle cramp, muscular weakness, myalgia, nausea, neutropenia, neutropenic colitis, neutropenic fever, obstipation, palpitation, pharyngitis, photosensitivity, pollakiuria, polydipsia, polyuria, postnasal drip, pruritus, rash, sensory disturbance, skin lesion, skin oily, sneezing, somnolence, staphylococcal infection, Stevens-Johnson syndrome, stomatitis, subileus, taste alteration, throat irritation, tinnitus, toxic epidermal necrolysis, urticaria, visual acuity decreased, vomiting, weight gain/loss, wheezing, xerostomia

Drug Interactions

Metabolism/Transport Effects Substrate of CYP1A2 (minor), CYP2C19 (minor), CYP3A4 (major); **Note:** Assignment of Major/Minor substrate status based on clinically relevant drug interaction potential; **Inhibits** CYP2C19 (weak), CYP2C9 (weak), CYP3A4 (weak); **Induces** CYP2C9 (weak/moderate), CYP3A4 (weak)

Avoid Concomitant Use

Avoid concomitant use of Fosaprepitant with any of the following: Astemizole; Cisapride; Conivaptan; Fusidic Acid (Systemic); Idelalisib; Pimozide; Terfenadine

Increased Effect/Toxicity

Fosaprepitant may increase the levels/effects of: Astemizole; Cisapride; Corticosteroids (Systemic); CYP3A4 Substrates; Diltiazem; Dofetilide; Flibanserin; Hydrocodone; Ifosfamide; Lomitapide; NiMODipine; Pimozide; Sirolimus; Terfenadine

The levels/effects of Fosaprepitant may be increased by: Aprepitant; Conivaptan; CYP3A4 Inhibitors (Moderate); CYP3A4 Inhibitors (Strong); Dasatinib; Diltiazem; Fusidic Acid (Systemic); Idelalisib; Ivacaftor; Luliconazole; Mifepristone; Netupitant; Osimertinib; Palbociclib; Simeprevir; Stiripentol

Decreased Effect

Fosaprepitant may decrease the levels/effects of: ARIPiprazole; Contraceptives (Estrogens); Contraceptives (Progestins); Hydrocodone; NiMODipine; PARoxetine; Saxagliptin; TOLBUTamide; Warfarin

The levels/effects of Fosaprepitant may be decreased by: Bosentan; CYP3A4 Inducers (Moderate); CYP3A4 Inducers (Strong); Dabrafenib; Deferasirox; Enzalutamide; Mitotane; Osimertinib; PARoxetine; Rifampin; Siltuximab; St Johns Wort; Tocilizumab

Food Interactions Aprepitant serum concentration may be increased when taken with grapefruit juice. Management: Avoid concurrent use.

Storage/Stability Store intact vials at 2°C to 8°C (36°F to 46°F). Solutions diluted to 1 mg/mL for infusion are stable for 24 hours at room temperature or at ≤25°C (≤77°F). Solutions diluted to a final volume of 250 mL (0.6 mg/mL) should be administered within 24 hours (data on file [Merck, 2013]).

Preparation for Administration Reconstitute vial with 5 mL of sodium chloride 0.9%, directing diluent down side of vial to avoid foaming; swirl gently. Add reconstituted contents of the 150 mg vial to 145 mL sodium chloride 0.9%, resulting in a final concentration of 1 mg/mL; gently invert bag to mix. Solutions may be diluted to a final volume of 250 mL (0.6 mg/mL) (data on file [Merck, 2013]).

Mechanism of Action Fosaprepitant is a prodrug of aprepitant, a substance P/neurokinin 1 (NK1) receptor antagonist. It is rapidly converted to aprepitant which prevents acute and delayed vomiting by inhibiting the substance P/neurokinin 1 (NK1) receptor; augments the antiemetic activity of the 5-HT$_3$ receptor antagonist and corticosteroid activity and inhibits chemotherapy-induced emesis.

Pharmacodynamics/Kinetics

Distribution: Fosaprepitant: ~5 L; Aprepitant: V_d: ~70 L; crosses the blood-brain barrier

Protein binding: Aprepitant: >95%

Metabolism:

Fosaprepitant: Hepatic and extrahepatic; rapidly (within 30 minutes after the end of infusion) converted to aprepitant (nearly complete conversion)

Aprepitant: Hepatic via CYP3A4 (major); CYP1A2 and CYP2C19 (minor); forms 7 weakly-active metabolites

Half-life elimination: Fosaprepitant: ~2 minutes; Aprepitant: ~9-13 hours

Time to peak, plasma: Fosaprepitant is converted to aprepitant within 30 minutes after the end of infusion

Excretion: Urine (57%); feces (45%)

Dosing

Adult & Geriatric Prevention of chemotherapy-induced nausea/vomiting: IV:

Single-dose regimen for highly-emetogenic chemotherapy: 150 mg ~30 minutes prior to chemotherapy on day 1 only (in combination with a 5-HT$_3$ antagonist on day 1 and dexamethasone on days 1 to 4)

Single-dose regimen for moderately-emetogenic chemotherapy: 150 mg ~30 minutes prior to chemotherapy on day 1 only (in combination with a 5-HT$_3$ antagonist and dexamethasone on day 1, and either a 5-HT$_3$ antagonist or dexamethasone on days 2 and 3) (NCCN Antiemesis guidelines v.1.2013)

◀ **Renal Impairment**
Mild, moderate, or severe impairment: No dosage adjustment necessary.
Dialysis-dependent end-stage renal disease (ESRD): No dosage adjustment necessary.

Hepatic Impairment
Mild or moderate impairment (Child-Pugh class A or B): No dosage adjustment necessary.
Severe impairment (Child-Pugh class C): Has not been evaluated; use with caution.

Administration 150 mg: Infuse over 20-30 minutes ~30 minutes prior to chemotherapy

Dosage Forms Excipient information presented when available (limited, particularly for generics); consult specific product labeling.
Solution Reconstituted, Intravenous:
Emend: 150 mg (1 ea) [contains disodium edta, polysorbate 80]

♦ **Fosaprepitant Dimeglumine** *see* Fosaprepitant *on page 759*

Foscarnet (fos KAR net)

Brand Names: US Foscavir
Brand Names: Canada Foscavir
Index Terms Foscavir; PFA; Phosphonoformate; Phosphonoformic Acid
Pharmacologic Category Antiviral Agent
Use
Cytomegalovirus retinitis: Treatment of cytomegalovirus (CMV) retinitis in persons with AIDS
Herpes simplex virus: Treatment of acyclovir-resistant mucocutaneous herpes simplex virus (HSV) infections in immunocompromised persons (eg, with advanced AIDS)
Pregnancy Risk Factor C
Dosing
Adult & Geriatric
Cytomegalovirus (CMV) retinitis: IV:
Induction treatment: 60 mg/kg/dose every 8 hours for 14 to 21 days **or** 90 mg/kg every 12 hours for 14 to 21 days
Maintenance therapy: 90 to 120 mg/kg/day as a single daily infusion; due to lower toxicity, begin with 90 mg/kg once daily, may escalate to 120 mg/kg once daily if lower dose tolerated or for retinitis progression
CMV infection (preemptive therapy) after allogeneic stem cell transplantation (off-label use; second-line therapy): IV:
<100 days posttransplant: Induction: 60 mg/kg every 12 hours for 7 to 14 days, followed by maintenance therapy: 90 mg/kg once daily if CMV is still detectable and declining, continue until indicator test is negative. Minimum total duration (induction and maintenance) is 2 weeks (Tomblyn 2009)
>100 days posttransplant: 60 mg/kg every 12 hours for 14 days, continue treatment with 90 mg/kg once daily for 7 to 14 days or until indicator test is negative (Tomblyn 2009)
CMV infection (prophylaxis) after allogeneic stem cell transplantation (off-label use; second-line therapy): IV: 60 mg/kg every 12 hours for 7 days, followed by 90 to 120 mg/kg once daily until day 100 after transplant (Tomblyn 2009)

CMV esophagitis or colitis in HIV-infected patients (alternative to preferred therapy) (off-label use): IV: 60 mg/kg/dose every 8 hours or 90 mg/kg/dose every 12 hours for 21 to 42 days or until symptom resolution (HHS [OI adult 2015])

CMV neurological disease in HIV-infected patients (off-label use): IV: 60 mg/kg/dose every 8 hours or 90 mg/kg/dose every 12 hours plus ganciclovir until symptoms improve followed by chronic maintenance suppression (secondary prophylaxis) (HHS [OI adult 2015])

Herpes simplex infections (acyclovir-resistant): Induction: IV: 40 mg/kg/dose every 8 to 12 hours for 14 to 21 days

Pediatric

Cytomegalovirus (CMV) infection (preemptive therapy) after allogeneic stem cell transplantation (off-label use; second-line therapy): IV:

<100 days posttransplant: Induction: 60 mg/kg every 12 hours for 7 to 14 days, followed by maintenance therapy: 90 mg/kg once daily if CMV is still detectable and declining, continue until indicator test is negative. Minimum total duration (induction and maintenance) is 2 weeks (Tomblyn 2009)

>100 days posttransplant: 60 mg/kg every 12 hours for 14 days, continue treatment with 90 mg/kg once daily for 7 to 14 days or until indicator test is negative (Tomblyn 2009)

CMV infection (prophylaxis) after allogeneic stem cell transplantation (off-label use; second-line therapy): IV: 60 mg/kg every 12 hours for 7 days, followed by 90 to 120 mg/kg once daily until day 100 after transplant (Tomblyn 2009)

CMV esophagitis or colitis in HIV-infected patients (alternative to preferred therapy) (off-label use): Adolescents: Refer to adult dosing.

CMV neurological disease in HIV-infected patients (off-label use): Adolescents: Refer to adult dosing

Renal Impairment See tables below and on next page.

Induction Dosing of Foscarnet in Patients With Abnormal Renal Function

CrCl (mL/min/kg)	HSV Equivalent to 40 mg/kg every 12 hours	HSV Equivalent to 40 mg/kg every 8 hours	CMV Equivalent to 60 mg/kg every 8 hours	CMV Equivalent to 90 mg/kg every 12 hours
<0.4	Not recommended	Not recommended	Not recommended	Not recommended
≥0.4-0.5	20 mg/kg every 24 hours	35 mg/kg every 24 hours	50 mg/kg every 24 hours	50 mg/kg every 24 hours
>0.5-0.6	25 mg/kg every 24 hours	40 mg/kg every 24 hours	60 mg/kg every 24 hours	60 mg/kg every 24 hours
>0.6-0.8	35 mg/kg every 24 hours	25 mg/kg every 12 hours	40 mg/kg every 12 hours	80 mg/kg every 24 hours
>0.8-1	20 mg/kg every 12 hours	35 mg/kg every 12 hours	50 mg/kg every 12 hours	50 mg/kg every 12 hours
>1-1.4	30 mg/kg every 12 hours	30 mg/kg every 8 hours	45 mg/kg every 8 hours	70 mg/kg every 12 hours
>1.4	40 mg/kg every 12 hours	40 mg/kg every 8 hours	60 mg/kg every 8 hours	90 mg/kg every 12 hours

◀ ## Maintenance Dosing of Foscarnet in Patients With Abnormal Renal Function

CrCl (mL/min/kg)	CMV Equivalent to 90 mg/kg every 24 hours	CMV Equivalent to 120 mg/kg every 24 hours
<0.4	Not recommended	Not recommended
≥0.4-0.5	50 mg/kg every 48 hours	65 mg/kg every 48 hours
>0.5-0.6	60 mg/kg every 48 hours	80 mg/kg every 48 hours
>0.6-0.8	80 mg/kg every 48 hours	105 mg/kg every 48 hours
>0.8-1	50 mg/kg every 24 hours	65 mg/kg every 24 hours
>1-1.4	70 mg/kg every 24 hours	90 mg/kg every 24 hours
>1.4	90 mg/kg every 24 hours	120 mg/kg every 24 hours

Hemodialysis:
Foscarnet is highly removed by hemodialysis (up to ~38% in 2.5 hours HD with high-flux membrane)
Doses of 50 mg/kg/dose posthemodialysis have been found to produce similar serum concentrations as doses of 90 mg/kg twice daily in patients with normal renal function
Doses of 60-90 mg/kg/dose loading dose (posthemodialysis) followed by 45-60 mg/kg/dose posthemodialysis (3 times/week) with the monitoring of weekly plasma concentrations to maintain peak plasma concentrations in the range of 400-800 μMolar have been recommended by some clinicians
Continuous arteriovenous or venovenous hemodiafiltration effects: Dose as for CrCl 10-50 mL/minute
Hepatic Impairment There are no dosage adjustments provided in manufacturer's labeling.
Additional Information Complete prescribing information should be consulted for additional detail.
Dosage Forms Excipient information presented when available (limited, particularly for generics); consult specific product labeling. [DSC] = Discontinued product
Solution, Intravenous, as sodium:
Generic: 24 mg/mL (500 mL [DSC])
Solution, Intravenous, as sodium [preservative free]:
Foscavir: 24 mg/mL (250 mL)
Generic: 24 mg/mL (250 mL [DSC])

◆ **5-FUDR** see Floxuridine on page 722

Fulvestrant (fool VES trant)

Related Information

Common Toxicity Criteria on page 2122

Safe Handling of Hazardous Drugs on page 2292

Brand Names: US Faslodex

Brand Names: Canada Faslodex

Index Terms ICI-182,780; ZD9238

Pharmacologic Category Antineoplastic Agent, Estrogen Receptor Antagonist

Use Breast cancer, metastatic: Treatment of hormone-receptor-positive metastatic breast cancer in postmenopausal women with disease progression following antiestrogen therapy

Labeled Contraindications Known hypersensitivity to fulvestrant or any component of the formulation

Pregnancy Considerations Adverse events were observed in animal reproduction studies. Fulvestrant is approved for use only in postmenopausal women. If used prior to confirmed menopause, women of reproductive potential should be advised not to become pregnant. Based on the mechanism of action, may cause fetal harm if administered during pregnancy.

Breast-Feeding Considerations Approved for use only in postmenopausal women. Because of the potential for serious adverse reactions in the nursing infant, a decision should be made to discontinue breast-feeding or the drug, taking into account the importance of treatment to the mother.

Warnings/Precautions Hazardous agent - use appropriate precautions for handling and disposal (NIOSH 2014 [group 1]). Exposure is increased and dosage adjustment is recommended in patients with moderate hepatic impairment. Safety and efficacy have not been established in severe hepatic impairment. Use with caution in patients with a history of bleeding disorders (including thrombocytopenia) and/or patients on anticoagulant therapy; bleeding/hematoma may occur from IM administration. Hypersensitivity reactions, including urticaria and angioedema, have been reported.

Benzyl alcohol and derivatives: Some dosage forms may contain benzyl alcohol; large amounts of benzyl alcohol (≥99 mg/kg/day) have been associated with a potentially fatal toxicity ("gasping syndrome") in neonates; the "gasping syndrome" consists of metabolic acidosis, respiratory distress, gasping respirations, CNS dysfunction (including convulsions, intracranial hemorrhage), hypotension and cardiovascular collapse (AAP ["Inactive" 1997]; CDC, 1982); some data suggests that benzoate displaces bilirubin from protein binding sites (Ahlfors 2001); avoid or use dosage forms containing benzyl alcohol with caution in neonates. See manufacturer's labeling.

Adverse Reactions Adverse reactions reported with 500 mg dose.

>10%:

Endocrine & metabolic: Hot flushes (7% to 13%)

Hepatic: Alkaline phosphatase increased (>15%; grades 3/4: 1% to 2%), transaminases increased (>15%; grades 3/4: 1% to 2%)

Local: Injection site pain (12% to 14%)

Neuromuscular & skeletal: Joint disorders (14% to 19%)

1% to 10%:

Cardiovascular: Ischemic disorder (1%)

Central nervous system: Fatigue (8%), headache (8%)

◄ Gastrointestinal: Nausea (10%), anorexia (6%), vomiting (6%), constipation (5%), weight gain (≤1%)

Genitourinary: Urinary tract infection (2% to 4%)

Neuromuscular & skeletal: Bone pain (9%), arthralgia (8%), back pain (8%), extremity pain (7%), musculoskeletal pain (6%), weakness (6%)

Respiratory: Cough (5%), dyspnea (4%)

<1%, postmarketing, and/or case reports (reported with 250 mg or 500 mg dose): Angioedema, bilirubin increased, GGT increased, hepatitis, hypersensitivity reactions, leukopenia, liver failure, myalgia, osteoporosis, thrombosis, urticaria, vaginal bleeding, vertigo

Drug Interactions

Metabolism/Transport Effects Substrate of CYP3A4 (minor); **Note:** Assignment of Major/Minor substrate status based on clinically relevant drug interaction potential

Avoid Concomitant Use There are no known interactions where it is recommended to avoid concomitant use.

Increased Effect/Toxicity There are no known significant interactions involving an increase in effect.

Decreased Effect There are no known significant interactions involving a decrease in effect.

Storage/Stability Store in original carton at 2°C to 8°C (36°F to 46°F). Protect from light.

Mechanism of Action Estrogen receptor antagonist; competitively binds to estrogen receptors on tumors and other tissue targets, producing a nuclear complex that causes a dose-related down-regulation of estrogen receptors and inhibits tumor growth.

Pharmacodynamics/Kinetics

Duration: IM: Steady state concentrations reached within first month, when administered with additional dose given 2 weeks following the initial dose; plasma levels maintained for at least 1 month

Distribution: V_d: ~3 to 5 L/kg

Protein binding: 99%; to plasma proteins (VLDL, LDL and HDL lipoprotein fractions)

Metabolism: Hepatic via multiple biotransformation pathways (CYP3A4 substrate involved in oxidation pathway, although relative contribution to metabolism unknown); metabolites formed are either less active or have similar activity to parent compound

Half-life elimination: 250 mg: ~40 days

Excretion: Feces (~90%); urine (<1%)

Dosing

Adult & Geriatric Breast cancer, metastatic (postmenopausal women): IM: Initial: 500 mg on days 1, 15, and 29; Maintenance: 500 mg once monthly. In studies, the 500 mg once monthly dose was administered at 28 days ± 3 days (Di Leo, 2014).

Breast cancer, advanced, second-line endocrine-based combination therapy (relapsed or progressive on prior endocrine therapy; off-label combination): Adults (females, HER-2 negative): IM: 500 mg every 14 days for 3 doses, then every 28 days (in combination with palbociclib [and goserelin if pre- or peri-menopausal]); continue until disease progression or unacceptable toxicity (Turner 2015).

Renal Impairment There are no dosage adjustments provided in the manufacturer's labeling (has not been studied). However, renal elimination of fulvestrant is negligible.

Hepatic Impairment

Mild impairment (Child-Pugh class A): No dosage adjustment is necessary.

Moderate impairment (Child-Pugh class B): Reduce initial doses and maintenance dose to 250 mg.

Severe impairment (Child-Pugh class C): There are no dosage adjustments provided in the manufacturer's labeling (use has not been evaluated).

Combination Regimens

Breast cancer: Palbociclib-Fulvestrant (Breast) on page 2057

Administration For IM administration only. Administer 500 mg dose as two 5 mL IM injections (one in each buttocks) slowly over 1 to 2 minutes per injection.

Hazardous agent; use appropriate precautions for handling and disposal (NIOSH 2014 [group 1]).

Dosage Forms Excipient information presented when available (limited, particularly for generics); consult specific product labeling.

Solution, Intramuscular:

Faslodex: 250 mg/5 mL (5 mL) [contains alcohol, usp, benzyl alcohol, benzyl benzoate]

♦ **Fungizone (Can)** see Amphotericin B (Conventional) on page 95

♦ **Fusilev** see LEVOleucovorin on page 1041

♦ **FXIII** see Factor XIII Concentrate (Human) on page 688

♦ **GA101** see Obinutuzumab on page 1220

♦ **^{67}Ga-Citrate** see Gallium Citrate Ga-67 on page 767

♦ **^{67}Ga-Gallium Citrate** see Gallium Citrate Ga-67 on page 767

Gallium Citrate Ga-67 (GAL ee um SIT rate jee aye SIX tee SEV en)

Index Terms ^{67}Ga-Citrate; ^{67}Ga-Gallium Citrate

Pharmacologic Category Radiopharmaceutical

Use Diagnostic imaging of Hodgkin's disease, lymphoma, bronchogenic carcinoma, and inflammatory lesions to identify fevers of unknown origin; nonbacterial infections

Pregnancy Risk Factor C

Dosing

Adult IV (based on 70 kg patient): 2-5 mCi (74-185 MBq). For tumors, dose may be 5-10 mCi (185-370 MBq).

Pediatric IV: 0.04-0.07 mCi/kg (1.5-2.6 MBq/kg)

Renal Impairment No dosage adjustment provided in manufacturer's labeling.

Hepatic Impairment No dosage adjustment provided in manufacturer's labeling.

Additional Information Complete prescribing information should be consulted for additional detail.

♦ **GamaSTAN S/D** see Immune Globulin on page 903

♦ **Gamastan S/D (Can)** see Immune Globulin on page 903

♦ **Gammagard** see Immune Globulin on page 903

♦ **Gammagard Liquid (Can)** see Immune Globulin on page 903

- ◆ **Gammagard S/D [DSC]** *see* Immune Globulin *on page 903*
- ◆ **Gammagard S/D (Can)** *see* Immune Globulin *on page 903*
- ◆ **Gammagard S/D Less IgA** *see* Immune Globulin *on page 903*
- ◆ **Gamma Globulin** *see* Immune Globulin *on page 903*
- ◆ **Gammaked** *see* Immune Globulin *on page 903*
- ◆ **Gammaphos** *see* Amifostine *on page 85*
- ◆ **Gammaplex** *see* Immune Globulin *on page 903*
- ◆ **Gamunex [DSC]** *see* Immune Globulin *on page 903*
- ◆ **Gamunex (Can)** *see* Immune Globulin *on page 903*
- ◆ **Gamunex-C** *see* Immune Globulin *on page 903*

Ganciclovir (Systemic) (gan SYE kloe veer)

Brand Names: US Cytovene
Brand Names: Canada Cytovene; Ganciclovir for Injection
Index Terms DHPG Sodium; GCV Sodium; Nordeoxyguanosine
Pharmacologic Category Antiviral Agent
Use Treatment of CMV retinitis in immunocompromised individuals, including patients with acquired immunodeficiency syndrome; prophylaxis of CMV infection in transplant patients
Pregnancy Risk Factor C
Dosing
Adult & Geriatric
CMV retinitis:
Manufacturer's labeling:
Induction therapy: IV (slow infusion): 5 mg/kg/dose every 12 hours for 14 to 21 days followed by maintenance therapy
Maintenance therapy: IV (slow infusion): 5 mg/kg/day as a single daily dose for 7 days/week or 6 mg/kg/day for 5 days/week
Alternate dosing (HHS [OI adult 2015]):
Peripheral lesions (alternative to preferred therapy): IV: Induction: 5 mg/kg/dose every 12 hours for 14 to 21 days followed by chronic maintenance (secondary prophylaxis)
Immediate sight-threatening lesions (adjacent to the optic nerve or fovea): Intravitreal injection (off-label route): Induction therapy: 2 mg of an extemporaneously prepared solution administered as intravitreal injections for 1 to 4 doses over a period of 7 to 10 days; administer with a concomitant systemically administered agent (oral valganciclovir preferred).
CMV disease, chronic maintenance (secondary prophylaxis) in HIV-infected patients (off-label use; alternative to preferred therapy): IV: 5 mg/kg/dose 5 to 7 times weekly; continue until sustained CD4 count >100 cells/mm^3 in response to ART for 3 to 6 months; discontinue only after consultation with an ophthalmologist (HHS [OI adult 2015]).
CMV disease, prophylaxis (secondary) in transplant patients: IV (slow infusion): 5 mg/kg/dose every 12 hours for 7 to 14 days, duration of maintenance therapy is dependent on clinical condition and degree of immunosuppression
CMV esophagitis or colitis in HIV-infected patients (off-label use): IV: 5 mg/kg/dose every 12 hours, then change to oral valganciclovir therapy once oral therapy is tolerated (HHS [OI adult 2015])

CMV neurological disease in HIV-infected patients (off-label use): IV: 5 mg/kg/dose every 12 hours plus foscarnet until symptoms improve (HHS [OI adult 2015])

Varicella-zoster: Acute retinal necrosis (ARN) in HIV-infected patients (off-label use): Intravitreal injection (off-label route): 2 mg of an extemporaneously prepared solution administered as an intravitreal injection twice weekly for 1 to 2 doses in combination with IV acyclovir for 10 to 14 days, followed by valacyclovir for 6 weeks (HHS [OI adult 2015])

Varicella-zoster: Progressive outer retinal necrosis in HIV-infected patients (off-label use): IV: 5 mg/kg/dose every 12 hours (with or without foscarnet IV) **plus** intravitreal ganciclovir and/or intravitreal foscarnet (HHS [OI adult 2015])

Pediatric

CMV retinitis:

Children: IV (slow infusion): Manufacturer's labeling:
  Induction therapy: 5 mg/kg/dose every 12 hours for 14 to 21 days followed by maintenance therapy
  Maintenance therapy: 5 mg/kg/day as a single daily dose for 7 days/week or 6 mg/kg/day for 5 days/week
Adolescents: Refer to adult dosing.

CMV disease, chronic maintenance (secondary prophylaxis) in HIV-exposed/-infected patients (off-label use):

Infants and Children: IV: 5 mg/kg/dose daily (CDC 2009)
Adolescents (alternative to preferred therapy): Refer to adult dosing.

CMV disease, prophylaxis (secondary) in transplant patients: Children: IV (slow infusion): Refer to adult dosing.

CMV esophagitis or colitis in HIV-infected patients (off-label use): Adolescents: Refer to adult dosing.

CMV neurological disease in HIV-exposed/-infected patients (off-label use): Infants, Children, and Adolescents: IV: Refer to adult dosing.

Varicella-zoster: Acute retinal necrosis (ARN) in HIV-infected patients (off-label use): Adolescents: Refer to adult dosing.

Varicella-zoster: Progressive outer retinal necrosis in HIV-exposed/-infected patients (off-label use):

Infants and Children: IV: 5 mg/kg/dose every 12 hours plus systemic foscarnet and intravitreal ganciclovir or intravitreal foscarnet (CDC 2009)
Adolescents: Refer to adult dosing.

Renal Impairment

IV (Induction):

CrCl 50 to 69 mL/minute: Administer 2.5 mg/kg/dose every 12 hours.
CrCl 25 to 49 mL/minute: Administer 2.5 mg/kg/dose every 24 hours.
CrCl 10 to 24 mL/minute: Administer 1.25 mg/kg/dose every 24 hours.
CrCl <10 mL/minute: Administer 1.25 mg/kg/dose 3 times/week following hemodialysis.

IV (Maintenance):

CrCl 50 to 69 mL/minute: Administer 2.5 mg/kg/dose every 24 hours.
CrCl 25 to 49 mL/minute: Administer 1.25 mg/kg/dose every 24 hours.
CrCl 10 to 24 mL/minute: Administer 0.625 mg/kg/dose every 24 hours
CrCl <10 mL/minute: Administer 0.625 mg/kg/dose 3 times/week following hemodialysis.

Intermittent hemodialysis (IHD) (administer after hemodialysis on dialysis days): Dialyzable (50%): CMV Infection: IV: Induction: 1.25 mg/kg every 48 to 72 hours; Maintenance: 0.625 mg/kg every 48 to 72 hours. **Note:** Dosing dependent on the assumption of 3 times/week, complete IHD sessions.

Peritoneal dialysis (PD): Dose as for CrCl <10 mL/minute.

Continuous renal replacement therapy (CRRT) (Heintz 2009; Trotman 2005): Drug clearance is highly dependent on the method of renal replacement, filter type, and flow rate. Appropriate dosing requires close monitoring of pharmacologic response, signs of adverse reactions due to drug accumulation, as well as drug concentrations in relation to target trough (if appropriate). The following are general recommendations only (based on dialysate flow/ultrafiltration rates of 1 to 2 L/hour and minimal residual renal function) and should not supersede clinical judgment: CMV Infection:

CVVH: IV: Induction: 2.5 mg/kg every 24 hours; Maintenance: 1.25 mg/kg every 24 hours

CVVHD/CVVHDF: IV: Induction: 2.5 mg/kg every 12 hours; Maintenance: 2.5 mg/kg every 24 hours

Hepatic Impairment No dosage adjustment provided in manufacturer's labeling.

Additional Information Complete prescribing information should be consulted for additional detail.

Dosage Forms Excipient information presented when available (limited, particularly for generics); consult specific product labeling.

Solution Reconstituted, Intravenous:

Cytovene: 500 mg (1 ea)

Generic: 500 mg (1 ea)

- ◆ **Ganciclovir for Injection (Can)** see Ganciclovir (Systemic) on page 768
- ◆ **Gardasil** see Papillomavirus (Types 6, 11, 16, 18) Vaccine (Human, Recombinant) on page 1330
- ◆ **Gardasil 9** see Papillomavirus (9-Valent) Vaccine (Human, Recombinant) on page 1328
- ◆ **Gazyva** see Obinutuzumab on page 1220
- ◆ **G-CSF** see Filgrastim on page 711
- ◆ **G-CSF (PEG Conjugate)** see Pegfilgrastim on page 1346
- ◆ **GCV Sodium** see Ganciclovir (Systemic) on page 768
- ◆ **GDC-0449** see Vismodegib on page 1771
- ◆ **GDC-0973** see Cobimetinib on page 357

Gefitinib (ge FI tye nib)
Related Information
Common Toxicity Criteria on page 2122

Management of Chemotherapy-Induced Nausea and Vomiting in Adults on page 2142

Management of EGFR Inhibitor Toxicities: Dermatologic, Ocular, and Gastrointestinal on page 2179

Prevention of Chemotherapy-Induced Nausea and Vomiting in Children on page 2203

Safe Handling of Hazardous Drugs on page 2292

Brand Names: US Iressa

Brand Names: Canada IRESSA
Index Terms ZD1839
Pharmacologic Category Antineoplastic Agent, Epidermal Growth Factor Receptor (EGFR) Inhibitor; Antineoplastic Agent, Tyrosine Kinase Inhibitor
Use

Non-small cell lung cancer:

US labeling: First-line treatment of metastatic non-small cell lung cancer (NSCLC) in tumors with epidermal growth factor receptor (EGFR) exon 19 deletions or exon 21 (L858R) substitution mutations as detected by an approved test.

Limitation of use: Safety and efficacy have not been established in patients with metastatic NSCLC whose tumors have EGFR mutations other than exon 19 deletions or exon 21 (L858R) substitution mutations

Canadian labeling: First-line treatment of locally advanced (nonresponsive to curative therapy) or metastatic NSCLC with activating mutations of the epidermal growth factor receptor tyrosine kinase (EGFR-TK).

Labeled Contraindications There are no contraindications listed in the manufacturer's US labeling.

Canadian labeling: Hypersensitivity to gefitinib or any component of the formulation.

Pregnancy Considerations Adverse events have been observed in animal reproduction studies. Gefitinib may cause fetal harm when administered to a pregnant woman. Women of reproductive potential should use effective contraception during and for at least 2 weeks following gefitinib treatment.

Breast-Feeding Considerations It is not known if gefitinib is excreted in breast milk. Due to the potential for serious adverse reactions in the nursing infant, breast-feeding is not recommended by the manufacturer.

Warnings/Precautions Hazardous agent - use appropriate precautions for handling and disposal (meets NIOSH 2014 criteria).

Interstitial lung disease (ILD) or ILD-like reactions (eg, acute respiratory distress syndrome, lung infiltration, pneumonitis, or pulmonary fibrosis) have occurred (rarely) with gefitinib; some cases were grade 3 or higher and some were fatal. Withhold gefitinib and promptly assess any patient with worsening respiratory symptoms (dyspnea, cough and fever); discontinue permanently if ILD is confirmed. Increased systemic gefitinib exposure is associated with an increased incidence of ILD. An increase in mortality was observed in patients with the following risk factors: Smoking, CT scan evidence of reduced normal lung (≤50%), preexisting ILD, increased age (≥65 years), and extensive areas adherent to pleura (≥50%).

Increases in ALT, AST, and bilirubin, including grade 3 or higher toxicity have been observed. Fatal hepatotoxicity has occurred rarely. Monitor liver functions tests periodically. Withhold gefitinib in patients with worsening liver function; discontinue for severe hepatic impairment. Gefitinib exposure is increased in patients with mild, moderate, and severe hepatic impairment due to cirrhosis. However, in a study of patients with liver metastases, patients with metastases and moderate impairment had similar systemic exposure as patients with metastases and normal hepatic function. Monitor for adverse reactions if administering to patients with moderate or severe hepatic impairment.

Gastrointestinal perforation has occurred (rarely); discontinue permanently if gastrointestinal perforation develops. Nausea, vomiting, decreased appetite, and stomatitis have also been reported. Diarrhea occurs in approximately one-third of patients; grade 3 or 4 diarrhea has been observed. Diarrhea symptoms should be managed as clinically indicated; avoid dehydration. Withhold gefitinib for severe or persistent (up to 14 days) diarrhea.

Ocular disorders, including keratitis, corneal erosion, abnormal eyelash growth, conjunctivitis, blepharitis, and dry eye have been reported; some events were grade 3. Recent corneal surgery and contact lens wearing may be risk factors for ocular toxicity. Advise patients to promptly report developing eye symptoms and promptly refer for ophthalmic evaluation if signs of keratitis (eg, acute or worsening of eye inflammation, lacrimation, blurred vision, pain, red eye, and/or light sensitivity). Interrupt gefitinib treatment or discontinue for severe or worsening ocular disorders. Skin reactions occurred in nearly one-half of patients taking gefitinib. Bullous skin disorders, including toxic epidermal necrolysis, Stevens Johnson syndrome, erythema multiforme, and dermatitis bullous have been reported. Interrupt gefitinib treatment or discontinue for development of severe bullous, blistering, or exfoliating dermatologic conditions.

Establish EGFR mutation status prior to treatment. Do not use in patients with EGFR mutation-negative tumors. Studies have demonstrated a subset of patients who are more likely to respond to gefitinib treatment. This subset includes patients of Asian origin, never-smokers, women, patients with bronchoalveolar adenocarcinoma, and patients with EGFR-mutated tumors. Deletion in exon 19 and mutation in exon 21 are the two most commonly found EGFR mutations; both mutations correlate with clinical response, resulting in increased response rates in patients with the mutation (Riely, 2006). Studies have compared gefitinib in treatment naïve patients to combination chemotherapy in the subsets of patients described above, resulting in a longer progression free survival in the gefitinib arm (Mok, 2009). Based on these data, the ASCO guidelines state that the first-line use of gefitinib may be recommended in stage IV disease with activating EGFR mutations (Azzoli, 2009; Azzoli, 2011). In patients with a KRAS mutation, however, EGFR-TKI therapy is not recommended.

Systemic exposure of gefitinib may be increased in CYP2D6 poor metabolizers; no dosage adjustment is recommended, although patients should be monitored closely for adverse reactions. Potentially significant drug-drug interactions may exist, requiring dose or frequency adjustment, additional monitoring, and/or selection of alternative therapy. Elevated gastric pH may reduce gefitinib plasma concentrations; if possible, avoid concomitant use with proton pump inhibitors. If proton pump inhibitor therapy is necessary, administer gefitinib 12 hours before or 12 hours after the proton pump inhibitor dose. May administer gefitinib 6 hours before or 6 hours after H_2-receptor antagonists or antacids. May contain lactose; consider intolerance risk in patients with galactose intolerance, Lapp lactase deficiency, or glucose-galactose malabsorption.

Adverse Reactions

>10%:

Central nervous system: Insomnia (15%), fatigue (14%)

Dermatologic: Dermatological reaction (58%; including pustular rash, itching, dry skin, skin fissures on an erythematous base), skin rash (52%), xeroderma (24%), pruritus (18%), paronychia (14%), acne vulgaris (11%), alopecia (5% to 11%)

Gastrointestinal: Diarrhea (35% to 47%), anorexia (19% to 20%), nausea (17% to 18%), vomiting (13% to 14%), stomatitis (11% to 13%), constipation (12%)

Hepatic: Increased serum ALT (11%)

Neuromuscular & skeletal: Weakness (18%)

1% to 10%:

Central nervous system: Hypoesthesia (4%), peripheral sensory neuropathy (4%), peripheral neuropathy (2%)

Dermatologic: Nail disease (8%), acneiform eruption (6%)

Endocrine & metabolic: Dehydration (2%; secondary to diarrhea, nausea, vomiting, or anorexia)

Gastrointestinal: Xerostomia (2%)

Genitourinary: Proteinuria (8%), cystitis (1%)

Hematologic & oncologic: Anemia (7%), pulmonary hemorrhage (4% to 5%), hemorrhage (4%; including epistaxis, hematuria), neutropenia (3%), leukopenia (2%), thrombocytopenia (1%)

Hepatic: Increased serum AST (8% to 9%), increased serum bilirubin (3%)

Neuromuscular & skeletal: Myalgia (8%), arthralgia (6%)

Ophthalmic: Eye disease (7%; including conjunctivitis, blepharitis, and dry eye)

Renal: Increased serum creatinine (2%)

Respiratory: Cough (9%), interstitial pulmonary disease (grades 3/4: 1% to 3%)

Miscellaneous: Fever (9%)

<1%, postmarketing, and/or case reports: Angioedema, bullous skin disease, corneal erosion (reversible; may be associated with aberrant eyelash growth), decreased white blood cell count, erythema multiforme, fulminant hepatitis, gastrointestinal perforation, hemorrhagic cystitis, hepatic failure, hepatitis, hypersensitivity angiitis, hypersensitivity reaction, keratitis, keratoconjunctivitis sicca, pancreatitis, renal failure, skin fissure, Stevens-Johnson syndrome, toxic epidermal necrolysis, urticaria

Drug Interactions

Metabolism/Transport Effects Substrate of BCRP, CYP2D6 (major), CYP3A4 (major); **Note:** Assignment of Major/Minor substrate status based on clinically relevant drug interaction potential; **Inhibits** BCRP, CYP2C19 (weak), CYP2D6 (weak)

Avoid Concomitant Use

Avoid concomitant use of Gefitinib with any of the following: Conivaptan; Fusidic Acid (Systemic); Idelalisib; PAZOPanib

Increased Effect/Toxicity

Gefitinib may increase the levels/effects of: ARIPiprazole; PAZOPanib; Topotecan; Vinorelbine; Vitamin K Antagonists

The levels/effects of Gefitinib may be increased by: Abiraterone Acetate; Aprepitant; Ceritinib; Cobicistat; Conivaptan; CYP2D6 Inhibitors (Moderate); CYP2D6 Inhibitors (Strong); CYP3A4 Inhibitors (Moderate); CYP3A4 Inhibitors (Strong); Darunavir; Dasatinib; Eltrombopag; Fosaprepitant; Fusidic Acid ▶

◀ (Systemic); Idelalisib; Ivacaftor; Luliconazole; Mifepristone; Netupitant; Osimertinib; Palbociclib; Panobinostat; Peginterferon Alfa-2b; Rolapitant; Simeprevir; Stiripentol; Teriflunomide

Decreased Effect

The levels/effects of Gefitinib may be decreased by: Antacids; Bosentan; CYP3A4 Inducers (Moderate); CYP3A4 Inducers (Strong); Dabrafenib; Deferasirox; Enzalutamide; H2-Antagonists; Mitotane; Osimertinib; Peginterferon Alfa-2b; Proton Pump Inhibitors; Siltuximab; St Johns Wort; Tocilizumab

Food Interactions Grapefruit juice may increase serum gefitinib concentrations. Management: Avoid concurrent use.

Storage/Stability Store at 20°C to 25°C (68°F to 77°F).

Mechanism of Action Gefitinib is a tyrosine kinase inhibitor (TKI) which reversibly inhibits kinase activity of wild-type and select activation mutations of epidermal growth factor receptor (EGFR). EGFR is expressed on cell surfaces of normal and cancer cells and has a role in cell growth and proliferation. Gefitinib prevents autophosphorylation of tyrosine residues associated with the EGFR receptor, which blocks downstream signaling and EGFR-dependent proliferation. Gefitinib has a higher binding affinity for EGFR exon 19 deletion and exon 21 (L858R) substitution mutation than for wild-type EGFR.

Pharmacodynamics/Kinetics

Absorption: Oral: Slow

Distribution: 1400 L

Protein binding: 90%, albumin and alpha$_1$-acid glycoprotein

Metabolism: Hepatic (extensive), primarily via CYP3A4, as well as CYP2D6; forms metabolites

Bioavailability: 60%

Half-life elimination: Oral: 41 hours

Time to peak, plasma: Oral: 3 to 7 hours

Excretion: Feces (86%); urine (<4%)

Dosing

Adult & Geriatric

Non-small cell lung cancer (NSCLC), metastatic, with EGFR exon 19 deletions or exon 21 (L858R) substitution mutations: Oral: 250 mg once daily until disease progression or unacceptable toxicity.

NSCLC, locally advanced or metastatic with EGFR mutations (Canadian labeling): Oral: 250 mg once daily.

Missed doses: Do not take a missed dose if it is within 12 hours of the next scheduled dose.

Dosage adjustment for concomitant therapy (US labeling): *Strong CYP3A4 inducers (eg, phenytoin, rifampin, or tricyclic antidepressants):* Increase gefitinib to 500 mg once daily (in the absence of severe adverse drug reactions); reduce gefitinib dose back to 250 mg once daily 7 days after discontinuing the strong CYP3A4 inducer.

Pediatric Non-small cell lung cancer (NSCLC), locally advanced or metastatic with EGFR mutations (Canadian labeling): Adolescents ≥17 years: Oral: Refer to Canadian adult dosing.

Renal Impairment

US labeling: There are no dosage adjustments provided in the manufacturer's labeling; however, due to minimal renal excretion (<4% of gefitinib and metabolites) the need for dosage adjustment is unlikely. Use has not been studied in patients with CrCl ≤20 mL/minute.

Canadian labeling: No dosage adjustment necessary. Use caution in severe impairment (CrCl ≤20 mL/minute).

Hepatic Impairment

Dosage adjustment for hepatic impairment at treatment initiation:

US labeling: There are no dosage adjustments provided in the manufacturer's labeling; systemic exposure is increased in hepatic impairment.

Canadian labeling: No dosage adjustment necessary. Use caution in moderate to severe impairment (Child-Pugh Class B or C) (systemic exposure may be increased); monitor closely.

Dosage adjustment for hepatotoxicity during treatment:

ALT and/or AST elevations (grade 2 or higher): Withhold treatment for up to 14 days; may resume treatment when fully resolved or improved to grade 1.

Severe hepatic impairment: Permanently discontinue.

Adjustment for Toxicity

Dermatologic toxicity:

Skin reactions (grade 3 or higher): Withhold treatment for up to 14 days; may resume treatment when fully resolved or improved to grade 1. *Canadian labeling:* Discontinue if unable to tolerate rechallenge following treatment interruption.

Severe bullous, blistering or exfoliating dermatologic conditions: Interrupt or discontinue treatment.

Gastrointestinal toxicity:

Diarrhea (grade 3 or higher): Withhold treatment for up to 14 days; may resume treatment when fully resolved or improved to grade 1. *Canadian labeling:* Discontinue if unable to tolerate rechallenge following treatment interruption.

Gastrointestinal perforation: Permanently discontinue.

Ocular toxicity:

Signs/symptoms of severe or worsening disorders, including keratitis: Withhold treatment for up to 14 days; may resume treatment when fully resolved or improved to grade 1. *Canadian labeling:* Discontinue if unable to tolerate rechallenge following treatment interruption.

Persistent ulcerative keratitis: Permanently discontinue.

Pulmonary toxicity:

Acute onset or worsening symptoms (dyspnea, cough, fever): Withhold treatment for up to 14 days; may resume treatment when fully resolved or improved to grade 1.

Interstitial lung disease (ILD), confirmed: Permanently discontinue.

Combination Regimens

Lung cancer (non-small cell): Gefitinib (NSCLC Regimen) on page 1989

Administration Oral: Administer with or without food.

For patients unable to swallow the tablet whole, place tablet in 120 to 240 mL water and stir for ~15 minutes; immediately drink the liquid or administer through a naso-gastric tube. Rinse the container with 120 to 240 mL water and immediately drink or administer through naso-gastric tube.

Hazardous agent; use appropriate precautions for handling and disposal (meets NIOSH 2014 criteria). When administering intact tablets, single gloves should be worn. If it is necessary to manipulate the tablets (eg, preparing an oral solution), it is recommended to double glove, wear a protective gown, and prepare in a controlled device (NIOSH, 2014).

Emetic Potential Children and Adults: Minimal (<10%)

Extemporaneous Preparations

Hazardous agent: Use appropriate precautions for handling and disposal (meets NIOSH 2014 criteria). When manipulating tablets, NIOSH recommends double gloving, a protective gown, and preparation in a controlled device; if not prepared in a controlled device, respiratory and eye protection as well as ventilated engineering controls are recommended (NIOSH 2014).

For patients unable to swallow the tablet whole, place tablet in 120 to 240 ml water and stir for ~15 minutes; immediately drink the liquid or administer through a naso-gastric tube. Rinse the container with 120 to 240 mL water and immediately drink or administer through naso-gastric tube.

Iressa (gefitinib) [prescribing information]. Wilmington, DE: AstraZeneca; July 2015.

Monitoring Parameters EGFR mutation status (prior to treatment initiation); liver function tests (ALT, AST, bilirubin at baseline and periodically thereafter); BUN, creatinine, and electrolytes (baseline and periodically thereafter); INR or prothrombin time (with concurrent warfarin treatment). Monitor for signs/symptoms of dermatologic toxicity, gastrointestinal perforation, ocular toxicity, and pulmonary toxicity; monitor closely for adverse reactions in CYP2D6 poor metabolizers and patients with hepatic impairment.

Dosage Forms Excipient information presented when available (limited, particularly for generics); consult specific product labeling.

Tablet, Oral:

Iressa: 250 mg

Dosage Forms: Canada Excipient information presented when available (limited, particularly for generics); consult specific product labeling.

Tablet, oral:

Iressa: 250 mg

◆ **Gelclair** see Mucosal Coating Agent on page 1175

Gemcitabine (jem SITE a been)

Related Information

Common Toxicity Criteria on page 2122

Management of Chemotherapy-Induced Nausea and Vomiting in Adults on page 2142

Management of Drug Extravasations on page 2159

Mucositis and Stomatitis on page 2186

Prevention of Chemotherapy-Induced Nausea and Vomiting in Children on page 2203

Safe Handling of Hazardous Drugs on page 2292

Brand Names: US Gemzar

Brand Names: Canada Gemcitabine For Injection; Gemcitabine For Injection Concentrate; Gemcitabine For Injection, USP; Gemcitabine Hydrochloride For Injection; Gemcitabine Injection; Gemcitabine Sun For Injection; Gemzar

Index Terms dFdC; dFdCyd; Difluorodeoxycytidine Hydrochlorothiazide; Gemcitabine Hydrochloride; LY-188011

Pharmacologic Category Antineoplastic Agent, Antimetabolite; Antineoplastic Agent, Antimetabolite (Pyrimidine Analog)

Use

Breast cancer: First-line treatment of metastatic breast cancer (in combination with paclitaxel) after failure of adjuvant chemotherapy which contained an anthracycline (unless contraindicated)

Non-small cell lung cancer (NSCLC): First-line treatment of inoperable, locally-advanced (stage IIIA or IIIB) or metastatic (stage IV) NSCLC (in combination with cisplatin)

Ovarian cancer: Treatment of advanced ovarian cancer (in combination with carboplatin) that has relapsed at least 6 months following completion of platinum-based chemotherapy

Pancreatic cancer: First-line treatment of locally-advanced (nonresectable stage II or III) or metastatic (stage IV) pancreatic adenocarcinoma

Labeled Contraindications Hypersensitivity to gemcitabine or any component of the formulation

Pregnancy Considerations Adverse events were observed in animal reproduction studies. May cause fetal harm if administered during pregnancy; adverse effects in reproduction are anticipated based on the mechanism of action.

Breast-Feeding Considerations It is not known if gemcitabine is excreted in breast milk. Due to the potential for serious adverse reactions in the nursing infant, the decision to discontinue gemcitabine or to discontinue breast-feeding should take into account the benefits of treatment to the mother.

Warnings/Precautions Hazardous agent - use appropriate precautions for handling and disposal (NIOSH 2014 [group 1]). Gemcitabine may suppress bone marrow function (neutropenia, thrombocytopenia, and anemia); myelosuppression is usually the dose-limiting toxicity; toxicity is increased when used in combination with other chemotherapy; monitor blood counts; dosage adjustments are frequently required.

Hemolytic uremic syndrome (HUS) has been reported; may lead to renal failure and dialysis (including fatalities); monitor for evidence of anemia with microangiopathic hemolysis (elevation of bilirubin or LDH, reticulocytosis, severe thrombocytopenia, and/or renal failure) and monitor renal function at baseline and periodically during treatment. Permanently discontinue if HUS or severe renal impairment occurs; renal failure may not be reversible despite discontinuation. Serious hepatotoxicity (including liver failure and death) has been reported (when used alone or in combination with other hepatotoxic medications); use in patients with hepatic impairment (history of cirrhosis, hepatitis, or alcoholism) or in patients with hepatic metastases may lead to exacerbation of hepatic impairment. Monitor hepatic function at baseline and periodically during treatment; consider dose adjustments with elevated bilirubin; discontinue if severe liver injury develops. Capillary leak syndrome (CLS) with serious consequences has been reported, both with single-agent gemcitabine and with combination chemotherapy; discontinue if CLS develops.

Pulmonary toxicity, including adult respiratory distress syndrome, interstitial pneumonitis, pulmonary edema, and pulmonary fibrosis, has been observed; may lead to respiratory failure (some fatal) despite discontinuation. Onset for symptoms of pulmonary toxicity may be delayed up to 2 weeks beyond the last dose. Discontinue for unexplained dyspnea (with or without bronchospasm) or other evidence or pulmonary toxicity. Posterior reversible encephalopathy syndrome (PRES) has been reported, both with single-agent therapy and with combination chemotherapy. PRES may manifest with blindness, confusion, headache, hypertension, lethargy, seizure, and other visual and neurologic disturbances. If PRES diagnosis is confirmed (by MRI), discontinue therapy. Not indicated for use with concurrent radiation therapy; radiation toxicity, including tissue injury, severe mucositis, esophagitis, or pneumonitis, has been reported with concurrent and nonconcurrent administration; may have radiosensitizing activity when gemcitabine and radiation therapy are given ≤7 days apart; radiation recall may occur when gemcitabine and radiation therapy are given >7 days apart. Potentially significant drug-drug interactions may exist, requiring dose or frequency adjustment, additional monitoring, and/or selection of alternative therapy.

Prolongation of the infusion duration >60 minutes or more frequent than weekly dosing have been shown to alter the half-life and increase toxicity (hypotension, flu-like symptoms, myelosuppression, weakness); a fixed-dose rate (FDR) infusion rate of 10 mg/m²/minute has been studied in adults in order to optimize the pharmacokinetics (off-label); prolonged infusion times increase the intracellular accumulation of the active metabolite, gemcitabine triphosphate (Ko, 2006; Tempero, 2003); patients who receive gemcitabine FDR experience more grade 3/4 hematologic toxicity (Ko, 2006; Poplin, 2009).

Adverse Reactions Frequency of adverse reactions reported for single-agent use of gemcitabine only; bone marrow depression is the dose-limiting toxicity.
>10%:
  Cardiovascular: Peripheral edema (20%), edema (13%)
  Central nervous system: Drowsiness (11%)
  Dermatologic: Skin rash (30%), alopecia (15%)
  Gastrointestinal: Nausea and vomiting (69%), diarrhea (19%), stomatitis (11%)
  Genitourinary: Proteinuria (45%), hematuria (35%)
  Hematologic & oncologic: Anemia (68%; grade 3: 7%; grade 4: 1%), neutropenia (63%; grade 3: 19%; grade 4: 6%), thrombocytopenia (24%; grade 3: 4%; grade 4: 1%), hemorrhage (17%; grade 3: <1%; grade 4: <1%)
  Hepatic: Increased serum ALT (68%; grade 3: 8%, grade 4: 2%), increased serum AST (67%; grade 3: 6%; grade 4: 2%), increased serum alkaline phosphatase (55%; grade 3: 7%; grade 4: 2%), increased serum bilirubin (13%; grade 3: 2%, grade 4: <1%)
  Infection: Infection (16%)
  Renal: Increased blood urea nitrogen (16%)
  Respiratory: Dyspnea (23%; grade 3: 3%; grade 4: <1%), flu-like symptoms (19%)
  Miscellaneous: Fever (41%)
1% to 10%:
  Central nervous system: Paresthesia (10%; grade 3: <1%)
  Local: Injection site reaction (4%)
  Renal: Increased serum creatinine (8%)
  Respiratory: Bronchospasm (<2%)
<1%, postmarketing, and/or case reports (reported with single-agent use or with combination therapy): Adult respiratory distress syndrome, anaphylactoid reaction, anorexia, arthralgia, bullous skin disease, capillary leak syndrome, cardiac arrhythmia, cardiac failure, cellulitis, cerebrovascular accident (Kuenen, 2002), constipation, desquamation, digital vasculitis, gangrene of skin or other tissue, hemolytic-uremic syndrome, hepatic failure, hepatic veno-occlusive disease, hepatotoxicity (rare), hyperglycemia, hypertension, hypocalcemia, hypotension, increased gamma-glutamyl transferase, interstitial pneumonitis, myocardial infarction, neuropathy, petechiae (Zupancic, 2007; Nishijima 2013), pruritus (Curtis, 2014), pulmonary edema, pulmonary fibrosis, radiation recall phenomenon, renal failure, respiratory failure, reversible posterior leukoencephalopathy syndrome, sepsis, supraventricular cardiac arrhythmia, thrombotic thrombocytopenic purpura (Zupancic, 2007; Nishijima, 2013)

Drug Interactions

Metabolism/Transport Effects None known.

Avoid Concomitant Use

Avoid concomitant use of Gemcitabine with any of the following: BCG (Intravesical); CloZAPine; Dipyrone; Natalizumab; Pimecrolimus; Tacrolimus (Topical); Tofacitinib; Vaccines (Live)

Increased Effect/Toxicity

Gemcitabine may increase the levels/effects of: Bleomycin; CloZAPine; Fingolimod; Fluorouracil (Systemic); Fluorouracil (Topical); Leflunomide; Natalizumab; Tofacitinib; Vaccines (Live); Warfarin

The levels/effects of Gemcitabine may be increased by: Denosumab; Dipyrone; Pimecrolimus; Roflumilast; Tacrolimus (Topical); Trastuzumab

Decreased Effect

Gemcitabine may decrease the levels/effects of: BCG (Intravesical); Coccidioides immitis Skin Test; Sipuleucel-T; Vaccines (Inactivated); Vaccines (Live)

The levels/effects of Gemcitabine may be decreased by: Echinacea

Storage/Stability

Lyophilized powder: Store intact vials at room temperature of 20°C to 25°C (68°F to 77°F); excursions permitted to 15°C to 30°C (59°F to 86°F). Reconstituted vials are stable for 24 hours at room temperature. Do not refrigerate (may form crystals).

Solution for injection: Store intact vials refrigerated at 2°C to 8°C (36°F to 46°F); do not freeze.

Solutions diluted for infusion in NS are stable for 24 hours at room temperature. Do not refrigerate.

Preparation for Administration

Hazardous agent; use appropriate precautions for handling and disposal (NIOSH 2014 [group 1]).

Reconstitute lyophilized powder with preservative free NS; add 5 mL to the 200 mg vial, add 25 mL to the 1000 mg vial, or add 50 mL to the 2000 mg vial, resulting in a reconstituted concentration of 38 mg/mL (solutions must be reconstituted to ≤40 mg/mL to completely dissolve). Gemcitabine is also supplied as a concentrated solution for injection in different concentrations (40 mg/mL [Canada only] and 38 mg/mL); verify product concentration prior to preparation for administration.

Further dilute reconstituted lyophilized powder or concentrated solution for injection in NS for infusion; to concentrations as low as 0.1 mg/mL.

Mechanism of Action A pyrimidine antimetabolite that inhibits DNA synthesis by inhibition of DNA polymerase and ribonucleotide reductase, cell cycle-specific for the S-phase of the cycle (also blocks cellular progression at G1/S-phase). Gemcitabine is phosphorylated intracellularly by deoxycytidine kinase to gemcitabine monophosphate, which is further phosphorylated to active metabolites gemcitabine diphosphate and gemcitabine triphosphate. Gemcitabine diphosphate inhibits DNA synthesis by inhibiting ribonucleotide reductase; gemcitabine triphosphate incorporates into DNA and inhibits DNA polymerase.

Pharmacodynamics/Kinetics

Distribution: Infusions <70 minutes: 50 L/m^2; Long infusion times (70-285 minutes): 370 L/m^2

Protein binding: Negligible

Metabolism: Metabolized intracellularly by nucleoside kinases to the active diphosphate (dFdCDP) and triphosphate (dFdCTP) nucleoside metabolites

Half-life elimination:

Gemcitabine: Infusion time ≤70 minutes: 42 to 94 minutes; infusion time 3 to 4 hours: 4 to 10.5 hours (affected by age and gender)

Metabolite (gemcitabine triphosphate), terminal phase: 1.7 to 19.4 hours

Time to peak, plasma: 30 minutes after completion of infusion

Excretion: Urine (92% to 98%; primarily as inactive uracil metabolite); feces (<1%)

Dosing

Adult & Geriatric Note: Prolongation of the infusion duration >60 minutes and administration more frequently than once weekly have been shown to increase toxicity.

Breast cancer, metastatic: IV: 1250 mg/m^2 over 30 minutes days 1 and 8; repeat cycle every 21 days (in combination with paclitaxel) **or** (off-label dosing; as a single agent) 800 mg/m^2 over 30 minutes days 1, 8, and 15 of a 28-day treatment cycle (Carmichael, 1995)

Non-small cell lung cancer, locally advanced or metastatic: IV: 1000 mg/m^2 over 30 minutes days 1, 8, and 15; repeat cycle every 28 days (in combination with cisplatin) **or** 1250 mg/m^2 over 30 minutes days 1 and 8; repeat cycle every 21 days (in combination with cisplatin) **or** (off-label dosing/combination) 1000 mg/m^2 over 30 minutes days 1 and 8; repeat cycle every 21 days (in combination with carboplatin) for up to 4 cycles (Grønberg, 2009) **or** (off-label combination) 1000 mg/m^2 over 30 minutes days 1, 8, and 15; repeat cycle every 28 days (in combination with carboplatin) for up to 4 cycles (Danson, 2003) **or** (off-label combination) 1000 mg/m^2 over 30 minutes days 1 and 8; repeat cycle every 21 days (in combination with docetaxel) for 8 cycles (Pujol, 2005) **or** (off-label combination) 1000 mg/m^2 days 1, 8, and 15; repeat cycle every 28 days (in combination with vinorelbine) for 6 cycles (Greco, 2007)

Ovarian cancer, advanced: IV: 1000 mg/m^2 over 30 minutes days 1 and 8; repeat cycle every 21 days (in combination with carboplatin) **or** (off-label dosing; as a single agent) 1000 mg/m^2 over 30-60 minutes days 1 and 8; repeat cycle every 21 days (Mutch, 2007)

Pancreatic cancer, locally advanced or metastatic: IV: Initial: 1000 mg/m^2 over 30 minutes once weekly for 7 weeks followed by 1 week rest; then once weekly for 3 weeks out of every 4 weeks **or** (off-label combinations) 1000 mg/m^2 over 30 minutes weekly for up to 7 weeks followed by 1 week rest; then weekly for 3 weeks out of every 4 weeks (in combination with erlotinib) (Moore, 2007) **or** 1000 mg/m^2 over 30 minutes days 1, 8, and 15 every 28 days (in combination with capecitabine) (Cunningham, 2009) **or** 1000 mg/m^2 over 30 minutes days 1 and 15 every 28 days (in combination with cisplatin) (Heinemann, 2006) **or** 1000 mg/m^2 infused at 10 mg/m^2/minute every 14 days (in combination with oxaliplatin) (Louvet, 2005) **or** 1000 mg/m^2 days 1, 8, and 15 every 28 days (in combination with paclitaxel [protein bound]) (Von Hoff, 2013)

Bladder cancer (off-label use):

Advanced or metastatic: IV: 1000 mg/m^2 over 30-60 minutes days 1, 8, and 15; repeat cycle every 28 days (in combination with cisplatin) (von der Maase, 2000) **or** 1000 mg/m^2 over 30 minutes days 1 and 8; repeat cycle every 21 days (in combination with carboplatin) until disease progression or unacceptable toxicity (De Santis, 2012)

Transitional cell carcinoma: Intravesicular instillation: 2000 mg (in 100 mL NS; retain for 1 hour) twice weekly for 3 weeks; repeat cycle every 4 weeks for at least 2 cycles (Dalbagni, 2006)

Cervical cancer, recurrent or persistent (off-label use): IV: 1000 mg/m^2 days 1 and 8; repeat cycle every 21 days (in combination with cisplatin) (Monk, 2009) **or** 1250 mg/m^2 over 30 minutes days 1 and 8; repeat cycle every 21 days (in combination with cisplatin) (Burnett, 2000) **or** 800 mg/m^2 over 30 minutes days 1, 8, and 15; repeat cycle every 28 days (as a single-agent) (Schilder, 2005) **or** 800 mg/m^2 days 1 and 8; repeat cycle every 28 days (in combination with cisplatin) (Brewer, 2006)

Head and neck cancer, nasopharyngeal (off-label use): IV: 1000 mg/m^2 over 30 minutes days 1, 8, and 15 every 28 days (Zhang, 2008) **or** 1000 mg/m^2 over 30 minutes days 1 and 8 every 21 days (in combination with vinorelbine) (Chen, 2012)

Hepatobiliary cancer, advanced (off-label use): IV: 1000 mg/m^2 over 30 minutes days 1 and 8; repeat cycle every 21 days (in combination with cisplatin) (Valle, 2010) **or** 1000 mg/m^2 over 30 minutes days 1 and 8; repeat cycle every 21 days (in combination with capecitabine) (Knox, 2005) **or** 1000 mg/m^2 infused at 10 mg/m^2/minute every 2 weeks (in combination with oxaliplatin) (Andre, 2004)

Hodgkin lymphoma, relapsed (off-label use): IV: 1000 mg/m^2 (800 mg/m^2 for post-transplant patients) over 30 minutes days 1 and 8; repeat cycle every 21 days (in combination with vinorelbine and doxorubicin liposomal) (Bartlett, 2007) **or** 800 mg/m^2 days 1 and 4; repeat cycle every 21 days (in combination with ifosfamide, mesna, vinorelbine, and prednisolone) (Santoro, 2007)

Malignant pleural mesothelioma (off-label use; in combination with cisplatin): IV: 1000 mg/m^2 over 30 minutes days 1, 8 and 15 every 28 days for up to 6 cycles (Nowak, 2002) **or** 1250 mg/m^2 over 30 minutes days 1 and 8 every 21 days for up to 6 cycles (van Haarst, 2002)

Non-Hodgkin lymphoma, refractory (off-label use): IV: 1000 mg/m^2 over 30 minutes days 1 and 8; repeat cycle every 21 days (in combination with cisplatin and dexamethasone) (Crump, 2004) **or** 1000 mg/m^2 every 15-21 days (in combination with oxaliplatin and rituximab) (Lopez, 2008)

Sarcoma (off-label uses): IV:

Ewing's sarcoma, refractory: 675 mg/m^2 over 90 minutes days 1 and 8; repeat cycle every 21 days (in combination with docetaxel) (Navid, 2008)

Osteosarcoma, refractory: 675 mg/m^2 over 90 minutes days 1 and 8; repeat cycle every 21 days (in combination with docetaxel) (Navid, 2008) **or** 1000 mg/m^2 weekly for 7 weeks followed by 1 week rest; then weekly for 3 weeks out of every 4 weeks (Merimsky, 2000)

Soft tissue sarcoma, advanced: 800 mg/m^2 over 90 minutes days 1 and 8; repeat cycle every 21 days (in combination with vinorelbine) (Dileo, 2007) **or** 675 mg/m^2 over 90 minutes days 1 and 8; repeat cycle every 21 days (in combination with docetaxel) (Leu, 2004) **or** 900 mg/m^2 over 90 minutes days 1 and 8; repeat cycle every 21 days (in combination with docetaxel) (Maki, 2007)

Small cell lung cancer, refractory or relapsed (off-label use): IV: 1000-1250 mg/m^2 over 30 minutes days 1, 8, and 15 every 28 days (as a single agent) (Masters, 2003)

Testicular cancer, refractory germ cell (off-label use): IV: 1000-1250 mg/m^2 over 30 minutes days 1 and 8 every 21 days (in combination with oxaliplatin) (DeGiorgi, 2006; Kohllmannsberger, 2004; Pectasides, 2004) **or** 1000 mg/m^2 over 30 minutes days 1, 8, and 15 every 28 days for up to 6 cycles (in combination with paclitaxel) (Hinton, 2002) **or** 800 mg/m^2 over 30 minutes days 1 and 8 every 21 days (in combination with oxaliplatin and paclitaxel) (Bokemeyer, 2008)

Unknown-primary, adenocarcinoma (off-label use): IV: 1250 mg/m^2 days 1 and 8 every 21 days (in combination with cisplatin) (Culine, 2003) **or** 1000 mg/m^2 over 30 minutes days 1 and 8 every 21 days for up to 6 cycles (in combination with docetaxel) (Pouessel, 2004)

Uterine cancer (off-label use): IV: 900 mg/m^2 over 90 minutes days 1 and 8 every 21 days (in combination with docetaxel) (Hensley, 2008) **or** 1000 mg/m^2 over 30 minutes days 1, 8, and 15 every 28 days (Look, 2004)

Pediatric Note: Prolongation of the infusion duration >60 minutes and administration more frequently than once weekly have been shown to increase toxicity. Refer to specific references for ages of populations studied:

Germ cell tumor, refractory (off-label use): IV: 1000 mg/m^2 over 30 minutes days 1, 8, and 15 every 28 days (in combination with paclitaxel) for up to 6 cycles (Hinton, 2002)

Hodgkin lymphoma, relapsed (off-label use): IV: 1000 mg/m^2 over 100 minutes days 1 and 8; repeat cycle every 21 days (in combination with vinorelbine) (Cole, 2009) **or** 800 mg/m^2 days 1 and 4; repeat cycle every 21 days (in combination with ifosfamide, mesna, vinorelbine, and prednisolone) (Santoro, 2007)

Sarcomas (off-label use): IV:

Ewing's sarcoma, refractory: 675 mg/m^2 over 90 minutes days 1 and 8; repeat cycle every 21 days (in combination with docetaxel) (Navid, 2008)

Osteosarcoma, refractory: 675 mg/m^2 over 90 minutes days 1 and 8; repeat cycle every 21 days (in combination with docetaxel) (Navid, 2008) **or** 1000 mg/m^2 weekly for 7 weeks followed by 1 week rest; then weekly for 3 weeks out of every 4 weeks (Merimsky, 2000)

Renal Impairment There are no dosage adjustments provided in the manufacturer's labeling; use with caution in patients with preexisting renal dysfunction. Discontinue if severe renal toxicity or hemolytic uremic syndrome (HUS) occur during gemcitabine treatment.

Mild-to-severe renal impairment: No dosage adjustment necessary (Janus, 2010; Li, 2007).

ESRD (on hemodialysis): Hemodialysis should begin 6-12 hours after gemcitabine infusion (Janus 2010; Li, 2007).

Hepatic Impairment There are no dosage adjustments provided in the manufacturer's labeling; use with caution. Discontinue if severe hepatotoxicity occurs during gemcitabine treatment. The following adjustments have been reported:

Transaminases elevated (with normal bilirubin): No dosage adjustment necessary (Venook, 2000).

Serum bilirubin >1.6 mg/dL: Use initial dose of 800 mg/m^2; may escalate if tolerated (Ecklund, 2005; Floyd, 2006; Venook, 2000).

Obesity *ASCO Guidelines for appropriate chemotherapy dosing in obese adults with cancer:* Utilize patient's actual body weight (full weight) for calculation of body surface area- or weight-based dosing, particularly when the intent of therapy is curative; manage regimen-related toxicities in the same manner as for nonobese patients; if a dose reduction is utilized due to

toxicity, consider resumption of full weight-based dosing with subsequent cycles, especially if cause of toxicity (eg, hepatic or renal impairment) is resolved (Griggs, 2012).

Adjustment for Toxicity

Nonhematologic toxicity (all indications):

Hold or decrease gemcitabine dose by 50% for the following: Severe (grade 3 or 4) nonhematologic toxicity until resolved (excludes nausea, vomiting, or alopecia [no dose modifications recommended])

Permanently discontinue gemcitabine for any of the following: Unexplained dyspnea (or other evidence of severe pulmonary toxicity), severe hepatotoxicity, hemolytic uremic syndrome (HUS), capillary leak syndrome (CLS), posterior reversible encephalopathy syndrome (PRES)

Hematologic toxicity:

Breast cancer:

Day 1:

Absolute granulocyte count (AGC) ≥1500/mm³ and platelet count ≥100,000/mm³: Administer 100% of full dose

AGC <1500/mm³ or platelet count <100,000/mm³: Hold dose

Day 8:

AGC ≥1200/mm³ and platelet count >75,000/mm³: Administer 100% of full dose

AGC 1000-1199/mm³ or platelet count 50,000-75,000/mm³: Administer 75% of full dose

AGC 700-999/mm³ and platelet count ≥50,000/mm³: Administer 50% of full dose

AGC <700/mm³ or platelet count <50,000/mm³: Hold dose

Non-small cell lung cancer (cisplatin dosage may also require adjustment):

AGC ≥1000/mm³ and platelet count ≥100,000/mm³: Administer 100% of full dose

AGC 500-999/mm³ or platelet count 50,000-99,999/mm³: Administer 75% of full dose

AGC <500/mm³ or platelet count <50,000/mm³: Hold dose

Ovarian cancer:

Day 1:

AGC ≥1500/mm³ and platelet count ≥100,000/mm³: Administer 100% of full dose

AGC <1500/mm³ or platelet count <100,000/mm³: Delay treatment cycle

Day 8:

AGC ≥1500/mm³ and platelet count ≥100,000/mm³: Administer 100% of full dose

AGC 1000-1499/mm³ or platelet count 75,000-99,999/mm³: Administer 50% of full dose

AGC <1000/mm³ or platelet count <75,000/mm³: Hold dose

Hematologic toxicity in previous cycle (dosing adjustment for subsequent cycles):

Initial occurrence: AGC <500/mm³ for >5 days, AGC <100/mm³ for >3 days, febrile neutropenia, platelet count <25,000/mm³, or cycle delay >1 week due to toxicity: Permanently reduce gemcitabine to 800 mg/m² on days 1 and 8.

Subsequent occurrence: AGC <500/mm^3 for >5 days, AGC <100/mm^3 for >3 days, neutropenic fever, platelet count <25,000/mm^3, or cycle delay >1 week due to toxicity: Permanently reduce gemcitabine to 800 mg/m^2 and administer on day 1 only.

Pancreatic cancer:

AGC ≥1000/mm^3 and platelet count ≥100,000/mm^3: Administer 100% of full dose

AGC 500-999/mm^3 or platelet count 50,000-99,999/mm^3: Administer 75% of full dose

AGC <500/mm^3 or platelet count <50,000/mm^3: Hold dose

Combination Regimens

Biliary adenocarcinoma:

Gemcitabine-Capecitabine (Biliary Cancer) on page 1990

Gemcitabine-Cisplatin (Biliary Cancer) on page 1991

GEMOX (Biliary Cancer) on page 1999

Bladder cancer:

Carboplatin-Gemcitabine (Bladder) on page 1867

Cisplatin-Docetaxel-Gemcitabine (Bladder) on page 1891

Cisplatin-Gemcitabine (Bladder) on page 1903

Gemcitabine-Paclitaxel (Bladder) on page 1995

PCG (Bladder) on page 2060

Bone sarcoma (Ewing sarcoma): Docetaxel-Gemcitabine (Ewing Sarcoma) on page 1942

Bone sarcoma (osteosarcoma): Docetaxel-Gemcitabine (Osteosarcoma) on page 1943

Breast cancer:

Gemcitabine (Breast Regimen) on page 1989

Gemcitabine-Paclitaxel (Breast) on page 1996

Cervical cancer:

Cisplatin-Gemcitabine (Cervical) on page 1904

Gemcitabine (Cervical Regimen) on page 1990

Head and neck cancer:

Gemcitabine (Head and Neck Regimen) on page 1993

Gemcitabine-Vinorelbine (Head and Neck) on page 1998

Lung cancer (non-small cell):

Bevacizumab-Cisplatin-Gemcitabine (NSCLC) on page 1840

Carboplatin-Gemcitabine (NSCLC) on page 1867

Cisplatin-Gemcitabine (NSCLC) on page 1905

Docetaxel-Gemcitabine (NSCLC) on page 1943

Gemcitabine-Vinorelbine (NSCLC) on page 1998

Lung cancer (small cell): Gemcitabine (Small Cell Lung Cancer Regimen) on page 1997

Lymphoma, Hodgkin:

GDP (Hodgkin) on page 1989

Gemcitabine-Dexamethasone-Carboplatin (Hodgkin) on page 1991

Gemcitabine (Hodgkin Regimen) on page 1993

GVD (Hodgkin) on page 2002

IGEV (Hodgkin) on page 2016

Lymphoma, non-Hodgkin (DLBCL):

Gemcitabine-Dexamethasone-Cisplatin (NHL-DLBCL) on page 1992

GEMOX-R (NHL-DLBCL) on page 2000

Rituximab-Gemcitabine-Dexamethasone-Carboplatin (NHL-DLBCL) on page 2081

Administration Infuse over 30 minutes; for off-label uses, infusion times may vary (refer to specific references). **Note:** Prolongation of the infusion time >60 minutes has been shown to increase toxicity. Gemcitabine has been administered at a fixed-dose rate (FDR) infusion rate of 10 mg/m^2/minute to optimize the pharmacokinetics (off-label); prolonged infusion times increase the intracellular accumulation of the active metabolite, gemcitabine triphosphate (Ko, 2006; Tempero, 2003). Patients who receive gemcitabine FDR experience more grade 3/4 hematologic toxicity (Ko, 2006; Poplin, 2009).

For intravesicular (bladder) instillation (off-label route), gemcitabine was diluted in 50 to 100 mL normal saline; patients were instructed to retain in the bladder for 1 hour (Addeo, 2010; Dalbaghi, 2006)

Hazardous agent; use appropriate precautions for handling and disposal (NIOSH 2014 [group 1]).

Vesicant/Extravasation Risk May be an irritant

Emetic Potential Children and Adults: Low (10% to 30%)

◄ **Monitoring Parameters** CBC with differential and platelet count (prior to each dose); hepatic and renal function (prior to initiation of therapy and periodically, thereafter); monitor electrolytes, including potassium, magnesium, and calcium (when in combination therapy with cisplatin); monitor pulmonary function; signs/symptoms of capillary leak syndrome and posterior reversible encephalopathy syndrome

Dosage Forms Excipient information presented when available (limited, particularly for generics); consult specific product labeling.

Solution, Intravenous:

Generic: 200 mg/5.26 mL (5.26 mL); 1 g/26.3 mL (26.3 mL); 2 g/52.6 mL (52.6 mL)

Solution Reconstituted, Intravenous:

Gemzar: 200 mg (1 ea); 1 g (1 ea)

Generic: 200 mg (1 ea); 1 g (1 ea); 2 g (1 ea)

Solution Reconstituted, Intravenous [preservative free]:

Generic: 200 mg (1 ea); 1 g (1 ea)

Dosage Forms: Canada Excipient information presented when available (limited, particularly for generics); consult specific product labeling.

Solution, Intravenous: 200 mg/5mL, 1 g/25 mL, 2 g/50 mL [40 mg/mL]

Solution, Intravenous: 200 mg/5.3 mL, 1 g/26.3 mL, 2 g/52.6 mL [38 mg/mL]

Solution Reconstituted, Intravenous: 200 mg, 1 g, 2 g

Gemtuzumab Ozogamicin (gem TOO zoo mab oh zog a MY sin)

Related Information

Management of Chemotherapy-Induced Nausea and Vomiting in Adults on page 2142

Prevention of Chemotherapy-Induced Nausea and Vomiting in Children on page 2203

Safe Handling of Hazardous Drugs on page 2292

Index Terms CMA-676; Mylotarg

Pharmacologic Category Antineoplastic Agent, Anti-CD33; Antineoplastic Agent, Antibody Drug Conjugate; Antineoplastic Agent, Monoclonal Antibody

Use Due to safety concerns, as well as lack of clinical benefit demonstrated in a post-approval clinical trial, gemtuzumab was withdrawn from the U.S. commercial market in 2010.

Labeled Contraindications Hypersensitivity to gemtuzumab ozogamicin, calicheamicin derivatives, or any component of the formulation; patients with anti-CD33 antibody

Pregnancy Considerations Teratogenic effects have been observed in animal reproduction studies. May cause fetal harm when administered to a pregnant woman. Women of childbearing potential should avoid becoming pregnant while receiving treatment.

Breast-Feeding Considerations It is not known if gemtuzumab ozogamicin is excreted in breast milk. Because human IgG is secreted in breast milk and the potential for serious adverse reactions in the nursing infant exists, a decision should be made whether to discontinue nursing or to discontinue the drug, taking into account the importance of treatment to the mother.

Warnings/Precautions Hazardous agent - use appropriate precautions for handling and disposal (NIOSH 2014 [group 1]).

Gemtuzumab has been associated with hepatotoxicity, including severe hepatic sinusoidal obstruction syndrome (SOS; formerly called veno-occlusive disease [VOD]). Symptoms of SOS include right upper quadrant pain, rapid weight gain, ascites, hepatomegaly, and bilirubin/transaminase elevations. Risk may be increased by combination chemotherapy, underlying hepatic disease, or hematopoietic stem cell transplant.

Severe hypersensitivity reactions (including anaphylaxis) and other infusion-related reactions may occur. Infusion-related events are common, generally reported to occur with the first dose after the end of the 2-hour intravenous infusion. These symptoms usually resolved after 2-4 hours with a supportive therapy of acetaminophen, diphenhydramine, and intravenous fluids. Other severe and potentially fatal infusion related pulmonary events (including dyspnea and hypoxia) have been reported infrequently. Symptomatic intrinsic lung disease or high peripheral blast counts may increase the risk of severe reactions. Fewer infusion-related events were observed after the second dose. Postinfusion reactions (may include fever, chills, hypotension, or dyspnea) may occur during the first 24 hours after administration. Consider discontinuation in patients who develop severe infusion-related reactions. In addition to infusion-related pulmonary events, gemtuzumab therapy is also associated with acute respiratory distress syndrome, pulmonary infiltrates, pleural effusion, noncardiogenic pulmonary edema, and pulmonary insufficiency.

Severe myelosuppression occurs in all patients at recommended dosages. Tumor lysis syndrome may occur as a consequence of leukemia treatment, adequate hydration and prophylactic allopurinol must be instituted prior to use. Other methods to lower WBC <30,000 cells/mm^3 may be considered (hydroxyurea or leukapheresis) to minimize the risk of tumor lysis syndrome, and/or severe infusion reactions. An increased number of deaths have been reported in patients receiving gemtuzumab in combination with chemotherapy, compared to those receiving chemotherapy alone.

Adverse Reactions Frequency not defined.

Cardiovascular: Cerebral hemorrhage, hyper-/hypotension, peripheral edema, tachycardia

Central nervous system: Anxiety, chills, depression, dizziness, fever, headache, insomnia, intracranial hemorrhage, pain

Dermatologic: Bruising, petechiae, pruritus, rash

Endocrine & metabolic: Hyperglycemia, hypocalcemia, hypokalemia, hypomagnesemia, hypophosphatemia

Gastrointestinal: Abdominal pain, anorexia, diarrhea, dyspepsia, gingival hemorrhage, melena, mucositis, nausea, stomatitis, vomiting

Genitourinary: Vaginal bleeding, vaginal hemorrhage

Hematologic: Anemia, disseminated intravascular coagulation (DIC), hemorrhage, leukopenia, lymphopenia, neutropenia (median recovery 40-51 days), neutropenic fever, thrombocytopenia (median recovery 36-51 days)

Hepatic: Alkaline phosphatase increased, ALT increased, ascites, AST increased, hyperbilirubinemia, LDH increased, prothrombin time increased, PTT increased, sinusoidal obstruction syndrome (SOS; veno-occlusive disease; higher frequency in patients with prior history of or subsequent hematopoietic stem cell transplant)

Local: Local reaction

Neuromuscular & skeletal: Arthralgia, back pain, myalgia, weakness

Renal: Creatinine increased, hematuria

Respiratory: Cough, dyspnea, epistaxis, hypoxia, pharyngitis, pneumonia, rhinitis

Miscellaneous: Cutaneous herpes simplex, infection, infusion reaction, sepsis

Infrequent and/or case reports: Acute respiratory distress syndrome, anaphylaxis, bradycardia, Budd-Chiari syndrome, gastrointestinal hemorrhage, hepatic failure, hepatosplenomegaly, hypersensitivity reactions, jaundice, neutropenic sepsis, noncardiogenic pulmonary edema, portal vain thrombosis, pulmonary hemorrhage, renal impairment, renal failure (including renal failure secondary to tumor lysis syndrome)

Drug Interactions

Metabolism/Transport Effects None known.

Avoid Concomitant Use

Avoid concomitant use of Gemtuzumab Ozogamicin with any of the following: BCG (Intravesical); Belimumab; CloZAPine; Dipyrone; Natalizumab; Pimecrolimus; Tacrolimus (Topical); Tofacitinib; Vaccines (Live)

Increased Effect/Toxicity

Gemtuzumab Ozogamicin may increase the levels/effects of: Belimumab; CloZAPine; Fingolimod; Leflunomide; Natalizumab; Tofacitinib; Vaccines (Live)

The levels/effects of Gemtuzumab Ozogamicin may be increased by: Denosumab; Dipyrone; Pimecrolimus; Roflumilast; Tacrolimus (Topical); Trastuzumab

Decreased Effect

Gemtuzumab Ozogamicin may decrease the levels/effects of: BCG (Intravesical); Coccidioides immitis Skin Test; Sipuleucel-T; Vaccines (Inactivated); Vaccines (Live)

The levels/effects of Gemtuzumab Ozogamicin may be decreased by: Echinacea

Storage/Stability Light sensitive; protect from light (including direct and indirect sunlight, and unshielded fluorescent light). The infusion container should be placed in a UV protectant bag immediately after preparation. Store intact vials under refrigeration at 2°C to 8°C (36°F to 46°F). Reconstituted solutions may be stored for up to 2 hours at room temperature or under refrigeration. Following dilution for infusion, solutions are stable for up to 16 hours at room temperature. Administration requires 2 hours; therefore, the maximum elapsed time from initial reconstitution to completion of infusion should be 20 hours.

Preparation for Administration Hazardous agent; use appropriate precautions for handling and disposal (NIOSH 2014 [group 1]). Protect from light during preparation (and administration). Prepare in biologic safety hood with shielded fluorescent light; (some institutions prepare in a darkened room with the lights in the biologic safety cabinet turned off). Allow to warm to room temperature prior to reconstitution. Reconstitute each 5 mg vial with sterile water for injection to a concentration of 1 mg/mL. Dilute in 100 mL of 0.9% sodium chloride injection.

Mechanism of Action Antibody to CD33 antigen, which is expressed on leukemic blasts in 80% of AML patients. Binds to the CD33 antigen, resulting in internalization of the antibody-antigen complex. Following internalization, the calicheamicin derivative is released inside the myeloid cell. The calicheamicin derivative binds to DNA resulting in double strand breaks and cell death. Pluripotent stem cells and nonhematopoietic cells are not affected.

Pharmacodynamics/Kinetics

Distribution: V_{ss}: Adults: Initial dose: 21 L; Repeat dose: 10 L

Half-life elimination: Total calicheamicin: Initial: 41-45 hours, Repeat dose: 60-64 hours; Unconjugated: 100-143 hours (no change noted in repeat dosing)

Dosing

Adult & Geriatric Note: Patients should receive diphenhydramine 50 mg orally and acetaminophen 650-1000 mg orally 1 hour prior to administration of each dose. Acetaminophen dosage should be repeated as needed every 4 hours for 2 additional doses. Pretreatment with methylprednisolone may ameliorate infusion-related symptoms.

Acute myeloid leukemia (off-label/investigational use): IV:

<60 years: 9 mg/m^2 infused over 2 hours. A full treatment course is a total of 2 doses administered with 14-28 days between doses (Larson, 2005).

≥60 years: 9 mg/m^2 infused over 2 hours. A full treatment course is a total of 2 doses administered with 14-28 days between doses (Larson, 2002; Larson, 2005).

Acute promyelocytic leukemia (off-label/investigational use): IV:

Single-agent therapy: 6 mg/m^2 infused over 2 hours on days 1 and 15; for patients testing PCR negative after 2 doses, a third dose was administered (LoCoco, 2004).

Combination therapy (high-risk patients; Ravandi, 2009):

Induction: 9 mg/m^2 as a single dose on day 1 (in combination with arsenic trioxide and tretinoin)

Post remission therapy (if arsenic trioxide or tretinoin discontinued due to toxicity): 9 mg/m^2 once every 4-5 weeks until 28 weeks after complete remission.

Renal Impairment No dosage adjustment provided in manufacturer's labeling (has not been studied).

Hepatic Impairment No dosage adjustment provided in manufacturer's labeling (has not been studied); use with caution.

Adjustment for Toxicity

Dyspnea or significant hypotension: Interrupt infusion; monitor

Anaphylaxis, pulmonary edema, acute respiratory distress syndrome: Strongly consider discontinuing treatment

Administration Do not administer as IV push or bolus. Administer via IV infusion, over at least 2 hours through a low protein-binding (0.2 to 1.2 micron) in-line filter. Protect from light during infusion. Premedicate with acetaminophen and diphenhydramine prior to each infusion.

Hazardous agent; use appropriate precautions for handling and disposal (NIOSH 2014 [group 1]).

Emetic Potential Children: Minimal (<10%)

◀ **Monitoring Parameters** Monitor vital signs during the infusion and for 4 hours following the infusion. Monitor for signs/symptoms of postinfusion reaction. Monitor electrolytes, liver function, CBC with differential and platelets frequently. Monitor for signs and symptoms of hepatic sinusoidal obstruction syndrome (SOS; veno-occlusive disease; weight gain, right upper quadrant abdominal pain, hepatomegaly, ascites).

Product Availability No longer commercially available in the US market for new patients. Available in Canada through a special access program.

Prescribing and Access Restrictions As of June 2010, gemtuzumab has been withdrawn from the U.S. market and is no longer commercially available to new patients; gemtuzumab is only available in the U.S. under an Investigational New Drug (IND) protocol.

In Canada, gemtuzumab is available through a special access program (access information is available from Health Canada).

◆ **Gemzar** see Gemcitabine on page 776

◆ **Gengraf** see CycloSPORINE (Systemic) on page 385

◆ **Gen-Hydroxyurea (Can)** see Hydroxyurea on page 839

◆ **Gen-Medroxy (Can)** see MedroxyPROGESTERone on page 1074

Gentamicin (Systemic) (jen ta MYE sin)

Brand Names: Canada Gentamicin Injection, USP

Index Terms Gentamicin Sulfate

Pharmacologic Category Antibiotic, Aminoglycoside

Use Treatment of susceptible bacterial infections, normally gram-negative organisms, including *Pseudomonas*, *Proteus*, *Serratia*, and gram-positive *Staphylococcus*; treatment of bone infections, respiratory tract infections, skin and soft tissue infections, as well as abdominal and urinary tract infections, and septicemia; treatment of infective endocarditis

Pregnancy Risk Factor D

Dosing

Adult & Geriatric Individualization is **critical** because of the low therapeutic index.

In underweight and nonobese patients, use of total body weight (TBW) instead of ideal body weight for determining the initial mg/kg/dose is widely accepted (Nicolau, 1995). Ideal body weight (IBW) also may be used to determine doses for patients who are neither underweight nor obese (Gilbert, 2009).

Initial and periodic plasma drug levels (eg, peak and trough with conventional dosing, post dose level at a prespecified time with extended-interval dosing) should be determined, particularly in critically-ill patients with serious infections or in disease states known to significantly alter aminoglycoside pharmacokinetics (eg, cystic fibrosis, burns, or major surgery).

Usual dosage ranges:

IM, IV:

Conventional: 1-2.5 mg/kg/dose every 8-12 hours; to ensure adequate peak concentrations early in therapy, higher initial dosage may be considered in selected patients when extracellular water is increased (edema, septic shock, postsurgical, or trauma)

Once daily: 4-7 mg/kg/dose once daily; some clinicians recommend this approach for all patients with normal renal function; this dose is at least as efficacious with similar, if not less, toxicity than conventional dosing

Intrathecal: 4-8 mg/day

Indication-specific dosing: IM, IV:

Brucellosis: 240 mg (IM) daily or 5 mg/kg (IV) daily for 7 days; either regimen recommended in combination with doxycycline

Cholangitis: 4-6 mg/kg once daily with ampicillin

Diverticulitis (complicated): 1.5-2 mg/kg every 8 hours (with ampicillin and metronidazole)

Endocarditis: Treatment: 3 mg/kg/day in 1-3 divided doses

Meningitis *Enterococcus* sp or *Pseudomonas aeruginosa*: IV: Loading dose 2 mg/kg, then 1.7 mg/kg/dose every 8 hours (administered with another bacteriocidal drug)

Pelvic inflammatory disease: Loading dose: 2 mg/kg, then 1.5 mg/kg every 8 hours

Alternate therapy: 4.5 mg/kg once daily

Plague *(Yersinia pestis)*: Treatment: 5 mg/kg/day, followed by postexposure prophylaxis with doxycycline

Pneumonia, hospital- or ventilator-associated: 7 mg/kg/day (with antipseudomonal beta-lactam or carbapenem)

Surgical (preoperative) prophylaxis (off-label use): IV: 5 mg/kg within 60 minutes prior to surgical incision with or without other antibiotics (procedure dependent). **Note:** Dose is based on actual body weight unless >20% above ideal body weight, then dosage requirement may best be estimated using a dosing weight of IBW + 0.4 (TBW - IBW) (Bratzler, 2013).

Synergy (for gram-positive infections): 3 mg/kg/day in 1-3 divided doses (with ampicillin)

Tularemia: 5 mg/kg/day divided every 8 hours for 1-2 weeks

Urinary tract infection: 1.5 mg/kg/dose every 8 hours

Pediatric Individualization is **critical** because of the low therapeutic index.

Use of ideal body weight (IBW) for determining the mg/kg/dose appears to be more accurate than dosing on the basis of total body weight (TBW).

Initial and periodic plasma drug levels (eg, peak and trough with conventional dosing) should be determined, particularly in critically-ill patients with serious infections or in disease states known to significantly alter aminoglycoside pharmacokinetics (eg, cystic fibrosis, burns, or major surgery).

Usual dosage ranges: IM, IV:

Infants and Children <5 years: 2.5 mg/kg/dose every 8 hours*

Children ≥5 years: 2-2.5 mg/kg/dose every 8 hours*

*Note: Higher individual doses and/or more frequent intervals (eg, every 6 hours) may be required in selected clinical situations (cystic fibrosis) or serum levels document the need.

Surgical (preoperative) prophylaxis (off-label use): Children ≥1 year: IV: 2.5 mg/kg within 60 minutes prior to surgical incision with or without other antibiotics (procedure dependent). **Note:** Dose is based on actual body weight unless >20% above ideal body weight, then dosage requirement may best be estimated using a dosing weight of IBW + 0.4 (TBW - IBW) (Bratzler, 2013).

◀ **Renal Impairment**

Conventional dosing:

CrCl ≥60 mL/minute: Administer every 8 hours

CrCl 40-60 mL/minute: Administer every 12 hours

CrCl 20-40 mL/minute: Administer every 24 hours

CrCl <20 mL/minute: Loading dose, then monitor levels

High-dose therapy: Interval may be extended (eg, every 48 hours) in patients with moderate renal impairment (CrCl 30-59 mL/minute) and/or adjusted based on serum level determinations.

Intermittent hemodialysis (IHD) (administer after hemodialysis on dialysis days) (Heintz, 2009): Dialyzable (~50%; variable; dependent on filter, duration, and type of IHD):

Loading dose of 2-3 mg/kg loading dose followed by:

Mild UTI or synergy: 1 mg/kg every 48-72 hours; consider redosing for pre-HD or post-HD concentrations <1 mg/L

Moderate-to-severe UTI: 1-1.5 mg/kg every 48-72 hours; consider redosing for pre-HD concentrations <1.5-2 mg/L or post-HD concentrations <1 mg/L

Systemic gram-negative rod infection: 1.5-2 mg/kg every 48-72 hours; consider redosing for pre-HD concentrations <3-5 mg/L or post-HD concentrations <2 mg/L

Note: Dosing dependent on the assumption of 3 times/week, complete IHD sessions.

Peritoneal dialysis (PD):

Administration via PD fluid:

Gram-positive infection (eg, synergy): 3-4 mg/L (3-4 mcg/mL) of PD fluid

Gram-negative infection: 4-8 mg/L (4-8 mcg/mL) of PD fluid

Administration via IV, IM route during PD: Dose as for CrCl <10 mL/minute and follow levels

Continuous renal replacement therapy (CRRT) (Heintz, 2009; Trotman, 2005): Drug clearance is highly dependent on the method of renal replacement, filter type, and flow rate. Appropriate dosing requires close monitoring of pharmacologic response, signs of adverse reactions due to drug accumulation, as well as drug concentrations in relation to target trough (if appropriate). The following are general recommendations only (based on dialysate flow/ultrafiltration rates of 1-2 L/hour and minimal residual renal function) and should not supersede clinical judgment:

CVVH/CVVHD/CVVHDF: Loading dose of 2-3 mg/kg followed by:

Mild UTI or synergy: 1 mg/kg every 24-36 hours (redose when concentration <1 mg/L)

Moderate-to-severe UTI: 1-1.5 mg/kg every 24-36 hours (redose when concentration <1.5-2 mg/L)

Systemic gram-negative infection: 1.5-2.5 mg/kg every 24-48 hours (redose when concentration <3-5 mg/L)

Hepatic Impairment Monitor plasma concentrations.

Obesity In moderate obesity (TBW/IBW ≥1.25) or greater (eg, morbid obesity [TBW/IBW >2]), initial dosage requirement may be estimated using a dosing weight of IBW + 0.4 (TBW - IBW) (Traynor, 1995).

Additional Information Complete prescribing information should be consulted for additional detail.

Dosage Forms Excipient information presented when available (limited, particularly for generics); consult specific product labeling.

Solution, Injection:

Generic: 10 mg/mL (2 mL); 40 mg/mL (2 mL, 20 mL)

Solution, Injection [preservative free]:

Generic: 10 mg/mL (2 mL)

Solution, Intravenous:

Generic: 60 mg (50 mL); 70 mg (50 mL); 80 mg (50 mL, 100 mL); 90 mg (100 mL); 100 mg (50 mL, 100 mL); 120 mg (100 mL); 10 mg/mL (6 mL, 8 mL, 10 mL)

◆ **Gentamicin Injection, USP (Can)** see Gentamicin (Systemic) on page 790

◆ **Gentamicin Sulfate** see Gentamicin (Systemic) on page 790

◆ **Gilotrif** see Afatinib on page 50

◆ **Giotrif (Can)** see Afatinib on page 50

◆ **Gleevec** see Imatinib on page 882

◆ **Gleostine** see Lomustine on page 1054

◆ **Gliadel Wafer** see Carmustine on page 284

◆ **Glivec** see Imatinib on page 882

Glucarpidase (gloo KAR pid ase)

Brand Names: US Voraxaze

Index Terms Carboxypeptidase-G2; CPDG2; CPG2; Voraxaze

Pharmacologic Category Antidote; Enzyme

Use Treatment of toxic plasma methotrexate concentrations (>1 micromole/L) in patients with delayed clearance due to renal impairment

Note: Due to the risk of subtherapeutic methotrexate exposure, glucarpidase is **NOT** indicated when methotrexate clearance is within expected range (plasma methotrexate concentration ≤2 standard deviations of mean methotrexate excretion curve specific for dose administered) **or** with normal renal function or mild renal impairment.

Labeled Contraindications There are no contraindications listed in the manufacturer's labeling.

Pregnancy Considerations Animal reproduction studies have not been conducted. If administered to a pregnant woman, the risk to the fetus is unknown; use only if clearly needed. In general, medications used as antidotes should take into consideration the health and prognosis of the mother.

Breast-Feeding Considerations Caution should be used if administered to a breast-feeding woman.

Warnings/Precautions Serious allergic reactions have been reported.

Leucovorin calcium administration should be continued after glucarpidase; the same dose as was given prior to glucarpidase should be continued for the first 48 hours after glucarpidase; after 48 hours, leucovorin doses should be based on methotrexate concentrations. A single methotrexate concentration should not determine when leucovorin should be discontinued; continue leucovorin until the methotrexate concentration remains below the threshold for leucovorin treatment for ≥3 days. Leucovorin calcium is a substrate for glucarpidase and may compete with methotrexate for binding sites; **do not administer leucovorin calcium within 2 hours before or after glucarpidase.** In addition to leucovorin, glucarpidase use should be accompanied with adequate hydration and urinary alkalinization. During the first 48 hours following glucarpidase administration, the only reliable method of measuring methotrexate concentrations is the chromatographic method. DAMPA, an inactive methotrexate metabolite with a half-life of 9 hours, may interfere with immunoassay and result in the overestimation of the methotrexate concentration (when collected within 48 hours of glucarpidase administration). Glucarpidase use for intrathecal methotrexate overdose (off-label route/use) should be used in conjunction with immediate lumbar drainage; concurrent dexamethasone (4 mg IV every 6 hours for 4 doses) may minimize methotrexate-induced chemical arachnoiditis; leucovorin calcium (100 mg IV every 6 hours for 4 doses) may prevent systemic methotrexate toxicity (Widemann, 2004).

Adverse Reactions

>10%: Immunologic: Antibody development (21%)

1% to 10%:

Cardiovascular: Flushing (2%), hypotension (1%)

Central nervous system: Headache (1%)

Gastrointestinal: Nausea/vomiting (2%)

Neuromuscular & skeletal: Paresthesia (2%)

<1%, postmarketing, and/or case reports: Blurred vision, diarrhea, hypersensitivity reaction, hypertension, localized warm feeling, skin rash, throat irritation, tremor

Drug Interactions

Metabolism/Transport Effects None known.

Avoid Concomitant Use There are no known interactions where it is recommended to avoid concomitant use.

Increased Effect/Toxicity There are no known significant interactions involving an increase in effect.

Decreased Effect

Glucarpidase may decrease the levels/effects of: Leucovorin Calcium-Levoleucovorin

Storage/Stability Store intact vials refrigerated at 2°C to 8°C (36°F to 46°F); do not freeze. Reconstituted solutions should be used immediately or may be stored for up to 4 hours under refrigeration.

Preparation for Administration

IV: Reconstitute each vial (1000 units/vial) with 1 mL normal saline. Mix gently by rolling or tilting vial; do not shake. Upon reconstitution, solution should be clear, colorless and free of particulate matter.

Intrathecal (off-label route/use): Reconstitute 2000 units with 12 mL preservative-free normal saline (Widemann, 2004)

Mechanism of Action Recombinant enzyme which rapidly hydrolyzes the carboxyl-terminal glutamate residue from extracellular methotrexate into inactive metabolites (DAMPA and glutamate), resulting in a rapid reduction of methotrexate concentrations independent of renal function

Pharmacodynamics/Kinetics

Onset of action: Methotrexate toxicity: Reduces methotrexate concentrations by ≥97% within 15 minutes of IV administration

Duration: Methotrexate toxicity: Maintains a >95% reduction of methotrexate concentrations for up to 8 days

Distribution: V_d: IV: 3.6 L; distribution restricted to plasma volume

Half-life elimination: IV: Normal renal function: 6-9 hours; impaired renal function (CrCl <30 mL/minute): 8-10 hours (Phillips, 2008)

Dosing

Adult & Geriatric

Methotrexate toxicity: IV: 50 units/kg (Buchen, 2005; Widemann, 1997; Widemann, 2010)

Intrathecal methotrexate overdose (off-label route/use): Intrathecal: 2000 units as soon as possible after accidental methotrexate overdose (Widemann, 2004)

Pediatric

Methotrexate toxicity: IV: Refer to adult dosing.

Intrathecal methotrexate overdose (off-label route/use): Intrathecal: Refer to adult dosing.

Renal Impairment No dosage adjustment necessary.

Hepatic Impairment There are no dosage adjustments provided in the manufacturer's labeling (has not been studied).

Administration

IV: Infuse over 5 minutes; flush IV line before and after glucarpidase administration

Intrathecal (for intrathecal methotrexate overdose; off-label route/use): Glucarpidase was administered within 3-9 hours of accidental intrathecal methotrexate overdose in conjunction with lumbar drainage or ventriculolumbar perfusion (Widemann, 2004). Administered over 5 minutes via lumbar route, ventriculostomy, Ommaya reservoir, or lumbar and ventriculostomy (O'Marcaigh, 1996; Widemann, 2004). In one case report, 1000 units was administered through the ventricular catheter over 5 minutes and another 1000 units was administered through the lumbar catheter (O'Marcaigh, 1996).

Monitoring Parameters

Serum methotrexate levels: Use chromatographic method if <48 hours from glucarpidase administration (DAMPA interferes with immunoassay results until >48 hours)

CBC with differential, bilirubin, ALT, AST, serum creatinine; evaluate for signs/symptoms of methotrexate toxicity

Test Interactions Methotrexate levels: During the first 48 hours following glucarpidase administration, the only reliable method of measuring methotrexate concentrations is the chromatographic method. DAMPA, an inactive methotrexate metabolite with a half-life of 9 hours, may interfere with immunoassay and result in the overestimation of the methotrexate concentration (when collected within 48 hours of glucarpidase administration).

Additional Information The utility of more than one glucarpidase dose in reducing plasma methotrexate levels was evaluated in a study of 100 patients with high-dose methotrexate-induced nephrotoxicity (Widemann, 2010). Glucarpidase 50 units/kg IV was administered either as a single dose (n=65), 2 doses given 24 hours apart (n=28), or 3 doses given at 4 hour intervals (n=7). Six of the 65 patients randomized to a single dose also received a second delayed glucarpidase dose (>24 hours later) due to persistent methotrexate concentrations ≥1 micromole/L in spite of a ≥90% decrease in the plasma methotrexate concentration after the initial dose. The use of scheduled second and third glucarpidase doses did not result in additional methotrexate concentration decreases; and only 2 of the 6 patients who received a second delayed glucarpidase dose (>24 hours later) experienced a ≥50% methotrexate concentration reduction.

◀ **Prescribing and Access Restrictions** Voraxaze® is distributed through ASD Healthcare; procurement information is available (24 hours a day; 365 days a year) at 1-855-7-VORAXAZE (1-855-786-7292). Voraxaze® is also commercially available in the U.S. through certain pharmacy wholesalers on a drop-ship basis; orders will only be processed during business hours for overnight delivery. For additional information, refer to http://www.btgplc.com/products/specialty-pharmaceuticals/voraxaze.

Dosage Forms Excipient information presented when available (limited, particularly for generics); consult specific product labeling.
Solution Reconstituted, Intravenous [preservative free]:
Voraxaze: 1000 units (1 ea)

◆ **GM-CSF** see Sargramostim on page 1515

◆ **GM-CSF-Encoding Oncolytic Herpes Simplex Virus** see Talimogene Laherparepvec on page 1590

◆ **GnRH Agonist** see Histrelin on page 816

Goserelin (GOE se rel in)

Related Information
Safe Handling of Hazardous Drugs on page 2292

Brand Names: US Zoladex

Brand Names: Canada Zoladex; Zoladex LA

Index Terms Goserelin Acetate; ICI-118630; ZDX

Pharmacologic Category Antineoplastic Agent, Gonadotropin-Releasing Hormone Agonist; Gonadotropin Releasing Hormone Agonist

Use

Breast cancer, advanced (3.6 mg only): Palliative treatment of advanced breast cancer in pre- and perimenopausal women (estrogen and progesterone receptor values may help to predict if goserelin is likely to be beneficial).

Endometrial thinning (3.6 mg only): Endometrial-thinning agent prior to endometrial ablation for dysfunctional uterine bleeding.

Endometriosis (3.6 mg only): Management of endometriosis, including pain relief and reduction of endometriotic lesions for the duration of therapy (goserelin experience for endometriosis has been limited to women 18 years and older treated for 6 months).

Prostate cancer, advanced: Palliative treatment of advanced carcinoma of the prostate.

Prostate cancer, stage B2 to C: Management of locally confined stage T2b to T4 (stage B2 to C) prostate cancer (in combination with flutamide); begin goserelin and flutamide 8 weeks prior to initiating radiation therapy and continue during radiation therapy.

Labeled Contraindications Hypersensitivity to goserelin, GnRH, GnRH agonist analogues, or any component of the formulation; pregnancy (except if using for palliative treatment of advanced breast cancer)

Pregnancy Considerations Adverse events were observed in animal reproduction studies. Goserelin induces hormonal changes which increase the risk for fetal loss and use is contraindicated in pregnancy unless being used for palliative treatment of advanced breast cancer.

Breast cancer: If used for the palliative treatment of breast cancer during pregnancy, the potential for increased fetal loss should be discussed with the patient.

Endometriosis, endometrial thinning: Use is contraindicated during pregnancy. Women of childbearing potential should not receive therapy until pregnancy has been excluded. Nonhormonal contraception is recommended for premenopausal women during therapy and for 12 weeks after therapy is discontinued. Although ovulation is usually inhibited and menstruation may stop, pregnancy prevention is not ensured during goserelin therapy. Changes in reproductive function may occur following chronic administration.

Breast-Feeding Considerations It is not known if goserelin is excreted in breast milk, although goserelin is inactivated when used orally. Due to the potential for serious adverse reactions in the breast-feeding infant, a decision should be made to discontinue breast-feeding or to discontinue the drug, taking into account the importance of treatment to the mother.

Warnings/Precautions Hazardous agent - use appropriate precautions for handling and disposal (NIOSH 2014 [group 1]). Transient increases in serum testosterone (in men with prostate cancer) and estrogen (in women with breast cancer) may result in a worsening of disease signs and symptoms (tumor flare) during the first few weeks of treatment. Some patients experienced a temporary worsening of bone pain, which may be managed symptomatically. Spinal cord compression and urinary tract obstruction have been reported when used for prostate cancer; closely observe patients for symptoms (eg, ureteral obstruction, weakness, paresthesias) in first few weeks of therapy. Manage with standard treatment; consider orchiectomy for extreme cases.

Androgen deprivation therapy may increase the risk for cardiovascular disease (Levine, 2010). An increased risk for MI, sudden cardiac death, and stroke has been observed. Monitor for signs/symptoms of cardiovascular disease; manage according to current clinical practice. Androgen deprivation therapy may cause prolongation of the QT/QTc interval; evaluate risk versus benefit in patients with congenital long QT syndrome, heart failure, frequent electrolyte abnormalities, and in patients taking medication known to prolong the QT interval. Correct electrolytes prior to initiation and consider periodic electrolyte and ECG monitoring. Hyperglycemia has been reported in males and may manifest as diabetes or worsening of preexisting diabetes (worsening glycemic control); monitor blood glucose and HbA$_{1c}$ and manage diabetes appropriately.

Injection site and vascular injury, including pain, hematoma, hemorrhage and hemorrhagic shock (requiring blood transfusions or surgical intervention) have been reported with goserelin. Use caution when administering to patients with a low BMI and/or to patients receiving full dose anticoagulation. Use caution while injecting goserelin into the anterior abdominal wall (due to the proximity of underlying inferior epigastric artery and its branches). Monitor for signs/symptoms of abdominal hemorrhage. Inform patient to immediately report abdominal pain, abdominal distention, dyspnea, dizziness, hypotension, and/or altered level of consciousness. Hypersensitivity reactions (including acute anaphylactic reactions) and antibody formation may occur; monitor. Hypercalcemia has been reported in prostate and breast cancer patients with bone metastases; initiate appropriate management if hypercalcemia occurs. Rare cases of pituitary apoplexy (frequently secondary to pituitary adenoma) have been observed with GnRH agonist administration (onset from 1 hour to usually <2 weeks); may present as sudden headache, vomiting, visual or mental status changes, and infrequently cardiovascular collapse; immediate medical attention required. A decreased AUC may be observed when using the 3-month implant in obese patients; monitor testosterone levels if desired clinical response is not observed. Use extra care when administering to patients with a ▶

low BMI. If implant removal is necessary, implant may be located by ultrasound.

Decreased bone density has been reported in women and may be irreversible; use caution if other risk factors are present; evaluate and institute preventive treatment if necessary. Cervical resistance may be increased; use caution when dilating the cervix for endometrial ablation. Women of childbearing potential should not receive therapy until pregnancy has been excluded. Nonhormonal contraception is recommended during therapy and for 12 weeks after therapy is discontinued. The 3-month implant currently has no approved indications for use in women. Chronic administration may result in effects on reproductive function due to antigonadotropic properties. Potentially significant drug-drug interactions may exist, requiring dose or frequency adjustment, additional monitoring, and/or selection of alternative therapy.

Adverse Reactions Some frequencies not defined. Percentages reported with the 1-month implant:

>10%:

Cardiovascular: Vasodilatation (females 57%), peripheral edema (females 21%)

Central nervous system: Headache (females 32% to 75%; males 1% to 5%), emotional lability (females 60%), depression (females 54%; males 1% to 5%), pain (8% to 17%), dyspareunia (females 14%), insomnia (5% to 11%)

Dermatologic: Diaphoresis (females 16% to 45%; males 6%), acne vulgaris (females 42%; usually within 1 month after starting treatment), seborrhea (females 26%)

Endocrine & metabolic: Hot flash (females 57% to 96%; males 64%), decreased libido (females 48% to 61%), increased libido (females 12%)

Gastrointestinal: Abdominal pain (females 7% to 11%), nausea (5% to 11%)

Genitourinary: Vaginitis (75%), breast atrophy (females 33%), sexual disorder (males 21%), breast hypertrophy (females 18%), decrease in erectile frequency (18%), pelvic symptoms (females 18%), genitourinary signs and symptoms (lower; males 13%)

Hematologic & oncologic: Tumor flare (females 23%; males: Incidence not reported)

Infection: Infection (females 13%; males: Incidence not reported)

Neuromuscular & skeletal: Decreased bone mineral density (females 23%; ~4% decrease from baseline in 6 months; male: Incidence not reported), weakness (females 11%)

1% to 10%:

Cardiovascular: Edema (females 5%; male 7%), hypertension (1% to 6%), cardiac failure (males 5%), cardiac arrhythmia (males >1% to <5%), cerebrovascular accident (males >1% to <5%), peripheral vascular disease (males >1% to <5%), varicose veins (males >1% to <5%), chest pain (1% to <5%), myocardial infarction (males <1% to <5%), palpitations, tachycardia (females)

Central nervous system: Lethargy (females ≤8%), migraine (females 1% to 7%), dizziness (females 6%; male 5%), malaise (females ≤5%), chills (males >1% to <5%), anxiety (1% to <5%), nervousness (females 3% to 5%), voice disorder (females 3%), abnormality in thinking, drowsiness, paresthesia

Dermatologic: Skin rash (males 6% to 8%; female frequency not reported), hair disease (females 4%), pruritus (females 2%), alopecia, skin discoloration, xeroderma

Endocrine & metabolic: Gynecomastia (males 8%), hirsutism (7%), gout (males >1% to <5%), hyperglycemia (males >1% to <5%), weight gain (>1% to <5%)

Gastrointestinal: Anorexia (1% to 5%), gastric ulcer (males >1% to <5%), constipation (1% to <5%), diarrhea (1% to <5%), vomiting (1% to <5%), increased appetite (females 2%), dyspepsia, flatulence, xerostomia

Genitourinary: Pelvic pain (females 9%; males 6%), mastalgia (>1% to 7%), uterine hemorrhage (6%), vulvovaginitis (5%), breast swelling (males >1% to <5%), urinary tract obstruction (males: >1% to <5%), urinary tract infection (1% to <5%), urinary frequency, vaginal hemorrhage

Hematologic & oncologic: Anemia (males >1% to <5%), bruise, hemorrhage

Hypersensitivity: Hypersensitivity reaction

Infection: Sepsis (males >1% to <5%)

Local: Application site reaction (females 6%)

Neuromuscular & skeletal: Myalgia (females 3%, males frequency not reported), leg cramps (females 2%, males frequency not reported), hypertonia (females 1%; male frequency not reported), arthralgia, arthropathy

Ophthalmic: Amblyopia, dry eye syndrome

Renal: Renal insufficiency (<1% to >5%)

Respiratory: Upper respiratory tract infection (males 7%), chronic obstructive pulmonary disease (males 5%), flu-like symptoms (females 5%, male frequency not reported), pharyngitis (females 5%), sinusitis (females ≥1%; male frequency not reported), bronchitis, cough, epistaxis, rhinitis

Miscellaneous: Fever

<1%, postmarketing, and/or case reports (with monthly or 3-month implant): Anaphylaxis, bone fracture, convulsions, decreased glucose tolerance, decreased HDL cholesterol, deep vein thrombosis, diabetes mellitus, hypercalcemia, hypercholesterolemia, hyperlipidemia, hypotension, increased HDL cholesterol, increased LDL cholesterol, increased serum ALT, increased serum AST, increased serum triglycerides, injection site reaction (including vascular injury, pain, hematoma, hemorrhage, hemorrhagic shock), osteoporosis, ovarian cyst, ovarian hyperstimulation syndrome, pituitary apoplexy, pituitary neoplasm (including adenoma), pulmonary embolism, psychotic reaction, transient ischemic attacks

Drug Interactions

Metabolism/Transport Effects None known.

Avoid Concomitant Use

Avoid concomitant use of Goserelin with any of the following: Corifollitropin Alfa; Highest Risk QTc-Prolonging Agents; Indium 111 Capromab Pendetide; Ivabradine; Mifepristone

Increased Effect/Toxicity

Goserelin may increase the levels/effects of: Corifollitropin Alfa; Highest Risk QTc-Prolonging Agents; Moderate Risk QTc-Prolonging Agents

The levels/effects of Goserelin may be increased by: Ivabradine; Mifepristone; QTc-Prolonging Agents (Indeterminate Risk and Risk Modifying)

Decreased Effect

Goserelin may decrease the levels/effects of: Antidiabetic Agents; Choline C 11; Indium 111 Capromab Pendetide

Storage/Stability Store at room temperature not to exceed 25°C (77°F).

◄ **Mechanism of Action** Goserelin (a gonadotropin-releasing hormone [GnRH] analog) causes an initial increase in luteinizing hormone (LH) and follicle stimulating hormone (FSH), chronic administration of goserelin results in a sustained suppression of pituitary gonadotropins. Serum testosterone falls to levels comparable to surgical castration. The exact mechanism of this effect is unknown, but may be related to changes in the control of LH or down-regulation of LH receptors.

Pharmacodynamics/Kinetics

Onset:

Females: Estradiol suppression reaches postmenopausal levels within 3 weeks and FSH and LH are suppressed to follicular phase levels within 4 weeks of initiation

Males: Testosterone suppression reaches castrate levels within 2 to 4 weeks after initiation

Duration:

Females: Estradiol, LH and FSH generally return to baseline levels within 12 weeks following the last monthly implant.

Males: Testosterone levels maintained at castrate levels throughout the duration of therapy.

Absorption: SubQ: Rapid and can be detected in serum in 30 to 60 minutes; 3.6 mg: released slowly in first 8 days, then rapid and continuous release for 28 days

Distribution: V_d: Male: 44.1 L; Female: 20.3 L

Protein binding: ~27%

Metabolism: Hepatic hydrolysis of the C-terminal amino acids

Time to peak, serum: SubQ: Male: 12 to 15 days, Female: 8 to 22 days

Excretion: Urine (>90%; 20% as unchanged drug)

Dosing

Adult

Prostate cancer, advanced: Males: SubQ:

28-day implant: 3.6 mg every 28 days

12-week implant: 10.8 mg every 12 weeks

Prostate cancer, stage B2 to C (in combination with an antiandrogen and radiotherapy); begin 8 weeks prior to radiotherapy): Males: SubQ:

Combination 28-day/12-week implant: 3.6 mg implant, followed in 28 days by 10.8 mg implant

28-day implant (alternate dosing): 3.6 mg; repeated every 28 days for a total of 4 doses

Breast cancer, advanced: Females: SubQ: 3.6 mg every 28 days

Endometriosis: Females: SubQ: 3.6 mg every 28 days for 6 months

Endometrial thinning: Females: SubQ: 3.6 mg every 28 days for 1 or 2 doses

Prevention of early menopause during chemotherapy for early stage hormone receptor negative breast cancer (off-label use): Females: SubQ: 3.6 mg every 28 days starting 1 week prior to the first chemotherapy dose; continue until within 2 weeks before or after the final chemotherapy dose (Moore, 2015).

Geriatric Males: Refer to adult dosing.

Renal Impairment No dosage adjustment necessary.

Hepatic Impairment No dosage adjustment necessary.

Administration SubQ: Administer implant by inserting needle at a 30 to 45 degree angle into the anterior abdominal wall below the navel line. Use caution while injecting goserelin into the anterior abdominal wall (due to the proximity of underlying inferior epigastric artery and its branches). Goserelin is an implant; therefore, do not attempt to eliminate air bubbles prior to injection (may displace implant). Do not attempt to aspirate prior to injection; if a large vessel is penetrated, blood will be visualized in the syringe chamber (if vessel is penetrated, withdraw needle and inject elsewhere with a new syringe). Do not penetrate into muscle or peritoneum. Implant may be detected by ultrasound if removal is required. Monitor for signs/symptoms of abdominal hemorrhage. Use extra care when administering goserelin to patients with a low BMI and/or to patients receiving full dose anticoagulation.

Hazardous agent; use appropriate precautions for handling and disposal (NIOSH 2014 [group 1]).

Monitoring Parameters Monitor blood glucose and HbA_{1c} (periodically), bone mineral density, serum calcium, cholesterol/lipids; monitor for signs/symptoms of abdominal hemorrhage following injection.

Prostate cancer: Consider periodic ECG and electrolyte monitoring. Monitor for weakness, paresthesias, tumor flare, urinary tract obstruction, and spinal cord compression in first few weeks of therapy.

Test Interactions Interferes with pituitary gonadotropic and gonadal function tests during and for up to 12 weeks after discontinued

Dosage Forms Excipient information presented when available (limited, particularly for generics); consult specific product labeling.

Implant, Subcutaneous:

Zoladex: 3.6 mg (1 ea); 10.8 mg (1 ea)

◆ **Goserelin Acetate** see Goserelin on page 796

◆ **GR38032R** see Ondansetron on page 1253

Granisetron (gra NI se tron)

Related Information

Management of Chemotherapy-Induced Nausea and Vomiting in Adults on page 2142

Prevention of Chemotherapy-Induced Nausea and Vomiting in Children on page 2203

Brand Names: US Granisol [DSC]; Sancuso

Brand Names: Canada Granisetron Hydrochloride Injection; Kytril

Index Terms BRL 43694; Granisetron Hydrochloride; Granisol; Kytril

Pharmacologic Category Antiemetic; Selective 5-HT$_3$ Receptor Antagonist

Use

Chemotherapy-associated nausea and vomiting: Prevention of nausea and vomiting associated with initial and repeat courses of emetogenic chemotherapy, including high-dose cisplatin (injection and tablets); prevention of nausea and vomiting associated with moderately and/or highly emetogenic chemotherapy regimens of up to 5 consecutive days of duration (transdermal).

Radiation-associated nausea and vomiting: Prevention of nausea and vomiting associated with radiation therapy, including total body radiation and fractionated abdominal radiation (tablets).

Labeled Contraindications Hypersensitivity to granisetron or any component of the formulation

◄ *Canadian labeling:* Additional contraindications (not in U.S. labeling): Concomitant use with apomorphine

Pregnancy Considerations Adverse events have not been observed in animal reproduction studies. Injection (1 mg/mL strength) may contain benzyl alcohol which may cross the placenta.

Breast-Feeding Considerations It is not known if granisetron is excreted in breast milk. The US manufacturer recommends that caution be exercised when administering granisetron to nursing women. The Canadian manufacturer does not recommend use in nursing women.

Warnings/Precautions Use with caution in patients with congenital long QT syndrome or other risk factors for QT prolongation (eg, medications known to prolong QT interval, electrolyte abnormalities, and cumulative high-dose anthracycline therapy). 5-HT$_3$ antagonists have been associated with a number of dose-dependent increases in ECG intervals (eg, PR, QRS duration, QT/QTc, JT), usually occurring 1 to 2 hours after IV administration. In general, these changes are not clinically relevant, however, when used in conjunction with other agents that prolong these intervals, arrhythmia may occur. When used with agents that prolong the QT interval (eg, Class I and III antiarrhythmics), clinically relevant QT interval prolongation may occur resulting in torsade de pointes. IV formulations of 5-HT$_3$ antagonists have more association with ECG interval changes, compared to oral formulations.

Antiemetics are most effective when used prophylactically (Roila 2010). If emesis occurs despite optimal antiemetic prophylaxis, re-evaluate emetic risk, disease, concurrent morbidities and medications to assure antiemetic regimen is optimized (Basch 2011).

Serotonin syndrome has been reported with 5-HT$_3$ receptor antagonists, predominantly when used in combination with other serotonergic agents (eg, SSRIs, SNRIs, MAOIs, mirtazapine, fentanyl, lithium, tramadol, and/or methylene blue). Some of the cases were fatal. The majority of serotonin syndrome reports due to 5-HT$_3$ receptor antagonist have occurred in a postanesthesia setting or in an infusion center. Serotonin syndrome has also been reported following overdose of another 5-HT$_3$ receptor antagonist. Monitor patients for signs of serotonin syndrome, including mental status changes (eg, agitation, hallucinations, delirium, coma); autonomic instability (eg, tachycardia, labile blood pressure, diaphoresis, dizziness, flushing, hyperthermia); neuromuscular changes (eg, tremor, rigidity, myoclonus, hyperreflexia, incoordination); gastrointestinal symptoms (eg, nausea, vomiting, diarrhea); and/or seizures. If serotonin syndrome occurs, discontinue 5-HT$_3$ receptor antagonist treatment and begin supportive management. Use with caution in patients allergic to other 5-HT$_3$ receptor antagonists; cross-reactivity has been reported. Does not stimulate gastric or intestinal peristalsis (should not be used instead of nasogastric suction); may mask progressive ileus and/or gastric distension. Potentially significant drug-drug interactions may exist, requiring dose or frequency adjustment, additional monitoring, and/or selection of alternative therapy.

Transdermal patch: Do not apply patch to red, irritated, or damaged skin. Application-site reactions have occurred with transdermal patch use; local reactions were generally mild and did not require discontinuation. If skin reaction is severe or generalized (allergic rash including erythematous, macular, or papular rash or pruritus), remove patch. Cover patch application site with clothing to protect from natural or artificial sunlight exposure while patch is applied and for 10 days following removal; granisetron may potentially be affected by natural or artificial sunlight. Do not apply heat (eg, heating pad) over or in area of the transdermal patch; avoid prolonged exposure to heat (may increase plasma concentrations).

Benzyl alcohol and derivatives: Some dosage forms may contain benzyl alcohol; large amounts of benzyl alcohol (≥99 mg/kg/day) have been associated with a potentially fatal toxicity ("gasping syndrome") in neonates; the "gasping syndrome" consists of metabolic acidosis, respiratory distress, gasping respirations, CNS dysfunction (including convulsions, intracranial hemorrhage), hypotension and cardiovascular collapse (AAP ["Inactive" 1997]; CDC 1982); some data suggests that benzoate displaces bilirubin from protein binding sites (Ahlfors 2001); avoid or use dosage forms containing benzyl alcohol with caution in neonates. See manufacturer's labeling.

Polysorbate 80: Some dosage forms may contain polysorbate 80 (also known as Tweens). Hypersensitivity reactions, usually a delayed reaction, have been reported following exposure to pharmaceutical products containing polysorbate 80 in certain individuals (Isaksson 2002; Lucente 2000; Shelley 1995). Thrombocytopenia, ascites, pulmonary deterioration, and renal and hepatic failure have been reported in premature neonates after receiving parenteral products containing polysorbate 80 (Alade 1986; CDC 1984). See manufacturer's labeling.

Adverse Reactions

>10%:

Central nervous system: Headache (oral and IV: 3% to 21%; transdermal: <1%)

Gastrointestinal: Nausea (20%), constipation (oral and IV: 3% to 18%; transdermal: 5%), vomiting (12%)

Neuromuscular & skeletal: Weakness (oral: 14% to 18%; IV: 5%)

1% to 10%:

Cardiovascular: Prolonged Q-T interval on ECG (1% to 3%; >450 milliseconds, not associated with any arrhythmias), hypertension (oral and IV: 1% to 2%)

Central nervous system: Dizziness (5%), insomnia (oral and IV: ≤5%), drowsiness (1% to 4%), anxiety (oral and IV: ≤2%), agitation (IV: <2%), central nervous system stimulation (IV: <2%)

Dermatologic: Alopecia (3%), skin rash (IV: 1%)

Gastrointestinal: Diarrhea (oral and IV: 4% to 9%), decreased appetite (6%), dyspepsia (oral: 6%), abdominal pain (4% to 6%), dysgeusia (IV: 2%)

Hematologic and oncologic: Leukopenia (9%), anemia (4%), thrombocytopenia (2%)

Hepatic: Increased serum ALT (>2 x ULN: 3% to 6%), increased serum AST (>2 x ULN: 3% to 5%)

Miscellaneous: Fever (3% to 9%)

<1%, postmarketing, and/or case reports: Angina pectoris, application site reaction (transdermal allergic rash including erythematous, macular, papular rash, or pruritus), atrial fibrillation, atrioventricular block (IV), cardiac arrhythmia, ECG abnormality (IV), extrapyramidal reaction (oral), hypersensitivity reaction (includes anaphylaxis, dyspnea, hypotension, urticaria), hypotension, serotonin syndrome, sinus bradycardia (IV), syncope, ventricular ectopy (IV; includes non-sustained tachycardia)

◄ **Drug Interactions**

Metabolism/Transport Effects Substrate of CYP3A4 (minor); **Note:** Assignment of Major/Minor substrate status based on clinically relevant drug interaction potential

Avoid Concomitant Use

Avoid concomitant use of Granisetron with any of the following: Apomorphine; Highest Risk QTc-Prolonging Agents; Ivabradine; Mifepristone

Increased Effect/Toxicity

Granisetron may increase the levels/effects of: Apomorphine; Highest Risk QTc-Prolonging Agents; Moderate Risk QTc-Prolonging Agents; Panobinostat; Serotonin Modulators

The levels/effects of Granisetron may be increased by: Ivabradine; Mifepristone; QTc-Prolonging Agents (Indeterminate Risk and Risk Modifying)

Decreased Effect

Granisetron may decrease the levels/effects of: Tapentadol; TraMADol

Storage/Stability

IV: Store at 15°C to 30°C (59°F to 86°F). Protect from light. Do not freeze vials. Stable when mixed in NS or D_5W for 7 days under refrigeration and for 3 days at room temperature.

Oral: Store tablet or oral solution at 15°C to 30°C (59°F to 86°F). Protect from light.

Transdermal patch: Store at 20°C to 25°C (68°F to 77°F). Keep patch in original packaging until immediately prior to use.

Mechanism of Action Selective $5\text{-}HT_3$-receptor antagonist, blocking serotonin, both peripherally on vagal nerve terminals and centrally in the chemoreceptor trigger zone

Pharmacodynamics/Kinetics

Duration: Oral, IV: Generally up to 24 hours

Absorption: Oral: Tablets and oral solution are bioequivalent; Transdermal patch: ~66% over 7 days

Distribution: V_d: 2 to 4 L/kg; widely throughout body

Protein binding: ~65%

Metabolism: Hepatic via N-demethylation, oxidation, and conjugation; some metabolites may have $5\text{-}HT_3$ antagonist activity

Half-life elimination: Oral: 6 hours; IV: ~9 hours

Time to peak, plasma: Transdermal patch: Maximum systemic concentrations: ~48 hours after application (range: 24 to 168 hours)

Excretion: Urine (12% as unchanged drug, 48% to 49% as metabolites); feces (34% to 38% as metabolites)

Dosing

Adult & Geriatric

Prevention of chemotherapy-associated nausea and vomiting:

Oral: 2 mg once daily up to 1 hour before chemotherapy or 1 mg twice daily; the first 1 mg dose should be given up to 1 hour before chemotherapy (with the second 1 mg dose 12 hours later). Administer only on the day(s) chemotherapy is given.

IV: 10 mcg/kg 30 minutes prior to chemotherapy; only on the day(s) chemotherapy is given.

Transdermal patch: Prophylaxis of chemotherapy-related emesis: Apply 1 patch at least 24 hours prior to chemotherapy; may be applied up to 48 hours before chemotherapy. Remove patch a minimum of 24 hours after chemotherapy completion. Maximum duration: Patch may be worn up to 7 days, depending on chemotherapy regimen duration.

Adult guideline recommendations:

American Society of Clinical Oncology (ASCO; Basch 2011): High emetic risk:

IV: 1 mg or 10 mcg/kg on the day(s) chemotherapy is administered (antiemetic regimen also includes dexamethasone and aprepitant or fosaprepitant)

Oral: 2 mg on the day(s) chemotherapy is administered (antiemetic regimen also includes dexamethasone and aprepitant or fosaprepitant)

Multinational Association of Supportive Care in Cancer (MASCC) and European Society of Medical Oncology (ESMO) (Roila 2010):

Highly emetic chemotherapy:

IV: 1 mg or 10 mcg/kg (antiemetic regimen includes dexamethasone and aprepitant/fosaprepitant) prior to chemotherapy on day 1

Oral: 2 mg (antiemetic regimen includes dexamethasone and aprepitant/fosaprepitant) prior to chemotherapy on day 1

Moderately emetic chemotherapy:

IV: 1 mg or 10 mcg/kg (antiemetic regimen includes dexamethasone [and aprepitant/fosaprepitant for AC chemotherapy regimen]) prior to chemotherapy on day 1

Oral: 2 mg (antiemetic regimen includes dexamethasone [and aprepitant/fosaprepitant for AC chemotherapy regimen]) prior to chemotherapy on day 1

Low emetic risk:

IV: 1 mg or 10 mcg/kg prior to chemotherapy on day 1

Oral: 2 mg prior to chemotherapy on day 1

Prophylaxis of radiation therapy-associated emesis: Oral: 2 mg once daily within 1 hour of radiation therapy.

Prevention of postoperative nausea and vomiting (off-label use): IV: 0.35 to 3 mg (5 to 20 **mcg**/kg) administered at the end of surgery (Gan 2014).

Pediatric

Prevention of chemotherapy-associated nausea and vomiting: Children ≥2 years and Adolescents: IV: 10 mcg/kg 30 minutes prior to chemotherapy; only on the day(s) chemotherapy is given.

Pediatric guideline recommendations:

Prevention of chemotherapy-induced nausea and vomiting (off-label dosing; Dupuis 2013):

Highly emetogenic chemotherapy: Infants ≥1 month and Children <12 years: IV: 40 mcg/kg as a single daily dose prior to chemotherapy. Antiemetic regimen also includes dexamethasone.

Highly emetogenic chemotherapy: Children ≥12 years and Adolescents: IV: 40 mcg/kg as a single daily dose prior to chemotherapy. Antiemetic regimen includes dexamethasone and (if no known or suspected drug interactions) aprepitant.

Moderately emetogenic chemotherapy: Infants ≥1 month, Children, and Adolescents:

IV: 40 mcg/kg as a single daily dose. Antiemetic regimen also includes dexamethasone

Oral: 40 mcg/kg every 12 hours. Antiemetic regimen also includes dexamethasone

Low emetogenic chemotherapy: Infants ≥1 month, Children, and Adolescents:

IV: 40 mcg/kg as a single daily dose.

Oral: 40 mcg/kg every 12 hours.

Renal Impairment No dosage adjustment necessary.

Hepatic Impairment Kinetic studies in patients with hepatic impairment showed that total clearance was approximately halved; however, standard doses were very well tolerated, and dose adjustments are not necessary.

Administration

Oral: Doses should be given up to 1 hour prior to initiation of chemotherapy/radiation

IV: Administer IV push over 30 seconds or as a 5- to 10-minute infusion

Transdermal (Sancuso): Apply patch to clean, dry, intact skin on upper outer arm. Do not use on red, irritated, or damaged skin. Remove patch from pouch immediately before application. Do not cut patch. Cover patch application site with clothing to protect from natural or artificial sunlight exposure while patch is applied and for 10 days following removal; granisetron may potentially be affected by natural or artificial sunlight. Do not apply heat (eg, heating pad) over or in area of the transdermal patch; avoid prolonged exposure to heat (may increase plasma concentrations).

Extemporaneous Preparations Note: Commercial oral solution is available (0.2 mg/mL)

A 0.2 mg/mL oral suspension may be made with tablets. Crush twelve 1 mg tablets in a mortar and reduce to a fine powder. Add 30 mL distilled water, mix well, and transfer to a bottle. Rinse the mortar with 10 mL cherry syrup and add to bottle. Add sufficient quantity of cherry syrup to make a final volume of 60 mL. Label "shake well". Stable 14 days at room temperature or refrigerated (Quercia 1997).

A 50 mcg/mL oral suspension may be made with tablets and one of three different vehicles (Ora-Sweet®, Ora-Plus®, or a mixture of methylcellulose 1% and Simple Syrup, N.F.). Crush one 1 mg tablet in a mortar and reduce to a fine powder. Add 20 mL of the chosen vehicle and mix to a uniform paste; transfer to a calibrated bottle. Label "shake well" and "refrigerate". Stable for 91 days refrigerated (Nahata 1998).

Nahata MC, Morosco RS, and Hipple TF, "Stability of Granisetron Hydrochloride in Two Oral Suspensions," *Am J Health Syst Pharm*, 1998, 55(23):2511-3.

Quercia RA, Zhang J, Fan C, et al, "Stability of Granisetron Hydrochloride in an Extemporaneously Prepared Oral Liquid," *Am J Health Syst Pharm*, 1997, 54(12):1404-6.

Dosage Forms Excipient information presented when available (limited, particularly for generics); consult specific product labeling. [DSC] = Discontinued product

Patch, Transdermal:

Sancuso: 3.1 mg/24 hr (1 ea)

Solution, Intravenous:

Generic: 0.1 mg/mL (1 mL); 1 mg/mL (1 mL); 4 mg/4 mL (4 mL)

Solution, Intravenous [preservative free]:

Generic: 0.1 mg/mL (1 mL); 1 mg/mL (1 mL)

Solution, Oral:
Granisol: 2 mg/10 mL (30 mL [DSC]) [contains fd&c yellow #6 (sunset yellow), sodium benzoate; orange flavor]
Tablet, Oral:
Generic: 1 mg
Dosage Forms: Canada Refer to Dosage Forms. **Note:** Transdermal patch is not available in Canada

♦ **Granisetron Hydrochloride** see Granisetron on page 801
♦ **Granisetron Hydrochloride Injection (Can)** see Granisetron on page 801
♦ **Granisol** see Granisetron on page 801
♦ **Granisol [DSC]** see Granisetron on page 801
♦ **Granix** see Filgrastim on page 711
♦ **Granulocyte Colony Stimulating Factor** see Filgrastim on page 711
♦ **Granulocyte Colony Stimulating Factor (PEG Conjugate)** see Pegfilgrastim on page 1346
♦ **Granulocyte-Macrophage Colony Stimulating Factor** see Sargramostim on page 1515
♦ **GS-1101** see Idelalisib on page 867
♦ **GSK-580299** see Papillomavirus (Types 16, 18) Vaccine (Human, Recombinant) on page 1332
♦ **GSK1120212** see Trametinib on page 1674
♦ **GSK2118436** see Dabrafenib on page 420
♦ **GW506U78** see Nelarabine on page 1191
♦ **GW572016** see Lapatinib on page 997
♦ **GW786034** see PAZOPanib on page 1334
♦ **h5G1.1** see Eculizumab on page 580
♦ **HAL** see Hexaminolevulinate on page 815
♦ **Halaven** see EriBULin on page 624
♦ **Haldol** see Haloperidol on page 807
♦ **Haldol Decanoate** see Haloperidol on page 807
♦ **Halichondrin B Analog** see EriBULin on page 624

Haloperidol (ha loe PER i dole)
Brand Names: US Haldol; Haldol Decanoate
Brand Names: Canada Apo-Haloperidol; Haloperidol Injection, USP; Haloperidol-LA; Haloperidol-LA Omega; Novo-Peridol; PMS-Haloperidol; PMS-Haloperidol LA
Index Terms Haloperidol Decanoate; Haloperidol Lactate
Pharmacologic Category First Generation (Typical) Antipsychotic
Use
Behavioral disorders (tablet, concentrate): Treatment of severe behavioral problems in children with combative, explosive hyperexcitability that cannot be accounted for by immediate provocation. Reserve for use in these children only after failure to respond to psychotherapy or medications other than antipsychotics.

◀ **Hyperactivity (tablet, concentrate):** Short-term treatment of hyperactive children who show excessive motor activity with accompanying conduct disorders consisting of some or all of the following symptoms: impulsivity, difficulty sustaining attention, aggression, mood lability, or poor frustration tolerance. Reserve for use in these children only after failure to respond to psychotherapy or medications other than antipsychotics.

Psychotic disorders (tablet, concentrate): Management of manifestations of psychotic disorders.

Schizophrenia:

IM, lactate: Treatment of schizophrenia.

IM, decanoate: Treatment of patients with schizophrenia who require prolonged parenteral antipsychotic therapy.

Tourette disorder (tablet, concentrate, IM lactate): Control of tics and vocal utterances in Tourette syndrome in adults and children.

Pregnancy Risk Factor C

Dosing

Adult

Psychosis:

Manufacturer's labeling: Oral: 0.5 to 5 mg 2 to 3 times daily; adjust dose based on response and tolerability. According to the manufacturer, daily dosages up to 100 mg may be necessary in some cases to achieve an optimal response; infrequently, doses >100 mg have been used in severely treatment resistant patients. Recommended dose range for schizophrenia: 5 to 20 mg/day (APA [Lehman 2004)].

Schizophrenia:

IM (as lactate): 2 to 5 mg; subsequent doses may be administered as often as every 60 minutes, although 4- to 8-hour intervals may be satisfactory.

IM (as decanoate): **Note**: Establish tolerance to oral haloperidol prior to changing to IM decanoate injection.

Initial: 10 to 20 times the daily oral dose. The initial dose should not exceed 100 mg regardless of previous antipsychotic requirements. If the initial dose conversion requires >100 mg, administer the dose in 2 injections (maximum of 100 mg for first injection) separated by 3 to 7 days.

Oral haloperidol ≤10 mg/day, elderly, or debilitated: Initiate dose at 10 to 15 times the daily oral dose

Oral haloperidol >10 mg/day or high risk of relapse: Initiate dose at 20 times the daily oral dose

Maintenance dose: 10 to 15 times the previous daily oral dose or 50 to 200 mg administer doses at 4-week intervals (Buchanan 2009; Hasan 2013).

Oral overlap: Following initial dose, taper the oral dose and discontinue after the first 2 or 3 injections (McEvoy 2006).

Alternative dosing regimen:

Loading dose regimen: Initial: 20 times the previous daily oral dose, divide total dose and give every 3 to 7 days, do not exceed 250 mg per injection; discontinue oral haloperidol prior to first injection. Reduce the dose by 25% each month, depending on clinical response, in months 2 to 4, and establish the maintenance dose.

Usual maintenance dose: 200 mg per month (Ereshefsky 1993)

Tourette syndrome: Oral: 0.5 to 5 mg 2 to 3 times daily; adjust dose based on response and tolerability. Tourette Canada Guidelines recommend a dosing range of 0.5 to 3 mg/day (Pringsheim 2012) and European Society for the Study of Tourette Syndrome recommend a dosing range of 0.25 to 15 mg/day (Roessner 2011). According to the manufacturer, daily dosages up to 100 mg may be necessary in some cases to achieve an optimal response; infrequently doses >100 mg have been used in severely treatment resistant patients.

Chemotherapy-induced nausea and vomiting (off-label use): Breakthrough nausea/vomiting: Oral, IV (off-label route): 0.5 to 1 mg every 6 hours as needed (Lohr 2008)

Delirium in the intensive care unit, treatment (off-label use): Note: The optimal dose and regimen of haloperidol for the treatment of severe agitation and/or delirium has not been established. Currently, there are no studies evaluating the role of haloperidol on duration or severity of delirium. Haloperidol has been used for symptomatic treatment (severe agitation) of delirious patients. Current guidelines do not advocate use of haloperidol for the treatment or prevention of delirium due to insufficient evidence (Barr 2013).

IV (off-label route): Initial: 0.5 to 10 mg depending on degree of agitation; if inadequate response, may repeat bolus dose (with sequential doubling of initial bolus dose) every 15 to 30 minutes until calm achieved, then administer 25% of the last bolus dose every 6 hours; monitor ECG and QTc interval. After the patient is controlled, haloperidol therapy should be tapered over several days. This strategy is based upon expert opinion; efficacy and safety have not been formally evaluated (Tesar 1988).

Note: Continuous infusions have also been used with doses in the range of 0.5 to 2 mg/hour with an optional loading dose of 2.5 mg (Reade 2009).

Delirium in the intensive care unit (patients at high risk of delirium), prevention (off-label use): Note: The optimal dose and regimen of haloperidol for prevention of ICU delirium has not been established. Current guidelines do not advocate use of haloperidol for the treatment or prevention of delirium due to insufficient evidence (Barr 2013). Haloperidol may decrease the incidence of delirium (Van den Boogaard 2013; Wang 2012).

IV (off-label route): 0.5 mg followed by a continuous infusion of 0.1 mg/hour for 12 hours (Wang 2012) **or** 0.5 to 1 mg every 8 hours (Van den Boogaard 2013)

Phencyclidine psychosis (off-label use): IM, IV (off-label route), Oral: 5 mg (Giannini 1984; MacNeal 2012). **Note:** Additional data may be necessary to further define the role of haloperidol in this condition.

Postoperative nausea and vomiting (PONV), prevention (off-label use): IM, IV (off-label route): 0.5 to 2 mg (Gan 2014)

Rapid tranquilization (agitation/aggression/violent behavior) (off-label use): IM (as lactate): 2.5 to 10 mg (Clinton 1987; MacDonald 2012; Powney 2012; Wilson 2012)

Geriatric

Psychosis: Oral: 0.5 to 2 mg 2 to 3 times daily; adjust dose based on response and tolerability. Maximum dosage per manufacturer's labeling: 100 mg/day. Recommended dose range for schizophrenia: 5 to 20 mg/day (APA [Lehman 2004]).

Psychosis/agitation related to Alzheimer disease and other dementias (off-label use): Initial: Oral: 0.25 to 0.5 mg/day (APA [Rabins 2007]; slowly increase dose based on response and tolerability every 4 to 7 days in increments of 0.25 to 1 mg (De Deyn 1999; Devanand 1998); usual maximum dose of 2 mg/day (APA [Rabins 2007]; Doses up to 6 mg/day in 1 to 2 divided doses were evaluated in clinical trials (Lonergan 2002).

Pediatric

Behavior disorders, nonpsychotic:

Children 3 to 12 years weighing 15 to 40 kg: Oral: Initial: 0.5 mg/day in 2 to 3 divided doses; may increase by 0.5 mg every 5 to 7 days to usual maintenance range of 0.05 to 0.075 mg/kg/day in 2 to 3 divided doses; maximum dose not established; children with severe, nonpsychotic disturbance may require higher doses; however, no improvement has been shown with doses >6 mg/day.

Children >40 kg and Adolescents (off-label dose): Oral: 0.5 to 15 mg/day in 2 to 3 divided doses; begin at lower end of the range and may increase as needed (no more frequently than every 5 to 7 days); maximum daily dose: 15 mg/day. **Note:** Higher doses may be necessary in severe or refractory cases (Kliegman 2011).

Psychosis:

Children 3 to 12 years weighing 15 to 40 kg: Oral: Initial: 0.5 mg/day in 2 to 3 divided doses; increase by 0.5 mg every 5 to 7 days to usual maintenance range of 0.05 to 0.15 mg/kg/day in 2 to 3 divided doses; higher doses may be necessary in severe or refractory cases; maximum dose not established; in adolescents, the maximum daily dose is 15 mg/day (Kliegman 2011)

Children >40 kg and Adolescents (off-label dose): Oral: 0.5 to 15 mg/day in 2 to 3 divided doses; begin at lower end of the range and may increase as needed (no more frequently than every 5 to 7 days); maximum daily dose: 15 mg/day (Kliegman 2011; Willner 1969). **Note:** Higher doses may be necessary in severe or refractory cases (Kliegman 2011).

Tourette syndrome:

Children 3 to 12 years weighing 15 to 40 kg: Oral:

Manufacturer's labeling: Initial: 0.5 mg/day in 2 to 3 divided doses; increase by 0.5 mg every 5 to 7 days to usual maintenance of 0.05 to 0.075 mg/kg/day in 2 to 3 divided doses; maximum dose not established; however, no improvement has been shown with doses >6 mg/day in patients with nonpsychotic disturbances

Alternate dosing: Initial: 0.25 to 0.5 mg/day in 2 to 3 divided doses titrated to a usual daily dose range of 1 to 4 mg/day (Roessner 2011; Scahill 2006)

Children >40 kg and Adolescents (off-label dose): Oral: 0.25 to 15 mg/day in 2 to 3 divided doses; begin at lower end of the range and may increase as needed (no more frequently than every 5 to 7 days) (Kleigman 2011; Roessner 2011); usual dose range: 1 to 4 mg/day (Roessner 2011; Scahill 2006); maximum dose not established; however, no improvement has been shown with doses >6 mg/day in patients with nonpsychotic disturbances

Renal Impairment There are no dosage adjustments provided in the manufacturer's labeling.

Hepatic Impairment There are no dosage adjustments provided in the manufacturer's labeling.

Additional Information Complete prescribing information should be consulted for additional detail.

Dosage Forms Excipient information presented when available (limited, particularly for generics); consult specific product labeling.

Concentrate, Oral, as lactate [strength expressed as base]:
Generic: 2 mg/mL (5 mL, 15 mL, 120 mL)

Solution, Intramuscular, as decanoate [strength expressed as base]:
Haldol Decanoate: 50 mg/mL (1 mL); 100 mg/mL (1 mL) [contains benzyl alcohol, sesame oil]
Generic: 50 mg/mL (1 mL, 5 mL); 100 mg/mL (1 mL, 5 mL)

Solution, Injection, as lactate [strength expressed as base]:
Haldol: 5 mg/mL (1 mL)
Generic: 5 mg/mL (1 mL, 10 mL)

Solution, Injection, as lactate [strength expressed as base, preservative free]:
Generic: 5 mg/mL (1 mL)

Tablet, Oral:
Generic: 0.5 mg, 1 mg, 2 mg, 5 mg, 10 mg, 20 mg

♦ **Haloperidol Decanoate** *see* Haloperidol *on page* 807

♦ **Haloperidol Injection, USP (Can)** *see* Haloperidol *on page* 807

♦ **Haloperidol-LA (Can)** *see* Haloperidol *on page* 807

♦ **Haloperidol Lactate** *see* Haloperidol *on page* 807

♦ **Haloperidol-LA Omega (Can)** *see* Haloperidol *on page* 807

♦ **Halotestin** *see* Fluoxymesterone *on page* 750

♦ **Hecoria [DSC]** *see* Tacrolimus (Systemic) *on page* 1576

♦ **Hedgehog Antagonist GDC-0449** *see* Vismodegib *on page* 1771

♦ **Helixate FS** *see* Antihemophilic Factor (Recombinant) *on page* 119

♦ **Hemofil M** *see* Antihemophilic Factor (Human) *on page* 117

Heparin (HEP a rin)

Brand Names: US Hep Flush-10

Brand Names: Canada Heparin Leo; Heparin Lock Flush; Heparin Sodium Injection, USP

Index Terms Heparin Calcium; Heparin Lock Flush; Heparin Sodium; Heparinized Saline

Pharmacologic Category Anticoagulant; Anticoagulant, Heparin

Use Anticoagulation: Prophylaxis and treatment of thromboembolic disorders. As an anticoagulant for extracorporeal and dialysis procedures

Note: Heparin lock flush solution is intended only to maintain patency of IV devices and is **not** to be used for systemic anticoagulant therapy.

Pregnancy Risk Factor C

Dosing

Adult Note: Many concentrations of heparin are available ranging from 1 unit/mL to 20,000 units/mL. Carefully examine each prefilled syringe or vial prior to use ensuring that the correct concentration is chosen. Heparin lock flush solution is intended only to maintain patency of IV devices and is not to be used for anticoagulant therapy.

Acute coronary syndromes (off-label use): IV infusion (weight-based dosing per institutional nomogram recommended):

STEMI: Adjunct to fibrinolysis (full-dose alteplase, reteplase, or tenecteplase) (Antman, 2008): Initial bolus of 60 units/kg (maximum: 4000 units), then 12 units/kg/hour (maximum: 1000 units/hour) as continuous infusion. Check aPTT every 4 to 6 hours; adjust to target of 1.5 to 2 times the upper limit of control (50 to 70 seconds). Continue for a minimum of 48 hours, and preferably for the duration of hospitalization (up to 8 days) or until revascularization (if performed) (ACCF/AHA [O'Gara, 2013]).

Unstable angina (UA)/non-ST-elevation myocardial infarction (NSTEMI): Initial bolus of 60 units/kg (maximum: 4000 units), followed by an initial infusion of 12 units/kg/hour (maximum: 1000 units/hour). Check aPTT every 4 to 6 hours; adjust to target of 1.5 to 2 times the upper limit of control (50 to 70 seconds). Optimal duration of therapy is unknown; however, most trials continued therapy for 2 to 5 days. Recommended duration is 48 hours or until percutaneous coronary intervention is performed (AHA/ACC [Amsterdam, 2014]).

Anticoagulation (Intermittent administration): IV: Initial: 10,000 units, then 50 to 70 units/kg (5000 to 10,000 units) every 4 to 6 hours

Atrial fibrillation (off-label use): Guidelines pertaining to peri-cardioversion use (ACCP [You, 2012]):

Patients with atrial fibrillation (for more than 48 hours or unknown duration) undergoing cardioversion: IV heparin to maintain an aPTT prolongation that corresponds to plasma heparin levels of 0.3 to 0.7 units/mL anti-Xa activity started at the time of transesophageal echocardiography (TEE) is recommended with cardioversion performed within 24 hours of the TEE if no thrombus is seen.

Patients with atrial fibrillation (for 48 hours or less) undergoing cardioversion: Cardioversion may be performed without prolonged anticoagulation. However, anticoagulation with IV heparin to maintain an aPTT prolongation that corresponds to plasma heparin levels of 0.3 to 0.7 units/mL anti-Xa activity should be started at presentation in patients with no contraindications to anticoagulation.

Emergency cardioversion in hemodynamically unstable patient: Cardioversion may be performed without prolonged anticoagulation. Anticoagulation with IV heparin to maintain an aPTT prolongation that corresponds to plasma heparin levels of 0.3 to 0.7 units/mL anti-Xa activity should be started prior to cardioversion in patients with no contraindications to anticoagulation.

Interstitial cystitis (bladder pain syndrome) (off-label use): Intravesical: **Note:** Various dosage regimens of heparin (20,000 to 50,000 units) alone or with alkalinized lidocaine (1% to 4%) have been used. When lidocaine and heparin are mixed, there is a risk of precipitation if proper alkalinization does not occur. Lidocaine stability and pH should be determined after the components have been mixed, prior to administration.

Single-dose regimen: Instill the combination of 50,000 units of heparin, lidocaine 200 mg, and sodium bicarbonate 420 mg in 15 mL of sterile water into the bladder via catheter and allow to dwell for 30 minutes before draining (Parsons, 2012).

Once-weekly dosing regimen: Instill the combination of 20,000 units of heparin, lidocaine 4% (5 mL), and sodium bicarbonate 7% (25 mL) into an empty bladder via catheter once weekly for 12 weeks and allow to dwell for 30 minutes before draining (Nomiya, 2013).

Twice-weekly dosing regimen: Instill 25,000 units of heparin (diluted with 5 mL of sterile water) into bladder via catheter twice weekly for 3 months (Kuo, 2001).

Maintenance of line patency (line flushing): When using daily flushes of heparin to maintain patency of single and double lumen central catheters, 10 units/mL is commonly used for younger infants (eg, <10 kg) while 100 units/mL is used for older infants, children, and adults. Capped PVC catheters and peripheral heparin locks require flushing more frequently (eg, every 6 to 8 hours). Volume of heparin flush is usually similar to volume of catheter (or slightly greater). Additional flushes should be given when stagnant blood is observed in catheter, after catheter is used for drug or blood administration, and after blood withdrawal from catheter.

Parenteral nutrition: Addition of heparin (0.5 to 3 unit/mL) to peripheral and central parenteral nutrition has not been shown to decrease catheter-related thrombosis. The final concentration of heparin used for TPN solutions may need to be decreased to 0.5 units/mL in small infants receiving larger amounts of volume in order to avoid approaching therapeutic amounts. Arterial lines are heparinized with a final concentration of 1 unit/mL.

Percutaneous coronary intervention (off-label use; Levine, 2011):
No prior anticoagulant therapy:

If no GPIIb/IIIa inhibitor use planned: Initial bolus of 70 to 100 units/kg (target ACT 250 to 300 seconds for HemoTec®, 300 to 350 seconds for Hemochron®)

or

If planning GPIIb/IIIa inhibitor use: Initial bolus of 50 to 70 units/kg (target ACT 200 to 250 seconds regardless of device)

Prior anticoagulant therapy:

If no GPIIb/IIIa inhibitor use planned: Additional heparin as needed (eg, 2000 to 5000 units) (target ACT 250 to 300 seconds for HemoTec®, 300 to 350 seconds for Hemochron®)

or

If planning GPIIb/IIIa inhibitor use: Additional heparin as needed (eg, 2000 to 5000 units) (target ACT 200 to 250 seconds regardless of device)

Thromboprophylaxis (low-dose heparin): SubQ: 5000 units every 8 to 12 hours. **Note:** The American College of Chest Physicians recommends a minimum of 10 to 14 days for patients undergoing total hip arthroplasty, total knee arthroplasty, or hip fracture surgery (Guyatt, 2012).

Venous thromboembolism (treatment): Note: Start warfarin on the first or second treatment day and continue heparin until INR is ≥2 for at least 24 hours (usually 5 to 7 days) (Guyatt, 2012).

DVT/PE (off-label dosing): IV: 80 units/kg (or alternatively 5000 units) IV push followed by continuous infusion of 18 units/kg/hour (or alternatively 1000 units/hour) (Guyatt, 2012)

or

DVT/PE (off-label dosing): SubQ: *Unmonitored dosing regimen:* Initial: 333 units/kg then 250 units/kg every 12 hours (Guyatt, 2012; Kearon, 2006)

Geriatric Patients >60 years of age may have higher serum levels and clinical response (longer aPTTs) as compared to younger patients receiving similar dosages. Lower dosages may be required.

◀ **Pediatric Note:** Many concentrations of heparin are available ranging from 1 unit/mL to 20,000 units/mL. Carefully examine each prefilled syringe or vial prior to use ensuring that the correct concentration is chosen. Heparin lock flush solution is intended only to maintain patency of IV devices and is not to be used for anticoagulant therapy.

Prophylaxis for cardiac catheterization (arterial approach): IV: Bolus: 100 units/kg (Freed, 1974; Monagle, 2012)

Systemic heparinization:

Intermittent IV: Initial: 50-100 units/kg, then 50-100 units/kg every 4 hours (**Note:** Continuous IV infusion is preferred)

IV infusion: Initial loading dose: 75 units/kg given over 10 minutes, then initial maintenance dose: 20 units/kg/hour; adjust dose to maintain aPTT of 60-85 seconds (assuming this reflects an antifactor Xa level of 0.35-0.7 units/mL); see table.

Pediatric Protocol For Systemic Heparin Adjustment

To be used after initial loading dose and maintenance IV infusion dose (see usual dosage listed above) to maintain aPTT of 60-85 seconds (assuming this reflects antifactor Xa level of 0.35-0.7 units/mL).

Obtain blood for aPTT 4 hours after heparin loading dose and 4 hours after every infusion rate change.

Obtain daily CBC and aPTT after aPTT is therapeutic.

aPTT (seconds)	Dosage Adjustment	Time to Repeat aPTT
<50	Give 50 units/kg bolus and increase infusion rate by 10%	4 h after rate change
50-59	Increase infusion rate by 10%	4 h after rate change
60-85	Keep rate the same	Next day
86-95	Decrease infusion rate by 10%	4 h after rate change
96-120	Hold infusion for 30 minutes and decrease infusion rate by 10%	4 h after rate change
>120	Hold infusion for 60 minutes and decrease infusion rate by 15%	4 h after rate change

Modified from Andrew M, et al, "Heparin Therapy in Pediatric Patients: A Prospective Cohort Study," *Pediatr Research*, 1994, 35(1):78-83.
Note: The aPTT range of 60-85 seconds corresponds to an anti-Xa level of 0.35-0.7 units/mL.

Note: Refer to adult dosing for notes on line flushing and TPN.

Renal Impairment No dosage adjustment required; adjust therapeutic heparin according to aPTT or anti-Xa activity.

Hepatic Impairment No dosage adjustment required; adjust therapeutic heparin according to aPTT or anti-Xa activity.

Additional Information Complete prescribing information should be consulted for additional detail.

Dosage Forms Excipient information presented when available (limited, particularly for generics); consult specific product labeling. [DSC] = Discontinued product

Solution, Injection, as sodium:

Generic: 1000 units (500 mL); 2000 units (1000 mL); 12,500 units (250 mL); 25,000 units (250 mL, 500 mL); 1000 units/mL (1 mL, 10 mL, 30 mL); 2500 units/mL (10 mL); 5000 units/mL (1 mL, 10 mL); 10,000 units/mL (1 mL, 4 mL, 5 mL); 20,000 units/mL (1 mL)

Solution, Injection, as sodium [preservative free]:
  Generic: 1000 units/mL (2 mL); 5000 units/0.5 mL (0.5 mL)
Solution, Intravenous, as sodium:
  Hep Flush-10: 10 units/mL (10 mL)
  Generic: 10,000 units (250 mL); 12,500 units (250 mL); 20,000 units (500 mL); 25,000 units (250 mL, 500 mL); 1 units/mL (1 mL, 2 mL, 2.5 mL, 3 mL, 5 mL, 10 mL); 2 units/mL (3 mL); 10 units/mL (1 mL, 2 mL, 2.5 mL, 3 mL, 5 mL, 10 mL, 30 mL); 100 units/mL (1 mL, 2 mL, 2.5 mL, 3 mL, 5 mL, 10 mL, 30 mL, 100 mL [DSC], 250 mL); 2000 units/mL (5 mL)
Solution, Intravenous, as sodium [preservative free]:
  Generic: 1 units/mL (3 mL); 10 units/mL (1 mL, 3 mL, 5 mL); 100 units/mL (1 mL, 3 mL, 5 mL)

◆ **Heparin Calcium** *see* Heparin *on page* 811
◆ **Heparinized Saline** *see* Heparin *on page* 811
◆ **Heparin Leo (Can)** *see* Heparin *on page* 811
◆ **Heparin Lock Flush** *see* Heparin *on page* 811
◆ **Heparin Sodium** *see* Heparin *on page* 811
◆ **Heparin Sodium Injection, USP (Can)** *see* Heparin *on page* 811
◆ **Hep Flush-10** *see* Heparin *on page* 811
◆ **Herceptin** *see* Trastuzumab *on page* 1685
◆ **Hexalen** *see* Altretamine *on page* 82
◆ **Hexamethylmelamine** *see* Altretamine *on page* 82

Hexaminolevulinate (hex a mee noe LEV ue lin ate)

Brand Names: US Cysview
Index Terms HAL; Hexaminolevulinate Hydrochloride
Pharmacologic Category Contrast Agent
Use Detection of non-muscle invasive papillary cancer of the bladder; used in conjunction with the Karl Storz D-Light C Photodynamic Diagnostic (PDD) system
Pregnancy Risk Factor C
Dosing
  Adult Cystoscopic examination: Intravesical instillation: 50 mL (100 mg) instilled into empty bladder via urinary catheter
  Renal Impairment No dosage adjustment provided in manufacturer's labeling.
  Hepatic Impairment No dosage adjustment provided in manufacturer's labeling.
Additional Information Complete prescribing information should be consulted for additional detail.
Dosage Forms Excipient information presented when available (limited, particularly for generics); consult specific product labeling.
Solution Reconstituted, Intravesical, as hydrochloride:
  Cysview: 100 mg (1 ea)

◆ **Hexaminolevulinate Hydrochloride** *see* Hexaminolevulinate *on page* 815
◆ **HHT** *see* Omacetaxine *on page* 1248
◆ **High-Molecular-Weight Iron Dextran (DexFerrum)** *see* Iron Dextran Complex *on page* 964

Histrelin (his TREL in)

Related Information
Safe Handling of Hazardous Drugs *on page 2292*

Brand Names: US Supprelin LA; Vantas

Brand Names: Canada Vantas

Index Terms GnRH Agonist; Histrelin Acetate; LH-RH Agonist

Pharmacologic Category Antineoplastic Agent, Gonadotropin-Releasing Hormone Agonist; Gonadotropin Releasing Hormone Agonist

Use

Central precocious puberty: Treatment of central precocious puberty (CPP) in children

Prostate cancer, advanced: Palliative treatment of advanced prostate cancer

Labeled Contraindications Hypersensitivity to histrelin acetate, gonadotropin releasing hormone (GnRH), GnRH-agonist analogs, or any component of the formulation; females who are or may become pregnant

Pregnancy Considerations Adverse events were observed in animal reproduction studies. May cause fetal harm or spontaneous abortion if administered during pregnancy. Histrelin is contraindicated for use during pregnancy or in women who may become pregnant.

Breast-Feeding Considerations It is not known if histrelin is excreted in breast milk. The products are not indicated for use in postpubertal women.

Warnings/Precautions Hazardous agent - use appropriate precautions for handling and disposal (meets NIOSH 2014 criteria). Proper surgical insertion technique is essential to avoid complications. Patients should keep arm dry for 24 hours and avoid heavy lifting/strenuous exertion of insertion arm for 7 days after implantation. Potentially significant drug-drug interactions may exist, requiring dose or frequency adjustment, additional monitoring, and/or selection of alternative therapy.

CPP: Transient increases in estradiol serum levels (female) or testosterone levels (female and male) may occur during the first week of use. Worsening symptoms may occur, however, manifestations of puberty should decrease within 4 weeks. If the implant breaks during removal, the remaining pieces should be removed; confirm the removal of the entire implant (refer to manufacturer's instructions for removal procedure).

Prostate cancer: Transient increases in testosterone serum levels occur during the first week of use (initial tumor flare), which may result in a worsening of disease signs and symptoms such as bone pain, hematuria, neuropathy, ureteral or bladder outlet obstruction, and spinal cord compression. Spinal cord compression may contribute to paralysis; close attention should be given during the first few weeks of therapy to both patients having metastatic vertebral lesions and/or urinary tract obstructions, and to any patients reporting weakness, paresthesias or poor urine output. Androgen-deprivation therapy (ADT) may increase the risk for cardiovascular disease (Levine, 2010); an increased risk of MI, sudden cardiac death, and stroke has been reported with GnRH agonist use in men; monitor for symptoms associated with cardiovascular disease. ADT may prolong the QT/QTc interval; consider the benefits of ADT versus the risk for QT prolongation in patients with a history of QTc prolongation, congenital long QT syndrome, heart failure, frequent electrolyte abnormalities, and in patients with medications known to prolong the QT interval, or with preexisting cardiac disease. Consider periodic monitoring of electrocardiograms and electrolytes in at-risk patients. Hyperglycemia has been reported with androgen deprivation therapy (in prostate cancer) and may manifest as diabetes or worsening of preexisting diabetes; monitor blood glucose and/or HbA_{1c}. Rare cases of pituitary apoplexy (frequently secondary to pituitary adenoma) have been observed with GnRH agonist administration (onset from 1 hour to usually <2 weeks); may present as sudden headache, vomiting, visual or mental status changes, and infrequently cardiovascular collapse; immediate medical attention required. Safety and efficacy have not been established in patients with hepatic dysfunction. In studies, the implant was not recovered in a small number of patients. Serum testosterone rose above castrate level and the implant was not palpable or visualized (via ultrasound); it was believed to have been extruded. Some patients had continued testosterone levels below castration level even though the implant was not palpable.

Adverse Reactions

CPP:

>10%: Local: Insertion site reaction (51%; includes bruising, discomfort, itching, pain, protrusion of implant area, soreness, swelling, tingling)

>2% to 10%:

Endocrine & metabolic: Metrorrhagia (4%)

Local: Keloid scar (6%), scar (6%), suture-related complication (6%), pain at the application site (4%), post procedural pain (4%)

≤2%, postmarketing, and/or case reports: Amblyopia, breast tenderness, cold feeling, disease progression, dysmenorrhea, epistaxis, erythema, flu-like syndrome, gynecomastia, headache, infection at the implant site, menorrhagia, migraine, mood swings, pituitary adenoma, pituitary apoplexy, pruritus, seizures, weight gain

Prostate cancer:

>10%:

Endocrine & metabolic: Hot flashes (66%)

Local: Implant site reaction (6% to 14%; includes bruising, erythema, pain, soreness, swelling, tenderness)

2% to 10%:

Central nervous system: Fatigue (10%), headache (3%), insomnia (3%)

Endocrine & metabolic: Gynecomastia (4%), sexual dysfunction (4%), libido decreased (2%)

Gastrointestinal: Constipation (4%), weight gain (2%)

Genitourinary: Expected pharmacological consequence of testosterone suppression: Testicular atrophy (5%)

Renal: Renal impairment (5%)

<2%: Abdominal discomfort, alopecia, anemia, appetite increased, arthralgia, AST increased, back pain, bone density decreased, bone pain, breast pain, breast tenderness, cold feeling, contusion, craving food, creatinine increased, depression, diaphoresis, dizziness, dyspnea (exertional), dysuria, fluid retention, flushing, genital pruritus, hematoma, hematuria, hepatic injury (severe), hypercalcemia, hypercholesterolemia, hyperglycemia, irritability, LDH increased, lethargy, limb pain, liver disorder, malaise, muscle twitching, myalgia, nausea, neck pain, night sweats, pain, palpitation, peripheral edema, prostatic acid phosphatase increased, pruritus, pituitary apoplexy, renal calculi, renal failure, stent occlusion, testosterone increased, tremor, urinary frequency, urinary retention, ventricular asystoles, weakness, weight loss

Drug Interactions

Metabolism/Transport Effects None known.

Avoid Concomitant Use
Avoid concomitant use of Histrelin with any of the following: Corifollitropin Alfa; Indium 111 Capromab Pendetide

Increased Effect/Toxicity
Histrelin may increase the levels/effects of: Corifollitropin Alfa; Highest Risk QTc-Prolonging Agents; Moderate Risk QTc-Prolonging Agents

The levels/effects of Histrelin may be increased by: Mifepristone

Decreased Effect
Histrelin may decrease the levels/effects of: Antidiabetic Agents; Choline C 11; Indium 111 Capromab Pendetide

Storage/Stability Upon delivery, separate contents of implant carton. Store implant under refrigeration at 2°C to 8°C (36°F to 46°F); excursions permitted to 25°C (77°F) for 7 days (if unused within 7 days, may return to proper refrigeration until product expiration date). Keep implant wrapped in the amber pouch for protection from light; do not freeze. The implantation insertion kit does not require refrigeration.

Preparation for Administration The implant may be slightly curved when removed from refrigerator; may roll implant (in sterile-gloved hands) a few times between fingers and thumb. If resistance is felt when inserting implant into insertion tool cannula, remove and manually manipulate or roll as needed and reinsert into cannula.

Hazardous agent; use appropriate precautions for handling and disposal (meets NIOSH 2014 criteria).

Mechanism of Action Potent inhibitor of gonadotropin secretion; continuous administration results in, after an initiation phase, the suppression of luteinizing hormone (LH), follicle-stimulating hormone (FSH), and a subsequent decrease in testosterone and dihydrotestosterone (males) and estrone and estradiol (premenopausal females). Testosterone levels are reduced to castrate levels in males (treated for prostate cancer) within 2 to 4 weeks. Additionally, in patients with CPP, linear growth velocity is slowed (improves chance of attaining predicted adult height).

Pharmacodynamics/Kinetics
Onset of action: Prostate cancer: Chemical castration: Within 2 to 4 weeks; CPP: Progression of sexual development stops and growth is decreased within 1 month

Duration: 12 months (plus a few additional weeks of histrelin release)

Distribution: Adults: V_d: ~58 L

Protein binding: Adults: 70% ± 9%

Metabolism: Hepatic via C-terminal dealkylation and hydrolysis

Bioavailability: Adults: 92%

Half-life elimination: Adults: Terminal: ~4 hours

Time to peak, serum: Adults: 12 hours

Dosing
Adult & Geriatric Prostate cancer, advanced (Vantas): SubQ: 50 mg implant surgically inserted every 12 months

Pediatric Central precocious puberty (CPP) (Supprelin LA): Children ≥2 years: SubQ: 50 mg implant surgically inserted every 12 months. Discontinue at the appropriate time for the onset of puberty.

Renal Impairment
Vantas: CrCl ≥15 mL/minute: No dosage adjustment necessary.

Supprelin LA: There are no dosage adjustments provided in the manufacturers' labeling.

Hepatic Impairment There are no dosage adjustments provided in the manufacturer's labeling (has not been studied).

Combination Regimens

Prostate cancer: Histrelin (Prostate Regimen) on page 2003

Administration SubQ: Surgical implantation (using a sterile field) into the inner portion of the upper arm requires the use of the implantation device provided. Use the patient's nondominant arm for placement; implant should be placed halfway between the shoulder and the elbow at the crease between the tricep and the bicep. Implant removal should occur after ~12 months; a replacement implant may be inserted if therapy is to be continued. Palpate area of incision to locate implant for removal. If not readily palpated, ultrasound, CT or MRI may be used to locate implant; plain films are not recommended because the implant is not radiopaque. Refer to manufacturer's labeling for full insertion and removal details.

Hazardous agent; use appropriate precautions for handling and disposal (meets NIOSH 2014 criteria).

Monitoring Parameters

CPP: LH, FSH, estradiol, or testosterone (after 1 month then every 6 months); height, bone age (every 6 to 12 months); tanner staging; monitor for clinical evidence of suppression of CPP manifestations

Prostate cancer: Serum testosterone levels, prostate specific antigen (PSA); bone mineral density; weakness, paresthesias, and urinary tract obstruction (especially during first few weeks of therapy); screen for diabetes; monitor for symptoms associated with cardiovascular disease. Consider periodic monitoring of electrocardiograms and electrolytes.

Test Interactions Results of diagnostic test of pituitary gonadotropic and gonadal functions may be affected during and after therapy

Dosage Forms Excipient information presented when available (limited, particularly for generics); consult specific product labeling.

Kit, Subcutaneous:

Supprelin LA: 50 mg

Vantas: 50 mg

- **HPV Vaccine (Bivalent)** *see* Papillomavirus (Types 16, 18) Vaccine (Human, Recombinant) *on page 1332*
- **HPV Vaccine (Quadrivalent)** *see* Papillomavirus (Types 6, 11, 16, 18) Vaccine (Human, Recombinant) *on page 1330*
- **HU** *see* Hydroxyurea *on page 839*
- **HuLuc63** *see* Elotuzumab *on page 585*
- **Humanized IgG1 Anti-CD52 Monoclonal Antibody** *see* Alemtuzumab *on page 62*
- **Human Normal Immunoglobulin** *see* Immune Globulin *on page 903*
- **Human Papillomavirus Vaccine (Bivalent)** *see* Papillomavirus (Types 16, 18) Vaccine (Human, Recombinant) *on page 1332*
- **Human Papillomavirus Vaccine (Quadrivalent)** *see* Papillomavirus (Types 6, 11, 16, 18) Vaccine (Human, Recombinant) *on page 1330*
- **Human Thyroid Stimulating Hormone** *see* Thyrotropin Alfa *on page 1645*
- **HuMax-CD20** *see* Ofatumumab *on page 1235*
- **HXM** *see* Altretamine *on page 82*

Hyaluronidase (hye al yoor ON i dase)

Related Information
Management of Drug Extravasations *on page 2159*

Brand Names: US Amphadase; Hylenex; Vitrase

Index Terms Wydase

Pharmacologic Category Antidote, Extravasation; Enzyme

Use
Absorption and dispersion of injected drugs: As an adjuvant to increase the absorption and dispersion of other injected drugs.

Subcutaneous fluid administration: As an adjuvant in subcutaneous fluid administration (hypodermoclysis) for achieving hydration.

Subcutaneous urography: As an adjunct in subcutaneous urography for improving resorption of radiopaque agents.

Labeled Contraindications Hypersensitivity to hyaluronidase or any component of the formulation

Pregnancy Considerations Adverse events have not been observed in animal reproduction studies (not conducted with all products). Administration during labor did not cause any increase in blood loss or differences in cervical trauma. It is not known whether it affects the fetus if used during labor. Hyaluronidase has been evaluated for use prior to intracytoplasmic sperm injection (ICSI) to increase male fertility (DeVos, 2008; Evison, 2009).

Breast-Feeding Considerations It is not known if hyaluronidase is excreted in breast milk. The manufacturer recommends that caution be exercised when administering hyaluronidase to nursing women.

Warnings/Precautions For labeled indications, do not administer intravenously (enzyme is rapidly inactivated and desired effects will not be produced); do not inject in or around infected or inflamed areas; may spread localized infection. Do not apply directly to the cornea; not for topical use. Hyaluronidase is ineffective for extravasation management of vasoconstrictors (eg, dopamine, epinephrine, norepinephrine, phenylephrine, vasopressin) or to reduce swelling of bites or stings; do not use in these settings. Use with caution in patients with reported history of bee sting allergy; hyaluronidase is an active component in bee venom. Discontinue if sensitization occurs (a skin test may be performed to determine hypersensitivity). Some products may contain albumin; albumin carries an extremely remote risk for transmission of viral diseases, Creutzfeldt-Jakob disease (CJD) and variant CJD (vCJD). No cases of transmission of viral diseases, CJD, or vCJD have been identified for licensed albumin or albumin contained in other licensed products. Potentially significant interactions may exist, requiring dose or frequency adjustment, additional monitoring, and/or selection of alternative therapy.

Adverse Reactions Frequency not defined.

Cardiovascular: Edema

Local: Injection site reaction

<1%, postmarketing, and/or case reports: Anaphylactic-like reactions (retrobulbar block or IV injections), anaphylaxis, angioedema, hypersensitivity reaction, urticaria

Drug Interactions

Metabolism/Transport Effects None known.

Avoid Concomitant Use

Avoid concomitant use of Hyaluronidase with any of the following: Phenylephrine (Systemic)

Increased Effect/Toxicity

Hyaluronidase may increase the levels/effects of: Alpha-/Beta-Agonists; DOPamine; Local Anesthetics; Phenylephrine (Systemic)

Decreased Effect

The levels/effects of Hyaluronidase may be decreased by: Antihistamines; Corticosteroids; Estrogen Derivatives; Salicylates

Storage/Stability

Amphadase, Hylenex: Store intact vials in refrigerator at 2°C to 8°C (36°F to 46°F); do not freeze.

Vitrase: Store intact vials in refrigerator at 2°C to 8°C (36°F to 46°F); do not freeze. Protect from light. If adding to other injectable solutions, store admixture at 15°C to 25°C (59°F to 77°F) and use within 6 hours.

Preparation for Administration Extravasation management (off-label use): To make a 15 units/mL concentration, mix 0.1 mL (of 150 units/mL) with 0.9 mL NS.

Mechanism of Action Enzymatically modifies the permeability of connective tissue through hydrolysis of hyaluronic acid, one of the chief components of tissue cement which offers resistance to diffusion of liquids through tissues; hyaluronidase increases the distribution/dispersion and absorption of locally injected or extravasated substances.

Pharmacodynamics/Kinetics

Onset of action: SubQ: Immediate; when used for extravasation, there is usually a reduction in swelling within 15-30 minutes after administration (Zenk, 1981b)

Duration: 24-48 hours (variable)

Dosing

Adult & Geriatric

Skin test: Intradermal: 0.02 mL (Amphadase 3 units, Hylenex 3 units, or Vitrase 4 units) of a 150 units/mL (Amphadase, Hylenex) or 200 units/mL (Vitrase) solution. Positive reaction consists of a wheal with pseudopods appearing within 5 minutes and persisting for 20-30 minutes with localized itching (transient erythema is not considered a positive reaction). Skin testing is not necessary prior to use for extravasation management.

◄ **Dehydration:** *Hypodermoclysis:* SubQ: 150 or 200 units followed by sub-cutaneous isotonic fluid administration ≥1000 mL **or** may be added to small volumes (≤200 mL) of subcutaneous replacement fluid. Rate and volume of a single clysis should not exceed those used for infusion of IV fluids.

Dispersion/absorption enhancement of injected drugs: SubQ: 50-300 units (usual dose: 150 units) either injected prior to drug administration or added to injection solution (consult compatibility reference prior to mixing)

Extravasation management (off-label use): Note: Administer as soon as extravasation is recognized. Do not use for extravasation of vasoconstric-tors (eg, dopamine, norepinephrine [manage with phentolamine]). For extravasation management, skin testing is not necessary prior to use. The concentration of doses used to manage extravasation ranges from **15 units/ mL to 150 units/mL**; refer to specific vesicant (below) for a description of doses/concentrations used in published case reports and/or reviews:

Aminophylline, calcium solutions, dextrose 10%, nafcillin, parenteral nutri-tion, potassium solutions, and radiocontrast media extravasation: Intra-dermal or SubQ: Inject a total of 1 mL (15 units/mL) as five separate 0.2 mL injections (using a 25-gauge needle) into area of extravasation at the leading edge in a clockwise manner (MacCara, 1983; Zenk, 1981b)

Contrast media extravasation: The injection of a total of 5 mL (150 units/ mL) as five separate 1 mL injections around the extravasation site has been also used successfully (Rowlett, 2012).

Dextrose 50% extravasation: Injection of a total of 1 mL (150 units/mL) as five separate 0.2 mL injections administered along the leading edge of erythema has also been used successfully for dextrose 50% extravasation (Wiegand, 2009).

Mannitol: SubQ: Administer multiple injections of 0.5-1 mL (15 units/mL) around the periphery of the extravasation (Kumar, 2003)

Paclitaxel: IV: Administer 1-6 mL (150 units/mL) into existing IV line, and/or, if needle/cannula has been removed, inject subcutaneously in a clockwise manner around area of extravasation; usual dose is 1 mL hyaluronidase for each 1 mL of extravasated drug; may repeat several times over the next 3-4 hours (Ener, 2004)

Sodium bicarbonate: SubQ: Administer 4-5 separate 0.2 mL injections (15 units/mL) around area of extravasation (Hurst, 2004)

Vinca alkaloid (vinblastine, vincristine, vindesine, vinorelbine) extravasation:
If needle/cannula still in place: IV: After gently aspirating to remove extravasated vesicant, administer 1-6 mL hyaluronidase (150 units/mL) into existing IV line; the usual dose is 1 mL hyaluronidase for each 1 mL of extravasated drug (Perez Fidalgo, 2012; Schulmeister, 2011).

If needle/cannula has been removed: SubQ: Inject 1-6 mL (150 units/mL) in a clock wise manner using 1 mL for every 1 mL of drug extravasated (Schulmeister, 2011) **or** administer 1 mL (150 units/mL) as 5 separate 0.2 mL injections (using a 25-gauge needle) into the extravasation site (Polovich, 2009).

Retrobulbar/peribulbar block (adjuvant in bupivacaine-lidocaine mix-ture) (off-label use): 3.75 units (150 units/mL concentration) or 7.5 units (150 units/mL concentration) for every 1 mL of a 1:1 mixture of bupivacaine 0.75% and lidocaine 2%; administer a total of 6-8 mL of mixture divided evenly between retrobulbar and peribulbar injections (Kallio, 2000).

Pediatric

Skin test: Children and Adolescents: Intradermal: 0.02 mL (Amphadase 3 units, Hylenex 3 units, or Vitrase 4 units) of a 150 units/mL (Amphadase, Hylenex) or 200 units/mL (Vitrase) solution. Positive reaction consists of a wheal with pseudopods appearing within 5 minutes and persisting for 20-30 minutes with localized itching (transient erythema is not considered a positive reaction). Skin testing is not necessary prior to use for extravasation management.

Dehydration: Hypodermoclysis: SubQ: 150 or 200 units followed by sub-cutaneous isotonic fluid administration ≥1000 mL **or** may be added to small volumes (≤200 mL) of subcutaneous replacement fluid

Premature Infants: Volume of a single clysis/day should not exceed 25 mL/kg and the rate of administration should not exceed 2 mL/minute

Children <3 years: Volume of a single clysis should not exceed 200 mL

Children ≥3 years and Adolescents: Rate and volume of a single clysis should not exceed those used for infusion of IV fluids

Dispersion/absorption enhancement of injected drugs: Children and Adolescents: SubQ: 50-300 units (usual dose: 150 units) either injected prior to drug administration or added to injection solution (consult compatibility reference prior to mixing)

Subcutaneous urography: Infants and Children: SubQ: 75 units over each scapula followed by injection of contrast medium at the same site; patient should be in the prone position during drug administration

Renal Impairment There are no dosage adjustments provided in the manufacturer's labeling.

Hepatic Impairment There are no dosage adjustments provided in the manufacturer's labeling.

Administration Do **not** administer IV for labeled uses (enzyme is rapidly inactivated and desired effects will not be produced).

Extravasation management (off-label use): Stop vesicant infusion immediately and disconnect IV line (leave needle/cannula in place); gently aspirate extravasated solution from the IV line (do **NOT** flush the line). Keep needle/cannula in place for vinca alkaloid extravasation, if appropriate, remove needle/cannula for other vesicants; elevate extremity.

Hyaluronidase administration:

Local administration (intradermal or subQ): Using a 150 units/mL concentration, mix 0.1 mL (of 150 units/mL) with 0.9 mL NS in 1 mL syringe to make final concentration of 15 units/mL; administer 5 x 0.2 mL (15 units/mL) intradermally and/or subcutaneously into area of extravasation (Mac-Cara, 1983).

Vinca alkaloids: If needle/cannula still in place, administer 1-6 mL hyaluronidase (150 units/mL) into the existing IV line; the usual dose is 1 mL hyaluronidase for each 1 mL of extravasated drug (Perez Fidalgo, 2012; Schulmeister, 2011). If needle/cannula has been removed, inject 1-6 mL (150 units/mL) subcutaneously in a clockwise manner using 1 mL for 1 mL of drug extravasated (Schulmeister, 2011) **or** administer 1 mL (150 units/mL) as 5 separate 0.2 mL injections (25-gauge needle) subcutaneously into the extravasation site (Polovich, 2009).

◀ Retrobulbar/peribulbar administration (off-label use): After combining hyaluronidase with a 1:1 mixture of bupivacaine 0.75% and lidocaine 2%, administer according to standard anesthetic technique (Kallio, 2000).

Monitoring Parameters Extravasation management (off-label use): Document and monitor extravasation site.

Additional Information
Amphadase: pH: 6.8 (solution in vial)
Hylenex: pH: 7 (solution in vial)
Vitrase: pH: 6.4-7.2 (solution in vial)

Dosage Forms Excipient information presented when available (limited, particularly for generics); consult specific product labeling. [DSC] = Discontinued product
Solution, Injection:
Amphadase: 150 units/mL (1 mL) [contains edetate disodium, thimerosal]
Solution, Injection [preservative free]:
Hylenex: 150 units/mL (1 mL [DSC]) [contains albumin human, edetate disodium]
Hylenex: 150 units/mL (1 mL) [contains albumin human, polysorbate 80]
Vitrase: 200 units/mL (1.2 mL)
Generic: 150 units/mL (1 mL)

♦ **Hycamptamine** see Topotecan on page 1653
♦ **Hycamtin** see Topotecan on page 1653
♦ **Hydeltra T.B.A. (Can)** see PrednisoLONE (Systemic) on page 1421
♦ **Hydrea** see Hydroxyurea on page 839

Hydrocortisone (Systemic) (hye droe KOR ti sone)

Related Information
Corticosteroids Systemic Equivalencies on page 2334
Management of EGFR Inhibitor Toxicities: Dermatologic, Ocular, and Gastrointestinal on page 2179
Prevention of Chemotherapy-Induced Nausea and Vomiting in Children on page 2203

Brand Names: US A-Hydrocort; Cortef; Solu-CORTEF
Brand Names: Canada Cortef; Solu-Cortef
Index Terms A-hydroCort; Compound F; Cortisol; Hydrocortisone Sodium Succinate
Pharmacologic Category Corticosteroid, Systemic
Use Primarily as an anti-inflammatory or immunosuppressant agent in the treatment of a variety of diseases including those of dermatologic, endocrine, GI, hematologic, allergic, inflammatory, neoplastic, neurologic, ophthalmic, renal, respiratory, and autoimmune origin.

Labeled Contraindications Hypersensitivity to hydrocortisone or any component of the formulation; systemic fungal infections; serious infections, except septic shock or tuberculous meningitis; viral, fungal, or tubercular skin lesions; IM administration contraindicated in idiopathic thrombocytopenia purpura; intrathecal administration of injection

Pregnancy Considerations Adverse events have been observed with corticosteroids in animal reproduction studies. Some studies have shown an association between first trimester systemic corticosteroid use and oral clefts (Park-Wyllie, 2000; Pradat, 2003). Systemic corticosteroids may also influence fetal growth (decreased birth weight); however, information is conflicting

(Lunghi, 2010). Hypoadrenalism may occur in newborns following maternal use of corticosteroids in pregnancy (monitor). When systemic corticosteroids are needed in pregnancy, it is generally recommended to use the lowest effective dose for the shortest duration of time, avoiding high doses during the first trimester (Leachman, 2006; Lunghi, 2010; Makol, 2011; Østensen, 2009).

Breast-Feeding Considerations Corticosteroids are excreted in breast milk. The manufacturer notes that when used systemically, maternal use of corticosteroids have the potential to cause adverse events in a nursing infant (eg, growth suppression, interfere with endogenous corticosteroid production). If there is concern about exposure to the infant, some guidelines recommend waiting 4 hours after the maternal dose of an oral systemic corticosteroid before breast-feeding in order to decrease potential exposure to the nursing infant (based on a study using prednisolone) (Bae, 2011; Leachman, 2006; Makol, 2011; Ost, 1985).

Warnings/Precautions Corticosteroids are not approved for epidural injection. Serious neurologic events (eg, spinal cord infarction, paraplegia, quadriplegia, cortical blindness, stroke), some resulting in death, have been reported with epidural injection of corticosteroids, with and without use of fluoroscopy. Avoid injection or leakage into the dermis; dermal and/or subdermal skin depression may occur at the site of injection. Avoid deltoid muscle injection; subcutaneous atrophy may occur.

Use with caution in patients with thyroid disease, hepatic impairment, renal impairment, heart failure, hypertension, diabetes, glaucoma, cataracts, myasthenia gravis, osteoporosis, seizures, or GI diseases (diverticulitis, intestinal anastomoses, peptic ulcer, ulcerative colitis) due to perforation risk. Avoid ethanol may enhance gastric mucosal irritation. Use caution following acute MI (corticosteroids have been associated with myocardial rupture). Because of the risk of adverse effects, systemic corticosteroids should be used cautiously in the elderly in the smallest possible effective dose for the shortest duration. May affect growth velocity; growth should be routinely monitored in pediatric patients. Withdraw therapy with gradual tapering of dose. Patients may require higher doses when subject to stress (ie, trauma, surgery, severe infection).

May cause hypercorticism or suppression of hypothalamic-pituitary-adrenal (HPA) axis, particularly in younger children or in patients receiving high doses for prolonged periods. HPA axis suppression may lead to adrenal crisis. Withdrawal and discontinuation of a corticosteroid should be done slowly and carefully. Particular care is required when patients are transferred from systemic corticosteroids to inhaled products due to possible adrenal insufficiency or withdrawal from steroids, including an increase in allergic symptoms. Adult patients receiving >20 mg per day of prednisone (or equivalent) may be most susceptible. Fatalities have occurred due to adrenal insufficiency in asthmatic patients during and after transfer from systemic corticosteroids to aerosol steroids; aerosol steroids do not provide the systemic steroid needed to treat patients having trauma, surgery, or infections.

Acute myopathy has been reported with high dose corticosteroids, usually in patients with neuromuscular transmission disorders; may involve ocular and/or respiratory muscles; monitor creatine kinase; recovery may be delayed. Corticosteroid use may cause psychiatric disturbances, including depression, euphoria, insomnia, mood swings, and personality changes. Preexisting psychiatric conditions may be exacerbated by corticosteroid use. Prolonged use of corticosteroids may increase the incidence of secondary infection, mask ▶

825

◀ acute infection (including fungal infections), prolong or exacerbate viral infections, or limit response to vaccines. Exposure to chickenpox should be avoided; corticosteroids should not be used to treat ocular herpes simplex. Corticosteroids should not be used for cerebral malaria, fungal infections, or viral hepatitis. Oral steroid treatment is not recommended for the treatment of acute optic neuritis. Close observation is required in patients with latent tuberculosis and/or TB reactivity; restrict use in active TB (only fulminating or disseminated TB in conjunction with antituberculosis treatment). Amebiasis should be ruled out in any patient with recent travel to tropic climates or unexplained diarrhea prior to initiation of corticosteroids. Prolonged treatment with corticosteroids has been associated with the development of Kaposi sarcoma (case reports); if noted, discontinuation of therapy should be considered. High-dose corticosteroids should not be used to manage acute head injury. Potentially significant drug-drug interactions may exist, requiring dose or frequency adjustment, additional monitoring, and/or selection of alternative therapy.

Benzyl alcohol and derivatives: Diluent for injection may contain benzyl alcohol and some dosage forms may contain sodium benzoate/benzoic acid; benzoic acid (benzoate) is a metabolite of benzyl alcohol; large amounts of benzyl alcohol (≥99 mg/kg/day) have been associated with a potentially fatal toxicity ("gasping syndrome") in neonates; the "gasping syndrome" consists of metabolic acidosis, respiratory distress, gasping respirations, CNS dysfunction (including convulsions, intracranial hemorrhage), hypotension and cardiovascular collapse (AAP ["Inactive" 1997]; CDC, 1982); some data suggests that benzoate displaces bilirubin from protein binding sites (Ahlfors, 2001); avoid or use dosage forms containing benzyl alcohol and/or benzyl alcohol derivative with caution in neonates. See manufacturer's labeling.

Adverse Reactions Frequency not defined.

Cardiovascular: Arrhythmias, bradycardia, cardiac arrest, cardiomegaly, circulatory collapse, congestive heart failure, edema, fat embolism, hypertension, hypertrophic cardiomyopathy (premature infants), myocardial rupture (post MI), syncope, tachycardia, thromboembolism, vasculitis

Central nervous system: Delirium, depression, emotional instability, euphoria, hallucinations, headache, insomnia, intracranial pressure increased, malaise, mood swings, nervousness, neuritis, neuropathy, personality changes, pseudotumor cerebri, psychic disorders, psychoses, seizure, vertigo

Dermatologic: Acne, allergic dermatitis, alopecia, bruising, burning/tingling, dry scaly skin, edema, erythema, hirsutism, hyper-/hypopigmentation, impaired wound healing, petechiae, rash, skin atrophy, skin test reaction impaired, sterile abscess, striae, urticaria

Endocrine & metabolic: Adrenal suppression, alkalosis, amenorrhea, carbohydrate intolerance increased, Cushing's syndrome, diabetes mellitus, glucose intolerance, growth suppression, hyperglycemia, hyperlipidemia, hypokalemia, hypokalemic alkalosis, menstrual irregularities, negative nitrogen balance, pituitary-adrenal axis suppression, potassium loss, protein catabolism, sodium and water retention, sperm motility increased/decreased, spermatogenesis increased/decreased

Gastrointestinal: Abdominal distention, appetite increased, bowel dysfunction (intrathecal administration), indigestion, nausea, pancreatitis, peptic ulcer, gastrointestinal perforation, ulcerative esophagitis, vomiting, weight gain

Genitourinary: Bladder dysfunction (intrathecal administration)

Hematologic: Leukocytosis (transient)

Hepatic: Hepatomegaly, transaminases increased

Local: Atrophy (at injection site), postinjection flare (intra-articular use), thrombophlebitis

Neuromuscular & skeletal: Arthralgia, necrosis (femoral and humoral heads), Charcot-like arthropathy, fractures, muscle mass loss, muscle weakness, myopathy, osteoporosis, tendon rupture, vertebral compression fractures

Ocular: Cataracts, exophthalmoses, glaucoma, intraocular pressure increased

Miscellaneous: Abnormal fat deposits, anaphylaxis, avascular necrosis, diaphoresis, hiccups, hypersensitivity reactions, infection, secondary malignancy

Drug Interactions

Metabolism/Transport Effects Substrate of CYP3A4 (minor), P-glycoprotein; **Note:** Assignment of Major/Minor substrate status based on clinically relevant drug interaction potential; **Induces** CYP3A4 (weak)

Avoid Concomitant Use

Avoid concomitant use of Hydrocortisone (Systemic) with any of the following: Aldesleukin; BCG (Intravesical); Indium 111 Capromab Pendetide; Mifepristone; Natalizumab; Pimecrolimus; Tacrolimus (Topical); Tofacitinib

Increased Effect/Toxicity

Hydrocortisone (Systemic) may increase the levels/effects of: Acetylcholinesterase Inhibitors; Amphotericin B; Androgens; Ceritinib; Deferasirox; Fingolimod; Leflunomide; Loop Diuretics; Natalizumab; Nicorandil; NSAID (COX-2 Inhibitor); NSAID (Nonselective); Quinolone Antibiotics; Thiazide Diuretics; Tofacitinib; Vaccines (Live); Warfarin

The levels/effects of Hydrocortisone (Systemic) may be increased by: Aprepitant; CYP3A4 Inhibitors (Strong); Denosumab; Estrogen Derivatives; Fosaprepitant; Indacaterol; Lumacaftor; Mifepristone; Neuromuscular-Blocking Agents (Nondepolarizing); P-glycoprotein/ABCB1 Inhibitors; Pimecrolimus; Ranolazine; Roflumilast; Salicylates; Tacrolimus (Topical); Telaprevir; Trastuzumab

Decreased Effect

Hydrocortisone (Systemic) may decrease the levels/effects of: Aldesleukin; Antidiabetic Agents; ARIPiprazole; BCG (Intravesical); Calcitriol (Systemic); Coccidioides immitis Skin Test; Corticorelin; Hyaluronidase; Hydrocodone; Indium 111 Capromab Pendetide; Isoniazid; NiMODipine; Salicylates; Saxagliptin; Sipuleucel-T; Telaprevir; Urea Cycle Disorder Agents; Vaccines (Inactivated); Vaccines (Live)

The levels/effects of Hydrocortisone (Systemic) may be decreased by: Antacids; Bile Acid Sequestrants; CYP3A4 Inducers (Strong); Echinacea; Lumacaftor; Mifepristone; Mitotane; P-glycoprotein/ABCB1 Inducers

Storage/Stability Store at controlled room temperature 20°C to 25°C (68°F to 77°F). Protect from light. Hydrocortisone sodium phosphate and hydrocortisone sodium succinate are clear, light yellow solutions which are heat labile.

Sodium succinate: After initial reconstitution, hydrocortisone sodium succinate solutions are stable for 3 days at room temperature or under refrigeration when protected from light. Stability of parenteral admixture (Solu-Cortef®) at room temperature (25°C) and at refrigeration temperature (4°C) is concentration-dependent:

Stability of concentration 1 mg/mL: 24 hours

Stability of concentration 2 mg/mL to 60 mg/mL: At least 4 hours

◀ **Preparation for Administration**

Sodium succinate: IV bolus or IM administration: Reconstitute 100 mg vials with bacteriostatic water or bacteriostatic sodium chloride (not >2 mL). Act-O-Vial (self-contained powder for injection plus diluent) may be reconstituted by pressing the activator to force diluent into the powder compartment. Following gentle agitation, solution may be withdrawn via syringe through a needle inserted into the center of the stopper. May be administered (IV or IM) without further dilution.

Solutions for IV infusion: Reconstituted solutions may be added to an appropriate volume of compatible solution for infusion. Concentration should generally not exceed 1 mg/mL. However, in cases where administration of a small volume of fluid is desirable, 100-3000 mg may be added to 50 mL of D_5W or NS (stability limited to 4 hours).

Mechanism of Action Short-acting corticosteroid with minimal sodium-retaining potential; decreases inflammation by suppression of migration of polymorphonuclear leukocytes and reversal of increased capillary permeability

Pharmacodynamics/Kinetics

Onset of action: Hydrocortisone sodium succinate (water soluble): Rapid

Absorption: Rapid

Metabolism: Hepatic

Half-life elimination: Biologic: 8 to 12 hours

Excretion: Urine (primarily as 17-hydroxysteroids and 17-ketosteroids)

Dosing

Adult & Geriatric Dose should be based on severity of disease and patient response.

Adrenal insufficiency (acute) (off-label dosing): IM, IV: 100 mg IV bolus, then 50-75 mg every 6 hours for 24 hours then slowly taper over the next 72 hours administering every 4-6 hours during taper. Alternatively, after the bolus dose, may administer as a continuous infusion at a rate of 10 mg/hour for the first 24 hours followed by a gradual reduction in dose over the next 72 hours. Once patient is stable, may change to an oral maintenance regimen. **Note:** Patients with primary adrenal insufficiency may require mineralocorticoid supplementation (eg, fludrocortisone) when shifting to an oral maintenance regimen (Gardner, 2011).

Adrenal insufficiency (chronic), physiologic replacement (off-label dosing): Oral: 15-25 mg/day in 2-3 divided doses. **Note:** Studies suggest administering one-half to two-thirds of the daily dose in the morning in order to mimic the physiological cortisol secretion pattern. If the twice-daily regimen is utilized, the second dose should be administered 6-8 hours following the first dose (Arlt, 2003).

Anti-inflammatory or immunosuppressive: Oral, IM, IV: 15-240 mg every 12 hours

Congenital adrenal hyperplasia (off-label dosing): Oral: 15-25 mg/day in 2-3 divided doses (Speiser, 2010)

Status asthmaticus: IV: 1-2 mg/kg/dose every 6 hours for 24 hours, then maintenance of 0.5-1 mg/kg every 6 hours

Stress dosing (surgery) in patients known to be adrenally-suppressed or on chronic systemic steroids: IV:

Minor stress (ie, inguinal herniorrhaphy): 25 mg/day for 1 day

Moderate stress (ie, joint replacement, cholecystectomy): 50-75 mg/day (25 mg every 8-12 hours) for 1-2 days

Major stress (pancreatoduodenectomy, esophagogastrectomy, cardiac surgery): 100-150 mg/day (50 mg every 8-12 hours) for 2-3 days

Septic shock (off-label use): IV: 50 mg every 6 hours (Annane, 2002; COIITSS Study Investigators, 2010). Practice guidelines suggest administering 200 mg daily as a continuous infusion over 24 hours to prevent adverse effects (eg, hyperglycemia) (Dellinger, 2013; Weber-Carstens, 2007); however, the impact of continuous infusion on patient outcomes has not been formally evaluated. Taper slowly (over several days) when vasopressors are no longer required; do not stop abruptly. **Note:** Hydrocortisone should be used alone (ie, without fludrocortisone) (Dellinger, 2013).

Thyroid storm (off-label use): IV: 300 mg loading dose, followed by 100 mg every 8 hours (Bahn, 2011)

Pediatric Dose should be based on severity of disease and patient response.

Anti-inflammatory or immunosuppressive:

Infants and Children:

Oral: 2.5-10 mg/kg/day **or** 75-300 mg/m²/day every 6-8 hours

IM, IV: 1-5 mg/kg/day **or** 30-150 mg/m²/day divided every 12-24 hours

Adolescents: Oral, IM, IV: 15-240 mg every 12 hours

Congenital adrenal hyperplasia (off-label dosing): Oral: **Note:** Doses must be individualized by monitoring growth, bone age, and hormonal levels.

Children: 10-15 mg/m²/day in 3 divided doses; higher initial doses may be required to achieve initial target hormone serum concentrations in infancy (Speiser, 2010)

Adolescents: Refer to adult dosing.

Physiologic replacement: Children: Oral: 8-10 mg/m²/day divided every 8 hours; up to 12 mg/m²/day in some patients (Ahmet, 2011; Gupta, 2008; Maguire, 2007)

Status asthmaticus: Children: IV: 1-2 mg/kg/dose every 6 hours for 24 hours, then maintenance of 0.5-1 mg/kg every 6 hours.

Septic shock (off-label use): Children: IV: Initial: 1-2 mg/kg/day (intermittent or as continuous infusion); may titrate up to 50 mg/kg/day for shock reversal (Brierley, 2009); alternative dosing suggests 50 mg/m²/day (Dellinger, 2008). **Note:** Use recommended only in fluid refractory, catecholamine-resistant shock, and suspected or proven absolute (classic) adrenal insufficiency.

Renal Impairment There are no dosage adjustments provided in the manufacturer's labeling; use with caution.

Hepatic Impairment There are no dosage adjustments provided in the manufacturer's labeling.

Combination Regimens

Lymphoma, non-Hodgkin (Burkitt):

CODOX-M/IVAC (NHL-Burkitt) on page 1920

CODOX-M (NHL-Burkitt) on page 1924

Administration

Oral: Administer with food or milk to decrease GI upset.

Parenteral: Hydrocortisone sodium succinate may be administered by IM or IV routes. Dermal and/or subdermal skin depression may occur at the site of injection. Avoid injection into deltoid muscle (high incidence of subcutaneous atrophy).

IV bolus: Administer over 30 seconds or over 10 minutes for doses ≥500 mg

IV intermittent infusion: Administer over 20-30 minutes

◀ **Extemporaneous Preparations** A 2.5 mg/mL oral suspension may be made with either tablets or powder and a vehicle containing sodium carboxymethylcellulose (1 g), syrup BP (10 mL), hydroxybenzoate 0.1% preservatives (0.1 g), polysorbate 80 (0.5 mL), citric acid (0.6 g), and water. To make the vehicle, dissolve the hydroxybenzoate, citric acid, and syrup BP in hot water. Cool solution and add the carboxymethylcellulose; leave overnight. Crush twelve-and-one-half 20 mg hydrocortisone tablets (or use 250 mg of powder) in a mortar and reduce to a fine powder while adding polysorbate 80. Add small portions of vehicle and mix to a uniform paste; mix while adding the vehicle in incremental proportions to **almost** 100 mL; transfer to a calibrated bottle, rinse mortar with vehicle, and add sufficient quantity of vehicle to make 100 mL. Label "shake well" and "refrigerate". Stable for 90 days.

Fawcett JP, Boulton DW, Jiang R, et al, "Stability of Hydrocortisone Oral Suspensions Prepared From Tablets and Powder," *Ann Pharmacother*, 1995, 29(10):987-90.

Monitoring Parameters Serum glucose, electrolytes; blood pressure, weight, presence of infection; monitor IOP with therapy >6 weeks; bone mineral density, growth in children

Test Interactions Interferes with skin tests

Dietary Considerations Systemic use of corticosteroids may require a diet with increased potassium, vitamins A, B_6, C, D, folate, calcium, zinc, phosphorus, and decreased sodium. Some products may contain sodium.

Dosage Forms Excipient information presented when available (limited, particularly for generics); consult specific product labeling.

Solution Reconstituted, Injection, as sodium succinate [strength expressed as base]:
A-Hydrocort: 100 mg (1 ea)
Solu-CORTEF: 100 mg (1 ea)

Solution Reconstituted, Injection, as sodium succinate [strength expressed as base, preservative free]:
Solu-CORTEF: 100 mg (1 ea); 250 mg (1 ea); 500 mg (1 ea); 1000 mg (1 ea)

Tablet, Oral, as base:
Cortef: 5 mg, 10 mg, 20 mg [scored]
Generic: 5 mg, 10 mg, 20 mg

◆ **Hydrocortisone Sodium Succinate** *see* Hydrocortisone (Systemic) *on page 824*

◆ **Hydromorph Contin (Can)** *see* HYDROmorphone *on page 830*

HYDROmorphone (hye droe MOR fone)

Brand Names: US Dilaudid; Dilaudid-HP; Exalgo

Brand Names: Canada Apo-Hydromorphone; Dilaudid; Dilaudid-HP; Hydromorph Contin; Hydromorphone HP; Hydromorphone HP 10; Hydromorphone HP 20; Hydromorphone HP 50; Hydromorphone HP Forte; Hydromorphone Hydrochloride Injection, USP; Jurnista; PMS-Hydromorphone; Teva-Hydromorphone

Index Terms Dihydromorphinone; Hydromorphone Hydrochloride; Palladone

Pharmacologic Category Analgesic, Opioid

Use

Pain:

Immediate-release formulations:

Tablet, liquid, injection: Management of pain in patients where an opioid analgesic is appropriate

HP injection: Management of moderate to severe pain in opioid-tolerant patients who require higher doses of opioids

Suppository: Management of moderate to severe pain

Extended-release formulations: Management of pain in opioid-tolerant patients severe enough to require daily, around-the-clock, long-term opioid treatment and for which alternative treatment options are inadequate

Limitations of use: Not indicated as an as-needed analgesic. Because of the risks of addiction, abuse, and misuse with opioids, even at recommended doses, and because of the greater risks of overdose and death with extended-release opioid formulations, reserve for use in patients for whom alternative treatment options (eg, nonopioid analgesics, immediate-release opioids) are ineffective, not tolerated, or would be otherwise inadequate to provide sufficient management of pain

Pregnancy Risk Factor C

Dosing

Adult

Acute pain (moderate to severe): Note: These are guidelines and do not represent the maximum doses that may be required in all patients. Doses should be titrated to provide adequate pain relief. When changing routes of administration, oral doses and parenteral doses are **NOT** equivalent; parenteral doses are up to 5 times more potent. Therefore, when administered parenterally, one-fifth of the oral dose will provide similar analgesia.

Oral: Immediate release: Initial: Opioid naive: 2 to 4 mg every 4 to 6 hours as needed (tablets) or 2.5 mg to 10 mg every 3 to 6 hours as needed (liquid); elderly/debilitated patients may require lower doses; patients with prior opioid exposure may require higher initial doses. **Note:** In adults with severe pain, the American Pain Society recommends an initial dose of 4 to 8 mg.

Therapy discontinuation (Canadian labeling): Decrease the previous daily dose by 50% (administered every 6 hours) for 2 days then decrease daily dose by 25% every 2 days.

IV: Initial: Opioid naive: 0.2 to 1 mg every 2 to 3 hours as needed; patients with prior opioid exposure may require higher initial doses. Dilaudid HP should **NOT** be used in opioid-naive patients.

Critically ill patients (off-label dosing): 0.2 to 0.6 mg every 1 to 2 hours as needed **or** 0.5 mg every 3 hours as needed (Barr 2013)

Continuous infusion: Usual dosage range: 0.5 to 3 mg/hour (Barr 2013)

Patient-controlled analgesia (PCA) (off-label dosing) (American Pain Society 2008): **Note:** Opioid naive: Consider lower end of dosing range. A continuous (basal) infusion is not recommended in opioid-naive patients (ISMP 2009):

Usual concentration: 0.2 mg/mL

Demand dose: Usual initial dose: 0.2 mg; range: 0.05 to 0.4 mg

Lockout interval: 5 to 10 minutes

Epidural PCA (off-label dosing) (de Leon-Casasola 1996; Liu 2010; Smith 2009):

Usual concentration: 0.01 mg/mL

Bolus dose: 0.4 to 1 mg

Infusion rate: 0.03 to 0.3 mg/**hour**

Demand dose: 0.02 to 0.05 mg

Lockout interval: 10 to 15 minutes

◀

    IM, SubQ: **Note:** IM use may result in variable absorption and lag time to peak effect; IM route not recommended for use (American Pain Society 2008). Equianalgesic doses: Morphine 10 mg IM = hydromorphone 1.5 mg IM.

        US labeling: Initial: 1 to 2 mg every 2 to 3 hours as needed; lower initial doses may be used in opioid-naive patients. Patients with prior opioid exposure may require higher initial doses.

        Canadian labeling: Opioid naive: 2 mg every 4 to 6 hours as needed; for severe pain, may administer 3 to 4 mg every 4 to 6 hours as needed. When discontinuation of therapy is necessary, decrease the previous daily dose by 50% (administered every 6 hours) for 2 days then decrease daily dose by 25% every 2 days. Hydromorphone HP or Hydromorphone HP Forte should **NOT** be used in opioid-naive patients.

    Rectal:

        US labeling: 3 mg (1 suppository) every 6 to 8 hours as needed

        Canadian labeling: 3 mg (1 suppository) at bedtime as needed

Chronic pain: Note: Patients taking opioids chronically may become tolerant and require doses higher than the usual dosage range to maintain the desired effect. Tolerance can be managed by appropriate dose titration. There is no optimal or maximal dose for hydromorphone in chronic pain. The appropriate dose is one that relieves pain throughout its dosing interval without causing unmanageable side effects.

    Controlled-release capsule (Hydromorph Contin [Canadian product]): Oral: **Note:** A patient's hydromorphone requirement should be established using prompt release formulations; conversion to long-acting products may be considered when chronic, continuous treatment is required. Higher dosages should be reserved for use only in opioid-tolerant patients. Capsule strengths ≥18 mg or a single dose >12 mg should be reserved for use only in opioid-tolerant patients requiring hydromorphone equivalent dosages ≥36 mg daily.

        Opioid naive or receiving low intermittent doses of weak opioids: Initial: 3 mg every 12 hours.

        Current therapy with other oral hydromorphone formulations: Initial: Initiate at same total daily hydromorphone dosage divided in 2 equal doses every 12 hours

        Current therapy with other opioids: Initial: Determine equivalent oral hydromorphone daily dosage and initiate in 2 equally divided doses every 12 hours. See table below for examples of equivalent dosing (refer to manufacturer labeling for additional equivalency dosing information).

Approximate Opioid Analgesic Equivalent Dosing (Oral)	
Hydromorphone	1 mg
Morphine	8 mg (5 to 7.5 mg with chronic dosing of morphine)
Oxycodone	4 mg
Codeine	~27 mg

    Extended-release tablet (Exalgo): **Note:** For use in opioid-tolerant patients only. Patients considered opioid tolerant are those who are receiving, for 1 week or longer, at least 60 mg of oral morphine daily, 25 mcg of transdermal fentanyl per hour, 30 mg of oral oxycodone daily, 8 mg of oral hydromorphone daily, 25 mg of oral oxymorphone daily, or an equianalgesic dose of another opioid.

Opioid-tolerant patients: Discontinue or taper all other extended-release opioids when starting therapy.

Individualization of dose: Suggested recommendations for converting to Exalgo from other analgesics are presented, but when selecting the initial dose, other characteristics (eg, patient status, degree of opioid tolerance, concurrent medications, type of pain, risk factors for addiction, abuse, and misuse) should also be considered. Pain relief and adverse events should be assessed frequently.

Conversion from other oral hydromorphone formulations to Exalgo: Start with the equivalent total daily dose of immediate-release hydromorphone administered once daily.

Conversion from other opioids to Exalgo: Discontinue all other around-the-clock opioids when therapy is initiated. Substantial interpatient variability exists in relative potency. Therefore, it is safer to underestimate a patient's daily oral hydromorphone requirement and provide breakthrough pain relief with rescue medication (eg, immediate release opioid) than to overestimate requirements. In general, start Exalgo at 50% of the calculated total daily dose every 24 hours (see Conversion Factors to Exalgo). The following conversion ratios may be used to convert from oral opioid therapy to Exalgo.

Conversion factors to Exalgo (see table): Select the opioid, sum the current total daily dose, multiply by the conversion factor on the table to calculate the approximate oral hydromorphone daily dose, then calculate the approximate starting dose for Exalgo at 50% of the calculated oral hydromorphone daily does; administer every 24 hours. Round down, if necessary, to the nearest strength available. For patients on a regimen of more than one opioid, calculate the approximate oral hydromorphone dose for each opioid and sum the totals to obtain the approximate total hydromorphone daily dose. For patients on a regimen of fixed-ratio opioid/nonopioid analgesic medications, only the opioid component of these medications should be used in the conversion. **Note:** The conversion factors in this conversion table are only to be used for the conversion from current oral opioid therapy to Exalgo. Conversion factors in this table cannot be used to convert from Exalgo to another oral opioid (doing so may lead to fatal overdose due to overestimation of the new opioid). This is not a table of equianalgesic doses.

Conversion Factors to Exalgo[1]

Previous Oral Opioid	Oral Conversion Factor
Hydromorphone	1
Codeine	0.06
Hydrocodone	0.4
Methadone[2]	0.6
Morphine	0.2
Oxycodone	0.4
Oxymorphone	0.6

[1] The conversion factors are only to be used for the conversion from current opioid therapy to Exalgo.

[2] Monitor closely; ratio between methadone and other opioid agonists may vary widely as a function of previous drug exposure. Methadone has a long half-life and may accumulate in the plasma.

Conversion from transdermal fentanyl to Exalgo: Treatment with Exalgo can be started 18 hours after the removal of the transdermal fentanyl patch. For every fentanyl 25 mcg/hour transdermal dose, the equianalgesic dose of Exalgo is 12 mg every 24 hours. An appropriate starting dose is 50% of the calculated total daily dose given every 24 hours. If necessary, round down to the appropriate Exalgo tablet strength available.

Titration and maintenance: Dose adjustments in 4 to 8 mg increments may occur every 3 to 4 days. In patients experiencing breakthrough pain, consider increasing the dose of Exalgo or providing rescue medication of an immediate-release analgesic at an appropriate dose. Do not administer Exalgo more frequently than every 24 hours.

Discontinuing Exalgo: Taper by gradually decreasing the dose by 25% to 50% every 2 to 3 days to a dose of 8 mg every 24 hours before discontinuing therapy.

Extended-release tablet: Jurnista [Canadian product]: **Note:** May be used in conjunction with usual doses of nonopioid analgesics and analgesic adjuvants. If appropriate, initiate therapy with an immediate-release opioid formulation to establish a safe and effective dosage, then convert to an equivalent daily dose of extended-release hydromorphone. Tablets ≥16 mg are intended only for opioid-tolerant patients requiring hydromorphone equivalent dosages ≥16 mg daily.

Initial:

Patients who are opioid naive or receiving low intermittent doses of weak opioid analgesics (eg, <40 mg daily oral morphine equivalents): Initial: 4 mg once daily (if clinically indicated, an initial dose of 8 mg may be used; maximum initial dose: 8 mg once daily); titrate dose in increments of 4 or 8 mg as needed but no sooner than every fourth dose (eg, if first dose is administered on Tuesday, increase no sooner than on Friday).

Patients receiving opioids regularly: Discontinue all other around-the-clock opioid analgesics; initial Jurnista dose is based on previous daily opioid dose. For opioids other than morphine, estimate the equivalent daily dose of morphine then determine the equivalent total daily dose of Jurnista by multiplying the equivalent morphine dose by a factor of 0.2. For example, morphine 60 mg daily multiplied by 0.2 is equivalent to hydromorphone 12 mg daily. If necessary, round down to nearest Jurnista dose available and administer once daily.

Maintenance: Dose is individualized based on response. May consider dose increases of 25% to 75% of current daily dose made no sooner than every 4th dose (eg, if first dose is administered on Tuesday, increase no sooner than on Friday). Reassess the need for around-the clock pain control periodically. Supplemental analgesia for breakthrough pain should typically not exceed 10% to 25% of the equivalent daily Jurnista dose.

Discontinuing Jurnista: Taper by gradually decreasing the dose by 50% every 2 days until lowest possible dose is reached and then discontinue. If signs of withdrawal occur during taper, stop taper and increase dose slightly until signs of withdrawal are no longer present. May then resume taper but with longer periods of time between each dose reduction, or before switching to an equianalgesic dose of another opioid to continue tapering.

Geriatric Doses should be titrated to appropriate analgesic effects. When changing routes of administration, oral doses and parenteral doses are **NOT** equivalent; parenteral doses are up to 5 times more potent. Therefore, when administered parenterally, one-fifth of the oral dose will provide similar analgesia.

Acute pain, opioid-naive:

Oral: Use with caution; initiation at the low end of dosage range is recommended. For patients >70 years, the American Pain Society recommends consideration to lowering initial doses by 25% to 50% followed by upward or downward titration (APS 2008).

IM, SubQ: Refer to adult dosing. Reduce initial doses as necessary.

IV: Reduce initial dose to 0.2 mg

Renal Impairment

Injectable:

US labeling: Initiate with 25% to 50% of the usual starting dose depending on the degree of impairment. Use with caution and monitor closely for respiratory and CNS depression.

Canadian labeling: There are no specific dosage adjustments provided in the manufacturer's labeling; however, a reduced initial dose is recommended for severe renal impairment. Use with caution and monitor closely for respiratory and CNS depression.

Oral (immediate release):

US labeling: There are no specific dosage adjustments provided in the manufacturer's labeling; however, a reduced initial dose is recommended for moderate impairment (CrCl ≤60 mL/minute) and an even lower initial dose is recommended for severe impairment (CrCl <30 mL/minute). Use with caution and monitor closely for respiratory and CNS depression.

Canadian labeling: There are no specific dosage adjustments provided in the manufacturer's labeling; however, a reduced initial dose is recommended for severe renal impairment. Use with caution and monitor closely for respiratory and CNS depression.

Oral (extended-release tablet):

Exalgo:

Mild impairment: There are no dosage adjustments provided in the manufacturer's labeling.

Moderate impairment (CrCl ≤60 mL/minute): Initiate with 50% of the usual starting dose for patients with normal renal function. Use with caution and monitor closely for respiratory and CNS depression.

Severe impairment (CrCl <30 mL/minute): Initiate with 25% of the usual starting dose for patients with normal renal function. Use with caution and monitor closely for respiratory and CNS depression. Consider use of an alternate analgesic with better dosing flexibility.

Jurnista [Canadian product]:

Mild impairment: There are no dosage adjustments provided in the manufacturer's labeling.

Moderate impairment: There are no specific dosage adjustments provided in the manufacturer's labeling; however, an initial dosage reduction is recommended. Use with caution and monitor closely for respiratory and CNS depression.

Severe impairment: There are no specific dosage adjustments provided in the manufacturer's labeling. Reduce initial dose and consider extending the dosing interval. Use with caution and monitor closely for respiratory and CNS depression.

Oral (extended-release capsule): Hydromorph contin [Canadian product]:

Mild impairment: There are no dosage adjustments provided in the manufacturer's labeling; use with caution and monitor closely for respiratory and CNS depression.

Moderate impairment: Initiate at 50% of initial dose for normal renal function; titrate cautiously. Monitor closely for respiratory and CNS depression following initiation of therapy and during titration.

Severe impairment: Initiate at 25% of initial dose for normal renal function; titrate cautiously. Monitor closely for respiratory and CNS depression following initiation of therapy and during titration.

Rectal suppository:

US labeling: There are no dosage adjustments provided in the manufacturer's labeling. Use with caution and monitor closely for respiratory and CNS depression.

Canadian labeling: There are no specific dosage adjustments provided in the manufacturer's labeling; however, an initial dosage reduction is recommended for severe renal impairment. Use with caution and monitor closely for respiratory and CNS depression

Hepatic Impairment

Injectable:

US labeling:

Mild impairment: There are no specific dosage adjustments provided in the manufacturer's labeling.

Moderate impairment: Initiate therapy with 25% to 50% of the usual initial dose. Use with caution and monitor closely for respiratory and CNS depression.

Severe impairment: There are no specific dosage adjustments provided in the manufacturer's labeling (has not been studied); however, further dose reductions (compared with those recommended for moderate impairment) are recommended. Use with caution and monitor closely for respiratory and CNS depression.

Canadian labeling: There are no specific dosage adjustments provided in the manufacturer's labeling; however, a reduced initial dose is recommended in severe hepatic impairment. Use with caution and monitor closely for respiratory and CNS depression.

There are no specific dosage adjustments provided in the manufacturer's labeling; however, an initial dosage reduction is recommended. Use with caution and monitor closely for respiratory and CNS depression.

Oral (immediate release):

US labeling:

Mild impairment: There are no specific dosage adjustments provided in the manufacturer's labeling.

Moderate impairment: There are no specific dosage adjustments provided in the manufacturer's labeling; however, an initial dosage reduction is recommended. Use with caution and monitor closely for respiratory and CNS depression.

Severe impairment: There are no specific dosage adjustments provided in the manufacturer's labeling (has not been studied); initial dose reduction is recommended. Use with caution and monitor closely for respiratory and CNS depression.

Canadian labeling: There are no specific dosage adjustments provided in the manufacturer's labeling; however, a reduced initial dose is recommended in severe hepatic impairment. Use with caution and monitor closely for respiratory and CNS depression.

Oral (extended-release tablet):

Exalgo:

Mild impairment: There are no dosage adjustments provided in the manufacturer's labeling.

Moderate impairment: Initiate with 25% of the usual starting dose for patients with normal hepatic function. Use with caution and monitor closely for respiratory and CNS depression.

Severe impairment: Use alternate analgesic.

Jurnista [Canadian product]:

Mild impairment: There are no dosage adjustments provided in the manufacturer's labeling.

Moderate impairment: There are no specific dosage adjustments provided in the manufacturer's labeling; however, a reduced initial dosage is recommended. Use with caution and monitor closely for respiratory and CNS depression.

Severe impairment: There are no specific dosage adjustments provided in the manufacturer's labeling; reduce initial dose and use with caution. Monitor closely for respiratory and CNS depression.

Oral (extended-release capsule): Hydromorph contin [Canadian product]:

Mild impairment: There are no dosage adjustments provided in the manufacturer's labeling; use with caution and monitor for respiratory and CNS depression.

Moderate impairment: Initiate at 25% of initial dose for normal hepatic function; titrate cautiously. Monitor closely for respiratory and CNS depression following initiation of therapy and during titration.

Severe impairment: Use is not recommended (has not been studied); consider alternative analgesics. If therapy with hydromorphone is initiated, the manufacturer recommends a more conservative dose than that recommended for moderate impairment but does not provide specific dosing recommendations. Monitor closely for respiratory and CNS depression.

Rectal suppository:

US labeling: There are no dosage adjustments provided in the manufacturer's labeling. Use with caution and monitor closely for respiratory and CNS depression.

Canadian labeling: There are no specific dosage adjustments provided in the manufacturer's labeling; however, an initial dosage reduction is recommended for severe hepatic impairment. Use with caution and monitor closely for respiratory and CNS depression.

Additional Information Complete prescribing information should be consulted for additional detail.

Prescribing and Access Restrictions Exalgo: As a requirement of the REMS program, healthcare providers who prescribe Exalgo need to receive training on the proper use and potential risks of Exalgo. For training, please refer to http://www.exalgorems.com. Prescribers will need retraining every 2 years or following any significant changes to the Exalgo REMS program.

Medication Guide Available Yes

Dosage Forms Excipient information presented when available (limited, particularly for generics); consult specific product labeling. [DSC] = Discontinued product

Liquid, Oral, as hydrochloride:
  Dilaudid: 1 mg/mL (473 mL) [contains methylparaben, propylparaben, sodium metabisulfite; sweet flavor]
  Generic: 1 mg/mL (473 mL)
Solution, Injection, as hydrochloride:
  Dilaudid: 1 mg/mL (1 mL [DSC]); 2 mg/mL (1 mL); 4 mg/mL (1 mL)
  Dilaudid-HP: 10 mg/mL (1 mL, 5 mL, 50 mL [DSC])
  Generic: 1 mg/mL (0.5 mL, 1 mL); 2 mg/mL (1 mL, 20 mL); 4 mg/mL (1 mL); 10 mg/mL (1 mL); 50 mg/5 mL (5 mL); 500 mg/50 mL (50 mL)
Solution, Injection, as hydrochloride [preservative free]:
  Generic: 10 mg/mL (1 mL); 50 mg/5 mL (5 mL); 500 mg/50 mL (50 mL)
Solution Prefilled Syringe, Intravenous:
  Generic: 10 mg/50 mL (50 mL)
Solution Reconstituted, Injection, as hydrochloride:
  Dilaudid-HP: 250 mg (1 ea [DSC])
Suppository, Rectal, as hydrochloride:
  Generic: 3 mg (6 ea)
Tablet, Oral, as hydrochloride:
  Dilaudid: 2 mg, 4 mg [contains fd&c yellow #10 aluminum lake, sodium metabisulfite]
  Dilaudid: 8 mg [scored; contains sodium metabisulfite]
  Generic: 2 mg, 4 mg, 8 mg
Tablet ER 24 Hour Abuse-Deterrent, Oral, as hydrochloride:
  Exalgo: 8 mg, 12 mg, 16 mg, 32 mg [contains sodium metabisulfite]
  Generic: 8 mg, 12 mg, 16 mg, 32 mg

Dosage Forms: Canada Excipient information presented when available (limited, particularly for generics); consult specific product labeling.

Capsule, controlled release:
  Hydromorph Contin: 3 mg, 4.5 mg, 6 mg, 9 mg, 12 mg, 18 mg, 24 mg, 30 mg
Tablet extended release 24 Hour, Oral, as hydrochloride:
  Jurnista: 4 mg, 8 mg, 16 mg, 32 mg (may contain traces of sodium metabisulfite)

Controlled Substance C-II

◆ **Hydromorphone HP (Can)** *see* HYDROmorphone *on page 830*
◆ **Hydromorphone HP 10 (Can)** *see* HYDROmorphone *on page 830*
◆ **Hydromorphone HP 20 (Can)** *see* HYDROmorphone *on page 830*
◆ **Hydromorphone HP 50 (Can)** *see* HYDROmorphone *on page 830*
◆ **Hydromorphone HP Forte (Can)** *see* HYDROmorphone *on page 830*
◆ **Hydromorphone Hydrochloride** *see* HYDROmorphone *on page 830*

- **Hydromorphone Hydrochloride Injection, USP (Can)** *see* HYDROmorphone *on page* 830
- **Hydroxycarbamide** *see* Hydroxyurea *on page* 839
- **Hydroxydaunomycin Hydrochloride** *see* DOXOrubicin (Conventional) *on page* 553
- **Hydroxyldaunorubicin Hydrochloride** *see* DOXOrubicin (Conventional) *on page* 553

Hydroxyurea (hye droks ee yoor EE a)

Related Information
Management of Chemotherapy-Induced Nausea and Vomiting in Adults *on page* 2142
Prevention of Chemotherapy-Induced Nausea and Vomiting in Children *on page* 2203
Safe Handling of Hazardous Drugs *on page* 2292

Brand Names: US Droxia; Hydrea

Brand Names: Canada Apo-Hydroxyurea; Gen-Hydroxyurea; Hydrea; Mylan-Hydroxyurea

Index Terms HU; Hydroxycarbamide; Hydurea

Pharmacologic Category Antineoplastic Agent, Miscellaneous

Use
Chronic myeloid leukemia: Treatment of refractory chronic myeloid leukemia (CML)

Head and neck cancer: Management (with concomitant radiation therapy) of locally advanced squamous cell head and neck cancer (excluding lip cancer)

Sickle cell anemia: Management of sickle cell anemia (to reduce the frequency of painful crises and to reduce the need for blood transfusions in patients with recurrent moderate to severe painful crises)

Labeled Contraindications Hypersensitivity to hydroxyurea or any component of the formulation

Pregnancy Considerations Animal reproduction studies have demonstrated teratogenicity and embryotoxicity at doses lower than the usual human dose (based on BSA). Hydroxyurea may cause fetal harm if administered during pregnancy. Women of childbearing potential should be advised to avoid becoming pregnant during treatment and should use effective contraception during and for at least 30 days after completion of therapy. Males of childbearing potential should use effective contraception during and for at least 1 year after therapy.

Breast-Feeding Considerations Hydroxyurea is excreted in breast milk. Due to the potential for serious adverse reactions in the nursing infant, breast-feeding is not recommended by the manufacturer.

Warnings/Precautions Hazardous agent - use appropriate precautions for handling and disposal (NIOSH 2014 [group 1]); to decrease risk of exposure, wear gloves when handling and wash hands before and after contact. **[US Boxed Warning]: Hydroxyurea may cause severe myelosuppression. Monitor blood counts at baseline and throughout treatment. Interrupt treatment and reduce dose as necessary.** Leukopenia and neutropenia commonly occur (thrombocytopenia and anemia are less common); leukopenia/neutropenia occur first. Severe or life-threatening myelosuppression may occur at the recommended dose. Hematologic toxicity reversible (rapid) with treatment interruption. Correct severe anemia prior to initiating treatment. Do not initiate therapy if bone marrow function is markedly reduced. Hydroxyurea should not be used in sickle cell anemia with severe bone marrow suppression (neutrophils <2,000/mm³, platelets <80,000/mm³, hemoglobin <4.5 g/dL, or reticulocytes <80,000/mm³ when hemoglobin <9 g/dL per manufacturer's labeling). Use with caution in patients with a history of prior chemotherapy or radiation therapy; myelosuppression is more common. Patients with a history of radiation therapy are also at risk for exacerbation of post irradiation erythema. Self-limiting macrocytosis/megaloblastic erythropoiesis may be seen early in treatment (may resemble pernicious anemia, but is unrelated to vitamin B_{12} or folic acid deficiency). Prophylactic folic acid supplementation is recommended. Plasma iron clearance may be delayed and iron utilization rate (by erythrocytes) may be reduced. Potentially significant drug-drug interactions may exist, requiring dose or frequency adjustment, additional monitoring, and/or selection of alternative therapy. When treated concurrently with hydroxyurea and antiretroviral agents (including didanosine and stavudine), HIV-infected patients are at higher risk for potentially fatal pancreatitis, hepatotoxicity, hepatic failure, and severe peripheral neuropathy; discontinue immediately if signs of these toxicities develop. Hyperuricemia may occur with antineoplastic treatment; adequate hydration and initiation or dosage adjustment of uricosuric agents (eg, allopurinol) may be necessary.

In patients with sickle cell anemia, Droxia is not recommended if neutrophils <2,000/mm³, platelets <80,000/mm³, hemoglobin <4.5 g/dL, or reticulocytes <80,000/mm³ when hemoglobin <9 g/dL per manufacturer's labeling. May cause macrocytosis, which can mask folic acid deficiency; prophylactic folic acid supplementation is recommended. **[US Boxed Warning]: Hydroxyurea is carcinogenic. Advise sun protection and monitor patients for malignancies.** Treatment of myeloproliferative disorders (eg, polycythemia vera, thrombocythemia) with long-term hydroxyurea is associated with secondary leukemia; it is unknown if this is drug-related or disease-related. Skin cancer has been reported with long-term hydroxyurea use. Monitor for signs/symptoms of secondary malignancies. Cutaneous vasculitic toxicities (vasculitic ulceration and gangrene) have been reported with hydroxyurea treatment, most often in patients with a history of or receiving concurrent interferon therapy; discontinue hydroxyurea and consider alternate cytoreductive therapy if cutaneous vasculitic toxicity develops. Use caution with renal dysfunction; may require dose reductions. Elderly patients may be more sensitive to the effects of hydroxyurea; may require lower doses.

Adverse Reactions Frequency not always defined.

Cardiovascular: Edema, hypersensitivity angiitis

Central nervous system: Chills, disorientation, dizziness, drowsiness (dose-related), hallucination, headache, malaise, peripheral neuropathy (HIV-infected patients), seizure, vasculitic ulcerations

Dermatologic: Eczema (infants and children 9 to 18 months: 13% [Thornburg 2012]), leg ulcer (7% [Hernández-Boluda 2011]), dermal ulcer (3% [Antonioli 2012]), nail discoloration (2% [Randi 2005]), alopecia (infrequent, [Hernández-Boluda 2011]), changes in nails (infrequent, [Hernández-Boluda 2011]), hyperpigmentation (infrequent, [Hernández-Boluda 2011]), atrophy of nail, dermatomyositis-like skin changes, desquamation, erythema (peripheral), facial erythema, gangrene of skin or other tissue, maculopapular rash, papule (violet), skin atrophy, skin carcinoma

Endocrine & metabolic: Increased uric acid

Gastrointestinal: Acute mucocutaneous toxicity (5% [Hernández-Boluda 2011]), diarrhea (infrequent, [Antonioli 2012]), gastric distress (infrequent, [Antonioli 2012]), nausea (infrequent, [Antonioli 2012]), oral mucosa ulcer (infrequent, [Hernández-Boluda 2011]), anorexia, BSP abnormality (retention), constipation, gastrointestinal irritation (potentiated with radiation therapy), mucositis (potentiated with radiation therapy), pancreatitis (HIV-infected patients), stomatitis, vomiting

Genitourinary: Dysuria

Hematologic & oncologic: Leukemia (4% [Hernández-Boluda 2011]; secondary; long-term use), leukopenia (2% [Hernández-Boluda 2011]), bone marrow depression (neutropenia [common], thrombocytopenia; hematologic recovery: within 2 weeks); abnormal erythropoiesis (megaloblastic; self-limiting), macrocytosis (MCV >97: 42% [Randi 2005]), reticulocytopenia (infants and children 9 to 18 months [Wang 2011])

Hepatic: Hepatic failure (HIV-infected patients), hepatotoxicity, increased liver enzymes

Neuromuscular & skeletal: Panniculitis (Antonioli 2012), weakness

Renal: Increased blood urea nitrogen, increased serum creatinine, renal tubular disease

Respiratory: Asthma (infants and children 9 to 18 months: 9% [Thornburg 2012]), dyspnea, pulmonary fibrosis (rare), pulmonary infiltrates (diffuse, rare)

<1%, postmarketing, and/or case reports: Actinic keratosis (Antonioli 2012), anemia (doses >20 mg/kg/day [Randi 2005]), basal cell carcinoma (Antonioli 2012), dermatitis (Antonioli 2012), fever (Antonioli 2012), hyperkeratosis (Antonioli 2012), lesion (dyschromic [Antonioli 2012]), malignant neoplasm (Wong 2014), mucous membrane lesion (Antonioli 2012), pneumonitis (Antonioli 2012), squamous cell carcinoma (Antonioli 2012)

Drug Interactions

Metabolism/Transport Effects None known.

Avoid Concomitant Use

Avoid concomitant use of Hydroxyurea with any of the following: BCG (Intravesical); CloZAPine; Didanosine; Dipyrone; Natalizumab; Pimecrolimus; Stavudine; Tacrolimus (Topical); Tofacitinib; Vaccines (Live)

Increased Effect/Toxicity

Hydroxyurea may increase the levels/effects of: CloZAPine; Didanosine; Fingolimod; Leflunomide; Natalizumab; Stavudine; Tofacitinib; Vaccines (Live)

The levels/effects of Hydroxyurea may be increased by: Denosumab; Didanosine; Dipyrone; Pimecrolimus; Roflumilast; Stavudine; Tacrolimus (Topical); Trastuzumab

Decreased Effect

Hydroxyurea may decrease the levels/effects of: BCG (Intravesical); Coccidioides immitis Skin Test; Sipuleucel-T; Vaccines (Inactivated); Vaccines (Live)

The levels/effects of Hydroxyurea may be decreased by: Echinacea

Storage/Stability Store at 25°C (77°F); excursions permitted between 15°C and 30°C (59°F and 86°F). Keep bottle tightly closed.

Mechanism of Action Antimetabolite which selectively inhibits ribonucleoside diphosphate reductase, preventing the conversion of ribonucleotides to deoxyribonucleotides, halting the cell cycle at the G1/S phase and therefore has radiation sensitizing activity by maintaining cells in the G_1 phase and interfering with DNA repair. In sickle cell anemia, hydroxyurea increases red blood cell

(RBC) hemoglobin F levels, RBC water content, deformability of sickled cells, and alters adhesion of RBCs to endothelium.

Pharmacodynamics/Kinetics

Onset: Sickle cell anemia: Fetal hemoglobin increase: 4 to 12 weeks

Absorption: Readily absorbed (≥80%)

Distribution: Distributes widely into tissues (including into the brain); estimated volume of distribution approximates total body water (Gwilt 1998); concentrates in leukocytes and erythrocytes

Metabolism: Up to 60% via hepatic and GI tract

Protein binding: 75% to 80% bound to serum proteins (Gwilt 1998)

Half-life elimination: 1.9 to 3.9 hours (Gwilt 1998); Children: Sickle cell anemia: 1.7 hours (range: 0.7 to 3 hours) (Ware 2011)

Time to peak: 1 to 4 hours

Excretion: Urine (sickle cell anemia: ~40% of administered dose)

Dosing

Adult Note: Doses should be based on ideal or actual body weight, whichever is less (per manufacturer). Prophylactic administration of folic acid is recommended.

Antineoplastic uses (chronic myeloid leukemia [CML], head and neck cancer): Oral: Initial: 15 mg/kg/day; individualize treatment based on tumor type, disease state, response to treatment, patient risk factors, and current clinical practice standards. May be used alone or in combination with other agents or radiation.

Sickle cell anemia: Oral:

Manufacturer's labeling: Initial: 15 mg/kg/day as a single dose; if blood counts are in an acceptable range, may increase by 5 mg/kg/day every 12 weeks until the maximum tolerated dose of 35 mg/kg/day is achieved or the dose that does not produce toxic effects over 24 consecutive weeks (do not increase dose if blood counts are between acceptable and toxic ranges). Monitor for toxicity every 2 weeks; if toxicity occurs, withhold treatment until the bone marrow recovers, then restart with a dose reduction of 2.5 mg/kg/day; if no toxicity occurs over the next 12 weeks, then the subsequent dose may be increased by 2.5 mg/kg/day every 12 weeks to a maximum tolerated dose (dose which does not produce hematologic toxicity for 24 consecutive weeks). If hematologic toxicity recurs a second time at a specific dose, do not retry that dose.

Acceptable hematologic ranges: Neutrophils ≥2,500/mm^3; platelets ≥95,000/mm^3; hemoglobin >5.3 g/dL, and reticulocytes ≥95,000/mm^3 if the hemoglobin concentration is <9 g/dL

Toxic hematologic ranges: Neutrophils <2,000/mm^3; platelets <80,000/mm^3; hemoglobin <4.5 g/dL; and reticulocytes <80,000/mm^3 if the hemoglobin concentration is <9 g/dL

Alternate recommendations (off-label dose): Initial: 15 mg/kg/day; if dosage escalation is warranted based on clinical/laboratory findings, may increase by 5 mg/kg/day increments every 8 weeks. Monitor for toxicity at least every 4 weeks when adjusting dose; aim for a target absolute neutrophils ≥2,000/mm^3 (younger patients with lower baseline counts may safely tolerate absolute neutrophils down to 1,250/mm^3; maintain platelet count ≥80,000/mm^3. Give until mild myelosuppression is achieved (absolute neutrophils: 2,000/mm^3 to 4,000/mm^3), up to a maximum dose of 35 mg/kg/day. If toxicity occurs (neutropenia or thrombocytopenia), withhold treatment until the bone marrow recovers (monitor weekly), then restart at a dose 5mg/kg/day lower than the dose given prior to onset of cytopenias (NHLBI 2014). **Note:** A clinical response to treatment may take 3 to 6 months; a 6 month trial on the maximum tolerated dose is recommended prior to considering discontinuation due to treatment failure; effectiveness of hydroxyurea depends upon daily dosing adherence. For patients who have a clinical response, long-term hydroxyurea therapy is indicated (NHLBI 2014)

Acute myeloid leukemia (AML), cytoreduction (off-label use): Oral: 50 to 100 mg/kg/day until WBC <100,000/mm^3 (Grund 1977) **or** 50 to 60 mg/kg/day until WBC <10,000 to 20,000/mm^3 (Dohner 2010)

Essential thrombocythemia, high-risk (off-label use): Oral: 500 to 1000 mg daily; adjust dose to maintain platelets <400,000/mm^3 (Harrison 2005)

Head and neck cancer (off-label dosing; with concurrent radiation therapy and fluorouracil): Oral: 1000 mg every 12 hours for 11 doses per cycle (Garden 2004)

Hypereosinophilic syndrome (off-label use): Oral: 1,000 to 3,000 mg/day (Klion 2006)

Meningioma (off-label use): Oral: 20 mg/kg once daily (Newton 2000; Rosenthal 2002)

Polycythemia vera, high-risk (off-label use): Oral: 15 to 20 mg/kg/day (Finazzi 2007)

Geriatric Refer to adult dosing. May require lower doses.

Pediatric Note: Doses should be based on ideal or actual body weight, whichever is less (per manufacturer). Prophylactic administration of folic acid is recommended.

Sickle cell anemia (off-label use): Infants ≥6 months, Children, and Adolescents: Oral: 20 mg/kg/dose once daily; increase by 5 mg/kg/**day** every 8 weeks until mild myelosuppression (neutrophils 2,000 to 4,000/mm^3) is achieved up to a maximum of 35 mg/kg/**day** (Hankins 2005; NHLBI 2014; Strouse 2012). If myelosuppression occurs (platelets <80,000/mm^3, neutrophils <2,000/mm^3; younger patients with lower baseline counts may safely tolerate ANC down to 1,250/mm^3), hold therapy until counts recover (monitor weekly); reinitiate at a dose 5 mg/kg/**day** lower than the dose given prior to onset of cytopenias (NHLBI 2014); some have recommended reinitiating at a dose 2.5 mg/kg/**day** lower (Hankins 2005; Heeney 2008; Wang 2001; Wang 2011; Zimmerman 2004). **Note:** A clinical response to treatment may take 3 to 6 months; a 6-month trial on the maximum tolerated dose is recommended prior to considering discontinuation due to treatment failure; effectiveness of hydroxyurea depends upon daily dosing adherence. For patients who have a clinical response, long-term hydroxyurea therapy is indicated (NHLBI 2014).

Renal Impairment

The manufacturer's labeling recommends the following adjustments:

Antineoplastic uses (CML, head and neck cancer):

CrCl ≥60 mL/minute: No dosage adjustment (of initial dose) necessary.

CrCl <60 mL/minute: Reduce initial dose by 50% to 7.5 mg/kg/day; titrate to response/avoidance of toxicity

End-stage renal diosorder (ESRD): Reduce initial dose by 50% to 7.5 mg/kg/dose (administer after dialysis on dialysis days); titrate to response/avoidance of toxicity

Sickle cell anemia:

CrCl ≥60 mL/minute: No dosage adjustment (of initial dose) necessary.

CrCl <60 mL/minute: Reduce initial dose to 7.5 mg/kg/day (Yan 2005); titrate to response/avoidance of toxicity (refer to usual dosing).

ESRD: Reduce initial dose to 7.5 mg/kg/dose (administer after dialysis on dialysis days); titrate to response/avoidance of toxicity.

The following adjustments have also been reported:

Aronoff 2007: Adults:

CrCl >50 mL/minute: No dosage adjustment necessary

CrCl 10 to 50 mL/minute: Administer 50% of dose.

CrCl <10 mL/minute: Administer 20% of dose.

Hemodialysis: Administer dose after dialysis on dialysis days.

Continuous renal replacement therapy (CRRT): Administer 50% of dose.

NHLBI 2014: Sickle cell anemia: Adults: Chronic kidney disease: Initial 5 to 10 mg/kg/day

Kintzel 1995:

CrCl 46 to 60 mL/minute: Administer 85% of dose.

CrCl 31 to 45 mL/minute: Administer 80% of dose.

CrCl <30 mL/minute: Administer 75% of dose.

Hepatic Impairment There are no dosage adjustments provided in the manufacturer's labeling; closely monitor for bone marrow toxicity.

Obesity *ASCO Guidelines for appropriate chemotherapy dosing in obese adults with cancer (solid tumors):* Utilize patient's actual body weight (full weight) for calculation of body surface area- or weight-based dosing, particularly when the intent of therapy is curative; manage regimen-related toxicities in the same manner as for nonobese patients; if a dose reduction is utilized due to toxicity, consider resumption of full weight-based dosing with subsequent cycles, especially if cause of toxicity (eg, hepatic or renal impairment) is resolved (Griggs 2012). **Note:** The manufacturer recommends dosing based on ideal or actual body weight, whichever is less.

Adjustment for Toxicity

Cutaneous vasculitic ulcerations: Discontinue

Pancreatitis: Discontinue permanently

Hematologic toxicity:

Antineoplastic uses (CML, head and neck cancer): Do not initiate therapy if bone marrow function is markedly reduced. Monitor blood counts prior to and during treatment; modify dose or discontinue hydroxyurea as needed.

Sickle cell anemia:

Manufacturer's labeling: Neutrophils <2,000/mm³, platelets <80,000/mm³, hemoglobin <4.5 g/dL, or reticulocytes <80,000/mm³ with hemoglobin <9 g/dL: Interrupt treatment; following recovery, may resume with a dose reduction of 2.5 mg/kg/day. If no toxicity occurs over the next 12 weeks, subsequent dose may be increased by 2.5 mg/kg/day every 12 weeks to a dose which does not produce hematologic toxicity for 24 consecutive weeks. If hematologic toxicity recurs a second time at a specific dose, do not retry that dose.

Alternate recommendations (off-label dose): Absolute neutrophils <2,000/mm³ (younger patients with lower baseline counts may safely tolerate absolute neutrophils down to 1,250/mm³), platelets <80,000/mm³; Interrupt treatment; following recovery, may restart at a dose 5mg/kg/day lower than the dose given prior to onset of cytopenias (NHLBI 2014).

Combination Regimens

Head and neck cancer: Fluorouracil-Hydroxyurea (Head and Neck Cancer) on page 1978

Leukemia, acute myeloid: Hydroxyurea (AML Regimen) on page 2003

Administration Administer at the same time each day.

Hazardous agent; use appropriate precautions for handling and disposal (NIOSH 2014 [group 1]). Impervious gloves should be worn when handling bottles containing hydroxyurea or when handling/administering intact capsules (single gloves are recommended). Wash hands with soap and water before and after contact with the bottle or capsules when handling. Avoid exposure to crushed or open capsules. If skin contact with crushed or opened capsules occurs, immediately wash the affected area thoroughly with soap and water. If eye(s) contact with crushed or opened capsules occurs, the affected area should be flushed thoroughly with water or isotonic eyewash designated for that purpose for at least 15 minutes. If the powder from the capsule is spilled, immediately wipe it up with a damp disposable towel and discard (along with the empty capsules) in a closed container, such as a plastic bag. The spill areas should then be cleaned 3 times using a detergent solution followed by clean water.

Although the manufacturer does not recommend opening the capsules, if it is necessary to manipulate the capsules (eg, to prepare an oral suspension or solution), it is recommended to double glove, wear a protective gown, and prepare in a controlled device (NIOSH 2014).

Emetic Potential Children and Adults: Minimal (<10%)

Extemporaneous Preparations Hazardous agent: Use appropriate precautions for handling and disposal (NIOSH 2014 [group 1]). When manipulating capsules, NIOSH recommends double gloving, a protective gown, and preparation in a controlled device; if not prepared in a controlled device, respiratory and eye protection as well as ventilated engineering controls are recommended (NIOSH 2014).

A 40 mg/mL oral suspension may be prepared with capsules and either a 1:1 mixture of Ora-Sweet® and Ora-Plus® or a 1:1 mixture of methylcellulose 1% and simple syrup NF. Empty the contents of eight 500 mg capsules into a mortar. Add small portions of chosen vehicle and mix to a uniform paste; mix while incrementally adding the vehicle to **almost** 100 mL; transfer to a calibrated bottle, rinse mortar with vehicle, and add sufficient quantity of vehicle to make 100 mL. Label "shake well" and "refrigerate". Store in plastic prescription bottles. Stable for 14 days at room temperature or refrigerated (preferred) (Nahata 2003).

A 100 mg/mL oral solution may be prepared with capsules. Mix the contents of twenty 500 mg capsules with enough room temperature sterile water (~50 mL) to initially result in a 200 mg/mL concentration. Stir vigorously using a magnetic stirrer for several hours, then filter to remove insoluble contents. Add 50 mL Syrpalta® (flavored syrup, HUMCO) to filtered solution, resulting in 100 mL of a 100 mg/mL hydroxyurea solution. Stable for 1 month at room temperature in amber plastic bottle (Heeney 2004).

Heeney MM, Whorton MR, Howard TA, et al, "Chemical and Functional Analysis of Hydroxyurea Oral Solutions," *J Pediatr Hematol Oncol* 2004, 26(3):179-84.

Nahata MC, Morosco RS, Boster EA, et al, "Stability of Hydroxyurea in Two Extemporaneously Prepared Oral Suspensions Stored at Two Temperatures," 2003, 38:P-161(E) [abstract from 2003 ASHP Midyear Clinical Meeting].

◀ **Monitoring Parameters** CBC with differential and platelets (once weekly for antineoplastic indications; every 2 weeks initially for sickle cell anemia), renal function and liver function tests, serum uric acid; hemoglobin F levels (sickle cell disease); monitor for cutaneous toxicities

Sickle cell disease: Monitor for toxicity every 2 weeks during dose escalation (neutrophils, platelets, hemoglobin, reticulocytes) (manufacturer's labeling) or at least every 4 weeks when adjusting the dose (CBC with WBC differential, reticulocytes) [NHLBI 2014]). Once on a stable dose, may monitor CBC with differential, reticulocyte count and platelets every 2 to 3 months (NHLBI 2014). Monitor RBC, MCV (mean corpuscular volume) and HbF (fetal hemoglobin) levels for evidence of consistent or progressive laboratory response (NHLBI 2014).

Test Interactions False-negative triglyceride measurement by a glycerol oxidase method. An analytical interference between hydroxyurea and enzymes (lactate dehydrogenase, urease, and uricase) may result in false elevations of lactic acid, urea, and uric acid.

Dietary Considerations Supplemental administration of folic acid is recommended; hydroxyurea may mask development of folic acid deficiency.

Dosage Forms Excipient information presented when available (limited, particularly for generics); consult specific product labeling.
Capsule, Oral:
  Droxia: 200 mg, 300 mg, 400 mg
  Hydrea: 500 mg
  Generic: 500 mg

Ibandronate (eye BAN droh nate)

Related Information
  Hypercalcemia of Malignancy on page 2241
Brand Names: US Boniva
Index Terms Ibandronate Sodium; Ibandronic Acid
Pharmacologic Category Bisphosphonate Derivative
Use Treatment and prevention of osteoporosis in postmenopausal females
Labeled Contraindications Hypersensitivity to ibandronate or any component of the formulation; hypocalcemia; oral tablets are also contraindicated in patients unable to stand or sit upright for at least 60 minutes and in patients with abnormalities of the esophagus which delay esophageal emptying, such as stricture or achalasia
Pregnancy Considerations Adverse effects were observed in animal reproduction studies. It is not known if bisphosphonates cross the placenta, but fetal exposure is expected (Djokanovic, 2008; Stathopoulos, 2011). Bisphosphonates are incorporated into the bone matrix and gradually released over time. The amount available in the systemic circulation varies by dose and duration of

therapy. Theoretically, there may be a risk of fetal harm when pregnancy follows the completion of therapy; however, available data have not shown that exposure to bisphosphonates during pregnancy significantly increases the risk of adverse fetal events (Djokanovic, 2008; Levy, 2009; Stathopoulos, 2011). Until additional data is available, most sources recommend discontinuing bisphosphonate therapy in women of reproductive potential as early as possible prior to a planned pregnancy; use in premenopausal women should be reserved for special circumstances when rapid bone loss is occurring (Bhalla, 2010; Pereira, 2012; Stathopoulos, 2011). Because hypocalcemia has been described following *in utero* bisphosphonate exposure, exposed infants should be monitored for hypocalcemia after birth (Djokanovic, 2008; Stathopoulos, 2011).

Breast-Feeding Considerations It is not known if ibandronate is excreted into breast milk. The manufacturer recommends caution be exercised when administering ibandronate to nursing women.

Warnings/Precautions Hypocalcemia must be corrected before therapy initiation. Ensure adequate calcium and vitamin D intake. Osteonecrosis of the jaw (ONJ) has been reported in patients receiving bisphosphonates. Risk factors include invasive dental procedures (eg, tooth extraction, dental implants, boney surgery); a diagnosis of cancer, with concomitant chemotherapy or corticosteroids; poor oral hygiene, ill-fitting dentures; and comorbid disorders (anemia, coagulopathy, infection, preexisting dental disease); risk may increase with duration of bisphosphonate use. Most reported cases occurred after IV bisphosphonate therapy; however, cases have been reported following oral therapy. A dental exam and preventive dentistry should be performed prior to placing patients with risk factors on chronic bisphosphonate therapy. The manufacturer's labeling states that discontinuing bisphosphonates in patients requiring invasive dental procedures may reduce the risk of ONJ. However, other experts suggest that there is no evidence that discontinuing therapy reduces the risk of developing ONJ (Assael, 2009). The benefit/risk must be assessed by the treating physician and/or dentist/surgeon prior to any invasive dental procedure. Patients developing ONJ while on bisphosphonates should receive care by an oral surgeon.

Atypical femur fractures have been reported in patients receiving bisphosphonates for treatment/prevention of osteoporosis. The fractures include subtrochanteric femur (bone just below the hip joint) and diaphyseal femur (long segment of the thigh bone). Some patients experience prodromal pain weeks or months before the fracture occurs. It is unclear if bisphosphonate therapy is the cause for these fractures, although the majority of cases have been reported in patients taking bisphosphonates. Patients receiving long-term (>3-5 years) therapy may be at an increased risk. Discontinue bisphosphonate therapy in patients who develop a femoral shaft fracture.

Infrequently, severe (and occasionally debilitating) bone, joint, and/or muscle pain have been reported during bisphosphonate treatment. The onset of pain ranged from a single day to several months. Discontinue intravenous ibandronate therapy in patients who experience severe symptoms; symptoms usually resolve upon discontinuation. Some patients experienced recurrence when rechallenged with same drug or another bisphosphonate; avoid use in patients with a history of these symptoms in association with bisphosphonate therapy.

Oral bisphosphonates may cause dysphagia, esophagitis, esophageal or gastric ulcer; risk may increase in patients unable to comply with dosing instructions; discontinue use if new or worsening symptoms develop. ▶

Intravenous bisphosphonates may cause transient decreases in serum calcium and have also been associated with renal toxicity.

Use not recommended with severe renal impairment (CrCl <30 mL/minute). In the management of osteoporosis, re-evaluate the need for continued therapy periodically; the optimal duration of treatment has not yet been determined. Consider discontinuing after 3-5 years of use in patients at low-risk for fracture; following discontinuation, re-evaluate fracture risk periodically. Potentially significant drug-drug interactions may exist, requiring dose or frequency adjustment, additional monitoring, and/or selection of alternative therapy.

Adverse Reactions Percentages vary based on frequency of administration (daily vs monthly). Unless specified, percentages are reported with oral use.

>10%:
  Gastrointestinal: Dyspepsia (4% to 12%)
  Neuromuscular & skeletal: Back pain (4% to 14%)
  Respiratory: Upper respiratory tract infection (2% to 34%)

1% to 10%:
  Cardiovascular: Hypertension (6% to 7%)
  Central nervous system: Headache (3% to 7%), dizziness (1% to 4%), fatigue (3%), insomnia (1% to 2%), depression (2%)
  Dermatologic: Skin rash (1% to 2%)
  Gastrointestinal: Abdominal pain (5% to 8%), diarrhea (2% to 7%), nausea (4% to 5%), dental disease (4%), constipation (3% to 4%), vomiting (3%), gastritis (3%), gastroenteritis (3%)
  Genitourinary: Urinary tract infection (2% to 6%), cystitis (3%)
  Hypersensitivity: Acute phase reaction-like symptoms (IV: 10%; oral: 3% to 9%), hypersensitivity reaction (3%)
  Infection: Influenza (4% to 8%)
  Local: Injection site reaction (<2%)
  Neuromuscular & skeletal: Limb pain (1% to 8%), arthralgia (4% to 9%), myalgia (1% to 6%), arthropathy (4%), weakness (4%), localized osteoarthritis (1% to 3%), muscle cramps (2%)
  Respiratory: Bronchitis (3% to 10%), pneumonia (6%), nasopharyngitis (3% to 4%), flu-like symptoms (1% to 3%), pharyngitis (3%)

Postmarketing and/or case reports: Acute renal failure, anaphylactic shock, anaphylaxis, angioedema, bronchospasm, bullous dermatitis, erythema multiforme, exacerbation of asthma, femur fracture (diaphyseal or subtrochanteric), hypocalcemia, iritis, musculoskeletal pain (bone, joint, or muscle; incapacitating), ophthalmic inflammation, osteonecrosis of the jaw, prolonged Q-T interval on ECG (Bonilla 2014), scleritis, Stevens-Johnson syndrome, uveitis

Drug Interactions

Metabolism/Transport Effects None known.

Avoid Concomitant Use There are no known interactions where it is recommended to avoid concomitant use.

Increased Effect/Toxicity

Ibandronate may increase the levels/effects of: Deferasirox; Highest Risk QTc-Prolonging Agents; Moderate Risk QTc-Prolonging Agents

The levels/effects of Ibandronate may be increased by: Aminoglycosides; Mifepristone; Nonsteroidal Anti-Inflammatory Agents; Systemic Angiogenesis Inhibitors

Decreased Effect

The levels/effects of Ibandronate may be decreased by: Antacids; Calcium Salts; Iron Salts; Magnesium Salts; Multivitamins/Minerals (with ADEK, Folate, Iron); Multivitamins/Minerals (with AE, No Iron); Proton Pump Inhibitors

Food Interactions Food may reduce absorption; mean oral bioavailability is decreased up to 90% when given with food. Management: Take with a full glass (6-8 oz) of plain water, at least 60 minutes prior to any food, beverages, or medications. Mineral water with a high calcium content should be avoided. Wait at least 60 minutes after taking ibandronate before taking anything else.

Storage/Stability Store at controlled room temperature of 25°C (77°F); excursions permitted to 15°C to 30°C (59°F to 86°F).

Mechanism of Action A bisphosphonate which inhibits bone resorption via actions on osteoclasts or on osteoclast precursors; decreases the rate of bone resorption, leading to an indirect increase in bone mineral density.

Pharmacodynamics/Kinetics

Distribution: Terminal V_d: 90 L; 40% to 50% of circulating ibandronate binds to bone

Protein binding: 85.7% to 99.5%

Metabolism: Not metabolized

Bioavailability: Oral: Minimal; reduced ~90% following standard breakfast

Half-life elimination:

Oral: 150 mg dose: Terminal: 37-157 hours

IV: Terminal: ~5-25 hours

Time to peak, plasma: Oral: 0.5-2 hours

Excretion: Urine (50% to 60% of absorbed dose, excreted as unchanged drug); feces (unabsorbed drug)

Dosing

Adult & Geriatric

Postmenopausal osteoporosis (treatment): Note: Consider discontinuing after 3-5 years of use for osteoporosis in patients at low-risk for fracture. Patients should receive supplemental calcium and vitamin D if dietary intake is inadequate.

Oral: 150 mg once monthly

IV: 3 mg every 3 months

Postmenopausal osteoporosis (prevention): Oral: 150 mg once monthly. **Note:** Patients should receive supplemental calcium and vitamin D if dietary intake is inadequate.

Hypercalcemia of malignancy (off-label use): IV: 2-6 mg over 1-2 hours (Pecherstorfer, 2003; Ralston, 1997)

Metastatic bone disease due to breast cancer (off-label use): IV: 6 mg every 3-4 weeks (Diel, 2004)

Missed doses:

Oral: If once-monthly oral dose is missed, it should be given the next morning after remembered if the next month's scheduled dose is >7 days away. If the next month's scheduled dose is within 7 days, wait until the next month's scheduled dose. May then return to the original monthly schedule (original scheduled day of the month). Do not give >150 mg within 7 days.

IV: If an IV dose is missed, it should be administered as soon as it can be rescheduled. Thereafter, it should be given every 3 months from the date of the last injection.

◀ **Renal Impairment**

Osteoporosis: Oral, IV:

CrCl ≥30 mL/minute: No dosage adjustment necessary.

CrCl <30 mL/minute: Use not recommended.

Oncologic uses (off-label): IV: CrCl <30 mL/minute: 2 mg every 3-4 weeks (von Moos, 2005)

Hepatic Impairment No dosage adjustment necessary (has not been studied); however, ibandronate does not undergo hepatic metabolism.

Administration

Oral: Administer 60 minutes before the first food or drink of the day (other than water) and prior to taking any oral medications or supplements (eg, calcium, antacids, vitamins). Ibandronate should be taken in an upright position with a full glass (6-8 oz) of plain water and the patient should avoid lying down for 60 minutes to minimize the possibility of GI side effects. Mineral water with a high calcium content should be avoided. The tablet should be swallowed whole; do not chew or suck. Do not eat or drink anything (except water) for 60 minutes following administration of ibandronate.

IV: Administer as a 15-30 second bolus intravenously; avoid paravenous or intraarterial administration (may cause tissue damage). Do not mix with calcium-containing solutions or other drugs. For osteoporosis, do not administer more frequently than every 3 months. Infuse over 1 hour for metastatic bone disease due to breast cancer (Diel, 2004) and over 1-2 hours for hypercalcemia of malignancy (Pecherstorfer, 2003; Ralston, 1997).

Monitoring Parameters

Osteoporosis: Bone mineral density (BMD) should be evaluated 1 to 2 years after initiating therapy and every 2 years thereafter (NOF [Cosman 2014]); annual measurements of height and weight, assessment of chronic back pain; serum calcium and 25(OH)D; may consider measuring biochemical markers of bone turnover

Serum creatinine prior to each IV dose

Test Interactions Bisphosphonates may interfere with diagnostic imaging agents such as technetium-99m-diphosphonate in bone scans.

Dietary Considerations

Ensure adequate calcium and vitamin D intake; if dietary intake is inadequate, dietary supplementation is recommended. Women and men should consume:

Calcium: 1,000 mg/day (men: 50 to 70 years) or 1,200 mg/day (women ≥51 years and men ≥71 years) (IOM, 2011; NOF [Cosman 2014])

Vitamin D: 800 to 1,000 int. units daily (men and women ≥50 years) (NOF [Cosman 2014]). Recommended Dietary Allowance (RDA): 600 int. units daily (men and women ≤70 years) or 800 int. units daily (men and women ≥71 years) (IOM, 2011).

Ibandronate tablet should be taken with a full glass (6 to 8 oz) of plain water, at least 60 minutes prior to any food, beverages, or medications. Mineral water with a high calcium content should be avoided.

Medication Guide Available Yes

Dosage Forms Excipient information presented when available (limited, particularly for generics); consult specific product labeling.

Solution, Intravenous:

Boniva: 3 mg/3 mL (3 mL)

Generic: 3 mg/3 mL (3 mL)

Solution, Intravenous [preservative free]:
  Generic: 3 mg/3 mL (3 mL)
Tablet, Oral:
  Boniva: 150 mg
  Generic: 150 mg

Ibritumomab (ib ri TYOO mo mab)

Related Information

Management of Drug Extravasations *on page 2159*

Brand Names: US Zevalin Y-90

Brand Names: Canada Zevalin

Index Terms Ibritumomab Tiuxetan; IDEC-Y2B8; Y-90 Ibritumomab; Y-90 Zevalin

Pharmacologic Category Antineoplastic Agent, Anti-CD20; Antineoplastic Agent, Monoclonal Antibody; Radiopharmaceutical

Use Non-Hodgkin lymphoma: Treatment of relapsed or refractory, low-grade or follicular B-cell non-Hodgkin lymphoma (NHL); treatment of previously untreated follicular NHL in patients who achieve a partial or complete response to first-line chemotherapy

Labeled Contraindications There are no contraindications listed within the manufacturer's labeling.

Pregnancy Considerations Animal reproduction studies have not been conducted. Based on the radioactivity, Y-90 ibritumomab may cause fetal harm if administered during pregnancy. IgG molecules are known to cross the placenta. Women of childbearing potential should avoid becoming pregnant during treatment with ibritumomab. Both males and females should use effective contraception for at least 12 months following treatment. The effect on future fertility is unknown.

Breast-Feeding Considerations It is not known whether ibritumomab is excreted in breast milk. Because many immunoglobulins are excreted in milk and the potential for serious adverse reactions in the nursing infant exists, the decision to either discontinue breast-feeding or to avoid ibritumomab use should take into account the potential benefits of treatment to the mother.

Warnings/Precautions Radiopharmaceutical; use appropriate precautions for handling, disposal, and minimizing exposure to patients and healthcare personnel. Use only under supervision of individuals with experience/training in the handling of radioactive materials approved by the applicable regulatory authority. **[US Boxed Warning]: Severe cutaneous and mucocutaneous skin reactions have been reported (with fatalities). Discontinue all components of the therapeutic regimen in patients experiencing severe cutaneous or mucocutaneous skin reactions,** including erythema multiforme, Stevens-Johnson syndrome, toxic epidermal necrolysis, bullous dermatitis, and exfoliative dermatitis. Onset may occur within days to 4 months following infusion.

To be used as part of the Zevalin therapeutic regimen (in combination with rituximab). **[US Boxed Warning]: Do not exceed the Y-90 ibritumomab maximum allowable dose of 32 mCi (1184 MBq).** Use should be reserved ▶

to physicians and other professionals qualified and experienced in the safe handling of radiopharmaceuticals, and in monitoring and emergency treatment of infusion reactions. The contents of the kit are not radioactive until radio-labeling occurs. During and after radiolabeling, adequate shielding should be used with this product, minimize radiation exposure (to patient and healthcare professionals) in accordance with institutional radiation safety practices.

[US Boxed Warning]: Serious fatal infusion reactions may occur with the rituximab component of the therapeutic regimen. Immediately stop infusion and discontinue all components of the therapeutic regimen in patients who develop severe infusion reactions. Fatalities due to ritux-imab infusion were associated with acute respiratory distress syndrome, hypoxia, pulmonary infiltrates, cardiogenic shock, MI, or ventricular fibrillation; 80% of fatalities occurred with the first rituximab infusion. Administer in a facility with immediate access to resuscitative measures. Infusion reactions typically occur with the first rituximab infusion (onset within 30 to 120 minutes). Reactions may also include hypotension, angioedema, bronchospasm, and urticaria. Less severe reactions may be managed by slowing or interrupting infusion.

[US Boxed Warning]: Delayed, prolonged, and severe cytopenias (throm-bocytopenia and neutropenia) are common. Do not administer to patients with ≥25% lymphoma marrow involvement, patients with impaired bone marrow reserve (eg, prior myeloablative treatment, platelet count <100,000/mm³, neutrophil count <1,500/mm³, hypocellular marrow), or to patients with prior stem cell collection failure. Cytopenias may persist beyond 12 weeks. Patients with mild baseline thrombocytopenia may experience higher incidences of severe neutropenia and thrombocytopenia. Hemorrhage may occur due to thrombocytopenia; avoid concomitant use of medications interfering with coagulation or platelet function. Monitor CBC and platelets weekly until recovery or as clinically indicated. Closely monitor patients for complications of cytopenias (eg, febrile neutropenia, hemorrhage) for up to 3 months after administration.

American Society of Clinical Oncology (ASCO) provisional clinical opinion update on hepatitis B virus screening recommendations (Hwang, 2015): Patients receiving anti-CD20 antibodies are at high risk for hepatitis B virus (HBV) reactivation. Screen for HBV infection with hepatitis B surface antigen (HBsAG) and hepatitis B core antibody (anti-HBc) tests prior to treatment initiation; either a total anti-HBc (with both IgG and IgM) or anti-HBc IgG test should be used to screen for chronic or unresolved HBV infection (do not use anti-HBc IgM as it may only confirm acute HBV infection). In addition, patients who have risk factors for HBV infection (eg, birthplace in a country with ≥2% HBV prevalence, household or sexual contact with HBV infected patients, high-risk behaviors [eg, IV drug use], and HIV infection) should also be screened prior to beginning therapy. Initiate prophylactic antiviral therapy (utilizing antivirals with low rates of viral resistance) for HBsAg positive/anti-HBc positive patients (without delaying cancer therapy) and continue the antivirals during and for ~6 to 12 months after completing treatment. HBsAg negative/anti-HBc positive patients should be monitored for HBV reactivation with HBV DNA and ALT testing approximately every 3 months during treat-ment; antiviral therapy may be initiated prophylactically or begun promptly at the first sign of HBV reactivation. Malignancies due to the radiation dose from therapeutic exposure may occur. Secondary malignancies (acute myeloge-nous leukemia and/or myelodysplastic syndrome) have been reported following use; the median time to diagnosis (secondary malignancy) following ibritumomab treatment was 1.9 years with a range of 0.4 to 6.3 years (Czuczman, 2007). Product contains albumin, which confers a theoretical risk of transmission of viral disease or Creutzfeldt-Jakob disease. The safety of immunization with live vaccines following ibritumomab therapy has not been studied; do not administer live viral vaccines to patients who have recently received ibritumomab treatment; the ability to generate a response to any vaccine after receiving treatment has not been studied. Potentially significant drug-drug interactions may exist, requiring dose or frequency adjustment, additional monitoring, and/or selection of alternative therapy. Infusion site erythema and ulceration have been reported following extravasation; monitor infusion site; promptly terminate infusion with symptoms/signs of extravasation (restart in another limb). There is a case report of (delayed) erythema and ulceration, which is described as radiation necrosis following yttrium-90-ibritumomab extravasation (Williams, 2006). Delayed (up to 1 month) radiation injury has occurred in or near areas of lymphomatous involvement. In a postmarketing registry of biodistribution images, biodistribution was altered in a limited number of patients.

Adverse Reactions

>10%:

Central nervous system: Fatigue (33%)

Gastrointestinal: Nausea (18%), abdominal pain (17%), diarrhea (11%)

Hematologic & oncologic: Thrombocytopenia (62% to 95%; grades 3/4: 51% to 63%; nadir: 49-53 days; median duration: 24 days; median time to recovery: 13 days), neutropenia (45% to 77%; grades 3/4: 41% to 60%; nadir: 61-62 days; median duration: 22 days; median time to recovery: 12 days), anemia (22% to 61%; grades 3/4: 5% to 17%; nadir: 68-69 days), leukopenia (43%; grades 3/4: 36%), lymphocytopenia (26%; grades 3/4: 18%), metastases (1% to 13%; includes acute myelogenous leukemia and myelodysplastic syndrome)

Infection: Infection (within first 3 months: 29%; serious: 1% to 3%; 3 months to 4 years after treatment: 6%)

Neuromuscular & skeletal: Weakness (15%)

Respiratory: Nasopharyngitis (19%), cough (11%)

1% to 10%:

Cardiovascular: Hypertension (7%)

Central nervous system: Dizziness (7%)

Dermatologic: Night sweats (8%), pruritus (7%), skin rash (7%)

Gastrointestinal: Anorexia (8%)

Genitourinary: Urinary tract infection (7%)

Hematologic & oncologic: Petechia (8%), bruise (7%), severe cytopenia (prolonged: 5%)

Immunologic: Antibody development (HAMA/HACA: 1% to 3%)

Neuromuscular & skeletal: Myalgia (9%)

Respiratory: Bronchitis (8%), flu-like symptoms (8%), rhinitis (8%), pharyngolaryngeal pain (7%), sinusitis (7%), epistaxis (5%)

Miscellaneous: Fever (10%), biodistribution altered (1%)

<1%, postmarketing, and/or case reports: Adult respiratory distress syndrome, angioedema, bullous dermatitis, cardiogenic shock, chills, dyspnea, erythema multiforme, exfoliative dermatitis, febrile neutropenia, headache, hypoxia, infusion-related reaction, injection site reaction (erythema/ulceration following extravasation), myocardial infarction, pain, pulmonary infiltrates, radiation injury (delayed [~1 month]; in tissues in or near areas of

◀ lymphomatous involvement), sepsis, Stevens-Johnson syndrome, tissue necrosis (following Yttrium-90-ibritumomab extravasation), toxic epidermal necrolysis, ventricular fibrillation, vomiting

Drug Interactions

Metabolism/Transport Effects None known.

Avoid Concomitant Use

Avoid concomitant use of Ibritumomab with any of the following: BCG (Intravesical); Belimumab; CloZAPine; Dipyrone; Natalizumab; Pimecrolimus; Tacrolimus (Topical); Tofacitinib; Vaccines (Live)

Increased Effect/Toxicity

Ibritumomab may increase the levels/effects of: Belimumab; CloZAPine; Fingolimod; Leflunomide; Natalizumab; Tofacitinib; Vaccines (Live)

The levels/effects of Ibritumomab may be increased by: Agents with Anti-platelet Properties; Anticoagulants; Denosumab; Dipyrone; Pimecrolimus; Roflumilast; Tacrolimus (Topical); Trastuzumab

Decreased Effect

Ibritumomab may decrease the levels/effects of: BCG (Intravesical); Coccidioides immitis Skin Test; Sipuleucel-T; Vaccines (Inactivated); Vaccines (Live)

The levels/effects of Ibritumomab may be decreased by: Echinacea

Storage/Stability Store kits at 2°C to 8°C (36°F to 46°F). Do not freeze. Administer Y-90 ibritumomab tiuxetan within 8 hours of radiolabeling.

Preparation for Administration Radiopharmaceutical; use appropriate precautions for handling and disposal. To prepare radiolabeled injection and determine radiochemical purity, follow detailed preparation guidelines provided by manufacturer. Use appropriate shielding during and after radiolabeling.

Mechanism of Action Ibritumomab is a monoclonal antibody directed against the CD20 antigen found on pre-B and mature B lymphocytes (normal and malignant). Ibritumomab binding induces apoptosis in B lymphocytes *in vitro*. It is combined with the chelator tiuxetan, which acts as a specific chelation site for Yttrium-90 (Y-90). The monoclonal antibody acts as a delivery system to direct the radioactive isotope to the targeted cells, however, binding has been observed in lymphoid cells throughout the body and in lymphoid nodules in organs such as the large and small intestines. Beta-emission induces cellular damage through the formation of free radicals (in both target cells and surrounding cells).

Pharmacodynamics/Kinetics

Duration: B cell recovery begins in ~12 weeks; generally in normal range within 9 months

Distribution: To lymphoid cells throughout the body and in lymphoid nodules in organs such as the large and small intestines, spleen, testes, and liver

Metabolism: Has not been characterized; the product of yttrium-90 radioactive decay is zirconium-90 (nonradioactive)

Half-life elimination: Y-90 ibritumomab: 30 hours; Yttrium-90 decays with a physical half-life of 64 hours

Excretion: A median of 7.2% of the radiolabeled activity was excreted in urine over 7 days

Dosing

Adult & Geriatric Note: Premedicate with oral acetaminophen 650 mg and oral diphenhydramine 50 mg prior to **each** rituximab infusion. Allow at least 6 weeks, but no more than 12 weeks following first-line chemotherapy before treatment initiation; platelets should recover to ≥150,000/mm^3 prior to initiation of treatment regimen.

Non-Hodgkin lymphoma: IV: Ibritumomab is administered **only** as part of the Zevalin therapeutic regimen (a combined treatment regimen with rituximab). The regimen consists of two steps:

Day 1:

Rituximab: 250 mg/m^2 at an initial rate of 50 mg/hour. If hypersensitivity or infusion-related events do not occur, increase infusion in increments of 50 mg/hour every 30 minutes, to a maximum of 400 mg/hour. Stop rituximab and discontinue regimen for severe infusion reaction. For less severe infusion reactions, temporarily slow or interrupt; the infusion may be resumed at one-half the previous rate upon improvement of symptoms.

Day 7, 8, or 9 of treatment:

Rituximab: 250 mg/m^2 at an initial rate of 100 mg/hour (50 mg/hour if infusion-related events occurred with the day 1 infusion). If hypersensitivity or infusion-related events do not occur, increase infusion in increments of 100 mg/hour every 30 minutes, to a maximum of 400 mg/hour, as tolerated (increase in 50 mg/hour increments every 30 minutes if initial infusion rate was 50 mg/hour).

Y-90 ibritumomab: Within 4 hours of completion of the rituximab infusion:

Platelet count ≥150,000 cells/mm^3: Inject 0.4 mCi/kg (14.8 MBq/kg) actual body weight over 10 minutes; maximum dose: 32 mCi (1184 MBq)

Platelet count between 100,000-149,000 cells/mm^3 (in relapsed or refractory patients): Inject 0.3 mCi/kg (11.1 MBq/kg) actual body weight over 10 minutes; maximum dose: 32 mCi (1184 MBq)

Platelet count <100,000 cells/mm^3: Do **not** administer

Maximum dose: The prescribed, measured, and administered dose of Y-90 ibritumomab must not exceed 32 mCi (1184 MBq), regardless of the patient's body weight

Renal Impairment No dosage adjustment provided in manufacturer's labeling.

Hepatic Impairment No dosage adjustment provided in manufacturer's labeling.

Administration

Rituximab: Administer the first infusion of rituximab at an initial rate of 50 mg/hour. If hypersensitivity or infusion-related events do not occur, escalate the infusion rate in 50 mg/hour increments every 30 minutes, to a maximum of 400 mg/hour. Immediately stop infusion for severe infusion reaction (discontinue ibritumomab regimen); less severe reactions may be managed by slowing or interrupting infusion. For less severe reactions, infusion may continue at one-half the previous rate upon improvement of patient symptoms. If infusion reaction did not occur in initial rituximab infusion, subsequent rituximab infusion can be administered at an initial rate of 100 mg/hour and increased in 100 mg/hour increments at 30-minute intervals, to a maximum of 400 mg/hour as tolerated. If infusion reaction occurred with initial rituximab infusion, initiate at 50 mg/hour with increases of 50 mg/hour increments every 30 minutes.

◀ Y-90 ibritumomab: Begin within 4 hours of completion of rituximab infusion. Inject slowly, over 10 minutes through a 0.22 micron low protein binding in-line filter (filter placed between syringe and infusion port) into a free-flowing IV line. After injection, flush line with at least 10 mL normal saline. Avoid extravasation; closely monitor infusion site; if signs or symptoms of extrav-asation occur, stop infusion and restart in another limb.

Radiopharmaceutical; use appropriate precautions for handling and disposal.

Vesicant/Extravasation Risk May be an irritant; there is an isolated case report of (delayed) erythema and ulceration, which is described as radiation necrosis following yttrium-90-ibritumomab extravasation (Williams, 2006).

Monitoring Parameters

CBC with differential and platelet counts weekly until recovery, or as clinically indicated. Platelet count must be obtained prior to day 7, 8, or 9; monitor for cytopenias (and related complications) for up to 3 months after use.

Hepatitis B virus screening recommendations (ASCO provisional clinical opinion update [Hwang, 2015]): Screen for hepatitis B virus (HBV) infection with hepatitis B surface antigen (HBsAG) and hepatitis B core antibody (anti-HBc) tests prior to treatment initiation; either a total anti-HBc (with both IgG and IgM) or anti-HBc IgG test should be used to screen for chronic or unresolved HBV infection (do not use anti-HBc IgM as it may only confirm acute HBV infection). HBsAg negative/anti-HBc positive patients should be monitored for HBV reactivation with HBV DNA and ALT testing approximately every 3 months during treatment.

Monitor for signs of active hepatitis B infection (during and for up to 12 months after therapy completion). Monitor for infusion-related allergic reactions (typically within 30 to 120 minutes of administration), for extravasation during ibritumomab infusion; and for severe cutaneous and mucocutaneous reactions.

Additional Information Ibritumomab tiuxetan is produced in Chinese hamster ovary cell cultures. Kit is not radioactive. Radiolabeling of ibritumomab with Yttrium-90 must be performed by appropriate personnel in a specialized facility.

Dosage Forms Excipient information presented when available (limited, particularly for generics); consult specific product labeling.

Kit, Intravenous [preservative free]:

Zevalin Y-90: 3.2 mg/2 mL [pyrogen free; contains albumin human]

◆ **Ibritumomab Tiuxetan** see Ibritumomab on page 851

Ibrutinib (eye BROO ti nib)

Related Information

Safe Handling of Hazardous Drugs on page 2292

Brand Names: US Imbruvica

Brand Names: Canada Imbruvica

Index Terms BTK inhibitor PCI-32765; CRA-032765; PCI-32765

Pharmacologic Category Antineoplastic Agent; Antineoplastic Agent, Bruton Tyrosine Kinase Inhibitor; Antineoplastic Agent, Tyrosine Kinase Inhibitor

Use

Chronic lymphocytic leukemia: Treatment of patients with chronic lymphocytic leukemia (CLL) who have received at least 1 prior therapy; treatment of CLL patients with 17p deletion.

Mantle cell lymphoma: Treatment of mantle cell lymphoma (MCL) in patients who have received at least 1 prior therapy

Waldenström macroglobulinemia: Treatment of patients with Waldenström macroglobulinemia

Labeled Contraindications

US labeling: There are no contraindications listed in the manufacturer's labeling.

Canadian labeling: Known hypersensitivity to ibrutinib or any component of the formulation.

Pregnancy Considerations Adverse events were observed in animal reproduction studies. The US labeling recommends women of reproductive potential avoid pregnancy during therapy. The Canadian labeling recommends women of reproductive potential use highly effective contraception during and for 3 months after completion of treatment; if using a hormonal method of contraception, add a barrier method; male patients should use a condom (during and for 3 months after completion of treatment) when engaging in sexual activity with a pregnant woman.

Breast-Feeding Considerations It is not known if ibrutinib is excreted in breast milk. Due to the potential for serious adverse reactions in the nursing infant, the manufacturer recommends a decision be made whether to discontinue nursing or to discontinue the drug, taking into account the importance of treatment to the mother.

Warnings/Precautions Hazardous agent – use appropriate precautions for handling and disposal (meets NIOSH 2014 criteria). Grade 3 and 4 neutropenia, thrombocytopenia, and anemia occurred commonly during clinical studies. Monitor blood counts monthly or as clinically necessary. Lymphocytosis (≥50% increase from baseline) may occur upon therapy initiation, generally within the first few weeks of therapy. The increase in lymphocytes is temporary, and resolves by a median of 8 weeks (mantle cell lymphoma) or 23 weeks (chronic lymphocytic leukemia). Some patients who developed lymphocytosis (lymphocytes >400,000/mcL) have developed intracranial hemorrhage, lethargy, headache, and gait instability (some cases may have been associated with disease progression). Monitor for leukostasis, particularly in patients experiencing a rapid increase in lymphocytes to >400,000/mcL. Grade 3 or higher bleeding events (subdural hematoma, gastrointestinal bleeding, hematuria, and postprocedural bleeding) have occurred; some events were fatal. Bleeding events of any grade, including bruising and petechiae have occurred in approximately half of patients receiving ibrutinib. Patients receiving concurrent antiplatelet or anticoagulant treatment may have an increased risk for bleeding. Evaluate the risk-benefit of withholding ibrutinib for 3 to 7 days prior to and after surgery, depending on the procedure type and risk of bleeding. Serious infections (some fatal) have been observed; monitor closely for fever and other signs/symptoms of infection. Evaluate promptly. Progressive multifocal encephalopathy (PML) has been observed; monitor closely and evaluate promptly. Patients treated with ibrutinib have developed second primary malignancies, including skin cancers and other carcinomas. Evaluate for sign/symptoms of malignancy during treatment.

Atrial fibrillation and atrial flutter have occurred, particularly in patients with cardiac risk factors, infections (acute), or with a history of atrial fibrillation. Monitor periodically for clinical symptoms of atrial fibrillation (eg, palpitations, lightheadedness); an ECG should be performed if symptoms or new onset dyspnea develop. For persistent atrial fibrillation, evaluate the risk-benefit of ibrutinib treatment and dose modification. Atrial fibrillation, hypertension, infections (eg, pneumonia, cellulitis, urinary tract infection), and gastrointestinal toxicity (eg, diarrhea and dehydration) were observed more frequently in

◄ elderly patients; maintain adequate hydration. Hyperviscosity may require plasmapheresis prior to or during ibrutinib treatment in patients with Waldenström macroglobulinemia; adjustment of ibrutinib dose due to plasmapheresis is not necessary. Use with caution in patients with preexisting renal impairment; has not been studied in those with severe impairment or in patients on dialysis. Renal failure has been reported with use; some cases were fatal. Clinical trials report serum creatinine increases of up to 3 times ULN; monitor renal function periodically and maintain hydration. Tumor lysis syndrome has been reported; increased uric acid levels have been observed, including grade 4 elevations. Monitor for tumor lysis syndrome in patients at risk (eg, high tumor burden). Ibrutinib is hepatically metabolized, and exposure is increased in patients with hepatic dysfunction. Dosage adjustment is recommended in patients with mild (Child-Pugh class A) impairment; avoid use in patients with moderate or severe (Child-Pugh class B or C) impairment. Monitor closely for toxicity. May cause dizziness, fatigue, and/or weakness which may impair physical or mental abilities; patients must be cautioned about performing tasks that require mental alertness (eg, operating machinery or driving). Potentially significant drug-drug/drug-food interactions may exist, requiring dose or frequency adjustment, additional monitoring, and/or selection of alternative therapy.

Adverse Reactions

Incidences combined for mantle cell lymphoma (MCL), chronic lymphocytic leukemia (CLL), Waldenström macroglobulinemia (WM) and unless otherwise specified.

>10%:

Cardiovascular: Peripheral edema (MCL: 35%, CLL: 23%; grades 3/4: MCL: 3%), hypertension (CLL: 17%; grades 3/4: CLL: 8%)

Central nervous system: Fatigue (MCL: 41%, CLL, WM: 21% to 31%; grades 3/4: CLL, MCL: 2% to 5%), dizziness (11% to 21%), headache (13% to 19%; grades 3/4: CLL: 1% to 2%), chills (CLL: 13%)

Dermatologic: Skin rash (22% to 27%; grades 3/4: CCL, MCL: 3%), skin infection (14% to 17%; grades 3/4: 2% to 6%), pruritus (WM: 11%)

Endocrine & metabolic: Increased uric acid (MCL: 40%; increased uric acid >10 mg/dL: MCL: 13%), hyperuricemia (MCL: 15%), dehydration (MCL: 12%; grades 3/4: MCL: 4%)

Gastrointestinal: Diarrhea (CLL, MCL: 48% to 63%, WM: 37%; grades 3/4: CCL, MCL: 4% to 5%), nausea (21% to 31%; grades 3/4: CLL: 2%), constipation (CLL, MCL: 15% to 25%; grades 3/4: CLL: 2%), abdominal pain (MCL: 24%, CLL: 15%; grades 3/4: MCL: 5%), vomiting (CLL, MCL: 14% to 23%; grades 3/4: CLL: ≤2%), decreased appetite (CLL, MCL: 17% to 21%; grades 3/4: CLL, MCL: 2%), stomatitis (16% to 21%; grades 3/4: CLL, MCL: 1%), gastroesophageal reflux disease (WM: 13%), dyspepsia (CLL, MCL: 11% to 13%)

Genitourinary: Urinary tract infection (CLL, MCL: 10% to 14%; grades 3/4: CLL, MCL: 3% to 4%)

Hematologic & oncologic: Decreased platelet count (CLL, MCL: 52% to 71%, WM: 43%; grades 3/4: 5% to 17%), bruise (11% to 54%; grades 3/4: CLL: 2%); neutropenia (44% to 54%; grades 3/4: 19% to 29%), decreased hemoglobin (CLL, MCL: 36% to 44%, WM: 13%; grades 3/4: MCL, WM: 8% to 9%), petechia (CLL, MCL: 11% to 17%), thrombocytopenia (5% to 17%), malignant neoplasm (secondary; 5% to 14%; includes one death due to histiocytic sarcoma), malignant neoplasm of skin (4% to 11%; nonmelanoma)

Infection: Infection (≥ grade 3: 14% to 26%)

Neuromuscular & skeletal: Musculoskeletal pain (CLL, MCL: 27% to 37%; grades 3/4: CLL: 2% to 6%; grades 3/4: MCL: 1%), arthralgia (CLL: 17% to 23%, MCL: 11%; grades 3/4: CLL: 1%), muscle spasm (14% to 21%; grades 3/4: CLL: 2%), weakness (CLL, MCL: 13% to 14%; grades 3/4: CLL, MCL: 3% to 4%), arthropathy (WM: 13%)

Respiratory: Upper respiratory tract infection (16% to 48%; grades 3/4: CLL: 1% to 2%), dyspnea (MCL: 27%, CLL: 10%; grades 3/4: MCL: 4%), sinusitis (11% to 21%; grades 3/4: CLL, MCL: 1% to 6%), cough (13% to 19%), oropharyngeal pain (CLL: 15%), pneumonia (10% to 15%; grades 3/4: 6% to 10%), epistaxis (MCL, WM: 11% to 19%)

Miscellaneous: Fever (CLL, MCL: 18% to 25%; grades 3/4: CLL, MCL: 1% to 2%)

1% to 10%:

Cardiovascular: Atrial fibrillation (≤6% to 9%), atrial flutter (≤6% to 9%)

Central nervous system: Anxiety (CLL: 10%), insomnia (CLL: 10%), peripheral neuropathy (CLL: 10%)

Hematologic & oncologic: Anemia (grades 3/4: ≤9%), hemorrhage (≤6%; grade 3 or higher bleeding events including gastrointestinal bleeding, hematuria, postprocedural bleeding, subdural hematoma), carcinoma (1% to 3%, other nonskin carcinoma)

Ophthalmic: Blurred vision (CLL: 10%)

Renal: Increased serum creatinine (1.5 to 3 x ULN: 9%)

Miscellaneous: Laceration (CLL: 10%; grades 3/4: CLL: 2%)

<1%, postmarketing, and/or case reports: Hypersensitivity (includes anaphylactic shock, angioedema, urticaria), progressive multifocal leukoencephalopathy, renal failure, tumor lysis syndrome

Drug Interactions

Metabolism/Transport Effects Substrate of CYP2D6 (minor), CYP3A4 (major); **Note:** Assignment of Major/Minor substrate status based on clinically relevant drug interaction potential; **Inhibits** BCRP, P-glycoprotein

Avoid Concomitant Use

Avoid concomitant use of Ibrutinib with any of the following: BCG (Intravesical); Bitter Orange; Bosutinib; CloZAPine; Conivaptan; CYP3A4 Inducers (Strong); CYP3A4 Inhibitors (Moderate); CYP3A4 Inhibitors (Strong); Dipyrone; Fusidic Acid (Systemic); Idelalisib; Natalizumab; PAZOPanib; Pimecrolimus; Silodosin; St Johns Wort; Tacrolimus (Topical); Tofacitinib; Topotecan; Vaccines (Live); VinCRIStine (Liposomal)

Increased Effect/Toxicity

Ibrutinib may increase the levels/effects of: Afatinib; Agents with Antiplatelet Properties; Anticoagulants; Bosutinib; Brentuximab Vedotin; CloZAPine; Colchicine; Dabigatran Etexilate; DOXOrubicin (Conventional); Edoxaban; Everolimus; Fingolimod; Ledipasvir; Leflunomide; Naloxegol; Natalizumab; PAZOPanib; P-glycoprotein/ABCB1 Substrates; Prucalopride; Ranolazine; Rifaximin; Silodosin; Tofacitinib; Topotecan; Vaccines (Live); VinCRIStine (Liposomal)

The levels/effects of Ibrutinib may be increased by: Bitter Orange; Conivaptan; CYP3A4 Inhibitors (Moderate); CYP3A4 Inhibitors (Strong); Dasatinib; Denosumab; Dipyrone; Flaxseed Oil; Fosaprepitant; Fusidic Acid (Systemic); Idelalisib; Ivacaftor; Luliconazole; Omega-3 Fatty Acids; Osimertinib; Palbociclib; Pimecrolimus; Roflumilast; Simeprevir; Stiripentol; Tacrolimus (Topical); Trastuzumab; Vitamin E; Vitamin E (Oral)

Decreased Effect

Ibrutinib may decrease the levels/effects of: BCG (Intravesical); Coccidioides immitis Skin Test; Sipuleucel-T; Vaccines (Inactivated); Vaccines (Live)

The levels/effects of Ibrutinib may be decreased by: CYP3A4 Inducers (Moderate); CYP3A4 Inducers (Strong); Dabrafenib; Deferasirox; Echinacea; Osimertinib; Siltuximab; St Johns Wort; Tocilizumab

Food Interactions Grapefruit and Seville oranges moderately inhibit CYP3A and may increase ibrutinib exposure. Management: Avoid grapefruit and Seville oranges during therapy.

Storage/Stability Store at 20°C to 25°C (68°F to 77°F); excursions are permitted between 15°C and 30°C (59°F and 86°F). Keep in original container until dispensing.

Mechanism of Action Ibrutinib is a potent and irreversible inhibitor of Bruton's tyrosine kinase (BTK), an integral component of the B-cell receptor (BCR) and cytokine receptor pathways. Constitutive activation of B-cell receptor signaling is important for survival of malignant B-cells; BTK inhibition results in decreased malignant B-cell proliferation and survival.

Pharmacodynamics/Kinetics

Distribution: ~10,000 L (Marostica 2015)

Bioavailability: Administration with food increased the C_{max} by ~2- to 4-fold and the AUC 2-fold (compared with overnight fasting). Administration under fasting conditions resulted in exposure of ~60% compared to when administered either 30 minutes before or after a meal, or 2 hours after a high-fat meal (de Jong 2015).

Protein binding: ~97%

Metabolism: Hepatic via CYP3A (major) and CYP2D6 (minor) to active metabolite PCI-45227

Half-life elimination: 4 to 6 hours

Time to peak: 1 to 2 hours (4 hours under fed conditions [de Jong 2015])

Excretion: Feces (80%; ~1% as unchanged drug); urine (<10%, as metabolites)

Dosing

Adult & Geriatric

Chronic lymphocytic leukemia (CLL), previously treated: Oral: 420 mg once daily (Byrd 2014).

CLL with 17p deletion: Oral: 420 mg once daily (Byrd 2014).

Mantle cell lymphoma (MCL), previously treated: Oral: 560 mg once daily (Wang 2013).

Waldenström macroglobulinemia (WM): Oral: 420 mg once daily (Treon 2015)

Missed doses: Administer as soon as the missed dose is remembered on the same day; return to normal scheduling the following day. Do not take extra capsules to make up for the missed dose.

Dosage adjustment for concomitant therapy:

Moderate or strong CYP3A inhibitors:

US labeling: Avoid concurrent use with moderate or strong CYP3A inhibitors which are taken chronically; consider an alternative agent with less CYP3A inhibition. If short term use (≤7 days) of a strong inhibitor is necessary, consider withholding ibrutinib therapy until the strong CYP3A inhibitor is discontinued. If concomitant use of a moderate inhibitor is necessary, reduce ibrutinib dose to 140 mg once daily. Monitor closely for toxicity during concomitant use.

Canadian labeling: Avoid concurrent use with moderate or strong CYP3A inhibitors; consider an alternative agent with less CYP3A inhibition. If use of a strong inhibitor is necessary, withhold ibrutinib temporarily until the strong CYP3A inhibitor is discontinued. If concomitant use of a moderate inhibitor is necessary, reduce ibrutinib dose to 140 mg once daily until the inhibitor is discontinued. Monitor closely for toxicity during concomitant use.

Strong CYP3A inducers: Avoid concurrent use with strong CYP3A inducers; consider alternative agents with less CYP3A induction.

Renal Impairment

Mild to moderate impairment (CrCl ≥25 mL/minute [US labeling] or CrCl >30 mL/minute [Canadian labeling]): There are no dosage adjustments provided in the manufacturer's labeling; however, renal excretion is minimal and drug exposure is not altered in patients with mild to moderate impairment.

Severe impairment (CrCl <25 mL/minute [US labeling] or CrCl ≤30 mL/minute [Canadian labeling]): There are no dosage adjustments provided in the manufacturer's labeling (has not been studied).

End-stage renal disease (ESRD) requiring dialysis: There are no dosage adjustments provided in the manufacturer's labeling (has not been studied).

Hepatic Impairment

US labeling:

Mild impairment (Child-Pugh class A): Reduce dose to 140 mg once daily.

Moderate and severe impairment (Child-Pugh class B and C): Avoid use.

Canadian labeling:

Mild impairment (Child-Pugh class A): May consider dose reduction to 140 mg once daily (based on preliminary data) only if clinically indicated; monitor closely.

Moderate and severe impairment (Child-Pugh class B and C): Avoid use.

Adjustment for Toxicity

Hematologic toxicity: ≥ Grade 3 neutropenia with infection or fever, or grade 4 toxicity: Interrupt therapy; upon improvement to grade 1 toxicity or baseline, resume dosing at the starting dose. If toxicity recurs, reduce daily dose by 140 mg. If toxicity recurs after first dose reduction, reduce daily dose by an additional 140 mg. If toxicity persists following 2 dose reductions, discontinue therapy.

Nonhematologic toxicity: ≥ Grade 3 toxicity: Interrupt therapy; upon improvement to grade 1 toxicity or baseline, resume dosing at the starting dose. If toxicity recurs, reduce daily dose by 140 mg. If toxicity recurs after first dose reduction, reduce daily dose by an additional 140 mg. If toxicity persists following 2 dose reductions, discontinue therapy.

Recommend dose reductions for toxicity (following recovery):

Chronic lymphocytic leukemia and Waldenström macroglobulinemia:

First occurrence: Restart at 420 mg once daily

Second occurrence: Restart at 280 mg once daily

Third occurrence: Restart at 140 mg once daily

Fourth occurrence: Discontinue

Mantle cell lymphoma:

First occurrence: Restart at 560 mg once daily

Second occurrence: Restart at 420 mg once daily

Third occurrence: Restart at 280 mg once daily

Fourth occurrence: Discontinue

Combination Regimens

Leukemia, chronic lymphocytic: Ibrutinib (CLL Regimen) on page 2012

Lymphoma, non-Hodgkin (Mantle Cell): Ibrutinib (NHL-Mantle Cell Regimen) on page 2013

Waldenstrom Macroglobulinemia: Ibrutinib (Waldenstrom Macroglobulinemia Regimen) on page 2013

Administration Administer orally with water at approximately the same time every day. Swallow capsules whole; do not open, break, or chew the capsules. Maintain adequate hydration during treatment. Hazardous agent; use appropriate precautions for handling and disposal (meets NIOSH 2014 criteria).

Based on an analysis of 3 pharmacokinetic studies, it is suggested that ibrutinib may be administered without regard to food (de Jong 2015).

Emetic Potential Low (10% to 30%)

Monitoring Parameters Monitor blood counts monthly or as clinically necessary; renal and hepatic function; uric acid levels as clinically necessary; sign/symptoms of bleeding, infections, progressive multifocal encephalopathy, tumor lysis syndrome, and second primary malignancies; signs/symptoms of atrial fibrillation; ECG prior to initiation (patients with cardiac risk factors or history of atrial fibrillation) and during therapy if clinically indicated.

Dietary Considerations Avoid grapefruit, grapefruit juice, and Seville oranges during therapy.

Dosage Forms Excipient information presented when available (limited, particularly for generics); consult specific product labeling.

Capsule, Oral:

Imbruvica: 140 mg

- ◆ **ICI-182,780** see Fulvestrant on page 765
- ◆ **ICI-46474** see Tamoxifen on page 1595
- ◆ **ICI-118630** see Goserelin on page 796
- ◆ **ICI-176334** see Bicalutamide on page 207
- ◆ **ICI-D1033** see Anastrozole on page 112
- ◆ **ICI-D1694** see Raltitrexed on page 1454
- ◆ **ICL670** see Deferasirox on page 478
- ◆ **Iclusig** see PONATinib on page 1403
- ◆ **ICRF-187** see Dexrazoxane on page 523
- ◆ **Idamycin PFS** see IDArubicin on page 862

IDArubicin (eye da ROO bi sin)

Related Information

Management of Chemotherapy-Induced Nausea and Vomiting in Adults on page 2142

Management of Drug Extravasations on page 2159

Prevention of Chemotherapy-Induced Nausea and Vomiting in Children on page 2203

Safe Handling of Hazardous Drugs on page 2292

Brand Names: US Idamycin PFS

Brand Names: Canada Idamycin PFS; Idarubicin Hydrochloride Injection

Index Terms 4-Demethoxydaunorubicin; 4-DMDR; Idarubicin Hydrochloride; IDR; IMI 30; SC 33428

Pharmacologic Category Antineoplastic Agent, Anthracycline; Antineoplastic Agent, Topoisomerase II Inhibitor

Use Acute myeloid leukemia: Treatment of acute myeloid leukemia (AML) in adults (in combination with other approved chemotherapy agents).

Labeled Contraindications Bilirubin >5 mg/dL

Documentation of allergenic cross-reactivity for drugs in this class is limited. However, because of similarities in chemical structure and/or pharmacologic actions, the possibility of cross-sensitivity cannot be ruled out with certainty.

Pregnancy Considerations Adverse events were observed in animal reproduction studies. Fetal fatality was noted in a case report following second trimester exposure in a pregnant woman. The manufacturer recommends that women of childbearing potential avoid pregnancy.

Breast-Feeding Considerations It is not known if idarubicin is excreted in breast milk. Due to the potential for serious adverse reactions in the nursing infant, breast-feeding is not recommended by the manufacturer.

Warnings/Precautions Hazardous agent - use appropriate precautions for handling and disposal (NIOSH 2014 [group 1]). **[US Boxed Warning]: May cause myocardial toxicity; may lead to heart failure. Cardiotoxicity is more common in patients who have previously received anthracyclines or have preexisting cardiac disease.** The risk of myocardial toxicity is also increased in patients with concomitant or prior mediastinal/pericardial irradiation, patients with anemia, bone marrow depression, infections, leukemic pericarditis or myocarditis. Patients with active or dormant cardiovascular disease, concurrent administration of cardiotoxic drugs, prior therapy with other anthracyclines or anthracenediones are also at increased risk for cardiotoxicity. Potentially fatal heart failure, acute arrhythmias (may be life-threatening) or other cardiomyopathies may also occur. Regular monitoring of LVEF and discontinuation at the first sign of impairment is recommended, especially in patients with cardiac risk factors or impaired cardiac function. The half-life of other cardiotoxic agents (eg, trastuzumab) must be considered. Avoid the use of anthracycline-based therapy for at least 5 half-lives after discontinuation of the cardiotoxic agent. Monitor cardiac function during treatment. Patients >60 years who were undergoing induction therapy experienced heart failure, serious arrhythmias, chest pain, MI, and asymptomatic declines in LVEF more frequently than younger patients.

[US Boxed Warning]: Vesicant; may cause severe local tissue damage and necrosis if extravasation occurs. For IV administration only. NOT for IM or SubQ administration. Administer through a rapidly flowing IV line. Ensure proper needle or catheter placement prior to and during infusion. Avoid extravasation.

[US Boxed Warning]: May cause severe myelosuppression when used at therapeutic doses. Patients are at risk of developing infection and bleeding (may be fatal) due to neutropenia and thrombocytopenia, respectively. Monitor blood counts frequently. Do not use in patients with preexisting bone marrow suppression unless the benefit outweighs the risk. **[US Boxed Warning]: Dosage reductions are recommended in patients with renal or hepatic impairment.** Do not use if bilirubin >5 mg/dL. Rapid lysis of leukemic cells may lead to hyperuricemia. Ensure adequate hydration and consider use of antihyperuricemic prophylaxis. Systemic infections should be controlled prior to initiation of treatment. **[US Boxed Warning]: Should be administered under the supervision of an experienced cancer chemotherapy physician.** Use in facilities with laboratory and supportive resources adequate to ▶

monitor drug tolerance and protect and maintain a patient compromised by drug toxicity. The physician and institution must be capable of responding rapidly and completely to severe hemorrhagic conditions and/or overwhelming infection. Idarubicin is associated with a moderate emetic potential; antiemetics are recommended to prevent nausea and vomiting (Basch, 2011; Dupuis, 2011; Roila, 2010). Abdominal pain, diarrhea, and mucositis may commonly occur. Potentially significant drug-drug interactions may exist, requiring dose or frequency adjustment, additional monitoring, and/or selection of alternative therapy.

Adverse Reactions

>10%:

Cardiovascular: CHF (dose related), transient ECG abnormalities (supraventricular tachycardia, S-T wave changes, atrial or ventricular extrasystoles); generally asymptomatic and self-limiting. The relative cardiotoxicity of idarubicin compared to doxorubicin is unclear. Some investigators report no increase in cardiac toxicity for adults at cumulative oral idarubicin doses up to 540 mg/m^2; other reports suggest a maximum cumulative intravenous dose of 150 mg/m^2.

Central nervous system: Headache

Dermatologic: Alopecia (25% to 30%), radiation recall, skin rash (11%), urticaria

Gastrointestinal: Nausea, vomiting (30% to 60%); diarrhea (9% to 22%); stomatitis (11%); GI hemorrhage (30%)

Genitourinary: Discoloration of urine (darker yellow)

Hematologic: Myelosuppression (nadir: 10-15 days; recovery: 21-28 days), primarily leukopenia; thrombocytopenia and anemia. Effects are generally less severe with oral dosing.

Hepatic: Bilirubin and transaminases increased (44%)

1% to 10%:

Central nervous system: Seizure

Neuromuscular & skeletal: Peripheral neuropathy

<1%, postmarketing, and/or case reports: Cardiomyopathy, hyperuricemia, myocarditis, neutropenic typhlitis

Drug Interactions

Metabolism/Transport Effects Substrate of P-glycoprotein

Avoid Concomitant Use

Avoid concomitant use of IDArubicin with any of the following: BCG (Intravesical); CloZAPine; Dipyrone; Natalizumab; Pimecrolimus; Tacrolimus (Topical); Tofacitinib; Vaccines (Live)

Increased Effect/Toxicity

IDArubicin may increase the levels/effects of: CloZAPine; Fingolimod; Leflunomide; Natalizumab; Tofacitinib; Vaccines (Live)

The levels/effects of IDArubicin may be increased by: Bevacizumab; Cyclophosphamide; Denosumab; Dipyrone; Lumacaftor; P-glycoprotein/ABCB1 Inhibitors; Pimecrolimus; Ranolazine; Roflumilast; Tacrolimus (Topical); Taxane Derivatives; Trastuzumab

Decreased Effect

IDArubicin may decrease the levels/effects of: BCG (Intravesical); Cardiac Glycosides; Coccidioides immitis Skin Test; Sipuleucel-T; Vaccines (Inactivated); Vaccines (Live)

The levels/effects of IDArubicin may be decreased by: Cardiac Glycosides; Echinacea; Lumacaftor; P-glycoprotein/ABCB1 Inducers

Storage/Stability Store intact vials of solution refrigerated at 2°C to 8°C (36°F to 46°F). Protect from light.

Preparation for Administration Hazardous agent; use appropriate precautions for handling and disposal (NIOSH 2014 [group 1]). May draw up 1 mg/mL solution into a syringe (for administration) or further dilute in NS or D_5W.

Mechanism of Action Similar to daunorubicin, idarubicin inhibits DNA and RNA synthesis by intercalation between DNA base pairs and by steric obstruction. Although the exact mechanism is unclear, it appears that direct binding to DNA (intercalation) and inhibition of DNA repair (topoisomerase II inhibition) result in blockade of DNA and RNA synthesis and fragmentation of DNA.

Pharmacodynamics/Kinetics

Distribution: V_{dss}: 1,500 L/m² (Robert, 1993); extensive tissue binding; CSF
Protein binding: 94% (idarubicinol) to 97% (idarubicin)
Metabolism: Hepatic to idarubicinol (active metabolite)
Half-life elimination: Terminal: 15 hours (idarubicin); >45 hours (idarubicinol)
Excretion: Primarily biliary; urine (8 to 10% as idarubicinol, ~2 to 5% as unchanged drug [Robert, 1993])

Dosing

Adult & Geriatric Idarubicin is associated with a moderate emetic potential; antiemetics are recommended to prevent nausea and vomiting (Basch, 2011; Roila, 2010).

Acute myeloid leukemia (AML): IV:
Manufacturer labeling: Induction: 12 mg/m²/day for 3 days (in combination with cytarabine); a second induction cycle may be administered if necessary.
Indication-specific dosing:
AML, relapsed/refractory: FLAG-IDA regimen: 10 mg/m²/day for 3 days (in combination with fludarabine, cytarabine, and filgrastim); a second course was given for consolidation upon hematologic recovery (Parker, 1997)
Acute promyelocytic leukemia (APL):
LPA 2005 (high-risk patients; Sanz, 2010):
Induction (all patients): 12 mg/m²/day on days 2, 4, 6, and 8 (day 8 dose was omitted in patients >70 years) in combination with ATRA (tretinoin) (Sanz, 2010)
Consolidation (patients ≤60 years): 5 mg/m²/day for 4 days in consolidation cycle 1 and 12 mg/m²/day for 1 day in consolidation cycle 3 (in combination with ATRA [tretinoin] and cytarabine) (Sanz, 2010)
APML4 protocol (Iland, 2012): Induction (age-adjusted dosing):
Age <60 years: 12 mg/m²/day on days 2, 4, 6, and 8 (in combination with ATRA [tretinoin] and arsenic trioxide)
Age 61 to 70 years: 9 mg/m²/day on days 2, 4, 6, and 8 (in combination with ATRA [tretinoin] and arsenic trioxide)
Age >70 years: 6 mg/m²/day on days 2, 4, 6, and 8 (in combination with ATRA [tretinoin] and arsenic trioxide)

Pediatric Note: Idarubicin is associated with a moderate emetic potential; antiemetics are recommended to prevent nausea and vomiting (Dupuis, 2011).

Acute myeloid leukemia (AML) (off-label use): IV:
Newly diagnosed (CCG-2961) (Lange, 2008):
Induction: IdaDCTER: Idarubicin 5 mg/m²/dose daily for 4 days on days 0 to 3 in combination with cytarabine, etoposide, thioguanine, and dexamethasone

Consolidation:

    IdaDCTER: Idarubicin 5 mg/m^2/dose daily for 4 days on days 0 to 3 in combination with cytarabine, etoposide, thioguanine, and dexamethasone

    or

    Idarubicin 12 mg/m^2/dose daily for 3 days on days 0 to 2 in combination with fludarabine and cytarabine

Relapsed/refractory: 12 mg/m^2 once daily for 3 days on days 0 to 2 in combination with fludarabine and cytarabine (Dinndorf, 1997; Leahey, 1997)

Renal Impairment There are no dosage adjustments provided in the manufacturer's labeling; however, it does recommend that dosage reductions be made. Patients with S$_{cr}$ ≥2 mg/dL did not receive treatment in many clinical trials. The following adjustments have been recommended (Aronoff, 2007):

Adults:

    CrCl >50 mL/minute: No dosage adjustment is necessary.

    CrCl 10 to 50 mL/minute: Administer 75% of dose.

    CrCl <10 mL/minute: Administer 50% of dose.

    Hemodialysis: Supplemental dose not needed.

    Continuous ambulatory peritoneal dialysis (CAPD): Supplemental dose not needed.

Infants, Children, and Adolescents:

    GFR >50 mL/minute/1.73 m^2: No dosage adjustment is necessary.

    GFR ≤50 mL/minute/1.73 m^2: Administer 75% of dose

    Intermittent hemodialysis: Administer 75% of dose

    Peritoneal dialysis (PD): Administer 75% of dose

    Continuous renal replacement therapy (CRRT): Administer 75% of dose

Hepatic Impairment

    Bilirubin 2.6 to 5 mg/dL: Administer 50% of dose (Perry, 2012)

    Bilirubin >5 mg/dL: Avoid use

Adjustment for Toxicity Manufacturer labeling: If patients experience severe mucositis during the first induction cycle, delay administration of the second cycle until mucositis has resolved; consider reducing the dose by 25%.

Combination Regimens

Leukemia, acute myeloid:

    5 + 2 (Cytarabine-Idarubicin) (AML Consolidation) on page 1816

    7 + 3 (Cytarabine-Idarubicin) (AML Induction) on page 1818

    FLAG-IDA (AML Induction) on page 1970

Leukemia, acute promyelocytic: Tretinoin-Idarubicin (APL) on page 2099

Administration Idarubicin is associated with a moderate emetic potential; antiemetics are recommended to prevent nausea and vomiting (Basch, 2011; Dupuis, 2011; Roila, 2010).

For IV administration only. Do not administer IM or SubQ; administer as slow injection over 10 to 15 minutes into a free-flowing IV solution of NS or D$_5$W. In some pediatric protocols (off label use), idarubicin was infused over 15 minutes or over at least 30 minutes (Lange, 2008; Leahy, 1997); refer to individual protocols for infusion rate details.

Vesicant; ensure proper needle or catheter placement prior to and during infusion; avoid extravasation.

Extravasation management: If extravasation occurs, stop infusion immediately and disconnect (leave cannula/needle in place); gently aspirate extravasated solution (do **NOT** flush the line); remove needle/cannula; elevate extremity. Initiate antidote (dexrazoxane or dimethyl sulfate [DMSO]). Apply dry cold compresses for 20 minutes 4 times daily for 1 to 2 days (Perez Fidalgo, 2012); withhold cooling beginning 15 minutes before dexrazoxane infusion; continue withholding cooling until 15 minutes after infusion is completed. Topical DMSO should not be administered in combination with dexrazoxane; may lessen dexrazoxane efficacy.

Dexrazoxane: Adults: 1000 mg/m^2 (maximum dose: 2000 mg) IV (administer in a large vein remote from site of extravasation) over 1 to 2 hours days 1 and 2, then 500 mg/m^2 (maximum dose: 1000 mg) IV over 1 to 2 hours day 3; begin within 6 hours of extravasation. Day 2 and day 3 doses should be administered at approximately the same time (± 3 hours) as the dose on day 1 (Mouridsen, 2007; Perez Fidalgo, 2012). **Note:** Reduce dexrazoxane dose by 50% in patients with moderate to severe renal impairment (CrCl <40 mL/minute).

DMSO: Children and Adults: Apply topically to a region covering twice the affected area every 8 hours for 7 days; begin within 10 minutes of extravasation; do not cover with a dressing (Perez Fidalgo, 2012).

Hazardous agent; use appropriate precautions for handling and disposal (NIOSH 2014 [group 1]).

Vesicant/Extravasation Risk Vesicant

Emetic Potential Children and Adults: Moderate (30% to 90%)

Monitoring Parameters CBC with differential and platelet count (frequently), cardiac function (LVEF; prior and during treatment), serum electrolytes, renal function (serum creatinine; prior to and during treatment), uric acid, liver function (ALT, AST, bilirubin; prior to and during treatment); monitor infusion site for signs of extravasation; monitor for gastrointestinal toxicity and infection

Dosage Forms Excipient information presented when available (limited, particularly for generics); consult specific product labeling.

Solution, Intravenous, as hydrochloride [preservative free]:

Idamycin PFS: 5 mg/5 mL (5 mL); 10 mg/10 mL (10 mL); 20 mg/20 mL (20 mL)

Generic: 5 mg/5 mL (5 mL); 10 mg/10 mL (10 mL); 20 mg/20 mL (20 mL)

♦ **Idarubicin Hydrochloride** *see* IDArubicin *on page 862*
♦ **Idarubicin Hydrochloride Injection (Can)** *see* IDArubicin *on page 862*
♦ **IDEC-C2B8** *see* RiTUXimab *on page 1482*
♦ **IDEC-Y2B8** *see* Ibritumomab *on page 851*

Idelalisib (eye del a LIS ib)

Related Information
Common Toxicity Criteria *on page 2122*
Safe Handling of Hazardous Drugs *on page 2292*
Brand Names: US Zydelig
Brand Names: Canada Zydelig
Index Terms CAL-101; GS-1101; PI$_3$K Delta Inhibitor CAL-101
Pharmacologic Category Antineoplastic Agent, Phosphatidylinositol 3-Kinase Inhibitor

Use

Chronic lymphocytic leukemia: Treatment of relapsed chronic lymphocytic leukemia (CLL) (in combination with rituximab) when rituximab alone is appropriate therapy due to other comorbidities

Follicular B-cell non-Hodgkin lymphoma: Treatment of relapsed follicular B-cell non-Hodgkin lymphoma after at least 2 prior systemic therapies

Small lymphocytic lymphoma: Treatment of relapsed small lymphocytic lymphoma (SLL) after at least 2 prior systemic therapies

Labeled Contraindications Serious hypersensitivity reactions, including anaphylaxis and toxic epidermal necrolysis, to idelalisib or any component of the formulation

Pregnancy Considerations Adverse events were observed in animal reproduction studies. Women of reproductive potential should use effective contraception during therapy and for at least 1 month after treatment discontinuation.

Breast-Feeding Considerations It is not known if idelalisib is excreted in breast milk. Due to the potential for serious adverse reactions in the nursing infant, the manufacturer recommends a decision be made whether to discontinue nursing or to discontinue the drug, taking into account the importance of treatment to the mother.

Warnings/Precautions Hazardous agent - use appropriate precautions for handling and disposal (meets NIOSH 2014 criteria). **[US Boxed Warning]: Serious hepatotoxicity (some fatal) has been observed. Monitor hepatic function at baseline and during therapy. May require treatment interruption and/or dosage reduction.** ALT/AST elevations >5 times ULN have occurred, and were generally observed during the first 12 weeks of therapy; transaminase elevations were reversible upon therapy interruption. Hepatotoxicity may recur upon rechallenge, even at a reduced dose; discontinue for recurrent hepatotoxicity. Avoid concomitant use with other hepatotoxic agents. Monitor ALT/AST at baseline and every 2 weeks for the first 3 months, every 4 weeks for the next 3 months, then every 1 to 3 months thereafter, or as clinically necessary. Increase monitoring to weekly if ALT or AST >3 times ULN until resolved. Interrupt therapy if ALT/AST >5 times ULN; monitor LFTs weekly until resolved. **[US Boxed Warning]: Serious and/or fatal diarrhea and colitis have been reported. Monitor closely; may require treatment interruption, dosage reduction, and/or discontinuation.** Grade 3 or higher diarrhea or colitis have been reported in clinical trials. Diarrhea may occur at any time during therapy and responds poorly to antidiarrheal (antimotility) medications. The median time to resolution of diarrhea was 1 week to 1 month (following therapy interruption); corticosteroids were used in some cases to manage toxicity. Avoid concomitant use with other promotility agents. **[US Boxed Warning]: Serious and fatal intestinal perforation may occur; discontinue permanently if perforation develops.** In some patients, perforation was preceded by moderate to severe diarrhea. Monitor closely for new or worsening abdominal pain, chills, fever, nausea, or vomiting.

[US Boxed Warning]: Serious and fatal pneumonitis may occur. Monitor for pulmonary symptoms and bilateral interstitial infiltrates. May require therapy interruption or discontinuation. Symptoms such as cough, dyspnea, hypoxia, interstitial infiltrates, or an oxygen saturation decrease of more than 5% should be promptly evaluated. Interrupt therapy for suspected pneumonitis; if diagnosis is confirmed, discontinue idelalisib and administer corticosteroids as appropriate. Serious allergic/hypersensitivity reactions, including anaphylaxis, have been reported. Discontinue permanently for serious reactions and manage appropriately.

Severe and/or life-threatening cutaneous reactions (grade 3 or higher), such as exfoliative dermatitis, rash (generalized, erythematous, macular-papular, pruritic, exfoliative), and skin disorder, have been observed. One case of toxic epidermal necrolysis (TEN) was reported when idelalisib was administered in combination with rituximab and bendamustine. Monitor closely for dermatologic toxicity and discontinue for severe reactions. Grade 3 or 4 neutropenia occurred in close to one-third of patients in clinical trials; thrombocytopenia and anemia (any grade) have also been reported. Monitor blood counts at least every 2 weeks for the first 3 months, and at least weekly in patients with neutropenia. May require treatment interruption and dosage reduction. Potentially significant interactions may exist, requiring dose or frequency adjustment, additional monitoring, and/or selection of alternative therapy. Consult drug interactions database for more detailed information.

Adverse Reactions As reported with monotherapy.

>10%:

Central nervous system: Fatigue (30%), insomnia (12%), headache (11%)

Dermatologic: Skin rash (21%; grade ≥3: 3%), night sweats (12%)

Gastrointestinal: Diarrhea (47%; grade ≥3: 14%), nausea (29%), abdominal pain (26%), decreased appetite (16%), vomiting (15%)

Hematologic & oncologic: Decreased neutrophils (53%; grade 3: 14%; grade 4: 11%), decreased hemoglobin (28%; grade 3: 2%), decreased platelet count (26%; grade 3: 3%; grade 4: 3%)

Hepatic: Increased serum ALT (50%; grade 3: 14%; grade 4: 5%), increased serum AST (41%; grade 3: 8%; grade 4: 4%), severe hepatotoxicity (14%)

Neuromuscular & skeletal: Weakness (12%)

Respiratory: Cough (29%), pneumonia (25%; grade ≥3: 16%), dyspnea (17%), upper respiratory tract infection (12%)

Miscellaneous: Fever (28%)

1% to 10%: Cardiovascular: Peripheral edema (10%)

Postmarketing and/or case reports (reported with mono- or combination therapy): Anaphylaxis, hypersensitivity reaction, intestinal perforation, toxic epidermal necrolysis

Drug Interactions

Metabolism/Transport Effects Substrate of CYP3A4 (major), P-glycoprotein, UGT1A4; **Note:** Assignment of Major/Minor substrate status based on clinically relevant drug interaction potential; **Inhibits** CYP2C19 (weak), CYP2C8 (weak), CYP3A4 (strong), UGT1A1

Avoid Concomitant Use

Avoid concomitant use of Idelalisib with any of the following: Ado-Trastuzumab Emtansine; Alfuzosin; Amodiaquine; Aprepitant; Astemizole; Avanafil; Axitinib; Barnidipine; BCG (Intravesical); Bosutinib; Bromocriptine; Cabozantinib; Ceritinib; Cobimetinib; Conivaptan; Crizotinib; CYP3A4 Inducers (Strong); CYP3A4 Substrates; Dabrafenib; Dapoxetine; Domperidone; Dronedarone; Eletriptan; Eplerenone; Everolimus; Flibanserin; Halofantrine; Ibrutinib; Isavuconazonium Sulfate; Ivabradine; Lapatinib; Lercanidipine; Lomitapide; Lovastatin; Lurasidone; Macitentan; Naloxegol; Natalizumab; Nilotinib; NiMODipine; Nisoldipine; Olaparib; Osimertinib; Palbociclib; Pimecrolimus; Pimozide; Ranolazine; Red Yeast Rice; Regorafenib; Salmeterol; Silodosin; Simeprevir; Simvastatin; Sonidegib; St Johns Wort; Suvorexant; Tacrolimus (Topical); Tamsulosin; Terfenadine; Ticagrelor; Tofacitinib; Tolvaptan; Toremifene; Trabectedin; Ulipristal; Vaccines (Live); Vemurafenib; VinCRIStine (Liposomal); Vorapaxar

Increased Effect/Toxicity

Idelalisib may increase the levels/effects of: Ado-Trastuzumab Emtansine; Alfuzosin; Almotriptan; Alosetron; Amodiaquine; Apixaban; Aprepitant; Astemizole; Avanafil; Axitinib; Barnidipine; Bedaquiline; Bortezomib; Bosentan; Bosutinib; Brentuximab Vedotin; Brinzolamide; Bromocriptine; Budesonide (Nasal); Budesonide (Oral Inhalation); Budesonide (Topical); Cabozantinib; Cannabis; Ceritinib; Cobimetinib; Conivaptan; Corticosteroids (Orally Inhaled); Corticosteroids (Systemic); Crizotinib; CYP3A4 Substrates; Dabrafenib; Dapoxetine; Dienogest; Dofetilide; Domperidone; Dronabinol; Dronedarone; Drospirenone; Dutasteride; Eletriptan; Eplerenone; Estazolam; Everolimus; Fingolimod; Flibanserin; Fluticasone (Nasal); Halofantrine; Ibrutinib; Iloperidone; Imatinib; Imidafenacin; Isavuconazonium Sulfate; Ivabradine; Lacosamide; Lapatinib; Leflunomide; Lercanidipine; Levobupivacaine; Lomitapide; Lovastatin; Lumefantrine; Lurasidone; Macitentan; Medroxy-PROGESTERone; MethylPREDNISolone; Naloxegol; Natalizumab; Nilotinib; NiMODipine; Nisoldipine; Olaparib; Osimertinib; Ospemifene; Oxybutynin; Palbociclib; Parecoxib; Paricalcitol; Pimozide; PONATinib; Pranlukast; PrednisoLONE (Systemic); PredniSONE; Propafenone; Ramelteon; Ranolazine; Red Yeast Rice; Regorafenib; Repaglinide; Retapamulin; Rilpivirine; RomiDEPsin; Salmeterol; Silodosin; Simeprevir; Simvastatin; Sonidegib; SORAfenib; Suvorexant; Tamsulosin; Tasimelteon; Terfenadine; Tetrahydrocannabinol; Ticagrelor; Tofacitinib; Tolvaptan; Toremifene; Trabectedin; TraMADol; Ulipristal; Vaccines (Live); Vemurafenib; Vilazodone; VinCRIStine (Liposomal); Vindesine; Vorapaxar; Zuclopenthixol

The levels/effects of Idelalisib may be increased by: CYP3A4 Inhibitors (Strong); Denosumab; Pimecrolimus; Roflumilast; Tacrolimus (Topical); Trastuzumab

Decreased Effect

Idelalisib may decrease the levels/effects of: BCG (Intravesical); Coccidioides immitis Skin Test; Ifosfamide; Prasugrel; Sipuleucel-T; Ticagrelor; Vaccines (Inactivated); Vaccines (Live)

The levels/effects of Idelalisib may be decreased by: Bosentan; CYP3A4 Inducers (Moderate); CYP3A4 Inducers (Strong); Deferasirox; Echinacea; Siltuximab; St Johns Wort; Tocilizumab

Storage/Stability Store at 20°C to 30°C (68°F to 86°F); excursions are permitted between 15°C and 30°C (59°F and 86°F). Dispense in the original container.

Mechanism of Action Potent small molecule inhibitor of the delta isoform of phosphatidylinositol 3-kinase (PI3Kδ), which is highly expressed in malignant lymphoid B-cells. PI3Kδ inhibition results in apoptosis of malignant tumor cells. In addition, idelalisib inhibits several signaling pathways, including B-cell receptor, CXCR4 and CXCR5 signaling which may play important roles in CLL pathophysiology (Furman, 2014).

Pharmacodynamics/Kinetics

Distribution: 23 L

Protein binding: >84%

Metabolism: Hepatic; primarily via aldehyde oxidase and CYP3A (to major metabolite GS-563117); minor metabolism via UGT1A4

Half-life elimination: ~8 hours

Time to peak: Median: 1.5 hours

Excretion: Feces (78%; 44% as GS-563117); urine (14%; 49% as GS-563117)

Dosing

Adult & Geriatric Note: The maximum recommended starting dose is 150 mg twice daily. Optimal duration and safety of therapy beyond several months is currently unknown.

Chronic lymphocytic leukemia, relapsed: Oral: 150 mg twice daily (in combination with rituximab); continue until disease progression or unacceptable toxicity (Furman, 2014)

Follicular B-cell non-Hodgkin lymphoma, relapsed: Oral: 150 mg twice daily; continue until disease progression or unacceptable toxicity (Gopal, 2014)

Small lymphocytic lymphoma, relapsed: Oral: 150 mg twice daily; continue until disease progression or unacceptable toxicity (Gopal, 2014)

Renal Impairment

US labeling:

CrCl ≥15 mL/minute: No dosage adjustment necessary.

CrCl <15 mL/minute: There are no dosage adjustments provided in the manufacturer's labeling (has not been studied).

Canadian labeling: No dosage adjustment necessary.

Hepatic Impairment

Preexisting hepatic impairment: Exposure is increased in patients with ALT/AST or bilirubin >ULN as compared to patients with normal hepatic function; patients with ALT/AST >2.5 times ULN or bilirubin >1.5 times ULN were excluded from some studies. Based on a pharmacokinetic study in patients with moderate and severe hepatic impairment, single oral doses of 150 mg were well tolerated; idelalisib and GS-563117 exposure differences were not considered clinically relevant (Jin, 2014). Monitor closely for toxicity. The Canadian labeling recommends no initial dosage adjustment for mild to moderate hepatic impairment; however, data are insufficient to make a dosing recommendation for severe impairment.

Hepatotoxicity during treatment:

US labeling:

ALT/AST >3 to 5 times ULN or bilirubin >1.5 to 3 times ULN: Continue current dose; monitor LFTs at least weekly until ALT/AST and/or bilirubin ≤1 times ULN.

ALT/AST >5 to 20 times ULN or bilirubin >3 to 10 times ULN: Temporarily interrupt therapy. Monitor LFTs at least weekly until ALT/AST and/or bilirubin ≤1 times ULN, then may reinitiate therapy at 100 mg twice daily.

ALT/AST >20 times ULN or bilirubin >10 times ULN: Discontinue permanently.

Recurrent hepatotoxicity: Discontinue.

Canadian labeling:

Grade 1 (ALT/AST ≤3 times ULN) or Grade 2 (ALT/AST >3 to 5 times ULN): Continue current dose; monitor LFTs at least weekly until ALT/AST ≤1 times ULN.

Grade 3 (ALT/AST >5 to 20 times ULN) or Grade 4 (ALT/AST >20 times ULN): Temporarily interrupt therapy. Monitor LFTs at least weekly until ALT/AST ≤1 times ULN, then may reinitiate therapy at 100 mg twice daily.

Recurrent hepatotoxicity: Discontinue.

◄ **Adjustment for Toxicity**

Anaphylaxis: Permanently discontinue.

Dermatologic toxicity:

Severe cutaneous reactions: Discontinue.

Rash (Canadian labeling):

Grade 1: Continue current dose

Grade 2: Temporarily interrupt therapy until resolved to ≤ grade 1.

Grade 3 or 4: Temporarily interrupt therapy; monitor at least weekly until resolved to ≤ grade 1 then reinitiate at 100 mg twice daily.

Hematologic toxicity:

Neutropenia:

ANC 1,000 to <1,500 cells/mm^3: Continue current dose.

ANC 500 to <1,000 cells/mm^3: Continue current dose; monitor blood counts at least weekly.

ANC <500 cells/mm^3: Temporarily interrupt therapy; monitor blood counts at least weekly until ANC ≥500 cells/mm^3, then may reinitiate therapy at 100 mg twice daily.

Thrombocytopenia:

US labeling:

Platelets 50,000 to <75,000 cells/mm^3: Continue current dose.

Platelets 25,000 to <50,000 cells/mm^3: Continue current dose; monitor platelet counts at least weekly.

Platelets <25,000 cells/mm^3: Temporarily interrupt therapy; monitor platelet counts at least weekly, may reinitiate therapy at 100 mg twice daily when platelets recover to ≥25,000 cells/mm^3.

Canadian labeling: There are no specific recommendations provided in the manufacturer's labeling.

Gastrointestinal toxicity:

US labeling:

Moderate diarrhea (increase of 4 to 6 stools/day over baseline): Continue current dose; monitor at least weekly until resolved.

Severe diarrhea (increase of ≥7 stools/day over baseline) or hospitalization: Temporarily interrupt therapy; monitor at least weekly until resolved, then may reinitiate therapy at 100 mg twice daily.

Life-threatening diarrhea: Discontinue permanently.

Canadian labeling:

Diarrhea/colitis:

Grade 1: Continue current dose; provide antidiarrheal (eg, loperamide)

Grade 2: Temporarily interrupt therapy; monitor at least weekly until resolved to ≤ grade 1.

Grade 3 or 4: Temporarily interrupt therapy and consider addition of anti-inflammatory drugs (eg, budesonide, sulfasalazine); monitor at least weekly until resolved to ≤ grade 1, then may reinitiate at 100 mg twice daily.

Ongoing inflammatory bowel disease: Use is not recommended.

Pulmonary toxicity: If pneumonitis is suspected, interrupt therapy and evaluate; discontinue for symptomatic pneumonitis of any severity thought to be associated with therapy (may also require corticosteroids). For patients in whom an infectious etiology has been established, the Canadian labeling recommends monitoring until resolved then reinitiate therapy at 100 mg twice daily.

Other toxicity (not listed above): If severe or life-threatening toxicities occur, interrupt therapy until toxicity is resolved. If the decision is made to resume therapy, reduce the dose to 100 mg twice daily. Discontinue permanently if severe or life-threatening toxicities recur upon rechallenge.

Combination Regimens

Leukemia, chronic lymphocytic: Idelalisib-Rituximab (CLL) on page 2014

Lymphoma, non-Hodgkin (Follicular): Idelalisib (NHL-Follicular Regimen) on page 2014

Administration Administer orally twice daily with or without food. Swallow tablets whole.

Missed doses: May administer a missed dose if within 6 hours of usual dosing time. If >6 hours, skip the missed dose and resume therapy with the next scheduled dose.

Hazardous agent; use appropriate precautions for handling and disposal (meets NIOSH 2014 criteria).

Emetic Potential Low (10% to 30%)

Monitoring Parameters Liver function tests at baseline and every 2 weeks for the first 3 months, every 4 weeks for the next 3 months, then every 1 to 3 months thereafter, or as clinically necessary; complete blood counts at least every 2 weeks for the first 3 months, and at least weekly in patients with neutropenia, or as clinically necessary; signs/symptoms of diarrhea/colitis, intestinal perforation, pneumonitis, dermatologic toxicity, and hypersensitivity reactions

Prescribing and Access Restrictions Available through specialty pharmacies. Further information may be obtained at http://www.zydeligaccessconnect. com/.

Dosage Forms Excipient information presented when available (limited, particularly for generics); consult specific product labeling.

Tablet, Oral:
Zydelig: 100 mg, 150 mg

◆ **IDR** see IDArubicin on page 862

◆ **Ifex** see Ifosfamide on page 873

Ifosfamide (eye FOSS fa mide)

Related Information

Management of Chemotherapy-Induced Nausea and Vomiting in Adults on page 2142

Management of Drug Extravasations on page 2159

Prevention of Chemotherapy-Induced Nausea and Vomiting in Children on page 2203

Safe Handling of Hazardous Drugs on page 2292

Brand Names: US Ifex

Brand Names: Canada Ifex; Ifosfamide for Injection

Index Terms Isophosphamide; Z4942

Pharmacologic Category Antineoplastic Agent, Alkylating Agent; Antineoplastic Agent, Alkylating Agent (Nitrogen Mustard)

Use

US labeling: Treatment (third-line) of germ cell testicular cancer (in combination with other chemotherapy drugs and with concurrent mesna)

◀ *Canadian labeling (not approved indications in the US):* Treatment of soft tissue sarcoma, pancreatic cancer (relapsed or refractory), cervical cancer (advanced or recurrent; as monotherapy or in combination with cisplatin and bleomycin)

Labeled Contraindications Hypersensitivity to ifosfamide or any component of the formulation; urinary outflow obstruction

Canadian labeling: Additional contraindications (not in U.S. labeling): Severe myelosuppression; severe renal or hepatic impairment; active infection (bacterial, fungal, viral); severe immunosuppression; urinary tract disease (eg, cystitis); advanced cerebral arteriosclerosis

Pregnancy Considerations Embryotoxic and teratogenic effects have been observed in animal reproduction studies. Fetal growth retardation and neonatal anemia have been reported with exposure to ifosfamide-containing regimens during human pregnancy. Male and female fertility may be affected (dose and duration dependent). Ifosfamide interferes with oogenesis and spermatogenesis; amenorrhea, azoospermia, and sterility have been reported and may be irreversible. Avoid pregnancy during treatment; male patients should not father a child for at least 6 months after completion of therapy.

Breast-Feeding Considerations Breast-feeding should be avoided during ifosfamide treatment. According to the manufacturer, due to the potential for serious adverse reactions in the nursing infant, a decision should be made to discontinue ifosfamide or to discontinue breast-feeding, taking into account the benefits of treatment to the mother.

Warnings/Precautions Hazardous agent: Use appropriate precautions for handling and disposal (NIOSH 2014 [group 1]). **[US Boxed Warning]: Hemorrhagic cystitis may occur (may be severe); concomitant mesna reduces the risk of hemorrhagic cystitis.** Hydration (at least 2 L/day in adults), dose fractionation, and/or mesna administration will reduce the incidence of hematuria and protect against hemorrhagic cystitis. Obtain urinalysis prior to each dose; if microscopic hematuria is detected, withhold until complete resolution. Exclude or correct urinary tract obstructions prior to treatment. Use with caution (if at all) in patients with active urinary tract infection. Hemorrhagic cystitis is dose-dependent and is increased with high single doses (compared with fractionated doses); past or concomitant bladder radiation or busulfan treatment may increase the risk for hemorrhagic cystitis. **[US Boxed Warning]: May cause severe nephrotoxicity, resulting in renal failure.** Acute and chronic renal failure as well as renal parenchymal and tubular necrosis (including acute) have been reported; tubular damage may be delayed and may persist. Renal manifestations include decreased glomerular rate, increased creatinine, proteinuria, enzymuria, cylindruria, aminoaciduria, phosphaturia, and glycosuria. Syndrome of inappropriate antidiuretic hormone (SIADH), renal rickets, and Fanconi syndrome have been reported. Evaluate renal function prior to and during treatment; monitor urine for erythrocytes and signs of urotoxicity.

[US Boxed Warning]: May cause CNS toxicity which may be severe, resulting in encephalopathy and death; monitor for CNS toxicity; discontinue for encephalopathy. Symptoms of CNS toxicity (somnolence, confusion, dizziness, disorientation, hallucinations, cranial nerve dysfunction, psychotic behavior, extrapyramidal symptoms, seizures, coma blurred vision, and/or incontinence) have been observed within a few hours to a few days after initial dose and generally resolve within 2-3 days of treatment discontinuation (although may persist longer); maintain supportive care until complete resolution. Risk factors may include hypoalbuminemia, renal dysfunction, and prior history of ifosfamide-induced encephalopathy. Concomitant centrally-acting medications may result in additive CNS effects. Peripheral neuropathy has been reported.

[US Boxed Warning]: Severe bone marrow suppression may occur (may be severe and lead to fatal infections); monitor blood counts before and after each cycle. Leukopenia, neutropenia, thrombocytopenia and anemia are associated with ifosfamide. Myelosuppression is dose dependent, increased with single high doses (compared to fractionated doses) and increased with decreased renal function. Severe myelosuppression may occur when administered in combination with other chemotherapy agents or radiation therapy. Use with caution in patients with compromised bone marrow reserve. Unless clinically necessary, avoid administering to patients with WBC <2000/mm^3 and platelets <50,000/mm^3. Antimicrobial prophylaxis may be necessary in some neutropenic patients; Administer antibiotics and/or antifungal agents for neutropenic fever. May cause significant suppression of the immune responses; may lead to serious infection, sepsis or septic shock; reported infections have included bacterial, viral, fungal, and parasitic; latent infections may be reactivated; use with caution with other immunosuppressants or in patients with infection.

Arrhythmias, ST-segment or T-wave changes, cardiomyopathy, pericardial effusion, pericarditis, and epicardial fibrosis have been observed; the risk for cardiotoxicity is dose-dependent; concomitant cardiotoxic agents (eg, anthracyclines), irradiation of the cardiac region, and renal impairment may also increase the risk; use with caution in patients with cardiac risk factors or preexisting cardiac disease. Interstitial pneumonitis, pulmonary fibrosis, and pulmonary toxicity leading to respiratory failure have been reported; monitor for signs and symptoms of pulmonary toxicity.

Anaphylactic/anaphylactoid reactions have been associated with ifosfamide; cross sensitivity with similar agents may occur. Hepatic sinusoidal obstruction syndrome (SOS), formerly called veno-occlusive disease (VOD), has been reported with ifosfamide-containing regimens. Secondary malignancies may occur; the risk for myelodysplastic syndrome (which may progress to acute leukemia) is increased with treatment. May interfere with wound healing. Potentially significant drug-drug interactions may exist, requiring dose or frequency adjustment, additional monitoring, and/or selection of alternative therapy. Use with caution in patients with prior radiation therapy. Ifosfamide is associated with a moderate emetic potential; antiemetics are recommended to prevent nausea and vomiting (Basch 2011; Dupuis 2011; Roila 2010).

Adverse Reactions
>10%:
  Central nervous system: CNS toxicity or encephalopathy (12% to 15%)
  Dermatologic: Alopecia (83% to 90%; 100% with combination therapy)
  Endocrine & metabolic: Metabolic acidosis (31%)
  Gastrointestinal: Nausea/vomiting (47% to 58%)
  Hematologic: Leukopenia (50% to ≤100%; grade 4: ≤50%; nadir: 8-14 days), anemia (38%), thrombocytopenia (20%; grades 3/4: ≤8%)
  Renal: Hematuria (6% to 92%; reduced with mesna; grade 2 [gross hematuria]: 8% to 12%)
1% to 10%:
  Central nervous system: Fever (1%)
  Gastrointestinal: Anorexia (1%)
  Hematologic: Neutropenic fever (1%)

Hepatic: Bilirubin increased (2% to 3%), liver dysfunction (2% to 3%), transaminases increased (2% to 3%)

Local: Phlebitis (2% to 3%)

Renal: Renal impairment (6%)

Miscellaneous: Infection (8% to 10%)

<1%, postmarketing, and/or case reports: Abdominal pain, acute renal failure, acute respiratory distress syndrome, acute tubular necrosis, agranulocytosis, alkaline phosphatase increased, allergic reaction, alveolitis (allergic), amenorrhea, aminoaciduria, amnesia, anaphylactic reaction, angina, angioedema, anuria, arrhythmia, arthralgia, asterixis, atrial ectopy, atrial fibrillation, atrial flutter, azoospermia, bladder irritation, bleeding, blurred vision, bone marrow failure, bradycardia, bradyphrenia, bronchospasm, bundle branch block, BUN increased, capillary leak syndrome, cardiac arrest, cardiogenic shock, cardiomyopathy, cardiotoxicity, catatonia, cecitis, chest pain, chills, cholestasis, chronic renal failure, coagulopathy, colitis, conjunctivitis, constipation, cough, creatinine clearance decreased/increased, creatinine increased, cylindruria, cytolytic hepatitis, delirium, delusion, dermatitis, diarrhea, disseminated intravascular coagulation, DVT, dysarthria, dysesthesia, dyspnea, dysuria, echolalia, edema, ejection fraction decreased, enterocolitis, enuresis, enzymuria, erythema, estrogen decreased, extrapyramidal disorder, facial swelling, Fanconi syndrome, fatigue, fecal incontinence, flushing, gait disturbance, gastrointestinal hemorrhage, GGT increased, glycosuria, gonadotropin increased, granulocytopenia, growth retardation (children), hearing loss, heart failure, hemolytic anemia, hemolytic uremic syndrome, hemorrhagic cystitis, hepatic failure, hepatic sinusoidal obstruction syndrome (SOS; formerly veno-occlusive disease [VOD]), hepatitis fulminant, hepatitis (viral), hepatorenal syndrome, herpes zoster, hyperglycemia, hyperhidrosis, hyper-/hypotension, hyperpigmentation, hypersensitivity reactions, hypesthesia, hypocalcemia, hypokalemia, hyponatremia, hypophosphatemia, hypoxia, ileus, immunosuppression, infertility, infusion site reactions (erythema, inflammation, pain, pruritus, swelling, tenderness), interstitial lung disease, interstitial pneumonitis, jaundice, LDH increased, leukoencephalopathy, limb pain, logorrhea, lymphopenia, malaise, mania, mental status change, methemoglobinemia, MI, mucosal inflammation/ulceration, multiorgan failure, muscle twitching, mutism, myalgia, myocardial hemorrhage, myocarditis, nail disorder, nephrogenic diabetes insipidus, neuralgia, neutropenia, oligospermia, oliguria, osteomalacia (adults), ovarian failure, ovulation disorder, pain, palmar-plantar erythrodysesthesia syndrome, pancreatitis, pancytopenia, panic attack, paranoia, paresthesia, pericardial effusion, pericarditis, peripheral neuropathy, petechiae, phosphaturia, physical deterioration (general), pleural effusion, *Pneumocystis jiroveci* pneumonia, pneumonia, pneumonitis, pollakiuria, polydipsia, polyneuropathy, polyuria, portal vein thrombosis, premature atrial contractions, premature menopause, progressive multifocal leukoencephalopathy, proteinuria, pruritus, pulmonary edema, pulmonary embolism, pulmonary fibrosis, pulmonary hypertension, QRS complex abnormal, radiation recall dermatitis, rash (including macular and papular), renal parenchymal damage, renal tubular acidosis, respiratory failure, reversible posterior leukoencephalopathy syndrome (RPLS), rhabdomyolysis, rickets, salivation, secondary malignancy (including ALL, AML, APL, lymphoma, MDS, RCC, sarcomas, thyroid cancer), seizures, sepsis, septic shock, SIADH, skin necrosis, spermatogenesis impaired, status epilepticus, sterility, Stevens-Johnson syndrome, stomatitis, ST-segment abnormal, supraventricular extrasystoles, tachycardia, tinnitus, toxic epidermal necrolysis, tubulointerstitial nephritis, tumor lysis syndrome,

T-wave inversion, uremia, urticaria, vasculitis, ventricular extrasystoles, ventricular failure, ventricular fibrillation, ventricular tachycardia, vertigo, visual impairment, wound healing impairment

Drug Interactions

Metabolism/Transport Effects Substrate of CYP2B6 (major), CYP2C19 (minor), CYP2C8 (minor), CYP2C9 (minor), CYP3A4 (minor); **Note:** Assignment of Major/Minor substrate status based on clinically relevant drug interaction potential; **Induces** CYP2C9 (weak/moderate)

Avoid Concomitant Use

Avoid concomitant use of Ifosfamide with any of the following: BCG (Intravesical); CloZAPine; Dipyrone; Natalizumab; Pimecrolimus; Tacrolimus (Topical); Tofacitinib; Vaccines (Live)

Increased Effect/Toxicity

Ifosfamide may increase the levels/effects of: CloZAPine; Fingolimod; Leflunomide; Natalizumab; Tofacitinib; Vaccines (Live); Vitamin K Antagonists

The levels/effects of Ifosfamide may be increased by: Aprepitant; Busulfan; CYP2B6 Inhibitors (Moderate); CYP3A4 Inducers (Moderate); CYP3A4 Inducers (Strong); Denosumab; Dipyrone; Fosaprepitant; Pimecrolimus; Quazepam; Roflumilast; Tacrolimus (Topical); Trastuzumab

Decreased Effect

Ifosfamide may decrease the levels/effects of: BCG (Intravesical); Coccidioides immitis Skin Test; Sipuleucel-T; Vaccines (Inactivated); Vaccines (Live)

The levels/effects of Ifosfamide may be decreased by: CYP2B6 Inducers (Strong); CYP3A4 Inducers (Moderate); CYP3A4 Inducers (Strong); CYP3A4 Inhibitors (Moderate); CYP3A4 Inhibitors (Strong); Dabrafenib; Echinacea; Lumacaftor

Storage/Stability Store intact vials of powder for injection at room temperature of 20°C to 25°C (68°F to 77°F); avoid temperatures >30°C (86°F). Store intact vials of solution under refrigeration at 2°C to 8°C (36°F to 46°F). Reconstituted solutions and solutions diluted for administration are stable for 24 hours refrigerated.

Preparation for Administration Hazardous agent; use appropriate precautions for handling and disposal (NIOSH 2014 [group 1]). Reconstitute powder with SWFI or bacteriostatic SWFI (1 g in 20 mL or 3 g in 60 mL) to a concentration of 50 mg/mL. Further dilution in 50-1000 mL D_5W, NS, or lactated Ringer's (to a final concentration of 0.6-20 mg/mL) is recommended for IV infusion (may also dilute in $D_{2.5}W$, $^1/_2$NS, or D_5NS).

Mechanism of Action Causes cross-linking of strands of DNA by binding with nucleic acids and other intracellular structures; inhibits protein synthesis and DNA synthesis

Pharmacodynamics/Kinetics Pharmacokinetics are dose dependent

Distribution: V_d: Approximates total body water; penetrates CNS, but not in therapeutic levels

Protein binding: Negligible

Metabolism: Hepatic to active metabolites isofosforamide mustard, 4-hydroxyifosfamide, acrolein, and inactive dichloroethylated and carboxy metabolites; acrolein is the agent implicated in development of hemorrhagic cystitis

Half-life elimination (increased in the elderly):

High dose (3,800 to 5,000 mg/m^2): ~15 hours

Lower dose (1,600 to 2,400 mg/m^2): ~7 hours

Excretion:
High dose (5,000 mg/m²): Urine (70% to 86%; 61% as unchanged drug)
Lower dose (1,600 to 2,400 mg/m²): Urine (12% to 18% as unchanged drug)

Dosing

Adult & Geriatric Note: To prevent bladder toxicity, ifosfamide should be given with the urinary protector mesna and hydration of at least 2 L of oral or IV fluid per day. Ifosfamide is associated with a moderate emetic potential; antiemetics are recommended to prevent nausea and vomiting (Basch 2011; Roila 2010).

Testicular cancer: IV:
US manufacturer's labeling; as part of combination chemotherapy and with mesna: 1,200 mg/m²/day for 5 days every 3 weeks or after hematologic recovery

VIP regimen: 1,200 mg/m²/day for 5 days every 3 weeks for 4 cycles (in combination with etoposide, mesna, and cisplatin) (Nichols 1998)

VeIP regimen: 1,200 mg/m²/day for 5 days every 3 weeks for 4 cycles (in combination with vinblastine, mesna, and cisplatin) (Loehrer 1998)

Canadian labeling: **Soft tissue sarcoma, cervical cancer (advanced or recurrent), pancreatic cancer (relapsed or refractory):** IV: 2,000 to 2,400 mg/m²/day for 5 consecutive days (with mesna), may repeat after 3 to 4 weeks (or longer depending on patient status) or if lower daily dosage or total dosage over a longer time period is indicated, administer every other day (eg, days 1, 3, 5, 7, 9) or over 10 consecutive days at reduced doses. High **single-dose** infusions of up to 5,000 to 8,000 mg/m²/24 hour with continuous mesna may also be feasible; may repeat after 3 to 4 weeks (or longer depending on patient's condition).

Adult off-label uses and/or dosing:

Testicular cancer: IV:
TIP regimen (off-label dosing): 1,500 mg/m²/day for 4 days (days 2 to 5) every 3 weeks for 4 cycles (in combination with paclitaxel, mesna, and cisplatin) (Kondagunta 2005)

TICE regimen (off-label dosing): 2,000 mg/m²/day for 3 days (days 2 to 4) over 4 hours every 2 weeks for 2 cycles (in combination with paclitaxel and mesna; followed by carboplatin and etoposide) (Kondagunta 2007)

Cervical cancer, recurrent or metastatic: IV: 1,500 mg/m²/day for 5 days every 3 weeks (with mesna) (Coleman 1986; Sutton 1993)

Hodgkin lymphoma, relapsed or refractory: IV:
ICE regimen: 5,000 mg/m² (over 24 hours) beginning on day 2 every 2 weeks for 2 cycles (in combination with mesna, carboplatin, and etoposide) (Moskowitz 2001)

IGEV regimen: 2,000 mg/m²/day for 4 days every 3 weeks for 4 cycles (in combination with mesna, gemcitabine, vinorelbine, and prednisolone) (Santoro 2007)

Non-Hodgkin lymphomas: IV:
CODOX-M/IVAC regimen:
Adults ≤65 years: Cycles 2 and 4 (IVAC): 1,500 mg/m²/day for 5 days (IVAC is combination with cytarabine, mesna, and etoposide; IVAC alternates with CODOX-M) (Mead 2008)

Adults >65 years: Cycles 2 and 4 (IVAC): 1,000 mg/m²/day for 5 days (IVAC is combination with cytarabine, mesna, and etoposide; IVAC alternates with CODOX-M) (Mead 2008)

RICE regimen: 5,000 mg/m² (over 24 hours) beginning on day 4 every 2 weeks for 3 cycles (in combination with mesna, carboplatin, etoposide, and rituximab) (Kewalramani 2004)

Ewing sarcoma: IV:

VAC/IE regimen: Adults ≤30 years: IE: 1,800 mg/m²/day for 5 days (in combination with mesna and etoposide) alternate with VAC (vincristine, doxorubicin, and cyclophosphamide) every 3 weeks for a total of 17 courses (Grier 2003)

VAIA regimen: 3,000 mg/m² day on days 1, 2, 22, 23, 43, and 44 for 4 courses (in combination with vincristine, doxorubicin, dactinomycin, and mesna) (Paulussen 2001) **or** Adults ≤35 years: 2,000 mg/m²/day for 3 days every 3 weeks for 14 courses (in combination with vincristine, doxorubicin, dactinomycin, and mesna) (Paulussen 2008)

VIDE regimen: Adults ≤50 years: 3,000 mg/m²/day over 1 to 3 hours for 3 days every 3 weeks for 6 cycles (in combination with vincristine, doxorubicin, etoposide, and mesna) (Juergens 2006)

IE regimen: 1,800 mg/m²/day over 1 hour for 5 days every 3 weeks for 12 cycles (in combination with etoposide and mesna) (Miser 1987)

ICE regimen: Adults ≤22 years: 1,800 mg/m²/day for 5 days every 3 weeks for up to 12 cycles (in combination with carboplatin and etoposide [and mesna]) (van Winkle 2005)

Osteosarcoma: IV:

Ifosfamide/cisplatin/doxorubicin/HDMT regimen: Adults <40 years: 3,000 mg/m²/day continuous infusion for 5 days during weeks 4 and 10 (preop) and during weeks 16, 25, and 34 (postop) (in combination with cisplatin, doxorubicin, methotrexate [high-dose], and mesna) (Bacci 2003)

Ifosfamide/cisplatin/epirubicin regimen: 2,000 mg/m²/day over 4 hours for 3 days (days 2, 3, and 4) every 3 weeks for 3 cycles (preop) and every 4 weeks for 3 cycles (postop) (in combination with cisplatin, epirubicin, and mesna) (Basaran 2007)

ICE regimen (adults ≤22 years): 1,800 mg/m²/day for 5 days every 3 weeks for up to 12 cycles (in combination with carboplatin and etoposide [and mesna]) (van Winkle 2005)

Soft tissue sarcoma: IV:

Single-agent ifosfamide: 3,000 mg/m²/day over 4 hours for 3 days every 3 weeks for at least 2 cycles or until disease progression (van Oosterom 2002)

ICE regimen: 1,500 mg/m²/day for 4 days every 4 weeks for 4 to 6 cycles (in combination with carboplatin, etoposide, and regional hyperthermia) (Nickenig 2009)

MAID regimen: 2,000 mg/m²/day continuous infusion for 3 days every 3 weeks (in combination with mesna, doxorubicin, and dacarbazine) (Antman 1993) **or** 2,500 mg/m²/day continuous infusion for 3 days every 3 weeks (in combination with mesna, doxorubicin, and dacarbazine); reduce ifosfamide to 1,500mg/m²/day if prior pelvic irradiation (Elias 1989)

Ifosfamide/epirubicin: 1,800 mg/m²/day over 1 hour for 5 days every 3 weeks for 5 cycles (in combination with mesna and epirubicin) (Frustaci 2001)

AIM regimens: 1,500 mg/m²/day over 2 hours for 4 days every 3 weeks for 4 to 6 cycles (in combination with mesna and doxorubicin) (Worden 2005) **or** 2,000 to 3,000 mg/m²/day over 3 hours for 3 days (in combination with mesna and doxorubicin) (Grobmyer 2004)

◄ **Pediatric Note:** To prevent bladder toxicity, ifosfamide should be given with the urinary protector mesna and hydration of at least 2 L of oral or IV fluid per day. Ifosfamide is associated with a moderate emetic potential; antiemetics are recommended to prevent nausea and vomiting (Dupuis 2011).

Ewing sarcoma (off-label use): IV:

VAC/IE regimen: IE: 1,800 mg/m^2/day for 5 days (in combination with mesna and etoposide) alternate with VAC (vincristine, doxorubicin, and cyclophosphamide) every 3 weeks for a total of 17 courses (Grier 2003)

ICE-CAV regimen: ICE: 1,800 mg/m^2/day for 5 days every 3 to 4 weeks for 2 courses (in combination with carboplatin and etoposide [and mesna]), followed by CAV (cyclophosphamide, doxorubicin, and vincristine) (Milano 2006)

VAIA regimen: 3,000 mg/m^2/day on days 1, 2, 22, 23, 43, and 44 for 4 courses (in combination with vincristine, doxorubicin, dactinomycin, and mesna) (Paulussen 2001) **or** 2,000 mg/m^2/day for 3 days every 3 weeks for 14 courses (in combination with vincristine, doxorubicin, dactinomycin, and mesna) (Paulussen 2008)

VIDE regimen: 3,000 mg/m^2/day over 1 to 3 hours for 3 days every 3 weeks for 6 courses (in combination with vincristine, doxorubicin, etoposide, and mesna) (Juergens 2006)

IE regimen: 1,800 mg/m^2/day over 1 hour for 5 days every 3 weeks for 12 cycles (in combination with etoposide and mesna) (Miser 1987)

ICE regimen: 1,800 mg/m^2/day for 5 days every 3 weeks for up to 12 cycles (in combination with carboplatin and etoposide [and mesna]) (van Winkle 2005)

Osteosarcoma (off-label use): IV:

Ifosfamide/cisplatin/doxorubicin/HDMT regimen: 3,000 mg/m^2/day continuous infusion for 5 days during weeks 4 and 10 (preop) and during weeks 16, 25, and 34 (postop) (in combination with cisplatin, doxorubicin, methotrexate [high-dose], and mesna) (Bacci 2003)

Ifosfamide/cisplatin/epirubicin regimen: Children ≥15 years: 2,000 mg/m^2/day over 4 hours for 3 days (days 2, 3, and 4) every 3 weeks for 3 cycles (preop) and every 4 weeks for 3 cycles (postop) (in combination with cisplatin, epirubicin, and mesna) (Basaran 2007)

IE regimen: 3,000 mg/m^2/day over 3 hours for 4 days every 3 to 4 weeks (in combination with etoposide and mesna) (Gentet 1997)

ICE regimen: Children ≥1 year: 1,800 mg/m^2/day for 5 days every 3 weeks for up to 12 cycles (in combination with carboplatin and etoposide [and mesna]) (van Winkle 2005)

Ifosfamide/HDMT/etoposide regimen: 3,000 mg/m^2/day over 3 hours for 4 days during weeks 4 and 9 (3 additional postop courses were administered in good responders) (in combination with methotrexate [high-dose], etoposide, and mesna) (Le Deley 2007)

Renal Impairment

US labeling: Consider dosage reduction in patients with renal impairment; however, there are no dosage adjustments provided in the manufacturer's labeling; ifosfamide (and metabolites) are excreted renally and may accumulate in patients with renal dysfunction. Ifosfamide and metabolites are dialyzable.

Canadian labeling:

Mild to moderate impairment: There are no dosage adjustments provided in the manufacturer's labeling.

Severe impairment: Use is contraindicated.

The following adjustments have also been recommended:

Aronoff 2007:

CrCl ≥10 mL/minute: Children and Adults: No dosage adjustment necessary.

CrCl <10 mL/minute: Children and Adults: Administer 75% of dose.

Hemodialysis (supplement for dialysis):

Children: 1 g/m^2 followed by hemodialysis 6 to 8 hours later

Adults: No supplemental dose needed

Kintzel 1995:

CrCl 46 to 60 mL/minute: Administer 80% of dose

CrCl 31 to 45 mL/minute: Administer 75% of dose

CrCl <30 mL/minute: Administer 70% of dose

Hepatic Impairment There are no dosage adjustments provided in the manufacturer's labeling; however, ifosfamide is extensively hepatically metabolized to both active and inactive metabolites; use with caution. The following adjustments have been recommended:

Floyd 2006: Bilirubin >3 mg/dL: Administer 25% of dose.

Canadian labeling:

Mild to moderate impairment: There are no dosage adjustments provided in the manufacturer labeling; use with caution.

Severe impairment: Use is contraindicated.

Obesity *ASCO Guidelines for appropriate chemotherapy dosing in obese adults with cancer:* Utilize patient's actual body weight (full weight) for calculation of body surface area- or weight-based dosing, particularly when the intent of therapy is curative; manage regimen-related toxicities in the same manner as for nonobese patients; if a dose reduction is utilized due to toxicity, consider resumption of full weight-based dosing with subsequent cycles, especially if cause of toxicity (eg, hepatic or renal impairment) is resolved (Griggs 2012).

Combination Regimens

Bone sarcoma (Ewing sarcoma):

Ifosfamide-Carboplatin-Etoposide (Ewing Sarcoma) on page 2014

Ifosfamide-Etoposide (Ewing Sarcoma) on page 2016

VAC Alternating With IE (Ewing Sarcoma) on page 2102

Bone sarcoma (osteosarcoma):

Ifosfamide-Carboplatin-Etoposide (Osteosarcoma) on page 2015

Ifosfamide-Cisplatin-Epirubicin (Osteosarcoma) on page 2015

Hepatoblastoma: IPA on page 2018

Lymphoma, Hodgkin:

ICE (Hodgkin) on page 2013

IGEV (Hodgkin) on page 2016

MINE-ESHAP (Hodgkin) on page 2036

VIM-D (Hodgkin) on page 2107

Lymphoma, non-Hodgkin:

ICE (Lymphoma, non-Hodgkin) on page 2013

R-ICE (NHL-DLBCL) on page 2076

Lymphoma, non-Hodgkin (Burkitt): CODOX-M/IVAC (NHL-Burkitt) on page 1920

Penile cancer: Paclitaxel-Ifosfamide-Cisplatin (Penile) on page 2052

Soft Tissue Sarcoma:

AIM (Soft Tissue Sarcoma) on page 1827

Epirubicin-Ifosfamide (Soft Tissue Sarcoma) on page 1957

MAID (Soft Tissue Sarcoma) on page 2031

Testicular cancer:
 TIP (Testicular) on page 2090
 VeIP (Testicular) on page 2106
 VIP (Testicular) on page 2110

Administration Ifosfamide is associated with a moderate emetic potential; antiemetics are recommended to prevent nausea and vomiting (Basch 2011; Dupuis 2011; Roila 2010).

Administer IV over at least 30 minutes (infusion times may vary by protocol; refer to specific protocol for infusion duration)

Hazardous agent; use appropriate precautions for handling and disposal (NIOSH 2014 [group 1]).

Vesicant/Extravasation Risk May be an irritant

Emetic Potential Children and Adults: Moderate (30% to 90%)

Monitoring Parameters CBC with differential (prior to each dose), urine output, urinalysis (prior to each dose), liver function, and renal function tests; signs and symptoms of neurotoxicity, pulmonary toxicity, and/or hemorrhagic cystitis

Dosage Forms Excipient information presented when available (limited, particularly for generics); consult specific product labeling.
Solution, Intravenous:
 Generic: 1 g/20 mL (20 mL); 3 g/60 mL (60 mL)
Solution, Intravenous [preservative free]:
 Generic: 1 g/20 mL (20 mL); 3 g/60 mL (60 mL)
Solution Reconstituted, Intravenous:
 Ifex: 1 g (1 ea); 3 g (1 ea)
 Generic: 1 g (1 ea); 3 g (1 ea)

◆ **Ifosfamide for Injection (Can)** see Ifosfamide on page 873

◆ **IG** see Immune Globulin on page 903

◆ **IGIM** see Immune Globulin on page 903

◆ **IGIV** see Immune Globulin on page 903

◆ **IGIVnex (Can)** see Immune Globulin on page 903

◆ **IGSC** see Immune Globulin on page 903

◆ **IL-2** see Aldesleukin on page 55

◆ **IL-11** see Oprelvekin on page 1262

Imatinib (eye MAT eh nib)

Related Information
Chemotherapy and Cancer Treatment During Pregnancy on page 2214
Common Toxicity Criteria on page 2122
Management of Chemotherapy-Induced Nausea and Vomiting in Adults on page 2142
Prevention of Chemotherapy-Induced Nausea and Vomiting in Children on page 2203
Principles of Anticancer Therapy on page 2261
Safe Handling of Hazardous Drugs on page 2292

Brand Names: US Gleevec
Brand Names: Canada ACT-Imatinib; Apo-Imatinib; Gleevec; Teva-Imatinib
Index Terms CGP-57148B; Glivec; Imatinib Mesylate; STI-571

Pharmacologic Category Antineoplastic Agent, BCR-ABL Tyrosine Kinase Inhibitor; Antineoplastic Agent, Tyrosine Kinase Inhibitor

Use

Acute lymphoblastic leukemia: Treatment of relapsed or refractory Philadelphia chromosome-positive (Ph+) acute lymphoblastic leukemia (ALL) in adults

Treatment of newly diagnosed Ph+ ALL in children (in combination with chemotherapy)

Aggressive systemic mastocytosis: Treatment of aggressive systemic mastocytosis without D816V c-Kit mutation (or c-Kit mutational status unknown) in adults

Chronic myeloid leukemia: Treatment of Ph+ chronic myeloid leukemia (CML) in chronic phase (newly diagnosed) in adults and children

Treatment of Ph+ CML in blast crisis, accelerated phase, or chronic phase after failure of interferon-alfa therapy

Dermatofibrosarcoma protuberans: Treatment with unresectable, recurrent, and/or metastatic dermatofibrosarcoma protuberans (DFSP) in adults

Gastrointestinal stromal tumors: Treatment of Kit (CD117)-positive unresectable and/or metastatic malignant gastrointestinal stromal tumors (GIST)

Adjuvant treatment of Kit (CD117)-positive GIST following complete gross resection

Hypereosinophilic syndrome and/or chronic eosinophilic leukemia: Treatment of hypereosinophilic syndrome (HES) and/or chronic eosinophilic leukemia (CEL) in adult patients who have the FIP1L1-platelet-derived growth factor (PDGF) receptor alpha fusion kinase (mutational analysis or fluorescent in situ hybridization [FISH] demonstration of CHIC2 allele deletion) and for patients with HES and/or CEL who are FIP1L1-PDGF receptor alpha fusion kinase negative or unknown

Myelodysplastic/Myeloproliferative diseases: Treatment of myelodysplastic syndrome/myeloproliferative diseases (MDS/MPD) associated with PDGF receptor gene rearrangements in adults

Canadian labeling (not an approved indication in the US): Treatment of newly diagnosed Ph+ ALL in adults as a single agent for induction therapy

Labeled Contraindications There are no contraindications listed in the manufacturer's US labeling.

Canadian labeling: Hypersensitivity to imatinib or any component of the formulation

Pregnancy Considerations Adverse events have been observed in animal reproduction studies. Women of childbearing potential are advised not to become pregnant (female patients and female partners of male patients); highly effective contraception is recommended. The Canadian labeling recommends women of childbearing potential have a negative pregnancy test (urine or serum) with a sensitivity of at least 25 milliunits/mL within 1 week prior to therapy initiation. Case reports of pregnancies while on therapy (both males and females) include reports of spontaneous abortion, minor abnormalities (hypospadias, pyloric stenosis, and small intestine rotation) at or shortly after birth, and other congenital abnormalities including skeletal malformations, hypoplastic lungs, exomphalos, kidney abnormalities, hydrocephalus, cerebellar hypoplasia, and cardiac defects.

Retrospective case reports of women with CML in complete hematologic response (CHR) with cytogenic response (partial or complete) who interrupted imatinib therapy due to pregnancy, demonstrated a loss of response in some patients while off treatment. At 18 months after treatment reinitiation following delivery, CHR was again achieved in all patients and cytogenic response was achieved in some patients. Cytogenetic response rates may not be at as high as compared to patients with 18 months of uninterrupted therapy (Ault, 2006; Pye, 2008).

Breast-Feeding Considerations Imatinib and its active metabolite are found in human breast milk; the milk/plasma ratio is 0.5 for imatinib and 0.9 for the active metabolite. Based on body weight, up to 10% of a therapeutic maternal dose could potentially be received by a breast-fed infant. Due to the potential for serious adverse reactions in the breast-feeding infant, the manufacturer recommends a decision be made to discontinue breast-feeding or to discontinue the drug, taking into account the importance of treatment to the mother.

Warnings/Precautions Hazardous agent - use appropriate precautions for handling and disposal (NIOSH 2014 [group 1]). Often associated with fluid retention, weight gain, and edema (risk increases with higher doses and age >65 years); occasionally serious and may lead to significant complications, including pleural effusion, pericardial effusion, pulmonary edema, and ascites. Monitor regularly for rapid weight gain or other signs/symptoms of fluid retention. Use with caution in patients where fluid accumulation may be poorly tolerated, such as in cardiovascular disease (heart failure [HF] or hypertension) and pulmonary disease. Severe HF and left ventricular dysfunction (LVD) have been reported occasionally, usually in patients with comorbidities and/or risk factors; carefully monitor patients with preexisting cardiac disease or risk factors for HF or history of renal failure. With initiation of imatinib treatment, cardiogenic shock and/or LVD have been reported in patients with hypereosinophilic syndrome and cardiac involvement (reversible with systemic steroids, circulatory support and temporary cessation of imatinib). Patients with high eosinophil levels and an abnormal echocardiogram or abnormal serum troponin level may benefit from prophylactic systemic steroids (for 1 to 2 weeks) with the initiation of imatinib.

Severe bullous dermatologic reactions (including erythema multiforme and Stevens-Johnson syndrome) have been reported; recurrence has been described with rechallenge. Case reports of successful resumption at a lower dose (with corticosteroids and/or antihistamine) have been described; however, some patients may experience recurrent reactions. Drug reaction with eosinophilia and systemic symptoms (DRESS) has been reported; if DRESS occurs, interrupt therapy and consider permanent discontinuation.

Hepatotoxicity may occur (may be severe); fatal hepatic failure and severe hepatic injury requiring liver transplantation have been reported with both short- and long-term use; monitor liver function prior to initiation and monthly or as needed thereafter; therapy interruption or dose reduction may be necessary. Transaminase and bilirubin elevations, and acute liver failure have been observed with imatinib in combination with chemotherapy. Use with caution in patients with preexisting hepatic impairment; dosage adjustment recommended in patients with severe impairment. Use with caution in renal impairment; dosage adjustment recommended for moderate and severe impairment. Tumor lysis syndrome (TLS), including fatalities, has been reported in patients with acute lymphoblastic leukemia (ALL), chronic myeloid leukemia (CML) eosinophilic leukemias, and gastrointestinal stromal tumors (GIST); risk for TLS is higher in patients with a high tumor burden or high proliferation rate; monitor closely; correct clinically significant dehydration and treat high uric acid levels prior to initiation of imatinib.

Imatinib is associated with a moderate emetic potential; antiemetics may be recommended to prevent nausea and vomiting (Dupuis, 2011; Roila, 2010). May cause GI irritation, severe hemorrhage (grades 3 and 4; including GI hemorrhage and/or tumor hemorrhage; hemorrhage incidence is higher in patients with GIST [GI tumors may have been hemorrhage source; gastric antral vascular ectasia has also been reported]), or hematologic toxicity (anemia, neutropenia, and thrombocytopenia; usually occurring within the first several months of treatment). Monitor blood counts weekly for the first month, biweekly for the second month, and as clinically necessary thereafter; median duration of neutropenia is 2 to 3 weeks; median duration of thrombocytopenia is 3 to 4 weeks. In CML, cytopenias are more common in accelerated or blast phase than in chronic phase. Hypothyroidism has been reported in patients who were receiving thyroid hormone replacement therapy prior to the initiation of imatinib; monitor thyroid function; the average onset for imatinib-induced hypothyroidism is 2 weeks; consider doubling levothyroxine doses upon initiation of imatinib (Hamnvik, 2011). Potentially significant drug-drug interactions may exist, requiring dose or frequency adjustment, additional monitoring, and/or selection of alternative therapy. Imatinib exposure may be reduced in patients who have had gastric surgery (eg, bypass, major gastrectomy, or resection); monitor imatinib trough concentrations (Liu, 2011; Pavlovsky, 2009; Yoo, 2010). Growth retardation has been reported in children receiving imatinib for the treatment of CML; generally where treatment was initiated in prepubertal children; growth velocity was usually restored as pubertal age was reached (Shima, 2011); monitor growth closely. The incidence of edema was increased with age older than 65 years in CML and GIST studies. Reports of accidents have been received but it is unclear if imatinib has been the direct cause in any case; advise patients regarding side effects such as dizziness, blurred vision, or somnolence; use caution when driving/operating motor vehicles and heavy machinery.

Adverse Reactions Adverse reactions listed as a composite of data across many trials, except where noted for a specific indication. Frequency not always defined.

>10%:

Cardiovascular: Edema (11% to 86%; grades 3/4: 3% to 13%; includes aggravated edema, anasarca, ascites, pericardial effusion, peripheral edema, pulmonary edema, and superficial edema), facial edema (≤17%), hypotension (Ph+ ALL [pediatric] grades 3/4: 11%), chest pain (7% to 11%)

Central nervous system: Fatigue (20% to 75%), pain (≤47%), headache (8% to 37%), dizziness (5% to 19%), insomnia (9% to 15%), depression (3% to 15%), taste disorder (≤13%), rigors (10% to 12%), anxiety (8% to 12%), paresthesia (≤12%), chills (≤11%)

Dermatologic: Skin rash (9% to 50%; grades 3/4: 1% to 9%), dermatitis (GIST ≤39%), pruritus (7% to 26%), night sweats (CML 13% to 17%), alopecia (7% to 15%), diaphoresis (GIST ≤13%)

Endocrine & metabolic: Increased lactate dehydrogenase (≤60%), hypokalemia (6% to 13%; Ph+ ALL [pediatric] grades 3/4: 34%), weight gain (5% to 32%), decreased serum albumin (≤21%; grades 3/4: ≤4%)

Gastrointestinal: Nausea (41% to 73%; Ph+ ALL [pediatric] grades 3/4: 16%), diarrhea (25% to 59%; Ph+ ALL [pediatric] grades 3/4: 9%), vomiting (11% to 58%), abdominal pain (3% to 57%), anorexia (≤36%), dyspepsia (11% to 27%), flatulence (≤25%), abdominal distension (≤19%), constipation (8% to 16%), stomatitis (≤16%)

◀ Hematologic & oncologic: Neutropenia (grades 3/4: 8% to 64%), thrombocytopenia (grades 3/4: 1% to 63%), anemia (grades 3/4: 3% to 53%),
hemorrhage (3% to 53%; grades 3/4: ≤19%), leukopenia (GIST 5% to
47%; grades 3/4: 2%), hypoproteinemia (≤32%)

Hepatic: Increased serum transaminases (Ph+ ALL [pediatric] grades 3/4:
57%), increased serum AST (≤38%; grades 3/4: ≤6%), increased serum
ALT (≤34%; grades 3/4:≤ 8%), increased alkaline phosphatase (≤17%;
grades 3/4: ≤6%), increased serum bilirubin (≤13%; grades 3/4: ≤4%)

Infection: Infection (Ph+ ALL [pediatric] grades 3/4: 53%; GIST ≤28%),
influenza (Ph+ CML ≤14%)

Neuromuscular & skeletal: Muscle cramps (16% to 62%), musculoskeletal
pain (children 21%; adults 38% to 49%), arthralgia (11% to 40%), myalgia
(9% to 32%), weakness (≤21%), back pain (≤17%), limb pain (≤16%),
ostealgia (≤11%)

Ophthalmic: Periorbital edema (15% to 74%), increased lacrimation (DFSP
25%; GIST ≤18%), eyelid edema (Ph+ CML 19%), blurred vision (≤11%)

Renal: Increased serum creatinine (≤44%; grades 3/4: ≤8%)

Respiratory: Nasopharyngitis (1% to 31%), cough (11% to 27%), upper
respiratory tract infection (3% to 21%), dyspnea (≤21%), pharyngolaryngeal
pain (≤18%), rhinitis (DFSP 17%), pharyngitis (CML 10% to 15%), flu-like
symptoms (1% to 14%), pneumonia (CML 4% to 13%), sinusitis (4%
to 11%)

Miscellaneous: Fever (6% to 41%)

1% to 10%:

Cardiovascular: Pleural effusion (Ph+ ALL [pediatric] grades 3/4: 7%),
palpitations (≤5%), hypertension (≤4%), cardiac failure (Ph+ CML 1%;
grades 3/4: <1%), flushing

Central nervous system: Cerebral hemorrhage (≤9%), hypoesthesia, peripheral neuropathy

Dermatologic: Skin photosensitivity (4% to 7%), xeroderma (≤7%), erythema,
nail disease

Endocrine & metabolic: Hypophosphatemia (10%), hyperglycemia (≤10%),
weight loss (≤10%), hypocalcemia (GIST ≤6%; Ph+ CML grades 3/4: <1%),
fluid retention (Ph+ CML 3%; pleural effusion, pericardial effusion, ascites,
or pulmonary edema 2%), hyperkalemia (1%)

Gastrointestinal: Decreased appetite (10%), gastroenteritis (≤10%), gastrointestinal hemorrhage (1% to 8%), increased serum lipase (CML grades 3/4:
4%), gastritis, gastroesophageal reflux, xerostomia

Hematologic & oncologic: Lymphocytopenia (≤10%; grades 3/4: 1% to 2%),
eosinophilia, febrile neutropenia, pancytopenia, purpura

Neuromuscular & skeletal: Joint swelling

Ophthalmic: Conjunctivitis (5% to 8%), conjunctival hemorrhage, dry eyes

Respiratory: Hypoxia (9%), pneumonitis (Ph+ ALL [pediatric] grades 3/4:
8%), oropharyngeal pain (Ph+ CML ≤6%), epistaxis

<1%, postmarketing, and/or case reports: Actinic keratosis, acute generalized
exanthematous pustulosis, anaphylactic shock, angina pectoris, angioedema, aplastic anemia, arthritis, ascites, atrial fibrillation, avascular necrosis
of bones, blepharitis, bullous rash, cardiac arrest, cardiac arrhythmia, cardiac
tamponade, cardiogenic shock, cataract, cellulitis, cerebral edema, cheilitis,
cold extremities, colitis, confusion, decreased libido, decreased linear skeletal growth rate (children), dehydration, diverticulitis, DRESS syndrome,
drowsiness, dyschromia, dysphagia, embolism, eructation, erythema multiforme, esophagitis, exfoliative dermatitis, folliculitis, fungal infection, gastric
ulcer, gastrointestinal obstruction, gastrointestinal perforation, glaucoma,

gout, gynecomastia, hearing loss, hematemesis, hematoma, hematuria, hemolytic anemia, hepatic failure, hepatic necrosis, hepatitis, hepatotoxicity, herpes simplex infection, herpes zoster, hypercalcemia, hypermenorrhea, hypersensitivity angiitis, hyperuricemia, hypomagnesemia, hyponatremia, hypothyroidism, IgA vasculitis, increased creatine phosphokinase, increased intracranial pressure, inflammatory bowel disease, interstitial pneumonitis, interstitial pulmonary disease, intestinal obstruction, jaundice, left ventricular dysfunction, lichen planus, lower respiratory tract infection, lymphadenopathy, macular edema, melena, memory impairment, menstrual disease, migraine, myocardial infarction, myopathy, onychoclasis, optic neuritis, oral mucosa ulcer, osteonecrosis (hip), ovarian cyst (hemorrhagic), palmar-plantar erythrodysesthesia, pancreatitis, papilledema, pericarditis, petechia, pleuritic chest pain, polyuria, psoriasis, pulmonary fibrosis, pulmonary hemorrhage, pulmonary hypertension, Raynaud's phenomenon, renal failure, respiratory failure, restless leg syndrome, retinal hemorrhage, rhabdomyolysis, ruptured corpus luteal cyst, sciatica, scrotal edema, seizure, sepsis, sexual disorder, Stevens-Johnson syndrome, subconjunctival hemorrhage, subdural hematoma, Sweet's syndrome, syncope, tachycardia, telangiectasia (gastric antral), thrombocythemia, thrombosis, tinnitus, toxic epidermal necrolysis, tremor, tumor hemorrhage (GIST), tumor lysis syndrome, urinary tract infection, urticaria, vertigo, vesicular eruption, vitreous hemorrhage

Drug Interactions

Metabolism/Transport Effects Substrate of CYP1A2 (minor), CYP2C19 (minor), CYP2C8 (minor), CYP2C9 (minor), CYP2D6 (minor), CYP3A4 (major), P-glycoprotein; **Note:** Assignment of Major/Minor substrate status based on clinically relevant drug interaction potential; **Inhibits** BCRP, CYP2C9 (weak), CYP2D6 (weak), CYP3A4 (moderate), P-glycoprotein

Avoid Concomitant Use

Avoid concomitant use of Imatinib with any of the following: Aprepitant; BCG (Intravesical); Bosutinib; CloZAPine; Cobimetinib; Dipyrone; Domperidone; Flibanserin; Ibrutinib; Ivabradine; Lomitapide; Naloxegol; Natalizumab; Olaparib; PAZOPanib; Pimecrolimus; Pimozide; Simeprevir; Tacrolimus (Topical); Tofacitinib; Tolvaptan; Trabectedin; Ulipristal; Vaccines (Live)

Increased Effect/Toxicity

Imatinib may increase the levels/effects of: Apixaban; Aprepitant; ARIPiprazole; Avanafil; Bosentan; Bosutinib; Brexpiprazole; Bromocriptine; Budesonide (Systemic); Budesonide (Systemic, Oral Inhalation); Budesonide (Topical); Cannabis; Cilostazol; CloZAPine; Cobimetinib; Colchicine; CycloSPORINE (Systemic); CYP3A4 Substrates; Dapoxetine; Dofetilide; Domperidone; DOXOrubicin (Conventional); Dronabinol; Eletriptan; Eliglustat; Eplerenone; Everolimus; FentaNYL; Fingolimod; Flibanserin; Halofantrine; Hydrocodone; Ibrutinib; Ivabradine; Ivacaftor; Leflunomide; Lomitapide; Lurasidone; Naloxegol; Natalizumab; NiMODipine; Olaparib; OxyCODONE; PAZOPanib; Pimozide; Propafenone; Ranolazine; Salmeterol; Saxagliptin; Simeprevir; Simvastatin; Sonidegib; Suvorexant; Tetrahydrocannabinol; Tofacitinib; Tolvaptan; Topotecan; Trabectedin; Ulipristal; Vaccines (Live); Vilazodone; Vindesine; Warfarin; Zopiclone; Zuclopenthixol

The levels/effects of Imatinib may be increased by: Acetaminophen; CYP3A4 Inhibitors (Moderate); CYP3A4 Inhibitors (Strong); Denosumab; Dipyrone; Lansoprazole; Osimertinib; P-glycoprotein/ABCB1 Inhibitors; Pimecrolimus; Propacetamol; Roflumilast; Tacrolimus (Topical); Trastuzumab

Decreased Effect

Imatinib may decrease the levels/effects of: BCG (Intravesical); Coccidioides immitis Skin Test; Fludarabine; Ifosfamide; Sipuleucel-T; Vaccines (Inactivated); Vaccines (Live)

The levels/effects of Imatinib may be decreased by: Bosentan; CYP3A4 Inducers (Moderate); CYP3A4 Inducers (Strong); Dabrafenib; Deferasirox; Dexamethasone (Systemic); Echinacea; Enzalutamide; Gemfibrozil; Ibuprofen; Mitotane; Osimertinib; P-glycoprotein/ABCB1 Inducers; Rifamycin Derivatives; Siltuximab; St Johns Wort; Tocilizumab

Food Interactions Food may reduce GI irritation. Grapefruit juice may increase imatinib plasma concentration. Management: Take with a meal and a large glass of water. Avoid grapefruit juice. Maintain adequate hydration, unless instructed to restrict fluid intake.

Storage/Stability Store at 25°C (77°F); excursions permitted between 15°C to 30°C (59°F to 86°F). Protect from moisture.

Mechanism of Action Inhibits Bcr-Abl tyrosine kinase, the constitutive abnormal gene product of the Philadelphia chromosome in chronic myeloid leukemia (CML). Inhibition of this enzyme blocks proliferation and induces apoptosis in Bcr-Abl positive cell lines as well as in fresh leukemic cells in Philadelphia chromosome positive CML. Also inhibits tyrosine kinase for platelet-derived growth factor (PDGF), stem cell factor (SCF), c-Kit, and cellular events mediated by PDGF and SCF.

Pharmacodynamics/Kinetics

Absorption: Rapid

Protein binding: Parent drug and metabolite: ~95% to albumin and alpha$_1$-acid glycoprotein

Metabolism: Hepatic via CYP3A4 (minor metabolism via CYP1A2, CYP2D6, CYP2C9, CYP2C19); primary metabolite (active): N-demethylated piperazine derivative (CGP74588); severe hepatic impairment (bilirubin >3 to 10 times ULN) increases AUC by 45% to 55% for imatinib and its active metabolite, respectively

Bioavailability: 98%; may be decreased in patients who have had gastric surgery (eg, bypass, total or partial resection) (Liu, 2011; Pavlovsky, 2009; Yoo, 2010)

Half-life elimination: Adults: Parent drug: ~18 hours; N-desmethyl metabolite: ~40 hours; Children: Parent drug: ~15 hours

Time to peak: 2 to 4 hours

Excretion: Feces (68% primarily as metabolites, 20% as unchanged drug); urine (13% primarily as metabolites, 5% as unchanged drug)

Dosing

Adult & Geriatric Note: Treatment may be continued until disease progression or unacceptable toxicity. The optimal duration of therapy for chronic myeloid leukemia (CML) in complete remission is not yet determined. Discontinuing CML treatment is not recommended unless part of a clinical trial (Baccarani, 2009). Imatinib is associated with a moderate emetic potential; antiemetics may be recommended to prevent nausea and vomiting (Roila, 2010).

Philadelphia chromosome-positive (Ph+) chronic myeloid leukemia (CML): Oral:

Chronic phase: 400 mg once daily; may be increased to 600 mg daily, if tolerated, for disease progression, lack of hematologic response after 3 months, lack of cytogenetic response after 6-12 months, or loss of previous hematologic or cytogenetic response. An increase to 800 mg daily has been used (Cortes, 2010; Hehlmann, 2014).

Canadian labeling: 400 mg once daily; may be increased to 600-800 mg daily

Accelerated phase or blast crisis: 600 mg once daily; may be increased to 800 mg daily (400 mg twice daily), if tolerated, for disease progression, lack of hematologic response after 3 months, lack of cytogenetic response after 6-12 months, or loss of previous hematologic or cytogenetic response

Ph+ acute lymphoblastic leukemia (ALL) (relapsed or refractory): Oral: 600 mg once daily

Gastrointestinal stromal tumors (GIST) (adjuvant treatment following complete resection): Oral: 400 mg once daily; recommended treatment duration: 3 years

GIST (unresectable and/or metastatic malignant): Oral: 400 mg once daily; may be increased up to 800 mg daily (400 mg twice daily), if tolerated, for disease progression. **Note:** Significant improvement (progression-free survival, objective response rate) was demonstrated in patients with KIT exon 9 mutation with 800 mg (versus 400 mg), although overall survival (OS) was not impacted. The higher dose did not demonstrate a difference in time to progression or OS patients with Kit exon 11 mutation or wild-type status (Debiec-Rychter, 2006; Heinrich, 2009).

Canadian labeling: 400-600 mg daily (depending on disease stage/progression); may be increased to 600-800 mg daily

Aggressive systemic mastocytosis (ASM) with eosinophilia: Oral: Initiate at 100 mg once daily; titrate up to a maximum of 400 mg once daily (if tolerated) for insufficient response to lower dose

ASM without D816V c-Kit mutation or c-Kit mutation status unknown: Oral: 400 mg once daily

Dermatofibrosarcoma protuberans (DFSP): Oral: 400 mg twice daily

Hypereosinophilic syndrome (HES) and/or chronic eosinophilic leukemia (CEL): Oral: 400 mg once daily

HES/CEL with FIP1L1-PDGFRα fusion kinase: Oral: Initiate at 100 mg once daily; titrate up to 400 mg once daily (if tolerated) if insufficient response to lower dose

Myelodysplastic/myeloproliferative disease (MDS/MPD): Oral: 400 mg once daily

Ph+ ALL (induction, newly diagnosed): *Canadian labeling (not an approved use in the US):* Oral: 600 mg once daily

Chordoma, progressive, advanced, or metastatic expressing PDGFRB and/or PDGFB (off-label use): Oral: 400 mg twice daily (Stacchiotti, 2012)

Desmoid tumors, unresectable and/or progressive (off-label use): Oral: 300 mg twice daily (BSA ≥1.5 m^2), 200 mg twice daily (BSA 1-1.49 m^2), 100 mg twice daily (BSA <1 m^2) (Chugh, 2010) **or** 400 mg once daily; may increase to 400 mg twice daily if progressive disease on 400 mg daily (Penel, 2011)

Melanoma, advanced or metastatic with C-KIT mutation (off-label use): Oral: 400 mg twice daily (Carvajal, 2011)

Stem cell transplant (SCT, off-label use) for CML (in patients who have not failed imatinib therapy prior to transplant): Oral:

Prophylactic use to prevent relapse post SCT: 400 mg daily starting after engraftment for 1 year post transplant (Carpenter, 2007) **or** 300 mg daily starting on day +35 post SCT (increased to 400 mg within 4 weeks) and continued until 12 months post transplant (Olavarria, 2007)

◄ *Relapse post SCT:* Initial: 400 mg daily; if inferior response after 3 months, dose may be increased to 600-800 mg daily (Hess, 2005) **or** 400-600 mg daily (chronic phase) **or** 600 mg daily (blast or accelerated phase) (DeAngelo, 2004)

Dosage adjustment with concomitant strong CYP3A4 inducers: Avoid concomitant use of strong CYP3A4 inducers (eg, dexamethasone, carbamazepine, phenobarbital, phenytoin, rifabutin, rifampin); if concomitant use cannot be avoided, increase imatinib dose by at least 50% with careful monitoring.

Pediatric Note: Treatment may be continued until disease progression or unacceptable toxicity. The optimal duration of therapy for CML in complete remission is not yet determined. Imatinib is associated with a moderate emetic potential; antiemetics may be recommended to prevent nausea and vomiting (Dupuis, 2011).

Philadelphia chromosome-positive (Ph+) acute lymphoblastic leukemia (ALL) (newly diagnosed): Children ≥1 year and Adolescents: Oral: 340 mg/m^2/day (in combination with chemotherapy); maximum: 600 mg daily

Ph+ chronic myeloid leukemia (CML), chronic phase, newly diagnosed: Children ≥1 year and Adolescents: Oral: 340 mg/m^2/day; maximum: 600 mg daily

Dosage adjustment with concomitant strong CYP3A4 inducers: Avoid concomitant use of strong CYP3A4 inducers (eg, dexamethasone, carbamazepine, phenobarbital, phenytoin, rifabutin, rifampin); if concomitant use cannot be avoided, increase imatinib dose by at least 50% with careful monitoring.

Dosage adjustment for hepatotoxicity: Refer to "Hepatic Impairment" dosing.

Dosage adjustment for hematologic adverse reactions: Refer to dosing adjustment for toxicity.

Dosage adjustment for nonhematologic adverse reactions: Refer to dosing adjustment for toxicity.

Renal Impairment

US labeling:

Mild impairment (CrCl 40-59 mL/minute): Maximum recommended dose: 600 mg.

Moderate impairment (CrCl 20-39 mL/minute): Decrease recommended starting dose by 50%; dose may be increased as tolerated; maximum recommended dose: 400 mg.

Severe impairment (CrCl <20 mL/minute): Use caution; a dose of 100 mg daily has been tolerated in a limited number of patients with severe impairment (Gibbons, 2008).

Canadian labeling:

Mild impairment (CrCl 40-59 mL/minute): Initial dose: 400 mg once daily (minimum effective dose); titrate to efficacy and tolerability.

Moderate impairment (CrCl 20-39 mL/minute): Initial dose: 400 mg once daily (minimum effective dose); titrate to efficacy and tolerability; the use of 800 mg dose is not recommended.

Severe impairment (CrCl <20 mL/minute): Use is not recommended.

Hepatic Impairment
US labeling:
Mild-to-moderate impairment: No dosage adjustment necessary.
Severe impairment: Reduce dose by 25%.
Canadian labeling:
Mild-to-moderate impairment: Initial dose: 400 mg once daily (minimum effective dose).
Severe impairment: Initial dose: 200 mg once daily; may increase up to 300 mg once daily in the absence of severe toxicity; decrease dose with unacceptable toxicity.

Dosage adjustment for hepatotoxicity (during therapy): If elevations of bilirubin >3 times ULN or transaminases >5 times ULN occur, withhold treatment until bilirubin <1.5 times ULN and transaminases <2.5 times ULN. Resume treatment at a reduced dose as follows (**Note:** The decision to resume treatment should take into consideration the initial severity of hepatotoxicity):
Adults:
If current dose 400 mg daily, reduce dose to 300 mg daily
If current dose 600 mg daily, reduce dose to 400 mg daily
If current dose 800 mg daily, reduce dose to 600 mg daily
Children ≥1 year and Adolescents: If current dose 340 mg/m^2/day, reduce dose to 260 mg/m^2/day

Adjustment for Toxicity
Hematologic toxicity:
Chronic phase CML (initial dose 400 mg daily in adults or 340 mg/m^2/day in children); ASM, MDS/MPD, and HES/CEL (initial dose 400 mg daily); or GIST (initial dose 400 mg daily [US labeling] or 400-600 mg daily [Canadian labeling]): If ANC <1 x 10^9/L and/or platelets <50 x 10^9/L: Withhold until ANC ≥1.5 x 10^9/L and platelets ≥75 x 10^9/L; resume treatment at original starting dose. For recurrent neutropenia and/or thrombocytopenia, withhold until recovery, and reinstitute treatment at a reduced dose as follows:
Children ≥1 year and Adolescents: If initial dose 340 mg/m^2/day, reduce dose to 260 mg/m^2/day.
Adults:
If initial dose 400 mg daily, reduce dose to 300 mg daily.
If initial dose 600 mg daily (Canadian labeling; not in US labeling), reduce dose to 400 mg daily.
CML (accelerated phase or blast crisis): Adults (initial dose 600 mg daily): If ANC <0.5 x 10^9/L and/or platelets <10 x 10^9/L, establish whether cytopenia is related to leukemia (bone marrow aspirate or biopsy). If unrelated to leukemia, reduce dose to 400 mg daily. If cytopenia persists for an additional 2 weeks, further reduce dose to 300 mg daily. If cytopenia persists for 4 weeks and is still unrelated to leukemia, withhold treatment until ANC ≥1 x 10^9/L and platelets ≥20 x 10^9/L, then resume treatment at 300 mg daily.
ASM associated with eosinophilia and HES/CEL with FIP1L1-PDGFRα fusion kinase: Adults (starting dose 100 mg daily): If ANC <1 x 10^9/L and/or platelets <50 x 10^9/L: Withhold until ANC ≥1.5 x 10^9/L and platelets ≥75 x 10^9/L; resume treatment at previous dose.
DFSP: Adults (initial dose 800 mg daily): If ANC <1 x 10^9/L and/or platelets <50 x 10^9/L, withhold until ANC ≥1.5 x 10^9/L and platelets ≥75 x 10^9/L; resume treatment at reduced dose of 600 mg daily. For recurrent neutropenia and/or thrombocytopenia, withhold until recovery, and reinstitute treatment with a further dose reduction to 400 mg daily.

◀ Ph+ ALL:

Pediatrics (Schultz, 2009): Hematologic toxicity requiring dosage adjustments was not observed in the study. No major toxicities were observed with imatinib at 340 mg/m^2/day in combination with intensive chemotherapy.

Adults (initial dose 600 mg daily): If ANC <0.5 x 10^9/L and/or platelets <10 x 10^9/L, establish whether cytopenia is related to leukemia (bone marrow aspirate or biopsy). If unrelated to leukemia, reduce dose to 400 mg daily. If cytopenia persists for an additional 2 weeks, further reduce dose to 300 mg daily. If cytopenia persists for 4 weeks and is still unrelated to leukemia, withhold treatment until ANC ≥1 x 10^9/L and platelets ≥20 x 10^9/L, then resume treatment at 300 mg daily.

Nonhematologic toxicity (eg, severe edema): Withhold treatment until toxicity resolves; may resume if appropriate (depending on initial severity of adverse event).

Combination Regimens

Leukemia, acute lymphocytic: Hyper-CVAD + Imatinib on page 2005
Leukemia, chronic myelogenous: Imatinib (CML Regimen) on page 2017
Soft tissue sarcoma (gastrointestinal stromal tumor [GIST]): Imatinib (GIST Regimen) on page 2017

Administration Imatinib is associated with a moderate emetic potential; antiemetics may be recommended to prevent nausea and vomiting (Dupuis, 2011; Roila, 2010).

Should be administered with a meal and a large glass of water. It is not recommended to crush or chew tablets due to bitter taste. Tablets may be dispersed in water or apple juice (using ~50 mL for 100 mg tablet, ~200 mL for 400 mg tablet); stir until dissolved and administer immediately. In adults, doses ≤600 mg may be given once daily; 800 mg dose should be administered as 400 mg twice daily. Dosing in children may be once or twice daily for chronic myeloid leukemia (CML) and once daily for Philadelphia chromosome–positive (Ph+) acute lymphoblastic leukemia (ALL). For daily dosing ≥800 mg, the 400 mg tablets should be used in order to reduce iron exposure.

Hazardous agent; use appropriate precautions for handling and disposal (NIOSH 2014 [group 1]). Avoid skin or mucous membrane contact with crushed tablets; if contact occurs, wash thoroughly. Avoid exposure to crushed tablets. If it is necessary to manipulate the tablets (eg, to prepare an oral solution), it is recommended to double glove, wear a protective gown, and prepare in a controlled device (NIOSH, 2014).

Emetic Potential Children and Adults: Moderate (30% to 60%)

Extemporaneous Preparations Hazardous agent: Use appropriate precautions for handling and disposal (NIOSH 2014 [group 1]). When manipulating tablets, NIOSH recommends double gloving, a protective gown, and preparation in a controlled device; if not prepared in a controlled device, respiratory and eye protection as well as ventilated engineering controls are recommended (NIOSH, 2014).

An oral suspension may be prepared by placing tablets (whole, do not crush) in a glass of water or apple juice. Use ~50 mL for 100 mg tablet, or ~200 mL for 400 mg tablet. Stir until tablets are disintegrated, then administer immediately. To ensure the full dose is administered, rinse the glass and administer residue.

Gleevec (imatinib) [prescribing information]. East Hanover, NJ: Novartis Pharmaceuticals; January 2015.

Monitoring Parameters CBC (weekly for first month, biweekly for second month, then periodically thereafter), liver function tests (at baseline and monthly or as clinically indicated; more frequently [at least weekly] in patients with moderate-to-severe hepatic impairment [Ramanathan, 2008]), renal function, serum electrolytes (including calcium, phosphorus, potassium and sodium levels); bone marrow cytogenetics (in CML; at 6-, 12-, and 18 months), pregnancy test (Canadian labeling recommends women of reproductive potential have a negative test [urine or serum] with a sensitivity of at least 25 milliunits/mL within 1 week prior to therapy initiation); fatigue, weight, and edema/fluid status; consider echocardiogram and serum troponin levels in patients with HES/CEL, and in patients with MDS/MPD or ASM with high eosinophil levels; in pediatric patients, also monitor serum glucose, albumin, and growth

Gastric surgery (eg, bypass, major gastrectomy, or resection) patients: Monitor imatinib trough concentrations (Liu, 2011; Pavlovsky, 2009; Yoo, 2010)

Thyroid function testing (Hamnvik, 2011):
  Preexisting levothyroxine therapy: Obtain baseline TSH levels, then monitor every 4 weeks until levels and levothyroxine dose are stable, then monitor every 2 months
  Without preexisting thyroid hormone replacement: TSH at baseline, then every 4 weeks for 4 months, then every 2-3 months

Monitor for signs/symptoms of CHF in patients with at risk for cardiac failure or patients with preexisting cardiac disease. In Canada, a baseline evaluation of left ventricular ejection fraction is recommended prior to initiation of imatinib therapy in all patients with known underlying heart disease or in elderly patients. Monitor for signs/symptoms of gastrointestinal irritation or perforation and dermatologic toxicities.

Dietary Considerations Avoid grapefruit juice.

Dosage Forms Excipient information presented when available (limited, particularly for generics); consult specific product labeling.
Tablet, Oral:
  Gleevec: 100 mg, 400 mg [scored]

Imipenem and Cilastatin (i mi PEN em & sye la STAT in)
Brand Names: US Primaxin I.V.

◀ **Brand Names: Canada** Imipenem and Cilastatin for Injection; Imipenem and Cilastatin for Injection, USP; Primaxin; RAN-Imipenem-Cilastatin

Index Terms Cilastatin and Imipenem; Imipemide; Primaxin I.M. [DSC]

Pharmacologic Category Antibiotic, Carbapenem

Use Treatment of lower respiratory tract, urinary tract, intra-abdominal, gynecologic, bone and joint, skin and skin structure, endocarditis (caused by *Staphylococcus aureus*) and polymicrobic infections as well as bacterial septicemia. Antibacterial activity includes gram-positive bacteria (methicillin-sensitive *S. aureus* and *Streptococcus* spp), resistant gram-negative bacilli (including extended spectrum beta-lactamase-producing *Escherichia coli* and *Klebsiella* spp, *Enterobacter* spp, and *Pseudomonas aeruginosa*), and anaerobes.

Pregnancy Risk Factor C

Dosing

Adult & Geriatric Doses based on **imipenem** content.

Usual dosage range: Weight ≥70 kg: 250-1000 mg every 6-8 hours; maximum: 4 g/day. **Note:** For adults weighing <70 kg, refer to Dosing Adjustment in Renal Impairment.

Indication-specific dosing:

Burkholderia pseudomallei **(melioidosis) (off-label use):** IV: Initial: 20 mg/kg every 8 hours for at least 10 days (White 2003) **or** 25 mg/kg (up to 1 g) every 6 hours for at least 10 days (Currie 2003); continue parenteral therapy until clinical improvement then switch to oral therapy if tolerated and/or appropriate.

Intra-abdominal infections: IV:

Mild infection: 250-500 mg every 6 hours

Severe infection: 500 mg every 6 hours **or** 1 g every 8 hours for 4-7 days (provided source controlled). **Note:** Not recommended for mild-to-moderate, community-acquired intra-abdominal infections due to risk of toxicity and the development of resistant organisms (Solomkin 2010)

Liver abscess (off-label use): IV: 500 mg every 6 hours for 4-6 weeks (Ulug 2010)

Moderate infections: IV:

Fully-susceptible organisms: 500 mg every 6-8 hours

Moderately-susceptible organisms: 500 mg every 6 hours or 1 g every 8 hours

Neutropenic fever (off-label use): IV: 500 mg every 6 hours (Paul 2006)

Pseudomonas **infections:** IV: 500 mg every 6 hours; **Note:** Higher doses may be required based on organism sensitivity.

Severe infections: IV:

Fully-susceptible organisms: 500 mg every 6 hours

Moderately-susceptible organisms: 1 g every 6-8 hours

Maximum daily dose should not exceed 50 mg/kg or 4 g/day, whichever is lower

Skin and soft tissue necrotizing infections (off-label use): IV: 1 g every 6 to 8 hours in combination with an agent effective against MRSA (eg, vancomycin, linezolid, daptomycin) for empiric therapy of polymicrobial [mixed] infections. Continue until further debridement is not necessary, patient has clinically improved, and patient is afebrile for 48 to 72 hours (IDSA [Stevens 2014]).

Surgical site infection (intestinal or genitourinary tract surgery) (off-label use): IV: 500 mg every 6 hours (IDSA [Stevens 2014]).

Urinary tract infection, uncomplicated: IV: 250 mg every 6 hours

Urinary tract infection, complicated: IV: 500 mg every 6 hours

Mild infections: Note: Rarely a suitable option in mild infections; normally reserved for moderate-severe cases: IV:

Fully-susceptible organisms: 250 mg every 6 hours

Moderately-susceptible organisms: 500 mg every 6 hours

Pediatric Dosage based on **imipenem** content:

Non-CNS infections: IV: Children: >3 months: 15-25 mg/kg every 6 hours
Maximum dosage: Susceptible infections: 2 g/day; moderately-susceptible organisms: 4 g/day

Burkholderia pseudomallei (melioidosis) (off-label use): IV: Initial: 20 mg/kg every 8 hours for at least 10 days (White 2003) **or** 25 mg/kg (up to 1 g) every 6 hours for at least 10 days (Currie 2003); continue parenteral therapy until clinical improvement, then switch to oral therapy if tolerated and/or appropriate

Cystic fibrosis: IV: Infants, Children, and Adolescents: Up to 100 mg/kg/day divided every 6 hours; maximum dose: 4 g daily has been used. **Note:** Efficacy in exacerbations may be limited due to rapid development of resistance (Zobell 2013).

Renal Impairment IV:

Patients with a CrCl ≤5 mL/minute/1.73 m² should not receive imipenem/cilastatin unless hemodialysis is instituted within 48 hours.

Patients weighing <30 kg with impaired renal function should not receive imipenem/cilastatin.

Reduced IV dosage regimen based on creatinine clearance and/or body weight: See table.

Intermittent hemodialysis (IHD) (administer after hemodialysis on dialysis days): Use the dosing recommendation for patients with a CrCl 6-20 mL/minute; administer dose after dialysis session and every 12 hours thereafter **or** 250-500 mg every 12 hours (Heintz 2009). **Note:** Dosing dependent on the assumption of 3 times/week, complete IHD sessions.

Peritoneal dialysis (off-label dosing): Dose as for CrCl 6-20 mL/minute (Somani 1988)

Continuous renal replacement therapy (CRRT) (Heintz 2009; Trotman 2005): Drug clearance is highly dependent on the method of renal replacement, filter type, and flow rate. Appropriate dosing requires close monitoring of pharmacologic response, signs of adverse reactions due to drug accumulation, as well as drug concentrations in relation to target trough (if appropriate). The following are general recommendations only (based on dialysate flow/ultrafiltration rates of 1-2 L/hour and minimal residual renal function) and should not supersede clinical judgment:

CVVH: Loading dose of 1 g followed by either 250 mg every 6 hours **or** 500 mg every 8 hours

CVVHD: Loading dose of 1 g followed by either 250 mg every 6 hours **or** 500 mg every 6-8 hours

CVVHDF: Loading dose of 1 g followed by either 250 mg every 6 hours **or** 500 mg every 6 hours

Note: Data suggest that 500 mg every 8-12 hours may provide sufficient time above MIC to cover organisms with MIC values ≤2 mg/L; however, a higher dose of 500 mg every 6 hours is recommended for resistant organisms (particularly *Pseudomonas* spp) with MIC ≥4 mg/L or deep-seated infections (Fish 2005).

◄ Reduced IV dosage regimen based on creatinine clearance and/or body weight:

U.S. labeling: See table.

Imipenem and Cilastatin Dosage in Renal Impairment

Reduced IV Dosage Regimen Based on Creatinine Clearance (mL/minute/1.73 m²) and/or Body Weight <70 kg					
	Body Weight (kg)				
	≥70	60	50	40	30
Total daily dose for normal renal function: 1 g/day					
CrCl ≥71	250 mg q6h	250 mg q8h	125 mg q6h	125 mg q6h	125 mg q8h
CrCl 41-70	250 mg q8h	125 mg q6h	125 mg q6h	125 mg q8h	125 mg q8h
CrCl 21-40	250 mg q12h	250 mg q12h	125 mg q8h	125 mg q12h	125 mg q12h
CrCl 6-20	250 mg q12h	125 mg q12h	125 mg q12h	125 mg q12h	125 mg q12h
Total daily dose for normal renal function: 1.5 g/day					
CrCl ≥71	500 mg q8h	250 mg q6h	250 mg q6h	250 mg q8h	125 mg q6h
CrCl 41-70	250 mg q6h	250 mg q8h	250 mg q8h	125 mg q6h	125 mg q8h
CrCl 21-40	250 mg q8h	250 mg q8h	250 mg q12h	125 mg q8h	125 mg q8h
CrCl 6-20	250 mg q12h	250 mg q12h	250 mg q12h	125 mg q12h	125 mg q12h
Total daily dose for normal renal function: 2 g/day					
CrCl ≥71	500 mg q6h	500 mg q8h	250 mg q6h	250 mg q6h	250 mg q8h
CrCl 41-70	500 mg q8h	250 mg q6h	250 mg q6h	250 mg q8h	125 mg q6h
CrCl 21-40	250 mg q6h	250 mg q8h	250 mg q8h	250 mg q12h	125 mg q8h
CrCl 6-20	250 mg q12h	250 mg q12h	250 mg q12h	250 mg q12h	125 mg q12h
Total daily dose for normal renal function: 3 g/day					
CrCl ≥71	1000 mg q8h	750 mg q8h	500 mg q6h	500 mg q8h	250 mg q6h
CrCl 41-70	500 mg q6h	500 mg q8h	500 mg q8h	250 mg q6h	250 mg q8h
CrCl 21-40	500 mg q8h	500 mg q8h	250 mg q6h	250 mg q8h	250 mg q8h
CrCl 6-20	500 mg q12h	500 mg q12h	250 mg q12h	250 mg q12h	250 mg q12h
Total daily dose for normal renal function: 4 g/day					
CrCl ≥71	1000 mg q6h	1000 mg q8h	750 mg q8h	500 mg q6h	500 mg q8h
CrCl 41-70	750 mg q8h	750 mg q8h	500 mg q6h	500 mg q8h	250 mg q6h
CrCl 21-40	500 mg q6h	500 mg q8h	500 mg q8h	250 mg q6h	250 mg q8h
CrCl 6-20	500 mg q12h	500 mg q12h	500 mg q12h	250 mg q12h	250 mg q12h

Canadian labeling: Reduced IV dosage regimen based on creatinine clearance (mL/minute/1.73 m²) and body weight ≥70 kg (**Note:** The manufacturer labeling recommends further proportionate dose reductions for patients <70 kg, but does not provide specific dosing recommendations):

Mild renal impairment (CrCl 31-70 mL/minute/1.73 m²):

Fully-susceptible organisms: Maximum dosage: 500 mg every 8 hours

Less susceptible organisms (primarily some *Pseudomonas* strains): Maximum dosage: 500 mg every 6 hours

Moderate renal impairment (CrCl 21-30 mL/minute/1.73 m²):

Fully-susceptible organisms: Maximum dosage: 500 mg every 12 hours

Less susceptible organisms (primarily some *Pseudomonas* strains): Maximum dosage: 500 mg every 8 hours

Severe renal impairment (CrCl 0-20 mL/minute/1.73 m^2):
Fully-susceptible organisms: Maximum dosage: 250 mg every 12 hours
Less susceptible organisms (primarily some *Pseudomonas* strains): Maximum dosage: 500 mg every 12 hours

Note: Patients with CrCl 6-20 mL/minute/1.73 m^2 should receive 250 mg every 12 hours or 3.5 mg/kg (whichever is lower) every 12 hours for most pathogens; seizure risk may increase with higher dosing.

Hepatic Impairment Hepatic dysfunction may further impair cilastatin clearance in patients receiving chronic renal replacement therapy; consider decreasing the dosing frequency.

Additional Information Complete prescribing information should be consulted for additional detail.

Dosage Forms Excipient information presented when available (limited, particularly for generics); consult specific product labeling.

Injection, powder for reconstitution: Imipenem 250 mg and cilastatin 250 mg; imipenem 500 mg and cilastatin 500 mg

Primaxin® I.V.: Imipenem 250 mg and cilastatin 250 mg [contains sodium 18.8 mg (0.8 mEq)]; imipenem 500 mg and cilastatin 500 mg [contains sodium 37.5 mg (1.6 mEq)]

◆ **Imipenem and Cilastatin for Injection (Can)** *see* Imipenem and Cilastatin *on page 893*

◆ **Imipenem and Cilastatin for Injection, USP (Can)** *see* Imipenem and Cilastatin *on page 893*

Imiquimod (i mi KWI mod)

Brand Names: US Aldara; Zyclara; Zyclara Pump

Brand Names: Canada Aldara P; Apo-Imiquimod; Vyloma; Zyclara

Pharmacologic Category Skin and Mucous Membrane Agent; Topical Skin Product

Use

Aldara®: Treatment of external genital and perianal warts/condyloma acuminata; nonhyperkeratotic, nonhypertrophic actinic keratosis on face or scalp; superficial basal cell carcinoma (sBCC) with a maximum tumor diameter of 2 cm located on the trunk (excluding anogenital skin), neck, or extremities (excluding hands or feet)

Vyloma™ (Canadian availability; not available in the U.S.): Treatment of external genital and perianal warts/condyloma acuminata

Zyclara®:
U.S. labeling: Treatment of external genital and perianal warts/condyloma acuminata (3.75% formulation); treatment of clinically typical visible or palpable, actinic keratoses on face or scalp (2.5% or 3.75% formulation)
Canadian labeling: Treatment of clinically typical visible or palpable, actinic keratoses on face or scalp

Labeled Contraindications

U.S. labeling: There are no contraindications listed within the approved manufacturer's labeling.

Canadian labeling: Hypersensitivity to imiquimod or any component of the formulation

Pregnancy Considerations Adverse events were observed in some animal reproduction studies following oral administration. Imiquimod may weaken condoms and vaginal diaphragms. Use in pregnant women is not recommended (CDC, 2010).

◀ **Breast-Feeding Considerations** It is not known if imiquimod is excreted in breast milk. The manufacturer recommends that caution be exercised when administering imiquimod to nursing women.

Warnings/Precautions Imiquimod is not intended for oral, nasal, intravaginal, or ophthalmic use. Topical imiquimod administration is not recommended until tissue is healed from any previous drug or surgical treatment. Treatment should not be prolonged beyond recommended period due to missed doses or rest periods. Imiquimod has the potential to exacerbate inflammatory conditions of the skin (including chronic graft-versus-host disease). Intense inflammatory reactions may occur, and may be accompanied by systemic symptoms (fever, malaise, myalgia); interruption of therapy should be considered. Severe inflammation of female external genitalia following topical application may lead to severe vulvar swelling and urinary retention; interruption or discontinuation of therapy may be necessary.

May increase sunburn susceptibility; in an animal study, topical imiquimod administration and concurrent ultraviolet radiation decreased the median time to skin tumor formation. Patients should protect themselves from the sun and artificial forms of sunlight. Safety and efficacy have not been established for immunosuppressed patients, or for basal cell nevus syndrome or xeroderma pigmentosum. Following 2 randomized, double-blind, placebo-controlled trials, efficacy of imiquimod was not established for molluscum contagiosum in children 2-12 years of age. Use with caution in patients with preexisting autoimmune disorders (onset or exacerbation of disease has been reported rarely with imiquimod).

Basal cell carcinoma: Use in basal cell carcinoma should be limited to superficial carcinomas with a maximum diameter of 2 cm. Safety and efficacy in treatment of sBCC lesions of the face, head, and anogenital area, or other subtypes of basal cell carcinoma (including nodular and morpheaform), have not been established.

Actinic keratosis: Safety and efficacy of repeated use of Aldara® or Zyclara® in a previously treated area have not been established. Prescribed course of therapy should be completed even if all lesions appear to be gone.

Genital warts: Safety and efficacy of Zyclara® 2.75% in the treatment of external genital warts have not been established. Imiquimod has not been evaluated for the treatment of urethral, intravaginal, cervical, rectal, or intra-anal human papilloma viral disease and is not recommended for these conditions.

Adverse Reactions Note: Frequency of reactions vary and are related to the degree of inflammation associated with the treated disease, number of weekly applications, product formulation, and individual sensitivity.
>10%:
Dermatologic: Localized erythema (58% to 100%; remote: 2%), xeroderma (local; including flaking, scaling; 18% to 93%; remote: 1%), crusted skin (local; 4% to 93%), skin sclerosis (local; 5% to 84%), dermal ulcer (local; 4% to 62%; remote: 2%), localized vesiculation (2% to 31%), excoriation (local; remote: 1%)
Infection: Fungal infection (2% to 11%)
Local: Localized edema (12% to 78%; remote: 1%), application site discharge (22% to 51%), local pruritus (3% to 32%), localized burning (9% to 26%)
Respiratory: Upper respiratory tract infection (15% to 33%)

1% to 10%:
Cardiovascular: Chest pain, localized blanching
Central nervous system: Headache (2% to 6%), fatigue (1% to 4%), dizziness (<1% to 3%), local discomfort (soreness; ≤3%), rigors (1%), anxiety, pain, tingling of skin (local)
Dermatologic: Skin pain (local; 1% to 8%), skin hypertrophy (local; 3%), skin infection (local; 1% to 3%), eczema (2%), cheilitis (≤2%), alopecia (1%), dermal hemorrhage (local), localized rash, papule (local), seborrhoeic keratosis, skin tenderness (local), stinging of the skin (local), tinea (cruris)
Endocrine & metabolic: Increased serum glucose
Gastrointestinal: Nausea (1% to 4%), diarrhea (1% to 3%), anorexia (≤3%), vomiting (1%), dyspepsia
Genitourinary: Bacterial vaginosis (3%), urinary tract infection (1%)
Hematologic & oncologic: Squamous cell carcinoma (4%), lymphadenopathy (2% to 3%)
Infection: Herpes simplex (≤3%)
Local: Local irritation (3% to 6%)
Neuromuscular & skeletal: Arthralgia (1% to 3%), myalgia (≥1%), back pain
Respiratory: Sinusitis (7%), flu-like symptoms (<1% to 4%), cough, pharyngitis, rhinitis
Miscellaneous: Fever (≤3%)
Postmarketing and/or case reports: Abdominal pain, acute exacerbations of multiple sclerosis, agitation, anemia, angioedema, atrial fibrillation, capillary leak syndrome, cardiac failure, cardiomyopathy, cellulitis (local), cerebrovascular accident, chills, depression, dermatitis, dyspnea, dysuria, erythema multiforme, erythema (scrotal), exacerbation of psoriasis, exacerbation of ulcerative colitis, exfoliative dermatitis, febrile seizures, Henoch-Schönlein purpura (IgA vasculitis), hepatic insufficiency, herpes zoster, hyperpigmentation, immune thrombocytopenia (ITP), insomnia, ischemia, lethargy, leukopenia, malignant lymphoma, myocardial infarction, pain (scrotal), palpitations, pancytopenia, paresis, proteinuria, psoriasis, pulmonary edema, scrotal edema, seizure, squamous cell carcinoma, supraventricular tachycardia, syncope, tachycardia, thrombocytopenia, thyroiditis, ulcerative colitis, ulcer (scrotal), urinary retention, urticaria, vertebral disk disease (spondylitis onset or exacerbated)

Drug Interactions
Metabolism/Transport Effects Substrate of CYP1A2 (minor), CYP3A4 (minor); Note: Assignment of Major/Minor substrate status based on clinically relevant drug interaction potential

Avoid Concomitant Use
Avoid concomitant use of Imiquimod with any of the following: BCG (Intravesical); Natalizumab; Pimecrolimus; Tacrolimus (Topical); Tofacitinib; Vaccines (Live)

Increased Effect/Toxicity
Imiquimod may increase the levels/effects of: Fingolimod; Leflunomide; Natalizumab; Tofacitinib; Vaccines (Live)

The levels/effects of Imiquimod may be increased by: Denosumab; Pimecrolimus; Roflumilast; Tacrolimus (Topical); Trastuzumab

◄ **Decreased Effect**
Imiquimod may decrease the levels/effects of: BCG (Intravesical); Cocci-dioides immitis Skin Test; Sipuleucel-T; Vaccines (Inactivated); Vaccines (Live)

The levels/effects of Imiquimod may be decreased by: Echinacea

Storage/Stability

Aldara®: Store at 4°C to 25°C (39°F to 77°F); do not freeze.

Vyloma™ (Canadian availability; not available in U.S.): Store at 15°C to 25°C (59°F to 77°F); do not freeze.

Zyclara®: Store at 25°C (77°F); excursions permitted to 15°C to 30°C (59°F to 86°F); do not freeze.

Mechanism of Action Precise mechanism of action is unknown; Toll-like receptor 7 agonist that induces cytokines, including interferon-alpha and others

Pharmacodynamics/Kinetics

Absorption: Minimal; systemic absorption more dependent upon surface area of application as opposed to dose

Time to peak: 9-12 hours

Excretion: Urine (≤2% of applied dose as imiquimod and metabolites)

Dosing

Adult & Geriatric Note: Imiquimod treatment should not be prolonged beyond recommended period due to missed doses or rest periods.

U.S. labeling:

Perianal warts/condyloma acuminata: Topical:

Aldara®: Apply a thin layer 3 times/week on alternative days prior to bedtime and leave on skin for 6-10 hours. Remove by washing with mild soap and water. Continue imiquimod treatment until there is total clearance of the genital/perianal warts or a maximum duration of therapy of 16 weeks.

Zyclara® 3.75%: Apply a thin layer using up to 1 packet or 1 full actuation of pump once daily prior to bedtime and leave on skin for ~8 hours. Remove with mild soap and water. Continue treatment until there is total clearance of the warts or a maximum duration of therapy of 8 weeks. Patient should not receive more than 56 packets or 2 x 7.5 g pumps or 1 x 15 g pump per course of treatment.

Actinic keratosis: Topical: **Note:** Prescribed course of therapy should be completed even if all lesions appear to be gone. Safety and efficacy of repeated use in a previously treated area has not been established.

Aldara®: Treatment should be limited to areas ≤25 cm^2; apply 2 times/week for 16 weeks to a treatment area on face or scalp (but not both concurrently); no more than 1 packet should be applied at each application and no more than 36 packets applied per 16 weeks; apply prior to bedtime and leave on skin for ~8 hours. Remove with mild soap and water.

Zyclara® 2.5%, 3.75%: Treatment consists of 2 cycles (14 days each) separated by 1 rest period (14 days) with no treatment. Apply up to 2 packets or 2 full actuations of pump once daily at bedtime to affected area on either face or balding scalp (but not both concurrently); leave on skin for ~8 hours. Remove with mild soap and water. Patient should not receive more than 56 packets or 2 x 7.5 g pumps or 1 x 15 g pump per 2 cycles of treatment.

Superficial basal cell carcinoma: Topical: Aldara®: Apply once daily prior to bedtime, 5 days/week for 6 weeks. No more than 36 packets should be used during the 6-week treatment period. Tumor treatment area should not exceed 3 cm (maximum of 2 cm tumor diameter plus a 1 cm margin of skin around the tumor). The diameter of cream droplet applied should range from 4 mm to 7 mm for tumor areas of 0.5 cm to 2 cm, respectively. Leave on skin for ~8 hours. Remove with mild soap and water. Safety and efficacy of repeated use in a previously treated area have not been established.

Canadian labeling:

Actinic keratosis: Topical: **Note:** Prescribed course of therapy should be completed even if all lesions appear to be gone; safety and efficacy of repeated use in a previously treated area have not been established.

Aldara®: Treatment should be limited to areas ≤25 cm²; apply 2 times/ week for 16 weeks to a treatment area on face or scalp (but not both concurrently); no more than 1 packet should be applied at each application; apply prior to bedtime and leave on skin for ~8 hours. Remove with mild soap and water.

Zyclara®: Treatment should be limited to an area <200 cm² on the face or scalp and consists of 2 cycles (14 days each) separated by 1 rest period (14 days) with no treatment. Apply up to 2 packets or 2 full actuations of pump once daily at bedtime to affected area on either face or balding scalp (but not both concurrently). Leave on skin for ~8 hours. Remove with mild soap and water. Patient should not receive more than 56 packets or 2 x 7.5 g pumps or 1 x 15 g pump per 2 cycles of treatment.

External genital and/or perianal warts/condyloma acuminata: Topical:

Aldara®: Apply a thin layer 3 times/week prior to bedtime and leave on skin for 6-10 hours. Remove with mild soap and water. Examples of 3 times/week application schedules are: Monday, Wednesday, Friday; or Tuesday, Thursday, Saturday. Continue treatment until there is total clearance of the warts or a maximum duration of therapy of 16 weeks.

Vyloma™: Apply a thin layer once daily prior to bedtime and leave on skin for ~8 hours. Remove with mild soap and water. Continue treatment until there is total clearance of the warts or maximum duration of therapy of 8 weeks.

Superficial basal cell carcinoma: Topical: Aldara®: Apply once daily prior to bedtime, 5 days/week for 6 weeks. Tumor treatment area should not exceed 3 cm (maximum of 2 cm tumor diameter plus a 1 cm margin of skin around the tumor). The diameter of cream droplet applied should range from 4 mm to 7 mm for tumor areas of 0.5 cm to 2 cm, respectively. Leave on skin for ~8 hours. Remove with mild soap and water. Safety and efficacy of repeated use in a previously treated area have not been established.

Common warts (off-label use): Topical (5% cream): Apply once daily prior to bedtime for 5 days/week for up to 16 weeks (Hengge, 2000) or apply twice daily for up to 24 weeks (Grussendorf-Conen, 2002)

Dosing adjustment for toxicity:

Local skin reactions (eg, erythema, edema, scabbing, etc): Temporarily interrupt treatment for up to several days for severe or intolerable reactions; may consider resuming therapy once reaction subsides.

Systemic/flu-like reactions (eg, malaise, fever, rigors, etc): Consider temporary interruption of therapy.

Vulvar swelling: Interrupt or discontinue therapy for severe vulvar swelling. ▶

◄ **Pediatric** Perianal warts/condyloma acuminata: Topical: Aldara®: Children ≥12 years: Refer to adult dosing.

Renal Impairment No dosage adjustment provided in manufacturer's labeling.

Hepatic Impairment No dosage adjustment provided in manufacturer's labeling.

Administration Topical: For all products, wash hands prior to and following application. Zyclara® pump should be primed prior to first use only by pressing top of pump completely down repeatedly until cream appears; discard cream obtained during priming. No further priming is required throughout therapy. Zyclara® pump should be discarded after a full course of therapy has been completed. Partially used packets of imiquimod cream should be discarded and not reused. Do not occlude the application site.

Actinic keratosis: The treatment area should be washed and thoroughly dried prior to application. Apply Aldara® over a single contiguous area (approximately 25 cm^2) on the face or scalp or Zyclara® over an area <200 cm^2 on the face or scalp. Both areas should not be treated concurrently. Apply a thin layer to the affected area and rub in until the cream is no longer visible. Avoid contact with the eyes, lips, and nostrils.

External genital warts: Instruct patients to apply to external or perianal warts; not for vaginal use. Apply a thin layer to the wart area and rub in until the cream is no longer visible. Avoid use of excessive amounts of cream. Nonocclusive dressings (such as cotton gauze or cotton underwear) may be used in the management of skin reactions.

Superficial basal cell carcinoma: Aldara®: Treatment area should have a maximum diameter no more than 2 cm on the trunk, neck, or extremities (excluding the hands, feet, and anogenital skin). Treatment area should include a 1 cm margin around the tumor. Wash and thoroughly dry treatment area prior to application; apply a thin layer to the affected area (and margin) and rub in until the cream is no longer visible. Avoid contact with the eyes, lips, and nostrils.

Monitoring Parameters Reduction in lesion size is indicative of a therapeutic response; signs and symptoms of hypersensitivity to imiquimod

Dosage Forms Excipient information presented when available (limited, particularly for generics); consult specific product labeling. [DSC] = Discontinued product

Cream, External:

Aldara: 5% (12 ea, 24 ea [DSC]) [contains benzyl alcohol, cetyl alcohol, methylparaben, propylparaben, sorbitan monostearate(sorbitan stearate)]

Zyclara: 3.75% (28 ea) [contains benzyl alcohol, cetyl alcohol, methylparaben, propylparaben]

Zyclara Pump: 2.5% (7.5 g); 3.75% (7.5 g) [contains benzyl alcohol, cetyl alcohol, methylparaben, propylparaben]

Generic: 5% (1 ea, 12 ea, 24 ea)

Dosage Forms: Canada Excipient information presented when available (limited, particularly for generics); consult specific product labeling.

Cream, topical:

Vyloma™: 3.75% (28s) [contains benzyl alcohol; 0.25 g/packet]

♦ **Imlygic** *see* Talimogene Laherparepvec *on page 1590*

♦ **Imlygic** *see* Talimogene Laherparepvec *on page 1590*

♦ **ImmuCyst (Can)** *see* BCG (Intravesical) *on page 174*

Immune Globulin (i MYUN GLOB yoo lin)

Related Information

Hematopoietic Stem Cell Transplantation *on page 2272*
Immune Globulin Product Comparison *on page 2335*
Prevention and Management of Infections *on page 2196*

Brand Names: US Bivigam; Carimune NF; Flebogamma DIF; Flebogamma [DSC]; GamaSTAN S/D; Gammagard; Gammagard S/D Less IgA; Gammagard S/D [DSC]; Gammaked; Gammaplex; Gamunex [DSC]; Gamunex-C; Hizentra; Hyqvia; Octagam; Privigen

Brand Names: Canada Gamastan S/D; Gammagard Liquid; Gammagard S/D; Gamunex; Hizentra; IGIVnex; Octagam 10%; Privigen

Index Terms Gamma Globulin; Human Normal Immunoglobulin; HyQvia; IG; IGIM; IGIV; IGSC; IMIG; Immune Globulin Subcutaneous (Human); Immune Serum Globulin; ISG; IV Immune Globulin; IVIG; Normal Immunoglobulin; Octagam 10%; Panglobulin; SCIG

Pharmacologic Category Blood Product Derivative; Immune Globulin

Use

Treatment of primary humoral immunodeficiency syndromes (congenital agammaglobulinemia, severe combined immunodeficiency syndromes [SCIDS], common variable immunodeficiency, X-linked immunodeficiency, Wiskott-Aldrich syndrome) (Bivigam, Carimune NF, Flebogamma DIF, HyQvia, Gammagard Liquid, Gammagard S/D, Gammaked, Gammaplex, Gamunex-C, Hizentra, Octagam 5%, Privigen)

Treatment of acute and chronic immune thrombocytopenia (ITP) (Carimune NF, Gammagard S/D, Gammaked, Gammaplex [chronic only], Gamunex-C, Octagam 10% [chronic only], Privigen [chronic only])

Treatment of chronic inflammatory demyelinating polyneuropathy (CIDP) (Gammaked, Gamunex-C)

Treatment of multifocal motor neuropathy (MMN) (Gammagard Liquid)

Prevention of coronary artery aneurysms associated with Kawasaki syndrome (in combination with aspirin) (Gammagard S/D)

Prevention of bacterial infection in patients with hypogammaglobulinemia and/or recurrent bacterial infections with B-cell chronic lymphocytic leukemia (CLL) (Gammagard S/D)

Provision of passive immunity in the following susceptible individuals (GamaSTAN S/D):

Hepatitis A: Pre-exposure prophylaxis; postexposure: within 14 days and/or prior to manifestation of disease

Measles: For use within 6 days of exposure in an unvaccinated person, who has not previously had measles

Rubella: Postexposure prophylaxis to reduce the risk of infection and fetal damage in exposed pregnant women who will not consider therapeutic abortion

Varicella: For immunosuppressed patients when varicella zoster immune globulin is not available

Labeled Contraindications Hypersensitivity to immune globulin or any component of the formulation; IgA deficiency (with anti-IgA antibodies and history of hypersensitivity); hyperprolinemia (Hizentra, Privigen); isolated IgA deficiency (GamaSTAN S/D); severe thrombocytopenia or coagulation disorders where IM injections are contraindicated (GamaSTAN S/D); hypersensitivity to corn (Octagam); hereditary intolerance to fructose (excluding Flebogamma); infants/neonates for whom sucrose or fructose tolerance has not been established (Gammaplex); hypersensitivity to hyaluronidase or recombinant human hyaluronidase (HyQvia)

Pregnancy Considerations Animal reproduction studies have not been conducted. Immune globulins cross the placenta in increased amounts after 30 weeks gestation. Intravenous immune globulin has been recommended for use in fetal-neonatal alloimmune thrombocytopenia and pregnancy-associated ITP (Anderson, 2007). Intravenous immune globulin is recommended to prevent measles in nonimmune women exposed during pregnancy (CDC, 2013). May also be used in postexposure prophylaxis for rubella to reduce the risk of infection and fetal damage in exposed pregnant women who will not consider therapeutic abortion (per GamaSTAN S/D product labeling; use for postexposure rubella prophylaxis is not currently recommended [CDC, 2013]).

HyQvia: Women who become pregnant during treatment are encouraged to enroll in the HyQvia Pregnancy Registry (1-866-424-6724).

Breast-Feeding Considerations It is not known if immune globulin from these preparations is excreted in breast milk. The manufacturer recommends that caution be exercised when administering immune globulin to nursing women. The manufacturer of HyQvia recommends administration to nursing women only if clearly indicated.

Warnings/Precautions [U.S. Boxed Warning]: IV administration only: Acute renal dysfunction (increased serum creatinine, oliguria, acute renal failure, osmotic nephrosis) can rarely occur and has been associated with fatalities; usually within 7 days of use (more likely with products stabilized with sucrose). Use with caution in the elderly, patients with renal disease, diabetes mellitus, overweight, hypovolemia, volume depletion, sepsis, paraproteinemia, and nephrotoxic medications due to risk of renal dysfunction. In patients at risk of renal dysfunction, ensure adequate hydration prior to administration; the dose, rate of infusion and concentration of solution should be minimized. Discontinue if renal function deteriorates.

[U.S. Boxed Warning]: Thrombosis may occur with immune globulin products even in the absence of risk factors for thrombosis. For patients at risk of thrombosis (eg, advanced age, history of atherosclerosis, impaired cardiac output, prolonged immobilization, hypercoagulable conditions, history of venous or arterial thrombosis, use of estrogens, indwelling central vascular catheters, hyperviscosity, and cardiovascular risk factors), administer at the minimum dose and infusion rate practicable. Ensure adequate hydration before administration. Monitor for signs and symptoms of thrombosis and assess blood viscosity in patients at risk for hyperviscosity such as those with cryoglobulins, fasting chylomicronemia/severe hypertriglyceridemia, or monoclonal gammopathies.

High-dose regimens (1 g/kg for 1 to 2 days) are not recommended for individuals with fluid overload or where fluid volume may be of concern. Hypersensitivity and anaphylactic reactions can occur (some severe); patients with anti-IgA antibodies are at greater risk; a severe fall in blood pressure may rarely occur with anaphylactic reaction; discontinue therapy and institute immediate treatment (including epinephrine 1:1000) should be available. Product of human plasma; may potentially contain infectious agents which could transmit disease, including unknown or emerging viruses and other pathogens. Screening of donors, as well as testing and/or inactivation or removal of certain viruses, reduces the risk. Infections thought to be transmitted by this product should be reported to the manufacturer. Aseptic meningitis may occur with high doses (≥1 g/kg) and/or rapid infusion; syndrome usually appears within several hours to 2 days following treatment; usually resolves within several days after product is discontinued; patients with a migraine history may be at higher risk for AMS. Increased risk of hypersensitivity, especially in patients with anti-IgA antibodies; use is contraindicated in patients with IgA deficiency (with antibodies against IgA and history of hypersensitivity) or isolated IgA deficiency (GamaSTAN S/D). Increased risk of hematoma formation when administered subcutaneously for the treatment of ITP.

Intravenous immune globulin has been associated with antiglobulin hemolysis (acute or delayed); monitor for signs of hemolytic anemia. Cases of hemolysis-related renal dysfunction/failure or disseminated intravascular coagulation (DIC) have been reported. Risk factors include high doses (≥2 g/kg) and non-O blood type (FDA, 2012). In chronic ITP, assess risk versus benefit of high-dose regimen in patients with increased risk of thrombosis, hemolysis, acute kidney injury, or volume overload.

Patients should be adequately hydrated prior to initiation of therapy. Hyperproteinemia, increased serum viscosity and hyponatremia may occur; distinguish hyponatremia from pseudohyponatremia to prevent volume depletion, a further increase in serum viscosity, and a higher risk of thrombotic events. Patients should be monitored for adverse events during and after the infusion. Stop administration with signs of infusion reaction (fever, chills, nausea, vomiting, and rarely shock). Risk may be increased with initial treatment, when switching brands of immune globulin, and with treatment interruptions of >8 weeks. Monitor for transfusion-related acute lung injury (TRALI); noncardiogenic pulmonary edema has been reported with immune globulin use. TRALI is characterized by severe respiratory distress, pulmonary edema, normal left ventricular function, hypoxemia, and fever (in the presence of normal left ventricular function) and usually occurs within 1 to 6 hours after infusion. Response to live vaccinations may be impaired. Some clinicians may administer intravenous immune globulin products as a subcutaneous infusion based on patient tolerability and clinical judgment. SubQ infusion should begin 1 week after the last IV dose; dose should be individualized based on clinical response and serum IgG trough concentrations; consider premedicating with acetaminophen and diphenhydramine.

Use with caution in the elderly; may be at increased risk for renal dysfunction/failure and thromboembolic events. Some products may contain maltose, which may result in falsely elevated blood glucose readings; maltose-containing products may be contraindicated in patients with an allergy to corn. Some products may contain sodium and/or sucrose. Some dosage forms may contain polysorbate 80 (also known as Tweens). Hypersensitivity reactions, usually a delayed reaction, have been reported following exposure to pharmaceutical products containing polysorbate 80 in certain individuals (Isaksson, 2002; Lucente 2000; Shelley, 1995). Thrombocytopenia, ascites, pulmonary deterioration, and renal and hepatic failure have been reported in premature neonates after receiving parenteral products containing polysorbate 80 (Alade, 1986; CDC, 1984). See manufacturer's labeling. Some products may contain sorbitol; do not use in patients with fructose intolerance. Hizentra and Privigen contain the stabilizer L-proline and are contraindicated in patients with hyperprolinemia. Packaging of some products may contain natural latex/natural rubber; skin testing should not be performed with GamaSTAN S/D as local irritation can occur and be misinterpreted as a positive reaction. Potentially ▶

◀ significant interactions may exist, requiring dose or frequency adjustment, additional monitoring, and/or selection of alternative therapy.

Adverse Reactions Frequency not defined. Adverse effects are reported as class effects rather than for specific products.

Cardiovascular: Chest tightness, edema, facial flushing, hypertension, hypotension, palpitations, tachycardia

Central nervous system: Anxiety, aseptic meningitis, chills, dizziness, drowsiness, fatigue, headache, lethargy, malaise, migraine, pain, rigors

Dermatologic: Dermatitis, diaphoresis, eczema, erythema, hyperhidrosis, pruritus, skin rash, urticaria

Endocrine & metabolic: Dehydration, increased lactate dehydrogenase

Gastrointestinal: Abdominal cramps, abdominal pain, diarrhea, dyspepsia, gastroenteritis, gastrointestinal distress, nausea, sore throat, toothache, vomiting

Genitourinary: Anuria, oliguria, osmotic nephrosis, proximal tubular nephropathy

Hematologic & oncologic: Anemia, bruise, decreased hematocrit, hematoma, hemolysis (mild), hemolytic anemia, hemorrhage, petechia, purpura, thrombocytopenia

Hepatic: Increased serum bilirubin

Hypersensitivity: Anaphylaxis, angioedema, hypersensitivity reaction

Local: Infusion site reaction (including erythema at injection site, irritation at injection site, itching at injection site, pain at injection site, swelling at injection site, warm sensation at injection site)

Neuromuscular & skeletal: Arthralgia, back pain, leg cramps, limb pain, muscle cramps, muscle spasm, myalgia, neck pain, weakness

Ophthalmic: Conjunctivitis

Otic: Otalgia

Renal: Acute renal failure, increased blood urea nitrogen, increased serum creatinine, renal tubular necrosis

Respiratory: Bronchitis, cough, dyspnea, epistaxis, exacerbation of asthma, flu-like symptoms, nasal congestion, oropharyngeal pain, pharyngitis, rhinitis, rhinorrhea, sinusitis, upper respiratory tract infection, wheezing

Miscellaneous: Fever, infusion related reaction

<1%, postmarketing, and/or case reports: Acute respiratory distress, adult respiratory distress syndrome, allergic dermatitis, antibody development (nonneutralizing antibodies to recombinant human hyaluronidase), apnea, blurred vision, bronchopneumonia, bronchospasm, bullous dermatitis, burning sensation, cardiac arrest, cerebrovascular accident, chest pain, circulatory shock, coma, cyanosis, decreased serum alkaline phosphatase, disseminated intravascular coagulation, epidermolysis, erythema multiforme, exacerbation of autoimmune pure red cell aplasia, hepatic insufficiency, hypoxemia, increased serum alkaline phosphatase, increased serum ALT, increased serum AST, insomnia, leukopenia, loss of consciousness, myocardial infarction, oxygen desaturation, pancytopenia, positive direct Coombs test, pulmonary edema, pulmonary embolism, renal insufficiency, respiratory distress, seizure, Stevens-Johnson syndrome, syncope, thromboembolism, thrombosis, transfusion-related acute lung injury, transient ischemic attack, tremor

Drug Interactions

Metabolism/Transport Effects None known.

Avoid Concomitant Use There are no known interactions where it is recommended to avoid concomitant use.

Increased Effect/Toxicity

The levels/effects of Immune Globulin may be increased by: Estrogen Derivatives

Decreased Effect

Immune Globulin may decrease the levels/effects of: Vaccines (Live)

Storage/Stability Stability is dependent upon the manufacturer and brand. Do not freeze (do not use if previously frozen). Do not shake. Do not heat (do not use if previously heated).

Bivigam: Store under refrigeration at 2°C to 8°C (36°F to 46°F). Dilution is not recommended.

Carimune NF: Prior to reconstitution, store at or below 30°C (86°F). Reconstitute with NS, D₅W, or SWFI. Following reconstitution in a sterile laminar air flow environment, store under refrigeration. Begin infusion within 24 hours.

Flebogamma DIF: Store at 2°C to 25°C (36°F to 77°F). Keep in original carton to protect from light. Do not freeze or use if solution has been frozen.

GamaSTAN S/D: Store under refrigeration at 2°C to 8°C (36°F to 46°F). The following stability information has also been reported for GamaSTAN S/D: May be exposed to room temperature for a cumulative 7 days (Cohen, 2007).

Gammagard Liquid: Prior to use, store at 2°C to 8°C (36°F to 46°F). May store at room temperature of 25°C (77°F) within the first 24 months of manufacturing. Storage time at room temperature varies with length of time previously refrigerated; refer to product labeling for details.

Gammagard S/D: Store at ≤25°C (≤77°F). May store diluted solution under refrigeration at 2°C to 8°C (36°F to 46°F) for up to 24 hours if originally prepared in a sterile laminar air flow environment.

Gammaked: Store at 2°C to 8°C (36°F to 46°F); may be stored at ≤25°C (≤77°F) for up to 6 months.

Gammaplex: Store at 2°C to 25°C (36°F to 77°F). Keep in original carton to protect from light. Do not freeze or use if solution has been frozen.

Gamunex-C: Store at 2°C to 8°C (36°F to 46°F); may be stored at ≤25°C (≤77°F) for up to 6 months.

Hizentra: Store at ≤25°C (≤77°F). Keep in original carton to protect from light.

HyQvia: Store at 2°C to 8°C (36°F to 46°F) for up to 36 months; may store at ≤25°C (≤77°F) for up to 3 months during the first 24 months from the date of manufacture (after 3 months at room temperature, discard); do not return vial to refrigerator after it has been stored at room temperature.

Octagam 5%: Store at 2°C to 25°C (36°F to 77°F).

Octagam 10%: Store at 2°C to 8°C (36°F to 46°F) for 24 months from the date of manufacture; within these first 12 months, may store up to 6 months at ≤25°C (77°F); after storage at ≤25°C (77°F), the product must be used or discarded.

Privigen: Store at ≤25°C (≤77°F). Protect from light.

Preparation for Administration Dilution is dependent upon the manufacturer and brand. Gently swirl; do not shake; avoid foaming. Do not heat. Do not mix products from different manufacturers together. Discard unused portion of vials.

Bivigam: Dilution is not recommended.

Carimune NF: In a sterile laminar air flow environment, reconstitute with NS, D₅W, or SWFI. Complete dissolution may take up to 20 minutes. Begin infusion within 24 hours.

Flebogamma DIF: Dilution is not recommended.

Gammagard Liquid: May dilute in D₅W only.

◀ Gammagard S/D: Reconstitute with SWFI.

Gammaked: May dilute in D_5W only.

Gamunex-C: May dilute in D_5W only.

HyQvia: Bring refrigerated product to room temperature before use. Do **not** mix hyaluronidase and immune globulin prior to administration.

Octagam 10%: Do not dilute. Bottles may be pooled into sterile infusion bags and infused within 8 hours after pooling.

Privigen: If necessary to further dilute, D_5W may be used.

Mechanism of Action Replacement therapy for primary and secondary immunodeficiencies, and IgG antibodies against bacteria, viral, parasitic and mycoplasma antigens; interference with F_c receptors on the cells of the reticuloendothelial system for autoimmune cytopenias and ITP; provides passive immunity by increasing the antibody titer and antigen-antibody reaction potential

Pharmacodynamics/Kinetics

Onset of action: IV: Provides immediate antibody levels

Duration: IM, IV: Immune effect: 3 to 4 weeks (variable)

Distribution: V_d: 0.05 to 0.13 L/kg

Intravascular portion (primarily): Healthy subjects: 41% to 57%; Patients with congenital humoral immunodeficiencies: ~70%

Half-life elimination: IM: ~23 days; SubQ: ~59 days (HyQvia); IV: IgG (variable among patients): Healthy subjects: 14 to 24 days; Patients with congenital humoral immunodeficiencies: 26 to 40 days; hypermetabolism associated with fever and infection have coincided with a shortened half-life

Time to peak:

Plasma: SubQ: Gammagard Liquid: 2.9 days; Hizentra: 2.9 days; HyQvia: ~5 days.

Serum: IM: ~48 hours

Dosing

Adult & Geriatric Note: Some clinicians may administer IGIV formulations FDA approved only for intravenous administration as a subcutaneous infusion based on clinical judgment and patient tolerability.

B-cell chronic lymphocytic leukemia (CLL) with hypogammaglobulinemia, prevention of bacterial infections (Gammagard S/D): IV: 400 mg/kg every 3 to 4 weeks

Chronic inflammatory demyelinating polyneuropathy (CIDP) (Gammaked, Gamunex-C): IV: Loading dose: 2,000 mg/kg (given in divided doses over 2 to 4 consecutive days); Maintenance: 1,000 mg/kg every 3 weeks. Alternatively, administer 500 mg/kg/day for 2 consecutive days every 3 weeks.

Hepatitis A (GamaSTAN S/D): IM:

Preexposure prophylaxis upon travel into endemic areas (hepatitis A vaccine preferred):

0.02 **mL**/kg for anticipated risk of exposure <3 months

0.06 **mL**/kg for anticipated risk of exposure ≥3 months; repeat every 4 to 6 months.

Postexposure prophylaxis: 0.02 **mL**/kg given within 14 days of exposure and/or prior to manifestation of disease; not needed if at least 1 dose of hepatitis A vaccine was given at ≥1 month before exposure (CDC 2006)

Immune thrombocytopenia (ITP):

Carimune NF: IV: Initial: 400 mg/kg/day for 2 to 5 consecutive days (6% solution recommended); Maintenance: 400 mg/kg (no more frequent than daily) as needed to maintain platelet count ≥30,000/mm³ and/or to control significant bleeding; may increase dose if needed (range: 800 to 1,000 mg/kg).

Gammagard S/D: IV: 1,000 mg/kg; up to 3 total doses may be given on alternate days based on patient response and/or platelet count.

Gammaked, Gamunex-C: IV: 1,000 mg/kg/day for 2 consecutive days (second dose may be withheld if adequate platelet response in 24 hours) **or** 400 mg/kg once daily for 5 consecutive days

Gammaplex, Octagam 10%, Privigen: IV: 1,000 mg/kg/day for 2 consecutive days

Measles:

GamaSTAN S/D: IM:

Immunocompetent: 0.25 **mL**/kg given within 6 days of exposure

Immunocompromised children: 0.5 **mL**/kg (maximum dose: 15 **mL**) immediately following exposure

Postexposure prophylaxis, any nonimmune person (off-label population): Patients ≤30 kg: 0.5 **mL**/kg (maximum dose: 15 **mL**) within 6 days of exposure. If patient >30 kg, patient will have lower titers than what is recommended due to the maximum volume that can be administered (CDC 2013)

Gammaked, Gamunex-C, Octagam 5%: IV:

Preexposure prophylaxis in patients with primary humoral immunodeficiency (**ONLY** if routine dose is <400 mg/kg): ≥400 mg/kg immediately before expected exposure followed by resumption of prior dosing in 3 to 4 weeks.

Postexposure prophylaxis in patients with primary humoral immunodeficiency: 400 mg/kg administered as soon as possible after exposure followed by resumption of prior dosing in 3 to 4 weeks.

Postexposure prophylaxis, any nonimmune person (off-label population): 400 mg/kg within 6 days of exposure (CDC 2013)

Hizentra: SubQ infusion:

Preexposure prophylaxis in patients with primary humoral immunodeficiency at risk of measles exposure (eg, during an outbreak; travel to endemic area):

Patients receiving weekly or more frequent dosing: Ensure total weekly dose of ≥200 mg/kg for 2 consecutive weeks followed by resumption of prior dosing schedule

Patients receiving biweekly dosing: Administer ≥400 mg/kg once followed by resumption of prior dosing schedule.

Postexposure prophylaxis in patients with primary humoral immunodeficiency regardless of prior dosing schedule (daily, weekly, or biweekly): 400 mg/kg administered as soon as possible after exposure followed by resumption of prior dosing schedule.

ACIP recommendations: The Advisory Committee on Immunization Practices (ACIP) recommends postexposure prophylaxis with immune globulin (IG) to any nonimmune person exposed to measles. The following patient groups are at risk for severe measles complications and should receive IG therapy: Infants <12 months of age, pregnant women without evidence of immunity; severely compromised persons (eg, persons with severe primary immunodeficiency; some bone marrow transplant patients; some ALL patients; and some patients with AIDS or HIV infection [refer to guidelines for additional details]). IGIM is recommended for infants <12 months of age. IGIV is recommended for pregnant women and immunocompromised persons. Although prophylaxis may be given to any nonimmune person, priority should be given to those at greatest risk for ▶

measles complications and also to persons exposed in settings with intense, prolonged, close contact (eg, households, daycare centers, classrooms). Following IG administration, any nonimmune person should then receive the measles mumps and rubella (MMR) vaccine if the person is ≥12 months of age at the time of vaccine administration and the vaccine is not otherwise contraindicated. MMR should not be given until 6 months following IGIM or 8 months following IGIV administration. If a person is already receiving IGIV therapy, a dose of 400 mg/kg IV within 3 weeks prior to exposure (or 200 mg/kg SubQ for 2 consecutive weeks prior to exposure if previously on SubQ therapy) should be sufficient to prevent measles infection. IG therapy is not indicated for any person who already received one dose of a measles-containing vaccine at ≥12 months of age unless they are severely immunocompromised (CDC 2013).

Multifocal motor neuropathy (MMN) (Gammagard Liquid): IV: 500 to 2400 mg/kg/**month** based upon response

Primary humoral immunodeficiency disorders:

IV infusion dosing:

Bivigam, Gammaplex: IV: 300 to 800 mg/kg every 3 to 4 weeks; dose adjusted based on monitored trough serum IgG concentrations and clinical response

Carimune NF: IV: 400 to 800 mg/kg every 3 to 4 weeks. **Note:** In previously untreated agammaglobulinemic or hypogammaglobulinemic patients use a 3% solution; may administer subsequent infusions with a higher concentration if patient tolerates lower concentration.

Flebogamma DIF 5%, Flebogamma DIF 10%, Gammagard Liquid, Gammagard S/D, Gammaked, Gamunex-C, Octagam 5%: IV: 300 to 600 mg/kg every 3 to 4 weeks; dose adjusted based on monitored trough serum IgG concentrations and clinical response

Privigen: IV: 200 to 800 mg/kg every 3 to 4 weeks; dose adjusted based on monitored trough serum IgG concentrations and clinical response

Switching to weekly subcutaneous infusion dosing:

Gammagard Liquid, Gammaked, Gamunex-C: SubQ infusion: Begin 1 week after last IV dose. Use the following equation to calculate initial dose:

Initial weekly dose (g) = [1.37 x IGIV dose (g)] divided by [IV dose interval (weeks)]

Note: For subsequent dose adjustments, refer to product labeling.

Hizentra: SubQ infusion: For weekly or frequent (up to daily) dosing, begin 1 week after last IV infusion or SubQ infusion. For biweekly (every 2 week) dosing, begin 1 or 2 weeks after last IV infusion or 1 week after the last SubQ weekly infusion. **Note:** Patient should have received an IV immune globulin routinely for at least 3 months before switching to SubQ. Use the following equation to calculate initial weekly dose:

Initial weekly dose (g) = [Previous IGIV dose (g)] divided by [IV dose interval (eg, 3 or 4 weeks)] then multiply by 1.37. To convert the dose (in g) to mL, multiply the calculated dose (in g) by 5.

Note: Provided the total weekly dose is maintained, any dosing interval from daily up to biweekly (every 2 weeks) may be used. For patients switching to Hizentra from a different SubQ formulation, the previous weekly SubQ dose should be used initially. Use the following calculations to calculate frequent or biweekly dosing:

Biweekly dosing (g) = multiply the calculated or previous weekly dose by 2.

Frequent (2 to 7 times per week) dosing (g) = divide the calculated or previous weekly dose by the desired number of times per week (eg, for 3 times per week dosing, divide weekly dose by 3)

Note: For subsequent dose adjustments, refer to product labeling.

SubQ infusion dosing:

HyQvia: SubQ: See manufacturer's labeling for initial ramp-up schedule (initiating treatment with a full monthly dose has not been evaluated); dose adjusted based on monitored trough serum IgG concentrations and clinical response after initial ramp-up. **Note:** For patients previously on another IgG treatment, administer the first dose ~1 week after the last infusion of previous treatment.

Patients naive to IgG therapy or switching from IG SubQ therapy: SubQ infusion: 300 to 600 mg/kg every 3 to 4 weeks, after the initial dose ramp-up

Patients switching from IGIV therapy: SubQ infusion: Administer the same dose and frequency as the previous IGIV therapy after the initial dose ramp-up. For subsequent dose adjustments, refer to product labeling.

Rubella (GamaSTAN S/D): IM: Postexposure prophylaxis during pregnancy: 0.55 mL/kg

Varicella (GamaSTAN S/D): IM: Prophylaxis: 0.6 to 1.2 mL/kg (varicella zoster immune globulin preferred) within 72 hours of exposure (Gershon 1978). **Note:** For patients at risk of thrombosis, administer at the lower end of the recommended dosage range.

Off-label uses: IV:

Acquired hypogammaglobulinemia secondary to malignancy (off-label use): 400 mg/kg/dose every 3 weeks; reevaluate every 4 to 6 months (Anderson 2007)

Dermatomyositis/polymyositis (refractory) (use in combination with other agents in patients with dermatomyositis) (off-label use): 2,000 mg/kg per treatment course administered in divided doses over 2 to 5 consecutive days (eg, 400 mg/kg/day for 5 days); maximum (per treatment course): 2,000 mg/kg (Feasby 2007).

Guillain-Barré syndrome (off-label use): A total dose of 2 g/kg per treatment course, given in divided doses over 2 to 5 consecutive days (eg, 400 mg/kg/day for 5 days) (Feasby 2007; Hughes 2014). European Federation of Neurological Societies (EFNS) guidelines recommend the 5-day treatment regimen (Elovaara, 2008).

Hematopoietic cell transplantation (HCT) with hypogammaglobulinemia (IgG <400 mg/dL), prevention of bacterial infection (off-label use): **Note:** Increase dose or frequency to maintain IgG concentration >400 mg/dL.

≤100 days post-HCT: 500 mg/kg/dose once weekly (Tomblyn 2009)

>100 days post-HCT: 500 mg/kg/dose every 3 to 4 weeks (Tomblyn 2009)

HIV-associated thrombocytopenia (off-label use): 1,000 mg/kg/day for 2 days (Anderson 2007)

Lambert-Eaton myasthenic syndrome (LEMS) (off-label use): 1,000 mg/kg/day for 2 days (Bain 1996; Patwa 2012)

Myasthenia gravis (acute exacerbation) (off-label use): Adjunctive therapy: 2 g/kg per treatment course, administered in divided doses over 2 to 5 consecutive days (eg, 400 mg/kg/day for 5 days) (Barth 2011; Feasby 2007; Zinman 2007). **Note:** A single dose of 1 g/kg may have similar efficacy to 1 g/kg given on 2 consecutive days (Gajdos 2005)

◀ **Relapsing-remitting multiple sclerosis (off-label use):** 1,000 mg/kg per month, with or without an induction of 400 mg/kg/day for 5 days (Feasby 2007). Optimal dosing has not been established.

Pediatric Note: Flebogamma DIF 10%, HyQvia, and Octagam 10% are **not** FDA-approved for use in children.

Children and Adolescents:

Hepatitis A: Refer to adult dosing.

Immune thrombocytopenia (ITP):

Carimune NF: IV: Initial: 400 mg/kg/day for 2 to 5 consecutive days (6% solution recommended); Maintenance: 400 mg/kg (no more frequent than daily) as needed to maintain platelet count ≥30,000/mm^3 and/or to control significant bleeding; may increase dose if needed (range: 800 to 1,000 mg/kg). For acute ITP, may discontinue after day 2 if platelet response is adequate (30,000 to 50,000/mm^3) after the first 2 doses.

Gammaked, Gamunex-C: IV: 1,000 mg/kg/day for 2 consecutive days (second dose may be withheld if adequate platelet response in 24 hours) **or** 400 mg/kg once daily for 5 consecutive days.

Privigen: IV: 1,000 mg/kg/day for 2 consecutive days (not approved for use in pediatric patients <15 years of age).

Kawasaki syndrome: IV:

Gammagard S/D: 1,000 mg/kg as a single dose **or** 400 mg/kg/day for 4 consecutive days. Begin within 7 days of onset of fever.

AHA guidelines (2004): 2,000 mg/kg as a single dose within 10 days of disease onset

Note: Must be used in combination with aspirin: 80 to 100 mg/kg/day orally, divided every 6 hours for up to 14 days (until fever resolves for at least 48 hours); then decrease dose to 3 to 5 mg/kg/day once daily. In patients without coronary artery abnormalities, give lower dose for 6 to 8 weeks. In patients with coronary artery abnormalities, low-dose aspirin should be continued indefinitely.

Measles: Refer to adult dosing.

Primary humoral immunodeficiency disorders:

IV infusion dosing:

Bivigam: IV: Children ≥6 years and Adolescents: 300 to 800 mg/kg every 3 to 4 weeks; dose adjusted based on monitored trough serum IgG concentrations and clinical response

Carimune NF: IV: Children and Adolescents: 400 to 800 mg/kg every 3 to 4 weeks. **Note:** In previously untreated agammaglobulinemic or hypogammaglobulinemic patients use a 3% solution; may administer subsequent infusions with a higher concentration if patient tolerates lower concentration.

Flebogamma DIF 5%: IV: Children ≥2 years, and Adolescents: 300 to 600 mg/kg every 3 to 4 weeks; dose adjusted based on monitored trough serum IgG concentrations and clinical response

Gammagard Liquid, Gammagard S/D: IV: Children ≥2 years and Adolescents: 300 to 600 mg/kg every 3 to 4 weeks; dose adjusted based on monitored trough serum IgG concentrations and clinical response.

Gammaked, Gamunex-C, Octagam 5%: IV: Children and Adolescents: 300 to 600 mg/kg every 3 to 4 weeks; dose adjusted based on monitored trough serum IgG concentrations and clinical response.

Gammaplex: IV: Children ≥2 years, and Adolescents: 300 to 800 mg/kg every 3 to 4 weeks; dose adjusted based on monitored trough serum IgG concentrations and clinical response.

Privigen: IV: Children ≥3 years and Adolescents: 200 to 800 mg/kg every 3 to 4 weeks; dose adjusted based on monitored trough serum IgG concentrations and clinical response

Switching to weekly subcutaneous infusion dosing:

Gammagard Liquid: Children ≥2 years and Adolescents:

SubQ infusion: Begin 1 week after last IV dose. Use the following equation to calculate initial dose:

Initial weekly dose (g) = [1.37 x IGIV dose (g)] divided by [IV dose interval (weeks)]

Note: For subsequent dose adjustments, refer to product labeling.

Hizentra: SubQ infusion: Children ≥2 years and Adolescents: For weekly or frequent (up to daily) dosing, begin 1 week after last IV infusion or SubQ infusion. For biweekly (every 2 week) dosing, begin 1 or 2 weeks after last IV infusion or 1 week after the last SubQ weekly infusion.

Note: Patient should have received an IV immune globulin routinely for at least 3 months before switching to SubQ. Use the following equation to calculate initial weekly dose:

Initial weekly dose (g) = [Previous IGIV dose (g)] divided by [IV dose interval (eg, 3 or 4 weeks)] then multiply by 1.37. To convert the dose (in g) to mL, multiply the calculated dose (in g) by 5.

Note: Provided the total weekly dose is maintained, any dosing interval from daily up to biweekly (every 2 weeks) may be used. For patients switching to Hizentra from a different SubQ formulation, the previous weekly SubQ dose should be used initially. Use the following calculations to calculate frequent or biweekly dosing:

Biweekly dosing (g) = multiply the calculated or previous weekly dose by 2.

Frequent (2 to 7 times per week) dosing (g) = divide the calculated or previous weekly dose by the desired number of times per week (eg, for 3 times per week dosing, divide weekly dose by 3).

Note: For subsequent dose adjustments, refer to product labeling.

Varicella: Refer to adult dosing.

Dermatomyositis/polymyositis (refractory) (use in combination with other agents in patients with dermatomyositis) (off-label use): IV: 2,000 mg/kg per treatment course administered in divided doses over 2 consecutive days (eg, 1,000 mg/kg/day for 2 days); maximum (per treatment course): 2,000 mg/kg (Feasby 2007)

Guillain-Barré syndrome (off-label use): Children and Adolescents: IV: 1,000 mg/kg/day for 2 days (Feasby 2007; Korinthenberg 2005) **or** 400 mg/kg/day for 5 days (El-Bayoumi 2011; Korinthenberg 2005). Two-day regimens have been associated with a higher incidence of early relapse (Korinthenberg 2005). American Academy of Neurology guidelines state optimal dosing has not been established (Patwa 2012).

Hematopoietic cell transplantation (HCT) with hypogammaglobulinemia (IgG <400 mg/dL), prevention of bacterial infection (off-label use) (Tomblyn 2009): IV: **Note:** Increase dose or frequency to maintain IgG concentration >400 mg/dL.

≤100 days post-HCT:

Infants and Children (Allogeneic HCT recipients): IV: 400 mg/kg/dose once monthly

Adolescents: IV: 500 mg/kg/dose once weekly

>100 days post-HCT: Infants, Children, and Adolescents: IV: 500 mg/kg/dose every 3 to 4 weeks

▶

Myasthenia gravis (acute exacerbation) (off-label use): Adolescents: Refer to adult dosing.

Renal Impairment

IV: Use with caution due to risk of immune globulin-induced renal dysfunction; the rate of infusion and concentration of solution should be minimized.

IM, SubQ infusion: There are no dosage adjustments provided in the manufacturer's labeling; risk of immune globulin-induced renal dysfunction has not been identified with IM and SubQ infusion administration.

Hepatic Impairment IM, IV, SubQ infusion: There are no dosage adjustments provided in manufacturer's labeling.

Obesity Some clinicians dose IGIV on ideal body weight or an adjusted ideal body weight in morbidly obese patients (Siegel 2010).

Administration Note: If plasmapheresis employed for treatment of condition, administer immune globulin **after** completion of plasmapheresis session.

IM: Administer IM in the anterolateral aspects of the upper thigh or deltoid muscle of the upper arm. Avoid gluteal region due to risk of injury to sciatic nerve. Divide doses >10 mL and inject in multiple sites.

GamaSTAN S/D is for IM administration only.

IV infusion: Infuse over 2 to 24 hours; administer in separate infusion line from other medications; if using primary line, flush with NS or D_5W (product specific; consult product prescribing information) prior to administration. Decrease dose, rate and/or concentration of infusion in patients who may be at risk of renal failure. Decreasing the rate or stopping the infusion may help relieve some adverse effects (flushing, changes in pulse rate, changes in blood pressure). Epinephrine should be available during administration. For initial treatment or in the elderly, a lower concentration and/or a slower rate of infusion should be used. Initial rate of administration and titration is specific to each IGIV product. Refrigerated product should be warmed to room temperature prior to infusion. Some products require filtration; refer to individual product labeling. Antecubital veins should be used, especially with concentrations ≥10% to prevent injection site discomfort.

Bivigam 10%: Primary humoral immunodeficiency: Initial (first 10 minutes): 0.5 mg/kg/minute (0.3 **mL**/kg/**hour**); Maintenance: Increase every 20 minutes (if tolerated) by 0.8 mg/kg/minute (0.48 **mL**/kg/**hour**) up to 6 mg/kg/minute (3.6 **mL**/kg/**hour**)

Carimune NF: Refer to product labeling.

Flebogamma DIF 5%: Primary humoral immunodeficiency: Initial: 0.5 mg/kg/minute (0.6 **mL**/kg/**hour**); Maintenance: Increase slowly (if tolerated) up to 5 mg/kg/minute (6 **mL**/kg/**hour**)

Flebogamma DIF 10%: Primary humoral immunodeficiency: Initial: 1 mg/kg/minute (0.6 **mL**/kg/**hour**); Maintenance: Increase slowly (if tolerated) up to 8 mg/kg/minute (4.8 **mL**/kg/**hour**)

Gammagard Liquid 10%:

Multifocal motor neuropathy (MMN): Initial: 0.8 mg/kg/minute (0.5 **mL**/kg/**hour**); Maintenance: Increase gradually (if tolerated) up to 9 mg/kg/minute (5.4 **mL**/kg/**hour**)

Primary humoral immunodeficiency: Initial (first 30 minutes): 0.8 mg/kg/minute (0.5 **mL**/kg/**hour**); Maintenance: Increase every 30 minutes (if tolerated) up to: 8 mg/kg/minute (5 **mL**/kg/**hour**)

Gammagard S/D: 5% solution: Initial: 0.5 **mL**/kg/**hour**; may increase (if tolerated) to a maximum rate of 4 **mL**/kg/**hour**. If 5% solution is tolerated at maximum rate, may administer 10% solution with an initial rate of 0.5 **mL**/kg/**hour**; may increase (if tolerated) to a maximum rate of 8 **mL**/kg/**hour**

Gammaked 10%:

   CIDP: Initial (first 30 minutes): 2 mg/kg/minute (1.2 **mL**/kg/**hour**); Maintenance: Increase gradually (if tolerated) up to 8 mg/kg/minute (4.8 **mL**/kg/**hour**)

   Primary humoral immunodeficiency or ITP: Initial (first 30 minutes): 1 mg/kg/minute (0.6 **mL**/kg/**hour**); Maintenance: Increase gradually (if tolerated) up to 8 mg/kg/minute (4.8 **mL**/kg/**hour**)

Gammaplex 5%: Primary humoral immunodeficiency or ITP: Initial (first 15 minutes): 0.5 mg/kg/minute (0.6 **mL**/kg/**hour**); Maintenance: Increase every 15 minutes (if tolerated) up to 4 mg/kg/minute (4.8 **mL**/kg/**hour**)

Gamunex-C 10%:

   CIDP: Initial (first 30 minutes): 2 mg/kg/minute (1.2 **mL**/kg/**hour**); Maintenance: Increase gradually (if tolerated) up to 8 mg/kg/minute (4.8 **mL**/kg/**hour**)

   Primary humoral immunodeficiency or ITP: Initial (first 30 minutes): 1 mg/kg/minute (0.6 **mL**/kg/**hour**); Maintenance: Increase gradually (if tolerated) up to 8 mg/kg/minute (4.8 **mL**/kg/**hour**)

Octagam 5%: Primary humoral immunodeficiency: Initial (first 30 minutes): 0.5 mg/kg/minute (0.6 **mL**/kg/**hour**); Maintenance: Double infusion rate (if tolerated) every 30 minutes up to a maximum rate of <3.33 mg/kg/minute (4.2 **mL**/kg/**hour**)

Octagam 10%: ITP: Initial (first 30 minutes):1 mg/kg/minute (0.6 **mL**/kg/**hour**); Maintenance: Double infusion rate (if tolerated) every 30 minutes up to a maximum rate of 12 mg/kg/minute (7.2 **mL**/kg/**hour**)

Privigen 10%:

   ITP: Initial: 0.5 mg/kg/minute (0.3 **mL**/kg/**hour**); Maintenance: Increase gradually (if tolerated) up to 4 mg/kg/minute (2.4 **mL**/kg/**hour**)

   Primary humoral immunodeficiency: Initial: 0.5 mg/kg/minute (0.3 **mL**/kg/**hour**); Maintenance: Increase gradually (if tolerated) up to 8 mg/kg/minute (4.8 **mL**/kg/**hour**)

SubQ infusion: Initial dose should be administered in a healthcare setting capable of providing monitoring and treatment in the event of hypersensitivity. Using aseptic technique, follow the infusion device manufacturer's instructions for filling the reservoir and preparing the pump. Remove air from administration set and needle by priming. For products excluding HyQvia, appropriate injection sites include the abdomen, thigh, upper arm, lower back, and/or lateral hip; dose may be infused into multiple sites (spaced ≥2 inches apart) simultaneously. HyQvia may be injected into the middle to upper abdomen or thigh (avoid bony prominences, or areas that are scarred, inflamed, or infected). If two sites are used simultaneously for HyQvia, the two infusion sites should be on opposite sides of the body. After the sites are clean and dry, insert subcutaneous needle and prime administration set. Attach sterile needle to administration set, gently pull back on the syringe to assure a blood vessel has not been inadvertently accessed (do not use needle and tubing if blood present). Repeat for each injection site; deliver the dose following instructions for the infusion device. Rotate the site(s) between successive infusions. Treatment may be transitioned to the home/home care setting in the absence of adverse reactions.

◀ Gammagard Liquid:
   Injection sites: ≤8 simultaneous injection sites
   Initial infusion rate:
      <40 kg: 15 mL/hour per injection site (maximum volume: 20 mL per injection site)
      ≥40 kg: 20 mL/hour per injection site (maximum volume: 30 mL per injection site)
   Maintenance infusion rate:
      <40 kg: 15 to 20 mL/hour per injection site (maximum volume: 20 mL per injection site)
      ≥40 kg: 20 to 30 mL/hour per injection site (maximum volume: 30 mL per injection site)
Gammaked, Gamunex-C:
   Injection sites: ≤8 simultaneous injection sites
   Recommended infusion rate: 20 mL/hour per injection site
Hizentra:
   Injection sites: ≤4 simultaneous injection sites or ≤12 sites consecutively per infusion
   Maximum infusion rate: First infusion: 15 mL/hour per injection site; subsequent infusions: 25 mL/hour per injection site
   Maximum infusion volume: First 4 infusions: 15 mL per injection site; subsequent infusions: 20 mL per injection site (maximum: 25 mL per site as tolerated)
HyQvia: Administer components of HyQvia (immune globulin and hyaluronidase) sequentially; do not use either component alone. Infusion pump capable of infusing rates up to 300 mL/hour/site required; must also have the ability to titrate the flow rate. Use a 24 gauge subcutaneous needle set labeled for high flow rates. Infuse the two components of HyQvia sequentially, beginning with the hyaluronidase. Initiate the infusion of the full dose of the immune globulin through the same subcutaneous needle set within ~10 minutes of hyaluronidase infusion. For each full or partial vial of immune globulin used, administer the entire contents of the hyaluronidase vial. A second site can be used based on tolerability and total volume; if a second site is used, administer half of total volume of the hyaluronidase in each site. Flush the infusion line with NS or D_5W if required.
   Injection sites:
      Volume per site:
         <40 kg: ≤300 mL per injection site
         ≥40 kg: ≤600 mL per injection site
   Infusion rate:
      Hyaluronidase: ~1 to 2 mL/minute, or as tolerated.
      Immune globulin:
         First 2 infusions:
            <40 kg: 5 mL/hour for 5 to 15 minutes; 10 mL/hour for 5 to 15 minutes; 20 mL/hour for 5 to 15 minutes; 40 mL/hour for 5 to 15 minutes; then 80 mL/hour for remainder of infusion
            ≥40 kg: 10 mL/hour for 5 to 15 minutes; 30 mL/hour for 5 to 15 minutes; 60 mL/hour for 5 to 15 minutes; 120 mL/hour for 5 to 15 minutes; then 240 mL/hour for remainder of infusion
         Next 2 or 3 infusions:
            <40 kg: 10 mL/hour for 5 to 15 minutes; 20 mL/hour for 5 to 15 minutes; 40 mL/hour for 5 to 15 minutes; 80 mL/hour for 5 to 15 minutes; then 160 mL/hour for remainder of infusion

≥40 kg: 10 mL/hour for 5 to 15 minutes; 30 mL/hour for 5 to 15 minutes; 120 mL/hour for 5 to 15 minutes; 240 mL/hour for 5 to 15 minutes; then 300 mL/hour for remainder of infusion

Monitoring Parameters Renal function, urine output, IgG concentrations, hemoglobin and hematocrit, platelets (in patients with ITP); infusion- or injection-related adverse reactions, anaphylaxis, signs and symptoms of hemolysis; blood viscosity (in patients at risk for hyperviscosity); presence of antineutrophil antibodies (if TRALI is suspected); volume status; neurologic symptoms (if AMS suspected); pulmonary adverse reactions; clinical response

For patients at high risk of hemolysis (dose ≥2 g/kg, given as a single dose or divided over several days, and non-O blood type): Hemoglobin or hematocrit prior to and 36 to 96 hours postinfusion.

SubQ infusion: Monitor IgG trough levels every 2 to 3 months before/after conversion from IV; subcutaneous infusions provide more constant IgG levels than usual IV immune globulin treatments.

Test Interactions Octagam 5% and Octagam 10% contain maltose. Falsely elevated blood glucose levels may occur when glucose monitoring devices and test strips utilizing the glucose dehydrogenase pyrroloquinolinequinone (GDH-PQQ) based methods are used. Glucose monitoring devices and test strips which utilize the glucose-specific method are recommended. Passively transferred antibodies may yield false-positive serologic testing results; may yield false-positive direct and indirect Coombs' test. Skin testing should not be performed with GamaSTAN S/D because local chemical irritation can occur and be misinterpreted as a positive reaction.

Dietary Considerations Some products may contain sodium.

Additional Information IM: When administering immune globulin for hepatitis A prophylaxis, use should be considered for the following close contacts of persons with confirmed hepatitis A: unvaccinated household and sexual contacts, persons who have shared illicit drugs, regular babysitters, staff and attendees of child care centers, food handlers within the same establishment (CDC, 2006).

For travelers, immune globulin is not an alternative to careful selection of foods and water; immune globulin can interfere with the antibody response to parenterally administered live virus vaccines. Frequent travelers should be tested for hepatitis A antibody, immune hemolytic anemia, and neutropenia (with ITP, IV route is usually used).

IgA content:
Bivigam: ≤200 mcg/mL
Carimune NF: 1000 to 2000 mcg/mL
Flebogamma 5% DIF: <50 mcg/mL
Flebogamma 10% DIF: <100 mcg/mL
Gammagard Liquid: 37 mcg/mL
Gammagard S/D 5% solution: <1 mcg/mL or <2.2 mcg/mL (product dependent) (see **Note**)
Gammaked: 46 mcg/mL
Gammaplex: <10 mcg/mL
Gamunex-C: 46 mcg/mL
Hizentra: ≤50 mcg/mL
Octagam 5%: ≤200 mcg/mL
Octagam 10%: 106 mcg/mL
Privigen: ≤25 mcg/mL

◀ **Note:** Manufacturer has discontinued Gammagard S/D 5% solution; however, the lower IgA product will remain available by special request for patients with known reaction to IgA or IgA deficiency with antibodies.

Dosage Forms Considerations

Carimune NF may contain a significant amount of sodium and also contains sucrose.

Gammagard S/D may contain a significant amount of sodium and also contains glucose.

Octagam contains maltose.

Hyqvia Kit is supplied with a Hyaluronidase (Human Recombinant) component intended for injection prior to Immune Globulin administration to improve dispersion and absorption of the Immune Globulin.

Dosage Forms Excipient information presented when available (limited, particularly for generics); consult specific product labeling. [DSC] = Discontinued product

Injectable, Intramuscular [preservative free]:

GamaSTAN S/D: 15% to 18% [150 to 180 mg/mL] (2 mL, 10 mL)

Kit, Subcutaneous:

Hyqvia: 2.5 g/25 mL, 5 g/50 mL, 10 g/100 mL, 20 g/200 mL, 30 g/300 mL [contains albumin human, edetate disodium dihydrate, mouse protein (murine) (hamster)]

Solution, Injection [preservative free]:

Gammagard: 1 g/10 mL (10 mL); 2.5 g/25 mL (25 mL); 5 g/50 mL (50 mL); 10 g/100 mL (100 mL); 20 g/200 mL (200 mL); 30 g/300 mL (300 mL) [latex free]

Gammaked: 1 g/10 mL (10 mL); 2.5 g/25 mL (25 mL); 5 g/50 mL (50 mL); 10 g/100 mL (100 mL); 20 g/200 mL (200 mL) [latex free]

Gamunex-C: 1 g/10 mL (10 mL); 2.5 g/25 mL (25 mL); 5 g/50 mL (50 mL); 10 g/100 mL (100 mL); 20 g/200 mL (200 mL); 40 g/400 mL (400 mL) [latex free]

Solution, Intravenous:

Gamunex: 10 g/100 mL (100 mL [DSC])

Solution, Intravenous [preservative free]:

Bivigam: 5 g/50 mL (50 mL); 10 g/100 mL (100 mL) [sugar free; contains polysorbate 80]

Flebogamma: 0.5 g/10 mL (10 mL [DSC])

Flebogamma DIF: 0.5 g/10 mL (10 mL); 2.5 g/50 mL (50 mL); 5 g/50 mL (50 mL); 5 g/100 mL (100 mL); 10 g/100 mL (100 mL); 10 g/200 mL (200 mL); 20 g/200 mL (200 mL); 20 g/400 mL (400 mL) [contains polyethylene glycol]

Gammaplex: 2.5 g/50 mL (50 mL); 5 g/100 mL (100 mL); 10 g/200 mL (200 mL); 20 g/400 mL (400 mL) [contains polysorbate 80]

Octagam: 1 g/20 mL (20 mL); 2 g/20 mL (20 mL); 2.5 g/50 mL (50 mL); 5 g/50 mL (50 mL); 5 g/100 mL (100 mL); 10 g/100 mL (100 mL); 10 g/200 mL (200 mL); 20 g/200 mL (200 mL); 25 g/500 mL (500 mL) [sucrose free]

Privigen: 5 g/50 mL (50 mL); 10 g/100 mL (100 mL); 20 g/200 mL (200 mL); 40 g/400 mL (400 mL)

Solution, Subcutaneous [preservative free]:

Hizentra: 1 g/5 mL (5 mL); 2 g/10 mL (10 mL); 4 g/20 mL (20 mL); 10 g/50 mL (50 mL) [contains polysorbate 80]

Solution Reconstituted, Intravenous [preservative free]:

Carimune NF: 3 g (1 ea [DSC]); 6 g (1 ea); 12 g (1 ea)

Gammagard S/D: 2.5 g (1 ea [DSC]); 5 g (1 ea [DSC]); 10 g (1 ea [DSC])

Gammagard S/D Less IgA: 5 g (1 ea); 10 g (1 ea)

◆ **Immune Globulin Subcutaneous (Human)** *see* Immune Globulin *on page 903*

◆ **Immune Serum Globulin** *see* Immune Globulin *on page 903*

◆ **Immunine VH (Can)** *see* Factor IX (Human) *on page 681*

◆ **INCB424** *see* Ruxolitinib *on page 1501*

◆ **INCB 18424** *see* Ruxolitinib *on page 1501*

◆ **Indium In-111 Pentetreotide Kit** *see* Indium In-111 Pentetreotide *on page 919*

Indium In-111 Pentetreotide

(IN dee um eye en won e LEV en pen te TREE oh tide)

Brand Names: US OctreoScan®

Index Terms ^{111}In-Pentetreotide; Indium In-111 Pentetreotide Kit; Octreo-Scan® (Prep Kit)

Pharmacologic Category Radiopharmaceutical

Use Scintigraphic localization of primary and metastatic neuroendocrine tumors with somatostatin receptors

Pregnancy Risk Factor C

Dosing

Adult

Planar imaging: IV: 3 mCi (111 MBq)

Single photon emission computed tomograph (SPECT) imaging: IV: 6 mCi (222 MBq)

Pediatric IV: 0.14 mCi/kg (5 MBq/kg)

Renal Impairment No dosage adjustment provided in manufacturer's labeling; use with caution.

Hepatic Impairment No dosage adjustment provided in manufacturer's labeling.

Additional Information Complete prescribing information should be consulted for additional detail.

Dosage Forms Excipient information presented when available (limited, particularly for generics); consult specific product labeling.

Kit, [preservative free]:

OctreoScan®:

Injection, powder for reconstitution: Pentetreotide 10 mcg

Injection, solution: Indium In-111 chloride 111 MBq (3.0 mCi) per 1 mL (1.1 mL)

◆ **INF-alpha 2** *see* Interferon Alfa-2b *on page 930*

◆ **Infed** *see* Iron Dextran Complex *on page 964*

◆ **Inflectra (Can)** *see* InFLIXimab *on page 919*

InFLIXimab (in FLIKS e mab)

Related Information

Hematopoietic Stem Cell Transplantation *on page 2272*

Brand Names: US Remicade

Brand Names: Canada Inflectra; Remicade; Remsima

Index Terms Avakine; Infliximab, Recombinant

Pharmacologic Category Antirheumatic, Disease Modifying; Gastrointestinal Agent, Miscellaneous; Immunosuppressant Agent; Monoclonal Antibody; Tumor Necrosis Factor (TNF) Blocking Agent

◀ **Use**

Ankylosing spondylitis: Treatment of adults with active ankylosing spondylitis (to reduce signs/symptoms)

Crohn disease: Treatment adults and children ≥6 years (US labeling) or ≥9 years (Canadian labeling) with moderately- to severely-active Crohn disease with inadequate response to conventional therapy (to reduce signs/symptoms and induce and maintain clinical remission) or to reduce the number of draining enterocutaneous and rectovaginal fistulas and maintain fistula closure

Plaque psoriasis: Treatment of adults with chronic severe (extensive and/or disabling) plaque psoriasis as an alternative to other systemic therapy

Psoriatic arthritis: Treatment of adults with psoriatic arthritis (to reduce signs/symptoms of active arthritis and inhibit progression of structural damage and improve physical function)

Rheumatoid arthritis: Treatment of adults with moderately- to severely-active rheumatoid arthritis (with methotrexate) (to reduce signs/symptoms of active arthritis and inhibit progression of structural damage and improve physical function)

Ulcerative colitis: Treatment of adults and children ≥6 years with moderately- to severely-active ulcerative colitis with inadequate response to conventional therapy (to reduce signs/symptoms and induce and maintain clinical remission, mucosal healing and eliminate corticosteroid use)

Note: Remsima and Inflectra [Canadian products] are biosimilar agents and are not approved for use in pediatric patients or in patients with Crohn disease or ulcerative colitis.

Labeled Contraindications

Hypersensitivity to infliximab, murine proteins, or any component of the formulation; doses >5 mg/kg in patients with moderate or severe heart failure (NYHA Class III/IV)

Canadian labeling: Additional contraindications (not in US labeling): Severe infections (eg, sepsis, abscesses, tuberculosis, and opportunistic infections); use in patients with moderate or severe heart failure (NYHA Class III/IV)

Pregnancy Considerations Animal reproduction studies have not been conducted. Infliximab crosses the placenta and can be detected in the serum of infants for up to 6 months following in utero exposure. A fatal outcome has been reported in an infant who received a live vaccine (BCG) after in utero exposure to infliximab; it is recommended to wait ≥6 months following birth before administering any live vaccine to infants exposed to infliximab in utero. If a biologic agent such as infliximab is needed to treat inflammatory bowel disease during pregnancy, it is recommended to hold therapy after 30 weeks gestation (Habal, 2012). The Canadian labeling recommends that women of childbearing potential use effective contraception during therapy and for at least 6 months after discontinuation.

Healthcare providers are also encouraged to enroll women exposed to infliximab during pregnancy in the MotherToBaby Autoimmune Diseases Study by contacting the Organization of Teratology Information Specialists (OTIS) (877-311-8972).

Breast-Feeding Considerations Small amounts of infliximab have been detected in breast milk. Information is available from three postpartum women who were administered infliximab 5 mg/kg 1-24 weeks after delivery. Infliximab was detected within 12 hours and the highest milk concentrations (0.09-0.105 mcg/mL) were seen 2-3 days after the dose. Corresponding maternal serum concentrations were 18-64 mcg/mL (Ben-Horin, 2011). Due to the potential for serious adverse reactions in the nursing infant, the manufacturer recommends a decision be made whether to discontinue nursing or to discontinue the drug, taking into account the importance of treatment to the mother.

Warnings/Precautions [US Boxed Warning]: **Patients receiving infliximab are at increased risk for serious infections which may result in hospitalization and/or fatality; infections usually developed in patients receiving concomitant immunosuppressive agents (eg, methotrexate or corticosteroids) and may present as disseminated (rather than local) disease. Active tuberculosis (or reactivation of latent tuberculosis), invasive fungal (including aspergillosis, blastomycosis, candidiasis, coccidioidomycosis, histoplasmosis, and pneumocystosis) and bacterial, viral or other opportunistic infections (including legionellosis and listeriosis) have been reported. Monitor closely for signs/symptoms of infection. Discontinue for serious infection or sepsis. Consider risks versus benefits prior to use in patients with a history of chronic or recurrent infection. Consider empiric antifungal therapy in patients who are at risk for invasive fungal infection and develop severe systemic illness.** Caution should be exercised when considering use the elderly or in patients with conditions that predispose them to infections (eg, diabetes) or residence/travel from areas of endemic mycoses (blastomycosis, coccidioidomycosis, histoplasmosis), or with latent or localized infections. Do not initiate infliximab therapy in patients with an active infection, including clinically important localized infection. Patients who develop a new infection while undergoing treatment should be monitored closely. Potentially significant drug interactions may exist, requiring dose or frequency adjustment, additional monitoring, and/or selection of alternative therapy.

[US Boxed Warning]: **Infliximab treatment has been associated with active tuberculosis (may be disseminated or extrapulmonary) or reactivation of latent infections; evaluate patients for tuberculosis risk factors and latent tuberculosis infection (with a tuberculin skin test) prior to and during therapy; treatment of latent tuberculosis should be initiated before use. Patients with initial negative tuberculin skin tests should receive continued monitoring for tuberculosis throughout treatment.** Most cases of reactivation have been reported within the first couple months of treatment. Caution should be exercised when considering the use of infliximab in patients who have been exposed to tuberculosis.

Patients should be brought up to date with all immunizations before initiating therapy. Live vaccines should not be given concurrently; there is no data available concerning secondary transmission of live vaccines in patients receiving therapy. A fatal outcome has been reported in an infant who received a live vaccine (BCG) after in utero exposure to infliximab; infliximab crosses the placenta and has been detected in infants' serum for up to 6 months. It is recommended to wait ≥6 months following birth before administering any live vaccine to infants exposed to infliximab in utero. Reactivation of hepatitis B virus (HBV) has occurred in chronic virus carriers (may be fatal); use with caution; evaluate prior to initiation and during treatment.

[US Boxed Warning]: **Lymphoma and other malignancies (may be fatal) have been reported in children and adolescent patients receiving TNF-blocking agents including infliximab.** Half the cases are lymphomas (Hodgkin's and non-Hodgkin's). [US Boxed Warning]: **Postmarketing cases of hepatosplenic T-cell lymphoma have been reported in patients treated** with infliximab. **Almost all patients had received and concurrent or prior treatment with azathioprine or mercaptopurine at or prior to diagnosis and the majority of reported cases occurred in adolescent and young adult males with Crohn disease or ulcerative colitis.** Malignancies occurred after a median of 30 months (range: 1 to 84 months) after the first dose of TNF blocker therapy; most patients were receiving concomitant immunosuppressants. The impact of infliximab on the development and course of malignancies is not fully defined. As compared to the general population, an increased risk of lymphoma has been noted in clinical trials; however, rheumatoid arthritis alone has been previously associated with an increased rate of lymphoma. Use caution in patients with a history of COPD, higher rates of malignancy were reported in COPD patients treated with infliximab. Psoriasis patients with a history of phototherapy had a higher incidence of nonmelanoma skin cancers. Melanoma and Merkel cell carcinoma have been reported in patients receiving TNF-blocking agents including infliximab. Perform periodic skin examinations in all patients during therapy, particularly those at increased risk for skin cancer.

Severe hepatic reactions (including hepatitis, jaundice, acute hepatic failure, and cholestasis) have been reported during treatment; reactions occurred between 2 weeks to >1 year after initiation of therapy and some cases were fatal or necessitated liver transplantation; discontinue with jaundice and/or marked increase in liver enzymes (≥5 times ULN). Use caution with heart failure; if a decision is made to use with heart failure, monitor closely and discontinue if exacerbated or new symptoms occur. Doses >5 mg/kg should not be administered in patients with moderate to severe heart failure (HF) (NYHA Class III/IV). The Canadian labeling contraindicates use in moderate or severe HF. Use caution with history of hematologic abnormalities; hematologic toxicities (eg, leukopenia, neutropenia, thrombocytopenia, pancytopenia) have been reported (may be fatal); discontinue if significant abnormalities occur. Positive antinuclear antibody titers have been detected in patients (with negative baselines). Rare cases of autoimmune disorder, including lupus-like syndrome, have been reported; monitor and discontinue if symptoms develop. Rare cases of optic neuritis and demyelinating disease (including multiple sclerosis, systemic vasculitis, and Guillain-Barré syndrome) have been reported; use with caution in patients with preexisting or recent onset CNS demyelinating disorders, or seizures; discontinue if significant CNS adverse reactions develop.

Acute infusion reactions may occur. Hypersensitivity reaction may occur within 2 hours of infusion. Medication and equipment for management of hypersensitivity reaction should be available for immediate use. Interruptions and/or reinstitution at a slower rate may be required (consult protocols). Pretreatment may be considered, and may be warranted in all patients with prior infusion reactions. Serum sickness-like reactions have occurred; may be associated with a decreased response to treatment. The development of antibodies to infliximab may increase the risk of hypersensitivity and/or infusion reactions; concomitant use of immunosuppressants may lessen the development of anti-infliximab antibodies. The risk of infusion reactions may be increased with re-treatment after an interruption or discontinuation of prior maintenance therapy. Re-treatment in psoriasis patients should be resumed as a scheduled maintenance regimen without any induction doses; use of an induction regimen should be used cautiously for re-treatment of all other patients.

Some dosage forms may contain polysorbate 80 (also known as Tweens). Hypersensitivity reactions, usually a delayed reaction, have been reported following exposure to pharmaceutical products containing polysorbate 80 in certain individuals (Isaksson, 2002; Lucente 2000; Shelley, 1995). Thrombocytopenia, ascites, pulmonary deterioration, and renal and hepatic failure have been reported in premature neonates after receiving parenteral products containing polysorbate 80 (Alade, 1986; CDC, 1984). See manufacturer's labeling.

Efficacy was not established in a study to evaluate infliximab use in juvenile idiopathic arthritis (JIA).

Adverse Reactions Although profile is similar, frequency of adverse effects may vary with disease state. Except where noted, percentages reported in adults with rheumatoid arthritis:

>10%:
  Central nervous system: Headache (18%)
  Gastrointestinal: Nausea (21%), diarrhea (12%), abdominal pain (Crohn's: 26%; other indications: 12%)
  Hepatic: Increased serum ALT (risk increased with concomitant methotrexate)
  Immunologic: Increased ANA titer (~50%), antibody development (double-stranded DNA, 20%), antibody development (anti-infliximab; variable; ~10% to 15% [range: 6% to 61%]; Mayer, 2006)
  Infection: Infection (36%), abscess (Crohn's patients with fistulizing disease: 15%)
  Respiratory: Upper respiratory tract infection (32%), sinusitis (14%), cough (12%), pharyngitis (12%)
  Miscellaneous: Infusion related reaction (20%; severe <1%)
5% to 10%:
  Cardiovascular: Hypertension (7%)
  Central nervous system: Fatigue (9%), pain (8%)
  Dermatologic: Skin rash (1% to 10%), pruritus (7%)
  Gastrointestinal: Dyspepsia (10%)
  Genitourinary: Urinary tract infection (8%)
  Infection: Candidiasis (5%)
  Neuromuscular & skeletal: Arthralgia (1% to 8%), back pain (8%)
  Respiratory: Bronchitis (10%), rhinitis (8%), dyspnea (6%)
  Miscellaneous: Fever (7%)
<5%: Abscess, adult respiratory distress syndrome, anemia, basal cell carcinoma, biliary colic, bradycardia, cardiac arrest, cardiac arrhythmia, cardiac failure, cellulitis, cerebral infarction, cholecystitis, cholelithiasis, circulatory shock, confusion, constipation, dehydration, delayed hypersensitivity (plaque psoriasis), diaphoresis, dizziness, edema, gastrointestinal hemorrhage, hemolytic anemia, hepatitis, herniated disk, hypersensitivity reaction, hypotension, intestinal obstruction, intestinal perforation, intestinal stenosis, leukopenia, lupus-like syndrome, lymphadenopathy, malignant lymphoma, malignant neoplasm, malignant neoplasm of breast, meningitis, menstrual disease, myalgia, myocardial infarction, nephrolithiasis, neuritis, pancreatitis, pancytopenia, peripheral neuropathy, peritonitis, pleural effusion, pleurisy, pulmonary edema, pulmonary embolism, rectal pain, renal failure, respiratory insufficiency, sarcoidosis, seizure, sepsis, serum sickness, suicidal tendencies, syncope, tachycardia, tendon disease, thrombocytopenia, thrombophlebitis (deep), ulcer

◀ **The following adverse events were reported in children with Crohn's disease and were found more frequently in children than adults:**

>10%:

Hepatic: Increased liver enzymes (18%; ≥5 times ULN: 1%)

Hematologic & oncologic: Anemia (11%)

Infection: Infection (56%; more common with every 8-week vs every 12-week infusions)

1% to 10%:

Cardiovascular: Flushing (9%)

Gastrointestinal: Bloody stools (10%)

Hematologic & oncologic: Leukopenia (9%), neutropenia (7%)

Hypersensitivity: Hypersensitivity reaction (respiratory, 6%)

Immunologic: Antibody development (anti-infliximab, 3%)

Infection: Viral infection (8%), bacterial infection (6%)

Neuromuscular & skeletal: Bone fracture (7%)

Postmarketing and/or case reports (adults or children): Agranulocytosis, anaphylactic shock, anaphylaxis, angina pectoris, angioedema, autoimmune hepatitis, bronchospasm, cardiac failure (worsening), cholestasis, demyelinating disease of the central nervous system (eg, multiple sclerosis, optic neuritis), demyelinating disease (peripheral; eg, Guillain-Barré syndrome, chronic inflammatory demyelinating polyneuropathy, multifocal motor neuropathy), dysgeusia, erythema multiforme, hepatic carcinoma, hepatic failure, hepatic injury, hepatitis B (reactivation), hepatotoxicity (idiosyncratic) (Chalasani, 2014), Hodgkin lymphoma, immune thrombocytopenia, interstitial fibrosis, interstitial pneumonitis, jaundice, laryngeal edema, leukemia, liver function tests increased, lupus-like syndrome (drug-induced), malignant lymphoma (hepatosplenic T-cell [HSTCL]), malignant melanoma, malignant neoplasm (leiomyosarcoma), Merkel cell carcinoma, neuropathy, numbness, opportunistic infection, pericardial effusion, pharyngeal edema, pneumonia, psoriasis (including new onset, palmoplantar, pustular, or exacerbation), reactivated tuberculosis, renal cell carcinoma, seizure, Stevens-Johnson syndrome, thrombotic thrombocytopenia purpura, tingling sensation, toxic epidermal necrolysis, transverse myelitis, tuberculosis, urticaria, vasculitis (systemic and cutaneous)

Drug Interactions

Metabolism/Transport Effects None known.

Avoid Concomitant Use

Avoid concomitant use of InFLIXimab with any of the following: Abatacept; Adalimumab; Anakinra; BCG (Intravesical); Belimumab; Canakinumab; Certolizumab Pegol; Etanercept; Golimumab; Natalizumab; Pimecrolimus; Rilonacept; Tacrolimus (Topical); Tocilizumab; Tofacitinib; Ustekinumab; Vaccines (Live); Vedolizumab

Increased Effect/Toxicity

InFLIXimab may increase the levels/effects of: Abatacept; Anakinra; Belimumab; Canakinumab; Certolizumab Pegol; Fingolimod; Leflunomide; Natalizumab; Rilonacept; Tofacitinib; Vaccines (Live); Vedolizumab

The levels/effects of InFLIXimab may be increased by: Adalimumab; Denosumab; Etanercept; Golimumab; Pimecrolimus; Roflumilast; Tacrolimus (Topical); Tocilizumab; Trastuzumab; Ustekinumab

Decreased Effect

InFLIXimab may decrease the levels/effects of: BCG (Intravesical); Coccidioides immitis Skin Test; Sipuleucel-T; Vaccines (Inactivated); Vaccines (Live)

The levels/effects of InFLIXimab may be decreased by: Echinacea

Storage/Stability Store intact vials at 2°C to 8°C (36°F to 46°F). The manufacturer recommends that diluted solutions for infusion should be used within 3 hours of preparation. However, a stability study of infliximab 0.4 mg/mL prepared in 0.9% sodium chloride in polyvinyl chloride (PVC) bags found no loss of biological activity when stored refrigerated at 4°C for up to 14 days (Ikeda 2012).

Preparation for Administration Reconstitute vials with 10 mL sterile water for injection (SWFI) with a 21-guage or smaller needle, directing the SWFI towards the wall of the vial. Swirl vial gently to dissolve powder; do not shake. Allow solution to stand for 5 minutes. Total dose of reconstituted product should be further diluted to 250 mL of 0.9% sodium chloride injection (add reconstituted infliximab slowly) to a final concentration of 0.4 to 4 mg/mL. Do not dilute reconstituted infliximab solution with any other diluent. Infusion should begin within 3 hours of preparation (see Storage/Stability for additional information).

Mechanism of Action Infliximab is a chimeric monoclonal antibody that binds to human tumor necrosis factor alpha (TNFα), thereby interfering with endogenous TNFα activity. Elevated TNFα levels have been found in involved tissues/fluids of patients with rheumatoid arthritis, ankylosing spondylitis, psoriatic arthritis, plaque psoriasis, Crohn disease and ulcerative colitis. Biological activities of TNFα include the induction of proinflammatory cytokines (interleukins), enhancement of leukocyte migration, activation of neutrophils and eosinophils, and the induction of acute phase reactants and tissue degrading enzymes. Animal models have shown TNFα expression causes polyarthritis, and infliximab can prevent disease as well as allow diseased joints to heal.

Pharmacodynamics/Kinetics

Onset of action: Crohn disease: ~2 weeks

Distribution: V_d: 3-6 L

Half-life elimination: 7-12 days

Dosing

Adult & Geriatric Note: Premedication with antihistamines (H_1-antagonist +/- H_2-antagonist), acetaminophen, and/or corticosteroids may be considered to prevent and/or manage infusion-related reactions. Remsima and Inflectra [Canadian products] are biosimilar agents and are not approved for use in Crohn disease or ulcerative colitis.

Ankylosing spondylitis: IV: 5 mg/kg at 0, 2, and 6 weeks, followed by 5 mg/kg every 6 weeks thereafter (Canadian labeling recommends every 6 to 8 weeks thereafter)

Crohn disease: IV: 5 mg/kg at 0, 2, and 6 weeks, followed by 5 mg/kg every 8 weeks thereafter; dose may be increased to 10 mg/kg in patients who respond but then lose their response. If no response by week 14, consider discontinuing therapy.

Plaque psoriasis: IV: 5 mg/kg at 0, 2, and 6 weeks, followed by 5 mg/kg every 8 weeks thereafter. **Note:** The Canadian labeling recommends discontinuing therapy at 14 weeks if response to therapy is inadequate.

◀ **Psoriatic arthritis (with or without methotrexate):** IV: 5 mg/kg at 0,2, and 6 weeks, followed by 5 mg/kg every 8 weeks thereafter. **Note:** The Canadian labeling recommends discontinuing therapy at 24 weeks in patients unresponsive to therapy.

Rheumatoid arthritis (in combination with methotrexate therapy): IV 3 mg/kg at 0, 2, and 6 weeks, followed by 3 mg/kg every 8 weeks thereafter; Remicade doses have ranged from 3 to 10 mg/kg repeated at 4- to 8-week intervals

Ulcerative colitis: IV: 5 mg/kg at 0, 2, and 6 weeks, followed by 5 mg/kg every 8 weeks thereafter. The Canadian labeling suggests that after assessment of infliximab trough levels and antibody titers, dose adjustment to 10 mg/kg may be considered in some patients to sustain response/remission.

Pustular psoriasis (off-label use): IV: 5 mg/kg at week 0, 2, and 6, followed by 5 mg/kg every 8 weeks for up to 46 weeks (Suguira 2014; Torii 2011)

Dosage adjustment with heart failure (HF): Weigh risk versus benefits for individual patient:

Mild HF (NYHA Class I/II):
  US labeling: No dosage adjustment necessary; use with caution and monitor closely for worsening of HF
  Canadian labeling: ≤5 mg/kg

Moderate to severe (NYHA Class III or IV):
  US labeling: ≤5 mg/kg
  Canadian labeling: Use is contraindicated.

Pediatric Note: Premedication with antihistamines (H_1-antagonist +/- H_2-antagonist), acetaminophen, and/or corticosteroids may be considered to prevent and/or manage infusion-related reactions. Remsima and Inflectra [Canadian products] are biosimilar agents and are not approved for use in pediatric patients.

Crohn disease: Children and Adolescents: US labeling ≥6 years, Canadian labeling ≥9 years: IV: 5 mg/kg at 0, 2, and 6 weeks, followed by 5 mg/kg every 8 weeks thereafter; if no response by week 14, consider discontinuing therapy

Ulcerative colitis: Children ≥6 years and Adolescents: IV: 5 mg/kg at 0, 2, and 6 weeks, followed by 5 mg/kg every 8 weeks thereafter

Juvenile idiopathic arthritis (off-label use): Children ≥4 years and Adolescents: IV: Initial: 3 mg/kg at 0, 2, and 6 weeks; then 3 to 6 mg/kg/dose every 8 weeks thereafter, in combination with methotrexate during induction and maintenance (Ruperto, 2010). Alternatively, some studies used 6 mg/kg starting at week 14 of a methotrexate induction regimen (weeks 0 to 13); repeat dose (6 mg/kg) at week 16 and 20, then every 8 weeks thereafter (Ruperto, 2007; Visvanathan, 2012).

Renal Impairment There are no dosage adjustments provided in the manufacturer's labeling.

Hepatic Impairment There are no dosage adjustments provided in the manufacturer's labeling.

Administration The infusion should begin within 3 hours of reconstitution and dilution. Infuse over at least 2 hours; do not infuse with other agents; use in-line low protein binding filter (≤1.2 micron). Temporarily discontinue or decrease infusion rate with infusion-related reactions. Antihistamines (H_1-antagonist +/- H_2-antagonist), acetaminophen and/or corticosteroids may be used to manage reactions. Infusion may be reinitiated at a lower rate upon resolution of mild to moderate symptoms.

Note: The Canadian labeling suggests that patients with rheumatoid arthritis who have tolerated 3 infusions over 2 hours (doses ≤6 mg/kg) may receive subsequent infusions at the same dose over not less than 1 hour. Safety of shortened infusion has not been studied with doses >6 mg/kg.

Guidelines for the treatment and prophylaxis of infusion reactions: (Note: Limited to adult patients and dosages used in Crohn disease; prospective data for other populations [pediatrics, other indications/dosing] are not available).

A protocol for the treatment of infusion reactions, as well as prophylactic therapy for repeat infusions, has been published (Mayer, 2006).

Treatment of infusion reactions: Medications for the treatment of hypersensitivity reactions should be available for immediate use. For mild reactions, the rate of infusion should be decreased to 10 mL/hour. Initiate a normal saline infusion (500 to 1,000 mL/hour) and appropriate symptomatic treatment (eg, acetaminophen and diphenhydramine); monitor vital signs every 10 minutes until normal. After 20 minutes, the infusion may be increased at 15-minute intervals, as tolerated, to completion (initial increase to 20 mL/hour, then 40 mL/hour, then 80 mL/hour, etc [maximum of 125 mL/hour]). For moderate reactions, the infusion should be stopped or slowed. Initiate a normal saline infusion (500 to 1,000 mL/hour) and appropriate symptomatic treatment. Monitor vital signs every 5 minutes until normal. After 20 minutes, the infusion may be reinstituted at 10 mL/hour; then increased at 15-minute intervals, as tolerated, to completion (initial increase 20 mL/hour, then 40 mL/hour, then 80 mL/hour, etc [maximum of 125 mL/hour]). For severe reactions, the infusion should be stopped with administration of appropriate symptomatic treatment (eg, hydrocortisone/methylprednisolone, diphenhydramine and epinephrine) and frequent monitoring of vitals (consult institutional policies, if available). Re-treatment after a severe reaction should only be done if the benefits outweigh the risks and with appropriate prophylaxis. Delayed infusion reactions typically occur 1 to 7 days after an infusion. Treatment should consist of appropriate symptomatic treatment (eg, acetaminophen, antihistamine, methylprednisolone).

Prophylaxis of infusion reactions: Premedication with acetaminophen and diphenhydramine 90 minutes prior to infusion may be considered in all patients with prior infusion reactions, and in patients with severe reactions corticosteroid administration is recommended. Steroid dosing may be oral (prednisone 50 mg orally every 12 hours for 3 doses prior to infusion) or intravenous (a single dose of hydrocortisone 100 mg or methylprednisolone 20 to 40 mg administered 20 minutes prior to the infusion). On initiation of the infusion, begin with a test dose at 10 mL/hour for 15 minutes. Thereafter, the infusion may be increased at 15-minute intervals, as tolerated, to completion (initial increase 20 mL/hour, then 40 mL/hour, then 80 mL/hour, etc). A maximum rate of 125 mL/hour is recommended in patients who experienced prior mild to moderate reactions and 100 mL/hour is recommended in patients who experienced prior severe reactions. In patients with cutaneous flushing, aspirin may be considered (Becker, 2004). For delayed infusion reactions, premedicate with acetaminophen and diphenhydramine 90 minutes prior to infusion. On initiation of the infusion, begin with a test dose at 10 mL/hour for 15 minutes. Thereafter, the infusion may be increased to infuse over 3 hours. Postinfusion therapy with acetaminophen for 3 days and an antihistamine for 7 days is recommended.

Monitoring Parameters Monitor improvement of symptoms and physical function assessments. During infusion, if reaction is noted, monitor vital signs every 2-10 minutes, depending on reaction severity, until normal. Latent TB screening prior to initiating and during therapy; signs/symptoms of infection (prior to, during, and following therapy); CBC with differential; signs/symptoms/worsening of heart failure; HBV screening prior to initiating (all patients), HBV carriers (during and for several months following therapy); signs and symptoms of hypersensitivity reaction; symptoms of lupus-like syndrome; LFTs (discontinue if >5 times ULN); signs and symptoms of malignancy (eg, splenomegaly, hepatomegaly, abdominal pain, persistent fever, night sweats, weight loss).

Psoriasis patients with history of phototherapy should be monitored for non-melanoma skin cancer.

Medication Guide Available Yes

Dosage Forms Considerations

Remicade contains sucrose 500 mg per vial

Dosage Forms Excipient information presented when available (limited, particularly for generics); consult specific product labeling.

Solution Reconstituted, Intravenous [preservative free]:

Remicade: 100 mg (1 ea) [contains polysorbate 80]

Dosage Forms: Canada Excipient information presented when available (limited, particularly for generics); consult specific product labeling.

Solution Reconstituted, Intravenous (preservative free):

Remicade: 100 mg (contains polysorbate 80, sucrose 500 mg)

Inflectra: 100 mg (contains polysorbate 80, sucrose 500 mg; biosimilar agent)

Remsima 100 mg (contains polysorbate 80, sucrose 500 mg; biosimilar agent)

- ◆ **Infliximab, Recombinant** see InFLIXimab on page 919
- ◆ **Infufer (Can)** see Iron Dextran Complex on page 964
- ◆ **Infumorph 200** see Morphine (Systemic) on page 1167
- ◆ **Infumorph 500** see Morphine (Systemic) on page 1167

Ingenol Mebutate (IN je nol MEB u tate)

Brand Names: US Picato

Index Terms Euphorbia peplus Derivative; PEP005

Pharmacologic Category Topical Skin Product

Use Actinic keratosis: Topical treatment of actinic keratosis

Labeled Contraindications Hypersensitivity to ingenol mebutate or any component of the formulation.

Pregnancy Considerations Adverse events were observed in some animal reproduction studies following IV administration of ingenol mebutate. Absorption is limited in humans following topical application.

Breast-Feeding Considerations Excretion into breast milk is unknown; absorption is limited following topical application

Warnings/Precautions Severe dermatologic reactions including erythema, crusting, swelling, vesiculation/pustulation, and erosion/ulceration can occur. Avoid treatment in the periocular area. Severe eye pain, chemical conjunctivitis, corneal burning, eyelid edema, eyelid ptosis, and periorbital edema can occur after exposure. Patients should wash hands immediately after applying and avoid transferring to the eye area. If accidental exposure occurs, patient should flush area with water and contact health care provider. Cases of hypersensitivity, including anaphylaxis and allergic contact dermatitis, have been reported. If anaphylaxis or other clinically significant hypersensitivity reaction occurs, discontinue immediately and manage as appropriate.

Apply to intact and nonirritated skin only. Instruct patients to wash hands well after applying and to avoid contact with the periocular area during and after application. Avoid touching the treated area for 6 hours after application. If inadvertent exposure to other area(s) occurs, flush the area with water and seek medical care as soon as possible. Avoid inadvertent transfer to other individuals. Administration of ingenol mebutate gel is not recommended until the skin is healed from any previous drug or surgical treatment. For topical use only; not for oral, ophthalmic, or intravaginal use.

Adverse Reactions

>10%: Dermatologic: Erythema (92% to 94%), desquamation (≤85% to 90%), exfoliation of skin (≤85% to 90%), crusted skin (74% to 80%), swelling of skin (64% to 79%), localized vesiculation (≤44% to 56%), local pustules (≤44% to 56%), dermal ulcer (≤26% to 32%), skin erosion (≤26% to 32%), application site pain (2% to 15%)

1% to 10%:

Central nervous system: Headache (2%)

Dermatologic: Application-site pruritus (8%), application site irritation (4%), skin infection (3%; at application site)

Ocular: Periorbital edema (3%)

Respiratory: Nasopharyngitis (2%)

<1%, postmarketing, and/or case reports: Conjunctivitis, eye injury (FDA Safety Alert, August 21, 2015), eyelid edema, eye pain, herpes zoster (FDA Safety Alert, August 21, 2015), severe hypersensitivity (FDA Safety Alert, August 21, 2015)

Drug Interactions

Metabolism/Transport Effects None known.

Avoid Concomitant Use There are no known interactions where it is recommended to avoid concomitant use.

Increased Effect/Toxicity There are no known significant interactions involving an increase in effect.

Decreased Effect There are no known significant interactions involving a decrease in effect.

Storage/Stability Store in a refrigerator at 2°C to 8°C (36°F to 46°F); excursions are permitted to 0°C to 15°C (32°F to 59°F); do not freeze. Discard tubes after single use.

Mechanism of Action Ingenol mebutate appears to induce primary necrosis of actinic keratosis with a subsequent neutrophil-mediated inflammatory response with antibody-dependent cytotoxicity of residual disease cells; killing residual disease cells may prevent future relapse (Ramsay 2011; Siller 2010).

Pharmacodynamics/Kinetics Absorption: Absorption through the skin is minimal (with proper use); expected systemic exposure is <0.1 ng/mL.

Dosing

Adult & Geriatric Actinic keratosis: Topical:

Face or scalp: Apply 0.015% gel once daily to affected area for 3 consecutive days

Trunk or extremities: Apply 0.05% gel once daily to affected area for 2 consecutive days

◀ **Renal Impairment** There are no dosage adjustments provided in the manufacturer's labeling. However, dosage adjustment unlikely due to low systemic absorption.

Hepatic Impairment There are no dosage adjustments provided in the manufacturer's labeling. However, dosage adjustment unlikely due to low systemic absorption.

Administration Apply topically to one contiguous affected area of skin using one unit-dose tube; one unit-dose tube will cover ~5 cm x 5 cm (~25 cm^2 or ~2 inch x 2 inch). Spread evenly then allow gel to dry for 15 minutes. Do not cover with bandages or occlusive dressings. Wash hands immediately after applying and avoid transferring gel to any other areas. Avoid washing or touching the treatment area for at least 6 hours, and following this period of time, patients may wash the area with a mild soap. Not for oral, ophthalmic, or intravaginal use. Avoid application near or around the mouth and lips. Avoid transfer of gel to the periocular area.

Dosage Forms Excipient information presented when available (limited, particularly for generics); consult specific product labeling.

Gel, External:

Picato: 0.015% (3 ea); 0.05% (2 ea) [contains benzyl alcohol, isopropyl alcohol]

◆ **Inlyta** see Axitinib on page 155

◆ **¹¹¹In-Pentetreotide** see Indium In-111 Pentetreotide on page 919

◆ **α-2-interferon** see Interferon Alfa-2b on page 930

◆ **Interferon Alfa-2b (PEG Conjugate)** see Peginterferon Alfa-2b on page 1350

Interferon Alfa-2b (in ter FEER on AL fa too bee)

Related Information

Malignant Pleural Effusions on page 2246

Management of Chemotherapy-Induced Nausea and Vomiting in Adults on page 2142

Prevention of Chemotherapy-Induced Nausea and Vomiting in Children on page 2203

Brand Names: US Intron A

Brand Names: Canada Intron A

Index Terms INF-alpha 2; Interferon Alpha-2b; rLFN-α2; α-2-interferon

Pharmacologic Category Antineoplastic Agent, Biological Response Modulator; Biological Response Modulator; Immunomodulator, Systemic; Interferon

Use

AIDS-related Kaposi sarcoma: Treatment of patients 18 years and older with AIDS-related Kaposi sarcoma

Chronic hepatitis B: Treatment of chronic hepatitis B in patients 1 year and older with compensated liver disease

Chronic hepatitis C: Treatment of chronic hepatitis C in patients 18 years and older with compensated liver disease who have a history of blood or blood-product exposure and/or are hepatitis C virus (HCV) antibody-positive; in combination with ribavirin for treatment of chronic hepatitis C in patients 3 years and older with compensated liver disease previously untreated with alpha interferon therapy and in patients 18 years and older who have relapsed following alpha interferon therapy

Condylomata acuminata: Treatment of patients 18 years and older with condylomata acuminata involving external surfaces of the genital and perianal areas

Follicular lymphoma: Initial treatment of clinically aggressive follicular non-Hodgkin lymphoma in conjunction with anthracycline-containing combination chemotherapy in patients 18 years and older

Hairy cell leukemia: Treatment of patients 18 years and older with hairy cell leukemia

Malignant melanoma: Adjuvant to surgical treatment in patients 18 years and older with malignant melanoma who are free of disease but at high risk for systemic recurrence, within 56 days of surgery

Labeled Contraindications

Hypersensitivity to interferon alfa or any component of the formulation; decompensated liver disease; autoimmune hepatitis

Combination therapy with interferon alfa-2b and ribavirin is also contraindicated in women who are pregnant, in males with pregnant partners; in patients with hemoglobinopathies (eg, thalassemia major, sickle-cell anemia); creatinine clearance <50 mL/minute; or hypersensitivity to ribavirin or any component of the formulation

Documentation of allergenic cross-reactivity for interferons is limited. However, because of similarities in chemical structure and/or pharmacologic actions, the possibility of cross-sensitivity cannot be ruled out with certainty.

Pregnancy Considerations Animal reproduction studies have demonstrated abortifacient effects. Disruption of the normal menstrual cycle was also observed in animal studies; therefore, the manufacturer recommends that reliable contraception is used in women of childbearing potential. Alfa interferon is endogenous to normal amniotic fluid. *In vitro* administration studies have reported that when administered to the mother, it does not cross the placenta. Case reports of use in pregnant women are limited. The Perinatal HIV Guidelines Working Group does not recommend that interferon-alfa be used during pregnancy. Interferon alfa-2b monotherapy should only be used in pregnancy when the potential benefit to the mother justifies the possible risk to the fetus. Combination therapy with ribavirin is contraindicated in pregnancy; two forms of contraception should be used during combination therapy and patients should have monthly pregnancy tests. A pregnancy registry has been established for women inadvertently exposed to ribavirin while pregnant (800-593-2214).

Breast-Feeding Considerations Breast milk samples obtained from a lactating mother prior to and after administration of interferon alfa-2b showed that interferon alfa is present in breast milk and administration of the medication did not significantly affect endogenous levels. Breast-feeding is not linked to the spread of hepatitis C virus; however, if nipples are cracked or bleeding, breast-feeding is not recommended. Mothers coinfected with HIV are discouraged from breast-feeding to decrease potential transmission of HIV.

Warnings/Precautions [US Boxed Warning]: May cause or aggravate fatal or life-threatening autoimmune disorders, neuropsychiatric symptoms (including depression and/or suicidal thoughts/behaviors), ischemic, and/or infectious disorders; monitor closely with clinical and laboratory evaluations (periodic); discontinue treatment for severe persistent or worsening symptoms; some cases may resolve with discontinuation.

Neuropsychiatric disorders: May cause neuropsychiatric events, including depression, psychosis, mania, suicidal behavior/ideation, attempts and completed suicides and homicidal ideation; may occur in patients with or without previous psychiatric symptoms. Effects are usually rapidly reversible upon therapy discontinuation, but have persisted up to three weeks. If psychiatric symptoms persist or worsen, or suicidal or homicidal ideation or aggressive behavior towards others is identified, discontinue treatment, and follow the patient closely. Careful neuropsychiatric monitoring is recommended during and for 6 months after treatment in patients who develop psychiatric disorders (including clinical depression). New or exacerbated neuropsychiatric or substance abuse disorders are best managed with early intervention. Use with caution in patients with a history of psychiatric disorders. Drug screening and periodic health evaluation (including monitoring of psychiatric symptoms) is recommended if initiating treatment in patients with coexisting psychiatric condition or substance abuse disorders. Suicidal ideation or attempts may occur more frequently in pediatric patients (eg, adolescents) when compared to adults. Higher doses, usually in elderly patients, may result in increased CNS toxicity (eg, obtundation and coma).

Hepatic disease: May cause hepatotoxicity; monitor closely if abnormal liver function tests develop. A transient increase in ALT (≥ 2 times baseline) may occur in patients treated with interferon alfa-2b for chronic hepatitis B. Therapy generally may continue; monitor. Worsening and potentially fatal liver disease, including jaundice, hepatic encephalopathy, and hepatic failure have been reported in patients receiving interferon alfa for chronic hepatitis B and C with decompensated liver disease, autoimmune hepatitis, history of autoimmune disease, and immunosuppressed transplant recipients; avoid use in these patients; use is contraindicated in decompensated liver disease. Patients with cirrhosis are at increased risk of hepatic decompensation. Therapy should be discontinued for any patient developing signs and symptoms of liver failure. Permanently discontinue for severe (grade 3) hepatic injury or hepatic decompensation (Child-Pugh class B and C [score >6]). Chronic hepatitis B or C patients with a history of autoimmune disease or who are immunosuppressed transplant recipients should not receive interferon alfa-2b.

Bone marrow suppression: Causes bone marrow suppression, including potentially severe cytopenias, and very rarely, aplastic anemia. Discontinue treatment for severe neutropenia (ANC <500/mm^3) or thrombocytopenia (platelets <25,000/mm^3). Hemolytic anemia (hemoglobin <10 g/dL) was observed when combined with ribavirin; anemia occurred within 1 to 2 weeks of initiation of therapy. Use caution in patients with preexisting myelosuppression and in patients with concomitant medications which cause myelosuppression.

Autoimmune disorders: Avoid use in patients with history of autoimmune disorders; development of autoimmune disorders (thrombocytopenia, vasculitis, Raynaud's disease, rheumatoid arthritis, lupus erythematosus and rhabdomyolysis) has been associated with use. Monitor closely; consider discontinuing. Worsening of psoriasis and sarcoidosis (and the development of new sarcoidosis) have been reported; use extreme caution.

Cardiovascular disease/coagulation disorders: Use caution and monitor closely in patients with cardiovascular disease (ischemic or thromboembolic), arrhythmias, hypertension, and in patients with a history of MI or prior therapy with cardiotoxic drugs. Patients with preexisting cardiac disease and/or advanced cancer should have baseline and periodic ECGs. May cause hypotension (during administration or delayed up to 2 days), arrhythmia, tachycardia (≥150 bpm), cardiomyopathy (~2% in AIDS-related Kaposi Sarcoma patients), and/or MI. Some experiencing cardiovascular adverse effects had no prior history of cardiac disease. Supraventricular arrhythmias occur rarely, and are associated with preexisting cardiac disease or prior therapy with cardiotoxic agents. Dose modification, discontinuation, and/or additional therapies may be necessary. Hemorrhagic cerebrovascular events have been observed with therapy. Use caution in patients with coagulation disorders.

Endocrine disorders: Thyroid disorders (possibly reversible) have been reported; use caution in patients with preexisting thyroid disease. TSH levels should be within normal limits prior to initiating interferon. Treatment should not be initiated in patients with preexisting thyroid disease who cannot be maintained in normal ranges by medication. Discontinue interferon use in patients who develop thyroid abnormalities during treatment and in patients with thyroid disease who subsequently cannot maintain normal ranges with thyroid medication. Discontinuation of interferon therapy may or may not reverse thyroid dysfunction. Diabetes mellitus has been reported; discontinue if cannot effectively manage with medication. Use with caution in patients with a history of diabetes mellitus, particularly if prone to DKA. Hypertriglyceridemia has been reported; discontinue if persistent and severe, and/or combined with symptoms of pancreatitis.

Pulmonary disease: Dyspnea, pulmonary infiltrates, pulmonary hypertension, interstitial pneumonitis, pneumonia, bronchiolitis obliterans, and sarcoidosis may be induced or aggravated by treatment, sometimes resulting in respiratory failure or fatality. Has been reported more in patients being treated for chronic hepatitis C, although has also occurred with use for oncology indications. Patients with fever, cough, dyspnea or other respiratory symptoms should be evaluated with a chest x-ray; monitor closely and consider discontinuing treatment with evidence of impaired pulmonary function. Use with caution in patients with a history of pulmonary disease.

Ophthalmic disorders: Decreased or loss of vision, macular edema, optic neuritis, retinal hemorrhages, cotton wool spots, papilledema, retinal detachment (serous), and retinal artery or vein thrombosis have occurred (or been aggravated) in patients receiving alpha interferons. Use caution in patients with preexisting eye disorders; monitor closely; a complete eye exam should be done promptly in patients who develop ocular symptoms; discontinue with new or worsening ophthalmic disorders.

Dental and periodontic disorders: In patients receiving combination interferon and ribavirin therapy, dental and periodontal disorders have been reported; additionally, dry mouth can damage teeth and mouth mucous membranes during chronic therapy.

Commonly associated with fever and flu-like symptoms; rule out other causes/ infection with persistent fever; use with caution in patients with debilitating conditions. Acute hypersensitivity reactions (eg, urticaria, angioedema, bronchoconstriction, anaphylaxis) have been reported (rarely) with alfa interferons. If an acute reaction develops, discontinue therapy immediately; transient rashes have occurred in some patients following injection, but have not necessitated treatment interruption. Do not treat patients with visceral AIDS-related Kaposi sarcoma associated with rapidly-progressing or life-threatening disease. Some formulations contain albumin, which may carry a remote risk of viral transmission. Due to differences in dosage, patients should not change brands of interferons without the concurrence of their healthcare provider. Combination therapy with ribavirin is associated with birth defects and/or fetal mortality and hemolytic anemia. Do not use combination therapy with ribavirin in patients with CrCl <50 mL/minute. Interferon alfa-2b at doses ≥10 million units/m^2 is associated with a moderate emetic potential; antiemetics may be recommended to prevent nausea and vomiting. Potentially significant drug-drug interactions may exist, requiring dose or frequency adjustment, additional monitoring, and/or selection of alternative therapy.

Some dosage forms may contain polysorbate 80 (also known as Tweens). Hypersensitivity reactions, usually a delayed reaction, have been reported following exposure to pharmaceutical products containing polysorbate 80 in certain individuals (Isaksson, 2002; Lucente 2000; Shelley 1995). Thrombocytopenia, ascites, pulmonary deterioration, and renal and hepatic failure have been reported in premature neonates after receiving parenteral products containing polysorbate 80 (Alade 1986; CDC 1984). See manufacturer's labeling.

Adverse Reactions Note: In a majority of patients, a flu-like symptom (fever, chills, tachycardia, malaise, myalgia, headache), occurs within 1-2 hours of administration; may last up to 24 hours and may be dose limiting.

>10%:
  Cardiovascular: Chest pain (≤28%)
  Central nervous system: Fatigue (8% to 96%), headache (21% to 62%), chills (≤54%), rigors (≤42%), depression (3% to 40%; grades 3/4: 2%), drowsiness (≤33%), dizziness (≤24%), irritability (≤22%), paresthesia (1% to 21%), pain (≤18%), right upper quadrant pain (≤15%), amnesia (≤14%), lack of concentration (≤14%), malaise (≤14%), confusion (≤12%), insomnia (≤12%)
  Dermatologic: Alopecia (≤38%), skin rash (≤25%), diaphoresis (1% to 21%), pruritus (≤11%)
  Endocrine & metabolic: Weight loss (<1% to 13%), amenorrhea (≤12%)
  Gastrointestinal: Anorexia (1% to 69%), nausea, (17% to 66%), diarrhea (2% to 45%), vomiting (children 27%; adults 2% to 32%), xerostomia (≤28%), dysgeusia (≤24%), abdominal pain (1% to 23%), constipation (≤14%), gingivitis (≤14%)
  Hematologic & oncologic: Neutropenia (≤92%; grade 4: 1% to 4%), leukopenia (≤68%), anemia (≤32%), thrombocytopenia (≤15%)
  Hepatic: Increased serum AST (≤63%; grades 3/4: 14%), increased serum ALT (≤15%), increased serum alkaline phosphatase (≤13%)
  Infection: Candidiasis (≤17%)
  Local: Injection site reaction (≤20%)
  Neuromuscular & skeletal: Myalgia (28% to 75%), weakness (≤63%), skeletal pain (≤21%), arthralgia (≤19%), back pain (≤19%)
  Renal: Increased blood urea nitrogen (≤12%)
  Respiratory: Flu-like symptoms (≤79%), dyspnea (≤34%), cough (≤31%), pharyngitis (≤31%), sinusitis (≤21%)
  Miscellaneous: Fever (34% to 94%; more common in children)
5% to 10%:
  Cardiovascular: Edema (≤10%), hypertension (≤9%)

Central nervous system: Hypoesthesia (≤10%), anxiety (≤9%), vertigo (≤8%), agitation (≤7%)

Dermatologic: Xeroderma (≤10%), dermatitis (≤8%)

Endocrine & metabolic: Decreased libido (≤5%)

Gastrointestinal: Loose stools (≤10%), dyspepsia (≤8%)

Genitourinary: Urinary tract infection (≤5%)

Hematologic & oncologic: Purpura (≤5%)

Infection: Infection (≤7%), herpes virus infection (≤5%)

Renal: Polyuria (≤10%), increased serum creatinine (≤6%)

Respiratory: Bronchitis (≤10%), nasal congestion (≤10%), epistaxis (≤7%)

<5%, postmarketing, and/or case reports:

Cardiovascular: Angina pectoris, arteritis, atrial fibrillation, bradycardia, cardiac arrhythmia, cardiac failure, cardiomegaly, cardiomyopathy, cerebrovascular accident, coronary artery disease, extrasystoles, flushing, heart valve disease, hypotension, myocardial infarction, palpitations, peripheral ischemia, periarteritis nodosa, pulmonary embolism, Raynaud's phenomenon, reduced ejection fraction, retinal vein occlusion, syncope, tachycardia, thrombosis, vasculitis

Central nervous system: Nervousness (≤3%), aggressive behavior, aphasia, ataxia, Bell's palsy, carpal tunnel syndrome, coma, dysphasia, extrapyramidal reaction, hallucination, homicidal ideation, hyporeflexia, hypothermia, mania, migraine, neuralgia, neuropathy, paranoia, peripheral neuropathy, psychoneurosis, psychosis, suicidal ideation, seizure

Dermatologic: Cellulitis, eczema, epidermal cyst, erythema, erythema multiforme, erythematous rash, exacerbation of psoriasis, folliculitis, lichenoid dermatitis, lipoma, maculopapular rash, psoriasis, skin photosensitivity, Stevens-Johnson syndrome, toxic epidermal necrolysis, urticaria

Endocrine & metabolic: Increased lactate dehydrogenase (≤1%), albuminuria, dehydration, diabetes mellitus, goiter, hirsutism, hot flash, hypercalcemia, hyperglycemia, hyperthyroidism, hypertriglyceridemia, hypothyroidism, pituitary insufficiency, menorrhagia

Gastrointestinal: Aphthous stomatitis, biliary colic, colitis, esophagitis, gastritis, gastrointestinal hemorrhage, mucositis, pancreatitis, stomatitis

Genitourinary: Cystitis, dysuria, hematuria, impotence, leukorrhea, mastitis, nephrotic syndrome, nocturia, pelvic pain, proteinuria, sexual disorder, urinary incontinence, uterine hemorrhage

Hematologic & oncologic: Aplastic anemia (rarely), exacerbation of sarcoidosis, granulocytopenia, hemolytic anemia, hypochromic anemia, immune thrombocytopenia, lipoma, lymphadenitis, lymphadenopathy, lymphocytopenia, lymphocytosis, pancytopenia, pure red cell aplasia, rectal hemorrhage, sarcoidosis, thrombotic thrombocytopenic purpura

Hepatic: Abnormal hepatic function tests, ascites, hepatic encephalopathy, hepatic failure, hepatitis, hepatotoxicity, hyperbilirubinemia, jaundice

Hypersensitivity: Anaphylaxis, angioedema, hypersensitivity reaction (acute)

Infection: Abscess, fungal infection, sepsis

Local: Tissue necrosis at injection site

Neuromuscular & skeletal: Amyotrophy, arthritis, leg cramps, myositis, rhabdomyolysis, rheumatoid arthritis, spondylitis, systemic lupus erythematosus, tendonitis, tremor

Ophthalmic: Blurred vision, conjunctivitis, macular edema, nystagmus, optic neuritis, papilledema, photophobia, retinal cotton-wool spot, retinal detachment (serous), retinal thrombosis, Vogt-Koyanagi-Harada syndrome

Otic: Auditory impairment, hearing loss

Renal: Renal failure, renal insufficiency

◀

Respiratory: Asthma, bronchiolitis obliterans, bronchoconstriction, broncho-spasm, cyanosis, hemoptysis, hypoventilation, interstitial pneumonitis, pleu-ral effusion, pneumonia, pneumothorax, pulmonary fibrosis, pulmonary hypertension, pulmonary infiltrates, respiratory insufficiency, upper respira-tory tract infection, wheezing

Miscellaneous: Abscess, alcohol intolerance

Drug Interactions

Metabolism/Transport Effects Inhibits CYP1A2 (weak)

Avoid Concomitant Use

Avoid concomitant use of Interferon Alfa-2b with any of the following: BCG (Intravesical); CloZAPine; Dipyrone; Telbivudine

Increased Effect/Toxicity

Interferon Alfa-2b may increase the levels/effects of: Aldesleukin; CloZAPine; Methadone; Ribavirin; Telbivudine; Theophylline Derivatives; TiZANidine; Zidovudine

The levels/effects of Interferon Alfa-2b may be increased by: Dipyrone

Decreased Effect

Interferon Alfa-2b may decrease the levels/effects of: BCG (Intravesical)

Storage/Stability Store intact vials under refrigeration at 2°C to 8°C (36°F to 46°F); do not freeze. After reconstitution of powder for injection, product should be used immediately, but may be stored under refrigeration for ≤24 hours.

Preparation for Administration Powder for injection: The manufacturer recommends reconstituting vial with the diluent provided (SWFI). When reconstituted with SWFI 1 mL, the 10 million unit vial concentration is 10 million units/mL, the 18 million unit vial concentration is 18 million units/mL, and the 50 million unit vial concentration is 50 million units/mL. Swirl gently. To prepare solution for infusion, further dilute appropriate dose in NS 100 mL. Final concentration should be ≥10 million units/100 mL.

Mechanism of Action Binds to a specific receptor on the cell wall to initiate intracellular activity; multiple effects can be detected including induction of gene transcription. Inhibits cellular growth, alters the state of cellular differ-entiation, interferes with oncogene expression, alters cell surface antigen expression, increases phagocytic activity of macrophages, and augments cytotoxicity of lymphocytes for target cells

Pharmacodynamics/Kinetics

Distribution: V_d: 31 L; but has been noted to be much greater (370-720 L) in leukemia patients receiving continuous infusion IFN; IFN does not penetrate the CSF

Metabolism: Primarily renal

Bioavailability: IM: 83%; SubQ: 90%

Half-life elimination: IV: ~2 hours; IM, SubQ: ~2-3 hours

Time to peak, serum: IM, SubQ: ~3-12 hours; IV: By the end of a 30-minute infusion

Dosing

Adult & Geriatric Consider premedication with acetaminophen prior to administration to reduce the incidence of some adverse reactions. Not all dosage forms and strengths are appropriate for all indications; refer to product labeling for details. Interferon alfa-2b at doses ≥10 million units/m^2 is associated with a moderate emetic potential; antiemetics may be recom-mended to prevent nausea and vomiting.

Hairy cell leukemia: IM, SubQ: 2 million units/m^2 3 times weekly for up to 6 months (may continue treatment with sustained treatment response); discontinue for disease progression or failure to respond after 6 months

Lymphoma (follicular): SubQ: 5 million units 3 times weekly for up to 18 months

Malignant melanoma: Induction: 20 million units/m^2 IV for 5 consecutive days per week for 4 weeks, followed by maintenance dosing of 10 million units/m^2 SubQ 3 times weekly for 48 weeks

AIDS-related Kaposi sarcoma: IM, SubQ: 30 million units/m^2 3 times weekly; continue until disease progression or until maximal response has been achieved after 16 weeks

Chronic hepatitis B: IM, SubQ: 5 million units/ daily or 10 million units 3 times weekly for 16 weeks

Chronic hepatitis C: IM, SubQ: 3 million units 3 times weekly. In patients with normalization of ALT at 16 weeks, continue treatment (if tolerated) for 18-24 months; consider discontinuation if normalization does not occur at 16 weeks. **Note:** May be used in combination therapy with ribavirin in previously untreated patients or in patients who relapse following alpha interferon therapy.

Condyloma acuminata: Intralesionally: 1 million units/lesion (maximum: 5 lesions per treatment) 3 times weekly (on alternate days) for 3 weeks. May administer a second course at 12-16 weeks.

Pediatric Consider premedication with acetaminophen prior to administration to reduce the incidence of some adverse reactions. Not all dosage forms and strengths are appropriate for all indications; refer to product labeling for details.

Note: The following dosing may also be used in **infants** in the setting of HIV-exposure/-infection (CDC 2009).

Chronic hepatitis B (including HIV coinfection): SubQ: Children and Adolescents 1 to 17 years: 3 million units/m^2 3 times weekly for 1 week, followed by 6 million units/m^2 3 times weekly (maximum: 10 million units per dose); total duration of therapy 16 to 24 weeks (treat for 24 weeks in HIV-exposure/-infection)

Chronic hepatitis C with HIV coinfection: IM, SubQ: Children and Adolescents 1 to 17 years: 3 to 5 million units/m^2 3 times weekly (maximum: 3 million units per dose) with ribavirin for 48 weeks, regardless of HCV genotype (CDC 2009)

Renal Impairment

Renal impairment at treatment initiation: Combination therapy with ribavirin (hepatitis C) is contraindicated in patients with CrCl <50 mL/minute; use combination therapy with ribavirin (hepatitis C) with caution in patients with impaired renal function and CrCl ≥50 mL/minute.

Renal toxicity during treatment: *Indication-specific adjustments:* Lymphoma (follicular): Serum creatinine >2 mg/dL: Permanently discontinue.

Hepatic Impairment

Hepatic impairment at treatment initiation: There are no dosage adjustments provided in the manufacturer's labeling. Contraindicated in patients with decompensated liver disease or autoimmune hepatitis.

Hepatotoxicity during treatment: Permanently discontinue for severe (grade 3) hepatic injury or hepatic decompensation (Child-Pugh class B and C [score >6]).

Indication-specific adjustments:

Lymphoma (follicular): AST >5 times ULN: Permanently discontinue.

Malignant melanoma (induction and maintenance):
ALT/AST >5 to 10 times ULN: Temporarily withhold; resume with a 50% dose reduction when adverse reaction abates
ALT/AST >10 times ULN: Permanently discontinue.

Adjustment for Toxicity

Hematologic toxicity (also refer to indication specified adjustments below): ANC <500/mm^3 or platelets <25,000/mm^3: Discontinue treatment.

Hypersensitivity reaction (acute, serious), ophthalmic disorders (new or worsening), thyroid abnormality development (which cannot be normalized with medication), signs or symptoms of liver failure: Discontinue treatment.

Liver function abnormality, pulmonary infiltrate development, evidence of pulmonary function impairment, or autoimmune disorder development, triglycerides >1,000 mg/dL: Monitor closely and discontinue if appropriate. Permanently discontinue for severe (grade 3) hepatic injury or hepatic decompensation (Child-Pugh class B and C [score >6]).

Neuropsychiatric disorders (during treatment):
Clinical depression or other psychiatric problem: Monitor closely during and for 6 months after treatment.
Severe depression or other psychiatric disorder: Discontinue treatment.
Persistent or worsening psychiatric symptoms, suicidal ideation, aggression towards others: Discontinue treatment and follow with appropriate psychiatric intervention.

Manufacturer-recommended adjustments, listed according to indication:
Lymphoma (follicular):
Neutrophils >1000/mm^3 to <1,500/mm^3: Reduce dose by 50%; may re-escalate to starting dose when neutrophils return to >1,500/mm^3
Severe toxicity (neutrophils <1000/mm^3 or platelets <50,000/mm^3): Temporarily withhold.
AST >5 times ULN or serum creatinine >2 mg/dL: Permanently discontinue.
Hairy cell leukemia:
Platelet count <50,000/mm^3: Do not administer intramuscularly (administer SubQ instead).
Severe toxicity: Reduce dose by 50% or temporarily withhold and resume with 50% dose reduction; permanently discontinue if persistent or recurrent severe toxicity is noted.
Chronic hepatitis B:
WBC <1,500/mm^3, granulocytes <750/mm^3, or platelet count <50,000/mm^3, or other laboratory abnormality or severe adverse reaction: Reduce dose by 50%; may re-escalate to starting dose upon resolution of hematologic toxicity. Discontinue for persistent intolerance.
WBC <1,000/mm^3, granulocytes <500/mm^3, or platelet count <25,000/mm^3: Permanently discontinue
Chronic hepatitis C: Severe toxicity: Reduce dose by 50% or temporarily withhold until subsides; permanently discontinue for persistent toxicities after dosage reduction.
AIDS-related Kaposi sarcoma: Severe toxicity: Reduce dose by 50% or temporarily withhold; may resume at reduced dose with toxicity resolution; permanently discontinue for persistent/recurrent toxicities.

Malignant melanoma (induction and maintenance):
Severe toxicity including neutrophils >250/mm^3 to <500/mm^3 or ALT/AST >5 to 10 times ULN: Temporarily withhold; resume with a 50% dose reduction when adverse reaction abates.
Neutrophils <250/mm^3, ALT/AST >10 times ULN, or severe/persistent adverse reactions: Permanently discontinue.

Combination Regimens

Lymphoma, non-Hodgkin: Fludarabine-Mitoxantrone-Dexamethasone-Rituximab on page 1975
Melanoma: CVD-Interleukin-Interferon (Melanoma) on page 1926
Renal cell cancer:
Bevacizumab-Interferon Alfa (RCC) on page 1844
Interleukin 2-Interferon Alfa-2 (RCC) on page 2018

Administration Administer dose in the evening (if possible) to enhance tolerability. Not all dosage forms are recommended for all administration routes; refer to manufacturer's labeling. Interferon alfa-2b at doses ≥10 million units/m^2 is associated with a moderate emetic potential; antiemetics may be recommended to prevent nausea and vomiting.

IM: Rotate injection sites; preferred sites for injection are anterior thigh, deltoid, and superolateral buttock. Some patients may be appropriate for self-administration with appropriate training. Allow to reach room temperature prior to injection. In hairy cell leukemia treatment, if platelets are <50,000/mm^3, do not administer intramuscularly (administer SubQ instead).
IV: Infuse over ~20 minutes
SubQ: Suggested for those who are at risk for bleeding or are thrombocytopenic. Rotate SubQ injection site; preferred sites for injection are abdomen (except around the navel), anterior thigh, and outer upper arm. Patient should be well hydrated. Some patients may be appropriate for self-administration with appropriate training. Allow to reach room temperature prior to injection.
Intralesional: Inject at an angle nearly parallel to the plane of the skin, directing the needle to center of the base of the wart to infiltrate the lesion core and cause a small wheal. Only infiltrate the keratinized layer; avoid administration which is too deep or shallow. Allow to reach room temperature prior to injection.

Emetic Potential

Children: Minimal (<10%)
Adults:
≥10 million units/m^2: Moderate (30% to 90%)
>5 to <10 million units/m^2: Low (10% to 30%)
≤5 million units/m^2: Minimal (<10%)

Monitoring Parameters

General monitoring parameters for *all indications*:
At baseline (repeat during therapy if clinically indicated): Chest x-ray, serum creatinine, albumin, prothrombin time, triglycerides.
At baseline and periodically thereafter: CBC with differential, platelets and hemoglobin, liver function tests, electrolytes and TSH; ophthalmic exam (or with new ocular symptoms); ECG (in patients with preexisting cardiac abnormalities or in advanced stages of cancer). Monitor serum bilirubin, ALT, AST, alkaline phosphatase and LDH at 2, 8 and 12 weeks following initiation, then every 6 months during treatment. Permanently discontinue for severe (grade 3) hepatic injury or hepatic decompensation (Child-Pugh class B and C [score >6]).

◄ During therapy: Weight; neuropsychiatric changes during and for 6 months after therapy.

Additional *indication-specific* monitoring parameters:

Chronic hepatitis B: CBC with differential and platelets and liver function tests: Baseline, weeks 1, 2, 4, 8, 12, and 16, at the end of treatment, and then 3 and 6 months post treatment

Chronic hepatitis C:

CBC with differential and platelets: Baseline, weeks 1 and 2, then monthly

Liver function: Every 3 months

TSH: Baseline and periodically during treatment; in patients with preexisting thyroid disorders also repeat at 3 months and 6 months

Condyloma acuminate (intralesional administration): Monitor CBC with differential, liver function tests (elevations have been reported).

Malignant melanoma: CBC with differential and platelets and liver function tests: Weekly during induction phase, then monthly during maintenance

Oncology patients: Thyroid function monitoring (Hamnvik 2011): TSH and anti-TPO antibodies at baseline; if TPO antibody positive, monitor TSH every 2 months; if TPO antibody negative, monitor TSH every 6 months

Medication Guide Available Yes

Dosage Forms Excipient information presented when available (limited, particularly for generics); consult specific product labeling.

Solution, Injection:

Intron A: 6,000,000 units/mL (3.8 mL); 10,000,000 units/mL (3.2 mL) [contains edetate disodium, metacresol, polysorbate 80]

Solution Reconstituted, Injection [preservative free]:

Intron A: 10,000,000 units (1 ea); 18,000,000 units (1 ea); 50,000,000 units (1 ea) [contains albumin human]

♦ **Interferon Alpha-2b** *see* Interferon Alfa-2b *on page 930*

♦ **Interleukin 2** *see* Aldesleukin *on page 55*

♦ **Interleukin-11** *see* Oprelvekin *on page 1262*

♦ **Intrapleural Talc** *see* Talc (Sterile) *on page 1588*

♦ **Intron A** *see* Interferon Alfa-2b *on page 930*

Iobenguane I 123 (eye oh BEN gwane eye one TWEN tee three)

Brand Names: US AdreView™

Index Terms 123 Meta-Iodobenzlyguanine Sulfate; 123I-Metaiodobenzyl-guanine (MIBG); I-123 MIBG; I^{123} Iobenguane; Iobenguane Sulfate I 123

Pharmacologic Category Radiopharmaceutical

Use As an adjunct to other diagnostic tests, in the detection of primary or metastatic pheochromocytoma or neuroblastoma; scintigraphic assessment of sympathetic myocardium innervation (by measurement of heart to mediastinum [H/M] ratio of radioactivity uptake) in patients with New York Heart Association class II or class III heart failure and LVEF ≤35% (may help identify lower 1 and 2 year mortality risks, indicated by H/M ratio ≥1.6)

Pregnancy Risk Factor C

Dosing

Adult & Geriatric Note: Thyroid protective agents (SSKI, Lugol's solution or potassium iodide), should be given at least 1 hour prior to administration (in patients at risk for accumulation in thyroid).

Radioimaging: IV: 10 mCi (370 MBq)

Heart failure: Adults: Begin anterior planar chest imaging 4 hours (± 10 minutes) following administration; single photon emission computed tomography (SPECT) may then be performed. Low-energy high-resolution is the recommended imaging collimator; the recommended matrix for planar images is 128x128; position camera to include entire heart and as much of upper chest as possible within field. Follow details within manufacturer's labeling to determine heart to mediastinum (H/M) ratio.

Pheochromocytoma and neuroblastoma: Perform whole body planar scintigraphy imaging 18-30 hours after iobenguane I 123 administration; SPECT may be performed following planar scintigraphy (as appropriate).

Pediatric Note: Thyroid protective agents (SSKI, Lugol's solution or potassium iodide), should be given at least 1 hour prior to administration (in patients at risk for accumulation in thyroid).

Radioimaging: *Pheochromocytoma and neuroblastoma:* Perform whole body planar scintigraphy imaging 18-30 hours after iobenguane I 123 administration; single photon emission computed tomography (SPECT) may be performed following planar scintigraphy (as appropriate). IV:

Children 1 month to 16 years and <70 kg: Dose according to body weight; see table.

Children <16 years and ≥70 kg: 10 mCi (370 MBq)

Children ≥16 years: Refer to adult dosing

Iobenguane I 123 Pediatric Dosing by Body Weight

(Children 1 Month to 16 Years and <70 kg)

Weight (kg)	mCi Dose	MBq Dose
3	1	37
4	1.4	52
6	1.9	70
8	2.3	85.1
10	2.7	99.9
12	3.2	118.4
14	3.6	133.2
16	4	148
18	4.4	162.8
20	4.6	170.2
22	5	185
24	5.3	196.1
26	5.6	207.2
28	5.8	214.6
30	6.2	229.4
32	6.5	240.5
34	6.8	251.6

(continued)

Iobenguane I 123 Pediatric Dosing by Body Weight (continued)

Weight (kg)	mCi Dose	MBq Dose
36	7.1	262.7
38	7.3	270.1
40	7.6	281.2
42	7.8	288.6
44	8	296
46	8.2	303.4
48	8.5	314.5
50	8.8	325.6
52-54	9	333
56-58	9.2	340.4
60-62	9.6	355.2
64-66	9.8	362.6
68	9.9	366.3

Renal Impairment No dosage adjustment provided in manufacturer's labeling (has not been studied). However, radiation exposure may be increased in patients with severe renal impairment, use with caution.

Hepatic Impairment No dosage adjustment provided in manufacturer's labeling.

Additional Information Complete prescribing information should be consulted for additional detail.

Dosage Forms Excipient information presented when available (limited, particularly for generics); consult specific product labeling.
Injection, solution:
  AdreView™: Iobenguane sulfate 0.08 mg and I 123 74 MBq (2 mCi) per mL (5 mL) [contains benzyl alcohol]

♦ **Iobenguane Sulfate I 123** *see* Iobenguane I 123 *on page 940*

♦ **Iodine I 131 Tositumomab and Tositumomab** *see* Tositumomab and Iodine I 131 Tositumomab *on page 1663*

♦ **Ionsys** *see* FentaNYL *on page 692*

Ipilimumab (ip i LIM u mab)

Related Information

Management of Chemotherapy-Induced Nausea and Vomiting in Adults *on page 2142*

Principles of Anticancer Therapy *on page 2261*

Brand Names: US Yervoy

Brand Names: Canada Yervoy

Index Terms MDX-010; MDX-CTLA-4; MOAB-CTLA-4

Pharmacologic Category Antineoplastic Agent, Monoclonal Antibody

Use

US labeling:

Melanoma, unresectable or metastatic: Treatment of unresectable or metastatic melanoma

Melanoma, adjuvant treatment: Adjuvant treatment of cutaneous melanoma in patients with pathologic involvement of regional lymph nodes of more than 1 mm who have undergone complete resection, including total lymphadenectomy

Canadian labeling:

Melanoma, unresectable or metastatic: Treatment of unresectable or metastatic melanoma

Labeled Contraindications There are no contraindications listed in the manufacturer's US labeling.

Canadian labeling: Hypersensitivity to ipilimumab or any component of the formulation; active life-threatening autoimmune disease, or with organ transplantation graft where further immune activation is potentially imminently life-threatening

Pregnancy Considerations Adverse effects were observed in animal reproduction studies. Ipilimumab is an IgG1 immunoglobulin and human IgG1 is known to cross the placenta, therefore, ipilimumab may be expected to reach the fetus. Ipilimumab may cause fetal harm if administered during pregnancy (based on the mechanism of action). Women of reproductive potential should use effective contraception during treatment and for 3 months following the last ipilimumab dose.

Breast-Feeding Considerations It is not known if ipilimumab is excreted in breast milk. The manufacturer recommends to discontinue breast-feeding during treatment and for 3 months following the final dose.

Warnings/Precautions [US Boxed Warning]: Severe and fatal immune-mediated adverse effects may occur. While any organ system may be involved, common severe effects include dermatitis (including toxic epidermal necrolysis), endocrinopathy, enterocolitis, hepatitis, and neuropathy. Reactions generally occur during treatment, although some reactions have occurred weeks to months after treatment discontinuation. Discontinue treatment (permanently) and initiate high-dose systemic corticosteroid treatment for severe immune mediated reactions. Evaluate liver function, adrenocorticotropic hormone (ACTH) level, and thyroid function tests at baseline and prior to each dose. Assess for signs and symptoms of enterocolitis, dermatitis, neuropathy, and endocrinopathy at baseline and prior to each dose. Initiate systemic corticosteroids (prednisone 1 to 2 mg/kg/day or equivalent) for severe reactions. Uncommon immune-mediated adverse effects reported include eosinophilia, hemolytic anemia, iritis, meningitis, myocarditis (fatal), nephritis, pancreatitis, pericarditis, pneumonitis, sarcoidosis, and uveitis. Other rare immune-mediated reactions reported in clinical trials include angiopathy, arthritis, autoimmune central neuropathy (encephalitis), autoimmune thyroiditis, blepharitis, conjunctivitis, episcleritis, erythema multiforme, leukocytoclastic vasculitis, myositis, neurosensory hypoacusis, ocular myositis, polymyalgia rheumatica, polymyositis, psoriasis, scleritis, temporal arteritis, and vasculitis, Administer corticosteroid ophthalmic drops in patients who develop episcleritis, iritis, or uveitis; permanently discontinue ipilimumab if unresponsive to topical ophthalmic immunosuppressive treatments. For severe immune-mediated episcleritis or uveitis, initiate systemic corticosteroids (prednisone 1 to 2 mg/kg/day or equivalent); taper over at least 1 month (Weber, 2012).

Immune-mediated enterocolitis (including fatal cases) may occur. The median time to onset of grade 3 to 5 enterocolitis was 1.1 to 1.7 months. Monitor for signs and symptoms of enterocolitis (abdominal pain, blood in stool, diarrhea, or mucous in stool; with or without fever) and intestinal perforation (peritoneal signs, ileus). If enterocolitis develops, infectious causes should be ruled out; consider endoscopy for persistent or severe symptoms. Withhold ipilimumab treatment and administer antidiarrheals for moderate enterocolitis (diarrhea with ≤6 stools over baseline abdominal pain, mucous or blood in stool); if persists for >1 week, initiate systemic corticosteroids (prednisone at 0.5 mg/kg/day or equivalent). If severe enterocolitis (diarrhea ≥7 stools above baseline, fever, ileus, peritoneal signs) develops, permanently discontinue ipilimumab and initiate systemic corticosteroids (prednisone 1 to 2 mg/kg/day or equivalent); when resolved to ≤ grade 1, taper corticosteroids slowly over ≥1 month (rapid tapering may cause recurrence or worsen symptoms). May consider adding anti-tumor necrosis factor (TNF) or other immunosuppressive therapy for management of immune-mediated enterocolitis unresponsive to 3 to 5 days of systemic corticosteroids or recurring after symptomatic improvement.

Severe, life-threatening or fatal hepatotoxicity and immune-mediated hepatitis have been observed. The median time to onset for grade 3 or 4 immune-mediated hepatitis in patients receiving ipilimumab for adjuvant treatment of melanoma was 2 months. Monitor liver function tests (LFTs) and evaluate for signs of hepatotoxicity prior to each dose; if hepatotoxicity develops, infectious or malignant causes should be ruled out and liver function should be monitored more frequently until resolves. Withhold treatment for grade 2 hepatotoxicity (ALT or AST 2.5 to 5 times ULN or total bilirubin 1.5 to 3 times ULN). If severe or grade 3 or 4 hepatotoxicity develops (ALT or AST >5 times ULN or total bilirubin >3 times ULN), permanently discontinue ipilimumab and initiate systemic corticosteroids (prednisone 1 to 2 mg/kg/day or equivalent). If transaminases do not decrease within 48 hours of steroid initiation, consider adding mycophenolate mofetil (Weber, 2012). May begin tapering corticosteroid (over 1 month) when LFTs show sustained improvement or return to baseline

Severe, life-threatening, or fatal immune-mediated dermatitis has been reported. The median time to onset for dermatologic toxicity is 2 to 3 weeks. Monitor for signs/symptoms of dermatitis, including rash and pruritus; dermatitis should be considered immune-mediated unless identified otherwise. Mild-to-moderate dermatitis (localized rash and pruritus) should be treated symptomatically; topical or systemic corticosteroids should be administered if not resolved within 1 week. Withhold treatment for moderate to severe dermatologic symptoms. Permanently discontinue ipilimumab and initiate systemic corticosteroid (prednisone 1 to 2 mg/kg/day or equivalent) for Stevens-Johnson syndrome, toxic epidermal necrolysis, or rash complicated by dermal ulceration (full thickness) or necrotic, bullous, or hemorrhagic manifestations; when dermatitis is controlled, taper corticosteroid over at least 1 month.

Severe or life-threatening endocrine disorders (hypophysitis, adrenal insufficiency [including adrenal crisis], hyperthyroidism and hypothyroidism) have been reported; may require hospitalization. Endocrine disorders of moderate severity (including hypothyroidism, adrenal insufficiency, hypopituitarism, and less commonly hyperthyroidism and Cushing's syndrome) which have required hormone replacement therapy or medical intervention have also been reported. The median onset for moderate-to-severe endocrine disorders was 2.2 to 2.5 months; long-term hormone replacement therapy has been required in many cases. Monitor thyroid function tests, adrenocorticotropic hormone (ACTH) level, and serum chemistries prior to each dose and as clinically necessary; also monitor for signs of hypophysitis, adrenal insufficiency and thyroid disorders (eg, abdominal pain, fatigue, headache, hypotension, mental status changes, unusual bowel habits); rule out other potential causes such as underlying disease or brain metastases. Endocrine disorders should be considered immune-mediated unless identified otherwise; consider endocrinology referral for further evaluation. If symptomatic, withhold ipilimumab treatment and initiate systemic corticosteroids (prednisone 1 to 2 mg/kg/day or equivalent) and appropriate hormone replacement therapy.

Immune-mediated neuropathies (some fatal) may occur. Severe peripheral motor neuropathy and fatal Guillain-Barré syndrome have been reported (rare). The median time to onset of grade 2 to 5 immune-mediated neuropathy in patients receiving ipilimumab for adjuvant treatment of melanoma was 1.4 to 27.4 months. Monitor for signs of motor or sensory neuropathy (unilateral or bilateral weakness, sensory changes or paresthesia). Withhold treatment in patients with neuropathy that does not interfere with daily activities (moderate neuropathy). Permanently discontinue for severe neuropathy (interferes with daily activities, including symptoms similar to Guillain-Barré syndrome) and treat accordingly. Consider initiating systemic corticosteroids (prednisone 1 to 2 mg/kg/day or equivalent) for severe neuropathies.

Adverse Reactions

>10%:
  Central nervous system: Fatigue (41%), headache (15% [Hodi 2010])
  Dermatologic: Pruritus (24% to 31% [Hodi 2010]), skin rash (19% to 29%; grades 3 to 5: 2% [Hodi 2010]), dermatitis (grade 2: 12%; grades 3 to 5: 2% to 3% [includes Stevens-Johnson syndrome, toxic epidermal necrolysis, dermal ulceration, necrotic, bullous or hemorrhagic dermatitis])
  Gastrointestinal: Nausea (35% [Hodi 2010]), diarrhea (32%; grades 3 to 5: 5%), decreased appetite (27% [Hodi 2010]), vomiting (24% [Hodi 2010]), constipation (21% [Hodi 2010]), abdominal pain (15% [Hodi 2010])
  Hematologic & oncologic: Anemia (12% [Hodi 2010])
  Respiratory: Cough (16% [Hodi 2010]), dyspnea (15% [Hodi 2010])
  Miscellaneous: Fever (12% [Hodi 2010])

1% to 10%:
  Dermatologic: Urticaria (2%), vitiligo (2% [Hodi 2010])
  Endocrine & metabolic: Pituitary insufficiency (4%; grade ≥2: ≤2%), hypophysitis (2% [Hodi 2010]), adrenal insufficiency (≤2% [Hodi 2010]), hypothyroidism (≤2% [Hodi 2010])
  Gastrointestinal: Colitis (8%; grades 3 to 5: 5%), enterocolitis (grade 2: 5%; grades 3 to 5: 7%), intestinal perforation (1%)
  Hematologic & oncologic: Eosinophilia (1%)
  Hepatic: Hepatotoxicity (grade 2: 3%; grades 3 to 5: 1% to 2%), ALT increased (≤2% [Hodi 2010])
  Immunologic: Antibody development (1%)
  Renal: Nephritis (≤1%)

<1%, postmarketing, and/or case reports: Acute respiratory distress, adrenocortical insufficiency (Hodi 2010), arthritis, blepharitis, bronchiolitis obliterans organizing pneumonia (Barjaktarevic 2013), capillary leak syndrome (Hodi 2010), conjunctivitis, Cushing's syndrome, DRESS syndrome, encephalitis, episcleritis, erythema multiforme, esophagitis, gastrointestinal ulcer, giant-cell arteritis, Guillain-Barré syndrome, hemolytic anemia, hepatic failure, hepatitis (immune-mediated), hypersensitivity angiitis, hyperthyroidism, hypoacusis (neurosensory), hypogonadism, increased serum AST, increased serum bilirubin, increased thyroid stimulating hormone level, infusion related reaction, iritis, meningitis, myasthenia gravis, myelofibrosis, myocarditis, myositis, myositis (ocular), neuropathy (sensory and motor), pancreatitis, pericarditis, peritonitis, pneumonitis, polymyalgia rheumatica, polymyositis, psoriasis,

renal failure, sarcoidosis, scleritis, sepsis, thyroiditis (autoimmune), uveitis, vascular disease, vasculitis

Drug Interactions

Metabolism/Transport Effects None known.

Avoid Concomitant Use There are no known interactions where it is recommended to avoid concomitant use.

Increased Effect/Toxicity

Ipilimumab may increase the levels/effects of: Vemurafenib

Decreased Effect There are no known significant interactions involving a decrease in effect.

Storage/Stability Store intact vials refrigerated at 2°C to 8°C (36°F to 46°C); do not freeze. Protect from light. Prior to preparation, allow vials to sit at room temperature for ~5 minutes. Solutions diluted for infusion are stable for up to 24 hours refrigerated or at room temperature.

Preparation for Administration Prior to preparation, allow vials to sit at room temperature for ~5 minutes. Inspect vial prior to use; solution may have a pale yellow color or may contain translucent or white amorphous ipilimumab particles; discard if cloudy or discolored. Withdraw appropriate ipilimumab volume and transfer to IV bag, dilute with NS or D5W to a final concentration between 1 to 2 mg/mL. Mix by gently inverting, do not shake.

Mechanism of Action Ipilimumab is a recombinant human IgG1 immunoglobulin monoclonal antibody which binds to the cytotoxic T-lymphocyte associated antigen 4 (CTLA-4). CTLA-4 is a down-regulator of T-cell activation pathways. Blocking CTLA-4 allows for enhanced T-cell activation and proliferation. In melanoma, ipilimumab may indirectly mediate T-cell immune responses against tumors.

Pharmacodynamics/Kinetics Half-life elimination: Terminal: 15.4 days

Dosing

Adult

Melanoma, unresectable or metastatic: IV: 3 mg/kg every 3 weeks for a maximum of 4 doses; doses may be delayed due to toxicity, but all doses must be administered within 16 weeks of the initial dose.

Melanoma, adjuvant treatment: IV: 10 mg/kg every 3 weeks for 4 doses, followed by 10 mg/kg every 12 weeks for up to 3 years; if toxicity occurs, doses are omitted (not delayed).

Melanoma, unresectable or metastatic, first-line combination therapy (off-label use): IV: 3 mg/kg every 3 weeks for 4 doses (in combination with nivolumab; with nivolumab continued until disease progression or unacceptable toxicity) (Larkin 2015)

Renal Impairment No dosage adjustment necessary.

Hepatic Impairment

Impairment at baseline:

Mild impairment (total bilirubin >1 to 1.5 x ULN **or** AST >ULN): No dosage adjustment necessary.

Moderate or severe impairment (total bilirubin >1.5 x ULN and any AST): There are no dosage adjustments provided in the manufacturer's labeling (has not been studied).

Impairment during treatment:

AST or ALT >2.5 to ≤5 x ULN or bilirubin >1.5 to ≤3 x ULN: Temporarily withhold treatment.

ALT or AST >5 times ULN, or total bilirubin >3 times ULN: Permanently discontinue; also administer systemic corticosteroids (prednisone 1 to 2 mg/kg/day or equivalent). May begin tapering corticosteroid (over 1 month) when LFTs show sustained improvement or return to baseline.

Adjustment for Toxicity

US labeling:

Dermatologic toxicity: Treat symptomatically for mild to moderate dermatitis (eg, localized rash and pruritus); topical or systemic corticosteroids should be administered if not resolved within 1 week. Withhold ipilimumab for moderate to severe dermatologic symptoms. Permanently discontinue for Stevens-Johnson syndrome, toxic epidermal necrolysis, or rash complicated by dermal ulceration (full thickness) or necrotic, bullous, or hemorrhagic manifestations; also initiate systemic corticosteroids (prednisone 1 to 2 mg/kg/day or equivalent). When dermatitis is controlled, taper corticosteroid over at least 1 month.

Endocrinopathy: Temporarily withhold ipilimumab for symptomatic endocrinopathy; initiate systemic corticosteroids (prednisone at 1 to 2 mg/kg/day or equivalent), and begin appropriate hormone replacement therapy. Resume treatment in patients with complete or partial resolution of toxicity (≤ grade 1) and who are receiving prednisone <7.5 mg daily (or equivalent). Permanently discontinue ipilimumab for symptomatic endocrinopathy lasting 6 weeks or longer, or if unable to reduce corticosteroid dose to prednisone ≤7.5 mg daily (or equivalent).

Gastrointestinal toxicity:

Moderate enterocolitis: Withhold ipilimumab and administer antidiarrheal treatment; if moderate enterocolitis persists for >1 week, initiate systemic corticosteroids (prednisone at 0.5 mg/kg/day or equivalent). May resume treatment in patients with complete or partial resolution of toxicity (≤ grade 1) and who are receiving prednisone <7.5 mg daily (or equivalent).

Severe enterocolitis: Permanently discontinue. Initiate systemic corticosteroids (prednisone 1 to 2 mg/kg/day or equivalent). Upon improvement to ≤ grade 1, taper corticosteroids slowly over ≥1 month (rapid tapering may cause recurrence or worsen symptoms). May consider adding anti-tumor necrosis factor (TNF) or other immunosuppressive therapy for management of immune-mediated enterocolitis unresponsive to 3 to 5 days of systemic corticosteroids or recurring after symptomatic improvement.

Neuropathy: Withhold therapy for moderate neuropathy (not interfering with daily activities). Permanently discontinue for severe neuropathy which interferes with daily activities, such as Guillain-Barré-like syndromes. Consider initiating systemic corticosteroids (prednisone 1 to 2 mg/kg/day or equivalent) for severe neuropathies.

Ophthalmologic toxicity: Administer corticosteroid eye drops for uveitis, iritis, or episcleritis. Permanently discontinue for grade 2 through 4 immune-mediated reactions which do not improve to ≤ grade 1 within 2 weeks while receiving topical therapy or which require systemic treatment.

Pancreatitis, immune-mediated: Permanent discontinuation is recommended for grades 3 or 4 amylase or lipase increases (Weber 2012)

◀ *Other toxicity:* Temporarily withhold ipilimumab for grade 2 adverse reactions. May resume treatment in patients (with grade 2 toxicity) with complete or partial resolution of toxicity (≤ grade 1) and who are receiving prednisone <7.5 mg daily (or equivalent). Initiate systemic corticosteroids (prednisone 1 to 2 mg/kg/day or equivalent) for severe immune-mediated adverse reactions. Permanently discontinue for clinically significant or severe immune-mediated adverse reactions, grade 2 reactions lasting 6 weeks or longer, grade 3 or 4 toxicity, or if unable to reduce corticosteroid dose to prednisone ≤7.5 mg daily (or equivalent).

Canadian labeling:

Temporarily withhold scheduled dose for the following:

Moderate immune-mediated reactions

Symptomatic endocrinopathy

Note: If receiving prednisone <7.5 mg daily (or equivalent), may resume with complete or partial resolution (to ≤ grade 1) of symptoms. Resume ipilimumab treatment at 3 mg/kg every 3 weeks until all 4 planned doses have been administered or until 16 weeks from initial dose, whichever occurs first.

Permanently discontinue for the following:

Failure to complete treatment course within 16 weeks of initial dose

Persistent moderate adverse reactions or unable to reduce corticosteroid dose to prednisone 7.5 mg daily (or equivalent)

Severe or life-threatening adverse reactions including:

Central nervous system or neuromuscular toxicity: Severe motor or sensory neuropathy, Guillain-Barré syndrome, or myasthenia gravis

Dermatologic toxicities: Stevens-Johnson syndrome, toxic epidermal necrolysis, or rash complicated by full thickness dermal ulceration, or necrotic, bullous, or hemorrhagic manifestations

Gastrointestinal toxicities: Colitis with abdominal pain, fever, ileus, or peritoneal symptoms, increase in stool frequency (≥7 over baseline), stool incontinence, require IV hydration for >24 hours, or GI hemorrhage or perforation; grades 3/4 amylase or lipase increases (Weber, 2012)

Ophthalmic toxicities: Immune-mediated ocular disease unresponsive to topical immunosuppressive treatment

Severe immune-mediated reactions involving any organ system (eg, myocarditis [noninfectious], nephritis, pancreatitis, pneumonitis)

Combination Regimens

Melanoma:

Ipilimumab (Melanoma Regimen) on page 2019

Ipilimumab-Nivolumab (Melanoma) on page 2019

Administration IV: Infuse over 90 minutes through a non-pyrogenic, low protein-binding in-line filter. Do not administer with other medications. Flush with NS or D5W at the end of infusion

Emetic Potential Minimal (<10%)

Monitoring Parameters Monitor liver function and evaluate for signs of hepatotoxicity prior to each dose; if hepatotoxicity develops, liver function should be monitored more frequently until resolves. If liver functions tests are >8 times ULN, monitor every other day until begin to fall, then weekly until normal (Weber, 2012). Monitor serum chemistries and adrenocorticotropic hormone (ACTH) prior to each dose. Monitor for signs of hypophysitis, adrenal insufficiency and thyroid disorders (eg, abdominal pain, fatigue, headache, hypotension, mental status changes, unusual bowel habits). Monitor TSH, free

T_4 and cortisol levels (morning) at baseline, prior to dose, and as clinically indicated. Monitor for signs and symptoms of enterocolitis (abdominal pain, blood or mucus in stool or diarrhea, and intestinal perforation (peritoneal signs, ileus). Monitor for rash and pruritus. Monitor for signs of motor or sensory neuropathy (unilateral or bilateral weakness, sensory changes or paresthesia). Monitor for ocular toxicity at baseline, then at 4 to 8 weeks with further evaluations as clinically indicated (Renouf, 2012).

Medication Guide Available Yes

Dosage Forms Excipient information presented when available (limited, particularly for generics); consult specific product labeling.

Solution, Intravenous [preservative free]:

Yervoy: 50 mg/10 mL (10 mL); 200 mg/40 mL (40 mL) [contains polysorbate 80]

♦ **Iressa** see Gefitinib on page 770
♦ **IRESSA (Can)** see Gefitinib on page 770

Irinotecan (Conventional) (eye rye no TEE kan con VEN sha nal)

Related Information

Chemotherapy and Obesity on page 2220

Management of Chemotherapy-Induced Nausea and Vomiting in Adults on page 2142

Management of Drug Extravasations on page 2159

Management of EGFR Inhibitor Toxicities: Dermatologic, Ocular, and Gastrointestinal on page 2179

Mucositis and Stomatitis on page 2186

Prevention of Chemotherapy-Induced Nausea and Vomiting in Children on page 2203

Safe Handling of Hazardous Drugs on page 2292

Brand Names: US Camptosar

Brand Names: Canada Camptosar; Irinotecan For Injection; Irinotecan Hydrochloride Injection; Irinotecan Hydrochloride Trihydrate For Injection; Irinotecan Hydrochloride Trihydrate Injection

Index Terms Camptothecin-11; Conventional Irinotecan; CPT-11; Irinotecan HCl; Irinotecan Hydrochloride

Pharmacologic Category Antineoplastic Agent, Camptothecin; Antineoplastic Agent, Topoisomerase I Inhibitor

Use Colorectal cancer, metastatic: Treatment of metastatic carcinoma of the colon or rectum

Labeled Contraindications Hypersensitivity to irinotecan or any component of the formulation

Pregnancy Considerations Adverse events were observed in animal reproduction studies. Information related to the use of irinotecan (conventional) during pregnancy is limited (Cirillo 2012; Taylor 2009). May cause fetal harm if administered during pregnancy. Women of childbearing potential should avoid becoming pregnant while receiving treatment.

Breast-Feeding Considerations It is not known if irinotecan is excreted in breast milk. Due to the potential for serious adverse reactions in the nursing infant, the manufacturer recommends a decision be made to discontinue nursing or to discontinue the drug, taking into account the importance of treatment to the mother.

Warnings/Precautions Hazardous agent - use appropriate precautions for handling and disposal (NIOSH 2014 [group 1]). Severe hypersensitivity reactions (including anaphylaxis) have occurred. Monitor closely; discontinue therapy if hypersensitivity occurs. Irinotecan is an irritant; avoid extravasation. If extravasation occurs, the manufacturer recommends flushing the external site with sterile water and applying ice.

[US Boxed Warning]: Severe diarrhea may be dose-limiting and potentially fatal; early-onset and late-onset diarrhea may occur. Early diarrhea occurs during or within 24 hours of receiving irinotecan and is characterized by cholinergic symptoms; may be prevented or treated with atropine. Late diarrhea may be life-threatening and should be promptly treated with loperamide. Antibiotics may be necessary if patient develops ileus, fever, or severe neutropenia. Interrupt treatment and reduce subsequent doses for severe diarrhea. Early diarrhea is generally transient and rarely severe; cholinergic symptoms may include increased salivation, rhinitis, miosis, diaphoresis, flushing, abdominal cramping, and lacrimation; bradycardia may also occur. Cholinergic symptoms may occur more frequently with higher irinotecan doses. Late diarrhea occurs more than 24 hours after treatment, which may lead to dehydration, electrolyte imbalance, or sepsis. Late diarrhea may be complicated by colitis, ulceration, bleeding, ileus, obstruction, or infection; cases of megacolon and intestinal perforation have been reported. The median time to onset for late diarrhea is 5 days with every-3-week irinotecan dosing and 11 days with weekly dosing. Advise patients to have loperamide readily available for the treatment of late diarrhea. Patients with diarrhea should be carefully monitored and treated promptly; may require fluid and electrolyte therapy. Bowel function should be returned to baseline for at least 24 hours prior to resumption of weekly irinotecan dosing. Avoid diuretics and laxatives in patients experiencing diarrhea. Patients >65 years of age are at greater risk for early and late diarrhea. A dose reduction is recommended for patients ≥70 years of age receiving the every-3-week regimen. Irinotecan is associated with a moderate emetic potential; antiemetics are recommended to prevent nausea and vomiting (Basch 2011; Dupuis 2011; Roila 2010).

[US Boxed Warning]: May cause severe myelosuppression. Deaths due to sepsis following severe neutropenia have been reported. Complications due to neutropenia should be promptly managed with antibiotics. Therapy should be temporarily withheld if neutropenic fever occurs or if the absolute neutrophil count is <1,000/mm^3; reduce the dose upon recovery to an absolute neutrophil count ≥1,000/mm^3. Patients who have previously received pelvic/abdominal radiation therapy have an increased risk of severe bone marrow suppression; the incidence of grade 3 or 4 neutropenia was higher in patients receiving weekly irinotecan who have previously received pelvic/abdominal radiation therapy. Concurrent radiation therapy is not recommended with irinotecan (based on limited data). Fatal cases of interstitial pulmonary disease (IPD)-like events have been reported with single-agent and combination therapy. Risk factors for pulmonary toxicity include preexisting lung disease, use of pulmonary toxic medications, radiation therapy, and colony-stimulating factors. Patients with risk factors should be monitored for respiratory symptoms before and during irinotecan treatment. Promptly evaluate progressive changes in baseline pulmonary symptoms or any new-onset pulmonary symptoms (eg, dyspnea, cough, fever). Discontinue all chemotherapy if IPD is diagnosed.

Patients with even modest elevations in total serum bilirubin levels (1 to 2 mg/dL) have a significantly greater likelihood of experiencing first-course grade 3 or 4 neutropenia than those with bilirubin levels that were <1 mg/dL. Patients with abnormal glucuronidation of bilirubin, such as those with Gilbert's syndrome, may also be at greater risk of myelosuppression when receiving therapy with irinotecan. Use caution when treating patients with known hepatic dysfunction or hyperbilirubinemia exposure to the active metabolite (SN-38) is increased; toxicities may be increased. Dosage adjustments should be considered.

Patients homozygous for the UGT1A1*28 allele are at increased risk of neutropenia; initial one-level dose reduction should be considered for both single-agent and combination regimens. Heterozygous carriers of the UGT1A1*28 allele may also be at increased neutropenic risk; however, most patients have tolerated normal starting doses. A test is available for clinical determination of UGT phenotype, although a dose reduction is already recommended in patients who have experienced toxicity.

Renal impairment and acute renal failure have been reported, possibly due to dehydration secondary to diarrhea. Use with caution in patients with renal impairment; not recommended in patients on dialysis. Patients with bowel obstruction should not be treated with irinotecan until resolution of obstruction. Contains sorbitol; do not use in patients with hereditary fructose intolerance. Thromboembolic events have been reported. Higher rates of hospitalization, neutropenic fever, thromboembolism, first-cycle discontinuation, and early mortality were observed in patients with a performance status of 2 than in patients with a performance status of 0 or 1. Except as part of a clinical trial, use in combination with fluorouracil and leucovorin administered for 4 or 5 consecutive days ("Mayo Clinic" regimen) is not recommended due to increased toxicity. Potentially significant interactions may exist, requiring dose or frequency adjustment, additional monitoring, and/or selection of alternative therapy. CYP3A4 enzyme inducers may decrease exposure to irinotecan and SN-38 (active metabolite); enzyme inhibitors may increase exposure; for use in patients with CNS tumors (off-label use), selection of antiseizure medications that are not enzyme inducers is preferred. Irinotecan (conventional) and irinotecan (liposomal) are **NOT** interchangeable. Dosing differs between formulations; verify intended product and dose prior to preparation and administration.

Adverse Reactions Frequency of adverse reactions reported for single-agent use of irinotecan only.

>10%:

Cardiovascular: Vasodilation (9% to 11%)

Central nervous system: Cholinergic toxicity (47% - includes rhinitis, increased salivation, miosis, lacrimation, diaphoresis, flushing and intestinal hyperperistalsis); fever (44% to 45%), pain (23% to 24%), dizziness (15% to 21%), insomnia (19%), headache (17%), chills (14%)

Dermatologic: Alopecia (46% to 72%), rash (13% to 14%)

Endocrine & metabolic: Dehydration (15%)

Gastrointestinal: Diarrhea, late (83% to 88%; grade 3/4: 14% to 31%), diarrhea, early (43% to 51%; grade 3/4: 7% to 22%), nausea (70% to 86%), abdominal pain (57% to 68%), vomiting (62% to 67%), cramps (57%), anorexia (44% to 55%), constipation (30% to 32%), mucositis (30%), weight loss (30%), flatulence (12%), stomatitis (12%)

◀ Hematologic: Anemia (60% to 97%; grades 3/4: 5% to 7%), leukopenia (63% to 96%, grades 3/4: 14% to 28%), thrombocytopenia (96%, grades 3/4: 1% to 4%), neutropenia (30% to 96%; grades 3/4: 14% to 31%)

Hepatic: Bilirubin increased (84%), alkaline phosphatase increased (13%)

Neuromuscular & skeletal: Weakness (69% to 76%), back pain (14%)

Respiratory: Dyspnea (22%), cough (17% to 20%), rhinitis (16%)

Miscellaneous: Diaphoresis (16%), infection (14%)

1% to 10%:

Cardiovascular: Edema (10%), hypotension (6%), thromboembolic events (5%)

Central nervous system: Somnolence (9%), confusion (3%)

Gastrointestinal: Abdominal fullness (10%), dyspepsia (10%)

Hematologic: Neutropenic fever (grades 3/4: 2% to 6%), hemorrhage (grades 3/4: 1% to 5%), neutropenic infection (grades 3/4: 1% to 2%)

Hepatic: AST increased (10%), ascites and/or jaundice (grades 3/4: 9%)

Respiratory: Pneumonia (4%)

<1%, postmarketing, and/or case reports: ALT increased, amylase increased, anaphylactoid reaction, anaphylaxis, angina, arterial thrombosis, bleeding, bradycardia, cardiac arrest, cerebral infarct, cerebrovascular accident, circulatory failure, colitis, deep thrombophlebitis, dysarthria, dysrhythmia, embolus, gastrointestinal bleeding, gastrointestinal obstruction, hepatomegaly, hiccups, hyperglycemia, hypersensitivity, hyponatremia, ileus, interstitial pulmonary disease (IPD), intestinal perforation, ischemic colitis, lipase increased, lymphocytopenia, megacolon, MI, muscle cramps, myocardial ischemia, neutropenic typhlitis, pancreatitis, paresthesia, peripheral vascular disorder, pulmonary embolus; pulmonary toxicity (dyspnea, fever, reticulo-nodular infiltrates on chest x-ray); renal failure (acute), renal impairment, syncope, thrombocytopenia (immune mediated), thrombophlebitis, thrombosis, typhlitis, ulceration, ulcerative colitis, vertigo

Note: In limited pediatric experience, dehydration (often associated with severe hypokalemia and hyponatremia) was among the most significant grade 3/4 adverse events, with a frequency up to 29%. In addition, grade 3/4 infection was reported in 24%.

Drug Interactions

Metabolism/Transport Effects Substrate of BCRP, CYP3A4 (major), P-glycoprotein, SLCO1B1, UGT1A1; **Note:** Assignment of Major/Minor substrate status based on clinically relevant drug interaction potential

Avoid Concomitant Use

Avoid concomitant use of Irinotecan (Conventional) with any of the following: BCG (Intravesical); CloZAPine; Conivaptan; CYP3A4 Inducers (Strong); CYP3A4 Inhibitors (Strong); Dipyrone; Fusidic Acid (Systemic); Idelalisib; Natalizumab; Pimecrolimus; St Johns Wort; Tacrolimus (Topical); Tofacitinib; UGT1A1 Inhibitors; Vaccines (Live)

Increased Effect/Toxicity

Irinotecan (Conventional) may increase the levels/effects of: CloZAPine; Fingolimod; Leflunomide; Natalizumab; Tofacitinib; Vaccines (Live)

The levels/effects of Irinotecan (Conventional) may be increased by: Aprepitant; Conivaptan; CYP3A4 Inhibitors (Moderate); CYP3A4 Inhibitors (Strong); Dasatinib; Denosumab; Dipyrone; Fosaprepitant; Fusidic Acid (Systemic); Idelalisib; Ivacaftor; Luliconazole; Mifepristone; Netupitant; Osimertinib; Palbociclib; P-glycoprotein/ABCB1 Inhibitors; Pimecrolimus; Ranolazine; Roflumilast; Rolapitant; Simeprevir; SORAfenib; Stiripentol; Tacrolimus (Topical); Teriflunomide; Trastuzumab; UGT1A1 Inhibitors

Decreased Effect

Irinotecan (Conventional) may decrease the levels/effects of: BCG (Intravesical); Coccidioides immitis Skin Test; Sipuleucel-T; Vaccines (Inactivated); Vaccines (Live)

The levels/effects of Irinotecan (Conventional) may be decreased by: Bosentan; CYP3A4 Inducers (Moderate); CYP3A4 Inducers (Strong); Dabrafenib; Deferasirox; Echinacea; Osimertinib; P-glycoprotein/ABCB1 Inducers; Siltuximab; St Johns Wort; Tocilizumab

Storage/Stability Store intact vials at 15°C to 30°C (59°F to 86°F). Protect from light; retain vials in original carton until use. Solutions diluted in NS may precipitate if refrigerated. Solutions diluted in D_5W are stable for 24 hours at room temperature or 48 hours under refrigeration at 2°C to 8°C (36°F to 46°F), although the manufacturer recommends use within 24 hours if refrigerated, or within 4 to 12 hours (manufacturer dependent; refer to specific prescribing information) at room temperature (including infusion time) only if prepared under strict aseptic conditions (eg, laminar flow hood). Do not freeze. Undiluted commercially available injectable solution prepared in oral syringes is stable for 21 days under refrigeration (Wagner 2010).

Preparation for Administration Hazardous agent; use appropriate precautions for handling and disposal (NIOSH 2014 [group 1]). Dilute in D_5W (preferred) or NS to a final concentration of 0.12 to 2.8 mg/mL.

Mechanism of Action Irinotecan and its active metabolite (SN-38) bind reversibly to topoisomerase I-DNA complex preventing religation of the cleaved DNA strand. This results in the accumulation of cleavable complexes and double-strand DNA breaks. As mammalian cells cannot efficiently repair these breaks, cell death consistent with S-phase cell cycle specificity occurs, leading to termination of cellular replication.

Pharmacodynamics/Kinetics

Protein binding, plasma: Predominantly albumin; Irinotecan: 30% to 68%, SN-38 (active metabolite): ~95%

Metabolism: Primarily hepatic to SN-38 (active metabolite) by carboxylesterase enzymes; may also undergo CYP3A4-mediated metabolism to inactive metabolites (one of which may be hydrolyzed to release SN-38). SN-38 undergoes conjugation by UDP-glucuronosyl transferase 1A1 (UGT1A1) to form a glucuronide metabolite. SN-38 is increased by UGT1A1*28 polymorphism (10% of North Americans are homozygous for UGT1A1*28 allele).

Half-life elimination: Irinotecan: 6 to 12 hours; SN-38: ~10 to 20 hours

Time to peak: SN-38: Following 90-minute infusion: ~1 hour

Excretion: Urine: Irinotecan (11% to 20%), metabolites (SN-38 <1%, SN-38 glucuronide, 3%)

Dosing

Adult

Note: A reduction in the starting dose by one dose level should be considered for prior pelvic/abdominal radiotherapy, performance status of 2, or known homozygosity for UGT1A1*28 allele (subsequent dosing/adjustments should be based on individual tolerance). Irinotecan (conventional) and irinotecan (liposomal) are **NOT** interchangeable. Dosing differs between formulations; verify intended product and dose prior to preparation and administration.

◄ **Premedications:** Consider premedication of atropine 0.25 to 1 mg IV or SubQ in patients with cholinergic symptoms (eg, increased salivation, rhinitis, miosis, diaphoresis, abdominal cramping) or early-onset diarrhea. Irinotecan is associated with a moderate emetic potential; antiemetics are recommended to prevent nausea and vomiting (Basch 2011; Dupuis 2011; Roila 2010).

Colorectal cancer, metastatic (single-agent therapy): IV:

Weekly regimen: 125 mg/m^2 over 90 minutes on days 1, 8, 15, and 22 of a 6-week treatment cycle (may adjust upward to 150 mg/m^2 if tolerated)

Adjusted dose level -1: 100 mg/m^2

Adjusted dose level -2: 75 mg/m^2

Further adjust to 50 mg/m^2 (in decrements of 25 to 50 mg/m^2) if needed

Once-every-3-week regimen: 350 mg/m^2 over 90 minutes, once every 3 weeks

Adjusted dose level -1: 300 mg/m^2

Adjusted dose level -2: 250 mg/m^2

Further adjust to 200 mg/m^2 (in decrements of 25 to 50 mg/m^2) if needed

Colorectal cancer, metastatic (in combination with fluorouracil and leucovorin): IV: Six-week (42-day) cycle:

Regimen 1: 125 mg/m^2 over 90 minutes on days 1, 8, 15, and 22; to be given in combination with bolus leucovorin and fluorouracil (leucovorin administered immediately following irinotecan; fluorouracil immediately following leucovorin)

Adjusted dose level -1: 100 mg/m^2

Adjusted dose level -2: 75 mg/m^2

Further adjust if needed in decrements of ~20%

Regimen 2: 180 mg/m^2 over 90 minutes on days 1, 15, and 29; to be given in combination with infusional leucovorin and bolus/infusion fluorouracil (leucovorin administered immediately following irinotecan; fluorouracil immediately following leucovorin)

Adjusted dose level -1: 150 mg/m^2

Adjusted dose level -2: 120 mg/m^2

Further adjust if needed in decrements of ~20%

Colorectal cancer, metastatic (off-label dosing): IV: FOLFOXIRI regimen: 165 mg/m^2 over 1 hour once every 2 weeks (in combination with oxaliplatin, leucovorin, and fluorouracil) (Falcone 2007)

Cervical cancer, recurrent or metastatic (off-label use): IV: 125 mg/m^2 over 90 minutes once weekly for 4 consecutive weeks followed by a 2-week rest during each 6 week treatment cycle (Verschraegen 1997)

CNS tumor, recurrent glioblastoma (off-label use): IV: 125 mg/m^2 over 90 minutes once every 2 weeks (in combination with bevacizumab). **NOTE:** In patients taking concurrent antiepileptic enzyme-inducing medications irinotecan dose was increased to 340 mg/m^2 (Friedman 2009; Vredenburgh 2007).

Esophageal cancer, metastatic or locally advanced (off-label use): IV: 65 mg/m^2 over 90 minutes days 1, 8, 15, and 22 of a 6-week treatment cycle (in combination with cisplatin) (Ajani 2002; Ilson 1999) **or** 180 mg/m^2 over 90 minutes every 2 weeks (in combination with leucovorin and fluorouracil) (Guimbaud 2014) **or** 250 mg/m^2 every 3 weeks (in combination with capecitabine) (Leary 2009; Moehler 2010)

Ewing sarcoma, recurrent or progressive (off-label use): IV: 20 mg/m^2 days 1 to 5 and days 8 to 12 every 3 weeks (in combination with temozolomide) (Casey 2009)

Gastric cancer, metastatic or locally advanced (off-label use): IV: 150 mg/m^2 (as a single agent) on days 1 and 15 of a 4-week treatment cycle (Hironaka 2013) **or** 65 mg/m^2 over 90 minutes days 1, 8, 15, and 22 of a 6-week treatment cycle (in combination with cisplatin) (Ajani 2002) **or** 70 mg/m^2 over 90 minutes on days 1 and 15 of a 4-week treatment cycle (in combination with cisplatin) for up to 6 cycles (Park 2005) **or** 180 mg/m^2 over 90 minutes every 2 weeks (in combination with leucovorin and fluorouracil) (Bouche 2004; Guimbaud 2014) **or** 250 mg/m^2 every 3 weeks (in combination with capecitabine) (Moehler 2010)

Non-small cell lung cancer, advanced (off-label use): IV: 60 mg/m^2 days 1, 8, and 15 every 4 weeks (in combination with cisplatin) (Ohe 2007)

Ovarian cancer, recurrent, platinum- and taxane-resistant (off-label use): IV: 100 mg/m^2 days 1, 8, and 15 every 4 weeks (as a single-agent) for up to 6 cycles (Matsumoto 2006)

Pancreatic cancer, advanced (off-label use): IV: FOLFIRINOX regimen: 180 mg/m^2 over 90 minutes every 2 weeks (in combination with oxaliplatin, leucovorin, and fluorouracil) (Conroy 2005; Conroy 2011)

Small cell lung cancer, extensive stage (off-label use): IV: 60 mg/m^2 days 1, 8, and 15 every 4 weeks (in combination with cisplatin) (Noda 2002) **or** 65 mg/m^2 days 1 and 8 every 3 weeks (in combination with cisplatin) (Hanna 2006) **or** 175 mg/m^2 day 1 every 3 weeks (in combination with carboplatin) (Hermes 2008) **or** 50 mg/m^2 days 1, 8 and 15 every 4 weeks (in combination with carboplatin) (Schmittel 2006)

Geriatric

Weekly dosing schedule: No dosing adjustment is recommended

Every 3-week dosing colorectal cancer schedule: Recommended initial dose is 300 mg/m^2/dose for patients ≥70 years

Pediatric See "Note" in adult dosing.

Ewing sarcoma, recurrent or progressive (off-label use): IV: Refer to adult dosing.

Rhabdomyosarcoma, relapsed/refractory (off-label use; Vassal 2007): IV:

Children <10 kg: 20 mg/kg once every 3 weeks

Children ≥10 kg and Adolescents: 600 mg/m^2 once every 3 weeks

Renal Impairment

Renal impairment: There are no dosage adjustments provided in the manufacturer's labeling (has not been studied); use with caution.

Dialysis: Use in patients with dialysis is not recommended by the manufacturer; however, literature suggests reducing weekly dose from 125 mg/m^2 to 50 mg/m^2 and administer after hemodialysis or on nondialysis days (Janus 2010).

Hepatic Impairment

Manufacturer's labeling:

Liver metastases with normal hepatic function: No dosage adjustment necessary.

Bilirubin >ULN to ≤2 mg/dL: Consider reducing initial dose by one dose level

Bilirubin >2 mg/dL: Use is not recommended

Alternate recommendations: The following adjustments have also been recommended:

Bilirubin 1.5 to 3 mg/dL: Administer 75% of dose (Floyd 2006)

Bilirubin 1.51 to 3 times ULN: Reduce dose from 350 mg/m^2 every 3 weeks to 200 mg/m^2 every 3 weeks (Raymond 2002)

Obesity *ASCO Guidelines for appropriate chemotherapy dosing in obese adults with cancer:* Utilize patient's actual body weight (full weight) for calculation of body surface area- or weight-based dosing, particularly when the intent of therapy is curative; manage regimen-related toxicities in the same manner as for nonobese patients; if a dose reduction is utilized due to toxicity, consider resumption of full weight-based dosing with subsequent cycles, especially if cause of toxicity (eg, hepatic or renal impairment) is resolved (Griggs 2012).

Adjustment for Toxicity It is recommended that new courses begin only after the granulocyte count recovers to ≥1,500/mm^3, the platelet counts recover to ≥100,000/mm^3, and treatment-related diarrhea has fully resolved. Depending on the patient's ability to tolerate therapy, doses should be adjusted in increments of 25 to 50 mg/m^2. Treatment should be delayed 1 to 2 weeks to allow for recovery from treatment-related toxicities. If the patient has not recovered after a 2-week delay, consider discontinuing irinotecan. See tables.

Colorectal Cancer: Single-Agent Schedule: Recommended Dosage Modifications[1]

Toxicity NCI Grade[2] (Value)	During a Cycle of Therapy	At Start of Subsequent Cycles of Therapy (After Adequate Recovery), Compared to Starting Dose in Previous Cycle[1]	
	Weekly	Weekly	Once Every 3 Weeks
No toxicity	Maintain dose level	↑ 25 mg/m^2 up to a maximum dose of 150 mg/m^2	Maintain dose level
Neutropenia			
Grade 1 (1,500 to 1,999/mm^3)	Maintain dose level	Maintain dose level	Maintain dose level
Grade 2 (1,000 to 1,499/mm^3)	↓ 25 mg/m^2	Maintain dose level	Maintain dose level
Grade 3 (500 to 999/mm^3)	Omit dose until resolved to ≤ grade 2, then ↓ 25 mg/m^2	↓ 25 mg/m^2	↓ 50 mg/m^2
Grade 4 (<500/mm^3)	Omit dose until resolved to ≤ grade 2, then ↓ 50 mg/m^2	↓ 50 mg/m^2	↓ 50 mg/m^2
Neutropenic Fever (grade 4 neutropenia and ≥ grade 2 fever)	Omit dose until resolved, then ↓ 50 mg/m^2	↓ 50 mg/m^2	↓ 50 mg/m^2
Other Hematologic Toxicities	Dose modifications for leukopenia, thrombocytopenia, and anemia during a course of therapy and at the start of subsequent courses of therapy are also based on NCI toxicity criteria and are the same as recommended for neutropenia above.		

(continued)

Colorectal Cancer: Single-Agent Schedule: Recommended Dosage Modifications[1] (continued)

Toxicity NCI Grade[2] (Value)	During a Cycle of Therapy	At Start of Subsequent Cycles of Therapy (After Adequate Recovery), Compared to Starting Dose in Previous Cycle[1]	
	Weekly	Weekly	Once Every 3 Weeks
Diarrhea			
Grade 1 (2 to 3 stools/day > pretreatment)	Maintain dose level	Maintain dose level	Maintain dose level
Grade 2 (4 to 6 stools/day > pretreatment)	↓ 25 mg/m²	Maintain dose level	Maintain dose level
Grade 3 (7 to 9 stools/day > pretreatment)	Omit dose until resolved to ≤ grade 2, then ↓ 25 mg/m²	↓ 25 mg/m²	↓ 50 mg/m²
Grade 4 (≥10 stools/day > pretreatment)	Omit dose until resolved to ≤ grade 2, then ↓ 50 mg/m²	↓ 50 mg/m²	↓ 50 mg/m²
Other Nonhematologic Toxicities[3]			
Grade 1	Maintain dose level	Maintain dose level	Maintain dose level
Grade 2	↓ 25 mg/m²	↓ 25 mg/m²	↓ 50 mg/m²
Grade 3	Omit dose until resolved to ≤ grade 2, then ↓ 25 mg/m²	↓ 25 mg/m²	↓ 50 mg/m²
Grade 4	Omit dose until resolved to ≤ grade 2, then ↓ 50 mg/m²	↓ 50 mg/m²	↓ 50 mg/m²

[1]All dose modifications should be based on the worst preceding toxicity.

[2]National Cancer Institute Common Toxicity Criteria (version 1.0).

[3]Excludes alopecia, anorexia, asthenia.

Colorectal Cancer: Combination Schedules: Recommended Dosage Modifications[1]

Toxicity NCI[2] Grade (Value)	During a Cycle of Therapy	At the Start of Subsequent Cycles of Therapy (After Adequate Recovery), Compared to the Starting Dose in the Previous Cycle[1]
No toxicity	Maintain dose level	Maintain dose level
Neutropenia		
Grade 1 (1,500 to 1,999/mm³)	Maintain dose level	Maintain dose level
Grade 2 (1,000 to 1,499/mm³)	↓ 1 dose level	Maintain dose level
Grade 3 (500 to 999/mm³)	Omit dose until resolved to ≤ grade 2, then ↓ 1 dose level	↓ 1 dose level
Grade 4 (<500/mm³)	Omit dose until resolved to ≤ grade 2, then ↓ 2 dose levels	↓ 2 dose levels

(continued) ▶

Colorectal Cancer: Combination Schedules: Recommended Dosage Modifications[1] *(continued)*

Toxicity NCI[2] Grade (Value)	During a Cycle of Therapy	At the Start of Subsequent Cycles of Therapy (After Adequate Recovery), Compared to the Starting Dose in the Previous Cycle[1]
Neutropenic Fever (grade 4 neutropenia and ≥ grade 2 fever)	Omit dose until resolved, then ↓ 2 dose levels	
Other Hematologic Toxicities	Dose modifications for leukopenia or thrombocytopenia during a course of therapy and at the start of subsequent courses of therapy are also based on NCI toxicity criteria and are the same as recommended for neutropenia above.	
Diarrhea		
Grade 1 (2 to 3 stools/day > pretreatment)	Delay dose until resolved to baseline, then give same dose	Maintain dose level
Grade 2 (4 to 6 stools/day > pretreatment)	Omit dose until resolved to baseline, then ↓ 1 dose level	Maintain dose level
Grade 3 (7 to 9 stools/day > pretreatment)	Omit dose until resolved to baseline, then ↓ by 1 dose level	↓ 1 dose level
Grade 4 (≥10 stools/day > pretreatment)	Omit dose until resolved to baseline, then ↓ 2 dose levels	↓ 2 dose levels
Other Nonhematologic Toxicities[3]		
Grade 1	Maintain dose level	Maintain dose level
Grade 2	Omit dose until resolved to ≤ grade 1, then ↓ 1 dose level	Maintain dose level
Grade 3	Omit dose until resolved to ≤ grade 2, then ↓ 1 dose level	↓ 1 dose level
Grade 4	Omit dose until resolved to ≤ grade 2, then ↓ 2 dose levels	↓ 2 dose levels
Mucositis and/or stomatitis	Decrease only 5-FU, not irinotecan	Decrease only 5-FU, not irinotecan

[1]All dose modifications should be based on the worst preceding toxicity.

[2]National Cancer Institute Common Toxicity Criteria (version 1.0).

[3]Excludes alopecia, anorexia, asthenia.

Combination Regimens

Bone sarcoma (Ewing sarcoma): Irinotecan-Temozolomide (Ewing Sarcoma) on page 2024
Brain tumors: Bevacizumab-Irinotecan (Glioblastoma) on page 1844
Cervical cancer: Irinotecan (Cervical Regimen) on page 2021
Colorectal cancer:
  Bevacizumab + FOLFIRI (Colorectal) on page 1842
  Cetuximab (Biweekly)-Irinotecan (Colorectal) on page 1879
  Cetuximab + FOLFIRI (Colorectal) on page 1882
  Cetuximab-Irinotecan (Colorectal) on page 1883
  Fluorouracil-Leucovorin-Irinotecan (Saltz Regimen) (Colorectal) on page 1981
  FOLFIRI (Colorectal) on page 1983

FOLFOXIRI (Colorectal) on page 1987
Irinotecan (Colorectal Regimen) on page 2022
Panitumumab + FOLFIRI (Colorectal) on page 2058
Ramucirumab-FOLFIRI (Colorectal) on page 2072
Ziv-Aflibercept + FOLFIRI (Colorectal) on page 2112
Esophageal cancer:
Irinotecan-Capecitabine (Esophageal Cancer) on page 2019
Irinotecan-Cisplatin (Esophageal Cancer) on page 2021
Irinotecan-Fluorouracil-Leucovorin (Esophageal Cancer) on page 2022
Gastric cancer:
Cisplatin-Irinotecan (Gastric) on page 1908
Irinotecan-Capecitabine (Gastric Cancer) on page 2020
Irinotecan-Leucovorin-Fluorouracil (Gastric Cancer) on page 2023
Lung cancer (non-small cell): Cisplatin-Irinotecan (NSCLC) on page 1908
Lung cancer (small cell):
Carboplatin-Irinotecan (Small Cell Lung Cancer) on page 1868
Cisplatin-Irinotecan (Small Cell Lung Cancer) on page 1908
Irinotecan (Small Cell Lung Cancer Regimen) on page 2024
Pancreatic cancer: FOLFIRINOX (Pancreatic) on page 1984

Administration Administer by IV infusion, usually over 90 minutes. Irinotecan is associated with a moderate emetic potential (Basch 2011; Dupuis 2011; Roila 2010); premedication with dexamethasone and a 5-HT$_3$ blocker is recommended 30 minutes prior to administration; prochlorperazine may be considered for subsequent use (if needed). Consider atropine 0.25 to 1 mg IV or SubQ as premedication for or treatment of cholinergic symptoms (eg, increased salivation, rhinitis, miosis, diaphoresis, abdominal cramping) or early onset diarrhea.

The recommended regimen to manage late diarrhea is loperamide 4 mg orally at onset of late diarrhea, followed by 2 mg every 2 hours (or 4 mg every 4 hours at night) until 12 hours have passed without a bowel movement. If diarrhea recurs, then repeat administration. Loperamide should not be used for more than 48 consecutive hours.

Hazardous agent; use appropriate precautions for handling and disposal (NIOSH 2014 [group 1]).

Vesicant/Extravasation Risk May be an irritant

Emetic Potential Children and Adults: Moderate (30% to 90%)

Monitoring Parameters CBC with differential, platelet count, and hemoglobin with each dose; bilirubin, electrolytes (with severe diarrhea); bowel movements and hydration status; signs/symptoms of pulmonary toxicity or hypersensitivity reactions; monitor infusion site for signs of inflammation and avoid extravasation

A test is available for genotyping of UGT1A1; however, use of the test is not widely accepted and a dose reduction is already recommended in patients who have experienced toxicity.

Dietary Considerations Contains sorbitol; do not use in patients with hereditary fructose intolerance.

Dosage Forms Excipient information presented when available (limited, particularly for generics); consult specific product labeling.
Solution, Intravenous, as hydrochloride:
Camptosar: 40 mg/2 mL (2 mL); 100 mg/5 mL (5 mL); 300 mg/15 mL (15 mL)
Generic: 40 mg/2 mL (2 mL); 100 mg/5 mL (5 mL); 500 mg/25 mL (25 mL)

Solution, Intravenous, as hydrochloride [preservative free]:
  Generic: 40 mg/2 mL (2 mL); 100 mg/5 mL (5 mL)

Irinotecan (Liposomal) (eye rye no TEE kan lye po SO mal)

Related Information
Common Toxicity Criteria *on page 2122*
Management of Chemotherapy-Induced Nausea and Vomiting in Adults *on page 2142*
Safe Handling of Hazardous Drugs *on page 2292*

Brand Names: US Onivyde

Index Terms Irinotecan Liposome; Liposomal Irinotecan; Liposome-Encapsulated Irinotecan Hydrochloride PEP02; MM-398; Onivyde

Pharmacologic Category Antineoplastic Agent, Camptothecin; Antineoplastic Agent, Topoisomerase I Inhibitor

Use
Pancreatic adenocarcinoma, metastatic: Treatment of metastatic adenocarcinoma of the pancreas (in combination with fluorouracil and leucovorin) disease progression following gemcitabine-based therapy.

Limitations of use: Irinotecan (liposomal) is not indicated as a single agent for the treatment of metastatic adenocarcinoma of the pancreas.

Labeled Contraindications Severe hypersensitivity to irinotecan (liposomal), irinotecan hydrochloride, or any component of the formulation

Pregnancy Considerations Animal reproduction studies have not been conducted with the liposomal formulation. Based on the mechanism of action as well as animal data using irinotecan (conventional), irinotecan (liposomal) may cause fetal harm if administered during pregnancy. Women of child-bearing potential should use effective contraception while receiving treatment and avoid pregnancy for one month following the last dose. Males with female partners of reproductive potential should use condoms during therapy and for four months following the last dose.

Breast-Feeding Considerations It is not known if irinotecan (liposomal) is excreted in breast milk. Due to the potential for serious adverse reactions in the nursing infant, the manufacturer does not recommend breast-feeding during therapy or for one month following the last dose.

Warnings/Precautions Hazardous agent - use appropriate precautions for handling and disposal (NIOSH 2014 [group 1]). **[US Boxed Warning]: Fatal neutropenic sepsis occurred in nearly 1% of patients receiving irinotecan (liposomal). Severe or life-threatening neutropenic fever or sepsis occurred in 3% and severe or life-threatening neutropenia occurred in 20% of patients receiving irinotecan (liposomal) in combination with fluorouracil and leucovorin. Withhold irinotecan (liposomal) for absolute neutrophil count below 1,500/mm³ or neutropenic fever. Monitor blood cell counts periodically during treatment** (days 1 and 8 of each cycle and more frequently if clinically necessary). May require therapy interruption, dose reduction, and/or discontinuation. Anemia, lymphopenia, and thrombocytopenia also commonly occur. The incidence of neutropenia was higher in Asian patients (compared to white patients).

[US Boxed Warning]: Severe diarrhea (may be life-threatening) occurred in 13% of patients receiving irinotecan (liposomal) in combination with fluorouracil and leucovorin. Do not administer irinotecan (liposomal) to patients with bowel obstruction. Withhold irinotecan (liposomal) for diarrhea of grade 2 to 4 severity. Administer loperamide for late diarrhea

of any severity. Administer atropine, if not contraindicated, for early diarrhea of any severity. Early onset diarrhea occurs within 24 hours of chemotherapy, and may cause other symptoms of cholinergic reaction. Late onset diarrhea occurs more than 24 hours following chemotherapy. Diarrhea may require therapy interruption, dosage reduction, and/or discontinuation. Nausea, vomiting and stomatitis commonly occur. The pharmacokinetics of irinotecan (liposomal) have not been studied in patients with hepatic impairment. However, exposure to the active metabolite (SN-38) is increased in patients with hepatic impairment receiving irinotecan (conventional); toxicities may be increased.

Irinotecan (conventional) may cause severe and fatal interstitial lung disease (ILD). Withhold irinotecan (liposomal) during diagnostic evaluation if new or progressive dyspnea, cough, or fever occurs during use. Discontinue therapy if ILD diagnosis is confirmed. Severe hypersensitivity reactions (including anaphylaxis) have occurred with irinotecan (conventional). Monitor closely; permanently discontinue irinotecan (liposomal) therapy if severe hypersensitivity occurs. Irinotecan (liposomal) and irinotecan (conventional) are NOT interchangeable. Dosing differs between formulations; verify intended product and dose prior to preparation and administration. Potentially significant interactions may exist, requiring dose or frequency adjustment, additional monitoring, and/or selection of alternative therapy. CYP3A4 enzyme inducers may decrease exposure to irinotecan and SN-38 (active metabolite); avoid concomitant use (substitute non-enzyme inducing therapies at least 2 weeks prior to irinotecan [liposomal] initiation). Enzyme inhibitors may increase exposure; avoid concomitant use (discontinue strong CYP3A4 inhibitors at least 1 week prior to irinotecan [liposomal] initiation).

Adverse Reactions Frequency not always defined. Percentages reported as part of combination chemotherapy regimens.

Cardiovascular: Septic shock (≥2%)

Central nervous system: Fatigue (≤56%)

Dermatologic: Alopecia (14%)

Endocrine & metabolic: Increased serum alanine aminotransferase (51%), hypoalbuminemia (43%), hypomagnesemia (35%), hypocalcemia (32%), hypokalemia (32%), hypophosphatemia (29%), hyponatremia (27%), weight loss (17%), dehydration (8%)

Gastrointestinal: Diarrhea (59%, grade 3/4: 13%; early onset 30%, grade 3/4: 3%; late onset 43%, grade 3/4: 9%), vomiting (52%), nausea (51%), decreased appetite (44%), stomatitis (32%), gastroenteritis (3%)

Hematologic & oncologic: Anemia (97%, grades 3/4: 6%), lymphopenia (81%, grades 3/4: 27%), neutropenia (52%, grades 3/4: 20%; incidence of neutropenia was higher among Asian patients), thrombocytopenia (41%, grades 3/4: 2%), neutropenic fever (≤3%, grades 3/4: ≤3%)

Hypersensitivity: Severe hypersensitivity

Infection: Sepsis (4%, grades 3/4: 3%), neutropenic sepsis (≤3%, grades 3/4: ≤3%)

Local: Catheter infection (3%)

Neuromuscular & skeletal: Weakness (≤56%)

Renal: Increased creatinine clearance (18%)

Respiratory: Pneumonia (≥2%), interstitial pulmonary disease

Renal: Acute renal failure (≥2%)

Miscellaneous: Fever (23%)

◀ **Drug Interactions**

Metabolism/Transport Effects Substrate of BCRP, CYP3A4 (major), P-glycoprotein, SLCO1B1, UGT1A1; **Note:** Assignment of Major/Minor substrate status based on clinically relevant drug interaction potential

Avoid Concomitant Use

Avoid concomitant use of Irinotecan (Liposomal) with any of the following: BCG (Intravesical); CloZAPine; Conivaptan; CYP3A4 Inducers (Strong); CYP3A4 Inhibitors (Strong); Dipyrone; Fusidic Acid (Systemic); Idelalisib; Natalizumab; Pimecrolimus; St Johns Wort; Tacrolimus (Topical); Tofacitinib; UGT1A1 Inhibitors; Vaccines (Live)

Increased Effect/Toxicity

Irinotecan (Liposomal) may increase the levels/effects of: CloZAPine; Fingolimod; Leflunomide; Natalizumab; Tofacitinib; Vaccines (Live)

The levels/effects of Irinotecan (Liposomal) may be increased by: Aprepitant; Conivaptan; CYP3A4 Inhibitors (Moderate); CYP3A4 Inhibitors (Strong); Dasatinib; Denosumab; Dipyrone; Fosaprepitant; Fusidic Acid (Systemic); Idelalisib; Ivacaftor; Luliconazole; Mifepristone; Netupitant; Osimertinib; Palbociclib; P-glycoprotein/ABCB1 Inhibitors; Pimecrolimus; Ranolazine; Roflumilast; Rolapitant; Simeprevir; SORAfenib; Stiripentol; Tacrolimus (Topical); Teriflunomide; Trastuzumab; UGT1A1 Inhibitors

Decreased Effect

Irinotecan (Liposomal) may decrease the levels/effects of: BCG (Intravesical); Coccidioides immitis Skin Test; Sipuleucel-T; Vaccines (Inactivated); Vaccines (Live)

The levels/effects of Irinotecan (Liposomal) may be decreased by: Bosentan; CYP3A4 Inducers (Moderate); CYP3A4 Inducers (Strong); Dabrafenib; Deferasirox; Echinacea; Osimertinib; P-glycoprotein/ABCB1 Inducers; Siltuximab; St Johns Wort; Tocilizumab

Storage/Stability Store intact vials at 2°C to 8°C (36°F to 46°F); do not freeze. Protect from light. Solution diluted for administration is stable for up to 4 hours when stored at room temperature, or up to 24 hours when refrigerated (administration should be completed within these time frames). Allow diluted solution to come to room temperature prior to administration.

Preparation for Administration Hazardous agent; use appropriate precautions for handling and disposal (NIOSH 2014 [group 1]). Withdraw appropriate dose from the vial and dilute in 500 mL D_5W or 0.9% sodium chloride injection. Mix by gentle inversion; protect diluted solution from light.

Mechanism of Action Irinotecan (liposomal) is a topoisomerase 1 inhibitor encapsulated in a lipid bilayer (liposome). Irinotecan and its active metabolite (SN-38) bind reversibly to topoisomerase I-DNA complex preventing re-ligation of the cleaved DNA strand. This results in the accumulation of cleavable complexes and double-strand DNA breaks. As mammalian cells cannot efficiently repair these breaks, cell death consistent with S-phase cell cycle specificity occurs, leading to termination of cellular replication.

Pharmacodynamics/Kinetics

Distribution: 4.1 L; 95% of irinotecan remains liposome-encapsulated

Protein binding: <1%

Metabolism: Irinotecan hydrochloride: Primarily hepatic to SN-38 (active metabolite) by carboxylesterase enzymes; may also undergo CYP3A4-mediated metabolism to inactive metabolites (one of which may be hydrolyzed to release SN-38). SN-38 undergoes conjugation by UDP-glucuronosyl transferase 1A1 (UGT1A1) to form a glucuronide metabolite. SN-38 is increased by UGT1A1*28 polymorphism (10% of North Americans are homozygous for UGT1A1*28 allele).

Half-life elimination: Total irinotecan: ~26 hours; SN-38: ~68 hours

Excretion: Urine: Irinotecan hydrochloride (11% to 20%), metabolites (SN-38 <1%, SN-38 glucuronide, 3%)

Dosing

Adult Note: Premedicate with a corticosteroid and an antiemetic 30 minutes prior to infusion. Irinotecan (liposomal) and irinotecan (conventional) are NOT interchangeable. Dosing differs between formulations; verify intended product and dose prior to preparation and administration.

Pancreatic adenocarcinoma, metastatic: IV: 70 mg/m² once every 2 weeks (in combination with fluorouracil and leucovorin). **Note:** Reduce initial starting dose to 50 mg/m² in patients known to be homozygous for the UGT1A1*28 allele; the dose may be increased to 70 mg/m² as tolerated in subsequent cycles.

Geriatric Refer to adult dosing

Renal Impairment

CrCl 30 to 89 mL/minute: There are no dosage adjustments provided in the manufacturer's labeling; however, a population pharmacokinetic analysis showed no effect on total SN-38 exposure in patients with mild to moderate renal impairment.

CrCl <30 mL/minute: There are no dosage adjustments provided in the manufacturer's labeling (insufficient data).

Hepatic Impairment Bilirubin >ULN: There are no dosage adjustments provided in the manufacturer's labeling.

Adjustment for Toxicity **Note:** Fluorouracil and leucovorin may also require dosage adjustment.

Hematologic toxicity: ANC <1,500/mm³ or neutropenic fever: Withhold treatment. Resume therapy when ANC ≥1,500/mm³ with a reduced dose for grade 3 or 4 neutropenia or neutropenic fever in subsequent cycles:

First occurrence: Reduce dose to 50 mg/m² (in patients receiving 70 mg/m²); reduce dose to 43 mg/m² in patients homozygous for UGT1A1*28 without previous increase to 70 mg/m²

Second occurrence: Reduce dose to 43 mg/m² (in patients receiving 50 mg/m²); reduce dose to 35 mg/m² in patients homozygous for UGT1A1*28 previously receiving 43 mg/m²

Third occurrence: Discontinue

Nonhematologic toxicity:

Anaphylactic reaction: Discontinue permanently

Diarrhea: Withhold therapy for grade 2 to 4 diarrhea. Administer IV or SubQ atropine 0.25 to 1 mg (unless clinically contraindicated) for early-onset diarrhea of any severity. Administer loperamide for late-onset diarrhea of any severity. Following recovery to ≤ grade 1 diarrhea, resume treatment at a reduced dose:

First occurrence: Reduce dose to 50 mg/m² (in patients receiving 70 mg/m²); reduce dose to 43 mg/m² in patients homozygous for UGT1A1*28 without previous increase to 70 mg/m²

Second occurrence: Reduce dose to 43 mg/m² (in patients receiving 50 mg/m²); reduce dose to 35 mg/m² in patients homozygous for UGT1A1*28 previously receiving 43 mg/m²

Third occurrence: Discontinue

Interstitial lung disease (ILD): Discontinue

Other grade 3 or 4 adverse reactions: Withhold therapy. Upon recovery to ≤ grade 1 toxicity, resume treatment at a reduced dose:

First occurrence: Reduce dose to 50 mg/m^2 (in patients receiving 70 mg/m^2); reduce dose to 43 mg/m^2 in patients homozygous for UGT1A1*28 without previous increase to 70 mg/m^2

Second occurrence: Reduce dose to 43 mg/m^2 (in patients receiving 50 mg/m^2); reduce dose to 35 mg/m^2 in patients homozygous for UGT1A1*28 previously receiving 43 mg/m^2

Third occurrence: Discontinue

Administration

Administer by IV infusion over 90 minutes. Premedicate with a corticosteroid and an antiemetic 30 minutes prior to infusion. Administer irinotecan (liposomal) prior to fluorouracil and leucovorin. Do not use in-line filters for administration.

Administer IV or SubQ atropine 0.25 to 1 mg (unless clinically contraindicated) for early onset diarrhea of any severity; initiate loperamide for late-onset diarrhea of any severity.

Hazardous agent; use appropriate precautions for handling and disposal (NIOSH 2014 [group 1]).

Emetic Potential Moderate (30% to 90%)

Monitoring Parameters
Complete blood counts on days 1 and 8 of each cycle and as clinically indicated; bilirubin, electrolytes (with severe diarrhea); bowel movements (diarrhea episodes) and hydration status; signs/symptoms of pulmonary toxicity or hypersensitivity reactions

Dosage Forms
Excipient information presented when available (limited, particularly for generics); consult specific product labeling.

Injectable, Intravenous:

Onivyde: 43 mg/10 mL (10 mL) [contains mpeg-2000-dspe (methoxy-terminated peg)]

♦ **Irinotecan For Injection (Can)** *see* Irinotecan (Conventional) *on page 949*

♦ **Irinotecan HCl** *see* Irinotecan (Conventional) *on page 949*

♦ **Irinotecan Hydrochloride** *see* Irinotecan (Conventional) *on page 949*

♦ **Irinotecan Hydrochloride Injection (Can)** *see* Irinotecan (Conventional) *on page 949*

♦ **Irinotecan Hydrochloride Trihydrate For Injection (Can)** *see* Irinotecan (Conventional) *on page 949*

♦ **Irinotecan Hydrochloride Trihydrate Injection (Can)** *see* Irinotecan (Conventional) *on page 949*

♦ **Irinotecan Liposome** *see* Irinotecan (Liposomal) *on page 960*

♦ **Iron (III) Hydroxide Sucrose Complex** *see* Iron Sucrose *on page 968*

♦ **Iron Dextran** *see* Iron Dextran Complex *on page 964*

Iron Dextran Complex (EYE ern DEKS tran KOM pleks)

Brand Names: US Dexferrum [DSC]; Infed

Brand Names: Canada Dexiron; Infufer

Index Terms High-Molecular-Weight Iron Dextran (DexFerrum); Imferon; Iron Dextran; Low-Molecular-Weight Iron Dextran (INFeD)

Pharmacologic Category Iron Salt

Use Iron deficiency: Treatment of iron deficiency in patients in whom oral administration is unsatisfactory or infeasible

Labeled Contraindications Hypersensitivity to iron dextran or any component of the formulation; any anemia not associated with iron deficiency

Pregnancy Considerations Adverse events have been observed in animal reproduction studies. It is not known if iron dextran (as iron dextran) crosses the placenta. It is recommended that pregnant women meet the dietary requirements of iron with diet and/or supplements in order to prevent adverse events associated with iron deficiency anemia in pregnancy. Treatment of iron deficiency anemia in pregnant women is the same as in nonpregnant women and in most cases, oral iron preparations may be used. Except in severe cases of maternal anemia, the fetus achieves normal iron stores regardless of maternal concentrations.

Breast-Feeding Considerations Trace amounts of iron dextran (as iron dextran) are found in human milk. Iron is normally found in breast milk. Breast milk or iron fortified formulas generally provide enough iron to meet the recommended dietary requirements of infants. The amount of iron in breast milk is generally not influenced by maternal iron status.

Warnings/Precautions [U.S. Boxed Warning]: Deaths associated with parenteral administration following anaphylactic-type reactions have been reported (use only where resuscitation equipment and personnel are available). A test dose should be administered to all patients prior to the first therapeutic dose. Fatal reactions have occurred even in patients who tolerated the test dose. Monitor patients for signs/symptoms of anaphylactic reactions during any iron dextran administration; fatalities have occurred with the test dose. A history of drug allergy (including multiple drug allergies) and/or the concomitant use of an ACE inhibitor may increase the risk of anaphylactic-type reactions. Adverse events (including life-threatening) associated with iron dextran usually occur with the high-molecular-weight formulation (Dexferrum), compared to low-molecular-weight (INFeD) (Chertow, 2006). Delayed (1-2 days) infusion reaction (including arthralgia, back pain, chills, dizziness, and fever) may occur with large doses (eg, total dose infusion) of IV iron dextran; usually subsides within 3-4 days. Delayed reaction may also occur (less commonly) with IM administration; subsiding within 3-7 days. Use with caution in patients with a history of significant allergies, asthma, serious hepatic impairment, preexisting cardiac disease (may exacerbate cardiovascular complications), and rheumatoid arthritis (may exacerbate joint pain and swelling). Avoid use during acute kidney infection.

In patients with chronic kidney disease (CKD) requiring iron supplementation, the IV route is preferred for hemodialysis patients; either oral iron or IV iron may be used for nondialysis and peritoneal dialysis CKD patients. In patients with cancer-related anemia (either due to cancer or chemotherapy-induced) requiring iron supplementation, the IV route is superior to oral therapy; IM administration is not recommended for parenteral iron supplementation.

[U.S. Boxed Warning]: Use only in patients where the iron deficient state is not amenable to oral iron therapy. Discontinue oral iron prior to initiating parenteral iron therapy. Exogenous hemosiderosis may result from excess iron stores; patients with refractory anemias and/or hemoglobinopathies may be prone to iron overload with unwarranted iron supplementation. Anemia in the elderly is often caused by "anemia of chronic disease" or associated with inflammation rather than blood loss. Iron stores are usually normal or ▶

increased, with a serum ferritin >50 ng/mL and a decreased total iron binding capacity. IV administration of iron dextran is often preferred over IM in the elderly secondary to a decreased muscle mass and the need for daily injections. Intramuscular injections of iron-carbohydrate complexes may have a risk of delayed injection site tumor development. Iron dextran products differ in chemical characteristics. The high-molecular-weight formulation (Dexferrum) and the low-molecular-weight formulation (INFeD) are not clinically interchangeable. Intramuscular iron dextran use in neonates may be associated with an increased incidence of gram-negative sepsis.

Adverse Reactions Frequency not defined. **Note:** Adverse event risk is reported to be higher with the high-molecular-weight iron dextran formulation.

Cardiovascular: Arrhythmia, bradycardia, cardiac arrest, chest pain, chest tightness, cyanosis, flushing, hyper-/hypotension, shock, syncope, tachycardia

Central nervous system: Chills, disorientation, dizziness, fever, headache, malaise, seizure, unconsciousness, unresponsiveness

Dermatologic: Pruritus, purpura, rash, urticaria

Gastrointestinal: Abdominal pain, diarrhea, nausea, taste alteration, vomiting

Genitourinary: Discoloration of urine

Hematologic: Leukocytosis, lymphadenopathy

Local: Injection site reactions (cellulitis, inflammation, pain, phlebitis, soreness, swelling), muscle atrophy/fibrosis (with IM injection), skin/tissue staining (at the site of IM injection), sterile abscess

Neuromuscular & skeletal: Arthralgia, arthritis/arthritis exacerbation, back pain, myalgia, paresthesia, weakness

Respiratory: Bronchospasm, dyspnea, respiratory arrest, wheezing

Renal: Hematuria

Miscellaneous: Anaphylactic reactions (sudden respiratory difficulty, cardiovascular collapse), diaphoresis

Postmarketing and/or case reports: Angioedema, tumor formation (at former injection site)

Drug Interactions

Metabolism/Transport Effects None known.

Avoid Concomitant Use

Avoid concomitant use of Iron Dextran Complex with any of the following: Dimercaprol

Increased Effect/Toxicity

The levels/effects of Iron Dextran Complex may be increased by: ACE Inhibitors; Dimercaprol

Decreased Effect There are no known significant interactions involving a decrease in effect.

Storage/Stability Store at 20°C to 25°C (68°F to 77°F); excursions permitted to 15°C to 30°C (59°F to 86°F).

Preparation for Administration Solutions for infusion should be diluted in 250-1000 mL NS.

Mechanism of Action The released iron, from the plasma, eventually replenishes the depleted iron stores in the bone marrow where it is incorporated into hemoglobin

Pharmacodynamics/Kinetics

Onset of action: IV: Serum ferritin peak: 7-9 days after dose

Absorption:

IM: 50% to 90% is promptly absorbed, balance is slowly absorbed over month

IV: Uptake of iron by the reticuloendothelial system appears to be constant at about 10-20 mg/hour

Excretion: Urine and feces via reticuloendothelial system

Dosing

Adult & Geriatric Note: A 0.5 mL test dose should be given prior to starting iron dextran therapy.

Iron-deficiency anemia: IM (INFeD), IV (Dexferrum, INFeD):

Dose (mL) = 0.0442 (desired hemoglobin - observed hemoglobin) x LBW + (0.26 x LBW)

Desired hemoglobin: Usually 14.8 g/dL

LBW = Lean body weight in kg

Iron replacement therapy for blood loss: (INFeD), IV (Dexferrum, INFeD):

Replacement iron (mg) = blood loss (mL) x Hct

Maximum daily dosage: Manufacturer's labeling. **Note:** Replacement of larger estimated iron deficits may be achieved by serial administration of smaller incremental dosages. Daily dosages should be limited to 100 mg iron (2 mL)

Cancer-/chemotherapy-associated anemia: IV: **Note:** Use the iron-deficiency anemia equation for determining a calculated dose, when applicable.

Weekly administration (off-label dosing; INFeD):

Weeks 1-3: Test dose of 25 mg (over 1-2 minutes), followed by 75 mg (bolus) once weekly

Weeks 4 and after: 100 mg over 5 minutes once weekly until the calculated dose is reached (Auerbach, 2004)

or

Week 1: Test dose of 25 mg (slow IV push), followed 1 hour later by 75 mg over 5 minutes

Weeks 2-10: 100 mg over 5 minutes once weekly for a total cumulative dose of 1000 mg (NCCN anemia guidelines v.2.2014)

Total dose infusion (off-label dosing; INFeD):

Test dose of 25 mg (over 1-2 minutes), followed 1 hour later by the balance of the calculated total dose mixed in 500 mL NS and infused at 175 mL/hour (Auerbach, 2004)

or

Test dose of 25 mg (slow IV push) followed 1 hour later by the balance of the total dose as a single infusion over several hours; if calculated dose exceeds 1000 mg, administer remaining dose in excess of 1000 mg after 4 weeks if inadequate hemoglobin response (NCCN anemia guidelines v.2.2014)

Pediatric Note: A 0.5 mL test dose (0.25 mL in infants) should be given prior to starting iron dextran therapy.

Iron-deficiency anemia: IM (INFeD), IV (Dexferrum, INFeD):

Children 5-15 kg: Should not normally be given in the first 4 months of life:

Dose (mL) = 0.0442 (desired hemoglobin - observed hemoglobin) x W + (0.26 x W)

Desired hemoglobin: Usually 12 g/dL

W = Total body weight in kg

Children >15 kg: Refer to adult dosing.

Iron replacement therapy for blood loss: Refer to adult dosing.

Maximum daily dose:

Children <5 kg: 25 mg iron (0.5 mL)

Children 5-10 kg: 50 mg iron (1 mL)

Children ≥10 kg: Refer to adult dosing.

Renal Impairment No dosage adjustment provided in manufacturer's labeling.

Hepatic Impairment No dosage adjustment provided in manufacturer's labeling.

Administration Note: A test dose should be given on the first day of therapy; patient should be observed for 1 hour for hypersensitivity reaction, then the remainder of the day's dose (dose minus test dose) should be given. Resuscitation equipment, medication, and trained personnel should be available. An uneventful test dose does not ensure an anaphylactic-type reaction will not occur during administration of the therapeutic dose.

IM (INFeD): Use Z-track technique (displacement of the skin laterally prior to injection); injection should be deep into the upper outer quadrant of buttock; alternate buttocks with subsequent injections. Administer test dose at same recommended site using the same technique.

IV: Test dose should be given gradually over at least 30 seconds (INFeD) or 5 minutes (Dexferrum), or over 1-2 minutes (INFeD) for cancer-/chemotherapy-associated anemia (Auerbach, 2004). Subsequent dose(s) may be administered by IV bolus undiluted at a rate not to exceed 50 mg/minute (maximum 100 mg). For total dose infusion in patients with cancer-/chemotherapy-associated anemia (off-label dose): 1 hour after the test dose, administer the balance of the dose diluted in 500 mL NS and infuse at 175 mL/hour (Auerbach, 2004) or administer over several hours (NCCN Anemia guidelines v.2.2104). Avoid dilutions with dextrose (increased incidence of local pain and phlebitis).

Monitoring Parameters Hemoglobin, hematocrit, reticulocyte count, serum ferritin, serum iron, TIBC; monitor for anaphylaxis/hypersensitivity reaction (during test dose and therapeutic dose)

Test Interactions May cause falsely elevated values of serum bilirubin and falsely decreased values of serum calcium. Residual iron dextran may remain in reticuloendothelial cells; may affect accuracy of examination of bone marrow iron stores. Bone scans with 99m Tc-labeled bone seeking agents may show reduced bony uptake, marked renal activity, and excess blood pooling and soft tissue accumulation following IV iron dextran infusion or with high serum ferritin levels. Following IM iron dextran, bone scans with 99m Tc-diphosphonate may show dense activity in the buttocks.

Dosage Forms Considerations

Strength of iron dextran complex is expressed as elemental iron.

Dosage Forms Excipient information presented when available (limited, particularly for generics); consult specific product labeling. [DSC] = Discontinued product

Solution, Injection:

Dexferrum: 50 mg/mL (1 mL [DSC], 2 mL [DSC])

Infed: 50 mg/mL (2 mL)

Iron Sucrose (EYE ern SOO krose)

Brand Names: US Venofer

Brand Names: Canada Venofer

Index Terms Iron (III) Hydroxide Sucrose Complex

Pharmacologic Category Iron Salt

Use Iron deficiency anemia: Treatment of iron-deficiency anemia in chronic kidney disease (CKD)

Labeled Contraindications Known hypersensitivity to iron sucrose or any component of the formulation

Pregnancy Considerations Teratogenic effects were not observed in animal studies. There are no adequate and well-controlled studies in pregnant women. Based on limited data, iron sucrose may be effective for the treatment of iron-deficiency anemia in pregnancy. It is recommended that pregnant women meet the dietary requirements of iron with diet and/or supplements in order to prevent adverse events associated with iron deficiency anemia in pregnancy. Treatment of iron deficiency anemia in pregnant women is the same as in nonpregnant women and in most cases, oral iron preparations may be used. Except in severe cases of maternal anemia, the fetus achieves normal iron stores regardless of maternal concentrations.

Breast-Feeding Considerations Iron is normally found in breast milk. Breast milk or iron fortified formulas generally provide enough iron to meet the recommended dietary requirements of infants. The amount of iron in breast milk is generally not influenced by maternal iron status.

Warnings/Precautions Hypersensitivity reactions, including rare postmarketing anaphylactic and anaphylactoid reactions (some fatal), have been reported; monitor patients during and for ≥30 minutes postadministration; discontinue immediately for signs/symptoms of a hypersensitivity reaction (shock, hypotension, loss of consciousness). Equipment for resuscitation and trained personnel experienced in handling medical emergencies should always be immediately available. Significant hypotension has been reported frequently in hemodialysis-dependent patients. Hypotension has also been reported in peritoneal dialysis and nondialysis patients. Hypotension may be related to total dose or rate of administration (avoid rapid IV injection), follow recommended guidelines. Withhold iron in the presence of tissue iron overload; periodic monitoring of hemoglobin, hematocrit, serum ferritin, and transferrin saturation is recommended.

Adverse Reactions Events and incidences are associated with use in adults unless otherwise specified.

>10%:

Cardiovascular: Hypotension (2% to 3%; children 2%; 39% in hemodialysis patients; may be related to total dose or rate of administration)

Central nervous system: Headache (3% to 13%; children 6%)

Gastrointestinal: Nausea (5% to 15%; children 3%)

Neuromuscular & skeletal: Muscle cramps (1% to 3%; 29% in hemodialysis patients)

Respiratory: Nasopharyngitis (2% to 16%), pharyngitis (2% to 16%), sinusitis (2% to 16%), upper respiratory infection (2% to 16%; children 4%)

1% to 10%:

Cardiovascular: Hypertension (7% to 8%; children 2%), peripheral edema (3% to 7%), chest pain (1% to 6%), arteriovenous fistula thrombosis (children 2%), heart failure (>1%)

Central nervous system: Dizziness (1% to 7%; children 4%), fever (1% to 3%; children 4%)

Dermatologic: Pruritus (2% to 4%)

Endocrine & metabolic: Hypoglycemia (≤4%), fluid overload (1% to 3%), gout (≤3%), hyperglycemia (≤3%)

Gastrointestinal: Vomiting (5% to 9%; children 4%), diarrhea (5% to 8%), taste perversion (≤8%), peritonitis (children 4%), abdominal pain (1% to 4%)

Local: Injection site reaction (≤6%)

Neuromuscular & skeletal: Extremity pain (3% to 6%), arthralgia (1% to 4%), myalgia (≤4%), weakness (1% to 3%), back pain (1% to 2%)

Ocular: Conjunctivitis (≤3%)

Otic: Ear pain (≤2%)

Respiratory: Dyspnea (1% to 6%), cough (1% to 3%; children 4%), nasal congestion (≤1%)

Miscellaneous: Graft complication (≤10%), sepsis (>1%)

<1%, postmarketing, and/or case reports: Anaphylactic shock, anaphylactoid reactions, angioedema, bradycardia, bronchospasm, cardiovascular collapse, confusion, facial rash, hyperhidrosis, hypersensitivity (including wheezing), hypoesthesia, injection site discoloration (following extravasation), joint swelling, lightheadedness, loss of consciousness, necrotizing enterocolitis (reported in premature infants, no causal relationship established), paresthesia, seizure, shock, urine discoloration, urticaria

Drug Interactions

Metabolism/Transport Effects None known.

Avoid Concomitant Use

Avoid concomitant use of Iron Sucrose with any of the following: Dimercaprol

Increased Effect/Toxicity

The levels/effects of Iron Sucrose may be increased by: Dimercaprol

Decreased Effect There are no known significant interactions involving a decrease in effect.

Storage/Stability Store intact vials at controlled room temperature of 20°C to 25°C (68°F to 77°F); excursions permitted to 15°C to 30°C (59°F to 86°F); do not freeze. Iron sucrose is stable for 7 days at room temperature (23°C to 27°C [73°F to 81°F]) or under refrigeration (2°C to 6°C [36°F to 43°F]) when undiluted in a plastic syringe or following dilution in normal saline in a plastic syringe (concentration 2-10 mg/mL) or for 7 days at room temperature (23°C to 27°C [73°F to 81°F]) following dilution in normal saline in an IV bag (concentration 1-2 mg/mL).

Preparation for Administration

Children: May administer undiluted or diluted in 25 mL of NS. Do not dilute to concentrations <1 mg/mL.

Adults: Doses ≤200 mg may be administered undiluted or diluted in a maximum of 100 mL NS. Doses >200 mg should be diluted in a maximum of 250 mL NS. Do not dilute to concentrations <1 mg/mL.

Mechanism of Action Iron sucrose is dissociated by the reticuloendothelial system into iron and sucrose. The released iron increases serum iron concentrations and is incorporated into hemoglobin.

Pharmacodynamics/Kinetics

Distribution: V_{dss}: Healthy adults: 7.9 L

Metabolism: Dissociated into iron and sucrose by the reticuloendothelial system

Half-life elimination: Healthy adults: 6 hours; Nondialysis-dependent adolescents: 8 hours

Excretion: Healthy adults: Urine (5%) within 24 hours

Dosing

Adult & Geriatric Doses expressed in mg of **elemental** iron. **Note:** Test dose: Product labeling does not indicate need for a test dose in product-naive patients.

Iron-deficiency anemia in chronic kidney disease (CKD): IV:

Hemodialysis-dependent patient: 100 mg administered during consecutive dialysis sessions to a cumulative total dose of 1000 mg (10 doses); may repeat treatment if clinically indicated.

Peritoneal dialysis-dependent patient: Two infusions of 300 mg administered 14 days apart, followed by a single 400 mg infusion 14 days later (total cumulative dose of 1000 mg in 3 divided doses); may repeat treatment if clinically indicated.

Nondialysis-dependent patient: 200 mg administered on 5 different occasions within a 14-day period (total cumulative dose: 1000 mg in 14-day period); may repeat treatment if clinically indicated. **Note:** Dosage has also been administered as 2 infusions of 500 mg on day 1 and day 14 (limited experience).

Chemotherapy-associated anemia (off-label use): IV: 200 mg once every 3 weeks for 5 doses (Bastit, 2008) or 100 mg once weekly during weeks 0 to 6, followed by 100 mg every other week from weeks 8 to 14 (Hedenus, 2007)

Pediatric Doses expressed in mg of **elemental** iron. **Note:** Test dose: Product labeling does not indicate need for a test dose in product-naive patients.

Iron-deficiency anemia in chronic kidney disease (CKD): Children ≥2 years and Adolescents: IV: **Note:** Not indicated for iron replacement treatment in children and adolescents.

Hemodialysis-dependent patient: Maintenance therapy: 0.5 mg/kg/dose (maximum: 100 mg) every 2 weeks for 6 doses; may repeat if clinically indicated.

Nondialysis-dependent patient: Maintenance therapy: 0.5 mg/kg/dose (maximum: 100 mg) every 4 weeks for 3 doses; may repeat if clinically indicated

Peritoneal dialysis-dependent patient: Maintenance therapy: 0.5 mg/kg/dose (maximum: 100 mg) every 4 weeks for 3 doses; may repeat if clinically indicated

Renal Impairment No dosage adjustment provided in manufacturer's labeling.

Hepatic Impairment No dosage adjustment provided in manufacturer's labeling.

Administration Administer intravenously as a slow IV injection (**not** for rapid IV injection) or as an IV infusion. Can be administered through dialysis line.

Children and Adolescents:

Slow IV injection: Administer undiluted over 5 minutes

Infusion: Infuse diluted solution over 5-60 minutes

Adults:

Slow IV injection: May administer doses ≤200 mg undiluted by slow IV injection over 2-5 minutes. When administering to hemodialysis-dependent patients, give iron sucrose early during the dialysis session.

Infusion: Infuse diluted doses ≤200 mg over at least 15 minutes; infuse diluted 300 mg dose over 1.5 hours; infuse diluted 400 mg dose over 2.5 hours; infuse diluted 500 mg dose over 3.5-4 hours (limited experience). When administering to hemodialysis-dependent patients, give iron sucrose early during the dialysis session.

Monitoring Parameters

CKD patients: Hematocrit, hemoglobin, serum ferritin, serum iron, transferrin, percent transferrin saturation, TIBC (takes ~4 weeks of treatment to see increased serum iron and ferritin, and decreased TIBC); iron status should be assessed ≥48 hours after last dose (due to rapid increase in values following administration); signs/symptoms of hypersensitivity reactions (during and ≥30 minutes following infusion); hypotension (following infusion)

◄ Chemotherapy-associated anemia (off-label use): Iron, total iron-binding capacity, transferrin saturation, or ferritin levels at baseline and periodically (Rizzo, 2011)

Dosage Forms Considerations Strength of iron sucrose is expressed as elemental iron.

Dosage Forms Excipient information presented when available (limited, particularly for generics); consult specific product labeling.

Solution, Intravenous [preservative free]:

Venofer: 20 mg/mL (2.5 mL, 5 mL, 10 mL)

◆ **Isavuconazole** see Isavuconazonium Sulfate on page 972

Isavuconazonium Sulfate (eye sa vue koe na ZOE nee um sul FATE)

Brand Names: US Cresemba

Index Terms BAL8557; Isavuconazole

Pharmacologic Category Antifungal Agent, Azole Derivative; Antifungal Agent, Oral; Antifungal Agent, Parenteral

Use

Aspergillosis: Treatment of invasive aspergillosis in adults

Mucormycosis: Treatment of invasive mucormycosis in adults

Pregnancy Risk Factor C

Dosing

Adult & Geriatric Note: Dosage expressed as milligrams of isavuconazonium sulfate; switching between the intravenous (IV) and oral formulations of isavuconazonium sulfate is acceptable; for maintenance dosing, it is not necessary to restart dosing with the initial dose regimen when switching between formulations.

Aspergillosis, invasive:

IV: Initial: 372 mg (isavuconazole 200 mg) every 8 hours for 6 doses; Maintenance: 372 mg (isavuconazole 200 mg) once daily. Start maintenance dose 12 to 24 hours after the last loading dose.

Oral: Initial: 372 mg (200 mg isavuconazole) every 8 hours for 6 doses; Maintenance: 372 mg (isavuconazole 200 mg) once daily. Start maintenance dose 12 to 24 hours after the last loading dose.

Mucormycosis, invasive:

IV: Initial: 372 mg (isavuconazole 200 mg) every 8 hours for 6 doses; Maintenance: 372 mg (isavuconazole 200 mg) once daily. Start maintenance dose 12 to 24 hours after the last loading dose.

Oral: Initial: 372 mg (isavuconazole 200 mg) every 8 hours for 6 doses; Maintenance: 372 mg (isavuconazole 200 mg) once daily. Start maintenance dose 12 to 24 hours after the last loading dose.

Renal Impairment No dosage adjustment necessary.

Hepatic Impairment

Mild or moderate impairment (Child-Pugh class A or B): No dosage adjustment necessary.

Severe impairment (Child-Pugh class C): There are no dosage adjustments provided in the manufacturer's labeling (has not been studied); use with caution.

Additional Information Complete prescribing information should be consulted for additional detail.

Dosage Forms Excipient information presented when available (limited, particularly for generics); consult specific product labeling.
Capsule, Oral:
  Cresemba: 186 mg [contains disodium edta]
Solution Reconstituted, Intravenous:
  Cresemba: 372 mg (1 ea)

◆ **ISG** see Immune Globulin on page 903

◆ **Isonipecaine Hydrochloride** see Meperidine on page 1086

◆ **Isophosphamide** see Ifosfamide on page 873

Isosulfan Blue (eye soe SUL fan bloo)

Brand Names: US Lymphazurin [DSC]
Pharmacologic Category Contrast Agent
Use Adjunct to lymphography for visualization of the lymphatic system; sentinel node identification
Pregnancy Risk Factor C
Dosing
  Adult Lymphography: SubQ: Inject 0.5 mL into 3 interdigital spaces of each extremity per study; maximum: 3 mL (30 mg)
  Renal Impairment No dosage adjustment provided in manufacturer's labeling.
  Hepatic Impairment No dosage adjustment provided in manufacturer's labeling.
Additional Information Complete prescribing information should be consulted for additional detail.
Dosage Forms Excipient information presented when available (limited, particularly for generics); consult specific product labeling. [DSC] = Discontinued product
Solution, Subcutaneous:
  Lymphazurin: 1% (5 mL [DSC])
Solution, Subcutaneous [preservative free]:
  Generic: 1% (5 mL)

ISOtretinoin (eye soe TRET i noyn)

Related Information
  Management of EGFR Inhibitor Toxicities: Dermatologic, Ocular, and Gastrointestinal on page 2179
  Safe Handling of Hazardous Drugs on page 2292
Brand Names: US Absorica; Amnesteem; Claravis; Myorisan; Zenatane
Brand Names: Canada Accutane; Clarus; Epuris
Index Terms 13-cis-Retinoic Acid; 13-cis-Vitamin A Acid; 13-CRA; Cis-Retinoic Acid; Accutane; Isotretinoinum
Pharmacologic Category Acne Products; Antineoplastic Agent, Retinoic Acid Derivative; Retinoic Acid Derivative
Use Treatment of severe recalcitrant nodular acne unresponsive to conventional therapy
Labeled Contraindications Hypersensitivity to isotretinoin or any component of the formulation; sensitivity to parabens, vitamin A, or other retinoids; pregnant women or those who may become pregnant

◀ **Pregnancy Considerations** Isotretinoin and its metabolites can be detected in fetal tissue following maternal use during pregnancy (Benifla, 1995; Kraft, 1989). **[U.S. Boxed Warnings]: Use of isotretinoin is contraindicated in females who are or may become pregnant. Birth defects (facial, eye, ear, skull, central nervous system, cardiovascular, thymus and parathyroid gland abnormalities) have been noted following isotretinoin exposure during pregnancy and the risk for severe birth defects is high, with any dose or even with short treatment duration. Low IQ scores have also been reported. The risk for spontaneous abortion and premature births is increased. Because of the high likelihood of teratogenic effects, all patients (male and female), prescribers, wholesalers, and dispensing pharmacists must register and be active in the iPLEDGE™ risk evaluation and mitigation strategy (REMS) program; do not prescribe isotretinoin for women who are or who are likely to become pregnant while using the drug. If pregnancy occurs during therapy, isotretinoin should be discontinued immediately and the patient referred to an obstetrician-gynecologist specializing in reproductive toxicity.** This medication is contraindicated in females of childbearing potential unless they are able to comply with the guidelines of the iPLEDGE™ pregnancy prevention program. Females of childbearing potential must have two negative pregnancy tests with a sensitivity of at least 25 milliunits/mL prior to beginning therapy and testing should continue monthly during therapy. Females of childbearing potential should not become pregnant during therapy or for 1 month following discontinuation of isotretinoin. Upon discontinuation of treatment, females of childbearing potential should have a pregnancy test after their last dose and again one month after their last dose. Two forms of contraception should be continued during this time. Any pregnancies should be reported to the iPLEDGE™ program (www.ipledgeprogram.com or 866-495-0654) and the FDA through MedWatch (800-FDA-1088).

Breast-Feeding Considerations It is not known if isotretinoin is excreted in breast milk. A case report describes a green discharge from the breast of a nonlactating woman which was determined to be iatrogenic galactorrhea due to isotretinoin (Larsen, 1985). Due to the potential for serious adverse reactions in the nursing infant, the manufacturer recommends a decision be made whether to discontinue nursing or to discontinue the drug, taking into account the importance of treatment to the mother.

Warnings/Precautions Hazardous agent - use appropriate precautions for handling and disposal (meets NIOSH 2014 criteria). This medication should only be prescribed by prescribers competent in treating severe recalcitrant nodular acne and experienced with the use of systemic retinoids. Anaphylaxis and other types of allergic reactions, including cutaneous reactions and allergic vasculitis, have been reported. **[U.S. Boxed Warnings]: Birth defects (facial, eye, ear, skull, central nervous system, cardiovascular, thymus and parathyroid gland abnormalities) have been noted following isotretinoin exposure during pregnancy and the risk for severe birth defects is high, with any dose or even with short treatment duration. Low IQ scores have also been reported. The risk for spontaneous abortion and premature births is increased. Because of the high likelihood of teratogenic effects, all patients (male and female), prescribers, wholesalers, and dispensing pharmacists must register and be active in the iPLEDGE risk evaluation and mitigation strategy (REMS) program; do not prescribe isotretinoin for women who are or who are likely to become pregnant while using the drug. If pregnancy occurs during therapy, isotretinoin should be**

discontinued immediately and the patient referred to an obstetrician-gynecologist specializing in reproductive toxicity (see Additional Information for details). Women of childbearing potential must be capable of complying with effective contraceptive measures. Patients must select and commit to two forms of contraception. Therapy is begun after two negative pregnancy tests; effective contraception must be used for at least 1 month before beginning therapy, during therapy, and for 1 month after discontinuation of therapy. Prescriptions should be written for no more than a 30-day supply, and pregnancy testing and counseling should be repeated monthly.

May cause depression, psychosis, aggressive or violent behavior, and changes in mood; use with extreme caution in patients with psychiatric disorders. Rarely, suicidal thoughts and actions have been reported during isotretinoin usage. All patients should be observed closely for symptoms of depression or suicidal thoughts. Discontinuation of treatment alone may not be sufficient, further evaluation may be necessary. Cases of pseudotumor cerebri (benign intracranial hypertension) have been reported, some with concomitant use of tetracycline (avoid using together). Patients with papilledema, headache, nausea, vomiting, and visual disturbances should be referred to a neurologist and treatment with isotretinoin discontinued. Hearing impairment, which can continue after therapy is discontinued, may occur. Clinical hepatitis, elevated liver enzymes, inflammatory bowel disease, skeletal hyperostosis, premature epiphyseal closure, vision impairment, corneal opacities, decreased tolerance to contact lenses (due to dry eyes), and decreased night vision have also been reported with the use of isotretinoin. Rare postmarketing cases of severe skin reactions (eg, Stevens-Johnson syndrome, erythema multiforme) have been reported with use.

Use with caution in patients with diabetes mellitus; impaired glucose control has been reported. Use caution in patients with hypertriglyceridemia; acute pancreatitis and fatal hemorrhagic pancreatitis (rare) have been reported. Instruct patients to avoid or limit ethanol; may increase triglyceride levels if taken in excess. Bone mineral density may decrease; use caution in patients with a genetic predisposition to bone disorders (ie, osteoporosis, osteomalacia) and with disease states or concomitant medications that can induce bone disorders. Patients may be at risk when participating in activities with repetitive impact (such as sports). Patients should be instructed not to donate blood during therapy and for 1 month following discontinuation of therapy due to risk of donated blood being given to a pregnant female. Safety of long-term use is not established and is not recommended. Some products may contain tartrazine (FD&C yellow no. 5), which may cause allergic reactions, including bronchial asthma, in certain individuals. Allergy is frequently seen in patients who also have an aspirin hypersensitivity.

Absorica: Absorption is ~83% greater than Accutane when administered under fasting conditions; they are bioequivalent when taken with a high-fat meal. Absorica is **not** interchangeable with other generic isotretinoin products. Isotretinoin and tretinoin (which is also known as all-*trans* retinoic acid, or ATRA) may be confused, while both products may be used in cancer treatment, they are **not** interchangeable; verify product prior to dispensing and administration to prevent medication errors.

Adverse Reactions Frequency not always defined.

Cardiovascular: Chest pain, edema, flushing, palpitation, stroke, syncope, tachycardia, vascular thrombotic disease

Central nervous system: Aggressive behavior, depression, dizziness, drowsiness, emotional instability, fatigue, headache, insomnia, lethargy, malaise, nervousness, paresthesia, pseudotumor cerebri, psychosis, seizure, stroke, suicidal ideation, suicide attempts, suicide, violent behavior

Dermatologic: Abnormal wound healing acne fulminans, alopecia, bruising, cheilitis, cutaneous allergic reactions, dry nose, dry skin, eczema, eruptive xanthomas, facial erythema, fragility of skin, hair abnormalities, hirsutism, hyperpigmentation, hypopigmentation, increased sunburn susceptibility, nail dystrophy, paronychia, peeling of palms, peeling of soles, photoallergic reactions, photosensitizing reactions, pruritus, purpura, rash

Endocrine & metabolic: Triglycerides increased (25%), abnormal menses, blood glucose increased, cholesterol increased, HDL decreased, hyperuricemia

Gastrointestinal: Bleeding and inflammation of the gums, colitis, esophagitis, esophageal ulceration, inflammatory bowel disease, nausea, nonspecific gastrointestinal symptoms, pancreatitis, weight loss, xerostomia

Genitourinary: Nonspecific urogenital findings

Hematologic: Agranulocytosis (rare), anemia, neutropenia, pyogenic granuloma, thrombocytopenia

Hepatic: Alkaline phosphatase increased, ALT increased, AST increased, GGTP increased, hepatitis, LDH increased

Neuromuscular & skeletal: Back pain (29% in pediatric patients), arthralgia, arthritis, bone abnormalities, bone mineral density decreased, calcification of tendons and ligaments, CPK increased, myalgia, premature epiphyseal closure, skeletal hyperostosis, tendonitis, weakness

Ocular: Conjunctivitis (4%), blepharitis (1%), chalazion (1%), hordeolum (1%), cataracts, color vision disorder, corneal opacities, eyelid inflammation, keratitis, night vision decreased, optic neuritis, photophobia, visual disturbances

Otic: Hearing impairment, tinnitus

Renal: Glomerulonephritis, hematuria, proteinuria, pyuria, vasculitis

Respiratory: Bronchospasms, epistaxis, respiratory infection, voice alteration, Wegener's granulomatosis

Miscellaneous: Allergic reactions, anaphylactic reactions, disseminated herpes simplex, diaphoresis, infection, lymphadenopathy

<1%, postmarketing, and/or case reports: Abnormal meibomian gland secretion, contact lens intolerance, dry eyes, erythema multiforme, eye pain, meibomian gland atrophy, myopia, ocular sicca, pseudotumor cerebri, rhabdomyolysis, Stevens-Johnson syndrome, tear osmolarity increased, toxic epidermal necrolysis, visual acuity decreased

Drug Interactions

Metabolism/Transport Effects None known.

Avoid Concomitant Use

Avoid concomitant use of ISOtretinoin with any of the following: Multivitamins/Fluoride (with ADE); Multivitamins/Minerals (with ADEK, Folate, Iron); Multivitamins/Minerals (with AE, No Iron); Tetracycline Derivatives; Vitamin A

Increased Effect/Toxicity

ISOtretinoin may increase the levels/effects of: Mipomersen; Porfimer; Verteporfin

The levels/effects of ISOtretinoin may be increased by: Alcohol (Ethyl); Multivitamins/Fluoride (with ADE); Multivitamins/Minerals (with ADEK, Folate, Iron); Multivitamins/Minerals (with AE, No Iron); Tetracycline Derivatives; Vitamin A

Decreased Effect

ISOtretinoin may decrease the levels/effects of: Contraceptives (Estrogens); Contraceptives (Progestins)

Food Interactions Isotretinoin bioavailability increased if taken with food or milk. Management: Administer orally with a meal (except Absorica™ which may be taken without regard to meals).

Storage/Stability Store at 20°C to 25°C (68°F to 77°F); excursions permitted between 15°C to 30°C (59°F to 86°F). Protect from light.

Mechanism of Action Reduces sebaceous gland size and reduces sebum production in acne treatment; in neuroblastoma, decreases cell proliferation and induces differentiation

Pharmacodynamics/Kinetics

Absorption: Enhanced with a high-fat meal; Absorica™ absorption is ~83% greater than Accutane® when administered under fasting conditions; they are bioequivalent when taken with a high-fat meal.

Protein binding: 99% to 100%; primarily albumin

Metabolism: Hepatic via CYP2B6, 2C8, 2C9, 2D6, 3A4; forms metabolites; major metabolite: 4-oxo-isotretinoin (active)

Half-life elimination: Terminal: Parent drug: 21 hours; Metabolite: 21-24 hours

Time to peak, serum: 3-5 hours

Excretion: Urine and feces (equal amounts)

Dosing

Adult & Geriatric

Acne, severe recalcitrant nodular: Oral: 0.5-1 mg/kg/day in 2 divided doses for 15-20 weeks; may discontinue earlier if the total cyst count decreases by 70%. Adults with very severe disease/scarring or primarily involves the trunk may require dosage adjustment up to 2 mg/kg/day. A second course of therapy may be initiated after a period of ≥2 months off therapy. A dose of ≤0.5 mg/kg/day may be used to minimize initial flaring (Strauss, 2007).

Acne, moderate (off-label use): Oral: 20 mg/day (~0.3-0.4 mg/kg/day) for 6 months (Amichai, 2006)

Pediatric

Acne, severe recalcitrant nodular: Children 12-17 years: Oral: 0.5-1 mg/kg/day in 2 divided doses for 15-20 weeks; may discontinue earlier if the total cyst count decreases by 70%. A second course of therapy may be initiated after a period of ≥2 months off therapy. A dose of ≤0.5 mg/kg/day may be used to minimize initial flaring (Strauss, 2007).

Acne, moderate (off-label use): Children 12-17 years: Oral: 20 mg/day (~0.3-0.4 mg/kg/day) for 6 months (Amichai, 2006)

Neuroblastoma, high-risk (off-label use): Children 1-17 years: Oral: 160 mg/m^2/day (in 2 divided doses) days 1 through 14 every 28 days for 6 cycles, beginning after continuation chemotherapy or transplantation (Matthay, 1999)

Renal Impairment No dosage adjustment provided in the manufacturer's labeling.

Hepatic Impairment

Hepatic impairment prior to treatment: No dosage adjustment provided in the manufacturer's labeling.

Hepatotoxicity during treatment: Liver enzymes may normalize with dosage reduction or with continued treatment; discontinue if normalization does not readily occur or if hepatitis is suspected.

◀ **Administration** Administer orally with a meal (except Absorica™ which may be taken without regard to meals). According to the manufacturers' labeling, capsules should be swallowed whole with a full glass of liquid. For patients unable to swallow capsule whole, an oral liquid may be prepared; may irritate esophagus if contents are removed from the capsule.

Hazardous agent; use appropriate precautions for handling and disposal (meets NIOSH 2014 criteria).

Extemporaneous Preparations Hazardous agent: Use appropriate precautions for handling and disposal of teratogenic capsule contents (meets NIOSH 2014 criteria).

For patients unable to swallow the capsules whole, an oral liquid may be prepared with softgel capsules (not recommended by the manufacturers) by one of the following methods:

Place capsules (softgel formulations only) in small container and add warm (~37°C [97°F]) water or milk to cover capsule(s); wait 2-3 minutes until capsule is softened and then drink the milk or water with the softened capsule, or swallow softened capsule.

Puncture capsule (softgel formulations only) with needle or cut with scissors; squeeze capsule contents into 5-10 mL of milk or tube feed formula; draw mixture up into oral syringe and administer via feeding tube; flush feeding tube with ≥30 mL additional milk or tube feeding formula.

Puncture capsule (softgel formulations only) with needle or cut with scissors and draw contents into oral syringe; add 1-5 mL of medium chain triglyceride, soybean, or safflower oil to the oral syringe; mix gently and administer via feeding tube; flush feeding tube with ≥30 mL milk or tube feeding formula.

Lam MS, "Extemporaneous Compounding of Oral Liquid Dosage Formulations and Alternative Drug Delivery Methods for Anticancer Drugs," *Pharmacotherapy*, 2011, 31(2):164-92.

Monitoring Parameters CBC with differential and platelet count, baseline sedimentation rate, glucose, CPK; signs of depression, mood alteration, psychosis, aggression, severe skin reactions

Pregnancy test (for all female patients of childbearing potential): Two negative tests with a sensitivity of at least 25 milliunits/mL prior to beginning therapy (the second performed at least 19 days after the first test and performed during the first 5 days of the menstrual period immediately preceding the start of therapy); monthly tests to rule out pregnancy prior to refilling prescription.

Lipids: Prior to treatment and at weekly or biweekly intervals until response to treatment is established. Test should not be performed <36 hours after consumption of ethanol.

Liver function tests: Prior to treatment and at weekly or biweekly intervals until response to treatment is established.

Dietary Considerations Should be taken with food, except Absorbica™ which may be taken without regard to meals. Limit intake of vitamin A; avoid use of other vitamin A products. Some formulations may contain soybean oil.

Additional Information All patients (male and female), must be registered in the iPLEDGE™ risk management program. Females of childbearing potential must receive oral and written information reviewing the hazards of therapy and the effects that isotretinoin can have on a fetus. Therapy should not begin without two negative pregnancy tests at least 19 days apart. Two forms of contraception (a primary and secondary form as described in the iPLEDGE™ program materials) must be used simultaneously beginning 1 month prior to treatment, during treatment, and for 1 month after therapy is discontinued; limitations to their use must be explained. Micro-dosed progesterone products that do not contain an estrogen ("mini-pills") are not an acceptable form of contraception during isotretinoin treatment. Prescriptions should be written for no more than a 30-day supply, and pregnancy testing and counseling should be repeated monthly. During therapy, pregnancy tests must be conducted by a CLIA-certified laboratory. Prescriptions must be filled and picked up from the pharmacy within 7 days of specimen collection for pregnancy test for women of childbearing potential. Prescriptions for males and females of nonchildbearing potential must be filled and picked up within 30 days of prescribing.

Any cases of accidental pregnancy should be reported to the iPLEDGE™ program or FDA MedWatch. All patients (male and female) must read and sign the informed consent material provided in the pregnancy prevention program.

Prescribing and Access Restrictions As a requirement of the REMS program, access to this medication is restricted. All patients (male and female), prescribers, wholesalers, and dispensing pharmacists must register and be active in the iPLEDGE™ risk management program, designed to eliminate fetal exposures to isotretinoin. This program covers all isotretinoin products (brand and generic). The iPLEDGE™ program requires that all patients meet qualification criteria and monthly program requirements (eg, pregnancy testing). Healthcare providers can only prescribe a maximum 30-day supply at each monthly visit and must counsel patients on the iPLEDGE™ program requirements and confirm counseling via the iPLEDGE™ automated system. Registration, activation, and additional information are provided at www.ipledgeprogram.com or by calling 866-495-0654.

Medication Guide Available Yes

Dosage Forms Excipient information presented when available (limited, particularly for generics); consult specific product labeling.

Capsule, Oral:

Absorica: 10 mg, 20 mg [contains soybean oil]

Absorica: 25 mg [contains brilliant blue fcf (fd&c blue #1), fd&c yellow #6 (sunset yellow), soybean oil, tartrazine (fd&c yellow #5)]

Absorica: 30 mg [contains soybean oil]

Absorica: 35 mg [contains fd&c blue #2 (indigotine), soybean oil]

Absorica: 40 mg [contains soybean oil]

Amnesteem: 10 mg, 20 mg, 40 mg [contains soybean oil]

Claravis: 10 mg [contains fd&c yellow #6 (sunset yellow), soybean oil]

Claravis: 20 mg [contains soybean oil]

Claravis: 30 mg

Claravis: 40 mg [contains fd&c yellow #6 (sunset yellow), soybean oil]

Myorisan: 10 mg, 20 mg [contains soybean oil]

Myorisan: 30 mg [contains edetate disodium, soybean oil]

Myorisan: 40 mg [contains fd&c yellow #6 (sunset yellow), soybean oil]

Zenatane: 10 mg [contains brilliant blue fcf (fd&c blue #1), edetate disodium, fd&c yellow #10 (quinoline yellow), methylparaben, propylparaben, soybean oil]

Zenatane: 20 mg [contains edetate disodium, methylparaben, propylparaben, soybean oil]

Zenatane: 30 mg [contains edetate disodium, fd&c blue #2 aluminum lake, fd&c yellow #10 (quinoline yellow), methylparaben, propylparaben, soybean oil]

◄ Zenatane: 40 mg [contains brilliant blue fcf (fd&c blue #1), edetate disodium, fd&c blue #2 (indigotine), fd&c yellow #10 (quinoline yellow), methylparaben, propylparaben, soybean oil]

♦ **Isotretinoinum** *see* ISOtretinoin *on page 973*

♦ **Istodax** *see* RomiDEPsin *on page 1494*

Itraconazole (i tra KOE na zole)

Brand Names: US Onmel; Sporanox; Sporanox Pulsepak
Brand Names: Canada Sporanox
Pharmacologic Category Antifungal Agent, Oral
Use

Aspergillosis (capsules): Treatment of pulmonary and extrapulmonary aspergillosis in immunocompromised and nonimmunocompromised patients who are intolerant of or refractory to amphotericin B therapy.

Blastomycosis (capsules): Treatment of pulmonary and extrapulmonary blastomycosis in immunocompromised and nonimmunocompromised patients.

Histoplasmosis (capsules): Treatment of histoplasmosis, including chronic cavitary pulmonary disease and disseminated, nonmeningeal histoplasmosis in immunocompromised and nonimmunocompromised patients.

Onychomycosis:

Capsules: Treatment of onychomycosis of the toenail, with or without fingernail involvement, and onychomycosis of the fingernail caused by dermatophytes (tinea unguium) in nonimmunocompromised patients

Tablets: Treatment of onychomycosis of the toenail caused by *Trichophyton rubrum* or *Trichophyton mentagrophytes* in nonimmunocompromised patients

Oropharyngeal/Esophageal candidiasis (oral solution): Treatment of oropharyngeal and esophageal candidiasis

Canadian labeling: Oral capsules: Additional indications (not in US labeling):

Candidiasis, oral and/or esophageal: Treatment of oral and/or esophageal candidiasis in immunocompromised and immunocompetent patients

Chromomycosis: Treatment of chromomycosis in immunocompromised and immunocompetent patients

Dermatomycoses: Treatment of dermatomycoses due to tinea pedis, tinea cruris, tinea corporis, and of pityriasis versicolor in patients for whom oral therapy is appropriate

Onychomycosis: Treatment of onychomycosis in immunocompromised and immunocompetent patients

Paracoccidioidomycosis: Treatment of paracoccidioidomycosis in immunocompromised and immunocompetent patients

Sporotrichosis: Treatment of cutaneous and lymphatic sporotrichosis in immunocompromised and immunocompetent patients

Pregnancy Risk Factor C
Dosing

Adult & Geriatric Note: Doses >200 mg daily should be administered in 2 divided doses.

Aspergillosis: Oral capsule: 200 to 400 mg daily. **Note:** For life-threatening infections, the US labeling recommends administering a loading dose of 200 mg 3 times daily (total: 600 mg daily) for the first 3 days of therapy.

Continue treatment for at least 3 months and until clinical and laboratory evidence suggest that infection has resolved.

Aspergillosis, invasive (salvage therapy; voriconazole-susceptible): Duration of therapy should be a minimum of 6 to 12 weeks or throughout period of immunosuppression: Oral capsule: 200 to 400 mg daily; **Note:** 2008 IDSA guidelines recommend 600 mg/day for 3 days, followed by 400 mg daily (Walsh, 2008).

Aspergillosis, allergic (ABPA, sinusitis): Oral: 200 mg daily; may be used in conjunction with corticosteroids (Andes, 2000; Walsh, 2008)

Blastomycosis: *Manufacturer labeling:* Oral capsule: Initial: 200 mg once daily; if no clinical improvement or evidence of progressive infection, may increase dose in increments of 100 mg up to maximum of 400 mg daily. **Note:** For life-threatening infections, the US labeling recommends administering a loading dose of 200 mg 3 times daily (total: 600 mg daily) for the first 3 days of therapy. Continue treatment for at least 3 months and until clinical and laboratory evidence suggest that infection has resolved.

Alternative dosing: 200 mg 3 times daily for 3 days, then 200 mg twice daily for 6 to 12 months; in moderately severe to severe infection, therapy should be initiated with ~2 weeks of amphotericin B (Chapman, 2008).

Candidiasis: Oral:

Esophageal:

US labeling: Oral solution: 100 to 200 mg once daily for a minimum of 3 weeks; continue dosing for 2 weeks after resolution of symptoms

Canadian labeling:

Oral solution: 100 to 200 mg once daily for a minimum of 3 weeks; continue dosing for 2 weeks after resolution of symptoms

Oral capsules: 100 mg once daily for 4 weeks; increase dose to 200 mg once daily in patients with AIDS and neutropenic patients

Alternate dosing: HIV-infected patients: Oral solution: 200 mg once daily for 14 to 21 days (HHS [OI adult 2015])

Oropharyngeal:

US labeling: Oral solution: 200 mg once daily for 1 to 2 weeks; in patients unresponsive or refractory to fluconazole: 100 mg twice daily (clinical response expected in 2 to 4 weeks)

Canadian labeling:

Oral solution: 200 mg once daily or in divided doses daily for 1 to 2 weeks

Oral capsules: 100 mg once daily for 2 weeks; increase dose to 200 mg once daily in patients with AIDS and neutropenic patients

Alternate dosing: HIV-infected patients (alternative to preferred therapy): Oral solution: 200 mg once daily for 7 to 14 days (HHS [OI adult 2015])

Vulvo-vaginal (uncomplicated) in HIV-infected patients (alternative to preferred therapy) (off-label use): Oral solution: 200 mg once daily for 3 to 7 days (HHS [OI adult 2015])

Chromomycosis: Canadian labeling (not in US labeling): Oral: 200 mg once daily for 6 months (when due to *Fonsecaea pedrosoi*) or 100 mg once daily for 3 months (when due to *Cladosporium carrioni*)

Coccidioidomycosis (nonprogressive, nondisseminated disease): 200 mg twice daily or 3 times daily (Galgiani 2005)

Coccidioidal pneumonia: Oral:

Mild to moderate: 200 mg twice daily (Galgiani 2005)

HIV-infected patients (focal pneumonia): 200 mg twice daily (HHS [OI adult 2015])

Coccidioidal meningitis: Oral: 400 to 600 mg daily (Galgiani 2005)

◀ **Coccidioidal meningitis in HIV-infected patients (off-label use; HHS [OI adult 2015]) (alternative to preferred therapy):** Oral:

Treatment: 200 mg 3 times daily for 3 days, then 200 mg twice daily, followed by chronic suppressive therapy

Chronic suppressive therapy: 200 mg twice daily continued indefinitely, even with increase in CD4 count on ART

Histoplasmosis:

Treatment:

Manufacturer's labeling: Oral capsule: Initial: 200 mg once daily; if no clinical improvement or evidence of progressive infection, may increase dose in increments of 100 mg up to maximum of 400 mg daily. **Note:** For life-threatening infections, the US labeling recommends administering a loading dose of 200 mg 3 times daily (total: 600 mg daily) for the first 3 days of therapy. Continue treatment for at least 3 months and until clinical and laboratory evidence suggest that infection has resolved.

Alternate dosing: 200 mg 3 times daily for 3 days, then 200 mg twice daily (or once daily in mild-moderate disease) for 6 to 12 weeks in mild-moderate disease or ≥12 months in progressive disseminated or chronic cavitary pulmonary histoplasmosis; in moderately-severe to severe infection, therapy should be initiated with ~2 weeks of a lipid formation of amphotericin B (Wheat, 2007). Duration of twice daily maintenance therapy should be at least 12 months in HIV-infected patients (HHS [OI adult 2015])

Prophylaxis (off-label use):

Primary prophylaxis in HIV-infected patients: 200 mg once daily; primary prophylaxis is indicated when CD4 count <150 cells/mm^3 and at increased risk of exposure (HHS [OI adult 2015])

Long-term suppression therapy (secondary prophylaxis) in HIV-infected patients: 200 mg once daily; long-term suppressive therapy is indicated in patients who relapse despite appropriate therapy or in patients with CNS or severe disseminated infection (HHS [OI adult 2015])

Microsporidiosis, disseminated (caused by *Trachipleistophora* or *Anncaliia*) in HIV-infected patients (off-label use): Oral: 400 mg once daily in combination with albendazole (HHS [OI adult 2015])

Onychomycosis (fingernail involvement only): Oral capsule: 200 mg twice daily for 1 week; repeat 1-week course after 3-week off-time

Onychomycosis (toenails due to *Trichophyton rubrum* or *T. mentagrophytes*): Oral tablet: 200 mg once daily for 12 consecutive weeks.

Onychomycosis (toenails with or without fingernail involvement): Oral capsule: 200 mg once daily for 12 consecutive weeks

Canadian labeling (not in US labeling): "Pulse-dosing": 200 mg twice daily for 1 week; repeat 1-week course twice with 3-week off-time between each course

Paracoccidioidomycosis: Canadian labeling (not in US labeling): Oral capsule: 100 mg once daily for 6 months

Penicilliosis in HIV-infected patients (off-label use; HHS [OI adult 2015]): Oral:

Primary prophylaxis: 200 mg once daily for patients with a CD4 count <100 cells/mm^3 who spend extensive time in northern Thailand, Vietnam, and Southern China, especially rural areas

Treatment: 200 mg twice daily for 8 weeks (mild disease) or 10 weeks (severe infections), then continue with maintenance therapy. In severely-ill patients, initiate therapy with 2 weeks of liposomal amphotericin B.

Chronic maintenance (secondary prophylaxis): 200 mg once daily until CD4 count >100 cells/mm^3 for ≥6 months in response to ART

Pityriasis versicolor: Canadian labeling (not in US labeling): Oral: 200 mg once daily for 7 days

Sporotrichosis: Oral:

Lymphocutaneous: 200 mg daily for 3 to 6 months (Kauffman, 2007)

Canadian labeling (not in US labeling): 100 mg once daily for 3 months

Osteoarticular and pulmonary: 200 mg twice daily for ≥1 years (may use amphotericin B initially for stabilization) (Kauffman, 2007)

Tinea corporis or tinea cruris: Canadian labeling (not in US labeling): Oral capsule: 100 mg once daily for 14 consecutive days or 200 mg once daily for 7 consecutive days. **Note:** Equivalency between regimens not established.

Tinea pedis: Canadian labeling (not in US labeling): Oral capsule: 100 mg once daily for 28 consecutive days or 200 mg twice daily for 7 consecutive days. **Note:** Equivalency between regimens not established. Patients with chronic resistant infection may benefit from lower dose and extended treatment time (100 mg once daily for 28 days).

Pediatric Note: Doses >200 mg daily should be administered in 2 divided doses.

Candidiasis:

Infants and Children (HIV-exposed/-positive; off-label use):

Oropharyngeal: Oral solution: 2.5 mg/kg/dose twice daily (maximum: 200 mg daily [400 mg daily if fluconazole-refractory]) for 7 to 14 days (CDC, 2009)

Esophageal: Oral solution: 5 mg/kg/day once daily or divided twice daily for 4 to 21 days (CDC, 2009)

Adolescents (off-label population): HIV-infected patients:

Esophageal: Oral solution: 200 mg once daily for 14 to 21 days (HHS [OI adult 2015])

Oropharyngeal (alternative to preferred therapy): Oral solution: 200 mg once daily for 7 to 14 days (HHS [OI adult 2015])

Vulvo-vaginal (uncomplicated) (off-label use): Refer to adult dosing.

Coccidioidomycosis: Infants and Children (HIV-exposed/-positive; off-label use):

Treatment: Oral: 5 to 10 mg/kg/dose twice daily for 3 days, followed by 2 to 5 mg/kg/dose orally twice daily (maximum: 400 mg daily) (CDC, 2009)

Relapse prevention: Oral: 2 to 5 mg/kg/dose twice daily (maximum: 400 mg daily) (CDC, 2009)

Coccidioidal meningitis in HIV-infected patients (off-label use) (alternative to preferred therapy): Adolescents: Refer to adult dosing.

Coccidioidal pneumonia (focal pneumonia) in HIV-infected patients (off-label use): Adolescents: Refer to adult dosing.

Cryptococcus: Infants and Children (HIV-exposed/-positive; off-label use):

Treatment, consolidation therapy: Oral solution (preferred): Initial: 2.5 to 5 mg/kg/dose 3 times daily (maximum daily dose: 600 mg daily) for 3 days (9 doses) followed by 5 to 10 mg/kg/day divided once or twice daily (maximum daily dose: 400 mg daily) for a minimum of 8 weeks (CDC, 2009)

Relapse prevention: Oral solution: 5 mg/kg/dose once daily (maximum: 200 mg daily) (CDC, 2009)

◀ **Histoplasmosis:**
　Infants and Children (HIV-exposed/-positive; off-label use):
　　Treatment of mild disseminated disease: Oral solution: 2 to 5 mg/kg/dose 3 times daily for 3 days (9 doses), followed by twice daily for 12 months (maximum: 200 mg per dose) (CDC, 2009)
　　Consolidation treatment for moderate-severe to severe disseminated disease, including CNS infection (following appropriate induction therapy): Oral solution: 2 to 5 mg/kg/dose 3 times daily for 3 days, followed by 2 to 5 mg/kg/dose (maximum: 200 mg per dose) twice daily for 12 months for non-CNS-disseminated disease or for ≥12 months for CNS infection (CDC, 2009)
　　Relapse prevention: Oral solution: 5 mg/kg/dose twice daily (maximum: 400 mg daily) (CDC, 2009)
　Adolescents (off-label population): HIV-positive patients:
　　Treatment (off-label dose): 200 mg 3 times daily for 3 days, then 200 mg twice daily. Duration of twice daily maintenance therapy should be at least 12 months (HHS [OI adult 2015])
　　Primary prophylaxis in HIV-infected patients (off-label use): Refer to adult dosing.
　　Long-term suppression therapy (secondary prophylaxis) (off-label use): Refer to adult dosing.
Microsporidiosis, disseminated (caused by *Trachipleistophora* or *Anncaliia*) in HIV-infected patients (off-label use): Adolescents: Refer to adult dosing.
Penicilliosis in HIV-infected patients (off-label use): Adolescents: Refer to adult dosing.
Renal Impairment The manufacturer's labeling states to use with caution in patients with renal impairment; dosage adjustment may be needed. Limited data suggest that no dosage adjustments are required in renal impairment; wide variations observed in plasma concentrations versus time profiles in patients with uremia, or receiving hemodialysis or continuous ambulatory peritoneal dialysis (Boelaert, 1988).
Hepatic Impairment There are no dosage adjustments provided in the manufacturer's labeling; however, use caution and monitor closely for signs/symptoms of toxicity.
Additional Information Complete prescribing information should be consulted for additional detail.
Dosage Forms Excipient information presented when available (limited, particularly for generics); consult specific product labeling.
Capsule, Oral:
　Sporanox: 100 mg [contains brilliant blue fcf (fd&c blue #1), d&c red #22 (eosine), fd&c blue #2 (indigotine)]
　Sporanox Pulsepak: 100 mg [contains brilliant blue fcf (fd&c blue #1), d&c red #22 (eosine), fd&c blue #2 (indigotine)]
　Generic: 100 mg
Solution, Oral:
　Sporanox: 10 mg/mL (150 mL) [contains propylene glycol, saccharin sodium]
Tablet, Oral:
　Onmel: 200 mg

◆ **IVIG** *see* Immune Globulin *on page 903*

◆ **IV Immune Globulin** *see* Immune Globulin *on page 903*

Ixabepilone (ix ab EP i lone)

Related Information

Chemotherapy-Induced Peripheral Neuropathy *on page 2116*
Common Toxicity Criteria *on page 2122*
Management of Chemotherapy-Induced Nausea and Vomiting in Adults *on page 2142*
Management of Drug Extravasations *on page 2159*
Prevention of Chemotherapy-Induced Nausea and Vomiting in Children *on page 2203*
Safe Handling of Hazardous Drugs *on page 2292*

Brand Names: US Ixempra Kit

Index Terms Azaepothilone B; BMS-247550; Epothilone B Lactam

Pharmacologic Category Antineoplastic Agent, Antimicrotubular; Antineoplastic Agent, Epothilone B Analog

Use Breast cancer: Treatment of metastatic or locally-advanced breast cancer resistant to treatment with an anthracycline and a taxane, or if taxane-resistant and further anthracycline therapy is contraindicated (in combination with capecitabine) or as monotherapy in tumors are resistant or refractory to anthracyclines, taxanes, and capecitabine.

Anthracycline resistance is defined as progression during treatment or within 3 months in the metastatic setting (within 6 months in the adjuvant setting). Taxane resistance is defined as progression during treatment within 4 months in the metastatic setting (within 12 months in the adjuvant setting).

Labeled Contraindications History of severe (grade 3 or 4) hypersensitivity to polyoxyethylated castor oil (Cremophor EL) or its derivatives; neutrophil count <1,500/mm^3 or platelet count <100,000/mm^3; combination therapy with ixabepilone and capecitabine in patients with AST or ALT >2.5 times ULN or bilirubin >1 times ULN

Pregnancy Considerations Adverse events were observed in animal reproduction studies. Women of childbearing potential should be advised to use effective contraception during treatment.

Breast-Feeding Considerations It is not known if ixabepilone is excreted in breast milk. Due to the potential for serious adverse reactions in the nursing infant, a decision should be made to discontinue breast-feeding or to discontinue the drug, taking into account the importance of treatment to the mother.

Warnings/Precautions Hazardous agent - use appropriate precautions for handling and disposal (NIOSH 2014 [group 1]). **[U.S. Boxed Warning]: Due to increased risk of toxicity and neutropenia-related mortality, combination therapy with capecitabine is contraindicated in patients with AST or ALT >2.5 times ULN or bilirubin >1 times ULN.** Use (as monotherapy) is not recommended if AST or ALT >10 times ULN or bilirubin >3 times ULN; use caution in patients with AST or ALT >5 times ULN. Toxicities and serious adverse reactions are increased (in mono- and combination therapy) with hepatic dysfunction; dosage reductions are necessary. Diluent contains polyoxyethylated castor oil (Cremophor EL), which is associated with hypersensitivity reactions; use is contraindicated in patients with a history of severe hypersensitivity to polyoxyethylated castor oil (Cremophor EL) or its derivatives. Medications for the treatment of reaction should be available for immediate use; reactions may also be managed with a reduction of infusion rate. Premedicate with an H$_1$- and H$_2$-antagonist 1 hour prior to infusion; patients who experience hypersensitivity (eg, bronchospasm, dyspnea, flushing, rash) should also be premedicated with a corticosteroid for all subsequent cycles if treatment is continued.

Dose-dependent myelosuppression, particularly neutropenia, may occur with mono- or combination therapy. Neutropenic fever and infection have been reported with use. The risk for neutropenia is increased with hepatic dysfunction, especially when used in combination with capecitabine. Severe neutropenia and/or thrombocytopenia may require dosage adjustment and/or treatment delay. Peripheral (sensory and motor) neuropathy occurs commonly; may require dose reductions, treatment delays or discontinuation. Usually occurs during the first 3 cycles. Use with caution in patients with preexisting neuropathy. Patients with diabetes may have an increased risk for severe peripheral neuropathy. Use with caution in patients with a history of cardiovascular disease; the incidence of MI, ventricular dysfunction, and supraventricular arrhythmias is higher when ixabepilone is used in combination with capecitabine (as compared to capecitabine alone). Consider discontinuing ixabepilone in patients who develop cardiac ischemia or impaired cardiac function.

Potentially significant drug-drug interactions may exist, requiring dose or frequency adjustment, additional monitoring, and/or selection of alternative therapy. Due to the ethanol content in the diluent, may cause cognitive impairment; patients must be cautioned about performing tasks which require mental alertness (eg, operating machinery or driving). Toxicities or serious adverse events with combination therapy may be increased in the elderly.

Adverse Reactions

Percentages reported with monotherapy:

>10%:

Central nervous system: Headache (11%)

Dermatologic: Alopecia (48%)

Gastrointestinal: Nausea (42%), vomiting (29%), mucositis/stomatitis (29%), diarrhea (22%), anorexia (19%), constipation (16%), abdominal pain (13%)

Hematologic: Leukopenia (grade 3: 36%; grade 4: 13%), neutropenia (grade 3: 31%; grade 4: 23%)

Neuromuscular & skeletal: Peripheral neuropathy (63%; grades 3/4: 14%; grade 3/4 median onset: cycle 4), sensory neuropathy (62%; grades 3/4: 14%), weakness (56%), myalgia/arthralgia (49%), musculoskeletal pain (20%)

1% to 10%:

Cardiovascular: Edema (9%), chest pain (5%)

Central nervous system: Fever (8%), pain (8%), dizziness (7%), insomnia (5%)

Dermatologic: Nail disorder (9%), rash (9%), palmar-plantar erythrodysesthesia/hand-and-foot syndrome (8%), pruritus (6%), skin exfoliation (2%), hyperpigmentation (2%)

Endocrine & metabolic: Hot flush (6%), dehydration (2%)

Gastrointestinal: Gastroesophageal reflux disease (6%), taste perversion (6%), weight loss (6%)

Hematologic: Anemia (grade 3: 6%; grade 4: 2%), neutropenic fever (3%; grade 3: 3%), thrombocytopenia (grade 3: 5%; grade 4: 2%)

Neuromuscular & skeletal: Motor neuropathy (10%; grade 3: 1%)

Ocular: Lacrimation increased (4%)

Respiratory: Dyspnea (9%), upper respiratory tract infection (6%), cough (2%)

Miscellaneous: Hypersensitivity (5%; grade 3: 1%), infection (5%)

Mono- and combination therapy: <1%, postmarketing, and/or case reports (limited to important or life-threatening): Alkaline phosphatase increased, angina, atrial flutter, autonomic neuropathy, cardiomyopathy, cerebral hemorrhage, coagulopathy, colitis, dysphagia, dysphonia, embolism, enterocolitis, erythema multiforme, gastrointestinal hemorrhage, gastroparesis, GGT increased, hemorrhage, hepatic failure (acute), hypokalemia, hyponatremia, hypotension, hypovolemia, hypovolemic shock, hypoxia, ileus, interstitial pneumonia, jaundice, left ventricular dysfunction, metabolic acidosis, MI, nephrolithiasis, neutropenic infection, orthostatic hypotension, pneumonia, pneumonitis, pulmonary edema (acute), radiation recall, renal failure, respiratory failure, sepsis, septic shock, supraventricular arrhythmia, syncope, thrombosis, transaminases increased, trismus, urinary tract infection, vasculitis

Drug Interactions

Metabolism/Transport Effects Substrate of CYP3A4 (major); **Note:** Assignment of Major/Minor substrate status based on clinically relevant drug interaction potential

Avoid Concomitant Use

Avoid concomitant use of Ixabepilone with any of the following: BCG (Intravesical); CloZAPine; Conivaptan; Dipyrone; Fusidic Acid (Systemic); Idelalisib; St Johns Wort

Increased Effect/Toxicity

Ixabepilone may increase the levels/effects of: CloZAPine

The levels/effects of Ixabepilone may be increased by: Aprepitant; Conivaptan; CYP3A4 Inhibitors (Moderate); CYP3A4 Inhibitors (Strong); Dasatinib; Dipyrone; Fosaprepitant; Fusidic Acid (Systemic); Idelalisib; Ivacaftor; Luliconazole; Mifepristone; Netupitant; Osimertinib; Palbociclib; Simeprevir; Stiripentol

Decreased Effect

Ixabepilone may decrease the levels/effects of: BCG (Intravesical)

The levels/effects of Ixabepilone may be decreased by: Bosentan; CYP3A4 Inducers (Moderate); CYP3A4 Inducers (Strong); Dabrafenib; Deferasirox; Dexamethasone (Systemic); Enzalutamide; Mitotane; Osimertinib; Siltuximab; St Johns Wort; Tocilizumab

Food Interactions Grapefruit juice may increase plasma concentrations of ixabepilone. Management: Avoid grapefruit juice.

Storage/Stability Store intact vials under refrigeration at 2°C to 8°C (36°F to 46°F); protect from light. Reconstituted solution (in the vial) is stable for up to 1 hour at room temperature; infusion solution diluted in appropriate solution for infusion is stable for 6 hours at room temperature if a pH range of 6 to 9 is maintained (infusion must be completed within 6 hours).

Preparation for Administration Hazardous agent; use appropriate precautions for handling and disposal (NIOSH 2014 [group 1]). Allow to reach room temperature for ~30 minutes prior to reconstitution. Diluent vial may contain a white precipitate which should dissolve upon reaching room temperature. **Reconstitute only with the provided diluent.** Dilute the 15 mg vial with 8 mL and the 45 mg vial with 23.5 mL (using provided diluent) to a concentration ▶

of 2 mg/mL (contains overfill). Gently swirl and invert vial until dissolved completely. Prior to administration, further dilute using a non-DEHP container (eg, glass, polypropylene or polyolefin), to a final concentration of 0.2 to 0.6 mg/mL in ~250 mL lactated Ringer's, adjusted sodium chloride 0.9% (pH adjusted prior to ixabepilone addition with 2 mEq sodium bicarbonate per 250 to 500 mL sodium chloride) or PLASMA-LYTE A Injection pH 7.4. Mix thoroughly.

Mechanism of Action Epothilone B analog; binds to the beta-tubulin subunit of the microtubule, stabilizing microtubular promoting tubulin polymerization and stabilizing microtubular function, thus arresting the cell cycle (at the G2/M phase) and inducing apoptosis. Activity in taxane-resistant cells has been demonstrated.

Pharmacodynamics/Kinetics

Distribution: >1,000 L

Protein binding: 67% to 77%

Metabolism: Extensively hepatic, via CYP3A4; >30 metabolites (inactive) formed

Half-life elimination: ~52 hours

Time to peak, plasma: At the end of infusion (3 hours)

Excretion: Feces (65%; 2% of the total dose as unchanged drug); urine (21%; 6% of the total dose as unchanged drug)

Dosing

Adult & Geriatric Note: Premedicate with an H_1-antagonist (eg, oral diphenhydramine 50 mg) and H_2-antagonist (eg, oral ranitidine 150 to 300 mg) ~1 hour prior to infusion. Patients with a history of hypersensitivity should also be premedicated with corticosteroids (dexamethasone 20 mg orally 1 hour before or IV 30 minutes before infusion). For dose calculation, body surface area (BSA) is capped at a maximum of 2.2 m^2.

Breast cancer (metastatic or locally advanced): IV: 40 mg/m^2/dose over 3 hours every 3 weeks (maximum dose: 88 mg) either as monotherapy or in combination with capecitabine

Dosage adjustment with concomitant strong CYP3A4 inhibitors/ inducers:

CYP3A4 inhibitors: Avoid concomitant administration with strong CYP3A4 inhibitors (eg, itraconazole, ketoconazole, voriconazole, clarithromycin, telithromycin, nefazodone, atazanavir, delavirdine, indinavir, nelfinavir, ritonavir, saquinavir); if concomitant administration with a strong CYP3A4 inhibitor cannot be avoided, consider a dose reduction to 20 mg/m^2. When a strong CYP3A4 inhibitor is discontinued, allow ~1 week to elapse prior to adjusting ixabepilone dose upward to the indicated dose.

CYP3A4 inducers: Avoid concomitant administration with strong CYP3A4 inducers (eg, dexamethasone, phenytoin, carbamazepine, rifampin, phenobarbital); if concomitant administration with a strong CYP3A4 inducer cannot be avoided and after maintenance on the strong CYP3A4 inducer is established, consider adjusting the ixabepilone dose gradually up to 60 mg/m^2 (as a 4-hour infusion), with careful monitoring. If the strong CYP3A4 enzyme inducer is discontinued, reduce ixabepilone dose to the dose used prior to initiation of the CYP3A4 inducer.

Renal Impairment There are no dosage adjustments provided in the manufacturer's labeling, however, renal excretion is minimal. Pharmacokinetics (monotherapy) are not affected in patients with mild-to-moderate renal insufficiency (CrCl >30 mL/minute); monotherapy has not been studied in patients with serum creatinine >1.5 times ULN. Combination therapy with capecitabine has not been studied in patients with CrCl <50 mL/minute.

Hepatic Impairment

Ixabepilone monotherapy (initial cycle; adjust doses for subsequent cycles based on toxicity):

AST and ALT ≤2.5 times ULN and bilirubin ≤1 times ULN: No dosage adjustment necessary

AST and ALT >2.5 to ≤10 times ULN and bilirubin >1 to ≤1.5 times ULN: Reduce dose to 32 mg/m²

AST and ALT ≤10 times ULN and bilirubin >1.5 to ≤3 times ULN: Reduce dose to 20 to 30 mg/m² (initiate treatment at 20 mg/m², may escalate up to a maximum of 30 mg/m² in subsequent cycles if tolerated)

AST or ALT >10 times ULN or bilirubin >3 times ULN: Use is not recommended

Combination therapy of ixabepilone with capecitabine:

AST and ALT ≤2.5 times ULN and bilirubin ≤1 times ULN: No dosage adjustment necessary

AST or ALT >2.5 times ULN or bilirubin >1 times ULN: Use is contraindicated

Obesity *ASCO Guidelines for appropriate chemotherapy dosing in obese adults with cancer:* In general, utilize patient's actual body weight (full weight) for calculation of body surface area- or weight-based dosing, particularly when the intent of therapy is curative; manage regimen-related toxicities in the same manner as for nonobese patients; if a dose reduction is utilized due to toxicity, consider resumption of full weight-based dosing with subsequent cycles, especially if cause of toxicity (eg, hepatic or renal impairment) is resolved (Griggs, 2012). **Note:** According to the manufacturer, patients with a body surface area (BSA) >2.2 m² should be dosed based upon a maximum BSA of 2.2 m²

Adjustment for Toxicity

Hematologic:

Neutrophils <500/mm³ for ≥7 days: Reduce ixabepilone dose by 20%

Neutropenic fever: Reduce ixabepilone dose by 20%

Platelets <25,000/mm³ (or <50,000/mm³ with bleeding): Reduce ixabepilone dose by 20%

Nonhematologic:

Neuropathy:

Grade 2 (moderate) for ≥7 days: Reduce ixabepilone dose by 20%

Grade 3 (severe) for <7 days: Reduce ixabepilone dose by 20%

Grade 3 (severe or disabling) for ≥7 days: Discontinue ixabepilone treatment

Grade 3 toxicity (severe; other than neuropathy): Reduce ixabepilone dose by 20%

Grade 3 arthralgia/myalgia or fatigue (transient): Continue ixabepilone at current dose

Grade 3 hand-foot syndrome: Continue ixabepilone at current dose

Grade 4 toxicity (disabling): Discontinue ixabepilone treatment

Note: Adjust dosage at the start of a cycle are based on toxicities (hematologic and nonhematologic) from the previous cycle; delay new cycles until neutrophils have recovered to ≥1,500/mm³, platelets have recovered to ≥100,000/mm³ and nonhematologic toxicities have resolved or improved to at least grade 1. If toxicities persist despite initial dose reduction, reduce dose an additional 20%.

▶

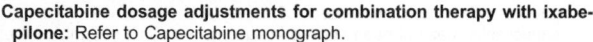

Capecitabine dosage adjustments for combination therapy with ixabepilone: Refer to Capecitabine monograph.

Combination Regimens

Breast cancer:

Capecitabine-Ixabepilone (Breast) on page 1858

Ixabepilone (Breast Regimen) on page 2024

Endometrial cancer: Ixabepilone (Endometrial Regimen) on page 2025

Administration IV: Infuse over 3 hours. Use non-DEHP administration set (eg, polyethylene); filter with a 0.2 to 1.2 micron inline filter. Administration should be completed within 6 hours of preparation. If the dose is increased (above 40 mg/m^2) due to concomitant CYP3A4 inducer use, infuse over 4 hours.

Hazardous agent; use appropriate precautions for handling and disposal (NIOSH 2014 [group 1]).

Vesicant/Extravasation Risk Irritant

Emetic Potential Children and Adults: Low (10% to 30%)

Monitoring Parameters CBC with differential; hepatic function (ALT, AST, bilirubin); monitor for hypersensitivity, signs/symptoms of neuropathy

Dietary Considerations Avoid grapefruit juice (may increase plasma concentrations of ixabepilone).

Dosage Forms Considerations Diluent supplied in Ixempra Kit contains polyoxyethylated castor oil (Cremophor EL)

Dosage Forms Excipient information presented when available (limited, particularly for generics); consult specific product labeling.

Solution Reconstituted, Intravenous:

Ixempra Kit: 15 mg (1 ea); 45 mg (1 ea) [contains alcohol, usp, cremophor el]

Ixazomib (ix AZ oh mib)

Index Terms Ninlaro

Pharmacologic Category Proteasome Inhibitor

Use Multiple myeloma: Treatment of multiple myeloma (in combination with lenalidomide and dexamethasone) in patients who have received at least one prior therapy

Labeled Contraindications There are no contraindications listed in the manufacturer's labeling.

Adverse Reactions Adverse reaction percentages reported as part of a combination regimen with lenalidomide and dexamethasone. Frequency not always defined.

>10%

Cardiovascular: Peripheral edema (25%)

Central nervous system: Peripheral neuropathy (28%; grade 3: 2%), peripheral sensory neuropathy (19%)

Dermatologic: Skin rash (19%; grade 3: 3%)

Gastrointestinal: Diarrhea (42%; grade 3: 6%), constipation (34%; grade 3: <1%), nausea (26%; grade 3: 2%), vomiting (22%; grade 3: 1%)

Hematologic & oncologic: Thrombocytopenia (78%; grades 3/4: 26%), neutropenia (67%; grades 3/4: 26%)

Neuromuscular & skeletal: Back pain (21%)

Ophthalmic: Eye disease (26%)

Respiratory: Upper respiratory tract infection (19%)

1% to 10%:

Hepatic: Hepatic insufficiency (6%)

Ophthalmic: Blurred vision (6%), conjunctivitis (6%), xerophthalmia (5%)

<1%, postmarketing, and/or case reports: Cholestatic hepatitis, hepatocellular hepatitis, hepatotoxicity, liver steatosis, peripheral motor neuropathy, reversible posterior leukoencephalopathy syndrome, Stevens-Johnson syndrome, Sweet's syndrome, thrombotic thrombocytopenic purpura, transverse myelitis, tumor lysis syndrome

Product Availability Ninlaro: Availability is currently unknown.

♦ **Ixempra Kit** see Ixabepilone on page 985

♦ **Ixinity** see Factor IX (Recombinant) on page 684

♦ **JAA-Prednisone (Can)** see PredniSONE on page 1426

♦ **Jadenu** see Deferasirox on page 478

♦ **Jakafi** see Ruxolitinib on page 1501

♦ **Jakavi (Can)** see Ruxolitinib on page 1501

♦ **JAMP-Allopurinol (Can)** see Allopurinol on page 73

♦ **JAMP-Anastrozole (Can)** see Anastrozole on page 112

♦ **JAMP-Bicalutamide (Can)** see Bicalutamide on page 207

♦ **JAMP-Ciprofloxacin (Can)** see Ciprofloxacin (Systemic) on page 327

♦ **JAMP-Letrozole (Can)** see Letrozole on page 1019

♦ **JAMP-Methotrexate (Can)** see Methotrexate on page 1104

♦ **JAMP-Mycophenolate (Can)** see Mycophenolate on page 1177

♦ **JAMP-Olanzapine ODT (Can)** see OLANZapine on page 1242

♦ **JAMP-Ondansetron (Can)** see Ondansetron on page 1253

♦ **JAMP-Tobramycin (Can)** see Tobramycin (Systemic) on page 1650

♦ **JAMP-Vancomycin (Can)** see Vancomycin on page 1720

♦ **Jevtana** see Cabazitaxel on page 250

♦ **JNJ-54767414** see Daratumumab on page 444

♦ **Jurnista (Can)** see HYDROmorphone on page 830

♦ **Kadcyla** see Ado-Trastuzumab Emtansine on page 43

♦ **Kadian** see Morphine (Systemic) on page 1167

♦ **Kaote DVI** see Antihemophilic Factor (Human) on page 117

♦ **Kemsol (Can)** see Dimethyl Sulfoxide on page 528

♦ **Keoxifene Hydrochloride** see Raloxifene on page 1451

♦ **Kepivance** see Palifermin on page 1304

♦ **Kepivance® (Can)** see Palifermin on page 1304

♦ **Keratinocyte Growth Factor, Recombinant Human** see Palifermin on page 1304

Ketoconazole (Systemic) (kee toe KOE na zole)

Brand Names: Canada Apo-Ketoconazole; Teva-Ketoconazole
Index Terms Nizoral
Pharmacologic Category Antifungal Agent, Imidazole Derivative; Antifungal Agent, Oral

◀ **Use Fungal infections:**
   U.S. labeling: Systemic fungal infections: Treatment of susceptible fungal infections, including blastomycosis, histoplasmosis, paracoccidioidomycosis, coccidioidomycosis, and chromomycosis in patients who have failed or who are intolerant to other antifungal therapies
   Canadian labeling: Treatment of serious or life-threatening systemic fungal infections (eg, systemic candidiasis, chronic mucocutaneous candidiasis, coccidioidomycosis, paracoccidioidomycosis, histoplasmosis, and chromomycosis) where alternate therapy is inappropriate or ineffective; may be considered for severe dermatophytoses unresponsive to other therapy

Pregnancy Risk Factor C

Dosing
  Adult & Geriatric
   Fungal infections: Oral: 200-400 mg once daily
     Therapy duration: Continue therapy until active fungal infection has resolved (based on clinical and laboratory parameters); some infections may require at least 6 months of therapy.
   Prostate cancer, advanced (off-label use): Oral: 400 mg 3 times daily (in combination with oral hydrocortisone) until disease progression (Ryan, 2007; Small, 2004)
  Pediatric Fungal infections: Children ≥2 years: Oral: 3.3-6.6 mg/kg once daily
     Therapy duration: Continue therapy until active fungal infection has resolved (based on clinical and laboratory parameters); some infections may require at least 6 months of therapy.
  Renal Impairment No dosage adjustment provided in manufacturer's labeling. Some clinicians suggest that no dosage adjustment is necessary in mild-to-severe impairment (Aronoff, 2007).
     Hemodialysis: Not dialyzable
  Hepatic Impairment No dosage adjustment provided in manufacturer's labeling; use with caution due to risks of hepatotoxicity.
     Hepatotoxicity during treatment:
     U.S. labeling: If ALT >ULN or 30% above baseline (or if patient is symptomatic), interrupt therapy and obtain full hepatic function panel. Upon normalization of liver function, may consider resuming therapy if benefit outweighs risk (hepatotoxicity has been reported on rechallenge).
     Canadian labeling: Discontinue therapy for liver function tests >3 times ULN or if abnormalities persist, worsen, or are associated with hepatotoxicity symptoms.
  Additional Information Complete prescribing information should be consulted for additional detail.

Medication Guide Available Yes

Dosage Forms Excipient information presented when available (limited, particularly for generics); consult specific product labeling.
   Tablet, Oral:
     Generic: 200 mg

♦ **Keytruda** *see* Pembrolizumab *on page 1362*

♦ **Khloditan** *see* Mitotane *on page 1155*

♦ **Kidrolase (Can)** *see* Asparaginase (*E. coli*) *on page 144*

♦ **Koate-DVI** *see* Antihemophilic Factor (Human) *on page 117*

♦ **Kogenate FS** *see* Antihemophilic Factor (Recombinant) *on page 119*

♦ **Kogenate FS Bio-Set** *see* Antihemophilic Factor (Recombinant) *on page 119*

♦ **KU-0059436** *see* Olaparib *on page 1245*

♦ **Kyprolis** *see* Carfilzomib *on page 278*

♦ **Kytril** *see* Granisetron *on page 801*

♦ **L-758,298** *see* Fosaprepitant *on page 759*

♦ **L 754030** *see* Aprepitant *on page 134*

♦ **Ladakamycin** *see* AzaCITIDine *on page 161*

♦ **L-AmB** *see* Amphotericin B (Liposomal) *on page 102*

♦ **Lambrolizumab** *see* Pembrolizumab *on page 1362*

Lanreotide (lan REE oh tide)

Brand Names: US Somatuline Depot
Brand Names: Canada Somatuline Autogel
Index Terms Lanreotide (Long-Acting Aqueous); Lanreotide Acetate; Lanreotide Autogel
Pharmacologic Category Somatostatin Analog
Use

US labeling:

Acromegaly: Long-term treatment of acromegalic patients who have had an inadequate response to surgery and/or radiotherapy, or for whom surgery and/or radiotherapy is not an option.

Gastroenteropancreatic neuroendocrine tumors: Treatment (to improve progression-free survival) of unresectable, well- or moderately-differentiated, locally advanced or metastatic gastroenteropancreatic neuroendocrine tumors (GEP-NETs).

Canadian labeling:

Acromegaly: Long-term treatment of patients with acromegaly due to pituitary tumors who have had an inadequate response to surgery and/or radiotherapy, or for whom surgery and/or radiotherapy is not an option; relief of symptoms associated with acromegaly.

Enteropancreatic neuroendocrine tumors: Treatment (to delay progression) of enteropancreatic neuroendocrine tumors in patients with grade 1 or a subset of grade 2 (equivalent to Ki67 <10%) unresectable, locally advanced, or metastatic disease.

Labeled Contraindications

US labeling: There are no contraindications listed in the manufacturer's labeling.

Canadian labeling: Hypersensitivity to lanreotide, somatostatin or related peptides, or any component of the formulation; complicated, untreated lithiasis of the bile ducts

Pregnancy Considerations Adverse events were observed in animal reproduction studies. Information related to the use of lanreotide in pregnancy is limited (deMenis, 1999) and it is recommended to discontinue therapy during pregnancy (Chandraharan 2003; Melmed 2012).

Breast-Feeding Considerations It is not known if lanreotide is excreted in breast milk. Due to the potential for serious adverse reactions in the breast-feeding infant, the manufacturer recommends a decision should be made to discontinue breast-feeding or to discontinue the drug, taking into account the importance of treatment to the mother.

◀ **Warnings/Precautions** Inhibition of insulin and glucagon secretion may affect glucose regulation, leading to hyper-/hypoglycemia, especially in patients with diabetes. Monitor serum glucose levels with the initiation of therapy and with dosage changes; dose adjustments in antidiabetic medications may be necessary. May reduce gall bladder motility, leading to cholelithiasis (may be dose- or duration-related); may require periodic monitoring (consider ultrasonography at baseline and periodically thereafter). Slight decreases in thyroid function have been observed during therapy; may require monitoring of thyroid function tests.

Bradycardia, sinus bradycardia, and hypertension have been observed with therapy; use with caution in patients with preexisting cardiac disease; monitor heart rate. Patients without preexisting cardiac disease may experience a decrease in heart rate though not to the level of bradycardia. Appropriate medical therapy should be initiated if patients develop symptomatic bradycardia. Use with caution in patients with moderate to severe renal and hepatic impairment; lower initial doses may be recommended. Diarrhea and loose stools may occur (may affect intestinal absorption of concurrently-administered medication); abdominal pain may also occur. Potentially significant drug-drug interactions may exist, requiring dose or frequency adjustment, additional monitoring, and/or selection of alternative therapy. Allergic reactions, including angioedema and anaphylaxis, have been reported (Somatuline Canadian labeling 2015).

Adverse Reactions

>10%:

Cardiovascular: Bradycardia (3% to 18%), hypertension (5% to 14%)

Central nervous system: Headache (5% to 16%)

Endocrine & metabolic: Weight loss (5% to 11%), dysglycemia (≤7%; includes diabetes, hyperglycemia, and hypoglycemia)

Gastrointestinal: Diarrhea (26% to 65%; dose related), abdominal pain (7% to 34%; dose related), vomiting (5% to 19%), flatulence (≤14%; dose related), nausea (9% to 11%)

Hematologic: Anemia (3% to 14%)

Hepatic: Cholelithiasis (2% to 27%), gall bladder sludge (20%)

Local: Injection site reaction (6% to 22%; induration 5%; pain 4%; mass 2%)

Neuromuscular & skeletal: Musculoskeletal pain (19%)

1% to 10%:

Cardiovascular: Sinus bradycardia (3% to 7%)

Central nervous system: Dizziness (9%), depression (7%)

Gastrointestinal: Loose stools (6% to 9%), constipation (5% to 8%)

Immunologic: Antibody development (<1% to 4%)

Neuromuscular & skeletal: Arthralgia (7% to 10%)

<1%, postmarketing, and/or case reports: Angioedema, cholecystitis, decreased heart rate, dysautonomia, hypersensitivity, hypothyroidism, injection site pruritus, pancreatitis, steatorrhea, valvular regurgitation (aortic, mitral)

Drug Interactions

Metabolism/Transport Effects None known.

Avoid Concomitant Use

Avoid concomitant use of Lanreotide with any of the following: Ceritinib

Increased Effect/Toxicity

Lanreotide may increase the levels/effects of: Bradycardia-Causing Agents; Bromocriptine; Ceritinib; Codeine; Hypoglycemia-Associated Agents; Ivabradine; Lacosamide; Pegvisomant

The levels/effects of Lanreotide may be increased by: Androgens; Antidiabetic Agents; Bretylium; Herbs (Hypoglycemic Properties); MAO Inhibitors; Pegvisomant; Quinolone Antibiotics; Ruxolitinib; Salicylates; Selective Serotonin Reuptake Inhibitors; Tofacitinib

Decreased Effect

Lanreotide may decrease the levels/effects of: Antidiabetic Agents; Cyclo-SPORINE (Systemic)

The levels/effects of Lanreotide may be decreased by: Quinolone Antibiotics

Storage/Stability Store under refrigeration 2°C to 8°C (36°F to 46°F). Protect from light.

Preparation for Administration Allow to reach room temperature by removing sealed pouch from refrigerator 30 minutes prior to administration; keep in sealed pouch until just prior to administration.

Mechanism of Action Synthetic octapeptide analogue of somatostatin which is a peptide inhibitor of multiple endocrine, neuroendocrine, and exocrine mechanisms. Displays a greater affinity for somatostatin type 2 (SSTR2) and type 5 (SSTR5) receptors found in pituitary gland, pancreas, and growth hormone (GH) secreting neoplasms of pituitary gland and a lesser affinity for somatostatin receptors 1, 3, and 4. Reduces GH secretion and also reduces the levels of insulin-like growth factor 1.

Pharmacodynamics/Kinetics

Distribution: V_{ss}: ~0.2 L/kg (Somatuline Canadian labeling 2015)

Protein binding: 79% to 83% (Somatuline Canadian labeling 2015)

Metabolism: Extensively within GI tract after biliary excretion (Somatuline Canadian labeling 2015)

Bioavailability: 69% to 78%

Half-life, elimination: *Depot:* 23 to 30 days

Time to peak, plasma: Mean: 7 to 12 hours (Somatuline Canadian labeling 2015)

Excretion: Urine (<5% as unchanged drug); feces (<0.5% as unchanged drug)

Dosing

Adult & Geriatric

US labeling:

Acromegaly: SubQ: Initial dose: 90 mg once every 4 weeks for 3 months; after initial 90 days of therapy, adjust dose based on clinical response of patient, growth hormone (GH) levels, and/or insulin-like growth factor 1 (IGF-1) levels as follows:

GH ≤1 ng/mL, IGF-1 normal, symptoms stable: 60 mg once every 4 weeks; once stabilized on 60 mg once every 4 weeks, may consider regimen of 120 mg once every 6 or 8 weeks (extended-interval dosing)

GH >1 to 2.5 ng/mL, IGF-1 normal, symptoms stable: 90 mg once every 4 weeks; once stabilized on 90 mg once every 4 weeks, may consider regimen of 120 mg once every 6 or 8 weeks (extended-interval dosing)

GH >2.5 ng/mL, IGF-1 elevated and/or uncontrolled symptoms: 120 mg once every 4 weeks

Gastroenteropancreatic neuroendocrine tumors (GEP-NETs): SubQ: 120 mg once every 4 weeks until disease progression or unacceptable toxicity

◄

Canadian labeling:

Acromegaly: SubQ: Initial dose: 90 mg once every 4 weeks for 3 months; after initial 90 days of therapy, adjust dose based on clinical response of patient, growth hormone (GH) levels, and/or insulin-like growth factor 1 (IGF-1) levels as follows:

GH ≤1 ng/mL, IGF-1 normal, symptoms stable: 60 mg once every 4 weeks; once stabilized on 60 mg once every 4 weeks, may consider regimen of 120 mg once every 6 or 8 weeks (extended-interval dosing)

GH >1 to 2.5 ng/mL, IGF-1 normal, symptoms stable: 90 mg once every 4 weeks; once stabilized on 90 mg once every 4 weeks, may consider regimen of 120 mg once every 6 or 8 weeks (extended-interval dosing)

GH >2.5 ng/mL, IGF-1 elevated and/or uncontrolled symptoms: 120 mg once every 4 weeks

Enteropancreatic neuroendocrine tumors (NETs): SubQ: 120 mg once every 4 weeks, continue until disease progression

Pediatric

Acromegaly: Adolescents ≥16 years (*Canadian labeling*): Refer to adult dosing.

Renal Impairment

Acromegaly:

Mild impairment (CrCl 60 to 89 mL/minute: No dosage adjustment necessary.

Moderate to severe impairment (CrCl ≤59 mL/minute): Initial dose: 60 mg once every 4 weeks for 3 months; adjust dose based on clinical response of patient, GH levels, and/or IGF-1 levels; use of an extended-interval dose of 120 mg once every 6 or 8 weeks should be done with caution.

Gastroenteropancreatic or enteropancreatic neuroendocrine tumors (GEP-NETs):

Mild to moderate impairment (CrCl ≥30 mL/minute): No dosage adjustment necessary.

Severe impairment (CrCl <30 mL/minute): There are no dosage adjustments provided in the manufacturer's labeling (has not been studied).

Hepatic Impairment

Acromegaly:

Mild impairment: No dosage adjustment necessary.

Moderate to severe impairment: Initial dose: 60 mg once every 4 weeks for 3 months; adjust dose based on clinical response of patient, GH levels, and/or IGF-1 levels; use of an extended-interval dose of 120 mg once every 6 or 8 weeks should be done with caution.

Gastroenteropancreatic or enteropancreatic neuroendocrine tumors (GEP-NETs): There are no dosage adjustments provided in the manufacturer's labeling (has not been studied).

Administration Administer by deep subcutaneous injection into superior outer quadrant of buttocks. Alternate injection sites between the right and left sides from one injection to the next. Remove sealed pouch from refrigerator 30 minutes prior to administration.

Monitoring Parameters Serum GH and IGF-1 at 3 months and as clinically indicated in acromegaly patients (obtain levels 6 weeks after dose adjustment when switching to extended-interval dosing), glucose levels, thyroid function (where clinically indicated); heart rate, consider gall bladder ultrasonography (baseline and periodically during therapy)

Dosage Forms Excipient information presented when available (limited, particularly for generics); consult specific product labeling.

Solution, Subcutaneous:

Somatuline Depot: 120 mg/0.5 mL (0.5 mL); 60 mg/0.2 mL (0.2 mL); 90 mg/ 0.3 mL (0.3 mL)

Dosage Forms: Canada Excipient information presented when available (limited, particularly for generics); consult specific product labeling.

Solution, Subcutaneous:

Somatuline Autogel: 60 mg/0.5 mL (0.5 mL); 90 mg/0.5 mL (0.5 mL); 120 mg/ 0.5 mL (0.5 mL)

♦ **Lanreotide Acetate** see Lanreotide on page 993

♦ **Lanreotide Autogel** see Lanreotide on page 993

♦ **Lanreotide (Long-Acting Aqueous)** see Lanreotide on page 993

♦ **Lanvis® (Can)** see Thioguanine on page 1637

Lapatinib (la PA ti nib)

Related Information

Common Toxicity Criteria on page 2122

Management of Chemotherapy-Induced Nausea and Vomiting in Adults on page 2142

Management of EGFR Inhibitor Toxicities: Dermatologic, Ocular, and Gastrointestinal on page 2179

Prevention of Chemotherapy-Induced Nausea and Vomiting in Children on page 2203

Principles of Anticancer Therapy on page 2261

Safe Handling of Hazardous Drugs on page 2292

Brand Names: US Tykerb

Brand Names: Canada Tykerb

Index Terms GW572016; Lapatinib Ditosylate

Pharmacologic Category Antineoplastic Agent, Anti-HER2; Antineoplastic Agent, Epidermal Growth Factor Receptor (EGFR) Inhibitor; Antineoplastic Agent, Tyrosine Kinase Inhibitor

Use

Breast cancer: Treatment of human epidermal growth receptor type 2 (HER2) overexpressing advanced or metastatic breast cancer (in combination with capecitabine) in patients who have received prior therapy (with an anthracycline, a taxane, and trastuzumab); HER2 overexpressing hormone receptor–positive metastatic breast cancer in postmenopausal women where hormone therapy is indicated (in combination with letrozole)

Limitations of use: Patients should have disease progression on trastuzumab prior to initiation of treatment with lapatinib in combination with capecitabine.

Labeled Contraindications Known severe hypersensitivity to lapatinib or any component of the formulation

Pregnancy Considerations Adverse events were demonstrated in animal reproduction studies. Lapatinib may cause fetal harm if administered during pregnancy. Women of childbearing potential should be advised to avoid pregnancy during treatment.

European Society for Medical Oncology (ESMO) guidelines for cancer during pregnancy recommend delaying treatment with HER-2 targeted agents until after delivery in pregnant patients with HER-2 positive disease (Peccatori 2013).

Breast-Feeding Considerations It is not known if lapatinib is excreted in breast milk. Due to the potential for serious adverse reactions in the nursing infant, the decision to discontinue lapatinib or discontinue breast-feeding during treatment should take in account the benefits of treatment to the mother.

Warnings/Precautions Hazardous agent - use appropriate precautions for handling and disposal (meets NIOSH 2014 criteria). Decreases in left ventricular ejection fraction (LVEF) have been reported (usually within the first 3 months of treatment); baseline and periodic LVEF evaluations are recommended; interrupt treatment with decreased LVEF ≥ grade 2 or LVEF <LLN; may reinitiate with a reduced dose after a minimum of 2 weeks if the LVEF recovers and the patient is asymptomatic. QTc prolongation has been observed; use caution in patients with a history of QTc prolongation or with medications known to prolong the QT interval; a baseline and periodic 12-lead ECG should be considered; correct electrolyte (potassium, calcium and magnesium) abnormalities prior to and during treatment. Use with caution in conditions which may impair left ventricular function and in patients with a history of or predisposed to (prior treatment with anthracyclines, chest wall irradiation) left ventricular dysfunction. Interstitial lung disease (ILD) and pneumonitis have been reported (with lapatinib monotherapy and with combination chemotherapy); monitor for pulmonary symptoms which may indicate ILD or pneumonitis; discontinue treatment for grade 3 (or higher) pulmonary symptoms indicative of ILD or pneumonitis (eg, dyspnea, dry cough).

[U.S. Boxed Warning]: Hepatotoxicity (ALT or AST >3 times ULN and total bilirubin >2 times ULN) has been reported with lapatinib; may be severe and/or fatal. Onset of hepatotoxicity may occur within days to several months after treatment initiation. Monitor (at baseline and every 4 to 6 weeks during treatment, and as clinically indicated); discontinue with severe changes in liver function; do not reinitiate. Use caution in patients with hepatic dysfunction; dose reductions should be considered in patients with preexisting severe (Child-Pugh class C) hepatic impairment. Potentially significant drug-drug interactions may exist, requiring dose or frequency adjustment, additional monitoring, and/or selection of alternative therapy. Patients who carry the HLA alleles DQA1*02:01 and DRB1*07:01 may experience a greater incidence of severe liver injury than patients who are noncarriers. These alleles are present in ~15% to 25% of Caucasian, Asian, African, and Hispanic patient populations and 1% in Japanese populations. May cause diarrhea (onset is generally within 6 days and duration is 4 to 5 days); may be severe and/or fatal; instruct patients to immediately report any bowel pattern changes. After first unformed stool, administer antidiarrheal agents; severe diarrhea may require hydration, electrolytes, antibiotics (if duration >24 hours, fever, or grade 3/4 neutropenia), and/or treatment interruption, dose reduction, or discontinuation. Severe cutaneous reactions have been reported with use. Discontinue therapy if life-threatening dermatologic reactions (eg, progressive skin rash with blisters or mucosal lesions) such as erythema multiforme, Stevens-Johnson syndrome, or toxic epidermal necrolysis occur.

Adverse Reactions Percentages reported for combination therapy.
>10%:
Central nervous system: Fatigue (≤20%), headache (14%)

Dermatologic: Palmar-plantar erythrodysesthesia (with capecitabine: 53%; grade 3: 12%), skin rash (28% to 44%), alopecia (13%), xeroderma (10% to 13%), pruritus (12%), nail disease (11%)

Gastrointestinal: Diarrhea (64% to 65%; grade 3: 9% to 13%; grade 4: ≤1%), nausea (31% to 44%), vomiting (17% to 26%), mucositis (15%), abdominal pain (≤15%), stomatitis (14%), anorexia (11%), dyspepsia (11%)

Hematologic: Decreased hemoglobin (with capecitabine: 56%; grade 3: <1%), decreased neutrophils (with capecitabine: 22%; grade 3: 3%; grade 4: <1%), decreased platelet count (with capecitabine: 18%; grade 3: <1%)

Hepatic: Increased serum AST (49% to 53%; grade 3: 2% to 6%; grade 4: <1%), increased serum ALT (37% to 46%; grade 3: 2% to 5%; grade 4: <1%), increased serum bilirubin (22% to 45%; grade 3: ≤4%; grade 4: <1%)

Neuromuscular & skeletal: Limb pain (12%), weakness (12%), back pain (11%)

Respiratory: Dyspnea (12%), epistaxis (11%)

1% to 10%: Central nervous system: Insomnia (10%)

<1%, postmarketing, and/or case reports: Anaphylaxis, hepatotoxicity, hypersensitivity, interstitial pulmonary disease, left ventricular ejection fraction, paronychia, pneumonitis, prolonged Q-T interval on ECG, severe dermatological reaction

Drug Interactions
Metabolism/Transport Effects **Substrate** of CYP3A4 (major), P-glycoprotein; **Note:** Assignment of Major/Minor substrate status based on clinically relevant drug interaction potential; **Inhibits** BCRP, CYP2C8 (moderate), CYP3A4 (weak), P-glycoprotein

Avoid Concomitant Use
Avoid concomitant use of Lapatinib with any of the following: Amodiaquine; Bosutinib; Conivaptan; CYP3A4 Inducers (Strong); CYP3A4 Inhibitors (Strong); Dexamethasone (Systemic); Fusidic Acid (Systemic); Grapefruit Juice; Idelalisib; PAZOPanib; Pimozide; Silodosin; St Johns Wort; Topotecan; VinCRIStine (Liposomal)

Increased Effect/Toxicity
Lapatinib may increase the levels/effects of: Afatinib; Amodiaquine; ARIPiprazole; Bosutinib; Brentuximab Vedotin; Colchicine; CYP2C8 Substrates; Dabigatran Etexilate; DOXOrubicin (Conventional); Edoxaban; Everolimus; Flibanserin; Highest Risk QTc-Prolonging Agents; Hydrocodone; Ledipasvir; Lomitapide; Moderate Risk QTc-Prolonging Agents; Naloxegol; NiMODipine; PAZOPanib; P-glycoprotein/ABCB1 Substrates; Pimozide; Prucalopride; Ranolazine; Rifaximin; Silodosin; Topotecan; VinCRIStine (Liposomal)

The levels/effects of Lapatinib may be increased by: Aprepitant; Conivaptan; CYP3A4 Inhibitors (Moderate); CYP3A4 Inhibitors (Strong); Dasatinib; Fosaprepitant; Fusidic Acid (Systemic); Grapefruit Juice; Idelalisib; Ivacaftor; Luliconazole; Mifepristone; Netupitant; Osimertinib; Palbociclib; P-glycoprotein/ABCB1 Inhibitors; Ranolazine; Simeprevir; Stiripentol

Decreased Effect
The levels/effects of Lapatinib may be decreased by: Bosentan; CYP3A4 Inducers (Moderate); CYP3A4 Inducers (Strong); Dabrafenib; Deferasirox; Dexamethasone (Systemic); Osimertinib; P-glycoprotein/ABCB1 Inducers; Siltuximab; St Johns Wort; Tocilizumab

◀ **Food Interactions** Systemic exposure of lapatinib is increased when administered with food (AUC three- to fourfold higher). Grapefruit juice may increase the levels/effects of lapatinib. Management: Administer once daily on an empty stomach, 1 hour before or 1 hour after a meal at the same time each day. Avoid grapefruit juice. Maintain adequate hydration, unless instructed to restrict fluid intake.

Storage/Stability Store at room temperature of 25°C (77°F); excursions permitted between 15°C and 30°C (59°F and 86°F).

Mechanism of Action Tyrosine kinase (dual kinase) inhibitor; inhibits EGFR (ErbB1) and HER2 (ErbB2) by reversibly binding to tyrosine kinase, blocking phosphorylation and activation of downstream second messengers (Erk1/2 and Akt), regulating cellular proliferation and survival in ErbB- and ErbB2-expressing tumors. Combination therapy with lapatinib and endocrine therapy may overcome endocrine resistance occurring in HER2+ and hormone receptor positive disease.

Pharmacodynamics/Kinetics

Absorption: Incomplete and variable

Protein binding: >99% to albumin and alpha$_1$-acid glycoprotein

Metabolism: Hepatic; extensive via CYP3A4 and 3A5, and to a lesser extent via CYP2C19 and 2C8 to oxidized metabolites

Half-life elimination: ~24 hours

Time to peak, plasma: ~4 hours (Burris, 2009)

Excretion: Feces (27% as unchanged drug; range 3% to 67%); urine (<2%)

Dosing

Adult & Geriatric

Breast cancer, metastatic, HER2+ (with prior anthracycline, taxane, and trastuzumab therapy): Oral: 1250 mg once daily (in combination with capecitabine) until disease progression or unacceptable toxicity (Geyer, 2006)

Breast cancer, metastatic, HER2+, hormonal therapy indicated: Oral: 1500 mg once daily (in combination with letrozole) until disease progression (Johnston, 2009)

Breast cancer, metastatic, HER2+ with brain metastases, first-line therapy (off-label use): Oral: 1250 mg once daily (in combination with capecitabine) until disease progression or unacceptable toxicity (Bachelot, 2013)

Breast cancer, metastatic, HER2+, with progression on prior trastuzumab therapy (off-label use): Oral: 1000 mg once daily (in combination with trastuzumab) (Blackwell, 2010; Blackwell, 2012)

Missed doses: If a dose is missed, resume with the next scheduled daily dose; do not double the dose the next day.

Dosage adjustment for concomitant CYP3A4 inhibitors/inducers:

CYP3A4 inhibitors: Avoid the use of concomitant strong CYP3A4 inhibitors. If concomitant use cannot be avoided, consider reducing lapatinib to 500 mg once daily with careful monitoring. When a strong CYP3A4 inhibitor is discontinued, allow ~1 week to elapse prior to adjusting the lapatinib dose upward.

CYP3A4 inducers: Avoid the use of concomitant strong CYP3A4 inducers.
  U.S. labeling: If concomitant use cannot be avoided, consider gradually titrating lapatinib from 1250 mg once daily up to 4500 mg daily (in combination with capecitabine) **or** from 1500 mg once daily up to 5500 mg daily (in combination with letrozole), based on tolerability and

with careful monitoring. If the strong CYP3A4 enzyme inducer is discontinued, reduce the lapatinib dose to the indicated dose.

Canadian labeling: If concomitant use cannot be avoided, titrate lapatinib dose gradually upward based on tolerability. If the strong CYP3A4 enzyme inducer is discontinued, reduce the lapatinib dose over 2 weeks.

Renal Impairment There are no dosage adjustments provided in the manufacturer's labeling (has not been studied); however, due to the minimal renal elimination (<2%), dosage adjustments may not be necessary.

Hepatic Impairment

Mild or moderate preexisting impairment (Child-Pugh class A or B): There are no dosage adjustments provided in the manufacturer's labeling.

Severe preexisting impairment (Child-Pugh class C):

US labeling: The following adjustments should be considered (and are predicted to normalize the AUC), however, there are no clinical data associated with the adjustments.

In combination with capecitabine: Reduce dose from 1250 mg once daily to 750 mg once daily.

In combination with letrozole: Reduce dose from 1500 mg once daily to 1000 mg once daily.

Canadian labeling: There are no specific dosage adjustments provided in the manufacturer's labeling; however, a dosage reduction is recommended based on pharmacokinetic modeling (safety and efficacy of dose reduction has not been demonstrated).

Severe hepatotoxicity during treatment: Discontinue permanently (do not rechallenge).

Adjustment for Toxicity

Cardiac toxicity: Discontinue treatment for at least 2 weeks for LVEF < LLN or decreased LVEF ≥ grade 2 (U.S. labeling) or decreased LVEF ≥ grade 3 (Canadian labeling); may be restarted at 1000 mg once daily (in combination with capecitabine) **or** 1250 mg once daily (in combination with letrozole) if LVEF recovers to normal and patient is asymptomatic.

Dermatologic toxicity: Discontinue treatment for suspected erythema multiforme, Stevens-Johnson syndrome, or toxic epidermal necrolysis.

Diarrhea:

Grade 3 diarrhea or grade 1 or 2 diarrhea with complicating features (moderate-to-severe abdominal cramping, grade 2 or higher nausea/vomiting, decreased performance status, fever, sepsis, neutropenia, frank bleeding, or dehydration):

U.S. labeling: Interrupt treatment; may restart at a reduced dose (from 1500 mg once daily to 1250 mg once daily or from 1250 mg once daily to 1000 mg once daily) when diarrhea resolves to ≤ grade 1.

Canadian labeling: Interrupt treatment; may restart at a reduced dose (from 1500 mg once daily to 1250 mg once daily or from 1250 mg once daily to 1000 mg once daily or from 1000 mg once daily to 750 mg once daily) when diarrhea resolves to ≤ grade 1.

Grade 4 diarrhea: Permanently discontinue.

Pulmonary toxicity: Discontinue treatment with pulmonary symptoms indicative of interstitial lung disease or pneumonitis which are ≥ grade 3

Other toxicities: Withhold for any toxicity (other than cardiac) ≥ grade 2 until toxicity resolves to ≤ grade 1 and reinitiate at the standard dose of 1250 or 1500 mg once daily; for persistent toxicity, reduce dosage to 1000 mg once daily (in combination with capecitabine) **or** 1250 mg once daily (in combination with letrozole)

Combination Regimens

Breast cancer:
Capecitabine + Lapatinib (Breast) on page 1858
Lapatinib-Letrozole (Breast) on page 2025
Lapatinib-Trastuzumab (Breast) on page 2025

Administration Administer once daily, on an empty stomach, 1 hour before or 1 hour after a meal. Take full dose at the same time each day; dividing dose throughout the day is not recommended.

Note: For combination treatment with capecitabine, capecitabine should be administered in 2 doses (approximately 12 hours apart) and taken with food or within 30 minutes after a meal.

Hazardous agent; use appropriate precautions for handling and disposal (meets NIOSH 2014 criteria).

Emetic Potential

Children: Minimal (<10%)
Adults: Low (10% to 30%)

Monitoring Parameters LVEF (baseline and periodic), CBC with differential, liver function tests, including transaminases, bilirubin, and alkaline phosphatase (baseline and every 4-6 weeks during treatment); electrolytes including calcium, potassium, magnesium; monitor for fluid retention; ECG monitoring if at risk for QTc prolongation; symptoms of ILD or pneumonitis; monitor for diarrhea and dermatologic toxicity

Dietary Considerations Avoid grapefruit juice.

Prescribing and Access Restrictions Lapatinib is available through specialty pharmacies only. Information is available at www.gskcta.com or 1-866-265-6491.

Dosage Forms Excipient information presented when available (limited, particularly for generics); consult specific product labeling.

Tablet, Oral:
Tykerb: 250 mg [contains fd&c yellow #6 (sunset yellow), fd&c yellow #6 aluminum lake]

◆ **Lapatinib Ditosylate** *see* Lapatinib *on page 997*

◆ **L-ASP** *see* Asparaginase (*E. coli*) *on page 144*

◆ **L-asparaginase (*E. coli*)** *see* Asparaginase (*E. coli*) *on page 144*

◆ **L-asparaginase (*Erwinia*)** *see* Asparaginase (*Erwinia*) *on page 150*

◆ **L-asparaginase with Polyethylene Glycol** *see* Pegaspargase *on page 1341*

◆ **Lazanda** *see* FentaNYL *on page 692*

◆ **LBH589** *see* Panobinostat *on page 1322*

◆ **LDE225** *see* Sonidegib *on page 1543*

◆ **LDK378** *see* Ceritinib *on page 305*

◆ **LDP-341** *see* Bortezomib *on page 223*

◆ **Lederle Leucovorin (Can)** *see* Leucovorin Calcium *on page 1023*

◆ **Lemtrada** *see* Alemtuzumab *on page 62*

Lenalidomide (le na LID oh mide)

Related Information

Chemotherapy and Cancer Treatment During Pregnancy *on page 2214*

Common Toxicity Criteria *on page 2122*

Management of Chemotherapy-Induced Nausea and Vomiting in Adults *on page 2142*

Prevention of Chemotherapy-Induced Nausea and Vomiting in Children *on page 2203*

Principles of Anticancer Therapy *on page 2261*

Safe Handling of Hazardous Drugs *on page 2292*

Brand Names: US Revlimid

Brand Names: Canada Revlimid

Index Terms CC-5013; IMid-1

Pharmacologic Category Angiogenesis Inhibitor; Antineoplastic Agent; Immunomodulator, Systemic

Use

US labeling:

Mantle cell lymphoma: Treatment of patients with mantle cell lymphoma that has relapsed or progressed after 2 prior therapies (one of which included bortezomib).

Multiple myeloma: Treatment of multiple myeloma (in combination with dexamethasone)

Myelodysplastic syndromes: Treatment of patients with transfusion-dependent anemia due to low- or intermediate-1-risk myelodysplastic syndromes (MDS) associated with a deletion 5q (del 5q) cytogenetic abnormality with or without additional cytogenetic abnormalities

Canadian labeling:

Multiple myeloma: Treatment of multiple myeloma (in combination with dexamethasone) in patients who have received at least one prior therapy

Myelodysplastic syndromes: Treatment of patients with transfusion-dependent anemia due to low- or intermediate-1-risk myelodysplastic syndromes (MDS) associated with a deletion 5q (del 5q) cytogenetic abnormality with or without additional cytogenetic abnormalities

Limitations of use: In the US and in Canada, lenalidomide is not indicated and is not recommended for the treatment of chronic lymphocytic leukemia (CLL) outside of controlled clinical trials.

Labeled Contraindications

Hypersensitivity (eg, angioedema, Stevens-Johnson syndrome, toxic epidermal necrolysis) to lenalidomide or any component of the formulation; pregnancy

Canadian labeling: Additional contraindications (not in US labeling): Platelet count <50,000/mm³ (in MDS patients); hypersensitivity to thalidomide or pomalidomide; women capable of becoming pregnant; breast-feeding women; male patients unable to follow or comply with required contraceptive measures

Pregnancy Considerations [US Boxed Warning]: Lenalidomide is an analogue of thalidomide (a human teratogen) and could potentially cause severe birth defects or embryo-fetal death; do not use during pregnancy (contraindication); avoid pregnancy while taking lenalidomide. Obtain 2 negative pregnancy tests prior to initiation of treatment; 2 forms of contraception (or abstain from heterosexual intercourse) must be used at least 4 weeks prior to, during, and for 4 weeks after lenalidomide

◄ **treatment (and during treatment interruptions). In order to decrease the risk of embryo-fetal exposure, lenalidomide is available only through a restricted distribution program (Revlimid REMS).** Animal reproduction studies with lenalidomide in nonhuman primates have demonstrated malformations similar to those observed in humans with thalidomide.

Women of childbearing potential should be treated only if they are able to comply with the conditions of the Revlimid REMS program. Women of reproductive potential must avoid pregnancy 4 weeks prior to therapy, during therapy, during therapy interruptions, and for ≥4 weeks after therapy is discontinued. Two forms of effective contraception (eg, tubal ligation, IUD, hormonal birth control methods, male latex or synthetic condom, diaphragm, or cervical cap) or total abstinence from heterosexual intercourse must be used by females who are not infertile or who have not had a hysterectomy. A negative pregnancy test (sensitivity of at least 50 milliunits/mL) 10 to 14 days prior to therapy, within 24 hours prior to beginning therapy, weekly during the first 4 weeks, and every 4 weeks (every 2 weeks for women with irregular menstrual cycles) thereafter is required for women of childbearing potential. Lenalidomide must be immediately discontinued for a missed period, abnormal pregnancy test or abnormal menstrual bleeding; refer patient to a reproductive toxicity specialist if pregnancy occurs during treatment.

Lenalidomide is also present in the semen of males. Males (including those vasectomized) should use a latex or synthetic condom during any sexual contact with women of childbearing age during treatment, during treatment interruptions, and for 4 weeks after discontinuation. Male patients should not donate sperm during, and for 4 weeks after treatment, and during therapy interruptions.

The parent or legal guardian for patients between 12 and 18 years of age must agree to ensure compliance with the required guidelines. Any suspected fetal exposure should be reported to the FDA via the MedWatch program (1-800-FDA-1088) and to Celgene Corporation (1-888-423-5436).

Breast-Feeding Considerations It is not known if lenalidomide is excreted in breast milk. Due to the potential for serious adverse reactions in the infant, a decision should be made to discontinue nursing or discontinue treatment. Use in breast-feeding women is contraindicated in the Canadian labeling.

Warnings/Precautions Hazardous agent - use appropriate precautions for handling and disposal (NIOSH 2014 [group 2]).

[US Boxed Warning]: Hematologic toxicity (neutropenia and thrombocytopenia) occurs in a majority of patients (grade 3/4: 80% in patients with del 5q myelodysplastic syndrome) and may require dose reductions and/or delays; the use of blood product support and/or growth factors may be needed. CBC should be monitored weekly for the first 8 weeks and at least monthly thereafter in patients being treated for del 5q myelodysplastic syndromes. In patients being treated for multiple myeloma, monitor CBC weekly for the first 2 cycles, every 2 weeks during cycle 3, and monthly thereafter. In patients receiving lenalidomide for mantle cell lymphoma (MCL), monitor CBC weekly for the first cycle, every 2 weeks during cycles 2 to 4, and monthly thereafter. Monitor for signs of infection, bleeding, or bruising; may require dosage adjustment. Lenalidomide use (≥4 cycles) may decrease the number of CD34+ cells collected for autologous stem cell transplant. Transplant eligible patients receiving lenalidomide should be referred to an appropriate transplant center in order to optimize the timing of stem cell collection.

Cyclophosphamide in combination with G-CSF or G-CSF in combination with a CXC chemokine receptor 4 inhibitor (eg, plerixafor) may be considered when CD34+ cell collection is impaired. **[US Boxed Warning]: Lenalidomide has been associated with a significant increase in risk for arterial and venous thromboembolic events in multiple myeloma patients treated with lenalidomide and dexamethasone combination therapy. Deep vein thrombosis (DVT), pulmonary embolism (PE), myocardial infarction, and stroke have occurred; monitor for signs and symptoms of thromboembolism (shortness of breath, chest pain, or arm or leg swelling) and seek prompt medical attention with development of these symptoms. Thromboprophylaxis is recommended; the choice of regimen should be based on assessment of the patient's underlying risk factors.** Erythropoietin-stimulating agents (ESAs) and estrogens may contribute to thromboembolic risk; use with caution. Patients with a prior history of arterial thromboembolic events may be at greater risk; minimize modifiable factors such as hyperlipidemia, hypertension, and smoking. Anticoagulant prophylaxis should be individualized and selected based on the thromboembolism risk of the combination treatment regimen, using the safest and easiest to administer (Palumbo, 2008).

In a clinical trial comparing lenalidomide versus chlorambucil single agent therapy in patients >65 years of age with chronic lymphocytic leukemia patients (not an FDA-approved indication), increased mortality was observed in the lenalidomide treatment arm. Atrial fibrillation, cardiac failure, and MI were observed more frequently in lenalidomide-treated patients; lenalidomide (alone or in combination) is not currently recommended for first-line treatment of CLL. Second primary malignancies (SPMs), including hematologic (AML, MDS, and B-cell malignancies, including Hodgkin lymphoma) and solid tumor malignancies, and skin cancers, have been reported with lenalidomide when used for the treatment of MDS and multiple myeloma; the incidence may be higher when lenalidomide is used in combination with an alkylating agent. Monitor for development of secondary malignancies.

Angioedema, Stevens-Johnson syndrome (SJS), and toxic epidermal necrolysis (TEN) have been reported; may be fatal. Consider interrupting or discontinuing treatment with grade 2 or 3 skin rash; discontinue and do not reinitiate treatment with grade 4 rash, exfoliative or bullous rash, or for suspected SJS or TEN. Patients with a history of grade 4 rash with thalidomide should not receive lenalidomide. Discontinue treatment with angioedema. Use caution in renal impairment; may experience an increased rate of toxicities (due to reduced clearance and increased half-life); initial dosage adjustments are recommended for moderate-to-severe and dialysis-dependent renal impairment. Tumor lysis syndrome (with fatalities) has been reported with lenalidomide; patients with a high tumor burden may be at risk for tumor lysis syndrome; monitor closely; institute appropriate management for hyperuricemia. Tumor flare reaction has been observed in studies of lenalidomide for the treatment of chronic lymphocytic leukemia (CLL) and lymphoma; clinical presentation includes low grade fever, pain, rash, and tender lymph node swelling. In patients with MCL, tumor flare may mimic disease progression; monitor closely. In clinical trials, the majority of tumor flare events occurred in the first cycle of therapy. Treatment with corticosteroids, nonsteroidal anti-inflammatory drugs (NSAIDs), and/or analgesics may be considered; therapy interruption may be necessary as well. Hepatic failure, including fatalities, has occurred in patients treated with combination lenalidomide and dexamethasone therapy; may have hepatocellular, cholestatic, or mixed characteristics. Risk factors may include preexisting viral liver disease, elevated liver enzymes at baseline, and concomitant medications. Monitor closely; interrupt therapy in patients with abnormal hepatic function tests. May consider resuming treatment at a lower dose upon return to baseline. Certain adverse reactions (DVT, pulmonary embolism, atrial fibrillation, renal failure) are more likely in elderly patients. Monitor renal function closely, and select dose accordingly.

[US Boxed Warning]: Lenalidomide is an analogue of thalidomide (a human teratogen) and could potentially cause severe birth defects or embryo-fetal death; do not use during pregnancy (contraindication); avoid pregnancy while taking lenalidomide. Obtain 2 negative pregnancy testes prior to initiation of treatment; 2 forms of contraception (or abstain from heterosexual intercourse) must be used at least 4 weeks prior to, during and for 4 weeks after lenalidomide treatment (and during treatment interruptions). Distribution is restricted; physicians, pharmacies, and patients must be registered with the Revlimid REMS program. In order to decrease the risk of embryo-fetal exposure, lenalidomide is available only through a restricted distribution program (Revlimid REMS). Prescribers and pharmacies must be certified with the program to prescribe or dispense lenalidomide. Males taking lenalidomide (even those vasectomized) must use a latex or synthetic condom during any sexual contact with women of childbearing potential and for up to 28 days following discontinuation of therapy. Males taking lenalidomide must not donate sperm. Patients should be advised not to donate blood during therapy and for 1 month following completion of therapy. May cause dizziness or fatigue; caution patients about performing tasks which require mental alertness (eg, operating machinery or driving). Potentially significant drug-drug interactions may exist, requiring dose or frequency adjustment, additional monitoring, and/or selection of alternative therapy. Formulation contains lactose; avoid use in patients with Lapp lactase deficiency, glucose-galactose malabsorption, or glucose intolerance. Lenalidomide should only be prescribed to patients (male and female) who can understand and comply with the conditions of the Revlimid REMS program. If used in patients between 12 to 18 years of age, the parent or legal guardian must agree to ensure compliance with the Revlimid REMS program.

Adverse Reactions Frequency not always defined; may vary based on indication and/or concomitant therapy.

Cardiovascular: Peripheral edema (8% to 26%), edema (10%), deep vein thrombosis (4% to 10%; grades 3/4: ≤8%), hypotension (7% to 10%), hypertension (6% to 8%), chest pain (5% to 8%), atrial fibrillation (3% to 7%; grades 3/4: ≤4%), palpitations (5%), myocardial infarction (1% to <5%), pulmonary embolism (2% to 4%; grades 3/4: 1% to 4%), syncope (grades 3/4: 1% to 3%), cerebrovascular tachycardia (grades 3/4: 2%), accident (≤2%), angina pectoris (≥1%), bradycardia (≥1%), cerebral ischemia (≥1%), cardiac failure (1%), cardiac arrest, cardiogenic shock, cardiomyopathy, cardiorespiratory arrest, cerebral infarction, increased cardiac enzymes (troponin I), ischemia, ischemic heart disease, septic shock, subarachnoid hemorrhage, supraventricular cardiac arrhythmia, tachyarrhythmia, thrombophlebitis, thrombosis, transiet ischemic attachs, ventricular dysfunction

Central nervous system: Fatigue (29% to 44%), insomnia (10% to 28%), dizziness (20% to 23%), headache (10% to 20%), depression (5% to 11%), chills (5% to 10%), falling (5% to 8%), hypoesthesia (7%), lethargy (7%), pain (7%), neuropathy (including peripheral, 5% to 7%), rigors (6%), noncardiac chest pain (3% to 6%), emotional lability (≥1%), glossalgia (≥1%), hallucination (≥1%), malaise (≥1%), abnormal gait, aphasia, cerebellar infarction, confusion, dysarthria, impaired consciousness, migraine, spinal cord compression, vertigo

Dermatologic: Pruritus (4% to 42%), skin rash (19% to 36%), xeroderma (9% to 14%), diaphoresis (7% to 10%), night sweats (8%), ecchymoses (5%), erythema (5%), cellulitis (≤5%), hyperpigmentation (≥1%), Sweet's syndrome

Endocrine & metabolic: Weight loss (9% to 20%), hypokalemia (7% to 17%), hyperglycemia (4% to 12%), hypocalcemia (3% to 11%), hypothyroidism (7%), hypomagnesemia (6% to 7%), dehydration (3% to 7%), diabetes mellitus (<5%), gout (<5%), hypophosphatemia (<5%, grades 3/4: ≤3%), hyponatremia (2% to <5%), hirsutism (≥1%), loss of libido (≥1%), Graves' disease, hypernatremia, hypoglycemia

Gastrointestinal: Diarrhea (17% to 49%), constipation (16% to 41%), nausea (24% to 30%), decreased appetite (7% to 23%), abdominal pain (8% to 21%), anorexia (10% to 16%), dysgeusia (4% to 15%), vomiting (10% to 12%), dyspepsia (5% to 11%), xerostomia (7%), loose stools (6%), gastroenteritis (2% to 6%), gastrointestinal hemorrhage (≥1%), biliary obstruction, cholecystitis, colonic polyps, diverticulitis, dysphagia, gastritis, gastroesophageal reflux disease, infection of mouth, inguinal hernia (obstructive), intestinal obstruction, intestinal perforation, irritable bowel syndrome, ischemic colitis, melena

Genitourinary: Urinary tract infection (4% to 14%), dysuria (7%), erectile dysfunction (≥1%), azotemia, hematuria, pelvic pain, perirectal obscess, urolithiasis, urosepsis

Hematologic & oncologic: Thrombocytopenia (19% to 62%; grades 3/4: 8% to 50%; MDS: Onset: 28 days [range: 8 to 290 days]; recovery: 22 days [range: 5 to 224 days]), neutropenia (33% to 61%; grades 3/4: 27% to 53%; MDS: Onset: 42 days [range: 14 to 411 days]; recovery: 17 days [range: 2 to 170 days]), anemia (12% to 44%; grades 3/4: 6% to 19%), leukopenia (8% to 15%; grades 3/4: 4% to 7%), tumor flare (10%), lymphocytopenia (5% to 7%; grades 3/4: 3% to 4%), bruise (3% to 6%), febrile neutropenia (1% to 6%; grades 3/4: 1% to 6%), second primary malignant neoplasms (≤5%, including AML, lymphomas, solid tumors), squamous cell carcinoma of skin (3% to <5%; grades 3/4: ≤3%), pancytopenia (<5%; grades 3/4: ≤2%), basal cell carcinoma (<5%; grades 3/4: <1%), granulocytopenia (grades 3/4: 2%), autoimmune hemolytic anemia (≥1%), acute leukemia, blood coagulation disorder, bone marrow depression, bronchogenic carcinoma, decreased hemoglobin, hemolysis, hemolytic anemia (including warm type), lung carcinoma, malignant lymphoma, myelocytic leukemia, neutropenic infection, pancreatitis, postoperative hemorrhage, prostate carcinoma, rectal hemorrhage, splenic infarction

Hepatic: Increased serum ALT (8%), abnormal hepatic function tests (≥1%), hepatic failure, hyperbilirubinemia

Hypersensitivity: Hypersensitivity reaction, transfusion reaction

Infection: Influenza (3% to 6%), sepsis (including *Enterobacter*, 3% to 6%; grades 3/4: 2% to 5%), bacteremia (1%), bacterial infection, clostridium infection, fungal infection, herpes virus infection, kidney infection, Klebsiella infection, localized infection, pseudomonas infection, staphylococcal infection

Local: Catheter infection

▶

◀ Neuromuscular & skeletal: Muscle cramps (18% to 33%), back pain (13% to 32%), weakness (14% to 28%), arthralgia (8% to 22%), tremor (21%), muscle spasm (11% to 21%), ostealgia (1% to 16%), limb pain (5% to 15%), musculoskeletal pain (7% to 13%), musculoskeletal chest pain (7% to 11%), myalgia (9%), myasthenia (5% to 8%), neck pain (2% to 8%), arthritis, bone fracture (femur, femoral neck, pelvis, hip, rib, spinal compression), calcium pyrophosphate deposition disease

Ophthalmic: Blurred vision (17%), cataract (≤14%; grades 3/4: ≤6%), subcapsular posterior cataract (<5%), blindness (≥1%), ocular hypertension (≥1%)

Otic: Otic infection

Renal: Renal failure (4% to 10%), increased serum creatinine

Respiratory: Cough (13% to 28%), upper respiratory tract infection (6% to 25%), dyspnea (17% to 24%), nasopharyngitis (6% to 23%), pneumonia (9% to 18%), bronchitis (6% to 17%), pharyngitis (14% to 16%), epistaxis (3% to 15%), oropharyngeal pain (3% to 10%), sinusitis (7% to 8%), pleural effusion (7%; grades 3/4: 1%), dyspnea on exertion (≤7%), respiratory tract infection (4% to 7%), rhinitis (3% to 7%), lower respiratory tract infection (2% to 6%), hypoxia (2%; grades 3/4: 1%), hoarseness (≥1%), pneumonitis (grades 3/4: 1%), pulmonary hypertension (grades 3/4: 1%), respiratory distress (1%; grades 3/4: 1% to 2%), chronic obstructive pulmonary disease, interstitial pulmonary disease, pulmonary edema, pulmonary infiltrates, respiratory failure, wheezing

Miscellaneous: Fever (14% to 28%), physical health deterioration (2%), multiorgan failure (grades 3/4: 1%), mass (renal), nodule

<1%, postmarketing, and/or case reports: Angioedema, atrial flutter, catheter infection, circulatory shock, desquamation, drug overdose, erythema multiforme, Fanconi's syndrome, hematologic disease (impaired stem cell mobilization), hemorrhage, hemorrhagic diathesis, hepatitis, intracranial hemorrhage, leukoencephalopathy, myopathy, nephrolithiasis, orthostatic hypotension, peripheral ischemia, pseudomembranous colitis, pseudomonas infection, pulmonary edema, pulmonary infiltrates, rectal hemorrhage, renal tubular necrosis, Stevens-Johnson syndrome, stomatitis, toxic epidermal necrolysis, tumor lysis syndrome, urinary retention, urticaria, viral infection

Drug Interactions

Metabolism/Transport Effects Substrate of P-glycoprotein

Avoid Concomitant Use

Avoid concomitant use of Lenalidomide with any of the following: Abatacept; Anakinra; BCG (Intravesical); Canakinumab; Certolizumab Pegol; CloZAPine; Dipyrone; Natalizumab; Pimecrolimus; Rilonacept; Tacrolimus (Topical); Tocilizumab; Tofacitinib; Vaccines (Live); Vedolizumab

Increased Effect/Toxicity

Lenalidomide may increase the levels/effects of: Abatacept; Anakinra; Bisphosphonate Derivatives; Canakinumab; Certolizumab Pegol; CloZAPine; Digoxin; Fingolimod; Leflunomide; Natalizumab; Rilonacept; Tofacitinib; Vaccines (Live); Vedolizumab

The levels/effects of Lenalidomide may be increased by: Denosumab; Dexamethasone (Systemic); Dipyrone; Erythropoiesis-Stimulating Agents; Estrogen Derivatives; Pimecrolimus; Roflumilast; Tacrolimus (Topical); Tocilizumab; Trastuzumab

Decreased Effect

Lenalidomide may decrease the levels/effects of: BCG (Intravesical); Coccidioides immitis Skin Test; Sipuleucel-T; Vaccines (Inactivated); Vaccines (Live)

The levels/effects of Lenalidomide may be decreased by: Echinacea

Storage/Stability Store at 20°C to 25°C (68°F to 77°F); excursions permitted to 15°C and 30°C (59°F and 86°F).

Mechanism of Action Immunomodulatory, antiangiogenic, and antineoplastic characteristics via multiple mechanisms. Selectively inhibits secretion of proinflammatory cytokines (potent inhibitor of tumor necrosis factor-alpha secretion); enhances cell-mediated immunity by stimulating proliferation of anti-CD3 stimulated T cells (resulting in increased IL-2 and interferon gamma secretion); inhibits trophic signals to angiogenic factors in cells. Inhibits the growth of myeloma cells by inducing cell cycle arrest and cell death.

Pharmacodynamics/Kinetics

Absorption: Rapid

Protein binding: ~30%

Half-life elimination: 3 to 5 hours; Moderate to severe renal impairment: Increased threefold; Hemodialysis patients: Increased ~4.5-fold

Time, to peak, plasma: MDS or myeloma patients: 0.5 to 6 hours

Excretion: Urine (~82%; as unchanged drug)

Hemodialysis effect: ~30% of the drug in body is removed in a 4-hour hemodialysis session

Dosing

Adult

Mantle cell lymphoma (MCL): Oral: 25 mg once daily for 21 days of a 28-day treatment cycle; continue until disease progression or unacceptable toxicity

Multiple myeloma: Oral: 25 mg once daily for 21 days of a 28-day treatment cycle (in combination with dexamethasone). In patients not eligible for autologous stem cell transplantation, continue until disease progression or unacceptable toxicity; in transplant eligible patients, hematopoietic stem cell mobilization should occur within 4 cycles.

Myelodysplastic syndrome (MDS) with deletion 5q: Oral:

US labeling: 10 mg once daily

Canadian labeling: 10 mg once daily for 21 days of 28-day treatment cycle; discontinue therapy if within 4 months of initiation, patient fails to achieve a rise in hemoglobin ≥1 g/dL (if not transfused) or ≥50% reduction in transfusion requirements.

Chronic lymphocytic leukemia (CLL), relapsed/refractory (off-label use): Oral: 10 mg once daily beginning on day 9 of cycle 1; administer continuously in combination with cyclic rituximab (Badoux, 2013)

Diffuse large B-cell lymphoma, relapsed/refractory (off-label use): Oral: 25 mg once daily for 21 days of a 28-day treatment cycle for up to 1 year (Wiernik, 2008)

Multiple myeloma, newly diagnosed (off-label combination): Oral: 25 mg once daily for 14 days of a 21-day cycle (in combination with bortezomib and dexamethasone) for 8 cycles (Kumar, 2012; Richardson, 2010)

Multiple myeloma, relapsed (off-label combination): Adults: Oral: 25 mg once daily for 21 days of 28-day cycle (in combination with carfilzomib and dexamethasone) until disease progression or unacceptable toxicity (Stewart, 2015)

◄ **Multiple myeloma, maintenance (following autologous stem cell transplant; off-label use):** Oral: 10 mg once daily for 3 months, then increased to 15 mg daily if tolerated; continue until relapse (Attal, 2012; McCarthy, 2012) **or** 10 mg once daily for 21 days of a 28-day treatment cycle until relapse (Palumbo, 2010)

Myelodysplastic syndrome (MDS), lower risk, without deletion 5q (off-label use): Oral: 10 mg once daily (Raza, 2008)

Systemic light chain amyloidosis (off-label use): Oral: 15 mg once daily for 21 days of a 28-day cycle (in combination with dexamethasone) (Nair, 2012; Sanchorawala, 2007)

Geriatric Refer to adult dosing. Due to the potential for decreased renal function in the elderly, select dose carefully and closely monitor renal function.

Renal Impairment

Recommended initial dose adjustment in the FDA-approved labeling; further individualize based on tolerance:

MCL:

CrCl >60 mL/minute: No adjustment required

CrCl 30 to 60 mL/minute: 10 mg once daily

CrCl <30 mL/minute (nondialysis dependent): 15 mg every 48 hours

ESRD: CrCl <30 mL/minute and dialysis dependent: 5 mg once daily (administer after dialysis on dialysis days)

MDS:

CrCl >60 mL/minute: No adjustment required

CrCl 30 to 60 mL/minute: 5 mg once daily

CrCl <30 mL/minute (nondialysis dependent): 2.5 mg once daily

ESRD: CrCl <30 mL/minute and dialysis dependent: 2.5 mg once daily (administer after dialysis on dialysis days)

Multiple myeloma:

CrCl >50 mL/minute: No adjustment required

CrCl 30 to 50 mL/minute: 10 mg once daily (may increase to 15 mg once daily after 2 cycles if nonresponsive but tolerating treatment; Chen, 2007)

CrCl <30 mL/minute (nondialysis dependent): 15 mg every 48 hours

ESRD: CrCl <30 mL/minute and dialysis dependent: 5 mg once daily (administer after dialysis on dialysis days)

Recommended adjustment in Canadian labeling:

MDS:

CrCl ≥60 mL/minute: No adjustment required

CrCl 30 to 59 mL/minute: 5 mg once daily

CrCl <30 mL/minute (nondialysis dependent): 5 mg every 48 hours

ESRD: CrCl <30 mL/minute and dialysis dependent: 5 mg 3 times weekly (administer after each dialysis)

Multiple myeloma:

CrCl ≥60 mL/minute: No adjustment required

CrCl 30 to 59 mL/minute: 10 mg once daily (may increase to 15 mg once daily after 2 cycles if nonresponsive but tolerating treatment; Chen, 2007)

CrCl <30 mL/minute (nondialysis dependent): 15 mg every 48 hours

ESRD: CrCl <30 mL/minute and dialysis dependent: 5 mg once daily (administer after dialysis on dialysis days)

Hepatic Impairment There are no dosage adjustments provided in the manufacturer's labeling (has not been studied). However, lenalidomide undergoes minimal hepatic metabolism.

Adjustment for Toxicity
NONHEMATOLOGIC toxicities:
Dermatologic toxicities:
Skin rash, grade 2 or 3: Consider interrupting or discontinuing treatment
Angioedema, grade 4 rash, exfoliative or bullous rash, or suspected Stevens-Johnson syndrome or toxic epidermal necrolysis: Discontinue treatment; do not rechallenge
Tumor flare reaction:
Grade 1 or 2: Continue therapy at physician's discretion; may consider symptom management with corticosteroids, nonsteroidal anti-inflammatory drugs (NSAIDs) and/or analgesic therapy.
Grade 3 or 4: Interrupt therapy until resolved to ≤ grade 1; consider symptom management with corticosteroids, nonsteroidal anti-inflammatory drugs (NSAIDs) and/or analgesic therapy.
Other toxicities: For additional treatment-related grade 3/4 toxicities, hold treatment and restart at next lower dose level when toxicity has resolved to ≤ grade 2.

HEMATOLOGIC toxicities:
Adjustment for thrombocytopenia in MCL:
Platelets <50,000/mm^3: Hold treatment, check CBC weekly
When platelets return to ≥50,000/mm^3: Resume treatment at 5 mg below previous dose; do not dose below 5 mg daily
Adjustment for neutropenia in MCL:
ANC <1000/mm^3 for at least 7 days or associated with fever (≥38.5°C [101°F]): Hold treatment, check CBC weekly
ANC <500/mm^3: Hold treatment, check CBC weekly
When ANC returns to ≥1000/mm^3: Resume treatment at 5 mg below previous dose; do not dose below 5 mg daily

Adjustment for thrombocytopenia in MDS:
Thrombocytopenia developing within 4 weeks of beginning treatment at 10 mg daily:
Baseline platelets ≥100,000/mm^3:
If platelets <50,000/mm^3: Hold treatment
When platelets return to ≥50,000/mm^3: Resume treatment at 5 mg daily
Baseline platelets <100,000/mm^3:
If platelets fall to 50% of baseline: Hold treatment
If baseline ≥60,000/mm^3 and platelet level returns to ≥50,000/mm^3: Resume at 5 mg daily
If baseline <60,000/mm^3 and platelet level returns to ≥30,000/mm^3: Resume at 5 mg daily
Thrombocytopenia developing after 4 weeks of beginning treatment at 10 mg daily:
Platelets <30,000/mm^3 **or** <50,000/mm^3 with platelet transfusions: Hold treatment
When platelets return to ≥30,000/mm^3 (without hemostatic failure): Resume at 5 mg daily
Thrombocytopenia developing with treatment at 5 mg daily:
Platelets <30,000/mm^3 **or** <50,000/mm^3 with platelet transfusions: Hold treatment
When platelets return to ≥30,000/mm^3 (without hemostatic failure):
US labeling: Resume at 2.5 mg once daily
Canadian labeling: Resume at 5 mg every other day

◀

Adjustment for neutropenia in MDS:
Neutropenia developing within 4 weeks of beginning treatment at 10 mg daily:
For baseline absolute neutrophil count (ANC) ≥1000/mm³:
ANC <750/mm³: Hold treatment
When ANC returns to ≥1000/mm³: Resume at 5 mg daily
For baseline absolute neutrophil count (ANC) <1000/mm³:
ANC <500/mm³: Hold treatment
When ANC returns to ≥500/mm³: Resume at 5 mg daily
Neutropenia developing after 4 weeks of beginning treatment at 10 mg daily:
ANC <500/mm³ for ≥7 days or associated with fever (≥38.5°C [101°F]): Hold treatment
When ANC returns to ≥500/mm³: Resume at 5 mg daily
Neutropenia developing with treatment at 5 mg daily:
ANC <500/mm³ for ≥7 days or associated with fever (≥38.5°C [101°F]): Hold treatment
When ANC returns to ≥500/mm³:
US labeling: Resume at 2.5 mg once daily
Canadian labeling: Resume at 5 mg every other day

Adjustment for thrombocytopenia in multiple myeloma:
US labeling:
Platelets <30,000/mm³: Hold treatment, check CBC weekly
When platelets return to ≥30,000/mm³: Resume at next lower dose; do not dose below 2.5 mg daily
Additional occurrence of platelets <30,000/mm³: Hold treatment
When platelets return to ≥30,000/mm³: Resume treatment at next lower dose; do not dose below 2.5 mg daily
Canadian labeling:
Platelets <30,000/mm³: Hold treatment, check CBC weekly
When platelets return to ≥30,000/mm³: Resume at 15 mg daily
Additional occurrence of platelets <30,000/mm³: Hold treatment
When platelets return to ≥30,000/mm³: Resume treatment at 5 mg less than previous dose; do not dose below 5 mg daily

Adjustment for neutropenia in multiple myeloma:
US labeling:
ANC <1000/mm³: Hold treatment, check CBC weekly
When ANC returns to ≥1000/mm³ (with neutropenia as only toxicity): Resume at 25 mg daily or initial starting dose
When ANC returns to ≥1000/mm³ (with additional toxicities): Resume at next lower dose; do not dose below 2.5 mg daily
Additional occurrence of ANC <1000/mm³: Hold treatment
When ANC returns to ≥1000/mm³: Resume treatment at next lower dose; do not dose below 2.5 mg daily
Canadian labeling:
ANC <1,000/mm³: Hold treatment, initiate granulocyte-colony stimulating factor (G-CSF), check CBC weekly
When ANC returns to ≥1,000/mm³ (with neutropenia as only toxicity): Resume at 25 mg daily
When ANC returns to ≥1,000/mm³ (with additional toxicities): Resume at 15 mg daily
Additional occurrence of ANC <1,000/mm³: Hold treatment

When ANC returns to ≥1,000/mm^3: Resume treatment at 5 mg less than previous dose; do not dose below 5 mg daily

Combination Regimens

Leukemia, chronic lymphocytic: Lenalidomide-Rituximab (CLL) on page 2029

Lymphoma, non-Hodgkin (DLBCL): Lenalidomide (NHL-DLBCL Regimen) on page 2029

Lymphoma, non-Hodgkin: (Mantle Cell): Lenalidomide (NHL-Mantle Cell Regimen) on page 2029

Multiple myeloma:

Bendamustine-Lenalidomide-Dexamethasone (Multiple Myeloma) on page 1834

Carfilzomib, Lenalidomide, Dexamethasone (Multiple Myeloma) on page 1875

Lenalidomide-Bortezomib-Dexamethasone (Multiple Myeloma) on page 2026

Lenalidomide-Dexamethasone (Multiple Myeloma) on page 2028

Administration Administer at about the same time each day with water; administer with or without food. Swallow capsule whole; do not break, open, or chew.

Missed doses: May administer a missed dose if within 12 hours of usual dosing time. If greater than 12 hours, patient should skip dose for that day and resume usual dosing the following day. Patient should **not** take 2 doses to make up for a missed dose.

Hazardous agent; use appropriate precautions for handling and disposal (NIOSH 2014 [group 2]).

Emetic Potential

Children: Minimal (<10%)

Adults: Low (10% to 30%)

Monitoring Parameters

CBC with differential (MCL - weekly for the first cycle, every 2 weeks during cycles 2 to 4; MDS - weekly for first 8 weeks; Multiple myeloma - weekly for the first 2 cycles, every 2 weeks during the third cycle), then monthly thereafter; serum creatinine, liver function tests, thyroid function tests (TSH at baseline then every 2 to 3 months during lenalidomide treatment [Hamnvik, 2011]); ECG when clinically indicated; monitor for signs and symptoms of infection (if neutropenic), secondary malignancies, thromboembolism, tumor lysis syndrome, or tumor flare reaction

Women of childbearing potential: Pregnancy test 10 to 14 days **and** 24 hours prior to initiating therapy, weekly during the first 4 weeks of treatment, then every 2 to 4 weeks through 4 weeks after therapy discontinued

Prescribing and Access Restrictions As a requirement of the REMS program, access to this medication is restricted. Lenalidomide is approved for marketing in the US only under a Food and Drug Administration (FDA) approved, restricted distribution program called Revlimid REMS (https://www.celgeneriskmanagement.com or 1-888-423-5436). Prescribers and pharmacies must be certified with the program to prescribe or dispense lenalidomide; patients must comply with the program requirements. No more than a 4-week supply should be dispensed. Prescriptions must be filled within 7 days (for females of reproductive potential) or within 30 days (for all other patients) after authorization number obtained. Subsequent prescriptions may be filled only if fewer than 7 days of therapy remain on the previous prescription. A new prescription is required for further dispensing (a telephone prescription may not

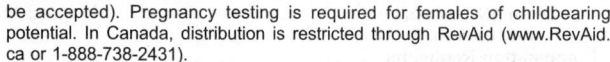

be accepted). Pregnancy testing is required for females of childbearing potential. In Canada, distribution is restricted through RevAid (www.RevAid. ca or 1-888-738-2431).

Medication Guide Available Yes

Dosage Forms Excipient information presented when available (limited, particularly for generics); consult specific product labeling.

Capsule, Oral:

Revlimid: 2.5 mg [contains fd&c blue #2 (indigotine)]

Revlimid: 5 mg

Revlimid: 10 mg, 15 mg, 20 mg [contains fd&c blue #2 (indigotine)]

Revlimid: 25 mg

Lenvatinib (len VA ti nib)

Related Information

Common Toxicity Criteria *on page 2122*

Management of Chemotherapy-Induced Nausea and Vomiting in Adults *on page 2142*

Principles of Anticancer Therapy *on page 2261*

Safe Handling of Hazardous Drugs *on page 2292*

Brand Names: US Lenvima 10 MG Daily Dose; Lenvima 14 MG Daily Dose; Lenvima 20 MG Daily Dose; Lenvima 24 MG Daily Dose

Index Terms E7080; Lenvatinib Mesylate

Pharmacologic Category Antineoplastic Agent, Tyrosine Kinase Inhibitor; Antineoplastic Agent, Vascular Endothelial Growth Factor (VEGF) Inhibitor

Use Thyroid cancer, differentiated: Treatment of locally recurrent or metastatic, progressive, radioactive iodine-refractory differentiated thyroid cancer (DTC)

Labeled Contraindications There are no contraindications listed in the manufacturer's labeling.

Pregnancy Considerations Adverse events were observed in animal reproduction studies. Based on the mechanism of action, lenvatinib may cause fetal harm if administered in pregnancy. Females of reproductive potential should use effective contraception during lenvatinib treatment and for at least 2 weeks after completion of therapy.

Breast-Feeding Considerations It is not known if lenvatinib is excreted into breast milk. The manufacturer recommends that breast-feeding be discontinued during therapy.

Warnings/Precautions Hazardous agent - use appropriate precautions for handling and disposal (meets NIOSH 2014 criteria). Hypertension, including grade 3 and 4 toxicity, occurred in ~75% of patients treated with lenvatinib in a clinical trial; the median time to onset of new or worsening hypertension was 16 days. Blood pressure should be controlled prior to initiating therapy; monitor frequently throughout treatment. Other cardiac events such as decreased left or right ventricular function, cardiac failure, or pulmonary edema were also reported. Decreased ejection fraction (EF) was the most commonly reported of these events; some patients experienced greater than 20% EF reduction. Monitor for signs/symptoms of cardiac decompensation. QT/QTc prolongation was also observed in lenvatinib-treated patients. Monitor and correct electrolyte abnormalities in all patients; obtain electrocardiograms in patients with congenital long QT syndrome, heart failure, bradyarrhythmias, or in those on concomitant medications known to prolong the QT interval. Cardiac effects may require therapy interruption, dosage reduction, or discontinuation. An increased incidence of hypocalcemia (including grade 3 events) was observed in lenvatinib-treated patients compared to the placebo group in a clinical trial. Calcium replacement therapy and dosage interruption or reduction generally corrected hypocalcemia. Monitor serum calcium levels at least monthly; replace calcium as necessary. May require therapy interruption or dosage reduction. Arterial thromboembolic events, including grade 3 events, have been reported. Discontinue treatment if arterial thrombosis occurs; the safety of resuming therapy after such an event has not been established. Lenvatinib has not been studied in patients who have had an arterial thromboembolic event within the preceding 6 months. Hemorrhagic events (most frequently epistaxis) occurred in over one-third of lenvatinib-treated patients. Monitor; may require therapy interruption, dosage reduction, or discontinuation.

Lenvatinib impairs exogenous thyroid suppression. In patients with a normal thyroid stimulating hormone (TSH) level at baseline, TSH elevations were observed in over half of lenvatinib-treated patients. Monitor TSH levels monthly; adjust thyroid hormone therapy as clinically necessary. Gastrointestinal perforation or fistula formation were reported in a small percentage of patients in a clinical trial. Discontinue use in patients who develop perforation or life-threatening fistula. Lenvatinib is associated with a moderate emetic potential; antiemetics are recommended to prevent nausea and vomiting. Nausea, vomiting, and diarrhea were commonly observed. Initiate appropriate management prior to therapy interruption or dosage reduction. Monitor closely; dehydration or hypovolemia due to diarrhea and vomiting are risk factors for renal toxicity. Reversible posterior leukoencephalopathy syndrome (RPLS) has occurred (rarely). If RPLS diagnosis is confirmed through MRI, interrupt treatment until fully resolved. Therapy may resume at a reduced dose or be discontinued, depending on the severity and persistence of neurologic symptoms. Palmar-plantar erythrodysesthesia (usually grades 1 to 2) was observed in nearly one-third of patients receiving lenvatinib.

Elevations in transaminases (including grade 3 or greater events) were observed. Hepatic failure (some fatal), as well as acute hepatitis have occurred rarely. Monitor liver function tests at baseline and throughout therapy. May require therapy interruption, dosage reduction, or discontinuation. If hepatic failure occurs, discontinue treatment. Proteinuria (including grade 3 toxicity) was commonly observed. Monitor for proteinuria at baseline and throughout therapy. If urine dipstick for proteinuria is 2+, obtain a 24-hour urine protein. If proteinuria ≥2 g/24 hours develops, withhold therapy and resume at a reduced dose when proteinuria is <2 g/24 hours. Discontinue for nephrotic syndrome. Renal impairment may also occur (may be grade 3 or higher); a primary risk factor for severe renal impairment is dehydration or hypovolemia due to diarrhea and vomiting. Monitor renal function throughout treatment; may require therapy interruption, dosage reduction, or discontinuation. Potentially significant drug-drug interactions may exist, requiring dose or frequency adjustment, additional monitoring, and/or selection of alternative therapy.

Adverse Reactions

>10%:

Cardiovascular: Hypertension (73%; grades 3/4: ≤44%), peripheral edema (21%; grades 3/4: <1%)

Central nervous system: Fatigue (67%; grades 3/4: 11%), headache (38%; grades 3/4: 3%), voice disorder (31%; grades 3/4: 1%), mouth pain (25%; grades 3/4: 1%), dizziness (15%; grades 3/4: <1%), insomnia (12%)

Dermatologic: Palmar-plantar erythrodysesthesia (32%; grades 3/4: 3%), skin rash (21%; grades 3/4: <1%), alopecia (12%)

◀

Endocrine & metabolic: Increased thyroid stimulating hormone level (57%), weight loss (51%; grades 3/4: 13%)

Hematologic & oncologic: Hemorrhage (35%)

Gastrointestinal: Diarrhea (67%; grades 3/4: 9%), decreased appetite (54%; grades 3/4: 7%), nausea (47%; grades 3/4: 2%), stomatitis (41%; grades 3/4: 5%), vomiting (36%; grades 3/4: 2%), abdominal pain (31%; grades 3/4: 2%), constipation (29%), dysgeusia (18%), xerostomia (17%; grades 3/4: <1%), dyspepsia (13%; grades 3/4: <1%), infection of mouth (10%; grades 3/4: 1%)

Genitourinary: Proteinuria (34%; grade 3: 11%), urinary tract infection (11%; grades 3/4: 1%)

Neuromuscular & skeletal: Arthralgia (≤62%; grades 3/4: ≤5%), myalgia (≤62%; grades 3/4: ≤5%)

Renal: Renal insufficiency (14%; grade 3 or higher: 3%)

Respiratory: Cough (24%), epistaxis (12%)

1% to 10%:

Cardiovascular: Hypotension (9%; grades 3/4: 2%), prolonged Q-T interval on ECG (9%; grades 3/4: 2%), thromboembolic complications (5%; grade 3 or higher: 3%; arterial events), pulmonary embolism (3%), reduced ejection fraction (2%; ejection fraction reduced by >20%)

Dermatologic: Hyperkeratosis (7%)

Endocrine & metabolic: Dehydration (9%; grades 3/4: 2%), hypocalcemia (grades 3/4: 9%), hypokalemia (grades 3/4: 6%), hypercalcemia (>5%), hypercholesterolemia (>5%), hyperkalemia (>5%), hypoalbuminemia (>5%), hypoglycemia (>5%), hypomagnesemia (>5%)

Gastrointestinal: Increased serum amylase (>5%), increased serum lipase (grades 3/4: 4%), gastrointestinal fistula (2%)

Hematologic & oncologic: Decreased platelet count (grades 3/4: 2%)

Hepatic: Hyperbilirubinemia (>5%), increased serum alkaline phosphatase (>5%), increased serum AST (grades 3 or higher: 5%), increased serum ALT (grades 3 or higher: 4%)

Renal: Increased serum creatinine (grades 3/4: 3%)

Respiratory: Pulmonary edema (7%; grade 3 or higher: 2%)

<1%, postmarketing, and/or case reports: Reversible posterior leukoencephalopathy syndrome

Drug Interactions

Metabolism/Transport Effects Substrate of BCRP, CYP3A4 (minor), P-glycoprotein; **Note:** Assignment of Major/Minor substrate status based on clinically relevant drug interaction potential; **Inhibits** BSEP, OAT1, OAT3, OCT1, OCT2, SLCO1B1, UGT1A1, UGT1A4

Avoid Concomitant Use

Avoid concomitant use of Lenvatinib with any of the following: Highest Risk QTc-Prolonging Agents; Irinotecan Products; Ivabradine; Mifepristone

Increased Effect/Toxicity

Lenvatinib may increase the levels/effects of: Highest Risk QTc-Prolonging Agents; Irinotecan Products; Moderate Risk QTc-Prolonging Agents

The levels/effects of Lenvatinib may be increased by: Ivabradine; Mifepristone; QTc-Prolonging Agents (Indeterminate Risk and Risk Modifying)

Decreased Effect There are no known significant interactions involving a decrease in effect.

Storage/Stability Store at 25°C (77°F); excursions are permitted between 15°C and 30°C (59°F and 86°F).

Mechanism of Action Lenvatinib is a multitargeted tyrosine kinase inhibitor of vascular endothelial growth factor (VEGF) receptors VEGFR1 (FLT1), VEGFR2 (KDR), VEGFR3 (FLT4), fibroblast growth factor (FGF) receptors FGFR1, 2, 3, and 4, platelet derived growth factor receptor alpha (PDGFRα), KIT, and RET. Inhibition of these receptor tyrosine kinases leads to decreased tumor growth and slowing of cancer progression.

Pharmacodynamics/Kinetics

Protein binding: 98% to 99%

Metabolism: Primarily enzymatic through CYP3A and aldehyde oxidase; non-enzymatic metabolism also occurs

Half-life elimination: ~28 hours

Time to peak: 1 to 4 hours

Excretion: Feces (~64%); urine (~25%)

Dosing

Adult & Geriatric Note: Lenvatinib is associated with a moderate emetic potential; antiemetics are recommended to prevent nausea and vomiting.

Thyroid cancer, differentiated: Oral: 24 mg once daily until disease progression or unacceptable toxicity (Schlumberger, 2015)

Missed doses: Do not take a missed dose within 12 hours of the next dose (if within 12 hours, skip the missed dose and return to regular administration time).

Renal Impairment

Preexisting renal impairment:

Mild or moderate impairment (CrCl ≥30 mL/minute): No dosage adjustment necessary.

Severe impairment (CrCl <30 mL/minute): 14 mg once daily

End-stage renal disease (ESRD): There are no dosage adjustments provided in the manufacturer's labeling (has not been studied).

Renal toxicity during treatment: Interrupt therapy if grade 3 or 4 renal failure or impairment develops. When improved to ≤ grade 1 or baseline, may either resume at a reduced dose or discontinue, depending on severity and persistence of toxicity.

Hepatic Impairment

Preexisting hepatic impairment:

Mild or moderate impairment (Child-Pugh class A or B): No dosage adjustment necessary.

Severe impairment (Child-Pugh class C): 14 mg once daily

Hepatotoxicity during treatment: Interrupt therapy if grade 3 or 4 hepatotoxicity develops. When improved to ≤ grade 1 or baseline, may either resume at a reduced dose or discontinue, depending on severity and persistence of toxicity. Discontinue for hepatic failure.

Adjustment for Toxicity

Recommended dose modifications for persistent and intolerable grade 2 or grade 3 adverse reactions or grade 4 laboratory abnormalities:

First occurrence: Interrupt therapy until resolved to ≤ grade 1 or baseline, then resume dosing at 20 mg once daily

Second occurrence (same or different toxicity): Interrupt therapy until resolved to ≤ grade 1 or baseline, then resume dosing at 14 mg once daily

Third occurrence (same or different toxicity): Interrupt therapy until resolved to ≤ grade 1 or baseline, then resume dosing at 10 mg once daily

Note: There are currently no recommendations for resuming therapy in patients who experience grade 4 clinical adverse reactions that resolve.

Arterial thrombotic event: Discontinue therapy.

◄ **Cardiac:**

Cardiac dysfunction: Temporarily interrupt therapy for a grade 3 event until improved to ≤ grade 1 or baseline; depending on severity and persistence of toxicity, may either resume therapy at a reduced dose or discontinue treatment. Discontinue for a grade 4 event.

Hypertension: Monitor blood pressure prior to and throughout therapy; initiate or adjust antihypertensive medication to control blood pressure. Temporarily interrupt therapy for grade 3 hypertension that persists despite optimal medical management. When hypertension is ≤ grade 2, resume therapy at a reduced dose. Discontinue therapy for life-threatening hypertension.

QT prolongation: Temporarily interrupt therapy for ≥ grade 3 QT prolongation. When improved to ≤ grade 1 or baseline, resume therapy at a reduced dose.

Gastrointestinal toxicity:

Nausea, vomiting, or diarrhea: Initiate medical management prior to interrupting dose or reducing therapy.

Perforation or fistula formation: Discontinue in patients who develop gastrointestinal perforation or life-threatening fistula.

Hemorrhage: Temporarily interrupt therapy for a grade 3 event until improved to ≤ grade 1 or baseline; depending on severity and persistence of toxicity, may either resume therapy at a reduced dose or discontinue treatment. Discontinue for a grade 4 event.

Hypocalcemia: Administer calcium replacement therapy as necessary; may require treatment interruption or dose reduction depending on the severity, presence of ECG changes, and persistence of hypocalcemia.

Nephrotic syndrome: Discontinue therapy.

Proteinuria: Temporarily interrupt therapy for ≥2 g proteinuria/24 hours; resume therapy at a reduced dose when improved to <2 g proteinuria/24 hours.

Reversible posterior leukoencephalopathy syndrome (RPLS): Interrupt therapy until fully resolved; depending on severity and persistence of neurologic symptoms, may either resume therapy at a reduced dose when resolved or discontinue treatment.

Combination Regimens

Thyroid cancer: Lenvatinib (Thyroid Regimen) on page 2030

Administration

Lenvatinib is associated with a moderate emetic potential; antiemetics are recommended to prevent nausea and vomiting.

Administer orally at the same time each day; may be taken without regards to meals. Hazardous agent; use appropriate precautions for handling and disposal (meets NIOSH 2014 criteria).

Emetic Potential Moderate (30% to 90%)

Monitoring Parameters Liver function tests (at baseline, every 2 weeks for 2 months, and at least monthly thereafter); renal function; electrolytes; serum calcium at least monthly; TSH levels at baseline and monthly or as clinically indicated; monitor for proteinuria at baseline and periodically during treatment (urine dipstick; if 2+ then 24-hour urine protein); monitor blood pressure after 1 week, then every 2 weeks for 2 months, and at least monthly thereafter; electrocardiogram in select patients; monitor for signs/symptoms of cardiac decompensation, arterial thrombosis, reversible posterior leukoencephalopathy syndrome, signs/symptoms of gastrointestinal perforation/fistula, and hemorrhagic events

Prescribing and Access Restrictions Lenvatinib is available only through specialty pharmacies. For further information on patient assistance, product availability, and prescribing instructions, please refer to the following website: http://www.lenvima.com/hcp/pharmacy-financial-options

Dosage Forms Considerations Each Lenvima Therapy Pack contains a 30 day supply of dosage units

Dosage Forms Excipient information presented when available (limited, particularly for generics); consult specific product labeling.

Capsule Therapy Pack, Oral:
Lenvima 10 MG Daily Dose: 10 mg (5 ea, 30 ea)
Lenvima 14 MG Daily Dose: 10 mg & 4 mg (10 ea, 60 ea)
Lenvima 20 MG Daily Dose: 2x10 mg (10 ea, 60 ea)
Lenvima 24 MG Daily Dose: 2x10 mg & 4 mg (15 ea, 90 ea)

◆ **Lenvatinib Mesylate** see Lenvatinib on page 1014
◆ **Lenvima 10 MG Daily Dose** see Lenvatinib on page 1014
◆ **Lenvima 14 MG Daily Dose** see Lenvatinib on page 1014
◆ **Lenvima 20 MG Daily Dose** see Lenvatinib on page 1014
◆ **Lenvima 24 MG Daily Dose** see Lenvatinib on page 1014

Letrozole (LET roe zole)

Related Information
Safe Handling of Hazardous Drugs on page 2292

Brand Names: US Femara

Brand Names: Canada ACH-Letrozole; Apo-Letrozole; Auro-Letrozole; Bio-Letrozole; Femara; JAMP-Letrozole; Mar-Letrozole; MED-Letrozole; Myl-Letrozole; Nat-Letrozole; PMS-Letrozole; RAN-Letrozole; Riva-Letrozole; Sandoz-Letrozole; Teva-Letrozole; Van-Letrozole; Zinda-Letrozole

Index Terms CGS-20267

Pharmacologic Category Antineoplastic Agent, Aromatase Inhibitor

Use Breast cancer in postmenopausal women: Adjuvant treatment of hormone receptor-positive early breast cancer, extended adjuvant treatment of early breast cancer after 5 years of tamoxifen; treatment of advanced breast cancer with disease progression following antiestrogen therapy; first-line treatment of hormone receptor–positive or hormone receptor-unknown, locally-advanced, or metastatic breast cancer

Labeled Contraindications Use in women who are or may become pregnant

Canadian labeling: Additional contraindications (not in U.S. labeling): Hypersensitivity to letrozole, other aromatase inhibitors, or any component of the formulation; use in patients <18 years of age; breast-feeding

Pregnancy Considerations Adverse events were observed in animal reproduction studies. Letrozole is FDA approved for postmenopausal women only (no clinical benefit for breast cancer has been demonstrated in premenopausal women). Use in women who are or who may become pregnant is contraindicated. Women who are perimenopausal or recently postmenopausal should use adequate contraception until postmenopausal status is fully established.

Breast-Feeding Considerations It is not known if letrozole is excreted in breast milk. Due to the potential for serious adverse reactions in the nursing infant, a decision should be made whether to discontinue nursing or to ▶

discontinue the drug, taking into account the importance of treatment to the mother. Use in nursing women is contraindicated in the Canadian labeling.

Warnings/Precautions Hazardous agent - use appropriate precautions for handling and disposal (NIOSH 2014 [group 1]). Not generally indicated for known hormone-receptor negative disease. Use caution with hepatic impairment; dose adjustment recommended in patients with cirrhosis or severe hepatic dysfunction. May cause dizziness, fatigue, and somnolence; patients should be cautioned before performing tasks which require mental alertness (eg, operating machinery or driving). May increase total serum cholesterol; in patients treated with adjuvant therapy and cholesterol levels within normal limits, an increase of ≥1.5 x ULN in total cholesterol has been demonstrated in 8.2% of letrozole-treated patients (25% requiring lipid-lowering medications) vs 3.2% of tamoxifen-treated patients (16% requiring medications); monitor cholesterol panel; may require antihyperlipidemics. May cause decreases in bone mineral density (BMD); a decrease in hip BMD by 3.8% from baseline in letrozole-treated patients vs 2% in placebo at 2 years has been demonstrated; however, there was no statistical difference in changes to the lumbar spine BMD scores; monitor BMD. Potentially significant drug-drug interactions may exist, requiring dose or frequency adjustment, additional monitoring, and/or selection of alternative therapy.

Adverse Reactions

>10%:

Cardiovascular: Edema (7% to 18%)

Central nervous system: Headache (4% to 20%), dizziness (3% to 14%), fatigue (8% to 13%)

Endocrine & metabolic: Hypercholesterolemia (3% to 52%), hot flashes (6% to 50%)

Gastrointestinal: Nausea (9% to 17%), weight gain (2% to 13%), constipation (2% to 11%)

Neuromuscular & skeletal: Weakness (4% to 34%), arthralgia (8% to 25%), arthritis (7% to 25%), bone pain (5% to 22%), back pain (5% to 18%), bone mineral density decreased/osteoporosis (5% to 15%), bone fracture (10% to 14%)

Respiratory: Dyspnea (6% to 18%), cough (6% to 13%)

Miscellaneous: Diaphoresis (≤24%), night sweats (15%)

1% to 10%:

Cardiovascular: Chest pain (6% to 8%), hypertension (5% to 8%), chest wall pain (6%), peripheral edema (5%); cerebrovascular accident including hemorrhagic stroke, thrombotic stroke (2% to 3%); thromboembolic event including venous thrombosis, thrombophlebitis, portal vein thrombosis, pulmonary embolism (2% to 3%); MI (1% to 2%), angina (1% to 2%), transient ischemic attack

Central nervous system: Insomnia (6% to 7%), pain (5%), anxiety (<5%), depression (<5%), vertigo (<5%), somnolence (3%)

Dermatologic: Rash (5%), alopecia (3% to 5%), pruritus (1%)

Endocrine & metabolic: Breast pain (2% to 7%), hypercalcemia (<5%)

Gastrointestinal: Diarrhea (5% to 8%), vomiting (3% to 7%), weight loss (6% to 7%), abdominal pain (6%), anorexia (1% to 5%), dyspepsia (3%)

Genitourinary: Urinary tract infection (6%), vaginal bleeding (5%), vaginal dryness (5%), vaginal hemorrhage (5%), vaginal irritation (5%)

Neuromuscular & skeletal: Limb pain (4% to 10%), myalgia (7% to 9%)

Ocular: Cataract (2%)

Renal: Renal disorder (5%)

Respiratory: Pleural effusion (<5%)

Miscellaneous: Infection (7%), influenza (6%), viral infection (6%), secondary malignancy (2% to 4%)

<1%, postmarketing, and/or case reports: Anaphylactic reaction, angioedema, appetite increased, arterial thrombosis, blurred vision, cardiac failure, carpal tunnel syndrome, dry skin, dysesthesia, endometrial cancer, endometrial hyperplasia, endometrial proliferation, erythema multiforme, eye irritation, fever, hepatitis, hypoesthesia, irritability, leukopenia, liver enzymes increased, memory impairment, nervousness, palpitations, paresthesia, stomatitis, tachycardia, taste disturbance, thirst, thrombocytopenia, toxic epidermal necrolysis, trigger finger, urinary frequency increased, urticaria, vaginal discharge, xerostomia

Drug Interactions

Metabolism/Transport Effects Substrate of CYP2A6 (minor), CYP3A4 (minor); **Note:** Assignment of Major/Minor substrate status based on clinically relevant drug interaction potential; **Inhibits** CYP2A6 (strong), CYP2C19 (weak)

Avoid Concomitant Use

Avoid concomitant use of Letrozole with any of the following: Artesunate; Tegafur

Increased Effect/Toxicity

Letrozole may increase the levels/effects of: Artesunate; CYP2A6 Substrates; Methadone

Decreased Effect

Letrozole may decrease the levels/effects of: Artesunate; Tegafur

The levels/effects of Letrozole may be decreased by: Tamoxifen

Storage/Stability Store at room temperature of 25°C (77°F); excursions permitted to 15°C to 30°C (59°F to 86°F).

Mechanism of Action Nonsteroidal competitive inhibitor of the aromatase enzyme system which binds to the heme group of aromatase, a cytochrome P450 enzyme which catalyzes conversion of androgens to estrogens (specifically, androstenedione to estrone and testosterone to estradiol). This leads to inhibition of the enzyme and a significant reduction in plasma estrogen (estrone, estradiol and estrone sulfate) levels. Does not affect synthesis of adrenal or thyroid hormones, aldosterone, or androgens.

Pharmacodynamics/Kinetics

Absorption: Rapid and well absorbed; not affected by food

Distribution: V_d: ~1.9 L/kg

Protein binding, plasma: Weak

Metabolism: Hepatic via CYP3A4 and 2A6 to an inactive carbinol metabolite

Half-life elimination: Terminal: ~2 days

Time to steady state, plasma: 2 to 6 weeks

Excretion: Urine (90%; 6% as unchanged drug, 75% as glucuronide carbinol metabolite, 9% as unidentified metabolites)

Dosing

Adult & Geriatric

Breast cancer, advanced (first- or second-line treatment): Females: Postmenopausal: Oral: 2.5 mg once daily; continue until tumor progression

Breast cancer, early (adjuvant treatment): Females: Postmenopausal: Oral: 2.5 mg once daily for a planned duration of 5 years; discontinue at relapse. **Note:** American Society of Clinical Oncology (ASCO) guidelines for Adjuvant Endocrine Therapy of Hormone Receptor–Positive Breast Cancer

◀ (Focused Update) recommend a maximum duration of 5 years of aromatase inhibitor therapy for postmenopausal women; aromatase inhibitors may be combined with tamoxifen for a total duration of up to 10 years of endocrine therapy. Refer to the guidelines for specific recommendations based on menopausal status and tolerability (Burstein 2014).

Breast cancer, early (extended adjuvant treatment): Females: Postmenopausal: Oral: 2.5 mg once daily for a planned duration of 5 years (after 5 years of tamoxifen); discontinue at relapse. In clinical trials, letrozole was initiated within 3 months of discontinuing tamoxifen (Goss 2003; Jin 2012).

Note: ASCO guidelines for Adjuvant Endocrine Therapy of Hormone Receptor-Positive Breast Cancer (Focused Update) recommend a maximum duration of 5 years of aromatase inhibitor therapy for postmenopausal women; aromatase inhibitors may be combined with tamoxifen for a total duration of up to 10 years of endocrine therapy. Refer to the guidelines for specific recommendations based on menopausal status and tolerability (Burstein 2014).

Off-label combinations:

Breast cancer, advanced, estrogen receptor-positive, HER2-negative: Females: Oral: 2.5 mg once daily (in combination with palbociclib) until disease progression or unacceptable toxicity (Finn 2015)

Breast cancer, metastatic, hormone receptor-positive, HER2-positive: Females: Oral: 2.5 mg once daily (in combination with lapatinib) until disease progression or unacceptable toxicity (Johnston 2009)

Infertility/ovulation stimulation in anovulatory women with polycystic ovarian syndrome (PCOS; off-label use): Oral: 2.5 to 7.5 mg daily on cycle days 3 to 7 (Franik 2014; Legro 2013; Legro 2014; Misso 2012). Up to 5 treatment cycles may be administered with the dose increased in subsequent cycles for nonresponse or poor ovulatory response as determined by progesterone levels; maximum dose: 7.5 mg daily (Legro 2014). Additional trials may be necessary to further define the routine use of letrozole in infertile women with PCOS.

Ovarian (epithelial) cancer (off-label use): Oral: 2.5 mg once daily; continue until disease progression (Ramirez 2008)

Renal Impairment

CrCl ≥10 mL/minute: No dosage adjustment necessary.

CrCl <10 mL/minute: There are no dosage adjustments provided in the manufacturer's labeling.

Hepatic Impairment

U.S. labeling:

Mild to moderate impairment (Child-Pugh class A or B): No dosage adjustment necessary.

Severe impairment (Child-Pugh class C) and cirrhosis: 2.5 mg every other day

Noncirrhotic patients with elevated bilirubin: There are no dosage adjustments provided in the manufacturer's labeling (effect has not been determined).

Canadian labeling:

Mild to moderate impairment (Child-Pugh class A or B): No dosage adjustment necessary.

Severe impairment (Child-Pugh class C): There are no dosage adjustments provided in the manufacturer's labeling (insufficient data). Monitor closely.

Combination Regimens

Breast cancer:
  Lapatinib-Letrozole (Breast) on page 2025
  Palbociclib-Letrozole (Breast) on page 2058

Administration Administer orally with or without food. Hazardous agent; use appropriate precautions for handling and disposal (NIOSH 2014 [group 1]).

Monitoring Parameters

Monitor periodically during therapy: Complete blood counts, thyroid function tests; serum electrolytes, cholesterol, transaminases, and creatinine; blood pressure; bone density

Canadian labeling recommends monitoring LH, FSH, and/or estradiol prior to initiating therapy and regularly for the first 6 months in women whose menopausal status is unclear or who become amenorrheic following chemotherapy. For infertility/ovarian stimulation (off-label use), a pregnancy test is recommended prior to initiation. Midluteal progestin concentrations (in a clinical study, nonresponse to treatment was defined as a progesterone concentration <3 ng/mL during the midluteal phase; poor ovulatory response was defined as progesterone concentrations indicating ovulation but just above the cutoff point) (Legro 2014).

Dietary Considerations Calcium and vitamin D supplementation are recommended.

Dosage Forms Excipient information presented when available (limited, particularly for generics); consult specific product labeling.

Tablet, Oral:
  Femara: 2.5 mg
  Generic: 2.5 mg

◆ **Leucovorin** see Leucovorin Calcium on page 1023

Leucovorin Calcium (loo koe VOR in KAL see um)

Related Information

Mucositis and Stomatitis on page 2186

Brand Names: Canada Lederle Leucovorin; Leucovorin Calcium Injection; Leucovorin Calcium Injection USP

Index Terms 5-Formyl Tetrahydrofolate; Calcium Folinate; Calcium Leucovorin; Citrovorum Factor; Folinate Calcium; Folinic Acid (error prone synonym); Leucovorin

Pharmacologic Category Antidote; Chemotherapy Modulating Agent; Rescue Agent (Chemotherapy); Vitamin, Water Soluble

Use

Methotrexate toxicity:
  Injection: Rescue agent after high-dose methotrexate treatment in osteosarcoma and to diminish the toxicity and counteract the effects of impaired methotrexate elimination and of inadvertent overdosage of folic acid antagonists.
  Oral: Rescue agent to diminish toxicity and counteract effects of impaired methotrexate elimination and inadvertent overdoses of folic acid antagonists.

Megaloblastic anemia: Injection: Treatment of megaloblastic anemias due to folic acid deficiency (when oral therapy is not feasible).

Advanced colorectal cancer: Injection: Palliative treatment of advanced colorectal cancer to prolong survival (in combination with 5-fluorouracil).

Labeled Contraindications Pernicious anemia and other megaloblastic anemias secondary to vitamin B_{12}-deficiency

Pregnancy Considerations Animal reproduction studies have not been conducted. Leucovorin is a biologically active form of folic acid. Adequate amounts of folic acid are recommended during pregnancy.

Breast-Feeding Considerations Leucovorin is a biologically active form of folic acid. Adequate amounts of folic acid are recommended in breast-feeding women.

Warnings/Precautions When used for the treatment of accidental folic acid antagonist overdose, administer as soon as possible. When used for the treatment of a methotrexate overdose, administer IV leucovorin as soon as possible. Monitoring of the serum methotrexate concentration is essential to determine the optimal dose/duration of leucovorin; however, do not wait for the results of a methotrexate level before initiating therapy. It is important to adjust the leucovorin dose once a methotrexate level is known. When used for methotrexate rescue therapy, methotrexate serum concentrations should be monitored to determine dose and duration of leucovorin therapy. The dose may need to be increased or administration prolonged in situations where methotrexate excretion may be delayed (eg, ascites, pleural effusion, renal insufficiency, inadequate hydration); **never administer leucovorin intrathecally**. Parenteral administration may be preferred to oral if vomiting or malabsorption is likely. Potentially significant drug-drug interactions may exist, requiring dose or frequency adjustment, additional monitoring, and/or selection of alternative therapy. Combination of leucovorin and sulfamethoxazole-trimethoprim for the acute treatment of PCP in patients with HIV infection has been reported to cause increased rates of treatment failure. Leucovorin may increase the toxicity of 5-fluorouracil; deaths from severe enterocolitis, diarrhea, and dehydration have been reported (in elderly patients); granulocytopenia and fever have also been reported. Hypersensitivity, including allergic reactions, anaphylactoid reactions, and urticaria have been reported with leucovorin.

Leucovorin is inappropriate treatment for pernicious anemia and other megaloblastic anemias secondary to a lack of vitamin B_{12}; a hematologic remission may occur while neurologic manifestations progress. Leucovorin is excreted renally; the risk for toxicities may be increased in patients with renal impairment.

Benzyl alcohol and derivatives: When doses >10 mg/m^2 are required using the powder for injection, reconstitute using sterile water for injection, not a solution containing benzyl alcohol; large amounts of benzyl alcohol ($\geq$99 mg/kg/day) have been associated with a potentially fatal toxicity ("gasping syndrome") in neonates; the "gasping syndrome" consists of metabolic acidosis, respiratory distress, gasping respirations, CNS dysfunction (including convulsions, intracranial hemorrhage), hypotension, and cardiovascular collapse (AAP ["Inactive" 1997]; CDC, 1982); some data suggests that benzoate displaces bilirubin from protein binding sites (Ahlfors, 2001); avoid or use dosage forms containing benzyl alcohol with caution in neonates. See manufacturer's labeling.

Injection: Due to calcium content, do not administer IV solutions at a rate >160 mg/minute. Not intended for intrathecal use.

Adverse Reactions Frequency not defined. Toxicities (especially gastrointestinal toxicity) of fluorouracil is higher when used in combination with leucovorin.

Dermatologic: Rash, pruritus, erythema, urticaria

Hematologic: Thrombocytosis

Respiratory: Wheezing

Miscellaneous: Allergic reactions, anaphylactoid reactions

Drug Interactions

Metabolism/Transport Effects None known.

Avoid Concomitant Use

Avoid concomitant use of Leucovorin Calcium with any of the following: Raltitrexed; Trimethoprim

Increased Effect/Toxicity

Leucovorin Calcium may increase the levels/effects of: Capecitabine; Fluorouracil (Systemic); Fluorouracil (Topical); Tegafur

Decreased Effect

Leucovorin Calcium may decrease the levels/effects of: Fosphenytoin; PHENobarbital; Phenytoin; Primidone; Raltitrexed; Trimethoprim

The levels/effects of Leucovorin Calcium may be decreased by: Glucarpidase

Storage/Stability

Powder for injection: Store at room temperature of 25°C (77°F). Protect from light. Solutions reconstituted with bacteriostatic water for injection U.S.P., must be used within 7 days. Solutions reconstituted with SWFI must be used immediately. Parenteral admixture is stable for 24 hours stored at room temperature (25°C) and for 4 days when stored under refrigeration (4°C).

Solution for injection: Prior to dilution, store vials under refrigeration at 2°C to 8°C (36°F to 46°F). Protect from light.

Tablet: Store at room temperature of 15°C to 30°C (59°F to 86°F).

Preparation for Administration

Powder for injection: Reconstitute with SWFI or BWFI; dilute in D_5W or NS for infusion. When doses >10 mg/m^2 are required, reconstitute using sterile water for injection, not a solution containing benzyl alcohol.

For methanol toxicity, dilute in D_5W (Barceloux, 2002).

Mechanism of Action A reduced form of folic acid, leucovorin supplies the necessary cofactor blocked by methotrexate. Leucovorin actively competes with methotrexate for transport sites, displaces methotrexate from intracellular binding sites, and restores active folate stores required for DNA/RNA synthesis. Stabilizes the binding of 5-dUMP and thymidylate synthetase, enhancing the activity of fluorouracil. When administered with pyrimethamine for the treatment of opportunistic infections, leucovorin reduces the risk for hematologic toxicity (HHS [OI adult 2015]).

Methanol toxicity treatment: Formic acid (methanol's toxic metabolite) is normally metabolized to carbon dioxide and water by 10-formyltetrahydrofolate dehydrogenase after being bound to tetrahydrofolate. Administering a source of tetrahydrofolate may aid the body in eliminating formic acid (Barceloux, 2002).

Pharmacodynamics/Kinetics

Absorption: Oral, IM: Well absorbed

Metabolism: Intestinal mucosa and hepatically to 5-methyl-tetrahydrofolate (5MTHF; active)

Bioavailability: Saturable at oral doses >25 mg; 25 mg (97%), 50 mg (75%), 100 mg (37%)

Half-life elimination: ~4-8 hours

Time to peak: Oral: ~2 hours; IV: Total folates: 10 minutes; 5MTHF: ~1 hour

Excretion: Urine (primarily); feces

◀ **Dosing**

Adult & Geriatric

Colorectal cancer (also refer to Combination Regimens): IV: 200 mg/m²/day over at least 3 minutes for 5 days every 4 weeks for 2 cycles, then every 4 to 5 weeks (in combination with fluorouracil) **or** 20 mg/m²/day for 5 days every 4 weeks for 2 cycles, then every 4 to 5 weeks (in combination with fluorouracil)

Folic acid antagonist (eg, trimethoprim, pyrimethamine) overdose: Oral: 5 to 15 mg once daily

Folate-deficient megaloblastic anemia: IM, IV: ≤1 mg once daily

High-dose methotrexate-rescue: Initial: Oral, IM, IV: 15 mg (~10 mg/m²); start 24 hours after beginning methotrexate infusion; continue every 6 hours for 10 doses, until methotrexate level is <0.05 micromolar. Adjust dose as follows:

Normal methotrexate elimination (serum methotrexate level ~10 micromolar at 24 hours after administration, 1 micromolar at 48 hours, and <0.2 micromolar at 72 hours): Oral, IM, IV: 15 mg every 6 hours for 60 hours (10 doses) beginning 24 hours after the start of methotrexate infusion

Delayed late methotrexate elimination (serum methotrexate level remaining >0.2 micromolar at 72 hours and >0.05 micromolar at 96 hours after administration): Continue leucovorin calcium 15 mg (oral, IM or IV) every 6 hours until methotrexate level is <0.05 micromolar

Delayed early methotrexate elimination and/or acute renal injury (serum methotrexate level ≥50 micromolar at 24 hours, or ≥5 micromolar at 48 hours, or a doubling of serum creatinine level at 24 hours after methotrexate administration): IV: 150 mg every 3 hours until methotrexate level is <1 micromolar, then 15 mg every 3 hours until methotrexate level is <0.05 micromolar

High-dose methotrexate overexposure: Leucovorin nomogram dosing for high-dose methotrexate overexposure (off-label dosing; generalized dosing derived from reference nomogram figures, refer to each reference [Bleyer, 1978; Bleyer, 1981; Widemann, 2006] or institution-specific nomogram for details):

At 24 hours:

For methotrexate levels of ≥100 micromolar at ~24 hours, leucovorin is initially dosed at 1,000 mg/m² every 6 hours

For methotrexate levels of ≥10 to <100 micromolar at 24 hours, leucovorin is initially dosed at 100 mg/m² every 3 or 6 hours

For methotrexate levels of ~1 to 10 micromolar at 24 hours, leucovorin is initially dosed at 10 mg/m² every 3 or 6 hours

At 48 hours:

For methotrexate levels of ≥100 micromolar at 48 hours, leucovorin is dosed at 1,000 mg/m² every 6 hours

For methotrexate levels of ≥10 to <100 micromolar at 48 hours, leucovorin is dosed at 100 mg/m² every 3 hours

For methotrexate levels of ~1 to 10 micromolar at 48 hours, leucovorin is dosed at 100 mg/m² every 6 hours **or** 10 to 100 mg/m² every 3 hours

At 72 hours:

For methotrexate levels of ≥10 micromolar at 72 hours, leucovorin is dosed at 100 to 1,000 mg/m² every 3 to 6 hours

For methotrexate levels of ~1 to 10 micromolar at 72 hours, leucovorin is dosed at 10 to 100 mg/m² every 3 hours

For methotrexate levels of ~0.1 to 1 micromolar at 72 hours, leucovorin is dosed at 10 mg/m^2 every 3 to 6 hours

If serum creatinine is increased more than 50% above baseline, increase the standard leucovorin dose to 100 mg/m^2 every 3 hours, then adjust according to methotrexate levels above.

Follow methotrexate levels daily, leucovorin may be discontinued when methotrexate level is <0.1 micromolar

Methotrexate overdose (inadvertent) (begin as soon as possible after overdose): Oral, IM, IV: 10 mg/m^2 every 6 hours until the methotrexate level is <0.01 micromolar. If serum creatinine is increased more than 50% above baseline 24 hours after methotrexate administration, if 24 hour methotrexate level is >5 micromolar, or if 48 hour methotrexate level is >0.9 micromolar, increase leucovorin dose to 100 mg/m^2 IV every 3 hours until the methotrexate level is <0.01 micromolar.

Do not administer leucovorin intrathecally; the use of intrathecal leucovorin is not advised (Jardine, 1996; Smith, 2008).

Cofactor therapy in methanol toxicity (off-label use): IV: 1 mg/kg (maximum dose: 50 mg) over 30-60 minutes every 4-6 hours. Therapy should continue until methanol and formic acid have been completely eliminated (Barceloux, 2002)

Pemetrexed toxicity (off-label dose): IV: 100 mg/m^2 once, followed by 50 mg/m^2 every 6 hours for 8 days (used in clinical trial for CTC grade 4 leukopenia ≥3 days; CTC grade 4 neutropenia ≥3 days; immediately for CTC grade 4 thrombocytopenia, bleeding associated with grade 3 thrombocytopenia, or grade 3 or 4 mucositis) (Alimta [prescribing information], 2013).

Prevention of pyrimethamine hematologic toxicity in HIV-infected patients (off-label use; HHS [OI adult 2015]): Oral:

Isosporiasis (*Isospora belli*):

Treatment: 10 to 25 mg once daily (in combination with pyrimethamine)

Chronic maintenance (secondary prophylaxis): 5 to 10 mg once daily (in combination with pyrimethamine)

Pneumocystis pneumonia (PCP): Prophylaxis (primary and secondary): 25 mg once weekly (in combination with pyrimethamine [with dapsone]) **or** 10 mg once daily (in combination with pyrimethamine [with atovaquone])

Toxoplasma gondii encephalitis:

Primary prophylaxis: 25 mg once weekly (in combination with pyrimethamine [with dapsone]) **or** 10 mg once daily (in combination with pyrimethamine [with atovaquone])

Treatment: 10 to 25 mg once daily (in combination with pyrimethamine [with either sulfadiazine, clindamycin, atovaquone, or azithromycin]). **Note:** May increase leucovorin to 50 to 100 mg/day in divided doses in cases of pyrimethamine toxicity (rash, nausea, bone marrow suppression).

Chronic maintenance (secondary prophylaxis): 10 to 25 mg once daily (in combination with pyrimethamine [with either sulfadiazine or clindamycin]) **or** 10 mg once daily (in combination with pyrimethamine [with atovaquone])

Pediatric

Folic acid antagonist (eg, trimethoprim, pyrimethamine) overdose: Refer to adult dosing.

Folate-deficient megaloblastic anemia: Refer to adult dosing.

◀ **High-dose methotrexate-rescue:** Refer to adult dosing.

Cofactor therapy in methanol toxicity (off-label use): Refer to adult dosing.

Prevention of pyrimethamine hematologic toxicity in HIV-exposed/-positive patients (off-label uses; CDC, 2009):

Infants and Children >1 month of age: **Note:** Leucovorin should continue for 1 week after pyrimethamine is discontinued.

Toxoplasmosis (*Toxoplasma gondii*):

Primary prophylaxis: Oral: 5 mg once every 3 days (in combination with pyrimethamine [with either dapsone or atovaquone])

Secondary prophylaxis: Oral: 5 mg once every 3 days (in combination with pyrimethamine [with either sulfadiazine, atovaquone, or clindamycin])

Treatment (congenital): Oral or IM: 10 mg with every pyrimethamine dose (in combination with either sulfadiazine or clindamycin); treatment duration: 12 months

Treatment (acquired): Oral: Acute induction: 10-25 mg once daily (in combination with pyrimethamine [with either sulfadiazine, clindamycin, or atovaquone]) for ≥6 weeks

Adolescents: Refer to adult dosing

Renal Impairment There are no dosage adjustments provided in manufacturer's labeling.

Hepatic Impairment There are no dosage adjustments provided in manufacturer's labeling.

Combination Regimens

Administration Due to calcium content, do not administer IV solutions at a rate >160 mg/minute; not intended for intrathecal use.

Refer to individual protocols. Should be administered IM, IV push, or IV infusion (15 minutes to 2 hours). Leucovorin should not be administered concurrently with methotrexate. It is commonly initiated 24 hours after the start of methotrexate. Toxicity to normal tissues may be irreversible if leucovorin is not initiated by ~40 hours after the start of methotrexate.

As a rescue after folate antagonists: Administer by IV bolus, IM, or orally.

Do not administer orally in the presence of nausea or vomiting. Doses >25 mg should be administered parenterally.

Combination therapy with fluorouracil: Fluorouracil is usually given after, or at the midpoint, of the leucovorin infusion. Leucovorin is usually administered by IV bolus injection or short (10-120 minutes) IV infusion. Other administration schedules have been used; refer to individual protocols.

For the treatment of methanol toxicity, infuse over 30 to 60 minutes (Barceloux, 2002)

Extemporaneous Preparations A 5 mg/mL oral suspension may be prepared with tablets, Cologel, and a 2:1 mixture of simple syrup and wild cherry syrup. Crush twenty-four 25 mg tablets in a glass mortar and reduce to a fine powder; transfer powder to amber bottle. Add 30 mL Cologel and shake mixture thoroughly. Add a quantity of syrup mixture sufficient to make 120 mL. Label "shake well" and "refrigerate". Stable for 28 days refrigerated.

Lam MS. Extemporaneous Compounding of Oral Liquid Dosage Formulations and Alternative Drug Delivery Methods for Anticancer Drugs. *Pharmacotherapy.* 2011;31(2):164-192.

Monitoring Parameters

High-dose methotrexate therapy: Plasma methotrexate concentration; leucovorin is continued until the plasma methotrexate level <0.05 micromolar. With 4- to 6-hour high-dose methotrexate infusions, plasma drug values in excess of 50 and 1 micromolar at 24 and 48 hours after starting the infusion, respectively, are often predictive of delayed methotrexate clearance.

Fluorouracil therapy: CBC with differential and platelets, liver function tests, electrolytes

Dietary Considerations Solutions for injection contain calcium 0.004 mEq per leucovorin 1 mg

Dosage Forms Excipient information presented when available (limited, particularly for generics); consult specific product labeling. [DSC] = Discontinued product

Solution, Injection [strength expressed as base]:
Generic: 100 mg/10 mL (10 mL [DSC]); 300 mg/30 mL (30 mL)

Solution Reconstituted, Injection [strength expressed as base]:
Generic: 100 mg (1 ea); 200 mg (1 ea); 350 mg (1 ea); 500 mg (1 ea)

Solution Reconstituted, Injection [strength expressed as base, preservative free]:
Generic: 50 mg (1 ea); 100 mg (1 ea); 200 mg (1 ea); 350 mg (1 ea)

Tablet, Oral [strength expressed as base]:
Generic: 5 mg, 10 mg, 15 mg, 25 mg

◆ **Leucovorin Calcium Injection (Can)** see Leucovorin Calcium on page 1023

◆ **Leucovorin Calcium Injection USP (Can)** see Leucovorin Calcium on page 1023

◆ **Leukeran** see Chlorambucil on page 317

◆ **Leukeran® (Can)** see Chlorambucil on page 317

◆ **Leukine** see Sargramostim on page 1515

Leuprolide (loo PROE lide)

Related Information

Safe Handling of Hazardous Drugs on page 2292

Brand Names: US Eligard; Lupron Depot; Lupron Depot-Ped

Brand Names: Canada Eligard; Lupron; Lupron Depot

Index Terms Abbott-43818; Leuprolide Acetate; Leuprorelin Acetate; TAP-144

Pharmacologic Category Antineoplastic Agent, Gonadotropin-Releasing Hormone Agonist; Gonadotropin Releasing Hormone Agonist

Use

Central precocious puberty: Treatment of children with central precocious puberty

Endometriosis: Management of endometriosis, including pain relief and reduction of endometriotic lesions

Prostate cancer: Palliative treatment of advanced prostate cancer

Uterine leiomyomata (fibroids): Treatment of anemia caused by uterine leiomyomata (fibroids)

Labeled Contraindications Hypersensitivity to leuprolide, GnRH, GnRH-agonist analogs, or any component of the formulation; undiagnosed abnormal vaginal bleeding (Lupron Depot 3.75 mg [monthly] and Lupron Depot 11.25 mg [3-month]); pregnancy; breast-feeding (Lupron Depot 3.75 mg [monthly] and Lupron Depot 11.25 mg [3-month])

Lupron Depot 22.5 mg, 30 mg, and 45 mg are also not indicated for use in women

Pregnancy Considerations Adverse events were observed in animal reproduction studies. Pregnancy must be excluded prior to the start of treatment. Although leuprolide usually inhibits ovulation and stops menstruation, contraception is not ensured and a nonhormonal contraceptive should be used. Use is contraindicated in pregnant women.

Breast-Feeding Considerations It is not known if leuprolide is excreted into breast milk; use is contraindicated in nursing women.

Warnings/Precautions Hazardous agent - use appropriate precautions for handling and disposal (NIOSH 2014 [group 1]). Transient increases in testosterone serum levels (~50% above baseline) occur at the start of treatment. Androgen-deprivation therapy (ADT) may increase the risk for cardiovascular disease (Levine, 2010); sudden cardiac death and stroke have been reported in men receiving GnRH agonists; ADT may prolong the QT/QTc interval; consider the benefits of ADT versus the risk for QT prolongation in patients with a history of QTc prolongation, congenital long QT syndrome, heart failure, frequent electrolyte abnormalities, and in patients with medications known to prolong the QT interval, or with preexisting cardiac disease. Consider periodic monitoring of electrocardiograms and electrolytes in at-risk patients. Tumor flare, bone pain, neuropathy, urinary tract obstruction, and spinal cord compression have been reported when used for prostate cancer; closely observe patients for weakness, paresthesias, hematuria, and urinary tract obstruction in first few weeks of therapy. Observe patients with metastatic vertebral lesions or urinary obstruction closely. Exacerbation of endometriosis or uterine leiomyomata may occur initially. Decreased bone density has been reported when used for ≥6 months; use caution in patients with additional risk factors for bone loss (eg, chronic alcohol use, corticosteroid therapy). In patients with prostate cancer, androgen deprivation therapy may increase the risk for cardiovascular disease, diabetes, insulin resistance, obesity, alterations in lipids, and fractures; monitor as clinically necessary. Use caution in patients with a history of psychiatric illness; alteration in mood, memory impairment, and depression have been associated with use. Rare cases of pituitary apoplexy (frequently secondary to pituitary adenoma) have been observed with GnRH agonist administration (onset from 1 hour to usually <2 weeks); may present as sudden headache, vomiting, visual or mental status changes, and infrequently cardiovascular collapse; immediate medical attention required. Convulsions have been observed in postmarketing reports; patients affected included both those with and without a history of cerebrovascular disorders, central nervous system anomalies or tumors, epilepsy, seizures, and those on concomitant medications which may lower the seizure threshold. If seizures occur, manage accordingly. Females treated for precocious puberty may experience menses or spotting during the first 2 months of treatment; notify healthcare provider if bleeding continues after the second month.

Benzyl alcohol and derivatives: Some dosage forms may contain benzyl alcohol; large amounts of benzyl alcohol (≥99 mg/kg/day) have been associated with a potentially fatal toxicity ("gasping syndrome") in neonates; the "gasping syndrome" consists of metabolic acidosis, respiratory distress, gasping respirations, CNS dysfunction (including convulsions, intracranial hemorrhage), hypotension, and cardiovascular collapse (AAP ["Inactive" 1997]; CDC, 1982); some data suggests that benzoate displaces bilirubin from protein binding sites (Ahlfors, 2001); avoid or use dosage forms containing benzyl alcohol with caution in neonates.

◄ Some dosage forms may contain polysorbate 80 (also known as Tweens). Hypersensitivity reactions, usually a delayed reaction, have been reported following exposure to pharmaceutical products containing polysorbate 80 in certain individuals (Isaksson, 2002; Lucente 2000; Shelley, 1995). Thrombocytopenia, ascites, pulmonary deterioration, and renal and hepatic failure have been reported in premature neonates after receiving parenteral products containing polysorbate 80 (Alade, 1986; CDC, 1984). See manufacturer's labeling.

Vehicle used in depot injectable formulations (polylactide-co-glycolide microspheres) has rarely been associated with retinal artery occlusion in patients with abnormal arteriovenous anastomosis. Due to different release properties, combinations of dosage forms or fractions of dosage forms should not be interchanged.

Adverse Reactions

Children (percentages based on 1-month and 3-month pediatric formulations combined):

>10%: Local: Pain at injection site (≤20%)

2% to 10%:

Cardiovascular: Vasodilatation (2%)

Central nervous system: Emotional lability (5%), mood changes (5%), headache (3% to 5%), pain (3%)

Dermatologic: Acne vulgaris (3%), seborrhea (3%), skin rash (3% including erythema multiforme)

Endocrine & metabolic: Weight gain (≤7%)

Genitourinary: Vaginal discharge (3%), vaginal hemorrhage (3%), vaginitis (3%)

Local: Injection site reaction (≤9%)

<2%: Abnormal gait, alopecia, arthralgia, asthma, body odor, bradycardia, cervix disease, constipation, cough, decreased appetite, decreased visual acuity, depression, dizziness, drowsiness, dysmenorrhea, dyspepsia, dysphagia, epistaxis, excessive crying, feminization, fever, flu-like symptoms, gingivitis, goiter, growth suppression, gynecomastia, hirsutism, hyperhidrosis, hyperkinesia, hypersensitivity reaction, hypertension, increased appetite, infection, lacrimation, leukoderma, limb pain, musculoskeletal pain, myalgia, myopathy, nausea, nervousness, obesity, pallor, peripheral edema, personality disorder, pharyngitis, precocious puberty, purpura, rhinitis, sinusitis, skin striae, syncope, urinary incontinence, vomiting, weakness

Adults: Note: For prostate cancer treatment, an initial rise in serum testosterone concentrations may cause "tumor flare" or worsening of symptoms, including bone pain, neuropathy, hematuria, or ureteral or bladder outlet obstruction during the first 2 weeks. Similarly, an initial increase in estradiol levels, with a temporary worsening of symptoms, may occur in women treated with leuprolide.

Delayed release formulations:

>10%:

Cardiovascular: Edema (≤14%)

Central nervous system: Headache (≤65%), pain (<2% to 33%), depression (≤31%), insomnia (≤31%), fatigue (≤17%), dizziness (≤16%)

Dermatologic: Allergic skin reaction (≤12%)

Endocrine & metabolic: Hot flash (25% to 98%), weight changes (≤13%), hyperlipidemia (≤12%), decreased libido (≤11%)

Gastrointestinal: Nausea and vomiting (≤25%), gastrointestinal disease (14%), change in bowel habits (≤14%)

Genitourinary: Vaginitis (11% to 28%), testicular atrophy (≤20%), genitourinary complaint (13% to 15%)

Local: Burning sensation at injection site burning (transient: ≤35%)

Neuromuscular & skeletal: Weakness (≤18%), arthropathy (≤12%)

Respiratory: Flu-like symptoms (≤12%), respiratory tract disease (11%)

1% to 10% (limited to important or life-threatening):

Cardiovascular: Angina pectoris (<5%), atrial fibrillation (<5%), bradycardia (<5%), cardiac arrhythmia (<5%), cardiac failure (<5%), deep thrombophlebitis (<5%), hyper-/hypotension (<5%), palpitations (<5%), syncope (<5%), tachycardia (<5%)

Central nervous system: Nervousness (≤8%), paresthesia (≤8%), anxiety (≤6%), agitation (<5%), confusion (<5%), delusions (<5%), dementia (<5%), neuropathy (<5%), paralysis (<5%), seizure (<5%), ostealgia (≤2%)

Dermatologic: Acne vulgaris (≤10%), alopecia (≤5%), diaphoresis (≤5%), cellulitis (<5%), hair disease (<5%), pruritus (≤3%), skin rash (≤2%)

Endocrine & metabolic: Dehydration (≤8%), gynecomastia (≤7%), decreased serum bicarbonate (≥5%), hypercholesterolemia (≥5%), hyperglycemia (≥5%), hyperphosphatemia (≥5%), hyperuricemia (≥5%), hypoalbuminemia (≥5%), hypocholesterolemia (≥5%), hypoproteinemia (≥5%), increased lactate dehydrogenase (≥5%), increased prostatic acid phosphatase (≥5%), menstrual disorder (≤2%), hirsutism (<2%)

Gastrointestinal: Anorexia (<5%), dysphagia (<5%), eructation (<5%), gastric ulcer (<5%), gastrointestinal hemorrhage (<5%), intestinal obstruction (<5%), peptic ulcer (<5%), constipation (≤3%), gastroenteritis (≤3%), diarrhea (≤2%)

Genitourinary: Mastalgia (≤6%), impotence (≤5%), balanitis (<5%), breast hypertrophy (<5%), lactation (<5%), penile disease (<5%), testicular disease (<5%), urinary incontinence (<5%), urinary tract infection (<5%), nocturia (≤4%), testicular pain (≤4%), dysuria (≤2%), bladder spasm (<2%), erectile dysfunction (<2%), hematuria (<2%), urinary retention (<2%), urinary urgency (<2%)

Hematologic & oncologic: Change in platelet count (increased; ≥5%), decreased prostatic acid phosphatase (≥5%), eosinophilia (≥5%), leukopenia (≥5%), bruise (≤5%), ecchymoses (<5%), lymphadenopathy (<5%), neoplasm (<5%), anemia, decreased hematocrit, decreased hemoglobin

Hepatic: Abnormal hepatic function tests (≥5%), increased serum AST (≥5%), prolonged partial thromboplastin time (≥5%), prolonged prothrombin time (≥5%), hepatomegaly (<5%)

Hypersensitivity: Hypersensitivity reaction (<5%)

Infection: Infection (5%)

Local: Pain at injection site (2% to 5%), injection site reaction (<5%), erythema at injection site (1% to 3%)

Neuromuscular & skeletal: Myalgia (≤8%), neuromuscular disease (<5%), pathological fracture (<5%), arthralgia (≤1%)

Renal: Decreased urine specific gravity (≥5%), increased blood urea nitrogen (≥5%), increased serum creatinine (≥5%), increased urine specific gravity (≥5%), polyuria (2% to 4%)

Respiratory: Emphysema (<5%), epistaxis (<5%), hemoptysis (<5%), increased bronchial secretions (<5%), pleural effusion (<5%), pulmonary edema (<5%), dyspnea (≤2%), cough (≤1%)

Miscellaneous: Fever (<5%)

Immediate release formulation:
>10%:
Cardiovascular: ECG changes (19%), peripheral edema (12%)
Central nervous system: Pain (13%)
Endocrine & metabolic: Hot flash (55%)
1% to 10% (limited to important or life-threatening):
Cardiovascular: Hypertension (8%), heart murmur (3%), thrombophlebitis (2%), cardiac failure (1%), angina pectoris, cardiac arrhythmia, myocardial infarction, pulmonary embolism, syncope
Central nervous system: Headache (7%), insomnia (7%), dizziness (5%), ostealgia (5%), anxiety, depression, fatigue, fever, nervousness, peripheral neuropathy
Dermatologic: Dermatitis (5%), alopecia, hyperpigmentation, pruritus, skin lesion
Endocrine & metabolic: Decreased libido, diabetes mellitus, goiter, gynecomastia, hypercalcemia, hypoglycemia
Gastrointestinal: Constipation (7%), anorexia (6%), nausea and vomiting (5%), diarrhea, dysphagia, gastrointestinal hemorrhage, peptic ulcer, rectal polyps
Genitourinary: Decreased testicular size (7%), hematuria (6%), urinary frequency (6%), impotence (4%), urinary tract infection (3%), bladder spasm, dysuria, incontinence, mastalgia, testicular pain, urinary tract obstruction
Hematologic & oncologic: Anemia (5%), bruise
Infection: Infection
Local: Injection site reaction
Neuromuscular & skeletal: Weakness (10%)
Ophthalmic: Blurred vision
Renal: Increased blood urea nitrogen, increased serum creatinine
Respiratory: Dyspnea (2%), cough, pneumonia, pulmonary fibrosis
Miscellaneous: Fever, inflammation

Children and Adults: *Any formulations:* Postmarketing and/or case reports: Abdominal pain, abscess at injection site, anaphylaxis, anaphylactoid reaction, asthma, bone fracture (spine), cerebrovascular accident, convulsions, coronary artery disease, decreased white blood cell count, diabetes mellitus, fibromyalgia syndrome (arthralgia/myalgia, headaches, GI distress), flushing, hemoptysis, hepatic injury, hepatic insufficiency, hepatotoxicity, hyperuricemia, hypokalemia, hypoproteinemia, induration at injection site, interstitial pulmonary disease, leukocytosis, myocardial infarction, osteopenia, paralysis, penile swelling, peripheral neuropathy, pituitary apoplexy (cardiovascular collapse, mental status altered, ophthalmoplegia, sudden headache, visual changes, vomiting), prolonged QT interval on ECG, prostate pain, pulmonary embolism, pulmonary infiltrates, retroperitoneal fibrosis (pelvic), seizure, skin photosensitivity, suicidal ideation (rare), tenosynovitis (symptoms), thrombocytopenia, transient ischemic attacks, urticaria

Drug Interactions
Metabolism/Transport Effects None known.
Avoid Concomitant Use
Avoid concomitant use of Leuprolide with any of the following: Corifollitropin Alfa; Highest Risk QTc-Prolonging Agents; Indium 111 Capromab Pendetide; Ivabradine; Mifepristone
Increased Effect/Toxicity
Leuprolide may increase the levels/effects of: Corifollitropin Alfa; Highest Risk QTc-Prolonging Agents; Moderate Risk QTc-Prolonging Agents

The levels/effects of Leuprolide may be increased by: Ivabradine; Mifepristone; QTc-Prolonging Agents (Indeterminate Risk and Risk Modifying)

Decreased Effect

Leuprolide may decrease the levels/effects of: Antidiabetic Agents; Choline C 11; Indium 111 Capromab Pendetide

Storage/Stability

Eligard: Store at 2°C to 8°C (36°F to 46°F). Allow to reach room temperature prior to using; once mixed, must be administered within 30 minutes.

Lupron Depot, Lupron Depot-Ped: Store at room temperature of 25°C (77°F); excursions permitted to 15°C to 30°C (59°F to 86°F). Upon reconstitution, the suspension does not contain a preservative and should be used immediately; discard if not used within 2 hours.

Leuprolide acetate 5 mg/mL solution: Store at 20°C to 25°C (68°F to 77°F); excursions permitted to 15°C to 30°C (59°F to 86°F). Protect from light and store vial in carton until use. Do not freeze.

Preparation for Administration Hazardous agent; use appropriate precautions for handling and disposal (NIOSH 2014 [group 1]).

Eligard: Packaged in two syringes; one contains the Atrigel polymer system and the second contains leuprolide acetate powder; follow package instructions for mixing

Lupron Depot, Lupron Depot-Ped: Reconstitute only with diluent provided

Mechanism of Action Leuprolide, is an agonist of gonadotropin releasing hormone (GnRH). Acting as a potent inhibitor of gonadotropin secretion; continuous administration results in suppression of ovarian and testicular steroidogenesis due to decreased levels of LH and FSH with subsequent decrease in testosterone (male) and estrogen (female) levels. In males, testosterone levels are reduced to below castrate levels. Leuprolide may also have a direct inhibitory effect on the testes, and act by a different mechanism not directly related to reduction in serum testosterone.

Pharmacodynamics/Kinetics

Onset of action: Following transient increase, testosterone suppression occurs in ~2-4 weeks of continued therapy

Distribution: Males: V_d: 27 L

Protein binding: 43% to 49%

Metabolism: Major metabolite, pentapeptide (M-1)

Bioavailability: SubQ: 94%

Excretion: Urine (<5% as parent and major metabolite)

Dosing

Adult & Geriatric

Prostate cancer, advanced:

IM:

Lupron Depot 7.5 mg (monthly): 7.5 mg every month **or**
Lupron Depot 22.5 mg (3 month): 22.5 mg every 12 weeks **or**
Lupron Depot 30 mg (4 month): 30 mg every 16 weeks **or**
Lupron Depot 45 mg (6 month): 45 mg every 24 weeks

SubQ:

Eligard: 7.5 mg monthly **or** 22.5 mg every 3 months **or** 30 mg every 4 months **or** 45 mg every 6 months

Leuprolide acetate 5 mg/mL solution: 1 mg daily

Endometriosis: IM: Initial therapy may be with leuprolide alone or in combination with norethindrone; if re-treatment for an additional 6 months is necessary, concomitant norethindrone should be used. Re-treatment is not recommended for longer than one additional 6-month course.

◄ *Lupron Depot:* 3.75 mg every month for up to 6 months **or**
Lupron Depot-3 month: 11.25 mg every 3 months for up to 2 doses (6 months total duration of treatment)

Uterine leiomyomata (fibroids): IM (in combination with iron):
Lupron Depot: 3.75 mg every month for up to 3 months **or**
Lupron Depot-3 month: 11.25 mg as a single injection

Breast cancer, premenopausal ovarian ablation (off-label use):
Lupron Depot: 3.75 mg every 28 days for up to 24 months (Boccardo, 1999) **or**
Lupron Depot-3 month: 11.25 mg every 3 months for up to 24 months (Boccardo, 1999; Schmid, 2007)

Treatment of paraphilia/hypersexuality (off-label use; Guay, 2009; Reilly, 2000): Males: IM:
Note: May cause an initial increase in androgen concentrations which may be treated with an antiandrogen (eg, flutamide, cyproterone) for 1-2 months (Guay, 2009). Avoid use in patients with osteoporosis or active pituitary pathology.
SubQ: Test dose: 1 mg (observe for hypersensitivity)
Depot IM: 3.75-7.5 mg monthly

Pediatric

Precocious puberty (consider discontinuing by age 11 for females and by age 12 for males):
IM:
Lupron Depot-Ped (monthly):
≤25 kg: 7.5 mg every month
>25-37.5 kg: 11.25 mg every month
>37.5 kg: 15 mg every month
Titrate dose upward in increments of 3.75 mg every 4 weeks if down-regulation is not achieved.
Lupron Depot-Ped (3 month): 11.25 mg or 30 mg every 12 weeks
SubQ (leuprolide acetate 5 mg/mL solution): Initial: 50 mcg/kg/day; titrate dose upward by 10 mcg/kg/day if down-regulation is not achieved. **Note:** Higher mg/kg doses may be required in younger children.

Renal Impairment There are no dosage adjustments provided in the manufacturer's labeling (has not been studied).

Hepatic Impairment There are no dosage adjustments provided in the manufacturer's labeling (has not been studied).

Administration

Do not use concurrently a fractional dose of the 3-, 4-, or 6-month depot formulation, or a combination of doses of the monthly depot formulation or any depot formulation due to different release characteristics. Do not use a combination of syringes to achieve a particular dose.

IM: Lupron Depot, Lupron Depot-Ped: Administer as a single injection into the gluteal area, anterior thigh, or deltoid. Vary injection site periodically

SubQ:
Eligard: Vary injection site; choose site with adequate subcutaneous tissue (eg, upper or mid-abdomen, upper buttocks); avoid areas that may be compressed or rubbed (eg, belt or waistband)
Leuprolide acetate 5 mg/mL solution: Vary injection site; if an alternate syringe from the syringe provided is required, insulin syringes should be used

Hazardous agent; use appropriate precautions for handling and disposal (NIOSH 2014 [group 1]).

Monitoring Parameters Bone mineral density

Precocious puberty: GnRH testing (blood LH and FSH levels), measurement of height and bone age every 6-12 months, testosterone in males and estradiol in females (IM [monthly] and SubQ formulations: 1-2 months after initiation of therapy or with dosage change; IM [3 month] formulation: 2-3 months after initiation of therapy, month 6, and as clinically indicated thereafter); Tanner staging

Prostatic cancer: LH and FSH levels, serum testosterone (~4 weeks after initiation of therapy), PSA; weakness, paresthesias, and urinary tract obstruction in first few weeks of therapy. Screen for diabetes (blood glucose and HbA_{1c}) and cardiovascular risk prior to initiating and periodically during treatment. Consider periodic monitoring of electrocardiograms and electrolytes.

Treatment of paraphilia/hypersexuality (off-label use; Reilly, 2000): CBC (baseline, monthly for 4 months then every 6 months); serum testosterone (baseline, monthly for 4 months then every 6 months); serum LH (baseline and every 6 months); FSH (baseline); serum BUN and creatinine and every 6 months); bone density (baseline and yearly); ECG (baseline)

Test Interactions Interferes with pituitary gonadotropic and gonadal function tests during and up to 3 months after monthly administration of leuprolide therapy.

Additional Information Eligard Atrigel: A nongelatin-based, biodegradable, polymer matrix

Oncology Comment: Guidelines from the American Society of Clinical Oncology (ASCO) for hormonal management of advanced prostate cancer which is androgen-sensitive (Loblaw, 2007) recommend either orchiectomy or luteinizing hormone-releasing hormone (LHRH) agonists as initial treatment for androgen deprivation.

Dosage Forms Excipient information presented when available (limited, particularly for generics); consult specific product labeling.

Kit, Injection, as acetate:
Generic: 1 mg/0.2 mL

Kit, Intramuscular, as acetate:
Lupron Depot: 7.5 mg, 45 mg [latex free; contains polysorbate 80]

Kit, Intramuscular, as acetate [preservative free]:
Lupron Depot: 3.75 mg, 11.25 mg, 22.5 mg, 30 mg [latex free; contains polysorbate 80]
Lupron Depot-Ped: 7.5 mg, 11.25 mg, 15 mg, 30 mg (Ped), 11.25 mg (Ped) [latex free; contains polysorbate 80]

Kit, Subcutaneous, as acetate:
Eligard: 7.5 mg, 22.5 mg, 30 mg, 45 mg

Levofloxacin (Systemic) (lee voe FLOKS a sin)

Brand Names: US Levaquin

Brand Names: Canada ACT Levofloxacin; APO-Levofloxacin; Levaquin; Levaquin in 5% Dextrose Injection; Mylan-Levofloxacin; PMS-Levofloxacin; Sandoz-Levofloxacin; Teva-Levofloxacin

Pharmacologic Category Antibiotic, Fluoroquinolone; Antibiotic, Respiratory Fluoroquinolone

Use Treatment of community-acquired pneumonia, including multidrug resistant strains of *S. pneumoniae* (MDRSP); nosocomial pneumonia; chronic bronchitis (acute bacterial exacerbation); acute bacterial rhinosinusitis (ABRS); prostatitis (chronic bacterial), urinary tract infection (uncomplicated or complicated); acute pyelonephritis; skin or skin structure infections (uncomplicated or complicated); reduce incidence or disease progression of inhalational anthrax (postexposure); prophylaxis and treatment of plague (pneumonic and septicemic) due to *Y. pestis*

Pregnancy Risk Factor C

Dosing

Adult & Geriatric Note: Sequential therapy (intravenous to oral) may be instituted based on prescriber's discretion.

Acute bacterial rhinosinusitis: Oral, IV:

Manufacturer's labeling: 750 mg every 24 hours for 5 days or 500 mg every 24 hours for 10-14 days

Alternate recommendations: 500 mg every 24 hours for 5-7 days (Chow 2012)

Anthrax (inhalational): Oral, IV: 500 mg every 24 hours for 60 days, beginning as soon as possible after exposure

Bite wounds (animal/human) (off-label use): Oral, IV: **Note:** Recommended as an alternative therapy for human bite wound in patients hypersensitive to beta-lactams: 750 mg once daily; in combination with metronidazole or clindamycin (IDSA [Stevens 2014])

***Chlamydia trachomatis* sexually transmitted infections (off-label use) (CDC 2010):** Oral: 500 mg every 24 hours for 7 days

Chronic bronchitis (acute bacterial exacerbation): Oral: 500 mg every 24 hours for 7 days; Canadian labeling (not in U.S. labeling) also includes a dosage regimen of 750 mg every 24 hours for 5 days

Diverticulitis, peritonitis (off-label use) (Solomkin, [IDSA] 2010): Oral, IV: 750 mg every 24 hours for 7-10 days; use adjunctive metronidazole therapy

Epididymitis, nongonococcal (off-label use) (CDC 2010): Oral: 500 mg once daily for 10 days

Gonococcal infection (off-label use) (CDC 2010): As of April 2007, the CDC no longer recommends the use of fluoroquinolones for the treatment of uncomplicated or more serious gonococcal disease, unless no other options exist and susceptibility can be confirmed via culture.

Intra-abdominal infection, complicated, community-acquired (in combination with metronidazole) (off-label use) (Solomkin, [IDSA] 2010): IV: 750 mg once daily for 4-7 days (provided source controlled). **Note:** Avoid using in settings where *E. coli* susceptibility to fluoroquinolones is <90%.

Pelvic inflammatory disease (off-label use) (CDC 2010): Oral: 500 mg once daily for 14 days with or without concomitant metronidazole; **Note:** The CDC recommends use as an alternative therapy only if standard parenteral cephalosporin therapy is not feasible and community prevalence of quinolone-resistant gonococcal organisms is low. Culture sensitivity must be confirmed.

Plague (prophylaxis and treatment): Oral, IV: 500 mg every 24 hours for 10-14 days, beginning as soon as possible after exposure. **Note:** Dose of 750 mg once daily may be considered if clinically warranted.

Pneumonia: Oral, IV:

Community-acquired (CAP): 500 mg every 24 hours for 7-14 days or 750 mg every 24 hours for 5 days (efficacy of 5-day regimen for MDRSP not established)

Healthcare-associated (HAP): 750 mg every 24 hours for 7-14 days

Prostatitis (chronic bacterial): Oral, IV: 500 mg every 24 hours for 28 days

Skin and skin structure infections: Oral, IV:

Uncomplicated: 500 mg every 24 hours for 7-10 days

Complicated: 750 mg every 24 hours for 7-14 days

Surgical (preoperative) prophylaxis (off-label use): IV: 500 mg within 120 minutes prior to surgical incision (Bratzler 2013)

Surgical site infections (intestinal or genitourinary tract; perineum or axilla) (off-label use): IV: 750 mg every 24 hours, in combination with metronidazole (IDSA [Stevens 2014])

Traveler's diarrhea (off-label use): Oral: 500 mg for one dose (Sanders 2007)

Tuberculosis, drug-resistant tuberculosis, or intolerance to first-line agents (off-label use): Oral: 500-1000 mg every 24 hours (CDC 2003)

Urethritis, nongonococcal (off-label use) (CDC 2010): Oral: 500 mg every 24 hours for 7 days

Urinary tract infections: Oral, IV:

Uncomplicated: 250 mg once daily for 3 days

Complicated, including pyelonephritis: 250 mg once daily for 10 days **or** 750 mg once daily for 5 days

Pediatric

Acute bacterial rhinosinusitis (off-label use): Oral, IV: 10-20 mg/kg/day divided every 12-24 hours for 10-14 days (maximum: 500 mg daily). **Note:** Recommended in patients with a type I penicillin allergy, after failure of initial therapy or in patients at risk for antibiotic resistance (eg, daycare attendance, age <2 years, recent hospitalization, antibiotic use within the past month) (Chow 2012).

Anthrax (inhalational, postexposure): Oral, IV

Infants ≥6 months and Children ≤50 kg: 8 mg/kg every 12 hours for 60 days (do not exceed 250 mg/dose), beginning as soon as possible after exposure

Children >50 kg: 500 mg every 24 hours for 60 days, beginning as soon as possible after exposure

Community-acquired pneumonia (CAP) (IDSA/PIDS 2011): Note: May consider addition of vancomycin or clindamycin to empiric therapy if community-acquired MRSA suspected; alternative to ceftriaxone or cefotaxime in patients not fully immunized for *H. influenzae* type b and *S. pneumoniae*, or significant local resistance to penicillin in invasive pneumococcal strains.

Infants ≥6 months and Children ≤4 years:

S. pneumoniae (MICs to penicillin ≤2.0 mcg/mL), mild infection or step-down therapy (alternative to amoxicillin): Oral: 8-10 mg/kg/dose every 12 hours (maximum: 750 mg daily)

S. pneumoniae (MICs to penicillin ≥4.0 mcg/mL):

Moderate-to-severe infection (alternative to ceftriaxone): IV: 8-10 mg/kg/dose every 12 hours (maximum: 750 mg daily)

◄

Mild infection, step-down therapy (preferred): Oral: 8-10 mg/kg/dose every 12 hours (maximum: 750 mg daily)

H. influenzae, moderate-to-severe infection (alternative to ampicillin, ceftriaxone, or cefotaxime): IV: 8-10 mg/kg/dose every 12 hours (maximum: 750 mg daily)

Atypical pathogens, moderate-to-severe infection (alternative to azithromycin) or empiric treatment (alternative to azithromycin +/- beta-lactam; should be limited to macrolide allergic/intolerant patients): Oral, IV: 8-10 mg/kg/dose every 12 hours (maximum: 750 mg daily)

Children 5-16 years:

S. pneumoniae (MICs to penicillin ≤2.0 mcg/mL), mild infection or step-down therapy (alternative to amoxicillin): Oral: 8-10 mg/kg/dose once daily (maximum: 750 mg daily)

S. pneumoniae (MICs to penicillin ≥4.0 mcg/mL):

Moderate-to-severe infection (alternative to ceftriaxone): IV: 8-10 mg/kg/dose once daily (maximum: 750 mg daily)

Mild infection, step-down therapy (preferred): Oral: 8-10 mg/kg/dose once daily (maximum: 750 mg daily)

H. influenzae, moderate-to-severe infection (alternative to ampicillin, ceftriaxone, or cefotaxime): IV: 8-10 mg/kg/dose once daily (maximum: 750 mg daily)

Atypical pathogens:

Moderate-to-severe infection (alternative to azithromycin): Oral, IV: 8-10 mg/kg/dose once daily (maximum: 750 mg daily)

Mild infection, step-down therapy (alternative to azithromycin in adolescents with skeletal maturity): Oral: 500 mg once daily

Plague (prophylaxis and treatment): Infants ≥6 months and Children: Oral, IV:

≤50 kg: 8 mg/kg every 12 hours for 10-14 days (do not exceed 250 mg/dose), beginning as soon as possible after exposure

>50 kg: 500 mg every 24 hours for 10-14 days, beginning as soon as possible after exposure. **Note:** Dose of 750 mg once daily may be considered if clinically warranted.

Surgical (preoperative) prophylaxis (off-label use): Children ≥1 year: IV: 10 mg/kg within 120 minutes prior to surgical incision (maximum: 500 mg) (Bratzler 2013)

Renal Impairment IV, Oral:

Normal renal function dosing of 250 mg daily:

CrCl 20-49 mL/minute: No dosage adjustment required.

CrCl 10-19 mL/minute: Administer 250 mg every 48 hours (except in uncomplicated UTI, where no dosage adjustment is required).

Hemodialysis/chronic ambulatory peritoneal dialysis (CAPD): No information available.

Normal renal function dosing of 500 mg daily:

CrCl 20-49 mL/minute: Administer 500 mg initial dose, followed by 250 mg every 24 hours.

CrCl 10-19 mL/minute: Administer 500 mg initial dose, followed by 250 mg every 48 hours.

Hemodialysis/chronic ambulatory peritoneal dialysis (CAPD): Administer 500 mg initial dose, followed by 250 mg every 48 hours; supplemental doses are not required following either hemodialysis or CAPD

Normal renal function dosing of 750 mg daily:
CrCl 20-49 mL/minute: Administer 750 mg every 48 hours.
CrCl 10-19 mL/minute: Administer 750 mg initial dose, followed by 500 mg every 48 hours.
Hemodialysis/chronic ambulatory peritoneal dialysis (CAPD): Administer 750 mg initial dose, followed by 500 mg every 48 hours; supplemental doses are not required following either hemodialysis or CAPD.
Normal renal function dosing of 750 or 1000 mg daily (treatment of tuberculosis **only**) (CDC 2003): CrCl <30 mL/minute: Administer 750 or 1000 mg 3 times per week (in hemodialysis patients administer after dialysis on dialysis days).
Continuous renal replacement therapy (CRRT) (Heintz 2009; Trotman 2005): Drug clearance is highly dependent on the method of renal replacement, filter type, and flow rate. Appropriate dosing requires close monitoring of pharmacologic response, signs of adverse reactions due to drug accumulation, as well as drug concentrations in relation to target trough (if appropriate). The following are general recommendations only (based on dialysate flow/ultrafiltration rates of 1-2 L/hour and minimal residual renal function) and should not supersede clinical judgment:
CVVH: Loading dose of 500-750 mg followed by 250 mg every 24 hours.
CVVHD: Loading dose of 500-750 mg followed by 250-500 mg every 24 hours.
CVVHDF: Loading dose of 500-750 mg followed by 250-750 mg every 24 hours.
Hepatic Impairment IV, Oral: No dosage adjustment provided in manufacturer's labeling (has not been studied). However, dosage adjustment unlikely due to limited hepatic metabolism.
Additional Information Complete prescribing information should be consulted for additional detail.
Medication Guide Available Yes
Dosage Forms Excipient information presented when available (limited, particularly for generics); consult specific product labeling. [DSC] = Discontinued product
Solution, Intravenous [preservative free]:
Levaquin: 250 mg/50 mL (50 mL [DSC]); 500 mg/100 mL (100 mL [DSC]); 750 mg/150 mL (150 mL [DSC])
Generic: 250 mg/50 mL (50 mL); 500 mg/100 mL (100 mL); 750 mg/150 mL (150 mL); 25 mg/mL (20 mL, 30 mL)
Solution, Oral:
Levaquin: 25 mg/mL (480 mL [DSC]) [contains propylene glycol]
Generic: 25 mg/mL (10 mL, 20 mL, 100 mL, 200 mL, 480 mL)
Tablet, Oral:
Levaquin: 250 mg, 500 mg, 750 mg
Generic: 250 mg, 500 mg, 750 mg

◆ **Levo-folinic Acid** see LEVOleucovorin on page 1041

LEVOleucovorin (lee voe loo koe VOR in)
Brand Names: US Fusilev
Index Terms 6S-leucovorin; Calcium Levoleucovorin; L-leucovorin; Levofolinic Acid; Levo-leucovorin; Levoleucovorin Calcium Pentahydrate; S-leucovorin

◀ **Pharmacologic Category** Antidote; Chemotherapy Modulating Agent; Rescue Agent (Chemotherapy)

Use

Colorectal cancer, metastatic: Palliative treatment of advanced, metastatic colorectal cancer (in combination with fluorouracil)

High-dose methotrexate rescue: Rescue agent after high-dose methotrexate therapy in osteosarcoma treatment

Folic acid antagonist overdose: Antidote for impaired methotrexate elimination and for inadvertent overdosage of folic acid antagonists

Limitations of use: Levoleucovorin is not approved for pernicious anemia and megaloblastic anemias secondary to the lack of vitamin B_{12} (improper use may result in hematologic remission with progressive neurologic manifestations)

Labeled Contraindications Previous allergic reaction to folic acid or leucovorin calcium (folinic acid)

Pregnancy Considerations Animal reproduction studies have not been conducted. Levoleucovorin is the levo isomeric form of racemic leucovorin, a biologically active form of folic acid. Adequate amounts of folic acid are recommended during pregnancy.

Breast-Feeding Considerations It is not known if levoleucovorin is excreted in breast milk. Due to the potential for serious adverse reactions in the nursing infant, a decision should be made to discontinue breast-feeding or to discontinue levoleucovorin, taking into account the importance of treatment to the mother. Levoleucovorin is the levo isomeric form of racemic leucovorin, a biologically active form of folic acid. Adequate amounts of folic acid are recommended in breast-feeding women.

Warnings/Precautions For IV administration only; do not administer intrathecally. Due to calcium content, do not administer IV solutions at a rate >160 mg levoleucovorin/minute. Methotrexate serum concentrations should be monitored to determine dose and duration of levoleucovorin therapy; dose may need to be increased or administration prolonged in situations where methotrexate excretion may be delayed (eg, ascites, pleural effusion, renal insufficiency, inadequate hydration). When used for the treatment of accidental folic acid antagonist overdose, administer as soon as possible.

Levoleucovorin and leucovorin calcium enhance the toxicity of fluorouracil. Deaths due to severe enterocolitis, diarrhea, and dehydration have been reported in elderly patients receiving weekly leucovorin calcium in combination with fluorouracil. Levoleucovorin is indicated in combination with fluorouracil for the palliative treatment of colorectal cancer; when administered together, the fluorouracil dose is reduced (compared to fluorouracil dosing without levoleucovorin). The typical fluorouracil gastrointestinal toxicities (eg, diarrhea, stomatitis) may be of greater severity or longer duration with fluorouracil and levoleucovorin combination therapy. Symptoms of gastrointestinal toxicity should be completely resolved prior to treatment. Elderly and/or debilitated patients are at higher risk for severe gastrointestinal toxicity. Concomitant use of leucovorin calcium and sulfamethoxazole-trimethoprim for the acute treatment of PCP in patients with HIV infection has been associated with increased rates of treatment failure and morbidity; may also occur with levoleucovorin. Seizures and/or syncope have been reported with leucovorin calcium; generally in patients with CNS metastases or other underlying risk factors. Potentially significant drug-drug interactions may exist, requiring dose or frequency adjustment, additional monitoring, and/or selection of alternative therapy.

Adverse Reactions Note: Adverse reactions reported with levoleucovorin either as a part of combination chemotherapy or following chemotherapy.
>10%:
  Central nervous system: Fatigue (≤29%)
  Dermatologic: Dermatitis (6% to 29%), alopecia (≤26%)
  Gastrointestinal: Stomatitis (38% to 72%; grades 3/4: 6% to 12%), diarrhea (6% to 70%; grades 3/4: ≤19%), nausea (19% to 62%), vomiting (38% to 40%), anorexia/appetite decreased (≤24%), abdominal pain (≤14%)
  Neuromuscular & skeletal: Weakness/malaise (≤29%)
1% to 10%:
  Central nervous system: Confusion (6%)
  Gastrointestinal: Dyspepsia (6%), taste perversion (6%), typhlitis (6%)
  Neuromuscular & skeletal: Neuropathy (6%)
  Renal: Renal function abnormal (6%)
  Respiratory: Dyspnea (6%)
<1%, postmarketing, and/or case reports: Allergic reactions, pruritus, rash, rigors, temperature changes

Drug Interactions

Metabolism/Transport Effects None known.

Avoid Concomitant Use
  Avoid concomitant use of LEVOleucovorin with any of the following: Raltitrexed; Trimethoprim

Increased Effect/Toxicity
  LEVOleucovorin may increase the levels/effects of: Capecitabine; Fluorouracil (Systemic); Fluorouracil (Topical); Tegafur

Decreased Effect
  LEVOleucovorin may decrease the levels/effects of: Fosphenytoin; PHENobarbital; Phenytoin; Primidone; Raltitrexed; Trimethoprim

  The levels/effects of LEVOleucovorin may be decreased by: Glucarpidase

Storage/Stability
  Lyophilized powder: Prior to reconstitution, store intact vials at 25°C (77°F); excursions permitted from 15°C to 30°C (59°F to 86°F). Protect from light. Initial reconstituted solution in the vial may be stored for 12 hours at room temperature. Solutions further diluted for infusion in NS are stable for 12 hours at room temperature. Solutions further diluted for infusion in D₅W are stable for 4 hours at room temperature.
  Injection solution: Store intact vials between 2°C and 8°C (36°F and 46°F). Protect from light. Store in carton until contents are used. Solutions further diluted for infusion in NS or D₅W are stable for up to 4 hours at room temperature.

Preparation for Administration
  Lyophilized powder: Reconstitute the 50 mg vial with 5.3 mL NS (preservative free) to a concentration of 10 mg/mL. Do not use if solution appears cloudy or contains a precipitate. May further dilute for infusion in NS or D₅W to a final concentration of 0.5 to 5 mg/mL.
  Injection solution: May further dilute for infusion in NS or D₅W to a concentration of 0.5 mg/mL.
  Do not prepare with other products in the same admixture; may cause precipitation.

Mechanism of Action Levoleucovorin counteracts the toxic (and therapeutic) effects of folic acid antagonists (eg, methotrexate) which act by inhibiting dihydrofolate reductase. Levoleucovorin is the levo isomeric and ▶

pharmacologic active form of leucovorin (levoleucovorin does not require reduction by dihydrofolate reductase). A reduced derivative of folic acid, leucovorin supplies the necessary cofactor blocked by methotrexate.

Leucovorin enhances the activity (and toxicity) of fluorouracil by stabilizing the binding of 5-fluoro-2'-deoxyuridine-5'-monophosphate (FdUMP; a fluorouracil metabolite) to thymidylate synthetase resulting in inhibition of this enzyme.

Pharmacodynamics/Kinetics

Metabolism: Converted to the active reduced form of folate, 5-methyl-tetrahydrofolate (5-methyl-THF; active)

Half-life elimination: Total-tetrahydrofolate: 5.1 hours; (6S)-5-methyl-5,6,7,8-tetrahydrofolate: 6.8 hours

Time to peak, serum: IV (healthy volunteers): 0.9 hours

Dosing

Adult & Geriatric Note: Levoleucovorin, when substituted in place of leucovorin calcium (the racemic form), is dosed at **one-half** the usual dose of leucovorin calcium:

Colorectal cancer, metastatic: IV: The following regimens have been used (in combination with fluorouracil; fluorouracil doses may need to be adjusted for toxicity; no adjustment is required for the levoleucovorin dose):

100 mg/m^2/day over at least 3 minutes (followed by fluorouracil 370 mg/m^2/day) for 5 days every 4 weeks for 2 cycles, then every 4 to 5 weeks depending on recovery from toxicities, **or**

10 mg/m^2/day (followed by fluorouracil 425 mg/m^2/day) for 5 days every 4 weeks for 2 cycles, then every 4 to 5 weeks depending on recovery from toxicities, **or**

Alternative dosing: Levoleucovorin, when substituted in place of leucovorin calcium within a chemotherapy regimen, is dosed at **one-half** the usual dose of leucovorin calcium (Goldberg 1997; Kovoor 2009)

High-dose methotrexate rescue: IV: Usual dose: 7.5 mg (~5 mg/m^2) every 6 hours for 10 doses, beginning 24 hours after the start of the methotrexate infusion (based on a methotrexate dose of 12 g/m^2 IV over 4 hours). Levoleucovorin (and hydration and urinary alkalinization) should be continued and/or adjusted until the methotrexate level is <0.05 micromolar (5 x 10^{-8} M) as follows:

Normal methotrexate elimination (serum methotrexate levels ~10 micromolar at 24 hours post administration, 1 micromolar at 48 hours and <0.2 micromolar at 72 hours post infusion): 7.5 mg IV every 6 hours for 10 doses

Delayed late methotrexate elimination (serum methotrexate levels >0.2 micromolar at 72 hours and >0.05 micromolar at 96 hours post methotrexate infusion): Continue 7.5 mg IV every 6 hours until methotrexate level is <0.05 micromolar

Delayed early methotrexate elimination and/or evidence of acute renal injury (serum methotrexate level ≥50 micromolar at 24 hours, ≥5 micromolar at 48 hours or a doubling or more of the serum creatinine level at 24 hours post methotrexate infusion): 75 mg IV every 3 hours until methotrexate level is <1 micromolar, followed by 7.5 mg IV every 3 hours until methotrexate level is <0.05 micromolar

Significant clinical toxicity in the presence of less severe abnormalities in methotrexate elimination or renal function (as described above): Extend levoleucovorin treatment for an additional 24 hours (total of 14 doses) in subsequent treatment cycles.

Delayed methotrexate elimination due to third space fluid accumulation, renal insufficiency, or inadequate hydration: May require higher levoleucovorin doses or prolonged administration.

Folic acid antagonist overdose: IV: 7.5 mg (~5 mg/m²) every 6 hours; continue until the methotrexate level is <0.01 micromolar (10^{-8} M). Initiate treatment as soon as possible after methotrexate overdose. Increase the levoleucovorin dose to 50 mg/m² IV every 3 hours if the 24-hour serum creatinine has increased 50% over baseline, or if the 24 hour methotrexate level is >5 micromolar (5×10^{-6} M), or if the 48-hour methotrexate level is >0.9 micromolar (9×10^{-7} M); continue levoleucovorin until the methotrexate level is <0.01 micromolar (10^{-8} M). Hydration (aggressive) and urinary alkalinization (with sodium bicarbonate) should also be maintained.

Pediatric Note: Levoleucovorin, when substituted in place of leucovorin calcium (the racemic form), is dosed at **one-half** the usual dose of leucovorin calcium:

High-dose methotrexate rescue: Refer to adult dosing.

Folic acid antagonist overdose: Refer to adult dosing.

Renal Impairment There are no dosage adjustments provided in the manufacturer's labeling.

Hepatic Impairment There are no dosage adjustments provided in the manufacturer's labeling.

Administration For IV administration only; do not administer intrathecally. Administer by slow IV push or infusion over at least 3 minutes, not to exceed 160 mg/minute (due to calcium content).

For colorectal cancer: Levoleucovorin has also been administered (off-label administration rate) as IV infusion over 2 hours (Comella 2000; Tournigand 2006).

Monitoring Parameters High-dose methotrexate therapy or methotrexate overdose (inadvertent): Serum methotrexate and creatinine levels at least once daily. Monitor fluid and electrolyte status in patients with delayed methotrexate elimination (likely to experience renal toxicity).

Dosage Forms Excipient information presented when available (limited, particularly for generics); consult specific product labeling.

Solution, Intravenous:

Generic: 175 mg/17.5 mL (17.5 mL)

Solution, Intravenous [preservative free]:

Generic: 175 mg/17.5 mL (17.5 mL); 250 mg/25 mL (25 mL)

Solution Reconstituted, Intravenous:

Fusilev: 50 mg (1 ea)

♦ **Levo-leucovorin** *see* LEVOleucovorin *on page 1041*

♦ **Levoleucovorin Calcium Pentahydrate** *see* LEVOleucovorin *on page 1041*

Levorphanol (lee VOR fa nole)

Index Terms Levo-Dromoran; Levorphan Tartrate; Levorphanol Tartrate

Pharmacologic Category Analgesic, Opioid

Use Relief of moderate-to-severe pain; preoperative sedation/analgesia; management of chronic pain (eg, cancer) requiring opioid therapy

Pregnancy Risk Factor C

Dosing

Adult & Geriatric Note: These are guidelines and do not represent the maximum doses that may be required in all patients. Doses should be titrated to pain relief/prevention.

◀ **Acute pain (moderate-to-severe):** *Oral:* Initial: Opioid-naive: 2 mg every 6-8 hours as needed; patients with prior opioid exposure may require higher initial doses; usual dosage range: 2-4 mg every 6-8 hours as needed

Note: The American Pain Society recommends an initial dose of 4 mg for severe pain in adults (APS, 6th ed)

Chronic pain: Patients taking opioids chronically may become tolerant and require doses higher than the usual dosage range to maintain the desired effect. Tolerance can be managed by appropriate dose titration. **There is no optimal or maximal dose for levorphanol in chronic pain. The appropriate dose is one that relieves pain throughout its dosing interval without causing unmanageable side effects.**

Renal Impairment Use with caution; initial dose should be reduced in severe renal impairment.

Hepatic Impairment Use with caution; initial dose should be reduced in severe hepatic impairment.

Additional Information Complete prescribing information should be consulted for additional detail.

Dosage Forms Excipient information presented when available (limited, particularly for generics); consult specific product labeling.

Tablet, Oral, as tartrate:

Generic: 2 mg

Controlled Substance C-II

- ◆ **Levorphanol Tartrate** *see* Levorphanol *on page 1045*
- ◆ **Levorphan Tartrate** *see* Levorphanol *on page 1045*
- ◆ **Levulan Kerastick** *see* Aminolevulinic Acid *on page 94*
- ◆ **LH-RH Agonist** *see* Histrelin *on page 816*

Lidocaine and Prilocaine (LYE doe kane & PRIL oh kane)

Brand Names: US EMLA; Livixil Pak; LP Lite Pak; Oraqix; Relador Pak

Brand Names: Canada EMLA; Oraqix

Index Terms Prilocaine and Lidocaine

Pharmacologic Category Local Anesthetic

Use

US labeling:

Cream: Topical anesthetic for use on normal intact skin to provide local analgesia; for use on genital mucous membranes for superficial minor surgery; and as pretreatment for infiltration anesthesia.

Periodontal gel: Topical anesthetic for use in periodontal pockets during scaling and/or root planing procedures

Canadian labeling:

Cream: Topical anesthetic for use on intact skin in connection with: IV cannulation or venipuncture; superficial surgical procedures (eg, split skin grafting, electrolysis, removal of molluscum contagiosum); laser treatment for superficial skin surgery (eg, telangiectasia, port wine stains, warts, moles, skin nodules, scar tissue); surgical procedures of genital mucosa (≤10 minutes) on small superficial localized lesions (eg, removal of condylomata by laser or cautery, biopsies); local infiltration anesthesia in genital mucous membranes; mechanical cleansing/debridement of leg ulcers; vaccination with measles-mumps-rubella (MMR), diphtheria-pertussis-tetanus-poliovirus (DPTP), *Haemophilus influenzae* b, and hepatitis B.

Patch: Topical anesthetic for use on intact skin in connection with IV cannulation or venipuncture; vaccination with measles-mumps-rubella (MMR), diphtheria-pertussis-tetanus-poliovirus (DPTP), *Haemophilus influenzae* b, and hepatitis B.

Periodontal gel: Topical anesthetic for use in periodontal pockets during scaling and/or root planing procedures

Pregnancy Risk Factor B

Dosing

Adult Anesthetic: Topical:

Cream (intact skin): **Note:** Apply a thick layer to intact skin and cover with an occlusive dressing. Dermal analgesia can be expected to increase for up to 3 hours under occlusive dressing and persist for 1 to 2 hours after removal of the cream.

US labeling:

Minor dermal procedures (eg, IV cannulation or venipuncture): Apply 2.5 g (1/2 of the 5 g tube) over 20 to 25 cm² of skin surface area) for at least 1 hour

Major dermal procedures (eg, more painful dermatological procedures involving a larger skin area such as split thickness skin graft harvesting): Apply 2 g per 10 cm² of skin and allow to remain in contact with the skin for at least 2 hours.

Adult male genital skin (eg, pretreatment prior to local anesthetic infiltration): Apply 1 g per 10 cm² to the skin surface for 15 minutes. Local anesthetic infiltration should be performed immediately after removal of cream.

Adult female genital mucous membranes: Minor procedures (eg, removal of condylomata acuminata, pretreatment for local anesthetic infiltration): Apply 5 to 10 g for 5 to 10 minutes. The local anesthetic infiltration or procedure should be performed immediately after removal of cream.

Canadian labeling:

Minor dermal procedures (eg, IV cannulation, venipuncture, surgical or laser treatment): Apply 2 g (~1/2 of the 5 g tube) over ~13.5 cm² for at least 1 hour but no longer than 5 hours

Major dermal procedures (eg, split-skin grafting): 1.5 to 2 g per 10 cm² (maximum: 60 g per 400 cm²) for at least 2 hours but no longer than 5 hours

Genital mucosa (eg, surgical procedures ≤10 minutes such as localized wart removal, and prior to local anesthetic infiltration): Apply 2 g (~1/2 of 5 g tube) per lesion (maximum: 10 g) for 5 to 10 minutes. Initiate procedure immediately after removing cream.

Leg ulcers (eg, mechanical cleansing/surgical debridement): Apply ~1 to 2 g per 10 cm² (maximum: 10 g) for at least 30 minutes and up to 60 minutes for necrotic tissue that is more difficult to penetrate. Initiate procedure immediately after removing cream.

Periodontal gel (Oraqix): Apply on gingival margin around selected teeth using the blunt-tipped applicator included in package. Wait 30 seconds, then fill the periodontal pockets using the blunt-tipped applicator until gel becomes visible at the gingival margin. Wait another 30 seconds before starting treatment. May reapply; maximum recommended dose: One treatment session: 5 cartridges (8.5 g)

Transdermal patch [Canadian product]: Minor procedures (eg, needle insertion): Apply 1 or more patches to intact skin surface area <10 cm² for at least 1 hour (maximum application time: 5 hours)

◀ **Geriatric** Smaller areas of treatment may be necessary depending on status of patient (eg, debilitated, impaired hepatic function). Refer to adult dosing.

Pediatric Although the incidence of systemic adverse effects is very low, caution should be exercised, particularly when applying over large areas and leaving on for >2 hours

Local anesthetic (procedures): Infants and Children (intact skin): Topical: **Note:** If a patient >3 months of age does not meet the minimum weight requirement, the maximum total dose should be restricted to the corresponding maximum based on patient weight.

Cream: Should **not** be used in neonates with a gestation age <37 weeks nor in infants <12 months of age who are receiving treatment with methemoglobin-inducing agents

Dosing is based on child's age and weight:

Age 0 to 3 months or <5 kg: Apply a maximum of 1 g over no more than 10 cm^2 of skin; leave on for no longer than 1 hour

Age 3 months to 12 months and >5 kg: Apply no more than a maximum 2 g total over no more than 20 cm^2 of skin; leave on for no longer than 4 hours

Age 1 to 6 years and >10 kg: Apply no more than a maximum of 10 g total over no more than 100 cm^2 of skin. US labeling recommends leaving on for no longer than 4 hours. Canadian labeling recommends leaving on for no longer than 5 hours.

Age 7 to 12 years and >20 kg: Apply no more than a maximum 20 g total over no more than 200 cm^2 of skin. US labeling recommends leaving on for no longer than 4 hours. Canadian labeling recommends leaving on for no longer than 5 hours.

Transdermal patch [Canadian product]: **Note:** Should not be used in neonates with a gestation age <37 weeks nor in infants <12 months of age who are receiving treatment with methemoglobin-inducing agents

Dosing is based on child's age and weight: Apply patch(es) to skin area(s) <10 cm^2:

Age 0 to 3 months or <5 kg: Apply 1 patch and leave on for ~1 hour (do not exceed 1-hour application time); do not apply more than 1 patch at same time; safety of repeated dosing not established

Age 3 months to 12 months and >5 kg: Apply 1 to 2 patches for ~1 hour (maximum application time: 4 hours); do not apply more than 2 patches at the same time

Age 1 to 6 years and >10 kg: Apply 1 or more patches for minimum of 1 hour (maximum application time: 5 hours); maximum dose: 10 patches

Age 7 to 12 years and >20 kg: Apply 1 or more patches for a minimum of 1 hour (maximum application time: 5 hours); maximum dose: 20 patches

Renal Impairment There are no dosage adjustments provided in the manufacturer labeling. Lidocaine and prilocaine primarily undergo hepatic metabolism and their pharmacokinetics are not expected to be changed significantly in renal impairment.

Hepatic Impairment Smaller areas of treatment are recommended for patients with severe hepatic impairment.

Additional Information Complete prescribing information should be consulted for additional detail.

Dosage Forms Excipient information presented when available (limited, particularly for generics); consult specific product labeling.

Cream, topical:

EMLA: Lidocaine 2.5% and prilocaine 2.5% (5 g, 30 g)

Livixil Pak: Lidocaine 2.5% and prilocaine 2.5% (3 x 30 g) [packaged with occlusive dressing]

LP Lite Pak: Lidocaine 2.5% and prilocaine 2.5% (2 x 30 g) [packaged with occlusive dressing]

Relador Pak: Lidocaine 2.5% and prilocaine 2.5% (3 x 30 g) [packaged with occlusive dressing]

Generic: Lidocaine 2.5% and prilocaine 2.5% (5 g, 30 g)

Gel, periodontal:

Oraqix: Lidocaine 2.5% and prilocaine 2.5% (1.7 g)

Dosage Forms: Canada Excipient information presented when available (limited, particularly for generics); consult specific product labeling.

Patch, transdermal:

EMLA Patch: Lidocaine 2.5% and prilocaine 2.5% per patch (2s, 20s) [active contact surface area of each 1 g patch: $10\ cm^2$; surface area of entire patch: $40\ cm^2$]

◆ Lilly CT-3231 *see* Vindesine *on page 1760*

Linezolid (li NE zoh lid)

Brand Names: US Zyvox

Brand Names: Canada Apo-Linezolid; Linezolid Injection; Sandoz-Linezolid; Zyvoxam

Pharmacologic Category Antibiotic, Oxazolidinone

Use

Enterococcal infections, vancomycin-resistant: Treatment of vancomycin-resistant *Enterococcus faecium* infections, including cases with concurrent bacteremia.

Pneumonia:

Community-acquired: Treatment of community-acquired pneumonia caused by *Streptococcus pneumoniae*, including cases with concurrent bacteremia, or *Staphylococcus aureus* (methicillin-susceptible isolates only).

Hospital-acquired or healthcare-associated: Treatment of hospital-acquired or healthcare-associated pneumonia caused by *S. aureus* (methicillin-susceptible and -resistant isolates), or *S. pneumoniae*.

Skin and skin structure infections:

Complicated: Treatment of complicated skin and skin structure infections, including diabetic foot infections, without concomitant osteomyelitis, caused by *S. aureus* (methicillin-susceptible and -resistant isolates), *Streptococcus pyogenes*, or *Streptococcus agalactiae*.

Uncomplicated: Treatment of uncomplicated skin and skin structure infections caused by *S. aureus* (methicillin-susceptible isolates) or *S. pyogenes*.

Limitations of use: Linezolid has not been studied in the treatment of decubitus ulcers. Linezolid is not indicated for treatment of gram-negative infections; if a concomitant gram-negative pathogen is documented or suspected, initiate specific therapy immediately.

Pregnancy Risk Factor C

Dosing

Adult & Geriatric

Usual dosage: Oral, IV: 600 mg every 12 hours

Indication-specific dosing:

Enterococcal infections,vancomycin-resistant, including concurrent bacteremia: Oral, IV: 600 mg every 12 hours for 14 to 28 days

◀

Pneumonia:

Community-acquired (CAP):

Manufacturer's labeling (includes concurrent bacteremia): Oral, IV: 600 mg every 12 hours for 10 to 14 days.

Alternate dosing (Liu 2011): Oral, IV: *S. aureus* (methicillin-resistant): 600 mg every 12 hours for 7 to 21 days

Hospital-acquired or healthcare-associated:

Manufacturer's labeling: Oral, IV: 600 mg every 12 hours for 10 to 14 days.

Note: May consider 7-day treatment course (versus manufacturer recommended 10 to 14 days) in patients with healthcare-, hospital-, and ventilator- associated pneumonia who have demonstrated good clinical response (ATS/IDSA 2005).

Alternate dosing (Liu 2011): Oral, IV: *S. aureus* (methicillin-resistant): 600 mg every 12 hours for 7 to 21 days

Skin and skin structure infections, complicated: Oral, IV: 600 mg every 12 hours for 10 to 14 days. **Note:** For diabetic foot infections, initial treatment duration is up to 4 weeks depending on severity of infection and response to therapy (Lipsky 2012).

Skin and skin structure infections, uncomplicated: Oral: 400 mg every 12 hours for 10 to 14 days. **Note:** 400 mg dose is recommended in the product labeling; however, 600 mg dose is commonly employed clinically; consider 5- to 10-day treatment course as opposed to the manufacturer recommended 10 to 14 days (Liu 2011; Stevens 2014). For diabetic foot infections, may extend treatment duration up to 4 weeks if slow to resolve (Lipsky 2012).

Brain abscess, subdural empyema, spinal epidural abscess (*S. aureus* [methicillin-resistant]) (off-label use) (Liu 2011): Oral, IV: 600 mg every 12 hours for 4 to 6 weeks

Meningitis (*S. aureus* [methicillin-resistant]) (off-label use) (Liu 2011): Oral, IV: 600 mg every 12 hours for 2 weeks

Osteomyelitis (*S. aureus* [methicillin-resistant]) (off-label use) (Liu 2011): Oral, IV: 600 mg every 12 hours for a minimum of 8 weeks (some experts combine with rifampin)

Prosthetic joint infection (off-label use):

Enterococcus spp (penicillin-susceptible or -resistant) (alternative treatment): Oral, IV: 600 mg every 12 hours for 4 to 6 weeks (consider adding an aminoglycoside) followed by an oral antibiotic suppressive regimen (Osmon 2013)

Staphylococci (oxacillin-sensitive or -resistant) (alternative treatment): Oral, IV: 600 mg every 12 hours for 2 to 6 weeks used in combination with rifampin followed by oral antibiotic treatment and suppressive regimens (Osmon 2013)

Septic arthritis (*S. aureus* [methicillin-resistant]) (off-label use) (Liu 2011): Oral, IV: 600 mg every 12 hours for 3 to 4 weeks

Septic thrombosis of cavernous or dural venous sinus (*S. aureus* [methicillin-resistant]) (off-label use) (Liu 2011): Oral, IV: 600 mg every 12 hours for 4 to 6 weeks

Pediatric

Usual dosage: Oral, IV:

Children ≤11 years: 10 mg/kg (maximum: 600 mg/dose) every 8 hours

Children ≥12 years and Adolescents: Refer to adult dosing.

Indication-specific dosing:

Enterococcal infections, vancomycin-resistant, including concurrent bacteremia: Oral, IV:

Infants and Children ≤11 years: 10 mg/kg every 8 hours for 14 to 28 days

Children ≥12 years and Adolescents: Refer to adult dosing.

Pneumonia:

Community-acquired (CAP):

Manufacturer's labeling (includes concurrent bacteremia): Oral, IV:

Infants and Children ≤11 years: 10 mg/kg/dose every 8 hours for 10 to 14 days

Children ≥12 years and Adolescents: Refer to adult dosing.

Alternate dosing:

Infants >3 months and Children ≤11 years (IDSA/PIDS 2011):

S. pneumoniae (MICs to penicillin ≤2.0 mcg/mL), mild infection or step-down therapy (alternative to amoxicillin): Oral: 10 mg/kg/dose every 8 hours

S. pneumoniae (MICs to penicillin ≥4.0 mcg/mL):

Severe infection (alternative to ceftriaxone): IV: 10 mg/kg/dose every 8 hours

Mild infection, step-down therapy (preferred): Oral: 10 mg/kg/dose every 8 hours

S. aureus (methicillin-resistant/clindamycin-susceptible):

Severe infection (alternative to vancomycin or clindamycin): IV: 10 mg/kg/dose every 8 hours

Mild infection, step-down therapy (alternative to clindamycin): Oral: 10 mg/kg/dose every 8 hours

S. aureus (methicillin- and clindamycin-resistant):

Severe infection (alternative to vancomycin): IV: 10 mg/kg/dose every 8 hours

Mild infection, step-down therapy (preferred): Oral: 10 mg/kg/dose every 8 hours

Children ≤11 years (Liu 2011): Oral, IV: *S. aureus* (methicillin-resistant): 10 mg/kg/dose every 8 hours for 7 to 21 days (maximum: 600 mg/dose)

Children ≥12 years and Adolescents (IDSA/PIDS 2011):

S. pneumoniae (MICs to penicillin ≤2.0 mcg/mL), mild infection or step-down therapy (alternative to amoxicillin): Oral: 10 mg/kg/dose every 12 hours

S. pneumoniae (MICs to penicillin ≥4.0 mcg/mL)

Severe infection (alternative to ceftriaxone): IV: 10 mg/kg/dose every 12 hours

Mild infection, step-down therapy (preferred): Oral: 10 mg/kg/dose every 12 hours

S. aureus (methicillin-resistant/clindamycin-susceptible):

Severe infection (alternative to vancomycin/clindamycin): IV: 10 mg/kg/dose every 12 hours

Mild infection, step-down therapy (alternative to clindamycin): Oral: 10 mg/kg/dose every 12 hours

S. aureus (methicillin- and clindamycin-resistant):

Severe infection (alternative to vancomycin): IV: 10 mg/kg/dose every 12 hours

Mild infection, step-down therapy (preferred): Oral: 10 mg/kg/dose every 12 hours

Children ≥12 years and Adolescents (Liu 2011): *S. aureus* (methicillin-resistant): Refer to adult dosing.

◄ Hospital-acquired or healthcare-associated: Oral, IV:

Manufacturer's labeling:

Infants and Children ≤11 years: 10 mg/kg every 8 hours for 10 to 14 days

Children ≥12 years and Adolescents: Refer to adult dosing.

Note: May consider 7-day treatment course (versus manufacturer recommended 10 to 14 days) in patients with healthcare-, hospital-, and ventilator-associated pneumonia who have demonstrated good clinical response (ATS/IDSA 2005).

Alternate dosing (Liu 2011): S. aureus (methicillin-resistant):

Infants and Children ≤11 years: 10 mg/kg/dose every 8 hours for 7 to 21 days (maximum: 600 mg/dose)

Children ≥12 years and Adolescents: Refer to adult dosing.

Skin and skin structure infections, complicated: Oral, IV:

Infants and Children ≤11 years: 10 mg/kg every 8 hours for 10 to 14 days

Children ≥12 years and Adolescents: Refer to adult dosing.

Skin and skin structure infections, uncomplicated: Oral:

Infants and Children <5 years: 10 mg/kg every 8 hours for 10 to 14 days

Children 5 to 11 years: 10 mg/kg every 12 hours for 10 to 14 days

Children ≥12 years and Adolescents: 600 mg every 12 hours for 10 to 14 days

Brain abscess, subdural empyema, spinal epidural abscess (*S. aureus* [methicillin-resistant]) (off-label use) (Liu 2011): Oral, IV: **Note:** The manufacturer does not recommend the use of linezolid for empiric treatment of pediatric CNS infections since therapeutic linezolid concentrations are not consistently achieved or maintained in the CSF of patients with ventriculoperitoneal shunts.

Children ≤11 years: 10 mg/kg every 8 hours for 4 to 6 weeks (maximum: 600 mg/dose)

Children ≥12 years and Adolescents: Refer to adult dosing.

Meningitis (*S. aureus* [methicillin-resistant]) (off-label use) (Liu 2011): Oral, IV:

Infants and Children ≤11 years: 10 mg/kg every 8 hours for 2 weeks (maximum: 600 mg/dose)

Children ≥12 years and Adolescents: Refer to adult dosing.

Osteomyelitis (*S. aureus* [methicillin-resistant]) (off-label use) (Liu 2011): Oral, IV:

Infants and Children ≤11 years: 10 mg/kg every 8 hours for a minimum of 4 to 6 weeks (maximum: 600 mg/dose)

Children ≥12 years and Adolescents: Refer to adult dosing.

Septic arthritis (*S. aureus* [methicillin-resistant]) (off-label use) (Liu 2011): Oral, IV:

Infants and Children ≤11 years: 10 mg/kg every 8 hours for 3 to 4 weeks (maximum: 600 mg/dose)

Children ≥12 years and Adolescents: Refer to adult dosing.

Septic thrombosis of cavernous or dural venous sinus (*S. aureus* [methicillin-resistant]) (off-label use) (Liu 2011): Oral, IV:

Children ≤11 years: 10 mg/kg every 8 hours for 4 to 6 weeks (maximum: 600 mg/dose)

Children ≥12 years and Adolescents: Refer to adult dosing.

Renal Impairment

Mild to severe impairment: No dosage adjustment necessary. The two primary metabolites may accumulate in patients with renal impairment but the clinical significance is unknown; use with caution.

End-stage renal disease (ESRD) on intermittent hemodialysis (IHD):
  Manufacturer's labeling: Dialyzable (~30% removed during 3-hour dialysis session): Administer after hemodialysis on dialysis days.
  Alternate dosing: If administration time is not immediately after dialysis session, may consider administration of a supplemental dose especially early in the treatment course to maintain levels above the MIC (Brier 2003). However, others have recommended no supplemental dose or dosage adjustment for patients on IHD (Heintz 2009; Trotman 2005)
  Peritoneal dialysis: No supplemental dose or dosage adjustment needed (Heintz 2009; Trotman 2005)
  Continuous renal replacement therapy (eg, CVVHD): No supplemental dose or dosage adjustment needed (Heintz 2009; Trotman 2005)

Hepatic Impairment
  Mild to moderate impairment (Child-Pugh class A or B): No dosage adjustment necessary.
  Severe impairment (Child-Pugh class C): There are no dosage adjustments provided in the manufacturer's labeling (has not been studied).

Additional Information Complete prescribing information should be consulted for additional detail.

Dosage Forms Excipient information presented when available (limited, particularly for generics); consult specific product labeling.
  Solution, Intravenous:
    Zyvox: 2 mg/mL (100 mL, 300 mL)
    Generic: 2 mg/mL (300 mL)
  Suspension Reconstituted, Oral:
    Zyvox: 100 mg/5 mL (150 mL) [orange flavor]
    Generic: 100 mg/5 mL (150 mL)
  Tablet, Oral:
    Zyvox: 600 mg
    Generic: 600 mg

Lomustine (loe MUS teen)

Related Information

Management of Chemotherapy-Induced Nausea and Vomiting in Adults *on page 2142*

Prevention of Chemotherapy-Induced Nausea and Vomiting in Children *on page 2203*

Safe Handling of Hazardous Drugs *on page 2292*

Brand Names: US CeeNU [DSC]; Gleostine

Brand Names: Canada CeeNU

Index Terms CCNU; CeeNU; Lomustinum

Pharmacologic Category Antineoplastic Agent, Alkylating Agent; Antineoplastic Agent, Alkylating Agent (Nitrosourea)

Use

Brain tumors: Treatment of primary and metastatic brain tumors (after appropriate surgical and/or radiotherapeutic procedures).

Hodgkin lymphoma: Treatment of relapsed or refractory Hodgkin lymphoma (secondary therapy) in combination with other chemotherapy agents; however, its use is limited in the management of Hodgkin lymphoma due to efficacy of other chemotherapy agents/regimens.

Labeled Contraindications Hypersensitivity to lomustine or any component of the formulation

Pregnancy Considerations Adverse effects have been observed in animal reproduction studies. May cause fetal harm when administered to a pregnant woman. Women of childbearing potential should be advised to avoid pregnancy during treatment with lomustine.

Breast-Feeding Considerations It is not known if lomustine is excreted in breast milk. Due to the potential for serious adverse reactions in the nursing infant, the decision to discontinue lomustine or to discontinue breast-feeding should take into account the importance of treatment to the mother.

Warnings/Precautions Hazardous agent - use appropriate precautions for handling and disposal (NIOSH 2014 [group 1]). **[U.S. Boxed Warnings]: Bone marrow suppression, particularly thrombocytopenia and leukopenia commonly occur and may be severe; may lead to bleeding and overwhelming infections in an already compromised patient. Hematologic toxicity may be delayed; monitor blood counts for at least 6 weeks after a dose. Do not administer courses more frequently than every 6 weeks due to delayed myelotoxicity. Because bone marrow toxicity is cumulative; dose adjustments should be based on nadir counts from prior dose.** Bone marrow suppression is dose-related. The onset of hematologic toxicity is ~4 to 6 weeks after administration; thrombocytopenia occurs at ~4 weeks and leukopenia occurs at 5 to 6 weeks; both persist for 1 to 2 weeks. Anemia may also be observed. Use with caution in patients with depressed platelet, leukocyte or erythrocyte counts.

May cause delayed pulmonary toxicity (infiltrates and/or fibrosis) which is rare and usually related to cumulative doses >1100 mg/m^2. May be delayed (may occur 6 months or later after treatment and has been reported up to 17 years after childhood administration in combination with radiation therapy). Patients with baseline below 70% of predicted forced vital capacity or carbon monoxide diffusing capacity are in increased risk. Long-term survivors who received nitrosoureas may have late reduction in pulmonary function; this fibrosis may be slowly progressive and has been fatal in some patients. Monitor pulmonary function tests at baseline and frequently throughout treatment. Lomustine is associated with a moderate emetic potential; antiemetics are recommended to prevent nausea and vomiting (Dupuis, 2011). Nausea and omitting may occur 3 to 6 hours after administration and the duration is generally <24 hours; may be reduced if administered on an empty stomach. Stomatitis has also been reported. Reversible hepatotoxicity (transaminase, alkaline phosphatase and bilirubin elevations) has been reported; periodically monitor liver function tests. Renal abnormalities, including azotemia (progressive), decreased kidney size, and renal failure have been reported with large cumulative doses and long-term use. Renal damage has also been observed with lower cumulative doses. Use with caution in patients with renal impairment; may require dosage adjustment; monitor renal function periodically during treatment.

Lomustine should only be administered as a single dose once every 6 weeks; serious and fatal adverse events have occurred when lomustine was inadvertently administered daily. The Institute for Safe Medication Practices (ISMP) recommends that prescribers only prescribe one dose at a time and pharmacies dispense only enough capsules for a single dose; in addition, patients should receive both verbal counseling and written instructions regarding proper dose and administration (ISMP, 2014). Long-term use of nitrosoureas may be associated with the development of secondary malignancies. Acute leukemias and bone marrow dysplasias have been reported follow chronic therapy. Potentially significant drug-drug interactions may exist, requiring dose or frequency adjustment, additional monitoring, and/or selection of alternative therapy. **[U.S. Boxed Warning]: Should be administered under the supervision of an experienced cancer chemotherapy physician.**

Adverse Reactions

>10%:

Gastrointestinal: Nausea and vomiting, (onset: 3-6 hours after oral administration; duration: <24 hours)

Hematologic: Myelosuppression (dose-limiting, delayed, cumulative); leukopenia (65%; nadir: 5-6 weeks; recovery 6-8 weeks); thrombocytopenia (nadir: 4 weeks; recovery 5-6 weeks)

Frequency not defined: Acute leukemia, alkaline phosphatase increased, alopecia, anemia, ataxia, azotemia (progressive), bilirubin increased, blindness, bone marrow dysplasia, disorientation, dysarthria, hepatotoxicity, kidney size decreased, lethargy, optic atrophy, pulmonary fibrosis, pulmonary infiltrates, renal damage, renal failure, stomatitis, transaminases increased, visual disturbances

Drug Interactions

Metabolism/Transport Effects Substrate of CYP2D6 (minor); **Note:** Assignment of Major/Minor substrate status based on clinically relevant drug interaction potential; **Inhibits** CYP2D6 (weak)

Avoid Concomitant Use

Avoid concomitant use of Lomustine with any of the following: BCG (Intravesical); CloZAPine; Dipyrone; Natalizumab; Pimecrolimus; Tacrolimus (Topical); Tofacitinib; Vaccines (Live)

Increased Effect/Toxicity

Lomustine may increase the levels/effects of: ARIPiprazole; CloZAPine; Fingolimod; Leflunomide; Natalizumab; Tofacitinib; Vaccines (Live)

The levels/effects of Lomustine may be increased by: Denosumab; Dipyrone; Pimecrolimus; Roflumilast; Tacrolimus (Topical); Trastuzumab

◀ **Decreased Effect**
Lomustine may decrease the levels/effects of: BCG (Intravesical); Coccidioides immitis Skin Test; Sipuleucel-T; Vaccines (Inactivated); Vaccines (Live)

The levels/effects of Lomustine may be decreased by: Echinacea

Storage/Stability Store at room temperature of 25°C (77°F); excursions permitted between 15°C and 30°C (59°F and 86°F). Avoid excessive heat (over 40°C [104°F]). Keep container closed tightly.

Mechanism of Action Inhibits DNA and RNA synthesis via carbamylation of DNA polymerase, alkylation of DNA, and alteration of RNA, proteins, and enzymes

Pharmacodynamics/Kinetics
Distribution: Crosses blood-brain barrier; CNS concentrations are ≥50% of plasma concentrations
Metabolism: Hepatic to active metabolites (Perry 2012)
Half-life elimination: Metabolites: 16 to 48 hours
Time to peak, serum: ~3 hours (Perry 2012)
Excretion: Urine (~50%, as metabolites)

Dosing
Adult & Geriatric Note: Dispense only enough capsules for a single dose; do not dispense more than one dose at a time (ISMP, 2014). Repeat courses should only be administered after adequate recovery of leukocytes to >4000/mm^3 and platelets to >100,000/mm^3. Doses should be rounded to the nearest 10 mg. Lomustine is associated with a moderate emetic potential; antiemetics are recommended to prevent nausea and vomiting.

Brain tumors: *Manufacturer's labeling:* Oral: 130 mg/m^2 as a single dose once every 6 weeks; reduce dose to 100 mg/m^2 as a single dose once every 6 weeks in patients with compromised bone marrow function (dosage reductions may be recommended for combination chemotherapy regimens).

Anaplastic oligodendroglioma: PCV regimen (off-label combination): Oral: 130 mg/m^2 on day 1 every 6 weeks for up to 4 cycles prior to radiation therapy (in combination with procarbazine and vincristine) (Cairncross, 2013; Cairncross, 2006).

Astrocytoma, high grade: POC regimen (off-label dosing): Adults ≤21 years: Oral: 100 mg/m^2 on day 1 every 6 weeks for 8 cycles (in combination with vincristine and prednisone) (Finlay, 1995).

Glioblastoma, recurrent:
PCV regimen (off-label dosing): Oral: 110 mg/m^2 on day 1 every 6 weeks for 7 cycles (in combination with procarbazine and vincristine) (Levin, 2000).
Single-agent therapy: Oral: 100 to 130 mg/m^2 every 6 weeks until disease progression or unacceptable toxicity (Wick, 2010).

Medulloblastoma (off-label dosing): Adults ≤21 years: Oral: 75 mg/m^2 on day 1 every 6 weeks for 8 cycles (in combination with cisplatin and vincristine) (Packer, 2006; Packer, 1999).

Hodgkin lymphoma: *Manufacturer's labeling:* Oral: 130 mg/m^2 as a single dose once every 6 weeks; reduce dose to 100 mg/m^2 as a single dose once every 6 weeks in patients with compromised bone marrow function (dosage reductions may be recommended for combination chemotherapy regimens).

Dosing adjustment (based on nadir) for subsequent cycles:
Leukocytes ≥3000/mm^3, platelets ≥75,000/mm^3: No dosage adjustment required
Leukocytes 2000 to 2999/mm^3, platelets 25,000 to 74,999/mm^3: Administer 70% of prior dose
Leukocytes <2000/mm^3, platelets <25,000/mm^3: Administer 50% of prior dose

Pediatric Note: Dispense only enough capsules for a single dose; do not dispense more than one dose at a time (ISMP, 2014). Repeat courses should only be administered after adequate recovery of leukocytes to >4,000/mm^3 and platelets to >100,000/mm^3. Doses should be rounded to the nearest 10 mg. Lomustine is associated with a moderate emetic potential; antiemetics are recommended to prevent nausea and vomiting (Dupuis, 2011).

Brain tumors: *Manufacturer's labeling:* Oral: 130 mg/m^2 as a single dose once every 6 weeks; reduce dose to 100 mg/m^2 as a single dose once every 6 weeks in patients with compromised bone marrow function (dosage reductions may be recommended for combination chemotherapy regimens)
Astrocytoma, high grade: POC regimen (off-label dosing): Children ≥18 months and Adolescents: Oral: 100 mg/m^2 on day 1 every 6 weeks for 8 cycles (in combination with vincristine and prednisone) (Finlay, 1995)
Medulloblastoma (off-label dosing): Children ≥3 years and Adolescents: Oral: 75 mg/m^2 once every 6 weeks for 8 cycles (in combination with cisplatin and vincristine) (Packer, 2006; Packer, 1999)

Hodgkin lymphoma: *Manufacturer's labeling:* Oral: 130 mg/m^2 as a single dose once every 6 weeks; reduce dose to 100 mg/m^2 as a single dose once every 6 weeks in patients with compromised bone marrow function (dosage reductions may be recommended for combination chemotherapy regimens)

Dosing adjustment (based on nadir) for subsequent cycles: Refer to adult dosing.

Renal Impairment
There are no dosage adjustments provided in the manufacturer's labeling. The following adjustments have been recommended:
Aronoff, 2007: Adults:
CrCl 10 to 50 mL/minute: Administer 75% of dose
CrCl <10 mL/minute: Administer 25% to 50% of dose
Hemodialysis: Supplemental dose is not necessary
Continuous ambulatory peritoneal dialysis (CAPD): Administer 25% to 50% of dose
Kintzel, 1995:
CrCl 46 to 60 mL/minute: Administer 75% of normal dose
CrCl 31 to 45 mL/minute: Administer 70% of normal dose
CrCl ≤30 mL/minute: Avoid use

Hepatic Impairment There are no dosage adjustments provided in the manufacturer's labeling. However, lomustine is hepatically metabolized and caution should be used in patients with hepatic dysfunction.

Obesity *ASCO Guidelines for appropriate chemotherapy dosing in obese adults with cancer:* Utilize patient's actual body weight (full weight) for calculation of body surface area- or weight-based dosing, particularly when the intent of therapy is curative; manage regimen-related toxicities in the same manner as for nonobese patients; if a dose reduction is utilized due to toxicity, consider resumption of full weight-based dosing with subsequent cycles, especially if cause of toxicity (eg, hepatic or renal impairment) is resolved (Griggs, 2012).

◀ **Combination Regimens**
Brain tumors:
PCV (Brain Tumor Regimen) on page 2061
POC on page 2067

Administration
Lomustine is associated with a moderate emetic potential; antiemetics are recommended to prevent nausea and vomiting (Dupuis, 2011).

Oral: Administer with fluids on an empty stomach; no food or drink for 2 hours after administration. Administering on an empty stomach will reduce the incidence of nausea and vomiting.

Varying strengths of capsules may be required to obtain necessary dose. Dispense only enough capsules for a single dose; do not dispense more than one dose at a time (ISMP, 2014). Do not break capsules.

Hazardous agent; use appropriate precautions for handling and disposal (NIOSH 2014 [group 1]). NIOSH recommends single gloving for administration of intact capsules (NIOSH 2014). Avoid exposure to broken capsules.

Emetic Potential Children and Adults: Moderate (30% to 90%)

Monitoring Parameters CBC with differential and platelet count (weekly for at least 6 weeks after a dose), hepatic and renal function tests (periodic), pulmonary function tests (baseline and periodic)

Dosage Forms Excipient information presented when available (limited, particularly for generics); consult specific product labeling. [DSC] = Discontinued product

Capsule, Oral:
CeeNU: 10 mg [DSC], 40 mg [DSC], 100 mg [DSC]
Gleostine: 5 mg, 10 mg, 40 mg, 100 mg
Generic: 10 mg, 40 mg, 100 mg

♦ **Lomustinum** see Lomustine on page 1054

♦ **Longastatin** see Octreotide on page 1226

♦ **Lonsurf** see Trifluridine and Tipiracil on page 1699

LORazepam (lor A ze pam)

Related Information
Management of Chemotherapy-Induced Nausea and Vomiting in Adults on page 2142
Palliative Care Medicine (Cancer) on page 2252
Prevention of Chemotherapy-Induced Nausea and Vomiting in Children on page 2203

Brand Names: US Ativan; LORazepam Intensol

Brand Names: Canada Apo-Lorazepam; Ativan; Dom-Lorazepam; Lorazepam Injection, USP; PHL-Lorazepam; PMS-Lorazepam; PRO-Lorazepam; Teva-Lorazepam

Pharmacologic Category Benzodiazepine

Use
Anxiety (oral): Management of anxiety disorders, short-term (≤4 months) relief of anxiety symptoms, or anxiety associated with depressive symptoms, or anxiety/stress-associated insomnia

Anesthesia premedication (parenteral): Anesthesia premedication to relieve anxiety or to produce amnesia (diminish recall) or sedation

Anesthesia premedication (sublingual): *Canadian labeling:* Anesthesia premedication to relieve anxiety prior to surgical procedures

Status epilepticus (parenteral): Treatment of status epilepticus

Labeled Contraindications

Hypersensitivity to lorazepam, any component of the formulation, or other benzodiazepines (cross-sensitivity with other benzodiazepines may exist); acute narrow-angle glaucoma; sleep apnea (parenteral); intra-arterial injection of parenteral formulation; severe respiratory insufficiency (except during mechanical ventilation)

Canadian labeling: Additional contraindications (not in U.S. labeling): Myasthenia gravis

Pregnancy Considerations Teratogenic effects have been observed in some animal reproduction studies. Lorazepam and its metabolite cross the human placenta. Teratogenic effects in humans have been observed with some benzodiazepines (including lorazepam); however, additional studies are needed. The incidence of premature birth and low birth weights may be increased following maternal use of benzodiazepines; hypoglycemia and respiratory problems in the neonate may occur following exposure late in pregnancy. Neonatal withdrawal symptoms may occur within days to weeks after birth and "floppy infant syndrome" (which also includes withdrawal symptoms) have been reported with some benzodiazepines (including lorazepam). Elimination of lorazepam in the newborn infant is slow; following *in utero* exposure, term infants may excrete lorazepam for up to 8 days (Bergman 1992; Iqbal 2002; Wikner 2007).

Breast-Feeding Considerations Lorazepam can be detected in breast milk. Drowsiness, lethargy, or weight loss in nursing infants have been observed in case reports following maternal use of some benzodiazepines (Iqbal 2002). Breast-feeding is not recommended by the manufacturer.

Warnings/Precautions Use with caution in elderly or debilitated patients, patients with hepatic disease (including alcoholics) or renal impairment. In older adults, benzodiazepines increase the risk of impaired cognition, delirium, falls, fractures, and motor vehicle accidents. Due to increased sensitivity in this age group, avoid use for treatment of insomnia, agitation, or delirium. (Beers Criteria). Use with caution in patients with respiratory disease (COPD or sleep apnea) or limited pulmonary reserve, or impaired gag reflex. Initial doses in elderly or debilitated patients should be at the lower end of the dosing range. May worsen hepatic encephalopathy.

Causes CNS depression (dose-related) resulting in sedation, dizziness, confusion, or ataxia which may impair physical and mental capabilities. Patients must be cautioned about performing tasks which require mental alertness (eg, operating machinery or driving). Effects may be potentiated when used with other sedative drugs or ethanol. Potentially significant drug-drug interactions may exist, requiring dose or frequency adjustment, additional monitoring, and/or selection of alternative therapy. Benzodiazepines have been associated with falls and traumatic injury and should be used with extreme caution in patients who are at risk of these events.

Lorazepam may cause anterograde amnesia. Paradoxical reactions, including hyperactive or aggressive behavior have been reported with benzodiazepines, particularly in adolescent/pediatric or psychiatric patients. Does not have analgesic, antidepressant, or antipsychotic properties.

◄ Preexisting depression may worsen or emerge during therapy. Not recommended for use in primary depressive or psychotic disorders. Should not be used in patients at risk for suicide without adequate antidepressant treatment. Risk of dependence increases in patients with a history of alcohol or drug abuse and those with significant personality disorders; use with caution in these patients. Tolerance, psychological and physical dependence may also occur with higher dosages and prolonged use. The risk of dependence is decreased with short-term treatment (2 to 4 weeks); evaluate the need for continued treatment prior to extending therapy duration. Benzodiazepines have been associated with dependence and acute withdrawal symptoms on discontinuation or reduction in dose. Acute withdrawal, including seizures, may be precipitated after administration of flumazenil to patients receiving long-term benzodiazepine therapy. Lorazepam is a short half-life benzodiazepine. Tolerance develops to the sedative, hypnotic, and anticonvulsant effects. It does not develop to the anxiolytic effects (Vinkers 2012). Chronic use of this agent may increase the perioperative benzodiazepine dose needed to achieve desired effect.

As a hypnotic agent, should be used only after evaluation of potential causes of sleep disturbance. Failure of sleep disturbance to resolve after 7 to 10 days may indicate psychiatric or medical illness. A worsening of insomnia or the emergence of new abnormalities of thought or behavior may represent unrecognized psychiatric or medical illness and requires immediate and careful evaluation.

Status epilepticus should not be treated with injectable benzodiazepines alone; requires close observation and management and possibly ventilatory support. When used as a component of preanesthesia, monitor for heavy sedation and airway obstruction; equipment necessary to maintain airway and ventilatory support should be available. Parenteral formulation of lorazepam contains polyethylene glycol which has resulted in toxicity during high-dose and/or longer-term infusions. Parenteral formulation also contains propylene glycol (PG); may be associated with dose-related toxicity and can occur ≥48 hours after initiation of lorazepam. Limited data suggest increased risk of PG accumulation at doses of ≥6 mg/hour for 48 hours or more (Nelson 2008). Monitor for signs of toxicity which may include acute renal failure, lactic acidosis, and/or osmol gap. May consider using enteral delivery of lorazepam tablets to decrease the risk of PG toxicity (Lugo 1999).

Benzyl alcohol and derivatives: Some dosage forms may contain benzyl alcohol; large amounts of benzyl alcohol (≥99 mg/kg/day) have been associated with a potentially fatal toxicity ("gasping syndrome") in neonates; the "gasping syndrome" consists of metabolic acidosis, respiratory distress, gasping respirations, CNS dysfunction (including convulsions, intracranial hemorrhage), hypotension, and cardiovascular collapse (AAP ["Inactive" 1997]; CDC 1982); some data suggests that benzoate displaces bilirubin from protein binding sites (Ahlfors 2001); avoid or use dosage forms containing benzyl alcohol with caution in neonates. See manufacturer's labeling.

Adverse Reactions Frequency not always defined.

Cardiovascular: Hypotension (≤2%)

Central nervous system: Sedation (≤16%), dizziness (≤7%), drowsiness (2% to 4%), unsteadiness (3%), headache (1%), coma (≤1%), stupor (≤1%), aggressive behavior, agitation, akathisia, amnesia, anxiety, central nervous system stimulation, disinhibition, disorientation, dysarthria, euphoria, excitement, extrapyramidal reaction, fatigue, hostility, hypothermia, irritability, mania, memory impairment, outbursts of anger, psychosis, seizures, sleep apnea (exacerbation), sleep disturbances, slurred speech, suicidal behavior, suicidal ideation, vertigo

Dermatologic: Alopecia, skin rash

Gastrointestinal: Changes in appetite, constipation

Endocrine & metabolic: Change in libido, hyponatremia, SIADH

Genitourinary: Impotence, orgasm disturbance

Hematologic & oncologic: Agranulocytosis, pancytopenia, thrombocytopenia

Hepatic: Increased serum alkaline phosphatase, increased serum bilirubin, increased serum transaminases, jaundice

Hypersensitivity: Anaphylaxis, anaphylactoid reaction, hypersensitivity reaction

Local: Pain at injection site (IM: 1% to 17%; IV: ≤2%), erythema at injection site (≤2%)

Neuromuscular & skeletal: Weakness (≤4%)

Ophthalmic: Visual disturbances (including diplopia and blurred vision)

Respiratory: Respiratory failure (1% to 2%), apnea (1%), hypoventilation (≤1%), exacerbation of obstructive pulmonary disease, nasal congestion, respiratory depression, worsening of sleep apnea

<1%, postmarketing, and/or case reports: Abnormal gait, abnormal hepatic function tests, abnormality in thinking, acidosis, cardiac arrhythmia, ataxia, blood coagulation disorder, bradycardia, cardiac arrest, cardiac failure, cerebral edema, chills, confusion, convulsions, cystitis, decreased mental acuity, delirium, depression, drug dependence (with prolonged use), drug toxicity (polyethylene glycol or propylene glycol poisoning [prolonged IV infusion]), excessive crying, gastrointestinal hemorrhage, hallucinations, hearing loss, heart block, hematologic abnormality, hepatotoxicity, hypertension, hyperventilation, hyporeflexia, infection, injection site reaction, myoclonus, nausea, nervousness, neuroleptic malignant syndrome, paralysis, pericardial effusion, pheochromocytoma (aggravation), pneumothorax, pulmonary edema, pulmonary hemorrhage, pulmonary hypertension, restlessness, seizure, sialorrhea, tachycardia, tremor, urinary incontinence, ventricular arrhythmia, vomiting, withdrawal syndrome

Drug Interactions

Metabolism/Transport Effects None known.

Avoid Concomitant Use

Avoid concomitant use of LORazepam with any of the following: Azelastine (Nasal); Methadone; OLANZapine; Orphenadrine; Paraldehyde; Sodium Oxybate; Thalidomide

Increased Effect/Toxicity

LORazepam may increase the levels/effects of: Alcohol (Ethyl); Azelastine (Nasal); Buprenorphine; CloZAPine; CNS Depressants; Fosphenytoin; Hydrocodone; Methadone; Methotrimeprazine; Metyrosine; Mirtazapine; Orphenadrine; Paraldehyde; Phenytoin; Pramipexole; ROPINIRole; Rotigotine; Selective Serotonin Reuptake Inhibitors; Sodium Oxybate; Suvorexant; Thalidomide; Zolpidem

The levels/effects of LORazepam may be increased by: Brimonidine (Topical); Cannabis; Doxylamine; Dronabinol; Droperidol; HydrOXYzine; Kava Kava; Loxapine; Magnesium Sulfate; Methotrimeprazine; Minocycline; Nabilone; OLANZapine; Perampanel; Probenecid; Rufinamide; Tapentadol; Teduglutide; Tetrahydrocannabinol; Valproate Products

◄ **Decreased Effect**
The levels/effects of LORazepam may be decreased by: Theophylline Derivatives; Yohimbine

Storage/Stability

Parenteral: Intact vials should be refrigerated (room temperature storage information may be available; contact product manufacturer to obtain current recommendations). Protect from light. Do not use discolored or precipitate-containing solutions. Parenteral admixture is stable at room temperature (25°C) for 24 hours.

Oral concentrate: Store at colder room temperature or refrigerate at 2°C to 8°C (36°F to 46°F). Discard open bottle after 90 days.

Oral tablet: Store at 25°C (77°F); excursions are permitted between 15°C and 30°C (59°F and 86°F).

Sublingual tablet [Canadian product]: Store at 15°C to 25°C (59°F to 77°F). Protect from light.

Preparation for Administration

IV injection: According to the manufacturer, dilute IV dose prior to use with an equal volume of compatible diluent (D_5W, NS, SWFI).

Infusion: Precipitation may occur upon dilution when preparing an infusion. Use 2 mg/mL injectable vial to prepare; there may be decreased stability when using 4 mg/mL vial. Dilute to ≤1 mg/mL with a compatible diluent in a non-PVC (eg, polyolefin, glass) container (consult parenteral admixture resource for additional detailed recommendations). Can also be administered undiluted (up to 4 mg/mL) via infusion into a central vein or into a peripheral vein with a running compatible maintenance IV solution (Johnson 2002).

IM: Administer undiluted.

Mechanism of Action Binds to stereospecific benzodiazepine receptors on the postsynaptic GABA neuron at several sites within the central nervous system, including the limbic system, reticular formation. Enhancement of the inhibitory effect of GABA on neuronal excitability results by increased neuronal membrane permeability to chloride ions. This shift in chloride ions results in hyperpolarization (a less excitable state) and stabilization. Benzodiazepine receptors and effects appear to be linked to the GABA-A receptors. Benzodiazepines do not bind to GABA-B receptors.

Pharmacodynamics/Kinetics

Duration: Anesthesia premedication: Adults: IM, IV: ~6 to 8 hours

Absorption: IM: Rapid and complete absorption; Oral: Readily absorbed

Distribution: IV: V_d: Neonates: 0.78 L/kg; Children and Adolescents: 1.9 L/kg; Adults: ~1.3 L/kg

Protein binding: ~85% to 93%; free fraction may be significantly higher in elderly (Greenblatt, 1981)

Metabolism: Hepatic; rapidly conjugated to lorazepam glucuronide (inactive)

Bioavailability: Oral: 90%

Half-life elimination:

IM: ~13 to 18 hours (Greenblatt, 1981)

IV: Neonates: ~42 hours; Children 2 to12 years: ~18 hours; Adolescents: ~28 hours; Adults: ~14 hours; End-stage renal disease (ESRD): ~18 hours

Oral: ~12 hours

Time to peak: IM: ≤3 hours; Oral: ~2 hours; Sublingual tablet [Canadian product]: 1 hour

Excretion: Urine (~88%; predominantly as inactive metabolites); feces (~7%)

Dosing
Adult

Anxiety disorder: Oral: Initial: 2 to 3 mg daily in 2 to 3 divided doses; usual dose: 2 to 6 mg daily in divided doses; however, daily dose may vary from 1 to 10 mg/day

Insomnia due to anxiety or stress: Oral: 2 to 4 mg at bedtime

Premedication for anesthesia:

IM: 0.05 mg/kg administered 2 hours before surgery (maximum dose: 4 mg)

IV: 0.044 mg/kg administered 15 to 20 minutes before surgery (usual dose: 2 mg; maximum dose: 4 mg). **Note:** Doses >2 mg should generally not be exceeded in patients >50 years.

Sublingual tablet [Canadian product]: 0.05 mg/kg 1 to 2 hours before surgery (maximum dose: 4 mg)

Status epilepticus: IV:

Neurocritical Care Society recommendation: 0.1 mg/kg (maximum dose: 4 mg) given at a maximum rate of 2 mg/minute; may repeat in 5 to 10 minutes (NCS [Brophy 2012]). **Note:** Dilute dose 1:1 with saline.

Manufacturer's labeling: 4 mg given slowly (2 mg/minute); may repeat in 10 to 15 minutes. May be given IM, but IV preferred.

Agitation in the ICU patient (off-label use): IV: Loading dose: 0.02 to 0.04 mg/kg (maximum single dose: 2 mg); Maintenance: 0.02 to 0.06 mg/kg every 2 to 6 hours as needed **or** 0.01 to 0.1 mg/kg/hour; maximum dose: ≤10 mg/hour (Barr 2013)

Alcohol withdrawal delirium (off-label use) (Mayo-Smith 2004):

IV: 1 to 4 mg every 5 to 15 minutes until calm, then every hour as needed to maintain light somnolence

IM: 1 to 4 mg every 30 to 60 minutes until calm, then every hour as needed to maintain light somnolence

Alcohol withdrawal syndrome (off-label use) (Mayo-Smith, 1997):

Oral, IM, IV (fixed-dose regimen): 2 mg every 6 hours for 4 doses, then 1 mg every 6 hours for 8 additional doses

Oral, IM, IV (symptom-triggered regimen): 2 to 4 mg every 1 hour as needed; dose determined by a validated severity assessment scale

Chemotherapy-associated nausea and vomiting (off-label use): Breakthrough nausea/vomiting or as adjunct to standard antiemetics: Oral, IV, Sublingual (off-label route): 0.5 to 2 mg every 6 hours as needed (Lohr 2008)

Partial complex seizures, refractory (off-label use): Oral: 1 mg twice daily; increase biweekly in increments of 1 mg twice daily until seizures stop or side effects occur (Walker, 1984); however, additional data may be necessary to further define the role of lorazepam in this condition

Psychogenic catatonia (off-label use):

IM, Sublingual (off-label route): 1 to 2 mg; repeat dose in 3 hours then again in another 3 hours if initial and subsequent doses, respectively, are ineffective (Rosebush, 1990; Rosebush 2010); however, additional data may be necessary to further define the role of lorazepam in this condition

or

Oral, IM, IV: Initial: 1 mg; may repeat in 5 minutes if necessary. If initial challenge is unsuccessful, may increase dose up to 4 to 8 mg per day; may continue treatment for up to 5 days (Bush, 1996); however, additional data may be necessary to further define the role of lorazepam in this condition

◀ **Rapid tranquilization of the agitated patient (off-label use):** Oral, IM: 1 to 3 mg administered every 30 to 60 minutes; may be administered with an antipsychotic (eg, haloperidol) (Allen 2005; Battaglia 2005; De Fruyt 2004). **Note:** When administering IM, may consider a lower initial dose (eg, 0.5 mg) (Allen 2005).

Dosage adjustment for lorazepam with concomitant medications: *Probenecid or valproic acid:* Reduce lorazepam dose by 50%

Geriatric Refer also to adult dosing. Dose selection should generally be on the low end of the dosage range (initial dose not to exceed 2 mg).

Anxiety disorder: Oral:

US labeling: Initial: 1 to 2 mg daily in divided doses; Beers Criteria: Avoid maintenance doses >3 mg daily

Canadian labeling: Initial: 0.5 mg daily; titrate cautiously as tolerated

Premedication for anesthesia: IM, IV: *Canadian labeling:* Reduce the initial dose by approximately 50% and adjust as needed and tolerated; IV dose should generally not exceed 2 mg in patients >50 years.

Pediatric

Chemotherapy-associated nausea and vomiting (off-label use):

Anticipatory nausea/vomiting (prevention and treatment): Infants ≥1 month, Children, and Adolescents: Oral: 0.04 to 0.08 mg/kg/dose (maximum dose: 2 mg) once at bedtime the evening prior to chemotherapy and once the next day before chemotherapy (Dupuis 2014)

Breakthrough nausea/vomiting: Children ≥2 years and Adolescents: IV: 0.025 to 0.05 mg/kg/dose (maximum dose: 2 mg) every 6 hours as needed (Dupuis 2003); however, additional data may be necessary to further define the role of lorazepam in children for chemotherapy-associated nausea and vomiting

Status epilepticus: Infants, Children, and Adolescents (off-label use):

Neurocritical Care Society recommendation: IV: 0.1 mg/kg (maximum dose: 4 mg) given at a maximum rate of 2 mg/minute; may repeat in 5 to 10 minutes (NCS [Brophy 2012]). **Note:** Dilute 1:1 with saline.

American Academy of Pediatrics recommendation: IV, IM: 0.05 to 0.1 mg/kg (maximum dose: 4 mg); may repeat dose every 10 to 15 minutes if seizure continues (AAP [Hegenbarth 2008])

Dosage adjustment for lorazepam with concomitant medications: *Probenecid or valproic acid:* Reduce lorazepam dose by 50%

Renal Impairment

Oral: No dosage adjustment necessary (Aronoff 2007).

IM, IV: Risk of propylene glycol toxicity. Monitor closely if using for prolonged periods of time or at high doses.

Mild-to-moderate disease: Use with caution.

Severe disease or failure: Use is not recommended.

Hepatic Impairment

Oral:

Mild-to-moderate disease: No dose adjustment necessary.

Severe insufficiency and/or encephalopathy: Use with caution; may require lower doses.

IM, IV:

Mild-to-moderate disease: Use with caution.

Severe disease or failure: Use is not recommended.

Administration

IM: Should be administered (undiluted) deep into the muscle mass.

IV injection: Dilute prior to use (according to the manufacturer). Do not exceed 2 mg/minute or 0.05 mg/kg over 2 to 5 minutes. Monitor IV site during administration. Avoid intra-arterial administration. Avoid extravasation.

Continuous IV infusion (off-label administration mode; Barr 2013) solutions should have an in-line filter and the solution should be checked frequently for possible precipitation (Grillo 1996).

Oral: Lorazepam oral concentrate: Use only the provided calibrated dropper to withdraw the prescribed dose. Mix the dose with liquid (eg, water, juice, soda, soda-like beverage) or semisolid food (eg, applesauce, pudding), and stir for a few seconds to blend completely. The prepared mixture should be administered immediately.

Sublingual tablet [Canadian product]: Place under tongue; patient should not swallow for at least 2 minutes.

Extemporaneous Preparations Note: Commercial oral solution is available (2 mg/mL)

Two different 1 mg/mL oral suspensions may be made from different generic lorazepam tablets (Mylan Pharmaceuticals or Watson Laboratories), sterile water, Ora-Sweet, and Ora-Plus.

Mylan tablets: Place one-hundred-eighty 2 mg tablets in a 12-ounce amber glass bottle; add 144 mL of sterile water to disperse the tablets; shake until slurry is formed. Add 108 mL Ora-Plus in incremental proportions; then add a quantity of Ora-Sweet sufficient to make 360 mL. Label "shake well" and "refrigerate". Stable for 91 days when stored in amber glass prescription bottles at room temperature or refrigerated (preferred).

Watson tablets: Place one-hundred-eighty 2 mg tablets in a 12-ounce amber glass bottle; add 48 mL sterile water to disperse the tablets; shake until slurry is formed. Add 156 mL of Ora-Plus in incremental proportions; then add a quantity of Ora-Sweet sufficient to make 360 mL. Label "shake well" and "refrigerate". Store in amber glass prescription bottles. Stable for 63 days at room temperature or 91 days refrigerated.

Lee ME, Lugo RA, Rusho WJ, et al, "Chemical Stability of Extemporaneously Prepared Lorazepam Suspension at Two Temperatures," *J Pediatr Pharmacol Ther*, 2004, 9(4):254-58.

Monitoring Parameters Respiratory and cardiovascular status, blood pressure, heart rate, symptoms of anxiety

CBC, liver function tests; clinical signs of propylene glycol toxicity (for continuous high-dose and/or long duration intravenous use) including serum creatinine, BUN, serum lactate, osmol gap

Critically-ill patients: Monitor depth of sedation with either the Richmond Agitation-Sedation Scale (RASS) or Sedation-Agitation Scale (SAS) (Barr 2013)

Dosage Forms Excipient information presented when available (limited, particularly for generics); consult specific product labeling.

Concentrate, Oral:

LORazepam Intensol: 2 mg/mL (30 mL) [alcohol free, dye free, sugar free; unflavored flavor]

Generic: 2 mg/mL (30 mL)

Solution, Injection:

Ativan: 2 mg/mL (1 mL, 10 mL); 4 mg/mL (1 mL, 10 mL) [contains benzyl alcohol, polyethylene glycol, propylene glycol]

Generic: 2 mg/mL (1 mL, 10 mL); 4 mg/mL (1 mL, 10 mL)

Tablet, Oral:
 Ativan: 0.5 mg
 Ativan: 1 mg, 2 mg [scored]
 Generic: 0.5 mg, 1 mg, 2 mg
Dosage Forms: Canada Excipient information presented when available (limited, particularly for generics); consult specific product labeling
 Tablet, Sublingual: 0.5 mg, 1 mg, 2 mg
Controlled Substance C-IV

- ◆ **Lorazepam Injection, USP (Can)** see LORazepam on page 1058
- ◆ **LORazepam Intensol** see LORazepam on page 1058
- ◆ **Lovenox** see Enoxaparin on page 594
- ◆ **Lovenox HP (Can)** see Enoxaparin on page 594
- ◆ **Lovenox With Preservative (Can)** see Enoxaparin on page 594
- ◆ **Low-Molecular-Weight Iron Dextran (INFeD)** see Iron Dextran Complex on page 964
- ◆ **L-PAM** see Melphalan on page 1080
- ◆ **L-Phenylalanine Mustard** see Melphalan on page 1080
- ◆ **LP Lite Pak** see Lidocaine and Prilocaine on page 1046
- ◆ **L-Sarcolysin** see Melphalan on page 1080
- ◆ **Lupron (Can)** see Leuprolide on page 1030
- ◆ **Lupron Depot** see Leuprolide on page 1030
- ◆ **Lupron Depot-Ped** see Leuprolide on page 1030
- ◆ **LY170053** see OLANZapine on page 1242
- ◆ **LY-188011** see Gemcitabine on page 776
- ◆ **LY231514** see PEMEtrexed on page 1368
- ◆ **LY303366** see Anidulafungin on page 116
- ◆ **Lymphazurin [DSC]** see Isosulfan Blue on page 973
- ◆ **Lymphocyte Immune Globulin** see Antithymocyte Globulin (Equine) on page 126
- ◆ **Lymphocyte Mitogenic Factor** see Aldesleukin on page 55
- ◆ **Lymphoseek** see Technetium Tc 99m Tilmanocept on page 1603
- ◆ **Lynparza** see Olaparib on page 1245
- ◆ **Lysodren** see Mitotane on page 1155
- ◆ **Lysteda** see Tranexamic Acid on page 1681
- ◆ **MabCampath (Can)** see Alemtuzumab on page 62
- ◆ **m-AMSA** see Amsacrine on page 105
- ◆ **Mar-Allopurinol (Can)** see Allopurinol on page 73
- ◆ **Mar-Anastrozole (Can)** see Anastrozole on page 112
- ◆ **Mar-Ciprofloxacin (Can)** see Ciprofloxacin (Systemic) on page 327
- ◆ **Marinol** see Dronabinol on page 577
- ◆ **Mar-Letrozole (Can)** see Letrozole on page 1019
- ◆ **Mar-Olanzapine (Can)** see OLANZapine on page 1242
- ◆ **Mar-Olanzapine ODT (Can)** see OLANZapine on page 1242
- ◆ **Mar-Ondansetron (Can)** see Ondansetron on page 1253

Mechlorethamine (Systemic) (me klor ETH a meen)

Related Information

Fertility and Cancer Therapy *on page 2137*

Management of Chemotherapy-Induced Nausea and Vomiting in Adults *on page 2142*

Management of Drug Extravasations *on page 2159*

Prevention of Chemotherapy-Induced Nausea and Vomiting in Children *on page 2203*

Safe Handling of Hazardous Drugs *on page 2292*

Brand Names: US Mustargen

Index Terms Chlorethazine; Chlorethazine Mustard; HN_2; Mechlorethamine Hydrochloride; Mustine; Nitrogen Mustard

Pharmacologic Category Antineoplastic Agent, Alkylating Agent; Antineoplastic Agent, Alkylating Agent (Nitrogen Mustard)

Use

Hodgkin lymphoma: Palliative treatment of Hodgkin lymphoma

Malignant effusion: Palliative treatment of effusions from metastatic carcinomas

Additional approved uses (manufacturer labeling): Treatment of lymphosarcoma, chronic myelocytic or chronic lymphocytic leukemia, polycythemia vera, mycosis fungoides, and bronchogenic carcinoma

Labeled Contraindications Hypersensitivity to mechlorethamine or any component of the formulation; presence of known infection

Pregnancy Considerations Adverse events have been observed in animal reproduction studies. Women of childbearing potential are advised not to become pregnant during treatment. **[U.S. Boxed Warning]: Avoid exposure during pregnancy.**

Breast-Feeding Considerations It is not known if mechlorethamine is excreted in human breast milk. Due to the potential for serious adverse reactions in the nursing infant, the decision to discontinue mechlorethamine or to discontinue breast-feeding should take into account the importance of treatment to the mother.

Warnings/Precautions Hazardous agent; use appropriate precautions for handling and disposal (NIOSH 2014 [group 1]). **[U.S. Boxed Warning]: Mechlorethamine is a highly toxic nitrogen mustard; avoid inhalation of vapors or dust; review and follow special handling procedures.** Avoid dust or vapor contact with skin or eyes. If accidental skin exposure occurs, wash/irrigate thoroughly with water for at least 15 minutes, followed by 2% sodium thiosulfate solution; remove and destroy any contaminated clothing. If exposure to eye(s) occurs, promptly irrigate for at least 15 minutes with copious amounts of water, normal saline, or balanced salt ophthalmic irrigating solution; obtain ophthalmology consultation. The manufacturer recommends neutralizing remaining unused mechlorethamine, empty or partial vials, gloves, tubing, glassware, etc., after mechlorethamine administration; soak in an aqueous solution containing equal volumes of sodium thiosulfate (5%) and sodium bicarbonate (5%) for 45 minutes; rinse with water; dispose of properly.

[U.S. Boxed Warning]: Mechlorethamine is a potent vesicant; extravasation results in painful inflammation with induration and sloughing. If extravasation occurs, promptly manage by infiltrating area with 1/6 molar sodium thiosulfate solution, followed by dry cold compresses for 6-12 hours. Ensure proper needle or catheter placement prior to and during infusion. Avoid extravasation.

Bone marrow suppression: May cause lymphopenia, leukopenia, granulocytopenia, thrombocytopenia and anemia. Agranulocytopenia may occur (rare); persistent pancytopenia has been reported. Monitor blood counts. Bleeding due to thrombocytopenia may occur. Use with caution in patients where neoplasm has bone marrow involvement or in those who have received prior myelosuppressive chemotherapy; marrow function may be further compromised (possibly fatal). Bone marrow function should recover after mechlorethamine administration prior to initiating radiation therapy or other chemotherapy regimens.

Hyperuricemia may occur, especially with lymphomas; ensure adequate hydration; consider antihyperuricemic therapy if appropriate. Mechlorethamine is associated with a high emetic potential (Basch, 2011; Dupuis, 2011; Roila, 2010); antiemetics are recommended to prevent nausea and vomiting. Hypersensitivity reactions, including anaphylaxis, have been reported. Mechlorethamine has immunosuppressant properties; may predispose patients to infections (bacterial, viral, or fungal). Alkylating agents, including mechlorethamine, are associated with in increased incidence of secondary malignancies; concurrent radiation therapy or combination chemotherapy may increase the risk. Potentially significant drug-drug interactions may exist, requiring dose or frequency adjustment, additional monitoring, and/or selection of alternative therapy.

[U.S. Boxed Warning]: Avoid exposure during pregnancy. Impaired spermatogenesis, azoospermia, and total germinal aplasia may occur in male patients treated with mechlorethamine, particularly when used in combination with other chemotherapy agents. Delayed menses, oligomenorrhea, or temporary or permanent amenorrhea may be observed in female patients treated with mechlorethamine.

Bone marrow failure and other toxicities are more common in chronic lymphocytic leukemia (CLL); in general, mechlorethamine is no longer used in the treatment of CLL. Bone and nervous system tumors typically respond poorly to treatment with mechlorethamine. The routine use of mechlorethamine in widely disseminated tumors is discouraged. **[U.S. Boxed Warning]: Should be administered under the supervision of an experienced cancer chemotherapy physician.**

Adverse Reactions Frequency not defined.

Central nervous system: Drowsiness, encephalopathy (high dose), fever, headache, lethargy, sedation, vertigo

Dermatologic: Alopecia, erythema multiforme, maculopapular rash, petechiae, rash

Endocrine & metabolic: Amenorrhea, hyperuricemia, oligomenorrhea, spermatogenesis decreased

Gastrointestinal: Anorexia, diarrhea, metallic taste, mucositis, nausea, vomiting

Hepatic: Jaundice

Hematologic: Agranulocytosis, granulocytopenia (onset 6-8 days, recovery 10-21 days), hemolytic anemia, leukopenia, lymphocytopenia, pancytopenia, secondary leukemias, thrombocytopenia

Local: Thrombophlebitis, tissue necrosis (extravasation)

Neuromuscular & skeletal: Weakness

Ocular: Lacrimation

Otic: Deafness, tinnitus

Miscellaneous: Anaphylaxis, diaphoresis, herpes zoster infection, hypersensitivity reactions

Drug Interactions

Metabolism/Transport Effects None known.

Avoid Concomitant Use

Avoid concomitant use of Mechlorethamine (Systemic) with any of the following: BCG (Intravesical); CloZAPine; Dipyrone; Natalizumab; Pimecrolimus; Tacrolimus (Topical); Tofacitinib; Vaccines (Live)

Increased Effect/Toxicity

Mechlorethamine (Systemic) may increase the levels/effects of: CloZAPine; Fingolimod; Leflunomide; Natalizumab; Tofacitinib; Vaccines (Live)

The levels/effects of Mechlorethamine (Systemic) may be increased by: Denosumab; Dipyrone; Pimecrolimus; Roflumilast; Tacrolimus (Topical); Trastuzumab

Decreased Effect

Mechlorethamine (Systemic) may decrease the levels/effects of: BCG (Intravesical); Coccidioides immitis Skin Test; Sipuleucel-T; Vaccines (Inactivated); Vaccines (Live)

The levels/effects of Mechlorethamine (Systemic) may be decreased by: Echinacea

Storage/Stability Store intact vials at room temperature of 15°C to 30°C (59°F to 86°F). Protect from light. Protect from humidity. **Must be prepared immediately before use;** degradation begins shortly after dilution.

Preparation for Administration Hazardous agent; use appropriate precautions for handling and disposal (NIOSH 2014 [group 1]). **Must be prepared immediately before use;** degradation begins shortly after dilution. Dilute powder with 10 mL SWFI or NS to a final concentration of 1 mg/mL. May be further diluted in 50-100 mL NS for intracavitary administration.

Mechanism of Action Bifunctional alkylating agent that inhibits DNA and RNA synthesis via formation of carbonium ions; produces interstrand and intrastrand cross-links in DNA resulting in miscoding, breakage, and failure of replication. Although not cell phase-specific *per se,* mechlorethamine effect is most pronounced in the S phase, and cell proliferation is arrested in the G_2 phase.

Pharmacodynamics/Kinetics

Metabolism: Rapid hydrolysis in the plasma to active metabolites (Perry, 2012)

Half-life elimination: 15-20 minutes (Perry, 2012)

Dosing

Adult & Geriatric Dosage should be based on ideal dry weight (evaluate the presence of edema or ascites so that dosage is based on actual weight unaugmented by edema/ascites). Mechlorethamine is associated with a high

◄   emetic potential (Basch, 2011; Roila, 2010); antiemetics are recommended to
prevent nausea and vomiting

Hodgkin lymphoma (off-label dosing): IV:

MOPP regimen: 6 mg/m^2 on days 1 and 8 of a 28-day treatment cycle for 6
to 8 cycles (Canelos, 1992; DeVita, 1970)

Stanford V regimen: 6 mg/m^2 as a single dose on day 1 in weeks 1, 5, and 9
(Horning, 2000; Horning, 2002)

Malignant effusion: Intracavitary: 0.4 mg/kg as a single dose; although
0.2 mg/kg (10-20 mg) as a single dose has been used by the *intraper-
icardial* route

Renal Impairment No dosage adjustment provided in manufacturer's labeling.

Hepatic Impairment No dosage adjustment provided in manufacturer's
labeling.

The following have also been reported:

Mild-to-moderate impairment: No dosage adjustment necessary
(Ecklund, 2005).

Severe liver impairment: No dosage adjustment necessary; concomitant
chemotherapy may require alteration until improvement in hepatic function
(Ecklund, 2005)

Obesity *ASCO Guidelines for appropriate chemotherapy dosing in obese
adults with cancer:* In general, utilize patient's actual body weight (full weight)
for calculation of body surface area- or weight-based dosing, particularly
when the intent of therapy is curative; manage regimen-related toxicities in
the same manner as for nonobese patients; if a dose reduction is utilized due
to toxicity, consider resumption of full weight-based dosing with subsequent
cycles, especially if cause of toxicity (eg, hepatic or renal impairment) is
resolved (Griggs, 2012). **Note:** The manufacturer recommends dosing be
based on ideal dry body weight and the presence of edema or ascites should
be considered so the dose will be based on unaugmented weight.

Combination Regimens

Lymphoma, Hodgkin:

MOPP/ABVD (Hodgkin) on page 2039

MOPP/ABV Hybrid (Hodgkin) on page 2040

MOPP (Hodgkin) on page 2041

Stanford V (Hodgkin) on page 2085

Administration

IV: Administer as a slow IV push over a few minutes into a free-flowing IV
solution. Mechlorethamine is associated with a high emetic potential (Basch,
2011; Dupuis, 2011; Roila, 2010); antiemetics are recommended to prevent
nausea and vomiting.

Intracavitary: May further dilute in 50-100 mL of normal saline prior to
instillation; rotate patient position every 5-10 minutes for 1 hour after
instillation to obtain uniform distribution.

Prepare immediately prior to administration.

Vesicant; ensure proper needle or catheter placement prior to and during
infusion; avoid extravasation.

Extravasation management: If extravasation occurs, stop infusion immediately and disconnect (leave cannula/needle in place); gently aspirate extravasated solution (do **NOT** flush the line); remove needle/cannula; elevate
extremity.

Sodium thiosulfate 1/6 M solution: Inject subcutaneously into extravasation area using 2 mL for each mg of mechlorethamine suspected to have extravasated (Perez Fidalgo, 2012; Polovich, 2009). Apply ice for 6-12 hours after sodium thiosulfate administration (Mustargen prescribing information, 2013; Polovich, 2009) **or** may apply dry cold compresses for 20 minutes 4 times daily for 1-2 days (Perez Fidalgo, 2012).

Hazardous agent; use appropriate precautions for handling and disposal (NIOSH 2014 [group 1]).

Vesicant/Extravasation Risk Vesicant

Emetic Potential Children and Adults: High (>90%)

Monitoring Parameters CBC with differential and platelet count; renal and hepatic function; signs/symptoms of hypersensitivity reactions, infection, and extravasation

Additional Information A topical gel is commercially approved for topical treatment of cutaneous T-cell lymphoma (mycosis fungoides type), please refer to Mechlorethamine (Topical) monograph.

Product Availability Mustargen: Mustargen was acquired by Recordati Rare Diseases in 2013; availability information is currently unknown.

Dosage Forms Excipient information presented when available (limited, particularly for generics); consult specific product labeling.
Solution Reconstituted, Injection, as hydrochloride:
   Mustargen: 10 mg (1 ea)

Mechlorethamine (Topical) (me klor ETH a meen)

Brand Names: US Valchlor

Index Terms Mechlorethamine HCl (Topical); Mechlorethamine Topical Gel

Pharmacologic Category Antineoplastic Agent, Alkylating Agent; Antineoplastic Agent, Alkylating Agent (Nitrogen Mustard)

Use Cutaneous T-cell lymphoma: Topical treatment of stage IA and IB mycosis fungoides-type cutaneous T-cell lymphoma in patients who have received prior skin-directed therapy

Labeled Contraindications Known severe hypersensitivity to mechlorethamine or any component of the formulation

Pregnancy Considerations Adverse events have been observed in animal reproduction studies. There have been case reports of teratogenic events following systemic use in humans. Pregnancy should be avoided if therapy is needed.

Breast-Feeding Considerations It is not known if mechlorethamine is excreted into breast milk following topical application. Due to the potential for serious adverse reactions in the nursing infant following topical or systemic exposure from the mother's skin, the manufacturer recommends a decision be made whether to discontinue nursing or to discontinue the drug, taking into account the importance of treatment to the mother.

Warnings/Precautions Hazardous agent – use appropriate precautions for handling and disposal (NIOSH 2014 [group 1]). Caregivers should wear nitrile gloves when applying to patients. Wash hands thoroughly with soap and water after handling/application. If accidental skin exposure occurs, wash thoroughly for at least 15 minutes with soap and water; remove any contaminated clothing. Eye exposure may result in pain, burning, inflammation, photophobia, and blurred vision. Blindness and severe anterior eye injury (irreversible) may occur. If exposure to eye(s) occurs, promptly irrigate for at least 15 minutes with copious amounts of water, normal saline, or balanced salt ophthalmic ▶

irrigating solution; obtain ophthalmology consultation. Exposure to mucous membranes may cause pain, redness, and ulceration; may be severe. If mucosal contact occurs, irrigate promptly for at least 15 minutes with copious amounts of water and obtain medical consultation.

Dermatitis commonly occurs; may be moderately severe or severe. Monitor for redness, swelling, itching, blistering, ulceration, and secondary skin infections. Facial, genitalia, anus and intertriginous skin areas are at increased risk for dermatitis. Dermatitis may require dosage reduction. Avoid direct contact with mechlorethamine (other than intended treatment areas for the patient). Secondary exposure risks include dermatitis, mucosal injury, and secondary malignancies. To prevent secondary exposure, follow recommended application procedures. In a clinical study, non-melanoma skin cancers developed during or within 1 year following treatment. Some instances occurred in patients who had received previous treatments that were associated with non-melanoma skin cancer. Monitor for non-melanoma skin cancers during and following treatment; may occur anywhere on the skin, including untreated areas.

Mechlorethamine gel contains alcohol and is flammable; follow recommended application procedures and avoid fire, flame, and smoking until mechlorethamine has dried.

Adverse Reactions

>10%:

Dermatologic: Dermatitis (56%; moderately severe or severe: 23%), pruritus (20%), bacterial skin infection (11%)

Hematologic & oncologic: Hematologic abnormality (decreased hemoglobin, neutrophils, or platelets; 13%)

1% to 10%:

Dermatologic: Dermal ulcer (6%), skin hyperpigmentation (5%)

Hematologic & oncologic: Malignant neoplasm (nonmelanoma skin cancer; 2%)

Postmarketing and/or case reports: Anaphylaxis, hypersensitivity reaction

Drug Interactions

Metabolism/Transport Effects None known.

Avoid Concomitant Use There are no known interactions where it is recommended to avoid concomitant use.

Increased Effect/Toxicity There are no known significant interactions involving an increase in effect.

Decreased Effect There are no known significant interactions involving a decrease in effect.

Storage/Stability Prior to dispensing, store in freezer at -25°C to -15°C (-13°F to 5°F). After dispensing, refrigerate at 2°C to 8°C (36°F to 46°F); apply immediately (or within 30 minutes) after removal from refrigerator; return to refrigerator promptly after each use. Discard unused product 60 days after opening.

Preparation for Administration Hazardous agent – use appropriate precautions for handling and disposal (NIOSH 2014 [group 1]).

Mechanism of Action Mechlorethamine is a nitrogen mustard alkylating agent which forms inter- and intra-strand DNA cross-links, resulting in inhibition of DNA synthesis. Topical application allows for skin-directed treatment while minimizing systemic nitrogen mustard exposure (Lessin, 2013).

Pharmacodynamics/Kinetics

Absorption: Topical: None detected (Lessin, 2013)

Distribution: Topical: No detectable systemic exposure in a clinical study (Lessin, 2013)

Dosing

Adult & Geriatric

Cutaneous T-cell lymphoma (mycosis fungoides-type): Topical: Apply a thin film once daily to affected areas of skin

Note: Concurrent use of topical or systemic corticosteroids was not allowed in the clinical study (Lessin, 2013).

Renal Impairment No dosage adjustment provided in the manufacturer's labeling; however, based on the lack of systemic exposure, dosage adjustment is likely not necessary.

Hepatic Impairment No dosage adjustment provided in the manufacturer's labeling; however, based on the lack of systemic exposure, dosage adjustment is likely not necessary.

Adjustment for Toxicity Skin ulceration (any grade), blistering, or dermatitis (moderately severe-to-severe): Withhold treatment; upon improvement, may reinitiate treatment with a reduced frequency of once every 3 days; if every 3-day application is tolerated for at least 1 week, may increase to every other day for at least 1 week, then (if tolerated) may increase to once daily.

Administration Apply a thin film topically to affected area. Apply immediately (or within 30 minutes) after removal from refrigerator; return to refrigerator promptly after each use. Apply to completely dry skin at least 4 hours before or 30 minutes after showering/washing. Allow treated area(s) to dry for 5-10 minutes after application before covering with clothing. May apply emollients (moisturizers) to treated area 2 hours before or 2 hours after mechlorethamine application. Do not use occlusive dressings over treatment areas. Avoid fire, flame, and smoking until mechlorethamine has dried.

Hazardous agent; use appropriate precautions for handling and disposal (NIOSH 2014 [group 1]). Caregivers should wear nitrile gloves when applying to patients. Wash hands thoroughly with soap and water after handling/application. If accidental skin exposure occurs, wash thoroughly for at least 15 minutes with soap and water; remove any contaminated clothing.

Monitoring Parameters Monitor for dermatologic toxicity (skin ulcers, blistering, dermatitis, secondary skin infections) and signs/symptoms of non-melanoma skin cancer.

Prescribing and Access Restrictions Valchlor is only available through a specialty pharmacy; information regarding prescribing and access may be found at www.valchlor.com.

Medication Guide Available Yes

Dosage Forms Considerations Valchlor 0.016% is equivalent to 0.02% mechlorethamine hydrochloride

Dosage Forms Excipient information presented when available (limited, particularly for generics); consult specific product labeling.

Gel, External:

Valchlor: 0.016% (60 g) [contains edetate disodium, isopropyl alcohol, menthol, propylene glycol]

◆ **Mechlorethamine HCl (Topical)** *see* Mechlorethamine (Topical) *on page 1071*

- ◆ **Mechlorethamine Hydrochloride** *see* Mechlorethamine (Systemic) *on page 1067*
- ◆ **Mechlorethamine Topical Gel** *see* Mechlorethamine (Topical) *on page 1071*
- ◆ **Med-Anastrozole (Can)** *see* Anastrozole *on page 112*
- ◆ **MED-Letrozole (Can)** *see* Letrozole *on page 1019*
- ◆ **Medrol** *see* MethylPREDNISolone *on page 1125*
- ◆ **Medrol Dose Pack** *see* MethylPREDNISolone *on page 1125*
- ◆ **Medrol (Pak)** *see* MethylPREDNISolone *on page 1125*
- ◆ **Medroxy (Can)** *see* MedroxyPROGESTERone *on page 1074*

MedroxyPROGESTERone (me DROKS ee proe JES te rone)

Brand Names: US Depo-Provera; Depo-SubQ Provera 104; Provera

Brand Names: Canada Alti-MPA; Apo-Medroxy; Depo-Prevera; Depo-Provera; Dom-Medroxyprogesterone; Gen-Medroxy; Medroxy; Medroxyprogesterone Acetate Injectable Suspension USP; Novo-Medrone; PMS-Medroxyprogesterone; Provera; Provera-Pak; Teva-Medroxyprogesterone

Index Terms Acetoxymethylprogesterone; Medroxyprogesterone Acetate; Methylacetoxyprogesterone; MPA

Pharmacologic Category Contraceptive; Progestin

Use

Abnormal uterine bleeding (tablet): Treatment of abnormal uterine bleeding due to hormonal imbalance in the absence of organic pathology, such as fibroids or uterine cancer.

Amenorrhea, secondary (tablet): Treatment of secondary amenorrhea due to hormonal imbalance in the absence of organic pathology, such as fibroids or uterine cancer.

Contraception (104 mg/0.65 mL and 150 mg/mL injection): Prevention of pregnancy in women of childbearing potential.

Endometrial hyperplasia (tablet): Prevention of endometrial hyperplasia in nonhysterectomized postmenopausal women receiving daily oral conjugated estrogens 0.625 mg.

Endometrial carcinoma (400 mg/mL injection): Adjunctive therapy and palliative treatment of inoperable, recurrent, and metastatic endometrial carcinoma.

Endometriosis (104 mg/0.65 mL injection): Management of endometriosis-associated pain.

Pregnancy Risk Factor X (tablet)

Dosing

Adult & Geriatric

Abnormal uterine bleeding: Oral: 5 or 10 mg daily for 5 to 10 days starting on day 16 or 21 of menstrual cycle. Secretory transformation of the endometrium will occur when adequately primed with endogenous or exogenous estrogen. Withdrawal bleeding may be expected within 3 to 7 days after discontinuing medroxyprogesterone.

Amenorrhea, secondary: Oral: 5 or 10 mg daily for 5 to 10 days. Therapy may be started at any time. Secretory transformation of the endometrium will occur when adequately primed with endogenous or exogenous estrogen. Withdrawal bleeding may be expected within 3 to 7 days after discontinuing medroxyprogesterone.

Contraception:
Depo-Provera Contraceptive: IM: 150 mg every 3 months (every 13 weeks)
depo-subQ provera 104: SubQ: 104 mg every 3 months (every 12 to 14 weeks)

Endometrial carcinoma, recurrent or metastatic (adjunctive/palliative treatment) (Depo-Provera): IM: Initial: 400 to 1,000 mg/week

Endometrial hyperplasia reduction: Oral: 5 or 10 mg daily for 12 to 14 consecutive days each month, starting on day 1 or day 16 of the cycle. When treating postmenopausal women, use for the shortest duration possible at the lowest effective dose consistent with treatment goals. Reevaluate patients as clinically appropriate to determine if treatment is still necessary. Consider use of an estrogen with a progestin in postmenopausal women with a uterus. Women who have had a hysterectomy generally do not need a progestin. Adjust dose based on patient response. Attempt to taper or discontinue at 3- to 6-month intervals.

Endometriosis (depo-subQ provera 104): SubQ: 104 mg every 3 months (every 12 to 14 weeks)

Paraphilia/hypersexuality (off-label use) (Reilly 2000): Males (**Note:** Avoid use if active pituitary pathology, hepatic failure, or thromboembolic disease): IM (Depo-Provera): 100 to 600 mg weekly
Oral: 100 to 500 mg daily

Pediatric Adolescents:

Abnormal uterine bleeding: Refer to adult dosing.

Amenorrhea, secondary: Refer to adult dosing.

Contraception: Refer to adult dosing.

Endometriosis: Refer to adult dosing.

Renal Impairment There are no dosage adjustments provided in the manufacturer's labeling (has not been studied).

Hepatic Impairment Medroxyprogesterone is extensively metabolized in the liver. Most products are contraindicated in patients with hepatic impairment. If needed for the palliative treatment metastatic endometrial carcinoma, monitor closely; withhold or discontinue treatment if liver dysfunction develops and do not resume until hepatic function has returned to normal.

Additional Information Complete prescribing information should be consulted for additional detail.

Dosage Forms Excipient information presented when available (limited, particularly for generics); consult specific product labeling.

Suspension, Intramuscular, as acetate:
Depo-Provera: 150 mg/mL (1 mL)
Depo-Provera: 150 mg/mL (1 mL) [contains methylparaben, polyethylene glycol, polysorbate 80, propylparaben]
Depo-Provera: 400 mg/mL (2.5 mL)
Generic: 150 mg/mL (1 mL)

Suspension, Subcutaneous, as acetate:
Depo-SubQ Provera 104: 104 mg/0.65 mL (0.65 mL) [contains methylparaben, propylparaben]

Tablet, Oral, as acetate:
Provera: 2.5 mg, 5 mg, 10 mg [scored]
Generic: 2.5 mg, 5 mg, 10 mg

◆ **Medroxyprogesterone Acetate** *see* MedroxyPROGESTERone
on page 1074

◆ **Medroxyprogesterone Acetate Injectable Suspension USP (Can)** *see* MedroxyPROGESTERone *on page* 1074

◆ **Megace ES** *see* Megestrol *on page* 1076

◆ **Megace Oral** *see* Megestrol *on page* 1076

◆ **Megace OS (Can)** *see* Megestrol *on page* 1076

Megestrol (me JES trole)

Related Information

Palliative Care Medicine (Cancer) *on page* 2252

Safe Handling of Hazardous Drugs *on page* 2292

Brand Names: US Megace ES; Megace Oral

Brand Names: Canada Megace OS; Megestrol

Index Terms 5071-1DL(6); Megestrol Acetate

Pharmacologic Category Antineoplastic Agent, Hormone; Appetite Stimulant; Progestin

Use

Anorexia or cachexia: *Suspension:* Treatment of anorexia, cachexia, or unexplained significant weight loss in patients with AIDS

Limitations of use: Treatment of AIDS-related weight loss should only be initiated after addressing the treatable causes (eg, malignancy, infection, malabsorption, endocrine disease, renal disease, psychiatric disorder) for weight loss. Megestrol is not intended to prevent weight loss.

Breast cancer: *Tablet:* Treatment (palliative) of advanced breast cancer

Endometrial cancer: *Tablet:* Treatment (palliative) of advanced endometrial carcinoma

Additional Canadian use (not an approved use in the U.S.): *Tablet:* Treatment of anorexia, cachexia, or weight loss secondary to metastatic cancer

Labeled Contraindications Hypersensitivity to megestrol or any component of the formulation; known or suspected pregnancy (suspension)

Pregnancy Considerations Adverse events were demonstrated in animal reproduction studies. May cause fetal harm if administered to a pregnant woman. Use during pregnancy is contraindicated (suspension) and appropriate contraception is recommended in women who may become pregnant. In clinical studies, megestrol was shown to cause breakthrough vaginal bleeding in women.

Breast-Feeding Considerations Megestrol is excreted into breast milk. Information is available from five nursing women, ~8 weeks postpartum, who were administered megestrol 4 mg in combination with ethinyl estradiol 50 mcg daily for contraception. Maternal serum and milk samples were obtained over 5 days, beginning 10 days after therapy began. The highest concentrations of megestrol were found at the samples taken 3 hours after the maternal dose. Mean concentrations of megestrol were 6.5 ng/mL (maternal serum; range: 3.7 to 10.8 ng/mL), 4.6 ng/mL (foremilk; range: 1.1 to 12.7 ng/mL), and 5.6 ng/mL (hindmilk; range: 1.2 to 18.5 ng/mL) (Nilsson, 1977). Due to the potential for adverse reaction in the newborn, the manufacturer recommends discontinuing breast-feeding while receiving megestrol. In addition, in the United States, where formula is accessible, affordable, safe, and sustainable, and the risk of infant mortality due to diarrhea and respiratory infections is low, complete avoidance of breast-feeding by HIV-infected women is recommended to decrease potential transmission of HIV (DHHS [perinatal], 2012).

Warnings/Precautions Hazardous agent - use appropriate precautions for handling and disposal (NIOSH 2014 [group 1]). May suppress hypothalamic-pituitary-adrenal (HPA) axis during chronic administration; consider the possibility of adrenal suppression in any patient receiving or being withdrawn from chronic therapy when signs/symptoms suggestive of hypoadrenalism are noted (during stress or in unstressed state). Laboratory evaluation and replacement/stress doses of rapid-acting glucocorticoid should be considered. Cushing syndrome has been reported with long-term use. New-onset diabetes and exacerbation of preexisting diabetes have been reported with long-term use. Use with caution in patients with a history of thromboembolic disease. Avoid use in older adults due to minimal effect on weight, and an increased risk of thrombosis and possibly death (Beers Criteria). Vaginal bleeding or discharge may occur in females. The effects on HIV viral replications are unknown in patients with AIDS-related cachexia. Potentially significant drug-drug interactions may exist, requiring dose or frequency adjustment, additional monitoring, and/or selection of alternative therapy.

Megace ES suspension is not equivalent to other formulations on a mg per mg basis; Megace ES suspension 625 mg/5 mL is equivalent to megestrol acetate suspension 800 mg/20 mL.

Benzyl alcohol and derivatives: Some dosage forms may contain sodium benzoate/benzoic acid; benzoic acid (benzoate) is a metabolite of benzyl alcohol; large amounts of benzyl alcohol (≥99 mg/kg/day) have been associated with a potentially fatal toxicity ("gasping syndrome") in neonates; the "gasping syndrome" consists of metabolic acidosis, respiratory distress, gasping respirations, CNS dysfunction (including convulsions, intracranial hemorrhage), hypotension, and cardiovascular collapse (AAP ["Inactive" 1997]; CDC, 1982); some data suggests that benzoate displaces bilirubin from protein binding sites (Ahlfors, 2001); avoid or use dosage forms containing benzyl alcohol derivative with caution in neonates. See manufacturer's labeling.

Adverse Reactions
Frequency not always defined.
Cardiovascular: Hypertension (4% to 8%), cardiomyopathy (1% to 3%), chest pain (1% to 3%), edema (1% to 3%), palpitations (1% to 3%), peripheral edema (1% to 3%), cardiac failure
Central nervous system: Headache (3% to 10%), pain (4% to 6%, similar to placebo), insomnia (1% to 6%), abnormality in thinking (1% to 3%), confusion (1% to 3%), convulsions (1% to 3%), depression (1% to 3%), hypoesthesia (1% to 3%), neuropathy (1% to 3%), paresthesia (1% to 3%), carpal tunnel syndrome, lethargy, malaise, mood changes
Dermatologic: Skin rash (6% to 12%), alopecia (1% to 3%), dermatological disease (1% to 3%), diaphoresis (1% to 3%), pruritus (1% to 3%), vesicobullous dermatitis (1% to 3%)
Endocrine & metabolic: Hyperglycemia (6%), decreased libido (1% to 5%), albuminuria (1% to 3%), gynecomastia (1% to 3%), increased lactate dehydrogenase (1% to 3%), adrenocortical insufficiency, amenorrhea, Cushing's syndrome, diabetes mellitus, hot flash, HPA-axis suppression, hypercalcemia, weight gain (not attributed to edema or fluid retention)
Gastrointestinal: Diarrhea (10%, similar to placebo), flatulence (6% to 10%), vomiting (4% to 6%), nausea (4% to 5%), dyspepsia (2% to 3%), abdominal pain (1% to 3%), constipation (1% to 3%), oral moniliasis (1% to 3%), sialorrhea (1% to 3%), xerostomia (1% to 3%)

◀ Genitourinary: Impotence (4% to 14%), urinary incontinence (1% to 3%), urinary tract infection (1% to 3%), urinary frequency (1% to 2%), breakthrough bleeding

Hematologic & oncologic: Leukopenia (1% to 3%), sarcoma (1% to 3%), tumor flare

Hepatic: Hepatomegaly (1% to 3%)

Infection: Candidiasis (1% to 3%), herpes virus infection (1% to 3%), infection (1% to 3%)

Neuromuscular & skeletal: Weakness (5% to 6%)

Ophthalmic: Amblyopia (1% to 3%)

Respiratory: Cough (1% to 3%), dyspnea (1% to 3%), pharyngitis (1% to 3%), pulmonary disorder (1% to 3%), pneumonia (1%), hyperventilation

Miscellaneous: Fever (1% to 6%)

Postmarketing and/or case reports: Decreased glucose tolerance, thromboembolic phenomena (including deep vein thrombosis, pulmonary embolism, thrombophlebitis)

Drug Interactions

Metabolism/Transport Effects None known.

Avoid Concomitant Use

Avoid concomitant use of Megestrol with any of the following: Dofetilide; Indium 111 Capromab Pendetide; Ulipristal

Increased Effect/Toxicity

Megestrol may increase the levels/effects of: C1 inhibitors; Dofetilide

The levels/effects of Megestrol may be increased by: Herbs (Progestogenic Properties)

Decreased Effect

Megestrol may decrease the levels/effects of: Anticoagulants; Antidiabetic Agents; Choline C 11; Indium 111 Capromab Pendetide; Ulipristal

The levels/effects of Megestrol may be decreased by: Ulipristal

Storage/Stability

Suspension: Store at 15°C to 25°C (59°F to 77°F); protect from heat. Store/dispense in a tight container.

Tablet: Store at 20°C to 25°C (68°F to 77°F); protect from light.

Mechanism of Action A synthetic progestin with antiestrogenic properties which disrupt the estrogen receptor cycle. Megestrol interferes with the normal estrogen cycle and results in a lower LH titer. May also have a direct effect on the endometrium. Megestrol is an antineoplastic progestin thought to act through an antileutenizing effect mediated via the pituitary. May stimulate appetite by antagonizing the metabolic effects of catabolic cytokines.

Pharmacodynamics/Kinetics

Metabolism: Hepatic (to free steroids and glucuronide conjugates)

Half-life elimination: Suspension: 20 to 50 hours; Tablet: 13 to 105 hours

Time to peak, serum: 1 to 3 hours

Excretion: Urine (57% to 78%; 5% to 8% as metabolites); feces (8% to 30%)

Dosing

Adult Note: Megace ES suspension is not equivalent to other formulations on a mg-per-mg basis.

Anorexia or cachexia associated with AIDS: Oral: Suspension:

U.S. labeling: Initial: 625 mg daily (of the 125 mg/mL suspension) or 800 mg daily (of the 40 mg/mL suspension); daily doses of 400 mg to 800 mg have been found to be effective

Canadian labeling: Usual dose: 400 to 800 mg once daily for at least 2 months

Breast cancer, advanced: Oral: Tablet:

U.S. labeling: 160 mg per day in divided doses of 40 mg 4 times daily for at least 2 months

Canadian labeling: 160 mg or 125 mg/m² daily (40 mg 4 times daily or 160 mg once daily) for at least 2 months

Endometrial cancer, advanced: Oral: Tablet:

U.S. labeling: 40 to 320 mg daily in divided doses for at least 2 months

Canadian labeling: 80 to 320 mg or 62.5 to 250 mg/m² daily in divided doses (40 to 80 mg 1 to 4 times daily or 160 to 320mg daily) for at least 2 months

Cancer-related cachexia: *Canadian labeling:* Oral: Tablet: 400 to 800 mg once daily for at least 2 months

Cancer-related cachexia (off-label use/dosing in U.S.): Oral: Doses ranging from 160 to 800 mg per day were effective in achieving weight gain, higher doses (>160 mg) were associated with more weight gain (Beller, 1997; Loprinzi, 1990; Loprinzi, 1993; Vadell, 1998); based on a meta-analysis, an optimal dose has not been determined (Ruiz Garcia, 2013)

Geriatric Use with caution; refer to adult dosing.

Renal Impairment There are no dosage adjustments provided in the manufacturer's labeling; however, the urinary excretion of megestrol acetate is substantial, use caution.

Hepatic Impairment There are no dosage adjustments provided in the manufacturer's labeling.

Administration Oral: Shake suspension well before use. Hazardous agent; use appropriate precautions for handling and disposal (NIOSH 2014 [group 1]).

Monitoring Parameters Observe for signs of thromboembolic events; blood pressure, weight; serum glucose

Dosage Forms Excipient information presented when available (limited, particularly for generics); consult specific product labeling. [DSC] = Discontinued product

Suspension, Oral, as acetate:

Megace ES: 625 mg/5 mL (150 mL) [contains alcohol, usp, sodium benzoate; lemon-lime flavor]

Megace Oral: 40 mg/mL (240 mL) [lemon-lime flavor]

Generic: 40 mg/mL (10 mL, 240 mL, 480 mL); 400 mg/10 mL (10 mL, 20 mL [DSC]); 625 mg/5 mL (150 mL)

Tablet, Oral, as acetate:

Generic: 20 mg, 40 mg

Dosage Forms: Canada Refer also to Dosage Forms. **Note:** Megace ES not available in Canada.

Excipient information presented when available (limited, particularly for generics); consult specific product labeling.

Tablet, Oral, as acetate: 160 mg

◆ **Megestrol Acetate** *see* Megestrol *on page* 1076

◆ **Mekinist** *see* Trametinib *on page* 1674

Melphalan (MEL fa lan)

Related Information

Chemotherapy and Obesity *on page 2220*

Hematopoietic Stem Cell Transplantation *on page 2272*

Management of Chemotherapy-Induced Nausea and Vomiting in Adults *on page 2142*

Management of Drug Extravasations *on page 2159*

Mucositis and Stomatitis *on page 2186*

Prevention of Chemotherapy-Induced Nausea and Vomiting in Children *on page 2203*

Safe Handling of Hazardous Drugs *on page 2292*

Brand Names: US Alkeran

Brand Names: Canada Alkeran

Index Terms L-PAM; L-Phenylalanine Mustard; L-Sarcolysin; Phenylalanine Mustard

Pharmacologic Category Antineoplastic Agent, Alkylating Agent; Antineoplastic Agent, Alkylating Agent (Nitrogen Mustard)

Use

Multiple myeloma: Palliative treatment of multiple myeloma (injection and tablets).

Ovarian carcinoma: Palliative treatment of nonresectable epithelial ovarian carcinoma (tablets)

Labeled Contraindications Hypersensitivity to melphalan or any component of the formulation; patients whose disease was resistant to prior melphalan therapy

Pregnancy Considerations Animal studies have demonstrated embryotoxicity and teratogenicity. Therapy may suppress ovarian function leading to amenorrhea. There are no adequate and well-controlled studies in pregnant women. May cause fetal harm if administered during pregnancy. Women of childbearing potential should be advised to avoid pregnancy while on melphalan therapy.

Breast-Feeding Considerations According to the manufacturer, melphalan should not be administered if breast-feeding.

Warnings/Precautions Hazardous agent; use appropriate precautions for handling and disposal (NIOSH 2014 [group 1]).

[U.S. Boxed Warning]: Bone marrow suppression is common; may be severe and result in infection or bleeding; has been demonstrated more with the IV formulation (compared to oral); myelosuppression is dose-related. Monitor blood counts; may require treatment delay or dose modification for thrombocytopenia or neutropenia. Use with caution in patients with prior bone marrow suppression, impaired renal function (consider dose reduction), or who have received prior (or concurrent) chemotherapy or irradiation. Myelotoxicity is generally reversible, although irreversible bone marrow failure has been reported. In patients who are candidates for autologous transplantation, avoid melphalan-containing regimens prior to transplant (due to the effects on stem cell reserve). Signs of infection, such as fever and WBC rise, may not occur; lethargy and confusion may be more prominent signs of infection.

[U.S. Boxed Warning]: Hypersensitivity reactions (including anaphylaxis) have occurred in ~2% of patients receiving IV melphalan, usually after multiple treatment cycles. Discontinue infusion and treat symptomatically.

Hypersensitivity may also occur (rarely) with oral melphalan. Do not readminister (oral or IV) in patients who experience hypersensitivity to melphalan.

Gastrointestinal toxicities, including nausea, vomiting, diarrhea and mucositis, are common. When administering high-dose melphalan in autologous transplantation, cryotherapy is recommended to prevent oral mucositis (Lalla, 2014). Melphalan is associated with a moderate emetic potential (depending on dose and/or administration route); antiemetics may be recommended to prevent nausea and vomiting (Dupuis, 2011). Abnormal liver function tests may occur; hepatitis and jaundice have also been reported; hepatic sinusoidal obstruction syndrome (SOS; formerly called veno-occlusive disease) has been reported with IV melphalan. Pulmonary fibrosis (some fatal) and interstitial pneumonitis have been observed with treatment. Dosage reduction is recommended with IV melphalan in patients with renal impairment; reduced initial doses may also be recommended with oral melphalan. Closely monitor patients with azotemia.

[U.S. Boxed Warning]: Produces chromosomal changes and is leukemogenic and potentially mutagenic; secondary malignancies (including acute myeloid leukemia, myeloproliferative disease, and carcinoma) have been reported reported (some patients were receiving combination chemotherapy or radiation therapy); the risk is increased with increased treatment duration and cumulative doses. Suppresses ovarian function and produces amenorrhea; may also cause testicular suppression.

Extravasation may cause local tissue damage; administration by slow injection into a fast running IV solution into an injection port or via a central line is recommended; do not administer directly into a peripheral vein. Some dosage forms may contain propylene glycol; large amounts are potentially toxic and have been associated hyperosmolality, lactic acidosis, seizures and respiratory depression; use caution (AAP, 1997; Zar, 2007). **[U.S. Boxed Warning]: Should be administered under the supervision of an experienced cancer chemotherapy physician.** Avoid vaccination with live vaccines during treatment if immunocompromised. Toxicity may be increased in elderly; start with lowest recommended adult doses. Potentially significant drug-drug interactions may exist, requiring dose or frequency adjustment, additional monitoring, and/ or selection of alternative therapy.

Adverse Reactions

>10%:

Gastrointestinal: Nausea/vomiting, diarrhea, oral ulceration

Hematologic: Myelosuppression, leukopenia (nadir: 14-21 days; recovery: 28-35 days), thrombocytopenia (nadir: 14-21 days; recovery: 28-35 days), anemia

Miscellaneous: Secondary malignancy (<2% to 20%; cumulative dose and duration dependent, includes acute myeloid leukemia, myeloproliferative syndrome, carcinoma)

1% to 10%: Miscellaneous: Hypersensitivity (IV: 2%; includes bronchospasm, dyspnea, edema, hypotension, pruritus, rash, tachycardia, urticaria)

Infrequent, frequency undefined, postmarketing, and/or case reports: Agranulocytosis, allergic reactions, alopecia, amenorrhea, anaphylaxis (rare), bleeding (with high-dose therapy), bone marrow failure (irreversible), BUN increased, cardiac arrest, cardiotoxicity (angina, arrhythmia, hypertension, MI; with high-dose therapy), encephalopathy, hemolytic anemia, hemorrhagic cystitis, hepatic sinusoidal obstruction syndrome (SOS; veno-occlusive disease; high-dose IV melphalan), hepatitis, infection, injection site reactions

◀ (ulceration, necrosis), interstitial pneumonitis, jaundice, mucositis (with high-dose therapy), ovarian suppression, paralytic ileus (with high-dose therapy), pruritus, pulmonary fibrosis, radiation myelopathy, rash (maculopapular), renal toxicity (with high-dose therapy), seizure (with high-dose therapy), sepsis, SIADH, skin hypersensitivity, sterility, stomatitis, testicular suppression, tingling sensation, transaminases increased, vasculitis, warmth sensation

Drug Interactions

Metabolism/Transport Effects None known.

Avoid Concomitant Use

Avoid concomitant use of Melphalan with any of the following: BCG (Intravesical); CloZAPine; Dipyrone; Nalidixic Acid; Natalizumab; Pimecrolimus; Tacrolimus (Topical); Tofacitinib; Vaccines (Live)

Increased Effect/Toxicity

Melphalan may increase the levels/effects of: Carmustine; CloZAPine; Cyclo-SPORINE (Systemic); Fingolimod; Leflunomide; Natalizumab; Tofacitinib; Vaccines (Live)

The levels/effects of Melphalan may be increased by: Denosumab; Dipyrone; Nalidixic Acid; Pimecrolimus; Roflumilast; Tacrolimus (Topical); Trastuzumab

Decreased Effect

Melphalan may decrease the levels/effects of: BCG (Intravesical); Coccidioides immitis Skin Test; Sipuleucel-T; Vaccines (Inactivated); Vaccines (Live)

The levels/effects of Melphalan may be decreased by: Echinacea

Food Interactions Food interferes with oral absorption. Management: Administer on an empty stomach.

Storage/Stability

Tablet: Store in refrigerator at 2°C to 8°C (36°F to 46°F). Protect from light.

Injection: Store intact vials at 20°C to 25°C (68°F to 77°F). Protect from light. The manufacturer recommends administration be completed within 60 minutes of reconstitution; **immediately** dilute dose in NS. Do not refrigerate solution; precipitation occurs.

Preparation for Administration Hazardous agent; use appropriate precautions for handling and disposal (NIOSH 2014 [group 1]).

Injection: Stability is limited; must be prepared fresh. **The time between reconstitution/dilution and administration of parenteral melphalan must be kept to a minimum (manufacturer recommends <60 minutes) because reconstituted and diluted solutions are unstable.** Dissolve powder initially with 10 mL of supplied diluent to a concentration of 5 mg/mL; shake immediately and vigorously to dissolve. **Immediately** dilute dose in NS to a concentration of ≤0.45 mg/mL (manufacturer recommended concentration). Do not refrigerate solution; precipitation occurs if stored at 5°C. The manufacturer recommends administration within 60 minutes of reconstitution.

Mechanism of Action Alkylating agent which is a derivative of mechlorethamine that inhibits DNA and RNA synthesis via formation of carbonium ions; cross-links strands of DNA; acts on both resting and rapidly dividing tumor cells.

Pharmacodynamics/Kinetics Note: Pharmacokinetics listed are for FDA-approved doses.

Absorption: Oral: Variable and incomplete

Distribution: V_d: 0.5 L/kg; low penetration into CSF

Protein binding: 53% to 92%; primarily to albumin (40% to 60%), ~20% to alpha$_1$-acid glycoprotein

Metabolism: Hepatic; chemical hydrolysis to monohydroxymelphalan and dihydroxymelphalan

Bioavailability: Oral: Variable; 56% to 93%; exposure is reduced with a high-fat meal

Half-life elimination: Terminal: IV: 75 minutes; Oral: 1 to 2 hours

Time to peak, serum: Oral: ~1 to 2 hours

Excretion: Oral: Feces (20% to 50%); urine (~10% as unchanged drug)

Dosing

Adult Note: Melphalan is associated with a moderate emetic potential (depending on dose and/or administration route); antiemetics may be recommended to prevent nausea and vomiting. Adjust dose based on patient response and weekly blood counts.

Multiple myeloma (palliative treatment): Note: Response is gradual; may require repeated courses to realize benefit:

Oral: Usual dose (as described in the manufacturer's labeling):

6 mg once daily for 2 to 3 weeks initially, followed by up to 4 weeks rest, then a maintenance dose of 2 mg daily as hematologic recovery begins **or**

10 mg daily for 7 to 10 days; institute 2 mg daily maintenance dose after WBC >4,000 cells/mm^3 and platelets >100,000 cells/mm^3 (~4 to 8 weeks); titrate maintenance dose to hematologic response **or**

0.15 mg/kg/day for 7 days, with a 2 to 6 week rest, followed by a maintenance dose of ≤0.05 mg/kg/day as hematologic recovery begins **or**

0.25 mg/kg/day for 4 days (or 0.2 mg/kg/day for 5 days); repeat at 4- to 6-week intervals as ANC and platelet counts return to normal

*Other dosing regimens in **combination therapy** (off-label doses):*

4 mg/m^2/day for 7 days every 4 weeks (in combination with prednisone **or** with prednisone and thalidomide) (Palumbo, 2006; Palumbo, 2008) **or**

6 mg/m^2/day for 7 days every 4 weeks (in combination with prednisone) (Palumbo, 2004) **or**

0.25 mg/kg/day for 4 days every 6 weeks (in combination with prednisone [Facon, 2006; Facon, 2007] **or** with prednisone and thalidomide [Facon, 2007]) **or**

9 mg/m^2/day for 4 days every 6 weeks (in combination with prednisone **or** with prednisone and bortezomib) (Dimopoulos, 2009; San Miguel, 2008)

IV: 16 mg/m^2 administered at 2-week intervals for 4 doses, then administer at 4-week intervals after adequate hematologic recovery.

Ovarian carcinoma: Oral: 0.2 mg/kg/day for 5 days, repeat every 4 to 5 weeks **or**

Off-label dosing: 7 mg/m^2/day in 2 divided doses for 5 days, repeat every 28 days (Wadler, 1996)

Amyloidosis, light chain (off-label use): Oral: 0.22 mg/kg/day for 4 days every 28 days (in combination with oral dexamethasone) (Palladini, 2004) **or** 10 mg/m^2/day for 4 days every month (in combination with oral dexamethasone) for 12 to 18 treatment cycles (Jaccard, 2007)

Hodgkin lymphoma, relapsed/refractory (off-label use): IV: 30 mg/m^2 on day 6 of combination chemotherapy (mini-BEAM) regimen (Colwill, 1995; Martin, 2001)

◀ **Conditioning regimen for autologous hematopoietic stem cell transplantation (off-label use):** IV:

200 mg/m² alone 2 days prior to transplantation (Fermand, 2005; Moreau, 2002) **or**

140 mg/m² 2 days prior to transplantation (combined with busulfan) (Fermand, 2005) **or**

140 mg/m² 2 days prior to transplantation (combined with total body irradiation [TBI]) (Moreau, 2002) **or**

140 mg/m² 5 days prior to transplantation (combined with TBI) (Barlogie, 2006)

Geriatric Refer to adult dosing. Use caution and begin at the lower end of dosing range.

Pediatric Note: Melphalan is associated with a moderate emetic potential (depending on dose and/or administration route); antiemetics may be recommended to prevent nausea and vomiting (Dupuis, 2011).

Conditioning regimen for autologous hematopoietic stem cell transplantation (off-label use): IV:

140 mg/m² 2 days prior to transplantation (combined with busulfan) (Canete, 2009; Oberlin, 2006) **or**

180 mg/m² (with pre- and posthydration) 12-30 hours prior to transplantation (Pritchard, 2005) **or**

45 mg/m²/day for 4 days starting 8 days prior to transplantation (combined with busulfan or etoposide and carboplatin) (Berthold, 2005)

Renal Impairment

The manufacturer's labeling contains the following adjustment recommendations (for approved dosing levels) based on route of administration:

Oral: Moderate-to-severe renal impairment: Consider a reduced dose initially.

IV: BUN ≥30 mg/dL: Reduce dose by up to 50%.

The following adjustments have also been recommended:

Aronoff, 2007: Adults: Oral (based on a 6 mg once-daily dose):

CrCl 10 to 50 mL/minute: Administer 75% of dose.

CrCl <10 mL/minute: Administer 50% of dose.

Hemodialysis: Administer dose after hemodialysis.

Continuous ambulatory peritoneal dialysis (CAPD): Administer 50% of dose.

Continuous renal replacement therapy (CRRT): Administer 75% of dose.

Carlson, 2005: Oral (for melphalan-prednisone combination therapy; based on a study evaluating toxicity with melphalan dosed at 0.25 mg/kg/day for 4 days/cycle):

CrCl >10 to <30 mL/minute: Administer 75% of dose

CrCl ≤10 mL/minute: Data is insufficient for a recommendation

Kintzel, 1995:

Oral: Adjust dose in the presence of hematologic toxicity

IV:

CrCl 46 to 60 mL/minute: Administer 85% of normal dose.

CrCl 31 to 45 mL/minute: Administer 75% of normal dose.

CrCl <30 mL/minute: Administer 70% of normal dose.

Badros, 2001: IV: Autologous stem cell transplant (single-agent conditioning regimen; no busulfan or irradiation): Serum creatinine >2 mg/dL: Reduce dose from 200 mg/m² over 2 days (as 100 mg/m²/day for 2 days) to 140 mg/m² given as a single-dose infusion

Hepatic Impairment Melphalan is hepatically metabolized; however, dosage adjustment does not appear to be necessary (King, 2001).

Obesity

*American Society of Clinical Oncology (ASCO) Guidelines for appropriate chemotherapy dosing in obese adults with cancer (**Note:** Excludes HSCT dosing):* Utilize patient's actual body weight (full weight) for calculation of body surface area- or weight-based dosing, particularly when the intent of therapy is curative; manage regimen-related toxicities in the same manner as for nonobese patients; if a dose reduction is utilized due to toxicity, consider resumption of full weight-based dosing with subsequent cycles, especially if cause of toxicity (eg, hepatic or renal impairment) is resolved (Griggs, 2012).

American Society for Blood and Marrow Transplantation (ASBMT) practice guideline committee position statement on chemotherapy dosing in obesity: Utilize actual body weight (full weight) for calculation of body surface area in melphalan dosing for hematopoietic stem cell transplant conditioning regimens in adults (Bubalo, 2014).

Adjustment for Toxicity

Oral:

WBC <3000/mm^3: Withhold treatment until recovery

Platelets <100,000/mm^3: Withhold treatment until recovery

IV: Adjust dose based blood cell count at the nadir and day of treatment

Combination Regimens

Lymphoma, Hodgkin:

Dexa-BEAM (Hodgkin) on page 1937

mini-BEAM (Hodgkin) on page 2037

Multiple myeloma:

Bortezomib-Melphalan-Prednisone-Thalidomide on page 1850

Melphalan-Prednisone-Bortezomib (Multiple Myeloma) on page 2033

Melphalan-Prednisone (Multiple Myeloma) on page 2034

Melphalan-Prednisone-Thalidomide (Multiple Myeloma) on page 2035

VBMCP (Multiple Myeloma) on page 2105

Administration Melphalan is associated with a moderate emetic potential (depending on dose and/or administration route); antiemetics may be recommended to prevent nausea and vomiting (Dupuis, 2011).

Oral: Administer on an empty stomach (Schmidt, 2002)

Parenteral: Due to limited stability, complete administration of IV dose should occur within 60 minutes of reconstitution

IV: Infuse over 15 to 20 minutes. Extravasation may cause local tissue damage; administration by slow injection into a fast running IV solution into an injection port or via a central line is recommended; do not administer by direct injection into a peripheral vein.

Hazardous agent; use appropriate precautions for handling and disposal (NIOSH 2014 [group 1]).

Vesicant/Extravasation Risk May be an irritant

Emetic Potential

Children:

IV: >50 mg/m^2: Moderate (30% to 90%)

IV (lower dose): Minimal (<10%)

Oral: Minimal (<10%)

◀ Adults:
　IV: Moderate (30% to 90%)
　Oral: Minimal (<10%)
Monitoring Parameters CBC with differential and platelet count, serum electrolytes, serum uric acid
Test Interactions False-positive Coombs' test [direct]
Dosage Forms Excipient information presented when available (limited, particularly for generics); consult specific product labeling.
　Solution Reconstituted, Intravenous:
　　Alkeran: 50 mg (1 ea) [contains alcohol, usp, propylene glycol]
　　Generic: 50 mg (1 ea)
　Tablet, Oral:
　　Alkeran: 2 mg

Meperidine (me PER i deen)

Brand Names: US Demerol; Meperitab
Brand Names: Canada Demerol
Index Terms Isonipecaine Hydrochloride; Meperidine Hydrochloride; Pethidine Hydrochloride
Pharmacologic Category Analgesic, Opioid
Use Management of moderate to severe pain; preoperative sedation, and obstetrical analgesia
Pregnancy Risk Factor C
Dosing
　Adult Note: The American Pain Society (2008) and ISMP (2007) do not recommend meperidine's use as an analgesic. If use in acute pain (in patients without renal or CNS disease) cannot be avoided, treatment should be limited to ≤48 hours and doses should not exceed 600 mg/24 hours. Oral route is not recommended for treatment of acute or chronic pain. If IV route is required, consider a reduced dose. Patients with prior opioid exposure may require higher initial doses.

　Pain, moderate to severe (analgesic): Oral, IM, SubQ: 50 to 150 mg every 3 to 4 hours as needed
　　Preoperatively: IM, SubQ: 50 to 100 mg given 30 to 90 minutes before the beginning of anesthesia
　　Obstetrical analgesia: IM, SubQ: 50 to 100 mg when pain becomes regular; may repeat at every 1- to 3-hour intervals
　Postoperative shivering (off-label use): IV: 25 to 50 mg once (Crowley 2008; Kranke 2002; Mercandante 1994; Wang 1999)
　Geriatric Avoid use (American Pain Society 2008; ISMP 2007).
　Pediatric Note: The American Pain Society (2008) and ISMP (2007) do not recommend meperidine's use as an analgesic. If use in acute pain (in patients without renal or CNS disease) cannot be avoided, treatment should be limited to ≤48 hours and doses should not exceed 600 mg/24 hours. Oral route is not recommended for treatment of acute or chronic pain. If IV route is required, consider a reduced dose. Patients with prior opioid exposure may require higher initial doses.

　Pain, moderate to severe (analgesic): Oral, IM, SubQ: 1.1 to 1.8 mg/kg/dose every 3 to 4 hours as needed (maximum: 50 to 150 mg/dose)
　　Preoperatively: IM, SubQ: 1.1 to 2.2 mg/kg given 30 to 90 minutes before the beginning of anesthesia (maximum: 50 to 100 mg/dose)

Renal Impairment Avoid use in renal impairment (American Pain Society 2008; ISMP 2007).

Hepatic Impairment Use with caution in severe hepatic impairment; consider a lower initial dose when initiating therapy. An increased opioid effect may be seen in patients with cirrhosis; dose reduction is more important for the oral than IV route.

Additional Information Complete prescribing information should be consulted for additional detail.

Dosage Forms Excipient information presented when available (limited, particularly for generics); consult specific product labeling.

Solution, Injection, as hydrochloride:

Demerol: 25 mg/mL (1 mL); 25 mg/0.5 mL (0.5 mL); 50 mg/mL (1 mL, 30 mL); 75 mg/1.5 mL (1.5 mL); 100 mg/2 mL (2 mL); 75 mg/mL (1 mL); 100 mg/mL (1 mL, 20 mL)

Generic: 10 mg/mL (30 mL); 25 mg/mL (1 mL); 50 mg/mL (1 mL); 100 mg/mL (1 mL)

Solution, Oral, as hydrochloride:

Generic: 50 mg/5 mL (500 mL)

Tablet, Oral, as hydrochloride:

Demerol: 50 mg [scored]

Demerol: 100 mg

Meperitab: 50 mg [scored]

Meperitab: 100 mg

Generic: 50 mg, 100 mg

Controlled Substance C-II

♦ **Meperidine Hydrochloride** *see* Meperidine *on page* 1086

♦ **Meperitab** *see* Meperidine *on page* 1086

♦ **Mercaptoethane Sulfonate** *see* Mesna *on page* 1094

Mercaptopurine (mer kap toe PURE een)

Related Information

Management of Chemotherapy-Induced Nausea and Vomiting in Adults *on page* 2142

Prevention of Chemotherapy-Induced Nausea and Vomiting in Children *on page* 2203

Safe Handling of Hazardous Drugs *on page* 2292

Brand Names: US Purinethol [DSC]; Purixan

Brand Names: Canada Purinethol

Index Terms 6-Mercaptopurine (error-prone abbreviation); 6-MP (error-prone abbreviation); Purinethol

Pharmacologic Category Antineoplastic Agent, Antimetabolite; Antineoplastic Agent, Antimetabolite (Purine Analog); Immunosuppressant Agent

Use Acute lymphoblastic leukemia: Treatment of acute lymphoblastic leukemia (ALL), as part of a combination chemotherapy regimen

Labeled Contraindications Hypersensitivity to mercaptopurine or any component of the formulation; patients whose disease showed prior resistance to mercaptopurine

Pregnancy Considerations May cause fetal harm if administered during pregnancy. Case reports of fetal loss have been noted with mercaptopurine administration during the first trimester; adverse effects have also been noted with second and third trimester use. Women of child bearing potential should avoid becoming pregnant during treatment.

Breast-Feeding Considerations Mercaptopurine is the active metabolite of azathioprine. Following administration of azathioprine, mercaptopurine can be detected in breast milk (Gardiner 2006). It is not known if/how much mercaptopurine is found in breast milk following oral administration. According to the manufacturer, the decision to discontinue mercaptopurine or discontinue breast-feeding during therapy should take into account the benefits of treatment to the mother.

Warnings/Precautions Hazardous agent - use appropriate precautions for handling and disposal (NIOSH 2014 [group 1]).

Hepatotoxicity has been reported, including jaundice, ascites, hepatic necrosis (may be fatal), intrahepatic cholestasis, parenchymal cell necrosis, and/or hepatic encephalopathy; may be due to direct hepatic cell damage or hypersensitivity. While hepatotoxicity or hepatic injury may occur at any dose, dosages exceeding the recommended dose are associated with a higher incidence. Signs of jaundice generally appear early in treatment, after ~1 to 2 months (range: 1 week to 8 years) and may resolve following discontinuation; recurrence with rechallenge has been noted. Monitor liver function tests, including transaminases, alkaline phosphatase, and bilirubin weekly with treatment initiation, then monthly thereafter (monitor more frequently if used in combination with other hepatotoxic drugs or in patients with preexisting hepatic impairment). Consider a reduced dose in patients with baseline hepatic impairment; monitor closely for toxicity. Withhold treatment for clinical signs of jaundice (hepatomegaly, anorexia, tenderness), deterioration in liver function tests, toxic hepatitis, or biliary stasis until hepatotoxicity is ruled out.

Dose-related leukopenia, thrombocytopenia, and anemia are common; however, may be indicative of disease progression. Hematologic toxicity may be delayed. Bone marrow may appear hypoplastic (could also appear normal). Monitor blood counts; dose may require adjusting for severe neutropenia or thrombocytopenia. Monitor for bleeding (due to thrombocytopenia) or infection (due to neutropenia). Profound severe or repeated hematologic toxicity may be indicative of TPMT deficiency. Patients with homozygous genetic defect of thiopurine methyltransferase (TPMT) are more sensitive to myelosuppressive effects; generally associated with rapid myelosuppression. Significant mercaptopurine dose reductions will be necessary (possibly with continued concomitant chemotherapy at normal doses). Patients who are heterozygous for TPMT defects will have intermediate activity; may have increased toxicity (primarily myelosuppression) although will generally tolerate normal mercaptopurine doses. Consider TPMT testing for severe toxicities/excessive myelosuppression. A germline variant in nucleoside diphophate-linked moiety X-type motif 15 (*NUDT15*) is strongly correlated with mercaptopurine intolerance in children receiving treatment for acute lymphoblastic leukemia (ALL). A genome-wide association study was performed in two prospective clinical childhood ALL trials, and showed that patients homozygous for the TT genotype were extremely sensitive to mercaptopurine, and achieved an average dose intensity of only 8.3%. The *NUDT15* genetic variant is most common in East Asian and Hispanic patients. In patients homozygous for either TPMT or *NUDT15* (or heterozygous for both), mercaptopurine dose reductions of ≥50% were required in 100% of patients (Yang 2015). Potentially significant drug-drug interactions may exist, requiring dose or frequency adjustment, additional monitoring, and/or selection of alternative therapy. Because azathioprine is metabolized to mercaptopurine, concomitant use with azathioprine may result in a significant increase in hematologic toxicity and profound myelosuppression; avoid concurrent use. Hematologic toxicity may be exacerbated by other medications which inhibit TPMT (eg, mesalamine, olsalazine, sulfasalazine) or by other myelosuppressive drugs.

Immunosuppressive agents, including mercaptopurine, are associated with the development of lymphoma and other malignancies including hepatosplenic T-cell lymphoma (HSTCL). Mercaptopurine is immunosuppressive; immune responses to infections may be impaired and the risk for infection is increased; common signs of infection, such as fever and leukocytosis may not occur; lethargy and confusion may be more prominent signs of infection. Immune response to vaccines may be diminished; live virus vaccines impose a risk for infection. Consider adjusting dosage in patients with renal impairment. Some renal adverse effects may be minimized with hydration and prophylactic antihyperuricemic therapy. To avoid potentially serious dosage errors, the terms "6-mercaptopurine" or "6-MP" should be avoided; use of these terms has been associated with six-fold overdosages.

Adverse Reactions Frequency not always defined.

Central nervous system: Malaise (5% to 20%), drug fever

Dermatologic: Skin rash (5% to 20%), hyperpigmentation (<5%), urticaria (<5%), alopecia

Endocrine & metabolic: Hyperuricemia (<5%)

Gastrointestinal: Anorexia (5% to 20%), diarrhea (5% to 20%), nausea (5% to 20%; minimal), vomiting (5% to 20%; minimal), oral lesion (<5%), pancreatitis (<5%), cholestasis, mucositis, sprue-like symptoms, stomach pain, ulcerative bowel lesion

Genitourinary: Oligospermia, renal toxicity, uricosuria

Hematologic & oncologic: Bone marrow depression (>20%; onset 7-10 days; nadir 14 days; recovery: 21 days), anemia, granulocytopenia, hemorrhage, hepatosplenic T-cell lymphomas, leukopenia, lymphocytopenia, metastases, neutropenia, thrombocytopenia

Hepatic: Hyperbilirubinemia (<5%), increased serum transaminases (<5%), ascites, hepatic encephalopathy, hepatic fibrosis, hepatic injury, hepatic necrosis, hepatomegaly, hepatotoxicity, intrahepatic cholestasis, jaundice, toxic hepatitis

Immunologic: Immunosuppression

Infection: Infection

Respiratory: Pulmonary fibrosis

Drug Interactions

Metabolism/Transport Effects None known.

Avoid Concomitant Use

Avoid concomitant use of Mercaptopurine with any of the following: AzaTHIOprine; BCG (Intravesical); CloZAPine; Dipyrone; Febuxostat; Natalizumab; Pimecrolimus; Tacrolimus (Topical); Tofacitinib

Increased Effect/Toxicity

Mercaptopurine may increase the levels/effects of: CloZAPine; Fingolimod; Leflunomide; Natalizumab; Tofacitinib; Vaccines (Live)

◀ *The levels/effects of Mercaptopurine may be increased by:* 5-ASA Derivatives; Allopurinol; AzaTHIOprine; Denosumab; Dipyrone; DOXOrubicin (Conventional); Febuxostat; Pimecrolimus; Roflumilast; Sulfamethoxazole; Tacrolimus (Topical); Trastuzumab; Trimethoprim

Decreased Effect

Mercaptopurine may decrease the levels/effects of: BCG (Intravesical); Coccidioides immitis Skin Test; Sipuleucel-T; Vaccines (Inactivated); Vaccines (Live); Vitamin K Antagonists

The levels/effects of Mercaptopurine may be decreased by: Echinacea

Food Interactions Absorption is variable with food. Management: Take on an empty stomach at the same time each day 1 hour before or 2 hours after a meal. Maintain adequate hydration, unless instructed to restrict fluid intake.

Storage/Stability

Tablets: Store at 15°C to 25°C (59°F to 77°F). Store in a dry place.

Suspension: Store at 15°C to 25°C (59°F to 77°F). Do not store above 25°C (77°F). Store in a dry place. Use within 6 weeks after opening.

Preparation for Administration Hazardous agent; use appropriate precautions for handling and disposal (NIOSH 2014 [group 1]).

Suspension: Wear disposable gloves when handling. Measure dose with an oral dosing syringe to assure proper dose is administered. Oral syringe provided by the manufacturer is intended to be reused, wash with warm soapy water and rinse well (hold syringe under water and move plunger several times to ensure inside of syringe is clean); allow to dry completely.

Mechanism of Action Mercaptopurine is a purine antagonist which inhibits DNA and RNA synthesis; acts as false metabolite and is incorporated into DNA and RNA, eventually inhibiting their synthesis; specific for the S phase of the cell cycle

Pharmacodynamics/Kinetics

Absorption: Variable and incomplete (~50% of a dose is absorbed); C_{max} of suspension is 34% higher than the tablet

Distribution: V_d: > total body water; CNS penetration is poor

Protein binding: ~19%

Metabolism: Hepatic and in GI mucosa; hepatically via xanthine oxidase and methylation via TPMT to sulfate conjugates, 6-thiouric acid, and other inactive compounds; first-pass effect

Half-life elimination (age dependent): ~2 hours

Excretion: Urine (46% as mercaptopurine and metabolites)

Dosing

Adult Note: Patients with minimal or no thiopurine S-methyltransferase (TPMT) activity are at increased risk for severe toxicity at conventional mercaptopurine doses and generally require dose reduction; consider TPMT gene polymorphism testing in patients who experience severe bone marrow suppression (homozygous deficient patients may require up to a 90% dosage reduction; heterozygous patients usually tolerate recommended doses, although some may require dosage reduction).

Acute lymphoblastic leukemia (ALL): Maintenance: Oral: 1.5 to 2.5 mg/kg once daily (50 to 75 mg/m² once daily); continue based on blood counts **or** *Off-label ALL dosing* (combination chemotherapy; refer to specific reference for combinations):

Early intensification (two 4-week courses): 60 mg/m²/day days 1 to 14 (Larson 1995; Larson 1998)

Interim maintenance (12-week course): 60 mg/m^2/day days 1 to 70 (Larson 1995; Larson 1998)

Maintenance (prolonged): 50 mg 3 times/day for 2 years (Kantarjian 2000) **or** 60 mg/m^2/day for 2 years from diagnosis (Larson 1995; Larson 1998)

Acute promyelocytic leukemia (APL) maintenance (off-label use): 60 mg/m^2/day for 1 year (in combination with tretinoin and methotrexate) (Powell 2010)

Crohn disease, remission maintenance or reduction of steroid use (off-label use): Oral: 1 to 1.5 mg/kg/day (Lichtenstein 2009)

Lymphoblastic lymphoma (off-label use): Maintenance (prolonged): 50 mg 3 times daily for 2 years (Kantarjian 2000; Thomas 2004)

Ulcerative colitis (off-label use): Oral:

Initial: 50 mg once daily; titrate dose up if clinical remission not achieved or down if leukopenia occurs (Lobel 2004) **or**

Initial: 50 mg (25 mg if heterozygous for TPMT activity) once daily; titrate up to goal of 1.5 mg/kg (0.75 mg/kg if heterozygous for TPMT activity) if WBC >4,000/mm^3 (and at least 50% of baseline) and LFTs and amylase are stable (Siegel 2005) **or**

Maintenance: 1 to 1.5 mg/kg/day (Carter 2004) **or**

Remission maintenance: 1.5 mg/kg/day (Danese 2011)

Dosage adjustment with concurrent allopurinol: Reduce mercaptopurine dosage to 25% to 33% of the usual dose.

Geriatric Due to renal decline with age, initiate treatment at the low end of recommended dose range.

Pediatric Note: Patients with minimal or no thiopurine S-methyltransferase (TPMT) activity are at increased risk for severe toxicity at conventional mercaptopurine doses and generally require dose reduction; consider TPMT gene polymorphism testing in patients who experience severe bone marrow suppression (homozygous deficient patients may require up to a 90% dosage reduction; heterozygous patients usually tolerate recommended doses, although some may require dosage reduction).

Acute lymphoblastic leukemia (ALL): Maintenance: Oral: 1.5 to 2.5 mg/kg once daily (50 to 75 mg/m^2 once daily); continue based on blood counts **or**

Off-label ALL dosing (combination chemotherapy; refer to specific reference for combinations): Adolescents ≥15 years:

Consolidation phase: 60 mg/m^2/day days 0 to 27 days (5-week course) (Stock 2008) **or** 60 mg/m^2/day days 0 to 13 and days 28 to 41 (9-week course) (Stock 2008)

Early intensification (two 4-week courses): 60 mg/m^2/day days 1 to 14 (Larson 1995; Larson 1998; Stock 2008)

Interim maintenance: 60 mg/m^2/day days 0-41 (8-week course) (Stock 2008) **or** 60 mg/m^2/day days 1 to 70 (12-week course) (Larson 1995; Larson 1998; Stock 2008)

Maintenance (prolonged): 50 mg 3 times/day for 2 years (Kantarjian 2000) **or** 60 mg/m^2/day for 2 years from diagnosis (Larson 1995; Larson 1998; Stock 2008) **or** 75 mg/m^2/day for 2 years (girls) or 3 years (boys) from first interim maintenance (Stock 2008)

Acute promyelocytic leukemia (APL) maintenance (off-label use): Oral: Adolescents ≥15 years: 60 mg/m^2/day for 1 year (in combination with tretinoin and methotrexate) (Powell 2010)

Autoimmune hepatitis (off-label use): Oral: 1.5 mg/kg/day (in combination with prednisone) (Manns 2010)

◄ **Crohn disease, remission maintenance (off-label use):** Doses range from 1 to 1.5 mg/kg/day (Grossman 2008; Markowitz 2000); children ≤6 years may require higher doses to achieve clinical improvement (Grossman 2008).

Lymphoblastic lymphoma (off-label use): Adolescents ≥15 years: Maintenance (prolonged): 50 mg 3 times daily for 2 years (Kantarjian 2000; Thomas 2004) **or** 60 mg/m^2/day for 2 years from diagnosis (Stock 2008) **or** 75 mg/m^2/day for 2 years (girls) or 3 years (boys) from first interim maintenance (Stock 2008)

Ulcerative colitis, remission maintenance (off-label use): Doses range from 1 to 1.5 mg/kg/day (Grossman 2008; Sandhu 2010); children ≤6 years may require higher doses to achieve clinical improvement (Grossman 2008); additional trials may be necessary to further define the role of mercaptopurine in pediatric patients with this condition.

Dosage adjustment with concurrent allopurinol: Reduce mercaptopurine dosage to 25% to 33% of the usual dose.

Renal Impairment The manufacturer's labeling recommends starting with reduced doses (starting at the low end of the dosing range) or increasing the dosing interval to every 36 to 48 hours in patients with renal impairment to avoid accumulation; however, no specific dosage adjustment is provided. The following adjustments have also been recommended (Aronoff 2007): Children:

CrCl ≤50 mL/minute/1.73 m^2: Administer every 48 hours

Hemodialysis: Administer every 48 hours

Continuous ambulatory peritoneal dialysis (CAPD): Administer every 48 hours

Continuous renal replacement therapy (CRRT): Administer every 48 hours

Hepatic Impairment The manufacturer's labeling recommends considering a reduced dose (starting at the low end of the dosing range) with close monitoring for toxicity dose in patients with baseline hepatic impairment; however, no specific dosage adjustment is provided.

Adjustment for Toxicity Adjust dosage for excessive hematologic toxicity.

Combination Regimens

Leukemia, acute lymphocytic:

CALGB 8811 Regimen (ALL) on page 1853

CALGB 9111 Regimen (ALL) on page 1854

Hyper-CVAD (Leukemia, Acute Lymphocytic) on page 2006

MTX/6-MP/VP (Maintenance) on page 2041

POMP on page 2068

PVA (POG 8602) on page 2069

Leukemia, acute promyelocytic:

Tretinoin-Daunorubicin (APL) on page 2096

Tretinoin-Daunorubicin-Cytarabine Induction, Consolidation, Maintenance (APL) on page 2097

Tretinoin-Idarubicin (APL) on page 2099

Administration Administer preferably on an empty stomach (1 hour before or 2 hours after meals)

ALL treatment in children (Schmiegelow 1997): Administration in the evening has demonstration superior outcome; administration with food did not significantly affect outcome.

Suspension: Shake well for at least 30 seconds to ensure suspension is mixed thoroughly (suspension is viscous). Measure dose with an oral dosing syringe (a 1 mL and a 5 mL oral dosing syringe are supplied by the manufacturer) to assure proper dose is administered. Patients and caregivers should be trained on appropriate measuring and administration, handling, storage, disposal, cleanup of accidental spills, and proper cleaning of oral dosing syringe. Use within 6 weeks after opening.

Hazardous agent; use appropriate precautions for handling and disposal (NIOSH 2014 [group 1]). Avoid exposure to crushed or broken tablets; if it is necessary to manipulate the tablets (eg, to prepare an oral solution), it is recommended to double glove, wear a protective gown, and prepare in a controlled device. Disposable gloves should be worn when handling tablets or suspension for administration; health care providers should also wear a protective gown (NIOSH 2014).

Emetic Potential Children and Adults: Minimal (<10%)

Extemporaneous Preparations Hazardous agent: Use appropriate precautions for handling and disposal (NIOSH 2014 [group 1]). When manipulating tablets, NIOSH recommends double gloving, a protective gown, and preparation in a controlled device; if not prepared in a controlled device, respiratory and eye protection as well as ventilated engineering controls are recommended (NIOSH 2014).

A 50 mg/mL oral suspension may be prepared in a vertical flow hood with tablets and a mixture of sterile water for injection (SWFI), simple syrup, and cherry syrup. Crush thirty 50 mg tablets in a mortar and reduce to a fine powder. Add ~5 mL SWFI and mix to a uniform paste; then add ~10 mL simple syrup; mix while continuing to add cherry syrup to make a final volume of 30 mL; transfer to a calibrated bottle. Label "shake well" and "caution chemotherapy". Stable for 35 days at room temperature.

Aliabadi HM, Romanick M, Desai, S, et al, "Effect of Buffer and Antioxidant on Stability of a Mercaptopurine Suspension," *Am J Health Syst Pharm* 2008, 65(5):441-7.

Monitoring Parameters CBC with differential (weekly initially, although clinical status may require increased frequency), bone marrow exam (to evaluate marrow status), liver function tests (transaminases, alkaline phosphatase, and bilirubin; weekly initially, then monthly; monitor more frequently if on concomitant hepatotoxic agents or in patients with preexisting hepatic impairment), renal function, urinalysis; consider TPMT genotyping to identify TPMT defect (if severe hematologic toxicity occurs)

For use as immunomodulatory therapy in CD or UC, monitor CBC with differential weekly for 1 month, then biweekly for 1 month, followed by monitoring every 1 to 2 months throughout the course of therapy. LFTs should be assessed every 3 months. Monitor for signs/symptoms of malignancy (eg, splenomegaly, hepatomegaly, abdominal pain, persistent fever, night sweats, weight loss).

Test Interactions TPMT testing: Recent transfusions may result in a misinterpretation of the actual TPMT activity. Concomitant drugs may influence TPMT activity in the blood.

Prescribing and Access Restrictions Distribution of Purixan is provided by the specialty pharmacy, AnovoRx. For ordering information, call 888-470-0904.

Dosage Forms Excipient information presented when available (limited, particularly for generics); consult specific product labeling. [DSC] = Discontinued product
Suspension, Oral:
Purixan: 2000 mg/100 mL (100 mL) [contains aspartame, methylparaben, propylparaben]
Tablet, Oral:
Purinethol: 50 mg [DSC] [scored]
Generic: 50 mg

◆ **6-Mercaptopurine (error-prone abbreviation)** *see* Mercaptopurine *on page* 1087

◆ **M-Eslon (Can)** *see* Morphine (Systemic) *on page* 1167

Mesna (MES na)

Brand Names: US Mesnex
Brand Names: Canada Mesna for injection; Uromitexan
Index Terms Mercaptoethane Sulfonate; Sodium 2-Mercaptoethane Sulfonate
Pharmacologic Category Antidote; Chemoprotective Agent
Use
Prevention of ifosfamide-induced hemorrhagic cystitis: Preventive agent to reduce the incidence of ifosfamide-induced hemorrhagic cystitis
Limitations of use: Mesna is not indicted to reduce the risk of hematuria due to other conditions such as thrombocytopenia
Labeled Contraindications Hypersensitivity to mesna or any component of the formulation
Pregnancy Considerations Adverse effects were not observed in animal reproduction studies. Use during pregnancy only if clearly needed.
Breast-Feeding Considerations It is not known if mesna is excreted in breast milk. Benzyl alcohol, a component in some formulations, does enter breast milk and may be absorbed by a nursing infant. Due to the potential for adverse reactions in the nursing infant, a decision should be made to discontinue breast-feeding or to discontinue mesna, taking into account the importance of treatment to the mother.
Warnings/Precautions Monitor urine for hematuria. Severe hematuria despite utilization of mesna may require ifosfamide dose reduction or discontinuation. Examine morning urine specimen for hematuria prior to ifosfamide or cyclophosphamide treatment; if hematuria (>50 RBC/HPF) develops, reduce the ifosfamide/cyclophosphamide dose or discontinue the drug; will not prevent hemorrhagic cystitis in all patients. Mesna will not reduce the risk of hematuria related to thrombocytopenia. Patients should receive adequate hydration during treatment. Mesna is intended for the prevention of hemorrhagic cystitis and will not prevent or alleviate other toxicities associated with ifosfamide or cyclophosphamide.

Hypersensitivity reactions have been reported; symptoms ranged from mild hypersensitivity to systemic anaphylactic reactions and may include fever, hypotension, tachycardia, acute renal impairment, hypoxia, respiratory distress, urticaria, angioedema, signs of disseminated intravascular coagulation, hematologic abnormalities, increased liver enzymes, nausea, vomiting, arthralgia, and myalgia. Reactions may occur with the first exposure, or after several months of treatment. Monitor for signs/symptoms of reactions. May require discontinuation. Patients with autoimmune disorders receiving cyclophosphamide and mesna may be at increased risk. Mesna is a thiol compound; it is unknown if the risk for reaction is increased in patients who have had a reaction to other thiol compounds (eg, amifostine). Drug rash with eosinophilia and systemic symptoms and bullous/ulcerative skin and mucosal reactions consistent with Stevens-Johnson syndrome (SJS) or toxic epidermal necrolysis (TEN) have been reported. The skin and mucosal reactions may be characterized by rash, pruritus, urticaria, erythema, burning sensation, angioedema, periorbital edema, flushing, and stomatitis. Reactions may occur with the first exposure, or after several months of treatment. May require discontinuation.

Benzyl alcohol and derivatives: Some dosage forms may contain benzyl alcohol; large amounts of benzyl alcohol (≥99 mg/kg/day) have been associated with a potentially fatal toxicity ("gasping syndrome") in neonates; the "gasping syndrome" consists of metabolic acidosis, respiratory distress, gasping respirations, CNS dysfunction (including convulsions, intracranial hemorrhage), hypotension, and cardiovascular collapse (AAP ["Inactive" 1997]; CDC, 1982); some data suggests that benzoate displaces bilirubin from protein binding sites (Ahlfors, 2001); avoid or use dosage forms containing benzyl alcohol with caution in neonates. See manufacturer's labeling.

Adverse Reactions

Mesna alone (frequency not defined):

Cardiovascular: Flushing

Central nervous system: Dizziness, fever, headache, hyperesthesia, somnolence

Dermatologic: Rash

Gastrointestinal: Anorexia, constipation, diarrhea, flatulence, nausea, taste alteration/bad taste (with oral administration), vomiting

Local: Injection site reactions

Neuromuscular: Arthralgia, back pain, rigors

Ocular: Conjunctivitis

Respiratory: Cough, pharyngitis, rhinitis

Miscellaneous: Flu-like syndrome

Mesna alone or in combination: Postmarketing and/or case reports: Allergic reaction, anaphylactic reaction, hypersensitivity, hyper-/hypotension, injection site erythema, injection site pain, limb pain, malaise, myalgia, platelets decreased, ST-segment increased, tachycardia, tachypnea, transaminases increased

Drug Interactions

Metabolism/Transport Effects None known.

Avoid Concomitant Use There are no known interactions where it is recommended to avoid concomitant use.

Increased Effect/Toxicity There are no known significant interactions involving an increase in effect.

Decreased Effect There are no known significant interactions involving a decrease in effect.

Storage/Stability Store intact vials and tablets at room temperature of 20°C to 25°C (68°F to 77°F); excursions are permitted between 15°C and 30°C (59°F and 86°F). Opened multidose vials may be stored and used for use up to 8 days after initial puncture. Solutions diluted for infusion stored at room temperature should be used within 24 hours. According to the manufacturer, mesna and ifosfamide may be mixed in the same bag if the final ifosfamide concentration is ≤50 mg/mL. Solutions of mesna and ifosfamide (1:1) in NS at a concentration of up to 20 mg/mL are stable for 14 days in PVC bags (Zhang,

2014). Solutions of mesna (0.5 to 3.2 mg/mL) and cyclophosphamide (1.8 to 10.8 mg/mL) in D_5W are stable for 48 hours refrigerated or 6 hours at room temperature (Menard, 2003). Mesna injection prepared for oral administration is stable for at least 9 days undiluted in polypropylene syringes and stored at 5°C, 24°C, 35°C; for 7 days when diluted 1:2 or 1:5 with syrups and stored at 24°C in capped tubes; or for 24 hours at 5°C when diluted to 1:2, 1:10, and 1:100 in orange or apple juice, milk, or carbonated beverages (Goren, 1991).

Preparation for Administration IV: Dilute in D_5W, NS, $D_5^1/_4NS$, $D_5^1/_3NS$, $D_5^1/_2NS$, or lactated Ringer's to a final concentration of 20 mg/mL.

Mechanism of Action In blood, mesna is oxidized to dimesna which in turn is reduced in the kidney back to mesna, supplying a free thiol group which binds to and inactivates acrolein, the urotoxic metabolite of ifosfamide and cyclophosphamide

Pharmacodynamics/Kinetics

Distribution: 0.65 ± 0.24 L/kg; distributed to total body water

Metabolism: Rapidly oxidized to mesna disulfide (dimesna)

Bioavailability: Oral: Free mesna: 58% (range: 45% to 71%); not affected by food

Half-life elimination: Mesna: ~22 minutes; Dimesna: ~70 minutes

Time to peak, plasma: Oral: Free mesna: 1.5 to 4 hours

Excretion: Urine (32% as mesna; 33% as dimesna)

Dosing

Adult & Geriatric Note: Mesna dosing schedule should be repeated each day ifosfamide is received. If ifosfamide dose is adjusted (decreased or increased), the mesna dose should also be modified to maintain the mesna-to-ifosfamide ratio.

Prevention of ifosfamide-induced hemorrhagic cystitis:

Standard-dose ifosfamide (manufacturer's labeling): IV: Mesna dose is equal to 20% of the ifosfamide dose given for 3 doses: With the ifosfamide dose, hour 4, and at hour 8 after the ifosfamide dose (total daily mesna dose is 60% of the ifosfamide dose)

Oral mesna (following IV mesna; for ifosfamide doses ≤2 g/m^2/day): Mesna dose (IV) is equal to 20% of the ifosfamide dose at hour 0, followed by mesna dose (orally) equal to 40% of the ifosfamide dose given 2 and 6 hours after the ifosfamide dose (total daily mesna dose is 100% of the ifosfamide dose). **Note:** If the oral mesna dose is vomited within 2 hours of administration, repeat the dose or administer IV mesna.

Short infusion standard-dose ifosfamide (<2.5 g/m^2/day): ASCO guidelines: IV: Total mesna dose is equal to 60% of the ifosfamide dose, in 3 divided doses (each mesna dose as 20% of ifosfamide dose), given 15 minutes before the ifosfamide dose, and 4 and 8 hours after each dose of ifosfamide (Hensley, 2009)

Continuous infusion standard-dose ifosfamide (<2.5 g/m^2/day): ASCO guidelines: IV: Mesna dose (as a bolus) is equal to 20% of the ifosfamide dose, followed by a continuous infusion of mesna at 40% of the ifosfamide dose; continue mesna infusion for 12-24 hours after completion of ifosfamide infusion (Hensley, 2009)

High-dose ifosfamide (>2.5 g/m^2/day): ASCO guidelines: Evidence for use is inadequate; more frequent and prolonged mesna administration regimens may be required (Hensley, 2009)

Other dosing strategies used in combination with ifosfamide (off-label dosing):

Mesna continuous infusion: IV: 1.8 g/m²/day to 5 g/m²/day as a continuous infusion (100% of the ifosfamide dose), repeated each day ifosfamide is received; see protocols for specific details (Bacci, 2003; Kolb, 2003; Moskowitz, 2011)

Mesna bolus followed by continuous infusion: IV: 1000 mg/m² 1 hour prior to ifosfamide on day 1, followed by 3000 mg/m²/day continuous infusion (continuous infusion is 100% of the ifosfamide dose) on days 1, 2, and 3 (with sufficient hydration) every 3 weeks for 6 courses (Juergens, 2006)

Prevention of cyclophosphamide-induced hemorrhagic cystitis (off-label use):

HDCAV/IE regimen for Ewing sarcoma: Children ≥4 years and Adults <40 years: IV: 2100 mg/m²/day continuous infusion (mesna dose is equivalent to the cyclophosphamide dose) for 2 days with cyclophosphamide infusion during cycles 1, 2, 3, and 6 (Kolb, 2003)

Hyper-CVAD regimen for ALL: Adults: IV: 600 mg/m²/day continuous infusion (mesna continuous infusion is same total dose as cyclophosphamide) on days 1, 2, and 3, beginning with cyclophosphamide and ending 6 hours after the last cyclophosphamide dose during odd-numbered cycles (cycles 1, 3, 5, 7) of an 8-cycle phase (Kantarjian, 2000)

Pediatric

Prevention of ifosfamide-induced hemorrhagic cystitis (off-label use):

Short infusion standard-dose ifosfamide (<2.5 g/m²/day): ASCO guidelines: Refer to adult dosing.

Continuous infusion standard-dose ifosfamide (<2.5 g/m²/day): ASCO guidelines: Refer to adult dosing.

Other dosing strategies used in combination with ifosfamide (off-label dosing):

Mesna continuous infusion: IV: 1.8 g/m²/day to 5 g/m²/day as a continuous infusion (100% of the ifosfamide dose), repeated each day ifosfamide is received; see protocols for specific details (Bacci, 2003; Kolb, 2003; Moskowitz, 2011)

Mesna bolus followed by continuous infusion: IV: 1000 mg/m² 1 hour prior to ifosfamide on day 1, followed by 3000 mg/m²/day continuous infusion (continuous infusion is 100% of the ifosfamide dose) on days 1, 2, and 3 (with sufficient hydration) every 3 weeks for 6 courses (Juergens, 2006)

Mesna (20% higher than ifosfamide) continuous infusion: IV: 3600 mg/m²/day continuous infusion for 4 days (mesna dose is 20% higher than ifosfamide), with hydration, during weeks 4 and 9 (3 additional postop courses were administered in good responders) (Le Deley, 2007)

Prevention of cyclophosphamide-induced hemorrhagic cystitis (off-label use): HDCAV/IE regimen for Ewing sarcoma: Children ≥4 years and Adults <40 years: IV: 2100 mg/m²/day continuous infusion (mesna dose is equivalent to the cyclophosphamide dose) for 2 days with cyclophosphamide infusion during cycles 1, 2, 3, and 6 (Kolb, 2003)

Renal Impairment There are no dosage adjustments provided in the manufacturer's labeling (has not been studied)

Hepatic Impairment There are no dosage adjustments provided in the manufacturer's labeling (has not been studied)

Combination Regimens

Bone sarcoma (osteosarcoma): Ifosfamide-Cisplatin-Epirubicin (Osteosarcoma) on page 2015

Leukemia, acute lymphocytic:
Lymphoma, Hodgkin:
Lymphoma, non-Hodgkin (Burkitt):
Testicular cancer:

Administration Maintain adequate hydration and urinary output during ifosfamide treatment

IV: Administer as an IV bolus (per manufacturer); may also be administered by
short infusion or continuous infusion (maintain continuous infusion for 12-24
hours after completion of ifosfamide infusion) (Hensley, 2009); refer to
specific protocol for administration rate/details

Oral: Administer orally in tablet formulation; patients who vomit within 2 hours
after taking oral mesna should repeat the dose or receive IV mesna. A
solution may be prepared from solution for injection by dilution in syrup,
juice, carbonate beverages, or milk (Goren, 1991); see Extemporaneous
Preparations section.

Extemporaneous Preparations An oral solution may be prepared from
mesna solution for injection. Dilute solution for injection to 20 mg/mL or
50 mg/mL with orange or grape syrup. Prior to administration, syrup-diluted
solutions may be diluted to a final concentration of 1, 10, or 50 mg/mL with any
of the following: carbonated beverages, apple juice, orange juice, or milk.
Mesna injection prepared for oral administration is stable for at least 9 days
undiluted in polypropylene syringes and stored at 5°C, 24°C, 35°C; for 7 days
when diluted 1:2 or 1:5 with syrups and stored at 24°C in capped tubes; or for
24 hours at 5°C when diluted to 1:2, 1:10, and 1:100 in orange or apple juice,
milk, or carbonated beverages. Dilution of mesna with diet or sugar-free
preparations has not been evaluated.

Goren MP, Lyman BA, Li JT. The stability of mesna in beverages and syrup for oral administration.
  Cancer Chemother Pharmacol. 1991;28(4):298-301.

Monitoring Parameters Monitor urine for hematuria; urine output and hydration status; monitor for signs/symptoms of hypersensitivity or dermatologic
toxicity

Test Interactions

Urinary ketones: False-positive tests for urinary ketones may occur in patients receiving mesna with the use of nitroprusside-based urine tests, including dipstick tests.

CPK activity: Mesna may interfere with enzymatic creatine kinase (CPK) activity tests which use a thiol compound (eg, N-acetylcysteine) for CPK reactivation; may result in a falsely low CPK level.

Ascorbic acid: Mesna may result in false-positive reactions in Tillman's reagent-based urine screening tests for ascorbic acid.

Additional Information Oncology Comment: Guidelines from the American Society of Clinical Oncology (ASCO) for the use of chemotherapy and radio-therapy protectants (Hensley, 2009 [update]; Schuchter, 2002) recommend mesna to decrease the incidence of ifosfamide-induced urotoxicity associated with short infusion and continuous infusion standard-dose ifosfamide (<2.5 g/m^2/day). Although evidence is inadequate regarding mesna's uroprotective effects in high-dose ifosfamide (>2.5 g/m^2/day), the guidelines suggest more frequent and prolonged mesna administration times may be required. For prevention of high-dose cyclophosphamide-induced urotoxicity (associated with stem cell transplantation), the guidelines recommend mesna in conjunction with saline diuresis (or forced saline diuresis alone).

Dosage Forms Excipient information presented when available (limited, particularly for generics); consult specific product labeling.

Solution, Intravenous:

Mesnex: 100 mg/mL (10 mL) [contains benzyl alcohol, edetate disodium]

Generic: 100 mg/mL (10 mL)

Tablet, Oral:

Mesnex: 400 mg [scored]

Dosage Forms: Canada Refer also to Dosage Forms. **Note:** Tablets are not available in Canada.

Excipient information presented when available (limited, particularly for generics); consult specific product labeling.

Solution, Intravenous:

Mesna for injection: 100 mg/mL (10 mL) [contains benzyl alcohol, edetate disodium]

Uromitexan: 100 mg/mL (4 mL, 10 mL) [contains edetate disodium]

Uromitexan: 100 mg/mL (10 mL, 50 mL) [contains benzyl alcohol, edetate disodium]

Methadone (METH a done)

Brand Names: US Dolophine; Methadone HCl Intensol; Methadose; Methadose Sugar-Free

Brand Names: Canada Metadol; Metadol-D; Methadose

Index Terms Methadone Hydrochloride

Pharmacologic Category Analgesic, Opioid

Use

Chronic pain (except for oral soluble tablets for suspension): Management of pain severe enough to require daily, around-the-clock, long-term opioid treatment and for which alternative treatment options are inadequate. Limitations of use: Because of the risks of addiction, abuse, and misuse with opioids, even at recommended doses, and because of the greater risks of overdose and death with long-acting opioids, reserve methadone for use in patients for whom alternative analgesic treatment options (eg, nonopioid analgesics, immediate-release opioid analgesics) are ineffective, not tolerated, or would be otherwise inadequate to provide sufficient management of pain. Methadone is not for use as an as-needed analgesic.

Detoxification: Detoxification and maintenance treatment of opioid addiction (heroin or other morphine-like drugs), in conjunction with appropriate social and medical services.

Pregnancy Risk Factor C

Dosing

Adult Regulations regarding methadone use may vary by state and/or country. Obtain advice from appropriate regulatory agencies and/or consult with pain management/palliative care specialists. **Note:** These are guidelines and do not represent the maximum doses that may be required. Consider total daily dose, potency, prior opioid use, degree of opioid experience and tolerance, conversion from previous opioid, patient's general condition, concurrent medications, and type and severity of pain during prescribing process. Other factors to consider:

- Interpatient variability in absorption, metabolism, and relative analgesic potency.
- Population-based equianalgesic conversion ratios between methadone and other opioids are not accurate when applied to individuals.
- Duration of analgesic action is much shorter than plasma elimination half-life.
- Steady-state plasma concentrations and full analgesic effects are not attained until at least 3 to 5 days after initiation, and may take longer in some patients.
- Methadone has a narrow therapeutic index, particularly when used concomitantly with other medications.

Chronic pain:

Manufacturer's labeling: Opioid-naive: Use as the first opioid analgesic:
Oral: Initial: 2.5 mg every 8 to 12 hours
IV: Initial: 2.5 to 10 mg every 8 to 12 hours; titrate slowly to effect; may also be administered by SubQ or IM injection (manufacturer's labeling)

Alternative recommendations: Opioid-naive: Oral:
Gradual titration (for chronic noncancer pain and situations where frequent monitoring is unnecessary): Initial: 2.5 mg every 8 hours; may increase dose by 2.5 mg per dose (Va/DoD, 2010) or 5 mg per day (Chou, 2014) every 5 to 7 days. Once a stable dose is reached, the dosing interval may be extended to every 8 to 12 hours, or longer (Va/DOD, 2010).
Faster titration (for cancer pain and situations where frequent monitoring is possible): Initial: 2.5 mg every 6 to 8 hours; may increase dose by 2.5 mg per dose as often as every day over about 4 days. Once a stable dose is reached, the dosing interval may be extended to every 8 to 12 hours, or longer (Va/DoD, 2010).

Conversion recommendations:
Manufacturer's labeling:

Conversion from oral opioids to oral methadone: Discontinue all other around-the-clock opioids when methadone therapy is initiated; fatalities have occurred in opioid-tolerant patients during conversion to methadone. Substantial interpatient variability exists in relative potency. Therefore, it is safer to underestimate a patient's daily oral methadone requirement and provide breakthrough pain relief with rescue medication (eg, immediate release opioid) than to overestimate requirements. Patient response to methadone needs to be monitored closely throughout the process of the conversion. Sum the current total daily dose of oral opioid, convert it to a morphine equivalent dose according to conversion factor for that specific opioid, then multiply the morphine equivalent dose by the corresponding percentage in the table to calculate the approximate oral methadone daily dose. Divide total daily methadone dose by intended dosing schedule (ie, divide by 3 for administration every 8 hours). Round down, if necessary, to the nearest strength available. For patients on a regimen of more than one opioid, calculate the approximate oral methadone dose for each opioid and sum the totals to obtain the approximate total methadone daily dose, and divide the total daily methadone dose by the intended dosing schedule (ie, divide by 3 for administration every 8 hours). For patients on a regimen of fixed-ratio opioid/nonopioid analgesic medications, only the opioid component of these medications should be used in the conversion. **Note:** Conversion factors in table are only for the conversion from another oral opioid analgesic to methadone. Table cannot be used to convert from methadone to another opioid (doing so may lead to fatal overdose due to overestimation of the new opioid). This is not a table of equianalgesic doses.

Daily oral morphine dose <100 mg: Estimated daily oral methadone dose: 20% to 30% of total daily morphine dose

Daily oral morphine dose 100 to 300 mg: Estimated daily oral methadone dose: 10% to 20% of total daily morphine dose

Daily oral morphine dose 300 to 600 mg: Estimated daily oral methadone dose: 8% to 12% of total daily morphine dose

Daily oral morphine dose 600 to 1000 mg: Estimated daily oral methadone dose: 5% to 10% of total daily morphine dose.

Daily oral morphine dose >1000 mg: Estimated daily oral methadone dose: <5% of total daily morphine dose.

Conversion from parenteral methadone to oral methadone: Initial dose: Parenteral: Oral ratio: 1:2 (eg, 5 mg parenteral methadone equals 10 mg oral methadone)

Alternative recommendations: Opioid-tolerant:

Conversion from oral morphine to oral methadone: 1) There is not a linear relationship when converting to methadone from oral morphine. The higher the daily morphine equivalent dose the more potent methadone is, and 2) conversion to methadone is more of a process than a calculation. In general, the starting methadone dose should not exceed 30 to 40 mg/day, even in patients on high doses of other opioids. Patient response to methadone needs to be monitored closely throughout the process of the conversion. There are several proposed ratios for converting from oral morphine to oral methadone (Ayonrinde, 2000; Mercadente, 2001; Ripamonti, 1998). The estimated total daily methadone dose should then be divided to reflect the intended dosing schedule (eg, divide by 3 and administer every 8 hours). Patients who have not taken an opioid for 1 to 2 weeks should be considered opioid naïve (Chou, 2014).

Titration and maintenance: Manufacturer's labeling: May adjust dosage every 3 to 5 days to a dose providing adequate analgesia and minimal adverse reactions. However, because of high interpatient variability, substantially longer periods between dose adjustments may be necessary in some patients (up to 12 days). Breakthrough pain may require a dose increase or rescue medication with an immediate-release analgesic. Some guidelines note that dose increases should not be more than 10 mg per day every 5 to 7 days (Chou, 2014).

Discontinuation: Manufacturer's labeling: When pain management is no longer required, do not abruptly discontinue. Reduce dose every 2 to 4 days to prevent signs or symptoms of withdrawal.

Critically-ill patients (off-label use; Barr, 2013): Note: May be used to slow development of tolerance when escalation with other opioids is required. Enteral methadone has also been used to wean prolonged continuous opioid infusions (Al Qadheeb, 2012)
Oral: 10 to 40 mg every 6 to 12 hours
IV: 2.5 to 10 mg every 8 to 12 hours

Detoxification: Oral:

Initial: A single dose of 20 to 30 mg is usually sufficient to suppress symptoms. Should not exceed 30 mg; lower doses should be considered in patients with low tolerance at initiation (eg, absence of opioids ≥5 days); an additional 5 to 10 mg of methadone may be provided if withdrawal symptoms have not been suppressed or if symptoms reappear after 2 to 4 hours; total daily dose on the first day should not exceed 40 mg. Do not increase dose without waiting for steady-state to be achieved. Levels will accumulate over the first few days; deaths have occurred in early treatment due to cumulative effects. Reassure the patient that duration of effect will increase as methadone accumulates.

Maintenance: Titrate to a dosage which prevents opioid withdrawal symptoms for 24 hours, prevents craving, attenuates euphoric effect of self-administered opioids, and tolerance to sedative effects of methadone. Usual range: 80 to 120 mg/day (titration should occur cautiously)

Withdrawal: Dose reductions should be <10% of the maintenance dose, every 10 to 14 days

Detoxification (short-term): Oral:

Initial: Titrate to ~40 mg/day in divided doses to achieve stabilization.

Maintenance: May continue 40 mg dose for 2 to 3 days.

Withdrawal: After 2 to 3 days of stabilization at 40 mg, gradually decrease the dose on a daily basis or at 2-day intervals. Keep dose at a level sufficient to keep withdrawal symptoms at a tolerable level. Hospitalized patients may tolerate a total daily dose decrease of 20%; ambulatory patients may require a slower reduction.

Dosage adjustment during pregnancy: Methadone dose may need to be increased or the dosing interval decreased when chronic doses are used during the second or third trimesters. Use is not appropriate for short term analgesia during labor and delivery.

Geriatric Oral, IM: 2.5 mg every 8 to 12 hours; refer to adult dosing.

Renal Impairment Off-label dosing (Aronoff, 2007): Adults:

CrCl ≥10 mL/minute: No dosage adjustment necessary

CrCl <10 mL/minute: Administer 50% to 75% of normal dose

Hepatic Impairment There are no dosage adjustments provided in the manufacturer's labeling; however, undergoes hepatic metabolism and systemic exposure may be increased after repeated dosing. Avoid in severe liver disease.

Adjustment for Toxicity

Excessive opioid-related adverse events: Reduce next dose. Assess and reduce both the maintenance dose and dosing interval if necessary. Some guidelines recommend holding the dose if there is evidence of sedation (Chou, 2014).

QTc prolongation (Chou, 2014):

QTc >450 to 499 msecs: Discuss potential risks and benefits. Evaluate and correct potential causes of QTc interval prolongation prior to initiating therapy. Consider alternative therapies or reduced methadone dose if QTc interval becomes ≥450 to 499 msecs during treatment.

QTc ≥500 msecs: Alternative therapies for opioid addiction or chronic pain are recommended. If QTc ≥500 msecs occurs during therapy, switch to an alternative therapy or immediately decrease the dose of methadone; correct any reversible causes of QTc interval prolongation and repeat ECG.

Additional Information Complete prescribing information should be consulted for additional detail.

Prescribing and Access Restrictions When used for treatment of opioid addiction: May only be dispensed in accordance to guidelines established by the Substance Abuse and Mental Health Services Administration's (SAMHSA) Center for Substance Abuse Treatment (CSAT). Regulations regarding methadone use may vary by state and/or country. Obtain advice from appropriate regulatory agencies and/or consult with pain management/palliative care specialists.

Note: Regulatory Exceptions to the General Requirement to Provide Opioid Agonist Treatment (per manufacturer's labeling):

1. During inpatient care, when the patient was admitted for any condition other than concurrent opioid addiction, to facilitate the treatment of the primary admitting diagnosis.

2. During an emergency period of no longer than 3 days while definitive care for the addiction is being sought in an appropriately licensed facility.

Medication Guide Available Yes

Dosage Forms Excipient information presented when available (limited, particularly for generics); consult specific product labeling.

Concentrate, Oral, as hydrochloride:

Methadone HCl Intensol: 10 mg/mL (30 mL) [unflavored flavor]

Methadose: 10 mg/mL (1000 mL) [cherry flavor]

Methadose Sugar-Free: 10 mg/mL (1000 mL) [dye free, sugar free; unflavored flavor]

Generic: 10 mg/mL (30 mL, 1000 mL)

Solution, Injection, as hydrochloride:

Generic: 10 mg/mL (20 mL)

Solution, Oral, as hydrochloride:

Generic: 5 mg/5 mL (500 mL); 10 mg/5 mL (500 mL)

Tablet, Oral, as hydrochloride:
  Dolophine: 5 mg, 10 mg [scored]
  Methadose: 10 mg [scored]
  Generic: 5 mg, 10 mg
Tablet Soluble, Oral, as hydrochloride:
  Methadose: 40 mg [scored]
  Generic: 40 mg
Dosage Forms: Canada Excipient information presented when available (limited, particularly for generics); consult specific product labeling.
Concentrate, Oral, as hydrochloride:
  Metadol: 10 mg/mL [unflavored]
  Methadose: 10 mg/mL [cherry flavor]
  Methadose Sugar-Free: 10 mg/mL [dye free, sugar free; unflavored]
Solution, Oral, as hydrochloride:
  Metadol: 1 mg/mL [unflavored]
Tablet, Oral, as hydrochloride:
  Metadol: 1 mg, 5 mg, 10 mg, 25 mg [scored]
Controlled Substance C-II

◆ **Methadone HCl Intensol** see Methadone on page 1099
◆ **Methadone Hydrochloride** see Methadone on page 1099
◆ **Methadose** see Methadone on page 1099
◆ **Methadose Sugar-Free** see Methadone on page 1099

Methotrexate (meth oh TREKS ate)

Related Information

Chemotherapy and Cancer Treatment During Pregnancy on page 2214
Hematopoietic Stem Cell Transplantation on page 2272
Management of Chemotherapy-Induced Nausea and Vomiting in Adults on page 2142
Mucositis and Stomatitis on page 2186
Prevention of Chemotherapy-Induced Nausea and Vomiting in Children on page 2203
Safe Handling of Hazardous Drugs on page 2292

Brand Names: US Otrexup; Rasuvo; Rheumatrex; Trexall
Brand Names: Canada Apo-Methotrexate; JAMP-Methotrexate; Methotrexate Injection USP; Methotrexate Injection, BP; Methotrexate Sodium Injection; Metoject; ratio-Methotrexate Sodium
Index Terms Amethopterin; Methotrexate Sodium; Methotrexatum; MTX (error-prone abbreviation)
Pharmacologic Category Antineoplastic Agent, Antimetabolite (Antifolate); Antirheumatic, Disease Modifying; Immunosuppressant Agent

Use

Oncology-related uses: Acute lymphoblastic leukemia (ALL) maintenance treatment, ALL meningeal leukemia (prophylaxis and treatment); treatment of trophoblastic neoplasms (gestational choriocarcinoma, chorioadenoma destruens and hydatidiform mole), breast cancer, head and neck cancer (epidermoid), cutaneous T-Cell lymphoma (advanced mycosis fungoides), lung cancer (squamous cell and small cell), advanced non-Hodgkin lymphomas (NHL), osteosarcoma

Nononcology uses: Treatment of psoriasis (severe, recalcitrant, disabling); severe, active rheumatoid arthritis (RA); active polyarticular-course juvenile idiopathic arthritis (pJIA)

Limitations of use: Otrexup and Rasuvo are not indicated for the treatment of neoplastic diseases.

Labeled Contraindications Known hypersensitivity to methotrexate or any component of the formulation; breast-feeding

Additional contraindications for patients with psoriasis or rheumatoid arthritis: Pregnancy, alcoholism, alcoholic liver disease or other chronic liver disease, immunodeficiency syndrome (overt or laboratory evidence); preexisting blood dyscrasias (eg, bone marrow hypoplasia, leukopenia, thrombocytopenia, significant anemia)

Pregnancy Considerations [U.S. Boxed Warning]: Methotrexate may cause fetal death and/or congenital abnormalities. Studies in animals and pregnant women have shown evidence of fetal abnormalities; therefore, the manufacturer classifies methotrexate as pregnancy category X (for psoriasis or RA). A pattern of congenital malformations associated with maternal methotrexate use is referred to as the aminopterin/methotrexate syndrome. Features of the syndrome include CNS, skeletal, and cardiac abnormalities. Low birth weight and developmental delay have also been reported. The use of methotrexate may impair fertility and cause menstrual irregularities or oligospermia during treatment and following therapy. Methotrexate is approved for the treatment of trophoblastic neoplasms (gestational choriocarcinoma, chorioadenoma destruens, and hydatidiform mole) and has been used for the medical management of ectopic pregnancy and the medical management of abortion. **[U.S. Boxed Warning]: Use is contraindicated for the treatment of psoriasis or RA in pregnant women.** Pregnancy should be excluded prior to therapy in women of childbearing potential. Use for the treatment of neoplastic diseases only when the potential benefit to the mother outweighs the possible risk to the fetus. Pregnancy should be avoided for ≥3 months following treatment in male patients and ≥1 ovulatory cycle in female patients. A registry is available for pregnant women exposed to autoimmune medications including methotrexate. For additional information contact the Organization of Teratology Information Specialists, OTIS Autoimmune Diseases Study, at 877-311-8972.

Breast-Feeding Considerations Low amounts of methotrexate are excreted into breast milk. Due to the potential for serious adverse reactions in a breast-feeding infant, use is contraindicated in nursing mothers.

Warnings/Precautions Hazardous agent - use appropriate precautions for handling and disposal (NIOSH 2014 [group 1]).

[US Boxed Warning]: Methotrexate has been associated with acute (elevated transaminases) and potentially fatal chronic (fibrosis, cirrhosis) hepatotoxicity. Risk is related to cumulative dose (≥1.5 g) and prolonged exposure. Monitor closely (with liver function tests, including serum albumin) for liver toxicities. Liver enzyme elevations may be noted, but may not be predictive of hepatic disease in long term treatment for psoriasis (but generally is predictive in rheumatoid arthritis [RA] treatment). With long-term use, liver biopsy may show histologic changes, fibrosis, or cirrhosis; periodic liver biopsy is recommended with long-term use for psoriasis patients with risk factors for hepatotoxicity and for persistent abnormal liver function tests in psoriasis patients without risk factors for hepatotoxicity and in RA patients; discontinue methotrexate with moderate-to-severe change in liver biopsy. Risk factors for hepatotoxicity include history of above moderate ethanol consumption, ▶

persistent abnormal liver chemistries, history of chronic liver disease (including hepatitis B or C), family history of inheritable liver disease, diabetes, obesity, hyperlipidemia, lack of folate supplementation during methotrexate therapy, cumulative methotrexate dose exceeding 1.5 g, continuous daily methotrexate dosing and history of significant exposure to hepatotoxic drugs. Use caution with preexisting liver impairment; may require dosage reduction. Use caution when used with other hepatotoxic agents (azathioprine, retinoids, sulfasalazine). **[US Boxed Warning]: Methotrexate elimination is reduced in patients with ascites and pleural effusions;** resulting in prolonged half-life and toxicity; may require dose reduction or discontinuation. Monitor closely for toxicity.

[US Boxed Warning]: May cause renal damage leading to acute renal failure, especially with high-dose methotrexate; monitor renal function and methotrexate levels closely, maintain adequate hydration and urinary alkalinization. Use caution in osteosarcoma patients treated with high-dose methotrexate in combination with nephrotoxic chemotherapy (eg, cisplatin). **[US Boxed Warning]: Methotrexate elimination is reduced in patients with renal impairment;** may require dose reduction or discontinuation; monitor closely for toxicity. **[US Boxed Warning]: Tumor lysis syndrome may occur in patients with high tumor burden;** use appropriate prevention and treatment.

[US Boxed Warning]: May cause potentially life-threatening pneumonitis (acute or chronic); may require treatment interruption; may be irreversible. Pulmonary symptoms may occur at any time during therapy and at any dosage; monitor closely for pulmonary symptoms, particularly dry, nonproductive cough. Other potential symptoms include fever, dyspnea, hypoxemia, or pulmonary infiltrate. **[US Boxed Warning]: Methotrexate elimination is reduced in patients with pleural effusions;** may require dose reduction or discontinuation. Monitor closely for toxicity.

[US Boxed Warning]: Bone marrow suppression may occur (sometimes fatal); aplastic anemia has been reported; anemia, pancytopenia, leukopenia, neutropenia, and/or thrombocytopenia may occur. Use caution in patients with preexisting bone marrow suppression. Discontinue treatment (immediately) in RA or psoriasis if a significant decrease in hematologic components is noted. **[US Boxed Warning]: Use of low-dose methotrexate has been associated with the development of malignant lymphomas;** may regress upon treatment discontinuation; treat lymphoma appropriately if regression is not induced by cessation of methotrexate. Discontinue methotrexate if lymphoma does not regress. Other secondary tumors have been reported.

[US Boxed Warning]: Gastrointestinal toxicity may occur; diarrhea and ulcerative stomatitis may require treatment interruption; hemorrhagic enteritis or intestinal perforation (with fatality) may occur. Use with caution in patients with peptic ulcer disease, ulcerative colitis. In children, doses ≥12 g/m^2 (IV) are associated with a high emetic potential; doses ≥250 mg/m^2 (IV) in adults and children are associated with moderate emetic potential (Dupuis, 2011). Antiemetics may be recommended to prevent nausea and vomiting.

May cause neurotoxicity including seizures (usually in pediatric ALL patients receiving intermediate-dose (1 g/m^2 methotrexate), leukoencephalopathy (usually in patients who have received cranial irradiation) and stroke-like encephalopathy (usually with high-dose regimens). Chemical arachnoiditis (headache, back pain, nuchal rigidity, fever) and myelopathy may result from intrathecal administration. Chronic leukoencephalopathy has been reported with high-dose and with intrathecal methotrexate; may be progressive and fatal. May cause dizziness and fatigue; may affect the ability to drive or operate heavy machinery.

[US Boxed Warning]: Any dose level, route of administration, or duration of therapy may cause severe and potentially fatal dermatologic reactions, including toxic epidermal necrolysis, Stevens-Johnson syndrome, exfoliative dermatitis, skin necrosis, and erythema multiforme. Recovery has been reported with treatment discontinuation. Radiation dermatitis and sunburn may be precipitated by methotrexate administration. Psoriatic lesions may be worsened by concomitant exposure to ultraviolet radiation.

Potentially significant drug-drug interactions may exist, requiring dose or frequency adjustment, additional monitoring, and/or selection of alternative therapy. **[US Boxed Warning]: Concomitant administration with NSAIDs may cause severe bone marrow suppression, aplastic anemia, and GI toxicity.** Do not administer NSAIDs prior to or during high-dose methotrexate therapy; may increase and prolong serum methotrexate levels. Doses used for psoriasis may still lead to unexpected toxicities; use caution when administering NSAIDs or salicylates with lower doses of methotrexate for RA. Methotrexate may increase the levels and effects of mercaptopurine; may require dosage adjustments. Vitamins containing folate may decrease response to systemic methotrexate; folate deficiency may increase methotrexate toxicity. Concomitant use of proton pump inhibitors with methotrexate (primarily high-dose methotrexate) may elevate and prolong serum methotrexate and metabolite (hydroxymethotrexate) levels; may lead to toxicities; use with caution. Immunization may be ineffective during methotrexate treatment. Immunization with live vaccines is not recommended; cases of disseminated vaccinia infections due to live vaccines have been reported. **[US Boxed Warning]: Concomitant methotrexate administration with radiotherapy may increase the risk of soft tissue necrosis and osteonecrosis.**

[US Boxed Warnings]: Should be administered under the supervision of a physician experienced in the use of antimetabolite therapy; serious and fatal toxicities have occurred at all dose levels. Immune suppression may lead to potentially fatal opportunistic infections, including *Pneumocystis jirovecii* pneumonia (PCP). Use methotrexate with extreme caution in patients with an active infection (contraindicated in patients with immunodeficiency syndrome). **[US Boxed Warnings]: For rheumatoid arthritis and psoriasis, immunosuppressive therapy should only be used when disease is active, severe, recalcitrant, and disabling; and where less toxic, traditional therapy is ineffective. Methotrexate formulations and/or diluents containing preservatives should not be used for intrathecal or high-dose methotrexate therapy. May cause fetal death or congenital abnormalities; do not use for psoriasis or RA treatment in pregnant women.** May cause impairment of fertility, oligospermia, and menstrual dysfunction. Toxicity from methotrexate or any immunosuppressive is increased in the elderly. Methotrexate injection may contain benzyl alcohol and should not be used in neonates. Errors have occurred (some resulting in death) when methotrexate was administered as a "daily" dose instead of a "weekly" dose intended for some indications. The ISMP Targeted Medication Safety Best Practices for Hospitals recommends hospitals use a weekly dosage regimen default for oral methotrexate orders, with a hard stop override requiring verification of appropriate oncology indication; manual systems ▶

should require verification of an oncology indication prior to dispensing oral methotrexate for daily administration. Pharmacists should provide patient education for patients discharged on weekly oral methotrexate; education should include written leaflets that contain clear instructions about the weekly dosing schedule and explain the danger of taking extra doses (ISMP, 2014).

When used for intrathecal administration, should not be prepared during the preparation of any other agents; after preparation, store intrathecal medications in an isolated location or container clearly marked with a label identifying as "intrathecal" use only; delivery of intrathecal medications to the patient should only be with other medications intended for administration into the central nervous system (Jacobson, 2009).

Benzyl alcohol and derivatives: Some dosage forms may contain benzyl alcohol; large amounts of benzyl alcohol (≥99 mg/kg/day) have been associated with a potentially fatal toxicity ("gasping syndrome") in neonates; the "gasping syndrome" consists of metabolic acidosis, respiratory distress, gasping respirations, CNS dysfunction (including convulsions, intracranial hemorrhage), hypotension, and cardiovascular collapse (AAP ["Inactive" 1997]; CDC, 1982); some data suggests that benzoate displaces bilirubin from protein binding sites (Ahlfors, 2001); avoid or use dosage forms containing benzyl alcohol with caution in neonates. See manufacturer's labeling.

Adverse Reactions Note: Adverse reactions vary by route and dosage. Frequency not always defined.

Cardiovascular: Arterial thrombosis, cerebral thrombosis, chest pain, deep vein thrombosis, hypotension, pericardial effusion, pericarditis, plaque erosion (psoriasis), pulmonary embolism, retinal thrombosis, thrombophlebitis, vasculitis

Central nervous system: Dizziness (≤3%), headache (pJIA 1%), abnormal cranial sensation, brain disease, chemical arachnoiditis (intrathecal; acute), chills, cognitive dysfunction (has been reported at low dosage), drowsiness, fatigue, leukoencephalopathy (intravenous administration after craniospinal irradiation or repeated high-dose therapy; may be chronic), malaise, mood changes (has been reported at low dosage), neurological signs and symptoms (at high dosages; including confusion, hemiparesis, transient blindness, seizures, and coma), severe neurotoxicity (reported with unexpectedly increased frequency among pediatric patients with acute lymphoblastic leukemia who were treated with intermediate-dose intravenous methotrexate), speech disturbance

Dermatologic: Alopecia (≤10%), burning sensation of skin (psoriasis 3% to 10%), skin photosensitivity (3% to 10%), skin rash (≤3%), dermatitis (rheumatoid arthritis 1% to 3%), pruritus (rheumatoid arthritis 1% to 3%), acne vulgaris, dermal ulcer, diaphoresis, ecchymoses, erythema multiforme, erythematous rash, exfoliative dermatitis, furunculosis, hyperpigmentation, hypopigmentation, skin abnormalities related to radiation recall, skin necrosis, Stevens-Johnson syndrome, telangiectasia, toxic epidermal necrolysis, urticaria

Endocrine & metabolic: Decreased libido, decreased serum albumin, diabetes mellitus, gynecomastia, menstrual disease

Gastrointestinal: Diarrhea (≤11%), nausea and vomiting (≤11%), stomatitis (2% to 10%), abdominal distress, anorexia, aphthous stomatitis, enteritis, gastrointestinal hemorrhage, gingivitis, hematemesis, intestinal perforation, melena

Genitourinary: Azotemia, cystitis, defective oogenesis, defective spermatogenesis, dysuria, hematuria, impotence, infertility, oligospermia, pancreatitis, proteinuria, severe renal disease, vaginal discharge

Hematologic & oncologic: Thrombocytopenia (rheumatoid arthritis 3% to 10%; platelet count <100,000/mm^3), leukopenia (1% to 3%; WBC <3000/mm^3), pancytopenia (rheumatoid arthritis 1% to 3%), agranulocytosis, anemia, aplastic anemia, bone marrow depression (nadir: 7-10 days), decreased hematocrit, eosinophilia, gastric ulcer, hypogammaglobulinemia, lymphadenopathy, lymphoma, lymphoproliferative disorder, neutropenia, non-Hodgkin's lymphoma (in patients receiving low-dose oral methotrexate), tumor lysis syndrome

Hepatic: Increased liver enzymes (14% to 15%), cirrhosis (chronic therapy), hepatic failure, hepatic fibrosis (chronic therapy), hepatitis (acute), hepatotoxicity

Hypersensitivity: Anaphylactoid reaction

Infection: Cryptococcosis, cytomegalovirus disease (including cytomegaloviral pneumonia, sepsis, nocardiosis), herpes simplex infection, herpes zoster, histoplasmosis, infection, pneumonia due to *pneumocystis jiroveci*, vaccinia (disseminated; following smallpox immunization)

Neuromuscular & skeletal: Arthralgia, myalgia, myelopathy (subacute), osteonecrosis (with radiotherapy), osteoporosis, stress fracture

Ophthalmic: Blurred vision, conjunctivitis, eye pain, visual disturbance

Otic: Tinnitus

Renal: Renal failure

Respiratory: Interstitial pneumonitis (rheumatoid arthritis 1%), chronic obstructive pulmonary disease, cough, epistaxis, pharyngitis, pneumonia, pulmonary alveolitis, pulmonary disease, pulmonary fibrosis, respiratory failure, upper respiratory tract infection

Miscellaneous: Fever, nodule, tissue necrosis

Drug Interactions

Metabolism/Transport Effects Substrate of BCRP, OAT3, P-glycoprotein, SLCO1B1

Avoid Concomitant Use

Avoid concomitant use of Methotrexate with any of the following: Acitretin; BCG (Intravesical); CloZAPine; Dipyrone; Foscarnet; Natalizumab; Pimecrolimus; Tacrolimus (Topical)

Increased Effect/Toxicity

Methotrexate may increase the levels/effects of: CloZAPine; CycloSPORINE (Systemic); Dipyrone; Fingolimod; Leflunomide; Loop Diuretics; Natalizumab; Tegafur; Theophylline Derivatives; Tofacitinib; Vaccines (Live)

The levels/effects of Methotrexate may be increased by: Acitretin; Alitretinoin (Systemic); Ciprofloxacin (Systemic); CycloSPORINE (Systemic); Denosumab; Dexketoprofen; Dipyrone; Eltrombopag; Foscarnet; Fosphenytoin-Phenytoin; Loop Diuretics; Lumacaftor; Mipomersen; Nonsteroidal Anti-Inflammatory Agents; Penicillins; P-glycoprotein/ABCB1 Inhibitors; Pimecrolimus; Probenecid; Proton Pump Inhibitors; Ranolazine; Roflumilast; Rolapitant; Salicylates; SulfaSALAzine; Sulfonamide Derivatives; Tacrolimus (Topical); Teriflunomide; Trastuzumab; Trimethoprim

◄ **Decreased Effect**
Methotrexate may decrease the levels/effects of: BCG (Intravesical); Coccidioides immitis Skin Test; Fosphenytoin-Phenytoin; Loop Diuretics; Sapropterin; Sipuleucel-T; Vaccines (Inactivated); Vaccines (Live)

The levels/effects of Methotrexate may be decreased by: Bile Acid Sequestrants; Echinacea; Lumacaftor; P-glycoprotein/ABCB1 Inducers

Food Interactions Methotrexate peak serum levels may be decreased if taken with food. Milk-rich foods may decrease methotrexate absorption. Management: Administer without regard to food.

Storage/Stability
Tablets: Store between 20°C and 25°C (68°F and 77°F); excursions are permitted between 15°C and 30°C (59°F and 86°F). Protect from light.

Injection: Store intact vials and autoinjectors between 20°C and 25°C (68°F and 77°F); excursions may be permitted between 15°C and 30°C (59°F and 86°F). Protect from light.

IV: Solution diluted in D_5W or NS is stable for 24 hours at room temperature (21°C to 25°C).

Intrathecal: Intrathecal dilutions are preservative free and should be used as soon as possible after preparation. After preparation, store intrathecal medications (until use) in an isolated location or container clearly marked with a label identifying as "intrathecal" use only.

Preparation for Administration Hazardous agent; use appropriate precautions for handling and disposal (NIOSH 2014 [group 1]). **Use preservative-free preparations for intrathecal or high-dose methotrexate administration.**

IV: Dilute powder with D_5W or NS to a concentration of ≤25 mg/mL (20 mg and 50 mg vials) and 50 mg/mL (1 g vial). May further dilute in D_5W or NS.

Intrathecal: Prepare intrathecal solutions with preservative-free NS, lactated Ringer's, or Elliot's B solution to a final volume of up to 12 mL (volume generally based on institution or practitioner preference). Intrathecal methotrexate concentrations may be institution specific or based on practitioner preference, generally ranging from a final concentration of 1 mg/mL (per prescribing information; Grossman, 1993; Lin, 2008) up to ~2 to 4 mg/mL (de Lemos, 2009; Glantz, 1999). For triple intrathecal therapy (methotrexate 12 mg/hydrocortisone 24 mg/cytarabine 36 mg), preparation to final volume of 12 mL is reported (Lin, 2008). Intrathecal medications should **NOT** be prepared during the preparation of any other agents.

Mechanism of Action Methotrexate is a folate antimetabolite that inhibits DNA synthesis, repair, and cellular replication. Methotrexate irreversibly binds to and inhibits dihydrofolate reductase, inhibiting the formation of reduced folates, and thymidylate synthetase, resulting in inhibition of purine and thymidylic acid synthesis, thus interfering with DNA synthesis, repair, and cellular replication. Methotrexate is cell cycle specific for the S phase of the cycle. Actively proliferative tissues are more susceptible to the effects of methotrexate.

The MOA in the treatment of rheumatoid arthritis is unknown, but may affect immune function. In psoriasis, methotrexate is thought to target rapidly proliferating epithelial cells in the skin.

In Crohn disease, it may have immune modulator and anti-inflammatory activity.

Pharmacodynamics/Kinetics
Onset of action: Antirheumatic: 3 to 6 weeks; additional improvement may continue longer than 12 weeks

Absorption:
Oral: Highly variable; dose dependent
IM injection: Complete

Distribution: Penetrates slowly into 3rd space fluids (eg, pleural effusions, ascites), exits slowly from these compartments (slower than from plasma); sustained concentrations retained in kidney and liver
V_d: IV: 0.18 L/kg (initial); 0.4 to 0.8 L/kg (steady state)

Protein binding: ~50%

Metabolism: Partially metabolized by intestinal flora (after oral administration) to DAMPA by carboxypeptidase; hepatic aldehyde oxidase converts methotrexate to 7-hydroxy methotrexate; polyglutamates are produced intracellularly and are just as potent as methotrexate; their production is dose- and duration-dependent and they are slowly eliminated by the cell once formed. Polyglutamated forms can be converted back to methotrexate.

Bioavailability: Oral: ~20% to 95%; in general, bioavailability is dose dependent and decreases as the dose increases (especially at doses >80 mg/m^2)

Half-life elimination: Low dose: 3 to 10 hours; High dose: 8 to 15 hours; Children: 1 to 6 hours

Time to peak, serum: Oral: 1 to 2 hours; IM: 30 to 60 minutes

Excretion: Dose and route dependent; IV: Urine (80% to 90% as unchanged drug; 5% to 7% as 7-hydroxy methotrexate); feces (<10%)

Dosing
Adult Note: Methotrexate doses between 100 to 500 mg/m^2 **may require** leucovorin calcium rescue. Doses >500 mg/m^2 **require** leucovorin calcium rescue (refer to Adjustment for Toxicity for leucovorin calcium dosing). Doses ≥250 mg/m^2 (IV) are associated with moderate emetic potential. Antiemetics may be recommended to prevent nausea and vomiting.

Acute lymphoblastic leukemia (ALL):
Meningeal leukemia prophylaxis or treatment: Intrathecal: Manufacturer's labeling: 12 mg (maximum 15 mg/dose) every 2 to 7 days; continue for 1 dose beyond CSF cell count normalization. **Note:** Optimal intrathecal chemotherapy dosing should be based on age rather than on body surface area (BSA); CSF volume correlates with age and not to BSA (Bleyer, 1983; Kerr, 2001).

CALGB 8811 regimen (Larson, 1995; combination therapy):
Early intensification: Intrathecal: 15 mg day 1 of early intensification phase, repeat in 4 weeks

CNS prophylaxis/interim maintenance phase:
Intrathecal: 15 mg day 1, 8, 15, 22, and 29
Oral: 20 mg/m^2 days 36, 43, 50, 57, and 64

Prolonged maintenance: Oral: 20 mg/m^2 days 1, 8, 15, and 22 every 4 weeks for 24 months from diagnosis

Dose-intensive regimen (Kantarjian, 2000; combination therapy):
IV: 200 mg/m^2 over 2 hours, followed by 800 mg/m^2 over 24 hours beginning day 1, (followed by leucovorin rescue) of even numbered cycles (in combination with cytarabine; alternates with Hyper-CVAD)

CNS prophylaxis: Intrathecal: 12 mg on day 2 of each cycle; duration depends on risk

Maintenance: IV: 10 mg/m^2/day for 5 days every month for 2 years (in combination with prednisone, vincristine, and mercaptopurine)

Breast cancer: IV: CMF regimen: 40 mg/m^2 days 1 and 8 every 4 weeks (in combination with cyclophosphamide and fluorouracil) for 6 to 12 cycles (Bonadonna, 1995; Levine, 1998)

Choriocarcinoma, chorioadenoma, gestational trophoblastic diseases: 15 to 30 mg oral or IM daily for a 5 day course; may repeat for 3 to 5 courses (manufacturer's labeling) **or** 100 mg/m^2 IV over 30 minutes followed by 200 mg/m^2 IV over 12 hours (with leucovorin 24 hours after the start of methotrexate), administer a second course if hCG levels plateau for 3 consecutive weeks (Garrett, 2002)

Head and neck cancer, advanced: IV: 40 mg/m^2 once weekly until disease progression or unacceptable toxicity (Forastiere, 1992; Guardiola, 2004; Stewart, 2009)

Lymphoma, non-Hodgkin: IV:

CODOX-M/IVAC regimen (Mead, 2008): Cycles 1 and 3 of CODOX-M (CODOX-M alternates with IVAC)

Adults ≤65 years: IV: 300 mg/m^2 over 1 hour (on day 10) followed by 2700 mg/m^2 over 23 hours (with leucovorin rescue)

Adults >65 years: IV: 100 mg/m^2 over 1 hour (on day 10) followed by 900 mg/m^2 over 23 hours (with leucovorin rescue)

Hyper-CVAD alternating with high-dose methotrexate/cytarabine regimen: IV: 1000 mg/m^2 over 24 hours on day 1 during even courses (2, 4, 6, and 8) of 21-day treatment cycles (Thomas, 2006) **or** 200 mg/m^2 bolus day 1 followed by 800 mg/m^2 over 24 hours during even courses (2, 4, 6, and 8) of 21-day treatment cycles (Khouri, 1998) with leucovorin rescue

Mycosis fungoides (cutaneous T-cell lymphoma): 5 to 50 mg once weekly or 15 to 37.5 mg twice weekly orally or IM for early stages (manufacturer's labeling) **or** 25 mg orally once weekly, may increase to 50 mg once weekly (Zackheim, 2003)

Osteosarcoma: Adults ≤30 years: IV: MAP regimen: 12 g/m^2 (maximum dose: 20 g) over 4 hours (followed by leucovorin rescue) for 4 doses during induction (before surgery) at weeks 3, 4, 8, and 9, and for 8 doses during maintenance (after surgery) at weeks 15, 16, 20, 21, 25, 26, 30, and 31 (in combination with doxorubicin and cisplatin) (Meyers, 2005); other combinations, intervals, age ranges, and doses (8 to 14 g/m^2/dose) have been described (with leucovorin rescue), refer to specific reference for details (Bacci, 2000; Bacci, 2003; Goorin, 2003; Le Deley, 2007; Meyers, 1992; Weiner, 1986; Winkler, 1988)

Psoriasis: Note: Some experts recommend concomitant folic acid 1 to 5 mg daily (except the day of methotrexate) to reduce hematologic, gastrointestinal, and hepatic adverse events related to methotrexate.

Oral: Initial: 2.5 to 5 mg/dose every 12 hours for 3 doses per week **or**

Oral, IM, IV, SubQ: Initial: 10 to 25 mg given once weekly; adjust dose gradually to optimal response (doses above 20 mg once weekly are associated with an increased incidence of toxicity); doses >30 mg per week should not be exceeded.

Note: An initial test dose of 2.5 to 5 mg is recommended in patients with risk factors for hematologic toxicity or renal impairment. (Kalb, 2009).

Rheumatoid arthritis: Note: Some experts recommend concomitant folic acid at a dose of least 5 mg per week (except the day of methotrexate) to reduce hematologic, gastrointestinal, and hepatic adverse events related to methotrexate.

Oral (manufacturer labeling): Initial: 7.5 mg once weekly or 2.5 mg every 12 hours for 3 doses per week; adjust dose gradually to optimal response (dosage exceeding 20 mg once weekly are associated with an increased incidence of toxicity; *alternatively*, 10 to 15 mg once weekly, increased by 5 mg every 2 to 4 weeks to a maximum of 20 to 30 mg once weekly has been recommended by some experts (Visser, 2009)

SubQ: Initial: 7.5 mg once weekly; adjust dose gradually to optimal response (doses above 20 mg once weekly are associated with an increased incidence of toxicity) **or** Initial: 15 mg once weekly; if insufficient response, after 16 weeks, may increase to 20 mg once weekly (Braun, 2008)

IM: 7.5 mg once weekly; adjust dose gradually to optimal response (doses above 20 mg once weekly are associated with an increased incidence of toxicity)

Off-label uses:

Bladder cancer (off-label use): IV:

Dose-dense MVAC regimen: 30 mg/m^2 day 1 every 2 weeks (in combination with vinblastine, doxorubicin, and cisplatin) (Sternberg, 2001)

CMV regimen: 30 mg/m^2 days 1 and 8 every 3 weeks for 3 cycles (in combination with cisplatin, vinblastine and leucovorin rescue) (Griffiths, 2011)

CNS Lymphoma (off-label use): IV: 8000 mg/m^2 over 4 hours (followed by leucovorin rescue) every 14 days until complete response or a maximum of 8 cycles; if complete response, follow with 2 consolidation cycles at the same dose every 14 days (with leucovorin rescue), followed by 11 maintenance cycles of 8000 mg/m^2 every 28 days with leucovorin rescue (Batchelor, 2003) **or** 2500 mg/m^2 over 2 to 3 hours every 14 days for 5 doses (in combination with vincristine, procarbazine, intrathecal methotrexate, leucovorin, dexamethasone, and cytarabine) (De Angelis, 2002) **or** 3500 mg/m^2 over 2 hours on day 2 every 2 weeks (in combination with rituximab, vincristine, procarbazine, and leucovorin [with intra-omaya methotrexate 12 mg between days 5 and 12 of each cycle if positive CSF cytology]) for 5 to 7 induction cycles (Shah, 2007)

Crohn disease, moderate/severe, corticosteroid-dependent or refractory (off-label use):

Remission induction or reduction of steroid use: IM, SubQ: 25 mg once weekly (Lichtenstein, 2009)

Remission maintenance: IM: 15 mg once weekly (Feagan, 2000; Lichtenstein, 2009)

Dermatomyositis/polymyositis (off-label uses):

Oral: Initial: 7.5 to 15 mg per week, often adjunctively with high-dose corticosteroid therapy; may increase in weekly 2.5 mg increments to target dose of 10 to 25 mg per week (**Note:** Administration of folate 5 to 7 mg per week has been used to reduce side effects) (Briemberg, 2003; Newman, 1995; Wiendl, 2008).

IV, IM: Doses of 20 to 60 mg/week have been employed if failure with oral therapy (doses >50 mg/week may require leucovorin calcium rescue) (Briemberg, 2003)

◄ **Ectopic pregnancy (off-label use): IM:**

Single-dose regimen: Methotrexate 50 mg/m^2 on day 1; Measure serum hCG levels on days 4 and 7; if needed, repeat dose on day 7 (Barnhart, 2009)

Two-dose regimen: Methotrexate 50 mg/m^2 on day 1; Measure serum hCG levels on day 4 and administer a second dose of methotrexate 50 mg/m^2; Measure serum hCG levels on day 7 and if needed, administer a third dose of 50 mg/m^2 (Barnhart, 2009)

Multidose regimen: Methotrexate 1 mg/kg on day 1; leucovorin calcium 0.1 mg/kg IM on day 2; measure serum hCG on day 2; methotrexate 1 mg/kg on day 3; leucovorin calcium 0.1 mg/kg on day 4; measure serum hCG on day 4; continue up to a total of 4 courses based on hCG concentrations (Barnhart, 2009)

Graft-versus-host disease, acute (aGVHD), prophylaxis: IV: 15 mg/m^2/dose on day 1 and 10 mg/m^2/dose on days 3 and 6 after allogeneic transplant (in combination with cyclosporine and prednisone) (Chao, 1993; Chao, 2000; Ross, 1999) **or** 15 mg/m^2/dose on day 1 and 10 mg/m^2/dose on days 3, 6, and 11 after allogeneic transplant (in combination with cyclosporine) (Chao, 2000) **or** 15 mg/m^2/dose on day 1 and 10 mg/m^2/dose on days 3, 6, and 11 after allogeneic transplant (in combination with cyclosporine, followed by leucovorin); may omit day 11 methotrexate for grade 2 or higher toxicity (Ruutu, 2013)

Nonleukemic meningeal cancer (off-label uses): Intrathecal: 12 mg/dose twice weekly for 4 weeks, then weekly for 4 doses, then monthly for 4 doses (Glantz, 1998) **or** 10 mg twice weekly for 4 weeks, then weekly for 1 month, then every 2 weeks for 2 months (Glantz, 1999) **or** 10 to 15 mg twice weekly for 4 weeks, then once weekly for 4 weeks, then a maintenance regimen of once a month (Chamberlain, 2010)

Soft tissue sarcoma (desmoid tumors, aggressive fibromatosis), advanced (off-label use): IV: 30 mg/m^2 every 7 to 10 days (dose usually rounded to 50 mg) in combination with vinblastine for 1 year (Azzarelli, 2001)

Systemic lupus erythematosus, moderate-to-severe (off-label use): Oral: Initial: 7.5 mg once weekly; may increase by 2.5 mg increments weekly (maximum: 20 mg once weekly), in combination with prednisone (Fortin, 2008)

Takayasu arteritis, refractory or relapsing disease (off-label use): Oral: Initial dose: 0.3 mg/kg/week (maximum: 15 mg per week), titrated by 2.5 mg increments every 1 to 2 weeks until reaching a maximum tolerated weekly dose of 25 mg (use in combination with a corticosteroid; Hoffman, 1994)

Geriatric Refer to adult dosing; adjust for renal impairment.

Breast cancer: Patients >60 years: IV: CMF regimen: 30 mg/m^2 days 1 and 8 every 4 weeks (in combination with cyclophosphamide and fluorouracil) for up to 12 cycles (Bonadonna, 1995)

Meningeal leukemia: Intrathecal: Consider a dose reduction (CSF volume and turnover may decrease with age)

Non-Hodgkin lymphoma: CODOX-M/IVAC regimen (Mead, 2008): Cycles 1 and 3 of CODOX-M (CODOX-M alternates with IVAC): IV: 100 mg over 1 hour (on day 10) followed by 900 mg over 23 hours (with leucovorin rescue)

Rheumatoid arthritis/psoriasis: Oral: Initial: 5 to 7.5 mg per week, not to exceed 20 mg per week

Pediatric Note: Methotrexate doses between 100 to 500 mg/m^2 **may require** leucovorin calcium rescue. Doses >500 mg/m^2 **require** leucovorin calcium rescue (refer to Adjustment for Toxicity for leucovorin calcium dosing). In children, doses ≥12 g/m^2 (IV) are associated with a high emetic potential; doses ≥250 mg/m^2 (IV) are associated with moderate emetic potential (Dupuis, 2011). Antiemetics may be recommended to prevent nausea and vomiting.

Polyarticular juvenile idiopathic arthritis (pJIA): Oral, IM, SubQ: Initial: 10 mg/m^2 once weekly, adjust gradually to optimum response; doses up to 20 to 30 mg/m^2 once weekly have been used (doses above 20 mg/m^2 once weekly may be associated with an increased risk of toxicity)

Acute lymphoblastic leukemia (ALL; intrathecal therapy is also administered [refer to specific reference]):

Consolidation/intensification phases (as part of a combination regimen): 1,000 mg/m^2 IV over 24 hours in week 1 of intensification and 20 mg/m^2 IM (use 50% dose reduction if on same day as intrathecal methotrexate) on day 1 of week 2 of intensification phase; Intensification repeats every 2 weeks for a total of 12 courses (Mahoney, 2000) **or** 5000 mg/m^2 IV over 24 hours days 8, 22, 36, and 50 of consolidation phase (Schrappe, 2000) with leucovorin rescue

Interim maintenance (as part of a combination regimen): 15 mg/m^2 orally days 0, 7, 14, 21, 28, and 35 of interim maintenance phase (Seibel, 2008) **or** 100 mg/m^2 (escalate dose by 50 mg/m^2 each dose) IV days 0, 10, 20, 30, and 40 of increased intensity interim maintenance phase (Seibel, 2008)

Maintenance (as part of a combination regimen): 20 mg/m^2 IM weekly on day 1 of weeks 25 to 130 (Mahoney, 2000) **or** 20 mg/m^2 orally days 7, 14, 21, 28, 35, 42, 49, 56, 63, 70, and 77 (Seibel, 2008)

T-cell acute lymphoblastic leukemia (Asselin, 2011; triple intrathecal therapy is also administered [refer to specific reference]):

Induction (weeks 1 to 6; as part of a combination regimen): IV:

Low dose: 40 mg/m^2 day 2

High dose: 500 mg/m^2 over 30 minutes followed by 4500 mg/m^2 over 23.5 hours (with leucovorin rescue) day 22

Consolidation (weeks 7 to 33; combination chemotherapy): IV: High dose: 500 mg/m^2 over 30 minutes followed by 4500 mg/m^2 over 23.5 hours (with leucovorin rescue) in weeks 7, 10, and 13 with leucovorin rescue

Continuation (weeks 34 to 108; combination chemotherapy): IV, IM: 30 mg/m^2 weekly until 2 years after documented complete remission

ALL, CNS prophylaxis triple intrathecal therapy (off-label dosing): Intrathecal: Age-based dosing (in combination with cytarabine and hydrocortisone): Days of administration vary based on risk status and protocol; refer to institutional protocols or reference for details (Matloub, 2006):

<2 years: 8 mg

2 to <3 years: 10 mg

3 to ≤8 years: 12 mg

>8 years: 15 mg

Meningeal leukemia, prophylaxis or treatment: Intrathecal: 6 to 12 mg/dose (based on age) every 2 to 7 days; continue for 1 dose beyond CSF cell count normalization. **Note:** Optimal intrathecal chemotherapy dosing should be based on age rather than on body surface area (BSA); CSF volume correlates with age and not to BSA (Bleyer, 1983; Kerr, 2001):

<1 year: 6 mg/dose
1 year: 8 mg/dose
2 years: 10 mg/dose
≥3 years: 12 mg/dose

Osteosarcoma: IV: MAP regimen: 12 g/m^2 (maximum dose: 20 g) over 4 hours (followed by leucovorin rescue) for 4 doses during induction (before surgery) at weeks 3, 4, 8, and 9, and for 8 doses during maintenance (after surgery) at weeks 15, 16, 20, 21, 25, 26, 30, and 31 (in combination with doxorubicin and cisplatin) (Meyers, 2005); other combinations, intervals, and doses (8 to 14 g/m^2/dose) have been described (with leucovorin rescue), refer to specific reference for details (Bacci, 2000; Bacci, 2003; Goorin, 2003; Le Deley, 2007; Meyers, 1992; Weiner, 1986; Winkler, 1988)

Crohn disease, induction and maintenance (off-label use): SubQ: 15 mg/m^2 once weekly; maximum dose: 25 mg (Rufo, 2012)

Dermatomyositis (off-label use): Oral, SubQ (preferred): The lesser of 15 mg/m^2 or 1 mg/kg once weekly (maximum dose: 40 mg/week) in combination with corticosteroids (Huber, 2010) **or** 15 mg/m^2 once weekly (range: 10 to 20 mg/m^2 once weekly; maximum dose: 25 mg/week) in combination with prednisone (Ramanan, 2005)

Graft-versus-host disease, acute (aGVHD) prophylaxis (off-label use): IV: Refer to adult dosing.

Renal Impairment There are no dosage adjustments provided in the manufacturer's labeling. The following adjustments have been recommended:

Aronoff, 2007:
Adults:
 CrCl 10 to 50 mL/minute: Administer 50% of dose
 CrCl <10 mL/minute: Avoid use
 Intermittent hemodialysis: Administer 50% of dose (post dialysis)
 Continuous renal replacement therapy (CRRT): Administer 50% of dose
Children:
 CrCl 10 to 50 mL/minute/1.73 m^2: Administer 50% of dose
 CrCl <10 mL/minute/1.73 m^2: Administer 30% of dose
 Intermittent hemodialysis: Administer 30% of dose (post dialysis)
 Continuous ambulatory peritoneal dialysis (CAPD): Administer 30% of dose
 Continuous renal replacement therapy (CRRT): Administer 50% of dose
Kintzel, 1995:
 CrCl 46 to 60 mL/minute: Administer 65% of normal dose
 CrCl 31 to 45 mL/minute: Administer 50% of normal dose
 CrCl <30 mL/minute: Avoid use
Hemodialysis patients with cancer (Janus, 2010): Administer 25% of dose after hemodialysis; monitor closely for toxicity

High-dose methotrexate, dose-intensive regimen for ALL (200 mg/m^2 over 2 hours, followed by 800 mg/m^2 over 24 hours with leucovorin rescue [Kant-arjian, 2000]):

Serum creatinine <1.5 mg/dL: No dosage adjustment necessary

Serum creatinine 1.5 to 2 mg/dL: Administer 75% of dose

Serum creatinine >2 mg/dL: Administer 50% of dose

Hepatic Impairment There are no dosage adjustments provided in the manufacturer's labeling; use with caution in patients with impaired hepatic function or preexisting hepatic damage. The following adjustments have been recommended (Floyd, 2006):

Bilirubin 3.1 to 5 mg/dL **or** transaminases >3 times ULN: Administer 75% of dose

Bilirubin >5 mg/dL: Avoid use

Obesity *ASCO Guidelines for appropriate chemotherapy dosing in obese adults with cancer:* Utilize patient's actual body weight (full weight) for calculation of body surface area- or weight-based dosing, particularly when the intent of therapy is curative; manage regimen-related toxicities in the same manner as for nonobese patients; if a dose reduction is utilized due to toxicity, consider resumption of full weight-based dosing with subsequent cycles, especially if cause of toxicity (eg, hepatic or renal impairment) is resolved (Griggs, 2012).

Adjustment for Toxicity

Methotrexate toxicities:

Nonhematologic toxicity: Diarrhea, stomatitis, or vomiting which may lead to dehydration: Discontinue until recovery

Hematologic toxicity:

Psoriasis, rheumatoid arthritis: Significant blood count decrease: Discontinue immediately.

Oncologic uses: Profound granulocytopenia and fever: Evaluate immediately; consider broad-spectrum parenteral antimicrobial coverage

Leucovorin calcium dosing (from methotrexate injection prescribing information; other leucovorin dosing/schedules may be specific to chemotherapy protocols):

Normal methotrexate elimination (serum methotrexate level ~10 micromolar at 24 hours after administration, 1 micromolar at 48 hours, and <0.2 micromolar at 72 hours): Leucovorin calcium 15 mg (oral, IM, or IV) every 6 hours for 60 hours (10 doses) beginning 24 hours after the start of methotrexate infusion

Delayed late methotrexate elimination (serum methotrexate level remaining >0.2 micromolar at 72 hours and >0.05 micromolar at 96 hours after administration): Continue leucovorin calcium 15 mg (oral, IM or IV) every 6 hours until methotrexate level is <0.05 micromolar

Delayed early methotrexate elimination and/or acute renal injury (serum methotrexate level ≥50 micromolar at 24 hours, or ≥5 micromolar at 48 hours, or a doubling of serum creatinine level at 24 hours after methotrexate administration): Leucovorin calcium 150 mg IV every 3 hours until methotrexate level is <1 micromolar, then 15 mg IV every 3 hours until methotrexate level <0.05 micromolar

◄ Leucovorin nomogram dosing for high-dose methotrexate overexposure (**generalized dosing** derived from reference nomogram figures, refer to each reference [Bleyer, 1978; Bleyer, 1981; Widemann, 2006] or institution-specific nomogram for details):

At 24 hours:
For methotrexate levels of ≥100 micromolar at ~24 hours, leucovorin is initially dosed at 1000 mg/m^2 every 6 hours
For methotrexate levels of ≥10 to <100 micromolar at 24 hours, leucovorin is initially dosed at 100 mg/m^2 every 3 or 6 hours
For methotrexate levels of ~1 to 10 micromolar at 24 hours, leucovorin is initially dosed at 10 mg/m^2 every 3 or 6 hours

At 48 hours:
For methotrexate levels of ≥100 micromolar at 48 hours, leucovorin is dosed at 1000 mg/m^2 every 6 hours
For methotrexate levels of ≥10 to <100 micromolar at 48 hours, leucovorin is dosed at 100 mg/m^2 every 3 hours
For methotrexate levels of ~1 to 10 micromolar at 48 hours, leucovorin is dosed at 100 mg/m^2 every 6 hours **or** 10 to 100 mg/m^2 every 3 hours

At 72 hours:
For methotrexate levels of ≥10 micromolar at 72 hours, leucovorin is dosed at 100 to 1000 mg/m^2 every 3 to 6 hours
For methotrexate levels of ~1 to 10 micromolar at 72 hours, leucovorin is dosed at 10 to 100 mg/m^2 every 3 hours
For methotrexate levels of ~0.1 to 1 micromolar at 72 hours, leucovorin is dosed at 10 mg/m^2 every 3 to 6 hours

If serum creatinine is increased more than 50% above baseline, increase the standard leucovorin dose to 100 mg/m^2 every 3 hours, then adjust according to methotrexate levels above.

Follow methotrexate levels daily, leucovorin may be discontinued when methotrexate level is <0.1 micromolar

Combination Regimens

Bladder cancer:
Bone sarcoma (osteosarcoma):
Breast cancer:
Gestational trophoblastic tumor:
Leukemia, acute lymphocytic:

Administration In children, doses ≥12 g/m^2 are associated with a high emetic potential; doses ≥250 mg/m^2 (IV) in adults and children are associated with moderate emetic potential (Dupuis, 2011). Antiemetics may be recommended to prevent nausea and vomiting.

Methotrexate may be administered orally, IM, IV, intrathecally, or SubQ; IV administration may be as slow push (10 mg/minute), bolus infusion, or 24-hour continuous infusion (route and rate of administration depend on indication and/or protocol; refer to specific references). Must use preservative-free formulation for intrathecal or high-dose methotrexate administration.

Specific dosing schemes vary, but high doses should be followed by leucovorin calcium rescue to prevent toxicity; refer to Additional Information.

Otrexup and Rasuvo are autoinjectors for once weekly subcutaneous use in the abdomen or thigh; patient may self-administer after appropriate training. All schedules should be continually tailored to the individual patient. An initial test dose may be given prior to the regular dosing schedule to detect any extreme sensitivity to adverse effects.

Hazardous agent; use appropriate precautions for handling and disposal (NIOSH 2014 [group 1]).

Emetic Potential
Children:
  IV:
    ≥12 g/m^2: High (>90%)
    ≥250 mg/m^2 to <12 g/m^2: Moderate (30% to 90%)
    >50 mg/m^2 to <250 mg/m^2: Low (10% to 30%)
    ≤50 mg/m^2: Minimal (<10%)
  Oral: Minimal (<10%)
Adults:
  IV:
    ≥250 mg/m^2: Moderate (30% to 90%)
    >50 to <250 mg/m^2: Low (10% to 30%)
    ≤50 mg/m^2: Minimal (<10%)
  Oral: Minimal (<10%)

◄ **Monitoring Parameters**

Oncologic uses: Baseline and frequently during treatment: CBC with differential and platelets, serum creatinine, BUN, liver function tests (LFTs); methotrexate levels and urine pH (with high-dose methotrexate); closely monitor fluid and electrolyte status in patients with impaired methotrexate elimination; chest x-ray (baseline); pulmonary function test (if methotrexate-induced lung disease suspected); monitor carefully for toxicities (due to impaired elimination) in patients with ascites, pleural effusion, decreased folate stores, renal impairment, and/or hepatic impairment

Psoriasis (Kalb, 2009; Menter, 2009):

CBC with differential and platelets (baseline, 7 to 14 days after initiating therapy or dosage increase, every 2 to 4 weeks for first few months, then every 1 to 3 months depending on leukocyte count and stability of patient) monitor more closely in patients with risk factors for hematologic toxicity (eg, renal insufficiency, advanced age, hypoalbuminemia); BUN and serum creatinine (baseline and every 2 to 3 months) calculate glomerular filtration rate if at risk for renal dysfunction; consider PPD for latent TB screening (baseline); LFTs (baseline, monthly for first 6 months, then every 1 to 2 months; more frequently if at risk for hepatotoxicity or if clinically indicated; liver function tests should be performed at least 5 days after the last dose); pregnancy test (if female of reproductive potential); chest x-ray (baseline if underlying lung disease); pulmonary function test (if methotrexate-induced lung disease suspected)

Liver biopsy for patients **with** risk factors for hepatotoxicity: Baseline or after 2 to 6 months of therapy and with each 1 to 1.5 g cumulative dose interval

Liver biopsy for patients **without** risk factors for hepatotoxicity: If persistent elevations in 5 of 9 AST levels during a 12-month period, or decline of serum albumin below the normal range with normal nutritional status. Consider biopsy after cumulative dose of 3.5 to 4 g and after each additional 1.5 g.

Rheumatoid arthritis (American College of Rheumatology Subcommittee, 2002; Kremer, 1994; Saag, 2008; Singh, 2012):

CBC with differential and platelets serum creatinine, and LFTs at baseline and every 2 to 4 weeks for 3 months after initiation or following dose increases, then every 8 to 12 weeks for 3 to 6 months, then every 12 weeks for 6 months; monitor more frequently if clinically indicated.

Chest x-ray (within 1 year prior to initiation), Hepatitis B and C serology (if at high risk); tuberculosis testing annually for patients who live, travel or work in areas with likely TB exposure

Liver biopsy: Baseline (if persistent abnormal baseline LFTs, history of alcoholism, or chronic hepatitis B or C) or during treatment if persistent LFT elevations (6 of 12 tests abnormal over 1 year or 5 of 9 results when LFTs performed at 6-week intervals)

Crohn disease (off-label use; Lichtenstein, 2009): CBC with differential and platelets (baseline and periodic) and liver function tests (baseline and every 1 to 2 months); baseline liver biopsy (in patients with abnormal baseline LFTs or with chronic liver disease); liver biopsy at 1 year if (over a 1-year span) AST consistently elevated or serum albumin consistently decreased; chest x-ray (baseline)

Ectopic pregnancy (off-label use; Barnhart, 2009): Prior to therapy, measure serum hCG, CBC with differential and platelets, liver function tests, serum creatinine. Serum hCG concentrations should decrease between treatment days 4 and 7. If hCG decreases by >15%, additional courses are not needed however, continue to measure hCG weekly until no longer detectable. If <15% decrease is observed, repeat dose per regimen.

Dietary Considerations Some products may contain sodium.

Additional Information Oncology Comment:

Glucarpidase: Methotrexate overexposure: The rescue agent, glucarpidase, is an enzyme which rapidly hydrolyzes extracellular methotrexate into inactive metabolites, resulting in a rapid reduction of methotrexate concentrations. Glucarpidase is approved for the treatment of toxic plasma methotrexate concentrations (>1 micromole/L) in patients with delayed clearance due to renal impairment. Glucarpidase has also been administered intrathecally (off-label use/route) for inadvertent intrathecal methotrexate overexposure. Refer to Glucarpidase monograph.

Dosage Forms Excipient information presented when available (limited, particularly for generics); consult specific product labeling. [DSC] = Discontinued product

Solution, Injection:
  Generic: 25 mg/mL (2 mL, 10 mL)
Solution, Injection [preservative free]:
  Generic: 25 mg/mL (2 mL, 4 mL, 8 mL, 10 mL, 40 mL); 50 mg/2 mL (2 mL); 100 mg/4 mL (4 mL); 200 mg/8 mL (8 mL [DSC]); 250 mg/10 mL (10 mL); 1 g/40 mL (40 mL)
Solution Auto-injector, Subcutaneous [preservative free]:
  Otrexup: 7.5 mg/0.4 mL (0.4 mL); 10 mg/0.4 mL (0.4 mL); 15 mg/0.4 mL (0.4 mL); 20 mg/0.4 mL (0.4 mL); 25 mg/0.4 mL (0.4 mL)
  Rasuvo: 7.5 mg/0.15 mL (0.15 mL); 10 mg/0.2 mL (0.2 mL); 12.5 mg/0.25 mL (0.25 mL); 15 mg/0.3 mL (0.3 mL); 17.5 mg/0.35 mL (0.35 mL); 20 mg/0.4 mL (0.4 mL); 22.5 mg/0.45 mL (0.45 mL); 25 mg/0.5 mL (0.5 mL); 27.5 mg/0.55 mL (0.55 mL); 30 mg/0.6 mL (0.6 mL)
Solution Reconstituted, Injection [preservative free]:
  Generic: 1 g (1 ea)
Tablet, Oral:
  Rheumatrex: 2.5 mg [scored]
  Trexall: 5 mg, 7.5 mg, 10 mg, 15 mg [scored]
  Generic: 2.5 mg

- ◆ **Methotrexate Injection, BP (Can)** see Methotrexate on page 1104
- ◆ **Methotrexate Injection USP (Can)** see Methotrexate on page 1104
- ◆ **Methotrexate Sodium** see Methotrexate on page 1104
- ◆ **Methotrexate Sodium Injection (Can)** see Methotrexate on page 1104
- ◆ **Methotrexatum** see Methotrexate on page 1104
- ◆ **Methylacetoxyprogesterone** see MedroxyPROGESTERone on page 1074

Methylene Blue (METH i leen bloo)

Index Terms Methylthionine Chloride; Methylthioninium Chloride

Pharmacologic Category Antidote

Use Methemoglobinemia: Treatment of drug-induced methemoglobinemia

Pregnancy Risk Factor X

◀ **Dosing**

Adult & Geriatric

Methemoglobinemia: IV: 1 to 2 mg/kg or 25 to 50 mg/m² over 5 to 10 minutes; may be repeated in 1 hour if necessary

Chromoendoscopy (off label use): Topical: 0.1% to 1% solution sprayed via catheter or directly applied onto gastrointestinal mucosa during procedure (Areia 2008; Ichimasa 2014; Kaminski 2014; Ngamruengphong 2009)

Ifosfamide-induced encephalopathy (off-label use): Oral, IV: **Note:** Treatment may not be necessary; encephalopathy may improve spontaneously (Patel 2006):

Prevention: 50 mg every 6 to 8 hours (Turner 2003)

Treatment: 50 mg as a single dose or every 4 to 8 hours until symptoms resolve (Patel 2006; Turner 2003)

Onychomycosis (toenail; off-label use): Topical: 2% solution applied to affected area(s) at 15 day intervals for 6 months; used in conjunction with photodynamic therapy (Figueiredo Souza 2014)

Sentinel node mapping in breast cancer surgery (off label use): Intraparenchymal: 5 mg in 3 to 5 mL NS administered once during procedure (Simmons 2001; Simmons 2003; Thevarajah 2005)

Vasoplegia syndrome associated with cardiac surgery (off-label use): IV: 1.5 to 2 mg/kg over 20 to 60 minutes administered once (Levin 2004; Leyh 2003). **Note:** Improvement of vasoplegia (eg, increased systemic vascular resistance, reduced vasopressor dosage) has been observed within 1 to 2 hours following methylene blue administration. Some have employed the use of continuous infusion (0.5 to 1 mg/kg/hour) after administration of the bolus dose; however, prospective clinical trials are necessary to validate this dosing schema (Grayling 2003; Omar 2014; Weiner 2013).

Pediatric Methemoglobinemia: Children and Adolescents: Refer to adult dosing.

Renal Impairment No dosage adjustment provided in manufacturer's labeling. However, use with caution in severe renal impairment.

Hepatic Impairment No dosage adjustment provided in manufacturer's labeling.

Additional Information Complete prescribing information should be consulted for additional detail.

Dosage Forms Excipient information presented when available (limited, particularly for generics); consult specific product labeling.

Solution, Injection:

Generic: 1% (1 mL, 10 mL)

◆ **Methylmorphine** see Codeine on page 363

Methylnaltrexone (meth il nal TREKS one)

Brand Names: US Relistor

Brand Names: Canada Relistor

Index Terms Methylnaltrexone Bromide; N-methylnaltrexone Bromide

Pharmacologic Category Gastrointestinal Agent, Miscellaneous; Opioid Antagonist, Peripherally-Acting

Use

Opioid-induced constipation with advanced illness: Treatment of opioid-induced constipation in adult patients with advanced illness (receiving palliative care) who have an inadequate response to conventional laxative regimens.

Opioid-induced constipation with chronic non-cancer pain: Treatment of opioid-induced constipation in adult patients with chronic non-cancer pain.

Labeled Contraindications

Known or suspected gastrointestinal obstruction; patients at increased risk of recurrent obstruction due to the potential for gastrointestinal perforation.

Canadian labeling: Additional contraindications (not in U.S. labeling): Hypersensitivity to methylnaltrexone or any component of the formulation

Pregnancy Considerations Adverse effects were not observed in animal reproduction studies. Maternal use of methylnaltrexone during pregnancy may precipitate opioid withdrawal effects in newborn.

Breast-Feeding Considerations It is not known if methylnaltrexone is excreted in breast milk. Due to the potential for serious adverse reactions in the nursing infant, the manufacturer recommends a decision be made whether to discontinue nursing or to discontinue the drug, taking into account the importance of treatment to the mother.

Warnings/Precautions Discontinue treatment for severe or persistent diarrhea. Gastrointestinal perforations have been reported in patients with advanced illnesses associated with impaired structural integrity of the GI wall (eg, Ogilvie's syndrome, peptic ulcer disease, diverticular disease, infiltrative GI tract malignancies, or peritoneal metastases). Use with caution in these patients or in patients with other conditions that may result in impaired integrity of the GI wall (eg, Crohn disease); Monitor for development of severe, persistent or worsening abdominal pain; discontinue therapy if this occurs. Use is contraindicated in patients with known or suspected GI obstruction or at increased risk of recurrent obstruction. Use with caution in patients with renal impairment; dosage adjustment recommended for severe renal impairment (CrCl <30 mL/minute). Has not been studied in patients with end-stage renal impairment requiring dialysis. May precipitate symptoms of opioid withdrawal (eg, abdominal pain, anxiety, chills, diarrhea, hyperhidrosis, and yawning). Use with caution in patients with disruptions to the blood-brain barrier; may increase the risk for withdrawal and/or reduced analgesia. Monitor for symptoms of opioid withdrawal in such patients. Discontinue methylnaltrexone if opioids are discontinued. Use beyond 4 months has not been studied.

Appropriate use for patients with opioid-induced constipation with chronic non-cancer pain: Efficacy has been established in patients who have taken opioids for ≥4 weeks; sustained exposure to opioids prior to initiation of methylnaltrexone may increase sensitivity to effects. All laxative maintenance therapy should be discontinued prior to initiation of therapy; laxative therapy may be added if a suboptimal response to therapy is noted after 3 days. When the opioid regimen has been changed, the patient should be re-evaluated for the need to continue methylnaltrexone therapy.

Adverse Reactions

>10%: Gastrointestinal: Abdominal pain (21% to 29%), flatulence (13%), nausea (9% to 12%)

1% to 10%:

Central nervous system: Dizziness (7%), chills (1%)

Dermatologic: Hyperhidrosis (6%)

Endocrine & metabolic: Hot flash (3%)

Gastrointestinal: Diarrhea (6%)

Neuromuscular & skeletal: Tremor (1%)

<1%, postmarketing, and/or case reports: Abdominal cramps, cerebrovascular accident, diaphoresis, flushing, gastrointestinal perforation, increased body temperature, malaise, muscle spasm, myocardial infarction, opioid with-drawal syndrome, pain, piloerection, syncope, vomiting

Drug Interactions

Metabolism/Transport Effects Substrate of CYP2D6 (minor); **Note:** Assignment of Major/Minor substrate status based on clinically relevant drug interaction potential

Avoid Concomitant Use

Avoid concomitant use of Methylnaltrexone with any of the following: Naloxegol; Opioid Antagonists

Increased Effect/Toxicity

Methylnaltrexone may increase the levels/effects of: Naloxegol; Opioid Antagonists

Decreased Effect There are no known significant interactions involving a decrease in effect.

Storage/Stability Store intact vials and prefilled syringes between 20°C and 25°C (68°F and 77°F); excursions are permitted between 15°C and 30°C (59°F and 86°F). Do not freeze. Protect from light. Solution withdrawn from the single use vial is stable in a syringe for 24 hours at room temperature. Do not remove the prefilled syringe from the tray until ready to administer.

Mechanism of Action An opioid receptor antagonist which blocks opioid binding at the mu receptor, methylnaltrexone is a quaternary derivative of naltrexone with restricted ability to cross the blood-brain barrier. It therefore functions as a peripheral acting opioid antagonist, including actions on the gastrointestinal tract to inhibit opioid-induced decreased gastrointestinal motility and delay in gastrointestinal transit time, thereby decreasing opioid-induced constipation. Does not affect opioid analgesic effects.

Pharmacodynamics/Kinetics

Onset of action: Usually within 30-60 minutes (in responding patients)

Absorption: SubQ: Rapid

Distribution: V_{dss}: ~1.1 L/kg

Protein binding: 11% to 15%

Metabolism: Metabolized to methyl-6-naltrexol isomers, methylnaltrexone sulfate, and other minor metabolites

Half-life elimination: Terminal: ~8 hours

Time to peak, plasma: SubQ: 30 minutes

Excretion: Urine (~54%, primarily as unchanged drug); feces (~17%, primarily as unchanged drug)

Dosing

Adult & Geriatric

Opioid-induced constipation with chronic non-cancer pain: SubQ: 12 mg once daily. **Note:** Discontinue all laxatives prior to use; if response is not optimal after 3 days, laxative therapy may be reinitiated.

Opioid-induced constipation with advanced illness: SubQ: Dosing is according to body weight: Administer 1 dose every other day as needed; maximum: 1 dose/24 hours

<38 kg: 0.15 mg/kg (round dose up to nearest 0.1 mL of volume)

38 to <62 kg: 8 mg

62 to 114 kg: 12 mg

>114 kg: 0.15 mg/kg (round dose up to nearest 0.1 mL of volume)

Renal Impairment

Mild-to-moderate impairment: No dosage adjustment necessary.

Severe impairment (CrCl <30 mL/minute): Administer 50% of normal dose.

End-stage renal impairment (dialysis-dependent): There are no dosing adjustments provided in the manufacturer's labeling (has not been studied).

Hepatic Impairment

Mild-to-moderate impairment (Child-Pugh class A or B): No dosage adjustment necessary.

Severe impairment: There are no dosing adjustments provided in the manufacturer's labeling (has not been studied).

Administration Administer by subcutaneous injection into the upper arm, abdomen, or thigh. Rotate injection sites at each dose. Toilet facilities should be nearby immediately following administration. Discard any unused medication that remains in the vial.

Monitoring Parameters Severe, persistent, or worsening abdominal pain; symptoms of opioid withdrawal; adequate analgesia; signs or symptoms of orthostatic hypotension.

Additional Information In some clinical trials, patients who received methylnaltrexone were on a palliative opioid therapy equivalent to a mean daily oral morphine dose of 172 mg, at a stable dose for ≥3 days. Constipation was defined as <3 bowel movements/week or no bowel movement for >2 days. Patients maintained their regular laxative regimen for at least 3 days prior to treatment and throughout the study.

Medication Guide Available Yes

Dosage Forms Excipient information presented when available (limited, particularly for generics); consult specific product labeling.

Kit, Subcutaneous:

Relistor: 12 mg/0.6 mL [contains edetate calcium disodium]

Solution, Subcutaneous:

Relistor: 8 mg/0.4 mL (0.4 mL); 12 mg/0.6 mL (0.6 mL) [contains edetate calcium disodium]

♦ **Methylnaltrexone Bromide** *see* Methylnaltrexone *on page 1122*

MethylPREDNISolone (meth il pred NIS oh lone)

Related Information

Corticosteroids Systemic Equivalencies *on page 2334*

Hematopoietic Stem Cell Transplantation *on page 2272*

Management of Chemotherapy-Induced Nausea and Vomiting in Adults *on page 2142*

Palliative Care Medicine (Cancer) *on page 2252*

Prevention and Management of Infections *on page 2196*

Brand Names: US A-Methapred; Depo-Medrol; Medrol; Medrol (Pak); Solu-MEDROL

Brand Names: Canada Depo-Medrol; Medrol; Methylprednisolone Acetate; Methylprednisolone Sodium Succinate For Injection; Methylprednisolone Sodium Succinate For Injection USP; Solu-Medrol

Index Terms 6-α-Methylprednisolone; A-Methapred; Medrol Dose Pack; Methylprednisolone Acetate; Methylprednisolone Sodium Succinate; Solumedrol

Pharmacologic Category Corticosteroid, Systemic

◀ **Use** Primarily as an anti-inflammatory or immunosuppressant agent in the treatment of a variety of diseases including those of dermatologic, endocrine, GI, hematologic, allergic, inflammatory, neoplastic, neurologic, ophthalmic, renal, respiratory, and autoimmune origin. Prevention and treatment of graft-versus-host disease following allogeneic bone marrow transplantation.

Labeled Contraindications Hypersensitivity to methylprednisolone or any component of the formulation; systemic fungal infection; administration of live virus vaccines; methylprednisolone formulations containing benzyl alcohol preservative are contraindicated in premature infants; IM administration in idiopathic thrombocytopenic purpura; intrathecal administration

Pregnancy Considerations Adverse events have been observed with corticosteroids in animal reproduction studies. Methylprednisolone crosses the placenta (Anderson 1981). Some studies have shown an association between first trimester systemic corticosteroid use and oral clefts (Park-Wyllie 2000; Pradat 2003). Systemic corticosteroids may also influence fetal growth (decreased birth weight); however, information is conflicting (Lunghi 2010). Hypoadrenalism may occur in newborns following maternal use of cortico-steroids in pregnancy; monitor.

When systemic corticosteroids are needed in pregnancy, it is generally recommended to use the lowest effective dose for the shortest duration of time, avoiding high doses during the first trimester (Leachman 2006; Lunghi 2010; Makol 2011; Østensen 2009). Inhaled corticosteroids are preferred for the treatment of asthma during pregnancy. Systemic corticosteroids such as methylprednisolone may be used for the treatment of severe persistent asthma if needed; the lowest dose administered on alternate days (if possible) should be used (NAEPP 2005).

Pregnant women exposed to methylprednisolone for antirejection therapy following a transplant may contact the National Transplantation Pregnancy Registry (NTPR) at 215-955-4820. Women exposed to methylprednisolone during pregnancy for the treatment of an autoimmune disease may contact the OTIS Autoimmune Diseases Study at 877-311-8972.

Breast-Feeding Considerations Corticosteroids are excreted in human milk. The manufacturer notes that when used systemically, maternal use of corticosteroids have the potential to cause adverse events in a nursing infant (eg, growth suppression, interfere with endogenous corticosteroid production) and therefore recommends a decision be made whether to discontinue nursing or to discontinue the drug, taking into account the importance of treatment to the mother. If there is concern about exposure to the infant, some guidelines recommend waiting 4 hours after the maternal dose of an oral systemic corticosteroid before breast-feeding in order to decrease potential exposure to the nursing infant (based on a study using prednisolone) (Bae 2011; Leachman 2006; Makol 2011; Ost 1985). Other guidelines note that maternal use of systemic corticosteroids is not a contraindication to breast-feeding (NAEPP 2005).

Warnings/Precautions Corticosteroids are not approved for epidural injection. Serious neurologic events (eg, spinal cord infarction, paraplegia, quad-riplegia, cortical blindness, stroke), some resulting in death, have been reported with epidural injection of corticosteroids, with and without use of fluoroscopy.

Use with caution in patients with thyroid disease, hepatic impairment, renal impairment, cardiovascular disease, diabetes, glaucoma, cataracts, myasthe-nia gravis, multiple sclerosis, osteoporosis, seizures, or GI diseases (diverticulitis, intestinal anastomoses, peptic ulcer, ulcerative colitis) due to perforation risk. Avoid ethanol may enhance gastric mucosal irritation. Not recommended for the treatment of optic neuritis; may increase frequency of new episodes. Use with caution in patients with a history of ocular herpes simplex; corneal perforation has occurred; do not use in active ocular herpes simplex, Use caution following acute MI (corticosteroids have been associated with myocardial rupture). Cardiomegaly and congestive heart failure have been reported following concurrent use of amphotericin B and hydrocortisone for the management of fungal infections.

Because of the risk of adverse effects, systemic corticosteroids should be used cautiously in the elderly in the smallest possible effective dose for the shortest duration. May affect growth velocity; growth should be routinely monitored in pediatric patients. Withdraw therapy with gradual tapering of dose. Patients may require higher doses when subject to stress (ie, trauma, surgery, severe infection).

May cause hypercorticism or suppression of hypothalamic-pituitary-adrenal (HPA) axis, particularly in younger children or in patients receiving high doses for prolonged periods. HPA axis suppression may lead to adrenal crisis. Withdrawal and discontinuation of a corticosteroid should be done slowly and carefully. Particular care is required when patients are transferred from systemic corticosteroids to inhaled products due to possible adrenal insufficiency or withdrawal from steroids, including an increase in allergic symptoms. Adult patients receiving >20 mg per day of prednisone (or equivalent) may be most susceptible. Fatalities have occurred due to adrenal insufficiency in asthmatic patients during and after transfer from systemic corticosteroids to aerosol steroids; aerosol steroids do not provide the systemic steroid needed to treat patients having trauma, surgery, or infections. Use in septic shock or sepsis syndrome may increase mortality in some populations (eg, patients with elevated serum creatinine, patients who develop secondary infections after use).

Acute myopathy has been reported with high dose corticosteroids, usually in patients with neuromuscular transmission disorders; may involve ocular and/or respiratory muscles; monitor creatine kinase; recovery may be delayed. Corticosteroid use may cause psychiatric disturbances, including depression, euphoria, insomnia, mood swings, and personality changes. Preexisting psychiatric conditions may be exacerbated by corticosteroid use. Prolonged use of corticosteroids may increase the incidence of secondary infection, cause activation of latent infections, mask acute infection (including fungal infections), prolong or exacerbate viral or parasitic infections, or limit response to vaccines. Exposure to chickenpox or measles should be avoided; corticosteroids should not be used to treat ocular herpes simplex. Corticosteroids should not be used for cerebral malaria, fungal infections, or viral hepatitis. Close observation is required in patients with latent tuberculosis and/or TB reactivity; restrict use in active TB (only fulminating or disseminated TB in conjunction with antituberculosis treatment). Amebiasis should be ruled out in any patient with recent travel to tropic climates or unexplained diarrhea prior to initiation of corticosteroids. Use with extreme caution in patients with *Strongyloides* infections; hyperinfection, dissemination and fatalities have occurred. Prolonged treatment with corticosteroids has been associated with the development of Kaposi's sarcoma (case reports); discontinuation may result in clinical improvement.

High-dose corticosteroids should not be used to manage acute head injury. Rare cases of anaphylactoid reactions have been observed in patients receiving corticosteroids. Avoid injection or leakage into the dermis; dermal and/or subdermal skin depression may occur at the site of injection. Avoid deltoid muscle injection; subcutaneous atrophy may occur. Potentially significant drug-drug interactions may exist, requiring dose or frequency adjustment, additional monitoring, and/or selection of alternative therapy.

Benzyl alcohol and derivatives: Methylprednisolone **acetate** IM injection (multiple-dose vial) and the diluent for methylprednisolone **sodium succinate** injection may contain benzyl alcohol; large amounts of benzyl alcohol (≥99 mg/kg/day) have been associated with a potentially fatal toxicity ("gasping syndrome") in neonates; the "gasping syndrome" consists of metabolic acidosis, respiratory distress, gasping respirations, CNS dysfunction (including convulsions, intracranial hemorrhage), hypotension, and cardiovascular collapse (AAP ["Inactive" 1997]; CDC 1982); some data suggests that benzoate displaces bilirubin from protein binding sites (Ahlfors 2001); avoid or use dosage forms containing benzyl alcohol with caution in neonates.

Some dosage forms may contain polysorbate 80 (also known as Tweens). Hypersensitivity reactions, usually a delayed reaction, have been reported following exposure to pharmaceutical products containing polysorbate 80 in certain individuals (Isaksson 2002; Lucente 2000; Shelley 1995). Thrombocytopenia, ascites, pulmonary deterioration, and renal and hepatic failure have been reported in premature neonates after receiving parenteral products containing polysorbate 80 (Alade 1986; CDC 1984). See manufacturer's labeling.

Adverse Reactions Frequency not defined.

Cardiovascular: Arrhythmias, bradycardia, cardiac arrest, cardiomegaly, circulatory collapse, congestive heart failure, edema, fat embolism, hypertension, hypertrophic cardiomyopathy in premature infants, myocardial rupture (post MI), syncope, tachycardia, thromboembolism, vasculitis

Central nervous system: Delirium, depression, emotional instability, euphoria, hallucinations, headache, intracranial pressure increased, insomnia, malaise, mood swings, nervousness, neuritis, personality changes, psychic disorders, pseudotumor cerebri (usually following discontinuation), seizure, vertigo

Dermatologic: Acne, allergic dermatitis, alopecia, dry scaly skin, ecchymoses, edema, erythema, hirsutism, hyper-/hypopigmentation, hypertrichosis, impaired wound healing, petechiae, rash, skin atrophy, sterile abscess, skin test reaction impaired, striae, urticaria

Endocrine & metabolic: Adrenal suppression, amenorrhea, carbohydrate intolerance increased, Cushing's syndrome, diabetes mellitus, fluid retention, glucose intolerance, growth suppression (children), hyperglycemia, hyperlipidemia, hypokalemia, hypokalemic alkalosis, menstrual irregularities, negative nitrogen balance, pituitary-adrenal axis suppression, protein catabolism, sodium and water retention

Gastrointestinal: Abdominal distention, appetite increased, bowel/bladder dysfunction (after intrathecal administration), gastrointestinal hemorrhage, gastrointestinal perforation, nausea, pancreatitis, peptic ulcer, perforation of the small and large intestine, ulcerative esophagitis, vomiting, weight gain

Hematologic: Leukocytosis (transient)

Hepatic: Hepatomegaly, transaminases increased

Local: Postinjection flare (intra-articular use), thrombophlebitis

Neuromuscular & skeletal: Arthralgia, arthropathy, aseptic necrosis (femoral and humoral heads), fractures, muscle mass loss, muscle weakness, myopathy (particularly in conjunction with neuromuscular disease or neuromuscular-blocking agents), neuropathy, osteoporosis, parasthesia, tendon rupture, vertebral compression fractures, weakness

Ocular: Cataracts, exophthalmoses, glaucoma, intraocular pressure increased

Renal: Glycosuria

Respiratory: Pulmonary edema

Miscellaneous: Abnormal fat disposition, anaphylactoid reaction, anaphylaxis, angioedema, avascular necrosis, diaphoresis, hiccups, hypersensitivity reactions, infections, secondary malignancy

<1%, postmarketing, and/or case reports: Venous thrombosis (Johannesdottir 2013)

Drug Interactions

Metabolism/Transport Effects Substrate of CYP3A4 (minor); **Note:** Assignment of Major/Minor substrate status based on clinically relevant drug interaction potential; **Inhibits** CYP2C8 (weak)

Avoid Concomitant Use

Avoid concomitant use of MethylPREDNISolone with any of the following: Aldesleukin; Amodiaquine; BCG (Intravesical); Indium 111 Capromab Pendetide; Mifepristone; Natalizumab; Pimecrolimus; Tacrolimus (Topical); Tofacitinib

Increased Effect/Toxicity

MethylPREDNISolone may increase the levels/effects of: Acetylcholinesterase Inhibitors; Amodiaquine; Amphotericin B; Androgens; CycloSPORINE (Systemic); Deferasirox; Fingolimod; Leflunomide; Loop Diuretics; Natalizumab; Nicorandil; NSAID (COX-2 Inhibitor); NSAID (Nonselective); Quinolone Antibiotics; Thiazide Diuretics; Tofacitinib; Vaccines (Live); Warfarin

The levels/effects of MethylPREDNISolone may be increased by: Aprepitant; CycloSPORINE (Systemic); CYP3A4 Inhibitors (Strong); Denosumab; Estrogen Derivatives; Fosaprepitant; Indacaterol; Mifepristone; Neuromuscular-Blocking Agents (Nondepolarizing); Pimecrolimus; Roflumilast; Salicylates; Tacrolimus (Topical); Telaprevir; Trastuzumab

Decreased Effect

MethylPREDNISolone may decrease the levels/effects of: Aldesleukin; Antidiabetic Agents; BCG (Intravesical); Calcitriol (Systemic); Coccidioides immitis Skin Test; Corticorelin; CycloSPORINE (Systemic); Hyaluronidase; Indium 111 Capromab Pendetide; Isoniazid; Salicylates; Sipuleucel-T; Telaprevir; Urea Cycle Disorder Agents; Vaccines (Inactivated); Vaccines (Live)

The levels/effects of MethylPREDNISolone may be decreased by: Antacids; Bile Acid Sequestrants; CYP3A4 Inducers (Strong); Echinacea; Mifepristone; Mitotane

Storage/Stability

Methylprednisolone acetate; tablets: Store at 20°C to 25°C (68°F to 77°F).

Methylprednisolone sodium succinate: Store intact vials at controlled room temperature of 20°C to 25°C (68°F to 77°F). Protect from light. Reconstituted solutions of methylprednisolone sodium succinate should be stored at room temperature of 20°C to 25°C (68°F to 77°F) and used within 48 hours. Stability of parenteral admixture at room temperature (25°C) and at refrigeration temperature (4°C) is 48 hours.

Preparation for Administration
Standard diluent (Solu-Medrol): 40 mg/50 mL D$_5$W; 125 mg/50 mL D$_5$W.
Minimum volume (Solu-Medrol): 50 mL D$_5$W.

Mechanism of Action In a tissue-specific manner, corticosteroids regulate gene expression subsequent to binding specific intracellular receptors and translocation into the nucleus. Corticosteroids exert a wide array of physiologic effects including modulation of carbohydrate, protein, and lipid metabolism and maintenance of fluid and electrolyte homeostasis. Moreover cardiovascular, immunologic, musculoskeletal, endocrine, and neurologic physiology are influenced by corticosteroids. Decreases inflammation by suppression of migration of polymorphonuclear leukocytes and reversal of increased capillary permeability.

Pharmacodynamics/Kinetics
Onset of action: Peak effect (route dependent): Oral: 1 to 2 hours; IM: 4 to 8 days; Intra-articular: 1 week; methylprednisolone sodium succinate is highly soluble and has a rapid effect by IM and IV routes

Duration (route dependent): Oral: 30 to 36 hours; IM: 1 to 4 weeks; Intra-articular: 1 to 5 weeks; methylprednisolone acetate has a low solubility and has a sustained IM effect

Distribution: V$_d$: 0.7 to 1.5 L/kg

Half-life elimination: 3 to 3.5 hours; reduced in obese

Excretion: Clearance: Reduced in obese

Dosing
Adult & Geriatric Only sodium succinate may be given IV; methylprednisolone sodium succinate is highly soluble and has a rapid effect by IM and IV routes. Methylprednisolone acetate has a low solubility and has a sustained IM effect.

Acute spinal cord injury (off-label use): IV (sodium succinate): 30 mg/kg over 15 minutes, followed in 45 minutes by a continuous infusion of 5.4 mg/kg/hour for 23 hours. **Note:** Due to insufficient evidence of clinical efficacy (ie, preserving or improving spinal cord function), the routine use of methylprednisolone in the treatment of acute spinal cord injury is no longer recommended. If used in this setting, methylprednisolone should not be initiated >8 hours after the injury; not effective in penetrating trauma (eg, gunshot) (Consortium for Spinal Cord Medicine 2008).

Allergic conditions: Oral: Tapered-dosage schedule (eg, dose-pack containing 21 x 4 mg tablets):

Day 1: 24 mg on day 1 administered as 8 mg (2 tablets) before breakfast, 4 mg (1 tablet) after lunch, 4 mg (1 tablet) after supper, and 8 mg (2 tablets) at bedtime **OR** 24 mg (6 tablets) as a single dose or divided into 2 or 3 doses upon initiation (regardless of time of day)

Day 2: 20 mg on day 2 administered as 4 mg (1 tablet) before breakfast, 4 mg (1 tablet) after lunch, 4 mg (1 tablet) after supper, and 8 mg (2 tablets) at bedtime

Day 3: 16 mg on day 3 administered as 4 mg (1 tablet) before breakfast, 4 mg (1 tablet) after lunch, 4 mg (1 tablet) after supper, and 4 mg (1 tablet) at bedtime

Day 4: 12 mg on day 4 administered as 4 mg (1 tablet) before breakfast, 4 mg (1 tablet) after lunch, and 4 mg (1 tablet) at bedtime

Day 5: 8 mg on day 5 administered as 4 mg (1 tablet) before breakfast and 4 mg (1 tablet) at bedtime

Day 6: 4 mg on day 6 administered as 4 mg (1 tablet) before breakfast

Anti-inflammatory or immunosuppressive:
Oral: 2 to 60 mg/day in 1 to 4 divided doses to start, followed by gradual reduction in dosage to the lowest possible level consistent with maintaining an adequate clinical response.

IM (sodium succinate): 10 to 80 mg/day once daily

IM (acetate): 10 to 80 mg every 1 to 2 weeks

IV (sodium succinate): 10 to 40 mg over a period of several minutes and repeated IV or IM at intervals depending on clinical response; when high dosages are needed, give 30 mg/kg over a period ≥30 minutes and may be repeated every 4 to 6 hours for 48 hours.

Arthritis: Intra-articular (acetate): Administer every 1 to 5 weeks.

Large joints (eg, knee, ankle): 20 to 80 mg

Medium joints (eg, elbow, wrist): 10 to 40 mg

Small joints: 4 to 10 mg

Asthma exacerbations, including status asthmaticus (emergency medical care or hospital doses): Oral, IV: 40 to 80 mg/day in 1 to 2 divided doses until peak expiratory flow is 70% of predicted or personal best (NAEPP 2007)

Asthma, severe persistent, long-term control: Oral: 7.5 to 60 mg/day (or on alternate days) (NAEPP 2007)

Bronchiolitis obliterans syndrome, prevention (off-label use): IV: 1000 mg daily for 3 days. **Note:** Many centers use 10 to 15 mg/kg/day for smaller patients (Meyer 2014).

Cadaveric organ recovery (hormonal resuscitation) (off-label use): IV: 15 mg/kg **or** 2,000 mg bolus administered to the brain-dead donor who is hemodynamically unstable requiring significant vasopressor support; give concomitantly with vasopressin, levothyroxine or liothyronine (preferred), dextrose (if bolus dose insulin used), and regular insulin (bolus dose or continuous infusion). If continuous infusion insulin is employed, maintain blood glucose 120 to 180 mg/dL (Rosendale 2003a; Rosendale 2003b; Rosengard 2002; Salim 2007; Zaroff 2002).

COPD exacerbation (off-label use): Note: Dose, frequency, and duration of therapy not established. GOLD guidelines recommend the use of oral prednisone; however, methylprednisolone may be used as an alternative (GOLD [Decramer 2014]). No comparative studies exist to examine safety and efficacy between low-, medium-, or high-dose regimens. While several clinical trials have examined the use of methylprednisolone in this setting, these trials included low numbers of patients, employed vastly different regimens, and/or examined different clinical outcomes (Albert 1980; Alía 2011; Niewoehner 1999; Sayiner 2001; Shortall 2002; Vrondracek 2006; Willaert 2002). Current dosing strategies are empiric and have not been established by clinical trials. Based on expert opinion, commonly used regimens ranging from 60 to 125 mg IV administered 1 to 4 times daily followed by oral therapy (eg, prednisone 40 mg once daily) for a total of 5 to 14 days of therapy may be employed; the shorter duration (ie, 5 days) may be preferred (Leuppi 2013); however, comparative prospective data does not exist. IV administration with a higher dose (eg, ≥60 mg) may be preferred for those patients with impending or actual acute respiratory failure; outcome trials not available for this approach.

Dermatitis, acute severe: IM (acetate): 80 to 120 mg as a single dose

Dermatitis, chronic: IM (acetate): 40 to 120 mg every 5 to 10 days

Dermatologic conditions (eg, keloids, lichen planus): Intralesional (acetate): 20 to 60 mg

◄ **Dermatomyositis/polymyositis:** IV (sodium succinate): 1 g/day for 3 to 5 days for severe muscle weakness, followed by conversion to oral prednisone (Drake 1996)

Gout, acute: IV, IM: Initial: 0.5 to 2 mg/kg; may be repeated as clinically indicated (ACR guidelines [Khanna 2012])

Lupus nephritis: High-dose "pulse" therapy: IV (sodium succinate): 0.5 to 1 g/day for 3 days (Ponticelli 2010)

Pneumocystis **pneumonia in AIDS patients:** IV: 30 mg twice daily for 5 days, then 30 mg once daily for 5 days, then 15 mg once daily for 11 days

Pediatric Dosing should be based on the lesser of ideal body weight or actual body weight. **Only sodium succinate may be given IV;** methylprednisolone sodium succinate is highly soluble and has a rapid effect by IM and IV routes. Methylprednisolone acetate has a low solubility and has a sustained IM effect.

Acute spinal cord injury (off-label use): IV (sodium succinate): 30 mg/kg over 15 minutes, followed in 45 minutes by a continuous infusion of 5.4 mg/kg/hour for 23 hours. **Note:** Due to insufficient evidence of clinical efficacy (ie, preserving or improving spinal cord function), the routine use of methylprednisolone in the treatment of acute spinal cord injury is no longer recommended. If used in this setting, methylprednisolone should not be initiated >8 hours after the injury; not effective in penetrating trauma (eg, gunshot) (Consortium for Spinal Cord Medicine 2008).

Anti-inflammatory or immunosuppressive: Oral, IM, IV (sodium succinate): 0.5 to 1.7 mg/kg/day **or** 5 to 25 mg/m²/day in divided doses every 6 to 12 hours; "Pulse" therapy: 15 to 30 mg/kg/dose over ≥30 minutes given once daily for 3 days

Asthma exacerbations, including status asthmaticus (emergency medical care or hospital doses) (NAEPP 2007): Children <12 years: Oral, IV: 1 to 2 mg/kg/day in 2 divided doses (maximum: 60 mg/day) until peak expiratory flow is 70% of predicted or personal best

Lupus nephritis: IV (sodium succinate): 30 mg/kg over ≥30 minutes every other day for 6 doses

Renal Impairment There are no dosage adjustments provided in the manufacturer's labeling; use with caution.

Hepatic Impairment There are no dosage adjustments provided in the manufacturer's labeling.

Combination Regimens

Leukemia, acute lymphocytic: Hyper-CVAD (Leukemia, Acute Lymphocytic) on page 2006

Lymphoma, Hodgkin:
ESHAP (Hodgkin) on page 1964
MINE-ESHAP (Hodgkin) on page 2036

Lymphoma, non-Hodgkin: ESHAP on page 1963

Administration

Administer with meals to decrease GI upset.

Parenteral: Methylprednisolone sodium succinate may be administered IM or IV; IV administration may be IVP over one to several minutes or IVPB or continuous IV infusion. **Acetate salt should not be given IV.** Avoid injection into the deltoid muscle due to a high incidence of subcutaneous atrophy. Avoid injection or leakage into the dermis; dermal and/or subdermal skin depression may occur at the site of injection.

IV: Succinate:

Low dose: ≤1.8 mg/kg or ≤125 mg/dose: IV push over 3 to 15 minutes
Moderate dose: ≥2 mg/kg or 250 mg/dose: IV over 15 to 30 minutes
High dose: 15 mg/kg or ≥500 mg/dose: IV over ≥30 minutes

Doses >15 mg/kg or ≥1 g: Administer over 1 hour

Do **not** administer high-dose IV push; hypotension, cardiac arrhythmia, and sudden death have been reported in patients given high-dose methyl-prednisolone IV push (>0.5 g over <10 minutes); intermittent infusion over 15 to 60 minutes; maximum concentration: IV push 125 mg/mL

IM: Avoid injection into the deltoid muscle due to a high incidence of subcutaneous atrophy. Avoid injection or leakage into the dermis; dermal and/or subdermal skin depression may occur at the site of injection. Do not inject into areas that have evidence of acute local infection.

Monitoring Parameters Blood pressure, blood glucose, electrolytes, growth in children

Test Interactions Interferes with skin tests

Dietary Considerations Take with meals to decrease GI upset; need diet rich in pyridoxine, vitamin C, vitamin D, folate, calcium, phosphorus, and protein.

Additional Information Sodium content of 1 g sodium succinate injection: 2.01 mEq; 53 mg of sodium succinate salt is equivalent to 40 mg of methyl-prednisolone base

Methylprednisolone acetate: Depo-Medrol
Methylprednisolone sodium succinate: Solu-Medrol

Dosage Forms Excipient information presented when available (limited, particularly for generics); consult specific product labeling. [DSC] = Discontinued product

Solution Reconstituted, Injection, as sodium succinate [strength expressed as base]:

A-Methapred: 40 mg (1 ea); 125 mg (1 ea) [contains benzyl alcohol]
Solu-MEDROL: 500 mg (1 ea); 1000 mg (1 ea)
Solu-MEDROL: 2 g (1 ea) [contains benzyl alcohol]
Generic: 40 mg (1 ea); 125 mg (1 ea); 500 mg (1 ea [DSC]); 1000 mg (1 ea); 1 g (1 ea [DSC])

Solution Reconstituted, Injection, as sodium succinate [strength expressed as base, preservative free]:

Solu-MEDROL: 40 mg (1 ea); 125 mg (1 ea); 500 mg (1 ea); 1000 mg (1 ea)

Suspension, Injection, as acetate:

Depo-Medrol: 20 mg/mL (5 mL); 40 mg/mL (5 mL, 10 mL) [contains benzyl alcohol, polyethylene glycol, polysorbate 80]
Depo-Medrol: 40 mg/mL (1 mL) [contains polyethylene glycol]
Depo-Medrol: 80 mg/mL (1 mL)
Depo-Medrol: 80 mg/mL (5 mL) [contains benzyl alcohol, polyethylene glycol, polysorbate 80]
Depo-Medrol: 80 mg/mL (1 mL) [contains polyethylene glycol]
Generic: 40 mg/mL (1 mL, 5 mL, 10 mL); 80 mg/mL (1 mL, 5 mL)

Suspension, Injection, as acetate [preservative free]:

Generic: 80 mg/mL (1 mL [DSC])

Tablet, Oral:

Medrol: 2 mg, 4 mg, 8 mg, 16 mg, 32 mg [scored]
Medrol (Pak): 4 mg [scored]
Generic: 4 mg, 8 mg, 16 mg, 32 mg

◆ **6-α-Methylprednisolone** see MethylPREDNISolone *on page 1125*

- ◆ **Methylprednisolone Acetate** *see* MethylPREDNISolone *on page 1125*
- ◆ **Methylprednisolone Sodium Succinate** *see* MethylPREDNISolone *on page 1125*
- ◆ **Methylprednisolone Sodium Succinate For Injection (Can)** *see* Methyl-PREDNISolone *on page 1125*
- ◆ **Methylprednisolone Sodium Succinate For Injection USP (Can)** *see* MethylPREDNISolone *on page 1125*
- ◆ **Methylthionine Chloride** *see* Methylene Blue *on page 1121*
- ◆ **Methylthioninium Chloride** *see* Methylene Blue *on page 1121*
- ◆ **3-methyl TTNEB** *see* Bexarotene (Systemic) *on page 200*

Metoclopramide (met oh KLOE pra mide)

Related Information

Management of Chemotherapy-Induced Nausea and Vomiting in Adults *on page 2142*

Palliative Care Medicine (Cancer) *on page 2252*

Brand Names: US Metozolv ODT; Reglan

Brand Names: Canada Apo-Metoclop; Metoclopramide Hydrochloride Injection; Metoclopramide Omega; Metonia; Nu-Metoclopramide; PMS-Metoclopramide

Index Terms Reglan

Pharmacologic Category Antiemetic; Gastrointestinal Agent, Prokinetic

Use

US labeling:

Injection:

Diabetic gastroparesis (diabetic gastric stasis): Relief of symptoms associated with acute and recurrent diabetic gastric stasis.

Prevention of nausea and vomiting associated with emetogenic cancer chemotherapy: Prophylaxis of vomiting associated with emetogenic cancer chemotherapy.

Prevention of postoperative nausea and vomiting: Prophylaxis of postoperative nausea and vomiting in circumstances where nasogastric suction is undesirable.

Radiological examination: To stimulate gastric emptying and intestinal transit of barium when delayed emptying interferes with radiological examination of the stomach and/or small intestine.

Small bowel intubation: To facilitate small bowel intubation in adults and pediatrics in whom the tube does not pass the pylorus with conventional maneuvers.

Oral:

Diabetic gastroparesis (diabetic gastric stasis): Relief of symptoms associated with acute and recurrent diabetic gastroparesis (gastric stasis) in adults.

Gastroesophageal reflux: Short-term (4 to 12 weeks) therapy for adults with documented symptomatic gastroesophageal reflux disease (GERD) who fail to respond to conventional therapy.

Limitations of use: Oral metoclopramide is indicated for adults only. Treatment should not exceed 12-week duration.

Canadian labeling:
Injection:

Gastroparesis: Adjunctive therapy in the management of gastroparesis associated with subacute and chronic gastritis and sequelae of surgical procedures (eg, vagotomy, pyloroplasty).

Prevention of vomiting associated with cancer chemotherapy regimens that include cisplatin: Prophylaxis of vomiting associated with cancer chemotherapy regimens that include cisplatin.

Prevention of postoperative nausea and vomiting: Prophylaxis of postoperative nausea and vomiting.

Small bowel intubation: To facilitate small bowel intubation.

Oral:

Gastroparesis: Adjunctive therapy in the management of gastroparesis associated with subacute and chronic gastritis and sequelae of surgical procedures (eg, vagotomy, pyloroplasty).

Prevention of postoperative vomiting: Prophylaxis of postoperative vomiting induced by narcotics.

Radiological examination: To stimulate gastric emptying and intestinal transit of barium when delayed emptying interferes with radiological examination of the stomach and/or small intestine.

Small bowel intubation: To facilitate small bowel intubation.

Limitations of use: Treatment should not exceed 12-week duration.

Labeled Contraindications Known sensitivity or intolerance to metoclopramide or any component of the formulation; situations where gastrointestinal (GI) motility may be dangerous, including mechanical GI obstruction, perforation, or hemorrhage; pheochromocytoma; history of seizure disorder (eg, epilepsy); concomitant use with other agents likely to increase extrapyramidal reactions

Canadian labeling: Additional contraindications (not in US labeling): Infants <1 year of age.

Pregnancy Considerations Adverse events were not observed in animal reproduction studies. Metoclopramide crosses the placenta and can be detected in cord blood and amniotic fluid (Arvela, 1983; Bylsma-Howell, 1983). Available evidence suggests safe use during pregnancy (Berkovitch, 2002; Matok, 2009; Sørensen, 2000). Metoclopramide may be used for the treatment of nausea and vomiting of pregnancy (ACOG, 2004; Levichek, 2002) and prophylaxis for nausea and vomiting associated with cesarean delivery (ASA, 2007; Mahadevan, 2006; Smith, 2011). Other agents are preferred for gastroesophageal reflux (Mahadevan, 2006).

Breast-Feeding Considerations Metoclopramide is excreted in breast milk. Information is available from studies conducted in mothers nursing preterm infants (n=14; delivered at 23-34 weeks gestation) or term infants (n=18) and taking metoclopramide 10 mg 3 times daily. The median concentration of metoclopramide in breast milk was ~45 ng/mL in the preterm infants and the mean concentration was ~48 ng/mL in the full term infants. The authors of both studies calculated the relative infant dose to be 3% to 5%, based on a therapeutic infant dose of 0.5 mg/kg/day. Metoclopramide was also detected in the serum of one nursing full term infant (Hansen, 2005; Kauppila, 1983). Metoclopramide may increase prolactin concentrations and cause galactorrhea and gynecomastia, but studies which evaluated its use to increase milk production for women who want to nurse have had mixed results. In addition, due to the potential for adverse events, nonpharmacologic measure should be considered prior to the use of medications as galactagogues (ABM, 2011). The ▶

manufacturer recommends that caution be used if administered to a nursing woman.

Warnings/Precautions [US Boxed Warning]: May cause tardive dyskinesia, a serious movement disorder which is often irreversible; the risk of developing tardive dyskinesia increases with duration of treatment and total cumulative dose. Discontinue metoclopramide in patients who develop signs/symptoms of tardive dyskinesia. There is no known treatment for tardive dyskinesia. In some patients, symptoms lessen or resolve after metoclopramide treatment is stopped. Avoid metoclopramide treatment longer than 12 weeks in all but rare cases in which therapeutic benefit is thought to outweigh the risk of developing tardive dyskinesia. Tardive dyskinesia is characterized by involuntary movements of the face, tongue, or extremities and may be disfiguring. An analysis of utilization patterns showed that ~20% of patients who used metoclopramide took it for longer than 12 weeks. Metoclopramide may mask underlying tardive disease by suppressing or partially suppressing tardive dyskinesia signs (metoclopramide should not be used to control tardive dyskinesia symptoms as the long-term course is unknown). The risk for tardive dyskinesia appears to be increased in the elderly, women, and diabetics, although it is not possible to predict which patients will develop tardive dyskinesia. There is no known effective treatment for established cases of tardive dyskinesia, although in some patients, tardive dyskinesia may remit (partially or completely) within several weeks to months after metoclopramide is withdrawn.

May cause extrapyramidal symptoms (EPS), generally manifested as acute dystonic reactions within the initial 24 to 48 hours of use at the usual adult dose (30 to 40 mg/day). Risk of these reactions is increased at higher doses, and in pediatric patients and adults <30 years of age. Symptoms may include involuntary limb movements, facial grimacing, torticollis, oculogyric crisis, rhythmic tongue protrusion, bulbar type speech, trismus, or dystonic reactions resembling tetanus. May also rarely present as stridor and dyspnea (may be due to laryngospasm). Dystonic symptoms may be managed with IM diphenhydramine or benztropine. Pseudoparkinsonism (eg, bradykinesia, tremor, rigidity, mask-like facies) may also occur (usually within first 6 months of therapy) and is generally reversible within 2 to 3 months following discontinuation. Symptoms of Parkinson disease may be exacerbated by metoclopramide; use with extreme caution (or avoid use) in patients with Parkinson disease.

Metoclopramide has been known to cause sinus arrest (usually with rapid IV administration or higher doses) (Bentsen, 2002; Malkoff 1995). The torsadogenic potential for metoclopramide is considered to be low (Claassen, 2005). Based on case reports, however, metoclopramide may cause QT prolongation and torsades de pointes in certain individuals (eg, heart failure patients with renal impairment); use with caution in these patients (Siddiquie, 2009). There is data in healthy male volunteers to show that metoclopramide actually shortens the QT interval while at the same time increasing QT variance (Ellidokuz, 2003). No human data other than case reports; however, has demonstrated a consistent QT prolonging effect with metoclopramide nor is there any substantiated evidence to show a direct association with the development of torsades de pointes.

Metoclopramide use may be associated (rarely) with neuroleptic malignant syndrome (NMS); may be fatal. Monitor for manifestations of NMS, which include hyperthermia, muscle rigidity, altered consciousness, and autonomic instability (irregular pulse or blood pressure, tachycardia, diaphoresis, and cardiac arrhythmias). Discontinue immediately if signs/symptoms of NMS appear and begin intensive symptomatic management and monitoring. Bromocriptine and dantrolene have been used to manage NMS, although effectiveness have not been established.

Mental depression has occurred (in patients with and without a history of depression), and symptoms range from mild to severe (suicidal ideation and suicide); use in patients with a history of depression only if anticipated benefits outweigh potential risks.

In a study in hypertensive patients, IV metoclopramide was associated with catecholamine release. Use with caution in patients with hypertension. There are reports of hypertensive crises in some patients with undiagnosed pheochromocytoma. Immediately discontinue with any rapid rise in blood pressure that is associated with metoclopramide. Hypertensive crises may be managed with phentolamine. Use with caution in patients who are at risk of fluid overload (HF, cirrhosis); metoclopramide causes a transient increase in serum aldosterone and increases the risk for fluid retention/overload; discontinue if adverse events or signs/symptoms appear.

Patients with NADH-cytochrome b5 reductase deficiency are at increased risk of methemoglobinemia and/or sulfhemoglobinemia. Use with caution in patients with renal impairment; dosage adjustment may be needed. Use with caution following surgical anastomosis/closure; promotility agents may theoretically increase pressure in suture lines.

For patients with diabetic gastroparesis, the usual manifestations of delayed gastric emptying (eg, nausea, vomiting, heartburn, persistent fullness after meals, anorexia) appear to respond to metoclopramide within different time intervals. Significant relief of nausea occurs early and continues to improve over a 3-week period; relief of vomiting and anorexia may precede the relief of abdominal fullness by a week or more. If gastroesophageal reflux symptoms are confined to particular situations, such as following the evening meal, consider use of metoclopramide as a single dose prior to the provocative situation, rather than using the drug throughout the day. Symptoms of postprandial and daytime heartburn respond better to metoclopramide, with less observed effect on nocturnal symptoms. Because there is no documented correlation between symptoms and healing of esophageal lesions, patients with documented lesions should be monitored endoscopically. Healing of esophageal ulcers and erosions has been endoscopically demonstrated at the end of a 12-week trial using a dosage of 15 mg 4 times daily.

Avoid use in older adults (except for diabetic gastroparesis) due to risk of extrapyramidal effects, including tardive dyskinesia; risk is potentially even greater in frail older adults (Beers Criteria). In addition, risk of tardive dyskinesia may be increased in older women. EPS are increased in pediatric patients. In neonates, prolonged clearance of metoclopramide may lead to increased serum concentrations. Neonates may also have decreased levels of NADH-cytochrome b5 reductase which increases the risk of methemoglobinemia. The Canadian labeling contraindicates use in infants <1 year of age and recommends avoiding use in children >1 year unless clearly necessary. Potentially significant drug-drug interactions may exist, requiring dose or frequency adjustment, additional monitoring, and/or selection of alternative therapy. CNS effects can be potentiated when used with other sedative drugs or ethanol. Abrupt discontinuation may (rarely) result in withdrawal symptoms (dizziness, headache, nervousness).

◀ Benzyl alcohol and derivatives: Some dosage forms may contain sodium benzoate/benzoic acid; benzoic acid (benzoate) is a metabolite of benzyl alcohol; large amounts of benzyl alcohol (≥99 mg/kg/day) have been associated with a potentially fatal toxicity ("gasping syndrome") in neonates; the "gasping syndrome" consists of metabolic acidosis, respiratory distress, gasping respirations, CNS dysfunction (including convulsions, intracranial hemorrhage), hypotension, and cardiovascular collapse (AAP ["Inactive" 1997]; CDC, 1982); some data suggest that benzoate displaces bilirubin from protein binding sites (Ahlfors, 2001); avoid or use dosage forms containing benzyl alcohol derivative with caution in neonates. See manufacturer's labeling.

Adverse Reactions Frequency not always defined.

Cardiovascular: Atrioventricular block, bradycardia, congestive heart failure, flushing (following high IV doses), hypertension, hypotension, supraventricular tachycardia

Central nervous system: Drowsiness (~10% to 70%; dose related), dystonic reaction (<1% to 25%; dose and age related), lassitude (~10%), restlessness (~10%), fatigue (2% to 10%), headache (4% to 5%), dizziness (1% to 4%), somnolence (2% to 3%), akathisia, confusion, depression, drug-induced Parkinson's disease, hallucination (rare), insomnia, neuroleptic malignant syndrome (rare), seizure, suicidal ideation, tardive dyskinesia

Dermatologic: Skin rash, urticaria

Endocrine & metabolic: Amenorrhea, fluid retention, galactorrhea, gynecomastia, hyperprolactinemia, porphyria

Gastrointestinal: Nausea (4% to 6%), vomiting (1% to 2%), diarrhea

Genitourinary: Impotence, urinary frequency, urinary incontinence

Hematologic & oncologic: Agranulocytosis, leukopenia, methemoglobinemia, neutropenia, sulfhemoglobinemia

Hepatic: Hepatotoxicity (rare)

Hypersensitivity: Angioedema (rare), hypersensitivity reaction

Neuromuscular & skeletal: Laryngospasm (rare)

Ophthalmic: Visual disturbance

Respiratory: Bronchospasm, laryngeal edema (rare)

Drug Interactions

Metabolism/Transport Effects Substrate of CYP1A2 (minor), CYP2D6 (minor); **Note:** Assignment of Major/Minor substrate status based on clinically relevant drug interaction potential; **Inhibits** CYP2D6 (weak)

Avoid Concomitant Use

Avoid concomitant use of Metoclopramide with any of the following: Antipsychotic Agents; Droperidol; Promethazine; Rivastigmine; Tetrabenazine; Trimetazidine

Increased Effect/Toxicity

Metoclopramide may increase the levels/effects of: Antipsychotic Agents; CycloSPORINE (Systemic); Highest Risk QTc-Prolonging Agents; Levosulpiride; Moderate Risk QTc-Prolonging Agents; Prilocaine; Promethazine; Selective Serotonin Reuptake Inhibitors; Serotonin/Norepinephrine Reuptake Inhibitors; Sodium Nitrite; Tetrabenazine; Tricyclic Antidepressants; Trimetazidine

The levels/effects of Metoclopramide may be increased by: Dapsone (Topical); Droperidol; Metyrosine; Mifepristone; Nitric Oxide; Rivastigmine; Serotonin Modulators

Decreased Effect

Metoclopramide may decrease the levels/effects of: Anti-Parkinson's Agents (Dopamine Agonist); Atovaquone; Posaconazole; Quinagolide

The levels/effects of Metoclopramide may be decreased by: Anticholinergic Agents

Storage/Stability

Injection: Store intact vials at 20°C to 25°C (68°F to 77°F); injection is photosensitive and should be protected from light during storage; parenteral admixtures in D_5W, $D_5^{1/2}NS$, NS, LR, or Ringer's injection are stable for up to 24 hours after preparation at normal light conditions or up to 48 hours if protected from light. When mixed with NS, can be stored frozen for up to 4 weeks; metoclopramide is degraded when admixed and frozen with D_5W.

Oral solution: Store at 20°C to 25°C (68°F to 77°F). Do not freeze. Dispense in tight, light-resistant container.

Tablet: Store at 20°C to 25°C (68°F to 77°F). Dispense in tight, light-resistant container.

Tablet, orally disintegrating: Store at 20°C to 25°C (68°F to 77°F). Keep in original packaging until just prior to use.

Preparation for Administration

Injection: Lower doses (≤10 mg): No dilution required; Higher doses (>10 mg): Dilute in 50 mL of compatible solution (preferably NS).

Mechanism of Action

Blocks dopamine receptors and (when given in higher doses) also blocks serotonin receptors in chemoreceptor trigger zone of the CNS; enhances the response to acetylcholine of tissue in upper GI tract causing enhanced motility and accelerated gastric emptying without stimulating gastric, biliary, or pancreatic secretions; increases lower esophageal sphincter tone

Pharmacodynamics/Kinetics

Onset of action: Oral: 30 to 60 minutes; IV: 1 to 3 minutes; IM: 10 to 15 minutes

Duration: Therapeutic: 1 to 2 hours, regardless of route

Absorption: Oral: Rapid, well absorbed

Distribution: V_d: ~3.5 L/kg

Protein binding: ~30%

Bioavailability: Oral: Range: 65% to 95%

Half-life elimination: Normal renal function: Pediatric: ~4 hours; Adults: 5 to 6 hours (may be dose dependent)

Time to peak, serum: Oral: 1 to 2 hours

Excretion: Urine (~85%)

Dosing

Adult

US labeling:

Diabetic gastroparesis:

Oral: 10 mg up to 4 times daily 30 minutes before meals or food and at bedtime for 2 to 8 weeks. Treatment >12 weeks is not recommended.

IM, IV (for severe symptoms): 10 mg over 1 to 2 minutes; 10 days of IV therapy may be necessary before symptoms are controlled to allow transition to oral administration.

Gastroparesis management, regardless of etiology (off-label use): American College of Gastroenterology Guidelines: Oral: Initial: 5 mg 3 times daily before meals. Dosage range: 5 to 10 mg 2 to 3 times daily before meals (maximum: 40 mg daily). Liquid formulation is preferred (to increase absorption) and the use of drug holidays or dose reductions (eg, 5 mg before the two main meals of the day) is also recommended when clinically possible (Camilleri, 2013).

Gastroesophageal reflux: Oral: 10 to 15 mg up to 4 times daily 30 minutes before meals and at bedtime; alternatively, single doses of up to 20 mg (rather than continuous treatment) may be administered prior to provoking situation if symptoms are intermittent. Treatment >12 weeks is not recommended.

Prevention of nausea and vomiting associated with emetogenic chemotherapy: IV: **Note:** Pretreatment with diphenhydramine will decrease risk of extrapyramidal reactions.

Highly emetogenic: Initial dose: 2 mg/kg over 15 minutes 30 minutes before chemotherapy; repeat every 2 hours for 2 doses, then every 3 hours for 3 doses

Less emetogenic: Initial dose: 1 mg/kg over 15 minutes 30 minutes before chemotherapy; repeat every 2 hours for 2 doses, then every 3 hours for 3 doses

Delayed-emesis prophylaxis (off-label): Oral: 20 to 40 mg (or 0.5 mg/kg/ dose) 2 to 4 times daily for 3 to 4 days in combination with dexamethasone (ASCO guidelines [Kris, 2006])

Refractory or intolerant to antiemetics with a higher therapeutic index (off-label; Hesketh, 2008):

IV: 1 to 2 mg/kg/dose before chemotherapy and repeat 2 hours after chemotherapy

Oral: 0.5 mg/kg every 6 hours on days 2 to 4

Prevention of postoperative nausea and vomiting: IM, IV (off-label route): Usual dose: 10 mg near end of surgery; some patients may require 20 mg. **Note:** Guidelines discourage use of 10 mg metoclopramide due to lack of effectiveness (Gan, 2007); comparative study indicates higher dose (20 mg) may be efficacious (Quaynor, 2002).

Radiological exam: IV: 10 mg as a single dose

Small bowel intubation (postpyloric feeding tube placement): IV: 10 mg as a single dose

Prevention of radiation therapy-induced nausea and vomiting (minimal emetic risk) (off-label use): Oral: 20 mg as rescue therapy; if rescue therapy is used, then administer prior to each fraction until the end of radiation therapy (Basch, 2011).

Canadian labeling:

Gastroparesis management (adjunctive therapy): Note: Total daily dose should not exceed 0.5 mg/kg.

IM, IV: 10 mg 2 to 3 times daily as needed by IM injection or by slow IV injection

Oral: 5 to 10 mg 3 to 4 times daily before meals based on response and weight

Prevention of vomiting associated with cancer chemotherapy regimens that include cisplatin: IV:

Cisplatin dose ≤100 mg/m^2: Metoclopramide 1 mg/kg over 15 minutes every 2 hours for 2 doses, then every 3 hours for 3 doses

Cisplatin dose >100 mg/m^2: Metoclopramide 2 mg/kg over 15 minutes every 2 hours for 2 doses, then every 3 hours for 3 doses

Prevention of postoperative vomiting: Note: Total daily dose should not exceed 0.5 mg/kg.

IM: 10 mg prior to end of surgical procedure and then every 4 to 6 hours as needed; dose may be increased to 20 mg for high-risk groups (eg, general anesthesia ≥2 hours, abdominal or pelvic surgery with visceral manipulation, absence of gastric suction)

Oral: 20 mg 2 hours prior to anesthesia

Radiological exam: Oral: 20 mg 5 to 10 minutes prior to barium swallow (total daily dose should not exceed 0.5 mg/kg)

Small bowel intubation (postpyloric feeding tube placement):

IV: 10 mg as a single dose by slow injection

Oral: 10 mg as single dose; may not be preferred route due to delayed onset of action when compared to IV route

Geriatric Initial: Dose at the lower end of the recommended range (may require only 5 mg/dose) and use the lowest effective dose. Refer to adult dosing.

Pediatric

US labeling: Children and Adolescents:

Small bowel intubation (postpyloric feeding tube placement): IV:

<6 years: 0.1 mg/kg as a single dose

6 to 14 years: 2.5 to 5 mg as a single dose

>14 years: Refer to adult dosing.

Canadian labeling: Children and Adolescents: **Note:** Total daily dose should not exceed 0.5 mg/kg.

Gastroparesis: Oral:

5 to 14 years: 2.5 mg to 5 mg 3 times daily before meals (based on body weight and response)

>14 years: Refer to adult dosing.

Small bowel intubation: IV:

5 to 14 years: 0.1 mg/kg as single dose by slow IV injection

>14 years: Refer to adult dosing.

Prevention of chemotherapy-associated nausea and vomiting (off-label use): IV: Moderately emetogenic chemotherapy (patients who cannot receive corticosteroids): IV: 1 mg/kg prior to chemotherapy, followed by Oral: 0.0375 mg/kg every 6 hours; regimen also includes ondansetron or granisetron; coadministration of diphenhydramine or benztropine is recommended to prevent metoclopramide-induced adverse effects (Dupuis, 2013).

Renal Impairment

CrCl <40 mL/minute: Administer 50% of normal dose.

Not dialyzable (0% to 5%); supplemental dose is not necessary (Aronoff, 2007).

Hepatic Impairment There are no dosage adjustments provided in the manufacturer's labeling. However, metoclopramide has been used safely in patients with advanced liver disease with normal renal function.

Administration

Injection: May be given IM, direct IV push, short infusion (at least 15 minutes), or continuous infusion; lower doses (≤10 mg) of metoclopramide can be given IV push undiluted over 1 to 2 minutes; higher doses (>10 mg) to be diluted in 50 mL of compatible solution (preferably NS) and given IVPB over at least 15 minutes. **Note:** Rapid IV administration may be associated with a transient (but intense) feeling of anxiety and restlessness, followed by drowsiness.

Tablets: When used for gastroparesis/reflux, administer 30 minutes prior to meals and at bedtime.

Orally disintegrating tablets: When used for gastroparesis/reflux, administer on an empty stomach at least 30 minutes prior to food and at bedtime (do not repeat if inadvertently taken with food). Do not remove from packaging until time of administration. If tablet breaks or crumbles while handling, discard ▶

◀ and remove new tablet. Using dry hands, place tablet on tongue and allow to dissolve (disintegrates within ~1 minute [range: 10 seconds to 14 minutes]). Swallow with saliva.

Oral solution: When used for gastroparesis/reflux, administer 30 minutes prior to meals and at bedtime.

Monitoring Parameters Signs of tardive dyskinesias, extrapyramidal symptoms; signs/symptoms of neuroleptic malignant syndrome

Medication Guide Available Yes

Dosage Forms Excipient information presented when available (limited, particularly for generics); consult specific product labeling. [DSC] = Discontinued product

Solution, Injection:

Reglan: 5 mg/mL (2 mL [DSC], 10 mL [DSC], 30 mL [DSC])

Generic: 5 mg/mL (2 mL)

Solution, Injection [preservative free]:

Generic: 5 mg/mL (2 mL)

Solution, Oral:

Generic: 5 mg/5 mL (10 mL, 473 mL); 10 mg/10 mL (10 mL)

Tablet, Oral:

Reglan: 5 mg [contains fd&c blue #1 aluminum lake, fd&c yellow #10 aluminum lake]

Reglan: 10 mg [dye free]

Generic: 5 mg, 10 mg

Tablet Dispersible, Oral:

Metozolv ODT: 5 mg, 10 mg [DSC]

Generic: 5 mg, 10 mg

◆ **Metoclopramide Hydrochloride Injection (Can)** *see* Metoclopramide *on page 1134*

◆ **Metoclopramide Omega (Can)** *see* Metoclopramide *on page 1134*

◆ **Metoject (Can)** *see* Methotrexate *on page 1104*

◆ **Metonia (Can)** *see* Metoclopramide *on page 1134*

◆ **Metozolv ODT** *see* Metoclopramide *on page 1134*

◆ **Metro** *see* MetroNIDAZOLE (Systemic) *on page 1142*

MetroNIDAZOLE (Systemic) (met roe NYE da zole)

Brand Names: US Flagyl; Flagyl ER; Metro

Brand Names: Canada Flagyl; Metronidazole Injection USP; Novo-Nidazol; PMS-Metronidazole

Index Terms Flagyl; Metronidazole Hydrochloride

Pharmacologic Category Amebicide; Antibiotic, Miscellaneous; Antiprotozoal; Nitroimidazole

Use

Amebiasis: Oral immediate release tablet and capsule: Treatment of acute intestinal amebiasis (amebic dysentery) and amebic liver abscess

Limitations of use (oral immediate-release tablet, capsule and injection): When used for amebic liver abscess, may be used concurrently with percutaneous needle aspiration when it is clinically indicated

Anaerobic bacterial infections (caused by *Bacteroides spp,* including the *B. fragilis* group): Oral immediate-release tablet, capsule, and injection:

Bacterial septicemia: Treatment of bacterial septicemia (also caused by *Clostridium spp*)

Bone and joint infections: Treatment (adjunctive therapy) of bone and joint infections

CNS Infections: Treatment of CNS infections, including meningitis and brain abscess

Endocarditis: Treatment of endocarditis

Gynecologic infections: Treatment of gynecologic infections including endometritis, endomyometritis, tubo-ovarian abscess, or postsurgical vaginal cuff infection (also caused by *Clostridium spp*, *Peptococcus spp*, *Peptostreptococcus spp*, and *Fusobacterium spp*)

Intra-abdominal infections: Treatment of intra-abdominal infections, including peritonitis, intra-abdominal abscess and liver abscess (also caused by *Clostridium spp*, *Eubacterium spp*, *Peptococcus spp*, and *Peptostreptococcus spp*)

Lower respiratory tract infections: Treatment of lower respiratory tract infections, including pneumonia, empyema and lung abscess

Skin and skin structure infections: Treatment of skin and skin structure infections (also caused by *Clostridium spp*, *Peptococcus spp*, *Peptostreptococcus spp*, and *Fusobacterium spp*)

Bacterial vaginosis: Oral extended-release tablet: Treatment of bacterial vaginosis in nonpregnant women

Surgical prophylaxis (colorectal surgery): Injection: Preoperative, intra-operative, and postoperative prophylaxis to reduce the incidence of postoperative infection in patients undergoing elective colorectal surgery classified as contaminated or potentially contaminated.

Trichomoniasis: Oral immediate-release tablet, capsule, and injection: Treatment of infections caused by *Trichomonas vaginalis*, including treatment of asymptomatic sexual partners

Pregnancy Risk Factor B

Dosing

Adult

Amebiasis (acute dysentery): Oral: Immediate-release tablets and capsules: 750 mg every 8 hours for 5 to 10 days

Amebic liver abscess: Oral:
Immediate-release tablets: 500 to 750 mg every 8 hours for 5 to 10 days
Capsules: 750 mg every 8 hours for 5 to 10 days

Anaerobic infections (diverticulitis, peritonitis, cholangitis, or abscess): Oral (immediate release), IV: 500 mg every 6 hours (maximum: 4 g/day); **Note:** Initial: 1 g IV loading dose may be administered

Bacterial vaginosis or vaginitis due to *Gardnerella, Mobiluncus:* Oral: Tablet:
Immediate release: 500 mg twice daily for 7 days (off-label use) (CDC 2010)
Extended release: 750 mg once daily for 7 days

Intra-abdominal infection:
Manufacturer's labeling: Oral (immediate release), IV: 500 mg every 6 hours (maximum: 4 g/day); **Note:** Initial: 1 g IV loading dose may be administered
Alternate dosing: Complicated, community-acquired, mild to moderate (in combination with cephalosporin or fluoroquinolone; off-label dosing): IV: 500 mg every 8 to 12 hours **or** 1.5 g every 24 hours for 4 to 7 days (provided source controlled) (Solomkin 2010)

Pelvic inflammatory disease (off-label dosing): Oral (immediate release): 500 mg twice daily for 14 days (in combination with a third generation parenteral cephalosporin and doxycycline) (CDC 2010)

◀ **Trichomoniasis (index case and sex partner):** Oral:
Immediate-release tablets:
Manufacturer's labeling: 250 mg every 8 hours for 7 days **or** 1 g twice daily for 2 doses (on same day) **or** 2 g as a single dose
Alternate dosing: 500 mg twice daily for 7 days (CDC 2010)
Capsules: 375 mg twice daily for 7 days

Trichomoniasis (failure of nitroimidazole [eg metronidazole] therapy in index case; treatment of sex partner; off-label dosing): Oral (immediate release): 500 mg twice daily for 7 days (CDC 2010)

Balantidiasis (off-label use): IV, Oral (immediate release): 750 mg 3 times daily for ≥5 days (Anagyrou 2003; Schuster 2008)

Bite wounds (animal/human) (off-label use) (IDSA [Stevens 2014]): Note: Use in combination with a second- or third-generation cephalosporin, levofloxacin, or sulfamethoxazole/trimethoprim for animal bites, or in combination with ciprofloxacin or levofloxacin for human bites.
Oral: 250 to 500 mg 3 times daily
IV: 500 mg every 8 hours

***Clostridium difficile*-associated diarrhea (CDAD) (off-label use):**
Mild to moderate infection: Oral (immediate release): 500 mg 3 times daily for 10 to 14 days (Cohen 2010; Surawicz 2013)
Severe complicated infection (no abdominal distention): IV: 500 mg 3 times daily with oral vancomycin for 10 to 14 days (Surawicz 2013)
Severe complicated infection (with ileus, toxic colitis, and/or abdominal distention): IV: 500 mg 3 times daily with oral and rectal vancomycin for 10 to 14 days (Surawicz 2013)
Note: Recent guideline recommends converting to oral vancomycin therapy if the patient does not show a clear clinical response after 5 to 7 days of metronidazole therapy (Surawicz 2013)

Crohn disease (off-label use): Oral (immediate release): 10 to 20 mg/kg/day; long-term (eg, several months) safety has not been established (Lichtenstein 2009). **Note:** Reserved for mild to moderate disease in patients not responsive to sulfasalazine and/or who have colonic involvement (eg, ileocolitis and colitis) (Lichtenstein 2009; Sutherland, 1991).

***Dientamoeba fragilis* infections (off-label use):** Oral (immediate release): 500 to 750 mg 3 times daily for 10 days (CDC 2012)

Giardiasis (off-label use): Oral (immediate release): 250 to 500 mg 3 times daily for 5 to 10 days (Granados 2012)

***Helicobacter pylori* eradication (off-label use):** Oral (immediate release):
Triple therapy: Metronidazole 500 mg twice daily for 10 to 14 days, in combination with clarithromycin and a proton pump inhibitor (Chey 2007)
Quadruple therapy: Metronidazole 250 mg 4 times daily for 10 to 14 days, in combination with bismuth subsalicylate, a tetracycline, and either ranitidine or a proton pump inhibitor (Chey 2007)

Periodontitis (associated with aggressive disease; off-label use): Oral (immediate release): 250 mg every 8 hours in combination with amoxicillin for 10 days; used in addition to scaling, root planing and pocket irrigation (Silva-Senem 2013)

Pouchitis (post ileal pouch-anal anastomosis, acute treatment; off-label use): Oral (immediate release): 400 to 500 mg three times daily for 7 days (Holubar 2010; Wall 2011)

Sexual assault (prophylaxis; off-label use): Oral (immediate release): 2 g as a single dose in combination with ceftriaxone and azithromycin or doxycycline (CDC 2010; CDC 2012)

Skin and soft tissue necrotizing infections (off-label use): IV: 500 mg every 6 hours, in combination with cefotaxime for empiric therapy of polymicrobial infections. Continue until further debridement is not necessary, patient has clinically improved, and patient is afebrile for 48 to 72 hours (IDSA [Stevens 2014]).

Surgical prophylaxis:

Manufacturer's labeling: IV: 15 mg/kg 1 hour prior to surgical incision; followed by 7.5 mg/kg 6 and 12 hours after initial dose

Alternate dosing:

IV: 500 mg within 60 minutes prior to surgical incision in combination with other antibiotics (Bratzler 2013). **Note:** Considered a recommended agent for select procedures other than colorectal surgery (off-label use) (Bratzler 2013).

Oral (for colorectal surgical prophylaxis only; immediate release; off-label use): 1 g every 3 to 4 hours for 3 doses, starting after mechanical bowel preparation the afternoon and evening before the procedure with or without additional oral antibiotics and with an appropriate IV antibiotic prophylaxis regimen (Bratzler 2013).

Surgical site infections (intestinal or GU tract; axilla or perineum) (off-label use): IV: 500 mg every 8 hours; in combination with ceftriaxone, ciprofloxacin, or levofloxacin (IDSA [Stevens 2014]).

Tetanus (*Clostridium tetani* infection; off-label use): Oral (immediate release): 500 mg every 6 hours for 7 to 10 days in combination with supportive therapy (Ahmadsyah, 1985)

Urethritis (for recurrent or persistent urethritis; off-label use): Oral: 2 g as a single dose with azithromycin. **Note:** Compliance with initial regimen and lack of re-exposure to an untreated sex partner should be excluded prior to use (CDC 2010)

Geriatric Refer to adult dosing.

Pediatric

Infants, Children, and Adolescents:

Amebiasis: Oral: 35 to 50 mg/kg/day in divided doses every 8 hours for 7 to 10 days (*Red Book* [AAP 2012])

Trichomoniasis: Oral: 15 mg/kg/day in divided doses every 8 hours for 7 days (*Red Book* [AAP 2012])

Anaerobic infections (off-label dosing):

Oral: 30 to 50 mg/kg/day in divided doses every 8 hours (maximum: 2,250 mg/day) (*Red Book* [AAP 2012])

IV: 22.5 to 40 mg/kg/day in divided doses every 8 hours (maximum: 1,500 mg/day) (*Red Book* [AAP 2012])

Balantidiasis (off-label use): Oral: 35 to 50 mg/kg/day in 3 divided doses for 5 days (*Red Book* [AAP 2012]; Schuster 2008)

***Clostridium difficile*-associated diarrhea (CDAD; off-label use):** Oral: 30 mg/kg/day divided every 6 hours for ≥10 days (maximum: 2 g/day) (*Red Book* [AAP 2012]; Schutze 2013). **Note:** Recommended agent for the initial treatment of mild to moderate disease and for first relapse (*Red Book* [AAP 2012]; Schutze 2013).

Giardiasis (off-label use): Oral: 15 mg/kg/day in divided doses every 8 hours for 5 to 10 days (Granados 2012; *Red Book* [AAP 2012])

***Helicobacter pylori* eradication (off-label use):** Oral: 20 mg/kg/day in 2 divided doses for 10 to 14 days in combination therapy with amoxicillin and either a proton pump inhibitor or bismuth subsalicylate daily or 20 mg/kg/day in 2 divided doses on days 6 through 10 in combination therapy with a proton pump inhibitor and clarithromycin (after treatment with amoxicillin and a proton pump inhibitor for days 1 through 5) (maximum: 1 g/day) (Koletzko 2011)

Skin and soft tissue necrotizing infections (off-label use): IV: 7.5 mg/kg every 6 hours, in combination with cefotaxime for empiric therapy of polymicrobial infections. Continue until further debridement is not necessary, patient has clinically improved, and patient is afebrile for 48 to 72 hours (IDSA [Stevens 2014]).

Surgical (preoperative) prophylaxis (off-label use):

Infants <1,200 g: IV: 7.5 mg/kg within 60 minutes prior to surgical incision in combination with other antibiotics (Bratzler 2013).

Infants ≥1,200 g and Children ≥1 year:

IV: 15 mg/kg within 60 minutes prior to surgical incision in combination with other antibiotics (maximum: 500 mg per dose) (Bratzler 2013).

Oral (for colorectal surgical prophylaxis only): 15 mg/kg (maximum: 1,000 mg) every 3 to 4 hours for 3 doses, starting after mechanical bowel preparation the afternoon and evening before the procedure, with or without additional oral antibiotics and with an appropriate IV antibiotic prophylaxis regimen (Bratzler 2013).

Tetanus (*Clostridium tetani* infection, off-label use): Oral, IV: 30 mg/kg per day in divided doses every 6 hours for 10 to 14 days in combination with tetanus immune globulin and supportive therapy (maximum: 4 g/day) (*Red Book* [AAP 2012])

Adolescents: Oral:

Pelvic inflammatory disease (off-label dosing): Refer to adult dosing

Sexual assault (prophylaxis; off-label use): Refer to adult dosing

Vaginal infections:

Vaginitis: (*Trichomonas vaginalis* ; off-label use): 2 g as a single dose (*Red Book* [AAP 2012])

Vaginosis (bacterial; off-label use): 500 mg twice daily for 7 days (*Red Book* [AAP 2012])

Renal Impairment

Manufacturer's labeling:

Mild, moderate, or severe impairment: There are no dosage adjustments provided in the manufacturer's labeling; however, decreased renal function does not alter the single-dose pharmacokinetics

End-stage renal disease (ESRD) requiring dialysis: Metronidazole metabolites may accumulate; monitor for adverse events. Accumulated metabolites may be rapidly removed by dialysis:

Intermittent hemodialysis (IHD): If administration cannot be separated from hemodialysis, consider supplemental dose following hemodialysis.

Peritoneal dialysis (PD): No dosage adjustment necessary.

Alternate dosing:

Intermittent hemodialysis (IHD) (administer after hemodialysis on dialysis days): Dialyzable (50% to 100%): 500 mg every 8 to 12 hours. **Note:** Dosing regimen highly dependent on clinical indication (trichomoniasis vs *C. difficile* colitis) (Heintz 2009). **Note:** Dosing dependent on the assumption of thrice weekly, complete IHD sessions.

Continuous renal replacement therapy (CRRT) (Heintz 2009; Trotman 2005): Drug clearance is highly dependent on the method of renal replacement, filter type, and flow rate. Appropriate dosing requires close monitoring of pharmacologic response, signs of adverse reactions due to drug accumulation, as well as drug concentrations in relation to target trough (if appropriate). The following are general recommendations only (based on dialysate flow/ultrafiltration rates of 1 to 2 L/hour and minimal residual renal function) and should not supersede clinical judgment:

CVVH/CVVHD/CVVHDF: 500 mg every 6 to 12 hours (or per clinical indication; dosage reduction generally not necessary)

Hepatic Impairment

Manufacturer's labeling:

Mild or moderate impairment (Child-Pugh class A or B): No dosage adjustment necessary; use with caution and monitor for adverse events

Severe impairment (Child-Pugh class C):

Extended-release tablets: Use is not recommended.

Immediate-release capsules:

Amebiasis: 375 mg 3 times daily

Trichomoniasis: 375 mg once daily

Immediate-release tablets, injection: Reduce dose by 50%

Alternate dosing: The pharmacokinetics of a single oral 500 mg dose were not altered in patients with cirrhosis; initial dose reduction is therefore not necessary (Daneshmend, 1982). In one study of IV metronidazole, patients with alcoholic liver disease (with or without cirrhosis), demonstrated a prolonged elimination half-life (eg, ~18 hours). The authors recommended the dose be reduced accordingly (clearance was reduced by ~62%) and the frequency may be prolonged (eg, every 12 hours instead of every 6 hours) (Lau, 1987). In another single IV dose study using metronidazole metabolism to predict hepatic function, patients classified as Child-Pugh class C demonstrated a half-life of ~21.5 hours (Muscara, 1995).

Additional Information Complete prescribing information should be consulted for additional detail.

Dosage Forms Considerations Parenteral solution contains 28 mEq of sodium/gram of metronidazole.

Dosage Forms Excipient information presented when available (limited, particularly for generics); consult specific product labeling.

Capsule, Oral:

Flagyl: 375 mg

Generic: 375 mg

Solution, Intravenous:

Metro: 500 mg (100 mL)

Generic: 500 mg (100 mL)

Solution, Intravenous [preservative free]:

Generic: 500 mg (100 mL)

Tablet, Oral:

Flagyl: 250 mg, 500 mg

Generic: 250 mg, 500 mg

Tablet Extended Release 24 Hour, Oral:

Flagyl ER: 750 mg

◆ **Metronidazole Hydrochloride** *see* MetroNIDAZOLE (Systemic) *on page 1142*

♦ **Metronidazole Injection USP (Can)** *see* MetroNIDAZOLE (Systemic) *on page 1142*

♦ **MET Tyrosine Kinase Inhibitor PF-02341066** *see* Crizotinib *on page 366*

♦ **Miacalcin** *see* Calcitonin *on page 259*

Micafungin (mi ka FUN gin)

Brand Names: US Mycamine

Brand Names: Canada Mycamine

Index Terms Micafungin Sodium

Pharmacologic Category Antifungal Agent, Parenteral; Echinocandin

Use

Candidemia, acute disseminated candidiasis, *Candida* peritonitis and abscesses: Treatment of candidemia, acute disseminated candidiasis, *Candida* peritonitis and abscesses

Esophageal candidiasis: Treatment of esophageal candidiasis

Prophylaxis of *Candida* infections: Prophylaxis of *Candida* infections in patients undergoing hematopoietic stem cell transplantation (HSCT)

Pregnancy Risk Factor C

Dosing

Adult & Geriatric

Aspergillosis (invasive) in HIV-infected patients (off-label use): IV: 100 to 150 mg once daily until infection resolution and CD4 count >200 cells/mm^3 (HHS [OI adult 2015])

Candidemia, acute disseminated candidiasis, and *Candida* peritonitis and abscesses: IV: 100 mg once daily; mean duration of therapy (from clinical trials) was 15 days (range: 10 to 47 days)

Esophageal candidiasis: IV: 150 mg once daily; mean duration of therapy (from clinical trials) was 15 days (range: 10 to 30 days)

Prophylaxis of *Candida* infection in hematopoietic stem cell transplantation: IV: 50 mg once daily; mean duration of therapy (from clinical trials) was 19 days (range: 6 to 51 days)

Pediatric

Aspergillosis (invasive) in HIV-infected patients (off-label use): IV: Adolescents: Refer to adult dosing.

Candidemia, acute disseminated candidiasis, and *Candida* peritonitis and abscesses: Infants ≥4 months, Children, and Adolescents: IV: 2 mg/kg once daily; maximum: 100 mg once daily

Esophageal candidiasis: Infants ≥4 months, Children, and Adolescents: IV: ≤30 kg: 3 mg/kg once daily
>30 kg: 2.5 mg/kg once daily; maximum: 150 mg once daily

Prophylaxis of *Candida* infection in hematopoietic stem cell transplantation: Infants ≥4 months, Children, and Adolescents: IV: 1 mg/kg once daily; maximum: 50 mg once daily

Primary antifungal prophylaxis in allogeneic HSCT (when fluconazole is contraindicated; off-label dosing/population; guideline recommendation): Infants ≥1 month, Children, and Adolescents <19 years: IV: 1 mg/kg once daily; maximum: 50 mg once daily (Science, 2014)

Renal Impairment

No dosage adjustment necessary.

Poorly dialyzed; no supplemental dose or dosage adjustment necessary, including patients on intermittent hemodialysis.

Hepatic Impairment No dosage adjustment necessary.

Additional Information Complete prescribing information should be consulted for additional detail.

Dosage Forms Excipient information presented when available (limited, particularly for generics); consult specific product labeling.
Solution Reconstituted, Intravenous, as sodium:
Mycamine: 50 mg (1 ea); 100 mg (1 ea)
Solution Reconstituted, Intravenous, as sodium [preservative free]:
Mycamine: 50 mg (1 ea); 100 mg (1 ea)

- ◆ **Micafungin Sodium** see Micafungin on page 1148
- ◆ **MICRhoGAM Ultra-Filtered Plus** see Rh$_o$(D) Immune Globulin on page 1471
- ◆ **Millipred** see PrednisoLONE (Systemic) on page 1421
- ◆ **Millipred DP** see PrednisoLONE (Systemic) on page 1421
- ◆ **Millipred DP 12-Day** see PrednisoLONE (Systemic) on page 1421
- ◆ **Minims Prednisolone Sodium Phosphate (Can)** see PrednisoLONE (Ophthalmic) on page 1424
- ◆ **Mint-Anastrozole (Can)** see Anastrozole on page 112
- ◆ **Mint-Ciproflox (Can)** see Ciprofloxacin (Systemic) on page 327
- ◆ **Mint-Ciprofloxacin (Can)** see Ciprofloxacin (Systemic) on page 327
- ◆ **Mint-Olanzapine ODT (Can)** see OLANZapine on page 1242
- ◆ **Mint-Ondansetron (Can)** see Ondansetron on page 1253
- ◆ **MITC** see MitoMYcin (Systemic) on page 1149
- ◆ **MITO** see MitoMYcin (Systemic) on page 1149
- ◆ **MITO-C** see MitoMYcin (Systemic) on page 1149
- ◆ **Mitomycin-X** see MitoMYcin (Systemic) on page 1149
- ◆ **Mitomycin-C** see MitoMYcin (Ophthalmic) on page 1153
- ◆ **Mitomycin-C** see MitoMYcin (Systemic) on page 1149

MitoMYcin (Systemic) (mye toe MYE sin)

Related Information

Management of Chemotherapy-Induced Nausea and Vomiting in Adults on page 2142
Management of Drug Extravasations on page 2159
Mucositis and Stomatitis on page 2186
Prevention of Chemotherapy-Induced Nausea and Vomiting in Children on page 2203
Safe Handling of Hazardous Drugs on page 2292

Brand Names: Canada Mitomycin For Injection; Mitomycin For Injection USP; Mutamycin®

Index Terms MITC; MITO; MITO-C; Mitomycin-C; Mitomycin-X; MMC; MTC; Mutamycin

Pharmacologic Category Antineoplastic Agent, Antibiotic

Use Treatment of adenocarcinoma of stomach or pancreas

Labeled Contraindications Hypersensitivity to mitomycin or any component of the formulation; thrombocytopenia; coagulation disorders, or other increased bleeding tendency

Pregnancy Considerations Teratogenic effects have been observed in animal reproduction studies.

▶

◀ **Breast-Feeding Considerations** It is not known if mitomycin is excreted in human milk; the manufacturer recommends against breast-feeding during treatment.

Warnings/Precautions Hazardous agent - use appropriate precautions for handling and disposal (NIOSH 2014 [group 1]). **[U.S. Boxed Warning]: Bone marrow suppression (thrombocytopenia and leukopenia) is common and may be severe and/or contribute to infections.** Fatalities due to sepsis have been reported; monitor for infections. Myelosuppression is dose-limiting, delayed in onset, and cumulative; therefore, monitor blood counts closely during and for ≥8 weeks following treatment; treatment delay or dosage adjustment may be required for significant thrombocytopenia (platelets <100,000/mm^3) or leukopenia (WBC<4000/mm^3) or a progressive decline in either value. Use with caution in patients who have received radiation therapy or in the presence of hepatobiliary dysfunction; reduce dosage in patients who are receiving radiation therapy simultaneously. Monitor for renal toxicity; do not administer if serum creatinine is >1.7 mg/dL. **[U.S. Boxed Warning]: Hemolytic-uremic syndrome (HUS) has been reported (incidence not defined); condition usually involves microangiopathic hemolytic anemia (hematocrit ≤5%), thrombocytopenia (≤100,000/mm^3), and irreversible renal failure (serum creatinine ≥1.6 mg/dL). HUS may occur at any time, is generally associated with single doses ≥60 mg, and HUS symptoms may be exacerbated by blood transfusion.** Other less common effects may include pulmonary edema, neurologic abnormalities, and hypertension. High mortality from HUS development has been reported, and is largely the result of renal failure. HUS may also be associated with cumulative doses ≥50 mg/m^2. Bladder fibrosis/contraction has been reported with intravesical administration (unapproved administration route). Mitomycin is a potent vesicant; ensure proper needle or catheter placement prior to and during infusion. Avoid extravasation. May cause necrosis and tissue sloughing; delayed erythema and/or ulceration have been reported.

Cases of acute respiratory distress syndrome (ARDS) have been reported in patients receiving mitomycin in combination with other chemotherapy who were maintained at FIO$_2$ concentrations >50% perioperatively; use caution to provide only enough oxygen to maintain adequate arterial saturation and avoid overhydration. Pulmonary toxicity has also been reported as dyspnea with nonproductive cough and appearance of pulmonary infiltrates on radiograph; discontinue therapy if pulmonary toxicity occurs and other potential etiologies have been ruled out. Shortness of breath and bronchospasm have been reported in patients receiving vinca alkaloids in combination with mitomycin or who received mitomycin previously; this acute respiratory distress has occurred within minutes to hours following the vinca alkaloid; may be managed with bronchodilators, steroids and/or oxygen. **[U.S. Boxed Warning]: Should be administered under the supervision of an experienced cancer chemotherapy physician.**

Adverse Reactions

>10%:

Central nervous system: Fever (14%)

Gastrointestinal: Nausea, vomiting, and anorexia (14%)

Hematologic: Myelosuppression (64%; onset: 4 weeks; recovery: 8-10 weeks)

Miscellaneous: Thrombotic thrombocytopenic purpura (TTP)/hemolytic uremic syndrome (HUS) (≤15%)

1% to 10%:
 Dermatologic: Alopecia, mucous membrane toxicity (4%)
 Gastrointestinal: Stomatitis (4%)
 Renal: Serum creatinine increased (2%)
<1%, postmarketing, and/or case reports: Adult respiratory distress syndrome (ARDS), bladder fibrosis/contraction (intravesical administration), dyspnea, extravasation reactions, heart failure, hepatic sinusoidal obstruction syndrome (SOS, veno-occlusive liver disease), interstitial fibrosis, malaise, nonproductive cough, pulmonary infiltrates, rash, renal failure (irreversible), weakness

Drug Interactions

Metabolism/Transport Effects Substrate of P-glycoprotein

Avoid Concomitant Use

Avoid concomitant use of MitoMYcin (Systemic) with any of the following: BCG (Intravesical); CloZAPine; Dipyrone; Natalizumab; Pimecrolimus; Tacrolimus (Topical); Tofacitinib; Vaccines (Live)

Increased Effect/Toxicity

MitoMYcin (Systemic) may increase the levels/effects of: CloZAPine; Fingolimod; Leflunomide; Natalizumab; Tofacitinib; Vaccines (Live)

The levels/effects of MitoMYcin (Systemic) may be increased by: Antineoplastic Agents (Vinca Alkaloids); Denosumab; Dipyrone; Lumacaftor; P-glycoprotein/ABCB1 Inhibitors; Pimecrolimus; Ranolazine; Roflumilast; Tacrolimus (Topical); Trastuzumab

Decreased Effect

MitoMYcin (Systemic) may decrease the levels/effects of: BCG (Intravesical); Coccidioides immitis Skin Test; Sipuleucel-T; Vaccines (Inactivated); Vaccines (Live)

The levels/effects of MitoMYcin (Systemic) may be decreased by: Echinacea; Lumacaftor; P-glycoprotein/ABCB1 Inducers

Storage/Stability Store intact vials at controlled room temperature; avoid exposure to temperatures >40°C (104°F). Reconstituted solution is stable for 7 days at room temperature and 14 days when refrigerated. Protect reconstituted solution from light. Solution of 0.5 mg/mL in a syringe is stable for 7 days at room temperature and 28 days when refrigerated and protected from light.
Further dilution to 20-40 mcg/mL:
 In normal saline: Stable for 12 hours at room temperature.
 In sodium lactate: Stable for 24 hours at room temperature.

Preparation for Administration Hazardous agent; use appropriate precautions for handling and disposal (NIOSH 2014 [group 1]). Dilute powder with SWFI to a concentration of 0.5 mg/mL. May further dilute in NS or sodium lactate to 20-40 mcg/mL.

Mechanism of Action Acts like an alkylating agent and produces DNA cross-linking (primarily with guanine and cytosine pairs); cell-cycle nonspecific; inhibits DNA and RNA synthesis; degrades preformed DNA, causes nuclear lysis and formation of giant cells. While not phase-specific *per se*, mitomycin has its maximum effect against cells in late G and early S phases.

Pharmacodynamics/Kinetics

Metabolism: Hepatic
Half-life elimination: 17-78 minutes; Terminal: 50 minutes
Excretion: Urine (~10% as unchanged drug)

◄ **Dosing**

Adult & Geriatric Details concerning dosing in combination regimens should also be consulted.

Stomach or pancreas adenocarcinoma (manufacturer's labeling): IV: 20 mg/m^2 every 6-8 weeks

Anal carcinoma (off-label use): IV: 10 mg/m^2 as an IV bolus on days 1 and 29 (maximum: 20 mg/dose) in combination with fluorouracil and radiation therapy (Ajani, 2008)

Bladder cancer, nonmuscle invasive (off-label use/route): Intravesicular instillation:

Low risk of recurrence (uncomplicated): 40 mg as a single dose post-operatively; retain in bladder for 2 hours (Hall, 2007)

Increased risk of recurrence: 20 mg weekly for 6 weeks, followed by 20 mg monthly for 3 years; retain in bladder for 1-2 hours (Friedrich, 2007)

Renal Impairment The manufacturer's labeling states to avoid use in patients with serum creatine >1.7 mg/dL, but no dosage adjustments are provided. The following adjustments have been used by some clinicians (Aronoff, 2007): Adults:

CrCl <10 mL/minute: Administer 75% of dose.

Continuous ambulatory peritoneal dialysis (CAPD): Administer 75% of dose.

Hepatic Impairment No dosage adjustment provided in manufacturer's labeling (has not been studied).

Obesity *ASCO Guidelines for appropriate chemotherapy dosing in obese adults with cancer:* Utilize patient's actual body weight (full weight) for calculation of body surface area- or weight-based dosing, particularly when the intent of therapy is curative; manage regimen-related toxicities in the same manner as for nonobese patients; if a dose reduction is utilized due to toxicity, consider resumption of full weight-based dosing with subsequent cycles, especially if cause of toxicity (eg, hepatic or renal impairment) is resolved (Griggs, 2012).

Adjustment for Toxicity

Leukocytes 2000 to <3000/mm^3: Hold therapy until leukocyte count ≥4000/mm^3; reduce to 70% of dose in subsequent cycles

Leukocytes <2000/mm^3: Hold therapy until leukocyte count ≥4000/mm^3; reduce to 50% of dose in subsequent cycles

Platelets 25,000 to <75,000/mm^3: Hold therapy until platelets ≥100,000/mm^3; reduce to 70% of dose in subsequent cycles

Platelets <25,000/mm^3: Hold therapy until platelets ≥100,000 mm^3; reduce to 50% of dose in subsequent cycles

Combination Regimens

Anal cancer: Fluorouracil-Mitomycin (Anal Cancer) on page 1983

Administration

IV: Administer slow IV push or by slow (15-30 minute) infusion via a freely-running saline infusion. Consider using a central venous catheter.

Vesicant; ensure proper needle or catheter placement prior to and during infusion; avoid extravasation.

Extravasation management: If extravasation occurs, stop infusion immediately and disconnect (leave cannula/needle in place); gently aspirate extravasated solution (do **NOT** flush the line); remove needle/cannula; elevate extremity. Initiate dimethyl sulfate (DMSO) antidote. Apply dry cold compress for 20 minutes 4 times/day for 1-2 days (Pérez Fidalgo, 2012).

DMSO: Apply topically to a region covering twice the affected area every 8 hours for 7 days; begin within 10 minutes of extravasation; do not cover with a dressing (Perez Fidalgo, 2012).

Intravesicular (off-label route): Instill into bladder and retain for up to 2 hours (Friedrich, 2007; Hall, 2007); rotate patient every 15-30 minutes

Hazardous agent; use appropriate precautions for handling and disposal (NIOSH 2014 [group 1]).

Vesicant/Extravasation Risk Vesicant

Emetic Potential Children and Adults: Low (10% to 30%)

Monitoring Parameters Monitor CBC with differential (repeatedly during therapy and for ≥8 weeks following therapy); serum creatinine; pulmonary function tests; monitor for signs/symptoms of HUS

Dosage Forms Excipient information presented when available (limited, particularly for generics); consult specific product labeling.

Solution Reconstituted, Intravenous:

Generic: 5 mg (1 ea); 20 mg (1 ea); 40 mg (1 ea)

MitoMYcin (Ophthalmic) (mye toe MYE sin)

Brand Names: US Mitosol

Index Terms Mitomycin-C; MMC

Pharmacologic Category Antineoplastic Agent, Antibiotic; Ophthalmic Agent, Miscellaneous

Use Adjunct to *ab externo* glaucoma surgery

Labeled Contraindications Hypersensitivity to mitomycin or any component of the formulation; pregnancy

Pregnancy Considerations Teratogenic effects have been observed in animal reproduction studies following parenteral administration. Reproduction studies using topical mitomycin have not been conducted. Use is contraindicated in pregnant women or women who may become pregnant during therapy.

Breast-Feeding Considerations It is not known if mitomycin can be detected in breast milk following topical application. Due to the potential for serious adverse reactions in a nursing infant, breast feeding is not recommended.

Warnings/Precautions Hazardous agent - use appropriate precautions for handling and disposal (NIOSH 2014 [group 1]). Solution should **not** be administered intraocularly; intraocular administration may result in cell death, potentially causing corneal and retinal infarction, and ciliary body atrophy. Therapy is only intended for topical application to the surgical site of glaucoma filtration surgery. Increased incidence of postoperative hypotony has been observed with use. Increased incidence of lenticular change and cataract formation has been correlated with use in phakic patients. Inadvertent corneal and/or scleral damage, including thinning or perforation, may occur with use of mitomycin solution in concentrations >0.2 mg/mL or for time periods >2 minutes. In addition, direct contact of the solution with the corneal endothelium will cause cell death. Use appropriate precautions for handling and disposal.

Adverse Reactions Frequency not defined: Ocular: Astigmatism induced, bleb (encapsulated/cystic/thin-walled), bleb leak (chronic), bleb ulceration, bleb-related infection, blebitis, capsule opacification, capsular constriction, capsulotomy rupture, cataract development, cataract progression, choroidal detachment, choroidal effusion, ciliary block, conjunctival necrosis, corneal endothelial damage, corneal vascularization, cystic conjunctival degeneration,

Descemet's detachment, disk hemorrhage, disk swelling, endophthalmitis, epithelial defect, fibrin reaction, glaucoma (malignant), hemiretinal vein occlusion, hyphema, hypotony, hypotony maculopathy, implants dislocated, intraocular lens capture, iritis, lacrimal drainage system obstruction, loss of vision (severe), macular edema, retinal detachment (serious and rhegatogenous), retinal hemorrhage, retinal pigment epithelial tear, retinal vein occlusion, sclera thinning/ulceration, subconjunctival hemorrhage, superficial punctuate keratitis, suprachoroidal effusion (including hypoechogenic), suprachoroidal hemorrhage, supraciliochoroidal fluid present, synechiae (anterior and posterior), upper eyelid retraction, visual acuity decreased, vitreal hemorrhage/clot, wound dehiscence (associated with blebitis and scleritis)

Drug Interactions

Metabolism/Transport Effects None known.

Avoid Concomitant Use There are no known interactions where it is recommended to avoid concomitant use.

Increased Effect/Toxicity There are no known significant interactions involving an increase in effect.

Decreased Effect There are no known significant interactions involving a decrease in effect.

Storage/Stability Store at 20°C to 25°C (68°F to 77°F). Protect from light. Reconstituted solution is stable for 1 hour at room temperature. Use appropriate precautions for handling and disposal.

Preparation for Administration Hazardous agent; use appropriate precautions for handling and disposal (NIOSH 2014 [group 1]). Kit should only be opened and reconstituted by sterile surgical scrub technician. To reconstitute, add 1 mL of SWFI; shake/swirl to dissolve (detailed instructions are available in the kit). If powder does not dissolve immediately, allow to stand at room temperature until it dissolves completely into solution.

Mechanism of Action Acts like an alkylating agent and produces DNA cross-linking (primarily with guanine and cytosine pairs); cell-cycle nonspecific; inhibits DNA and RNA synthesis; degrades preformed DNA, causes nuclear lysis and formation of giant cells. While not phase-specific per se, mitomycin has its maximum effect against cells in late G and early S phases.

During use in trabeculectomy (filtration surgery) for glaucoma, mitomycin topical application is believed to alter conjunctival vascular endothelium and inhibit fibroblast proliferation.

Pharmacodynamics/Kinetics

Absorption: Systemic absorption following ocular administration is unknown; however, systemic concentrations are expected to be of multiple orders of magnitude lower than concentrations produced following parenteral administration.

Metabolism: Cleared from ophthalmic tissue following topical administration and irrigation; systemic metabolism primarily occurs in the liver

Dosing

Adult & Geriatric Glaucoma surgery, adjunctive therapy: Topical ophthalmic: 0.2 mg solution is aseptically applied via saturated sponges to surgical site of glaucoma filtration surgery for 2 minutes

Administration The inner tray and the contents of the kit are sterile and should only be handled, opened and assembled by a sterile surgical scrub technician. Use within 1 hour of reconstitution. Technician should fully saturate sponges provided in the kit with the entire reconstituted solution (0.2 mg). Allow saturated sponges to remain undisturbed in kit for 60 seconds. Saturated sponges should be applied aseptically with the use of surgical forceps in a single layer to a treatment area ~10 mm x 6 mm (± 2 mm); sponges should be removed from the treatment area after 2 minutes. Following removal of sponges from eye, the surgical site should be copiously irrigated. Saturated sponges should be returned to the provided tray for ultimate disposal into chemotherapy waste bag. Consult product labeling for additional details. Solution is **not** intended for intraocular administration.

Hazardous agent; use appropriate precautions for handling and disposal (NIOSH 2014 [group 1]).

Dosage Forms Excipient information presented when available (limited, particularly for generics); consult specific product labeling.
Kit, Ophthalmic:
Mitosol: 0.2 mg

♦ **Mitomycin For Injection (Can)** see MitoMYcin (Systemic) on page 1149
♦ **Mitomycin For Injection USP (Can)** see MitoMYcin (Systemic) on page 1149
♦ **Mitosol** see MitoMYcin (Ophthalmic) on page 1153

Mitotane (MYE toe tane)

Related Information

Management of Chemotherapy-Induced Nausea and Vomiting in Adults on page 2142
Prevention of Chemotherapy-Induced Nausea and Vomiting in Children on page 2203
Safe Handling of Hazardous Drugs on page 2292

Brand Names: US Lysodren
Brand Names: Canada Lysodren
Index Terms Chloditan; Chlodithane; Khloditan; Mytotan; o,p'-DDD; Ortho, para-DDD
Pharmacologic Category Antineoplastic Agent, Miscellaneous
Use Adrenocortical carcinoma: Treatment of inoperable adrenocortical carcinoma (both functional and non-functional types)
Labeled Contraindications Hypersensitivity to mitotane or any component of the formulation
Pregnancy Considerations Animal reproduction studies have not been conducted. May cause fetal harm if administered during pregnancy; adverse outcomes have been reported. Women of reproductive potential should use effective contraception during treatment and after treatment until plasma levels are no longer detected.
Breast-Feeding Considerations Mitotane has been detected in human breast milk. Due to the potential for serious adverse reactions in the nursing infant, breast-feeding should be discontinued until plasma levels are no longer detected.
Warnings/Precautions Hazardous agent - use appropriate precautions for handling and disposal (NIOSH 2014 [group 1]). Patients treated with mitotane may develop adrenal insufficiency; steroid replacement with glucocorticoid, and sometimes mineralocorticoid, is necessary. It has been recommended that steroid replacement therapy be initiated at the start of therapy, rather than waiting for evidence of adrenal insufficiency. **[U.S. Boxed Warning]: Because the primary action of mitotane is through adrenal suppression, discontinue mitotane temporarily with onset of shock or severe trauma;** ▶

◀ **administer appropriate steroid coverage.** Because mitotane can increase the metabolism of exogenous steroids, higher than usual replacement steroid doses may be required. Mitotane increases hormone binding proteins; monitor free cortisol and corticotropin levels for optimal replacement. Surgically remove tumor tissues from metastatic masses prior to initiation of treatment; rapid cytotoxic effect may cause tumor hemorrhage. Long-term (>2 years) use may lead to brain damage or functional impairment; observe patients for neurotoxicity (neurologic and behavior) regularly. Plasma concentrations >20 mcg/mL are associated with an increased incidence of higher-grade neurotoxicity. Neurologic impairment may reverse upon discontinuation. Use caution with hepatic impairment (other than metastatic lesions from adrenal cortex); metabolism may be decreased. Other CNS adverse effects, including lethargy, sedation, and vertigo may occur; patients must be cautioned about performing tasks which require mental alertness (eg, operating machinery or driving). CNS effects may be potentiated when used with other sedative drugs or ethanol. The manufacturer recommends initiating treatment within a hospital environment until a stabilized dose is achieved. Continue treatment as long as clinical benefit (maintenance of clinical status or metastatic lesion grown slowing) is observed. Clinical benefit is usually observed within 3 months at maximum tolerated dose, although 10% of patients may require more than 3 months for benefit. Continuous treatment at the maximum tolerated dose is generally the best approach. Some patients have been treated intermittently, restarting when severe symptoms reappear, although often response is no longer observed after 3 or 4 courses of intermittent treatment. Potentially significant drug-drug interactions may exist, requiring dose or frequency adjustment, additional monitoring, and/or selection of alternative therapy. Prolonged bleeding time may occur; consider bleeding possibility prior to any surgical intervention. **[U.S. Boxed Warnings]: Should be administered under the supervision of an experienced cancer chemotherapy physician.** Mitotane is associated with a moderate emetic potential; antiemetics may be needed to prevent nausea and vomiting.

Adverse Reactions The majority of adverse events are dose-dependent.

>10%:

Central nervous system: Central nervous system depression (32%), lethargy/ drowsiness (25%), dizziness/vertigo (15%)

Dermatologic: Skin rash (15%)

Gastrointestinal: Anorexia (24%), nausea (39%), vomiting (37%), diarrhea (13%)

Neuromuscular & skeletal: Weakness (12%)

1% to 10%:

Central nervous system: Headache (5%), confusion (3%)

Neuromuscular & skeletal: Tremor (3%)

<1%, postmarketing, and/or case reports: Abnormal thyroid function test, adrenocortical insufficiency, albuminuria, anemia, ataxia, autoimmune hepatitis, blurred vision, brain damage (may be reversible) cataract, decreased protein-bound iodine, diplopia, dysarthria, flushing, generalized aches, growth suppression, gynecomastia, hematuria, hemorrhagic cystitis, hepatitis, hypercholesterolemia, hyperpyrexia, hypertension, hypertriglyceridemia, hypogonadism (primary), hypouricemia, increased gamma-glutamyl transferase, increased liver enzymes, increased serum transaminases, increased serum triglycerides, increased sex hormone binding globulin, leukopenia, macular edema, maculopathy, memory impairment, mental deficiency, mucositis, myalgia, neuropathy, neutropenia, orthostatic hypotension, prolonged

bleeding time, psychological disturbances (neuro), retinopathy (toxic), thrombocytopenia

Drug Interactions

Metabolism/Transport Effects Induces CYP3A4 (strong)

Avoid Concomitant Use

Avoid concomitant use of Mitotane with any of the following: Abiraterone Acetate; Antihepaciviral Combination Products; Apixaban; Apremilast; Aprepitant; Artemether; Axitinib; Bedaquiline; Boceprevir; Bortezomib; Bosutinib; Cabozantinib; Cariprazine; Ceritinib; CloZAPine; Cobimetinib; Crizotinib; Dabrafenib; Daclatasvir; Dienogest; Dronedarone; Eliglustat; Enzalutamide; Everolimus; Flibanserin; Ibrutinib; Idelalisib; Irinotecan Products; Isavuconazonium Sulfate; Itraconazole; Ivabradine; Ivacaftor; Lapatinib; Lumefantrine; Lurasidone; Macitentan; Mifepristone; Naloxegol; Netupitant; NIFEdipine; Nilotinib; NiMODipine; Nisoldipine; Olaparib; Osimertinib; Palbociclib; Panobinostat; PAZOPanib; Perampanel; PONATinib; Praziquantel; Ranolazine; Regorafenib; Rivaroxaban; Roflumilast; RomiDEPsin; Simeprevir; Sonidegib; SORAfenib; Suvorexant; Tasimelteon; Telaprevir; Ticagrelor; Tofacitinib; Tolvaptan; Toremifene; Trabectedin; Ulipristal; Vandetanib; Vemurafenib; VinCRIStine (Liposomal); Vorapaxar

Increased Effect/Toxicity

Mitotane may increase the levels/effects of: Clarithromycin; Ifosfamide

The levels/effects of Mitotane may be increased by: Clarithromycin; MAO Inhibitors

Decreased Effect

Mitotane may decrease the levels/effects of: Abiraterone Acetate; Antihepaciviral Combination Products; Apixaban; Apremilast; Aprepitant; ARIPiprazole; ARIPiprazole Lauroxil; Artemether; Axitinib; Bedaquiline; Boceprevir; Bortezomib; Bosutinib; Brentuximab Vedotin; Brexpiprazole; Cabozantinib; Cannabidiol; Cannabis; Cariprazine; Ceritinib; Clarithromycin; CloZAPine; Cobimetinib; Corticosteroids (Systemic); Crizotinib; CYP3A4 Substrates; Dabrafenib; Daclatasvir; Dasatinib; Dexamethasone (Systemic); Dienogest; DOXOrubicin (Conventional); Dronabinol; Dronedarone; Eliglustat; Enzalutamide; Erlotinib; Etoposide; Etoposide Phosphate; Everolimus; Exemestane; FentaNYL; Flibanserin; Gefitinib; GuanFACINE; Ibrutinib; Idelalisib; Ifosfamide; Imatinib; Irinotecan Products; Isavuconazonium Sulfate; Itraconazole; Ivabradine; Ivacaftor; Ixabepilone; Lapatinib; Linagliptin; Lumefantrine; Lurasidone; Macitentan; Maraviroc; MethylPREDNISolone; Mifepristone; Naloxegol; Netupitant; NIFEdipine; Nilotinib; NiMODipine; Nisoldipine; Olaparib; Osimertinib; Palbociclib; Panobinostat; PAZOPanib; Perampanel; PONATinib; Praziquantel; Propafenone; QUEtiapine; Ranolazine; Regorafenib; Rivaroxaban; Roflumilast; Rolapitant; RomiDEPsin; Saxagliptin; Simeprevir; Sonidegib; SORAfenib; SUNItinib; Suvorexant; Tadalafil; Tasimelteon; Telaprevir; Tetrahydrocannabinol; Ticagrelor; Tofacitinib; Tolvaptan; Toremifene; Trabectedin; Ulipristal; Vandetanib; Vemurafenib; Vilazodone; VinCRIStine (Liposomal); Vorapaxar; Vortioxetine; Zaleplon; Zuclopenthixol

The levels/effects of Mitotane may be decreased by: Spironolactone

Storage/Stability Store at 25°C (77°F); excursions are permitted between 15°C and 30°C (59°F and 86°F).

Mechanism of Action Adrenolytic agent which causes adrenal cortical atrophy; affects mitochondria in adrenal cortical cells and decreases production of cortisol; also alters the peripheral metabolism of steroids

Pharmacodynamics/Kinetics
Duration: Blood levels undetectable in most patients after 6-9 weeks.
Absorption: Oral: ~40%
Distribution: Stored mainly in fat tissue but is found in all body tissues
Metabolism: Hepatic and other tissues
Half-life elimination: 18-159 days
Time to peak, serum: 3-5 hours
Excretion: Urine (~10%, as metabolites); feces (1% to 17%, as metabolites)

Dosing
Adult & Geriatric Note: Mitotane is associated with a moderate emetic potential; antiemetics may be needed to prevent nausea and vomiting.

Adrenocortical carcinoma: Oral: Initial: 2 to 6 g daily in 3 to 4 divided doses, then increase incrementally to 9 to 10 g daily in 3 to 4 divided doses (maximum tolerated range: 2 to 16 g daily, usually 9 to 10 g daily; maximum dose studied: 18 to 19 g daily); continue as long as clinical benefit is demonstrated

Off-label dosing: Initial 1 to 2 g daily; increase by 1 to 2 g daily at 1 to 2 week intervals as tolerated to a maximum of 6 to 10 g daily; usual dose 4 to 5 g daily (Veytsman, 2009)

Cushing syndrome (off-label use): Oral: Initial dose: 500 mg 3 times daily; maximum dose: 3 g 3 times daily (Biller, 2008)

Renal Impairment No dosage adjustment provided in manufacturer's labeling.

Hepatic Impairment No dosage adjustment provided in manufacturer's labeling. However, drug accumulation may occur in patients with liver disease; use with caution.

Adjustment for Toxicity
Severe side effects: Reduce dose until a maximum tolerated dose is achieved.
Significant neuropsychiatric adverse effects: Withhold treatment for at least 1 week and restart at a lower dose (Allolio, 2006).

Administration Note: Mitotane is associated with a moderate emetic potential; antiemetics may be needed to prevent nausea and vomiting.

Oral: Administer in 3 to 4 divided doses/day. Do not crush tablets. Mitotane is associated with a moderate emetic potential; antiemetics may be needed to prevent nausea and vomiting.

Hazardous agent; use appropriate precautions for handling and disposal (NIOSH 2014 [group 1]). Wear impervious gloves when handling; avoid exposure to crushed or broken tablets.

Emetic Potential Moderate (30% to 90%)

Monitoring Parameters
Adrenal function; neurologic assessments (including behavioral) at regular intervals with chronic (>2 years) use.
Monitor mitotane levels (gas chromatography-flame ionization assay) every 4-8 weeks until levels at 10-14 mg/L are attained, then monitor every 3 months; urinary free cortisol levels; TSH and free thyroxine every few months (Veytsman, 2009)

Dosage Forms Excipient information presented when available (limited, particularly for generics); consult specific product labeling.
Tablet, Oral:
Lysodren: 500 mg [scored]

MitoXANtrone (mye toe ZAN trone)

Related Information

Hematopoietic Stem Cell Transplantation *on page 2272*

Management of Chemotherapy-Induced Nausea and Vomiting in Adults *on page 2142*

Management of Drug Extravasations *on page 2159*

Prevention of Chemotherapy-Induced Nausea and Vomiting in Children *on page 2203*

Safe Handling of Hazardous Drugs *on page 2292*

Brand Names: Canada Mitoxantrone Injection; Mitoxantrone Injection USP

Index Terms CL-232315; DHAD; DHAQ; Dihydroxyanthracenedione; Dihydroxyanthracenedione Dihydrochloride; Mitoxantrone Dihydrochloride; Mitoxantrone HCl; Mitoxantrone Hydrochloride; Mitozantrone; Novantrone

Pharmacologic Category Antineoplastic Agent, Anthracenedione; Antineoplastic Agent, Topoisomerase II Inhibitor

Use Initial treatment of acute nonlymphocytic leukemias (ANLL [includes myelogenous, promyelocytic, monocytic and erythroid leukemias]); treatment of advanced hormone-refractory prostate cancer; secondary progressive or relapsing-remitting multiple sclerosis (MS)

Canadian labeling: Additional uses (not in U.S. labeling): Treatment of metastatic breast cancer, relapsed leukemia (adults), lymphoma, and hepatocellular carcinoma

Labeled Contraindications Hypersensitivity to mitoxantrone or any component of the formulation

Canadian labeling: Additional contraindications (not in U.S. labeling): Prior hypersensitivity to anthracyclines; prior substantial anthracycline exposure and abnormal cardiac function prior to initiation of mitoxantrone therapy; presence of severe myelosuppression due to prior chemo- and/or radiotherapy; severe hepatic impairment; intrathecal administration

Pregnancy Considerations Adverse events have been observed in animal reproduction studies. Based on the mechanism of action, mitoxantrone may cause fetal harm if administered during pregnancy. Use of effective contraception during therapy is recommended. Information related to pregnancy outcomes following maternal use of mitoxantrone in pregnancy is limited (Amato 2015; Houtchens 2013; NTP 2013).

Infertility and amenorrhea have been reported in women with MS using mitoxantrone (Amato 2015; Houtchens 2013). Women with multiple sclerosis who are of reproductive potential should have a pregnancy test prior to each dose. Women who wish to become pregnant should discontinue therapy at least 2 to 3 months prior to conception (Houtchens 2013).

The European Society for Medical Oncology has published guidelines for diagnosis, treatment, and follow-up of cancer during pregnancy. The guidelines recommend referral to a facility with expertise in cancer during pregnancy and encourage a multidisciplinary team (obstetrician, neonatologist, oncology team). In general, if chemotherapy is indicated, it should be avoided in the first trimester, there should be a 3-week time period between the last chemotherapy dose and anticipated delivery, and chemotherapy should not be administered beyond week 33 of gestation (Peccatori 2013).

◀ **Breast-Feeding Considerations** Mitoxantrone is excreted in human milk and significant concentrations (18 ng/mL) have been reported for 28 days after the last administration. Due to the potential for serious adverse reactions in the nursing infant, the manufacturer recommends that breast-feeding be discontinued before starting treatment.

Warnings/Precautions Hazardous agent - use appropriate precautions for handling and disposal (NIOSH 2014 [group 1]).

[U.S. Boxed Warning]: Usually should not be administered if baseline neutrophil count <1500 cells/mm³ (except for treatment of ANLL). Monitor blood counts and monitor for infection due to neutropenia. Treatment may lead to severe myelosuppression; unless the expected benefit outweighs the risk, use is generally not recommended in patients with preexisting myelosuppression from prior chemotherapy.

[U.S. Boxed Warning]: May cause myocardial toxicity and potentially-fatal heart failure (HF); risk increases with cumulative dosing. Effects may occur during therapy or may be delayed (months or years after completion of therapy). Predisposing factors for mitoxantrone-induced cardiotoxicity include prior anthracycline or anthracenedione therapy, prior cardiovascular disease, concomitant use of cardiotoxic drugs, and mediastinal/pericardial irradiation, although may also occur in patients without risk factors. Prior to therapy initiation, evaluate all patients for cardiac-related signs/symptoms, including history, physical exam, and ECG; and evaluate baseline left ventricular ejection fraction (LVEF) with echocardiogram or multigated radionuclide angiography (MUGA) or MRI. Not recommended for use in MS patients when LVEF <50%, or baseline LVEF below the lower limit of normal (LLN). Evaluate for cardiac signs/symptoms (by history, physical exam, and ECG) and evaluate LVEF (using same method as baseline LVEF) in MS patients prior to each dose and if signs/symptoms of HF develop. Use in MS should be limited to a cumulative dose of ≤140 mg/m², and discontinued if LVEF falls below LLN or a significant decrease in LVEF is observed; decreases in LVEF and HF have been observed in patients with MS who have received cumulative doses <100 mg/m². Patients with MS should undergo annual LVEF evaluation following discontinuation of therapy to monitor for delayed cardiotoxicity.

[U.S. Boxed Warning]: For IV administration only, into a free-flowing IV; may cause severe local tissue damage if extravasation occurs; do not administer subcutaneously, intramuscularly, or intra-arterially. Do not administer intrathecally; may cause serious and permanent neurologic damage. Irritant with vesicant-like properties; extravasation resulting in burning, erythema, pain, swelling and skin discoloration (blue) has been reported; may result in tissue necrosis and require debridement for skin graft. Ensure proper needle or catheter placement prior to and during infusion. Avoid extravasation. May cause urine, saliva, tears, and sweat to turn blue-green for 24 hours postinfusion. Whites of eyes may have blue-green tinge. [U.S. Boxed Warning]: Treatment with mitoxantrone increases the risk of developing secondary acute myelogenous leukemia (AML) in patients with cancer and in patients with MS; acute promyelocytic leukemia (APL) has also been observed. Symptoms of acute leukemia include excessive bruising, bleeding and recurrent infections. The risk for secondary leukemia is increased in patients who are heavily pretreated, with higher doses, and with combination chemotherapy.

[U.S. Boxed Warning]: Should be administered under the supervision of a physician experienced in cancer chemotherapy agents. Dosage should be reduced in patients with impaired hepatobiliary function (clearance is reduced). Canadian labeling contraindicates use in severe hepatic impairment. Not for treatment of multiple sclerosis in patients with concurrent hepatic impairment. Not for treatment of primary progressive multiple sclerosis. Rapid lysis of tumor cells may lead to hyperuricemia.

Adverse Reactions Includes events reported with any indication; incidence varies based on treatment, dose, and/or concomitant medications

>10%:

Cardiovascular: Edema (10% to 30%), arrhythmia (3% to 18%), cardiac function changes (≤18%), ECG changes (≤11%)

Central nervous system: Fever (6% to 78%), pain (8% to 41%), fatigue (≤39%), headache (6% to 13%)

Dermatologic: Alopecia (20% to 61%), nail bed changes (≤11%), petechiae/bruising (6% to 11%)

Endocrine & metabolic: Menstrual disorder (26% to 61%), amenorrhea (28% to 53%), hyperglycemia (10% to 31%)

Gastrointestinal: Nausea (26% to 76%), vomiting (6% to 72%), diarrhea (14% to 47%), mucositis (10% to 29%; onset: ≤1 week), stomatitis (8% to 29%; onset: ≤1 week), anorexia (22% to 25%), weight gain/loss (13% to 17%), constipation (10% to 16%), GI bleeding (2% to 16%), abdominal pain (9% to 15%), dyspepsia (5% to 14%)

Genitourinary: Urinary tract infection (7% to 32%), abnormal urine (5% to 11%)

Hematologic: Neutropenia (79% to 100%; onset: ≤3 weeks; grade 4: 23% to 54%), leukopenia (9% to 100%), lymphopenia (72% to 95%), anemia/hemoglobin decreased (5% to 75%) thrombocytopenia (33% to 39%; grades 3/4: 3% to 4%), neutropenic fever (≤11%)

Hepatic: Alkaline phosphatase increased (≤37%), transaminases increased (5% to 20%), GGT increased (3% to 15%)

Neuromuscular & skeletal: Weakness (≤24%)

Renal: BUN increased (≤22%), creatinine increased (≤13%), hematuria (≤11%)

Respiratory: Upper respiratory tract infection (7% to 53%), pharyngitis (≤19%), dyspnea (6% to 18%), cough (5% to 13%)

Miscellaneous: Infection (4% to 60%), sepsis (ANLL 31% to 34%), fungal infection (9% to 15%)

1% to 10%:

Cardiovascular: CHF (≤5%), ischemia (≤5%), LVEF decreased (≤5%), hypertension (≤4%)

Central nervous system: Chills (≤5%), anxiety (5%), depression (5%), seizure (2% to 4%)

Dermatologic: Cutaneous mycosis (≤10%), skin infection (≤5%)

Endocrine & metabolic: Hypocalcemia (10%), hypokalemia (7% to 10%), hyponatremia (9%), menorrhagia (7%)

Gastrointestinal: Aphthosis (≤10%)

Genitourinary: Impotence (≤7%), sterility (≤5%)

Hematologic: Granulocytopenia (6%), hemorrhage (5% to 6%), secondary acute leukemias (≤3%; includes AML, APL)

Hepatic: Jaundice (3% to 7%)

Neuromuscular & skeletal: Back pain (6% to 8%), myalgia (≤5%), arthralgia (≤5%)

Ocular: Conjunctivitis (≤5%), blurred vision (≤3%)

Renal: Renal failure (≤8%), proteinuria (≤6%)

Respiratory: Rhinitis (10%), pneumonia (≤9%), sinusitis (≤6%)

Miscellaneous: Systemic infection (≤10%), diaphoresis (≤9%)

<1%, postmarketing, and/or case reports: Allergic reaction, anaphylactoid reactions, anaphylaxis, chest pain, dehydration; extravasation at injection site (may result in burning, erythema, pain, skin discoloration, swelling, or tissue necrosis); interstitial pneumonitis (with combination chemotherapy), hyperuricemia, hypotension, phlebitis at the infusion site, rash, sclera discoloration (blue); tachycardia, urine discoloration (blue-green), urticaria

Drug Interactions

Metabolism/Transport Effects Substrate of BCRP

Avoid Concomitant Use

Avoid concomitant use of MitoXANtrone with any of the following: BCG (Intravesical); CloZAPine; Dipyrone; Natalizumab; Pimecrolimus; Tacrolimus (Topical); Tofacitinib; Vaccines (Live)

Increased Effect/Toxicity

MitoXANtrone may increase the levels/effects of: CloZAPine; Fingolimod; Leflunomide; Natalizumab; Tofacitinib; Vaccines (Live)

The levels/effects of MitoXANtrone may be increased by: CycloSPORINE (Systemic); Denosumab; Dipyrone; Eltrombopag; Pimecrolimus; Roflumilast; Rolapitant; Tacrolimus (Topical); Teriflunomide; Trastuzumab

Decreased Effect

MitoXANtrone may decrease the levels/effects of: BCG (Intravesical); Coccidioides immitis Skin Test; Sipuleucel-T; Vaccines (Inactivated); Vaccines (Live)

The levels/effects of MitoXANtrone may be decreased by: Echinacea

Storage/Stability Store intact vials at 15°C to 25°C (59°F to 77°F); do not freeze. Opened vials may be stored at room temperature for 7 days or under refrigeration for up to 14 days. Solutions diluted for administration are stable for 7 days at room temperature or under refrigeration, although the manufacturer recommends immediate use.

Preparation for Administration Hazardous agent; use appropriate precautions for handling and disposal (NIOSH 2014 [group 1]). Dilute in at least 50 mL of NS or D_5W.

Mechanism of Action Related to the anthracyclines, mitoxantrone intercalates into DNA resulting in cross-links and strand breaks; binds to nucleic acids and inhibits DNA and RNA synthesis by template disordering and steric obstruction; replication is decreased by binding to DNA topoisomerase II and seems to inhibit the incorporation of uridine into RNA and thymidine into DNA; active throughout entire cell cycle (cell-cycle nonspecific)

Pharmacodynamics/Kinetics

Absorption: Oral: Poor

Distribution: V_d: 14 L/kg; V_{dss}: >1000 L/m²; distributes extensively into tissue (pleural fluid, kidney, thyroid, liver, heart) and red blood cells

Protein binding: 78%

Metabolism: Hepatic; pathway not determined

Half-life elimination: Terminal: 23-215 hours (median: ~75 hours); may be prolonged with hepatic impairment

Excretion: Feces (25%); urine (6% to 11%; 65% as unchanged drug)

Dosing

Adult & Geriatric Details concerning dosing in combination regimens should also be consulted.

U.S. labeling:

Acute nonlymphocytic leukemias (ANLL):

Acute myeloid leukemia (AML) induction: 12 mg/m^2 once daily for 3 days (in combination with cytarabine); for incomplete response, may repeat (7-10 days later) at 12 mg/m^2 once daily for 2 days (in combination with cytarabine) (Arlin, 1990)

AML consolidation (beginning ~6 weeks after initiation of the final induction course): 12 mg/m^2 once daily for 2 days (in combination with cytarabine), repeat in 4 weeks (Arlin, 1990)

Multiple sclerosis: 12 mg/m^2 every 3 months (maximum lifetime cumulative dose: 140 mg/m^2; discontinue use with LVEF <50% or clinically significant reduction in LVEF)

Prostate cancer (advanced, hormone-refractory): 12-14 mg/m^2 every 3 weeks (in combination with corticosteroids)

Canadian labeling:

Acute nonlymphocytic leukemias (ANLL):

AML induction: 10-12 mg/m^2 once daily for 3 days (in combination with cytarabine); for incomplete response, may repeat at 10-12 mg/m^2 once daily for 2 days (in combination with cytarabine)

AML consolidation (beginning ~6 weeks after initiation of the final induction course): 12 mg/m^2 once daily for 2 days (in combination with cytarabine), repeat in 4 weeks

Acute leukemias (relapsed): Induction: 12 mg/m^2 once daily for 5 consecutive days; may repeat once if needed (at the same dose and duration)

Breast cancer (metastatic), lymphoma: Initial: Single agent: 14 mg/m^2 every 21 days; reduce initial dose to ≤12 mg/m^2 for myelosuppression due to previous treatment or for poor general health. When used in combination with other agents, reduce initial dose to 10-12 mg/m^2

Hepatocellular cancer: Initial: Single agent: 14 mg/m^2 every 21 days; reduce initial dose to ≤12 mg/m^2 for myelosuppression due to previous treatment or for poor general health

Adult off-label uses and/or dosing:

AML, refractory:

CLAG-M regimen: 10 mg/m^2 once daily for 3 days (in combination with cladribine, cytarabine, and filgrastim), may repeat once if needed (Wierzbowska, 2008)

MEC or EMA regimen: 6 mg/m^2 once daily for 6 days (in combination with cytarabine and etoposide) (Amadori, 1991)

Mitoxantrone/Etoposide: 10 mg/m^2 once daily for 5 days (in combination with etoposide) (Ho, 1988)

APL consolidation phase (second course): 10 mg/m^2 once daily for 5 days (Sanz, 2004)

Hodgkin lymphoma, refractory:

MINE-ESHAP regimen: 10 mg/m^2 on day 1 every 28 days for up to 2 cycles (MINE is combination with mesna, ifosfamide, mitoxantrone, and etoposide; MINE alternates with ESHAP for up to 2 cycles of each) (Fernandez, 2010)

VIM-D regimen: 10 mg/m^2 on day 1 every 28 days (in combination with etoposide, ifosfamide, mesna, and dexamethasone) (Phillips, 1990)

◀ **Non-Hodgkin lymphoma (as part of combination chemotherapy regimens):**
CNOP regimen: 10 mg/m^2 every 21 days (Bessell, 2003)
FCMR regimen: 8 mg/m^2 every 28 days (Forstpointner, 2004)
FMR regimen: 10 mg/m^2 every 21 days (Zinzani, 2004)
FND regimen: 10 mg/m^2 every 28 days (Tsimberidou, 2002)
MINE-ESHAP regimen: 8 mg/m^2 every 21 days for 6 cycles (MINE is combination with mesna, ifosfamide, mitoxantrone, and etoposide; followed by ESHAP) (Rodriguez, 1995)

Stem cell transplantation, autologous: 60 mg/m^2 administered 4-5 days prior to autografting (as 3 divided doses over 1 hour each at 1-2 hour intervals on the same day; in combination with other chemotherapeutic agent[s]) (Oyan, 2006; Tarella, 2001)

Pediatric Details concerning dosing in combination regimens should also be consulted.

Acute nonlymphocytic leukemias: IV:
Acute myeloid leukemia (AML) consolidation phase (second course; off-label use): 10 mg/m^2 once daily for 5 days (in combination with cytarabine) (Stevens, 1998)
Acute promyelocytic leukemia (APL) consolidation phase (second course; off-label use): 10 mg/m^2 once daily for 5 days (Ortega, 2005; Sanz, 2004)

Renal Impairment No dosage adjustment provided in manufacturer's labeling (has not been studied).
Hemodialysis: Supplemental dose is not necessary
Peritoneal dialysis: Supplemental dose is not necessary
Elderly: Clearance is decreased in elderly patients; use with caution

Hepatic Impairment
U.S. labeling: No dosage adjustment provided in the manufacturer's labeling; however, clearance is reduced in hepatic dysfunction. Patients with severe hepatic dysfunction (bilirubin >3.4 mg/dL) have an AUC of 3 times greater than patients with normal hepatic function; consider dose adjustments. **Note:** MS patients with hepatic impairment should not receive mitoxantrone.
Canadian labeling:
Mild-to-moderate impairment: No specific dosage adjustment provided; consider dose adjustments and monitor closely.
Severe impairment: Use is contraindicated.

Obesity *ASCO Guidelines for appropriate chemotherapy dosing in obese adults with cancer:* Utilize patient's actual body weight (full weight) for calculation of body surface area- or weight-based dosing, particularly when the intent of therapy is curative; manage regimen-related toxicities in the same manner as for nonobese patients; if a dose reduction is utilized due to toxicity, consider resumption of full weight-based dosing with subsequent cycles, especially if cause of toxicity (eg, hepatic or renal impairment) is resolved (Griggs, 2012).

Adjustment for Toxicity
ANLL patients: Severe or life-threatening nonhematologic toxicity: Withhold treatment until toxicity resolves
MS patients:
Neutrophils <1500/mm^3: Use is not recommended.
Signs/symptoms of HF: Evaluate for cardiac signs/symptoms and LVEF.
LVEF <50% or baseline LVEF below the lower limit of normal (LLN): Use is not recommended.

Canadian labeling (not in U.S. labeling): **Hepatocellular cancer, lymphoma, or breast cancer (metastatic):**

WBC nadir >1500/mm³ **and** platelet nadir >50,000/mm³ and recovery ≤21 days: Repeat previous dose or increase dose by 2 mg/m² if myelosuppression is inadequate.

WBC nadir >1500/mm³ **and** platelet nadir >50,000/mm³ and recovery >21 days: Withhold treatment until recovery then resume at previous dose.

WBC nadir <1500/mm³ **or** platelet nadir <50,000/mm³ (regardless of recovery time): Withhold treatment until recovery then decrease previous dose by 2 mg/m².

WBC nadir <1000/mm³ **or** platelet nadir <25,000/mm³ (regardless of recovery time): Withhold treatment until recovery then decrease previous dose by 4 mg/m².

Combination Regimens

Leukemia, acute myeloid:
5 + 2 (Cytarabine-Mitoxantrone) (AML Consolidation) on page 1816
7 + 3 (Cytarabine-Mitoxantrone) (AML Induction) on page 1818
CLAG-M (AML Induction) on page 1917
MEC-G (AML Induction) on page 2032
Mitoxantrone-Etoposide (AML Induction) on page 2037
Mitoxantrone-Etoposide-Cytarabine (AML) on page 2038

Leukemia, acute promyelocytic: Tretinoin-Idarubicin (APL) on page 2099

Lymphoma, Hodgkin:
MINE-ESHAP (Hodgkin) on page 2036
VIM-D (Hodgkin) on page 2107

Lymphoma, non-Hodgkin:
Fludarabine-Cyclophosphamide-Mitoxantrone-Rituximab on page 1972
Fludarabine-Mitoxantrone-Dexamethasone (NHL) on page 1975
Fludarabine-Mitoxantrone-Dexamethasone-Rituximab on page 1975

Prostate cancer: Mitoxantrone-Prednisone (Prostate) on page 2038

Administration For IV administration only; do not administer intrathecally, subcutaneously, intramuscularly or intra-arterially. Must be diluted prior to use. Usually administered as a short IV infusion over 5-15 minutes; do not infuse over <3-5 minutes.

High doses for bone marrow transplant (off-label use) are usually given as 3 divided doses over 1 hour each at 1-2 hour intervals on the same day (Oyan, 2006; Tarella, 2001).

Irritant with vesicant-like properties; ensure proper needle or catheter placement prior to and during infusion; avoid extravasation.

Extravasation management: If extravasation occurs, stop infusion immediately and disconnect (leave cannula/needle in place); gently aspirate extravasated solution (do **NOT** flush the line); remove needle/cannula; elevate extremity. Initiate antidote (dexrazoxane or dimethyl sulfate [DMSO]). Apply dry cold compresses for 20 minutes 4 times daily for 1-2 days (Perez Fidalgo, 2012); withhold cooling beginning 15 minutes before dexrazoxane infusion; continue withholding cooling until 15 minutes after infusion is completed. Topical DMSO should not be administered in combination with dexrazoxane; may lessen dexrazoxane efficacy.

Dexrazoxane: Adults: 1000 mg/m² (maximum dose: 2000 mg) IV (administer in a large vein remote from site of extravasation) over 1-2 hours days 1 and 2, then 500 mg/m² (maximum dose: 1000 mg) IV over 1-2 hours day 3; begin within 6 hours of extravasation. Day 2 and day 3 doses should be ▶

administered at approximately the same time (±3 hours) as the dose on day 1 (Mouridsen, 2007; Perez Fidalgo, 2012). **Note:** Reduce dexrazoxane dose by 50% in patients with moderate to severe renal impairment (CrCl <40 mL/minute).

DMSO: Children and Adults: Apply topically to a region covering twice the affected area every 8 hours for 7 days; begin within 10 minutes of extravasation; do not cover with a dressing (Perez Fidalgo, 2012).

Hazardous agent; use appropriate precautions for handling and disposal (NIOSH 2014 [group 1]).

Vesicant/Extravasation Risk Vesicant; see Management of Drug Extravasations on page 2159.

Emetic Potential Children and Adults: Low (10% to 30%)

Monitoring Parameters CBC with differential, serum uric acid (for leukemia treatment), liver function tests; for the treatment of multiple sclerosis, obtain pregnancy test; monitor injection site for extravasation

Cardiac monitoring: Prior to initiation, evaluate all patients for cardiac-related signs/symptoms, including history, physical exam, and ECG; evaluate baseline and periodic left ventricular ejection fraction (LVEF) with echocardiogram or multigated radionuclide angiography (MUGA) or MRI. In patients with MS, evaluate for cardiac signs/symptoms (by history, physical exam, and ECG) and evaluate LVEF (using same method as baseline LVEF) prior to each dose and if signs/symptoms of HF develop. Patients with MS should undergo annual LVEF evaluation following discontinuation of therapy to monitor for delayed cardiotoxicity.

Medication Guide Available Yes

Dosage Forms Excipient information presented when available (limited, particularly for generics); consult specific product labeling.

Concentrate, Intravenous:

Generic: 20 mg/10 mL (10 mL); 25 mg/12.5 mL (12.5 mL); 30 mg/15 mL (15 mL)

◆ **MoAb CD52** *see* Alemtuzumab *on page* 62

◆ **MOAB Ch14.18** *see* Dinutuximab *on page* 530

◆ **MOAB-CTLA-4** *see* Ipilimumab *on page* 942

◆ **MOAB HER2** *see* Trastuzumab *on page* 1685

◆ **Moi-Stir® [OTC]** *see* Saliva Substitute *on page* 1511

◆ **Monicure (Can)** *see* Fluconazole *on page* 725

◆ **Monoclate-P** *see* Antihemophilic Factor (Human) *on page* 117

◆ **Monoclonal Antibody 2C4** *see* Pertuzumab *on page* 1380

◆ **Monoclonal Antibody 5G1.1** *see* Eculizumab *on page* 580

◆ **Monoclonal Antibody ABX-EGF** *see* Panitumumab *on page* 1316

◆ **Monoclonal Antibody Anti-C5** *see* Eculizumab *on page* 580

◆ **Monoclonal Antibody Campath-1H** *see* Alemtuzumab *on page* 62

◆ **Monoclonal Antibody CD52** *see* Alemtuzumab *on page* 62

◆ **Mononine** *see* Factor IX (Human) *on page* 681

◆ **Moroctocog Alfa** *see* Antihemophilic Factor (Recombinant) *on page* 119

◆ **MorphaBond** *see* Morphine (Systemic) *on page* 1167

Morphine (Systemic) (MOR feen)

Brand Names: US Astramorph; AVINza [DSC]; Duramorph; Infumorph 200; Infumorph 500; Kadian; MS Contin; Oramorph SR [DSC]

Brand Names: Canada Doloral; Kadian; M-Eslon; M.O.S. 10; M.O.S. 20; M.O.S. 30; M.O.S.-SR; M.O.S.-Sulfate; Morphine Extra Forte Injection; Morphine Forte Injection; Morphine HP; Morphine LP Epidural; Morphine SR; Morphine-EPD; MS Contin; MS Contin SRT; MS-IR; Novo-Morphine SR; PMS-Morphine Sulfate SR; ratio-Morphine; ratio-Morphine SR; Sandoz-Morphine SR; Statex; Teva-Morphine SR

Index Terms MorphaBond; MS (error-prone abbreviation and should not be used); MSO$_4$ (error-prone abbreviation and should not be used); Oramorph SR; Roxanol

Pharmacologic Category Analgesic, Opioid

Use

Immediate-release oral products: Relief of moderate to severe acute and chronic pain for which use of an opioid analgesic is appropriate.

Injection: Relief of severe pain, such as myocardial infarction and severe injuries; relief of dyspnea of acute left ventricular failure and pulmonary edema; preanesthetic medication

Preservative-free injectable solution:

Infumorph: Used in continuous microinfusion devices for intrathecal or epidural administration in treatment of intractable chronic pain

Duramorph: For intravenous, epidural, or intrathecal administration in the management of pain for extended periods without attendant loss of motor, sensory, or sympathetic function. **Note:** Not for use in continuous microinfusion devices.

Extended-release oral products: Management of pain severe enough to require daily, around-the-clock, long-term opioid treatment and for which alternative treatment options are inadequate.

▶

◀ Limitations of use: Because of the risks of addiction, abuse, and misuse with opioids, even at recommended doses, and because of the greater risks of overdose and death with extended-release formulations, reserve extended-release formulations for use in patients for whom alternative treatment options (eg, nonopioid analgesics, immediate-release opioids) are ineffective, not tolerated, or would be otherwise inadequate to provide sufficient management of pain. MS Contin, Kadian, and Avinza are not indicated as as-needed analgesics.

Pregnancy Risk Factor C
Dosing

Adult These are guidelines and do not represent the doses that may be required in all patients. Doses and dosage intervals should be titrated to pain relief/prevention.

Acute pain (moderate to severe):

Oral (immediate-release formulations): Opioid naive: Initial: **Note:** Usual dosage range: 10 to 30 mg every 4 hours as needed. Patients with prior opioid exposure may require higher initial doses.
Solution: 10 to 20 mg every 4 hours as needed
Tablet: 15 to 30 mg every 4 hours as needed

IM, SubQ: **Note:** Repeated SubQ administration causes local tissue irritation, pain, and induration. The use of IM injections is no longer recommended especially for repeated administration due to painful administration, variable absorption and lag time to peak effect; other routes are more reliable and less painful (APS, 2008).
Initial: Opioid naive: 5 to 10 mg every 4 hours as needed; usual dosage range: 5 to 15 mg every 4 hours as needed. Patients with prior opioid exposure may require higher initial doses.

IV: Initial: Opioid naive: 2.5 to 5 mg every 3 to 4 hours; patients with prior opioid exposure may require higher initial doses. **Note:** Administration of 2 to 3 mg every 5 minutes until pain relief or if associated sedation, oxygen saturation <95%, or serious adverse event occurs may be appropriate in treating acute moderate to severe pain in settings such as the immediate postoperative period or the emergency department (Aubrun, 2012; Lvovschi, 2008); dose reduction in the immediate postoperative period (postanesthesia care unit) in the elderly is usually not necessary (Aubrun, 2002). A maximum cumulative dose (eg, 10 mg) prompting reevaluation of continued morphine use and/or dose should be included as part of any medication order intended for short-term use (eg, PACU orders). Refer to institution-specific protocols as appropriate.
Acute myocardial infarction, analgesia (off-label use): Initial management: 4 to 8 mg (lower doses in elderly patients); subsequently may give 2 to 8 mg every 5 to 15 minutes as needed (O'Gara, 2012)
Critically ill patients, analgesia (off-label dose): 2 to 4 mg every 1 to 2 hours **or** 4 to 8 mg every 3 to 4 hours as needed (Barr, 2013)

IV, SubQ continuous infusion: 0.8 to 10 mg/hour; usual range: Up to 80 mg/hour. **Note:** May administer a loading dose (amount administered should depend on severity of pain) prior to initiating the infusion. A continuous (basal) infusion is not recommended in an opioid-naive patient (ISMP, 2009)
Continuous infusion for critically ill patients: Usual dosage range: 2 to 30 mg/hour (Barr, 2013)

Patient-controlled analgesia (PCA) (APS, 2008): **Note:** In opioid-naive patients, consider lower end of dosing range:
Usual concentration: 1 mg/mL
Demand dose: Usual: 1 mg; range: 0.5 to 2.5 mg
Lockout interval: 5 to 10 minutes

Epidural: Pain management: **Note: Must be preservative free.** Administer with extreme caution and in reduced dosage to geriatric or debilitated patients. Vigilant monitoring is particularly important in these patients.
Single dose: **Lumbar region:** Astramorph/PF, Duramorph: 30 to 100 mcg/kg (optimal range: 2.5 to 3.75 mg; may depend upon patient comorbidities; Bujedo, 2012; Sultan, 2011)
Continuous infusion (may be combined with bupivacaine): 0.2 to 0.4 mg/hour (Bujedo, 2012)
Continuous microinfusion (Infumorph):
Opioid naive: Initial: 3.5 to 7.5 mg over 24 hours
Opioid tolerant: Initial: 4.5 to 10 mg over 24 hours, titrate to effect; usual maximum is ~30 mg per 24 hours

Intrathecal: **Note: Must be preservative free.** Administer with extreme caution and in reduced dosage to geriatric or debilitated patients. Intrathecal dose is usually $1/10$ (one-tenth) that of epidural dosage.
Opioid naive: Single dose: Lumbar region: Astramorph/PF, Duramorph: 0.1 to 0.3 mg (may provide adequate relief for up to 24 hours; APS, 2008); repeat doses are **not** recommended. If pain recurs within 24 hours of administration, use of an alternate route of administration is recommended. **Note:** Although product labeling recommends doses up to 1 mg, an analgesic ceiling exists with doses >0.3 mg and the risk of respiratory depression is higher with doses >0.3 mg (Rathmell, 2005).
Continuous microinfusion (Infumorph): Lumbar region: After initial in-hospital evaluation of response to single-dose injections (Astramorph/PF, Duramorph) the initial dose of Infumorph is 0.2 to 1 mg over 24 hours
Opioid tolerant: Continuous microinfusion (Infumorph): Lumbar region: Dosage range: 1 to 10 mg over 24 hours, titrate to effect; usual maximum is ~20 mg over 24 hours
Rectal: 10 to 20 mg every 3 to 4 hours

Chronic pain: Note: Patients taking opioids chronically may become tolerant and require doses higher than the usual dosage range to maintain the desired effect. Tolerance can be managed by appropriate dose titration. There is no optimal or maximal dose for morphine in chronic pain. The appropriate dose is one that relieves pain throughout its dosing interval without causing unmanageable side effects. Consider total daily dose, potency, prior opioid use, degree of opioid experience and tolerance, conversion from previous opioid (including opioid formulation), patient's general condition, concurrent medications, and type and severity of pain during prescribing process. Opioid tolerance is defined as: Patients already taking at least 60 mg of oral morphine daily, 25 mcg transdermal fentanyl per hour, 30 mg of oral oxycodone daily, 8 mg oral hydromorphone daily, 25 mg of oral oxymorphone daily, or an equivalent dose of another opioid for at least 1 week.

Oral (extended-release formulations): A patient's morphine requirement should be established using immediate-release formulations. Conversion to long-acting products may be considered when chronic, continuous treatment is required. Higher dosages should be reserved for use only in opioid-tolerant patients.

Capsules, extended release (Avinza): Daily dose administered once daily (for best results, administer at same time each day). **Note:** Avinza 90 mg and 120 mg are only indicated for use in opioid-tolerant patents.

Use as the first opioid analgesic or use in patients who are **not** opioid tolerant: Initial: 30 mg once daily

Conversion from other oral morphine formulations to Avinza: Total daily morphine dose given as once daily. The first dose of Avinza may be taken with the last dose of the immediate-release morphine. Maximum: 1600 mg daily due to fumaric acid content.

Conversion from other opioids to Avinza: Discontinue all other around-the-clock opioids when Avinza is initiated. Initial dose: 30 mg once daily; there are no established conversion ratios from other opioids to Avinza. Substantial interpatient variability exists in relative potency. Therefore, it is safer to underestimate a patient's daily oral morphine requirement and provide rescue medication (eg, immediate-release morphine) than to overestimate requirements. The first dose of Avinza may be taken with the last dose of the immediate-release opioid.

Titration and maintenance: Adjust in increments ≤30 mg daily every 3 to 4 days. Maximum: 1600 mg daily due to fumaric acid content.

Discontinuation of Avinza: Gradually titrate dose downward every 2 to 4 days. Do not discontinue abruptly.

Capsules, extended release (Kadian): **Note:** Kadian 100 mg, 130 mg, 150 mg, and 200 mg are only indicated for use in opioid-tolerant patients.

Use as the first opioid analgesic: Has not been evaluated. Use an immediate-release morphine formulation and then convert patients to Kadian in the same fashion as initiating therapy in a nonopioid-tolerant patient.

Use in patients who are **not** opioid tolerant: Initial: 30 mg once daily.

Conversion from other oral morphine formulations to Kadian: Total daily oral morphine dose may be either administered once daily or in 2 divided doses daily (every 12 hours).

Conversion from other opioids to Kadian: Discontinue all other around-the-clock opioids when Kadian is initiated. Initial dose: 30 mg once daily; there are no established conversion ratios from other opioids to Kadian. Substantial interpatient variability exists in relative potency. Therefore, it is safer to underestimate a patient's daily oral morphine requirement and provide rescue medication (eg, immediate-release morphine) than to overestimate requirements.

Titration and maintenance: Dose adjustments may be done every 1 to 2 days.

Discontinuation of Kadian: Gradually titrate dose downward every 2 to 4 days. Do not discontinue abruptly.

Tablets, extended release (MS Contin): **Note:** MS Contin 100 mg and 200 mg tablets are only indicated for use in opioid-tolerant patients.

Use as the first opioid analgesic: Initial: 15 mg every 8 to 12 hours

Use in patients who are **not** opioid tolerant: Initial: 15 mg every 12 hours.

Conversion from other oral morphine formulations to MS Contin: Total daily oral morphine dose may be either administered in 2 divided doses daily (every 12 hours) **or** in 3 divided doses (every 8 hours).

Conversion from other opioids to MS Contin: Discontinue all other around-the-clock opioids when MS Contin is initiated. Initial: 15 mg every 8 to 12 hours; there are no established conversion ratios from other opioids to MS Contin. Substantial interpatient variability exists in relative potency. Therefore, it is safer to underestimate a patient's daily oral morphine requirement and provide rescue medication (eg, immediate-release morphine) than to overestimate requirements.

Titration and maintenance: Dose adjustments may be done every 1 to 2 days.

Discontinuation of MS Contin: Gradually titrate dose downward. Do not discontinue abruptly.

Conversion from parenteral morphine or other opioids to extended-release formulations: Substantial interpatient variability exists in relative potency. Therefore, it is safer to underestimate a patient's daily oral morphine requirement and provide breakthrough pain relief with immediate-release morphine than to overestimate requirements. Consider the parenteral to oral morphine ratio or other oral or parenteral opioids to oral morphine conversions.

Parenteral to oral morphine ratio: Between 2 to 6 mg of oral morphine may be required for analgesia equivalent to 1 mg of parenteral morphine. An oral dose 3 times the daily parenteral dose may be sufficient in chronic pain settings.

Other parenteral or oral nonmorphine opioids to oral morphine: Specific recommendations are not available; refer to published relative potency data realizing that such ratios are only approximations. In general, it is safest to administer half of the estimated daily morphine requirement as the initial dose, and to manage inadequate analgesia by supplementation with immediate-release morphine.

Conversion from methadone to extended-release formulations: Close monitoring is required when converting methadone to another opioid. Ratio between methadone and other opioid agonists varies widely according to previous dose exposure. Methadone has a long half-life and can accumulate in the plasma.

Geriatric Refer to adult dosing. Use with caution; may require reduced dosage in the elderly and debilitated patients.

Pediatric These are guidelines and do not represent the doses that may be required in all patients. Doses and dosage intervals should be titrated to pain relief/prevention.

Acute pain (moderate to severe): Children >6 months and <50 kg:

Oral (immediate release formulations): 0.15 to 0.3 mg/kg every 3 to 4 hours as needed. **Note:** The American Pain Society recommends an initial dose of 0.3 mg/kg for children with severe pain (American Pain Society [APS], 2008)

IM, SubQ: 0.1 to 0.2 mg/kg; **Note:** Repeated SubQ administration causes local tissue irritation, pain, and induration. The use of IM injections is no longer recommended especially for repeated administration due to painful administration, variable absorption and lag time to peak effect.

IV: 0.05 to 0.3 mg/kg every 3 to 4 hours as needed, not to exceed 10 mg per dose

Continuous infusion: Initial: 10 to 30 **mcg/kg/hour**; titrate as needed to control pain

◀   *Patient-controlled analgesia (PCA)* (APS, 2008): **Note:** Opioid-naive: Consider lower end of dosing range:
    Usual concentration: 1 mg/mL
    Demand dose: Usual: 0.02 mg/kg/dose; range: 0.01 to 0.03 mg/kg/dose
    Lockout interval: 8 to 10 minutes
    Usual basal rate: 0 to 0.03 mg/kg/hour

Renal Impairment
  CrCl 10 to 50 mL/minute: Children and Adults: Administer at 75% of normal dose.
  CrCl <10 mL/minute: Children and Adults: Administer at 50% of normal dose.
  Intermittent HD:
    Adults: Administer 50% of normal dose. No supplemental dose necessary.
    Children: Administer 50% of normal dose.
  Peritoneal dialysis: Children: Administer 50% of normal dose.
  CRRT: Children and Adults: Administer 75% of normal dose, titrate.

Hepatic Impairment No dosage adjustment provided in manufacturer's labeling. Pharmacokinetics unchanged in mild liver disease; substantial extrahepatic metabolism may occur. In cirrhosis, increases in half-life and AUC suggest dosage adjustment required.

Additional Information Complete prescribing information should be consulted for additional detail.

Product Availability MorphaBond (morphine sulfate extended-release tablets): FDA approved October 2015; anticipated availability is currently unknown. Information pertaining to this product within the monograph is pending revision. Consult prescribing information for additional information.

Medication Guide Available Yes

Dosage Forms Excipient information presented when available (limited, particularly for generics); consult specific product labeling. [DSC] = Discontinued product

Capsule Extended Release 24 Hour, Oral, as sulfate:
  AVINza: 30 mg [DSC] [contains fd&c yellow #10 (quinoline yellow), fumaric acid]
  AVINza: 45 mg [DSC] [contains fd&c blue #2 (indigotine)]
  AVINza: 60 mg [DSC] [contains fumaric acid]
  AVINza: 75 mg [DSC]
  AVINza: 90 mg [DSC] [contains fd&c red #40, fumaric acid]
  AVINza: 120 mg [DSC] [contains brilliant blue fcf (fd&c blue #1), fumaric acid]
  Kadian: 10 mg [contains brilliant blue fcf (fd&c blue #1)]
  Kadian: 20 mg [contains fd&c yellow #10 (quinoline yellow)]
  Kadian: 30 mg [contains brilliant blue fcf (fd&c blue #1)]
  Kadian: 40 mg [contains brilliant blue fcf (fd&c blue #1), fd&c yellow #10 (quinoline yellow)]
  Kadian: 50 mg, 60 mg [contains brilliant blue fcf (fd&c blue #1), fd&c red #40]
  Kadian: 70 mg [DSC] [contains brilliant blue fcf (fd&c blue #1)]
  Kadian: 80 mg [contains brilliant blue fcf (fd&c blue #1), fd&c red #40, fd&c yellow #6 (sunset yellow)]
  Kadian: 100 mg [contains brilliant blue fcf (fd&c blue #1), fd&c yellow #10 (quinoline yellow)]
  Kadian: 130 mg [DSC] [contains brilliant blue fcf (fd&c blue #1), fd&c red #40, fd&c yellow #6 (sunset yellow)]
  Kadian: 150 mg [DSC] [contains brilliant blue fcf (fd&c blue #1), fd&c yellow #10 (quinoline yellow)]
  Kadian: 200 mg

Generic: 10 mg, 20 mg, 30 mg, 45 mg, 50 mg, 60 mg, 75 mg, 80 mg, 90 mg, 100 mg, 120 mg

Device, Intramuscular, as sulfate:
Generic: 10 mg/0.7 mL (0.7 mL)

Solution, Injection, as sulfate:
Astramorph: 1 mg/mL (10 mL [DSC])
Generic: 2 mg/mL (1 mL); 4 mg/mL (1 mL); 5 mg/mL (1 mL); 8 mg/mL (1 mL); 10 mg/mL (1 mL, 10 mL [DSC]); 15 mg/mL (1 mL, 20 mL [DSC])

Solution, Injection, as sulfate [preservative free]:
Astramorph: 0.5 mg/mL (2 mL, 10 mL [DSC]); 1 mg/mL (2 mL)
Duramorph: 0.5 mg/mL (10 mL); 1 mg/mL (10 mL)
Infumorph 200: 200 mg/20 mL (10 mg/mL) (20 mL) [antioxidant free]
Infumorph 500: 500 mg/20 mL (25 mg/mL) (20 mL) [antioxidant free]
Generic: 0.5 mg/mL (10 mL); 1 mg/mL (10 mL)

Solution, Intravenous, as sulfate:
Generic: 1 mg/mL (10 mL, 30 mL, 250 mL [DSC]); 5 mg/mL (30 mL [DSC]); 25 mg/mL (4 mL, 10 mL); 50 mg/mL (20 mL, 50 mL)

Solution, Intravenous, as sulfate [preservative free]:
Generic: 1 mg/mL (30 mL); 2 mg/mL (1 mL); 4 mg/mL (1 mL); 150 mg/30 mL (30 mL); 8 mg/mL (1 mL); 10 mg/mL (1 mL); 15 mg/mL (1 mL); 25 mg/mL (10 mL)

Solution, Oral, as sulfate:
Generic: 10 mg/5 mL (5 mL, 15 mL, 100 mL, 500 mL); 20 mg/5 mL (5 mL, 100 mL, 500 mL); 100 mg/5 mL (15 mL, 30 mL, 120 mL, 240 mL)

Suppository, Rectal, as sulfate:
Generic: 5 mg (12 ea); 10 mg (12 ea); 20 mg (12 ea); 30 mg (12 ea)

Tablet, Oral, as sulfate:
Generic: 15 mg, 30 mg

Tablet Extended Release, Oral, as sulfate:
MS Contin: 15 mg, 30 mg, 60 mg, 100 mg, 200 mg
Oramorph SR: 15 mg [DSC], 30 mg [DSC], 60 mg [DSC], 100 mg [DSC]
Generic: 15 mg, 30 mg, 60 mg, 100 mg, 200 mg

Dosage Forms: Canada Excipient information presented when available (limited, particularly for generics); consult specific product labeling.
Solution, oral, as hydrochloride:
Doloral: 1 mg/mL (10 mL, 250 mL, 500 mL); 5 mg/mL (10 mL, 250 mL, 500 mL)

Controlled Substance C-II

Morphine (Liposomal) (MOR feen)

Brand Names: US DepoDur

Index Terms Extended Release Epidural Morphine; Liposomal Morphine; MS (error-prone abbreviation and should not be used); MSO$_4$ (error-prone abbreviation and should not be used)

Pharmacologic Category Analgesic, Opioid

Use Epidural (lumbar) single-dose management of surgical pain

Pregnancy Risk Factor C

Dosing

Adult Surgical anesthesia: Epidural: Single-dose (extended release, Depo-Dur®): Lumbar epidural only; not recommended in patients <18 years of age:
Cesarean section: 10 mg (after clamping umbilical cord)
Lower abdominal/pelvic surgery: 10-15 mg

◀

Major orthopedic surgery of lower extremity: 15 mg; **Note:** Some patients may benefit from a 20 mg dose; however, the incidence of adverse effects may be increased.

To minimize the pharmacokinetic interaction resulting in higher peak serum concentrations of morphine, administer the test dose of the local anesthetic at least 15 minutes prior to administration. Use with epidural local anesthetics has not been studied. Other medications should not be administered into the epidural space for at least 48 hours after administration.

Geriatric Refer to adult dosing. Use with caution; may require reduced dosage in the elderly and debilitated patients.

Renal Impairment No dosage adjustment necessary.

Hepatic Impairment No dosage adjustment necessary.

Additional Information Complete prescribing information should be consulted for additional detail.

Dosage Forms Excipient information presented when available (limited, particularly for generics); consult specific product labeling.

Suspension, Epidural, as sulfate:

DepoDur: 10 mg/mL (1 mL); 15 mg/1.5 mL (1.5 mL)

Controlled Substance C-II

Mucosal Coating Agent (myoo KOH sul KOH ting AY gent)

Brand Names: US Episil; Gelclair; Mucotrol; MuGard; Orafate; ProThelial

Index Terms Mucosal Adherent Agent; Mucosal Barrier Agent; Mucosal Barrier Gel; Mucosal Bioadherent Agent; Mucosal Protective Agent; Oral Wound Care Products

Pharmacologic Category Gastrointestinal Agent, Miscellaneous

Use Mucosal protection: Management of oral mucosal pain and protection from further irritation caused by oral mucositis/stomatitis (resulting from chemotherapy or radiation therapy); irritation; lesions, periodontal and gingival inflammation, tooth extractions, and wounds due to oral surgery; chafing; minor lesions; traumatic ulcers, and abrasions caused by braces/ill-fitting dentures or disease; diffuse aphthous ulcers (canker sores).

Labeled Contraindications Hypersensitivity to any component of the formulation

Additional product-specific contraindications: Episil: Hypersensitivity to peanuts, soya, or peppermint oil

Warnings/Precautions May decrease absorption of sublingually administered medications. Episil contains alcohol (may cause irritation when applied), propylene glycol (may cause skin irritation), soy, and peppermint oil (may cause allergic reaction). Avoid eating or drinking for at least 1 hour (Mucotrol, MuGard, Orafate, ProThelial) or 30-60 minutes (Gelclair) following use. Consult a health care provider if no improvement is seen after 7 days of use. Orafate and ProThelial are safe if swallowed; however, evaluate swallowing capability prior to use to minimize incidental ingestion. Orafate and ProThelial may cause constipation if swallowed.

Adverse Reactions Postmarketing and/or case reports: Burning sensation in the mouth, mild inflammation and stinging of the oral cavity

Drug Interactions

Metabolism/Transport Effects None known.

Avoid Concomitant Use There are no known interactions where it is recommended to avoid concomitant use.

Increased Effect/Toxicity There are no known significant interactions involving an increase in effect.

Decreased Effect There are no known significant interactions involving a decrease in effect.

◀ **Storage/Stability** Store at room temperature. Protect from direct sunlight.

Episil: Store bottle in outer carton; use within 1 month of first use.

Gelclair: Use immediately after mixing with water.

Mucotrol: Do not refrigerate. Protect from moisture.

MuGard: Tightly seal bottle after use.

Preparation for Administration

Episil, Orafate, ProThelial: Does not require reconstitution.

Gelclair: Pour 15 mL (the contents of a single-use packet) into a glass and mix with water (refer to product information for details). Stir well and use immediately.

MuGard: Dilution prior to use is not recommended.

Mechanism of Action Adheres to the mucosal surface of mouth forming a protective film or coating over the irritated areas and lesions, protecting the lesion from further irritation and pain.

Dosing

Adult & Geriatric

Mucosal protection: Oral:

Episil: Apply 1-3 pumps to the oral cavity 2-3 times daily, or as needed; maximum duration for continuous use: 30 days

Gelclair: Rinse, gargle, and spit 15 mL (1 single-use packet) mixed in water 3 times daily, or as needed.

Mucotrol: Slowly dissolve 1 wafer by swishing around in the mouth, 3 times daily, or as needed

MuGard: Rinse with 5 mL 4-6 times daily or as needed; may use up to 10 mL if needed to fully coat inside of mouth

Orafate:

General dental use: Use 2 times daily for the first day or as directed and then for 1-4 weeks thereafter (maximum: 40 mL daily).

Following dental cleaning (scaling/root planing): Brush 1.25 mL into gingival pocket twice daily for a week (maximum: 40 mL daily)

Following tooth extraction: Place 1.25-2.5 mL into wound 3 times daily, then twice daily or as instructed (maximum: 40 mL daily)

Following tonsillectomy or uvuloplasty: Place 2.5-5 mL into tongue and swish, gargle, then spit as instructed (maximum: 40 mL daily)

ProThelial: 2.5-5 mL every 8 hours on the first day; 2.5-5 mL every 12 hours thereafter (maximum: 40 mL daily)

Administration

Episil: Remove protective cap from pump and prime pump by pumping into a paper cloth until an even liquid stream develops; firmly press pump (1-3 times) to apply liquid stream to oral cavity, distribute to affected areas of mouth and wait for gel and protective film to form. Do not swallow. Wait 5 minutes after use before eating and drinking.

Gelclair: Use before meals or as directed. Add 15 mL (1 single use packet) to water and stir (refer to product information for details); rinse around the mouth for a minimum of 1 minute (as long as possible) to coat the tongue, palate, throat, inside of cheeks, and all oral tissue thoroughly. Mixture should be gargled and spit out. Avoid eating or drinking for at least 30-60 minutes following treatment. If unable to rinse and gargle, apply directly to mouth using a sponge or swab. No adverse effects are anticipated is accidently swallowed.

Mucotrol: Wafer should be swished around the mouth and allowed to slowly dissolve. Avoid eating or drinking for at least 1 hour following treatment.

MuGard: Gently pour 5 mL into mouth and rinse entire oral cavity for at least 1 minute (if rinsing is painful, spread throughout mouth by gently rotating head); may use up to 10 mL to coat entire oral cavity if needed. May spit or swallow excess rinse. Avoid eating or drinking for at least 1 hour following treatment.

Orafate: Apply in any of the following ways: Brushed alone or with toothpaste over affected tooth-gum line area; mix with equal portions of dentifrice (tooth paste, powder, gel) and layer over areas of teeth cleaned by the dentist; dab directly on to affected gum margin; layer onto affected gum area; or place in mouth and suck back and forth through spaces between teeth. Safe if swallowed. Avoid eating or drinking for at least 1 hour following use.

ProThelial: Scoop paste from jar and place in mouth for 30 seconds. Use tongue to apply paste throughout mouth. Can be swished and then expectorated or swallowed. May also be applied with cotton swab to affected areas of the oral mucosa. Avoid eating or drinking for at least 1 hour following use.

Monitoring Parameters Monitor mucositis/stomatitis symptoms/severity

Dosage Forms Excipient information presented when available (limited, particularly for generics); consult specific product labeling. [DSC] = Discontinued product

Gel, Mouth/Throat:
  Gelclair: 15 mL/packet (15 mL)
Liquid, Mouth/Throat:
  Episil: (10 mL)
  MuGard: (5 mL, 240 mL) [contains benzyl alcohol]
Paste, Mouth/Throat:
  Orafate: 10% (30 mL) [contains methylparaben, propylparaben, saccharin sodium; strawberry flavor]
  ProThelial: 10% (125 mL, 250 mL, 500 mL) [contains methylparaben, propylparaben, saccharin sodium]
Wafer, Mouth/Throat:
  Mucotrol: (21 ea, 45 ea) [sugar free; mild licorice flavor]

♦ **Mucosal Protective Agent** see Mucosal Coating Agent on page 1175

♦ **Mucotrol** see Mucosal Coating Agent on page 1175

♦ **MuGard** see Mucosal Coating Agent on page 1175

♦ **Mustargen** see Mechlorethamine (Systemic) on page 1067

♦ **Mustine** see Mechlorethamine (Systemic) on page 1067

♦ **Mutamycin** see MitoMYcin (Systemic) on page 1149

♦ **Mutamycin® (Can)** see MitoMYcin (Systemic) on page 1149

♦ **Mycamine** see Micafungin on page 1148

♦ **Mycelex** see Clotrimazole (Oral) on page 356

Mycophenolate (mye koe FEN oh late)

Related Information

Hematopoietic Stem Cell Transplantation on page 2272
Safe Handling of Hazardous Drugs on page 2292

Brand Names: US CellCept; CellCept Intravenous; Myfortic

Brand Names: Canada Ach-Mycophenolate; Apo-Mycophenolate; CellCept; CellCept I.V.; CO Mycophenolate; JAMP-Mycophenolate; Myfortic; Mylan-Mycophenolate; Novo-Mycophenolate; Sandoz-Mycophenolate Mofetil

Index Terms MMF; MPA; Mycophenolate Mofetil; Mycophenolate Sodium; Mycophenolic Acid

◄ **Pharmacologic Category** Immunosuppressant Agent

Use Prophylaxis of organ rejection concomitantly with cyclosporine and corticosteroids in patients receiving allogeneic renal (CellCept, Myfortic), cardiac (CellCept), or hepatic (CellCept) transplants

Labeled Contraindications Hypersensitivity to mycophenolate mofetil, mycophenolic acid, mycophenolate sodium, or any component of the formulation

Cellcept: Intravenous formulation is also contraindicated in patients who are allergic to polysorbate 80

Pregnancy Considerations [US Boxed Warning]: Mycophenolate is associated with an increased risk of congenital malformations and first trimester pregnancy loss when used by pregnant women. Females of reproductive potential must be counseled about pregnancy prevention and planning. Alternative agents should be considered for women planning a pregnancy. Adverse events have been reported in animal reproduction studies. In humans, the following congenital malformations have been reported: external ear abnormalities, cleft lip and palate, anomalies of the distal limbs, heart, esophagus, kidney, and nervous system. Spontaneous abortions have also been noted. Females of reproductive potential (girls who have entered puberty, women with a uterus who have not passed through clinically confirmed menopause) should have a negative pregnancy test with a sensitivity of ≥25 milliunits/mL immediately before therapy and the test should be repeated 8 to 10 days later. Pregnancy tests should be repeated during routine follow-up visits. Acceptable forms of contraception should be used during treatment and for 6 weeks after therapy is discontinued. The effectiveness of hormonal contraceptive agents may be affected by mycophenolate. For women with lupus nephritis taking mycophenolate and who are planning a pregnancy, mycophenolate should be discontinued at least 6 weeks prior to trying to conceive (Hahn, 2012).

Healthcare providers should report female exposures to mycophenolate during pregnancy or within 6 weeks of discontinuing therapy to the Mycophenolate Pregnancy Registry (800-617-8191). The National Transplantation Pregnancy Registry (NTPR, Temple University) is a registry for pregnant women taking immunosuppressants following any solid organ transplant. The NTPR encourages reporting of all immunosuppressant exposures during pregnancy in transplant recipients at 877-955-6877.

Breast-Feeding Considerations It is unknown if mycophenolate is excreted in human milk. Due to potentially serious adverse reactions, the decision to discontinue the drug or discontinue breast-feeding should be considered. Breast-feeding is not recommended during therapy or for 6 weeks after treatment is complete.

Warnings/Precautions Hazardous agent - use appropriate precautions for handling and disposal (NIOSH 2014 [group 2]).

[US Boxed Warning]: Risk for bacterial, viral, fungal, and protozoal infections, including opportunistic infections, is increased with immunosuppressant therapy; infections may be serious and potentially fatal. Due to the risk of oversuppression of the immune system, which may increase susceptibility to infection, combination immunosuppressant therapy should be used with caution. Polyomavirus associated nephropathy (PVAN), JC virus-associated progressive multifocal leukoencephalopathy (PML), cytomegalovirus (CMV) infections, reactivation of hepatitis B (HBV) or hepatitis C (HCV), have been reported with use. A reduction in immunosuppression should be considered for patients with new or reactivated viral infections; however, in transplant recipients, the risk that reduced immunosuppression presents to the functioning graft should also be considered. PVAN, primarily from activation of BK virus, may lead to the deterioration of renal function and/ or renal graft loss. PML, a potentially fatal condition, commonly presents with hemiparesis, apathy, ataxia, cognitive deficiencies, confusion, and hemiparesis. Risk factors for development of PML include treatment with immunosuppressants and immune function impairment; consultation with a neurologist should be considered in any patient with neurological symptoms receiving immunosuppressants. Risk of CMV viremia or disease is increased in transplant recipients CMV seronegative at the time of transplant who receive a graft from a CMV seropositive donor. In patients infected with HBV or HCV, viral reactivation may occur; these patients should be monitored for signs of active HBV or HCV. **[US Boxed Warning]: Risk of development of lymphoma and skin malignancy is increased.** The risk for malignancies is related to intensity/duration of therapy. Patients should be monitored appropriately, instructed to limit exposure to sunlight/UV light to decrease the risk of skin cancer, and given supportive treatment should these conditions occur. Post-transplant lymphoproliferative disorder related to EBV infection has been reported in immunosuppressed organ transplant patients; risk is highest in EBV seronegative patients (including many young children). Neutropenia (including severe neutropenia) may occur, requiring dose reduction or interruption of treatment (risk greater from day 31-180 post-transplant). Use may rarely be associated with gastric or duodenal ulcers, GI bleeding and/or perforation. Use caution in patients with active serious digestive system disease; patients with active peptic ulcers were not included in clinical studies. Use caution in renal impairment as toxicity may be increased; may require dosage adjustment in severe impairment.

[US Boxed Warning]: Mycophenolate is associated with an increased risk of congenital malformations and first trimester pregnancy loss when used by pregnant women. Females of reproductive potential must be counseled about pregnancy prevention and planning. Alternative agents should be considered for women planning a pregnancy. Females of reproductive potential should have a negative pregnancy test with a sensitivity of ≥25 milliunits/mL immediately before therapy and the test should be repeated 8-10 days later. Pregnancy tests should be repeated during routine follow-up visits. Acceptable forms of contraception should be used during treatment and for 6 weeks after therapy is discontinued. Females of childbearing potential should have a negative pregnancy test within 1 week prior to beginning therapy. Two reliable forms of contraception should be used beginning 4 weeks prior to, during, and for 6 weeks after therapy. Because mycophenolate mofetil has demonstrated teratogenic effects in rats and rabbits, tablets should not be crushed, and capsules should not be opened or crushed. Avoid inhalation or direct contact with skin or mucous membranes of the powder contained in the capsules and the powder for oral suspension. Caution should be exercised in the handling and preparation of solutions of intravenous mycophenolate. Avoid skin contact with the intravenous solution and reconstituted suspension. If such contact occurs, wash thoroughly with soap and water, rinse eyes with plain water.

Theoretically, use should be avoided in patients with the rare hereditary deficiency of hypoxanthine-guanine phosphoribosyltransferase (such as Lesch-Nyhan or Kelley-Seegmiller syndrome). Intravenous solutions should

◀ be given over at least 2 hours; never administer intravenous solution by rapid or bolus injection. Live attenuated vaccines should be avoided during use; vaccinations may be less effective during therapy. **[US Boxed Warning]: Should be administered under the supervision of a physician experienced in immunosuppressive therapy.**

Note: CellCept and Myfortic dosage forms should not be used interchangeably due to differences in absorption. Some dosage forms may contain phenylalanine. Some dosage forms may contain polysorbate 80 (also known as Tweens). Hypersensitivity reactions, usually a delayed reaction, have been reported following exposure to pharmaceutical products containing polysorbate 80 in certain individuals (Isaksson, 2002; Lucente 2000; Shelley, 1995). Thrombocytopenia, ascites, pulmonary deterioration, and renal and hepatic failure have been reported in premature neonates after receiving parenteral products containing polysorbate 80 (Alade, 1986; CDC, 1984). See manufacturer's labeling.

Adverse Reactions Data for incidence >20% as reported in adults following oral dosing of CellCept alone in renal, cardiac, and hepatic allograft rejection studies. Profile in 3% to <20% range reflects use in combination with cyclosporine and corticosteroids. In general, lower doses used in renal rejection patients had less adverse effects than higher doses. Rates of adverse effects were similar for each indication, except for those unique to the specific organ involved. The type of adverse effects observed in pediatric patients was similar to those seen in adults, with the exception of abdominal pain, anemia, diarrhea, fever, hypertension, infection, pharyngitis, respiratory tract infection, sepsis, and vomiting; lymphoproliferative disorder was the only type of malignancy observed. Percentages of adverse reactions were similar in studies comparing CellCept to Myfortic in patients following renal transplant.

>20%:
  Cardiovascular: Hypertension (28% to 78%), hypotension (33%), peripheral edema (27% to 64%), edema (27% to 28%), chest pain (26%), tachycardia (20% to 22%)
  Central nervous system: Pain (31% to 76%), headache (16% to 54%), insomnia (41% to 52%), fever (21% to 52%), dizziness (29%), anxiety (28%)
  Dermatologic: Rash (22%)
  Endocrine & metabolic: Hyperglycemia (44% to 47%), hypercholesterolemia (41%), hypomagnesemia (39%), hypokalemia (32% to 37%), hypocalcemia (30%), hyperkalemia (22%)
  Gastrointestinal: Abdominal pain (25% to 63%), nausea (20% to 55%), diarrhea (31% to 51%), constipation (19% to 41%), vomiting (33% to 34%), anorexia (25%), dyspepsia (22%)
  Genitourinary: Urinary tract infection (37%)
  Hematologic: Leukopenia (23% to 46%), anemia (26% to 43%; hypochromic 25%), leukocytosis (22% to 41%), thrombocytopenia (24% to 38%)
  Hepatic: Liver function tests abnormal (25%), ascites (24%)
  Neuromuscular & skeletal: Back pain (35% to 47%), weakness (35% to 43%), tremor (24% to 34%), paresthesia (21%)
  Renal: Creatinine increased (39%), BUN increased (35%), kidney function abnormal (22% to 26%)
  Respiratory: Dyspnea (31% to 37%), respiratory tract infection (22% to 37%), pleural effusion (34%), cough (31%), lung disorder (22% to 30%), sinusitis (26%)

Miscellaneous: Infection (18% to 27%), sepsis (27%), lactate dehydrogenase increased (23%), *Candida* (17% to 22%), herpes simplex (10% to 21%)

3% to <20%:

Cardiovascular: Angina, arrhythmia, arterial thrombosis, atrial fibrillation, atrial flutter, bradycardia, cardiac arrest, cardiac failure, CHF, extrasystole, facial edema, hyper-/hypovolemia, orthostatic hypotension, pallor, palpitation, pericardial effusion, peripheral vascular disorder, supraventricular extrasystoles, supraventricular tachycardia, syncope, thrombosis, vasodilation, vasospasm, venous pressure increased, ventricular extrasystole, ventricular tachycardia

Central nervous system: Agitation, chills with fever, confusion, delirium, depression, emotional lability, hallucinations, hypoesthesia, malaise, nervousness, psychosis, seizure, somnolence, thinking abnormal, vertigo

Dermatologic: Acne, alopecia, bruising, cellulitis, fungal dermatitis, hirsutism, petechia, pruritus, skin carcinoma, skin hypertrophy, skin ulcer, vesiculobullous rash

Endocrine & metabolic: Acidosis, alkalosis, Cushing's syndrome, dehydration, diabetes mellitus, gout, hypercalcemia, hyper-hypophosphatemia, hyperlipemia, hyperuricemia, hypochloremia, hypoglycemia, hyponatremia, hypoproteinemia, hypothyroidism, parathyroid disorder

Gastrointestinal: Abdomen enlarged, dysphagia, esophagitis, flatulence, gastritis, gastroenteritis, gastrointestinal hemorrhage, gastrointestinal moniliasis, gingivitis, gum hyperplasia, ileus, melena, mouth ulceration, oral moniliasis, stomach disorder, stomach ulcer, stomatitis, xerostomia, weight gain/loss

Genitourinary: Impotence, nocturia, pelvic pain, prostatic disorder, scrotal edema, urinary frequency, urinary incontinence, urinary retention, urinary tract disorder

Hematologic: Coagulation disorder, hemorrhage, neutropenia, pancytopenia, polycythemia, prothrombin time increased, thromboplastin time increased

Hepatic: Alkaline phosphatase increased, bilirubinemia, cholangitis, cholestatic jaundice, GGT increased, hepatitis, jaundice, liver damage, transaminases increased

Local: Abscess

Neuromuscular & skeletal: Arthralgia, hypertonia, joint disorder, leg cramps, myalgia, myasthenia, neck pain, neuropathy, osteoporosis

Ocular: Amblyopia, cataract, conjunctivitis, eye hemorrhage, lacrimation disorder, vision abnormal

Otic: Deafness, ear disorder, ear pain, tinnitus

Renal: Albuminuria, creatinine increased, dysuria, hematuria, hydronephrosis, oliguria, pyelonephritis, renal failure, renal tubular necrosis

Respiratory: Apnea, asthma, atelectasis, bronchitis, epistaxis, hemoptysis, hiccup, hyperventilation, hypoxia, respiratory acidosis, pharyngitis, pneumonia, pneumothorax, pulmonary edema, pulmonary hypertension, respiratory moniliasis, rhinitis, sputum increased, voice alteration

Miscellaneous: *Candida* (mucocutaneous 16% to 18%), CMV viremia/syndrome (12% to 14%), CMV tissue invasive disease (6% to 12%), herpes zoster cutaneous disease (4% to 10%), cyst, diaphoresis, flu-like syndrome, healing abnormal, hernia, ileus infection, neoplasm, peritonitis, thirst

<1%, postmarketing and/or case reports: Atypical mycobacterial infection, BK virus-associated nephropathy, bronchiectasis (Boddana 2011, Rook 2006), colitis, gastrointestinal perforation, hypogammaglobulinemia (Boddana 2011; Keven 2003; Robertson 2009), infectious endocarditis, interstitial lung disorder, intestinal villous atrophy, lymphoma, lymphoproliferative disease,

malignancy, meningitis, pancreatitis, progressive multifocal leukoencephal-opathy (sometimes fatal), pulmonary fibrosis (fatal), pure red cell aplasia, tuberculosis

Drug Interactions

Metabolism/Transport Effects Substrate of OAT3, SLCO1B1, SLCO1B3, UGT1A10, UGT1A8, UGT1A9, UGT2B7

Avoid Concomitant Use

Avoid concomitant use of Mycophenolate with any of the following: BCG (Intravesical); Bile Acid Sequestrants; Cholestyramine Resin; Natalizumab; Pimecrolimus; Rifamycin Derivatives; Tacrolimus (Topical); Tofacitinib; Vaccines (Live)

Increased Effect/Toxicity

Mycophenolate may increase the levels/effects of: Acyclovir-Valacyclovir; Fingolimod; Ganciclovir-Valganciclovir; Leflunomide; Natalizumab; Tofacitinib; Vaccines (Live)

The levels/effects of Mycophenolate may be increased by: Acyclovir-Valacyclovir; Denosumab; Ganciclovir-Valganciclovir; Isavuconazonium Sulfate; Pimecrolimus; Probenecid; Roflumilast; Tacrolimus (Topical); Teriflunomide; Trastuzumab

Decreased Effect

Mycophenolate may decrease the levels/effects of: BCG (Intravesical); Coccidioides immitis Skin Test; Contraceptives (Estrogens); Contraceptives (Progestins); Sipuleucel-T; Vaccines (Inactivated); Vaccines (Live)

The levels/effects of Mycophenolate may be decreased by: Antacids; Bile Acid Sequestrants; Cholestyramine Resin; CycloSPORINE (Systemic); Echinacea; Magnesium Salts; MetroNIDAZOLE (Systemic); Penicillins; Proton Pump Inhibitors; Quinolone Antibiotics; Rifamycin Derivatives; Sevelamer

Food Interactions Food decreases C_{max} of MPA by 40% following CellCept administration and 33% following Myfortic use; the extent of absorption is not changed. Management: Take CellCept or Myfortic on an empty stomach to decrease variability; however, Cellcept may be taken with food if necessary in stable renal transplant patients.

Storage/Stability

Capsules: Store at 25°C (77°F); excursions permitted to 15°C to 30°C (59°F to 86°F).

Tablets: Store at 25°C (77°F); excursions permitted to 15°C to 30°C (59°F to 86°F). Protect from moisture and light.

Oral suspension: Store powder for oral suspension at 25°C (77°F); excursions permitted to 15°C to 30°C (59°F to 86°F). Once reconstituted, the oral solution may be stored at room temperature or under refrigeration. Do not freeze. The mixed suspension is stable for 60 days.

Injection: Store intact vials and diluted solutions at 25°C (77°F); excursions permitted to 15°C to 30°C (59°F to 86°F). Begin infusion within 4 hours of reconstitution.

Preparation for Administration Hazardous agent; use appropriate precautions for handling and disposal (NIOSH 2014 [group 2]).

Oral suspension: Should be constituted prior to dispensing to the patient and **not** mixed with any other medication. Add 47 mL of water to the bottle and shake well for ~1 minute. Add another 47 mL of water to the bottle and shake well for an additional minute. Final concentration is 200 mg/mL of mycophenolate mofetil.

IV: Reconstitute the contents of each vial with 14 mL of 5% dextrose injection; dilute the contents of a vial with 5% dextrose in water to a final concentration of 6 mg mycophenolate mofetil per mL. **Note:** Vial is vacuum-sealed; if a lack of vacuum is noted during preparation, the vial should not be used.

Mechanism of Action MPA exhibits a cytostatic effect on T and B lymphocytes. It is an inhibitor of inosine monophosphate dehydrogenase (IMPDH) which inhibits *de novo* guanosine nucleotide synthesis. T and B lymphocytes are dependent on this pathway for proliferation.

Pharmacodynamics/Kinetics

Onset of action: Peak effect: Correlation of toxicity or efficacy is still being developed, however, one study indicated that 12-hour AUCs >40 mcg/mL/ hour were correlated with efficacy and decreased episodes of rejection

Absorption: AUC values for MPA are lower in the early post-transplant period versus later (>3 months) post-transplant period. The extent of absorption in pediatrics is similar to that seen in adults, although there was wide variability reported.

Oral: Myfortic: 93%

Distribution:

CellCept: MPA: Oral: 4 L/kg; IV: 3.6 L/kg

Myfortic: MPA: Oral: 54 L (at steady state); 112 L (elimination phase)

Protein binding: MPA: >97%, MPAG 82%

Metabolism: Hepatic and via GI tract; CellCept is completely hydrolyzed in the liver to mycophenolic acid (MPA; active metabolite); enterohepatic recirculation of MPA may occur; MPA is glucuronidated to MPAG (inactive metabolite)

Bioavailability: Oral: CellCept: 94%; Myfortic: 72%

Half-life elimination:

CellCept: MPA: Oral: 18 hours; IV: 17 hours

Myfortic: MPA: Oral: 8-16 hours; MPAG: 13-17 hours

Time to peak, plasma: Oral: MPA:

CellCept: 1-1.5 hours

Myfortic: 1.5-2.75 hours

Excretion:

CellCept: MPA: Urine (<1%), feces (6%); MPAG: Urine (87%)

Myfortic: MPA: Urine (3%), feces; MPAG: Urine (>60%)

Dosing

Adult Note: May be used IV for up to 14 days; transition to oral therapy as soon as tolerated.

Renal transplant:

CellCept:

Oral: 1 g twice daily. Doses >2 g daily are not recommended.

IV: 1 g twice daily

Myfortic: Oral: 720 mg twice daily (total daily dose: 1440 mg)

Cardiac transplantation: *CellCept:*

Oral: 1.5 g twice daily

IV: 1.5 g twice daily

Hepatic transplantation: *CellCept:*

Oral: 1.5 g twice daily

IV: 1 g twice daily

Autoimmune hepatitis, refractory (off-label use): *CellCept:* Oral: 2 g daily (Manns, 2010)

◄ **Lupus nephritis (off-label use):** CellCept: Oral:

Induction: 1 g twice daily for 6 months in combination with a glucocorticoid (Ong, 2005) **or** 2-3 g daily for 6 months in combination with glucocorticoids (Hahn, 2012)

Maintenance: 0.5-3 g daily (Contreras, 2004) **or** 1 g twice daily (Dooley, 2011) **or** 1-2 g daily (Hahn, 2012)

Myasthenia gravis (off-label use): *CellCept:* Oral: 1 g twice daily (range: 1-3 g daily) (Cahoon, 2006; Ciafaloni, 2001; Merriggioli, 2003)

Psoriasis, moderate-to-severe (off-label use): *CellCept:* Oral: 2-3 g daily (Menter, 2009)

Geriatric Dosage is the same as younger patients, however, dosing should be cautious due to possibility of increased hepatic, renal, or cardiac dysfunction. Elderly patients may be at an increased risk of certain infections, gastrointestinal hemorrhage, and pulmonary edema, as compared to younger patients.

Pediatric

Renal transplant: Oral:

CellCept: Infants ≥3 months, Children, and Adolescents: *Cellcept suspension:* 600 mg/m^2/dose twice daily; maximum dose: 1 g twice daily

Alternatively, may use Cellcept solid dosage forms according to BSA as follows:

BSA 1.25-1.5 m^2: 750 mg capsule twice daily

BSA >1.5 m^2: 1 g capsule or tablet twice daily

Myfortic: Children ≥5 years and Adolescents: Usual dosage: 400 mg/m^2/dose twice daily; maximum dose: 720 mg twice daily

BSA <1.19 m^2: Use of this formulation is not recommended

BSA 1.19-1.58 m^2: 540 mg twice daily (maximum: 1080 mg daily)

BSA >1.58 m^2: 720 mg twice daily (maximum: 1440 mg daily)

Renal Impairment

Renal transplant: GFR <25 mL/minute/1.73 m^2 in patients outside the immediate post-transplant period:

CellCept: Doses of >1 g administered twice daily should be avoided; patients should also be carefully observed; no dose adjustments are needed in renal transplant patients experiencing delayed graft function postoperatively

Myfortic: No dose adjustments are needed in renal transplant patients experiencing delayed graft function postoperatively; however, monitor carefully for potential concentration dependent adverse events

Cardiac or liver transplant: No data available; mycophenolate may be used in cardiac or hepatic transplant patients with severe chronic renal impairment if the potential benefit outweighs the potential risk.

Autoimmune disease (off-label use): There have been no specific dosage adjustments identified, although use of lower doses may be required. MPA exposure appears to be inversely related to renal function (Abd Rahman, 2013); monitor closely for efficacy and adverse effects, especially in patients with end-stage renal disease (Haubitz, 2002; MacPhee, 2000).

Hemodialysis: Not removed; supplemental dose is not necessary.

Peritoneal dialysis: Supplemental dose is not necessary.

Hepatic Impairment No dosage adjustment is recommended for renal patients with severe hepatic parenchymal disease; however, it is not currently known whether dosage adjustments are necessary for hepatic disease with other etiologies.

Adjustment for Toxicity Neutropenia (ANC <1.3 x 10³/μL): Dosing should be interrupted or the dose reduced, appropriate diagnostic tests performed and patients managed appropriately

Administration

Oral dosage formulations (tablet, capsule, suspension) should be administered on an empty stomach (1 hour before or 2 hours after meals) to avoid variability in MPA absorption. The oral solution may be administered via a nasogastric tube (minimum 8 French, 1.7 mm interior diameter); oral suspension should not be mixed with other medications. Delayed release tablets should not be crushed, cut, or chewed. Cellcept may be administered with food in stable renal transplant patients when necessary. If a dose is missed, administer as soon as it is remembered. If it is close to the next scheduled dose, skip the missed dose and resume at next regularly scheduled time; do not double a dose to make up for a missed dose.

Intravenous solutions should be administered over at least 2 hours (either peripheral or central vein); do **not** administer intravenous solution by rapid or bolus injection.

Hazardous agent; use appropriate precautions for handling and disposal (NIOSH 2014 [group 2]).

Extemporaneous Preparations Hazardous agent; use appropriate precautions for handling and disposal (NIOSH 2014 [group 2]).

A 50 mg/mL oral suspension may be made with mycophenolate mofetil capsules, Ora-Plus, and cherry syrup. In a vertical flow hood, empty six 250 mg capsules into a mortar; add 7.5 mL Ora-Plus and mix to a uniform paste. Mix while adding 15 mL of cherry syrup in incremental proportions; transfer to a calibrated bottle, rinse mortar with cherry syrup, and add sufficient quantity of cherry syrup to make 30 mL. Label "shake well". Stable for 210 days at 5°C, for 28 days at 25°C to 37°C, and for 11 days at 45°C.

Venkataramanan R, McCombs JR, Zuckerman S, et al, "Stability of Mycophenolate Mofetil as an Extemporaneous Suspension," *Ann Pharmacother,* 1998, 32(7-8):755-7.

Monitoring Parameters Complete blood count (weekly for first month, twice monthly during months 2 and 3, then monthly thereafter through the first year); renal and liver function; signs and symptoms of organ rejection; signs and symptoms of bacterial, fungal, protozoal, new or reactivated viral, or opportunistic infections; neurological symptoms (eg, hemiparesis, confusion, cognitive deficiencies, ataxia) suggestive of PML, pregnancy test (immediately prior to initiation and 8-10 days later in females of childbearing potential, followed by repeat tests during therapy); monitor skin (for lesions suspicious of skin cancer); monitor for signs of lymphoma

Dietary Considerations Oral dosage formulations should be taken on an empty stomach to avoid variability in MPA absorption. However, in stable renal transplant patients, Cellcept may be administered with food if necessary. Some products may contain phenylalanine.

Additional Information Females of reproductive potential are required to have contraceptive counseling and use acceptable birth control unless heterosexual intercourse is completely avoided. Use of an intrauterine device (IUD), tubal sterilization, or vasectomy of the female patient's partner are acceptable contraceptive methods that can be used alone. If a hormonal contraceptive is used (eg, combination oral contraceptive pills, transdermal patches, vaginal rings, or progestin only products), then one barrier method must also be used (eg, diaphragm or cervical cap with spermicide, contraceptive sponge, male or female condom). Alternatively, the use of two barrier methods is also acceptable (eg, diaphragm or cervical cap with spermicide, or contraceptive sponge **PLUS** male or female condom). Refer to manufacturer's labeling for full details.

Medication Guide Available Yes

Dosage Forms Considerations Single dose pharmacokinetic studies in adult renal transplant patients suggest that bioavailability is similar between oral mycophenolate mofetil (1000 mg) and delayed release mycophenolic acid (720 mg) (Arns, 2005). In clinical trials, comparative efficacy and safety profiles have been observed in adult renal transplant patients randomized to either oral mycophenolate mofetil (1000 mg twice daily) or delayed release mycophenolic acid (720 mg twice daily) (Budde, 2004; Salvadori, 2003).

Dosage Forms Excipient information presented when available (limited, particularly for generics); consult specific product labeling.

Capsule, Oral, as mofetil:
CellCept: 250 mg [contains fd&c blue #2 (indigotine)]
Generic: 250 mg [imprints], 250 mg
Solution Reconstituted, Intravenous, as mofetil hydrochloride:
CellCept Intravenous: 500 mg (1 ea)
Suspension Reconstituted, Oral, as mofetil:
CellCept: 200 mg/mL (160 mL) [contains aspartame, methylparaben, soybean lecithin; mixed fruit flavor]
Generic: 200 mg/mL (160 mL)
Tablet, Oral, as mofetil:
CellCept: 500 mg [contains fd&c blue #2 aluminum lake]
Generic: 500 mg
Tablet Delayed Release, Oral, as mycophenolic acid:
Myfortic: 180 mg [contains fd&c blue #2 (indigotine)]
Myfortic: 360 mg
Generic: 180 mg, 360 mg

- **Mycophenolate Mofetil** see Mycophenolate on page 1177
- **Mycophenolate Sodium** see Mycophenolate on page 1177
- **Mycophenolic Acid** see Mycophenolate on page 1177
- **Myfortic** see Mycophenolate on page 1177
- **Mylan-Acyclovir (Can)** see Acyclovir (Systemic) on page 35
- **Mylan-Anagrelide (Can)** see Anagrelide on page 109
- **Mylan-Anastrozole (Can)** see Anastrozole on page 112
- **Mylan-Bicalutamide (Can)** see Bicalutamide on page 207
- **Mylan-Ciprofloxacin (Can)** see Ciprofloxacin (Systemic) on page 327
- **Mylan-Fentanyl Matrix Patch (Can)** see FentaNYL on page 692
- **Mylan-Fluconazole (Can)** see Fluconazole on page 725
- **Mylan-Hydroxyurea (Can)** see Hydroxyurea on page 839
- **Mylan-Levofloxacin (Can)** see Levofloxacin (Systemic) on page 1038
- **Mylan-Mycophenolate (Can)** see Mycophenolate on page 1177
- **Mylan-Olanzapine (Can)** see OLANZapine on page 1242
- **Mylan-Olanzapine ODT (Can)** see OLANZapine on page 1242
- **Mylan-Ondansetron (Can)** see Ondansetron on page 1253
- **Mylan-Tamoxifen (Can)** see Tamoxifen on page 1595
- **Mylan-Valacyclovir (Can)** see ValACYclovir on page 1712

♦ **Myleran** *see* Busulfan *on page 242*

♦ **Myl-Letrozole (Can)** *see* Letrozole *on page 1019*

♦ **Mylotarg** *see* Gemtuzumab Ozogamicin *on page 786*

♦ **Myocet (Can)** *see* DOXOrubicin (Liposomal) *on page 565*

♦ **Myorisan** *see* ISOtretinoin *on page 973*

♦ **Mytotan** *see* Mitotane *on page 1155*

Nabilone (NA bi lone)

Related Information

Management of Chemotherapy-Induced Nausea and Vomiting in Adults *on page 2142*

Brand Names: US Cesamet

Brand Names: Canada ACT Nabilone; Cesamet; PMS-Nabilone; RAN™-Nabilone; Teva-Nabilone

Pharmacologic Category Antiemetic

Use Treatment of refractory nausea and vomiting associated with cancer chemotherapy

Labeled Contraindications Hypersensitivity to nabilone, other cannabinoids, or any component of the formulation

Pregnancy Considerations Adverse events have been observed in animal reproduction studies.

Breast-Feeding Considerations Because some cannabinoids are excreted in breast milk, use in breast-feeding is not recommended.

Warnings/Precautions May cause tachycardia and orthostatic hypotension; use caution with cardiovascular disease. May affect CNS function (dizziness, drowsiness, ataxia, depression, hallucinations, and psychosis have been reported); use with caution in the elderly and those with preexisting CNS depression. May cause additive CNS effects with sedatives, hypnotics, or other psychoactive agents; patients must be cautioned about performing tasks which require mental alertness (eg, operating machinery or driving). Use caution in patients with mania, depression, or schizophrenia; cannabinoid use may reveal symptoms of psychiatric disorders. Careful psychiatric monitoring is recommended; psychiatric adverse reactions may persist for up to 3 days after discontinuing treatment. Has potential for abuse and or dependence, use caution in patients with substance abuse history or potential.

Adverse Reactions

>10%:

Central nervous system: Drowsiness (52% to 66%), dizziness (59%), vertigo (52% to 59%), euphoria (11% to 38%), ataxia (13% to 14%), depression (14%), concentration decreased (12%), sleep disturbance (11%)

Gastrointestinal: Xerostomia (22% to 36%)

Ocular: Visual disturbance (13%)

1% to 10%:

Cardiovascular: Hypotension (8%)

Central nervous system: Dysphoria (9%), headache (6% to 7%), sedation (3%), depersonalization (2%), disorientation (2%)

Gastrointestinal: Anorexia (8%), nausea (4%), appetite increased (2%)

Neuromuscular & skeletal: Weakness (8%)

<1%, postmarketing, or frequency not reported: Abdominal pain, abnormal dreams, akathisia, allergic reaction, amblyopia, anemia, anhydrosis, anxiety, apathy, aphthous ulcer, arrhythmia, back pain, cerebral vascular accident, ▶

chest pain, chills, confusion, constipation, cough, diaphoresis, diarrhea, dyspepsia, dyspnea, dystonia, emotional disorder, emotional lability, epistaxis, equilibrium dysfunction, eye irritation, fatigue, fever, flushing, gastritis, hallucinations, hot flashes, hyperactivity, hypertension, infection, insomnia, joint pain, leukopenia, lightheadedness, malaise, memory disturbance, mood swings, mouth irritation, muscle pain, nasal congestion, neck pain, nervousness, neurosis (phobic), numbness, orthostatic hypotension, pain, palpitation, panic disorder, paranoia, paresthesia, perception disturbance, pharyngitis, photophobia, photosensitivity, polyuria, pruritus, psychosis (including toxic), pupil dilation, rash, seizure, sinus headache, speech disorder, stupor, syncope, tachycardia, taste perversion, thirst, thought disorder, tinnitus, tremor, urination decreased/increased, urinary retention, visual field defect, voice change, vomiting, wheezing, withdrawal, xerophthalmia

Drug Interactions

Metabolism/Transport Effects None known.

Avoid Concomitant Use There are no known interactions where it is recommended to avoid concomitant use.

Increased Effect/Toxicity

Nabilone may increase the levels/effects of: Alcohol (Ethyl); CNS Depressants; Sympathomimetics

The levels/effects of Nabilone may be increased by: Anticholinergic Agents; Cocaine

Decreased Effect There are no known significant interactions involving a decrease in effect.

Storage/Stability Store at 25°C (77°F); excursion permitted to 15°C and 30°C (59°F and 86°F).

Mechanism of Action Antiemetic activity may be due to effect on cannabinoid receptors (CB1) within the central nervous system.

Pharmacodynamics/Kinetics

Absorption: Rapid and complete

Distribution: ~12.5 L/kg

Metabolism: Extensively metabolized to several active metabolites by oxidation and stereospecific enzyme reduction; CYP450 enzymes may also be involved

Half-life elimination: Parent compound: ~2 hours; Metabolites: ~35 hours

Time to peak, serum: Within 2 hours

Excretion: Feces (~60%); renal (~24%)

Dosing

Adult Nausea and vomiting associated with cancer chemotherapy: Oral: 1-2 mg twice daily (maximum: 6 mg divided in 3 doses daily); begin with the lower dose in the range and increase if needed. May administer 2 or 3 times per day during the entire chemotherapy course; continue for up to 48 hours after the last chemotherapy dose. A dose of 1-2 mg the night before chemotherapy may also be of benefit.

Geriatric Refer to adult dosing. Use the lower end of the dosing range (to minimize adverse events).

Pediatric Nausea and vomiting associated with cancer chemotherapy (off-label use; Dupuis, 2003): Oral: Children >4 years:

<18 kg: 0.5 mg every 12 hours

18-30 kg: 1 mg every 12 hours

>30 kg: 1 mg every 8-12 hours

Renal Impairment No dosage adjustment provided in manufacturer's labeling (has not been studied).

Hepatic Impairment No dosage adjustment provided in manufacturer's labeling (has not been studied).

Administration Initial dose should be given 1-3 hours before chemotherapy.

Monitoring Parameters Blood pressure, heart rate; signs and symptoms of excessive use, abuse, or misuse

Dosage Forms Excipient information presented when available (limited, particularly for generics); consult specific product labeling.

Capsule, Oral:

Cesamet: 1 mg [contains fd&c blue #2 (indigotine)]

Controlled Substance C-II

◆ **nab-Paclitaxel** *see* PACLitaxel (Protein Bound) *on page* 1292

Nafcillin (naf SIL in)

Brand Names: US Nallpen in Dextrose

Index Terms Ethoxynaphthamido Penicillin Sodium; Nafcillin Sodium; Nallpen; Sodium Nafcillin

Pharmacologic Category Antibiotic, Penicillin

Use Treatment of infections such as osteomyelitis, bacteremia, septicemia, endocarditis, and CNS infections caused by susceptible strains of *Staphylococcus* species

Pregnancy Risk Factor B

Dosing

Adult & Geriatric

Endocarditis: Methicillin-susceptible *Staphylococcus aureus* (MSSA): IV:

Native valve: 12 g/24 hours in 4-6 divided doses (ie, 2 g every 4 hours or 3 g every 6 hours) for 6 weeks. **Note:** Dosing intended for ***complicated*** right-sided infective endocarditis (IE) or left-sided IE. For ***uncomplicated*** right-sided IE, 2 weeks of therapy may be adequate (Baddour 2005). The British Society for Antimicrobial Chemotherapy (BSAC) recommends 4 weeks of therapy with a penicillinase-resistant penicillin for all patients with native valve IE due to MSSA unless patient has intracardiac prostheses, secondary lung abscesses, or osteomyelitis, then extend treatment to ≥6 weeks (Gould 2012).

Prosthetic valve: 12 g/24 hours in 6 divided doses (ie, 2 g every 4 hours) for ≥6 weeks (use with rifampin for entire course and gentamicin for first 2 weeks) (Baddour 2005)

Skin and soft tissue infections(IDSA [Stevens 2014]):

Due to methicillin-susceptible Staphylococcus aureus (MSSA): IV: 1 to 2 g every 4 hours for 7 to 14 days

Necrotizing infection due to MSSA (off-label use): IV: 1 to 2 g every 4 hours; continue until further debridement is not necessary, patient has clinically improved, and patient is afebrile for 48 to 72 hours

Streptococcal skin infections (off-label use): IV: 1 to 2 g every 4 to 6 hours (IDSA [Stevens 2014])

Surgical site infections (trunk or extremity [away from axilla or perineum]) (off-label use): IV: 2 g every 6 hours (IDSA [Stevens 2014])

Pediatric

Mild-to-moderate infections: IM, IV: 100-150 mg/kg/day in divided doses every 6 hours (maximum dose: 4000 mg daily)

◄ **Severe infections:** IM, IV: 150-200 mg/kg/day in divided doses every 4-6 hours; for life-threatening infection (eg, meningitis) daily doses up to 200 mg/kg are used (maximum dose: 12 g daily)

Skin and soft tissue infections (IDSA [Stevens 2014]):
Due to methicillin-susceptible Staphylococcus aureus (MSSA): IV: 100 to 150 mg/kg/day in divided doses every 6 hours for 7 to 14 days
Necrotizing infection due to MSSA (off-label use): IV: 200 mg/kg/day in divided doses every 6 hours; continue until further debridement is not necessary, patient has clinically improved, and patient is afebrile for 48 to 72 hours

Streptococcal skin infections (off-label use): IV: 200 mg/kg/day in divided doses every 6 hours (IDSA [Stevens 2014])

Renal Impairment No dosage adjustment is necessary unless in the setting of concomitant hepatic impairment; however, manufacturer labeling does not provide specific dosage adjustments.
Poorly dialyzed. No supplemental dose or dosage adjustment necessary, including patients on intermittent hemodialysis, peritoneal dialysis, or continuous renal replacement therapy (eg, CVVHD) (Aronoff 2007; Heintz 2009).

Hepatic Impairment No specific dosage adjustments provided in manufacturer's labeling; however, dosage adjustment may be necessary particularly in the setting of concomitant renal impairment; nafcillin primarily undergoes hepatic metabolism. In patients with both hepatic and renal impairment, monitoring of serum drug levels and modification of dosage may be necessary.

Additional Information Complete prescribing information should be consulted for additional detail.

Dosage Forms Excipient information presented when available (limited, particularly for generics); consult specific product labeling.
Solution, Intravenous:
Nallpen in Dextrose: 1 g/50 mL (50 mL); 2 g/100 mL (100 mL)
Solution Reconstituted, Injection:
Generic: 1 g (1 ea); 2 g (1 ea); 10 g (1 ea)
Solution Reconstituted, Injection [preservative free]:
Generic: 1 g (1 ea); 2 g (1 ea); 10 g (1 ea)
Solution Reconstituted, Intravenous:
Generic: 1 g (1 ea); 2 g (1 ea)

Necitumumab (ne si TOOM oo mab)

Index Terms Portrazza

Pharmacologic Category Antineoplastic Agent, Epidermal Growth Factor Receptor (EGFR) Inhibitor; Antineoplastic Agent, Monoclonal Antibody

Use

Non-small cell lung cancer (squamous), metastatic: First-line treatment of metastatic squamous non-small cell lung cancer in combination with gemcitabine and cisplatin

Limitations of use: Not indicated for treatment of non-squamous cell lung cancer.

Labeled Contraindications There are no contraindications listed in the manufacturer's labeling.

Product Availability Portrazza: FDA approved November 2015; anticipated availability is currently unknown.

Nelarabine (nel AY re been)

Related Information

Common Toxicity Criteria *on page 2122*

Management of Chemotherapy-Induced Nausea and Vomiting in Adults *on page 2142*

Prevention and Management of Infections *on page 2196*

Prevention of Chemotherapy-Induced Nausea and Vomiting in Children *on page 2203*

Safe Handling of Hazardous Drugs *on page 2292*

Brand Names: US Arranon

Brand Names: Canada Atriance

Index Terms 2-Amino-6-Methoxypurine Arabinoside; 506U78; GW506U78

Pharmacologic Category Antineoplastic Agent, Antimetabolite; Antineoplastic Agent, Antimetabolite (Purine Analog)

Use T-cell acute lymphoblastic leukemia/lymphoma: Treatment of relapsed or refractory T-cell acute lymphoblastic leukemia/lymphoma following at least 2 chemotherapy regimens.

Labeled Contraindications

There are no contraindications listed in the US labeling.

Canadian labeling: Hypersensitivity to nelarabine or any component of the formulation.

Pregnancy Considerations Adverse effects were observed in animal reproduction studies and nelarabine may cause fetal harm if administered during pregnancy. Women of childbearing potential should be advised to use effective contraception and avoid becoming pregnant during therapy.

The European Society for Medical Oncology has published guidelines for diagnosis, treatment, and follow-up of cancer during pregnancy. The guidelines recommend referral to a facility with expertise in cancer during pregnancy and encourage a multidisciplinary team (obstetrician, neonatologist, oncology team). In general, if chemotherapy is indicated, it should be avoided during the first trimester, there should be a 3-week time period between the last chemotherapy dose and anticipated delivery, and chemotherapy should not be administered beyond week 33 of gestation. Specific use of nelarabine is not discussed (Peccatori 2013).

◀ **Breast-Feeding Considerations** It is not known if nelarabine or ara-G are excreted in breast milk. Due to the potential for serious adverse reactions in the nursing infant, the manufacturer recommends a decision be made whether to discontinue nursing or to discontinue the drug taking into account the importance of treatment to the mother.

Warnings/Precautions Hazardous agent - use appropriate precautions for handling and disposal (NIOSH 2014 [group 1]). **[US Boxed Warning]: Severe neurotoxicities, including mental status changes, severe somnolence, seizures, and peripheral neuropathy (ranging from numbness and paresthesias to motor weakness and paralysis), have been reported. Observe closely for signs and symptoms of neurotoxicity; discontinue if ≥ grade 2. Adverse reactions associated with demyelination and ascending peripheral neuropathies similar to Guillain-Barré syndrome have also been reported. Neurologic toxicities may not fully return to baseline after treatment cessation.** Neurologic toxicity is dose-limiting. Risk of neurotoxicity may increase in patients with concurrent or previous intrathecal chemotherapy or history of craniospinal irradiation. Fatal neurological outcomes have been reported following concurrent use of nelarabine with intrathecal chemotherapy. The Canadian labeling does not recommend concurrent use with intrathecal therapy and/or craniospinal radiation. Tumor lysis syndrome (TLS) may occur as a consequence of leukemia treatment. May lead to life threatening acute renal failure; adequate hydration and prophylactic allopurinol should be instituted prior to treatment to prevent hyperuricemia and TLS; monitor closely. Bone marrow suppression, including leukopenia, thrombocytopenia, anemia, neutropenia and febrile neutropenia are associated with treatment; monitor blood counts regularly. Use caution in patients with renal impairment; ara-G clearance may be reduced with renal dysfunction. Use caution with severe hepatic impairment; risk of adverse reactions may be higher with severe hepatic dysfunction. Avoid administration of live vaccines. Potentially significant drug-drug interactions may exist, requiring dose or frequency adjustment, additional monitoring, and/or selection of alternative therapy.

Adverse Reactions Note: Pediatric adverse reactions fell within a range similar to adults except where noted.

>10%:

Cardiovascular: Peripheral edema (15%), edema (11%)

Central nervous system: Fatigue (50%), fever (23%), somnolence (7% to 23%; grades 2-4: 1% to 6%), dizziness (21%; grade 2: 8% adults), headache (15% to 17%; grades 2-4: 4% to 8%), hypoesthesia (6% to 17%; grades 2/3: children 5%, adults 12%), pain (11%)

Dermatologic: Petechiae (12%)

Endocrine & metabolic: Hypokalemia (11%)

Gastrointestinal: Nausea (41%), diarrhea (22%), vomiting (10% to 22%), constipation (21%)

Hematologic: Anemia (95% to 99%; grade 4: 10% to 14%), neutropenia (81% to 94%; grade 4: children 62%, adults 49%), thrombocytopenia (86% to 88%; grade 4: 22% to 32%), leukopenia (38%; grade 4: 7%), neutropenic fever (12%; grade 4: 1%)

Hepatic: Transaminases increased (12%; grade 3: 4%)

Neuromuscular & skeletal: Peripheral neuropathy (12% to 21%; grades 2/3: 11% to 14%), weakness (6% to 17%; grade 4: 1%), paresthesia (4% to 15%; grades 2/3: 3% to 4%), myalgia (13%)

Respiratory: Cough (25%), dyspnea (7% to 20%)

1% to 10%:

Cardiovascular: Hypotension (8%), sinus tachycardia (8%), chest pain (5%)

Central nervous system: Ataxia (2% to 9%; grades 2/3: children 1%, adults 8%), confusion (8%), insomnia (7%), depressed level of consciousness (6%; grades 2-4: 2%), depression (6%), seizure (grade 3: 1% adults; grade 4: 6% children), motor dysfunction (4%; grades 2/3: 2%), amnesia (3%; grade 2: 1%), balance disorder (2%; grade 2: 1%), sensory loss (1% to 2%), aphasia (grade 3: 1%), attention disturbance (1%), cerebral hemorrhage (grade 4: 1%), coma (grade 4: 1%), encephalopathy (grade 4: 1%), hemiparesis (grade 3: 1%), hydrocephalus (1%), intracranial hemorrhage (grade 4: 1%), lethargy (1%), leukoencephalopathy (grade 4: 1%), loss of consciousness (grade 3: 1%), mental impairment (1%), nerve paralysis (1%), neuropathic pain (1%), nerve palsy (1%), paralysis (1%), sciatica (1%), sensory disturbance (1%), speech disorder (1%)

Endocrine & Metabolic: Hypocalcemia (8%), dehydration (7%), hyper-/hypoglycemia (6%), hypomagnesemia (6%)

Gastrointestinal: Abdominal pain (9%), anorexia (9%), stomatitis (8%), abdominal distension (6%), taste perversion (3%)

Hepatic: Albumin decreased (10%), bilirubin increased (10%; grade 3: 7%, grade 4: 2%), AST increased (6%)

Neuromuscular & skeletal: Arthralgia (9%), back pain (8%), muscle weakness (8%), rigors (8%), limb pain (7%), abnormal gait (6%), noncardiac chest pain (5%), tremor (4% to 5%; grade 2: 2% to 3%), dysarthria (1%), hyporeflexia (1%), hypertonia (1%), incoordination (1%)

Ocular: Blurred vision (4%), nystagmus (1%)

Renal: Creatinine increased (6%)

Respiratory: Pleural effusion (10%), epistaxis (8%), pneumonia (8%), sinusitis (7%), wheezing (5%), sinus headache (1%)

Miscellaneous: Infection (5% to 9%)

<1%, postmarketing, and/or case reports: CPK increased, craniospinal demyelination, neuropathy (peripheral) (similar to Guillain-Barré syndrome), opportunistic infection, pneumothorax, progressive multifocal leukoencephalopathy (PML), respiratory arrest, rhabdomyolysis, tumor lysis syndrome

Drug Interactions

Metabolism/Transport Effects None known.

Avoid Concomitant Use

Avoid concomitant use of Nelarabine with any of the following: BCG (Intravesical); CloZAPine; Dipyrone; Natalizumab; Pentostatin; Pimecrolimus; Tacrolimus (Topical); Tofacitinib; Vaccines (Live)

Increased Effect/Toxicity

Nelarabine may increase the levels/effects of: CloZAPine; Fingolimod; Leflunomide; Natalizumab; Tofacitinib; Vaccines (Live)

The levels/effects of Nelarabine may be increased by: Denosumab; Dipyrone; Pimecrolimus; Roflumilast; Tacrolimus (Topical); Trastuzumab

Decreased Effect

Nelarabine may decrease the levels/effects of: BCG (Intravesical); Coccidioides immitis Skin Test; Sipuleucel-T; Vaccines (Inactivated); Vaccines (Live)

The levels/effects of Nelarabine may be decreased by: Echinacea; Pentostatin

◀ **Storage/Stability** Store unopened vials at 25°C (77°F); excursions permitted to 15°C to 30°C (59°F to 86°F). Stable in plastic (PVC) or glass containers for up to 8 hours at room temperature.

Preparation for Administration Hazardous agent; use appropriate precautions for handling and disposal (NIOSH 2014 [group 1]). Reconstitution is not required; do not dilute; the appropriate dose should be added to empty plastic (PVC) bag or glass container.

Mechanism of Action Nelarabine, a prodrug of ara-G, is demethylated by adenosine deaminase to ara-G and then converted to ara-GTP. Ara-GTP is incorporated into the DNA of the leukemic blasts, leading to inhibition of DNA synthesis and inducing apoptosis. Ara-GTP appears to accumulate at higher levels in T-cells, which correlates to clinical response.

Pharmacodynamics/Kinetics

Distribution: V_{ss}:
  Nelarabine: Children: ~213 L/m^2; Adults: ~197 L/m^2
  Ara-G: Children: ~33 L/m^2; Adults: ~50 L/m^2

Protein binding: Nelarabine and ara-G: <25%

Metabolism: Hepatic; demethylated by adenosine deaminase to form ara-G (active); also hydrolyzed to form methylguanine. Both ara-G and methylguanine metabolized to guanine. Guanine is deaminated into xanthine, which is further oxidized to form uric acid, which is then oxidized to form allantoin.

Half-life elimination: Children: Nelarabine: 13 minutes, Ara-G: 2 hours; Adults: Nelarabine: 18 minutes, Ara-G: 3 hours

Time to peak: Ara-G: Adults: 3 to 25 hours (of day 1)

Excretion: Urine (nelarabine 5% to 10%, ara-G 20% to 30%)

Dosing

Adult & Geriatric T-cell acute lymphoblastic leukemia/lymphoma: IV: 1,500 mg/m^2/dose on days 1, 3, and 5; repeat every 21 days until a transplant candidate, disease progression, or unacceptable toxicity.

Pediatric T-cell acute lymphoblastic leukemia/lymphoma: IV: 650 mg/m^2/dose on days 1 through 5; repeat every 21 days until a transplant candidate, disease progression, or unacceptable toxicity.

Renal Impairment

CrCl ≥50 mL/minute: No dosage adjustment necessary.

CrCl <50 mL/minute: There are no dosage adjustments provided in the manufacturer's labeling, (although ARA-G clearance is decreased as renal function declines, data is insufficient for a dosing recommendation); monitor closely.

Hepatic Impairment There are no dosage adjustments provided in the manufacturer's labeling (has not been studied); closely monitor with severe impairment (total bilirubin >3 times ULN).

Adjustment for Toxicity

Neurologic toxicity ≥ grade 2: Discontinue treatment.

Hematologic or other (non-neurologic) toxicity: Consider treatment delay.

Administration Adequate IV hydration recommended to prevent tumor lysis syndrome; allopurinol may be used if hyperuricemia is anticipated.

IV:
  Children: Infuse over 1 hour daily for 5 consecutive days
  Adults: Infuse over 2 hours on days 1, 3, and 5

Hazardous agent; use appropriate precautions for handling and disposal (NIOSH 2014 [group 1]).

Emetic Potential Children and Adults: Minimal (<10%)

Monitoring Parameters CBC with differential, liver and kidney function; monitor closely for neurologic toxicity (severe somnolence, seizure, peripheral neuropathy, confusion, ataxia, paresthesia, hypoesthesia, coma, or craniospinal demyelination); signs and symptoms of tumor lysis syndrome; hydration status

Dosage Forms Excipient information presented when available (limited, particularly for generics); consult specific product labeling.
Solution, Intravenous:
Arranon: 5 mg/mL (50 mL)

Dosage Forms: Canada Excipient information presented when available (limited, particularly for generics); consult specific product labeling.
Injection, solution:
Atriance: 5 mg/mL (50 mL)

- **Neoral** see CycloSPORINE (Systemic) *on page 385*
- **Neosar** see Cyclophosphamide *on page 372*
- **NEPA** see Netupitant and Palonosetron *on page 1195*
- **NESP** see Darbepoetin Alfa *on page 448*

Netupitant and Palonosetron (net UE pi tant & pal oh NOE se tron)

Related Information
Management of Chemotherapy-Induced Nausea and Vomiting in Adults *on page 2142*

Brand Names: US Akynzeo

Index Terms NEPA; Palonosetron and Netupitant

Pharmacologic Category Antiemetic; Selective 5-HT$_3$ Receptor Antagonist; Substance P/Neurokinin 1 Receptor Antagonist

Use Chemotherapy-induced nausea and vomiting: Prevention of acute and delayed nausea and vomiting associated with initial and repeat courses of cancer chemotherapy, including, but not limited to, highly emetogenic chemotherapy.

Labeled Contraindications There are no contraindications listed in the manufacturer's labeling.

Pregnancy Considerations Adverse events were observed in some animal reproduction studies using the components of this combination product.

Breast-Feeding Considerations It is not known if netupitant or palonosetron are excreted in breast milk. Due to the potential for serious adverse reactions in the nursing infant, the manufacturer recommends a decision be made whether to discontinue nursing or to discontinue the drug, taking into account the importance of treatment to the mother.

Warnings/Precautions Serotonin syndrome has been reported with 5-HT$_3$ receptor antagonists, predominantly when used in combination with other serotonergic agents (eg, SSRIs, SNRIs, MAOIs, mirtazapine, fentanyl, lithium, tramadol, and methylene blue). Some of the cases have been fatal. The majority of serotonin syndrome reports with 5-HT$_3$ receptor antagonists occurred in a postanesthesia setting or in an infusion center. Serotonin syndrome has also been reported following overdose of another 5-HT$_3$ receptor antagonist. Monitor patients for signs of serotonin syndrome, including mental status changes (eg, agitation, hallucinations, delirium, coma); autonomic instability (eg, tachycardia, labile blood pressure, diaphoresis, dizziness, flushing, hyperthermia); neuromuscular changes (eg, tremor, rigidity, myoclonus, hyperreflexia, incoordination); gastrointestinal symptoms (eg, ▶

nausea, vomiting, diarrhea); and/or seizures. If serotonin syndrome occurs, discontinue 5-HT$_3$ receptor antagonist treatment and begin supportive management.

Hypersensitivity (including anaphylaxis) has been reported with or without known hypersensitivity to other 5-HT$_3$ receptor antagonists. Avoid use in severe hepatic impairment; dosage adjustment not necessary in mild or moderate impairment. Avoid use in severe renal impairment or end stage renal disease; dosage adjustment not necessary in mild or moderate impairment. Potentially significant drug-drug interactions may exist, requiring dose or frequency adjustment, additional monitoring, and/or selection of alternative therapy. Use caution when dosing elderly patients due to a higher frequency of decreased hepatic, renal, cardiac function, and concomitant disease or drug therapy.

Adverse Reactions 1% to 10%:

Central nervous system: Headache (9%), fatigue (4% to 7%)

Dermatologic: Erythema (3%)

Gastrointestinal: Dyspepsia (4%), constipation (3%)

Neuromuscular & skeletal: Weakness (8%)

Drug Interactions

Metabolism/Transport Effects Refer to individual components.

Avoid Concomitant Use

Avoid concomitant use of Netupitant and Palonosetron with any of the following: Apomorphine; Aprepitant; Bosutinib; Cobimetinib; CYP3A4 Inducers (Strong); Domperidone; Flibanserin; Ibrutinib; Ivabradine; Lomitapide; Naloxegol; Olaparib; Pimozide; Simeprevir; Tolvaptan; Trabectedin; Ulipristal

Increased Effect/Toxicity

Netupitant and Palonosetron may increase the levels/effects of: Apixaban; Apomorphine; Aprepitant; ARIPiprazole; Avanafil; Bosentan; Bosutinib; Brexpiprazole; Bromocriptine; Budesonide (Systemic); Budesonide (Systemic, Oral Inhalation); Budesonide (Topical); Cannabis; Cilostazol; Cobimetinib; Colchicine; CYP3A4 Substrates; Dapoxetine; Dexamethasone (Systemic); Dofetilide; Domperidone; DOXOrubicin (Conventional); Dronabinol; Eletriptan; Eliglustat; Eplerenone; Everolimus; FentaNYL; Flibanserin; Halofantrine; Hydrocodone; Ibrutinib; Imatinib; Ivabradine; Ivacaftor; Lomitapide; Lurasidone; Naloxegol; NiMODipine; Olaparib; OxyCODONE; Pimecrolimus; Pimozide; Propafenone; Ranolazine; Salmeterol; Saxagliptin; Serotonin Modulators; Simeprevir; Sonidegib; Suvorexant; Tetrahydrocannabinol; Tolvaptan; Trabectedin; Ulipristal; Vilazodone; Vindesine; Zopiclone; Zuclopenthixol

The levels/effects of Netupitant and Palonosetron may be increased by: Osimertinib

Decreased Effect

Netupitant and Palonosetron may decrease the levels/effects of: Ifosfamide; Tapentadol; TraMADol

The levels/effects of Netupitant and Palonosetron may be decreased by: Bosentan; CYP3A4 Inducers (Moderate); CYP3A4 Inducers (Strong); Dabrafenib; Deferasirox; Osimertinib; Siltuximab; St Johns Wort; Tocilizumab

Storage/Stability Store at 20°C to 25°C (68°F to 77°F); excursions are permitted between 15°C and 30°C (59°F and 86°F)

Mechanism of Action Netupitant is a selective substance P/neurokinin (NK_1) receptor antagonist, which augments the antiemetic activity of $5\text{-}HT_3$ receptor antagonists and corticosteroids to inhibit acute and delayed chemotherapy-induced emesis. Palonosetron is a selective $5\text{-}HT_3$ receptor antagonist, which blocks serotonin, both on vagal nerve terminals in the periphery and centrally in the chemoreceptor trigger zone. Palonosetron inhibits the cross-talk between the $5\text{-}HT_3$ and NK_1 receptors. The combination of palonosetron and netupitant works synergistically to inhibit substance P response to a greater extent than either agent alone (Aapro, 2014).

Pharmacodynamics/Kinetics

Netupitant:

Absorption: Within 15 minutes to 3 hours

Distribution: V_d: 1,982 ± 906 L

Protein binding: >99.5% for netupitant; >97% for major metabolites

Metabolism: Extensively hepatic via CYP3A4 (major), CYP2C9 (minor) and CYP2D6 (minor); forms active metabolites M1, M2, and M3

Half-life elimination: 80 ± 29 hours

Time to peak: ~5 hours

Excretion: Feces (~71%); urine (~4%)

Palonosetron:

Absorption: Well absorbed

Distribution: V_d: 8.3 ± 2.5 L/kg

Protein binding: ~62%

Metabolism: ~50% metabolized to relatively inactive metabolites (N-oxide-palonosetron and 6-S-hydroxy-palonosetron); CYP2D6, 3A4, and 1A2 contribute to metabolism

Half-life elimination: 48 ± 19 hours

Time to peak: ~5 hours

Excretion: Feces (5% to 8%); urine (85% to 93%; 40% as unchanged drug)

Dosing

Adult

Highly-emetogenic chemotherapy (including cisplatin-based): Oral: One capsule ~1 hour prior to initiation of chemotherapy on day 1 (Gralla, 2014). **Note:** Antiemetic regimen also includes dexamethasone 12 mg orally ~30 minutes prior to initiation of chemotherapy on day 1, and 8 mg orally once daily on days 2 to 4.

Anthracycline and cyclophosphamide-based chemotherapy and chemotherapy not considered highly emetogenic: Oral: One capsule ~1 hour prior to initiation of chemotherapy on day 1 (Gralla, 2014). **Note:** Antiemetic regimen also includes dexamethasone 12 mg orally ~30 minutes prior to chemotherapy on day 1.

Geriatric No dosage adjustment necessary. Refer to adult dosing.

Renal Impairment

Mild or moderate impairment: No dosage adjustment is necessary.

Severe impairment or ESRD: Avoid use.

Hepatic Impairment

Mild or moderate impairment (Child-Pugh score 5 to 8): No dosage adjustment is necessary.

Severe impairment (Child-Pugh score >9): Avoid use.

Administration Oral: May administer with or without food.

NETUPITANT AND PALONOSETRON

Dosage Forms Excipient information presented when available (limited, particularly for generics); consult specific product labeling.
Capsule, Oral:
Akynzeo: Netupitant 300 mg and palonosetron 0.5 mg

- ◆ **Neulasta** see Pegfilgrastim on page 1346
- ◆ **Neulasta Delivery Kit** see Pegfilgrastim on page 1346
- ◆ **Neulasta Onpro kit** see Pegfilgrastim on page 1346
- ◆ **Neumega [DSC]** see Oprelvekin on page 1262
- ◆ **Neupogen** see Filgrastim on page 711
- ◆ **NeutraSal®** see Saliva Substitute on page 1511
- ◆ **NexAVAR** see SORAfenib on page 1547
- ◆ **Nexavar (Can)** see SORAfenib on page 1547
- ◆ **Niastase (Can)** see Factor VIIa (Recombinant) on page 676
- ◆ **Niastase RT (Can)** see Factor VIIa (Recombinant) on page 676
- ◆ **Niftolid** see Flutamide on page 751
- ◆ **Nilandron** see Nilutamide on page 1205

Nilotinib (nye LOE ti nib)

Related Information
Common Toxicity Criteria on page 2122
Management of Chemotherapy-Induced Nausea and Vomiting in Adults on page 2142
Principles of Anticancer Therapy on page 2261
Safe Handling of Hazardous Drugs on page 2292

Brand Names: US Tasigna

Brand Names: Canada Tasigna

Index Terms AMN107; Nilotinib Hydrochloride Monohydrate

Pharmacologic Category Antineoplastic Agent, BCR-ABL Tyrosine Kinase Inhibitor; Antineoplastic Agent, Tyrosine Kinase Inhibitor

Use Chronic myelogenous leukemia:
Treatment of adults with newly diagnosed Philadelphia chromosome-positive chronic myelogenous leukemia (CML) in chronic phase.
Treatment of chronic- and accelerated-phase Philadelphia chromosome-positive CML in adults resistant or intolerant to prior therapy that included imatinib.

Labeled Contraindications
Hypokalemia, hypomagnesemia, or long QT syndrome
Canadian labeling: Additional contraindication (not in US labeling): Hypersensitivity to nilotinib or any component of the formulation; persistent QTc >480 msec

Pregnancy Considerations Adverse effects were observed in animal reproduction studies. May cause fetal harm if administered during pregnancy. Women of childbearing potential should be advised to use effective contraception during treatment. The Canadian labeling recommends that women of childbearing potential and/or male patients receiving nilotinib use highly effective contraception during treatment and for at least 4 weeks after completion of therapy.

Breast-Feeding Considerations It is not known if nilotinib is excreted in breast milk. Due to the potential for serious adverse reactions in the nursing infant, the decision to discontinue breast-feeding during therapy or to discontinue nilotinib should take into account the benefits of treatment to the mother.

Warnings/Precautions Hazardous agent - use appropriate precautions for handling and disposal (NIOSH 2014 [group 1]). **[US Boxed Warnings]: May prolong the QT interval; sudden deaths have been reported. Use in patients with hypokalemia, hypomagnesemia, or long QT syndrome is contraindicated. Correct hypomagnesemia and hypokalemia prior to initiating therapy; monitor electrolytes periodically. Monitor ECG and QTc (baseline, at 7 days, with dose change, and periodically). Avoid the use of QT-prolonging agents.** Avoid concurrent use with antiarrhythmics and other drugs which may prolong QT interval; may increase the risk of potentially-fatal arrhythmias. Sudden deaths appear to be related to dose-dependent ventricular repolarization abnormalities. Prolonged QT interval may result in torsade de pointes, which may cause syncope, seizure, and/or death. Patients with uncontrolled or significant cardiovascular disease were excluded from studies. **[US Boxed Warning]: Administer on an empty stomach, at least 1 hour before and 2 hours after food;** administration with food may prolong the QTc. Nilotinib solubility is decreased at higher pH; concurrent use with proton pump inhibitors is not recommended. If necessary, H_2-receptor blockers may be administered ~10 hours before and 2 hours after a nilotinib dose. Antacids (eg, aluminum hydroxide, magnesium hydroxide, simethicone) may be administered ~2 hours before or 2 hours after nilotinib. Potentially significant drug-drug/drug-food interactions may exist, requiring dose or frequency adjustment, additional monitoring, and/or selection of alternative therapy. **[US Boxed Warning]: Avoid concurrent use with strong CYP3A4 inhibitors.**

Cardiovascular events such as ischemic heart disease-related events, arterial vascular occlusive events, peripheral arterial occlusive disease, and ischemic cerebrovascular accident have been reported. Use caution in patients with preexisting risk factors, and monitor for new or worsening symptoms suggestive of cardiovascular events. Fluid retention, including pleural and pericardial effusions, ascites, and pulmonary edema were reported; may be severe. Monitor closely for signs/symptoms of fluid retention (eg, rapid weight gain or swelling) and for symptoms of respiratory or cardiac distress (eg, shortness of breath). Evaluate promptly and manage as appropriate. In a clinical study comparing nilotinib and imatinib in the treatment of newly diagnosed Ph+ chronic phase CML, hemorrhagic events (eg, gastrointestinal hemorrhage, including grade 3 or 4 events) occurred more frequently in the nilotinib arm.

Dosage reduction is recommended in patients with hepatic impairment, along with close monitoring of the QT interval. Nilotinib metabolism is primarily hepatic (exposure is increased in patients with hepatic impairment). May cause hepatotoxicity, including dose-limiting elevations in bilirubin, transaminases, and alkaline phosphatase; monitor liver function. UGT1A1 polymorphisms may be a risk factor for increased toxicity (eg, hyperbilirubinemia) (Shibata, 2013).

Reversible myelosuppression, including grades 3 and 4 thrombocytopenia, neutropenia, and anemia may occur; may require dose reductions and/or treatment delay; monitor blood counts. Use with caution in patients with a history of pancreatitis, may cause dose-limiting elevations of serum lipase and amylase; monitor. In patients with abdominal symptoms in conjunction with lipase increases, withhold treatment and consider diagnostics to exclude ▶

◄ pancreatitis. Tumor lysis syndrome (TLS) has been reported in patients with resistant or intolerant CML; the majority of cases had malignant disease progression, high WBC counts, and/or dehydration; maintain adequate hydration and treat high uric acid levels prior to nilotinib. Consider alternative therapy or a dosage increase (with more frequent monitoring) in patients with total gastrectomy (nilotinib exposure is reduced). Capsules contain lactose; do not use with galactose intolerance, severe lactase deficiency, or glucose-galactose malabsorption syndromes.

Adverse Reactions

>10%:

Cardiovascular: Peripheral edema (≤15%; grade 3/4: <1%), hypertension (10% to 11%)

Central nervous system: Headache (20% to 35%), fatigue (21% to 32%), insomnia (7% to 12%), dizziness (≤12%)

Dermatologic: Skin rash (≤38%; grades 3/4: ≤2%), pruritus (20% to 32%), night sweats (12% to 27%), alopecia (11% to 13%), xeroderma (>5% to 12%)

Endocrine & metabolic: Increased serum glucose (50%), hyperglycemia (≤50%; grades 3/4: 7% to 12%), increased serum cholesterol (28%), hypophosphatemia (≥10%; grades 3/4: 5% to 17%)

Gastrointestinal: Nausea (20% to 37%), vomiting (11% to 29%), diarrhea (14% to 28%), increased serum lipase (28%; grades 3/4: 9% to 18%), constipation (17% to 26%), upper abdominal pain (12% to 18%; grade 3/4: <1%), abdominal pain (15% to 16%), decreased appetite (including anorexia 15%)

Hematologic & oncologic: Neutropenia (grades 3/4: 12% to 42%; median duration: 15 days), thrombocytopenia (grades 3/4: 10% to 42%; median duration: 22 days), anemia (grades 3/4: 4% to 27%)

Hepatic: Hepatic: Increased serum ALT (10% to 72%; grades 3/4: 4%), increased serum AST (10% to 47%; grades 3/4: 1% to 3%), hyperbilirubinemia (≥10%; grades 3/4: 4% to 9%), increased serum ALT (≥10%; grades 3/4: 4%), increased serum AST (≥10%; grades 3/4: 1% to 3%)

Infection: Influenza (≤13%)

Neuromuscular & skeletal: Arthralgia (16% to 26%), limb pain (11% to 20%), myalgia (14% to 19%), back pain (15% to 19%), weakness (11% to 16%), ostealgia (14% to 15%), muscle spasm (11% to 15%), musculoskeletal pain (11% to 12%)

Respiratory: Cough (14% to 27%), nasopharyngitis (≤27%), upper respiratory tract infection (≤17%), dyspnea (9% to 15%), oropharyngeal pain (≤12%), flu-like symptoms (11%)

Miscellaneous: Fever (11% to 28%)

1% to 10%:

Cardiovascular: Peripheral arterial disease (3% to 4%), cerebral ischemia (1% to 3%), ischemic heart disease (5% to 9%), pericardial effusion (≤2%; grades 3/4: ≤1%), angina pectoris, cardiac arrhythmia (including AV block, atrial fibrillation, bradycardia, cardiac flutter, extrasystoles, and tachycardia), chest discomfort, chest pain (including noncardiac), flushing, palpitations, prolonged Q-T interval on ECG

Central nervous system: Anxiety, depression, flank pain, hypoesthesia, malaise, myasthenia, pain, paresthesia, peripheral neuropathy, vertigo, voice disorder

Dermatologic: Acne vulgaris, dermatitis (including allergic and acneiform), eczema, erythema, folliculitis, hyperhidrosis, urticaria

Endocrine & metabolic: Hypokalemia (grades 3/4: ≤9%), hyponatremia (grades 3/4: ≤7%), hyperkalemia (grades 3/4: 2% to 6%), hypocalcemia (grades 3/4: ≤5%), decreased serum albumin (grades 3/4: ≤4%), fluid retention (grades 3/4: 3% to 4%), diabetes mellitus, hypercalcemia, hypercholesterolemia, hyperlipidemia, hyperphosphatemia, hypertriglyceridemia, hypomagnesemia, increased gamma-glutamyl transferase, increased HDL cholesterol, increased VLDL, weight gain, weight loss

Gastrointestinal: Dyspepsia (4% to 10%), gastrointestinal hemorrhage (≤5%), abdominal distension, abdominal distress, dysgeusia, flatulence, increased serum amylase, pancreatitis

Genitourinary: Pollakiuria

Hematologic & oncologic: Hemorrhage (grades 3/4: 1% to 2%), bruise, cutaneous papilloma, decreased hemoglobin, eosinophilia, febrile neutropenia, hemophthalmos, leukopenia, lymphocytopenia, pancytopenia

Hepatic: Ascites (≤2%; grades 3/4: ≤1%), increased serum alkaline phosphatase (grades 3/4: ≤1%), hepatic insufficiency

Immunologic: Decreased serum globulins

Neuromuscular & skeletal: Increased creatine phosphokinase, neck pain

Ophthalmic: Eyelid edema (1%), conjunctivitis, eye pruritus, periorbital edema, xerophthalmia

Respiratory: Pleural effusion (≤2%; grades 3/4: ≤1%), pulmonary edema (≤2%; grades 3/4: ≤1%), dyspnea (exertional), epistaxis

<1%, postmarketing, and/or case reports: Abscess, amnesia, aortic valve sclerosis, arteriosclerosis, arthritis, auditory impairment, blepharitis, blurred vision, breast induration, bronchitis, candidiasis, cardiac failure, cardiomegaly, cerebral edema, cerebral infarction, chills, cholestasis, chorioretinopathy, confusion, conjunctival hemorrhage, coronary artery disease, cyanosis, decreased visual acuity, dehydration, dermal cyst, dermal ulcer, diplopia, disorientation, drug eruption, dysesthesia, dysphoria, dysuria, ecchymoses, enterocolitis, erectile dysfunction, erythema multiforme, erythema nodosum, esophageal pain, exfoliative dermatitis, eye irritation, eye pain, facial edema, furuncle, gastric ulcer, gastric ulcer perforation, gastritis, gastroenteritis, gastroesophageal reflux disease, gingivitis, gout, gynecomastia, heart murmur, hematemesis, hematoma, hematuria, hemorrhagic shock, hemorrhoids, hepatitis, hepatomegaly, hepatotoxicity, herpes simplex infection, hiatal hernia, hyperemia (scleral, conjunctival, ocular), hyperesthesia, hyperinsulinemia, hyperkeratosis, hypermenorrhea, hyperparathyroidism (secondary), hypersensitivity, hypertensive crisis, hyperthyroidism, hyperuricemia, hypoglycemia, hypoinsulinemia, hypotension, hypothyroidism, increased appetite, increased blood urea nitrogen, increased lactate dehydrogenase, increased parathyroid hormone, increased serum creatinine, insulin C-peptide decreased, interstitial pulmonary disease, intracranial hemorrhage, jaundice, joint swelling, lack of concentration, lethargy, leukocytosis, local alterations in temperature sensations, localized edema, loss of consciousness, mastalgia, melena, mesenteric artery occlusion, migraine, myocardial infarction, nipple swelling, nocturia, nonhemorrhagic stroke, optic neuritis, oral mucosa ulcer, oral papilloma, otalgia, palmar-plantar erythrodysesthesia, papilledema, paraproteinemia, pericarditis, petechiae, pharyngolaryngeal pain, photophobia, photopsia, pleurisy, pleuritic chest pain, pneumonia, psoriasis, pulmonary hypertension, rectal hemorrhage, reduced ejection fraction, renal failure, restless leg syndrome, retroperitoneal hemorrhage, sebaceous hyperplasia, sensitive teeth, sepsis, sinusitis, skin atrophy, skin blister, skin discoloration, skin hyperpigmentation, skin hypertrophy, skin pain, skin photosensitivity, stiffness, stomatitis, stricture of artery (basilar, coronary, peripheral), subileus,

swelling of eye, syncope, throat irritation, thrombocythemia, thrombosis, thyroiditis, tinea pedis, tinnitus, transient ischemic attacks, tremor, troponin increased, tumor lysis syndrome, ulcerative esophagitis, urinary incontinence, urinary tract infection, urinary urgency, urine discoloration, vasculitis, ventricular dysfunction, wheezing, xerostomia

Drug Interactions

Metabolism/Transport Effects Substrate of CYP3A4 (major), P-glycoprotein; **Note:** Assignment of Major/Minor substrate status based on clinically relevant drug interaction potential; **Inhibits** CYP2C8 (moderate), CYP2C9 (weak), CYP2D6 (moderate), CYP3A4 (moderate), P-glycoprotein, UGT1A1; **Induces** CYP2B6 (weak/moderate), CYP2C8 (weak/moderate), CYP2C9 (weak/moderate)

Avoid Concomitant Use

Avoid concomitant use of Nilotinib with any of the following: Amodiaquine; Aprepitant; BCG (Intravesical); Bosutinib; CloZAPine; Cobimetinib; Conivaptan; CYP3A4 Inducers (Strong); CYP3A4 Inhibitors (Strong); Dexamethasone (Systemic); Dipyrone; Domperidone; Flibanserin; Fusidic Acid (Systemic); Highest Risk QTc-Prolonging Agents; Ibrutinib; Idelalisib; Irinotecan Products; Ivabradine; Lomitapide; Mifepristone; Moderate Risk QTc-Prolonging Agents; Naloxegol; Natalizumab; Olaparib; PAZOPanib; Pimecrolimus; Pimozide; Silodosin; Simeprevir; St Johns Wort; Tacrolimus (Topical); Thioridazine; Tofacitinib; Tolvaptan; Topotecan; Trabectedin; Ulipristal; Vaccines (Live); VinCRIStine (Liposomal)

Increased Effect/Toxicity

Nilotinib may increase the levels/effects of: Afatinib; Amodiaquine; Apixaban; Aprepitant; Avanafil; Bosentan; Bosutinib; Brentuximab Vedotin; Brexpiprazole; Bromocriptine; Budesonide (Systemic); Budesonide (Systemic, Oral Inhalation); Budesonide (Topical); Cannabis; Cilostazol; CloZAPine; Cobimetinib; Colchicine; CYP2C8 Substrates; CYP2D6 Substrates; CYP3A4 Substrates; Dabigatran Etexilate; Dapoxetine; Domperidone; DOXOrubicin (Conventional); Dronabinol; Edoxaban; Eletriptan; Eplerenone; Everolimus; FentaNYL; Fesoterodine; Fingolimod; Flibanserin; Highest Risk QTc-Prolonging Agents; Hydrocodone; Ibrutinib; Imatinib; Irinotecan Products; Ivabradine; Ivacaftor; Ledipasvir; Leflunomide; Lomitapide; Lurasidone; Metoprolol; Naloxegol; Natalizumab; Nebivolol; NiMODipine; Nintedanib; Olaparib; OxyCODONE; PAZOPanib; P-glycoprotein/ABCB1 Substrates; Pimozide; Prucalopride; Ranolazine; Rifaximin; Rivaroxaban; Saxagliptin; Silodosin; Simeprevir; Sonidegib; Suvorexant; Tetrahydrocannabinol; Thioridazine; Tofacitinib; Tolvaptan; Topotecan; Trabectedin; Ulipristal; Vaccines (Live); Vilazodone; VinCRIStine (Liposomal); Vindesine; Zopiclone

The levels/effects of Nilotinib may be increased by: Conivaptan; CYP3A4 Inhibitors (Moderate); CYP3A4 Inhibitors (Strong); Denosumab; Dipyrone; Fosaprepitant; Fusidic Acid (Systemic); Idelalisib; Ivabradine; Luliconazole; Mifepristone; Moderate Risk QTc-Prolonging Agents; Netupitant; Palbociclib; Pimecrolimus; QTc-Prolonging Agents (Indeterminate Risk and Risk Modifying); Roflumilast; Stiripentol; Tacrolimus (Topical); Trastuzumab

Decreased Effect

Nilotinib may decrease the levels/effects of: Antidiabetic Agents; BCG (Intravesical); Coccidioides immitis Skin Test; Codeine; Ifosfamide; Sipuleucel-T; Tamoxifen; TraMADol; Vaccines (Inactivated); Vaccines (Live)

The levels/effects of Nilotinib may be decreased by: Antacids; Bosentan; CYP3A4 Inducers (Moderate); CYP3A4 Inducers (Strong); Dabrafenib; Deferasirox; Dexamethasone (Systemic); Echinacea; H2-Antagonists; Proton Pump Inhibitors; Siltuximab; St Johns Wort; Tocilizumab

Food Interactions Grapefruit juice may result in increased concentrations of nilotinib and potentiate QT prolongation. Management: Avoid grapefruit juice.

Storage/Stability Store at 25°C (77°F); excursions are permitted between 15°C and 30°C (59°F and 86°F).

Mechanism of Action Selective tyrosine kinase inhibitor that targets BCR-ABL kinase, c-KIT and platelet derived growth factor receptor (PDGFR); does not have activity against the SRC family. Inhibits BCR-ABL mediated proliferation of leukemic cell lines by binding to the ATP-binding site of BCR-ABL and inhibiting tyrosine kinase activity. Nilotinib has activity in imatinib-resistant BCR-ABL kinase mutations.

Pharmacodynamics/Kinetics

Protein binding: ~98%

Metabolism: Hepatic; oxidation and hydroxylation, via CYP3A4 to primarily inactive metabolites

Bioavailability: Capsule: ~50% (when compared to oral solution with pH of 1.2 to 1.3); two 200 mg capsules sprinkled on applesauce was determined to be bioequivalent to two 200 mg intact capsules; bioavailability is increased 82% when administered 30 minutes after a high-fat meal

Half-life elimination: ~15 to 17 hours

Time to peak: 3 hours

Excretion: Feces (93%; 69% as parent drug)

Dosing

Adult & Geriatric Note: If clinically indicated, may be administered in combination with hematopoietic growth factors (eg, erythropoietin, filgrastim) and with hydroxyurea or anagrelide.

Chronic myeloid leukemia (CML), Ph+, newly-diagnosed in chronic phase: Oral: 300 mg twice daily

CML, Ph+, resistant or intolerant in chronic or accelerated phase: Oral: 400 mg twice daily

Gastrointestinal stromal tumor (GIST), refractory (off-label use): Oral: 400 mg twice daily until disease progression or unacceptable toxicity (Reichardt, 2012)

Missed doses: If a dose is missed, do not make up, resume with next scheduled dose.

Dosage adjustment for concomitant CYP3A4 inhibitors/inducers:

CYP3A4 inhibitors: Avoid the concomitant use of a strong CYP3A4 inhibitor with nilotinib. If a strong CYP3A4 inhibitor is required, interruption of nilotinib treatment is recommended.

If therapy cannot be interrupted and concurrent use with a strong CYP3A4 inhibitor cannot be avoided:

US labeling: Consider reducing the nilotinib dose to 300 mg once daily in patients with resistant or intolerant Ph+ CML (chronic or accelerated phase) or to 200 mg once daily in newly-diagnosed chronic phase Ph+ CML, with careful monitoring, especially of the QT interval. When a strong CYP3A4 inhibitor is discontinued, allow a washout period prior to adjusting nilotinib dose upward.

Canadian labeling: There are no dosage adjustments provided in the manufacturer's labeling; use caution and monitor QT interval closely

◄   *CYP3A4 inducers:* Avoid the concomitant use of a strong CYP3A4 inducer
with nilotinib (based on pharmacokinetic parameters, an increased nilotinib
dose is not likely to compensate for decreased exposure).

Renal Impairment There are no dosage adjustments provided in the
manufacturer's labeling (has not been studied in patients with serum creatinine >1.5 times ULN); however, nilotinib and its metabolites have minimal
renal excretion; dosage adjustments for renal dysfunction may not be
necessary.

Hepatic Impairment

For hepatic impairment at treatment initiation: **Note:** Consider alternative
therapies first if possible; recommendations vary by indication

  US labeling:

    Newly-diagnosed Ph+ CML in chronic phase: Mild-to-severe impairment
(Child-Pugh class A, B, or C): Initial: 200 mg twice daily; may increase to
300 mg twice daily based on patient tolerability

    Resistant or intolerant Ph+ CML in chronic or accelerated phase:

      Mild-to-moderate impairment (Child-Pugh class A or B): Initial: 300 mg
twice daily; may increase to 400 mg twice daily based on patient
tolerability

      Severe impairment (Child-Pugh class C): Initial: 200 mg twice daily; may
increase to 300 mg twice daily and then further increase to 400 mg
twice daily based on patient tolerability

  Canadian labeling: No dosage adjustment necessary; use caution and
monitor (including QT interval) closely.

For hepatotoxicity during treatment:

  If bilirubin >3 times ULN (≥ grade 3): Withhold treatment, monitor bilirubin,
resume treatment at 400 mg once daily when bilirubin returns to ≤1.5
times ULN (≤ grade 1)

  If ALT or AST >5 times ULN (≥ grade 3): Withhold treatment, monitor
transaminases, resume treatment at 400 mg once daily when ALT or
AST returns to ≤2.5 times ULN (≤ grade 1)

Adjustment for Toxicity

**Dosage adjustment for hematologic toxicity unrelated to underlying
leukemia:**

  ANC <1000/mm³ and/or platelets <50,000/mm³: Withhold treatment, monitor blood counts

  If ANC >1000/mm³ and platelets >50,000/mm³ within 2 weeks: Resume at
prior dose

  If ANC <1000/mm³ and/or platelets <50,000/mm³ for >2 weeks: Reduce
dose to 400 mg once daily

Dosage adjustment for nonhematologic toxicity:

  Amylase or lipase >2 times ULN (≥ grade 3): Withhold treatment, monitor
serum amylase or lipase, resume treatment at 400 mg once daily when
lipase or amylase returns to ≤1.5 times ULN (≤ grade 1)

  Lipase increases in conjunction with abdominal symptoms: Withhold treatment and consider diagnostics to exclude pancreatitis.

  Clinically-significant moderate or severe nonhematologic toxicity: Withhold
treatment, upon resolution of toxicity, resume at 400 mg once daily; may
escalate back to initial dose (300 mg twice daily or 400 mg twice daily
depending on indication) if clinically appropriate.

Dosage adjustment for QT prolongation: Note: Repeat ECG ~7 days after
any dosage adjustment.

QTc >480 msec: Withhold treatment, monitor and correct potassium and magnesium levels; review concurrent medications.

If QT_cF returns to <450 msec and to within 20 msec of baseline within 2 weeks: Resume at prior dose.

If QT_cF returns to 450 to 480 msec after 2 weeks: Reduce dose to 400 mg once daily.

If QT_cF >480 msec after dosage reduction to 400 mg once daily: Discontinue treatment.

Combination Regimens

Leukemia, chronic myelogenous: Nilotinib (CML Regimen) on page 2043

Soft tissue sarcoma (gastrointestinal stromal tumor [GIST]): Nilotinib (GIST Regimen) on page 2044

Administration Administer twice daily with doses ~12 hours apart. Administer on an empty stomach, at least 1 hour before or 2 hours after food. Capsules should be swallowed whole with water. If unable to swallow whole, may empty contents into 5 mL applesauce and administer within 15 minutes (do not save for later use).

Hazardous agent; use appropriate precautions for handling and disposal (NIOSH 2014 [group 1]).

Emetic Potential Children and Adults: Low (10% to 30%)

Monitoring Parameters CBC with differential (every 2 weeks for first 2 months, then monthly); electrolytes (including potassium, calcium, and magnesium; baseline and periodic); lipid profile and glucose (baseline and periodically during the first year, then at least yearly), hepatic function (ALT/AST, bilirubin, alkaline phosphatase; baseline and monthly or as clinically indicated); serum lipase/amylase (baseline and monthly or as clinically indicated), uric acid (baseline); bone marrow assessments; ECG and QTc (baseline, 7 days after treatment initiation or dosage adjustments, and periodically thereafter); signs/symptoms of cardiovascular events, hemorrhage, or fluid retention; additional baseline and/or periodic monitoring recommended by Canadian labeling include CPK, creatinine, lactate dehydrogenase, and weight.

Thyroid function testing (Hamnvik, 2011):

Preexisting levothyroxine therapy: Obtain baseline TSH levels, then monitor every 4 weeks until levels and levothyroxine dose are stable, then monitor every 2 months

Without preexisting thyroid hormone replacement: TSH at baseline, then monthly for 4 months, then every 2 to 3 months

Dietary Considerations The bioavailability of nilotinib is increased with food. Take on an empty stomach, at least 1 hour before or 2 hours after food. Avoid grapefruit juice.

Medication Guide Available Yes

Dosage Forms Excipient information presented when available (limited, particularly for generics); consult specific product labeling.

Capsule, Oral:

Tasigna: 150 mg, 200 mg [contains lactose]

◆ **Nilotinib Hydrochloride Monohydrate** see Nilotinib on page 1198

Nilutamide (ni LOO ta mide)

Related Information

Safe Handling of Hazardous Drugs on page 2292

Brand Names: US Nilandron

◄ **Brand Names: Canada** Anandron

Index Terms RU-23908

Pharmacologic Category Antineoplastic Agent, Antiandrogen

Use Prostate cancer, metastatic: Treatment of metastatic prostate cancer (in combination with surgical castration)

Labeled Contraindications Hypersensitivity to nilutamide or any component of the formulation; severe hepatic impairment; severe respiratory insufficiency

Pregnancy Considerations Animal reproduction studies have not been conducted. Not indicated for use in women.

Breast-Feeding Considerations Not indicated for use in women.

Warnings/Precautions Hazardous agent - use appropriate precautions for handling and disposal (meets NIOSH 2014 criteria). **[U.S. Boxed Warning]: Interstitial pneumonitis has been reported in 2% of patients exposed to nilutamide. An increased incidence has been observed in one small study of Japanese patients. Symptoms typically include exertional dyspnea, cough, chest pain and fever; interstitial changes (including pulmonary fibrosis) leading to hospitalization and fatalities have been reported (rarely). Most cases occurred within the first 3 months of treatment and generally reversed after discontinuation. X-rays showed interstitial or alveolo-interstitial changes; pulmonary function tests revealed a restrictive pattern with decreased DLco. Perform chest x-ray prior to treatment initiation and consider baseline pulmonary function testing. Instruct patients to report new or worsening dyspnea. Discontinue nilutamide immediately if signs and/or symptoms of interstitial pneumonitis are observed until a causal effect can be ruled out.**

Androgen-deprivation therapy may increase the risk for cardiovascular disease (Levine, 2010). Androgen deprivation therapy with other antiandrogen agents has resulted in prolongation of the QT/QTc interval (Garnick, 2004). Correct electrolytes prior to initiation and consider periodic electrolyte and ECG monitoring in patients at risk for QT prolongation. The Canadian labeling recommends avoiding use in patients with congenital long QT syndrome and to discontinue therapy in patients developing QT prolongation during therapy.

Hepatitis or marked increases in liver enzymes leading to drug discontinuation occurred in 1% of patients receiving nilutamide; rare cases of hospitalization or deaths due to severe liver injury have been reported, with hepatotoxicity generally being reported within first 3 to 4 months of therapy. Discontinue treatment for jaundice or ALT >2 times the upper limit of normal (ULN) (US labeling) or ALT >3 times the ULN (Canadian labeling). Approximately 5% of patients experience intolerance (facial flushing, hypotension, malaise) when ethanol is combined with nilutamide. Instruct patients to avoid ethanol. Hyperglycemia has been observed; use with caution in diabetic patients and monitor for loss of glucose control. Prolonged use of antiandrogen therapy is associated with decreased bone mineral density and an increased risk of osteoporosis and fracture (Smith, 2003). Anemia may occur with testosterone suppression.

A delay in adaptation to dark has been reported; in clinical studies, this was reported by 13% to 57% of patients; the delay ranged from seconds to a few minutes after passing from a light to a dark area (this may not abate with continued treatment although may be alleviated by wearing tinted sunglasses); caution patients who experience adaptation delay about driving at night or through tunnels. Not indicated for use in women and pediatric patients.

Patients with disease progression while receiving antiandrogen therapy may experience clinical improvement with discontinuation of the antiandrogen. The Canadian labeling recommends that patients with prostate specific antigen (PSA) progression during therapy discontinue therapy immediately and be monitored for a withdrawal response for 6 to 8 weeks following discontinuation prior to proceeding with alternative prostate cancer therapy. Potentially significant drug-drug interactions may exist, requiring dose or frequency adjustment, additional monitoring, and/or selection of alternative therapy.

Adverse Reactions

>10%:
- Central nervous system: Insomnia (16%), headache (14%)
- Endocrine & metabolic: Hot flashes (28% to 67%)
- Gastrointestinal: Nausea (10% to 24%), constipation (7% to 20%), anorexia (11%), abdominal pain (10%)
- Genitourinary: Testicular atrophy (16%), libido decreased (11%)
- Hepatic: AST increased (8% to 13%), ALT increased (8% to 9%)
- Ocular: Impaired dark adaptation (13% to 57%)
- Respiratory: Dyspnea (6% to 11%)

1% to 10%:
- Cardiovascular: Hypertension (5% to 9%), chest pain (7%), heart failure (3%), angina (2%), edema (2%), syncope (2%)
- Central nervous system: Dizziness (7% to 10%), depression (9%), hypoesthesia (5%), malaise (2%), nervousness (2%)
- Dermatologic: Alopecia (6%), dry skin (5%), rash (5%), pruritus (2%)
- Endocrine & metabolic: Alcohol intolerance (5%), hyperglycemia (4%)
- Gastrointestinal: Vomiting (6%), diarrhea (2%), GI hemorrhage (2%), melena (2%), weight loss (2%), xerostomia (2%), dyspepsia
- Genitourinary: Nocturia (7%)
- Hematologic: Anemia (7%), haptoglobin increased (2%), leukopenia (2%)
- Hepatic: Alkaline phosphatase increased (3%)
- Neuromuscular & skeletal: Bone pain (6%), arthritis (2%), paresthesia (2%)
- Ocular: Chromatopsia (9%), impaired light adaptation (8%), abnormal vision (6% to 7%), cataract (2%), photophobia (2%)
- Renal: Hematuria (8%), BUN increased (2%), creatinine increased (2%)
- Respiratory: Pneumonia (5%), cough (2%), interstitial pneumonitis (2%), rhinitis (2%)
- Miscellaneous: Flu-like syndrome (7%), diaphoresis (6%)

<1%, postmarketing, and/or case reports: Aplastic anemia, hepatitis

Drug Interactions

Metabolism/Transport Effects Substrate of CYP2C19 (major); **Note:** Assignment of Major/Minor substrate status based on clinically relevant drug interaction potential; **Inhibits** CYP2C19 (weak)

Avoid Concomitant Use
Avoid concomitant use of Nilutamide with any of the following: Alcohol (Ethyl); Indium 111 Capromab Pendetide

Increased Effect/Toxicity
Nilutamide may increase the levels/effects of: Alcohol (Ethyl)

The levels/effects of Nilutamide may be increased by: CYP2C19 Inhibitors (Moderate); CYP2C19 Inhibitors (Strong); Luliconazole

Decreased Effect
Nilutamide may decrease the levels/effects of: Choline C 11; Indium 111 Capromab Pendetide

The levels/effects of Nilutamide may be decreased by: CYP2C19 Inducers (Strong); Dabrafenib; Enzalutamide; Lumacaftor

Storage/Stability Store at room temperature of 25°C (77°F); excursions permitted between 15°C to 30°C (59°F to 86°F). Protect from light.

Mechanism of Action Nonsteroidal antiandrogen which blocks testosterone effects at the androgen receptor level, preventing androgen response.

Pharmacodynamics/Kinetics

Absorption: Rapid and complete

Metabolism: Hepatic (extensive), forms active metabolites

Half-life elimination: Terminal: 38 to 59 hours; Metabolites: 59 to 126 hours

Excretion: Urine (62%; <2% as unchanged drug); feces (1% to 7%)

Dosing

Adult & Geriatric Prostate cancer, metastatic: Oral: 300 mg once daily (starting the same day or day after surgical castration) for 30 days, followed by 150 mg once daily. Consider therapy discontinuation in patients with evidence of disease progression.

Renal Impairment There are no dosage adjustments provided in the manufacturer's labeling.

Hepatic Impairment

Hepatic impairment at treatment initiation:

Mild or moderate impairment: There are no dosage adjustments provided in the manufacturer's labeling.

Severe impairment: Use is contraindicated.

Hepatotoxicity during treatment:

US labeling: ALT >2 times ULN or jaundice: Discontinue treatment.

Canadian labeling: Transaminases >3 times ULN: Interrupt treatment.

Administration Administer without regard to meals. Hazardous agent; use appropriate precautions for handling and disposal (meets NIOSH 2014 criteria).

Monitoring Parameters CBC (periodic), liver function tests (baseline and repeated regularly during the first 4 months of treatment, and periodically thereafter; more frequently if clinically indicated), electrolytes, serum testosterone, PSA, blood glucose and/or glycosylated hemoglobin (HbA1c) in patients with diabetes; chest x-ray (baseline); consider pulmonary function testing (baseline); bone-mineral density (as clinically indicated in patients at risk of osteoporosis); ECG; signs and symptoms of liver dysfunction; vision changes. If initiating nilutamide in patients who are on warfarin, closely monitor prothrombin time.

Dosage Forms Excipient information presented when available (limited, particularly for generics); consult specific product labeling.

Tablet, Oral:

Nilandron: 150 mg

Dosage Forms: Canada Excipient information presented when available (limited, particularly for generics); consult specific product labeling.

Tablet, Oral:

Anandron: 50 mg

♦ **Ninlaro** see Ixazomib *on page 990*

♦ **Nipent** see Pentostatin *on page 1375*

♦ **Nitrogen Mustard** see Mechlorethamine (Systemic) *on page 1067*

Nivolumab (nye VOL ue mab)

Related Information

Common Toxicity Criteria *on page 2122*

Management of Chemotherapy-Induced Nausea and Vomiting in Adults *on page 2142*

Principles of Anticancer Therapy *on page 2261*

Brand Names: US Opdivo

Brand Names: Canada Opdivo

Index Terms Anti-PD-1 human monoclonal antibody MDX-1106; BMS-936558; MDX-1106; ONO-4538

Pharmacologic Category Antineoplastic Agent, Anti-PD-1 Monoclonal Antibody; Antineoplastic Agent, Monoclonal Antibody

Use

US labeling:

Melanoma, unresectable or metastatic: Treatment (as a single agent) of unresectable or metastatic melanoma with disease progression following ipilimumab and (if BRAF V600 mutation positive) a BRAF inhibitor; treatment of BRAF V600 wild-type, unresectable, or metastatic melanoma (in combination with ipilimumab)

Non-small cell lung cancer, metastatic: Treatment of metastatic non-small cell lung cancer (NSCLC) that has progressed on or after platinum-based chemotherapy. Patients with EGFR or ALK genomic tumor aberrations should have disease progression (on approved EGFR- or ALK-directed therapy) prior to receiving nivolumab.

Canadian labeling:

Melanoma, unresectable or metastatic: Treatment of unresectable or metastatic BRAF V600 wild-type melanoma in previously untreated adults.

Labeled Contraindications

There are no contraindications listed in the manufacturer's US labeling.

Canadian labeling: Hypersensitivity to nivolumab or any component of the formulation.

Pregnancy Considerations Adverse events were observed in animal reproduction studies. Nivolumab may be expected to cross the placenta; effects to the fetus may be greater in the second and third trimesters. Based on its mechanism of action, nivolumab is expected to cause fetal harm if used during pregnancy. Women of reproductive potential should use highly effective contraception during therapy and for at least 5 months after nivolumab treatment has been discontinued.

Breast-Feeding Considerations It is not known if nivolumab is excreted into breast milk. Due to the potential for serious adverse reactions in the nursing infant, the manufacturer recommends a decision be made to discontinue nursing or to discontinue the drug, taking into account the importance of treatment to the mother.

Warnings/Precautions Immune-mediated pneumonitis (severe pneumonitis or interstitial lung disease) has been observed, including cases which were fatal. Immune-mediated pneumonitis is defined as no other clear etiology and requiring corticosteroid use. The median time to development was 2.2 to 7.2 months (range: 25 days to 13.1 months) across several clinical trials. Some cases developed after nivolumab was discontinued for other reasons. With high-dose systemic corticosteroids (followed by a corticosteroid taper), all patients improved to grade 0 or 1; some patients with grade 2 or 3 pneumonitis had complete resolution (after completing corticosteroid therapy) and ▶

nivolumab was reinitiated without recurrence in some patients. Monitor for signs (with radiographic imaging) and symptoms of pneumonitis. May require treatment interruption, corticosteroid therapy, and/or permanent discontinuation. Grade 2 or higher pneumonitis should be managed with prednisone 1 to 2 mg/kg daily (or equivalent) followed by a corticosteroid taper. Withhold treatment until resolution for moderate (grade 2) immune-mediated pneumonitis; permanently discontinue for severe (grade 3) or life-threatening (grade 4) immune-mediated pneumonitis.

Diarrhea or colitis occurred commonly in patients receiving nivolumab (some cases were fatal). Immune-mediated colitis (defined as no other clear etiology and requiring corticosteroid use) including cases of grades 2 and 3 colitis occurred in some patients. The median time to onset of colitis was 1.4 to 2.7 months (range: 6 days to 19 months) from nivolumab initiation; some cases developed after nivolumab was discontinued for other reasons. In studies, the median duration of high-dose systemic corticosteroid therapy was 2.9 weeks to 1.4 months (range: 1 day to 6 months). Most patients with grade 2 or 3 immune-related colitis had complete resolution (improvement to grade 0); after resolution, nivolumab was reinitiated in some patients without recurrence, although was permanently discontinued in other patients. Monitor for signs and symptoms of colitis. May require treatment interruption, corticosteroid therapy, and/or permanent discontinuation. Severe colitis (grade 3) or life-threatening colitis (grade 4) should be managed with prednisone 1 to 2 mg/kg daily (or equivalent) followed by a corticosteroid taper. Moderate colitis (grade 2) of >5 days duration should be managed with prednisone 0.5 to 1 mg/kg daily (or equivalent) followed by a corticosteroid taper; may increase to prednisone 1 to 2 mg/kg daily (or equivalent) if colitis worsens or does not improve despite corticosteroid therapy. Permanently discontinue nivolumab for grade 4 colitis or diarrhea, or colitis that recurs upon reinitiation (single-agent therapy) or for severe or life-threatening colitis (grade 3 or 4) or for colitis that recurs upon reinitiation (in combination with ipilimumab).

ALT, AST, alkaline phosphatase, and total bilirubin elevations have occurred in nivolumab-treated patients. Immune-mediated hepatitis (defined as no other clear etiology and requiring corticosteroid use) occurred in patients receiving nivolumab; most cases included grade 2 and grade 3 hepatitis, although grade 4 toxicity also occurred. The time to onset ranged from ~3 weeks to ~8 months after nivolumab initiation (one case developed after nivolumab was discontinued for other reasons). Immune-mediated hepatitis was managed with high-dose systemic corticosteroids; liver function tests improved to grade 1 within 15 days of corticosteroid initiation in one trial. Immune-mediated hepatitis resolved and did not recur with continued corticosteroid use in some patients, although some patients experienced grade 3 recurrence and permanently discontinued treatment in a trial utilizing nivolumab as single-agent therapy. When used in combination with ipilimumab, several patients had complete resolution of hepatitis after completion of steroid therapy, and some patients had recurrence or worsening hepatitis when nivolumab and ipilimumab were restarted. Immune-mediated hepatitis recurred following nivolumab reinitiation in a NSCLC trial, leading to permanent nivolumab discontinuation. Monitor liver function at baseline and periodically for changes. Initiate prednisone 1 to 2 mg/kg daily (or equivalent) for grade 2 or higher transaminase elevations (with or without total bilirubin elevations). Withhold treatment for moderate (grade 2) immune-mediated hepatitis; permanently discontinue for severe (grade 3) or life-threatening (grade 4) immune-mediated hepatitis.

Creatinine elevations have occurred with nivolumab therapy. Immune-mediated nephritis (defined as ≥ grade 2 creatinine elevations with no other clear etiology and requiring corticosteroid use) may occur with nivolumab treatment. The time to onset for grade 2 or higher events ranged from ~1 week to 7 months after nivolumab initiation; patients received high-dose systemic corticosteroids and treatment was withheld and discontinued. In clinical trials with single-agent nivolumab, immune-mediated nephritis resolved and did not recur with continued corticosteroid use in some patients, although other patients experienced ongoing renal dysfunction. In a clinical trial of nivolumab and ipilimumab combination therapy for the treatment of metastatic melanoma, immune-mediated renal dysfunction resolved with systemic corticosteroid use and interruption of nivolumab in one patient; another patient died with persistent renal dysfunction. Monitor serum creatinine at baseline and periodically during treatment. Initiate prednisone 1 to 2 mg/kg daily (or equivalent) followed by a corticosteroid taper for life-threatening (grade 4) serum creatinine elevation and permanently discontinue nivolumab. Withhold treatment for moderate (grade 2) and severe (grade 3) creatinine elevations and administer prednisone 0.5 to 1 mg/kg daily (or equivalent) followed by a corticosteroid taper; if toxicity worsens or does not improve, permanently discontinue and increase to prednisone 1 to 2 mg/kg daily (or equivalent).

In clinical trials, immune-mediated rash (including grade 2, 3, and 4 toxicity) was observed in patients receiving nivolumab (as a single agent or in combination with ipilimumab, although the incidence was higher with combination therapy). In one study (combination therapy with ipilimumab), the median time to onset of rash was 2.4 weeks (range: 1 day to 6.5 months). Among the patients with grade 3 rash who received nivolumab in combination with ipilimumab, several received systemic corticosteroid treatment and some patients had combination therapy withheld then reinitiated (with no recurrence of high-grade rash); all had resolution to ≤ grade 1 with no further corticosteroid requirements. Monitor closely; administer prednisone 1 to 2 mg/kg/day (or equivalent) for severe (grade 3) or life-threatening (grade 4) rash. Withhold treatment for grade 3 rash and permanently discontinue for life-threatening rash.

Immune-mediated encephalitis with both single-agent and combination nivolumab therapy may occur (rarely); may be fatal. Withhold nivolumab for new-onset moderate to severe neurologic signs/symptoms; evaluate to rule out infection or other neurologic causes. Brain MRI and/or lumbar puncture may be necessary. For confirmed immune-mediated encephalitis felt to be caused by nivolumab, administer prednisone 1 to 2 mg/kg/day (or equivalent), followed by a corticosteroid taper. Permanently discontinue if immune-mediated encephalitis occurs.

Hypophysitis may occur; over 10% of patients receiving nivolumab in combination with ipilimumab for metastatic melanoma developed grade 2 and 3 toxicity. The median time to onset was ~3 months (range: 1.4 to 5.5 months). Most patients received corticosteroids; combination therapy was restarted for the majority of the patients without worsening hypophysitis (several patients continued on corticosteroid therapy). Monitor for signs/symptoms of hypophysitis. Administer prednisone 1 mg/kg/day (or equivalent) for grade 2 or higher toxicity. Withhold nivolumab for moderate (grade 2) or severe (grade 3) and permanently discontinue treatment for life-threatening (grade 4) hypophysitis. Adrenal insufficiency may occur; ~9% of patients receiving nivolumab in combination with ipilimumab developed adrenal insufficiency (including grade 3 toxicity). The median time to onset was 3 months (range: 1.2 to 5.6 months). Adrenal insufficiency occurred after treatment discontinuation in some patients. Toxicity resolved in several patients, some of whom remained on corticosteroid therapy; in two patients, combination therapy with nivolumab and ipilimumab was restarted and adrenal insufficiency did not recur. Monitor for signs/symptoms of adrenal insufficiency both during and after treatment. Administer prednisone 1 to 2 mg/kg/day (or equivalent) for severe (grade 3) or life-threatening (grade 4) adrenal insufficiency. Withhold nivolumab for moderate (grade 2) and permanently discontinue for severe (grade 3) or life-threatening (grade 4) toxicity.

Immune-mediated hyperthyroidism and hypothyroidism have occurred, mostly grades 1 and 2 hyper-/hypothyroidism (one patient receiving nivolumab in combination with ipilimumab experienced grade 3 autoimmune thyroiditis). The median onset for hyperthyroidism was ~1 to 2 months (range: Up to 3.3 months); most cases resolved (may require medical management, including corticosteroids and methimazole). Hypothyroidism occurred with a median onset of ~2 to 3 months (range: 1 day to 11.8 months). Most patients received subsequent nivolumab treatment (with or without ipilimumab) while continuing thyroid replacement therapy; in some patients, hypothyroidism completely resolved and levothyroxine was discontinued. Monitor thyroid function at baseline and for changes periodically during treatment (in one study patients were evaluated at baseline, treatment day 1, and every 6 weeks). Isolated hypothyroidism may be managed with hormone replacement therapy; initiate medical management to control hyperthyroidism. There are case reports of patients receiving nivolumab in combination with ipilimumab who developed hypothyroidism after resolution of grade 1 hyperthyroidism.

Other clinically relevant other immune-mediated disorders may occur; may develop after discontinuation of nivolumab. Immune-mediated adverse reactions observed included abducens nerve paresis, autoimmune neuropathy, demyelination, diabetic ketoacidosis, duodenitis, facial nerve paralysis, gastritis, Guillain-Barré syndrome, hypopituitarism, motor dysfunction, myasthenic syndrome, pancreatitis, polymyalgia rheumatic, sarcoidosis, uveitis, and vasculitis. If an immune-mediated adverse event is suspected, evaluate to exclude other causes. Based on symptom severity, withhold nivolumab, administer high-dose corticosteroids, and if appropriate, initiate hormone-replacement therapy. Upon improvement to grade 0 or 1, begin corticosteroid taper (over at least 1 month). After corticosteroid taper is completed and based on the severity of the reaction, may consider reinitiating nivolumab. Potentially significant drug-drug interactions may exist, requiring dose or frequency adjustment, additional monitoring, and/or selection of alternative therapy.

Adverse Reactions Frequency not always defined.

>10%:

Cardiovascular: Edema (17%; grade 3/4: 2%), chest pain (13%)

Central nervous system: Fatigue (50%; grade 3/4: 7%)

Dermatologic: Skin rash (16%; grade 3/4: <1%), pruritus (11%; grade 3/4: <1%)

Endocrine & metabolic: Hyponatremia (38%; grade 3/4: 10%), hypokalemia (20%; grade 3/4: 3%), hypomagnesemia (20%), hypercalcemia (20%; grade 3/4: 3%), hyperkalemia (18%; grade 3/4: 4%), hypocalcemia (18%; grade 3/4: 2%), weight loss (13%; grade 3/4: <1%)

Gastrointestinal: Decreased appetite (35%; grade 3/4: 3%), nausea (29%; grade 3/4: 2%), constipation (24%), colitis (≤21%, grades 3/4: 2%), diarrhea (18% to 21%; grade 3/4: 3%), vomiting (19%; grade 3/4: <1%), abdominal pain (16%; grade 3/4: 2%)

Hematologic & oncologic: Lymphocytopenia (47%; grade 3/4: 16%), anemia (28%; grade 3/4: 3%), thrombocytopenia (14%)

Hepatic: Increased serum AST (16%; grade 3/4: <1%), increased serum alkaline phosphatase (14%), increased serum ALT (12%)

Neuromuscular & skeletal: Musculoskeletal pain (36%; grade 3/4: 6%), weakness (19%; grade 3/4: 2%), arthralgia (13%)

Renal: Increased serum creatinine (22%)

Respiratory: Dyspnea (38%; grade 3/4: 9%), cough (32%; grade 3/4: 2%), pneumonia (10%; grade 3/4: 5%)

Miscellaneous: Fever (17%)

1% to 10%:

Cardiovascular: Vasculitis (<2%)

Central nervous system: Pain (10%; grade 3/4: 3%), peripheral sensory neuropathy (<10%), motor dysfunction (<2%), sixth nerve palsy (<2%), Guillain-Barre syndrome, myasthenia

Endocrine & metabolic: Hypothyroidism (4%), hyperthyroidism (2%), adreno-cortical insufficiency (<2%), diabetic ketoacidosis, hypophysitis, pituitary insufficiency

Gastrointestinal: Pancreatitis (<2%)

Hepatic: Increased serum bilirubin (3%)

Neuromuscular & skeletal: Lambert-Eaton syndrome

Ophthalmic: Uveitis (<2%)

Respiratory: Bronchitis (<10%), upper respiratory tract infection (<10%), pneumonitis (6%)

<1%, postmarketing, and/or case reports: Renal insufficiency

Drug Interactions

Metabolism/Transport Effects None known.

Avoid Concomitant Use

Avoid concomitant use of Nivolumab with any of the following: Belimumab

Increased Effect/Toxicity

Nivolumab may increase the levels/effects of: Belimumab

Decreased Effect There are no known significant interactions involving a decrease in effect.

Storage/Stability Store intact vials refrigerated at 2°C to 8°C (36°F to 46°F); do not freeze. Protect from light. Do not shake. After preparation, store the infusion solution at room temperature for no more than 4 hours (including infusion time) or refrigerated at 2°C to 8°C (36°F to 46°F) for up to 24 hours (including infusion time). Infusion must be completed within 24 hours of preparation. Do not freeze solutions prepared for infusion.

Preparation for Administration Withdraw the required volume and transfer into an IV container. Dilute with either NS or D5W to a final concentration of 1 to 10 mg/mL. Mix by gentle inversion; do not shake.

◄ **Mechanism of Action**

Nivolumab is a fully human immunoglobulin G4 (IgG4) monoclonal antibody that selectively inhibits programmed cell death-1 (PD-1) activity by binding to the PD-1 receptor to block the ligands PD-L1 and PD-L2 from binding. The negative PD-1 receptor signaling that regulates T-cell activation and proliferation is therefore disrupted (Robert 2015). This releases PD-1 pathway-mediated inhibition of the immune response, including the antitumor immune response.

Combining nivolumab (anti-PD-1) with ipilimumab (anti-CTLA-4) results in enhanced T-cell function that is greater than that of either antibody alone, resulting in improved anti-tumor responses in metastatic melanoma.

Pharmacodynamics/Kinetics

Distribution: V_d: ~8 L (single-agent and combination therapy with ipilimumab)

Half-life elimination: ~27 days (single agent); ~25 days (combination therapy with ipilimumab)

Dosing

Adult & Geriatric

US labeling:

Melanoma, unresectable or metastatic: IV: 3 mg/kg once every 2 weeks (as a single agent) until disease progression or unacceptable toxicity (Weber 2015).

Melanoma, unresectable or metastatic, first-line combination therapy: IV: 1 mg/kg once every 3 weeks (in combination with ipilimumab) for 4 doses, followed by 3 mg/kg once every 2 weeks (nivolumab monotherapy) until disease progression or unacceptable toxicity (Larkin 2015). **Note:** If nivolumab therapy is withheld, ipilimumab should also be withheld.

Non-small cell lung cancer, metastatic: IV: 3 mg/kg once every 2 weeks until disease progression or unacceptable toxicity (Borghaei 2015; Brahmer 2015).

Canadian labeling: **Melanoma, unresectable or metastatic (BRAF V600 wild-type), first-line therapy:** IV: 3 mg/kg once every 2 weeks (as a single agent), continue as long as benefiting clinically or until unacceptable toxicity occurs.

Melanoma, unresectable or metastatic (without a BRAF mutation), first-line therapy (off-label use in the US): IV: 3 mg/kg once every 2 weeks (as a single agent) until disease progression or unacceptable toxicity (Robert 2015).

Renal cell cancer, clear cell, advanced (off-label use; second- or third-line therapy): IV: 3 mg/kg once every 2 weeks, continue as long as benefiting clinically or until unacceptable toxicity occurs (Motzer 2015).

Renal Impairment

*Renal impairment **prior to** treatment initiation:*

US labeling: No dosage adjustment necessary.

Canadian labeling:

Mild to moderate impairment: No dosage adjustment necessary.

Severe impairment: There is no dosage adjustment provided in the manufacturer's labeling (insufficient data).

*Renal toxicity **during** treatment:*

US labeling:

Creatinine >1.5 to 6 times ULN or >1.5 times baseline: Withhold treatment; administer prednisone 0.5 to 1 mg/kg daily (or equivalent) followed by a corticosteroid taper; may resume therapy upon recovery to grade 0 or 1 toxicity. If toxicity worsens or does not improve, permanently discontinue and increase corticosteroid dose to prednisone 1 to 2 mg/kg daily (or equivalent).

Creatinine >6 times ULN or life-threatening: Permanently discontinue; initiate high-dose systemic corticosteroids (prednisone 1 to 2 mg/kg daily or equivalent) followed by a corticosteroid taper.

Canadian labeling:

Creatinine >1.5 to 3 times baseline or >1.5 to 3 times ULN: Withhold treatment and manage with corticosteroids (0.5 to 1 mg/kg methylprednisolone equivalent) followed by a taper; may resume therapy upon recovery to baseline and corticosteroid management is complete. If toxicity worsens or does not improve, permanently discontinue and increase corticosteroid dose (1 to 2 mg/kg methylprednisolone equivalent).

Creatinine >3 times baseline or >3 times ULN: Permanently discontinue; initiate high-dose systemic corticosteroids (1 to 2 mg/kg methylprednisolone equivalent).

Hepatic Impairment

*Hepatic impairment **prior to** treatment initiation:*

Mild impairment (total bilirubin ≤ ULN and AST > ULN or total bilirubin <1 to 1.5 times ULN and any AST): No dosage adjustment necessary.

Moderate (total bilirubin >1.5 to 3 times ULN and any AST) to severe (total bilirubin >3 times ULN and any AST) impairment: There are no dosage adjustments provided in the manufacturer's labeling (has not been studied).

*Hepatotoxicity **during** treatment:*

AST or ALT >3 to 5 times ULN or total bilirubin >1.5 to 3 times ULN: Withhold treatment; may resume therapy upon recovery to grade 0 or 1 toxicity.

AST or ALT >5 times ULN or total bilirubin >3 times ULN: Permanently discontinue.

Immune-mediated hepatitis:

Grade 2 or higher transaminase elevations (with or without total bilirubin elevations): Withhold treatment and initiate high-dose systemic corticosteroids (prednisone 1 to 2 mg/kg daily or equivalent)

Severe (grade 3) or life-threatening (grade 4): Permanently discontinue treatment and initiate high-dose systemic corticosteroids (prednisone 1 to 2 mg/kg daily or equivalent)

Adjustment for Toxicity

Withhold treatment for any of the following (may resume upon recovery to grade 0 or 1 toxicity):

Note: If receiving combination therapy with ipilimumab, when nivolumab is withheld, ipilimumab should also be withheld.

Adrenal insufficiency (grade 2)

◀ Colitis:

Grade 2 colitis or diarrhea; for grade 2 colitis with a duration >5 days; also administer systemic corticosteroids (prednisone 0.5 to 1 mg/kg daily or equivalent) followed by a corticosteroid taper; may increase to prednisone 1 to 2 mg/kg daily (or equivalent) if colitis worsens or does not improve despite corticosteroid use

Grade 3 colitis or diarrhea (single-agent nivolumab); also administer systemic corticosteroids (prednisone 1 to 2 mg/kg daily or equivalent) followed by a corticosteroid taper

Hypophysitis (grade 2 or 3 [US labeling] or grade 2 [Canadian labeling]); also administer high-dose systemic corticosteroids (prednisone 1 mg/kg daily or equivalent)

Neurologic toxicity, new onset (moderate or severe)

Pneumonitis (grade 2); also administer high-dose systemic corticosteroids (prednisone 1 to 2 mg/kg daily or equivalent) followed by a corticosteroid taper

Rash (grade 3); also administer high-dose systemic corticosteroids (prednisone 1 to 2 mg/kg daily or equivalent)

Other immune-mediated toxicities; also administer high-dose systemic corticosteroids followed by a corticosteroid taper (over 1 month)

Other treatment-related toxicity (severe or grade 3, first occurrence)

Permanently discontinue for:

Adrenal insufficiency (grade 3 or 4); also administer high-dose systemic corticosteroids (prednisone 1 to 2 mg/kg daily or equivalent)

Colitis or diarrhea (grade 3, if in combination with ipilimumab) or colitis or diarrhea (grade 4); also administer high-dose systemic corticosteroids (prednisone 1 to 2 mg/kg daily or equivalent) followed by a corticosteroid taper

Colitis (recurrent)

Encephalitis (immune mediated); also administer high-dose systemic corticosteroids (prednisone 1 to 2 mg/kg daily or equivalent) followed by a corticosteroid taper

Hypophysitis (grade 4 [US labeling] or grade 3 or 4 [Canadian labeling]); also administer high-dose systemic corticosteroids (prednisone 1 mg/kg daily or equivalent)

Pneumonitis (grade 3 or 4); also administer high-dose systemic corticosteroids (prednisone 1 to 2 mg/kg daily or equivalent) followed by a corticosteroid taper

Rash (grade 4); also administer high-dose systemic corticosteroids (prednisone 1 to 2 mg/kg daily or equivalent)

Inability to reduce corticosteroid dose to prednisone ≤10 mg/day (or equivalent) within 12 weeks.

Other adverse reactions that are life-threatening or grade 4, severe or grade 3 adverse reactions that recur, or persistent grade 2 or 3 treatment-related toxicity lasts beyond 12 weeks.

Infusion-related reaction:

Mild or moderate reaction: Interrupt or slow the infusion rate

Severe or life-threatening reaction: Discontinue

Thyroid disorder (hyperthyroidism or hypothyroidism):

US labeling: There are no recommended dosage modifications.

Canadian labeling: Grade 4 hyperthyroidism: Permanently discontinue.

Combination Regimens

Lung cancer (non-small cell): Nivolumab (NSCLC Regimen) on page 2045
Melanoma:

Ipilimumab-Nivolumab (Melanoma) on page 2019
Nivolumab (Melanoma Regimen) on page 2044

Administration IV: Administer over 60 minutes through a line with a sterile, nonpyrogenic, low protein binding 0.2 to 1.2 micrometer in-line filter. Do not administer other medications through the same IV line. Flush IV line at the end of the infusion. When administered in combination with ipilimumab, infuse nivolumab first followed by ipilimumab on the same day. Use separate infusion bags and filters for each infusion. If nivolumab therapy is withheld, ipilimumab should also be withheld.

Emetic Potential Minimal (<10%)

Monitoring Parameters Hepatic and renal function tests (baseline and periodic), thyroid function (baseline and periodically [eg, at treatment day 1 and every 6 weeks]). Monitor for signs/symptoms of adrenal insufficiency, hypophysitis, thyroid disorders, immune-mediated colitis, pneumonitis, rash, encephalitis; monitor for infusion reactions

Medication Guide Available Yes

Dosage Forms Excipient information presented when available (limited, particularly for generics); consult specific product labeling.
Solution, Intravenous [preservative free]:
Opdivo: 40 mg/4 mL (4 mL); 100 mg/10 mL (10 mL) [contains polysorbate 80]

◆ **Nizoral** see Ketoconazole (Systemic) on page 991

◆ **N-Methylhydrazine** see Procarbazine on page 1436

◆ **N-methylnaltrexone Bromide** see Methylnaltrexone on page 1122

◆ **Nocdurna (Can)** see Desmopressin on page 505

◆ **Nolvadex** see Tamoxifen on page 1595

◆ **Nolvadex-D (Can)** see Tamoxifen on page 1595

◆ **Nordeoxyguanosine** see Ganciclovir (Systemic) on page 768

◆ **Normal Immunoglobulin** see Immune Globulin on page 903

◆ **Novantrone** see MitoXANtrone on page 1159

◆ **Novel Erythropoiesis-Stimulating Protein** see Darbepoetin Alfa on page 448

◆ **Novo-Benzydamine (Can)** see Benzydamine on page 190

◆ **Novo-Cyproterone (Can)** see Cyproterone on page 402

◆ **Novoeight** see Antihemophilic Factor (Recombinant) on page 119

◆ **Novo-Fluconazole (Can)** see Fluconazole on page 725

◆ **Novo-Medrone (Can)** see MedroxyPROGESTERone on page 1074

◆ **Novo-Morphine SR (Can)** see Morphine (Systemic) on page 1167

◆ **Novo-Mycophenolate (Can)** see Mycophenolate on page 1177

◆ **Novo-Nidazol (Can)** see MetroNIDAZOLE (Systemic) on page 1142

◆ **Novo-Ofloxacin (Can)** see Ofloxacin (Systemic) on page 1240

◆ **Novo-Peridol (Can)** see Haloperidol on page 807

◆ **Novo-Prednisolone (Can)** see PrednisoLONE (Systemic) on page 1421

◆ **Novo-Purol (Can)** see Allopurinol on page 73

◆ **NovoSeven RT** see Factor VIIa (Recombinant) on page 676

Nystatin (Oral) (nye STAT in)

Brand Names: US Bio-Statin
Brand Names: Canada PMS-Nystatin
Pharmacologic Category Antifungal Agent, Oral Nonabsorbed
Use Treatment of susceptible cutaneous, mucocutaneous, and oral cavity fungal infections normally caused by the *Candida* species
Pregnancy Risk Factor C
Dosing
Adult & Geriatric
Oral candidiasis: Suspension (swish and swallow): 400,000-600,000 units 4 times/day; swish in the mouth and retain for as long as possible (several minutes) before swallowing
Intestinal infections: Oral tablets: 500,000-1,000,000 units every 8 hours
Note: Powder for compounding: 1/8 teaspoon (500,000 units) to equal approximately 1/2 cup of water; give 4 times/day
Pediatric Oral candidiasis:
Suspension:
Premature infants: 100,000 units 4 times/day; paint suspension into recesses of the mouth
Infants: 200,000 units 4 times/day or 100,000 units to each side of mouth 4 times/day; paint suspension into recesses of the mouth
Children: 400,000-600,000 units 4 times/day; swish in the mouth and retain for as long as possible (several minutes) before swallowing
Powder for compounding: Children: Refer to adult dosing.
Renal Impairment No dosage adjustment provided in manufacturer's labeling.
Hepatic Impairment No dosage adjustment provided in manufacturer's labeling.
Additional Information Complete prescribing information should be consulted for additional detail.
Dosage Forms Excipient information presented when available (limited, particularly for generics); consult specific product labeling.
Capsule, Oral [preservative free]:
Bio-Statin: 500,000 units, 1,000,000 units [dye free]
Powder, Oral:
Bio-Statin: (1 ea)
Generic: (1 ea)

Suspension, Mouth/Throat:
  Generic: 100,000 units/mL (5 mL, 60 mL, 473 mL, 480 mL)
Tablet, Oral:
  Generic: 500,000 units

Nystatin (Topical) (nye STAT in)

Brand Names: US Nyamyc; Nystop; Pedi-Dri [DSC]; Pediaderm AF Complete
Brand Names: Canada Nyaderm; Ratio-Nystatin
Pharmacologic Category Antifungal Agent, Topical
Use Fungal infections (cutaneous and mucocutaneous): Treatment of cutaneous and mucocutaneous fungal infections caused by *Candida albicans* and other susceptible *Candida* species.
Pregnancy Risk Factor C
Dosing
  Adult & Geriatric Fungal infections (cutaneous and mucocutaneous):
    Topical: **Note:** Cream is usually preferred to ointment for intertriginous areas; very moist lesions are best treated with topical powder
    Cream, ointment: Apply to the affected areas twice daily or as indicated until healing is complete
    Powder: Apply to the affected areas 2 to 3 times daily until healing is complete
  Pediatric Fungal infections (cutaneous and mucocutaneous): Infants, Children, and Adolescents: Topical: Refer to adult dosing.
  Renal Impairment There are no dosage adjustments provided in the manufacturer's labeling. However, dosage adjustment unlikely due to low systemic absorption
  Hepatic Impairment There are no dosage adjustments provided in the manufacturer's labeling. However, dosage adjustment unlikely due to low systemic absorption
  Additional Information Complete prescribing information should be consulted for additional detail.
  Dosage Forms Excipient information presented when available (limited, particularly for generics); consult specific product labeling. [DSC] = Discontinued product
  Cream, External:
    Generic: 100,000 units/g (15 g, 30 g)
  Kit, External:
    Pediaderm AF Complete: 100,000 units/g [contains methylparaben, propylene glycol, propylparaben]
  Ointment, External:
    Generic: 100,000 units/g (15 g, 30 g)
  Powder, External:
    Nyamyc: 100,000 units/g (15 g, 30 g, 60 g)
    Nystop: 100,000 units/g (15 g, 30 g, 60 g)
    Pedi-Dri: 100,000 units/g (56.7 g [DSC])
    Generic: 100,000 units/g (15 g, 30 g, 60 g)
  Tablet, Vaginal:
    Generic: 100,000 units [DSC]

◆ **Nystop** see Nystatin (Topical) on page 1219
◆ **Oasis®** see Saliva Substitute on page 1511

Obinutuzumab (oh bi nue TOOZ ue mab)

Related Information
Prevention and Management of Infections *on page 2196*

Brand Names: US Gazyva

Brand Names: Canada Gazyva

Index Terms GA101; R05072759; R7159

Pharmacologic Category Antineoplastic Agent, Anti-CD20; Antineoplastic Agent, Monoclonal Antibody

Use Chronic lymphocytic leukemia: Treatment of patients with previously untreated chronic lymphocytic leukemia (CLL) in combination with chlorambucil

Labeled Contraindications
US labeling: There are no contraindications listed in the manufacturer's labeling.

Canadian labeling: Known hypersensitivity (IgE mediated) to obinutuzumab or any component of the formulation.

Pregnancy Considerations Adverse effects were observed in animal reproduction studies. Monoclonal antibodies are known to cross the placenta. Based on the mechanism of action and on animal data, if exposure occurs during pregnancy, B-cell counts may be depleted and immunologic function may be affected in the neonate after birth. Administration of live vaccines to neonates and infants exposed *in utero* should be avoided until after B-cell recovery. The Canadian labeling recommends that women of child bearing potential use effective contraception during therapy and for 18 months after the last treatment.

Breast-Feeding Considerations It is not known if obinutuzumab is excreted into breast milk. However, endogenous human immunoglobulin can be detected in milk. Although antibodies in breast milk may not enter the nursing infant's circulations in substantial amounts, the US labeling recommends the decision to breast-feed during therapy should take into account the risk of exposure to the infant and the benefits of treatment to the mother. The Canadian labeling recommends discontinuing nursing during therapy and for 18 months after the last treatment.

Warnings/Precautions [US Boxed Warning]: Hepatitis B virus (HBV) reactivation may occur with use of CD20-directed cytolytic antibodies (including obinutuzumab) and may result in fulminant hepatitis, hepatic failure, and death. Screen all patients for HBV infection by measuring hepatitis B surface antigen (HBsAg) and hepatitis B core antibody (anti-HBc) prior to therapy initiation; monitor patients for clinical and laboratory signs of hepatitis or HBV during and for several months after treatment. Discontinue obinutuzumab (and concomitant chemotherapy) if viral hepatitis develops and initiate appropriate antiviral therapy. Reactivation has occurred in patients who are HBsAg positive as well as in those who are HBsAg negative but are anti-HBc positive; HBV reactivation has also been observed in patients who had previously resolved HBV infection. HBV reactivation has been reported for other CD20-directed antibodies after therapy discontinuation. Reactivation of HBV replication is often followed by hepatitis. Use cautiously in patients who show evidence of prior HBV infection (eg, HBsAg positive [regardless of antibody status] or HBsAG negative but anti-HBc positive); consult with appropriate clinicians regarding monitoring and consideration of antiviral therapy before and/or during obinutuzumab treatment. The safety of resuming obinutuzumab treatment following HBV reactivation is not known; discuss reinitiation of therapy in patients with resolved HBV reactivation with physicians experienced in HBV management. American Society of Clinical Oncology (ASCO) provisional clinical opinion update on HBV screening recommendations (Hwang 2015): Patients receiving anti-CD20 antibodies are at high risk for HBV reactivation. Screen for HBV infection with HBsAG and anti-HBc tests prior to treatment initiation; either a total anti-HBc (with both immunoglobulin [IgG] and immunoglobulin [IgM]) or anti-HBc IgG test should be used to screen for chronic or unresolved HBV infection (do not use anti-HBc IgM as it may only confirm acute HBV infection). In addition, patients who have risk factors for HBV infection (eg, birthplace in a country with ≥2% HBV prevalence, household or sexual contact with HBV-infected patients, high-risk behaviors [eg, intravenous drug use], and HIV infection) should also be screened prior to beginning therapy. Initiate prophylactic antiviral therapy (utilizing antivirals with low rates of viral resistance) for HBsAg-positive/anti-HBc–positive patients (without delaying cancer therapy) and continue the antivirals during and for ~6 to 12 months after completing treatment. HBsAg-negative/anti-HBc–positive patients should be monitored for HBV reactivation with HBV DNA and ALT testing approximately every 3 months during treatment; antiviral therapy may be initiated prophylactically or begun promptly at the first sign of HBV reactivation.

[US Boxed Warning]: Progressive multifocal leukoencephalopathy (PML) resulting in death may occur with treatment. PML is due to JC virus infection. Consider PML in any patient with new onset or worsening neurological symptoms and if PML is suspected, discontinue obinutuzumab (consider discontinuation or dose reduction of any concomitant chemotherapy or immunosuppressive therapy) and evaluate promptly.

May cause severe and life-threatening infusion reactions; reactions may include bronchospasm, dyspnea, tachycardia, larynx and throat irritation, wheezing, laryngeal edema, flushing, hypertension, hypotension, fever, nausea, vomiting, diarrhea, headache and/or chills. Infusion reactions occur more frequently with the first 1,000 mg infused. Delayed reactions (up to 24 hours later) and reactions with subsequent infusions have occurred. Premedicate with acetaminophen, an antihistamine, and an IV glucocorticoid (dexamethasone or methylprednisolone) prior to infusion. Hydrocortisone has not been effective in reducing the rate of infusion reactions and is not recommended). Infusion reactions may require rate reduction, interruption of therapy, or treatment discontinuation. Monitor during the entire infusion; monitor patients with preexisting cardiac or pulmonary conditions closely. Due to the risk for hypotension, consider temporarily withholding antihypertensive therapies for 12 hours prior to, during, and for 1 hour after administration. Administer in a facility with immediate access to resuscitative measures (eg, glucocorticoids, epinephrine, bronchodilators, and/or oxygen). Serious cardiovascular events (some fatal) have been reported.

In clinical trials, grade 3 and 4 neutropenia and thrombocytopenia occurred when used in combination with chlorambucil. Neutropenia may have a late onset (>28 days after therapy completion) and/or be prolonged (duration >28 days). Monitor for signs/symptoms of infection; antimicrobial prophylaxis is recommended in neutropenic patients. Antiviral and/or antifungal prophylaxis should also be considered. In a small percentage of patients, thrombocytopenia occurred acutely (within 24 hours) after obinutuzumab administration; platelet transfusions may be necessary. Fatal hemorrhagic events during the first cycle have been reported; monitor frequently for thrombocytopenia and bleeding episodes, particularly during the initial cycle. Thrombocytopenia may require dose delays of obinutuzumab and chlorambucil and/or dose reductions of chlorambucil. Consider withholding platelet inhibitors, anticoagulants, or other medications which may increase bleeding risk (especially during the first cycle). Leukopenia and lymphopenia commonly occur. Monitor blood counts frequently throughout therapy. Bacterial, fungal, and new or reactivated viral infections may occur during and/or following therapy; fatal infections have been reported. Do not administer to patients with an active infection. Patients with a history of recurrent or chronic infections may be at increased risk. Tumor lysis syndrome (TLS) has been reported with obinutuzumab (some cases fatal). Acute renal failure, hyperkalemia, hypocalcemia, hyperuricemia, and/or hyperphosphatemia may occur. Administer prophylaxis (antihyperuricemic therapy [eg, allopurinol or rasburicase] and hydration) in patients at high risk (high circulating lymphocyte counts [>25,000/mm³], high tumor burden, or renal impairment) prior to initiating obinutuzumab therapy (administer prior to each subsequent cycle if needed). Monitor lab parameters during initial treatment days in patients at risk for TLS. Correct electrolyte abnormalities; monitor renal function and hydration status, and administer supportive care, including dialysis as indicated. Administration of live virus vaccines during treatment (and until B-cell recovery) is not recommended; the safety and efficacy of immunization with live or attenuated viral vaccines during or after obinutuzumab therapy has not been determined. If obinutuzumab exposure occurs during pregnancy, the safety and timing of live virus vaccinations for the infant should be evaluated. Potentially significant drug-drug interactions may exist, requiring dose or frequency adjustment, additional monitoring, and/or selection of alternative therapy.

Adverse Reactions Adverse reactions reported in combination with chlorambucil. Frequency not always defined.

>10%:

Endocrine & metabolic: Hypocalcemia (37% to 38%; grades 3/4: 3%), hyperkalemia (14% to 33%; grades 3/4: 1 to 5%), hyponatremia (26% to 30%; grades 3/4: 7% to 8%), hypoalbuminemia (23%; grades 3/4: <1%), hypokalemia (15%; grade 3/4: 1%)

Hematologic & oncologic: Leukopenia (6% to 84%; grades 3/4: 4% to 37%), lymphocytopenia (80%; grades 3/4: 39% to 40%), neutropenia (38% to 78%; grades 3/4: 33% to 48%; onset ≥28 days after completion of treatment: 16%), thrombocytopenia (11% to 48%; grades 3/4: 10% to 13% onset within 24 hours of infusion: 4%), anemia (12% to 39%; grades 3/4: 5% to 10%)

Hepatic: Increased serum AST (27% to 29%; grades 3/4: 1% to 2%), increased serum ALT (27% to 28%; grades 3/4: 2%), increased serum alkaline phosphatase (18%)

Infection: Infection (38%; grades 3/4: 11%)

Neuromuscular & skeletal: Musculoskeletal signs and symptoms (18%; including pain)

Renal: Increased serum creatinine (30%; grades 3/4: <1%)

Miscellaneous: Infusion related reaction (initial infusion: 65% to 69%; grades 3/4: 20% to 21%; second infusion: 3%; subsequent infusions: <1%)

1% to 10%:

Cardiovascular: Thrombohemorrhagic event (4%), exacerbation of cardiac disease, flushing, hypertension, hypotension, tachycardia

Central nervous system: Chills, headache, progressive multifocal leukoencephalopathy

Endocrine & metabolic: Hyperphosphatemia, hyperuricemia

Gastrointestinal: Diarrhea (10%; grades 3/4: 2%), constipation (8%), vomiting

Genitourinary: Urinary tract infection (5% to 6%; grades 3/4: 1% to 2%)

Hematologic & oncologic: Tumor lysis syndrome (grades 3/4: 2%)

Hepatic: Increased liver enzymes (4%; may be secondary or exacerbated by premedications)

Infection: JCV (John Cunningham virus) infection, reactivation of HBV, viral infection (new or reactivation)

Neuromuscular & skeletal: Back pain (5%; grade 3/4: <1%)

Renal: Acute renal failure

Respiratory: Cough (10%), nasopharyngitis (6%; grades: <1%), broncho-spasm, dyspnea, laryngeal edema, throat irritation, wheezing

Miscellaneous: Fever (9% to 10%; grades 3/4: <1%)

Drug Interactions

Metabolism/Transport Effects None known.

Avoid Concomitant Use

Avoid concomitant use of Obinutuzumab with any of the following: BCG (Intravesical); Belimumab; CloZAPine; Dipyrone; Natalizumab; Pimecrolimus; Tacrolimus (Topical); Tofacitinib; Vaccines (Live)

Increased Effect/Toxicity

Obinutuzumab may increase the levels/effects of: Belimumab; CloZAPine; Fingolimod; Leflunomide; Natalizumab; Tofacitinib; Vaccines (Live)

The levels/effects of Obinutuzumab may be increased by: Agents with Antiplatelet Properties; Anticoagulants; Antihypertensives; Denosumab; Dipyrone; Pimecrolimus; Roflumilast; Tacrolimus (Topical); Trastuzumab

Decreased Effect

Obinutuzumab may decrease the levels/effects of: BCG (Intravesical); Coc-cidioides immitis Skin Test; Sipuleucel-T; Vaccines (Inactivated); Vaccines (Live)

The levels/effects of Obinutuzumab may be decreased by: Echinacea

Storage/Stability Store intact vials at 2°C to 8°C (36°F to 46°F); do not freeze or shake. Protect from light. Diluted solutions for infusion should be used immediately. If not used immediately, the diluted solutions may be stored up to 24 hours at 2°C to 8°C (36°F to 46°F) followed by 48 hours (including infusion time) at room temperature of ≤30°C (≤86°F).

Preparation for Administration

Cycle 1, day 1 and 2 doses (100 mg and 900 mg, respectively): Withdraw 40 mL of obinutuzumab solution from vial. Dilute 4 mL into a 100 mL infusion bag of NS (100 mg dose; use immediately). Dilute remaining 36 mL into a 250 mL NS infusion bag (900 mg dose, for use on day 2); store at 2°C to 8°C (36°F to 46°F) for up to 24 hours; use immediately after reaching room temperature. Gently invert to mix; do not shake or freeze.

Cycle 1 (day 8 and 15 doses) and cycles 2 through 6 (1000 mg): Withdraw 40 mL of obinutuzumab solution from vial. Dilute into a 250 mL NS infusion bag. Gently invert to mix; do not shake or freeze.

Do not use other diluents (eg, dextrose) to prepare the infusion. Final concentration for administration should be 0.4 to 4 mg/mL. May use PVC or non-PVC infusion bags.

Mechanism of Action Obinutuzumab is a glycoengineered type II anti-CD20 monoclonal antibody. The CD20 antigen is expressed on the surface of pre B- and mature B-lymphocytes; upon binding to CD20, obinutuzumab activates complement-dependent cytotoxicity, antibody-dependent cellular cytotoxicity and antibody-dependent cellular phagocytosis, resulting in cell death (Sehn 2012).

Pharmacodynamics/Kinetics

Distribution: V_d: ~3.9 L

Half-life elimination: ~29.7 days

Dosing

Adult & Geriatric Note: Premedication with acetaminophen, an antihistamine, and a glucocorticoid (dexamethasone or methylprednisolone) 30 to 60 minutes prior to treatment may be necessary (see Administration). Antihyperuricemic prophylaxis and adequate hydration are recommended for patients at risk for tumor lysis syndrome. Antimicrobial, antiviral, and antifungal prophylaxis may be considered in certain patients.

Chronic lymphocytic leukemia (CLL): IV:

Cycle 1: 100 mg on day 1, followed by 900 mg on day 2, followed by 1,000 mg weekly for 2 doses (days 8 and 15)

Cycles 2 through 6: 1,000 mg on day 1 every 28 days for 5 doses

Missed doses: Administer the missed dose as soon as possible; adjust dosing schedule accordingly. In some cases, patients who do not complete the day 1 cycle 1 dose may proceed to the day 2 cycle 1 treatment (if appropriate).

Renal Impairment

CrCl ≥30 mL/minute: There are no dosage adjustments provided in the US manufacturer's labeling; however, pharmacokinetics are not affected (based on pharmacokinetic analysis). The Canadian labeling recommends that no dosage adjustment is necessary.

CrCl <30 mL/minute: There are no dosage adjustments provided in the manufacturer's labeling (has not been studied)

Hepatic Impairment There are no dosage adjustments provided in the manufacturer's labeling (has not been studied)

Adjustment for Toxicity

Hematologic: Grade 3 or 4 cytopenia: Consider treatment interruption

Infusion reactions:

Mild-to-moderate (Grades 1 and 2): Reduce infusion rate or interrupt infusion and manage symptoms as appropriate. Upon symptom resolution, continue or resume infusion. If no further infusion reaction symptoms occur, may resume infusion rate escalation as appropriate for the treatment cycle dose. Day 1 (cycle 1) infusion rate may be increased back up to a maximum of 25 mg/hour after 1 hour.

Severe (Grade 3): Interrupt therapy; manage symptoms as appropriate. Upon symptom resolution, may reinitiate infusion at no more than 50% of the rate at which the reaction occurred. If no further infusion reaction symptoms occur, may resume infusion rate escalation as appropriate for the treatment cycle dose. Day 1 (cycle 1) infusion rate may be increased back up to a maximum of 25 mg/hour after 1 hour. Permanently discontinue if ≥ grade 3 infusion-related symptoms occur upon rechallenge.

Life-threatening (Grade 4): Discontinue infusion immediately; permanently discontinue therapy.

Infection: Consider treatment interruption.

Other toxicity: Consider treatment interruption for ≥ grade 2 nonhematologic toxicity.

Combination Regimens

Leukemia, chronic lymphocytic: Chlorambucil-Obinutuzumab (CLL) on page 1884

Administration For IV infusion only. Do not administer IV push or as a bolus. Administer through a dedicated IV line; do not mix with or infuse with other medications. May use PVC or non-PVC administration sets. Premedication with acetaminophen, an antihistamine, and a glucocorticoid (dexamethasone or methylprednisolone) may be required to prevent infusion reactions (see below). In patients with neutropenia, antimicrobial prophylaxis is strongly recommended throughout the treatment period; antiviral and antifungal prophylaxis should be considered.

Premedication to prevent infusion reactions:

Cycle 1 (days 1 and 2): All patients should receive acetaminophen (650 to 1,000 mg) and an antihistamine (eg, diphenhydramine 50 mg) at least 30 minutes prior to infusion. In addition, an IV glucocorticoid (dexamethasone 20 mg or methylprednisolone 80 mg) should be administered at least 1 hour prior to infusion.

Cycle 1 (days 8 and 15), and cycles 2 through 6: All patients should receive acetaminophen 650 to 1,000 mg at least 30 minutes prior to infusion.

If patients experienced grade 1 or higher infusion-related reaction with previous infusion: Administer an antihistamine (eg, diphenhydramine 50 mg) in addition to acetaminophen at least 30 minutes prior to infusion.

If patients experienced a grade 3 infusion-related reaction with previous infusion **or** have a lymphocyte count >25,000 cells/mm^3 prior to next treatment: Administer an IV glucocorticoid (dexamethasone 20 mg or methylprednisolone 80 mg) at least 1 hour prior to infusion, in addition to acetaminophen and an antihistamine at least 30 minutes prior to infusion.

Infusion rate:

Cycle 1 (day 1): Infuse at 25 mg/hour over 4 hours; do not increase the infusion rate

Cycle 1 (day 2): If no reaction to previous infusion, initiate infusion at 50 mg/hour for 30 minutes; if tolerated, may escalate rate in increments of 50 mg/hour every 30 minutes to a maximum rate of 400 mg/hour.

Cycle 1 (days 8 and 15), and cycles 2 through 6: If no reaction to previous infusion, initiate infusion at 100 mg/hour for 30 minutes; if tolerated, may escalate infusion rate in increments of 100 mg/hour every 30 minutes to a maximum rate of 400 mg/hour.

Emetic Potential Minimal (<10%)

Monitoring Parameters

CBC with differential (at regular intervals), renal function, electrolytes, uric acid (if at risk for tumor lysis syndrome); hepatitis B screening in all patients (HBsAG and anti-HBc measurements) prior to therapy initiation. Hepatitis B virus (HBV) screening recommendations (American Society of Clinical Oncology provisional clinical opinion update [Hwang 2015]): Screen for HBV infection with hepatitis B surface antigen (HBsAG) and hepatitis B core antibody (anti-HBc) tests prior to treatment initiation; either a total anti-HBc (with both immunoglobulin G [IgG] and immunoglobulin M [IgM]) or anti-HBc IgG test should be used to screen for chronic or unresolved HBV infection (do not use anti-HBc IgM as it may only confirm acute HBV infection). HBsAg-negative/anti-HBc–positive patients should be monitored for HBV reactivation with HBV DNA and ALT testing approximately every 3 months during treatment.

◄ Monitor for signs of active hepatitis B infection (during and for up to 12 months after therapy completion). Monitor for signs or symptoms of infusion reaction; signs of infection; fluid status; signs/symptoms of progressive multifocal leukoencephalopathy (PML; focal neurologic deficits, which may present as hemiparesis, visual field deficits, cognitive impairment, aphasia, ataxia, and/or cranial nerve deficits); evaluate for PML with brain MRI, lumbar puncture, and neurologist consultation.

Dosage Forms Excipient information presented when available (limited, particularly for generics); consult specific product labeling.
Solution, Intravenous [preservative free]:
Gazyva: 1000 mg/40 mL (40 mL)

◆ **Obizur** see Antihemophilic Factor (Recombinant [Porcine Sequence]) on page 123

◆ **Ocphyl (Can)** see Octreotide on page 1226

◆ **Octacog Alfa** see Antihemophilic Factor (Recombinant) on page 119

◆ **Octagam** see Immune Globulin on page 903

◆ **Octagam 10%** see Immune Globulin on page 903

◆ **Octostim (Can)** see Desmopressin on page 505

◆ **OctreoScan®** see Indium In-111 Pentetreotide on page 919

◆ **OctreoScan® (Prep Kit)** see Indium In-111 Pentetreotide on page 919

Octreotide (ok TREE oh tide)

Related Information
Management of EGFR Inhibitor Toxicities: Dermatologic, Ocular, and Gastrointestinal on page 2179

Brand Names: US SandoSTATIN; SandoSTATIN LAR Depot

Brand Names: Canada Ocphyl; Octreotide Acetate Omega; Octreotide Injection; Sandostatin; Sandostatin LAR

Index Terms Longastatin; Octreotide Acetate

Pharmacologic Category Antidiarrheal; Antidote; Somatostatin Analog

Use

Acromegaly:
Injection solution: To reduce blood levels of growth hormone (GH) and insulin-like growth factor 1 (IGF-1) in patients with inadequate response to or who cannot be treated with surgical resection, pituitary irradiation, and bromocriptine mesylate at maximally tolerated doses; goal of therapy is to achieve normalization of GH and IGF-1 levels.

LAR depot suspension: Long-term maintenance treatment of acromegaly in patients with an inadequate response to surgery and/or radiotherapy (or for whom surgery/radiotherapy are not options) with a goal of therapy to reduce GH and IGF-1 levels to normal.

Carcinoid tumors:
Injection solution: Management of symptoms (diarrhea and flushing) in patients with metastatic carcinoid tumors.

LAR depot suspension: Long-term treatment of severe diarrhea and flushing episodes associated with metastatic carcinoid tumors.

Vasoactive intestinal peptide-secreting tumors:
Injection solution: Treatment of profuse watery diarrhea associated with vasoactive intestinal peptide-secreting tumors (VIPomas).

LAR depot suspension: Long-term treatment of profuse watery diarrhea associated with VIPomas.

Limitations of use: The effects of octreotide (injection solution and LAR depot suspension) on tumor size, rate of growth, and development of metastases in patients with carcinoid syndrome and VIPomas have not been determined.

Labeled Contraindications Hypersensitivity to octreotide or any component of the formulation

Pregnancy Considerations Adverse events have not been observed in animal reproduction studies. Octreotide crosses the placenta and can be detected in the newborn at delivery (Caron 1995; Fassnacht 2001; Maffei 2010); data concerning use in pregnancy is limited. In case reports of acromegalic women who received normal doses of octreotide during pregnancy, no congenital malformations were reported. Because normalization of IGF-1 and GH may restore fertility in women with acromegaly, women of childbearing potential should use adequate contraception during treatment. Long-acting formulations should be discontinued ~2 months prior to a planned pregnancy; use short acting octreotide as needed until conception. Octreotide therapy may be considered in pregnant women with worsening symptoms if needed. Monitoring of IGF-1 and/or GH is not recommended during pregnancy (Katznelson 2014).

Breast-Feeding Considerations Octreotide is excreted in breast milk. In a case report, a woman was taking octreotide SubQ in doses up to 2400 mcg/day prior to and throughout pregnancy. Octreotide was measurable in the colostrum in concentrations similar to those in the maternal serum (Maffei 2010); however, oral absorption of octreotide is considered to be poor (Battershill, 1989). The manufacturer recommends that caution be exercised when administering octreotide to nursing women.

Warnings/Precautions May impair gallbladder function; monitor patients for cholelithiasis. The incidence of gallbladder stone or biliary sludge increases with a duration of therapy of ≥12 months. Prophylactic cholecystectomy is recommended in patients with gastrointestinal or pancreatic neuroendocrine tumors undergoing abdominal surgery if octreotide treatment is planned (Oberg 2004). Use with caution in patients with renal and/or hepatic impairment; dosage adjustment may be required in patients receiving dialysis and in patients with established cirrhosis. Somatostatin analogs may affect glucose regulation. In type I diabetes, severe hypoglycemia may occur; in type II diabetes or patients without diabetes, hyperglycemia may occur. Insulin and other hypoglycemic medication requirements may change. Octreotide may worsen hypoglycemia in patients with insulinomas; use with caution. Do not use depot formulation for the treatment of sulfonylurea-induced hypoglycemia. Bradycardia, conduction abnormalities, and arrhythmia have been observed in acromegalic and carcinoid syndrome patients; use caution with CHF or concomitant medications that alter heart rate or rhythm. Cardiovascular medication requirements may change. Octreotide may enhance the adverse/toxic effects of other QTc-prolonging agents. May alter absorption of dietary fats; monitor for pancreatitis. May reduce excessive fluid loss in patients with conditions that cause such loss; monitor for elevations in zinc levels in such patients that are maintained on total parenteral nutrition (TPN). Chronic treatment has been associated with abnormal Schillings test; monitor vitamin B_{12} levels. Suppresses secretion of TSH; monitor for hypothyroidism.

◄ Postmarketing cases of serious and fatal events, including hypoxia and necrotizing enterocolitis, have been reported with octreotide use in children (usually with serious underlying conditions), particularly in children <2 years of age. In studies with octreotide depot, the incidence of cholelithiasis in children is higher than the reported incidences for adults and efficacy was not demonstrated. Therapy may restore fertility; females of childbearing potential should use adequate contraception. Dosage adjustment may be necessary in the elderly; significant increases in elimination half-life have been observed in older adults. Vehicle used in depot injection (polylactide-co-glycolide microspheres) has rarely been associated with retinal artery occlusion in patients with abnormal arteriovenous anastomosis. Therapy with immediate release octreotide (solution) should be withheld 24 hours prior to administration of radiolabeled somatostatin analogs; the IM (depot) formulation should be withheld at least 2 months before administration of radiolabeled somatostatin analogs (Oberg 2004). Potentially significant drug-drug interactions may exist, requiring dose or frequency adjustment, additional monitoring, and/or selection of alternative therapy.

Adverse Reactions Adverse reactions vary by route of administration and dosage form. Frequency of cardiac, endocrine, and gastrointestinal adverse reactions was generally higher in acromegalics.

>16%:

Cardiovascular: Sinus bradycardia (19% to 25%), chest pain (≤20%; non-depot formulations)

Central nervous system: Fatigue (1% to 32%), headache (6% to 30%), malaise (16% to 20%), fever (16% to 20%), dizziness (5% to 20%)

Dermatologic: Pruritus (≤18%)

Endocrine & metabolic: Hyperglycemia (2% to 27%)

Gastrointestinal: Abdominal pain (5% to 61%), loose stools (5% to 61%), nausea (5% to 61%), diarrhea (34% to 61%), flatulence (≤38%), cholelithiasis (13% to 38%; length of therapy dependent), biliary sludge (24%; length of therapy dependent), constipation (9% to 21%), vomiting (4% to 21%), biliary duct dilatation (12%)

Local: Injection site pain (2% to 50%; dose and formulation related)

Neuromuscular & skeletal: Back pain (1% to 27%), arthropathy (8% to 19%), myalgia (≤18%)

Respiratory: Upper respiratory infection (10% to 23%), dyspnea (≤20%; non-depot formulations)

Miscellaneous: Antibodies to octreotide (up to 25%; no efficacy change), flu symptoms (1% to 20%)

5% to 15%:

Cardiovascular: Hypertension (≤13%), conduction abnormalities (9% to 10%), arrhythmia (3% to 9%), palpitation, peripheral edema

Central nervous system: Pain (4% to 15%), anxiety, confusion, hypoesthesia, insomnia

Dermatologic: Rash (15%; depot formulation), alopecia (≤13%)

Endocrine & metabolic: Hypothyroidism (≤12%; non-depot formulations), goiter (≤8%; non-depot formulations)

Gastrointestinal: Dyspepsia (4% to 6%), feces discoloration (4% to 6%), steatorrhea (4% to 6%), tenesmus (4% to 6%), anorexia, cramping

Hematologic: Anemia (≤15%; non-depot formulations: <1%)

Neuromuscular & skeletal: Arthralgia, myalgia, paresthesia, rigors, weakness

Otic: Earache

Renal: Renal calculus

Respiratory: Cough, pharyngitis, rhinitis, sinusitis

Miscellaneous: Allergy, diaphoresis

1% to 4%:

Cardiovascular: Angina, cardiac failure, edema, flushing, hematoma, phlebitis

Central nervous system: Abnormal gait, amnesia, depression, dysphonia, hallucinations, nervousness, neuralgia, somnolence, vertigo

Dermatologic: Acne, bruising, cellulitis

Endocrine & metabolic: Hypoglycemia (2% to 4%), hypokalemia, hypoproteinemia, gout, cachexia, breast pain, impotence

Gastrointestinal: Colitis, diverticulitis, dysphagia, fat malabsorption, gastritis, gastroenteritis, gingivitis, glossitis, melena, stomatitis, taste perversion, xerostomia

Genitourinary: Incontinence, pollakiuria (non-depot formulations), urinary tract infection

Local: Injection site hematoma

Neuromuscular & skeletal: Hyperkinesia, hypertonia, joint pain, neuropathy, tremor

Ocular: Blurred vision, visual disturbance

Otic: Tinnitus

Renal: Albuminuria, renal abscess

Respiratory: Bronchitis, epistaxis

Miscellaneous: Bacterial infection, cold symptoms, moniliasis

<1%, postmarketing, and/or case reports: Amenorrhea, anaphylactic shock, anaphylactoid reactions, aneurysm, aphasia, appendicitis, arthritis, ascending cholangitis, ascites, atrial fibrillation, basal cell carcinoma, Bell's palsy, biliary obstruction, breast carcinoma, cardiac arrest, cerebral vascular disorder, CHF, cholecystitis, cholestatic hepatitis, CK increased, creatinine increased, deafness, diabetes insipidus, diabetes mellitus, facial edema, fatty liver, galactorrhea, gallbladder polyp, GI bleeding, GI hemorrhage, GI ulcer, glaucoma, gynecomastia, hearing impairment, hematuria, hemiparesis, hemorrhoids, hepatitis, hyperesthesia, hypertensive reaction, hypoadrenalism, hypoxia (children), intestinal obstruction, intracranial hemorrhage, intraocular pressure increased, iron deficiency, ischemia, jaundice, joint effusion, LFTs increased, libido decreased, malignant hyperpyrexia, MI, migraine, necrotizing enterocolitis (neonates), nephrolithiasis, neuritis, oligomenorrhea, orthostatic hypotension, pancreatitis, pancytopenia, paranoia, paresis, petechiae, pituitary apoplexy, pleural effusion, pneumonia, pneumothorax, polymenorrhea, pulmonary embolism, pulmonary hypertension, pulmonary nodule, QT prolongation, Raynaud's syndrome, rectal bleeding, renal failure, renal insufficiency, retinal vein thrombosis, scotoma, seizures, status asthmaticus, suicide attempt, syncope, tachycardia, thrombocytopenia, thrombophlebitis, thrombosis, urticaria, vaginitis, visual field defect, vitamin B_{12} deficiency, weight loss, wheal/erythema

Drug Interactions

Metabolism/Transport Effects None known.

Avoid Concomitant Use

Avoid concomitant use of Octreotide with any of the following: Ceritinib

Increased Effect/Toxicity

Octreotide may increase the levels/effects of: Bradycardia-Causing Agents; Bromocriptine; Ceritinib; Codeine; Highest Risk QTc-Prolonging Agents; Hypoglycemia-Associated Agents; Ivabradine; Lacosamide; Moderate Risk QTc-Prolonging Agents; Pegvisomant

◄ *The levels/effects of Octreotide may be increased by:* Androgens; Antidiabetic Agents; Bretylium; Herbs (Hypoglycemic Properties); MAO Inhibitors; Mifepristone; Pegvisomant; Quinolone Antibiotics; Ruxolitinib; Salicylates; Selective Serotonin Reuptake Inhibitors; Tofacitinib

Decreased Effect

Octreotide may decrease the levels/effects of: Antidiabetic Agents; Cyclo-SPORINE (Systemic)

The levels/effects of Octreotide may be decreased by: Quinolone Antibiotics

Food Interactions Octreotide may alter absorption of dietary fats. Management: Administer injections between meals to decrease GI effects.

Storage/Stability

Injection solution: Octreotide is a clear solution and should be stored at refrigerated temperatures between 2°C and 8°C (36°F and 46°F). Protect from light. May be stored at room temperature of 20°C to 30°C (68°F and 86°F) for up to 14 days when protected from light. Stable as a parenteral admixture in NS or D_5W for 24 hours. Discard multidose vials within 14 days after initial entry.

LAR depot suspension: Prior to dilution, store at refrigerated temperatures between 2°C and 8°C (36°F and 46°F). Protect from light. Additionally, the manufacturer reports that octreotide suspension may be stored at room temperature of 20°C to 25°C (68°F and 77°F) for up to 10 days when protected from light (data on file [Novartis 2011]). Depot drug product kit may be at room temperature for 30 to 60 minutes prior to use. Use suspension immediately after preparation.

Mechanism of Action Mimics natural somatostatin by inhibiting serotonin release, and the secretion of gastrin, VIP, insulin, glucagon, secretin, motilin, and pancreatic polypeptide. Decreases growth hormone and IGF-1 in acromegaly. Octreotide provides more potent inhibition of growth hormone, glucagon, and insulin as compared to endogenous somatostatin. Also suppresses LH response to GnRH, secretion of thyroid-stimulating hormone and decreases splanchnic blood flow.

Pharmacodynamics/Kinetics

Duration: SubQ: 6 to 12 hours

Absorption: SubQ: Rapid and complete; IM (depot formulation): Released slowly (via microsphere degradation in the muscle)

Distribution: V_d: 14 L (13 to 30 L in acromegaly)

Protein binding: 65%, primarily to lipoprotein (41% in acromegaly)

Metabolism: Extensively hepatic

Bioavailability: SubQ: 100%; IM: 60% to 63% of SubQ dose

Half-life elimination: 1.7 to 1.9 hours; Increased in elderly patients; Cirrhosis: Up to 3.7 hours; Fatty liver disease: Up to 3.4 hours; Renal impairment: Up to 3.1 hours

Time to peak, plasma: SubQ: 0.4 hours (0.7 hours acromegaly); IM: 1 hour

Excretion: Urine (32% as unchanged drug)

Dosing

Adult

Acromegaly:

SubQ, IV: Initial: 50 mcg 3 times/day; titrate to achieve growth hormone levels <5 ng/mL or IGF-I (somatomedin C) levels <1.9 units/mL in males and <2.2 units/mL in females. Usual effective dose: 100 mcg 3 times/day; range: 300 to 1,500 mcg/day. Doses above 300 mcg/day rarely result in additional benefit; if increased dose fails to provide additional benefit, the dose should be reduced. **Note:** Should be withdrawn yearly for a 4-week interval (8 weeks for depot injection) in patients who have received irradiation. Resume if levels increase and signs/symptoms recur.

IM depot injection: Patients must be stabilized on subcutaneous octreotide for at least 2 weeks before switching to the long-acting depot. Upon switch: 20 mg IM intragluteally every 4 weeks for 3 months, then the dose may be modified based upon response.

Dosage adjustment for acromegaly: After 3 months of depot injections, the dosage may be continued or modified as follows:

GH ≤1 ng/mL, IGF-1 normal, and symptoms controlled: Reduce octreotide depot to 10 mg IM every 4 weeks

GH ≤2.5 ng/mL, IGF-1 normal, and symptoms controlled: Maintain octreotide depot at 20 mg IM every 4 weeks

GH >2.5 ng/mL, IGF-1 elevated, and/or symptoms uncontrolled: Increase octreotide depot to 30 mg IM every 4 weeks

Note: Patients not adequately controlled at a dose of 30 mg may increase dose to 40 mg every 4 weeks. Dosages >40 mg are not recommended.

Carcinoid tumors:

SubQ, IV: Initial 2 weeks: 100 to 600 mcg/day in 2 to 4 divided doses; usual range: 50 to 750 mcg/day (some patients may require up to 1,500 mcg/day); experience with doses above 750 mcg/day is limited.

IM depot injection: Patients must be stabilized on subcutaneous octreotide for at least 2 weeks before switching to the long-acting depot. Upon switch: 20 mg IM intragluteally every 4 weeks for 2 months, then the dose may be modified based upon response.

Note: Patients should continue to receive their SubQ injections for the first 2 weeks at the same dose in order to maintain therapeutic levels (some patients may require 3 to 4 weeks of continued SubQ injections). Patients who experience periodic exacerbations of symptoms may require temporary SubQ injections in addition to depot injections (at their previous SubQ dosing regimen) until symptoms have resolved.

Dosage adjustment for carcinoid tumors: After 2 months of depot injections, the dosage may be continued or modified as follows:

Increase to 30 mg IM every 4 weeks if symptoms are inadequately controlled

Decrease to 10 mg IM every 4 weeks, for a trial period, if initially responsive to 20 mg dose

Dosage >30 mg is not recommended

Vasoactive intestinal peptide tumors (VIPomas):

SubQ, IV: Initial 2 weeks: 200 to 300 mcg/day in 2 to 4 divided doses; titrate dose based on response/tolerance. Range: 150 to 750 mcg/day (doses >450 mcg/day are rarely required)

IM depot injection: Patients must be stabilized on subcutaneous octreotide for at least 2 weeks before switching to the long-acting depot. Upon switch: 20 mg IM intragluteally every 4 weeks for 2 months, then the dose may be modified based upon response.

Note: Patients receiving depot injection should continue to receive their SubQ injections for the first 2 weeks at the same dose in order to maintain therapeutic levels (some patients may require 3 to 4 weeks of continued SubQ injections). Patients who experience periodic exacerbations of symptoms may require temporary SubQ injections in addition to depot injections (at their previous SubQ dosing regimen) until symptoms have resolved.

Dosage adjustment for VIPomas: After 2 months of depot injections, the dosage may be continued or modified as follows:

Increase to 30 mg IM every 4 weeks if symptoms are inadequately controlled

Decrease to 10 mg IM every 4 weeks, for a trial period, if initially responsive to 20 mg dose

Dosage >30 mg is not recommended

Carcinoid crisis, prevention (off-label use): Immediate release octreotide solution (Oberg 2004):

Patients controlled with octreotide IM (depot) 20 to 30 mg: SubQ: 250 to 500 mcg within 1 to 2 hours prior to procedure.

Emergency surgery in somatostatin analog-naïve patients with functional neuroendocrine tumors:

IV bolus: 500 to 1000 mcg 1 to 2 hours prior to procedure **or**

SubQ: 500 mcg 1 to 2 hours prior to procedure

Intraoperative use for carcinoid crisis with hypotension: IV: 500 to 1,000 mcg bolus, repeat at 5 minute intervals until symptoms are controlled or IV: 500 to 1,000 mcg bolus followed by 50 to 200 mcg/hour continuous infusion during the procedure.

Postoperative dose (if supplemental doses required during procedure): IV: 50 to 200 mcg/hour continuous infusion for 24 hours, followed by resumption of the preoperative treatment schedule.

Diarrhea (off-label use): IV: Initial: 50 to 100 mcg every 8 hours; increase by 100 mcg/dose at 48-hour intervals; maximum dose: 500 mcg every 8 hours

Diarrhea (refractory) associated with chemotherapy (off-label use):

Low grade or uncomplicated: SubQ: 100 to 150 mcg every 8 hours (Benson 2004; Kornblau 2000)

Severe: Initial: SubQ: 100 to 150 mcg every 8 hours; may increase to 500 to 1500 mcg IV or SubQ every 8 hours (Kornblau 2000)

Complicated: IV, SubQ: Initial: 100 to 150 mcg 3 times/day or IV Infusion: 25 to 50 mcg/hour; may escalate to 500 mcg 3 times/day until controlled (Benson 2004)

Diarrhea associated with acute graft-versus-host disease (GVHD) (off-label use): IV: 500 mcg every 8 hours; discontinue within 24 hours of diarrhea resolution to avoid ileus; Maximum duration of therapy if diarrhea is not resolved: 7 days (Kornblau 2000)

Esophageal varices bleeding (off-label use): IV bolus: 25 to 100 mcg (usual bolus dose: 50 mcg) followed by continuous IV infusion of 25 to 50 mcg/hour for 2 to 5 days; may repeat bolus in first hour if hemorrhage not controlled (Corley 2001; Erstad 2001; Garcia-Tsao 2010)

Gastroenteropancreatic neuroendocrine tumors (off-label use):

IM (depot): 30 mg every 4 weeks until tumor progression or death (Rinke 2009) **or**

SubQ: Initial: 100 to 500 mcg 2 to 4 times daily (usually 150 mcg 3 times daily), may increase to response (symptom control) by doubling the dose every 3 to 4 days or a continuous subQ infusion of 1,000 to 2,000 mcg/day (Oberg 2004) **or**

IM (depot): Assure tolerability by initiating with the SubQ formulation for 3 to 7 days (and continue with SubQ for the first ~14 days after the initial IM depot dose). Then initiate IM (depot): 20 to 30 mg every 28 days (SubQ doses of 200 to 600 mcg/day should receive 20 mg IM and SubQ doses of 750 to 1,500 mcg/day should receive 30 mg IM); IM (depot) range: 20 to 60 mg every 28 days (Oberg 2004).

Malignant bowel obstruction (off-label use): SubQ: 200 to 900 mcg/day in 2 to 3 divided doses (Mercadante 2007; Mercadante 2012) or 300 mcg/day by continuous SubQ infusion (Mercadante 2000)

Sulfonylurea-induced hypoglycemia (off-label use): Note: Although octreotide use has been advocated as a first line therapy, indications and dosing for octreotide are not firmly established (Glatstein 2012). Octreotide may reduce the incidence of recurrent hypoglycemia seen with dextrose-alone therapy (Fasano 2008). In addition, although subcutaneous administration is the preferred route, administration via intravenous bolus and intravenous infusion have also been described in the literature (Barkin 2013; Braatvedt 1997; Carr 2002; Crawford 2004; Dougherty 2010; Dougherty 2013; Fasano 2008; Graudins 1997; Green 2003; Hung 1997; McLaughlin 2000; Mordel 1998). Optimal care decisions should be made based upon patient-specific details. Repeat dosing, dose escalation, or initiation of a continuous infusion may be required in patients who experience recurrent hypoglycemia. Duration of treatment may exceed 24 hours.

SubQ: 50 to 75 mcg; repeat every 6 hours as needed based upon blood glucose concentrations (Fasano 2008; Howland 2011)

IV: Doses up to 125 mcg/hour have been used successfully (McLaughlin 2000)

Thymoma/thymic malignancies, advanced (off-label use): SubQ: 500 mcg 3 times daily; evaluate after 2 months, patients with remission (complete or partial) continued octreotide for up to a maximum of 12 months; patients with stable disease continued octreotide and also received prednisone for up to 12 months or until disease progression or unacceptable toxicity (Loehrer 2004).

Geriatric Refer to adult dosing. Elimination half-life is increased by 46% and clearance is decreased by 26%; dose adjustment may be required. Dosing should generally begin at the lower end of dosing range.

Pediatric Infants and Children:

Congenital hyperinsulinism (off-label use): SubQ: Initial: 2 to 10 mcg/kg/day; up to 40 mcg/kg/day have been used (Stanley 1997).

Secretory diarrhea (off-label use): IV, SubQ: Doses of 1 to 10 mcg/kg every 12 hours have been used in children beginning at the low end of the range and increasing by 0.3 mcg/kg/dose at 3-day intervals. Suppression of growth hormone (animal data) is of concern when used as long-term therapy.

Sulfonylurea-induced hypoglycemia (off-label use): Note: Although octreotide use has been advocated as a first line therapy, indications and dosing for octreotide are not firmly established (Glatstein 2012). Octreotide may reduce the incidence of recurrent hypoglycemia seen with dextrose-alone therapy (Fasano 2008). In addition, although subcutaneous administration is the preferred route, administration via intravenous bolus and intravenous infusion have also been described in the literature (Barkin 2013; Braatvedt 1997; Carr 2002; Crawford 2004; Dougherty 2010; Dougherty 2013; Fasano 2008; Graudins 1997; Green 2003; Hung 1997; McLaughlin 2000; Mordel 1998). Optimal care decisions should be made based upon patient-specific details. Repeat dosing, dose escalation, or initiation of a continuous infusion may be required in patients who experience recurrent hypoglycemia. Duration of treatment may exceed 24 hours. SubQ: 1 to 1.25 mcg/kg; repeat in 6 hours as needed based upon blood glucose concentrations (Howland 2011). Children generally need only a single dose (Dougherty 2013).

◄ **Renal Impairment**

Regular injection:

Mild to severe impairment: There are no dosage adjustments provided in the manufacturer's labeling.

Dialysis-dependent impairment: There are no specific dosage adjustments provided in the manufacturer's labeling; however, a dosage adjustment may be needed since clearance is reduced by ~50%.

Depot injection:

Mild to severe impairment: No dosage adjustment necessary.

Dialysis-dependent impairment: Initial dose: 10 mg IM every 4 weeks; titrate based upon response (clearance is reduced by ~50%)

Hepatic Impairment

Regular injection: There are no dosage adjustments provided in the manufacturer's labeling. Half-life is prolonged and total body clearance is decreased in patients with cirrhosis and fatty liver disease.

Depot injection: Patients with established cirrhosis of the liver: Initial dose: 10 mg IM every 4 weeks; titrate based upon response.

Usual Infusion Concentrations: Adult IV infusion: 500 mcg in 250 mL (concentration: 2 **mcg**/mL) of D_5W or NS

Administration

Regular injection formulation (do not use if solution contains particles or is discolored): Administer SubQ or IV; IV administration may be IV push (undiluted over 3 minutes), intermittent IV infusion (over 15 to 30 minutes), or continuous IV infusion (off-label route). In emergency situations (eg, carcinoid crisis), octreotide may be given as a rapid IV bolus.

SubQ: Use the concentration with smallest volume to deliver dose to reduce injection site pain. Rotate injection site; may bring to room temperature prior to injection.

Depot formulation: Administer IM intragluteal (avoid deltoid administration); alternate gluteal injection sites to avoid irritation. **Do not** administer Sandostatin LAR® intravenously or subcutaneously; must be administered immediately after mixing.

Monitoring Parameters

Acromegaly: Growth hormone, somatomedin C (IGF-1)

Carcinoid: 5-HIAA, plasma serotonin and plasma substance P

VIPomas: Vasoactive intestinal peptide

Chronic therapy: Thyroid function (baseline and periodic), vitamin B_{12} level, blood glucose, glycemic control and antidiabetic regimen (patients with diabetes mellitus), cardiac function (heart rate, ECG), zinc level (patients with excessive fluid loss maintained on TPN)

Dietary Considerations Schedule injections between meals to decrease GI effects. May alter absorption of dietary fats.

Dosage Forms Excipient information presented when available (limited, particularly for generics); consult specific product labeling.

Kit, Intramuscular:

SandoSTATIN LAR Depot: 10 mg, 20 mg, 30 mg

Solution, Injection:

SandoSTATIN: 50 mcg/mL (1 mL); 100 mcg/mL (1 mL)

SandoSTATIN: 200 mcg/mL (5 mL) [contains phenol]

SandoSTATIN: 500 mcg/mL (1 mL)

SandoSTATIN: 1000 mcg/mL (5 mL) [contains phenol]

Generic: 50 mcg/mL (1 mL); 100 mcg/mL (1 mL); 200 mcg/mL (5 mL); 1000 mcg/5 mL (5 mL); 500 mcg/mL (1 mL); 1000 mcg/mL (5 mL)

Solution, Injection [preservative free]:
Generic: 100 mcg/mL (1 mL); 500 mcg/mL (1 mL)

◆ **Octreotide Acetate** see Octreotide on page 1226
◆ **Octreotide Acetate Omega (Can)** see Octreotide on page 1226
◆ **Octreotide Injection (Can)** see Octreotide on page 1226
◆ **Odomzo** see Sonidegib on page 1543

Ofatumumab (oh fa TOOM yoo mab)

Related Information
Management of Chemotherapy-Induced Nausea and Vomiting in Adults on page 2142
Prevention and Management of Infections on page 2196
Principles of Anticancer Therapy on page 2261

Brand Names: US Arzerra
Brand Names: Canada Arzerra
Index Terms HuMax-CD20
Pharmacologic Category Antineoplastic Agent, Anti-CD20; Antineoplastic Agent, Monoclonal Antibody

Use
Chronic lymphocytic leukemia (CLL), previously untreated: Treatment of previously untreated CLL (in combination with chlorambucil) when fludarabine-based therapy is considered inappropriate

Chronic lymphocytic leukemia (CLL), refractory: Treatment of CLL refractory to fludarabine and alemtuzumab

Labeled Contraindications
U.S. labeling: There are no contraindications listed in the manufacturer's labeling.

Canadian labeling: Hypersensitivity to ofatumumab or any component of the formulation; presence or history of progressive multifocal leukoencephalopathy.

Pregnancy Considerations Teratogenicity was not observed in animal reproduction studies, although prolonged depletion of circulating B cells was observed in animal offspring. The Canadian labeling recommends women of childbearing potential avoid pregnancy during and for 6 months after the last treatment.

Breast-Feeding Considerations It is not known if ofatumumab is excreted in human milk. However, human IgG is excreted in breast milk, and therefore, ofatumumab may also be excreted in milk. The effects of local GI and systemic exposure are unknown, therefore caution should be used in nursing women receiving ofatumumab.

Warnings/Precautions [US Boxed Warning]: Hepatitis B virus (HBV) reactivation may occur in patients receiving CD20-directed antibody treatment, including ofatumumab; may result in fulminant hepatitis, hepatic failure, and death. Fatal cases of HBV have also occurred in patients not previously infected with HBV. Prior to initiating therapy, obtain hepatitis B surface antigen (HBsAg) and hepatitis B core antibody (anti-HBc) measurements in all patients; monitor for clinical and laboratory signs of hepatitis or HBV during and for several months after treatment. HBV reactivation has been reported up to 12 months after therapy discontinuation. Discontinue ofatumumab (and concomitant medications) if viral hepatitis develops and initiate appropriate antiviral therapy. Reactivation has occurred in patients who are

HBsAg positive as well as in those who are HBsAg negative but are anti-HBc positive; HBV reactivation has also been observed in patients who had previously resolved HBV infection. Use cautiously in patients who show evidence of prior HBV infection (eg, HBsAg positive [regardless of antibody status] or HBsAG negative but anti-HBc positive); consult with appropriate clinicians regarding monitoring and consideration of antiviral therapy before and/or during ofatumumab treatment. The safety of resuming ofatumumab treatment following HBV reactivation is not known; discuss reinitiation of therapy in patients with resolved HBV reactivation with physicians experienced in HBV management. Bacterial, fungal, and other new or reactivated viral infections may occur during and/or following therapy; monitor closely for signs/symptoms of infection. Discontinue therapy for serious infections and treat appropriately.

American Society of Clinical Oncology (ASCO) provisional clinical opinion update on hepatitis B virus screening [Hwang, 2015]) recommendations: Patients receiving anti-CD20 antibodies are at high risk for hepatitis B virus (HBV) reactivation. Screen for HBV infection with hepatitis B surface antigen (HBsAG) and hepatitis B core antibody (anti-HBc) tests prior to treatment initiation; either a total anti-HBc (with both IgG and IgM) or anti-HBc IgG test should be used to screen for chronic or unresolved HBV infection (do not use anti-HBc IgM as it may only confirm acute HBV infection). In addition, patients who have risk factors for HBV infection (eg, birthplace in a country with ≥2% HBV prevalence, household or sexual contact with HBV infected patients, high-risk behaviors [eg, intravenous drug use], and HIV infection) should also be screened prior to beginning therapy. Initiate prophylactic antiviral therapy (utilizing antivirals with low rates of viral resistance) for HBsAg positive/anti-HBc positive patients (without delaying cancer therapy) and continue the antivirals during and for ~6 to 12 months after completing treatment. HBsAg negative/anti-HBc positive patients should be monitored for HBV reactivation with HBV DNA and ALT testing approximately every 3 months during treatment; antiviral therapy may be initiated prophylactically or begun promptly at the first sign of HBV reactivation.

May cause serious infusion reaction (some fatal); reactions may include bronchospasm, dyspnea, laryngeal edema, pulmonary edema, flushing, hypertension, hypotension, syncope, cardiac ischemia/infarction, acute coronary syndrome, arrhythmia, bradycardia, back pain, abdominal pain, fever, rash, urticaria, angioedema, cytokine release syndrome, and/or anaphylactoid/anaphylactic reactions. Infusion reactions occur more frequently with the first 2 infusions and may occur despite premedication. Premedicate prior to infusion with acetaminophen, an antihistamine, and a corticosteroid. Interrupt infusion for reaction of any severity and institute appropriate treatment; may require subsequent rate modification. Discontinue immediately and permanently if anaphylactic reaction occurs. Bowel obstruction and abdominal pain have been reported; patients presenting with abdominal pain should be assessed for presence of obstruction and treated appropriately.

[US Boxed Warning]: Progressive multifocal leukoencephalopathy (PML) resulting in death may occur with CD20-directed antibody treatment, including ofatumumab. Consider PML in any patient with new onset or worsening neurological symptoms, and if suspected, discontinue ofatumumab and evaluate promptly. Severe and prolonged (≥1 week) cytopenias (neutropenia, thrombocytopenia, and anemia) may occur. Grade 3 or 4 late-onset neutropenia (onset ≥42 days after last treatment dose) and/or prolonged neutropenia (not resolved 24 to 42 days after last dose) has been reported. Pancytopenia, agranulocytosis, and fatal neutropenic sepsis have occurred when used in combination with chlorambucil. Monitor blood counts regularly during and after treatment; more frequently if grade 3 or 4 cytopenias develop. Tumor lysis syndrome (TLS) has occurred in patients receiving ofatumumab; patients with a high tumor burden and/or high circulating lymphocyte counts (>25,000/mm^3) are at increased risk for TLS. Administer prophylactic antihyperuricemic therapy and aggressive hydration beginning 12 to 24 hours prior to ofatumumab treatment. Correct electrolyte abnormalities; monitor renal function and hydration status.

Potentially significant drug-drug interactions may exist, requiring dose or frequency adjustment, additional monitoring, and/or selection of alternative therapy. Live vaccines should not be given to patients who have recently received ofatumumab; there is no data concerning secondary transmission; the ability to generate an immune response to any vaccine following treatment is unknown. Patients ≥65 years experienced a higher incidence of adverse reactions (compared with younger patients).

Adverse Reactions

>10%:

Central nervous system: Fatigue (15%)

Dermatologic: Skin rash (14%)

Gastrointestinal: Diarrhea (18%), nausea (11%)

Hematologic & oncologic: Neutropenia (≥ grade 3: 42%; grade 4: 18%; may be prolonged >2 weeks), anemia (16%; grades 3/4: 5%)

Infection: Infection (70%; includes bacterial, fungal, or viral; ≥ grade 3: 29%)

Respiratory: Pneumonia (23%), cough (19%), dyspnea (14%), bronchitis (11%), upper respiratory tract infection (11%)

Miscellaneous: Infusion related reaction (first infusion [300 mg]: 44%; second infusion [2000 mg]: 29%), fever (20%)

1% to 10%:

Cardiovascular: Peripheral edema (9%), hypertension (5%), hypotension (5%), tachycardia (5%)

Central nervous system: Chills (8%), insomnia (7%), headache (6%)

Dermatologic: Urticaria (8%), hyperhidrosis (5%)

Infection: Sepsis (8%), herpes zoster (6%)

Neuromuscular & skeletal: Back pain (8%), muscle spasm (5%)

Respiratory: Nasopharyngitis (8%), sinusitis (5%)

<1%, postmarketing, and/or case reports: Abdominal pain, angina pectoris, bacteremia, hemolytic anemia, hepatitis B (new onset or reactivation), hepatitis (cytolytic), hypoxia, interstitial pulmonary disease (infectious), intestinal obstruction, laryngeal edema, peritonitis, pharyngolaryngeal pain, progressive multifocal leukoencephalopathy (PML), pruritus, rigors, sepsis (neutropenic), septic shock, throat tightness, thrombocytopenia

Drug Interactions

Metabolism/Transport Effects None known.

Avoid Concomitant Use

Avoid concomitant use of Ofatumumab with any of the following: BCG (Intravesical); Belimumab; Natalizumab; Pimecrolimus; Tacrolimus (Topical); Tofacitinib; Vaccines (Live)

Increased Effect/Toxicity

Ofatumumab may increase the levels/effects of: Belimumab; Fingolimod; Leflunomide; Natalizumab; Tofacitinib; Vaccines (Live)

The levels/effects of Ofatumumab may be increased by: Denosumab; Pimecrolimus; Roflumilast; Tacrolimus (Topical); Trastuzumab

Decreased Effect

Ofatumumab may decrease the levels/effects of: BCG (Intravesical); Coccidioides immitis Skin Test; Sipuleucel-T; Vaccines (Inactivated); Vaccines (Live)

The levels/effects of Ofatumumab may be decreased by: Echinacea

Storage/Stability Store intact vials at 2°C to 8°C (36°F to 46°F); do not freeze. Protect from light. Diluted solutions for infusion must be started within 12 hours of preparation (may store at 2°C to 8°C [36°F to 46°F] if not used immediately); discard any remaining solution 24 hours after preparation.

Preparation for Administration Prepare all doses in 1000 mL NS. Begin infusion within 12 hours of preparation.

300 mg dose: Withdraw 15 mL from a 1000 mL NS bag. Add contents of 3 ofatumumab 100 mg vials to NS bag. Gently invert to mix; do not shake.

1000 mg dose: Withdraw 50 mL from a 1000 mL NS bag. Add contents of 1 ofatumumab 1000 mg vial. Gently invert to mix; do not shake.

2000 mg dose: Withdraw 100 mL from a 1000 mL NS bag. Add contents of 2 ofatumumab 1000 mg vials to NS bag. Gently invert to mix; do not shake.

Mechanism of Action Ofatumumab is a monoclonal antibody which binds specifically the extracellular (large and small) loops of the CD20 molecule (which is expressed on normal B lymphocytes and in B-cell CLL) resulting in potent complement-dependent cell lysis and antibody-dependent cell-mediated toxicity in cells that overexpress CD20.

Pharmacodynamics/Kinetics

Distribution: V_{dss}: 5.7 L (following repeated infusions)

Half-life elimination: 15.6 days (following repeated infusions)

Dosing

Adult & Geriatric Note: Premedicate with acetaminophen, an antihistamine, and a corticosteroid 30 to 120 minutes prior to treatment (see Administration).

Chronic lymphocytic leukemia (CLL), previously untreated: IV: Cycle 1 (cycle is 28 days): 300 mg on day 1, followed by 1000 mg on day 8; Subsequent cycles: 1000 mg on day 1 every 28 days; continue for at least 3 cycles until best response or a maximum of 12 cycles (in combination with chlorambucil)

CLL, refractory: IV: Initial dose: 300 mg week 1, followed 1 week later by 2000 mg once weekly for 7 doses (doses 2 to 8), followed 4 weeks later by 2000 mg once every 4 weeks for 4 doses (doses 9 to 12; for a total of 12 doses)

Renal Impairment

Mild or moderate impairment: There are no dosage adjustments provided in the U.S. manufacturer's labeling; however, there were no clinically relevant pharmacokinetic effects observed in patients with baseline CrCl ≥30 mL/minute. The Canadian labeling recommends that no dosage adjustment is necessary for CrCl >30 mL/minute.

Severe impairment: There are no dosage adjustments provided in the manufacturer's labeling.

Hepatic Impairment There are no dosage adjustments provided in the manufacturer's labeling (has not been studied).

Adjustment for Toxicity Infusion reaction: Interrupt infusion for infusion reaction (any severity). If the reaction resolves or remains at ≤ grade 2, resume with the following modifications (based on the grade of the initial reaction):

Grade 1 or 2 infusion reaction:

U.S. labeling: Resume at one-half of the previous rate; may increase (see Administration) based on patient tolerance.

Canadian labeling: Resume at one-half of the previous rate; may increase (see Administration) based on patient tolerance. If the infusion rate had not been increased above 12 mL/hour prior to interrupting therapy, resume infusion at 12 mL/hour; may then increase based on patient tolerance.

Grade 3 or 4 infusion reaction: Resume infusion at 12 mL/hour; may increase (see Administration) based on patient tolerance.

If reaction severity does not resolve to ≤ grade 2 despite management: Consider permanent discontinuation

Anaphylactic reaction: Discontinue permanently

Combination Regimens

Leukemia, chronic lymphocytic:

Chlorambucil-Ofatumumab (CLL) on page 1885

Ofatumumab (CLL Regimen) on page 2046

Administration Do not administer IV push, IV bolus, or as a subcutaneous injection. Premedicate with acetaminophen, an antihistamine, and a corticosteroid 30 to 120 minutes prior to administration. Infuse in an environment equipped to monitor for and manage infusion reactions. Administer with infusion pump and administration set. Do not exceed infusion rates below. Do not mix with or infuse with other medications. Flush line before and after infusion with NS. Begin infusion within 12 hours of preparation. Interrupt infusion for any severity of infusion reaction; if the reaction resolves or remains at ≤ grade 2, may resume infusion (see Adjustment for Toxicity).

Previously untreated chronic lymphocytic leukemia:

Premedication: Premedicate with oral acetaminophen (1000 mg) or equivalent, an oral or IV antihistamine (eg, diphenhydramine 50 mg or cetirizine 10 mg orally or equivalent), and an IV corticosteroid (prednisolone 50 mg or equivalent). Full dose corticosteroid is recommended for the first 2 infusions; in the absence of infusion reaction ≥ grade 3, may gradually reduce or omit corticosteroid dose for subsequent infusions.

Cycle 1, day 1: Initiate infusion at 12 mL/hour for 30 minutes, if tolerated (no infusion reaction) increase to 25 mL/hour for 30 minutes, if tolerated, increase to 50 mL/hour for 30 minutes, if tolerated, increase to 100 mL/hour for 30 minutes, if tolerated, increase to 200 mL/hour for 30 minutes, if tolerated increase to 300 mL/hour for 30 minutes, if tolerated, increase to 400 mL/hour for remainder of infusion. Median duration of infusion: 5.2 hours.

Cycle 1, day 8 and cycles 2 to 12 (if no reaction to previous infusion): Initiate infusion at 25 mL/hour for 30 minutes, if tolerated (no infusion reaction) increase to 50 mL/hour for 30 minutes, if tolerated, increase to 100 mL/hour for 30 minutes, if tolerated, increase to 200 mL/hour for 30 minutes, if tolerated, increase to 400 mL/hour for remainder of infusion. Median duration of infusion: 4.2 to 4.4 hours.

◀ **Refractory chronic lymphocytic leukemia:**

Premedication: Premedicate with oral acetaminophen (1000 mg) or equivalent, an oral or IV antihistamine (eg, diphenhydramine 50 mg or cetirizine 10 mg orally or equivalent), and an IV corticosteroid (prednisolone 100 mg or equivalent). Full dose corticosteroid is recommended for doses 1, 2, and 9; in the absence of infusion reaction ≥ grade 3, may gradually reduce or omit corticosteroid dose for doses 3 to 8; administer full or half corticosteroid dose with doses 10 to 12 if ≥ grade 3 reaction did not occur with dose 9.

Doses 1 and 2: Initiate infusion at 12 mL/hour for 30 minutes, if tolerated (no infusion reaction) increase to 25 mL/hour for 30 minutes, if tolerated, increase to 50 mL/hour for 30 minutes, if tolerated, increase to 100 mL/hour for 30 minutes, if tolerated, increase to 200 mL/hour for remainder of infusion. Median duration of infusion: 6.8 hours.

Doses 3 to 12: Initiate infusion at 25 mL/hour for 30 minutes, if tolerated (no infusion reaction) increase to 50 mL/hour for 30 minutes, if tolerated, increase to 100 mL/hour for 30 minutes, if tolerated, increase to 200 mL/hour for 30 minutes, if tolerated, increase to 400 mL/hour for remainder of infusion. Median duration of infusion: 4.2 to 4.4 hours.

Emetic Potential Minimal (<10%)

Monitoring Parameters CBC with differential, renal function, electrolytes

Hepatitis B virus screening recommendations (ASCO provisional clinical opinion update [Hwang, 2015]): Screen for hepatitis B virus (HBV) infection with hepatitis B surface antigen (HBsAG) and hepatitis B core antibody (anti-HBc) tests prior to treatment initiation; either a total anti-HBc (with both IgG and IgM) or anti-HBc IgG test should be used to screen for chronic or unresolved HBV infection (do not use anti-HBc IgM as it may only confirm acute HBV infection). HBsAg negative/anti-HBc positive patients should be monitored for HBV reactivation with HBV DNA and ALT testing approximately every 3 months during treatment.

Signs of active hepatitis B infection (during and for up to 12 months after therapy completion); signs or symptoms of infusion reaction; signs of infection; fluid status; signs/symptoms of intestinal obstruction (eg, abdominal pain, repeated vomiting); signs/symptoms of progressive multifocal leukoencephalopathy (focal neurologic deficits, which may present as hemiparesis, visual field deficits, cognitive impairment, aphasia, ataxia, and/or cranial nerve deficits).

Dosage Forms Excipient information presented when available (limited, particularly for generics); consult specific product labeling.

Concentrate, Intravenous [preservative free]:

Arzerra: 100 mg/5 mL (5 mL); 1000 mg/50 mL (50 mL) [contains edetate disodium, mouse protein (murine) (hamster), polysorbate 80]

Ofloxacin (Systemic) (oh FLOKS a sin)

Brand Names: Canada Apo-Oflox; Novo-Ofloxacin

Pharmacologic Category Antibiotic, Fluoroquinolone

Use Quinolone antibiotic for the treatment of acute exacerbations of chronic bronchitis, community-acquired pneumonia, skin and skin structure infections (uncomplicated), urethral and cervical gonorrhea (acute, uncomplicated), urethritis and cervicitis (nongonococcal), mixed infections of the urethra and cervix, pelvic inflammatory disease (acute), cystitis (uncomplicated), urinary tract infections (complicated), prostatitis

Note: As of April 2007, the CDC no longer recommends the use of fluoroquinolones for the treatment of gonococcal disease.

Pregnancy Risk Factor C

Dosing

Adult

Cervicitis/urethritis (nongonococcal): Oral:

Nongonococcal: 300 mg every 12 hours for 7 days

Gonococcal (acute, uncomplicated): 400 mg as a single dose; **Note:** As of April 2007, the CDC no longer recommends the use of fluoroquinolones for the treatment of uncomplicated gonococcal disease.

Chronic bronchitis (acute exacerbation), community-acquired pneumonia, skin and skin structure infections (uncomplicated): Oral: 400 mg every 12 hours for 10 days

Pelvic inflammatory disease (acute): Oral: 400 mg every 12 hours for 10 to 14 days; **Note:** The CDC recommends use only if standard cephalosporin therapy is not feasible and community prevalence of quinolone-resistant gonococcal organisms is low. Culture sensitivity must be confirmed.

Prostatitis: Oral:

Acute: 400 mg for 1 dose, then 300 mg twice daily for 10 days

Chronic: 200 mg every 12 hours for 6 weeks

UTI: Oral:

Uncomplicated: 200 mg every 12 hours for 3 to 7 days

Complicated: 200 mg every 12 hours for 10 days

Epididymitis, nongonococcal (off-label use): Oral: 300 mg twice daily for 10 days (CDC, 2010); 200 mg twice daily for 14 days (Canadian STI Guidelines, 2008)

Leprosy (multibacillary) (off-label use): Oral: 400 mg once daily (in combination with dapsone and rifampin) for 12 months (WHO, 2012) **or** alternatively, 400 mg once monthly (in combination with monthly rifampin and minocycline) for 24 months (Villahermosa, 2004; WHO, 1998; WHO, 2012).

Leprosy (paucibacillary) (off-label use):

Multiple-dose regimen: 400 mg once daily (in combination with rifampin) for 4 weeks (Balagon 2010).

Single-dose regimen: 400 mg as a single dose (in combination with single doses of rifampin and minocycline) (Manickam 2012). **Note:** Found to be less effective than standard WHO multiple drug therapy (WHO-MDT) for paucibacillary leprosy; should only be used if close follow-up of relapse is possible (Manickam, 2012; Setia, 2011).

Traveler's diarrhea (off-label use): Oral: 200 mg twice daily for 3 days (Hill, 2006)

Geriatric Oral: 200 to 400 mg every 12 to 24 hours (based on estimated renal function) for 7 days to 6 weeks depending on indication.

Renal Impairment Adults: Oral: After a normal initial dose, adjust as follows:

CrCl 20 to 50 mL/minute: Administer usual dose every 24 hours

CrCl <20 mL/minute: Administer half the usual dose every 24 hours

Continuous arteriovenous or venovenous hemodiafiltration effects: Administer 300 mg every 24 hours

Hepatic Impairment Severe impairment: Maximum dose: 400 mg/day

Additional Information Complete prescribing information should be consulted for additional detail.

Medication Guide Available Yes

◀ **Dosage Forms** Excipient information presented when available (limited, particularly for generics); consult specific product labeling. [DSC] = Discontinued product
Tablet, Oral:
Generic: 200 mg [DSC], 300 mg [DSC], 400 mg

OLANZapine (oh LAN za peen)

Brand Names: US ZyPREXA; ZyPREXA Relprevv; ZyPREXA Zydis
Brand Names: Canada Abbott-Olanzapine ODT; Accel-Olanzapine; ACT Olanzapine; ACT Olanzapine ODT; Apo-Olanzapine; Apo-Olanzapine ODT; JAMP-Olanzapine ODT; Mar-Olanzapine; Mar-Olanzapine ODT; Mint-Olanzapine ODT; Mylan-Olanzapine; Mylan-Olanzapine ODT; Olanzapine for injection; Olanzapine ODT; PHL-Olanzapine; PHL-Olanzapine ODT; PMS-Olanzapine; PMS-Olanzapine ODT; RAN-Olanzapine; RAN-Olanzapine ODT; Riva-Olanzapine; Riva-Olanzapine ODT; Sandoz-Olanzapine; Sandoz-Olanzapine ODT; Teva-Olanzapine; Teva-Olanzapine OD; Zyprexa; Zyprexa Intramuscular; Zyprexa Zydis
Index Terms LY170053; Olanzapine Pamoate; Zyprexa Zydis
Pharmacologic Category Antimanic Agent; Second Generation (Atypical) Antipsychotic
Use
Oral: Treatment of the manifestations of schizophrenia; treatment of acute or mixed mania episodes associated with bipolar I disorder (as monotherapy or in combination with lithium or valproate); maintenance treatment of bipolar I disorder; in combination with fluoxetine for treatment-resistant or bipolar I depression
IM, extended-release (Zyprexa Relprevv): Treatment of schizophrenia
IM, short-acting (Zyprexa IntraMuscular): Treatment of acute agitation associated with schizophrenia and bipolar I mania
Pregnancy Risk Factor C
Dosing
Adult & Geriatric
Schizophrenia:
Oral: Initial: 5 to 10 mg once daily (increase to 10 mg once daily within 5 to 7 days); thereafter, adjust by 5 mg daily at 1-week intervals, up to a recommended maximum of 20 mg daily. Maintenance: 10 to 20 mg once daily. Doses up to 60 mg daily have been used in treatment-resistant schizophrenia; however, supporting evidence is limited (APA [Lehman, 2004]).
Special risk patients: Initial: 5 mg once daily is recommended in patients who are debilitated, who have a predisposition to hypotensive reactions, who exhibit a combination of factors that may result in slower metabolism of olanzapine (eg, nonsmoking female patients ≥65 years), or who may be more pharmacodynamically sensitive to olanzapine; increase dose with caution as clinically indicated.
Extended-release IM injection: **Note:** Establish tolerance to oral olanzapine prior to changing to extended-release IM injection. Maximum dose: 300 mg/2 weeks or 405 mg/4 weeks
Patients established on oral olanzapine 10 mg daily: Initial dose: 210 mg every 2 weeks for 4 doses or 405 mg every 4 weeks for 2 doses; Maintenance dose: 150 mg every 2 weeks or 300 mg every 4 weeks

Patients established on oral olanzapine 15 mg daily: Initial dose: 300 mg every 2 weeks for 4 doses; Maintenance dose: 210 mg every 2 weeks or 405 mg every 4 weeks

Patients established on oral olanzapine 20 mg daily: Initial and maintenance dose: 300 mg every 2 weeks

Special risk patients: Initial: 150 mg every 4 weeks is recommended in patients who are debilitated, who have a predisposition to hypotensive reactions, who exhibit a combination of factors that may result in slower metabolism of olanzapine (eg, nonsmoking female patients ≥65 years), or who may be more pharmacodynamically sensitive to olanzapine; increase dose with caution as clinically indicated.

Bipolar I (acute mixed or manic episodes: Oral:

Monotherapy: Initial: 10 to 15 mg once daily; increase by 5 mg daily at intervals of not less than 24 hours. Maintenance: 5 to 20 mg daily; recommended maximum dose: 20 mg daily.

Combination therapy (with lithium or valproate): Initial: 10 mg once daily; dosing range: 5 to 20 mg daily

Agitation (acute, associated with bipolar disorder or schizophrenia): Short-acting IM injection: Initial dose: 10 mg (a lower dose of 5 to 7.5 mg may be considered when clinical factors warrant); additional doses (up to 10 mg) may be considered; however, 2 hours after the initial dose and 4 hours after the second dose should be allowed between doses to evaluate response (maximum total daily dose: 30 mg)

Special risk patients: Consider a lower dose of 2.5 mg in patients who are debilitated, who have a predisposition to hypotensive reactions, or who may be more pharmacodynamically sensitive to olanzapine.

Depression:

Depression associated with bipolar disorder (in combination with fluoxetine): Oral: Initial: 5 mg in the evening; adjust as tolerated to usual range of 5 to 12.5 mg daily. See **"Note"**

Treatment-resistant depression (in combination with fluoxetine): Oral: Initial: 5 mg in the evening; adjust as tolerated to range of 5 to 20 mg daily. See **"Note"**

Note (olanzapine/fluoxetine combination [Symbyax]): When using individual components of fluoxetine with olanzapine rather than fixed dose combination product (Symbyax), approximate dosage correspondence is as follows:

Olanzapine 2.5 mg + fluoxetine 20 mg = Symbyax 3/25

Olanzapine 5 mg + fluoxetine 20 mg = Symbyax 6/25

Olanzapine 12.5 mg + fluoxetine 20 mg = Symbyax 12/25

Olanzapine 5 mg + fluoxetine 50 mg = Symbyax 6/50

Olanzapine 12.5 mg + fluoxetine 50 mg = Symbyax 12/50

Special risk patients: Initial: 2.5 to 5 mg once daily is recommended in patients who have a predisposition to hypotensive reactions, who have hepatic impairment, who exhibit a combination of factors that may result in slower metabolism of olanzapine (eg, female, elderly, nonsmoking status), or who may be more pharmacodynamically sensitive to olanzapine; increase dose with caution as clinically indicated.

Delirium (off-label use): Oral: 5 mg once daily for up to 5 days (NICE, 2010)

Post-traumatic stress disorder (off-label use): Oral: Initial: 5 to 10 mg daily; adjust dose based on response and tolerability every 1 to 2 weeks, up to 20 mg daily (Carey, 2012; Stein, 2002).

◄ **Prevention of chemotherapy-associated delayed nausea or vomiting (off-label use; in combination with a corticosteroid and serotonin [5-HT₃] antagonist):** Oral: 10 mg once daily for 3 to 5 days, beginning on day 1 of chemotherapy **or** 5 mg once daily for 2 days before chemotherapy, followed by 10 mg once daily (beginning on the day of chemotherapy) for 3 to 8 days

Tourette syndrome (off-label use): Initial: 2.5 to 5 mg daily; increase gradually based on response and tolerability to a usual dosage range of 2.5 to 20 mg daily (Pringsheim, 2012; Roessner, 2011). After initial dosage, increments of 2.5 to 5 mg weekly or biweekly were commonly used for dosage adjustments in clinical trials up to a maximum dosage of 20 mg/day (Budman, 2001; Onofrj, 2000; Stamenkovic, 2000).

Pediatric

Bipolar I (acute mixed or manic episodes): Adolescents ≥13 years: Oral: Initial: 2.5 to 5 mg once daily; adjust by 2.5 to 5 mg daily to target dose of 10 mg daily; dosing range: 2.5 to 20 mg daily

Depression associated with bipolar I disorder (in combination with fluoxetine): Children and Adolescents 10 to 17 years: Oral: Initial: 2.5 mg once daily in the evening (in combination with fluoxetine); adjust dose, if needed, as tolerated; safety of doses >12 mg of olanzapine in combination with fluoxetine doses >50 mg has not been studied in pediatrics. Refer to adult dosing for **"Note"** for olanzapine/fluoxetine combination (Symbyax).

Schizophrenia: Adolescents ≥13 years: Oral: Initial: 2.5 to 5 mg once daily; adjust by 2.5 to 5 mg daily to target dose of 10 mg daily; dosing range: 2.5 to 20 mg daily

Tourette syndrome (off-label use): Children and Adolescents: Initial: 2.5 to 5 mg once daily; increase gradually based on response and tolerability to a usual dosage of 2.5 to 12.5 mg once daily (AACAP [Murphy 2013]; Pringsheim 2012). After initial dosage, increments of 2.5 to 5 mg weekly or biweekly were used for dosage adjustments in clinical trials up to a maximum dosage of 20 mg/day (McCracken 2008; Stephens 2004)

Renal Impairment No dosage adjustment necessary. Not removed by dialysis.

Hepatic Impairment There are no dosage adjustments provided in the manufacturer's labeling except when used in combination with fluoxetine (as separate components) the initial olanzapine dose should be limited to 2.5 to 5 mg daily. Use with caution (cases of hepatitis and liver injury have been reported with olanzapine use).

Additional Information Complete prescribing information should be consulted for additional detail.

Prescribing and Access Restrictions As a requirement of the REMS program, only prescribers, healthcare facilities, and pharmacies registered with the Zyprexa Relprevv Patient Care Program are able to prescribe, distribute, or dispense Zyprexa Relprevv for patients who are enrolled in and meet all conditions of the program. Zyprexa Relprevv must be administered at a registered healthcare facility. Prescribers will need to be recertified every 3 years. Contact the Zyprexa Relprevv Patient Care Program at 1-877-772-9390.

Medication Guide Available Yes

Dosage Forms Excipient information presented when available (limited, particularly for generics); consult specific product labeling.

Solution Reconstituted, Intramuscular:

ZyPREXA: 10 mg (1 ea) [contains tartaric acid]

Generic: 10 mg (1 ea)
Suspension Reconstituted, Intramuscular:
ZyPREXA Relprevv: 210 mg (1 ea); 300 mg (1 ea); 405 mg (1 ea) [contains polysorbate 80]
Tablet, Oral:
ZyPREXA: 2.5 mg, 5 mg, 7.5 mg, 10 mg
ZyPREXA: 15 mg [contains fd&c blue #2 aluminum lake]
ZyPREXA: 20 mg
Generic: 2.5 mg, 5 mg, 7.5 mg, 10 mg, 15 mg, 20 mg
Tablet Dispersible, Oral:
ZyPREXA Zydis: 5 mg, 10 mg, 15 mg, 20 mg [contains aspartame, methyl-paraben sodium, propylparaben sodium]
Generic: 5 mg, 10 mg, 15 mg, 20 mg

Dosage Forms: Canada Note: Refer to Dosage Forms. ZyPREXA Relprevv is not available in Canada.

- ◆ **Olanzapine for injection (Can)** *see* OLANZapine *on page 1242*
- ◆ **Olanzapine ODT (Can)** *see* OLANZapine *on page 1242*
- ◆ **Olanzapine Pamoate** *see* OLANZapine *on page 1242*

Olaparib (oh LAP a rib)

Related Information
Common Toxicity Criteria *on page 2122*
Management of Chemotherapy-Induced Nausea and Vomiting in Adults *on page 2142*
Principles of Anticancer Therapy *on page 2261*
Safe Handling of Hazardous Drugs *on page 2292*
Brand Names: US Lynparza
Index Terms AZD2281; KU-0059436; PARP inhibitor AZD2281
Pharmacologic Category Antineoplastic Agent, PARP Inhibitor
Use Ovarian cancer, advanced: Treatment (monotherapy) of deleterious or suspected deleterious germline BRCA mutated (as detected by an approved test) advanced ovarian cancer in patients who have been treated with 3 or more prior lines of chemotherapy
Labeled Contraindications There are no contraindications listed in the manufacturer's labeling.
Pregnancy Considerations Adverse events were observed in animal reproduction studies at doses less than human exposure. Based on its mechanism of action, olaparib may be expected to cause adverse events to the fetus. Women of reproductive potential should use highly effective contraception during therapy and for at least one month after treatment is discontinued.
Breast-Feeding Considerations It is not known if olaparib is excreted into breast milk. Due to the potential for serious adverse reactions in the nursing infant, the manufacturer recommends a decision be made to discontinue nursing or to discontinue the drug, taking into account the importance of treatment to the mother.
Warnings/Precautions Hazardous agent - use appropriate precautions for handling and disposal (meets NIOSH 2014 criteria). Anemia, neutropenia, thrombocytopenia and lymphopenia have been reported. Monitor complete blood counts at baseline and monthly thereafter; do not initiate olaparib until any hematologic toxicity caused by previous chemotherapy has resolved to ≤ grade 1. Myelodysplastic syndrome/acute myeloid leukemia (MDS/AML) has

been reported (rarely) in a clinical trial of patients with deleterious or suspected deleterious germline BRCA-mutated advanced cancers receiving olaparib monotherapy. Most MDS/AML cases were fatal. The duration of therapy prior to development of the secondary cancers ranged from less than 6 months to greater than 2 years; all patients had received prior chemotherapy with platinum agents and/or other DNA-damaging medications. If prolonged hematologic toxicity occurs during therapy, interrupt treatment and monitor blood counts weekly until recovered; if counts do not recover to ≤ grade 1 after 4 weeks, further evaluation (including bone marrow and cytogenetic analyses) is necessary. If MDS/AML is confirmed, discontinue therapy.

Pneumonitis (including some fatalities) has occurred rarely. Interrupt treatment for new or worsening respiratory symptoms such as cough, dyspnea, fever, wheezing, or radiologic abnormalities; evaluate promptly. Discontinue treatment if pneumonitis is confirmed. Olaparib is associated with a moderate emetic potential; antiemetics are recommended to prevent nausea and vomiting. Potentially significant drug-drug interactions may exist, requiring dose or frequency adjustment, additional monitoring, and/or selection of alternative therapy.

Adverse Reactions

Note: Frequency not always defined

≥10%:

Cardiovascular: Peripheral edema (10% to <20%)

Central nervous system: Fatigue (including weakness; 66% to 68%), headache (10% to 25%), dizziness (10% to <20%)

Dermatologic: Skin rash (10% to 25%)

Gastrointestinal: Nausea (64% to 75%), abdominal pain (43%), vomiting (32% to 43%), diarrhea (28% to 31%), dyspepsia (25%), decreased appetite (22% to 25%), dysgeusia (10% to 21%), constipation (10% to <20%)

Genitourinary: Urinary tract infection (10% to <20%)

Hematologic & oncologic: Decreased hemoglobin (85% to 90%; grades 3/4: 8% to 15%), increased MCV (57% to 85%), decreased absolute lymphocyte count (56%; grades 3/4: 17%), anemia (25% to 34%; grades 3/4: 4% to 18%), decreased neutrophils (25% to 32%; grades 3/4: 7% to 8%), decreased platelet count (26% to 30%; grades 3/4: 3% to 6%)

Neuromuscular & skeletal: Musculoskeletal pain (21% to 32%), myalgia (22% to 25%), back pain (10% to 25%)

Renal: Increased serum creatinine (26% to 30%)

Respiratory: Upper respiratory tract infection (26% to 43%), cough (10% to 21%), dyspnea (10% to <20%)

1% to ≤10%:

Cardiovascular: Hypertension, venous thrombosis (including pulmonary embolism)

Central nervous system: Anxiety, depression, insomnia, peripheral neuropathy

Dermatologic: Pruritus, xeroderma (including eczema)

Endocrine & metabolic: Hot flash, hyperglycemia, hypomagnesemia

Gastrointestinal: Stomatitis

Genitourinary: Dysuria, urinary incontinence, vulvovaginal disease

Hematologic & oncologic: Myelodysplastic syndrome (acute myeloid leukemia; 2%), leukopenia

Miscellaneous: Fever

<1%, postmarketing, and/or case reports: Pneumonitis

Drug Interactions

Metabolism/Transport Effects Substrate of CYP3A4 (major), P-glycoprotein; **Note:** Assignment of Major/Minor substrate status based on clinically relevant drug interaction potential

Avoid Concomitant Use

Avoid concomitant use of Olaparib with any of the following: BCG (Intravesical); Bitter Orange; CloZAPine; Conivaptan; CYP3A4 Inducers (Moderate); CYP3A4 Inducers (Strong); CYP3A4 Inhibitors (Moderate); CYP3A4 Inhibitors (Strong); Dipyrone; Fusidic Acid (Systemic); Idelalisib

Increased Effect/Toxicity

Olaparib may increase the levels/effects of: CloZAPine

The levels/effects of Olaparib may be increased by: Bitter Orange; Conivaptan; CYP3A4 Inhibitors (Moderate); CYP3A4 Inhibitors (Strong); Dasatinib; Dipyrone; Fosaprepitant; Fusidic Acid (Systemic); Idelalisib; Ivacaftor; Luliconazole; Osimertinib; Palbociclib; Simeprevir; Stiripentol

Decreased Effect

Olaparib may decrease the levels/effects of: BCG (Intravesical)

The levels/effects of Olaparib may be decreased by: CYP3A4 Inducers (Moderate); CYP3A4 Inducers (Strong); Deferasirox; Osimertinib; Siltuximab; Tocilizumab

Food Interactions Coadministration with grapefruit or Seville oranges may increase olaparib plasma concentrations. Management: Avoid concomitant administration with grapefruit or Seville oranges.

Storage/Stability Store at 25°C (77°F); excursions permitted from 15°C to 30°C (59°F to 86°F). Do not expose capsules to temperatures >40°C (104°F).

Mechanism of Action Olaparib is a poly (ADP-ribose) polymerase (PARP) enzyme inhibitor, including PARP1, PARP2, and PARP3. PARP enzymes are involved in DNA transcription, cell cycle regulation, and DNA repair. Olaparib is a potent oral PARP inhibitor which induces synthetic lethality in BRCA1/2 deficient tumor cells through the formation of double-stranded DNA breaks which cannot be accurately repaired, which leads to disruption of cellular homeostasis and cell death (Ledermann, 2012).

Pharmacodynamics/Kinetics

Absorption: Rapid; delayed with a high-fat meal (extent of absorption not significantly altered)

Distribution: 167 ± 196 L

Protein binding: ~82%

Metabolism: Primarily hepatic via CYP3A4; the majority of metabolism is through oxidation with some metabolites undergoing subsequent glucuronide or sulfate conjugation

Half-life elimination, terminal: 11.9 ± 4.8 hours

Time to peak: 1 to 3 hours

Excretion: Urine (44%, mostly metabolites); feces (42%, mostly metabolites)

Dosing

Adult & Geriatric Note: Administer only to patients with deleterious or suspected deleterious germline BRCA mutations, as detected by an approved test. Olaparib is associated with a moderate emetic potential; antiemetics are recommended to prevent nausea and vomiting.

Ovarian cancer, advanced: Oral: 400 mg twice daily until disease progression or unacceptable toxicity

◄ *Missed doses:* If a dose is missed, administer the next dose at its scheduled time.

Dosage adjustment for concomitant therapy with CYP3A inhibitors: Avoid concomitant use with moderate or strong CYP3A inhibitors. Reduce dose to 200 mg twice daily if coadministration with a **moderate** CYP3A inhibitor cannot be avoided; reduce dose to 150 mg twice daily if coadministration with a **strong** CYP3A inhibitor cannot be avoided.

Renal Impairment

Mild impairment (CrCl 50 to 80 mL/minute): No dosage adjustment necessary; monitor closely for toxicity, as an increase in mean AUC has been observed in patients with mild impairment.

Moderate or severe impairment (CrCl <50 mL/minute): There are no dosage adjustments provided in the manufacturer's labeling (has not been studied).

Dialysis: There are no dosage adjustments provided in the manufacturer's labeling (has not been studied).

Hepatic Impairment There are no dosage adjustments provided in the manufacturer's labeling (has not been studied). Patients with bilirubin >1.5 times ULN and AST/ALT ≥2.5 times ULN (≥5 times ULN in the presence of liver metastases) were excluded from clinical trials.

Adjustment for Toxicity

Consider therapy interruption or dose reduction if adverse reactions occur. The recommended dose reduction is to 200 mg twice daily; if further reduction is required, reduce dose to 100 mg twice daily.

Pneumonitis: Discontinue

Secondary AML/MDS: Discontinue

Administration Olaparib is associated with a moderate emetic potential; antiemetics are recommended to prevent nausea and vomiting.

Oral: Swallow capsule whole; do not chew, dissolve, or open capsule. Do not administer if capsules appear deformed or show evidence of leakage.

Hazardous agent; use appropriate precautions for handling and disposal (meets NIOSH 2014 criteria).

Emetic Potential Moderate (30% to 90%)

Monitoring Parameters Complete blood count at baseline and monthly thereafter, or as clinically indicated (weekly until recovery for prolonged hematologic toxicity); monitor for signs/symptoms of AML/MDS and pneumonitis

Dietary Considerations Avoid grapefruit or Seville oranges.

Prescribing and Access Restrictions Olaparib is available only through the designated specialty pharmacy Biologics, Inc. For further information on patient assistance, product availability, and prescribing instructions, please refer to the following website: http://myaccess360.com/hcp/reimbursement/Oncology.aspx?product=lynparza or call 1-844-275-2360.

Medication Guide Available Yes

Dosage Forms Excipient information presented when available (limited, particularly for generics); consult specific product labeling.

Capsule, Oral:

Lynparza: 50 mg

Omacetaxine (oh ma se TAX een)

Related Information

Safe Handling of Hazardous Drugs *on page 2292*

Brand Names: US Synribo

Index Terms CGX-625; HHT; Homoharringtonine; Omacetaxine Mepesuccinate

Pharmacologic Category Antineoplastic Agent, Cephalotaxine; Antineoplastic Agent, Protein Synthesis Inhibitor

Use Chronic myeloid leukemia: Treatment of chronic or accelerated phase chronic myeloid leukemia (CML) in adult patients resistant and/or intolerant to ≥2 tyrosine kinase inhibitors

Labeled Contraindications There are no contraindications listed in the manufacturer's labeling.

Pregnancy Considerations Adverse events were observed in animal reproduction studies at doses less than the equivalent human dose (based on BSA). Based on the mechanism of action, omacetaxine may cause fetal harm if administered during pregnancy. Women of reproductive potential should avoid pregnancy during therapy. Omacetaxine may impair fertility in males.

Breast-Feeding Considerations It is not known if omacetaxine is excreted in breast milk. Due to the potential for serious adverse reactions in the nursing infant, the decision to discontinue omacetaxine or to discontinue breast-feeding should take into account the importance of treatment to the mother.

Warnings/Precautions Hazardous agent: Use appropriate precautions for handling and disposal (NIOSH 2014 [group 1]). Grade 3/4 neutropenia, thrombocytopenia, and anemia commonly occur; generally reversible, although may require treatment delay and/or a reduction in the number of treatment days with future cycles. Myelosuppression may rarely be fatal. Monitor blood counts (in induction and maintenance cycles). Neutropenia may increase the risk for infection. Thrombocytopenia may increase the risk of bleeding; cerebrovascular hemorrhages have been reported (some fatal); gastrointestinal hemorrhages have occurred. Due to the increased risk of bleeding, avoid the use of anticoagulants, aspirin, and NSAIDs when the platelet count is <50,000/mm^3. Patients ≥65 years of age are more likely to experience hematologic toxicity. Omacetaxine may induce glucose intolerance; hyperglycemia has been observed; hyperosmolar nonketotic hyperglycemia has been reported (case report). Monitor blood glucose frequently, especially in patients with diabetes or with risk factors for diabetes. Avoid use in patients with poorly controlled diabetes; may initiate after glycemic control has been established. Potentially significant interactions may exist, requiring dose or frequency adjustment, additional monitoring, and/or selection of alternative therapy.

Adverse Reactions

>10%:

Cardiovascular: Peripheral edema (16%)

Central nervous system: Fatigue (29% to 31%), headache (13% to 20%), chills (13%), insomnia (12%)

Dermatologic: Alopecia (15%), skin rash (11%)

Endocrine & metabolic: Uric acid increased (grades 3/4: 56% to 57%), hyperglycemia (grades 3/4: 10% to 15%; hyperosmolar nonketotic hyperglycemia <1%)

Gastrointestinal: Diarrhea (35% to 41%), nausea (29% to 35%), abdominal pain (16% to 23%), vomiting (12% to 15%), constipation (14%), anorexia (10% to 13%)

Hematologic: Thrombocytopenia (58% to 76%; grades 3/4: 49% to 88%), anemia 51% to 61%; grades 3/4: 36% to 80%), neutropenia (20% to 53%; grades 3/4: 18% to 81%), leukocytes decreased (grades 3/4: 61% to 72%), neutropenic fever (10% to 20%; grades 3/4: 10% to 16%), lymphopenia (17%; grades 3/4: 16%)

Local: Injection site reactions (22% to 35%; includes infusion related reaction, erythema, hematoma, hemorrhage, hypersensitivity, induration, inflammation, irritation, mass, edema, pruritus, and rash)

Neuromuscular & skeletal: Weakness (23% to 24%), arthralgia (19%), limb pain (11% to 13%), back pain (12%), myalgia (11%)

Renal: Creatinine increased (grades 3/4: 9% to 16%)

Respiratory: Epistaxis (11% to 17%), cough (≤16%), dyspnea (11%)

Miscellaneous: Infection (46% to 56%; grades 3/4: 11% to 20%), fever (25% to 29%)

1% to 10%:

Cardiovascular: Acute coronary syndrome, angina pectoris, arrhythmia, bradycardia, cerebral hemorrhage, chest pain, edema, hypertension, hypotension, palpitations, tachycardia, ventricular extrasystoles

Central nervous system: Anxiety, agitation, confusion, depression, dizziness, dysphonia, hyperthermia, hypoesthesia, lethargy, malaise, mental status change, pain, seizures

Dermatologic: Bruising, burning sensation, dry skin, erythema, hyperhidrosis, hyperpigmentation, petechiae, pruritus, purpura, skin exfoliation, skin lesions, skin ulceration

Endocrine & metabolic: Glucose decreased (grades 3/4: 6% to 8%), dehydration, diabetes mellitus, gout, hot flashes

Gastrointestinal: Abdominal distension, abnormal taste, anal fissure, aphthous stomatitis, appetite decreased, dyspepsia, dysphagia, gastritis, gastroesophageal reflux disease, GI bleeding, gingival bleeding, gingival pain, gingivitis, hemorrhoids, melena, mouth ulceration, mouth hemorrhage, mucosal inflammation, oral pain, stomatitis, xerostomia

Genitourinary: Dysuria

Hematologic: Bone marrow failure (10%; grades 3/4: 10%), hematoma

Hepatic: Bilirubin increased (grades 3/4: 6% to 9%), ALT increased (grades 3/4: 2% to 6%)

Neuromuscular & skeletal: Bone pain, muscle spasms, muscle weakness, musculoskeletal chest pain, musculoskeletal discomfort, musculoskeletal pain, paresthesia, sciatica, stiffness, tremor

Ocular: Blurred vision, cataract, conjunctival hemorrhage, conjunctivitis, diplopia, dry eyes, eye pain, eyelid edema, lacrimation increased

Otic: Ear hemorrhage, ear pain, tinnitus

Respiratory: Hemoptysis, nasal congestion, pharyngolaryngeal pain, rales, rhinorrhea, sinus congestion

Miscellaneous: Flu-like syndrome, hypersensitivity reactions, night sweats, transfusion reaction

Drug Interactions

Metabolism/Transport Effects Substrate of P-glycoprotein

Avoid Concomitant Use

Avoid concomitant use of Omacetaxine with any of the following: Anticoagulants; Aspirin; BCG (Intravesical); Natalizumab; Nonsteroidal Anti-Inflammatory Agents; Pimecrolimus; Tacrolimus (Topical); Tofacitinib; Vaccines (Live)

Increased Effect/Toxicity

Omacetaxine may increase the levels/effects of: Fingolimod; Leflunomide; Natalizumab; Tofacitinib; Vaccines (Live)

The levels/effects of Omacetaxine may be increased by: Anticoagulants; Aspirin; Denosumab; Nonsteroidal Anti-Inflammatory Agents; Pimecrolimus; Roflumilast; Tacrolimus (Topical); Trastuzumab

Decreased Effect

Omacetaxine may decrease the levels/effects of: Antidiabetic Agents; BCG (Intravesical); Coccidioides immitis Skin Test; Sipuleucel-T; Vaccines (Inactivated); Vaccines (Live)

The levels/effects of Omacetaxine may be decreased by: Echinacea

Storage/Stability Store intact vials at 20°C to 25°C (68°F to 77°F); excursions are permitted between 15°C and 30°C (59°F and 86°F). Protect from light (intact vial and reconstituted solutions). Reconstituted solution should be used within 12 hours if stored at room temperature or within 6 days (144 hours) if refrigerated at 2°C to 8°C (36°F to 46°F).

Preparation for Administration Hazardous agent: Use appropriate precautions for handling and disposal (NIOSH 2014 [group 1]). Avoid skin and eye contact; wear protective eyewear and gloves during handling and administration. Reconstitute each 3.5 mg vial with sodium chloride 0.9% (NS) 1 mL, resulting in a concentration of 3.5 mg/mL. Gently swirl until solution is clear (lyophilized powder dissolves completely in <1 minute).

Mechanism of Action Omacetaxine is a reversible protein synthesis inhibitor which binds to the A-site cleft of the ribosomal subunit to interfere with chain elongation and inhibit protein synthesis. It acts independently of BCR-ABL1 kinase-binding activity, and has demonstrated activity against tyrosine kinase inhibitor-resistant BCR-ABL mutations.

Pharmacodynamics/Kinetics

Onset:

Chronic phase CML: Mean time to major cytogenetic response: 3.5 months

Accelerated phase CML: Mean time to response: 2.3 months

Duration:

Chronic phase CML: Median duration of major cytogenetic response: 12.5 months

Accelerated phase CML: Median duration of major hematologic response: 4.7 months

Absorption: SubQ: Rapid (Nemunaitis, 2013)

Distribution: V_{dss}: 141 ± 93 L

Protein binding: ≤50%

Metabolism: Hydrolyzed by plasma esterases to 4'-DMHHT; minimal hepatic metabolism

Half-life elimination: ~6 hours

Time to peak: SubQ: ~30 minutes

Excretion: Urine (<15%)

Dosing

Adult & Geriatric Chronic myeloid leukemia (CML), chronic or accelerated phase: SubQ:

Induction: 1.25 mg/m² twice daily for 14 consecutive days of a 28-day treatment cycle; continue until hematologic response is achieved

Maintenance: 1.25 mg/m² twice daily for 7 consecutive days of a 28-day treatment cycle; continue until no longer achieving clinical treatment benefit

◄ *Missed doses:* If a dose is missed, skip that dose and resume with the next regularly scheduled dose. Do not administer 2 doses at the same time to make up for a missed dose.

Renal Impairment There are no dosage adjustments provided in the manufacturer's labeling (has not been studied). Based on the minimal amount of unchanged drug excreted in the urine, dosage adjustment is not likely necessary (Nemunaitis, 2013).

Hepatic Impairment There are no dosage adjustments provided in the manufacturer's labeling (has not been studied).

Adjustment for Toxicity

Hematologic toxicity: May delay treatment cycles and/or reduce the number of treatment days during a cycle for hematologic toxicities.

Neutropenia grade 4 (ANC <500/mm^3) or thrombocytopenia ≥ grade 3 (platelets <50,000/mm^3) during a cycle: Delay the start of the next cycle until ANC ≥1000/mm^3 and platelets ≥50,000/mm^3 **AND** reduce the number of treatment days by 2 days (eg, reduce from 14 days to 12 days or reduce from 7 days to 5 days)

Nonhematologic toxicity: Manage symptomatically; interrupt and/or delay treatment until toxicity resolves.

Combination Regimens

Leukemia, chronic myelogenous: Omacetaxine (CML Regimen) on page 2046

Administration Administer subcutaneously at approximately 12 hour intervals. If home administration is to occur, advise patient on proper handling, storage conditions, administration, disposal, and clean-up of accidental spillage; ensure that the patient or patient's caregiver is an appropriate candidate for home administration.

Hazardous agent: Use appropriate precautions for handling and disposal (NIOSH 2014 [group 1]). Avoid skin and eye contact; wear protective eyewear and gloves during handling and administration.

Emetic Potential Low (10% to 30%)

Monitoring Parameters CBC with differential and platelets (weekly during induction and initial maintenance cycles, then every 2 weeks or as clinically indicated after initial maintenance cycles); blood glucose (frequently); signs/symptoms of infection; signs of bleeding

Medication Guide Available Yes

Dosage Forms Excipient information presented when available (limited, particularly for generics); consult specific product labeling.

Solution Reconstituted, Subcutaneous, as mepesuccinate [preservative free]:
Synribo: 3.5 mg (1 ea)

◆ **Omacetaxine Mepesuccinate** *see* Omacetaxine *on page 1248*

◆ **Omnipred** *see* PrednisoLONE (Ophthalmic) *on page 1424*

◆ **Omnitarg** *see* Pertuzumab *on page 1380*

◆ **Oncaspar** *see* Pegaspargase *on page 1341*

◆ **Oncotice (Can)** *see* BCG (Intravesical) *on page 174*

◆ **OncoVEX GM-CSF** *see* Talimogene Laherparepvec *on page 1590*

◆ **Oncovin** *see* VinCRIStine *on page 1746*

Ondansetron (on DAN se tron)

Related Information

Management of Chemotherapy-Induced Nausea and Vomiting in Adults *on page 2142*

Brand Names: US Zofran; Zofran ODT; Zuplenz

Brand Names: Canada ACT Ondansetron; Apo-Ondansetron; Ava-Ondansetron; Dom-Ondansetron; JAMP-Ondansetron; Mar-Ondansetron; Mint-Ondansetron; Mylan-Ondansetron; NAT-Ondansetron; Ondansetron Hydrochloride Dihydrate Injection; Ondansetron Injection; Ondansetron Injection USP; Ondansetron-Odan; Ondansetron-Omega; Ondissolve ODF; PHL-Ondansetron; PMS-Ondansetron; RAN-Ondansetron; ratio-Ondansetron; Sandoz-Ondansetron; Septa-Ondansetron; Teva-Ondansetron; Zofran; Zofran ODT

Index Terms GR38032R; Ondansetron Hydrochloride

Pharmacologic Category Antiemetic; Selective 5-HT$_3$ Receptor Antagonist

Use

Cancer chemotherapy-induced nausea and vomiting:

IV: Prevention of nausea and vomiting associated with initial and repeat courses of emetogenic cancer chemotherapy (including high-dose cisplatin)

Oral:

Prevention of nausea and vomiting associated with highly emetogenic cancer chemotherapy (including cisplatin ≥50 mg/m^2).

Prevention of nausea and vomiting associated with initial and repeat courses of moderately emetogenic cancer chemotherapy.

Radiotherapy-associated nausea and vomiting: Oral: Prevention of nausea and vomiting associated with radiotherapy in patients receiving either total body irradiation, single high-dose fraction to the abdomen, or daily fractions to the abdomen.

Postoperative nausea and/or vomiting: IV and Oral: Prevention of postoperative nausea and/or vomiting (PONV). If nausea/vomiting occur in a patient who had not received prophylactic ondansetron, IV ondansetron may be administered to prevent further episodes.

Limitations of use: Routine prophylaxis for PONV in patients with minimal expectation of nausea and/or vomiting is not recommended, although use is recommended in patients when nausea and vomiting must be avoided in the postoperative period, even if the incidence of PONV is low.

Canadian labeling: Additional use (not in U.S. labeling): IV: Treatment of PONV

Labeled Contraindications Hypersensitivity to ondansetron or any component of the formulation; concomitant use of apomorphine

Pregnancy Considerations Teratogenic effects were not observed in animal reproduction studies. Ondansetron readily crosses the human placenta in the first trimester of pregnancy and can be detected in fetal tissue (Siu, 2006). The use of ondansetron for the treatment of nausea and vomiting of pregnancy (NVP) has been evaluated. Although a significant increase in birth defects has not been described in case reports and some studies (Ferreira, 2012; Pasternak, 2013), other studies have shown a possible association with ondansetron exposure and adverse fetal events (Anderka, 2012; Einarson, 2004). Additional studies are needed to determine safety to the fetus, particularly during the first trimester. Based on available data, use is generally reserved for severe NVP (hyperemesis gravidarum) or when conventional treatments are not effective (ACOG, 2004; Koren, 2012; Levicheck, 2002; Tan, 2011). Because a dose-dependent QT-interval prolongation occurs with

1253

use, the manufacturer recommends ECG monitoring in patients with electrolyte abnormalities (which can be associated with some cases of NVP; Koren, 2012). An international consensus panel recommends that 5-HT$_3$ antagonists (including ondansetron) should not be withheld in pregnant patients receiving chemotherapy for the treatment of gynecologic cancers, when chemotherapy is given according to general recommendations for chemotherapy use during pregnancy (Amant, 2010).

Breast-Feeding Considerations It is not known if ondansetron is excreted into breast milk. The U.S. manufacturer labeling recommends caution be used if administered to nursing women. The Canadian labeling recommends avoiding nursing during ondansetron treatment.

Warnings/Precautions Antiemetics are most effective when used prophylactically (Roila, 2010). If emesis occurs despite optimal antiemetic prophylaxis, reevaluate emetic risk, disease, concurrent morbidities and medications to assure antiemetic regimen is optimized (Basch, 2011). Does not stimulate gastric or intestinal peristalsis; may mask progressive ileus and/or gastric distension. Use with caution in patients allergic to other 5-HT$_3$ receptor antagonists; cross-reactivity has been reported.

Dose-dependent QT interval prolongation occurs with ondansetron use. Cases of torsade de pointes have also been reported to the manufacturer. Selective 5-HT$_3$ antagonists, including ondansetron, have been associated with a number of dose-dependent increases in ECG intervals (eg, PR, QRS duration, QT/QTc, JT), usually occurring 1 to 2 hours after IV administration. Single doses >16 mg ondansetron IV are no longer recommended due to the potential for an increased risk of QT prolongation. In most patients, these changes are not clinically relevant; however, when used in conjunction with other agents that prolong these intervals or in those at risk for QT prolongation, arrhythmia may occur. When used with agents that prolong the QT interval (eg, Class I and III antiarrhythmics) or in patients with cardiovascular disease, clinically relevant QT interval prolongation may occur resulting in torsade de pointes. Avoid ondansetron use in patients with congenital long QT syndrome. Use caution and monitor ECG in patients with other risk factors for QT prolongation (eg, medications known to prolong QT interval, electrolyte abnormalities [hypokalemia or hypomagnesemia], heart failure, bradyarrhythmias, and cumulative high-dose anthracycline therapy). IV formulations of 5-HT$_3$ antagonists have more association with ECG interval changes, compared to oral formulations. Dose limitations are recommended for patients with severe hepatic impairment (Child-Pugh class C); use with caution in mild-moderate hepatic impairment; clearance is decreased and half-life increased in hepatic impairment.

Serotonin syndrome has been reported with 5-HT$_3$ receptor antagonists, predominantly when used in combination with other serotonergic agents (eg, SSRIs, SNRIs, MAOIs, mirtazapine, fentanyl, lithium, tramadol, and/or methylene blue). Some of the cases have been fatal. The majority of serotonin syndrome reports due to 5-HT$_3$ receptor antagonist have occurred in a postanesthesia setting or in an infusion center. Serotonin syndrome has also been reported following overdose of ondansetron. Monitor patients for signs of serotonin syndrome, including mental status changes (eg, agitation, hallucinations, delirium, coma); autonomic instability (eg, tachycardia, labile blood pressure, diaphoresis, dizziness, flushing, hyperthermia); neuromuscular changes (eg, tremor, rigidity, myoclonus, hyperreflexia, incoordination); gastrointestinal symptoms (eg, nausea, vomiting, diarrhea); and/or seizures. If serotonin syndrome occurs, discontinue 5-HT$_3$ receptor antagonist treatment and begin supportive management. Potentially significant drug-drug interactions may exist, requiring dose or frequency adjustment, additional monitoring, and/or selection of alternative therapy. Orally disintegrating tablets contain phenylalanine.

Benzyl alcohol and derivatives: Some dosage forms may contain sodium benzoate/benzoic acid; benzoic acid (benzoate) is a metabolite of benzyl alcohol; large amounts of benzyl alcohol (≥99 mg/kg/day) have been associated with a potentially fatal toxicity ("gasping syndrome") in neonates; the "gasping syndrome" consists of metabolic acidosis, respiratory distress, gasping respirations, CNS dysfunction (including convulsions, intracranial hemorrhage), hypotension, and cardiovascular collapse (AAP ["Inactive" 1997]; CDC, 1982); some data suggests that benzoate displaces bilirubin from protein binding sites (Ahlfors, 2001); avoid or use dosage forms containing benzyl alcohol derivative with caution in neonates. See manufacturer's labeling.

Adverse Reactions Note: Percentages reported in adult patients unless otherwise specified.

>10%:

Central nervous system: Headache (oral: 9% to 27%; IV: 17%), fatigue (oral: ≤9% to 13%), malaise (oral: ≤9% to 13%)

Gastrointestinal: Constipation (6% to 11%)

1% to 10%:

Central nervous system: Drowsiness (IV: ≤8%), sedation (IV: ≤8%), (dizziness (7%), agitation (oral: ≤6%), anxiety (oral: ≤6%), paresthesia (IV: 2%), sensation of cold (IV: 2%)

Dermatologic: Pruritus (2% to 5%), skin rash (1%)

Gastrointestinal: Diarrhea (oral: 6% to 7%; IV: Children 1 to 24 months of age: 2%)

Genitourinary: Gynecologic disease (oral: 7%), urinary retention (oral: 5%)

Hepatic: Increased serum ALT (>2 times ULN: 1% to 5%; transient), increased serum AST (>2 times ULN: 1% to 5%; transient)

Local: Injection site reaction (IV: 4%; includes burning sensation at injection site, erythema at injection site, injection site pain)

Respiratory: Hypoxia (oral: 9%)

Miscellaneous: Fever (2% to 8%)

<1%, postmarketing, and/or case reports: Abdominal pain, accommodation disturbance, anaphylactoid reaction, anaphylaxis, angina pectoris, angioedema, atrial fibrillation, bradycardia, bronchospasm, bullous skin disease, cardiac arrhythmia, cardiorespiratory arrest (IV), chest pain, chills, depression of ST segment on ECG, dyspnea, dystonic reaction, ECG changes, extrapyramidal reaction (IV), flushing, hepatic failure (when used with other hepatotoxic medications), hiccups, hypersensitivity reaction, hypokalemia, hypotension, ischemic heart disease, laryngeal edema, laryngospasm (IV), liver enzyme disorder, mucosal tissue reaction, myocardial infarction, neuroleptic malignant syndrome, oculogyric crisis, palpitations, positive lymphocyte transformation test, prolonged Q-T interval on ECG (dose dependent), second-degree atrioventricular block, serotonin syndrome, shock (IV), Stevens-Johnson syndrome, stridor, supraventricular tachycardia, syncope, tachycardia, tonic-clonic seizures, torsades de pointes, toxic epidermal necrolysis, transient blindness (lasted ≤48 hours), transient blurred vision (following infusion), urticaria, vascular occlusive events, ventricular premature contractions, ventricular tachycardia, weakness, xerostomia

◀ **Drug Interactions**
Metabolism/Transport Effects Substrate of CYP1A2 (minor), CYP2C9 (minor), CYP2D6 (minor), CYP2E1 (minor), CYP3A4 (major), P-glycoprotein; **Note:** Assignment of Major/Minor substrate status based on clinically relevant drug interaction potential; **Inhibits** CYP1A2 (weak), CYP2C9 (weak), CYP2D6 (weak)

Avoid Concomitant Use
Avoid concomitant use of Ondansetron with any of the following: Apomorphine; Highest Risk QTc-Prolonging Agents; Ivabradine; Mifepristone

Increased Effect/Toxicity
Ondansetron may increase the levels/effects of: Apomorphine; ARIPiprazole; Highest Risk QTc-Prolonging Agents; Moderate Risk QTc-Prolonging Agents; Panobinostat; Serotonin Modulators; TiZANidine

The levels/effects of Ondansetron may be increased by: Ivabradine; Mifepristone; P-glycoprotein/ABCB1 Inhibitors; QTc-Prolonging Agents (Indeterminate Risk and Risk Modifying); Ranolazine

Decreased Effect
Ondansetron may decrease the levels/effects of: Tapentadol; TraMADol

The levels/effects of Ondansetron may be decreased by: Bosentan; CYP3A4 Inducers (Moderate); CYP3A4 Inducers (Strong); Dabrafenib; Deferasirox; Enzalutamide; Mitotane; P-glycoprotein/ABCB1 Inducers; Siltuximab; St Johns Wort; Tocilizumab

Food Interactions Tablet: Food slightly increases the extent of absorption. Management: Administer without regard to meals.

Storage/Stability
Oral soluble film: Store between 20°C and 25°C (68°F and 77°F). Store pouches in cartons; keep film in individual pouch until ready to use.
Oral solution: Store between 15°C and 30°C (59°F and 86°F). Protect from light.
Tablet: Store between 2°C and 30°C (36°F and 86°F).
Vial: Store between 2°C and 30°C (36°F and 86°F). Protect from light. Stable when mixed in D_5W or NS for 48 hours at room temperature.
Premixed bag in D_5W: Store at 20°C to 25°C (68°F to 77°F), excursions permitted from 15°C to 30°C (59°F to 86°F); may refrigerate; avoid freezing and excessive heat; protect from light.

Preparation for Administration Prior to IV infusion, dilute in 50 mL D_5W or NS.

Mechanism of Action Selective $5\text{-}HT_3$-receptor antagonist, blocking serotonin, both peripherally on vagal nerve terminals and centrally in the chemoreceptor trigger zone

Pharmacodynamics/Kinetics
Onset of action: ~30 minutes
Absorption: Oral: Well absorbed from GI tract
Distribution: V_d: Children: 1.9 to 3.7 L/kg
Protein binding, plasma: 70% to 76%
Metabolism: Extensively hepatic via hydroxylation, followed by glucuronide or sulfate conjugation; CYP1A2, CYP2D6, and CYP3A4 substrate; some demethylation occurs
Bioavailability: Oral: ~56% (some first pass metabolism)
Half-life elimination: Children <15 years: 2 to 7 hours; Adults: 3 to 6 hours
Mild-to-moderate hepatic impairment (Child-Pugh classes A and B): Adults: 12 hours

Severe hepatic impairment (Child-Pugh class C): Adults: 20 hours
Time to peak: Oral: ~2 hours; Oral soluble film: ~1 hour
Excretion: Urine (44% to 60% as metabolites, ~5% as unchanged drug); feces (~25%)

Dosing
Adult
Prevention of chemotherapy-induced nausea and vomiting:
U.S. labeling:
Prevention of nausea and vomiting associated with emetogenic chemotherapy: IV: 0.15 mg/kg/dose (maximum: 16 mg/dose) administered over 15 minutes for 3 doses, beginning 30 minutes prior to chemotherapy, followed by subsequent doses 4 and 8 hours after the first dose

Prevention of nausea and vomiting associated with highly emetogenic chemotherapy: Oral: 24 mg 30 minutes prior to the start of single-day chemotherapy

Prevention of nausea and vomiting associated with moderately emetogenic chemotherapy: Oral: 8 mg beginning 30 minutes before chemotherapy; repeat dose 8 hours after initial dose, then 8 mg every 12 hours for 1 to 2 days after chemotherapy completed

Canadian labeling:
Prevention of nausea and vomiting associated with highly emetogenic chemotherapy:
IV: 8 to 16 mg (maximum: 16 mg/dose) administered over 15 minutes at least 30 minutes prior to chemotherapy; may administer an additional 8 mg dose at 4 and 8 hours after the initial dose. May convert to oral therapy after the first 24 hours.
Oral: 8 mg every 8 hours for up to 5 days following chemotherapy; oral therapy is initiated after receiving 24 hours of IV ondansetron.

Prevention of nausea and vomiting associated with less emetogenic chemotherapy:
IV: 8 mg administered over 15 minutes at least 30 minutes prior to chemotherapy; may convert to oral therapy twice daily
Oral: 8 mg administered 1-2 hours prior to chemotherapy, followed by 8 mg orally twice daily for up to 5 days following chemotherapy

Guideline recommendations: Prevention of chemotherapy-induced nausea and vomiting:
American Society of Clinical Oncology (ASCO; Basch, 2011):
High emetic risk: Day(s) chemotherapy is administered (antiemetic regimen also includes dexamethasone and aprepitant or fosaprepitant):
IV: 8 mg or 0.15 mg/kg. **Note:** Single IV doses >16 mg are no longer recommended by the manufacturer due to the potential for QT prolongation.
Oral: 8 mg twice daily
Multinational Association of Supportive Care in Cancer (MASCC) and European Society of Medical Oncology (ESMO) (Roila, 2010):
Highly emetic chemotherapy (antiemetic regimen includes dexamethasone and aprepitant/fosaprepitant):
IV: 8 mg or 0.15 mg/kg as a single dose prior to chemotherapy. **Note:** Single IV doses >16 mg are no longer recommended by the manufacturer due to the potential for QT prolongation
Oral: 24 mg as a single dose prior to chemotherapy

Moderately emetic chemotherapy (antiemetic regimen includes dexamethasone [and aprepitant/fosaprepitant for AC chemotherapy regimen]):

IV: 8 mg or 0.15 mg/kg as a single dose prior to chemotherapy. **Note:** Single IV doses >16 mg are no longer recommended by the manufacturer due to the potential for QT prolongation.

Oral: 16 mg (as 8 mg twice daily)

Low emetic risk: Ondansetron (dose not specified) prior to chemotherapy on day 1

Prevention of radiation therapy-induced nausea and vomiting:

U.S. labeling:

Total body irradiation: Oral: 8 mg administered 1 to 2 hours before each daily fraction of radiotherapy

Single high-dose fraction radiotherapy to abdomen: Oral: 8 mg administered 1 to 2 hours before irradiation, then 8 mg every 8 hours after first dose for 1 to 2 days after completion of radiotherapy

Daily fractionated radiotherapy to abdomen: Oral: 8 mg administered 1 to 2 hours before irradiation, then 8 mg every 8 hours after first dose for each day of radiotherapy

Canadian labeling: Oral: 8 mg 1 to 2 hours prior to radiation followed by 8 mg every 8 hours for up to 5 days after a course of treatment

American Society of Clinical Oncology Antiemetic Guideline recommendations (Basch, 2011): Give before each fraction throughout radiation therapy for high emetic risk (continue for at least 24 hours after completion) and for moderate emetic risk. For low emetic risk, may give either as prevention or rescue; for minimal emetic risk, give as rescue (if rescue used for either low or minimal emetic risk, then prophylaxis should be given until the end of radiation therapy).

IV (off-label route/dosing): 8 mg or 0.15 mg/kg. **Note:** Single IV doses >16 mg are no longer recommended by the manufacturer due to the potential for QT prolongation.

Prevention of postoperative nausea and vomiting (PONV):

IM, IV (U.S. labeling) or IV (Canadian labeling): 4 mg as a single dose (over 2 to 5 minutes if giving IV) administered ~30 minutes before the end of anesthesia (see **Note** below) or as treatment if vomiting occurs after surgery (Gan, 2007).

Note: The manufacturer recommends administration immediately before induction of anesthesia; however, this has been shown not to be as effective as administration at the end of surgery (Sun, 1997). Repeat doses given in response to inadequate control of nausea/vomiting from preoperative doses are generally ineffective.

Oral: 16 mg administered 1 hour prior to induction of anesthesia

Treatment of postoperative nausea and vomiting (Canadian labeling):

IV: 4 mg as a single dose (preferably over 2 to 5 minutes, but not less than 30 seconds)

Treatment of severe or refractory hyperemesis gravidum (off-label use):

IV: 8 mg administered over 15 minutes every 12 hours (ACOG, 2004)

Oral: 8 mg every 12 hours (Levichek, 2002)

Geriatric

U.S. labeling: Oral, IV: No dosing adjustment required; refer to adult dosing.

Canadian labeling:

IV: Refer to adult dosing. **Note:** Not approved for post operative nausea/vomiting in elderly patients. In the prevention of nausea and vomiting associated with emetogenic chemotherapy, ECG monitoring should be considered in patients 65 to 74 years receiving higher initial dosing (eg, 16 mg); in patients ≥75 years, the initial dose should not exceed 8 mg; per usual adult dosing, may give 2 additional IV doses of 8 mg at least 4 hours apart (if third dose is needed, consider ECG monitoring).

Oral: No dosage adjustment required; refer to adult dosing.

Pediatric

Prevention of chemotherapy-induced nausea and vomiting:

U.S. labeling:

Prevention of nausea and vomiting associated with emetogenic chemotherapy: Infants ≥6 months, Children, and Adolescents: IV: 0.15 mg/kg/dose (maximum: 16 mg/dose) over 15 minutes for 3 doses, beginning 30 minutes prior to chemotherapy, followed by subsequent doses administered 4 and 8 hours after the first dose

Prevention of nausea and vomiting associated with moderately-emetogenic chemotherapy: Oral:

Children 4 to 11 years: 4 mg 30 minutes before chemotherapy; repeat 4 and 8 hours after initial dose, then 4 mg every 8 hours for 1 to 2 days after chemotherapy completed

Children ≥12 years: Refer to adult dosing.

Canadian labeling:

Prevention of nausea and vomiting associated with emetogenic chemotherapy: Children 4 to 12 years:

IV: 3 to 5 mg/m^2 over 15 minutes at least 30 minutes prior to chemotherapy, then convert to oral therapy; continue for up to 5 days following chemotherapy

Oral: 4 mg every 8 hours for up to 5 days following chemotherapy; oral therapy is started after an IV dose is given prior to chemotherapy

Pediatric guideline recommendations:

Prevention of chemotherapy-induced nausea and vomiting (off-label dosing; Dupuis, 2013):

Highly emetogenic chemotherapy: Infants ≥1 month and Children <12 years: IV, Oral: 0.15 mg/kg/dose (5 mg/m^2/dose) prior to chemotherapy and then every 8 hours; maximum recommended IV dose: 16 mg. Antiemetic regimen also includes dexamethasone

Highly emetogenic chemotherapy: Children ≥12 years and Adolescents: IV, Oral: 0.15 mg/kg/dose (5 mg/m^2/dose) prior to chemotherapy and then every 8 hours; maximum recommended IV dose: 16 mg. Antiemetic regimen includes dexamethasone and if no known or suspected drug interactions, aprepitant.

Moderately emetogenic chemotherapy: Infants ≥1 month, Children, and Adolescents: IV, Oral: 0.15 mg/kg/dose (5 mg/m^2/dose; maximum: 8 mg dose); prior to chemotherapy and then every 12 hours. Antiemetic regimen also includes dexamethasone.

Low emetogenicity chemotherapy: Infants ≥1 month, Children, and Adolescents: IV, Oral: 0.3 mg/kg/dose (10 mg/m^2/dose; maximum IV dose: 16 mg) prior to chemotherapy

Prevention of postoperative nausea and vomiting (PONV): U.S. labeling:

Infants ≥1 month and Children ≤12 years: IV:

≤40 kg: 0.1 mg/kg as a single dose over 2 to 5 minutes

>40 kg: 4 mg as a single dose over 2 to 5 minutes

Renal Impairment No dosage adjustment necessary (there is no experience for oral ondansetron beyond day 1)

◄ **Hepatic Impairment**
U.S. labeling:
Mild to moderate impairment: No dosage adjustment necessary.
Severe impairment (Child-Pugh class C):
IV: Day 1: Maximum daily dose: 8 mg (there is no experience beyond day 1)
Oral: Maximum daily dose: 8 mg
Canadian labeling:
Mild impairment: No dosage adjustment necessary.
Moderate to severe impairment: Maximum daily dose: 8 mg

Administration

Oral: Oral dosage forms should be administered 30 minutes prior to chemotherapy; 1 to 2 hours before radiotherapy; 1 hour prior to the induction of anesthesia

Orally-disintegrating tablets: Do not remove from blister until needed. Peel backing off the blister, do not push tablet through. Using dry hands, place tablet on tongue and allow to dissolve. Swallow with saliva.

Oral soluble film: Do not remove from pouch until immediately before use. Using dry hands, place film on top of tongue and allow to dissolve (4 to 20 seconds). Swallow with or without liquid. If using more than one film, each film should be allowed to dissolve completely before administering the next film.

IM: Should be administered undiluted.

IV:

IVPB: Infuse diluted solution over 15 to 30 minutes; 24-hour continuous infusions have been reported, but are rarely used.

Chemotherapy-induced nausea and vomiting: Give first dose 30 minutes prior to beginning chemotherapy.

IV push: Prevention of postoperative nausea and vomiting: Single doses may be administered IV injection as undiluted solution over at least 30 seconds but preferably over 2 to 5 minutes

Extemporaneous Preparations Note: Commercial oral solution is available (0.8 mg/mL)

If commercial oral solution is unavailable, a 0.8 mg/mL syrup may be made with ondansetron tablets, Ora-Plus® (Paddock), and any of the the following syrups: Cherry syrup USP, Syrpalta® (HUMCO), Ora-Sweet® (Paddock), or Ora-Sweet® Sugar-Free (Paddock). Crush ten 8 mg tablets in a mortar and reduce to a fine powder (flaking of the tablet coating occurs). Add 50 mL Ora-Plus® in 5 mL increments, mixing thoroughly; mix while adding the chosen syrup in incremental proportions to **almost** 100 mL; transfer to a calibrated bottle, rinse mortar with syrup, and add sufficient quantity of syrup to make 100 mL. Label "shake well" and "refrigerate". Stable for 42 days refrigerated (Trissel, 1996).

Rectal suppositories: Calibrate a suppository mold for the base being used. Determine the displacement factor (DF) for ondansetron for the base being used (Fattibase® = 1.1; Polybase® = 0.6). Weigh the ondansetron tablet(s). Divide the tablet weight by the DF; this result is the weight of base displaced by the drug. Subtract the weight of base displaced from the calculated weight of base required for each suppository. Grind the ondansetron tablets in a mortar and reduce to a fine powder. Weigh out the appropriate weight of suppository base. Melt the base over a water bath (<55°C). Add the ondansetron powder to

the suppository base and mix well. Pour the mixture into the suppository mold and cool. Stable for at least 30 days refrigerated (Tenjarla, 1998).

Tenjarla SN, Ward ES, and Fox JL, "Ondansetron Suppositories: Extemporaneous Preparation, Drug Release, Stability and Flux Through Rabbit Rectal Membrane," *Int J Pharm Compound*, 1998, 2(1):83-8.

Trissel LA, *Trissel's Stability of Compounded Formulations*, Washington, DC: American Pharmaceutical Association, 1996.

Monitoring Parameters ECG (if applicable in high-risk or elderly patients); potassium, magnesium

Dietary Considerations Some products may contain phenylalanine.

Dosage Forms Excipient information presented when available (limited, particularly for generics); consult specific product labeling. [DSC] = Discontinued product

Film, Oral:
Zuplenz: 4 mg (1 ea, 10 ea); 8 mg (1 ea, 10 ea)
Solution, Injection:
Zofran: 40 mg/20 mL (20 mL) [contains methylparaben, propylparaben]
Generic: 4 mg/2 mL (2 mL); 40 mg/20 mL (20 mL)
Solution, Injection [preservative free]:
Generic: 4 mg/2 mL (2 mL)
Solution, Intravenous [preservative free]:
Generic: 32 mg (50 mL [DSC])
Solution, Oral:
Zofran: 4 mg/5 mL (50 mL) [strawberry flavor]
Generic: 4 mg/5 mL (50 mL)
Tablet, Oral:
Zofran: 4 mg, 8 mg
Generic: 4 mg, 8 mg, 24 mg
Tablet Dispersible, Oral:
Zofran ODT: 4 mg, 8 mg [contains aspartame, methylparaben sodium, propylparaben sodium; strawberry flavor]
Generic: 4 mg, 8 mg

Dosage Forms: Canada Refer to Dosage Forms. **Note:** Oral Film is not available in Canada.

◆ **Ondansetron Hydrochloride** see Ondansetron on page 1253

◆ **Ondansetron Hydrochloride Dihydrate Injection (Can)** see Ondansetron on page 1253

◆ **Ondansetron Injection (Can)** see Ondansetron on page 1253

◆ **Ondansetron Injection USP (Can)** see Ondansetron on page 1253

◆ **Ondansetron-Odan (Can)** see Ondansetron on page 1253

◆ **Ondansetron-Omega (Can)** see Ondansetron on page 1253

◆ **Ondissolve ODF (Can)** see Ondansetron on page 1253

◆ **Onivyde** see Irinotecan (Liposomal) on page 960

◆ **Onmel** see Itraconazole on page 980

◆ **ONO-4538** see Nivolumab on page 1209

◆ **Onsolis [DSC]** see FentaNYL on page 692

◆ **Onxyl** see PACLitaxel (Conventional) on page 1284

◆ **Opana** see Oxymorphone on page 1281

◆ **Opana ER** see Oxymorphone on page 1281

◆ **o,p'-DDD** see Mitotane on page 1155

◆ **Opdivo** *see* Nivolumab *on page 1209*

Oprelvekin (oh PREL ve kin)

Brand Names: US Neumega [DSC]

Index Terms IL-11; Interleukin-11; Recombinant Human Interleukin-11; Recombinant Interleukin-11; rhIL-11

Pharmacologic Category Biological Response Modulator; Human Growth Factor

Use Thrombocytopenia: Prevention of severe thrombocytopenia and to reduce the need for platelet transfusions following myelosuppressive chemotherapy for nonmyeloid malignancy in adults who are at high risk for thrombocytopenia

Labeled Contraindications Hypersensitivity to oprelvekin or any component of the formulation

Pregnancy Considerations Adverse events have been observed in animal reproduction studies

Breast-Feeding Considerations It is not known if oprelvekin is excreted in breast milk. Due to the potential for serious adverse reactions in breast-feeding infants, the manufacturer recommends a decision be made to discontinue breast-feeding or the drug, taking into account the importance of treatment to the mother.

Warnings/Precautions [US Boxed Warning]: Allergic or hypersensitivity reactions, including anaphylaxis, have been reported. Permanently discontinue in any patient developing an allergic or hypersensitivity reaction. Reaction may occur with the first or with subsequent doses. Allergic reactions included facial/tongue/larynx edema, dyspnea, wheezing, chest pain, hypotension (including shock), rash, urticaria, flushing, fever, loss of consciousness, mental status changes, and/or dysarthria.

Arrhythmias, pulmonary edema, and cardiac arrest have been reported; use in patients with a history of atrial arrhythmia only if the potential benefit exceeds possible risks. Stroke has been reported in patients who develop atrial fibrillation/flutter while receiving oprelvekin. Ventricular arrhythmia has also been reported, occurring within 2 to 7 days of treatment initiation. May cause serious fluid retention, which may result in peripheral edema, dyspnea, pulmonary edema, capillary leak syndrome, atrial arrhythmias, and exacerbation of preexisting pleural effusion. Serious fluid retention (sometimes fatal) has been reported. Use with caution in patients with clinically evident heart failure or who may be susceptible to developing heart failure, patients receiving aggressive hydration, patients with a history of heart failure who are well compensated and receiving appropriate medical therapy, and patients who may develop fluid retention as a result of associated medical conditions or whose medical condition may be exacerbated by fluid retention. Monitor fluid and electrolyte status; preexisting fluid collections, including pericardial effusions or ascites, should also be monitored. Dilutional anemia may occur due to increased plasma volume; presenting as moderate decreases in hemoglobin concentration, hematocrit, and red blood cells without a decrease in red blood cell mass; effect generally appears within 3 to 5 days of initiation of therapy and resolves over approximately 1 week following oprelvekin discontinuation.

Papilledema has occurred, usually following repeated cycles. The incidence of papilledema occurred more frequently in children. Use with caution in patients with preexisting papilledema or with CNS tumors; may worsen or develop during treatment. Patients experiencing oprelvekin-related papilledema may be at risk for visual acuity changes and/or visual field defects ranging from blurred vision to blindness. Use with caution in patients with renal impairment (oprelvekin is renally eliminated); dosage adjustment required in severe renal impairment.

Begin 6 to 24 hours following completion of chemotherapy; safety and efficacy of oprelvekin administered immediately before or during cytotoxic chemotherapy or initiated at the time of expected nadir has not been established. Not indicated following myeloablative chemotherapy; increased toxicities (hypotension, tachycardia, edema, and conjunctival bleeding) were reported and efficacy was not demonstrated. A higher incidence of adverse events (fluid retention/overload, facial/pulmonary edema, capillary leak syndrome) has also been reported when used following bone marrow transplantation. Efficacy has not been evaluated with chemotherapy regimens >5 days' duration or with regimens associated with delayed myelosuppression (eg, nitrosoureas, mitomycin). Safety and efficacy have not been established with chronic administration.

Adverse Reactions

>10%:

Cardiovascular: Tachycardia (children 84%; adults 20%), edema (59%), cardiomegaly (children 21%), vasodilation (19%), atrial arrhythmia (12% to 15%), palpitation (14%), syncope (13%)

Central nervous system: Neutropenic fever (48%), headache (41%), dizziness (38%), fever (36%), insomnia (33%)

Dermatologic: Rash (25%)

Endocrine & metabolic: Fluid retention

Gastrointestinal: Nausea/vomiting (77%), diarrhea (43%), mucositis (43%), oral moniliasis (14%), weight gain (due to fluid retention)

Hematologic: Anemia (dilutional; onset: 3-5 days; duration: ≤1 week)

Neuromuscular & skeletal: Weakness (severe 14%), periostitis (children 11%), arthralgia

Ocular: Conjunctival injection/redness/swelling (children 57%; adults 19%), papilledema (children 16%; adults 1%)

Respiratory: Dyspnea (48%), rhinitis (42%), cough (29%), pharyngitis (25%)

1% to 10%: Respiratory: Pleural effusion (10%)

<1%, postmarketing, and/or case reports: Allergic reaction, amblyopia, anaphylaxis/anaphylactoid reactions, blindness, blurred vision, capillary leak syndrome, cardiac arrest, chest pain, dehydration, dysarthria, exfoliative dermatitis, eye hemorrhage, facial edema, fibrinogen increased, fluid overload, HF, hypoalbuminemia, hypocalcemia, hypokalemia, hypotension, injection site reactions (dermatitis, pain, discoloration), loss of consciousness, mental status changes, optic neuropathy, paresthesia, pericardial effusion, peripheral edema, pneumonia, pulmonary edema, renal failure, shock, skin discoloration, stroke, urticaria, ventricular arrhythmia, visual acuity changes, visual field defect, von Willebrand factor concentration increased, wheezing

Drug Interactions

Metabolism/Transport Effects None known.

Avoid Concomitant Use There are no known interactions where it is recommended to avoid concomitant use.

Increased Effect/Toxicity There are no known significant interactions involving an increase in effect.

Decreased Effect There are no known significant interactions involving a decrease in effect.

Storage/Stability Store intact vials (and prefilled diluent syringe) refrigerated between 2°C and 8°C (36°F and 46°F); do not freeze. Protect from light. Store reconstituted solution in the vial at either 2°C to 8°C (36°F to 46°F) or room temperature of ≤25°C (77°F); use within 3 hours of reconstitution. Do not freeze or shake reconstituted solution.

Preparation for Administration Reconstitute with 1 mL provided sterile water for injection (without preservative) to a final concentration of 5 mg/mL; direct diluent down side of vial; swirl gently, avoid excessive or vigorous agitation.

Mechanism of Action Oprelvekin is a thrombopoietic growth factor that stimulates megakaryocytopoiesis and thrombopoiesis, resulting in proliferation of megakaryocyte progenitors and megakaryocyte maturation, thereby increasing platelet production.

Pharmacodynamics/Kinetics
Bioavailability: >80%
Half-life elimination: Terminal: 6.9 ± 1.7 hours
Time to peak, serum: 3.2 ± 2.4 hours
Excretion: Urine (primarily; predominantly as metabolites)

Dosing
Adult & Geriatric
Thrombocytopenia: SubQ: 50 mcg/kg once daily until postnadir platelet count ≥50,000/mm^3. Begin ~6 to 24 hours after the end of chemotherapy. In studies, doses were administered for 10 to 21 days (do not administer for more than 21 days). Discontinue at least 2 days prior to the next planned chemotherapy cycle.

Renal Impairment For dosage adjustment purposes, renal function may be estimated using the Cockcroft-Gault formula.
CrCl ≥30 mL/minute: No dosage adjustment necessary.
CrCl <30 mL/minute: Reduce dose to 25 mcg/kg once daily.

Hepatic Impairment There are no dosage adjustments provided in the manufacturer's labeling.

Administration For subcutaneous administration in the abdomen, thigh, or hip; outer upper arm may also be used (if not self-injecting). Rotate injection sites each day.

Monitoring Parameters Monitor electrolytes and fluid balance during therapy (including persisting fluid collections [pericardial effusions or ascites]); obtain a complete blood cell count (CBC) at baseline and at regular intervals during therapy; monitor platelet counts during the time of expected nadir and until adequate recovery has occurred; renal function (at baseline)

Dosage Forms Excipient information presented when available (limited, particularly for generics); consult specific product labeling. [DSC] = Discontinued product
Solution Reconstituted, Subcutaneous [preservative free]:
Neumega: 5 mg (1 ea [DSC])

◆ **Orafate** see Mucosal Coating Agent on page 1175
◆ **Oral Wound Care Products** see Mucosal Coating Agent on page 1175
◆ **Oramorph SR** see Morphine (Systemic) on page 1167
◆ **Oramorph SR [DSC]** see Morphine (Systemic) on page 1167
◆ **Oraprep [DSC]** see PrednisoLONE (Systemic) on page 1421
◆ **Oraprep ODT** see PrednisoLONE (Systemic) on page 1421
◆ **Oraqix** see Lidocaine and Prilocaine on page 1046

- ◆ **Ortho,para-DDD** *see* Mitotane *on page 1155*
- ◆ **Orzel** *see* Tegafur and Uracil *on page 1604*
- ◆ **OSI-774** *see* Erlotinib *on page 628*

Osimertinib (oh si mer ti nib)

Related Information

Safe Handling of Hazardous Drugs *on page 2292*

Brand Names: US Tagrisso

Index Terms AZD9291; Tagrisso

Pharmacologic Category Antineoplastic Agent, Epidermal Growth Factor Receptor (EGFR) Inhibitor; Antineoplastic Agent, Tyrosine Kinase Inhibitor

Use Non-small cell lung cancer, metastatic: Treatment of metastatic epidermal growth factor receptor (EGFR) T790M mutation-positive non-small cell lung cancer (NSCLC), as detected by an approved test, in patients who have progressed on or after EGFR tyrosine kinase inhibitor (TKI) therapy

Labeled Contraindications There are no contraindications listed in the manufacturer's labeling.

Pregnancy Considerations Based on data from animal reproduction studies and the mechanism of action, use during pregnancy is expected to cause fetal harm. Women of reproductive potential should use effective contraception during therapy and for 6 weeks after the last dose. Males with female partners of reproductive potential should also use effective contraception during therapy and for 4 months after the last dose.

Breast-Feeding Considerations It is not known if osimertinib is excreted into breast milk. Because of the potential for serious adverse reactions in the nursing infant, breast-feeding is not recommended by the manufacturer during therapy or for 2 weeks after the last dose.

Warnings/Precautions Hazardous agent – use appropriate precautions for handling and disposal (meets NIOSH 2014 criteria).

Interstitial lung disease (ILD) and pneumonitis was observed in clinical studies; some events were fatal. Withhold treatment with worsening respiratory symptoms (dyspnea, cough, fever) which may be indicative of ILD; permanently discontinue if ILD is confirmed.

Cardiomyopathy (cardiac failure, pulmonary edema, decreased ejection fraction, or stress cardiomyopathy) has been observed; some events were fatal. In patients who had baseline and at least one follow up assessment, a left ventricular ejection fraction (LVEF) decline of >10% and a drop to below 50% was noted. Assess LVEF (by echocardiogram or multigated acquisition [MUGA] scan) prior to treatment and then every 3 months while on treatment. Withhold treatment if ejection fraction decreases by 10% from baseline and is <50%. Permanently discontinue for symptomatic heart failure or persistent, asymptomatic left ventricular dysfunction that does not resolve within 4 weeks. Prolongation of the QTc interval may occur; QTc >500 msec and an increase from baseline of >60 msec have been reported. Patients with a baseline QTc of ≥470 were excluded from clinical trials. Monitor ECG and electrolytes periodically in patients with a history of long QTc syndrome, heart failure, electrolyte abnormalities, and/or those taking concurrent medications known to prolong the QTc interval. Permanently discontinue in patients who develop QTc interval prolongation with signs/symptoms of life-threatening arrhythmia.

Lymphopenia, thrombocytopenia, neutropenia, and anemia may occur (usually grades 1 and 2) with osimertinib. Diarrhea (usually grades 1 and 2) was observed in almost half the patients receiving osimertinib. Skin reactions, including rash, dry skin, and itching may occur. Nail toxicity may also occur). Potentially significant drug-drug interactions may exist, requiring dose or frequency adjustment, additional monitoring, and/or selection of alternative therapy. Confirm the presence of a T790M epidermal growth factor receptor (EGFR) mutation prior to treatment initiation. Information on diagnostic tests approved for detection of T790M EGFR mutations may be found at www.fda. gov/companiondiagnostics.

Adverse Reactions

>10%:

Central nervous system: Fatigue (14%), headache (10%)

Dermatologic: Skin rash (41%, including erythematous rash, macular rash, maculopapular rash, papular rash, pustular rash, erythema, folliculitis, acne vulgaris, dermatitis, dermatitis acneiform), xeroderma (31%), nail disease (25%), pruritus (14%)

Endocrine & metabolic: Hyponatremia (26%), hypermagnesemia (20%)

Gastrointestinal: Diarrhea (42%), nausea (17%), decreased appetite (16%), constipation (15%), stomatitis (12%)

Hematologic & oncologic: Lymphopenia (63%, grades 3/4: 3%), thrombocytopenia (54%, grades 3/4: 1%), anemia (44%, grades 3/4: <1%), neutropenia (33%, grades 3/4: 3%)

Neuromuscular & skeletal: Back pain (13%)

Ophthalmic: Eye disorder (19%, including dry eyes, blurred vision, keratitis, cataract, eye irritation, blepharitis, eye pain, increased lacrimation, vitreous floaters, <1% other ocular toxicity)

Respiratory: Cough (14%)

1% to 10%:

Cardiovascular: Venous thromboembolism (7%, including deep vein thrombosis, internal jugular thrombosis), cerebrovascular accident (3%), prolonged Q-T interval on EKG (≤3%; prolonged from baseline), pulmonary embolism (≤2%), reduced ejection fraction (<2%), cardiomyopathy (≤1%)

Respiratory: Pneumonia (≤4%; grade 3/4: 2%), interstitial pneumonitis (3%)

Drug Interactions

Metabolism/Transport Effects Substrate of BCRP, CYP3A4 (minor), P-glycoprotein; **Note:** Assignment of Major/Minor substrate status based on clinically relevant drug interaction potential; **Inhibits** BCRP

Avoid Concomitant Use

Avoid concomitant use of Osimertinib with any of the following: CYP3A4 Inducers (Strong); CYP3A4 Inhibitors (Strong); Highest Risk QTc-Prolonging Agents; Ivabradine; Mifepristone; St Johns Wort

Increased Effect/Toxicity

Osimertinib may increase the levels/effects of: CYP3A4 Substrates; Highest Risk QTc-Prolonging Agents; Moderate Risk QTc-Prolonging Agents

The levels/effects of Osimertinib may be increased by: CYP3A4 Inhibitors (Strong); Ivabradine; Mifepristone; QTc-Prolonging Agents (Indeterminate Risk and Risk Modifying)

Decreased Effect

Osimertinib may decrease the levels/effects of: CYP1A2 Substrates; CYP3A4 Substrates

The levels/effects of Osimertinib may be decreased by: CYP3A4 Inducers (Strong); St Johns Wort

Storage/Stability Store at 25°C (77°F); excursions are permitted between 15°C and 30°C (59°F and 86°F).

Preparation for Administration

Hazardous agent; use appropriate precautions for handling and disposal (meets NIOSH 2014 criteria). For patients who have difficulty swallowing tablets, disperse tablet in ~50 mL of noncarbonated water (only), stir until tablet is completely dispersed and use immediately; rinse container with 120 to 240 mL water and drink or administer immediately. Do not crush, heat, or ultrisonicate during preparation. When it is necessary to manipulate the tablets (eg, to prepare an oral liquid), it is recommended to double glove, wear a protective gown, and prepare in a controlled device (NIOSH 2014).

Mechanism of Action Osimertinib is an irreversible epidermal growth factor receptor (EGFR) tyrosine kinase inhibitor which binds to select mutant forms of EGFR, including T790M, L858R, and exon 19 deletion at lower concentrations than wild-type. Osimertinib is selective for sensitizing mutations and the T790M resistance mutation, which is the most common mechanism of resistance to EGFR tyrosine kinase inhibitors (Janne 2015).

Pharmacodynamics/Kinetics

Distribution: V_{ss}/F: 986 L

Protein binding: Binding is likely high

Metabolism: Hepatic; predominantly oxidation (via CYP3A4) and dealkylation to 2 active metabolites (AZ5550 and AZ5104)

Bioavailability: AUC is increased by 19% with a high-fat, high-calorie meal

Half-life, elimination: Mean (estimated): 48 hours

Time to peak: Median: 6 hours (range: 3 to 24 hours)

Excretion: Feces (68%; ~2% as unchanged drug); Urine (14%; ~2% as unchanged drug)

Dosing

Adult & Geriatric Note: T790M EGFR mutation status of tumor specimen should be confirmed prior to treatment initiation.

Non-small cell lung cancer, metastatic (T790M EGFR mutation-positive):
Oral: 80 mg once daily until disease progression or unacceptable toxicity
Missed doses: If a dose is missed, do not make up the missed dose, take the next dose as scheduled.

Renal Impairment

CrCl 30 to 89 mL/minute: No dosage adjustment necessary.

CrCl <30 mL/minute and end stage renal disease: There are no dosage adjustments provided in the manufacturer's labeling (has not been studied).

Hepatic Impairment

Mild impairment (total bilirubin <ULN and AST 1 to 1.5 times ULN **or** total bilirubin 1 to 1.5 times ULN and any AST): No dosage adjustment necessary.

Moderate (total bilirubin 1.5 to 3 times ULN and any AST) or severe impairment (total bilirubin 3 to 10 times ULN and any AST): There are no dosage adjustments provided in the manufacturer's labeling (has not been studied).

Adjustment for Toxicity

Cardiotoxicity:

QTc interval >500 msec on at least 2 separate ECGs: Withhold treatment until QTc interval is <481 msec or recovers to baseline (if baseline QTc ≥481 msec) and then resume at a dose of 40 mg once daily.

QTc interval prolongation with signs/symptoms of life-threatening arrhythmia: Permanently discontinue.

Asymptomatic absolute decrease in left ventricular ejections fraction (LVEF) of 10% from baseline and below 50%: Withhold treatment for up to 4 weeks. If improved to baseline, resume treatment; if not improved to baseline, permanently discontinue.

Symptomatic heart failure: Permanently discontinue.

Pulmonary toxicity: Interstitial lung disease/pneumonitis: Permanently discontinue.

Other toxicities: Grade 3 or higher adverse reaction: Withhold treatment for up to 3 weeks. If improves to grade 2 or lower within 3 weeks, resume at either 80 mg once daily or 40 mg once daily. If not improved within 3 weeks, permanently discontinue.

Administration

Oral: May be administered with or without food.

For patients who have difficulty swallowing tablets, disperse tablet in ~50 mL of noncarbonated water (only), stir until tablet is completely dispersed and immediately swallow or administer through NG tube. Rinse container with 120 to 240 mL water and immediately drink or administer through NG tube. Do not crush, heat, or ultrasonicate during preparation.

Hazardous agent; use appropriate precautions for handling and disposal (meets NIOSH 2014 criteria). NIOSH recommends single gloving for administration of intact tablets (NIOSH 2014). Avoid exposure to crushed tablets. When it is necessary to manipulate the tablets (eg, to prepare an oral liquid), it is recommended to double glove, wear a protective gown, and prepare in a controlled device (NIOSH 2014).

Monitoring Parameters T790M epidermal growth factor receptor (EGFR) mutation status (prior to treatment). Monitor ECG and electrolytes periodically (in patients with a history of long QTc syndrome, heart failure, electrolyte abnormalities, and/or those taking concurrent medications known to prolong the QTc interval). Assess LVEF (by echocardiogram or multigated acquisition [MUGA] scan) prior to treatment and then every 3 months while on treatment. Monitor for signs/symptoms of interstitial lung disease or pneumonitis, dermatologic, and gastrointestinal toxicity.

Prescribing and Access Restrictions Available through specialty pharmacies and distributors. Further information may be obtained from the manufacturer, Astra Zeneca, at 1-844-275-2360 or at https://www.tagrisso.com.

Dosage Forms Excipient information presented when available (limited, particularly for generics); consult specific product labeling.

Tablet, Oral:

Tagrisso: 40 mg, 80 mg

◆ **OTFC (Oral Transmucosal Fentanyl Citrate)** see FentaNYL on page 692

◆ **Otrexup** see Methotrexate on page 1104

◆ **Oxalatoplatin** see Oxaliplatin on page 1269

◆ **Oxalatoplatinum** see Oxaliplatin on page 1269

Oxaliplatin (ox AL i pla tin)

Related Information

Chemotherapy-Induced Peripheral Neuropathy *on page 2116*
Common Toxicity Criteria *on page 2122*
Management of Chemotherapy-Induced Nausea and Vomiting in Adults *on page 2142*
Management of Drug Extravasations *on page 2159*
Mucositis and Stomatitis *on page 2186*
Prevention of Chemotherapy-Induced Nausea and Vomiting in Children *on page 2203*
Safe Handling of Hazardous Drugs *on page 2292*

Brand Names: US Eloxatin

Brand Names: Canada Eloxatin

Index Terms Diaminocyclohexane Oxalatoplatinum; L-OHP; Oxalatoplatin; Oxalatoplatinum

Pharmacologic Category Antineoplastic Agent, Alkylating Agent; Antineoplastic Agent, Platinum Analog

Use

Colon cancer, stage III (adjuvant therapy): Adjuvant treatment of stage III colon cancer (in combination with infusional fluorouracil and leucovorin) after complete resection of primary tumor.

Colorectal cancer, advanced: Treatment of advanced colorectal cancer (in combination with infusional fluorouracil and leucovorin).

Labeled Contraindications

Hypersensitivity to oxaliplatin, other platinum-containing compounds, or any component of the formulation

Canadian labeling: Additional contraindications (not in US labeling): Pregnancy, breast-feeding; severe renal impairment (CrCl <30 mL/minute)

Pregnancy Considerations Adverse events were observed in animal reproduction studies at one-tenth the equivalent human dose. Women of childbearing potential should be advised to avoid pregnancy and use effective contraception during treatment.

Canadian labeling: Use in pregnant women is contraindicated in the Canadian labeling. Males should be advised not to father children during and for up to 6 months following therapy. May cause permanent infertility in males. Prior to initiating therapy, advise males desiring to father children, to seek counseling on sperm storage.

Breast-Feeding Considerations It is not known if oxaliplatin is excreted in breast milk. Due to the potential for serious adverse reactions in the breast-feeding infant, the decision to discontinue breast-feeding or to discontinue oxaliplatin should take into account the benefits of treatment to the mother.

Warnings/Precautions Hazardous agent - use appropriate precautions for handling and disposal (NIOSH 2014 [group 1]). **[US Boxed Warning]: Anaphylactic/anaphylactoid reactions have been reported with oxaliplatin (may occur within minutes of administration); symptoms may be managed with epinephrine, corticosteroids, antihistamines,** and discontinuation; oxygen and bronchodilators have also been used (Kim 2009). Grade 3 or 4 hypersensitivity has been observed. Allergic reactions are similar to reactions reported with other platinum analogs, and may occur with any cycle. Reactions typically occur after multiple cycles; in retrospective reviews, reaction occurred at a median of 7 to 9 cycles, with an onset of 5 to 70 minutes (Kim

2009; Polyzos 2009). Symptoms may include bronchospasm (rare), erythema, hypotension (rare), pruritus, rash, and/or urticaria; previously-untreated patients have also experienced flushing, diaphoresis, diarrhea, shortness of breath, chest pain, hypotension, syncope, and disorientation. According to the manufacturer, rechallenge is contraindicated (deaths due to anaphylaxis have been associated with platinum derivatives). In patients rechallenged after mild hypersensitivity, reaction recurred at a higher level of severity; for patients with severe hypersensitivity, rechallenge (with 2 to 3 days of antihistamine and corticosteroid premedication, and prolongation of infusion time) allowed for 2 to 4 additional oxaliplatin cycles; however, rechallenge was not feasible in nearly two-thirds of patients due to the severity of the initial reaction (Polyzos 2009).

Two different types of peripheral sensory neuropathy may occur: First, an acute (within hours to 1 to 2 days), reversible (resolves within 14 days), with primarily peripheral symptoms that are often exacerbated by cold (may include pharyngolaryngeal dysesthesia; commonly recur with subsequent doses; avoid mucositis prophylaxis with ice chips, exposure to cold temperatures, or consumption of cold food/beverages during or within hours after oxaliplatin infusion. Cold-triggered neuropathy may last up to 7 days after oxaliplatin administration (Grothey 2011). Secondly, a more persistent (>14 days) presentation that often interferes with daily activities (eg, writing, buttoning, swallowing), these symptoms may improve in some patients upon discontinuing treatment. In a retrospective evaluation of patients treated with oxaliplatin for colorectal cancer, the incidence of peripheral sensory neuropathy was similar between diabetic and nondiabetic patients (Ramanathan 2010). Several retrospective studies (as well as a small, underpowered randomized trial) have suggested calcium and magnesium infusions before and after oxaliplatin administration may reduce incidence of cumulative sensory neuropathy; however, a recent abstract of an ongoing randomized, placebo-controlled, double-blind study in patients with colorectal cancer suggests there is no benefit of calcium and magnesium in preventing sensory neuropathy or in decreasing oxaliplatin discontinuation rates (Loprinzi 2013).

Grade 3 and 4 neutropenia occurs commonly with oxaliplatin in combination with fluorouracil and leucovorin; sepsis, neutropenic sepsis, and septic shock have been reported (some fatal). Delay treatment until neutrophils are $\geq 1500/mm^3$; withhold treatment for sepsis or septic shock. Reduce the dose after recovery from grade 4 neutropenia or neutropenic fever. QT prolongation and ventricular arrhythmias, including fatal torsades de pointes have been reported in postmarketing surveillance. ECG monitoring is recommend in patients with heart failure, bradyarrhythmias, concomitant medications known to cause QT prolongation (including class Ia and III antiarrhythmics), and electrolyte abnormalities. Avoid use in patients with congenital long QT syndrome. Monitor potassium and magnesium prior to and periodically during treatment; correct hypokalemia and hypomagnesemia prior to treatment initiation.

Oxaliplatin is associated with a moderate emetic potential; antiemetics are recommended to prevent nausea and vomiting (Basch 2011; Dupuis 2011; Roila 2010). Cases of reversible posterior leukoencephalopathy syndrome (RPLS) have been reported. Signs/symptoms include headache, mental status changes, seizure, blurred vision, blindness and/or other vision changes; may be associated with hypertension; diagnosis is confirmed with brain imaging. May cause pulmonary fibrosis; withhold treatment for unexplained pulmonary symptoms (eg, crackles, dyspnea, nonproductive cough, pulmonary infiltrates) until interstitial lung disease or pulmonary fibrosis are excluded. Hepatotoxicity (including rare cases of hepatitis and hepatic failure) has been reported. Liver biopsy has revealed peliosis, nodular regenerative hyperplasia, sinusoidal alterations, perisinusoidal fibrosis, and veno-occlusive lesions; the presence of hepatic vascular disorders (including veno-occlusive disease) should be considered, especially in individuals developing portal hypertension or who present with increased liver function tests. Rhabdomyolysis (including fatal cases) has been reported with oxaliplatin; discontinue if signs/symptoms of rhabdomyolysis occur. Use caution with renal dysfunction; increased toxicity may occur; reduce initial dose in severe impairment. The Canadian labeling contraindicates use in severe renal impairment (CrCl <30 mL/minute). Potentially significant drug-drug interactions may exist, requiring dose or frequency adjustment, additional monitoring, and/or selection of alternative therapy. Elderly patients are more sensitive to some adverse events including diarrhea, dehydration, hypokalemia, leukopenia, fatigue and syncope. Oxaliplatin is an irritant with vesicant-like properties; ensure proper needle or catheter placement prior to and during infusion; avoid extravasation.

Adverse Reactions Percentages reported with monotherapy.

>10%:

Central nervous system: Peripheral neuropathy (may be dose limiting; 76% to 92%; acute 65%; grades 3/4: 5%; persistent 43%; grades 3/4: 3%), fatigue (61%), pain (14%), headache (13%), insomnia (11%)

Gastrointestinal: Nausea (64%), diarrhea (46%), vomiting (37%), abdominal pain (31%), constipation (31%), anorexia (20%), stomatitis (14%)

Hematologic & oncologic: Anemia (64%; grades 3/4: 1%), thrombocytopenia (30%; grades 3/4: 3%), leukopenia (13%)

Hepatic: Increased serum AST (54%; grades 3/4: 4%), increased serum ALT (36%; grades 3/4: 1%), increased serum bilirubin (13%; grades 3/4: 5%)

Neuromuscular & skeletal: Back pain (11%)

Respiratory: Dyspnea (13%), cough (11%)

Miscellaneous: Fever (25%)

1% to 10%:

Cardiovascular: Edema (10%), chest pain (5%), peripheral edema (5%), flushing (3%), thromboembolism (2%)

Central nervous system: Rigors (9%), dizziness (7%)

Dermatologic: Skin rash (5%), alopecia (3%), palmar-plantar erythrodysesthesia (1%)

Endocrine & metabolic: Dehydration (5%), hypokalemia (3%)

Gastrointestinal: Dyspepsia (7%), dysgeusia (5%), flatulence (3%), hiccups (2%), mucositis (2%), gastroesophageal reflux disease (1%), dysphagia (acute 1% to 2%)

Genitourinary: Dysuria (1%)

Hematologic & oncologic: Neutropenia (7%)

Hypersensitivity: Hypersensitivity reaction (3%; includes urticaria, pruritus, facial flushing, shortness of breath, bronchospasm, diaphoresis, hypotension, syncope: grades 3/4: 2% to 3%)

Local: Injection site reaction (9%; redness/swelling/pain)

Neuromuscular & skeletal: Arthralgia (7%)

Ocular: Abnormal lacrimation (1%)

Renal: Increased serum creatinine (5% to 10%)

Respiratory: Upper respiratory tract infection (7%), rhinitis (6%), epistaxis (2%), pharyngitis (2%), pharyngolaryngeal dysesthesia (grades 3/4: 1% to 2%)

<1%, postmarketing, and/or case reports (reported with mono- and combination therapy): Abnormal gait, acute renal failure, anaphylaxis, anaphylactic shock, anaphylactoid reaction, angioedema, aphonia, ataxia, blepharoptosis, cerebral hemorrhage, colitis, cranial nerve palsy, decreased deep tendon reflex, deafness, decreased visual acuity, diplopia, dysarthria, eosinophilic pneumonitis, fasciculations, febrile neutropenia, hematuria, hemolysis, hemolytic anemia (immuno-allergic), hemolytic-uremic syndrome, hemorrhage, hepatic failure, hepatic sinusoidal obstruction syndrome (SOS; veno-occlusive disease), hepatitis, hepatotoxicity, hypertension, hypomagnesemia, hypoxia, idiopathic noncirrhotic portal hypertension (nodular regenerative hyperplasia), increased INR, increased serum alkaline phosphatase, infusion related reaction (extravasation [including necrosis]), interstitial nephritis (acute), interstitial pulmonary disease, intestinal obstruction, laryngospasm, Lhermittes' sign, metabolic acidosis, muscle spasm, myoclonus, neutropenic enterocolitis, neutropenic infection (sepsis), optic neuritis, pancreatitis, prolonged prothrombin time, purpura, rectal hemorrhage, renal tubular necrosis, reversible posterior leukoencephalopathy syndrome (RPLS), rhabdomyolysis, seizure, sepsis, temporary vision loss, thrombocytopenia (immuno-allergic), trigeminal neuralgia, visual field loss, voice disorder

Drug Interactions

Metabolism/Transport Effects Substrate of OCT2

Avoid Concomitant Use

Avoid concomitant use of Oxaliplatin with any of the following: BCG (Intravesical); CloZAPine; Dipyrone; Natalizumab; Pimecrolimus; Tacrolimus (Topical); Tofacitinib; Vaccines (Live)

Increased Effect/Toxicity

Oxaliplatin may increase the levels/effects of: CloZAPine; Fingolimod; Highest Risk QTc-Prolonging Agents; Leflunomide; Moderate Risk QTc-Prolonging Agents; Natalizumab; Taxane Derivatives; Tofacitinib; Topotecan; Vaccines (Live)

The levels/effects of Oxaliplatin may be increased by: BuPROPion; Denosumab; Dipyrone; Mifepristone; Pimecrolimus; Roflumilast; Tacrolimus (Topical); Trastuzumab

Decreased Effect

Oxaliplatin may decrease the levels/effects of: BCG (Intravesical); Coccidioides immitis Skin Test; Fosphenytoin-Phenytoin; Sipuleucel-T; Vaccines (Inactivated); Vaccines (Live)

The levels/effects of Oxaliplatin may be decreased by: Echinacea

Storage/Stability Store intact vials at room temperature of 25°C (77°F); excursions permitted to 15°C to 30°C (59°F to 86°F); do not freeze. Protect concentrated solution from light (store in original outer carton). According to the manufacturer, solutions diluted for infusion are stable up to 6 hours at room temperature of 20°C to 25°C (68°F to 77°F) or up to 24 hours under refrigeration at 2°C to 8°C (36°F to 46°F). Oxaliplatin solution diluted with D_5W to a final concentration of 0.7 mg/mL (polyolefin container) has been shown to retain >90% of the original concentration for up to 30 days when stored at room temperature or refrigerated; artificial light did not affect the concentration (Andre 2007). As this study did not examine sterility, refrigeration would be preferred to limit microbial growth. Solutions diluted for infusion do not require protection from light.

Preparation for Administration Hazardous agent; use appropriate precautions for handling and disposal (NIOSH 2014 [group 1]).

Do not prepare using a chloride-containing solution such as NaCl due to rapid conversion to monochloroplatinum, dichloroplatinum, and diaquoplatinum; all highly reactive in sodium chloride (Takimoto 2007). Do not use needles or administration sets containing aluminum during preparation.

Aqueous solution: Dilution with D_5W (250 or 500 mL) is required prior to administration.

Lyophilized powder: Use only SWFI or D_5W to reconstitute powder. To obtain final concentration of 5 mg/mL add 10 mL of diluent to 50 mg vial or 20 mL diluent to 100 mg vial. Gently swirl vial to dissolve powder. Dilution with D_5W (250 or 500 mL) is required prior to administration. Discard unused portion of vial.

Mechanism of Action Oxaliplatin, a platinum derivative, is an alkylating agent. Following intracellular hydrolysis, the platinum compound binds to DNA forming cross-links which inhibit DNA replication and transcription, resulting in cell death. Cytotoxicity is cell-cycle nonspecific.

Pharmacodynamics/Kinetics

Distribution: V_d: 440 L

Protein binding: >90% primarily albumin and gamma globulin (irreversible binding to platinum)

Metabolism: Nonenzymatic (rapid and extensive), forms active and inactive derivatives

Half-life elimination: Terminal: 391 hours

Excretion: Urine (~54%); feces (~2%)

Dosing

Adult Note: Oxaliplatin is associated with a moderate emetic potential; antiemetics are recommended to prevent nausea and vomiting (Basch 2011; Dupuis 2011; Roila 2010).

Colorectal cancer (advanced): IV: 85 mg/m² every 2 weeks until disease progression or unacceptable toxicity (in combination with infusional fluorouracil/leucovorin)

Colon cancer, stage III (adjuvant therapy): IV: 85 mg/m² every 2 weeks for 6 months (12 cycles; in combination with infusional fluorouracil/leucovorin)

Colon/colorectal cancer (off-label doses or combinations): IV: 85 mg/m²/dose on days 1, 15, and 29 of an 8-week treatment cycle in combination with fluorouracil/leucovorin (Kuebler 2007) **or** 85 mg/m² every 2 weeks in combination with fluorouracil/leucovorin/irinotecan (Falcone 2007) **or** 130 mg/m² every 3 weeks in combination with capecitabine (Cassidy 2008; Haller 2011)

Biliary adenocarcinoma, advanced (off-label use): IV:

GEMOX regimen: 100 mg/m² on day 2 every 2 weeks (in combination with gemcitabine) until disease progression or unacceptable toxicity (Andre 2004) **or**

CAPOX regimen: 130 mg/m² on day 1 every 3 weeks (in combination with capecitabine) until disease progression or unacceptable toxicity (Nehls 2008)

Chronic lymphocytic leukemia, fludarabine-refractory (off-label use): IV: OFAR regimen: 25 mg/m²/day for 4 days every 4 weeks (in combination with fludarabine, cytarabine, and rituximab) for up to 6 cycles (Tsimberidou 2008)

Esophageal/gastric cancers (off-label use): IV: 130 mg/m² on day 1 every 3 weeks (in combination with epirubicin and either capecitabine or fluorouracil) for up to 8 cycles (Cunningham 2008) **or** 85 mg/m² on day 1 every

◀ 2 weeks (in combination with docetaxel, leucovorin, and fluorouracil) for up to 8 cycles (Al-Batran 2008) **or** 85 mg/m² on day 1 every 2 weeks (in combination with leucovorin and fluorouracil; FOLFOX4) for 6 cycles (Conroy 2010)

or

Gastric cancer: IV: 130 mg/m² on day 1 every 3 weeks (in combination with capecitabine) for 8 cycles (Bang 2012)

Non-Hodgkin lymphoma, relapsed/refractory (off-label use): IV: 100 mg/m² on day 1 every 3 weeks (in combination with gemcitabine and rituximab) (Lopez 2008; Rodriguez 2007) **or** 130 mg/m² on day 1 every 3 weeks (in combination with cytarabine and dexamethasone) (Chau 2001)

Ovarian cancer, advanced (off-label use): IV: 130 mg/m² once every 3 weeks until disease progression or unacceptable toxicity (Dieras 2002; Piccart 2000)

Pancreatic cancer, advanced (off-label use): IV: 85 mg/m² every 2 weeks (in combination with fluorouracil, leucovorin, and irinotecan; FOLFIRINOX regimen) for up to 6 months (Conroy 2011) **or** 110 to 130 mg/m² on day 1 every 3 weeks (in combination with capecitabine) until disease progression or unacceptable toxicity (Xiong 2008)

Testicular cancer, refractory (off-label use): IV: 130 mg/m² every 3 weeks in combination with gemcitabine (De Georgi 2006; Kollmannsberger 2004; Pectasides 2004) **or** 130 mg/m² on day 1 every 3 weeks (in combination with gemcitabine and paclitaxel) for up to 8 cycles (Bokemeyer 2008)

Geriatric No dosage adjustment necessary. Refer to adult dosing.

Renal Impairment

Manufacturer's labeling:

US labeling:

CrCl ≥30 mL/minute: No dosage adjustment necessary.

CrCl <30 mL/minute: Reduce dose from 85 mg/m² to 65 mg/m².

Canadian labeling:

CrCl ≥50 mL/minute: No dosage adjustment necessary.

CrCl 30 to <50 mL/minute: No dosage adjustment necessary; monitor closely and reduce dose if toxicities occur.

CrCl <30 mL/minute: Use is contraindicated.

Alternate recommendations: CrCl ≥20 mL/minute: In a study with a limited number of patients with mild to moderate impairment, defined by the authors as CrCl 20 to 59 mL/minute (determined using 24-hour urine collection), oxaliplatin was well tolerated, suggesting a dose reduction may not be necessary in patients with CrCl ≥20 mL/minute receiving every-3-week dosing (dose range: 80 to 130 mg/m² every 3 weeks) (Takimoto 2003).

Hepatic Impairment Mild, moderate, or severe impairment: No dosage adjustment necessary (Doroshow 2003; Synold 2007).

Obesity *ASCO Guidelines for appropriate chemotherapy dosing in obese adults with cancer:* Utilize patient's actual body weight (full weight) for calculation of body surface area- or weight-based dosing, particularly when the intent of therapy is curative; manage regimen-related toxicities in the same manner as for nonobese patients; if a dose reduction is utilized due to toxicity, consider resumption of full weight-based dosing with subsequent cycles, especially if cause of toxicity (eg, hepatic or renal impairment) is resolved (Griggs 2012).

Adjustment for Toxicity Acute toxicities: Longer infusion time (6 hours) may mitigate acute toxicities (eg, pharyngolaryngeal dysesthesia).

Neurosensory events:

Persistent (>7 days) grade 2 neurosensory events:

Adjuvant treatment of stage III colon cancer: Reduce dose to 75 mg/m²

Advanced colorectal cancer: Reduce dose to 65 mg/m²

Consider withholding oxaliplatin for grade 2 neuropathy lasting >7 days despite dose reduction.

Persistent (>7 days) grade 3 neurosensory events:

US labeling: Consider discontinuing oxaliplatin.

Canadian labeling:

Adjuvant treatment of stage III colon cancer: Discontinue oxaliplatin.

Advanced colorectal cancer: Reduce dose to 65 mg/m²; if not resolved prior to next cycle, then discontinue.

Persistent grade 4 neurosensory events (Canadian labeling): Advanced colorectal cancer: Discontinue oxaliplatin

Gastrointestinal toxicity (grade 3/4) occurring despite prophylactic treatment:

Adjuvant treatment of stage III colon cancer: Delay next dose until recovery from toxicity, then reduce dose to 75 mg/m².

Advanced colorectal cancer: Delay next dose until recovery from toxicity, then reduce dose to 65 mg/m².

Hematologic toxicity (grade 4 neutropenia [Canadian labeling: grade 3 or 4 neutropenia], febrile neutropenia, or grade 3/4 thrombocytopenia):

Adjuvant treatment of stage III colon cancer: Delay next dose until neutrophils recover to ≥1500/mm³ and platelets recover to ≥75,000/mm³, then reduce dose to 75 mg/m².

Advanced colorectal cancer: Delay next dose until neutrophils recover to ≥1500/mm³ and platelets recover to ≥75,000/mm³, then reduce dose to 65 mg/m².

Pulmonary toxicity (unexplained respiratory symptoms including nonproductive cough, dyspnea, crackles, pulmonary infiltrates): Discontinue until interstitial lung disease or pulmonary fibrosis have been excluded.

Rhabdomyolysis: Discontinue for signs/symptoms of rhabdomyolysis.

Sepsis or septic shock: Withhold treatment.

Combination Regimens

Biliary adenocarcinoma: GEMOX (Biliary Cancer) on page 1999

Colorectal cancer:

Bevacizumab FOLFOX (Colorectal) on page 1842

Bevacizumab + XELOX (Colorectal) on page 1846

FLOX (Colorectal) on page 1970

FOLFOX1 (Colorectal) on page 1984

FOLFOX2 (Colorectal) on page 1985

FOLFOX3 (Colorectal) on page 1985

FOLFOX4 (Colorectal) on page 1985

FOLFOX6 and mFOLFOX6 (Colorectal) on page 1986

FOLFOX7 (Colorectal) on page 1987

FOLFOXIRI (Colorectal) on page 1987

Panitumumab + FOLFOX4 (Colorectal) on page 2059

XELOX (Colorectal) on page 2111

Esophageal cancer:

Docetaxel-Oxaliplatin-Leucovorin-Fluorouracil (Esophageal Cancer) on page 1946

Epirubicin-Oxaliplatin-Capecitabine (Gastric/Esophageal) on page 1957

Administration Administer as IV infusion over 2 hours; extend infusion time to 6 hours for acute toxicities. Flush infusion line with D_5W prior to administration of any concomitant medication. Avoid mucositis prophylaxis with ice chips, exposure to cold temperatures, or consumption of cold food/beverages during or within hours after oxaliplatin infusion (may exacerbate acute neurological symptoms). Do not use needles or administration sets containing aluminum. When used in combination with a fluoropyrimidine (eg, 5-FU), infuse oxaliplatin first.

Oxaliplatin is associated with a moderate emetic potential; antiemetics are recommended to prevent nausea and vomiting (Basch 2011; Dupuis 2011; Roila 2010).

Irritant with vesicant-like properties; ensure proper needle or catheter placement prior to and during infusion. Avoid extravasation; monitor IV site for redness, swelling, or pain.

Extravasation management: If extravasation occurs, stop infusion immediately and disconnect (leave cannula/needle in place); gently aspirate extravasated solution (do **NOT** flush the line); remove needle/cannula; elevate extremity. Information conflicts regarding use of warm or cold compresses. Cold compresses could potentially precipitate or exacerbate peripheral neuropathy (de Lemos 2005).

Hazardous agent; use appropriate precautions for handling and disposal (NIOSH 2014 [group 1]).

Vesicant/Extravasation Risk Irritant with vesicant-like properties

Cold compress may cause local vasoconstriction and reduce cellular injury; however, may cause or exacerbate peripheral neuropathy; warm compresses may increase local drug removal, although may also increase cellular uptake and injury (de Lemos 2005).

Emetic Potential Children and Adults: Moderate (30% to 90%)

Monitoring Parameters CBC with differential, blood chemistries, including serum creatinine, ALT, AST, and bilirubin (prior to each cycle), electrolytes, including potassium and magnesium (prior to and periodically during treatment); INR and prothrombin time (in patients on oral anticoagulant therapy); neurologic evaluation prior to each dose and periodically thereafter; hypersensitivity; respiratory effects; RPLS

Dosage Forms Excipient information presented when available (limited, particularly for generics); consult specific product labeling. [DSC] = Discontinued product

Solution, Intravenous [preservative free]:
Eloxatin: 50 mg/10 mL (10 mL [DSC]); 100 mg/20 mL (20 mL [DSC]); 200 mg/40 mL (40 mL)
Generic: 50 mg/10 mL (10 mL); 100 mg/20 mL (20 mL)
Solution Reconstituted, Intravenous [preservative free]:
Generic: 50 mg (1 ea); 100 mg (1 ea)

◆ **Oxaydo** see OxyCODONE on page 1277
◆ **Oxecta** see OxyCODONE on page 1277
◆ **Oxecta [DSC]** see OxyCODONE on page 1277

OxyCODONE (oks i KOE done)

Brand Names: US Oxaydo; Oxecta [DSC]; OxyCONTIN; Roxicodone
Brand Names: Canada ACT Oxycodone CR; Apo-Oxycodone CR; Oxy.IR; OxyNEO; PMS-Oxycodone; PMS-Oxycodone CR; Supeudol
Index Terms Dihydrohydroxycodeinone; Oxaydo; Oxecta; Oxycodone Hydrochloride
Pharmacologic Category Analgesic, Opioid
Use

Pain management:

Immediate release formulations: Management of moderate to severe pain where the use of an opioid analgesic is appropriate.

Extended release formulation: Management of pain severe enough to require daily, around-the-clock, long-term opioid treatment and for which alternative treatment options are inadequate.

Limitations of use: Because of the risks of addiction, abuse, and misuse with opioids, even at recommended doses, and because of the greater risks of overdose and death with extended-release opioid formulations, reserve oxycodone ER for use in patients for whom alternative treatment options (eg, nonopioid analgesics, immediate-release opioids) are ineffective, not tolerated, or would be otherwise inadequate to provide sufficient management of pain. Oxycodone ER is not indicated as an as-needed analgesic.

Pregnancy Risk Factor B/C (manufacturer specific)

◀ **Dosing**

Adult Pain management: Oral: **Note:** All doses should be titrated to appropriate effect. Reduced initial doses may be necessary in patients with adrenocortical insufficiency (eg, Addison disease), hypothyroidism, myxedema, severe respiratory impairment, toxic psychosis, prostatic hypertrophy or urethral stricture:

Immediate release: Initial: 5 to 15 mg every 4 to 6 hours as needed; dosing range: 5 to 20 mg per dose (APS 6th edition). For severe chronic pain, administer on a regularly scheduled basis, every 4 to 6 hours, at the lowest dose that will achieve adequate analgesia.

Extended release: **Note:** Oxycodone ER 60 mg and 80 mg strengths, a single dose >40 mg, or a total dose of >80 mg daily are for use only in opioid-tolerant patients. Opioid tolerance is defined as: Patients already taking at least 60 mg of oral morphine daily, 25 mcg of transdermal fentanyl per hour, 30 mg of oral oxycodone daily, 8 mg oral hydromorphone daily, or an equivalent dose of another opioid for at least 1 week.

Opioid naive (use as the first opioid analgesic or use in patients who are **not** opioid tolerant): Initial: 10 mg every 12 hours

Conversion from other oral oxycodone formulations to extended release oxycodone: Initiate extended release oxycodone with one-half the total daily oral oxycodone daily dose (mg/day) administered every 12 hours.

Conversion from other opioids to extended release oxycodone:

US labeling: Discontinue all other around-the-clock opioids when extended release oxycodone is initiated. Initiate with 10 mg every 12 hours. Substantial interpatient variability exists in relative potency. Therefore, it is safer to underestimate a patient's daily oral oxycodone requirement and provide breakthrough pain relief with rescue medication (eg, immediate release opioid) than to overestimate requirements.

Canadian labeling: Discontinue all other around-the-clock opioids when extended release oxycodone is initiated. Determine oral oxycodone equivalent daily dose (refer to manufacturer labeling for equivalent dosing conversion). Divide total daily oxycodone dose into 2 equal doses and administer every 12 hours.

Conversion from transdermal fentanyl to extended release oxycodone: For each 25 mcg/hour transdermal dose, substitute 10 mg extended release oxycodone every 12 hours; should be initiated 18 hours after the removal of the transdermal fentanyl patch

Conversion from methadone to extended release oxycodone: Close monitoring is required when converting methadone to another opioid. Ratio between methadone and other opioid agonists varies widely according to previous dose exposure. Methadone has a long half-life and can accumulate in the plasma.

Conversion from fixed-dose oxycodone/nonopioid combinations to extended release oxycodone: *Canadian labeling:*

If previous total daily dose of oxycodone in combination product was 5 to 25 mg, begin oxycodone extended release 10 to 20 mg every 12 hours.

If previous total daily dose of oxycodone in combination product was 30 to 45 mg, begin oxycodone extended release 20 to 30 mg every 12 hours.

If previous total daily dose of oxycodone in combination product was 50 to 60 mg, begin oxycodone extended release 30 to 40 mg every 12 hours.

If previous total daily dose of oxycodone in combination product was >60 mg, base dose on total daily dose of oxycodone.

Dose adjustment: Doses may be adjusted every 1 to 2 days; the total daily oxycodone dose may be increased by 25% to 50%. The total daily dose should be administered in divided doses every 12 hours. **Note:** Some clinicians have reported that in certain chronic pain patients, more frequent dosing (ie, every 8 hours) is required for effective pain relief (Gallagher 2007; Marcus 2004; Nicholson 2006), although dosing more frequently than every 12 hours is not recommended by the manufacturer, and safety and efficacy has not been established.

Dosage adjustment for concomitant therapy: Concomitant CNS depressants: Reduce usual initial oxycodone dose by 33% to 50%.

Discontinuation of therapy:

US labeling:

Immediate release: Decrease previous daily dose by 25% to 50% each day; monitor for signs/symptoms of withdrawal. If patient displays withdrawal symptoms, increase dose to previous dose and then reduce dose more slowly by increasing interval between dose reductions, decreasing amount of daily dose reduction, or both.

Extended release: Gradually titrate dose downward to prevent withdrawal signs/symptoms. Do not abruptly discontinue.

Canadian labeling: Decrease previous daily dose by 50% (administer in divided doses every 6 hours for 2 days [immediate release] or every 12 hours for 2 days [extended release]), then decrease dose by 25% every 2 days.

Dosage adjustment in debilitated patients (nonopioid tolerant):

Immediate release: Initial

US labeling: There are no dosage adjustments provided in the manufacturer's labeling; use caution.

Canadian labeling: There are no specific dosage adjustments provided in the manufacturer's labeling; however, a reduced dosage is recommended; use caution.

Extended release: Initial:

US labeling: Decrease dose by 33% to 50% of usual starting dose

Canadian labeling: There are no specific dosage adjustments provided in the manufacturer's labeling; however, a reduced dosage is recommended; use caution.

Geriatric Refer to adult dosing. Initiate therapy at low end of dosing range and use caution.

Pediatric Pain management: Children (off-label use): Oral: Immediate release, initial dose: 0.1 to 0.2 mg/kg/dose (moderate pain) or 0.2 mg/kg/dose (severe pain) (APS 6th edition). For severe chronic pain, administer on a regularly scheduled basis, every 4 to 6 hours, at the lowest dose that will achieve adequate analgesia.

Renal Impairment

US labeling: There are no dosage adjustments provided in the manufacturer's labeling. Serum concentrations are increased ~50% in patients with CrCl <60 mL/minute; adjust dose as clinically indicated.

Canadian labeling: Initial: Decrease dose to 33% to 50% of usual initial dose; titrate carefully.

Hepatic Impairment

Immediate release:

US labeling: Reduced initial doses may be necessary (use a conservative approach to initial dosing); adjust dose based on clinical situation.

◀   *Canadian labeling:* Initial: Decrease dose to 33% to 50% of usual initial dose; titrate carefully.

Extended release: Initial: Decrease dose to 33% to 50% of usual starting dose; titrate carefully.

Additional Information Complete prescribing information should be consulted for additional detail.

Product Availability

Oxaydo: FDA approved immediate-release oxycodone product formulated to discourage abuse via snorting; availability anticipated in the third quarter of 2015.

Oxaydo is indicated for the management of acute and chronic moderate to severe pain where the use of an opioid analgesic is appropriate. Oxaydo is formerly known as Oxecta (Pfizer).

Prescribing and Access Restrictions As a requirement of the REMS program, healthcare providers who prescribe OxyContin need to receive training on the proper use and potential risks of OxyContin. For training, please refer to http://www.oxycontinrems.com.

Medication Guide Available Yes

Dosage Forms Excipient information presented when available (limited, particularly for generics); consult specific product labeling. [DSC] = Discontinued product

Capsule, Oral, as hydrochloride:
 Generic: 5 mg

Concentrate, Oral, as hydrochloride:
 Generic: 20 mg/mL (30 mL); 100 mg/5 mL (15 mL, 30 mL)

Solution, Oral, as hydrochloride:
 Generic: 5 mg/5 mL (5 mL, 15 mL, 473 mL, 500 mL)

Tablet, Oral, as hydrochloride:
 Roxicodone: 5 mg [DSC]
 Roxicodone: 5 mg [scored]
 Roxicodone: 15 mg [scored; contains fd&c blue #2 (indigotine), fd&c yellow #10 (quinoline yellow)]
 Roxicodone: 30 mg [DSC]
 Roxicodone: 30 mg [scored]
 Generic: 5 mg, 10 mg, 15 mg, 20 mg, 30 mg

Tablet Abuse-Deterrent, Oral, as hydrochloride:
 Oxaydo: 5 mg, 7.5 mg
 Oxecta: 5 mg [DSC], 7.5 mg [DSC]

Tablet ER 12 Hour Abuse-Deterrent, Oral, as hydrochloride:
 OxyCONTIN: 10 mg, 15 mg, 20 mg, 30 mg, 40 mg, 60 mg
 OxyCONTIN: 80 mg [contains fd&c blue #2 aluminum lake]
 Generic: 10 mg, 20 mg, 40 mg, 80 mg

Dosage Forms: Canada Note: Refer also to Dosage Forms. Excipient information presented when available (limited, particularly for generics); consult specific product labeling.

Tablet, Oral, as hydrochloride:
 Oxy IR: 5 mg, 10 mg, 20 mg
 Supeudol: 5 mg, 10 mg, 20 mg

Tablet Controlled Release, Oral, as hydrochloride
 OxyNeo: 10 mg, 15 mg, 20 mg, 30 mg, 40 mg, 60 mg, 80 mg

Controlled Substance C-II

♦ **Oxycodone Hydrochloride** *see* OxyCODONE *on page 1277*

♦ **OxyCONTIN** *see* OxyCODONE *on page 1277*

♦ **Oxy.IR (Can)** *see* OxyCODONE *on page 1277*

Oxymorphone (oks i MOR fone)

Brand Names: US Opana; Opana ER

Index Terms Oxymorphone Hydrochloride

Pharmacologic Category Analgesic, Opioid

Use Pain management:

Parenteral: Management of moderate-to-severe acute pain; analgesia during labor; preoperative medication; anesthesia support; relief of anxiety in patients with dyspnea associated with pulmonary edema secondary to acute left ventricular failure

Oral, regular release: Management of moderate-to-severe acute pain

Oral, extended release: Management of pain severe enough to require daily, around-the-clock, long-term opioid treatment and for which alternative treatment options are inadequate

Limitations of use: Because of the risks of addiction, abuse, and misuse with opioids, even at recommended doses, and because of the greater risks of overdose and death with ER opioid formulations, reserve oxymorphone ER for use in patients for whom alternative treatment options (eg, nonopioid analgesics, immediate-release opioids) are ineffective, not tolerated, or would be otherwise inadequate to provide sufficient pain management. Not indicated as an as-needed analgesic.

Pregnancy Risk Factor C

Dosing

Adult Analgesia: Note: Dosage must be individualized.

IM, SubQ: Initial: 1 to 1.5 mg; may repeat every 4 to 6 hours as needed

Labor analgesia: IM: 0.5 to 1 mg

IV: Initial: 0.5 mg

Oral:

Immediate release: Acute pain:

Opioid-naive: Initial: 5 to 10 mg every 4 to 6 hours as needed (American Pain Society [Miaskowski, 2008]). Dosage adjustment should be based on level of analgesia, side effects, pain intensity, and patient comorbidities.

Currently on stable dose of parenteral oxymorphone: Approximately 10 times the total daily parenteral requirement. The calculated total oral daily amount should be given in 4 to 6 equally divided doses.

Currently on other opioids: Use standard conversion chart to convert total daily dose of current opioid to oxymorphone equivalent. Generally start with one-half ($^1/_2$) the calculated total daily oxymorphone dosage and administer in divided doses every 4 to 6 hours.

Extended release: Chronic pain:

Opioid-naive (use as the first opioid analgesic or in patients who are not opioid tolerant): Initial: 5 mg every 12 hours.

Note: Opioid tolerance is defined as: Patients already taking at least 60 mg of oral morphine daily, 25 mcg of transdermal fentanyl per hour, 30 mg of oral oxycodone daily, 8 mg oral hydromorphone daily, 25 mg oral oxymorphone daily, or an equivalent dose of another opioid for at least 1 week.

Conversion from stable dose of parenteral oxymorphone to extended-release oxymorphone: Approximately 10 times the total daily parenteral requirement should be given in 2 divided doses as oxymorphone extended-release tablets (eg, [IV dose x 10] divided by 2). Due to patient variability, closely monitor patient for analgesia and adverse reactions upon conversion.

Conversion of stable dose of immediate-release oxymorphone to extended-release oxymorphone: Use same total daily dose. Administer one-half (1/2) of the daily dose of immediate-release oxymorphone as the extended-release formulation every 12 hours

Conversion from other oral opioids to extended-release oxymorphone: Discontinue all other around-the-clock opioids when extended release oxymorphone is initiated. Substantial interpatient variability exists in relative potency of opioids. Therefore, it is safer to underestimate a patient's daily oral oxymorphone requirement and provide breakthrough pain relief with rescue medication (eg, immediate release opioid) than to overestimate requirements. The conversion factors, per the manufacturer, in the chart (see table) provide an estimate to convert the daily dose of current opioid to an oxymorphone equivalent. Select the prior oral opioid, sum the current total daily dose, multiply by the conversion factor on the table to calculate the approximate oral oxymorphone daily dose, then divide daily dose by 2 to administer every 12 hours as oxymorphone extended release. Round down, if necessary, to the nearest strength available. For patients on a regimen of more than one opioid, calculate the approximate oral oxymorphone dose for each opioid and sum the totals to obtain the approximate total oxymorphone daily dose. For patients on a regimen of fixed-ratio opioid/nonopioid analgesic medications, only the opioid component of these medications should be used in the conversion. **Note:** The conversion factors in this conversion table are only to be used for the conversion from current opioid therapy to oxymorphone ER. Conversion factors in this table cannot be used to convert from oxymorphone ER to another opioid (doing so may lead to fatal overdose due to overestimation of the new opioid). This is not a table of equianalgesic doses. When converting from methadone to extended release oxymorphone, close monitoring is required. Ratio between methadone and other opioid agonists varies widely according to previous dose exposure. Methadone has a long half-life and can accumulate in the plasma.

Conversion Factors to Oxymorphone ER

Prior Oral Opioid	Approximate Oral Conversion Factor
Oxymorphone	1
Hydrocodone	0.5
Oxycodone	0.5
Methadone	0.5
Morphine	0.333

Titration and maintenance: Adjust therapy incrementally by 5 to 10 mg every 12 hours at intervals of every 3 to 7 days. Breakthrough pain may require a dose increase or rescue medication with an immediate-release analgesic.

Discontinuation of therapy: Gradually titrate dose downward every 2 to 4 days to prevent withdrawal signs/symptoms. Do not abruptly discontinue.

Geriatric Refer to adult dosing. **Note:** Initiate dosing at the lower end of the dosage range.

Renal Impairment CrCl <50 mL/minute: Reduce initial dosage of oral and parenteral formulations (bioavailability increased 57% to 65%). Begin therapy at lowest dose and titrate slowly with careful monitoring.

Hepatic Impairment

Mild impairment: Initiate with lowest possible dose and titrate slowly with careful monitoring.

Moderate to severe impairment: Use is contraindicated.

Additional Information Complete prescribing information should be consulted for additional detail.

Medication Guide Available Yes

Dosage Forms Excipient information presented when available (limited, particularly for generics); consult specific product labeling. [DSC] = Discontinued product

Solution, Injection, as hydrochloride:

Opana: 1 mg/mL (1 mL)

Tablet, Oral, as hydrochloride:

Opana: 5 mg [contains fd&c blue #2 aluminum lake]

Opana: 10 mg [contains d&c red #30 aluminum lake]

Generic: 5 mg, 10 mg

Tablet ER 12 Hour Abuse-Deterrent, Oral, as hydrochloride:

Opana ER: 5 mg, 7.5 mg

Opana ER: 10 mg [contains fd&c yellow #6 (sunset yellow)]

Opana ER: 15 mg

Opana ER: 20 mg [contains brilliant blue fcf (fd&c blue #1), fd&c yellow #10 (quinoline yellow), fd&c yellow #6 (sunset yellow)]

Opana ER: 30 mg

Opana ER: 40 mg [contains fd&c yellow #10 (quinoline yellow), fd&c yellow #6 (sunset yellow)]

Tablet Extended Release 12 Hour, Oral, as hydrochloride:

Opana ER: 5 mg [DSC] [contains methylparaben, polysorbate 80]

Opana ER: 10 mg [DSC] [contains fd&c yellow #6 (sunset yellow), methylparaben, polysorbate 80]

Opana ER: 20 mg [DSC] [contains brilliant blue fcf (fd&c blue #1), fd&c yellow #10 (quinoline yellow), fd&c yellow #6 (sunset yellow), methylparaben, polysorbate 80]

Opana ER: 30 mg [DSC] [contains methylparaben, polysorbate 80]

Opana ER: 40 mg [DSC] [contains fd&c yellow #10 (quinoline yellow), fd&c yellow #6 (sunset yellow), methylparaben]

Generic: 5 mg, 7.5 mg, 10 mg, 15 mg, 20 mg, 30 mg, 40 mg

Controlled Substance C-II

◆ **Oxymorphone Hydrochloride** see Oxymorphone on page 1281

◆ **OxyNEO (Can)** see OxyCODONE on page 1277

PACLitaxel (Conventional) (pac li TAKS el con VEN sha nal)

Related Information

Chemotherapy and Obesity *on page 2220*

Chemotherapy-Induced Peripheral Neuropathy *on page 2116*

Chronic Pain Management (Cancer) *on page 2229*

Management of Chemotherapy-Induced Nausea and Vomiting in Adults *on page 2142*

Management of Drug Extravasations *on page 2159*

Mucositis and Stomatitis *on page 2186*

Prevention of Chemotherapy-Induced Nausea and Vomiting in Children *on page 2203*

Principles of Anticancer Therapy *on page 2261*

Safe Handling of Hazardous Drugs *on page 2292*

Brand Names: Canada Apo-Paclitaxel; Paclitaxel for Injection; Paclitaxel Injection USP

Index Terms Conventional Paclitaxel; Onxyl; Taxol

Pharmacologic Category Antineoplastic Agent, Antimicrotubular; Antineoplastic Agent, Taxane Derivative

Use

Breast cancer: Adjuvant treatment of node-positive breast cancer; treatment of metastatic breast cancer after failure of combination chemotherapy or relapse within 6 months of adjuvant chemotherapy (prior therapy should have included an anthracycline)

Kaposi sarcoma (AIDS-related): Second-line treatment of AIDS-related Kaposi sarcoma

Non-small cell lung cancer: First-line treatment of non-small cell lung cancer (in combination with cisplatin) in patients who are not candidates for potentially curative surgery and/or radiation therapy

Ovarian cancer: Subsequent therapy for treatment of advanced ovarian cancer; first-line therapy of ovarian cancer (in combination with cisplatin)

Labeled Contraindications Hypersensitivity to paclitaxel, polyoxyl 35/polyoxyethylated castor oil (Cremophor EL), or any component of the formulation; treatment of solid tumors in patients with baseline neutrophil counts <1,500/mm³; treatment of Kaposi sarcoma in patients with baseline neutrophil counts <1,000/mm³.

Pregnancy Considerations Adverse events (embryotoxicity, fetal toxicity, and maternal toxicity) have been observed in animal reproduction studies at doses less than the recommended human dose. An *ex vivo* human placenta perfusion model illustrated that paclitaxel crossed the placenta at term. Placental transfer was low and affected by the presence of albumin; higher albumin concentrations resulted in lower paclitaxel placental transfer (Berveiller, 2012). Some pharmacokinetic properties of paclitaxel may be altered in pregnant women (van Hasselt, 2014). Women of childbearing potential should be advised to avoid becoming pregnant. A pregnancy registry is available for all cancers diagnosed during pregnancy at Cooper Health (877-635-4499).

Breast-Feeding Considerations Paclitaxel is excreted in breast milk (case report). The mother (3 months postpartum) was treated with paclitaxel 30 mg/m² (56.1 mg) and carboplatin once weekly for papillary thyroid cancer. Milk samples were obtained 4-316 hours after the infusion given at the sixth and final week of therapy. The average paclitaxel milk concentration over the testing interval was 0.78 mg/L. Although maternal serum concentrations were not noted in the report, the relative infant dose to a nursing infant was calculated to be ~17% of the maternal dose. Paclitaxel continued to be detected in breast milk when sampled at 172 hours after the dose and was below the limit of detection when sampled at 316 hours after the infusion (Griffin, 2012). Due to the potential for serious adverse reactions in a nursing infant, breast-feeding is not recommended.

Warnings/Precautions Hazardous agent - use appropriate precautions for handling and disposal (NIOSH 2014 [group 1]). **[US Boxed Warning]: Anaphylaxis and severe hypersensitivity reactions (dyspnea requiring bronchodilators, hypotension requiring treatment, angioedema, and/or generalized urticaria) have occurred in 2% to 4% of patients in clinical studies; premedicate with corticosteroids, diphenhydramine, and H$_2$ antagonists prior to infusion. Some reactions have been fatal despite premedication. If severe hypersensitivity occurs, stop infusion and do not rechallenge.** Minor hypersensitivity reactions (flushing, skin reactions, dyspnea, hypotension, or tachycardia) do not require interruption of treatment. Infusion-related hypotension, bradycardia, and/or hypertension may occur; frequent monitoring of vital signs is recommended, especially during the first hour of the infusion. Conventional paclitaxel formulations contain polyoxyl 35/polyoxyethylated castor oil (Cremophor EL) which is associated with hypersensitivity reactions. Formulations also contain dehydrated alcohol which may cause adverse CNS effects.

[US Boxed Warning]: Bone marrow suppression (primarily neutropenia; may be severe or result in infection) may occur. Monitor blood counts frequently. Do not administer if baseline neutrophil count is <1,500/mm^3 (for solid tumors) or <1,000/mm^3 (for patients with AIDS-related Kaposi sarcoma). Bone marrow suppression (usually neutropenia) is dose-dependent and is the dose-limiting toxicity; neutrophil nadir is usually at a median of 11 days. Subsequent cycles should not be administered until neutrophils are >1,500/mm^3 (for solid tumors) and 1,000/mm^3 (for Kaposi sarcoma); platelets should recover to 100,000/mm^3. Reduce future doses by 20% for severe neutropenia (<500/mm^3 for 7 days or more) and consider the use of supportive therapy, including growth factor treatment.

Use extreme caution with hepatic dysfunction (myelotoxicity may be worsened in patients with total bilirubin >2 times ULN); dose reductions are recommended. Peripheral neuropathy may commonly occur; patients with preexisting neuropathies from prior chemotherapy or coexisting conditions (eg, diabetes mellitus) may be at a higher risk; reduce dose by 20% for severe neuropathy. Rare but severe conduction abnormalities have been reported; conduct continuous cardiac monitoring during subsequent infusions for these patients. Elderly patients have an increased risk of toxicity (neutropenia, neuropathy, and cardiovascular events); use with caution. Intraperitoneal administration of paclitaxel is associated with a higher incidence of chemotherapy-related toxicity (Armstrong, 2006).

Paclitaxel is an irritant with vesicant-like properties; ensure proper needle or catheter placement prior to and during infusion; avoid extravasation. Injection site reactions are generally mild (skin discoloration, tenderness, erythema, or swelling) and occur more commonly with an extended infusion duration (eg, 24 hours); injection site reactions may be delayed (7 to 10 days). More severe reactions (phlebitis, cellulitis, skin exfoliation, necrosis, fibrosis, and induration) have also been reported. Recall skin reactions may occur despite administering through a different IV site. **[US Boxed Warning]: Should be administered under the supervision of an experienced cancer chemotherapy**

◄ physician; **administer in a facility sufficient to appropriately diagnose and manage complications.** Potentially significant drug-drug interactions may exist, requiring dose or frequency adjustment, additional monitoring, and/or selection of alternative therapy.

Adverse Reactions Percentages reported with single-agent therapy. **Note:** Myelosuppression is dose related, schedule related, and infusion-rate dependent (increased incidences with higher doses, more frequent doses, and longer infusion times) and, in general, rapidly reversible upon discontinuation.

>10%:

Cardiovascular: Flushing (28%), ECG abnormal (14% to 23%), edema (21%), hypotension (4% to 12%)

Dermatologic: Alopecia (87%), rash (12%)

Gastrointestinal: Nausea/vomiting (52%), diarrhea (38%), mucositis (17% to 35%; grades 3/4: up to 3%), stomatitis (15%; most common at doses >390 mg/m^2), abdominal pain (with intraperitoneal paclitaxel)

Hematologic: Neutropenia (78% to 98%; grade 4: 14% to 75%; onset 8-10 days, median nadir 11 days, recovery 15-21 days), leukopenia (90%; grade 4: 17%), anemia (47% to 90%; grades 3/4: 2% to 16%), thrombocytopenia (4% to 20%; grades 3/4: 1% to 7%), bleeding (14%)

Hepatic: Alkaline phosphatase increased (22%), AST increased (19%)

Local: Injection site reaction (erythema, tenderness, skin discoloration, swelling: 13%)

Neuromuscular & skeletal: Peripheral neuropathy (42% to 70%; grades 3/4: up to 7%), arthralgia/myalgia (60%), weakness (17%)

Renal: Creatinine increased (observed in KS patients only: 18% to 34%; severe: 5% to 7%)

Miscellaneous: Hypersensitivity reaction (31% to 45%; grades 3/4: up to 2%), infection (15% to 30%)

1% to 10%:

Cardiovascular: Bradycardia (3%), tachycardia (2%), hypertension (1%), rhythm abnormalities (1%), syncope (1%), venous thrombosis (1%)

Dermatologic: Nail changes (2%)

Hematologic: Febrile neutropenia (2%)

Hepatic: Bilirubin increased (7%)

Respiratory: Dyspnea (2%)

<1%, postmarketing, and/or case reports: Anaphylaxis, arrhythmia, ataxia, atrial fibrillation, AV block, back pain, cardiac conduction abnormalities, cellulitis, CHF, chills, conjunctivitis, dehydration, enterocolitis, extravasation recall, hepatic encephalopathy, hepatic necrosis, induration, intestinal obstruction, intestinal perforation, interstitial pneumonia, ischemic colitis, lacrimation increased, maculopapular rash, malaise, MI, myocardial ischemia, necrotic changes and ulceration following extravasation, neuroencephalopathy, neutropenic enterocolitis, neutropenic typhlitis, ototoxicity (tinnitus and hearing loss), pancreatitis, paralytic ileus, phlebitis, pneumonitis, pruritus, pulmonary embolism, pulmonary fibrosis, radiation recall, radiation pneumonitis, renal insufficiency, scleroderma exacerbation, seizure, skin edema (diffuse), skin exfoliation, skin fibrosis, skin necrosis, skin sclerosis, skin thickening, Stevens-Johnson syndrome, supraventricular tachycardia, toxic epidermal necrolysis, ventricular tachycardia (asymptomatic), visual disturbances (scintillating scotomata)

Drug Interactions

Metabolism/Transport Effects Substrate of CYP2C8 (major), CYP3A4 (major), P-glycoprotein; **Note:** Assignment of Major/Minor substrate status based on clinically relevant drug interaction potential; **Induces** CYP3A4 (weak)

Avoid Concomitant Use

Avoid concomitant use of PACLitaxel (Conventional) with any of the following: Atazanavir; BCG (Intravesical); CloZAPine; Conivaptan; Dipyrone; Fusidic Acid (Systemic); Idelalisib; Natalizumab; Pimecrolimus; SORAfenib; Tacrolimus (Topical); Tofacitinib; Vaccines (Live)

Increased Effect/Toxicity

PACLitaxel (Conventional) may increase the levels/effects of: Antineoplastic Agents (Anthracycline, Systemic); Bexarotene (Systemic); CloZAPine; DOXOrubicin (Conventional); Fingolimod; Leflunomide; Natalizumab; Tofacitinib; Trastuzumab; Vaccines (Live); Vinorelbine

The levels/effects of PACLitaxel (Conventional) may be increased by: Abiraterone Acetate; Aprepitant; Atazanavir; Conivaptan; CYP2C8 Inhibitors (Moderate); CYP2C8 Inhibitors (Strong); CYP3A4 Inhibitors (Moderate); CYP3A4 Inhibitors (Strong); Dasatinib; Deferasirox; Denosumab; Dipyrone; Fosaprepitant; Fusidic Acid (Systemic); Idelalisib; Ivacaftor; Luliconazole; Mifepristone; Netupitant; Osimertinib; Palbociclib; P-glycoprotein/ABCB1 Inhibitors; Pimecrolimus; Platinum Derivatives; Ranolazine; Roflumilast; Simeprevir; SORAfenib; Stiripentol; Tacrolimus (Topical)

Decreased Effect

PACLitaxel (Conventional) may decrease the levels/effects of: ARIPiprazole; BCG (Intravesical); Coccidioides immitis Skin Test; Hydrocodone; NiMODipine; Saxagliptin; Sipuleucel-T; Vaccines (Inactivated); Vaccines (Live)

The levels/effects of PACLitaxel (Conventional) may be decreased by: Bexarotene (Systemic); Bosentan; CYP2C8 Inducers (Strong); CYP3A4 Inducers (Moderate); CYP3A4 Inducers (Strong); Dabrafenib; Deferasirox; Echinacea; Enzalutamide; Mitotane; Osimertinib; P-glycoprotein/ABCB1 Inducers; Siltuximab; St Johns Wort; Tocilizumab; Trastuzumab

Storage/Stability Store intact vials at room temperature of 20°C to 25°C (68°F to 77°F). Protect from light. Solutions diluted for infusion in D$_5$W and NS are stable for up to 27 hours at ambient temperature (~25°C).

Paclitaxel should be dispensed in either glass or non-PVC containers (eg, Excel/PAB). Use **nonpolyvinyl** (non-PVC) tubing (eg, polyethylene) to minimize leaching. Formulated in a vehicle known as polyoxyl 35/polyoxyethylated castor oil (Cremophor EL), which has been found to leach the plasticizer DEHP from polyvinyl chloride infusion bags or administration sets. Contact of the undiluted concentrate with plasticized polyvinyl chloride (PVC) equipment or devices is not recommended.

Preparation for Administration Hazardous agent; use appropriate precautions for handling and disposal (NIOSH 2014 [group 1]). Dilute for infusion in 250 to 1,000 mL D$_5$W, D$_5$LR, D$_5$NS, or NS to a concentration of 0.3 to 1.2 mg/mL, use a non-PVC container (glass or polyethylene). Chemotherapy dispensing devices (eg, Chemo Dispensing Pin) should not be used to withdraw paclitaxel from the vial; closed system transfer devices may not be compatible with undiluted paclitaxel.

PACLITAXEL (CONVENTIONAL)

◄ **Mechanism of Action** Paclitaxel promotes microtubule assembly by enhancing the action of tubulin dimers, stabilizing existing microtubules, and inhibiting their disassembly, interfering with the late G_2 mitotic phase, and inhibiting cell replication. In addition, the drug can distort mitotic spindles, resulting in the breakage of chromosomes. Paclitaxel may also suppress cell proliferation and modulate immune response.

Pharmacodynamics/Kinetics

V_{dss}: 24-hour infusion: 227 to 688 L/m^2; widely distributed into body fluids and tissues; affected by dose and duration of infusion

Protein binding: 89% to 98%

Metabolism: Hepatic via CYP2C8 and 3A4; forms metabolites (primarily 6α-hydroxypaclitaxel)

Half-life elimination:

3-hour infusion: Mean (terminal): ~13 to 20 hours

24-hour infusion: Mean (terminal): ~16 to 53 hours

Excretion: Feces (~71%; ~5% as unchanged drug); urine (~14%)

Dosing

Adult & Geriatric Note: Premedication with dexamethasone (20 mg orally at 12 and 6 hours prior to the dose [reduce dexamethasone dose to 10 mg orally with advanced HIV disease]), diphenhydramine (50 mg IV 30 to 60 minutes prior to the dose), and cimetidine, famotidine, or ranitidine (IV 30 to 60 minutes prior to the dose) is recommended.

Breast cancer, adjuvant treatment: IV: 175 mg/m^2 over 3 hours every 3 weeks for 4 cycles (administer sequentially following an anthracycline-containing regimen)

Breast cancer, metastatic or relapsed: IV: 175 mg/m^2 over 3 hours every 3 weeks

Non-small cell lung cancer: IV: 135 mg/m^2 over 24 hours every 3 weeks (in combination with cisplatin)

Ovarian cancer, advanced:

Previously treated: IV: 135 or 175 mg/m^2 over 3 hours every 3 weeks

Previously untreated: IV: 175 mg/m^2 over 3 hours every 3 weeks (in combination with cisplatin) or 135 mg/m^2 over 24 hours administered every 3 weeks (in combination with cisplatin)

Intraperitoneal (off-label route): 60 mg/m^2 on day 8 of a 21-day treatment cycle for 6 cycles, in combination with IV paclitaxel (135 mg/m^2 over 24 hours on day 1) and intraperitoneal cisplatin (Armstrong, 2006). **Note:** Administration of intraperitoneal paclitaxel should include the standard paclitaxel premedication regimen.

Previously untreated (off-label combination): IV: 175 mg/m^2 over 3 hours every 3 weeks (in combination with carboplatin) for 6 cycles, or 60 mg/m^2 over 1 hour weekly (in combination with carboplatin) for 18 weeks (Pignata, 2014)

Kaposi sarcoma, AIDS related: IV: 135 mg/m^2 over 3 hours every 3 weeks **or** 100 mg/m^2 over 3 hours every 2 weeks (due to dose-related toxicity, the 100 mg/m^2 dose should be used for patients with a lower performance status). **Note:** Reduce the dexamethasone premedication dose to 10 mg.

Bladder cancer, advanced or metastatic (off-label use): IV: 150 mg/m^2 every 2 weeks (in combination with gemcitabine) (Sternberg, 2001) **or** 200 mg/m^2 over 1 hour every 3 weeks (in combination with gemcitabine) for 6 cycles (Meluch, 2001)

Cervical cancer, advanced (off-label use): IV: 135 or 175 mg/m^2 every 3 weeks (in combination with bevacizumab and cisplatin) until disease progression or unacceptable toxicity (Tewari, 2014) **or** 175 mg/m^2 every 3 weeks (in combination with bevacizumab and topotecan) until disease progression or unacceptable toxicity (Tewari, 2014) **or** 135 mg/m^2 over 24 hours every 3 weeks (in combination with cisplatin) for 6 cycles (Monk, 2009; Moore, 2004).

Esophageal/gastric cancer, preoperative chemoradiation (off-label use): IV: 50 mg/m^2 on days 1, 8, 15, 22, and 29 (in combination with carboplatin and radiation therapy) followed by surgery within 4 to 6 weeks (van Hagen, 2012)

Head and neck cancers, advanced (off-label use): IV: 175 mg/m^2 over 3 hours every 3 weeks (in combination with cisplatin) for at least 6 cycles (Gibson, 2005)

Penile cancer, metastatic (off-label use): IV: 175 mg/m^2 over 3 hours every 3 to 4 weeks (in combination with ifosfamide and cisplatin) for 4 cycles (Pagliaro, 2010)

Small cell lung cancer, relapsed/refractory (off-label use): IV: 175 mg/m^2 over 3 hours every 3 weeks (as a single agent) for up to 5 cycles (Smit, 1998) **or** 80 mg/m^2 over 1 hour weekly for 6 weeks of an 8-week treatment cycle (as a single agent) until disease progression or unacceptable toxicity (Yamamoto, 2006)

Soft tissue sarcoma (angiosarcoma), advanced/unresectable (off-label use): IV: 80 mg/m^2 over 1 hour on days 1, 8, and 15 of a 4-week treatment cycle (as a single agent) for up to 6 cycles (Penel, 2008) **or** 135 to 175 mg/m^2 over 3 hours every 3 weeks (as a single agent) (Schlemmer, 2008) **or** 75 to 100 mg/m^2 once weekly (as a single agent) (Schlemmer, 2008)

Testicular germ cell tumors, relapsed/refractory (off-label use): IV: 80 mg/m^2 over 1 hour on days 1 and 8 of a 3-week treatment cycle (in combination with gemcitabine and oxaliplatin) for 2 cycles beyond best response and up to a maximum of 8 cycles (Bokemeyer, 2008) **or** 250 mg/m^2 over 24 hours on day 1 of a 3-week treatment cycle (in combination with ifosfamide, mesna, cisplatin, and filgrastim) for 4 cycles (Kondagunta, 2005) **or** 100 mg/m^2 over 1 hour on days 1, 8, and 15 of a 4-week treatment cycle (in combination with gemcitabine) for up to 6 cycles (Einhorn, 2007)

Thymoma/thymic carcinoma, advanced (off-label use): IV: 225 mg/m^2 over 3 hours every 3 weeks (in combination with carboplatin) for up to 6 cycles (Lemma, 2011)

Unknown primary adenocarcinoma (off-label use): IV: 200 mg/m^2 over 3 hours every 3 weeks (in combination with carboplatin) for 6 to 8 cycles (Briasoulis, 2000) **or** 200 mg/m^2 over 1 hour every 3 weeks (in combination with carboplatin and etoposide) for 4 to 8 cycles (Greco, 2000)

Renal Impairment There are no dosage adjustments provided in the manufacturer's labeling. Aronoff (2007) recommends no dosage adjustment necessary for adults with CrCl <50 mL/minute.

Hepatic Impairment Note: The manufacturer's labeling recommendations are based upon the patient's first course of therapy where the usual dose would be 135 mg/m^2 dose over 24 hours or the 175 mg/m^2 dose over 3 hours in patients with normal hepatic function. Dosage in subsequent courses should be based upon individual tolerance. Adjustments for other regimens are not available.

24-hour infusion:

Transaminases <2 times upper limit of normal (ULN) and bilirubin level ≤1.5 mg/dL: 135 mg/m²

Transaminases 2 to <10 times ULN and bilirubin level ≤1.5 mg/dL: 100 mg/m²

Transaminases <10 times ULN and bilirubin level 1.6 to 7.5 mg/dL: 50 mg/m²

Transaminases ≥10 times ULN or bilirubin level >7.5 mg/dL: Avoid use

3-hour infusion:

Transaminases <10 times ULN and bilirubin level ≤1.25 times ULN: 175 mg/m²

Transaminases <10 times ULN and bilirubin level 1.26 to 2 times ULN: 135 mg/m²

Transaminases <10 times ULN and bilirubin level 2.01 to 5 times ULN: 90 mg/m²

Transaminases ≥10 times ULN or bilirubin level >5 times ULN: Avoid use

Obesity *ASCO Guidelines for appropriate chemotherapy dosing in obese adults with cancer:* Utilize patient's actual body weight (full weight) for calculation of body surface area- or weight-based dosing, particularly when the intent of therapy is curative; manage regimen-related toxicities in the same manner as for nonobese patients; if a dose reduction is utilized due to toxicity, consider resumption of full weight-based dosing with subsequent cycles, especially if cause of toxicity (eg, hepatic or renal impairment) is resolved (Griggs, 2012).

Adjustment for Toxicity

Dosage modification for toxicity (solid tumors, including ovary, breast, and lung carcinoma): Courses of paclitaxel should not be repeated until the neutrophil count is ≥1,500/mm³ and the platelet count is ≥100,000/mm³; reduce dosage by 20% for patients experiencing severe peripheral neuropathy or severe neutropenia (neutrophil <500/mm³ for a week or longer)

Dosage modification for immunosuppression in advanced HIV disease: Paclitaxel should not be given to patients with HIV if the baseline or subsequent neutrophil count is <1000 cells/mm³. Additional modifications include: Reduce dosage of dexamethasone in premedication to 10 mg orally; reduce dosage by 20% in patients experiencing severe peripheral neuropathy or severe neutropenia (neutrophil <500/mm³ for a week or longer); initiate concurrent hematopoietic growth factor (G-CSF) as clinically indicated

Combination Regimens

Bladder cancer:

Gemcitabine-Paclitaxel (Bladder) on page 1995

PCG (Bladder) on page 2060

Breast cancer:

AC (Dose-Dense) followed by Paclitaxel (Dose-Dense) (Breast) on page 1822

AC (Dose-Dense) followed by Paclitaxel (Dose-Dense)-Trastuzumab (Breast) on page 1823

AC (Dose-Dense) followed by Paclitaxel Weekly (Breast) on page 1824

AC followed by Paclitaxel-Trastuzumab (Breast) on page 1825

AC followed by Paclitaxel Weekly (Breast) on page 1825

Bevacizumab-Paclitaxel (Breast) on page 1844

Carboplatin-Paclitaxel-Trastuzumab (Breast) on page 1872

FEC followed by Paclitaxel Weekly (Breast) on page 1967

Gemcitabine-Paclitaxel (Breast) on page 1996
Paclitaxel (Breast Regimen) on page 2049
Paclitaxel-Pertuzumab-Trastuzumab (Breast) on page 2054
Paclitaxel-Trastuzumab (Breast) on page 2056

Cervical cancer:
Bevacizumab-Cisplatin-Paclitaxel (Cervical) on page 1841
Bevacizumab-Paclitaxel-Topotecan (Cervical) on page 1845
Carboplatin-Paclitaxel (Cervical Cancer) on page 1868
Cisplatin-Paclitaxel (Cervical Cancer) on page 1909

Endometrial cancer:
Carboplatin-Paclitaxel (Endometrial) on page 1869
Cisplatin-Doxorubin-Paclitaxel (Endometrial) on page 1893

Esophageal cancer:
Paclitaxel-Carboplatin (Esophageal Cancer) on page 2050
Paclitaxel-Cisplatin (Esophageal Cancer) on page 2050
Paclitaxel-Cisplatin-Fluorouracil (Esophageal Cancer) on page 2051
Paclitaxel-Fluorouracil (Esophageal Cancer) on page 2052

Gastric cancer: Paclitaxel-Ramucirumab (Gastric) on page 2056

Head and neck cancer:
Cisplatin-Paclitaxel (Head and Neck Cancer) on page 1909
Paclitaxel-Cetuximab on page 2050

Lung cancer (non-small cell):
Bevacizumab-Carboplatin-Paclitaxel (NSCLC) on page 1839
Carboplatin-Paclitaxel (NSCLC) on page 1870
Cisplatin-Paclitaxel (NSCLC) on page 1910

Lung cancer (small cell): Paclitaxel (Small Cell Lung Cancer Regimen) on page 2056

Ovarian cancer:
Bevacizumab-Paclitaxel (Ovarian) on page 1845
Carboplatin-Paclitaxel (Ovarian) on page 1871
Cisplatin-Paclitaxel Intraperitoneal (Ovarian) on page 1910
Cisplatin-Paclitaxel (Ovarian) on page 1910
Paclitaxel (Ovarian Regimen) on page 2053

Penile cancer: Paclitaxel-Ifosfamide-Cisplatin (Penile) on page 2052
Soft tissue sarcoma (angiosarcoma): Paclitaxel (Angiosarcoma Regimen) on page 2048

Testicular cancer:
Gemcitabine-Oxaliplatin-Paclitaxel (Testicular) on page 1994
Gemcitabine-Paclitaxel (Testicular) on page 1996
TIP (Testicular) on page 2090

Thymoma/Thymic carcinoma: Carboplatin-Paclitaxel (Thymoma/Thymic) on page 1872

Unknown primary, adenocarcinoma:
Carboplatin-Etoposide-Paclitaxel (Unknown Primary, Adenocarcinoma) on page 1864
Carboplatin-Paclitaxel (Unknown Primary, Adenocarcinoma) on page 1873

Unknown primary, squamous cell: Cisplatin-Fluorouracil-Paclitaxel (Unknown Primary, Squamous Cell) on page 1903

Administration

IV: Infuse over 3 or 24 hours (depending on indication/protocol); some off-label protocols use a 1-hour infusion. Infuse through a 0.22-micron in-line filter and polyethylene-lined (non-PVC) administration set. When administered as a part of a combination chemotherapy regimen, sequence of administration

◀

may vary by regimen; refer to specific protocol for sequence recommendation.

Premedication with dexamethasone (20 mg orally or IV at 12 and 6 hours before the dose; reduce to 10 mg with advanced HIV disease), diphenhydramine (50 mg IV 30 to 60 minutes prior to the dose), and cimetidine 300 mg, famotidine 20 mg, or ranitidine 50 mg (IV 30 to 60 minutes prior to the dose) is recommended.

Irritant with vesicant-like properties; avoid extravasation. Ensure proper needle or catheter position prior to administration.

Extravasation management: If extravasation occurs, stop infusion immediately and disconnect (leave cannula/needle in place); gently aspirate extravasated solution (do **NOT** flush the line); remove needle/cannula; initiate antidote (hyaluronidase); remove needle/cannula; elevate extremity. Information conflicts regarding the use of warm or cold compresses (Perez Fidalgo, 2012; Polovich, 2009).

Hyaluronidase: If needle/cannula still in place: Administer 1 to 6 mL (150 units/mL) into existing IV line; usual dose is 1 mL for each 1 mL of extravasated drug; if needle/cannula has been removed, inject subcutaneously in a clockwise manner around area of extravasation; may repeat several times over the next 3 to 4 hours (Ener, 2004).

Intraperitoneal (off-label route): Solution was prepared in warmed saline and infused as rapidly as possible through an implantable intraperitoneal catheter (Armstrong, 2006).

Hazardous agent; use appropriate precautions for handling and disposal (NIOSH 2014 [group 1]).

Vesicant/Extravasation Risk Irritant with vesicant-like properties

Emetic Potential Children and Adults: Low (10% to 30%)

Monitoring Parameters CBC with differential and platelet count, liver and kidney function; monitor for hypersensitivity reactions, vital signs (frequently during the first hour of infusion), continuous cardiac monitoring (patients with conduction abnormalities); monitor infusion site during infusion.

Dosage Forms Considerations

Paclitaxel injection contains polyoxyl 35/olyoxyethylated castor oil (Cremophor EL)

Dosage Forms Excipient information presented when available (limited, particularly for generics); consult specific product labeling.

Concentrate, Intravenous:

Generic: 100 mg/16.7 mL (16.7 mL); 30 mg/5 mL (5 mL); 150 mg/25 mL (25 mL); 300 mg/50 mL (50 mL)

Concentrate, Intravenous [preservative free]:

Generic: 100 mg/16.7 mL (16.7 mL); 30 mg/5 mL (5 mL); 300 mg/50 mL (50 mL)

PACLitaxel (Protein Bound) (pac li TAKS el PROE teen bownd)

Related Information

Management of Drug Extravasations *on page 2159*

Prevention of Chemotherapy-Induced Nausea and Vomiting in Children *on page 2203*

Safe Handling of Hazardous Drugs *on page 2292*

Brand Names: US Abraxane

Brand Names: Canada Abraxane for Injectable Suspension

Index Terms ABI-007; Albumin-Bound Paclitaxel; Albumin-Stabilized Nano-particle Paclitaxel; nab-Paclitaxel; Nanoparticle Albumin-Bound Paclitaxel; Paclitaxel (Nanoparticle Albumin Bound); Paclitaxel, Albumin-Bound; Protein-Bound Paclitaxel

Pharmacologic Category Antineoplastic Agent, Antimicrotubular; Antineo-plastic Agent, Taxane Derivative

Use

Breast cancer, metastatic: Treatment of refractory (metastatic) or relapsed (within 6 months of adjuvant therapy) breast cancer after failure of combina-tion chemotherapy (including anthracycline-based therapy unless clinically contraindicated)

Non-small cell lung cancer (NSCLC): First-line treatment of locally advanced or metastatic NSCLC (in combination with carboplatin) in patients ineligible for curative surgery or radiation therapy

Pancreatic adenocarcinoma: First-line treatment of metastatic adenocarci-noma of the pancreas (in combination with gemcitabine)

Labeled Contraindications Baseline neutrophil count of <1500/mm^3; severe hypersensitivity reaction to paclitaxel (protein bound) or any component of the formulation

Pregnancy Considerations Adverse events were observed in animal repro-duction studies. An *ex vivo* human placenta perfusion model illustrated that paclitaxel (non-protein bound preparation) crossed the placenta at term. Placental transfer was low and affected by the presence of albumin; higher albumin concentrations resulted in lower paclitaxel placental transfer (Berveil-ler 2012). Women of childbearing potential should be advised to avoid becoming pregnant during therapy; may cause fetal harm if administered during pregnancy. Additionally, testicular atrophy/degeneration was observed in animal studies; males should be advised to not father a child during therapy. A pregnancy registry is available for all cancers diagnosed during pregnancy at Cooper Health (877-635-4499).

Breast-Feeding Considerations Paclitaxel (non-protein bound) is excreted in breast milk (case report). The mother (3 months postpartum) was treated with paclitaxel 30 mg/m^2 (56.1 mg) and carboplatin once weekly for papillary thyroid cancer. Milk samples were obtained 4-316 hours after the infusion given at the sixth and final week of therapy. The average paclitaxel milk concentration over the testing interval was 0.78 mg/L. Although maternal serum concentrations were not noted in the report, the relative infant dose to a nursing infant was calculated to be ~17% of the maternal dose. Paclitaxel continued to be detected in breast milk when sampled at 172 hours after the dose and was below the limit of detection when sampled at 316 hours after the infusion (Griffin 2012).

Due to the potential for serious adverse reactions in the nursing infant, the decision to discontinue the drug or to discontinue breast-feeding should take into consideration the benefit of treatment to the mother.

Warnings/Precautions Hazardous agent - use appropriate precautions for handling and disposal (NIOSH 2014 [group 1]).

[US Boxed Warning]: Paclitaxel (protein-bound) is not interchangeable with other forms of paclitaxel, including Cremophor-based or unbound paclitaxel.

PACLITAXEL (PROTEIN BOUND)

[US Boxed Warning]: **Bone marrow suppression, primarily neutropenia, may occur; monitor peripheral blood counts frequently. Baseline neutrophils should be ≥1500/mm³ for administration** on day 1 of each cycle; platelets should recover to >100,000/mm³ prior to day 1 of the next treatment cycle. Hematologic toxicity is dose-dependent and dose-limiting. For severe neutropenia, dose reductions may be recommended for subsequent cycles. Dose- and schedule-related cumulative sensory neuropathy is common; severe sensory neuropathy may occur. If ≥ grade 3 sensory neuropathy occurs, withhold therapy until resolution to grade 1 or 2 (breast cancer) or ≤ grade 1 (non-small cell lung cancer [NSCLC] and pancreatic cancer). Upon recovery, subsequent cycles should be dose reduced. Prior therapy with neurotoxic agents may influence the frequency and severity of neurologic toxicity. Severe hypersensitivity reactions (including anaphylaxis) have been reported; do not rechallenge after severe hypersensitivity reaction. Premedication is not generally necessary prior to paclitaxel (protein bound), but may be needed in patient's with prior mild-to-moderate hypersensitivity reactions. Use has not been studied in patients with a prior hypersensitivity reaction to conventional paclitaxel or to albumin.

Pneumonitis (including fatal cases) was observed in clinical trials when used in combination with gemcitabine. Monitor for signs/symptoms of pneumonitis; interrupt therapy during diagnostic process. If pneumonitis is confirmed, permanently discontinue. Sepsis was observed in both neutropenic and non-neutropenic patients treated with paclitaxel (protein bound) in combination with gemcitabine for pancreatic cancer; biliary obstruction and/or the presence of a biliary stent may be risk factors for severe and/or fatal sepsis. Treat promptly with broad spectrum antibiotics if fever occurs (regardless of neutrophil count). May require therapy interruption and/or dosage reduction.

Exposure may be increased in patients with hepatic impairment; monitor closely; the risk of toxicities (particularly myelosuppression) is increased. Reduced initial dosages are recommended for breast cancer and NSCLC patients with moderate and severe hepatic impairment; use is not recommended in pancreatic patients with moderate or severe impairment (bilirubin >1.5 times ULN and AST ≤10 times ULN). Use is not recommended in patients with AST >10 times ULN or total bilirubin >5 times ULN. Product contains albumin, which confers a remote risk of viral disease transmission and a theoretical risk of transmission of Creutzfeldt-Jakob disease. Certain adverse events (myelosuppression, peripheral neuropathy, arthralgia, diarrhea, decreased appetite, dehydration, fatigue, and epistaxis) occurred more frequently in older adults ≥65 years compared to younger adults.

Adverse Reactions Frequency may vary based on indication and/or concomitant therapy.

>10%:
Cardiovascular: ECG abnormality (60%; 35% in patients with a normal baseline), peripheral edema (10% to 46%)
Central nervous system: Peripheral sensory neuropathy (71%; grades 3/4: 10%; dose dependent; cumulative), fatigue (25% to 59%), peripheral neuropathy (48% to 54%; grade 3: 3% to 17%), headache (14%), depression (12%)
Dermatologic: Alopecia (50% to 90%), skin rash (10% to 30%)
Endocrine & metabolic: Dehydration (21%), increased gamma-glutamyl transferase (grades 3/4: 14%), hypokalemia (12%)

Gastrointestinal: Nausea (27% to 54%; grades 3/4: 3% to 6%), diarrhea (15% to 44%; grades 3/4: ≤6%), decreased appetite (17% to 36%), vomiting (12% to 36%; grades 3/4: 4% to 6%), constipation (16%), dysgeusia (16%)

Genitourinary: Urinary tract infection (11%)

Hematologic & oncologic: Anemia (33% to 98%; grades 3/4: 1% to 28%), neutropenia (73% to 85%; grades 3/4: 34% to 47%), thrombocytopenia (2% to 74%; grades 3/4: <1% to 18%), bone marrow depression (dose-related)

Hepatic: Increased serum AST (39%), increased serum alkaline phosphatase (36%)

Infection: Infection (24%; primarily included oral candidiasis, respiratory tract infection, and pneumonia)

Neuromuscular & skeletal: Weakness (16% to 47%; severe: 8%), musculoskeletal pain (10% to 44%; myalgia/arthralgia), limb pain (11%)

Ophthalmic: Visual disturbance (13%; severe [keratitis, blurred vision]: 1%)

Renal: Increased serum creatinine (11%; severe 1%)

Respiratory: Cough (7% to 17%), epistaxis (7% to 15%), dyspnea (12%)

Miscellaneous: Fever (41%)

1% to 10%:

Cardiovascular: Edema (10%), cardiac failure (<10%), hypotension (5%), significant cardiovascular event (grades 3/4: 3%; included chest pain, cardiac arrest, supraventricular tachycardia, thrombosis, pulmonary thromboembolism, pulmonary emboli, and hypertension)

Gastrointestinal: Mucositis (7% to 10%; grades 3/4: ≤1%)

Hematologic & oncologic: Hemorrhage (2%), febrile neutropenia (2%)

Hepatic: Increased serum bilirubin (7%)

Hypersensitivity: Hypersensitivity reaction (4%, includes anaphylactic reactions, chest pain, dyspnea, flushing, hypotension; severe: <1%)

Infection: Sepsis (5%)

Ophthalmic: Cystoid macular edema (<10%)

Respiratory: Pneumonitis (4%)

<1%, postmarketing, and/or case reports: Atrioventricular block, autonomic neuropathy, bradycardia, cardiac arrhythmia, cerebrovascular accident, cranial nerve palsy, decreased visual acuity, embolism, erythema, hepatic encephalopathy, hepatic necrosis, injection site reaction (mild), intestinal obstruction, intestinal perforation, ischemic colitis, ischemic heart disease, left ventricular dysfunction, maculopapular rash, myocardial infarction, nail discoloration, neutropenic sepsis, optic nerve damage (rare), palmar-plantar erythrodysesthesia (in patients previously exposed to capecitabine), pancreatitis, pancytopenia, paralytic ileus, peripheral motor neuropathy, pneumonia, pneumothorax, pruritus, pulmonary embolism, radiation pneumonitis (with concurrent radiation therapy), radiation recall phenomenon, skin photosensitivity, Stevens-Johnson syndrome, thrombosis, toxic epidermal necrolysis, transient ischemic attacks, ventricular dysfunction, vocal cord paralysis

Drug Interactions

Metabolism/Transport Effects Substrate of CYP2C8 (major), CYP3A4 (major), P-glycoprotein; **Note:** Assignment of Major/Minor substrate status based on clinically relevant drug interaction potential; **Induces** CYP3A4 (weak)

Avoid Concomitant Use

Avoid concomitant use of PACLitaxel (Protein Bound) with any of the following: BCG (Intravesical); CloZAPine; Conivaptan; Dipyrone; Fusidic Acid (Systemic); Idelalisib; Natalizumab; Pimecrolimus; Tacrolimus (Topical); Tofacitinib; Vaccines (Live)

◀ **Increased Effect/Toxicity**

PACLitaxel (Protein Bound) may increase the levels/effects of: Antineoplastic Agents (Anthracycline, Systemic); CloZAPine; DOXOrubicin (Conventional); Fingolimod; Leflunomide; Natalizumab; Tofacitinib; Vaccines (Live); Vinorelbine

The levels/effects of PACLitaxel (Protein Bound) may be increased by: Abiraterone Acetate; Aprepitant; Conivaptan; CYP2C8 Inhibitors (Moderate); CYP2C8 Inhibitors (Strong); CYP3A4 Inhibitors (Moderate); CYP3A4 Inhibitors (Strong); Dasatinib; Deferasirox; Denosumab; Dipyrone; Fosaprepitant; Fusidic Acid (Systemic); Idelalisib; Ivacaftor; Luliconazole; Mifepristone; Netupitant; Osimertinib; Palbociclib; P-glycoprotein/ABCB1 Inhibitors; Pimecrolimus; Platinum Derivatives; Ranolazine; Roflumilast; Simeprevir; Stiripentol; Tacrolimus (Topical); Trastuzumab

Decreased Effect

PACLitaxel (Protein Bound) may decrease the levels/effects of: ARIPiprazole; BCG (Intravesical); Coccidioides immitis Skin Test; Hydrocodone; NiMODipine; Saxagliptin; Sipuleucel-T; Vaccines (Inactivated); Vaccines (Live)

The levels/effects of PACLitaxel (Protein Bound) may be decreased by: Bosentan; CYP2C8 Inducers (Strong); CYP3A4 Inducers (Moderate); CYP3A4 Inducers (Strong); Dabrafenib; Deferasirox; Echinacea; Enzalutamide; Mitotane; Osimertinib; P-glycoprotein/ABCB1 Inducers; Siltuximab; St Johns Wort; Tocilizumab

Food Interactions Paclitaxel (protein bound) serum concentrations may be increased when taken with grapefruit or grapefruit juice. Management: Avoid concurrent use.

Storage/Stability Store intact vials at 20°C to 25°C (68°F to 77°F) and protect from bright light. Freezing or refrigerating do not adversely affect the stability of intact vials. Reconstituted solution in the vial as well as solution in infusion container for administration may be stored under refrigeration at 2°C to 8°C (36°F to 46°F) for up to 24 hours, although the manufacturer recommends immediate use. Protect solution from light. The total combined refrigerated storage time of both reconstituted solution in the vial and administration bag is 24 hours; solution may then be stored at room temperature (~25°C [77°F]) and ambient light for up to 4 hours.

Preparation for Administration Hazardous agent; use appropriate precautions for handling and disposal (NIOSH 2014 [group 1]). Reconstitute vial with 20 mL NS to a concentration of 5 mg/mL. Add NS slowly (over a minimum of 1 minute), directing it along inside vial wall; allow vial to sit for 5 minutes, then gently swirl for 2 minutes; avoid foaming. If foaming or clumping occurs, allow solution to stand for at least 15 minutes until foaming subsides. Reconstituted solution will appear milky and homogenous without visible particulates; if particulates or settling are visible, gently invert vial to re-suspend. Discard reconstituted suspension if precipitates are observed. Draw calculated dose slowly into syringe, then place without further dilution into an empty sterile container. **Note:** Use of DEHP-free containers or administration sets is not necessary. Do not use syringes or IV bags containing silicone oil as a lubricant; may result in formation of proteinaceous strands.

Mechanism of Action Albumin-bound paclitaxel nanoparticle formulation; paclitaxel promotes microtubule assembly by enhancing the action of tubulin dimers, stabilizing existing microtubules, and inhibiting their disassembly, interfering with the late G_2 mitotic phase, and inhibiting cell replication. May also distort mitotic spindles, resulting in the breakage of chromosomes.

Paclitaxel may also suppress cell proliferation and modulate immune response.

Pharmacodynamics/Kinetics

Distribution: V_d: 1741 L (extensive extravascular distribution and/or tissue binding)

Protein binding: 94%

Metabolism: Hepatic primarily via CYP2C8 to 6-alpha-hydroxypaclitaxel; also to minor metabolites via CYP3A4

Half-life elimination: Terminal: 13 to 27 hours

Excretion: Feces (~20%); urine (4% as unchanged drug, <1% as metabolites)

Dosing

Adult & Geriatric Note: When administered as part of a combination chemotherapy regimen, sequence of administration may vary by regimen; refer to specific protocol for sequence of administration. Premedication is not generally necessary prior to paclitaxel (protein bound), but may be needed in patients with prior mild-to-moderate hypersensitivity reactions.

Breast cancer, metastatic: IV: 260 mg/m² every 3 weeks (Gradishar 2005)
Off-label dosing: IV: 100 to 150 mg/m² on days 1, 8, and 15 of a 28-day cycle (Gradishar 2009)

Non-small cell lung cancer (NSCLC), locally advanced or metastatic: IV: 100 mg/m² on days 1, 8, and 15 of each 21-day cycle (in combination with carboplatin) (Socinski 2012)

Pancreatic adenocarcinoma, metastatic: IV: 125 mg/m² on days 1, 8, and 15 of a 28-day cycle (in combination with gemcitabine) (Von Hoff 2013)

Melanoma, metastatic (off-label use): IV:
Previously treated patients: 100 mg/m² on days 1, 8, and 15 of a 28-day cycle; if tolerated, may increase dose by 25 mg/m² in cycle 2 and beyond (Hersh 2010)
Previously untreated patients: 150 mg/m² on days 1, 8, and 15 of a 28-day cycle (Hersh 2010)

Ovarian, fallopian tube, or primary peritoneal cancer, recurrent (off-label use): IV: 260 mg/m² on day 1 of a 21-day cycle for 6 to 8 cycles (Teneriello 2009) **or** 100 mg/m² on days 1, 8, and 15 of a 28-day cycle until disease progression or unacceptable toxicity (Coleman 2011)

Renal Impairment There are no dosage adjustments provided in the manufacturer's labeling (has not been studied).

Hepatic Impairment

Dosage adjustment for hepatic impairment at treatment initiation:
Breast cancer (every 3 week regimen):
Mild impairment (AST ≤10 times ULN and bilirubin >1 to ≤1.5 times ULN): No dosage adjustment is necessary.
Moderate impairment (AST ≤10 times ULN and bilirubin >1.5 to ≤3 times ULN): Reduce dose to 200 mg/m²; may increase up to 260 mg/m² if the reduced dose is tolerated for 2 cycles
Severe impairment:
AST ≤10 times ULN and bilirubin >3 to ≤5 times ULN: Reduce dose to 200 mg/m²; may increase up to 260 mg/m² in subsequent cycles if the reduced dose is tolerated for 2 cycles
AST >10 times ULN or bilirubin >5 times ULN: Use is not recommended (has not been studied).

Non-small cell lung cancer (NSCLC) regimen:
Mild impairment (AST ≤10 times ULN and bilirubin >1 to ≤1.5 times ULN): No dosage adjustment is necessary.

Moderate impairment (AST ≤10 times ULN and bilirubin >1.5 to ≤3 times ULN): Reduce dose to 80 mg/m²; may increase up to 100 mg/m² in subsequent cycles if the reduced dose is tolerated for 2 cycles

Severe impairment:

AST ≤10 times ULN and bilirubin >3 to ≤5 times ULN: Reduce dose to 80 mg/m²; may increase up to 100 mg/m² in subsequent cycles if the reduced dose is tolerated for 2 cycles

AST >10 times ULN or bilirubin >5 times ULN: Use is not recommended (has not been studied).

Pancreatic adenocarcinoma:

Mild impairment (AST ≤10 times ULN and bilirubin >1 to ≤1.5 times ULN): No dosage adjustment is necessary.

Moderate impairment (AST ≤10 times ULN and bilirubin >1.5 to ≤3 times ULN): Use is not recommended.

Severe impairment:

AST ≤10 times ULN and bilirubin >3 to ≤5 times ULN: Use is not recommended.

AST >10 times ULN or bilirubin >5 times ULN: Use is not recommended.

Dosage adjustment for hepatic impairment during treatment: AST >10 times ULN or bilirubin >5 times ULN: Withhold treatment

Obesity *ASCO Guidelines for appropriate chemotherapy dosing in obese adults with cancer:* Utilize patient's actual body weight (full weight) for calculation of body surface area- or weight-based dosing, particularly when the intent of therapy is curative; manage regimen-related toxicities in the same manner as for nonobese patients; if a dose reduction is utilized due to toxicity, consider resumption of full weight-based dosing with subsequent cycles, especially if cause of toxicity (eg, hepatic or renal impairment) is resolved (Griggs 2012).

Adjustment for Toxicity

Breast cancer (every 3 week regimen):

Severe neutropenia (<500 cells/mm³) ≥1 week: Reduce dose to 220 mg/m² for subsequent courses

Recurrent severe neutropenia: Reduce dose to 180 mg/m² for subsequent courses

Sensory neuropathy

Grade 1 or 2: Dosage adjustment generally not required

Grade 3: Hold treatment until resolved to grade 1 or 2, then resume with reduced dose for all subsequent cycles

Severe sensory neuropathy: Reduce dose to 220 mg/m² for subsequent courses

Recurrent severe sensory neuropathy: Reduce dose to 180 mg/m² for subsequent courses

Non-small cell lung cancer (NSCLC):

Neutropenia: ANC <1500 cells/mm³: Withhold therapy until ANC is ≥1500 cells/mm³ on day 1 or ≥500 cells/mm³ on days 8 or 15. Reduce dose upon therapy reinitiation if:

Neutropenic fever (ANC <500 cells/mm³ with fever >38°C) **or** delay of next cycle by >7 days due to ANC <1500 cells/mm³ **or** ANC <500 cells/mm³ for >7 days:

First occurrence: Permanently reduce dose to 75 mg/m²

Second occurrence: Permanently reduce dose to 50 mg/m²

Third occurrence: Discontinue therapy.

Thrombocytopenia: Platelet count <100,000 cells/mm^3: Withhold therapy until platelet count is ≥100,000 cells/mm^3 on day 1 or ≥50,000 cells/mm^3 on days 8 or 15. Reduce dose upon therapy reinitiation if:

Platelet count <50,000 cells/mm^3:

First occurrence: Permanently reduce dose to 75 mg/m^2

Second occurrence: Discontinue therapy.

Sensory neuropathy: Withhold therapy for grade 3 or 4 peripheral neuropathy. Resume therapy at reduced doses when neuropathy resolves completely or improves to grade 1:

First occurrence: Permanently reduce dose to 75 mg/m^2

Second occurrence: Permanently reduce dose to 50 mg/m^2

Third occurrence: Discontinue therapy.

Pancreatic adenocarcinoma:

Note: Dose level reductions for toxicity:

Full dose: 125 mg/m^2

First dose reduction: 100 mg/m^2

Second dose reduction: 75 mg/m^2

If additional dose reduction is necessary: Discontinue.

Hematologic toxicity (neutropenia and/or thrombocytopenia):

Day 1: If ANC is <1500 cells/mm^3 or platelet count is <100,000 cells/mm^3: Withhold therapy until ANC is ≥1500 cells/mm^3 and platelet count is ≥100,000 cells/mm^3

Day 8:

If ANC is 500 to <1000 cells/mm^3 **or** platelet count is 50,000 to <75,000 cells/mm^3: Reduce 1 dose level

If ANC is <500 cells/mm^3 **or** platelet count is <50,000 cells/mm^3: Withhold day 8 dose

Day 15 (if day 8 doses were reduced or given without modification):

If ANC is 500 to <1000 cells/mm^3 **or** platelet count is 50,000 to <75,000 cells/mm^3: Reduce 1 dose level from day 8

If ANC is <500 cells/mm^3 **or** platelet count is <50,000 cells/mm^3: Withhold day 15 dose

Day 15 (if day 8 doses were withheld):

If ANC is ≥1000 cells/mm^3 **or** platelet count is ≥75,000 cells/mm^3: Reduce 1 dose level from day 1

If ANC is 500 to <1000 cells/mm^3 **or** platelet count is 50,000 to <75,000 cells/mm^3: Reduce 2 dose levels from day 1

If ANC is <500 cells/mm^3 **or** platelet count is <50,000 cells/mm^3: Withhold day 15 dose

Neutropenic fever: Withhold therapy for grade 3 or 4 fever. Resume therapy at next lower dose level when fever resolves and ANC is ≥1500 cells/mm^3.

Peripheral neuropathy: Withhold therapy for grade 3 or 4 peripheral neuropathy. Resume therapy at next lower dose level when neuropathy improves to ≤ grade 1.

Dermatologic toxicity: For grade 2 or 3 toxicity, reduce dose to next lower dose level; if toxicity persists, discontinue.

Gastrointestinal toxicity: Withhold therapy for grade 3 mucositis or diarrhea. Resume therapy at next lower dose level when improves to ≤ grade 1.

Combination Regimens

Breast cancer: Paclitaxel (Protein Bound) (Breast Regimen) on page 2054

Lung cancer (non-small cell):

Carboplatin-Paclitaxel (Protein Bound) (NSCLC) on page 1872

Paclitaxel (Protein Bound) (NSCLC Regimen) on page 2055

Ovarian cancer: Paclitaxel (Protein Bound) (Ovarian Regimen) on page 2055
Pancreatic cancer: Gemcitabine-Paclitaxel (Protein Bound) (Pancreatic) on page 1996

Administration IV: Administer over 30 minutes (breast cancer and NSCLC) or over 30 to 40 minutes (pancreatic cancer); limiting the infusion rate to 30 minutes reduces the risk for infusion-related reaction. Monitor infusion site; avoid extravasation. When given on a weekly (off-label) schedule, infusions were administered over ~30 minutes (Gradishar 2009; Hersh 2010; Rizvi 2008). When administered as part of a combination chemotherapy regimen, sequence of administration may vary by regimen; refer to specific protocol for sequence of administration. According to the manufacturer, paclitaxel (protein bound should be given first, followed immediately by carboplatin (NSCLC) or gemcitabine (pancreatic cancer).

Hazardous agent; use appropriate precautions for handling and disposal (NIOSH 2014 [group 1]).

Vesicant/Extravasation Risk May be an irritant

Emetic Potential Children and Adults: Low (10% to 30%)

Monitoring Parameters CBC with differential (prior to day 1 of cycle for metastatic breast cancer and prior to days 1, 8, and 15 for NSCLC); hepatic function; monitor infusion site; monitor for neuropathy and signs/symptoms of pneumonitis and sepsis

Dosage Forms Excipient information presented when available (limited, particularly for generics); consult specific product labeling.
Suspension Reconstituted, Intravenous:
   Abraxane: 100 mg (1 ea)

◆ **Paclitaxel, Albumin-Bound** *see* PACLitaxel (Protein Bound) *on page 1292*

◆ **Paclitaxel for Injection (Can)** *see* PACLitaxel (Conventional) *on page 1284*

◆ **Paclitaxel Injection USP (Can)** *see* PACLitaxel (Conventional) *on page 1284*

◆ **Paclitaxel (Nanoparticle Albumin Bound)** *see* PACLitaxel (Protein Bound) *on page 1292*

Palbociclib (pal boe SYE klib)

Related Information
Common Toxicity Criteria *on page 2122*
Principles of Anticancer Therapy *on page 2261*
Safe Handling of Hazardous Drugs *on page 2292*

Brand Names: US Ibrance

Index Terms Palbociclib Isethionate; PD 0332991; PD-0332991; PD-332991

Pharmacologic Category Antineoplastic Agent, Cyclin-Dependent Kinase Inhibitor

Use Breast cancer, advanced (initial endocrine-based therapy): Treatment of estrogen receptor (ER)-positive, human epidermal growth factor receptor 2 (HER2)-negative advanced breast cancer (in combination with letrozole) in postmenopausal women as initial endocrine-based therapy for metastatic disease

Labeled Contraindications There are no contraindications listed in the manufacturer's labeling.

Pregnancy Considerations Adverse events were observed in animal reproduction studies. Women of reproductive potential should use effective contraception during treatment and for at least 2 weeks after the last dose. Although not indicated for use in men, animal data suggests that palbociclib may affect male fertility.

Breast-Feeding Considerations It is not known if palbociclib is excreted into breast milk. Due to the potential for serious adverse reactions in the nursing infant, breast-feeding is not recommended by the manufacturer.

Warnings/Precautions Hazardous agent: Use appropriate precautions for handling and disposal (meets NIOSH 2014 criteria).

Neutropenia was commonly observed in clinical studies, including grades 3 and 4 neutropenia. The median time to the first neutropenia episode (any grade) was 15 days (range: 13 to 117 days); the median duration of grade 3 or higher neutropenia was 7 days. Leukopenia, anemia, lymphocytopenia, thrombocytopenia, and neutropenic fever have also been reported. Monitor blood counts; treatment interruption, delay, or dose reduction is recommended for grade 3 or 4 neutropenia.

Infections (including grades 3 and 4) were reported more frequently in patients receiving palbociclib and letrozole compared with those receiving only letrozole. Monitor for signs/symptoms of infection and manage appropriately. Pulmonary embolism was observed more frequently in patients receiving palbociclib and letrozole, compared to those receiving letrozole alone. Monitor for signs/symptoms of pulmonary embolism and manage appropriately. Nausea, vomiting, diarrhea, and stomatitis (generally grade 1 or 2) were reported from clinical studies. Potentially significant drug-drug interactions may exist, requiring dose or frequency adjustment, additional monitoring, and/or selection of alternative therapy.

Adverse Reactions Frequency not always defined.

>10%:
Central nervous system: Fatigue (41%; grade 3/4: 2%), peripheral neuropathy (13%)

Dermatologic: Alopecia (22%)

Gastrointestinal: Nausea (25%; grade 3: 2%), stomatitis (25%), diarrhea (21%; grade 3: 4%), decreased appetite (16%; grade 3: 1%), vomiting (15%)

Hematologic & oncologic: Abnormal absolute lymphocyte count (81%; grade 3: 17%; grade 4: 1%; decreased lymphocytes), neutropenia (75%; grade 3: 48%; grade 4: 6%), leukopenia (43%; grade 3: 19%), anemia (35%; grade 3: 5%; grade 4: 1%), thrombocytopenia (17%; grade 3: 2%)

Infection: Infection (55%; grade 3/4: 5%)

Neuromuscular & skeletal: Weakness (13%; grade 3: 2%)

Respiratory: Epistaxis (11%)

1% to 10%:
Cardiovascular: Pulmonary embolism (4% to 5%)

Respiratory: Upper respiratory tract infection (31%; grade 3: 1%)

Drug Interactions

Metabolism/Transport Effects Substrate of CYP3A4 (major); **Note:** Assignment of Major/Minor substrate status based on clinically relevant drug interaction potential; **Inhibits** CYP3A4 (weak)

Avoid Concomitant Use

Avoid concomitant use of Palbociclib with any of the following: BCG (Intravesical); CloZAPine; Conivaptan; CYP3A4 Inducers (Moderate); CYP3A4 Inducers (Strong); CYP3A4 Inhibitors (Strong); Dipyrone; Fusidic Acid

◀ (Systemic); Grapefruit Juice; Idelalisib; Natalizumab; Pimecrolimus; Pimozide; Tacrolimus (Topical); Tofacitinib; Vaccines (Live)

Increased Effect/Toxicity

Palbociclib may increase the levels/effects of: ARIPiprazole; CloZAPine; CYP3A4 Substrates; Dofetilide; Fingolimod; Flibanserin; Hydrocodone; Leflunomide; Lomitapide; Natalizumab; NiMODipine; Pimozide; Tofacitinib; Vaccines (Live)

The levels/effects of Palbociclib may be increased by: Aprepitant; Conivaptan; CYP3A4 Inhibitors (Moderate); CYP3A4 Inhibitors (Strong); Dasatinib; Denosumab; Dipyrone; Fosaprepitant; Fusidic Acid (Systemic); Grapefruit Juice; Idelalisib; Ivacaftor; Luliconazole; Mifepristone; Netupitant; Osimertinib; Pimecrolimus; Roflumilast; Simeprevir; Stiripentol; Tacrolimus (Topical); Trastuzumab

Decreased Effect

Palbociclib may decrease the levels/effects of: BCG (Intravesical); Coccidioides immitis Skin Test; Sipuleucel-T; Vaccines (Inactivated); Vaccines (Live)

The levels/effects of Palbociclib may be decreased by: CYP3A4 Inducers (Moderate); CYP3A4 Inducers (Strong); Deferasirox; Echinacea; Osimertinib; Siltuximab; Tocilizumab

Food Interactions Coadministration with grapefruit may increase palbociclib plasma concentrations. Management: Avoid concomitant administration with grapefruit.

Storage/Stability Store at 20°C to 25°C (68°F to 77°F); excursions are permitted between 15°C and 30°C (59°F and 86°F).

Mechanism of Action Palbociclib is a reversible small molecule cyclin-dependent kinase (CDK) inhibitor which is selective for CDK 4 and 6. CDKs have a role in regulating progression through the cell cycle at the G1/S phase by blocking retinoblastoma (Rb) hyperphosphorylation (Finn, 2015). Palbociclib reduces proliferation of breast cancer cell lines by preventing progression from the G1 to the S cell cycle phase. The combination of palbociclib and letrozole provides for increased inhibition of Rb phosphorylation, downstream signaling, and tumor growth compared with each agent alone.

Pharmacodynamics/Kinetics

Absorption: Increased with high-fat, high-calorie food

Distribution: V_d (mean): 2,583 L

Protein binding: ~85%

Metabolism: Extensively hepatic; Major pathways: Oxidation and sulfonation, primarily by CYP3A and sulfotransferase (SULT) enzyme SULT2A1; Minor pathways: Acylation and glucuronidation

Bioavailability: Mean absolute bioavailability: 46%

Half-life elimination: 29 ± 5 hours

Time to peak: 6 to 12 hours

Excretion: Feces (~74%, primarily as metabolites); Urine (~18%; primarily as metabolites)

Dosing

Adult & Geriatric

Breast cancer, advanced, initial endocrine-based therapy: Females (HER-2 negative): Oral: 125 mg once daily for 21 days, followed by a 7-day rest period to complete a 28-day treatment cycle (in combination with continuous letrozole); continue until disease progression or unacceptable toxicity (Finn 2015).

Breast cancer, advanced, second-line endocrine-based therapy (off-label use): Females (HER-2 negative): Oral: 125 mg once daily for 21 days, followed by 7 days off, repeat every 28 days (in combination with fulvestrant [and goserelin if pre- or peri-menopausal]); continue until disease progression or unacceptable toxicity (Turner 2015).

Missed/vomited doses: If a dose is vomited or missed, an additional dose should not be taken that day. Resume dosing with the next scheduled daily dose.

Dosage adjustment for concomitant therapy:

Strong CYP3A4 inhibitors: Avoid concomitant use with strong CYP3A4 inhibitors (eg, azole antifungals, clarithromycin, nefazodone, protease inhibitors, telithromycin, verapamil, grapefruit or grapefruit juice) and consider alternatives with no or minimal CYP3A4 inhibition. If coadministration with a strong CYP3A4 inhibitor cannot be avoided, reduce palbociclib dose to 75 mg once daily. If the strong inhibitor is discontinued, increase palbociclib dose (after 3 to 5 inhibitor half-lives have elapsed) to the dose used prior to initiating the strong CYP3A4 inhibitor.

CYP3A4 inducers: Avoid concomitant use with moderate or strong CYP3A4 inducers.

Renal Impairment

Mild to moderate impairment (CrCl 30 to <90 mL/minute): There are no dosage adjustments provided in the manufacturer's labeling, although palbociclib exposure is not increased.

Severe impairment (CrCl <30 mL/minute): There are no dosage adjustments provided in the manufacturer's labeling (has not been studied).

Hepatic Impairment

Mild impairment (total bilirubin ≤ULN and AST >ULN or total bilirubin >1 to 1.5 times ULN and any AST): There are no dosage adjustments provided in the manufacturer's labeling, although palbociclib exposure is not increased.

Moderate to severe impairment (total bilirubin >1.5 times ULN and any AST): There are no dosage adjustments provided in the manufacturer's labeling (has not been studied).

Adjustment for Toxicity May require treatment interruption/delay, dose reduction, or discontinuation for some adverse reactions. The recommended dose reduction (based on individual safety and tolerance) is to 100 mg daily; if further reduction is required, reduce dose to 75 mg daily. If dose reduction below 75 mg daily is required, discontinue treatment.

Hematologic toxicity (according to Common Toxicity Criteria for Adverse Events Version 4):

Grade 1 or 2: No dosage adjustment required.

Grade 3 (except lymphopenia unless associated with clinical events [eg, opportunistic infection]): No dosage adjustment required. Consider repeating CBC with differential one week later. Withhold initiation of the next cycle until ≤ grade 2.

Grade 3 (ANC 500/mm³ to <1,000/mm³) plus fever ≥38.5°C and/or infection: Withhold palbociclib treatment (and initiation of the next cycle) until resolved to ≤ grade 2. Resume at next lower dose upon restarting.

Grade 4 (except lymphopenia unless associated with clinical events [eg, opportunistic infection]): Withhold palbociclib treatment (and initiation of the next cycle) until resolved to ≤ grade 2. After resolution, resume at next lower dose.

◀ *Nonhematologic toxicity (according to Common Toxicity Criteria for Adverse Events Version 4):*
  Grade 1 or 2: No dosage adjustment required.
  Grade 3 or higher (if persistent despite medical management): Withhold palbociclib until symptoms resolve to ≤ grade 1 or ≤ grade 2 (if toxicity is not a safety risk); after resolution, resume at the next lower dose.

Combination Regimens
  Breast cancer:
    Palbociclib-Fulvestrant (Breast) on page 2057
    Palbociclib-Letrozole (Breast) on page 2058

Administration Oral: Administer with food. Take at approximately the same time each day. Swallow whole, do not crush, chew, or open capsules prior to swallowing (do not ingest if capsules are broken, cracked, or not fully intact). Hazardous agent; use appropriate precautions for handling and disposal (meets NIOSH 2014 criteria).

Emetic Potential Low (10% to 30%)

Monitoring Parameters CBC with differential (prior to treatment initiation, every 2 weeks for first 2 cycles, then prior to each cycle, or as clinically indicated); monitor for signs/symptoms of infection and pulmonary embolism.

Dietary Considerations Avoid grapefruit.

Prescribing and Access Restrictions Palbociclib is available through specialty pharmacies. For more information, refer to http://www.ibrance.com/getting-ibrance

Dosage Forms Excipient information presented when available (limited, particularly for generics); consult specific product labeling.
  Capsule, Oral:
    Ibrance: 75 mg, 100 mg, 125 mg

◆ **Palbociclib Isethionate** *see* Palbociclib *on page 1300*

Palifermin (pal ee FER min)

Related Information
  Mucositis and Stomatitis *on page 2186*
  Safe Handling of Hazardous Drugs *on page 2292*

Brand Names: US Kepivance

Brand Names: Canada Kepivance®

Index Terms AMJ 9701; Keratinocyte Growth Factor, Recombinant Human; rhKGF; rhu Keratinocyte Growth Factor; rHu-KGF

Pharmacologic Category Chemoprotective Agent; Keratinocyte Growth Factor

Use Decrease the incidence and duration of severe oral mucositis associated with hematologic malignancies in patients receiving myelotoxic therapy requiring hematopoietic stem cell support (when the preparative regimen is expected to result in mucositis ≥ grade 3 in most patients)

Note: Use (safety and efficacy) is not established for nonhematologic malignancies; use is not recommended with conditioning regimens containing melphalan 200 mg/m^2

Labeled Contraindications There are no contraindications listed within the manufacturer's U.S. product labeling.

Canadian labeling: Hypersensitivity to palifermin, *E. coli*-derived proteins, or any component of the formulation

Pregnancy Considerations Palifermin has been shown to be embryotoxic in animal reproduction studies at doses also associated with maternal toxicity. Use in pregnancy only if the potential benefit outweighs the potential risk for the fetus.

Breast-Feeding Considerations According to the manufacturer labeling, the decision to discontinue palifermin or discontinue breast-feeding during treatment should take into account the benefits of treatment to the mother.

Warnings/Precautions Hazardous agent - use appropriate precautions for handling and disposal (NIOSH 2014 [group 2]).

Edema, erythema, pruritus, rash, oral/perioral dysesthesia, taste alteration, tongue discoloration, and tongue thickening may occur (median onset of cutaneous toxicities following initial dose is 6 days; median duration is 5 days); instruct patients to report mucocutaneous effects. Safety and efficacy have not been established with nonhematologic malignancies; effect on the growth of keratinocyte growth factor (KGF) receptor expressing, nonhematopoietic human tumors is not known. Palifermin has been shown to enhance epithelial tumor cell lines *in vitro*. Do not administer within 24 hours before, during, or after myelotoxic chemotherapy. If administered during or within 24 hours of (before or after) chemotherapy, palifermin may increase the severity and duration of mucositis due to the increased sensitivity of rapidly-dividing epithelial cells.

Adverse Reactions
>10%:
  Cardiovascular: Edema (28%)
  Central nervous system: Fever (39%); pain (16%); dysesthesia (oral hyperesthesia, hypoesthesia, and paresthesia 12%)
  Dermatologic: Rash (62%; grade 3: 3%), pruritus (35%), erythema (32%)
  Gastrointestinal: Serum amylase increased (62%, grades 3/4: 38%), serum lipase increased (28%, grades 3/4: 11%), mouth/tongue discoloration or thickness (17%), taste alteration (16%)
1% to 10%:
  Neuromuscular & skeletal: Arthralgia (10%)
  Miscellaneous: Antibody formation (2%)
<1%, postmarketing, and/or case reports: Cataracts, cough, flexural hyperpigmentation, palmar-plantar erythrodysesthesia syndrome (hand-foot syndrome), perianal pain, rhinitis, vaginal edema, vaginal erythema

Drug Interactions

Metabolism/Transport Effects None known.

Avoid Concomitant Use There are no known interactions where it is recommended to avoid concomitant use.

Increased Effect/Toxicity
  The levels/effects of Palifermin may be increased by: Heparin; Heparin (Low Molecular Weight)

Decreased Effect There are no known significant interactions involving a decrease in effect.

Storage/Stability Store intact vials under refrigeration at 2°C to 8°C (36°F to 46°F). Protect from light. Although the manufacturer recommends immediate use, reconstituted vials are stable for up to 24 hours refrigerated. Bring to room temperature for up to 1 hour prior to administration; however, do not use if left at room temperature >1 hour. Protect reconstituted solution from light. Do not freeze reconstituted product.

◄ **Preparation for Administration** Hazardous agent; use appropriate precautions for handling and disposal (NIOSH 2014 [group 2]).

To reconstitute, slowly add 1.2 mL SWFI, to a final concentration of 5 mg/mL. Swirl gently; do not shake or vigorously agitate. May take up to 3 minutes to dissolve; reconstituted solution should be clear and colorless. Do not filter during preparation or administration.

Mechanism of Action Palifermin is a recombinant keratinocyte growth factor (KGF) produced in *E. coli*. Endogenous KGF is produced by mesenchymal cells in response to epithelial tissue injury. KGF binds to the KGF receptor resulting in proliferation, differentiation and migration of epithelial cells in multiple tissues, including (but not limited to) the tongue, buccal mucosa, esophagus, and salivary gland.

Pharmacodynamics/Kinetics

Onset of action: Epithelial cell proliferation (dose-dependent): 48 hours

Half-life elimination: 4.5 hours (range: 3.3-5.7 hours)

Dosing

Adult & Geriatric Oral mucositis associated with hematopoietic stem cell transplant (HSCT) conditioning regimens: IV: 60 mcg/kg/day for 3 consecutive days before and 3 consecutive days after myelotoxic therapy; total of 6 doses (Spielberger, 2004)

Note: Administer first 3 doses prior to myelotoxic therapy, with the 3rd dose given 24-48 hours before beginning the myelotoxic conditioning regimen. Administer the last 3 doses after completion of the conditioning regimen, with the first of these doses after but on the same day as HSCT infusion and at least 4 days after the most recent dose of palifermin.

Renal Impairment No dosage adjustment necessary.

Hepatic Impairment No dosage adjustment provided in the manufacturer's labeling (has not been studied).

Administration Administer by IV bolus. If heparin is used to maintain the patency of the IV line, flush line with saline prior to and after palifermin administration. Do not administer palifermin during or within 24 hours before or after chemotherapy. Allow solution to reach room temperature prior to administration; do not use if at room temperature >1 hour. Do not filter.

Hazardous agent; use appropriate precautions for handling and disposal (NIOSH 2014 [group 2]).

Monitoring Parameters Monitor for oral mucositis

Additional Information Oncology Comment: The Multinational Association of Supportive Care in Cancer and the International Society for Oral Oncology (MASCC/ISOO) guidelines for the prevention and treatment of mucositis recommend palifermin (at the FDA-approved dose) for the prevention of oral mucositis in patients with hematologic malignancies who are receiving high-dose chemotherapy and total body irradiation with autologous stem cell transplantation (Keefe, 2007).

Guidelines from the American Society of Clinical Oncology (ASCO) for the use of chemotherapy and radiotherapy protectants (Hensley, 2008) recommend the use of palifermin to decrease the incidence of severe mucositis in patients undergoing autologous stem-cell transplantation with a total body irradiation (TBI) conditioning regimen. According to the ASCO guidelines, data are insufficient to recommend palifermin when the conditioning regimen is chemotherapy only. Palifermin may be considered in patients undergoing myeloablative allogeneic stem-cell transplantation with a TBI conditioning regimen, however data are again insufficient to recommend palifermin when the conditioning regimen is chemotherapy only. Due to a lack of appropriate data, the guidelines also do not recommend palifermin use in non-stem-cell transplantation treatment regimens or for use when treating solid tumors.

Dosage Forms Excipient information presented when available (limited, particularly for generics); consult specific product labeling.

Solution Reconstituted, Intravenous [preservative free]:

Kepivance: 6.25 mg (1 ea)

◆ **Palladone** see HYDROmorphone on page 830

Palonosetron (pal oh NOE se tron)

Related Information

Management of Chemotherapy-Induced Nausea and Vomiting in Adults on page 2142

Brand Names: US Aloxi

Index Terms Palonosetron Hydrochloride; RS-25259; RS-25259-197

Pharmacologic Category Antiemetic; Selective 5-HT$_3$ Receptor Antagonist

Use

Chemotherapy-induced nausea and vomiting: Prevention of acute and delayed nausea and vomiting associated with initial and repeat courses in patients treated with moderately emetogenic cancer chemotherapy in adults; prevention of acute nausea and vomiting associated with initial and repeat courses in patients treated with highly emetogenic cancer chemotherapy in adults; prevention of acute nausea and vomiting associated with initial and repeat courses of emetogenic cancer chemotherapy (including highly emetogenic chemotherapy) in pediatric patients 1 month to <17 years.

Postoperative nausea and vomiting: Prevention of postoperative nausea and vomiting (PONV) for up to 24 hours following surgery in adults.

Limitations of use: Routine prophylaxis for PONV in patients with minimal expectation of nausea and/or vomiting is not recommended, although use is recommended in patients when nausea and vomiting must be avoided in the postoperative period, even if the incidence of PONV is low.

Labeled Contraindications Hypersensitivity to palonosetron or any component of the formulation

Pregnancy Considerations Adverse events have not been observed in animal reproduction studies. Use during pregnancy only if clearly needed.

Breast-Feeding Considerations It is not known if palonosetron is excreted in breast milk. Due to the potential for adverse reactions in the nursing infant, the manufacturer recommends a decision be made whether to discontinue nursing or to discontinue palonosetron, taking into account the importance of treatment to the mother.

Warnings/Precautions Hypersensitivity (including anaphylaxis) has been reported in patients with or without known hypersensitivity to other 5-HT$_3$ receptor antagonists. Serotonin syndrome has been reported with 5-HT$_3$ receptor antagonists, predominantly when used in combination with other serotonergic agents (eg, SSRIs, SNRIs, MAOIs, mirtazapine, fentanyl, lithium, tramadol, and/or methylene blue). Some of the cases have been fatal. The majority of serotonin syndrome reports due to 5-HT$_3$ receptor antagonists have occurred in a post-anesthesia setting or in an infusion center. Serotonin syndrome has also been reported following overdose of another 5-HT$_3$ receptor antagonist. Monitor patients for signs of serotonin syndrome, including mental status changes (eg, agitation, hallucinations, delirium, coma);

◀ autonomic instability (eg, tachycardia, labile blood pressure, diaphoresis, dizziness, flushing, hyperthermia); neuromuscular changes (eg, tremor, rigidity, myoclonus, hyperreflexia, incoordination); gastrointestinal symptoms (eg, nausea, vomiting, diarrhea); and/or seizures. If serotonin syndrome occurs, discontinue 5-HT$_3$ receptor antagonist treatment and begin supportive management.

Although other selective 5-HT$_3$ receptor antagonists have been associated with dose-dependent increases in ECG intervals (eg, PR, QRS duration, QT/QTc, JT), palonosetron has not been shown to significantly affect the QT/QTc interval (Gonullu, 2012; Morganroth, 2008). Reduction in heart rate may occur with the 5-HT$_3$ antagonists, including palonosetron (Gonullu, 2012). Antiemetics are most effective when used prophylactically (Roila, 2010). Potentially significant drug-drug interactions may exist, requiring dose or frequency adjustment, additional monitoring, and/or selection of alternative therapy. If emesis occurs despite optimal antiemetic prophylaxis, re-evaluate emetic risk, disease, concurrent morbidities and medications to assure antiemetic regimen is optimized (Basch, 2011). For postoperative nausea and vomiting (PONV), may use for low expectation of PONV if it is essential to avoid nausea and vomiting in the postoperative period; use is not recommended if there is little expectation of nausea and vomiting.

Adverse Reactions Frequencies reported for both indications (chemotherapy-associated nausea and vomiting and postoperative nausea and vomiting) and in adults unless otherwise noted.

1% to 10%:

Cardiovascular: Prolonged Q-T interval on ECG (PONV 1% to 5%; chemotherapy-associated <1%), bradycardia (chemotherapy-associated 1%), sinus bradycardia (PONV: 1%), tachycardia (may be nonsustained; 1%), hypotension (≤1%)

Central nervous system: Headache (chemotherapy-associated: Adults 9%; infants, children, and adolescents <1%), anxiety (chemotherapy-associated: 1%), dizziness (infants, children, adolescents, and adults ≤1%)

Dermatologic: Pruritus (PONV: 1%)

Endocrine & metabolic: Hyperkalemia (chemotherapy-associated: 1%)

Gastrointestinal: Constipation (chemotherapy-associated: 5%), diarrhea (≤1%), flatulence (≤1%)

Genitourinary: Urinary retention (≤1%)

Hepatic: Increased serum ALT (≤1%; may be transient), increased serum AST (≤1%; may be transient)

Neuromuscular & skeletal: Weakness (chemotherapy-associated: 1%)

<1%, postmarketing, and/or case reports: Abdominal pain, allergic dermatitis, amblyopia, anaphylactic shock (very rare), anaphylaxis (very rare), anasarca, anemia, anorexia, arthralgia, cardiac arrhythmia, chills, decreased appetite, decreased blood pressure, decreased gastrointestinal motility, decreased platelet count, dermatological disease (infants, children, and adolescents), distended vein, drowsiness, dyskinesia (infants, children, and adolescents), dyspepsia, electrolyte disturbance, epistaxis, erythema, euphoria, extrasystoles, eye irritation, fatigue, fever, flattened T wave on ECG, flu-like symptoms, glycosuria, hiccups, hot flash, hyperglycemia, hypersensitivity (very rare), hypersomnia, hypertension, hypokalemia, hypoventilation, increased bilirubin (transient), increased liver enzymes, infusion site pain (infants, children, and adolescents), injection site reaction (very rare; includes burning sensation at injection site, discomfort at injection site, induration at injection site, pain at injection site), insomnia, ischemic heart disease, laryngospasm,

limb pain, metabolic acidosis, motion sickness, paresthesia, serotonin syndrome, sialorrhea, sinus arrhythmia, sinus tachycardia, skin rash, supraventricular extrasystole, tinnitus, vein discoloration, ventricular premature contractions, xerostomia

Drug Interactions

Metabolism/Transport Effects Substrate of CYP1A2 (minor), CYP2D6 (minor), CYP3A4 (minor); **Note:** Assignment of Major/Minor substrate status based on clinically relevant drug interaction potential

Avoid Concomitant Use

Avoid concomitant use of Palonosetron with any of the following: Apomorphine

Increased Effect/Toxicity

Palonosetron may increase the levels/effects of: Apomorphine; Serotonin Modulators

Decreased Effect

Palonosetron may decrease the levels/effects of: Tapentadol; TraMADol

Storage/Stability Store intact vials at 20°C to 25°C (68°F to 77°F); excursions permitted to 15°C to 30°C (59°F to 86°F). Do not freeze. Protect from light. Solutions of 5 mcg/mL and 30 mcg/mL in NS, D_5W, $D_5^{1/2}NS$, and D_5LR injection are stable for 48 hours at room temperature and 14 days under refrigeration (Trissel, 2004a).

Mechanism of Action Selective 5-HT$_3$ receptor antagonist, blocking serotonin, both on vagal nerve terminals in the periphery and centrally in the chemoreceptor trigger zone

Pharmacodynamics/Kinetics

Distribution: V_d: 8.3 ± 2.5 L/kg

Protein binding: ~62%

Metabolism: ~50% metabolized via CYP enzymes (and likely other pathways) to relatively inactive metabolites (N-oxide-palonosetron and 6-S-hydroxy-palonosetron); CYP1A2, 2D6, and 3A4 contribute to its metabolism

Half-life elimination: IV: Adults: ~40 hours; Children: ~20 to 30 hours

Excretion: Urine (80%; 40% as unchanged drug)

Dosing

Adult

Prevention of chemotherapy-induced nausea and vomiting: IV: 0.25 mg beginning ~30 minutes prior to the start of chemotherapy

Prevention of postoperative nausea and vomiting: IV: 0.075 mg immediately prior to anesthesia induction

Geriatric No dosage adjustment necessary. Refer to adult dosing.

Pediatric Prevention of chemotherapy-induced nausea and vomiting: Infants ≥1 month, Children, and Adolescents <17 years: IV: 20 **mcg**/kg (maximum dose: 1.5 **mg**) beginning ~30 minutes prior to the start of chemotherapy

Renal Impairment No dosage adjustment is necessary.

Hepatic Impairment No dosage adjustment is necessary.

Administration Flush IV line with NS prior to and following administration.

Prevention of chemotherapy-induced nausea and vomiting:

Children: Infuse over 15 minutes, beginning ~30 minutes prior to the start of chemotherapy

Adults: Infuse over 30 seconds, beginning ~30 minutes prior to the start of chemotherapy

◀ Prevention of postoperative nausea and vomiting: Infuse over 10 seconds immediately prior to anesthesia induction

Dosage Forms Excipient information presented when available (limited, particularly for generics); consult specific product labeling.
Solution, Intravenous:
Aloxi: 0.25 mg/5 mL (5 mL) [contains edetate disodium]

♦ **Palonosetron and Netupitant** *see* Netupitant and Palonosetron *on page 1195*

♦ **Palonosetron Hydrochloride** *see* Palonosetron *on page 1307*

Pamidronate (pa mi DROE nate)

Related Information
Chronic Pain Management (Cancer) *on page 2229*
Hypercalcemia of Malignancy *on page 2241*
Safe Handling of Hazardous Drugs *on page 2292*

Brand Names: Canada Aredia; Pamidronate Disodium; Pamidronate Disodium Omega; PMS-Pamidronate

Index Terms Pamidronate Disodium

Pharmacologic Category Bisphosphonate Derivative

Use
Hypercalcemia of malignancy: Treatment of moderate or severe hypercalcemia associated with malignancy, with or without bone metastases, in conjunction with adequate hydration.

Osteolytic bone metastases of breast cancer and osteolytic lesions of multiple myeloma: Treatment of osteolytic bone metastases of breast cancer and osteolytic lesions of multiple myeloma in conjunction with standard antineoplastic therapy.

Paget disease: Treatment of patients with moderate to severe Paget disease of bone.

Labeled Contraindications Hypersensitivity to pamidronate, other bisphosphonates, or any component of the formulation

Pregnancy Considerations Adverse events were observed in animal reproduction studies. It is not known if bisphosphonates cross the placenta, but fetal exposure is expected (Djokanovic, 2008; Stathopoulos, 2011). Bisphosphonates are incorporated into the bone matrix and gradually released over time. The amount available in the systemic circulation varies by dose and duration of therapy. Theoretically, there may be a risk of fetal harm when pregnancy follows the completion of therapy; however, available data have not shown that exposure to bisphosphonates during pregnancy significantly increases the risk of adverse fetal events (Djokanovic, 2008; Levy, 2009; Stathopoulos, 2011). Until additional data is available, most sources recommend discontinuing bisphosphonate therapy in women of reproductive potential as early as possible prior to a planned pregnancy; use in premenopausal women should be reserved for special circumstances when rapid bone loss is occurring (Bhalla, 2010; Pereira, 2012; Stathopoulos, 2011). Because hypocalcemia has been described following *in utero* bisphosphonate exposure, exposed infants should be monitored for hypocalcemia after birth (Djokanovic, 2008; Stathopoulos, 2011).

Breast-Feeding Considerations It is not known if pamidronate is excreted in breast milk. Pamidronate was not detected in the milk of a nursing woman receiving pamidronate 30 mg IV monthly (therapy started ~6 months postpartum). Following the first infusion, milk was pumped and collected for 0-24 hours and 25-48 hours, and each day pooled for analysis. Pamidronate readings were below the limit of quantification (<0.4 micromole/L). During therapy, breast milk was pumped and discarded for the first 48 hours following each infusion prior to resuming nursing. The infant was breast-fed >80% of the time; adverse events were not observed in the nursing infant (Simonoski, 2000). Monitoring the serum calcium concentrations of nursing infants is recommended (Stathopoulos, 2011). Due to the potential for serious adverse reactions in the nursing infant, the manufacturer recommends a decision be made whether to discontinue nursing or to discontinue the drug, taking into account the importance of treatment to the mother.

Warnings/Precautions Hazardous agent - use appropriate precautions for handling and disposal (meets NIOSH 2014 criteria). Osteonecrosis of the jaw (ONJ) has been reported in patients receiving bisphosphonates. Risk factors include invasive dental procedures (eg, tooth extraction, dental implants, boney surgery); a diagnosis of cancer, with concomitant chemotherapy, radiotherapy, or corticosteroids; poor oral hygiene, ill-fitting dentures; and comorbid disorders (anemia, coagulopathy, infection, preexisting dental disease). Most reported cases occurred after IV bisphosphonate therapy; however, cases have been reported following oral therapy. A dental exam and preventive dentistry should be performed prior to placing patients with risk factors on chronic bisphosphonate therapy. There is no evidence that discontinuing therapy reduces the risk of developing ONJ (Assael, 2009). The benefit/risk must be assessed by the treating physician and/or dentist/surgeon prior to any invasive dental procedure. Patients developing ONJ while on bisphosphonates should receive care by an oral surgeon.

Atypical femur fractures (after minimal or no trauma) have been reported. The fractures include subtrochanteric femur (bone just below the hip joint) and diaphyseal femur (long segment of the thigh bone). Some patients experience prodromal pain weeks or months before the fracture occurs. It is unclear if bisphosphonate therapy is the cause for these fractures. Patients receiving long-term (>3 to 5 years) bisphosphonate therapy may be at an increased risk. Consider discontinuing pamidronate in patients with a suspected femoral shaft fracture. Patients who present with thigh or groin pain in the absence of trauma should be evaluated. Infrequently, severe (and occasionally debilitating) musculoskeletal (bone, joint, and/or muscle) pain have been reported during bisphosphonate treatment. The onset of pain ranged from a single day to several months. Consider discontinuing therapy in patients who experience severe symptoms; symptoms usually resolve upon discontinuation. Some patients experienced recurrence when rechallenged with same drug or another bisphosphonate; avoid use in patients with a history of these symptoms in association with bisphosphonate therapy.

Initial or single doses have been associated with renal deterioration, progressing to renal failure and dialysis. Withhold pamidronate treatment (until renal function returns to baseline) in patients with evidence of renal deterioration. Glomerulosclerosis (focal segmental) with or without nephrotic syndrome has also been reported. Longer infusion times (>2 hours) may reduce the risk for renal toxicity, especially in patients with preexisting renal insufficiency. Single pamidronate doses should not exceed 90 mg. Patients with serum creatinine

>3 mg/dL were not studied in clinical trials; limited data are available in patients with CrCl <30 mL/minute. Evaluate serum creatinine prior to each treatment. For the treatment of bone metastases, use is not recommended in patients with severe renal impairment; for renal impairment in indications other than bone metastases, use clinical judgment to determine if benefits outweigh potential risks.

Use has been associated with asymptomatic electrolyte abnormalities (including hypophosphatemia, hypokalemia, hypomagnesemia, and hypocalcemia). Rare cases of symptomatic hypocalcemia, including tetany have been reported. Patients with a history of thyroid surgery may have relative hypoparathyroidism; predisposing them to pamidronate-related hypocalcemia. Patients with preexisting anemia, leukopenia, or thrombocytopenia should be closely monitored during the first 2 weeks of treatment.

Hypercalcemia of malignancy (HCM): Adequate hydration is required during treatment (urine output ~2 L/day); avoid overhydration, especially in patients with heart failure.

Multiple myeloma: Patients with Bence-Jones proteinuria and dehydration should be adequately hydrated prior to therapy. The American Society of Clinical Oncology (ASCO) has also published guidelines on bisphosphonates use for prevention and treatment of bone disease in multiple myeloma (Kyle, 2007). Bisphosphonate (pamidronate or zoledronic acid) use is recommended in multiple myeloma patients with lytic bone destruction or compression spine fracture from osteopenia. Bisphosphonates may also be considered in patients with pain secondary to osteolytic disease, adjunct therapy to stabilize fractures or impending fractures, and for multiple myeloma patients with osteopenia but no radiographic evidence of lytic bone disease. Bisphosphonates are not recommended in patients with solitary plasmacytoma, smoldering (asymptomatic) or indolent myeloma, or monoclonal gammopathy of undetermined significance. The guidelines recommend monthly treatment for a period of 2 years. At that time, consider discontinuing in responsive and stable patients, and reinitiate if a new-onset skeletal-related event occurs. The ASCO guidelines are in alignment with the prescribing information for dosing, renal dose adjustments, infusion times, prevention and management of osteonecrosis of the jaw, and monitoring of laboratory parameter recommendations. According to the guidelines, in patients with extensive bone disease with existing severe renal disease (a serum creatinine >3 mg/dL or CrCl <30 mL/minute) pamidronate at a dose of 90 mg over 4 to 6 hours should be used (unless preexisting renal disease in which case a reduced initial dose should be considered). Monitor for albuminuria every 3 to 6 months; in patients with unexplained albuminuria >500 mg/24 hours, withhold the dose until level returns to baseline, then recheck every 3 to 4 weeks. Pamidronate may be reinitiated at a dose not to exceed 90 mg every 4 weeks with a longer infusion time of at least 4 hours.

Breast cancer (metastatic): The American Society of Clinical Oncology (ASCO) updated guidelines on the role of bone-modifying agents (BMAs) in the prevention and treatment of skeletal-related events for metastatic breast cancer patients (Van Poznak, 2011). The guidelines recommend initiating a BMA (denosumab, pamidronate, zoledronic acid) in patients with metastatic breast cancer to the bone. There is currently no literature indicating the superiority of one particular BMA. Optimal duration is not yet defined; however, the guidelines recommend continuing therapy until substantial decline in patient's performance status. The ASCO guidelines are in alignment with prescribing information for dosing, renal dose adjustments, infusion times, prevention and management of osteonecrosis of the jaw, and monitoring of laboratory parameter recommendations. BMAs are not the first-line therapy for pain. BMAs are to be used as adjunctive therapy for cancer-related bone pain associated with bone metastasis, demonstrating a modest pain control benefit. BMAs should be used in conjunction with agents such as NSAIDS, opioid and nonopioid analgesics, corticosteroids, radiation/surgery, and interventional procedures.

Adverse Reactions Note: Actual percentages may vary by indication and duration of infusion; treatment for multiple myeloma is associated with higher percentage.

>10%:

Central nervous system: Fatigue (≤37%), headache (≤26%), insomnia (≤22%)

Endocrine & metabolic: Hypophosphatemia (≤18%), hypokalemia (4% to 18%), hypocalcemia (≤3% to 17%), hypomagnesemia (10% to 12%)

Gastrointestinal: Nausea (≤54%), vomiting (≤36%), anorexia (≤26%), abdominal pain (≤23%), dyspepsia (≤23%)

Genitourinary: Urinary tract infection (≤19%)

Hematologic & oncologic: Anemia (≤43%), metastases (21% to 31%), granulocytopenia (≤20%)

Local: Infusion site reaction (≤18%; includes induration, pain, redness, and swelling)

Neuromuscular & skeletal: Myalgia (≤26%), weakness (≤22%), arthralgia (≤14%), osteonecrosis of the jaw (cancer patients: 1% to 11%)

Renal: Increased serum creatinine (≤19%)

Respiratory: Dyspnea (≤30%), cough (≤26%), upper respiratory tract infection (≤24%), sinusitis (≤16%), pleural effusion (≤11%)

Miscellaneous: Fever (18% to 39%; transient)

1% to 10%:

Cardiovascular: Atrial fibrillation (≤6%), hypertension (≤6%), syncope (≤6%), tachycardia (≤6%), atrial flutter (≤1%), cardiac failure (≤1%), edema (≤1%)

Central nervous system: Drowsiness (≤6%), psychosis (≤4%), seizure (≤2%)

Endocrine & metabolic: Hypothyroidism (≤6%)

Gastrointestinal: Constipation (≤6%), gastrointestinal hemorrhage (≤6%), diarrhea (≤1%), stomatitis (≤1%)

Genitourinary: Uremia (≤4%)

Hematologic & oncologic: Leukopenia (≤4%), neutropenia (≤1%), thrombocytopenia (≤1%)

Infection: Candidiasis (≤6%)

Neuromuscular & skeletal: Back pain, ostealgia

Respiratory: Rales (≤6%), rhinitis (≤6%)

<1%, postmarketing, and/or case reports: Acute renal failure, anaphylactic shock, angioedema, bronchospasm, cardiac failure, confusion, conjunctivitis, electrolyte disturbance, episcleritis, flu-like symptoms, focal segmental glomerulosclerosis (including collapsing variant), hallucination (visual), hematuria, herpes virus infection (reactivation), hyperkalemia, hypernatremia, hypersensitivity reaction, hypervolemia, hypotension, inflammation at injection site, injection site phlebitis, iridocyclitis, iritis, left heart failure, lymphocytopenia, malaise, mineral abnormalities, nephrotic syndrome, osteonecrosis (other than jaw), paresthesia, pruritus, renal failure, renal insufficiency, scleritis, skin rash, tetany, uveitis, xanthopsia

◀ **Drug Interactions**

Metabolism/Transport Effects None known.

Avoid Concomitant Use There are no known interactions where it is recommended to avoid concomitant use.

Increased Effect/Toxicity

Pamidronate may increase the levels/effects of: Deferasirox

The levels/effects of Pamidronate may be increased by: Aminoglycosides; Nonsteroidal Anti-Inflammatory Agents; Systemic Angiogenesis Inhibitors; Thalidomide

Decreased Effect

The levels/effects of Pamidronate may be decreased by: Proton Pump Inhibitors

Storage/Stability

Powder for reconstitution: Store at 20°C to 25°C (68°F to 77°F). The reconstituted solution is stable for 24 hours stored under refrigeration at 2°C to 8°C (36°F to 46°F). The diluted solution for infusion is stable at room temperature for up to 24 hours.

Solution for injection: Store at 20°C to 25°C (68°F to 77°F). The diluted solution for infusion is stable at room temperature for up to 24 hours.

Preparation for Administration Hazardous agent; use appropriate precautions for handling and disposal (meets NIOSH 2014 criteria).

Powder for injection: Reconstitute by adding 10 mL of SWFI to each vial of lyophilized powder, the resulting solution will be 30 mg/10 mL or 90 mg/10 mL.

Pamidronate may be further diluted in 250 to 1000 mL of 0.45% or 0.9% sodium chloride or 5% dextrose. (The manufacturers recommend dilution in 1000 mL for hypercalcemia of malignancy, 500 mL for Paget's disease and bone metastases of myeloma, and 250 mL for bone metastases of breast cancer.)

Mechanism of Action Nitrogen-containing bisphosphonate; inhibits bone resorption and decreases mineralization by disrupting osteoclast activity (Gralow, 2009; Rogers, 2011)

Pharmacodynamics/Kinetics

Onset of action:

Hypercalcemia of malignancy (HCM): ≤24 hours for decrease in albumin-corrected serum calcium; maximum effect: ≤7 days

Paget disease: ~1 month for ≥50% decrease in serum alkaline phosphatase

Duration: HCM: 7 to 14 days; Paget disease: 1 to 372 days

Distribution: 38% to 70% over 120 hours

Metabolism: Not metabolized

Half-life elimination: 21 to 35 hours

Excretion: Biphasic; urine (30% to 62% as unchanged drug; lower in patients with renal dysfunction) within 120 hours

Dosing

Adult Note: Single doses should not exceed 90 mg.

Hypercalcemia of malignancy: IV:

Moderate cancer-related hypercalcemia (corrected serum calcium: 12 to 13.5 mg/dL): 60 to 90 mg, as a single dose over 2 to 24 hours

Severe cancer-related hypercalcemia (corrected serum calcium: >13.5 mg/dL): 90 mg, as a single dose over 2 to 24 hours

Re-treatment in patients who show an initial complete or partial response (allow at least 7 days to elapse prior to re-treatment): May re-treat at the same dose if serum calcium does not return to normal or does not remain normal after initial treatment.

Multiple myeloma, osteolytic bone lesions: IV: 90 mg over 4 hours once monthly:

Lytic disease: American Society of Clinical Oncology (ASCO) guidelines: 90 mg over at least 2 hours once every 3 to 4 weeks for 2 years; discontinue after 2 years in patients with responsive and/or stable disease; resume therapy with new-onset skeletal-related events (Kyle, 2007)

Newly-diagnosed, symptomatic (off-label dose): 30 mg over 2.5 hours once monthly for at least 3 years (Gimsing, 2010)

Breast cancer, osteolytic bone metastases: IV: 90 mg over 2 hours once every 3 to 4 weeks

Paget's disease (moderate-to-severe): IV: 30 mg over 4 hours once daily for 3 consecutive days (total dose = 90 mg); may re-treat at initial dose if clinically indicated

Prevention of androgen deprivation-induced osteoporosis (off-label use): Males: IV: 60 mg over 2 hours once every 3 months (Smith, 2001)

Geriatric Refer to adult dosing. Begin at lower end of adult dosing range.

Renal Impairment Patients with serum creatinine >3 mg/dL were excluded from clinical trials; there are only limited pharmacokinetic data in patients with CrCl <30 mL/minute.

Manufacturer recommends the following guidelines:

Treatment of bone metastases: Use is not recommended in patients with severe renal impairment.

Renal impairment in indications other than bone metastases: Use clinical judgment to determine if benefits outweigh potential risks.

Multiple myeloma: American Society of Clinical Oncology (ASCO) guidelines (Kyle, 2007):

Severe renal impairment (serum creatinine >3 mg/dL **or** CrCl <30 mL/minute) and extensive bone disease: 90 mg over 4 to 6 hours. However, a reduced initial dose should be considered if renal impairment was preexisting.

Albuminuria >500 mg/24 hours (unexplained): Withhold dose until returns to baseline, then recheck every 3 to 4 weeks; consider reinitiating at a dose not to exceed 90 mg every 4 weeks and with a longer infusion time of at least 4 hours

Dosing adjustment in renal toxicity: In patients with bone metastases, treatment should be withheld for deterioration in renal function (increase of serum creatinine ≥0.5 mg/dL in patients with normal baseline [serum creatinine <1.4 mg/dL] or ≥1 mg/dL in patients with abnormal baseline [serum creatinine ≥1.4 mg/dL]). Resumption of therapy may be considered when serum creatinine returns to within 10% of baseline.

Hepatic Impairment

Mild to moderate impairment: No dosage adjustment necessary.

Severe impairment: There are no dosage adjustments provided in the manufacturer's labeling (has not been studied).

Administration IV: Infusion rate varies by indication. Longer infusion times (>2 hours) may reduce the risk for renal toxicity, especially in patients with preexisting renal insufficiency. The manufacturer recommends infusing over 2 to 24 hours for hypercalcemia of malignancy; over 2 hours for osteolytic bone lesions with metastatic breast cancer; and over 4 hours for Paget's disease

◀

and for osteolytic bone lesions with multiple myeloma. The ASCO guidelines for bisphosphonate use in multiple myeloma recommend infusing pamidronate over at least 2 hours; if therapy is withheld due to renal toxicity, infuse over at least 4 hours upon reintroduction of treatment after renal recovery (Kyle, 2007).

Hazardous agent; use appropriate precautions for handling and disposal (meets NIOSH 2014 criteria).

Monitoring Parameters Serum creatinine (prior to each treatment); serum electrolytes, including calcium, phosphate, magnesium, and potassium; CBC with differential; monitor for hypocalcemia for at least 2 weeks after therapy; dental exam and preventive dentistry prior to therapy for patients at risk of osteonecrosis, including all cancer patients; patients with preexisting anemia, leukopenia, or thrombocytopenia should be closely monitored during the first 2 weeks of treatment; in addition, monitor urine albumin every 3 to 6 months in multiple myeloma patients

Test Interactions Bisphosphonates may interfere with diagnostic imaging agents such as technetium-99m-diphosphonate in bone scans.

Dietary Considerations Multiple myeloma or metastatic bone lesions from solid tumors or Paget's disease: Take adequate daily calcium and vitamin D supplement (if patient is not hypercalcemic).

Dosage Forms Excipient information presented when available (limited, particularly for generics); consult specific product labeling.
Solution, Intravenous, as disodium:
 Generic: 30 mg/10 mL (10 mL); 90 mg/10 mL (10 mL)
Solution, Intravenous, as disodium [preservative free]:
 Generic: 30 mg/10 mL (10 mL); 6 mg/mL (10 mL); 90 mg/10 mL (10 mL)
Solution Reconstituted, Intravenous, as disodium:
 Generic: 30 mg (1 ea); 90 mg (1 ea)

◆ **Pamidronate Disodium** *see* Pamidronate *on page 1310*

◆ **Pamidronate Disodium Omega (Can)** *see* Pamidronate *on page 1310*

◆ **Panglobulin** *see* Immune Globulin *on page 903*

Panitumumab (pan i TOOM yoo mab)

Related Information

Management of Chemotherapy-Induced Nausea and Vomiting in Adults *on page 2142*

Management of EGFR Inhibitor Toxicities: Dermatologic, Ocular, and Gastro-intestinal *on page 2179*

Prevention of Chemotherapy-Induced Nausea and Vomiting in Children *on page 2203*

Principles of Anticancer Therapy *on page 2261*

Brand Names: US Vectibix

Brand Names: Canada Vectibix

Index Terms ABX-EGF; MOAB ABX-EGF; Monoclonal Antibody ABX-EGF; rHuMAb-EGFr

Pharmacologic Category Antineoplastic Agent, Epidermal Growth Factor Receptor (EGFR) Inhibitor; Antineoplastic Agent, Monoclonal Antibody

Use
Colorectal cancer, metastatic: Treatment of patients with wild-type *KRAS* (exon 2 in codons 12 or 13) metastatic colorectal cancer (mCRC), either as first-line therapy in combination with FOLFOX (fluorouracil, leucovorin, and oxaliplatin) or as a single agent following disease progression after prior treatment with fluoropyrimidine-, oxaliplatin-, and irinotecan-containing chemotherapy regimens

Limitations of use: Panitumumab is not indicated for the treatment of patients with *RAS*-mutant mCRC or for whom *RAS* mutation status is unknown.

Labeled Contraindications
There are no contraindications listed in the manufacturer's US labeling.

Canadian labeling: History of severe or life-threatening hypersensitivity reactions to panitumumab or any component of the formulation.

Pregnancy Considerations Animal reproduction studies have demonstrated adverse fetal effects. Based on animal studies, panitumumab may disrupt normal menstrual cycles. IgG is known to cross the placenta; therefore, it is possible the developing fetus may be exposed to panitumumab. Because panitumumab inhibits epidermal growth factor (EGF), a component of fetal development, adverse effects on pregnancy would be expected. Men and women of childbearing potential should use effective contraception during and for 6 months after treatment. In the US and Canada, women who become pregnant during panitumumab treatment are encouraged to enroll in Amgen's Pregnancy Surveillance Program (US: 1-800-772-6436; Canada: 1-866-512-6436).

Breast-Feeding Considerations It is not known if panitumumab is excreted in breast milk. The decision to discontinue panitumumab or discontinue breast-feeding should take into account the benefits of treatment to the mother. If breast-feeding is interrupted for panitumumab treatment, based on the half-life, breast-feeding should not be resumed for at least 2 months following the last dose. In the US and Canada, women who nurse during panitumumab treatment are encouraged to enroll in Amgen's Lactation Surveillance Program (US: 1-800-772-6436; Canada: 1-866-512-6436).

Warnings/Precautions [US Boxed Warning]: Dermatologic toxicities have been reported in 90% of patients receiving single agent panitumumab and were severe (grade 3 or higher) in 15% of patients); may include dermatitis acneiform, pruritus, erythema, rash, skin exfoliation, paronychia, dry skin, and skin fissures. Severe skin toxicities may be complicated by infection, sepsis, necrotizing fasciitis, or abscesses. The median time to development of skin (or ocular) toxicity was 2 weeks, with resolution ~12 weeks after discontinuation. Monitor all dermatologic toxicities for development of inflammation or infection. Rare cases of Stevens-Johnson syndrome and toxic epidermal necrolysis have been reported; bullous mucocutaneous disease (life-threatening/fatal) have been observed. Withhold treatment for severe or life-threatening dermatologic or soft tissue toxicities associated with severe/life-threatening inflammatory or infectious complications; dermatologic toxicity may require dose reduction or permanent discontinuation. The severity of dermatologic toxicity is predictive for response; grades 2 to 4 skin toxicity correlates with improved progression free survival and overall survival, compared to grade 1 skin toxicity (Peeters, 2009; Van Cutsem, 2007). Patients should minimize sunlight exposure and wear sunscreen and protective clothing/hat; sunlight may exacerbate skin reactions. Keratitis and ulcerative keratitis (known risk factors for corneal perforation) have occurred. Monitor for evidence of ocular toxicity; interrupt or discontinue treatment for acute or worsening keratitis. Gastric mucosal and nail toxicities have also been reported.

Severe infusion reactions (bronchospasm, dyspnea, fever, chills, and hypotension) have been reported in ~1% of patients; fatal infusion reactions have been reported with postmarketing surveillance. Discontinue infusion for severe reactions; permanently discontinue in patients with persistent severe infusion reactions. Appropriate medical support for the management of infusion reactions should be readily available. Mild-to-moderate infusion reactions are managed by slowing the infusion rate.

Pulmonary fibrosis and interstitial lung disease have been observed (rarely) in clinical trials; fatalities have been reported. Interrupt treatment for acute onset or worsening of pulmonary symptoms; permanently discontinue treatment if interstitial lung disease is confirmed. Patients with a history of or evidence of interstitial pneumonitis or pulmonary fibrosis were excluded from most clinical trials; consider the benefits of therapy versus the risk of pulmonary complications in such patients. May cause diarrhea; the incidence and severity of chemotherapy-induced diarrhea and other toxicities (rash, electrolyte abnormalities, stomatitis) is increased with combination chemotherapy; severe diarrhea and dehydration (which may lead to acute renal failure) has been observed with panitumumab in combination with chemotherapy. In a study of bevacizumab with combination chemotherapy ± panitumumab, the use of panitumumab resulted in decreased progression-free and overall survival and significantly increased toxicity compared to regimens without panitumumab (Hecht, 2009). Toxicities included rash/acneiform dermatitis, diarrhea/dehydration, electrolyte disturbances, mucositis/stomatitis, and an increased incidence of pulmonary embolism. Magnesium and/or calcium depletion may occur during treatment (may be delayed; hypomagnesemia occurred ≥8 weeks after completion of panitumumab) and after treatment is discontinued; electrolyte repletion may be necessary; monitor for hypomagnesemia and hypocalcemia during treatment and for at least 8 weeks after completion. Hypokalemia has also been reported. Patients >65 years of age receiving panitumumab plus FOLFOX experienced a higher incidence of serious adverse events including severe diarrhea.

Patients with colorectal cancer with tumors with codons 12 and 13 (exon 2), codons 59 and 61 (exon 3), or codons 117 and 146 (exon 4) RAS (KRAS or NRAS) mutations are unlikely to benefit from EGFR inhibitor therapy. Panitumumab is not indicated patients with RAS mutation-positive metastatic colorectal cancer or patients in which RAS mutation status is unknown. Utilizing an anti-EGFR-directed antibody in patients whose tumors contain RAS mutations resulted in increased toxicity without clinical benefit. In a study of FOLFOX4 (fluorouracil, leucovorin and oxaliplatin) ± panitumumab, patients with a KRAS mutation who received panitumumab with FOLFOX4 experienced a significantly shortened progression-free survival (Douillard, 2010). In addition, a subset analysis of patients with wild-type KRAS identified additional RAS (KRAS [exons 3 and 4] or NRAS [exons 2, 3, 4]) mutations; progression-free survival and overall survival were significantly shortened in patients with RAS mutations who received FOLFOX4 in combination with panitumumab (Douillard, 2013). The American Society of Clinical Oncology (ASCO) provisional clinical opinion (Allegra, 2009) recommends genotyping tumor tissue for KRAS mutation in all patients with metastatic colorectal cancer (genotyping may be done on archived specimens). An updated ASCO provisional clinical opinion recommends that all patients with metastatic colorectal cancer who are candidates for anti-EGFR therapy should be tested (in a certified lab) for mutations in both *KRAS* and *NRAS* exon 2 (codons 12 and 13), exon 3 (codons 59 and 61), and exon 4 (codons 117 and 146); anti-EGFR monoclonal antibody therapy should only be considered in patients whose tumors lack mutations after extended *RAS* testing (Allegra, 2015). Panitumumab is also reported to be ineffective in patients with BRAF V600E mutation (Di Nicolantonio, 2008).

Adverse Reactions

Monotherapy:

>10%:

Central nervous system: Fatigue (26%)

Dermatologic: Skin toxicity (90%; grades 3/4: 15%), erythema (66%; grades 3/4: 6%), pruritus (58%; grades 3/4: 3%), acneiform eruption (57%; grades 3/4: 7%), paronychia (25%; grades 3/4: 2%), rash (22%; grades 3/4: 1%), skin fissure (20%; grades 3/4: 1%), exfoliative dermatitis (18%; grades 3/4: 2%), acne vulgaris (14%; grades 3/4: 1%)

Endocrine & metabolic: Hypomagnesemia (grades 3/4: 7%)

Gastrointestinal: Nausea (23%), diarrhea (21%; grades 3/4: 2%), vomiting (19%)

Ophthalmic: Ocular toxicity (16%)

Respiratory: Dyspnea (18%), cough (15%)

Miscellaneous: Fever (17%)

1% to 10%:

Cardiovascular: Pulmonary embolism (1%)

Central nervous system: Chills (3%)

Dermatologic: Nail toxicity (10%), xeroderma (10%), desquamation (9%; grades 3/4: <1%), dermal ulcer (6%; grades 3/4: <1%), pustular rash (4%), papular rash (2%)

Endocrine & metabolic: Dehydration (3%)

Gastrointestinal: Mucositis (7%), stomatitis (7%), xerostomia (5%)

Immunologic: Antibody formation (≤5%)

Ophthalmic: Abnormal eyelash growth (6%), conjunctivitis (5%)

Respiratory: Epistaxis (4%), interstitial pulmonary disease (1%)

Miscellaneous: Infusion related reaction (3%; grades 3/4: <1%)

<1%: Hypersensitivity reaction, pulmonary fibrosis

Combination therapy with FOLFOX:

>10%:

Dermatologic: Skin rash (56%; grades 3/4: 17% to 26%), acneiform eruption (32%; grades 3/4: 10%), pruritus (23%; grades 3/4: <1%), paronychia (21%; grades 3/4: 3%), xeroderma (21%; grades 3/4: 2%), erythema (16%; grades 3/4: 2%), skin fissure (16%; grades 3/4: <1%), alopecia (15%), acne vulgaris (14%; grades 3/4: 3%)

Endocrine & metabolic: Hypomagnesemia (30%), hypokalemia (21%), weight loss (18%)

Gastrointestinal: Diarrhea (62%), anorexia (36%), abdominal pain (28%), stomatitis (27%), mucosal inflammation (25%)

Neuromuscular & skeletal: Weakness (25%)

Ophthalmic: Conjunctivitis (18%)

Respiratory: Epistaxis (14%)

1% to 10%:

Cardiovascular: Deep vein thrombosis (5%)

Central nervous system: Fatigue (≥1%), paresthesia (≥1%)

◄

Dermatologic: Nail disorder (10%; grades 3/4: 1%), palmar-plantar eryth-rodysesthesia (9%; grades 3/4: 1%), cellulitis (3%)

Endocrine & metabolic: Dehydration (8%), hypocalcemia (6%)

Hypersensitivity: Hypersensitivity (≥1%)

Local: Localized infection (4%)

<1%: Antibody development

Postmarketing and/or case reports (mono- and combination therapy): Abscess, angioedema, bullous skin disease (mucocutaneous), corneal ulcer, keratitis, necrotizing fasciitis, sepsis, skin necrosis, Stevens-Johnson syndrome, toxic epidermal necrolysis

Drug Interactions

Metabolism/Transport Effects None known.

Avoid Concomitant Use There are no known interactions where it is recommended to avoid concomitant use.

Increased Effect/Toxicity

Panitumumab may increase the levels/effects of: Porfimer; Verteporfin

Decreased Effect There are no known significant interactions involving a decrease in effect.

Storage/Stability Store intact vials in the original cartons under refrigeration at 2°C to 8°C (36°F to 46°F) until the time of use. Do not freeze; do not shake; protect from direct sunlight. Solution diluted for infusion should be used within 6 hours of preparation if stored at room temperature or within 24 hours of dilution if stored at 2°C to 8°C (36°F to 46°F); do not freeze.

Preparation for Administration Inspect vial prior to use; solution is colorless but may contain a small amount of translucent-to-white amorphous panitumumab protein particles (will be removed with administration filter). Dilute in 100 mL (for doses ≤1000 mg) or 150 mL (doses >1000 mg) of normal saline to a final concentration of ≤10 mg/mL. Gently invert to mix; do not shake. Discard any unused portion remaining in the vial.

Mechanism of Action Recombinant human IgG2 monoclonal antibody which binds specifically to the epidermal growth factor receptor (EGFR, HER1, c-ErbB-1) and competitively inhibits the binding of epidermal growth factor (EGF) and other ligands. Binding to the EGFR blocks phosphorylation and activation of intracellular tyrosine kinases, resulting in inhibition of cell survival, growth, proliferation and transformation. EGFR signal transduction may result in *KRAS* and *NRAS* wild-type activation; cells with *RAS* mutations appear to be unaffected by EGFR inhibition.

Pharmacodynamics/Kinetics Half-life elimination: ~7.5 days (range: 4 to 11 days)

Dosing

Adult & Geriatric

Colorectal cancer, metastatic, *KRAS* wild-type: IV: 6 mg/kg every 14 days as a single agent (Van Cutsem, 2007) or in combination with FOLFOX (fluorouracil, leucovorin, and oxaliplatin) (Douillard, 2010; Douillard, 2013); continue until disease progression or unacceptable toxicity (Douillard, 2010; Van Cutsem, 2007)

Colorectal cancer, metastatic, *KRAS* wild-type in combination with FOLFIRI (fluorouracil, leucovorin, and irinotecan; off-label combination): IV: 6 mg/kg every 14 days; continue until disease progression or unacceptable toxicity (Peeters, 2010)

Missed dose (Canadian labeling): Doses should be administered within 3 days before or after the scheduled dose (unless withheld for toxicity). If a dose is missed, administer as soon as possible; the next dose then should be administered on a new every 2 week schedule based on the day of the most recently administered dose.

Renal Impairment There are no dosage adjustments provided in the manufacturer's labeling (has not been studied).

Hepatic Impairment There are no dosage adjustments provided in the manufacturer's labeling (has not been studied).

Adjustment for Toxicity

Infusion reactions, mild-to-moderate (grade 1 or 2): Reduce the infusion rate by 50% for the duration of infusion.

Infusion reactions, severe (grade 3 or 4): Stop infusion; consider permanent discontinuation (depending on severity or persistence of reaction).

Dermatologic toxicity:

Grade 3 toxicity (first occurrence): Withhold 1 to 2 doses; if reaction improves to <grade 3, resume therapy at initial dose.

Grade 3 toxicity (second occurrence): Withhold 1 to 2 doses; if reaction improves to <grade 3, resume therapy at 80% of initial dose.

Grade 3 toxicity (third occurrence): Withhold 1 to 2 doses; if reaction improves to <grade 3, resume therapy at 60% of initial dose.

Grade 3 toxicity (fourth occurrence), grade 3 toxicity that does not recover to <grade 3 after withholding 1 or 2 doses, or grade 4 toxicity: Permanently discontinue.

Ocular toxicity (acute or worsening keratitis): Interrupt or discontinue treatment.

Pulmonary toxicity:

Acute onset or worsening pulmonary symptoms: Interrupt treatment.

Interstitial lung disease: Permanently discontinue treatment.

Combination Regimens

Colorectal cancer:

Panitumumab (Colorectal Regimen) on page 2058

Panitumumab + FOLFIRI (Colorectal) on page 2058

Panitumumab + FOLFOX4 (Colorectal) on page 2059

Administration IV: Administer via infusion pump; do not administer IV push or as a bolus. Doses ≤1000 mg, infuse over 1 hour; if first infusion is tolerated, subsequent doses may be administered over 30 to 60 minutes. Doses >1000 mg, infuse over 90 minutes. Administer through a low protein-binding 0.2 or 0.22 micrometer in-line filter. Flush line with NS before and after infusion; do not mix or administer with other medications. Reduce infusion rate by 50% for mild-to-moderate infusion reactions (grades 1 and 2); stop infusion for severe infusion reactions (grades 3 and 4) and consider permanent discontinuation. Appropriate medical support for the management of infusion reactions should be readily available.

Emetic Potential

Children: Minimal (<10%)

Adults: Low (10% to 30%)

Monitoring Parameters *KRAS* genotyping of tumor tissue. Monitor serum electrolytes, including magnesium and calcium (periodically during and for at least 8 weeks after therapy), and potassium. Monitor vital signs and temperature before, during, and after infusion. Monitor for skin toxicity, for evidence of ocular toxicity, and for acute onset or worsening pulmonary symptoms.

◀ **Dosage Forms** Excipient information presented when available (limited, particularly for generics); consult specific product labeling.

Solution, Intravenous [preservative free]:

Vectibix: 100 mg/5 mL (5 mL); 400 mg/20 mL (20 mL)

Panobinostat (pan oh BIN oh stat)

Related Information

Management of Chemotherapy-Induced Nausea and Vomiting in Adults *on page 2142*

Principles of Anticancer Therapy *on page 2261*

Safe Handling of Hazardous Drugs *on page 2292*

Brand Names: US Farydak

Index Terms Faridak; LBH589; Panobinostat Lactate

Pharmacologic Category Antineoplastic Agent, Histone Deacetylase (HDAC) Inhibitor

Use Multiple myeloma: Treatment of multiple myeloma (in combination with bortezomib and dexamethasone) in patients who have received at least 2 prior regimens, including bortezomib and an immunomodulatory agent.

Labeled Contraindications There are no contraindications listed in the manufacturer's labeling.

Pregnancy Considerations Adverse events were observed in animal reproduction studies. Pregnancy should be ruled out prior to treatment. Women of reproductive potential should avoid pregnancy and use an effective contraceptive during therapy and for 1 month after treatment. Males should use condoms during therapy and for 3 months after treatment.

Breast-Feeding Considerations It is not known if panobinostat is excreted into breast milk. Due to the potential for serious adverse reactions in the nursing infant, the manufacturer recommends a decision be made to discontinue nursing or to discontinue the drug, taking into account the importance of treatment to the mother.

Warnings/Precautions Hazardous agent; use appropriate precautions for handling and disposal (meets NIOSH 2014 criteria).

[US Boxed Warning]: Severe diarrhea occurred in one-fourth of panobinostat treated patients. Monitor for symptoms, institute antidiarrheal treatment, interrupt panobinostat, and then reduce dose or discontinue panobinostat. Any grade diarrhea was reported in over two-thirds of patients, and may occur at any time. Monitor hydration status and serum electrolytes (including magnesium, potassium, and phosphate). Patients should have antidiarrheal medications available for use; begin antidiarrheal medications at the first sign of diarrhea, loose stools, or abdominal cramping. Interrupt panobinostat treatment for moderate diarrhea (4 to 6 stools per day). Panobinostat is associated with nausea and vomiting (moderate emetic potential); consider antiemetics to prevent nausea and vomiting. Some antiemetics known to prolong the QT interval (eg, dolasetron or ondansetron) may be used with frequent ECG monitoring.

[US Boxed Warning]: Severe and fatal cardiac ischemic events, severe arrhythmias, and ECG changes have occurred in patients receiving panobinostat. Arrhythmias may be exacerbated by electrolyte abnormalities. Obtain ECG and electrolytes at baseline and periodically during treatment as clinically indicated. ECG abnormalities including ST-segment depression and T-wave abnormalities have been observed. Monitor and correct electrolyte abnormalities as needed. Panobinostat may prolong the

QT interval. Do not initiate treatment in patients with a QTcF >450 msec or with clinically significant baseline ST-segment or T-wave abnormalities. Interrupt treatment if QTcF increases to ≥480 msec; correct electrolyte abnormalities; if QT prolongation does not resolve, permanently discontinue panobinostat. Concomitant use with mediations known to prolong the QT interval is not recommended. Do not initiate panobinostat treatment in patients with a history of recent MI or unstable angina.

Severe thrombocytopenia, neutropenia and anemia have occurred; may require treatment interruption, dosage modification, discontinuation, transfusion or granulocyte colony-stimulating factor support. Monitor CBC with differential at baseline and during treatment; patients >65 years may require more frequent monitoring. Serious and fatal hemorrhage has occurred, including grade 3 and 4 hemorrhage. All patients with hemorrhage also experienced thrombocytopenia at the time of hemorrhage. Localized and systemic infections (including pneumonia, bacterial infections, invasive fungal infections, and viral infections) have been observed; infections may be severe (or fatal). Do not initiate treatment in patients with active infections. Monitor for sings/symptoms of infections during treatment. If infection occurs, begin appropriate management and consider interrupting or discontinuing panobinostat.

Hepatic dysfunction (transaminase and total bilirubin elevations) has been reported. Monitor liver function prior to and during treatment. If liver function tests are abnormal, consider dosage adjustments and monitor until liver function returns to normal or baseline. Initial dose should be reduced in patients with mild-to-moderate hepatic impairment; avoid use in patients with severe impairment. Potentially significant drug-drug/drug-food interactions may exist, requiring dose or frequency adjustment, additional monitoring, and/or selection of alternative therapy.

Adverse Reactions Frequency not always defined.

>10%:

Cardiovascular: Abnormal T waves on ECG (40%), peripheral edema (29%; grades 3/4: 2%), depression of ST segment on ECG (22%), cardiac arrhythmia (12%; grades 3/4: 3%)

Central nervous system: Fatigue (≤60%, grades 3/4: ≤25%), lethargy (≤60%; grades 3/4: ≤25%), malaise (≤60%; grades 3/4: ≤25%)

Endocrine & metabolic: Hypocalcemia (67%; grades 3/4: 5%), hypoalbuminemia (63%; grades 3/4: 2%), hypophosphatemia (63%; grades 3/4: 20%), hypokalemia (52%; grades 3/4: 18%), hyponatremia (49%; grades 3/4: 13%), hyperphosphatemia (29%; grades 3/4: 2%), hypermagnesemia (27%; grades 3/4: 5%), weight loss (12%; grades 3/4: 2%)

Gastrointestinal: Diarrhea (68%; grades 3/4: 25%), nausea (36%; grades 3/4: 6%), decreased appetite (28%; grades 3/4: 3%), vomiting (26%; grades 3/4: 7%)

Hematologic & oncologic: Thrombocytopenia (97%; grades 3/4: 67%), lymphocytopenia (82%; grades 3/4: 53%), leukopenia (81%; grades 3/4: 23%), neutropenia (75%; grades 3/4: 34%), anemia (62%; grades 3/4: 18%)

Hepatic: Hyperbilirubinemia (21%; grades 3/4: 1%)

Infection: Severe infection (31%; includes bacterial, fungal, and viral infections)

Neuromuscular & skeletal: Weakness (≤60%; grades ≥3: ≤25%)

Renal: Increased serum creatinine (41%; grades 3/4: 1%)

Miscellaneous: Fever (26%)

◀ 1% to 10%:

Cardiovascular: Hypertension (>2% to <10%), hypotension (>2% to <10%), orthostatic hypotension (>2% to <10%), palpitations (>2% to <10%), syncope (>2% to <10%), ischemic heart disease (4%), ECG changes, prolonged Q-T interval on ECG

Central nervous system: Chills (>2% to <10%), dizziness (>2% to <10%), headache (>2% to <10%), insomnia (>2% to <10%)

Dermatologic: Cheilitis (>2% to <10%), erythema (>2% to <10%), skin lesion (>2% to <10%), skin rash (>2% to <10%)

Endocrine & metabolic: Dehydration (>2% to <10%), fluid retention (>2% to <10%), hyperglycemia (>2% to <10%), hyperuricemia (>2% to <10%), hypomagnesemia (>2% to <10%), hypothyroidism (>2% to <10%)

Gastrointestinal: Abdominal distention (>2% to <10%), abdominal pain (>2% to <10%), colitis (>2% to <10%), dysgeusia (>2% to <10%), dyspepsia (>2% to <10%), flatulence (>2% to <10%), gastritis (>2% to <10%), gastrointestinal pain (>2% to <10%), xerostomia (>2% to <10%), gastrointestinal toxicity

Genitourinary: Urinary incontinence (>2% to <10%)

Hematologic & oncologic: Hemorrhage (grades 3/4: 4%)

Hepatic: Hepatitis B (>2% to <10%), increased serum alkaline phosphatase (>2% to <10%), increased aminotransferases, increased serum bilirubin

Infection: Sepsis (6%)

Neuromuscular & skeletal: Joint swelling (>2% to <10%), tremor (>2% to <10%)

Renal: Increased blood urea nitrogen (>2% to <10%), mean glomerular filtration rate decreased (>2% to <10%), renal failure (>2% to <10%)

Respiratory: Cough (>2% to <10%), dyspnea (>2% to <10%), rales (>2% to <10%), respiratory failure (>2% to <10%), wheezing (>2% to <10%)

Drug Interactions

Metabolism/Transport Effects Substrate of CYP2C19 (minor), CYP2D6 (minor), CYP3A4 (major), P-glycoprotein; **Note:** Assignment of Major/Minor substrate status based on clinically relevant drug interaction potential; **Inhibits** CYP2D6 (moderate)

Avoid Concomitant Use

Avoid concomitant use of Panobinostat with any of the following: BCG (Intravesical); Conivaptan; CYP3A4 Inducers (Strong); Fusidic Acid (Systemic); Grapefruit Juice; Highest Risk QTc-Prolonging Agents; Idelalisib; Ivabradine; Mifepristone; Natalizumab; Pimecrolimus; Pomegranate; Star Fruit; Tacrolimus (Topical); Thioridazine; Tofacitinib; Vaccines (Live)

Increased Effect/Toxicity

Panobinostat may increase the levels/effects of: CYP2D6 Substrates; DOXOrubicin (Conventional); Fesoterodine; Fingolimod; Highest Risk QTc-Prolonging Agents; Leflunomide; Metoprolol; Moderate Risk QTc-Prolonging Agents; Natalizumab; Nebivolol; Thioridazine; Tofacitinib; Vaccines (Live)

The levels/effects of Panobinostat may be increased by: Aprepitant; Conivaptan; CYP3A4 Inhibitors (Moderate); CYP3A4 Inhibitors (Strong); Dasatinib; Denosumab; Dolasetron; Fosaprepitant; Fusidic Acid (Systemic); Granisetron; Grapefruit Juice; Idelalisib; Ivabradine; Ivacaftor; Luliconazole; Mifepristone; Netupitant; Ondansetron; Palbociclib; Pimecrolimus; Pomegranate; QTc-Prolonging Agents (Indeterminate Risk and Risk Modifying); Roflumilast; Simeprevir; Star Fruit; Stiripentol; Tacrolimus (Topical); Trastuzumab

Decreased Effect

Panobinostat may decrease the levels/effects of: BCG (Intravesical); Coccidioides immitis Skin Test; Codeine; Sipuleucel-T; Tamoxifen; TraMADol; Vaccines (Inactivated); Vaccines (Live)

The levels/effects of Panobinostat may be decreased by: Bosentan; CYP3A4 Inducers (Moderate); CYP3A4 Inducers (Strong); Dabrafenib; Deferasirox; Echinacea; Siltuximab; St Johns Wort; Tocilizumab

Food Interactions Star fruit, pomegranate or pomegranate juice, and grapefruit or grapefruit juice may interfere with panobinostat metabolism. Management: Avoid star fruit, pomegranate or pomegranate juice, and grapefruit or grapefruit juice.

Storage/Stability Store at 20°C to 25°C (68°F to 77°F); excursions are permitted between 15°C and 30°C (59°F and 86°F). Store blister pack in original carton. Protect from light.

Mechanism of Action Panobinostat is a histone deacetylase (HDAC) inhibitor; inhibits enzymatic activity of HDACs resulting in increased acetylation of histone proteins. Accumulation of acetylated histones and other proteins induces cell cycle arrest and/or apoptosis of some transformed cells. Panobinostat has minimal activity in multiple myeloma as a single-agent; however, synergistic activity is demonstrated when combined with bortezomib and dexamethasone (San-Miguel 2014).

Pharmacodynamics/Kinetics

Protein binding: ~90% to plasma proteins

Metabolism: Extensive via reduction, hydrolysis, oxidation, and glucuronidation; CYP3A4 accounts for ~40% of elimination, CYP2D6 and CYP2C19 are minor pathways.

Bioavailability: ~21%; AUC is 16% lower (compared with fasting) when administered with a high-fat meal.

Half-life elimination: ~37 hours

Time to peak: Within 2 hours

Excretion: Feces (44% to 77%; <4% as unchanged drug); Urine (29% to 51%; <3% as unchanged drug)

Dosing

Adult & Geriatric Determine QTcF prior to the start of therapy and verify that QTcF <450 msec prior to panobinostat initiation. Baseline ANC should be at least 1,500/mm³ and platelets at least 100,000/mm³ prior to treatment. Panobinostat is associated with a moderate emetic potential; consider antiemetics to prevent nausea and vomiting.

Multiple myeloma: Adults: Oral: 20 mg once every other day for 3 doses each week during weeks 1 and 2 of a 21-day treatment cycle (eg, Monday, Wednesday, and Friday of weeks 1 and 2 only, rest during week 3) for up to 8 cycles (in combination with bortezomib and dexamethasone); treatment may continue (the same schedule for panobinostat; bortezomib and dexamethasone schedules are modified) for an additional 8 cycles in patients experiencing clinical benefit and acceptable toxicity (San-Miguel 2014). The total duration of therapy may be up to 16 cycles (48 weeks).

Missed doses: Missed doses may be taken up to 12 hours after the scheduled time. Do not repeat the dose if vomiting occurs; patients should take the next usual scheduled dose.

◄ **Dosage adjustment for concomitant therapy:**

CYP2D6 substrates: Avoid coadministration with sensitive CYP2D6 substrates (eg, atomoxetine, desipramine, dextromethorphan, metoprolol, nebivolol, perphenazine, tolterodine, venlafaxine) or CYP2D6 substrates that have a narrow therapeutic index (eg, thioridazine, pimozide).

Strong CYP3A inducers: Avoid concomitant use with strong CYP3A inducers.

Strong CYP3A inhibitors: Reduce the starting panobinostat dose to 10 mg with strong CYP3A inhibitors (eg, boceprevir, clarithromycin, conivaptin, indinavir, itraconazole, ketoconazole, lopinavir/ritonavir, nefazodone, nelfinavir, posaconazole, ritonavir, saquinavir, telaprevir, telithromycin, voriconazole).

Renal Impairment

Mild to severe impairment (CrCl <80 mL/minute): There are no dosage adjustments provided in the manufacturer's labeling. However, based on a pharmacokinetic study of a single 30 mg dose, renal impairment does not appear to impact panobinostat exposure in patients with mild, moderate, and severe renal impairment (excluding dialysis patients), and initial dosage adjustment is not necessary (Sharma 2015).

End-stage renal disease (ESRD) and ESRD on dialysis: There are no dosage adjustments provided in the manufacturer's labeling (has not been studied). The dialyzability of panobinostat is unknown.

Hepatic Impairment

Hepatic impairment *prior to* treatment:

Mild impairment (bilirubin ≤1 times ULN and AST >1 times ULN or bilirubin >1 to 1.5 times ULN and any AST): Reduce initial dose to 15 mg; monitor frequently for adverse events and adjust dose as needed for toxicity.

Moderate impairment (bilirubin >1.5 to 3 times ULN and any AST): Reduce initial dose to 10 mg; monitor frequently for adverse events and adjust dose as needed for toxicity.

Severe impairment: Avoid use.

Hepatic impairment *during* treatment: If liver function tests are abnormal, consider dosage adjustments and monitor until liver function returns to normal or baseline.

Adjustment for Toxicity If dose reductions are necessary, keep the same treatment schedule and reduce panobinostat dose in increments of 5 mg (from 20 mg to 15 mg, from 15 mg to 10 mg); if dose reduction below 10 mg 3 times a week is necessary, discontinue treatment.

Hematologic toxicity:

Thrombocytopenia:

Grade 3 (platelets <50,000/mm^3): No dosage adjustments are necessary; monitor platelets weekly.

Grade 3 (platelets <50,000/mm^3) with bleeding: Interrupt panobinostat treatment, monitor platelets weekly until platelets ≥50,000/mm^3 and then restart panobinostat at a reduced dose. (Interrupt bortezomib until platelets ≥75,000/mm^3; if only 1 dose omitted, restart bortezomib at the same dose; if ≥2 consecutive doses or doses within the same cycle are omitted, then restart bortezomib at a reduced dose.)

Grade 4 (platelets <25,000/mm^3): Interrupt panobinostat treatment, monitor platelets weekly until platelets ≥50,000/mm^3 and then restart panobinostat at a reduced dose. (Interrupt bortezomib until platelets ≥75,000/mm^3; if only 1 dose omitted, restart bortezomib at the same dose; if ≥2 consecutive doses or doses within the same cycle are omitted, then restart bortezomib at a reduced dose.)

Severe thrombocytopenia: Consider platelet transfusions. Discontinue panobinostat if thrombocytopenia does not improve despite treatment modifications or if repeated platelet transfusions are required.

Neutropenia:

Grade 3 (ANC 750 to 1,000/mm^3): No dosage adjustments are necessary.

Grade 3 (ANC 500 to 750/mm^3 [2 or more occurrences]): Interrupt panobinostat treatment until ANC ≥1,000/mm^3 and then restart at the same dose. (Bortezomib dosage adjustment is not necessary.)

Grade 3 (ANC <1,000/mm^3) with neutropenic fever: Interrupt panobinostat treatment until neutropenic fever resolves and ANC ≥1,000/mm^3 and then restart at a reduced dose. (Interrupt bortezomib until neutropenic fever resolves and ANC ≥1,000/mm^3; if only 1 dose omitted, restart bortezomib at the same dose; if ≥2 consecutive doses or doses within the same cycle are omitted, then restart bortezomib at a reduced dose.)

Grade 4 (ANC <500/mm^3): Interrupt panobinostat treatment until ANC ≥1,000/mm^3 and then restart at a reduced dose. (Interrupt bortezomib until ANC ≥1,000/mm^3; if only 1 dose omitted, restart bortezomib at the same dose; if ≥2 consecutive doses or doses within the same cycle are omitted, then restart bortezomib at a reduced dose.)

Neutropenia, grade 3 or 4: Consider growth factor support or dose modification; if neutropenia does not improve or if severe infection occurs despite dose modification or growth factor support, discontinue panobinostat.

Anemia: Grade 3 (hemoglobin <8 g/dL): Interrupt panobinostat until hemoglobin ≥10 g/dL and then restart at a reduced dose.

Nonhematologic toxicity:

Cardiovascular: QTcF increase to ≥480 msec: Interrupt panobinostat treatment; correct electrolyte abnormalities. If QT prolongation does not resolve then permanently discontinue panobinostat.

Diarrhea:

First sign of abdominal cramping, loose stools, or onset of diarrhea: Begin antidiarrheal medication (eg, loperamide).

Grade 2 (moderate diarrhea; 4 to 6 stools per day): Interrupt panobinostat until resolved and then restart at the same dose. (Consider interruption of bortezomib until resolved and then restart at the same dose.)

Grade 3 (severe diarrhea; ≥7 stools per day, IV fluids or hospitalization required): Interrupt panobinostat treatment until resolved and then restart at a reduced dose. (Interrupt bortezomib until resolved and then restart at a reduced dose.)

Grade 4 (life-threatening): Permanently discontinue panobinostat. (Permanently discontinue bortezomib.)

Infection: Consider interrupting or discontinuing panobinostat.

Nausea or vomiting (panobinostat is associated with nausea and vomiting; consider prophylactic antiemetics):

Severe nausea (grades 3/4): Interrupt panobinostat treatment until resolved and then restart at a reduced dose.

Severe/life-threatening vomiting (grades 3/4): Interrupt panobinostat treatment until resolved and then restart at a reduced dose.

Other toxicities:

Grade 3 or 4 toxicity or recurrent grade 2 toxicity: Withhold panobinostat treatment until recovery to grade 1 or less and then restart at a reduced dose.

Recurrent grade 3 or 4 toxicity: Withhold panobinostat treatment until recovery to grade 1 or less and then restart at a reduced dose.

Combination Regimens

Multiple myeloma: Panobinostat-Bortezomib-Dexamethasone (Multiple Myeloma) on page 2059

Administration Panobinostat is associated with a moderate emetic potential; consider antiemetics to prevent nausea and vomiting. Administer orally at approximately the same time on scheduled days. May administer with or without food. Swallow capsule whole with a cup of water. Do not open, crush, or chew the capsules.

Hazardous agent; use appropriate precautions for handling and disposal (meets NIOSH 2014 criteria). Avoid exposure to crushed and/or broken capsules. Avoid direct skin or mucous membrane contact with powder inside the capsules; if contact occurs, wash thoroughly.

Emetic Potential Moderate (30% to 90%)

Monitoring Parameters CBC with differential and platelets (prior to treatment initiation then weekly or more often if clinically indicated during treatment); serum electrolytes, including potassium and magnesium prior to treatment and during treatment (in the clinical trial, electrolytes were monitored prior to the start of each cycle, after the fifth panobinostat dose in week 2 through cycle 8 and then at the beginning of cycles 9 to 16); liver function tests at baseline and regularly during treatment; pregnancy test (in women of reproductive potential, rule out pregnancy prior to and intermittently during treatment); ECG (prior to treatment initiation and periodically as clinically indicated during treatment); hydration status; monitor for gastrointestinal toxicity (eg, diarrhea, nausea, vomiting), signs/symptoms of hemorrhage and/or infection.

Dietary Considerations Avoid star fruit, pomegranate or pomegranate juice, and grapefruit or grapefruit juice.

Medication Guide Available Yes

Dosage Forms Excipient information presented when available (limited, particularly for generics); consult specific product labeling.

Capsule, Oral:

Farydak: 10 mg [contains brilliant blue fcf (fd&c blue #1)]

Farydak: 15 mg, 20 mg

◆ **Panobinostat Lactate** see Panobinostat on page 1322

◆ **Panretin** see Alitretinoin (Topical) on page 73

Papillomavirus (9-Valent) Vaccine (Human, Recombinant)

(pap ih LO ma VYE rus nine VAY lent vak SEEN YU man ree KOM be nant)

Brand Names: US Gardasil 9

Index Terms HPV9

Pharmacologic Category Vaccine; Vaccine, Inactivated (Viral)

Use

Prevention of human papillomavirus infection:

Females 9 to 26 years of age:

For the prevention of the following diseases:

Cervical, vulvar, vaginal, and anal cancer caused by human papillomavirus (HPV) types 16, 18, 31, 33, 45, 52, and 58

Genital warts (condyloma acuminata) caused by HPV types 6 and 11

For the prevention of the following precancerous or dysplastic lesions caused by HPV types 6, 11, 16, 18, 31, 33, 45, 52, and 58:

Cervical intraepithelial neoplasia (CIN) grades 1, 2, and 3

Cervical adenocarcinoma in situ (AIS)

Vulvar intraepithelial neoplasia (VIN) grades 2 and 3

Vaginal intraepithelial neoplasia (VaIN) grades 2 and 3

Anal intraepithelial neoplasia (AIN) grades 1, 2, and 3

Males 9 through 15 years of age:

For the prevention of the following diseases:

Anal cancer caused by HPV types 16, 18, 31, 33, 45, 52, and 58

Genital warts (condyloma acuminata) caused by HPV types 6 and 11

For the prevention of the following precancerous or dysplastic lesions caused by HPV types 6, 11, 16, 18, 31, 33, 45, 52, and 58:

Anal intraepithelial neoplasia (AIN) grades 1, 2, and 3

The Advisory Committee on Immunization Practices (ACIP) recommends routine vaccination for females and males 11 to 12 years of age; can be administered as young as 9 years; catch-up vaccination is recommended for females 13 to 26 years of age and males 13 to 21 years of age. Vaccination for males 22 through 26 years of age is recommended if immunocompromised (including HIV) and for men who have sex with men and may be considered for any other male in this age group (CDC/ACIP [Petrosky 2015]).

Pregnancy Risk Factor B

Dosing

Adult

Immunization: IM: Females ≤26 years: 0.5 mL at 0, 2, and 6 months

CDC/ACIP recommended immunization schedule: 0.5 mL per dose for a total of 3 doses; administer the second and third doses at 2 and 6 months after initial dose. There should be a 1-month minimum interval between the first and second dose; a 3-month minimum interval between the second and third dose; a 6-month minimum interval between the first and third dose. Begin series in females ≤26 years or males ≤21 years if not previously vaccinated or completed the 3-dose series (typically administer first dose at age 11 to 12 years). Vaccination for males 22 through 26 years of age is recommended if immunocompromised (including HIV) and for men who have sex with men and may be considered for any other male in this age group. Second and third doses may be given after age 26 years to complete a previously initiated series (CDC/ACIP [Petrosky 2015]).

Pediatric

Immunization: IM:

Females: Children ≥9 years and Adolescents: 0.5 mL at 0, 2, and 6 months

Males: Children ≥9 years and, Adolescents ≤15 years: 0.5 mL at 0, 2, and 6 months

◀ CDC/ACIP recommended immunization schedule: Children ≥9 years and Adolescents: IM: 0.5 mL per dose for a total of 3 doses administered as follows: Initial dose followed by a second dose at 1 to 2 months after initial and third doses at 6 months after the initial. Administer first dose at age 11 to 12 years although series may be initiated as early as 9 years of age. Minimum interval between first and second doses is 4 weeks; the minimum interval between the second and third dose is 12 weeks; the minimum interval between first and third doses is 24 weeks; begin series in females ages 13 to 26 years or males 13 to 21 years if not previously vaccinated or who have not completed the 3-dose series. Males may also be vaccinated 22 through 26 years of age. Second and third doses may be given after age 26 years to complete a previously initiated series (CDC/ACIP [Petrosky 2015]).

Renal Impairment There are no dosage adjustments provided in the manufacturer's labeling.

Hepatic Impairment There are no dosage adjustments provided in the manufacturer's labeling.

Additional Information Complete prescribing information should be consulted for additional detail.

Dosage Forms Excipient information presented when available (limited, particularly for generics); consult specific product labeling.

Suspension, Intramuscular [preservative free]:

Gardasil 9: (0.5 mL) [contains polysorbate 80, yeast extract]

Suspension Prefilled Syringe, Intramuscular [preservative free]:

Gardasil 9: (0.5 mL) [contains polysorbate 80, yeast extract]

Papillomavirus (Types 6, 11, 16, 18) Vaccine (Human, Recombinant)

(pap ih LO ma VYE rus typs six e LEV en SIX teen AYE teen vak SEEN YU man ree KOM be nant)

Brand Names: US Gardasil

Brand Names: Canada Gardasil

Index Terms HPV Vaccine (Quadrivalent); HPV4; Human Papillomavirus Vaccine (Quadrivalent); Papillomavirus Vaccine, Recombinant; Quadrivalent Human Papillomavirus Vaccine

Pharmacologic Category Vaccine; Vaccine, Inactivated (Viral)

Use

Prevention of human papillomavirus infection:

US labeling:

Females 9 to 26 years of age:

For the prevention of the following diseases: Cervical, vulvar, vaginal, and anal cancer caused by HPV types 16 and 18; genital warts (condyloma acuminatum) caused by HPV types 6 and 11

For the prevention of the following precancerous or dysplastic lesions caused by HPV types 6, 11, 16, and 18: Cervical intraepithelial neoplasia (CIN) grade 2/3 and cervical adenocarcinoma in situ; CIN grade 1; vulvar intraepithelial neoplasia grade 2 and 3; vaginal intraepithelial neoplasia grade 2 and 3; and anal intraepithelial neoplasia grades 1, 2, and 3.

Males 9 through 26 years of age:

For the prevention of the following diseases: anal cancer caused by HPV types 16 and 18; genital warts (condyloma acuminata) caused by HPV types 6 and 11

For the prevention of anal intraepithelial neoplasia grades 1, 2, and 3 caused by HPV types 6, 11, 16, and 18.

Limitations of use: Does not provide protection against vaccine HPV types to which a person has already been previously exposed, or HPV types not contained in the vaccine; does not prevent CIN grade 2/3 or worse in women >26 years of age. Not intended for the treatment of active external genital lesions or cervical, vulvar, vaginal, and anal cancers.

Canadian labeling:

Females ≥9 years and ≤26 years of age: Prevention of anal cancer caused by HPV types 16 and 18; anal intraepithelial neoplasia caused by HPV types 6, 11, 16, and 18

Females ≥9 years and ≤45 years of age: Prevention of cervical, vulvar, and vaginal cancer caused by HPV types 16 and 18; genital warts caused by HPV types 6 and 11; cervical adenocarcinoma *in situ*, vulvar, vaginal, or cervical intraepithelial neoplasia caused by HPV types 6, 11, 16, and 18

Males ≥9 years and ≤26 years of age: Prevention of anal cancer caused by HPV types 16 and 18; anal intraepithelial neoplasia caused by HPV types 6, 11, 16, and 18; genital warts caused by HPV types 6 and 11

The Advisory Committee on Immunization Practices (ACIP) recommends routine vaccination for females and males 11 to 12 years of age; can be administered as young as 9 years; catch-up vaccination is recommended for females 13 to 26 years of age and males 13 to 21 years of age. Vaccination for males 22 through 26 years of age is recommended if immunocompromised (including HIV) and for men who have sex with men and may be considered for any other male in this age group (CDC/ACIP [Markowitz 2014]; CDC/ACIP [Strikas 2015]).

Pregnancy Risk Factor B

Dosing

Adult Immunization regimen:

US labeling: IM: Adults ≤26 years: 0.5 mL per dose for a total of 3 doses; administer the second and third doses at 2 and 6 months after initial dose

Canadian labeling: IM: Adults ≤45 years: 0.5 mL per dose for a total of 3 doses; administer the second and third doses at 2 and 6 months after initial dose

CDC/ACIP recommended immunization schedule: 0.5 mL per dose for a total of 3 doses; administer the second and third doses at 1 to 2 and 6 months after initial dose. There should be a 4-week minimum interval between the first and second dose; a 12-weeks minimum interval (16 weeks preferred) between the second and third dose; a 24-week minimum interval between the first and third dose. Begin series in females ≤26 years or males ≤21 years if not previously vaccinated or completed the 3-dose series (typically administer first dose at age 11 to 12 years). Vaccination for males 22 through 26 years of age is recommended if immunocompromised (including HIV) and for men who have sex with men and may be considered for any other male in this age group. Second and third doses may be given after age 26 years to complete a previously initiated series. The HPV vaccine series should be completed with the same product whenever possible (CDC/ACIP [Kim 2015]; CDC/ACIP [Markowitz 2014]).

◄ **Pediatric**

Immunization: IM:

US labeling: Children ≥9 years and Adolescents: 0.5 mL per dose for a total of 3 doses; administer the second and third doses at 2 and 6 months after initial dose

Canadian labeling: Children ≥9 years and Adolescents: 0.5 mL per dose for a total of 3 doses; administer the second and third doses at 2 and 6 months after initial dose

CDC/ACIP recommended immunization schedule: 0.5 mL per dose for a total of 3 doses; administer the second and third doses at 1 to 2 and 6 months after initial dose. There should be a 4-week minimum interval between the first and second dose; a 12-weeks minimum interval (16 weeks preferred) between the second and third dose; a 24-week minimum interval between the first and third dose. Typically, administer first dose at age 11 to 12 years but may administer as young as 9 years; begin series in adolescents (≥13 years) if not previously vaccinated or who have not completed the 3-dose series (CDC/ACIP [Markowitz 2014]; CDC/ACIP [Strikas 2015]).

Renal Impairment There are no dosage adjustments provided in the manufacturer's labeling.

Hepatic Impairment There are no dosage adjustments provided in the manufacturer's labeling.

Additional Information Complete prescribing information should be consulted for additional detail.

Medication Guide Available Yes

Dosage Forms Excipient information presented when available (limited, particularly for generics); consult specific product labeling.

Injection, suspension [preservative free]:

Gardasil: HPV 6 L1 protein 20 mcg, HPV 11 L1 protein 40 mcg, HPV 16 L1 protein 40 mcg, and HPV 18 L1 protein 20 mcg per 0.5 mL (0.5 mL) [contains aluminum, polysorbate 80; manufactured using *S. cerevisiae* (baker's yeast)]

Papillomavirus (Types 16, 18) Vaccine (Human, Recombinant)

(pap ih LO ma VYE rus typs SIX teen AYE teen vak SEEN YU man ree KOM be nant)

Brand Names: US Cervarix

Brand Names: Canada Cervarix

Index Terms Bivalent Human Papillomavirus Vaccine; GSK-580299; HPV 16/18 L1 VLP/AS04 VAC; HPV Vaccine (Bivalent); HPV2; Human Papillomavirus Vaccine (Bivalent); Papillomavirus Vaccine, Recombinant

Pharmacologic Category Vaccine; Vaccine, Inactivated (Viral)

Use

Prevention of human papillomavirus infection:

US labeling: Prevention in females 9 to 25 years of age of the following diseases caused by oncogenic HPV types 16 and 18: Cervical cancer, cervical intraepithelial neoplasia (CIN) grade 2 or higher and adenocarcinoma in situ, and CIN grade 1.

The Advisory Committee on Immunization Practices (ACIP) recommends routine vaccination for females 11 to 12 years of age; can be administered as young as 9 years; catch-up vaccination is recommended for females 13 to 26 years of age (CDC/ACIP [Markowitz, 2014]; CDC/ACIP [Strikas, 2015]).

Canadian labeling: Females 9 through 45 years of age: Prevention of cervical cancer, cervical adenocarcinoma *in situ*, and cervical intraepithelial neoplasia caused by human papillomavirus (HPV) types 16, 18

The National Advisory Committee on Immunization (NACI) recommends routine vaccination for females between 9 and 26 years of age. It should not be administered in females <9 years but may be administered to females >26 years who are at ongoing risk of exposure (NACI [CCDR, 2012]).

Pregnancy Risk Factor B

Dosing

Adult Immunization: IM:

US labeling: Females ≤25 years: 0.5 mL at 0, 1, and 6 months

CDC/ACIP recommended immunization schedule: 0.5 mL per dose for a total of 3 doses; administer the second and third doses at 1 to 2 and 6 months after initial dose. There should be a 4-week minimum interval between the first and second dose; a 12-weeks minimum interval (16 weeks preferred) between the second and third dose; a 24-week minimum interval between the first and third dose. Begin series in females ≤26 years if not previously vaccinated or who have not completed the 3 dose series (typically administer first dose at age 11 to 12 years). If a female reaches 27 years of age before the vaccination series is complete, the remaining doses can be administered after age 26 years. Inadequate doses or doses received following a shorter than recommended dosing interval should be repeated. The HPV vaccine series should be completed with the same product whenever possible (CDC/ACIP [Kim, 2015]; CDC/ACIP [Markowitz, 2014]).

Canadian labeling: Females ≤45 years: 0.5 mL per dose for a total of 3 doses; administer the second and third doses at 1 and 6 months after initial dose; if necessary, may administer the second and third doses at 1 to 2.5 months and 5 to 12 months respectively after the initial dose.

Pediatric Immunization: IM:

US labeling: Children ≥9 years and Adolescents: Females: 0.5 mL per dose for a total of 3 doses; administer the second and third doses at 1 and 6 months after initial dose

CDC/ACIP recommended immunization schedule: 0.5 mL per dose for a total of 3 doses; administer the second and third doses at 1 to 2 and 6 months after initial dose. There should be a 4-week minimum interval between the first and second dose; a 12-weeks minimum interval (16 weeks preferred) between the second and third dose; a 24-week minimum interval between the first and third dose. Typically administer first dose to females at age 11 to 12 years but may administer as young as 9 years; begin series in female adolescents (≥13 years) if not previously vaccinated or who have not completed the 3-dose series. Inadequate doses or doses received following a shorter than recommended dosing interval should be repeated. The HPV vaccine series should be completed with the same product whenever possible (CDC/ACIP [Markowitz, 2014]; CDC/ACIP [Strikas, 2015]).

Canadian labeling: Children ≥9 years and Adolescents: Females: 0.5 mL per dose for a total of 3 doses; administer the second and third doses at 1 and 6 months after initial dose; if necessary, may administer the second and third doses at 1 to 2.5 months and 5 to 12 months respectively after the initial dose.

◄ **Renal Impairment** There are no dosage adjustments provided in the manufacturer's labeling.

Hepatic Impairment There are no dosage adjustments provided in the manufacturer's labeling.

Additional Information Complete prescribing information should be consulted for additional detail.

Medication Guide Available Yes

Dosage Forms Excipient information presented when available (limited, particularly for generics); consult specific product labeling.

Injection, suspension [preservative free]:

Cervarix: HPV 16 L1 protein 20 mcg and HPV 18 L1 protein 20 mcg per 0.5 mL (0.5 mL) [contains aluminum, natural rubber/natural latex in prefilled syringe; manufactured using *Trichoplusia ni* (insect cells)]

♦ **Papillomavirus Vaccine, Recombinant** see Papillomavirus (Types 6, 11, 16, 18) Vaccine (Human, Recombinant) *on page 1330*

♦ **Papillomavirus Vaccine, Recombinant** see Papillomavirus (Types 16, 18) Vaccine (Human, Recombinant) *on page 1332*

♦ **Paraplatin** see CARBOplatin *on page 270*

♦ **PARP inhibitor AZD2281** see Olaparib *on page 1245*

PAZOPanib (paz OH pa nib)

Related Information

Management of Chemotherapy-Induced Nausea and Vomiting in Adults *on page 2142*

Principles of Anticancer Therapy *on page 2261*

Safe Handling of Hazardous Drugs *on page 2292*

Brand Names: US Votrient

Brand Names: Canada Votrient

Index Terms GW786034; Pazopanib Hydrochloride

Pharmacologic Category Antineoplastic Agent, Tyrosine Kinase Inhibitor; Antineoplastic Agent, Vascular Endothelial Growth Factor (VEGF) Inhibitor

Use

Renal cell carcinoma, advanced: Treatment of advanced renal cell carcinoma

Soft tissue sarcoma, advanced: Treatment of advanced soft tissue sarcoma (in patients who have received prior chemotherapy)

Limitations of use: The efficacy of pazopanib for the treatment of adipocytic soft tissue sarcoma or gastrointestinal stromal tumors has not been demonstrated.

Labeled Contraindications

There are no contraindications listed in the manufacturer's US labeling.

Canadian labeling: Hypersensitivity to pazopanib or any component of the formulation; use in pediatric patients <2 years of age (due to the antiangiogenic effects)

Pregnancy Considerations Adverse effects were observed in animal reproduction studies. Based on its mechanism of action, pazopanib would be expected to cause fetal harm if administered to a pregnant woman. Women of childbearing potential should avoid becoming pregnant during treatment.

Breast-Feeding Considerations It is not known if pazopanib is excreted in breast milk. According to the manufacturer, the decision to continue or discontinue breast-feeding during therapy should take into account the risk of exposure to the infant and the benefits of treatment to the mother.

Warnings/Precautions Hazardous agent - use appropriate precautions for handling and disposal (NIOSH 2014 [group 1]). **[US Boxed Warning]: Severe and fatal hepatotoxicity (transaminase and bilirubin elevations) has been observed in studies. Monitor hepatic function and interrupt treatment, reduce dose, or discontinue as recommended.** Liver function testes should be monitored at baseline; at weeks 3, 5, 7, and 9; at months 3 and 4; and as clinically necessary, then periodically (after month 4). Transaminase elevations usually occur early in the treatment course. Use is not recommended in patients with preexisting severe hepatic impairment (bilirubin >3 times ULN with any ALT level); dosage reductions is recommended for preexisting moderate hepatic impairment (bilirubin >1.5 to 3 times ULN). Mild indirect (unconjugated) hyperbilirubinemia may occur in patients with Gilbert's syndrome; for patients with known Gilbert syndrome (only a mild indirect bilirubin elevation) and ALT >3 times ULN, follow isolated ALT elevation dosage modification recommendations.

Venous and arterial thromboembolism have been reported. DVT, pulmonary embolism, angina, transient ischemic attack, MI, and ischemic stroke were observed more frequently in the pazopanib group (versus placebo) in clinical trials. Fatalities were observed. Monitor for signs/symptoms of venous thrombotic events and pulmonary embolism. Use with caution in patients with a history of or an increased risk for these events. Use in patients with recent arteriothrombotic event (within 6 months) has not been studied and is not recommended. Thrombotic microangiopathy (TMA), including thrombotic thrombocytopenic purpura (TTP) and hemolytic uremic syndrome (HUS), has been observed in clinical studies. TMA has occurred with pazopanib monotherapy or when used in combination with bevacizumab or topotecan (off-label use); it typically occurs within 90 days of treatment initiation. Monitor for signs/symptoms and permanently discontinue in patients who develop TMA. Hemorrhagic events (including fatal events) have been reported. In clinical studies, the most common events in renal cell carcinoma patients were hematuria, epistaxis, hemoptysis, and rectal hemorrhage. Epistaxis, mouth hemorrhage, and anal hemorrhage were most common in soft tissue sarcoma patients. Use is not recommended in patients with a history of hemoptysis, cerebral hemorrhage or clinically significant gastrointestinal hemorrhage within 6 months (these populations were excluded from clinical trials).

May cause and/or worsen hypertension (hypertensive crisis has been observed); monitor frequently; blood pressure should be controlled prior to treatment initiation; antihypertensive therapy should be used if needed. Hypertension usually occurs early in the treatment course. Dosage reduction may be necessary for hypertension that is persistent despite management with antihypertensive therapy; discontinue for hypertensive crisis, or for severe and persistent hypertension which is refractory to dose reduction and antihypertensive therapy. May cause new-onset or worsening of existing heart failure; baseline and periodic LVEF monitoring is recommended in patients at increased risk of heart failure (eg, prior anthracycline treatment). Concurrent hypertension may increase the risk for cardiac dysfunction. Monitor for signs/symptoms of heart failure. QTc prolongation, including torsade de pointes, has been observed; use caution in patients with a history of QTc prolongation, with ▶

medications known to prolong the QT interval, or with preexisting cardiac disease. Obtain baseline and periodic ECGs; correct electrolyte (potassium, calcium, and magnesium) abnormalities prior to and during treatment.

Gastrointestinal perforation and fistula (including fatal events) have been reported; monitor for symptoms of gastrointestinal perforation and fistula. Proteinuria has been reported with use. Obtain baseline and periodic urinalysis and 24-hour urine protein when clinically indicated. Dosage reduction may be necessary for significant proteinuria (≥3 g/24 hours); discontinue for recurrent proteinuria. Interstitial lung disease (ILD)/pneumonitis has been reported with pazopanib; may be fatal. Monitor for pulmonary symptoms which could indicate ILD/pneumonitis; discontinue if ILD or pneumonitis develop. Hypothyroidism has been reported with use; monitor thyroid function tests. Vascular endothelial growth factor (VEGF) receptor inhibitors are associated with impaired wound healing. Discontinue treatment at least 7 days prior to scheduled surgery; treatment reinitiation should be guided by clinical judgment. Discontinue if wound dehiscence occurs.

Patients with mild-to-moderate renal impairment (CrCl ≥30 mL/minute) were included in trials. There are no pharmacokinetic data in patients with severe renal impairment undergoing dialysis (peritoneal and hemodialysis); however, renal impairment is not expected to significantly influence pazopanib pharmacokinetics or exposure. Potentially significant drug-drug interactions may exist, requiring dose or frequency adjustment, additional monitoring, and/or selection of alternative therapy. Increased toxicity and mortality has been observed in trials evaluating concurrent use of pazopanib with other chemotherapeutic agents (pemetrexed, lapatinib). Pazopanib is not approved for use in combination with other chemotherapy.

Hand-foot skin reaction (HFSR) observed with tyrosine kinase inhibitors (TKIs) is distinct from hand-foot syndrome (palmar-plantar erythrodysesthesia) associated with traditional chemotherapy agents. HFSR due to TKIs is localized with defined hyperkeratotic lesions; symptoms include burning, dysesthesia, paresthesia, or tingling of the palms/soles, and generally occur within the first 2 to 4 weeks of treatment. Pressure and flexor areas may develop blisters (callus-like), dry/cracked skin, edema, erythema, desquamation, or hyperkeratosis. The incidence of hand-foot skin reaction (HFSR) is lower with pazopanib (compared to other tyrosine kinase inhibitors). Examine skin at baseline (remove calluses with pedicure prior to treatment) and with each visit; apply an emollient based moisturizer twice daily during treatment. If HSFR develops, consider changing moisturizer to a urea-based product; topical steroids may be utilized for the anti-inflammatory effect; avoid excessive friction or pressure to affected areas and avoid restrictive footwear. Temporary dose reduction or treatment interruption may be necessary (Appleby 2011).

Reversible posterior leukoencephalopathy syndrome (RPLS) has been reported (rarely); may be fatal. Monitor for neurological changes or symptoms (blindness, confusion, headache, lethargy, seizure, visual or neurologic disturbances); permanently discontinue pazopanib in patients who develop RPLS. Serious, including fatal, infections have been reported; monitor for signs and symptoms of infection. Temporarily or permanently discontinue therapy for serious infections as clinically indicated. Patients >60 years of age may be at greater risk for transaminase elevations (ALT >3 time ULN). Patients ≥65 years of age experienced increased incidences of grade 3 or 4 fatigue, hypertension, decreased appetite, and transaminase elevations and are at increased risk for hepatotoxicity. Pazopanib is not approved for use in pediatric patients. Based on its mechanism of action, organ growth and maturation during early postnatal development may be affected. May potentially cause serious adverse effects on organ development, particularly in children <2 years of age.

Adverse Reactions Frequency not always defined.

Cardiovascular: Hypertension (40% to 42%; grade 3: 4% to 7%, early in treatment), bradycardia (2% to 19%), peripheral edema (STS: 14%), cardiac insufficiency (11% to 13%), chest pain (5% to 10%; STS, grade 3: 2%), left ventricular systolic dysfunction (STS: 8%), venous thrombosis (1% to 5%), ischemia (2%), myocardial infarction (2%), prolonged Q-T interval on ECG (2%), facial edema (1%), transient ischemic attacks (1%), decreased left ventricular ejection fraction, hypertensive crisis

Central nervous system: Fatigue (19%, grade 3: 2%; STS: 65%, grades 3/4: 1% to 13%), tumor pain (STS: 29%, grade 3: 8%), headache (10%; STS: 23%, grade 3: 1%), dizziness (11%), insomnia (STS: 9%), voice disorder (4% to 8%), chills (STS: 5%), reversible posterior leukoencephalopathy syndrome

Dermatologic: Hair discoloration (38% to 39%, grade 3: <1%), exfoliative dermatitis (STS: 18%, grade 3: <1%), skin rash (8%), alopecia (8% to 12%), dermatological disease (STS: 11%, grade 3: 2%), hypopigmentation (STS, skin: 11%), palmar-plantar erythrodysesthesia (6%), skin depigmentation (3%), xeroderma (STS: 6%), nail disease (STS: 5%)

Endocrine & metabolic: Weight loss (9%, STS: 48%, grade 3: 4%), increased serum glucose (41% to 45%, grade 3: <1%), increased thyroid-stimulating hormone (TSH), decreased serum albumin (STS: 34%, grade 3: 1%), decreased serum phosphate (34%, grade 3: 4%), decreased serum sodium (31%, grade 3: 1% to 4%), decreased serum magnesium (26%, grades 3/4: ≤1%), decreased serum glucose (17%, grade 4: <1%), increased serum potassium (STS: 16%, grade 3: 1%), hypothyroidism (4% to 8%)

Gastrointestinal: Diarrhea (52% to 59%; grades 3/4: ≤5%), nausea (26%, grade 3: <1%; STS: 56%, grade 3: 3%), decreased appetite (STS: 40%, grade 3: 6%), anorexia (22%, grade 3: 2%), vomiting (21%, grades 3/4: ≤2%; STS: 33%, grade 3: 3%), dysgeusia (8%, STS: 28%), increased serum lipase (27%, grades 3/4: 4%), gastrointestinal pain (STS: 23%, grade 3: 3%), abdominal pain (11%, grade 3: 2%), mucositis (STS: 12%, grade 3: 2%), stomatitis (STS: 11%, grade 3: <1%), dyspepsia (5% to 7%), anal hemorrhage (2%), gastrointestinal perforation (1%)

Genitourinary: Proteinuria (1% to 9%), hematuria (4%)

Hematologic & oncologic: Leukopenia (37% to 44%; STS, grade 3: 1%), lymphocytopenia (31%; grades 3/4: ≤4%; STS: 43%, grade 3: 10%), thrombocytopenia (32% to 36%; grades 3/4: ≤3%; grade 4: ≤1%), neutropenia (33% to 34%; grades 3/4: ≤4%), hemorrhage (13% to 22%, including pulmonary, gastrointestinal, and genitourinary, grade 4: 1%, including intracranial, subarachnoid, and peritoneal), oral hemorrhage (3%), rectal hemorrhage (1%), hemolytic-uremic syndrome, thrombotic thrombocytopenic purpura

Hepatic: Increased serum AST (51% to 53%; grades 3/4: ≤7%), increased serum ALT (4% to 53%; grades 3/4: 2% to 10%), increased serum bilirubin (29% to 36%; grades 3/4: ≤3%), increased serum alkaline phosphatase (STS: 32%, grade 3: 3%), hepatotoxicity, severe hepatotoxicity

Infection: Serious infection

1337

◀ Neuromuscular & skeletal: Musculoskeletal pain (STS: 23%, grade 3: 2%), myalgia (STS: 23%, grade 3: 2%), weakness (14%, grade 3: 3%), arthralgia, muscle spasm

Ophthalmic: Blurred vision (STS: 5%)

Respiratory: Dyspnea (STS: 20%, grades 3/4: ≤5%), cough (STS: 17%), epistaxis (2% to 8%), pneumothorax (≤3%), hemoptysis (2%)

Miscellaneous: Tumor pain (29%), fistula (1%)

<1%, postmarketing, and/or case reports: Cardiac disease, cerebral hemorrhage, cerebrovascular accident, congestive heart failure, nephrotic syndrome, pancreatitis, retinal detachment, torsade de pointes

Drug Interactions

Metabolism/Transport Effects Substrate of BCRP, CYP1A2 (minor), CYP2C8 (minor), CYP3A4 (major), P-glycoprotein; **Note:** Assignment of Major/Minor substrate status based on clinically relevant drug interaction potential; **Inhibits** CYP2C8 (weak), CYP2D6 (weak), CYP3A4 (weak), SLCO1B1, UGT1A1

Avoid Concomitant Use

Avoid concomitant use of PAZOPanib with any of the following: Amodiaquine; BCG (Intravesical); BCRP/ABCG2 Inhibitors; Conivaptan; CYP3A4 Inducers (Strong); Fusidic Acid (Systemic); Grapefruit Juice; H2-Antagonists; Highest Risk QTc-Prolonging Agents; Idelalisib; Irinotecan Products; Ivabradine; Lapatinib; Mifepristone; Natalizumab; P-glycoprotein/ABCB1 Inhibitors; Pimecrolimus; Pimozide; Proton Pump Inhibitors; Tacrolimus (Topical); Tofacitinib; Vaccines (Live)

Increased Effect/Toxicity

PAZOPanib may increase the levels/effects of: Amodiaquine; ARIPiprazole; Bisphosphonate Derivatives; Fingolimod; Highest Risk QTc-Prolonging Agents; Hydrocodone; Irinotecan Products; Leflunomide; Moderate Risk QTc-Prolonging Agents; Natalizumab; NiMODipine; Pimozide; Tofacitinib; Vaccines (Live)

The levels/effects of PAZOPanib may be increased by: Aprepitant; BCRP/ABCG2 Inhibitors; Conivaptan; CYP3A4 Inhibitors (Moderate); CYP3A4 Inhibitors (Strong); Dasatinib; Denosumab; Fosaprepitant; Fusidic Acid (Systemic); Grapefruit Juice; HMG-CoA Reductase Inhibitors; Idelalisib; Ivabradine; Lapatinib; Luliconazole; Mifepristone; Netupitant; Palbociclib; P-glycoprotein/ABCB1 Inhibitors; Pimecrolimus; QTc-Prolonging Agents (Indeterminate Risk and Risk Modifying); Roflumilast; Stiripentol; Tacrolimus (Topical); Trastuzumab

Decreased Effect

PAZOPanib may decrease the levels/effects of: BCG (Intravesical); Coccidioides immitis Skin Test; Sipuleucel-T; Vaccines (Inactivated); Vaccines (Live)

The levels/effects of PAZOPanib may be decreased by: Antacids; Bosentan; CYP3A4 Inducers (Moderate); CYP3A4 Inducers (Strong); Deferasirox; Echinacea; H2-Antagonists; P-glycoprotein/ABCB1 Inducers; Proton Pump Inhibitors; Siltuximab; St Johns Wort; Tocilizumab

Food Interactions Systemic exposure of pazopanib is increased when administered with food (AUC twofold higher with a meal). Grapefruit juice may increase the levels/effects of pazopanib. Management: Take on an empty stomach 1 hour before or 2 hours after a meal. Maintain adequate nutrition and hydration, unless instructed to restrict fluid intake. Avoid grapefruit/grapefruit juice.

Storage/Stability Store at 20°C to 25°C (68°F to 77°F); excursions are permitted between 15°C and 30°C (59°F and 86°F).

Mechanism of Action Tyrosine kinase (multikinase) inhibitor; limits tumor growth via inhibition of angiogenesis by inhibiting cell surface vascular endothelial growth factor receptors (VEGFR-1, VEGFR-2, VEGFR-3), platelet-derived growth factor receptors (PDGFR-alpha and -beta), fibroblast growth factor receptor (FGFR-1 and -3), cytokine receptor (cKIT), interleukin-2 receptor inducible T-cell kinase, leukocyte-specific protein tyrosine kinase (Lck), and transmembrane glycoprotein receptor tyrosine kinase (c-Fms)

Pharmacodynamics/Kinetics

Protein binding: >99%

Metabolism: Hepatic; primarily via CYP3A4, minor metabolism via CYP1A2 and CYP2C8

Bioavailability: Rate and extent of bioavailability are increased with food and increased if tablets are crushed (do not crush tablets)

Half-life elimination: ~31 hours

Time to peak, plasma: 2 to 4 hours

Excretion: Feces (primarily); urine (<4%)

Dosing

Adult & Geriatric

Renal cell carcinoma (RCC), advanced: Oral: 800 mg once daily (Sternberg 2010)

Soft tissue sarcoma (STS), advanced: Oral: 800 mg once daily (Van Der Graaf 2012)

Thyroid cancer, advanced differentiated (off-label use): Oral: 800 mg once daily until disease progression or unacceptable toxicity (Bible 2010; Bible 2014)

Missed doses: If a dose is missed, do not take if <12 hours until the next dose.

Concomitant CYP3A4 inhibitors/inducers:
CYP3A4 inhibitors: Avoid concomitant strong CYP3A4 inhibitors (may increase pazopanib concentrations). If pazopanib must be administered concomitantly with a potent enzyme inhibitor, reduce pazopanib to 400 mg once daily with careful monitoring; further dosage reductions may be needed if adverse events occur.

CYP3A4 inducers: Avoid concomitant strong CYP3A4 inducers (may decrease pazopanib concentrations); use of pazopanib is not recommended in situations where the chronic use of a strong CYP3A4 inducer is required.

Renal Impairment No dosage adjustment necessary.

Hepatic Impairment

Preexisting impairment:
Mild (bilirubin ≤1.5 times ULN or ALT >ULN): No dosage adjustment required (Shibata 2013).

Moderate (bilirubin >1.5 to 3 times ULN): Consider alternative therapy or reduce to 200 mg once daily (maximum tolerated dose in patients with moderate hepatic impairment) (Shibata 2013).

Severe (bilirubin >3 times ULN with any ALT level): Use is not recommended.

During treatment:
Isolated ALT elevations 3 to 8 times ULN: Continue treatment, monitor liver function weekly until ALT returns to grade 1 or baseline.

◄ Isolated ALT elevations >8 times ULN: Interrupt treatment until ALT returns to grade 1 or baseline. If therapy benefit is greater than the risk of hepatotoxicity, may reinitiate treatment at ≤400 mg once daily (with liver function monitored weekly for 8 weeks); permanently discontinue if ALT >3 times ULN occurs with reinitiation.

ALT >3 times ULN concurrently with bilirubin >2 times ULN: Permanently discontinue; monitor until resolution.

Gilbert syndrome with mild indirect bilirubin elevation and ALT >3 times ULN: Refer to isolated ALT elevations dosage recommendations above.

Adjustment for Toxicity

Initial dosage reduction: Note: Prior to dose reduction, temporarily discontinue therapy if 24-hour urine protein ≥3 g or for other toxicities when clinically indicated.

RCC: Reduce to 400 mg once daily

STS: Reduce to 600 mg once daily

Further modification: *RCC, STS:* Adjust dose in 200 mg increments or decrements based on individual tolerance; maximum dose: 800 mg

Hypertension: Manage as appropriate with antihypertensive therapy and interrupt treatment or reduce dose as clinically warranted.

Hypertension (severe, persistent, and refractory to antihypertensives and dose reduction) or evidence of hypertensive crisis: Discontinue treatment.

Infection, serious: Consider treatment interruption or discontinuation.

Proteinuria (24-hour urine protein ≥3 g): Interrupt treatment and reduce the dose.

Proteinuria (recurrent 24-hour urine protein ≥3 g refractory to dose reduction): Discontinue treatment.

Pulmonary toxicity: Interstitial lung disease (ILD) or pneumonitis: Discontinue treatment.

Reversible posterior leukoencephalopathy syndrome (RPLS): Permanently discontinue.

Thrombotic microangiopathy (TMA): Permanently discontinue.

Wound dehiscence: Discontinue treatment.

Combination Regimens

Renal cell cancer: Pazopanib (RCC Regimen) on page 2060

Soft tissue sarcoma: Pazopanib (Soft Tissue Sarcoma Regimen) on page 2060

Thyroid cancer: Pazopanib (Thyroid Regimen) on page 2060

Administration Administer on an empty stomach, 1 hour before or 2 hours after a meal. Do not crush tablet (rate of absorption may be increased; may affect systemic exposure).

Hazardous agent; use appropriate precautions for handling and disposal (NIOSH 2014 [group 1]).

Emetic Potential Minimal (<10%)

Monitoring Parameters Monitor liver function tests at baseline; at weeks 3, 5, 7, and 9; at months 3 and 4; and as clinically necessary, then periodically after month 4 (US labeling) or at weeks 2, 4, 6, and 8 (Canadian labeling); months 3 and 4, and periodically thereafter (monitor more frequently if clinically indicated); serum electrolytes (eg, calcium, magnesium, potassium); urinalysis (for proteinuria; baseline and periodic), 24-hour urine protein (if clinically indicated); thyroid function (TSH and T_4 at baseline and TSH every 6 to 8 weeks during treatment [Appleby 2011]); blood pressure; ECG (baseline and periodic); LVEF (if at risk for cardiac dysfunction; baseline and periodic); signs/symptoms of gastrointestinal perforation or fistula, venous thrombotic events, pulmonary embolism, interstitial lung disease (ILD)/pneumonitis, infection, heart failure, or neurological changes.

Dietary Considerations Avoid grapefruit juice.

Medication Guide Available Yes

Dosage Forms Excipient information presented when available (limited, particularly for generics); consult specific product labeling.

Tablet, Oral:

Votrient: 200 mg

♦ **Pazopanib Hydrochloride** see PAZOPanib on page 1334

♦ **PCB** see Procarbazine on page 1436

♦ **PCC (Caution: Confusion-prone synonym)** see Factor IX Complex (Human) [(Factors II, IX, X)] on page 677

♦ **PCI-32765** see Ibrutinib on page 856

♦ **PCZ** see Procarbazine on page 1436

♦ **PD 0332991** see Palbociclib on page 1300

♦ **PDX** see PRALAtrexate on page 1417

♦ **Pediaderm AF Complete** see Nystatin (Topical) on page 1219

♦ **Pediapred** see PrednisoLONE (Systemic) on page 1421

♦ **Pedi-Dri [DSC]** see Nystatin (Topical) on page 1219

♦ **PEG-L-asparaginase** see Pegaspargase on page 1341

♦ **PEG-ASP** see Pegaspargase on page 1341

♦ **PEG-asparaginase** see Pegaspargase on page 1341

Pegaspargase (peg AS par jase)

Related Information

Management of Chemotherapy-Induced Nausea and Vomiting in Adults on page 2142

Prevention of Chemotherapy-Induced Nausea and Vomiting in Children on page 2203

Brand Names: US Oncaspar

Index Terms L-asparaginase with Polyethylene Glycol; PEG-ASP; PEG-asparaginase; PEG-L-asparaginase; PEGLA; Polyethylene Glycol-L-asparaginase

Pharmacologic Category Antineoplastic Agent, Enzyme; Antineoplastic Agent, Miscellaneous

Use

Acute lymphoblastic leukemia and hypersensitivity to asparaginase: Treatment of acute lymphoblastic leukemia (ALL) in patients with hypersensitivity to native forms of L-asparaginase (as a component of a multiagent chemotherapy regimen)

Acute lymphoblastic leukemia, first-line: First-line treatment of ALL (as a component of a multiagent chemotherapy regimen)

Labeled Contraindications History of serious allergic reactions to pegaspargase or any component of the formulation; history of any of the following with prior L-asparaginase treatment: serious thrombosis, pancreatitis, and/or serious hemorrhagic events

Pregnancy Considerations Animal reproduction studies have not been conducted with pegaspargase.

◄ **Breast-Feeding Considerations** It is not known if pegaspargase is excreted in breast milk. Due to the potential for serious adverse reactions in the nursing infant, the manufacturer recommends a decision be made to discontinue nursing or to discontinue the drug, taking into account the importance of treatment to the mother.

Warnings/Precautions Anaphylaxis and serious allergic reactions (eg, bronchospasm, hypotension, laryngeal edema, local erythema or swelling, systemic rash, urticaria) may occur; discontinue in patients with serious allergic reaction. The risk of serious allergic reactions is increased in patients with a history of hypersensitivity reactions to other L-asparaginase products. Observe patients for 1 hour after administration; equipment and immediate treatment for hypersensitivity reactions should be available during administration.

Serious thrombotic events, including sagittal sinus thrombosis may occur; discontinue with serious thrombotic event. Anticoagulation prophylaxis during therapy may be considered in some patients (Farge 2013). Pancreatitis may occur; promptly evaluate patients with abdominal pain. The manufacturer recommends discontinuing pegaspargase if pancreatitis occurs during treatment. May consider continuing therapy for asymptomatic chemical pancreatitis (amylase or lipase >3 times ULN) or only radiologic abnormalities; monitor closely for rising amylase and/or lipase levels (Stock 2011). Discontinue permanently for clinical pancreatitis (eg, vomiting, severe abdominal pain) with amylase/lipase elevation >3 times ULN for >3 days and/or development of a pancreatic pseudocyst. Avoid alcohol use (Stock 2011). May cause glucose intolerance; irreversible in some cases; use with caution in patients with hyperglycemia, or diabetes. Monitor serum glucose. Increased prothrombin time, increased partial thromboplastin time, and hypofibrinogenemia may occur. Severe or symptomatic coagulopathy may require treatment with fresh-frozen plasma; use with caution in patients with underlying coagulopathy or previous hematologic complications from asparaginase. Monitor coagulation parameters at baseline and periodically during and after therapy. Altered liver function tests (eg, increased AST, ALT, alkaline phosphatase, bilirubin [direct and indirect], and decreased serum albumin, plasma fibrinogen) may occur with therapy. Use with caution in patients with preexisting hepatic impairment. Monitor liver function tests at baseline and periodically during treatment. Potentially significant drug-drug interactions may exist, requiring dose or frequency adjustment, additional monitoring, and/or selection of alternative therapy. Do not interchange pegaspargase for asparaginase (*E. coli*) or asparaginase (*Erwinia*); ensure the proper asparaginase formulation, route of administration, and dose prior to administration.

Adverse Reactions

>10%:

  Hepatic: Increased serum transaminases (ALT, AST; grades 3/4: 3% to 11%)

  Hypersensitivity: Hypersensitivity reaction (grades 3/4: 1%, includes anaphylaxis, bronchospasm, erythema, hives, hypotension, laryngeal edema, skin rash, swelling, urticaria; relapsed acute lymphoblastic leukemia [ALL] with no prior asparaginase hypersensitivity: 10%; relapsed ALL with prior asparaginase hypersensitivity: 32%)

1% to 10%:

  Cardiovascular: Thrombosis (4%)

  Central nervous system: Cerebral thrombosis (or hemorrhage of the brain: 2%; grades 3/4: 3%)

  Endocrine & metabolic: Hyperglycemia (3% [some patients required insulin therapy]; grades 3/4: 5%)

Gastrointestinal: Pancreatitis (1%; grades 3/4: 2% [includes 3 deaths])
Hematologic: Blood coagulation disorder (grades 3/4: 2% to 7%; includes prolonged prothrombin time or partial thromboplastin time or decreased serum fibrogen)
Hepatic: Abnormal hepatic function tests (grades 3/4: 5%), hyperbilirubinemia (grades 3/4: 1% to 2%)
Immunologic: Hypersensitivity to L-asparaginase (grades 3/4: 2%)
<1%, postmarketing, case reports, and/or frequency not defined: Abdominal pain, anemia, anorexia, antithrombin III deficiency, arthralgia, ascites, bacteremia, bronchospasm, bruise, chest pain, chills, coagulation time increased, colitis, confusion, constipation, cough, deep vein thrombosis, disseminated intravascular coagulation, dizziness, dyspnea, edema, emotional lability, endocarditis, epistaxis, facial edema, fatigue, fever, gastrointestinal pain, headache, hematuria, hemolytic anemia, hemorrhagic cystitis, hepatic failure, hepatomegaly, hyperammonemia, hypertension, hyperuricemia, hypoalbuminemia, hypoglycemia, hyponatremia, increased blood urea nitrogen, increased serum amylase, increased serum creatinine, increased serum lipase, increased thirst, injection site pain, jaundice, leukopenia, lip edema, liver steatosis, malaise, metabolic acidosis, myalgia, nausea, night sweats, osteoalgia, pancytopenia, paresthesia, petechial rash, prolonged prothrombin time, proteinuria, purpura, renal failure, renal function abnormality, sagittal sinus thrombosis, seizure, sepsis, septic shock, subacute bacterial endocarditis, superficial venous thrombosis, tachycardia, thrombocytopenia, uric acid nephropathy, urticaria, vomiting

Drug Interactions
Metabolism/Transport Effects None known.
Avoid Concomitant Use
Avoid concomitant use of Pegaspargase with any of the following: BCG (Intravesical); Natalizumab; Pimecrolimus; Tacrolimus (Topical); Tofacitinib; Vaccines (Live)
Increased Effect/Toxicity
Pegaspargase may increase the levels/effects of: Fingolimod; Leflunomide; Natalizumab; Tofacitinib; Vaccines (Live)

The levels/effects of Pegaspargase may be increased by: Denosumab; Pimecrolimus; Roflumilast; Tacrolimus (Topical); Trastuzumab
Decreased Effect
Pegaspargase may decrease the levels/effects of: BCG (Intravesical); Coccidioides immitis Skin Test; Sipuleucel-T; Vaccines (Inactivated); Vaccines (Live)

The levels/effects of Pegaspargase may be decreased by: Echinacea; Pegloticase
Storage/Stability Store intact vials at 2°C to 8°C (36°F to 46°F); do not freeze. Do not shake; protect from light. Discard vial if previously frozen, stored at room temperature for >48 hours, excessively shaken/agitated, or if cloudy, discolored, or if precipitate is present. If not used immediately, solutions for infusion should be protected from light, refrigerated at 2°C to 8°C (36°F to 46°F) and used within 48 hours (including administration time).
Preparation for Administration IV: Dilute in 100 mL NS or D_5W.
Mechanism of Action Pegaspargase is a modified version of L-asparaginase, conjugated with polyethylene glycol. In leukemic cells, asparaginase hydrolyzes L-asparagine to ammonia and L-aspartic acid, leading to depletion of asparagine. Leukemia cells, especially lymphoblasts, require exogenous

asparagine; normal cells can synthesize asparagine. Asparagine depletion in leukemic cells leads to inhibition of protein synthesis and apoptosis. Asparaginase is cycle-specific for the G_1 phase of the cell cycle.

Pharmacodynamics/Kinetics

Onset: Asparagine depletion: IM: Within 4 days

Duration: Asparagine depletion: IV (in asparaginase naive adults): 2 to 4 weeks (Douer 2007); IM: ~21 days

Absorption: IM: Slow

Distribution: IV: Adults (asparaginase naive): 2.4 L/m^2 (Douer 2007)

Metabolism: Systemically degraded

Half-life elimination: IM: ~6 days; half-life decreased to ~3 days (range: 1.4 to 5 days) in patients with previous hypersensitivity to native L-asparaginase; IV: Adults (asparaginase naive): 7 days (Douer 2007)

Time to peak: IM: 3 to 4 days

Dosing

Adult & Geriatric Acute lymphoblastic leukemia (ALL): IM, IV: 2500 units/ m^2 (as part of a combination chemotherapy regimen), do not administer more frequently than every 14 days

Pediatric Acute lymphoblastic leukemia (ALL): IM, IV: Refer to adult dosing.

Renal Impairment There are no dosage adjustments provided in the manufacturer's labeling.

Hepatic Impairment There are no initial dosage adjustments provided in the manufacturer's labeling. The following adjustments have been recommended (Stock 2011):

ALT/AST >3 to 5 times ULN: Continue therapy.

ALT/AST >5 to 20 times ULN: Delay next dose until transaminases <3 times ULN.

ALT/AST >20 times ULN: Discontinue therapy if it takes longer than 1 week for transaminases to return to <3 times ULN.

Direct bilirubin <3 mg/dL: Continue therapy.

Direct bilirubin 3.1 to 5 mg/dL: Hold pegaspargase and resume when direct bilirubin <2 mg/dL; consider switching to alternate asparaginase product.

Direct bilirubin >5 mg/dL: Discontinue pegaspargase; do not substitute other asparaginase products; do not make up for missed doses.

Adjustment for Toxicity The following adjustments have been recommended (Stock 2011):

Hyperammonemia-related fatigue: Continue therapy for grade 2 toxicity. If grade 3 toxicity occurs, reduce dose by 25%; resume full dose when toxicity ≤ grade 2 (make up for missed doses). If grade 4 toxicity occurs, reduce dose by 50%; resume full dose when toxicity ≤ grade 2 (make up for missed doses).

Hyperglycemia: Continue therapy for uncomplicated hyperglycemia. If hyperglycemia requires insulin therapy, hold pegaspargase (and any concomitant corticosteroids) until blood glucose controlled; resume dosing at prior dose level. For life-threatening hyperglycemia or toxicity requiring urgent intervention, hold pegaspargase (and corticosteroids) until blood glucose is controlled with insulin; resume pegaspargase and do not make up for missed doses.

Hypersensitivity reactions: May continue dosing for urticaria without bronchospasm, hypotension, edema, or need for parenteral intervention. If wheezing or other symptomatic bronchospasm with or without urticaria, angioedema, hypotension, and/or life-threatening hypersensitivity reactions occur, discontinue pegaspargase. Replace pegaspargase with asparaginase (Erwinia).

Hypertriglyceridemia: If serum triglyceride level <1,000 mg/dL, continue pegaspargase but monitor closely for pancreatitis. If triglyceride level >1,000 mg/dL, hold pegaspargase and monitor; resume therapy at prior dose level after triglyceride level returns to baseline.

Pancreatitis:

Asymptomatic amylase or lipase >3 times ULN (chemical pancreatitis) or radiologic abnormalities only: Continue pegaspargase and monitor levels closely.

Clinical pancreatitis (abdominal pain with amylase or lipase >3 times ULN for >3 days and/or development of pancreatic pseudocyst): Permanently discontinue pegaspargase.

Thrombosis and bleeding, CNS:

Thrombosis: Continue therapy for abnormal laboratory findings without a clinical correlate. If grade 3 toxicity occurs, discontinue therapy; if CNS signs/symptoms are fully resolved and further pegaspargase doses are required, may resume therapy at a lower dose and/or longer intervals between doses. Discontinue therapy for grade 4 toxicity.

Hemorrhage: Discontinue therapy; do not withhold therapy for abnormal laboratory findings without a clinical correlate. If grade 3 toxicity occurs, discontinue therapy; if CNS signs/symptoms are fully resolved and further pegaspargase doses are required, may resume therapy at a lower dose and/or longer intervals between doses. Discontinue therapy for grade 4 toxicity.

Thrombosis and bleeding, non-CNS:

Thrombosis: Continue therapy for abnormal laboratory findings without a clinical correlate. If grade 3 or 4 toxicity occurs, withhold therapy until acute toxicity and clinical signs resolve and anticoagulant therapy is stable or completed. Do not withhold therapy for abnormal laboratory findings without clinical correlate.

Hemorrhage: If grade 2 bleeding in conjunction with hypofibrinogenemia occurs, withhold therapy until bleeding ≤ grade 1. Do not withhold therapy for abnormal laboratory findings without clinical correlate. For grade 3 or 4 bleeding, withhold therapy until bleeding ≤ grade 1 and until acute toxicity and clinical signs resolve and coagulant replacement therapy is stable or completed.

Combination Regimens

Leukemia (acute lymphocytic): Hyper-CVAD (Leukemia, Acute Lymphocytic) on page 2006

Administration Have available appropriate agents for maintenance of an adequate airway and treatment of a hypersensitivity reaction (antihistamine, epinephrine, oxygen, IV corticosteroids). Be prepared to treat anaphylaxis at each administration.

IM: Must only be administered as a deep intramuscular injection into a large muscle. Do not exceed 2 mL per injection site; use multiple injection sites for IM injection volume >2 mL.

IV: Administer over 1 to 2 hours through a running IV infusion line; **do not administer IV push.**

Emetic Potential Children and Adults: Minimal (<10%)

Monitoring Parameters CBC with differential, platelets, amylase/lipase, liver function tests (baseline and periodically during treatment), fibrinogen, PT, PTT (coagulation parameters [baseline and periodically during and after treatment]), renal function tests; urine glucose, blood glucose; triglycerides; vital signs during administration; monitor for onset of abdominal pain; observe for allergic reaction (for 1 hour after administration); signs/symptoms of thrombosis or bleeding

Dosage Forms Excipient information presented when available (limited, particularly for generics); consult specific product labeling.

Solution, Injection [preservative free]:

Oncaspar: 750 units/mL (5 mL)

Pegfilgrastim (peg fil GRA stim)

Brand Names: US Neulasta; Neulasta Delivery Kit

Brand Names: Canada Neulasta

Index Terms G-CSF (PEG Conjugate); Granulocyte Colony Stimulating Factor (PEG Conjugate); Neulasta Onpro kit; Pegylated G-CSF; SD/01

Pharmacologic Category Colony Stimulating Factor; Hematopoietic Agent

Use

Prevention of chemotherapy-induced neutropenia: To decrease the incidence of infection (as manifested by febrile neutropenia), in patients with nonmyeloid malignancies receiving myelosuppressive cancer chemotherapy associated with a clinically significant incidence of febrile neutropenia.

Limitation of use: Pegfilgrastim is not indicated for mobilization of peripheral blood progenitor cells for hematopoietic stem cell transplant.

Labeled Contraindications Hypersensitivity (serious allergic reaction) to pegfilgrastim, filgrastim, or any component of the formulation

Pregnancy Considerations Adverse events were observed in some animal reproduction studies.

Women who are exposed to Neulasta during pregnancy are encouraged to enroll in the Amgen Pregnancy Surveillance Program (800-772-6436).

Breast-Feeding Considerations It is not known if pegfilgrastim is excreted in breast milk. The manufacturer recommends that caution be exercised when administering pegfilgrastim to nursing women.

Warnings/Precautions Do not use pegfilgrastim in the period 14 days before to 24 hours after administration of cytotoxic chemotherapy because of the potential sensitivity of rapidly dividing myeloid cells to cytotoxic chemotherapy. Safety and efficacy have not been established with dose-dense chemotherapy regimens (Smith 2006). Not indicated for peripheral blood progenitor cell (PBPC) mobilization for hematopoietic stem cell transplantation.

Serious allergic reactions (including anaphylaxis) may occur, usually with the initial dose; may recur within days after discontinuation of initial antiallergic treatment. Permanently discontinue for severe reactions. Do not administer in patients with a history of serious allergic reaction to pegfilgrastim or filgrastim. Acute respiratory distress syndrome (ARDS) has been reported with use; evaluate patients with pulmonary symptoms such as fever, pulmonary infiltrates, or respiratory distress for ARDS. Discontinue pegfilgrastim if ARDS occurs. Rare cases of splenic rupture have been reported (some fatal); patients must be instructed to report left upper abdominal pain or shoulder pain. May precipitate sickle cell crises in patients with sickle cell disorders (severe and sometimes fatal sickle cell crises have occurred with filgrastim). The granulocyte-colony stimulating factor (G-CSF) receptor through which pegfilgrastim (and filgrastim) work has been located on tumor cell lines. May potentially act as a growth factor for any tumor type, including myeloid malignancies and myelodysplasia (pegfilgrastim is not approved for myeloid malignancies). Capillary leak syndrome (CLS), characterized by hypotension, hypoalbuminemia, edema, and hemoconcentration, may occur in patients receiving human granulocyte colony-stimulating factors (G-CSF), including pegfilgrastim. CLS episodes vary in frequency and severity. If CLS develops, monitor closely and manage symptomatically (may require intensive care). CLS may be life-threatening if treatment is delayed.

Leukocytosis (WBC ≥100,000/mm^3) has been reported in patients receiving pegfilgrastim. Monitor complete blood counts during therapy. Glomerulonephritis has occurred, and generally resolved after pegfilgrastim dose reduction or discontinuation. Diagnosis was made by the presence of azotemia, microscopic and macroscopic hematuria, proteinuria, and renal biopsy. Evaluate if glomerulonephritis is suspected; if felt due to pegfilgrastim, consider dose reduction or therapy interruption.

The On-body injector contains an acrylic adhesive; may result in a significant reaction in patients who react to acrylic adhesives. A health care provider must fill the On-body injector prior to applying to the patient's skin. The On-body delivery system may be applied on the same day as chemotherapy administration as long as pegfilgrastim is delivered no less than 24 hours after chemotherapy is administered. The prefilled syringe provided in the On-body kit contains overfill to compensate for loss during delivery; do not use for manual subcutaneous injection (will result in higher than recommended dose). Do not use prefilled syringe intended for manual injection to fill the On-body injector; may result in lower than intended dose. The On-body injector is only for use with pegfilgrastim; do not use to deliver other medications. Do not expose the On-body injector to oxygen-rich environments (eg, hyperbaric chambers), MRI, x-ray (including airport x-ray), CT scan, or ultrasound (may damage injector system). Keep the On-body injector at least 4 inches away from electrical equipment, including cell phones, cordless phones, microwaves, and other common appliances (injector may not work properly).

Colony-stimulating factors may be considered in cancer patients with febrile neutropenia who are at high risk for infection-associated complications or who have prognostic factors indicative of a poor clinical outcome (eg, prolonged and severe neutropenia, age >65 years, hypotension, pneumonia, sepsis syndrome, presence of invasive fungal infection, uncontrolled primary disease, hospitalization at the time of fever development) (Freifeld 2011; Smith 2006). Colony-stimulating factors should not be routinely used for patients with neutropenia who are afebrile. Dose-dense regimens that require colony-stimulating factors should only be used within the context of a clinical trial or if supported by convincing evidence. The safety/efficacy of pegfilgrastim in the setting of dose-dense therapy has not been fully established (Smith 2015).

ASCO guidelines recommend that prophylactic colony-stimulating factors be used in patients ≥65 years with diffuse aggressive lymphoma treated with curative chemotherapy (eg, rituximab, cyclophosphamide, doxorubicin, vincristine, prednisone), especially if patients have comorbid conditions (Smith 2015). The 6 mg fixed dose should not be used in infants, children, and adolescents weighing <45 kg. CSF use in pediatric patients is typically directed by clinical pediatric protocols. ASCO Recommendations for the Use of WBC Growth Factors Clinical Practice Guideline Update states that CSFs may be reasonable as primary prophylaxis in pediatric patients when chemotherapy regimens with a high likelihood of febrile neutropenia are employed. Likewise, secondary CSF prophylaxis should be limited to high-risk patients. In pediatric cancers in which dose-intense chemotherapy (with a survival benefit) is used, CSFs should be given to facilitate chemotherapy administration. CSFs should not be used in the pediatric population for non-relapsed acute lymphoblastic or myeloid leukemia when no infection is present (Smith 2015).The packaging (needle cover) contains latex.

Adverse Reactions

Neuromuscular & skeletal: Ostealgia (31%), limb pain (9%)

<1%, postmarketing, and/or case reports: Acute respiratory distress syndrome (ARDS), alopecia, anaphylaxis, antibody development, arthralgia, back pain, bruising at injection site, capillary leak syndrome, chest pain, constipation, diarrhea, erythema, fatigue, fever, flushing, headache, hypersensitivity angiitis, hypertonia, increased serum alkaline phosphatase, increased uric acid, influenza, injection site reaction, leukocytosis, musculoskeletal pain, myalgia, neck pain, pain, pain at injection site, periorbital edema, peripheral edema, polyarthralgia, polymyalgia rheumatica, rhinitis, severe sickle cell crisis, skeletal pain, splenic rupture, splenomegaly, Sweet's syndrome, urticaria, vomiting, weakness

Drug Interactions

Metabolism/Transport Effects None known.

Avoid Concomitant Use There are no known interactions where it is recommended to avoid concomitant use.

Increased Effect/Toxicity There are no known significant interactions involving an increase in effect.

Decreased Effect

The levels/effects of Pegfilgrastim may be decreased by: Pegloticase

Storage/Stability Store under refrigeration at 2°C to 8°C (36°F to 46°F); do not freeze. If syringe for manual injection is inadvertently frozen, allow to thaw in refrigerator; discard if frozen more than one time. Protect from light. Do not shake. Allow to reach room temperature prior to injection. Prefilled syringe for manual injection may be kept at room temperature for up to 48 hours. The On-body injector kit should not be held at room temperature for longer than 12 hours prior to use (discard if stored at room temperature for >12 hours).

Preparation for Administration

On-body injector: A health care provider must fill the On-body injector prior to applying to the patient's skin. The On-body delivery system may be applied on the same day as chemotherapy administration as long as pegfilgrastim is delivered no less than 24 hours after chemotherapy is administered.

The prefilled syringe provided in the On-body kit contains overfill to compensate for loss during delivery; do not use for manual subcutaneous injection (will result in higher than recommended dose). Do not use prefilled syringe intended for manual injection to fill the On-body injector; may result in lower than intended dose.

Mechanism of Action Stimulates the production, maturation, and activation of neutrophils, pegfilgrastim activates neutrophils to increase both their migration and cytotoxicity. Pegfilgrastim has a prolonged duration of effect relative to filgrastim and a reduced renal clearance.

Pharmacodynamics/Kinetics Half-life elimination: SubQ: Adults: 15 to 80 hours; Children (100 mcg/kg dose): ~20 to 30 hours. Pharmacokinetics were comparable between manual subcutaneous injection and the On-body injector system.

Dosing

Adult & Geriatric Note: Do not administer in the period between 14 days before and 24 hours after administration of cytotoxic chemotherapy.

Prevention of chemotherapy-induced neutropenia: SubQ: 6 mg once per chemotherapy cycle, beginning at least 24 hours after completion of chemotherapy

Pediatric Note: Do not administer in the period between 14 days before and 24 hours after administration of cytotoxic chemotherapy.

Prevention of chemotherapy-induced neutropenia (solid tumors): Children and Adolescents (off-label use): SubQ: 100 mcg/kg (maximum dose: 6 mg) once per chemotherapy cycle, beginning 24 to 72 hours after completion of chemotherapy (Andre 2007; Borinstein 2009)

Renal Impairment No dosage adjustment necessary.

Hepatic Impairment There are no dosage adjustments provided in the manufacturer's labeling (has not been studied).

Combination Regimens

Bone sarcoma (Ewing sarcoma): Docetaxel-Gemcitabine (Ewing Sarcoma) on page 1942

Bone sarcoma (osteosarcoma): Docetaxel-Gemcitabine (Osteosarcoma) on page 1943

Breast cancer: AC (Dose-Dense) followed by Paclitaxel (Dose-Dense)-Trastuzumab (Breast) on page 1823

Endometrial cancer: Cisplatin-Doxorubin-Paclitaxel (Endometrial) on page 1893

Lymphoma, non-Hodgkin (Mantle Cell): Cladribine-Rituximab (NHL-Mantle Cell) on page 1916

Soft tissue sarcoma: Docetaxel-Gemcitabine (Soft Tissue Sarcoma) on page 1943

Uterine sarcoma: Docetaxel-Gemcitabine (Uterine Leiomyosarcoma) on page 1944

Administration Administer subcutaneously. Do not use 6 mg fixed dose in infants, children, or adolescents <45 kg (Smith 2006). Pegfilgrastim is available in prefilled syringes for manual subcutaneous administration or as a kit for use with the On-body injector.

Manual subcutaneous administration: Administer to outer upper arms, abdomen (except within 2 inches of navel), front middle thigh, or upper outer buttocks. Engage/activate needle guard following use to prevent accidental needlesticks

On-body injector: A health care provider must fill the On-body injector prior to applying to the patient's skin. Apply to intact, nonirritated skin on the back of the arm or abdomen (only use the back of the arm if caregiver is available to monitor On-body injection status). The On-body injector system will deliver pegfilgrastim over ~45 minutes approximately 27 hours after application. The On-body delivery system may be applied on the same day as chemotherapy administration as long as pegfilgrastim is delivered at least 24 hours after chemotherapy is administered. Keep the On-body injector dry for ~3 hours before dose delivery. A missed dose may occur if the On-body injector fails or leaks; if a dose is missed, administer a new dose by manual subcutaneous injection as soon as possible after discovery of missed dose. Do not expose the On-body injector to oxygen-rich environments (eg, hyperbaric chambers), MRI, x-ray (including airport x-ray), CT-scan, or ultrasound (may damage injector system). Keep the On-body injector at least 4 inches away from

◄ electrical equipment, including cell phones, cordless phones, microwaves, and other common appliances (injector may not work properly). Refer to prescribing information for further details.

The prefilled syringe provided in the On-body kit contains overfill to compensate for loss during delivery; do not use for manual subcutaneous injection (will result in higher than recommended dose). Do not use prefilled syringe intended for manual injection to fill the On-body injector; may result in lower than intended dose. The On-body injector is only for use with pegfilgrastim; do not use to deliver other medications.

Monitoring Parameters Complete blood count (with differential) and platelet count should be obtained prior to chemotherapy and as clinically necessary. Monitor platelets and hematocrit regularly. Evaluate fever, pulmonary infiltrates, and respiratory distress; evaluate for left upper abdominal pain, shoulder tip pain, or splenomegaly. Monitor for signs/symptoms of glomerulonephritis (azotemia, hematuria, proteinuria) and capillary leak syndrome (hypotension, hypoalbuminemia, edema and hemoconcentration). Monitor for sickle cell crisis (in patients with sickle cell anemia).

Test Interactions May interfere with bone imaging studies; increased hematopoietic activity of the bone marrow may appear as transient positive bone imaging changes

Dosage Forms Excipient information presented when available (limited, particularly for generics); consult specific product labeling.
Solution, Subcutaneous [preservative free]:
Neulasta: 6 mg/0.6 mL (0.6 mL)
Neulasta Delivery Kit: 6 mg/0.6 mL (0.6 mL)

◆ **PEG-IFN Alfa-2b** see Peginterferon Alfa-2b on page 1350

Peginterferon Alfa-2b (peg in ter FEER on AL fa too bee)
Related Information
Common Toxicity Criteria on page 2122
Management of Chemotherapy-Induced Nausea and Vomiting in Adults on page 2142
Prevention of Chemotherapy-Induced Nausea and Vomiting in Children on page 2203

Brand Names: US Peg-Intron; Peg-Intron Redipen; Peg-Intron Redipen Pak 4; PegIntron; Sylatron

Brand Names: Canada PegIntron

Index Terms Interferon Alfa-2b (PEG Conjugate); PEG-IFN Alfa-2b; Pegylated Interferon Alfa-2b; Polyethylene Glycol Interferon Alfa-2b

Pharmacologic Category Antineoplastic Agent, Biological Response Modulator; Biological Response Modulator; Immunomodulator, Systemic; Interferon

Use
Chronic hepatitis C (CHC): Peg-Intron: Treatment of chronic hepatitis C (CHC) in compensated liver disease:
Combination therapy with ribavirin and an approved hepatitis C virus [HCV] NS3/4A protease inhibitor in adult patients with HCV genotype 1 infection.
Combination therapy with ribavirin in adult patients with HCV genotypes other than 1, in pediatric patients (3 to 17 years), or in patients with HCV genotype 1 with contraindications or intolerance to HCV NS3/4A protease inhibitor use.
Monotherapy in adult patients with contraindications or significant intolerance to ribavirin if previously untreated.

Limitations of use: Combination therapy with ribavirin provides substantially better response rates than monotherapy

Melanoma: Sylatron: Adjuvant treatment of melanoma (with microscopic or gross nodal involvement within 84 days of definitive surgical resection, including complete lymphadenectomy)

Labeled Contraindications

Hypersensitivity (including urticaria, angioedema, bronchoconstriction, anaphylaxis, Stevens Johnson syndrome, and toxic epidermal necrolysis) to peginterferon alfa-2b, interferon alfa-2b, other alfa interferons, or any component of the formulation; autoimmune hepatitis; decompensated liver disease (Child-Pugh score >6, classes B and C)

Documentation of allergic cross-reactivity for interferons is limited. However, because of similarities in chemical structure and/or pharmacologic actions, the possibility of cross-sensitivity cannot be ruled out with certainty

Combination therapy with peginterferon alfa-2b and ribavirin is also contraindicated in pregnancy, women who may become pregnant, males with pregnant partners; hemoglobinopathies (eg, thalassemia major, sickle-cell anemia); renal dysfunction (CrCl <50 mL/minute)

Pregnancy Considerations Reproduction studies with pegylated interferon alfa have not been conducted. Animal reproduction studies with nonpegylated interferon alfa-2b have demonstrated abortifacient effects. Disruption of the normal menstrual cycle was also observed in animal studies; therefore, the manufacturer recommends that reliable contraception is used in women of childbearing potential. Alfa interferon is endogenous to normal amniotic fluid (Lebon, 1982). In vitro administration studies have reported that when administered to the mother, it does not cross the placenta (Waysbort, 1993). Case reports of use in pregnant women are limited. The DHHS Perinatal HIV Guidelines do not recommend that peginterferon alfa be used during pregnancy (DHHS [perinatal], 2012). **[U.S. Boxed Warning]: Combination therapy with ribavirin may cause birth defects and/or fetal mortality; avoid pregnancy in females and female partners of male patients;** combination therapy with ribavirin is contraindicated in pregnancy. Two forms of contraception should be used along with monthly pregnancy tests during combination therapy and for 6 months after therapy has been discontinued.

A pregnancy registry has been established for women inadvertently exposed to ribavirin while pregnant (800-593-2214).

Breast-Feeding Considerations Breast milk samples obtained from a lactating mother prior to and after administration of interferon alfa-2b showed that interferon alfa is present in breast milk and administration of the medication did not significantly affect endogenous levels (Kumar, 2000). Breast-feeding is not linked to the spread of hepatitis C virus (ACOG, 2007); however, if nipples are cracked or bleeding, breast-feeding is not recommended (CDC, 2010). Mothers coinfected with HIV are discouraged from breast-feeding to decrease potential transmission of HIV (DHHS [perinatal], 2012).

Warnings/Precautions [U.S. Boxed Warnings]: May cause or aggravate severe depression or other neuropsychiatric adverse events (including suicide and suicidal ideation) in patients with and without a history of psychiatric disorder; monitor closely with clinical evaluations (periodic); discontinue treatment with worsening or persistently severe signs/symptoms of neuropsychiatric disorders (eg, depression, encephalopathy, psychosis). Many cases resolve upon discontinuation, although some cases may persist. May cause or aggravate fatal or life-threatening autoimmune disorders, infectious disorders, ischemic disorders;

◀ **monitor closely with clinical evaluations (periodic); discontinue treatment in patients with worsening or persistently severe signs/symptoms of infectious disorders; may resolve with discontinuation.** May also cause hemorrhagic cerebrovascular events.

Neuropsychiatric disorders: Neuropsychiatric effects may occur in patients with and without a history of psychiatric disorder; addiction relapse, aggression, depression, homicidal ideation and suicidal behavior/ideation have been observed with peginterferon alfa-2b; bipolar disorder, encephalopathy, hallucinations, mania, and psychosis have been observed with other alfa interferons. Onset may be delayed (up to 6 months after discontinuation). Higher doses may be associated with the development of encephalopathy (higher risk in elderly patients). Use with caution in patients with a history of psychiatric disorders, including depression or substance abuse history. New or exacerbated neuropsychiatric or substance abuse disorders are best managed with early intervention. Drug screening and periodic health evaluation (including monitoring of psychiatric symptoms) is recommended if initiating treatment in patients with coexisting psychiatric condition or substance abuse disorders. Monitor all patients for evidence of depression and other psychiatric symptoms; patients being treated for melanoma should be monitored for depression and psychiatric symptoms every 3 weeks during the first 8 weeks of treatment and every 6 months thereafter; permanently discontinue treatment if psychiatric symptoms persist, worsen or if suicidal behavior develops. Patients should continue to be monitored for 6 months after completion of therapy.

Bone marrow suppression: Causes bone marrow suppression, including potentially severe cytopenias; alfa interferons may (rarely) cause aplastic anemia. Use with caution in patients who are chronically immunosuppressed, with low peripheral blood counts or myelosuppression, including concurrent use of myelosuppressive therapy. Dosage modification may be necessary for hematologic toxicity. Combination therapy with ribavirin may potentiate the neutropenic effects of alfa interferons. When used in combination with ribavirin, an increased incidence of anemia was observed when using ribavirin weight-based dosing, as compared to flat-dose ribavirin.

Hepatic disease: Use is contraindicated in patients with hepatic decompensation or autoimmune hepatitis. Discontinue treatment immediately with hepatic decompensation (Child Pugh score >6) or evidence of severe hepatic injury. Patients with chronic hepatitis C (CHC) with cirrhosis receiving peginterferon alfa-2b are at risk for hepatic decompensation. CHC patients coinfected with human immunodeficiency virus (HIV) are at increased risk for hepatic decompensation when receiving highly active antiretroviral therapy (HAART); monitor closely. A transient increase in ALT (2-5 times above baseline) which is not associated with deterioration of liver function may occur with peginterferon alfa-2b use (for the treatment of chronic hepatitis C); therapy generally may continue with monitoring. Instruct patients to avoid alcohol; may increase hepatic effects.

Gastrointestinal disorders: Pancreatitis (including fatal cases) has been observed with alfa interferon therapy; discontinue therapy if known or suspected pancreatitis develops. Ulcerative or hemorrhagic/ischemic colitis has been observed with alfa interferons (within 12 weeks of initiation); withhold treatment for suspected pancreatitis; discontinue therapy for known pancreatitis. Ulcerative or hemorrhagic/ischemic colitis has been observed with alfa interferons; discontinue therapy if signs of colitis (abdominal pain, bloody diarrhea, fever) develop; symptoms typically resolve within 1-3 weeks.

Autoimmune disorders: Thyroiditis, thrombotic thrombocytopenic purpura, immune thrombocytopenia (ITP), rheumatoid arthritis, interstitial nephritis, systemic lupus erythematosus, and psoriasis have been reported with therapy; use with caution in patients with autoimmune disorders.

Cardiovascular disease: Use with caution in patients with cardiovascular disease or a history of cardiovascular disease; hypotension, arrhythmia, bundle branch block, tachycardia, cardiomyopathy, angina pectoris and MI have been observed with treatment. Patients with preexisting cardiac abnormalities should have baseline ECGs prior to combination treatment with ribavirin; closely monitor patients with a history of MI or arrhythmia. Patients with a history of significant or unstable cardiac disease should not receive combination treatment with ribavirin. Discontinue treatment (permanently) for new-onset ventricular arrhythmia or cardiovascular decompensation.

Endocrine disorders: Diabetes mellitus (including new-onset type I diabetes), hyperglycemia, and thyroid disorders have been reported; discontinue peginterferon alfa-2b if cannot be effectively managed with medication. Use caution in patients with a history of diabetes mellitus, particularly if prone to DKA. Use with caution in patients with thyroid disorders; may cause or aggravate hyper- or hypothyroidism.

Pulmonary disease: May cause or aggravate dyspnea, pulmonary infiltrates, pneumonia, bronchiolitis obliterans, interstitial pneumonitis, pulmonary hypertension, and sarcoidosis which may result in respiratory failure; may recur upon rechallenge with treatment; monitor closely. Use with caution in patients with existing pulmonary disease (eg, chronic obstructive pulmonary disease). Withhold combination therapy with ribavirin for development of pulmonary infiltrate or pulmonary function impairment.

Ophthalmic disorders: Ophthalmologic disorders (including decreased visual acuity, blindness, macular edema, retinal hemorrhages, optic neuritis, papilledema, cotton wool spots, retinal detachment [serous], and retinal artery or vein thrombosis) have occurred with peginterferon alfa-2b and/or with other alfa interferons. Prior to start of therapy, ophthalmic exams are recommended for all patients; patients with diabetic or hypertensive retinopathy should have periodic ophthalmic exams during treatment; a complete eye exam should be done promptly in patients who develop ocular symptoms. Permanently discontinue treatment with new or worsening ophthalmic disorder.

[U.S. Boxed Warning]: Combination treatment with ribavirin may cause birth defects and/or fetal mortality (avoid pregnancy in females and female partners of male patients); hemolytic anemia (which may worsen cardiac disease), genotoxicity, mutagenicity, and may possibly be carcinogenic. Potentially significant drug-drug interactions may exist, requiring dose or frequency adjustment, additional monitoring, and/or selection of alternative therapy. Peripheral neuropathy has been reported with alpha interferons when used in combination with telbivudine. Interferon therapy is commonly associated with flu-like symptoms, including fever; rule out other causes/infection with persistent or high fever. Acute hypersensitivity reactions (eg, urticaria, angioedema, bronchoconstriction, anaphylaxis) and cutaneous reactions (eg, Stevens-Johnson syndrome, toxic epidermal necrolysis) have been reported (rarely) with alfa interferons; prompt discontinuation is recommended; transient rashes do not require interruption of therapy. Hyper-triglyceridemia has been reported (may result in pancreatitis); periodically monitor and manage with appropriate treatment; consider discontinuing peginterferon if persistent and severe (triglycerides >1000 mg/dL), particularly if combined with symptoms of pancreatitis. Interferons are commonly associated with flu-like symptoms. Use with caution in patients with debilitating conditions. Use with caution in patients with renal impairment (CrCl <50 mL/minute); monitor closely for signs of interferon toxicity. For the treatment of chronic hepatitis C, dosage adjustments are recommended with monotherapy in patients with moderate-to-severe impairment; do not use combination therapy with ribavirin in adult patients renal dysfunction (CrCl <50 mL/minute); discontinue if serum creatinine >2 mg/dL in children. Dosage adjustment is also recommended when used for the treatment of melanoma. Serum creatinine increases have been reported in patients with renal insufficiency. Use with caution in the elderly; the potential adverse effects (eg, neuropsychiatric events, cardiac events, systemic effects) may be more pronounced. Encephal-opathy has also been observed in primarily elderly patients treated with higher doses of peginterferon alfa-2b. For the treatment of hepatitis, elderly patients generally do not respond to interferon treatment as well as younger patients. When used in combination with ribavirin, closely monitor adults >50 years of age for the development of anemia. Dental/periodontal disorders have been reported with combination therapy; dry mouth may affect teeth and mucous membranes; instruct patients to brush teeth twice daily; encourage regular dental exams; rinse mouth thoroughly after vomiting.

Combination therapy with ribavirin is preferred over monotherapy for the treatment of chronic hepatitis C. Safety and efficacy have not been established in patients who have received organ transplants or are coinfected with HIV or hepatitis B. Patients with significant bridging fibrosis or cirrhosis, genotype 1 infection or who have not responded to prior therapy, including previous pegylated interferon treatment are less likely to benefit from combination therapy with peginterferon alfa-2b and ribavirin. Growth velocity (height and weight) was decreased in children on combination treatment with ribavirin during the length of treatment. Severely inhibited growth velocity has been noted. Long-term follow-up data indicate that combination therapy may inhibit growth, resulting in reduced adult height in some patients. Growth should be closely monitored in pediatric patients during therapy and posttreatment. **[U.S. Boxed Warning]: Combination therapy with ribavirin is contraindicated in pregnancy.** Due to differences in dosage, patients should not change brands of interferon. Some dosage forms may contain polysorbate 80 (also known as Tweens). Hypersensitivity reactions, usually a delayed reaction, have been reported following exposure to pharmaceutical products containing polysor-bate 80 in certain individuals (Isaksson, 2002; Lucente 2000; Shelley, 1995). Thrombocytopenia, ascites, pulmonary deterioration, and renal and hepatic failure have been reported in premature neonates after receiving parenteral products containing polysorbate 80 (Alade, 1986; CDC, 1984). See manufac-turer's labeling.

Adverse Reactions

Antiviral:

>10%:

Central nervous system: Headache (56%), fatigue (including asthenia; ≤52%), depression (29%), anxiety (≤28%), emotional lability (≤28%), irritability (≤28%), insomnia (23%), rigors (23%), dizziness (12%)

Dermatologic: Alopecia (22%), pruritus (12%)

Endocrine & metabolic: Weight Loss (11%)

Gastrointestinal: Nausea (26%), anorexia (20%), diarrhea (18%), abdominal pain (15%)

Infection: Viral infection (11%)

Local: Inflammation at injection site (47%), injection site reaction (47%)

Neuromuscular & skeletal: Myalgia (54%), weakness (52%), musculoskeletal pain (28%), arthralgia (23%)

Miscellaneous: Fever (22%)

1 to 10%:

Cardiovascular: Chest pain (6%), flushing (6%)

Central nervous system: Lack of concentration (10%), right upper quadrant pain (8%), malaise (7%), nervousness (4%), agitation (2%), suicidal ideation (≤2%)

Dermatologic: Diaphoresis (6%), skin rash (6%)

Endocrine & metabolic: Hypothyroidism (5%), menstrual disease (4%), hyperthyroidism (3%)

Gastrointestinal: Vomiting (7%), dyspepsia (6%), xerostomia (6%), constipation (1%)

Hematologic & oncologic: Thrombocytopenia (7%), neutropenia (6%)

Hepatic: Increased serum ALT (10%), hepatomegaly (6%)

Local: Pain at injection site (2% to 3%)

Ophthalmic: Conjunctivitis (4%), blurred vision (2%)

Respiratory: Pharyngitis (10%), cough (8%), sinusitis (7%), dyspnea (4%), rhinitis (2%)

Antineoplastic:

>10%:

Central nervous system: Fatigue (94%), headache (70%), chills (63%), depression (59%, grades 3/4: 7%), dizziness (35%), neuropathy (olfactory) (23%), paresthesia (21%)

Dermatologic: Exfoliative rash (36%), alopecia (34%)

Endocrine & metabolic: Weight loss (11%)

Gastrointestinal: Anorexia (69%), nausea (64%), dysgeusia (38%), diarrhea (37%), vomiting (26%)

Hepatic: Increased serum ALT (≤77%, grades 3/4: ≤11%), increased serum AST (≤77%, grades 3/4: ≤11%), increased serum alkaline phosphatase (23%)

Local: Injection site reaction (62%)

Neuromuscular & skeletal: Myalgia (68%), arthralgia (51%)

Miscellaneous: Fever (75%)

1 to 10%:

Cardiovascular: Bundle branch block (≤4%), myocardial infarction (≤4%), supraventricular cardiac arrhythmia (≤4%), ventricular tachycardia (≤4%)

Endocrine & metabolic: Increased gamma-glutamyl transferase (8%, grades 3/4: 4%)

Genitourinary: Proteinuria (7%)

Hematologic & oncologic: Anemia (6%)

Respiratory: Dyspnea (6%), cough (5%)

<1%, postmarketing, and/or case reports: Aggressive behavior, amnesia, anaphylaxis, angina pectoris, angioedema, aphthous stomatitis, aplastic anemia, auditory impairment, bacterial infection, bipolar mood disorder, brain disease (including exacerbations), bronchiolitis obliterans, bronchoconstriction, cardiac arrest, cardiac arrhythmia, cardiomyopathy, cerebrovascular accident, colitis, cytopenia, dehydration, diabetes mellitus, diabetic

ketoacidosis, drug dependence (including relapse), drug overdose, dysgeusia, erythema multiforme, exacerbation of autoimmune disease, exacerbation of renal failure (increases in serum creatinine), fungal infection, hallucination, hearing loss, hemorrhagic colitis, homicidal ideation, hyperglycemia, hypersensitivity reaction, hypertension, hypertriglyceridemia, hypotension, immune thrombocytopenia, interstitial nephritis, interstitial pneumonitis, ischemic colitis, leukopenia, lupus-like syndrome, macular edema, mania, migraine, myositis, optic neuritis, palpitations, pancreatitis, papilledema, paresthesia, peripheral neuropathy, pneumonia, psoriasis, pulmonary fibrosis, pulmonary hypertension, pulmonary infiltrates, pure red cell aplasia, renal failure, renal insufficiency, retinal cotton-wool spot, retinal detachment, retinal hemorrhage, retinal thrombosis, retinopathy, rhabdomyolysis, rheumatoid arthritis, sarcoidosis, seizure, sepsis, Stevens-Johnson syndrome, systemic lupus erythematosus, tachycardia, thrombotic thrombocytopenic purpura, thyroiditis, toxic epidermal necrolysis, ulcerative colitis, urticaria, vertigo, vision loss, visual disturbance, Vogt-Koyanagi-Harada syndrome

Drug Interactions

Metabolism/Transport Effects Inhibits CYP1A2 (weak), CYP2D6 (weak)

Avoid Concomitant Use

Avoid concomitant use of Peginterferon Alfa-2b with any of the following: BCG (Intravesical); CloZAPine; Dipyrone; Telbivudine

Increased Effect/Toxicity

Peginterferon Alfa-2b may increase the levels/effects of: Aldesleukin; ARIPiprazole; CloZAPine; CYP1A2 Substrates; CYP2D6 Substrates; Methadone; Ribavirin; Telbivudine; TiZANidine; Zidovudine

The levels/effects of Peginterferon Alfa-2b may be increased by: Dipyrone

Decreased Effect

Peginterferon Alfa-2b may decrease the levels/effects of: BCG (Intravesical); CYP2D6 Substrates; FLUoxetine

The levels/effects of Peginterferon Alfa-2b may be decreased by: Pegloticase

Storage/Stability Prior to reconstitution, store Redipen at 2°C to 8°C (36°F to 46°F). Store intact vials at 25°C (77°F); excursions permitted to 15°C to 30°C (59°F to 86°F). Do not freeze. Once reconstituted each product should be used immediately or may be stored for ≤24 hours at 2°C to 8°C (36°F to 46°F); do not freeze. Do not shake. Keep away from heat. Products do not contain preservative (single use; do not reuse).

Preparation for Administration

Redipen: Hold cartridge upright and press the two halves together until there is a "click". Gently invert to mix; do not shake; do not reuse (single use).

Peg-Intron (vial): Add 0.7 mL sterile water for injection, USP (supplied single-use diluent; discard unused portion) to the vial. Gently swirl. Do not re-enter vial after dose removed.

Sylatron (vial): Add 0.7 mL sterile water for injection and swirl gently (do not shake), resulting in the following concentrations (do not withdraw more than 0.5 mL from each vial):

296 mcg vial: 40 mcg/0.1 mL

444 mcg vial: 60 mcg/0.1 mL

888 mcg vial: 120 mcg/0.1 mL

Mechanism of Action Alpha interferons are a family of proteins, produced by nucleated cells, that have antiviral, antiproliferative, and immune-regulating activity. There are 16 known subtypes of alpha interferons. Interferons interact with cells through high affinity cell surface receptors. Following activation, multiple effects can be detected including induction of gene transcription. Inhibits cellular growth, alters the state of cellular differentiation, interferes with oncogene expression, alters cell surface antigen expression, increases phagocytic activity of macrophages, and augments cytotoxicity of lymphocytes for target cells.

Pharmacodynamics/Kinetics

Bioavailability: Increases with chronic dosing

Half-life elimination: CHC: ~40 hours (range: 22 to 60 hours); Melanoma: ~43 to 51 hours

Time to peak: CHC: 15 to 44 hours

Excretion: Urine (~30%)

Dosing

Adult & Geriatric

Melanoma: SubQ: Initial: 6 mcg/kg/week for 8 doses; Maintenance: 3 mcg/kg/week for up to 5 years. **Note:** Premedicate with acetaminophen (500-1000 mg orally) 30 minutes prior to the first dose and as needed for subsequent doses thereafter.

Chronic hepatitis C (CHC): SubQ:

Manufacturer's labeling: **Note:** Discontinue after 12 weeks in patients with HCV (genotype 1) if HCV RNA does not decrease by at least 2 log (compared to pretreatment) or if detectable HCV RNA present at 24. Discontinuation is also recommended in patients who previously failed therapy (regardless of genotype) if detectable HCV RNA present at 12 or 24 weeks.

Combination therapy with ribavirin (treatment duration is 48 weeks for genotype 1, 24 weeks for genotypes 2 and 3, or 48 weeks for patients who previously failed therapy [regardless of genotype]): Initial dose (based on an average weekly dose of 1.5 mcg/kg):

<40 kg: 50 mcg once weekly (with ribavirin 800 mg/day)
40 to 50 kg: 64 mcg once weekly (with ribavirin 800 mg/day)
51 to 60 kg: 80 mcg once weekly (with ribavirin 800 mg/day)
61 to 65 kg: 96 mcg once weekly (with ribavirin 800 mg/day)
66 to 75 kg: 96 mcg once weekly (with ribavirin 1000 mg/day)
76 to 80 kg: 120 mcg once weekly (with ribavirin 1000 mg/day)
81 to 85 kg: 120 mcg once weekly (with ribavirin 1200 mg/day)
86 to 105 kg: 150 mcg once weekly (with ribavirin 1200 mg/day)
>105 kg: 1.5 mcg/kg once weekly (with ribavirin 1400 mg/day)

Monotherapy (duration of treatment is 1 year): Initial dose (based on average weekly dose of 1 mcg/kg):

≤45 kg: 40 mcg once weekly
46 to 56 kg: 50 mcg once weekly
57 to 72 kg: 64 mcg once weekly
73 to 88 kg: 80 mcg once weekly
89 to 106 kg: 96 mcg once weekly
107 to 136 kg: 120 mcg once weekly
137 to 160 kg: 150 mcg once weekly

Alternative dosing: **Note:** Current AASLD/IDSA recommendations do not specify a particular peginterferon (eg, 2a or 2b); however, guideline recommendations are based on clinical trials that used peginterferon alfa-2a. It is not known whether peginterferon alfa 2b could be used interchangeably. Please refer to http://www.hcvguidelines.org for additional information.

◄ **Pediatric Chronic hepatitis C (CHC):**

Manufacturer labeling: Children 3 to 17 years: SubQ: Combination therapy with ribavirin: 60 mcg/m² once weekly; **Note:** Children who reach their 18th birthday during treatment should remain on the pediatric regimen. Treatment duration is 48 weeks for genotype 1, 24 weeks for genotypes 2 and 3. Discontinue combination therapy in patients with HCV (genotype 1) at 12 weeks if HCV-RNA does not decrease by at least 2 log (compared to pretreatment) or if detectable HCV-RNA present at 24 weeks.

American Association for the Study of Liver Diseases (AASLD) guideline recommendations (Ghany, 2009): Children 2-17 years: SubQ: Treatment of choice: Peginterferon alfa-2b 60 mcg/m² once weekly in combination with oral ribavirin 15 mg/kg/day for 48 weeks

Renal Impairment Chronic hepatitis C:

Peginterferon alfa-2b combination with ribavirin:

Adults: CrCl <50 mL/minute: Combination therapy with ribavirin is not recommended.

Children: Serum creatinine >2 mg/dL: Discontinue treatment.

Peginterferon alfa-2b monotherapy:

CrCl 30 to 50 mL/minute: Reduce dose by 25%

CrCl 10 to 29 mL/minute: Reduce dose by 50%

Hemodialysis: Reduce dose by 50%

Discontinue use if renal function declines during treatment.

Melanoma:

CrCl >50 mL/minute/1.73 m²: No dosage adjustment is necessary.

CrCl 30 to 50 mL/minute/1.73 m²: Reduce initial dose to 4.5 mcg/kg/week; reduce maintenance dose to 2.25 mcg/kg/week

CrCl <30 mL/minute/1.73 m² and ESRD on dialysis: Reduce initial dose to 3 mcg/kg/week; reduce maintenance dose to 1.5 mcg/kg/week

Hemodialysis: Following a single 1 mcg/kg/ dose, no clinically meaningful amount of peginterferon alfa-2b was removed during hemodialysis.

Hepatic Impairment

Decompensated liver disease or autoimmune hepatitis: Use is contraindicated.

Hepatic decompensation or severe hepatic injury during treatment (Child-Pugh score >6 [class B or C]): Discontinue immediately.

Adjustment for Toxicity

Melanoma:

Discontinue for any of the following: Persistent or worsening severe neuropsychiatric disorders (depression, psychosis, encephalopathy), grade 4 nonhematologic toxicity, new or worsening retinopathy, new-onset ventricular arrhythmia or cardiovascular decompensation, evidence of hepatic injury (severe) or hepatic decompensation (Child-Pugh score >6 [Class B or C]), development of hyper- or hypothyroidism or diabetes that cannot be effectively managed with medication, or inability to tolerate a dose of 1 mcg/kg/week

Temporarily withhold for any of the following: ANC <500/mm³, platelets <50,000/mm³, ECOG performance status (PS) ≥2, nonhematologic toxicity ≥ grade 3

May reinitiate at a reduced dose once ANC ≥500/mm³, platelets ≥50,000/mm³, ECOG PS at 0 to 1, and nonhematologic toxicity completely resolved or improved to grade 1.

Reduced dose schedule, Weeks 1 to 8:
First dose reduction (if prior dose 6 mcg/kg/week): 3 mcg/kg/week
Second dose reduction (if prior dose 3 mcg/kg/week): 2 mcg/kg/week
Third dose reduction (if prior dose 2 mcg/kg/week): 1 mcg/kg/week
Discontinue permanently if unable to tolerate 1 mcg/kg/week

Reduced dose schedule, Weeks 9 to 260:
First dose reduction (if prior dose 3 mcg/kg/week): 2 mcg/kg/week
Second dose reduction (if prior dose 2 mcg/kg/week): 1 mcg/kg/week
Discontinue permanently if unable to tolerate 1 mcg/kg/week

Chronic hepatitis C: Dosage adjustment for depression (severity based upon DSM-IV criteria):

Mild depression: No dosage adjustment required; evaluate once weekly by visit/phone call. If depression remains stable, continue weekly visits. If depression improves, resume normal visit schedule. For worsening depression, see "Moderate depression" or "Severe depression" below.

Moderate depression: **Note:** Evaluate once weekly (visit or phone) with an office visit at least every other week. If depression remains stable, consider psychiatric evaluation and continue with reduced dosing. If symptoms improve and remain stable for 4 weeks, resume normal visit schedule; continue reduced dosing or return to normal dose. For worsening depression, see "Severe depression" below.

Children: Decrease peginterferon alfa-2b dose to 40 mcg/m^2/week, may further decrease to 20 mcg/m^2/week if needed

Adults:
Peginterferon alfa-2b combination therapy: Refer to adult weight-based dosage reduction with combination therapy for depression below
Peginterferon alfa-2b monotherapy: Refer to adult weight-based dosage reduction with monotherapy for depression below

Severe depression: Discontinue peginterferon alfa-2b and ribavirin permanently. Obtain immediate psychiatric consultation. Utilize followup psychiatric therapy as needed.

Chronic hepatitis C: Dosage adjustment in hematologic toxicity:

Children:
Hemoglobin decrease ≥2 g/dL in any 4-week period and stable cardiac disease: Decrease peginterferon alfa-2b dose by 50%; decrease ribavirin dose by 200 mg daily (regardless of the patient's initial dose); monitor and evaluate weekly. If hemoglobin <8.5 g/dL any time after dose reduction or <12 g/dL after 4 weeks of dose reduction, permanently discontinue both peginterferon alfa-2b and ribavirin.

Hemoglobin 8.5 to <10 g/dL and no history of cardiac disease: Decrease ribavirin dose to 12 mg/kg/day; may further reduce to 8 mg/kg/day; no dosage adjustment necessary for peginterferon alfa-2b.

WBC 1000 to <1500/mm^3, neutrophils 500 to <750/mm^3, or platelets 50,000 to <70,000/mm^3: Reduce peginterferon alfa-2b dose to 40 mcg/m^2/week; may further reduce to 20 mcg/m^2/week

Hemoglobin <8.5 g/dL, WBC <1000/mm^3, neutrophils <500/mm^3, or platelets <50,000/mm^3: Permanently discontinue peginterferon alfa-2b and ribavirin

◀

Adults:

Hemoglobin decrease ≥2 g/dL in any 4-week period and stable cardiac disease: Decrease peginterferon alfa-2b dose by 50%; decrease ribavirin dose by 200 mg daily. If hemoglobin <8.5 g/dL any time after dose reduction or <12 g/dL after 4 weeks of dose reduction, permanently discontinue both peginterferon alfa-2b and ribavirin.

Hemoglobin 8.5 to <10 g/dL and no history of cardiac disease: Decrease ribavirin dose by 200 mg daily (patients receiving 1400 mg daily should decrease dose by 400 mg daily [ie, first dose reduction to 1000 mg daily]); may further reduce ribavirin dose by additional 200 mg daily if needed. No dosage adjustment necessary for peginterferon alfa-2b.

WBC 1000 to <1500/mm^3, neutrophils 500 to <750/mm^3, or platelets 25,000 to <50,000/mm^3:

Peginterferon alfa-2b combination therapy: Refer to adult weight-based dosage reduction with combination therapy for hematologic toxicity below.

Peginterferon alfa-2b monotherapy: Refer to adult weight-based dosage reduction monotherapy for hematologic toxicity below.

Hemoglobin <8.5 g/dL, WBC <1000/mm^3, neutrophils <500/mm^3, or platelets <25,000/mm^3: Permanently discontinue peginterferon alfa-2b and ribavirin.

Chronic hepatitis C: **Adult weight-based dosage reduction for depression or hematologic toxicity:**

Peginterferon alfa-2b combination therapy: Initially reduce to average weekly dose of 1 mcg/kg; may further reduce to average weekly dose of 0.5 mcg/kg if needed as follows:

<40 kg: 35 mcg once weekly; may further reduce to 20 mcg once weekly if needed

40 to 50 kg: 45 mcg once weekly; may further reduce to 25 mcg once weekly if needed

51 to 60 kg: 50 mcg once weekly; may further reduce to 30 mcg once weekly if needed

61 to 75 kg: 64 mcg once weekly; may further reduce to 35 mcg once weekly if needed

76 to 85 kg: 80 mcg once weekly; may further reduce to 45 mcg once weekly if needed

86 to 104 kg: 96 mcg once weekly; may further reduce to 50 mcg once weekly if needed

105 to 125 kg: 108 mcg once weekly; may further reduce to 64 mcg once weekly if needed

>125 kg: 135 mcg once weekly; may further reduce to 72 mcg once weekly if needed

Peginterferon alfa-2b monotherapy: Reduce to average weekly dose of 0.5 mcg/kg as follows:

≤45 kg: 20 mcg once weekly

46 to 56 kg: 25 mcg once weekly

57 to 72 kg: 30 mcg once weekly

73 to 88 kg: 40 mcg once weekly

89 to 106 kg: 50 mcg once weekly

107 to 136 kg: 64 mcg once weekly

≥137 kg: 80 mcg once weekly

Administration For SubQ administration; rotate injection site; thigh, outer surface of upper arm, and abdomen are preferred injection sites; do not inject near navel or waistline; patients who are thin should only use thigh or upper arm. Do not inject into bruised, infected, irritated, red, or scarred skin. The weekly dose may be administered at bedtime to reduce flu-like symptoms. For the treatment of CHC, the administration volume depends on the patient's weight and the peginterferon concentration used.

Emetic Potential Children and Adults: Minimal (<10%)

Monitoring Parameters Baseline and periodic TSH (for patients being treated for melanoma, obtain baseline within 4 weeks prior to treatment initiation, and then at 3 and 6 months, and every 6 months thereafter during treatment); CBC with differential and platelets; serum chemistries, liver function tests (for patients with melanoma, monitor serum bilirubin, ALT, AST, alkaline phosphatase, and LDH at 2 and 8 weeks, and 2 and 3 months following initiation, then every 6 months during therapy), renal function, triglycerides; serum glucose or HbA$_{1c}$ (for patients with diabetes mellitus). Clinical studies (for combination therapy) tested as follows: CBC (including hemoglobin, WBC, and platelets) and chemistries (including liver function tests and uric acid) measured at weeks 2, 4, 8, and 12, and then every 6 weeks; TSH measured every 12 weeks during treatment. ECG at baseline for patients with preexisting cardiac abnormalities (for combination therapy with ribavirin).

Hepatitic C: Serum HCV RNA levels (pretreatment, 12 and 24 weeks after therapy initiation, 24 weeks after completion of therapy). **Note:** Discontinuation of therapy may be considered after 12 weeks in patients with HCV (genotype 1) who fail to achieve an early virologic response (EVR) (defined as ≥2-log decrease in HCV RNA compared to pretreatment) or after 24 weeks with detectable HCV RNA. Treat patients with HCV (genotypes 2,3) for 24 weeks (if tolerated) and then evaluate HCV RNA levels (Ghany, 2009).

Evaluate for depression and other psychiatric symptoms before and after initiation of therapy; patients being treated for melanoma should be monitored for depression and psychiatric symptoms every 3 weeks during the first eight weeks of treatment and every 6 months thereafter, and continued monitoring for 6 months after the last dose; baseline ophthalmic eye examination; periodic ophthalmic exam in patients with diabetic or hypertensive retinopathy; baseline ECG in patients with cardiac disease; serum glucose or HbA$_{1c}$ (for patients with diabetes mellitus). In combination therapy with ribavirin, pregnancy tests (for women of childbearing age who are receiving treatment or who have male partners who are receiving treatment), continue monthly up to 6 months after discontinuation of therapy. In pediatric patients, growth velocity and weight should also be monitored during and periodically after treatment discontinuation.

Medication Guide Available Yes

Dosage Forms Excipient information presented when available (limited, particularly for generics); consult specific product labeling. [DSC] = Discontinued product

Kit, Subcutaneous:

Sylatron: 4 x 200 mcg, 4 x 300 mcg, 4 x 600 mcg [DSC] [contains polysorbate 80]

◀ Kit, Subcutaneous [preservative free]:
Peg-Intron: 50 mcg/0.5 mL, 80 mcg/0.5 mL, 120 mcg/0.5 mL, 150 mcg/0.5 mL
Peg-Intron Redipen: 50 mcg/0.5 mL, 80 mcg/0.5 mL, 120 mcg/0.5 mL, 150 mcg/0.5 mL
Peg-Intron Redipen Pak 4: 50 mcg/0.5 mL [DSC], 80 mcg/0.5 mL [DSC], 120 mcg/0.5 mL, 150 mcg/0.5 mL [DSC]
PegIntron: 50 mcg/0.5 mL, 80 mcg/0.5 mL, 120 mcg/0.5 mL, 150 mcg/0.5 mL [contains polysorbate 80]
Sylatron: 200 mcg, 300 mcg, 600 mcg [contains polysorbate 80]

Pembrolizumab (pem broe LIZ ue mab)

Brand Names: US Keytruda

Brand Names: Canada Keytruda

Index Terms Anti-PD-1 Monoclonal Antibody MK-3475; Lambrolizumab; MK-3475; SCH 90045

Pharmacologic Category Antineoplastic Agent, Anti-PD-1 Monoclonal Antibody; Antineoplastic Agent, Monoclonal Antibody

Use

US labeling:

Melanoma, unresectable or metastatic: Treatment of unresectable or metastatic melanoma with disease progression following ipilimumab and a BRAF inhibitor (if BRAF V600 mutation positive).

Non-small cell lung cancer, metastatic: Treatment of metastatic non-small cell lung cancer in patients with PD-L1-expressing tumors (as determined by an approved test) who have disease progression on or after platinum-containing chemotherapy. Patients with EGFR or ALK genomic tumor aberrations should have disease progression (on approved EGFR- or ALK-directed therapy) prior to receiving pembrolizumab.

Canadian labeling: **Melanoma:** Treatment of unresectable or metastatic melanoma with disease progression following ipilimumab and if BRAF V600 mutation positive, a BRAF inhibitor or MEK inhibitor.

Labeled Contraindications

There are no contraindications listed in the US labeling.

Canadian labeling: Hypersensitivity to pembrolizumab or any component of the formulation.

Pregnancy Considerations Animal reproduction studies have not been conducted. Immunoglobulins are known to cross the placenta; therefore fetal exposure to pembrolizumab is expected. Based on the mechanism of action, pembrolizumab may cause fetal harm if administered during pregnancy; an alteration in the immune response or immune mediated disorders may develop following in utero exposure. Women of reproductive potential should use highly effective contraception during therapy and for at least 4 months after treatment is complete.

Breast-Feeding Considerations It is not known if pembrolizumab is excreted into breast milk. The manufacturer recommends that breast-feeding be discontinued during therapy and for 4 months following the final dose. Immunoglobulins are excreted in breast milk; therefore pembrolizumab may be expected to appear in breast milk.

Warnings/Precautions Immune-mediated pneumonitis has been observed, including fatal cases. For patients with melanoma, the median time to development was 5 months (range: ~2 days to ~10 months) and the median duration was ~5 months (range: 1 week to 14.4 months). Some patients required initial management with high-dose systemic corticosteroids (median initial prednisone dose of 63.4 mg/day or equivalent), the median duration of initial corticosteroid therapy was 3 days (range: 1 to 34 days) followed by a corticosteroid taper. For patients with NSCLC, the median time to development was 1.7 months (range: ~1 week to ~13 months) and the median duration was 1.2 months (range: ~1 week to ~12 months). Some patients had complete resolution of pneumonitis. May require treatment interruption, corticosteroid therapy (prednisone 1 to 2 mg/kg /day [or equivalent] followed by a taper, for grade 2 or higher pneumonitis), and/or permanent discontinuation. Monitor for signs and symptoms of pneumonitis; if pneumonitis is suspected, evaluate with radiographic imaging and administer systemic corticosteroids for grade 2 or higher pneumonitis. For NSCLC, pneumonitis occurred more frequently in patients with a history of asthma, COPD, or prior thoracic radiation.

Immune-mediated colitis (including microscopic colitis) has occurred, including cases of grade 2 or 3 colitis. The median time to onset of colitis was 6.5 months (range: ~2 to 10 months) and the mediation duration was 2.6 months (range: 4 days to 3.6 months) in patients with melanoma. In patients with NSCLC, the median time to onset was 1.6 months (range: ~1 to ~2 months) and the median duration was 16 days (range: 1 to ~6 weeks). In melanoma patients, grade 2 or 3 colitis was managed with high-dose systemic corticosteroids (prednisone ≥40 mg/day [median initial dose 70 mg/day] or equivalent) with a median duration of initial corticosteroid therapy of 7 days (range: 4 to 41 days), followed by a corticosteroid taper. Most patients with colitis experienced complete resolution. May require treatment interruption, systemic corticosteroid therapy, and/or permanent discontinuation. Monitor for signs and symptoms of colitis; administer systemic corticosteroids for grade 2 or higher colitis.

Hepatitis, including autoimmune hepatitis, occurred (case reports, including 1 case of grade 4 hepatitis). The median onset for grade 4 hepatitis was 22 days; the duration was 1.1 months. Administer corticosteroids (prednisone 0.5 to 1 mg/kg/day [or equivalent] for grade 2, and prednisone 1 to 2 mg/kg/day [or equivalent] for grade 3, each followed a taper), and withhold or discontinue therapy based on the severity of liver enzyme elevations. Grade 4 hepatitis occurred in a patient with melanoma and was managed with high-dose systemic corticosteroids (prednisone ≥40 mg/day or equivalent), followed a corticosteroid taper. Monitor for liver function changes. May require treatment ▶

interruption, systemic corticosteroids (for grade 2 or higher toxicity), and/or permanent discontinuation.

Immune-mediated hypophysitis occurred (1 case each of grades 2, 3, and 4). The time to onset ranged from 1.3 to 3.7 months. Hypophysitis was managed with high-dose systemic corticosteroids (prednisone ≥40 mg/day or equivalent), followed by a corticosteroid taper. Patients then remained on physiologic corticosteroid replacement. Monitor for signs/symptoms of hypophysitis (eg, hypopituitarism, adrenal insufficiency). May require treatment interruption, systemic corticosteroids (for grade 2 or higher toxicity), hormone replacement, and/or permanent discontinuation.

Nephritis, including case reports of autoimmune nephritis and interstitial nephritis with renal failure, has occurred. The onset for autoimmune nephritis in melanoma patients was 11.6 months after the first dose and 5 months after the last dose, and duration was 3.2 months. Acute interstitial nephritis was confirmed by renal biopsy in 2 patients with grades 3/4 renal failure. Grade 2 or higher nephritis should be managed with systemic corticosteroids (prednisone initial dose of 1 to 2 mg/kg/day [or equivalent], followed by a taper). Monitor for renal function changes. May require treatment interruption, systemic corticosteroids (for grade 2 or higher toxicity), and/or permanent discontinuation.

Immune-mediated hyperthyroidism and hypothyroidism have occurred. The median onset for hyperthyroidism was 1.5 to 1.8 months (range: 2 days to ~3 months), and the median duration was 2.8 to 4.5 months (range: 1 to ~8 months). May require management with high-dose systemic corticosteroids (prednisone ≥40 mg/day or equivalent), followed by a corticosteroid taper. Hyperthyroidism resolved in all cases observed in one clinical trial. Hypothyroidism occurred with a median onset of 3.5 to ~4 months (range: 5 days to 19 months). Hypothyroidism was generally managed with long-term thyroid hormone replacement therapy, although some patients only required short-term replacement therapy. Hypothyroidism did not require systemic corticosteroid therapy or discontinuation. Thyroid disorders may occur at any point in pembrolizumab therapy. Monitor for changes in thyroid function (at baseline, periodically during treatment and as clinically indicated) and for signs/symptoms of thyroid disorder. Administer thionamides and beta-blockers for hyperthyroidism as appropriate; may require treatment interruption and/or permanent discontinuation. Isolated hypothyroidism may be managed with replacement therapy (without corticosteroids and treatment interruption). Type 1 diabetes mellitus has occurred (including diabetic ketoacidosis). Insulin therapy may be required; if severe hyperglycemia is observed, administer antihyperglycemics and withhold pembrolizumab treatment until glucose control has been accomplished.

Other clinically relevant immune-mediated disorders have been observed, including rash, exfoliative dermatitis, uveitis, arthritis, vasculitis, myositis, pancreatitis, hemolytic anemia, serum sickness, myasthenia gravis, and partial seizures (in a patient with inflammatory foci in brain parenchyma). Bullous pemphigoid and Guillain-Barre syndrome have also been observed in patients receiving pembrolizumab. If an immune-mediated adverse event is suspected, evaluate appropriately to confirm or exclude other causes; withhold treatment and administer systemic corticosteroids based on severity of reaction. Upon resolution to grade 0 or 1, initiate corticosteroid taper (continue tapering over at least 1 month). When reaction remains at grade 1 or less during taper may reinitiate pembrolizumab. Discontinue permanently for severe or grade 3 immune-mediated adverse event that is recurrent or life-threatening. Infusion-related reactions (including severe and life-threatening cases) have occurred. Interrupt infusion for severe (grade 3) or life-threatening (grade 4) reactions; and permanently discontinue for severe (grade 3) or life-threatening (grade 4) infusion-related reactions.

Adverse Reactions

>10%:

Cardiovascular: Peripheral edema (17%; grade 3: 1%)

Central nervous system: Fatigue (47%; grade 3: 7%), headache (16%), chills (14%), insomnia (14%), dizziness (11%)

Dermatologic: Pruritus (30%), skin rash (29%), vitiligo (11%)

Endocrine & metabolic: Hyperglycemia (40%; grade 3: 1%; grade 4: 1%), hyponatremia (35%; grade 3: 9%), hypoalbuminemia (34%), hypertriglyceridemia (25%), hypocalcemia (24%; grade 3: 1%)

Gastrointestinal: Nausea (30%), decreased appetite (26%), constipation (21%), diarrhea (20%), vomiting (16%), abdominal pain (12%)

Hematologic & oncologic: Anemia (14% to 55%; grade 3: 5% to 7%; grade 4: 1%)

Hepatic: Increased serum AST (24%; grade 3: 1%; grade 4: 1%)

Neuromuscular & skeletal: Arthralgia (20%), limb pain (18%; grade 3: 1%), myalgia (14%; grade 3: 1%), back pain (12%; grade 3: 1%)

Respiratory: Cough (30%; grade 3: 1%), dyspnea (18%; grade 3: 2%), upper respiratory tract infection (11%; grade 3: 1%)

Miscellaneous: Fever (11%)

1% to 10%:

Dermatologic: Cellulitis (≥2%)

Endocrine & metabolic: Hypothyroidism (immune-mediated; 8%; grade 3: <1%), hyperthyroidism (immune-mediated; 1%; grade 2: <1%; grade 3: <1%)

Gastrointestinal: Colitis (including microscopic colitis: 1%; grade 2: <1%, grade 3: <1%)

Infection: Sepsis (≤10%)

Renal: Renal failure (≥2%)

Respiratory: Pneumonitis (3%; grade 2: 2%; grade 3: <1%), pneumonia (≥2%)

<1%, postmarketing, and/or case reports: Adrenocortical insufficiency (immune-mediated), arthritis (immune-mediated), bullous pemphigoid, diabetic ketoacidosis, exfoliative dermatitis (immune-mediated), hemolytic anemia (immune-mediated), hepatitis (including autoimmune hepatitis; grade 4: <1%), hypophysitis (grade 2: <1%; grade 4: <1%), infusion related reaction, interstitial nephritis (with renal failure; grade 3: <1%; grade 4: <1%), Lambert-Eaton syndrome (immune-mediated), myositis (immune-mediated), nephritis (grade 2 autoimmune: <1%), optic neuritis (immune-mediated), pancreatitis (immune-mediated), partial epilepsy (immune-mediated; in a patient with inflammatory foci in brain parenchyma), rhabdomyolysis (immune-mediated), severe dermatitis, type 1 diabetes mellitus, uveitis (immune-mediated)

Drug Interactions

Metabolism/Transport Effects None known.

Avoid Concomitant Use There are no known interactions where it is recommended to avoid concomitant use.

Increased Effect/Toxicity There are no known significant interactions involving an increase in effect.

◀ **Decreased Effect** There are no known significant interactions involving a decrease in effect.

Storage/Stability Lyophilized powder (50 mg vial) and injection solution (100 mg/4 mL vial): Store intact vials refrigerated at 2°C to 8°C (36°F to 46°F); protect injection solution vials from light and do not shake or freeze. Reconstituted solutions and solutions diluted for infusion may be stored at room temperature for up to 6 hours (infusion must be completed within 6 hours of reconstitution) or refrigerated at 2°C to 8°C (36°F to 46°F) for no more than 24 hours from the time of reconstitution. Do not freeze. If refrigerated, allow to reach room temperature prior to administration.

Preparation for Administration

Injection solution (100 mg/4 mL vial): Withdraw appropriate volume from vial and transfer to IV bag containing 0.9% sodium chloride or D_5W; final concentration should be between 1 to 10 mg/mL. Mix by gently inverting bag. Discard unused portion of the vial.

Lyophilized powder (50 mg vial): Reconstitute by adding 2.3 mL SWFI along the vial wall (do not add directly to lyophilized powder); resulting vial concentration is 25 mg/mL. Slowly swirl vial; do not shake. Allow up to 5 minutes for bubbles to dissipate. Reconstituted solution is a clear to slightly opalescent and colorless to slightly yellow solution; discard if visible particles present. Withdraw appropriate volume from vial and transfer to IV bag containing 0.9% sodium chloride or D_5W final concentration should be between 1 to 10 mg/mL. Mix by gently inverting bag. Discard unused portion of the vial.

Mechanism of Action Highly selective anti-PD-1 humanized monoclonal antibody which inhibits programmed cell death-1 (PD-1) activity by binding to the PD-1 receptor on T-cells to block PD-1 ligands (PD-L1 and PD-L2) from binding. Blocking the PD-1 pathway inhibits the negative immune regulation caused by PD-1 receptor signaling (Hamid, 2013). Anti-PD-1 antibodies (including pembrolizumab) reverse T-cell suppression and induce antitumor responses (Robert, 2014).

Pharmacodynamics/Kinetics

V_{dss}: 7.75 L

Half-life elimination: 28 days

Dosing

Adult & Geriatric

Melanoma, unresectable or metastatic: IV: 2 mg/kg once every 3 weeks until disease progression or unacceptable toxicity.

Non-small cell lung cancer, metastatic: IV: 2 mg/kg once every 3 weeks until disease progression or unacceptable toxicity.

Renal Impairment

US labeling: No dosage adjustment necessary. In a pharmacokinetic study, no difference in clearance was noted for patients with mild, moderate, or severe impairment (eGFR ≥15 mL/minute to 89 mL/minute) when compared to patients with normal renal function (eGFR ≥90 mL/minute); patients with eGFR <15 mL/minute were not studied.

Canadian labeling:

Mild or moderate impairment: eGFR ≥30 mL/minute/1.73 m^2 to <90 mL/minute/1.73 m^2: No dosage adjustment necessary.

Severe impairment: There are no dosage adjustments provided in the manufacturer's labeling.

Hepatic Impairment

*Hepatic impairment **prior** to treatment initiation:*

Mild impairment (total bilirubin ≤ULN and AST >ULN or total bilirubin >1 to 1.5 times ULN and any AST): No dosage adjustment necessary.

Moderate (total bilirubin >1.5 to 3 times ULN and any AST) to severe (total bilirubin >3 times ULN and any AST) impairment: There are no dosage adjustments provided in the manufacturer's labeling (has not been studied).

*Hepatotoxicity **during** treatment:* **Note:** For patients with baseline grade 2 ALT or AST abnormalities due to liver metastases, permanently discontinue if AST or ALT increases by ≥50% (relative to baseline) and persists at least 1 week.

AST or ALT >3 to 5 times ULN or total bilirubin >1.5 to 3 times ULN: Withhold treatment; may resume therapy upon recovery to grade 0 or 1 toxicity. Also administer corticosteroids (prednisone 0.5 to 1 mg/kg/day [or equivalent] followed by a taper).

AST or ALT >5 times ULN or total bilirubin >3 times ULN: Permanently discontinue. Also administer corticosteroids (prednisone 1 to 2 mg/kg/day [or equivalent] followed a taper).

Adjustment for Toxicity

Withhold treatment for any of the following (may resume upon recovery to grade 0 or 1 toxicity):

Colitis, moderate (grade 2) or severe (grade 3); also administer corticosteroids (prednisone 1 to 2 mg/kg/day [or equivalent] followed by a taper).

Endocrinopathies:

Hyperthyroidism, severe (grade 3) or life threatening (grade 4); manage with thionamides and beta-blockers as appropriate.

Hypophysitis, grade 2 (symptomatic); also administer corticosteroids (followed by a taper) and hormone replacement therapy if appropriate.

Nephritis, grade 2; also administer corticosteroids (prednisone 1 to 2 mg/kg/day [or equivalent] followed by a taper).

Pneumonitis, moderate (grade 2); also administer corticosteroids (prednisone 1 to 2 mg/kg/day [or equivalent] followed by a taper).

Other treatment-related toxicity, severe or grade 3; may require corticosteroids (≥40 mg/day of prednisone or equivalent, based on severity). Upon improvement to grade 0 or 1, initiate corticosteroid taper and continue to taper over at least 1 month. Restart pembrolizumab if the adverse reaction remains at grade 0 or 1.

Withhold (may resume upon recovery to grade 0 or 1 toxicity) or discontinue for:

Hyperthyroidism, severe (grade 3) or life-threatening (grade 4); manage with thionamides and beta-blockers as appropriate.

Hypophysitis, severe (grade 3) or life-threatening (grade 4); also administer corticosteroids and hormone replacement as appropriate.

Permanently discontinue for:

Adverse reactions that are life-threatening, persistent grade 2 or 3 adverse reaction (excluding endocrinopathies controlled with hormone replacement therapy) that does not recover to grade 0 or 1 within 12 weeks after the last pembrolizumab dose, or any recurrent severe or grade 3 treatment-related adverse reaction. Also administer corticosteroids (≥40 mg/day of prednisone or equivalent).

Colitis, life-threatening (grade 4); also administer corticosteroids (prednisone 1 to 2 mg/kg/day [or equivalent] followed by a taper).

Immune mediated adverse reactions: Discontinue permanently if unable to reduce corticosteroid dose to prednisone ≤10 mg/day (or equivalent) within 12 weeks.

Infusion-related reaction, grade 3 or 4.

Nephritis, severe (grade 3) or life-threatening (grade 4); also administer corticosteroids (prednisone 1 to 2 mg/kg/day [or equivalent] followed by a taper).

Pneumonitis, severe (grade 3), life-threatening (grade 4), or moderate (grade 2) that recurs; also administer corticosteroids (prednisone 1 to 2 mg/kg/day [or equivalent] followed by a taper).

Administration IV: Infuse over 30 minutes through a 0.2 to 5 micron sterile, nonpyrogenic, low-protein binding inline or add-on filter. Do not infuse other medications through the same infusion line.

Emetic Potential Minimal (<10%)

Monitoring Parameters PD-L1 expression status in patients with NSCLC; liver function tests (AST, ALT, and total bilirubin); renal function; thyroid function (at baseline, periodically during treatment and as clinically indicated); glucose; signs/symptoms of colitis, hypophysitis, thyroid disorders, pneumonitis, infusion reactions.

Medication Guide Available Yes

Dosage Forms Excipient information presented when available (limited, particularly for generics); consult specific product labeling.

Solution, Intravenous [preservative free]:

Keytruda: 100 mg/4 mL (4 mL) [contains polysorbate 80]

Solution Reconstituted, Intravenous [preservative free]:

Keytruda: 50 mg (1 ea) [contains polysorbate 80]

PEMEtrexed (pem e TREKS ed)

Related Information

Common Toxicity Criteria *on page 2122*

Management of Chemotherapy-Induced Nausea and Vomiting in Adults *on page 2142*

Prevention of Chemotherapy-Induced Nausea and Vomiting in Children *on page 2203*

Safe Handling of Hazardous Drugs *on page 2292*

Brand Names: US Alimta

Brand Names: Canada Alimta

Index Terms LY231514; Pemetrexed Disodium

Pharmacologic Category Antineoplastic Agent, Antimetabolite; Antineoplastic Agent, Antimetabolite (Antifolate)

Use

Mesothelioma: Treatment of unresectable malignant pleural mesothelioma (in combination with cisplatin)

Non-small cell lung cancer (NSCLC), nonsquamous: Treatment of locally advanced or metastatic **non**squamous NSCLC (as initial treatment in combination with cisplatin, as single-agent maintenance treatment after 4 cycles of initial platinum-based double therapy, and single-agent treatment after prior chemotherapy)

Limitation of use: Not indicated for the treatment of **squamous** cell NSCLC

Labeled Contraindications Severe hypersensitivity to pemetrexed or any component of the formulation

Canadian labeling (additional contraindications; not in U.S. labeling): Concomitant yellow fever vaccine

Pregnancy Considerations Adverse effects (embryotoxicity, fetotoxicity and teratogenicity) were observed in animal reproduction studies. Based on the mechanism of action, may cause fetal harm if administered to a pregnant woman. Women of childbearing potential should have a negative serum pregnancy test prior to treatment and should use effective contraceptive measures to avoid becoming pregnant during treatment. Irreversible infertility has been reported in males; prior to receiving treatment, males should be counseled on sperm storage. The Canadian labeling recommends that males receiving therapy use effective contraceptive measures and not father a child during, and for up to 6 months after therapy.

Breast-Feeding Considerations According to the manufacturer, the decision to continue or discontinue breast-feeding during therapy should take into account the risk of exposure to the infant and the benefits of treatment to the mother.

Warnings/Precautions Hazardous agent - use appropriate precautions for handling and disposal (NIOSH 2014 [group 1]). Hypersensitivity (including anaphylaxis) has been reported with use. May cause bone marrow suppression (anemia, neutropenia, thrombocytopenia and/or pancytopenia); frequent laboratory monitoring is necessary (myelosuppression is often dose-limiting). Dose reductions in subsequent cycles may be required. Prophylactic folic acid and vitamin B_{12} supplements are necessary to reduce hematologic and gastrointestinal toxicity and infection; initiate supplementation 1 week before the first dose of pemetrexed. Pretreatment with dexamethasone is necessary to reduce the incidence and severity of cutaneous reactions. Rarely, Stevens-Johnson syndrome and toxic epidermal necrolysis have been reported. Although the effect of third space fluid is not fully defined, studies have determined pemetrexed concentrations in patients with mild-to-moderate ascites/pleural effusions were similar to concentrations in trials of patients without third space fluid accumulation. Drainage of fluid from ascites/effusions may be considered, but is not likely necessary. Use caution with hepatic dysfunction not due to metastases; may require dose adjustment. Interstitial pneumonitis with respiratory insufficiency has been observed with use; interrupt therapy and evaluate promptly with progressive dyspnea and cough.

The manufacturer does not recommend use in patients with CrCl <45 mL/minute. Decreased renal function results in increased toxicity. Potentially significant drug-drug interactions may exist, requiring dose or frequency adjustment, additional monitoring, and/or selection of alternative therapy. Use caution in patients receiving concurrent nephrotoxins; may result in delayed pemetrexed clearance. NSAIDs may reduce the clearance of pemetrexed. In patients with CrCl 45-79 mL/minute, interruption of NSAID therapy may be necessary prior to, during, and immediately after pemetrexed therapy. Not indicated for use in patients with squamous cell NSCLC.

Adverse Reactions

>10%:

Central nervous system: Fatigue (18% to 34%; dose-limiting)

Dermatologic: Rash/desquamation (10% to 14%)

Gastrointestinal: Nausea (12% to 31%), anorexia (19% to 22%), vomiting (6% to 16%), stomatitis (5% to 15%), diarrhea (5% to 13%)

Hematologic: Anemia (15% to 19%; grades 3/4: 3% to 5%), leukopenia (6% to 12%; grades 3/4: 2% to 4%), neutropenia (6% to 11%; grades 3/4: 3% to 5%; dose-limiting; nadir: 8-10 days; recovery: 4-8 days after nadir)

Respiratory: Pharyngitis (15%)

1% to 10%:

Cardiovascular: Edema (1% to 5%)

Central nervous system: Fever (1% to 8%)

Dermatologic: Pruritus (1% to 7%), alopecia (1% to 6%), erythema multiforme (≤5%)

Gastrointestinal: Constipation (1% to 6%), weight loss (1%), abdominal pain (≤5%)

Hematologic: Thrombocytopenia (1% to 8%; grades 3/4: 2%; dose-limiting), febrile neutropenia (grades 3/4: 2%)

Hepatic: ALT increased (8% to 10%; grades 3/4: ≤2%), AST increased (7% to 8%; grades 3/4: ≤1%)

Neuromuscular & skeletal: Sensory neuropathy (≤9%), motor neuropathy (≤5%)

Ocular: Conjunctivitis (≤5%), lacrimation increased (≤5%)

Renal: Creatinine increased/creatinine clearance decreased (1% to 5%)

Miscellaneous: Allergic reaction/hypersensitivity (≤5%), infection (≤5%), sepsis (1%)

<1%, postmarketing, and/or case reports: Arrhythmia, chest pain, colitis, dehydration, depression, esophagitis, gastrointestinal obstruction, GGT increased, hemolytic anemia, hepatobiliary failure, hypertension, interstitial pneumonitis, pain, pancreatitis, pancytopenia, peripheral ischemia, pulmonary embolism, radiation recall (median onset: 6 days; range: 1-35 days), renal failure, Stevens-Johnson syndrome, supraventricular arrhythmia, syncope, thrombosis/embolism, toxic epidermal necrolysis, ventricular tachycardia

Drug Interactions

Metabolism/Transport Effects None known.

Avoid Concomitant Use

Avoid concomitant use of PEMEtrexed with any of the following: BCG (Intravesical); CloZAPine; Dipyrone; Natalizumab; Pimecrolimus; Tacrolimus (Topical); Tofacitinib; Vaccines (Live)

Increased Effect/Toxicity

PEMEtrexed may increase the levels/effects of: CloZAPine; Fingolimod; Leflunomide; Natalizumab; Tofacitinib; Vaccines (Live)

The levels/effects of PEMEtrexed may be increased by: Denosumab; Dipyrone; NSAID (Nonselective); Pimecrolimus; Roflumilast; Tacrolimus (Topical); Trastuzumab

Decreased Effect

PEMEtrexed may decrease the levels/effects of: BCG (Intravesical); Coccidioides immitis Skin Test; Sipuleucel-T; Vaccines (Inactivated); Vaccines (Live)

The levels/effects of PEMEtrexed may be decreased by: Echinacea

Storage/Stability Store intact vials at room temperature of 25°C (77°F); excursions permitted to 15°C to 30°C (59°F to 86°F). Reconstituted solution in NS and infusion solutions (in D₅W or NS) are stable for 24 hours when refrigerated at 2°C to 8°C (36°F to 46°F). Concentrations at 25 mg/mL are stable in polypropylene syringes for 2 days at room temperature (23°C) (Zhang, 2005).

Preparation for Administration Hazardous agent; use appropriate precautions for handling and disposal (NIOSH 2014 [group 1]). Reconstitute with NS (preservative free); add 4.2 mL to the 100 mg vial and 20 mL to the 500 mg vial, resulting in a 25 mg/mL concentration. Gently swirl. Solution may be colorless to green-yellow. Further dilute in 100 mL NS prior to infusion (the manufacturer recommends a total volume of 100 mL); may also dilute in D_5W (Zhang, 2006), although the manufacturer recommends NS.

Mechanism of Action Antifolate; disrupts folate-dependent metabolic processes essential for cell replication. Inhibits thymidylate synthase (TS), dihydrofolate reductase (DHFR), glycinamide ribonucleotide formyltransferase (GARFT), and aminoimidazole carboxamide ribonucleotide formyltransferase (AICARFT), the enzymes involved in folate metabolism and DNA synthesis, resulting in inhibition of purine and thymidine nucleotide and protein synthesis.

Pharmacodynamics/Kinetics

Distribution: V_{dss}: 16.1 L

Protein binding: ~73% to 81%

Metabolism: Minimal

Half-life elimination: Normal renal function: 3.5 hours; CrCl 40 to 59 mL/minute: 5.3 to 5.8 hours

Excretion: Urine (70% to 90% as unchanged drug)

Dosing

Adult & Geriatric Note: Start vitamin supplements 1 week before initial pemetrexed dose: Folic acid 400 to 1000 mcg daily orally (begin 7 days prior to treatment initiation; continue daily during treatment and for 21 days after last pemetrexed dose) and vitamin B_{12} 1000 mcg IM 7 days prior to treatment initiation and then every 3 cycles. Give dexamethasone 4 mg orally twice daily for 3 days, beginning the day before treatment to minimize cutaneous reactions. New treatment cycles should not begin unless ANC ≥1500/mm³, platelets ≥100,000/mm³, and CrCl ≥45 mL/minute.

Malignant pleural mesothelioma: IV: 500 mg/m² on day 1 of each 21-day cycle (in combination with cisplatin) **or** (off-label) in combination with carboplatin (Castagneto, 2008; Ceresoli, 2006) **or** (off-label) as single-agent therapy (Jassem, 2008; Taylor, 2008)

Non-small cell lung cancer, nonsquamous: IV:

Initial treatment: 500 mg/m² on day 1 of each 21-day cycle (in combination with cisplatin)

Maintenance or second-line treatment: 500 mg/m² on day 1 of each 21-day cycle (as a single-agent)

Bladder cancer, metastatic (off-label use): IV: 500 mg/m² on day 1 of each 21-day cycle until disease progression or unacceptable toxicity (Sweeney, 2006)

Cervical cancer, persistent or recurrent (off-label use): IV: 500 mg/m² on day 1 of each 21-day cycle until disease progression or unacceptable toxicity occurs (Lorusso, 2010) **or** 900 mg/m² on day 1 of each 21-day cycle (Miller, 2008)

Ovarian cancer, platinum-resistant (off-label use): IV: 500 mg/m² on day 1 of each 21-day cycle (Vergote, 2009)

Thymic malignancies, metastatic (off-label use): IV: 500 mg/m² on day 1 of each 21-day cycle for 6 cycles or until disease progression or unacceptable toxicity occurs (Loehrer, 2006)

◄ **Renal Impairment**

Renal function may be estimated using the Cockcroft-Gault formula (using actual body weight) or glomerular filtration rate (GFR) measured by Tc99m-DPTA serum clearance.

CrCl ≥45 mL/minute: No dosage adjustment necessary.

CrCl <45 mL/minute: Use is not recommended (an insufficient number of patients have been studied for dosage recommendations).

Concomitant NSAID use with renal dysfunction:

CrCl ≥80 mL/minute: No dosage adjustment necessary.

CrCl 45 to 79 mL/minute and NSAIDs with short half-lives (eg, ibuprofen, indomethacin, ketoprofen, ketorolac): Avoid NSAID for 2 days before, the day of, and for 2 days following a dose of pemetrexed.

Any creatinine clearance and NSAIDs with long half-lives (eg, nabumetone, naproxen, oxaprozin, piroxicam): Avoid NSAID for 5 days before, the day of, and 2 days following a dose of pemetrexed.

Hepatic Impairment Grade 3 (5.1 to 20 times ULN) **or** 4 (>20 times ULN) transaminase elevation during treatment: Reduce pemetrexed dose to 75% of previous dose (and cisplatin).

Obesity *ASCO Guidelines for appropriate chemotherapy dosing in obese adults with cancer:* Utilize patient's actual body weight (full weight) for calculation of body surface area- or weight-based dosing, particularly when the intent of therapy is curative; manage regimen-related toxicities in the same manner as for nonobese patients; if a dose reduction is utilized due to toxicity, consider resumption of full weight-based dosing with subsequent cycles, especially if cause of toxicity (eg, hepatic or renal impairment) is resolved (Griggs, 2012).

Adjustment for Toxicity

Toxicity: Discontinue if patient develops grade 3 or 4 toxicity after two dose reductions or immediately if grade 3 or 4 neurotoxicity develops

Hematologic toxicity: Upon recovery, reinitiate therapy

Nadir ANC <500/mm³ and nadir platelets ≥50,000/mm³: Reduce dose to 75% of previous dose of pemetrexed (and cisplatin)

Nadir platelets <50,000/mm³ **without bleeding** (regardless of nadir ANC): Reduce dose to 75% of previous dose of pemetrexed (and cisplatin)

Nadir platelets <50,000/mm³ **with bleeding** (regardless of nadir ANC): Reduce dose to 50% of previous dose of pemetrexed (and cisplatin)

Nonhematologic toxicity ≥ grade 3 (excluding neurotoxicity): Withhold treatment until recovery to baseline; upon recovery, reinitiate therapy as follows:

Grade 3 or 4 toxicity (excluding mucositis): Reduce dose to 75% of previous dose of pemetrexed (and cisplatin)

Grade 3 or 4 diarrhea or any diarrhea requiring hospitalization: Reduce dose to 75% of previous dose of pemetrexed (and cisplatin)

Grade 3 or 4 mucositis: Reduce pemetrexed dose to 50% of previous dose (continue cisplatin at 100% of previous dose)

Neurotoxicity:

Grade 0 to 1: Continue pemetrexed at 100% of previous dose (and cisplatin)

Grade 2: Continue pemetrexed at 100% of previous dose; reduce cisplatin dose to 50% of previous dose

Combination Regimens

Bladder cancer: Pemetrexed (Bladder Cancer Regimen) on page 2062

Cervical cancer: Pemetrexed (Cervical Regimen) on page 2063

Lung cancer (non-small cell):
Malignant pleural mesothelioma:

Administration IV: Infuse over 10 minutes. Hazardous agent; use appropriate precautions for handling and disposal (NIOSH 2014 [group 1]).

Emetic Potential Children and Adults: Low (10% to 30%)

Monitoring Parameters CBC with differential and platelets (before each dose; monitor for nadir and recovery); serum creatinine, creatinine clearance, BUN, total bilirubin, ALT, AST (periodic); signs/symptoms of mucositis and diarrhea

Dietary Considerations Initiate folic acid supplementation 1 week before first dose of pemetrexed, continue for full course of therapy, and for 21 days after last dose. Institute vitamin B_{12} 1 week before the first dose; administer every 9 weeks thereafter.

Dosage Forms Excipient information presented when available (limited, particularly for generics); consult specific product labeling.
Solution Reconstituted, Intravenous:
Alimta: 100 mg (1 ea); 500 mg (1 ea)

♦ **Pemetrexed Disodium** see PEMEtrexed on page 1368

♦ **Pentahydrate** see Sodium Thiosulfate on page 1540

♦ **Pentam** see Pentamidine (Systemic) on page 1373

Pentamidine (Systemic) (pen TAM i deen)

Brand Names: US Pentam

Index Terms Pentamidine Isethionate

Pharmacologic Category Antifungal Agent; Antiprotozoal

Use Treatment of pneumonia caused by *Pneumocystis jirovecii* pneumonia (PCP)

Pregnancy Risk Factor C

Dosing

Adult & Geriatric

Pneumocystis jirovecii **pneumonia (PCP), treatment:**
Manufacturer labeling: IM, IV: 4 mg/kg once daily for 14 to 21 days
HIV-infected patients (alternative to preferred therapy): IV: 4 mg/kg/dose once daily for 21 days; may reduce to 3 mg/kg/dose once daily if toxicity occurs (HHS [OI adult 2015])

Trypanosomiasis (off-label use): IM, IV: 4 mg/kg once daily for 7 to 10 days (CDC 2013)

◄ **Pediatric**

Pneumocystis jirovecii **pneumonia (PCP), prophylaxis (primary and secondary) in oncology patients (including HSCT recipients) (off-label use): Note:** For patients intolerant to sulfamethoxazole and trimethoprim: Children ≥2 years and Adolescents: IV: 4 mg/kg/dose once a month (Kim 2008; Prasad 2007); in HSCT recipient, doses have been administered every 2 to 4 weeks (Tomblyn [CDC/IDSA 2009])

Pneumocystis jirovecii **pneumonia (PCP), treatment (moderate-severe disease): Note:** For patients who cannot tolerate or who fail to respond to 5 to 7 days of sulfamethoxazole and trimethoprim.

Manufacturer's labeling: Infants ≥5 months, Children, and Adolescents: IM, IV: 4 mg/kg/dose once daily for 14 to 21 days

HIV-exposed/-positive:

Infants and Children: IV: 4 mg/kg/dose once daily; if clinical improvement after 7 to 10 days of therapy, may change to an oral regimen to complete a 21-day course (HHS [OI pediatric 2013])

Adolescents: IV: Refer to adult dosing.

Non-HIV-exposed/-positive: Infants, Children, and Adolescents: IV: 3 to 4 mg/kg/dose once daily for 21 days (Bradley 2015)

Trypanosomiasis, treatment (non-CNS disease) (off-label use): Infants, Children, Adolescents, and Adults: IM, IV: 4 mg/kg/dose once daily for 7 to 10 days (Bradley 2015; CDC 2013; *Red Book* [AAP 2015])

Renal Impairment IV: The FDA-approved labeling recommends that caution should be used in patients with renal impairment; however, no specific dosage adjustment guidelines are available. The following guidelines have been used by some clinicians (Aronoff 2007):

Adults:

CrCl ≥10 mL/minute: No dosage adjustment necessary.

CrCl <10 mL/minute: Administer 4 mg/kg every 24 to 36 hours.

Children:

CrCl >30 mL/minute: No dosage adjustment necessary.

CrCl 10 to 30 mL/minute: Administer 4 mg/kg every 36 hours.

CrCl <10 mL/minute and peritoneal dialysis: Administer 4 mg/kg every 48 hours.

Hemodialysis: Administer 4 mg/kg every 48 hours, after dialysis on dialysis days.

Hepatic Impairment There are no dosage adjustments provided in the manufacturer's labeling (has not been studied). Use with caution.

Additional Information Complete prescribing information should be consulted for additional detail.

Dosage Forms Excipient information presented when available (limited, particularly for generics); consult specific product labeling.

Solution Reconstituted, Injection, as isethionate:

Pentam: 300 mg (1 ea)

Pentamidine (Oral Inhalation) (pen TAM i deen)

Brand Names: US Nebupent

Index Terms Pentamidine Isethionate

Pharmacologic Category Antifungal Agent; Antiprotozoal

Use Prevention of *Pneumocystis jirovecii* pneumonia (PCP) in high-risk, HIV-infected patients either with a history of PCP or with a CD4+ count ≤200/mm^3

Pregnancy Risk Factor C

Dosing

Adult & Geriatric

***Pneumocystis jirovecii* pneumonia (PCP), prevention:** Primary or secondary prophylaxis (alternative to preferred therapy): Inhalation: 300 mg once every 4 weeks via Respirgard II nebulizer (HHS [OI adult 2015])

Pediatric

***Pneumocystis jirovecii* pneumonia (PCP), prevention:**

Children ≥5 years (off-label population): Inhalation: 300 mg once every 4 weeks via Respirgard II nebulizer (HHS [OI pediatric 2013]; *Redbook* [AAP 2015]; Tomblyn 2009)

Adolescents (off-label population): Refer to adult dosing.

Renal Impairment There are no dosage adjustments provided in manufacturer's labeling (has not been studied). Use with caution.

Hepatic Impairment There are no dosage adjustments provided in manufacturer's labeling (has not been studied). Use with caution.

Additional Information Complete prescribing information should be consulted for additional detail.

Dosage Forms Excipient information presented when available (limited, particularly for generics); consult specific product labeling.

Solution Reconstituted, Inhalation, as isethionate:

Nebupent: 300 mg (1 ea)

♦ **Pentamidine Isethionate** *see* Pentamidine (Oral Inhalation) *on page 1374*

♦ **Pentamidine Isethionate** *see* Pentamidine (Systemic) *on page 1373*

Pentostatin (pen toe STAT in)

Related Information

Hematopoietic Stem Cell Transplantation *on page 2272*

Management of Chemotherapy-Induced Nausea and Vomiting in Adults *on page 2142*

Prevention of Chemotherapy-Induced Nausea and Vomiting in Children *on page 2203*

Safe Handling of Hazardous Drugs *on page 2292*

Brand Names: US Nipent

Brand Names: Canada Nipent

Index Terms 2'-Deoxycoformycin; Co-Vidarabine; dCF; Deoxycoformycin

Pharmacologic Category Antineoplastic Agent, Antimetabolite; Antineoplastic Agent, Antimetabolite (Purine Analog)

Use Hairy cell leukemia: Treatment (as a single-agent) of untreated and interferon-refractory hairy cell leukemia in patients with active disease (clinically significant anemia, neutropenia, thrombocytopenia, or disease-related symptoms)

Labeled Contraindications Hypersensitivity to pentostatin or any component of the formulation

Pregnancy Considerations Adverse events were observed in animal reproduction studies. Women of childbearing potential should be advised to avoid becoming pregnant during treatment.

Breast-Feeding Considerations It is not known if pentostatin is excreted in breast milk. Due to the potential for serious adverse reactions in nursing the infant, a decision should be made to discontinue pentostatin or to discontinue breast feeding, taking into account the importance of treatment to the mother.

◀ **Warnings/Precautions** Hazardous agent; use appropriate precautions for handling and disposal (NIOSH 2014 [group 1]). **[U.S. Boxed Warnings]: Severe renal, liver, pulmonary, and CNS toxicities have occurred with doses higher than recommended; do not exceed the recommended dose.** May cause elevations (usually reversible) in liver function tests. Withhold treatment or discontinue for CNS toxicity. Serum creatinine elevations occurring at recommended doses are usually minor and reversible. Withhold treatment for elevated serum creatinine and determine creatinine clearance. May require dosage adjustment or therapy discontinuation. Use with caution in patients with renal dysfunction (CrCl <60 mL/minute); the terminal half-life is prolonged; may require dosage adjustment.

Myelosuppression may occur, primarily early in treatment (first few courses). Neutropenia may worsen during initial courses for the treatment of hairy cell leukemia. If severe neutropenia persists beyond early cycles, evaluate for disease status. Monitor blood counts during treatment (more frequently in the initial cycles). In patients who present with infections prior to treatment, infections should be resolved, if possible, prior to initiation of treatment; preexisting infections may worsen with pentostatin treatment. Treatment should be temporarily withheld for active infections during therapy. Use in patients with infections only if the potential benefit justifies the potential risk.

Severe rashes may occur and worsen with therapy continuation; may require treatment interruption or discontinuation. Potentially significant drug-drug interactions may exist, requiring dose or frequency adjustment, additional monitoring, and/or selection of alternative therapy. **[U.S. Boxed Warnings]: Do not administer concurrently with fludarabine; concomitant use has resulted in serious or fatal pulmonary toxicity.** Fatal pulmonary edema and hypotension have been reported in patients treated with pentostatin in combination with carmustine, etoposide, or high-dose cyclophosphamide as part of a myeloablative regimen for bone marrow transplant. **[U.S. Boxed Warning]: Should be administered under the supervision of an experienced cancer chemotherapy physician.**

Adverse Reactions

>10%:
Central nervous system: Fever (42% to 46%), fatigue (29% to 42%), pain (8% to 20%), chills (11% to 19%), headache (13% to 17%), CNS toxicity (1% to 11%)

Dermatologic: Rash (26% to 43%), pruritus (10% to 21%), skin disorder (4% to 17%)

Gastrointestinal: Nausea/vomiting (22% to 63%), diarrhea (15% to 17%), anorexia (13% to 16%), abdominal pain (4% to 16%), stomatitis (5% to 12%)

Hematologic: Myelosuppression (nadir: 7 days; recovery: 10-14 days), leukopenia (22% to 60%), anemia (8% to 35%), thrombocytopenia (6% to 32%)

Hepatic: Transaminases increased (2% to 19%)

Neuromuscular & skeletal: Myalgia (11% to 19%), weakness (10% to 12%)

Respiratory: Cough (17% to 20%), upper respiratory infection (13% to 16%), rhinitis (10% to 11%), dyspnea (8% to 11%)

Miscellaneous: Infection (7% to 36%), allergic reaction (2% to 11%)

1% to 10%:

Cardiovascular: Chest pain (3% to 10%), facial edema (3% to 10%), hypotension (3% to 10%), peripheral edema (3% to 10%), angina (<3%), arrhythmia (<3%), AV block (<3%), bradycardia (<3%), cardiac arrest (<3%), deep thrombophlebitis (<3%), heart failure (<3%), hypertension (<3%), pericardial effusion (<3%), sinus arrest (<3%), syncope (<3%), tachycardia (<3%), vasculitis (<3%), ventricular extrasystoles (<3%)

Central nervous system: Anxiety (3% to 10%), confusion (3% to 10%), depression (3% to 10%), dizziness (3% to 10%), insomnia (3% to 10%), nervousness (3% to 10%), somnolence (3% to 10%), abnormal dreams/thinking (<3%), amnesia (<3%), ataxia (<3%), emotional lability (<3%), encephalitis (<3%), hallucination (<3%), hostility (<3%), meningism (<3%), neuritis (<3%), neurosis (<3%), seizure (<3%), vertigo (<3%)

Dermatologic: Cellulitis (6%), furunculosis (4%), dry skin (3% to 10%), urticaria (3% to 10%), acne (<3%), alopecia (<3%), eczema (<3%), petechial rash (<3%), photosensitivity (<3%), abscess (2%)

Endocrine & metabolic: Amenorrhea (<3%), hypercalcemia (<3%), hyponatremia (<3%), gout (<3%), libido decreased/loss (<3%)

Gastrointestinal: Dyspepsia (3% to 10%) flatulence (3% to 10%), gingivitis (3% to 10%), constipation (<3%), dysphagia (<3%), glossitis (<3%), ileus (<3%), taste perversion (<3%), oral moniliasis (2%)

Genitourinary: Urinary tract infection (3%), impotence (<3%)

Hematologic: Agranulocytosis (3% to 10%), hemorrhage (3% to 10%), acute leukemia (<3%), aplastic anemia (<3%), hemolytic anemia (<3%)

Local: Phlebitis (<3%)

Neuromuscular & skeletal: Arthralgia (3% to 10%), paresthesia (3% to 10%), arthritis (<3%), dysarthria (<3%), hyperkinesia (<3%), neuralgia (<3%), neuropathy (<3%), paralysis (<3%), twitching (<3%), osteomyelitis (1%)

Ocular: Conjunctivitis (4%), amblyopia (<3%), eyes nonreactive (<3%), lacrimation disorder (<3%), photophobia (<3%), retinopathy (<3%), vision abnormal (<3%), watery eyes (<3%), xerophthalmia (<3%)

Otic: Deafness (<3%), earache (<3%), labyrinthitis (<3%), tinnitus (<3%)

Renal: Creatinine increased (3% to 10%), nephropathy (<3%), renal failure (<3%), renal insufficiency (<3%), renal function abnormal (<3%), renal stone (<3%)

Respiratory: Pharyngitis (8% to 10%), sinusitis (6%), pneumonia (5%), asthma (3% to 10%), bronchitis (3%), bronchospasm (<3%), laryngeal edema (<3%), pulmonary embolus (<3%)

Miscellaneous: Diaphoresis (8% to 10%), herpes zoster (8%), viral infection (≤8%), bacterial infection (5%), herpes simplex (4%), sepsis (3%), flu-like syndrome (<3%)

<1%, postmarketing, and/or case reports: Dysuria, fungal infection (skin), hematuria, lethargy, pulmonary edema, pulmonary toxicity (fatal; in combination with fludarabine), uveitis/vision loss

Drug Interactions

Metabolism/Transport Effects None known.

Avoid Concomitant Use

Avoid concomitant use of Pentostatin with any of the following: BCG (Intravesical); CloZAPine; Dipyrone; Fludarabine; Natalizumab; Nelarabine; Pegademase Bovine; Pimecrolimus; Tacrolimus (Topical); Tofacitinib; Vaccines (Live)

Increased Effect/Toxicity

Pentostatin may increase the levels/effects of: CloZAPine; Cyclophosphamide; Fingolimod; Fludarabine; Leflunomide; Natalizumab; Tofacitinib; Vaccines (Live)

The levels/effects of Pentostatin may be increased by: Denosumab; Dipyrone; Fludarabine; Pimecrolimus; Roflumilast; Tacrolimus (Topical); Trastuzumab

Decreased Effect

Pentostatin may decrease the levels/effects of: BCG (Intravesical); Coccidioides immitis Skin Test; Nelarabine; Pegademase Bovine; Sipuleucel-T; Vaccines (Inactivated); Vaccines (Live)

The levels/effects of Pentostatin may be decreased by: Echinacea; Pegademase Bovine

Storage/Stability Store intact vials under refrigeration at 2°C to 8°C (36°F to 46°F). Reconstituted vials and solutions diluted for infusion (in D_5W or NS) may be stored at room temperature for 8 hours.

Preparation for Administration Hazardous agent; use appropriate precautions for handling and disposal (NIOSH 2014 [group 1]). Reconstitute with 5 mL SWFI to a concentration of 2 mg/mL. The solution may be further diluted in 25 to 50 mL NS or D_5W for infusion. When diluted for infusion in D_5W or NS at concentrations of 0.18 to 0.33 mg/mL, pentostatin is compatible with PVC containing infusion bags and infusion sets.

Mechanism of Action Pentostatin is a purine antimetabolite that inhibits adenosine deaminase, preventing the deamination of adenosine to inosine. Accumulation of deoxyadenosine (dAdo) and deoxyadenosine 5'-triphosphate (dATP) results in a reduction of purine metabolism which blocks DNA synthesis and leads to cell death.

Pharmacodynamics/Kinetics

Distribution: V_d: IV: 20 L/m^2 (Lathia, 2002)

Protein binding: ~4%

Half-life elimination: Terminal: ~6 hours; Renal impairment (CrCl <50 mL/minute): 18 hours (range: 11 to 23 hours [Lathia, 2002])

Excretion: Urine (~90%, as unchanged drug)

Dosing

Adult & Geriatric

Hairy cell leukemia: IV: 4 mg/m^2 every 2 weeks. **Note:** The optimal duration has not been determined; in the absence of unacceptable toxicity, may continue until complete response is achieved or until 2 doses after complete response. Discontinue after 6 months if partial or complete response is not achieved.

Acute graft-versus-host disease (GVHD), steroid-refractory (off-label use): IV:

Initial therapy: 1.5 mg/m^2 days 1 to 3 and days 15 to 17 (in combination with corticosteroids) (Alousi, 2009)

Steroid-refractory disease: 1.5 mg/m^2 daily for 3 days; may repeat after 2 weeks if needed (Bolanos-Meade, 2005)

Chronic graft-versus-host disease (GVHD), steroid-refractory (off-label use): IV: 4 mg/m^2 once every 2 weeks; discontinue after 6 months for sustained objective response, or continue every 2 to 4 weeks for up to 12 months if still improving (Jacobsohn, 2007; Jacobsohn, 2009) **or** 4 mg/m^2 once every 2 weeks for 3 months (Wolff, 2011)

Chronic lymphocytic leukemia (CLL; off-label use): IV:

Previously treated: 4 mg/m^2 once every 3 weeks (in combination with cyclophosphamide and rituximab) for 6 cycles (Lamanna, 2006)

Previously untreated: 2 mg/m^2 once every 3 weeks (in combination with cyclophosphamide and rituximab) for 6 cycles (Kay, 2007)

Cutaneous T-cell lymphoma, mycosis fungoides/Sezary syndrome (off-label use): IV: 4 mg/m^2 once weekly for 3 weeks, then every 2 weeks for 6 weeks, then once monthly for a maximum of 6 months (Ho, 1999)

T-cell prolymphocytic leukemia, refractory (off-label use): IV: 4 mg/m^2 once weekly for 4 weeks then every 2 weeks until optimum response is achieved (Mercieca, 1994) **or** 4 mg/m^2 once weekly for 4 weeks then every 2 weeks (in combination with alemtuzumab) until complete or best response or up to a total of 14 doses (Ravandi, 2009)

Pediatric

Chronic graft-versus-host disease (GVHD), steroid-refractory: IV: 4 mg/m^2 once every 2 weeks; discontinue after 6 months for sustained objective response, or continue every 2 to 4 weeks for up to 12 months if still improving (Jacobsohn, 2007; Jacobsohn, 2009) **or** 4 mg/m^2 once every 2 weeks for 3 months (Wolff, 2011)

Renal Impairment There are no dosage adjustments provided in the manufacturer's labeling; although not adequately studied, two patients with CrCl 50 to 60 mL/minute achieved responses when treated with 2 mg/m^2/dose. For renal toxicity *during* treatment, withhold for elevated serum creatinine and determine creatinine clearance. The following adjustments have also been recommended:

Kintzel, 1995:

CrCl 46 to 60 mL/minute: Administer 70% of dose

CrCl 31 to 45 mL/minute: Administer 60% of dose

CrCl <30 mL/minute: Consider use of alternative drug

Lathia, 2002:

CrCl ≥60 mL/minute: Administer 4 mg/m^2/dose

CrCl 40 to 59 mL/minute: Administer 3 mg/m^2/dose

CrCl 20 to 39 mL/minute: Administer 2 mg/m^2/dose

Alousi, 2009; Jacobsohn, 2009; Poi, 2013 (for GVHD treatment):

CrCl 30 to 50 mL/minute/1.73 m^2: Reduce dose by 50%

CrCl <30 mL/minute/1.73 m^2: Withhold dose

Lamanna, 2006 (for previously treated CLL): Serum creatinine >2 mg/dL or 20% above patient's baseline: Withhold treatment until serum creatinine ≤2 mg/dL or returns to baseline, or until CrCl ≥50 mL/minute

Hepatic Impairment There are no dosage adjustments provided in the manufacturer's labeling.

Obesity

American Society of Clinical Oncology (ASCO) Guidelines for appropriate chemotherapy dosing in obese adults with cancer: Utilize patient's actual body weight (full weight) for calculation of body surface area- or weight-based dosing, particularly when the intent of therapy is curative; manage regimen-related toxicities in the same manner as for nonobese patients; if a dose reduction is utilized due to toxicity, consider resumption of full weight-based dosing with subsequent cycles, especially if cause of toxicity (eg, hepatic or renal impairment) is resolved (Griggs, 2012).

◄

American Society for Blood and Marrow Transplantation (ASBMT) practice guideline committee position statement on chemotherapy dosing in obesity: Utilize actual body weight (full weight) for calculation of body surface area in pentostatin dosing for hematopoietic stem cell transplant conditioning regimens in adults (Bubalo, 2014).

Adjustment for Toxicity

ANC <200/mm^3 (with baseline ANC >500/mm^3): Temporarily interrupt treatment until ANC returns to pre-dose levels.

CNS toxicity: Withhold treatment or discontinue.

Infection, active: Interrupt treatment until infection is controlled.

Rash: Severe rashes may require treatment interruption or discontinuation.

Other severe adverse reactions: Withhold treatment or discontinue.

Combination Regimens

Leukemia, chronic lymphocytic: Pentostatin-Cyclophosphamide-Rituximab (CLL) on page 2065

Administration Administer IV over 20 to 30 minutes or as a bolus infusion. Hydrate with 500 to 1,000 mL fluid prior to infusion and 500 mL after infusion.

Hazardous agent; use appropriate precautions for handling and disposal (NIOSH 2014 [group 1]).

Emetic Potential

Children: Minimal (<10%)

Adults: Low (10% to 30%)

Monitoring Parameters CBC with differential and platelet count (prior to each dose; more frequently during initial cycles), peripheral blood smears (periodically for hairy cells and to assess treatment response), liver function, serum uric acid, renal function (serum creatinine and/or creatinine clearance at baseline, and serum creatinine prior to each dose), bone marrow evaluation, signs/symptoms of pulmonary and CNS toxicity

Dosage Forms Excipient information presented when available (limited, particularly for generics); consult specific product labeling. [DSC] = Discontinued product

Solution Reconstituted, Intravenous:

Nipent: 10 mg (1 ea)

Solution Reconstituted, Intravenous [preservative free]:

Generic: 10 mg (1 ea [DSC])

♦ **PEP005** see Ingenol Mebutate on page 928

♦ **Periactin** see Cyproheptadine on page 400

♦ **Perjeta** see Pertuzumab on page 1380

Pertuzumab (per TU zoo mab)

Related Information

Management of Chemotherapy-Induced Nausea and Vomiting in Adults on page 2142

Safe Handling of Hazardous Drugs on page 2292

Brand Names: US Perjeta

Brand Names: Canada Perjeta

Index Terms 2C4 Antibody; MOAB 2C4; Monoclonal Antibody 2C4; Omnitarg; rhuMAb-2C4

Pharmacologic Category Antineoplastic Agent, Anti-HER2; Antineoplastic Agent, Monoclonal Antibody

Use

Breast cancer, metastatic: Treatment of human epidermal growth factor receptor 2 (HER2)-positive metastatic breast cancer (in combination with trastuzumab and docetaxel) in patients who have not received prior anti-HER2 therapy or chemotherapy to treat metastatic disease

Breast cancer, neoadjuvant treatment: Neoadjuvant treatment of locally advanced, inflammatory, or early stage HER2-positive, breast cancer (either greater than 2 cm in diameter or node positive) in combination with trastuzumab and docetaxel (as part of a complete treatment regimen for early breast cancer).

Limitations of use: The safety of pertuzumab as part of a doxorubicin-containing regimen has not been established; the safety of pertuzumab administered for more than 6 cycles for early breast cancer has not been established.

Labeled Contraindications Hypersensitivity to pertuzumab or any component of the formulation

Pregnancy Considerations May cause fetal harm if administered during pregnancy. **[US Boxed Warning]: Pertuzumab exposure during pregnancy may result in embryo-fetal mortality and birth defects. Oligohydramnios, delayed fetal kidney development, and embryo-fetal death have been observed in animal reproduction studies. Advise patients of the risks and the need for effective contraception.** Verify pregnancy status prior to treatment initiation. Effective contraception should be used during therapy and for 7 months after the last dose (of pertuzumab in combination with trastuzumab) for women of childbearing potential. Advise patients to immediately report to healthcare provider if pregnancy is suspected during treatment. Effects during pregnancy are likely to occur in all 3 trimesters. If pertuzumab exposure occurs during pregnancy or exposure to pertuzumab in combination with trastuzumab occurs within 7 months prior to conception, healthcare providers should report the exposure to the Genentech Adverse Event Line (888-835-2555); monitor for oligohydramnios (if oligohydramnios occurs, fetal testing is indicated). Women exposed to pertuzumab during pregnancy or exposed to pertuzumab in combination with trastuzumab within 7 months prior to conception are encouraged to enroll in MotHER Pregnancy Registry (1-800-690-6720).

European Society for Medical Oncology (ESMO) guidelines for cancer during pregnancy recommend delaying treatment with HER2-targeted agents until after delivery in pregnant patients with HER2-positive disease (Peccatori 2013).

Breast-Feeding Considerations It is not known if pertuzumab is excreted in human milk. Because many immunoglobulins are excreted in human milk, and the potential for serious adverse reactions in the nursing infant exists, the decision to discontinue breast-feeding or to discontinue pertuzumab should take into account the benefits of treatment to the mother. The extended half-life should be considered for decisions regarding breast-feeding after treatment is completed.

Warnings/Precautions Hazardous agent - use appropriate precautions for handling and disposal (meets NIOSH 2014 criteria). **[US Boxed Warning]: May result in cardiac failure (clinical and subclinical). Assess left ventricular ejection fraction (LVEF) in all patients at baseline and during treatment. Discontinue for confirmed clinically significant decline in left ventricular function.** Decreases in LVEF are associated with HER-2 inhibitors, including pertuzumab. Patients who received prior anthracycline therapy or chest irradiation may be at an increased risk for cardiotoxicity. In studies of

◄ pertuzumab (versus placebo) in combination with trastuzumab and docetaxel for the treatment of metastatic breast cancer, the rate of cardiotoxicity (LVEF decline or symptomatic LV systolic dysfunction) was not increased in the pertuzumab group when compared to placebo. In the neoadjuvant setting, the incidence of LV dysfunction was higher in patients treated with pertuzumab. In a study of pertuzumab, trastuzumab and docetaxel, compared with trastuzumab and docetaxel, the incidence of LVEF decline (of >10% decrease from baseline or to <50%) was 8.4% and 1.9%., respectively; LVEF recovered to ≥50% in all patients. In another neoadjuvant study, LVEF declines (of >10% decrease from baseline or to <50%) were noted in 6.9% to 16% of patients receiving various combinations and sequences of pertuzumab plus trastuzumab with FEC (fluorouracil, epirubicin, and cyclophosphamide), docetaxel, and/or carboplatin; LVEF recovered to ≥50% in most patients. Of note, patients with pretreatment LVEF ≤50%, CHF, LVEF decreases to <50% during prior trastuzumab treatment, or conditions which could impair LV function (eg, uncontrolled hypertension, recent MI, serious arrhythmia requiring treatment, or cumulative lifetime anthracycline exposure >360 mg/m^2 doxorubicin or its equivalent) were excluded from studies. Assess LVEF at baseline, every 3 months during treatment (metastatic patients) or every 6 weeks during treatment (neoadjuvant setting), and every 6 months after therapy discontinuation up to 24 months after the last dose of pertuzumab and/or trastuzumab. Withhold pertuzumab and trastuzumab if LVEF <45% **or** 45% to 49% with a ≥10% absolute decline from baseline; repeat LVEF assessment in ~3 weeks; discontinue if LVEF has not improved or has declined further (unless potential benefits outweigh risks).

Infusion reactions (either during or on the day of infusion) have been associated with pertuzumab; commonly described as fever, chills, fatigue, headache, weakness, myalgia, hypersensitivity, abnormal taste or vomiting. The incidence of hypersensitivity/anaphylaxis was slightly higher in the group receiving pertuzumab (compared to placebo) in combination with trastuzumab and docetaxel. Monitor for 1 hour after the first infusion and for 30 minutes after subsequent infusions. For significant infusion reactions, interrupt or slow infusion rate; for severe infusion reactions, consider permanently discontinuing. Medications and equipment for the treatment of hypersensitivity should be available for immediate use during infusion. May cause fetal harm is administered during pregnancy. **[US Boxed Warning]: Pertuzumab exposure during pregnancy may result in embryo-fetal mortality and birth defects. Oligohydramnios, delayed fetal kidney development, and embryo-fetal death have been observed in animal reproduction studies. Advise patients of the risks and the need for effective contraception.** Verify pregnancy status prior to treatment initiation. Effective contraception should be used by all patients receiving pertuzumab during therapy and for 7 months after the last dose (of pertuzumab in combination with trastuzumab) in women of childbearing potential. Effects during pregnancy are likely to occur in any trimester.

Establish HER2 status prior to treatment; has only been studied in patients with evidence of HER2 overexpression, either as 3+ IHC (Dako Herceptest™) or FISH amplification ratio ≥2 (Dako *HER2* FISH pharmDx™ test). Safety of combination or sequential therapy with doxorubicin-containing regimens has not been established. For early breast cancer, the safety of treatment beyond 6 cycles has not been determined.

Adverse Reactions Note: Reactions reported in combination therapy with trastuzumab and docetaxel unless otherwise noted.

>10%:

Central nervous system: Fatigue (26% to 38%), headache (11% to 21%), decreased left ventricular ejection fraction (8% to 16%), insomnia (8% to 13%), dizziness (3% to 13%)

Dermatologic: Alopecia (52% to 65%), skin rash (11% to 34%; grades 3/4: <1%), pruritus (4% to 14%), palmar-plantar erythrodysesthesia (11%), xeroderma (9% to 11%)

Gastrointestinal: Diarrhea (46% to 67%; grades 3/4: 5% to 8%), nausea (39% to 53%; monotherapy 24%), vomiting (13% to 36%; monotherapy 15%), decreased appetite (11% to 29%), constipation (23%), mucositis (20% to 28%), stomatitis (17% to 19%), dysgeusia (13% to 18%), abdominal pain (monotherapy 12%)

Hematologic & oncologic: Neutropenia (47% to 53%; grades 3/4: 43% to 49%), anemia (3% to 23%; grades 3/4: 3% to 4%), leukopenia (9% to 16%; grades 3/4: 5% to 12%), febrile neutropenia (8% to 14%; grades 3/4: 9% to 13%)

Hypersensitivity: Hypersensitivity (1% to 11%; grades 3/4: 2%)

Neuromuscular & skeletal: Weakness (15% to 26%), myalgia (11% to 23%), arthralgia (10% to 12%)

Respiratory: Upper respiratory tract infection (4% to 17%; grades 3/4: <1%), epistaxis (11%)

Miscellaneous: Fever (9% to 19%; grades 3/4: 1%), infusion reactions (13%; grades 3/4: <1%)

1% to 10%:

Cardiovascular: Left ventricular dysfunction (3% to 4%), peripheral edema (3% to 4%)

Central nervous system: Peripheral sensory neuropathy (8%; grades 3/4: 1%), peripheral neuropathy (1%)

Dermatologic: Nail disease (7%), paronychia (1% to 7%)

Gastrointestinal: Dyspepsia (8%), anorexia (monotherapy 5%)

Hematologic & oncologic: Thrombocytopenia (1%)

Hepatic: Increased serum ALT (3%)

Ophthalmic: Increased lacrimation (4% to 5%)

Respiratory: Dyspnea (5% to 8%), nasopharyngitis (7%), oropharyngeal pain (7%), cough (5%)

<1%, postmarketing, and/or case reports with combination therapy: Heart failure, pleural effusion, sepsis

Drug Interactions

Metabolism/Transport Effects None known.

Avoid Concomitant Use

Avoid concomitant use of Pertuzumab with any of the following: Belimumab

Increased Effect/Toxicity

Pertuzumab may increase the levels/effects of: Belimumab

Decreased Effect There are no known significant interactions involving a decrease in effect.

Storage/Stability Store intact vials at 2°C to 8°C (36°F to 46°F) until time of use. Protect from light. Do not freeze. Do not shake. Solutions diluted for infusion should be used immediately; if not used immediately, maybe stored at 2°C to 8°C (36°F to 46°F) for up to 24 hours.

◀ **Preparation for Administration** Hazardous agent; use appropriate precautions for handling and disposal (meets NIOSH 2014 criteria). Dilute in 250 mL NS only (do not use dextrose 5% solutions) in PVC or non-PVC (polyolefin) bags. Gently invert to mix; do not shake. Do not mix with other medications.

Mechanism of Action Pertuzumab is a recombinant humanized monoclonal antibody which targets the extracellular human epidermal growth factor receptor 2 protein (HER2) dimerization domain. Inhibits HER2 dimerization and blocks HER downstream signaling halting cell growth and initiating apoptosis. Pertuzumab binds to a different HER2 epitope than trastuzumab so that when pertuzumab is combined with trastuzumab, a more complete inhibition of HER2 signaling occurs (Baselga, 2012).

Pharmacodynamics/Kinetics

Distribution: V_d: 5.12 L (Gianni, 2010)

Half-life elimination: Terminal: 18 days

Dosing

Adult & Geriatric Note: For pertuzumab, trastuzumab, and docetaxel combination regimens, pertuzumab and trastuzumab may be administered in any order; however, docetaxel should be given after pertuzumab and trastuzumab. Observe patients for 30 to 60 minutes after each pertuzumab infusion and before subsequent infusions of trastuzumab or docetaxel.

Breast cancer, metastatic HER2+: IV: 840 mg over 60 minutes followed by a maintenance dose of 420 mg over 30 to 60 minutes every 3 weeks until disease progression or unacceptable toxicity (in combination with trastuzumab and docetaxel) (Baselga, 2012; Swain, 2015).

Breast cancer, neoadjuvant treatment HER2+: Adults: IV: 840 mg over 60 minutes followed by a maintenance dose of 420 mg over 30 to 60 minutes every 3 weeks for 3 to 6 cycles; may be administered as one of the regimens below. Postoperatively, continue trastuzumab to complete 1 year of treatment.

Four preoperative cycles of pertuzumab, trastuzumab, and docetaxel, followed by 3 postoperative cycles of fluorouracil, epirubicin, and cyclophosphamide (FEC) (Gianni, 2012) **or**

Three preoperative cycles of FEC (alone) followed by 3 preoperative cycles of pertuzumab, trastuzumab, and docetaxel (Schneeweiss, 2013) **or**

Six preoperative cycles of pertuzumab, trastuzumab, docetaxel, and carboplatin (Schneeweiss, 2013)

Missed doses or delays: If <6 weeks has elapsed, administer the 420 mg maintenance dose; do not wait until the next planned dose. If ≥6 weeks has elapsed, readminister the 840 mg initial dose (over 60 minutes), and then follow with a maintenance dose of 420 mg (over 30 to 60 minutes) every 3 weeks.

Renal Impairment

CrCl ≥30 mL/minute: No dosage adjustment necessary.

CrCl <30 mL/minute: There are no dosage adjustments provided in the manufacturer's labeling (has not been studied).

Hepatic Impairment There are no dosage adjustments provided in the manufacturer's labeling (has not been studied).

Adjustment for Toxicity Note: Dose reductions are not recommended for pertuzumab; if trastuzumab is withheld, pertuzumab should also be withheld; if trastuzumab is discontinued, pertuzumab should be discontinued; pertuzumab and trastuzumab may be continued if docetaxel is discontinued.

Infusion-related reaction: Slow or interrupt the infusion

Serious hypersensitivity: Discontinue immediately

Cardiotoxicity: Left ventricular ejection fraction (LVEF) declines to <45% **or** LVEF between 45% to 49% with ≥10% absolute decrease below pretreatment values: Withhold treatment (pertuzumab and trastuzumab) for at least 3 weeks; may resume if LVEF returns to >49% **or** to 45% to 49% with <10% absolute decrease below pretreatment values. If after a repeat assessment within ~3 weeks, LVEF has not improved (or has declined further), discontinue pertuzumab and trastuzumab (unless the benefit of treatment outweighs risks).

Combination Regimens

Breast cancer:

Paclitaxel-Pertuzumab-Trastuzumab (Breast) on page 2054

Pertuzumab-Trastuzumab-Docetaxel (Metastatic Breast) on page 2066

Pertuzumab-Trastuzumab-Docetaxel (Neoadjuvant Breast) on page 2067

Administration For IV infusion only, as a short infusion; infuse initial dose (840 mg) over 60 minutes; infuse maintenance dose (420 mg) over 30 to 60 minutes. Do not administer IV push or as a rapid bolus. Do not mix with other medications. For pertuzumab, trastuzumab, and docetaxel combination regimens, pertuzumab and trastuzumab may be administered in any order; however, docetaxel should be given after pertuzumab and trastuzumab. Observe patients for 30 to 60 minutes after each pertuzumab infusion and before subsequent infusions of trastuzumab or docetaxel.

Hazardous agent; use appropriate precautions for handling and disposal (meets NIOSH 2014 criteria).

Emetic Potential Minimal (<10%)

Monitoring Parameters HER2 expression (either as 3+ IHC [Dako Herceptest™] or FISH amplification ratio ≥2 [Dako *HER2* FISH pharmDx™ test]); pregnancy test; assess LVEF at baseline, every 3 months during treatment (more frequently for declines) in metastatic treatment and every 6 weeks for neoadjuvant treatment, and every 6 months following discontinuation for up to 24 months from the last dose of pertuzumab and/or trastuzumab); monitor for infusion reaction and hypersensitivity

Dosage Forms Excipient information presented when available (limited, particularly for generics); consult specific product labeling.

Solution, Intravenous [preservative free]:

Perjeta: 420 mg/14 mL (14 mL) [contains mouse protein (murine) (hamster)]

◆ **Pethidine Hydrochloride** *see* Meperidine *on page 1086*

◆ **PF-02341066** *see* Crizotinib *on page 366*

◆ **PFA** *see* Foscarnet *on page 762*

◆ **pFVIII** *see* Antihemophilic Factor (Recombinant [Porcine Sequence]) *on page 123*

◆ **Pharixia (Can)** *see* Benzydamine *on page 190*

◆ **Pharmorubicin (Can)** *see* EPIrubicin *on page 608*

◆ **Phenylalanine Mustard** *see* Melphalan *on page 1080*

◆ **PHL-Bicalutamide (Can)** *see* Bicalutamide *on page 207*

◆ **PHL-Ciprofloxacin (Can)** *see* Ciprofloxacin (Systemic) *on page 327*

◆ **PHL-Dexamethasone (Can)** *see* Dexamethasone (Systemic) *on page 513*

◆ **PHL-Fluconazole (Can)** *see* Fluconazole *on page 725*

◆ **PHL-Lorazepam (Can)** *see* LORazepam *on page 1058*

- ◆ **PHL-Olanzapine (Can)** *see* OLANZapine *on page 1242*
- ◆ **PHL-Olanzapine ODT (Can)** *see* OLANZapine *on page 1242*
- ◆ **PHL-Ondansetron (Can)** *see* Ondansetron *on page 1253*
- ◆ **PHL-Valacyclovir (Can)** *see* ValACYclovir *on page 1712*
- ◆ **Phosphonoformate** *see* Foscarnet *on page 762*
- ◆ **Phosphonoformic Acid** *see* Foscarnet *on page 762*
- ◆ **Photofrin** *see* Porfimer *on page 1409*
- ◆ **PI₃K Delta Inhibitor CAL-101** *see* Idelalisib *on page 867*
- ◆ **Picato** *see* Ingenol Mebutate *on page 928*
- ◆ **Pidorubicin** *see* EPIrubicin *on page 608*
- ◆ **Pidorubicin Hydrochloride** *see* EPIrubicin *on page 608*

Pilocarpine (Systemic) (pye loe KAR peen)

Related Information

Mucositis and Stomatitis *on page 2186*

Brand Names: US Salagen

Brand Names: Canada Salagen®

Index Terms Pilocarpine Hydrochloride

Pharmacologic Category Cholinergic Agonist

Use Symptomatic treatment of xerostomia caused by salivary gland hypofunction resulting from radiotherapy for cancer of the head and neck or Sjögren's syndrome

Labeled Contraindications Hypersensitivity to pilocarpine or any component of the formulation; uncontrolled asthma; angle-closure glaucoma, severe hepatic impairment

Pregnancy Considerations Adverse events were observed in some animal reproduction studies.

Breast-Feeding Considerations It is not known if pilocarpidine systemic is excreted in breast milk. Due to the potential for serious adverse reactions in the nursing infant, a decision should be made whether to discontinue nursing or to discontinue the drug, taking into account the importance of treatment to the mother.

Warnings/Precautions Use caution with cardiovascular disease; patients may have difficulty compensating for transient changes in hemodynamics or rhythm induced by pilocarpine. Use caution with controlled asthma, chronic bronchitis, or COPD; may increase airway resistance, bronchial smooth muscle tone, and bronchial secretions. Use caution with cholelithiasis, biliary tract disease, and nephrolithiasis; adjust dose with moderate hepatic impairment.

Adverse Reactions

>10%:

Cardiovascular: Flushing (8% to 13%)

Central nervous system: Chills (3% to 15%), dizziness (5% to 12%), headache (11%)

Gastrointestinal: Nausea (6% to 15%)

Genitourinary: Urinary frequency (9% to 12%)

Neuromuscular & skeletal: Weakness (2% to 12%)

Respiratory: Rhinitis (5% to 14%)

Miscellaneous: Diaphoresis (29% to 68%)

1% to 10%:

Cardiovascular: Edema (<1% to 5%), facial edema, hypertension (3%), palpitation, tachycardia

Central nervous system: Pain (4%), fever, somnolence

Dermatologic: Pruritus, rash

Gastrointestinal: Diarrhea (4% to 7%), dyspepsia (7%), vomiting (3% to 4%), constipation, flatulence, glossitis, salivation increased, stomatitis, taste perversion

Genitourinary: Vaginitis, urinary incontinence

Neuromuscular & skeletal: Myalgias, tremor

Ocular: Lacrimation (6%), amblyopia (4%), abnormal vision, blurred vision, conjunctivitis

Otic: Tinnitus

Respiratory: Cough increased, dysphagia, epistaxis, sinusitis

Miscellaneous: Allergic reaction, voice alteration

<1%: Abnormal dreams, abnormal thinking, alopecia, angina pectoris, anorexia, anxiety, aphasia, appetite increased, arrhythmia, arthralgia, arthritis, bilirubinemia, body odor, bone disorder, bradycardia, breast pain, bronchitis, cataract, cholelithiasis, colitis, confusion, contact dermatitis, cyst, deafness, depression, dry eyes, dry mouth, dry skin, dyspnea, dysuria, ear pain, ECG abnormality, eczema, emotional lability, eructation, erythema nodosum, esophagitis, exfoliative dermatitis, eye hemorrhage, eye pain, gastritis, gastroenteritis, gastrointestinal disorder, gingivitis, glaucoma, hematuria, hepatitis, herpes simplex, hiccup, hyperkinesias, hypoesthesia, hypoglycemia, hypotension, hypothermia, insomnia, intracranial hemorrhage, laryngismus, laryngitis, leg cramps, leukopenia, liver function test abnormal, lymphadenopathy, mastitis, melena, menorrhagia, metrorrhagia, migraine, moniliasis, myasthenia, MI, neck pain, photosensitivity reaction, nervousness, ovarian disorder, pancreatitis, paresthesia, parotid gland enlargement, peripheral edema, platelet abnormality, pneumonia, pyuria, salivary gland enlargement, salpingitis, seborrhea, skin ulcer, speech disorder, sputum increased, stridor, syncope, taste loss, tendon disorder, tenosynovitis, thrombocythemia, thrombocytopenia, thrombosis, tongue disorder, twitching, urethral pain, urinary impairment, urinary urgency, vaginal hemorrhage, vaginal moniliasis, vesiculobullous rash, WBC abnormality, yawning

Drug Interactions

Metabolism/Transport Effects Inhibits CYP2A6 (weak), CYP2E1 (weak)

Avoid Concomitant Use There are no known interactions where it is recommended to avoid concomitant use.

Increased Effect/Toxicity

The levels/effects of Pilocarpine (Systemic) may be increased by: Acetylcholinesterase Inhibitors; Beta-Blockers

Decreased Effect

Pilocarpine (Systemic) may decrease the levels/effects of: Cimetropium

Food Interactions Fat decreases the rate of absorption, maximum concentration and increases the time it takes to reach maximum concentration. Management: Avoid administering with a high-fat meal.

Storage/Stability Store at controlled room temperature of 15°C to 30°C (59°F to 86°F).

Pharmacodynamics/Kinetics

Onset of action: 20 minutes

Duration: 3-5 hours

◀ Half-life elimination: 0.76-1.35 hours; increased with hepatic impairment
Excretion: Urine

Dosing

Adult & Geriatric Xerostomia: Oral:

Following head and neck cancer: 5 mg 3 times/day, titration up to 10 mg 3 times/day may be considered for patients who have not responded adequately; do not exceed 2 tablets/dose

Sjögren's syndrome: 5 mg 4 times/day

Renal Impairment No dosage adjustment necessary.

Hepatic Impairment

Mild impairment (Child-Pugh score 5-6): No dosage adjustment necessary.

Moderate impairment (Child-Pugh score 7-9): 5 mg twice daily regardless of indication; adjust dose based on response and tolerability

Severe impairment (Child-Pugh score >10): Not recommended.

Administration Avoid administering with high-fat meal.

Monitoring Parameters Intraocular pressure, funduscopic exam, visual field testing

Dietary Considerations Avoid taking with a high-fat meal.

Dosage Forms Excipient information presented when available (limited, particularly for generics); consult specific product labeling.

Tablet, Oral, as hydrochloride:

Salagen: 5 mg

Salagen: 7.5 mg [contains fd&c blue #2 aluminum lake]

Generic: 5 mg, 7.5 mg

◆ **Pilocarpine Hydrochloride** *see* Pilocarpine (Systemic) *on page 1386*

Piperacillin and Tazobactam (pi PER a sil in & ta zoe BAK tam)

Brand Names: US Zosyn

Brand Names: Canada AJ-PIP/TAZ; Piperacillin and Tazobactam for Injection; Tazocin

Index Terms Piperacillin and Tazobactam Sodium; Piperacillin Sodium and Tazobactam Sodium; Tazobactam and Piperacillin

Pharmacologic Category Antibiotic, Penicillin

Use

Moderate to severe bacterial infections: For the treatment of patients with moderate to severe infections caused by susceptible isolates of the designated bacteria in the following conditions.

Community-acquired pneumonia: Treatment of moderate severity community-acquired pneumonia (CAP) caused by beta-lactamase-producing strains of *Haemophilus influenzae*. IDSA/ATS guidelines only recommend piperacillin/tazobactam for CAP caused by *P. aeruginosa* or due to aspiration (Mandell 2007).

Intra-abdominal infections: Treatment of appendicitis complicated by rupture or abscess and peritonitis caused by beta-lactamase-producing strains of *Escherichia coli*, *Bacteroides fragilis*, *Bacteroides ovatus*, *Bacteroides thetaiotaomicron*, or *Bacteroides vulgatus*.

Nosocomial pneumonia: Treatment of moderate to severe nosocomial pneumonia caused by beta-lactamase-producing strains of *Staphylococcus aureus* and by piperacillin/tazobactam-susceptible *Acinetobacter baumanii*, *H. influenzae*, *Klebsiella pneumoniae*, and *Pseudomonas aeruginosa* (nosocomial pneumonia caused by *P. aeruginosa* should be treated in combination with an aminoglycoside).

Pelvic infections: Treatment of postpartum endometriosis or pelvic inflammatory disease caused by beta-lactamase-producing strains of *E. coli*.

Skin and skin structure infections: Treatment of skin and skin structure infections, including cellulitis, cutaneous abscesses, and ischemic/diabetic foot infections caused by beta-lactamase-producing strains of *S. aureus*.

Pregnancy Risk Factor B

Dosing

Adult & Geriatric Note: Dosing presented is based on traditional infusion method (IV infusion over 30 minutes) unless otherwise specified as the extended infusion method (IV infusion over 4 hours [off-label method]).

Usual dosage range: IV: 3.375 g every 6 hours or 4.5 g every 6 to 8 hours; maximum: 18 g daily

Extended infusion method (off-label dosing): 3.375 to 4.5 g IV over 4 hours every 8 hours (Kim 2007; Shea 2009); an alternative regimen of 4.5 g IV over 3 hours every 6 hours has also been described (Kim 2007)

Indication-specific dosing:

Appendicitis, diverticulitis, intra-abdominal abscess, peritonitis: IV: 3.375 g every 6 hours for 7 to 10 days

Pneumonia:

Community-acquired pneumonia (CAP): IV: 3.375 g every 6 hours for 7 to 10 days. **Note:** IDSA/ATS guidelines only recommend piperacillin/tazobactam for CAP caused by *P. aeruginosa* or due to aspiration (Mandell 2007).

Nosocomial pneumonia: IV: 4.5 g every 6 hours for 7 to 14 days (when used empirically, combination with an aminoglycoside or antipseudomonal fluoroquinolone is recommended; consider discontinuation of additional agent if *P. aeruginosa* is not isolated) (ATS 2005).

Skin and soft tissue infection: IV: 3.375 g every 6 hours for 7 to 10 days. **Note:** For severe diabetic foot infections, recommended treatment duration is up to 4 weeks depending on severity of infection and response to therapy (Lipsky 2012).

Necrotizing infections (off-label use): IV:3.375 g every 6 to 8 hours (in combination with vancomycin for empiric therapy); continue until further debridement is not necessary, patient has clinically improved, and patient is afebrile for 48 to 72 hours (IDSA [Stevens 2014]).

Bite wounds (animal) (off-label use): IV: 3.375 g every 6 to 8 hours (IDSA [Stevens 2014])

Intra-abdominal infection, complicated (off-label use): IV: 3.375 g every 6 hours for 4 to 7 days (provided source controlled). **Note:** Increase to 3.375 g every 4 hours or 4.5 g every 6 hours if *P. aeruginosa* is suspected. Not recommended for mild-to-moderate, community-acquired intra-abdominal infections due to risk of toxicity and the development of resistant organisms (Solomkin 2010).

Surgical (perioperative) prophylaxis (off-label use): IV: 3.375 g within 60 minutes prior to surgery. Doses may be repeated in 2 hours if procedure is lengthy or if there is excessive blood loss (Bratzler 2013).

Surgical site infections (intestinal or genitourinary tract) (off-label use): IV: 3.375 g every 6 hours or 4.5 g every 8 hours (IDSA [Stevens 2014])

Pediatric Note: Piperacillin and tazobactam is a combination product; each 3.375 g vial contains 3 g piperacillin sodium and 0.375 g tazobactam sodium in an 8:1 ratio. Dosage recommendations in **pediatric** patients are based on the **piperacillin** component. Dosing presented is based on traditional infusion method (IV infusion over 30 minutes) unless otherwise specified as the extended infusion method (IV infusion over 4 hours [off-label method]).

Usual dosage range: IV:

Infants 2 to 9 months: 80 mg piperacillin/kg/dose every 8 hours (Red Book [AAP] 2012):

Infants >9 months, Children, and Adolescents: 100 mg piperacillin/kg/dose every 8 hours (maximum dose: 16 g piperacillin/day) (Red Book [AAP] 2012):

Children and Adolescents: Extended-infusion method: Limited data available: 100 mg piperacillin/kg/dose infused over 4 hours 3 times daily. Dosing based on a prospective, observational study (n=332) in a single children's hospital comparing the extended interval method to traditional dosing (Nichols 2012).

Indication-specific dosing: Infants, Children, and Adolescents: **Note:** In pediatric patients, dosage recommendations are based on the **piperacillin** component. Dosing is presented in mg/kg/**dose** and mg/kg/**day**; use caution.

Appendicitis, peritonitis:

Infants 2 to 9 months: IV: 80 mg piperacillin/kg/dose every 8 hours

Infants >9 months, Children, and Adolescents ≤40 kg: IV: 100 mg piperacillin/kg/dose every 8 hours (maximum: 3,000 mg piperacillin/dose)

Children and Adolescents >40 kg: Refer to adult dosing.

Cystic fibrosis, pseudomonal lung infections (off-label use):

Standard dosing: IV: 240 to 400 mg piperacillin/kg/**day** divided every 8 hours (Kliegman, 2011); others have used 350 to 400 mg/kg/**day** divided every 4 hours in early piperacillin trials (Zobell, 2013)

High-dose: Limited data available: IV: 450 mg piperacillin/kg/**day** every 4 to 6 hours or 600 mg piperacillin/kg/**day** divided every 4 hours has been described from early studies of piperacillin alone; usual maximum daily dose: 18 to 24 g piperacillin/**day**. **Note:** Piperacillin doses >600 mg/kg/day or an extended duration of therapy (>14 days) have been associated with dose-related adverse effects including serum sickness, immune-mediated hemolytic anemia and bone marrow suppression (Zobell 2013).

Intra-abdominal infection, complicated (off-label use): IV: 200 to 300 mg piperacillin/kg/day divided every 6 to 8 hours (maximum dose: 12 g piperacillin/day) (Solomkin, 2010).

Skin and soft tissue necrotizing infections (off-label use): IV: 60 to 75 mg piperacillin/kg every 6 hours (in combination with vancomycin for empiric therapy); continue until further debridement is not necessary, patient has clinically improved, and patient is afebrile for 48 to 72 hours. (IDSA [Stevens 2014])

Surgical (perioperative) prophylaxis (off-label use): Note: Doses may be repeated in 2 hours if procedure is lengthy or if there is excessive blood loss (Bratzler 2013): IV:

Infants 2 to 9 months: 80 mg piperacillin/kg within 60 minutes prior to surgical incision (maximum: 3,000 mg piperacillin/dose)

Infants >9 months, Children, and Adolescents ≤40 kg: 100 mg piperacillin/kg within 60 minutes prior to surgical incision (maximum: 3,000 mg piperacillin/dose).

Children and Adolescents >40 kg: Refer to adult dosing.

Renal Impairment

Adults:

Traditional infusion method (ie, IV infusion over 30 minutes): Manufacturer's labeling:

CrCl >40 mL/minute: No dosage adjustment necessary.

CrCl 20 to 40 mL/minute: Administer 2.25 g every 6 hours (3.375 g every 6 hours for nosocomial pneumonia)

CrCl <20 mL/minute: Administer 2.25 g every 8 hours (2.25 g every 6 hours for nosocomial pneumonia)

Note: Some clinicians suggest adjusting the dose at CrCl ≤20 mL/minute (rather than CrCl <40 mL/minute) in patients receiving either traditional or extended-infusion methods, particularly if treating serious gram-negative infections (empirically or definitively) (Patel 2010).

Extended infusion method (off-label dosing): CrCl ≤20 mL/minute: 3.375 g IV over 4 hours every 12 hours (Patel 2010)

End-stage renal disease (ESRD):

Intermittent hemodialysis (IHD): 2.25 g every 12 hours (2.25 g every 8 hours for nosocomial pneumonia). **Note:** Dosing dependent on the assumption of 3 times/week, complete IHD sessions. Administer scheduled doses after hemodialysis on dialysis days; if next regularly scheduled dose is not due right after dialysis session, administer an additional dose of 0.75 g after the dialysis session.

Peritoneal dialysis (PD): 2.25 g every 12 hours (2.25 g every 8 hours for nosocomial pneumonia).

Continuous renal replacement therapy (CRRT) (Heintz 2009; Trotman 2005): Drug clearance is highly dependent on the method of renal replacement, filter type, and flow rate. Appropriate dosing requires close monitoring of pharmacologic response, signs of adverse reactions due to drug accumulation, as well as drug concentrations in relation to target trough (if appropriate). The following are general recommendations only (based on dialysate flow/ultrafiltration rates of 1 to 2 L/hour and minimal residual renal function) and should not supersede clinical judgment (Trotman 2005):

CVVH: 2.25 to 3.375 g every 6 to 8 hours

CVVHD: 2.25 to 3.375 g every 6 hours

CVVHDF: 3.375 g every 6 hours

Note: Higher dose of 3.375 g should be considered when treating resistant pathogens (especially *Pseudomonas* spp); alternative recommendations suggest dosing of 4.5 g every 8 hours (Valtonen 2001); regardless of regimen, there is some concern of tazobactam (TAZ) accumulation, given its lower clearance relative to piperacillin (PIP). Some clinicians advocate dosing with PIP to alternate with PIP/TAZ, particularly in CVVH-dependent patients, to lessen this concern.

Infants, Children, and Adolescents: There are no dosage adjustments provided in the manufacturer's labeling; however, the following adjustments have been recommended (Aronoff, 2007): Dosing based on a usual dose of 200 to 300 mg piperacillin/kg/day in divided doses every 6 hours.

GFR >50 mL/minute/1.73 m^2: No dosage adjustment necessary.

GFR 30 to 50 mL/minute/1.73 m^2: 35 to 50 mg piperacillin/kg/dose every 6 hours

GFR <30 mL/minute/1.73 m^2: 35 to 50 mg piperacillin/kg/dose every 8 hours

End-stage renal disease (ESRD) on intermittent hemodialysis (IHD): Hemodialysis removes 30% to 40% of a piperacillin/tazobactam dose: 50 to 75 mg piperacillin/kg/dose every 12 hours

Peritoneal dialysis (PD): Peritoneal dialysis removes 21% of tazobactam and 6% of piperacillin: 50 to 75 mg piperacillin/kg/dose every 12 hours

Continuous renal replacement therapy (CRRT): 35 to 50 mg piperacillin/kg/dose every 8 hours

Hepatic Impairment No dosage adjustment necessary.

Additional Information Complete prescribing information should be consulted for additional detail.

Dosage Forms Excipient information presented when available (limited, particularly for generics); consult specific product labeling.

Note: 8:1 ratio of piperacillin sodium/tazobactam sodium

Infusion [premixed iso-osmotic solution]:

Zosyn: 2.25 g: Piperacillin 2 g and tazobactam 0.25 g (50 mL) [contains edetate disodium, sodium 130 mg (5.68 mEq)]

Zosyn: 3.375 g: Piperacillin 3 g and tazobactam 0.375 g (50 mL) [contains edetate disodium, sodium 195 mg (8.52 mEq)]

Zosyn: 4.5 g: Piperacillin 4 g and tazobactam 0.5 g (100 mL) [contains edetate disodium, sodium 260 mg (11.36 mEq)]

Injection, powder for reconstitution: 2.25 g: Piperacillin 2 g and tazobactam 0.25 g; 3.375 g: Piperacillin 3 g and tazobactam 0.375 g; 4.5 g: Piperacillin 4 g and tazobactam 0.5 g; 40.5 g: Piperacillin 36 g and tazobactam 4.5 g

Zosyn: 2.25 g: Piperacillin 2 g and tazobactam 0.25 g [contains edetate disodium, sodium 130 mg (5.68 mEq)]

Zosyn: 3.375 g: Piperacillin 3 g and tazobactam 0.375 g [contains edetate disodium, sodium 195 mg (8.52 mEq)]

Zosyn: 4.5 g: Piperacillin 4 g and tazobactam 0.5 g [contains edetate disodium, sodium 260 mg (11.36 mEq)]

Zosyn: 40.5 g: Piperacillin 36 g and tazobactam 4.5 g [contains edetate disodium, sodium 2340 mg (102.24 mEq); bulk pharmacy vial]

♦ **Piperacillin and Tazobactam for Injection (Can)** *see* Piperacillin and Tazobactam *on page 1388*

♦ **Piperacillin and Tazobactam Sodium** *see* Piperacillin and Tazobactam *on page 1388*

♦ **Piperacillin Sodium and Tazobactam Sodium** *see* Piperacillin and Tazobactam *on page 1388*

♦ **Platinol** *see* CISplatin *on page 334*

♦ **Platinol-AQ** *see* CISplatin *on page 334*

Plerixafor (pler IX a fore)

Related Information

Hematopoietic Stem Cell Transplantation *on page 2272*

Safe Handling of Hazardous Drugs *on page 2292*

Brand Names: US Mozobil

Brand Names: Canada Mozobil

Index Terms AMD3100; LM3100

Pharmacologic Category Hematopoietic Agent; Hematopoietic Stem Cell Mobilizer

Use Peripheral stem cell mobilization: Mobilization of hematopoietic stem cells (HSC) for collection and subsequent autologous transplantation (in combination with filgrastim) in patients with non-Hodgkin lymphoma (NHL) and multiple myeloma (MM)

Labeled Contraindications History of hypersensitivity to plerixafor or any component of the formulation (anaphylactic shock has occurred).

Pregnancy Considerations Adverse effects have been observed in animal reproduction studies. May cause fetal harm if administered to pregnant women. Women of childbearing potential should use effective contraceptive measures to avoid becoming pregnant during treatment.

Breast-Feeding Considerations It is not known if plerixafor is excreted in breast milk. Due to the potential for serious adverse reactions in the nursing infant, a decision should be made to discontinue plerixafor or to discontinue breast-feeding, taking into account the importance of treatment to the mother.

Warnings/Precautions Hazardous agent - use appropriate precautions for handling and disposal (NIOSH 2014 [group 3]). Serious hypersensitivity reactions, including anaphylactic-type reactions (may be life-threatening with serious hypotension and shock) have been reported. Observe patients for hypersensitivity symptoms during, for 30 minutes after administration, and until clinically stable. Medication, personnel, and equipment for hypersensitivity management should be available. Mild-to-moderate allergic reactions may also occur, usually within 30 minutes of administration. Increases circulating leukocytes when used in conjunction with filgrastim; monitor WBC counts. Thrombocytopenia has been observed; monitor platelet counts. Not intended for mobilization in patients with leukemia; may contaminate apheresis product by mobilizing leukemic cells. When used in combination with filgrastim, tumor cells released from marrow could be collected in leukapheresis product; potential effect of tumor cell reinfusion is unknown. Splenomegaly and splenic rupture have been reported (rarely) with filgrastim use; instruct patients to report left upper quadrant pain or scapular/shoulder tip pain; promptly evaluate in any patient who report these symptoms.

Primary route of elimination is renal; dosage reduction is recommended in patients with moderate-to-severe renal impairment (CrCl ≤50 mL/minute). Medications that may reduce renal function or compete for active tubular secretion may increase serum concentrations of plerixafor. Use has not been studied in patients weighing >175% of ideal body weight.

Adverse Reactions Adverse reactions reported with filgrastim combination therapy.

>10%:

Central nervous system: Fatigue (27%), headache (22%), dizziness (11%)

Gastrointestinal: Diarrhea (37%), nausea (34%)

Local: Injection site reaction (34%, including edema, erythema, hematoma, hemorrhage, induration, inflammation, irritation, pain, paresthesia, pruritus, skin rash, urticaria)

Neuromuscular & skeletal: Arthralgia (13%)

5% to 10%:

Central nervous system: Insomnia (7%)

Gastrointestinal: Vomiting (10%), flatulence (7%)

Hematologic & oncologic: Hyperleukocytosis (7%)

<5%, postmarketing, and/or case reports: Abdominal distension, abdominal distress, abdominal pain, abnormal dreams, anaphylaxis, constipation, diaphoresis, dyspepsia, dyspnea, hypersensitivity reaction, hypoxia, leukocytosis, malaise, musculoskeletal pain, nightmares, oral hypoesthesia, orthostatic hypotension, periorbital swelling, syncope, thrombocytopenia, xerostomia

Drug Interactions

Metabolism/Transport Effects None known.

Avoid Concomitant Use There are no known interactions where it is recommended to avoid concomitant use.

Increased Effect/Toxicity There are no known significant interactions involving an increase in effect.

Decreased Effect There are no known significant interactions involving a decrease in effect.

Storage/Stability Store at 25°C (77°F); excursions permitted to 15°C to 30°C (59°F to 86°F).

Mechanism of Action Reversibly inhibits binding of stromal cell-derived factor-1-alpha (SDF-1α), expressed on bone marrow stromal cells, to the CXC chemokine receptor 4 (CXCR4), resulting in mobilization of hematopoietic stem and progenitor cells from bone marrow into peripheral blood. Plerixafor used in combination with filgrastim results in synergistic increase in CD34+ cell mobilization. Mobilized CD34+ cells are capable of engrafting with extended repopulating capacity.

Pharmacodynamics/Kinetics

Onset of action: Peak CD34+ mobilization (healthy volunteers): Plerixafor monotherapy: 6 to 9 hours after administration; Plerixafor + filgrastim: 10 to 14 hours

Duration: Sustained elevation in CD34+ cells (healthy volunteers): 4 to 18 hours after administration

Absorption: SubQ: Rapid; exposure using the mg/kg dosing increases with increasing body weight; the fixed dosing (20 mg) results in higher exposure than the mg/kg dose, but the median time to reach the target cell count is the same for both dosing regimens

Distribution: 0.3 L/kg; primarily to extravascular fluid space

Protein binding: ≤58%

Metabolism: Not metabolized

Half-life elimination: Terminal: 3 to 5 hours

Time to peak, plasma: SubQ: 30 to 60 minutes

Excretion: Urine (~70%; as parent drug)

Dosing

Adult & Geriatric Note: Dosing is based on actual body weight. Begin plerixafor after patient has received filgrastim (10 mcg/kg once daily) for 4 days; plerixafor, filgrastim, and apheresis should be continued daily until sufficient cell collection up to a maximum of 4 days.

Hematopoietic stem cell mobilization (in non-Hodgkin lymphoma and multiple myeloma): SubQ: Administer ~11 hours prior to apheresis
US labeling:
  Patients ≤83 kg: 20 mg fixed dose **or** 0.24 mg/kg once daily for up to 4 consecutive days
  Patients >83 kg: 0.24 mg/kg once daily for up to 4 consecutive days; maximum dose: 40 mg daily
Canadian labeling: 0.24 mg/kg once daily for up to 4 consecutive days; maximum dose: 40 mg daily

Renal Impairment Note: Creatinine clearance estimate based on Cockcroft-Gault formula:

US labeling:

CrCl >50 mL/minute: No dosage adjustment necessary.

CrCl ≤50 mL/minute:

Patients ≤83 kg: 13 mg fixed dose **or** 0.16 mg/kg once daily

Patients >83 kg and <160 kg: 0.16 mg/kg once daily; maximum dose: 27 mg daily

Hemodialysis: There are no dosage adjustments provided in the manufacturer's labeling (has not been studied).

Canadian labeling:

CrCl >50 mL/minute: No dosage adjustment necessary

CrCl 20 to 50 mL/minute: 0.16 mg/kg once daily; maximum dose: 27 mg daily

CrCl <20 mL/minute and hemodialysis: There are no dosage adjustments provided in the manufacturer's labeling (has not been studied).

Hepatic Impairment There are no dosage adjustments provided in the manufacturer's labeling.

Obesity The manufacturer recommends calculating the dose based on actual weight for patients weighing up to 175% of ideal body weight (maximum dose: 40 mg daily). Dosing in patients >175% of ideal body weight has not been studied.

Administration Administer subcutaneously, ~11 hours prior to initiation of apheresis. In some clinical trials, plerixafor administration began in the evening prior to apheresis; filgrastim was begun on day 1, plerixafor initiated in the evening on day 4 and apheresis in the morning on day 5; with filgrastim, plerixafor, and apheresis then continued daily until sufficient cell collection for autologous transplant (DiPersio, 2009a; DiPersio, 2009b).

Hazardous agent; use appropriate precautions for handling and disposal (NIOSH 2014 [group 3]).

Monitoring Parameters CBC with differential and platelets; signs/symptoms of hypersensitivity (during, for 30 minutes after administration, and until clinically stable); signs/symptoms of splenomegaly

Dosage Forms Excipient information presented when available (limited, particularly for generics); consult specific product labeling.

Solution, Subcutaneous [preservative free]:

Mozobil: 24 mg/1.2 mL (1.2 mL)

- ◆ **PMS-Fentanyl MTX (Can)** *see* FentaNYL *on page 692*
- ◆ **PMS-Fluconazole (Can)** *see* Fluconazole *on page 725*
- ◆ **PMS-Flutamide (Can)** *see* Flutamide *on page 751*
- ◆ **PMS-Haloperidol (Can)** *see* Haloperidol *on page 807*
- ◆ **PMS-Haloperidol LA (Can)** *see* Haloperidol *on page 807*
- ◆ **PMS-Hydromorphone (Can)** *see* HYDROmorphone *on page 830*
- ◆ **PMS-Letrozole (Can)** *see* Letrozole *on page 1019*
- ◆ **PMS-Levofloxacin (Can)** *see* Levofloxacin (Systemic) *on page 1038*
- ◆ **PMS-Lorazepam (Can)** *see* LORazepam *on page 1058*
- ◆ **PMS-Medroxyprogesterone (Can)** *see* MedroxyPROGESTERone *on page 1074*
- ◆ **PMS-Metoclopramide (Can)** *see* Metoclopramide *on page 1134*
- ◆ **PMS-Metronidazole (Can)** *see* MetroNIDAZOLE (Systemic) *on page 1142*
- ◆ **PMS-Morphine Sulfate SR (Can)** *see* Morphine (Systemic) *on page 1167*
- ◆ **PMS-Nabilone (Can)** *see* Nabilone *on page 1187*
- ◆ **PMS-Nystatin (Can)** *see* Nystatin (Oral) *on page 1218*
- ◆ **PMS-Olanzapine (Can)** *see* OLANZapine *on page 1242*
- ◆ **PMS-Olanzapine ODT (Can)** *see* OLANZapine *on page 1242*
- ◆ **PMS-Ondansetron (Can)** *see* Ondansetron *on page 1253*
- ◆ **PMS-Oxycodone (Can)** *see* OxyCODONE *on page 1277*
- ◆ **PMS-Oxycodone CR (Can)** *see* OxyCODONE *on page 1277*
- ◆ **PMS-Pamidronate (Can)** *see* Pamidronate *on page 1310*
- ◆ **PMS-Prednisolone Sodium Phosphate Forte (Can)** *see* PrednisoLONE (Ophthalmic) *on page 1424*
- ◆ **PMS-Prochlorperazine (Can)** *see* Prochlorperazine *on page 1441*
- ◆ **PMS-Raloxifene (Can)** *see* Raloxifene *on page 1451*
- ◆ **PMS-Tamoxifen (Can)** *see* Tamoxifen *on page 1595*
- ◆ **PMS-Valacyclovir (Can)** *see* ValACYclovir *on page 1712*
- ◆ **PMS-Vancomycin (Can)** *see* Vancomycin *on page 1720*
- ◆ **PN401** *see* Uridine Triacetate *on page 1709*
- ◆ **Polyethylene Glycol-L-asparaginase** *see* Pegaspargase *on page 1341*
- ◆ **Polyethylene Glycol Interferon Alfa-2b** *see* Peginterferon Alfa-2b *on page 1350*

Pomalidomide (poe ma LID oh mide)

Related Information

Common Toxicity Criteria *on page 2122*
Safe Handling of Hazardous Drugs *on page 2292*

Brand Names: US Pomalyst
Brand Names: Canada Pomalyst
Index Terms CC-4047
Pharmacologic Category Angiogenesis Inhibitor; Antineoplastic Agent; Immunomodulator, Systemic

Use Multiple myeloma, relapsed/refractory: Treatment of multiple myeloma (in combination with dexamethasone) in patients who have received at least 2 prior therapies, including lenalidomide and a proteasome inhibitor, and have demonstrated disease progression on or within 60 days of completion of the last therapy.

Labeled Contraindications Pregnancy

Canadian labeling: Additional contraindications (not in US labeling): Hypersensitivity to pomalidomide, thalidomide, lenalidomide, or any component of the formulation; breast-feeding; women of childbearing potential not using 2 effective means of contraception; male patients unable to comply with required contraceptive measures

Pregnancy Considerations [US Boxed Warning]: Pomalidomide is an analogue of thalidomide (a known human teratogen) and may cause severe birth defects or embryo-fetal death if taken during pregnancy. Pomalidomide cannot be used in women who are pregnant or may become pregnant during therapy. Obtain 2 negative pregnancy tests prior to initiation of treatment; 2 forms of contraception (or abstain from heterosexual intercourse) must be used at least 4 weeks prior to, during, and for ≥4 weeks after pomalidomide treatment (and during treatment interruptions) in females of reproductive potential. In order to decrease the risk of embryo-fetal exposure, pomalidomide is available only through a restricted distribution program (Pomalyst REMS). In Canada, distribution is restricted to physicians, pharmacists, and patients registered with the RevAid program.

Studies in animals have shown evidence of fetal abnormalities and use is contraindicated in women who are or may become pregnant. Women of childbearing potential should be treated only if they are able to comply with the conditions of the Pomalyst REMS Program (US) or RevAid program (Canada). Reliable contraception is required even with a history of infertility (unless due to hysterectomy or if ≥24 consecutive months postmenopausal (natural). Reliable methods of birth control include one highly effective method (eg, tubal ligation, IUD, hormonal [birth control pills, injections, hormonal patches, vaginal rings, or implants], or partner's vasectomy) and one additional effective method (eg, male latex or synthetic condom, diaphragm, or cervical cap). Pregnancy tests should be performed 10 to 14 days (US labeling) or 7 to 14 days (Canadian labeling) and 24 hours prior to beginning therapy; weekly for the first 4 weeks and then every 4 weeks (every 2 weeks if menstrual cycle irregular) thereafter and during therapy interruptions for at least 4 weeks after discontinuation. Pomalidomide must be immediately discontinued for a missed period, abnormal pregnancy test or abnormal menstrual bleeding; refer patient to a reproductive toxicity specialist if pregnancy occurs during treatment. Pomalidomide is present in the semen of males taking this medication. Males (including those vasectomized) should use a latex or synthetic condom during any sexual contact with women of childbearing age during treatment, during treatment interruptions, and for 28 days after discontinuation. Male patients should not donate sperm. Any suspected fetal exposure should be reported in the US to the FDA via the MedWatch program (1-800-332-1088) and to Celgene Corporation (1-888-423-5436) and in Canada to Celgene (1-888-738-2341).

Breast-Feeding Considerations It is not known if pomalidomide is excreted into breast milk. Due to the potential for serious adverse reactions in the nursing infant, a decision should be made to discontinue nursing or to discontinue treatment with pomalidomide, taking into account the importance of treatment to the mother.

Warnings/Precautions Hazardous agent - use appropriate precautions for handling and disposal (meets NIOSH 2014 criteria). Due to the embryo-fetal risk, pomalidomide is only available through a restricted program under the Pomalyst REMS program. Pomalidomide should only be prescribed to patients who can understand and comply with the conditions of the Pomalyst REMS program. Prescribers and pharmacies must be certified with the REMS program. In Canada, pomalidomide is only available through the restricted RevAid program. Prescribers and pharmacists must be registered with the program to prescribe and dispense pomalidomide; patients must also be registered and meet all conditions of the program.

[US Boxed Warning]: Pomalidomide is a thalidomide (human teratogen) analog and may cause severe life-threatening birth defects or embryo-fetal deaths; use is contraindicated in pregnancy. Pregnancy must be excluded prior to therapy initiation with 2 negative pregnancy tests; prevent pregnancy during therapy with 2 reliable forms of contraception (or abstain from heterosexual intercourse) beginning 4 weeks prior to, during and for 4 weeks after pomalidomide therapy (and during treatment interruptions) in females of reproductive potential. In order to decrease the risk of embryo-fetal exposure, pomalidomide is available only through a restricted distribution program (Pomalyst REMS). Reliable methods of birth control include one highly effective method (eg, tubal ligation, IUD, hormonal [birth control pills, injections, hormonal patches, vaginal rings, or implants], or partner's vasectomy) or one additional effective method (eg, male latex or synthetic condom, diaphragm, or cervical cap). Males taking pomalidomide must use a latex or synthetic condom during any sexual contact with a woman of childbearing potential during therapy and for up to 28 days after treatment discontinuation, even if successfully vasectomized. Patients should not donate blood during pomalidomide treatment and for 1 month after therapy discontinuation; male patients receiving pomalidomide must not donate sperm.

Neutropenia, anemia, and thrombocytopenia were frequently reported in clinical trials; neutropenia was the most frequently reported grade 3/4 adverse event, followed by anemia and thrombocytopenia. Neutropenic fever has also been reported. Monitor complete blood counts weekly for the first 8 weeks of therapy and monthly or as clinically indicated thereafter; may require therapy interruption, reduction and/or discontinuation. Acute myelogenous leukemia (AML) as a secondary malignancy has been reported in patients receiving pomalidomide in the investigational treatment of condition(s) other than multiple myeloma. **[US Boxed Warning]: Venous and arterial thromboembolic events such as deep vein thrombosis (DVT), pulmonary embolism (PE), MI, and stroke have occurred during pomalidomide therapy. Clinical trials utilized antithrombotic prophylaxis. Thromboprophylaxis is recommended; and should be based on assessment of the patient's underlying risk factors.** Arterial thrombotic events also included cerebrovascular ischemia and ischemic heart disease. Monitor for signs/symptoms of thromboembolism (shortness of breath, chest pain, or arm or leg swelling) and advise patients to promptly seek medical attention should symptoms occur. May cause dizziness and/or confusion; caution patients to avoid tasks that require mental alertness (eg, operating machinery or driving). Avoid concomitant medications which may exacerbate dizziness and confusion. Angioedema and severe dermatologic reactions have been reported. Discontinue (permanently) for angioedema, skin exfoliation, bullae, or any other severe dermatologic toxicity. Use with caution in patients with a prior history of serious hypersensitivity reactions to thalidomide or lenalidomide; such patients were excluded from pomalidomide clinical trials and may therefore be at risk for hypersensitivity reactions when administered pomalidomide. Peripheral and sensory neuropathy occurred in clinical trials, including some cases of grade 3 neuropathy, although no cases of grade 4 neuropathy were observed. Monitor closely for signs/symptoms of neuropathy; may require therapy interruption, dose modification and/or discontinuation.

Safety and efficacy have not been evaluated in patients with renal or hepatic impairment. Pomalidomide is hepatically metabolized; avoid use in patients with serum bilirubin >2 mg/dL and AST/ALT >3 times ULN (has not been studied). Hepatic failure (with fatalities) has been reported; elevated bilirubin and ALT have also been observed; monitor liver function tests; interrupt treatment and reduce dose if liver enzymes are elevated. Pomalidomide and its metabolites are excreted by the kidneys; avoid use in patients with serum creatinine >3 mg/dL (has not been studied). The Canadian labeling recommends avoiding use if CrCl <45 mL/minute. Patients with a high tumor burden may be at risk for tumor lysis syndrome; monitor closely; institute appropriate management for hyperuricemia. Potentially significant drug-drug interactions may exist, requiring dose or frequency adjustment, additional monitoring, and/or selection of alternative therapy. Cigarette smoking may induce CYP1A2 mediated metabolism of pomalidomide, potentially reducing its systemic exposure and efficacy.

Adverse Reactions Frequency not always defined.

Cardiovascular: Peripheral edema (25%), angina pectoris, congestive cardiac failure, hypotension, myocardial infarction, septic shock, syncope

Central nervous system: Fatigue (≤58%), peripheral neuropathy (22%), dizziness (22%; grades 3/4: <5%), neuropathy (18%; grades 3/4: 2%), headache (15%), anxiety (13%), confusion (12%; grades 3/4: 6%), chills (10%), insomnia (7%), pain (6%), altered mental status, depression, falling, noncardiac chest pain

Dermatologic: Skin rash (21%), pruritus (15%), xeroderma (9%), hyperhidrosis (8%), cellulitis

Endocrine & metabolic: Hypercalcemia (22%; grades 3/4: 10%), hypokalemia (12%; grades 3/4: <5%), hyperglycemia (11%; grades 3/4: <5%), hyponatremia (11%; grades 3/4: <5%), dehydration (<10%; grade 3/4: 5%), hypocalcemia (6%), weight gain (≤5%)

Gastrointestinal: Constipation (36%), nausea (36%), diarrhea (35%), decreased appetite (23%), weight loss (15%), vomiting (14%), weight loss (15%), abdominal pain, *clostridium difficile*, increased serum alanine aminotransferase

Genitourinary: Urinary tract infection (10%, grades 3/4: 2%), urosepsis

Hematologic & oncologic: Neutropenia (53%; grades 3/4: 48%), anemia (38%; grades 3/4: 23%), thrombocytopenia (26%; grades 3/4: 22%), leukopenia (13%; grades 3/4: 7%), febrile neutropenia (<10%), lymphocytopenia (4%; grades 3/4: 2%), decreased hemoglobin

Infection: Sepsis (<10%), bacteremia, pneumonia due to *Streptococcal* species, viral infection

◀ Neuromuscular & skeletal: Weakness (≤58%), back pain (35%), musculoskeletal chest pain (23%), muscle spasm (22%), arthralgia (17%), myasthenia (14%), musculoskeletal pain (12%), ostealgia (12%), tremor (10%), limb pain (8%), fracture, vertebral compression fracture

Renal: Increased serum creatinine (19%), renal failure (15%)

Respiratory: Upper respiratory tract infection (37%), dyspnea (36%), pneumonia (28%), epistaxis (17%), cough (17%), productive cough (9%), oropharyngeal pain (6%), bronchospasm, lobar pneumonia, pulmonary infection

Miscellaneous: Fever (23%), night sweats (5%), failure to thrive, multi-organ failure, physical health deterioration

<1%, postmarketing, and/or case reports: Acute myelocytic leukemia, hepatic failure, hyperbilirubinemia, hyperkalemia, hypersensitivity reaction, increased liver enzymes, increased serum ALT, interstitial pulmonary disease, neutropenic sepsis, pancytopenia, pelvic pain, *Pneumocystis jiroveci* pneumonia, respiratory syncytial virus infection, tumor lysis syndrome, urinary retention, vertigo

Drug Interactions

Metabolism/Transport Effects Substrate of CYP1A2 (major), CYP2C19 (minor), CYP2D6 (minor), CYP3A4 (minor), P-glycoprotein; **Note:** Assignment of Major/Minor substrate status based on clinically relevant drug interaction potential

Avoid Concomitant Use

Avoid concomitant use of Pomalidomide with any of the following: Abatacept; Anakinra; Azelastine (Nasal); BCG (Intravesical); Canakinumab; Certolizumab Pegol; CloZAPine; CYP1A2 Inhibitors (Strong); Dipyrone; Natalizumab; Orphenadrine; Paraldehyde; Pimecrolimus; Rilonacept; Tacrolimus (Topical); Thalidomide; Tocilizumab; Tofacitinib; Vaccines (Live); Vedolizumab

Increased Effect/Toxicity

Pomalidomide may increase the levels/effects of: Abatacept; Alcohol (Ethyl); Anakinra; Azelastine (Nasal); Bisphosphonate Derivatives; Buprenorphine; Canakinumab; Certolizumab Pegol; CloZAPine; CNS Depressants; Fingolimod; Hydrocodone; Leflunomide; Methotrimeprazine; Metyrosine; Mirtazapine; Natalizumab; Orphenadrine; Paraldehyde; Pramipexole; Rilonacept; ROPINIRole; Rotigotine; Selective Serotonin Reuptake Inhibitors; Suvorexant; Thalidomide; Tofacitinib; Vaccines (Live); Vedolizumab; Zolpidem

The levels/effects of Pomalidomide may be increased by: Abiraterone Acetate; Brimonidine (Topical); Cannabis; CYP1A2 Inhibitors (Moderate); CYP1A2 Inhibitors (Strong); Deferasirox; Denosumab; Dipyrone; Doxylamine; Dronabinol; Droperidol; HydrOXYzine; Kava Kava; Magnesium Sulfate; Methotrimeprazine; Minocycline; Nabilone; Peginterferon Alfa-2b; Perampanel; Pimecrolimus; Roflumilast; Rufinamide; Sodium Oxybate; Tacrolimus (Topical); Tapentadol; Tetrahydrocannabinol; Tocilizumab; Trastuzumab; Vemurafenib

Decreased Effect

Pomalidomide may decrease the levels/effects of: BCG (Intravesical); Coccidioides immitis Skin Test; Sipuleucel-T; Vaccines (Inactivated); Vaccines (Live)

The levels/effects of Pomalidomide may be decreased by: Cannabis; CYP1A2 Inducers (Strong); Cyproterone; Echinacea; Osimertinib; Teriflunomide

Storage/Stability Store at 20°C to 25°C (68°F to 77°F); excursions permitted to 15°C to 30°C (59°F to 86°F).

Mechanism of Action Induces cell cycle arrest and apoptosis directly in multiple myeloma cells; enhances T cell- and natural killer (NK) cell-mediated cytotoxicity; inhibits production of proinflammatory cytokines tumor necrosis factor-α (TNF-α), IL-1, IL-6, and IL-12; inhibits angiogenesis (Zhu 2013)

Pharmacodynamics/Kinetics

Absorption: Rapid; slowed by food. Canadian labeling suggests that the overall effect of food on extent of absorption is minimal (AUC decreased 8%).

Distribution: V_{dss}: 62 to 138 L; semen distribution is ~67% of plasma levels

Protein binding: 12% to 44%

Metabolism: Hepatic via CYP1A2 and CYP3A4; CYP2C19 and CYP2D6 (minor)

Half-life elimination: ~9.5 hours (healthy subjects); ~7.5 hours (multiple myeloma patients)

Time to peak: 2 to 3 hours

Excretion: Urine (73%; 2% as unchanged drug); feces (15%; 8% as unchanged drug)

Dosing

Adult Note: ANC should be ≥500 cells/mm³ (US labeling) or ≥1,000 cells/mm³ (Canadian labeling) and platelets ≥50,000 cells/mm³ prior to initiating new cycles of therapy.

Multiple myeloma, relapsed/refractory: Oral:

4 mg once daily on days 1 to 21 of 28-day cycles (in combination with dexamethasone); continue until disease progression or unacceptable toxicity (Richardson 2014; San Miguel 2013).

Dosage adjustment for concomitant therapy with strong CYP1A2 inhibitors in the presence of strong CYP3A4 and P-gp inhibitors: Avoid concomitant use of strong CYP1A2 inhibitors. If concomitant use of strong CYP1A2 inhibitors in the presence of strong CYP3A4 and P-gp inhibitors cannot be avoided, reduce the pomalidomide dose by 50%.

Geriatric Refer to adult dosing. The Canadian labeling recommends reducing the dosage of concurrent dexamethasone by 50% in patients >75 years of age.

Renal Impairment Serum creatinine >3 mg/dL (US labeling) or CrCl <45 mL/minute (Canadian labeling): Avoid use (has not been studied).

Hepatic Impairment

*Hepatic impairment **prior** to treatment:* Bilirubin >2 mg/dL and AST/ALT >3 times ULN: Avoid use (has not been studied).

*Hepatic impairment **during** treatment:* If liver enzymes are elevated, stop pomalidomide and evaluate; after liver enzymes return to baseline, may consider restarting at a lower dose.

Adjustment for Toxicity

Hematologic:

If ANC <500 cells/mm³ (or ANC <1,000 cells/mm³ with fever ≥38.5°C) and/or platelets <25,000 cells/mm³: Interrupt therapy and follow weekly CBCs. When ANC ≥500 cells/mm³ (US labeling) or ≥1,000 cells/mm³ (Canadian labeling) and/or platelets ≥50,000 cells/mm³: Resume dosing at 3 mg once daily.

For each subsequent drop of ANC <500 cells/mm³ and/or platelets <25,000 cells/mm³: Interrupt therapy. When ANC ≥500 cells/mm³ (US labeling) or ≥1,000 cells/mm³ (Canadian labeling) and/or platelets ≥50,000 cells/mm³: Resume dosing at 1 mg less than the previous dose. If toxicities occur at 1 mg daily dose, discontinue treatment.

Nonhematologic: If grade 3 or 4 toxicity occurs, interrupt therapy until resolved to ≤ grade 2; if appropriate, may restart therapy at 1 mg less than the previous dose. If toxicities occur at 1 mg daily dose, discontinue treatment.

Dermatologic toxicity:

Angioedema, skin exfoliation, bullae, or any other severe dermatologic toxicity: Permanently discontinue.

Canadian labeling: Grade 2 to 3 skin rash: Consider treatment interruption or discontinuation; may consider reinitiation only if potential benefits outweigh potential risks.

Combination Regimens

Multiple myeloma: Pomalidomide-Dexamethasone (Multiple Myeloma) on page 2068

Administration Swallow whole; do not break, chew, or open the capsules.

US labeling: Administer on an empty stomach with water (at least 2 hours before or 2 hours after a meal).

Canadian labeling: Administer without regard to meals.

Missed doses: May administer a missed dose if within 12 hours of usual dosing time. If >12 hours, skip the dose for that day and resume usual dosing the following day. Do not take 2 doses to make up for a skipped dose.

Hazardous agent; use appropriate precautions for handling and disposal (meets NIOSH 2014 criteria).

Emetic Potential Minimal (<10%)

Monitoring Parameters CBC with differential and platelets weekly for the first 8 weeks and monthly or as clinically necessary thereafter; renal function (ie, serum creatinine, creatinine clearance); liver function tests (monthly); monitor for signs/symptoms of thromboembolism and neuropathy. Consider thyroid function tests (TSH recommended at baseline and every 2 to 3 months during treatment for structurally similar medications [Hamnvik 2011]).

Women of childbearing potential: Pregnancy test 10 to 14 days (US labeling) or 7 to 14 days (Canadian labeling) **and** 24 hours prior to initiating therapy, weekly during the first month, then monthly thereafter in women with regular menstrual cycles or every 2 weeks in women with irregular menstrual cycles. Pregnancy tests should be continued for at least 4 weeks after discontinuation.

Prescribing and Access Restrictions As a requirement of the REMS program, access to this medication is restricted. Pomalidomide is approved for marketing in the US only under a Food and Drug Administration (FDA) approved, restricted distribution program called Pomalyst REMS (celgeneriskmanagement.com or 1-888-423-5436). Prescribers and pharmacies must be certified with the program to prescribe or dispense pomalidomide; patients must comply with the program requirements. No more than a 4-week supply should be dispensed. Prescriptions must be filled within 7 days (for females of reproductive potential) or within 30 days (for all other patients) after the authorization number is obtained. Subsequent prescriptions may be filled only if fewer than 7 days of therapy remain on the previous prescription. A new prescription is required for further dispensing (a telephone prescription may not be accepted). Pregnancy testing with a sensitivity of at least 50 milliunits/mL is required for females of childbearing potential.

In Canada, pomalidomide is only available through a restricted distribution program called RevAid. Only physicians and pharmacists registered with the program are authorized to prescribe or dispense pomalidomide. Patients must also be registered and meet all conditions of the program. Two negative pregnancy tests with a sensitivity of at least 25 milliunits/mL are required prior to initiating therapy in women of childbearing potential. Further information is available at 1-888-738-2431 or www.RevAid.ca.

Medication Guide Available Yes

Dosage Forms Excipient information presented when available (limited, particularly for generics); consult specific product labeling.

Capsule, Oral:

Pomalyst: 1 mg, 2 mg, 3 mg [contains fd&c blue #2 (indigotine)]

Pomalyst: 4 mg [contains brilliant blue fcf (fd&c blue #1), fd&c blue #2 (indigotine)]

♦ **Pomalyst** see Pomalidomide on page 1396

PONATinib (poe NA ti nib)

Related Information

Safe Handling of Hazardous Drugs on page 2292

Brand Names: US Iclusig

Index Terms AP24534; Ponatinib Hydrochloride

Pharmacologic Category Antineoplastic Agent, BCR-ABL Tyrosine Kinase Inhibitor; Antineoplastic Agent, Tyrosine Kinase Inhibitor

Use

Acute lymphoblastic leukemia: Treatment of Philadelphia chromosome-positive acute lymphoblastic leukemia (Ph+ ALL) for whom no other tyrosine kinase inhibitor therapy is indicated or who are T315I positive

Chronic myeloid leukemia: Treatment of chronic myeloid leukemia (CML) in chronic, accelerated, or blast phase for whom no other tyrosine kinase inhibitor therapy is indicated or who are T315I positive

Labeled Contraindications There are no contraindications listed in the manufacturer's labeling.

Pregnancy Considerations Adverse events were observed in animal reproduction studies when administered in doses lower than or equivalent to the normal human dose. Based on its mechanism of action, adverse effects on pregnancy would be expected. Women of childbearing potential should be advised to avoid pregnancy during therapy.

Breast-Feeding Considerations It is not known if ponatinib is excreted in breast milk. Due to the potential for serious adverse reactions in the nursing infant, a decision should be made whether to discontinue nursing or to discontinue the drug, taking into account the importance of treatment to the mother.

Warnings/Precautions Hazardous agent - use appropriate precautions for handling and disposal (meets NIOSH 2014 criteria). **[U.S. Boxed Warning]: Arterial and venous thrombosis and occlusions have occurred in ponatinib-treated patients. Events included fatal myocardial infarction (MI), stroke, stenosis of large arterial vessels of the brain, severe peripheral vascular disease, and the need for urgent revascularization procedures; incidents were observed in patients with and without cardiovascular risk factors (including patients ≤50 years of age). Monitor closely for thromboembolism/vascular occlusion; interrupt or discontinue therapy immediately for vascular occlusion. Consider benefit:risk ratio when deciding**

◀ **to restart therapy.** Fatal and life-threatening vascular occlusion may occur within 2 weeks of therapy initiation and is not dose dependent (events have occurred at doses as low as 15 mg daily), and may cause recurrent or multisite occlusion. Increasing age and a prior history of ischemia, hypertension, diabetes, or hyperlipidemia are risk factors for development of ponatinib-associated vascular occlusion. Many patients required a revascularization procedure (cerebrovascular, coronary, and peripheral arterial) due to serious arterial thrombosis/occlusion. MI and coronary artery occlusion may result in heart failure due to myocardial ischemia. Peripheral arterial occlusive events, including fatal mesenteric artery occlusion and life-threatening peripheral arterial disease, have occurred. Some patients have required amputation due to digital or distal extremity necrosis. Venous thromboembolism, including deep vein thrombosis, pulmonary embolism, superficial thrombophlebitis, and retinal vein thrombosis, have been reported. May require dosage adjustment or discontinuation. Monitor for signs/symptoms of arterial or venous thromboembolism.

[U.S. Boxed Warning]: Serious heart failure (HF) or left ventricular dysfunction, including fatalities, were reported in clinical trials. Monitor for signs/symptoms of HF; interrupt or discontinue ponatinib therapy for new or worsening HF. Treat as clinically warranted if HF develops. Consider ponatinib discontinuation in the event of serious HF. Cardiac arrhythmias (bradyarrhythmias and tachyarrhythmias) have also been reported. Symptomatic bradyarrhythmia which required pacemaker implantation occurred in a few patients; other rhythms identified were complete heart block, sick sinus syndrome, and atrial fibrillation with bradycardia and pauses. Tachyarrhythmias reported include atrial fibrillation (most common), atrial flutter, supraventricular tachycardia, and atrial tachycardia; some events required hospitalization. Monitor for sign/symptoms of bradycardia (fainting, dizziness, chest pain) and tachycardia (palpitations, dizziness). May require therapy interruption. Treatment-emergent hypertension developed in over half of ponatinib-treated patients; symptomatic hypertension or hypertensive crisis were reported in several patients, requiring urgent intervention. Blood pressure may worsen in patients with preexisting hypertension. Monitor blood pressure closely, and manage elevated pressures as clinically indicated. May require therapy interruption, dosage reduction, or discontinuation if hypertension is resistant to medical management.

[U.S. Boxed Warning]: Liver failure and death resulting from ponatinib-induced hepatotoxicity were observed; monitor liver function prior to and at least monthly (or as clinically indicated) during treatment. Hepatotoxicity may require treatment interruption (followed by dose reduction) or discontinuation. One case of fulminant hepatic failure leading to death occurred within 1 week of therapy initiation; acute liver failure has also occurred. Treatment may result in ALT and/or AST elevations, and may be irreversible. A single-dose (30 mg) pharmacokinetic study found that ponatinib exposure was not increased in patients with hepatic impairment (Child-Pugh class A, B, or C) as compared to patients with normal hepatic function. While generally well tolerated, patients with hepatic impairment did have an increased overall incidence of adverse reactions (eg, gastrointestinal disorders, pancreatitis). Monitor closely when administering to patients with impaired hepatic function. The starting dose should be reduced in patients with hepatic impairment.

Severe myelosuppression (grade 3 or 4) was commonly observed in clinical trials, and the incidence was greater in patients with accelerated or blast phase CML and Ph+ ALL. Monitor blood counts closely; may require therapy interruption and/or dosage reduction. Hemorrhagic events occurred commonly in ponatinib-treated patients, including serious events such as cerebral and gastrointestinal hemorrhages; fatalities were reported. Serious bleeding episodes occurred more frequently in patients with accelerated or blast phase CML, and Ph+ ALL; most patients had grade 4 thrombocytopenia. Monitor platelet levels closely and for signs/symptoms of bleeding, and interrupt therapy if necessary.

Treatment-related lipase elevations and clinical pancreatitis occurred in clinical studies; the majority of cases resolved within 2 weeks of therapy interruption or dose reduction. Monitor serum lipase every 2 weeks for the first 2 months and monthly thereafter or as clinically indicated; more frequent monitoring may be considered in patients with a history of pancreatitis or alcohol abuse. Monitor for clinical signs of pancreatitis, such as abdominal symptoms; interrupt therapy if necessary. Do not reinitiate treatment until complete resolution of symptoms and lipase level is <1.5 times ULN. Serious gastrointestinal perforation (fistula) occurred very rarely; monitor for signs/symptoms of perforation and/or fistula. Serious fluid retention events, including fatality due to brain edema (very rare), were observed in ponatinib-treated patients. Peripheral edema, pleural effusions, and pericardial effusions were commonly seen; effusions and ascites were less common. Monitor patients for fluid retention; may require therapy interruption, dosage reduction, or discontinuation.

Peripheral and cranial neuropathy have been reported. Peripheral neuropathy, paresthesia, hypoesthesia, and hyperesthesia occurred most frequently; cranial neuropathy occurred rarely. In one-third of patients who experienced symptoms, neuropathy developed during the first month of therapy. Monitor for signs/symptoms of neuropathy; consider interrupting treatment if neuropathy develops. Serious ocular events such as blindness and blurred vision have occurred with ponatinib use. Macular edema, retinal vein occlusion, and retinal hemorrhage have been reported in a small percentage of patients; conjunctival or corneal irritation, dry eye, or eye pain occurred more frequently. Other toxicities include cataracts, glaucoma, iritis, iridocyclitis, and ulcerative keratitis. Perform comprehensive ophthalmic exams prior to therapy initiation and periodically during treatment.

Hyperuricemia and serious tumor lysis syndrome (rare) were reported. Patients should receive adequate hydration and be monitored for elevated uric acid levels and/or the development of tumor lysis syndrome. Correct elevated uric acid levels prior to initiating therapy. As ponatinib inhibits VEGF activity, therapy may impair wound healing. Hold therapy for at least 1 week prior to major surgery; resume therapy post procedure based on clinical judgment of appropriate wound healing. Potentially significant drug-drug interactions may exist, requiring dose or frequency adjustment, additional monitoring, and/or selection of alternative therapy. Patients ≥65 years of age may be more likely to experience weakness, decreased appetite, dyspnea, increased lipase, muscle spasms, peripheral edema, and thrombocytopenia; monitor closely. Cautious dose selection is recommended based on greater frequency of decreased hepatic, renal, or cardiac function, and of concomitant disease or other drug therapy.

◀ **Adverse Reactions**

>10%:

Cardiovascular: Hypertension (53% to 71%), peripheral edema (13% to 22%; grades 3/4: ≤1%), arterial ischemia (3% to 20%; grades 3/4: ≤11%; including cardiac, cerebrovascular, and peripheral-vascular ischemia), cardiac failure (6% to 15%; including congestive heart failure, reduced ejection fraction, pulmonary edema, cardiogenic shock, cardiorespiratory arrest, right ventricular failure), myocardial infarction (12%)

Central nervous system: Fatigue or weakness (31% to 39%), headache (25% to 39%), pain (6% to 16%), chills (7% to 13%), insomnia (7% to 12%), dizziness (3% to 11%)

Dermatologic: Skin rash (34% to 54%), xeroderma (24% to 39%), cellulitis (≤11%)

Endocrine & metabolic: Increased serum glucose (58%), decreased serum phosphate (57%), decreased serum calcium (52%), decreased serum sodium (29%), decreased serum glucose (24%), decreased serum potassium (16%), increased serum potassium (15%), decreased serum bicarbonate (11%)

Gastrointestinal: Abdominal pain (34% to 49%), constipation (24% to 47%), increased serum lipase (41%; grades 3/4: 15%), nausea (22% to 32%), decreased appetite (8% to 31%), diarrhea (13% to 26%), vomiting (13% to 24%), stomatitis (9% to 23%), weight loss (5% to 13%), gastrointestinal hemorrhage (2% to 11%; grades 3/4: ≤6%)

Genitourinary: Urinary tract infection (≤12%)

Hematologic & oncologic: Neutropenia (grades 3/4: 24% to 63%), leukopenia (grades 3/4: 14% to 63%), thrombocytopenia (grades 3/4: 36% to 57%), anemia (grades 3/4: 9% to 55%), bone marrow depression (severe grade 3 or 4: 48%), lymphocytopenia (grades 3/4: 10% to 37%), febrile neutropenia (1% to 25%), hemorrhage (24%; including cerebral hemorrhage and gastrointestinal hemorrhage)

Hepatic: Increased serum ALT (53%; grades 3/4: 8%), increased serum AST (41%; grades 3/4: 4%), increased serum alkaline phosphatase (37%), decreased serum albumin (28%), increased serum bilirubin (19%)

Infection: Sepsis (1% to 22%)

Miscellaneous: Fever (23% to 32%)

Neuromuscular & skeletal: Arthralgia (13% to 31%), myalgia (6% to 22%), limb pain (9% to 17%), back pain (11% to 16%), peripheral neuropathy (6% to 16%; including burning sensation), muscle spasm (5% to 13%), osteoalgia (9% to 12%)

Respiratory: Dyspnea (6% to 21%), pleural effusion (3% to 19%; grades 3/4: ≤3%), cough (6% to 18%), pneumonia (3% to 13%), nasopharyngitis (3% to 12%), upper respiratory tract infection (≤11%)

1% to 10%:

Cardiovascular: Peripheral ischemia (8%), supraventricular tachycardia (5%), venous thromboembolism (5%); atrial fibrillation (4%), pericardial effusion (1% to 3%), cerebral hemorrhage (2%), bradycardia (1%; symptomatic)

Endocrine & metabolic: Increased serum sodium (10%), hyperuricemia (7%), increased serum calcium (5%), increased serum triglycerides (3%)

Gastrointestinal: Pancreatitis (6%; grade 3: 5%), increased serum amylase (3%)

Ophthalmic: Blurred vision (6%), retinal toxicity (3%, including macular edema, retinal vein occlusion, retinal hemorrhage)

Renal: Increased serum creatinine (7%)

Frequency not defined:

Cardiovascular: Cerebrovascular accident

Gastrointestinal: Mouth pain, oral mucosa ulcer, oropharyngeal pain, throat ulcer, tongue ulcer

Ophthalmic: Cataract, conjunctival irritation, corneal ulcer, dry eye syndrome, eye pain, glaucoma, iridocyclitis, iritis, keratitis

<1%, postmarketing, and/or case reports: Acute hepatic failure, ascites, atrial flutter, atrial tachycardia, cerebral edema, complete atrioventricular block, gastrointestinal fistula, gastrointestinal perforation, mesenteric artery occlusion, pulmonary embolism, retinal vein thrombosis, sick sinus syndrome, tumor lysis syndrome (serious)

Drug Interactions

Metabolism/Transport Effects **Substrate** of BCRP, CYP2C8 (minor), CYP2D6 (minor), CYP3A4 (minor), P-glycoprotein; **Note:** Assignment of Major/Minor substrate status based on clinically relevant drug interaction potential; **Inhibits** BCRP, BSEP, P-glycoprotein

Avoid Concomitant Use

Avoid concomitant use of PONATinib with any of the following: BCG (Intravesical); CloZAPine; CYP3A4 Inducers (Strong); Dipyrone; St Johns Wort

Increased Effect/Toxicity

PONATinib may increase the levels/effects of: CloZAPine

The levels/effects of PONATinib may be increased by: CYP3A4 Inhibitors (Strong); Dipyrone; Grapefruit Juice

Decreased Effect

PONATinib may decrease the levels/effects of: BCG (Intravesical)

The levels/effects of PONATinib may be decreased by: CYP3A4 Inducers (Strong); St Johns Wort

Storage/Stability Store at 20°C to 25°C (68°F to 77°F); excursions permitted between 15°C to 30°C (59°F to 86°F).

Mechanism of Action Ponatinib is a pan-BCR-ABL tyrosine kinase inhibitor with *in vitro* activity against cells expressing native or mutant BCR-ABL (including T315I); it also inhibits VEGFR, FGFR, PDGFR, EPH, and SRC kinases, as well as KIT, RET, TIE2, and FLT3.

Pharmacodynamics/Kinetics

Absorption: Plasma concentrations not affected by food

Distribution: V_d: 1223 L

Protein binding: >99% to plasma proteins

Metabolism: Primarily hepatic through CYP3A4; CYP2C8, CYP2D6, and CYP3A5 are also involved in metabolism. Phase II metabolism occurs via esterases and/or amidases.

Half-life elimination: ~24 hours (range: 12 to 66 hours)

Time to peak: ≤6 hours

Excretion: Feces (~87%); urine (~5%)

Dosing

Adult & Geriatric Note: The optimal ponatinib dose has not been identified. Consider discontinuing therapy if no response has occurred by 3 months of therapy.

Acute lymphoblastic leukemia (ALL), Philadelphia chromosome-positive (Ph+), in patients for whom no other tyrosine kinase inhibitor therapy is indicated or who are T315I-positive: Oral: Initial: 45 mg once daily

◀ **Chronic myeloid leukemia (CML; chronic, accelerated, or blast phase), in patients for whom no other tyrosine kinase inhibitor therapy is indicated or who are T315I-positive:** Oral: Initial: 45 mg once daily; consider reducing the dose for patients in chronic or accelerated phase who have achieved a major cytogenetic response

Dosage adjustment for strong CYP3A inhibitors: Reduce ponatinib dose to 30 mg once daily when administered with concomitant strong CYP3A inhibitors (eg, boceprevir, clarithromycin, conivaptan, grapefruit juice, indinavir, itraconazole, ketoconazole, lopinavir/ritonavir, nefazodone, nelfinavir, posaconazole, ritonavir, saquinavir, telaprevir, telithromycin, voriconazole).

Renal Impairment There are no dosage adjustments provided in the manufacturer's labeling (has not been studied); although renal excretion is not a major excretion route for ponatinib.

Hepatic Impairment

Hepatic impairment prior to treatment initiation: Mild-to-severe impairment (Child-Pugh class A, B, or C): Initial: 30 mg once daily; monitor closely for toxicity.

Hepatotoxicity during treatment:

AST or ALT >3 times ULN (≥ grade 2): If toxicity occurs at a dose of 45 mg daily, interrupt therapy; upon recovery to ≤ grade 1 (<3 times ULN), resume therapy at 30 mg daily. If toxicity occurs at a dose of 30 mg daily, interrupt therapy; upon recovery to ≤ grade 1, resume therapy at 15 mg daily. If toxicity occurs at a dose of 15 mg daily, discontinue therapy.

ALT or AST ≥3 times ULN with bilirubin >2 times ULN and alkaline phosphatase <2 times ULN: Discontinue therapy.

Adjustment for Toxicity

Hematologic: ANC <1000/mm³ or platelets <50,000/mm³:

First occurrence: Interrupt therapy; upon recovery of ANC to ≥1500/mm³ and platelets to ≥75,000/mm³, resume therapy at 45 mg daily.

Second occurrence: Interrupt therapy; upon recovery of ANC to ≥1500/mm³ and platelets to ≥75,000/mm³, resume therapy at a reduced dose of 30 mg daily.

Third occurrence: Interrupt therapy; upon recovery of ANC to ≥1500/mm³ and platelets to ≥75,000/mm³, resume therapy at a reduced dose of 15 mg daily.

Nonhematologic toxicity:

Arterial or venous occlusive reactions: Interrupt therapy; do not resume ponatinib in the event of serious occlusive events unless the potential benefit of therapy outweighs the risk of recurrent occlusions and other treatment options are not available.

Pancreatitis and lipase elevations:

Asymptomatic grade 1 or 2 serum lipase elevation: Consider interrupting therapy or dose reduction.

Asymptomatic grade 3 or 4 serum lipase elevation (>2 times ULN) or asymptomatic radiologic pancreatitis (grade 2): If toxicity occurs at a dose of 45 mg daily, interrupt therapy; upon recovery to ≤ grade 1 (<1.5 times ULN), resume therapy at a reduced dose of 30 mg daily. If toxicity occurs at a dose of 30 mg daily, interrupt therapy; upon recovery to ≤ grade 1, resume therapy at a reduced dose of 15 mg daily. If toxicity occurs at a dose of 15 mg daily, discontinue therapy.

Symptomatic grade 3 pancreatitis: If toxicity occurs at a dose of 45 mg daily, interrupt therapy; upon recovery of serum lipase elevation to ≤ grade 1 and complete symptom resolution, resume therapy at a reduced dose of 30 mg daily. If toxicity occurs at a dose of 30 mg daily, interrupt therapy; upon recovery of serum lipase elevation to ≤ grade 1 and complete symptom resolution, resume therapy at a reduced dose of 15 mg daily. If toxicity occurs at a dose of 15 mg daily, discontinue therapy.

Grade 4 pancreatitis: Discontinue therapy.

Other nonhematologic toxicities: For serious reactions (other than arterial or venous occlusion), do not restart therapy until symptom resolution or unless the benefit of therapy outweighs the risk of recurrent toxicity.

Combination Regimens
Leukemia, Acute Promyelocytic: Ponatinib (ALL Regimen) on page 2068
Leukemia, chronic myelogenous: Ponatinib (CML Regimen) on page 2069

Administration Administer with or without food. Swallow tablets whole (do not crush or dissolve). Hazardous agent; use appropriate precautions for handling and disposal (meets NIOSH 2014 criteria).

Emetic Potential Minimal (<10%)

Monitoring Parameters CBC with differential and platelets every 2 weeks for the first 3 months, then monthly or as clinically needed; liver function tests at baseline and at least monthly thereafter or more frequently if clinically warranted; serum lipase every 2 weeks for the first 2 months and monthly thereafter (more frequently in patients with a history of pancreatitis or alcohol abuse); serum electrolytes and uric acid; monitor cardiac function, blood pressure, signs/symptoms of arterial/venous occlusion or thromboembolism, hemorrhage, fluid retention, pancreatitis (clinical signs), gastrointestinal perforation/fistula, hepatotoxicity (jaundice, anorexia, bleeding, bruising); comprehensive ocular exam at baseline and periodically; signs/symptoms of neuropathy

Dietary Considerations May be taken without regard to food. Avoid grapefruit juice.

Prescribing and Access Restrictions Patient access and support is available through the ARIAD PASS program. Information regarding program enrollment may be found at http://www.ariadpass.com or by calling 1-855-447-PASS (7277).

Medication Guide Available Yes

Dosage Forms Excipient information presented when available (limited, particularly for generics); consult specific product labeling.
Tablet, Oral:
Iclusig: 15 mg, 45 mg

♦ **Ponatinib Hydrochloride** see PONATinib on page 1403

Porfimer (POR fi mer)
Related Information
Safe Handling of Hazardous Drugs on page 2292
Brand Names: US Photofrin
Brand Names: Canada Photofrin
Index Terms CL-184116; Dihematoporphyrin Ether; Porfimer Sodium
Pharmacologic Category Antineoplastic Agent, Miscellaneous

◀ **Use**

Barrett esophagus: Ablation of high-grade dysplasia in Barrett esophagus (in patients who do not undergo esophagectomy)

Endobronchial cancer: Treatment of microinvasive endobronchial non-small cell lung cancer (NSCLC) in patients for whom surgery and radiation therapy are not indicated; reduction of obstruction and symptom palliation in patients with obstructing (partial or complete) endobronchial NSCLC

Esophageal cancer: Palliation of obstructing (partial or complete) esophageal cancer (in patients who cannot be treated satisfactorily with laser therapy)

Canadian labeling: Additional use (not in US labeling: Second-line treatment of recurrent, superficial papillary bladder cancer

Labeled Contraindications Porphyria

Photodynamic therapy (PDT) is contraindicated in patients with current tracheoesophageal or bronchoesophageal fistula; tumors eroding into a major blood vessel; emergency treatment of severe acute respiratory distress when caused by endobronchial lesion; esophageal or gastric varices; esophageal ulcers >1 cm in diameter

Canadian labeling: Additional contraindications (not in US labeling: Hypersensitivity to porphyrins; photodynamic therapy is contraindicated in patients with papillary bladder cancer who have received prior total bladder radiation or whose functional bladder capacity is <200 mL and in patients with coexisting bladder tumors of stage greater than stage 1 (T1) who have invasive cancer

Pregnancy Considerations Adverse events were observed in animal reproduction studies. Effective contraception is recommended for women of childbearing potential.

Breast-Feeding Considerations It is not known if porfimer is excreted in breast milk. Due to the potential for serious adverse reactions in the nursing infant, a decision should be made to discontinue breast-feeding or not administer porfimer photodynamic therapy, taking into account the importance of treatment to the mother.

Warnings/Precautions Hazardous agent - use appropriate precautions for handling and disposal (meets NIOSH 2014 criteria). Treatment-induced inflammation may obstruct airway; use with caution in patients with endobronchial tumors, especially if in areas where main airway may be obstructed (long or surrounding tumors); necrotic debris or mucositis may also cause airway obstruction; monitor closely between laser therapy and debridement for respiratory distress; may require urgent bronchoscopy to remove secretions or debris. Not suited for treatment of patients with esophageal or gastric varices due to the high risk for hemorrhage; patients with esophageal varices or tumors eroding into pulmonary blood vessels are at increased risk for hemorrhage, including fatal massive pulmonary hemoptysis (FMH); other risk factors for FMH include large, centrally-located tumors, cavitating tumors, or extensive tumor extrinsic to the bronchus. In patients with Barrett esophagus, conduct rigorous surveillance (endoscopic biopsy every 3 months until 4 consecutive negative results for high-grade dysplasia followed by further follow-up per physician judgment); the long-term effects of photodynamic therapy in patients with Barrett esophagus is not known. Esophageal strictures may occur, usually within 6 months of treatment; esophageal dilation may be required; the risk for strictures is increased with nodule pretreatment or with retreatment of the same area. Serious and potentially fatal gastrointestinal and esophageal necrosis and perforation may occur following treatment; due to the high risk for fistula, do not use in patients with esophageal tumors eroding into the trachea or bronchial tree/wall; use is contraindicated in patients with existing tracheoesophageal or bronchoesophageal fistula.

Photosensitivity reactions are common in patients are exposed to direct sunlight or bright indoor light (eg, fluorescent lights, unshaded light bulbs, examination/operating lights). Photosensitivity may last 30 to 90 days or more. Encourage ambient indoor light exposure (aids in gradually inactivating residual porfimer); re-exposure to general sunlight should be gradual (expose small area of skin [not the face] for 10 minutes, if no photosensitivity (eg, edema, erythema, blistering) occurs after 24 hours, may gradually resume normal outdoor activities; if photosensitivity occurs then wait 2 weeks and retest). Ocular discomfort has been reported with sun or bright light exposure; for at least 30 days (and until ocular sensitivity resolves), when outdoors, patients should wear dark sunglasses which have an average white light transmittance of <4%. Patients should be educated to test for residual photosensitivity before resuming exposure to direct sunlight. Conventional sunscreens are **not** protective against photosensitivity reactions caused by visible light. Allow 2 to 4 weeks to elapse after phototherapy prior to initiating radiation therapy; 4 weeks should elapse after radiation therapy prior to initiating phototherapy. Concurrent use with other photosensitizing agents may increase the risk for photosensitivity reactions. Avoid extravasation; if occurs, protect affected area from light.

Thromboembolic events may occur, generally in patients with additional risk factors for thromboembolism (eg, advanced cancer, prolonged immobilization, cardiovascular disease, or following major surgery). Inflammatory responses within the treatment area may result in substernal chest pain. Avoid extravasation; if occurs, protect affected area from light; use of antidotes is of unknown benefit. Elimination may be prolonged in hepatic and renal impairment; toxicities may be increased; photosensitivity may be increased beyond 90 days in patients mild-to-severe hepatic impairment and in patients with severe renal impairment.

Adverse Reactions
>10%:
  Cardiovascular: Chest pain (5% to 31%), edema (3% to 18%)
  Central nervous system: Fever (8% to 31%), pain (1% to 22%), insomnia (5% to 14%)
  Dermatologic: Photosensitivity reaction (19% to 69%)
  Gastrointestinal: Esophageal stricture/stenosis (6% to 38%), nausea (24% to 37%), vomiting (17% to 31%), constipation (5% to 24%), dysphagia (10% to 24%), mucositis (≤20%), abdominal pain (5% to 20%)
  Hematologic: Anemia (32% in esophageal cancer patients)
  Neuromuscular & skeletal: Back pain (3% to 11%)
  Respiratory: Pleural effusion (5% to 32%), dyspnea (7% to 30%), bronchial obstruction/mucus plug (21%), pneumonia (6% to 18%), hemoptysis (7% to 16%), cough (5% to 15%), bronchostenosis (11%), pharyngitis (11%)
5% to 10%:
  Cardiovascular: Atrial fibrillation, cardiac failure (esophageal cancer), hyper-/hypotension, tachycardia
  Central nervous system: Anxiety, confusion, dysphonia
  Endocrine & metabolic: Dehydration

◀

Gastrointestinal: Anorexia, diarrhea, dyspepsia, eructation, esophageal edema, esophageal pain, esophagitis, hematemesis, melena, odynophagia, weight loss

Genitourinary: Urinary tract infection

Neuromuscular & skeletal: Weakness

Respiratory: Bronchial ulceration, bronchitis, fatal massive hemoptysis, respiratory insufficiency, tracheoesophageal fistula

Miscellaneous: Hiccups, moniliasis, tumor hemorrhage, surgical complication

Common adverse reactions observed in papillary bladder cancer (Canadian labeling; not an approved use in the U.S.):

Cardiovascular: Peripheral edema

Central nervous system: Anxiety, insomnia, pain

Gastrointestinal: Constipation, nausea

Genitourinary: Bladder contracture (irreversible), dysuria, genital edema, micturition frequency, nocturia, suprapubic pain, urinary incontinence, urinary tract infection, urinary urgency

Renal: Hematuria

<5%, postmarketing, and/or case reports (limited to important or life-threatening): Abnormal vision, airway obstruction, angina, bradycardia, bronchospasm, cardiac failure, cataracts, cerebrovascular accident, diplopia, dizziness, erythema, esophageal perforation, eye pain, fluid imbalance, gastric ulcer, gastroesophageal fistula/perforation, hair growth increased, hemorrhage, ileus, infusion reactions, jaundice, laryngotracheal edema, lung abscess, MI, ocular sensitivity, peritonitis, photophobia, pneumonitis, pruritus, pseudoporphyria state, pulmonary edema, pulmonary embolism, pulmonary hemorrhage, pulmonary thrombosis, respiratory distress/failure, sepsis, sick sinus syndrome, skin blistering, skin discoloration, skin fragility, skin nodules, skin wrinkles, stridor, supraventricular tachycardia, thromboembolic events, urticaria

Drug Interactions

Metabolism/Transport Effects None known.

Avoid Concomitant Use There are no known interactions where it is recommended to avoid concomitant use.

Increased Effect/Toxicity

The levels/effects of Porfimer may be increased by: Photosensitizing Agents

Decreased Effect There are no known significant interactions involving a decrease in effect.

Storage/Stability Store intact vials at 20°C to 25°C (68°F to 77°F). Reconstituted solutions should be protected from light and used immediately after preparation.

Preparation for Administration Hazardous agent; use appropriate precautions for handling and disposal (meets NIOSH 2014 criteria).

U.S. labeling: Reconstitute each 75 mg vial with 31.8 mL of either D₅W or NS injection resulting in a final concentration of 2.5 mg/mL.

Canadian labeling: Reconstitute each 75 mg vial with 31.8 mL of D₅W (only) resulting in a final concentration of 2.5 mg/mL. Reconstitute each 15 mg vial with 6.6 mL of D₅W only resulting in a final concentration of 2.5 mg/mL.

Shake well until dissolved. Protect the reconstituted product from bright light and use immediately. Use appropriate precautions for handling and disposal.

Mechanism of Action Porfimer's cytotoxic activity is dependent on light and oxygen. Following administration, the drug is selectively retained in neoplastic tissues. Exposure of the drug to laser light at wavelengths >630 nm results in the production of oxygen free-radicals. Release of thromboxane A_2, leading to vascular occlusion and ischemic necrosis, may also occur.

Pharmacodynamics/Kinetics

Distribution: V_{dss}: 0.49 L/kg

Protein binding, plasma: ~90%

Half-life elimination: First dose: 17 days; Second dose: 30 days

Dosing

Adult & Geriatric

Photodynamic therapy in esophageal cancer or endobronchial non-small cell lung cancer: IV: 2 mg/kg, followed by endoscopic exposure to the appropriate laser light and debridement; repeat courses must be separated by at least 30 days (delay subsequent treatment for insufficient healing) for a maximum of 3 courses

Photodynamic therapy in Barrett esophagus dysplasia: IV: 2 mg/kg, followed by endoscopic exposure to the appropriate laser light; repeat courses must be separated by at least 90 days (delay subsequent treatment for insufficient healing) for a maximum of 3 courses

Photodynamic therapy in papillary bladder cancer (Canadian labeling; not in U.S. labeling): IV: 2 mg/kg, followed by cystoscopic exposure to the appropriate laser light. **Note:** Repeat dosing is not recommended due to increased risk of bladder contracture.

Renal Impairment There are no dosage adjustments provided in the manufacturer's labeling (has not been studied).

Hepatic Impairment There are no dosage adjustments provided in the manufacturer's labeling (has not been studied).

Administration Administer slow IV injection over 3 to 5 minutes. Avoid contact with skin during administration. Avoid extravasation (if extravasation occurs, protect area from light and sunlight). Hazardous agent; use appropriate precautions for handling and disposal (meets NIOSH 2014 criteria).

Monitoring Parameters Monitor injection site during infusion (for extravasation); monitor in between laser and for evidence of respiratory distress in patients with endobronchial tumors; monitor for signs/symptoms of photosensitivity, hemorrhage, thromboembolic events, gastroesophageal fistulas/perforation, esophageal strictures.

Dosage Forms Excipient information presented when available (limited, particularly for generics); consult specific product labeling.

Solution Reconstituted, Intravenous, as sodium [preservative free]:

Photofrin: 75 mg (1 ea)

Dosage Forms: Canada Excipient information presented when available (limited, particularly for generics); consult specific product labeling.

Injection, powder for reconstitution, as sodium:

Photofrin®: 15 mg

◆ **Porfimer Sodium** see Porfimer on page 1409

◆ **Portrazza** see Necitumumab on page 1191

Posaconazole (poe sa KON a zole)

Brand Names: US Noxafil

Brand Names: Canada Posanol

Index Terms SCH 56592

◄ **Pharmacologic Category** Antifungal Agent, Oral
Use

Prophylaxis of invasive *Aspergillus* and *Candida* infections: Suspension and delayed-release tablets (13 years and older) and injection (18 years and older): Prophylaxis of invasive *Aspergillus* and *Candida* infections in patients who are at high risk of developing these infections due to being severely immunocompromised (eg, hematopoietic stem cell transplant [HSCT] recipients with graft-versus-host disease [GVHD] or those with prolonged neutropenia secondary to chemotherapy for hematologic malignancies).

Oropharyngeal candidiasis: Suspension (13 years and older): Treatment of oropharyngeal candidiasis (including patients refractory to itraconazole and/or fluconazole)

Canadian labeling: Additional use (not in US labeling): **Invasive *Aspergillus* and *Candida* infections:** Suspension and delayed-release tablets (13 years and older) and injection (18 years and older): Treatment of invasive aspergillosis in patients refractory to or intolerant of itraconazole or amphotericin B

Pregnancy Risk Factor C
Dosing

Adult & Geriatric Note: The delayed-release tablet and oral suspension are not to be used interchangeably due to dosing differences for each formulation.

Aspergillosis, invasive:
Prophylaxis:
Oral:
Suspension: 200 mg 3 times daily; duration of therapy is based on recovery from neutropenia or immunosuppression. In patients with acute myelogenous leukemia (AML) or myelodysplastic syndromes (MDS), posaconazole was initiated at the time of chemotherapy initiation (or if receiving anthracyclines, 24 hours after the last anthracycline dose) and was continued until recovery from neutropenia, until complete remission, or for up to 12 weeks, whichever occurred first (Cornely 2007). The Canadian labeling recommends initiating posaconazole in patients with AML or MDS several days before the anticipated onset of neutropenia and continuing for 7 days after the neutrophil count rises above 500/mm^3. In patients with graft-versus-host disease (GVHD) receiving immunosuppressive therapy, posaconazole was continued for 112 days (Ullmann 2007), although the optimal duration in GVHD has not been fully defined (Tomblyn 2009).
Tablets (delayed release): Initial: 300 mg twice daily on day 1; Maintenance dose: 300 mg once daily on day 2 and thereafter. Duration is based on recovery from neutropenia or immunosuppression. The Canadian labeling recommends initiating posaconazole in patients with AML or MDS several days before the anticipated onset of neutropenia and continuing for 7 days after the neutrophil count rises above 500/mm^3.
Missed doses: Take as soon as remembered. If it is <12 hours until the next dose, skip the missed does and return to the regular schedule. Do not double doses.
IV: Loading dose: 300 mg twice a day on day 1; maintenance dose: 300 mg once daily on day 2 and thereafter. Duration is based on recovery from neutropenia or immunosuppression. The Canadian labeling recommends initiating posaconazole in patients with AML or MDS

several days before the anticipated onset of neutropenia and continuing for 7 days after the neutrophil count rises above 500/mm³.

Treatment (refractory to or intolerant of conventional therapy):

US off-label use: Oral: Suspension: 200 mg 4 times daily initially; after disease stabilization, may decrease frequency to 400 mg twice daily (Walsh 2007). **Note:** Duration of therapy should be a minimum of 6 to 12 weeks or throughout period of immunosuppression and until lesions have resolved (Walsh 2008). Duration of therapy in HIV-infected patients should be until infection resolution and CD4 count >200 cells/mm³ (HHS [OI adult 2015])

Canadian labeling:

Oral:

Suspension: 400 mg twice daily; in patients unable to tolerate food or nutritional supplement, administer 200 mg 4 times daily; duration of therapy is based on severity of underlying disease, recovery from immunosuppression, and clinical response.

Tablets (delayed release): Initial: 300 mg twice daily on day 1; Maintenance dose: 300 mg once daily; duration of therapy is based on disease severity, recovery from immunosuppression, and clinical response.

IV: Loading dose: 300 mg twice daily on day 1; Maintenance dose: 300 mg once daily on day 2 and thereafter. Duration of therapy is based on disease severity, recovery from immunosuppression, and clinical response.

Candidal infections:

US labeling:

Prophylaxis:

Oral:

Suspension: 200 mg 3 times daily; duration of therapy is based on recovery from neutropenia or immunosuppression

Tablets (delayed release): Oral: Initial: 300 mg twice daily on day 1; Maintenance dose: 300 mg once daily on day 2 and thereafter; duration of therapy is based on recovery from neutropenia or immunosuppression

Missed doses: Take as soon as remembered. If it is <12 hours until the next dose, skip the missed does and return to the regular schedule. Do not double doses.

IV: Initial: 300 mg twice daily on day 1; Maintenance dose: 300 mg once daily on day 2 and thereafter; duration of therapy is based on recovery from neutropenia or immunosuppression.

Treatment: Oral: Suspension:

Oropharyngeal infection: Initial: 100 mg twice daily on day 1; Maintenance: 100 mg once daily on day 2 and thereafter for 13 days

Refractory oropharyngeal infection:

Manufacturer's labeling: 400 mg twice daily; duration of therapy is based on underlying disease and clinical response

Alternate dosing: HIV-infected patients (alternative to fluconazole or azole refractory): 400 mg twice daily on day 1, then 400 mg once daily for 7 to 14 days for initial episodes (continue for 28 days in azole refractory patients) (HHS [OI adult 2015])

Esophageal infection in HIV-infected patients (azole refractory) (off-label use): 400 mg twice daily for 28 days. **Note:** If patient has frequent or severe recurrences, may continue for suppressive therapy; consider discontinuing when CD4 >200/mm³ (HHS [OI adult 2015])

Canadian labeling:

Prophylaxis: **Note:** Initiate posaconazole in patients with AML or MDS several days before the anticipated onset of neutropenia and continue therapy for 7 days after the neutrophil count rises above 500/mm^3.
Oral:

Suspension: 200 mg 3 times daily; duration of therapy is based on recovery from neutropenia or immunosuppression.

Tablets (delayed release): Initial: 300 mg twice daily on day 1; Maintenance dose: 300 mg once daily on day 2 and thereafter; duration of therapy is based on recovery from neutropenia or immunosuppression.

Injection: IV: Initial: 300 mg twice daily on day 1; Maintenance dose: 300 mg once daily on day 2 and thereafter; duration of therapy is based on recovery from neutropenia or immunosuppression.

Treatment: Oral: Suspension: Oropharyngeal infection: Initial: 100 mg twice daily for 1 day; Maintenance: 100 mg once daily for 13 days

Coccidioidomycosis in HIV-infected patients (alternative to preferred therapy) (off-label use; HHS [OI adult 2015]): Oral:

Mild infections (eg, focal pneumonia): 200 to 400 mg twice daily; patients who complete initial therapy should be considered for lifelong suppressive therapy.

Chronic suppressive therapy: 200 mg twice daily

Mucormycosis (off-label use): Suspension: Oral: 800 mg daily in 2 or 4 divided doses; duration of therapy is based on response and risk of relapse due to immunosuppression (Greenberg 2006)

Cryptococcal infections:

Pulmonary, nonimmunosuppressed (off-label use): 400 mg twice daily. **Note:** Fluconazole is considered first-line treatment (Perfect 2010).

Salvage treatment of relapsed infection (off-label use): 400 mg twice daily (or 200 mg 4 times daily) for 10 to 12 weeks. **Note:** Salvage treatment should only be started after an appropriate course of an induction regimen (Perfect 2010).

Pediatric Note: The delayed-release tablet and oral suspension are not to be used interchangeably due to dosing differences for each formulation.

Aspergillosis, invasive (prophylaxis): Oral: Adolescents ≥13 years: Refer to adult dosing.

Candidal infections: Oral: Adolescents ≥13 years: Refer to adult dosing.

Coccidioidomycosis in HIV-infected patients (alternative to preferred therapy) (off-label use): Adolescents: Oral: Refer to adult dosing.

Primary antifungal prophylaxis in allogeneic HSCT with grades 2 to 4 acute graft-versus-host-disease (GVHD) or chronic extensive GVHD (guideline recommendation): Adolescents ≥13 years: Oral: Suspension: 200 mg 3 times daily beginning with GVHD diagnosis, continue until GVHD resolves (Science 2014)

Primary antifungal prophylaxis in AML or MDS in centers with a high local incidence of mold infections (alternative to fluconazole; guideline recommendation): Adolescents ≥13 years: Oral: Suspension: 200 mg 3 times daily during chemotherapy-associated neutropenia (Science 2014)

Renal Impairment

Delayed-release tablets and oral suspension:

eGFR 20 to 80 mL/minute/1.73 m^2: No dosage adjustment necessary.

eGFR <20 mL/minute/1.73 m^2: No dosage adjustment necessary; however, monitor for breakthrough fungal infections due to variability in posaconazole exposure.

Intravenous infusion:

eGFR ≥50 mL/minute/1.73 m^2: No dosage adjustment recommended

eGFR <50 mL/minute/1.73 m^2: Avoid use unless risk/benefit has been assessed; the intravenous vehicle (cyclodextrin) may accumulate. Monitor serum creatinine levels; if increases occur, consider oral therapy.

Hepatic Impairment

US labeling: Mild-to-severe insufficiency (Child-Pugh class A, B, or C): No dosage adjustment necessary. **Note:** if patient shows clinical signs and symptoms of liver disease due to posaconazole, consider discontinuing therapy. Hepatic impairment studies were only conducted with oral suspension; however, recommendations also apply to patients receiving injection or delayed-release tablets.

Canadian labeling: There are no dosage adjustments provided in the manufacturer's labeling; use with caution in severe impairment.

Additional Information Complete prescribing information should be consulted for additional detail.

Dosage Forms Excipient information presented when available (limited, particularly for generics); consult specific product labeling.

Solution, Intravenous:

Noxafil: 300 mg/16.7 mL (16.7 mL) [contains edetate disodium]

Suspension, Oral:

Noxafil: 40 mg/mL (105 mL) [contains polysorbate 80, sodium benzoate; cherry flavor]

Tablet Delayed Release, Oral:

Noxafil: 100 mg

◆ **Posanol (Can)** *see* Posaconazole *on page 1413*

◆ **PR-171** *see* Carfilzomib *on page 278*

PRALAtrexate (pral a TREX ate)

Related Information

Management of Chemotherapy-Induced Nausea and Vomiting in Adults *on page 2142*

Safe Handling of Hazardous Drugs *on page 2292*

Brand Names: US Folotyn

Index Terms PDX

Pharmacologic Category Antineoplastic Agent, Antimetabolite; Antineoplastic Agent, Antimetabolite (Antifolate)

Use Peripheral T-cell lymphoma: Treatment of relapsed or refractory peripheral T-cell lymphoma (PTCL)

Labeled Contraindications There are no contraindications listed in the manufacturer's labeling.

Pregnancy Considerations Adverse effects were observed in animal reproduction studies. May cause fetal harm if administered to a pregnant woman.

Breast-Feeding Considerations It is not known if pralatrexate is excreted in breast milk. Due to the potential for serious adverse reactions in the nursing infant, a decision should be made to discontinue breast-feeding or to discontinue pralatrexate, taking into account the benefits of treatment to the mother.

Warnings/Precautions Hazardous agent - use appropriate precautions for handling and disposal (NIOSH 2014 [group 1]). May cause bone marrow suppression (thrombocytopenia, neutropenia and anemia); may require dosage modification; monitor blood counts. Mucositis, including stomatitis or mucosal inflammation of gastrointestinal and genitourinary tracts, may occur; monitor weekly; may require dosage modification. Prophylactic folic acid and vitamin B_{12} supplements are necessary to reduce hematologic toxicity and treatment-related mucositis. Severe and potentially fatal dermatologic reactions, including skin exfoliation, ulceration, and toxic epidermal necrolysis (TEN) have been reported. Skin reaction may be progressive; severity may increase with continued treatment; may also involve skin and subcutaneous tissues which are affected by lymphoma; monitor all dermatologic reactions closely; withhold or discontinue treatment for severe dermatologic reaction.

Pralatrexate may cause tumor lysis syndrome (TLS); monitor closely, if TLS develops, treat for associated complications. Use with caution in patients with moderate-to-severe renal impairment (has not been studied in patients with renal impairment); monitor renal function and for systemic toxicity due to increased exposure. Concurrent use with drugs with substantial renal clearance (eg, NSAIDs, sulfamethoxazole/trimethoprim) may result in delayed pralatrexate clearance. Liver function test abnormalities have been observed with use; monitor liver function; persistent abnormalities may indicate hepatotoxicity and may require dosage modification or discontinuation.

Patients with moderate-to-severe renal impairment are at risk for increased exposure and toxicity. Avoid use in patients with end-stage renal disease (ESRD), including patients undergoing dialysis (unless the potential benefit outweighs potential risks); serious adverse reactions, including toxic epidermal necrolysis and mucositis were reported in patients with ESRD undergoing dialysis. Monitor renal function and for systemic toxicity due to increased exposure. Potentially significant drug-drug interactions may exist, requiring dose or frequency adjustment, additional monitoring, and/or selection of alternative therapy.

Adverse Reactions

>10%:

Cardiovascular: Edema (30%)

Central nervous system: Fatigue (36%), fever (32%)

Dermatologic: Rash (15%; grades 3/4: 0%), pruritus (14%; grade 3: 2%; grade 4: 0%)

Endocrine & metabolic: Hypokalemia (15%)

Gastrointestinal: Mucositis (70%; grade 3: 17%; grade 4: 4%), nausea (40%), constipation (33%), vomiting (25%), diarrhea (21%), anorexia (15%), abdominal pain (12%)

Hematologic: Thrombocytopenia (41%; grade 3: 14%; grade 4: 19%), anemia (34%; grade 3: 15%; grade 4: 2%), neutropenia (24%; grade 3: 13%; grade 4: 7%), leukopenia (11%; grade 3: 3%; grade 4: 4%)

Hepatic: Transaminases increased (13%; grade 3: 5%; grade 4: 0%)

Neuromuscular & skeletal: Limb pain (12%), back pain (11%)

Respiratory: Cough (28%), epistaxis (26%), dyspnea (19%), pharyngolaryngeal pain (14%)

Miscellaneous: Night sweats (11%), infection

1% to 10%:

Cardiovascular: Tachycardia (10%)

Endocrine & metabolic: Dehydration (serious >3%)

Hematologic: Neutropenic fever (serious >3%)

Neuromuscular & skeletal: Weakness (10%)

Respiratory: Upper respiratory infection (10%)

Miscellaneous: Sepsis (serious >3%)

<1%, postmarketing, and/or case reports: Bowel obstruction, cardiopulmonary arrest, lymphopenia, odynophagia, pancytopenia, skin exfoliation, skin ulceration, toxic epidermal necrolysis (TEN), tumor lysis syndrome (TLS)

Drug Interactions

Metabolism/Transport Effects Substrate of BCRP

Avoid Concomitant Use

Avoid concomitant use of PRALAtrexate with any of the following: BCG (Intravesical); Natalizumab; Pimecrolimus; Tacrolimus (Topical); Tofacitinib; Vaccines (Live)

Increased Effect/Toxicity

PRALAtrexate may increase the levels/effects of: Fingolimod; Leflunomide; Natalizumab; Tofacitinib; Vaccines (Live)

The levels/effects of PRALAtrexate may be increased by: Denosumab; Nonsteroidal Anti-Inflammatory Agents; Pimecrolimus; Probenecid; Roflumilast; Salicylates; Sulfamethoxazole; Tacrolimus (Topical); Trastuzumab; Trimethoprim

Decreased Effect

PRALAtrexate may decrease the levels/effects of: BCG (Intravesical); Coccidioides immitis Skin Test; Sapropterin; Sipuleucel-T; Vaccines (Inactivated); Vaccines (Live)

The levels/effects of PRALAtrexate may be decreased by: Echinacea

Storage/Stability Store intact vials refrigerated at 2°C to 8°C (36°F to 46°F). Store in original carton to protect from light until use. Unopened vials (stored in the original carton) are stable for up to 72 hours at room temperature (discard after 72 hours).

Preparation for Administration Hazardous agent; use appropriate precautions for handling and disposal (NIOSH 2014 [group 1]). Withdraw into syringe for administration; do not dilute (manufacturer recommends immediate use after placing in syringe). Discard unused portion in the vial.

Mechanism of Action Antifolate analog; inhibits DNA, RNA, and protein synthesis by selectively entering cells expressing reduced folate carrier (RFC-1), is polyglutamylated by folylpolyglutamate synthetase (FPGS) and then competes for the DHFR-folate binding site to inhibit dihydrofolate reductase (DHFR)

Pharmacodynamics/Kinetics

Distribution: *S*-diastereomer: 105 L; *R*-diastereomer: 37 L

Protein binding: ~67%

Half-life elimination: 12 to 18 hours

Excretion: Urine (~34% as unchanged drug)

◄ **Dosing**

Adult & Geriatric Note: Initiate vitamin supplements before initial pralatrexate dose: Folic acid 1 to 1.25 mg/day orally beginning 10 days prior to initial pralatrexate dose; continue during treatment and for 30 days after last pralatrexate dose; vitamin B_{12} 1,000 mcg IM within 10 weeks prior to initial pralatrexate dose and every 8 to 10 weeks thereafter (after initial dose, B_{12} may be administered on the same day as pralatrexate).

Prior to administering any dose, mucositis should be ≤ grade 1 and absolute neutrophil count (ANC) should be ≥1,000/mm^3; platelets should be ≥100,000/mm^3 for the first dose and ≥50,000/mm^3 for subsequent doses

Peripheral T-cell lymphoma (PTCL), relapsed or refractory: IV: 30 mg/m^2 once weekly for 6 weeks of a 7-week treatment cycle; continue until disease progression or unacceptable toxicity (O'Connor, 2011)

Cutaneous T-cell lymphoma, relapsed or refractory (off-label use): IV: 15 mg/m^2 once weekly for 3 weeks of a 4-week treatment cycle (Horwitz, 2012)

Renal Impairment

Moderate-to-severe renal impairment: Exposure and toxicities may be increased; monitor for toxicities and adjust dose accordingly.

End-stage renal disease (ESRD), including dialysis-dependent: Avoid use (unless the potential benefit outweighs risks).

Hepatic Impairment Patients with total bilirubin >1.5 mg/dL, AST or ALT >2.5 times the upper limit of normal (ULN), or ALT or AST >5 times ULN if documented hepatic lymphoma involvement were excluded from clinical trials. Persistent abnormalities may indicate hepatotoxicity requiring dosage modification:

Grade 3 (AST or ALT >5 to 20 times ULN or bilirubin >3 to 10 times ULN): Omit dose; decrease to 20 mg/m^2 when recovers to ≤ grade 2

Grade 4 (AST or ALT >20 times ULN or bilirubin >10 times ULN): Discontinue treatment.

Obesity *ASCO Guidelines for appropriate chemotherapy dosing in obese adults with cancer:* Utilize patient's actual body weight (full weight) for calculation of body surface area- or weight-based dosing, particularly when the intent of therapy is curative; manage regimen-related toxicities in the same manner as for nonobese patients; if a dose reduction is utilized due to toxicity, consider resumption of full weight-based dosing with subsequent cycles, especially if cause of toxicity (eg, hepatic or renal impairment) is resolved (Griggs, 2012).

Adjustment for Toxicity Severe or intolerable adverse events may require dose omission, reduction or interruption. Do not make up omitted doses at the end of a cycle; do not re-escalate dose after a reduction due to toxicity.

Hematologic toxicity:

Platelets:

<50,000/mm^3 (for 1-week duration): Omit dose; continue at previous dose if platelets recover within 1 week

<50,000/mm^3 (for 2-week duration): Omit dose; decrease to 20 mg/m^2 if platelets recover within 2 weeks

<50,000/mm^3 (for 3-week duration): Discontinue treatment.

ANC:

500 to 1,000/mm^3 without fever (for 1-week duration): Omit dose; continue at previous dose if ANC recovers within 1 week

500 to 1,000/mm^3 with fever **or** ANC <500/mm^3 (for 1-week duration): Omit dose, give filgrastim or sargramostim support; continue at previous dose (with growth factor support) if ANC recovers within 1 week

500 to 1,000/mm^3 with fever **or** ANC <500/mm^3 (recurrent or for 2-week duration): Omit dose and give filgrastim or sargramostim support; decrease to 20 mg/m^2 (with growth factor support) if ANC recovers within 2 weeks

500 to 1,000/mm^3 with fever **or** ANC <500/mm^3 (second recurrence or for 3 week duration): Discontinue treatment.

Nonhematologic toxicity: Mucositis (on day of treatment):

Grade 2: Omit dose; continue at previous dose when recovers to ≤ grade 1

Grade 3 or recurrent grade 2: Omit dose and decrease to 20 mg/m^2 when recovers to ≤ grade 1

Grade 4: Discontinue treatment.

Nonhematologic toxicity (other than mucositis):

Grade 3: Omit dose; decrease to 20 mg/m^2 when recovers to ≤ grade 2

Grade 4: Discontinue treatment.

Administration Administer IV push (undiluted) over 3 to 5 minutes into the line of a free-flowing normal saline IV

Hazardous agent; use appropriate precautions for handling and disposal (NIOSH 2014 [group 1]).

Emetic Potential Low (10% to 30%)

Monitoring Parameters CBC with differential (baseline and weekly); serum chemistries, including renal and liver function tests (prior to the first and fourth doses in each cycle); mucositis severity (baseline and weekly); monitor for signs of tumor lysis syndrome and for dermatologic reactions

Dosage Forms Excipient information presented when available (limited, particularly for generics); consult specific product labeling.

Solution, Intravenous [preservative free]:

Folotyn: 20 mg/mL (1 mL); 40 mg/2 mL (2 mL)

♦ **Pred Forte** *see* PrednisoLONE (Ophthalmic) *on page 1424*

♦ **Pred Mild** *see* PrednisoLONE (Ophthalmic) *on page 1424*

PrednisoLONE (Systemic) (pred NISS oh lone)

Brand Names: US AsmalPred Plus [DSC]; AsmalPred [DSC]; Flo-Pred; Millipred; Millipred DP; Millipred DP 12-Day; Orapred ODT; Orapred [DSC]; Pediapred; Prelone; Veripred 20

Brand Names: Canada Hydeltra T.B.A.; Novo-Prednisolone; Pediapred

Index Terms Prednisolone Sodium Phosphate; Prelone

Pharmacologic Category Corticosteroid, Systemic

Use Treatment of endocrine disorders, rheumatic disorders, collagen diseases, allergic states, respiratory diseases, hematologic disorders, neoplastic diseases, edematous states, and gastrointestinal diseases; resolution of acute exacerbations of multiple sclerosis; management of fulminating or disseminated tuberculosis and trichinosis; acute or chronic solid organ rejection

Pregnancy Risk Factor C/D (manufacturer specific)

◀ **Dosing**

Adult Dose depends upon condition being treated and response of patient. Oral dosage expressed in terms of prednisolone base. Consider alternate day therapy for long-term therapy. Discontinuation of long-term therapy requires gradual withdrawal by tapering the dose. Patients undergoing unusual stress while receiving corticosteroids, should receive increased doses prior to, during, and after the stressful situation.

Usual dose (range): Oral: 5 to 60 mg daily

Asthma exacerbations:

Global Initiative for Asthma guidelines (GINA 2015): Management in primary care or acute care facility: 1 mg/kg/day (maximum: 50 mg daily) as a single daily dose usually given for 5 to 7 days

National Asthma Education and Prevention Program guidelines (NAEPP 2007):

Asthma exacerbations (emergency care or hospital doses): 40 to 80 mg/day in a single dose or in 2 divided doses until peak expiratory flow is 70% of predicted or personal best

Short-course outpatient "burst" (acute asthma): 40 to 60 mg/day in a single dose or in 2 divided doses for 5 to 10 days. **Note:** Burst should be continued until symptoms resolve and peak expiratory flow is at least 80% of personal best; usually requires 3 to 10 days of treatment; longer treatment may be required

Long-term treatment: 7.5 to 60 mg daily given as a single dose in the morning or every other day as needed for asthma control

Rheumatoid arthritis: Oral: Initial: 5 to 7.5 mg daily, adjust dose as necessary

Multiple sclerosis: Oral: 200 mg daily for 1 week followed by 80 mg every other day for 1 month

Acute exacerbations of chronic obstructive pulmonary disease (COPD) (off-label use): Oral: 30 to 40 mg daily for 10 to 14 days (GOLD guidelines 2013)

Bell's palsy (off-label use): Oral: 60 mg once daily for 5 days, then taper dose downward by 10 mg daily for 5 days (total treatment duration: 10 days) (Engstrom 2008; Berg 2012) **or** 50 mg daily (in 1 or 2 divided doses) for 10 days (begin within 72 hours of onset of symptoms) (Baugh 2013; Sullivan 2007)

Severe alcoholic hepatitis (Maddrey Discriminant Function [MDF] score ≥32) (off-label use): Oral: 40 mg daily for 28 days, followed by a 2-week taper (O'Shea 2010)

Dosing adjustment in hyperthyroidism: Prednisolone dose may need to be increased to achieve adequate therapeutic effects.

Geriatric Use lowest effective adult dose. Dose depends upon condition being treated and response of patient; alternate day dosing may be attempted in some disease states.

Pediatric Dose depends upon condition being treated and response of patient; dosage for infants and children should be based on severity of the disease and response of the patient rather than on strict adherence to dosage indicated by age, weight, or body surface area. Oral dosage expressed in terms of prednisolone base. Consider alternate day therapy for long-term therapy. Discontinuation of long-term therapy requires gradual withdrawal by tapering the dose. Patients undergoing unusual stress while receiving corticosteroids, should receive increased doses prior to, during, and after the stressful situation.

Asthma exacerbations:

Global Initiative for Asthma guidelines (GINA 2015): Management in primary care or acute care facility:

Children ≤2 years: 1 to 2 mg/kg/day (maximum: 20 mg daily) for up to 5 days

Children 3 to 5 years: 1 to 2 mg/kg/day (maximum: 30 mg daily) for up to 5 days

Children 6 to 11 years: 1 to 2 mg/kg/day (maximum: 40 mg daily) usually given for 3 to 5 days

Children ≥12 years and Adolescents: Refer to adult dosing.

National Asthma Education and Prevention Program guidelines (NAEPP 2007):

Children <12 years:

Asthma exacerbations (emergency care or hospital doses): 1 to 2 mg/kg/day in 2 divided doses (maximum: 60 mg/day) until peak expiratory flow is 70% of predicted or personal best

Short-course "burst" (acute asthma): 1 to 2 mg/kg/day in single dose or 2 divided doses for 3 to 10 days; maximum dose: 60 mg/day. **Note:** Burst should be continued until symptoms resolve or patient achieves peak expiratory flow 80% of personal best; usually requires 3 to 10 days of treatment; longer treatment may be required

Long-term treatment: 0.25 to 2 mg/kg/day given as a single dose in the morning or every other day as needed for asthma control; maximum dose: 60 mg/day

Children ≥12 years and Adolescents: Refer to adult dosing.

Anti-inflammatory or immunosuppressive dose: Oral: 0.1 to 2 mg/kg/day in divided doses 1 to 4 times daily

Nephrotic syndrome: Oral:

Initial (first 3 episodes): 2 mg/kg/day **or** 60 mg/m^2/day (maximum: 80 mg daily) in divided doses 3 to 4 times daily until urine is protein free for 3 consecutive days (maximum: 28 days); followed by 1 to 1.5 mg/kg/dose **or** 40 mg/m^2/dose given every other day for 4 weeks

Maintenance (for frequent relapses): 0.5 to 1 mg/kg/dose given every other day for 3-6 months

Bell's palsy (off-label use): Adolescents ≥16 years: Oral: 50 mg daily (in 1 or 2 divided doses) for 10 days; treatment should begin within 72 hours of onset of symptoms (Baugh 2013; Sullivan 2007)

Dosing adjustment in hyperthyroidism: Refer to adult dosing.

Renal Impairment No dosage adjustment provided in manufacturer's labeling. Use with caution.

Hemodialysis: Slightly dialyzable (5% to 20%); administer dose posthemodialysis

Peritoneal dialysis: Supplemental dose is not necessary

Hepatic Impairment No dosage adjustment provided in manufacturer's labeling.

Additional Information Complete prescribing information should be consulted for additional detail.

◀ **Dosage Forms Considerations**

Orapred oral solution contains fructose.

Orapred ODT dispersible tablets contain sucrose.

Prelone oral syrup contains sucrose.

Dosage Forms Excipient information presented when available (limited, particularly for generics); consult specific product labeling. [DSC] = Discontinued product

Solution, Oral, as base:

Generic: 15 mg/5 mL (240 mL, 480 mL)

Solution, Oral, as sodium phosphate [strength expressed as base]:

AsmalPred: 15 mg/5 mL (89 mL [DSC]) [contains alcohol, usp, sodium benzoate]

AsmalPred Plus: 15 mg/5 mL (237 mL [DSC]) [contains alcohol, usp, sodium benzoate]

Millipred: 10 mg/5 mL (237 mL) [alcohol free; dye free; contains edetate disodium, methylparaben, saccharin sodium; grape flavor]

Orapred: 15 mg/5 mL (20 mL [DSC], 237 mL [DSC]) [dye free; contains alcohol, usp, sodium benzoate; grape flavor]

Pediapred: 5 mg/5 mL (120 mL) [alcohol free, dye free, sugar free; contains edetate disodium, methylparaben; raspberry flavor]

Veripred 20: 20 mg/5 mL (237 mL) [alcohol free, dye free; contains edetate disodium, methylparaben, saccharin sodium; grape flavor]

Generic: 15 mg/5 mL (237 mL, 473 mL [DSC]); 25 mg/5 mL (237 mL); 5 mg/5 mL (120 mL)

Suspension, Oral, as acetate [strength expressed as base]:

Flo-Pred: 15 mg/5 mL (30 mL) [contains butylparaben, disodium edta, propylene glycol; cherry flavor]

Syrup, Oral, as base:

Prelone: 15 mg/5 mL (240 mL) [contains alcohol, usp, benzoic acid, brilliant blue fcf (fd&c blue #1), fd&c red #40, propylene glycol, saccharin sodium; cherry flavor]

Generic: 15 mg/5 mL (240 mL, 480 mL)

Tablet, Oral, as base:

Millipred: 5 mg [scored; contains fd&c yellow #10 (quinoline yellow), fd&c yellow #6 (sunset yellow), sodium benzoate]

Millipred DP: 5 mg [scored; contains fd&c yellow #10 (quinoline yellow), fd&c yellow #6 (sunset yellow), sodium benzoate]

Millipred DP 12-Day: 5 mg [scored; contains fd&c yellow #10 (quinoline yellow), fd&c yellow #6 (sunset yellow), sodium benzoate]

Tablet Dispersible, Oral, as sodium phosphate [strength expressed as base]:

Orapred ODT: 10 mg, 15 mg, 30 mg [grape flavor]

Generic: 10 mg, 15 mg, 30 mg

PrednisoLONE (Ophthalmic) (pred NISS oh lone)

Brand Names: US Omnipred; Pred Forte; Pred Mild

Brand Names: Canada Minims Prednisolone Sodium Phosphate; PMS-Prednisolone Sodium Phosphate Forte; Pred Forte; Pred Mild; Ratio-Prednisolone; Sandoz Prednisolone

Index Terms Econopred; Prednisolone Acetate, Ophthalmic; Prednisolone Sodium Phosphate, Ophthalmic

Pharmacologic Category Corticosteroid, Ophthalmic

Use

Corneal injury: Treatment of corneal injury from chemical or thermal burns (excluding Pred Forte) or to radiation burns or penetration of foreign bodies (excluding Pred Forte, Pred Mild).

Ophthalmic inflammatory conditions: Treatment of steroid-responsive inflammatory conditions of the palpebral and bulbar conjunctiva, cornea, and anterior segment of the globe such as acne rosacea, allergic conjunctivitis, cyclitis, herpes zoster keratitis, iritis, superficial punctate keratitis, and selected infective conjunctivitis.

Pregnancy Risk Factor C

Dosing

Adult & Geriatric

Ophthalmic inflammatory conditions/corneal injury: Ophthalmic:

Prednisolone acetate: Instill 1 to 2 drops in the affected eye(s) 2 to 4 times daily. During the initial 24 to 48 hours, the dosing frequency may be increased if necessary. If signs and symptoms fail to improve after 2 days, re-evaluate. Do not discontinue therapy prematurely; withdraw therapy with gradual tapering of dose in chronic conditions.

Prednisolone sodium phosphate: Instill 1 to 2 drops into conjunctival sac every hour during the day and every 2 hours at night until satisfactory response is obtained, then use 1 drop every 4 hours; subsequent reduction to 1 drop 3 to 4 times daily may be adequate. Do not discontinue therapy prematurely; withdraw therapy with gradual tapering of dose in chronic conditions.

Pediatric Ophthalmic inflammation, treatment: Children and Adolescents (off-label use): Ophthalmic: Prednisolone acetate 1%: Limited data available: Instill 1 to 2 drops into conjunctival sac 3 to 6 times daily. If signs and symptoms fail to improve after 2 days, re-evaluate. Initiate with more frequent dosing, and decrease as clinically indicated. If signs and symptoms fail to improve after 2 days, re-evaluate (Wilson, 2009).

Renal Impairment There are no dosage adjustments provided in the manufacturer's labeling.

Hepatic Impairment There are no dosage adjustments provided in the manufacturer's labeling.

Additional Information Complete prescribing information should be consulted for additional detail.

Dosage Forms Excipient information presented when available (limited, particularly for generics); consult specific product labeling.

Solution, Ophthalmic, as sodium phosphate:

Generic: 1% (10 mL)

Suspension, Ophthalmic, as acetate:

Omnipred: 1% (5 mL, 10 mL) [contains benzalkonium chloride, edetate disodium, polysorbate 80]

Pred Forte: 1% (1 mL, 5 mL, 10 mL, 15 mL) [contains benzalkonium chloride, edetate disodium, polysorbate 80, sodium bisulfite]

Pred Mild: 0.12% (5 mL, 10 mL)

Generic: 1% (5 mL, 10 mL, 15 mL)

◆ **Prednisolone Acetate, Ophthalmic** see PrednisoLONE (Ophthalmic) on page 1424

◆ **Prednisolone Sodium Phosphate** see PrednisoLONE (Systemic) on page 1421

♦ **Prednisolone Sodium Phosphate, Ophthalmic** *see* PrednisoLONE (Ophthalmic) *on page 1424*

PredniSONE (PRED ni sone)

Related Information

Corticosteroids Systemic Equivalencies *on page 2334*
Palliative Care Medicine (Cancer) *on page 2252*

Brand Names: US Deltasone; PredniSONE Intensol; Rayos

Brand Names: Canada Apo-Prednisone; JAA-Prednisone; Teva-Prednisone; Winpred

Index Terms Deltacortisone; Deltadehydrocortisone; Deltasone

Pharmacologic Category Corticosteroid, Systemic

Use

Allergic states: Control of severe or incapacitating allergic conditions intractable to adequate trials of conventional treatment in drug hypersensitivity reactions, seasonal or perennial allergic rhinitis; serum sickness.

Dermatologic diseases: Atopic dermatitis; bullous dermatitis herpetiformis; contact dermatitis; exfoliative dermatitis/erythroderma; mycosis fungoides; pemphigus; severe erythema multiforme (Stevens-Johnson syndrome). *Immediate-release only:* Severe psoriasis, severe seborrheic dermatitis.

Endocrine disorders: Congenital adrenal hyperplasia; hypercalcemia of malignancy; nonsuppurative thyroiditis; primary or secondary adrenocortical insufficiency (hydrocortisone or cortisone is the first choice; synthetic analogues may be used in conjunction with mineralocorticoids where applicable; in infancy, mineralocorticoid supplementation is of particular importance).

GI diseases: During acute episodes in regional enteritis (Crohn disease) and ulcerative colitis.

Hematologic disorders: Acquired (autoimmune) hemolytic anemia; congenital (erythroid) hypoplastic anemia/Diamond-Blackfan anemia; idiopathic thrombocytopenic purpura in adults; secondary thrombocytopenia in adults. *Delayed-release only:* Pure red cell aplasia. *Immediate-release only:* Erythroblastopenia (red blood cell anemia).

Neoplastic diseases:
Delayed-release only: Treatment of acute leukemia and aggressive lymphomas.
Immediate-release only: Palliative management of leukemias and lymphomas in adults; acute leukemia of childhood.

Nervous system (delayed-release only): Acute exacerbations of multiple sclerosis; cerebral edema associated with primary or metastatic brain tumor, craniotomy, or head injury.

Ophthalmic diseases:
Delayed-release only: Severe acute and chronic allergic and inflammatory processes involving the eye and its adnexa, such as sympathetic ophthalmia; uveitis and ocular inflammatory conditions unresponsive to topical steroids.
Immediate-release only: Severe acute and chronic allergic and inflammatory processes involving the eye and its adnexa, such as allergic conjunctivitis, allergic corneal marginal ulcers, anterior segment inflammation, chorioretinitis, diffuse posterior uveitis and choroiditis, herpes zoster ophthalmicus, iridocyclitis, iritis, keratitis, optic neuritis, sympathetic ophthalmia.

Renal diseases: To induce a diuresis or remission of proteinuria in the nephrotic syndrome, without uremia, of the idiopathic type or that is caused by lupus erythematosus.

Respiratory diseases: Aspiration pneumonitis; asthma; fulminating or disseminated pulmonary tuberculosis when used concurrently with appropriate chemotherapy; symptomatic sarcoidosis.

Delayed-release only: Acute exacerbations of chronic obstructive pulmonary disease (COPD); allergic bronchopulmonary aspergillosis; hypersensitivity pneumonitis; idiopathic bronchiolitis obliterans with organizing pneumonia; idiopathic eosinophilic pneumonias; idiopathic pulmonary fibrosis; *Pneumocystis carinii* pneumonia (PCP) associated with hypoxemia occurring in an HIV-positive individual who is also under treatment with appropriate anti-PCP antibiotics.

Immediate-release only: Berylliosis; Loeffler syndrome not manageable by other means.

Rheumatic disorders:

Maintenance therapy:

Delayed-release only: During an exacerbation or as maintenance therapy in selected cases of ankylosing spondylitis, dermatomyositis/polymyositis, polymyalgia rheumatica, psoriatic arthritis, relapsing polychondritis, rheumatoid arthritis including juvenile rheumatoid arthritis, Sjögren syndrome, systemic lupus erythematosus, vasculitis.

Immediate-release only: During an exacerbation or as maintenance therapy in selected cases of acute rheumatic carditis, systemic dermatomyositis (polymyositis), systemic lupus erythematosus.

Short-term therapy:

Delayed release only: As adjunctive therapy for short-term administration in acute gouty arthritis.

Immediate-release only: As adjunctive therapy for short-term administration in acute and subacute bursitis; acute gouty arthritis; acute nonspecific tenosynovitis; ankylosing spondylitis; epicondylitis; posttraumatic osteoarthritis; psoriatic arthritis; rheumatoid arthritis including juvenile rheumatoid arthritis; synovitis of osteoarthritis.

Miscellaneous: Trichinosis with neurologic or myocardial involvement; tuberculous meningitis with subarachnoid block or impending block when used concurrently with appropriate antituberculous chemotherapy.

Delayed-release only: Acute or chronic solid organ rejection.

Labeled Contraindications Hypersensitivity to prednisone or any component of the formulation; administration of live or live attenuated vaccines with immunosuppressive doses of prednisone; systemic fungal infections

Documentation of allergenic cross-reactivity for corticosteroids is limited. However, because of similarities in chemical structure and/or pharmacologic actions, the possibility of cross-sensitivity cannot be ruled out with certainty.

Pregnancy Considerations Adverse events have been observed with corticosteroids in animal reproduction studies. Prednisone and its metabolite, prednisolone, cross the human placenta. In the mother, prednisone is converted to the active metabolite prednisolone by the liver. Prior to reaching the fetus, prednisolone is converted by placental enzymes back to prednisone. As a result, the level of prednisone remaining in the maternal serum and reaching the fetus are similar; however, the amount of prednisolone reaching the fetus is ~8-10 times lower than the maternal serum concentration (healthy women at term) (Beitins, 1972). Some studies have shown an association between first trimester systemic corticosteroid use and oral clefts (Park-Wyllie 2000; Pradat 2003). Systemic corticosteroids may also influence fetal growth (decreased birth weight); however, information is conflicting (Lunghi 2010).

◀ Hypoadrenalism may occur in newborns following maternal use of cortico-steroids in pregnancy; monitor.

When systemic corticosteroids are needed in pregnancy, it is generally recommended to use the lowest effective dose for the shortest duration of time, avoiding high doses during the first trimester (Leachman 2006; Lunghi 2010; Makol 2011; Østensen 2009). Inhaled corticosteroids are preferred for the treatment of asthma during pregnancy. Oral corticosteroids, such as prednisone, may be used for the treatment of severe persistent asthma if needed; the lowest dose administered on alternate days (if possible) should be used (NAEPP 2005). Prednisone may be used to treat lupus nephritis in pregnant women who have active nephritis or substantial extrarenal disease activity (Hahn 2012).

Pregnant women exposed to prednisone for antirejection therapy following a transplant may contact the National Transplantation Pregnancy Registry (NTPR) at 215-955-4820. Women exposed to prednisone during pregnancy for the treatment of an autoimmune disease (eg, rheumatoid arthritis) may contact the OTIS Autoimmune Diseases Study at 877-311-8972.

Breast-Feeding Considerations Prednisone and its metabolite, predniso-lone, are found in low concentrations in breast milk. Following a maternal dose of 10 mg (n=1), milk concentrations were measured ~2 hours after the maternal dose (prednisone 0.0016 mcg/mL; prednisolone 0.0267 mcg/mL) (Katz, 1975). In a study which included six mother/infant pairs, adverse events were not observed in nursing infants (maternal prednisone dose not provided) (Ito, 1993).

The manufacturer notes that when used systemically, maternal use of cortico-steroids have the potential to cause adverse events in a nursing infant (eg, growth suppression, interfere with endogenous corticosteroid production) and therefore, a decision should be made whether to discontinue nursing or to discontinue the drug, taking into account the importance of treatment to the mother. If there is concern about exposure to the infant, some guidelines recommend waiting 4 hours after the maternal dose of an oral systemic corticosteroid before breast-feeding in order to decrease potential exposure to the nursing infant (based on a study using prednisolone) (Bae 2011; Leachman 2006; Makol 2011; Ost, 1985). Other guidelines note that maternal use of prednisone is not a contraindication to breast-feeding (NAEPP 2005).

Warnings/Precautions May cause hypercorticism or suppression of hypo-thalamic-pituitary-adrenal (HPA) axis, particularly in younger children or in patients receiving high doses for prolonged periods. HPA axis suppression may lead to adrenal crisis. Withdrawal and discontinuation of a corticosteroid should be done slowly and carefully. Particular care is required when patients are transferred from systemic corticosteroids to inhaled products due to possible adrenal insufficiency or withdrawal from steroids, including an increase in allergic symptoms. Patients receiving >20 mg per day of predni-sone (or equivalent) may be most susceptible. Fatalities have occurred due to adrenal insufficiency in asthmatic patients during and after transfer from systemic corticosteroids to aerosol steroids; aerosol steroids do **not** provide the systemic steroid needed to treat patients having trauma, surgery, or infections.

Acute myopathy has been reported with high dose corticosteroids, usually in patients with neuromuscular transmission disorders; may involve ocular and/or respiratory muscles; monitor creatine kinase; recovery may be delayed.

Prolonged use of corticosteroids may increase the incidence of secondary infection, mask acute infection (including fungal infections), prolong or exacerbate viral infections, or limit response to inactivated vaccines. Exposure to chickenpox or measles should be avoided. Corticosteroids should not be used to treat viral hepatitis or cerebral malaria. Close observation is required in patients with latent tuberculosis and/or TB reactivity; restrict use in active TB (only fulminating or disseminated TB in conjunction with antituberculosis treatment). Amebiasis should be ruled out in any patient with recent travel to tropic climates or unexplained diarrhea prior to initiation of corticosteroids. Prolonged treatment with corticosteroids has been associated with the development of Kaposi sarcoma (case reports); if noted, discontinuation of therapy should be considered (Goedert 2002). Use with caution in patients with cataracts and/or glaucoma; increased intraocular pressure, open-angle glaucoma, and cataracts have occurred with prolonged use. Use with caution in patients with a history of ocular herpes simplex; corneal perforation has occurred; do not use in active ocular herpes simplex. Consider routine eye exams in chronic users. Corticosteroid use may cause psychiatric disturbances, including severe depression, euphoria, insomnia, mood swings, and personality changes, to frank psychotic manifestations. Preexisting psychiatric conditions may be exacerbated by corticosteroid use. Rare cases of anaphylactoid reactions have been observed in patients receiving corticosteroids.

Use with caution in patients with HF, hypertension, diabetes, GI diseases (diverticulitis, fresh intestinal anastomoses, active or latent peptic ulcer, ulcerative colitis [nonspecific]), hepatic impairment, myasthenia gravis, MI, patients with or who are at risk for osteoporosis, renal impairment, seizure disorders or thyroid disease. May affect growth velocity; growth and development should be routinely monitored in pediatric patients. Because of the risk of adverse effects, systemic corticosteroids should be used cautiously in the elderly in the smallest possible effective dose for the shortest duration.

Withdraw therapy with gradual tapering of dose. Increased mortality was observed in patients receiving high-dose IV methylprednisolone; high-dose corticosteroids should not be used for the management of head injury. Potentially significant drug-drug interactions may exist, requiring dose or frequency adjustment, additional monitoring, and/or selection of alternative therapy.

Benzyl alcohol and derivatives: Some dosage forms may contain sodium benzoate/benzoic acid; benzoic acid (benzoate) is a metabolite of benzyl alcohol; large amounts of benzyl alcohol (≥99 mg/kg/day) have been associated with a potentially fatal toxicity ("gasping syndrome") in neonates; the "gasping syndrome" consists of metabolic acidosis, respiratory distress, gasping respirations, CNS dysfunction (including convulsions, intracranial hemorrhage), hypotension, and cardiovascular collapse (AAP ["Inactive" 1997]; CDC, 1982); some data suggests that benzoate displaces bilirubin from protein binding sites (Ahlfors 2001); avoid or use dosage forms containing benzyl alcohol derivative with caution in neonates. See manufacturer's labeling.

Propylene glycol: Some dosage forms may contain propylene glycol; large amounts are potentially toxic and have been associated hyperosmolality, lactic acidosis, seizures, and respiratory depression; use caution (AAP ["Inactive" 1997]; Zar 2007).

◀ **Adverse Reactions** Frequency not defined.

Cardiovascular: Congestive heart failure (in susceptible patients), hypertension

Central nervous system: Emotional instability, headache, intracranial pressure increased (with papilledema), psychic derangements (including euphoria, insomnia, mood swings, personality changes, severe depression), seizure, vertigo

Dermatologic: Bruising, facial erythema, petechiae, thin fragile skin, urticaria, wound healing impaired

Endocrine & metabolic: Adrenocortical and pituitary unresponsiveness (in times of stress), carbohydrate intolerance, Cushing's syndrome, diabetes mellitus, fluid retention, growth suppression (in children), hypokalemic alkalosis, hypothyroidism enhanced, menstrual irregularities, negative nitrogen balance due to protein catabolism, potassium loss, sodium retention

Gastrointestinal: Abdominal distension, pancreatitis, peptic ulcer (with possible perforation and hemorrhage), ulcerative esophagitis

Hepatic: ALT increased, AST increased, alkaline phosphatase increased

Neuromuscular & skeletal: Aseptic necrosis of femoral and humeral heads, muscle mass loss, muscle weakness, osteoporosis, pathologic fracture of long bones, steroid myopathy, tendon rupture (particularly Achilles tendon), vertebral compression fractures

Ocular: Exophthalmos, glaucoma, intraocular pressure increased, posterior subcapsular cataracts

Miscellaneous: Allergic reactions, anaphylactic reactions, diaphoresis, hypersensitivity reactions, infections, Kaposi's sarcoma

<1%, postmarketing, and/or case reports: Venous thrombosis (Johannesdottir, 2013)

Drug Interactions

Metabolism/Transport Effects Substrate of CYP3A4 (minor); **Note:** Assignment of Major/Minor substrate status based on clinically relevant drug interaction potential; **Induces** CYP2C19 (weak/moderate), CYP3A4 (weak)

Avoid Concomitant Use

Avoid concomitant use of PredniSONE with any of the following: Aldesleukin; BCG (Intravesical); Indium 111 Capromab Pendetide; Mifepristone; Natalizumab; Pimecrolimus; Tacrolimus (Topical); Tofacitinib

Increased Effect/Toxicity

PredniSONE may increase the levels/effects of: Acetylcholinesterase Inhibitors; Amphotericin B; Androgens; Ceritinib; CycloSPORINE (Systemic); Deferasirox; Fingolimod; Leflunomide; Loop Diuretics; Natalizumab; Nicorandil; NSAID (COX-2 Inhibitor); NSAID (Nonselective); Quinolone Antibiotics; Thiazide Diuretics; Tofacitinib; Vaccines (Live); Warfarin

The levels/effects of PredniSONE may be increased by: Aprepitant; Boceprevir; CycloSPORINE (Systemic); CYP3A4 Inhibitors (Strong); Denosumab; Estrogen Derivatives; Fluconazole; Fosaprepitant; Indacaterol; Mifepristone; Neuromuscular-Blocking Agents (Nondepolarizing); Pimecrolimus; Ritonavir; Roflumilast; Salicylates; Tacrolimus (Topical); Telaprevir; Trastuzumab

Decreased Effect

PredniSONE may decrease the levels/effects of: Aldesleukin; Antidiabetic Agents; ARIPiprazole; BCG (Intravesical); Calcitriol (Systemic); Coccidioides immitis Skin Test; Corticorelin; CycloSPORINE (Systemic); Hyaluronidase; Hydrocodone; Indium 111 Capromab Pendetide; Isoniazid; NiMODipine; Salicylates; Saxagliptin; Sipuleucel-T; Telaprevir; Urea Cycle Disorder Agents; Vaccines (Inactivated); Vaccines (Live)

The levels/effects of PredniSONE may be decreased by: Antacids; Bile Acid Sequestrants; CYP3A4 Inducers (Strong); Echinacea; Mifepristone; Mitotane; Somatropin; Tesamorelin

Storage/Stability

Store at 25°C (77°F); excursions permitted to 15°C to 30°C (59°F to 86°F). Protect from light and moisture.

Oral solution, concentrate: Discard opened bottle after 90 days.

Mechanism of Action

Decreases inflammation by suppression of migration of polymorphonuclear leukocytes and reversal of increased capillary permeability; suppresses the immune system by reducing activity and volume of the lymphatic system; suppresses adrenal function at high doses. Antitumor effects may be related to inhibition of glucose transport, phosphorylation, or induction of cell death in immature lymphocytes. Antiemetic effects are thought to occur due to blockade of cerebral innervation of the emetic center via inhibition of prostaglandin synthesis.

Pharmacodynamics/Kinetics

Absorption: 50% to 90% (may be altered in hepatic failure, chronic renal failure, inflammatory bowel disease, hyperthyroidism, and in the elderly) (Frey 1990)

Protein binding (concentration dependent): <50% (Frey 1990)

Metabolism: Hepatic to metabolite prednisolone (active)

Half-life elimination: 2 to 3 hours

Time to peak: Oral:

Immediate-release tablet: 2 hours; Delayed-release tablet: 6 to 6.5 hours

Excretion: Urine (as conjugates)

Dosing

Adult General dosing range: Oral: Initial: 5 to 60 mg daily. **Note:** Dose depends upon condition being treated and response of patient. Consider alternate day therapy for long-term therapy. Discontinuation of long-term therapy requires gradual withdrawal by tapering the dose.

Prednisone taper (other regimens also available):

Day 1: 30 mg divided as 10 mg before breakfast, 5 mg at lunch, 5 mg at dinner, 10 mg at bedtime

Day 2: 5 mg at breakfast, 5 mg at lunch, 5 mg at dinner, 10 mg at bedtime

Day 3: 5 mg 4 times daily (with meals and at bedtime)

Day 4: 5 mg 3 times daily (breakfast, lunch, bedtime)

Day 5: 5 mg 2 times daily (breakfast, bedtime)

Day 6: 5 mg before breakfast

Indication-specific dosing:

Acute asthma (NAEPP 2007): Oral: 40 to 60 mg per day for 3 to 10 days; administer as single or 2 divided doses

Acute exacerbations of chronic obstructive pulmonary disease (COPD) (off-label use for immediate release products; off-label dose): Oral: 40 mg once daily for 5 days (GOLD 2014).

Acute gout (ACR guidelines [Khanna 2012]): Oral: Initial: ≥0.5 mg/kg for 5 to 10 days

Anaphylaxis, adjunctive treatment (Lieberman 2005): Oral: 0.5 mg/kg

Antineoplastic: Oral: Usual range: 10 mg daily to 100 mg/m^2/day (depending on indication). **Note:** Details concerning dosing in combination regimens should also be consulted.

Autoimmune hepatitis (off-label use; Czaja 2002): Oral: Initial treatment: 60 mg daily for 1 week, *followed by* 40 mg daily for 1 week, *then* 30 mg daily for 2 weeks, *then* 20 mg daily. Half this dose should be given when used in combination with azathioprine

◀ **Bell palsy (off-label use):** Oral: 60 mg daily for 5 days, followed by a 5-day taper. Treatment should begin within 72 hours of onset of symptoms (Baugh 2013).

Crohn disease, moderate/severe (off-label use): Oral: 40 to 60 mg daily until resolution of symptoms and resumption of weight gain (usual duration: 7 to 28 days) (Lichtenstein 2009)

Dermatomyositis/polymyositis: Oral: 1 mg/kg daily (range: 0.5 to 1.5 mg/kg/day), often in conjunction with steroid-sparing therapies; depending on response/tolerance, consider slow tapering after 2 to 8 weeks depending on response; taper regimens vary widely, but often involve 5 to 10 mg decrements per week and may require 6 to 12 months to reach a low once-daily or every-other-day dose to prevent disease flare (Briemberg 2003; Hengstman 2009; Iorizzo 2008; Wiendl 2008)

Giant cell arteritis (off-label use): Oral: Initial: 40 to 60 mg daily; typically requires 1 to 2 years of treatment, but may begin to taper after 2 to 3 months; alternative dosing of 30 to 40 mg daily has demonstrated similar efficacy (Hiratzka 2010)

Graves ophthalmopathy prophylaxis (off-label use): Oral: 0.4 to 0.5 mg/kg/day, starting 1 to 3 days after radioactive iodine treatment, and continued for 1 month, then gradually taper over 2 months (Bahn 2011)

Herpes zoster (off-label use; Dworkin 2007): Oral: 60 mg daily for 7 days, *followed by* 30 mg daily for 7 days, *then* 15 mg daily for 7 days

Immune thrombocytopenia (ITP) (American Society of Hematology, 1997): Oral: 1 to 2 mg/kg/day

Lupus nephritis, induction (Hahn 2012): Oral:

Class III-IV lupus nephritis: 0.5 to 1 mg/kg/day (after glucocorticoid pulse) tapered after a few weeks to lowest effective dose, in combination with an immunosuppressive agent

Class V lupus nephritis: 0.5 mg/kg/day for 6 months in combination mycophenolate mofetil; if not improved after 6 months, use 0.5 to 1 mg/kg/day (after a glucocorticoid pulse) for an additional 6 months in combination with cyclophosphamide

Multiple sclerosis, acute exacerbations: Oral: 200 mg daily for 1 week, followed by 80 mg every other day for 1 month.

***Pneumocystis* pneumonia (adjunctive therapy) in HIV-infected patients (off-label dose):** Oral: 40 mg twice daily for 5 days beginning as early as possible and within 72 hours of PCP therapy, followed by 40 mg once daily on days 6 through 10, followed by 20 mg once daily on days 11 through 21 (HHS [OI adult 2015])

Polymyalgia rheumatica (off-label dose): Oral: Evidence to support an optimal dose and duration are lacking; recommendations provided are general guidelines only. Individualize therapy using the minimum effective dose and duration (Dejaco [EULAR/ACR 2015]):

Initial: Dosage range: 12.5 to 25 mg daily; consider higher doses within this range for patients at high risk of relapse and low risk of adverse events; consider lower doses within this range for patients with high risk factors for side effects (eg, diabetes, osteoporosis, glaucoma). Single daily doses are preferred over divided daily doses. Avoid initial doses ≤7.5 mg/day or >30 mg/day.

Tapering: For initial dosing, taper to a dose of 10 mg/day within 4 to 8 weeks. If relapse occurs, increase dosing to the prerelapse dose and gradually taper back to the dose which relapse occurred within 4 to 8 weeks. Once remission is achieved (initial or relapse therapy), taper daily dose by 1 mg every 4 weeks (or by 1.25 mg decrements if using schedules such as 10 mg and 7.5 mg on alternate days) until discontinuation.

Prostate cancer, metastatic (off-label use): Oral: 5 mg twice daily (in combination with abiraterone) until disease progression or unacceptable toxicity (de Bono 2011; Ryan 2015) **or** 10 mg once daily (in combination with cabazitaxel) for up to 10 cycles (de Bono 2010) **or** 5 mg twice daily (in combination with docetaxel) for up to 10 cycles (Berthold 2008; Tannock 2004).

Rheumatoid arthritis (American College of Rheumatology 2002): Oral: ≤10 mg daily

Subacute thyroiditis (off-label use): Oral: 40 mg daily for 1 to 2 weeks; gradually taper over 2 to 4 weeks or longer depending on clinical response. **Note:** NSAIDs should be considered first-line therapy in such patients (Bahn 2011).

Takayasu arteritis (off-label use): Oral: Initial: 40 to 60 mg daily; taper to lowest effective dose when ESR and CRP levels are normal; usual duration: 1 to 2 years (Hiratzka 2010)

Thyrotoxicosis (type II amiodarone-induced; off-label use): Oral: 40 mg daily for 14 to 28 days; gradually taper over 2 to 3 months depending on clinical response (Bahn 2011)

Tuberculosis, severe, paradoxical reactions (off-label dose, AIDS*info* guidelines 2008): Oral: 1 mg/kg/day, gradually reduce after 1 to 2 weeks

Geriatric Refer to adult dosing; use the lowest effective dose.

Pediatric

General dosing range: Oral: Refer to adult dosing. **Note:** Dose depends upon condition being treated and response of patient; dosage for infants and children should be based on severity of the disease and response of the patient rather than on strict adherence to dosage indicated by age, weight, or body surface area. Consider alternate day therapy for long-term therapy. Discontinuation of long-term therapy requires gradual withdrawal by tapering the dose.

Indication-specific dosing:

Acute asthma (NAEPP 2007): Oral:

0 to 11 years 1 to 2 mg/kg/day for 3 to 10 days (maximum: 60 mg daily)

≥12 years: Refer to Adults dosing

Autoimmune hepatitis (off-label use; Czaja 2002): Oral: Initial treatment: 2 mg/kg/day for 2 weeks (maximum: 60 mg daily), followed by a taper over 6 to 8 weeks to a dose of 0.1 to 0.2 mg/kg/day or 5 mg daily

Bell palsy (off-label use): Adolescents ≥16 years: Oral: 60 mg daily for 5 days, followed by a 5-day taper. Treatment should begin within 72 hours of onset of symptoms (Baugh 2013).

Nephrotic syndrome (Pediatric Nephrology Panel recommendations [Hogg 2000]): Oral: Initial: 2 mg/kg daily or 60 mg/m^2/day given every day in 1 to 3 divided doses (maximum: 80 mg daily) until urine is protein free or for 4 to 6 weeks; followed by maintenance dose: 2 mg/kg/dose or 40 mg/m^2/dose given every other day in the morning; gradually taper and discontinue after 4 to 6 weeks. **Note:** No definitive treatment guidelines exist. Dosing is dependent on institution protocols and individual response.

◄ ***Pneumocystis* pneumonia (adjunctive therapy) in HIV-infected patients (off-label dose; AIDS*info* guidelines 2008):** Oral:

Children: 1 mg/kg twice daily for 5 days, *followed by* 0.5 to 1 mg/kg twice daily for 5 days, *followed by* 0.5 mg/kg once daily for 11 to 21 days

Adolescents: Refer to adult dosing.

Renal Impairment Dosing adjustment in renal impairment: There are no dosage adjustments provided in the manufacturer's labeling.

Hemodialysis effects: Supplemental dose is not necessary.

Hepatic Impairment There are no dosage adjustments provided in the manufacturer's labeling.

Combination Regimens Note: In the US, prednisone is the preferred corticosteroid. However, in the British literature, prednisolone is often used. The oral doses of these two agents are equivalent (ie, 1 mg prednisone = 1 mg prednisolone). Also, early clinical trials gave prednisone only with the first and fourth cycles. Some clinicians give prednisone with every cycle.

Multiple myeloma:

Bortezomib-Melphalan-Prednisone-Thalidomide on page 1850

Melphalan-Prednisone-Bortezomib (Multiple Myeloma) on page 2033

Melphalan-Prednisone (Multiple Myeloma) on page 2034

Melphalan-Prednisone-Thalidomide (Multiple Myeloma) on page 2035

VBMCP (Multiple Myeloma) on page 2105

Prostate cancer:

Abiraterone-Prednisone (Prostate) on page 1820

Cabazitaxel-Prednisone (Prostate) on page 1852

Docetaxel-Prednisone (Prostate) on page 1946

Mitoxantrone-Prednisone (Prostate) on page 2038

Waldenstrom Macroglobulinemia: R-CHOP (Waldenstrom Macroglobulinemia) on page 2072

Administration
Administer after meals or with food or milk to decrease GI upset. May administer antacids between meals to help prevent peptic ulcers.

Delayed-release tablets: Swallow whole; do not break, divide, crush, or chew.

Oral solution, concentrate: Administer only with provided calibrated dropper.

Monitoring Parameters Blood pressure; weight; serum glucose; electrolytes; growth in pediatric patients; presence of infection, bone mineral density; assess HPA axis suppression (eg, ACTH stimulation test, morning plasma cortisol test, urinary free cortisol test); Hgb, occult blood loss; chest x-ray (at regular intervals during prolonged therapy); IOP with therapy >6 weeks.

Test Interactions Decreased response to skin tests

Dietary Considerations May require increased dietary intake of pyridoxine, vitamin C, vitamin D, folate, calcium, and phosphorus; may require decreased dietary intake of sodium and potassium supplementation

Additional Information Tapering of corticosteroids after a short course of therapy (<7-10 days) is generally not required unless the disease/inflammatory process is slow to respond. Tapering after prolonged exposure is dependent upon the individual patient, duration of corticosteroid treatments, and size of steroid dose. Recovery of the HPA axis may require several months. Subtle but important HPA axis suppression may be present for as long as several months after a course of as few as 10-14 days duration. Testing of HPA axis (cosyntropin) may be required, and signs/symptoms of adrenal insufficiency should be monitored in patients with a history of use.

Dosage Forms Excipient information presented when available (limited, particularly for generics); consult specific product labeling.

Concentrate, Oral:

PrediSONE Intensol: 5 mg/mL (30 mL) [contains alcohol, usp; unflavored flavor]

Solution, Oral:

Generic: 5 mg/5 mL (5 mL, 120 mL, 500 mL)

Tablet, Oral:

Deltasone: 20 mg [scored; contains fd&c yellow #10 aluminum lake, fd&c yellow #6 aluminum lake]

Generic: 1 mg, 2.5 mg, 5 mg, 10 mg, 20 mg, 50 mg

Tablet Delayed Release, Oral:

Rayos: 1 mg, 2 mg, 5 mg

◆ **PrediSONE Intensol** *see* PrediSONE *on page 1426*

◆ **Prelone** *see* PrednisoLONE (Systemic) *on page 1421*

◆ **Prialt** *see* Ziconotide *on page 1785*

- **Prilocaine and Lidocaine** *see* Lidocaine and Prilocaine *on page 1046*
- **Primaxin (Can)** *see* Imipenem and Cilastatin *on page 893*
- **Primaxin I.M. [DSC]** *see* Imipenem and Cilastatin *on page 893*
- **Primaxin I.V.** *see* Imipenem and Cilastatin *on page 893*
- **Privigen** *see* Immune Globulin *on page 903*
- **PRO-Bicalutamide (Can)** *see* Bicalutamide *on page 207*

Procarbazine (proe KAR ba zeen)

Related Information
Chemotherapy and Cancer Treatment During Pregnancy *on page 2214*
Fertility and Cancer Therapy *on page 2137*
Management of Chemotherapy-Induced Nausea and Vomiting in Adults *on page 2142*
Prevention of Chemotherapy-Induced Nausea and Vomiting in Children *on page 2203*
Safe Handling of Hazardous Drugs *on page 2292*

Brand Names: US Matulane

Brand Names: Canada Matulane; Natulan

Index Terms Benzmethyzin; Ibenzmethyzin; N-Methylhydrazine; PCB; PCZ; Procarbazine Hydrochloride

Pharmacologic Category Antineoplastic Agent, Alkylating Agent

Use Treatment of Hodgkin lymphoma

Labeled Contraindications Hypersensitivity to procarbazine or any component of the formulation; inadequate bone marrow reserve

Pregnancy Considerations Adverse events were observed in animal reproduction studies. There are case reports of fetal malformations in the offspring of pregnant women exposed to procarbazine as part of a combination chemotherapy regimen. Women of reproductive potential should avoid becoming pregnant during treatment.

Breast-Feeding Considerations It is not known if procarbazine is excreted in breast milk. Due to the potential for serious adverse reactions in the nursing infant, nursing is not recommended during treatment with procarbazine.

Warnings/Precautions Hazardous agent - use appropriate precautions for handling and disposal (NIOSH 2014 [group 1]). Hematologic toxicity (leukopenia and thrombocytopenia) may occur 2-8 weeks after treatment initiation. Allow ≥1 month interval between radiation therapy or myelosuppressive chemotherapy and initiation of procarbazine treatment. Withhold treatment for leukopenia (WBC <4000/mm^3) or thrombocytopenia (platelets <100,000/mm^3). Monitor for infections due to neutropenia. May cause hemolysis and/or production of Heinz inclusion bodies in erythrocytes. Procarbazine is associated with a high emetic potential; antiemetics are recommended to prevent nausea and vomiting (Dupuis, 2011; Roila, 2010). May cause diarrhea and stomatitis; withhold treatment for diarrhea or stomatitis. Withhold treatment for CNS toxicity, hemorrhage, or hypersensitivity. Azoospermia and infertility have been reported with procarbazine when used in combination with other chemotherapy agents. Possibly carcinogenic; acute myeloid leukemia and lung cancer have been reported following use.

Use with caution in patients with hepatic or renal impairment. Potentially significant drug-drug interactions may exist, requiring dose or frequency adjustment, additional monitoring, and/or selection of alternative therapy. Possesses MAO inhibitor activity and has potential for severe drug and food interactions; follow MAOI diet (avoid tyramine-containing foods). Avoid ethanol consumption, may cause disulfiram-like reaction. **[U.S. Boxed Warning]: Should be administered under the supervision of an experienced cancer chemotherapy physician.**

Adverse Reactions Frequency not always defined.

Cardiovascular: Edema, flushing, hypotension, syncope, tachycardia

Central nervous system: Apprehension, ataxia, chills, coma, confusion, depression, dizziness, drowsiness, falling, fatigue, hallucination, headache, hyporeflexia, insomnia, lethargy, nervousness, neuropathy, nightmares, pain, paresthesia, seizure, slurred speech, unsteadiness

Dermatologic: Alopecia, dermatitis, diaphoresis, hyperpigmentation, pruritus, skin rash, urticaria

Endocrine & metabolic: Gynecomastia (in prepubertal and early pubertal males)

Gastrointestinal: Nausea and vomiting (60% to 90%; increasing the dose in a stepwise fashion over several days may minimize), abdominal pain, anorexia, constipation, diarrhea, dysphagia, hematemesis, melena, stomatitis, xerostomia

Genitourinary: Reduced fertility (>10%), azoospermia (reported with combination chemotherapy), hematuria, nocturia

Hematologic & oncologic: Malignant neoplasm (2% to 15%; secondary; nonlymphoid; reported with combination therapy), anemia, bone marrow depression, eosinophilia, hemolysis (in patients with G6PD deficiency), hemolytic anemia, pancytopenia, petechia, purpura, thrombocytopenia

Hepatic: Hepatic insufficiency, jaundice

Hypersensitivity: Hypersensitivity reaction

Infection: Herpes virus infection, increased susceptibility to infection

Neuromuscular & skeletal: Arthralgia, foot-drop, myalgia, tremor, weakness

Ophthalmic: Accommodation disturbance, diplopia, nystagmus, papilledema, photophobia, retinal hemorrhage

Otic: Hearing loss

Renal: Polyuria

Respiratory: Cough, epistaxis, hemoptysis, hoarseness, pleural effusion, pneumonitis, pulmonary toxicity (<1%)

Miscellaneous: Fever

Drug Interactions

Metabolism/Transport Effects Inhibits Monoamine Oxidase

Avoid Concomitant Use

Avoid concomitant use of Procarbazine with any of the following: Alpha-/Beta-Agonists (Indirect-Acting); Alpha1-Agonists; Amphetamines; Anilidopiperidine Opioids; Antidepressants (Serotonin Reuptake Inhibitor/Antagonist); Apraclonidine; AtoMOXetine; Atropine (Ophthalmic); BCG (Intravesical); Bezafibrate; Buprenorphine; BuPROPion; BusPIRone; CarBAMazepine; CloZAPine; Cyclobenzaprine; Cyproheptadine; Dapoxetine; Dexmethylphenidate; Dextromethorphan; Diethylpropion; Dipyrone; Hydrocodone; HYDROmorphone; Isometheptene; Levonordefrin; Linezolid; Maprotiline; Meperidine; Mequitazine; Methyldopa; Methylene Blue; Methylphenidate; Mianserin; Mirtazapine; Moclobemide; Morphine (Liposomal); Morphine (Systemic); Natalizumab; Oxymorphone; Pholcodine; Pimecrolimus; Pizotifen; Selective Serotonin Reuptake Inhibitors; Serotonin 5-HT1D Receptor Agonists; Serotonin/Norepinephrine Reuptake Inhibitors; Tacrolimus (Topical); Tapentadol; Tetrabenazine; Tetrahydrozoline (Nasal); Tianeptine; Tofacitinib; Tricyclic Antidepressants; Tryptophan; Vaccines (Live)

◀ **Increased Effect/Toxicity**

Procarbazine may increase the levels/effects of: Alpha-/Beta-Agonists (Indirect-Acting); Alpha1-Agonists; Amphetamines; Antidepressants (Serotonin Reuptake Inhibitor/Antagonist); Antihypertensives; Antipsychotic Agents; Apraclonidine; AtoMOXetine; Atropine (Ophthalmic); Beta2-Agonists; Betahistine; Bezafibrate; Blood Glucose Lowering Agents; Brimonidine (Ophthalmic); Brimonidine (Topical); BuPROPion; Carbocisteine; CloZAPine; Cyproheptadine; Dexmethylphenidate; Dextromethorphan; Diethylpropion; Domperidone; Doxapram; EPINEPHrine (Nasal); Epinephrine (Racemic); EPINEPHrine (Systemic, Oral Inhalation); Fingolimod; Hydrocodone; HYDROmorphone; Isometheptene; Leflunomide; Levonordefrin; Levosulpiride; Linezolid; Lithium; Meperidine; Mequitazine; Methadone; Methyldopa; Methylene Blue; Methylphenidate; Metoclopramide; Mianserin; Mirtazapine; Moclobemide; Morphine (Liposomal); Morphine (Systemic); Natalizumab; Norepinephrine; Orthostatic Hypotension Producing Agents; OxyCODONE; Pizotifen; Reserpine; Selective Serotonin Reuptake Inhibitors; Serotonin 5-HT1D Receptor Agonists; Serotonin Modulators; Serotonin/Norepinephrine Reuptake Inhibitors; Tetrahydrozoline (Nasal); Tofacitinib; Tricyclic Antidepressants; Vaccines (Live)

The levels/effects of Procarbazine may be increased by: Altretamine; Anilidopiperidine Opioids; Antiemetics (5HT3 Antagonists); Antipsychotic Agents; Buprenorphine; BusPIRone; CarBAMazepine; COMT Inhibitors; Cyclobenzaprine; Dapoxetine; Denosumab; Dipyrone; Levodopa; MAO Inhibitors; Maprotiline; Metaxalone; Oxymorphone; Pholcodine; Pimecrolimus; Roflumilast; Tacrolimus (Topical); Tapentadol; Tedizolid; Tetrabenazine; Tianeptine; TraMADol; Trastuzumab; Tryptophan

Decreased Effect

Procarbazine may decrease the levels/effects of: BCG (Intravesical); Coccidioides immitis Skin Test; Domperidone; Sipuleucel-T; Vaccines (Inactivated); Vaccines (Live)

The levels/effects of Procarbazine may be decreased by: Cyproheptadine; Domperidone; Echinacea

Food Interactions

Ethanol: Ethanol may cause a disulfiram reaction. Management: Avoid ethanol.

Food: Concurrent ingestion of foods rich in tyramine, dopamine, tyrosine, phenylalanine, tryptophan, or caffeine may cause sudden and severe high blood pressure (hypertensive crisis or serotonin syndrome). Management: Avoid tyramine-containing foods (aged or matured cheese, air-dried or cured meats including sausages and salamis; fava or broad bean pods, tap/draft beers, Marmite concentrate, sauerkraut, soy sauce, and other soybean condiments). Food's freshness is also an important concern; improperly stored or spoiled food can create an environment in which tyramine concentrations may increase. Avoid foods containing dopamine, tyrosine, phenylalanine, tryptophan, or caffeine.

Storage/Stability Protect from light.

Mechanism of Action Inhibits DNA, RNA, and protein synthesis by inhibiting transmethylation of methionine into transfer RNA; may also damage DNA directly through alkylation.

Pharmacodynamics/Kinetics

Absorption: Rapid and complete

Distribution: Crosses blood-brain barrier; equilibrates between plasma and CSF

Metabolism: Oxidized to active metabolites methylazoxy-procarbazine and benzylazoxy-procarbazine, then further metabolized to inactive metabolites (Kintzel, 1995)

Half-life elimination: ~1 hour

Time to peak, plasma: ≤1 hour

Excretion: Urine (70% as inactive metabolites [Kintzel, 1995])

Dosing

Adult Note: Procarbazine is associated with a high emetic potential; antiemetics are recommended to prevent nausea and vomiting (Roila, 2010). The manufacturer suggests that an estimated lean body mass be used in obese patients and patients with rapid weight gain due to edema, ascites, or abnormal fluid retention.

Hodgkin lymphoma:

MOPP regimen: While procarbazine is approved as part of the MOPP regimen, the MOPP regimen is generally no longer used due to improved toxicity profiles with other combination regimens used in the treatment of Hodgkin lymphoma.

BEACOPP, standard or escalated regimen (off-label dosing): Oral: 100 mg/m^2 days 1 to 7 every 21 days (in combination with bleomycin, etoposide, doxorubicin, cyclophosphamide, vincristine, and prednisone) for 8 cycles (Diehl, 2003)

Non-Hodgkin lymphomas (NHL; off-label use):

CEPP regimen: Oral: 60 mg/m^2 days 1 to 10 every 28 days (in combination with cyclophosphamide, etoposide and prednisone) (Chao, 1990)

PEP-C regimen: Oral: 50 mg daily at bedtime (length of induction cycle depends on phase of treatment and blood counts; frequency may vary based on tolerance in maintenance cycle; in combination with prednisone, etoposide, and cyclophosphamide) (Coleman, 2008)

CNS tumors, anaplastic oligodendroglioma/oligoastrocytoma (off-label use): *PCV regimen:* Oral: 60 mg/m^2 days 8 to 21 every 6 weeks (in combination with lomustine and vincristine) for 6 cycles (van den Bent, 2006) **or** 75 mg/m^2 days 8-21 every 6 weeks (in combination with lomustine and vincristine) for up to 4 cycles (Cairncross, 2006).

Primary CNS lymphoma (off-label use): Oral: 100 mg/m^2 for 7 days in cycles 1, 3, and 5 (in combination with methotrexate [high-dose], vincristine, methotrexate [intrathecal], leucovorin, dexamethasone, cytarabine [high-dose], and whole brain radiation) (DeAngelis, 2002).

Geriatric Refer to adult dosing; use with caution.

Pediatric Note: Procarbazine is associated with a high emetic potential; antiemetics are recommended to prevent nausea and vomiting (Dupuis, 2011). The manufacturer suggests that an estimated lean body mass be used in obese patients and patients with rapid weight gain due to edema, ascites, or abnormal fluid retention.

Hodgkin lymphoma:

MOPP regimen: While procarbazine is approved as part of the MOPP regimen, the MOPP regimen is generally no longer used due to improved toxicity profiles with other combination regimens used in the treatment of Hodgkin lymphoma.

BEACOPP regimen (off-label dosing): Oral: 100 mg/m² days 0 to 6 of a 21-day treatment cycle (in combination with bleomycin, etoposide, doxorubicin, cyclophosphamide, vincristine, and prednisone) for 4 cycles (Kelley, 2011).

Renal Impairment No dosage adjustment provided in manufacturer's labeling; use with caution; may result in increased toxicity. However, because predominantly inactive metabolites are excreted via the kidneys, dosage adjustment is not necessary (Kintzel, 1995).

Hepatic Impairment No dosage adjustment provided in manufacturer's labeling; use with caution; may result in increased toxicity. The following adjustments have been reported in literature:

Floyd, 2006:

Transaminases 1.6-6 times ULN: Administer 75% of dose

Transaminases >6 times ULN: Use clinical judgment

Serum bilirubin >5 mg/dL or transaminases >3 times ULN: Avoid use

King, 2001: Serum bilirubin >5 mg/dL or transaminases >180 units/L: Avoid use

Obesity *ASCO Guidelines for appropriate chemotherapy dosing in obese adults with cancer:* Utilize patient's actual body weight (full weight) for calculation of body surface area- or weight-based dosing, particularly when the intent of therapy is curative; manage regimen-related toxicities in the same manner as for nonobese patients; if a dose reduction is utilized due to toxicity, consider resumption of full weight-based dosing with subsequent cycles, especially if cause of toxicity (eg, hepatic or renal impairment) is resolved (Griggs, 2012). **Note:** The manufacturer suggests that an estimated lean body mass be used in obese patients and patients with rapid weight gain due to edema, ascites, or abnormal fluid retention.

Adjustment for Toxicity Withhold treatment (promptly) for any of the following: CNS toxicity (eg, paresthesia, confusion, neuropathy), hematologic toxicity (WBC <4000/mm³ or platelets <100,000/mm³), hypersensitivity, gastrointestinal toxicities (stomatisis, diarrhea), and hemorrhage or bleeding.

Combination Regimens

Brain tumors: PCV (Brain Tumor Regimen) on page 2061

Lymphoma, Hodgkin:

BEACOPP-14 (Hodgkin) on page 1829

BEACOPP Escalated (Hodgkin) on page 1830

BEACOPP Escalated Plus Standard (Hodgkin) on page 1830

BEACOPP Standard (Hodgkin) on page 1832

ChlVPP (Hodgkin) on page 1886

C-MOPP/ABV Hybrid (Hodgkin) on page 1919

MOPP/ABVD (Hodgkin) on page 2039

MOPP/ABV Hybrid (Hodgkin) on page 2040

MOPP (Hodgkin) on page 2041

Lymphoma, non-Hodgkin: PEP-C (NHL) on page 2066

Lymphoma, non-Hodgkin (DLBCL): CEPP (NHL-DLBCL) on page 1878

Administration Oral: May be given as a single daily dose or in 2 to 3 divided doses. Procarbazine is associated with a high emetic potential; antiemetics are recommended to prevent nausea and vomiting (Dupuis, 2011; Roila, 2010).

Hazardous agent; use appropriate precautions for handling and disposal (NIOSH 2014 [group 1]).

Emetic Potential Children and Adults: High (>90%)

Extemporaneous Preparations Hazardous agent: Use appropriate precautions for handling and disposal (NIOSH 2014 [group 1]).

A 10 mg/mL oral suspension may be prepared using capsules, glycerin, and strawberry syrup. Empty the contents of ten 50 mg capsules into a mortar. Add 2 mL glycerin and mix to a thick uniform paste. Add 10 mL strawberry syrup in incremental proportions; mix until uniform. Transfer the mixture to an amber glass bottle and rinse mortar with small amounts of strawberry syrup; add rinses to the bottle in sufficient quantity to make 50 mL. Label "shake well" and "protect from light". Stable for 7 days at room temperature.

Matulane® data on file, Sigma Tau Pharmaceuticals, Inc.

Monitoring Parameters CBC with differential, platelet and reticulocyte count, urinalysis, liver function test, renal function test. Monitor for infections, CNS toxicity, and gastrointestinal toxicities.

Dietary Considerations Avoid tyramine-containing foods/beverages. Some examples include aged or matured cheese, air-dried or cured meats (including sausages and salamis), fava or broad bean pods, tap/draft beers, Marmite concentrate, sauerkraut, soy sauce and other soybean condiments.

Dosage Forms Excipient information presented when available (limited, particularly for generics); consult specific product labeling.

Capsule, Oral, as hydrochloride:

Matulane: 50 mg

♦ **Procarbazine Hydrochloride** see Procarbazine on page 1436

Prochlorperazine (proe klor PER a zeen)

Related Information

Management of Chemotherapy-Induced Nausea and Vomiting in Adults on page 2142

Brand Names: US Compazine; Compro

Brand Names: Canada Apo-Prochlorperazine; Nu-Prochlor; PMS-Prochlorperazine; Sandoz-Prochlorperazine

Index Terms Chlormeprazine; Compazine; Prochlorperazine Edisylate; Prochlorperazine Maleate; Prochlorperazine Mesylate

Pharmacologic Category Antiemetic; First Generation (Typical) Antipsychotic

Use Management of severe nausea and vomiting; psychotic disorders, including schizophrenia and anxiety (**Note:** Not a recommended therapy by schizophrenia treatment guidelines [Hasan 2012; Lehman 2004]); nonpsychotic anxiety

Labeled Contraindications

Hypersensitivity to prochlorperazine or any component of the formulation (cross-reactivity between phenothiazines may occur); coma or presence of large amounts of CNS depressants (eg, alcohol, opioids, barbiturates); postoperative management of nausea/vomiting following pediatric surgery; use in infants and children <2 years or <9 kg; pediatric conditions for which dosage has not been established

Documentation of allergenic cross-reactivity for phenothiazines is limited. However, because of similarities in chemical structure and/or pharmacologic actions, the possibility of cross-sensitivity cannot be ruled out with certainty.

Canadian labeling: Additional contraindications (not in US labeling): Presence of circulatory collapse; severe cardiovascular disorders; altered state of consciousness; concomitant use of high dose hypnotics; severe depression; presence of blood dyscrasias, hepatic or renal impairment, or

◀ pheochromocytoma; suspected or established subcortical brain damage with or without hypothalamic damage

Pregnancy Considerations Jaundice or hyper- or hyporeflexia have been reported in newborn infants following maternal use of phenothiazines. Antipsychotic use during the third trimester of pregnancy has a risk for abnormal muscle movements (extrapyramidal symptoms [EPS]) and withdrawal symptoms in newborns following delivery. Symptoms in the newborn may include agitation, feeding disorder, hypertonia, hypotonia, respiratory distress, somnolence, and tremor; these effects may be self-limiting or require hospitalization. Use may interfere with pregnancy tests, causing false positive results. Prochlorperazine has been used for the treatment of nausea and vomiting associated with pregnancy (Levicheck 2002; Mahadevan 2006); however, other agents may be preferred (ACOG 2004).

Breast-Feeding Considerations Other phenothiazines are excreted in human milk; excretion of prochlorperazine is not known.

Warnings/Precautions [US Boxed Warning]: Elderly patients with dementia-related psychosis treated with antipsychotics are at an increased risk of death (compared to placebo). This was based on analyses of 17 placebo-controlled trials (duration ~10 weeks), predominantly in patients taking atypical antipsychotics which revealed a risk of death in drug-treated patients between 1.6 and 1.7 times the risk of death in placebo-treated patients. Over the course of a typical 10-week controlled trial, the rate of death in drug-treated patients was ~4.5% compared with ~2.6% in the placebo group. Although the causes of death varied, most deaths appeared to be either cardiovascular (eg, heart failure, sudden death) or infectious (eg, pneumonia) in nature. Observational studies suggest that, similar to atypical antipsychotic drugs, treatment with conventional antipsychotic drugs may increase mortality, although the extent to which increased mortality may be attributed to the antipsychotic drug as opposed to some characteristic(s) of the patients is not clear. Prochlorperazine is not approved for the treatment of dementia-related psychosis.

Prochlorperazine may cause extrapyramidal symptoms (EPS), including pseudoparkinsonism, acute dystonic reactions, akathisia, and tardive dyskinesia. Risk of dystonia (and possibly other EPS) may be greater with increased doses, use of conventional antipsychotics, males, and younger patients. Risk of tardive dyskinesia and potential for irreversibility often associated with total cumulative dose and therapy duration and may also be increased in elderly patients (particularly elderly women); antipsychotics may also mask signs/symptoms of tardive dyskinesia. Consider therapy discontinuation with signs/symptoms of tardive dyskinesia. Antipsychotic use has been associated with esophageal dysmotility and aspiration; use with caution in patients at risk of pneumonia (ie, Alzheimer's disease).

May be sedating and impair physical or mental abilities; use with caution in disorders where CNS depression is a feature. Use with caution in Parkinson's disease; hemodynamic instability; predisposition to seizures; subcortical brain damage; and in severe cardiac, hepatic, or renal disease. Canadian labeling contraindicates use in patients with severe cardiac disease, hepatic or renal impairment, subcortical brain damage, and circulatory collapse. May alter temperature regulation, obscure intestinal obstruction or brain tumor or mask toxicity of other drugs. May alter cardiac conduction. Hypotension may occur following administration, particularly when parenteral form is used or in high dosages. May cause orthostatic hypotension; use with caution in patients at risk of this effect or in those who would not tolerate transient hypotensive episodes (cerebrovascular disease, cardiovascular disease, hypovolemia, or concurrent medication use which may predispose to hypotension/bradycardia).

Leukopenia, neutropenia, and agranulocytosis (sometimes fatal) have been reported in clinical trials and postmarketing reports with antipsychotic use; presence of risk factors (eg, preexisting low WBC or history of drug-induced leuko-/neutropenia) should prompt periodic blood count assessment. Discontinue therapy at first signs of blood dyscrasias or if absolute neutrophil count <1000/mm^3.

Due to its potent anticholinergic effects, may be inappropriate in older adults depending on comorbidities (eg, dementia, delirium) (Beers Criteria). Use with caution in patients with decreased gastrointestinal motility, urinary retention, BPH, xerostomia, visual problems, or narrow-angle glaucoma (screening is recommended). Use caution with exposure to heat. May cause pigmentary retinopathy, and lenticular and corneal deposits, particularly with prolonged therapy. Use associated with increased prolactin levels; clinical significance of hyperprolactinemia in patients with breast cancer or other prolactin-dependent tumors is unknown. Avoid use in patients with signs/symptoms suggestive of Reye's syndrome. Children with acute illness or dehydration are more susceptible to neuromuscular reactions; use cautiously. May be associated with neuroleptic malignant syndrome (NMS). Some dosage forms may contain sodium sulfite.

Benzyl alcohol and derivatives: Some dosage forms may contain benzyl alcohol; large amounts of benzyl alcohol (≥99 mg/kg/day) have been associated with a potentially fatal toxicity ("gasping syndrome") in neonates; the "gasping syndrome" consists of metabolic acidosis, respiratory distress, gasping respirations, CNS dysfunction (including convulsions, intracranial hemorrhage), hypotension, and cardiovascular collapse (AAP ["Inactive" 1997]; CDC 1982); some data suggests that benzoate displaces bilirubin from protein binding sites (Ahlfors 2001); avoid or use dosage forms containing benzyl alcohol with caution in neonates. See manufacturer's labeling. Potentially significant drug-drug interactions may exist, requiring dose or frequency adjustment, additional monitoring, and/or selection of alternative therapy.

Adverse Reactions Reported with prochlorperazine or other phenothiazines. Frequency not defined.

Cardiovascular: Cardiac arrest, cerebral edema, hypotension, peripheral edema, Q-wave distortions, sudden death, T-wave distortions

Central nervous system: Agitation, altered cerebrospinal fluid proteins, catatonia, coma, cough reflex suppressed, dizziness, drowsiness, fever (mild [IM]), headache, hyperpyrexia, impairment of temperature regulation, insomnia, neuroleptic malignant syndrome (NMS), oculogyric crisis, opisthotonos, restlessness, seizure, somnolence, tremulousness

Dermatologic: Angioedema, contact dermatitis, epithelial keratopathy, erythema, eczema, exfoliative dermatitis, itching, photosensitivity, skin pigmentation, urticaria

Endocrine & metabolic: Amenorrhea, galactorrhea, gynecomastia, glucosuria, hyper-/hypoglycemia, lactation, libido (changes in), menstrual irregularity

Gastrointestinal: Appetite increased, atonic colon, constipation, ileus, nausea, obstipation, vomiting, weight gain, xerostomia

Genitourinary: Ejaculating dysfunction, ejaculatory disturbances, impotence, priapism, urinary retention

◄ Hematologic: Agranulocytosis, aplastic anemia, eosinophilia, hemolytic anemia, leukopenia, pancytopenia, thrombocytopenic purpura

Hepatic: Biliary stasis, cholestatic jaundice, hepatotoxicity

Neuromuscular & skeletal: Dystonias (torticollis, carpopedal spasm, trismus, protrusion of tongue); extrapyramidal symptoms (pseudoparkinsonism, akathisia, dystonias, tardive dyskinesia, hyperreflexia); SLE-like syndrome, tremor

Ocular: Blurred vision, lenticular/corneal deposits, miosis, mydriasis, pigmentary retinopathy

Respiratory: Asthma, laryngeal edema, nasal congestion

Miscellaneous: Allergic reactions, asphyxia, diaphoresis

Drug Interactions

Metabolism/Transport Effects None known.

Avoid Concomitant Use

Avoid concomitant use of Prochlorperazine with any of the following: Aclidinium; Amisulpride; Azelastine (Nasal); Cimetropium; Dofetilide; Eluxadoline; Glucagon; Glycopyrrolate; Ipratropium (Oral Inhalation); Levosulpiride; Metoclopramide; Orphenadrine; Paraldehyde; Potassium Chloride; Sulpiride; Thalidomide; Tiotropium; Umeclidinium

Increased Effect/Toxicity

Prochlorperazine may increase the levels/effects of: AbobotulinumtoxinA; Alcohol (Ethyl); Amisulpride; Analgesics (Opioid); Anticholinergic Agents; Antidepressants (Serotonin Reuptake Inhibitor/Antagonist); Azelastine (Nasal); Beta-Blockers; Buprenorphine; Cimetropium; CNS Depressants; Dofetilide; Eluxadoline; Glucagon; Glycopyrrolate; Hydrocodone; Mequitazine; Methotrimeprazine; Methylphenidate; Metyrosine; Mirabegron; Mirtazapine; OnabotulinumtoxinA; Orphenadrine; Paraldehyde; Porfimer; Potassium Chloride; Ramosetron; RimabotulinumtoxinB; Selective Serotonin Reuptake Inhibitors; Serotonin Modulators; Sulpiride; Suvorexant; Thalidomide; Thiazide Diuretics; Thiopental; Tiotropium; Topiramate; Verteporfin; Zolpidem

The levels/effects of Prochlorperazine may be increased by: Acetylcholinesterase Inhibitors (Central); Aclidinium; Antidepressants (Serotonin Reuptake Inhibitor/Antagonist); Antimalarial Agents; Beta-Blockers; Brimonidine (Topical); Cannabis; Deferoxamine; Doxylamine; Dronabinol; Droperidol; HydrOXYzine; Ipratropium (Oral Inhalation); Kava Kava; Lithium; Magnesium Sulfate; Methotrimeprazine; Methylphenidate; Metoclopramide; Metyrosine; Mianserin; Minocycline; Nabilone; Perampanel; Pramlintide; Rufinamide; Serotonin Modulators; Sodium Oxybate; Tapentadol; Tetrabenazine; Tetrahydrocannabinol; Umeclidinium

Decreased Effect

Prochlorperazine may decrease the levels/effects of: Acetylcholinesterase Inhibitors; Amphetamines; Anti-Parkinson's Agents (Dopamine Agonist); Gastrointestinal Agents (Prokinetic); Itopride; Levosulpiride; Quinagolide; Secretin

The levels/effects of Prochlorperazine may be decreased by: Acetylcholinesterase Inhibitors; Antacids; Anti-Parkinson's Agents (Dopamine Agonist); Lithium

Storage/Stability

Injection:

Edisylate: Store at 20°C to 25°C (68°F to 77°F); do not freeze. Protect from light. Clear or slightly yellow solutions may be used.

Mesylate (Canadian availability; not available in US): Store at 15°C to 30°C (59°F to 86°F). Protect from light. Do not use if solution is discolored or hazy.

IV infusion: Injection may be diluted in 50 to 100 mL NS or D_5W.

Suppository: Store at 20°C to 25°C (68°F to 77°F). Do not remove from wrapper until ready to use.

Tablet: Store at 20°C to 25°C (68°F to 77°F). Protect from light.

Mechanism of Action Prochlorperazine is a piperazine phenothiazine antipsychotic which blocks postsynaptic mesolimbic dopaminergic D_1 and D_2 receptors in the brain, including the chemoreceptor trigger zone; exhibits a strong alpha-adrenergic and anticholinergic blocking effect and depresses the release of hypothalamic and hypophyseal hormones; believed to depress the reticular activating system, thus affecting basal metabolism, body temperature, wakefulness, vasomotor tone and emesis

Pharmacodynamics/Kinetics

Onset of action: Oral: 30 to 40 minutes; IM: 10 to 20 minutes; Rectal: ~60 minutes

Peak antiemetic effect: IV: 30 to 60 minutes

Duration: Rectal: 3 to 12 hours; IM, Oral: 3 to 4 hours

Distribution: V_d: 1400 to 1548 L (Taylor 1987)

Metabolism: Primarily hepatic; N-desmethyl prochlorperazine (major active metabolite)

Bioavailability: Oral: 12.5% (Isah 1991)

Half-life elimination: Oral: 6 to 10 hours (single dose), 14 to 22 hours (repeated dosing) (Isah 1991); IV: 6 to 10 hours (Isah 1991; Taylor 1987)

Excretion: Mainly in feces

Dosing

Adult Note: Injection solution mesylate formulation has Canadian availability (not available in US).

Antiemetic:

Oral (tablet): 5 to 10 mg 3 to 4 times/day; usual maximum: 40 mg/day; larger doses may rarely be required

IM (as edisylate): 5 to 10 mg every 3 to 4 hours; usual maximum: 40 mg/day

IM (as mesylate): 5 to 10 mg 2 to 3 times/day; usual maximum: 40 mg/day

IV (as edisylate): 2.5 to 10 mg; maximum: 10 mg/dose or 40 mg/day; may repeat dose every 3 to 4 hours as needed

Rectal:

US labeling: 25 mg twice daily

Canadian labeling: 5 to 10 mg 3 to 4 times/day

Surgical nausea/vomiting: Note: Should not exceed 40 mg/day

IM (as edisylate): 5 to 10 mg 1 to 2 hours before anesthesia induction or to control symptoms during or after surgery; may repeat once if necessary

IM (as mesylate): 5 to 10 mg 1 to 2 hours before anesthesia induction; may repeat once if needed during surgery; postoperatively: 5 to 10 mg every 3 to 4 hours as needed up to maximum of 40 mg daily

IV (as edisylate): 5 to 10 mg 15 to 30 minutes before anesthesia induction or to control symptoms during or after surgery; may repeat once if necessary

IV (as mesylate): 20 mg/L of IV solution during surgery or postoperatively; usual maximum: 30 mg daily

Rectal (off-label use; Golembiewski 2005): 25 mg

◀ **Antipsychotic:**

Oral: 5 to 10 mg 3 to 4 times/day; titrate dose slowly every 2 to 3 days; doses up to 150 mg/day may be required in some patients for treatment of severe disturbances

IM (as edisylate): Initial: 10 to 20 mg; if necessary repeat initial dose every 2 to 4 hours to gain control; more than 3 to 4 doses are rarely needed. If parenteral administration is still required; give 10 to 20 mg every 4 to 6 hours; convert to oral therapy as soon as possible.

IM (as mesylate): Initial: 10 to 20 mg; if necessary repeat initial dose every 2 to 4 hours to gain control; more than 3 to 4 doses are rarely needed; convert to oral therapy as soon as possible.

Nonpsychotic anxiety: *Oral (tablet):* Usual dose: 5 mg 3 to 4 times/day; do not exceed 20 mg/day or administer >12 weeks

Geriatric Initiate at lower end of dosage range; titrate slowly and cautiously. Refer to adult dosing.

Pediatric Note: Injection solution mesylate formulation has Canadian availability (not available in US).

Use is contraindicated in children <9 kg or <2 years.

Antiemetic:

Oral (therapy >1 day usually not required):

9 to 13 kg: 2.5 mg 1 to 2 times/day as needed (maximum: 7.5 mg/day)

>13 to 18 kg: 2.5 mg 2 to 3 times/day as needed (maximum: 10 mg/day)

>18 to 39 kg: 2.5 mg 3 times/day or 5 mg 2 times/day as needed (maximum: 15 mg/day)

IM (as edisylate): 0.13 mg/kg/dose; convert to oral therapy as soon as possible

IM (as mesylate): 0.14 mg/kg/dose; convert to oral therapy at equivalent or greater dose (if necessary) as soon as possible

Antipsychotic: Children 2 to 12 years:

Oral: 2.5 mg 2 to 3 times/day; do not give more than 10 mg the first day; increase dosage as needed to maximum daily dose of 20 mg for 2 to 5 years and 25 mg for 6 to 12 years

IM (as edisylate): 0.13 mg/kg/dose; convert to oral therapy as soon as possible

IM (as mesylate): 0.14 mg/kg/dose; convert to oral therapy at equivalent or greater dose (if necessary) as soon as possible

Renal Impairment

US labeling: There are no dosage adjustments provided in the manufacturer's labeling.

Canadian labeling: Use is contraindicated.

Hepatic Impairment

US labeling: There are no dosage adjustments provided in the manufacturer's labeling; systemic exposure may be increased as drug undergoes hepatic metabolism.

Canadian labeling: Use is contraindicated.

Administration

IM: Inject by deep IM into outer quadrant of buttocks.

IV: May be administered by slow IV push at a rate not exceeding 5 mg/minute or by IV infusion. Do not administer as a bolus injection. To reduce the risk of hypotension, patients receiving IV prochlorperazine must remain lying down and be observed for at least 30 minutes following administration. Avoid skin contact with injection solution, contact dermatitis has occurred. Do not dilute with any diluent containing parabens as a preservative.

Oral: Administer tablet without regard to meals.

Rectal: Do not remove from wrapper until ready to use.

Monitoring Parameters Mental status; vital signs (as clinically indicated); weight, height, BMI, waist circumference (baseline; at every visit for the first 6 months; quarterly with stable antipsychotic dose); CBC (as clinically indicated; monitor frequently during the first few months of therapy in patients with preexisting low WBC or history of drug-induced leukopenia/neutropenia); electrolytes and liver function (annually and as clinically indicated); fasting plasma glucose level/HbA$_{1c}$ (baseline, then yearly; in patients with diabetes risk factors or if gaining weight repeat 4 months after starting antipsychotic, then yearly); lipid panel (baseline; repeat every 2 years if LDL level is normal; repeat every 6 months if LDL level is >130 mg/dL); changes in menstruation, libido, development of galactorrhea, erectile and ejaculatory function (at each visit for the first 12 weeks after the antipsychotic is initiated or until the dose is stable, then yearly); abnormal involuntary movements or parkinsonian signs (baseline; repeat weekly until dose stabilized for at least 2 weeks after introduction and for 2 weeks after any significant dose increase); tardive dyskinesia (every 6 months; high-risk patients every 3 months); visual changes (inquire yearly); ocular examination (yearly in patients >40 years; every 2 years in younger patients) (ADA 2004; Lehman 2004; Marder 2004).

Test Interactions False-positives for phenylketonuria, pregnancy

Dietary Considerations Increase dietary intake of riboflavin; should be administered with food or water. Rectal suppositories may contain coconut and palm oil.

Additional Information Not recommended as an antipsychotic due to inferior efficacy compared to other phenothiazines.

Dosage Forms Excipient information presented when available (limited, particularly for generics); consult specific product labeling.

Solution, Injection, as edisylate [strength expressed as base]:
  Generic: 5 mg/mL (2 mL, 10 mL)
Suppository, Rectal:
  Compazine: 25 mg (12 ea)
  Compro: 25 mg (12 ea)
  Generic: 25 mg (12 ea, 1000 ea)
Tablet, Oral, as maleate [strength expressed as base]:
  Compazine: 5 mg, 10 mg
  Generic: 5 mg, 10 mg

Dosage Forms: Canada Excipient information presented when available (limited, particularly for generics); consult specific product labeling.

Injection, solution, as mesylate [strength expressed as base]: 5 mg/mL (2 mL)
Suppository, rectal: 10 mg (10s)

- **Profilnine SD** see Factor IX Complex (Human) [(Factors II, IX, X)] on page 677
- **PRO-Fluconazole (Can)** see Fluconazole on page 725
- **Prograf** see Tacrolimus (Systemic) on page 1576
- **Prokine** see Sargramostim on page 1515
- **Proleukin** see Aldesleukin on page 55
- **Prolia** see Denosumab on page 499
- **PRO-Lorazepam (Can)** see LORazepam on page 1058
- **Promacta** see Eltrombopag on page 585
- **Proquin XR** see Ciprofloxacin (Systemic) on page 327
- **Prostate Cancer Vaccine, Cell-Based** see Sipuleucel-T on page 1528
- **Protein-Bound Paclitaxel** see PACLitaxel (Protein Bound) on page 1292
- **ProThelial** see Mucosal Coating Agent on page 1175
- **Prothrombin Complex Concentrate (Caution: Confusion-prone synonym)** see Factor IX Complex (Human) [(Factors II, IX, X)] on page 677
- **Protrin DF (Can)** see Sulfamethoxazole and Trimethoprim on page 1560
- **PRO-Valacyclovir (Can)** see ValACYclovir on page 1712
- **Provenge** see Sipuleucel-T on page 1528
- **Provera** see MedroxyPROGESTERone on page 1074
- **Provera-Pak (Can)** see MedroxyPROGESTERone on page 1074
- **PS-341** see Bortezomib on page 223
- **PTG** see Teniposide on page 1622
- **Purinethol** see Mercaptopurine on page 1087
- **Purinethol [DSC]** see Mercaptopurine on page 1087
- **Purixan** see Mercaptopurine on page 1087
- **PXD101** see Belinostat on page 178
- **Quadramet** see Samarium Sm 153 Lexidronam on page 1513
- **Quadrivalent Human Papillomavirus Vaccine** see Papillomavirus (Types 6, 11, 16, 18) Vaccine (Human, Recombinant) on page 1330
- **R7159** see Obinutuzumab on page 1220
- **R05072759** see Obinutuzumab on page 1220
- **223Ra** see Radium Ra 223 Dichloride on page 1448
- **RAD001** see Everolimus on page 656
- **Radium-223 Chloride** see Radium Ra 223 Dichloride on page 1448
- **Radium-223 Dichloride** see Radium Ra 223 Dichloride on page 1448

Radium Ra 223 Dichloride
(RAY dee um R A two twenty-three dye KLOR ide)

Related Information
Safe Handling of Hazardous Drugs on page 2292

Brand Names: US Xofigo

Index Terms 223Ra; Alpharadin; BAY88-8223; Radium-223 Chloride; Radium-223 Dichloride

Pharmacologic Category Radiopharmaceutical

Use Prostate cancer: Treatment of patients with castration-resistant prostate cancer (CRPC), symptomatic bone metastases and no known visceral metastatic disease

Labeled Contraindications Use in women who are or may become pregnant

Pregnancy Considerations Based on the mechanism of action, radiopharmaceuticals have the potential to cause fetal harm if administered during pregnancy. Use is contraindicated in women who are or may become pregnant; not indicated for use in women. Men who are sexually active should use condoms during and for 6 months after completing treatment; their female partners of reproductive potential should use a highly effective contraceptive method during and for 6 months after treatment is completed.

Breast-Feeding Considerations It is not known if radium Ra 223 dichloride is excreted in breast milk. Not indicated for use in women.

Warnings/Precautions Radiopharmaceutical; use appropriate precautions for handling, disposal, and minimizing exposure to patients and healthcare personnel. Use only under supervision of individuals with experience/training in the handling of radioactive materials approved by the applicable regulatory authority.

Hematologic toxicity, including anemia, lymphocytopenia, thrombocytopenia, leukopenia, and neutropenia commonly occur; monitor blood counts at baseline and prior to each dose. Bone marrow failure occurred in 2% of patients receiving radium Ra 223 dichloride in clinical studies (did not occur in patients who received placebo). Bone marrow failure may be prolonged and fatal (rare); may require blood transfusion support. Vascular hemorrhage due to thrombocytopenia has been reported. Infection may occur due to neutropenia. Prior to initial dose, ANC should be ≥1500/mm^3, platelets ≥100,000/mm^3, and hemoglobin ≥10 g/dL; prior to subsequent doses, ANC should be ≥1000/mm^3 and platelets ≥50,000/mm^3. Neutrophils and platelet nadirs typically occurred 2-3 weeks after administration; recovery generally occurred ~6-8 weeks after administration. If recovery does not occur within 6-8 weeks from the last dose (despite supportive care), treatment should be discontinued. Closely monitor patients with compromised bone marrow reserve; discontinue if life-threatening complications occur despite supportive care.

The safety and efficacy of concurrent chemotherapy have not been established. Due to the potential for additive bone marrow toxicity, concurrent use with chemotherapy is not recommended outside of a clinical trial. If chemotherapy, other systemic radioisotopes, or external radiotherapy are required, radium Ra 223 dichloride should be discontinued. Although fewer malignancies were reported for radium Ra 223 dichloride than for placebo (from clinical studies), long-term cumulative radiation exposure may increase the risk for malignancies (onset may be delayed). Dehydration may occur due to gastrointestinal adverse events (diarrhea, nausea, vomiting); monitor oral intake, hydration status, and urine output.

Adverse Reactions

>10%:

Cardiovascular: Peripheral edema (13%)

Gastrointestinal: Nausea (36%), diarrhea (25%), vomiting (19%)

Hematologic & oncologic: Anemia (93%; grades 3/4: 6%), lymphocytopenia (72%; grades 3/4: 20%), leukopenia (35%; grades 3/4: 3%), thrombocytopenia (31%; grades 3/4: 1% to 6%), neutropenia (18%; grades 3/4: 1% to 3%)

1% to 10%:
Endocrine & metabolic: Dehydration (3%)
Hematologic & oncologic: Pancytopenia (2%; grades 3/4: 1%)
Local: Injection site reactions (erythema, pain, swelling: 1%)
Renal: Renal failure/insufficiency (3%)
<1%: Aplastic anemia

Storage/Stability Store at room temperature <40°C (104°F). Keep in original container or equivalent radiation shielding.

Preparation for Administration Do not dilute or mix with any solutions. Radiopharmaceutical; use appropriate precautions for handling and disposal. Wear gloves and use adequate shielding for handling and administration.

Mechanism of Action Alpha particle-emitting isotope; emits high energy, short-range alpha particles which target bone metastases; mimics calcium to form complexes with bone mineral in areas with increased bone turnover. Alpha emission induces double strand DNA breaks in adjacent cells, which results in an antitumor effect on the bone metastases.

Pharmacodynamics/Kinetics

Onset: A significant response in pain index was seen at week 2 (Nilsson, 2012).
Duration: Mean duration of pain relief: 44 days (Nilsson, 2012)
Distribution: Primarily to the bone or excreted in to intestine
Metabolism: Decays (is not metabolized)
Half-life elimination: 11.4 days (Nilsson, 2007)
Excretion: Feces (13%); urine (2%)

Dosing

Adult & Geriatric Note: Calculate administration volume using patient weight, radioactivity content (at the reference date), and decay correction factor; determine net patient dose immediately before and after administration with an appropriate radioisotope dose calibrator; refer to product labeling for further details. Prior to initial dose, ANC should be ≥1500/mm^3, platelets ≥100,000/mm^3, and hemoglobin ≥10 g/dL.

Prostate cancer, castration-resistant with symptomatic bone metastases: Males: IV: 50 kBq/kg (1.35 microcurie/kg) every 4 weeks for 6 doses.

Renal Impairment

Mild (CrCl 60-89 mL/minute) or moderate (CrCl 30-59 mL/minute) impairment: No dosage adjustment necessary.
Severe impairment (CrCl <30 mL/minute): No dosage adjustment provided in manufacturer's labeling, (has not been studied).

Hepatic Impairment

Mild impairment: No dosage adjustment necessary.
Moderate-to-severe impairment: No dosage adjustment provided in manufacturer's labeling (has not been studied); however, dosage adjustment is not likely needed because not metabolized hepatically or eliminated in bile.

Adjustment for Toxicity

ANC <1000/mm^3 or platelets <50,000/mm^3 (prior to subsequent doses): Withhold treatment until hematologic recovery; if recovery does not occur within 6-8 weeks from the last dose (despite supportive care), discontinue treatment.
Compromised bone marrow reserve: Closely monitor; discontinue if life-threatening complications occur despite supportive care

Administration Administer as a slow IV injection over 1 minute. Flush IV line or cannula before and after administration with saline. Radiopharmaceutical; use appropriate precautions for handling and disposal.

Monitoring Parameters CBC with differential at baseline and prior to each dose. Monitor fluid intake, hydration status, and urine output.

Additional Information Patients and caregivers should use the following precautions to minimize exposure:

1. When handling bodily fluids, wear gloves and wash hands after handling.
2. Wash any clothing soiled with radium Ra 223 dichloride promptly and separately from other clothing.
3. Where a normal toilet is available, use in preference to a urinal.
4. Flush toilet several times after use.
5. Wash hands thoroughly after urination.

Dosage Forms Considerations Xofigo contains 1000 kBq/mL (27 microcurie/mL)

Dosage Forms Excipient information presented when available (limited, particularly for generics); consult specific product labeling.

Solution, Intravenous:

Xofigo: 27 MCCI/ML (1 ea)

◆ **rAHF** see Antihemophilic Factor (Recombinant) on page 119

◆ **rAHF** see Antihemophilic Factor (Recombinant [Porcine Sequence]) on page 123

◆ **Ralivia (Can)** see TraMADol on page 1672

Raloxifene (ral OKS i feen)

Related Information

Safe Handling of Hazardous Drugs on page 2292

Brand Names: US Evista

Brand Names: Canada ACT Raloxifene; Apo-Raloxifene; Evista; PMS-Raloxifene; Teva-Raloxifene

Index Terms Keoxifene Hydrochloride; Raloxifene Hydrochloride

Pharmacologic Category Selective Estrogen Receptor Modulator (SERM)

Use Prevention and treatment of osteoporosis in postmenopausal women; risk reduction for invasive breast cancer in postmenopausal women with osteoporosis and in postmenopausal women with high risk for invasive breast cancer

Labeled Contraindications History of or current venous thromboembolic disorders (including DVT, PE, and retinal vein thrombosis); pregnancy or women who could become pregnant; breast-feeding

Pregnancy Considerations Adverse events were observed in in animal reproduction studies. Raloxifene is contraindicated for use in women who are or may become pregnant.

Breast-Feeding Considerations It is not known if raloxifene is excreted into breast milk. Breast-feeding is contraindicated by the manufacturer.

Warnings/Precautions Hazardous agent - use appropriate precautions for handling and disposal (NIOSH 2014 [group 2]).

[U.S. Boxed Warning]: May increase the risk for DVT or PE; use contraindicated in patients with history of or current venous thromboembolic disorders. Use with caution in patients at high risk for venous thromboembolism; the risk for DVT and PE are higher in the first 4 months of treatment. Discontinue at least 72 hours prior to and during prolonged immobilization (postoperative recovery or prolonged bedrest). **[U.S. Boxed Warning]: The risk of death due to stroke may be increased in women with coronary heart disease or in women at risk for coronary events;** use with caution in patients with cardiovascular disease. Not be used for the prevention of ▶

◄ cardiovascular disease. Use caution with moderate-to-severe renal dysfunction, hepatic impairment, unexplained uterine bleeding, and in women with a history of elevated triglycerides in response to treatment with oral estrogens (or estrogen/progestin). Safety with concomitant estrogen therapy has not been established. Safety and efficacy in premenopausal women or men have not been established. Not indicated for treatment of invasive breast cancer, to reduce the risk of recurrence of invasive breast cancer or to reduce the risk of noninvasive breast cancer. The efficacy (for breast cancer risk reduction) in women with inherited BRCA1 and BRCA1 mutations has not been established.

Adverse Reactions Note: Raloxifene has been associated with increased risk of thromboembolism (DVT, PE) and superficial thrombophlebitis; risk is similar to reported risk of HRT

>10%:

  Cardiovascular: Peripheral edema (3% to 14%)

  Endocrine & metabolic: Hot flashes (8% to 29%)

  Neuromuscular & skeletal: Arthralgia (11% to 16%), leg cramps/muscle spasm (6% to 12%)

  Miscellaneous: Flu syndrome (14% to 15%), infection (11%)

1% to 10%:

  Cardiovascular: Chest pain (3%), venous thromboembolism (1% to 2%)

  Central nervous system: Insomnia (6%)

  Dermatologic: Rash (6%)

  Endocrine & metabolic: Breast pain (4%)

  Gastrointestinal: Weight gain (9%), abdominal pain (7%), vomiting (5%), flatulence (2% to 3%), cholelithiasis (≤3%), gastroenteritis (≤3%)

  Genitourinary: Vaginal bleeding (6%), leukorrhea (3%), urinary tract disorder (3%), uterine disorder (3%), vaginal hemorrhage (3%), endometrial disorder (≤3%)

  Neuromuscular & skeletal: Myalgia (8%), tendon disorder (4%)

  Respiratory: Bronchitis (10%), sinusitis (10%), pharyngitis (8%), pneumonia (3%), laryngitis (≤2%)

  Miscellaneous: Diaphoresis (3%)

<1%, postmarketing, and/or case reports: Apolipoprotein A-1 increased, apolipoprotein B decreased, death related to VTE, fibrinogen decreased, hypertriglyceridemia (in women with a history of increased triglycerides in response to oral estrogens), intermittent claudication, LDL cholesterol decreased, lipoprotein decreased, retinal vein occlusion, stroke related to VTE, superficial thrombophlebitis, total serum cholesterol decreased

Drug Interactions

Metabolism/Transport Effects None known.

Avoid Concomitant Use

  Avoid concomitant use of Raloxifene with any of the following: Ospemifene

Increased Effect/Toxicity

  Raloxifene may increase the levels/effects of: Ospemifene

Decreased Effect

  Raloxifene may decrease the levels/effects of: Levothyroxine; Ospemifene

  The levels/effects of Raloxifene may be decreased by: Bile Acid Sequestrants

Storage/Stability Store at controlled room temperature of 20°C to 25°C (68°F to 77°F); excursions permitted to 15°C to 30°C (59°F to 86°F).

Mechanism of Action A selective estrogen receptor modulator (SERM), meaning that it affects some of the same receptors that estrogen does, but not all, and in some instances, it antagonizes or blocks estrogen; it acts like estrogen to prevent bone loss and has the potential to block some estrogen effects in the breast and uterine tissues. Raloxifene decreases bone resorption, increasing bone mineral density and decreasing fracture incidence.

Pharmacodynamics/Kinetics

Onset of action: 8 weeks

Absorption: Rapid; ~60%

Distribution: 2348 L/kg

Protein binding: >95% to albumin and α-glycoprotein; does not bind to sex-hormone-binding globulin

Metabolism: Hepatic, extensive first-pass effect; metabolized to glucuronide conjugates

Bioavailability: ~2%

Half-life elimination: 28-33 hours

Excretion: Primarily feces; urine (<0.2% as unchanged drug; <6% as glucuronide conjugates)

Dosing

Adult & Geriatric

Osteoporosis: Females: Oral: 60 mg once daily

Invasive breast cancer risk reduction: Female: Oral: 60 mg once daily for 5 years per ASCO guidelines (Visvanathan, 2009)

Renal Impairment No dosage adjustment provided in manufacturer's labeling. Use caution in moderate-to-severe impairment.

Hepatic Impairment No dosage adjustment provided in manufacturer's labeling (has not been studied). Use with caution.

Administration May be administered without regard to meals.

Hazardous agent; use appropriate precautions for handling and disposal (NIOSH 2014 [group 2]).

Monitoring Parameters Lipid profile; adequate diagnostic measures, including endometrial sampling, if indicated, should be performed to rule out malignancy in all cases of undiagnosed abnormal vaginal bleeding

Osteoporosis: Bone mineral density (BMD) should be evaluated 1 to 2 years after initiating therapy and every 2 years thereafter (NOF [Cosman 2014]); annual measurements of height and weight; serum calcium and 25(OH)D; may consider monitoring biochemical markers of bone turnover

Dietary Considerations May be taken without regard to meals. Osteoporosis prevention or treatment: Ensure adequate calcium and vitamin D intake; if dietary intake is inadequate, dietary supplementation is recommended. Women and men should consume:

Calcium: 1000 mg/day (men: 50 to 70 years) **or** 1200 mg/day (women ≥51 years and men ≥71 years) (IOM, 2011; NOF [Cosman 2014])

Vitamin D: 800 to 1000 int. units daily (men and women ≥50 years) (NOF [Cosman 2014]). Recommended Dietary Allowance (RDA): 600 int. units daily (men and women ≤70 years) **or** 800 int. units daily (men and women ≥71 years) (IOM, 2011).

Additional Information The decrease in estrogen-related adverse effects with the selective estrogen-receptor modulators in general and raloxifene in particular should improve compliance and decrease the incidence of cardiovascular events and fractures while not increasing breast cancer.

◄ **Oncology Comment:** The American Society of Clinical Oncology (ASCO) guidelines for breast cancer risk reduction (Visvanathan, 2009) recommend raloxifene (for 5 years) as an option to reduce the risk of ER-positive invasive breast cancer in postmenopausal women with a 5-year projected risk (based on NCI trial model) of ≥1.66%, or with lobular carcinoma *in situ*. Raloxifene should not be used in premenopausal women. Women with osteoporosis may use raloxifene beyond 5 years of treatment. According to the NCCN breast cancer risk reduction guidelines (v.2.2009), raloxifene is only recommended for postmenopausal women (≥35 years of age), and is equivalent to tamoxifen although, raloxifene has a better adverse event profile; however, tamoxifen is superior in reducing the risk on noninvasive breast cancer.

Medication Guide Available Yes

Dosage Forms Excipient information presented when available (limited, particularly for generics); consult specific product labeling.

Tablet, Oral, as hydrochloride:

Evista: 60 mg

Generic: 60 mg

◆ **Raloxifene Hydrochloride** *see Raloxifene on page 1451*

Raltitrexed (ral ti TREX ed)

Related Information

Safe Handling of Hazardous Drugs *on page 2292*

Brand Names: Canada Tomudex

Index Terms D1694; ICI-D1694; Raltitrexed Disodium; TDX; ZD1694

Pharmacologic Category Antineoplastic Agent, Antimetabolite; Antineoplastic Agent, Antimetabolite (Antifolate)

Use Note: Not approved in the US

Treatment of advanced colorectal cancer

Labeled Contraindications Hypersensitivity to raltitrexed or any component of the formulation; severe renal or hepatic impairment; pregnancy or breast-feeding

Pregnancy Considerations Use is contraindicated in women who are or may become pregnant during treatment. Pregnancy should be excluded prior to treatment, and should be avoided during treatment and for 6 months following treatment (including women with male partners receiving treatment). Pregnant women should not handle this medication.

Breast-Feeding Considerations Use in nursing women is contraindicated by the manufacturer.

Warnings/Precautions Hazardous agent - use appropriate precautions for handling and disposal (meets NIOSH 2014 criteria). Neutropenia, leukopenia, anemia, and thrombocytopenia may occur. Use with caution in patients with preexisting marrow suppression. Nausea, vomiting and diarrhea are common; mucositis and stomatitis may also occur. Severe diarrhea with concomitant hematologic toxicity (neutropenia) may be life-threatening and may require discontinuation or subsequent dose reduction.

Use caution in elderly, mild-to-moderate hepatic or renal dysfunction (use in severe hepatic or renal impairment is contraindicated). Use is not recommended in clinical jaundice or decompensated hepatic disease. Therapy interruption is required in patients with hepatotoxicity; may reintroduce therapy only with decrease in hepatic enzymes to grade 2. Asymptomatic and self-limiting increases (reversible) in ALT and AST may occur. Use caution in patients who have received prior radiation therapy.

Folinic acid (leucovorin calcium), folic acid, or folate-containing medications (eg, multivitamins) may interfere with raltitrexed; do not administer immediately prior to or concurrently with raltitrexed. May cause malaise/weakness (caution patients concerning operation of machinery/driving). Use in pediatric patients is not recommended by the manufacturer.

Adverse Reactions

>10%:

Central nervous system: Fever (2% to 23%)

Dermatologic: Rash (14%)

Gastrointestinal: Nausea (58%; grades 3/4: 12%), diarrhea (38%; grades 3/4: 11%), vomiting (38%; grades 3/4: 12%), anorexia (26% to 28%), abdominal pain (18%), constipation (13% to 15%), mucositis/stomatitis (12%; grades 3/4: 2%)

Hematologic: Leukopenia (20% to 22%; grade 3/4: 12% to 13%; nadir within 7-14 days, recovery by 21 days); anemia (15% to 18%; grades 3/4: 7% to 8%)

Hepatic: Transaminases increased (14% to 18%; grades 3/4: 10%)

Neuromuscular & skeletal: Weakness (46% to 49%)

1% to 10%:

Cardiovascular: Peripheral edema (10%), arrhythmias (3%), CHF (2%)

Central nervous system: Headache (6%), dizziness (4% to 5%), chills (4%), malaise (4%), pain (4%), insomnia (3% to 4%), depression (3%)

Dermatologic: Alopecia (6%), cellulitis (3%), pruritus (3%)

Endocrine & metabolic: Dehydration (6% to 7%), hypokalemia (2%)

Gastrointestinal: Dyspepsia (6%), taste perversion (6%), weight loss (6%), flatulence (2% to 3%), xerostomia (2% to 3%)

Genitourinary: Urinary tract infection (3%)

Hematologic: Thrombocytopenia (5% to 6%; grades 3/4: 4%)

Hepatic: Alkaline phosphatase increased (2% to 3%), bilirubin increased (2% to 3%; grades 3/4: 2%)

Neuromuscular & skeletal: Paresthesia (2% to 3%), myalgia (3%), arthralgia (<2%), hypertonia (<2%)

Ocular: Conjunctivitis (2% to 3%)

Renal: Serum creatinine increased (2% to 3%)

Respiratory: Cough (5%), dyspnea (4% to 5%), pharyngitis (4% to 5%)

Miscellaneous: Flu-like syndrome (6% to 8%), diaphoresis (3% to 4%), infection (3%), sepsis (2% to 3%)

<1%: Desquamation

Drug Interactions

Metabolism/Transport Effects None known.

Avoid Concomitant Use

Avoid concomitant use of Raltitrexed with any of the following: BCG (Intravesical); CloZAPine; Dipyrone; Folic Acid; Leucovorin Calcium-Levoleucovorin; Levomefolate; Methylfolate; Multivitamins/Minerals (with ADEK, Folate, Iron)

Increased Effect/Toxicity

Raltitrexed may increase the levels/effects of: CloZAPine

The levels/effects of Raltitrexed may be increased by: Dipyrone

◄ **Decreased Effect**
Raltitrexed may decrease the levels/effects of: BCG (Intravesical)

The levels/effects of Raltitrexed may be decreased by: Folic Acid; Leucovorin Calcium-Levoleucovorin; Levomefolate; Methylfolate; Multivitamins/Minerals (with ADEK, Folate, Iron)

Storage/Stability Intact vials should be refrigerated at 2°C to 25°C (36°F to 77°F). Protect from light. Reconstituted and subsequent IV admixture solutions (saline or dextrose) are stable for up to 24 hours under refrigeration at 2°C to 8°C (36°F to 46°F), although the manufacturer recommends use as soon as possible after preparation.

Preparation for Administration Hazardous agent; use appropriate precautions for handling and disposal (meets NIOSH 2014 criteria). Reconstitute 2 mg vial with 4 mL SWFI to produce 0.5 mg/mL solution; volume required for dose should be further diluted by adding to 50-250 mL NS or D_5W.

Mechanism of Action Raltitrexed is a folate analogue that inhibits thymidylate synthase, blocking purine synthesis. This results in an overall inhibition of DNA synthesis.

Pharmacodynamics/Kinetics

Distribution: V_{ss}: 548 L

Protein binding: 93%

Metabolism: Undergoes extensive intracellular metabolism to active polyglutamate forms; appears to be little or no systemic metabolism of the drug

Half-life elimination: Triphasic; Beta: 2 hours; Terminal: 198 hours

Excretion: Urine (~50% as unchanged drug); feces (~15%)

Dosing

Adult & Geriatric Note: Treatment should be administered only if WBC >4000/mm^3, ANC >2000/mm^3, and platelets >100,000/mm^3

Colorectal cancer, advanced: IV: 3 mg/m^2 every 3 weeks

Malignant pleural mesothelioma (off-label use): IV: 3 mg/m^2 every 3 weeks (in combination with cisplatin) (van Meerbeeck, 2005)

Renal Impairment

CrCl >65 mL/minute: No dosage adjustment necessary.

CrCl 55-65 mL/minute: Administer 75% of dose every 4 weeks

CrCl 25-54 mL/minute: Administer percentage of dose equivalent to CrCl every 4 weeks (eg, 25% of dose for CrCl of 25 mL/minute)

CrCl <25 mL/minute: Do not administer (use is contraindicated in severe renal impairment)

Hepatic Impairment Use is not recommended in clinical jaundice or decompensated liver disease. Patients who develop hepatic toxicity should have treatment held until returns to grade 2.

Mild-to-moderate impairment: No dosage adjustment necessary.

Severe impairment: Use is contraindicated.

Obesity *ASCO Guidelines for appropriate chemotherapy dosing in obese adults with cancer:* Utilize patient's actual body weight (full weight) for calculation of body surface area- or weight-based dosing, particularly when the intent of therapy is curative; manage regimen-related toxicities in the same manner as for nonobese patients; if a dose reduction is utilized due to toxicity, consider resumption of full weight-based dosing with subsequent cycles, especially if cause of toxicity (eg, hepatic or renal impairment) is resolved (Griggs, 2012).

Adjustment for Toxicity Delay dose in subsequent cycles until recovery from toxicity.

Grade 4 gastrointestinal toxicity (diarrhea or mucositis) or grade 3 gastrointestinal toxicity in combination with grade 4 hematologic toxicity: Discontinue therapy and manage with supportive measures.

Grade 3 hematologic toxicity (neutropenia or thrombocytopenia) or grade 2 gastrointestinal toxicity (diarrhea or mucositis): Reduce dose by 25%.

Grade 4 hematologic toxicity (neutropenia or thrombocytopenia) or grade 3 gastrointestinal toxicity (diarrhea or mucositis): Reduce dose by 50%.

Combination Regimens

Malignant pleural mesothelioma: Cisplatin-Raltitrexed (Mesothelioma) on page 1911

Administration Administer via IV infusion over 15 minutes. Hazardous agent; use appropriate precautions for handling and disposal (meets NIOSH 2014 criteria).

Monitoring Parameters CBC with differential (at baseline, prior to each treatment, or weekly if GI toxicity observed); hepatic function tests and serum creatinine (at baseline and prior to each treatment); signs of GI toxicity

Dietary Considerations Avoid folic acid, folinic acid (leucovorin calcium), and multivitamins with folic acid close to and during administration.

Product Availability Not available in the US

Dosage Forms: Canada Excipient information presented when available (limited, particularly for generics); consult specific product labeling.

Injection, powder for reconstitution, as disodium:

Tomudex®: 2 mg

♦ **Raltitrexed Disodium** see Raltitrexed on page 1454

Ramucirumab (ra mue SIR ue mab)

Related Information

Common Toxicity Criteria on page 2122

Brand Names: US Cyramza

Brand Names: Canada Cyramza

Index Terms IMC-1121B

Pharmacologic Category Antineoplastic Agent, Monoclonal Antibody; Antineoplastic Agent, Vascular Endothelial Growth Factor (VEGF) Inhibitor; Antineoplastic Agent, Vascular Endothelial Growth Factor Receptor 2 (VEGFR2) Inhibitor

Use

US labeling:

Colorectal cancer, metastatic: Treatment (in combination with FOLFIRI [irinotecan, leucovorin, and fluorouracil]) of metastatic colorectal cancer (mCRC) in patients with disease progression on or after prior therapy with bevacizumab, oxaliplatin, and a fluoropyrimidine.

Gastric cancer, advanced or metastatic: Treatment (single-agent or in combination with paclitaxel) of advanced or metastatic gastric or gastroesophageal junction adenocarcinoma in patients with disease progression on or following fluoropyrimidine- or platinum-containing chemotherapy

Non-small cell lung cancer, metastatic: Treatment (in combination with docetaxel) of metastatic non-small cell lung cancer (NSCLC) in patients with disease progression on or after platinum-based chemotherapy. Patients with EGFR or ALK genomic tumor aberrations should have disease progression on FDA-approved therapy for these aberrations prior to receiving ramucirumab.

◄ *Canadian labeling:* **Gastric cancer, advanced or metastatic:** Treatment (single-agent or in combination with paclitaxel) of advanced or metastatic gastric or gastroesophageal junction adenocarcinoma in patients with disease progression on or following fluoropyrimidine- or platinum-containing chemotherapy.

Labeled Contraindications

There are no contraindications listed in the manufacturer's US labeling.

Canadian labeling: Hypersensitivity to ramucirumab or any component of the formulation.

Pregnancy Considerations Ramucirumab inhibits angiogenesis, which is of critical importance to human fetal development. Based on the mechanism of action, ramucirumab may cause fetal harm if administered during pregnancy. Women of reproductive potential should use effective contraception during and for at least 3 months after the last ramucirumab dose. Ramucirumab may impair fertility in women.

Breast-Feeding Considerations It is not known if ramucirumab is excreted in breast milk. Immunoglobulins are excreted in breast milk, and it is assumed that ramucirumab may appear in breast milk. Due to the potential for serious adverse reactions in the nursing infant, breast-feeding is not recommended by the manufacturer.

Warnings/Precautions **[US Boxed Warning]: Ramucirumab is associated with an increased risk of hemorrhage and gastrointestinal hemorrhage, which may be severe or sometimes fatal. Discontinue ramucirumab permanently in patients who experience serious bleeding.** Patients receiving NSAIDs were excluded from some clinical trials; the risk of gastric hemorrhage in patients with gastric tumors receiving NSAIDs is not known. In addition, NSCLC patients receiving therapeutic anticoagulation or chronic NSAID or other antiplatelet therapy (other than aspirin), or with radiograph evidence of major airway or blood vessel involvement or intratumor cavitation were also excluded from the clinical study; the risk of pulmonary hemorrhage in such patients is not known. Serious and fatal arterial thrombotic events, including MI, cardiac arrest, cerebrovascular accident, and cerebral ischemia, have occurred with ramucirumab. Discontinue permanently in patients who experience serious arterial thrombotic events.

Ramucirumab is associated with infusion-related reactions (may be severe), generally occurring with the first or second dose. Symptoms of infusion reactions have included chills, flushing, hypotension, bronchospasm, dyspnea, hypoxia, wheezing, chest pain/tightness, supraventricular tachycardia, back pain/spasms, rigors/tremors, and/or paresthesia. Monitor for infusion reaction symptoms during infusion; discontinue immediately and permanently for grade 3 or 4 reactions. Administer in a facility equipped to manage infusion reactions. May cause and/or worsen hypertension; the incidence of severe hypertension is increased with ramucirumab. Blood pressure (BP) should be controlled prior to treatment initiation. Monitor BP every 2 weeks (more frequently if indicated) during treatment. If severe hypertension occurs, temporarily withhold until medically controlled. Discontinue permanently if medically significant hypertension cannot be controlled with antihypertensive therapy or in patients with hypertensive crisis or hypertensive encephalopathy. Ramucirumab is associated with proteinuria (may be severe). Monitor proteinuria during treatment by urine dipstick and/or urinary protein creatinine ratio for the development of and/or worsening of proteinuria. Withhold treatment for urine protein levels ≥2 grams/24 hours. Discontinue permanently for urine protein >3 grams/24 hours or for nephrotic syndrome.

[US Boxed Warning]: Ramucirumab may increase the risk of gastro-intestinal perforation, a potentially fatal event. Discontinue permanently in patients who experience a gastrointestinal perforation. Cases of reversible posterior leukoencephalopathy syndrome (RPLS) have been reported (may be fatal). Symptoms of RPLS include headache, seizure, confusion, lethargy, blindness and/or other vision, or neurologic disturbances. Confirm diagnosis of RPLS with MRI; discontinue ramucirumab with confirmed RPLS diagnosis. Resolution of symptoms may occur within days after discontinuation, although neurologic sequelae may remain in some patients. **[US Boxed Warning]: Impaired wound healing can occur with antibodies inhibiting the VEGF pathway. Discontinue ramucirumab in patients with impaired wound healing. Withhold ramucirumab prior to surgery and discontinue in patients who develop wound healing complications.** Following surgery, use clinical judgment to resume based on adequate wound healing. If wound healing complications develop during treatment, withhold ramucirumab until wound is fully healed. Ramucirumab was not studied in patients with serious or nonhealing wounds. Clinical deterioration, including new onset or worsening encephalopathy, ascites, or hepatorenal syndrome has been reported in patients with Child-Pugh class B or C cirrhosis receiving ramucirumab. Use in patients with Child-Pugh class B or C cirrhosis only if the potential benefits outweigh the potential risks. Hypothyroidism has been observed; monitor thyroid function during treatment.

A higher incidence of neutropenia and thrombocytopenia were observed when ramucirumab was used in combination with paclitaxel (compared to paclitaxel with placebo); monitor CBC with differential when used in combination with paclitaxel. Antiangiogenic medications may increase the risk for heart failure (HF); events consistent with HF have been reported with ramucirumab. Use with caution in patients with known (or at risk of) coronary artery disease. Ramucirumab may enhance the cardiotoxicity of other chemotherapy with cardiotoxic potential (Cyramza Canadian labeling 2015).

Adverse Reactions As reported with monotherapy. Frequency not always defined.

Cardiovascular: Hypertension (16%; grades 3/4: 8%), arterial thrombosis (including myocardial infarction, cardiac arrest, cerebrovascular accident, and cerebral ischemia; 2%)

Central nervous system: Headache (9%)

Dermatologic: Skin rash (4%)

Endocrine & metabolic: Hyponatremia (6%)

Gastrointestinal: Diarrhea (14%), intestinal obstruction (2%)

Genitourinary: Proteinuria (8% to 17%; grade ≥3: 1%)

Hematologic & oncologic: Decreased red blood cells (requiring transfusion; 11%), neutropenia (5%), anemia (4%), hemorrhage (2% to 4%)

Immunologic: Antibody development (3%; neutralizing: 1%)

Respiratory: Epistaxis (5%)

Miscellaneous: Infusion related reaction (≤16%; reactions minimized with premedications)

<1% and frequency not defined: Gastrointestinal perforation, reversible posterior leukoencephalopathy syndrome

Drug Interactions

Metabolism/Transport Effects None known.

Avoid Concomitant Use

Avoid concomitant use of Ramucirumab with any of the following: Belimumab ▶

◀ **Increased Effect/Toxicity**
Ramucirumab may increase the levels/effects of: Belimumab; Bisphospho-nate Derivatives

Decreased Effect There are no known significant interactions involving a decrease in effect.

Storage/Stability Store intact vials at 2°C to 8°C (36°F to 46°F); do not freeze. Retain in original carton to protect from light. Do not shake. Solutions diluted for infusion may be stored at 2°C to 8°C (36°F to 46°F) for no longer than 24 hours (do not freeze) or may be stored for 4 hours at room temperature (below 25°C [77°F]); do not shake diluted product.

Preparation for Administration Dilute total dose in NS 250 mL prior to administration (the manufacturer recommends a final volume of 250 mL). Do not use dextrose containing solutions. Invert gently to mix thoroughly; do not shake. Discard unused portion of the vial.

Mechanism of Action Ramucirumab is a recombinant monoclonal antibody which inhibits vascular endothelial growth factor receptor 2 (VEGFR2). Ramu-cirumab has a high affinity for VEGFR2 (Spratlin, 2010), binding to it and blocking binding of VEGFR ligands, VEGF-A, VEGF-C, and VEGF-D to inhibit activation of VEGFR2, thereby inhibiting ligand-induced proliferation and migration of endothelial cells. VEGFR2 inhibition results in reduced tumor vascularity and growth (Fuchs, 2014).

Pharmacodynamics/Kinetics Half-life elimination: 14 days

Dosing

Adult & Geriatric Note: Premedicate prior to infusion with an IV H_1 antagonist (for patients who experienced a grade 1 or 2 infusion reaction with a prior infusion, also premedicate with dexamethasone or equivalent and acetaminophen).

US labeling:

Colorectal cancer, metastatic: IV: 8 mg/kg every 2 weeks in combination with FOLFIRI (irinotecan, leucovorin, and fluorouracil); continue until disease progression or unacceptable toxicity.

Gastric cancer, advanced or metastatic: IV: 8 mg/kg every 2 weeks as a single agent or in combination with paclitaxel; continue until disease progression or unacceptable toxicity.

Non-small cell lung cancer, metastatic: IV: 10 mg/kg on day 1 every 21 days in combination with docetaxel; continue until disease progression or unacceptable toxicity

Canadian labeling: **Gastric cancer, advanced or metastatic:** Adults: IV: 8 mg/kg every 2 weeks as a single agent or in combination with paclitaxel; continue until disease progression or unacceptable toxicity.

Renal Impairment No dosage adjustment necessary.

Hepatic Impairment

Mild impairment (normal bilirubin with AST > ULN **or** total bilirubin >1 to 1.5 times ULN and any AST): No dosage adjustment necessary.

Moderate impairment (total bilirubin >1.5 to 3 times ULN and any AST): No dosage adjustment necessary.

Severe impairment (total bilirubin >3 times ULN and any AST): There are no dosage adjustments provided in the manufacturer's labeling (has not been studied). Use in patients with Child-Pugh class B or C cirrhosis only if the potential benefits outweigh the potential risks.

Adjustment for Toxicity

Infusion-related reaction:

Grade 1 or 2: Reduce infusion rate by 50%

Grade 3 or 4: Permanently discontinue

Hypertension:

Severe hypertension: Interrupt infusion until controlled with medical management

Severe hypertension, uncontrolled: Permanently discontinue

Proteinuria:

Urine protein ≥2 g/24 hours (first dose reduction): Withhold treatment; when urine protein returns to <2 g/24 hours, reinitiate at a reduced dose of 6 mg/kg (if initial dose was 8 mg/kg) or 8 mg/kg (if initial dose was 10 mg/kg)

Recurrent urine protein ≥2 g/24 hours (second dose reduction): Withhold treatment; when urine protein returns to <2 g/24 hours, reinitiate at a reduced dose of 5 mg/kg (if first dose reduction was to 6 mg/kg) or 6 mg/kg (if first dose reduction was to 8 mg/kg)

Urine protein >3 g/24 hours: Discontinue permanently

Nephrotic syndrome: Discontinue permanently

Arterial thrombotic events: Discontinue permanently

Bleeding, grade 3 or 4: Discontinue permanently

Gastrointestinal perforation: Discontinue permanently

Reversible posterior leukoencephalopathy syndrome (RPLS): Discontinue permanently for confirmed diagnosis

Wound healing complications: Withhold treatment prior to surgery; do not reinitiate until the surgical wound is fully healed. If wound healing complications develop during treatment, withhold ramucirumab until the wound is fully healed.

Combination Regimens

Colorectal cancer: Ramucirumab-FOLFIRI (Colorectal) on page 2072

Gastric cancer:

Paclitaxel-Ramucirumab (Gastric) on page 2056

Ramucirumab (Gastric Regimen) on page 2072

Lung cancer (non-small cell): Docetaxel-Ramucirumab (NSCLC) on page 1946

Administration Premedicate prior to infusion with an IV H_1 antagonist; for patients who experienced a grade 1 or 2 infusion reaction with a prior infusion, also premedicate with dexamethasone (or equivalent) and acetaminophen.

Infuse over 60 minutes through a separate infusion line using an infusion pump; the use of a 0.22 micron protein sparing filter is recommended. Do not administer as an IV push or bolus. Flush the line with NS after infusion is complete. Do not infuse in the same IV line with electrolytes or other medications. Administer ramucirumab prior to docetaxel, paclitaxel, or FOLFIRI if administering in combination. Monitor for infusion reaction; reduce infusion rate (by 50%) for grade 1 or 2 infusion reaction; discontinue permanently for grade 3 or 4 infusion reaction.

Emetic Potential Minimal (<10%)

Monitoring Parameters Liver function tests; urine protein (by urine dipstick and/or urinary protein creatinine ratio); thyroid function; CBC with differential (when used as a part of combination chemotherapy); blood pressure (every 2 weeks; more frequently if indicated); signs/symptoms of infusion-related reactions (during infusion); signs/symptoms of arterial thromboembolic events,

◀ bleeding/hemorrhage, gastrointestinal perforation, wound healing impairment, and reversible posterior leukoencephalopathy syndrome

Dosage Forms Excipient information presented when available (limited, particularly for generics); consult specific product labeling.

Solution, Intravenous [preservative free]:

Cyramza: 100 mg/10 mL (10 mL); 500 mg/50 mL (50 mL) [contains polysorbate 80]

- ◆ **RAN-Anastrozole (Can)** *see* Anastrozole *on page 112*
- ◆ **RAN-Bicalutamide (Can)** *see* Bicalutamide *on page 207*
- ◆ **RAN-Ciproflox (Can)** *see* Ciprofloxacin (Systemic) *on page 327*
- ◆ **RAN-Fentanyl Matrix Patch (Can)** *see* FentaNYL *on page 692*
- ◆ **RAN-Imipenem-Cilastatin (Can)** *see* Imipenem and Cilastatin *on page 893*
- ◆ **RAN-Letrozole (Can)** *see* Letrozole *on page 1019*
- ◆ **RAN™-Nabilone (Can)** *see* Nabilone *on page 1187*
- ◆ **RAN-Olanzapine (Can)** *see* OLANZapine *on page 1242*
- ◆ **RAN-Olanzapine ODT (Can)** *see* OLANZapine *on page 1242*
- ◆ **RAN-Ondansetron (Can)** *see* Ondansetron *on page 1253*
- ◆ **Rapamune** *see* Sirolimus *on page 1531*
- ◆ **Rapamycin** *see* Sirolimus *on page 1531*

Rasburicase (ras BYOOR i kayse)

Brand Names: US Elitek

Brand Names: Canada Fasturtec

Index Terms Recombinant Urate Oxidase; Urate Oxidase

Pharmacologic Category Enzyme; Enzyme, Urate-Oxidase (Recombinant)

Use

Hyperuricemia associated with malignancy: Initial management of uric acid levels in pediatric and adult patients with leukemia, lymphoma, and solid tumor malignancies receiving chemotherapy expected to result in tumor lysis and elevation of plasma uric acid

Limitations of use: Indicated only for a single course of treatment

Labeled Contraindications History of anaphylaxis or severe hypersensitivity to rasburicase or any component of the formulation; history of hemolytic reaction or methemoglobinemia associated with rasburicase; glucose-6-phosphatase dehydrogenase (G6PD) deficiency

Pregnancy Considerations Adverse effects were observed in animal reproduction studies. Use during pregnancy only if the benefit to the mother outweighs the potential risk to the fetus.

Breast-Feeding Considerations It is not known if rasburicase is excreted in breast milk. Due to the potential for serious adverse reactions in the nursing infant, a decision should be made to discontinue breast-feeding or the drug, taking into account the benefits of treatment to the mother. The Canadian labeling does not recommend use in breast-feeding women.

Warnings/Precautions [US Boxed Warning]: Severe hypersensitivity reactions (including anaphylaxis) have been reported; immediately and permanently discontinue in patients developing serious hypersensitivity reaction; reactions may occur at any time during treatment, including the initial dose. Signs and symptoms of hypersensitivity may include bronchospasm, chest pain/tightness, dyspnea, hypotension, hypoxia, shock, or urticaria. The safety and efficacy of more than one course of administration has not been established. **[US Boxed Warning]: Due to the risk for hemolysis (<1%), rasburicase is contraindicated in patients with G6PD deficiency; discontinue immediately and permanently in any patient developing hemolysis. Patients at higher risk for G6PD deficiency (eg, African or Mediterranean descent) should be screened prior to therapy;** severe hemolytic reactions occurred within 2 to 4 days of rasburicase initiation. **[US Boxed Warning]: Methemoglobinemia has been reported (<1%). Discontinue immediately and permanently in any patient developing methemoglobinemia;** initiate appropriate treatment (eg, transfusion, methylene blue) if methemoglobinemia occurs.

[US Boxed Warning]: Enzymatic degradation of uric acid in blood samples will occur if left at room temperature, which may interfere with serum uric acid measurements; specific guidelines for the collection of plasma uric acid samples must be followed, including collection in prechilled tubes with heparin anticoagulant, immediate ice water bath immersion and assay within 4 hours. Patients at risk for tumor lysis syndrome should receive appropriate IV hydration as part of uric acid management; however, alkalinization (with sodium bicarbonate) concurrently with rasburicase is not recommended (Coiffier 2008). Rasburicase is immunogenic and can elicit an antibody response; efficacy may be reduced with subsequent courses of therapy.

Adverse Reactions

>10%:
  Cardiovascular: Peripheral edema (50%)
  Central nervous system: Headache (26%), anxiety (24%)
  Dermatologic: Rash (13%; serious: <1%)
  Endocrine & metabolic: Hypophosphatemia (17%), hypervolemia (12%)
  Gastrointestinal: Nausea (27% to 58%), vomiting (38% to 50%), abdominal pain (20% to 22%), constipation (20%), diarrhea (20%), mucositis (15%)
  Hepatic: Hyperbilirubinemia (16%), increased serum ALT (11%)
  Immunologic: Antibody development (children: 11%; IgE: 6%), development of IgG antibodies (18%; neutralizing 8%)
  Infection: Sepsis (12%; serious: 5%)
  Respiratory: Pharyngolaryngeal pain (14%)
  Miscellaneous: Fever (46%)
1% to 10%:
  Cardiovascular: Ischemic heart disease (≥2%), supraventricular arrhythmia (≥2%)
  Endocrine & metabolic: Hyperphosphatemia (10%)
  Gastrointestinal: Gastrointestinal infection (≥2%)
  Hematologic & oncologic: Pulmonary hemorrhage (≥2%)
  Hypersensitivity: Hypersensitivity (4%)
  Infection: Infection (abdominal, ≥2%)
  Respiratory: Respiratory failure (≥2%)
<1%, postmarketing, and/or case reports: Anaphylaxis, hemolysis, methemoglobinemia, muscle spasm, seizure

Drug Interactions

Metabolism/Transport Effects None known.

Avoid Concomitant Use There are no known interactions where it is recommended to avoid concomitant use.

Increased Effect/Toxicity There are no known significant interactions involving an increase in effect.

◀ **Decreased Effect** There are no known significant interactions involving a decrease in effect.

Storage/Stability The lyophilized drug product and the diluent for reconstitution should be stored at 2°C to 8°C (36°F to 46°F); do not freeze. Protect from light. Reconstituted solution and solution diluted for infusion may be stored for up to 24 hours at 2°C to 8°C (36°F to 46°F). Discard unused product.

Preparation for Administration Reconstitute with provided diluent (use 1 mL diluent for the 1.5 mg vial and 5 mL diluent for the 7.5 mg vial). Mix by gently swirling; do **not** shake or vortex. Discard if discolored or containing particulate matter. Total dose should be further diluted in NS to a final volume of 50 mL. Do not use filters during reconstitution or administration.

Mechanism of Action Rasburicase is a recombinant urate-oxidase enzyme, which converts uric acid to allantoin (an inactive and soluble metabolite of uric acid); it does not inhibit the formation of uric acid.

Pharmacodynamics/Kinetics

Onset: Uric acid levels decrease within 4 hours of initial administration

Distribution: Children: 110 to 127 mL/kg; Adults: 76 to 138 mL/kg

Half-life elimination: ~16 to 23 hours

Dosing

Adult & Geriatric Hyperuricemia associated with malignancy: IV: 0.2 mg/kg once daily for up to 5 days (US labeling [use beyond 5 days or administration of more than 1 course is not recommended]) or up to 7 days (Canadian labeling) **or**

Alternate dosing (off-label; Coiffier 2008): 0.05 to 0.2 mg/kg once daily for 1 to 7 days (average of 2 to 3 days) with the duration of treatment dependent on plasma uric acid levels and clinical judgment (patients with significant tumor burden may require an increase to twice daily); the following dose levels are recommended based on risk of tumor lysis syndrome (TLS):

High risk: 0.2 mg/kg once daily (duration is based on plasma uric acid levels)

Intermediate risk: 0.15 mg/kg once daily (duration is based on plasma uric acid levels)

Low risk: 0.1 mg/kg once daily (duration is based on clinical judgment); a dose of 0.05 mg/kg was used effectively in one trial

Single-dose rasburicase (off-label; based on limited data): 0.15 mg/kg (Campara 2009; Liu 2005) **or** 3 to 7.5 mg as a single dose (Hutcherson 2006; McBride 2013; McDonnell 2006; Reeves 2008; Trifilio 2006); repeat doses (1.5 to 6 mg) may be needed based on serum uric acid levels

Prevention in high-risk patients with hematologic malignancies (off-label dosing): 3 mg as a single dose (Jones, 2015)

Pediatric Hyperuricemia associated with malignancy: IV: 0.2 mg/kg once daily for up to 5 days (US labeling [use beyond 5 days or administration of more than 1 course is not recommended]) or up to 7 days (Canadian labeling) **or**

Alternate dosing (off-label; Coiffier 2008): 0.05 to 0.2 mg/kg once daily for 1 to 7 days (average of 2 to 3 days) with the duration of treatment dependent on plasma uric acid levels and clinical judgment (patients with significant tumor burden may require an increase to twice daily); the following dose levels are recommended based on risk of tumor lysis syndrome (TLS):

High risk: 0.2 mg/kg once daily (duration is based on plasma uric acid levels)

Intermediate risk: 0.15 mg/kg once daily (duration is based on plasma uric acid levels); may consider managing initially with a single dose

Low risk: 0.1 mg/kg once daily (duration is based on clinical judgment); a dose of 0.05 mg/kg was used effectively in one trial

Single-dose rasburicase (off-label dosing; based on limited data): 0.15 mg/kg; additional doses may be needed based on serum uric acid levels (Liu 2005)

Prevention in high-risk patients with hematologic malignancies (off-label dosing): 0.2 mg/kg as a single dose (Jones, 2015)

Renal Impairment There are no dosage adjustments provided in the manufacturer's labeling.

Hepatic Impairment There are no dosage adjustments provided in the manufacturer's labeling.

Administration

IV infusion over 30 minutes; do **not** administer as a bolus infusion. Do **not** filter during infusion. If not possible to administer through a separate line, IV line should be flushed with at least 15 mL saline prior to and following rasburicase infusion.

The optimal timing of rasburicase administration (with respect to chemotherapy administration) is not specified in the US labeling. In some studies, chemotherapy was administered 4 to 24 hours after the first rasburicase dose (Cortes 2010; Kikuchi 2009; Vadhan-Raj 2012); however, rasburicase generally may be administered irrespective of chemotherapy timing. The Canadian labeling recommends initiating chemotherapy as soon as 4 hours after rasburicase administration.

Monitoring Parameters Plasma uric acid levels (4 hours after rasburicase administration, then every 6 to 8 hours until TLS resolution), CBC, G6PD deficiency screening (in patients at high risk for deficiency); monitor for hypersensitivity

Test Interactions Specific handling procedures must be followed to prevent the degradation of uric acid in plasma samples. Blood must be collected in prechilled tubes containing heparin anticoagulant. Samples must then be **immediately** immersed and maintained in an ice water bath. Prepare samples by centrifugation in a precooled centrifuge (4°C). Samples must be analyzed within 4 hours of collection.

Dosage Forms Excipient information presented when available (limited, particularly for generics); consult specific product labeling.

Solution Reconstituted, Intravenous:

Elitek: 1.5 mg (1 ea); 7.5 mg (1 ea)

- ◆ **Rayos** *see* PredniSONE *on page 1426*
- ◆ **Reclast** *see* Zoledronic Acid *on page 1790*
- ◆ **Recombinant Factor XIII A-Subunit** *see* Factor XIII A-Subunit (Recombinant) *on page 687*
- ◆ **Recombinant Granulocyte-Macrophage Colony Stimulating Factor** *see* Sargramostim *on page 1515*
- ◆ **Recombinant Human Interleukin-2** *see* Aldesleukin *on page 55*
- ◆ **Recombinant Human Interleukin-11** *see* Oprelvekin *on page 1262*
- ◆ **Recombinant Human Thyrotropin** *see* Thyrotropin Alfa *on page 1645*
- ◆ **Recombinant Interleukin-11** *see* Oprelvekin *on page 1262*
- ◆ **Recombinant Urate Oxidase** *see* Rasburicase *on page 1462*
- ◆ **Recombinate** *see* Antihemophilic Factor (Recombinant) *on page 119*
- ◆ **Reglan** *see* Metoclopramide *on page 1134*

Regorafenib (re goe RAF e nib)

Related Information
Common Toxicity Criteria *on page 2122*
Management of Chemotherapy-Induced Nausea and Vomiting in Adults *on page 2142*
Safe Handling of Hazardous Drugs *on page 2292*

Brand Names: US Stivarga

Brand Names: Canada Stivarga

Index Terms BAY 73-4506

Pharmacologic Category Antineoplastic Agent, Tyrosine Kinase Inhibitor; Antineoplastic Agent, Vascular Endothelial Growth Factor (VEGF) Inhibitor

Use

Colorectal cancer, metastatic: Treatment of metastatic colorectal cancer in patients previously treated with fluoropyrimidine-, oxaliplatin-, and irinotecan-based chemotherapy, anti-VEGF therapy, and anti-EGFR therapy (if *KRAS* wild type)

Gastrointestinal stromal tumors: Treatment of locally-advanced, unresectable, or metastatic gastrointestinal stromal tumor (GIST) in patients previously treated with imatinib and sunitinib

Labeled Contraindications There are no contraindications listed in the manufacturer's US labeling.

Canadian labeling: Hypersensitivity to regorafenib, any component of the formulation, or sorafenib.

Pregnancy Considerations In animal reproduction studies, teratogenic effects were observed with doses less than the equivalent human dose. Based on the mechanism of action, regorafenib may cause fetal harm if administered during pregnancy. Patients (male and female) should use effective contraception during therapy and for at least 2 months following treatment.

Breast-Feeding Considerations It is not known if regorafenib is excreted into breast milk. Due to the potential for serious adverse reactions in the nursing infant, a decision should be made to discontinue regorafenib or to discontinue breast-feeding during therapy, taking into account the benefits of treatment to the mother.

Warnings/Precautions Hazardous agent - use appropriate precautions for handling and disposal (meets NIOSH 2014 criteria). Myocardial ischemia and infarction were observed at a higher incidence than placebo in a clinical trial.

Interrupt therapy in patients who develop new or acute onset ischemia or infarction; resume only if the benefit of therapy outweighs the cardiovascular risk. Hand-foot skin reaction (HFSR), also known as palmar-plantar erythrodysesthesia (PPE), and rash were commonly seen in clinical trials; erythema multiforme and Stevens Johnson syndrome were also observed more frequently in regorafenib-treated patients. Toxic epidermal necrolysis occurred rarely. Onset of dermatologic toxicity typically occurs in the first cycle of treatment. Therapy interruptions, dosage reductions, and/or discontinuation may be necessary depending on the severity and persistence. Supportive treatment may be of benefit for symptomatic relief. Gastrointestinal perforation or fistula has occurred in a small number of patients treated with regorafenib; some cases were fatal. Monitor for signs/symptoms of perforation (fever, abdominal pain with constipation, and/or nausea/vomiting); permanently discontinue therapy if perforation or fistula develop. The incidence of hemorrhage was increased with regorafenib. Hemorrhage of the respiratory, gastrointestinal, or genitourinary tracts was observed in trials; some cases were fatal. Permanently discontinue in patients who experience severe or life-threatening bleeding. In patients receiving concomitant warfarin, monitor INR frequently.

[U.S. Boxed Warning]: Severe and sometimes fatal hepatotoxicity has been observed in clinical trials. Monitor hepatic function at baseline and during treatment. Interrupt therapy for hepatotoxicity; dose reductions or discontinuation are necessary depending on the severity and persistence. Hepatocyte necrosis with lymphocyte infiltration has been demonstrated with liver biopsy. Regorafenib is primarily eliminated hepatically. Closely monitor for adverse effects in patients with mild or moderate impairment; use is not recommended in severe hepatic impairment.

Elevated blood pressure was observed in clinical trials (onset typically in the first cycle of therapy); ensure blood pressure is adequately controlled prior to initiation. Monitor blood pressure weekly for the first 6 weeks and monthly thereafter or as clinically indicated; if hypertension develops, interrupt therapy or permanently discontinue for severe or uncontrolled hypertension. Hypertensive crisis has occurred in some patients. Reversible posterior leukoencephalopathy syndrome (RPLS) occurred very rarely in regorafenib-treated patients; evaluate promptly if symptoms (eg, seizures, headache, visual disturbances, confusion, or altered mental function) occur. Discontinue if diagnosis is confirmed. Regorafenib inhibits vascular endothelial growth factor, which may lead to impaired wound healing. Stop therapy at least 2 weeks prior to scheduled surgery; resume regorafenib postsurgery based on clinical judgment of wound healing; discontinue therapy if wound dehiscence occurs.

Potentially significant drug-drug or drug-food interactions may exist, requiring dose or frequency adjustment, additional monitoring, and/or selection of alternative therapy.

Adverse Reactions

>10%:

Cardiovascular: Hypertension (30% to 59%; grade ≥3: 8% to 28%)

Central nervous system: Fatigue (52% to 64%), voice disorder (30% to 39%), pain (29%), headache (10% to 16%)

Dermatologic: Palmar-plantar erythrodysesthesia (45% to 67%; grade ≥3: 17% to 22%), skin rash (26% to 30%; grade ≥3: 6% to 7%), alopecia (8% to 24%)

Endocrine & metabolic: Hypocalcemia (17% to 59%), hypophosphatemia (55% to 57%), weight loss (14% to 32%), hyponatremia (30%), increased amylase (26%), hypokalemia (21% to 26%), hypothyroidism (4% to 18%)

Gastrointestinal: Diarrhea (43% to 47%), decreased appetite (31% to 47%), increased serum lipase (14% to 46%), mucositis (33% to 40%), nausea (20%), vomiting (17%)

Hematologic & oncologic: Anemia (79%; grade 3: 5%; grade 4: 1%), lymphocytopenia (30% to 54%; grade 3: 8% to 9%), thrombocytopenia (13% to 41%; grade 3: 1% to 2%; grade 4: <1%), increased INR (24%), hemorrhage (11% to 21%; grade ≥3: 2% to 4%), neutropenia (3% to 16%; grade 3: 1%)

Hepatic: Increased serum AST (58% to 65%; grade 3: 5%; grade 4: 1%), increased serum ALT (45%; grade 3: 4% to 5%; grade 4: 1%), hyperbilirubinemia (33% to 45%)

Infection: Infection (31% to 32%; grade ≥3: 5% to 9%)

Neuromuscular & skeletal: Stiffness (14%)

Renal: Proteinuria (33% to 60%)

Miscellaneous: Fever (21% to 28%)

1% to 10%:

Cardiovascular: Ischemic heart disease (≤1%), myocardial infarction (≤1%)

Gastrointestinal: Dysgeusia (8%), xerostomia (5%), gastrointestinal fistula (≤2%), gastrointestinal perforation (≤2%), gastroesophageal reflux disease (1%)

Hepatic: Hepatic failure (≤2%)

Neuromuscular & skeletal: Tremor (2%)

Respiratory: Dyspnea (2%)

<1%, postmarketing, and/or case reports: Bradycardia, erythema multiforme, hepatic injury (severe), hypersensitivity reaction, hypertensive crisis, reversible posterior leukoencephalopathy syndrome (RPLS), Stevens-Johnson syndrome, toxic epidermal necrolysis

Drug Interactions

Metabolism/Transport Effects **Substrate** of CYP3A4 (major), UGT1A9; **Note:** Assignment of Major/Minor substrate status based on clinically relevant drug interaction potential; **Inhibits** BCRP, P-glycoprotein, UGT1A1, UGT1A9

Avoid Concomitant Use

Avoid concomitant use of Regorafenib with any of the following: Conivaptan; CYP3A4 Inducers (Strong); CYP3A4 Inhibitors (Strong); Fusidic Acid (Systemic); Grapefruit Juice; Idelalisib; Irinotecan Products; St Johns Wort

Increased Effect/Toxicity

Regorafenib may increase the levels/effects of: Beta-Blockers; Bisphosphonate Derivatives; Calcium Channel Blockers (Nondihydropyridine); Digoxin; Irinotecan Products; Ivabradine

The levels/effects of Regorafenib may be increased by: Aprepitant; Conivaptan; CYP3A4 Inhibitors (Moderate); CYP3A4 Inhibitors (Strong); Dasatinib; Fosaprepitant; Fusidic Acid (Systemic); Grapefruit Juice; Idelalisib; Ivacaftor; Luliconazole; Mifepristone; Netupitant; Osimertinib; Palbociclib; Simeprevir; Stiripentol; Warfarin

Decreased Effect

The levels/effects of Regorafenib may be decreased by: Bosentan; CYP3A4 Inducers (Moderate); CYP3A4 Inducers (Strong); Dabrafenib; Deferasirox; Osimertinib; Siltuximab; St Johns Wort; Tocilizumab

Food Interactions Regorafenib serum concentrations may be altered when taken with grapefruit or grapefruit juice. Management: Avoid concurrent use.

Storage/Stability Store at 25°C (77°F); excursions permitted to 15°C to 30°C (59°F to 86°F). Store tablets in the original bottle and protect from moisture (do not remove the desiccant); keep container tightly closed. Discard any unused tablets 7 weeks after opening the bottle.

Mechanism of Action Regorafenib is a multikinase inhibitor; it targets kinases involved with tumor angiogenesis, oncogenesis, and maintenance of the tumor microenvironment which results in inhibition of tumor growth. Specifically, it inhibits VEGF receptors 1-3, KIT, PDGFR-alpha, PDGFR-beta, RET, FGFR1 and 2, TIE2, DDR2, TrkA, Eph2A, RAF-1. BRAF, BRAF^{V600E}, SAPK2, PTK5, and Abl.

Pharmacodynamics/Kinetics

Absorption: A high-fat meal increased the mean AUC of the parent drug by 48% compared to the fasted state and decreased the mean AUC of the M-2 (N-oxide) and M-5 (N-oxide and N-desmethyl) active metabolites by 20% and 51%, respectively. A low-fat meal increased the mean AUC of regorafenib, M-2, and M-5 by 36%, 40% and 23%, respectively (as compared to the fasted state).

Protein binding: 99.5% (active metabolites M-2 and M-5 are also highly protein bound)

Metabolism: Hepatic via CYP3A4 and UGT1A9, primarily to active metabolites M-2 (N-oxide) and M-5 (N-oxide and N-desmethyl)

Bioavailability: Tablets: 69%; Oral solution: 83%

Half-life elimination: Regorafenib: 28 hours (range: 14 to 58 hours); M-2 metabolite: 25 hours (range: 14 to 32 hours); M-5 metabolite: 51 hours (range: 32 to 70 hours)

Time to peak: 4 hours

Excretion: Feces (71%; 47% as parent compound); 24% as metabolites); Urine (19%)

Dosing

Adult & Geriatric

Colorectal cancer, metastatic: Oral: 160 mg once daily for the first 21 days of each 28-day cycle; continue until disease progression or unacceptable toxicity (Grothey, 2013)

Gastrointestinal stromal tumor (GIST), locally-advanced, unresectable, or metastatic: Oral: 160 mg once daily for the first 21 days of each 28-day cycle; continue until disease progression or unacceptable toxicity (Demetri, 2013)

Missed doses: Do not administer 2 doses on the same day to make up for a missed dose from the previous day.

Renal Impairment

Preexisting mild impairment (CrCl 60 to 89 mL/minute): No dosage adjustment necessary.

Preexisting moderate impairment (CrCl 30 to 59 mL/minute): There are no dosage adjustments provided in the manufacturer's labeling (limited pharmacokinetic data available).

Preexisting severe impairment (CrCl <30 mL/minute): There are no dosage adjustments provided in the manufacturer's labeling (has not been studied).

Hepatic Impairment

Preexisting mild or moderate impairment (Child-Pugh Class A or B): No dosage adjustment necessary; closely monitor for adverse effects.

Preexisting severe impairment (Child-Pugh Class C): Use is not recommended (has not been studied).

◄ Hepatotoxicity during treatment:

Grade 3 AST and/or ALT elevation: Withhold dose until recovery. If benefit of treatment outweighs toxicity risk, resume therapy at a reduced dose of 120 mg once daily.

AST or ALT >20 times ULN: Discontinue permanently.

AST or ALT >3 times ULN **and** bilirubin >2 times ULN: Discontinue permanently.

Recurrence of AST or ALT >5 times ULN despite dose reduction to 120 mg: Discontinue permanently.

Adjustment for Toxicity

Dermatologic:

Grade 2 hand-foot skin reaction (HFSR; palmar-plantar erythrodysesthesia [PPE]) of any duration: Reduce dose to 120 mg once daily for first occurrence. If grade 2 HFSR recurs at this dose, further reduce the dose to 80 mg once daily. Interrupt therapy for grade 2 HFSR that is recurrent or fails to improve within 7 days in spite of dosage reduction.

Grade 3 HFSR: Interrupt therapy for a minimum of 7 days. Upon recovery, reduce dose to 120 mg once daily. If grade 2 to 3 toxicity recurs at this dose, further reduce dose to 80 mg once daily upon recovery. Interrupt therapy for grade 2 to 3 HFSR that is recurrent or fails to improve within 7 days in spite of dosage reduction.

Recurrent or persistent HFSR at 80 mg once daily: Discontinue treatment.

Hypertension: Grade 2 (symptomatic): Interrupt therapy.

Other toxicity: Any grade 3 or 4 adverse reaction (other than hepatotoxicity): Interrupt therapy; upon recovery, reduce dose to 120 mg once daily. If any grade 3 or 4 adverse reaction occurs while on this reduced dose, may further reduce dose to 80 mg once daily upon recovery. For any grade 4 adverse reaction, only resume therapy if the benefit outweighs the risk. Permanently discontinue therapy if unable to tolerate 80 mg once daily.

Gastrointestinal perforation/fistula: Discontinue permanently.

Hemorrhage (severe or life-threatening): Discontinue permanently.

Reversible posterior leukoencephalopathy syndrome (RPLS): Discontinue.

Wound dehiscence: Discontinue.

Combination Regimens

Colorectal cancer: Regorafenib (Colorectal Regimen) on page 2075

Soft tissue sarcoma (gastrointestinal stromal tumor [GIST]): Regorafenib (GIST Regimen) on page 2075

Administration Take at the same time each day. Swallow tablet whole with water after a low-fat meal (containing <600 calories and <30% fat). Hazardous agent; use appropriate precautions for handling and disposal (meets NIOSH 2014 criteria).

Emetic Potential Minimal (<10%)

Monitoring Parameters Monitor for hand-foot skin reaction (HFSR)/palmar-plantar erythrodysesthesia (PPE); signs/symptoms of cardiac ischemia or infarction; bleeding; signs/symptoms of GI perforation or fistula; signs/symptoms of reversible posterior leukoencephalopathy syndrome (severe headaches, seizure, confusion, or change in vision). Monitor for impaired wound healing. Obtain liver function tests at baseline, every 2 weeks during the first 2 months of treatment, then monthly or more frequently if clinically necessary (weekly until improvement if liver function tests are elevated). Monitor blood pressure weekly for the first 6 weeks of therapy and with every subsequent cycle, or more frequently if indicated. CBC with differential and platelets and serum electrolytes (baseline and periodic). Monitor INR more frequently if receiving warfarin.

Dietary Considerations Take with a low-fat breakfast (<30% fat)

Prescribing and Access Restrictions Regorafenib is available only through the REACH support program. Information regarding program enrollment may be found at http://www.stivarga-us.com/hcp/mcrc/support.html or by calling 1-866-639-2827.

Dosage Forms Excipient information presented when available (limited, particularly for generics); consult specific product labeling.

Tablet, Oral:

Stivarga: 40 mg [contains soybean lecithin]

◆ **Relador Pak** see Lidocaine and Prilocaine on page 1046

◆ **Relistor** see Methylnaltrexone on page 1122

◆ **Remicade** see InFLIXimab on page 919

◆ **Remsima (Can)** see InFLIXimab on page 919

◆ **Revlimid** see Lenalidomide on page 1003

◆ **Revolade** see Eltrombopag on page 585

◆ **rFVIIa** see Factor VIIa (Recombinant) on page 676

◆ **rFXIII** see Factor XIII A-Subunit (Recombinant) on page 687

◆ **RG7204** see Vemurafenib on page 1734

◆ **rhAT** see Antithrombin on page 124

◆ **rhATIII** see Antithrombin on page 124

◆ **Rheumatrex** see Methotrexate on page 1104

◆ **RhIG** see Rh$_o$(D) Immune Globulin on page 1471

◆ **rhIL-11** see Oprelvekin on page 1262

◆ **rhKGF** see Palifermin on page 1304

◆ **Rho(D) Immune Globulin (Human)** see Rh$_o$(D) Immune Globulin on page 1471

Rh$_o$(D) Immune Globulin (ar aych oh (dee) i MYUN GLOB yoo lin)

Brand Names: US HyperRHO S/D; MICRhoGAM Ultra-Filtered Plus; Rho-GAM Ultra-Filtered Plus; Rhophylac; WinRho SDF

Brand Names: Canada WinRho SDF

Index Terms Anti-D Immunoglobulin; RhIG; Rho(D) Immune Globulin (Human); RhoGIV; RhoIVIM

Pharmacologic Category Blood Product Derivative; Immune Globulin

Use

Immune thrombocytopenia (ITP):

Rhophylac: To increase platelet counts in Rh$_o$ (D) positive nonsplenectomized adults with chronic ITP.

WinRho SDF: To increase platelet counts in Rho (D) positive nonsplenectomized patients with the following conditions: acute ITP (children), chronic ITP (adults and children), or ITP secondary to HIV infection (adults and children).

◄ **Pregnancy and other obstetric conditions:**

Prevention of rhesus (Rh) isoimmunization in an Rh-incompatible pregnancy. All products are for use in Rh$_O$(D) negative mothers who are not already sensitized to the Rh$_O$(D) factor. An Rh-incompatible pregnancy is assumed if the fetus/baby is either Rh$_O$(D) positive or Rh$_O$(D) unknown or if the father is either Rh$_O$(D) positive or Rh$_O$(D) unknown. Use is not needed if the father or baby is conclusively Rh$_O$(D) negative. Product specific indications are as follows based on the above criteria:

HyperRHO S/D Full Dose: For antepartum prophylaxis at ~28 weeks gestation; for administration within 72 hours of birth for the prevention of hemolytic disease of the newborn; for administration within 72 hours of spontaneous or induced abortion, ruptured tubal pregnancy, amniocentesis or abdominal trauma.

HyperRHO S/D Mini Dose: For administration within 3 hours (or as soon as possible) of spontaneous or induced abortion up to 12 weeks' gestation.

MICRhoGAM Ultra-Filtered Plus: For administration within 72 hours of actual or threatened termination of pregnancy (spontaneous or induced) up to and including 12 weeks' gestation.

RhoGAM Ultra-Filtered Plus: For antepartum prophylaxis at 26 to 28 weeks' gestation; for administration within 72 hours of birth for prevention of hemolytic disease of the newborn; for administration within 72 hours of amniocentesis, chorionic villus sampling (CVS), percutaneous umbilical blood sampling (PUBS), abdominal trauma or obstetrical manipulation, ectopic pregnancy, threatened pregnancy loss after 12 weeks' gestation (with continuation of pregnancy), pregnancy termination (spontaneous or induced) after 12 weeks' gestation.

Rhophylac: For antepartum prophylaxis at 28 to 30 weeks' gestation; for administration within 72 hours of birth for the prevention of hemolytic disease of the newborn; for administration within 72 hours of obstetric complications including miscarriage, abortion, threatened abortion, ectopic pregnancy or hydatiform mole, transplacental hemorrhage resulting from antepartum hemorrhage; for administration within 72 hours of invasive procedures during pregnancy including amniocentesis, chorionic biopsy, or obstetric manipulative procedures such as external version or abdominal trauma.

WinRho SDF: For antepartum prophylaxis at 28 weeks' gestation; for administration within 72 hours of birth for the prevention of hemolytic disease of the newborn; for administration following obstetric complications including miscarriage, abortion, threatened abortion, ectopic pregnancy or hydatiform mole, transplacental hemorrhage resulting from antepartum hemorrhage; for administration following invasive procedures during pregnancy including amniocentesis, chorionic biopsy, or obstetric manipulative procedures such as external version or abdominal trauma.

Transfusion:

HyperRHO S/D Full Dose, MICRhoGAM Ultra-Filtered Plus, RhoGAM Ultra-Filtered Plus, Rhophylac, and WinRho SDF: To prevent isoimmunization in Rh$_O$(D) negative individuals who have been transfused with Rh$_O$(D) positive red blood cells or blood components containing red blood cells.

Labeled Contraindications

HyperRHO S/D Full Dose, HyperRHO S/D Mini Dose: There are no contraindications listed in the manufacturer's labeling.

MICRhoGAM Ultra-Filtered Plus, RhoGAM Ultra-Filtered Plus: Use in Rh-positive individuals.

Rhophylac: Anaphylactic or severe systemic reaction to a previous dose of human immune globulin; use in IgA-deficient patients with antibodies to IgA and a history of hypersensitivity; administration to the neonate of a mother who received Rhophylac postpartum.

WinRho SDF: Anaphylactic or severe systemic reaction to a previous dose of human immune globulin; use in IgA-deficient patients with antibodies to IgA and a history of hypersensitivity; autoimmune hemolytic anemia; preexisting hemolysis or at high risk for hemolysis; suppression of $Rh_o(D)$ isoimmunization in infants.

WinRho SDF Canadian labeling: Additional contraindications (not in US labeling): All uses: Use in IgA-deficient patients; hypersensitivity to $Rh_o(D)$ immune globulin or any component of the formulation.

Rh Immunization prophylaxis: Use in $Rh_o(D)$-positive women; $Rh_o(D)$ negative women who are Rh immunized.

Immune thrombocytopenia (ITP): $Rh_o(D)$-negative patients; splenectomized patients; ITP secondary to other conditions including leukemia, lymphoma, or active viral infections with EBV or HCV; elderly patients with underlying cardiac, renal, or hepatic comorbidities that would predispose them to acute hemolytic reactions (AHR) complications; autoimmune hemolytic anemia (Evan syndrome); systemic lupus erythematosus (SLE); antiphospholipid antibody syndrome.

Documentation of allergenic cross-reactivity for immune globulins is limited. However, because of similarities in chemical structure and/or pharmacologic actions, the possibility of cross-sensitivity cannot be ruled out with certainty.

Pregnancy Considerations Animal reproduction studies have not been conducted.

$Rh_o(D)$ immune globulin (RhIG) is administered to pregnant women to prevent alloimmunization of $Rh_o(D)$ negative mothers who may potentially have a fetus who is $Rh_o(D)$ positive. Administration of the immune globulin prevents the mother from developing antibodies to the D antigen and the development of hemolytic anemia in the newborn. Current guidelines recommend administration of RhIG to pregnant women who are $Rh_o(D)$ negative and who are not already $Rh_o(D)$ alloimmunized at ~28 weeks gestation (unless the father is known to be $Rh_o(D)$ negative), within 72 hours of delivery of an $Rh_o(D)$ positive infant, after a first trimester pregnancy loss, or after invasive procedures such as amniocentesis, chorionic villus sampling (CVS), or fetal blood sampling (ACOG 1999). Available evidence suggests that $Rh_o(D)$ immune globulin administration during pregnancy does not harm the fetus or affect future pregnancies.

In pregnant women who require treatment for ITP, other agents are preferred. RhIG for this indication in pregnancy is limited to case reports and small studies (Neunert 2011).

Breast-Feeding Considerations Adverse events in the nursing infant have not been observed when administered to women for the suppression of Rh isoimmunization. The manufacturer recommends that caution be used if administered to nursing women. The purified immune globulin in these products is obtained from human donors; the $Rh_o(D)$ antibodies are endogenous to human plasma.

Warnings/Precautions Rhophylac, WinRho SDF: **[US Boxed Warning]: May cause fatal intravascular hemolysis (IVH) in $Rh_o(D)$-positive patients treated with intravenous (IV) $Rh_o(D)$ immune globulin for immune thrombocytopenia (ITP). IVH may result in clinically compromising anemia and** ▶

◀ multiorgan system failure including acute respiratory distress syndrome. Acute renal insufficiency, renal failure, severe anemia, and disseminated intravascular coagulation (DIC) have also been reported. Patients should be closely monitored for at least 8 hours after administration. Alert patients to, and monitor them for back pain, shaking chills, fever, and discolored urine or hematuria. Absence of these signs and/or symptoms within 8 hours does not indicate IVH cannot occur subsequently. If signs and/or symptoms of intravascular hemolysis are present or suspected, perform post-treatment laboratory tests, including plasma hemoglobin, haptoglobin, LDH, and plasma bilirubin (direct and indirect). Previous administration of IV Rh$_o$(D) immune globulin does not preclude the possibility of IVH. Transfuse patients with hemolysis and clinically compromising anemia after receiving Rh$_o$(D) immune globulin; use Rh$_o$(D)-negative packed red blood cells.

Severe hypersensitivity reactions may occur. Immediate treatment (including epinephrine 1:1000) for anaphylactoid and/or hypersensitivity reactions should be available during use. Some products are specifically contraindicated in patients with a previous anaphylactic or severe systemic reaction to an immune globulin. If symptoms of allergic or early signs of hypersensitivity reactions occur, discontinue immediately and institute appropriate treatment. Use with caution in patients with IgA deficiency, may contain trace amounts of IgA; patients with known antibodies to IgA have a greater risk of developing potentially anaphylactic reactions. Some products are specifically contraindicated in patients with antibodies against IgA.

Acute renal dysfunction/failure, osmotic nephropathy, and death may occur with IGIV products. Use with caution and administer at the minimum infusion rate possible in patients at risk for renal disease (eg, diabetes mellitus, >65 years of age, volume depletion, sepsis, paraproteinemia, concomitant use of nephrotoxic medications); ensure adequate hydration prior to administration in these patients. Thrombotic events have been reported with administration of intravenous immune globulins (IVIG); use with caution in patients with a history of atherosclerosis or cardiovascular and/or thrombotic risk factors or patients with known/suspected hyperviscosity. Consider a baseline assessment of blood viscosity in patients at risk for hyperviscosity. Administer at the minimum practical infusion rate. Monitor for adverse pulmonary events including transfusion-related acute lung injury (TRALI); noncardiogenic pulmonary edema has been reported with IVIG use. TRALI is characterized by severe respiratory distress, pulmonary edema, hypoxemia, and fever in the presence of normal left ventricular function and usually occurs within 1 to 6 hours after infusion; may be managed with oxygen and respiratory support.

Use with caution in patients with thrombocytopenia or coagulation disorders; bleeding/hematoma may occur from IM administration. Use with caution in patients with renal impairment or those at risk for renal disease (eg, diabetes mellitus, advanced age [>65 years], volume depletion, sepsis, paraproteinemia, concomitant use of nephrotoxic medications). In patients at risk of renal dysfunction, ensure adequate hydration prior to administration; administer at the minimum practical infusion rate. Product of human plasma; may potentially contain infectious agents which could transmit disease. Screening of donors, as well as testing and/or inactivation or removal of certain viruses, reduces the risk. Infections thought to be transmitted by this product should be reported to the manufacturer.

Some products may contain maltose, which may result in falsely elevated blood glucose readings. Some dosage forms may contain polysorbate 80 (also known as Tweens). Hypersensitivity reactions, usually a delayed reaction, have been reported following exposure to pharmaceutical products containing polysorbate 80 in certain individuals (Isaksson 2002; Lucente 2000; Shelley 1995). Thrombocytopenia, ascites, pulmonary deterioration, and renal and hepatic failure have been reported in premature neonates after receiving parenteral products containing polysorbate 80 (Alade 1986; CDC 1984). See manufacturer's labeling.

Immune globulin deficiency syndromes: Not for replacement therapy in immune globulin deficiency syndromes.

ITP: Appropriate use: Safety and efficacy of WinRho not established in Rh$_o$(D) negative, non-ITP thrombocytopenia, or splenectomized patients; safety and efficacy of Rhophylac not established in patients with preexisting anemia (may increase the severity of preexisting anemia). Dose adjustment may be required with decreased hemoglobin. Do not administer IM or SubQ; administer dose IV only. Although Rh$_o$(D) immune globulin is not the preferred pharmacologic agent for the management of ITP, a single dose may be used in nonsplenectomized children who are Rh$_o$(D) positive and require treatment, or in adults when corticosteroids are contraindicated (Neunert 2011).

Rh$_o$(D) suppression: For use in the mother; do not administer to the neonate. If Rh$_o$(D) antibodies are already present in the mother, use of the Rh$_o$(D) immune globulin is not beneficial. In addition, if the father is known to be Rh$_o$(D) negative, administration of the immune globulin is not needed. When treatment is indicated, administration should be within the time frame recommended. However, there may still be benefit if therapy is given as late as 28 days postpartum. The longer treatment is delayed, the less protection will be provided (ACOG 1999).

Adverse Reactions Frequency not defined.

Cardiovascular: Hyper-/hypotension, pallor, vasodilation

Central nervous system: Chills, dizziness, fever, headache, malaise, somnolence

Dermatologic: Pruritus, rash

Gastrointestinal: Abdominal pain, diarrhea, nausea, vomiting

Hematologic: Haptoglobin decreased, hemoglobin decreased (patients with ITP), intravascular hemolysis (patients with ITP)

Hepatic: Bilirubin increased, LDH increased

Local: Injection site reaction: Discomfort, induration, mild pain, redness, swelling

Neuromuscular & skeletal: Arthralgia, back pain, hyperkinesia, myalgia, weakness

Renal: Acute renal insufficiency

Miscellaneous: Anaphylaxis, diaphoresis, infusion-related reactions, positive anti-C antibody test (transient), shivering

Postmarketing and/or case reports: Anemia (clinically-compromising), anuria, ARDS, cardiac arrest, cardiac failure, chest pain, chromaturia, DIC, edema, erythema, fatigue, hematuria, hemoglobinemia, hemoglobinuria (transient in patients with ITP), hyperhidrosis, hypersensitivity, injection site irritation, jaundice, myocardial infarction, muscle spasm, nausea, pain in extremities, renal failure, renal impairment, tachycardia, transfusion-related acute lung injury

◀ **Drug Interactions**

Metabolism/Transport Effects None known.

Avoid Concomitant Use There are no known interactions where it is recommended to avoid concomitant use.

Increased Effect/Toxicity There are no known significant interactions involving an increase in effect.

Decreased Effect

Rho(D) Immune Globulin may decrease the levels/effects of: Vaccines (Live)

Storage/Stability

Store at 2°C to 8°C (35°F to 46°F); do not freeze.

Rhophylac: Store at 2°C to 8°C (35°F to 46°F); do not freeze. Protect from light.

Preparation for Administration

Rhophylac: Bring prefilled syringe to room temperature before use.

WinRho SDF: ITP: May dilute in NS prior to IV administration if needed; do not dilute with D$_5$W.

Mechanism of Action

Rh suppression: Not completely characterized; prevents isoimmunization by suppressing the immune response and antibody formation by Rh$_O$(D)-negative individuals to Rh$_O$(D)-positive red blood cells. When administered within 72 hours of a full term delivery, the incidence of Rh isoimmunization decreases from 12% to 13% to 1% to 2%. The rate further decreases to <1% with administration at both 28 weeks' gestation and postpartum.

ITP: Not completely characterized; Rh$_O$(D) immune globulin is thought to form anti-D-coated red blood cell complexes which bind to macrophage Fc receptors within the reticuloendothelial system (RES); blocks or saturates the RES ability to clear antibody-coated cells, including platelets. Thus, platelets are spared from destruction.

Pharmacodynamics/Kinetics

Onset of platelet increase: ITP: WinRho: Platelets should rise within 1 to 2 days

Peak effect: WinRho: In 7 to 14 days

Duration: Suppression of Rh isoimmunization: Rhophylac 300 mcg dose: Rh$_O$(D) immune globulin titers detected up to and at least 9 weeks; WinRho SDF 120 mcg dose: ≤6 weeks; Treatment of ITP: 30 days (variable)

Distribution: V$_d$: IM: RhoGAM Ultra Filtered Plus: 7.3 ± 1.5 L

Bioavailability: IM: Rhophylac: 69%

Half-life elimination: RhoGAM Ultra Filtered Plus: 30.9 ± 13.8 days (IM); Rhophylac: 16 ± 4 days (IV), 18 ± 5 days (IM); WinRho SDF ~24 days (IV), ~30 days (IM)

Time to peak, plasma: RhoGAM Ultra Filtered Plus: 4 days (IM); Rhophylac: 2 to 7 days (IM); WinRho SDF: ≤2 hours (IV), 5 to 10 days (IM)

Dosing

Adult

Note: Rh$_O$(D) immune globulin 300 mcg has traditionally been referred to as a "full dose". Potency and dosing recommendations may also be expressed in international units by comparison to the WHO anti-Rh$_O$(D) standard where 1 mcg = 5 international units

Immune thrombocytopenia (ITP):

Rhophylac: IV: 50 mcg/kg

WinRho SDF: IV:

Initial: 50 mcg/kg as a single injection, or can be given as a divided dose on separate days. If hemoglobin is <10 g/dL: Dose should be reduced to 25 to 40 mcg/kg.

Subsequent dosing: 25 to 60 mcg/kg can be used if required to increase platelet count; frequency of dosing is dependent upon clinical response

Maintenance dosing if patient **did respond** to initial dosing: 25 to 60 mcg/kg based on platelet count and hemoglobin concentration

Maintenance dosing if patient **did not respond** to initial dosing:

Hemoglobin <8 g/dL: Alternative treatment should be used

Hemoglobin 8 to 10 g/dL: Redose between 25 to 40 mcg/kg

Hemoglobin >10 g/dL: Redose between 50 to 60 mcg/kg

Rh$_o$(D) suppression: Note: In general, a 300 mcg dose will suppress the immune response to a fetal-maternal hemorrhage with ≤15 mL of Rh-positive RBC. If exposure to >15 mL of Rh-positive RBC is suspected, an appropriate dose should be calculated. If the first dose is administered early in pregnancy, additional doses may be needed to ensure adequate levels of passively acquired anti-D at delivery (ACOG 1999). If delivery occurs within 3 weeks after the last antepartum dose, a postpartum dose may be withheld, but testing for fetal-maternal hemorrhage of >15 mL should be performed (ACOG 1999).

Pregnancy prophylaxis: Note: if antepartum prophylaxis is indicated, the mother may also need a postpartum dose if the infant is Rh-positive.

Antepartum prophylaxis:

HyperRHO S/D Full Dose: IM: 300 mcg at ~28 weeks' gestation.

RhoGAM: IM: 300 mcg at 26 to 28 weeks' gestation; if delivery does not occur within 12 weeks after the dose, a second 300 mcg dose is recommended. If the first dose is prior to 26 weeks' gestation, administer every 12 weeks to ensure adequate levels of passively acquired anti-D. If delivery occurs within 3 weeks after the last antepartum dose, a postpartum dose may be withheld, but testing for fetal-maternal hemorrhage of >15 mL should be performed.

Rhophylac: IM, IV: 300 mcg at 28 to 30 weeks' gestation.

WinRho SDF: IM, IV: 300 mcg at 28 weeks' gestation. If the first dose is administered early in pregnancy, administer every 12 weeks to ensure adequate levels of passively acquired anti-D.

Postpartum prophylaxis:

HyperRHO S/D Full Dose: IM: 300 mcg provides sufficient antibody if volume of Rh-positive RBC exposure is ≤15 mL. If exposure to >15 mL of Rh-positive RBC is suspected, an appropriate dose should be calculated (see dosing for excessive fetomaternal hemorrhage). The dose should be administered within 72 hours of delivery, but may provide some benefit if given later.

RhoGAM: IM: 300 mcg provides sufficient antibody if volume of Rh-positive RBC exposure is ≤15 mL. If exposure to >15 mL of Rh-positive RBC is suspected, an appropriate dose should be calculated. The dose should be administered within 72 hours of delivery.

Rhophylac: IM, IV: 300 mcg provides sufficient antibody if volume of Rh-positive RBC exposure is ≤15 mL. If exposure to >15 mL of Rh-positive RBC is suspected, an appropriate dose should be calculated (see dosing for excessive fetomaternal hemorrhage). The dose should be administered within 72 hours of delivery.

WinRho SDF: IM, IV: 120 mcg. The dose should be administered within 72 hours of delivery but may be given up to 28 days after delivery.

◄ **Other pregnancy/obstetric conditions:**
Abdominal trauma:
HyperRHO S/D Full Dose: IM: 300 mcg following abdominal trauma in the second or third trimester. If exposure to >15 mL of Rh-positive RBC is suspected, an appropriate dose should be calculated (see dosing for excessive fetomaternal hemorrhage).
RhoGam: IM: 300 mcg within 72 hours following abdominal trauma or obstetrical manipulation occurring at ≥13 weeks' gestation. If exposure to >15 mL of Rh-positive RBC is suspected, an appropriate dose should be calculated.
Rhophylac: IV, IM: 300 mcg within 72 hours of complication. If exposure to >15 mL of Rh-positive RBC is suspected, an appropriate dose should be calculated (see dosing for excessive fetomaternal hemorrhage).
Amniocentesis:
HyperRHO S/D Full Dose: IM: 300 mcg at 15 to 18 weeks' gestation or during the third trimester. If exposure to >15 mL of Rh-positive RBC is suspected, an appropriate dose should be calculated (see dosing for excessive fetomaternal hemorrhage).
RhoGam: IM: 300 mcg within 72 hours of a procedure occurring at ≥13 weeks' gestation. If exposure to >15 mL of Rh-positive RBC is suspected, an appropriate dose should be calculated.
Rhophylac: IV, IM: 300 mcg within 72 hours of procedure. If exposure to >15 mL of Rh-positive RBC is suspected, an appropriate dose should be calculated (see dosing for excessive fetomaternal hemorrhage).
WinRho SDF: IV, IM: 300 mcg immediately after amniocentesis occurring before 34 weeks' gestation; repeat dose every 12 weeks during pregnancy. Administer 120 mcg within 72 hours of amniocentesis occurring after 34 weeks' gestation.
Ectopic pregnancy:
HyperRHO S/D Full Dose: IM: 300 mcg for complications occurring at ≥13 weeks' gestation. If exposure to >15 mL of Rh-positive RBC is suspected, an appropriate dose should be calculated (see dosing for excessive fetomaternal hemorrhage).
RhoGam: IM: 300 mcg within 72 hours of complications occurring at ≥13 weeks' gestation. If exposure to >15 mL of Rh-positive RBC is suspected, an appropriate dose should be calculated.
Rhophylac: IV, IM: 300 mcg within 72 hours of complication. If exposure to >15 mL of Rh-positive RBC is suspected, an appropriate dose should be calculated (see dosing for excessive fetomaternal hemorrhage).
Termination of pregnancy (spontaneous or induced):
HyperRHO S/D Mini Dose: IM: 50 mcg within 3 hours or as soon as possible following spontaneous or induced abortion occurring <13 weeks' gestation; administer within 72 hours of termination if prompt administration is not possible.
HyperRHO S/D Full Dose: IM: 300 mcg following miscarriage or abortion occurring ≥13 weeks' gestation. If exposure to >15 mL of Rh-positive RBC is suspected, an appropriate dose should be calculated (see dosing for excessive fetomaternal hemorrhage).
MICRhoGAM: IM: 50 mcg within 72 hours of actual or threatened termination occurring <13 weeks' gestation.
RhoGAM: IM: 300 mcg within 72 hours following spontaneous or induced termination occurring ≥13 weeks' gestation. If exposure to >15 mL of Rh-positive RBC is suspected, an appropriate dose should be calculated.

Rhophylac: IV, IM: 300 mcg within 72 hours of miscarriage or abortion. If exposure to >15 mL of Rh-positive RBC is suspected, an appropriate dose should be calculated (see dosing for excessive fetomaternal hemorrhage).

WinRho SDF: IV, IM: 120 mcg within 72 hours of abortion occurring after 34 weeks' gestation.

Threatened pregnancy loss with continuation of pregnancy:

HyperRHO S/D Full Dose: IM: 300 mcg following threatened loss at any time during pregnancy; administer as soon as possible. If exposure to >15 mL of Rh-positive RBC is suspected, an appropriate dose should be calculated (see dosing for excessive fetomaternal hemorrhage).

RhoGAM: IM: 300 mcg within 72 hours following threatened loss ≥13 weeks' gestation. If exposure to >15 mL of Rh-positive RBC is suspected, an appropriate dose should be calculated.

Rhophylac: IV, IM: 300 mcg within 72 hours of threatened abortion. If exposure to >15 mL of Rh-positive RBC is suspected, an appropriate dose should be calculated (see dosing for excessive fetomaternal hemorrhage).

WinRho SDF: IV, IM: 300 mcg immediately following a threatened abortion occurring any time during pregnancy

Additional invasive/manipulative procedures or obstetric complications:

RhoGam: IM: 300 mcg within 72 hours of chorionic villus sampling or percutaneous umbilical blood sampling ≥13 weeks' gestation. If exposure to >15 mL of Rh-positive RBC is suspected, an appropriate dose should be calculated.

Rhophylac: IV, IM: 300 mcg within 72 hours of procedures such as chorionic biopsy or external version, or within 72 hours of complications such as hydatidiform mole, or transplacental hemorrhage resulting from antepartum hemorrhage. If exposure to >15 mL of Rh-positive RBC is suspected, an appropriate dose should be calculated (see dosing for excessive fetomaternal hemorrhage).

WinRho SDF: IV, IM: 300 mcg immediately after chorionic villus sampling before 34 weeks' gestation; repeat dose every 12 weeks during pregnancy. Administer 120 mcg within 72 hours of manipulation occurring after 34 weeks' gestation.

Dosing for excessive fetomaternal hemorrhage:

HyperRHO S/D Full Dose: IM: When exposure to >15 mL Rh-positive RBC or >30 mL whole blood is suspected, a fetal red cell count should be calculated. The fetal RBC volume is then divided by 15 mL, providing the number of 300 mcg doses (vials/syringes) to administer. If the dose calculated results in a fraction, round up to the next higher whole 300 mcg dose (vial/syringe).

Rhophylac: IV, IM: When exposure to >15 mL Rh-positive RBC, administer 300 mcg; in addition, administer 20 mcg per mL fetal RBC in excess of 15 mL if bleeding can be quantified or an additional 300 mcg if excess bleeding cannot be quantified. Total dose should be administered within 72 hours of complication.

Transfusion: Note: Actual dose is based upon volume of blood/blood product exposure.

WinRho SDF: Administer within 72 hours after exposure of incompatible blood transfusion.

IV: Calculate dose as follows; administer 600 mcg every 8 hours until the total dose is administered:

Exposure to Rh₀(D) positive whole blood: 9 mcg/mL blood

Exposure to Rh₀(D) positive red blood cells: 18 mcg/mL cells

IM: Calculate dose as follows; administer 1,200 mcg every 12 hours until the total dose is administered:

Exposure to Rh₀(D) positive whole blood: 12 mcg/mL blood

Exposure to Rh₀(D) positive red blood cells: 24 mcg/mL cells

HyperRHO S/D Full Dose: IM: Multiply the volume of Rh-positive whole blood administered by the hematocrit of the donor unit to equal the volume of RBCs transfused. The volume of RBCs is then divided by 15 mL, providing the number of 300 mcg doses (vials/syringes) to administer. If the dose calculated results in a fraction, round up to the next higher whole 300 mcg dose (vial/syringe). Administer as soon as possible and within 72 hours after an incompatible transfusion.

MICRhoGAM: IM: <2.5 mL of Rh-positive red blood cell exposure: 50 mcg. Administer within 72 hours after an incompatible transfusion.

RhoGAM: IM:

2.5 to 15 mL Rh-positive red blood cell exposure: 300 mcg. Administer within 72 hours after an incompatible transfusion.

>15 mL Rh-positive red blood cell exposure: 20 mcg per mL of Rh-positive red blood cell exposure. Multiple doses may be given at the same time or spaced at intervals; total dose must be given within 72 hours of exposure.

Rhophylac: IM, IV: 20 mcg per 2 mL transfused blood or 20 mcg per mL erythrocyte concentrate. Administer within 72 hours after an incompatible transfusion.

Geriatric Refer to adult dosing. Patients >65 years of age with a concurrent comorbid condition may be at increased risk of developing acute hemolytic reactions. Fatal outcomes associated with IVH have occurred most frequently in those >65 years. Use with caution; consider starting at lower doses.

Pediatric Immune thrombocytopenia (ITP): Children and Adolescents: WinRho SDF: Refer to adult dosing.

Renal Impairment There are no dosage adjustments provided in the manufacturer's labeling.

Hepatic Impairment There are no dosage adjustments provided in the manufacturer's labeling.

Administration

When used for the prevention of rhesus (Rh) isoimmunization in an Rh-incompatible pregnancy, the dose is administered to the mother, not the neonate.

HyperRHO S/D Full Dose, HyperRHO S/D Mini Dose, MICRhoGAM Ultra-Filtered Plus and RhoGAM Ultra-Filtered Plus are for IM administration only.

Rhophylac and WinRho SDF may be administered IM or IV (based on indication). Do not administer Rhophylac subcutaneously into the fatty tissue. There have been reports of lack of effect in patients with a BMI ≥30 kg/m² when Rhophylac was administered IM.

IM: Administer into the deltoid muscle of the upper arm or anterolateral aspect of the upper thigh; avoid gluteal region due to risk of sciatic nerve injury. If large doses (>5 mL) are needed, administration in divided doses at different sites is recommended. **Note:** Do not administer IM Rh₀(D) immune globulin for ITP.

IV:

Rhophylac: ITP: Infuse at 2 mL per 15 to 60 seconds

WinRho SDF: Infuse at 2 mL per 5 to 15 seconds when used for the prevention of rhesus (Rh) isoimmunization or over 3 to 5 minutes when used for the treatment of ITP.

Monitoring Parameters

Immune thrombocytopenia (ITP): Signs and symptoms of intravascular hemolysis (IVH), including anemia, renal insufficiency, back pain, shaking, chills, discolored urine, or hematuria; observe patient for 8 hours following administration. In addition, CBC (prior to therapy and 1 to 3 days after first infusion); differential and peripheral blood smear (prior to therapy), direct antiglobulin test and antibody screen (prior to therapy); reticulocyte count (prior to therapy); urinalysis (prior to therapy and 1 to 2 hours after treatment [product labeling specifies dipstick urinalysis at baseline and 2, and 4 hours prior to the end of the monitoring period]); serum creatinine and BUN (prior to therapy; monitor after therapy if post treatment hemoglobin decreases by >1 g/dL) (Despotovic 2012). For patients with suspected IVH, monitor plasma hemoglobin, haptoglobin, LDH, and plasma bilirubin (direct and indirect).

Pregnancy/obstetric conditions: Monitor for systemic reactions for 20 minutes after administration

Transfusion: Signs and symptoms of hemolytic reaction

Test Interactions Rhₒ(D) immune globulin may affect the results of blood typing, the antibody screening test, and the direct antiglobulin (Coombs') test in the mother and neonate. Fetal-maternal hemorrhage may cause false blood-typing result in the mother; when there is any doubt to the patients' Rh type, Rhₒ(D) immune globulin should be administered. WinRho SDF liquid contains maltose; may result in falsely elevated blood glucose levels with dehydrogenase pyrroloquinolinequinone or glucose-dye-oxidoreductase testing methods. WinRho SDF also contains trace amounts of anti-A, B, C, and E; may alter Coombs' tests. Rhophylac can contain antibodies to other Rh antigens (eg, anti-C antibodies), which might be detected by sensitive serological tests.

Dosage Forms Excipient information presented when available (limited, particularly for generics); consult specific product labeling. [DSC] = Discontinued product

Solution, Injection:

WinRho SDF: 2500 units/2.2 mL (2.2 mL); 5000 units/4.4 mL (4.4 mL); 1500 units/1.3 mL (1.3 mL); 15,000 units/13 mL (13 mL)

Solution, Injection [preservative free]:

WinRho SDF: 2500 units/2.2 mL (2.2 mL); 5000 units/4.4 mL (4.4 mL); 1500 units/1.3 mL (1.3 mL); 15,000 units/13 mL (13 mL) [contains polysorbate 80]

Solution Prefilled Syringe, Injection [preservative free]:

Rhophylac: 1500 units/2 mL (2 mL)

Solution Prefilled Syringe, Intramuscular:

HyperRHO S/D: 250 units (1 ea [DSC])

Solution Prefilled Syringe, Intramuscular [preservative free]:

HyperRHO S/D: 250 units (1 ea); 1500 units (1 ea) [latex free]

MICRhoGAM Ultra-Filtered Plus: 250 units (1 ea) [latex free, thimerosal free; contains polysorbate 80]

RhoGAM Ultra-Filtered Plus: 1500 units (1 ea) [latex free, thimerosal free; contains polysorbate 80]

◆ **RhoGAM Ultra-Filtered Plus** see Rhₒ(D) Immune Globulin *on page 1471*

◆ **RhoIGIV** see Rhₒ(D) Immune Globulin *on page 1471*

RiTUXimab (ri TUK si mab)

Related Information

Common Toxicity Criteria *on page* 2122

Hematopoietic Stem Cell Transplantation *on page* 2272

Management of Chemotherapy-Induced Nausea and Vomiting in Adults *on page* 2142

Prevention and Management of Infections *on page* 2196

Prevention of Chemotherapy-Induced Nausea and Vomiting in Children *on page* 2203

Principles of Anticancer Therapy *on page* 2261

Brand Names: US Rituxan

Brand Names: Canada Rituxan

Index Terms Anti-CD20 Monoclonal Antibody; C2B8 Monoclonal Antibody; IDEC-C2B8

Pharmacologic Category Antineoplastic Agent, Anti-CD20; Antineoplastic Agent, Monoclonal Antibody; Antirheumatic Miscellaneous; Immunosuppressant Agent; Monoclonal Antibody

Use

Treatment of CD20-positive non-Hodgkin lymphomas (NHL):

Relapsed or refractory, low-grade or follicular B-cell NHL (as a single agent)

Follicular B-cell NHL, previously untreated (in combination with first-line chemotherapy, and as single-agent maintenance therapy if response to first-line rituximab with chemotherapy)

Nonprogressing, low-grade B-cell NHL (as a single agent after first-line CVP treatment)

Diffuse large B-cell NHL, previously untreated (in combination with CHOP chemotherapy [or other anthracycline-based regimen])

Treatment of CD20-positive chronic lymphocytic leukemia (CLL) (in combination with fludarabine and cyclophosphamide)

Treatment of moderately- to severely-active rheumatoid arthritis (in combination with methotrexate) in adult patients with inadequate response to one or more TNF antagonists

Treatment of granulomatosis with polyangiitis (GPA; Wegener's granulomatosis) (in combination with glucocorticoids)

Treatment of microscopic polyangiitis (MPA) (in combination with glucocorticoids)

Labeled Contraindications There are no contraindications listed in the FDA-approved manufacturer's labeling.

Canadian labeling (not in U.S. labeling): Type 1 hypersensitivity or anaphylactic reaction to murine proteins, Chinese Hamster Ovary (CHO) cell proteins, or any component of the formulation; patients who have or have had progressive multifocal leukoencephalopathy (PML)

Pregnancy Considerations Animal reproduction studies have demonstrated adverse effects including decreased (reversible) B-cells and immunosuppression. Rituximab crosses the placenta and can be detected in the newborn. In one infant born at 41 weeks gestation, *in utero* exposure occurred from week 16-37; rituximab concentrations were higher in the neonate at birth (32,095 ng/mL) than the mother (9750 ng/mL) and still measurable at 18 weeks of age (700 ng/mL infant; 500 ng/mL mother) (Friedrichs, 2006).

B-cell lymphocytopenia lasting <6 months may occur in exposed infants. Limited information is available following maternal use of rituximab for the treatment of lymphomas and hematologic disorders (Ton, 2011). Retrospective case reports of inadvertent pregnancy during rituximab treatment collected by the manufacturer (often combined with concomitant teratogenic therapies) describe premature births and infant hematologic abnormalities and infections; no specific pattern of birth defects has been observed (limited data) (Chakravarty, 2010). Use is not recommended to treat non-life-threatening maternal conditions (eg, rheumatoid arthritis) during pregnancy (Makol, 2011; Østensen, 2008) and other agents are preferred for treating lupus nephritis in pregnant women (Hahn, 2012).

Effective contraception should be used during and for 12 months following treatment. Healthcare providers are encouraged to enroll women with rheumatoid arthritis exposed to rituximab during pregnancy in the MotherToBabyAutoImmune Diseases Study by contacting the Organization of Teratology Information Specialists (OTIS) (877-311-8972).

Breast-Feeding Considerations It is not known if rituximab is excreted in human milk. However, human IgG is excreted in breast milk, and therefore, rituximab may also be excreted in milk. Although rituximab would not be expected to enter the circulation of a nursing infant in significant amounts, the decision to discontinue rituximab or discontinue breast-feeding should take into account the benefits of treatment to the mother.

Warnings/Precautions [U.S. Boxed Warning]: Severe (occasionally fatal) infusion-related reactions have been reported, usually with the first infusion; fatalities have been reported within 24 hours of infusion; monitor closely during infusion; discontinue for severe reactions and provide medical intervention for grades 3 or 4 infusion reactions. Reactions usually occur within 30-120 minutes and may include hypotension, angioedema, bronchospasm, hypoxia, urticaria, and in more severe cases pulmonary infiltrates, acute respiratory distress syndrome, myocardial infarction, ventricular fibrillation, cardiogenic shock and/or anaphylaxis. Risk factors associated with fatal outcomes include chronic lymphocytic leukemia, female gender, mantle cell lymphoma, or pulmonary infiltrates. Closely monitor patients with a history of prior cardiopulmonary reactions or with preexisting cardiac or pulmonary conditions and patients with high numbers of circulating malignant cells (>25,000/mm^3). Prior to infusion, premedicate patients with acetaminophen and an antihistamine (and methylprednisolone for patients with RA). Discontinue infusion for severe reactions; treatment is symptomatic. Medications for the treatment of hypersensitivity reactions (eg, bronchodilators, epinephrine, antihistamines, corticosteroids) should be available for immediate use. Discontinue infusion for serious or life-threatening cardiac arrhythmias. Perform cardiac monitoring during and after the infusion in patients who develop clinically significant arrhythmias or who have a history of arrhythmia or angina. Mild-to-moderate infusion-related reactions (eg, chills, fever, rigors) occur frequently and are typically managed through slowing or interrupting the infusion. Infusion may be resumed at a 50% infusion rate reduction upon resolution of symptoms. Due to the potential for hypotension, consider withholding antihypertensives 12 hours prior to treatment.

[U.S. Boxed Warning]: Hepatitis B virus (HBV) reactivation may occur with use and may result in fulminant hepatitis, hepatic failure, and death. Screen all patients for HBV infection by measuring hepatitis B surface antigen (HBsAG) and hepatitis B core antibody (anti-HBc) prior to therapy initiation; monitor patients for clinical and laboratory signs of hepatitis or HBV during and for several months after treatment. Discontinue rituximab (and concomitant medications) if viral hepatitis develops and initiate appropriate antiviral therapy. Reactivation has occurred in patients who are HBsAg positive as well as in those who are HBsAg negative but are anti-HBc positive; HBV reactivation has also been observed in patients who had previously resolved HBV infection. HBV reactivation has been reported up to 24 months after therapy discontinuation. Use cautiously in patients who show evidence of prior HBV infection (eg, HBsAg positive [regardless of antibody status] or HBsAG negative but anti-HBc positive); consult with appropriate clinicians regarding monitoring and consideration of antiviral therapy before and/or during rituximab treatment. The safety of resuming rituximab treatment following HBV reactivation is not known; discuss reinitiation of therapy in patients with resolved HBV reactivation with physicians experienced in HBV management.

[U.S. Boxed Warning]: Progressive multifocal leukoencephalopathy (PML) due to JC virus infection has been reported with rituximab use; may be fatal. Cases were reported in patients with hematologic malignancies receiving rituximab either with combination chemotherapy, or with hematopoietic stem cell transplant. Cases were also reported in patients receiving rituximab for autoimmune diseases who had received prior or concurrent immunosuppressant therapy. Onset may be delayed, although most cases were diagnosed within 12 months of the last rituximab dose. A retrospective analysis of patients (n=57) diagnosed with PML following rituximab therapy, found a median of 16 months (following rituximab initiation), 5.5 months (following last rituximab dose), and 6 rituximab doses preceded PML diagnosis. Clinical findings included confusion/disorientation, motor weakness/hemiparesis, altered vision/speech, and poor motor coordination with symptoms progressing over weeks to months (Carson, 2009). Promptly evaluate any patient presenting with neurological changes; consider neurology consultation, brain MRI and lumbar puncture for suspected PML. Discontinue rituximab in patients who develop PML; consider reduction/discontinuation of concurrent chemotherapy or immunosuppressants. Avoid use if severe active infection is present. Serious and potentially fatal bacterial, fungal, and either new or reactivated viral infections may occur during treatment and after completing rituximab. Infections have been observed in patients with prolonged hypogammaglobulinemia, defined as hypogammaglobulinemia >11 months after rituximab exposure; monitor immunoglobulin levels as necessary. Associated new or reactivated viral infections have included cytomegalovirus, herpes simplex virus, parvovirus B19, varicella zoster virus, West Nile virus, and hepatitis B and C. Discontinue rituximab in patients who develop other serious infections and initiate appropriate anti-infective treatment.

Tumor lysis syndrome leading to acute renal failure requiring dialysis (some fatal) may occur 12-24 hours following the first dose when used as a single agent in the treatment of NHL. Hyperkalemia, hypocalcemia, hyperuricemia, and/or hyperphosphatemia may occur. Administer prophylaxis (antihyperuricemic therapy, hydration) in patients at high risk (high numbers of circulating malignant cells $\geq 25,000/mm^3$ or high tumor burden). May cause fatal renal toxicity in patients with hematologic malignancies. Patients who received combination therapy with cisplatin and rituximab for NHL experienced renal toxicity during clinical trials; this combination is not an approved treatment regimen. Monitor for signs of renal failure; discontinue rituximab with increasing serum creatinine or oliguria. Correct electrolyte abnormalities; monitor hydration status.

[U.S. Boxed Warning]: Severe and sometimes fatal mucocutaneous reactions (lichenoid dermatitis, paraneoplastic pemphigus, Stevens-Johnson syndrome, toxic epidermal necrolysis and vesiculobullous dermatitis) have been reported; onset has been variable but has occurred as early as the first day of exposure. Discontinue in patients experiencing severe mucocutaneous skin reactions; the safety of re-exposure following mucocutaneous reactions has not been evaluated. Use caution with preexisting cardiac or pulmonary disease, or prior cardiopulmonary events. Rheumatoid arthritis patients are at increased risk for cardiovascular events; monitor closely during and after each infusion. Elderly patients are at higher risk for cardiac (supraventricular arrhythmia) and pulmonary adverse events (pneumonia, pneumonitis). Abdominal pain, bowel obstruction, and perforation (rarely fatal) have been reported with an average onset of symptoms of ~6 days (range: 1-77 days); complaints of abdominal pain or repeated vomiting should be evaluated, especially if early in the treatment course. Live vaccines should not be given concurrently with rituximab; there is no data available concerning secondary transmission of live vaccines with or following rituximab treatment. RA patients should be brought up to date with nonlive immunizations (following current guidelines) at least 4 weeks before initiating therapy; evaluate risks of therapy delay versus benefit (of nonlive vaccines) for NHL patients. Safety and efficacy of rituximab in combination with biologic agents or disease-modifying antirheumatic drugs (DMARDs) other than methotrexate have not been established. Rituximab is not recommended for use in RA patients who have not had prior inadequate response to TNF antagonists. Safety and efficacy of re-treatment for RA have not been established. The safety of concomitant immunosuppressants other than corticosteroids has not been evaluated in patients with granulomatosis with polyangiitis (GPA; Wegener's granulomatosis) or microscopic polyangiitis (MPA) after rituximab-induced B-cell depletion. There are only limited data on subsequent courses of rituximab for GPA or MPA; safety and efficacy of re-treatment have not been established. ▶

◀ Some dosage forms may contain polysorbate 80 (also known as Tweens). Hypersensitivity reactions, usually a delayed reaction, have been reported following exposure to pharmaceutical products containing polysorbate 80 in certain individuals (Isaksson, 2002; Lucente 2000; Shelley, 1995). Thrombocytopenia, ascites, pulmonary deterioration, and renal and hepatic failure have been reported in premature neonates after receiving parenteral products containing polysorbate 80 (Alade, 1986; CDC, 1984). See manufacturer's labeling.

Adverse Reactions Note: Patients treated with rituximab for rheumatoid arthritis (RA) may experience fewer adverse reactions.

>10%:

Cardiovascular: Peripheral edema (8% to 16%), hypertension (6% to 12%)

Central nervous system: Fever (5% to 53%), fatigue (13% to 39%), chills (3% to 33%), headache (17% to 19%), insomnia (≤14%), pain (12%)

Dermatologic: Rash (10% to 17%; grades 3/4: 1%), pruritus (5% to 17%), angioedema (11%; grades 3/4: 1%)

Gastrointestinal: Nausea (8% to 23%), diarrhea (10% to 17%), abdominal pain (2% to 14%), weight gain (11%)

Hematologic: Cytopenias (grades 3/4: ≤48%; may be prolonged), lymphopenia (48%; grades 3/4: 40%; median duration: 14 days), anemia (8% to 35%; grades 3/4: 3%), leukopenia (NHL: 14%; grades 3/4: 4%; CLL: grades 3/4: 23%; GPA/MPA: 10%), neutropenia (NHL: 14%; grades 3/4: 4% to 6%; median duration 13 days; CLL: grades 3/4: 30% to 49%), neutropenic fever (CLL: grades 3/4: 9% to 15%), thrombocytopenia (12%; grades 3/4: 2% to 11%)

Hepatic: ALT increased (≤13%)

Neuromuscular & skeletal: Neuropathy (≤30%), weakness (2% to 26%), muscle spasm (≤17%), arthralgia (6% to 13%)

Respiratory: Cough (13%), rhinitis (3% to 12%), epistaxis (≤11%)

Miscellaneous: Infusion-related reactions (lymphoma: First dose 77%; decreases with subsequent infusions; may include angioedema, bronchospasm, chills, dizziness, fever, headache, hyper-/hypotension, myalgia, nausea, pruritus, rash, rigors, urticaria, and vomiting; reactions reported are lower [first infusion: 32%] in RA; CLL: 59%; grades 3/4: 7% to 9%; GPA/MPA: 12%); infection (19% to 62%; grades 3/4: 4%; bacterial: 19%; viral 10%; fungal: 1%), human antichimeric antibody (HACA) positive (1% to 23%), night sweats (15%)

1% to 10%:

Cardiovascular: Hypotension (10%; grades 3/4: 2%), flushing (5%)

Central nervous system: Dizziness (10%), anxiety (2% to 5%), migraine (RA: 2%)

Dermatologic: Urticaria (2% to 8%)

Endocrine & metabolic: Hyperglycemia (9%)

Gastrointestinal: Vomiting (10%), dyspepsia (RA: 3%)

Neuromuscular & skeletal: Back pain (10%), myalgia (10%), paresthesia (2%)

Respiratory: Dyspnea (≤10%), throat irritation (2% to 9%), bronchospasm (8%), dyspnea (7%), upper respiratory tract infection (RA: 7%), sinusitis (6%)

Miscellaneous: LDH increased (7%)

Postmarketing and/or case reports: Acute renal failure, anaphylactoid reaction/ anaphylaxis, angina, aplastic anemia, ARDS, arrhythmia, bowel obstruction/ perforation, bronchiolitis obliterans, cardiac failure, cardiogenic shock, disease progression (Kaposi's sarcoma), encephalomyelitis, fatal infusion-related reactions, fulminant hepatitis, gastrointestinal perforation, hemolytic anemia, hepatic failure, hepatitis, hepatitis B reactivation, hyperviscosity syndrome (in Waldenström's macroglobulinemia), hypogammaglobulinemia (prolonged), hypoxia, interstitial pneumonitis, laryngeal edema, lichenoid dermatitis, lupus-like syndrome, marrow hypoplasia, MI, mucositis, mucocutaneous reaction, neutropenia (late-onset occurring >40 days after last dose), optic neuritis, pancytopenia (prolonged), paraneoplastic pemphigus (uncommon), pleuritis, pneumonia, pneumonitis, polyarticular arthritis, polymyositis, posterior reversible encephalopathy syndrome (PRES), progressive multifocal leukoencephalopathy (PML), pure red cell aplasia, renal toxicity, reversible posterior leukoencephalopathy syndrome (RPLS), serum sickness, Stevens-Johnson syndrome, supraventricular arrhythmia, systemic vasculitis, toxic epidermal necrolysis, tuberculosis reactivation, tumor lysis syndrome, uveitis, vasculitis with rash, ventricular fibrillation, ventricular tachycardia, vesiculobullous dermatitis, viral reactivation (includes JC virus, cytomegalovirus, herpes simplex virus, parvovirus B19, varicella zoster virus, West Nile virus, and hepatitis C), wheezing

Drug Interactions

Metabolism/Transport Effects None known.

Avoid Concomitant Use

Avoid concomitant use of RiTUXimab with any of the following: Abatacept; BCG (Intravesical); Belimumab; Certolizumab Pegol; CloZAPine; Dipyrone; Natalizumab; Pimecrolimus; Tacrolimus (Topical); Tofacitinib; Vaccines (Live)

Increased Effect/Toxicity

RiTUXimab may increase the levels/effects of: Abatacept; Belimumab; Certolizumab Pegol; CloZAPine; Fingolimod; Leflunomide; Natalizumab; Tofacitinib; Vaccines (Live)

The levels/effects of RiTUXimab may be increased by: Antihypertensives; Denosumab; Dipyrone; Pimecrolimus; Roflumilast; Tacrolimus (Topical); Trastuzumab

Decreased Effect

RiTUXimab may decrease the levels/effects of: BCG (Intravesical); Coccidioides immitis Skin Test; Sipuleucel-T; Vaccines (Inactivated); Vaccines (Live)

The levels/effects of RiTUXimab may be decreased by: Echinacea

Storage/Stability Store intact vials refrigerated at 2°C to 8°C (36°F to 46°F); do not freeze. Do not shake. Protect vials from direct sunlight. Solutions for infusion are stable at 2°C to 8°C (36°F to 46°F) for 24 hours and at room temperature for an additional 24 hours.

Preparation for Administration Withdraw necessary amount of rituximab and dilute to a final concentration of 1-4 mg/mL with 0.9% sodium chloride or 5% dextrose in water. Gently invert the bag to mix the solution. Do not shake.

Mechanism of Action Rituximab is a monoclonal antibody directed against the CD20 antigen on B-lymphocytes. CD20 regulates cell cycle initiation; and, possibly, functions as a calcium channel. Rituximab binds to the antigen on the cell surface, activating complement-dependent B-cell cytotoxicity; and to human Fc receptors, mediating cell killing through an antibody-dependent cellular toxicity. B-cells are believed to play a role in the development and progression of rheumatoid arthritis. Signs and symptoms of RA are reduced by targeting B-cells and the progression of structural damage is delayed.

Pharmacodynamics/Kinetics

Duration: Detectable in serum 3-6 months after completion of treatment; B-cell recovery begins ~6 months following completion of treatment; median B-cell levels return to normal by 12 months following completion of treatment

Absorption: IV: Immediate and results in a rapid and sustained depletion of circulating and tissue-based B cells

Distribution: RA: 3.1 L; GPA/MPA: 4.5 L

Half-life elimination:

CLL: Median terminal half-life: 32 days (range: 14-62 days)

NHL: Median terminal half-life: 22 days (range: 6-52 days)

RA: Mean terminal half-life: 18 days (range: 5-78 days)

GPA/MPA: 23 days (range: 9-49 days)

Excretion: Uncertain; may undergo phagocytosis and catabolism in the reticuloendothelial system (RES)

Dosing

Adult & Geriatric Note: Details concerning dosing in combination regimens should also be consulted. Pretreatment with acetaminophen and an antihistamine is recommended for all indications. For oncology uses, antihyperuricemic therapy and aggressive hydration are recommended for patients at risk for tumor lysis syndrome (high tumor burden or lymphocytes >25,000/mm^3). In patients with CLL, *Pneumocystis jirovecii* pneumonia (PCP) and antiherpetic viral prophylaxis is recommended during treatment (and for up to 12 months following treatment). In patients with granulomatosis with polyangiitis (GPA) and microscopic polyangiitis (MPA), PCP prophylaxis is recommended during and for 6 months after rituximab treatment. For patients with RA, premedication with methylprednisolone 100 mg IV (or equivalent) is recommended 30 minutes prior to each dose.

Chronic lymphocytic leukemia (CLL): IV infusion: 375 mg/m^2 on the day prior to fludarabine/cyclophosphamide in cycle 1, then 500 mg/m^2 on day 1 (every 28 days) of cycles 2-6

Granulomatosis with polyangiitis (GPA; Wegener's granulomatosis): IV infusion: 375 mg/m^2 once weekly for 4 doses (in combination with methylprednisolone IV for 1-3 days followed by daily prednisone)

Non-Hodgkin lymphoma (NHL; relapsed/refractory, low-grade or follicular CD20-positive, B-cell): IV infusion: 375 mg/m^2 once weekly for 4 or 8 doses

Re-treatment following disease progression: 375 mg/m^2 once weekly for 4 doses

NHL (diffuse large B-cell): IV infusion: 375 mg/m^2 given on day 1 of each chemotherapy cycle for up to 8 doses

NHL (follicular, CD20-positive, B-cell, previously untreated): IV infusion: 375 mg/m^2 given on day 1 of each chemotherapy cycle for up to 8 doses

Maintenance therapy (as a single agent, in patients with partial or complete response to rituximab plus chemotherapy; begin 8 weeks after completion of combination chemotherapy): IV infusion: 375 mg/m^2 every 8 weeks for 12 doses

NHL (nonprogressing, low-grade, CD20-positive, B-cell, after 6-8 cycles of first line CVP are completed): IV infusion: 375 mg/m^2 once weekly for 4 doses every 6 months for a maximum of 16 doses

NHL: Combination therapy with ibritumomab: IV infusion: 250 mg/m^2 IV day 1; repeat in 7-9 days with ibritumomab (also see Ibritumomab monograph)

Canadian labeling: **NHL, low grade or follicular:** IV infusion:

Initial: 375 mg/m^2 once weekly for 4 doses (as a single agent) **or** 375 mg/m^2 on day 1 of each 21-day cycle for 8 cycles (in combination with CVP chemotherapy)

Maintenance (responding to induction therapy): 375 mg/m^2 every 3 months until disease progression or up to a maximum of 2 years

Rheumatoid arthritis: IV infusion: 1000 mg on days 1 and 15 in combination with methotrexate; subsequent courses may be administered every 24 weeks (based on clinical evaluation), if necessary may be repeated no sooner than every 16 weeks

Microscopic polyangiitis (MPA): IV infusion: 375 mg/m^2 once weekly for 4 doses (in combination with methylprednisolone IV for 1-3 days followed by daily prednisone)

Chronic graft-versus-host disease (GVHD), refractory (off-label use): IV infusion: 375 mg/m^2 once weekly for 4 doses (Cutler, 2006)

Idiopathic thrombocytopenic purpura (ITP; off-label use): IV infusion: 375 mg/m^2 once weekly for 4 doses (Arnold, 2007; Godeau, 2008)

Hodgkin lymphoma (off-label use): IV infusion: 375 mg/m^2 once weekly for 4 weeks (Ekstrand, 2003; Schulz, 2008)

Idiopathic membranous nephropathy (IMN), resistant (off-label use): IV infusion: 375 mg/m^2 once weekly for 4 doses with re-treatment at 6 months (Fervenza, 2010) **or** 1000 mg on days 1 and 15 (Fervenza, 2008) **or** 375 mg/m^2 single doses titrated to B cell response (Cravedi, 2007)

Lupus nephritis, refractory (off-label use): IV infusion: 375 mg/m^2 once weekly for 4 doses (Melander, 2009) **or** 500-1000 mg on days 1 and 15 (Vigna-Perez, 2006)

Pemphigus vulgaris, refractory (off-label use): IV infusion: 375 mg/m^2 once weekly of weeks 1, 2, and 3 of a 4-week cycle, repeat for 1 additional cycle, then 1 dose per month for 4 months (total of 10 doses in 6 months) (Ahmed, 2006)

Post-transplant lymphoproliferative disorder (off-label use): IV infusion: 375 mg/m^2 once weekly for 4 doses (Choquet, 2006)

Thrombotic thrombocytopenic purpura (TTP), relapsed/refractory (off-label use): IV infusion: 375 mg/m^2 once weekly for 4 doses (Scully, 2007; Scully, 2011)

Waldenström's macroglobulinemia (off-label use): IV infusion: 375 mg/m^2 once weekly for 4 weeks (Dimopoulos, 2002)

Pediatric Note: Pretreatment with acetaminophen and an antihistamine is recommended.

Autoimmune hemolytic anemia (AIHA; off-label use): IV infusion: 375 mg/m^2 once weekly for 2-4 doses (Zecca, 2003)

Chronic immune thrombocytopenia (ITP; off-label use): IV infusion: 375 mg/m^2 once weekly for 4 doses (Parodi, 2009; Wang, 2005)

Nephrotic syndrome, severe, refractory (off-label use): IV infusion: 375 mg/m^2 once weekly for 1-4 doses has been used in small case series, case reports, and retrospective analyses, including reports of successful remission induction of severe or refractory nephrotic syndromes that are poorly responsive to standard therapies (Dello Strologo, 2009; Fujinaga, 2010; Guigonis, 2008; Prytula, 2010)

Renal Impairment No dosage adjustment provided in manufacturer's labeling (has not been studied).

Hepatic Impairment No dosage adjustment provided in manufacturer's labeling (has not been studied).

▶

◄ **Combination Regimens**

Leukemia, chronic lymphocytic:

Lymphoma, non-Hodgkin:

Lymphoma, non-Hodgkin (Burkitt): Hyper-CVAD Alternating With High-Dose Methotrexate-Cytarabine + Rituximab + CNS Prophylaxis (NHL-Burkitt) on

Lymphoma, non-Hodgkin (DLBCL):

Lymphoma, non-Hodgkin (Follicular):

Lymphoma, non-Hodgkin (Mantle Cell):

Primary CNS Lymphoma: Temozolomide-Rituximab (CNS Lymphoma) on

Waldenstrom Macroglobulinemia:

Administration Note: Some pediatric protocols utilize an alternate rituximab administration rate. Refer to specific protocol for administration rate guidelines.

Do **not** administer IV push or bolus. If a reaction occurs, slow or stop the infusion. If the reaction abates, restart infusion at 50% of the previous rate. Discontinue infusion in the event of serious or life-threatening cardiac arrhythmias.

IV: Initial infusion: Start rate of 50 mg/hour; if there is no reaction, increase the rate by 50 mg/hour increments every 30 minutes, to a maximum rate of 400 mg/hour.

Subsequent infusions:

Standard infusion rate: If patient tolerated initial infusion, start at 100 mg/hour; if there is no reaction, increase the rate by 100 mg/hour increments every 30 minutes, to a maximum rate of 400 mg/hour.

Accelerated infusion rate (90 minutes): For patients with previously untreated follicular NHL and diffuse large B-cell NHL who are receiving a corticosteroid as part of their combination chemotherapy regimen, have a circulating lymphocyte count <5000/mm^3, or have no significant cardiovascular disease. After tolerance has been established (no grade 3 or 4 infusion-related event) at the recommended infusion rate in cycle 1, a rapid infusion rate may be used beginning with cycle 2. The daily corticosteroid, acetaminophen, and diphenhydramine are administered prior to treatment, then the rituximab dose is administered over 90 minutes, with 20% of the dose administered over the first 30 minutes and the remaining 80% is given over 60 minutes (Sehn, 2007). If the 90-minute infusion in cycle 2 is tolerated, the same rate may be used for the remainder of the treatment regimen (through cycles 6 or 8).

Emetic Potential Children and Adults: Minimal (<10%)

Monitoring Parameters CBC with differential and platelets (obtain at weekly to monthly intervals and more frequently in patients with cytopenias, or at 2-4 month intervals in rheumatoid arthritis patients, GPA and MPA), peripheral CD20$^+$ cells; HAMA/HACA titers (high levels may increase the risk of allergic reactions); renal function, fluid balance; vital signs; monitor for infusion reactions, cardiac monitoring during and after infusion in rheumatoid arthritis patients and in patients with preexisting cardiac disease or if arrhythmias develop during or after subsequent infusions.

Screen all patients for HBV infection prior to therapy initiation (eg, HBsAG and anti-HBc measurements). In addition, carriers and patients with evidence of current infection or recovery from prior hepatitis B infection should be monitored closely for clinical and laboratory signs of HBV reactivation and/or infection during therapy and for up to 2 years following completion of treatment. High-risk patients should be screened for hepatitis C (per NCCN NHL guidelines v.2.2013).

Complaints of abdominal pain, especially early in the course of treatment, should prompt a thorough diagnostic evaluation and appropriate treatment. Signs or symptoms of progressive multifocal leukoencephalopathy (focal neurologic deficits, which may present as hemiparesis, visual field deficits, cognitive impairment, aphasia, ataxia, and/or cranial nerve deficits). If PML is suspected, obtain brain MRI scan and lumbar puncture.

Medication Guide Available Yes

Dosage Forms Excipient information presented when available (limited, particularly for generics); consult specific product labeling.

Solution, Intravenous [preservative free]:

Rituxan: 10 mg/mL (10 mL, 50 mL) [contains polysorbate 80]

◆ **Riva-Anastrozole (Can)** see Anastrozole on page 112

◆ **Riva-Ciprofloxacin (Can)** see Ciprofloxacin (Systemic) on page 327

◆ **Riva-Fluconazole (Can)** see Fluconazole on page 725

◆ **Riva-Letrozole (Can)** see Letrozole on page 1019

- ◆ **Riva-Olanzapine (Can)** *see* OLANZapine *on page 1242*
- ◆ **Riva-Olanzapine ODT (Can)** *see* OLANZapine *on page 1242*
- ◆ **Riva-Valacyclovir (Can)** *see* ValACYclovir *on page 1712*
- ◆ **Rixubis** *see* Factor IX (Recombinant) *on page 684*
- ◆ **rLFN-α2** *see* Interferon Alfa-2b *on page 930*
- ◆ **Ro 5488** *see* Tretinoin (Systemic) *on page 1692*
- ◆ **RO5185426** *see* Vemurafenib *on page 1734*
- ◆ **Rocephin** *see* CefTRIAXone *on page 299*

Rolapitant (roe LA pi tant)

Related Information

Management of Chemotherapy-Induced Nausea and Vomiting in Adults *on page 2142*

Brand Names: US Varubi

Index Terms Rolapitant Hydrochloride; Rolapitant Monohydrate Hydrochloride; SCH-619734

Pharmacologic Category Antiemetic; Substance P/Neurokinin 1 Receptor Antagonist

Use Chemotherapy-induced nausea and vomiting (CINV), prevention: Prevention of delayed nausea and vomiting associated with initial and repeat courses of emetogenic cancer chemotherapy, including, but not limited to, highly-emetogenic chemotherapy in adults (in combination with other antiemetic agents).

Labeled Contraindications Concurrent use of thioridazine (a CYP2D6 substrate)

Pregnancy Considerations Adverse events were observed in some animal reproduction studies.

Breast-Feeding Considerations It is not known if rolapitant is excreted into breast milk. According to the manufacturer, the decision to breast-feed during therapy should take into account the risk of exposure to the infant and the benefits of treatment to the mother.

Warnings/Precautions Avoid use in patients with severe hepatic impairment; if use cannot be avoided, monitor for adverse reactions related to rolapitant. Potentially significant drug-drug interactions may exist, requiring dose or frequency adjustment, additional monitoring, and/or selection of alternative therapy. Rolapitant's inhibitory effect on CYP2D6 may persist for at least 7 days (or longer); increased plasma concentrations of certain CYP2D6 substrates may result in QT prolongation and torsades de pointes. Monitor for adverse reactions if concomitant use with CYP2D6 substrates with a narrow therapeutic index cannot be avoided. Avoid concurrent use with pimozide; concurrent use with thioridazine is contraindicated.

Adverse Reactions Clinical trials were conducted in patients receiving combination therapy with a 5-HT3 receptor antagonist and dexamethasone. It is not possible to correlate frequency of adverse events with rolaprepitant alone.

1% to 10%:

Central nervous system: Dizziness (6%)

Gastrointestinal: Decreased appetite (9%), hiccups (5%), dyspepsia (4%), stomatitis (4%), abdominal pain (3%)

Genitourinary: Urinary tract infection (4%)

Hematologic & oncologic: Neutropenia (7% to 9%), anemia (3%)

Drug Interactions

Metabolism/Transport Effects Substrate of CYP3A4 (major); **Note:** Assignment of Major/Minor substrate status based on clinically relevant drug interaction potential; **Inhibits** BCRP, CYP2B6 (weak), CYP2C8 (weak), CYP2D6 (moderate), P-glycoprotein

Avoid Concomitant Use

Avoid concomitant use of Rolapitant with any of the following: Amodiaquine; Bosutinib; PAZOPanib; Pimozide; Silodosin; Thioridazine; Topotecan; VinCRIStine (Liposomal)

Increased Effect/Toxicity

Rolapitant may increase the levels/effects of: Afatinib; Amodiaquine; ARIPiprazole; BCRP/ABCG2 Substrates; Bosutinib; Brentuximab Vedotin; Brexpiprazole; Colchicine; CYP2D6 Substrates; Dabigatran Etexilate; DOXOrubicin (Conventional); Edoxaban; Eliglustat; Everolimus; Fesoterodine; Ledipasvir; Metoprolol; Naloxegol; Nebivolol; PAZOPanib; P-glycoprotein/ABCB1 Substrates; Pimozide; Prucalopride; Ranolazine; Rifaximin; Silodosin; Thioridazine; Topotecan; VinCRIStine (Liposomal)

The levels/effects of Rolapitant may be increased by: Osimertinib; Propafenone

Decreased Effect

Rolapitant may decrease the levels/effects of: Codeine; Tamoxifen; TraMADol

The levels/effects of Rolapitant may be decreased by: Bosentan; CYP3A4 Inducers (Moderate); CYP3A4 Inducers (Strong); Dabrafenib; Deferasirox; Enzalutamide; Mitotane; Osimertinib; Siltuximab; St Johns Wort; Tocilizumab

Storage/Stability Store at 20°C to 25°C (68°F to 77°F); excursions are permitted between 15°C and 30°C (59°F and 86°F)

Mechanism of Action Rolapitant prevents delayed nausea and vomiting associated with emetogenic chemotherapy by selectively and competitively inhibiting the substance P/neurokinin 1 (NK$_1$) receptor.

Pharmacodynamics/Kinetics

Distribution: V$_d$/F: 387 L

Protein binding: 99.8%

Metabolism: Hepatic; primarily by CYP3A4 to form active metabolite M19 (major)

Half-life elimination: ~7 days (range: 169 to 183 hours)

Time to peak: ~4 hours

Excretion: Feces (73%); urine (~14%; primarily as metabolites)

Dosing

Adult & Geriatric

Chemotherapy-induced nausea and vomiting (prevention): Oral: **Note:** Do not administer rolapitant at less than 2-week intervals. No dosage adjustment for concomitant dexamethasone is required.

Highly emetogenic chemotherapy (cisplatin-based): 180 mg administered ~1 to 2 hours prior to chemotherapy on day 1 only (in combination with dexamethasone given on days 1, 2, 3, and 4 and a 5-HT$_3$ receptor antagonist given on day 1)

Moderately emetogenic chemotherapy and anthracycline/cyclophosphamide combinations: 180 mg administered ~1 to 2 hours prior to chemotherapy on day 1 only (in combination with dexamethasone given on day 1 and a 5-HT$_3$ receptor antagonist given as appropriate based the agent selected)

◀ ### Renal Impairment

CrCl 30 to 90 mL/minute: There are no dosage adjustments provided in the manufacturer's labeling; however, based on pharmacokinetics, dosage adjustment is not likely necessary.

CrCl <30 ml/minute and end-stage renal disease (ESRD): There are no dosage adjustments provided in the manufacturer's labeling (has not been studied).

Hepatic Impairment

Child-Pugh classes A and B: No dosage adjustment is necessary.

Child-Pugh class C: Avoid use if possible (has not been studied); if use cannot be avoided, monitor closely for adverse reactions related to rolapitant.

Administration Administer orally ~1 to 2 hours prior to each chemotherapy cycle (on day 1 only). May be administered without regard to meals.

Monitoring Parameters If concomitant use with CYP2D6 substrates with a narrow therapeutic index cannot be avoided, monitor for adverse reactions.

Dosage Forms Excipient information presented when available (limited, particularly for generics); consult specific product labeling.

Tablet, Oral:

Varubi: 90 mg [contains fd&c blue #2 aluminum lake]

◆ **Rolapitant Hydrochloride** see Rolapitant on page 1492

◆ **Rolapitant Monohydrate Hydrochloride** see Rolapitant on page 1492

RomiDEPsin (roe mi DEP sin)

Related Information

Common Toxicity Criteria on page 2122

Management of Chemotherapy-Induced Nausea and Vomiting in Adults on page 2142

Principles of Anticancer Therapy on page 2261

Safe Handling of Hazardous Drugs on page 2292

Brand Names: US Istodax

Index Terms Depsipeptide; FK228; FR901228

Pharmacologic Category Antineoplastic Agent, Histone Deacetylase (HDAC) Inhibitor

Use

Cutaneous T-cell lymphoma: Treatment of cutaneous T-cell lymphoma (CTCL) in patients who have received at least one systemic prior therapy

Peripheral T-cell lymphoma: Treatment of peripheral T-cell lymphoma (PTCL) in patients who have received at least one prior therapy

Labeled Contraindications There are no contraindications listed in the manufacturer's labeling.

Pregnancy Considerations Adverse events were observed in animal reproduction studies. Based on the mechanism of action, romidepsin may cause fetal harm if administered during pregnancy.

Breast-Feeding Considerations It is not known if romidepsin is excreted in breast milk. Due to the potential for serious adverse reactions in the nursing infant, the manufacturer recommends a decision be made whether to discontinue nursing or to discontinue the drug, taking into account the importance of treatment to the mother.

Warnings/Precautions Hazardous agent - use appropriate precautions for handling and disposal (NIOSH 2014 [group 1]). Anemia, leukopenia, neutropenia, lymphopenia and thrombocytopenia may occur; may require dosage modification; monitor blood counts during treatment. Serious infections (occasionally fatal), including pneumonia, sepsis, and viral reactivation (eg, Epstein Barr and hepatitis B) have occurred during or within 30 days of treatment. Monitor patients with a history of hepatitis B infections closely for viral reactivation; consider antiviral prophylaxis. Epstein Barr reactivation leading to liver failure has also been reported, with ganciclovir antiviral prophylaxis failure in one case. The risk of life-threatening infection may be increased in patients who have received prior with antilymphocytic monoclonal antibodies or who have disease involvement in the bone marrow. QTc prolongation has been observed; use caution in patients with a history of QTc prolongation, congenital long QT syndrome, with medications known to prolong the QT interval, or with preexisting cardiac disease. Obtain baseline and periodic ECG (12-lead); monitor and correct electrolyte (potassium, magnesium, and calcium) abnormalities prior to and during treatment. T-wave and ST-segment changes have also been reported. Use with caution in patients with moderate-to-severe hepatic impairment or end-stage renal disease. Tumor lysis syndrome (TLS) has been observed; closely monitor patients with advanced disease and/or with a high tumor burden (risk of TLS may be higher); if TLS occurs, initiate appropriate treatment. Potentially significant drug-drug interactions may exist, requiring dose or frequency adjustment, additional monitoring, and/or selection of alternative therapy.

Adverse Reactions

>10%:

Cardiovascular: ST-T wave changes (2% to 63%), hypotension (7% to 23%)

Central nervous system: Fatigue (53% to 77%), fever (20% to 47%), headache (15% to 34%), chills (11% to 17%)

Dermatologic: Pruritus (7% to 31%), dermatitis/exfoliative dermatitis (4% to 27%)

Endocrine & metabolic: Hypocalcemia (4% to 52%), hyperglycemia (2% to 51%), hypoalbuminemia (3% to 48%), hyperuricemia (≤33%), hypomagnesemia (22% to 28%), hypermagnesemia (≤27%), hypophosphatemia (≤27%), hypokalemia (6% to 20%), hyponatremia (≤20%)

Gastrointestinal: Nausea (56% to 86%; grades 3/4: 2% to 6%), anorexia (23% to 54%), vomiting (34% to 52%; grades 3/4: ≤10%), taste alteration (15% to 40%), constipation (12% to 40%), diarrhea (20% to 36%), weight loss (10% to 15%), abdominal pain (13% to 14%)

Hematologic: Anemia (19% to 72%; grades 3/4: 3% to 28%), thrombocytopenia (17% to 72%; grades 3/4: ≤36%), neutropenia (11% to 66%; grades 3/4: 4% to 47%), lymphopenia (4% to 57%; grades 3/4: ≤37%), leukopenia (4% to 55%; grades 3/4: ≤45%)

Hepatic: AST increased (3% to 28%), ALT increased (3% to 22%)

Neuromuscular & skeletal: Weakness (53% to 77%)

Respiratory: Cough (18% to 21%), dyspnea (13% to 21%)

Miscellaneous: Infection (46% to 54%; grades 3/4: 11% to 33%)

1% to 10%:

Cardiovascular: Peripheral edema (6% to 10%), tachycardia (≤10%), chest pain, DVT, edema, QT prolongation, supraventricular arrhythmia, syncope, ventricular arrhythmia

Dermatologic: Cellulitis

Endocrine & metabolic: Dehydration

Gastrointestinal: Stomatitis (6% to 10%)

Hematologic: Neutropenic fever

Hepatic: Hyperbilirubinemia

Respiratory: Hypoxia, pneumonia, pneumonitis, pulmonary embolism

Miscellaneous: Central line infection, hypersensitivity, sepsis, tumor lysis syndrome (1% to 2%)

<1%, postmarketing, and/or case reports: Acute renal failure, acute respiratory distress syndrome, atrial fibrillation, bacteremia, candida infection, cardiopulmonary failure, cardiogenic shock, Epstein-Barr virus reactivation, multiorgan failure, myocardial ischemia, septic shock

Drug Interactions

Metabolism/Transport Effects Substrate of CYP3A4 (major), P-glycoprotein; **Note:** Assignment of Major/Minor substrate status based on clinically relevant drug interaction potential; **Inhibits** BSEP

Avoid Concomitant Use

Avoid concomitant use of RomiDEPsin with any of the following: BCG (Intravesical); CloZAPine; CYP3A4 Inducers (Strong); Dexamethasone (Systemic); Dipyrone; Natalizumab; Pimecrolimus; Rifampin; St Johns Wort; Tacrolimus (Topical); Tofacitinib; Vaccines (Live)

Increased Effect/Toxicity

RomiDEPsin may increase the levels/effects of: CloZAPine; Fingolimod; Highest Risk QTc-Prolonging Agents; Leflunomide; Moderate Risk QTc-Prolonging Agents; Natalizumab; Tofacitinib; Vaccines (Live); Warfarin

The levels/effects of RomiDEPsin may be increased by: CYP3A4 Inhibitors (Strong); Denosumab; Dipyrone; Mifepristone; Osimertinib; P-glycoprotein/ABCB1 Inhibitors; Pimecrolimus; Ranolazine; Rifampin; Roflumilast; Tacrolimus (Topical); Trastuzumab

Decreased Effect

RomiDEPsin may decrease the levels/effects of: BCG (Intravesical); Coccidioides immitis Skin Test; Sipuleucel-T; Vaccines (Inactivated); Vaccines (Live)

The levels/effects of RomiDEPsin may be decreased by: Bosentan; CYP3A4 Inducers (Moderate); CYP3A4 Inducers (Strong); Dabrafenib; Deferasirox; Dexamethasone (Systemic); Echinacea; Osimertinib; P-glycoprotein/ABCB1 Inducers; Siltuximab; St Johns Wort; Tocilizumab

Food Interactions Grapefruit juice may increase the levels/effects of romidepsin. Management: Avoid grapefruit juice.

Storage/Stability Store intact vials at room temperature of 20°C to 25°C (68°F to 77°F); excursions are permitted between 15°C and 30°C (59°F and 86°F). The reconstituted solution is stable for 8 hours at room temperature. Solutions diluted for infusion are stable for 24 hours at room temperature; however, the manufacturer recommends use as soon as possible after dilution.

Preparation for Administration Hazardous agent; use appropriate precautions for handling and disposal (NIOSH 2014 [group 1]). Reconstitute each 10 mg vial with 2 mL of supplied diluent to a reconstituted concentration of 5 mg/mL; swirl until dissolved. (**Note:** Although the reconstituted vial contains a final volume of 2 mL, due to the viscosity of the reconstituted solution, a total volume <2 mL [usually ~1.6-1.8 mL] can be withdrawn from each vial.) Further dilute in 500 mL normal saline; compatible with polyvinyl chloride (PVC), ethylene vinyl acetate (EVA), polyethylene (PE) and glass infusion containers.

Mechanism of Action Histone deacetylase inhibitor; catalyzes acetyl group removal from protein lysine residues (including histone and transcription factors). Inhibition of histone deacetylase results in accumulation of acetyl groups, leading to alterations in chromatin structure and transcription factor activation causing termination of cell growth (induces arrest in cell cycle at G_1 and G_2/M phases) leading to cell death.

Pharmacodynamics/Kinetics

Protein binding: 92% to 94%; primarily to α_1-acid glycoprotein

Metabolism: Hepatic, primarily via CYP3A4, minor metabolism from CYP3A5, 1A1, 2B6, and 2C19

Half-life elimination: ~3 hours

Dosing

Adult & Geriatric

Cutaneous T-cell lymphoma: IV: 14 mg/m^2 days 1, 8, and 15 of a 28-day treatment cycle; repeat cycle as long as benefit continues and treatment is tolerated.

Peripheral T-cell lymphoma: IV: 14 mg/m^2 days 1, 8, and 15 of a 28-day treatment cycle; repeat cycle as long as benefit continues and treatment is tolerated.

Renal Impairment There are no dosage adjustments provided in the manufacturer's labeling (has not been studied). However, dosage adjustment is not likely necessary since pharmacokinetics are unaffected by renal impairment. Use with caution in patients with end-stage renal disease (has not been studied).

Hepatic Impairment

Mild impairment: There are no dosage adjustments provided in the manufacturer's labeling. However, mild hepatic impairment does not significantly influence the pharmacokinetics of romidepsin.

Moderate or severe impairment: There are no dosage adjustments provided in the manufacturer's labeling. Use with caution.

Obesity *American Society of Clinical Oncology (ASCO) Guidelines for appropriate chemotherapy dosing in obese adults with cancer:* Utilize patient's actual body weight (full weight) for calculation of body surface area- or weight-based dosing, particularly when the intent of therapy is curative; manage regimen-related toxicities in the same manner as for nonobese patients; if a dose reduction is utilized due to toxicity, consider resumption of full weight-based dosing with subsequent cycles, especially if cause of toxicity (eg, hepatic or renal impairment) is resolved (Griggs, 2012).

Adjustment for Toxicity

Nonhematologic toxicity (excluding alopecia):

Grade 2 or 3: Delay treatment until toxicity returns to ≤ grade 1 or baseline, may restart at 14 mg/m^2

Grade 4 or recurrent grade 3 toxicity: Delay treatment until toxicity returns to ≤ grade 1 or baseline, permanently reduce dose to 10 mg/m^2

Recurrent grade 3 or 4 toxicity despite dosage reduction: Discontinue treatment

Hematologic toxicity:

Grade 3 or 4 neutropenia or thrombocytopenia: Delay treatment until ANC ≥1500/mm^3 and/or platelets ≥75,000/mm^3 or baseline, may restart at 14 mg/m^2

Grade 4 febrile neutropenia or thrombocytopenia requiring platelet transfusion: Delay treatment until toxicity returns to ≤ grade 1 or baseline, permanently reduce dose to 10 mg/m^2

◄ **Administration** Infuse over 4 hours. Although romidepsin has a low emetic potential, antiemetics to prevent nausea and vomiting were used in clinical trials (Piekarz, 2009; Piekarz, 2011).

Hazardous agent; use appropriate precautions for handling and disposal (NIOSH 2014 [group 1]).

Emetic Potential Low (10% to 30%)

Monitoring Parameters Serum electrolytes (baseline and periodic; especially potassium and magnesium); CBC with differential and platelets, ECG (baseline and periodic; in patients with significant cardiovascular disease, congenital long QT syndrome, and in patients taking QT-prolonging medications); signs/ symptoms of infection or tumor lysis syndrome

Dietary Considerations Avoid grapefruit juice.

Dosage Forms Excipient information presented when available (limited, particularly for generics); consult specific product labeling.
Solution Reconstituted, Intravenous:
Istodax: 10 mg (1 ea) [contains alcohol, usp, propylene glycol]

RomiPLOStim (roe mi PLOE stim)

Brand Names: US Nplate
Brand Names: Canada Nplate
Index Terms AMG 531
Pharmacologic Category Colony Stimulating Factor; Hematopoietic Agent; Thrombopoietic Agent

Use
Chronic immune thrombocytopenia: Treatment of thrombocytopenia in patients with chronic immune thrombocytopenia (ITP) who have had insufficient response to corticosteroids, immune globulin, or splenectomy
Limitations of use: Should be used only when the degree of thrombocytopenia and clinical condition increase the risk for bleeding; should not be used in attempt to normalize platelet counts; **not** indicated for the treatment of thrombocytopenia due to myelodysplastic syndrome or any cause of thrombocytopenia other than chronic ITP.

Labeled Contraindications
There are no contraindications listed in the US labeling.
Canadian labeling: Hypersensitivity to romiplostim or any component of the formulation; known history of sensitivity or allergy to any *E. coli*-derived product.

Pregnancy Considerations Adverse events have been observed in animal reproduction studies. Use during pregnancy only if the potential benefit to the mother outweighs the potential risk to the fetus.

Women exposed to romiplostim during pregnancy are encouraged to enroll in the Nplate pregnancy (1-800-772-6436). In Canada, women who become pregnant during treatment are encouraged to enroll in Amgen's Pregnancy Surveillance Program (1-866-512-6436).

Breast-Feeding Considerations It is not known if romiplostim is excreted in breast milk. Due to the potential for serious adverse reactions in the nursing infant, the manufacturer recommends a decision be made to discontinue breast-feeding or to discontinue romiplostim, taking into account the importance of treatment to the mother. In Canada, women who nurse during treatment are encouraged to enroll in Amgen's Lactation Surveillance Program (1-866-512-6436).

Warnings/Precautions May increase the risk for bone marrow reticulin formation or progression; this formation may improve upon discontinuation of therapy. Thromboembolism or thrombotic complications may occur with increased platelets; follow dosage adjustment recommendations to minimize the risk for thrombotic or thromboembolic complications; use with caution in patients with a history of cerebrovascular disease. Progression from existing myelodysplastic syndrome (MDS) to acute myeloid leukemia (AML) has been observed in clinical trials studying romiplostim for severe thrombocytopenia associated with MDS (not an approved indication); a higher percentage of patients receiving romiplostim experienced transformation to AML (compared to placebo). An increase in the percentage of circulating myeloblasts in peripheral blood counts was also noted (both in patients who progressed to AML and in those who did not); blast cells decreased to baseline after discontinuation in some patients.

Indicated only when the degree of thrombocytopenia and clinical conditions increase the risk for bleeding; use the lowest dose necessary to achieve and maintain platelet count ≥50,000/mm³. Do not use to normalize platelet counts. Discontinue if platelet count does not respond to a level to avoid clinically important bleeding after 4 weeks at the maximum recommended dose. May be used in combination with other therapies for ITP, including corticosteroids, danazol, azathioprine, immune globulin, or Rho(D) immune globulin; not indicated for the treatment of thrombocytopenia due to any cause other than chronic ITP. Reduce dose or discontinue ITP medications when platelet count ≥50,000/mm³. Lack of response or failure to maintain platelet response should trigger investigation in to causative factors, including neutralizing antibodies to romiplostim.

Overdose may result in thrombotic/thromboembolic complications due to excessive platelet levels; underdose may result in lack of platelet response and potential for bleeding. Use caution when calculating dose and appropriate volume for administration (volume may be very small; administer with syringe that allows for 0.01 mL graduations).

Upon discontinuation of therapy, rebound thrombocytopenia and risk of bleeding may develop. Severity may be greater than pretreatment level; monitor CBCs and platelet counts weekly for at least 2 weeks after discontinuation.

Use with caution in patients with chronic liver disease; portal vein thrombosis has been reported in these patients.

Adverse Reactions
>10%:
Central nervous system: Headache (35%), dizziness (17%), insomnia (16%)
Gastrointestinal: Abdominal pain (11%)
Hematologic: Circulating myeloblasts increased (MDS patients: 17%)
Neuromuscular & skeletal: Arthralgia (26%), myalgia (14%), limb pain (13%)
1% to 10%:
Gastrointestinal: Dyspepsia (7%)
Hematologic: Rebound thrombocytopenia (7%), AML (MDS patients: 4% to 6%), bone marrow reticulin formation/deposition (4%)
Neuromuscular & skeletal: Shoulder pain (8%), paresthesia (6%)
Miscellaneous: Antibody formation (romiplostim 6%; TPO 4%)
<1%, postmarketing, and/or case reports: Angioedema, erythromelalgia, hypersensitivity, marrow fibrosis with collagen, thromboembolism, thrombotic complications

◀ **Drug Interactions**

Metabolism/Transport Effects None known.

Avoid Concomitant Use There are no known interactions where it is recommended to avoid concomitant use.

Increased Effect/Toxicity There are no known significant interactions involving an increase in effect.

Decreased Effect There are no known significant interactions involving a decrease in effect.

Storage/Stability Store intact vials refrigerated at 2°C to 8°C (36°F to 46°F); do not freeze. Protect from light. Store in original carton until use. Reconstituted solution may be stored at room temperature of 25°C (77°F) or refrigerated at 2°C to 8°C (36°F to 46°F) for up to 24 hours prior to administration. Protect reconstituted solution from light; discard any unused portion.

Preparation for Administration Reconstitute with only preservative free SWFI (add 0.72 mL to 250 mcg vial or 1.2 mL to 500 mcg vial). Do not use bacteriostatic water for injection. Gently invert vial and swirl; do not shake. Usually dissolves within 2 minutes.

Mechanism of Action Thrombopoietin (TPO) peptide mimetic which increases platelet counts in ITP by binding to and activating the human TPO receptor.

Pharmacodynamics/Kinetics

Onset of action: Platelet count increase: SubQ: 4 to 9 days (Wang, 2004); Peak platelet count increase: Days 12 to 16 (Wang, 2004)

Duration: Platelet counts return to baseline by day 28 (Wang, 2004)

Absorption: SubQ: Slow (Wang, 2004)

Half-life elimination: Median: 3.5 days (range: 1 to 34 days)

Time to peak, plasma: SubQ: Median: 14 hours (range: 7 to 50 hours)

Dosing

Adult & Geriatric Note: Initial dose is based on actual body weight. Use the lowest dose sufficient to maintain platelet count ≥50,000/mm^3 as necessary to reduce the risk of bleeding. Adjust dose based on platelet count response; discontinue if platelet count does not respond to a level that avoids clinically important bleeding after 4 weeks at the maximum recommended dose. Do not use to normalize platelet counts.

Chronic immune thrombocytopenia (ITP): SubQ: Initial: 1 mcg/kg once weekly; adjust dose by 1 mcg/kg/week increments to achieve platelet count ≥50,000/mm^3 and to reduce the risk of bleeding; Maximum dose: 10 mcg/kg/week (median dose needed to achieve response in clinical trials: 2 mcg/kg)

Dosage adjustment recommendations:

Platelet count <50,000/mm^3:

US labeling: Increase weekly dose by 1 mcg/kg

Canadian labeling: Increase weekly dose by 1 mcg/kg every 1 to 2 weeks

Platelet count >200,000/mm^3 for 2 consecutive weeks: Reduce weekly dose by 1 mcg/kg

Platelet count >400,000/mm^3: Withhold dose; assess platelet count weekly; when platelet count <200,000/mm^3, resume with the weekly dose reduced by 1 mcg/kg

Renal Impairment There are no dosage adjustments provided in the manufacturer's labeling (has not been studied).

Hepatic Impairment There are no dosage adjustments provided in the manufacturer's labeling (has not been studied).

Administration Administer SubQ. Administration volume may be small; use appropriate syringe (with graduations to 0.01 mL) for administration. Verify calculations, final concentration, and volume drawn up for administration.

Monitoring Parameters CBC with differential and platelets (baseline, during treatment [weekly until platelet response stable for at least 4 weeks then monthly] and weekly for at least 2 weeks following discontinuation or completion of treatment)

Evaluate for neutralizing antibodies in patients with inadequate response (blood samples may be submitted to the manufacturer for assay [1-800-772-6436]).

Dietary Considerations Some products may contain sucrose.

Additional Information Restricted access to Nplate was previously a REMS requirement via the Nplate NEXUS (Network of Experts Understanding and Supporting Nplate and Patients) program. Patients, prescribers, and pharmacies were required to be enrolled in this program. However, the FDA eliminated this REMS requirement in December 2011. There is currently no restricted access to obtaining Nplate.

Medication Guide Available Yes

Dosage Forms Excipient information presented when available (limited, particularly for generics); consult specific product labeling.
Solution Reconstituted, Subcutaneous [preservative free]:
Nplate: 250 mcg (1 ea); 500 mcg (1 ea)

♦ **Roxanol** see Morphine (Systemic) on page 1167

♦ **Roxicodone** see OxyCODONE on page 1277

♦ **RP-6976** see DOCEtaxel on page 535

♦ **rpFVIII** see Antihemophilic Factor (Recombinant [Porcine Sequence]) on page 123

♦ **RPR-116258A** see Cabazitaxel on page 250

♦ **RS-25259** see Palonosetron on page 1307

♦ **RS-25259-197** see Palonosetron on page 1307

♦ **RU-23908** see Nilutamide on page 1205

♦ **Rubidomycin Hydrochloride** see DAUNOrubicin (Conventional) on page 463

Ruxolitinib (rux oh LI ti nib)

Related Information

Management of Chemotherapy-Induced Nausea and Vomiting in Adults on page 2142

Safe Handling of Hazardous Drugs on page 2292

Brand Names: US Jakafi

Brand Names: Canada Jakavi

Index Terms INCB 18424; INCB018424; INCB424; Ruxolitinib Phosphate

Pharmacologic Category Antineoplastic Agent, Janus Associated Kinase Inhibitor; Antineoplastic Agent, Tyrosine Kinase Inhibitor; Janus Associated Kinase Inhibitor

◄ **Use**
  US labeling:
    Myelofibrosis: Treatment of intermediate or high-risk myelofibrosis, includ-
    ing primary myelofibrosis, post-polycythemia vera (post-PV) myelofibrosis
    and post-essential thrombocythemia (post-ET) myelofibrosis
    Polycythemia vera: Treatment of polycythemia vera with an inadequate
    response to or intolerance to hydroxyurea
  Canadian labeling:
    Myelofibrosis: Treatment of splenomegaly and/or its associated symptoms
    in adult patients with primary myelofibrosis, post-PV myelofibrosis or post-
    ET myelofibrosis

Labeled Contraindications
  There are no contraindications listed in the manufacturer's U.S. labeling.
  Canadian labeling: Hypersensitivity to ruxolitinib or any component of the
  formulation or container; history of or current progressive multifocal leukoencephalopathy

Pregnancy Considerations Increased resorptions (late) and reduced fetal
  weights were observed in animal reproduction studies. The Canadian labeling
  recommends avoiding use during pregnancy and that women of childbearing
  potential and male patients use effective contraception during therapy.

Breast-Feeding Considerations It is not known if ruxolitinib is excreted in
  breast milk. According to the manufacturer, due to the potential for serious
  adverse reactions in the nursing infant, a decision should be made to
  discontinue ruxolitinib or to discontinue breast-feeding during therapy, taking
  into account the benefits of treatment to the mother.

Warnings/Precautions Hazardous agent - use appropriate precautions for
  handling and disposal (meets NIOSH 2014 criteria). Hematologic toxicity,
  including thrombocytopenia, anemia and neutropenia may occur; may require
  dosage modification; monitor complete blood counts at baseline, every 2 to 4
  weeks during dose stabilization, and then as clinically necessary. Thrombocytopenia is generally reversible with treatment interruption or dose reduction;
  platelet transfusions may be administered during treatment if clinically indicated. Anemia may require blood transfusion; may consider dose modification.
  Neutropenia (ANC <500/mm^3) is generally reversible and managed by treatment interruption.

Serious bacterial, mycobacterial (including tuberculosis), fungal, or viral infections have occurred. Active serious infections should be resolved prior to
  treatment initiation. Monitor for infections (including signs/symptoms of active
  tuberculosis and herpes zoster) during treatment. Prompt treatment is recommended if symptoms of active tuberculosis and/or herpes zoster infection
  develop. Evaluate for tuberculosis risk factors prior to treatment initiation;
  patients at higher risk for tuberculosis (prior residence/travel to countries with
  a high tuberculosis prevalence, close contacts with active tuberculosis, or
  history of latent or active tuberculosis where adequate treatment course cannot
  be confirmed) should be tested for latent infection. For patients with evidence
  of tuberculosis (active or latent), decide risk-benefit of continuing treatment.
  Progressive multifocal leukoencephalopathy (PML) has been reported; discontinue and evaluate if suspected. May require initial dosage reduction for
  hepatic impairment; in patients with myelofibrosis, avoid use if platelets
  <50,000/mm^3 and with hepatic impairment (any degree). May require initial
  dosage reduction for renal impairment. Avoid use in patients with ESRD not
  requiring dialysis; in patients with myelofibrosis, avoid use if platelets
  <50,000/mm^3 and with moderate-to-severe renal impairment. Ruxolitinib is

not removed by dialysis, however, some active metabolites may be removed. On dialysis days, patients are advised to take their dose following dialysis sessions. Potentially significant drug-drug interactions may exist, requiring dose or frequency adjustment, additional monitoring, and/or selection of alternative therapy. Discontinue treatment in myelofibrosis patients after 6 months if no reduction in spleen size or no improvement in symptoms. Consider gradually tapering off if discontinuing for reasons other than thrombocytopenia. Within ~1 week after discontinuation, symptoms of myelofibrosis generally return to pretreatment levels. Acute relapse of myelofibrosis symptoms (eg, fever, respiratory distress, hypotension, DIC, multiorgan failure), splenomegaly, worsening cytopenias, hemodynamic compensation, and septic shock-like syndrome have been reported with treatment tapering or discontinuation (Tefferi, 2011). Symptoms generally return over approximately 1 week. Evaluate and treat any intercurrent illness and consider restarting or increasing dose. Consider gradually tapering off if discontinuing for reasons other than thrombocytopenia or neutropenia. Patients should not interrupt/discontinue treatment without consulting healthcare provider.

Non-melanoma skin cancers (basal cell, squamous cell, and Merkel cell carcinoma) have been reported in patients who have received ruxolitinib; periodic skin examinations should be performed. Use with caution in patients with a history of bradycardia, conduction disturbances, ischemic heart disease, heart failure and/or receiving other drugs that also affect heart rate/conduction; decreased heart rate (mean change 6 to 8 bpm) and prolongation of the PR interval (mean change 6 to 9 msec) and of the QT interval (mean 4 to 5 msec) were observed during some clinical trials. Canadian labeling recommends obtaining an ECG at baseline and periodically; monitor heart rate and blood pressure during treatment.

Adverse Reactions

>10%:
  Central nervous system: Dizziness (15% to 18%), headache (15% to 16%), fatigue (15%), insomnia (12%) (Verstovsek 2012)
  Dermatologic: Bruise (23%), pruritus (14%)
  Endocrine & metabolic: Increased serum cholesterol (17% to 35%), hypertriglyceridemia (15%)
  Gastrointestinal: Diarrhea (15%), abdominal pain (15%)
  Hematologic & oncologic: Anemia (72% to 96%; grade 3: ≤34%; grade 4: ≤11%), thrombocytopenia (27% to 70%; grade 3: 5% to 9%; grade 4: ≤4%), neutropenia (3% to 19%; grade 3: 5%; grade 4: ≤2%)
  Hepatic: Increased serum ALT (25%; grade 3: <1%), increased serum AST (17% to 23%)
  Neuromuscular & skeletal: Muscle spasm (12%)
  Respiratory: Dyspnea (13%)
1% to 10%:
  Cardiovascular: Edema (8%), hypertension (<6%)
  Endocrine & metabolic: Weight gain (≤7%)
  Gastrointestinal: Constipation (8%), nausea (6%), flatulence (5%), vomiting
  Genitourinary: Urinary tract infection (≤9%)
  Infection: Herpes zoster (2% yo 6%)
  Neuromuscular & skeletal: Weakness (7%)
  Respiratory: Nasopharyngitis (9%), cough (8%), epistaxis (6%)

◀ <1%, postmarketing, and/or case reports: Bradycardia, disseminated intra-vascular coagulation, fever, hemorrhagic diathesis, hypotension, multi-organ failure, myelofibrosis (symptom exacerbation), progressive multifocal leu-koencephalopathy, prolonged Q-T interval on ECG, respiratory distress, systolic hypertension, tuberculosis, withdrawal syndrome

Drug Interactions

Metabolism/Transport Effects Substrate of CYP3A4 (major); **Note:** Assignment of Major/Minor substrate status based on clinically relevant drug interaction potential

Avoid Concomitant Use

Avoid concomitant use of Ruxolitinib with any of the following: BCG (Intra-vesical); CloZAPine; Conivaptan; Dipyrone; Fusidic Acid (Systemic); Idelali-sib; Natalizumab; Pimecrolimus; Tacrolimus (Topical); Tofacitinib; Vaccines (Live)

Increased Effect/Toxicity

Ruxolitinib may increase the levels/effects of: Bradycardia-Causing Agents; CloZAPine; Fingolimod; Leflunomide; Natalizumab; Tofacitinib; Vaccines (Live)

The levels/effects of Ruxolitinib may be increased by: Aprepitant; Coniva-ptan; CYP3A4 Inhibitors (Moderate); CYP3A4 Inhibitors (Strong); Dasatinib; Denosumab; Dipyrone; Fluconazole; Fosaprepitant; Fusidic Acid (Systemic); Grapefruit Juice; Idelalisib; Ivacaftor; Luliconazole; Mifepristone; Netupitant; Osimertinib; Palbociclib; Pimecrolimus; Roflumilast; Simeprevir; Stiripentol; Tacrolimus (Topical); Trastuzumab

Decreased Effect

Ruxolitinib may decrease the levels/effects of: BCG (Intravesical); Cocci-dioides immitis Skin Test; Sipuleucel-T; Vaccines (Inactivated); Vaccines (Live)

The levels/effects of Ruxolitinib may be decreased by: Bosentan; CYP3A4 Inducers (Moderate); CYP3A4 Inducers (Strong); Dabrafenib; Deferasirox; Echinacea; Enzalutamide; Mitotane; Osimertinib; Siltuximab; St Johns Wort; Tocilizumab

Food Interactions Grapefruit juice may increase the effects of ruxolitinib. Management: Avoid grapefruit juice.

Storage/Stability Store at 20°C to 25°C (68°F to 77°F); excursions are permitted between 15°C and 30°C (59°F and 86°F).

Mechanism of Action Kinase inhibitor which selectively inhibits Janus Associated Kinases (JAKs), JAK1 and JAK2. JAK1 and JAK2 mediate signal-ing of cytokine and growth factors responsible for hematopoiesis and immune function; JAK mediated signaling involves recruitment of STATs (signal trans-ducers and activators of transcription) to cytokine receptors which leads to modulation of gene expression. In myelofibrosis and polycythemia vera, JAK1/2 activity is dysregulated; ruxolitinib modulates the affected JAK1/2 activity.

Pharmacodynamics/Kinetics

Absorption: Rapid

Distribution: V_d: Myelofibrosis: 72 L; Polycythemia vera: 75 L

Protein binding: ~97%; primarily to albumin

Metabolism: Hepatic, primarily via CYP3A4 (and minimally CYP2C9); forms active metabolites responsible for 20% to 50% of activity

Half-life elimination: Ruxolitinib: 2.8 to 3 hours (hepatic impairment: 4 to 5 hours); Ruxolitinib + metabolites: ~6 hours

Time to peak: Within 1 to 2 hours

Excretion: Urine (74%, <1% as unchanged drug); feces (22%, <1% as unchanged drug)

Dosing

Adult Note: Consider gradually tapering off (by 5 mg twice daily each week) if discontinuing for reasons other than thrombocytopenia.

Myelofibrosis: Oral: Initial dose (based on platelet count, titrate dose thereafter based on efficacy and safety):

Platelets >200,000/mm^3: 20 mg twice daily

Platelets 100,000 to 200,000/mm^3: 15 mg twice daily

Platelets 50,000 to <100,000/mm^3: 5 mg twice daily

Dosage modification based on response in patients with baseline platelet count ≥100,000/mm^3 prior to initial treatment with ruxolitinib: For insufficient response (with adequate platelet and neutrophil counts), may increase the dose in 5 mg twice daily increments to a maximum dose of 25 mg twice daily. Do not increase during initial 4 weeks and no more frequently than every 2 weeks. Discontinue treatment after 6 months if no reduction in spleen size or no improvement in symptoms. When discontinuing for reasons other than thrombocytopenia, consider gradually tapering by ~5 mg twice daily per week.

Dose increases may be considered if meet all of the following situations:
- Failure to achieve either a 50% reduction (from baseline) in palpable spleen length or a 35% reduction (from baseline) in spleen volume (measured by CT or MRI)
- Platelet count >125,000/mm^3 at 4 weeks (and never <100,000/mm^3)
- Absolute neutrophil count (ANC) >750/mm^3

Dosage modification for bleeding requiring intervention (regardless of platelet count): Interrupt treatment until bleeding resolved; may consider resuming at the prior dose if the underlying cause of bleeding has resolved or at a reduced dose if the underlying cause of bleeding persists.

Dosage modification based on response in patients with baseline platelet 50,000 to <100,000/mm^3 prior to initial treatment with ruxolitinib: For insufficient response (with adequate platelet and neutrophil counts), may increase the dose in 5 mg daily increments to a maximum dose of 10 mg twice daily. Do not increase during initial 4 weeks and no more frequently than every 2 weeks. Discontinue treatment after 6 months if no reduction in spleen size or no improvement in symptoms.

Dose increases may be considered if meet all of the following situations:
- Platelet count remains ≥40,000/mm^3 and did not decrease more than 20% in prior 4 weeks
- Absolute neutrophil count (ANC) >1,000/mm^3
- No adverse event or hematological toxicity resulting in dose reduction or interruption occurred in prior 4 weeks

Polycythemia vera: Oral: Initial dose: 10 mg twice daily (titrate dose based on efficacy and safety)

◄

Dose modification due to insufficient response: If response is insufficient and platelet, hemoglobin, and neutrophil counts are adequate, the dose may be increased in 5 mg twice daily increments to a maximum of 25 mg twice daily, Do not increase dose in the first 4 weeks of treatment and not more frequently than every 2 weeks. Consider dose increases in patients who meet all of the following conditions:

- Inadequate efficacy demonstrated by one or more of the following: Continued need for phlebotomy, WBC >ULN of normal range, platelet count >ULN of normal range, or palpable spleen that is reduced by <25% from baseline.
- Platelet count ≥140,000/mm^3
- Hemoglobin ≥12 g/dL
- ANC ≥1,500/mm^3

Dosage adjustment with concomitant strong CYP3A4 inhibitors (eg, azole antifungals, clarithromycin, conivaptin, grapefruit juice, mibefradil, nefazodone, protease inhibitors, telithromycin) and fluconazole (≤200 mg):

US labeling: **Note:** Avoid concomitant use with fluconazole doses >200 mg daily.

Myelofibrosis: Initial dose:

Platelets ≥100,000/mm^3: 10 mg twice daily.

Platelets 50,000/mm^3 to <100,000/mm^3: 5 mg once daily.

Polycythemia vera: Initial dose: 5 mg twice daily

Patients stabilized on ruxolitinib ≥10 mg twice daily: Reduce dose by 50% (rounded up to the closest available tablet strength).

Patients stabilized on ruxolitinib 5 mg twice daily: Reduce dose to 5 mg once daily.

Patients stabilized on ruxolitinib 5 mg once daily: Avoid strong CYP3A4 inhibitors or fluconazole or interrupt treatment for the duration of strong CYP3A4 inhibitor or fluconazole use.

Monitor closely and further adjust dose based on safety and efficacy.

Dosage adjustment with concomitant strong CYP3A4 inhibitors or concomitant moderate CYP2C9 and CYP3A4 inhibitors (Canadian labeling): Initial dose: 10 mg twice daily (~50% of the dose, rounded to the closest available strength); monitor hematologic parameters more frequently (eg, twice weekly) and titrate dose based on safety and efficacy. Avoid concomitant use if platelets <100,000/mm^3. If used concomitantly with fluconazole, do not exceed fluconazole 200 mg/day.

Renal Impairment

U.S. labeling:

Myelofibrosis:

CrCl 15 to 59 mL/minute and platelets >150,000/mm^3: No dosage adjustment is necessary.

CrCl 15 to 59 mL/minute and platelets 100,000 to 150,000/mm^3: Initial dose: 10 mg twice daily; additional dose adjustments should be made with careful monitoring.

CrCl 15 to 59 mL/minute and platelets 50,000 to <100,000/mm^3: Initial dose: 5 mg once daily; additional dose adjustments should be made with careful monitoring.

CrCl 15 to 59 mL/minute and platelets <50,000/mm^3: Avoid use.

End-stage renal disease (ESRD) on dialysis and platelets 100,000 to 200,000/mm^3: Initial dose: 15 mg once after dialysis; administer subsequent doses after dialysis on dialysis days. Additional dose adjustments should be made with frequent monitoring.

ESRD on dialysis and platelets >200,000/mm^3: Initial dose: 20 mg once after dialysis; administer subsequent doses after dialysis on dialysis days. Additional dose adjustments should be made with frequent monitoring.

ESRD not requiring dialysis: Avoid use.

Polycythemia vera:

CrCl 15 to 59 mL/minute and any platelet count: Initial: 5 mg twice daily. Additional dose adjustments should be made with frequent monitoring.

End-stage renal disease (ESRD) on dialysis: Initial dose: 10 mg once after dialysis; additional dose adjustments should be made with careful monitoring

ESRD not requiring dialysis: Avoid use.

Canadian labeling:

CrCl <50 mL/minute and platelets ≥100,000/mm^3: Initial dose: 10 mg twice daily; additional dose adjustments should be made with careful monitoring

CrCl <50 mL/minute and platelets <100,000/mm^3: Avoid use

ESRD on dialysis and platelets 100,000 to 200,000/mm^3: Initial dose: 15 mg; administer subsequent doses after dialysis on dialysis days. Additional dose adjustments should be made with careful monitoring.

ESRD on dialysis and platelets >200,000/mm^3: Initial dose: 20 mg; administer subsequent doses after dialysis on dialysis days. Additional dose adjustments should be made with careful monitoring.

Hepatic Impairment

U.S. labeling:

Myelofibrosis:

Mild-to-severe impairment (Child-Pugh class A, B, or C) and platelets >150,000/mm^3: No dosage adjustment is necessary.

Mild-to-severe impairment (Child-Pugh class A, B, or C) and platelets 100,000 to 150,000/mm^3: Initial dose: 10 mg twice daily; additional dose adjustments should be made with careful monitoring.

Mild-to-severe impairment (Child-Pugh class A, B, or C) and platelets 50,000 to <100,000/mm^3: Initial dose: 5 mg once daily; additional dose adjustments should be made with careful monitoring.

Mild-to-severe impairment (Child-Pugh class A, B, or C) and platelets <50,000/mm^3: Avoid use.

Polycythemia vera: Mild-to-severe impairment (Child-Pugh class A, B, or C) and any platelet count: Initial dose: 5 mg twice daily; additional dose adjustments should be made with careful monitoring.

Canadian labeling:

Hepatic impairment and platelets ≥100,000/mm³: Initial dose: 10 mg twice daily; additional dose adjustments should be made with careful monitoring.

Hepatic impairment and platelets <100,000/mm³: Avoid use.

Adjustment for Toxicity

Myelofibrosis:

Dosage modification for treatment interruption:

U.S. labeling:

If baseline platelet count ≥100,000/mm³ prior to initial treatment with ruxolitinib and:

Platelets <50,000/mm³ and ANC <500/mm³: Interrupt treatment; upon platelet recovery (to ≥50,000/mm³) or ANC recovery (to ≥750/mm³), dosing may be restarted or increased based on the following platelet or ANC levels

Platelets ≥125,000/mm³: Dose should be at least 5 mg twice daily below the dose at treatment interruption, up to a maximum of 20 mg twice daily

Platelets 100,000 to <125,000/mm³: Dose should be at least 5 mg twice daily below the dose at treatment interruption, up to a maximum of 15 mg twice daily

Platelets 75,000 to <100,000/mm³: Dose should be at least 5 mg twice daily below the dose at treatment interruption, up to a maximum of 10 mg twice daily for at least 2 weeks; may increase to 15 mg twice daily if stable

Platelets 50,000 to <75,000/mm³: 5 mg twice daily for at least 2 weeks; may increase to 10 mg twice daily if stable

Platelets <50,000/mm³: Continue to withhold treatment

ANC ≥750/mm³: Resume at 5 mg once daily or 5 mg twice daily below the largest dose in the week prior to treatment interruption, whichever is greater

Note: Long-term maintenance at 5 mg twice daily has not demonstrated responses; limit use of the dose level to patients where the benefits outweigh risks

If baseline platelet count 50,000 to <100,000/mm³ prior to initial treatment with ruxolitinib and:

Platelets <25,000/mm³ and ANC <500/mm³: Interrupt treatment; upon platelet recovery (to ≥35,000/mm³) or ANC recovery (to ≥750/mm³), resume at 5 mg once daily or 5 mg twice daily below the largest dose in the week prior to treatment interruption, whichever is greater

Note: Long-term maintenance at 5 mg twice daily has not demonstrated responses; limit use of the dose level to patients where the benefits outweigh risks

Canadian labeling: Platelets <50,000/mm³ or ANC <500 mm³: Interrupt treatment; upon recovery of platelets to ≥50,000/mm³ or ANC to ≥500/mm³, dosing may be restarted at 5 mg twice daily and then gradually titrated based on blood cell counts.

Dosage reduction for thrombocytopenia in patients with baseline platelet count ≥100,000/mm³ prior to initial treatment with ruxolitinib:

Platelet Count	Dose at Time of Thrombocytopenia				
	25 mg twice/day	20 mg twice/day	15 mg twice/day	10 mg twice/day	5 mg twice/day
	New Dose	New Dose	New Dose	New Dose	New Dose
100,000 to <125,000/mm³	20 mg twice/day	15 mg twice/day	No change	No change	No change
75,000 to <100,000/mm³	10 mg twice/day	10 mg twice/day	10 mg twice/day	No change	No change
50,000 to <75,000/mm³	5 mg twice/day	5 mg twice/day	5 mg twice/day	5 mg twice/day	No change
<50,000/mm³	Hold dose	Hold dose	Hold dose	Hold dose	Hold dose

Note: Long-term maintenance at 5 mg twice daily has not demonstrated responses; limit use of the dose level to patients where the benefits outweigh risks

Dosage reduction for thrombocytopenia in patients with baseline platelet 50,000 to <100,000/mm³ prior to initial treatment with ruxolitinib:
Platelets 25,000 to <35,000/mm³ **and** platelet count decreased <20% during prior 4 weeks:
  If current daily dose >5 mg: Reduce dose by 5 mg once daily
  If current dose 5 mg once daily: Continue 5 mg once daily
Platelets 25,000 to <35,000/mm³ **and** platelet count decreased ≥20% during prior four weeks:
  If current daily dose >10 mg: Reduce dose by 5 mg twice daily
  If current dose 5 mg twice daily: Reduce dose to 5 mg once daily
  If current dose 5 mg once daily: Continue 5 mg once daily
Platelets <25,000 mm³: Continue to withhold treatment
Note: Long-term maintenance at 5 mg twice daily has not demonstrated responses; limit use of the dose level to patients where the benefits outweigh risks

Polycythemia vera:
Hematologic toxicity:
  Hemoglobin ≥12 g/dL AND platelets ≥100,000/mm³: No dosage adjustment necessary.
  Hemoglobin 10 to <12 g/dL AND platelets 75,000 to <100,000/mm³: Consider dosage adjustment to avoid dose interruptions due to anemia and thrombocytopenia.
  Hemoglobin 8 to <10 g/dL OR platelets 50,000 to <75,000/mm³: Reduce dose by 5 mg twice daily; for patients currently receiving 5 mg twice daily, reduce dose to 5 mg once daily.
  Hemoglobin <8 g/dL OR platelets <50,000/mm³ OR ANC <1,000/mm³: Interrupt dosing.
  Dosage reduction following treatment interruption (use the most severe category of hemoglobin, platelets or ANC to determine reinitiation dose):
  Hemoglobin <8 g/dL OR platelets <50,000/mm³ OR ANC <1,000/mm³: Continue to hold.

Hemoglobin 8 to <10 g/dL OR platelets 50,000 to <75,000/mm^3 OR ANC 1,000 to <1,500/mm^3: Restart at a maximum of 5 mg twice daily (continue treatment for at least 2 weeks, if stable, then may increase dose by 5 mg twice daily) or no more than 5 mg twice daily less than the dose that resulted in dose interruption

Hemoglobin 10 to <12 g/dL OR platelets 75,000 to <100,000/mm^3 OR ANC 1,500 to <2,000/mm^3: Restart at a maximum of 10 mg twice daily (continue treatment for at least 2 weeks, if stable, then may increase dose by 5 mg twice daily) or no more than 5 mg twice daily less than the dose that resulted in dose interruption

Hemoglobin ≥12 g/dL OR platelets ≥100,000/mm^3 OR ANC ≥2,000/mm^3: Restart at a maximum of 15 mg twice daily (continue treatment for at least 2 weeks, if stable, then may increase dose by 5 mg twice daily) or no more than 5 mg twice daily less than the dose that resulted in dose interruption

Note: If dose interruption was required while receiving 5 mg twice daily, may restart at 5 mg twice daily or 5 mg once daily (but not higher) once hemoglobin is ≥10 g/dL, platelets are ≥75,000/mm^3, and ANC is ≥1,500/mm^3

Dose management after restarting treatment: After restarting following a dose interruption, the dose may be titrated, although the maximum total daily dose should not exceed 5 mg less than the dose resulting in the interruption (unless dose interruption following phlebotomy-associated anemia, in which case the maximum total daily dose is not limited).

Administration Oral:

U.S. labeling: May be administered orally with or without food. If a dose is missed, return to the usual dosing schedule and do **not** administer an additional dose.

If unable to ingest tablets, may administer through a nasogastric (NG) tube (≥8 Fr): Suspend 1 tablet in ~40 mL water and stir for ~10 minutes and administer (within 6 hours after dispersion) with appropriate syringe; rinse NG tube with ~75 mL water (effect of enteral tube feeding on ruxolitinib exposure has not been evaluated)

Canadian labeling: May be administered orally with or without food. Tablet should be swallowed whole and not be cut, broken, dissolved, crushed, or chewed. If a dose is missed, return to the usual dosing schedule and do not administer an additional dose.

Hazardous agent; use appropriate precautions for handling and disposal (meets NIOSH 2014 criteria).

Emetic Potential Minimal (<10%)

Extemporaneous Preparations Hazardous agent; use appropriate precautions for handling and disposal (meets NIOSH 2014 criteria).

A suspension for nasogastric administration may be prepared with tablets. Place one tablet in ~40 mL water; stir for approximately 10 minutes. Administer within 6 hour after preparation.

Jakafi (ruxolitinib) [prescribing information]. Wilmington, DE: Incyte Corporation; December 2014.

Monitoring Parameters CBC (baseline, every 2 to 4 weeks until dose stabilized, then as clinically indicated), renal function, hepatic function. Perform periodic skin examinations monitor for signs/symptoms of infection. Additional Canadian labeling recommendations include tuberculin skin test and/or interferon-gamma release assay prior to initiation and ECG at baseline and then periodically during therapy; monitor heart rate and blood pressure during therapy

Dietary Considerations Avoid grapefruit juice (may increase the effects of ruxolitinib).

Prescribing and Access Restrictions Available through specialty/network pharmacies. Further information may be obtained from the manufacturer, Incyte, at 1-855-452-5234 or at www.Jakafi.com.

Dosage Forms Excipient information presented when available (limited, particularly for generics); consult specific product labeling.
Tablet, Oral:
Jakafi: 5 mg, 10 mg, 15 mg, 20 mg, 25 mg

♦ **Ruxolitinib Phosphate** see Ruxolitinib on page 1501

♦ **Rybix ODT [DSC]** see TraMADol on page 1672

♦ **Ryzolt** see TraMADol on page 1672

♦ **Ryzolt [DSC]** see TraMADol on page 1672

♦ **SAHA** see Vorinostat on page 1780

♦ **Salagen** see Pilocarpine (Systemic) on page 1386

♦ **Salagen® (Can)** see Pilocarpine (Systemic) on page 1386

♦ **Salcatonin** see Calcitonin on page 259

Saliva Substitute (sa LYE va SUB stee tute)

Brand Names: US Aquoral™; Biotene® Moisturizing Mouth Spray [OTC]; Biotene® Oral Balance® [OTC]; Caphosol®; Entertainer's Secret® [OTC]; Moi-Stir® [OTC]; Mouth Kote® [OTC]; NeutraSal®; Numoisyn™; Oasis®; Saliva-Sure™ [OTC]

Index Terms Artificial Saliva

Pharmacologic Category Gastrointestinal Agent, Miscellaneous

Use Relief of dry mouth and throat in xerostomia or hyposalivation; adjunct to standard oral care in relief of symptoms associated with chemotherapy or radiation therapy-induced mucositis

Labeled Contraindications
Numoisyn™ liquid: Hypersensitivity to saliva substitute or any component of the formulation.
Numoisyn™ lozenges: Fructose intolerance

Adverse Reactions Frequency not defined.
Central nervous system: Altered speech
Gastrointestinal: Abnormal taste, digestive problems (minor), dysphagia

Drug Interactions
Metabolism/Transport Effects None known.
Avoid Concomitant Use There are no known interactions where it is recommended to avoid concomitant use.
Increased Effect/Toxicity There are no known significant interactions involving an increase in effect.
Decreased Effect There are no known significant interactions involving a decrease in effect.

Storage/Stability Store at room temperature.
Caphosol®: Do not refrigerate. Use immediately after mixing.
NeutraSal®: Avoid excess heat or moisture. Use immediately after mixing.
Numoisyn™ liquid: Do not refrigerate. Use within 3 months after opening.

◀ **Preparation for Administration**

Caphosol®: Mix contents of 1 blue (A) and 1 clear (B) ampul in clean container; use immediately after mixing.

NeutraSal®: Mix contents of packet with 1 ounce of water in clean container; use immediately after mixing.

Mechanism of Action Protein or electrolyte mixtures which restore/replace saliva, lubricate, moisten, clean, and/or provide a coating on oral mucosa

Dosing

Adult & Geriatric

Mucositis (due to high-dose chemotherapy or radiation therapy): Oral:

Caphosol®, NeutraSal®: Swish and spit 4-10 doses daily (use for the duration of chemo- or radiation therapy)

Xerostomia: Oral: Use as needed, or product-specific dosing:

Aquoral™: 2 sprays 3-4 times daily

Biotene® Oral Balance® gel: Apply one-half inch length onto tongue and spread evenly; repeat as often as needed

Caphosol®, NeutraSal®: Swish and spit 2-10 doses daily

Entertainer's Secret®: Spray as often as needed

Mouth Kote® spray: Spray 3-5 times, swish for 8-10 seconds, then spit or swallow; use as often as needed

Numoisyn™ liquid: Use 2 mL as needed

Numoisyn™ lozenges: Dissolve 1 lozenge slowly; maximum 16 lozenges daily

Oasis® mouthwash: Rinse mouth with ~30 mL twice daily or as needed; do not swallow

Oasis® spray: 1-2 sprays as needed; maximum 60 sprays daily

SalivaSure™: Dissolve 1 lozenge slowly as needed; for severe symptoms, 1 lozenge per hour is recommended

Administration Oral:

Biotene® Oral Balance® gel: Apply on tongue and spread evenly.

Biotene® spray: Spray directly into mouth; spray is safe to swallow.

Caphosol®: Swish mixed solution thoroughly with ½ of mixture (15 mL) for 1 minute and spit; repeat. Avoid eating or drinking for at least 15 minutes after use.

Entertainer's Secret®: Tilt head back and spray into throat or nostril while inhaling sharply.

Mouth Kote® spray: Spray into mouth and swirl for 8-10 seconds; spray may be swallowed or spit out.

NeutraSal®: For each dose, swish ½ the prepared solution around the mouth for 1 minute and spit out; repeat with the remaining solution. Avoid eating or drinking for at least 15 minutes after use.

Numoisyn™ liquid: Rinse in mouth before swallowing.

Numoisyn™ lozenges: Dissolve slowly in mouth; move lozenge around mouth for optimal effect.

Oasis® mouthwash: Rinse for 30 seconds.

Oasis® spray: Spray into mouth holding bottle upright; do not rinse.

SalivaSure® lozenges: Allow lozenge to move around and slowly dissolve in mouth.

Dietary Considerations

Caphosol®: Contains sodium 75 mg/30 mL dose

Moi-Stir®: Contains sodium: 6.47 mEq/120 mL, potassium: 1.93 mEq/120 mL, magnesium: 0.128 mEq/120 mL

Dosage Forms Excipient information presented when available (limited, particularly for generics); consult specific product labeling.

Liquid, oral:

Biotene® Oral Balance®: Water, starch, sunflower oil, propylene glycol, xylitol, glycerine, purified milk extract (45 mL) [sugar-free]

Numoisyn™: Water, sorbitol, linseed extract, *Chondrus crispus*, methylparaben, sodium benzoate, potassium sorbate, dipotassium phosphate, propylparaben (300 mL)

Lozenge, oral:

Numoisyn™: Sorbitol 0.3 g/lozenge, polyethylene glycol, malic acid, sodium citrate, calcium phosphate dibasic, hydrogenated cottonseed oil, citric acid, magnesium stearate, silicon dioxide (100s)

SalivaSure™: Xylitol, citric acid, apple acid, sodium citrate dihydrate, sodium carboxymethylcellulose, dibasic calcium phosphate, silica colloidal, magnesium stearate, stearic acid (90s)

Powder, for reconstitution, oral:

NeutraSal®: Sodium, phosphates, calcium, chloride, bicarbonate (30s, 120s)

Solution, oral:

Caphosol®: Dibasic sodium phosphate 0.032%, monobasic sodium phosphate 0.009%, calcium chloride 0.052%, sodium chloride 0.569%, purified water (30 mL) [packaged in two 15 mL ampuls when mixed together provide one 30 mL dose]

Entertainer's Secret®: Sodium carboxymethylcellulose, aloe vera gel, glycerin (60 mL) [ethanol free; honey-apple flavor]

Solution, oral [mouthwash/gargle]:

Oasis®: Water, glycerin, sorbitol, poloxamer 338, PEG-60, hydrogenated castor oil, copovidone, sodium benzoate, carboxymethylcellulose (473 mL) [ethanol free, sugar free; mild mint flavor]

Solution, oral [spray]:

Aquoral™: Oxidized glycerol triesters and silicon dioxide (40 mL) [contains aspartame; delivers 400 sprays, citrus flavor]

Biotene® Moisturizing Mouth Spray: Water, polyglycitol, propylene glycol, sunflower oil, xylitol, milk protein extract, potassium sorbate, acesulfame K, potassium thiocyanate, lysozyme, lactoferrin, lactoperoxidase (45 mL)

Moi-Stir®: Water, sorbitol, sodium carboxymethylcellulose, methylparaben, propylparaben, potassium chloride, dibasic sodium phosphate, calcium chloride, magnesium chloride, sodium chloride (120 mL)

Mouth Kote®: Water, xylitol, sorbitol, yerba santa, citric acid, ascorbic acid, sodium saccharin, sodium benzoate (5 mL, 60 mL, 240 mL) [ethanol free, sugar free; lemon-lime flavor]

Oasis®: Glycerin, cetylpyridinium, copovidone (30 mL) [ethanol free, sugar free; contains sodium benzoate; delivers ~150 sprays, mild mint flavor]

◆ SalivaSure™ [OTC] *see* Saliva Substitute *on page 1511*

Samarium Sm 153 Lexidronam

(sa MAR ee um es em won fif tee three lex ID roe nam)

Brand Names: US Quadramet

Index Terms ¹⁵³Sm-Lexidronam

Pharmacologic Category Radiopharmaceutical

Use Relief of pain associated with osteoblastic metastatic bone lesions that demonstrate increased localization on radionuclide bone scans

Pregnancy Risk Factor D

◄ **Dosing**

Adult Palliation of osteoblastic metastatic bone lesions: IV: 1 mCi/kg (37 MBq/kg)

Renal Impairment No dosage adjustment provided in manufacturer's labeling (has not been studied).

Hepatic Impairment No dosage adjustment provided in manufacturer's labeling. However, dosage adjustment unlikely since studies have not revealed hepatic excretion.

Additional Information Complete prescribing information should be consulted for additional detail.

Dosage Forms Excipient information presented when available (limited, particularly for generics); consult specific product labeling.

Solution, Intravenous:

Quadramet: 1850 MBq/mL (3 mL)

♦ **Sancuso** *see* Granisetron *on page 801*

♦ **SandIMMUNE** *see* CycloSPORINE (Systemic) *on page 385*

♦ **Sandimmune I.V. (Can)** *see* CycloSPORINE (Systemic) *on page 385*

♦ **SandoSTATIN** *see* Octreotide *on page 1226*

♦ **Sandostatin (Can)** *see* Octreotide *on page 1226*

♦ **Sandostatin LAR (Can)** *see* Octreotide *on page 1226*

♦ **SandoSTATIN LAR Depot** *see* Octreotide *on page 1226*

♦ **Sandoz-Anagrelide (Can)** *see* Anagrelide *on page 109*

♦ **Sandoz-Anastrozole (Can)** *see* Anastrozole *on page 112*

♦ **Sandoz-Bicalutamide (Can)** *see* Bicalutamide *on page 207*

♦ **Sandoz-Ciprofloxacin (Can)** *see* Ciprofloxacin (Systemic) *on page 327*

♦ **Sandoz-Cyclosporine (Can)** *see* CycloSPORINE (Systemic) *on page 385*

♦ **Sandoz-Famciclovir (Can)** *see* Famciclovir *on page 689*

♦ **Sandoz Fentanyl Patch (Can)** *see* FentaNYL *on page 692*

♦ **Sandoz-Letrozole (Can)** *see* Letrozole *on page 1019*

♦ **Sandoz-Levofloxacin (Can)** *see* Levofloxacin (Systemic) *on page 1038*

♦ **Sandoz-Linezolid (Can)** *see* Linezolid *on page 1049*

♦ **Sandoz-Morphine SR (Can)** *see* Morphine (Systemic) *on page 1167*

♦ **Sandoz-Mycophenolate Mofetil (Can)** *see* Mycophenolate *on page 1177*

♦ **Sandoz-Olanzapine (Can)** *see* OLANZapine *on page 1242*

♦ **Sandoz-Olanzapine ODT (Can)** *see* OLANZapine *on page 1242*

♦ **Sandoz-Ondansetron (Can)** *see* Ondansetron *on page 1253*

♦ **Sandoz Prednisolone (Can)** *see* PrednisoLONE (Ophthalmic) *on page 1424*

♦ **Sandoz-Prochlorperazine (Can)** *see* Prochlorperazine *on page 1441*

♦ **Sandoz-Tacrolimus (Can)** *see* Tacrolimus (Systemic) *on page 1576*

♦ **Sandoz-Voriconazole (Can)** *see* Voriconazole *on page 1775*

Sargramostim (sar GRAM oh stim)

Related Information

Hematopoietic Stem Cell Transplantation *on page 2272*

Mucositis and Stomatitis *on page 2186*

Brand Names: US Leukine

Brand Names: Canada Leukine

Index Terms GM-CSF; GMCSF; Granulocyte-Macrophage Colony Stimulating Factor; Prokine; Recombinant Granulocyte-Macrophage Colony Stimulating Factor; rhuGM-CSF

Pharmacologic Category Colony Stimulating Factor; Hematopoietic Agent

Use

Acute myeloid leukemia (AML; following induction chemotherapy): To shorten time to neutrophil recovery and to reduce the incidence of severe and life-threatening infections and infections resulting in death following induction chemotherapy in older adults (≥55 years of age)

Bone marrow transplant (allogeneic or autologous) failure or engraftment delay: For graft failure or engraftment delay in patients who have undergone allogeneic or autologous bone marrow transplantation, to prolong survival (survival benefit may be greater in patients with autologous bone marrow transplant failure or engraftment delay, no previous total body irradiation, malignancy other than leukemia, or multiple organ failure score ≤2)

Myeloid reconstitution after allogeneic bone marrow transplantation: To accelerate myeloid recovery in patients undergoing allogeneic bone marrow transplant from HLA-matched related donors (safe and effective in accelerating myeloid engraftment, reducing the incidence of bacteremia and other culture-positive infections, and shortening the median hospitalization duration)

Myeloid reconstitution after autologous bone marrow transplantation: To accelerate myeloid recovery following transplantation in non-Hodgkin lymphoma (NHL), acute lymphoblastic leukemia (ALL), Hodgkin lymphoma patients undergoing autologous bone marrow transplant (safe and effective in accelerating myeloid engraftment, reducing the median duration of antibiotic administration, reducing the median duration of infectious episodes, and shortening the median hospitalization duration)

Peripheral stem cell transplantation (autologous), mobilization and post-transplant: Mobilization of hematopoietic progenitor cells for collection by leukapheresis (increases the number of progenitor cells capable of engraftment and may lead to more rapid engraftment); to accelerate myeloid reconstitution following peripheral blood progenitor cell transplantation

Labeled Contraindications Hypersensitivity to sargramostim, yeast-derived products, or any component of the formulation; concurrent (24 hours preceding/following) use with myelosuppressive chemotherapy or radiation therapy; patients with excessive (≥10%) leukemic myeloid blasts in bone marrow or peripheral blood

Pregnancy Considerations Animal reproduction studies have not been conducted.

Breast-Feeding Considerations It is not known if sargramostim is excreted in breast milk. Breast-feeding is not recommended by the manufacturer.

◄ **Warnings/Precautions** Simultaneous administration or administration 24 hours preceding/following cytotoxic chemotherapy or radiotherapy is contraindicated due to the sensitivity of rapidly dividing hematopoietic progenitor cells. If there is a rapid increase in blood counts (ANC >20,000/mm³, WBC >50,000/mm³, or platelets >500,000/mm³), decrease the dose by 50% or discontinue therapy. Excessive blood counts should fall to normal within 3 to 7 days after the discontinuation of therapy. Monitor CBC with differential twice weekly during treatment. Limited response to sargramostim may be seen in patients who have received bone marrow purged by chemical agents which do not preserve an adequate number of responsive hematopoietic progenitors (eg, <1.2 x 10⁴/kg progenitors). In patients receiving autologous bone marrow transplant, response to sargramostim may be limited if extensive radiotherapy to the abdomen or chest or multiple myelotoxic agents were administered prior to transplantation. May potentially act as a growth factor for any tumor type, particularly myeloid malignancies; caution should be exercised when using in any malignancy with myeloid characteristics. Discontinue use if disease progression occurs during treatment.

Anaphylaxis or other serious allergic reactions have been reported; discontinue immediately and initiate appropriate therapy if a serious allergic or anaphylactic reaction occurs. A "first-dose effect", characterized by respiratory distress, hypoxia, flushing, hypotension, syncope, and/or tachycardia, may occur (rarely) with the first dose of a cycle and resolve with appropriate symptomatic treatment; symptoms do not usually occur with subsequent doses within that cycle. Sequestration of granulocytes in pulmonary circulation and dyspnea have been reported; monitor respiratory symptoms during and following IV infusion. Decrease infusion rate by 50% if dyspnea occurs; discontinue the infusion if dyspnea persists despite reduction in the rate of administration. Subsequent doses may be administered at the standard rate with careful monitoring. Use with caution in patients with hypoxia or preexisting pulmonary disease. Edema, capillary leak syndrome, pleural and/or pericardial effusion have been reported; fluid retention has been shown to be reversible with dosage reduction or discontinuation of sargramostim with or without concomitant use of diuretics. Use with caution in patients with preexisting fluid retention, pulmonary infiltrates, or congestive heart failure; may exacerbate fluid retention.

Use with caution in patients with preexisting cardiac disease. Reversible transient supraventricular arrhythmias have been reported, especially in patients with a history of arrhythmias. Use with caution in patients with hepatic impairment (hyperbilirubinemia and elevated transaminases have been observed) or renal impairment (serum creatinine elevations have been observed). Monitor hepatic and renal function at least every other week in patients with history of impairment.

Benzyl alcohol and derivatives: Some dosage forms may contain benzyl alcohol; large amounts of benzyl alcohol (≥99 mg/kg/day) have been associated with a potentially fatal toxicity ("gasping syndrome") in neonates; the "gasping syndrome" consists of metabolic acidosis, respiratory distress, gasping respirations, CNS dysfunction (including convulsions, intracranial hemorrhage), hypotension, and cardiovascular collapse (AAP ["Inactive" 1997]; CDC, 1982); some data suggests that benzoate displaces bilirubin from protein binding sites (Ahlfors, 2001); avoid or use dosage forms containing benzyl alcohol with caution in neonates. See manufacturer's labeling.

Adverse Reactions

>10%:

Cardiovascular: Hypertension (34%), edema (13% to 25%), pericardial effusion (4% to 25%), thrombosis (19%), chest pain (15%), peripheral edema (11%), tachycardia (11%)

Central nervous system: Malaise (57%), headache (26%), chills (25%), anxiety (11%), insomnia (11%)

Dermatologic: Skin rash (44% to 77%), pruritus (23%)

Endocrine & metabolic: Weight loss (37%), hyperglycemia (25%), hypercholesterolemia (17%), hypomagnesemia (15%)

Gastrointestinal: Diarrhea (81% to 89%), nausea (58% to 70%), vomiting (46% to 70%), gastric ulcer (50%), abdominal pain (38%), anorexia (13%), hematemesis (13%), dysphagia (11%), gastrointestinal hemorrhage (11%)

Hepatic: Hyperbilirubinemia (30%)

Neuromuscular & skeletal: Weakness (66%), ostealgia (21%), arthralgia (11% to 21%), myalgia (18%)

Ophthalmic: Retinal hemorrhage (11%)

Renal: Increased blood urea nitrogen (23%), increased serum creatinine (15%)

Respiratory: Pharyngitis (23%), epistaxis (17%), dyspnea (15%)

Miscellaneous: Fever (81%)

1% to 10%:

Immunologic: Antibody development (2%)

Respiratory: Pleural effusion (1%)

<1%, postmarketing, and/or case reports: Anaphylaxis, capillary leak syndrome, cardiac arrhythmia, dizziness, eosinophilia, flushing, hypotension, hypoxia, injection site reaction, lethargy, leukocytosis, liver function impairment (transient), pain, pericarditis, prolonged prothrombin time, respiratory distress, rigors, sore throat, supraventricular cardiac arrhythmia, syncope, thrombocythemia, thrombophlebitis

Drug Interactions

Metabolism/Transport Effects None known.

Avoid Concomitant Use There are no known interactions where it is recommended to avoid concomitant use.

Increased Effect/Toxicity

Sargramostim may increase the levels/effects of: Bleomycin

The levels/effects of Sargramostim may be increased by: Cyclophosphamide

Decreased Effect There are no known significant interactions involving a decrease in effect.

Storage/Stability

Store intact vials at 2°C to 8°C (36°F to 46°F); do not freeze. Do not shake.

Solution for injection: May be stored for up to 20 days at 2°C to 8°C (36°F to 46°F) once the vial has been entered. Discard remaining solution after 20 days.

Powder for injection: Preparations made with SWFI should be administered as soon as possible, and discarded within 6 hours of reconstitution. Solutions reconstituted with bacteriostatic water may be stored for up to 20 days at 2°C to 8°C (36°F to 46°F); do not freeze. When combining previously reconstituted solutions with freshly reconstituted solutions, administer within 6 hours following preparation; the contents of vials reconstituted with different diluents should not be mixed together.

◀ **Preparation for Administration**

Powder for injection: May be reconstituted with 1 mL of preservative free SWFI or bacteriostatic water for injection. Direct the diluent toward the side of the vial and gently swirl to reconstitute; do not shake. Do not mix the contents of vials which have been reconstituted with different diluents.

SubQ: May be administered without further dilution.

IV: Further dilution with NS is required. If the final sargramostim concentration is <10 mcg/mL, 1 mg of human albumin per 1 mL of NS should be added (eg, add 1 mL of 5% human albumin per 50 mL of NS).

Mechanism of Action Stimulates proliferation, differentiation and functional activity of neutrophils, eosinophils, monocytes, and macrophages.

Pharmacodynamics/Kinetics

Duration: WBCs return to baseline within 1 to 2 weeks of discontinuing drug

Half-life elimination: IV: ~60 minutes; SubQ: ~2.7 hours

Time to peak, serum: SubQ: 1 to 3 hours

Dosing

Adult & Geriatric Note: May round the dose to the nearest vial size (Ozer, 2000).

Acute myeloid leukemia (following induction chemotherapy): Adults ≥55 years: IV: 250 mcg/m^2/day (infused over 4 hours) starting approximately on day 11 or 4 days following the completion of induction chemotherapy (if day 10 bone marrow is hypoplastic with <5% blasts), continue until ANC >1500/mm^3 for 3 consecutive days or a maximum of 42 days. If WBC >50,000/mm^3 and/or ANC >20,000/mm^3, interrupt treatment or reduce the dose by 50%.

If a second cycle of chemotherapy is necessary, administer ~4 days after the completion of chemotherapy if the bone marrow is hypoplastic with <5% blasts

Discontinue sargramostim immediately if leukemic regrowth occurs. If a severe adverse reaction occurs, reduce the dose by 50% or temporarily discontinue the dose until the reaction abates.

Bone marrow transplantation (allogeneic or autologous) failure or engraftment delay: IV: 250 mcg/m^2/day (infused over 2 hours) for 14 days; If engraftment has not occurred after 7 days off sargramostim, may repeat. If engraftment still has not occurred after 7 days off sargramostim, a third course of 500 mcg/m^2/day for 14 days may be attempted. If there is still no improvement, it is unlikely that further dose escalation will be of benefit.

If a severe adverse reaction occurs, reduce the dose by 50% or temporarily discontinue the dose until the reaction abates

If blast cells appear or disease progression occurs, discontinue treatment

If WBC >50,000/mm^3 and/or ANC >20,000 cells/mm^3, interrupt treatment or reduce the dose by 50%.

Myeloid reconstitution after allogeneic or autologous bone marrow transplantation: IV: 250 mcg/m^2/day (infused over 2 hours), begin 2 to 4 hours after the marrow infusion and ≥24 hours after chemotherapy or radiotherapy, when the post marrow infusion ANC is <500 /mm^3, and continue until ANC >1500 /mm^3 for 3 consecutive days. If WBC >50,000/mm^3 and/or ANC >20,000/mm^3, interrupt treatment or reduce the dose by 50%.

If a severe adverse reaction occurs, reduce dose by 50% or temporarily discontinue the dose until the reaction abates

If blast cells appear or progression of the underlying disease occurs, discontinue treatment

Peripheral stem cell transplantation (autologous), mobilization: IV, SubQ: 250 mcg/m^2/day IV (infused over 24 hours) or SubQ once daily; continue the same dose throughout peripheral blood progenitor cell collection. If WBC >50,000/mm^3, reduce the dose by 50%.

Note: The optimal schedule for peripheral blood progenitor cell collection has not been established (usually begun by day 5 and performed daily until protocol specified targets are achieved). If adequate numbers of progenitor cells are not collected, consider other mobilization therapy.

Peripheral stem cell transplantation (autologous), post-transplant: IV, SubQ: 250 mcg/m^2/day IV (infused over 24 hours) or SubQ once daily beginning immediately following infusion of progenitor cells; continue until ANC is >1500/mm^3 for 3 consecutive days.

Primary prophylaxis of neutropenia in patients receiving chemotherapy (outside transplant and AML) or who are at high risk for neutropenic fever (off-label use): SubQ: 250 mcg/m^2/day (may round to the nearest vial size [Ozer, 2000]) beginning at least 24 hours after chemotherapy administration; continue until ANC >2000 to 3000/mm^3 (Smith, 2006).

Treatment of radiation-induced myelosuppression of the bone marrow (off-label use): SubQ: 250 mcg/m^2/day; continue until ANC >1000/mm^3 (Smith, 2006; Waselenko, 2004).

Renal Impairment There are no dosage adjustments provided in the manufacturer's labeling.

Hepatic Impairment There are no dosage adjustments provided in the manufacturer's labeling.

Combination Regimens

Leukemia, acute myeloid: MEC-G (AML Induction) on page 2032

Lymphoma, non-Hodgkin (Burkitt): CODOX-M/IVAC (NHL-Burkitt) on page 1920

Administration Sargramostim is administered as a subcutaneous injection or intravenous infusion.

IV: Infuse over 2 hours, 4 hours or 24 hours (indication specific). An in-line membrane filter should **NOT** be used for intravenous administration.

SubQ: Administer undiluted; rotate injection sites, avoiding navel/waistline.

Monitoring Parameters CBC with differential (twice weekly during treatment), renal/liver function tests (at least every 2 weeks in patients displaying renal or hepatic dysfunction prior to treatment initiation); pulmonary function; vital signs; hydration status; weight

Test Interactions May interfere with bone imaging studies; increased hematopoietic activity of the bone marrow may appear as transient positive bone imaging changes

Dosage Forms Excipient information presented when available (limited, particularly for generics); consult specific product labeling. [DSC] = Discontinued product

Solution, Injection:

Leukine: 500 mcg/mL (1 mL [DSC]) [contains benzyl alcohol]

Solution Reconstituted, Intravenous [preservative free]:

Leukine: 250 mcg (1 ea)

◆ **SB-497115** *see* Eltrombopag *on page 585*

◆ **SB-497115-GR** *see* Eltrombopag *on page 585*

◆ **SC 33428** *see* IDArubicin *on page 862*

◆ **SCH 13521** *see* Flutamide *on page 751*

Scopolamine (Systemic) (skoe POL a meen)

Related Information

Hospice (End of Life) Care *on page* 2238

Management of Chemotherapy-Induced Nausea and Vomiting in Adults *on page* 2142

Brand Names: US Transderm-Scop

Brand Names: Canada Buscopan; Scopolamine Hydrobromide Injection; Transderm-V

Index Terms Hyoscine Butylbromide; Scopolamine Base; Scopolamine Butylbromide; Scopolamine Hydrobromide

Pharmacologic Category Anticholinergic Agent

Use

Scopolamine base: Transdermal: Prevention of nausea/vomiting associated with motion sickness and recovery from anesthesia and surgery

Scopolamine hydrobromide: Injection: Preoperative medication to produce amnesia, sedation, tranquilization, antiemetic effects, and decrease salivary and respiratory secretions

Scopolamine butylbromide [Canadian product]: Oral/injection: Treatment of smooth muscle spasm of the genitourinary or gastrointestinal tract; injection may also be used prior to radiological/diagnostic procedures to prevent spasm

Labeled Contraindications

Transdermal, oral: Hypersensitivity to scopolamine, other belladonna alkaloids, or any component of the formulation; narrow-angle glaucoma

Injection: Hypersensitivity to scopolamine, other belladonna alkaloids, or any component of the formulation; narrow-angle glaucoma; chronic lung disease (repeated administration)

Canadian labeling: Additional contraindications (not in U.S. labeling):

Oral: Glaucoma, megacolon, myasthenia gravis, obstructive prostatic hypertrophy

Injection:

Hyoscine butylbromide: Untreated narrow-angle glaucoma; megacolon, prostatic hypertrophy with urinary retention; stenotic lesions of the GI tract; myasthenia gravis; tachycardia, angina, or heart failure; IM administration in patients receiving anticoagulant therapy

Scopolamine hydrobromide: Glaucoma or predisposition to narrow-angle glaucoma; paralytic ileus; prostatic hypertrophy; pyloric obstruction; tachycardia secondary to cardiac insufficiency or thyrotoxicosis

Pregnancy Considerations Adverse events were observed in some animal reproduction studies. Scopolamine crosses the placenta; may cause respiratory depression and/or neonatal hemorrhage when used during pregnancy. Transdermal scopolamine has been used as an adjunct to epidural anesthesia for cesarean delivery without adverse CNS effects on the newborn. Parenteral administration does not increase the duration of labor or affect uterine contractions. Except when used prior to cesarean section, use during pregnancy only if the benefit to the mother outweighs the potential risk to the fetus.

Breast-Feeding Considerations Scopolamine is excreted into breast milk. The manufacturer recommends caution be used if scopolamine is administered to a nursing woman.

Warnings/Precautions Use with caution in patients with coronary artery disease, tachyarrhythmias, heart failure, hypertension, or hyperthyroidism; evaluate tachycardia prior to administration. Use caution in hepatic or renal impairment; adverse CNS effects occur more often in these patients. Use injectable and transdermal products with caution in patients with prostatic hyperplasia or urinary retention. Discontinue if patient reports unusual visual disturbances or pain within the eye. Use caution in GI obstruction, hiatal hernia, reflux esophagitis, and ulcerative colitis. Use with caution in patients with a history of seizure or psychosis; may exacerbate these conditions. Lower doses (0.1mg) may have vagal mimetic effects (eg, increase vagal tone causing paradoxical bradycardia).

Anaphylaxis including episodes of shock has been reported following parenteral administration; observe for signs/symptoms of hypersensitivity following parenteral administration. Patients with a history of allergies or asthma may be at increased risk of hypersensitivity reactions. Adverse events (including dizziness, headache, nausea, vomiting) may occur following abrupt discontinuation of large doses or in patients with Parkinson's disease; adverse events may also occur following removal of the transdermal patch although symptoms may not appear until ≥24 hours after removal.

Idiosyncratic reactions may rarely occur; patients may experience acute toxic psychosis, agitation, confusion, delusions, hallucinations, paranoid behavior, and rambling speech. May cause CNS depression, which may impair physical or mental abilities; patients must be cautioned about performing tasks which require mental alertness (eg, operating machinery or driving). Effects with other sedative drugs or ethanol may be potentiated.

Transdermal patch may contain conducting metal (eg, aluminum); remove patch prior to MRI. Use of the transdermal product in patients with open-angle glaucoma may necessitate adjustments in glaucoma therapy.

Scopolamine (hyoscine) hydrobromide should not be interchanged with scopolamine butylbromide formulations; dosages are not equivalent.

Avoid use in the elderly due to potent anticholinergic adverse effects and uncertain effectiveness (Beers Criteria). Use with caution in infants and children since they may be more susceptible to adverse effects of scopolamine. Tablets may contain sucrose; avoid use of tablets in patients who are fructose intolerant.

Adverse Reactions Frequency not defined.

Cardiovascular: Bradycardia, flushing, orthostatic hypotension, tachycardia

Central nervous system: Acute toxic psychosis (rare), agitation (rare), ataxia, confusion, delusion (rare), disorientation, dizziness, drowsiness, fatigue, hallucination (rare), headache, irritability, loss of memory, paranoid behavior (rare), restlessness, sedation

Dermatologic: Drug eruptions, dry skin, dyshidrosis, erythema, pruritus, rash, urticaria

Endocrine & metabolic: Thirst

Gastrointestinal: Constipation, diarrhea, dry throat, dysphagia, nausea, vomiting, xerostomia

◀ Genitourinary: Dysuria, urinary retention

Neuromuscular & skeletal: Tremor, weakness

Ocular: Accommodation impaired, blurred vision, conjunctival infection, cycloplegia, dryness, glaucoma (narrow-angle), increased intraocular pain, itching, photophobia, pupil dilation, retinal pigmentation

Respiratory: Dry nose, dyspnea

Miscellaneous: Anaphylaxis (rare), anaphylactic shock (rare), angioedema, diaphoresis decreased, heat intolerance, hypersensitivity reactions

Drug Interactions

Metabolism/Transport Effects None known.

Avoid Concomitant Use

Avoid concomitant use of Scopolamine (Systemic) with any of the following: Aclidinium; Azelastine (Nasal); Cimetropium; Eluxadoline; Glucagon; Glycopyrrolate; Ipratropium (Oral Inhalation); Levosulpiride; Orphenadrine; Paraldehyde; Potassium Chloride; Thalidomide; Tiotropium; Umeclidinium

Increased Effect/Toxicity

Scopolamine (Systemic) may increase the levels/effects of: AbobotulinumtoxinA; Alcohol (Ethyl); Analgesics (Opioid); Anticholinergic Agents; Azelastine (Nasal); Buprenorphine; Cimetropium; CNS Depressants; Eluxadoline; Glucagon; Glycopyrrolate; Hydrocodone; Methotrimeprazine; Metyrosine; Mirabegron; Mirtazapine; OnabotulinumtoxinA; Orphenadrine; Paraldehyde; Potassium Chloride; Pramipexole; Ramosetron; RimabotulinumtoxinB; ROPINIRole; Rotigotine; Selective Serotonin Reuptake Inhibitors; Suvorexant; Thalidomide; Thiazide Diuretics; Tiotropium; Topiramate; Zolpidem

The levels/effects of Scopolamine (Systemic) may be increased by: Aclidinium; Brimonidine (Topical); Cannabis; Doxylamine; Dronabinol; Droperidol; HydrOXYzine; Ipratropium (Oral Inhalation); Kava Kava; Magnesium Sulfate; Methotrimeprazine; Mianserin; Minocycline; Nabilone; Perampanel; Pramlintide; Rufinamide; Sodium Oxybate; Tapentadol; Tetrahydrocannabinol; Umeclidinium

Decreased Effect

Scopolamine (Systemic) may decrease the levels/effects of: Acetylcholinesterase Inhibitors; Gastrointestinal Agents (Prokinetic); Itopride; Levosulpiride; Secretin

The levels/effects of Scopolamine (Systemic) may be decreased by: Acetylcholinesterase Inhibitors

Storage/Stability

Solution for injection:

Butylbromide [Canadian product]: Store at room temperature. Do not freeze. Protect from light and heat. Stable in D_5W, $D_{10}W$, NS, Ringer's solution, and LR for up to 8 hours.

Hydrobromide: Store at room temperature of 20°C to 25°C (68°F to 77°F). Protect from light. Avoid acid solutions; hydrolysis occurs at pH <3.

Tablet [Canadian product]: Store at room temperature. Protect from light and heat.

Transdermal system: Store at 20°C to 25°C (68°F to 77°F).

Preparation for Administration Solution for injection:

IM: Butylbromide: No dilution required.

IV:

Butylbromide: No dilution is necessary prior to injection.

Hydrobromide: Dilute with an equal volume of sterile water.

Mechanism of Action Blocks the action of acetylcholine at parasympathetic sites in smooth muscle, secretory glands and the CNS; increases cardiac output, dries secretions, antagonizes histamine and serotonin; at usual recommended doses, causes blockade of muscarinic receptors at the cardiac SA-node and is parasympatholytic (ie, blocks vagal activity increasing heart rate)

Pharmacodynamics/Kinetics

Onset of action: Oral, IM: 0.5 to 1 hour; IV: 10 minutes; Transdermal: 6 to 8 hours

Duration: IM, IV, SubQ: 4 hours

Absorption: IM, SubQ: Rapid; Oral: Quaternary salts (butylbromide) are poorly absorbed (local concentrations in the GI tract following oral dosing may be high)

Distribution: V_d: Butylbromide: 128 L

Protein binding: Butylbromide: ~4% (albumin)

Metabolism: Hepatic

Bioavailability: Oral: 8%

Half-life elimination: Butylbromide: ~5 to 11 hours; Hydrobromide: ~1 to 4 hours; Scopolamine base: 9.5 hours

Time to peak: Hydrobromide: IM: ~20 minutes, SubQ: ~15 minutes; Butylbromide: Oral: ~2 hours; Scopolamine base: Transdermal: 24 hours

Excretion: Urine (<10%, as parent drug and metabolites); IV: Butylbromide: Urine (42% to 61% [half as parent drug]), feces (28% to 37%)

Dosing

Adult Note: Scopolamine injection is no longer available in the US.

Note: Scopolamine (hyoscine) hydrobromide should not be interchanged with scopolamine butylbromide formulations. Dosages are not equivalent.

Scopolamine base:

Preoperative: Transdermal patch: Apply 1 patch to hairless area behind ear the night before surgery or 1 hour prior to cesarean section (apply no sooner than 1 hour before surgery to minimize newborn exposure); remove 24 hours after surgery

Motion sickness: Transdermal patch: Apply 1 patch to hairless area behind the ear at least 4 hours prior to exposure and every 3 days as needed; effective if applied as soon as 2 to 3 hours before anticipated need, best if 12 hours before

Chemotherapy-induced nausea and vomiting, breakthrough (off-label use): Apply 1 patch every 72 hours (NCCN Antiemesis guidelines v.1.2012)

Scopolamine hydrobromide:

Antiemetic: SubQ: 0.6 to 1 mg

Preoperative: IM, IV, SubQ: 0.3 to 0.65 mg

Sedation, tranquilization: IM, IV, SubQ:

U.S. labeling: 0.6 mg 3 to 4 times/day

Canadian labeling: 0.3 to 0.6 mg 3 to 4 times/day

Scopolamine butylbromide [Canadian product]: *Gastrointestinal/genitourinary spasm:*

Oral: Acute therapy: 10 to 20 mg daily (1 to 2 tablets); prolonged therapy: 10 mg (1 tablet) 3 to 5 times/day; maximum: 60 mg/day

IM, IV, SubQ: 10 to 20 mg; maximum: 100 mg/day

Geriatric Lower dosages may be required. Refer to adult dosing.

Pediatric Note: Scopolamine injection is no longer available in the US.

Scopolamine hydrobromide:

Antiemetic: SubQ: 0.006 mg/kg

◀ *Preoperative:* IM, IV, SubQ:
  Children 6 months to 3 years: 0.1 to 0.15 mg
  Children 3 to 6 years: 0.2-0.3 mg

Renal Impairment No dosage adjustment provided in manufacturer's labeling. However, caution is recommended due to increased risks of adverse effects.

Hepatic Impairment No dosage adjustment provided in manufacturer's labeling. However, caution is recommended due to increased risks of adverse effects.

Administration Note: Butylbromide or hydrobromide may be administered by IM, IV, or SubQ injection.

IM: **Butylbromide:** Intramuscular injections should be administered 10-15 minutes prior to radiological/diagnostic procedures.

IV:

  Butylbromide: No dilution is necessary prior to injection; inject at a rate of 1 mL/minute

  Hydrobromide: Dilute with an equal volume of sterile water and administer by direct IV; inject over 2-3 minutes

Oral: Tablet should be swallowed whole and taken with a full glass of water.

Transdermal: Apply to hairless area of skin behind the ear. Wash hands before and after applying the disc to avoid drug contact with eyes. Do not use any patch that has been damaged, cut, or manipulated in any way. Topical patch is programmed to deliver 1 mg over 3 days. Once applied, do not remove the patch for 3 full days (motion sickness). When used postoperatively for nausea/vomiting, the patch should be removed 24 hours after surgery. If patch becomes displaced, discard and apply a new patch. Dispose of used or unused patches in the trash out of reach from children and pets.

Monitoring Parameters Body temperature, heart rate, urinary output, intraocular pressure

Test Interactions Interferes with gastric secretion test

Product Availability Scopolamine injection is no longer available in the US.

Dosage Forms Excipient information presented when available (limited, particularly for generics); consult specific product labeling.

Patch 72 Hour, Transdermal:
  Transderm-Scop: 1.5 mg (1 ea, 4 ea, 10 ea, 24 ea)
Solution, Injection, as hydrobromide:
  Generic: 0.4 mg/mL (1 mL)

Dosage Forms: Canada

Note: Refer also to Dosage Forms

Excipient information presented when available (limited, particularly for generics); consult specific product labeling.

Tablet, oral, as butylbromide:
  Buscopan: 10 mg
Solution, Injection, as butylbromide:
  Buscopan: 20 mg/mL (1 mL)

♦ **Scopolamine Base** *see* Scopolamine (Systemic) *on page 1520*

♦ **Scopolamine Butylbromide** *see* Scopolamine (Systemic) *on page 1520*

♦ **Scopolamine Hydrobromide** *see* Scopolamine (Systemic) *on page 1520*

♦ **Scopolamine Hydrobromide Injection (Can)** *see* Scopolamine (Systemic) *on page 1520*

♦ **SD/01** *see* Pegfilgrastim *on page 1346*

- ◆ **SDX-105** *see* Bendamustine *on page 182*
- ◆ **Sensipar** *see* Cinacalcet *on page 324*
- ◆ **Septa-Ciprofloxacin (Can)** *see* Ciprofloxacin (Systemic) *on page 327*
- ◆ **Septa-Ondansetron (Can)** *see* Ondansetron *on page 1253*
- ◆ **Septra** *see* Sulfamethoxazole and Trimethoprim *on page 1560*
- ◆ **Septra Injection (Can)** *see* Sulfamethoxazole and Trimethoprim *on page 1560*
- ◆ **SGN-35** *see* Brentuximab Vedotin *on page 237*
- ◆ **SH 714** *see* Cyproterone *on page 402*

Siltuximab (sil TUX i mab)

Brand Names: US Sylvant
Brand Names: Canada Sylvant
Index Terms CNTO 328
Pharmacologic Category Antineoplastic Agent, Monoclonal Antibody; Interleukin-6 Receptor Antagonist
Use
Castleman disease: Treatment of patients with multicentric Castleman disease (MCD) who are human immunodeficiency virus (HIV) negative and human herpesvirus-8 (HHV-8) negative
Limitations of use: Has not been studied in patients with MCD who are HIV positive or HHV-8 positive because in a nonclinical study, siltuximab did not bind to virally produced IL-6
Labeled Contraindications Severe hypersensitivity to siltuximab or any component of the formulation
Pregnancy Considerations Adverse events were not observed in animal reproduction studies. However, decreased globulin levels were detected in the pregnant animals and their offspring. Infants born to pregnant women treated with siltuximab may be at increased risk for infection. Use during pregnancy only if the potential benefit outweighs the possible risk to the fetus. Women of childbearing potential should use effective contraception during and for 3 months following treatment discontinuation.
Breast-Feeding Considerations It is not known if siltuximab is excreted in breast milk. Because many immunoglobulins are excreted in breast milk and the potential for adverse reactions in the nursing infant exists, the manufacturer recommends a decision be made whether to discontinue nursing or to discontinue the drug, taking into account the importance of treatment to the mother.
Warnings/Precautions Discontinue infusion immediately if signs of anaphylaxis occur; do not reinitiate therapy. If a mild to moderate infusion reaction develops, temporarily discontinue the infusion; if the reaction resolves, may reinitiate at a lower rate. Consider premedication with acetaminophen, antihistamines, and corticosteroids. If infusion-related reactions recur despite appropriate premedication and infusion rate reduction, discontinue therapy. Administer in a setting equipped to provide resuscitation equipment; medications for the treatment of hypersensitivity reactions (eg, bronchodilators, epinephrine, antihistamines, and corticosteroids) should be readily available. Siltuximab may mask signs and symptoms of infection, including signs of acute inflammation (eg, fever, C-reactive protein elevation). Do not administer to patients with severe infections; monitor closely for infections and initiate appropriate antibiotic therapy if needed. If infection develops, withhold therapy

◀ until resolved. Siltuximab administration may result in elevated hemoglobin levels in patients with multicentric Castleman disease; monitor blood counts prior to each dose for the first 12 months and every 3 dosing cycles thereafter, or as clinically necessary. May require therapy interruption. Gastrointestinal perforation has been observed in clinical trials. Use with caution in patients at risk for perforation; promptly evaluate concerning symptoms. Do not administer live vaccines to patients receiving siltuximab; IL-6 inhibition may interfere with immune response to vaccination. Approved for use only in patients who are HIV negative and HHV-8 negative. Siltuximab was not studied in patients positive for these disease states due to the lack of drug binding to virally produced IL-6 in a nonclinical study.

Adverse Reactions

>10%:
Cardiovascular: Peripheral edema (16%)
Central nervous system: Fatigue (21%; long-term exposure)
Dermatologic: Pruritus (28%), skin rash (28%)
Endocrine & metabolic: Weight gain (19%), hyperuricemia (11%)
Gastrointestinal: Diarrhea (32%; long-term exposure), abdominal pain (12%)
Neuromuscular & skeletal: Arthralgia (21%; long-term exposure), limb pain (21%; long-term exposure)
Respiratory: Upper respiratory tract infection (26%; long-term exposure: 63%)
1% to 10%:
Cardiovascular: Hypotension (4% to 6%; grades 3/4: 2% [anaphylactic reaction])
Central nervous system: Headache (8%)
Dermatologic: Eczema (4%), psoriasis (4%), skin hyperpigmentation (4%), xeroderma (4%)
Endocrine & metabolic: Hypertriglyceridemia (8%), dehydration (4%), hypercholesterolemia (4%)
Gastrointestinal: Constipation (8%), decreased appetite (4%)
Hematologic & oncologic: Thrombocytopenia (9%)
Renal: Renal insufficiency (8%)
Respiratory: Lower respiratory tract infection (8%), oropharyngeal pain (8%)
Miscellaneous: Infusion related reaction (5%)
<1%: Anaphylaxis, antibody development (non-neutralizing)

Drug Interactions

Metabolism/Transport Effects None known.

Avoid Concomitant Use

Avoid concomitant use of Siltuximab with any of the following: BCG (Intravesical); Belimumab; Natalizumab; Pimecrolimus; Tacrolimus (Topical); Tofacitinib; Vaccines (Live)

Increased Effect/Toxicity

Siltuximab may increase the levels/effects of: Belimumab; Fingolimod; Leflunomide; Natalizumab; Tofacitinib; Vaccines (Live)

The levels/effects of Siltuximab may be increased by: Denosumab; Pimecrolimus; Roflumilast; Tacrolimus (Topical); Trastuzumab

Decreased Effect

Siltuximab may decrease the levels/effects of: BCG (Intravesical); Coccidioides immitis Skin Test; CYP3A4 Substrates; Sipuleucel-T; Vaccines (Inactivated); Vaccines (Live)

The levels/effects of Siltuximab may be decreased by: Echinacea

Storage/Stability Store intact vials at 2°C to 8°C (36°F to 46°F); protect from light. Reconstituted solution should be further diluted for infusion within 2 hours; complete infusion within 4 hours of dilution of the reconstituted solution to the infusion bag. Discard any unused portion of the reconstituted solution or solution diluted for infusion.

Preparation for Administration Allow intact vials to come to room temperature (~30 minutes). Reconstitute with 5.2 mL (100 mg vial) or 20 mL (400 mg vial) SWFI to a final concentration of 20 mg/mL; gently swirl to fully dissolve powder. Do not shake or swirl vigorously. Must further dilute within 2 hours to 250 mL with D_5W (infusion bag must be made of polyvinyl chloride (PVC) with di-[2-ethylhexyl]phthalate (DEHP) or polyolefin). Remove a volume equal to the total calculated dose volume of reconstituted siltuximab from the bag of D_5W; slowly add the appropriate volume of reconstituted siltuximab solution to the infusion bag and gently invert to mix. Complete infusion within 4 hours of dilution of the reconstituted solution to the infusion bag.

Mechanism of Action Chimeric monoclonal antibody which binds with high affinity and specificity to IL-6; prevents IL-6 from binding to both soluble and membrane-bound IL-6 receptors. Overproduction of IL-6 may lead to systemic manifestations in multicentric Castleman disease (MCD) patients by inducing C-reactive protein (CRP) synthesis (Kurzrock, 2010). Lowering serum IL-6 levels may improve systemic symptoms of Castleman disease.

Pharmacodynamics/Kinetics
Distribution: 4.5 L

Half-life elimination: ~21 days (range: 14.2 to 29.7 days)

Dosing
Adult & Geriatric Note: Consider delaying first dose if ANC <1000/mm^3, platelets <75,000/mm^3, and hemoglobin ≥17 g/dL; subsequent doses may be delayed if ANC <1000/mm^3, platelets <50,000/mm^3, and hemoglobin ≥17 g/dL. Do not reduce dose.

Castleman disease, multicentric (in patients who are HIV negative and HHV-8 negative): IV: 11 mg/kg over 1 hour every 3 weeks until treatment failure

Renal Impairment
CrCl ≥15 mL/minute: No initial dosage adjustment is necessary.

CrCl <15 mL/minute: There are no dosage adjustments provided in the manufacturer's labeling (has not been studied).

End-stage renal disease (ESRD): There are no dosage adjustments provided in the manufacturer's labeling (has not been studied).

Hepatic Impairment
Mild to moderate impairment (Child Pugh class A or B): No initial dosage adjustment is necessary.

Severe impairment (Child Pugh class C): There are no dosage adjustments provided in the manufacturer's labeling (has not been studied).

Adjustment for Toxicity
Hematologic toxicity: ANC <1000/mm^3, platelets <50,000/mm^3, and hemoglobin ≥17 g/dL: Consider delaying treatment until ANC ≥1000/mm^3, platelets ≥50,000/mm^3, and hemoglobin <17 g/dL

Anaphylaxis, cytokine release syndromes, and/or severe infusion-related or allergic reactions: Discontinue permanently.

Infection, severe: Withhold treatment until infection resolves.

Administration Administer IV over 1 hour using administration sets lined with polyvinyl chloride (PVC) with di-[2-ethylhexyl]phthalate (DEHP) or polyurethane (PU) which contain a 0.2 micron inline polyethersulfone (PES) filter. Do not infuse in the same line with other medications. Complete infusion within 4 hours of dilution of the reconstituted solution to the infusion bag.

Emetic Potential Minimal (<10%)

Monitoring Parameters Monitor complete blood count with differential prior to each dose for the first 12 months and every 3 dosing cycles thereafter, or as clinically necessary; monitor for anaphylaxis and signs/symptoms of infusion-related, allergic, or cytokine release reactions; monitor for infection and signs/symptoms of gastrointestinal perforation.

Dosage Forms Excipient information presented when available (limited, particularly for generics); consult specific product labeling.

Solution Reconstituted, Intravenous [preservative free]:
  Sylvant: 100 mg (1 ea); 400 mg (1 ea) [contains mouse protein (murine) (hamster), polysorbate 80]

◆ **Simulect** see Basiliximab on page 170

Sipuleucel-T (si pu LOO sel tee)

Brand Names: US Provenge

Index Terms APC8015; Prostate Cancer Vaccine, Cell-Based

Pharmacologic Category Cellular Immunotherapy, Autologous

Use Prostate cancer, metastatic: Treatment of asymptomatic or minimally symptomatic metastatic castrate-resistant (hormone-refractory) prostate cancer.

Labeled Contraindications There are no contraindications listed in the manufacturer's labeling.

Pregnancy Considerations Animal reproduction studies have not been conducted. Not indicated for use in women.

Breast-Feeding Considerations Not indicated for use in women.

Warnings/Precautions For autologous use only; patient identity must be matched to the patient identifiers on the infusion bag and on the Final Product Disposition Notification (provided by manufacturer) prior to infusion; confirmation of product release must be received from the manufacturer prior to infusion.

Acute infusion reactions may occur within 1 day of infusion and are usually mild or moderate for most patients; the incidence of severe reaction may be higher with the second infusion, while the third infusion is associated with a decrease in the incidence of severe reactions. Premedication with oral acetaminophen and diphenhydramine is recommended. Depending on the severity of infusion reaction, interrupt or slow infusion rate; in clinical trials, acetaminophen, intravenous (IV) H_1 and/or H_2 antagonists, and low-dose meperidine were used to manage acute symptoms. Symptoms of acute infusion reaction may include chills, rigor, fever, bronchospasm, dyspnea, hypoxia, hypertension, tachycardia, syncope, hypotension, joint or muscle aches, nausea, vomiting, dizziness, fatigue, headache, and weakness; fever and chills usually resolved within 2 days. Observe patient for at least 30 minutes after infusion.

Cerebrovascular (hemorrhagic and ischemic stroke) and cardiovascular events (myocardial infarction [MI]) have occurred; transient ischemic attacks have been reported following infusion (postmarketing reports). Such events usually occurred in patients with multiple risk factors for cerebrovascular or cardiovascular incidents. Deep venous thrombosis (DVT) and pulmonary embolism occurred following sipuleucel-T infusion (postmarketing reports), usually in patients with multiple risk factors for thromboembolism. Use with caution in patients at risk for thromboembolic events. Closely monitor during infusion in patients with cardiac or pulmonary conditions. Concurrent use with immunosuppressives (eg, corticosteroids) has not been studied; may alter the efficacy and/or safety of sipuleucel-T. Carefully evaluate patients for appropriateness of reducing or discontinuing immunosuppressive agents prior to treatment. Concurrent use with chemotherapy has not been studied. In clinical trials, patients who had androgen deprivation therapy without prior bilateral orchiectomy were continued on gonadal suppression with a luteinizing hormone-releasing hormone (LHRH) agonist (Higano, 2009).

Apply universal precautions for product handling; sipuleucel-T is not routinely tested for transmissible infectious diseases; patient specific leukapheresis collection and activated product may have a risk for infectious disease transmission. Preliminary sterility testing is done based on a 2-day incubation period; final (7-day incubation) testing is not available until after administration; physicians will be notified if 7-day sterility tests are positive for microbial contamination. If unable to receive a scheduled reinfusion, an additional leukapheresis procedure may be required; advise patients of this possibility before treatment initiation.

Adverse Reactions Note: Initial infusion-related events usually present within the first 24 hours after administration.

>10%:
  Central nervous system: Chills (53%; grades ≥3: 2%), fatigue (41%; grades ≥3: 1%), headache (18%; grades ≥3: <1%), dizziness (12%; grades ≥3: <1%), pain (12%)
  Gastrointestinal: Nausea (22%; grades ≥3: <1%), vomiting (13% grades ≥3: <1%), constipation (12%; grades ≥3: <1%)
  Hematologic: Anemia (13%)
  Hypersensitivity: Severe infusion related reaction (71%; grade 3: 4%)
  Neuromuscular & skeletal: Back pain (30%; grades ≥3: 3%), myalgia (12%; grades ≥3: <1%), weakness (11%; grades ≥3: 1%)
  Miscellaneous: Fever (31%; grades ≥3: 1%), citrate toxicity (15%)
1% to 10%:
  Cardiovascular: Hypertension (8% grades ≥3: <1%), hemorrhagic stroke (4%)
  Dermatologic: Diaphoresis (5%; grades ≥3: <1%), skin rash (5%)
  Gastrointestinal: Anorexia (7%), acute ischemic stroke (4%)
  Genitourinary: Hematuria (8%)
  Neuromuscular & skeletal: Musculoskeletal pain (9%; grades ≥3: <1%), muscle spasm (8%; grades ≥3: <1%), neck pain (6%), tremor (5%)
  Renal: Hematuria (8%)
  Respiratory: Flu-like symptoms (10%), dyspnea (9%; grades ≥3: 2%)
<1%, postmarketing, and/or case reports: Cerebrovascular accident, eosinophilia, hypotension, myasthenia gravis, myocardial infarction, myositis, paresthesia (grades ≥3), pulmonary embolism, rhabdomyolysis, sepsis, syncope, transient ischemic attacks, tumor flare, venous thrombosis

Drug Interactions

  Metabolism/Transport Effects None known.

  Avoid Concomitant Use There are no known interactions where it is recommended to avoid concomitant use.

◄ **Increased Effect/Toxicity** There are no known significant interactions involving an increase in effect.

Decreased Effect

The levels/effects of Sipuleucel-T may be decreased by: Immunosuppressants

Storage/Stability Do not remove the infusion bag from the insulated polyurethane container within the shipping box until administration (do not remove the insulated container from the shipping box, or open the lid of the insulated container, until administration). Product may only remain at room temperature for ≤3 hours once removed from shipping container; after removal from shipping container, do not return product to container. Infusion must begin prior to product expiration.

Preparation for Administration Sipuleucel-T will arrive as a prepared patient-specific 250 mL suspension in lactated Ringer's injection. Contents may appear clear to opaque and will be a white to red color, including shades of off-white, cream, light yellow, and orange. If clumps or clots are present, gently mix to resuspend. Do not administer if the bag leaks during handling, is damaged, or if clumps remain.

Mechanism of Action Autologous cellular immunotherapy which stimulates an immune response against an antigen (PAP) expressed in most prostate cancer tissues. Peripheral blood is collected (~3 days prior to infusion) from the patient via leukapheresis, from which peripheral blood mononuclear cells (PBMCs) are isolated. Antigen presenting cell (APC) precursors, consisting of CD54-positive cells that include dendritic cells, are isolated from the PBMCs. The APCs are then activated (*in vitro*) with a recombinant human fusion protein, PAP-GM-CSF (also termed PA2024), composed of an antigen specific for prostate cancer, prostatic acid phosphatase (PAP) linked to granulocyte-macrophage colony-stimulating factor (GM-CSF) and cultured for ~40 hours. The final product, sipuleucel-T, is reinfused into the patient, inducing T-cell immunity to tumors that express PAP.

Dosing

Adult & Geriatric Note: Premedicate with oral acetaminophen 650 mg and an antihistamine (eg, diphenhydramine 50 mg) ~30 minutes prior to infusion. For autologous use only. Do not infuse until confirmation of product release has been received from the company.

Prostate cancer, metastatic: IV: Each dose contains ≥50 million autologous CD54+ cells (obtained through leukapheresis) activated with PAP-GM-CSF; administer doses at ~2-week intervals for a total of 3 doses (Kantoff, 2010). If unable to receive a scheduled infusion, an additional leukapheresis procedure will be necessary prior to continuing a course of treatment.

Renal Impairment There are no dosage adjustments provided in the manufacturer's labeling.

Hepatic Impairment There are no dosage adjustments provided in the manufacturer's labeling.

Adjustment for Toxicity Acute infusion reaction: Interrupt or slow infusion rate (depending on the severity of infusion reaction); may require acetaminophen, IV H_1 and/or H_2 antagonists, or low-dose meperidine to manage acute symptoms.

Administration For autologous use only; the identity of the patient must be matched to the patient identifiers on the infusion bag and on the "Final Product Disposition Notification" prior to infusion. Do not infuse until confirmation of product release is received from the company. Keep the sealed infusion bag in the insulated polyurethane container inside the shipping box until ready for administration. Prior to infusion, inspect bag for signs of leaks (do not administer if leaking) or damage. Gently mix to resuspend contents; inspect for clumps or clotting; small clumps should disperse with the gentle mixing; do not administer if clumps remain. Infusion must begin prior to the expiration date and time; do **NOT** infuse if expired.

For IV infusion only. Infuse over ~60 minutes; infuse the entire contents of the bag. Do **NOT** use a cell filter for infusion. For acute infusion reaction, interrupt or slow infusion rate (depending on the severity of infusion reaction); may require acetaminophen, IV H_1 and/or H_2 antagonists, or low-dose meperidine to manage acute symptoms. If infusion is interrupted, keep infusion bag at room temperature; do not resume if bag is retained at room temperature for >3 hours. Observe patient for at least 30 minutes after infusion.

Monitoring Parameters Monitor for infusion reaction during and for at least 30 minutes after infusion; monitor closely during infusion for patients with cardiovascular and pulmonary disease; monitor for thromboembolic and vascular events.

Prescribing and Access Restrictions Patients may receive Sipuleucel-T at a participating site. Physicians must go through an inservice and register to prescribe the treatment; patients must also complete an enrollment form. Information on registration and enrollment is available at 1-877-336-3736.

Dosage Forms Excipient information presented when available (limited, particularly for generics); consult specific product labeling.
Suspension, Intravenous [preservative free]:
Provenge: (250 mL)

Sirolimus (sir OH li mus)

Related Information
Hematopoietic Stem Cell Transplantation on page 2272
Safe Handling of Hazardous Drugs on page 2292
Brand Names: US Rapamune
Brand Names: Canada Rapamune
Index Terms Rapamycin
Pharmacologic Category Immunosuppressant Agent; mTOR Kinase Inhibitor
Use

Lymphangioleiomyomatosis: Treatment of lymphangioleiomyomatosis. Therapeutic drug monitoring is recommended for all patients receiving sirolimus.

Renal transplantation: Prophylaxis of organ rejection in patients receiving renal transplants (in low-to-moderate immunologic risk patients in combination with cyclosporine and corticosteroids with cyclosporine withdrawn 2 to 4 months after transplant, and in high immunologic risk patients in combination with cyclosporine and corticosteroids for the first year after transplant). Therapeutic drug monitoring is recommended for all patients receiving sirolimus. High immunologic risk renal transplant patients are defined (per the manufacturer's labeling) as Black transplant recipients and/or repeat renal transplant recipients who lost a previous allograft based on an immunologic process and/or patients with high PRA (panel-reactive antibodies; peak PRA level >80%).

◄ Limitations of use (renal transplantation): Cyclosporine withdrawal has not been studied in patients with Banff grade 3 acute rejection or vascular rejection prior to cyclosporine withdrawal, patients who are dialysis-dependent, patients with serum creatinine >4.5 mg/dL, Black patients, patients with multiorgan transplants or secondary transplants, or those with high levels of PRA. In patients at high immunologic risk, the safety and efficacy of sirolimus used in combination with cyclosporine and corticosteroids have not been studied beyond 1 year; therefore, after the first 12 months following transplantation, consider any adjustments to the immunosuppressive regimen on the basis of the clinical status of the patient. The safety and efficacy of sirolimus have not been established in patients younger than 13 years or in pediatric renal transplant patients younger than 18 years who are considered at high immunologic risk. The safety and efficacy of de novo use of sirolimus without cyclosporine have not been established in renal transplant patients. The safety and efficacy of conversion from calcineurin inhibitors to sirolimus in maintenance renal transplant patients have not been established.

Labeled Contraindications Hypersensitivity to sirolimus or any component of the formulation

Pregnancy Considerations Adverse events have been observed in animal reproduction studies. Effective contraception must be initiated before therapy with sirolimus and continued for 12 weeks after discontinuation.

The National Transplantation Pregnancy Registry (NTPR, Temple University) is a registry for pregnant women taking immunosuppressants following any solid organ transplant. The NTPR encourages reporting of all immunosuppressant exposures during pregnancy in transplant recipients at 1-877-955-6877.

Breast-Feeding Considerations It is not known if sirolimus is excreted in breast milk. Due to the potential for serious adverse reactions in the nursing infant, the manufacturer recommends a decision be made whether to discontinue nursing or to discontinue the drug, taking into account the importance of treatment to the mother.

Warnings/Precautions Hazardous agent - use appropriate precautions for handling and disposal (NIOSH 2014 [group 2]).

[US Boxed Warning]: Immunosuppressive agents, including sirolimus, increase the risk of infection and may be associated with the development of lymphoma. Immune suppression may also increase the risk of opportunistic infections including activation of latent viral infections (including BK virus-associated nephropathy), fatal infections, and sepsis. Prophylactic treatment for *Pneumocystis jirovecii* pneumonia (PCP) should be administered for 1 year post-transplant; prophylaxis for cytomegalovirus (CMV) should be taken for 3 months post-transplant in patients at risk for CMV. Progressive multifocal leukoencephalopathy (PML), an opportunistic CNS infection caused by reactivation of the JC virus, has been reported in patients receiving immunosuppressive therapy, including sirolimus. Clinical findings of PML include apathy, ataxia, cognitive deficiency, confusion, and hemiparesis; promptly evaluate any patient presenting with neurological changes; consider decreasing the degree of immunosuppression with consideration to the risk of organ rejection in transplant patients.

[US Boxed Warning]: Sirolimus is not recommended for use in liver or lung transplantation. Bronchial anastomotic dehiscence cases have been reported in lung transplant patients when sirolimus was used as

part of an immunosuppressive regimen; most of these reactions were fatal. Studies indicate an association with an increased risk of hepatic artery thrombosis (HAT), graft failure, and increased mortality (with evidence of infection) in liver transplant patients when sirolimus is used in combination with cyclosporine and/or tacrolimus. Most cases of HAT occurred within 30 days of transplant.

In renal transplant patients, *de novo* use without cyclosporine has been associated with higher rates of acute rejection. Sirolimus should be used in combination with cyclosporine (and corticosteroids) initially when used in renal transplant patients. Cyclosporine may be withdrawn in low-to-moderate immunologic risk patients after 2 to 4 months, in conjunction with an increase in sirolimus dosage. In high immunologic risk patients, use in combination with cyclosporine and corticosteroids is recommended for the first year. Safety and efficacy of combination therapy with cyclosporine in high immunologic risk patients has not been studied beyond 12 months of treatment; adjustment of immunosuppressive therapy beyond 12 months should be considered based on clinical judgment. Monitor renal function closely when combined with cyclosporine; consider dosage adjustment or discontinue in patients with increasing serum creatinine.

May increase serum creatinine and decrease GFR. Use caution when used concurrently with medications which may alter renal function. May delay recovery of renal function in patients with delayed allograft function. Increased urinary protein excretion has been observed when converting renal transplant patients from calcineurin inhibitors to sirolimus during maintenance therapy. A higher level of proteinuria prior to sirolimus conversion correlates with a higher degree of proteinuria after conversion. In some patients, proteinuria may reach nephrotic levels; nephrotic syndrome (new onset) has been reported. Increased risk of BK viral-associated nephropathy which may impair renal function and cause graft loss; consider decreasing immunosuppressive burden if evidence of deteriorating renal function.

Use caution with hepatic impairment; a reduction in the maintenance dose is recommended. Has been associated with an increased risk of fluid accumulation and lymphocele; peripheral edema, lymphedema, ascites, and pleural and pericardial effusions (including significant effusions and tamponade) were reported; use with caution in patients in whom fluid accumulation may be poorly tolerated, such as in cardiovascular disease (heart failure or hypertension) and pulmonary disease. Cases of interstitial lung disease (ILD) (eg, pneumonitis, bronchiolitis obliterans organizing pneumonia [BOOP], pulmonary fibrosis) have been observed (some fatal); may be associated with pulmonary hypertension (including pulmonary arterial hypertension) and risk may be increased with higher trough levels. ILD may resolve with dose reduction or discontinuation of therapy. Potentially significant drug-drug interactions may exist, requiring dose or frequency adjustment, additional monitoring, and/or selection of alternative therapy. Concurrent use with a calcineurin inhibitor (cyclosporine, tacrolimus) may increase the risk of calcineurin inhibitor-induced hemolytic uremic syndrome/thrombotic thrombocytopenic purpura/thrombotic microangiopathy (HUS/TTP/TMA). Immunosuppressants may affect response to vaccination. Therefore, during treatment with sirolimus, vaccination may be less effective. The use of live vaccines should be avoided. ▶

◄ Hypersensitivity reactions, including anaphylactic/anaphylactoid reactions, angioedema, exfoliative dermatitis, and hypersensitivity vasculitis have been reported. Concurrent use with other drugs known to cause angioedema (eg, ACE inhibitors) may increase risk. Immunosuppressant therapy is associated with an increased risk of skin cancer; limit sun and ultraviolet light exposure; use appropriate sun protection. May increase serum lipids (cholesterol and triglycerides); use with caution in patients with hyperlipidemia; monitor cholesterol/lipids; if hyperlipidemia occurs, follow current guidelines for management (diet, exercise, lipid lowering agents); antihyperlipidemic therapy may not be effective in normalizing levels. May be associated with wound dehiscence and impaired healing; use caution in the perioperative period. Patients with a body mass index (BMI) >30 kg/m^2 are at increased risk for abnormal wound healing.

Sirolimus tablets and oral solution are not bioequivalent, due to differences in absorption. Clinical equivalence was seen using 2 mg tablet and 2 mg solution. It is not known if higher doses are also clinically equivalent. Monitor sirolimus levels if changes in dosage forms are made. Some dosage forms may contain propylene glycol; large amounts are potentially toxic and have been associated hyperosmolality, lactic acidosis, seizures, and respiratory depression; use caution (AAP, 1997; Zar 2007). **[US Boxed Warning]: Should only be used by physicians experienced in immunosuppressive therapy and management of transplant patients. Adequate laboratory and supportive medical resources must be readily available.** Sirolimus concentrations are dependent on the assay method (eg, chromatographic and immunoassay) used; assay methods are not interchangeable. Variations in methods to determine sirolimus whole blood concentrations, as well as interlaboratory variations, may result in improper dosage adjustments, which may lead to subtherapeutic or toxic levels. Determine the assay method used to assure consistency (or accommodations if changes occur), and for monitoring purposes, be aware of alterations to assay method or reference range and that values from different assays may not be interchangeable.

Adverse Reactions Incidence of many adverse effects is dose related. Reported events exclusive to renal transplant patients unless otherwise noted. Frequency not always defined.

Cardiovascular: Peripheral edema (≥20% to 58%, LAM and renal transplants), hypertension (49%), edema (18% to 20%), chest pain (LAM), deep vein thrombosis, pulmonary embolism, tachycardia

Central nervous system: Headache (≥20% to 34%, LAM and renal transplants), pain (29% to 33%), dizziness (LAM)

Dermatologic: Acne vulgaris (≥20% to 22%, LAM and renal transplants), skin rash (10% to 20%)

Endocrine & metabolic: Hypertriglyceridemia (45% to 57%), hypercholesterolemia (≥20% to 46%, LAM and renal transplants), amenorrhea, diabetes mellitus, hypermenorrhea, hypervolemia, hypokalemia, increased lactate dehydrogenase, menstrual disease, ovarian cyst

Gastrointestinal: Constipation (36% to 38%), abdominal pain (≥20% to 36%, LAM and renal transplants), diarrhea (≥20% to 35%, LAM and renal transplants), nausea (≥20% to 31%, LAM and renal transplants), stomatitis (3% to >20%)

Genitourinary: Urinary tract infection (33%)

Hematologic & oncologic: Anemia (23% to 33%), thrombocytopenia (14% to 30%), lymphoproliferative disorder (≤3%; including lymphoma), skin carcinoma (≤3%; includes basal cell carcinoma, squamous cell carcinoma, melanoma), hemolytic-uremic syndrome, leukopenia, lymphocele, thrombotic thrombocytopenic purpura

Infection: Herpes simplex infection, herpes zoster, sepsis

Neuromuscular & skeletal: Arthralgia (25% to 31%), myalgia (LAM), osteonecrosis

Renal: Increased serum creatinine (39% to 40%), pyelonephritis

Respiratory: Nasopharyngitis (LAM), epistaxis, pneumonia, upper respiratory tract infection (LAM)

Miscellaneous: Wound healing impairment

<3%, postmarketing, and/or case reports: Abnormal hepatic function tests, anaphylactoid reaction, anaphylaxis, angioedema, ascites, azoospermia, cardiac tamponade, cytomegalovirus, dehiscence (fascial), Epstein-Barr infection, exfoliative dermatitis, fluid retention, focal segmental glomerulosclerosis, gingival hyperplasia, hepatic necrosis, hepatotoxicity, hyperglycemia, hypersensitivity angiitis, hypersensitivity reaction, hypophosphatemia, incisional hernia, increased serum ALT, increased serum AST, increased susceptibility to infection (including opportunistic), interstitial pulmonary disease (dose related; includes pneumonitis, pulmonary fibrosis, and bronchiolitis obliterans organizing pneumonia with no identified infectious etiology), joint disorders, lymphedema, mycobacterium infection, nephrotic syndrome, neutropenia, pancreatitis, pancytopenia, pericardial effusion, pleural effusion, pneumonia due to *Pneumocystis carinii*, progressive multifocal leukoencephalopathy, proteinuria, pseudomembranous colitis, pulmonary alveolitis, pulmonary hemorrhage, renal disease (BK virus-associated), reversible posterior leukoencephalopathy syndrome, tuberculosis, weight loss, wound dehiscence

Drug Interactions

Metabolism/Transport Effects Substrate of CYP3A4 (major), P-glycoprotein; **Note:** Assignment of Major/Minor substrate status based on clinically relevant drug interaction potential

Avoid Concomitant Use

Avoid concomitant use of Sirolimus with any of the following: BCG (Intravesical); CloZAPine; Conivaptan; Crizotinib; Dipyrone; Enzalutamide; Fusidic Acid (Systemic); Idelalisib; Mifepristone; Natalizumab; Pimecrolimus; Posaconazole; Tacrolimus (Systemic); Tacrolimus (Topical); Tofacitinib; Vaccines (Live); Voriconazole

Increased Effect/Toxicity

Sirolimus may increase the levels/effects of: ACE Inhibitors; CloZAPine; CycloSPORINE (Systemic); Fingolimod; Leflunomide; Natalizumab; Tacrolimus (Systemic); Tacrolimus (Topical); Tofacitinib; Vaccines (Live)

The levels/effects of Sirolimus may be increased by: Aprepitant; Boceprevir; Clotrimazole (Topical); Conivaptan; Crizotinib; CycloSPORINE (Systemic); CYP3A4 Inhibitors (Moderate); CYP3A4 Inhibitors (Strong); Dasatinib; Denosumab; Dipyrone; Fluconazole; Fosaprepitant; Fusidic Acid (Systemic); Idelalisib; Itraconazole; Ivacaftor; Ketoconazole (Systemic); Luliconazole; Macrolide Antibiotics; Mifepristone; Nelfinavir; Netupitant; Ombitasvir, Paritaprevir, Ritonavir, and Dasabuvir; Osimertinib; Palbociclib; P-glycoprotein/ABCB1 Inhibitors; Pimecrolimus; Posaconazole; Ranolazine; Roflumilast; Stiripentol; Tacrolimus (Systemic); Tacrolimus (Topical); Telaprevir; Trastuzumab; Voriconazole

◀ **Decreased Effect**

Sirolimus may decrease the levels/effects of: Antidiabetic Agents; BCG (Intravesical); Coccidioides immitis Skin Test; Sipuleucel-T; Tacrolimus (Systemic); Vaccines (Inactivated); Vaccines (Live)

The levels/effects of Sirolimus may be decreased by: Bosentan; CYP3A4 Inducers (Moderate); CYP3A4 Inducers (Strong); Dabrafenib; Deferasirox; Echinacea; Efavirenz; Enzalutamide; Fosphenytoin; Mitotane; Osimertinib; P-glycoprotein/ABCB1 Inducers; Phenytoin; Rifampin; Siltuximab; St Johns Wort; Tocilizumab

Food Interactions Grapefruit juice may decrease clearance of sirolimus. Ingestion with high-fat meals decreases peak concentrations but increases AUC by 23% to 35%. Management: Avoid grapefruit juice. Take consistently (either with or without food) to minimize variability.

Storage/Stability

Oral solution: Store at 2°C to 8°C (36°F to 46°F). Protect from light. A slight haze may develop in refrigerated solutions, but the quality of the product is not affected. After opening, solution should be used within 1 month. If necessary, may be stored at temperatures up to 25°C (77°F) for ≤15 days after opening. Product may be stored in amber syringe for a maximum of 24 hours (at room temperature or refrigerated). Discard syringe after single use. Solution should be used immediately following dilution.

Tablet: Store at 20°C to 25°C (68°F to 77°F). Protect from light.

Mechanism of Action Sirolimus inhibits T-lymphocyte activation and proliferation in response to antigenic and cytokine stimulation and inhibits antibody production. Its mechanism differs from other immunosuppressants. Sirolimus binds to FKBP-12, an intracellular protein, to form an immunosuppressive complex which inhibits the regulatory kinase, mTOR (mechanistic target of rapamycin). This inhibition suppresses cytokine mediated T-cell proliferation, halting progression from the G1 to the S phase of the cell cycle. It inhibits acute rejection of allografts and prolongs graft survival.

In lymphangioleiomyomatosis, the mTOR signaling pathway is activated through the loss of the tuberous sclerosis complex (TSC) gene function (resulting in cellular proliferation and release of lymphangiogenic growth factors). By inhibiting the mTOR pathway, sirolimus prevents the proliferation of lymphangioleiomyomatosis cells.

Pharmacodynamics/Kinetics

Absorption: Rapid

Distribution: 12 L/kg (range: 4 to 20 L/kg)

Protein binding: ~92%, primarily to albumin

Metabolism: Extensive; in intestinal wall via P-glycoprotein and hepatic via CYP3A4 to 7 major metabolites

Bioavailability: Oral solution: 14%; Oral tablet: 18%

Half-life elimination: Mean: 62 hours (range: 46 to 78 hours); extended in hepatic impairment (Child-Pugh class A or B) to 113 hours

Time to peak: Oral solution: 1 to 3 hours; Tablet: 1 to 6 hours

Excretion: Feces (91% due to P-glycoprotein-mediated efflux into gut lumen); urine (2%)

Dosing
Adult & Geriatric
Low-to-moderate immunologic risk renal transplant patients: Oral:

<40 kg: Loading dose: 3 mg/m^2 on day 1, followed by maintenance dosing of 1 mg/m^2 once daily

≥40 kg: Loading dose: 6 mg on day 1; maintenance: 2 mg once daily

High immunologic risk renal transplant patients: Oral: Loading dose: Up to 15 mg on day 1; maintenance: 5 mg/day; obtain trough concentration between days 5 to 7 and adjust accordingly. Continue concurrent cyclosporine/sirolimus/corticosteroid therapy for 1 year following transplantation. Further adjustment of the regimen must be based on clinical status.

Dosage adjustment for renal transplantation: Sirolimus dosages should be adjusted to maintain trough concentrations within desired range based on risk and concomitant therapy. Maximum daily dose: 40 mg. Dosage should be adjusted at intervals of 7 to 14 days to account for the long half-life of sirolimus. In general, dose proportionality may be assumed. New sirolimus dose **equals** current dose **multiplied by** (target concentration **divided by** current concentration). **Note:** If large dose increase is required, consider loading dose calculated as:

Loading dose **equals** (new maintenance dose **minus** current maintenance dose) **multiplied by** 3

Maximum dose in 1 day: 40 mg; if required dose is >40 mg (due to loading dose), divide loading dose over 2 days. Whole blood concentrations should not be used as the sole basis for dosage adjustment (monitor clinical signs/symptoms, tissue biopsy, and laboratory parameters).

Maintenance therapy after withdrawal of cyclosporine: Cyclosporine withdrawal is not recommended in high immunological risk patients. Following 2 to 4 months of combined therapy, withdrawal of cyclosporine may be considered in low-to-moderate immunologic risk patients. Cyclosporine should be discontinued over 4 to 8 weeks, and a necessary increase in the dosage of sirolimus (up to fourfold) should be anticipated due to removal of metabolic inhibition by cyclosporine and to maintain adequate immunosuppressive effects. Dose-adjusted trough target concentrations are typically 16 to 24 ng/mL for the first year post-transplant and 12 to 20 ng/mL thereafter (measured by chromatographic methodology).

Lymphangioleiomyomatosis: Adults: Oral: Initial: 2 mg once daily. Obtain trough concentration in 10 to 20 days; adjust dose to maintain a target concentration of 5 to 15 ng/mL.

Dosage adjustment for lymphangioleiomyomatosis: Once the maintenance dose is adjusted, further adjustments should be made at 7 to 14 day intervals to account for the long half-life of sirolimus. In general, dose proportionality may be assumed. New sirolimus dose **equals** current dose **multiplied by** (target concentration **divided by** current concentration). Once a stable dose is achieved, trough concentrations should be assessed at least every 3 months.

Graft-versus-host disease (GVHD): Oral:

GVHD prophylaxis (off-label use): 12 mg loading dose on day -3, followed by 4 mg daily (target trough level: 3 to 12 ng/mL); taper off after 6 to 9 months (Armand 2008; Cutler 2007)

Treatment of refractory acute GVHD (off-label use): 4 to 5 mg/m^2 for 14 days (no loading dose) (Benito 2001)

◄ **Treatment of chronic GVHD (off-label use):** 6 mg loading dose, followed by 2 mg daily (target trough level: 7 to 12 ng/mL) for 6 to 9 months (Couriel 2005)

Heart transplantation (off-label use): Oral: **Note:** The use of sirolimus in the immediate post-cardiac transplant period (ie, *de novo* heart transplant) as a primary immunosuppressant has fallen out of favor due to adverse effects (eg, impaired wound healing and infection); however, patients may be converted to sirolimus from a calcineurin inhibitor (after at least 6 months from time of transplant [Costanzo 2010]) or may have sirolimus added to a calcineurin inhibitor to prevent or minimize further transplant related vasculopathy or renal toxicity due to calcineurin inhibitor use.

Conversion from a calcineurin inhibitor (CNI) (ie, cyclosporine, tacrolimus): Reduce cyclosporine by 25 mg twice daily or tacrolimus by 1 mg twice daily followed by initiation of sirolimus 1 mg once daily; adjust sirolimus dose to target trough level of 8 to 14 ng/mL, withdraw CNI, repeat biopsy 2 weeks after CNI withdrawal (Topilsky 2012). Alternatively, maintain CNI concentrations and initiate sirolimus 1 mg once daily for 1 week; adjust sirolimus to target trough levels of 10 to 15 ng/mL over 2 weeks, then reduce CNI to target 50% of therapeutic concentrations and after 2 weeks evaluate for rejection. If no rejection, continue same regimen for an additional month, then reduce CNI to 25% of therapeutic concentrations with repeat biopsy 2 weeks later; if no rejection, may discontinue CNI after 2 weeks and continue to maintain sirolimus trough levels of 10 to 15 ng/mL (usual doses required to maintain target levels: 1 to 8 mg daily) (Kushwaha 2005).

Conversion from antiproliferative drug (ie, azathioprine or mycophenolate) while maintaining calcineurin inhibitor: Upon discontinuation of antiproliferative, administer sirolimus 6 mg loading dose followed by 2 mg once daily titrated to a target trough level of 4 to 15 ng/mL (Mancini 2003) or 4 to 12 ng/mL per ISHLT recommendations (Costanzo 2010).

Renal angiomyolipoma (off-label use): Oral: Initial: 0.5 mg/m^2 once daily titrated to a target trough level of 3 to 6 ng/mL (may increase to target trough level of 6 to 10 ng/mL if <10% reduction in lesion diameters at 2 months) for 2 years (Davies 2011)

Pediatric Low-to-moderate immunologic risk renal transplant patients: Adolescents ≥13 years: Oral: Refer to adult dosing.

Renal Impairment No dosage adjustment is necessary. However, adjustment of regimen (including discontinuation of therapy) should be considered when used concurrently with cyclosporine and elevated or increasing serum creatinine is noted.

Hepatic Impairment

Loading dose: No dosage adjustment is necessary.

Maintenance dose:

Mild to moderate impairment (Child-Pugh classes A and B): Reduce maintenance dose by ~33%.

Severe impairment (Child-Pugh class C): Reduce maintenance dose by ~50%.

Administration Initial dose should be administered as soon as possible after transplant. Sirolimus should be taken 4 hours after oral cyclosporine (Neoral or Gengraf). Should be administered consistently (either with or without food).

Solution: Mix (by stirring vigorously) with at least 2 ounces of water or orange juice. No other liquids should be used for dilution. Patient should drink diluted solution immediately. The cup should then be refilled with an additional 4 ounces of water or orange juice, stirred vigorously, and the patient should drink the contents at once.

Tablet: Do not crush, split, or chew.

Hazardous agent; use appropriate precautions for handling and disposal (NIOSH 2014 [group 2]).

Monitoring Parameters Monitor LFTs and CBC during treatment. Monitor sirolimus levels in all patients (especially in pediatric patients, patients ≥13 years of age weighing <40 kg, patients with hepatic impairment, or on concurrent potent inhibitors or inducers of CYP3A4 or P-gp, and/or if cyclosporine dosing is markedly reduced or discontinued), and when changing dosage forms of sirolimus. Also monitor serum cholesterol and triglycerides, blood pressure, serum creatinine, and urinary protein. Serum drug concentrations should be determined 3 to 4 days after loading doses and 7 to 14 days after dosage adjustments for renal transplant patients; however, these concentrations should not be used as the sole basis for dosage adjustment, especially during withdrawal of cyclosporine (monitor clinical signs/symptoms, tissue biopsy, and laboratory parameters). Monitor serum trough concentration 10 to 20 days after initiating therapy for lymphangioleiomyomatosis and 7 to 14 days after dosage adjustments. Once a stable dose is achieved, trough concentrations should be assessed at least every 3 months. **Note:** Concentrations and ranges are dependent on and will vary with assay methodology (chromatographic or immunoassay); assay methods are not interchangeable.

Medication Guide Available Yes

Dosage Forms Excipient information presented when available (limited, particularly for generics); consult specific product labeling.

Solution, Oral:
  Rapamune: 1 mg/mL (60 mL) [contains alcohol, usp]
Tablet, Oral:
  Rapamune: 0.5 mg, 1 mg, 2 mg
  Generic: 0.5 mg, 1 mg, 2 mg

Sodium Thiosulfate (SOW dee um thye oh SUL fate)

Related Information

Management of Drug Extravasations *on page 2159*

Index Terms Disodium Thiosulfate Pentahydrate; Pentahydrate; Sodium Hyposulfate; Sodium Thiosulphate; Thiosulfuric Acid Disodium Salt

Pharmacologic Category Antidote; Antidote, Extravasation

Use Cyanide poisoning: Treatment of acute, life-threatening cyanide poisoning in combination with sodium nitrite. Consider consultation with a poison control center at 1-800-222-1222.

Labeled Contraindications There are no contraindications listed within the manufacturer's labeling.

Pregnancy Considerations Teratogenic effects were not observed in animal reproduction studies of sodium thiosulfate. In general, medications used as antidotes should take into consideration the health and prognosis of the mother; antidotes should be administered to pregnant women if there is a clear indication for use and should not be withheld because of fears of teratogenicity (Bailey 2003).

Breast-Feeding Considerations It is not known if sodium thiosulfate is excreted in breast milk. Because sodium thiosulfate may be used as an antidote in life-threatening situations, breast-feeding is not a contraindication to use. It is not known when breast-feeding may safely be restarted following administration; the manufacturer recommends caution be used following administration to nursing women.

Warnings/Precautions Due to the risk for serious adverse effects, use with caution in patients where the diagnosis of cyanide poisoning is uncertain. However, if clinical suspicion of cyanide poisoning is high, treatment should not be delayed. Treatment of cyanide poisoning should include external decontamination and supportive therapy. Collection of pretreatment blood cyanide concentrations does not preclude administration and should not delay administration in the emergency management of highly suspected or confirmed cyanide toxicity. Pretreatment levels may be useful as postinfusion levels may be inaccurate. Monitor patients for return of symptoms for 24-48 hours; repeat treatment (one-half the original dose) should be administered if symptoms return. Fire victims may present with both cyanide and carbon monoxide poisoning. In these patients, the induction of methemoglobinemia with amyl nitrite or sodium nitrite is contraindicated until carbon monoxide levels return to normal due to the risk of tissue hypoxia. Methemoglobinemia decreases the oxygen-carrying capacity of hemoglobin and the presence of carbon monoxide prevents hemoglobin from releasing oxygen to the tissues. In this scenario, sodium thiosulfate may be used alone to promote the clearance of cyanide. Hydroxocobalamin, however, should be considered to avoid the nitrite-related problems and because sodium thiosulfate has a slow onset of action. Hydroxocobalamin, however, should be considered to avoid the nitrite-related problems and because sodium thiosulfate has a slow onset of action. Consider consultation with a poison control center at 1-800-222-1222.

The presence of sulfite hypersensitivity should not preclude the use of this medication.

Adverse Reactions Frequency not defined

Cardiovascular: Hypotension

Central nervous system: Disorientation, headache

Gastrointestinal: Nausea, salty taste, vomiting

Hematologic: Bleeding time prolonged

Miscellaneous: Warmth

Drug Interactions

Metabolism/Transport Effects None known.

Avoid Concomitant Use There are no known interactions where it is recommended to avoid concomitant use.

Increased Effect/Toxicity There are no known significant interactions involving an increase in effect.

Decreased Effect There are no known significant interactions involving a decrease in effect.

Storage/Stability Store at 20°C to 25°C (68°F to 77°F); excursions permitted to 15°C to 30°C (59°F to 86°F). Protect from light. Do not freeze.

Extravasation management (off-label use/route): Store the 1/6 M solution for SubQ administration at 15°C to 30°C (59°F to 86°F) (Polovich 2009).

Preparation for Administration

Calciphylaxis (off-label use): May dilute dose in 100 mL of NS (Nigwekar 2013)

Extravasation management (off-label use/route): To prepare a 1/6 M solution for SubQ administration (off-label route), add 4 mL of a 10% sodium thiosulfate solution to 6 mL SWFI or 1.6 mL of a 25% sodium thiosulfate solution to 8.4 mL SWFI (Polovich 2009).

Mechanism of Action

Cyanide toxicity: Serves as a sulfur donor in rhodanese-catalyzed formation of thiocyanate (much less toxic than cyanide)

Extravasation management: Neutralizes the reactive species of mechlorethamine; reduces the formation of hydroxyl radicals which cause tissue injury

Pharmacodynamics/Kinetics

Half-life elimination: Thiosulfate: ~3 hours; Thiocyanate: ~3 days; Renal impairment: ≤9 days

Excretion: Urine (~20% to 50% as unchanged drug)

Dosing

Adult

Cyanide poisoning: IV: **Note:** Administer in conjunction with sodium nitrite. Administer sodium nitrite first, followed immediately by the administration of sodium thiosulfate: 12.5 g (50 mL of a 25% solution); may repeat at one-half the original dose if symptoms of cyanide toxicity return

Note: Monitor the patient for 24 to 48 hours; if symptoms return, repeat both sodium nitrite and sodium thiosulfate at one-half the original doses.

Calciphylaxis (off-label use): IV: **Note:** Optimal dose is not established.

Dialysis patients: 25 g administered 3 times per week during the last hour of or after the hemodialysis session. Therapy should continue until there is complete resolution of symptoms (Ackermann 2007; Auriemma 2011; Cicone 2004; Nigwekar 2013;Subramaniam 2008).

Patients not on dialysis (normal renal function or mildly reduced GFR): 25 g administered 3 times per week (Baker 2007; Hackett 2011).

Extravasation management (off-label use):

Mechlorethamine: SubQ (off-label route): Inject 2 mL of a 1/6 M (~4%) sodium thiosulfate solution (into the extravasation site) for each mg of mechlorethamine suspected to have extravasated (Pérez Fidalgo 2012; Polovich 2009)

Cisplatin, concentrated: Inject 2 mL of a 1/6 M (~4%) sodium thiosulfate solution into existing IV line for each 100 mg of cisplatin extravasated; consider also injecting 1 mL of a 1/6 M (~4%) sodium thiosulfate solution as 0.1 mL subcutaneous injections (clockwise) into the area around the extravasation, may repeat subcutaneous injections several times over the next 3-4 hours (Ener 2004)

Bendamustine: SubQ: Bendamustine extravasation may be managed with 1/6 M (~4%) sodium thiosulfate solution in the same manner as mechlorethamine extravasation (Schulmeister 2011)

Geriatric Refer to adult dosing; use with caution due to likelihood of decreased renal function.

Pediatric Cyanide poisoning: IV: **Note:** Administer in conjunction with sodium nitrite. Administer sodium nitrite first, followed immediately by the administration of sodium thiosulfate. 250 mg/kg (1 mL/kg or ~30 to 40 mL/m^2 of a 25% solution) or 500 mg/kg (2 mL/kg of a 25% solution) (Howland 2011); maximum dose: 12.5 g (50 mL of a 25% solution); may repeat at one-half the original dose if symptoms of cyanide toxicity return

Note: Monitor the patient for 24-48 hours; if symptoms return, repeat both sodium nitrite and sodium thiosulfate at one-half the original doses.

Renal Impairment

No dosage adjustment provided in manufacturer's labeling; however, renal elimination is significant and risk of adverse effects may be increased in patients with renal impairment.

Calciphylaxis (off-label use): No dosage adjustment necessary. When used for patients not on dialysis (normal renal function or mildly reduced GFR), because sodium thiosulfate is cleared by the kidney, dose may be adjusted based on appearance of adverse effects (eg, metabolic acidosis, hypotension) (Hackett 2011; Nigwekar 2013).

Hepatic Impairment No dosage adjustment provided in the manufacturer's labeling (has not been studied).

Administration

IV: Cyanide poisoning: Administer by IV infusion over 10 to 30 minutes immediately after the administration of sodium nitrite (Howland 2011). Decrease rate of infusion in the event of significant hypotension.

Calciphylaxis (off-label use): Administer by IV infusion over 30 to 60 minutes (Cicone 2004; Nigwekar 2013).

Extravasation management (off-label use): Stop vesicant infusion immediately and disconnect IV line (leave needle/cannula in place); gently aspirate extravasated solution from the IV line (do **NOT** flush the line); remove needle/cannula (temporarily keep in place for cisplatin extravasation to allow for sodium thiosulfate administration through the needle/cannula); elevate extremity.

Mechlorethamine: Inject subcutaneously (off-label route) into the extravasation site using ≤25-gauge needle; change needle with each injection (Pérez Fidalgo 2012; Polovich 2009).

Cisplatin, concentrated: Inject into the existing IV line; consider also injecting 1 mL as 0.1 mL subcutaneous injections (clockwise) into the area around the extravasation using a new 25- or 27-gauge needle for each injection (Ener 2004).

Bendamustine: SubQ: Bendamustine extravasation may be managed with sodium thiosulfate in the same manner as mechlorethamine extravasation (Schulmeister 2011).

Monitoring Parameters

Cyanide poisoning: Monitor for at least 24-48 hours after administration; blood pressure and heart rate during and after infusion; hemoglobin/hematocrit; cooximetry; serum lactate levels; venous-arterial PO_2 gradient; serum methemoglobin and oxyhemoglobin. Pretreatment cyanide levels may be useful diagnostically.

Extravasation management: Monitor and document extravasation site for pain, blister formation, skin sloughing, arm/hand swelling/stiffness; monitor for fever, chills, or worsening pain

Dosage Forms Excipient information presented when available (limited, particularly for generics); consult specific product labeling. [DSC] = Discontinued product

Solution, Intravenous:

Generic: 10% [100 mg/mL] (10 mL [DSC]); 25% [250 mg/mL] (50 mL)

♦ **Sodium Thiosulphate** see Sodium Thiosulfate on page 1540

♦ **Soliris** see Eculizumab on page 580

♦ **Soltamox** see Tamoxifen on page 1595

♦ **Solu-CORTEF** see Hydrocortisone (Systemic) on page 824

♦ **Solu-Cortef (Can)** see Hydrocortisone (Systemic) on page 824

♦ **Solumedrol** see MethylPREDNISolone on page 1125

♦ **Solu-MEDROL** see MethylPREDNISolone on page 1125

♦ **Solu-Medrol (Can)** see MethylPREDNISolone on page 1125

♦ **Somatuline Autogel (Can)** see Lanreotide on page 993

♦ **Somatuline Depot** see Lanreotide on page 993

Sonidegib (soe ni DEG ib)

Related Information

Common Toxicity Criteria on page 2122

Principles of Anticancer Therapy on page 2261

Safe Handling of Hazardous Drugs on page 2292

Brand Names: US Odomzo

Index Terms Erismodegib; LDE225; NVP-LDE225; Sonidegib Phosphate

Pharmacologic Category Antineoplastic Agent, Hedgehog Pathway Inhibitor

Use Basal cell carcinoma, locally advanced: Treatment of adult patients with locally advanced basal cell carcinoma (BCC) that has recurred following surgery or radiation therapy, or those who are not candidates for surgery or radiation therapy.

Labeled Contraindications There are no contraindications listed in the manufacturer's labeling.

Pregnancy Considerations [US Boxed Warning]: Sonidegib can cause embryo-fetal death or severe birth defects when administered to a pregnant woman. Sonidegib is embryotoxic, fetotoxic, and teratogenic in animals. Verify the pregnancy status of females of reproductive potential prior to initiating therapy. Advise females of reproductive potential to use effective contraception during treatment with sonidegib and for at least 20 months after the last dose. Advise males of the potential risk of exposure through semen and to use condoms with a pregnant partner or a female partner of reproductive potential during treatment with sonidegib and for at least 8 months after the last dose. It is not known if sonidegib is present in semen. Males with female partners of reproductive potential should use condoms even following a vasectomy. Advise male patients not to donate sperm during sonidegib treatment and for at least 8 months after the last sonidegib dose.

Health care providers should notify the manufacturer of pregnancies which may occur following exposure to sonidegib (888-669-6682).

Breast-Feeding Considerations It is not known if sonidegib is excreted in breast milk. Due to the potential for serious adverse reactions in the nursing infant, breast-feeding is not recommended by the manufacturer during therapy and for 20 months after treatment.

Warnings/Precautions Hazardous agent - use appropriate precautions for handling and disposal (meets NIOSH 2014 criteria). **[US Boxed Warning]: Sonidegib can cause embryo-fetal death or severe birth defects when administered to a pregnant woman. Sonidegib is embryotoxic, fetotoxic, and teratogenic in animals. Verify the pregnancy status of females of reproductive potential prior to initiating therapy. Advise females of reproductive potential to use effective contraception during treatment with sonidegib and for at least 20 months after the last dose. Advise males of the potential risk of exposure through semen and to use condoms with a pregnant partner or a female partner of reproductive potential during treatment with sonidegib and for at least 8 months after the last dose.** It is not known if sonidegib is present in semen. Advise patients not to donate sperm during sonidegib treatment and for at least 8 months after the last sonidegib dose. Amenorrhea lasting for at least 18 months was observed in women of reproductive potential. Advise patients not to donate blood or blood products during sonidegib treatment and for at least 20 months after the last sonidegib dose.

Musculoskeletal toxicity occurred in more than two-thirds of patients treated with sonidegib (including grade 3 and 4 events). Muscle spasms, musculoskeletal pain, and myalgia were the most frequently reported musculoskeletal adverse reactions. Increased serum creatine kinase (CK) levels were also commonly observed (some events were grade 3 or 4); CK elevations were usually preceded by musculoskeletal pain and myalgia. When CK elevations were grade 2 or higher, the median time to symptom onset was ~13 weeks (range: 2 to 39 weeks), and the median time to resolution (to ≤ grade 1) was 12 days. More than one-quarter of patients required medical management for musculoskeletal toxicity (eg, magnesium supplementation, muscle relaxants, and analgesics/narcotics); several patients required intravenous hydration or hospitalization. Rhabdomyolysis was observed in 1 patient in clinical trials (at a dose higher than the FDA-approved dose). Monitor serum CK levels and serum creatinine at baseline and periodically during therapy (more frequently if muscle symptoms are reported or if clinically indicated). Advise patients to promptly report new unexplained muscle pain, tenderness, or weakness (either occurring during therapy or persisting after discontinuation). May require therapy interruption or discontinuation. Increased serum creatinine was observed in the majority of patients receiving sonidegib, although the measurement remained within the normal range in more than 75% of patients. While dosage adjustment is not required in patients with renal impairment, monitor serum creatinine at baseline and periodically, particularly if patients present with musculoskeletal toxicity. Potentially significant interactions may exist, requiring dose or frequency adjustment, additional monitoring, and/or selection of alternative therapy.

Adverse Reactions

>10%:

Central nervous system: Fatigue (41%), headache (15%), pain (14%)

Dermatologic: Alopecia (53%)

Endocrine & metabolic: Hyperglycemia (51%), weight loss (30%), increased serum ALT (19%), increased serum AST (19%), increased amylase (16%)

Gastrointestinal: Dysgeusia (46%), increased serum lipase (43%), nausea (39%), diarrhea (32%), decreased appetite (23%), abdominal pain (18%), vomiting (11%)

Hematologic & oncologic: Anemia (32%), lymphocytopenia (28%, grades 3/4: 3%)

Neuromuscular & skeletal: Increased creatine phosphokinase (61%, grades 3/4: 8%), muscle spasm (54%; grade 3: 3%), musculoskeletal pain (32%, grade 3: 1%), myalgia (19%)

Renal: Increased serum creatinine (92%)

1% to 10%:

Dermatologic: Pruritus (10%)

<1%, postmarketing, and/or case reports: Amenorrhea, rhabdomyolysis

Drug Interactions

Metabolism/Transport Effects Substrate of CYP3A4 (major); **Note:** Assignment of Major/Minor substrate status based on clinically relevant drug interaction potential; **Inhibits** BCRP

Avoid Concomitant Use

Avoid concomitant use of Sonidegib with any of the following: Conivaptan; CYP3A4 Inducers (Moderate); CYP3A4 Inducers (Strong); CYP3A4 Inhibitors (Strong); Fusidic Acid (Systemic); Idelalisib

Increased Effect/Toxicity

The levels/effects of Sonidegib may be increased by: Conivaptan; CYP3A4 Inhibitors (Moderate); CYP3A4 Inhibitors (Strong); Dasatinib; Fosaprepitant; Fusidic Acid (Systemic); Idelalisib; Ivacaftor; Luliconazole; Mifepristone; Osimertinib; Palbociclib; Simeprevir; Stiripentol

Decreased Effect

The levels/effects of Sonidegib may be decreased by: CYP3A4 Inducers (Moderate); CYP3A4 Inducers (Strong); Deferasirox; Osimertinib; Siltuximab; Tocilizumab

Food Interactions Taking sonidegib with a high-fat meal (~1,000 calories with 50% fat content) will increase systemic exposure (7- to 8-fold). Management: Do not administer with food; must be taken on an empty stomach, at least 1 hour before and 2 hours after food.

Storage/Stability Store at 25°C (77°F); excursions permitted to 15°C to 30°C (59°F to 86°F).

Mechanism of Action Basal cell cancer is associated with mutations in Hedgehog pathway components. Hedgehog regulates cell growth and differentiation in embryogenesis; while generally not active in adult tissue, Hedgehog mutations associated with basal cell cancer can activate the pathway resulting in unrestricted proliferation of skin basal cells (Von Hoff, 2009). Sonidegib is a selective Hedgehog pathway inhibitor which binds to and inhibits Smoothened homologue (SMO), the transmembrane protein involved in Hedgehog signal transduction.

Pharmacodynamics/Kinetics

Absorption: AUC_{inf} and C_{max} are increased by 7.4- to 7.8-fold, respectively, when administered with a high-fat meal (~1,000 calories with 50% fat content)

Distribution: 9,166 L

Protein binding: >97%

Metabolism: Primarily hepatic through CYP3A

Bioavailability: <10% of an oral dose is absorbed

Half-life elimination: ~28 days

Time to peak: 2 to 4 hours

Excretion: Feces (~70%); urine (30%)

Dosing

Adult & Geriatric Note: Verify pregnancy status of females of reproductive potential prior to therapy initiation. Measure serum creatine kinase (CK) levels and renal function tests in all patients prior to starting treatment.

Basal cell carcinoma, locally advanced: Oral: 200 mg once daily until disease progression or unacceptable toxicity (Migden, 2015)

Missed doses: If a dose is missed, skip the missed dose and resume dosing with the next scheduled dose.

Renal Impairment No dosage adjustment is necessary.

Hepatic Impairment

Mild impairment (total bilirubin ≤ULN and AST >ULN or total bilirubin >1 to 1.5 times ULN): No dosage adjustment is necessary.

Moderate or severe impairment: There are no dosage adjustments provided in the manufacturer's labeling (has not been studied).

Adjustment for Toxicity

Withhold treatment for any of the following (may resume at 200 mg daily upon resolution of toxicity):

Creatine kinase (CK) serum elevation between 2.5 and 10 times ULN (first occurrence) or between 2.5 and 5 times ULN (recurrent)

Musculoskeletal toxicity, severe or intolerable

Permanently discontinue therapy for:

CK serum elevation >2.5 times ULN with worsening renal function

CK serum elevation >10 times ULN

CK serum elevation >5 times ULN (recurrent)

Musculoskeletal toxicity, severe or intolerable (recurrent)

Combination Regimens

Basal cell carcinoma: Sonidegib (Basal Cell Regimen) on page 2083

Administration Administer orally on an empty stomach at least 1 hour before or 2 hours after a meal. Hazardous agent; use appropriate precautions for handling and disposal (meets NIOSH 2014 criteria)

Monitoring Parameters Serum creatine kinase (CK) and serum creatinine (baseline, periodically during treatment, and at least weekly with musculoskeletal toxicity and CK elevations >2.5 times ULN until resolution), liver function, pregnancy status, signs/symptoms of musculoskeletal toxicity.

Medication Guide Available Yes

Dosage Forms Excipient information presented when available (limited, particularly for generics); consult specific product labeling.

Capsule, Oral:

Odomzo: 200 mg

◆ **Sonidegib Phosphate** see Sonidegib on page 1543

SORAfenib (sor AF e nib)

Related Information

Common Toxicity Criteria *on page 2122*

Management of Chemotherapy-Induced Nausea and Vomiting in Adults *on page 2142*

Prevention of Chemotherapy-Induced Nausea and Vomiting in Children *on page 2203*

Principles of Anticancer Therapy *on page 2261*

Safe Handling of Hazardous Drugs *on page 2292*

Brand Names: US NexAVAR

Brand Names: Canada Nexavar

Index Terms BAY 43-9006; Sorafenib Tosylate

Pharmacologic Category Antineoplastic Agent, Tyrosine Kinase Inhibitor; Antineoplastic Agent, Vascular Endothelial Growth Factor (VEGF) Inhibitor

Use

Hepatocellular cancer: Treatment of unresectable hepatocellular cancer (HCC)

Renal cell cancer, advanced: Treatment of advanced renal cell cancer (RCC)

Thyroid cancer, differentiated: Treatment of locally recurrent or metastatic, progressive, differentiated thyroid cancer (refractory to radioactive iodine treatment)

Labeled Contraindications Known severe hypersensitivity to sorafenib or any component of the formulation; use in combination with carboplatin and paclitaxel in patients with squamous cell lung cancer

Pregnancy Considerations Animal reproduction studies have demonstrated teratogenicity and fetal loss. Based on its mechanism of action and because sorafenib inhibits angiogenesis, a critical component of fetal development, adverse effects on pregnancy would be expected. Women of childbearing potential should be advised to avoid pregnancy. Men and women of reproductive potential should use effective birth control during treatment and for at least 2 weeks after treatment is discontinued.

Breast-Feeding Considerations It is not known if sorafenib is excreted in human milk. Due to the potential for serious adverse reactions in the nursing infant, the decision to discontinue sorafenib or to discontinue breast-feeding during therapy should take into account the benefits of treatment to the mother.

Warnings/Precautions Hazardous agent - use appropriate precautions for handling and disposal (NIOSH 2014 [group 1]). May cause hypertension (generally mild-to-moderate), especially in the first 6 weeks of treatment; monitor; use caution in patients with underlying or poorly-controlled hypertension; consider discontinuing (temporary or permanent) in patients who develop severe or persistent hypertension while on appropriate antihypertensive therapy. May cause cardiac ischemia or infarction; consider discontinuing (temporarily or permanently) in patients who develop these conditions; use in patients with unstable coronary artery disease or recent myocardial infarction has not been studied. QT prolongation has been observed; may increase the risk for ventricular arrhythmia. Avoid use in patients with congenital long QT syndrome; monitor electrolytes and ECG in patients with heart failure, bradyarrhythmias, and concurrent medications known to prolong the QT interval; correct electrolyte (calcium, magnesium, potassium) imbalances; interrupt treatment for QTc interval >500 msec or for ≥60 msec increase from baseline.

◄ Serious bleeding events may occur (consider permanently discontinuing if serious); monitor PT/INR in patients on warfarin therapy. Fatal bleeding events have been reported. Thyroid cancer patients with tracheal, bronchial, and esophageal infiltration should be treated with local therapy prior to administering sorafenib due to the potential bleeding risk. May complicate wound healing; temporarily withhold treatment for patients undergoing major surgical procedures (the appropriate timing for reinitiation after surgical procedures has not been determined). Gastrointestinal perforation has been reported (rare); monitor patients for signs/symptoms (abdominal pain, constipation, or vomiting); discontinue treatment if gastrointestinal perforation occurs. Potentially significant drug-drug interactions may exist, requiring dose or frequency adjustment, additional monitoring, and/or selection of alternative therapy. Avoid concurrent use with strong CYP3A4 inducers (eg, carbamazepine, dexamethasone, phenobarbital, phenytoin, rifampin, St John's wort); may decrease sorafenib levels/effects. Use caution when administering sorafenib with compounds that are metabolized predominantly via UGT1A1 (eg, irinotecan). Use in combination with carboplatin and paclitaxel in patients with squamous cell lung cancer is contraindicated.

Hand-foot skin reaction and rash (generally grades 1 or 2) are the most common drug-related adverse events, and typically appear within the first 6 weeks of treatment; usually managed with topical treatment, treatment delays, and/or dose reductions. Consider permanently discontinuing with severe or persistent dermatological toxicities. The risk for hand-foot skin reaction increased with cumulative doses of sorafenib (Azad, 2009). The incidence of hand-foot syndrome is also increased in patients treated with sorafenib plus bevacizumab in comparison to those treated with sorafenib monotherapy (Azad, 2009). Severe dermatologic toxicities, including Stevens-Johnson syndrome (SJS) and toxic epidermal necrolysis (TEN) have been reported; may be life-threatening; discontinue sorafenib for suspected SJS or TEN.

Sorafenib impairs exogenous thyroid suppression; TSH level elevations were commonly observed in the thyroid cancer study; monitor TSH levels monthly and as clinically necessary, and adjust thyroid replacement as needed. Sorafenib levels in patients with mild-to-moderate hepatic impairment (Child-Pugh classes A and B) were similar to levels observed in patients without hepatic impairment; has not been studied in patients with severe hepatic impairment. In a small study of Asian patients with advanced HCC, sorafenib demonstrated efficacy with adequate tolerability in a hepatitis B-endemic area (Yau, 2009). There have been reports of sorafenib-induced hepatitis (including hepatic failure and death) which is characterized by hepatocellular liver damage and transaminase increases (significant); increased bilirubin and INR may also occur. Monitor hepatic function regularly; discontinue sorafenib for unexplained significant transaminase increases.

Adverse Reactions
>10%:

Cardiovascular: Hypertension (9% to 41%; grade 3: 3% to 4%; grade 4: <1%; grades 3/4: 10%, onset: ~3 weeks)

Central nervous system: Fatigue (37% to 46%), headache (≤10% to 17%), mouth pain (14%), voice disorder (13%), peripheral sensory neuropathy (≤13%), pain (11%)

Dermatologic: Palmar-plantar erythrodysesthesia (21% to 69%; grade 3: 6% to 8%; grades 3/4: 19%), alopecia (14% to 67%), skin rash (including desquamation; 19% to 40%; grade 3: ≤1%; grades 3/4: 5%), pruritus (14% to 20%), xeroderma (10% to 13%), erythema (≥10%)

Endocrine & metabolic: Hypoalbuminemia (≤59%), weight loss (10% to 49%), hypophosphatemia (35% to 45%; grade 3: 11% to 13%; grade 4: <1%), increased thyroid stimulating hormone level (>0.5 mU/L: 41%; due to impairment of exogenous thyroid suppression), hypocalcemia (12% to 36%), increased amylase (30% to 34% [usually transient])

Gastrointestinal: Diarrhea (43% to 68%; grade 3: 2% to 10%; grade 4: <1%), increased serum lipase (40% to 41% [usually transient]), abdominal pain (11% to 31%), decreased appetite (30%), anorexia (16% to 29%), stomatitis (24%), nausea (21% to 24%), constipation (14% to 16%), vomiting (11% to 16%)

Hematologic & oncologic: Lymphocytopenia (23% to 47%; grades 3/4: ≤13%), thrombocytopenia (12% to 46%; grades 3/4: 1% to 4%), increased INR (≤42%), neutropenia (≤18%; grades 3/4: ≤5%), hemorrhage (15% to 17%; grade 3: 2%), leukopenia

Hepatic: Increased serum ALT (59%; grades 3/4: 4%), increased serum AST (54%; grades 3/4: 2%), hepatic insufficiency (≤11%; grade 3: 2%; grade 4: 1%)

Infection: Infection

Neuromuscular & skeletal: Limb pain (15%), weakness (12%), myalgia

Respiratory: Dyspnea (≤14%), cough (≤13%)

Miscellaneous: Fever (11%)

1% to 10%:

Cardiovascular: Ischemic heart disease (including myocardial infarction; ≤3%), cardiac failure (2%, congestive), flushing

Central nervous system: Depression, glossalgia

Dermatologic: Hyperkeratosis (7%), acne vulgaris, exfoliative dermatitis, folliculitis

Endocrine & metabolic: Hypokalemia (5% to 10%), hyponatremia, hypothyroidism

Gastrointestinal: Dysgeusia (6%), dyspepsia, dysphagia, gastroesophageal reflux disease, mucositis, xerostomia

Genitourinary: Erectile dysfunction, proteinuria

Hematologic & oncologic: Squamous cell carcinoma of skin (3%; grades 3/4: 3%), anemia

Hepatic: Increased serum transaminases (transient)

Neuromuscular & skeletal: Muscle spasm (10%), arthralgia (≤10%), myalgia

Renal: Renal failure

Respiratory: Epistaxis (7%), flu-like symptoms, hoarseness, rhinorrhea

<1%, postmarketing, and/or case reports: Acute renal failure, anaphylaxis, angioedema, aortic dissection, amyotrophy, cardiac arrhythmia, cardiac failure, cerebral hemorrhage, cholangitis, cholecystitis, dehydration, eczema, erythema multiforme, gastritis, gastrointestinal hemorrhage, gastrointestinal perforation, gynecomastia, hepatic failure, hepatitis, hypersensitivity reaction (skin reaction, urticaria), hypertensive crisis, hyperthyroidism, increased serum alkaline phosphatase, increased serum bilirubin, interstitial pulmonary disease (acute respiratory distress, interstitial pneumonia, lung inflammation, pneumonitis, pulmonitis, radiation pneumonitis), jaundice, malignant neoplasm of skin (keratoacanthomas), nephrotic syndrome, ostealgia, osteonecrosis of the jaw, pancreatitis, pleural effusion, prolonged QT interval on ECG, respiratory tract hemorrhage, reversible posterior leukoencephalopathy ▶

◀ syndrome, rhabdomyolysis, Stevens-Johnson syndrome, thromboembolism, tinnitus, toxic epidermal necrolysis, transient ischemic attacks, tumor lysis syndrome, tumor pain

Drug Interactions

Metabolism/Transport Effects Substrate of CYP3A4 (minor), UGT1A9; **Note:** Assignment of Major/Minor substrate status based on clinically relevant drug interaction potential; **Inhibits** BSEP, CYP2B6 (moderate), CYP2C8 (weak), CYP2C9 (moderate), UGT1A9

Avoid Concomitant Use

Avoid concomitant use of SORAfenib with any of the following: Amodiaquine; BCG (Intravesical); CARBOplatin; Cholic Acid; CloZAPine; CYP3A4 Inducers (Strong); Dipyrone; Natalizumab; PACLitaxel (Conventional); Pimecrolimus; St Johns Wort; Tacrolimus (Topical); Tofacitinib; Vaccines (Live)

Increased Effect/Toxicity

SORAfenib may increase the levels/effects of: Acetaminophen; Amodiaquine; Bisphosphonate Derivatives; Bosentan; BuPROPion; Cannabis; CARBOplatin; Carvedilol; Cholic Acid; CloZAPine; CYP2B6 Substrates; CYP2C9 Substrates; DOCEtaxel; DOXOrubicin (Conventional); Dronabinol; Fingolimod; Fluorouracil (Systemic); Fluorouracil (Topical); Highest Risk QTc-Prolonging Agents; Irinotecan Products; Leflunomide; Moderate Risk QTc-Prolonging Agents; Natalizumab; PACLitaxel (Conventional); Propacetamol; Tetrahydrocannabinol; Tofacitinib; Vaccines (Live); Warfarin

The levels/effects of SORAfenib may be increased by: Acetaminophen; Bevacizumab; CYP3A4 Inhibitors (Strong); Denosumab; Dipyrone; Mifepristone; Pimecrolimus; Roflumilast; Tacrolimus (Topical); Trastuzumab

Decreased Effect

SORAfenib may decrease the levels/effects of: BCG (Intravesical); Coccidioides immitis Skin Test; Dacarbazine; Fluorouracil (Systemic); Fluorouracil (Topical); Sipuleucel-T; Vaccines (Inactivated); Vaccines (Live)

The levels/effects of SORAfenib may be decreased by: CYP3A4 Inducers (Strong); Echinacea; Neomycin; St Johns Wort

Food Interactions Bioavailability is decreased 29% with a high-fat meal (bioavailability is similar to fasting state when administered with a moderate-fat meal). Management: Administer on an empty stomach 1 hour before or 2 hours after eating.

Storage/Stability Store at 25°C (77°F); excursions are permitted between 15°C and 30°C (59°F and 86°F). Protect from moisture.

Mechanism of Action Multikinase inhibitor; inhibits tumor growth and angiogenesis by inhibiting intracellular Raf kinases (CRAF, BRAF, and mutant BRAF), and cell surface kinase receptors (VEGFR-1, VEGFR-2, VEGFR-3, PDGFR-beta, cKIT, FLT-3, RET, and RET/PTC)

Pharmacodynamics/Kinetics

Protein binding: 99.5%

Metabolism: Hepatic, via CYP3A4 (primarily oxidated to the pyridine N-oxide; active, minor) and UGT1A9 (glucuronidation)

Bioavailability: 38% to 49%; reduced by 29% when administered with a high-fat meal

Half-life elimination: 25 to 48 hours

Time to peak, plasma: ~3 hours

Excretion: Feces (77%, 51% of dose as unchanged drug); urine (19%, as metabolites)

Dosing

Adult & Geriatric Note: Interrupt treatment (temporarily) in patients undergoing major surgical procedures.

Hepatocellular cancer (HCC): Oral: 400 mg twice daily; continue until no longer clinically benefiting or until unacceptable toxicity occurs (Llovet, 2008)

Renal cell cancer (RCC), advanced: Oral: 400 mg twice daily; continue until no longer clinically benefiting or until unacceptable toxicity occurs (Escudier, 2007; Escudier, 2009)

Thyroid cancer, differentiated: Oral: 400 mg twice daily; continue until no longer clinically benefiting or until unacceptable toxicity occurs (Brose, 2013)

Angiosarcoma (off-label use): Oral: 400 mg twice daily (Maki, 2009)

Gastrointestinal stromal tumor (GIST) (off-label use): Oral: 400 mg twice daily (Wiebe, 2008)

Renal Impairment

Manufacturer's labeling: No dosage adjustment is necessary for mild, moderate, or severe impairment (not dependent on dialysis); has not been studied in dialysis patients.

The following adjustments have also been reported: Safety and pharmacokinetics were studied in varying degrees of renal dysfunction with the following empiric dose levels recommended based on patient tolerance (Miller, 2009):

Mild renal dysfunction (CrCl 40 to 59 mL/minute): 400 mg twice daily
Moderate renal dysfunction (CrCl 20 to 39 mL/minute): 200 mg twice daily
Severe renal dysfunction (CrCl <20 mL/minute): Data inadequate to define dose
Hemodialysis (any CrCl): 200 mg once daily

Hepatic Impairment

Hepatic impairment at baseline:

Manufacturer's labeling:

Mild to moderate (Child-Pugh class A and B) impairment: No dosage adjustment is necessary.

Severe impairment (Child-Pugh class C): There are no dosage adjustments provided in the manufacturer's labeling (has not been studied).

The following adjustments have also been reported: Safety and pharmacokinetics were studied in varying degrees of hepatic dysfunction with the following empiric dose levels recommended based on patient tolerance (Miller, 2009):

Mild hepatic dysfunction (bilirubin >1 to ≤1.5 times ULN and/or AST >ULN): 400 mg twice daily
Moderate hepatic dysfunction (bilirubin >1.5 to ≤3 times ULN; any AST): 200 mg twice daily
Severe hepatic dysfunction:
Bilirubin >3 to 10 x ULN (any AST): 200 mg every 3 days was **not** tolerated
Albumin <2.5 g/dL (any bilirubin and any AST): 200 mg once daily

Drug-induced liver injury during treatment: Unexplained (eg, not due to viral hepatitis or progressive underlying malignancy) significantly increased transaminases: Discontinue treatment.

Adjustment for Toxicity Temporary interruption and/or dosage reduction may be necessary for management of adverse drug reactions.

◀ **Cardiovascular toxicity:**
   Cardiac ischemia or infarction: Consider temporary interruption or perma-
   nent discontinuation.
   Hypertension, severe or persistent (despite antihypertensive therapy): Con-
   sider temporary interruption or permanent discontinuation.
   QT prolongation (QTc interval >500 msec or ≥60 msec increase from
   baseline): Interrupt treatment.
Gastrointestinal perforation: Permanently discontinue.
Hemorrhage requiring medical intervention: Consider permanent discon-
   tinuation.
Dermatologic toxicity: If Stevens-Johnson syndrome or toxic epidermal
   necrolysis is suspected, discontinue therapy.
   U.S. labeling:
   RCC and HCC: If dosage reductions are necessary, decrease dose to
      400 mg once daily. If further reductions are needed, decrease dose to
      400 mg every other day.
      Grade 1 (numbness, dysesthesia, paresthesia, tingling, painless swel-
         ling, erythema, or discomfort of the hands or feet which do not disrupt
         normal activities): Continue sorafenib and consider symptomatic treat-
         ment with topical therapy.
      Grade 2 (painful erythema and swelling of the hands or feet and/or
         discomfort affecting normal activities):
         First occurrence: Continue sorafenib and consider symptomatic treat-
            ment with topical therapy. **Note:** If no improvement within 7 days, see
            dosing for second or third occurrence.
         Second or third occurrence (or no improvement after 7 days of 1st
            occurrence): Hold treatment until resolves to grade 0-1; resume treat-
            ment with dose reduced by one dose level (400 mg daily or 400 mg
            every other day).
         Fourth occurrence: Discontinue treatment.
      Grade 3 (moist desquamation, ulceration, blistering, or severe pain of the
         hands or feet or severe discomfort that prevents working or performing
         daily activities):
         First or second occurrence: Hold treatment until resolves to grade 0-1;
            resume treatment with dose reduced by one dose level (400 mg daily
            or 400 mg every other day).
         Third occurrence: Discontinue treatment.
   Thyroid cancer:
      First dose level reduction: Reduce to 600 mg daily (in 2 divided doses, as
         400 mg and 200 mg, separated by 12 hours).
      Second dose level reduction: Reduce dose to 200 mg twice daily.
      Third dose level reduction: Reduce dose to 200 mg once daily.
      Grade 1 (numbness, dysesthesia, paresthesia, tingling, painless swel-
         ling, erythema, or discomfort of the hands or feet which do not disrupt
         normal activities): Continue sorafenib treatment.
      Grade 2 (painful erythema and swelling of the hands or feet and/or
         discomfort affecting normal activities):
         First occurrence: Decrease dose to 600 mg daily (in divided doses).
            Note: If no improvement within 7 days, see dosing for second
            occurrence.
         Second occurrence (or no improvement after 7 days of the reduced
            dose after 1st occurrence): Hold treatment until resolved or improved
            to grade 1; if resumed, decrease the dose by 1 dose level.

Third occurrence: Hold treatment until resolved or improved to grade 1; if resumed, decrease the dose by 1 dose level.

Fourth occurrence: Permanently discontinue.

Grade 3 (moist desquamation, ulceration, blistering, or severe pain of the hands or feet or severe discomfort that prevents working or performing daily activities):

First occurrence: Hold treatment until resolved or improved to grade 1; if resumed, decrease by 1 dose level.

Second occurrence: Hold treatment until resolved or improved to grade 1; if resumed, decrease by 2 dose levels.

Third occurrence: Permanently discontinue.

Following improvement of grade 2 or 3 dermatologic toxicity to grade 0 or 1 after at least 28 days of a reduced dose, the sorafenib dose may be increased 1 dose level from the reduced dose (~50% of patients requiring dose reduction for dermatologic toxicity may meet the criteria for increased dosing; and half of those patients may tolerate the increased dose without recurrent grade 2 or higher dermatologic toxicity).

Canadian labeling: RCC and HCC:

Grade 1 (any occurrence): Initiate supportive treatment immediately and continue sorafenib.

Grade 2:

First occurrence: Initiate supportive treatment immediately and consider a dose reduction to 400 mg daily for 28 days. If toxicity resolves to ≤ grade 1 after 28 days with dose reduction, increase dose to 400 mg twice daily. If toxicity does not resolve to ≤ grade 1 despite dose reduction, withhold treatment for a minimum of 7 days until toxicity resolves to ≤ grade 1, then resume treatment at reduced dose of 400 mg daily for 28 days. If toxicity remains ≤ grade 1 at the reduced dose for 28 days, increase dose to 400 mg twice daily.

Second or third occurrence: Follow procedure for first occurrence; however, when resuming treatment, decrease dose to 400 mg daily (indefinitely).

Fourth occurrence: Treatment discontinuation should be considered based on clinical assessment and patient preference.

Grade 3:

First occurrence: Initiate supportive measures immediately and withhold treatment for a minimum of 7 days and until toxicity ≤ grade 1. Resume at reduced dose of 400 mg daily for 28 days. If toxicity remains ≤ grade 1 at the reduced dose for 28 days, increase dose to 400 mg twice daily.

Second occurrence: Follow procedure for first occurrence; however, when resuming treatment, decrease dose to 400 mg daily (indefinitely).

Third occurrence: Treatment discontinuation should be considered based on clinical assessment and patient preference.

Combination Regimens

Hepatocellular: Sorafenib (Hepatocellular Regimen) on page 2084

Renal cell cancer: Sorafenib (RCC Regimen) on page 2084

Soft tissue sarcoma (angiosarcoma): Sorafenib (Angiosarcoma Regimen) on page 2083

Soft tissue sarcoma (gastrointestinal stromal tumor [GIST]): Sorafenib (GIST Regimen) on page 2083

Thyroid cancer: Sorafenib (Thyroid Regimen) on page 2084

Administration Administer on an empty stomach (1 hour before or 2 hours after eating).

Hazardous agent; use appropriate precautions for handling and disposal (NIOSH 2014 [group 1]).

Emetic Potential Children and Adults: Minimal (<10%)

Extemporaneous Preparations Hazardous agent: Use appropriate precautions for handling and disposal (NIOSH 2014 [group 1]).

An oral suspension may be prepared with tablets. Place two 200 mg tablets into a glass containing 60 mL (2 oz) water; let stand 5 minutes before stirring. Stir until tablets are completely disintegrated, forming a uniform suspension. Administer within 1 hour after preparation. Stir suspension again immediately before administration. To ensure the full dose is administered, rinse glass several times with a total of 180 mL (6 oz) water and administer residue. **Note:** Brown tablet coating may initially form a thin film but has no effect on the dosing accuracy.

Nexavar data on file, Bayer Healthcare Pharmaceuticals.

Monitoring Parameters

CBC with differential, electrolytes (magnesium, potassium, calcium), phosphorus, lipase and amylase levels; liver function tests; blood pressure (baseline, weekly for the first 6 weeks, then periodic); monitor for hand-foot skin reaction and other dermatologic toxicities; monitor ECG in patients at risk for prolonged QT interval; signs/symptoms of bleeding; signs/symptoms of GI perforation. Additionally the Canadian labeling recommends considering monitoring of left ventricular ejection fraction at baseline and periodically during treatment.

Thyroid function testing:

Patients with differentiated thyroid cancer: Monitor TSH monthly.

Patients with RCC and HCC (Hamnvik, 2011):

Preexisting levothyroxine therapy: Obtain baseline TSH levels, then monitor every 4 weeks until levels and levothyroxine dose are stable, then monitor every 2 weeks

Without preexisting thyroid hormone replacement: TSH at baseline, then every 4 weeks for 4 months, then every 2 to 3 months

Additional Information Hand-foot skin reaction (HFSR) management (Lacouture, 2008): The following treatments may be used in addition to the recommended dosage modifications. Prior to treatment initiation, a pedicure is recommended to remove hyperkeratotic areas/calluses, which may predispose to HFSR; avoid vigorous exercise/activities which may stress hands or feet. During therapy, patients should reduce exposure to hot water (may exacerbate hand-foot symptoms); avoid constrictive footwear and excessive skin friction. Patients may also wear thick cotton gloves or socks and should wear shoes with padded insoles. Grade 1 HFSR may be relieved with moisturizing creams, cotton gloves and socks (at night) and/or keratolytic creams such as urea (20% to 40%) or salicylic acid (6%). Apply topical steroid (eg, clobetasol ointment) twice daily to erythematous areas of Grade 2 HFSR; topical anesthetics (eg, lidocaine 2%) and then systemic analgesics (if appropriate) may be used for pain control. Resolution of acute erythema may result in keratotic areas which may be softened with keratolytic agents.

Prescribing and Access Restrictions Available from specialty pharmacies. Further information may be obtained at 1-866-639-2827 or www.nexavar-us.com.

Dosage Forms Excipient information presented when available (limited, particularly for generics); consult specific product labeling.
Tablet, Oral:
  NexAVAR: 200 mg

♦ **Sorafenib Tosylate** *see* SORAfenib *on page 1547*

♦ **Sporanox** *see* Itraconazole *on page 980*

♦ **Sporanox Pulsepak** *see* Itraconazole *on page 980*

♦ **Sprycel** *see* Dasatinib *on page 455*

♦ **SR-89** *see* Strontium-89 *on page 1558*

♦ **Statex (Can)** *see* Morphine (Systemic) *on page 1167*

♦ **Sterile Talc** *see* Talc (Sterile) *on page 1588*

♦ **Sterile Talc Powder** *see* Talc (Sterile) *on page 1588*

♦ **Sterile Vancomycin Hydrochloride, USP (Can)** *see* Vancomycin *on page 1720*

♦ **STI-571** *see* Imatinib *on page 882*

♦ **Stimate** *see* Desmopressin *on page 505*

♦ **Stivarga** *see* Regorafenib *on page 1466*

Streptozocin (strep toe ZOE sin)

Related Information
  Management of Chemotherapy-Induced Nausea and Vomiting in Adults *on page 2142*
  Management of Drug Extravasations *on page 2159*
  Prevention of Chemotherapy-Induced Nausea and Vomiting in Children *on page 2203*
  Safe Handling of Hazardous Drugs *on page 2292*
Brand Names: US Zanosar
Brand Names: Canada Zanosar
Index Terms Streptozotocin
Pharmacologic Category Antineoplastic Agent, Alkylating Agent; Antineoplastic Agent, Alkylating Agent (Nitrosourea)
Use Treatment of metastatic islet cell carcinoma of the pancreas (symptomatic or progressive disease)
Labeled Contraindications There are no contraindications listed within the manufacturer's labeling.
Pregnancy Considerations Teratogenic events have been observed in animal reproduction studies.
Breast-Feeding Considerations It is not known if streptozocin is excreted in breast milk. Due to the potential for serious adverse reactions in the nursing infant, breast-feeding is not recommended.
Warnings/Precautions Hazardous agent - use appropriate precautions for handling and disposal (NIOSH 2014 [group 1]).

[U.S. Boxed Warning]: Renal toxicity is dose-related and cumulative; may be severe or fatal. Azotemia, anuria, hypophosphatemia, glycosuria and renal tubular acidosis have been reported. Adequate hydration may reduce the risk for nephrotoxicity. Monitor renal function (BUN, serum creatinine, and serial urinalysis) and serum electrolytes prior to, weekly during, and after each treatment course. Mild proteinuria is an early sign of renal toxicity; if proteinuria

◀ is detected with urinalysis, obtain 24-hour urine collection. Avoid use in combination with other nephrotoxic medications. Use with caution in patients with preexisting renal disease. **[U.S. Boxed Warning]: Liver dysfunction has been observed;** hepatotoxicity may be characterized by elevated transaminases and LDH, or by hypoalbuminemia; monitor liver function weekly; may require dosage reduction or discontinuation.

[U.S. Boxed Warning]: Hematologic toxicity has been observed; mild bone marrow suppression (rare) may occur; monitor blood counts weekly; may require dosage reduction or discontinuation. May cause confusion, lethargy or depression; caution patients about performing tasks that require mental alertness (eg, operating machinery or driving). **[U.S. Boxed Warning]: Diarrhea has been observed. May cause severe nausea and vomiting.** Streptozocin is associated with a high emetic potential; antiemetics are recommended to prevent nausea and vomiting (Basch, 2011; Dupuis, 2011; Roila, 2010). Mild to moderate glucose intolerance may occur; generally is reversible.

[U.S. Boxed Warning]: Streptozocin is mutagenic; parenteral use is tumorigenic and carcinogenic in animals. [U.S. Boxed Warning]: Should be administered under the supervision of an experienced cancer chemotherapy physician. Administer in a facility with sufficient access to lab and supportive resources for monitoring toxicities. Streptozocin is an irritant with vesicant-like properties; avoid extravasation. Local tissue irritation or inflammation (burning, edema, erythema, tenderness) may occur but usually resolves within a few days.

Adverse Reactions

Frequency not defined:

Endocrine & metabolic: Glucose intolerance, hyper-/hypoglycemia, hypoalbuminemia, hypophosphatemia

Gastrointestinal: Diarrhea, nausea, vomiting

Hepatic: LDH increased, transaminases increased

Local: Injection site reactions (burning, edema, erythema, inflammation, irritation, tenderness)

Renal: Anuria, azotemia, BUN increased, creatinine increased, glycosuria, nephrotoxicity, proteinuria, renal dysfunction, renal tubular acidosis

Infrequent, postmarketing, and/or case reports: Anemia, confusion, depression, diabetes insipidus, lethargy, leukopenia, myelosuppression (nadir: at 2-3 weeks), secondary malignancies, thrombocytopenia, liver dysfunction, secondary malignancy

Drug Interactions

Metabolism/Transport Effects None known.

Avoid Concomitant Use

Avoid concomitant use of Streptozocin with any of the following: BCG (Intravesical); CloZAPine; Dipyrone; Natalizumab; Pimecrolimus; Tacrolimus (Topical); Tofacitinib; Vaccines (Live)

Increased Effect/Toxicity

Streptozocin may increase the levels/effects of: CloZAPine; Fingolimod; Leflunomide; Natalizumab; Tofacitinib; Vaccines (Live)

The levels/effects of Streptozocin may be increased by: Denosumab; Dipyrone; Pimecrolimus; Roflumilast; Tacrolimus (Topical); Trastuzumab

Decreased Effect

Streptozocin may decrease the levels/effects of: BCG (Intravesical); Coccidioides immitis Skin Test; Sipuleucel-T; Vaccines (Inactivated); Vaccines (Live)

The levels/effects of Streptozocin may be decreased by: Echinacea

Storage/Stability Store intact vials refrigerated at 2°C to 8°C (36°F to 46°F). Protect from light. The manufacturer recommends use within 12 hours of reconstitution; vial does not contain a preservative.

Preparation for Administration Hazardous agent; use appropriate precautions for handling and disposal (NIOSH 2014 [group 1]). Reconstitute powder with 9.5 mL D_5W or NS to a concentration of 100 mg/mL. May further dilute for infusion in D_5W or NS.

Mechanism of Action Inhibits DNA synthesis by alkylation and cross-linking the strands of DNA, and by possible protein modification; cell cycle nonspecific

Pharmacodynamics/Kinetics

Onset: 1500 mg/m^2 once weekly: Onset of response: 17 days; median time to maximum response: 35 days

Distribution: Concentrates in liver, kidney, and pancreatic beta cells

Metabolism: Rapid; primarily hepatic

Half-life elimination: <1 hour

Excretion: Urine (primarily; as parent drug and metabolites)

Dosing

Adult Note: Streptozocin is associated with a high emetic potential; antiemetics are recommended to prevent nausea and vomiting (Basch, 2011; Roila, 2010).

Pancreatic islet cell carcinoma, metastatic: IV:

Daily schedule: 500 mg/m^2/day for 5 consecutive days every 6 weeks until maximum benefit or until unacceptable toxicity

Weekly schedule: 1000 mg/m^2 once weekly; if therapeutic response not achieved after 2 weeks, may escalate dose to a maximum of 1500 mg/m^2 weekly

Off-label dosing: 1000 mg/m^2 once every 3 weeks for up to 6 cycles (in combination with leucovorin, fluorouracil and cisplatin) (Turner, 2010) **or** 400 mg/m^2 days 1 to 5 every 4 weeks (in combination with fluorouracil and doxorubicin) until disease progression or unacceptable toxicity (Kouvaraki, 2004)

Adrenal carcinoma, metastatic (off-label use): IV: 1000 mg once daily for 5 days (cycle 1) followed by 2000 mg on day 1 (subsequent cycles) every 3 weeks (in combination with mitotane) (Fassnacht, 2012; Khan 2000)

Geriatric Refer to adult dosing. Select dose cautiously, beginning at the lower end of dosing range.

Renal Impairment No dosage adjustment provided in the manufacturer's labeling; however, it is recommended to use clinical judgment weighing benefit vs risk of renal toxicity in patients with preexisting renal impairment. The following dosing adjustments have been recommended (Aronoff, 2007): Adults (based on a usual dose of 500 mg/m^2):

CrCl >50 mL/minute: No dosage adjustment necessary.

CrCl 10-50 mL/minute: Administer 75% of dose

CrCl <10 mL/minute: Administer 50% of dose

Hepatic Impairment No dosage adjustment provided in the manufacturer's labeling. However, streptozocin is rapidly hepatically metabolized; dose should be decreased in patients with severe liver disease.

◄ **Obesity** *ASCO Guidelines for appropriate chemotherapy dosing in obese adults with cancer:* Utilize patient's actual body weight (full weight) for calculation of body surface area- or weight-based dosing, particularly when the intent of therapy is curative; manage regimen-related toxicities in the same manner as for nonobese patients; if a dose reduction is utilized due to toxicity, consider resumption of full weight-based dosing with subsequent cycles, especially if cause of toxicity (eg, hepatic or renal impairment) is resolved (Griggs, 2012).

Adjustment for Toxicity *Bone marrow suppression or hepatic dysfunction:* May require dosage reduction or discontinuation.

Administration Streptozocin is associated with a high emetic potential; antiemetics are recommended to prevent nausea and vomiting (Basch, 2011; Dupuis, 2011; Roila, 2010).

Administer as either a rapid IV injection **or** as short or prolonged infusion.

Irritant with vesicant-like properties; ensure proper needle or catheter placement prior to and during infusion; avoid extravasation.

Extravasation management: If extravasation occurs, stop infusion immediately and disconnect (leave cannula/needle in place); gently aspirate extravasated solution (do **NOT** flush the line); remove needle/cannula; elevate extremity.

Hazardous agent; use appropriate precautions for handling and disposal (NIOSH 2014 [group 1]).

Vesicant/Extravasation Risk Irritant with vesicant-like properties

Emetic Potential Children and Adults: High (>90%)

Monitoring Parameters Renal function tests, including BUN, serum creatinine, and serial urinalysis, and serum electrolytes (at baseline, weekly during, and for 4 weeks after treatment); 24-hour urine collection if proteinuria is detected on urinalysis; liver function tests (weekly), CBC with differential and platelets (weekly), blood glucose; monitor infusion site

Dosage Forms Excipient information presented when available (limited, particularly for generics); consult specific product labeling.
Solution Reconstituted, Intravenous:
  Zanosar: 1 g (1 ea)

♦ **Streptozotocin** *see* Streptozocin *on page 1555*
♦ **Strontium-89 Chloride** *see* Strontium-89 *on page 1558*

Strontium-89 (STRON shee um atey nine)

Related Information
  Chronic Pain Management (Cancer) *on page 2229*
  Safe Handling of Hazardous Drugs *on page 2292*

Brand Names: US Metastron

Brand Names: Canada Metastron®

Index Terms SR-89; Sr89; Strontium Chloride SR 89; Strontium-89 Chloride

Pharmacologic Category Radiopharmaceutical

Use Relief of bone pain in patients with skeletal metastases

Labeled Contraindications There are no contraindications listed within the manufacturer's labeling.

Pregnancy Considerations May cause fetal harm if administered during pregnancy. Women of childbearing potential should avoid becoming pregnant.

Breast-Feeding Considerations It is not known whether this drug is excreted in human milk. Because strontium acts as a calcium analog, secretion of Strontium-89 into human milk is likely. It is recommended that nursing be discontinued by mothers about to receive intravenous Strontium-89.

Warnings/Precautions Radiopharmaceutical; use appropriate precautions for handling and disposal. Use appropriate precautions for handling, disposal, and minimizing exposure to patients and healthcare personnel. Use only under supervision of individuals with experience/training in the handling of radioactive materials approved by the applicable regulatory authority.

Bone marrow suppression (thrombocytopenia and leukopenia) is likely to occur. Use is not recommended in patients with seriously compromised bone marrow function from prior therapies or from disease infiltration (unless potential benefit outweighs risks). Monitor CBC weekly. Use with caution in patients whose platelet counts fall <60,000/mm^3 or whose white blood cell counts fall <2400/mm^3. Carefully evaluate bone marrow status and toxicity of initial treatment if considering repeat administration. Incontinent patients may require urinary catheterization (to minimize radioactive contamination). Body fluids may remain radioactive up to one week after injection. Not indicated for use in patients with cancer not involving bone or in patients with a short life expectancy (due to delayed onset of pain relief). A small number of patients have experienced a transient increase in bone pain at 36-72 hours postdose; this reaction is generally mild and self-limiting. Patients may experience a flushing sensation following rapid (<30 seconds) injection. Primarily eliminated renally; possible risk versus benefit should be evaluated in patients with renal impairment.

Adverse Reactions Frequency not defined.
Cardiovascular: Flushing (after rapid injection)
Hematologic: Leukopenia, thrombocytopenia (nadir: 12-16 weeks; recovery: 6 months)
Neuromuscular & skeletal: Bone pain (transient increase; duration: 36-72 hours)
Postmarketing and/or case reports: Chills, fever, hot flash, septicemia

Drug Interactions
Metabolism/Transport Effects None known.
Avoid Concomitant Use There are no known interactions where it is recommended to avoid concomitant use.
Increased Effect/Toxicity There are no known significant interactions involving an increase in effect.
Decreased Effect There are no known significant interactions involving a decrease in effect.
Storage/Stability Store vial and its contents inside its transportation container at room temperature of 15°C to 25°C (59°F to 77°F).
Mechanism of Action Selectively (locally) irradiates primary and metastatic bone lesions to reduce pain.
Pharmacodynamics/Kinetics
Onset: Pain relief: 7-20 days
Distribution: Retained in bone mineral (preferentially to metastatic bone lesions)
Excretion: In patients with bone metastases: Urine (67%); feces (33%)
Dosing
Adult & Geriatric Note: Measure dose by a suitable radioactivity calibration system immediately prior to administration.

◄ **Bone pain due to skeletal metastases:** IV: 148 megabecquerel (4 millicurie) or 1.5-2.2 megabecquerel (40-60 microcurie)/kg; repeat doses are generally not recommended at intervals <90 days

Renal Impairment No dosage adjustment provided in manufacturer's labeling. However, consider benefit versus risk due to extensive renal excretion.

Hepatic Impairment No dosage adjustment provided in manufacturer's labeling.

Administration Administer intravenously slowly over 1-2 minutes. Radiopharmaceutical; use appropriate precautions for handling and disposal.

Monitoring Parameters CBC with differential (every other week)

Additional Information Patients should the following precautions (Silberstein, 2003):

1. Avoid soiling underclothing or areas around toilet bowls for 2 weeks after injection.
2. Wash any underclothing separately if significantly stained with urine.
3. Where a normal toilet is available, use in preference to a urinal.
4. Flush toilet twice after use.
5. Wash hands thoroughly after urination.

Dosage Forms Excipient information presented when available (limited, particularly for generics); consult specific product labeling.

Solution, Intravenous, as chloride [preservative free]:

Metastron: 1 mCi/mL (4 mL) [pyrogen free]

♦ **Strontium Chloride SR 89** see Strontium-89 on page 1558

♦ **SU011248** see SUNItinib on page 1567

♦ **Suberoylanilide Hydroxamic Acid** see Vorinostat on page 1780

♦ **Subsys** see FentaNYL on page 692

Sulfamethoxazole and Trimethoprim
(sul fa meth OKS a zole & trye METH oh prim)

Brand Names: US Bactrim; Bactrim DS; Sulfatrim Pediatric

Brand Names: Canada Apo-Sulfatrim; Apo-Sulfatrim DS; Apo-Sulfatrim Pediatric; Protrin DF; Septra Injection; Teva-Trimel; Teva-Trimel DS; Trisulfa; Trisulfa DS; Trisulfa S

Index Terms Co-Trimoxazole; Septra; SMX-TMP; SMZ-TMP; Sulfatrim; TMP-SMX; TMP-SMZ; Trimethoprim and Sulfamethoxazole

Pharmacologic Category Antibiotic, Miscellaneous; Antibiotic, Sulfonamide Derivative

Use

Oral: Treatment of urinary tract infections due to *E. coli*, *Klebsiella* and *Enterobacter* sp, *M. morganii*, *P. mirabilis* and *P. vulgaris*; acute otitis media; acute exacerbations of chronic bronchitis due to susceptible strains of *H. influenzae* or *S. pneumoniae*; treatment and prophylaxis of *Pneumocystis* pneumonia (PCP); traveler's diarrhea due to enterotoxigenic *E. coli*; treatment of enteritis caused by *Shigella flexneri* or *Shigella sonnei*

IV: Treatment of *Pneumocystis* pneumonia (PCP); treatment of enteritis caused by *Shigella flexneri* or *Shigella sonnei*; treatment of severe or complicated urinary tract infections due to *E. coli*, *Klebsiella* and *Enterobacter* spp, *M. morganii*, *P. mirabilis*, and *P. vulgaris*

Pregnancy Risk Factor D

Dosing

Adult & Geriatric Dosage recommendations are based on the trimethoprim component. double-strength tablets are equivalent to sulfamethoxazole 800 mg and trimethoprim 160 mg.

General dosing guidelines:

Oral: 1 to 2 double-strength tablets (sulfamethoxazole 800 mg; trimethoprim 160 mg) every 12 to 24 hours

IV: 8 to 20 mg TMP/kg/day divided every 6 to 12 hours

Bite wounds (animal) (off-label use) (IDSA [Stevens 2014]):

Oral: One double-strength tablet twice daily; in combination with clindamycin or metronidazole

IV: 5 to 10 mg TMP/kg/day in divided doses every 6 to 12 hours in combination with clindamycin or metronidazole

Chronic bronchitis (acute): Oral: One double-strength tablet every 12 hours for 10 to 14 days

Cyclosporiasis (off-label use): Oral, IV: 160 mg TMP twice daily for 7 to 10 days. **Note:** AIDS patients: Oral: One double-strength tablet 2 to 4 times/ day for 10 days, then 1 double-strength tablet 3 times/week for 10 weeks (Pape 1994; Verdier 2000).

Granuloma inguinale (donovanosis) (off-label use): Oral: One double-strength tablet every 12 hours for at least 3 weeks and until lesions have healed (CDC 2010)

Isosporiasis (*Isospora belli* infection) in HIV-infected patients (off-label use; HHS [OI adult 2015]):

Treatment: Oral, IV: 160 mg TMP 4 times/day for 10 days **or** 160 mg TMP 2 times/day for 7 to 10 days. May start with twice daily regimen and increase dose and/or duration up to 3 to 4 weeks if symptoms worsen or persist.

Chronic maintenance therapy (secondary prophylaxis) in patients with CD4 count <200 cells/mm^3: Oral: 160 mg TMP 3 times/week (preferred) or alternatively, 160 mg TMP daily or 320 mg TMP 3 times/week.

Melioidosis (*Burkholderia pseudomallei*) (off-label use) (Lipsitz 2012): Oral, IV:

Severe, acute phase involving brain, prostate, bone, or joint: Administer as 2 divided doses; given with ceftazidime or a carbapenem for ≥10 days followed by eradication therapy:

Adults <40 kg: 320 mg TMP daily

Adults 40 to 60 kg: 480 mg TMP daily

Adults >60 kg: 640 mg TMP daily

Eradication therapy: Administer as 2 divided doses for ≥12 weeks:

Adults <40 kg: 320 mg TMP daily

Adults 40 to 60 kg: 480 mg TMP daily

Adults >60 kg: 640 mg TMP daily

Postexposure prophylaxis: Administer as 2 divided doses for 21 days:

Adults <40 kg: 320 mg TMP daily

Adults 40 to 60 kg: 480 mg TMP daily

Adults >60 kg: 640 mg TMP daily

Meningitis (bacterial): IV: 10 to 20 mg TMP/kg/day in divided doses every 6-12 hours

◄   *Nocardia* (off-label use): Oral, IV:

    Cutaneous infections: 5 to 10 mg TMP/kg/day in 2 to 4 divided doses

    Severe infections (pulmonary/cerebral): 15 mg TMP/kg/day in 2 to 4 divided doses for 3 to 4 weeks, then 10 mg TMP/kg/day in 2 to 4 divided doses. Treatment duration is controversial; an average of 7 months has been reported.

    Note: Therapy for severe infection may be initiated IV and converted to oral therapy (frequently converted to approximate dosages of oral solid dosage forms: 2 DS tablets every 8 to 12 hours). Although not widely available, sulfonamide levels should be considered in patients with questionable absorption, at risk for dose-related toxicity, or those with poor therapeutic response.

Osteomyelitis due to MRSA (off-label use): Oral, IV: 3.5 to 4 mg TMP/kg/dose every 8 to 12 hours for a minimum of 8 weeks with rifampin 600 mg once daily (Liu 2011)

Pneumocystis **pneumonia (PCP):**

    Manufacturer's labeling:

      Oral:

        Prophylaxis: 160 mg TMP daily

        Treatment: 15 to 20 mg TMP/kg/day divided every 6 hours for 14 to 21 days

      IV: Treatment: 15 to 20 mg TMP/kg/day divided every 6 to 8 hours for up to 14 days

    Alternate dosing in HIV-infected patients (off-label dose; HHS [OI adult 2015]):

      Primary or secondary prophylaxis: Oral: 80 or 160 mg TMP daily **or** alternatively, 160 mg TMP 3 times/week

      Duration of prophylaxis: May discontinue primary or secondary prophylaxis if CD4 count increases from <200 cells/mm^3 to ≥200 cells/mm^3 for at least 3 months in response to ART; therapy must be restarted if CD4 count <200 cells/mm^3

      Treatment:

        Mild to moderate: Oral: 15 to 20 mg TMP/kg/day in 3 divided doses for 21 days **or** alternatively, 320 mg TMP 3 times/day for 21 days

        Moderate to severe: IV: 15 to 20 mg TMP/kg/day in 3 to 4 divided doses for 21 days; may switch to oral therapy after clinical improvement

Prosthetic joint infection (off-label use): Oral phase treatment (after completion of pathogen-specific IV therapy) following debridement and prosthesis retention or 1-stage exchange:

    Total ankle, elbow, hip, or shoulder arthroplasty: 160 mg TMP 2 times daily for 3 months. **Note:** Must be used in combination with rifampin (Cordero-Ampuero 2007; Osmon 2013).

    Total knee arthroplasty: Adults: 160 mg TMP 2 times daily for 6 months. **Note:** Must be used in combination with rifampin (Cordero-Ampuero 2007; Osmon 2013).

Q fever (off-label use): Oral:

    Acute (in pregnant women) (CDC 2013): 160 mg TMP twice daily throughout pregnancy but not beyond 32 weeks gestation. **Note:** Discontinue therapy for the final 8 weeks of pregnancy due to hyperbilirubinemia risk

    Chronic: Infectious Disease consult recommended for treatment of chronic Q fever

Sepsis: IV: 20 mg TMP/kg/day divided every 6 hours

Septic arthritis due to MRSA (off-label use): Oral, IV: 3.5 to 4 mg TMP/kg/
dose every 8 to 12 hours for 3 to 4 weeks (some experts combine with
rifampin) (Liu 2011)

Shigellosis: Note: Due to reported widespread resistance, empiric therapy
with sulfamethoxazole and trimethoprim is not recommended (CDC-
NARMS 2010; WHO 2005).

Oral: One double-strength tablet every 12 hours for 5 days

IV: 8-10 mg TMP/kg/day in divided doses every 6, 8, or 12 hours for up to
5 days

Skin/soft tissue infection due to MSSA or MRSA (off-label use): Oral: 1 to
2 double-strength tablets every 12 hours for 5 to 10 days (Lui 2011) or 7 to
14 days (IDSA [Stevens 2014]); **Note:** If beta-hemolytic *Streptococcus* spp
are also suspected, a beta-lactam antibiotic should be added to the regimen
(Liu 2011)

Spontaneous bacterial peritonitis (prevention) (off-label use): Oral: Long-
term prophylaxis: One double-strength (trimethoprim 160 mg/sulfamethox-
azole 800 mg) tablet once daily (preferred) (Lontos 2014). Daily dosing for 5
days per week has been studied (Alvarez 2005; Singh 1995), but concerns
regarding bacterial resistance with intermittent dosing limit use (AASLD
[Runyon 2012]). American Association for the Study of Liver Diseases
(AASLD) guidelines note that intermittent dosing (ie, 5 days/week, once
weekly) of antibiotics, although shown to be effective in SBP prevention,
may be inferior to daily dosing due to development of bacterial resistance.
Daily dosing regimens are preferred (AASLD [Runyon 2012]).

***Stenotrophomonas maltophilia* (ventilator-associated pneumonia) (off-
label use):** IV: Most clinicians have utilized 12 to 15 mg TMP/kg/day for the
treatment of VAP caused by *Stenotrophomonas maltophilia*. Higher doses
(up to 20 mg TMP/kg/day) have been mentioned for treatment of severe
infection in patients with normal renal function (Looney 2009; Vartivarian
1989; Wood 2010)

**Surgical site infections (trunk or extremity [away from axilla or peri-
neum]) (off-label use):** Oral: One double-strength tablet every 6 hours
(IDSA [Stevens 2014])

***Toxoplasma gondii* encephalitis in HIV-infected patients (off-label use;
HHS [OI adult 2015]):** Oral:

Primary prophylaxis: Oral: 160 mg TMP daily (preferred) **or** 160 mg TMP 3
times/week **or** 80 mg TMP daily; primary prophylaxis is indicated for
Toxoplasma IgG-positive patients with CD4 count <100 cells/mm^3

Treatment (alternative to preferred therapy): Oral, IV: 5 mg/kg TMP twice
daily for at least 6 weeks; longer duration may be needed if clinical or
radiologic disease is extensive or response is incomplete at 6 weeks.

Chronic maintenance therapy (alternative to preferred therapy): Oral:
160 mg TMP twice daily; may discontinue when asymptomatic and CD4
count >200 cells/mm^3 for 6 months in response to ART

Travelers' diarrhea: Oral: One double-strength tablet every 12 hours for
5 days

Urinary tract infection:

Oral: One double-strength tablet every 12 hours

Duration of therapy: Uncomplicated: 3 to 5 days; Complicated: 7 to
10 days

Pyelonephritis: 14 days

Prostatitis: Acute: 2 weeks; Chronic: 2 to 3 months

IV: 8 to 10 mg TMP/kg/day in divided doses every 6, 8, or 12 hours for up to
14 days with severe infections

◀ **Pediatric** Recommendations are based on the trimethoprim component.
General dosing guidelines: Children >2 months: Manufacturer's labeling:
Mild-to-moderate infections: Oral: 8 mg TMP/kg/day in divided doses every 12 hours
Serious infection:
Oral: 15 to 20 mg TMP/kg/day in divided doses every 6 hours
IV: 8 to 12 mg TMP/kg/day in divided doses every 6 to 12 hours

Indication specific dosing:
Acute otitis media: Infants >2 months and Children: Oral: 8 mg TMP/kg/day in divided doses every 12 hours for 10 days. **Note:** Recommended by the American Academy of Pediatrics as an alternative agent in penicillin allergic patients at a dose of 6 to 10mg TMP/kg/day (AOM guidelines 2004).
Cyclosporiasis (off-label use): Infants >2 months and Children: Oral, IV: 5 mg TMP/kg twice daily for 7 to 10 days (*Red Book* 2009)
Isosporiasis (*Isospora belli* infection) in HIV-infected patients (off-label use): Adolescents: Refer to adult dosing.
Melioidosis (*Burkholderia pseudomallei*) (off-label use; Lipsitz 2012): Oral, IV:
Severe, acute phase involving brain, prostate, bone, or joint: Administer as 2 divided doses; given with ceftazidime or a carbapenem for ≥10 days followed by eradication therapy:
Children: 16 mg TMP/kg/day (maximum: 640 mg TMP daily)
Adolescents: Refer to adult dosing
Eradication therapy: Administer as 2 divided doses for ≥12 weeks:
Children: 16 mg TMP/kg/day (maximum: 640 mg TMP daily)
Adolescents: Refer to adult dosing
Postexposure prophylaxis: Administer as 2 divided doses for 21 days:
Children: 16 mg TMP/kg/day (maximum: 640 mg TMP daily)
Adolescents: Refer to adult dosing
Pneumocystis pneumonia (PCP):
Infants >2 months and Children:
Treatment: Manufacturer's labeling:
Oral: 15 to 20 mg TMP/kg/day in divided doses every 6 hours for 14 to 21 days
IV: 15 to 20 mg TMP/kg/day in divided doses every 6 to 8 hours for up to 14 days
Prophylaxis: Oral:
Manufacturer's labeling: 150 mg TMP/m^2/day in divided doses every 12 hours and administered for 3 days/week on consecutive (maximum: trimethoprim 320 mg and sulfamethoxazole 1,600 mg/day)
Alternate dosing: HIV-exposed/-infected patients: 150 mg TMP/m^2/day in 2 divided doses daily (CDC 2009)
Adolescents: HV-infected patients (off-label dose; HHS [OI adult 2015]):
Primary prophylaxis: Oral: 80 to 160 mg TMP daily or alternatively, 160 mg TMP 3 times/week
Secondary prophylaxis: Oral: 80 to 160 mg TMP daily or alternatively, 160 mg TMP 3 times/week
Duration of prophylaxis: May discontinue primary or secondary prophylaxis if CD4 count increases from <200 cells/mm^3 to ≥200 cells/mm^3 for at least 3 months in response to ART; therapy must be restarted if CD4 count <200 cells/mm^3

Treatment:

Mild-to-moderate: Oral: 15 to 20 mg TMP/kg/day in 3 divided doses for 21 days or alternatively, 320 mg TMP 3 times/day for 21 days

Moderate-to-severe: IV: 15 to 20 mg TMP/kg/day in 3 to 4 divided doses for 21 days; may switch to oral therapy after clinical improvement

Q fever (off-label use): Oral:

Acute: Infants ≥2 months and Children <8 years with mild or uncomplicated illness (if patient remains febrile past 5 days of doxycycline treatment): 4 to 20 mg TMP/kg/day in divided doses every 12 hours (maximum: trimethoprim 320 mg daily) (CDC 2013). **Note:** Some clinicians may recommend initial treatment with sulfamethoxazole and trimethoprim for children <8 years with mild or uncomplicated illness (CDC 2013; Hartzell 2008).

Chronic: Infectious Disease consult recommended for treatment of chronic Q fever (CDC 2013)

Shigellosis: Note: Due to reported widespread resistance, empiric therapy with sulfamethoxazole and trimethoprim is not recommended (CDC-NARMS 2010; WHO 2005).

Oral:

Manufacturer's labeling: 8 mg TMP/kg/day in divided doses every 12 hours for 5 days

Alternate recommendations (off-label dose): 10 mg TMP/kg/day in divided doses every 12 hours for 5 days (Ashkenazi 1993)

IV: 8 to 10 mg TMP/kg/day in divided doses every 6, 8, or 12 hours for up to 5 days

Skin/soft tissue infection due to MSSA or MRSA (off-label use): Note: If beta-hemolytic *Streptococcus* spp are also suspected, a beta-lactam antibiotic should be added to the regimen (Liu 2011)

Oral: 8 to 12 mg TMP/kg/day in divided doses every 12 hours for 5 to 10 days (IDSA [Liu 2011] or 7 to 14 days (IDSA [Stevens 2014])

IV: 8 to 12 mg TMP/kg/day in divided doses every 6 hours for 7 to 14 days (IDSA [Stevens 2014])

***Toxoplasma gondii* encephalitis in HIV-exposed/-infected patients (off-label use):**

Primary prophylaxis:

Infants ≥2 months and Children: Oral: 150 mg TMP/m^2/day for 3 to 7 days of every week; total daily dose may be given in divided doses every 12 hours for 3 consecutive or alternating days, in divided doses every 12 hours every day or as a single daily dose for 3 consecutive days (HHS [OI pediatric 2013])

Adolescents: Oral: Refer to adult dosing.

Treatment (alternative to preferred therapy): Adolescents: Oral, IV: Refer to adult dosing.

Chronic maintenance therapy (alternative to preferred therapy): Adolescents: Oral: Refer to adult dosing.

Urinary tract infection: Infants >2 months and Children:

Treatment:

Oral: Manufacturer's labeling: 8 mg TMP/kg/day in divided doses every 12 hours for 10 days

IV: Manufacturer's labeling: 8 to 10 mg TMP/kg/day in divided doses every 6, 8, or 12 hours for up to 14 days with serious infections

Prophylaxis: Oral: 2 mg TMP/kg/dose daily or 5 mg TMP/kg/dose twice weekly

◀ **Renal Impairment** Oral, IV:

Manufacturer's labeling: Children and Adults:

CrCl >30 mL/minute: No dosage adjustment required

CrCl 15-30 mL/minute: Administer 50% of recommended dose

CrCl <15 mL/minute: Use is not recommended

Alternate recommendations:

CrCl 15-30 mL/minute:

Treatment: Administer full daily dose (divided every 12 hours) for 24-48 hours, then decrease daily dose by 50% and administer every 24 hours (**Note:** For serious infections including *Pneumocystis jirovecii* pneumonia [PCP], full daily dose is given in divided doses every 6-8 hours for 2 days, followed by reduction to 50% daily dose divided every 12 hours) (Nahata 1995).

PCP prophylaxis: One-half single-strength tablet (40 mg trimethoprim) daily **or** 1 single-strength tablet (80 mg trimethoprim) daily or 3 times weekly (Masur 2002).

CrCl <15 mL/minute:

Treatment: Administer full daily dose every 48 hours (Nahata 1995)

PCP prophylaxis: One-half single-strength tablet (40 mg trimethoprim) daily **or** 1 single-strength tablet (80 mg trimethoprim) 3 times weekly (Masur 2002). While the guidelines do acknowledge the alternative of giving 1 single-strength tablet daily, this may be inadvisable in the uremic/ESRD patient.

GFR <10 mL/minute/1.73 m^2: Children: Use is not recommended, but if required, administer 5-10 mg trimethoprim/kg every 24 hours (Aronoff 2007).

Intermittent Hemodialysis (IHD) (administer after hemodialysis on dialysis days):

Adults: 2.5-10 mg/kg trimethoprim every 24 hours or 5-20 mg/kg trimethoprim 3 times weekly after IHD. **Note:** Dosing is highly dependent upon indication for use (eg, treatment of cystitis versus treatment of PCP pneumonia (Heinz 2009).

PCP prophylaxis: One single-strength tablet (80 mg trimethoprim) after each dialysis session (Masur 2002)

Note: Dosing dependent on the assumption of 3 times/week, complete IHD sessions.

Children: Use is not recommended, but if required, administer 5-10 mg trimethoprim/kg every 24 hours (Aronoff 2007).

Peritoneal dialysis (PD):

Use CrCl <15 mL/minute dosing recommendations. Not significantly removed by PD; supplemental dosing is not required (Aronoff 2007):

GFR <10 mL/minute/1.73 m^2: Children: Use is not recommended, but if required 5-10 mg TMP/kg every 24 hours.

Exit-site and tunnel infections: Oral: One single-strength tablet daily (Li 2010)

Intraperitoneal: Loading dose: TMP-SMX 320/1600 mg/L; Maintenance: TMP-SMX 80/400 mg/L (Aronoff 2007; Warady 2000)

Peritonitis: Oral: One double-strength tablet twice daily (Li 2010)

Continuous renal replacement therapy (CRRT) (Heintz 2009; Trotman 2005): Drug clearance is highly dependent on the method of renal replacement, filter type, and flow rate. Appropriate dosing requires close monitoring of pharmacologic response, signs of adverse reactions due to drug accumulation, as well as drug concentrations in relation to target trough (if appropriate). The following are general recommendations only (based on dialysate flow/ultrafiltration rates of 1-2 L/hour and minimal residual renal function) and should not supersede clinical judgment:

CVVH/CVVHD/CVVHDF: 2.5-7.5 mg/kg of TMP every 12 hours. **Note:** Dosing regimen dependent on clinical indication. Critically-ill patients with *P. jirovecii* pneumonia receiving CVVHDF may require up to 10 mg/kg every 12 hours (Heintz 2009).

Hepatic Impairment There are no dosage adjustments provided in manufacturer's labeling. Use with caution; use is contraindicated in cases of marked hepatic damage.

Additional Information Complete prescribing information should be consulted for additional detail.

Dosage Forms Considerations

The 5:1 ratio (SMX:TMP) remains constant in all dosage forms.

Dosage Forms Excipient information presented when available (limited, particularly for generics); consult specific product labeling.

Solution, Intravenous:

Generic: Sulfamethoxazole 80 mg and trimethoprim 16 mg per mL (5 mL, 10 mL, 30 mL)

Suspension, Oral:

Sulfatrim Pediatric: Sulfamethoxazole 200 mg and trimethoprim 40 mg per 5 mL (473 mL) [contains alcohol, usp, fd&c red #40, fd&c yellow #6 (sunset yellow), methylparaben, polysorbate 80, propylene glycol, propylparaben, saccharin sodium; cherry flavor]

Generic: Sulfamethoxazole 200 mg and trimethoprim 40 mg per 5 mL (20 mL, 473 mL)

Tablet, Oral:

Bactrim: Sulfamethoxazole 400 mg and trimethoprim 80 mg [scored; contains sodium benzoate]

Bactrim DS: Sulfamethoxazole 800 mg and trimethoprim 160 mg [scored; contains sodium benzoate]

Generic: Sulfamethoxazole 400 mg and trimethoprim 80 mg, Sulfamethoxazole 800 mg and trimethoprim 160 mg

♦ **Sulfatrim** see Sulfamethoxazole and Trimethoprim on page 1560

♦ **Sulfatrim Pediatric** see Sulfamethoxazole and Trimethoprim on page 1560

♦ **Sulfur Colloid** see Technetium Tc 99m Sulfur Colloid on page 1602

SUNItinib (su NIT e nib)

Related Information

Management of Chemotherapy-Induced Nausea and Vomiting in Adults on page 2142

Prevention of Chemotherapy-Induced Nausea and Vomiting in Children on page 2203

Principles of Anticancer Therapy on page 2261

Safe Handling of Hazardous Drugs on page 2292

Brand Names: US Sutent

Brand Names: Canada Sutent

◄ **Index Terms** SU011248; SU11248; Sunitinib Malate

Pharmacologic Category Antineoplastic Agent, Tyrosine Kinase Inhibitor; Antineoplastic Agent, Vascular Endothelial Growth Factor (VEGF) Inhibitor; Vascular Endothelial Growth Factor (VEGF) Inhibitor

Use

Gastrointestinal stromal tumor: Treatment of gastrointestinal stromal tumor (GIST) after disease progression on or intolerance to imatinib

Pancreatic neuroendocrine tumors, advanced: Treatment of progressive, well-differentiated pancreatic neuroendocrine tumors in patients with unresectable locally advanced or metastatic disease

Renal cell carcinoma, advanced: Treatment of advanced renal cell carcinoma

Labeled Contraindications There are no contraindications listed in the manufacturer's US labeling.

Canadian labeling: Hypersensitivity to sunitinib or any component of the formulation; pregnancy

Pregnancy Considerations Animal reproduction studies have demonstrated teratogenicity, embryotoxicity, and fetal loss. Because sunitinib inhibits angiogenesis, a critical component of fetal development, adverse effects on pregnancy would be expected. Women of childbearing potential should be advised to avoid pregnancy if receiving sunitinib.

Breast-Feeding Considerations It is not known if sunitinib is excreted in human milk. Due to the potential for serious adverse reactions in the nursing infant, the decision to discontinue breast-feeding or discontinue sunitinib should take into account the benefits of treatment to the mother.

Warnings/Precautions Hazardous agent - use appropriate precautions for handling and disposal (NIOSH 2014 [group 1]). **[U.S. Boxed Warning]: Hepatotoxicity, which may be severe and/or fatal, has been observed in clinical trials and in postmarketing surveillance.** Signs of liver failure include jaundice, elevated transaminases, and/or hyperbilirubinemia, in conjunction with encephalopathy, coagulopathy and/or renal failure. Monitor liver function tests at baseline, with each treatment cycle, and if clinically indicated. Withhold treatment for grade 3 or 4 hepatotoxicity; discontinue if hepatotoxicity does not resolve. Do not reinitiate in patients with severe changes in liver function tests or other signs/symptoms of liver failure. Sunitinib has not been studied in patients with ALT or AST >2.5 times ULN (or >5 times ULN if due to liver metastases).

Cardiovascular events (some fatal), including heart failure, cardiomyopathy, myocardial ischemia and myocardial infarction (MI) have been reported. Use with caution in patients at risk for cardiovascular events. May cause a decrease in left ventricular ejection fraction (LVEF), including some grade 3 reductions. Obtain LVEF evaluation prior to treatment. Discontinue with clinical signs and symptoms of heart failure. Interrupt therapy and/or decrease dose with LVEF <50% and >20% reduction from baseline in patients without clinical heart failure signs/symptoms. Patients with cardiac events (MI, bypass grafts, symptomatic heart failure, cerebrovascular accident, transient ischemic attack, and pulmonary embolism) within the previous 12 months were excluded from clinical trials and it is not known if the risk for left ventricular dysfunction is increased in patient with these conditions; assess risks versus benefits; monitor for clinical signs/symptoms of heart failure, in addition to baseline, also obtain periodic LVEF evaluation.

May cause hypertension; monitor and control with antihypertensives if needed; interrupt therapy until hypertension is controlled for severe hypertension. Use caution and closely monitor in patients with underlying or poorly controlled hypertension. Potentially significant drug-drug interactions may exist, requiring dose or frequency adjustment, additional monitoring, and/or selection of alternative therapy.

Hemorrhagic events have been reported including epistaxis, rectal, gingival, upper GI, urinary tract, genital, brain, wound bleeding, tumor-related, and hemoptysis/pulmonary hemorrhage; may be serious and/or fatal. Proteinuria and nephrotic syndrome have been reported; some cases have led to renal failure and fatal outcomes. Monitor for new onset or worsening proteinuria with baseline and periodic urinalysis and follow up with 24-hour urine protein if clinically indicated. If urine protein is ≥3 g/24 hours, interrupt treatment and reduce the dose. Discontinue treatment in patients with nephrotic syndrome or persistent urine protein ≥3 g/24 hours despite dose reductions. The safety of continuing treatment with sunitinib in patients with moderate to severe proteinuria has not been evaluated. Thrombotic microangiopathy (including thrombotic thrombocytopenic purpura and hemolytic uremic syndrome), sometimes leading to renal failure or fatality, has been reported with sunitinib, both as monotherapy and in combination with bevacizumab. Discontinue if thrombotic microangiopathy develops; effects may be reversible after discontinuation. Impaired wound healing has been reported with sunitinib; temporarily withhold treatment for patients undergoing major surgical procedures; the optimal time to resume treatment after a procedure has not been determined. Serious and fatal GI complications, including GI perforation, have occurred (rarely). Pancreatitis has been observed in RCC patients; discontinue sunitinib if symptoms are present. Thyroid dysfunction (eg, hypothyroidism, hyperthyroidism, and thyroiditis) may occur; the risk for hypothyroidism appears to increase with therapy duration; hyperthyroidism, sometimes followed by hypothyroidism has also been reported; monitor thyroid function at baseline. Patients not receiving thyroid hormone replacement therapy at sunitinib initiation should be monitored (TSH) every 4 weeks for 4 months and then every 2 to 3 months; those already receiving levothyroxine prior to initiating sunitinib should have TSH monitored every 4 weeks until levels and levothyroxine dose are stable, then monitor every 2 months (Hamnvik, 2011). Adrenal function abnormalities have been reported; monitor for adrenal insufficiency in patients with stress such as trauma, severe infection, or who are undergoing surgery. Symptomatic hypoglycemia has been associated with sunitinib; may result in loss of consciousness or require hospitalization. Hypoglycemia occurred infrequently in patients with renal cell cancer and gastrointestinal stromal tumors (GIST); however, the incidence is higher (~10%) in patients with pancreatic neuroendocrine tumors (PNET); preexisting glucose homeostasis abnormalities were not always present in hypoglycemic patients with PNET. Blood glucose decreases may be worse in patients with diabetes. Monitor blood glucose levels regularly during and following discontinuation of treatment. Dose modifications of antidiabetic medications may be necessary to minimize the risk of hypoglycemia.

Severe cutaneous reactions, including erythema multiforme (EM), Stevens-Johnson syndrome (SJS), and toxic epidermal necrolysis (TEN) have been reported (some fatal); if signs/symptoms of EM, SJS, or TEN (progressive skin rash, often with blisters or mucosal lesions) are present, discontinue sunitinib. Do not restart treatment if SJS or TEN are suspected. Necrotizing fasciitis (with ▶

◀ fatalities) has been reported, including perineum necrotizing fasciitis and fasciitis secondary to fistula formation. Discontinue sunitinib in patients who develop necrotizing fasciitis. Sunitinib may cause skin and/or hair depigmentation or discoloration. Hand-foot skin reaction (HFSR) observed with tyrosine kinase inhibitors (TKIs) is distinct from hand-foot syndrome (palmar-plantar erythrodysesthesia) associated with traditional chemotherapy agents; HFSR due to TKIs is localized with defined hyperkeratotic lesions; symptoms include burning, dysesthesia, paresthesia, or tingling on the palms/soles, and generally occur within the first 2 to 4 weeks of treatment; pressure and flexor areas may develop blisters (callus-like), dry/cracked skin, edema, erythema, desquamation, or hyperkeratosis (Appleby, 2011). The following treatments may be used in addition to the recommended dosage modifications (Lacouture, 2008). Prior to treatment initiation, a pedicure is recommended to remove hyperkeratotic areas/calluses, which may predispose to HFSR; avoid vigorous exercise/activities that may stress hands or feet. During therapy, patients should reduce exposure to hot water (may exacerbate hand-foot symptoms); avoid constrictive footwear and excessive skin friction. Patients may also wear thick cotton gloves or socks and should wear shoes with padded insoles. Grade 1 HFSR may be relieved with moisturizing creams, cotton gloves and socks (at night) and/or keratolytic creams such as urea (20% to 40%) or salicylic acid (6%). Apply topical steroid (eg, clobetasol ointment) twice daily to erythematous areas of grade 2 HFSR; topical anesthetics (eg, lidocaine 2%) and then systemic analgesics (if appropriate) may be used for pain control. Resolution of acute erythema may result in keratotic areas which may be softened with keratolytic agents. Reversible posterior leukoencephalopathy syndrome (RPLS) has been reported (rarely, some fatal); symptoms include confusion, headache, hypertension, lethargy, seizure, blindness and/or other vision, or neurologic disturbances; interrupt treatment and begin hypertension management. Tumor lysis syndrome (TLS), including fatalities, has been reported, predominantly in patients with RCC or GIST; risk for TLS is higher in patients with a high tumor burden prior to treatment; monitor closely; correct clinically significant dehydration and treat high uric acid levels prior to initiation of treatment. An increased incidence of fatigue, thyroid dysfunction and treatment-induced hypertension was reported in patients with renal insufficiency (CrCl ≤60 mL/minute) who received sunitinib for the treatment of renal cell cancer (Gupta, 2011). Osteonecrosis of the jaw (ONJ) has been observed with sunitinib; concurrent bisphosphonate use or dental disease may increase the risk for ONJ. If possible, avoid invasive dental procedures in patients with current or prior bisphosphonate use. Consider a dental exam and appropriate prophylactic dentistry prior to treatment initiation Dosing schedules vary by indication; some treatment regimens are continuous daily dosing; other treatment schedules are daily dosing for 4 weeks of a 6-week cycle (4 weeks on, 2 weeks off).

Adverse Reactions

>10%:

Cardiovascular: Hypertension (27% to 34%, GIST: 8% to 15%; grade 3: 10% to 13%, GIST: 4%), decreased left ventricular ejection fraction (RCC: 16% to 27%, grade 3: 3% to 7%; GIST: 11%, grade 3: 1%), peripheral edema (RCC: 24%), chest pain (RCC: 13%), severe hypertension (4% to 10%; >200 mmHg systolic or 110 mmHg diastolic)

Central nervous system: Fatigue (RCC: 62%, pNET: 33%), glossalgia (pNET: ≤48%; RCC: 11%), mouth pain (pNET: ≤48%; RCC: 6% to 14%), headache (18% to 23%), insomnia (15% to 18%), chills (RCC: 14%), depression (RCC: 11%), dizziness (RCC: 11%)

Dermatologic: Skin discoloration (≤25% to 30%; yellow color), hair discoloration (20% to 29%; GIST: 7%), palmar-plantar erythrodysesthesia (23% to 29%, GIST: 14%; grades 3/4: 4% to 8%), xeroderma (15% to 23%), skin rash (14% to 18%; RCC: 29%), alopecia (5% to 14%), erythema (RCC: 12%), pruritus (RCC: 12%)

Endocrine & metabolic: Increased uric acid (RCC: 46%), decreased serum calcium (34% to 42%), decreased serum albumin (pNET: 41%, RCC: 28%), decreased serum phosphate (31% to 36%), increased serum glucose (RCC: 23%), decreased serum potassium (12% to 21%), decreased serum sodium (RCC: 20%), decreased serum magnesium (pNET: 19%), increased serum potassium (16% to 18%), hypothyroidism (4% to 7%; RCC: 16%), increased serum calcium (RCC: 13%), increased serum sodium (10% to 13%)

Gastrointestinal: Diarrhea (59% to 66%; GIST: 40%), nausea (RCC: 58%; pNET: 45%), increased serum lipase (17% to 25%; RCC: 56%; grades 3/4: 5% to 18%), anorexia (RCC: 48%; GIST: 33%), mucositis (47% to 48%, GIST: 29%; includes aphthous stomatitis, dry mucous membranes, gingival pain, gingivitis, glossitis, oral discomfort, oral mucosal ulcer, stomatitis, tongue ulceration), dysgeusia (21%; RCC: 47%), vomiting (34% to 39%), abdominal pain (30% to 39%), increased serum amylase (17% to 20%; RCC: 35%; grades 3/4: 4% to 6%), dyspepsia (RCC: 34%; pNET: 15%), constipation (20% to 23%), weight loss (16%), flatulence (RCC: 14%), xerostomia (RCC: 13%), gastroesophageal reflux disease (RCC: 12%)

Hematologic & oncologic: Decreased hemoglobin (RCC: 79%, pNET: 65%, GIST: 26%; grades 3/4: ≤8%), leukocyte disorder (decreased leukocytes; RCC: 78%; grades 3/4: 8%), decreased neutrophils (71% to 77%, GIST: 53%; grades 3/4: 10% to 17%), abnormal absolute lymphocyte count (decreased; RCC: 68%, pNET: 56%, GIST: 38%; grades 3/4: RCC: 18%, pNET: 7%), decreased platelet count (60% to 68%, GIST: 38%, GIST and RCC: grades 3/4: 5% to 9%), hemorrhage (18% to 22%; RCC: 37%; RCC and GIST, grades 3/4: 3% to 4%; includes hematemesis, hematochezia, hematoma, hemoptysis, melena, metrorrhagia)

Hepatic: Increased serum AST (pNET: 72%, RCC: 56%, GIST: ≤39%; grades 3/4: ≤2% to 5%), increased serum ALT (pNET: 61%; RCC: 51%; GIST: ≤39%; grades 3/4: ≤2% to 4%), increased serum alkaline phosphatase (RCC: 46%; GIST: 24%; grades 3/4: 2% to 4%), increased serum bilirubin (16% to 20%; pNET: 37%; RCC and GIST, grades 3/4: 1%), increased indirect serum bilirubin (RCC and GIST: 10% to 13%; grades 3/4: ≤1%)

Neuromuscular & skeletal: Increased creatine phosphokinase (RCC: 49%), limb pain (RCC: 40%; GIST: ≤14%), weakness (22% to 34%), arthralgia (RCC: 30%; pNET: 15%), back pain (RCC: 28%), myalgia (GIST: ≤14%)

Renal: Increased serum creatinine (RCC: 70%; GIST: 12%)

Respiratory: Cough (RCC: 27%), dyspnea (RCC: 26%), epistaxis (pNET: 20%), nasopharyngitis (RCC: 14%), oropharyngeal pain (RCC: 14%), upper respiratory tract infection (RCC: 11%)

Miscellaneous: Fever (RCC: 22%)

1% to 10%:

Cardiovascular: Deep vein thrombosis (≤3%), pulmonary embolism (≤3%)

Endocrine & metabolic: Hypoglycemia (2%; pNET: 10%)

Gastrointestinal: Hemorrhoids (RCC: 10%), pancreatitis (1%)

◄ Respiratory: Flu-like symptoms (RCC: 5%)

<1%, postmarketing, and/or case reports: Acute renal failure, adrenocortical insufficiency, arterial thrombosis (includes cerebral infarction, cerebrovascular accident, transient ischemic attack), cardiac failure, cardiomyopathy, cerebral hemorrhage, cholecystitis (particularly acalculous), erythema multiforme, esophagitis, fistula (sometimes associated with tumor necrosis and/or regression), fulminant necrotizing fasciitis (including of the perineum), gastrointestinal hemorrhage, gastrointestinal perforation, hemolytic uremic syndrome, hepatic failure, hepatotoxicity, hypersensitivity (includes angioedema), hyperthyroidism, ischemic heart disease, myocardial infarction, myopathy (with/without acute renal failure), nephrotic syndrome, neutropenic infection, osteonecrosis of the jaw, preeclampsia (like syndrome with proteinuria and reversible hypertension) (Gallucci 2013; Patel 2008), prolonged Q-T interval on ECG (dose dependent), proteinuria, pulmonary hemorrhage, pyoderma gangrenosum (including positive dechallenges), renal insufficiency, respiratory tract hemorrhage, respiratory tract infection (may be serious), reversible posterior leukoencephalopathy syndrome, rhabdomyolysis (with/without acute renal failure), seizure, sepsis, septic shock, skin infection (may be serious), Stevens-Johnson syndrome, thrombotic thrombocytopenic purpura, thyroiditis (Feldt 2012), torsades de pointes, toxic epidermal necrolysis, tumor hemorrhage, tumor lysis syndrome, urinary tract hemorrhage, urinary tract infection (may be serious), ventricular arrhythmia, wound healing impairment

Drug Interactions

Metabolism/Transport Effects Substrate of CYP3A4 (major); **Note:** Assignment of Major/Minor substrate status based on clinically relevant drug interaction potential; **Inhibits** BCRP, P-glycoprotein

Avoid Concomitant Use

Avoid concomitant use of SUNItinib with any of the following: BCG (Intravesical); Bevacizumab; Bosutinib; Conivaptan; Fusidic Acid (Systemic); Idelalisib; Natalizumab; PAZOPanib; Pimecrolimus; Silodosin; St Johns Wort; Tacrolimus (Topical); Temsirolimus; Tofacitinib; Topotecan; Vaccines (Live); VinCRIStine (Liposomal)

Increased Effect/Toxicity

SUNItinib may increase the levels/effects of: Afatinib; Bevacizumab; Bisphosphonate Derivatives; Bosutinib; Brentuximab Vedotin; Colchicine; Dabigatran Etexilate; DOXOrubicin (Conventional); Edoxaban; Everolimus; Fingolimod; Highest Risk QTc-Prolonging Agents; Hypoglycemia-Associated Agents; Ledipasvir; Leflunomide; Moderate Risk QTc-Prolonging Agents; Naloxegol; Natalizumab; PAZOPanib; P-glycoprotein/ABCB1 Substrates; Prucalopride; Ranolazine; Rifaximin; Silodosin; Tofacitinib; Topotecan; Vaccines (Live); VinCRIStine (Liposomal)

The levels/effects of SUNItinib may be increased by: Androgens; Antidiabetic Agents; Antifungal Agents (Azole Derivatives, Systemic); Aprepitant; Bevacizumab; Conivaptan; CYP3A4 Inhibitors (Moderate); CYP3A4 Inhibitors (Strong); Dasatinib; Denosumab; Fosaprepitant; Fusidic Acid (Systemic); Herbs (Hypoglycemic Properties); Idelalisib; Ivacaftor; Luliconazole; MAO Inhibitors; Mifepristone; Netupitant; Osimertinib; Palbociclib; Pegvisomant; Pimecrolimus; Quinolone Antibiotics; Roflumilast; Salicylates; Selective Serotonin Reuptake Inhibitors; Simeprevir; Stiripentol; Tacrolimus (Topical); Temsirolimus; Trastuzumab

Decreased Effect

SUNItinib may decrease the levels/effects of: BCG (Intravesical); Coccidioides immitis Skin Test; Sipuleucel-T; Vaccines (Inactivated); Vaccines (Live)

The levels/effects of SUNItinib may be decreased by: Bosentan; CYP3A4 Inducers (Moderate); CYP3A4 Inducers (Strong); Dabrafenib; Deferasirox; Dexamethasone (Systemic); Echinacea; Enzalutamide; Mitotane; Osimertinib; Quinolone Antibiotics; Siltuximab; St Johns Wort; Tocilizumab

Food Interactions Grapefruit juice may increase the levels/effects of sunitinib. Food has no effect on the bioavailability of sunitinib. Management: Avoid grapefruit juice.

Storage/Stability Store at 25°C (77°F); excursions are permitted between 15°C to 30°C (59°F to 86°F).

Mechanism of Action Exhibits antitumor and antiangiogenic properties by inhibiting multiple receptor tyrosine kinases, including platelet-derived growth factors (PDGFRα and PDGFRβ), vascular endothelial growth factors (VEGFR1, VEGFR2, and VEGFR3), FMS-like tyrosine kinase-3 (FLT3), colony-stimulating factor type 1 (CSF-1R), and glial cell-line-derived neurotrophic factor receptor (RET).

Pharmacodynamics/Kinetics

Distribution: V_d/F: 2230 L

Protein binding: Sunitinib: 95%; SU12662: 90%

Metabolism: Hepatic; primarily metabolized by CYP3A4 to the N-desethyl metabolite SU12662 (active)

Half-life elimination: Terminal: Sunitinib: 40 to 60 hours; SU12662: 80 to 110 hours

Time to peak, plasma: 6 to 12 hours

Excretion: Feces (61%); urine (16%)

Dosing

Adult & Geriatric Note: Dosage modifications should be done in increments or decrements of 12.5 mg; individualize based on safety and tolerability.

Gastrointestinal stromal tumor (GIST): Oral: 50 mg once daily for 4 weeks of a 6-week treatment cycle (4 weeks on, 2 weeks off)

GIST off-label dosing: Oral: 37.5 mg once daily, continuous daily dosing (George, 2009, *EJC*)

Pancreatic neuroendocrine tumors, advanced (PNET): Oral: 37.5 mg once daily, continuous daily dosing (maximum daily dose used in clinical trials: 50 mg)

Renal cell cancer, advanced (RCC): Oral: 50 mg once daily for 4 weeks of a 6-week treatment cycle (4 weeks on, 2 weeks off)

Soft tissue sarcoma, non-GIST (off-label use): Oral: 37.5 mg once daily, continuous daily dosing (George, 2009, *JCO*)

Thyroid cancer, refractory (off-label use): Oral: 50 mg once daily for 4 weeks of a 6-week treatment cycle (4 weeks on, 2 weeks off) (Cohen, 2008; Ravaud, 2008)

Dosage adjustment with concurrent CYP3A4 inhibitor: Avoid concomitant administration with strong CYP3A4 inhibitors (eg, clarithromycin, erythromycin, itraconazole, ketoconazole, nefazodone, protease inhibitors, telithromycin, voriconazole); if concomitant administration with a strong CYP3A4 inhibitor cannot be avoided, consider a dose reduction to a minimum of 37.5 mg/day (GIST, RCC) or 25 mg/day (PNET).

◄ *Dosage adjustment with concurrent CYP3A4 inducer:* Avoid concomitant administration with strong CYP3A4 inducers (eg, carbamazepine, dexamethasone, phenobarbital, phenytoin, rifampin, St John's wort); if concomitant administration with a strong CYP3A4 inducer cannot be avoided, consider a dosage increase (with careful monitoring for toxicity) to a maximum of 87.5 mg/day (GIST, RCC) or 62.5 mg/day (PNET).

Renal Impairment

Mild, moderate, or severe impairment: No initial adjustment required; subsequent adjustments may be needed based on safety and tolerance.

ESRD on hemodialysis: No initial adjustment required; subsequent dosage **increases** (up to twofold) may be required due to reduced (47%) exposure

Hepatic Impairment

Preexisting hepatic impairment: No adjustment is necessary with mild-to-moderate (Child-Pugh class A or B) hepatic impairment; not studied in patients with severe (Child-Pugh class C) hepatic impairment. Studies excluded patients with ALT or AST >2.5 x ULN, or if due to liver metastases, ALT or AST >5 x ULN.

Hepatotoxicity during treatment: Hepatic adverse events ≥ grade 3 or 4: Withhold treatment; discontinue if hepatotoxicity does not resolve. Do not reinitiate in patients with severe changes in liver function tests or other signs/symptoms of liver failure.

Adjustment for Toxicity Dosage modifications should be done in increments or decrements of 12.5 mg; individualize based on safety and tolerability.

Cardiac toxicity:

Ejection fraction <50% and >20% below baseline without evidence of CHF: Interrupt treatment and/or reduce dose.

LV dysfunction with CHF clinical manifestations: Discontinue treatment.

Dermatologic toxicity:

Signs/symptoms of erythema multiforme (EM), Stevens-Johnson syndrome (SJS), and toxic epidermal necrolysis (TEN), including progressive skin rash, often with blisters or mucosal lesions: Discontinue sunitinib; do not restart treatment if SJS or TEN are suspected.

Necrotizing fasciitis: Discontinue sunitinib.

Hypertension, severe: Temporarily interrupt treatment until hypertension is controlled.

Nephrotic syndrome: Discontinue treatment.

Pancreatitis: Discontinue treatment.

Proteinuria:

Urine protein ≥3 g/24 hours: Interrupt treatment and reduce the dose.

Persistent urine protein ≥3 g/24 hours despite dose reductions: Discontinue treatment.

Reversible posterior leukoencephalopathy (RPLS): Temporarily withhold treatment; after resolution, may resume with discretion.

Thrombotic microangiopathy: Discontinue treatment.

Combination Regimens

Renal cell cancer: Sunitinib (RCC Regimen) on page 2086

Soft tissue sarcoma: Sunitinib (Soft Tissue Sarcoma Regimen) on page 2086

Soft tissue sarcoma (gastrointestinal stromal tumor [GIST]): Sunitinib (GIST Regimen) on page 2086

Administration May be administered with or without food. Hazardous agent; use appropriate precautions for handling and disposal (NIOSH 2014 [group 1]). Avoid contact with broken or leaking capsules; if contact occurs, wash immediately with soap and water. If it is necessary to manipulate the capsules (eg, to prepare an oral suspension), it is recommended to double glove, wear a protective gown, and prepare in a controlled device (NIOSH, 2014).

Emetic Potential
Children: Minimal (<10%)
Adults: Low (10% to 30%)

Extemporaneous Preparations Hazardous agent: Use appropriate precautions for handling and disposal (NIOSH 2014 [group 1]). When manipulating capsules, NIOSH recommends double gloving, a protective gown, and preparation in a controlled device; if not prepared in a controlled device, respiratory and eye protection as well as ventilated engineering controls are recommended (NIOSH, 2014).

A 10 mg/mL sunitinib oral suspension may be made with capsules and a 1:1 mixture of Ora-Sweet and Ora-Plus. Empty the contents of three 50 mg sunitinib capsules into a mortar; add small portions of vehicle and mix to a uniform paste. Mix while adding vehicle in incremental proportions to 15 mL. Transfer to amber plastic bottle and label "shake well". This suspension maintains an average concentration of 96% to 106% (of the original concentration) at room temperature or refrigerated for up to 60 days in plastic amber prescription bottles.

Navid F, Christensen R, Minkin P, et al, "Stability of Sunitinib in Oral Suspension," *Ann Pharmacother*, 2008, 42(7):962-6.

Monitoring Parameters LVEF, baseline (and periodic with cardiac risk factors), ECG (12-lead; baseline and periodic), blood pressure; adrenal function CBC with differential and platelets (prior to each treatment cycle), liver function tests (baseline, with each cycle and if clinically indicated), serum chemistries including magnesium, phosphate, and potassium (prior to each treatment cycle), blood glucose levels (regularly during and following discontinuation of treatment), urinalysis (for proteinuria development or worsening); consider dental exam prior to treatment initiation; symptoms of hypothyroidism, hyperthyroidism, or thyroiditis; signs/symptoms of hypoglycemia
Thyroid function testing (Hamnvik, 2011):
  Preexisting levothyroxine therapy: Obtain baseline TSH levels, then monitor every 4 weeks until levels and levothyroxine dose are stable, then monitor every 2 months
  Without preexisting thyroid hormone replacement: TSH at baseline, then every 4 weeks for 4 months, then every 2-3 months

Dietary Considerations Avoid grapefruit juice.

Medication Guide Available Yes

Dosage Forms Excipient information presented when available (limited, particularly for generics); consult specific product labeling.
Capsule, Oral:
  Sutent: 12.5 mg, 25 mg, 37.5 mg, 50 mg

◆ **Sunitinib Malate** see SUNItinib *on page 1567*

◆ **Supeudol (Can)** see OxyCODONE *on page 1277*

◆ **Supprelin LA** see Histrelin *on page 816*

◆ **Sutent** see SUNItinib *on page 1567*

◆ **Sylatron** see Peginterferon Alfa-2b *on page 1350*

- ◆ **Sylvant** *see* Siltuximab *on page 1525*
- ◆ **Synapryn FusePaq** *see* TraMADol *on page 1672*
- ◆ **Synribo** *see* Omacetaxine *on page 1248*
- ◆ **Tabloid** *see* Thioguanine *on page 1637*

Tacrolimus (Systemic) (ta KROE li mus)

Related Information
Hematopoietic Stem Cell Transplantation *on page 2272*
Management of EGFR Inhibitor Toxicities: Dermatologic, Ocular, and Gastrointestinal *on page 2179*
Safe Handling of Hazardous Drugs *on page 2292*

Brand Names: US Astagraf XL; Envarsus XR; Hecoria [DSC]; Prograf
Brand Names: Canada Advagraf; Prograf; Sandoz-Tacrolimus
Index Terms FK506
Pharmacologic Category Calcineurin Inhibitor; Immunosuppressant Agent
Use Organ rejection prophylaxis:

US labeling:
Astagraf XL: Prevention of organ rejection in kidney transplant recipients
Envarsus XR: Prevention of organ rejection in kidney transplant recipients converted from tacrolimus immediate-release formulation.
Hecoria and Prograf: Prevention of organ rejection in heart, kidney, and liver transplant recipients

Canadian labeling:
Advagraf: Prevention of organ rejection in kidney and liver transplant recipients
Prograf: Prevention of organ rejection in heart, kidney, or liver transplant recipients; treatment of refractory rejection in kidney or liver transplant recipients; treatment of active rheumatoid arthritis in adult patients nonresponsive to disease-modifying antirheumatic drug (DMARD) therapy or when DMARD therapy is inappropriate

Labeled Contraindications Hypersensitivity to tacrolimus, polyoxyl 60 hydrogenated castor oil (HCO-60), or any other component of the formulation.

Pregnancy Considerations Adverse events were observed in animal reproduction studies. Tacrolimus crosses the human placenta and is measurable in the cord blood, amniotic fluid, and newborn serum. Tacrolimus concentrations in the placenta may be higher than the maternal serum (Jain 1997). Infants with lower birth weights have been found to have higher tacrolimus concentrations (Bramham 2013). Transient neonatal hyperkalemia and renal dysfunction have been reported.

Tacrolimus pharmacokinetics are altered during pregnancy. Whole blood concentrations decrease as pregnancy progresses; however, unbound concentrations increase. Measuring unbound concentrations may be preferred, especially in women with anemia or hypoalbuminemia. If unbound concentration measurement is not available, interpretation of whole blood concentrations should account for RBC count and serum albumin concentration (Hebert 2013; Zheng 2012).

In general, women who have had a kidney transplant should be instructed that fertility will be restored following the transplant but that pregnancy should be avoided for ~2 years. Tacrolimus may be used as an immunosuppressant during pregnancy. The risk of infection, hypertension, and pre-eclampsia may be increased in pregnant women who have had a kidney transplant (EPBG 2002).

The National Transplantation Pregnancy Registry (NTPR) is a registry which follows pregnancies which occur in maternal transplant recipients or those fathered by male transplant recipients. The NTPR encourages reporting of pregnancies following solid organ transplant by contacting them at 877-955-6877.

Breast-Feeding Considerations Tacrolimus is excreted into breast milk; concentrations are variable and lower than that of the maternal serum. The low bioavailability of tacrolimus following oral absorption may also decrease the amount of exposure to a nursing infant (Bramham 2013; French 2003; Gardiner 2006). In one study, tacrolimus serum concentrations in the infants did not differ between those who were bottle fed or breast-fed (all infants were exposed to tacrolimus throughout pregnancy) (Bramham 2013). Available information suggests that tacrolimus exposure to the nursing infant is ≤0.5% of the weight-adjusted maternal dose (Bramham 2013; French 2003; Gardiner 2006). The manufacturer recommends that nursing be discontinued, taking into consideration the importance of the drug to the mother.

Warnings/Precautions Hazardous agent - use appropriate precautions for handling and disposal (NIOSH 2014 [group 2]).

[US Boxed Warning]: Risk of developing infections (including bacterial, viral [including CMV], fungal, and protozoal infections [including opportunistic infections]) is increased. Latent viral infections may be activated, including BK virus (associated with polyoma virus-associated nephropathy [PVAN]) and JC virus (associated with progressive multifocal leukoencephalopathy [PML]); may result in serious adverse effects. Immunosuppression increases the risk for CMV viremia and/or CMV disease; the risk of CMV disease is increased for patients who are CMV-seronegative prior to transplant and receive a graft from a CMV-seropositive donor. Consider reduction in immunosuppression if PVAN, PML, CMV viremia and/or CMV disease occurs.

[US Boxed Warning]: Immunosuppressive therapy may result in the development of lymphoma and other malignancies (predominantly skin malignancies). The risk for new-onset diabetes and insulin-dependent posttransplant diabetes mellitus (PTDM) is increased with tacrolimus use after transplantation, including in patients without pretransplant history of diabetes mellitus; insulin dependence may be reversible; monitor blood glucose frequently; risk is increased in African-American and Hispanic kidney transplant patients. Nephrotoxicity (acute or chronic) occur when used in high doses, in patients with impaired renal function, or with other nephrotoxic drugs (eg, sirolimus, cyclosporine). Monitor renal function and consider dosage reduction in nephrotoxicity occurs. Neurotoxicity may occur especially when used in high doses; tremor headache, coma and delirium have been reported and are associated with serum concentrations. Seizures may also occur. Posterior reversible encephalopathy syndrome (PRES) has been reported; symptoms (altered mental status, headache, hypertension, seizures, and visual disturbances) are reversible with dose reduction or discontinuation of therapy; stabilize blood pressure and reduce dose with suspected or confirmed PRES diagnosis.

Pure red cell aplasia (PRCA) has been reported in patients receiving tacrolimus. Use with caution in patients with risk factors for PRCA including parvovirus B19 infection, underlying disease, or use of concomitant medications associated with PRCA (eg, mycophenolate). Discontinuation of therapy ▶

should be considered with diagnosis of PRCA. Monitoring of serum concentrations (trough for oral therapy) is essential to prevent organ rejection and reduce drug-related toxicity. Use caution in renal or hepatic dysfunction, dosing adjustments may be required. Delay initiation of therapy in kidney transplant patients if postoperative oliguria occurs; begin therapy no sooner than 6 hours and within 24 hours post-transplant, but may be delayed until renal function has recovered. Mild-to-severe hyperkalemia may occur; monitor serum potassium levels. Hypertension may commonly occur; antihypertensive treatment may be necessary; avoid use of potassium-sparing diuretics due to risk of hyperkalemia; concurrent use of calcium channel blockers may require tacrolimus dosage adjustment. Gastrointestinal perforation may occur; all reported cases were considered to be a complication of transplant surgery or accompanied by infection, diverticulum, or malignant neoplasm. Myocardial hypertrophy has been reported (rare). Prolongation of the QT/QTc and torsade de pointes may occur; avoid use in patients with congenital long QT syndrome. Consider obtaining electrocardiograms and monitoring electrolytes (magnesium, potassium, calcium) periodically during treatment in patients with congestive heart failure, bradyarrhythmias, those taking certain antiarrhythmic medications or other medicinal products that lead to QT prolongation, and those with electrolyte disturbances such as hypokalemia, hypocalcemia, or hypomagnesemia. Potentially significant drug-drug/drug-food interactions may exist, requiring dose or frequency adjustment, additional monitoring, and/or selection of alternative therapy. In liver transplantation, the tacrolimus dose and target range should be reduced to minimize the risk of nephrotoxicity when used in combination with everolimus. Extended release tacrolimus in combination with sirolimus is not recommended in renal transplant patients; the safety and efficacy of immediate release tacrolimus in combination with sirolimus has not been established in this patient population. Concomitant use was associated with increased mortality, graft loss, and hepatic artery thrombosis in liver transplant patients, as well as increased risk of renal impairment, wound healing complications, and PTDM in heart transplant recipients.

Immediate release and extended release capsules are NOT interchangeable or substitutable. The extended release formulation is a once daily preparation; and immediate release is intended for twice daily administration. Serious adverse events, including organ rejection may occur if inadvertently substituted. **[US Boxed Warning]: Astagraf XL was associated with increased mortality in female liver transplant recipients; the use of extended release tacrolimus is not recommended in liver transplantation.** Mortality at 12 months was 18% in females who received extended release tacrolimus compared to 8% for females who received regular release tacrolimus. Each mL of injection contains polyoxyl 60 hydrogenated castor oil (HCO-60) (200 mg) and dehydrated alcohol USP 80% v/v.

Hypersensitivity reactions, including anaphylaxis, have been reported with tacrolimus injection. Tacrolimus injection contains polyoxyl 60 hydrogenated castor oil (HCO-60), a castor oil derivative. HCO-60 is a solubilizer similar to polyoxyethylated castor oil (also known as polyoxyl 35 castor oil or Cremophor EL); polyoxyethylated castor oil is associated with hypersensitivity reactions (Nicolai 2012). Tacrolimus intravenous (IV) use should be limited to patients unable to take oral capsules. Monitor patient for a minimum of 30 minutes after initiation of infusion and then at frequent intervals; discontinue infusion if anaphylaxis occurs. Patients should be transitioned from IV to oral tacrolimus as soon as the patient can tolerate oral administration. Patients should not be immunized with live vaccines during or shortly after treatment and should avoid close contact with recently vaccinated (live vaccine) individuals. Oral formulations contain lactose; the Canadian labeling does not recommend use of these products in patients who may be lactose intolerant (eg, Lapp lactase deficiency, glucose-galactose malabsorption, galactose intolerance). **[US Boxed Warning]: Should be administered under the supervision of a physician experienced in immunosuppressive therapy and organ transplantation in a facility appropriate for monitoring and managing therapy.**

Adverse Reactions As reported for kidney, liver, and heart transplantation:

≥15%:

Cardiovascular: Hypertension (13% to 89%), peripheral edema (11% to 36%), chest pain (19%), edema (<15% to 18%), pericardial effusion (heart transplant 15%; Astagraf XL <15%)

Central nervous system: Headache (10% to 64%), insomnia (9% to 64%), pain (24% to 63%), paresthesia (<15% to 40%), dizziness (<15% to 19%), fatigue (2% to 16%)

Dermatologic: Pruritus (<15% to 36%), skin rash (10% to 24%)

Endocrine & metabolic: Diabetes mellitus (post-transplant; kidney transplant 20% to 75%; heart transplant 13% to 22%; liver transplant 11% to 18%), hyperglycemia (16% to 70%), hypertriglyceridemia (65%), hypoglycemia (<15% to 61%), hypercholesterolemia (<15% to 57%), hypophosphatemia (5% to 49%), hypomagnesemia (3% to 48%), hyperkalemia (13% to 45%), hyperlipidemia (7% to 34%), hypokalemia (13% to 29%)

Gastrointestinal: Diarrhea (25% to 72%), abdominal pain (29% to 59%; Astagraf XL <15%), nausea (13% to 46%), constipation (14% to 40%), anorexia (7% to 34%), vomiting (13% to 29%), dyspepsia (18% to 28%; Astagraf XL <15%)

Genitourinary: Urinary tract infection (1% to 34%), oliguria (<15% to 19%)

Hematologic & oncologic: Anemia (5% to 50%; hemoglobin <10 g/dL 65%), leukopenia (11% to 48%), leukocytosis (8% to 32%), thrombocytopenia (14% to 24%)

Hepatic: Abnormal hepatic function tests (6% to 36%), ascites (7% to 27%)

Infection: Infection (15% to 45%), bacterial infection (8% to 41%), cytomegalovirus disease (heart transplant 32%; kidney transplant 6% to 12%), serious infection (19% to 24%)

Local: Postoperative wound complication (kidney transplant 28%)

Neuromuscular & skeletal: Tremor (15% to 56%; heart transplant 15%), weakness (11% to 52%), back pain (17% to 30%), arthralgia (25%; Astagraf XL <15%)

Renal: Renal function abnormality (36% to 56%), increased serum creatinine (16% to 45%), increased blood urea nitrogen (12% to 30%)

Respiratory: Pleural effusion (30% to 36%), respiratory tract infection (22% to 34%), dyspnea (5% to 29%), atelectasis (5% to 28%), cough (<15% to 18%), bronchitis (17%)

Miscellaneous: Fever (19% to 48%), postoperative pain (kidney transplant 29%), graft complications (kidney transplant 14% to 24%)

<15%:

Cardiovascular: Angina pectoris, atrial fibrillation, atrial flutter, bradycardia, cardiac arrest, cardiac arrhythmia, cardiac failure, cardiorespiratory arrest, cerebral infarction, cerebral ischemia, decreased heart rate, deep vein thrombophlebitis, deep vein thrombosis, ECG abnormality (QRS or ST segment or T wave), flushing, hemorrhagic stroke, hypertrophic cardiomyopathy, hypotension, ischemic heart disease, myocardial infarction, orthostatic hypotension, peripheral vascular disease, phlebitis, syncope, tachycardia, thrombosis, vasodilatation, ventricular premature contractions

Central nervous system: Abnormal dreams, abnormality in thinking, agitation, amnesia, anxiety, aphasia, ataxia, brain disease, carpal tunnel syndrome, chills, confusion, convulsions, depression, drowsiness, emotional lability, excessive crying, falling, flaccid paralysis, hallucination, hypertonia, hypoesthesia, mental status changes, mood elevation, myasthenia, myoclonus, nervousness, neurotoxicity, nightmares, paresis, peripheral neuropathy, psychosis, seizure, vertigo, voice disorder, writing difficulty

Dermatologic: Acne vulgaris, alopecia, bruise, cellulitis, condyloma acuminatum, dermal ulcer, dermatitis (including fungal), dermatological reaction, diaphoresis, exfoliative dermatitis, hypotrichosis, skin discoloration, skin photosensitivity

Endocrine & metabolic: Acidosis, albuminuria, alkalosis, anasarca, Cushing's syndrome, decreased serum bicarbonate, decreased serum iron, dehydration, gout, hirsutism, hypercalcemia, hyperphosphatemia, hyperuricemia, hypervolemia, hypocalcemia, hyponatremia, increased gamma-glutamyl transferase, increased lactate dehydrogenase, weight changes

Gastrointestinal: Gastroenteritis (2% to 7%), aphthous stomatitis, cholangitis, colitis, delayed gastric emptying, duodenitis, dysphagia, enlargement of abdomen, esophagitis (including ulcerative), flatulence, gastric ulcer, gastritis, gastroesophageal reflux disease, gastrointestinal hemorrhage, gastrointestinal perforation, hernia, hiccups, increased appetite, intestinal obstruction, oral candidiasis, pancreatic disease (pseudocyst), pancreatitis (including hemorrhagic and necrotizing), peritonitis, rectal disease, stomach cramps, stomatitis

Genitourinary: Anuria, bladder spasm, cystitis, dysuria, hematuria, nocturia, proteinuria, toxic nephrosis, urinary frequency, urinary incontinence, urinary retention, urinary urgency, vaginitis

Hematologic & oncologic: Blood coagulation disorder, decreased prothrombin time, hemolytic anemia, hemorrhage, hypochromic anemia, hypoproteinemia, increased hematocrit, increased INR, Kaposi's sarcoma, malignant neoplasm of bladder, malignant neoplasm of thyroid (papillary), neutropenia, pancytopenia, polycythemia, skin neoplasm

Hepatic: Cholestatic jaundice, hepatic injury, hepatitis (including acute, chronic, and granulomatous), hyperbilirubinemia, increased liver enzymes, increased serum alkaline phosphatase, jaundice

Hypersensitivity: Hypersensitivity reaction

Infection: Polyoma virus infection (≤5%), abscess, Epstein Barr virus infection, herpes simplex infection, sepsis, tinea versicolor

Local: Localized phlebitis

Neuromuscular & skeletal: Arthropathy, leg cramps, muscle spasm, muscle weakness of the extremities, myalgia, neuropathy (including compression), osteopenia, osteoporosis

Ophthalmic: Amblyopia, blurred vision, conjunctivitis, visual disturbance

Otic: Hearing loss, otalgia, otitis externa, otitis media, tinnitus

Renal: Acute renal failure, hydronephrosis, renal disease (BK nephropathy), renal tubular necrosis

Respiratory: Allergic rhinitis, asthma, emphysema, flu-like symptoms, pharyngitis, pneumonia, pneumothorax, pulmonary disease, pulmonary edema, pulmonary infiltrates, respiratory depression, respiratory failure, rhinitis, sinusitis

Miscellaneous: Wound healing impairment

Postmarketing and/or case reports: Adult respiratory distress syndrome, agranulocytosis, anaphylactoid reaction, anaphylaxis, angioedema, basal cell carcinoma, biliary tract disease (stenosis), blindness, cerebrovascular accident, coma, deafness, decreased serum fibrinogen, delirium, disseminated intravascular coagulation, dysarthria, graft versus host disease (acute and chronic), hemiparesis, hemolytic-uremic syndrome, hemorrhagic cystitis, hepatic cirrhosis, hepatic failure, hepatic necrosis, hepatic veno-occlusive disease, hepatosplenic T-cell lymphomas, hepatotoxicity, hyperpigmentation, interstitial pulmonary disease, leukemia, leukoencephalopathy, liver steatosis, lymphoproliferative disorder (post-transplant or related to EBV), malignant lymphoma, malignant melanoma, multiorgan failure, mutism, optic atrophy, osteomyelitis, photophobia, polyarthritis, progressive multifocal leukoencephalopathy (PML), prolonged partial thromboplastin time, prolonged Q-T interval on ECG, pulmonary hypertension, pure red cell aplasia, quadriplegia, reversible posterior leukoencephalopathy syndrome, rhabdomyolysis, septicemia, squamous cell carcinoma, status epilepticus, Stevens-Johnson syndrome, supraventricular extrasystole, supraventricular tachycardia, thrombocytopenic purpura, thrombotic thrombocytopenic purpura, torsades de pointes, toxic epidermal necrolysis, urticaria, venous thrombosis, ventricular fibrillation

Note: Calcineurin inhibitor-induced hemolytic uremic syndrome/thrombotic thrombocytopenic purpura/thrombotic microangiopathy (HUS/TTP/TMA) have been reported (with concurrent sirolimus).

Drug Interactions

Metabolism/Transport Effects Substrate of CYP3A4 (major), P-glycoprotein; **Note:** Assignment of Major/Minor substrate status based on clinically relevant drug interaction potential; **Inhibits** P-glycoprotein

Avoid Concomitant Use

Avoid concomitant use of Tacrolimus (Systemic) with any of the following: BCG (Intravesical); Bosutinib; CloZAPine; Conivaptan; Crizotinib; CycloSPORINE (Systemic); Dipyrone; Enzalutamide; Eplerenone; Foscarnet; Fusidic Acid (Systemic); Grapefruit Juice; Idelalisib; Mifepristone; Natalizumab; Nelfinavir; PAZOPanib; Pimecrolimus; Potassium-Sparing Diuretics; Silodosin; Sirolimus; Tacrolimus (Topical); Temsirolimus; Tofacitinib; Topotecan; Vaccines (Live); VinCRIStine (Liposomal)

Increased Effect/Toxicity

Tacrolimus (Systemic) may increase the levels/effects of: Afatinib; Bosutinib; Brentuximab Vedotin; CloZAPine; Colchicine; CycloSPORINE (Systemic); Dabigatran Etexilate; DOXOrubicin (Conventional); Dronedarone; Edoxaban; Everolimus; Fenofibrate and Derivatives; Fingolimod; Fosphenytoin; Highest Risk QTc-Prolonging Agents; Ledipasvir; Leflunomide; Moderate Risk QTc-Prolonging Agents; Naloxegol; Natalizumab; PAZOPanib; P-glycoprotein/ABCB1 Substrates; Phenytoin; Prucalopride; Rifaximin; Silodosin; Sirolimus; Temsirolimus; Tofacitinib; Topotecan; Vaccines (Live); VinCRIStine (Liposomal)

◀ *The levels/effects of Tacrolimus (Systemic) may be increased by:* Alcohol (Ethyl); Antidepressants (Serotonin Reuptake Inhibitor/Antagonist); Aprepitant; Boceprevir; Calcium Channel Blockers (Dihydropyridine); Calcium Channel Blockers (Nondihydropyridine); Chloramphenicol; Clotrimazole (Oral); Clotrimazole (Topical); Conivaptan; Crizotinib; CycloSPORINE (Systemic); CYP3A4 Inhibitors (Moderate); CYP3A4 Inhibitors (Strong); Danazol; Dasatinib; Denosumab; Dipyrone; Dronedarone; Efonidipine; Eplerenone; Ertapenem; Fluconazole; Fosaprepitant; Foscarnet; Fusidic Acid (Systemic); Grapefruit Juice; Idelalisib; Itraconazole; Ivacaftor; Ketoconazole (Systemic); Levofloxacin (Systemic); Luliconazole; Macrolide Antibiotics; Mifepristone; Nelfinavir; Netupitant; Nonsteroidal Anti-Inflammatory Agents; Ombitasvir, Paritaprevir, and Ritonavir; Ombitasvir, Paritaprevir, Ritonavir, and Dasabuvir; Osimertinib; Palbociclib; P-glycoprotein/ABCB1 Inhibitors; Pimecrolimus; Posaconazole; Potassium-Sparing Diuretics; Protease Inhibitors; Proton Pump Inhibitors; Ranolazine; Ritonavir; Roflumilast; Schisandra; Sirolimus; Stiripentol; Tacrolimus (Topical); Telaprevir; Temsirolimus; Trastuzumab; Voriconazole

Decreased Effect

Tacrolimus (Systemic) may decrease the levels/effects of: Antidiabetic Agents; BCG (Intravesical); Coccidioides immitis Skin Test; Sipuleucel-T; Vaccines (Inactivated); Vaccines (Live)

The levels/effects of Tacrolimus (Systemic) may be decreased by: Bosentan; Caspofungin; Cinacalcet; CYP3A4 Inducers (Moderate); CYP3A4 Inducers (Strong); Dabrafenib; Deferasirox; Echinacea; Efavirenz; Enzalutamide; Fosphenytoin; Mitotane; Osimertinib; P-glycoprotein/ABCB1 Inducers; Phenytoin; Rifamycin Derivatives; Sevelamer; Siltuximab; Sirolimus; St Johns Wort; Temsirolimus; Tocilizumab

Food Interactions

Ethanol: Alcohol may increase the rate of release of extended-release tacrolimus and adversely affect tacrolimus safety and/or efficacy. Management: Avoid alcohol.

Food: Food decreases rate and extent of absorption. High-fat meals have most pronounced effect (37% and 25% decrease in AUC, respectively, and 77% and 25% decrease in C_{max}, respectively, for immediately release and extended release formulations). Grapefruit juice, a CYP3A4 inhibitor, may increase serum level and/or toxicity of tacrolimus. Management: Administer with or without food (immediate release), but be consistent. Administer extended release on an empty stomach. Avoid concurrent use of grapefruit juice.

Storage/Stability

Injection: Prior to dilution, store at 5°C to 25°C (41°F to 77°F). Following dilution, stable for 24 hours in D_5W or NS in glass or polyethylene containers. Do not store in polyvinyl chloride containers since the polyoxyl 60 hydrogenated castor oil injectable vehicle may leach phthalates from polyvinyl chloride containers.

Capsule, tablet:

Astagraf XL, Envarsus XR, Prograf: Store at 25°C (77°F); excursions permitted between 15°C and 30°C (59°F and 86°F).

Hecoria: Store at 20°C to 25°C (68°F to 77°F).

Preparation for Administration Hazardous agent; use appropriate precautions for handling and disposal (NIOSH 2014 [group 2]).

Injection: Dilute with 5% dextrose injection or 0.9% sodium chloride injection to a final concentration between 0.004 mg/mL and 0.02 mg/mL.

Mechanism of Action Suppresses cellular immunity (inhibits T-lymphocyte activation), by binding to an intracellular protein, FKBP-12 and complexes with calcineurin dependent proteins to inhibit calcineurin phosphatase activity

Pharmacodynamics/Kinetics

Absorption: Better in resected patients with a closed stoma; unlike cyclosporine, clamping of the T-tube in liver transplant patients does not alter trough concentrations or AUC; Oral: Incomplete and variable; the rate and extent of absorption is decreased by food (particularly a high-fat meal). Oral absorption may be variable in stem cell transplant patients with mucositis due to the conditioning regimen.

Distribution: V_d: Children: 0.5 to 4.7 L/kg; Adults: 0.55 to 2.47 L/kg

Protein binding: ~99% primarily to albumin and alpha$_1$-acid glycoprotein

Metabolism: Extensively hepatic via CYP3A4 to eight possible metabolites (major metabolite, 31-demethyl tacrolimus, shows same activity as tacrolimus *in vitro*)

Bioavailability: Oral: Children: 7% to 55%, Adults: 7% to 32%; Absolute: Unknown

Half-life elimination:

Immediate release: Variable, 23 to 46 hours in healthy volunteers; 2.1 to 36 hours in transplant patients

Extended release: 23 to 41 hours

Time to peak: 0.5 to 6 hours

Excretion: Feces (~93%); urine (<1% as unchanged drug)

Dosing

Adult & Geriatric

Prevention of organ rejection in transplant recipients: Note: The initial postoperative dose of tacrolimus (immediate release) should begin no sooner than 6 hours after liver and heart transplant and within 24 hours of kidney transplant (but may be delayed until renal function has recovered); titrate to target trough concentrations. Adjunctive therapy with corticosteroids is recommended early post-transplant. IV route should only be used in patients not able to take oral medications and continued only until oral medication can be tolerated; anaphylaxis has been reported with IV administration. If switching from IV to oral, the oral dose should be started 8 to 12 hours after stopping the infusion.

Liver transplant:

Oral:

Immediate release: Initial: 0.1 to 0.15 mg/kg/day in 2 divided doses, given every 12 hours (titrate to target trough concentrations)

Extended release: Canadian labeling (Advagraf): 0.1 to 0.2 mg/kg once daily in combination with corticosteroids; initiate within 12 to 18 hours of transplantation. Titrate to target trough concentrations.

Conversion from immediate release to extended release: Patients stable on immediate release tacrolimus may be converted to extended release by initiating extended-release treatment in a 1:1 ratio (mg:mg) using previously established total daily dose of immediate-release product. Administer once daily.

IV: Initial: 0.03 to 0.05 mg/kg/day as a continuous infusion

◀ **Heart transplant:** Use in combination with azathioprine or mycophenolate mofetil is recommended.

Oral: Immediate release: Initial: 0.075 mg/kg/day in 2 divided doses, given every 12 hours (titrate to target trough concentrations)

IV: Initial: 0.01 mg/kg/day as a continuous infusion

Kidney transplant: Use in combination with azathioprine or mycophenolate mofetil is recommended. **Note:** African-American patients may require larger doses to attain trough concentration.

Oral:

US labeling:

Immediate release (Hecoria, Prograf): Initial: 0.2 mg/kg/day in combination with azathioprine or 0.1 mg/kg/day in combination with mycophenolate mofetil; titrate to target trough concentrations. Administer in 2 divided doses, given every 12 hours.

Extended release (Astagraf XL):

With basiliximab induction (prior to or within 48 hours of transplant completion): 0.15 mg/kg once daily (in combination with corticosteroids and mycophenolate); titrate to target trough concentrations

Without basiliximab induction: Preoperative dose (administer within 12 hours prior to reperfusion): 0.1 mg/kg

Without basiliximab induction: Postoperative dosing (administer at least 4 hours after preoperative dose and within 12 hours of reperfusion): 0.2 mg/kg once daily (in combination with corticosteroids and mycophenolate); titrate to target trough concentrations

Conversion from IV to extended release: Administer the first oral extended release dose 8 to 12 hours after discontinuation of IV tacrolimus

Conversion from immediate release to extended release: Initiate extended release treatment in a 1:1 ratio (mg:mg) using previously established total daily dose of immediate release (Van Hooff 2012). Administer once daily.

Extended release (Envarsus XR): Conversion from immediate release to extended release: Initiate extended-release treatment with a once-daily dose that is 80% of the total daily dose of the immediate-release tacrolimus

Canadian labeling:

Immediate release (Prograf): Initial: 0.2 to 0.3 mg/kg/day in 2 divided doses, given every 12 hours in combination with corticosteroids and other immunosuppressive agents; titrate to target trough concentrations

Extended release (Advagraf): Initial: 0.15 to 0.2 mg/kg once daily; titrate to target trough concentrations. Administer in combination with corticosteroids and mycophenolate mofetil (MMF) in *de novo* kidney transplant recipients. Antibody induction therapy should also be used.

Conversion from immediate release to extended release: Initiate extended release treatment in a 1:1 ratio (mg:mg) using previously established total daily dose of immediate release. Administer once daily.

IV: Initial: 0.03 to 0.05 mg/kg/day as a continuous infusion

Graft-versus-host disease (GVHD) (off-label use):

Prevention:

Oral: Convert from IV to immediate release oral dose (1:4 ratio): Multiply total daily IV dose times 4 and administer in 2 divided oral doses per day, every 12 hours (Uberti 1999; Yanik 2000).

IV: Initial: 0.03 mg/kg/day (based on lean body weight) as continuous infusion. Treatment should begin at least 24 hours prior to stem cell infusion and continued only until oral medication can be tolerated (Przepiorka 1999; Yanik 2000).

Treatment:

Oral: Immediate release: 0.06 mg/kg twice daily (Furlong 2000; Przepiorka 1999)

IV: Initial: 0.03 mg/kg/day (based on lean body weight) as continuous infusion (Furlong 2000; Przepiorka 1999)

Lung transplant (off-label use):

Oral, nasogastric: Immediate release: 0.05 to 0.3 mg/kg/day in 2 divided doses, given every 12 hours (usual dose: 0.05 mg/kg every 12 hours); titrate to target trough concentrations (Treede 2001; Treede 2012; Zuckermann 2003). May also be administered sublingually at ~50% of the oral/NG dose (Doligalski 2014; Watkins 2012).

Note: May convert from twice-daily dosing to once-daily dosing (on a mg per mg basis) using the extended-release formulation (Astagraf XL [US] or Advagraf [Canada]) in stable lung transplant recipients (Mendez 2014).

IV: 0.01 to 0.05 mg/kg over 24 hours as a continuous IV infusion; titrate to target trough concentrations (Treede 2001; Treede 2012; Zuckermann 2003). For patients receiving the initial dose of tacrolimus intravenously, may begin immediately after transplantation, or up to 2 days postoperatively depending on renal function and hemodynamic stability (Treede 2001; Treede 2012; Witt 2013; Zuckermann 2003). When patient is able to take oral medication, may switch to an oral maintenance regimen (typically transitioned after extubation).

Rheumatoid arthritis: Canadian labeling (not in US labeling): Oral: Immediate release: 3 mg once daily; carefully monitor serum creatinine during therapy

Pediatric

Liver transplant:

Oral: Immediate release: Initial: 0.15-0.20 mg/kg/day in 2 divided doses, given every 12 hours (titrate to target trough concentrations)

IV: Initial: 0.03-0.05 mg/kg/day as a continuous infusion

Note: The initial postoperative dose of tacrolimus should begin no sooner than 6 hours after liver and heart transplant and within 24 hours of kidney transplant (but may be delayed until renal function has recovered). Adjunctive therapy with corticosteroids is recommended early post-transplant. IV route should only be used in patients not able to take oral medications and continued only until oral medication can be tolerated; anaphylaxis has been reported with IV administration. If switching from IV to oral, the oral dose should be started 8-12 hours after stopping the infusion. Patients without preexisting renal or hepatic dysfunction have required (and tolerated) higher doses than adults to achieve similar blood concentrations. It is recommended that therapy be initiated at the **high end** of the recommended adult IV and oral dosing ranges; dosage adjustments may be required.

Prevention of graft-vs-host disease (GVHD) (off-label use): Oral, IV: Refer to adult dosing.

◀ **Renal Impairment** Evidence suggests that lower doses should be used; patients should receive doses at the lowest value of the recommended IV and oral dosing ranges; further reductions in dose below these ranges may be required. May also require dose reductions due to nephrotoxicity.

Kidney transplant: Tacrolimus therapy in patients with postoperative oliguria should begin no sooner than 6 hours and within 24 hours (immediate release) or 48 hours (extended release) post-transplant, but may be delayed until renal function displays evidence of recovery.

Hemodialysis: Not removed by hemodialysis; supplemental dose is not necessary.

Peritoneal dialysis: Significant drug removal is unlikely based on physio-chemical characteristics.

Hepatic Impairment Use of tacrolimus in liver transplant recipients experiencing post-transplant hepatic impairment may be associated with increased risk of developing renal insufficiency related to high whole blood levels of tacrolimus. The presence of moderate-to-severe hepatic dysfunction (serum bilirubin >2 mg/dL; Child-Pugh score ≥10) appears to affect the metabolism of tacrolimus. The half-life of the drug was prolonged and the clearance reduced after IV administration. The bioavailability of tacrolimus was also increased after oral administration. The higher plasma concentrations as determined by ELISA, in patients with severe hepatic dysfunction are probably due to the accumulation of metabolites of lower activity. These patients should be monitored closely and dosage adjustments should be considered. Some evidence indicates that lower doses could be used in these patients.

Administration

IV: If IV administration is necessary, administer by continuous infusion only. Do not use PVC tubing when administering diluted solutions. Tacrolimus is usually intended to be administered as a continuous infusion over 24 hours. Do not mix with solutions with a pH ≥9 (eg, acyclovir or ganciclovir) due to chemical degradation of tacrolimus (use different ports in multilumen lines). Do not alter dose with concurrent T-tube clamping. Adsorption of the drug to PVC tubing may become clinically significant with low concentrations.

Oral:

Immediate release: Administer with or without food; be consistent with timing and composition of meals if GI intolerance occurs and administration with food becomes necessary (per manufacturer). If dosed once daily, administer in the morning. If dosed twice daily, doses should be 12 hours apart. If the morning and evening doses differ, the larger dose (differences are never >0.5-1 mg) should be given in the morning. If dosed 3 times daily, separate doses by 8 hours.

Combination therapy with everolimus for liver transplantation: Administer tacrolimus at the same time as everolimus.

Extended release: Administer on an empty stomach at least 1 hour before or 2 hours after a meal. Advagraf [Canadian product] labeling suggests that the capsule may be taken with food if necessary but should be administered consistently with or without food. Swallow whole, do not chew, crush, or divide. Take once daily in the morning at a consistent time each day. Missed doses may be taken up to 14 hours (15 hours for Envarsus XR) after scheduled time; if >14 hours (>15 hours for Enbarsus XR), resume at next regularly scheduled time; do not double a dose to make up for a missed dose.

Nasogastric tube: In patients unable to swallow capsules, contents of immediate release capsule(s) may be mixed with water and flushed through a nasogastric tube; clamp nasogastric tube for 30 to 60 minutes after administration (Taylor 2001).

Sublingual: In patients unable to swallow capsules, tacrolimus may be administered sublingually (at a reduced dose) by opening the immediate-release capsules and placing the contents of the capsule(s) under the tongue allowing contents to completely dissolve; avoid food, beverages, or mechanical suctioning for at least 30 minutes after administration (Doligalski 2014; Watkins 2012).

Hazardous agent; use appropriate precautions for handling and disposal (NIOSH 2014 [group 2]). Avoid contact with broken capsules. If it is necessary to manipulate capsules (eg, to open capsules or prepare an oral suspension), it is recommended to double glove, wear a protective gown, and prepare in a controlled device (NIOSH 2014).

Extemporaneous Preparations Hazardous agent; use appropriate precautions for handling and disposal (NIOSH 2014 [group 2]). When manipulating capsules, NIOSH recommends double gloving, a protective gown, and preparation in a controlled device; if not prepared in a controlled device, respiratory and eye protection as well as ventilated engineering controls are recommended (NIOSH 2014).

A 0.5 mg/mL tacrolimus oral suspension may be made with immediate release capsules and a 1:1 mixture of Ora-Plus and Simple Syrup, N.F. Mix the contents of six 5 mg tacrolimus capsules with quantity of vehicle sufficient to make 60 mL. Store in glass or plastic amber prescription bottles; label "shake well". Stable for 56 days at room temperature (Esquivel 1996; Foster 1996).

A 1 mg/mL tacrolimus oral suspension may be made with immediate release capsules, sterile water, Ora-Plus, and Ora-Sweet. Pour the contents of six 5 mg capsules into a plastic amber prescription bottle. Add ~5 mL of sterile water and agitate bottle until drug disperses into a slurry. Add equal parts Ora-Plus and Ora-Sweet in sufficient quantity to make 30 mL. Store in plastic amber prescription bottles; label "shake well". Stable for 4 months at room temperature (Elefante 2006).

Elefante A, Muindi J, West K, et al, "Long-Term Stability of a Patient-Convenient 1 mg/mL Suspension of Tacrolimus for Accurate Maintenance of Stable Therapeutic Levels," *Bone Marrow Transplant*. 2006, 37(8):781-4.

Esquivel C, So S, McDiarmid S, Andrews W, and Colombani PM, "Suggested Guidelines for the Use of Tacrolimus in Pediatric Liver Transplant Patients," *Transplantation*, 1996, 61(5):847-8.

Foster JA, Jacobson PA, Johnson CE, et al, "Stability of Tacrolimus in an Extemporaneously Compounded Oral Liquid (Abstract of Meeting Presentation)," *American Society of Health-System Pharmacists Annual Meeting*, 1996, 53:P-52(E).

Monitoring Parameters Renal function, hepatic function, serum electrolytes (calcium, magnesium, potassium), glucose and blood pressure, measure 3 times/week for first few weeks, then gradually decrease frequency as patient stabilizes. Whole blood concentrations should be used for monitoring (trough for oral therapy); frequency varies depending on transplant type, time since transplantation, and clinical situation. Signs/symptoms of anaphylactic reactions during IV infusion should also be monitored. Patients should be monitored for hypersensitivity during the first 30 minutes of the infusion, and frequently thereafter. Monitor for QT prolongation; consider echocardiographic evaluation in patients who develop renal failure, electrolyte abnormalities, or clinical manifestations of ventricular dysfunction.

◄ Tacrolimus serum levels may be falsely elevated in infected liver transplant patients due to interference from β-galactosidase antibodies.

Dietary Considerations Capsule: Administer immediate release with or without food; be consistent with timing and composition of meals, food decreases bioavailability. Administer extended release on an empty stomach 1 hour before or 2 hours after a meal. Avoid grapefruit and grapefruit juice. Avoid alcohol.

Medication Guide Available Yes

Dosage Forms Considerations Prograf injection contains polyoxyl 60 hydrogenated castor oil (HCO-60)

Dosage Forms Excipient information presented when available (limited, particularly for generics); consult specific product labeling. [DSC] = Discontinued product

Capsule, Oral:

  Hecoria: 0.5 mg [DSC], 1 mg [DSC], 5 mg [DSC]

  Prograf: 0.5 mg, 1 mg, 5 mg

  Generic: 0.5 mg, 1 mg, 5 mg

Capsule Extended Release 24 Hour, Oral:

  Astagraf XL: 0.5 mg, 1 mg, 5 mg

Solution, Intravenous:

  Prograf: 5 mg/mL (1 mL) [contains alcohol, usp, cremophor el]

Tablet Extended Release 24 Hour, Oral:

  Envarsus XR: 0.75 mg, 1 mg, 4 mg

Dosage Forms: Canada Note: Also refer to Dosage Forms

Excipient information presented when available (limited, particularly for generics); consult specific product labeling.

Capsule Extended Release 24 Hour, Oral:

  Advagraf: 0.5 mg, 1 mg, 3 mg, 5 mg

◆ **Tafinlar** see Dabrafenib on page 420

◆ **Tagrisso** see Osimertinib on page 1265

◆ **Talc** see Talc (Sterile) on page 1588

◆ **Talc for Pleurodesis** see Talc (Sterile) on page 1588

Talc (Sterile) (talk STARE il)

Related Information

  Malignant Pleural Effusions on page 2246

Brand Names: US Sclerosol Intrapleural; Sterile Talc Powder

Index Terms Intrapleural Talc; Sterile Talc; Talc; Talc for Pleurodesis

Pharmacologic Category Sclerosing Agent

Use Pleural effusion, malignant: Sclerosing agent to decrease or prevent the recurrence of malignant pleural effusion in symptomatic patients (following maximal drainage of pleural effusion)

Labeled Contraindications There are no contraindications listed in the manufacturer's labeling.

Pregnancy Considerations Adverse events were not observed in animal reproduction studies. Use during pregnancy only if clearly needed.

Breast-Feeding Considerations It is not known if sterile talc is excreted in breast milk.

Warnings/Precautions Acute pneumonitis and acute respiratory distress syndrome (ARDS), including fatalities have been reported with intrapleural talc administration; most cases of ARDS occurred with talc doses of 10 g via a chest tube. Products are for intrapleural use only; IV administration (not recommended) is associated with pulmonary hypertension and lung parenchymal disease. Silicosis or asbestosis-like conditions (chronic bronchitis, bronchogenic carcinoma, and pleural plaques) are associated with inhaled talc. Should not be used for potentially curable malignancies where systemic therapy would be more appropriate (sterile talc does not have antineoplastic activity). Clinicians should evaluate need for future diagnostic or surgical procedures before use; sclerosis of pleural space may preclude or complicate subsequent procedures (eg, pneumonectomy for transplantation). Sclerosol contents under pressure and should be kept away from any heat source or open flame; do not puncture canister.

Adverse Reactions Frequency not defined.

Cardiovascular: Asystolic arrest, chest pain, hypotension (transient), hypovolemia, MI, tachycardia

Central nervous system: Fever (generally lasting <24 hours)

Local: Bleeding (localized), infection at administration site, pain

Respiratory: ARDS, bronchopleural fistula, dyspnea, empyema, hemoptysis, hypoxemia, pneumonia, pulmonary edema, pulmonary embolism, subcutaneous emphysema

Storage/Stability

Sclerosol Intrapleural Aerosol: Store at 20°C to 25°C (68°F to 77°F); excursions are permitted between 15°C and 30°C (59°F and 86°F); do not expose to temperatures above 49°C (120°F). Do not freeze. Protect from sunlight.

Sterile Talc Powder: Store at 25°C (77°F); excursions are permitted between 15°C and 30°C (59°F and 86°F). Protect from sunlight. If not used immediately after mixing, refrigerate and use within 12 hours of preparation.

Preparation for Administration

Sclerosol Intrapleural Aerosol: Shake well.

Sterile Talc Powder: Vent bottle with needle; slowly add NS 50 mL to bottle using aseptic technique. Swirl the bottle to disperse talc and avoid settling. Divide the contents of bottle into two 60 mL syringes (25 mL of talc suspension in each). Add an additional NS 25 mL to each syringe for a total of 50 mL (2.5 g/50 mL). Draw syringe back to add 10 mL air to facilitate mixing prior to administration. Shake well to resuspend prior to use. If not used immediately, label "For pleurodesis only; **NOT for IV administration**."

Mechanism of Action Induces an inflammatory reaction, promoting adherence of the visceral to the parietal pleura, therefore, preventing reaccumulation of pleural fluid.

Pharmacodynamics/Kinetics Absorption: Not well studied; systemic exposure may be influenced by integrity of visceral pleura

Dosing

Adult

Pleural effusion, malignant:

Intrapleural aerosol: 4 to 8 g (1 to 2 cans) as a single dose

Intrapleural suspension: 5 g

Renal Impairment There are no dosage adjustments provided in the manufacturer's labeling.

Hepatic Impairment There are no dosage adjustments provided in the manufacturer's labeling.

◀ **Administration** For intrapleural administration. Administer after adequate drainage of the effusion.

Sclerosol Intrapleural Aerosol: Shake well and attach delivery tube. Insert delivery tube through pleural trocar, manually press on actuator button of canister to release; point in several different directions to distribute to all pleural surfaces. Keep canister in an upright position for optimal distribution. Rate of delivery is 1.2 g per second.

Sterile Talc Powder: Administer as a suspension. Shake well before instillation. Vent the10 mL air headspace and empty contents of each syringe into chest cavity through the chest tube by gently applying pressure to syringe plunger. After administration, clamp the chest tube for 1 to 2 hours and then drain the pleural fluid; the chest tube can be removed when drainage is <100 to 150 mL/24 hours (Dresler, 2005; Kvale, 2002). For intrapleural use only; **not for IV administration.**

Dosage Forms Excipient information presented when available (limited, particularly for generics); consult specific product labeling.

Aerosol Powder, Intrapleural:

Sclerosol Intrapleural: 4 g (30 g) [contains dichlorodifluoromethane]

Suspension Reconstituted, Intrapleural:

Sterile Talc Powder: 5 g (1 ea)

Talimogene Laherparepvec (tal IM oh jeen la her pa REP vek)

Related Information

Safe Handling of Hazardous Drugs *on page 2292*

Brand Names: US Imlygic

Index Terms GM-CSF-Encoding Oncolytic Herpes Simplex Virus; Imlygic; OncoVEX GM-CSF; T-VEC; Talminogene Laherparepvec

Pharmacologic Category Antineoplastic Agent, Oncolytic Virus

Use

Melanoma, unresectable: Treatment (local) of unresectable cutaneous, subcutaneous, and nodal lesions in patients with melanoma recurrent after initial surgery

Limitations of use: Has not been shown to improve overall survival or have an effect on visceral metastases.

Labeled Contraindications Immunocompromised patients, including those with a history of primary or acquired immunodeficient states, leukemia, lymphoma, AIDS or other clinical manifestations of infection with human immunodeficiency viruses, and those on immunosuppressive therapy; pregnancy

Pregnancy Considerations Use is contraindicated in pregnant women.

Women of reproductive potential should use effective contraception during therapy. Talimogene laherparepvec is a live, attenuated, genetically modified herpes simplex virus type 1 (HSV-1). HSV-1 is known to cross the placenta, can be transmitted during birth, and produce infections in the fetus or neonate. It is not known if this can occur following exposure to talimogene laherparepvec. Pregnant women should not prepare or administer this medication. Pregnant women who are in close contact of patients treated with talimogene laherparepvec should not change dressings or clean injection sites, and should avoid direct contact with the injection site, dressings, or body fluids of patients.

Breast-Feeding Considerations It is not known if talimogene laherparepvec is excreted in breast milk. The manufacturer recommends a decision be made to discontinue nursing or to discontinue the drug, taking into account the importance of treatment to the mother.

Warnings/Precautions Hazardous agent - use appropriate precautions for handling and disposal (meets NIOSH 2014 criteria). Health care providers who are immunocompromised or pregnant should not prepare or administer talimogene laherparepvec. Accidental talimogene laherparepvec exposure may lead to herpetic infection. Health care providers, close contacts (eg, household members, caregivers, sex partners, or persons sharing the same bed), pregnant women, and newborns should avoid direct contact with injected lesions, dressings, or body fluids of patients treated with talimogene laherparepvec. Protective gloves should be worn when assisting patients with dressing changes; safely dispose of used dressings, gloves, and cleaning materials. Needle stick and/or splashback to the eyes have been reported during talimogene laherparepvec preparation and administration. If accidently exposed to talimogene laherparepvec, clean the affected area thoroughly with soap and water and/or a disinfectant. Contact a health care provider if signs/symptoms of herpetic infection develop. Counsel patients to avoid touching or scratching injection site(s) or the dressings (may lead to inadvertent transfer of drug to other parts of the body).

Herpetic infections (eg, cold sores and herpetic keratitis) have been reported; disseminated herpetic infection may occur in immunocompromised patients. If herpes-like lesions develop, follow standard practice to prevent viral transmission; contact a health care provider for evaluation. Suspected herpetic lesions should be reported to Amgen at 1-855-465-9442. Talimogene laherparepvec is sensitive to acyclovir. Acyclovir (or other antiviral medications) may interfere with the efficacy of talimogene laherparepvec; consider the risks and benefits of treatment prior to administering antiviral agents. Immune-mediated events (eg, glomerulonephritis, pneumonitis, vasculitis, vitiligo, and worsening psoriasis) have been reported in clinical studies. Consider risk/benefit ratio of initiating treatment in patients with underlying autoimmune disease or prior to continuing talimogene laherparepvec treatment in patients who develop immune-mediated events.

Injection-site complications, such as necrosis, tumor tissue ulceration, and impaired healing may occur during treatment with talimogene laherparepvec. Cellulitis and system bacterial infection have been observed. Monitor wounds carefully; infection precautions are recommended, particularly if tissue necrosis results in open wounds. Patients with underlying risk factors for impaired wound healing (eg, previous radiation at the injection site or lesions in poorly vascularized areas) may be at risk for complications. One patient had a lower extremity amputation 6 months after talimogene laherparepvec administration due to an infected non-healing wound. Monitor closely. Consider risk/benefit of continued treatment in patients with persistent infection or impaired wound healing at injection site(s). In one clinical study, a patient with smoldering multiple myeloma developed a plasmacytoma near the talimogene laherparepvec injection site. Consider the risks/benefits of talimogene laherparepvec therapy in patients with multiple myeloma or in those who develop plasmacytoma during treatment. Potentially significant interactions may exist, requiring dose or frequency adjustment, additional monitoring, and/or selection of alternative therapy. Talimogene laherparepvec is available in two different dose strengths: 10^6 (1 million) plaque-forming units (PFU) per mL (initial dose only), and 10^8 (100 million) PFU per mL (all subsequent doses). Verify appropriate dose and vial prior to preparation and administration.

◄ **Adverse Reactions** Frequency not always defined. Most reactions resolved within 72 hours.

Cardiovascular: Vasculitis

Central nervous system: Fatigue (50%), chills (49%), headache (19%), dizziness (10%)

Dermatologic: Cellulitis, exacerbation of psoriasis, vitiligo

Endocrine & metabolic: Weight loss (6%)

Gastrointestinal: Nausea (36%), vomiting (21%), diarrhea (19%), constipation (12%), abdominal pain (9%), oral herpes

Infection: Bacterial infection (systemic), herpes virus infection

Local: Pain at injection site (28%), inflammation at injection site (tumor tissue ulceration), injection site lesion (plasmacytoma), injection site reaction (impaired healing; previous radiation or poorly vascularized lesion may increase risk), tissue necrosis at injection site

Neuromuscular & skeletal: Myalgia (18%), arthralgia (17%), pain in extremity (16%)

Renal: Glomerulonephritis

Respiratory: Flu-like symptoms (31%), oropharyngeal pain (6%), pneumonitis

Miscellaneous: Fever (43%)

Drug Interactions

Metabolism/Transport Effects None known.

Avoid Concomitant Use There are no known interactions where it is recommended to avoid concomitant use.

Increased Effect/Toxicity There are no known significant interactions involving an increase in effect.

Decreased Effect

The levels/effects of Talimogene Laherparepvec may be decreased by: Antiherpetic Antivirals

Storage/Stability Store intact vials at -90°C to -70°C (-130°F to -94°F); protect from light. Store vials in the carton until use. Thaw vials immediately prior to administration. If not used immediately, may store (in the original vial and carton) refrigerated at 2°C to 8°C (36°F to 46°F) for up to 12 hours (for the 10^6 [1 million] PFU per mL strength) or up to 48 hours (for the 10^8 [100 million] PFU per mL strength). Do not refreeze vials after thawing; discard any vial left in the refrigerator if longer than the specified times. After thawed, do not shake.

Preparation for Administration Hazardous agent; use appropriate precautions for handling and disposal (meets NIOSH 2014 criteria). Health care providers who are immunocompromised or pregnant should not prepare or administer talimogene laherparepvec and should not handle injection sites, dressings, or body fluids of treated patients. Personal protective equipment (eg, gown or laboratory coat, safety glasses or face shield, and gloves) should be worn during preparation or administration. Cover any exposed wounds prior to handling talimogene laherparepvec. If accidental exposure occurs through an eye splash or a splash to mucous membranes, flush the area with clean water for at least 15 minutes. If exposure to broken skin or a needle stick occurs, clean the affected area thoroughly with soap and water and/or a disinfectant. Treat spills with virucidal agent such as sodium hypochlorite 1% and blot using absorbent materials. Dispose of all materials that may have come into contact with talimogene laherparepvec in compliance with universal biohazard precautions.

Thaw vials at room temperature until talimogene laherparepvec is liquid (~30 minutes); do not thaw at higher temperatures. Keep vial in the original carton during thawing. Swirl gently; do not shake. Administer immediately after thawing or store in the refrigerator for 12 to 48 hours (vial strength dependent; see Storage/Stability for details). Do not refreeze after thawing. Withdraw the vial contents (using a detachable needle of 18 to 26 gauge) into the syringe (note the total volume). Avoid generating aerosols; use a biologic safety cabinet if available.

Mechanism of Action Talimogene laherparepvec is a genetically modified attenuated herpes simplex virus 1 (HSV) oncolytic virus which selectively replicates in and lyses tumor cells (Andtbacka 2015). Talimogene laherparepvec is modified through deletion of two nonessential viral genes. Deletion of the herpes virus neurovirulence factor gene ICP34.5 diminishes viral pathogenicity and increases tumor-selective replication; deletion of the ICP47 gene reduces virally mediated suppression of antigen presentation and increases the expression of the HSV US11 gene (Andtback, 2015). Virally derived GM-CSF recruits and activates antigen-presenting cells, leading to an antitumor immune response.

Pharmacodynamics/Kinetics Time to peak: Peak levels of talimogene laherparepvec were detected in the urine on the day of treatment

Dosing

Adult & Geriatric Note: Administer by intralesional injection into cutaneous, subcutaneous, and/or nodal lesions that are visible, palpable, or detectable by ultrasound. It may not be possible to inject all lesions at each treatment visit or over the full course of treatment. Previously injected and/or uninjected lesion(s) may be treated at subsequent visits.

Melanoma, unresectable: Intralesional: Maximum volume (per treatment visit, for all injected lesions combined): 4 mL. Continue treatment for at least 6 months unless other therapy is necessary or until there are no injectable lesions to treat. Reinitiate treatment if new unresectable lesions appear after a previous complete response.

Use the following to determine the volume of talimogene laherparepvec to be injected (lesion size is based on longest dimension; when lesions are clustered together, inject them as a single lesion):
- If the lesion size is >5 cm, inject up to 4 mL
- If the lesion size is >2.5 cm to 5 cm, inject up to 2 mL
- If the lesion size is >1.5 cm to 2.5 cm, inject up to 1 mL
- If the lesion size is >0.5 cm to 1.5 cm, inject up to 0.5 mL
- If the lesion size is ≤0.5 cm, inject up to 0.1 mL

Initial treatment visit: Inject up to 4 mL at a concentration of 10^6 (1 million) PFU/mL. Inject largest lesion(s) first; inject remaining lesion(s) based on lesion size until maximum injection volume is reached or all lesions have been treated.

Second treatment visit (3 weeks after initial treatment): Inject up to 4 mL at a concentration of 10^8 (100 million) PFU/mL. Inject any new lesion(s) that have developed since initial treatment first; inject remaining lesion(s) based on lesion size until maximum injection volume is reached or all lesions have been treated.

◄ *All subsequent treatment visits, including reinitiation (2 weeks after previous treatment):* Inject up to 4 mL at a concentration of 10^8 (100 million) PFU/mL. Inject any new lesion(s) that have developed since previous treatment first; inject remaining lesion(s) based on lesion size until maximum injection volume is reached or all lesions have been treated.

Renal Impairment Dosage adjustment for renal impairment: There are no dosage adjustments provided in the manufacturer's labeling (has not been studied).

Hepatic Impairment Dosage adjustment for hepatic impairment: There are no dosage adjustments provided in the manufacturer's labeling (has not been studied).

Administration Administer by intralesional injection into cutaneous, subcutaneous, and/or nodal lesions that are visible, palpable, or detectable by ultrasound. Clean the lesion and surrounding areas with alcohol and allow to dry. If necessary, treat the injection site with a topical or local anesthetic agent (but do not inject the anesthetic directly into the lesion [inject around periphery of lesion]). Using a single insertion point, inject talimogene laherparepvec (using a 22 to 26 gauge needle) along multiple tracks as far as the needle allows within the lesion to achieve dispersion; multiple lesion points may be used if a lesion is larger than the radial reach of the needle.

Inject talimogene laherparepvec evenly and completely within the lesion by pulling the needle back without removing it from the lesion. Redirect the needle as necessary while injecting the remainder of the dose; continue until the full dose is evenly and completely dispersed. Remove the needle from the lesion slowly to avoid leakage. Repeat steps for other lesions to be treated. Use a new needle if the needle is completely removed from a lesion and each time a different lesion is injected. Apply pressure with sterile gauze for at least 30 seconds after the injection is completed; swab the injection site(s) and surrounding areas with alcohol. Change gloves, then cover lesion(s) with an absorbent pad and dry occlusive dressing, and wipe the exterior of the dressing with alcohol. The injection site should be covered for at least the first week after each treatment or longer if the injection site is weeping or oozing (replace dressing if it falls off).

Hazardous agent; use appropriate precautions for handling and disposal (meets NIOSH 2014 criteria).. Immunocompromised or pregnant health care providers should not prepare or administer talimogene laherparepvec and should have direct contact with injections sites, dressings, or body fluids of treated patients. Avoid accidental exposure; follow biohazard precautions (personal protective equipment) for administration. Patients should place used dressings and cleaning materials in a sealed plastic bag and dispose of with household waste

Monitoring Parameters Monitor for signs/symptoms of herpetic infections (eg, cold sores and herpetic keratitis), injection-site complications, and immune-mediated events

Medication Guide Available Yes

Dosage Forms Excipient information presented when available (limited, particularly for generics); consult specific product labeling.
Suspension, Intralesional [preservative free]:
Imlygic: 10^6 (1 million) PFU/mL (1 mL); 10^8 (100 million) PFU/mL (1 mL) [contains bovine serum]

◆ **Talminogene Laherparepvec** *see* Talimogene Laherparepvec *on page 1590*

Tamoxifen (ta MOKS i fen)

Related Information
Chemotherapy and Cancer Treatment During Pregnancy *on page 2214*
Hypercalcemia of Malignancy *on page 2241*
Safe Handling of Hazardous Drugs *on page 2292*

Brand Names: US Soltamox

Brand Names: Canada Apo-Tamox; Mylan-Tamoxifen; Nolvadex-D; PMS-Tamoxifen; Teva-Tamoxifen

Index Terms ICI-46474; Nolvadex; Tamoxifen Citras; Tamoxifen Citrate

Pharmacologic Category Antineoplastic Agent, Estrogen Receptor Antagonist; Selective Estrogen Receptor Modulator (SERM)

Use Treatment of metastatic (female and male) breast cancer; adjuvant treatment of breast cancer after primary treatment with surgery and radiation; reduce risk of invasive breast cancer in women with ductal carcinoma *in situ* (DCIS) after surgery and radiation; reduce the incidence of breast cancer in women at high risk

Labeled Contraindications Hypersensitivity to tamoxifen or any component of the formulation; concurrent warfarin therapy or history of deep vein thrombosis or pulmonary embolism (when tamoxifen is used for breast cancer risk reduction in women at high risk for breast cancer or with ductal carcinoma *in situ* [DCIS])

Pregnancy Considerations Animal reproduction studies have demonstrated fetal adverse effects and fetal loss. There have been reports of vaginal bleeding, birth defects and fetal loss in pregnant women. Tamoxifen use during pregnancy may have a potential long term risk to the fetus of a DES-like syndrome. For sexually-active women of childbearing age, initiate during menstruation (negative β-hCG immediately prior to initiation in women with irregular cycles). Tamoxifen may induce ovulation. Barrier or nonhormonal contraceptives are recommended. Pregnancy should be avoided during treatment and for 2 months after treatment has been discontinued.

Breast-Feeding Considerations It is not known if tamoxifen is excreted in breast milk, however, it has been shown to inhibit lactation. Due to the potential for adverse reactions, women taking tamoxifen should not breast-feed.

Warnings/Precautions Hazardous agent - use appropriate precautions for handling and disposal (NIOSH 2014 [group 1]). **[U.S. Boxed Warning]: Serious and life-threatening events (some fatal), including stroke, pulmonary emboli, and uterine or endometrial malignancies, have occurred at an incidence greater than placebo during use for breast cancer risk reduction in women at high-risk for breast cancer and in women with ductal carcinoma *in situ* (DCIS). In women already diagnosed with breast cancer, the benefits of tamoxifen treatment outweigh risks; evaluate risks versus benefits (and discuss with patients) when used for breast cancer risk reduction.** An increased incidence of thromboembolic events, including DVT and pulmonary embolism, has been associated with use for breast cancer; risk is increased with concomitant chemotherapy; use with caution in individuals with a history of thromboembolic events. Thrombocytopenia and/or leukopenia may occur; neutropenia and pancytopenia have been reported rarely. Although the relationship to tamoxifen therapy is uncertain, rare hemorrhagic episodes have occurred in patients with significant thrombocytopenia. Use with caution in patients with hyperlipidemias; infrequent postmarketing cases of hyperlipidemias have been reported. Decreased visual acuity, retinal vein thrombosis, retinopathy, corneal changes, color perception changes, and

◀ increased incidence of cataracts (and the need for cataract surgery), have been reported. Hypercalcemia has occurred in some patients with bone metastasis, usually within a few weeks of therapy initiation; institute appropriate hypercalcemia management; discontinue if severe. Local disease flare and increased bone and tumor pain may occur in patients with metastatic breast cancer; may be associated with (good) tumor response.

Potentially significant drug-drug interactions may exist, requiring dose or frequency adjustment, additional monitoring, and/or selection of alternative therapy. Decreased efficacy and an increased risk of breast cancer recurrence has been reported with concurrent moderate or strong CYP2D6 inhibitors (Aubert, 2009; Dezentje, 2009). Concomitant use with select SSRIs may result in decreased tamoxifen efficacy. Strong CYP2D6 inhibitors (eg, fluoxetine, paroxetine) and moderate CYP2D6 inhibitors (eg, sertraline) are reported to interfere with transformation to the active metabolite endoxifen; when possible, select alternative medications with minimal or no impact on endoxifen levels (NCCN Breast Cancer Risk Reduction Guidelines v.1.2013; Sideras, 2010). Weak CYP2D6 inhibitors (eg, venlafaxine, citalopram) have minimal effect on the conversion to endoxifen (Jin, 2005; NCCN Breast Cancer Risk Reduction Guidelines v.1.2013); escitalopram is also a weak CYP2D6 inhibitor. In a retrospective analysis of breast cancer patients taking tamoxifen and SSRIs, concomitant use of paroxetine and tamoxifen was associated with an increased risk of death due to breast cancer (Kelly, 2010). Lower plasma concentrations of endoxifen have been observed in patients associated with reduced CYP2D6 activity (Jin, 2005; Schroth, 2009) and may be associated with reduced efficacy, although data is conflicting. Routine CYP2D6 testing is not recommended at this time in order to determine optimal endocrine therapy (NCCN Breast Cancer Guidelines v.2.2013; Visvanathan, 2009).

Tamoxifen use may be associated with changes in bone mineral density (BMD) and the effects may be dependent upon menstrual status. In postmenopausal women, tamoxifen use is associated with a protective effect on bone mineral density (BMD), preventing loss of BMD which lasts over the 5-year treatment period. In premenopausal women, a decline (from baseline) in BMD mineral density has been observed in women who continued to menstruate; may be associated with an increased risk of fractures. Liver abnormalities such as cholestasis, fatty liver, hepatitis, and hepatic necrosis have occurred. Hepatocellular carcinomas have been reported in some studies; relationship to treatment is unclear. Tamoxifen is associated with an increased incidence of uterine or endometrial cancers. Endometrial hyperplasia, polyps, endometriosis, uterine fibroids, and ovarian cysts have occurred. Monitor and promptly evaluate any report of abnormal vaginal bleeding. Amenorrhea and menstrual irregularities have been reported with tamoxifen use.

Adverse Reactions
>10%:
    Cardiovascular: Vasodilation (41%), flushing (33%), hypertension (11%), peripheral edema (11%)
    Central nervous system: Mood changes (12% to 18%), pain (3% to 16%), depression (2% to 12%)
    Dermatologic: Skin changes (6% to 19%), rash (13%)
    Endocrine & metabolic: Hot flashes (3% to 80%), fluid retention (32%), altered menses (13% to 25%), amenorrhea (16%)
    Gastrointestinal: Nausea (5% to 26%), weight loss (23%), vomiting (12%)
    Genitourinary: Vaginal discharge (13% to 55%), vaginal bleeding (2% to 23%)

Neuromuscular & skeletal: Weakness (18%), arthritis (14%), arthralgia (11%)

Respiratory: Pharyngitis (14%)

Miscellaneous: Lymphedema (11%)

1% to 10%:

Cardiovascular: Chest pain (5%), venous thrombotic events (5%), edema (4%), cardiovascular ischemia (3%), angina (2%), deep venous thrombus (≤2%), MI (1%)

Central nervous system: Insomnia (9%), dizziness (8%), headache (8%), anxiety (6%), fatigue (4%)

Dermatologic: Alopecia (≤5%)

Endocrine & metabolic: Oligomenorrhea (9%), breast pain (6%), menstrual disorder (6%), breast neoplasm (5%), hypercholesterolemia (4%)

Gastrointestinal: Abdominal pain (9%), weight gain (9%), constipation (4% to 8%), diarrhea (7%), dyspepsia (6%), throat irritation (oral solution 5%), abdominal cramps (1%), anorexia (1%)

Genitourinary: Urinary tract infection (10%), leukorrhea (9%), vaginal hemorrhage (6%), vaginitis (5%), vulvovaginitis (5%), ovarian cyst (3%)

Hematologic: Thrombocytopenia (≤10%), anemia (5%)

Hepatic: AST increased (5%), serum bilirubin increased (2%)

Neuromuscular & skeletal: Back pain (10%), bone pain (6% to 10%), osteoporosis (7%), fracture (7%), arthrosis (5%), joint disorder (5%), myalgia (5%), paresthesia (5%), musculoskeletal pain (3%)

Ocular: Cataract (7%)

Renal: Serum creatinine increased (≤2%)

Respiratory: Cough (4% to 9%), dyspnea (8%), bronchitis (5%), sinusitis (5%)

Miscellaneous: Infection/sepsis (≤9%), diaphoresis (6%), flu-like syndrome (6%), cyst (5%), neoplasm (5%), allergic reaction (5%)

<1%, infrequent, or frequency not defined: Cholestasis, corneal changes, endometriosis, endometrial cancer, endometrial hyperplasia, endometrial polyps, fatty liver, hepatic necrosis, hepatitis, hypercalcemia, hyperlipidemia, lightheadedness, phlebitis, pruritus vulvae, pulmonary embolism, retinal vein thrombosis, retinopathy, second primary tumors, stroke, superficial phlebitis, taste disturbances, tumor pain and local disease flare (including increase in lesion size and erythema) during treatment of metastatic breast cancer (generally resolves with continuation), uterine fibroids, vaginal dryness

Postmarketing and/or case reports: Angioedema, bullous pemphigoid, erythema multiforme, hypersensitivity reactions, hypertriglyceridemia, impotence (males), interstitial pneumonitis, loss of libido (males), pancreatitis, Stevens-Johnson syndrome, visual color perception changes

Drug Interactions

Metabolism/Transport Effects Substrate of CYP2A6 (minor), CYP2B6 (minor), CYP2C9 (major), CYP2D6 (major), CYP2E1 (minor), CYP3A4 (major); **Note:** Assignment of Major/Minor substrate status based on clinically relevant drug interaction potential; **Inhibits** CYP2B6 (weak), CYP2C8 (moderate), CYP2C9 (weak), P-glycoprotein

Avoid Concomitant Use

Avoid concomitant use of Tamoxifen with any of the following: Amodiaquine; Bosutinib; Conivaptan; CYP2D6 Inhibitors (Strong); Fusidic Acid (Systemic); Idelalisib; Ospemifene; PAZOPanib; Silodosin; Topotecan; VinCRIStine (Liposomal); Vitamin K Antagonists

◀ **Increased Effect/Toxicity**

Tamoxifen may increase the levels/effects of: Afatinib; Amodiaquine; Bosutinib; Brentuximab Vedotin; Colchicine; CYP2C8 Substrates; Dabigatran Etexilate; DOXOrubicin (Conventional); Edoxaban; Everolimus; Highest Risk QTc-Prolonging Agents; Ledipasvir; Mipomersen; Moderate Risk QTc-Prolonging Agents; Naloxegol; Ospemifene; PAZOPanib; P-glycoprotein/ABCB1 Substrates; Prucalopride; Ranolazine; Rifaximin; Silodosin; Topotecan; VinCRIStine (Liposomal); Vitamin K Antagonists

The levels/effects of Tamoxifen may be increased by: Abiraterone Acetate; Conivaptan; CYP2C9 Inhibitors (Moderate); CYP2C9 Inhibitors (Strong); CYP3A4 Inhibitors (Moderate); CYP3A4 Inhibitors (Strong); Dasatinib; Fosaprepitant; Fusidic Acid (Systemic); Idelalisib; Ivacaftor; Luliconazole; Mifepristone; Netupitant; Osimertinib; Palbociclib; Panobinostat; Peginterferon Alfa-2b; Simeprevir

Decreased Effect

Tamoxifen may decrease the levels/effects of: Anastrozole; Letrozole; Ospemifene

The levels/effects of Tamoxifen may be decreased by: Bexarotene (Systemic); Bosentan; CYP2C9 Inducers (Strong); CYP2D6 Inhibitors (Moderate); CYP2D6 Inhibitors (Strong); CYP3A4 Inducers (Moderate); CYP3A4 Inducers (Strong); Dabrafenib; Deferasirox; Enzalutamide; Mitotane; Osimertinib; Peginterferon Alfa-2b; Rifamycin Derivatives; Siltuximab; St Johns Wort; Tocilizumab

Food Interactions Grapefruit juice may decrease the metabolism of tamoxifen. Management: Avoid grapefruit juice.

Storage/Stability

Oral solution: Store at ≤25°C (77°F); do not freeze or refrigerate. Protect from light. Discard opened bottle after 3 months.

Tablets: Store at 20°C to 25°C (68°F to 77°F). Protect from light.

Mechanism of Action Competitively binds to estrogen receptors on tumors and other tissue targets, producing a nuclear complex that decreases DNA synthesis and inhibits estrogen effects; nonsteroidal agent with potent antiestrogenic properties which compete with estrogen for binding sites in breast and other tissues; cells accumulate in the G_0 and G_1 phases; therefore, tamoxifen is cytostatic rather than cytocidal.

Pharmacodynamics/Kinetics

Absorption: Well absorbed

Distribution: High concentrations found in uterus, endometrial and breast tissue

Protein binding: 99%

Metabolism: Hepatic; via CYP2D6 to 4-hydroxytamoxifen and via CYP3A4/5 to N-desmethyl-tamoxifen. Each is then further metabolized into endoxifen (4-hydroxy-tamoxifen via CYP3A4/5 and N-desmethyl-tamoxifen via CYP2D6); both 4-hydroxy-tamoxifen and endoxifen are 30- to 100-fold more potent than tamoxifen

Half-life elimination: Tamoxifen: ~5-7 days; N-desmethyl tamoxifen: ~14 days

Time to peak, serum: ~5 hours

Excretion: Feces (26% to 51%); urine (9% to 13%)

Dosing

Adult & Geriatric Note: For the treatment of breast cancer, patients receiving both tamoxifen and chemotherapy should receive treatment sequentially, with tamoxifen following completion of chemotherapy.

Breast cancer treatment: Oral:

Adjuvant therapy (females): 20 mg once daily for 5 years

Premenopausal women: Duration of treatment is 5 years (Burstein, 2010; NCCN Breast Cancer guidelines v.2.2013)

Postmenopausal women: Duration of tamoxifen treatment is 2-3 years followed by an aromatase inhibitor (AI) to complete 5 years; may take tamoxifen for the full 5 years (if contraindications or intolerance to AI) or extended therapy: 4.5-6 years of tamoxifen followed by 5 years of an AI (Burstein, 2010; NCCN Breast Cancer guidelines v.2.2013)

ER-positive early breast cancer: Extended duration: Duration of treatment of 10 years demonstrated a reduced risk of recurrence and mortality (Davies, 2012)

Metastatic (males and females): 20-40 mg daily (doses >20 mg should be given in 2 divided doses). **Note:** Although the FDA-approved labeling recommends dosing up to 40 mg daily, clinical benefit has not been demonstrated with doses above 20 mg daily (Bratherton, 1984).

Ductal carcinoma in situ (DCIS) (females), to reduce the risk for invasive breast cancer: 20 mg once daily for 5 years

Breast cancer risk reduction (pre- and postmenopausal high-risk females): Oral: 20 mg once daily for 5 years

Endometrial carcinoma, recurrent, metastatic, or high-risk (endometrioid histologies only) (off-label use): Oral:

Monotherapy: 20 mg twice daily until disease progression or unacceptable toxicity (Thigpen, 2001)

Combination therapy: 20 mg twice daily for 3 weeks (alternating with megestrol acetate every 3 weeks); continue alternating until disease progression or unacceptable toxicity) (Fiorica, 2004)

Induction of ovulation (off-label use): Oral: 20 mg once daily (range: 20-80 mg once daily) for 5 days (Steiner, 2005)

Ovarian cancer, advanced and/or recurrent (off-label use): Oral: 20 mg twice daily (Hatch, 1991; Markman, 1996)

Paget's disease of the breast (risk reduction; with DCIS or without associated cancer): Oral: 20 mg once daily for 5 years (NCCN Breast Cancer Guidelines, v.2.2013)

Dosage adjustment for DVT, pulmonary embolism, cerebrovascular accident, or prolonged immobilization: Discontinue tamoxifen (NCCN Breast Cancer Risk Reduction Guidelines, v.1.2013)

Pediatric Females: Precocious puberty secondary to McCune-Albright syndrome (off-label use): Oral: A dose of 20 mg daily has been reported in patients 2-10 years of age; safety and efficacy have not been established for treatment of longer than 1 year duration (Eugster, 2003)

Renal Impairment No dosage adjustment provided in manufacturer's labeling.

Chronic dialysis: No dosage adjustment necessary (Janus, 2013).

Hepatic Impairment No dosage adjustment provided in manufacturer's labeling (has not been studied).

Administration Administer tablets or oral solution orally with or without food. Use supplied dosing cup for oral solution.

Hazardous agent; use appropriate precautions for handling and disposal (NIOSH 2014 [group 1]).

◀ **Extemporaneous Preparations** Hazardous agent: Use appropriate precautions for handling and disposal (NIOSH 2014 [group 1]).

A 0.5 mg/mL oral suspension may be prepared with tablets. Place two 10 mg tablets into 40 mL purified water and let stand ~2-5 minutes. Stir until tablets are completely disintegrated (dispersion time for each 10 mg tablet is ~2-5 minutes). Administer immediately after preparation. To ensure the full dose is administered, rinse glass several times with water and administer residue.
Lam MS, "Extemporaneous Compounding of Oral Liquid Dosage Formulations and Alternative Drug Delivery Methods for Anticancer Drugs," *Pharmacotherapy*, 2011, 31(2):164-92.

Monitoring Parameters CBC with platelets, serum calcium, LFTs; triglycerides and cholesterol (in patients with preexisting hyperlipidemias); INR and PT (in patients on vitamin K antagonists); abnormal vaginal bleeding; breast and gynecologic exams (baseline and routine), mammogram (baseline and routine); signs/symptoms of DVT (leg swelling, tenderness) or PE (shortness of breath); ophthalmic exam (if vision problem or cataracts); bone mineral density (premenopausal women)

Test Interactions T_4 elevations (which may be explained by increases in thyroid-binding globulin) have been reported; not accompanied by clinical hyperthyroidism

Dietary Considerations Tablets and oral solution may be taken with or without food. Avoid grapefruit and grapefruit juice.

Additional Information Estrogen receptor status may predict if adjuvant treatment with tamoxifen is of benefit. In metastatic breast cancer, patients with estrogen receptor positive tumors are more likely to benefit from tamoxifen treatment. With tamoxifen use to reduce the incidence of breast cancer in high risk-women, high risk is defined as women ≥35 years of age with a 5 year NCI Gail model predicted risk of breast cancer ≥1.67%.

Oncology Comment: The American Society of Clinical Oncology (ASCO) guidelines for adjuvant endocrine therapy in postmenopausal women with HR-positive breast cancer (Burstein, 2010) recommend considering aromatase inhibitor (AI) therapy at some point in the treatment course (primary, sequentially, or extended). Optimal duration at this time is not known; however, treatment with an AI should not exceed 5 years in primary and extended therapies, and 2-3 years if followed by tamoxifen in sequential therapy (total of 5 years). If initial therapy with AI has been discontinued before the 5 years, consideration should be taken to receive tamoxifen for a total of 5 years. The optimal time to switch to an AI is also not known; but data supports switching after 2-3 years of tamoxifen (sequential) or after 5 years of tamoxifen (extended). If patient becomes intolerant or has poor adherence, consideration should be made to switch to another AI or initiate tamoxifen.

Recent data suggest that continuing tamoxifen for 10 years (rather than stopping after 5 years of therapy) may provide a further reduction in breast cancer recurrence and mortality in women with early stage disease (Davies, 2012). The Adjuvant Tamoxifen: Longer Against Shorter (ATLAS) trial randomized 6846 patients with estrogen receptor positive disease to continue tamoxifen for a total of 10 years of treatment or to stop after 5 years. Breast cancer recurrence was observed in 617 patients in the 10-year arm versus 711 recurrences in the 5-year arm (p=0.002). Breast cancer mortality was significantly reduced with 10 years of tamoxifen therapy versus 5 years (331 deaths vs 397 deaths, respectively; p=0.01) (Davies, 2012).

The adjuvant endocrine therapy of choice is tamoxifen for men with breast cancer and for pre- or perimenopausal women at diagnosis. CYP2D6 genotyping is not recommended, however, due to the potential for drug-drug interactions use caution and consider avoiding concomitant therapy with tamoxifen and known CYP2D6 inhibitors.

Medication Guide Available Yes

Dosage Forms Excipient information presented when available (limited, particularly for generics); consult specific product labeling.

Solution, Oral:

Soltamox: 10 mg/5 mL (150 mL) [sugar free; contains alcohol, usp, propylene glycol; licorice-aniseed flavor]

Tablet, Oral:

Generic: 10 mg, 20 mg

- ◆ **Tamoxifen Citras** see Tamoxifen on page 1595
- ◆ **Tamoxifen Citrate** see Tamoxifen on page 1595
- ◆ **Tantum (Can)** see Benzydamine on page 190
- ◆ **TAP-144** see Leuprolide on page 1030
- ◆ **Tarceva** see Erlotinib on page 628
- ◆ **Targretin** see Bexarotene (Systemic) on page 200
- ◆ **Targretin** see Bexarotene (Topical) on page 205
- ◆ **Taro-Anastrozole (Can)** see Anastrozole on page 112
- ◆ **Taro-Ciprofloxacin (Can)** see Ciprofloxacin (Systemic) on page 327
- ◆ **Taro-Fluconazole (Can)** see Fluconazole on page 725
- ◆ **Taro-Zoledronic Acid (Can)** see Zoledronic Acid on page 1790
- ◆ **Taro-Zoledronic Acid Concentrate (Can)** see Zoledronic Acid on page 1790
- ◆ **TAS-102** see Trifluridine and Tipiracil on page 1699
- ◆ **Tasigna** see Nilotinib on page 1198
- ◆ **Taxol** see PACLitaxel (Conventional) on page 1284
- ◆ **Taxotere** see DOCEtaxel on page 535
- ◆ **Tazicef** see CefTAZidime on page 296
- ◆ **Tazidime** see CefTAZidime on page 296
- ◆ **Tazobactam and Piperacillin** see Piperacillin and Tazobactam on page 1388
- ◆ **Tazocin (Can)** see Piperacillin and Tazobactam on page 1388
- ◆ **Tbo-Filgrastim** see Filgrastim on page 711
- ◆ **Tc99m Sestamibi** see Technetium Tc 99m Sestamibi on page 1602
- ◆ **Tc99m-Sulfur Colloid** see Technetium Tc 99m Sulfur Colloid on page 1602
- ◆ **Tc99m Tilmanocept** see Technetium Tc 99m Tilmanocept on page 1603
- ◆ **T-Cell Growth Factor** see Aldesleukin on page 55
- ◆ **TCGF** see Aldesleukin on page 55
- ◆ **T-DM1** see Ado-Trastuzumab Emtansine on page 43
- ◆ **TDX** see Raltitrexed on page 1454
- ◆ **Technetium (99mTc) Sestamibi** see Technetium Tc 99m Sestamibi on page 1602

- ◆ **Technetium (99mTc) Sulfur Colloid** *see* Technetium Tc 99m Sulfur Colloid *on page 1602*
- ◆ **Technetium (99mTc) Tilmanocept** *see* Technetium Tc 99m Tilmanocept *on page 1603*
- ◆ **Technetium Sestamibi (99mTc)** *see* Technetium Tc 99m Sestamibi *on page 1602*
- ◆ **Technetium Sulfur Colloid (^{99m}Tc)** *see* Technetium Tc 99m Sulfur Colloid *on page 1602*

Technetium Tc 99m Sestamibi

(tek NEE shee um tee see nyne tee nyne em ses ta MIB ee)

Brand Names: US Cardiolite

Index Terms 99m Technetium Sestamibi; 99mTc-Sestamibi; Tc99m Sestamibi; Technetium (99mTc) Sestamibi; Technetium Sestamibi (99mTc)

Pharmacologic Category Radiopharmaceutical

Use Imaging agent: Myocardial perfusion agent used in detection of coronary artery disease in conjunction with exercise stress testing or pharmacologic stress testing to identify reversible myocardial ischemia with or without myocardial infarction; planar breast imaging after mammography to assist in evaluation of breast lesions in patients with abnormal mammogram or palpable breast mass (second-line)

Pregnancy Risk Factor C

Dosing

Adult

Breast imaging: IV (based on 70 kg patient): 20 to 30 mCi (740 to 1,110 MBq)

Myocardial imaging: IV (based on 70 kg patient): 10 to 30 mCi (370 to 1,110 MBq)

Geriatric Refer to adult dosing.

Renal Impairment There are no dosage adjustments provided in the manufacturer's labeling.

Hepatic Impairment There are no dosage adjustments provided in the manufacturer's labeling.

Additional Information Complete prescribing information should be consulted for additional detail.

Dosage Forms Excipient information presented when available (limited, particularly for generics); consult specific product labeling.

Kit, for Injection:

Cardiolite: 2-methoxy isobutyl isonitrile (MIBI) copper tetrafluoroborate 1 mg (2s, 5s, 20s) [to be combined with sodium pertechnetate Tc99m injection solution (not included)]

Generic: 2-methoxy isobutyl isonitrile (MIBI) copper tetrafluoroborate 1 mg (5s, 30s) [to be combined with sodium pertechnetate Tc99m injection solution (not included)]

Technetium Tc 99m Sulfur Colloid

(tek NEE shee um tee see nyne tee nyne em SUL fyoor ko LOYD)

Brand Names: US CIS-SULFUR COLLOID

Index Terms ^{99m}Tc-Sulfur Colloid; Sulfur Colloid; Tc^{99m}-Sulfur Colloid; Technetium (99mTc) Sulfur Colloid; Technetium (^{99m}Tc) Sulfur Colloid; Technetium Sulfur Colloid (^{99m}Tc)

Pharmacologic Category Radiopharmaceutical

Use Imaging agent: Localization of lymph nodes draining a primary tumor in patients with breast cancer or malignant melanoma (when used with a handheld gamma counter); reticuloendothelial cell imaging agent (liver, spleen, bone marrow); evaluation of peritoneovenous shunt patency; esophageal transit studies, gastroesophageal reflux scintigraphy, detection of pulmonary aspiration of gastric contents

Pregnancy Risk Factor C

Dosing

Adult & Geriatric

Breast cancer or malignant melanoma, lymph node localization: SubQ: 3.7-37 MBq (0.1-1 mCi) in volumes ranging from 0.1 to 1 mL

Peritoneovenous shunt patency evaluation:

Intraperitoneal injection: 37-111 MBq (1-3 mCi)

Percutaneous transtubal (efferent limb) injection: 12-37 MBq (0.3-1 mCi) in a maximum volume of 0.5 mL

Reticuloendothelial cell imaging:

Bone marrow: IV: 111-444 MBq (3-12 mCi)

Liver/spleen: IV: 37-296 MBq (1-8 mCi)

Esophageal transit studies, gastroesophageal reflux scintigraphy, pulmonary aspiration imaging:

Gastroesophageal studies: Oral: 5.55-11.1 MBq (0.15-0.3 mCi)

Pulmonary aspiration studies: Oral: 11.1-18.5 MBq (0.3-0.5 mCi)

Pediatric

Reticuloendothelial cell imaging:

Bone marrow: Pediatrics: IV: 1.11-5.55 MBq/**kg** (0.03-0.15 mCi/**kg**)

Liver/spleen:

Newborns: IV: 7.4-18.5 MBq (0.2-0.5 mCi)

Children: IV: 0.56-2.78 MBq/**kg** (0.015-0.075 mCi/**kg**)

Esophageal transit studies, gastroesophageal reflux scintigraphy, pulmonary aspiration imaging: *Gastroesophageal studies or pulmonary aspiration studies:* Pediatrics: Oral or nasogastric tube: 3.7-11.1 MBq (0.1-0.3 mCi)

Renal Impairment No dosage adjustment provided in manufacturer's labeling.

Hepatic Impairment No dosage adjustment provided in manufacturer's labeling.

Additional Information Complete prescribing information should be consulted for additional detail.

Technetium Tc 99m Tilmanocept
(tek NEE shee um tee see nyne tee nyne em til MAN oh sept)

Brand Names: US Lymphoseek

Index Terms 99mTc-Tilmanocept; Tc99m Tilmanocept; Technetium (99mTc) Tilmanocept; Technetium Tilmanocept (99mTc)

Pharmacologic Category Radiopharmaceutical

Use

Diagnostic imaging: Radioactive diagnostic agent indicated with or without scintigraphic imaging (using a handheld gamma counter) for:

- Lymphatic mapping to locate lymph nodes draining a primary tumor site in patients with solid tumors for which this procedure is a component of intraoperative management.

- Guiding sentinel lymph node biopsy in patients with clinically node negative squamous cell carcinoma of the oral cavity, breast cancer, or melanoma.

◄ **Pregnancy Risk Factor** C

Dosing

Adult & Geriatric Note: The route of administration, number of injections, and total injection volume per patient will vary depending on cancer and planned injection technique.

Breast cancer lymphatic mapping: Intradermal, SubQ, subareolar, or peritumoral: 18.5 MBq (0.5 mCi) as radioactivity dose and 50 mcg as a mass dose at least 15 minutes prior to intraoperative lymphatic mapping

Melanoma lymphatic mapping: Intradermal or SubQ: 18.5 MBq (0.5 mCi) as radioactivity dose and 50 mcg as a mass dose at least 15 minutes prior to intraoperative lymphatic mapping

Oral cavity squamous cell carcinoma sentinel lymph node biopsy: Peritumoral: 18.5 MBq (0.5 mCi) as radioactivity dose and 50 mcg as a mass dose at least 15 minutes prior to intraoperative sentinel node biopsy

Renal Impairment There are no dosage adjustments provided in the manufacturer's labeling.

Hepatic Impairment There are no dosage adjustments provided in the manufacturer's labeling.

Additional Information Complete prescribing information should be consulted for additional detail.

Prescribing and Access Restrictions Lymphoseek may only be obtained through Cardinal Health's Nuclear Pharmacy Services.

Dosage Forms Excipient information presented when available (limited, particularly for generics); consult specific product labeling.

Injection, powder for reconstitution [kit]:

Lymphoseek: Tilmanocept 250 mcg (5s) [vial contents to be combined with Technetium Tc 99m pertechnetate sodium (not included)]

◆ **Technetium Tilmanocept (99mTc)** *see* Technetium Tc 99m Tilmanocept *on page 1603*

Tegafur and Uracil (TEG a fur & URE a sil)

Related Information

Management of Chemotherapy-Induced Nausea and Vomiting in Adults *on page 2142*

Safe Handling of Hazardous Drugs *on page 2292*

Index Terms Ftorafur and Uracil; Orzel; Tegafur Uracil; UFT; Uftoral; Uracil and Ftorafur; Uracil and Tegafur; Uracil and Tetrahydrofuranyl-5-Fluorouracil

Pharmacologic Category Antineoplastic Agent, Antimetabolite; Antineoplastic Agent, Antimetabolite (Pyrimidine Analog)

Use

European labeling: Treatment (first-line) of metastatic colorectal cancer (in combination with leucovorin calcium)

Singapore labeling: Treatment of head and neck, gastric, colorectal, hepatocellular, hepatobiliary, pancreatic, lung, breast, bladder, and uterine/cervical cancers

Labeled Contraindications

European labeling: Hypersensitivity to tegafur and uracil, fluorouracil, or any component of the formulation; use in women who are or may become pregnant; women who are breast-feeding; use in infants, children, or adolescents; severe hepatic impairment; evidence of bone marrow suppression from prior radiation therapy or prior chemotherapy; known deficiency of hepatic CYP2A6; known or suspected dihydropyrimidine dehydrogenase (DPD) deficiency; concurrent or recent treatment with DPD inhibitors

Singapore labeling: Hypersensitivity to tegafur and uracil, fluorouracil, or any component of the formulation; concurrent use (or within 7 days) of tegafur/gimeracil/oteracil; use in women who are or may become pregnant

Pregnancy Considerations Use is contraindicated in women who are or may become pregnant; may cause fetal harm if administered during pregnancy. Both men and women of childbearing potential should use effective contraception during and for 3 months following cessation of treatment. May cause irreversible infertility. Male patients who wish to father a child during or after treatment should seek advice regarding sperm cryopreservation prior to treatment initiation.

Breast-Feeding Considerations It is not known if tegafur/uracil is excreted in breast milk. Use is contraindicated in women who are breast-feeding.

Warnings/Precautions Hazardous agent - use appropriate precautions for handling and disposal (meets NIOSH 2014 criteria). Anemia, leukopenia, neutropenia, and thrombocytopenia are commonly observed; may require dosage modification. Monitor blood counts as clinically necessary. Neutropenic fever may occur. Monitor for signs/symptoms of infections (due to neutropenia) and bleeding (due to thrombocytopenia). Cardiovascular adverse effects including MI have been reported with tegafur and uracil. Use with caution in patients with a history of significant cardiac disease; myocardial ischemia and angina have been observed with other fluoropyrimidine-based treatments.

May cause diarrhea (generally mild); if severe diarrhea occurs, monitor carefully for electrolyte imbalance or dehydration. Withhold treatment for grade 2 or higher diarrhea. Use with caution in patients with signs/symptoms of bowel obstruction. Nausea, vomiting, anorexia, stomatitis, and abdominal pain commonly occur. Hepatotoxicity, including fatal fulminant hepatitis, has been reported. If signs/symptoms of hepatitis or other liver impairment occur, evaluate hepatic function. Long-term administration may lead to hepatic cirrhosis without remarkable increase in transaminases; discontinue if prolonged prothrombin time or decreased albumin occur (Singapore labeling). Patients with mild-to-moderate hepatic impairment should be monitored closely. Use is contraindicated in severe hepatic impairment (European labeling). Use with caution in patients with renal impairment; has not been studied.

Administration to patients with genetic dihydropyrimidine dehydrogenase (DPD) deficiency has been associated with prolonged clearance and increased and potentially fatal toxicity (diarrhea, neutropenia, and neurotoxicity). Administration to patients with known or suspected DPD deficiency or with concurrent or recent treatment with DPD inhibitors is contraindicated (European labeling). Potentially significant drug-drug interactions may exist, requiring dose or frequency adjustment, additional monitoring, and/or selection of alternative therapy.

Adverse Reactions

>10%:

Gastrointestinal: Diarrhea (20%; may be dose limiting), abdominal pain (12%), nausea and vomiting (12%), anorexia, stomatitis

Hematologic & oncologic: Anemia, leukopenia, neutropenia (may be dose limiting), thrombocytopenia

Hepatic: Increased serum alkaline phosphatase, increased serum ALT, increased serum AST, increased serum bilirubin

Neuromuscular & skeletal: Weakness

◀ 1% to 10%:

Cardiovascular: Deep vein thrombophlebitis, peripheral edema

Central nervous system: Ageusia, chills, confusion, depression, dizziness, drowsiness, headache, insomnia, malaise, pain, paresthesia

Dermatologic: Alopecia, diaphoresis, exfoliative dermatitis, nail disease, pruritus, skin rash, skin discoloration, skin photosensitivity, xeroderma

Endocrine & metabolic: Cachexia, dehydration, weight loss

Gastrointestinal: Constipation, dysgeusia, dyspepsia, eructation, flatulence, intestinal obstruction, mucositis, xerostomia

Hematologic & oncologic: Blood coagulation disorder, febrile neutropenia

Infection: Candidiasis

Neuromuscular & skeletal: Arthralgia, back pain, myalgia

Ophthalmic: Conjunctivitis, lacrimation

Respiratory: Cough, dyspnea, pharyngitis

Miscellaneous: Fever

<1%, postmarketing, and/or case reports: Abnormal gait, acute myelocytic leukemia (including promyelocytic), acute pancreatitis, acute renal failure, agranulocytosis, altered sense of smell, amnesia, angina pectoris, anosmia, ascites, cardiac arrest, cardiac arrhythmia, cardiac failure, chest pain, dermatological reaction (including blistering, dermatitis), disseminated intravascular coagulation, duodenal ulcer, enteritis, enterocolitis, extrapyramidal reaction, fatigue, fulminant hepatitis, gastric ulcer, gastritis, hematuria, hemolytic anemia, hepatic cirrhosis, hepatic failure, hepatic fibrosis, hepatitis, hypoesthesia, ileitis, impaired consciousness, impotence, increased susceptibility to infection, intestinal perforation, ischemic colitis, jaundice, leukoencephalopathy, lupus erythematous-like rash (discoid), movement disorder, multi-organ failure, myelodysplastic syndrome, myocardial infarction, nephrotic syndrome, palmar-plantar erythrodysesthesia, pancytopenia, paralysis (extremities), paralytic ileus, pneumonia, pulmonary embolism, renal insufficiency, sepsis, shock, speech disturbance, Stevens-Johnson syndrome, urinary incontinence, urinary retention, urticaria

Drug Interactions

Metabolism/Transport Effects Refer to individual components.

Avoid Concomitant Use

Avoid concomitant use of Tegafur and Uracil with any of the following: Allopurinol; BCG (Intravesical); CloZAPine; CYP2A6 Inhibitors (Moderate); CYP2A6 Inhibitors (Strong); Dipyrone; Gimeracil; Natalizumab; Pimecrolimus; Tacrolimus (Topical); Tofacitinib; Vaccines (Live)

Increased Effect/Toxicity

Tegafur and Uracil may increase the levels/effects of: Bosentan; Carvedilol; CloZAPine; CYP2C9 Substrates; Diclofenac (Systemic); Dronabinol; Fingolimod; Fosphenytoin-Phenytoin; Lacosamide; Leflunomide; Natalizumab; Ospemifene; Parecoxib; Ramelteon; Tetrahydrocannabinol; Tofacitinib; Vaccines (Live); Vitamin K Antagonists

The levels/effects of Tegafur and Uracil may be increased by: Cannabis; Cimetidine; Denosumab; Dipyrone; Gimeracil; Leucovorin Calcium-Levoleucovorin; Methotrexate; MetroNIDAZOLE (Systemic); Pimecrolimus; Roflumilast; Tacrolimus (Topical); Trastuzumab

Decreased Effect

Tegafur and Uracil may decrease the levels/effects of: BCG (Intravesical); Coccidioides immitis Skin Test; Sipuleucel-T; Vaccines (Inactivated); Vaccines (Live)

The levels/effects of Tegafur and Uracil may be decreased by: Allopurinol; CYP2A6 Inducers (Strong); CYP2A6 Inhibitors (Moderate); CYP2A6 Inhibitors (Strong); Echinacea

Storage/Stability Store at ≤25°C (77°F).

Mechanism of Action Tegafur is a prodrug of fluorouracil. It is converted *in vivo* to fluorouracil through hepatic microsomal cytochrome P450, and also via thymidine phosphorylase and spontaneous anabolic conversion. Uracil is a competitive inhibitor of dihydropyrimidine dehydrogenase (DPD), the enzyme responsible for catabolism of approximately 85% of fluorouracil to fluoro-β alanine.

Pharmacodynamics/Kinetics

Absorption: Rapid

Distribution: V_d: Tegafur: 59 L; Uracil: 474 L

Protein binding: Tegafur: 52%; Uracil: Negligible

Metabolism: Hepatic (via oxidation, partially by CYP2A6) and hydrolysis by cytosolic enzymes

Half-life elimination: Tegafur: 11 hours; Uracil: 20-40 minutes

Time to peak: ~1-2 hours

Excretion: Tegafur: Urine (<20% as parent drug)

Dosing

Adult & Geriatric

European labeling: **Colorectal cancer, metastatic:** Oral: 300 mg/m²/day (tegafur component) and 672 mg/m²/day (uracil component) in 3 divided doses (every 8 hours) days 1 through 28 every 35 days (in combination with oral leucovorin calcium); begin subsequent cycles after the 7-day break

Dose based on BSA (number of tegafur and uracil [UFT] capsules required):

Tegafur and Uracil (UFT) BSA-Based Dosing (Number of Capsules Required)

BSA	UFT capsules daily	Daily Schedule		
		Morning	Midday	Evening
<1.17	3	1	1	1
1.17-1.49	4	2	1	1
1.5-1.83	5	2	2	1
>1.83	6	2	2	2

Singapore labeling:

Head and neck, gastric, colorectal, hepatocellular, hepatobiliary, pancreatic, lung, breast, and bladder cancer: Oral: 300-600 mg (based on tegafur component) daily in 2-3 divided doses

Uterine/cervical cancers: Oral: 600 mg (based on tegafur component) daily in 2-3 divided doses

Renal Impairment No dosage adjustment provided in the manufacturer's labeling (has not been studied); monitor closely for toxicities.

Hepatic Impairment

Mild-to-moderate impairment: No dosage adjustment provided in the manufacturer's labeling (has not been studied).

Severe impairment: Use is contraindicated (European labeling).

Obesity *ASCO Guidelines for appropriate chemotherapy dosing in obese adults with cancer:* Utilize patient's actual body weight (full weight) for calculation of body surface area- or weight-based dosing, particularly when the intent of therapy is curative; manage regimen-related toxicities in the same manner as for nonobese patients; if a dose reduction is utilized due to toxicity, consider resumption of full weight-based dosing with subsequent cycles, especially if cause of toxicity (eg, hepatic or renal impairment) is resolved (Griggs, 2012).

Adjustment for Toxicity *European labeling:* **Note:** Do not make up doses that are withheld during the 28 days of consecutive treatment. If tegafur and uracil treatment is withheld, leucovorin calcium should also be withheld. Do not reduce leucovorin calcium dose if tegafur and uracil dose is reduced.

Nonhematologic toxicity:

Grade 1: No change in treatment.

Grade 2: Withhold treatment until resolved to ≤ grade 1; resume at previous dose.

Grades 3 and 4: Withhold treatment until resolved to ≤ grade 1; resume with the dose reduced by 1 capsule daily for current and future cycles.

Hematologic toxicity:

First incident:

Grade 1: No change in treatment

Grades 2 to 4: Withhold treatment until granulocytes ≥1500/mm^3 and platelets ≥100,000/mm^3

Subsequent incidents:

Grades 1 and 2: No change in treatment.

Grades 3 and 4: Decrease subsequent doses by 1 capsule daily for current and future cycles.

Administration Take at least 1 hour before or 1 hour after meals. Hazardous agent; use appropriate precautions for handling and disposal (meets NIOSH 2014 criteria).

Emetic Potential Low (10% to 30%)

Monitoring Parameters CBC with differential (at least monthly for first 2 months [Singapore labeling]); liver function; prothrombin time (with long-term use); albumin (with long-term use); renal function; signs/symptoms of gastrointestinal toxicity (diarrhea, nausea, vomiting, stomatitis, abdominal pain) and cardiovascular toxicity (myocardial ischemia/infarction, angina)

Dosage Forms Excipient information presented when available (limited, particularly for generics); consult specific product labeling.

Capsule, Oral: Tegafur 100 mg and uracil 224 mg

◆ **Tegafur Uracil** see Tegafur and Uracil on page 1604

◆ **Temodal (Can)** see Temozolomide on page 1608

◆ **Temodar** see Temozolomide on page 1608

Temozolomide (te moe ZOE loe mide)

Related Information

Common Toxicity Criteria on page 2122

Management of Chemotherapy-Induced Nausea and Vomiting in Adults on page 2142

Prevention of Chemotherapy-Induced Nausea and Vomiting in Children on page 2203

Safe Handling of Hazardous Drugs on page 2292

Brand Names: US Temodar

Brand Names: Canada ACH-Temozolomide; ACT Temozolomide; Temodal

Index Terms SCH 52365; TMZ

Pharmacologic Category Antineoplastic Agent, Alkylating Agent (Triazene)

Use

Anaplastic astrocytoma: Treatment of refractory anaplastic astrocytoma (refractory to a regimen containing a nitrosourea and procarbazine)

Glioblastoma multiforme: Treatment of newly-diagnosed glioblastoma multiforme (initially in combination with radiotherapy, then as maintenance treatment)

Canadian labeling: Treatment of newly-diagnosed glioblastoma multiforme (initially in combination with radiotherapy, then as maintenance treatment), treatment of recurrent or progressive glioblastoma multiforme or anaplastic astrocytoma

Labeled Contraindications

Hypersensitivity (eg, allergic reaction, anaphylaxis, urticaria, Stevens-Johnson syndrome, toxic epidermal necrolysis) to temozolomide or any component of the formulation; hypersensitivity to dacarbazine (both drugs are metabolized to MTIC)

Canadian labeling: Additional contraindications (not in U.S. labeling): Not recommended in patients with severe myelosuppression

Pregnancy Considerations Adverse events were observed in animal reproduction studies. May cause fetal harm when administered to pregnant women. Male and female patients should avoid pregnancy while receiving temozolomide. The Canadian labeling recommends that male and female patients also avoid pregnancy for 6 months after discontinuation of therapy.

Breast-Feeding Considerations It is not known if temozolomide is excreted in breast milk. Due to the potential for serious adverse reactions in the nursing infant, the manufacturer recommends a decision be made whether to discontinue nursing or to discontinue the drug, taking into account the importance of treatment to the mother.

Warnings/Precautions Hazardous agent - use appropriate precautions for handling and disposal (NIOSH 2014 [group 1]). *Pneumocystis jirovecii* pneumonia (PCP) may occur; risk is increased in those receiving steroids or longer dosing regimens; monitor all patients for development of PCP (particularly if also receiving corticosteroids); PCP prophylaxis is required in patients receiving radiotherapy in combination with the 42-day temozolomide regimen. Myelosuppression may occur; may require treatment interruption, dose reduction, and/or discontinuation; monitor blood counts; an increased incidence has been reported in geriatric and female patients. Prolonged pancytopenia resulting in aplastic anemia has been reported (may be fatal); concurrent use of temozolomide with medications associated with aplastic anemia (eg, carbamazepine, co-trimoxazole, phenytoin) may obscure assessment for development of aplastic anemia. ANC should be ≥1,500/mm^3 and platelets ≥100,000/mm^3 prior to treatment. Rare cases of myelodysplastic syndrome and secondary malignancies, including acute myeloid leukemia, have been reported. Use caution in patients with severe hepatic or renal impairment; has not been studied in dialysis patients. Hepatotoxicity has been reported; may be severe or fatal. Monitor liver function tests at baseline, halfway through the first cycle, prior to each subsequent cycle, and at ~2 to 4 weeks after the last dose. Postmarketing reports of hepatotoxicity have included liver function abnormalities, hepatitis, hepatic failure, cholestasis, hepatitis cholestasis, jaundice, cholelithiasis, hepatic steatosis, hepatic necrosis, hepatic lesion, and hepatic encephalopathy (Sarganas 2012).

◀ Temozolomide is associated with a moderate emetic potential (Dupuis 2011; Roila 2010); antiemetics are recommended to prevent nausea and vomiting. Increased MGMT (O-6-methylguanine-DNA methyltransferase) activity/levels within tumor tissue is associated with temozolomide resistance. Glioblastoma patients with decreased levels (due to methylated MGMT promoter) may be more likely to benefit from the combination of radiation therapy and temozolomide (Hegi 2008; Stupp 2009). Determination of MGMT status may be predictive for response to alkylating agents. Potentially significant drug-drug interactions may exist, requiring dose or frequency adjustment, additional monitoring, and/or selection of alternative therapy. Bioequivalence has only been established when IV temozolomide is administered over 90 minutes; shorter or longer infusion times may result in suboptimal dosing.

Polysorbate 80: Some dosage forms may contain polysorbate 80 (also known as Tweens). Hypersensitivity reactions, usually a delayed reaction, have been reported following exposure to pharmaceutical products containing polysorbate 80 in certain individuals (Isaksson 2002; Lucente 2000; Shelley 1995). Thrombocytopenia, ascites, pulmonary deterioration, and renal and hepatic failure have been reported in premature neonates after receiving parenteral products containing polysorbate 80 (Alade 1986; CDC 1984). See manufacturer's labeling.

Adverse Reactions Note: With CNS malignancies, it may be difficult to distinguish between CNS adverse events caused by temozolomide versus the effects of progressive disease.

>10%:

Cardiovascular: Peripheral edema (11%)

Central nervous system: Fatigue (34% to 61%), headache (23% to 41%), convulsions (6% to 23%), hemiparesis (18%), dizziness (5% to 12%), ataxia (8% to 11%)

Dermatologic: Alopecia (55%), skin rash (8% to 13%)

Gastrointestinal: Nausea (49% to 53%; grades 3/4: 1% to 10%), vomiting (29% to 42%; grades 3/4: 2% to 6%), constipation (22% to 33%), anorexia (9% to 27%), diarrhea (10% to 16%)

Hematologic & oncologic: Lymphocytopenia (grades 3/4: 55%), thrombocytopenia (grades 3/4: adults: 4% to 19%; children: 25%), neutropenia (grades 3/4: adults: 8% to 14%; children: 20%), leukopenia (grades 3/4: 11%)

Infection: Viral infection (11%)

Neuromuscular & skeletal: Weakness (7% to 13%)

Miscellaneous: Fever (13%)

1% to 10%:

Central nervous system: Amnesia (10%), insomnia (4% to 10%), drowsiness (9%), paresthesia (9%), paresis (8%), anxiety (7%), memory impairment (7%), abnormal gait (6%), depression (6%), confusion (5%)

Dermatologic: Pruritus (5% to 8%), xeroderma (5%), erythema (1%)

Endocrine & metabolic: Hypercorticoidism (8%), weight gain (5%)

Gastrointestinal: Stomatitis (9%), abdominal pain (5% to 9%), dysphagia (7%), dysgeusia (5%)

Genitourinary: Urinary incontinence (8%), urinary tract infection (8%), mastalgia (females 6%), urinary frequency (6%)

Hematologic & oncologic: Anemia (grades 3/4: 4%)

Hypersensitivity: Hypersensitivity reaction (≤3%)

Neuromuscular & skeletal: Back pain (8%), arthralgia (6%), myalgia (5%)

Ophthalmic: Blurred vision (5% to 8%), diplopia (5%), visual disturbance (visual deficit/vision changes 5%)

Respiratory: Pharyngitis (8%), upper respiratory tract infection (8%), cough (5% to 8%), sinusitis (6%), dyspnea (5%)

Miscellaneous: Radiation injury (2% maintenance phase after radiotherapy)

<1%, postmarketing, and/or case reports (limited to important or life-threatening): Agitation, anaphylaxis, apathy, aplastic anemia, cholestasis, cytomegalovirus disease (reactivation), diabetes insipidus, emotional lability, erythema multiforme, febrile neutropenia, flu-like symptoms, hallucination, hematoma, hemorrhage, hepatitis, hepatitis B (reactivation), hepatotoxicity, herpes simplex infection, herpes zoster, hyperbilirubinemia, hyperglycemia, hypersensitivity pneumonitis, hypokalemia, increased serum alkaline phosphatase, increased serum transaminases, injection site reaction (erythema, irritation, pain, pruritus, swelling, warmth), interstitial pneumonitis, metastases (including myeloid leukemia), myelodysplastic syndrome, neuropathy, opportunistic infection (including pneumocystosis), oral candidiasis, pancytopenia (may be prolonged), peripheral neuropathy, petechia, pneumonitis, pulmonary fibrosis, Stevens-Johnson syndrome, toxic epidermal necrolysis, weight loss

Drug Interactions

Metabolism/Transport Effects None known.

Avoid Concomitant Use

Avoid concomitant use of Temozolomide with any of the following: BCG (Intravesical); CloZAPine; Dipyrone; Natalizumab; Pimecrolimus; Tacrolimus (Topical); Tofacitinib; Vaccines (Live)

Increased Effect/Toxicity

Temozolomide may increase the levels/effects of: CloZAPine; Fingolimod; Leflunomide; Natalizumab; Tofacitinib; Vaccines (Live)

The levels/effects of Temozolomide may be increased by: Denosumab; Dipyrone; Pimecrolimus; Roflumilast; Tacrolimus (Topical); Trastuzumab; Valproate Products

Decreased Effect

Temozolomide may decrease the levels/effects of: BCG (Intravesical); Coccidioides immitis Skin Test; Sipuleucel-T; Vaccines (Inactivated); Vaccines (Live)

The levels/effects of Temozolomide may be decreased by: Echinacea

Food Interactions Food reduces rate and extent of absorption. Management: Administer consistently either with food or without food (was administered in studies under fasting and nonfasting conditions).

Storage/Stability

Capsule: Store at room temperature of 25°C (77°F); excursions permitted to 15°C to 30°C (59°F to 86°F).

Injection: Store intact vials refrigerated at 2°C to 8°C (36°F to 46°F). Reconstituted vials may be stored for up to 14 hours at room temperature of 25°C (77°F); infusion must be completed within 14 hours of reconstitution.

Preparation for Administration Hazardous agent; use appropriate precautions for handling and disposal (NIOSH 2014 [group 1]). Bring to room temperature prior to reconstitution. Reconstitute each 100 mg vial with 41 mL sterile water for injection to a final concentration of 2.5 mg/mL. Swirl gently; do not shake. Place dose without further dilution into a 250 mL empty sterile infusion bag. Infusion must be completed within 14 hours of reconstitution.

◄ **Mechanism of Action** Temozolomide is a prodrug which is rapidly and nonenzymatically converted to the active alkylating metabolite MTIC [(methyl-triazene-1-yl)-imidazole-4-carboxamide]; this conversion is spontaneous, nonenzymatic, and occurs under physiologic conditions in all tissues to which it distributes. The cytotoxic effects of MTIC are manifested through alkylation (methylation) of DNA at the O^6, N^7 guanine positions which lead to DNA double strand breaks and apoptosis. Non-cell cycle specific.

Pharmacodynamics/Kinetics

Absorption: Oral: Rapid and complete

Distribution: V_d: Parent drug: 0.4 L/kg; penetrates blood-brain barrier; CSF levels are ~35% to 39% of plasma levels (Yung 1999)

Protein binding: 15%

Metabolism: Prodrug, hydrolyzed to the active form, MTIC; MTIC is eventually eliminated as CO_2 and 5-aminoimidazole-4-carboxamide (AIC), a natural constituent in urine; CYP isoenzymes play only a minor role in metabolism (of temozolomide and MTIC)

Bioavailability: Oral: 100% (on a mg-per-mg basis, IV temozolomide, infused over 90 minutes, is bioequivalent to an oral dose)

Half-life elimination: Mean: Parent drug: 1.8 hours

Time to peak: Oral: Empty stomach: 1 hour; with food (high-fat meal): 2.25 hours

Excretion: Urine (~38%; parent drug 6%); feces <1%

Dosing

Adult Note: Temozolomide is associated with a moderate emetic potential (Roila 2010); antiemetics are recommended to prevent nausea and vomiting. Prior to dosing, ANC should be ≥1,500/mm³ and platelets ≥100,000/mm³.

Anaplastic astrocytoma (refractory): Oral, IV: Initial dose: 150 mg/m² once daily for 5 consecutive days of a 28-day treatment cycle. If ANC ≥1,500/mm³ and platelets ≥100,000/mm³, on day 1 of subsequent cycles, may increase to 200 mg/m² once daily for 5 consecutive days of a 28-day treatment cycle. May continue until disease progression.

Dosage modification for toxicity:

ANC <1,000/mm³ or platelets <50,000/mm³ on day 22 or day 29 (day 1 of next cycle): Postpone therapy until ANC >1,500/mm³ and platelets >100,000/mm³; reduce dose by 50 mg/m²/day (but not below 100 mg/m²) for subsequent cycle

ANC 1,000 to 1,500/mm³ or platelets 50,000-100,000/mm³ on day 22 or day 29 (day 1 of next cycle): Postpone therapy until ANC >1,500/mm³ and platelets >100,000/mm³; maintain initial dose

Glioblastoma multiforme (newly diagnosed, high-grade glioma): Oral, IV:
Concomitant phase: 75 mg/m² once daily for 42 days with focal radiotherapy (60 Gy administered in 30 fractions). **Note:** PCP prophylaxis is required during concomitant phase and should continue in patients who develop lymphocytopenia until lymphocyte recovery to ≤ grade 1. Obtain weekly CBC.

Continue at 75 mg/m² once daily throughout the 42-day concomitant phase (up to 49 days) as long as ANC ≥1,500/mm³, platelet count ≥100,000/mm³, and nonhematologic toxicity ≤ grade 1 (excludes alopecia, nausea/vomiting)

Dosage modification for toxicity:

ANC ≥500/mm^3 but <1,500/mm^3 **or** platelet count ≥10,000/mm^3 but <100,000/mm^3 **or** grade 2 nonhematologic toxicity (excludes alopecia, nausea/vomiting): Interrupt therapy

ANC <500/mm^3 **or** platelet count <10,000/mm^3 **or** grade 3/4 nonhematologic toxicity (excludes alopecia, nausea/vomiting): Discontinue therapy

Maintenance phase (consists of 6 treatment cycles): Begin 4 weeks after concomitant phase completion. **Note:** Each subsequent cycle is 28 days (consisting of 5 days of drug treatment followed by 23 days without treatment). Draw CBC on day 22 (or within 48 hours of day 22); hold next cycle and do weekly CBC until ANC >1,500/mm^3 and platelet count >100,000/mm^3; dosing modification should be based on lowest blood counts and worst nonhematologic toxicity during the previous cycle.

Cycle 1: 150 mg/m^2 once daily for 5 days of a 28-day treatment cycle

Cycles 2 to 6: May increase to 200 mg/m^2 once daily for 5 days; repeat every 28 days (if ANC ≥1,500/mm^3, platelets ≥100,000/mm^3 and nonhematologic toxicities for cycle 1 are ≤ grade 2 [excludes alopecia, nausea/vomiting]); **Note:** If dose was not escalated at the onset of cycle 2, do not increase for cycles 3 to 6)

Dosage modification (during maintenance phase) for toxicity:

ANC <1,000/mm^3, platelet count <50,000/mm^3, or grade 3 nonhematologic toxicity (excludes alopecia, nausea/vomiting) during previous cycle: Decrease dose by 1 dose level (by 50 mg/m^2/day for 5 days), unless dose has already been lowered to 100 mg/m^2/day, then discontinue therapy.

If dose reduction <100 mg/m^2/day is required or grade 4 nonhematologic toxicity (excludes alopecia, nausea/vomiting), or if the same grade 3 nonhematologic toxicity occurs after dose reduction: Discontinue therapy

Glioblastoma multiforme (recurrent glioma): *Canadian labeling (off-label use in the U.S.):* 200 mg/m^2 once daily for 5 days every 28 days; if previously treated with chemotherapy, initiate at 150 mg/m^2 once daily for 5 days every 28 days and increase to 200 mg/m^2 once daily for 5 days every 28 days with cycle 2 if no hematologic toxicity (Brada 2001; Yung 2000)

Cutaneous T-cell lymphoma, advanced (mycosis fungoides [MF] and Sézary syndrome [SS]; off-label use): Oral: 200 mg/m^2 once daily for 5 days every 28 days for up to 1 year (Querfeld 2011)

Ewing's sarcoma, recurrent or progressive (off-label use): Oral: 100 mg/m^2/dose days 1 to 5 every 21 days (in combination with irinotecan) (Casey 2009). Additional data may be necessary to further define the role of temozolomide in this condition

Melanoma, advanced or metastatic (off-label use): Oral: 200 mg/m^2 once daily for 5 days every 28 days (for up to 12 cycles). For subsequent cycles reduce dose to 75% of the original dose for grade 3/4 hematologic toxicity and reduce the dose to 50% of the original dose for grade 3/4 nonhematologic toxicity (Middleton 2000).

Neuroendocrine tumors, advanced (off-label use): Oral: 150 mg/m^2 once daily for 7 days every 14 days (in combination with thalidomide) until disease progression (Kulke 2006) **or** 200 mg/m^2 once daily (at bedtime) days 10 to 14 of a 28-day treatment cycle (in combination with capecitabine) (Strosberg 2011)

◄ **Primary CNS lymphoma, refractory (off-label use):** Oral: 150 mg/m² once daily for 5 days every 28 days, initially in combination with rituximab (for 4 cycles), followed by temozolomide monotherapy: 150 mg/m² once daily for 5 days every 28 days for 8 cycles (Wong 2004) **or** 150 mg/m² once daily on days 1 to 7 and 15 to 21 every 28 days (initially in combination with rituximab for 1 or 2 cycles), followed by temozolomide maintenance monotherapy: 150 mg/m² once daily for 5 days every 28 days (Enting 2004). However, additional data may be necessary to further define the role of temozolomide in this condition.

Soft tissue sarcoma (off-label use): Oral:

Soft tissue sarcoma, metastatic or unresectable: 75 mg/m² once daily for 6 weeks (Garcia del Muro 2005)

Hemangiopericytoma/solitary fibrous tumor: 150 mg/m² once daily days 1 to 7 and days 15 to 21 of a 28-day treatment cycle (in combination with bevacizumab) (Park 2011). Additional data may be necessary to further define the role of temozolomide in this condition

Geriatric Refer to adult dosing. **Note:** Patients ≥70 years of age in the anaplastic astrocytoma study had a higher incidence of grade 4 neutropenia and thrombocytopenia in the first cycle of therapy than patients <70 years of age.

Pediatric Note: Temozolomide is associated with a moderate emetic potential (Dupuis 2011); antiemetics are recommended to prevent nausea and vomiting.

Ewing's sarcoma, recurrent or progressive (off-label use): Children and Adolescents: Oral: Refer to adult dosing.

Neuroblastoma, relapsed or refractory (off-label use):

Children and Adolescents: Oral: 100 mg/m²/dose days 1 to 5 every 21 days (in combination with irinotecan) for up to 6 cycles (Bagatell 2011)

Children ≥6 months and Adolescents: Oral: 150 mg/m²/dose days 1 to 5 every 28 days (in combination with topotecan) until disease progression or unacceptable toxicity (Di Giannatale 2014)

Renal Impairment Oral:

CrCl ≥36 mL/minute/m²: There are no dosage adjustments provided in the manufacturer's labeling; however, dosage adjustment is not likely needed as no effect on temozolomide clearance was demonstrated.

Severe renal impairment (CrCl <36 mL/minute/m²): There are no dosage adjustments provided in the manufacturer's labeling; use with caution (has not been studied).

Dialysis patients: There are no dosage adjustments provided in the manufacturer's labeling (has not been studied).

Hepatic Impairment

Mild to moderate impairment: There are no dosage adjustments provided in the manufacturer's labeling; however, pharmacokinetics are similar to patients with normal hepatic function.

Severe hepatic impairment: There are no dosage adjustments provided in the manufacturer's labeling; use with caution (has not been studied).

Obesity *ASCO Guidelines for appropriate chemotherapy dosing in obese adults with cancer:* Utilize patient's actual body weight (full weight) for calculation of body surface area- or weight-based dosing, particularly when the intent of therapy is curative; manage regimen-related toxicities in the same manner as for nonobese patients; if a dose reduction is utilized due to toxicity, consider resumption of full weight-based dosing with subsequent cycles, especially if cause of toxicity (eg, hepatic or renal impairment) is resolved (Griggs 2012).

Combination Regimens

Bone sarcoma (Ewing sarcoma): Irinotecan-Temozolomide (Ewing Sarcoma) on page 2024

Primary CNS Lymphoma: Temozolomide-Rituximab (CNS Lymphoma) on page 2087

Administration Temozolomide is associated with a moderate emetic potential (Dupuis 2011; Roila 2010); antiemetics are recommended to prevent nausea and vomiting.

Oral:

US labeling: Swallow capsules whole with a glass of water. Absorption is affected by food; therefore, administer consistently either with food or without food (was administered in studies under fasting and nonfasting conditions). May administer on an empty stomach and/or at bedtime to reduce nausea and vomiting. Do not repeat dose if vomiting occurs after dose is administered; wait until the next scheduled dose. Do not open or chew capsules; avoid contact with skin or mucous membranes if capsules are accidentally opened or damaged.

Canadian labeling: Administer on an empty stomach at least one hour before a meal. Swallow capsules whole with a glass of water. Do not repeat dose if vomiting occurs after dose is administered; wait until the next scheduled dose. Do not open or chew capsules; avoid contact with skin or mucous membranes if capsules are accidentally opened or damaged.

IV: Infuse over 90 minutes. Flush line before and after administration. May be administered through the same IV line as sodium chloride 0.9%; do not administer other medications through the same IV line.

Hazardous agent; use appropriate precautions for handling and disposal (NIOSH 2014 [group 1]). NIOSH recommends single gloving for administration of intact capsules. Although the manufacturer does not recommend opening capsules, if necessary to manipulate the capsules (eg, to prepare an oral suspension), it is recommended to double glove, wear a protective gown, and prepare in a controlled device (NIOSH 2014).

Emetic Potential Children and Adults: IV and Oral: Moderate (30% to 90%)

Extemporaneous Preparations Hazardous agent: Use appropriate precautions for handling and disposal (NIOSH 2014 [group 1]). When manipulating capsules, NIOSH recommends double gloving, a protective gown, and preparation in a controlled device; if not prepared in a controlled device, respiratory and eye protection as well as ventilated engineering controls are recommended (NIOSH 2014).

A 10 mg/mL temozolomide oral suspension may be compounded in a vertical flow hood. Mix the contents of ten 100 mg capsules and 500 mg of povidone K-30 powder in a glass mortar; add 25 mg anhydrous citric acid dissolved in 1.5 mL purified water and mix to a uniform paste; mix while adding 50 mL Ora-Plus in incremental proportions. Transfer to an amber plastic bottle, rinse mortar 4 times with small portions of either Ora-Sweet or Ora-Sweet SF, and add quantity of Ora-Sweet or Ora-Sweet SF sufficient to make 100 mL. Store in plastic amber prescription bottles; label "shake well" and "refrigerate"; include the beyond-use date. Stable for 7 days at room temperature or 60 days refrigerated (preferred).

Trissel LA, Yanping Z, and Koontz SE, "Temozolomide Stability in Extemporaneously Compounded Oral Suspension," *Int J Pharm Compound*, 2006, 10(5):396-9.

◀ **Monitoring Parameters** CBC with differential and platelets (prior to each cycle; weekly during glioma concomitant phase treatment; at or within 48 hours of day 22 and weekly until ANC >1,500/mm³ and platelets >100,000/mm³ for glioma maintenance and astrocytoma treatment). Monitor liver function tests at baseline, halfway through the first cycle, prior to each subsequent cycle, and at ~2 to 4 weeks after the last dose. The Canadian labeling additionally recommends HBV screening at baseline (all patients) and monitoring for hepatitis or HBV reactivation during therapy and for several months after discontinuation (patients with evidence of current or prior HBV infection).

Dietary Considerations The incidence of nausea/vomiting is decreased when taken on an empty stomach. Take capsules consistently either with food or without food (absorption is affected by food). The Canadian labeling recommends taking capsules on an empty stomach one hour before a meal.

Dosage Forms Excipient information presented when available (limited, particularly for generics); consult specific product labeling.

Capsule, Oral:

Temodar: 5 mg [contains fd&c blue #2 (indigotine)]

Temodar: 20 mg, 100 mg

Temodar: 140 mg [contains fd&c blue #2 (indigotine)]

Temodar: 180 mg, 250 mg

Generic: 5 mg, 20 mg, 100 mg, 140 mg, 180 mg, 250 mg

Solution Reconstituted, Intravenous:

Temodar: 100 mg (1 ea) [pyrogen free; contains polysorbate 80]

Temsirolimus (tem sir OH li mus)

Related Information

Common Toxicity Criteria *on page 2122*

Management of Chemotherapy-Induced Nausea and Vomiting in Adults *on page 2142*

Prevention of Chemotherapy-Induced Nausea and Vomiting in Children *on page 2203*

Principles of Anticancer Therapy *on page 2261*

Safe Handling of Hazardous Drugs *on page 2292*

Brand Names: US Torisel

Brand Names: Canada Torisel

Index Terms CCI-779

Pharmacologic Category Antineoplastic Agent, mTOR Kinase Inhibitor

Use Renal cell carcinoma, advanced: Treatment of advanced renal cell carcinoma (RCC)

Labeled Contraindications Bilirubin >1.5 times the upper limit of normal (ULN)

Canadian labeling: Additional contraindications (not in U.S. labeling): History of anaphylaxis after exposure to temsirolimus, sirolimus, or any component of the formulation

Pregnancy Considerations Adverse events have been observed in animal reproduction studies. Based on its mechanism of action, temsirolimus may cause fetal harm if administered to a pregnant woman. Women of childbearing potential should be advised to avoid pregnancy. Men and women should use effective birth control during temsirolimus treatment, and continue for 3 months after temsirolimus discontinuation.

Breast-Feeding Considerations It is not known if temsirolimus is excreted in breast milk. Due to the potential for serious adverse reactions in the nursing infant, a decision should be made to discontinue breast-feeding or to discontinue temsirolimus, taking into account the importance of treatment to the mother.

Warnings/Precautions Hazardous agent - use appropriate precautions for handling and disposal (NIOSH 2014 [group 1]).

Hypersensitivity/infusion reactions (eg, anaphylaxis, apnea, dyspnea, flushing, loss of consciousness, hypotension, and/or chest pain) have been reported. Infusion reaction may occur during the initial infusion (early in infusion) or with subsequent infusions. Premedicate with an antihistamine (H_1 antagonist) prior to infusion; monitor throughout infusion (appropriate supportive care should be available); interrupt infusion for hypersensitivity reaction and observe patient for 30-60 minutes. With discretion, treatment may be resumed at a slower infusion rate; administer an H_1 antagonist (if not given as premedication) and/or an IV H_2 antagonist ~30 minutes prior to resuming infusion. For severe infusion reactions, assess risk versus benefit of continued treatment. Use with caution in patients with hypersensitivity temsirolimus, sirolimus (a metabolite), or polysorbate 80. Angioneurotic edema has been reported; concurrent use with other drugs known to cause angioedema (eg, ACE inhibitors) may increase risk.

Temsirolimus is predominantly cleared by the liver; use with caution and reduce dose in patients with mild hepatic impairment (bilirubin >1 to 1.5 x ULN or AST >ULN with bilirubin ≤ULN). Toxicities were increased in patients with baseline bilirubin >1.5 x ULN. Use is contraindicated in patients with moderate-to-severe hepatic impairment (bilirubin >1.5 x ULN).

Potentially significant interactions may exist, requiring dose or frequency adjustment, additional monitoring, and/or selection of alternative therapy. Avoid concomitant use with strong CYP3A4 inhibitors and strong CYP3A4 inducers; consider alternative agents that avoid or lessen the potential for CYP-mediated interactions. Patients should not be immunized with live, viral vaccines during or shortly after treatment and should avoid close contact with recently vaccinated (live vaccine) individuals. Patients who are receiving anticoagulant therapy or those with CNS tumors/metastases may be at increased risk for developing intracerebral bleeding (may be fatal). Combination therapy with temsirolimus and sunitinib has resulted in dose-limiting toxicities, including grade 3 or 4 rash, gout, and/or cellulitis.

Some dosage forms may contain polysorbate 80 (also known as Tweens). Hypersensitivity reactions, usually a delayed reaction, have been reported following exposure to pharmaceutical products containing polysorbate 80 in certain individuals (Isaksson, 2002; Lucente 2000; Shelley, 1995). Thrombocytopenia, ascites, pulmonary deterioration, and renal and hepatic failure have been reported in premature neonates after receiving parenteral products containing polysorbate 80 (Alade, 1986; CDC, 1984). See manufacturer's labeling.

Increases in serum glucose commonly occur during treatment; initiation or alteration of insulin and/or oral hypoglycemic therapy may be required; monitor serum glucose before and during treatment; use with caution in patients with diabetes. Use with caution in patients with hyperlipidemia; may increase serum lipids (cholesterol and triglycerides); initiation or dosage adjustment of anti-hyperlipidemic agents may be required; monitor cholesterol/triglyceride panel at baseline and periodically during treatment. Treatment may result in immunosuppression, may increase risk of opportunistic infections and/or sepsis. Pneumocystis jiroveci pneumonia (PCP) has been reported; some cases were fatal. Development of PCP may be associated with the use of concomitant corticosteroids or other immunosuppressive agents; consider PCP prophylaxis in patients receiving concomitant immunosuppressive or corticosteroid therapy. Interstitial lung disease (ILD), sometimes fatal, has been reported; symptoms include dyspnea, cough, hypoxia, and/or fever, although asymptomatic or mild cases may present; promptly evaluate worsening respiratory symptoms. If symptoms develop, consider withholding temsirolimus until symptom recovery and radiographic improvement occur. Consider empiric treatment with corticosteroids and/or antibiotic therapy; baseline chest radiographic assessment (CT scan or x-ray) is recommended; follow periodically, even in the absence of clinical pulmonary symptoms. Cases of bowel perforation (fatal) have occurred (usually presenting with abdominal pain, bloody stools, diarrhea, fever, or metabolic acidosis); promptly evaluate any new or worsening abdominal pain or bloody stools. Temsirolimus may be associated with impaired wound healing; use caution in the perioperative period. Cases of acute renal failure with rapid progression have been reported (unrelated to disease progression), including cases unresponsive to dialysis. An increased incidence of rash, infection and dose interruptions have been reported in patients with renal insufficiency (CrCl ≤60 mL/minute) who received mTOR inhibitors for the treatment of renal cell cancer (Gupta, 2011). Elderly patients may be more likely to experience adverse reactions, including diarrhea, edema, and pneumonia.

Adverse Reactions

>10%:

Cardiovascular: Edema (35%), chest pain (16%)

Central nervous system: Pain (28%), headache (15%), insomnia (12%)

Dermatologic: Skin rash (47%), pruritus (19%), nail disease (14%), xeroderma (11%)

Endocrine & metabolic: Increased serum glucose (89%; grades 3/4: 16%), increased serum cholesterol (87%; grades 3/4: 2%), hypertriglyceridemia (83%; grades 3/4: 44%), hypophosphatemia (49%; grades 3/4: 18%), hyperglycemia (26%), hyperlipidemia (≥30%), hypokalemia (21%; grades 3/4: 5%), weight loss (19%)

Gastrointestinal: Mucositis (41%), nausea (37%), anorexia (32%), diarrhea (27%), abdominal pain (21%; grades 3/4: 4%), constipation (20%), dysgeusia (20%), stomatitis (20%), vomiting (19%)

Genitourinary: Urinary tract infection (15%)

Hematologic & oncologic: Decreased hemoglobin (94%; grades 3/4: 20%), lymphocytopenia (53%; grades 3/4: 16%), thrombocytopenia (40%; grades 3/4: 1%; dose-limiting toxicity), decreased white blood cell count (32%; grades 3/4: 1%), anemia (≥30%), decreased neutrophils (19%; grades 3/4: 5%)

Hepatic: Increased serum alkaline phosphatase (68%; grades 3/4: 3%), increased serum AST (38%; grades 3/4: 2%)

Infection: Infection (20%; grades 3/4: 3%; includes abscess, bronchitis, cellulitis, herpes simplex, herpes zoster)

Neuromuscular & skeletal: Weakness (51%), back pain (20%), arthralgia (18%)

Renal: Increased serum creatinine (57%; grades 3/4: 3%)

Respiratory: Dyspnea (28%), cough (26%), epistaxis (12%), pharyngitis (12%)

Miscellaneous: Fever (24%; grades 3/4: 1%)

1% to 10%:

Cardiovascular: Hypertension (7%), venous thromboembolism (2%; includes deep vein thrombosis and pulmonary embolism), pericardial effusion (1%), thrombophlebitis (1%)

Central nervous system: Chills (8%), depression (4%), convulsions (1%)

Dermatologic: Acne vulgaris (10%)

Endocrine & metabolic: Diabetes mellitus (5%)

Gastrointestinal: Gastrointestinal hemorrhage (1%)

Hematologic & oncologic: Rectal hemorrhage (1%)

Hepatic: Hyperbilirubinemia (8%)

Infection: Sepsis (1%), wound infection (1%)

Neuromuscular & skeletal: Myalgia (8%)

Ophthalmic: Conjunctivitis (8%; including lacrimation disorder)

Respiratory: Rhinitis (10%), pneumonia (8%), upper respiratory tract infection (7%), pleural effusion (4%)

Miscellaneous: Wound healing impairment (1%)

<1%, postmarketing, and/or case reports: Acute renal failure, angioedema, causalgia, cholecystitis, cholelithiasis, decreased glucose tolerance, extravasation reactions (with pain, swelling, warmth, erythema), hypersensitivity reaction, interstitial pulmonary disease, intestinal perforation, pancreatitis, pneumonitis, rhabdomyolysis, seizure, Stevens-Johnson syndrome

Drug Interactions

Metabolism/Transport Effects Substrate of CYP3A4 (major), P-glycoprotein; **Note:** Assignment of Major/Minor substrate status based on clinically relevant drug interaction potential; **Inhibits** CYP2D6 (weak)

Avoid Concomitant Use

Avoid concomitant use of Temsirolimus with any of the following: BCG (Intravesical); CloZAPine; Conivaptan; Dipyrone; Fusidic Acid (Systemic); Idelalisib; Natalizumab; Pimecrolimus; SUNItinib; Tacrolimus (Systemic); Tacrolimus (Topical); Tofacitinib; Vaccines (Live)

Increased Effect/Toxicity

Temsirolimus may increase the levels/effects of: ACE Inhibitors; ARIPiprazole; CloZAPine; CycloSPORINE (Systemic); Fingolimod; Leflunomide; Natalizumab; SUNItinib; Tacrolimus (Systemic); Tacrolimus (Topical); Tofacitinib; Vaccines (Live)

The levels/effects of Temsirolimus may be increased by: Aprepitant; Conivaptan; CYP3A4 Inhibitors (Moderate); CYP3A4 Inhibitors (Strong); Dasatinib; Denosumab; Dipyrone; Fluconazole; Fosaprepitant; Fusidic Acid (Systemic); Idelalisib; Itraconazole; Ivacaftor; Ketoconazole (Systemic); Luliconazole; Macrolide Antibiotics; Mifepristone; Netupitant; Osimertinib; Palbociclib; P-glycoprotein/ABCB1 Inhibitors; Pimecrolimus; Posaconazole; Protease Inhibitors; Ranolazine; Roflumilast; Simeprevir; Stiripentol; Tacrolimus (Systemic); Tacrolimus (Topical); Trastuzumab

Decreased Effect

Temsirolimus may decrease the levels/effects of: Antidiabetic Agents; BCG (Intravesical); Coccidioides immitis Skin Test; Sipuleucel-T; Tacrolimus (Systemic); Vaccines (Inactivated); Vaccines (Live)

◄ *The levels/effects of Temsirolimus may be decreased by:* Bosentan; CarBA-
Mazepine; CYP3A4 Inducers (Moderate); CYP3A4 Inducers (Strong); Dabrafenib; Deferasirox; Echinacea; Enzalutamide; Fosphenytoin; Mitotane;
Osimertinib; P-glycoprotein/ABCB1 Inducers; Phenytoin; Rifamycin Derivatives; Siltuximab; St Johns Wort; Tocilizumab

Food Interactions Grapefruit and grapefruit juice may increase the levels/
effects of sirolimus. Management: Avoid grapefruit and grapefruit juice.

Storage/Stability Store intact vials refrigerated at 2°C to 8°C (36°F to 46°F).
Diluted solution in the vial (10 mg/mL) is stable for 24 hours at room temperature (below 25°C [77°F]). Solutions diluted for infusion (in NS) must be
infused within 6 hours of preparation. Protect from light during storage,
preparation, and handling.

Preparation for Administration Hazardous agent; use appropriate precautions for handling and disposal (NIOSH 2014 [group 1]). Preparation requires a
two-step dilution process (do not add undiluted temsirolimus to aqueous
solution; addition to aqueous solution prior to step 1 will result in precipitation).
Step 1: Total amount in undiluted vial is 30 mg/1.2 mL (25 mg/mL concentration); contains overfill. Vials should initially be diluted with 1.8 mL of provided
diluent to a concentration of 10 mg/mL. Once diluted with provided diluent, mix
by inverting vial. *Step 2:* After allowing air bubbles to subside, the intended
dose should be withdrawn from the 10 mg/mL diluted vial (ie, 2.5 mL for a
25 mg dose) and further diluted in 250 mL of NS in a non-DEHP/non-PVC
container (glass, polyolefin, or polypropylene). Mix by inverting bottle or bag;
avoid excessive shaking (may result in foaming).

Mechanism of Action Temsirolimus and its active metabolite, sirolimus, are
targeted inhibitors of mTOR (mechanistic target of rapamycin) kinase activity.
Temsirolimus (and sirolimus) bind to FKBP-12, an intracellular protein, to form
a complex which inhibits mTOR signaling, halting the cell cycle at the G1
phase in tumor cells. Inhibition of mTOR blocks downstream phosphorylation
of p70S6k and S6 ribosomal proteins. In renal cell carcinoma, mTOR inhibition
also exhibits anti-angiogenesis activity by reducing levels of HIF-1 and HIF-2
alpha (hypoxia inducible factors) and vascular endothelial growth factor
(VEGF).

Pharmacodynamics/Kinetics

Distribution: V_{dss}: 172 L

Metabolism: Hepatic; via CYP3A4 to sirolimus (primary active metabolite) and
4 minor metabolites

Half-life elimination: Temsirolimus: ~17 hours; Sirolimus: ~55 hours

Time to peak, plasma: Temsirolimus: At end of infusion; Sirolimus: 0.5 to 2
hours after temsirolimus infusion

Excretion: Feces (78%); urine (<5%)

Dosing

Adult & Geriatric Note: For infusion reaction prophylaxis, premedicate with
an H_1 antagonist (eg, diphenhydramine 25 to 50 mg IV) ~30 minutes prior to
infusion.

Renal cell cancer (RCC), advanced: IV: 25 mg once weekly; continue until
disease progression or unacceptable toxicity

Dosage adjustment for concomitant CYP3A4 inhibitors/inducers:

CYP3A4 inhibitors: Avoid concomitant administration with strong CYP3A4
inhibitors (eg, clarithromycin, itraconazole, ketoconazole, nefazodone,
protease inhibitors, telithromycin, voriconazole); if concomitant administration with a strong CYP3A4 inhibitor cannot be avoided, consider a dose
reduction to 12.5 mg once weekly. When a strong CYP3A4 inhibitor is

discontinued; allow ~1 week to elapse prior to adjusting the temsirolimus upward to the dose used prior to initiation of the CYP3A4 inhibitor.

CYP3A4 inducers: Avoid concomitant administration with strong CYP3A4 inducers (eg, carbamazepine, dexamethasone, phenobarbital, phenytoin, rifabutin, rifampin, St John's wort); if concomitant administration with a strong CYP3A4 inducer cannot be avoided, consider adjusting temsirolimus dose up to 50 mg once weekly. If the strong CYP3A4 enzyme inducer is discontinued, reduce the temsirolimus to the dose used prior to initiation of the CYP3A4 inducer.

Renal Impairment No dosage adjustment necessary.

Hemodialysis: There are no dosage adjustments provided in the manufacturer's labeling (has not been studied).

Hepatic Impairment

Mild hepatic impairment (bilirubin >1 to 1.5 x ULN or AST >ULN with bilirubin ≤ULN): Reduce dose to 15 mg once weekly.

Moderate-to-severe hepatic impairment (bilirubin >1.5 x ULN): Use is contraindicated.

Adjustment for Toxicity

Hematologic toxicity: ANC <1000/mm^3 or platelets <75,000/mm^3: Withhold treatment until resolves and reinitiate treatment with the dose reduced by 5 mg weekly; minimum dose: 15 mg weekly if adjustment for toxicity is needed.

Nonhematologic toxicity: Any toxicity ≥ grade 3: Withhold treatment until resolves to ≤ grade 2; reinitiate treatment with the dose reduced by 5 mg weekly; minimum dose: 15 mg weekly if adjustment for toxicity is needed.

Infusion/hypersensitivity reaction: Interrupt infusion and observe for 30 to 60 minutes; treatment may be resumed with discretion at a slower infusion rate (up to 60 minutes); administer an H$_1$ antagonist (if not given as premedication) and/or an IV H$_2$ antagonist 30 minutes prior to resuming infusion.

Interstitial lung disease: Consider withholding treatment for clinically significant respiratory symptoms until after recovery of symptoms or radiographic improvement.

Combination Regimens

Renal cell cancer: Temsirolimus (RCC Regimen) on page 2088

Administration Infuse over 30 to 60 minutes via an infusion pump (preferred). Use polyethylene-lined non-DEHP administration tubing. Administer through an inline polyethersulfone filter ≤5 micron; if set does not contain an inline filter, a polyethersulfone end filter (0.2 to 5 micron) should be added (do not use both an inline and an end filter). Premedicate with an H$_1$ antagonist (eg, diphenhydramine 25 to 50 mg IV) ~30 minutes prior to infusion. Monitor during infusion; interrupt infusion for hypersensitivity/infusion reaction; monitor for 30 to 60 minutes; may reinitiate at a reduced infusion rate (over 60 minutes) with discretion, 30 minutes after administration of a histamine H$_1$ antagonist and/or a histamine H$_2$ antagonist (eg, famotidine or ranitidine). Administration should be completed within 6 hours of admixture.

Hazardous agent; use appropriate precautions for handling and disposal (NIOSH 2014 [group 1]).

Emetic Potential

Children: Minimal (<10%)

Adults: Low (10% to 30%)

◀ **Monitoring Parameters** CBC with differential and platelets (weekly), serum chemistries including glucose (baseline and every other week), serum cholesterol and triglycerides (baseline and periodic), liver function (baseline and periodic), renal function tests (baseline and periodic)

Monitor for infusion reactions; infection; symptoms of ILD (or radiographic changes), symptoms of hyperglycemia (excessive thirst, polyuria); symptoms of bowel perforation

Dietary Considerations Avoid grapefruit juice (may increase the levels of the major metabolite, sirolimus).

Dosage Forms Excipient information presented when available (limited, particularly for generics); consult specific product labeling.

Solution, Intravenous:

Torisel: 25 mg/mL (1 mL) [contains alcohol, usp, polyethylene glycol, polysorbate 80, propylene glycol]

Teniposide (ten i POE side)

Related Information

Management of Chemotherapy-Induced Nausea and Vomiting in Adults *on page 2142*

Management of Drug Extravasations *on page 2159*

Prevention of Chemotherapy-Induced Nausea and Vomiting in Children *on page 2203*

Safe Handling of Hazardous Drugs *on page 2292*

Brand Names: US Vumon [DSC]

Brand Names: Canada Vumon

Index Terms EPT; PTG; VM-26

Pharmacologic Category Antineoplastic Agent, Podophyllotoxin Derivative; Antineoplastic Agent, Topoisomerase II Inhibitor

Use Acute lymphoblastic leukemia, refractory: Treatment of refractory childhood acute lymphoblastic leukemia (ALL) in combination with other chemotherapy

Labeled Contraindications Hypersensitivity to teniposide, polyoxyl 35/polyoxyethylated castor oil (Cremophor EL), or any component of the formulation

Pregnancy Considerations Adverse effects were observed in animal reproduction studies. May cause fetal harm if administered during pregnancy. Women of childbearing potential should avoid becoming pregnant during teniposide treatment.

Breast-Feeding Considerations It is not known if teniposide is excreted in breast milk. Due to the potential for serious adverse reactions in the nursing infant, a decision should be made to discontinue teniposide or to discontinue breast-feeding, taking into account the importance of treatment to the mother.

Warnings/Precautions Hazardous agent - use appropriate precautions for handling and disposal (NIOSH 2014 [group 1]).

[US Boxed Warning]: Severe myelosuppression resulting in infection or bleeding may occur; may be dose-limiting; monitor blood counts. Patients with Down syndrome and leukemia may be more sensitive to the myelosuppressive effects; reduced initial doses are recommended. Contains polyoxyl 35/polyoxyethylated castor oil (Cremophor EL), which is associated with hypersensitivity reactions. [US Boxed Warning]: Hypersensitivity reactions, including anaphylaxis-like reactions, have been reported; may occur with initial dosing or with repeated exposure to teniposide. Epinephrine, with

or without corticosteroids and antihistamines, has been employed to alleviate hypersensitivity reaction symptoms. Hypersensitivity reactions may include bronchospasm, dyspnea, hypertension, hypotension, tachycardia, flushing, chills, fever, or urticaria. Monitor closely during infusion (observe continuously for first 60 minutes, frequently thereafter). Stop infusion for signs of anaphylaxis; immediate treatment for anaphylactic reaction should be available during administration (may require treatment with epinephrine, corticosteroids, antihistamines, pressors, or volume expanders). Patients experiencing prior hypersensitivity are at risk for recurrence; re-treat only if the potential benefit outweighs the risk of hypersensitivity; premedication (with corticosteroids and antihistamines) is recommended for re-treatment. Hypotension may occur with rapid infusion; infuse slowly over at least 30 to 60 minutes; discontinue for clinically significant hypotension; if infusion is restarted after being withheld for hypotension, reinitiate at a slower infusion rate.

Use with caution in patients with renal or hepatic impairment; may require dosage reduction in patients with significant impairment. Teniposide is considered an irritant (Perez Fidalgo, 2012). For IV use only; ensure proper catheter/needle position prior to infusion; monitor infusion site; may cause local tissue necrosis and/or thrombophlebitis if extravasation occurs. Since teniposide is highly bound to plasma proteins, carefully monitor patients with hypoalbuminemia. Product contains about 43% alcohol. Acute CNS depression, hypotension and metabolic acidosis have been reported; these events occurred in patients who received high-dose teniposide (investigation protocol) and were premedicated with antiemetics, which along with the alcohol content of teniposide, may have contributed to the CNS depression. **[US Boxed Warning]: Should be administered under the supervision of an experienced cancer chemotherapy physician. Appropriate management of therapy and complications is possible only when adequate treatment facilities are readily available.** Potentially significant drug-drug interactions may exist, requiring dose or frequency adjustment, additional monitoring, and/or selection of alternative therapy.

Benzyl alcohol and derivatives: Some dosage forms may contain benzyl alcohol; large amounts of benzyl alcohol (≥99 mg/kg/day) have been associated with a potentially fatal toxicity ("gasping syndrome") in neonates; the "gasping syndrome" consists of metabolic acidosis, respiratory distress, gasping respirations, CNS dysfunction (including convulsions, intracranial hemorrhage), hypotension, and cardiovascular collapse (AAP ["Inactive" 1997]; CDC, 1982); some data suggests that benzoate displaces bilirubin from protein binding sites (Ahlfors, 2001); avoid or use dosage forms containing benzyl alcohol with caution in neonates. See manufacturer's labeling.

N,N-dimethylacetamide: Teniposide contains N,N-dimethylacetamide, which is incompatible with many closed system transfer devices (CSTDs); the plastic components of CSTDs may dissolve and result in subsequent leakage and potential infusion of dissolved plastic into the patient (ISMP [Smetzer 2015]).

Adverse Reactions

>10%:

Gastrointestinal: Mucositis (76%), diarrhea (33%), nausea/vomiting (29%; mild to moderate)

Hematologic: Neutropenia (95%), leukopenia (89%), anemia (88%), thrombocytopenia (85%), myelosuppression (75%)

Miscellaneous: Infection (12%)

1% to 10%:

Cardiovascular: Hypotension (2%; associated with rapid [<30 minutes] infusions)

Central nervous system: Fever (3%)

Dermatologic: Alopecia (9%; usually reversible), rash (3%)

Hematologic: Bleeding (5%)

Miscellaneous: Hypersensitivity reactions (5%; includes bronchospasm, chills, dyspnea, fever, flushing, hyper-/hypotension, tachycardia, or urticaria)

1% (Limited to important or life-threatening): Arrhythmia, CNS depression, confusion, headache, hepatic dysfunction, intractable hypotension, metabolic abnormality, metabolic acidosis, neuropathy (severe), neurotoxicity, renal dysfunction, thrombophlebitis, tissue necrosis (upon extravasation), weakness

Drug Interactions

Metabolism/Transport Effects Substrate of CYP3A4 (major), P-glycoprotein; **Note:** Assignment of Major/Minor substrate status based on clinically relevant drug interaction potential; **Inhibits** CYP2C9 (weak)

Avoid Concomitant Use

Avoid concomitant use of Teniposide with any of the following: BCG (Intravesical); CloZAPine; Conivaptan; Dipyrone; Fusidic Acid (Systemic); Idelalisib; Natalizumab; Pimecrolimus; Tacrolimus (Topical); Tofacitinib; Vaccines (Live)

Increased Effect/Toxicity

Teniposide may increase the levels/effects of: CloZAPine; Fingolimod; Leflunomide; Natalizumab; Tofacitinib; Vaccines (Live); VinCRIStine; VinCRIStine (Liposomal)

The levels/effects of Teniposide may be increased by: Aprepitant; Conivaptan; CYP3A4 Inhibitors (Moderate); CYP3A4 Inhibitors (Strong); Dasatinib; Denosumab; Dipyrone; Fosaprepitant; Fusidic Acid (Systemic); Idelalisib; Ivacaftor; Luliconazole; Mifepristone; Netupitant; Osimertinib; Palbociclib; P-glycoprotein/ABCB1 Inhibitors; Pimecrolimus; Ranolazine; Roflumilast; Simeprevir; Stiripentol; Tacrolimus (Topical); Trastuzumab

Decreased Effect

Teniposide may decrease the levels/effects of: BCG (Intravesical); Coccidioides immitis Skin Test; Sipuleucel-T; Vaccines (Inactivated); Vaccines (Live)

The levels/effects of Teniposide may be decreased by: Barbiturates; Bosentan; CYP3A4 Inducers (Moderate); CYP3A4 Inducers (Strong); Dabrafenib; Deferasirox; Echinacea; Enzalutamide; Fosphenytoin; Mitotane; Osimertinib; P-glycoprotein/ABCB1 Inducers; Phenytoin; Siltuximab; St Johns Wort; Tocilizumab

Storage/Stability Store ampuls in refrigerator at 2°C to 8°C (36°F to 46°F). Protect from light. Solutions diluted for infusion to a concentration of 0.1, 0.2, or 0.4 mg/mL are stable at room temperature for up to 24 hours after preparation; solutions diluted to 1 mg/mL should be used within 4 hours of preparation. Because precipitation may occur at any concentration, the manufacturer recommends administrating as soon as possible after preparation. Use appropriate precautions for handling and disposal. Do not refrigerate solutions prepared for infusion.

Preparation for Administration Hazardous agent; use appropriate precautions for handling and disposal (NIOSH 2014 [group 1]). Precipitation may occur at any concentration. Teniposide must be diluted with either D_5W or 0.9% sodium chloride solutions to a final concentration of 0.1, 0.2, 0.4, or 1 mg/mL. **Solutions should be prepared in non-DEHP-containing containers such as glass or polyolefin containers.** The use of polyvinyl chloride (PVC) containers is not recommended. Because precipitation may occur at any concentration, the manufacturer recommends administrating as soon as possible after preparation. Teniposide contains N,N-dimethylacetamide, which is incompatible with many closed system transfer devices (CSTDs); the plastic components of CSTDs may dissolve and result in subsequent leakage and potential infusion of dissolved plastic into the patient (ISMP [Smetzer 2015]).

Mechanism of Action Teniposide does not inhibit microtubular assembly; it has been shown to delay transit of cells through the S phase and arrest cells in late S or early G_2 phase, preventing cells from entering mitosis. Teniposide is a topoisomerase II inhibitor, and appears to cause DNA strand breaks by inhibition of strand-passing and DNA ligase action.

Pharmacodynamics/Kinetics

Distribution: V_{dss}: Adults: 8 to 44 L/m^2; Children: 3 to 11 L/m^2; crosses blood-brain barrier to a limited extent

Protein binding: >99%

Metabolism: Extensively hepatic

Half-life elimination: Children: 5 hours

Excretion: Urine (44%, 4% to 12% as unchanged drug); feces (≤10%)

Dosing

Adult Note: Patients with Down syndrome and leukemia may be more sensitive to the myelosuppressive effects; administer the first course at half the usual dose and adjust dose in subsequent cycles upward based on degree of toxicities (myelosuppression and mucositis) in the previous course(s).

Acute lymphoblastic leukemia (ALL) consolidation treatment (off-label use; combination chemotherapy): IV: 165 mg/m^2/dose days 1, 4, 8, and 11 of alternating consolidation cycles (Linker, 1991)

Pediatric Note: Patients with Down syndrome and leukemia may be more sensitive to the myelosuppressive effects; administer the first course at half the usual dose and adjust dose in subsequent cycles upward based on degree of toxicities (myelosuppression and mucositis) in the previous course(s).

Acute lymphoblastic leukemia (ALL), refractory (combination chemotherapy): IV: 165 mg/m^2 twice weekly for 8 to 9 doses (in combination with cytarabine) **or** 250 mg/m^2 weekly for 4 to 8 weeks (in combination with vincristine and prednisone)

Renal Impairment There are no specific dosage adjustments provided in the manufacturer's labeling (has not been studied). However, dosage adjustment may be necessary in patients with significant renal impairment.

Hepatic Impairment There are no specific dosage adjustments provided in the manufacturer's labeling (has not been studied). However, dosage adjustment may be necessary in patients with significant hepatic impairment.

Combination Regimens

Leukemia, acute lymphocytic: Linker Protocol (ALL) on page 2030 ▶

◄ **Administration** IV; must be administered slowly (over at least 30-60 minutes); do not administer by rapid IV injection. Administer through non-DEHP-containing administration sets. Incompatible with heparin; flush infusion line with D_5W or NS before and after infusion. Precipitation may occur at any concentration; administer as soon as possible after preparation; inspect solution prior to administration. Observe patient continuously for at least the first 60 minutes after the start of the infusion, observe frequently thereafter. Stop infusion for signs of anaphylaxis (may require treatment with epinephrine, corticosteroids, antihistamines, pressors, or volume expanders); discontinue for clinically significant hypotension during infusion; if infusion is restarted after being withheld for hypotension, reinitiate at a slower infusion rate.

Teniposide contains N, N-dimethylacetamide, which is incompatible with many closed system transfer devices (CSTDs); the plastic components of CSTDs may dissolve and result in subsequent leakage and potential infusion of dissolved plastic into the patient (ISMP [Smetzer 2015]).

Hazardous agent; use appropriate precautions for handling and disposal (NIOSH 2014 [group 1]).

Vesicant/Extravasation Risk Irritant

Emetic Potential Children: Low (10% to 30%)

Monitoring Parameters CBC with differential and platelet count, renal and hepatic function tests; blood pressure; monitor for hypersensitivity reaction (observe continuously for first 60 minutes of infusion, frequently thereafter)

Dosage Forms Considerations Injectable solution may contain alcohol, benzyl alcohol, or polyoxyl 35/polyoxyethylated castor oil (Cremophor EL)

Dosage Forms Excipient information presented when available (limited, particularly for generics); consult specific product labeling. [DSC] = Discontinued product

Solution, Intravenous:
  Vumon: 10 mg/mL (5 mL [DSC]) [contains alcohol, usp, benzyl alcohol, cremophor el, dimethylacetamide]
  Generic: 10 mg/mL (5 mL)

- **Teva-Levofloxacin (Can)** *see* Levofloxacin (Systemic) *on page 1038*
- **Teva-Lorazepam (Can)** *see* LORazepam *on page 1058*
- **Teva-Medroxyprogesterone (Can)** *see* MedroxyPROGESTERone *on page 1074*
- **Teva-Morphine SR (Can)** *see* Morphine (Systemic) *on page 1167*
- **Teva-Nabilone (Can)** *see* Nabilone *on page 1187*
- **Teva-Olanzapine (Can)** *see* OLANZapine *on page 1242*
- **Teva-Olanzapine OD (Can)** *see* OLANZapine *on page 1242*
- **Teva-Ondansetron (Can)** *see* Ondansetron *on page 1253*
- **Teva-Prednisone (Can)** *see* PredniSONE *on page 1426*
- **Teva-Raloxifene (Can)** *see* Raloxifene *on page 1451*
- **Teva-Tamoxifen (Can)** *see* Tamoxifen *on page 1595*
- **Teva-Trimel (Can)** *see* Sulfamethoxazole and Trimethoprim *on page 1560*
- **Teva-Trimel DS (Can)** *see* Sulfamethoxazole and Trimethoprim *on page 1560*
- **Teva-Voriconazole (Can)** *see* Voriconazole *on page 1775*
- **TG** *see* Thioguanine *on page 1637*
- **6-TG (error-prone abbreviation)** *see* Thioguanine *on page 1637*

Thalidomide (tha LI doe mide)
Related Information
Chemotherapy and Cancer Treatment During Pregnancy *on page 2214*
Chemotherapy-Induced Peripheral Neuropathy *on page 2116*
Common Toxicity Criteria *on page 2122*
Hematopoietic Stem Cell Transplantation *on page 2272*
Management of Chemotherapy-Induced Nausea and Vomiting in Adults *on page 2142*
Prevention of Chemotherapy-Induced Nausea and Vomiting in Children *on page 2203*
Principles of Anticancer Therapy *on page 2261*
Safe Handling of Hazardous Drugs *on page 2292*
Brand Names: US Thalomid
Brand Names: Canada Thalomid
Pharmacologic Category Angiogenesis Inhibitor; Antineoplastic Agent; Immunomodulator, Systemic
Use
US labeling:
Erythema nodosum leprosum: Acute treatment of cutaneous manifestations of moderate to severe erythema nodosum leprosum; maintenance treatment for prevention and suppression of cutaneous manifestations of erythema nodosum leprosum recurrence
Limitation of use: Thalidomide is not indicated as monotherapy for erythema nodosum leprosum treatment in the presence of moderate to severe neuritis.
Multiple myeloma: Treatment of newly diagnosed multiple myeloma (in combination with dexamethasone)

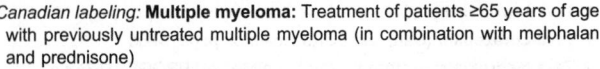

Canadian labeling: **Multiple myeloma:** Treatment of patients ≥65 years of age with previously untreated multiple myeloma (in combination with melphalan and prednisone)

Labeled Contraindications

Hypersensitivity to thalidomide or any component of the formulation; pregnancy

Canadian labeling: Additional contraindications (not in US labeling): Hypersensitivity to lenalidomide or pomalidomide; both females at risk of becoming pregnant and male patients who are unable to follow or comply with conditions for use (refer to manufacturer labeling); breast-feeding

Pregnancy Considerations [US Boxed Warning]: Thalidomide may cause severe birth defects or embryo-fetal death if taken during pregnancy. Thalidomide cannot be used in women who are pregnant or may become pregnant during therapy as even a single dose may cause severe birth defects. In order to decrease the risk of fetal exposure, thalidomide is available only through a special restricted distribution program (Thalomid REMS). Reproduction studies in animals and data from pregnant women have shown evidence of fetal abnormalities; use is contraindicated in women who are or may become pregnant. Anomalies observed in humans include amelia, phocomelia, bone defects, ear and eye abnormalities, facial palsy, congenital heart defects, urinary and genital tract malformations; mortality in ~40% of infants at or shortly after birth has also been reported.

Women of reproductive potential must avoid pregnancy 4 weeks prior to therapy, during therapy, during therapy interruptions, and for ≥4 weeks after therapy is discontinued. Two forms of effective contraception or total abstinence from heterosexual intercourse must be used by females who are not infertile or who have not had a hysterectomy. A negative pregnancy test (sensitivity of at least 50 milliunits/mL) 10 to 14 days prior to therapy, within 24 hours prior to beginning therapy, weekly during the first 4 weeks, and every 4 weeks (every 2 weeks for women with irregular menstrual cycles) thereafter is required for women of childbearing potential. Thalidomide must be immediately discontinued for a missed period, abnormal pregnancy test or abnormal menstrual bleeding; refer patient to a reproductive toxicity specialist if pregnancy occurs during treatment.

Females of reproductive potential (including health care workers and caregivers) must also avoid contact with thalidomide capsules.

Thalidomide is also present in the semen of males. Males (even those vasectomized) must use a latex or synthetic condom during any sexual contact with women of childbearing potential and for up to 28 days following discontinuation of therapy. Males taking thalidomide must not donate sperm.

The parent or legal guardian for patients between 12 to 18 years of age must agree to ensure compliance with the required guidelines.

If pregnancy occurs during treatment, thalidomide must be immediately discontinued and the patient referred to a reproductive toxicity specialist. Any suspected fetal exposure to thalidomide must be reported to the FDA via the MedWatch program (1-800-FDA-1088) and to Celgene Corporation (1-888-423-5436). In Canada, thalidomide is available only through a restricted-distribution program called RevAid (1-888-738-2431).

Breast-Feeding Considerations It is not known if thalidomide is excreted in breast milk. Due to the potential for serious adverse reactions in the infant, a decision should be made to discontinue nursing or discontinue treatment with thalidomide, taking into account the importance of treatment to the mother. Use in breast-feeding women is contraindicated in the Canadian labeling.

Warnings/Precautions Hazardous agent - use appropriate precautions for handling and disposal (NIOSH 2014 [group 2]). Avoid exposure to nonintact capsules and body fluids of patients receiving thalidomide. If exposure occurs, wash area with soap and water. Wear gloves to prevent cutaneous exposure.

[US Boxed Warning]: Thalidomide use for the treatment of multiple myeloma is associated with an increased risk for venous thromboembolism (VTE), including deep vein thrombosis (DVT) and pulmonary embolism (PE); the risk is increased when used in combination with standard chemotherapy agents, including dexamethasone. In one controlled study, the incidence of VTE was 22.5% in patients receiving thalidomide in combination with dexamethasone, compared to 4.9% for dexamethasone alone. Monitor for signs and symptoms of thromboembolism (shortness of breath, chest pain, or arm or leg swelling) and instruct patients to seek prompt medical attention with development of these symptoms. Consider thromboprophylaxis based on risk factors. Ischemic heart disease, including MI and stroke, also occurred at a higher rate (compared to placebo) in myeloma patients receiving thalidomide plus dexamethasone who had not received prior treatment. Assess individual risk factors for thromboembolism and consider thromboprophylaxis. The American Society of Clinical Oncology guidelines for VTE prophylaxis and treatment recommend thromboprophylaxis for patients receiving thalidomide in combination with chemotherapy and/or dexamethasone; either aspirin or low molecular weight heparin (LMWH) are recommended for lower risk patient and LMWH is recommended for higher risk patients (Lyman 2013). Anticoagulant prophylaxis should be individualized and selected based on the venous thromboembolism risk of the combination treatment regimen, using the safest and easiest to administer (Palumbo 2008). The Canadian labeling recommends anticoagulant prophylaxis for at least the first 5 months of thalidomide-based therapy. Monitor for signs/symptoms of thromboembolism and advise patients to seek immediate care if symptoms (shortness of breath, chest pain, arm/leg swelling) develop. Other medications that are also associated with thromboembolism should be used with caution.

May cause leukopenia and neutropenia; avoid initiating therapy if ANC <750/mm^3. Persistent neutropenia may require treatment interruption. Thrombocytopenia (including grades 3 and 4) has been reported; may require dose reduction, treatment delay, or discontinuation. Monitor for signs and symptoms of bleeding (including petechiae, epistaxis, and gastrointestinal bleeding), especially if concomitant medication may increase the risk of bleeding. Monitor CBC with differential and platelets. Anemia has also been observed. May cause bradycardia; use with caution when administering concomitantly with medications that may also decrease heart rate. May require thalidomide dose reduction or discontinuation. Stevens-Johnson syndrome (SJS) and toxic epidermal necrolysis (TEN) have been reported (may be fatal); withhold therapy and evaluate if skin rash occurs; permanently discontinue if rash is exfoliative, purpuric, bullous or if SJS or TEN is suspected. Hypersensitivity, including erythematous macular rash, possibly associated with fever, tachycardia and hypotension has been reported. May require treatment interruption for severe reactions; discontinue if recurs with rechallenge. Abnormal liver function tests have been reported. Hepatotoxicity (including some serious and fatal cases of hepatic injury) has been observed usually within the first 2 months of treatment (Thalomid Canadian labeling 2015); most events resolved without intervention after discontinuing thalidomide.

Increased incidence of second primary malignancies (SPMs), including acute myeloid leukemia (AML) and myelodysplastic syndrome (MDS), has been observed in previously untreated multiple myeloma patients receiving thalidomide in combination with melphalan, and prednisone. In addition to AML and MDS, solid tumors have been reported with thalidomide maintenance treatment for multiple myeloma (Usmani, 2012). Carefully evaluate patients for SPMs prior to and during treatment and manage as clinically indicated.

Thalidomide is commonly associated with peripheral neuropathy; may be irreversible. Neuropathy generally occurs following chronic use (over months), but may occur with short-term use; onset may be delayed. Use caution with other medications that may also cause peripheral neuropathy. Monitor for signs/symptoms of neuropathy monthly for the first 3 months of therapy and regularly thereafter. Electrophysiological testing may be considered at baseline and every 6 months to detect asymptomatic neuropathy. To limit further damage, immediately discontinue (if clinically appropriate) in patients who develop neuropathy. Reinitiate therapy only if neuropathy returns to baseline; may require dosage reduction or permanent discontinuation. Seizures (including grand mal convulsions) have been reported in postmarketing data; monitor closely for clinical changes indicating potential seizure activity in patients with a history of seizures, concurrent therapy with drugs that alter seizure threshold, or conditions that predispose to seizures. May cause dizziness, drowsiness, and/or somnolence; caution patients about performing tasks that require mental alertness (eg, operating machinery or driving). Avoid ethanol and concomitant medications that may exacerbate these symptoms; dose reductions may be necessary for excessive drowsiness or somnolence. May cause orthostatic hypotension; use with caution in patients who would not tolerate transient hypotensive episodes. When arising from a recumbent position, advise patients to sit upright for a few minutes prior to standing. Constipation may commonly occur. May require treatment interruption or dosage reduction. Certain adverse reactions (constipation, fatigue, weakness, nausea, hypokalemia, hyperglycemia, DVT, pulmonary embolism, atrial fibrillation) are more likely in elderly patients. In studies conducted prior to the use of highly active antiretroviral therapy, thalidomide use was associated with increased viral loads in HIV infected patients. Monitor viral load after the 1st and 3rd months of therapy and every 3 months thereafter. Patients with a high tumor burden may be at risk for tumor lysis syndrome; monitor closely; institute appropriate management for hyperuricemia.

Potentially significant drug-drug interactions may exist, requiring dose or frequency adjustment, additional monitoring, and/or selection of alternative therapy. Patients should not donate blood during thalidomide treatment and for 1 month after therapy discontinuation

[US Boxed Warning]: Thalidomide may cause severe birth defects or embryo-fetal death if taken during pregnancy. Thalidomide cannot be used in women who are pregnant or may become pregnant during therapy as even a single dose may cause severe birth defects. In order to decrease the risk of fetal exposure, thalidomide is available only

through a special restricted distribution program (Thalomid REMS). Use is contraindicated in women who are or may become pregnant. Pregnancy must be excluded prior to therapy initiation with 2 negative pregnancy tests. Women of reproductive potential must avoid pregnancy 4 weeks prior to therapy, during therapy, during therapy interruptions, and for ≥4 weeks after therapy is discontinued; two reliable methods of birth control, or abstinence from heterosexual intercourse, must be used. Males taking thalidomide (even those vasectomized) must use a latex or synthetic condom during any sexual contact with women of childbearing potential and for up to 28 days following discontinuation of therapy. Males taking thalidomide must not donate sperm. Some forms of contraception may not be appropriate in certain patients. An intrauterine device (IUD) or implantable contraceptive may increase the risk of infection or bleeding; estrogen containing products may increase the risk of thromboembolism.

Due to the embryo-fetal risk, thalidomide is only available through a restricted program under the Thalomid REMS program. Prescribers and pharmacies must be certified with the program to prescribe or dispense thalidomide. Patients must sign an agreement and comply with the REMS program requirements.

Adverse Reactions

>10%:

Cardiovascular: Edema (57%), thrombosis/embolism (23%; grade 3: 13%, grade 4: 9%), hypotension (16%)

Central nervous system: Fatigue (79%; grade 3: 14%, grade 4: 3%), somnolence (36% to 38%), dizziness (4% to 20%), sensory neuropathy (54%), confusion (28%), anxiety/agitation (9% to 26%), fever (19% to 23%), motor neuropathy (22%), headache (13% to 19%)

Dermatologic: Rash/desquamation (21% to 30%; grade 3: 4%), dry skin (21%), maculopapular rash (4% to 19%), acne (3% to 11%)

Endocrine & metabolic: Hypocalcemia (72%)

Gastrointestinal: Constipation (3% to 55%), nausea (4% to 28%), anorexia (3% to 28%), weight loss (23%), weight gain (22%), diarrhea (4% to 19%), oral moniliasis (4% to 11%)

Hematologic: Leukopenia (17% to 35%), neutropenia (31%), anemia (6% to 13%), lymphadenopathy (6% to 13%)

Hepatic: AST increased (3% to 25%), bilirubin increased (14%)

Neuromuscular & skeletal: Muscle weakness (40%), tremor (4% to 26%), weakness (6% to 22%), myalgia (17%), paresthesia (6% to 16%), arthralgia (13%)

Renal: Hematuria (11%)

Respiratory: Dyspnea (42%)

Miscellaneous: Diaphoresis (13%)

1% to 10%:

Cardiovascular: Peripheral edema (3% to 8%), facial edema (4%)

Central nervous system: Insomnia (9%), nervousness (3% to 9%), malaise (8%), vertigo (8%), pain (3% to 8%)

Dermatologic: Dermatitis (fungal 4% to 9%), pruritus (3% to 8%), nail disorder (3% to 4%)

Endocrine & metabolic: Hyperlipemia (6% to 9%)

Gastrointestinal: Xerostomia (8% to 9%), flatulence (8%), tooth pain (4%)

Genitourinary: Impotence (3% to 8%)

Hepatic: LFTs abnormal (9%)

◀ Neuromuscular & skeletal: Neuropathy (8%), back pain (4% to 6%), neck pain (4%), neck rigidity (4%)
Renal: Albuminuria (3% to 8%)
Respiratory: Pharyngitis (4% to 8%), rhinitis (4%), sinusitis (3% to 8%)
Miscellaneous: Infection (6% to 8%)

Postmarketing and/or case reports (limited to important or life-threatening): Acute renal failure, alkaline phosphatase increased, ALT increased, amenorrhea, angioedema, aphthous stomatitis, arrhythmia, atrial fibrillation, bile duct obstruction, bradycardia, BUN increased, carpal tunnel, cerebral vascular accident, CML, creatinine clearance decreased, creatinine increased, deafness, depression, diplopia, dysesthesia, ECG abnormalities, enuresis, eosinophilia, epistaxis, erythema multiforme, erythema nodosum, erythroleukemia, exfoliative dermatitis, febrile neutropenia, foot drop, galactorrhea, granulocytopenia, gynecomastia, hearing loss, hepatomegaly, Hodgkin lymphoma, hypercalcemia, hyper-/hypokalemia, hypersensitivity, hypertension, hyper-/hypothyroidism, hypersensitivity, hyperuricemia, hypomagnesemia, hyponatremia, hypoproteinemia, intestinal obstruction, intestinal perforation, interstitial pneumonitis, LDH increased, lethargy, leukocytosis, loss of consciousness, lymphedema, lymphopenia, mental status changes, metrorrhagia, MI, myxedema, nystagmus, oliguria, orthostatic hypotension, pancytopenia, paresthesia, petechiae, peripheral neuritis, photosensitivity, pleural effusion, prothrombin time changes, psychosis, pulmonary embolus, pulmonary hypertension, purpura, Raynaud syndrome, renal failure, secondary malignancy (AML, MDS, solid tumors), seizure, sepsis, septic shock, sexual dysfunction, sick sinus syndrome, status epilepticus, Stevens-Johnson syndrome, stomach ulcer, stupor, suicide attempt, syncope, tachycardia, thrombocytopenia, toxic epidermal necrolysis, transient ischemic attack, tumor lysis syndrome, urticaria

Drug Interactions
Metabolism/Transport Effects None known.
Avoid Concomitant Use
Avoid concomitant use of Thalidomide with any of the following: Abatacept; Anakinra; Azelastine (Nasal); BCG (Intravesical); Canakinumab; Certolizumab Pegol; CloZAPine; CNS Depressants; Dipyrone; Natalizumab; Orphenadrine; Paraldehyde; Pimecrolimus; Rilonacept; Tacrolimus (Topical); Tocilizumab; Tofacitinib; Vaccines (Live); Vedolizumab
Increased Effect/Toxicity
Thalidomide may increase the levels/effects of: Abatacept; Alcohol (Ethyl); Anakinra; Azelastine (Nasal); Bisphosphonate Derivatives; Canakinumab; Certolizumab Pegol; CloZAPine; Fingolimod; Leflunomide; Metyrosine; Natalizumab; Orphenadrine; Pamidronate; Paraldehyde; Pramipexole; Rilonacept; ROPINIRole; Rotigotine; Selective Serotonin Reuptake Inhibitors; Tofacitinib; Vaccines (Live); Vedolizumab; Zoledronic Acid

The levels/effects of Thalidomide may be increased by: Brimonidine (Topical); Cannabis; CNS Depressants; Contraceptives (Estrogens); Contraceptives (Progestins); Denosumab; Dexamethasone (Systemic); Dipyrone; Dronabinol; Erythropoiesis-Stimulating Agents; Estrogen Derivatives; Kava Kava; Magnesium Sulfate; Minocycline; Nabilone; Pimecrolimus; Roflumilast; Rufinamide; Tacrolimus (Topical); Tetrahydrocannabinol; Tocilizumab; Trastuzumab

Decreased Effect

Thalidomide may decrease the levels/effects of: BCG (Intravesical); Coccidioides immitis Skin Test; Sipuleucel-T; Vaccines (Inactivated); Vaccines (Live)

The levels/effects of Thalidomide may be decreased by: Echinacea

Storage/Stability Store at 20°C to 25°C (68°F to 77°F); excursions are permitted between 15°C and 30°C (59°F and 86°F). Protect from light. Keep in original package.

Mechanism of Action Immunomodulatory and antiangiogenic characteristics; immunologic effects may vary based on conditions; may suppress excessive tumor necrosis factor-alpha production in patients with ENL, yet may increase plasma tumor necrosis factor-alpha levels in HIV-positive patients. In multiple myeloma, thalidomide is associated with an increase in natural killer cells and increased levels of interleukin-2 and interferon gamma. Other proposed mechanisms of action include suppression of angiogenesis, prevention of free-radical-mediated DNA damage, increased cell mediated cytotoxic effects, and altered expression of cellular adhesion molecules.

Pharmacodynamics/Kinetics

Absorption: Slow, good

Protein binding: 55% to 66%

Metabolism: Minimal (unchanged drug is the predominant circulating component)

Half-life elimination: 5.5 to 7.3 hours

Time to peak, plasma: ~2 to 5 hours

Excretion: Urine (92%; <4% of the dose as unchanged drug); feces (<2%)

Dosing

Adult & Geriatric

Erythema nodosum leprosum, acute cutaneous: Oral: Initial: 100 to 300 mg once daily at bedtime, continue until signs/symptoms subside (usually ~2 weeks), then taper off in 50 mg decrements every 2 to 4 weeks. For severe cases with moderate to severe neuritis, corticosteroids may be initiated with thalidomide (taper off and discontinue corticosteroids when neuritis improves).

Patients weighing <50 kg: Initiate at lower end of the dosing range

Severe cutaneous reaction or patients previously requiring high doses: May be initiated at up to 400 mg once daily at bedtime or in divided doses

Erythema nodosum leprosum, maintenance (prevention/suppression, or with flares during tapering attempts): Oral: Maintain on the minimum dosage necessary to control the reaction; efforts to taper off should be attempted every 3 to 6 months, in decrements of 50 mg every 2 to 4 weeks.

Multiple myeloma, newly diagnosed: Oral:

US labeling: 200 mg once daily at bedtime (in combination with dexamethasone)

Canadian labeling: Adults ≥65 years: 200 mg once daily; maximum: 12 six-week cycles (in combination with melphalan and prednisone)

Multiple myeloma (off-label dosing):

In combination with bortezomib and dexamethasone (off-label combination): Induction therapy: 100 mg once daily for the first 14 days, then 200 mg once daily for 3 (21-day) cycles (Cavo, 2010) **or** 100 mg once daily for up to 8 (21-day) cycles (Kaufman, 2010)

In combination with melphalan and prednisone (off-label combination in US): 200 to 400 mg once daily (Facon, 2007) **or** 100 mg once daily (Palumbo, 2008)

Multiple myeloma, maintenance (following autologous stem cell transplant; off-label use): Oral: 200 mg once daily starting 3 to 6 months after transplant; continue until disease progression or unacceptable toxicity (Brinker, 2006) or 100 mg once daily starting 42 to 60 days following transplant; increase to 200 mg once daily after 2 weeks if tolerated; continue for up to 12 months (in combination with prednisolone) (Spencer, 2009)

Multiple myeloma, salvage therapy: Initial: 200 mg once daily at bedtime; may increase daily dose by 200 mg every 2 weeks for 6 weeks (if tolerated) to a maximum of 800 mg once daily at bedtime (Singhal, 1999) **or** 100 mg once daily (in combination with dexamethasone) (Palumbo, 2001) **or** 200 mg once daily (in combination with bortezomib and dexamethasone) for 1 year (Garderet, 2012) **or** 400 mg once daily at bedtime (in combination with dexamethasone, cisplatin, doxorubicin, cyclophosphamide and etoposide) (Lee, 2003)

AIDS-related aphthous stomatitis (off-label use): Oral: 200 mg once daily at bedtime for up to 8 weeks, if no response, then 200 mg twice daily for 4 weeks (Jacobson, 1997)

Chronic graft-versus-host disease (refractory), treatment (off-label second-line use; optimum dose not determined): Oral: Initial: 100 mg once daily at bedtime, with dose escalation up to 400 mg daily in 3 to 4 divided doses (Wolff, 2010) **or** Initial: 50 to 100 mg 3 times daily; maximum dose: 600 to 1,200 mg daily (Kulkarni, 2003) **or** 200 mg 4 times daily (dose adjusted to goal thalidomide concentration of ≥5 mcg/mL 2 hours postdose) (Vogelsang, 1992) **or** 100 to 300 mg 4 times daily (Parker, 1995)

Systemic light chain amyloidosis (off-label use): Oral: 200 mg once daily (starting dose 50 to 100 mg once daily; titrate at 4-week intervals) in combination with cyclophosphamide and dexamethasone (Wechalekar, 2007)

Waldenström macroglobulinemia (off-label use): Oral: ≤200 mg once daily for up to 52 weeks (in combination with rituximab) (Treon, 2008)

Pediatric

Erythema nodosum leprosum, acute cutaneous: Children ≥12 years: Oral: Refer to adult dosing.

Erythema nodosum leprosum, maintenance (prevention/suppression, or with flares during tapering attempts): Children ≥12 years: Oral: Refer to adult dosing.

Chronic graft-versus-host disease (refractory), treatment (off-label second-line use; limited data): Children ≥3 years: Oral: 3 mg/kg 4 times daily (dose adjusted to goal thalidomide concentration of ≥5 mcg/mL 2 hours postdose) (Vogelsang 1992) **or** Initial: 3 to 6 mg/kg/day in 2 to 4 divided doses; target dose 12 mg/kg/day; Maximum daily dose: 800 mg (Rovelli, 1998)

Renal Impairment No dosage adjustment necessary for patients with renal impairment and on dialysis (per manufacturer). In a study of 6 patients with end-stage renal disease on dialysis, although clearance was increased by dialysis, a supplemental dose was not needed (Eriksson, 2003).

Multiple myeloma: An evaluation of 29 newly diagnosed myeloma patients with renal failure (serum creatinine ≥2 mg/dL) treated with thalidomide and dexamethasone (some also received cyclophosphamide) found that toxicities and efficacy were similar to patients with normal renal function (Seol, 2010). A study evaluating induction therapy with thalidomide and dexamethasone in 31 newly diagnosed myeloma patients with renal failure (CrCl <50 mL/minute), including 16 patients with severe renal impairment (CrCl <30 mL/minute) and 7 patients on chronic hemodialysis found that toxicities were similar to patients without renal impairment and that thalidomide and dexamethasone could be administered safely (Tosi, 2009).

Hepatic Impairment There are no dosage adjustments provided in the manufacturer's labeling (has not been studied). However, thalidomide does not appear to undergo significant hepatic metabolism.

Adjustment for Toxicity

ANC ≤750/mm³: Withhold treatment if clinically appropriate

Grade 3 or 4 adverse reactions: Consider dose reduction, delay or discontinuation (based on clinical judgment).

Multiple myeloma:

US labeling: Constipation, oversedation, peripheral neuropathy: Temporarily withhold or continue with a reduced dose

Canadian labeling:

ANC <1,500/mm³: Withhold melphalan and prednisone for 1 week; resume melphalan and prednisone after 1 week if ANC >1,500/mm³ **or** if ANC 1,000 to 1,500/mm³ reduce melphalan dose by 50% **or** if ANC <1,000/mm³ adjust chemotherapy dose based on clinical status of patient.

Constipation, oversedation: Temporarily withhold thalidomide treatment or continue with a reduced dose

Peripheral neuropathy, Grade 1 (paresthesia, weakness and/or loss of reflexes) without loss of function): Evaluate patient and consider dose reduction with worsening of symptoms; symptom improvement may not follow dose reduction, however.

Peripheral neuropathy, Grade 2 (interferes with function but not with daily activities), Grade 3 (interferes with daily activities), or Grade 4 (disabling neuropathy): Discontinue thalidomide treatment

Thromboembolic events: Withhold therapy and initiate standard anticoagulant treatment; may resume thalidomide therapy at original dose following stabilization of patient and resolution of thromboembolic event; maintain anticoagulant treatment for duration of thalidomide therapy

Off-label dosage adjustment (Richardson, 2012): Peripheral neuropathy:

Grade 1: Reduce dose by 50%

Grade 2: Temporarily interrupt therapy; once resolved to ≤ grade 1, resume therapy with a 50% dosage reduction (if clinically appropriate)

Grade 3 or higher: Discontinue therapy

Combination Regimens

Multiple myeloma:

Bortezomib-Melphalan-Prednisone-Thalidomide on page 1850

DTPACE on page 1952

Melphalan-Prednisone-Thalidomide (Multiple Myeloma) on page 2035

Thalidomide-Dexamethasone (MM) on page 2088

Administration Oral: Swallow capsules whole with water. Do not open or crush capsules. Avoid extensive handling of capsules; capsules should remain in blister pack until ingestion.

◄   *US labeling:* Administer orally, preferably at bedtime once daily, at least 1 hour after the evening meal. Doses >400 mg/day may be given in divided doses at least 1 hour after meals.

Canadian labeling: Administer orally as a single dose at the same time each day (preferably at bedtime to decrease somnolence); may be taken without regard to meals.

Missed doses: For missed doses, if <12 hours patient may receive dose; if >12 hours wait until next dose due.

Hazardous agent; use appropriate precautions for handling and disposal (NIOSH 2014 [group 2]). Wear gloves to prevent cutaneous exposure. If exposed to the powder content from broken capsules or body fluids from patients receiving thalidomide, the exposed area should be washed with soap and water. Although the manufacturer does not recommend opening the capsules, if it is necessary to manipulate the capsules (eg, to prepare an oral suspension), it is recommended to double glove, wear a protective gown, and prepare in a controlled device (NIOSH 2014).

Emetic Potential

Children: Minimal (<10%)

Adults: Low (10% to 30%)

Extemporaneous Preparations Hazardous agent; use appropriate precautions for handling and disposal (NIOSH 2014 [group 2]). When manipulating capsules, NIOSH recommends double gloving, a protective gown, and preparation in a controlled device; if not prepared in a controlled device, respiratory and eye protection, as well as ventilated engineering controls, are recommended (NIOSH, 2014).

A 20 mg/mL oral suspension may be prepared with capsules and a 1:1 mixture of Ora-Sweet and Ora-Plus. Empty the contents of twelve 100 mg capsules into a glass mortar. Add small portions of the vehicle and mix to a uniform paste; mix while adding the vehicle in incremental proportions to almost 60 mL; transfer to an amber calibrated bottle, rinse mortar with vehicle, and add quantity of vehicle sufficient to make 60 mL. Label "shake well," "protect from light," and "refrigerate". Stable for 35 days refrigerated.

Kraft S, Johnson CE, and Tyler RP, "Stability of an Extemporaneously Prepared Thalidomide Suspension," *Am J Health Syst Pharm,* 2011, 69(1):56-8.

Monitoring Parameters CBC with differential, platelets; thyroid function tests (TSH at baseline then every 2 to 3 months during thalidomide treatment [Hamnvik 2011]). Hepatic function tests (periodic; particularly with preexisting hepatic dysfunction or concomitant use of drugs associated with hepatotoxicity). In HIV-seropositive patients: viral load after 1 and 3 months, then every 3 months. Pregnancy testing (sensitivity of at least 50 milliunits/mL) is required within 24 hours prior to initiation of therapy, weekly during the first 4 weeks, then every 4 weeks in women with regular menstrual cycles or every 2 weeks in women with irregular menstrual cycles. Signs of neuropathy monthly for the first 3 months, then periodically during treatment; consider monitoring of sensory nerve application potential amplitudes (at baseline and every 6 months) to detect asymptomatic neuropathy. Monitor for signs and symptoms of thromboembolism (shortness of breath, chest pain, arm/leg swelling), tumor lysis syndrome, bradycardia and syncope; monitor for clinical changes indicating potential seizure activity (in patients with a history of seizure).

Prescribing and Access Restrictions US: As a requirement of the REMS program, access to this medication is restricted. Thalidomide is approved for marketing only under a special distribution program, the Thalomid REMS (https://www.celgeneriskmanagement.com or 1-888-423-5436), which has been approved by the FDA. Prescribers, patients, and pharmacies must be certified with the program to prescribe or dispense thalidomide. No more than a 4-week supply should be dispensed. Blister packs should be dispensed intact (do not repackage capsules). Prescriptions must be filled within 7 days (for females of reproductive potential) or within 30 days (for all other patients) after authorization number obtained. Subsequent prescriptions may be filled only if fewer than 7 days of therapy remain on the previous prescription. A new prescription is required for further dispensing (a telephone prescription may not be accepted.) Pregnancy testing is required for females of childbearing potential.

Canada: Access to thalidomide is restricted through a controlled distribution program called RevAid. Only physicians and pharmacists enrolled in this program are authorized to prescribe or dispense thalidomide. Patients must be enrolled in the program by their physicians. Further information is available at www.RevAid.ca or by calling 1-888-738-2431.

Medication Guide Available Yes

Dosage Forms Excipient information presented when available (limited, particularly for generics); consult specific product labeling.

Capsule, Oral:

Thalomid: 50 mg, 100 mg

Thalomid: 150 mg, 200 mg [contains fd&c blue #2 (indigotine)]

- ◆ **Thalomid** see Thalidomide on page 1627
- ◆ **THC** see Dronabinol on page 577
- ◆ **TheraCys** see BCG (Intravesical) on page 174

Thioguanine (thye oh GWAH neen)

Related Information

Chemotherapy and Cancer Treatment During Pregnancy on page 2214

Management of Chemotherapy-Induced Nausea and Vomiting in Adults on page 2142

Prevention of Chemotherapy-Induced Nausea and Vomiting in Children on page 2203

Safe Handling of Hazardous Drugs on page 2292

Brand Names: US Tabloid

Brand Names: Canada Lanvis®

Index Terms 2-Amino-6-Mercaptopurine; 6-TG (error-prone abbreviation); 6-Thioguanine (error-prone abbreviation); TG; Tioguanine

Pharmacologic Category Antineoplastic Agent, Antimetabolite; Antineoplastic Agent, Antimetabolite (Purine Analog)

Use Treatment of acute myelogenous (nonlymphocytic) leukemia (AML)

Labeled Contraindications Prior resistance to thioguanine (or mercaptopurine)

Canadian labeling: Additional contraindications (not in US labeling): Hypersensitivity to thioguanine or any component of the formulation

Pregnancy Considerations Animal studies have demonstrated adverse effects. There are no adequate and well-controlled studies in pregnant women. May cause fetal harm if administered during pregnancy. Women of childbearing potential should avoid becoming pregnant during treatment.

THIOGUANINE

◀ **Breast-Feeding Considerations** Due to the potential for serious adverse reactions in the nursing infant, the manufacturer recommends to discontinue breast-feeding during therapy.

Warnings/Precautions Hazardous agent - use appropriate precautions for handling and disposal (NIOSH 2014 [group 1]).

Not recommended for maintenance therapy or long-term continuous treatment; long-term continuous therapy or maintenance treatment is associated with a high risk for hepatotoxicity, hepatic sinusoidal obstruction syndrome (SOS; formerly called veno-occlusive disease), or portal hypertension; monitor liver function carefully for liver toxicity and discontinue in patients with evidence of hepatic SOS (eg, hyperbilirubinemia, hepatomegaly [tender], and weight gain due to ascites and fluid retention) or portal hypertension (eg, splenomegaly, thrombocytopenia, esophageal varices); hepatotoxicity with or without transaminase elevations may occur; pathologic findings of hepatotoxicity include hepatoportal sclerosis, nodular regenerative hyperplasia, peliosis hepatitis, and periportal fibrosis. Advise patients to avoid alcohol; may increase the risk for hepatotoxicity.

Myelosuppression (anemia, leukopenia, and/or thrombocytopenia) is a common dose-related toxicity (may be delayed); monitor for infection (due to leukopenia) or bleeding(due to thrombocytopenia); withhold treatment with abnormally significant drop in blood counts. Patients with genetic enzyme deficiency of thiopurine methyltransferase (TPMT) or who are receiving drugs which inhibit this enzyme (mesalazine, olsalazine, sulfasalazine) may be highly sensitive to myelosuppressive effects and may require substantial dose reductions.

Hyperuricemia occurs commonly with treatment; institute adequate hydration and prophylactic allopurinol. Thioguanine is potentially carcinogenic. Cross resistance with mercaptopurine generally occurs. Avoid vaccination with live vaccines during treatment.

Adverse Reactions Frequency not defined.

Endocrine & metabolic: Fluid retention, hyperuricemia (common)

Gastrointestinal: Anorexia, intestinal necrosis, intestinal perforation, nausea, splenomegaly, stomatitis, vomiting, weight gain

Hematologic: Anemia (may be delayed), bleeding, granulocytopenia, leukopenia (common; may be delayed), marrow hypoplasia, pancytopenia, thrombocytopenia (common; may be delayed)

Hepatic: Ascites, esophageal varices, hepatic necrosis (centrilobular), hepatic sinusoidal obstruction syndrome (SOS; veno-occlusive disease), hepatitis, hepatomegaly [tender], hepatoportal sclerosis, hepatotoxicity, hyperbilirubinemia, jaundice, LFTs increased, nodular regenerative hyperplasia, peliosis hepatitis, periportal fibrosis, portal hypertension

Miscellaneous: Infection

Drug Interactions

Metabolism/Transport Effects None known.

Avoid Concomitant Use

Avoid concomitant use of Thioguanine with any of the following: BCG (Intravesical); CloZAPine; Dipyrone; Natalizumab; Pimecrolimus; Tacrolimus (Topical); Tofacitinib; Vaccines (Live)

Increased Effect/Toxicity
Thioguanine may increase the levels/effects of: CloZAPine; Fingolimod; Leflunomide; Natalizumab; Tofacitinib; Vaccines (Live)

The levels/effects of Thioguanine may be increased by: 5-ASA Derivatives; Denosumab; Dipyrone; Pimecrolimus; Roflumilast; Tacrolimus (Topical); Trastuzumab

Decreased Effect
Thioguanine may decrease the levels/effects of: BCG (Intravesical); Coccidioides immitis Skin Test; Sipuleucel-T; Vaccines (Inactivated); Vaccines (Live)

The levels/effects of Thioguanine may be decreased by: Echinacea

Storage/Stability Store tablet at room temperature at 15°C to 25°C (59°F to 77°F). Protect from moisture.

Mechanism of Action Purine analog that is incorporated into DNA and RNA resulting in the blockage of synthesis and metabolism of purine nucleotides

Pharmacodynamics/Kinetics
Absorption: ~30% (range: 14% to 46%; highly variable)

Distribution: Does not reach therapeutic concentrations in the CSF

Metabolism: Hepatic; rapidly and extensively via thiopurine methyltransferase (TPMT) to 2-amino-6-methylthioguanine (MTG; active) and inactive compounds

Half-life elimination: Terminal: 5-9 hours

Time to peak, serum: Within 8 hours; predominantly metabolite(s)

Dosing
Pediatric Pediatric ALL (off-label use; combination therapy): Oral: Delayed intensification treatment phase: 60 mg/m^2/day for 14 days (Lange, 2002; Nachman, 1998)

Renal Impairment
Adults: There are no dosage adjustments provided in manufacturer's labeling.

Children: No adjustment required (Aronoff, 2007).

Hepatic Impairment
Deterioration in transaminases, alkaline phosphatase or bilirubin, toxic hepatitis, biliary stasis, clinical jaundice, evidence of hepatic sinusoidal obstruction syndrome (veno-occlusive disease), or evidence of portal hypertension: Discontinue treatment.

Combination Regimens
Leukemia, acute lymphocytic:
CALGB 8811 Regimen (ALL) on page 1853
CALGB 9111 Regimen (ALL) on page 1854

Administration Administer orally; total daily dose can be given at one time. Hazardous agent; use appropriate precautions for handling and disposal (NIOSH 2014 [group 1]).

Emetic Potential Children and Adults: Minimal (<10%)

Extemporaneous Preparations Hazardous agent: Use appropriate precautions for handling and disposal (NIOSH 2014 [group 1]).

A 20 mg/mL oral suspension may be made with tablets, methylcellulose 1%, and simple syrup NF. Crush fifteen 40 mg tablets in a mortar and reduce to a fine powder. Add 10 mL methylcellulose 1% in incremental proportions and mix to a uniform paste. Transfer to a graduated cylinder, rinse mortar with simple syrup, and add quantity of simple syrup sufficient to make 30 mL. Label "shake well" and "refrigerate". Stable for 84 days refrigerated (preferred) or at room temperature.

Dressman JB and Poust RI, "Stability of Allopurinol and Five Antineoplastics in Suspension," *Am J Hosp Pharm*, 1983, 40(4):616-8.

Nahata MC, Pai VB, and Hipple TF, *Pediatric Drug Formulations*, 5th ed, Cincinnati, OH: Harvey Whitney Books Co, 2004.

Monitoring Parameters CBC with differential and platelet count; liver function tests (weekly when beginning therapy then monthly, more frequently in patients with liver disease or concurrent hepatotoxic drugs); serum uric acid; some laboratories offer testing for TPMT deficiency

Hepatotoxicity may present with signs of portal hypertension (splenomegaly, esophageal varices, thrombocytopenia) or sinusoidal obstruction syndrome (veno-occlusive disease; fluid retention, ascites, hepatomegaly with tenderness, or hyperbilirubinemia)

Dosage Forms Excipient information presented when available (limited, particularly for generics); consult specific product labeling. [DSC] = Discontinued product

Tablet, Oral:

Tabloid: 40 mg

Tabloid: 40 mg [DSC] [scored]

♦ **6-Thioguanine (error-prone abbreviation)** *see* Thioguanine *on page 1637*

♦ **Thiophosphoramide** *see* Thiotepa *on page 1640*

♦ **Thioplex** *see* Thiotepa *on page 1640*

♦ **Thiosulfuric Acid Disodium Salt** *see* Sodium Thiosulfate *on page 1540*

Thiotepa (thye oh TEP a)

Related Information

Chemotherapy and Obesity *on page 2220*

Management of Chemotherapy-Induced Nausea and Vomiting in Adults *on page 2142*

Management of Drug Extravasations *on page 2159*

Prevention of Chemotherapy-Induced Nausea and Vomiting in Children *on page 2203*

Safe Handling of Hazardous Drugs *on page 2292*

Index Terms TESPA; Thiophosphoramide; Thioplex; Triethylenethiophosphoramide; TSPA

Pharmacologic Category Antineoplastic Agent, Alkylating Agent

Use Treatment of superficial papillary bladder cancer; palliative treatment of adenocarcinoma of breast or ovary; controlling intracavitary effusions caused by metastatic tumors

Labeled Contraindications Hypersensitivity to thiotepa or any component of the formulation

Note: May be contraindicated in certain circumstances of hepatic, renal, and/or bone marrow failure; evaluate on an individual basis as lower dose treatment (with close monitoring) may still be appropriate if the potential benefit outweighs the risks

Pregnancy Considerations Adverse events were observed in animal reproduction studies. May cause harm if administered during pregnancy. Effective contraception is recommended for men and women of childbearing potential.

Breast-Feeding Considerations It is not known if thiotepa is excreted in breast milk. Due to the potential for serious adverse reactions in the nursing infant, the manufacturer recommends a decision be made whether to discontinue nursing or to discontinue the drug, taking into account the importance of treatment to the mother.

Warnings/Precautions Hazardous agent - use appropriate precautions for handling and disposal (NIOSH 2014 [group 1]). Myelosuppression is common; use with caution in patients with bone marrow damage, dosage reduction recommended. Use may be contraindicated with existing marrow damage and should be limited to cases where benefit outweighs risk. Monitor for infection or bleeding; death due to septicemia and hemorrhage has occurred. Myelosuppression (including fatal cases) has also been reported with intravesicular administration (due to systemic absorption). Monitor blood counts closely. Potentially teratogenic, mutagenic, and carcinogenic; myelodysplastic syndrome and acute myeloid leukemia (AML) have been reported. Reduce dosage and use extreme caution in patients with hepatic, renal, or bone marrow damage. Use may be contraindicated with impairment/damage and should be limited to cases where benefit outweighs risk. In children, thiotepa is associated with a high emetic potential at doses ≥300 mg/m^2; antiemetics are recommended to prevent nausea and vomiting (Dupuis, 2011).

When used for intrathecal administration (off-label route), should not be prepared during the preparation of any other agents; after preparation, keep intrathecal medications in an isolated location or container clearly marked with a label identifying as "intrathecal" use only; delivery of intrathecal medications to the patient should only be with other medications intended for administration into the central nervous system (Jacobson, 2009). Potentially significant drug-drug interactions may exist, requiring dose or frequency adjustment, additional monitoring, and/or selection of alternative therapy.

Due to the shortage of the U.S. generic product, the FDA is allowing temporary importation of a European product (brand name Tepadina) to fulfill clinical need. Indications and dosing vary greatly between the U.S. and European products; verify product, dosing, and preparation instructions prior to dispensation and administration.

Adverse Reactions

Frequency not defined:

Central nervous system: Chills, dizziness, fatigue, fever, headache

Dermatologic: Alopecia, contact dermatitis, depigmentation (with topical treatment), dermatitis, rash, urticaria

Endocrine & metabolic: Amenorrhea, spermatogenesis inhibition

Gastrointestinal: Abdominal pain, anorexia, nausea, vomiting

Genitourinary: Dysuria, urinary retention

Hematologic: Anemia, bleeding, leukopenia, thrombocytopenia

Local: Injection site pain

Neuromuscular & skeletal: Weakness

Ocular: Blurred vision, conjunctivitis

Renal: Hematuria

Respiratory: Asthma, epistaxis, laryngeal edema, wheezing

Miscellaneous: Allergic reaction, anaphylactic shock, infection

Infrequent, postmarketing, and/or case reports: Acute myeloid leukemia (AML), chemical cystitis (bladder instillation), hemorrhagic cystitis (bladder instillation), myelodysplastic syndrome

◄ **Drug Interactions**

Metabolism/Transport Effects Inhibits CYP2B6 (moderate)

Avoid Concomitant Use

Avoid concomitant use of Thiotepa with any of the following: BCG (Intravesical); CloZAPine; Dipyrone; Natalizumab; Pimecrolimus; Tacrolimus (Topical); Tofacitinib; Vaccines (Live)

Increased Effect/Toxicity

Thiotepa may increase the levels/effects of: BuPROPion; CloZAPine; CYP2B6 Substrates; Fingolimod; Leflunomide; Natalizumab; Tofacitinib; Vaccines (Live)

The levels/effects of Thiotepa may be increased by: Denosumab; Dipyrone; Pimecrolimus; Roflumilast; Tacrolimus (Topical); Trastuzumab

Decreased Effect

Thiotepa may decrease the levels/effects of: BCG (Intravesical); Coccidioides immitis Skin Test; Sipuleucel-T; Vaccines (Inactivated); Vaccines (Live)

The levels/effects of Thiotepa may be decreased by: Echinacea

Storage/Stability Note: Due to drug shortage in the United States, the FDA is allowing temporary importation of a European product (Tepadina). Verify product, storage, and preparation instructions prior to dispensation and administration. Refer to specific product labeling for details.

Tepadina: Store intact vials under refrigeration at 2°C to 8°C (36°F to 46°F). Protect from light; do not freeze. Reconstituted solution (10 mg/mL) is stable for 8 hours when stored at 2°C to 8°C (36°F to 46°F). Solution further diluted for infusion is stable for 24 hours when stored at 2°C to 8°C (36°F to 46°F), or for 4 hours when stored at 25°C (77°F).

Generic product labeling (U.S.): Store intact vials under refrigeration at 2°C to 8°C (36°F to 46°F). Protect from light. Reconstituted solutions (10 mg/mL) are stable for up to 8 hours when stored under refrigeration. Solutions further diluted for infusion should be used immediately.

After preparation, keep intrathecal medications in an isolated location or container clearly marked with a label identifying as "intrathecal" use only.

Preparation for Administration

Hazardous agent; use appropriate precautions for handling and disposal (NIOSH 2014 [group 1]). **Note:** Due to drug shortage in the U.S., the FDA is allowing temporary importation of a European product (Tepadina). Verify product, storage, and preparation instructions prior to dispensation and administration. Refer to specific product labeling for details.

Tepadina: Reconstitute each 15 mg vial with 1.5 mL SWFI, or each 100 mg vial with 10 mL SWFI, to a concentration of 10 mg/mL. Gently mix by repeated inversions. Solution may be clear or opalescent; do not use if particulate matter is present. Further dilute reconstituted solution for IV infusion in 500 mL NS (1000 mL NS if dose >500 mg). If dose is <250 mg, dilute in an appropriate volume of NS to achieve a final concentration of 0.5 to 1 mg/mL.

Generic product labeling (US): Reconstitute each 15 mg vial with 1.5 mL SWFI to a concentration of 10 mg/mL. Solutions for IV use should be further diluted in NS injection prior to infusion. Filter through a 0.22 micron filter (polysulfone membrane [eg, Sterile Aerodisc®] or triton-free cellulose mixed ester [eg, Millex®-GS]) prior to administration; do not use solutions which precipitate or remain opaque after filtering. Solutions for intravesicular administration should be diluted in 30 to 60 mL NS.

Solutions for intrathecal administration (off-label use) should be diluted to a concentration of 1 mg/mL in preservative-free buffered solution (Grossman, 1993). Intrathecal medications should not be prepared during the preparation of any other agents.

Mechanism of Action Alkylating agent that reacts with DNA phosphate groups to produce cross-linking of DNA strands leading to inhibition of DNA, RNA, and protein synthesis; mechanism of action has not been explored as thoroughly as the other alkylating agents, it is presumed that the aziridine rings open and react as nitrogen mustard; reactivity is enhanced at a lower pH

Pharmacodynamics/Kinetics

Absorption: Intracavitary instillation: Unreliable (10% to 100%) through bladder mucosa

Metabolism: Extensively hepatic; major metabolite (active): TEPA

Half-life elimination: Terminal (dose-dependent clearance): ~2 hours

Excretion: Urine (as metabolites and unchanged drug)

Dosing

Adult & Geriatric

Bladder cancer: Intravesical: 60 mg in 30 to 60 mL NS retained for 2 hours once weekly for 4 weeks

Ovarian, breast cancer: IV: 0.3 to 0.4 mg/kg every 1 to 4 weeks

Effusions: Intracavitary: 0.6 to 0.8 mg/kg

Leptomeningeal metastases (off-label use/route): Intrathecal: 10 mg twice a week (on days 1 and 4 each week) for 8 weeks (Grossman, 1993)

Hematopoietic stem cell transplant (HSCT) for CNS malignancy (off-label use; combination chemotherapy): IV: 250 mg/m^2/day for 3 days beginning 9 days prior to transplant (Soussain, 2008) **or** 150 mg/m^2/dose every 12 hours for 6 doses, followed by stem cell reinfusion 96 hours after completion of thiotepa (Abrey, 2006)

Pediatric Note: In children, thiotepa is associated with a high emetic potential at doses ≥300 mg/m^2; antiemetics are recommended to prevent nausea and vomiting (Dupuis, 2011).

Hematopoietic stem cell transplant (HSCT) for CNS malignancy (off-label use; combination chemotherapy): *IV:* 300 mg/m^2/day for 3 days beginning 8 days prior to transplant (Gilheeney, 2010) **or** 300 mg/m^2/day for 3 days beginning 5 days prior to transplant (Dunkel, 2010; Grodman, 2009)

Renal Impairment There are no dosage adjustments provided in the manufacturer's labeling. Use with caution; reduced dose may be warranted. Use may be contraindicated with existing renal impairment and should be limited to cases where benefit outweighs risk.

Hepatic Impairment There are no dosage adjustments provided in the manufacturer's labeling. Use with caution; reduced dose may be warranted. Use may be contraindicated with existing hepatic impairment and should be limited to cases where benefit outweighs risk.

Obesity

*American Society of Clinical Oncology (ASCO) Guidelines for appropriate chemotherapy dosing in obese adults with cancer (**Note: Excludes HSCT dosing**):* Utilize patient's actual body weight (full weight) for calculation of body surface area- or weight-based dosing, particularly when the intent of therapy is curative; manage regimen-related toxicities in the same manner as for nonobese patients; if a dose reduction is utilized due to toxicity, consider resumption of full weight-based dosing with subsequent cycles, especially if cause of toxicity (eg, hepatic or renal impairment) is resolved (Griggs, 2012).

American Society for Blood and Marrow Transplantation (ASBMT) practice guideline committee position statement on chemotherapy dosing in obesity: Utilize actual body weight (full weight) for calculation of body surface area in thiotepa dosing for hematopoietic stem cell transplant conditioning regimens in adult patients weighing ≤120% of their ideal body weight (IBW). In patients weighing >120% IBW, utilize adjusted body weight 40% (ABW40) to calculate BSA (Bubalo, 2014).

ABW40: Adjusted wt (kg) = Ideal body weight (kg) + 0.4 [actual wt (kg) - ideal body weight (kg)]

Adjustment for Toxicity IV: **Note:** Use may be contraindicated with preexisting marrow damage and should be limited to cases where benefit outweighs risk.

WBC ≤3000/mm^3: Discontinue treatment

Platelets ≤150,000/mm^3: Discontinue treatment

Administration In children, thiotepa is associated with a high emetic potential at doses ≥300 mg/m^2; antiemetics are recommended to prevent nausea and vomiting (Dupuis, 2011).

IV: Administer as a rapid injection. Infusion times may be longer for high-dose (off-label use) treatment; refer to specific protocols. *Tepadina:* Administer using a 0.2 micron in-line filter; flush line prior to and after infusion with ~5 mL NS.

Intravesical instillation: Instill directly into the bladder and retain for 2 hours; patient should be repositioned every 15 to 30 minutes for maximal exposure

Intrathecal route (off-label use/route): Was administered in 10 mL (preservative free) buffered solutions (Grossman, 1993)

Hazardous agent; use appropriate precautions for handling and disposal (NIOSH 2014 [group 1]).

Vesicant/Extravasation Risk May be an irritant

Emetic Potential

Children:

≥300 mg/m^2: High (>90%)

<300 mg/m^2: Low (10% to 30%)

Adults: Low (10% to 30%)

Monitoring Parameters CBC with differential and platelet count (monitor weekly during treatment and for at least 3 weeks after treatment); renal and liver function tests; uric acid, urinalysis

Dosage Forms Excipient information presented when available (limited, particularly for generics); consult specific product labeling.

Solution Reconstituted, Injection:

Generic: 15 mg (1 ea)

- ◆ **Thorazine** *see* ChlorproMAZINE *on page 322*
- ◆ **Three-Factor PCC** *see* Factor IX Complex (Human) [(Factors II, IX, X)] *on page 677*
- ◆ **Thrombate III** *see* Antithrombin *on page 124*
- ◆ **Thrombate III® (Can)** *see* Antithrombin *on page 124*
- ◆ **Thymocyte Stimulating Factor** *see* Aldesleukin *on page 55*
- ◆ **Thymoglobulin** *see* Antithymocyte Globulin (Rabbit) *on page 130*
- ◆ **Thyrogen** *see* Thyrotropin Alfa *on page 1645*

Thyrotropin Alfa (thye roe TROH pin AL fa)

Brand Names: US Thyrogen

Brand Names: Canada Thyrogen

Index Terms Human Thyroid Stimulating Hormone; Recombinant Human Thyrotropin; Rh-TSH; Thyrotropin Alpha; TSH

Pharmacologic Category Diagnostic Agent

Use

Diagnostic imaging: Adjunctive diagnostic tool for serum thyroglobulin (Tg) testing (with or without radioiodine imaging) in follow up of patients with well-differentiated thyroid cancer who have previously undergone thyroidectomy. Limitations of use: Thyrotropin alfa-stimulated Tg levels are generally lower than and do not correlate with Tg levels after thyroid hormone withdrawal; even when thyrotropin alfa-stimulated Tg testing is performed in combination with radioiodine imaging, there is a risk of missing a thyroid cancer diagnosis or of underestimating disease extent; anti-Tg antibodies may confound Tg assay and render Tg levels uninterpretable, in such cases, even with a negative or low-stage thyrotropin alfa radioiodine scan, consider further patient evaluation.

Thyroid tissue remnant ablation: Adjunctive treatment for radioiodine ablation of thyroid tissue remnants after total or near-total thyroidectomy in patients with well-differentiated thyroid cancer without evidence of metastatic disease

Limitations of use: The effect of thyrotropin alfa on long-term thyroid cancer outcomes has not been determined. Due to relatively small clinical experience, it is not possible to conclude if long-term thyroid cancer outcomes would be equivalent after thyrotropin alfa use or withholding thyroid hormone for TSH elevation prior to remnant ablation.

Labeled Contraindications

U.S. labeling: There are no contraindications listed in the manufacturer's labeling.

Canadian labeling: Hypersensitivity to thyrotropin alfa or any component of the formulation.

Pregnancy Considerations Animal reproduction studies have not been conducted. Effects on the fetus or pregnant woman are unknown.

Breast-Feeding Considerations It is not known if thyrotropin alfa is excreted in breast milk. The manufacturer recommends that caution be exercised when administering thyrotropin alfa to nursing women.

Warnings/Precautions Thyrotropin alfa use may cause a transient (over 7 to 14 days) and significant rise in serum thyroid hormone concentration in patients with substantial *in situ* thyroid tissue or with functional thyroid cancer metastases. Thyrotropin alfa-induced hyperthyroidism may result in serious complications in patients with certain risk factors (heart disease, extensive metastatic disease or with underlying serious illness); consider hospitalization for administration and subsequent observation. Deaths within 24 hours of thyrotropin alfa administration have been reported. Elderly patients with residual thyroid disease and patients with a known history of heart disease in the presence of significant residual thyroid tissue are at increased risk for thyrotropin alfa-induced hyperthyroidism.

Postmarketing reports of stroke or symptoms suggestive of stroke (eg, unilateral weakness) have occurred within 3 days of administration in patients without known central nervous system metastases. A majority of these patients had risk factors for stroke (eg, smokers or history of migraine) or were young women taking oral contraceptives. Patients should be well hydrated prior to administration. Sudden, rapid, and painful growth of residual thyroid tissue or distant metastases may occur following thyrotropin alfa administration. Symptoms are associated with tissue location and include acute hemiplegia, hemiparesis, and vision loss 1 to 3 days after administration. Laryngeal edema, pain at site of distant metastases, and respiratory distress requiring tracheotomy have also been reported. Consider glucocorticoid premedication in patients where local tumor enlargement may compromise vital structures (trachea, CNS, or extensive macroscopic lung metastases). Thyrotropin alfa elimination is significantly reduced in dialysis-dependent end-stage renal impairment, leading to prolonged elevation of TSH levels.

Adverse Reactions

>10%:

Gastrointestinal: Nausea (3% to 12%)

1% to 10%:

Central nervous system: Headache (1% to 7%), dizziness (≤3%), fatigue (1% to 3%), insomnia (≤2%), paresthesia (≤2%)

Endocrine & metabolic: Hypercholesterolemia (≤3%), blood cholesterol abnormal (≤1%)

Gastrointestinal: Vomiting (1% to 3%), diarrhea (≤1%)

Neuromuscular & skeletal: Weakness (≤2%)

Respiratory: Nasopharyngitis (≤1%)

Adverse reactions that may be related to local edema or hemorrhage at metastatic sites: Exacerbation of papillary carcinoma (enlargement of locally-recurring papillary carcinoma, accompanied by dyspnea, stridor, or dysphonia), hemiparesis, hemiplegia, laryngeal edema (with respiratory distress), pain, sudden blindness

<1%, postmarketing, and/or case reports: Ageusia, antibody development to thyrotropin alfa, atrial arrhythmia, cerebrovascular accident, flu-like symptoms (arthralgia, chills, fever, myalgia, shivering), hypersensitivity reaction (eg, dyspnea, flushing, pruritus, skin rash, urticaria), hyperthyroidism, myocardial infarction, pain, weakness (unilateral)

Drug Interactions

Metabolism/Transport Effects None known.

Avoid Concomitant Use There are no known interactions where it is recommended to avoid concomitant use.

Increased Effect/Toxicity There are no known significant interactions involving an increase in effect.

Decreased Effect There are no known significant interactions involving a decrease in effect.

Storage/Stability Store intact vials at 2°C to 8°C (36°F to 46°F). Protect from light. May store reconstituted solution for up to 24 hours between 2°C and 8°C (36°F and 46°F); avoid microbial contamination. If reconstituted solution is not refrigerated, use within 3 hours. Discard unused portion of the vial.

Preparation for Administration Reconstitute each vial with 1.2 mL of sterile water for injection to a concentration of 0.9 mg/mL. Gently swirl vial until dissolved; do not shake. Reconstituted solution should be clear and colorless; do not use if cloudy or discolored.

Mechanism of Action Thyrotropin alfa, derived from a recombinant DNA source, has the identical amino acid sequence as endogenous human thyroid stimulating hormone (TSH). As a diagnostic tool in conjunction with serum thyroglobulin (Tg) testing, thyrotropin alfa stimulates the secretion of Tg from any remaining thyroid tissues (remnants). Under conditions of successful thyroidectomy and complete ablation, very little serum Tg should be detected under TSH stimulatory conditions; conversely, elevated Tg levels suggest the presence of remnant thyroid tissues. Since the source of TSH is exogenous, stimulation of Tg synthesis can be achieved in euthyroid patients, avoiding the need for thyroid hormone withdrawal.

As an adjunctive agent for radioiodine ablation treatment of thyroid cancer tissue remnants, thyrotropin alfa binds to TSH receptors on these tissues, stimulating the uptake and organification of iodine, including radiolabeled iodine (I^{131}). Cancerous tissue is destroyed via gamma emission from the radioiodine concentrated in these tissues.

Pharmacodynamics/Kinetics
Half-life elimination: 25 ± 10 hours
Time to peak: Median: 10 hours (range: 3-24 hours)

Dosing
Adult & Geriatric Note: Consider pretreatment with glucocorticoids for patients in whom local tumor expansion may compromise vital anatomic structures (such as trachea, CNS, or extensive macroscopic lung metastases).
   Diagnostic imaging: IM: 0.9 mg, followed 24 hours later by a second 0.9 mg dose; obtain serum Tg sample 72 hours after the second thyrotropin alfa injection
   Thyroid tissue remnant ablation: IM: 0.9 mg, followed 24 hours later by a second 0.9 mg dose.
   Radioiodine administration should be given 24 hours following the second thyrotropin alfa injection (for diagnostic scanning and remnant ablation). Perform diagnostic scanning 48 hours after radioiodine administration (72 hours after the second thyrotropin alfa injection). Post-therapy scanning may be delayed (additional days) to allow decline of background activity.
Renal Impairment There are no dosage adjustments provided in the manufacturer's labeling; however, elimination is significantly slower in dialysis-dependent end-stage renal impairment and TSH level elevation may be prolonged.
Hepatic Impairment There are no dosage adjustments provided in the manufacturer's labeling (has not been studied).
Administration Administer only by IM injection into the buttock. Do **not** administer intravenously.
Monitoring Parameters Neurologic adverse events (hemiplegia, hemiparesis, stroke, weakness); dyspnea, dysphonia, stridor or other symptoms of local tumor growth
Test Interactions Thyroglobulin assay may be confounded by thyroglobulin antibodies, possibly leading to misinterpreted or difficult to interpret thyroglobulin levels. Routine measurement of TSH levels after thyrotropin alfa use is not recommended.
Dosage Forms Excipient information presented when available (limited, particularly for generics); consult specific product labeling.
Solution Reconstituted, Intramuscular:
   Thyrogen: 1.1 mg (1 ea)

◆ **Thyrotropin Alpha** *see* Thyrotropin Alfa *on page 1645*

Ticarcillin and Clavulanate Potassium
(tye kar SIL in & klav yoo LAN ate poe TASS ee um)
   Brand Names: US Timentin [DSC]

◀ **Index Terms** Ticarcillin and Clavulanic Acid
Pharmacologic Category Antibiotic, Penicillin
Use

Bone and joint infections: Treatment of bone and joint infections caused by beta-lactamase-producing isolates of *Staphylococcus aureus*.

Endometritis: Treatment of endometritis caused by beta-lactamase-producing isolates of *Prevotella melaninogenicus*, *Enterobacter* species (including *E. cloacae*), *Klebsiella pneumoniae*, *Escherichia coli*, *S. aureus*, or *Staphylococcus epidermidis*.

Lower respiratory tract infections: Treatment of lower respiratory tract infections caused by beta-lactamase-producing isolates of *S. aureus*, *Haemophilus influenzae*, or *Klebsiella* species.

Peritonitis: Treatment of peritonitis caused by beta-lactamase-producing isolates of *E. coli*, *K. pneumonia*, or *Bacteroides fragilis* group.

Septicemia: Treatment of septicemia (including bacteremia) caused by beta-lactamase-producing isolates of *Klebsiella* species, *E. coli*, *S. aureus*, or *Pseudomonas aeruginosa* (or other *Pseudomonas* species).

Skin and skin structure infections: Treatment of skin and skin structure infections caused by beta-lactamase-producing isolates of *S. aureus*, *Klebsiella* species, or *E. coli*.

Urinary tract infections: Treatment of complicated and uncomplicated urinary tract infections caused by beta-lactamase-producing isolates of *E. coli*, *Klebsiella* species, *P. aeruginosa* (and other *Pseudomonas* species), *Citrobacter* species, *Enterobacter cloacae*, *Serratia marcescens*, or *S. aureus*.

Pregnancy Risk Factor B
Dosing

Adult Note: Timentin (ticarcillin/clavulanate) is a combination product; each 3.1 g dosage form contains 3 g ticarcillin disodium and 0.1 g clavulanic acid.

Gynecologic infections (eg, endometritis): IV:
Moderate infections: 200 mg ticarcillin/kg/day in divided doses every 6 hours (maximum: 12 g daily)
Severe infections: 300 mg ticarcillin/kg/day in divided doses every 4 hours (maximum: 18 g daily)

Systemic infections: IV:
<60 kg: 200-300 mg ticarcillin/kg/day in divided doses every 4-6 hours (maximum: 18 g daily)
≥60 kg: 3.1 g every 4-6 hours

Urinary tract infections: IV:
<60 kg: 200-300 mg ticarcillin/kg/day in divided doses every 4-6 hours (maximum: 18 g daily)
≥60 kg: 3.1 g every 4-6 hours

Intra-abdominal infection, complicated, community-acquired, mild-to-moderate (off-label use): IV: 3.1 g every 6 hours for 4-7 days (provided source controlled) (Solomkin, 2010)

Geriatric Refer to adult dosing

Pediatric Note: Timentin (ticarcillin/clavulanate) is a combination product; each 3.1 g dosage form contains 3 g ticarcillin disodium and 0.1 g clavulanic acid.

Mild to moderate infections: Infants ≥3 months, Children, and Adolescents: IV:
<60 kg: 200 mg ticarcillin/kg/day in divided doses every 6 hours (maximum: 12 g daily)
≥60 kg: 3.1 g every 6 hours

Severe infections: Infants ≥3 months, Children, and Adolescents: IV:
  <60 kg: 300 mg ticarcillin/kg/day in divided doses every 4 hours. (maximum: 18 g daily)
  ≥60 kg: 3.1 g every 4 hours

Cystic fibrosis (off-label use): Infants, Children, and Adolescents: IV: 400 mg ticarcillin/kg/day in divided doses every 6 hours; higher doses have been used: 400-750 mg ticarcillin/kg/day in divided doses every 6 hours (maximum: 24-30 g ticarcillin daily) (Zobell, 2013)

Intra-abdominal infection, complicated (off-label use): Infants, Children, and Adolescents: IV: 200-300 mg ticarcillin/kg/day in divided every 4-6 hours (Solomkin, 2010)

Renal Impairment

Loading dose: IV: 3.1 g one dose, followed by maintenance dose based on creatinine clearance:
  CrCl 30-60 mL/minute: Administer 2 g of ticarcillin component every 4 hours
  CrCl 10-30 mL/minute: Administer 2 g of ticarcillin component every 8 hours
  CrCl <10 mL/minute: Administer 2 g of ticarcillin component every 12 hours
  CrCl <10 mL/minute with concomitant hepatic dysfunction: 2 g of ticarcillin component every 24 hours

Intermittent hemodialysis (IHD) (administer after hemodialysis on dialysis days): Dialyzable (20% to 50%): 2 g of ticarcillin component every 12 hours; supplemented with 3.1 g (ticarcillin/clavulanate) after each dialysis session. Alternatively, administer 2 g every 8 hours without a supplemental dose for deep-seated infections (Heintz, 2009). **Note:** Dosing dependent on the assumption of 3 times/week, complete IHD sessions.

Peritoneal dialysis (PD): 3.1 g every 12 hours

Continuous renal replacement therapy (CRRT) (Heintz, 2009; Trotman, 2005): Drug clearance is highly dependent on the method of renal replacement, filter type, and flow rate. Appropriate dosing requires close monitoring of pharmacologic response, signs of adverse reactions due to drug accumulation, as well as drug concentrations in relation to target trough (if appropriate). The following are general recommendations only (based on dialysate flow/ultrafiltration rates of 1-2 L/hour and minimal residual renal function) and should not supersede clinical judgment:
  CVVH: Loading dose of 3.1g followed by 2 g every 6-8 hours
  CVVHD: Loading dose of 3.1 g followed by 3.1 g every 6-8 hours
  CVVHDF: Loading dose of 3.1 g followed by 3.1 g every 6 hours
  Note: Do not administer in intervals exceeding every 8 hours. Clavulanate component is hepatically eliminated; extending the dosing interval beyond 8 hours may result in loss of beta-lactamase inhibition.

Hepatic Impairment With concomitant renal dysfunction (CrCl <10 mL/minute): 2 g of ticarcillin component every 24 hours.

Additional Information Complete prescribing information should be consulted for additional detail.

Product Availability Not available in the US

Dosage Forms Excipient information presented when available (limited, particularly for generics); consult specific product labeling. [DSC] = discontinued product

Infusion [premixed, frozen]:
  Timentin: Ticarcillin 3 g and clavulanic acid 0.1 g (100 mL [DSC]) [contains sodium 4.51 mEq and potassium 0.15 mEq per g]

◀   Injection, powder for reconstitution:
Timentin: Ticarcillin 3 g and clavulanic acid 0.1 g (3.1 g [DSC], 31 g [DSC])
[contains sodium 4.51 mEq and potassium 0.15 mEq per g]

- ◆ **Ticarcillin and Clavulanic Acid** *see* Ticarcillin and Clavulanate Potassium *on page 1647*

- ◆ **Tice BCG** *see* BCG (Intravesical) *on page 174*

- ◆ **Tigan** *see* Trimethobenzamide *on page 1702*

- ◆ **Timentin [DSC]** *see* Ticarcillin and Clavulanate Potassium *on page 1647*

- ◆ **Tioguanine** *see* Thioguanine *on page 1637*

- ◆ **Tipiracil and Trifluridine** *see* Trifluridine and Tipiracil *on page 1699*

- ◆ **TMP-SMX** *see* Sulfamethoxazole and Trimethoprim *on page 1560*

- ◆ **TMP-SMZ** *see* Sulfamethoxazole and Trimethoprim *on page 1560*

- ◆ **TMZ** *see* Temozolomide *on page 1608*

Tobramycin (Systemic) (toe bra MYE sin)

Brand Names: Canada JAMP-Tobramycin; Tobramycin For Injection; Tobramycin For Injection, USP; Tobramycin Injection; Tobramycin Injection, USP
Index Terms Tobramycin Sulfate
Pharmacologic Category Antibiotic, Aminoglycoside
Use Treatment of documented or suspected infections caused by susceptible gram-negative bacilli, including *Pseudomonas aeruginosa.*
Pregnancy Risk Factor D
Dosing

Adult Note: Individualization is **critical** because of the low therapeutic index.
In underweight and nonobese patients, use of total body weight (TBW) instead of ideal body weight for determining the initial mg/kg/dose is widely accepted (Nicolau, 1995). Ideal body weight (IBW) also may be used to determine doses for patients who are neither underweight nor obese (Gilbert, 2009).

Initial and periodic plasma drug levels (eg, peak and trough with conventional dosing, post dose level at a prespecified time with extended-interval dosing) should be determined, particularly in critically-ill patients with serious infections or in disease states known to significantly alter aminoglycoside pharmacokinetics (eg, cystic fibrosis, burns, or major surgery).

Severe life-threatening infections: IM, IV:
Conventional: 1 to 2.5 mg/kg/dose every 8 to 12 hours; to ensure adequate peak concentrations early in therapy, higher initial dosage may be considered in selected patients when extracellular water is increased (edema, septic shock, postsurgical, and/or trauma)
Once-daily: 4 to 7 mg/kg/dose once daily; some clinicians recommend this approach for all patients with normal renal function; this dose is at least as efficacious with similar, if not less, toxicity than conventional dosing.
Brucellosis: IM, IV: 240 mg (IM) daily or 5 mg/kg (IV) daily for 7 days; either regimen recommended in combination with doxycycline
Cholangitis: IM, IV: 4 to 6 mg/kg once daily with ampicillin
CNS shunt infection: Intrathecal (off-label route): 5 to 20 mg/day (Tunkel, 2004)
Diverticulitis, complicated: IM, IV: 1.5 to 2 mg/kg every 8 hours (with ampicillin and metronidazole)

Infective endocarditis (*Pseudomonas aeruginosa*) (off-label use): IM, IV: 8 mg/kg once daily (in combination with an extended-spectrum penicillin, or ceftazidime or cefepime) for a minimum of 6 weeks; adjust doses to maintain peak concentrations of 15 to 20 mcg/mL and trough concentrations ≤2 mcg/mL (AHA/IDSA [Baddour, 2005]; Rybak, 1986)

Meningitis *(Enterococcus or Pseudomonas aeruginosa)*: IV: 5 mg/kg/day in divided doses every 8 hours (administered with another bacteriocidal drug)

Pelvic inflammatory disease: IM, IV: Loading dose: 2 mg/kg, then 1.5 mg/kg every 8 hours **or** 4.5 mg/kg once daily

Plague *(Yersinia pestis)*: IM, IV: Treatment: 5 mg/kg/day, followed by postexposure prophylaxis with doxycycline

Pneumonia, hospital- or ventilator-associated: IM, IV: 7 mg/kg/day (with antipseudomonal beta-lactam or carbapenem)

Prophylaxis against endocarditis (dental, oral, upper respiratory procedures, GI/GU procedures): IM, IV: 1.5 mg/kg with ampicillin (50 mg/kg) 30 minutes prior to procedure. **Note:** AHA guidelines now recommend prophylaxis only in patients undergoing invasive procedures and in whom underlying cardiac conditions may predispose to a higher risk of adverse outcomes should infection occur. As of April 2007, routine prophylaxis no longer recommended by the AHA.

Tularemia: IM, IV: 5 mg/kg/day divided every 8 hours for 1 to 2 weeks

Urinary tract infection: IM, IV: 1.5 mg/kg/dose every 8 hours

Geriatric Dosage should be based on an estimate of ideal body weight.

IM, IV: 1.5 to 5 mg/kg/day in 1 to 2 divided doses

IV: Once daily or extended interval: 5 to 7 mg/kg/dose given every 24, 36, or 48 hours based on creatinine clearance

Pediatric Individualization is **critical** because of the low therapeutic index

Use of ideal body weight (IBW) for determining the mg/kg/dose appears to be more accurate than dosing on the basis of total body weight (TBW).

Usual dosage range: IM, IV:

Infants and Children <5 years: 2.5 mg/kg/dose every 8 hours

Children >5 years: 2 to 2.5 mg/kg/dose every 8 hours

CNS shunt infection: Intrathecal (off-label route): Refer to adult dosing.

Cystic fibrosis: IM, IV: 2.5 to 3.3 mg/kg every 6 to 8 hours. **Note:** Some patients may require larger or more frequent doses if serum levels document the need (eg, cystic fibrosis or febrile granulocytopenic patients).

Renal Impairment IM, IV:

Conventional dosing:

CrCl ≥60 mL/minute: Administer every 8 hours.

CrCl 40 to 60 mL/minute: Administer every 12 hours.

CrCl 20 to 40 mL/minute: Administer every 24 hours.

CrCl 10 to 20 mL/minute: Administer every 48 hours.

CrCl <10 mL/minute: Administer every 72 hours.

High-dose therapy: Interval may be extended (eg, every 48 hours) in patients with moderate renal impairment (CrCl 30 to 59 mL/minute) and/or adjusted based on serum level determinations.

◄ Intermittent hemodialysis (IHD) (administer after hemodialysis on dialysis days) (Heintz, 2009): Dialyzable (25% to 70%; variable; dependent on filter, duration, and type of HD): IV:

Loading dose of 2 to 3 mg/kg, followed by:

Mild UTI or synergy: IV: 1 mg/kg every 48 to 72 hours; consider redosing for pre-HD or post-HD concentrations <1 mg/L

Moderate-to-severe UTI: IV: 1 to 1.5 mg/kg every 48 to 72 hours; consider redosing for pre-HD concentrations <1.5 to 2 mg/L or post-HD concentrations <1 mg/L

Systemic gram-negative infection: IV: 1.5 to 2 mg/kg every 48 to 72 hours; consider redosing for pre-HD concentrations <3 to 5 mg/L or post-HD concentrations <2 mg/L

Note: Dosing dependent on the assumption of 3 times/week, complete IHD sessions.

Peritoneal dialysis (PD):

Administration via peritoneal dialysis (PD) fluid:

Gram-negative infection: 4 to 8 mg/L (4 to 8 mcg/mL) of PD fluid

Gram-positive infection (ie, synergy): 3 to 4 mg/L (3 to 4 mcg/mL) of PD fluid

Administration IVPB/IM: Dose as for CrCl <10 mL/minute and follow levels

Continuous renal replacement therapy (CRRT) (Heintz, 2009; Trotman, 2005): Drug clearance is highly dependent on the method of renal replacement, filter type, and flow rate. Appropriate dosing requires close monitoring of pharmacologic response, signs of adverse reactions due to drug accumulation, as well as drug concentrations in relation to target trough (if appropriate). The following are general recommendations only (based on dialysate flow/ultrafiltration rates of 1 to 2 L/hour and minimal residual renal function) and should not supersede clinical judgment:

CVVH/CVVHD/CVVHDF: IV: Loading dose of 2 to 3 mg/kg, followed by:

Mild UTI or synergy: IV 1 mg/kg every 24 to 36 hours (redose when concentration <1 mg/L)

Moderate-severe UTI: IV: 1 to 1.5 mg/kg every 24 to 36 hours (redose when concentration <1.5 to 2 mg/L)

Systemic gram-negative infection: IV: 1.5 to 2.5 mg/kg every 24 to 48 hours (redose when concentration <3 to 5 mg/L)

Hepatic Impairment No dosage adjustment necessary; does not undergo hepatic metabolism.

Obesity In moderate obesity (TBW/IBW ≥1.25) or greater, (eg, morbid obesity [TBW/IBW >2]), initial dosage requirement may be estimated using a dosing weight of IBW + 0.4 (TBW - IBW) (Traynor, 1995).

Additional Information Complete prescribing information should be consulted for additional detail.

Dosage Forms Excipient information presented when available (limited, particularly for generics); consult specific product labeling.

Solution, Injection:

Generic: 10 mg/mL (2 mL); 80 mg/2 mL (2 mL); 1.2 g/30 mL (30 mL); 2 g/50 mL (50 mL)

Solution, Intravenous:

Generic: 80 mg (100 mL)

Solution Reconstituted, Injection:

Generic: 1.2 g (1 ea)

Solution Reconstituted, Injection [preservative free]:

Generic: 1.2 g (1 ea)

Topotecan (toe poe TEE kan)

Related Information

Brand Names: US Hycamtin

Brand Names: Canada Hycamtin; Topotecan For Injection; Topotecan Hydrochloride For Injection

Index Terms Hycamptamine; SKF 104864; SKF 104864-A; Topotecan Hydrochloride

Pharmacologic Category Antineoplastic Agent, Camptothecin; Antineoplastic Agent, Topoisomerase I Inhibitor

Use

Cervical cancer, recurrent or resistant: Treatment of recurrent or resistant (stage IVB) cervical cancer (in combination with cisplatin) which is not amenable to curative treatment

Ovarian cancer, metastatic: Treatment of metastatic ovarian cancer (as a single agent) after disease progression on or after initial or subsequent chemotherapy

Small cell lung cancer, relapsed:

Injection: Treatment of small cell lung cancer (as a single agent) in patients with platinum-sensitive disease which has progressed at least 60 days after initiation of first-line chemotherapy

Oral: Treatment of relapsed small cell lung cancer in patients with a prior complete or partial response and who are at least 45 days from the end of first-line chemotherapy

Labeled Contraindications

Hypersensitivity to topotecan or any component of the formulation

Canadian labeling: Additional contraindications (not in U.S. labeling): Severe renal impairment (CrCl <20 mL/minute); pregnancy; breast-feeding; severe bone marrow depression

Pregnancy Considerations Adverse effects were observed in animal reproduction studies. May cause fetal harm in pregnant women. Women of childbearing potential should use highly effective contraception to prevent pregnancy during treatment and for at least 1 month after therapy

◀ discontinuation. Males with female partners of childbearing potential should use highly effective contraception during treatment and for 3 months after therapy discontinuation. Topotecan may have both acute and long-term effects on fertility in women; fertility in males may be impaired due to effects on spermatogenesis.

Breast-Feeding Considerations It is not known if topotecan is excreted in breast milk. Due to the potential for serious adverse reactions in the nursing infant, the manufacturer recommends to discontinue breast-feeding in women who are receiving topotecan.

Warnings/Precautions Hazardous agent - use appropriate precautions for handling and disposal (NIOSH 2014 [group 1]). **[US Boxed Warning]: May cause severe myelosuppression. Monitor blood counts frequently. Do NOT administer to patients with baseline neutrophils <1500/mm^3 and platelets <100,000/mm^3.** The dose-limiting toxicity is bone marrow suppression (primarily neutropenia); may also cause thrombocytopenia and anemia. Grade 3 and 4 events were common. Severe myelotoxicity has also been reported when used in combination with cisplatin. Neutropenia is not cumulative overtime. The median duration of neutropenia and thrombocytopenia was 7 days and 5 days, respectively. Nadir neutrophil and platelet counts occurred at a median of 15 days (when administered orally). In a clinical study comparing IV to oral topotecan, G-CSF support was administered in a higher percentage of patients receiving oral topotecan (Eckardt 2007). Bone marrow suppression may require dosage reduction and/or growth factor support. Topotecan-induced neutropenia may lead to typhlitis (neutropenic enterocolitis), including fatalities; should be considered in patients presenting with neutropenia, fever, and abdominal pain.

Diarrhea has been reported with oral topotecan; may be severe (requiring hospitalization); incidence may be higher in the elderly; educate patients on early recognition and proper management, including diet changes, increase in fluid intake, antidiarrheals, and antibiotics. The median time to onset of diarrhea (grade 2 or worse) was 9 days. The incidence of diarrhea may be higher in the elderly. Do not administer in patients with grade 3 or 4 diarrhea; reduce dose upon recovery to ≤ grade 1 toxicity. Interstitial lung disease (ILD) (with fatalities) has been reported; discontinue use in patients with confirmed ILD diagnosis; risk factors for ILD include a history of ILD, pulmonary fibrosis, lung cancer, thoracic radiation, and the use of colony-stimulating factors or medication with pulmonary toxicity; monitor pulmonary symptoms (cough, fever, dyspnea, and/or hypoxia). Use caution in renal impairment; may require dose adjustment (use in severe renal impairment is contraindicated in the Canadian labeling). Potentially significant drug-drug interactions may exist, requiring dose or frequency adjustment, additional monitoring, and/or selection of alternative therapy. Topotecan exposure is increased when oral topotecan is used concurrently with P-glycoprotein inhibitors; avoid concurrent use. Topotecan overdoses have been reported; potential causes include omission of the leading zero and missing the decimal point when prescribing, preparing, and administering. Recommended intravenous doses should generally not exceed 4 mg in adults; verify dose prior to administration. Extravasation injuries have been reported (some severe); if extravasation occurs, discontinue infusion immediately and manage appropriately. Ensure proper needle or catheter placement prior to and during infusion. Avoid extravasation.

Adverse Reactions

>10%:

Central nervous system: Fatigue (oral: 11% to 19%)

Dermatologic: Alopecia (oral: 10% to 20%)

Gastrointestinal: Nausea (oral: 27% to 33%), anorexia (intravenous: 32%; oral: 7% to 14%), diarrhea (oral: 14% to 22%, grade 3: 4%, grade 4: ≤1%; intravenous: grades 3/4: 6%), vomiting (oral: 19% to 21%)

Hematologic & oncologic: Anemia (oral: 94% to 98%; grades 3/4: 25%; grade 3: 15% to 18%; grade 4: 7% to 10%; intravenous: grades 3/4: 37% to 42%), neutropenia (oral: 83% to 91%; grade 3: 24% to 28%; grade 4: 32% to 33%; intravenous: grade 4: 70% to 80%; nadir 12 to 15 days; duration: 7 days), thrombocytopenia (oral: 81%; grade 3: 29% to 30%; grade 4: 6% to 7%; intravenous: grade 4: 27% to 29%; nadir: 15 days; duration: 3 to 5 days), febrile neutropenia (intravenous: grade 3/4: 23% to 28%; oral: grade 4: 4%), neutropenic infection (13% to 17%)

1% to 10%:

Gastrointestinal: Abdominal pain (intravenous: grades 3/4: 5% to 6%)

Hepatic: Increased liver enzymes (intravenous: 8%; transient)

Neuromuscular & skeletal: Weakness (3% to 7%)

Respiratory: Dyspnea (intravenous: 6% to 9%)

Miscellaneous: Fever (oral: 5% to 7%), sepsis (intravenous: grades 3/4: 5%; oral: 2%)

<1%, postmarketing, and/or case reports: Anaphylactoid reactions, angioedema, arthralgia, chest pain, cough, dermatitis (severe), extravasation, headache, hemorrhage (severe, associated with thrombocytopenia), hypersensitivity reaction, interstitial pulmonary disease, leukopenia, myalgia, neutropenic enterocolitis, pancytopenia, paresthesia, pruritus (severe), skin rash, stomatitis, typhlitis

Drug Interactions

Metabolism/Transport Effects Substrate of BCRP

Avoid Concomitant Use

Avoid concomitant use of Topotecan with any of the following: BCG (Intravesical); CloZAPine; Dipyrone; Natalizumab; P-glycoprotein/ABCB1 Inhibitors; Pimecrolimus; Tacrolimus (Topical); Tofacitinib; Vaccines (Live)

Increased Effect/Toxicity

Topotecan may increase the levels/effects of: CloZAPine; Fingolimod; Leflunomide; Natalizumab; Tofacitinib; Vaccines (Live)

The levels/effects of Topotecan may be increased by: BCRP/ABCG2 Inhibitors; Denosumab; Dipyrone; Filgrastim; P-glycoprotein/ABCB1 Inhibitors; Pimecrolimus; Platinum Derivatives; Roflumilast; Tacrolimus (Topical); Trastuzumab

Decreased Effect

Topotecan may decrease the levels/effects of: BCG (Intravesical); Coccidioides immitis Skin Test; Sipuleucel-T; Vaccines (Inactivated); Vaccines (Live)

The levels/effects of Topotecan may be decreased by: Echinacea; Fosphenytoin-Phenytoin

Storage/Stability

IV:

Solution for injection: Store intact vials at 2°C to 8°C (36°F to 45°F). Protect from light. Single-use vials should be discarded after initial vial entry.

◀ Stability of solutions diluted for infusion is variable; refer to specific product information for details.

Lyophilized powder: Store intact vials at 20°C to 25°C (68°F to 77°F). Protect from light. Reconstituted solution is stable for up to 28 days at 20°C to 25°C (68°F to 77°F), although the manufacturer recommends use immediately after reconstitution. Solutions diluted in D_5W or NS are stable for 24 hours at room temperature (manufacturer's labeling) or up to 7 days under refrigeration (Craig 1997). Reconstituted solution for injection (reconstituted with bacteriostatic SWFI to 1 mg/mL) for oral administration is stable for 14 days at 4°C in plastic syringes (Daw 2004).

Oral: Store at 2°C to 8°C (36°F to 46°F). Protect from light.

Preparation for Administration Hazardous agent; use appropriate precautions for handling and disposal (NIOSH 2014 [group 1]). Reconstitute lyophilized powder with 4 mL SWFI. Reconstituted lyophilized powder and solution for injection should be further diluted in D_5W or NS for infusion.

Mechanism of Action Binds to topoisomerase I and stabilizes the cleavable complex so that religation of the cleaved DNA strand cannot occur. This results in the accumulation of cleavable complexes and single-strand DNA breaks. Topotecan acts in S phase of the cell cycle.

Pharmacodynamics/Kinetics

Absorption: Oral: Rapid

Distribution: V_d: 25 to 75 L/m^2 (Hartmann 2006)

Protein binding: ~35%

Metabolism: Undergoes a rapid, pH-dependent hydrolysis of the lactone ring to yield a relatively inactive hydroxy acid in plasma; metabolized in the liver to N-demethylated metabolite

Bioavailability: Oral: ~40%

Half-life elimination: IV: 2 to 3 hours; renal impairment: ~5 hours; Oral: 3 to 6 hours

Time to peak, plasma: Oral: 1 to 2 hours; delayed with high-fat meal (3 to 4 hours)

Excretion:

IV: Urine (51%; ~3% as N-desmethyl topotecan); feces (18%; ~2% as N-desmethyl topotecan)

Oral: Urine (20%; 2% as N-desmethyl topotecan); feces (33%; <2% as N-desmethyl topotecan)

Dosing

Adult & Geriatric Note: Baseline neutrophil count should be ≥1500/mm^3 and platelets should be ≥100,000/mm^3 prior to treatment; for re-treatment, neutrophil count should be >1000/mm^3; platelets >100,000/mm^3 and hemoglobin ≥9 g/dL. Intravenous doses should generally not exceed 4 mg; verify dose prior to administration.

Cervical cancer, recurrent or resistant: IV: 0.75 mg/m^2/day for 3 days (in combination with cisplatin on day 1 only, [with hydration]) every 21 days

Ovarian cancer, metastatic: IV: 1.5 mg/m^2/day for 5 consecutive days every 21 days **or** (off-label dosing) 1.25 mg/m^2/day for 5 days every 21 days until disease progression or unacceptable toxicity or a maximum of 12 months (Sehouli 2011) **or** (weekly administration; off-label dosing) 4 mg/m^2 on days 1, 8, and 15 every 28 days until disease progression or unacceptable toxicity or a maximum of 12 months (Sehouli 2011)

Small cell lung cancer (SCLC), relapsed:
IV: 1.5 mg/m^2/day for 5 consecutive days every 21 days
Oral: 2.3 mg/m^2/day for 5 consecutive days every 21 days (round dose to the nearest 0.25 mg); if patient vomits after dose is administered, do not give a replacement dose.

Ewing's sarcoma, relapsed/refractory or metastatic (off-label use): IV: 0.75 mg/m^2/day for 5 consecutive days every 21 days (in combination with cyclophosphamide) (Hunold 2006; Saylors 2001)

Primary CNS lymphoma, relapsed or refractory (off-label use): IV: 1.5 mg/m^2 for 5 days every 21 days for a maximum of 10 cycles or until disease progression or unacceptable toxicity (Voloschin 2008). Additional data may be necessary to further define the role of topotecan in this condition.

Rhabdomyosarcoma, metastatic (off-label use): Adults <21 years: IV: 0.75 mg/m^2/day for 5 consecutive days every 21 days for 2 cycles (window therapy; in combination with cyclophosphamide); if objective response occurred by week 6, follow with alternating cycles of vincristine, topotecan, and cyclophosphamide (VTC) with vincristine, dactinomycin, and cyclophosphamide (VAC) (Walterhouse 2004)

Pediatric Note: Baseline neutrophil count should be ≥1500/mm^3 and platelets should be ≥100,000/mm^3 prior to treatment; for re-treatment, neutrophil count should be >1000/mm^3; platelets >100,000/mm^3 and hemoglobin ≥9 g/dL. Intravenous doses should generally not exceed 4 mg; verify dose prior to administration.

CNS malignancy, relapsed/refractory (off-label use; based on limited data): Oral: 0.8 mg/m^2/day for 21 consecutive days every 4 weeks for ≥12 cycles (Minturn 2011); additional data may be necessary to further define the role of topotecan in this condition

Ewing's sarcoma, relapsed/refractory or metastatic (off-label use): IV: 0.75 mg/m^2/day for 5 consecutive days every 21 days (in combination with cyclophosphamide) (Hunold 2006; Saylors 2001)

Neuroblastoma, relapsed/refractory (off-label use): IV: 0.75 mg/m^2/day for 5 days every 21 days (in combination with cyclophosphamide) (Ashraf 2013; London 2010) **or** 2 mg/m^2/day for 5 days every 21 days (monotherapy) (London 2010)

Rhabdomyosarcoma, metastatic (off-label use): IV: 0.75 mg/m^2/day for 5 consecutive days every 21 days for 2 cycles (window therapy; in combination with cyclophosphamide); if objective response occurred by week 6, follow with alternating cycles of vincristine, topotecan, and cyclophosphamide (VTC) with vincristine, dactinomycin, and cyclophosphamide (VAC) (Walterhouse 2004)

Renal Impairment
Manufacturer's labeling:
IV (single agent topotecan):
CrCl ≥40 mL/minute: No dosage adjustment necessary.
CrCl 20 to 39 mL/minute: Reduce dose to 0.75 mg/m^2/dose
CrCl <20 mL/minute: There are no dosage adjustments provided in manufacturer's U.S. labeling (insufficient data available for dosing recommendation); use is contraindicated in the Canadian labeling.

◄ Oral:

CrCl ≥50 mL/minute: No dosage adjustment necessary.

CrCl 30 to 49 mL/minute: Reduce dose to 1.5 mg/m^2/day; may increase after the 1st cycle by 0.4 mg/m^2/day if no severe hematologic or gastrointestinal toxicities occur.

CrCl <30 mL/minute: Reduce dose to 0.6 mg/m^2/day; may increase after the 1st cycle by 0.4 mg/m^2/day if no severe hematologic or gastrointestinal toxicities occur.

Alternate recommendations:

Aronoff 2007: IV:

Adults:

CrCl >50 mL/minute: Administer 75% of dose

CrCl 10 to 50 mL/minute: Administer 50% of dose

CrCl <10 mL/minute: Administer 25% of dose

Hemodialysis: Avoid use

Continuous ambulatory peritoneal dialysis (CAPD): Avoid use

Continuous renal replacement therapy (CRRT): 0.75 mg/m^2

Children:

CrCl 30 to 50 mL/minute: Administer 75% of dose

CrCl 10 to 29 mL/minute: Administer 50% of dose

CrCl <10 mL/minute: Administer 25% of dose

Continuous renal replacement therapy (CRRT): Administer 50% of dose

Kintzel 1995: IV:

CrCl 46 to 60 mL/minute: Administer 80% of dose

CrCl 31 to 45 mL/minute: Administer 75% of dose

CrCl ≤30 mL/minute: Administer 70% of dose

Hepatic Impairment Manufacturer's labeling:

IV:

US labeling: Bilirubin 1.7 to 15 mg/dL: There are no dosage adjustments provided in the manufacturer's labeling, although clearance is reduced up to 33%.

Canadian labeling: Bilirubin >1.5 to <10 mg/dL: No dosage adjustment is necessary (the half-life is increased slightly; usual doses are generally tolerated).

Oral: There is no dosage adjustment provided in the manufacturer's labeling; however, dosage adjustment is likely not necessary as the pharmacokinetics of topotecan do not differ significantly based on serum bilirubin, ALT, or AST.

Obesity *ASCO Guidelines for appropriate chemotherapy dosing in obese adults with cancer:* Utilize patient's actual body weight (full weight) for calculation of body surface area- or weight-based dosing, particularly when the intent of therapy is curative; manage regimen-related toxicities in the same manner as for nonobese patients; if a dose reduction is utilized due to toxicity, consider resumption of full weight-based dosing with subsequent cycles, especially if cause of toxicity (eg, hepatic or renal impairment) is resolved (Griggs 2012).

Adjustment for Toxicity

Cervical cancer (cisplatin may also require dosage adjustment): IV: Severe febrile neutropenia (<1000/mm^3 with temperature of ≥38°C) or platelet count <25,000/mm^3: Reduce topotecan to 0.6 mg/m^2/day for subsequent cycles (may consider G-CSF support [beginning on day 4] prior to instituting dose reduction for neutropenic fever).

If necessary, may further reduce dose to 0.45 mg/m²/day for subsequent cycles.

Ovarian cancer: IV: Dosage adjustment for hematological effects: Severe neutropenia (<500/mm³) or platelet count <25,000/mm³: Reduce dose to 1.25 mg/m²/day for subsequent cycles (may consider G-CSF support [beginning on day 6] prior to instituting dose reduction for severe neutropenia). **Note:** The Canadian labeling states that the dose may be further reduced to 1 mg/m²/day if necessary.

Small cell lung cancer (SCLC):

IV: Dosage adjustment for hematological effects: Severe neutropenia (<500/mm³) or platelet count <25,000/mm³: Reduce dose to 1.25 mg/m²/day for subsequent cycles (may consider G-CSF support [beginning on day 6] prior to instituting dose reduction for severe neutropenia). **Note:** The Canadian labeling states that the dose may be further reduced to 1 mg/m²/day if necessary.

Oral:

Severe neutropenia (neutrophils <500/mm³ associated with fever or infection or lasting ≥7 days) or prolonged neutropenia (neutrophils 500/mm³ to 1000/mm³ lasting beyond day 21) or platelets <25,000/mm³: Reduce dose by 0.4 mg/m²/day for subsequent cycles.

Diarrhea (grade 3 or 4): Do not administer to patients with grade 3 or 4 diarrhea. Upon recovery to ≤ grade 1 toxicity, reduce dose by 0.4 mg/m²/day for subsequent cycles.

Combination Regimens

Bone sarcoma (Ewing sarcoma): Cyclophosphamide-Topotecan (Ewing Sarcoma) on page 1930

Cervical cancer:

Bevacizumab-Paclitaxel-Topotecan (Cervical) on page 1845

Cisplatin-Topotecan (Cervical Cancer) on page 1912

Lung cancer, small cell:

Topotecan Intravenous (Small Cell Lung Cancer Regimen) on page 2091

Topotecan Oral (Small Cell Lung Cancer Regimen) on page 2091

Neuroblastoma: Cyclophosphamide-Topotecan (Neuroblastoma) on page 1930

Ovarian cancer:

Bevacizumab-Topotecan Daily (Ovarian) on page 1845

Bevacizumab-Topotecan Weekly (Ovarian) on page 1846

Topotecan (Ovarian Cancer Regimen) on page 2091

Topotecan Weekly (Ovarian Cancer Regimen) on page 2092

Soft tissue sarcoma (rhabdomyosarcoma): Cyclophosphamide-Topotecan (Rhabdomyosarcoma) on page 1931

Administration

IV: Administer IVPB over 30 minutes. For combination chemotherapy with cisplatin, administer pretreatment hydration.

Oral: Administer without regard to meals. Swallow whole; do not open, crush, chew, or divide capsule. If vomiting occurs after dose, do not take replacement dose. For patients unable to swallow capsules whole, reconstituted topotecan solution for injection (1 mg/mL concentration) may be mixed with up to 30 mL of acidic fruit juice (eg, apple, orange, grape) immediately prior to oral administration (Daw 2004).

Hazardous agent; use appropriate precautions for handling and disposal (NIOSH 2014 [group 1]).

Vesicant/Extravasation Risk Irritant

◄ **Emetic Potential** Children and Adults: Low (10% to 30%)

Extemporaneous Preparations

Hazardous agent; use appropriate precautions for handling and disposal (NIOSH 2014 [group 1]). When compounding an oral solution, NIOSH recommends double gloving, a protective gown, and preparation in a controlled device; if not prepared in a controlled device, respiratory and eye protection as well as ventilated engineering controls are recommended (NIOSH 2014).

For patients unable to swallow capsules whole, reconstituted topotecan solution for injection (1 mg/mL concentration) may be mixed with up to 30 mL of acidic fruit juice (eg, apple, orange, grape) immediately prior to oral administration.

Daw NC, Santana VM, Iacono LC, et al. Phase I and pharmacokinetic study of topotecan administered orally once daily for 5 days for 2 consecutive weeks to pediatric patients with refractory solid tumors. *J Clin Oncol.* 2004;22(5):829-837.

Monitoring Parameters CBC with differential and platelet count, renal function tests, bilirubin; monitor for symptoms of interstitial lung disease; diarrhea symptoms/hydration status

Dosage Forms Excipient information presented when available (limited, particularly for generics); consult specific product labeling.

Capsule, Oral:

Hycamtin: 0.25 mg, 1 mg

Solution, Intravenous:

Generic: 4 mg/4 mL (4 mL)

Solution, Intravenous [preservative free]:

Generic: 4 mg/4 mL (4 mL)

Solution Reconstituted, Intravenous:

Hycamtin: 4 mg (1 ea)

Generic: 4 mg (1 ea)

Solution Reconstituted, Intravenous [preservative free]:

Generic: 4 mg (1 ea)

◆ **Topotecan For Injection (Can)** see Topotecan on page 1653

◆ **Topotecan Hydrochloride** see Topotecan on page 1653

◆ **Topotecan Hydrochloride For Injection (Can)** see Topotecan on page 1653

Toremifene (tore EM i feen)

Related Information

Safe Handling of Hazardous Drugs on page 2292

Brand Names: US Fareston

Brand Names: Canada Fareston

Index Terms FC1157a; Toremifene Citrate

Pharmacologic Category Antineoplastic Agent, Estrogen Receptor Antagonist; Selective Estrogen Receptor Modulator (SERM)

Use Breast cancer, metastatic: Treatment of metastatic breast cancer in postmenopausal women with estrogen receptor positive or estrogen receptor status unknown tumors

Labeled Contraindications Known hypersensitivity to toremifene or any component of the formulation; long QT syndrome (congenital or acquired QT prolongation), uncorrected hypokalemia, uncorrected hypomagnesemia

Pregnancy Considerations Adverse events were observed in animal reproduction studies. Based on the mechanism of action, may cause fetal harm if administered during pregnancy. Toremifene is only approved for use in postmenopausal women; however, if prescribed in premenopausal women, effective non-hormonal contraception should be used.

Breast-Feeding Considerations It is not known if toremifene is excreted in breast milk. Due to the potential for serious adverse reactions in the nursing infant, the manufacturer recommends a decision be made to discontinue nursing or to discontinue the drug, taking into account the importance of treatment to the mother.

Warnings/Precautions Hazardous agent - use appropriate precautions for handling and disposal (NIOSH 2014 [group 1]).

[US Boxed Warning]: May prolong the QT interval; QTc prolongation is dose-dependent and concentration dependent. QT prolongation may lead to a form of ventricular tachycardia called torsades de pointes, which may result in syncope, seizure and/or sudden death. Use is contraindicated in patients with congenital or acquired QT prolongation (long QT syndrome), uncorrected hypokalemia, or uncorrected hypomagnesemia. Avoid use with other medications known to prolong the QT interval and with strong CYP3A4 inhibitors. Use with caution in patients with heart failure, hepatic impairment, or electrolyte abnormalities. Monitor electrolytes; correct hypokalemia and hypomagnesemia prior to treatment. Obtain ECG at baseline and as clinically indicated in patients at risk for QT prolongation.

Hypercalcemia and tumor flare have been reported during the first weeks of treatment in some breast cancer patients with bone metastases; monitor closely for hypocalcemia. Institute appropriate measures if hypercalcemia occurs, and if severe, discontinue treatment. Medications that decrease renal calcium excretion (eg, thiazide diuretics) may increase the risk of hypercalcemia in patients receiving toremifene. Tumor flare consists of diffuse musculoskeletal pain and erythema with initial increased size of tumor lesions that later regress; is often accompanied by hypercalcemia. Tumor flare does not imply treatment failure or represent tumor progression. Leukopenia and thrombocytopenia have been reported rarely; monitor leukocyte and platelet counts in patients with leukopenia and thrombocytopenia. Endometrial hyperplasia has been reported; some patients have developed endometrial cancer, although a role of toremifene in endometrial cancer development has not been established. Avoid long-term use in patients with preexisting endometrial hyperplasia. Use with caution in patients with hepatic failure. Avoid use in patients with a history of thromboembolic disease. Potentially significant drug-drug/drug-food interactions may exist, requiring dose or frequency adjustment, additional monitoring, and/or selection of alternative therapy.

Adverse Reactions

>10%:

Endocrine & metabolic: Hot flashes (35%)

Gastrointestinal: Nausea (14%)

Genitourinary: Vaginal discharge (13%)

Hepatic: Alkaline phosphatase increased (8% to 19%), AST increased (5% to 19%)

Miscellaneous: Diaphoresis (20%)

◀ 1% to 10%:
   Cardiovascular: Edema (5%), arrhythmia (≤2%), CVA/TIA (≤2%), thrombosis
      (≤2%), cardiac failure (≤1%), MI (≤1%)
   Central nervous system: Dizziness (9%)
   Endocrine & metabolic: Hypercalcemia (≤3%)
   Gastrointestinal: Vomiting (4%)
   Genitourinary: Vaginal bleeding (2%)
   Hepatic: Bilirubin increased (1% to 2%)
   Local: Thrombophlebitis (≤2%)
   Ocular: Cataracts (≤10%), xerophthalmia (≤9%), visual field abnormal (≤4%),
      corneal keratopathy (≤2%), glaucoma (≤2%), vision abnormal/diplo-
      pia (≤2%)
   Respiratory: Pulmonary embolism (≤2%)
   <1%, postmarketing, and/or case reports: Alopecia, angina, anorexia, arthritis,
   ataxia, blurred vision, constipation, corneal opacity (reversible), corneal
   verticulata, depression, dermatitis, dyspnea, endometrial cancer, endometrial
   hyperplasia, fatigue, hepatitis (toxic), incoordination, ischemic attack, jaundice, lethargy, leukopenia, paresis, pruritus, QT prolongation, rigors, skin
   discoloration, thrombocytopenia, tremor, tumor flare, vertigo, weakness

Drug Interactions
   Metabolism/Transport Effects Substrate of CYP1A2 (minor), CYP3A4
   (major); **Note:** Assignment of Major/Minor substrate status based on clinically
   relevant drug interaction potential

Avoid Concomitant Use
   Avoid concomitant use of Toremifene with any of the following: CYP3A4
   Inducers (Strong); CYP3A4 Inhibitors (Strong); Grapefruit Juice; Highest Risk
   QTc-Prolonging Agents; Ivabradine; Mifepristone; Moderate Risk QTc-Pro-
   longing Agents; Ospemifene

Increased Effect/Toxicity
   Toremifene may increase the levels/effects of: Highest Risk QTc-Prolonging
   Agents; Ospemifene; Vitamin K Antagonists

   The levels/effects of Toremifene may be increased by: CYP3A4 Inhibitors
   (Strong); Grapefruit Juice; Ivabradine; Mifepristone; Moderate Risk QTc-
   Prolonging Agents; QTc-Prolonging Agents (Indeterminate Risk and Risk
   Modifying); Thiazide Diuretics

Decreased Effect
   Toremifene may decrease the levels/effects of: Ospemifene; Sugammadex

   The levels/effects of Toremifene may be decreased by: Bosentan; CYP3A4
   Inducers (Moderate); CYP3A4 Inducers (Strong); Dabrafenib; Deferasirox;
   Siltuximab; St Johns Wort; Tocilizumab

Food Interactions Grapefruit juice may increase toremifene levels. Management: Avoid grapefruit juice.

Storage/Stability Store at 25°C (77°F); excursions permitted to 15°C to 30°C
(59°F to 86°F); protect from heat. Protect from light.

Mechanism of Action Nonsteroidal, triphenylethylene derivative with potent
antiestrogenic properties (also has estrogenic effects). Competitively binds to
estrogen receptors on tumors and inhibits the growth stimulating effects of
estrogen.

Pharmacodynamics/Kinetics
   Absorption: Well absorbed
   Distribution: V_d: 580 L
   Protein binding, plasma: >99.5%, primarily to albumin

Metabolism: Extensively hepatic, principally by CYP3A4 to N-demethyltoremifene (a weak antiestrogen)

Bioavailability: Not affected by food

Half-life elimination: Toremifene: ~5 days, ~7 days (females >60 years); N-demethyltoremifene: 6 days

Time to peak, serum: ≤3 hours

Excretion: Primarily feces; urine (~10%) during a 1-week period

Dosing

Adult & Geriatric

Breast cancer, metastatic: Postmenopausal women: Oral: 60 mg once daily, continue until disease progression.

Soft tissue sarcoma (desmoid tumors) (off-label use): Oral: 180 mg once daily until disease progression or unacceptable toxicity (Fiore, 2011) **or** 200 mg daily; in some patients with tumor progression, the dose was increased to 400 to 600 mg daily (Brooks, 1992). Additional data may be necessary to further define the role of toremifene in this condition.

Renal Impairment There are no dosage adjustments listed in the manufacturer's labeling. However, pharmacokinetics in patients with renal impairment are similar to those in patients with normal renal function and dosage adjustment is unlikely to be necessary.

Hepatic Impairment There are no dosage adjustments provided in the manufacturer's labeling. However, hepatic impairment increases the half-life of toremifene.

Administration Administer with or without food.

Hazardous agent; use appropriate precautions for handling and disposal (NIOSH 2014 [group 1]).

Monitoring Parameters CBC with differential (periodically), electrolytes (magnesium and potassium prior to and periodically during treatment; calcium periodically), hepatic function (periodically). Obtain ECG (baseline and periodically during treatment) in patients at risk for QT prolongation. In patients with bone metastases, monitor closely for hypercalcemia during the first few weeks of treatment.

Dietary Considerations Avoid grapefruit juice.

Dosage Forms Excipient information presented when available (limited, particularly for generics); consult specific product labeling.

Tablet, Oral:

Fareston: 60 mg

◆ **Toremifene Citrate** see Toremifene on page 1660

◆ **Torisel** see Temsirolimus on page 1616

◆ **Tositumomab I-131** see Tositumomab and Iodine I 131 Tositumomab on page 1663

Tositumomab and Iodine I 131 Tositumomab

(toe si TYOO mo mab & EYE oh dyne eye one THUR tee one toe si TYOO mo mab)

Brand Names: US Bexxar [DSC]

Brand Names: Canada Bexxar

Index Terms 131 I Anti-B1 Antibody; 131 I-Anti-B1 Monoclonal Antibody; Anti-CD20-Murine Monoclonal Antibody I-131; Iodine I 131 Tositumomab and Tositumomab; Tositumomab I-131

Pharmacologic Category Antineoplastic Agent, Anti-CD20; Antineoplastic Agent, Monoclonal Antibody; Radiopharmaceutical

◄ **Use** Treatment of relapsed or refractory CD20 positive, low-grade, follicular, or transformed non-Hodgkin's lymphoma (NHL), with progression during or after rituximab treatment

Pregnancy Risk Factor D

Dosing

Adult & Geriatric Non-Hodgkin's lymphoma (NHL), relapsed or refractory: IV: Dosing consists of four components administered in 2 steps. Refer to manufacturer's labeling for additional details. Indicated for a single treatment course. Thyroid protective agents (SSKI, Lugol's solution or potassium iodide) should be administered beginning at least 24 hours prior to Step 1. Premedicate with acetaminophen 650 mg and diphenhydramine 50 mg orally 30 minutes prior to step 1 and step 2.

Step 1: Dosimetric step (Day 0):
Tositumomab 450 mg administered over 60 minutes
Iodine I 131 tositumomab (containing I-131 5 mCi and tositumomab 35 mg) administered over 20 minutes

Note: Whole body dosimetry and biodistribution should be determined on Day 0; days 2, 3, or 4; and day 6 or 7 prior to administration of Step 2. If biodistribution is not acceptable, do not administer the therapeutic step. On day 6 or 7, calculate the patient specific activity of iodine I 131 tositumomab to deliver 75 cGy total body dose (TBD) or 65 cGy TBD (in mCi).

Step 2: Therapeutic step (one dose administered 7-14 days after step 1):
Tositumomab 450 mg administered over 60 minutes
Iodine I 131 tositumomab:
Platelets ≥150,000/mm^3: Iodine I 131 calculated to deliver 75 cGy total body irradiation and tositumomab 35 mg over 20 minutes
Platelets ≥100,000/mm^3 and <150,000/mm^3: Iodine I 131 calculated to deliver 65 cGy total body irradiation and tositumomab 35 mg over 20 minutes

Renal Impairment No specific dosage adjustment provided in manufacturer's labeling (has not been studied). However, greater exposure to I-131 Tositumomab may occur in patients with renal impairment.

Hepatic Impairment No dosage adjustment provided in manufacturer's labeling.

Adjustment for Toxicity
Infusion-related toxicity (with tositumomab or iodine I-131 tositumomab):
Mild-to-moderate: Reduce infusion rate by 50%
Severe: Interrupt infusion; after complete resolution, resume with previous infusion rate reduced by 50%
Serious allergic reaction: Discontinue infusion.

Additional Information Complete prescribing information should be consulted for additional detail.

Product Availability Bexxar: Manufacturing and sales discontinued (in the US and Canada) February 2014. In the United States, the last day to schedule dosing is February 11, 2014; the final day for patient availability is February 20, 2014.

Dosage Forms Excipient information presented when available (limited, particularly for generics); consult specific product labeling. [DSC] = Discontinued product
Note: Not all components are shipped from the same facility. When ordering, ensure that all will arrive on the same day.

Kit [dosimetric package]: Tositumomab 225 mg/16.1 mL [2 vials], tositumomab 35 mg/2.5 mL [1 vial], and iodine I 131 tositumomab 0.1 mg/mL and 0.61mCi/mL (20 mL) [1 vial] [DSC]

Kit [therapeutic package]: Tositumomab 225 mg/16.1 mL [2 vials], tositumomab 35 mg/2.5 mL [1 vial], and iodine I 131 tositumomab 1.1 mg/mL and 5.6 mCi/mL (20 mL) [1 or 2 vials] [DSC]

◆ **Totect** see Dexrazoxane on page 523
◆ **tPA** see Alteplase on page 78
◆ **tRA** see Tretinoin (Systemic) on page 1692

Trabectedin (tra BEK te din)

Related Information
Common Toxicity Criteria on page 2122
Management of Drug Extravasations on page 2159
Safe Handling of Hazardous Drugs on page 2292
Brand Names: US Yondelis
Brand Names: Canada Yondelis
Index Terms Ecteinascidin; Ecteinascidin 743; ET-743
Pharmacologic Category Antineoplastic Agent, Miscellaneous
Use
US labeling:
Soft tissue sarcoma: Treatment of unresectable or metastatic soft tissue sarcoma (liposarcoma or leiomyosarcoma) in patients who have received a prior anthracycline-containing regimen.
Canadian labeling:
Ovarian cancer: Treatment of relapsed platinum-sensitive ovarian cancer (in combination with doxorubicin liposomal)
Soft tissue sarcoma: Treatment of metastatic soft tissue sarcoma (liposarcoma or leiomyosarcoma) after failure of prior anthracycline and ifosfamide chemotherapy
Labeled Contraindications
Hypersensitivity (including anaphylaxis) to trabectedin or any component of the formulation
Canadian labeling: Additional contraindications: Active serious or uncontrolled infection; breast-feeding
Pregnancy Considerations Animal reproduction studies have not been conducted. Based on the mechanism of action, trabectedin may cause fetal harm if administered during pregnancy. Women of reproductive potential should use effective contraception during and for at least 2 months after treatment (Canadian labeling: 3 months). Males with partners of reproductive potential should use effective contraception during and for at least 5 months following treatment. Trabectedin may cause decreased fertility in males and females. The Canadian labeling recommends that male patients who wish to father a child during or after treatment should seek advice regarding sperm cryopreservation prior to treatment initiation.
Breast-Feeding Considerations It is not known if trabectedin is excreted in human milk. Due to the potential for serious adverse reactions in the nursing infant, the manufacturer recommends discontinuing nursing during trabectedin treatment. Breast-feeding is contraindicated during and for 3 months after treatment in the Canadian labeling.

Warnings/Precautions Hazardous agent - use appropriate precautions for handling and disposal (meets NIOSH 2014 criteria). Anemia, neutropenia, and thrombocytopenia commonly occur; neutropenic fever and neutropenic sepsis (with fatalities) have been reported. The median onset for first occurrence of grade 3/4 neutropenia was 16 days (range: 8 days to ~10 months) and median time to recovery was 13 days (range: 3 days to ~2 months). Monitor neutrophil count prior to each dose and periodically throughout treatment cycle. Withhold treatment for neutrophil count <1,500/mm^3. Reduce dose (permanently) for life-threatening or prolonged severe neutropenia in the preceding cycle.

Trabectedin may cause rhabdomyolysis and musculoskeletal toxicity (some fatal). Creatine phosphokinase (CPK) elevations occurred in nearly one-third of patients receiving trabectedin; grade 3 and 4 CPK elevations, some complicated by renal failure, occurred. The median time to first occurrence of grade 3 or 4 CPK elevation was 2 months (range: 1 to 11.5 months) and the median time to complete resolution was 14 days (range: 5 to 30 days). Monitor CPK levels prior to each dose; withhold treatment for CPK levels >2.5 times upper limit of normal (ULN); discontinue permanently if rhabdomyolysis occurs.

Cardiomyopathy, including heart failure, decreased ejection fraction, diastolic dysfunction, or right ventricular dysfunction, has been observed; some events were grades 3 and 4. The median time to development of grades 3 and 4 cardiomyopathy was ~5 months (range: 1 to 15 months). Monitor left ventricular ejection fraction (LVEF) by echocardiogram or MUGA scan prior to treatment initiation and every 2 to 3 months until trabectedin is discontinued. Withhold treatment if LVEF is below the lower limit of normal (LLN); permanently discontinue for symptomatic cardiomyopathy or persistent ventricular dysfunction that does not recover to LLN within 3 weeks. Patients with a history of New York Heart Association class II, III, or IV heart failure or abnormal LVEF were excluded from the sarcoma study. QTc prolongation has been reported (single case report). Pulmonary embolism has been reported.

Hepatotoxicity (including hepatic failure) may occur with trabectedin. Grade 3 and 4 liver function test (LFT) elevations (AST, ALT, total bilirubin, or alkaline phosphatase) occurred in over one-third of patients. The median onset for grade 3/4 ALT or AST elevations was 29 days (range: 3 days to 11.5 months) and the median time to resolution was 13 days (range: 4 days to ~4 months). Drug-induced liver injury (ALT or AST elevation >3 times ULN, alkaline phosphatase <2 times ULN, and total bilirubin ≥2 times ULN) and ALT or AST elevations >8 times ULN have been reported. Monitor LFTs prior to each dose; may require treatment interruption, dose reduction, and/or discontinuation (based on severity and duration). Premedication with dexamethasone appears to reduce the frequency and severity of transaminase elevations (Yondelis Canadian labeling 2014). Trabectedin should only be used in patients with a normal bilirubin and AST or ALT ≤2.5 times ULN. Patients with bilirubin above the ULN or AST or ALT >2.5 times the ULN were excluded from the sarcoma clinical trial. Use is also not recommended in the Canadian labeling if alkaline phosphatase (nonosseous origin) >2.5 times ULN, albumin <25 g/L, or in patients with clinically relevant liver disease (eg, active chronic hepatitis). Serious hypersensitivity reactions have been reported (Yondelis Canadian labeling 2014). The Canadian labeling recommends to avoid use in patients with CrCl <30 mL/minute and for combination therapy with doxorubicin liposomal; use is not recommended in patients with CrCl <60 mL/minute; monitor renal function.

Vesicant; ensure proper needle or catheter placement prior to and during infusion. Infuse through a central line. Avoid extravasation. Extravasation of trabectedin with subsequent tissue necrosis requiring debridement has been reported; evidence of necrosis may be delayed up to 1 week after extravasation. Nausea and vomiting are common; corticosteroid premedication (eg, dexamethasone) is recommended; other antiemetics may also be needed. Constipation and diarrhea (generally mild) also commonly occur. Potentially significant drug-drug interactions may exist, requiring dose or frequency adjustment, additional monitoring, and/or selection of alternative therapy.

Adverse Reactions Note: Adverse reactions as reported for monotherapy and combination therapy with doxorubicin liposomal.

>10%:

Central nervous system: Fatigue (46% to 53%), fever (5% to 20%), headache (15% to 16%), paresthesia (monotherapy: 11%)

Dermatologic: Palmar-Plantar erythrodysesthesia (24%), alopecia (3% to 12%), skin rash (11%)

Endocrine & metabolic: Hypokalemia (5% to 42%), hypophosphatemia (34%)

Gastrointestinal: Nausea (72% to 74%; grade 3: 4% to 10%), vomiting (39% to 56%; grade 3: 2% to 12%; grade 4: <1%), anorexia (19% to 32%), constipation (18% to 32%), diarrhea (15% to 26%), abdominal pain (5% to 20%), stomatitis (20%), weight gain (monotherapy: 20%), dyspepsia (5% to 13%), mucosal inflammation (12%)

Hematologic: Anemia (27% to 97%; grade 3: 1% to 13%; grade 4: ≤6%), leukopenia (12% to 95%; grade 3: 3% to 45%; grade 4: 2% to 18%), neutropenia (49% to 92%; grade 3: 22% to 30%; grade 4: 13% to 42%), thrombocytopenia (20% to 64%; grade 3: 8% to 12%, grade 4: 2% to 11%), decreased neutrophils (12%; grade 3: 6%; grade 4: 3%)

Hepatic: Increased ALT (54% to 96%; grade 3: 37% to 46%; grade 4: 2% to 5%), increased AST (47% to 89%, grade 3: 12% to 23%; grade 4: ≤2%), increased alkaline phosphatase (28% to 61%; grade 3: 2%), hyperbilirubinemia (8% to 25%; grade 3:≤1%)

Local: Phlebitis (monotherapy: 15%), injection/catheter site reactions (14%)

Neuromuscular & skeletal: Increased CPK (2% to 26%; grade 3: 1% to 4%, grade 4: 1% to 4%), weakness (15% to 17%), arthralgia (5% to 12%)

Renal: Increased serum creatinine (28%: grade 3: <1%; grade 4: <1%)

Respiratory: Dyspnea (5% to 15%), cough (12%)

1% to 10%:

Cardiovascular: Peripheral edema (5% to 9%), palpitation (4%), edema (3%), syncope (2%), chest pain (1%), left ventricular dysfunction (1%; grade 3: <1%)

Central nervous system: Insomnia (6% to 10%), dizziness (5%)

Dermatologic: Hyperpigmentation (6%)

Endocrine & metabolic: Dehydration (5%)

Gastrointestinal: Decreased appetite (6%), dysgeusia (5% to 8%)

Hematologic: Bleeding complications (9%), febrile neutropenia (2% to 8%, grade 3: 6%, grade 4: 2%), decreased white blood cell count (7%; grade 3: 3%), decreased hemoglobin (5%), decreased platelet count (5%; grade 3: 1%), bone marrow failure (2%), granulocytopenia (2%), pancytopenia (2%), neutropenic infection (1%; grade 3: 1%)

Hepatic: Increased serum transaminases (5%; grade 3: 2%), hepatotoxicity (2%; grade 3: 1%)

Hypersensitivity: Hypersensitivity (2%)

◄ Local: Catheter site pain (3%), catheter site erythema (2%), catheter site inflammation (2%)

Neuromuscular & skeletal: Myalgia (5% to 10%), peripheral neuropathy (5%), musculoskeletal pain (4%)

Renal: Renal failure (2%; grade 3: 1%; grade 4: <1%)

Respiratory: Pulmonary embolism (5%), pulmonary edema (1%)

Miscellaneous: Neutropenic sepsis (1%; grade 3: <1%; grade 4: <1%)

<1%, postmarketing, and/or case reports: Extravasation (with tissue necrosis, requiring debridement), hepatic failure, hepatomegaly, increased heart rate (transient), jaundice, liver pain, multiorgan failure, prolonged QT interval on ECG, rhabdomyolysis, septic shock

Drug Interactions

Metabolism/Transport Effects Substrate of CYP3A4 (major), P-glycoprotein; **Note:** Assignment of Major/Minor substrate status based on clinically relevant drug interaction potential

Avoid Concomitant Use

Avoid concomitant use of Trabectedin with any of the following: Alcohol (Ethyl); BCG (Intravesical); CloZAPine; Conivaptan; CYP3A4 Inducers (Strong); CYP3A4 Inhibitors (Moderate); CYP3A4 Inhibitors (Strong); Dipyrone; Fusidic Acid (Systemic); Idelalisib; Natalizumab; Pimecrolimus; St Johns Wort; Tacrolimus (Topical); Tofacitinib; Vaccines (Live)

Increased Effect/Toxicity

Trabectedin may increase the levels/effects of: CloZAPine; Fingolimod; Leflunomide; Natalizumab; Tofacitinib; Vaccines (Live)

The levels/effects of Trabectedin may be increased by: Alcohol (Ethyl); Conivaptan; CYP3A4 Inhibitors (Moderate); CYP3A4 Inhibitors (Strong); Dasatinib; Denosumab; Dipyrone; Fosaprepitant; Fusidic Acid (Systemic); HMG-CoA Reductase Inhibitors; Idelalisib; Ivacaftor; Luliconazole; Osimertinib; Palbociclib; P-glycoprotein/ABCB1 Inhibitors; Pimecrolimus; Ranolazine; Roflumilast; Simeprevir; Stiripentol; Tacrolimus (Topical); Trastuzumab

Decreased Effect

Trabectedin may decrease the levels/effects of: BCG (Intravesical); Coccidioides immitis Skin Test; Sipuleucel-T; Vaccines (Inactivated); Vaccines (Live)

The levels/effects of Trabectedin may be decreased by: Bosentan; CYP3A4 Inducers (Moderate); CYP3A4 Inducers (Strong); Dabrafenib; Deferasirox; Echinacea; Osimertinib; P-glycoprotein/ABCB1 Inducers; Siltuximab; St Johns Wort; Tocilizumab

Food Interactions Coadministration with grapefruit or grapefruit juice may increase trabectedin plasma concentrations. Management: Avoid concomitant administration with grapefruit or grapefruit juice.

Storage/Stability Store intact vials at 2°C to 8°C (36°F to 46°F). Solutions diluted for infusion should be used within 30 hours of reconstitution (infusion should be completed within that 30 hours).

Preparation for Administration Hazardous agent; use appropriate precautions for handling and disposal (meets NIOSH 2014 criteria). Reconstitute the 1 mg vial with 20 mL SWFI resulting in a reconstituted concentration of 0.05 mg/mL. Shake until completely dissolved. Immediately after reconstitution, further dilute for infusion in 500 mL sodium chloride 0.9% or D_5W. Diluted solution is compatible in type I glass, polyvinyl chloride (PVC) and polyethylene (PE) bags and tubing, PE and polypropylene (PP) mixture bags, polyethersulfone (PES) inline filters, titanium, platinum, or plastic ports, silicone and polyurethane catheters, and pumps with PVC, PE, or PE/PP contact surfaces. Do not mix with other medications.

Mechanism of Action Trabectedin is a marine-derived compound which blocks the cell cycle at the G_2/M phase by covalently binding to the minor DNA groove, bending the helix toward the major groove and altering DNA transcription (Garcia-Carbonero 2005). Also alters DNA repair mechanism.

Pharmacodynamics/Kinetics

Distribution: V_d: >5,000 L

Protein binding: ~97%; to plasma proteins

Metabolism: Extensively hepatic; via CYP3A4

Half-life elimination: ~175 hours

Excretion: Feces (58%; only negligible amounts as unchanged drug); urine (6%; only negligible amounts as unchanged drug)

Dosing

Adult & Geriatric Note: Prior to each treatment cycle, ANC should be ≥1500/mm^3, platelets ≥100,000/mm^3 total bilirubin ≤ULN, and alkaline phosphatase, ALT, AST, and CPK ≤2.5 times ULN.

Premedications: Administer dexamethasone 20 mg IV 30 minutes prior to each infusion. Additional antiemetics may be necessary.

Soft tissue sarcoma, unresectable/metastatic: IV: 1.5 mg/m^2 continuous infusion over 24 hours once every 3 weeks, continue until disease progression or unacceptable toxicity (Demetri 2015)

Ovarian cancer, relapsed, platinum sensitive (Canadian labeling; not an approved use in the US): IV: 1.1 mg/m^2 over 3 hours every 3 weeks (in combination with doxorubicin liposomal), continue as long as clinical benefit is demonstrated (Monk 2010; Monk 2012; Poveda 2011)

Renal Impairment

US labeling:

CrCl ≥30 mL/minute: No dosage adjustment is necessary.

CrCl <30 mL/minute or ESRD: There is no dosage adjustment provided in the manufacturer's labeling (has not been studied).

Canadian labeling:

Mild to moderate impairment: Renal impairment should have minimal impact on pharmacokinetics/elimination.

CrCl <30 mL/minute or serum creatinine >1.5 mg/dL: Avoid use (has not been studied).

CrCl <60 mL/minute: Combination therapy with doxorubicin liposomal is not recommended (has not been studied).

Hepatic Impairment

Hepatic impairment prior to treatment:

US labeling:

Bilirubin within normal limits and AST or ALT ≤2.5 times ULN: No dosage adjustment necessary.

Bilirubin >ULN: There is no dosage adjustment provided in the manufacturer's labeling (has not been studied).

Canadian labeling: Bilirubin >ULN, alkaline phosphatase (nonosseous origin) >2.5 times ULN, ALT and AST >2.5 times ULN, albumin <25 g/L, or clinically relevant liver disease (eg, active chronic hepatitis): Use is not recommended (has not been studied).

Hepatotoxicity during treatment: US labeling:

Total bilirubin >ULN: Delay dose for up to 3 weeks and reduce the next dose by one dose level

ALST or ALT >2.5 times ULN: Delay dose for up to 3 weeks

ALST or ALT >5 times ULN: Reduce the next dose by one dose level

Alkaline phosphatase >2.5 times ULN: Delay dose for up to 3 weeks and reduce the next dose by one dose level

Severe liver dysfunction (bilirubin 2 times ULN and AST or ALT 3 times ULN with alkaline phosphatase <2 times ULN in prior treatment cycle): Permanently discontinue

Obesity *ASCO Guidelines for appropriate chemotherapy dosing in obese adults with cancer:* Utilize patient's actual body weight (full weight) for calculation of body surface area- or weight-based dosing, particularly when the intent of therapy is curative; manage regimen-related toxicities in the same manner as for nonobese patients; if a dose reduction is utilized due to toxicity, consider resumption of full weight-based dosing with subsequent cycles, especially if cause of toxicity (eg, hepatic or renal impairment) is resolved (Griggs 2012).

Adjustment for Toxicity

US labeling: Soft tissue sarcoma:

Recommended dose reduction levels (once a dose is reduced it should not be increased in subsequent cycles):

First dose reduction: 1.2 mg/m² once every 3 weeks

Second dose reduction: 1 mg/m² once every 3 weeks

Hematologic toxicity:

ANC <1,500/mm³: Delay dose for up to 3 weeks

ANC <1,000/mm³ with fever or infection or <500/mm³ lasting >5 days: Reduce the next dose by one dose level

Platelets <100,000/mm³: Delay dose for up to 3 weeks

Platelets <25,000/mm³: Reduce the next dose by one dose level

Nonhematologic toxicity:

Creatine phosphokinase: >2.5 times ULN: Delay dose for up to 3 weeks

Creatine phosphokinase: >5 times ULN: Reduce the next dose by one dose level

Decreased left ventricular ejection fraction (LVEF): Less than the lower limit of normal (LLN) or clinical evidence of cardiomyopathy: Delay dose for up to 3 weeks

Decreased LVEF: Absolute decrease of 10% or more from baseline and less than the LLN or clinical evidence of cardiomyopathy: Reduce the next dose by one dose level

Other nonhematologic toxicity: Grade 3 or 4: Delay dose for up to 3 weeks and reduce the next dose by one dose level

Adverse reactions with trabectedin administered at 1 mg/m² and requiring further dose reduction: Permanently discontinue

Persistent adverse events requiring a delay of more than 3 weeks: Permanently discontinue.

Canadian labeling:

Delay the next treatment cycle for up to 3 weeks if ANC <1,500/mm³, platelets <100,000/mm³, hemoglobin <9 g/dL, bilirubin >ULN; alkaline phosphatase (nonosseous origin), ALT, and AST >2.5 times ULN; albumin <25 g/L, creatinine clearance <30 mL/minute (single-agent therapy), serum creatinine >1.5 mg/dL or creatinine clearance <60 mL/minute (combination therapy with doxorubicin liposomal); if persists beyond 3 weeks, consider discontinuing treatment.

Reduce dose if the following occur in between cycles: ANC <500/mm^3 for >5 days or associated with fever or infection, platelets <25,000/mm^3, bilirubin >ULN, alkaline phosphatase (nonosseous origin) >2.5 times ULN, ALT or AST >2.5 times ULN (single-agent therapy) or >5 times ULN (combination therapy with doxorubicin liposomal) which has not recovered by day 21, or any other grade 3 or 4 adverse reaction (eg, nausea, vomiting, fatigue):

Ovarian cancer:

First occurrence: Reduce trabectedin dose to 0.9 mg/m^2 (also reduce doxorubicin liposomal dose)

Second occurrence: Reduce trabectedin dose to 0.75 mg/m^2 (also reduce doxorubicin liposomal dose)

Third occurrence: Consider treatment discontinuation.

Soft tissue sarcoma (liposarcoma or leiomyosarcoma):

First occurrence: Reduce trabectedin dose to 1.2 mg/m^2

Second occurrence: Reduce trabectedin dose to 1 mg/m^2

Third occurrence: Consider treatment discontinuation.

CPK >2.5 times ULN: Withhold treatment until full recovery.

Combination Regimens

Ovarian cancer: Trabectedin-Doxorubicin (Liposomal) (Ovarian Cancer) on page 2092

Administration Infuse through a central line with a 0.2 micron polyethersulfone filter. Infusion must be completed within 30 hours of reconstitution. Premedicate with a corticosteroid (eg, dexamethasone IV) 30 minutes prior to treatment; additional antiemetics may be needed.

Soft tissue sarcoma: Single-agent therapy: Infuse as a continuous infusion over 24 hours

Ovarian cancer: Canadian labeling: Combination therapy with doxorubicin liposomal: Administer doxorubicin liposomal first, flush line with D$_5$W, then follow with trabectedin infusion over 3 hours.

Vesicant; ensure proper needle or catheter placement prior to and during infusion; avoid extravasation.

Extravasation management: If extravasation occurs, stop infusion immediately and disconnect (leave cannula/needle in place); gently aspirate extravasated solution (do **NOT** flush the line); remove needle/cannula; elevate extremity.

Hazardous agent; use appropriate precautions for handling and disposal (meets NIOSH 2014 criteria).

Vesicant/Extravasation Risk Vesicant

Monitoring Parameters CBC with differential (baseline and periodically during treatment cycles); total bilirubin (prior to each cycle), ALT, AST, and alkaline phosphatase (prior to each cycle); renal function (baseline and during treatment); CPK (prior to each treatment cycle), evaluate LVEF via MUGA or echocardiogram (baseline and every 2 to 3 months); monitor infusion site for signs/symptoms of extravasation

Dietary Considerations Avoid grapefruit and grapefruit juice.

Product Availability Yondelis: FDA approved October 2015; anticipated availability is currently unknown.

Dosage Forms Excipient information presented when available (limited, particularly for generics); consult specific product labeling.

Solution Reconstituted, Intravenous:

Yondelis: 1 mg (1 ea)

◀ **Dosage Forms: Canada** Excipient information presented when available (limited, particularly for generics); consult specific product labeling.

Injection, powder for reconstitution:

Yondelis: 1 mg [contains sucrose]

TraMADol (TRA ma dole)

Brand Names: US Active-Tramadol; ConZip; EnovaRX-Tramadol; Rybix ODT [DSC]; Ryzolt [DSC]; Synapryn FusePaq; Ultram; Ultram ER

Brand Names: Canada Apo-Tramadol; Durela; Ralivia; Tridural; Ultram; Zytram XL

Index Terms Ryzolt; Tramadol Hydrochloride

Pharmacologic Category Analgesic, Opioid

Use Relief of moderate to moderately-severe pain

Extended release formulations are indicated for patients requiring around-the-clock management of moderate to moderately-severe pain for an extended period of time

Pregnancy Risk Factor C

Dosing

Adult Moderate-to-severe pain: Oral:

Immediate release: 50-100 mg every 4-6 hours (not to exceed 400 mg/day). For patients not requiring rapid onset of effect, tolerability may be improved by starting dose at 25 mg/day and titrating dose by 25 mg every 3 days, until reaching 25 mg 4 times/day. The total daily dose may then be increased by 50 mg every 3 days as tolerated, to reach dose of 50 mg 4 times/day. After titration, 50-100 mg may be given every 4-6 hours as needed up to a maximum 400 mg/day.

Orally-disintegrating tablet (Rybix™ ODT): 50-100 mg every 4-6 hours (not to exceed 400 mg/day); for patients not requiring rapid onset of effect, tolerability may be improved by starting dose at 50 mg/day and titrating dose by 50 mg every 3 days, until reaching 50 mg 4 times/day. After titration, 50-100 mg may be given every 4-6 hours as needed up to a maximum 400 mg/day.

Extended release:

U.S. labeling: ConZip™, Ultram® ER:

Patients not currently on immediate-release tramadol: 100 mg once daily; titrate every 5 days (ConZip™, Ultram® ER); maximum dose: 300 mg daily

Patients currently on immediate-release tramadol: Calculate 24-hour immediate release total dose and initiate total extended release daily dose (round dose to the next lowest 100 mg increment); titrate as tolerated to desired effect (maximum: 300 mg daily)

Canadian labeling: **Note:** Patients currently on immediate-release tramadol: When switching to extended release, initiate at the same or lowest nearest total daily tramadol dose. Not to exceed recommended maximum daily dosing.

Durela™, Ralivia™, Tridural™: Patients not currently on immediate-release tramadol or opioids: Initial: 100 mg once daily; titrate every 5 days (Durela™, Ralivia™) or every 2 days (Tridural™) as needed based on clinical response and severity of pain (maximum: 300 mg daily)

Zytram® XL: Patients not currently on immediate-release tramadol or opioids: 150 mg once daily; if pain relief is not achieved may titrate by increasing dosage incrementally, with sufficient time to evaluate effect of increased dosage; generally not more often than every 7 days (maximum: 400 mg daily)

Geriatric Elderly >65 years: Oral: Use caution and initiate at the lower end of the dosing range. Refer to adult dosing.

Elderly >75 years:

Immediate release: Do not exceed 300 mg/day; see dosing adjustments for renal and hepatic impairment.

Extended release: Use with great caution; see dosing for adults, renal, and hepatic impairment.

Pediatric Moderate-to-severe pain: Oral: Children ≥17 years: Refer to adult dosing.

Renal Impairment

Immediate release: CrCl <30 mL/minute: Administer 50-100 mg dose every 12 hours (maximum: 200 mg/day).

Extended release: Should not be used in patients with CrCl <30 mL/minute.

Hepatic Impairment

Immediate release: Cirrhosis: Recommended dose: 50 mg every 12 hours.

Extended release: Should not be used in patients with severe (Child-Pugh class C) hepatic dysfunction.

Additional Information Complete prescribing information should be consulted for additional detail.

Dosage Forms Considerations

ConZip extended release capsules are formulated as a biphasic product, providing immediate and extended release components:

100 mg: 25 mg (immediate release) and 75 mg (extended release)

200 mg: 50 mg (immediate release) and 150 mg (extended release)

300 mg: 50 mg (immediate release) and 250 mg (extended release)

EnovaRX-Tramadol and Active-Tramadol creams are compounded from kits. Refer to manufacturer's labeling for compounding instructions.

Synapryn FusePaq is a compounding kit for the preparation of an oral suspension. Refer to manufacturer's labeling for compounding instructions.

Dosage Forms Excipient information presented when available (limited, particularly for generics); consult specific product labeling. [DSC] = Discontinued product

Capsule Extended Release 24 Hour, Oral, as hydrochloride:

ConZip: 100 mg, 200 mg, 300 mg [contains fd&c blue #2 aluminum lake, fd&c yellow #10 aluminum lake]

Generic: 100 mg, 150 mg, 200 mg, 300 mg

Cream, External, as hydrochloride:

Active-Tramadol: 8% (120 g) [contains chlorocresol (chloro-m-cresol)]

EnovaRX-Tramadol: 5% (60 g, 120 g) [contains cetyl alcohol]

Suspension Reconstituted, Oral, as hydrochloride:

Synapryn FusePaq: 10 mg/mL (500 mL) [contains saccharin sodium, sodium benzoate]

Tablet, Oral, as hydrochloride:

Ultram: 50 mg [scored]

Generic: 50 mg

Tablet Dispersible, Oral, as hydrochloride:

Rybix ODT: 50 mg [DSC] [contains aspartame]

Tablet Extended Release 24 Hour, Oral, as hydrochloride:
Ryzolt: 100 mg [DSC], 200 mg [DSC], 300 mg [DSC]
Ultram ER: 100 mg, 200 mg, 300 mg
Generic: 100 mg, 200 mg, 300 mg
Dosage Forms: Canada Excipient information presented when available (limited, particularly for generics); consult specific product labeling.
Capsule Extended Release 24 Hour, Oral, as hydrochloride:
Durela: 100 mg, 200 mg, 300 mg
Tablet Extended Release 24 Hour, Oral, as hydrochloride
Ralivia: 100 mg, 200 mg, 300 mg
Tridural: 100 mg, 200 mg, 300 mg
Zytram XL: 75 mg, 150 mg, 200 mg, 300 mg, 400 mg
Controlled Substance C-IV

♦ **Tramadol Hydrochloride** *see* TraMADol *on page 1672*

Trametinib (tra ME ti nib)

Brand Names: US Mekinist
Brand Names: Canada Mekinist
Index Terms GSK1120212; Trametinib Dimethyl Sulfoxide
Pharmacologic Category Antineoplastic Agent, MEK Inhibitor
Use Melanoma: Treatment of unresectable or metastatic melanoma in patients with a BRAF V600E or BRAF V600K mutation (as detected by an approved test), either as a single-agent or in combination with dabrafenib. **Note:** Trametinib as a single-agent is not recommended in patients who have received prior BRAF-inhibitor therapy.
Labeled Contraindications There are no contraindications listed in the manufacturer's U.S. labeling.
Canadian labeling: Hypersensitivity to trametinib or any component of the formulation.
Pregnancy Considerations Adverse effects were observed in animal reproduction studies. Based on its mechanism of action, trametinib would be expected to cause fetal harm if administered to a pregnant woman. Females of reproductive potential should use a highly effective contraceptive during therapy and for 4 months after treatment is complete. When trametinib is used in combination with dabrafenib, a highly effective nonhormonal contraceptive method should be used (dabrafenib may diminish efficacy of hormonal contraceptives). Fertility may also be impaired in females. Due to a risk for impaired spermatogenesis, males who may want to father a child should seek fertility/family planning counseling prior to initiating combination therapy with dabrafenib.
Breast-Feeding Considerations It is not known if trametinib is excreted into breast milk. Due to the potential for serious adverse reactions in the nursing infant, the manufacturer recommends a decision be made whether to discontinue nursing or to discontinue the drug, taking into account the importance of treatment to the mother.
Warnings/Precautions Hazardous agent - use appropriate precautions for handling and disposal (meets NIOSH 2014 criteria). Cardiac events such as heart failure, left ventricular dysfunction, or decreased left ventricular ejection fraction (LVEF) were observed in clinical trials (for single-agent trametinib and when used in combination with dabrafenib); the median time to onset of cardiomyopathy for single-agent trametinib was ~2 months (range: 16 to 156 days) and ~3 months (range: 27 to 253 days) when used in combination with

dabrafenib. Assess LVEF (by echocardiogram or MUGA scan) prior to therapy initiation, at one month, and then at 2- to 3-month intervals while on therapy. Cardiac dysfunction may require treatment interruption, dosage reduction, or discontinuation; such measures resulted in resolution of cardiomyopathy in some patients. May cause hypertension; monitor blood pressure. Venous thromboembolism events (some fatal) may occur when trametinib is used in combination with dabrafenib. DVT and PE occurred at an increased incidence with combination therapy. Patients should seek immediate medical attention with symptoms of DVT or PE (shortness of breath, chest pain, arm/leg swelling). Withhold trametinib for uncomplicated DVT or PE; may resume at a lower dose if improves within 3 weeks; permanently discontinue trametinib (and dabrafenib) for life-threatening PE. Interstitial lung disease (ILD) and pneumonitis were observed in clinical trials; median time to initial presentation was 160 days (range: 60 to 172 days). Monitor for new or progressive pulmonary symptoms (eg, cough, dyspnea, hypoxia, pleural effusion, infiltrates); withhold treatment if symptoms occur; permanently discontinue with diagnosis of ILD or pneumonitis.

Dermatologic toxicity (eg, rash, dermatitis, acneiform rash, palmar-plantar erythrodysesthesia syndrome, and erythema) was commonly observed in trametinib-treated patients (either as a single-agent or when used in combination with dabrafenib); some patients required hospitalization for severe toxicity or for secondary skin infections. The median time to onset and resolution of skin toxicity for single-agent trametinib was 15 days (range: 1 to 221 days) and 48 days (range: 1 to 282 days), respectively. The median time to onset and resolution of skin toxicity for combination therapy was 37 days (range: 1 to 225 days) and 33 days (range: 3 to 421 days), respectively. Monitor for dermatologic toxicity and signs/symptoms of secondary infections. Treatment interruption, dose reductions, and/or therapy discontinuation may be necessary. New primary cutaneous malignancies (which are associated with dabrafenib as single-agent therapy) may occur at a higher rate when trametinib is given in combination with dabrafenib. The incidence of basal cell carcinoma (BCC) is 9% for combination therapy versus 2% for single-agent dabrafenib. The time to BCC diagnosis ranged from 28 to 249 days for patients receiving combination therapy. Cutaneous squamous cell carcinomas (SCC), including keratoacanthoma, occurred at a lower rate for combination therapy compared to single-agent dabrafenib (7% vs 19%, respectively), with a time to diagnosis ranging from 136 to 197 days for combination therapy. Dermatologic exams should be performed prior to initiation of combination therapy, every 2 months while receiving combination treatment, and for up to 6 months following discontinuation.

Retinal pigment epithelial detachments (RPED) and retinal vein occlusion were seen in clinical trials (rare). Detachments were typically bilateral and multifocal and occurred in the macular area of the retina. RPED resolution occurred after a median of 11.5 days (range: 3 to 71 days) following therapy interruption, although some visual disturbances persisted beyond 1 month. Retinal vein occlusion may lead to macular edema, degeneration, decreased visual function, neovascularization, and glaucoma. Promptly refer patients for ophthalmological evaluations if loss of vision or other visual disturbances occur. In clinical trials, ophthalmic exams (including retinal evaluation) were performed prior to and regularly during treatment. Interrupt trametinib therapy for RPED; may resume at a lower dose if resolves within 3 weeks; discontinue if not resolved within 3 weeks. Permanently discontinue if retinal vein occlusion develops.

◄ Uveitis and iritis have been reported when trametinib is used in combination with dabrafenib and are managed symptomatically with ophthalmic steroid and mydriatic drops (does not require alteration in trametinib therapy).

Serious febrile reactions and fever (any severity) accompanied by hypotension, rigors/chills, dehydration, or renal failure may occur when trametinib is used in combination with dabrafenib. The incidence and severity were higher with combination therapy than with single-agent dabrafenib; the median time to onset of fever was 30 days and duration was 6 days for patients receiving combination therapy. Withhold trametinib for fever >104°F (if using in combination, withhold dabrafenib for fever ≥101.3°F) or for any fever with rigors/chills, hypotension, dehydration, or renal failure (evaluate for infection); may require prophylactic antipyretics upon therapy resumption. Hemorrhage, including symptomatic bleeding in a critical area/organ, may occur when trametinib is used in combination with dabrafenib. Major bleeding events (some fatal) included intracranial or gastrointestinal hemorrhage; may require treatment interruption and dosage reduction; permanently discontinue trametinib (and dabrafenib) for all grade 4 hemorrhagic events and any grade 3 event that does not improve with therapy interruption. While not reported with single-agent trametinib, hyperglycemia may occur while on combination therapy with dabrafenib; may require initiation of insulin or oral hypoglycemic agent therapy (or an increased dose if already taking); monitor serum glucose as clinically necessary, particularly in patients with preexisting diabetes or hyperglycemia. Instruct patients to report symptoms of severe hyperglycemia (eg, polydipsia, polyuria).

Prior to initiating therapy, confirm BRAF mutation status with an approved test; approved for use in patients with BRAF V600K and BRAF V600E mutations. Current data regarding use in patients with BRAF V600K mutation is limited; compared to BRAF V600E mutation, lower response rates have been observed with BRAF V600K mutation. Data regarding other less common BRAF V600 mutations is lacking. There are case reports of noncutaneous malignancies, including pancreatic cancer (KRAS mutation-positive), colorectal cancer (recurrent NRAS mutation-positive), hand and neck cancer, and glioblastoma, with combination therapy; monitor for signs/symptoms of noncutaneous malignancies. No trametinib dosage modification is necessary for new primary cutaneous and noncutaneous malignancies; dabrafenib should be permanently discontinued if RAS mutation-positive noncutaneous malignancies develop. Serious adverse reactions (tumor promotion, hemolytic anemia), which occur with single-agent dabrafenib, may also occur when trametinib is administered in combination with dabrafenib. Potentially significant drug-drug interactions may exist, requiring dose or frequency adjustment, additional monitoring, and/or selection of alternative therapy.

Adverse Reactions

Adverse reactions reported with monotherapy:

>10%:

Cardiovascular: Hypertension (15%; grade 3/4: 12%), cardiomyopathy (7% to 11%; defined as cardiac failure, decreased left ventricular ejection fraction, or left ventricular dysfunction)

Dermatologic: Skin toxicity (87%, most commonly dermatitis acneiform rash, erythema, skin rash; severe: 12%; severe toxicity and secondary skin infection requiring hospitalization: 3%), skin rash (57%; grades 3/4: 8%), acneiform eruption (19%; grades 3/4: <1%), xeroderma (11%)

Endocrine & metabolic: Hypoalbuminemia (42%)

Gastrointestinal: Diarrhea (43%), stomatitis (15%), abdominal pain (13%)

Hematologic & oncologic: Anemia (38%; grades 3/4: 2%), lymphedema (32%; includes edema, peripheral edema; grade 3/4: 1%), hemorrhage (13%; includes epistaxis, gingival bleeding, hematochezia, rectal hemorrhage, melena, vaginal hemorrhage, hemorrhoidal hemorrhage, hematuria, conjunctival hemorrhage; grade 3/4: <1%)

Hepatic: Increased serum AST (60%), increased serum ALT (39%), increased serum alkaline phosphatase (24%)

1% to 10%:

Cardiovascular: Decreased left ventricular ejection fraction (5%, ≥20% below baseline), bradycardia

Central nervous system: Dizziness

Dermatologic: Paronychia (10%), pruritus (10%; grade 3/4: 2%), cellulitis, folliculitis, pustular rash

Gastrointestinal: Dysgeusia, xerostomia

Neuromuscular & skeletal: Rhabdomyolysis

Ophthalmic: Blurred vision, dry eye syndrome

Respiratory: Interstitial lung disease (or pneumonitis: 2%)

<1%, postmarketing, case reports, and frequency not defined: Palmar-plantar erythrodysesthesia, retinal detachment, retinal vein occlusion

Adverse reactions reported with dual therapy (trametinib plus dabrafenib):

>10%

Cardiovascular: Peripheral edema (28% to 31%; includes edema and lymphedema), prolonged Q-T Interval on ECG (13% QTcF increased >60 msec; 4% QTcF prolongation to >500 msec)

Central nervous system: Chills (50% to 58%; grade 3/4: 2%), fatigue (53% to 57%), headache (29% to 37%), insomnia (11% to 18%), dizziness (13% to 16%)

Dermatologic: Skin toxicity (65%; any skin toxicity), skin rash (43% to 45%; includes generalized rash, pruritic rash, erythematous rash, papular rash, vesicular rash, macular rash, maculopapular rash; grade 3/4: ≤2%), night sweats (15% to 24%), xeroderma (9% to 18%), acneiform eruption (11% to 16%), erythema (6% to 15%), pruritus (11%)

Endocrine & metabolic: Hyperglycemia (58% to 67%; grade 3/4: 5% or 6%), increased gamma-glutamyl transferase (54% to 56%), hyponatremia (48% to 55%), hypoalbuminemia (43% to 53%), hypophosphatemia (41% to 47%), hypokalemia (15% to 29%), hyperkalemia (18% to 22%), hypocalcemia (13% to 20%), hypercalcemia (15% to 19%), hypomagnesemia (2% to 18%), dehydration (6% to 11%; grade 3/4: ≤2%)

Gastrointestinal: Nausea (44% to 46%; grade 3/4: 2% or 6%), vomiting (40% to 43%), diarrhea (26% to 36%; grade 3/4: ≤2%), abdominal pain (24% to 33%), decreased appetite (22% to 30%), constipation (17% to 22%), xerostomia (11%)

Genitourinary: Urinary tract infection (6% to 13%)

Hematologic & oncologic: Leukopenia (46% to 62%; grade 3/4: 4% or 5%), lymphocytopenia (55% to 59%; grade 3/4: 19% to 22%), anemia (46% to 55%; grade 3/4: 4% to 7%), neutropenia (37% to 55%; grade 3/4: 2% to 13%), thrombocytopenia (31%; grade 3/4: 2% to 4%), hemorrhage (11% to 16%); includes brain stem hemorrhage, cerebral hemorrhage, epistaxis, eye hemorrhage, gastric hemorrhage, gingival hemorrhage, hematuria, intracranial hemorrhage, vaginal hemorrhage, vitreous hemorrhage; grade 3/4: ≤5%)

◀ Hepatic: Increased serum alkaline phosphatase (60% to 67%), increased serum AST (54% to 60%), increased serum ALT (35% to 42%), hyperbilirubinemia (7% to 15%)

Infection: Actinic keratosis (7% to 15%)

Neuromuscular & skeletal: Arthralgia (27% to 44%), myalgia (22% to 24%), back pain (11% to 18%), limb pain (11% to 16%), muscle spasm (2% to 16%)

Renal: Increased serum creatinine (20% to 24%)

Respiratory: Cough (11% to 29%), oropharyngeal pain (7% to 13%)

Miscellaneous: Fever (57% to 71%; grade 3/4: 5% to 9%), febrile reaction (complicated with chills/rigors: 51%, accompanied by hypotension, rigors or chills: 25%, complicated with dehydration: 9%, complicated with renal failure: 4%, complicated with syncope: 4%)

1% to 10%

Cardiovascular: Cardiomyopathy (8% to 9%), hypertension

Dermatologic: Cellulitis, folliculitis, hyperhidrosis, hyperkeratosis, palmar-plantar erythrodysesthesia, paronychia, pustular rash

Gastrointestinal: Pancreatitis, stomatitis

Hematologic & oncologic: Basal cell carcinoma (9%), squamous cell carcinoma of skin (7%; including keratoacanthoma), major hemorrhage (5%; gastric or intracranial hemorrhage), cutaneous papilloma

Neuromuscular & skeletal: Weakness

Ophthalmic: Uveitis (1%), blurred vision, transient blindness

Renal: Renal failure (2% to 7%; includes acute renal failure; grade 3/4: ≤7%)

<1%, postmarketing, case reports, and frequency not defined: Deep vein thrombosis, pulmonary embolism

Drug combination trials:

Cardiovascular: Decreased left ventricular ejection fraction (2%; ≥20% below baseline)

Drug Interactions

Metabolism/Transport Effects Inhibits CYP2C8 (weak); **Induces** CYP3A4 (weak)

Avoid Concomitant Use

Avoid concomitant use of Trametinib with any of the following: Amodiaquine

Increased Effect/Toxicity

Trametinib may increase the levels/effects of: Amodiaquine; Dabrafenib

Decreased Effect

Trametinib may decrease the levels/effects of: ARIPiprazole; Hydrocodone; NiMODipine; Saxagliptin

Food Interactions Administration with a high-fat, high-calorie meal decreased AUC by 24%, C_{max} by 70%, and delayed T_{max} by ~4 hours. Management: Administer 1 hour before or 2 hours after a meal.

Storage/Stability Store refrigerated at 2°C to 8°C (36°F to 46°F); do not freeze. Dispense in original bottle; do not remove desiccant. Protect from light and moisture. Do not transfer to pill boxes.

Mechanism of Action Reversibly and selectively inhibits mitogen-activated extracellular kinase (MEK) 1 and 2 activation and kinase activity. MEK is a downstream effector of the protein kinase B-raf (BRAF); BRAF V600 mutations result in constitutive activation of the BRAF pathway (including MEK1 and MEK2). Through inhibition of MEK 1 and 2 kinase activity, trametinib causes decreased cellular proliferation, cell cycle arrest, and increased apoptosis (Kim, 2013). The combination of trametinib and dabrafenib allows for greater inhibition of the MAPK pathway, resulting in BRAF V600 melanoma cell death (Flaherty, 2012).

Pharmacodynamics/Kinetics

Absorption: Rapid; decreased with a high-fat, high-calorie meal

Distribution: 214 L

Protein binding: ~97% to plasma proteins

Metabolism: Predominantly deacetylation (via hydrolytic enzymes) alone or with mono-oxygenation or in combination with glucuronidation

Bioavailability: 72%

Half-life elimination: 4-5 days

Time to peak: 1.5 hours; delayed with a high-fat, high-calorie meal

Excretion: Feces (>80%); urine (<20% with <0.1% as unchanged drug)

Dosing

Adult

Melanoma, metastatic or unresectable (with BRAF V600E or BRAF V600K mutations): Oral: 2 mg once daily (either as a single-agent or in combination with dabrafenib), continue until disease progression or unacceptable toxicity

Missed doses: Do not take a missed dose within 12 hours of the next dose.

Renal Impairment

Mild to moderate impairment (GFR ≥30 mL/minute/1.73 m^2): No dosage adjustment necessary.

Severe impairment (GFR <30 mL/minute/1.73 m^2): No dosage adjustment provided in manufacturer's labeling (has not been studied); however, renal excretion is low and is unlikely to affect drug exposure.

Hepatic Impairment

Mild impairment (total bilirubin ≤ ULN and AST > ULN **or** total bilirubin >1-1.5 times ULN with any AST): No dosage adjustment necessary.

Moderate to severe impairment: No dosage adjustment provided in manufacturer's labeling (has not been studied).

Adjustment for Toxicity

Recommended trametinib dose reductions for toxicity:

First dose reduction: 1.5 mg once daily

Second dose reduction: 1 mg once daily

Subsequent modification (if unable to tolerate 1 mg once daily): Permanently discontinue

Note: If using combination therapy, refer to Dabrafenib monograph for recommended dabrafenib dose reductions

Cardiac:

Asymptomatic, 10% or greater absolute decrease in LVEF from baseline and LVEF is below institutional lower limits of normal (LLN) from pretreatment value: Interrupt trametinib therapy for up to 4 weeks. If LVEF improves to normal within 4 weeks following therapy interruption, resume at a lower dose level. If LVEF does not improve to normal within 4 weeks following therapy interruption, permanently discontinue trametinib.

>20% absolute decrease in LVEF from baseline and LVEF is below institutional LLN: Permanently discontinue trametinib.

Symptomatic heart failure: Permanently discontinue trametinib.

Dermatologic:

Intolerable Grade 2 skin toxicity or Grade 3 or 4 skin toxicity: Interrupt trametinib therapy for up to 3 weeks. If toxicity improves within 3 weeks, resume at a lower dose level. If toxicity does not improve within 3 weeks following therapy interruption, permanently discontinue trametinib.

◀ New primary cutaneous malignancies: No trametinib dosage modification is necessary.

Fever: Fever >40°C (104°F) or fever (any severity) complicated by rigors, hypotension, dehydration, or renal failure: Interrupt trametinib therapy until fever resolves, then resume at the same or a lower dose level. May require prophylactic antipyretics upon resumption.

Hemorrhage:

Grade 3 hemorrhage: Interrupt trametinib therapy for up to 3 weeks. If hemorrhage improves within 3 weeks, resume at a lower dose level. If hemorrhage does not improve within 3 weeks following therapy interruption, permanently discontinue trametinib.

Grade 4 hemorrhage: Permanently discontinue trametinib.

Ocular:

Uveitis and iritis: No trametinib dosage modification necessary.

Grade 2 or 3 retinal pigment epithelial detachments (RPED): Interrupt trametinib therapy for up to 3 weeks. If improves to ≤ grade 1 within 3 weeks following therapy interruption, resume at a lower dose level. If RPED does not improve within 3 weeks following therapy interruption, permanently discontinue trametinib.

Recurrence of RPED (any grade) after dose reduction/therapy interruption: *Canadian labeling (not in U.S. labeling):* Permanently discontinue trametinib.

Retinal vein occlusion: Permanently discontinue trametinib.

Pulmonary: Interstitial lung disease or pneumonitis: Permanently discontinue trametinib.

Venous thromboembolism:

Uncomplicated DVT or PE: Interrupt trametinib therapy for up to 3 weeks. If improves to ≤ grade 1 within 3 weeks following therapy interruption, resume at a lower dose level. If toxicity does not improve within 3 weeks following therapy interruption, permanently discontinue trametinib.

Life-threatening PE: Permanently discontinue trametinib.

Other toxicity:

Intolerable Grade 2 adverse reaction or any Grade 3 adverse reaction: Interrupt therapy for up to 3 weeks. If toxicity improves to ≤ grade 1 within 3 weeks following therapy interruption, resume at a lower dose level. If toxicity does not improve within 3 weeks following therapy interruption, permanently discontinue trametinib.

Grade 4 adverse reaction, first occurrence: Interrupt trametinib therapy until improves to ≤ grade 1, then resume at a lower dose level **or** permanently discontinue trametinib.

Grade 4 adverse reaction, recurrent: Permanently discontinue trametinib.

New primary noncutaneous malignancy: No trametinib dosage modification is necessary.

Combination Regimens

Melanoma:

Dabrafenib-Trametinib (Melanoma) on page 1934

Trametinib (Melanoma Regimen) on page 2092

Administration Administer at least 1 hour before or 2 hours after a meal. Do not take a missed dose within 12 hours of the next dose. When administered in combination with dabrafenib, take the once daily trametinib dose at the same time each day with either the morning or evening dose of dabrafenib.

Hazardous agent; use appropriate precautions for handling and disposal (meets NIOSH 2014 criteria).

Emetic Potential Minimal (<10%)

Monitoring Parameters CBC and liver function tests at baseline and periodically; assess LVEF (by echocardiogram or MUGA scan) at baseline, 1 month after therapy initiation, and then at 2- to 3-month intervals; ophthalmological evaluation as necessary (if reports of visual disturbance); monitor for signs/symptoms of pulmonary toxicity (eg, cough dyspnea, hypoxia, pleural effusion, or infiltrates); monitor for dermatologic toxicity and secondary skin infections; blood pressure; diarrhea; signs/symptoms of bleeding.

For patients receiving combination therapy with dabrafenib: Blood glucose; dermatologic exams should be performed prior to treatment initiation, every 2 months while receiving combination treatment, and for up to 6 months following therapy discontinuation. Monitor for signs/symptoms of cutaneous and noncutaneous malignancies and uveitis/iritis.

Dietary Considerations Take at least 1 hour before or 2 hours after a meal.

Dosage Forms Excipient information presented when available (limited, particularly for generics); consult specific product labeling.

Tablet, Oral:
Mekinist: 0.5 mg, 2 mg

♦ **Trametinib Dimethyl Sulfoxide** see Trametinib on page 1674

Tranexamic Acid (tran eks AM ik AS id)

Brand Names: US Cyklokapron; Lysteda

Brand Names: Canada Cyklokapron; Tranexamic Acid Injection BP

Index Terms Cyklokapron

Pharmacologic Category Antifibrinolytic Agent; Antihemophilic Agent; Hemostatic Agent; Lysine Analog

Use

Tooth extraction in patients with hemophilia (injection): Short-term use (2 to 8 days) in hemophilia patients to reduce or prevent hemorrhage and reduce need for replacement therapy during and following tooth extraction

Cyclic heavy menstrual bleeding (oral): Treatment of cyclic heavy menstrual bleeding

Pregnancy Risk Factor B

Dosing

Adult & Geriatric

Elective cesarean section, blood loss reduction (off-label use): IV: 1000 mg over 5 minutes at least 10 minutes prior to skin incision (Gungorduk 2011)

Hereditary angioedema (HAE) (off-label use):

Long-term prophylaxis: Oral: 1000-1500 mg 2-3 times daily; reduce to 500 mg/dose once or twice daily when frequency of attacks reduces (Gompels 2005; Levy 2010) **or** 25 mg/kg/dose administered 2-3 times daily (Bowen 2004)

Short-term prophylaxis (eg, for dental work): Oral: 75 mg/kg/day divided 2-3 times daily for 5 days before and 2 days after the event (Bowen 2004) **or** 1000 mg 4 times daily for 48 hours before and after procedure (Gompels 2005)

Treatment of acute HAE attack: Oral, IV: 25 mg/kg/dose (maximum single dose: 1000 mg) every 3-4 hours (maximum: 75 mg/kg/day) (Bowen 2004) **or** 1000 mg 4 times daily for 48 hours (Gompels 2005)

Hip fracture surgery, blood conservation (off-label use): 15 mg/kg administered at the time of skin incision followed by a second dose (15 mg/kg) 3 hours later (Zufferey 2010). Additional data may be necessary to further define the role of tranexamic acid in this setting.

Menorrhagia: Oral: 1300 mg 3 times daily (3900 mg daily) for up to 5 days during monthly menstruation

Orthognathic surgery, blood loss reduction (off-label use): IV: 20 mg/kg over 15 minutes prior to incision (Choi 2009)

Perioperative blood loss reduction in *bilateral* total knee arthroplasty (off-label use):

Three-dose regimen: 10 mg/kg administered as a slow IV infusion 30 minutes before tourniquet deflation for the first operation, 30 minutes before tourniquet deflation for the second operation, and 3 hours after commencement of the second dose (Kim 2014).

Two-dose regimen: 10 or 15 mg/kg administered over 10 minutes before deflation of the first tourniquet, with the second dose administered 3 hours after the first dose (MacGillivray 2011).

Perioperative blood loss reduction in *unilateral* total knee arthroplasty (off-label use):

Intra- and postoperative regimen: 10 mg/kg at least 10 to 30 minutes prior to tourniquet release (deflation) and 10 mg/kg at 3 hours after the first dose (Alvarez 2008; Camarasa 2006; Maniar 2012). Instead of the second dose, a postoperative infusion may be administered at 1 mg/kg/hour for 6 hours (Alvarez 2008).

Pre- and intraoperative regimen: 10 mg/kg at least 20 minutes or immediately before tourniquet inflation and repeated at least 15 minutes prior to deflation or immediately after release of tourniquet (Lozano 2008; Maniar 2012).

Pre-, intra-, and postoperative regimen: 10 mg/kg at least 20 minutes before tourniquet inflation, repeated at least 15 minutes prior to deflation and postoperatively at 3 hours after the second dose (Maniar 2012).

Prevention of dental procedure bleeding in patients on oral anticoagulant therapy (off-label use): Oral rinse: 4.8% solution: Hold 10 mL in mouth and rinse for 2 minutes then spit out. Repeat 4 times daily for 2 days after procedure. **Note:** Patient should not eat or drink for 1 hour after using oral rinse (Carter 2003).

Prevention of perioperative bleeding associated with cardiac surgery (off-label use): IV: Loading dose of 30 mg/kg over 30 minutes (total loading dose includes a test dose administered over the first 10 minutes followed by the remainder of dose) prior to incision, followed by 16 mg/kg/hour until sternal closure; add an additional 2 mg/kg to cardiopulmonary bypass circuit (Fergusson 2008)

or

Loading dose of 10 mg/kg over 20 minutes prior to incision followed by 2 mg/kg/hour continued for 2 hours after transfer to ICU; add a prime dose of 50 mg for a 2.5 L cardiopulmonary bypass circuit; maintenance infusion adjusted for renal insufficiency (Nuttall 2008)

or

Loading dose of 10-15 mg/kg over 10 to 15 minutes, followed by 1-1.5 mg/kg/hour. The authors suggest adding 2-2.5 mg/kg to cardiopulmonary bypass circuit; however, amounts have varied widely in clinical trials (Gravlee 2008).

Prevention of perioperative bleeding associated with spinal surgery (eg, spinal fusion) (off-label use): IV: 2000 mg over 20 minutes prior to incision followed by 100 mg/hour during surgery and for 5 hours postoperatively (Elwatidy 2008) **or** 10 mg/kg prior to incision followed by 1 mg/kg/hour for the remainder of the surgery; discontinue at time of wound closure (Wong 2008)

Tooth extraction in patients with hemophilia (in combination with appropriate factor replacement therapy): IV: 10 mg/kg immediately before surgery, then 10 mg/kg/dose 3-4 times daily; may be used for 2-8 days

Total hip replacement surgery, blood conservation (off-label use): 10 to 15 mg/kg (or 1000 mg) administered over 5-10 minutes immediately before the operation or 15 minutes before skin incision; the preoperative dose may be followed by 10 mg/kg administered 3 to 12 hours after the operation. Postoperative doses ranged from a 10 mg/kg IV bolus (or 1000 mg) to a 1 mg/kg/hour infusion over 10 hours (Gandhi 2013; Oremus 2014).
Note: Multiple regimens have been evaluated in varying degrees of evidence quality. The regimen listed here reflects the more commonly used dosing based on a number of prospective randomized controlled trials (Johansson 2005; McConnell 2011; Niskanen 2005; Oremus 2014). Metaanalyses have also been conducted demonstrating significant reduction in blood loss perioperatively without an increased risk of thromboembolic events (Gandhi 2013; Sukeik 2011; Zhou 2013). The use of *intra-articular* tranexamic acid (ie, 1000 mg/50 mL of NaCl 0.9% sprayed into the wound at the end of the procedure) has also been evaluated demonstrating effectiveness (Alshryda 2014a; Alshryda 2014b).

Transurethral prostatectomy, blood loss reduction (off-label use): Oral: 2000 mg 3 times daily on the operative and first postoperative day (Rannikko 2004)

Trauma-associated hemorrhage (off-label use): IV: Loading dose: 1000 mg over 10 minutes, followed by 1000 mg over the next 8 hours.
Note: Clinical trial included patients with significant hemorrhage (SBP <90 mm Hg, heart rate >110 bpm, or both) or those at risk of significant hemorrhage. Treatment began within 8 hours of injury (CRASH-2 Trial Collaborators 2010).

Traumatic hyphema (off-label use): Oral: 25 mg/kg administered 3 times daily for 5-7 days (Rahmani, 1999; Vangsted, 1983; Varnek, 1980). **Note:** This same regimen may also be used for secondary hemorrhage after an initial traumatic hyphema event.

Pediatric

Menorrhagia: Children ≥12 years and Adolescents: Oral: 1300 mg 3 times daily (3900 mg daily) for up to 5 days during monthly menstruation

Hereditary angioedema (HAE) (off-label use): Oral:
Long-term prophylaxis: 20-40 mg/kg/day in 2-3 divided doses (maximum dose: 3000 mg daily) (Farkas 2007) **or** 50 mg/kg/day (or 1000-2000 mg daily; depending on age and size of patient); may consider alternate-day regimen or twice-weekly regimen when frequency of attacks reduces; diarrhea may be a dose-limiting side effect (Gompels 2005)
Short-term prophylaxis: 20-40 mg/kg/day in 2-3 divided doses (maximum dose: 3000 mg daily) (Farkas 2007) **or** 500 mg 4 times daily (Gompels 2005). **Note:** For short-term prophylaxis (eg, dental work), initiate 2-5 days before and continue for 2 days after the procedure (Bowen 2004; Gompels 2005).

◄ **Prevention of perioperative bleeding associated with cardiac surgery (off-label use):** IV: 10 mg/kg given over 30 minutes prior to incision, 10 mg/kg while on cardiopulmonary bypass, and 10 mg/kg administered after protamine reversal (Chauhan 2004a; Chauhan 2004b)

or

Loading dose of 100 mg/kg over 15 minutes prior to incision, followed by 10 mg/kg/hour infusion (continued until ICU transport); add 100 mg/kg to pump reservoir when cardiopulmonary bypass initiated (Reid, 1997)

Prevention of perioperative bleeding associated with craniosynostosis surgery (off-label use): IV: Loading dose of 50 mg/kg over 15 minutes prior to incision, followed by 5 mg/kg/hour (Goobie 2011) **or** 15 mg/kg over 15 minutes prior to incision, followed by 10 mg/kg/hour until skin closure (Dadure 2011)

Prevention of perioperative bleeding associated with spinal surgery (eg, spinal fusion) (off-label use): Children and Adolescents: IV: 10 mg/kg given over 15 minutes prior to incision followed by 1 mg/kg/hour for the remainder of the surgery; discontinue at time of wound closure (Neilipovitz 2001; Verma 2010)

or

100 mg/kg over 15 minutes prior to incision followed by 10 mg/kg/hour until skin closure (Sethna 2005)

or

30 mg/kg over 20 minutes prior to incision followed by 1 mg/kg/hour during surgery and for 5 hours postoperatively (Elwatidy 2008)

Tooth extraction in patients with hemophilia (in combination with appropriate factor replacement therapy): Children and Adolescents: IV: Refer to adult dosing.

Traumatic hyphema (off-label use): Oral: Refer to adult dosing.

Renal Impairment

IV formulation:

Tooth extraction in patients with hemophilia:

Serum creatinine 1.36-2.83 mg/dL: Maintenance dose of 10 mg/kg/dose twice daily

Serum creatinine 2.83-5.66 mg/dL: Maintenance dose of 10 mg/kg/dose once daily

Serum creatinine >5.66 mg/dL: Maintenance dose of 10 mg/kg/dose every 48 hours **or** 5 mg/kg/dose once daily

Cardiac surgery (the following dose adjustments have been recommended [Nuttall 2008]):

Serum creatinine 1.6-3.3 mg/dL: Reduce maintenance infusion to 1.5 mg/kg/hour (based on a 25% reduction from 2 mg/kg/hour)

Serum creatinine 3.3-6.6 mg/dL: Reduce maintenance infusion to 1 mg/kg/hour (based on a 50% reduction from 2 mg/kg/hour)

Serum creatinine >6.6 mg/dL: Reduce maintenance infusion to 0.5 mg/kg/hour (based on a 75% reduction from 2 mg/kg/hour)

Oral formulation: Cyclic heavy menstrual bleeding:

Serum creatinine >1.4-2.8 mg/dL: 1300 mg twice daily (2600 mg daily) for up to 5 days

Serum creatinine 2.9-5.7 mg/dL: 1300 mg once daily for up to 5 days

Serum creatinine >5.7 mg/dL: 650 mg once daily for up to 5 days

Hepatic Impairment No dosage adjustment is necessary.

Additional Information Complete prescribing information should be consulted for additional detail.

Dosage Forms Excipient information presented when available (limited, particularly for generics); consult specific product labeling.
Solution, Intravenous:
Cyklokapron: 100 mg/mL (10 mL)
Generic: 100 mg/mL (10 mL)
Solution, Intravenous [preservative free]:
Generic: 100 mg/mL (10 mL)
Tablet, Oral:
Lysteda: 650 mg
Generic: 650 mg

◆ **Tranexamic Acid Injection BP (Can)** *see* Tranexamic Acid *on page 1681*
◆ **Transderm-V (Can)** *see* Scopolamine (Systemic) *on page 1520*
◆ **Transderm-Scop** *see* Scopolamine (Systemic) *on page 1520*
◆ ***trans*-Retinoic Acid** *see* Tretinoin (Systemic) *on page 1692*
◆ ***trans* Vitamin A Acid** *see* Tretinoin (Systemic) *on page 1692*

Trastuzumab (tras TU zoo mab)

Related Information
Management of Chemotherapy-Induced Nausea and Vomiting in Adults *on page 2142*
Prevention of Chemotherapy-Induced Nausea and Vomiting in Children *on page 2203*
Principles of Anticancer Therapy *on page 2261*
Safe Handling of Hazardous Drugs *on page 2292*

Brand Names: US Herceptin

Brand Names: Canada Herceptin

Index Terms anti-c-erB-2; anti-ERB-2; Conventional Trastuzumab; MOAB HER2; rhuMAb HER2; Trastuzumab (Conventional)

Pharmacologic Category Antineoplastic Agent, Anti-HER2; Antineoplastic Agent, Monoclonal Antibody

Use

Breast cancer, adjuvant treatment: Treatment (adjuvant) of human epidermal growth receptor 2 (HER2)-overexpressing node positive or node negative (estrogen receptor/progesterone receptor negative or with 1 high risk feature) breast cancer as part of a treatment regimen consisting of doxorubicin, cyclophosphamide, and either paclitaxel or docetaxel; with docetaxel and carboplatin; or as a single agent following multimodality anthracycline-based therapy.

Breast cancer, metastatic: First-line treatment of HER2-overexpressing metastatic breast cancer (in combination with paclitaxel); single agent treatment of HER2-overexpressing breast cancer in patients who have received 1 or more chemotherapy regimens for metastatic disease.

Gastric cancer, metastatic: Treatment of HER2-overexpressing metastatic gastric or gastroesophageal junction adenocarcinoma (in combination with cisplatin and either capecitabine or 5-fluorouracil) in patients who have not received prior treatment for metastatic disease.

Labeled Contraindications
There are no contraindications listed in the manufacturer's US labeling.
Canadian labeling: Hypersensitivity to trastuzumab, Chinese hamster ovary (CHO) cell proteins, or any component of the formulation

◀ **Pregnancy Considerations** Trastuzumab inhibits HER2 protein, which has a role in embryonic development. **[US Boxed Warning]: Trastuzumab exposure during pregnancy may result in oligohydramnios and oligohydramnios sequence (pulmonary hypoplasia, skeletal malformations and neonatal death).** Oligohydramnios (reversible in some cases) has been reported with trastuzumab use alone or with combination chemotherapy. If trastuzumab exposure occurs during pregnancy, monitor for oligohydramnios. Women of reproductive potential should use effective contraception during treatment and for at least 7 months after the last trastuzumab dose. If trastuzumab is administered during pregnancy, or if a patient becomes pregnant during or within 7 months after treatment, report exposure to Genentech Adverse Events at 1-888-835-2555. Women exposed to trastuzumab during pregnancy (or within 7 months of conception) are encouraged to enroll in MotHER (the Herceptin Pregnancy Registry; 1-800-690-6720).

European Society for Medical Oncology (ESMO) guidelines for cancer during pregnancy recommend delaying treatment with trastuzumab (and other HER-2 targeted agents) until after delivery in pregnant patients with HER-2 positive disease (Peccatori 2013).

Breast-Feeding Considerations It is not known whether trastuzumab is secreted in human milk. Because many immunoglobulins are secreted in milk, and the potential for serious adverse reactions in the nursing infant exists, the decision to discontinue trastuzumab or discontinue breast-feeding during treatment should take in account the benefits of treatment to the mother. The extended half-life should also be considered for decisions regarding breast-feeding after therapy completion.

Warnings/Precautions Hazardous agent - use appropriate precautions for handling and disposal (meets NIOSH 2014 criteria). **[US Boxed Warning]: Trastuzumab is associated with symptomatic and asymptomatic reductions in left ventricular ejection fraction (LVEF) and heart failure (HF); the incidence is highest in patients receiving trastuzumab with an anthracycline-containing chemotherapy regimen. Evaluate LVEF in all patients prior to and during treatment; discontinue for cardiomyopathy.** Extreme caution should be used in patients with preexisting cardiac disease or dysfunction. Prior or concurrent exposure to anthracyclines or radiation therapy significantly increases the risk of cardiomyopathy; other potential risk factors include advanced age, high or low body mass index, smoking, diabetes, hypertension, and hyper-/hypothyroidism. Patients who receive anthracyclines after completion or discontinuation of trastuzumab are at increased risk of cardiac dysfunction (anthracyclines should be avoided for at least 7 months after the last trastuzumab dose, and then monitor cardiac function closely if anthracyclines are used). Discontinuation should be strongly considered in patients who develop a clinically significant reduction in LVEF during therapy; treatment with HF medications (eg, ACE inhibitors, beta-blockers) should be initiated. Withhold treatment for ≥16% decrease from pretreatment levels or LVEF below normal limits and ≥10% decrease from baseline (see dosage adjustment for cardiotoxicity). Cardiomyopathy due to trastuzumab is generally reversible over a period of 1 to 3 months after discontinuation. Long term (8 years) follow up in the adjuvant setting (trastuzumab for 1 or 2 years administered sequentially following chemotherapy and radiation therapy) has demonstrated a low incidence of cardiac events, which were generally reversible in most patients (de Azambuja, 2014). Trastuzumab is also associated with arrhythmias, hypertension, mural thrombus formation, stroke, and even cardiac death.

[US Boxed Warning]: Serious adverse events, including hypersensitivity reaction (anaphylaxis), infusion reactions (including fatalities), and pulmonary events (including acute respiratory distress syndrome [ARDS]) have been associated with trastuzumab. Discontinue for anaphylaxis, angioedema, ARDS or interstitial pneumonitis. Most of these events occur with the first infusion; pulmonary events may occur during or within 24 hours of the first infusion; delayed reactions have occurred. Interrupt infusion for dyspnea or significant hypotension; monitor until symptoms resolve. Infusion reactions may consist of fever and chills, and may also include nausea, vomiting, pain, headache, dizziness, dyspnea, hypotension, rash, and weakness. Re-treatment of patients who experienced severe hypersensitivity reactions has been attempted (with premedication). Some patients tolerated re-treatment, while others experienced a second severe reaction. When used in combination with myelosuppressive chemotherapy, trastuzumab may increase the incidence of neutropenia (moderate-to-severe) and febrile neutropenia; the incidence of anemia may be higher when trastuzumab is added to chemotherapy. Rare cases of nephrotic syndrome with evidence of glomerulopathy have been reported, with an onset of 4 to 18 months from trastuzumab initiation; complications may include volume overload and HF. The incidence of renal impairment was increased in metastatic gastric cancer patients when trastuzumab is added to chemotherapy.

May cause serious pulmonary toxicity (dyspnea, hypoxia, interstitial pneumonitis, pulmonary infiltrates, pleural effusion, noncardiogenic pulmonary edema, pulmonary insufficiency, acute respiratory distress syndrome, and/or pulmonary fibrosis); use caution in patients with preexisting pulmonary disease or patients with extensive pulmonary tumor involvement. Establish HER2 status prior to treatment; has only been studied in patients with evidence of HER2 protein overexpression, either by validated immunohistochemistry (IHC) assay or fluorescence in situ hybridization (FISH) assay. Tests appropriate for the specific tumor type (breast or gastric) should be used to assess HER2 status. [US Boxed Warning]: Trastuzumab exposure during pregnancy may result in oligohydramnios and oligohydramnios sequence (pulmonary hypoplasia, skeletal malformations and neonatal death). Effective contraception is recommended in women of childbearing potential during treatment and for at least 7 months after the last trastuzumab dose. Conventional trastuzumab and ado-trastuzumab emtansine are **not** interchangeable; verify product label prior to reconstitution and administration to prevent medication errors. Dosing and treatment schedules between conventional trastuzumab (Herceptin) and ado-trastuzumab emtansine (Kadcyla) are different; confusion between the products may potentially cause harm to the patient. Potentially significant drug-drug interactions may exist, requiring dose or frequency adjustment, additional monitoring, and/or selection of alternative therapy.

Adverse Reactions Note: Percentages reported with single-agent therapy.
>10%:
　Cardiovascular: Decreased left ventricular ejection fraction (4% to 22%)
　Central nervous system: Pain (47%), chills (5% to 32%), headache (10% to 26%), insomnia (14%), dizziness (4% to 13%)
　Dermatologic: Skin rash (4% to 18%)
　Gastrointestinal: Nausea (6% to 33%), diarrhea (7% to 25%), vomiting (4% to 23%), abdominal pain (2% to 22%), anorexia (14%)
　Infection: Infection (20%)
　Neuromuscular & skeletal: Weakness (4% to 42%), back pain (5% to 22%)

Respiratory: Cough (5% to 26%), dyspnea (3% to 22%), rhinitis (2% to 14%), pharyngitis (12%)

Miscellaneous: Infusion related reaction (21% to 40%, chills and fever most common; severe: 1%), fever (6% to 36%)

1% to 10%:

Cardiovascular: Peripheral edema (5% to 10%), edema (8%), cardiac failure (2% to 7%; severe: <1%), tachycardia (5%), hypertension (4%), arrhythmia (3%), palpitations (3%)

Central nervous system: Paresthesia (2% to 9%), depression (6%), peripheral neuritis (2%), neuropathy (1%)

Dermatologic: Acne vulgaris (2%), nail disease (2%), pruritus (2%)

Gastrointestinal: Constipation (2%), dyspepsia (2%)

Genitourinary: Urinary tract infection (3% to 5%)

Hematologic & oncologic: Anemia (4%; grade 3: <1%), leukopenia (3%)

Hypersensitivity: Hypersensitivity reaction (3%)

Infection: Influenza (4%), herpes simplex infection (2%)

Neuromuscular & skeletal: Arthralgia (6% to 8%), ostealgia (3% to 7%), myalgia (4%), muscle spasm (3%)

Respiratory: Flu-like symptoms (2% to 10%), sinusitis (2% to 9%), nasopharyngitis (8%), upper respiratory tract infection (3%), epistaxis (2%), pharyngolaryngeal pain (2%)

Miscellaneous: Accidental injury (6%)

<1%, postmarketing, and/or case reports (as a single-agent or with combination chemotherapy): Abnormality in thinking, adult respiratory distress syndrome, amblyopia, anaphylactic shock, anaphylactoid reaction, anaphylaxis, angioedema, apnea, ascites, asthma, ataxia, blood coagulation disorder, bradycardia, bronchitis, bronchospasm, cardiac arrest, cardiogenic shock, cardiomyopathy, cellulitis, cerebral edema, cerebrovascular accident, cerebrovascular disease, chest discomfort, colitis, coma, confusion, cystitis, deafness, dermal ulcer, dermatitis, dysuria, erysipelas, esophageal ulcer, febrile neutropenia, focal segmental glomerulosclerosis, gastritis, gastroenteritis, glomerulonephritis (membraneous, focal and fibrillary), glomerulopathy, hematemesis, hemorrhage, hemorrhagic cystitis, hepatic failure, hepatic injury, hepatitis, herpes zoster, hiccups, hydrocephalus, hydronephrosis, hypercalcemia, hypervolemia, hypoprothrombinemia, hypotension, hypothyroidism, hypoxia, intestinal obstruction, interstitial pneumonitis, jaundice, laryngeal edema, laryngitis, lethargy, leukemia (acute), limb pain, lymphangitis, madarosis, mania, mastalgia, meningitis, musculoskeletal pain, myopathy, nephrotic syndrome, neutropenia, neutropenic sepsis, oligohydramnios, onychoclasis, osteonecrosis, oxygen desaturation, pancreatitis, pancytopenia, paresis, paroxysmal nocturnal dyspnea, pathological fracture, pericardial effusion, pericarditis, pleural effusion, pneumonitis, pneumothorax, pulmonary edema (noncardiogenic), pulmonary fibrosis, pulmonary hypertension, pulmonary infiltrates, pyelonephritis, radiation injury, renal failure, respiratory distress, respiratory failure, seizure, sepsis, shock, syncope, stomatitis, thrombosis (including mural), thyroiditis (autoimmune), urticaria, vertigo, ventricular dysfunction, wheezing

Drug Interactions

Metabolism/Transport Effects None known.

Avoid Concomitant Use

Avoid concomitant use of Trastuzumab with any of the following: Belimumab

Increased Effect/Toxicity

Trastuzumab may increase the levels/effects of: Antineoplastic Agents (Anthracycline, Systemic); Belimumab; Immunosuppressants

The levels/effects of Trastuzumab may be increased by: PACLitaxel (Conventional)

Decreased Effect

Trastuzumab may decrease the levels/effects of: PACLitaxel (Conventional)

Storage/Stability Prior to reconstitution, store intact vials under refrigeration at 2°C to 8°C (36°F to 46°F). Following reconstitution with bacteriostatic SWFI, the solution in the vial is stable refrigerated for 28 days from the date of reconstitution; do not freeze. Solutions reconstituted with sterile water for injection without preservatives must be used immediately. The solution diluted in 250 mL NS for infusion may be stored refrigerated for up to 24 hours prior to use; do not freeze.

Preparation for Administration Hazardous agent; use appropriate precautions for handling and disposal (meets NIOSH 2014 criteria). Check vial labels to assure appropriate product is being reconstituted (conventional trastuzumab and ado-trastuzumab emtansine are different products and are **NOT** interchangeable).

Reconstitute each vial with 20 mL of bacteriostatic sterile water for injection to a concentration of 21 mg/mL. Swirl gently; do not shake. Allow vial to rest for ~5 minutes. If the patient has a known hypersensitivity to benzyl alcohol, trastuzumab may be reconstituted with sterile water for injection without preservatives, which must be used immediately. Further dilute the appropriate volume for the trastuzumab dose in 250 mL NS prior to administration. Gently invert bag to mix.

Mechanism of Action Trastuzumab is a monoclonal antibody which binds to the extracellular domain of the human epidermal growth factor receptor 2 protein (HER-2); it mediates antibody-dependent cellular cytotoxicity by inhibiting proliferation of cells which overexpress HER-2 protein.

Pharmacodynamics/Kinetics Note: In most patients, trastuzumab concentrations will decrease to ~3% (~97% washout) by 7 months following discontinuation.

Dosing

Adult & Geriatric Note: Do **NOT** substitute conventional trastuzumab for or with ado-trastuzumab emtansine; products are different and are **NOT** interchangeable. Details concerning dosing in combination regimens should also be consulted.

Breast cancer, adjuvant treatment, HER2+: IV: **Note:** Extending adjuvant treatment beyond 1 year is not recommended
With concurrent paclitaxel or docetaxel:
Initial loading dose: 4 mg/kg infused over 90 minutes, followed by
Maintenance dose: 2 mg/kg infused over 30 minutes weekly for total of 12 weeks, followed 1 week later (when concurrent chemotherapy completed) by 6 mg/kg infused over 30 to 90 minutes every 3 weeks for total therapy duration of 52 weeks

With concurrent docetaxel/carboplatin:
Initial loading dose: 4 mg/kg infused over 90 minutes, followed by
Maintenance dose: 2 mg/kg infused over 30 minutes weekly for total of 18 weeks, followed 1 week later (when concurrent chemotherapy completed) by 6 mg/kg infused over 30 to 90 minutes every 3 weeks for total therapy duration of 52 weeks
Following completion of multi-modality anthracycline-based chemotherapy:
Initial loading dose: 8 mg/kg infused over 90 minutes, followed by
Maintenance dose: 6 mg/kg infused over 30 to 90 minutes every 3 weeks for total therapy duration of 52 weeks

Breast cancer, metastatic, HER2+ (either as a single agent or in combination with paclitaxel): IV:
Initial loading dose: 4 mg/kg infused over 90 minutes, followed by
Maintenance dose: 2 mg/kg infused over 30 minutes weekly until disease progression

Gastric cancer, metastatic, HER2+ (in combination with cisplatin and either capecitabine or fluorouracil for 6 cycles followed by trastuzumab monotherapy; Bang, 2010): IV:
Initial loading dose: 8 mg/kg infused over 90 minutes, followed by
Maintenance dose: 6 mg/kg infused over 30 to 90 minutes every 3 weeks until disease progression

Missed doses: If a dose is missed by ≤1 week, the usual maintenance dose should be administered as soon as possible (do not wait until the next planned cycle) and subsequent maintenance doses should be administered 7 or 21 days later (based on patient's maintenance dose/schedule); if a dose is missed by >1 week, then a re-loading dose (4 mg/kg if patient receives trastuzumab weekly; 8 mg/kg if on an every-3-week schedule) should be administered, followed by the usual maintenance dose administered 7 or 21 days later (based on patient's maintenance dose/schedule).

Breast cancer (early stage, locally advanced, or inflammatory), neoadjuvant treatment, HER2+ (off-label use): IV: Trastuzumab, pertuzumab, and docetaxel (in patients with operable disease who had received no prior chemotherapy): Initial: 8 mg/kg (cycle 1) followed by 6 mg/kg every 3 weeks for a total of 4 neoadjuvant cycles; postoperatively, administer 3 cycles of adjuvant FEC [fluorouracil, epirubicin, and cyclophosphamide] chemotherapy and continue trastuzumab to complete 1 year of treatment (Gianni, 2012)

Breast cancer, metastatic, HER2+ (off-label combinations): IV: **Note:** There are multiple trastuzumab-containing regimens for the treatment of HER2+ metastatic breast cancer; commonly used regimens are listed below:
Trastuzumab, pertuzumab, and docetaxel (in patients with no prior anti-HER2 therapy or chemotherapy to treat metastatic disease): Initial: 8 mg/kg followed by a maintenance dose of 6 mg/kg every 3 weeks until disease progression or unacceptable toxicity (Baselga, 2012)
Trastuzumab, pertuzumab, and weekly paclitaxel: Initial: 8 mg/kg followed by a maintenance dose of 6 mg/kg every 3 weeks until disease progression (Dang, 2015)
Trastuzumab and lapatinib (in patients with progression on prior trastuzumab containing therapy): Initial: 4 mg/kg followed by a maintenance dose of 2 mg/kg every week (Blackwell, 2010; Blackwell, 2012)

Other trastuzumab combinations: Initial: 8 mg/kg followed by a maintenance dose of 6 mg/kg every 3 weeks until disease progression or unacceptable toxicity (in combination with docetaxel **or** vinorelbine) (Andersson, 2011) **or** 4 mg/kg loading dose followed by a maintenance dose of 2 mg/kg weekly until disease progression (in combination with docetaxel) (Marty, 2005)

Renal Impairment There are no dosage adjustments provided in the manufacturer's labeling, although data suggest that the disposition of trastuzumab is not altered based on serum creatinine (up to 2 mg/dL).

Hepatic Impairment There are no dosage adjustments provided in the manufacturer's labeling.

Adjustment for Toxicity

Cardiotoxicity: LVEF ≥16% decrease from baseline or LVEF below normal limits and ≥10% decrease from baseline: Withhold treatment for at least 4 weeks and repeat LVEF every 4 weeks. May resume trastuzumab treatment if LVEF returns to normal limits within 4 to 8 weeks and remains at ≤15% decrease from baseline value. Discontinue permanently for persistent (>8 weeks) LVEF decline or for >3 incidents of treatment interruptions for cardiomyopathy.

Infusion-related events:

Mild-moderate infusion reactions: Decrease infusion rate.

Dyspnea, clinically significant hypotension: Interrupt infusion.

Severe or life-threatening infusion reactions: Discontinue.

Combination Regimens

Breast cancer:

Administration Check label to ensure appropriate product is being administered (conventional trastuzumab and ado-trastuzumab emtansine are different products and are **NOT** interchangeable).

Administered by IV infusion; loading doses are infused over 90 minutes; maintenance doses may be infused over 30 minutes if tolerated. Do not administer with D$_5$W. **Do not administer IV push or by rapid bolus. Do not mix with any other medications.**

◀ Observe patients closely during the infusion for fever, chills, or other infusion-related symptoms. Treatment with acetaminophen, diphenhydramine, and/or meperidine is usually effective for managing infusion-related events.

Hazardous agent; use appropriate precautions for handling and disposal (meets NIOSH 2014 criteria).

Emetic Potential
Children: Minimal (<10%)
Adults: Low (10% to 30%)

Monitoring Parameters Assessment for HER2 overexpression and HER2 gene amplification by validated immunohistochemistry (IHC) or fluorescence *in situ* hybridization (FISH) methodology (pretherapy); test should be specific for cancer type (breast vs gastric cancer). Pregnancy test (prior to treatment). Monitor vital signs during infusion; signs and symptoms of cardiac dysfunction; LVEF (baseline, every 3 months during treatment, upon therapy completion and if component of adjuvant therapy, every 6 months for at least 2 years; if treatment is withheld for significant LVEF dysfunction, monitor LVEF at 4-week intervals); signs and symptoms of infusion reaction or pulmonary toxicity; if pregnancy inadvertently occurs during treatment, monitor amniotic fluid volume

Dosage Forms Excipient information presented when available (limited, particularly for generics); consult specific product labeling.
Solution Reconstituted, Intravenous:
   Herceptin: 440 mg (1 ea) [contains benzyl alcohol, mouse protein (murine) (hamster)]

♦ **Trastuzumab-MCC-DM1** see Ado-Trastuzumab Emtansine *on page 43*

♦ **Trastuzumab (Conventional)** see Trastuzumab *on page 1685*

♦ **Trastuzumab-DM1** see Ado-Trastuzumab Emtansine *on page 43*

♦ **Trastuzumab Emtansine** see Ado-Trastuzumab Emtansine *on page 43*

♦ **Treanda** see Bendamustine *on page 182*

♦ **Trelstar** see Triptorelin *on page 1703*

♦ **Trelstar Mixject** see Triptorelin *on page 1703*

Tretinoin (Systemic) (TRET i noyn)
Related Information
Chemotherapy and Cancer Treatment During Pregnancy *on page 2214*
Management of Chemotherapy-Induced Nausea and Vomiting in Adults *on page 2142*
Management of EGFR Inhibitor Toxicities: Dermatologic, Ocular, and Gastro-intestinal *on page 2179*
Prevention of Chemotherapy-Induced Nausea and Vomiting in Children *on page 2203*
Principles of Anticancer Therapy *on page 2261*
Safe Handling of Hazardous Drugs *on page 2292*

Brand Names: Canada Vesanoid
Index Terms *trans* Vitamin A Acid; *trans*-Retinoic Acid; All-*trans* Retinoic Acid; All-*trans* Vitamin A Acid; ATRA; Ro 5488; tRA; Tretinoinum; Vesanoid
Pharmacologic Category Antineoplastic Agent, Retinoic Acid Derivative; Retinoic Acid Derivative
Use Induction of remission in patients with acute promyelocytic leukemia (APL), French American British (FAB) classification M3 (including the M3 variant) characterized by t(15;17) translocation and/or PML/RARα gene presence

Labeled Contraindications Hypersensitivity to tretinoin, other retinoids, parabens, or any component of the formulation

Pregnancy Considerations Adverse events were observed in animal reproduction studies. **[U.S. Boxed Warning]: High risk of teratogenicity; if treatment with tretinoin is required in women of childbearing potential, two reliable forms of contraception should be used simultaneously during and for 1 month after treatment, unless abstinence is the chosen method. Within 1 week prior to starting therapy, serum or urine pregnancy test (sensitivity at least 50 milliunits/mL) should be collected. If possible, delay therapy until results are available. Repeat pregnancy testing and contraception counseling monthly throughout the period of treatment.** Contraception must be used even when there is a history of infertility or menopause, unless a hysterectomy has been preformed. Tretinoin was detected in the serum of a neonate at birth following maternal use of standard doses during pregnancy (Takitani, 2005). Use in humans for the treatment of acute promyelocytic leukemia (APL) is limited and exposure occurred after the first trimester in most cases (Valappil, 2007). However, major fetal abnormalities and spontaneous abortions have been reported with other retinoids; some of these abnormalities were fatal. If the clinical condition of a patient presenting with APL during pregnancy warrants immediate treatment, tretinoin use should be avoided in the first trimester; treatment with tretinoin may be considered in the second and third trimester with careful fetal monitoring, including cardiac monitoring (Sanz, 2009).

Breast-Feeding Considerations It is not known if tretinoin is excreted in breast milk. Due to the potential for serious adverse reactions in the nursing infant, breast-feeding should be discontinued prior to treatment initiation.

Warnings/Precautions Hazardous agent: Use appropriate precautions for handling and disposal (NIOSH 2014 [group 3]).

[U.S. Boxed Warning]: About 25% of patients with APL treated with tretinoin have experienced APL differentiation syndrome (DS) (formerly called retinoic-acid-APL [RA-APL] syndrome), which is characterized by fever, dyspnea, acute respiratory distress, weight gain, radiographic pulmonary infiltrates and pleural or pericardial effusions, edema, and hepatic, renal, and/or multiorgan failure. DS usually occurs during the first month of treatment, with some cases reported following the first dose. DS has been observed with or without concomitant leukocytosis and has occasionally been accompanied by impaired myocardial contractility and episodic hypotension; endotracheal intubation and mechanical ventilation have been required in some cases due to progressive hypoxemia, and several patients have expired with multiorgan failure. About one-half of DS cases are severe, which is associated with increased mortality. Management has not been defined, although high-dose steroids given at the first suspicion appear to reduce morbidity and mortality. Regardless of the leukocyte count, at the first signs suggestive of DS, immediately initiate steroid therapy with dexamethasone 10 mg IV every 12 hours for 3-5 days; taper off over 2 weeks. Most patients do not require termination of tretinoin therapy during treatment of DS.

[U.S. Boxed Warning]: During treatment, ~40% of patients will develop rapidly evolving leukocytosis. A high WBC at diagnosis increases the risk for further leukocytosis and may be associated with a higher risk of life-threatening complications. If signs and symptoms of the APL-DS syndrome are present together with leukocytosis, initiate treatment with high-dose steroids immediately. Consider adding full-dose chemotherapy (including an

◀ anthracycline, if not contraindicated) to the tretinoin therapy on day 1 or 2 for patients presenting with a WBC count of >5 x 10⁹/L. Consider adding chemotherapy immediately in patients who presented with a WBC count of <5 x 10⁹/L, yet the WBC count reaches ≥6 x 10⁹/L by day 5, or ≥10 x 10⁹/L by day 10, or ≥15 x 10⁹/L by day 28.

[U.S. Boxed Warning]: High risk of teratogenicity; if treatment with tretinoin is required in women of childbearing potential, two reliable forms of contraception should be used during and for 1 month after treatment. Microdosed progesterone products ("minipill") may provide inadequate pregnancy protection. Repeat pregnancy testing and contraception counseling monthly throughout the period of treatment. If possible, initiation of treatment with tretinoin should be delayed until negative pregnancy test result is confirmed.

Retinoids have been associated with pseudotumor cerebri (benign intracranial hypertension), especially in children. Concurrent use of other drugs associated with this effect (eg, tetracyclines) may increase risk. Early signs and symptoms include papilledema, headache, nausea, vomiting, visual disturbances, intracranial noises, or pulsate tinnitus.

Up to 60% of patients experienced hypercholesterolemia or hypertriglyceridemia, which were reversible upon completion of treatment. Venous thrombosis and MI have been reported in patient without risk factors for thrombosis or MI; the risk for thrombosis (arterial and venous) is increased during the first month of treatment. Use with caution with antifibrinolytic agents; thrombotic complications have been reported (rarely) with concomitant use. Elevated liver function test results occur in 50% to 60% of patients during treatment. Carefully monitor liver function test results during treatment and give consideration to a temporary withdrawal of tretinoin if test results reach >5 times the upper limit of normal. Most liver function test abnormalities will resolve without interruption of treatment or after therapy completion. May cause headache, malaise, and/or dizziness; caution patients about performing tasks which require mental alertness (eg, operating machinery or driving). Effects may be potentiated when used with other sedative drugs or ethanol. Patients with APL are at high risk and can have severe adverse reactions to tretinoin. **[U.S. Boxed Warning]: Should be administered under the supervision of an experienced cancer chemotherapy physician.** Tretinoin treatment for APL should be initiated early, discontinue if pending cytogenetic analysis does not confirm APL by t(15;17) translocation or the presence of the PML/RARα fusion protein (caused by translocation of the promyelocytic [PML] gene on chromosome 15 and retinoic acid receptor [RAR] alpha gene on chromosome 17).

Tretinoin (which is also known as all-*trans* retinoic acid, or ATRA) and isotretinoin may be confused, while both products may be used in cancer treatment, they are **not** interchangeable; verify product prior to dispensing and administration to prevent medication errors.

Adverse Reactions Most patients will experience drug-related toxicity, especially headache, fever, weakness and fatigue. These are seldom permanent or irreversible and do not typically require therapy interruption.
>10%:
  Cardiovascular: Peripheral edema (52%), chest discomfort (32%), edema (29%), arrhythmias (23%), flushing (23%), hypotension (14%), hypertension (11%)

Central nervous system: Headache (86%), fever (83%), malaise (66%), pain (37%), dizziness (20%), anxiety (17%), depression (14%), insomnia (14%), confusion (11%)

Dermatologic: Skin/mucous membrane dryness (77%), rash (54%), pruritus (20%), alopecia (14%), skin changes (14%)

Endocrine & metabolic: Hypercholesterolemia and/or hypertriglyceridemia (≤60%)

Gastrointestinal: Nausea/vomiting (57%), GI hemorrhage (34%), abdominal pain (31%), mucositis (26%), diarrhea (23%), weight gain (23%), anorexia (17%), constipation (17%), weight loss (17%), dyspepsia (14%), abdominal distention (11%)

Hematologic: Hemorrhage (60%), leukocytosis (40%), disseminated intravascular coagulation (DIC) (26%)

Hepatic: Liver function tests increased (50% to 60%)

Local: Phlebitis (11%)

Neuromuscular & skeletal: Bone pain (77%), paresthesia (17%), myalgia (14%)

Ocular: Ocular disorder (17%), visual disturbances (17%)

Otic: Earache/ear fullness (23%)

Renal: Renal insufficiency (11%)

Respiratory: Upper respiratory tract disorders (63%), dyspnea (60%), respiratory insufficiency (26%), pleural effusion (20%), expiratory wheezing (14%), pneumonia (14%), rales (14%)

Miscellaneous: Shivering (63%), infections (58%), retinoic acid-acute promyelocytic leukemia syndrome differentiation syndrome (≤25%), diaphoresis (20%)

1% to 10%:

Cardiovascular: Cerebral hemorrhage (9%), cardiac failure (6%), facial edema (6%), pallor (6%), cardiac arrest (3%), cardiomyopathy (3%), heart enlarged (3%), heart murmur (3%), ischemia (3%), MI (3%), myocarditis (3%), pericarditis (3%), stroke (3%)

Central nervous system: Agitation (9%), intracranial hypertension (9%), hallucination (6%), aphasia (3%), cerebellar edema (3%), CNS depression (3%), coma (3%), dementia (3%), encephalopathy (3%), facial paralysis (3%), forgetfulness (3%), hypotaxia (3%), hypothermia (3%), light reflex absent (3%), seizure (3%), slow speech (3%), somnolence (3%), spinal cord disorder (3%), unconsciousness (3%)

Dermatologic: Cellulitis (8%)

Endocrine & metabolic: Fluid imbalance (6%), acidosis (3%)

Gastrointestinal: Hepatosplenomegaly (9%), ulcer (3%)

Genitourinary: Dysuria (9%), micturition frequency (3%), prostate enlarged (3%)

Hepatic: Ascites (3%), hepatitis (3%)

Neuromuscular & skeletal: Flank pain (9%), abnormal gait (3%), asterixis (3%), bone inflammation (3%), dysarthria (3%), hemiplegia (3%), hyporeflexia (3%), leg weakness (3%), tremor (3%)

Ocular: Visual acuity change (6%), agnosia (3%), visual field deficit (3%)

Otic: Hearing loss (6%)

Renal: Acute renal failure (3%), renal tubular necrosis (3%)

Respiratory: Lower respiratory tract disorders (9%), pulmonary infiltration (6%), bronchial asthma (3%), larynx edema (3%), pulmonary hypertension (3%)

Miscellaneous: Lymph disorder (6%)

<1%, postmarketing, and/or case reports: Arterial thrombosis, basophilia, erythema nodosum, genital ulceration, hypercalcemia, hyperhistaminemia, irreversible hearing loss, myositis, organomegaly, pancreatitis, pseudotumor cerebri, renal infarct, Sweet's syndrome, thrombocytosis, vasculitis (skin), venous thrombosis

Drug Interactions

Metabolism/Transport Effects Substrate of CYP2A6 (minor), CYP2B6 (minor), CYP2C8 (major), CYP2C9 (minor); **Note:** Assignment of Major/Minor substrate status based on clinically relevant drug interaction potential; **Inhibits** CYP2C9 (weak); **Induces** CYP2E1 (weak/moderate)

Avoid Concomitant Use

Avoid concomitant use of Tretinoin (Systemic) with any of the following: BCG (Intravesical); Multivitamins/Fluoride (with ADE); Multivitamins/Minerals (with ADEK, Folate, Iron); Multivitamins/Minerals (with AE, No Iron); Natalizumab; Pimecrolimus; Tacrolimus (Topical); Tetracycline Derivatives; Tofacitinib; Vaccines (Live); Vitamin A

Increased Effect/Toxicity

Tretinoin (Systemic) may increase the levels/effects of: Antifibrinolytic Agents; Fingolimod; Leflunomide; Natalizumab; Porfimer; Tofacitinib; Vaccines (Live); Verteporfin

The levels/effects of Tretinoin (Systemic) may be increased by: Abiraterone Acetate; CYP2C8 Inhibitors (Moderate); CYP2C8 Inhibitors (Strong); Deferasirox; Denosumab; Lumacaftor; Mifepristone; Multivitamins/Fluoride (with ADE); Multivitamins/Minerals (with ADEK, Folate, Iron); Multivitamins/Minerals (with AE, No Iron); Pimecrolimus; Roflumilast; Tacrolimus (Topical); Tetracycline Derivatives; Trastuzumab; Vitamin A

Decreased Effect

Tretinoin (Systemic) may decrease the levels/effects of: BCG (Intravesical); Coccidioides immitis Skin Test; Contraceptives (Estrogens); Contraceptives (Progestins); Sipuleucel-T; Vaccines (Inactivated); Vaccines (Live)

The levels/effects of Tretinoin (Systemic) may be decreased by: CYP2C8 Inducers (Strong); Dabrafenib; Echinacea; Lumacaftor

Food Interactions Absorption of retinoids has been shown to be enhanced when taken with food. Management: Administer with a meal.

Storage/Stability Store capsule at 20°C to 25°C (68°F to 77°F). Protect from light.

Mechanism of Action Tretinoin appears to bind one or more nuclear receptors and decreases proliferation and induces differentiation of APL cells; initially produces maturation of primitive promyelocytes and repopulates the marrow and peripheral blood with normal hematopoietic cells to achieve complete remission

Pharmacodynamics/Kinetics

Absorption: Well absorbed

Protein binding: >95%, predominantly to albumin

Metabolism: Hepatic via CYP; primary metabolite: 4-oxo-all-*trans*-retinoic acid; displays autometabolism

Half-life elimination: Terminal: Parent drug: 0.5-2 hours

Time to peak, serum: 1-2 hours

Excretion: Urine (63%); feces (30%)

Dosing

Adult & Geriatric Details concerning dosing in combination regimens should also be consulted. **Note:** Induction treatment of APL with tretinoin should be initiated early; discontinue if pending cytogenetic analysis does not confirm t(15;17) translocation or the presence of the PML/RARα fusion protein.

Acute promyelocytic leukemia (APL): Oral:

Remission induction (in combination with an anthracycline ± cytarabine; off-label use): 45 mg/m^2/day in 2 equally divided doses until complete remission or 90 days (Powell, 2010) or until complete hematologic remission (Ades, 2008; Sanz, 2008; Sanz, 2010)

Remission induction (in combination with arsenic trioxide; off-label use): 45 mg/m^2/day in 2 equally divided doses until <5% blasts in marrow and no abnormal promyelocytes or up to 85 days (Estey, 2006; Ravandi, 2009)

Consolidation therapy (off-label use): 45 mg/m^2/day in 2 equally divided doses for 15 days each month for 3 months (in combination with chemotherapy) (Lo-Coco, 2010; Sanz 2010) **or** 45 mg/m^2/day for 14 days every 4 weeks for 7 cycles (in combination with arsenic trioxide) (Ravandi, 2009)

Maintenance therapy, intermediate- and high-risk patients (off-label use): 45 mg/m^2/day in 2 equally divided doses for 15 days every 3 months for 2 years (Sanz, 2004)

Pediatric Details concerning dosing in combination regimens should also be consulted. **Note:** Induction treatment of APL with tretinoin should be initiated early; discontinue if pending cytogenetic analysis does not confirm t(15;17) translocation or the presence of the PML/RARα fusion protein.

Acute promyelocytic leukemia (APL): Oral:

Remission induction: 45 mg/m^2/day in 2 equally divided doses until documentation of complete remission (CR); discontinue 30 days after CR or after 90 days of treatment, whichever occurs first

Remission induction (in combination with an anthracycline; off-label use): 25 mg/m^2/day in 2 equally divided doses until complete remission or 90 days (Ortega, 2005)

Consolidation therapy, intermediate- and high-risk patients (off-label use): 25 mg/m^2/day in 2 equally divided doses for 15 days each month for 3 months (Ortega, 2005)

Maintenance therapy, intermediate- and high-risk patients (off-label use): 25 mg/m^2/day in 2 equally divided doses for 15 days every 3 months for 2 years (Ortega, 2005)

Renal Impairment No dosage adjustment provided in the manufacturer's labeling (has not been studied).

Hepatic Impairment No dosage adjustment provided in the manufacturer's labeling (has not been studied).

Obesity *ASCO Guidelines for appropriate chemotherapy dosing in obese adults with cancer:* Utilize patient's actual body weight (full weight) for calculation of body surface area- or weight-based dosing, particularly when the intent of therapy is curative; manage regimen-related toxicities in the same manner as for nonobese patients; if a dose reduction is utilized due to toxicity, consider resumption of full weight-based dosing with subsequent cycles, especially if cause of toxicity (eg, hepatic or renal impairment) is resolved (Griggs, 2012).

◀ **Adjustment for Toxicity**

APL differentiation syndrome: Initiate dexamethasone 10 mg IV every 12 hours for 3-5 days; consider interrupting tretinoin until resolution of hypoxia

Liver function tests >5 times the upper limit of normal: Consider temporarily withholding treatment

Combination Regimens

Leukemia, acute promyelocytic:

Tretinoin-Arsenic Trioxide (APL) on page 2095

Tretinoin-Daunorubicin (APL) on page 2096

Tretinoin-Daunorubicin-Cytarabine Induction, Consolidation, Maintenance (APL) on page 2097

Tretinoin-Idarubicin (APL) on page 2099

Administration Administer orally with a meal; do not crush capsules.

Although the manufacturer does not recommend the use of the capsule contents to extemporaneously prepare tretinoin suspension, there are limited case reports of use in patients who are unable to swallow the capsules whole. In a patient with a nasogastric (NG) tube, tretinoin capsules were cut open, with partial aspiration of the contents into a glass syringe, the residual capsule contents were mixed with soy bean oil and aspirated into the same syringe and administered (Shaw, 1995). Tretinoin capsules have also been mixed with sterile water (~20 mL) and heated in a water bath (37°C) to melt the capsules and create an oily suspension for NG tube administration (Bargetzi, 1996). Tretinoin has also been administered sublingually by squeezing the capsule contents beneath the tongue (Kueh, 1999). Low plasma concentrations have been reported when tretinoin has been administered through a feeding tube, although patient-specific impaired absorption or a lack of excipient (eg, soybean oil) may have been a contributing factor (Takitani, 2004).

Hazardous agent - use appropriate precautions for handling and disposal (NIOSH 2014 [group 3]).

Emetic Potential Children and Adults: Low (10% to 30%)

Extemporaneous Preparations Hazardous agent: Use appropriate precautions for handling and disposal (NIOSH 2014 [group 3]).

Although the manufacturer does not recommend the use of the capsule contents to extemporaneously prepare a suspension of tretinoin (due to reports of low plasma levels) (Vesanoid® data on file), there are limited case reports of use in patients who are unable to swallow the capsules whole. In a patient with a nasogastric (NG) tube, tretinoin capsules were cut open, with partial aspiration of the contents aspirated into a glass syringe. The residual capsule contents were mixed with soybean oil, aspirated into the syringe, and administered (Shaw, 1995). Tretinoin capsules have also been mixed with sterile water (~20 mL) and heated in a water bath to melt the capsules and create an oily suspension for NG tube administration (Bargetzi, 1996). Tretinoin has also been administered sublingually by squeezing the capsule contents beneath the tongue (Kueh, 1999).

Bargetzi MJ, Tichelli A, Gratwohl A, et al, "Oral All-Transretinoic Acid Administration in Intubated Patients With Acute Promyelocytic Leukemia," *Schweiz Med Wochenschr,* 1996, 126 (45):1944-5.

Kueh YK, Liew PP, Ho PC, et al, "Sublingual Administration of All-*Trans*-Retinoic Acid to a Comatose Patient With Acute Promyelocytic Leukemia," *Ann Pharmacother,* 1999, 33(4):503-5.

Shaw PJ, Atkins MC, Nath CE, et al, "ATRA Administration in the Critically Ill Patient," *Leukemia,* 1995, 9(7):1288.

Vesanoid® data on file, Roche Pharmaceuticals

Monitoring Parameters Bone marrow cytology to confirm t(15;17) translocation or the presence of the PML/RARα fusion protein (do not withhold treatment initiation for results); monitor CBC with differential, coagulation profile, liver function test results, and triglyceride and cholesterol levels frequently; monitor closely for signs of APL differentiation syndrome (eg, monitor volume status, pulmonary status, temperature, respiration)

Dietary Considerations The absorption of retinoids (as a class) is enhanced when taken with food. Capsule contains soybean oil.

Dosage Forms Excipient information presented when available (limited, particularly for generics); consult specific product labeling.
Capsule, Oral:
Generic: 10 mg

♦ **Tretinoinum** *see* Tretinoin (Systemic) *on page 1692*
♦ **Tretten** *see* Factor XIII A-Subunit (Recombinant) *on page 687*
♦ **Trexall** *see* Methotrexate *on page 1104*
♦ **Triacetyluridine** *see* Uridine Triacetate *on page 1709*
♦ **Tridural (Can)** *see* TraMADol *on page 1672*
♦ **Triethylenethiophosphoramide** *see* Thiotepa *on page 1640*

Trifluridine and Tipiracil (trye FLURE i deen & tye PIR a sil)
Related Information
Common Toxicity Criteria *on page 2122*
Safe Handling of Hazardous Drugs *on page 2292*
Brand Names: US Lonsurf
Index Terms TAS-102; Tipiracil and Trifluridine; Trifluridine and Tipiracil Hydrochloride
Pharmacologic Category Antineoplastic Agent, Antimetabolite; Antineoplastic Agent, Antimetabolite (Pyrimidine Analog); Thymidine Phosphorylase Inhibitor
Use Colorectal cancer, metastatic: Treatment of metastatic colorectal cancer in patients who have been previously treated with fluoropyrimidine-, oxaliplatin- and irinotecan-based chemotherapy, an anti-VEGF biological therapy, and if RAS wild-type, an anti-EGFR therapy.
Labeled Contraindications There are no contraindications listed in the manufacturer's labeling.
Pregnancy Considerations Based on the mechanism of action, use of trifluridine/tipiracil would be expected to cause fetal harm when used during pregnancy. Females of reproductive potential should use effective contraception during therapy. Males who have female partners of reproductive potential should use condoms during therapy and for ≥3 months following the final dose.
Breast-Feeding Considerations It is not known if trifluridine or tipiracil are excreted in breast milk. Due to the potential for serious adverse reactions in the nursing infant, breast-feeding is not recommended by the manufacturer during therapy and for one day following the last dose.
Warnings/Precautions Hazardous agent – use appropriate precautions for handling and disposal (meets NIOSH 2014 criteria). Severe and life-threatening bone marrow suppression (anemia, neutropenia, thrombocytopenia) has occurred, including a fatality related to neutropenic infection. In one clinical trial, close to 10% of patients received growth factor support. Monitor blood counts prior to the start of each cycle as well as on day 15, or more frequently if ▶

clinically necessary. May require therapy interruption and/or dose reduction. Nausea, vomiting, diarrhea, and abdominal pain have been commonly reported. Stomatitis may also occur. Advise patients to report severe gastrointestinal toxicity to their health care provider. Patients with moderate (total bilirubin >1.5 to 3 times ULN and any AST) or severe (total bilirubin >3 times ULN and any AST) were excluded from the clinical trial; use with caution in patients with moderate or severe hepatic impairment. Use with caution in patients with renal impairment; dosage adjustments due to toxicities may be necessary in patients with moderate impairment. Patients with severe renal impairment (CrCl <30 mL/minute) or end-stage renal disease (ESRD) were excluded from the clinical trial. Patients ≥65 years experienced a higher incidence of grade 3 and grade 4 neutropenia and thrombocytopenia, as well as increased grade 3 anemia compared to younger patients. Trifluridine/tipiracil is available in two tablet strengths (trifluridine 15 mg/tipiracil 6.14 mg and trifluridine 20 mg/tipiracil 8.19 mg); both tablet strengths may be necessary to provide the correct dose. Read labels carefully in order to ensure the appropriate dose is administered. Dosing is based on the trifluridine component. The manufacturer recommends rounding doses to the nearest 5 mg increment.

Adverse Reactions

>10%:

Central nervous system: Fatigue (≤52%)

Gastrointestinal: Nausea (48%), decreased appetite (39%), diarrhea (32%), vomiting (28%), abdominal pain (21%)

Hematologic & oncologic: Anemia (77%; grade 3: 18%), neutropenia (67%; grade 3: 27%; grade 4: 11%), thrombocytopenia (42%; grade 3: 5%; grade 4: 1%)

Neuromuscular & skeletal: Weakness (≤52%)

Miscellaneous: Fever (19%)

1% to 10%:

Cardiovascular: Pulmonary embolism (2%)

Dermatologic: Alopecia (7%)

Gastrointestinal: Stomatitis (8%), dysgeusia (7%)

Genitourinary: Urinary tract infection (4%)

Respiratory: Nasopharyngitis (4%)

<1%, postmarketing, and/or case reports: Lung disease

Drug Interactions

Metabolism/Transport Effects None known.

Avoid Concomitant Use

Avoid concomitant use of Trifluridine and Tipiracil with any of the following: BCG (Intravesical); CloZAPine; Dipyrone; Natalizumab; Pimecrolimus; Tacrolimus (Topical); Tofacitinib; Vaccines (Live)

Increased Effect/Toxicity

Trifluridine and Tipiracil may increase the levels/effects of: CloZAPine; Fingolimod; Highest Risk QTc-Prolonging Agents; Leflunomide; Moderate Risk QTc-Prolonging Agents; Natalizumab; Tofacitinib; Vaccines (Live)

The levels/effects of Trifluridine and Tipiracil may be increased by: Denosumab; Dipyrone; Mifepristone; Pimecrolimus; Roflumilast; Tacrolimus (Topical); Trastuzumab

Decreased Effect

Trifluridine and Tipiracil may decrease the levels/effects of: BCG (Intravesical); Coccidioides immitis Skin Test; Sipuleucel-T; Vaccines (Inactivated); Vaccines (Live)

The levels/effects of Trifluridine and Tipiracil may be decreased by: Echinacea

Storage/Stability Store at 20°C to 25°C (68°F to 77°F); excursions are permitted to 15°C to 30°C (59°F to 86°F). If stored outside the original bottle, discard tablets after 30 days.

Mechanism of Action Trifluridine, the active cytotoxic component of trifluridine/tipiracil, is a thymidine-based nucleic acid analogue; the triphosphate form of trifluridine is incorporated into DNA which interferes with DNA synthesis and inhibits cell proliferation. Tipiracil is a potent thymidine phosphorylase inhibitor which prevents the rapid degradation of trifluridine, allowing for increased trifluridine exposure (Mayer 2015).

Pharmacodynamics/Kinetics

Protein binding: Trifluridine: >96% (primarily to albumin); Tipiracil: <8%

Metabolism: Trifluridine and tipiracil are not metabolized by cytochrome P450 (CYP) enzymes. Trifluridine is mainly eliminated by metabolism via thymidine phosphorylase to form an inactive metabolite, 5-(trifluoromethyl) uracil (FTY)

Half-life elimination: Trifluridine: 2.1 hours (at steady state); Tipiracil: 2.4 hours (at steady state)

Time to peak, plasma: ~2 hours

Excretion: Trifluridine: Urine (<2% [as unchanged drug]; ~19% [as inactive metabolite FTY]); Tipiracil: Urine (~29% [as unchanged drug])

Dosing

Adult & Geriatric Note: Obtain blood counts prior to starting each cycle and on day 15 of each cycle. Do not initiate a cycle until ANC ≥1,500/mm^3 or febrile neutropenia is resolved, platelets are ≥75,000/mm^3, and/or grade 3 or 4 nonhematologic reactions are ≤ grade 1.

Colorectal cancer, metastatic: Oral: 35 mg/m^2 (based on the trifluridine component) twice daily on days 1 to 5 and days 8 to 12 of a 28-day cycle (maximum per dose: trifluridine 80 mg); continue until disease progression or unacceptable toxicity (Mayer 2015). The manufacturer recommends rounding each dose to the nearest 5 mg increment.

Missed dose: Do not take additional doses to make up for missed or held doses.

Renal Impairment

CrCl ≥30 mL/minute: No initial dosage adjustment is necessary. Monitor closely; patients with moderate impairment (CrCl 30 to 59 mL/minute) may experience greater toxicity and may require dose reduction during treatment.

CrCl <30 mL/minute and ESRD: There are no dosage adjustments provided in the manufacturer's labeling (has not been studied).

Hepatic Impairment

Mild impairment (total bilirubin ≤ULN and AST >ULN or total bilirubin <1 to 1.5 times ULN and any AST): No dosage adjustment necessary.

Moderate impairment (total bilirubin >1.5 to 3 times ULN and any AST) or severe impairment (total bilirubin >3 times ULN and any AST): There are no dosage adjustments provided in the manufacturer's labeling (has not been studied).

◀ **Adjustment for Toxicity** A maximum of 3 dose reductions are allowed (to a minimum dose of 20 mg/m^2). Do not re-escalate dose after it has been reduced.

Hematologic toxicity:

ANC <500/mm^3 (uncomplicated or resulting in >1 week delay in the start of the next cycle) or febrile neutropenia: Interrupt therapy; following recovery to ANC ≥1,500/mm^3 or resolution of febrile neutropenia, may resume therapy with the dose reduced by 5 mg/m^2/dose from the previous dose

Platelets <50,000/mm^3 (or resulting in >1 week delay in the start of the next cycle): Interrupt therapy; following recovery to platelets ≥75,000/mm^3, may resume therapy with the dose reduced by 5 mg/m^2/dose from the previous dose

Nonhematologic toxicity: Grade 3 or 4 toxicity: Interrupt therapy until recovery to ≤ grade 1; following recovery, may resume with the dose reduced by 5 mg/m^2/dose from the previous dose (excludes dose reduction for grade 3 nausea and/or vomiting controlled by antiemetic therapy or grade 3 diarrhea responsive to antidiarrheal treatment).

Administration

Hazardous agent: Use appropriate precautions for handling and disposal (meets NIOSH 2014 criteria). Wash hands after handling tablets; caregivers should wear gloves when handling. NIOSH recommends single gloving for administration of intact tablets (NIOSH 2014).

Administer orally twice daily within 1 hour of completion of morning and evening meals.

Monitoring Parameters Complete blood counts prior to each cycle and on day 15 of each cycle (or more frequently if clinically necessary); signs/symptoms of gastrointestinal toxicity.

Dosage Forms Excipient information presented when available (limited, particularly for generics); consult specific product labeling.

Tablet, Oral:

Lonsurf: Trifluridine 15 mg and tipiracil 6.14 mg, Trifluridine 20 mg and tipiracil 8.19 mg

♦ **Trifluridine and Tipiracil Hydrochloride** *see* Trifluridine and Tipiracil *on page 1699*

Trimethobenzamide (trye meth oh BEN za mide)

Brand Names: US Tigan

Brand Names: Canada Tigan

Index Terms Trimethobenzamide HCl; Trimethobenzamide Hydrochloride

Pharmacologic Category Antiemetic

Use Nausea and vomiting: Treatment of postoperative nausea and vomiting; treatment of nausea associated with gastroenteritis

Dosing

Adult

Nausea/vomiting:

Oral: 300 mg 3 or 4 times daily

IM: 200 mg 3 or 4 times daily

Geriatric According to the manufacturer, consider dosage reduction or increasing the dosing interval in elderly patients with renal impairment, although use should be avoided in this age group due to the risk of EPS adverse effects combined with lower efficacy, as compared to other antiemetics (Beers Criteria).

Renal Impairment CrCl ≤70 mL/minute/1.73 m^2: Although no specific dosage adjustment provided in the manufacturer's labeling, dosage reduction or increasing the dosing interval is recommended.

Hepatic Impairment No dosage adjustment provided in the manufacturer's labeling.

Additional Information Complete prescribing information should be consulted for additional detail.

Dosage Forms Excipient information presented when available (limited, particularly for generics); consult specific product labeling. [DSC] = Discontinued product

Capsule, Oral, as hydrochloride:
Tigan: 300 mg
Generic: 300 mg
Solution, Intramuscular, as hydrochloride:
Tigan: 100 mg/mL (2 mL)
Tigan: 100 mg/mL (20 mL) [contains phenol]
Generic: 100 mg/mL (2 mL [DSC], 20 mL [DSC])

- **Trimethobenzamide HCl** *see* Trimethobenzamide *on page 1702*
- **Trimethobenzamide Hydrochloride** *see* Trimethobenzamide *on page 1702*
- **Trimethoprim and Sulfamethoxazole** *see* Sulfamethoxazole and Trimethoprim *on page 1560*

Triptorelin (trip toe REL in)

Related Information
Safe Handling of Hazardous Drugs *on page 2292*

Brand Names: US Trelstar; Trelstar Mixject

Brand Names: Canada Decapeptyl; Trelstar

Index Terms AY-25650; CL-118,532; D-Trp(6)-LHRH; Detryptoreline; Triptorelin Embonate; Triptorelin Pamoate; Tryptoreline

Pharmacologic Category Gonadotropin Releasing Hormone Agonist

Use

Advanced prostate cancer: Palliative treatment of advanced prostate cancer

Assisted reproductive technologies: Decapeptyl [Canadian product]: Adjunctive therapy in women undergoing controlled ovarian hyperstimulation for assisted reproductive technologies (ART)

Labeled Contraindications Hypersensitivity to triptorelin or any component of the formulation, other GnRH agonists or GnRH; pregnancy

Canadian labeling: Additional contraindications (not in U.S. labeling): Breast-feeding women

Pregnancy Considerations Use is contraindicated in pregnant women. When used for ART, pregnancy must be ruled out prior to therapy and nonhormonal contraception should be used until menses occurs. Due to the short half-life of triptorelin (formulations used for ART), it is not expected to be present in the maternal serum at the time of embryo transfer. In case reports, spontaneous abortion, congenital anomalies, and other adverse events have been reported following triptorelin (Decapeptyl) exposure during pregnancy.

Breast-Feeding Considerations It is not known if triptorelin is excreted in breast milk. Trelstar is not indicated for use in women. Use of Decapeptyl [Canadian product] in nursing women is contraindicated.

◀ **Warnings/Precautions** Hazardous agent - use appropriate precautions for handling and disposal (NIOSH 2014 [group 1]). Transient increases in testosterone can lead to worsening symptoms (bone pain, hematuria, bladder outlet obstruction, neuropathy) of prostate cancer during the first few weeks of therapy. Androgen-deprivation therapy (ADT) may increase the risk for decreased bone mineral density. Hyperglycemia and an increased risk of developing diabetes has been reported with therapy and may manifest as diabetes or worsening of glycemic control in patients with diabetes; monitor blood glucose and/or glycosylated hemoglobin (HbA_{1c}) as clinically necessary. Cases of spinal cord compression, which may contribute to weakness or paralysis (possible fatal complications), have been reported. Closely observe (during the first 2 weeks of treatment) patients with metastatic vertebral lesions or urinary tract obstruction. Hypersensitivity reactions including angioedema and anaphylactic shock have occurred; discontinue if severe reaction occurs. Patients with preexisting depression should be monitored closely during therapy; mood changes including depression have been reported with use (Trelstar Canadian product monograph, 2013). Rare cases of pituitary apoplexy (frequently secondary to pituitary adenoma) have been observed with GnRH agonist administration (onset from 1 hour to usually <2 weeks); may present as sudden headache, vomiting, visual or mental status changes, and infrequently cardiovascular collapse; immediate medical attention required.

ADT may increase the risk for cardiovascular disease (Levine, 2010). Myocardial infarction, sudden cardiac death and stroke have been reported in men receiving GnRH agonists. ADT may prolong the QT/QTc interval; consider the benefits of ADT versus the risk for QT prolongation in patients with a history of QTc prolongation, congenital long QT syndrome, heart failure, frequent electrolyte abnormalities, and in patients with medications known to prolong the QT interval. Consider periodic monitoring of electrocardiograms and electrolytes in at-risk patients.

Decapeptyl [Canadian product]: Ovarian hyperstimulation syndrome (OHSS), an exaggerated response to ovulation induction therapy, is characterized by an increase in vascular permeability which causes a fluid shift from intravascular space to third space compartments (eg, peritoneal cavity, thoracic cavity) (ASRM, 2008; SOGC-CFAS, 2011). This syndrome may begin within 24 hours of treatment, but may become most severe 7 to 10 days after therapy (SOGC-CFAS, 2011). OHSS is typically self-limiting with spontaneous resolution, although it may be more severe and protracted if pregnancy occurs (ASRM, 2008). Symptoms of mild/moderate OHSS may include abdominal distention/discomfort, diarrhea, nausea, and/or vomiting. Severe OHSS symptoms may include abdominal pain that is severe, acute respiratory distress syndrome, anuria/oliguria, ascites, dyspnea, hypotension, nausea/vomiting (intractable), pericardial effusions, tachycardia, or thromboembolism. Decreased creatinine clearance, hemoconcentration, hypoproteinemia, elevated liver enzymes, elevated WBC, and electrolyte imbalances may also be present (ASRM, 2008; Fiedler, 2012; SOGC-CFAS, 2011). If severe OHSS occurs, stop treatment and consider hospitalizing the patient (ASRM, 2008; SOGC-CFAS, 2011). Treatment is primarily symptomatic and includes fluid and electrolyte management, analgesics, and prevention of thromboembolic complications (ASRM, 2008; SOGC-CFAS, 2011). The ascitic, pleural, and pericardial fluids may be removed if needed to relieve symptoms (eg, pulmonary distress or cardiac tamponade) (ASRM, 2008; SOGC-CFAS, 2011). Women with OHSS should avoid pelvic examination and/or intercourse (ASRM, 2008; SOGC-CFAS, 2011).

Adverse Reactions Prostate cancer: As reported with all strengths; frequency of effect may vary by strength:

>10%:

Endocrine & metabolic: Hot flash (59% to 72%), increased serum glucose, increased testosterone (peak: days 2-4; decline to low levels by weeks 3-4)

Hematologic & oncologic: Decreased hemoglobin, decreased red blood cells

Hepatic: Increased serum alkaline phosphatase (2% to >10%), increased serum ALT, increased serum AST

Neuromuscular & skeletal: Musculoskeletal pain (12% to 13%)

Renal: Increased blood urea nitrogen

1% to 10%:

Cardiovascular: Lower extremity edema (6%), hypertension (≤4%), chest pain (2%), dependent edema (2%), peripheral edema (≤1%)

Central nervous system: Headache (2% to 7%), pain (2% to 3%), dizziness (1% to 3%), fatigue (2%), insomnia (1% to ≤2%), emotional lability (1%)

Dermatologic: Skin rash (2%), pruritus (1%)

Endocrine & metabolic: Decreased libido (2%), gynecomastia (2%)

Gastrointestinal: Nausea (3%), anorexia (2%), constipation (2%), dyspepsia (2%), mastalgia (2%), vomiting (2%), abdominal pain (1%), diarrhea (1%)

Genitourinary: Erectile dysfunction (10%), testicular atrophy (8%), impotence (2% to 7%), dysuria (5%), urinary retention (≤1%), urinary tract infection (≤1%)

Hematologic & oncologic: Anemia (1%)

Local: Pain at injection site (4%)

Neuromuscular & skeletal: Leg pain (2% to 5%), back pain (≤3%), leg cramps (2%), arthralgia (≤2%), myalgia (1%), weakness (1%)

Ophthalmic: Conjunctivitis (1%), eye pain (1%)

Respiratory: Cough (2%), dyspnea (1%), pharyngitis (1%)

Reproductive studies:

>10%:

Central nervous system: Headache (4% to 27%)

Gastrointestinal: Abdominal pain (9% to 15%)

Genitourinary: Vaginal hemorrhage (2% to 24%)

Local: Inflammation at injection site (10% to 12%)

1% to 10%:

Cardiovascular: Flushing (4%)

Central nervous system: Dizziness (4% to 5%), fatigue (3% to 4%), malaise (2%)

Endocrine & metabolic: Spontaneous abortion (7%), dysmenorrhea (2% to 6%), ovarian hyperstimulation syndrome (3%), hot flash (2%), ovarian cyst (1%)

Gastrointestinal: Nausea (3% to 10%), vomiting (3%), abdominal distension (2%), diarrhea (2%)

Genitourinary: Pelvic pain (6%), gynecological pain (adnexa uteri, 2%), leukorrhea (2%)

Local: Pain at injection site (4% to 7%), bruising at injection site (3%), injection site reaction (2% to 3%)

Neuromuscular & skeletal: Postoperative pain (3% to 4%), back pain (3%)

Respiratory: Upper respiratory tract infection (4%), flu-like symptoms (3%), pharyngitis (3%), dyspnea (2%), rhinitis (2%)

◀ Postmarketing and/or case reports (all indications): Anaphylactic shock, anaphylaxis, angioedema, bladder outflow obstruction, blurred vision, cerebrovascular accident, circulatory shock, deep vein thrombosis, dyspareunia, exacerbation of depression, hematuria, hypersensitivity reaction, increased appetite, limb pain, myocardial infarction, neuropathy, ostealgia, pituitary apoplexy, prolonged Q-T interval on ECG, pulmonary embolism, renal insufficiency, seizure, sleep disorder, spinal cord compression, thrombophlebitis, tissue necrosis at injection site, transient ischemic attacks, tumor flare, urethral obstruction, vaginal dryness

Drug Interactions

Metabolism/Transport Effects None known.

Avoid Concomitant Use

Avoid concomitant use of Triptorelin with any of the following: Corifollitropin Alfa; Indium 111 Capromab Pendetide

Increased Effect/Toxicity

Triptorelin may increase the levels/effects of: Corifollitropin Alfa; Highest Risk QTc-Prolonging Agents; Moderate Risk QTc-Prolonging Agents

The levels/effects of Triptorelin may be increased by: Mifepristone

Decreased Effect

Triptorelin may decrease the levels/effects of: Antidiabetic Agents; Choline C 11; Indium 111 Capromab Pendetide

Storage/Stability

Trelstar:

U.S. labeling: Store at 20°C to 25°C (68°F to 77°F). Do not freeze MIXJECT system. Administer immediately after reconstitution.

Canadian labeling:

Trelstar with MIXJECT system: Store at 20°C to 25°C (68°F to 77°F). Protect from light. Do not freeze MIXJECT system. Administer immediately after reconstitution.

Trelstar vials without MIXJECT system: Store at 4°C to 25°C (39°F to 77°F); do not freeze. Protect from light.

Decapeptyl [Canadian product]: Store at 2°C to 8°C (36°F to 46°F); do not freeze. Protect from light.

Preparation for Administration Hazardous agent; use appropriate precautions for handling and disposal (NIOSH 2014 [group 1]).

Trelstar: Reconstitute with 2 mL sterile water for injection. Shake well to obtain a uniform suspension. Solution will appear milky. Administer immediately after reconstitution.

MIXJECT System: Follow manufacturer's instructions for mixing prior to use.

Mechanism of Action Triptorelin is an agonist analog of gonadotropin releasing hormone (GnRH) and causes suppression of ovarian and testicular steroidogenesis due to decreased levels of LH and FSH with subsequent decrease in testosterone (male) and estrogen (female) levels. After chronic and continuous administration, usually 2 to 4 weeks after initiation, a sustained decrease in LH and FSH secretion occurs. When used for ART, prevents premature LH surge in women undergoing controlled ovarian hyperstimulation.

Pharmacodynamics/Kinetics

Distribution: V_d: 30 to 33 L

Protein binding: None

Metabolism: Unknown; unlikely to involve CYP; no known metabolites

Half-life elimination: 2.8 ± 1.2 hours
  Moderate-to-severe renal impairment: 6.6 to 7.7 hours
  Hepatic impairment: 7.6 hours
Time to peak: 1 to 3 hours
Excretion: Urine (42% as intact peptide); hepatic

Dosing

Adult & Geriatric

Advanced prostate carcinoma: IM:
  3.75 mg once every 4 weeks **or**
  11.25 mg once every 12 weeks **or**
  22.5 mg once every 24 weeks

Controlled ovarian hyperstimulation for assisted reproductive technologies (ART) (adjunctive therapy): *Decapeptyl [Canadian product]):* Females: SubQ: Usual dose: 0.1 mg once daily initiated on day 2 or 3 or days 21 to 23 of menstrual cycle (or 5 to 7 days prior to expected onset of menses). Dose may be adjusted according to ovarian response as measured by ovarian ultrasound with or without serum estradiol levels. Treatment is continued until follicles achieve suitable size (typically 4 to 7 weeks).

Treatment of paraphilia/hypersexuality (off-label use; Guay, 2009; Thibaut, 1993): Males:
  Note: May cause an initial increase in androgen concentrations which may be treated with an antiandrogen (eg, flutamide, cyproterone) for 1 to 2 months (Guay, 2009). Avoid use in patients with osteoporosis or active pituitary pathology.
  SubQ: Test dose: 1 mg (observe for hypersensitivity)
  IM: 3.75 mg monthly

Renal Impairment There are no dosage adjustments provided in the manufacturer's labeling. However, renal impairment increases systemic exposure to triptorelin.

Hepatic Impairment There are no dosage adjustments provided in the manufacturer's labeling. However, hepatic impairment increases systemic exposure to triptorelin.

Administration

Administer by IM injection into the buttock; alternate injection sites. Administer immediately after reconstitution.

Decapeptyl [Canadian product] is administered by subcutaneous injection into the lower abdomen; alternate injection sites. If a dose is missed, it can be administered on the same day; however, do not double doses.

Hazardous agent; use appropriate precautions for handling and disposal (NIOSH 2014 [group 1]).

Monitoring Parameters

Serum testosterone levels, prostate-specific antigen, glucose and HbA$_{1c}$ (periodically), bone density, signs and symptoms of emerging cardiovascular disease; consider periodic monitoring of electrocardiograms and electrolytes.

Decapeptyl [Canadian product]: Negative pregnancy test prior to initiation of therapy; signs/symptoms of allergic reaction for 30 minutes after administration; ultrasound and/or estradiol levels to assess follicle development; ultrasound to assess number and size of follicles

◀

OHSS: Monitoring of hospitalized patients should include abdominal circumference, albumin, cardiorespiratory status, electrolytes, fluid balance, hematocrit, hemoglobin, serum creatinine, urine output, urine specific gravity, vital signs, weight (daily or as necessary) and liver enzymes (weekly) (ASRM, 2008; SOGC-CFAS, 2011).

Treatment of paraphilia/hypersexuality (off-label use): The following monitoring has been recommended for other GnRH agonists: CBC (baseline, monthly for 4 months then every 6 months); serum testosterone (baseline, monthly for 4 months then every 6 months); serum LH (baseline and every 6 months), FSH (baseline), serum BUN and creatinine (baseline and every 6 months); bone density (baseline and yearly); ECG (baseline) (Reilly, 2000)

Test Interactions Pituitary-gonadal function may be suppressed with chronic administration and for up to 8 weeks after triptorelin therapy has been discontinued.

Dosage Forms Excipient information presented when available (limited, particularly for generics); consult specific product labeling.

Suspension Reconstituted, Intramuscular:

Trelstar: 3.75 mg (1 ea); 11.25 mg (1 ea) [contains polysorbate 80]

Trelstar Mixject: 3.75 mg (1 ea); 11.25 mg (1 ea); 22.5 mg (1 ea) [contains polysorbate 80]

Dosage Forms: Canada Refer also to Dosage Forms. Excipient information presented when available (limited, particularly for generics); consult specific product labeling.

Injection, solution, as acetate [preservative free]:

Decapeptyl: 100 mcg/mL (equivalent to 95.6 mcg triptorelin free base) (1 mL) [prefilled syringe]

Uridine Triacetate (URE i deen trye AS e tate)

Index Terms PN401; Triacetyluridine; Vistonuridine; Xuriden

Pharmacologic Category Antidote

Use Hereditary orotic aciduria: Treatment of hereditary orotic aciduria

Labeled Contraindications There are no contraindications listed in the manufacturer's labeling.

Pregnancy Considerations Adverse events were not observed in animal reproduction studies. Information related to the use of uridine triacetate for the treatment of hereditary orotic aciduria during pregnancy is limited; monitor closely, dose adjustments may be required (Bensen 1991). In general, medications used as antidotes should take into consideration the health and prognosis of the mother; antidotes should be administered to pregnant women if there is a clear indication for use and should not be withheld because of fears of teratogenicity (Bailey 2003).

Breast-Feeding Considerations It is not known if uridine triacetate is excreted into breast milk. According to the manufacturer, the decision to breast-feed during therapy should take into account the risk of exposure to the infant and the benefits of treatment to the mother.

Warnings/Precautions There are no warnings listed in the manufacturer's labeling.

Adverse Reactions There are no adverse reactions listed in the manufacturer's labeling.

Drug Interactions

Metabolism/Transport Effects Inhibits P-glycoprotein

Avoid Concomitant Use There are no known interactions where it is recommended to avoid concomitant use.

Increased Effect/Toxicity There are no known significant interactions involving an increase in effect.

Decreased Effect There are no known significant interactions involving a decrease in effect.

Storage/Stability Store at 25°C (77°F); excursions permitted to 15°C to 30°C (59°F to 86°F). If administering in food (applesauce, pudding, or yogurt), use immediately after preparation.

◀ **Preparation for Administration** Measure the dose using either a scale accurate to at least 0.1 g, or a graduated teaspoon, accurate to the fraction of the dose to be administered; discard the unused portion of granule packet (do not use granules left in the open packet).

Administration with food: Place 3 to 4 ounces of applesauce, pudding or yogurt in a small clean container. Mix the measured amount of granules in the applesauce, pudding or yogurt.

Administration in milk or infant formula: May be mixed with milk or infant formula for patients receiving a dose of up to 2 g (³/₄ teaspoon). After weighing/measuring the dose, pour 5 mL of milk or infant formula into a 30 mL medicine cup. Insert the tip of an oral syringe into medicine cup and draw up 5 mL of milk/infant formula into syringe. Hold the syringe with the tip pointing upward, pull down on the plunger until the plunger reaches 10 mL (this will add air to the syringe). Place the cap over the tip of the syringe. Then invert the syringe so the syringe tip is pointing down, and remove the plunger. Pour the measured amount of uridine triacetate granules into the syringe barrel and reinsert the syringe plunger. Do not push up on the plunger. Gently swirl the syringe to mix the uridine triacetate granules with the liquid. Turn the syringe so the syringe tip is pointing up. Then remove the syringe cap and push up on the plunger until plunger reaches the 5 mL mark to remove air from the syringe. Place the tip of the syringe in the patient's mouth between the cheek and gum at the back of the mouth. Gently push the plunger all the way down. Refill the syringe with another 5 mL of milk/infant formula. Gently swirl the syringe to rinse remaining uridine triacetate granules from the syringe barrel. Place the tip of the syringe in the patient's mouth between the cheek and gum at the back of the mouth. Gently push the plunger all the way down. May follow with a bottle of milk or infant formula.

Mechanism of Action Uridine triacetate is an acetylated form of uridine which is deacetylated following administration to provide circulating uridine in patients with hereditary orotic aciduria. In patients with fluorouracil overdose or over-exposure (off-label use), uridine triacetate is a direct chemical antagonist against fluorouracil toxicity (Bamat 2013). Uridine reduces incorporation of fluorouridine triphosphate (FUTP; a fluorouracil metabolite) into RNA of hematopoietic progenitor cells and gastrointestinal mucosal cells to reduce fluorouracil toxicity in normal tissues (Hidalgo 2000).

Pharmacodynamics/Kinetics

Onset: Oral exogenous uridine improves hematologic abnormalities of hereditary orotic aciduria within 2 to 3 weeks; urinary orotic acid reduced within 1 to 2 weeks of initiating therapy.

Duration of action: Hematologic abnormalities and orotic aciduria return within days up to 2 to 3 weeks after discontinuation or dose reduction.

Distribution: Distributes into cells; crosses the blood brain barrier

Metabolism: Deacetylated (by nonspecific esterases) to uridine and free acetate (Hidalgo 2000)

Half-life elimination: 2 to 2.5 hours

Time to peak: 2 to 3 hours

Excretion: Urine; also catabolic metabolism in tissues.

Dosing
Adult & Geriatric
Hereditary orotic aciduria: Oral: Initial: 60 mg/kg once daily; increase to 120 mg/kg (maximum: 8 g) for insufficient efficacy (eg, urine orotic acid levels remaining above normal or increasing above the usual/expected range for the patient; lab values affected by orotic acid [red or white blood cell indices] worsening; worsening disease signs/symptoms).

Uridine Triacetate Daily Dose Based on Weight (kg)

Patient weight	60 mg/kg[1] dose Dose in grams (dose in teaspoons[2])	120 mg/kg[1] dose Dose in grams (dose in teaspoons[2])
≤5 kg	0.4 g (1/8 tsp)	0.8 g (1/4 tsp)
6 to 10 kg	0.4 to 0.6 g (1/4 tsp)	0.8 to 1.2 g (1/2 tsp)
11 to 15 kg	0.7 to 0.9 g (1/2 tsp)	1.4 to 1.8 g (3/4 tsp or 1 entire packet)
16 to 20 kg	1 to 1.2 g (1/2 tsp)	2 to 2.4 g (1 tsp)
21 to 25 kg	1.3 to 1.5 g (1/2 tsp)	2.6 to 3 g (1 tsp)
26 to 30 kg	1.6 to 1.8 g (3/4 tsp or 1 entire packet)	3.2 to 3.6 g (1 1/4 tsp)
31 to 35 kg	1.9 to 2.1 g (3/4 tsp or 1 entire packet)	3.8 to 4.2 g (1 1/2 tsp or 2 entire packets)
36 to 40 kg	2.2 to 2.4 g (1 tsp)	4.4 to 4.8 g (1 3/4 tsp)
41 to 45 kg	2.5 to 2.7 g (1 tsp)	5 to 5.4 g (2 tsp or 3 entire packets)
46 to 50 kg	2.8 to 3 g (1 tsp)	5.6 to 6 g (2 tsp or 3 entire packets)
51 to 55 kg	3.1 to 3.3 g (1 1/4 tsp)	6.2 to 6.6 g (2 1/4 tsp)
56 to 60 kg	3.4 to 3.6 g (1 1/4 tsp)	6.8 to 7.2 g (2 1/2 tsp)
61 to 65 kg	3.7 to 3.9 g (1 1/2 tsp or 2 entire packets)	7.4 to 7.8 g (2 1/2 tsp)
66 to 70 kg	4 to 4.2 g (1 1/2 tsp or 2 entire packets)	8 g (2 3/4 tsp or 4 entire packets)
71 to 75 kg	4.3 to 4.5 g (1 1/2 tsp or 2 entire packets)	8 g (2 3/4 tsp or 4 entire packets)
>75 kg	6 g (2 tsp or 3 entire packets)	8 g (2 3/4 tsp or 4 entire packets)

Note: One packet contains uridine triacetate 2 g.

[1]Doses rounded (by the manufacturer) by weight category to achieve approximate dose level

[2]A 2 gram uridine triacetate packet contains approximately 3/4 tsp

◀ **Fluorouracil overdose/overexposure (off-label use):** Adults: Oral: 10 g every 6 hours for 20 doses beginning as soon as possible (8 to 96 hours) after fluorouracil overdose/overexposure (Bamat, 2013; von Borstel, 2009)

Pediatric Hereditary orotic aciduria: Infants, Children, and Adolescents: Oral: Refer to adult dosing.

Renal Impairment There are no dosage adjustments provided in the manufacturer's labeling.

Hepatic Impairment There are no dosage adjustments provided in the manufacturer's labeling.

Administration

Granules: Measure the prescribed dose using either a scale accurate to at least 0.1 gram, or a graduated teaspoon, accurate to the fraction of the dose to be administered. Discard the unused portion of granule packet after measuring out the dose. Do not chew granules. May be administered without regard to meals (food does not have an effect on uridine exposure).

Administration with food: May be mixed in food (ie, 3 to 4 ounces of applesauce, pudding, or yogurt) and administered immediately, followed by drinking at least 120 mL water. Do not chew the granules. Do not save for later use.

Administration in milk or infant formula: May be mixed with milk or infant formula for patients receiving a dose of up to 2 grams (¾ teaspoon). See Preparation for Administration for oral syringe preparation instructions. Place the tip of the oral syringe in the patient's mouth between the cheek and gum at the back of the mouth. Gently push the plunger all the way down. Refill the syringe with another 5 mL of milk/infant formula. Gently swirl the syringe to rinse remaining uridine triacetate granules from the syringe barrel. Place the tip of the syringe in the patient's mouth between the cheek and gum at the back of the mouth. Gently push the plunger all the way down. May follow with a bottle of milk or infant formula.

Fluorouracil overdose/overexposure (off-label use): Administer orally; begin as soon as possible (within 8 to 96 hours) following fluorouracil overdose/overexposure (Bamat 2013; von Borstel 2009).

Monitoring Parameters Fluorouracil overdose/overexposure (off-label use): CBC with differential; gastrointestinal toxicity (Hidalgo 2000).

Product Availability Xuriden: FDA approved September 2015; availability anticipated in early 2016. Xuriden is FDA approved for the treatment of hereditary orotic aciduria. Consult prescribing information for additional information.

Prescribing and Access Restrictions Fluorouracil accidental overdose/overexposure: Uridine triacetate (formerly called vistonuridine) is supplied for emergency use under an expanded access protocol and FDA emergency treatment provisions. Procurement information is available from Wellstat Therapeutics at 1-443-831-5626.

♦ **Uromitexan (Can)** *see* Mesna *on page 1094*

ValACYclovir (val ay SYE kloe veer)

Brand Names: US Valtrex

Brand Names: Canada Apo-Valacyclovir; CO Valacyclovir; DOM-Valacyclovir; Mylan-Valacyclovir; PHL-Valacyclovir; PMS-Valacyclovir; PRO-Valacyclovir; Riva-Valacyclovir; Valtrex

Index Terms Valacyclovir Hydrochloride

Pharmacologic Category Antiviral Agent; Antiviral Agent, Oral

Use Treatment of herpes zoster (shingles) in immunocompetent patients; treatment of first-episode and recurrent genital herpes; suppression of recurrent genital herpes and reduction of transmission of genital herpes in immunocompetent patients; suppression of genital herpes in HIV-infected individuals; treatment of herpes labialis (cold sores); chickenpox in immunocompetent children

Pregnancy Risk Factor B

Dosing

Adult & Geriatric

CMV prophylaxis in allogeneic HSCT recipients (off-label use): 2 g 4 times daily

Herpes labialis (cold sores): Oral: 2 g twice daily for 1 day (separate doses by ~12 hours)

Herpes labialis (cold sores) in HIV-infected patients (off-label use): Oral: 1 g twice daily for 5 to 10 days (HHS [OI adult 2015])

Herpes zoster (shingles): Oral:

Immunocompetent patients: 1 g 3 times daily for 7 days

HIV-infected patients (off-label use): 1 g 3 times daily for 7 to 10 days; consider longer duration if lesions resolve slowly.

HSV, VZV in cancer patients (off-label use):

Prophylaxis: 500 mg 2-3 times daily

Treatment: 1 g 3 times daily

Herpes simplex virus, genital infection: Oral:

Manufacturer's labeling:

Initial episode: Immunocompetent patients: 1 g twice daily for 10 days

Recurrent episode: Immunocompetent patients: 500 mg twice daily for 3 days

Reduction of transmission: 500 mg once daily (source partner)

Suppressive therapy:

Immunocompetent patients: 1 g once daily (500 mg once daily in patients with ≤9 recurrences per year)

HIV-infected patients (CD4 ≥100 cells/mm^3): 500 mg twice daily

Alternate dosing: HIV-infected patients:

Initial or recurrent episodes (off-label use): 1 g twice daily for 5 to 14 days (HHS [OI adult 2015])

Chronic suppressive therapy: 500 mg twice daily; continue indefinitely regardless of CD4 count in patients with severe recurrences or in patients who want to minimize frequency of recurrences (HHS [OI adult 2015])

Varicella (chickenpox) in HIV-infected patients (off-label use): 1 g 3 times daily for 5 to 7 days in uncomplicated cases (HHS [OI adult 2015])

Pediatric

Herpes labialis (cold sores): Oral: Children ≥12 years and Adolescents: Refer to adult dosing.

Herpes labialis (cold sores) in HIV-infected patients (off-label use): Adolescents: Refer to adult dosing.

Herpes simplex virus, genital infection in HIV-infected patients: Adolescents (off-label population): Oral:

Initial or recurrent episodes (off-label use): 1 g twice daily for 5 to 14 days (HHS [OI adult 2015])

Chronic suppressive therapy (off-label dose): 500 mg twice daily; continue indefinitely regardless of CD4 count in patients with severe recurrences or in patients who want to minimize frequency of recurrences (HHS [OI adult 2015])

Herpes zoster (shingles) in HIV-infected patients (off-label use): Adolescents: Refer to adult dosing.

Varicella (chickenpox): Oral:

Immunocompetent patients: Children ≥2 years and Adolescents: 20 mg/kg/dose 3 times daily for 5 days (maximum: 1 g 3 times daily)

HIV-infected patients (off-label use): Adolescents: Refer to adult dosing.

Renal Impairment

Herpes zoster: Adults:

CrCl 30 to 49 mL/minute: 1 g every 12 hours

CrCl 10 to 29 mL/minute: 1 g every 24 hours

CrCl <10 mL/minute: 500 mg every 24 hours

Genital herpes: Adults:

U.S. labeling:

Initial episode:

CrCl 10 to 29 mL/minute: 1 g every 24 hours

CrCl <10 mL/minute: 500 mg every 24 hours

Recurrent episode: CrCl <29 mL/minute: 500 mg every 24 hours

Suppressive therapy: CrCl <29 mL/minute:

For usual dose of 1 g every 24 hours, decrease dose to 500 mg every 24 hours

For usual dose of 500 mg every 24 hours, decrease dose to 500 mg every 48 hours

HIV-infected patients: 500 mg every 24 hours

Canadian labeling:

Initial episode:

CrCl 10 to 29 mL/minute: 1 g every 24 hours

CrCl <10 mL/minute: 500 mg every 24 hours

Recurrent episode:

CrCl 10 to 29 mL/minute: 500 mg every 24 hours

CrCl <10 mL/minute: 500 mg every 24 hours

Suppressive therapy:

CrCl 10 to 29 mL/minute:

Immunocompetent or HIV-infected patients: 500 mg every 24 hours

Immunocompetent patients with ≤9 recurrences/year: 500 mg every 48 hours

CrCl <10 mL/minute:

Immunocompetent or HIV-infected patients: 500 mg every 24 hours

Immunocompetent patients with ≤9 recurrences/year: 500 mg every 48 hours

Herpes labialis: Adolescents and Adults *(U.S. labeling)* or Adults *(Canadian labeling)*:

CrCl 30 to 49 mL/minute: 1 g every 12 hours for 2 doses

CrCl 10 to 29 mL/minute: 500 mg every 12 hours for 2 doses

CrCl <10 mL/minute: 500 mg as a single dose

Hemodialysis: Dialyzable (~33% removed during 4-hour session); administer dose postdialysis

Chronic ambulatory peritoneal dialysis/continuous arteriovenous hemofiltration dialysis: Pharmacokinetic parameters are similar to those in patients with ESRD; supplemental dose not needed following dialysis

Hepatic Impairment No dosage adjustment necessary.

Additional Information Complete prescribing information should be consulted for additional detail.

Dosage Forms Excipient information presented when available (limited, particularly for generics); consult specific product labeling.

Tablet, Oral:

Valtrex: 500 mg [contains fd&c blue #2 aluminum lake]

Valtrex: 1 g [scored; contains fd&c blue #2 aluminum lake]

Generic: 500 mg, 1 g

◆ **Valacyclovir Hydrochloride** see ValACYclovir on page 1712

◆ **Valchlor** see Mechlorethamine (Topical) on page 1071

◆ **Valcyte** see ValGANciclovir on page 1715

ValGANciclovir (val gan SYE kloh veer)

Brand Names: US Valcyte

Brand Names: Canada Apo-Valganciclovir; Valcyte

Index Terms Valganciclovir Hydrochloride

Pharmacologic Category Antiviral Agent

Use

CMV disease (prophylaxis):

Prevention of CMV disease in high-risk adult patients (donor CMV seropositive/recipient CMV seronegative) undergoing kidney, heart, or kidney/pancreas transplantation

Prevention of CMV disease in high risk pediatric patients undergoing kidney transplant (age 4 months to 16 years) or heart transplant (age 1 month to 16 years)

Cytomegalovirus (CMV) retinitis (treatment): Treatment of cytomegalovirus (CMV) retinitis in patients with acquired immunodeficiency syndrome (AIDS)

Dosing

Adult & Geriatric Note: Manufacturer recommends that adult patients should use tablet formulation, NOT the oral solution.

CMV retinitis (treatment): Oral:

Induction: 900 mg twice daily for 21 days

Maintenance: Following induction treatment, or for patients with inactive CMV retinitis who require maintenance therapy: 900 mg once daily

CMV disease (prophylaxis): 900 mg once daily beginning within 10 days of transplantation; continue therapy until 100 days (heart or kidney-pancreas transplant) or 200 days (kidney transplant) post-transplantation

Pediatric

Infants, Children, and Adolescents 1 month to 16 years:

CMV disease (prophylaxis) following heart transplantation: Oral: Dose (mg) = 7 x body surface area x creatinine clearance (see calculation on next page) once daily beginning within 10 days of transplantation; continue therapy until 100 days post-transplantation. Doses should be rounded to the nearest 10 mg increment; maximum dose: 900 mg daily.

Infants, Children, and Adolescents 4 months to 16 years:

CMV disease (prophylaxis) following kidney transplantation: Oral: Dose (mg) = 7 x body surface area x creatinine clearance (see calculation on next page) once daily beginning within 10 days of transplantation; continue therapy until 200 days post-transplantation. Doses should be rounded to the nearest 10 mg increment; maximum dose: 900 mg daily.

Calculation of creatinine clearance: CrCl (mL/minute/1.73 m^2) = [k x Height (cm)] divided by serum creatinine (mg/dL)

Note: If the calculated CrCl is >150 mL/minute/1.73 m^2, then a maximum value of 150 mL/minute/1.73 m^2 should be used to calculate the dose.

Note: Calculated using *modified* Schwartz formula where k is as follows:

Infants with low birth weight for gestational age: k = 0.33

Infants with birth weight appropriate for gestational age: k = 0.45

Children 1 to <2 years: k = 0.45

Girls 2 to 16 years: k = 0.55

Boys 2 to <13 years: k = 0.55

Boys 13 to 16 years: k = 0.7

Adolescents >16 years: Oral: Refer to adult dosing

Renal Impairment

Infants, Children, and Adolescents 1 month to 16 years: No dosage adjustment necessary; calculation for pediatric dosing adjusts for renal function.

Adolescents >16 years and Adults:

Induction dose:

CrCl ≥60 mL/minute: No dosage adjustment necessary

CrCl 40 to 59 mL/minute: 450 mg twice daily

CrCl 25 to 39 mL/minute: 450 mg once daily

CrCl 10 to 24 mL/minute: 450 mg every 2 days

CrCl <10 mL/minute:

Manufacturer labeling: Use not recommended; ganciclovir (with appropriately specified renal dosage adjustment) should be used instead of valganciclovir

Alternate dosing: HIV-1 infected persons: Consider valganciclovir solution 200 mg 3 times weekly (Lucas, 2014)

End stage renal disease (ESRD) on intermittent hemodialysis (IHD):

Manufacturer labeling: Use not recommended; ganciclovir (with appropriately specified renal dosage adjustment) should be used instead of valganciclovir.

Alternate dosing: HIV-1 infected persons: Consider valganciclovir solution 200 mg 3 times weekly (Lucas, 2014); valganciclovir is dialyzable and should be administered following dialysis.

Maintenance/prevention dose:

CrCl ≥60 mL/minute: No dosage adjustment necessary

CrCl 40 to 59 mL/minute: 450 mg once daily

CrCl 25 to 39 mL/minute: 450 mg every 2 days

CrCl 10 to 24 mL/minute: 450 mg twice weekly

CrCl <10 mL/minute:

Manufacturer labeling: Use not recommended; ganciclovir (with appropriately specified renal dosage adjustment) should be used instead of valganciclovir

Alternate dosing: HIV infected persons: Consider valganciclovir solution 100 mg 3 times weekly (Lucas, 2014)

End stage renal disease (ESRD) on intermittent hemodialysis (IHD):

Manufacturer labeling: Use not recommended; ganciclovir (with appropriately specified renal dosage adjustment) should be used instead of valganciclovir.

Alternate dosing: HIV-1 infected persons: Consider valganciclovir solution: 100 mg 3 times weekly (Lucas, 2014); valganciclovir is dialyzable and should be administered following dialysis.

Hepatic Impairment There are no dosage adjustments provided in the manufacturer labeling (has not been studied).

Additional Information Complete prescribing information should be consulted for additional detail.

Dosage Forms Excipient information presented when available (limited, particularly for generics); consult specific product labeling.

Solution Reconstituted, Oral:

Valcyte: 50 mg/mL (88 mL) [contains saccharin sodium, sodium benzoate; tutti-frutti flavor]

Tablet, Oral:

Valcyte: 450 mg

Generic: 450 mg

◆ **Valganciclovir Hydrochloride** see ValGANciclovir on page 1715

Valrubicin (val ROO bi sin)

Related Information

Management of Chemotherapy-Induced Nausea and Vomiting in Adults on page 2142

Prevention of Chemotherapy-Induced Nausea and Vomiting in Children on page 2203

Safe Handling of Hazardous Drugs on page 2292

Brand Names: US Valstar

Brand Names: Canada Valtaxin

Index Terms N-trifluoroacetyladriamycin-14-valerate; AD32

Pharmacologic Category Antineoplastic Agent, Anthracycline; Antineoplastic Agent, Topoisomerase II Inhibitor

Use Bladder cancer: Intravesical treatment of BCG-refractory bladder carcinoma in situ of the urinary bladder when cystectomy would be associated with unacceptable morbidity or mortality.

Labeled Contraindications Known hypersensitivity to anthracyclines, polyoxyl castor oil, or any component of the formulation; concurrent urinary tract infection; small bladder capacity (unable to tolerate a 75 mL instillation)

Pregnancy Considerations Adverse effects were observed in animal reproduction studies. Systemic exposure (eg, with bladder perforation) during human pregnancy may result in fetal harm. Women of childbearing potential should avoid becoming pregnant during treatment. All patients of reproductive age should use an effective method of contraception during the treatment period.

Breast-Feeding Considerations It is not known if valrubicin is excreted in breast milk. Due to the potential for serious adverse reactions in the nursing infant, breast-feeding should be discontinued prior to initiation of therapy.

Warnings/Precautions Hazardous agent - use appropriate precautions for handling and disposal (NIOSH 2014 [group 1]). Delay valrubicin therapy for at least 2 weeks after transurethral resection and/or fulguration. Evaluate bladder status prior to instillation; do not administer if mucosal integrity of bladder has been compromised or bladder perforation is present (delay treatment until restoration of bladder integrity). Use aseptic technique to prevent urinary tract infection or traumatizing urinary mucosa. Although clamping of the urinary catheter after administration is not recommended, use caution and appropriate medical supervision if performed. Irritable bladder symptoms may occur during instillation and retention, and for a brief time after voiding. Use caution in patients with severe irritable bladder symptoms. Red-tinged urine is typical for the first 24 hours after instillation. Prolonged symptoms or discoloration should prompt contact with the physician.

Contains polyoxyl castor oil which may be associated with hypersensitivity reactions; use is contraindicated in patients with hypersensitivity to polyoxyl castor oil. Delaying cystectomy for intravesical treatment may lead to meta-static bladder cancer; the risk for metastatic disease increases with delay duration; reconsider cystectomy for recurrence or if complete response to treatment does not occur within 3 months.

Adverse Reactions Note: In general, local adverse reactions occur during or shortly after instillation and resolve within 1 to 7 days.

> >10%: Genitourinary: Bladder irritation (88%), urinary frequency (61%), urinary urgency (57%), dysuria (56%), bladder spasm (31%), hematuria (29%; gross: 1%), bladder pain (28%), urinary incontinence (22%), cystitis (15%), urinary tract infection (15%), urine red-tinged

1% to 10%:
Cardiovascular: Chest pain (3%), vasodilation (2%), peripheral edema (1%)
Central nervous system: Headache (4%), malaise (4%), dizziness (3%), fever (2%)
Dermatologic: Rash (3%)
Endocrine & metabolic: Hyperglycemia (1%)
Gastrointestinal: Abdominal pain (5%), nausea (5%), diarrhea (3%), vomiting (2%), flatulence (1%)
Genitourinary: Nocturia (7%), burning symptoms (5%), urinary retention (4%), urethral pain (3%), pelvic pain (1%), hematuria (microscopic) (3%)
Hematologic: Anemia (2%)
Neuromuscular & skeletal: Weakness (4%), back pain (3%), myalgia (1%)
Respiratory: Pneumonia (1%)

> <1%, postmarketing, and/or case reports: Hematologic toxicity (following instillation into perforated bladder), nonprotein nitrogen increased, pruritus, skin irritation (local), taste loss, tenesmus, urine flow decreased, urethritis

Drug Interactions

Metabolism/Transport Effects None known.

Avoid Concomitant Use There are no known interactions where it is recommended to avoid concomitant use.

Increased Effect/Toxicity There are no known significant interactions involving an increase in effect.

Decreased Effect There are no known significant interactions involving a decrease in effect.

Storage/Stability Store intact vials at 2°C to 8°C (36°F to 48°F). Do not freeze. Solutions diluted in 0.9% sodium chloride are stable for 12 hours at room temperature.

Preparation for Administration Hazardous agent; use appropriate precau-tions for handling and disposal (NIOSH 2014 [group 1]). Allow vials to slowly warm to room temperature (do not heat) prior to use. A waxy precipitate (due to polyoxyl castor oil) may form at temperatures <4°C, warm vial in the hand until solution is clear (do not use vial if particulate still present). Dilute 800 mg (20 mL) with 55 mL NS (total volume of 75 mL). Use non-PVC containers (glass, polyolefin, or polypropylene) and administration sets to avoid leaching of DEHP plasticizers. Stable for 12 hours at room temperature when diluted in 0.9% sodium chloride. Do not mix with other drugs.

Mechanism of Action Blocks function of DNA topoisomerase II; inhibits DNA synthesis, causes extensive chromosomal damage, and arrests cell development (G_2 phase); unlike other anthracyclines, does not appear to intercalate DNA; readily penetrates cells.

Pharmacodynamics/Kinetics

Absorption: Intravesical: Penetrates into bladder wall; negligible systemic absorption (dependent on bladder wall condition; trauma to mucosa may increase absorption, bladder wall perforation may significantly increase absorption and systemic myelotoxicity).

Metabolism: Negligible after intravesical instillation and 2-hour retention

Excretion: Urine (post 2-hour retention): 98.6% as intact drug; 0.4% as *N*-trifluoroacetyladriamycin)

Dosing

Adult & Geriatric Note: Delay for at least 2 weeks after transurethral resection and/or fulguration.

Bladder cancer: Intravesical: 800 mg once weekly (retain for 2 hours) for 6 weeks

Renal Impairment There are no dosage adjustments provided in the manufacturer's labeling. However, dosage adjustment unlikely due to low systemic absorption.

Hepatic Impairment There are no dosage adjustments provided in the manufacturer's labeling. However, dosage adjustment unlikely due to low systemic absorption.

Adjustment for Toxicity In clinical trials (Steinberg 2000), treatment was delayed for 1 week for the following adverse events: Grade 3 dysuria (not controlled with phenazopyridine), frequency/urgency lasting >24 hours, grade 2 gross hematuria (without clots) lasting >48 hours, grade 3 hematuria (with clots) lasting >48 hours. For local toxicities <grade 4 (eg, dysuria [not controlled with phenazopyridine] or severe bladder spasm), anticholinergic therapy (systemic or topical) or topical anesthesia was administered prior to subsequent instillations.

Administration For intravesical use only; not for IV or IM use.

Intravesicular bladder instillation: Insert urinary catheter, empty bladder prior to instillation, slowly by gravity flow, instill 800 mg/75 mL (in 0.9% sodium chloride injection), remove catheter. Retain in the bladder for 2 hours, then void. Administer through non-PVC tubing due to the polyoxyl castor oil component. Maintain adequate hydration following treatment.

Hazardous agent; use appropriate precautions for handling and disposal (NIOSH 2014 [group 1]). Use appropriate protective gown, goggles, and gloves during administration.

Emetic Potential Children and Adults: Minimal (<10%)

Monitoring Parameters Cystoscopy, biopsy, and urine cytology every 3 months for recurrence or progression

Dosage Forms Excipient information presented when available (limited, particularly for generics); consult specific product labeling.

Solution, Intravesical [preservative free]:

Valstar: 40 mg/mL (5 mL) [contains alcohol, usp, cremophor® el]

◆ **Vancocin** *see* Vancomycin *on page* 1720

◆ **Vancocin HCl** *see* Vancomycin *on page* 1720

Vancomycin (van koe MYE sin)

Brand Names: US First-Vancomycin 25; First-Vancomycin 50; Vancocin HCl; Vancomycin+SyrSpend SF PH4

Brand Names: Canada JAMP-Vancomycin; PMS-Vancomycin; Sterile Vancomycin Hydrochloride, USP; Val-Vancomycin; Vancocin; Vancomycin Hydrochloride for Injection; Vancomycin Hydrochloride for Injection, USP

Index Terms Vancocin; Vancomycin Hydrochloride

Pharmacologic Category Glycopeptide

Use

IV: Treatment of patients with infections caused by staphylococcal species and streptococcal species

Oral: Treatment of *C. difficile*-associated diarrhea and treatment of enterocolitis caused by *Staphylococcus aureus* (including methicillin-resistant strains)

Pregnancy Risk Factor B (oral); C (injection)

Dosing

Adult & Geriatric

Usual dosage range: Note: Initial intravenous dosing should be based on actual body weight; subsequent dosing adjusted based on serum trough vancomycin concentrations.

IV:

Manufacturer's labeling: Usual dose: 500 mg every 6 hours **or** 1,000 mg every 12 hours

Alternate recommendations: 15 to 20 mg/kg/dose every 8 to 12 hours (ASHP/IDSA/SIDP [Rybak, 2009]); **Note:** Dose requires adjustment in renal impairment.

Complicated infections in seriously ill patients: A loading dose of 25 to 30 mg/kg (based on actual body weight) may be used to rapidly achieve target concentrations (ASHP/IDSA/SIDP [Rybak, 2009]).

Oral: 500 to 2,000 mg daily in divided doses every 6 hours. **Note:** Not appropriate for systemic infections due to low absorption.

Indication-specific dosing:

Bacteremia (*S. aureus* [methicillin-resistant]) (off-label use): IV: 15 to 20 mg/kg/dose (based on actual body weight) every 8 to 12 hours for 2 to 6 weeks depending on severity. A loading dose of 25 to 30 mg/kg (based on actual body weight) may be used to rapidly achieve target concentrations in seriously ill patients (ASHP/IDSA/SIDP [Rybak, 2009]; IDSA [Liu, 2011]).

Brain abscess, subdural empyema, spinal epidural abscess (*S. aureus* [methicillin-resistant]) (off-label use): IV: 15 to 20 mg/kg/dose (based on actual body weight) every 8 to 12 hours for 4 to 6 weeks (with or without rifampin). A loading dose of 25 to 30 mg/kg (based on actual body weight) may be used to rapidly achieve target concentrations in seriously ill patients (ASHP/IDSA/SIDP [Rybak, 2009]; IDSA [Liu, 2011]).

Catheter-related infections: Antibiotic lock technique (Mermel, 2009): 2 mg/mL ± 10 units heparin/mL **or** 2.5 mg/mL ± 2,500 **or** 5,000 units heparin/mL **or** 5 mg/mL ± 5,000 units heparin/mL (preferred regimen); instill into catheter port with a volume sufficient to fill the catheter (2 to 5 mL). **Note:** May use SWFI/NS or D_5W as diluents. Do not mix with any other solutions. Dwell times generally should not exceed 48 hours before renewal of lock solution. Remove lock solution prior to catheter use, then replace.

C. difficile-associated diarrhea (CDAD): Oral:

Manufacturer's labeling: 125 mg 4 times daily for 10 days

Alternate dosing:

HIV-infected patients: 125 mg 4 times daily for 10 to 14 days (HHS [OI adult 2015])

Mild to moderate disease unresponsive to metronidazole: 125 mg 4 times daily for 10 days (ACG [Surawicz, 2013])

Severe disease (defined as serum albumin <3 g/dL and either WBC ≥15,000 or abdominal tenderness): 125 mg 4 times daily for 10 days (ACG [Surawicz, 2013])

Severe, complicated infection without abdominal distention: 125 mg 4 times daily with IV metronidazole (ACG [Surawicz, 2013])

Severe, complicated infection: 500 mg every 6 hours for 10 to 14 days with or without concurrent IV metronidazole. May consider vancomycin retention enema (in patients with complete ileus) (SHEA/IDSA [Cohen, 2010])

Severe, complicated infection with significant abdominal distention, ileus, and/or toxic colon: 500 mg 4 times daily plus rectal vancomycin in combination with IV metronidazole (ACG [Surawicz, 2013])

Recurrent, severe infection (if initial regimen did not include vancomycin): 125 mg 4 times daily for 10 days (ACG [Surawicz, 2013])

Rectal (off-label route): Retention enema:

Severe, complicated infection in patients with ileus: 500 mg every 6 hours (in 100 mL 0.9% sodium chloride) with oral vancomycin with or without concurrent IV metronidazole (SHEA/IDSA [Cohen, 2010])

Severe and complicated disease with abdominal distention, ileus, and/or toxic colon: 500 mg 4 times daily (in 500 mL NS) in combination with oral vancomycin and IV metronidazole (ACG [Surawicz, 2013])

Endocarditis:

Native valve (*Enterococcus*, vancomycin MIC ≤4 mg/L) (off-label use): IV: 15 to 20 mg/kg/dose (based on actual body weight) every 8 to 12 hours. A loading dose of 25 to 30 mg/kg (based on actual body weight) may be used to rapidly achieve target concentrations in seriously ill patients (ASHP/IDSA/SIDP [Rybak, 2009]) **or** 1,000 mg every 12 hours for 4 to 6 weeks (combine with gentamicin for 4 to 6 weeks) (BSAC [Gould, 2012]).

Native valve (*S. aureus* [methicillin-resistant]) (off-label use): IV: 15 to 20 mg/kg/dose (based on actual body weight) every 8 to 12 hours for 6 weeks. A loading dose of 25 to 30 mg/kg (based on actual body weight) may be used to rapidly achieve target concentrations in seriously ill patients (ASHP/IDSA/SIDP [Rybak, 2009]; IDSA [Liu, 2011]). **Note:** European guidelines support the entire duration of therapy to be 4 weeks and in combination with rifampin (BSAC [Gould, 2012]).

Native or prosthetic valve (streptococcal [penicillin MIC >0.5 mg/L or patient intolerant to penicillin]) (off-label use): IV: 15 to 20 mg/kg/dose (based on actual body weight) every 8 to 12 hours for 6 weeks. A loading dose of 25 to 30 mg/kg (based on actual body weight) may be used to rapidly achieve target concentrations in seriously ill patients (AHA [Baddour, 2005]; ASHP/IDSA/SIDP [Rybak, 2009]) **or** 1,000 mg every 12 hours for 4 to 6 weeks (combine with gentamicin for at least the first 2 weeks). **Note:** The longer duration of treatment (ie, 6 weeks) should be used for patients with prosthetic valve endocarditis (BSAC [Gould, 2012]).

◄ **Prosthetic valve (*Enterococcus*, vancomycin MIC ≤4 mg/L) (off-label use):** IV: Adults: 15 to 20 mg/kg/dose (based on actual body weight) every 8 to 12 hours for 6 weeks. A loading dose of 25 to 30 mg/kg (based on actual body weight) may be used to rapidly achieve target concentrations in seriously ill patients (AHA [Baddour, 2005]; ASHP/IDSA/SIDP [Rybak, 2009]) **or** 1,000 mg every 12 hours for 6 weeks (combine with gentamicin for 6 weeks) (BSAC [Gould, 2012]).

Prosthetic valve (*S. aureus* [methicillin-resistant]) (off-label use): IV: 15 to 20 mg/kg/dose (based on actual body weight) every 8 to 12 hours for at least 6 weeks (combine with rifampin for the entire duration of therapy and gentamicin for the first 2 weeks). A loading dose of 25 to 30 mg/kg (based on actual body weight) may be used to rapidly achieve target concentrations in seriously ill patients (ASHP/IDSA/SIDP [Rybak, 2009]; IDSA [Liu, 2011]).

Endophthalmitis (off-label use): Intravitreal: Usual dose: 1 mg/0.1 mL NS instilled into vitreum; may repeat administration, if necessary, in 2 to 3 days, usually in combination with ceftazidime or an aminoglycoside (Kelsey, 1995). **Note:** Based on concerns for retinotoxicity, some clinicians have recommended using a lower dose of 0.2 mg/0.1mL; may repeat in 3 to 4 days, if necessary (Gan, 2001).

Enterocolitis (*S. aureus*): Oral: 500 to 2,000 mg/day in 3 to 4 divided doses for 7 to 10 days (usual dose: 125 to 500 mg every 6 hours)

Group B streptococcus (neonatal prophylaxis): IV: 1,000 mg every 12 hours until delivery. **Note:** Reserved for penicillin allergic patients at high risk for anaphylaxis if organism is resistant to clindamycin or where no susceptibility data are available (CDC, 2010).

Meningitis:
IV: 15 to 20 mg/kg/dose (based on actual body weight) every 8 to 12 hours (for empiric therapy, use in combination with a third-generation cephalosporin; for patients >50 years, include ampicillin); duration of therapy should be individualized based upon clinical response (in general, 10 to 21 days). A loading dose of 25 to 30 mg/kg (based on actual body weight) may be used to rapidly achieve target concentration in seriously ill patients (ASHP/IDSA/SIDP [Rybak, 2009]; IDSA [Tunkel, 2004]). **Note:** For PCN-resistant *Streptococcus pneumoniae* (MIC ≥2 mcg/mL), combine with a third-generation cephalosporin (IDSA [Tunkel, 2004]). For methicillin-resistant S. aureus, treat for 2 weeks (with or without rifampin) (IDSA [Liu, 2011]).
Intrathecal, intraventricular (off-label route): 5 to 20 mg/day (IDSA [Tunkel, 2004])

Osteomyelitis (*S. aureus* [methicillin-resistant]) (off-label use): IV: 15 to 20 mg/kg/dose (based on actual body weight) every 8 to 12 hours for a minimum of 8 weeks (with or without rifampin). A loading dose of 25 to 30 mg/kg (based on actual body weight) may be used to rapidly achieve target concentrations in seriously ill patients (ASHP/IDSA/SIDP [Rybak, 2009]; IDSA [Liu, 2011]).

Pneumonia: IV:
Community-acquired pneumonia (CAP): S. aureus (methicillin-resistant): 15 to 20 mg/kg/dose (based on actual body weight) every 8 to 12 hours for 7 to 21 days depending on severity. A loading dose of 25 to 30 mg/kg (based on actual body weight) may be used to rapidly achieve target concentrations in seriously ill patients (ASHP/IDSA/SIDP [Rybak, 2009]; IDSA [Liu, 2011]).

Healthcare-associated pneumonia (HAP): S. aureus (methicillin-resistant): 15 to 20 mg/kg/dose (based on actual body weight) every 8 to 12 hours for 7 to 21 days depending on severity. A loading dose of 25 to 30 mg/kg (based on actual body weight) may be used to rapidly achieve target concentrations in seriously ill patients (ASHP/IDSA/SIDP [Rybak, 2009]; IDSA [Liu, 2011]).

Prophylaxis against infective endocarditis: IV:

Dental, oral, or upper respiratory tract surgery: 1,000 mg 1 hour before surgery. **Note:** AHA guidelines now recommend prophylaxis only in patients undergoing invasive procedures and in whom underlying cardiac conditions may predispose to a higher risk of adverse outcomes should infection occur

GI/GU procedure: 1,000 mg plus 1.5 mg/kg gentamicin 1 hour prior to surgery. **Note:** As of April 2007, routine prophylaxis no longer recommended by the AHA.

Prosthetic joint infection (off-label use): IV:

Enterococcus spp (penicillin-susceptible or -resistant), Propionibacterium acnes, streptococci (beta-hemolytic): 15 mg/kg every 12 hours for 4 to 6 weeks, followed by an oral antibiotic suppressive regimen (IDSA [Osman, 2013]).

Note: For penicillin-susceptible or -resistant *Enterococcus* spp, consider addition of an aminoglycoside; in penicillin-susceptible *Enterococcus*, beta-hemolytic streptococcus or *Propionibacterium acnes* infections, only use vancomycin if patient has penicillin allergy (IDSA [Osman, 2013]).

Staphylococci (oxacillin-susceptible or -resistant): 15 mg/kg every 12 hours for 2 to 6 weeks in combination with rifampin followed by oral antibiotic treatment and suppressive regimens (IDSA [Osman, 2013]).

Sepsis/Septic shock (empiric treatment or treatment for specific sensitive organism): IV: 15 to 20 mg/kg/dose (based on actual body weight) every 8 to 12 hours. A loading dose of 25 to 30 mg/kg (based on actual body weight) may be used to rapidly achieve target concentrations in seriously ill patients (ASHP/IDSA/SIDP [Rybak, 2009]). The Society of Critical Care Medicine recommends administration of empiric antibiotics within 1 hour of identifying severe sepsis (SCCM [Dellinger, 2013]).

Septic arthritis (*S. aureus* [methicillin-resistant]) (off-label use): IV: 15 to 20 mg/kg/dose (based on actual body weight) every 8 to 12 hours for 3 to 4 weeks. A loading dose of 25 to 30 mg/kg (based on actual body weight) may be used to rapidly achieve target concentrations in seriously ill patients (ASHP/IDSA/SIDP [Rybak, 2009]; IDSA [Liu, 2011]).

Septic thrombosis of cavernous or dural venous sinus (*S. aureus* [methicillin-resistant]) (off-label use): IV: 15 to 20 mg/kg/dose (based on actual body weight) every 8 to 12 hours for 4 to 6 weeks (with or without rifampin). A loading dose of 25 to 30 mg/kg (based on actual body weight) may be used to rapidly achieve target concentrations in seriously ill patients (ASHP/IDSA/SIDP [Rybak, 2009]; IDSA [Liu, 2011]).

Skin and skin structure infections (*S. aureus* [methicillin-resistant]) (off-label use): IV: 15 to 20 mg/kg/dose every 8 to 12 hours for 7 to 14 days (IDSA [Liu 2011; Stevens 2014]). A loading dose of 25 to 30 mg/kg (based on actual body weight) may be used to rapidly achieve target concentrations in seriously ill patients (ASHP/IDSA/SIDP [Rybak 2009]; IDSA [Liu 2011]).

◀ **Skin and soft tissue necrotizing infections due to *S. aureus* (resistant strains) or polymicrobial (mixed) (off-label use):** IV: 15 mg/kg/dose every 12 hours. **Note:** Give in combination with piperacillin/tazobactam for empiric therapy of polymicrobial [mixed] infections. Continue until further debridement is not necessary, patient has clinically improved, and patient is afebrile for 48 to 72 hours (IDSA [Stevens, 2014]).

Surgical (perioperative) prophylaxis (off-label use): IV: 15 mg/kg within 120 minutes prior to surgical incision. May be administered in combination with other antibiotics depending upon the surgical procedure (ASHP/IDSA/SIS/SHEA [Bratzler, 2013]).

Note: For patients known to be colonized with methicillin-resistant *S. aureus*, a single 15 mg/kg preoperative dose may be added to other recommended agents for the specific procedure (ASHP/IDSA/SIS/SHEA [Bratzler, 2013]).

The Society of Thoracic Surgeons recommends 1,000 to 1,500 mg or 15 mg/kg over 60 minutes with completion within 1 hour of skin incision. Although not well established, a second dose of 7.5 mg/kg may be considered during cardiopulmonary bypass (STS [Engelman, 2007]).

Surgical site infections (trunk or extremity [away from axilla or perineum]) (unlabeled use): IV: 15 mg/kg/dose every 12 hours (IDSA [Stevens 2014])

Pediatric

Usual dosage range: Note: Initial IV dosing should be based on actual body weight; subsequent dosing adjusted based on serum trough vancomycin concentrations.

Infants >1 month, Children, and Adolescents: IV:
Manufacturer's labeling: 10 mg/kg/dose every 6 hours
Alternate recommendations: 15 mg/kg/dose (maximum: 2,000 mg/dose) every 6 hours (IDSA [Liu, 2011])

Indication-specific dosing:

Bacteremia (*S. aureus* [methicillin-resistant]) (off-label use): Children and Adolescents: IV: 15 mg/kg/dose every 6 hours for 2 to 6 weeks depending on severity (IDSA [Liu, 2011])

Brain abscess, subdural empyema, spinal epidural abscess (*S. aureus* [methicillin-resistant]) (off-label use): Children and Adolescents: IV: 15 mg/kg/dose every 6 hours for 4 to 6 weeks (with or without rifampin) (IDSA [Liu, 2011])

***C. difficile*-associated diarrhea (CDAD):** Infants >1 month, Children, and Adolescents: Oral:
Manufacturer's labeling: 40 mg/kg/day in 3 to 4 divided doses for 7 to 10 days (maximum: 2,000 mg/day)
Alternate dosing: Adolescents: HIV-infected patients: 125 mg 4 times daily for 10 to 14 days (HHS [OI adult 2015])

Endocarditis:

Native valve (*S. aureus* [methicillin-resistant]) (off-label use): Children and Adolescents: IV: 15 mg/kg/dose every 6 hours for 6 weeks (IDSA [Liu, 2011])

Prosthetic valve (*S. aureus* [methicillin-resistant]) (off-label use): Children and Adolescents: IV: 15 mg/kg/dose every 6 hours for at least 2 to 6 weeks depending on source, presence of endovascular infection, and metastatic foci of infection (IDSA [Liu, 2011]).

Enterocolitis *(S. aureus):* Infants >1 months, Children, and Adolescents: Oral: 40 mg/kg/day in 3 to 4 divided doses for 7 to 10 days (maximum: 2,000 mg/day)

Meningitis: Infants >1 month, Children, and Adolescents:

IV: 15 mg/kg/dose every 6 hours (for empiric therapy, use in combination with a third-generation cephalosporin); duration of therapy should be individualized based upon clinical response (in general, 10 to 21 days) (IDSA [Tunkel, 2004]). For methicillin-resistant *S. aureus*, treat for 2 weeks (with or without rifampin) (IDSA [Liu, 2011]).

Intrathecal, intraventricular (off-label route): 5 to 20 mg/day (IDSA [Tunkel, 2004])

Osteomyelitis *(S. aureus* [methicillin-resistant]) (off-label use): Children and Adolescents: IV: 15 mg/kg/dose every 6 hours for 4 to 6 weeks (IDSA [Liu, 2011]).

Pneumonia:

Community-acquired pneumonia (CAP) (IDSA/PIDS, 2011): Infants >3 months, Children, and Adolescents: IV: **Note:** In children ≥5 years, a macrolide antibiotic should be added if atypical pneumonia cannot be ruled out. Also consider if community-acquired MRSA suspected.

Group A *Streptococcus* (alternative to ampicillin or penicillin in beta-lactam allergic patients): 40 to 60 mg/kg/day divided every 6 to 8 hours

Presumed bacterial (in addition to recommended antibiotic therapy), *S. pneumoniae*, moderate to severe infection (MICs to penicillin ≤2.0 mcg/mL) (alternative to ampicillin or penicillin): 40 to 60 mg/kg/day divided every 6 to 8 hours

S. aureus (methicillin-susceptible) (alternative to cefazolin/oxacillin): 40 to 60 mg/kg/day divided every 6 to 8 hours

S. aureus, moderate to severe infection (methicillin-resistant +/- clindamycin susceptible) (preferred): 40 to 60 mg/kg/day divided every 6 to 8 hours **or** dosing to achieve AUC/MIC >400

Alternate regimen: 60 mg/kg/day divided every 6 hours for 7 to 21 days, depending on severity (Liu, 2011)

S. pneumoniae, moderate to severe infection (MICs to penicillin ≥4.0 mcg/mL) (alternative to ceftriaxone in beta-lactam allergic patients): 40 to 60 mg/kg/day divided every 6 to 8 hours

Healthcare-associated pneumonia (HAP), S. aureus (methicillin-resistant): IV: Infants, Children, and Adolescents: 60 mg/kg/day divided every 6 hours for 7 to 21 days depending on severity (IDSA [Liu, 2011])

Prophylaxis against infective endocarditis: Children and Adolescents: IV: Dental, oral, or upper respiratory tract surgery: 20 mg/kg/dose administered 1 hour prior to the procedure. **Note:** American Heart Association (AHA) guidelines recommend prophylaxis only in patients undergoing invasive procedures and in whom underlying cardiac conditions may predispose to a higher risk of adverse outcomes should infection occur.

GI/GU procedure: 20 mg/kg (plus gentamicin 1.5 mg/kg) administered 1 hour prior to surgery. **Note:** Routine prophylaxis no longer recommended by the AHA.

Septic arthritis *(S. aureus* [methicillin-resistant]) (off-label use): Children and Adolescents: IV: 15 mg/kg/dose every 6 hours for minimum of 3 to 4 weeks (IDSA [Liu, 2011])

Septic thrombosis of cavernous or dural venous sinus *(S. aureus* [methicillin-resistant]) (off-label use): Children and Adolescents: IV: 15 mg/kg/dose every 6 hours for 4 to 6 weeks (with or without rifampin) (IDSA [Liu, 2011])

◄   **Skin and skin structure infections (*S. aureus* [methicillin-resistant]) (off-label use):** Children and Adolescents: IV: 10 to 15 mg/kg/dose every 6 hours for 7 to 14 days (IDSA [Liu 2011; Stevens 2014])

Skin and soft tissue necrotizing infections due to *S. aureus* (resistant strains) or polymicrobial (mixed) (off-label use): Children and Adolescents: IV: 15 mg/kg/dose every 6 hours. **Note:** Give in combination with piperacillin/tazobactam for empiric therapy of polymicrobial [mixed] infections. Continue until further debridement is not necessary, patient has clinically improved, and patient is afebrile for 48 to 72 hours (IDSA [Stevens 2014])

Surgical (perioperative) prophylaxis (off-label use): Children and Adolescents: IV: 15 mg/kg/dose within 120 minutes prior to surgical incision. May be administered in combination with other antibiotics depending upon the surgical procedure (ASHP/IDSA/SIS/SHEA [Bratzler, 2013]).

Note: for patients known to be colonized with methicillin-resistant *S. aureus*, a single 15 mg/kg preoperative dose may be added to other recommended agents for the specific procedure (ASHP/IDSA/SIS/SHEA [Bratzler, 2013]).

Renal Impairment

Oral: No dosage adjustment provided in manufacturer's labeling, However, dosage adjustment unlikely due to low systemic absorption.

IV: Vancomycin levels should be monitored in patients with any renal impairment:

CrCl >50 mL/minute: Start with 15 to 20 mg/kg/dose (usual: 750 to 1,500 mg) every 8 to 12 hours

CrCl 20 to 49 mL/minute: Start with 15 to 20 mg/kg/dose (usual: 750 to 1,500 mg) every 24 hours

CrCl <20 mL/minute: Will need longer intervals; determine by serum concentration monitoring

Note: In the critically-ill patient with renal insufficiency, the initial loading dose (25 to 30 mg/kg) should not be reduced. However, subsequent dosage adjustments should be made based on renal function and trough serum concentrations.

Poorly dialyzable by intermittent hemodialysis (0% to 5%); however, use of high-flux membranes and continuous renal replacement therapy (CRRT) increases vancomycin clearance, and generally requires replacement dosing.

Intermittent hemodialysis (IHD) (administer after hemodialysis on dialysis days): Following loading dose of 15 to 25 mg/kg, give either 500 to 1,000 mg **or** 5 to 10 mg/kg after each dialysis session (Heintz, 2009). **Note:** Dosing dependent on the assumption of 3 times/week, complete IHD sessions.

Redosing based on pre-HD concentrations:
    <10 mg/L: Administer 1,000 mg after HD
    10 to 25 mg/L: Administer 500 to 750 mg after HD
    >25 mg/L: Hold vancomycin

Redosing based on post-HD concentrations: <10 to 15 mg/L: Administer 500 to 1,000 mg

Peritoneal dialysis (PD):
    Administration via PD fluid: 15 to 30 mg/L (15 to 30 mcg/mL) of PD fluid
    Systemic: Loading dose of 1,000 mg, followed by 500 to 1,000 mg every 48 to 72 hours with close monitoring of levels

Continuous renal replacement therapy (CRRT) (Heintz, 2009; Trotman, 2005): Drug clearance is highly dependent on the method of renal replacement, filter type, and flow rate. Appropriate dosing requires close monitoring of pharmacologic response, signs of adverse reactions due to drug accumulation, as well as drug concentrations in relation to target trough (if appropriate). The following are general recommendations only (based on dialysate flow/ultrafiltration rates of 1 to 2 L/hour and minimal residual renal function) and should not supersede clinical judgment:

CVVH: Loading dose of 15 to 25 mg/kg, followed by either 1,000 mg every 48 hours **or** 10 to 15 mg/kg every 24 to 48 hours

CVVHD: Loading dose of 15 to 25 mg/kg, followed by either 1,000 mg every 24 hours **or** 10 to 15 mg/kg every 24 hours

CVVHDF: Loading dose of 15 to 25 mg/kg, followed by either 1,000 mg every 24 hours **or** 7.5 to 10 mg/kg every 12 hours

Note: Consider redosing patients receiving CRRT for vancomycin concentrations <10 to 15 mg/L.

Hepatic Impairment

Oral: No dosage adjustment provided in the manufacturer's labeling. However, dosage adjustment unlikely due to low systemic absorption.

IV: No dosage adjustment provided in manufacturer's labeling. However, degrees of hepatic dysfunction do not affect the pharmacokinetics of vancomycin (Marti, 1996).

Additional Information Complete prescribing information should be consulted for additional detail.

Dosage Forms Considerations First-Vancomycin oral solution and Vancomycin+SyrSpend SF oral suspension are compounding kits. Refer to manufacturer's labeling for compounding instructions.

Dosage Forms Excipient information presented when available (limited, particularly for generics); consult specific product labeling.

Capsule, Oral:
Vancocin HCl: 125 mg, 250 mg [contains fd&c blue #2 (indigotine)]
Generic: 125 mg, 250 mg

Solution, Intravenous:
Generic: 500 mg/100 mL (100 mL); 750 mg/150 mL (150 mL); 1 g/200 mL (200 mL)

Solution, Oral:
First-Vancomycin 25: 25 mg/mL (150 mL, 300 mL) [contains fd&c red #40, fd&c yellow #10 (quinoline yellow), sodium benzoate; white grape flavor]
First-Vancomycin 50: 50 mg/mL (150 mL, 210 mL, 300 mL) [contains fd&c red #40, fd&c yellow #10 (quinoline yellow), sodium benzoate; white grape flavor]

Solution Reconstituted, Intravenous:
Generic: 500 mg (1 ea); 750 mg (1 ea); 1000 mg (1 ea); 5000 mg (1 ea); 10 g (1 ea)

Solution Reconstituted, Intravenous [preservative free]:
Generic: 1000 mg (1 ea); 5000 mg (1 ea); 10 g (1 ea)

Suspension, Oral:
Vancomycin+SyrSpend SF PH4: 50 mg/mL (1 ea)

◆ **Vancomycin Hydrochloride** *see* Vancomycin *on page 1720*

◆ **Vancomycin Hydrochloride for Injection (Can)** *see* Vancomycin *on page 1720*

- **Vancomycin Hydrochloride for Injection, USP (Can)** *see* Vancomycin *on page 1720*
- **Vancomycin+SyrSpend SF PH4** *see* Vancomycin *on page 1720*

Vandetanib (van DET a nib)

Related Information
Management of Chemotherapy-Induced Nausea and Vomiting in Adults *on page 2142*
Management of EGFR Inhibitor Toxicities: Dermatologic, Ocular, and Gastrointestinal *on page 2179*
Principles of Anticancer Therapy *on page 2261*
Safe Handling of Hazardous Drugs *on page 2292*

Brand Names: US Caprelsa
Brand Names: Canada Caprelsa
Index Terms AZD6474; Zactima; ZD6474; Zictifa
Pharmacologic Category Antineoplastic Agent, Epidermal Growth Factor Receptor (EGFR) Inhibitor; Antineoplastic Agent, Tyrosine Kinase Inhibitor; Antineoplastic Agent, Vascular Endothelial Growth Factor (VEGF) Inhibitor
Use Thyroid cancer: Treatment of metastatic or unresectable locally-advanced medullary thyroid cancer (symptomatic or progressive)
Labeled Contraindications Congenital long QT syndrome

Canadian labeling: Additional contraindications (not in U.S. labeling): Hypersensitivity to vandetanib or any component of the formulation; persistent Fridericia-corrected QT interval (QTcF) ≥500 ms; uncorrected hypokalemia, hypomagnesemia, or hypocalcemia; uncontrolled hypertension

Pregnancy Considerations Animal reproduction studies have demonstrated teratogenic effects and fetal loss. Because vandetanib inhibits angiogenesis, a critical component of fetal development, adverse effects on pregnancy would be expected. Women of childbearing potential should be advised to avoid pregnancy and use effective contraception during and for 4 months following treatment with vandetanib. Canadian labeling recommends that nonsterile males employ reliable contraceptive methods (barrier method in conjunction with spermicide) during and for 2 months after vandetanib treatment.

Breast-Feeding Considerations It is not known if vandetanib is excreted in human breast milk. Due to the potential for serious adverse reactions in the nursing infant, a decision should be made to discontinue vandetanib or to discontinue breast-feeding, taking into account the importance of treatment to the mother.

Warnings/Precautions Hazardous agent - use appropriate precautions for handling and disposal (NIOSH 2014 [group 1]). **[U.S. Boxed Warning]: May prolong the QT interval; torsade de pointes and sudden death have been reported. Do not use in patients with hypocalcemia, hypokalemia, hypomagnesemia, or long QT syndrome. Correct electrolyte imbalance prior to initiating therapy. Monitor electrolytes and ECG (to monitor QT interval) at baseline, at 2-4 weeks, at 8-12 weeks, and every 3 months thereafter; monitoring (at the same frequency) is required following dose reductions for QT prolongation or with dose interruptions >2 weeks. Avoid the use of QT-prolonging agents; if concomitant use with QT prolonging agents cannot be avoided, monitor ECG more frequently. Vandetanib has a long half-life (19 days), therefore, adverse reactions (including QT prolongation) may resolve slowly; monitor appropriately.** Ventricular tachycardia has also been reported. The potential for QT prolongation is dose-dependent. Do not initiate treatment unless QT interval, Fridericia-corrected QT interval (QTcF) is <450 msec. During treatment, if QTcF >500 msec, withhold vandetanib and resume at a reduced dose when QTcF is <450 msec. Do not use in patients with a history of torsade de pointes, congenital long QT syndrome, bradyarrhythmias or uncompensated heart failure. Patients with ventricular arrhythmias or recent MI were excluded from clinical trials. To reduce the risk of QT prolongation, maintain serum calcium and magnesium within normal limits and maintain serum potassium ≥4 mEq/L. Heart failure (HF) has been reported; monitor for signs and symptoms of HF; may require discontinuation (HF may not be reversible upon discontinuation). Hypertension and hypertensive crisis have been observed with vandetanib; monitor blood pressure and initiate or adjust antihypertensive therapy as needed; may require vandetanib dosage adjustment or treatment interruption; discontinue vandetanib (permanently) if blood pressure cannot be adequately controlled. Canadian labeling contraindicates use in uncontrolled hypertension.

Diarrhea has been reported with use; may cause electrolyte imbalance (closely monitor electrolytes and ECGs to detect QT prolongation resulting from dehydration); routine antidiarrheals are recommended; withhold vandetanib treatment until resolution for severe diarrhea; dose reduction is recommended when treatment is resumed. Stevens-Johnson syndrome and other serious skin reactions (including fatal) have been reported. Mild-to-moderate skin reactions, including acne, dermatitis, dry skin, palmar-plantar erythrodysesthesia syndrome, pruritus, and rash have also been reported. Withhold treatment for dermatologic toxicity of grade 3 or higher; consider a reduced dose or permanent discontinuation upon improvement in symptoms. Consider discontinuation for severe dermatologic toxicity. Mild-to-moderate toxicity has responded to corticosteroids (systemic or topical), oral antihistamines, and antibiotics (topical or systemic). Increased risk of photosensitivity is associated with use; effective sunscreen and protective clothing are recommended during and for at least 4 months after treatment discontinuation.

Reversible posterior leukoencephalopathy syndrome (RPLS) been observed with vandetanib; symptoms of RPLS include altered mental function, confusion, headache, seizure, or visual disturbances; generally associated with hypertension; consider discontinuing treatment if RPLS occurs. Serious and sometimes fatal hemorrhagic events have been reported with use; discontinue in patients with severe hemorrhage; do not administer in patients with a recent history of hemoptysis with ≥2.5 mL of red blood. Ischemic cerebrovascular events (some fatal) have been observed with vandetanib; discontinue treatment in patients with severe ischemic events (the safety of resuming treatment after an ischemic event has not been studied). Interstitial lung disease (ILD) or pneumonitis (including fatalities) has been reported with vandetanib. Patients should be advised to report any new or worsening respiratory symptoms; ILD should be suspected with nonspecific respiratory symptoms such as hypoxia, pleural effusion, cough or dyspnea. Interrupt therapy for acute or worsening pulmonary symptoms; discontinue if ILD diagnosis is confirmed.

Increased doses of thyroid replacement therapy have been required in patients with prior thyroidectomy; obtain TSH at baseline, at 2-4 weeks, 8-12 weeks, and every 3 months after vandetanib initiation; if signs and symptoms of hypothyroidism occur during treatment, evaluate thyroid hormone levels and adjust replacement therapy if needed. Dosage reduction is recommended in patients with moderate-to-severe renal impairment. Exposure is increased in

◄ patients with impaired renal function; closely monitor QT interval; has not been studied in patients with end stage renal disease requiring dialysis. Not recommended for use in patients with moderate-to-severe hepatic impairment. Potentially significant drug-drug interactions may exist, requiring dose or frequency adjustment, additional monitoring, and/or selection of alternative therapy. Due to the risk for serious treatment-related adverse events, use in patients whose disease is not progressive or symptomatic should be only be undertaken after careful consideration. **[U.S. Boxed Warning]: Vandetanib is only available through a restricted access program; prescribers and pharmacies must be certified with the restricted distribution program to prescribe and dispense vandetanib.**

Adverse Reactions

>10%:

Cardiovascular: Hypertension (33%; grades 3/4: 9%), prolonged Q-T interval on ECG (14%; grades 3/4: 8%)

Central nervous system: Headache (26%; grades 3/4: 1%), fatigue (24%; grades 3/4: 6%), insomnia (13%)

Dermatologic: Skin rash (53%; grades 3/4: 5%), acne vulgaris (35%; grades 3/4: 1%), xeroderma (15%), skin photosensitivity (13%; grades 3/4: 2%), pruritus (11%; grades 3/4: 1%)

Endocrine & metabolic: Hypocalcemia (11% to 57%; grades 3/4: 2%), hypoglycemia (24%)

Gastrointestinal: Pseudomembranous colitis (57%; grades 3/4: 11%), nausea (33%; grades 3/4: 1%), abdominal pain (21%; grades 3/4: 3%), decreased appetite (21%; grades 3/4: 1% to 4%), vomiting (15%; grades 3/4: 1%), dyspepsia (11%)

Hematologic & oncologic: Leukopenia (19%), hemorrhage (13% to 14%), anemia (13%; grades 3/4: <1%)

Hepatic: Increased serum ALT (51%), increased serum bilirubin (13%)

Neuromuscular & skeletal: Weakness (15%)

Ophthalmic: Corneal changes (13%; corneal edema, corneal opacity, corneal dystrophy, iris hyperpigmentation, keratopathy, arcus lipoides, corneal deposits, acquired corneal dystrophy)

Renal: Increased serum creatinine (16%)

Respiratory: Upper respiratory tract infection (23%), cough (11%), nasopharyngitis (11%)

1% to 10%:

Cardiovascular: Cardiac failure (2%), cerebral ischemia (1%)

Central nervous system: Depression (10%; grades 3/4: 2%)

Dermatologic: Nail disease (9%; inflammation, tenderness, paronychia), alopecia (8%)

Endocrine & metabolic: Weight loss (10%), hypercalcemia (7%), hypomagnesemia (7%), hyperkalemia (6%), hypokalemia (6%), hypothyroidism (6%), hyperglycemia (5%), hypermagnesemia (3%)

Gastrointestinal: Xerostomia (9%), dysgeusia (8%)

Genitourinary: Proteinuria (10%)

Hematologic & oncologic: Neutropenia (10%; grades 3/4: <1%), thrombocytopenia (9%)

Infection: Sepsis (2%)

Neuromuscular & skeletal: Muscle spasm (6%)

Ophthalmic: Blurred vision (9%)

Respiratory: Aspiration pneumonia (2%), respiratory arrest (2%), respiratory failure (2%)

<1%, postmarketing, and/or case reports: Arthralgia, cardiorespiratory arrest, fever, interstitial pulmonary disease, palmar-plantar erythrodysesthesia, pancreatitis, pneumonitis, reversible posterior leukoencephalopathy syndrome, Stevens-Johnson syndrome, torsades de pointes, ventricular tachycardia

Drug Interactions

Metabolism/Transport Effects Substrate of CYP3A4 (major); **Note:** Assignment of Major/Minor substrate status based on clinically relevant drug interaction potential; **Inhibits** BCRP, P-glycoprotein

Avoid Concomitant Use

Avoid concomitant use of Vandetanib with any of the following: Bosutinib; CYP3A4 Inducers (Strong); Highest Risk QTc-Prolonging Agents; Ivabradine; Mifepristone; Moderate Risk QTc-Prolonging Agents; PAZOPanib; Silodosin; St Johns Wort; Topotecan; VinCRIStine (Liposomal)

Increased Effect/Toxicity

Vandetanib may increase the levels/effects of: Afatinib; Bisphosphonate Derivatives; Bosutinib; Brentuximab Vedotin; Colchicine; Dabigatran Etexilate; Digoxin; DOXOrubicin (Conventional); Edoxaban; Everolimus; Highest Risk QTc-Prolonging Agents; Ledipasvir; MetFORMIN; Naloxegol; PAZOPanib; P-glycoprotein/ABCB1 Substrates; Prucalopride; Rifaximin; Silodosin; Topotecan; VinCRIStine (Liposomal)

The levels/effects of Vandetanib may be increased by: Ivabradine; Mifepristone; Moderate Risk QTc-Prolonging Agents; QTc-Prolonging Agents (Indeterminate Risk and Risk Modifying)

Decreased Effect

The levels/effects of Vandetanib may be decreased by: Bosentan; CYP3A4 Inducers (Moderate); CYP3A4 Inducers (Strong); Dabrafenib; Deferasirox; Siltuximab; St Johns Wort; Tocilizumab

Storage/Stability Store at 25°C (77°F); excursions permitted to 15°C to 30°C (59°F to 86°F).

Mechanism of Action Multikinase inhibitor; inhibits tyrosine kinases including epidermal growth factor reception (EGFR), vascular endothelial growth factor (VEGF), rearranged during transfection (RET), protein tyrosine kinase 6 (BRK), TIE2, EPH kinase receptors and SRC kinase receptors, selectively blocking intracellular signaling, angiogenesis and cellular proliferation

Pharmacodynamics/Kinetics

Absorption: Slow

Protein binding: ~90%; to albumin and alpha 1-acid-glycoprotein

Distribution: V_d: ~7450 L

Metabolism: Hepatic, via CYP3A4 to N-desmethyl vandetanib and via flavin-containing monooxygenase enzymes to vandetanib-N-oxide

Bioavailability: Not affected by food

Half life, elimination: 19 days

Time to peak: 6 hours (range: 4-10 hours)

Excretion: Feces (~44%); urine (~25%)

Dosing

Adult & Geriatric Note: Do not initiate treatment unless QTcF <450 msec. Avoid concomitant use of QT-prolonging agents and strong CYP3A4 inducers. To reduce the risk of QT prolongation, maintain serum calcium and magnesium within normal limits and maintain serum potassium ≥4 mEq/L.

◄ **Medullary thyroid cancer, locally-advanced or metastatic:** Oral: 300 mg once daily, continue treatment until no longer clinically benefiting or until unacceptable toxicity

Renal Impairment

CrCl ≥50 mL/minute: No dosage adjustment necessary.

CrCl <50 mL/minute: Reduce initial dose to 200 mg once daily; closely monitor QT interval.

Hepatic Impairment

Mild impairment (Child-Pugh class A): No dosage adjustment provided in manufacturer's labeling.

Moderate and severe impairment (Child-Pugh class B or C): Use is not recommended.

Adjustment for Toxicity

Toxicity ≥ grade 3: Interrupt dose until resolves or improves to grade 1, then resume at a reduced dose

Dosage reduction: Reduce from 300 mg once daily to 200 mg once daily, further reduce if needed to 100 mg once daily. For recurrent toxicities, reduce dose to 100 mg once daily after symptom improvement to ≤ grade 1 toxicity, if continued treatment is warranted.

Management of specific toxicities:

Cardiac: QTcF >500 msec: Withhold dose until QTcF returns to <450 msec, then resume at a reduced dose

Diarrhea (severe): Withhold treatment until resolution. Dose reduction is recommended when treatment is resumed. Routine antidiarrheals are recommended. Closely monitor electrolytes and ECGs to detect QT prolongation resulting from dehydration.

Heart failure: May require discontinuation.

Hemorrhage (severe): Discontinue.

Hypertension: Initiate or adjust antihypertensive therapy as needed; may require vandetanib dosage adjustment or treatment interruption; discontinue permanently if blood pressure cannot be adequately controlled.

Interstitial lung disease (ILD)/pneumonitis: Interrupt therapy for acute or worsening pulmonary symptoms. Discontinue if ILD diagnosis is confirmed.

Ischemic cerebrovascular events (severe): Discontinue treatment (safety of resuming treatment after an ischemic event has not been studied).

Reversible posterior leukoencephalopathy syndrome (RPLS): Discontinue treatment.

Skin reactions: Withhold treatment for dermatologic toxicity of grade 3 or higher. Consider a reduced dose or permanent discontinuation upon improvement in symptoms. Consider permanent discontinuation for severe dermatologic toxicity. Mild-to-moderate toxicity has responded to corticosteroids (systemic or topical), oral antihistamines, and antibiotics (topical or systemic).

Combination Regimens

Thyroid cancer: Vandetanib (Thyroid Regimen) on page 2105

Administration May be administered with or without food. Missed doses should be omitted if within 12 hours of the next scheduled dose. Do not crush tablet. If unable to swallow tablet whole or if nasogastric or gastrostomy tube administration is necessary, disperse one tablet in 2 ounces of water (noncarbonated only) and stir for 10 minutes to disperse (will not dissolve completely) and administer immediately. Rinse residue in glass with additional 4 ounces of water (noncarbonated only) and administer.

Hazardous agent; use appropriate precautions for handling and disposal (NIOSH 2014 [group 1]).

Emetic Potential Low (10% to 30%)

Extemporaneous Preparations Hazardous agent: Use appropriate precautions for handling and disposal (NIOSH 2014 [group 1]).

An oral solution may be prepared using the tablet. Disperse one tablet in 2 ounces of water (noncarbonated only) and stir for 10 minutes to disperse (will not dissolve completely) and administer immediately. Rinse residue in glass with additional 4 ounces of water (noncarbonated only) and administer.

Monitoring Parameters Monitor electrolytes (calcium, magnesium, potassium), TSH, and ECG (QT interval) at baseline, at 2-4 weeks, at 8-12 weeks, and every 3 months thereafter; also monitor QT interval at same frequency for dose reduction due to QT interval or treatment delays >2 weeks (monitor electrolytes and ECG more frequently if diarrhea). Monitor renal function, hepatic function, blood pressure; monitor for signs and symptoms of heart failure, reversible posterior leukoencephalopathy syndrome (RPLS), pulmonary and skin toxicities

Dietary Considerations May be taken with or without food.

Prescribing and Access Restrictions As a requirement of the REMS program, access to vandetanib is restricted. Vandetanib is approved for marketing under a Food and Drug Administration (FDA) approved, risk management program, and through a restricted distribution program, the Vandetanib REMS Program (1-800-236-9933). Prescribers and pharmacies must be certified with the program to prescribe or dispense vandetanib.

In Canada, vandetanib is available only through the CAPRELSA Restricted Distribution Program. Prescribers and pharmacies must be certified with the program to prescribe or dispense vandetanib. Further information may be obtained at 1-800-668-6000.

Medication Guide Available Yes

Dosage Forms Excipient information presented when available (limited, particularly for generics); consult specific product labeling. [DSC] = Discontinued product
Tablet, Oral:
  Caprelsa: 100 mg, 300 mg
  Generic: 100 mg [DSC], 300 mg [DSC]

◆ **Van-Letrozole (Can)** see Letrozole on page 1019

◆ **Vantas** see Histrelin on page 816

◆ **Varubi** see Rolapitant on page 1492

◆ **Vascular Endothelial Growth Factor Trap** see Ziv-Aflibercept (Systemic) on page 1785

◆ **VDS** see Vindesine on page 1760

◆ **Vectibix** see Panitumumab on page 1316

◆ **VEGF Trap** see Ziv-Aflibercept (Systemic) on page 1785

◆ **VEGF Trap R1R2** see Ziv-Aflibercept (Systemic) on page 1785

◆ **Velban** see VinBLAStine on page 1740

◆ **Velcade** see Bortezomib on page 223

Vemurafenib (vem ue RAF e nib)

Related Information

Management of Chemotherapy-Induced Nausea and Vomiting in Adults *on page 2142*

Principles of Anticancer Therapy *on page 2261*

Safe Handling of Hazardous Drugs *on page 2292*

Brand Names: US Zelboraf

Brand Names: Canada Zelboraf

Index Terms BRAF(V600E) Kinase Inhibitor RO5185426; PLX4032; RG7204; RO5185426

Pharmacologic Category Antineoplastic Agent, BRAF Kinase Inhibitor

Use Melanoma:

US labeling: Treatment of unresectable or metastatic melanoma in patients with a BRAFV600E mutation (as detected by an approved test).

Canadian labeling: Treatment of unresectable or metastatic melanoma in patients with a BRAFV600 mutation (as identified by a validated test).

Limitations of use: Vemurafenib is not indicated in patients with wild-type BRAF melanoma.

Labeled Contraindications There are no contraindications listed in the manufacturer's labeling.

Canadian labeling: Hypersensitivity to vemurafenib or any component of the formulation.

Pregnancy Considerations Adverse effects were not demonstrated in animal reproduction studies. Based on the mechanism of action, vemurafenib may cause fetal harm if administered during pregnancy or in patients who become pregnant during treatment. Women of childbearing potential and men of reproductive potential should use adequate contraception methods during and for at least 2 months after treatment (Canadian labeling recommends during and for at least 6 months after treatment).

Breast-Feeding Considerations It is not known if vemurafenib is excreted in breast milk. Due to the potential for serious adverse reactions in the nursing infant, the manufacturer recommends a decision be made to discontinue nursing or to discontinue the drug, taking into account the importance of treatment to the mother.

Warnings/Precautions Hazardous agent - use appropriate precautions for handling and disposal (NIOSH 2014 [group 1]). Only patients with a BRAFV600 mutation-positive melanoma (including BRAFV600E) will benefit from treatment; mutation must be detected and confirmed by an approved test prior to treatment. The cobas 4800 BRAF V600 Mutation Test was used in clinical trials and is FDA-approved to detect BRAFV600E mutation.

Cutaneous squamous cell carcinomas (cuSCC), keratoacanthomas, and melanoma have been reported (at a higher rate in patients receiving vemurafenib compared to control). Cutaneous SCC generally occurs early in the treatment course (median onset: 7 to 8 weeks) and is managed with excision (while continuing vemurafenib treatment). Approximately one-third of patients experienced >1 cuSCC occurrence and the median time between occurrences was 6 weeks. Potential risk factors for cuSCC include age ≥65 years, history of skin cancer, or chronic sun exposure. Monitor for skin lesions (with dermatology evaluation) at baseline and every 2 months during treatment; consider continued monitoring for 6 months after treatment. Noncutaneous squamous cell carcinomas (SCC) of the head and neck have also been observed; monitor closely for signs/symptoms. Vemurafenib may promote malignancies correlated with RAS activation; monitor for signs/symptoms of other malignancies.

Dermatologic reactions have been observed, including case reports of Stevens-Johnson syndrome and toxic epidermal necrolysis; discontinue (permanently) for severe dermatologic toxicity. Photosensitivity ranging from mild to severe has been reported. Advise patients to avoid sun exposure and wear protective clothing and use effective UVA/UVB sunscreen and lip balm (SPF ≥30) when outdoors. Dosage modifications are recommended for intolerable photosensitivity consisting of erythema ≥10% to 30% of body surface area. Uveitis (including iritis), blurred vision, and photophobia may occur; monitor for signs and symptoms. Uveitis may be managed with corticosteroid and mydriatic eye drops. Retinal vein occlusion has been reported in clinical trials. Radiation sensitization and recall (some cases may be severe or involve cutaneous and visceral organs) have been reported in patients treated with radiation prior to, during, or after treatment with vemurafenib. Monitor closely when vemurafenib is administered concomitantly or sequentially with radiation treatment.

QT prolongation (dose-dependent) has been observed; may lead to increased risk for ventricular arrhythmia, including torsade de pointes. Monitor electrolytes (calcium, magnesium and potassium) at baseline and with dosage adjustments. Monitor ECG at baseline, 15 days after initiation, then monthly for 3 months, then every 3 months thereafter (more frequently if clinically appropriate); also monitor with dosage adjustments. Do not initiate treatment if baseline QTc >500 msec. During treatment, if QTc >500 msec, temporarily interrupt treatment; correct electrolytes and control other risk factors for QT prolongation. May reinitiate with a dose reduction once QTc falls to <500 msec. Discontinue (permanently), if after correction of risk factors, both the QTc continues to increase >500 msec and there is >60 msec change above baseline. Do not initiate treatment in patients with electrolyte abnormalities which are not correctable, long QT syndrome, or taking concomitant medication known to prolong the QT interval.

Liver injury has been reported with use, and may cause functional impairment such as coagulopathy or other organ dysfunction. Monitor transaminases, alkaline phosphatase and bilirubin at baseline and monthly during therapy, or as clinically necessary. May require dosage reduction, therapy interruption, or discontinuation. Anaphylaxis and severe hypersensitivity may occur during treatment or upon reinitiation. Serious reactions have included generalized rash, erythema, hypotension, and drug rash with eosinophilia and systemic symptoms (DRESS syndrome). Discontinue (permanently) with severe hypersensitivity reaction. Pancreatitis has been reported (case reports), with onset generally occurring within 2 weeks of initiation (Muluneh, 2013; Zelboraf Canadian product monograph, 2015); exacerbation of pancreatitis has also occurred upon rechallenge. Patients with unexplained abdominal pain should be promptly evaluated for pancreatitis (eg, serum lipase and amylase; abdominal CT) as clinically indicated. Elderly patients may be at increased risk for adverse effects; in clinical trials, there was an increased incidence of cuSCC and keratoacanthoma, atrial fibrillation, peripheral edema, and nausea/decreased appetite in patients ≥65 years of age. Potentially significant drug-drug interactions may exist, requiring dose or frequency adjustment, additional monitoring, and/or selection of alternative therapy.

◀ **Adverse Reactions**

>10%:

Cardiovascular: Peripheral edema (17% to 23%)

Central nervous system: Fatigue (38% to 54%; grade 3: 2% to 4%), headache (23% to 27%)

Dermatologic: Skin rash (37% to 52%; grade 3: 7% to 8%), skin photosensitivity (33% to 49%; grade 3: 3%), alopecia (36% to 45%), pruritus (23% to 30%; grade 3: 2%), hyperkeratosis (24% to 28%; actinic: 8% to 17%; seborrheic: 10% to 14%; pilaris: ≤10%), maculopapular rash (9% to 21%; grade 3: 2% to 6%), xeroderma (16% to 19%), sunburn (10% to 14%), erythema (8% to 14%), papular rash (5% to 13%)

Gastrointestinal: Nausea (35% to 37%; grade 3: 2%), diarrhea (28% to 29%; grade 3: <1%), vomiting (18% to 26%; grade 3: 1% to 2%), decreased appetite (18% to 21%), constipation (12% to 16%), dysgeusia (11% to 14%)

Hematologic & oncologic: Cutaneous papilloma (21% to 30%), squamous cell carcinoma of skin (24%; grade 3: 22% to 24%)

Hepatic: Increased gamma-glutamyl transferase (5% to 15%)

Neuromuscular & skeletal: Arthralgia (53% to 67%; grade 3: 4% to 8%), myalgia (13% to 24%; grade 3: <1%), limb pain (9% to 18%), back pain (8% to 11%; grade 3: <1%), musculoskeletal pain (8% to 11%), weakness (2% to 11%)

Respiratory: Cough (8% to 12%)

Miscellaneous: Fever (17% to 19%)

1% to 10%:

Cardiovascular: Atrial fibrillation, hypotension, prolonged Q-T interval on ECG, retinal vein occlusion, vasculitis

Central nervous system: Cranial nerve palsy (facial), dizziness, peripheral neuropathy

Dermatologic: Erythema nodosum, folliculitis, palmar-plantar erythrodysesthesia, Stevens-Johnson syndrome, toxic epidermal necrolysis

Endocrine & metabolic: Weight loss

Hematologic & oncologic: Basal cell carcinoma, malignant melanoma (new primary), squamous cell carcinoma (oropharyngeal)

Hepatic: Increased serum alkaline phosphatase, increased serum ALT, increased serum AST, increased serum bilirubin

Hypersensitivity: Anaphylaxis, hypersensitivity

Neuromuscular & skeletal: Arthritis

Ophthalmic: Blurred vision, iritis, photophobia, uveitis

Renal: Increased serum creatinine

<1%, postmarketing, and/or case reports: Chronic myelomonocytic leukemia with NRAS mutation (progression of preexisting condition), drug reaction with eosinophilia and systemic symptoms (DRESS syndrome), febrile neutropenia, hepatic failure, neutropenia, pancreatitis, panniculitis, recall skin sensitization

Drug Interactions

Metabolism/Transport Effects Substrate of BCRP, CYP3A4 (major), P-glycoprotein; **Note:** Assignment of Major/Minor substrate status based on clinically relevant drug interaction potential; **Inhibits** BCRP, CYP1A2 (moderate), CYP2D6 (weak), P-glycoprotein; **Induces** CYP3A4 (weak)

Avoid Concomitant Use

Avoid concomitant use of Vemurafenib with any of the following: Bosutinib; Conivaptan; CYP3A4 Inducers (Strong); CYP3A4 Inhibitors (Strong); Fusidic Acid (Systemic); Highest Risk QTc-Prolonging Agents; Idelalisib; Ivabradine;

Mifepristone; Moderate Risk QTc-Prolonging Agents; PAZOPanib; Silodosin; TiZANidine; Topotecan; VinCRIStine (Liposomal)

Increased Effect/Toxicity

Vemurafenib may increase the levels/effects of: Afatinib; Bosutinib; Brentuximab Vedotin; Colchicine; CYP1A2 Substrates; Dabigatran Etexilate; Digoxin; DOXOrubicin (Conventional); Edoxaban; Everolimus; Highest Risk QTc-Prolonging Agents; Ledipasvir; Naloxegol; PAZOPanib; P-glycoprotein/ABCB1 Substrates; Pirfenidone; Porfimer; Prucalopride; Rifaximin; Silodosin; TiZANidine; Topotecan; Verteporfin; VinCRIStine (Liposomal); Warfarin

The levels/effects of Vemurafenib may be increased by: Aprepitant; Conivaptan; CYP3A4 Inhibitors (Moderate); CYP3A4 Inhibitors (Strong); Fosaprepitant; Fusidic Acid (Systemic); Idelalisib; Ipilimumab; Ivabradine; Ivacaftor; Luliconazole; Mifepristone; Moderate Risk QTc-Prolonging Agents; Netupitant; Palbociclib; P-glycoprotein/ABCB1 Inhibitors; QTc-Prolonging Agents (Indeterminate Risk and Risk Modifying); Simeprevir; Stiripentol

Decreased Effect

Vemurafenib may decrease the levels/effects of: ARIPiprazole; Hydrocodone; NiMODipine; Saxagliptin

The levels/effects of Vemurafenib may be decreased by: Bosentan; CYP3A4 Inducers (Moderate); CYP3A4 Inducers (Strong); Dabrafenib; Deferasirox; P-glycoprotein/ABCB1 Inducers; Siltuximab; St Johns Wort; Tocilizumab

Storage/Stability Store at room temperature of 20°C to 25°C (68°F to 77°F); excursions permitted to 15°C and 30°C (59°F and 86°F). Store in the original container with the lid tightly closed.

Mechanism of Action BRAF kinase inhibitor (potent) which inhibits tumor growth in melanomas by inhibiting kinase activity of certain mutated forms of BRAF, including BRAF with V600E mutation, thereby blocking cellular proliferation in melanoma cells with the mutation. Does not have activity against cells with wild-type BRAF. BRAFV600E activating mutations are present in ~50% of melanomas; V600E mutation involves the substitution of glutamic acid for valine at amino acid 600. The cobas 4800 BRAF V600 mutation test is approved to detect BRAFV600E mutation.

Pharmacodynamics/Kinetics

Distribution: V_d: ~106 L

Protein binding: >99%, to albumin and α_1-acid glycoprotein

Half-life, elimination: 57 hours (range: 30 to 120 hours)

Time to peak: ~3 hours

Excretion: Feces (~94%); urine (~1%)

Dosing

Adult & Geriatric

US labeling: **Melanoma, metastatic or unresectable (with BRAFV600E mutation):** Oral: 960 mg every 12 hours; continue until disease progression or unacceptable toxicity.

Canadian labeling: **Melanoma, metastatic or unresectable (with BRAFV600 mutation):** Oral: 960 mg twice daily; continue until disease progression or unacceptable toxicity.

Missed doses: A missed dose may be taken up to 4 hours prior to the next scheduled dose. If it is within 4 hours of the next scheduled dose, administer the next dose at the regular schedule. If vomiting occurs after a dose is taken, do not take an additional dose; continue with the next scheduled dose.

◄ **Renal Impairment**
US labeling:
Mild to moderate impairment (preexisting): No dosage adjustment necessary.
Severe impairment (preexisting): There are no dosage adjustments provided in the manufacturer's labeling (data are insufficient to determine if dosage adjustment is necessary); use with caution.
Canadian labeling: There are no dosage adjustments provided in the manufacturer's labeling.

Hepatic Impairment
Mild to moderate impairment (preexisting): No dosage adjustment necessary.
Severe impairment (preexisting): There are no dosage adjustments provided in manufacturer's labeling (data are insufficient to determine if dosage adjustment is necessary); use with caution.
Hepatotoxicity/lab abnormalities during treatment: Refer to Dosage Adjustment for Toxicity and manage with dose reduction, treatment interruption, or discontinuation.

Adjustment for Toxicity Note: Do not dose reduce below 480 mg twice daily. NCI Common Terminology Criteria for Adverse Events (CTC-AE) version 4.0 used for adverse event grades.
Grade 1 or grade 2 (tolerable) toxicity: No dosage adjustment recommended.
Grade 2 (intolerable) or grade 3 toxicity:
First incident: Interrupt treatment until toxicity returns to grade 0 or 1, then resume at 720 mg twice daily
Second incident: Interrupt treatment until toxicity returns to grade 0 or 1, then resume at 480 mg twice daily
Third incident: Discontinue permanently.
Grade 4 toxicity:
First incident: Interrupt treatment until toxicity returns to grade 0 or 1, then resume at 480 mg twice daily **or** discontinue permanently
Second incident: Discontinue permanently.
Specific toxicities:
Severe hypersensitivity or severe dermatologic toxicity: Discontinue permanently.
QTc interval changes:
US labeling:
QTc >500 msec (grade ≥3): Temporarily withhold treatment, correct electrolytes and control risk factors for QT prolongation; may reinitiate with a dose reduction once QTc ≤500 msec.
QTc persistently >500 msec and >60 msec above baseline: Discontinue permanently.
Canadian labeling:
QTc >500 msec during treatment and ≤60 msec change from baseline:
First incident: Interrupt treatment until QTc <500 msec, then resume at 720 mg twice daily or 480 mg twice daily if dose previously reduced.
Second incident: Interrupt treatment until QTc <500 msec, then resume at 480 mg twice daily or discontinue permanently if dose previously reduced to 480 mg twice daily.
Third incident: Discontinue permanently.
QTc >500 msec during treatment and >60 msec above baseline: Discontinue permanently.

Combination Regimens

Melanoma: Vemurafenib (Melanoma Regimen) on page 2107

Administration Doses should be administered orally in the morning and evening, ~12 hours apart. May be taken with or without a meal. If vomiting occurs after a dose is taken, do not take an additional dose; continue with the next scheduled dose.

Swallow whole with a glass of water; do not crush or chew. There are case reports of vemurafenib administration after crushing (Janson, 2013; Khimani, 2014), however vemurafenib is nearly insoluble in water and is manufactured as a microprecipitated bulk powder core (to improve solubility/bioavailability) within a film coated tablet (Shah, 2013). Pharmacokinetics and efficacy of administration other than swallowing tablets whole have not been determined.

Hazardous agent; use appropriate precautions for handling and disposal (NIOSH 2014 [group 1]). Although crushing of the tablets is not recommended, if it is necessary to manipulate tablets, it is recommended to double glove, wear a protective gown, and prepare in a controlled device (NIOSH 2014).

Emetic Potential Minimal (<10%)

Monitoring Parameters Liver transaminases, alkaline phosphatase and bilirubin at baseline and monthly during treatment (or as clinically appropriate). Electrolytes (calcium, magnesium and potassium) at baseline and after dosage modification. ECG at baseline, 15 days after initiation, then monthly for 3 months, then every 3 months thereafter (more frequently if clinically appropriate) and with dosage adjustments. Dermatology evaluation (for new skin lesions) at baseline and every 2 months during treatment; also consider continued monitoring for 6 months after completion of treatment. Signs/symptoms of hypersensitivity reactions, uveitis, and malignancies; signs of radiation sensitization and recall.

Prescribing and Access Restrictions Available through specialty pharmacies. Further information may be obtained from the manufacturer, Genentech, at 1-888-249-4918, or at http://www.zelboraf.com.

Medication Guide Available Yes

Dosage Forms Excipient information presented when available (limited, particularly for generics); consult specific product labeling.

Tablet, Oral:

Zelboraf: 240 mg

- ◆ **Venofer** see Iron Sucrose on page 968
- ◆ **VePesid** see Etoposide on page 641
- ◆ **Vepesid (Can)** see Etoposide on page 641
- ◆ **Veripred 20** see PrednisoLONE (Systemic) on page 1421
- ◆ **Vesanoid** see Tretinoin (Systemic) on page 1692
- ◆ **Vfend** see Voriconazole on page 1775
- ◆ **VFEND (Can)** see Voriconazole on page 1775
- ◆ **Vfend IV** see Voriconazole on page 1775
- ◆ **VFEND For Injection (Can)** see Voriconazole on page 1775
- ◆ **Vidaza** see AzaCITIDine on page 161

VinBLAStine (vin BLAS teen)

Related Information

Management of Chemotherapy-Induced Nausea and Vomiting in Adults *on page 2142*

Management of Drug Extravasations *on page 2159*

Prevention of Chemotherapy-Induced Nausea and Vomiting in Children *on page 2203*

Safe Handling of Hazardous Drugs *on page 2292*

Brand Names: Canada Vinblastine Sulphate Injection

Index Terms Velban; Vinblastine Sulfate; Vincaleukoblastine; VLB

Pharmacologic Category Antineoplastic Agent, Antimicrotubular; Antineoplastic Agent, Vinca Alkaloid

Use Treatment of Hodgkin lymphoma; lymphocytic lymphoma; histiocytic lymphoma; mycosis fungoides; testicular cancer; Kaposi sarcoma; histiocytosis X (Letterer-Siwe disease); has also been used for the treatment of refractory/resistant breast cancer and choriocarcinoma

Labeled Contraindications Significant granulocytopenia (unless as a result of condition being treated); presence of bacterial infection

Pregnancy Considerations Adverse effects were observed in animal reproduction studies. May cause fetal harm if administered during pregnancy. Women of childbearing potential should avoid becoming pregnant during vinblastine treatment. Aspermia has been reported in males who have received treatment with vinblastine.

Breast-Feeding Considerations It is not known if vinblastine is excreted in breast milk. Due to the potential for serious adverse reactions in the nursing infant, a decision should be made whether to discontinue vinblastine or to discontinue breast-feeding, taking into account the importance of treatment to the mother.

Warnings/Precautions Hazardous agent - use appropriate precautions for handling and disposal (NIOSH 2014 [group 1]). Avoid eye contamination (exposure may cause severe irritation). **[US Boxed Warning]: For IV use only. Intrathecal administration may result in death.** To prevent administration errors, the Institute for Safe Medication Practices (ISMP) Targeted Medication Safety Best Practices for Hospitals initiative strongly recommends dispensing vinblastine diluted in a minibag (ISMP, 2014). **If not dispensed in a minibag, affix an auxiliary label stating "For intravenous use only - fatal if given by other routes" and also place in an overwrap labeled "Do not remove covering until moment of injection."** Vinblastine should **NOT** be prepared during the preparation of any intrathecal medications. After preparation, keep vinblastine in a location **away** from the separate storage location recommended for intrathecal medications. Vinblastine should **NOT** be delivered to the patient at the same time with any medications intended for central nervous system administration.

[US Boxed Warning]: Vinblastine is a vesicant; ensure proper needle or catheter placement prior to and during infusion. Avoid extravasation. Extravasation may cause significant irritation. Individuals administering should be experienced in vinblastine administration. If extravasation occurs, discontinue immediately and initiate appropriate extravasation management, including local injection of hyaluronidase and moderate heat application to the affected area. Use a separate vein to complete administration.

Leukopenia commonly occurs; granulocytopenia may be severe with higher doses. The leukocyte nadir generally occurs 5 to 10 days after administration; recovery typically occurs 7 to 14 days later. Monitor for infections if WBC <2,000/mm³. Leukopenia may be more pronounced in cachectic patients and patients with skin ulceration and may be less pronounced with lower doses used for maintenance therapy. Leukocytes and platelets may fall considerably with moderate doses when marrow is infiltrated with malignant cells (further use in this situation is not recommended). Thrombocytopenia and anemia may occur rarely.

May rarely cause disabling neurotoxicity; usually reversible. Seizures and severe and permanent CNS damage has occurred with higher then recommended doses and/or when administered more frequently than recommended. Acute shortness of breath and severe bronchospasm have been reported, most often in association with concurrent administration of mitomycin; may occur within minutes to several hours following vinblastine administration or up to 14 days following mitomycin administration; use caution in patients with preexisting pulmonary disease. Use with caution in patients with hepatic impairment; toxicity may be increased; may require dosage modification. Use with caution in patients with ischemic heart disease. Stomatitis may occur (rare); may be disabling, but is usually reversible.

Potentially significant drug-drug interactions may exist, requiring dose or frequency adjustment, additional monitoring, and/or selection of alternative therapy. **[US Boxed Warning]: Should be administered under the supervision of an experienced cancer chemotherapy physician.**

Benzyl alcohol and derivatives: Some dosage forms may contain benzyl alcohol; large amounts of benzyl alcohol (≥99 mg/kg/day) have been associated with a potentially fatal toxicity ("gasping syndrome") in neonates; the "gasping syndrome" consists of metabolic acidosis, respiratory distress, gasping respirations, CNS dysfunction (including convulsions, intracranial hemorrhage), hypotension, and cardiovascular collapse (AAP ["Inactive" 1997]; CDC, 1982); some data suggests that benzoate displaces bilirubin from protein binding sites (Ahlfors, 2001); avoid or use dosage forms containing benzyl alcohol with caution in neonates. See manufacturer's labeling.

Adverse Reactions Frequency not defined.
Common:
Cardiovascular: Hypertension
Central nervous system: Malaise
Dermatologic: Alopecia
Gastrointestinal: Constipation
Hematologic: Myelosuppression, leukopenia/granulocytopenia (nadir: 5-10 days; recovery: 7-14 days; dose-limiting toxicity)
Neuromuscular & skeletal: Bone pain, jaw pain, tumor pain
Less common:
Cardiovascular: Angina, cerebrovascular accident, coronary ischemia, ECG abnormalities, limb ischemia, MI, myocardial ischemia, Raynaud's phenomenon
Central nervous system: Depression, dizziness, headache, neurotoxicity (duration: >24 hours), seizure, vertigo

Dermatologic: Dermatitis, photosensitivity (rare), rash, skin blistering

Endocrine & metabolic: Aspermia, hyperuricemia, SIADH

Gastrointestinal: Abdominal pain, anorexia, diarrhea, gastrointestinal bleeding, hemorrhagic enterocolitis, ileus, metallic taste, nausea (mild), paralytic ileus, rectal bleeding, stomatitis, toxic megacolon, vomiting (mild)

Genitourinary: Urinary retention

Hematologic: Anemia, thrombocytopenia (recovery within a few days), thrombotic thrombocytopenic purpura

Local: Cellulitis (with extravasation), irritation, phlebitis (with extravasation), radiation recall

Neuromuscular & skeletal: Deep tendon reflex loss, myalgia, paresthesia, peripheral neuritis, weakness

Ocular: Nystagmus

Otic: Auditory damage, deafness, vestibular damage

Renal: Hemolytic uremic syndrome

Respiratory: Bronchospasm, dyspnea, pharyngitis

Drug Interactions

Metabolism/Transport Effects Substrate of CYP2D6 (minor), CYP3A4 (major), P-glycoprotein; **Note:** Assignment of Major/Minor substrate status based on clinically relevant drug interaction potential; **Inhibits** CYP2D6 (weak); **Induces** P-glycoprotein

Avoid Concomitant Use

Avoid concomitant use of VinBLAStine with any of the following: BCG (Intravesical); CloZAPine; Conivaptan; Dabigatran Etexilate; Dipyrone; Fusidic Acid (Systemic); Idelalisib; Ledipasvir; Natalizumab; Pimecrolimus; Sofosbuvir; Tacrolimus (Topical); Tofacitinib; Vaccines (Live); VinCRIStine (Liposomal)

Increased Effect/Toxicity

VinBLAStine may increase the levels/effects of: ARIPiprazole; CloZAPine; Fingolimod; Leflunomide; MitoMYcin (Systemic); Natalizumab; Tofacitinib; Tolterodine; Vaccines (Live)

The levels/effects of VinBLAStine may be increased by: Aprepitant; Conivaptan; CYP3A4 Inhibitors (Moderate); CYP3A4 Inhibitors (Strong); Dasatinib; Denosumab; Dipyrone; Fosaprepitant; Fusidic Acid (Systemic); Idelalisib; Itraconazole; Ivacaftor; Lopinavir; Luliconazole; Macrolide Antibiotics; MAO Inhibitors; Mifepristone; Netupitant; Osimertinib; Palbociclib; P-glycoprotein/ABCB1 Inhibitors; Pimecrolimus; Posaconazole; Ranolazine; Ritonavir; Roflumilast; Simeprevir; Stiripentol; Tacrolimus (Topical); Trastuzumab; Voriconazole

Decreased Effect

VinBLAStine may decrease the levels/effects of: Afatinib; BCG (Intravesical); Brentuximab Vedotin; Coccidioides immitis Skin Test; Dabigatran Etexilate; DOXOrubicin (Conventional); Ledipasvir; Linagliptin; P-glycoprotein/ABCB1 Substrates; Sipuleucel-T; Sofosbuvir; Vaccines (Inactivated); Vaccines (Live); VinCRIStine (Liposomal)

The levels/effects of VinBLAStine may be decreased by: Bosentan; CYP3A4 Inducers (Moderate); CYP3A4 Inducers (Strong); Dabrafenib; Deferasirox; Echinacea; Enzalutamide; Mitotane; Osimertinib; P-glycoprotein/ABCB1 Inducers; Siltuximab; St Johns Wort; Tocilizumab

Storage/Stability Note: Dispense in an overwrap which bears the statement "Do not remove covering until the moment of injection. Fatal if given intrathecally. For IV use only." If dispensing in a syringe (minibag is preferred) should be labeled: "Fatal if given intrathecally. For IV use only."

Store intact vials under refrigeration at 2°C to 8°C (36°F to 46°F). Protect from light.

Preparation for Administration Hazardous agent; use appropriate precautions for handling and disposal (NIOSH 2014 [group 1]). For infusion, may dilute in 25 to 50 mL NS or D$_5$W; dilution in larger volumes (≥100 mL) of IV fluids is not recommended. **Note:** In order to prevent inadvertent intrathecal administration, the Institute for Safe Medication Practices (ISMP) strongly recommends dispensing vinblastine in a minibag (**NOT** in a syringe).

Mechanism of Action Vinblastine binds to tubulin and inhibits microtubule formation, therefore, arresting the cell at metaphase by disrupting the formation of the mitotic spindle; it is specific for the M and S phases. Vinblastine may also interfere with nucleic acid and protein synthesis by blocking glutamic acid utilization.

Pharmacodynamics/Kinetics

Metabolism: Hepatic (via CYP3A) to active metabolite

Half-life elimination: Terminal: ~25 hours

Excretion: Feces (30% to 36%); urine (12% to 17%)

Dosing

Adult & Geriatric Note: Frequency and duration of therapy may vary by indication, concomitant combination chemotherapy and hematologic response. **For IV use only.** In order to prevent inadvertent intrathecal administration, the Institute for Safe Medication Practices (ISMP) strongly recommends dispensing vinblastine in a minibag (**NOT** a syringe).

Hodgkin lymphoma, lymphocytic lymphoma, histiocytic lymphoma, mycosis fungoides, testicular cancer, Kaposi sarcoma, histiocytosis X (Letterer-Siwe disease): *Manufacturer's labeling:* IV: 3.7 mg/m^2; adjust dose every 7 days (based on white blood cell response) up to 5.5 mg/m^2 (second dose); 7.4 mg/m^2 (third dose); 9.25 mg/m^2 (fourth dose); and 11.1 mg/m^2 (fifth dose); do not administer more frequently than every 7 days. Usual dosage range: 5.5 to 7.4 mg/m^2 every 7 days; Maximum dose: 18.5 mg/m^2; dosage adjustment goal is to reduce white blood cell count to ~3,000/mm^3

Off-label and/or indication-specific dosing:

Hodgkin lymphoma (off-label dosing): IV:

ABVD regimen: 6 mg/m^2 days 1 and 15 of a 28-day cycle (in combination with doxorubicin, bleomycin, and dacarbazine) for 2 cycles (early/favorable disease) or for 4 cycles (unfavorable disease) (Eich, 2010; Engert, 2007)

Stanford V regimen: 6 mg/m^2 weeks 1, 3, 5, 7, 9, and 11 (in combination with doxorubicin, mechlorethamine, vincristine, bleomycin, etoposide, and prednisone) (Bartlett, 1995; Horning, 2002)

Testicular cancer (off-label dosing): VelP regimen: IV: 0.11 mg/kg daily for 2 days every 21 days (in combination with ifosfamide, cisplatin, and mesna) for 4 cycles (Loehrer, 1988; Loehrer, 1988 [correction]; Loehrer, 1998)

◄ **Bladder cancer (off-label use):** IV:

Metastatic disease:

Dose-dense MVAC regimen: 3 mg/m^2 day 2 every 14 days (in combination with methotrexate, doxorubicin, and cisplatin) until disease progression or unacceptable toxicity (Sternberg, 2001; Sternberg, 2006)

MVAC regimen: 3 mg/m^2 days 2, 15, and 22 every 28 days (in combination with methotrexate, doxorubicin, and cisplatin) for up to 6 cycles (von der Maase, 2000) **or** 3 mg/m^2 days 2, 15, and 22 every 28 days (in combination with methotrexate, doxorubicin, and cisplatin) until disease progression or unacceptable toxicity (Sternberg, 2001; Sternberg, 2006) **or** 3 mg/m^2 days 1, 15, and 22 every 28 days (in combination with methotrexate, doxorubicin, and cisplatin) for up to 6 cycles (Bamias, 2004)

Neoadjuvant treatment:

MVAC regimen: 3 mg/m^2 days 2, 15, and 22 every 28 days (in combination with methotrexate, doxorubicin, and cisplatin) for 3 cycles (Grossman, 2003)

CMV regimen: 4 mg/m^2 days 1 and 8 every 21 days (in combination with methotrexate, cisplatin, and leucovorin) for 3 cycles (Griffiths, 2011)

Melanoma, metastatic (off-label use): IV:

CVD regimen: 2 mg/m^2 days 1 to 4 and 22 to 25 of a 6-week treatment cycle (in combination with cisplatin and dacarbazine); may repeat if tumor response (Eton, 2002)

CVD + immunotherapy regimen: 1.5 mg/m^2 days 1 to 4 and 22 to 25 of a 6-week treatment cycle (in combination with cisplatin, dacarbazine, aldesleukin, and interferon alfa-2b); may repeat if tumor response (Eton, 2002)

Non-small cell lung cancer (off-label use): IV:

Adjuvant treatment after complete resection: 4 mg/m^2 days 1, 8, 15, 22, and 29, then every 2 weeks (in combination with cisplatin) until last cisplatin dose (Arriagada, 2004)

Concurrent radiation: 5 mg/m^2 days 1, 8, 15, 22, and 29 (in combination with cisplatin and concurrent radiation therapy) (Curran, 2011)

Soft tissue sarcoma (desmoid tumors, aggressive fibromatosis), advanced (off-label use): IV: 6 mg/m^2 every 7 to 10 days (dose usually rounded to 10 mg) in combination with methotrexate for 1 year (Azzarelli, 2001)

Pediatric Note: Frequency and duration of therapy may vary by indication, concomitant combination chemotherapy and hematologic response. **For IV use only.** In order to prevent inadvertent intrathecal administration, the Institute for Safe Medication Practices (ISMP) strongly recommends dispensing vinblastine in a minibag (**NOT** a syringe).

Hodgkin lymphoma: IV: Initial dose: 6 mg/m^2; do not administer more frequently than every 7 days **or** ABVD regimen (off-label dosing): IV: 6 mg/m^2 days 1 and 15 of a 28-day cycle (in combination with doxorubicin, bleomycin, and dacarbazine) for 6 cycles (Hutchinson, 1998)

Letterer-Siwe disease: IV: Initial dose: 6.5 mg/m^2; do not administer more frequently than every 7 days

Testicular cancer: IV: Initial dose: 3 mg/m^2; do not administer more frequently than every 7 days

Renal Impairment No dosage adjustment necessary.

Hepatic Impairment

The manufacturer's labeling recommends the following adjustment: Serum bilirubin >3 mg/dL: Administer 50% of dose

The following adjustments have also been recommended (Floyd, 2006; Superfin, 2007):

Serum bilirubin 1.5 to 3 mg/dL or transaminases 2 to 3 times ULN: Administer 50% of dose

Serum bilirubin >3 times ULN: Avoid use.

Obesity *ASCO Guidelines for appropriate chemotherapy dosing in obese adults with cancer:* Utilize patient's actual body weight (full weight) for calculation of body surface area- or weight-based dosing, particularly when the intent of therapy is curative; manage regimen-related toxicities in the same manner as for nonobese patients; if a dose reduction is utilized due to toxicity, consider resumption of full weight-based dosing with subsequent cycles, especially if cause of toxicity (eg, hepatic or renal impairment) is resolved (Griggs, 2012).

Combination Regimens

Bladder cancer:

CMV (Bladder) on page 1920

Dose Dense MVAC (Bladder Cancer) on page 1948

MVAC (Bladder) on page 2042

Lung cancer (non-small cell): Cisplatin-Vinblastine (NSCLC) on page 1913

Lymphoma, Hodgkin:

ABVD Early Stage (Hodgkin) on page 1820

ABVD (Hodgkin) on page 1821

ChlVPP (Hodgkin) on page 1886

C-MOPP/ABV Hybrid (Hodgkin) on page 1919

MOPP/ABVD (Hodgkin) on page 2039

MOPP/ABV Hybrid (Hodgkin) on page 2040

Stanford V (Hodgkin) on page 2085

VAMP (Hodgkin) on page 2104

Vinblastine (Hodgkin Regimen) on page 2107

Melanoma:

Cisplatin-Vinblastine-Dacarbazine (Melanoma) on page 1912

CVD-Interleukin-Interferon (Melanoma) on page 1926

Soft tissue sarcoma: Methotrexate-Vinblastine (Soft Tissue Sarcoma) on page 2036

Testicular cancer: VeIP (Testicular) on page 2106

Administration In order to prevent inadvertent intrathecal administration, the Institute for Safe Medication Practices (ISMP) strongly recommends dispensing vinblastine in a minibag (NOT in a syringe). For IV administration only. **Fatal if given intrathecally.** The preferred administration is as a short infusion in a 25 to 50 mL minibag. If administration via a minibag is not possible, may also be administered as an undiluted 1-minute infusion into a free flowing IV line to prevent venous irritation/extravasation. Prolonged administration times (≥30 to 60 minutes) and/or increased administration volumes may increase the risk of vein irritation and extravasation.

Vesicant; ensure proper needle or catheter placement prior to and during infusion. Avoid extravasation.

Extravasation management: If extravasation occurs, stop infusion immediately and disconnect (leave cannula/needle in place); gently aspirate extravasated solution (do **NOT** flush the line); initiate hyaluronidase antidote; remove needle/cannula; apply dry warm compresses for 20 minutes 4 times a day for 1-2 days; elevate extremity (Perez Fidalgo, 2012). Remaining portion of the vinblastine dose should be infused through a separate vein.

Hyaluronidase: If needle/cannula still in place, administer 1-6 mL hyaluronidase (150 units/mL) into the existing IV line; the usual dose is 1 mL hyaluronidase for each 1 mL of extravasated drug (Perez Fidalgo, 2012; Schulmeister, 2011). If needle/cannula was removed, inject 1-6 mL (150 units/mL) subcutaneously in a clockwise manner using 1 mL for each 1 mL of drug extravasated (Schulmeister, 2011) **or** administer 1 mL (150 units/mL) as 5 separate 0.2 mL injections (using a 25-gauge needle) subcutaneously into the extravasation site (Polovich, 2009).

Hazardous agent; use appropriate precautions for handling and disposal (NIOSH 2014 [group 1]).

Vesicant/Extravasation Risk Vesicant

Emetic Potential Children and Adults: Minimal (<10%)

Monitoring Parameters CBC with differential and platelet count, serum uric acid, hepatic function tests

Dosage Forms Excipient information presented when available (limited, particularly for generics); consult specific product labeling.
Solution, Intravenous, as sulfate:
  Generic: 1 mg/mL (10 mL)
Solution Reconstituted, Intravenous, as sulfate:
  Generic: 10 mg (1 ea)

◆ **Vinblastine Sulfate** *see* VinBLAStine *on page 1740*
◆ **Vinblastine Sulphate Injection (Can)** *see* VinBLAStine *on page 1740*
◆ **Vincaleukoblastine** *see* VinBLAStine *on page 1740*
◆ **Vincasar PFS** *see* VinCRIStine *on page 1746*

VinCRIStine (vin KRIS teen)

Related Information
Chemotherapy and Cancer Treatment During Pregnancy *on page 2214*
Chemotherapy and Obesity *on page 2220*
Chronic Pain Management (Cancer) *on page 2229*
Management of Chemotherapy-Induced Nausea and Vomiting in Adults *on page 2142*
Management of Drug Extravasations *on page 2159*
Prevention of Chemotherapy-Induced Nausea and Vomiting in Children *on page 2203*
Safe Handling of Hazardous Drugs *on page 2292*

Brand Names: US Vincasar PFS

Brand Names: Canada Vincristine Sulfate Injection; Vincristine Sulfate Injection USP

Index Terms Conventional Vincristine; Leurocristine Sulfate; Oncovin; Vincristine (Conventional); Vincristine Sulfate

Pharmacologic Category Antineoplastic Agent, Antimicrotubular; Antineoplastic Agent, Vinca Alkaloid

Use Treatment of acute lymphocytic leukemia (ALL), Hodgkin lymphoma, non-Hodgkin lymphomas, Wilms' tumor, neuroblastoma, rhabdomyosarcoma

Labeled Contraindications Patients with the demyelinating form of Charcot-Marie-Tooth syndrome

Pregnancy Considerations Animal reproduction studies have demonstrated teratogenicity and fetal loss. May cause fetal harm if administered during pregnancy. Women of childbearing potential should avoid becoming pregnant during treatment.

Breast-Feeding Considerations It is not known if vincristine is excreted in breast milk. Due to the potential for serious adverse reactions in the nursing infant, the decision to discontinue vincristine or to discontinue breast-feeding should take into account the benefits of treatment to the mother.

Warnings/Precautions Hazardous agent - use appropriate precautions for handling and disposal (NIOSH 2014 [group 1]); avoid eye contamination.

[U.S. Boxed Warning]: For IV administration only; inadvertent intrathecal administration usually results in death. To prevent administration errors, the Institute for Safe Medication Practices (ISMP) Targeted Medication Safety Best Practices for Hospitals initiative and the World Health Organization strongly recommend dispensing vincristine diluted in a minibag (ISMP, 2014; WHO, 2007), **if not dispensed in a minibag, affix an auxiliary label stating "For intravenous use only - fatal if given by other routes" and also place in an overwrap labeled "Do not remove covering until moment of injection."** Vincristine should **NOT** be prepared during the preparation of any intrathecal medications. After preparation, keep vincristine in a location **away** from the separate storage location recommended for intrathecal medications. Vincristine should **NOT** be delivered to the patient at the same time with any medications intended for central nervous system administration.

[U.S. Boxed Warning]: Vincristine is a vesicant; ensure proper needle or catheter placement prior to and during infusion. Avoid extravasation. Individuals administering should be experienced in vincristine administration. Extravasation may cause significant irritation. If extravasation occurs, discontinue immediately and initiate appropriate extravasation management, including local injection of hyaluronidase and moderate heat application to the affected area. Use a separate vein to complete administration.

Neurotoxicity, including alterations in mental status such as depression, confusion, or insomnia may occur; neurologic effects are dose-limiting (may require dosage reduction) and may be additive with those of other neurotoxic agents and spinal cord irradiation. Use with caution in patients with preexisting neuromuscular disease and/or with concomitant neurotoxic agents. Constipation, paralytic ileus, intestinal necrosis and/or perforation may occur; constipation may present as upper colon impaction with an empty rectum (may require flat film of abdomen for diagnosis); generally responds to high enemas and laxatives. All patients should be on a prophylactic bowel management regimen.

Potentially significant drug-drug interactions may exist, requiring dose or frequency adjustment, additional monitoring, and/or selection of alternative therapy. Acute shortness of breath and severe bronchospasm have been reported with vinca alkaloids, usually when used in combination with mitomycin. Onset may be several minutes to hours after vincristine administration and up to 2 weeks after mitomycin. Progressive dyspnea may occur. Permanently discontinue vincristine if pulmonary dysfunction occurs.

◄ Use with caution in patients with hepatic impairment; dosage modification required. May be associated with hepatic sinusoidal obstruction syndrome (SOS; formerly called veno-occlusive disease), increased risk in children <3 years of age; use with caution in hepatobiliary dysfunction. Monitor for signs or symptoms of hepatic SOS, including bilirubin >1.4 mg/dL, unexplained weight gain, ascites, hepatomegaly, or unexplained right upper quadrant pain (Arndt, 2004). Acute uric acid nephropathy has been reported with vincristine. Use with caution in the elderly; may cause or exacerbate syndrome of inappropriate antidiuretic hormone secretion or hyponatremia; monitor sodium closely with initiation or dosage adjustments in older adults (Beers Criteria).

Adverse Reactions Frequency not defined.

Cardiovascular: Edema, hyper-/hypotension, MI, myocardial ischemia

Central nervous system: Ataxia, coma, cranial nerve dysfunction (auditory damage, extraocular muscle impairment, laryngeal muscle impairment, paralysis, paresis, vestibular damage, vocal cord paralysis), dizziness, fever, headache, neurotoxicity (dose-related), neuropathic pain (common), seizure, vertigo

Dermatologic toxicity: Alopecia (common), rash

Endocrine & metabolic: Hyperuricemia, parotid pain, SIADH (rare)

Gastrointestinal: Abdominal cramps, abdominal pain, anorexia, constipation (common), diarrhea, intestinal necrosis, intestinal perforation, nausea, oral ulcers, paralytic ileus, vomiting, weight loss

Genitourinary: Bladder atony, dysuria, polyuria, urinary retention

Hematologic: Anemia (mild), leukopenia (mild), thrombocytopenia (mild), thrombotic thrombocytopenic purpura

Hepatic: Hepatic sinusoidal obstruction syndrome (SOS; veno-occlusive liver disease)

Local: Phlebitis, tissue irritation/necrosis (if infiltrated)

Neuromuscular & skeletal: Back pain, bone pain, deep tendon reflex loss, difficulty walking, foot drop, gait changes, jaw pain, limb pain, motor difficulties, muscle wasting, myalgia, paralysis, paresthesia, peripheral neuropathy (common), sensorimotor dysfunction, sensory loss

Ocular: Cortical blindness (transient), nystagmus, optic atrophy with blindness

Otic: Deafness

Renal: Acute uric acid nephropathy, hemolytic uremic syndrome

Respiratory: Bronchospasm, dyspnea, pharyngeal pain

Miscellaneous: Allergic reactions (rare), anaphylaxis (rare), hypersensitivity (rare)

Drug Interactions

Metabolism/Transport Effects Substrate of CYP3A4 (major), P-glycoprotein; **Note:** Assignment of Major/Minor substrate status based on clinically relevant drug interaction potential

Avoid Concomitant Use

Avoid concomitant use of VinCRIStine with any of the following: BCG (Intravesical); Conivaptan; Fusidic Acid (Systemic); Idelalisib; Natalizumab; Pimecrolimus; Tacrolimus (Topical); Tofacitinib; Vaccines (Live)

Increased Effect/Toxicity

VinCRIStine may increase the levels/effects of: Fingolimod; Leflunomide; MitoMYcin (Systemic); Natalizumab; Tofacitinib; Vaccines (Live)

The levels/effects of VinCRIStine may be increased by: Aprepitant; Conivaptan; CYP3A4 Inhibitors (Moderate); CYP3A4 Inhibitors (Strong); Dasatinib; Denosumab; Fosaprepitant; Fusidic Acid (Systemic); Idelalisib; Itraconazole; Ivacaftor; Lopinavir; Luliconazole; Macrolide Antibiotics; MAO

Inhibitors; Mifepristone; Netupitant; NIFEdipine; Osimertinib; Palbociclib; P-glycoprotein/ABCB1 Inhibitors; Pimecrolimus; Posaconazole; Ranolazine; Ritonavir; Roflumilast; Simeprevir; Stiripentol; Tacrolimus (Topical); Teniposide; Trastuzumab; Voriconazole

Decreased Effect

VinCRIStine may decrease the levels/effects of: BCG (Intravesical); Coccidioides immitis Skin Test; Fosphenytoin; Phenytoin; Sipuleucel-T; Vaccines (Inactivated); Vaccines (Live)

The levels/effects of VinCRIStine may be decreased by: Bosentan; CYP3A4 Inducers (Moderate); CYP3A4 Inducers (Strong); Dabrafenib; Deferasirox; Echinacea; Enzalutamide; Fosphenytoin; Mitotane; Osimertinib; P-glycoprotein/ABCB1 Inducers; Phenytoin; Siltuximab; St Johns Wort; Tocilizumab

Storage/Stability Store intact vials refrigerated at 2°C to 8°C (36°F to 46°F). Protect from light.

IV solution: Diluted in 25 to 50 mL NS or D$_5$W, stable for 7 days under refrigeration, or 2 days at room temperature. In ambulatory pumps, solution is stable for 7 days at room temperature. After preparation, keep vincristine in a location away from the separate storage location recommended for intrathecal medications.

Preparation for Administration Hazardous agent; use appropriate precautions for handling and disposal (NIOSH 2014 [group 1]).

Solutions for IV infusion may be mixed in NS or D$_5$W. **Note:** In order to prevent inadvertent intrathecal administration the World Health Organization (WHO) and the Institute for Safe Medication Practices (ISMP) strongly recommend dispensing vincristine in a minibag (**NOT** in a syringe). Vincristine should **NOT** be prepared during the preparation of any intrathecal medications. If dispensing vincristine in a syringe, affix an auxiliary label stating **"For intravenous use only - fatal if given by other routes"** to the syringe, and the syringe must also be packaged in the manufacturer-provided overwrap which bears the statement **"Do not remove covering until the moment of injection. For intravenous use only. Fatal if given intrathecally."**

Mechanism of Action Binds to tubulin and inhibits microtubule formation, therefore, arresting the cell at metaphase by disrupting the formation of the mitotic spindle; it is specific for the M and S phases. Vincristine may also interfere with nucleic acid and protein synthesis by blocking glutamic acid utilization.

Pharmacodynamics/Kinetics

Distribution: Rapidly removed from bloodstream and tightly bound to tissues; penetrates blood-brain barrier poorly

Metabolism: Extensively hepatic, via CYP3A4

Half-life elimination: Terminal: 85 hours (range: 19-155 hours)

Excretion: Feces (~80%); urine (10% to 20%; <1% as unchanged drug)

Dosing

Adult & Geriatric Note: Doses may be capped at a maximum of 2 mg/dose. Dosing and frequency may vary by protocol and/or treatment phase; refer to specific protocol. In order to prevent inadvertent intrathecal administration, the World Health Organization (WHO) and the Institute for Safe Medication Practices (ISMP) strongly recommend dispensing vincristine in a minibag (**NOT** a syringe).

Doses in the manufacturer's U.S. labeling: IV: 1.4 mg/m^2/dose; frequency may vary based on protocol

◀ Additional dosing in combination therapy; indication-specific and/or off-label dosing:

Acute lymphocytic leukemia (ALL): IV:

Hyper-CVAD regimen: 2 mg/dose days 4 and 11 during odd-numbered cycles (cycles 1, 3, 5, 7) of an 8-cycle phase, followed by maintenance treatment (if needed) of 2 mg monthly for 2 years (Kantarjian, 2004)

CALBG 8811 regimen: Induction phase: 2 mg/dose days 1, 8, 15, and 22 (4-week treatment cycle); Early intensification phase: 2 mg/dose days 15, and 22 (4-week treatment cycle, repeat once); Late intensification phase: 2 mg/dose days 1, 8, 15 (8-week treatment cycle); Maintenance phase: 2 mg/dose day 1 every 4 weeks until 24 months from diagnosis (Larson, 1995)

Central nervous system tumors: IV: PCV regimen: 1.4 mg/m^2/dose (maximum dose: 2 mg) on days 8 and 29 of a 6-week treatment cycle for a total of 6 cycles (van de Bent, 2006) **or** 1.4 mg/m^2/dose (no maximum dose) on days 8 and 29 of a 6-week treatment cycle for up to 4 cycles (Cairncross, 2006)

Hodgkin lymphoma: IV:

BEACOPP regimen: 1.4 mg/m^2/dose (maximum dose: 2 mg) on day 8 of a 21-day treatment cycle (Diehl, 2003)

Stanford-V regimen: 1.4 mg/m^2/dose (maximum dose: 2 mg) in weeks 2, 4, 6, 8, 10, and 12 (Horning, 2000; Horning, 2002)

Non-Hodgkin lymphoma: IV:

Burkitt lymphoma:

CODOX-M/IVAC: Cycles 1 and 3 (CODOX-M): 1.5 mg/m^2 (no maximum dose) days 1 and 8 of cycle 1 and days 1, 8, and 15 of cycle 3 (Magrath, 1996) **or** 1.5 mg/m^2 (maximum dose: 2 mg) days 1 and 8 of cycles 1 and 3 (Mead 2002; Mead 2008); CODOX-M is in combination with cyclophosphamide, doxorubicin, methotrexate, and CNS prophylaxis and alternates with IVAC (etoposide, ifosfamide, mesna, cytarabine, and CNS prophylaxis) for a total of 4 cycles

Hyper-CVAD: 2 mg (flat dose) days 4 and 11 of courses 1, 3, 5, and 7 (in combination with cyclophosphamide, doxorubicin, and dexamethasone) and alternates with even courses 2, 4, 6, and 8 (methotrexate and cytarabine) (Thomas, 2006)

Follicular lymphoma: CVP regimen: 1.4 mg/m^2/dose (maximum dose: 2 mg) on day 1 of a 21-day treatment cycle (in combination with cyclophosphamide and prednisone) for 8 cycles (Marcus, 2005)

Large B-cell lymphoma:

CHOP regimen: 1.4 mg/m^2/dose (maximum dose: 2 mg) on day 1 of a 21-day treatment cycle for 8 cycles (Coiffier, 2002)

EPOCH regimen: 0.4 mg/m^2/day continuous infusion for 4 days (over 96 hours) (total 1.6 mg/m^2/cycle; dose not usually capped) of a 21-day treatment cycle (Wilson, 2002)

Ewing's sarcoma (off-label use): IV: VAC/IE regimen: VAC: 2 mg/m^2 (maximum dose: 2 mg) on day 1 of a 21-day treatment cycle (in combination with doxorubicin and cyclophosphamide), alternates with IE (ifosfamide and etoposide) for a total of 17 cycles (Grier, 2003)

Gestational trophoblastic tumors, high-risk (off-label use): IV: EMA/CO regimen: 1 mg/m^2 on day 8 of 2-week treatment cycle (in combination with etoposide methotrexate, dactinomycin, and cyclophosphamide), continue for at least 2 treatment cycles after a normal hCG level (Escobar, 2003)

Multiple myeloma (off-label use): IV:

DVD regimen: 1.4 mg/m²/dose (maximum dose: 2 mg) on day 1 of a 28-day treatment cycle (Rifkin, 2006)

VAD regimen: 0.4 mg/day continuous infusion for 4 days (over 96 hours) (total 1.6 mg/cycle) of a 28-day treatment cycle (Rifkin, 2006)

Ovarian cancer (off-label use): IV: VAC regimen: 1.5 mg/m²/dose (maximum dose: 2 mg) weekly for 8-12 weeks (Slayton, 1985)

Small cell lung cancer (off-label use): IV: CAV regimen: 1.4 mg/m²/dose day 1 of a 21-day treatment cycle (Hong, 1989) **or** 2 mg/dose on day 1 of a 21-day treatment cycle (von Pawel, 1999)

Thymoma, advanced (off-label use): IV: ADOC regimen: 0.6 mg/m² on day 3 every 3 weeks (in combination with cisplatin, doxorubicin, and cyclophosphamide) (Fornasiero, 1991)

Pediatric Note: Doses may be capped at a maximum of 2 mg/dose. Dosing and frequency may vary by protocol and/or treatment phase; refer to specific protocol. In order to prevent inadvertent intrathecal administration, the World Health Organization (WHO) and the Institute for Safe Medication Practices (ISMP) strongly recommend dispensing vincristine in a minibag (**NOT** in a syringe).

Doses in the manufacturer's U.S. labeling: IV:

Children ≤10 kg: 0.05 mg/kg/dose once weekly

Children >10 kg: 1.5-2 mg/m²/dose; frequency may vary based on protocol

Additional dosing in combination therapy; indication-specific and/or off-label dosing:

Acute lymphocytic lymphoma (ALL): IV: Induction phase: 1.5 mg/m²/dose days 0, 7, 14, and 21; Consolidation phase: 1.5 mg/m²/dose days 0, 28, and 56; Delayed intensification phase: 1.5 mg/m²/dose days 0, 7, and 14; Maintenance phase: 1.5 mg/m²/dose days 0, 28, and 56 (Bostrom, 2003) **or** Induction phase: 1.5 mg/m²/dose days 0, 7, 14, and 21; Consolidation phase: 1.5 mg/m²/dose days 0, 28, and 56; Interim maintenance phases: 1.5 mg/m²/dose days 0 and 28; Delayed intensification phase: 1.5 mg/m²/dose days 0, 7, and 14; Maintenance phase: 1.5 mg/m²/dose every 4 weeks (Avramis, 2002)

Burkitt lymphoma and B-cell ALL: IV: 1.5 mg/m² (maximum dose: 2 mg) on days 4 and 11 of initial phase cycle (initial phase is in combination with cyclophosphamide, doxorubicin, and CNS prophylaxis; alternates with secondary phase) for a total of 4 cycles of each phase (Bowman, 1996) **or** 1.5 mg/m² (maximum dose: 2 mg) on day 1 of cycle AA (in combination with dexamethasone, ifosfamide, methotrexate, cytarabine, etoposide and CNS prophylaxis) and on day 1 of cycle BB (in combination with dexamethasone, cyclophosphamide, methotrexate, doxorubicin, and CNS prophylaxis) (Reiter, 1999)

Ewing's sarcoma (off-label use): IV: 2 mg/m²/dose (maximum dose: 2 mg) on day 1 of a 21-day cycle, administer either every cycle or during odd-numbered cycles (Grier, 2003) **or** 0.67 mg/m²/day continuous infusion days 1, 2, and 3 (total 2 mg/m²/cycle; maximum dose/cycle: 2 mg) during cycles 1, 2, 3, and 6 (Kolb, 2003)

Hodgkin lymphoma: IV: BEACOPP regimen: 2 mg/m²/dose (maximum dose: 2 mg) on day 7 of a 21-day treatment cycle (Kelly, 2002)

Neuroblastoma: IV:

CE-CAdO regimen: 1.5 mg/m² (maximum dose: 2 mg) days 1 and 5 every 21 days for 2 cycles (Rubie, 1998) **or** 0.05 mg/kg days 1 and 5 for 2 cycles (Rubie, 2001)

◄

CAV-P/VP regimen (off-label dosing): 0.033 mg/kg/day continuous infusion days 1, 2, and 3, then 1.5 mg/m² bolus day 9 of courses 1, 2, 4, and 6 (Kushner, 1994)

Retinoblastoma (off-label use): IV:

Children: 0.05 mg/kg on day 1 every 21 days (in combination with carboplatin) for 8 cycles (Rodriguez-Galindo, 2003)

or

Children ≤36 months: 0.05 mg/kg on day 0 every 28 days (in combination with carboplatin and etoposide) for 6 cycles (Freidman, 2000)

or

Children >36 months: 1.5 mg/m² (maximum dose: 2 mg) on day 0 every 28 days (in combination with carboplatin and etoposide) for 6 cycles (Friedman, 2000)

Rhabdomyosarcoma: IV:

VA regimen: 1.5 mg/m²/dose (maximum dose: 2 mg) weeks 1-8, weeks 13-20, and weeks 25-32 (Crist, 2001)

VAC regimen: 1.5 mg/m²/dose (maximum dose: 2 mg) weeks 0-12, week 16, weeks 20-25; Continuation therapy: Weeks 29-34, and weeks 38-43 (Crist, 2001)

Wilms' tumor: IV:

Children <1 year: 0.75 mg/m²/dose weekly for 10-11 weeks, then every 3 weeks for 15 additional weeks (total 25-26 weeks) (Pritchard, 1995)

Children ≥1 year: 1.5 mg/m²/dose weekly for 10-11 weeks, then every 3 weeks for 15 additional weeks (total 25-26 weeks) (Pritchard, 1995)

or

Children ≤30 kg: 0.05 mg/kg/dose (maximum dose: 2 mg) weeks 1, 2, 4, 5, 6, 7, 8, 10, and 11, followed by 0.067 mg/kg/dose (maximum dose: 2 mg) weeks 12, 13, 18, and 24 (Green, 2007)

Children >30 kg: 1.5 mg/m²/dose (maximum dose: 2 mg) weeks 1, 2, 4, 5, 6, 7, 8, 10, and 11, followed by 2 mg/m²/dose (maximum dose: 2 mg) weeks 12, 13, 18, and 24 (Green, 2007)

Renal Impairment No dosage adjustment necessary (Kintzel, 1995).

Hepatic Impairment The manufacturer's labeling recommends the following adjustment: Serum bilirubin >3 mg/dL: Administer 50% of normal dose.

The following adjustments have also been recommended:

Floyd, 2006: Serum bilirubin 1.5-3 mg/dL or transaminases 2-3 times ULN or alkaline phosphatase increased: Administer 50% of dose.

Superfin, 2007:

Serum bilirubin 1.5-3 mg/dL: Administer 50% of dose.

Serum bilirubin >3 mg/dL: Avoid use.

Obesity *ASCO Guidelines for appropriate chemotherapy dosing in obese adults with cancer:* Dose should be capped at a maximum of 2 mg due to neurotoxicity concerns (Griggs, 2012)

Combination Regimens

Bone sarcoma (Ewing Sarcoma): VAC Alternating With IE (Ewing Sarcoma) on page 2102

Brain tumors:

COPE on page 1926

PCV (Brain Tumor Regimen) on page 2061

POC on page 2067

Gestational trophoblastic tumor: EMA/CO (Gestational Trophoblastic Tumor) on page 1954

◀ Soft tissue sarcoma (rhabdomyosarcoma):
VAC Pulse on page 2103
VAC (Rhabdomyosarcoma) on page 2103
Waldenstrom Macroglobulinemia: R-CHOP (Waldenstrom Macroglobulinemia)
on page 2072
Wilms' tumor:
EE-4A (Wilms' Tumor) on page 1953
DD-4A (Wilms' Tumor) on page 1936
Regimen I (Wilms' Tumor) on page 2074
VAD (Wilms' Tumor) on page 2104

Administration For IV administration only. **FATAL IF GIVEN INTRATHE-CALLY.**

In order to prevent inadvertent intrathecal administration, the World Health Organization (WHO) and the Institute for Safe Medication Practices (ISMP) strongly recommend dispensing vincristine in a minibag (NOT in a syringe). Vincristine should **NOT** be delivered to the patient at the same time with any medications intended for central nervous system administration.

IV: Preferred administration is as a short 5- to 10-minute infusion in a 25 to 50 mL minibag. If administration via minibag is not possible, may also be administered as a slow (1-minute) push. Some protocols utilize a 24-hour continuous infusion.

Vesicant; ensure proper needle or catheter placement prior to and during infusion. Avoid extravasation.

Extravasation management: If extravasation occurs, stop infusion immediately and disconnect (leave cannula/needle in place); gently aspirate extravasated solution (do **NOT** flush the line); initiate hyaluronidase antidote; remove needle/cannula; apply dry warm compresses for 20 minutes 4 times a day for 1 to 2 days; elevate (Perez Fidalgo, 2012). Remaining portion of the vincristine dose should be infused through a separate vein.

Hyaluronidase: If needle/cannula still in place, administer 1 to 6 mL hyaluronidase (150 units/mL) into the existing IV line; the usual dose is 1 mL hyaluronidase for each 1 mL of extravasated drug (Perez Fidalgo, 2012; Schulmeister, 2011). If needle/cannula was removed, inject 1 to 6 mL (150 units/mL) subcutaneously in a clockwise manner using 1 mL for each 1 mL of drug extravasated (Schulmeister, 2011) **or** administer 1 mL (150 units/mL) as 5 separate 0.2 mL injections (using a 25-gauge needle) subcutaneously into the extravasation site (Polovich, 2009).

Hazardous agent; use appropriate precautions for handling and disposal (NIOSH 2014 [group 1]).

Vesicant/Extravasation Risk Vesicant

Emetic Potential Children and Adults: Minimal (<10%)

Monitoring Parameters Serum electrolytes (sodium), hepatic function tests, CBC with differential, serum uric acid; monitor infusion site; neurologic examination, monitor for constipation/ileus and for signs/symptoms of peripheral neuropathy

Dosage Forms Excipient information presented when available (limited, particularly for generics); consult specific product labeling.

Solution, Intravenous, as sulfate:

Vincasar PFS: 1 mg/mL (1 mL, 2 mL)

Solution, Intravenous, as sulfate [preservative free]:

Generic: 1 mg/mL (1 mL, 2 mL)

VinCRIStine (Liposomal) (vin KRIS teen lye po SO mal)

Related Information

Common Toxicity Criteria *on page 2122*

Management of Chemotherapy-Induced Nausea and Vomiting in Adults *on page 2142*

Safe Handling of Hazardous Drugs *on page 2292*

Brand Names: US Marqibo

Index Terms Liposomal Vincristine; Liposome Vincristine; Vincristine Liposome; Vincristine Sulfate Liposome; VSLI

Pharmacologic Category Antineoplastic Agent, Antimicrotubular; Antineoplastic Agent, Vinca Alkaloid

Use Treatment of relapsed Philadelphia chromosome-negative (Ph-) acute lymphoblastic leukemia (ALL) in adult patients whose disease has progressed after two or more antileukemic therapies

Labeled Contraindications Hypersensitivity to vincristine, liposomal vincristine, or any component of the formulation; patients with Charcot-Marie-Tooth syndrome or other demyelinating conditions; administration via the intrathecal route

Pregnancy Considerations Adverse events (fetal malformations, decreased fetal weight, and fetal loss) were observed in animal reproduction studies at doses less than the recommended human dose. Given the mechanism of action, adverse fetal events would be expected to occur with use in pregnant women. Women of childbearing potential should avoid becoming pregnant during therapy.

Breast-Feeding Considerations Due to the potential for adverse reactions in the nursing infant, the decision to discontinue breast-feeding or to discontinue liposomal vincristine should take into account the benefits of treatment to the mother.

Warnings/Precautions Hazardous agent - use appropriate precautions for handling and disposal (NIOSH 2014 [group 1]). **[US Boxed Warning]: For IV administration only. Intrathecal administration is contraindicated; inadvertent intrathecal administration has resulted in death.** Liposomal vincristine should **NOT** be prepared during the preparation of any intrathecal medications. After preparation, keep liposomal vincristine in a location **away** from the separate storage location recommended for intrathecal medications. Liposomal vincristine should **NOT** be delivered to the patient at the same time with any medications intended for central nervous system administration.

[US Boxed Warning]: Vincristine LIPOSOME and conventional vincristine are NOT interchangeable. Dosing differs between formulations; verify intended product and dose prior to preparation and administration to avoid overdoses. Avoid extravasation of liposomal vincristine (conventional vincristine is a vesicant). Only individuals experienced with vesicant administration should administer liposomal vincristine. Check for proper needle placement; if extravasation occurs, discontinue liposomal vincristine infusion immediately and institute appropriate extravasation management procedures.

Grade 3 and greater neutropenia, anemia, and thrombocytopenia were observed in clinical trials. Monitor blood counts closely and adjust dose or withhold therapy if necessary. Constipation, ileus, bowel obstruction, and colonic pseudo-obstruction have occurred with liposomal vincristine. Patients should be initiated on a prophylactic bowel regimen including a stool softener, dietary fiber, and hydration; laxative treatments may be considered. Severe ▶

fatigue was noted in clinical trials; treatment delay, dosage adjustment, or discontinuation may be necessary.

Neuropathies (sensory and motor) are common and cumulative. Neuropathy symptoms may include paresthesia, hyper-/hypoesthesia, hyporeflexia or areflexia, neuralgia, jaw pain, cranial neuropathy, ileus, arthralgia, myalgia, muscle spasm, and/or weakness. Evaluate neurologic status of patients closely prior to liposomal vincristine administration; neurologic toxicity risk is greater when given to patients with preexisting neuromuscular conditions or when used concomitantly with other neurotoxic agents. Treatment delay, dosage adjustment, and/or discontinuation may be necessary. Tumor lysis syndrome may occur as a consequence of therapy; monitor closely for signs and symptoms and manage accordingly.

Hepatotoxicity (including fatal cases) and increased AST have been reported. Monitor hepatic function tests; reduce dose or interrupt therapy if necessary. Use caution in patients with hepatic impairment; liposomal vincristine has not been studied in patients with severe hepatic impairment. In a study in a limited number of melanoma patients with moderate (Child-Pugh class B) hepatic impairment secondary to liver metastases, C_{max} and AUC were comparable to those in patients with normal hepatic function; patients with hepatic impairment received a dose of 1 mg/m² every 2 weeks versus 2 mg/m² in subjects with normal hepatic function (Bedikian, 2011). Potentially significant drug-drug interactions may exist, requiring dose or frequency adjustment, additional monitoring, and/or selection of alternative therapy. Avoid concomitant therapy with strong CYP3A4 or P-glycoprotein (P-gp) inducers or inhibitors. Use with caution in the elderly patient population; conventional vincristine may cause or exacerbate hyponatremia or syndrome of inappropriate antidiuretic hormone secretion; monitor sodium closely with therapy initiation or dosage adjustments (Beers Criteria).

Adverse Reactions

>10%:
  Central nervous system: Fever (43%), fatigue (41%), insomnia (32%)
  Gastrointestinal: Constipation (57%), nausea (52%), diarrhea (37%), appetite decreased (33%)
  Hematologic: Neutropenic fever (38%; grades 3/4: 31%), anemia (34%; grades 3/4: 17%), neutropenia (grades 3/4: 18%), thrombocytopenia (grades 3/4: 17%)
  Hepatic: AST increased (grades 3/4: 6% to 11%)
  Neuromuscular & skeletal: Peripheral neuropathy (39%; grades 3/4: 17%)
1% to 10%:
  Cardiovascular: Cardiac arrest (grades 3/4: 6%), hypotension (grades 3/4: 6%)
  Central nervous system: Pain (grades 3/4: 8%), mental status changes (grades 3/4: 4%)
  Gastrointestinal: Abdominal pain (grades 3/4: 8%), ileus (grades 3/4: 6%)
  Neuromuscular & skeletal: Weakness (grades 3/4: 5%), muscle weakness (grades 3/4: 1%)
  Respiratory: Pneumonia (grades 3/4: 8%), respiratory distress (grades 3/4: 6%), respiratory failure (grades 3/4: 5%)
  Miscellaneous: Septic shock (grades 3/4: 6%), staphylococcal bacteremia (grades 3/4: 6%)

Drug Interactions

Metabolism/Transport Effects Substrate of CYP3A4 (major), P-glycoprotein; **Note:** Assignment of Major/Minor substrate status based on clinically relevant drug interaction potential

Avoid Concomitant Use

Avoid concomitant use of VinCRIStine (Liposomal) with any of the following: BCG (Intravesical); CloZAPine; Conivaptan; CYP3A4 Inducers (Strong); CYP3A4 Inhibitors (Strong); Dexamethasone (Systemic); Dipyrone; Fusidic Acid (Systemic); Idelalisib; Natalizumab; P-glycoprotein/ABCB1 Inducers; P-glycoprotein/ABCB1 Inhibitors; Pimecrolimus; St Johns Wort; Tacrolimus (Topical); Tofacitinib; Vaccines (Live)

Increased Effect/Toxicity

VinCRIStine (Liposomal) may increase the levels/effects of: CloZAPine; Fingolimod; Leflunomide; MitoMYcin (Systemic); Natalizumab; Tofacitinib; Vaccines (Live)

The levels/effects of VinCRIStine (Liposomal) may be increased by: Aprepitant; Conivaptan; CYP3A4 Inhibitors (Moderate); CYP3A4 Inhibitors (Strong); Dasatinib; Denosumab; Dipyrone; Fosaprepitant; Fusidic Acid (Systemic); Idelalisib; Luliconazole; Macrolide Antibiotics; MAO Inhibitors; Mifepristone; Netupitant; NIFEdipine; Osimertinib; Palbociclib; P-glycoprotein/ABCB1 Inhibitors; Pimecrolimus; Roflumilast; Stiripentol; Tacrolimus (Topical); Teniposide; Trastuzumab

Decreased Effect

VinCRIStine (Liposomal) may decrease the levels/effects of: BCG (Intravesical); Coccidioides immitis Skin Test; Sipuleucel-T; Vaccines (Inactivated); Vaccines (Live)

The levels/effects of VinCRIStine (Liposomal) may be decreased by: Bosentan; CYP3A4 Inducers (Moderate); CYP3A4 Inducers (Strong); Dabrafenib; Deferasirox; Dexamethasone (Systemic); Echinacea; Osimertinib; P-glycoprotein/ABCB1 Inducers; Siltuximab; St Johns Wort; Tocilizumab

Storage/Stability Store intact kit (containing vincristine vial, sphingomyelin/cholesterol liposome vial, and sodium phosphate vial) refrigerated at 2°C to 8°C (36°F to 46°F); do not freeze. Use appropriate precautions for handling and disposal. Once prepared, liposomal vincristine is stable for no more than 12 hours at room temperature. After preparation, keep liposomal vincristine in a location away from the separate storage location recommended for intrathecal medications.

Preparation for Administration Hazardous agent; use appropriate precautions for handling and disposal (NIOSH 2014 [group 1]). Vincristine liposome preparation requires 60-90 minutes of dedicated time utilizing the manufacturer supplied kit. Do not reuse kit components with future doses.

1). Outside the sterile area, fill a water bath to a depth of at least 8 cm (3.2 inches); water should be heated to and maintained at **63°C to 67°C** (145.4°F to 152.6°F) for the entire procedure (use calibrated thermometer to monitor temperature). Maintain water depth of at least 8 cm (3.2 inches) throughout process. Water bath must remain outside the sterile area.

2). In a biological safety cabinet, vent the sodium phosphate vial with a sterile venting needle (with a 0.2 micron filter or other suitable venting device). Venting needle should always be kept above liquid level. Remove 1 mL of sphingomyelin/cholesterol liposome injection and inject into the sodium phosphate vial. Withdraw 5 mL of vincristine sulfate injection and inject into the sodium phosphate vial. Remove the venting needle and gently invert the

◀ sodium phosphate vial 5 times to mix (do **not** shake). Place flotation ring on the sodium phosphate vial.

3). Confirm the water bath is maintained between **63°C to 67°C** (145.4°F to 152.6°F). Outside the sterile area, place constituted sodium phosphate vial in the water bath for 10 minutes. Record constitution start and stop time, as well as starting and ending water temperature. After 10 minutes, remove the vial (with tongs), remove flotation ring, then dry the vial, affix vial overlabel, and gently invert 5 times to mix (do **not** shake). Allow the vial to equilibrate for at least 30 minutes at room temperature of 15°C to 30°C (59°F to 86°F), but for no longer than 12 hours. Once prepared, vincristine sulfate liposome concentration is 5 mg/31 mL (0.16 mg/mL).

4). Return vial to biologic safety cabinet. Calculate patient's vincristine liposome dose (based on actual BSA); remove corresponding volume from 100 mL NS or D_5W infusion bag. Inject vincristine liposome dose into the infusion bag (final volume of 100 mL). Do not use if a precipitate or other foreign matter is present in the vial or infusion bag. The amount contained in each vial may exceed the prescribed dose; use care with dosage and volume calculations. Discard unused portion of the vial. After preparation, keep liposomal vincristine in a location away from the separate storage location recommended for intrathecal medications.

Mechanism of Action Vincristine is a cell cycle specific agent which binds to tubulin, leading to microtubule depolymerization and cellular apoptosis. The liposomal formulation increases the half-life, allowing for enhanced cytotoxic activity in tumor cells.

Pharmacodynamics/Kinetics

Distribution: V_{dss}: 2.7 L (Bedikian, 2006)

Metabolism: Primarily hepatic

Half-life elimination: 45 hours (urinary half-life); dependent on rate of vincristine release from sphingosome (Bedikian, 2006)

Excretion: Feces (69%); urine (<8%)

Dosing

Adult & Geriatric Note: Vincristine liposomal and conventional vincristine are **NOT** interchangeable. Dosing differs between formulations; verify intended product and dose prior to preparation and administration. The liposomal vincristine dose is based on actual body surface area (BSA) and was not capped in studies (O'Brien, 2009; Rodriguez, 2009; Silverman, 2010).

Acute lymphoblastic leukemia (ALL; Philadelphia chromosome-negative), relapsed: IV: 2.25 mg/m^2 once every 7 days

Renal Impairment No dosage adjustment provided in manufacturer's labeling (has not been studied); however, liposomal vincristine is minimally excreted by the kidney and like the conventional formulation, likely does not require dosage adjustment in renal impairment.

Hepatic Impairment

Moderate impairment (Child-Pugh class B): In a study in a limited number of melanoma patients with moderate (Child-Pugh class B) hepatic impairment secondary to liver metastases, C_{max} and AUC were comparable to those in patients with normal hepatic function; patients with hepatic impairment received a dose of 1 mg/m^2 every 2 weeks versus 2 mg/m^2 in subjects with normal hepatic function (Bedikian, 2011).

Severe impairment (Child-Pugh class C): No dosage adjustment provided in manufacturer's labeling (has not been studied).

Hepatotoxicity during treatment: Reduce dose or interrupt treatment.

Adjustment for Toxicity

Fatigue, severe: Consider dose delay, reduction, or therapy discontinuation.

Hematologic toxicity: Grade 3 or 4 neutropenia, thrombocytopenia, or anemia: Consider dose reduction or modification.

Hepatic toxicity: Reduce dose or interrupt treatment.

Peripheral neuropathy:

Grade 3 or persistent grade 2 toxicity: Interrupt therapy until recovery to grade 1 or 2, then reduce dose to 2 mg/m^2. If grade 3 toxicity persists or if grade 4 toxicity occurs, discontinue liposomal vincristine.

Persistent grade 2 toxicity after first dose reduction to 2 mg/m^2: Interrupt therapy for up to 7 days until recovery to grade 1, then reduce dose to 1.825 mg/m^2. If neuropathy increases to grade 3 or 4, discontinue liposomal vincristine.

Persistent grade 2 toxicity after second dose reduction to 1.825 mg/m^2: Interrupt therapy for up to 7 days until recovery to grade 1, then reduce dose to 1.5 mg/m^2. If neuropathy increases to grade 3 or 4, discontinue liposomal vincristine.

Preexisting neuropathy, severe: Assess treatment benefit versus risk.

Administration Conventional vincristine is a vesicant. Limited information is available regarding liposomal vincristine extravasation, but may cause inflammation if extravasated; avoid extravasation. **For IV administration only. FATAL IF GIVEN INTRATHECALLY.** Liposomal vincristine should **NOT** be delivered to the patient at the same time as any medications intended for central nervous system administration.

IV: Infuse over 1 hour. Do not administer IV push or bolus; do not use with in-line filters. Infusion must be completed within 12 hours of preparation.

Hazardous agent; use appropriate precautions for handling and disposal (NIOSH 2014 [group 1]).

Emetic Potential Minimal (<10%)

Monitoring Parameters CBC with differential and platelets; hepatic function; signs/symptoms of peripheral neuropathy or other neurologic toxicities; sodium (in elderly patients; conventional vincristine may cause or exacerbate hyponatremia or syndrome of inappropriate antidiuretic hormone secretion); signs/symptoms of tumor lysis syndrome; symptoms of constipation; monitor infusion site for extravasation

Additional Information The liposomal formulation of vincristine consists of vincristine encapsulated in sphingosomes, which are composed of sphingomyelin and cholesterol (Bedikian, 2006).

Dosage Forms Excipient information presented when available (limited, particularly for generics); consult specific product labeling.

Suspension, Intravenous, as sulfate:

Marqibo: 5 mg/31 mL (1 ea)

- ◆ **Vincristine (Conventional)** *see* VinCRIStine *on page 1746*
- ◆ **Vincristine Liposome** *see* VinCRIStine (Liposomal) *on page 1755*
- ◆ **Vincristine Sulfate** *see* VinCRIStine *on page 1746*
- ◆ **Vincristine Sulfate Injection (Can)** *see* VinCRIStine *on page 1746*
- ◆ **Vincristine Sulfate Injection USP (Can)** *see* VinCRIStine *on page 1746*
- ◆ **Vincristine Sulfate Liposome** *see* VinCRIStine (Liposomal) *on page 1755*

Vindesine (VIN de seen)

Related Information
Management of Drug Extravasations *on page 2159*
Safe Handling of Hazardous Drugs *on page 2292*

Index Terms DAVA; Deacetyl Vinblastine Carboxamide; Desacetyl Vinblastine Amide; DVA; Eldisine; Lilly CT-3231; VDS; Vindesine Sulfate

Pharmacologic Category Antineoplastic Agent, Antimicrotubular; Antineoplastic Agent, Vinca Alkaloid

Use Note: Not approved in the US and/or Canada

Acute lymphoblastic leukemia: Treatment of resistant childhood acute lymphoblastic leukemia

Breast cancer: Treatment of advanced breast cancer unresponsive to appropriate endocrine surgery and/or hormonal therapy (if indicated)

Chronic myeloid leukemia: Treatment of blast crisis of chronic myeloid leukemia

Melanoma, malignant: Treatment of unresponsive malignant melanoma

Labeled Contraindications Hypersensitivity to vindesine sulphate or any component of the formulation; intrathecal administration (fatal); demyelinating form of Charcot-Marie-Tooth syndrome; severe granulocytopenia (<1500/mm^3) or severe thrombocytopenia; severe bacterial infection

Pregnancy Considerations Animal reproduction studies suggest teratogenic effects. Women of childbearing potential and men with female partners of childbearing potential should use effective contraception to prevent pregnancy during treatment.

Breast-Feeding Considerations Use during breast-feeding is not recommended.

Warnings/Precautions Hazardous agent - use appropriate precautions for handling and disposal (meets NIOSH 2014 criteria). Avoid eye contamination; severe irritation or corneal ulceration may occur. **For IV use only. Intrathecal administration may be fatal.** To prevent administration errors, the World Health Organization strongly recommends dispensing vinca alkaloids diluted in a minibag (WHO 2007), **if not dispensed in a minibag, affix an auxiliary label stating "For intravenous use only - fatal if given by other routes" and also place in an overwrap labeled "Do not remove covering until moment of injection."** Vindesine should be administered by individuals experienced in administering vinca alkaloids. Vinca alkaloids should **NOT** be prepared during the preparation of any intrathecal medications. After preparation, keep vindesine in a location **away** from the separate storage location recommended for intrathecal medications. Vindesine should **NOT** be delivered to the patient at the same time with any medications intended for central nervous system administration (Jacobson 2009).

Vindesine is a vesicant; ensure proper needle or catheter placement prior to and during infusion. Avoid extravasation. Extravasation may cause significant irritation. If extravasation occurs, discontinue immediately and initiate appropriate extravasation management, including local injection of hyaluronidase and moderate heat application to the affected area. Use a separate vein to complete administration.

Vindesine has been reported to have cross-resistance with vincristine. Neurotoxicity (eg, paresthesias, jaw pain, loss of deep tendon reflexes, foot drop, headache, and convulsions) may occur; may require dose reduction. Use with caution in patients with neuromuscular disease; neurotoxicity may be additive.

Neurotoxicity associated with vindesine may typically be less severe/progressive than that seen with other vinca alkaloids. Nausea, vomiting, constipation, ileus, stomatitis, diarrhea, and/or abdominal pain may occur. Monitor for acute abdominal pain (paralytic ileus may be a risk if further doses are administered). Patients should be on a prophylactic bowel regimen to prevent obstipation. Granulocytopenia is the dose-limiting toxicity; the nadir is generally 3 to 5 days after administration and recovery is rapid and usually complete within 7 to 10 days after the dose. Monitor for infection if granulocytes are <1,000/mm^3. Thrombocytopenia may occur if administered more frequently than once weekly, although platelets are usually unaffected or may increase when vindesine is administered weekly; thrombocytopenia is more likely when platelets are already low prior to treatment. Mild anemia may occur (rare). Acute shortness of breath and severe bronchospasm have been reported with vinca alkaloids, usually when used in combination with mitomycin (may be severe in patients with preexisting pulmonary toxicity). Onset may be several minutes to hours after vinca administration and up to 2 weeks after mitomycin. Progressive dyspnea may occur. Permanently discontinue vindesine if pulmonary dysfunction occurs.

Use with caution (if at all) in patients with hepatic impairment. Dosage reduction may be necessary for significant hepatic or biliary impairment. If radiation therapy is through portals which include the liver, delay the use of vindesine until after completion of radiation therapy. Potentially significant drug-drug interactions may exist, requiring dose or frequency adjustment, additional monitoring, and/or selection of alternative therapy.

Adverse Reactions
>10%:
Central nervous system: Pyrexia, malaise (up to 60%)
Dermatologic: Alopecia (6% to 92%)
Gastrointestinal: Mild nausea and vomiting (7% to 27%), constipation (10% to 17%) - related to the neurotoxicity
Hematologic: Leukopenia (50%) and thrombocytopenia (14% to 26%), may be dose limiting; thrombocytosis (20% to 28%)
Nadir: 6-12 days
Recovery: Days 14-18
Neuromuscular & skeletal: Paresthesia (40% to 70%); loss of deep tendon reflexes (35% to 60%, may be dose limiting); myalgia (up to 60%)
1% to 10%:
Dermatologic: Rashes
Gastrointestinal: Loss of taste
Hematologic: Anemia
Local: Phlebitis
Neuromuscular & skeletal: Facial paralysis
<1%: Acute chest pain, ECG changes, paralytic ileus, jaw pain, photophobia

Drug Interactions
Metabolism/Transport Effects Substrate of CYP3A4 (minor); **Note:** Assignment of Major/Minor substrate status based on clinically relevant drug interaction potential

Avoid Concomitant Use
Avoid concomitant use of Vindesine with any of the following: BCG (Intravesical); CloZAPine; Dipyrone; Natalizumab; Pimecrolimus; Tacrolimus (Topical); Tofacitinib; Vaccines (Live)

◀ **Increased Effect/Toxicity**

Vindesine may increase the levels/effects of: CloZAPine; Fingolimod; Leflunomide; MitoMYcin (Systemic); Natalizumab; Tofacitinib; Vaccines (Live)

The levels/effects of Vindesine may be increased by: CYP3A4 Inhibitors (Moderate); CYP3A4 Inhibitors (Strong); Denosumab; Dipyrone; Macrolide Antibiotics; Pimecrolimus; Posaconazole; Roflumilast; Tacrolimus (Topical); Trastuzumab; Voriconazole

Decreased Effect

Vindesine may decrease the levels/effects of: BCG (Intravesical); Coccidioides immitis Skin Test; Phenytoin; Sipuleucel-T; Vaccines (Inactivated); Vaccines (Live)

The levels/effects of Vindesine may be decreased by: Echinacea

Storage/Stability Store intact vials at 2°C to 8°C (36°F to 46°F). Solutions reconstituted in preservative-free sodium chloride 0.9% (NS) may be stored for up to 24 hours refrigerated. Solutions reconstituted with NS containing 2% benzyl alcohol may be stored for up to 28 days refrigerated.

Preparation for Administration Hazardous agent; use appropriate precautions for handling and disposal (meets NIOSH 2014 criteria). Reconstitute powder with 5 mL sodium chloride 0.9% (NS) to a concentration of 1 mg/mL. Reconstitute with NS preserved with 2% benzyl alcohol if planning to retain reconstituted vindesine beyond 24 hours. May further dilute for infusion with dextrose 5% in water or sodium chloride. Dispensing in a mini bag is preferred (WHO 2007). Do not mix with other medications.

Mechanism of Action Vindesine is a semisynthetic vinca alkaloid derived from vinblastine; works by binding to and stabilizing tubulin disrupting the formation of the mitotic spindle to arrest the cell cycle at metaphase.

Pharmacodynamics/Kinetics

Metabolism: Hepatic

Excretion: Feces; urine

Dosing

Adult & Geriatric

Breast cancer, advanced: Adults: IV: Initial: 3 mg/m^2; if no toxicity and granulocyte count is acceptable (avoid sustained granulocyte counts <2,500/mm^3), may increase dose in 0.5 mg/m^2 increments at weekly intervals (do not increase dose if granulocyte count <1,500/mm^3, platelet count <100,000/mm^3, or if acute abdominal pain is present). Usual range: 3 to 4 mg/m^2; maximum dose/week: 4 mg/m^2.

Chronic myeloid leukemia (blast crisis): Adults: IV: Initial: 3 mg/m^2; if no toxicity and granulocyte count is acceptable (avoid sustained granulocyte counts <2,500/mm^3), may increase dose in 0.5 mg/m^2 increments at weekly intervals (do not increase dose if granulocyte count <1,500/mm^3, platelet count <100,000/mm^3, or if acute abdominal pain is present). Usual range: 3 to 4 mg/m^2; maximum dose/week: 4 mg/m^2.

Melanoma, malignant, unresponsive: Adults: IV: Initial: 3 mg/m^2; if no toxicity and granulocyte count is acceptable (avoid sustained granulocyte counts <2,500/mm^3), may increase dose in 0.5 mg/m^2 increments at weekly intervals (do not increase dose if granulocyte count <1,500/mm^3, platelet count <100,000/mm^3, or if acute abdominal pain is present). Usual range: 3 to 4 mg/m^2; maximum dose/week: 4 mg/m^2.

Non-Hodgkin lymphoma, diffuse large B-cell (off-label use):

Adults ≤59 years: IV: 2 mg/m² on days 1 and 5 every 2 weeks (in combination with doxorubicin, cyclophosphamide, bleomycin, prednisone, and rituximab [R-ACVBP regimen]) for 4 cycles (with growth factor support), followed by sequential consolidation therapy (Molina 2014; Recher 2011).

Adults <61 years: IV: 2 mg/m² on days 1 and 5 every 2 weeks (in combination with doxorubicin, cyclophosphamide, bleomycin, and prednisone [ACVBP regimen]) for 3 cycles, followed by sequential consolidation therapy (Reyes 2005).

T-cell leukemia/lymphoma (off-label use): Adults: IV: 2.4 mg/m² on day 15 (as part of the VCAP-AMP-VECP multi-agent chemotherapy regimen) (Tsukasaki 2007).

Pediatric

Acute lymphoblastic leukemia, resistant: Children: IV: Initial: 4 mg/m²; if no toxicity and granulocyte count is acceptable (avoid sustained granulocyte counts <2,500/mm³), may increase dose in 0.5 mg/m² increments at weekly intervals (do not increase dose if granulocyte count <1,500/mm³, platelet count <100,000/mm³, or if acute abdominal pain is present). Usual range: 4 to 5 mg/m².

Renal Impairment There are no dosage adjustments provided in the manufacturer's labeling.

Hepatic Impairment Dosage reductions may be necessary for significant hepatic or biliary impairment, however the manufacturer's labeling does not provide specific adjustment recommendations.

Obesity ASCO Guidelines for appropriate chemotherapy dosing in obese adults with cancer: Utilize patient's actual body weight (full weight) for calculation of body surface area- or weight-based dosing, particularly when the intent of therapy is curative; manage regimen-related toxicities in the same manner as for nonobese patients; if a dose reduction is utilized due to toxicity, consider resumption of full weight-based dosing with subsequent cycles, especially if cause of toxicity (eg, hepatic or renal impairment) is resolved (Griggs 2012).

Adjustment for Toxicity

Gastrointestinal toxicity (acute abdominal pain): Withhold dose. After treatment is resumed, do not increase dose above the dose where acute abdominal pain occurred.

Neurotoxicity: May require dose reduction or temporary discontinuation.

Pulmonary toxicity (progressive dyspnea requiring chronic therapy): Discontinue (do not readminister).

Administration For IV administration only. **Fatal if given intrathecally. In order to prevent inadvertent intrathecal administration, the World Health Organization (WHO) strongly recommends dispensing vinca alkaloids in a minibag (NOT in a syringe).** Vindesine should **NOT** be delivered to the patient at the same time with any medications intended for central nervous system administration.

Administer as a rapid IV push over 1 to 3 minutes into a free flowing IV line.

Vesicant; ensure proper needle or catheter placement prior to and during infusion; avoid extravasation.

◀

Extravasation management: If extravasation occurs, stop infusion immediately and disconnect (leave cannula/needle in place); gently aspirate extravasated solution (do **NOT** flush the line); initiate hyaluronidase antidote; remove needle/cannula; apply dry warm compresses for 20 minutes 4 times a day for 1 to 2 days; elevate extremity (Perez Fidalgo 2012). Remaining portion of the vindesine dose should be infused through a separate vein.

Hyaluronidase: If needle/cannula still in place, administer 1 to 6 mL hyaluronidase (150 units/mL) into the existing IV line; the usual dose is 1 mL hyaluronidase for each 1 mL of extravasated drug (Perez Fidalgo 2012; Schulmeister 2011). If needle/cannula was removed, inject 1 to 6 mL (150 units/mL) subcutaneously in a clockwise manner using 1 mL for each 1 mL of drug extravasated (Schulmeister 2011) **or** administer 1 mL (150 units/mL) as 5 separate 0.2 mL injections (using a 25-gauge needle) subcutaneously into the extravasation site (Polovich 2009).

Hazardous agent; use appropriate precautions for handling and disposal (meets NIOSH 2014 criteria).

Vesicant/Extravasation Risk Vesicant

Monitoring Parameters CBC with differential, liver function tests; monitor infusion site, monitor for infection, neurotoxicity, or pulmonary toxicity.

Product Availability Not available in the US.

Dosage Forms Excipient information presented when available (limited, particularly for generics); consult specific product labeling.

Solution Reconstituted, Injection, as sulphate: Eldisine: 5 mg [contains mannitol]

♦ **Vindesine Sulfate** *see* Vindesine *on page 1760*

Vinorelbine (vi NOR el been)

Related Information

Chemotherapy and Obesity *on page 2220*

Management of Chemotherapy-Induced Nausea and Vomiting in Adults *on page 2142*

Management of Drug Extravasations *on page 2159*

Prevention of Chemotherapy-Induced Nausea and Vomiting in Children *on page 2203*

Safe Handling of Hazardous Drugs *on page 2292*

Brand Names: US Navelbine

Brand Names: Canada Navelbine; Vinorelbine Injection, USP; Vinorelbine Tartrate for Injection

Index Terms Dihydroxydeoxynorvinkaleukoblastine; Vinorelbine Tartrate

Pharmacologic Category Antineoplastic Agent, Antimicrotubular; Antineoplastic Agent, Vinca Alkaloid

Use Treatment of non-small cell lung cancer (NSCLC)

Labeled Contraindications Pretreatment granulocyte counts <1000/mm^3

Pregnancy Considerations Animal reproduction studies have demonstrated embryotoxicity, fetotoxicity, decreased fetal weight, and delayed ossification. May cause fetal harm if administered during pregnancy. Women of childbearing potential should avoid becoming pregnant during vinorelbine treatment.

Breast-Feeding Considerations It is not known if vinorelbine is excreted in breast milk. Due to the potential for serious adverse reactions in the nursing infant, breast-feeding should be discontinued during treatment.

Warnings/Precautions Hazardous agent - use appropriate precautions for handling and disposal (NIOSH 2014 [group 1]). **[U.S. Boxed Warning]: For IV use only; intrathecal administration of other vinca alkaloids has resulted in death. If dispensed in a syringe, should be labeled "for intravenous use only - fatal if given intrathecally". [U.S. Boxed Warning]: Vesicant; ensure proper needle or catheter placement prior to and during infusion. Avoid extravasation. Extravasation may cause local tissue necrosis and/or thrombophlebitis. [U.S. Boxed Warning]: Severe granulocytopenia may occur with treatment (may lead to infection); granulocyte counts should be ≥1000 cells/mm³ prior to treatment initiation; dosage adjustment may be required based on blood counts (monitor blood counts prior to each dose).** Granulocytopenia is a dose-limiting toxicity; nadir is generally 7-10 days after administration and recovery occurs within the following 7-14 days. Monitor closely for infections and/or fever in patients with severe granulocytopenia. Use with extreme caution in patients with compromised marrow reserve due to prior chemotherapy or radiation therapy.

Fatal cases of interstitial pulmonary changes and ARDS have been reported (with single-agent therapy (mean onset of symptoms: 1 week); promptly evaluate changes in baseline pulmonary symptoms or any new onset pulmonary symptoms (eg, dyspnea, cough, hypoxia). Acute shortness of breath and severe bronchospasm have been reported with vinca alkaloids; usually associated with the concurrent administration of mitomycin.

Vinorelbine should **NOT** be prepared during the preparation of any intrathecal medications. After preparation, keep vinorelbine in a location **away** from the separate storage location recommended for intrathecal medications. Elimination is predominantly hepatic; while there is no evidence that toxicity is enhanced in patients with elevated transaminases, use with caution in patients with severe hepatic injury or impairment; dosage modification required for elevated total bilirubin. May cause new onset or worsening of preexisting neuropathy; use with caution in patients with neuropathy; monitor for new or worsening sign/symptoms of neuropathy; dosage adjustment required. May cause severe constipation (grade 3-4), paralytic ileus, intestinal obstruction, necrosis, and/or perforation; some events were fatal. Oral vinorelbine (not available in the U.S.) is associated with a moderate antiemetic potential; antiemetics are recommended to prevent nausea/vomiting (Dupuis, 2011; Roila, 2010); IV vinorelbine has a minimal emetic potential (Dupuis, 2011; Roila, 2010). Potentially significant drug-drug interactions may exist, requiring dose or frequency adjustment, additional monitoring, and/or selection of alternative therapy. May have radiosensitizing effects with prior or concurrent radiation therapy; radiation recall reactions may occur in patients who have received prior radiation therapy. Avoid eye contamination (exposure may cause severe irritation). **[U.S. Boxed Warning]: Should be administered under the supervision of an experienced cancer chemotherapy physician.**

◀ **Adverse Reactions Note:** Reported with single-agent therapy.

>10%:

Central nervous system: Fatigue (27%)

Dermatologic: Alopecia (12% to 30%)

Gastrointestinal: Nausea (31% to 44%; grade 3: 1% to 2%), constipation (35%; grade 3: 3%), vomiting (20% to 31%; grade 3: 1% to 2%), diarrhea (12% to 17%)

Hematologic: Leukopenia (83% to 92%; grade 4: 6% to 15%), granulocytopenia (90%; grade 4: 36%; nadir: 7-10 days; recovery 14-21 days), neutropenia (85%; grade 4: 28%), anemia (83%; grades 3/4: 9%)

Hepatic: AST increased (67%; grade 3: 5%; grade 4: 1%), total bilirubin increased (5% to 13%; grade 3: 4%; grade 4: 3%)

Local: Injection site reaction (22% to 28%; includes erythema, vein discoloration), injection site pain (16%)

Neuromuscular & skeletal: Weakness (36%), peripheral neuropathy (25%; grade 3: 1%; grade 4: <1%)

Renal: Creatinine increased (13%)

1% to 10%:

Cardiovascular: Chest pain (5%)

Dermatologic: Rash (<5%)

Gastrointestinal: Paralytic ileus (1%)

Hematologic: Neutropenic fever/sepsis (8%; grade 4: 4%), thrombocytopenia (3% to 5%; grades 3/4: 1%)

Local: Phlebitis (7% to 10%)

Neuromuscular & skeletal: Loss of deep tendon reflexes (<5%), myalgia (<5%), arthralgia (<5%), jaw pain (<5%)

Otic: Ototoxicity (≤1%)

Respiratory: Dyspnea (7%)

<1%, postmarketing, and/or case reports: Abdominal pain, allergic reactions, anaphylaxis, angioedema, back pain, DVT, dysphagia, esophagitis, flushing, gait instability, headache, hemolytic uremic syndrome, hemorrhagic cystitis, hyper-/hypotension, hyponatremia, intestinal necrosis, intestinal obstruction, intestinal perforation, interstitial pulmonary changes, local rash, local urticaria, MI (rare), mucositis, muscle weakness, myocardial ischemia, pancreatitis, paralytic ileus, pneumonia, pruritus, pulmonary edema, pulmonary embolus, radiation recall (dermatitis, esophagitis), skin blistering, syndrome of inappropriate ADH secretion, tachycardia, thromboembolic events, thrombotic thrombocytopenic purpura, tumor pain, urticaria, vasodilation

Drug Interactions

Metabolism/Transport Effects Substrate of CYP2D6 (minor), CYP3A4 (major); **Note:** Assignment of Major/Minor substrate status based on clinically relevant drug interaction potential; **Inhibits** CYP2D6 (weak)

Avoid Concomitant Use

Avoid concomitant use of Vinorelbine with any of the following: BCG (Intravesical); CloZAPine; Conivaptan; Dipyrone; Fusidic Acid (Systemic); Idelalisib; Natalizumab; Pimecrolimus; Tacrolimus (Topical); Tofacitinib; Vaccines (Live)

Increased Effect/Toxicity

Vinorelbine may increase the levels/effects of: ARIPiprazole; CloZAPine; Fingolimod; Leflunomide; MitoMYcin (Systemic); Natalizumab; Tofacitinib; Vaccines (Live)

The levels/effects of Vinorelbine may be increased by: Aprepitant; CISplatin; Conivaptan; CYP3A4 Inhibitors (Moderate); CYP3A4 Inhibitors (Strong); Dasatinib; Denosumab; Dipyrone; Fosaprepitant; Fusidic Acid (Systemic); Gefitinib; Idelalisib; Itraconazole; Ivacaftor; Luliconazole; Macrolide Antibiotics; Mifepristone; Netupitant; Osimertinib; PACLitaxel (Conventional); PACLitaxel (Protein Bound); Palbociclib; Pimecrolimus; Posaconazole; Roflumilast; Simeprevir; Stiripentol; Tacrolimus (Topical); Trastuzumab; Voriconazole

Decreased Effect

Vinorelbine may decrease the levels/effects of: BCG (Intravesical); Coccidioides immitis Skin Test; Sipuleucel-T; Vaccines (Inactivated); Vaccines (Live)

The levels/effects of Vinorelbine may be decreased by: Bosentan; CYP3A4 Inducers (Moderate); CYP3A4 Inducers (Strong); Dabrafenib; Deferasirox; Echinacea; Enzalutamide; Mitotane; Osimertinib; Siltuximab; St Johns Wort; Tocilizumab

Storage/Stability Store intact vials refrigerated at 2°C to 8°C (36°F to 46°F); do not freeze. Protect from light. Intact vials are stable at room temperature of 25°C (77°F) for up to 72 hours. Solutions diluted for infusion in polypropylene syringes or polyvinyl chloride bags are stable for 24 hours at 5°C to 30°C (41°F to 86°F). After preparation, keep vinorelbine in a location **away** from the separate storage location recommended for intrathecal medications.

Preparation for Administration Hazardous agent; use appropriate precautions for handling and disposal (NIOSH 2014 [group 1]). Dilute in D_5W or NS to a final concentration of 1.5-3 mg/mL (for syringe) or D_5W, NS, $1/2NS$, $D_51/2NS$, LR, or Ringer's to a final concentration of 0.5-2 mg/mL (for IV bag). Vinorelbine should **NOT** be prepared during the preparation of any intrathecal medications.

Mechanism of Action Semisynthetic vinca alkaloid which binds to tubulin and inhibits microtubule formation, therefore, arresting the cell at metaphase by disrupting the formation of the mitotic spindle; it is specific for the M and S phases. Vinorelbine may also interfere with nucleic acid and protein synthesis by blocking glutamic acid utilization.

Pharmacodynamics/Kinetics

Distribution: V_d: 25-40 L/kg; binds extensively to human platelets and lymphocytes (80% to 91%)

Protein binding: 80% to 91%

Metabolism: Extensively hepatic, via CYP3A4, to two metabolites, deacetylvinorelbine (active) and vinorelbine N-oxide

Half-life elimination: Triphasic: Terminal: 28-44 hours

Excretion: Feces (46%); urine (18%, 10% to 12% as unchanged drug)

Dosing

Adult & Geriatric

Non-small cell lung cancer (NSCLC): IV:

Single-agent therapy: 30 mg/m² every 7 days until disease progression or unacceptable toxicity

Combination therapy: 25-30 mg/m² every 7 days (in combination with cisplatin)

Off-label dosing: 25 mg/m² days 1 and 8 every 21 days (in combination with cisplatin and cetuximab) for up to 6 cycles (Pirker, 2009) **or** 25-30 mg/m² days 1, 8, and 15 every 28 days (in combination with gemcitabine) for 6 cycles **or** until disease progression or unacceptable toxicity (Herbst, 2002; Greco, 2007)

Breast cancer, metastatic (off-label use): IV: 25 mg/m^2 every 7 days (as a single agent) until disease progression or unacceptable toxicity (Zelek, 2001) **or** 30 mg/m^2 every 7 days (as a single agent); after 13 weeks, may administer every 14 days for patient convenience, continue until disease progression or unacceptable toxicity (Vogel, 1999) **or** 25 mg/m^2 every 7 days (in combination with trastuzumab) until disease progression or unacceptable toxicity (Burstein, 2001; Burstein 2007) **or** 30 or 35 mg/m^2 days 1 and 8 every 21 days (in combination with trastuzumab) until disease progression or unacceptable toxicity (Andersson, 2011)

Cervical cancer (off-label use): IV: 30 mg/m^2 days 1 and 8 of a of a 21-day treatment cycle (Muggia, 2004; Muggia, 2005)

Hodgkin lymphoma, relapsed or refractory (off-label use): IV:

GVD regimen: 15 mg/m^2 (post-transplant patients) or 20 mg/m^2 (transplant-naïve patients) on days 1 and 8 of a 21-day cycle (in combination with gemcitabine and doxorubicin liposomal) for 2 to 6 cycles (Bartlett, 2007)

IGEV regimen: 20 mg/m^2 on day 1 of a 21-day cycle (in combination with ifosfamide, mesna, gemcitabine, and prednisolone) for 4 cycles (Santoro, 2007)

Malignant pleural mesothelioma (off-label use): IV: 30 mg/m^2 (maximum dose: 60 mg) every 7 days per 6-week treatment cycle, continue until disease progression (Stebbing, 2009) **or** 30 mg/m^2 (maximum dose: 60 mg) every 7 days for 6 weeks, off 2 weeks, then repeat cycle (Muers, 2008)

Ovarian cancer, relapsed (off-label use): IV: 25 mg/m^2 every 7 days (Bajetta, 1996) **or** 30 mg/m^2 days 1 and 8 of a 21-day treatment cycle (Rothenberg, 2004) until disease progression or unacceptable toxicity

Salivary gland cancer, recurrent (off-label use): IV: 25 mg/m^2 on days 1 and 8 of a 21-day cycle (in combination with cisplatin) for a minimum of 3 cycles and for up to 6 cycles (Airoldi, 2001) **or** 30 mg/m^2 every 7 days (monotherapy) for a minimum of 9 weeks and for up to 6 cycles (Airoldi, 2001)

Small cell lung cancer, refractory (off-label use): IV: 25 or 30 mg/m^2 every 7 days until disease progression or unacceptable toxicity (Furuse, 1996; Jessem, 1993)

Soft tissue sarcoma, advanced (off-label use): IV: 25 mg/m^2 days 1 and 8 of a 21-day treatment cycle (in combination with gemcitabine) until disease progression or unacceptable toxicity (Dileo, 2007)

Renal Impairment

Renal insufficiency: No dosage adjustment necessary.

Hemodialysis: Initial: IV: Reduce dose to 20 mg/m^2/week; administer either after dialysis (on dialysis days) or on nondialysis days (Janus, 2010)

Hepatic Impairment Note: In patients with concurrent hematologic toxicity and hepatic impairment, administer the lower of the doses determined from the adjustment recommendations.

Administer with caution in patients with hepatic insufficiency. In patients who develop hyperbilirubinemia during treatment with vinorelbine, the dose should be adjusted for total bilirubin as follows:

Serum bilirubin ≤2 mg/dL: Administer 100% of dose

Serum bilirubin 2.1-3 mg/dL: Administer 50% of dose (Ecklund, 2005; Floyd, 2006; Superfin, 2006)

Serum bilirubin >3 mg/dL: Administer 25% of dose (Ecklund, 2005; Floyd, 2006; Superfin, 2006)

Patients (breast cancer) with extensive liver metastases (>75% of liver volume): Administer 50% of dose (Ecklund, 2005; Superfin, 2006)

Obesity *ASCO Guidelines for appropriate chemotherapy dosing in obese adults with cancer:* Utilize patient's actual body weight (full weight) for calculation of body surface area- or weight-based dosing, particularly when the intent of therapy is curative; manage regimen-related toxicities in the same manner as for nonobese patients; if a dose reduction is utilized due to toxicity, consider resumption of full weight-based dosing with subsequent cycles, especially if cause of toxicity (eg, hepatic or renal impairment) is resolved (Griggs, 2012).

Adjustment for Toxicity Note: In patients with concurrent hematologic toxicity and hepatic impairment, administer the lower of the doses determined from the adjustment recommendations.

Dosage adjustment in hematological toxicity (based on granulocyte counts):

Granulocytes ≥1500 cells/mm³ on day of treatment: Administer 100% of starting dose.

Granulocytes 1000-1499 cells/mm³ on day of treatment: Administer 50% of starting dose.

Granulocytes <1000 cells/mm³ on day of treatment: Do not administer. Repeat granulocyte count in 1 week. If 3 consecutive doses are held because granulocyte count is <1000 cells/mm³, discontinue vinorelbine.

Adjustment: For patients who, during treatment, have experienced fever or sepsis while granulocytopenic or had 2 consecutive weekly doses held due to granulocytopenia, subsequent doses of vinorelbine should be:
75% of starting dose for granulocytes ≥1500 cells/mm³
37.5% of starting dose for granulocytes 1000-1499 cells/mm³

Dosage adjustment for neurotoxicity: Neurotoxicity ≥ grade 2: Discontinue treatment

Dosage adjustment for other adverse events: Severe adverse events: Reduce dose or discontinue treatment

Combination Regimens

Breast cancer: Trastuzumab-Vinorelbine (Breast) on page 2095
Cervical cancer:
  Cisplatin-Vinorelbine (Cervical Cancer) on page 1914
  Vinorelbine (Cervical Regimen) on page 2108
Head and neck cancer: Gemcitabine-Vinorelbine (Head and Neck) on page 1998
Lung cancer (non-small cell):
  Cetuximab-Cisplatin-Vinorelbine (NSCLC) on page 1881
  Cisplatin-Vinorelbine (Adjuvant NSCLC) on page 1914
  Cisplatin-Vinorelbine (Metastatic NSCLC) on page 1915
  Gemcitabine-Vinorelbine (NSCLC) on page 1998
  Vinorelbine (NSCLC Regimen) on page 2109
Lung cancer (small cell): Vinorelbine (Small Cell Lung Cancer Regimen) on page 2110
Lymphoma, Hodgkin:
  GVD (Hodgkin) on page 2002
  IGEV (Hodgkin) on page 2016
  Vinorelbine (Hodgkin Regimen) on page 2109
Malignant pleural mesothelioma: Vinorelbine (Mesothelioma Regimen) on page 2109

◀ Ovarian cancer: Vinorelbine (Ovarian Regimen) on page 2109
Soft tissue sarcoma: Gemcitabine-Vinorelbine (Soft Tissue Sarcoma) on page 1999

Administration For IV use only; **FATAL IF GIVEN INTRATHECALLY.** Administer as a direct intravenous push or rapid bolus, over 6-10 minutes (up to 30 minutes). Longer infusions may increase the risk of pain and phlebitis. Intravenous doses should be followed by at least 75-125 mL of saline or D_5W to reduce the incidence of phlebitis and inflammation.

Vesicant; ensure proper needle or catheter position prior to administration. Avoid extravasation.

Extravasation management: If extravasation occurs, stop infusion immediately and disconnect (leave cannula/needle in place); gently aspirate extravasated solution (do **NOT** flush the line); initiate hyaluronidase antidote; remove needle/cannula; apply dry warm compresses for 20 minutes 4 times a day for 1-2 days; elevate extremity (Perez Fidalgo, 2012). Remaining portion of the vinorelbine dose should be infused through a separate vein.

Hyaluronidase: If needle/cannula still in place, administer 1-6 mL hyaluronidase (150 units/mL) into the existing IV line; the usual dose is 1 mL hyaluronidase for each 1 mL of extravasated drug (Perez Fidalgo, 2012; Schulmeister, 2011). If needle/cannula was removed, inject 1-6 mL (150 units/mL) subcutaneously in a clockwise manner using 1mL for each 1 mL of drug extravasated (Schulmeister, 2011) **or** administer 1 mL (150 units/mL) as 5 separate 0.2 mL injections (using a 25-gauge needle) subcutaneously into the extravasation site (Polovich, 2009).

Hazardous agent; use appropriate precautions for handling and disposal (NIOSH 2014 [group 1]).

Vesicant/Extravasation Risk Vesicant.

Emetic Potential
Children and Adults:
IV: Minimal (<10%)
Oral (not available in the U.S.): Moderate (30% to 90%)

Monitoring Parameters CBC with differential and platelet count (prior to each dose, and after treatment), hepatic function tests; monitor for new-onset pulmonary symptoms (or worsening from baseline); monitor for neuropathy (new or worsening symptoms; monitor infusion site; monitor for signs symptoms of constipation/ileus

Dosage Forms Excipient information presented when available (limited, particularly for generics); consult specific product labeling.
Solution, Intravenous:
Navelbine: 10 mg/mL (1 mL); 50 mg/5 mL (5 mL)
Generic: 10 mg/mL (1 mL); 50 mg/5 mL (5 mL)
Solution, Intravenous [preservative free]:
Generic: 10 mg/mL (1 mL); 50 mg/5 mL (5 mL)

◆ **Vinorelbine Injection, USP (Can)** *see* Vinorelbine *on page* 1764

◆ **Vinorelbine Tartrate** *see* Vinorelbine *on page* 1764

◆ **Vinorelbine Tartrate for Injection (Can)** *see* Vinorelbine *on page* 1764

Vismodegib (vis moe DEG ib)

Related Information

Common Toxicity Criteria *on page 2122*

Management of Chemotherapy-Induced Nausea and Vomiting in Adults *on page 2142*

Safe Handling of Hazardous Drugs *on page 2292*

Brand Names: US Erivedge

Brand Names: Canada Erivedge

Index Terms GDC-0449; Hedgehog Antagonist GDC-0449

Pharmacologic Category Antineoplastic Agent, Hedgehog Pathway Inhibitor

Use Basal cell carcinoma, metastatic or locally advanced: Treatment of metastatic basal cell carcinoma, or locally-advanced basal cell carcinoma that has recurred following surgery or in patients who are not candidates for surgery, and not candidates for radiation therapy

Labeled Contraindications

US labeling: There are no contraindications listed in the manufacturer's labeling.

Canadian labeling: Hypersensitivity to vismodegib or any component of the formulation; pregnancy or females at risk of becoming pregnant; breast-feeding; male patients or female patients of childbearing potential who do not comply with the Erivedge Pregnancy Prevention Program; children and adolescents <18 years of age.

Pregnancy Considerations [US Boxed Warning]: May result in severe birth defects or embryo-fetal death. Teratogenic effects (severe midline defects, missing digits, and other irreversible malformations), embryotoxic, and fetotoxic events were observed in animal reproduction studies when administered in doses less than the normal human dose. Based on its mechanism of action adverse effects on pregnancy would be expected. **[US Boxed Warning]: Verify pregnancy status (in females of reproductive potential) within 7 days prior to initiating treatment and advise patients (female and male) of the risk of birth defects, the need for contraception and risk of exposure through semen and to use condoms with a pregnant partner or a female partner of childbearing potential.** In females of childbearing potential, obtain pregnancy test within 7 days prior to treatment initiation; after the negative pregnancy test, initiate highly effective contraception prior to the first vismodegib dose and continue during and for 7 months after treatment. During treatment (including treatment interruptions) and for 3 months after treatment, male patients should not donate sperm and should use condoms with spermicide (even after vasectomy) if their partner is of childbearing potential.

Women exposed to vismodegib during pregnancy (directly or via seminal fluid) are encouraged to participate in the Erivedge Pregnancy Pharmacovigilance program by contacting the Genentech Adverse Event Line (1-888-835-2555). Pregnancies occurring during or within 7 months after treatment should be reported to the Genentech Adverse Event Line.

The Canadian labeling recommends that females of childbearing potential use 2 simultaneous forms of effective contraception beginning at least 4 weeks prior to treatment initiation, during treatment (including treatment interruptions), and for 24 months after discontinuation. Pregnancy testing should be performed within 7 days prior to treatment initiation, monthly during treatment (including treatment interruptions) and for 24 months after discontinuation. For

◀ females of child bearing potential, a new prescription is required each month to allow for monthly pregnancy testing. Any suspected exposure (directly or via seminal fluid) during pregnancy should be immediately reported to the Erivedge Pregnancy Prevention Program (EPPP) at 1-888-748-8926.

Breast-Feeding Considerations It is not known if vismodegib is excreted in breast milk. Due to the potential for serious adverse reactions in the nursing infant, breast-feeding is not recommended by the manufacturer during therapy and for 7 months after treatment. The Canadian labeling contraindicates use in women who are nursing and recommends that women abstain from nursing for 24 months after discontinuation of therapy.

Warnings/Precautions Hazardous agent - use appropriate precautions for handling and disposal (meets NIOSH 2014 criteria). **[U.S. Boxed Warnings]: May result in severe birth defects or embryo-fetal death. Teratogenic effects (severe midline defects, missing digits, and other irreversible malformations), embryotoxic, and fetotoxic events were observed in animal reproduction studies. Verify pregnancy status (in females of reproductive potential) within 7 days prior to initiating treatment and advise patients (female and male) of the risk of birth defects, the need for contraception and risk of exposure through semen and to use condoms with a pregnant partner or a female partner of childbearing potential.** Amenorrhea was observed in women of reproductive potential; it is unknown if this is reversible.

Cardiac events (eg, cardiac failure, atrial fibrillation, left ventricular dysfunction, restrictive cardiomyopathy, myocardial infarction) have been observed during treatment. All events ≥ grade 3 occurred in patients with a history of significant cardiac disease. Cases of cutaneous squamous cell cancer (cuSCC) have been reported. Patients with advanced basal cell carcinoma are at risk for developing cuSCC; monitor during treatment. Vismodegib is associated with a moderate emetic potential; antiemetics may be needed to prevent nausea and vomiting. Diarrhea, constipation, abdominal pain, and decreased appetite may also occur.

Vismodegib metabolism is primarily hepatic. Elevated liver function tests (ALT, AST, total bilirubin, and alkaline phosphatase) have been observed; cases of cholestasis, hepatitis, and hepatocellular injury have also been reported. Monitor liver function tests; may require treatment interruption or discontinuation (Erivedge Canadian product monograph, 2015). Population pharmacokinetic analyses demonstrate that creatinine clearance (range: 30 to 80 mL/minute) does not have a clinically meaningful effect on systemic exposure; urinary excretion is <5%.

Advise patients not to donate blood or blood products during vismodegib treatment and for at least 7 months after the last vismodegib dose. The Canadian labeling recommends patients not donate blood or blood products during treatment (including treatment interruptions) and for 24 months after discontinuation. Vismodegib is present in semen, although the amount of drug in semen that may cause embryotoxicity and/or fetotoxicity is not known. Advise patients not to donate sperm during vismodegib treatment and for 3 months after the last vismodegib dose. In a study of vismodegib in patients with basal cell nevus syndrome (not an approved use), with discontinuation of vismodegib treatment, taste alteration and muscle cramps abated within 1 month, and scalp and body hair began to regrow within 3 months (Tang 2012). Potentially significant drug-drug interactions may exist, requiring dose or frequency adjustment, additional monitoring, and/or selection of alternative therapy.

Adverse Reactions

>10%:

Central nervous system: Fatigue (40%)

Dermatologic: Alopecia (64%)

Endocrine & metabolic: Amenorrhea (30%)

Gastrointestinal: Dysgeusia (55%), weight loss (45%), nausea (30%), diarrhea (29%), decreased appetite (25%), constipation (21%), vomiting (14%), ageusia (11%)

Neuromuscular & skeletal: Muscle spasm (72%), arthralgia (16%)

1% to 10%:

Endocrine & metabolic: Hyponatremia (grade 3: 4%), hypokalemia (grade 3: 1%)

Renal: Azotemia (grade 3: 2%)

<1%, postmarketing, and/or case reports: Cholestasis, hepatic injury, hepatitis, rhabdomyolysis

Drug Interactions

Metabolism/Transport Effects Substrate of CYP2C9 (minor), CYP3A4 (minor), P-glycoprotein; **Note:** Assignment of Major/Minor substrate status based on clinically relevant drug interaction potential; **Inhibits** BCRP, CYP2C19 (weak), CYP2C9 (weak)

Avoid Concomitant Use There are no known interactions where it is recommended to avoid concomitant use.

Increased Effect/Toxicity There are no known significant interactions involving an increase in effect.

Decreased Effect There are no known significant interactions involving a decrease in effect.

Storage/Stability Store at 20°C to 25°C (68°F to 77°F); excursions permitted to 15°C to 30°C (59°F to 86°F).

Mechanism of Action Basal cell cancer is associated with mutations in Hedgehog pathway components. Hedgehog regulates cell growth and differentiation in embryogenesis; while generally not active in adult tissue, Hedgehog mutations associated with basal cell cancer can activate the pathway resulting in unrestricted proliferation of skin basal cells. Vismodegib is a selective Hedgehog pathway inhibitor which binds to and inhibits Smoothened homologue (SMO), the transmembrane protein involved in Hedgehog signal transduction.

Pharmacodynamics/Kinetics

Distribution: V_d: 16.4 to 26.6 L

Males: In a small pharmacokinetic study, the average vismodegib concentration in semen was 6.5% of the average steady state plasma concentration on day 8

Protein binding: >99%; primarily to serum albumin and alpha$_1$ acid glycoprotein (AAG)

Metabolism: Metabolized by oxidation, glucuronidation, and pyridine ring cleavage, although >98% of circulating components are as the parent drug

Bioavailability: ~32%

Half-life, elimination: Continuous daily dosing: ~4 days; Single dose: ~12 days

Time to peak: ~2.4 days (Graham, 2011)

Excretion: Feces (82%); urine (4%)

◀ **Dosing**

Adult Note: Vismodegib is associated with a moderate emetic potential; antiemetics may be needed to prevent nausea and vomiting.

Basal cell carcinoma, metastatic or locally advanced: Oral: 150 mg once daily until disease progression or unacceptable toxicity.

Missed doses: If a dose is missed, do not make up; resume dosing with the next scheduled dose.

Renal Impairment No dosage adjustment necessary.

Hepatic Impairment No dosage adjustment necessary.

Adjustment for Toxicity In clinical trials, no dosage reductions were allowed for toxicities, however, treatment interruptions up to 4 to 8 weeks were allowed for toxicity recovery (Basset-Seguin 2015; Sekulik 2012).

Combination Regimens

Basal cell carcinoma: Vismodegib (Basal Cell Regimen) on page 2111

Administration Oral: May be taken with or without food. Swallow capsules whole; do not open or crush. Vismodegib is associated with a moderate emetic potential; antiemetics may be needed to prevent nausea and vomiting. Hazardous agent; use appropriate precautions for handling and disposal (meets NIOSH 2014 criteria).

Emetic Potential Moderate (30% to 90%)

Monitoring Parameters Pregnancy test within 1 week prior to treatment initiation.

Canadian labeling: Pregnancy testing (minimum sensitivity of 25 milliunits/mL) within 1 week prior to treatment initiation, monthly during treatment (including during treatment interruptions), and for 24 months after discontinuation; CBC with differential and comprehensive metabolic panel at baseline and every 4 weeks thereafter; liver function tests; skin examination routinely during therapy.

Prescribing and Access Restrictions

U.S.: Available at specialty pharmacies through the Erivedge Access Solutions program. Further information may be obtained from the manufacturer, Genentech, at 1-888-249-4918, or at www.ErivedgeAccessSolutions.com

Canada: Available through a controlled distribution program called Erivedge Pregnancy Prevention Program (EPPP). Registration with the program is required for participating prescribers and pharmacies. Patients must also be registered with the program and meet all necessary requirements to receive vismodegib. Consult product monograph for detailed information regarding program requirements. Further information may also be obtained at 1-888-748-8926 or at www.erivedge.ca.

Medication Guide Available Yes

Dosage Forms Excipient information presented when available (limited, particularly for generics); consult specific product labeling.

Capsule, Oral:

Erivedge: 150 mg

♦ **Vistonuridine** see Uridine Triacetate on page 1709

♦ **Vitrase** see Hyaluronidase on page 820

♦ **VLB** see VinBLAStine on page 1740

♦ **VM-26** see Teniposide on page 1622

♦ **Voraxaze** see Glucarpidase on page 793

Voriconazole (vor i KOE na zole)

Brand Names: US Vfend; Vfend IV

Brand Names: Canada Apo-Voriconazole; Sandoz-Voriconazole; Teva-Voriconazole; VFEND; VFEND For Injection; Voriconazole For Injection

Index Terms UK109496

Pharmacologic Category Antifungal Agent, Oral; Antifungal Agent, Parenteral

Use Treatment of fungal infections: Treatment of invasive aspergillosis; treatment of esophageal candidiasis; treatment of candidemia (in non-neutropenic patients); treatment of disseminated *Candida* infections of the skin and abdomen, kidney, bladder wall and wounds; treatment of serious fungal infections caused by *Scedosporium apiospermum* and *Fusarium* spp (including *Fusarium solani*) in patients intolerant of, or refractory to, other therapy in children >12 years of age, adolescents and adults

Pregnancy Risk Factor D

Dosing

Adult & Geriatric Note: Actual body weight should be used for all weight-based dosing calculations.

Aspergillosis, invasive, including disseminated and extrapulmonary infection: Duration of therapy should be a minimum of 6-12 weeks or throughout period of immunosuppression (Walsh 2008); duration of therapy in HIV-positive patients should be until resolution of infection and CD4 count >200 cells/mm^3 (HHS [OI adult 2015]):

IV:

Initial: 6 mg/kg every 12 hours for 2 doses

Maintenance dose: 4 mg/kg every 12 hours

Oral: Maintenance dose:

Manufacturer's labeling: **Note:** If patient has inadequate clinical response, titrate in 50 mg/dose increments for weight <40 kg and 100 mg/dose increments for weight ≥40 kg.

Weight <40 kg: 100 mg every 12 hours

Weight ≥40 kg: 200 mg every 12 hours

IDSA recommendations (Walsh 2008): May consider oral therapy in place of IV with dosing of 4 mg/kg (rounded up to convenient tablet dosage form) every 12 hours; however, IV administration is preferred in serious infections since comparative efficacy with the oral formulation has not been established.

Candidemia in non-neutropenic patients and disseminated *Candida* infections in skin, and infections in abdomen, kidney, bladder wall and wounds: Treatment should continue for a minimum of 14 days following resolution of symptoms or following last positive culture, whichever is longer.

IV:

Initial: 6 mg/kg every 12 hours for 2 doses

Maintenance: 3 to 4 mg/kg every 12 hours

Oral:

Manufacturer's labeling: Maintenance dose: **Note:** If patient has inadequate clinical response, titrate in 50 mg/dose increments for weight <40 kg and 100 mg/dose increments for weight ≥40 kg

Weight <40 kg: 100 mg every 12 hours

Weight ≥40 kg: 200 mg every 12 hours

◀ Alternate recommendations (Pappas 2009):
Initial: 400 mg every 12 hours for 2 doses
Maintenance: 200 mg every 12 hours

Coccidioidomycosis in HIV-infected patients (alternative to preferred therapy) (off-label use; HHS [OI adult 2015]): Oral:

Mild infections (eg, focal pneumonia): 200 mg twice daily; patients who complete initial therapy should be considered for lifelong suppressive therapy.

Chronic suppressive therapy: 200 mg twice daily

Esophageal candidiasis:

Manufacturer's labeling: Oral: Treatment should continue for a minimum of 14 days, and for at least 7 days following resolution of symptoms. **Note:** If patient has inadequate clinical response, titrate in 50 mg/dose increments for weight <40 kg and 100 mg/dose increments for weight ≥40 kg

Weight <40 kg: 100 mg every 12 hours; maximum: 300 mg daily

Weight ≥40 kg: 200 mg every 12 hours; maximum: 600 mg daily

Alternative dosing: HIV-positive patients (alternative to preferred therapy):

Oral, IV: 200 mg twice daily for 14 to 21 days (HHS [OI adult 2015])

Scedosporiosis, fusariosis:

IV:

Initial: 6 mg/kg every 12 hours for 2 doses

Maintenance dose: 4 mg/kg every 12 hours for >7 days

Oral: Maintenance dose: **Note:** If patient has inadequate clinical response, titrate in 50 mg/dose increments for weight <40 kg and 100 mg/dose increments for weight ≥40 kg.

Weight <40 kg: 100 mg every 12 hours.

Weight ≥40 kg: 200 mg every 12 hours.

Endophthalmitis, fungal (off-label use; Pappas 2009): IV: 6 mg/kg every 12 hours for 2 doses, then 3 to 4 mg/kg every 12 hours.

Infection prophylaxis in graft-versus-host disease (GVHD) (high-risk patients) (off-label use; Maertens 2011; Tomblyn 2009; Wingard 2010): Note: The optimal duration of prophylaxis in GVHD has not been determined.

Oral: Weight >40 kg: 200 mg every 12 hours

IV: Weight >40 kg: 4 mg/kg every 12 hours

Infection prophylaxis in standard- or high-risk patients with allogeneic hematopoietic stem cell transplant (HSCT) or certain autologous HSCT (off-label use; Castagna 2012; Maertens 2011; Tomblyn 2009; Wingard 2010): Note: Begin prophylaxis at the start of chemotherapy or the day of transplantation. The ASBMT recommends continuing prophylaxis until engraftment (ie, 30 days) or for 7 days after the ANC reaches >1000 cells/mm³ (Tomblyn 2009). The IDSA recommends anti-mold prophylaxis in allograft HSCT patients "through the neutropenic period and beyond," based on a demonstrated survival advantage in patients receiving prophylaxis for 75 days post-HSCT, or until cessation of immunosuppressive therapy (Freifeld 2011).

Oral: Weight >40 kg: 200 mg every 12 hours

IV: Weight >40 kg: 4 mg/kg every 12 hours.

Meningitis (secondary to contaminated [eg, *Exserohilum rostratum*] steroid products) (off-label use) (CDC [parameningeal] 2012; Kauffman 2013): Note: Consult an infectious disease specialist and current CDC guidelines for specific treatment recommendations. Therapy duration is ≥3 months; trough serum concentrations must be maintained between 2 to 5 mcg/mL.

IV: 6 mg/kg every 12 hours. If patient does not improve or has severe disease, consider adding amphotericin B (liposomal).

Oral (only in mild disease in adherent patients whose trough concentrations/ response to therapy can be closely monitored): 6 mg/kg every 12 hours (CDC [parameningeal] 2012).

Osteoarticular infection involving the spine, discitis, epidural abscess or vertebral osteomyelitis (secondary to contaminated [eg, *Exserohilum rostratum*] steroid products) (off-label use) (CDC [osteoarticular] 2012; Kauffman 2013): IV: 6 mg/kg every 12 hours for ≥3 months. **Note:** Consult an infectious disease specialist and current CDC guidelines for specific treatment recommendations. Trough serum concentrations must be maintained between 2 to 5 mcg/mL. If patient has severe disease, consider adding amphotericin B (liposomal). Patients may be switched to oral therapy if condition has improved or stabilized.

Osteoarticular infection not involving the spine (secondary to contaminated [eg, *Exserohilum rostratum*] steroid products) (off-label use) (CDC [osteoarticular] 2012; Kauffman 2013): Note: Consult an infectious disease specialist and current CDC guidelines for specific treatment recommendations. Therapy duration is ≥3 months. Trough serum concentrations must be maintained between 2 to 5 mcg/mL.

IV: 6 mg/kg every 12 hours for 2 doses, then 4 mg/kg every 12 hours. If patient has severe disease, consider adding amphotericin B (liposomal)

Oral (only in mild disease in adherent patients whose trough concentrations/ response to therapy can be closely monitored): 6 mg/kg every 12 hours for 2 doses, then 4 mg/kg every 12 hours

***Penicillium marneffei* infection in HIV-infected patients (off-label use; HHS [OI adult 2015]):**

Acute infection in severely ill patients: 6 mg/kg IV every 12 hours for 2 doses, then 4 mg/kg IV every 12 hours for at least 3 days, followed by 200 mg orally twice daily for a maximum of 12 weeks; follow with itraconazole chronic maintenance therapy

Mild disease: Oral: 400 mg twice daily for 2 doses, then 200 mg twice daily for a maximum of 12 weeks; follow with itraconazole chronic maintenance therapy

Dosage adjustment in patients with inadequate response:

IV: Maintenance dose may be increased from 3 mg/kg every 12 hours to 4 mg/kg every 12 hours, depending upon condition.

Oral: Maintenance dose may be increased from 200 mg every 12 hours to 300 mg every 12 hours in patients weighing ≥40 kg (or to 150 mg every 12 hours in patients <40 kg), depending upon condition.

Dosage adjustment in patients unable to tolerate treatment:

IV: Maintenance dose may be reduced from 4 mg/kg every 12 hours to 3 mg/kg every 12 hours, depending upon condition.

Oral: Maintenance dose may be reduced in 50 mg decrements to a minimum dosage of 200 mg every 12 hours in patients weighing ≥40 kg (or to 100 mg every 12 hours in patients <40 kg), depending upon condition.

Dosage adjustment in patients receiving concomitant CYP450 enzyme inducers or substrates:

Efavirenz: Oral: Increase maintenance dose of voriconazole to 400 mg every 12 hours and reduce efavirenz dose to 300 mg once daily; upon discontinuation of voriconazole, return to the initial dose of efavirenz.

◄ Phenytoin:

IV: Increase voriconazole maintenance dose to 5 mg/kg every 12 hours.

Oral: Increase voriconazole maintenance dose to 400 mg every 12 hours in patients ≥40 kg (200 mg every 12 hours in patients <40 kg).

Pediatric Note: Actual body weight should be used for all weight-based dosing calculations.

Aspergillosis, invasive including disseminated and extrapulmonary infection treatment (off-label use):

Children >2 to <12 years (<40 kg): Duration of therapy should be a minimum of 6 to 12 weeks or throughout period of immunosuppression (Walsh 2008):

IV: **Note:** Data suggest higher doses (mg/kg) are required; consider using a loading dose: 9 mg/kg/dose every 12 hours for 2 doses on day 1, followed by a maintenance dose: 8 to 9 mg/kg/dose every 12 hours; maximum dose: 350 mg. Monitoring of concentrations may be warranted (Driscoll 2011; *Red Book* [AAP 2012]).

Non-HIV-exposed/-positive (Walsh 2008): 5 to 7 mg/kg/dose every 12 hours; see **Note** regarding higher dose recommendations

HIV-exposed/-positive (CDC 2009): See **Note** regarding higher dose recommendations.

Initial: 6 to 8 mg/kg/dose (maximum: 400 mg/dose) every 12 hours for 2 doses on day 1

Maintenance: 7 mg/kg/dose (maximum: 200 mg/dose) every 12 hours; change to oral administration when able; duration of therapy (IV and oral combined): ≥12 weeks but should be individualized

Oral suspension: May consider oral therapy once the patient is stable

Non-HIV-exposed/-positive (Red Book [AAP 2012]): 9 mg/kg/dose every 12 hours

HIV-exposed/-positive (CDC 2009): **Note:** Data suggest higher doses (mg/kg) are required (9 mg/kg every 12 hours) (*Red Book* [AAP 2012])

Initial: 8 mg/kg/dose (maximum: 400 mg/dose) every 12 hours for 2 doses on day 1

Maintenance: 7 mg/kg/dose (maximum: 200 mg/dose) every 12 hours

Children ≥12 years and Adolescents: Refer to adult dosing.

Candidiasis or other serious fungal infection, treatment (off-label use; Driscoll 2011; *Red Book* [AAP 2012]):

Children >2 to <12 years: IV: Loading dose: 9 mg/kg/dose every 12 hours for 2 doses on day 1, followed by a maintenance dose: 8 to 9 mg/kg/dose every 12 hours; maximum dose: 350 mg

Children ≥12 years and Adolescents: Refer to adult dosing.

Catheter-related bloodstream infections due to *Malassezia furfur* (off-label use; Mermel 2009):

Children >2 to <12 years: IV: **Note:** Recent data suggest higher doses (mg/kg) than described in the guideline may be required (Driscoll 2011):

Initial: 6 mg/kg every 12 hours for 2 doses.

Maintenance: 4 mg/kg every 12 hours.

Children ≥12 years and Adolescents: Refer to adult dosing.

Coccidioidomycosis in HIV-infected patients (alternative to preferred therapy) (off-label use; HHS [OI adult 2015]): Adolescents: Oral: Refer to adult dosing.

Esophageal candidiasis:

Manufacturer's labeling: Children ≥12 years and Adolescents: Refer to adult dosing.

Alternative dosing: HIV-infected patients (alternative to preferred therapy): Adolescents: Refer to adult dosing.

Infection prophylaxis in graft-versus-host disease (GVHD) (off-label use; Tombyln 2009; Wingard 2010):
Children >2 to <12 years: **Note:** The optimal duration of prophylaxis in GVHD has not been determined.
IV: 4 mg/kg every 12 hours (maximum dose not to exceed weight-based oral dose)
Oral:
Weight <20 kg: 50 mg every 12 hours
Weight ≥20 kg: 100 mg every 12 hours
Children ≥12 years and Adolescents: Refer to adult dosing.

Infection prophylaxis in standard- or high-risk patients with allogeneic hematopoietic stem cell transplant (HSCT) or certain autologous HSCT (off-label use): Adolescents (>40 kg): Refer to adult dosing.

Penicillium marneffei infection in HIV-infected patients (off-label use; HHS [OI adult 2015]): Refer to adult dosing.

Renal Impairment
IV:
CrCl ≥50 mL/minute: There are no dosage adjustments provided in the manufacturer's labeling.
CrCl <50 mL/minute: There are no specific dosage adjustments provided in the manufacturer's labeling. Due to accumulation of the intravenous vehicle (cyclodextrin), the manufacturer recommends the use of oral voriconazole in these patients unless an assessment of the benefit:risk justifies the use of IV voriconazole; if IV therapy is used, closely monitor serum creatinine and change to oral voriconazole when possible. IV therapy has been used in select patients with CrCl <50 mL/minute using varying doses (median duration of treatment 7 to 10 days) (Neofytos 2012; Oude Lashof 2012).
Oral:
Mild to severe impairment: No dosage adjustment necessary.
Dialysis: Poorly dialyzed; no supplemental dose or dosage adjustment necessary, including patients on intermittent hemodialysis (IHD) with thrice weekly sessions or peritoneal dialysis.
Continuous renal replacement therapy (CRRT) (Heintz 2009): Drug clearance is highly dependent on the method of renal replacement, filter type, and flow rate. Appropriate dosing requires close monitoring of pharmacologic response, signs of adverse reactions due to drug accumulation, as well as drug concentrations in relation to target trough (if appropriate). The following are general recommendations only (based on dialysate flow/ultrafiltration rates of 1 to 2 L/hour and minimal residual renal function) and should not supersede clinical judgment:
CVVH, CVVHD, and CVVHDF: Loading dose of 400 mg every 12 hours for 2 doses, followed by 200 mg every 12 hours.

Hepatic Impairment
Mild to moderate impairment (Child-Pugh class A or B): Following standard loading dose, reduce maintenance dosage by 50%
Severe impairment (Child-Pugh class C): There are no dosage adjustments provided in the manufacturer's labeling (has not been studied). Should only be used if benefit outweighs risk; monitor closely for toxicity

Additional Information Complete prescribing information should be consulted for additional detail.

◀ **Dosage Forms** Excipient information presented when available (limited, particularly for generics); consult specific product labeling.
Solution Reconstituted, Intravenous:
Generic: 200 mg (1 ea)
Solution Reconstituted, Intravenous [preservative free]:
Vfend IV: 200 mg (1 ea) [latex free]
Vfend IV: 200 mg (1 ea)
Suspension Reconstituted, Oral:
Vfend: 40 mg/mL (75 mL) [contains sodium benzoate; orange flavor]
Generic: 40 mg/mL (75 mL)
Tablet, Oral:
Vfend: 50 mg, 200 mg
Generic: 50 mg, 200 mg

◆ **Voriconazole For Injection (Can)** see Voriconazole on page 1775

Vorinostat (vor IN oh stat)

Related Information

Hematopoietic Stem Cell Transplantation on page 2272
Management of Chemotherapy-Induced Nausea and Vomiting in Adults on page 2142
Prevention of Chemotherapy-Induced Nausea and Vomiting in Children on page 2203
Principles of Anticancer Therapy on page 2261
Safe Handling of Hazardous Drugs on page 2292

Brand Names: US Zolinza

Brand Names: Canada Zolinza

Index Terms SAHA; Suberoylanilide Hydroxamic Acid

Pharmacologic Category Antineoplastic Agent, Histone Deacetylase (HDAC) Inhibitor

Use Cutaneous T-cell lymphoma: Treatment of cutaneous manifestations of cutaneous T-cell lymphoma (CTCL) with progressive, persistent, or recurrent disease on or following 2 systemic treatments

Labeled Contraindications There are no contraindications in the manufacturer's U.S. labeling.

Canadian labeling: Hypersensitivity to vorinostat or any component of the formulation; severe hepatic impairment (total bilirubin ≥3 times ULN)

Pregnancy Considerations Adverse events were observed in animal reproduction studies. Based on the mechanism of action, may cause fetal harm if administered during pregnancy. Inform patient of potential hazard if used during pregnancy or if pregnancy occurs during treatment.

Breast-Feeding Considerations It is not known if vorinostat is excreted in breast milk. Due to the potential for serious adverse reactions in the nursing infant, the decision to discontinue vorinostat or to discontinue breast-feeding should take into account the benefits of treatment to the mother.

Warnings/Precautions Hazardous agent - use appropriate precautions for handling and disposal (NIOSH 2014 [group 1]). Pulmonary embolism and deep vein thrombosis (DVT) have been reported; monitor for signs/symptoms; use caution in patients with a history of thrombotic events. Dose-related thrombocytopenia and/or anemia may occur; may require dosage adjustments or discontinuation; monitor blood counts (every 2 weeks for 2 months, then monthly). Gastrointestinal bleeding due to severe thrombocytopenia has been reported in patients receiving vorinostat in combination with other histone deacetylase inhibitors (eg, valproic acid); monitor platelet counts more frequently in patients receiving concomitant histone deacetylase inhibitor therapy. QTc prolongation has been observed; baseline and periodic ECGs were done in clinical trials (Duvic, 2007; Olsen, 2007). Correct electrolyte abnormalities prior to treatment and monitor and correct potassium, calcium, and magnesium levels during therapy. Use caution in patients with a history of QTc prolongation or with medications known to prolong the QT interval. May cause hyperglycemia (may be severe); monitor serum glucose and use with caution in diabetics; may require diet and/or therapy modifications. Nausea, vomiting, and diarrhea may occur; antiemetics and antidiarrheals may be required; control preexisting nausea, vomiting, and diarrhea prior to treatment initiation; replace fluids and electrolytes to avoid dehydration. Adverse anastomotic healing events have occurred in patients recovering from bowel surgery; use with caution in the perioperative period in patients requiring bowel surgery. May cause dizziness or fatigue; caution patients about performing tasks which require mental alertness (eg, operating machinery or driving). Use with caution in patients with hepatic impairment; dose reductions are recommended (elimination is predominantly hepatic). The Canadian labeling does not recommend use in patients with moderate hepatic impairment (total bilirubin 1.5 to 3 times ULN) and contraindicates use in severe hepatic impairment (bilirubin ≥3 times ULN). Potentially significant drug-drug interactions may exist, requiring dose or frequency adjustment, additional monitoring, and/or selection of alternative therapy.

Adverse Reactions

>10%:

Cardiovascular: Peripheral edema (13%)

Central nervous system: Fatigue (52%), chills (16%), dizziness (15%), headache (12%), fever (11%)

Dermatologic: Alopecia (19%), pruritus (12%)

Endocrine & metabolic: Hyperglycemia (8% to 69%; grade 3: 5%), dehydration (1% to 16%)

Gastrointestinal: Diarrhea (52%), nausea (41%), taste alteration (28%), anorexia (24%), weight loss (21%), xerostomia (16%), constipation (15%), vomiting (15%), appetite decreased (14%)

Hematologic: Thrombocytopenia (26%; grades 3/4: 6%), anemia (14%; grades 3/4: 2%)

Neuromuscular & skeletal: Muscle spasm (20%)

Renal: Proteinuria (51%), creatinine increased (16% to 47%)

Respiratory: Cough (11%), upper respiratory infection (11%)

1% to 10%:

Cardiovascular: QTc prolongation (3% to 4%)

Dermatologic: Squamous cell carcinoma (4%)

Respiratory: Pulmonary embolism (5%)

<1%, postmarketing, and/or case reports: Abdominal pain, angioneurotic edema, blurred vision, chest pain, cholecystitis, deafness, diverticulitis, dysphagia, DVT, enterococcal infection, exfoliative dermatitis, gastrointestinal bleeding, gastrointestinal hemorrhage, Guillain-Barré syndrome, hemoptysis, hypertension, hypokalemia, hyponatremia, infection, lethargy, leukopenia, MI, neutropenia, pneumonia, renal failure, sepsis, spinal cord injury, streptococcal bacteremia, stroke (ischemic), syncope, T-cell lymphoma, tumor hemorrhage, ureteric obstruction, ureteropelvic junction obstruction, urinary retention, vasculitis, weakness

◀ **Drug Interactions**

Metabolism/Transport Effects None known.

Avoid Concomitant Use

Avoid concomitant use of Vorinostat with any of the following: BCG (Intravesical); CloZAPine; Dipyrone

Increased Effect/Toxicity

Vorinostat may increase the levels/effects of: CloZAPine; Highest Risk QTc-Prolonging Agents; Moderate Risk QTc-Prolonging Agents; Vitamin K Antagonists

The levels/effects of Vorinostat may be increased by: Dipyrone; Mifepristone; Valproate Products

Decreased Effect

Vorinostat may decrease the levels/effects of: Antidiabetic Agents; BCG (Intravesical)

Storage/Stability Store at 20°C to 25°C (68°F to 77°F); excursions permitted to 15°C to 30°C (59°F to 86°F).

Mechanism of Action Inhibits histone deacetylase enzymes, HDAC1, HDAC2, HDAC3, and HDAC6, which catalyze acetyl group removal from protein lysine residues (including histones and transcription factors). Histone deacetylase inhibition results in accumulation of acetyl groups, which alters chromatin structure and transcription factor activation; cell growth is terminated and apoptosis occurs.

Pharmacodynamics/Kinetics

Protein binding: ~71%

Metabolism: Glucuronidated and hydrolyzed (followed by beta-oxidation) to inactive metabolites

Bioavailability: Fasting: ~43%

Half-life elimination: ~2 hours

Time to peak, plasma: With high-fat meal: ~4 hours (range: 2 to 10 hours)

Excretion: Urine: 52% (~52% as inactive metabolites; <1% as unchanged drug)

Dosing

Adult & Geriatric Cutaneous T-cell lymphoma (CTCL): Oral: 400 mg once daily until disease progression or unacceptable toxicity

Renal Impairment There are no dosage adjustments provided in the manufacturer's labeling (has not been studied). However, based on the minimal renal elimination, adjustment not expected. Use with caution.

Hepatic Impairment

U.S. labeling: Initial:

Mild-to-moderate impairment (total bilirubin 1-3 times ULN **or** AST >ULN): 300 mg once daily

Severe impairment (total bilirubin >3 times ULN): There are no dosage adjustments provided in the manufacturer's labeling (evidence is insufficient for a starting dose recommendation). Doses of 100 to 200 mg once daily were studied in a limited number of patients with severe impairment (Ramalingam, 2010); according to the manufacturer, the maximum dose used was 200 mg once daily.

Canadian labeling:
  Mild impairment (total bilirubin >1 to 1.5 times ULN or total bilirubin ≤ULN and AST >ULN): 300 mg once daily
  Moderate impairment (total bilirubin 1.5-3 times ULN): Use is not recommended
  Severe impairment (total bilirubin ≥3 times ULN): Use is contraindicated

Adjustment for Toxicity
  U.S. labeling: Intolerance: Reduce dose to 300 mg once daily; if needed, may further reduce to 300 mg daily for 5 consecutive days per week
  Canadian labeling: Grade 3 or 4 toxicity: Interrupt therapy until resolves to ≤ grade 1 (excluding grade 3 anemia and thrombocytopenia). Upon recovery, may reduce dose to 300 mg once daily. If necessary, may further reduce dose to 300 mg once daily for 5 consecutive days per week.
  Additionally, in clinical trials, **dose reductions** were instituted for the following adverse events: Increased serum creatinine, decreased appetite, hypokalemia, leukopenia, nausea, neutropenia, thrombocytopenia, and vomiting. Vorinostat was **discontinued** for the following adverse events: Anemia, angioneurotic edema, weakness, chest pain, exfoliative dermatitis, DVT, ischemic stroke, lethargy, pulmonary embolism, and spinal cord injury.
  Treatment was withheld in clinical trials for grade 4 anemia or thrombocytopenia or other grade 3 or 4 drug related toxicity, until resolved to ≤ grade 1. Treatment was reinitiated with dose reduction (Olsen, 2007).

Combination Regimens
Lymphoma, non-Hodgkin (CTCL): Vorinostat (NHL-CTCL Regimen) on page 2111

Administration
Administer with food. Do not open, crush, break, or chew capsules. Maintain adequate hydration (≥2 L/day fluids) during treatment.

Hazardous agent; use appropriate precautions for handling and disposal (NIOSH 2014 [group 1]). Avoid direct skin or mucous membrane contact with crushed or broken capsules and/or capsule contents.

Emetic Potential
Children and Adults: Low (10% to 30%)

Extemporaneous Preparations
Hazardous agent: Use appropriate precautions for handling and disposal (NIOSH 2014 [group 1]).

Although not recommended by the manufacturer, a 50 mg/mL oral suspension may be prepared with capsules. Add 20 mL Ora-Plus® into a glass bottle (≥4 oz). Add the contents of twenty 100 mg capsules and shake thoroughly to disperse (may take up to 3 minutes). Add 20 mL Ora-Sweet® and shake to disperse. Label "shake well". Stable for 14 days at room temperature.

Fouladi M, Park JR, Stewart CF, et al, "Pediatric Phase I Trial and Pharmacokinetic Study of Vorinostat: A Children's Oncology Group Phase I Consortium Report," *J Clin Oncol*, 2010, 28 (22):3623-9.

Monitoring Parameters
CBC with differential and serum chemistries, including calcium, magnesium, potassium, glucose and creatinine (baseline, then every 2 weeks for 2 months, then monthly, or as clinically necessary), hepatic function, INR (if on concomitant warfarin therapy), fluid status, signs/symptoms of thromboembolism. Baseline and periodic ECGs were done in clinical trials (and are recommended in the Canadian labeling).

Dosage Forms
Excipient information presented when available (limited, particularly for generics); consult specific product labeling.
Capsule, Oral:
  Zolinza: 100 mg

♦ **Votrient** *see* PAZOPanib *on page 1334*

- ◆ **Zevalin (Can)** see Ibritumomab on page 851
- ◆ **Zevalin Y-90** see Ibritumomab on page 851

Ziconotide (zi KOE no tide)

Brand Names: US Prialt

Pharmacologic Category Analgesic, Nonopioid; Calcium Channel Blocker, N-Type

Use Management of severe chronic pain in patients requiring intrathecal therapy and who are intolerant or refractory to other therapies

Pregnancy Risk Factor C

Dosing

Adult Chronic pain: Intrathecal: Initial dose: ≤2.4 mcg/day (0.1 mcg/hour)

Dose may be titrated by ≤2.4 mcg/day (0.1 mcg/hour) at intervals ≤2-3 times/ week to a maximum dose of 19.2 mcg/day (0.8 mcg/hour) by day 21; average dose at day 21: 6.9 mcg/day (0.29 mcg/hour). A faster titration should be used only if the urgent need for analgesia outweighs the possible risk to patient safety.

Geriatric Refer to adult dosing. Use with caution.

Renal Impairment No dosage adjustment provided in manufacturer's labeling (has not been studied).

Hepatic Impairment No dosage adjustment provided in manufacturer's labeling (has not been studied).

Adjustment for Toxicity

Cognitive impairment: Reduce dose or discontinue. Effects are generally reversible within 3-15 days of discontinuation.

Reduced level of consciousness: Discontinue until event resolves.

CK elevation with neuromuscular symptoms: Consider dose reduction or discontinuation.

Additional Information Complete prescribing information should be consulted for additional detail.

Dosage Forms Excipient information presented when available (limited, particularly for generics); consult specific product labeling.

Solution, Intrathecal, as acetate [preservative free]:

Prialt: 500 mcg/20 mL (20 mL); 100 mcg/mL (1 mL); 500 mcg/5 mL (5 mL)

- ◆ **Zictifa** see Vandetanib on page 1728
- ◆ **Zinda-Anastrozole (Can)** see Anastrozole on page 112
- ◆ **Zinda-Letrozole (Can)** see Letrozole on page 1019
- ◆ **Zinecard** see Dexrazoxane on page 523

Ziv-Aflibercept (Systemic) (ziv a FLIB er sept)

Brand Names: US Zaltrap

Index Terms Aflibercept I.V.; Vascular Endothelial Growth Factor Trap; VEGF Trap; VEGF Trap R1R2

Pharmacologic Category Antineoplastic Agent; Vascular Endothelial Growth Factor (VEGF) Inhibitor

Use Colorectal cancer, metastatic: Treatment of metastatic colorectal cancer (in combination with fluorouracil, leucovorin, and irinotecan [FOLFIRI]) in patients who are resistant to or have progressed on an oxaliplatin-based regimen

Labeled Contraindications There are no contraindications listed in the manufacturer's labeling.

▶

◀ **Pregnancy Considerations** Adverse events were observed in animal reproduction studies with doses providing systemic exposure equivalent to ~30% of a human dose. The incidence of fetal malformations increased with increasing doses. Patients (male and female) should use effective contraception during therapy and for at least 3 months following treatment.

Breast-Feeding Considerations It is not known if ziv-aflibercept is excreted into breast milk. Due to the potential for serious adverse reactions in the nursing infant, the manufacturer recommends a decision to be made whether to discontinue nursing or to discontinue aflibercept, taking into account the importance of treatment to the mother.

Warnings/Precautions The risk for hemorrhage is increased with ziv-aflibercept. **[U.S. Boxed Warning]: Severe and occasionally fatal hemorrhage, including gastrointestinal (GI) bleeding, has been reported with ziv-aflibercept/FOLFIRI. Monitor for signs and symptoms of GI and other severe bleeding events; do not administer to patients with severe hemorrhage; discontinue if severe hemorrhage develops.** Hemorrhagic events have also included hematuria, postprocedural hemorrhage, intracranial hemorrhage, and pulmonary hemorrhage/hemoptysis.

[U.S. Boxed Warning]: Severe or fatal GI perforation is a possibility; discontinue ziv-aflibercept if GI perforation occurs; monitor for signs/symptoms of GI perforation. The risk for GI and non-GI fistulas is increased with ziv-aflibercept; fistula sites have included anal, enterovesical, enterocutaneous, colovaginal and intestinal; discontinue in patients who develop fistula. Severe diarrhea and dehydration have been reported; the incidence of diarrhea is increased in patients ≥65 years of age; monitor elderly patients closely for diarrhea.

Proteinuria, nephrotic syndrome, and thrombotic microangiopathy (TMA) have been associated with ziv-aflibercept. Evaluate for proteinuria during treatment with urine dipstick and/or urinary protein creatinine ratio (UPCR); if dipstick ≥2+ for protein or UPCR >1, obtain 24-hour urine collection. Withhold ziv-aflibercept for proteinuria ≥2 g per 24 hours; for recurrent proteinuria, withhold treatment until <2 g per 24 hours and then resume with permanent dose reduction. Discontinue treatment for nephrotic syndrome or TMA.

The risk for grades 3/4 hypertension is increased; onset is generally within the first 2 treatment cycles. Monitor blood pressure every 2 weeks (more frequently if clinically indicated); treat with appropriate antihypertensive therapy (may require adjustment of existing antihypertensives); temporarily withhold treatment with uncontrolled hypertension; may reinitiate with permanent dose reduction when controlled. Discontinue for hypertensive crisis or encephalopathy. Patients with NYHA class III or IV heart failure were excluded from clinical trials.

[U.S. Boxed Warning]: Severely compromised wound healing may occur with ziv-aflibercept/FOLFIRI. Discontinue ziv-aflibercept with compromised wound healing. Withhold ziv-aflibercept at least 4 weeks prior to elective surgery. Do not resume ziv-aflibercept treatment until at least 4 weeks after major surgery AND until the surgical wound is completely healed. For minor surgeries (eg, central venous access port placement, biopsy, or tooth extraction), ziv-aflibercept may be resumed or initiated as soon as the surgical wound is fully healed.

A higher incidence of neutropenia and complications due to neutropenia (neutropenic fever and infection) occurred in patients receiving ziv-aflibercept; leukopenia and thrombocytopenia were also observed in clinical trials; monitor CBC with differential (baseline and prior to each cycle); delay treatment until ANC is ≥1,500/mm³. Cases of reversible posterior leukoencephalopathy syndrome (RPLS) have been reported; confirm diagnosis with MRI; discontinue ziv-aflibercept if verified; symptoms generally resolve or improve within days, although persistent neurologic symptoms and death have been reported. Arterial thrombotic events (ATE), including transient ischemic attack, cerebrovascular accidents, and angina have occurred. Discontinue ziv-aflibercept in patients who experience ATEs. Certain adverse events, such as diarrhea, dizziness, weakness, weight loss, and dehydration, occurred at a higher incidence in elderly compared to younger adults; monitor closely during treatment.

Adverse Reactions Note: Reactions reported in combination therapy with fluorouracil, leucovorin, and irinotecan (FOLFIRI).

>10%:

Cardiovascular: Hypertension (41%; grades 3/4: 19%)

Central nervous system: Fatigue (48%), dysphonia (25%), headache (22%)

Dermatologic: Palmar-plantar erythrodysesthesia (11%)

Gastrointestinal: Diarrhea (69%), stomatitis (50%), appetite decreased (32%), weight loss (32%), abdominal pain (27%), upper abdominal pain (11%)

Hematologic: Leukopenia (78%; grades 3/4: 16%), neutropenia (67%; grades 3/4: 37%), thrombocytopenia (48%; grades 3/4: 3%), bleeding (38%; grades 3/4: 3%)

Hepatic: AST increased (62%), ALT increased (50%)

Neuromuscular & skeletal: Weakness (18%)

Renal: Proteinuria (62%; grades 3/4: 8%), creatinine increased (23%)

Respiratory: Epistaxis (28%), dyspnea (12%)

Miscellaneous: Infection (46%)

1% to 10%:

Cardiovascular: Venous thromboembolic events (9%), arterial thromboembolic events (3%; grades 3/4: 2%)

Central nervous system: Reversible posterior encephalopathy syndrome (RPLS) (1%)

Dermatologic: Hyperpigmentation (8%)

Endocrine & metabolic: Dehydration (9%)

Gastrointestinal: Hemorrhoids (6%), proctalgia (5%), rectal hemorrhage (5%), gastrointestinal perforation (1%)

Genitourinary: Urinary tract infection (9%)

Hematologic: Neutropenic fever (grades 3/4: 4%), neutropenic infection/sepsis (grades 3/4: 2%)

Renal: Nephrotic syndrome (1%)

Respiratory: Oropharyngeal pain (8%), rhinorrhea (6%), pulmonary embolism (5%)

Miscellaneous: Antibody formation (3%), fistula formation (2%; grades 3/4: <1%)

<1%: Hypersensitivity reactions, thrombotic microangiopathy, wound healing impaired

◀ **Drug Interactions**

Metabolism/Transport Effects None known.

Avoid Concomitant Use

Avoid concomitant use of Ziv-Aflibercept (Systemic) with any of the following: BCG (Intravesical); CloZAPine; Dipyrone

Increased Effect/Toxicity

Ziv-Aflibercept (Systemic) may increase the levels/effects of: Bisphosphonate Derivatives; CloZAPine

The levels/effects of Ziv-Aflibercept (Systemic) may be increased by: Dipyrone

Decreased Effect

Ziv-Aflibercept (Systemic) may decrease the levels/effects of: BCG (Intravesical)

Storage/Stability Store intact vials refrigerated at 2°C to 8°C (36°F to 46°F). Protect from light (store in original outer carton).

Solutions diluted for infusion may be stored in refrigerator for up to 24 hours, or at 20°C to 25°C (68°F to 77°F) for up to 8 hours.

Preparation for Administration Prior to infusion, dilute in D_5W or NS to a final concentration of 0.6-8 mg/mL. Use polyvinyl chloride (PVC) infusion bags containing DEHP or polyolefin bags. After initial vial puncture, do not re-enter; discard any unused portion of the vial. Do not mix with other medications.

Mechanism of Action Also known as VEGF-trap, ziv-aflibercept is a recombinant fusion protein which is comprised of portions of binding domains for vascular endothelial growth factor (VEGF) receptors 1 and 2, attached to the Fc portion of human IgG1. Ziv-aflibercept acts as a decoy receptor for VEGF-A, VEGF-B, and placental growth factor (PlGF) which prevent VEGF receptor binding/activation to their receptors (an action critical to angiogenesis), thus leading to antiangiogenesis and tumor regression.

Pharmacodynamics/Kinetics Half-life elimination: ~6 days (range: 4 to 7 days)

Dosing

Adult & Geriatric Colorectal cancer, metastatic: IV: 4 mg/kg every 2 weeks (in combination with fluorouracil, leucovorin, and irinotecan [FOLFIRI]), continue until disease progression or unacceptable toxicity

Renal Impairment There are no dosage adjustments provided in the manufacturer's labeling; however, need for adjustment is not likely because exposure in patients with mild, moderate, and severe impairment was similar to that of patients with normal renal function.

Hepatic Impairment

Mild (total bilirubin >1 to 1.5 times ULN) to moderate (total bilirubin >1.5 to 3 times ULN) impairment: There are no dosage adjustments provided in the manufacturer's labeling; however, need for adjustment is not likely because exposure was similar to that of patients with normal hepatic function.

Severe impairment (total bilirubin >3 times ULN): There are no dosage adjustments provided in the manufacturer's labeling (no data available).

Adjustment for Toxicity

Arterial thrombotic events: Discontinue treatment.

Fistula formation: Discontinue treatment.

Gastrointestinal perforation: Discontinue treatment.

Hemorrhage, severe: Discontinue treatment.

Hypertension:
Recurrent or severe hypertension: Temporarily withhold treatment until controlled and then resume with a permanent dose reduction to 2 mg/kg every 2 weeks.
Hypertensive crisis or hypertensive encephalopathy: Discontinue treatment.
Neutropenia: Temporarily withhold treatment until ANC is ≥1500/mm³.
Renal effects:
Proteinuria (≥2 g/24 hours): Temporarily withhold treatment until proteinuria <2 g/24 hours and then resume at previous dose.
Recurrent proteinuria: Temporarily withhold treatment until proteinuria <2 g/24 hours and then resume with a permanent dose reduction to 2 mg/kg every 2 weeks.
Nephrotic syndrome or thrombotic microangiopathy: Discontinue treatment
Reversible posterior leukoencephalopathy syndrome (RPLS): Discontinue treatment.
Surgery/wound healing impairment:
Elective surgery: Temporarily withhold treatment for at least 4 weeks prior to elective surgery; do not resume until at least 4 weeks after major surgery AND until wound is fully healed; for minor surgery (eg, biopsy, central venous port placement, tooth extraction), may be resumed after wound is fully healed.
Wound healing impaired: Discontinue treatment.
Note: For toxicities related to FOLFIRI, refer to individual Fluorouracil or Irinotecan monographs.

Combination Regimens
Colorectal cancer: Ziv-Aflibercept + FOLFIRI (Colorectal) on page 2112

Administration IV: Infuse over 1 hour. Do not administer as an IV push or bolus. Administer prior to any FOLFIRI component. Do not administer other medications through the same intravenous line.

Infuse via a 0.2 micron polyethersulfone filter; do not use filters made of polyvinylidene fluoride (PVDF) or nylon. Administer with one of the following types of infusion sets: Polyvinyl chloride (PVC) containing DEHP, DEHP-free PVC containing trioctyl-trimellitate (TOTM), polypropylene, polyethylene lined PVC, or polyurethane.

Emetic Potential Low (10% to 30%)

Monitoring Parameters CBC with differential (baseline and prior to each cycle); urine protein (dipstick analysis and/or urinary protein creatinine ratio [UPCR], obtain 24-hour urine collection if dipstick ≥2+ for protein or UPCR >1); blood pressure (every 2 weeks; more frequently if clinically indicated); monitor for signs/symptoms of hemorrhage or GI perforation; monitor elderly patients closely for diarrhea and/or dehydration. Monitor wounds for healing impairment.

Dosage Forms Excipient information presented when available (limited, particularly for generics); consult specific product labeling.
Solution, Intravenous [preservative free]:
Zaltrap: 100 mg/4 mL (4 mL); 200 mg/8 mL (8 mL) [contains mouse protein (murine) (hamster)]

◆ **Zofran** see Ondansetron *on page 1253*
◆ **Zofran ODT** see Ondansetron *on page 1253*
◆ **Zol 446** see Zoledronic Acid *on page 1790*
◆ **Zoladex** see Goserelin *on page 796*

♦ **Zoladex LA (Can)** *see* Goserelin *on page* 796
♦ **Zoledronate** *see* Zoledronic Acid *on page* 1790

Zoledronic Acid (zoe le DRON ik AS id)

Related Information

Chronic Pain Management (Cancer) *on page* 2229
Hypercalcemia of Malignancy *on page* 2241
Safe Handling of Hazardous Drugs *on page* 2292

Brand Names: US Reclast; Zometa

Brand Names: Canada Aclasta; Taro-Zoledronic Acid; Taro-Zoledronic Acid Concentrate; Zoledronic Acid Injection; Zoledronic Acid for Injection; Zoledronic Acid Z; Zometa Concentrate

Index Terms CGP-42446; Zol 446; Zoledronate

Pharmacologic Category Bisphosphonate Derivative

Use

Glucocorticoid-induced osteoporosis (Reclast, Aclasta [Canadian product]): Treatment and prevention of glucocorticoid-induced osteoporosis in men and women who are initiating or continuing systemic glucocorticoids in a daily dose equivalent to 7.5 mg or more of prednisone and who are expected to remain on glucocorticoids for at least 12 months.

Hypercalcemia of malignancy (Zometa): Treatment of hypercalcemia (albumin-corrected serum calcium ≥12 mg/dL) of malignancy.

Multiple myeloma and bone metastases from solid tumors (Zometa): Treatment of patients with multiple myeloma and patients with documented bone metastases from solid tumors, in conjunction with standard antineoplastic therapy.

Osteoporosis in men (Reclast, Aclasta [Canadian product]): To increase bone mass in men with osteoporosis.

Paget disease of bone (Reclast, Aclasta [Canadian product]): Treatment of Paget disease of bone in men and women. **Note:** In patients without contraindications, zoledronic acid is recommended as the treatment of choice per Endocrine Society guidelines (Singer, 2014).

Postmenopausal osteoporosis (Reclast, Aclasta [Canadian product]): Treatment and prevention of osteoporosis in postmenopausal women.

Labeled Contraindications

U.S. labeling:

Hypersensitivity to zoledronic acid or any component of the formulation; hypocalcemia (Reclast only); CrCl <35 mL/minute and in those with evidence of acute renal impairment (Reclast only).

Documentation of allergenic cross-reactivity for bisphosphonates is limited. However, because of similarities in chemical structure and/or pharmacologic actions, the possibility of cross-sensitivity cannot be ruled out with certainty.

Canadian labeling:

All indications: Hypersensitivity to zoledronic acid or other bisphosphonates, or any component of the formulation; uncorrected hypocalcemia at the time of infusion; pregnancy; breast-feeding

Nononcology uses: Additional contraindications: Use in patients with CrCl <35 mL/minute and use in patients with evidence of acute renal impairment due to an increased risk of renal failure

Pregnancy Considerations Adverse events were observed in animal reproduction studies. It is not known if bisphosphonates cross the placenta, but fetal exposure is expected (Djokanovic, 2008; Stathopoulos, 2011).

Bisphosphonates are incorporated into the bone matrix and gradually released over time. The amount available in the systemic circulation varies by dose and duration of therapy. Theoretically, there may be a risk of fetal harm when pregnancy follows the completion of therapy; however, available data have not shown that exposure to bisphosphonates during pregnancy significantly increases the risk of adverse fetal events (Djokanovic, 2008; Levy, 2009; Stathopoulos, 2011). Until additional data is available, most sources recommend discontinuing bisphosphonate therapy in women of reproductive potential as early as possible prior to a planned pregnancy; use in premenopausal women should be reserved for special circumstances when rapid bone loss is occurring (Bhalla, 2010; Pereira, 2012; Stathopoulos, 2011). Because hypocalcemia has been described following *in utero* bisphosphonate exposure, exposed infants should be monitored for hypocalcemia after birth (Djokanovic, 2008; Stathopoulos, 2011). Use in pregnant women is contraindicated per the Canadian labeling.

Breast-Feeding Considerations It is not known if zoledronic acid is excreted into breast milk. Due to the potential for serious adverse reactions in the nursing infant, the U.S. manufacturer recommends a decision be made whether to discontinue nursing or to discontinue the drug, taking into account the importance of treatment to the mother. Use in nursing women is contraindicated per the Canadian labeling.

Warnings/Precautions Hazardous agent - use appropriate precautions for handling and disposal (NIOSH 2014 [group 3]).

Osteonecrosis of the jaw (ONJ) has been reported in patients receiving bisphosphonates. Risk factors include invasive dental procedures (eg, tooth extraction, dental implants, boney surgery); a diagnosis of cancer, with concomitant chemotherapy (including antiangiogenesis treatment), radiotherapy, or corticosteroids; poor oral hygiene, ill-fitting dentures; and comorbid disorders (anemia, coagulopathy, infection, preexisting dental disease). Most reported cases occurred after IV bisphosphonate therapy; however, cases have been reported following oral therapy. A dental exam and preventive dentistry should be performed prior to placing patients with risk factors on chronic bisphosphonate therapy. The manufacturer's labeling states that there are no data to suggest whether discontinuing bisphosphonates in patients requiring invasive dental procedures reduces the risk of ONJ. However, other experts suggest that there is no evidence that discontinuing therapy reduces the risk of developing ONJ (Assael, 2009). The benefit/risk must be assessed by the treating physician and/or dentist/surgeon prior to any invasive dental procedure. Patients developing ONJ while on bisphosphonates should receive care by an oral surgeon.

Atypical, low-energy, or low-trauma femur fractures have been reported in patients receiving bisphosphonates. The fractures include subtrochanteric femur (bone just below the hip joint) and diaphyseal femur (long segment of the thigh bone). Some patients experience prodromal pain weeks or months before the fracture occurs. It is unclear if bisphosphonate therapy is the cause for these fractures; atypical femur fractures have also been reported in patients not taking bisphosphonates, and in patients receiving glucocorticoids. Patients receiving long-term (>3 to 5 years) bisphosphonate therapy may be at an increased risk. Patients presenting with thigh or groin pain with a history of receiving bisphosphonates should be evaluated for femur fracture. Consider interrupting bisphosphonate therapy in patients who develop a femoral shaft fracture; assess for fracture in the contralateral limb.

Infrequently, severe (and occasionally debilitating) musculoskeletal (bone, joint, and/or muscle) pain have been reported during bisphosphonate treatment. The onset of pain ranged from a single day to several months. Consider discontinuing therapy in patients who experience severe symptoms; symptoms usually resolve upon discontinuation. Some patients experienced recurrence when rechallenged with same drug or another bisphosphonate; avoid use in patients with a history of these symptoms in association with bisphosphonate therapy.

Hypocalcemia (including severe and life-threatening cases) has been reported with use; patients with Paget disease may be at significant risk for hypocalcemia after treatment with zoledronic acid (because pretreatment rate of bone turnover may be elevated); severe and life-threatening hypocalcemia has also been reported with oncology-related uses. Measure serum calcium prior to treatment initiation. Correct preexisting hypocalcemia before initiation of therapy in patients with Paget disease, osteoporosis, or oncology indications. Use with caution with other medications known to cause hypocalcemia (severe hypocalcemia may develop). Ensure adequate calcium and vitamin D supplementation during therapy. Use caution in patients with disturbances of calcium and mineral metabolism (eg, hypoparathyroidism, thyroid/parathyroid, surgery, malabsorption syndromes, excision of small intestine).

Nononcology indications: Use is contraindicated in patients with CrCl <35 mL/minute and in patients with evidence of acute renal impairment due to an increased risk of renal failure. Obtain serum creatinine and calculate creatinine clearance (using actual body weight) with the Cockcroft-Gault formula prior to each administration. In the management of osteoporosis, reevaluate the need for continued therapy periodically; the optimal duration of treatment has not yet been determined. Consider discontinuing after 3 to 5 years of use in patients at low risk for fracture; following discontinuation, reevaluate fracture risk periodically.

Oncology indications: Use caution in mild to moderate renal dysfunction; dosage adjustment required. In cancer patients, renal toxicity has been reported with doses >4 mg or infusions administered over 15 minutes. Risk factors for renal deterioration include preexisting renal insufficiency and repeated doses of zoledronic acid and other bisphosphonates. Dehydration and the use of other nephrotoxic drugs which may contribute to renal deterioration should be identified and managed. Use is not recommended in patients with severe renal impairment (serum creatinine >3 mg/dL or CrCl <30 mL/minute) and bone metastases (limited data); use in patients with hypercalcemia of malignancy and severe renal impairment (serum creatinine >4.5 mg/dL for hypercalcemia of malignancy) should only be done if the benefits outweigh the risks. Diuretics should not be used before correcting hypovolemia. Renal deterioration, resulting in renal failure and dialysis has occurred in patients treated with zoledronic acid after single and multiple infusions at recommended doses of 4 mg over 15 minutes. Assess renal function prior to treatment and withhold for renal deterioration [increase in serum creatinine of 0.5 mg/dL (if baseline level normal) or increase of 1 mg/dL (if baseline level abnormal)]; treatment should be withheld until renal function returns to within 10% of baseline.

Adequate hydration is required during treatment (urine output ~2 L/day); avoid overhydration, especially in patients with heart failure. Preexisting renal compromise, severe dehydration, and concurrent use with diuretics or other nephrotoxic drugs may increase the risk for renal impairment. Single and multiple infusions in patients with both normal and impaired renal function have been associated with renal deterioration, resulting in renal failure and dialysis or death (rare). Patients with underlying moderate to severe renal impairment, increased age, concurrent use of nephrotoxic or diuretic medications, or severe dehydration prior to or after zoledronic acid administration may have an increased risk of acute renal impairment or renal failure. Others with increased risk include patients with renal impairment or dehydration secondary to fever, sepsis, gastrointestinal losses, or diuretic use. If history or physical exam suggests dehydration, treatment should not be given until the patient is normovolemic. Transient increases in serum creatinine may be more pronounced in patients with impaired renal function; consider monitoring creatinine clearance in at-risk patients taking other renally eliminated drugs.

Conjunctivitis, uveitis, episcleritis, iritis, scleritis, and orbital inflammation have been reported (infrequently) with use; further ophthalmic evaluation (and possibly therapy discontinuation) may be necessary in patients with complicated infection. Use caution in patients with aspirin-sensitive asthma (may cause bronchoconstriction) and elderly patients (because decreased renal function occurs more commonly in elderly patients). Rare cases of urticaria and angioedema and very rare cases of anaphylactic reactions/shock have been reported. Do not administer Zometa and Reclast (Aclasta [Canadian product]) to the same patient for different indications.

Breast cancer (metastatic): The American Society of Clinical Oncology (ASCO) updated guidelines on the role of bone-modifying agents (BMAs) in the prevention and treatment of skeletal-related events for metastatic breast cancer patients (Van Poznak, 2011). The guidelines recommend initiating a BMA (denosumab, pamidronate, zoledronic acid) in patients with metastatic breast cancer to the bone. There is currently no literature indicating the superiority of one particular BMA. Optimal duration is not yet defined; however, the guidelines recommend continuing therapy until substantial decline in patient's performance status. The ASCO guidelines are in alignment with prescribing information for dosing, renal dose adjustments, infusion times, prevention and management of osteonecrosis of the jaw, and monitoring of laboratory parameter recommendations. BMAs are not the first-line therapy for pain. BMAs are to be used as adjunctive therapy for cancer-related bone pain associated with bone metastasis, demonstrating a modest pain control benefit. BMAs should be used in conjunction with agents such as NSAIDS, opioid and nonopioid analgesics, corticosteroids, radiation/surgery, and interventional procedures.

Multiple myeloma: The American Society of Clinical Oncology (ASCO) has published guidelines on bisphosphonate use for prevention and treatment of bone disease in multiple myeloma (Kyle, 2007). Bisphosphonate (pamidronate or zoledronic acid) use is recommended in multiple myeloma patients with lytic bone destruction or compression spine fracture from osteopenia. Bisphosphonates may also be considered in patients with pain secondary to osteolytic disease, adjunct therapy to stabilize fractures or impending fractures, and for multiple myeloma patients with osteopenia but no radiographic evidence of lytic bone disease. Bisphosphonates are not recommended in patients with solitary plasmacytoma, smoldering (asymptomatic) or indolent myeloma, or monoclonal gammopathy of undetermined significance. The guidelines recommend monthly treatment for a period of 2 years. At that time, consider discontinuing in responsive and stable patients, and reinitiate if a new-onset ▶

skeletal-related event occurs. The ASCO guidelines are in alignment with prescribing information for dosing, renal dose adjustments, infusion times, prevention and management of osteonecrosis of the jaw, and monitoring of laboratory parameter recommendations. According to the guidelines, in patients with a serum creatinine >3 mg/dL or CrCl <30 mL/minute or extensive bone disease, an alternative bisphosphonate (pamidronate) should be used. Monitor for albuminuria every 3 to 6 months; in patients with unexplained albuminuria >500 mg/24 hours, withhold the dose until level returns to baseline, then recheck every 3 to 4 weeks. Upon reinitiation, the guidelines recommend considering increasing the zoledronic acid infusion time to at least 30 minutes; however, one study has demonstrated that extending the infusion to 30 minutes did not change the safety profile (Berenson, 2011).

Adverse Reactions Note: An acute reaction (eg, arthralgia, fever, flu-like symptoms, myalgia) may occur within the first 3 days following infusion in up to 44% of patients; usually resolves within 3-4 days of onset, although may take up to 14 days to resolve. The incidence may be decreased with acetaminophen (prior to infusion and for 72 hours postinfusion).

Oncology indications:
>10%:
Cardiovascular: Lower extremity edema (5% to 21%), hypotension (11%)
Central nervous system: Fatigue (39%), headache (5% to 19%), dizziness (18%), insomnia (15% to 16%), anxiety (11% to 14%), depression (14%), agitation (13%), confusion (7% to 13%), hypoesthesia (12%), rigors (11%)
Dermatologic: Alopecia (12%), dermatitis (11%)
Endocrine & metabolic: Dehydration (5% to 14%), hypophosphatemia (13%), hypokalemia (12%), hypomagnesemia (11%)
Gastrointestinal: Nausea (29% to 46%), vomiting (14% to 32%), constipation (27% to 31%), diarrhea (17% to 24%), anorexia (9% to 22%), abdominal pain (14% to 16%), weight loss (16%), decreased appetite (13%)
Genitourinary: Urinary tract infection (12% to 14%)
Hematologic & oncologic: Anemia (22% to 33%), progression of cancer (16% to 20%), neutropenia (12%)
Infection: Candidiasis (12%)
Neuromuscular & skeletal: Ostealgia (55%), weakness (5% to 24%), myalgia (23%), arthralgia (5% to 21%), back pain (15%), paresthesia (15%), limb pain (14%), skeletal pain (12%)
Renal: Renal insufficiency (8% to 17%; up to 40% in patients with abnormal baseline creatinine)
Respiratory: Dyspnea (22% to 27%), cough (12% to 22%)
Miscellaneous: Fever (32% to 44%)
1% to 10%:
Cardiovascular: Chest pain (5% to 10%)
Central nervous system: Somnolence (5% to 10%)
Endocrine & metabolic: Hypocalcemia (5% to 10%; grades 3/4: ≤1%), hypermagnesemia (grade 3: 2%)
Gastrointestinal: Dyspepsia (5% to 10%), dysphagia (5% to 10%), mucositis (5% to 10%), stomatitis (8%), sore throat (8%)
Hematologic & oncologic: Granulocytopenia (5% to 10%), pancytopenia (5% to 10%), thrombocytopenia (5% to 10%)
Infection: Infection (nonspecific; 5% to 10%)
Renal: Increased serum creatinine (grades 3/4: ≤2%)
Respiratory: Upper respiratory tract infection (10%)

Nononcology indications:

>10%:

Cardiovascular: Hypertension (5% to 13%)

Central nervous system: Pain (2% to 24%), fever (9% to 22%), headache (4% to 20%), chills (2% to 18%), fatigue (2% to 18%)

Endocrine & metabolic: Hypocalcemia (≤3%; Paget's disease 21%)

Gastrointestinal: Nausea (5% to 18%)

Immunologic: Infusion related reaction (4% to 25%)

Neuromuscular & skeletal: Arthralgia (9% to 27%), myalgia (5% to 23%), back pain (4% to 18%), limb pain (3% to 16%), musculoskeletal pain (≤12%)

Respiratory: Flu-like symptoms (1% to 11%)

1% to 10%:

Cardiovascular: Chest pain (1% to 8%), peripheral edema (3% to 6%), atrial fibrillation (1% to 3%), palpitations (≤3%)

Central nervous system: Dizziness (2% to 9%), rigors (8%), malaise (1% to 7%), hypoesthesia (≤6%), lethargy (3% to 5%), vertigo (1% to 4%), paresthesia (2%), hyperthermia (≤2%)

Dermatologic: Skin rash (2% to 3%), hyperhidrosis (≤3%)

Gastrointestinal: Abdominal pain (1% to 9%), diarrhea (5% to 8%), vomiting (2% to 8%), constipation (6% to 7%), dyspepsia (2% to 7%), abdominal discomfort (1% to 2%), anorexia (1% to 2%)

Hematologic & oncologic: Change in serum protein (C-reactive protein increased; ≤5%)

Neuromuscular & skeletal: Ostealgia (3% to 9%), arthritis (2% to 9%), shoulder pain (≤7%), neck pain (1% to 7%), weakness (2% to 6%), muscle spasm (2% to 6%), stiffness (1% to 5%), jaw pain (2% to 4%), joint swelling (≤3%)

Ophthalmic: Eye pain (≤2%)

Renal: Increased serum creatinine (2%)

Respiratory: Dyspnea (5% to 7%)

All indications: <1%, postmarketing, and/or case reports: Acute renal failure (requiring hospitalization/dialysis), acute renal tubular necrosis (toxic), anaphylactic shock, anaphylaxis, angioedema, arthralgia (sometimes severe and/or incapacitating), blurred vision, bradycardia, bronchoconstriction, cardiac arrhythmia, conjunctivitis, diaphoresis, dysgeusia, episcleritis, exacerbation of asthma, femur fracture (diaphyseal or subtrochanteric), hematuria, hyperesthesia, hyperkalemia, hypernatremia, hyperparathyroidism, hypersensitivity, hypertension, injection site reaction (eg, itching, pain, redness), interstitial lung disease, iridocyclitis, iritis, muscle cramps, myalgia (sometimes severe and/or incapacitating), numbness, osteonecrosis (primarily of the jaws), periorbital edema, periorbital swelling, prolonged QT interval on ECG, proteinuria, pruritus, renal insufficiency, scleritis, seizure, skin rash, Stevens-Johnson syndrome, tetany, toxic epidermal necrolysis, tremor, urticaria, uveitis, weight gain, xerostomia

Drug Interactions

Metabolism/Transport Effects None known.

Avoid Concomitant Use There are no known interactions where it is recommended to avoid concomitant use.

◀ **Increased Effect/Toxicity**

Zoledronic Acid may increase the levels/effects of: Deferasirox

The levels/effects of Zoledronic Acid may be increased by: Aminoglycosides; Calcitonin; Nonsteroidal Anti-Inflammatory Agents; Systemic Angiogenesis Inhibitors; Thalidomide

Decreased Effect

The levels/effects of Zoledronic Acid may be decreased by: Proton Pump Inhibitors

Storage/Stability Solution for injection:

Aclasta [Canadian product]: Store at room temperature of 15°C to 30°C (59°F to 86°F). Keep sealed in original package until administration.

Reclast: Store at room temperature of 25°C (77°F); excursions permitted to 15°C to 30°C (59°F to 86°F). After opening, stable for 24 hours at 2°C to 8°C (36°F to 46°F). If refrigerated, allow the refrigerated solution to reach room temperature before administration.

Zometa: Store concentrate vials and ready-to-use bottles at 25°C (77°F); excursions permitted to 15°C to 30°C (59°F to 86°F). Diluted solutions for infusion which are not used immediately after preparation should be refrigerated at 2°C to 8°C (36°F to 46°F). Infusion of solution must be completed within 24 hours of preparation. The ready-to-use bottles are for single use only; if any preparation is necessary (preparing reduced dosage for patients with renal impairment), the prepared, diluted solution may be refrigerated at 2°C to 8°C (36°F to 46°F) if not used immediately. Infusion of solution must be completed within 24 hours of preparation. The previously withdrawn volume from the ready-to-use solution should be discarded; do not store or reuse.

Preparation for Administration Hazardous agent; use appropriate precautions for handling and disposal (NIOSH 2014 [group 3]).

Solution for injection:

Reclast, Aclasta [Canadian product]: No further preparation is necessary.

Zometa concentrate vials: Further dilute in 100 mL NS or D_5W prior to administration.

Zometa ready-to-use bottles: No further preparation is necessary. If reduced doses are required for patients with renal impairment, withdraw the appropriate volume of solution and replace with an equal amount of NS or D_5W.

Mechanism of Action A bisphosphonate which inhibits bone resorption via actions on osteoclasts or on osteoclast precursors; inhibits osteoclastic activity and skeletal calcium release induced by tumors. Decreases serum calcium and phosphorus, and increases their elimination. In osteoporosis, zoledronic acid inhibits osteoclast-mediated resorption, therefore reducing bone turnover.

Pharmacodynamics/Kinetics

Distribution: Binds to bone

Protein binding: 23% to 53%

Metabolism: Primarily eliminated intact via the kidney; metabolism not likely

Half-life elimination: Triphasic; Terminal: 146 hours

Excretion: Urine (39% ± 16% as unchanged drug) within 24 hours; feces (<3%)

Dosing

Adult & Geriatric Note: Acetaminophen administration after the infusion may reduce symptoms of acute-phase reactions. Patients treated for multiple myeloma and Paget disease should receive a daily calcium and vitamin D supplement, and patients with osteoporosis should receive calcium and vitamin D supplementation if dietary intake is inadequate.

Hypercalcemia of malignancy (albumin-corrected serum calcium ≥12 mg/dL) (Zometa): IV: 4 mg (maximum) given as a single dose. Wait at least 7 days before considering re-treatment.

Multiple myeloma or metastatic bone lesions from solid tumors (Zometa): IV: 4 mg once every 3 to 4 weeks

Osteoporosis, glucocorticoid-induced, treatment and prevention (Reclast, Aclasta [Canadian product]): IV: 5 mg once a year

Osteoporosis, prevention: IV:

Reclast: 5 mg once every 2 years

Aclasta [Canadian product]: 5 mg as a single (one-time) dose

Osteoporosis, treatment (Reclast, Aclasta [Canadian product]): IV: 5 mg once a year; consider discontinuing after 3 to 5 years of use in patients at low risk for fracture

Paget disease: IV:

Reclast, Aclasta [Canadian product]: 5 mg as a single dose.

Re-treatment:

Reclast: Data concerning retreatment is not available; retreatment may be considered for relapse (increase in alkaline phosphatase) if appropriate, for inadequate response, or in patients who are symptomatic.

Aclasta [Canadian product]: Data concerning retreatment is limited; retreatment with 5 mg (single dose) may be considered for relapse after an interval of at least 1 year from initial treatment.

The Endocrine Society guidelines suggest re-treatment is seldom required within 5 years (Singer, 2014).

Prevention of aromatase inhibitor-induced bone loss in breast cancer (off-label use): IV: 4 mg once every 6 months for 5 years (Brufsky, 2012)

Prevention of androgen deprivation-induced bone loss in nonmetastatic prostate cancer (off-label use): IV: 4 mg once every 3 months for 1 year (Smith, 2003) or 4 mg every 12 months (Michaelson, 2007)

Renal Impairment Note: Prior to each dose, obtain serum creatinine and calculate the creatinine clearance using the Cockcroft-Gault formula.

Nononcology uses: **Note:** Use actual body weight in the Cockcroft-Gault formula when calculating clearance for nononcology uses.

CrCl ≥35 mL/minute: No dosage adjustment is necessary.

CrCl <35 mL/minute: Use is contraindicated.

Oncology uses:

Multiple myeloma and bone metastases:

CrCl >60 mL/minute: 4 mg (no dosage adjustment is necessary)

CrCl 50 to 60 mL/minute: Reduce dose to 3.5 mg

CrCl 40 to 49 mL/minute: Reduce dose to 3.3 mg

CrCl 30 to 39 mL/minute: Reduce dose to 3 mg

CrCl <30 mL/minute: Use is not recommended.

Hypercalcemia of malignancy:

Mild to moderate impairment: No dosage adjustment is necessary.

Severe impairment (serum creatinine >4.5 mg/dL):

U.S. labeling: Evaluate risk versus benefit

Canadian labeling: Use is not recommended.

Dosage adjustment for renal toxicity (during treatment):

Hypercalcemia of malignancy: Evidence of renal deterioration: Evaluate risk versus benefit.

◀ Multiple myeloma and bone metastases: Evidence of renal deterioration: Withhold dose until renal function returns to within 10% of baseline; renal deterioration defined as follows:

Normal baseline creatinine: Increase of 0.5 mg/dL

Abnormal baseline creatinine: Increase of 1 mg/dL

Reinitiate therapy at the same dose administered prior to treatment interruption.

Multiple myeloma: Albuminuria >500 mg/24 hours (unexplained): Withhold dose until return to baseline, then reevaluate every 3 to 4 weeks; consider reinitiating with a longer infusion time of at least 30 minutes (Kyle, 2007).

Hepatic Impairment There are no dosage adjustments provided in the manufacturer's labeling (has not been studied); however, zoledronic acid is not metabolized hepatically.

Administration

If refrigerated, allow solution to reach room temperature before administration. Infuse over at least 15 minutes. Flush IV line with 10 mL NS flush following infusion. Infuse in a line separate from other medications. Patients must be appropriately hydrated prior to treatment. Acetaminophen after administration may reduce the incidence of acute reaction (eg, arthralgia, fever, flu-like symptoms, myalgia).

Multiple myeloma: If treatment is withheld for unexplained albuminuria, consider increasing the infusion time to at least 30 minutes upon reinitiation (Kyle, 2007).

Hazardous agent; use appropriate precautions for handling and disposal (NIOSH 2014 [group 3]).

Monitoring Parameters Prior to initiation of therapy, dental exam and preventive dentistry for patients at risk for osteonecrosis, including all cancer patients

Nononcology uses: Serum creatinine prior to each dose, especially in patients with risk factors, calculate creatinine clearance before each treatment (consider interim monitoring in patients at risk for acute renal failure), evaluate fluid status and adequately hydrate patients prior to and following administration.

Osteoporosis: Bone mineral density (BMD) should be evaluated 1 to 2 years after initiating therapy and every 2 years thereafter (NOF [Cosman 2014]); in patients with combined zoledronic acid and glucocorticoid treatment, BMD should be made at initiation of therapy and repeated after 6 to 12 months; serum calcium and 25(OH)D; annual measurements of height and weight, assessment of chronic back pain; serum calcium and 25(OH)D; phosphorus and magnesium; may consider monitoring biochemical markers of bone turnover

Paget disease: Alkaline phosphatase at 6 to 12 weeks for initial response to treatment (when bone turnover will have shown a substantial decline) and potentially at 6 months (maximal suppression of high bone turnover); following treatment completion, monitor at ~1- to 2-year intervals (Singer, 2014); monitoring more specific biochemical markers of bone turnover (eg, serum P1NP, NTX, serum beta-CTx) is generally only warranted in patients with Paget disease who have abnormal liver or biliary tract function or when early assessment of response to treatment is needed (eg, spinal compression, very active disease) (Singer, 2014); serum calcium and 25(OH)D; phosphorus and magnesium; symptoms of hypocalcemia, pain

Oncology uses: Serum creatinine prior to each dose; serum electrolytes, phosphate, magnesium, and hemoglobin/hematocrit should be evaluated regularly. Monitor serum calcium to assess response and avoid overtreatment. In patients with multiple myeloma, monitor urine every 3 to 6 months for albuminuria.

Test Interactions Bisphosphonates may interfere with diagnostic imaging agents such as technetium-99m-diphosphonate in bone scans.

Dietary Considerations

Multiple myeloma or metastatic bone lesions from solid tumors: Take daily calcium supplement (500 mg) and daily multivitamin (with 400 units vitamin D).

Osteoporosis: Ensure adequate calcium and vitamin D intake; if dietary intake is inadequate, dietary supplementation is recommended. Women and men should consume:

Calcium: 1,000 mg/day (men: 50 to 70 years) **or** 1200 mg/day (women ≥51 years and men ≥71 years) (IOM, 2011; NOF [Cosman 2014])

Vitamin D: 800 to 1,000 int. units/day (men and women ≥50 years) (NOF, 2014). Recommended Dietary Allowance (RDA): 600 int. units/day (men and women ≤70 years) **or** 800 int. units/day (men and women ≥71 years) (IOM, 2011).

Paget disease: Take elemental calcium 1500 mg/day (750 mg twice daily or 500 mg 3 times/day) and vitamin D 800 units/day, particularly during the first 2 weeks after administration.

Medication Guide Available Yes

Dosage Forms Excipient information presented when available (limited, particularly for generics); consult specific product labeling.

Concentrate, Intravenous:
Zometa: 4 mg/5 mL (5 mL)
Generic: 4 mg/5 mL (5 mL)
Concentrate, Intravenous [preservative free]:
Generic: 4 mg/5 mL (5 mL)
Solution, Intravenous:
Reclast: 5 mg/100 mL (100 mL)
Zometa: 4 mg/100 mL (100 mL)
Generic: 5 mg/100 mL (100 mL)
Solution, Intravenous [preservative free]:
Generic: 4 mg/100 mL (100 mL); 5 mg/100 mL (100 mL)
Solution Reconstituted, Intravenous:
Generic: 4 mg (1 ea)

Dosage Forms: Canada Excipient information presented when available (limited, particularly for generics); consult specific product labeling.

Concentrate, Intravenous:
Zometa: 4 mg/5 mL (5 mL)
Infusion, Solution [premixed]:
Aclasta: 5 mg/100 mL (100 mL)

◆ **Zoledronic Acid for Injection (Can)** see Zoledronic Acid on page 1790
◆ **Zoledronic Acid Injection (Can)** see Zoledronic Acid on page 1790
◆ **Zoledronic Acid Z (Can)** see Zoledronic Acid on page 1790
◆ **Zolinza** see Vorinostat on page 1780
◆ **Zometa** see Zoledronic Acid on page 1790
◆ **Zometa Concentrate (Can)** see Zoledronic Acid on page 1790

- **Zortress** *see* Everolimus *on page 656*
- **Zosyn** *see* Piperacillin and Tazobactam *on page 1388*
- **Zovirax** *see* Acyclovir (Systemic) *on page 35*
- **Zovirax** *see* Acyclovir (Topical) *on page 42*
- **Zuplenz** *see* Ondansetron *on page 1253*
- **Zyclara** *see* Imiquimod *on page 897*
- **Zyclara Pump** *see* Imiquimod *on page 897*
- **Zydelig** *see* Idelalisib *on page 867*
- **Zykadia** *see* Ceritinib *on page 305*
- **Zyloprim** *see* Allopurinol *on page 73*
- **ZyPREXA** *see* OLANZapine *on page 1242*
- **Zyprexa (Can)** *see* OLANZapine *on page 1242*
- **Zyprexa Intramuscular (Can)** *see* OLANZapine *on page 1242*
- **ZyPREXA Relprevv** *see* OLANZapine *on page 1242*
- **Zyprexa Zydis** *see* OLANZapine *on page 1242*
- **ZyPREXA Zydis** *see* OLANZapine *on page 1242*
- **Zytiga** *see* Abiraterone Acetate *on page 30*
- **Zytram XL (Can)** *see* TraMADol *on page 1672*
- **Zyvox** *see* Linezolid *on page 1049*
- **Zyvoxam (Can)** *see* Linezolid *on page 1049*

CHEMOTHERAPY REGIMEN INDEX

CHEMOTHERAPY REGIMEN INDEX

GASTROINTESTINAL

Anal Cancer

Biliary Adenocarcinoma

GENITOURINARY

GYNECOLOGIC

LUNG CANCER

LYMPHOMA

Hodgkin Lymphoma

◀ # UNKNOWN PRIMARY (ADENOCARCINOMA)

UNKNOWN PRIMARY (SQUAMOUS CELL)

WALDENSTROM MACROGLOBULINEMIA

ALPHABETICAL LISTING OF CHEMOTHERAPY REGIMENS

5 + 2 (Cytarabine-Daunorubicin) (AML Induction)

Index Terms Cytarabine-Daunorubicin (5 + 2) (AML); Daunorubicin-Cytarabine (5 + 2) (AML)

Use Leukemia, acute myeloid

Regimen

Cytarabine: IV: 100 mg/m^2/day continuous infusion days 1 to 5
[total dose/cycle = 500 mg/m^2]
Daunorubicin: IV: 45 mg/m^2/day IV bolus days 1 and 2
[total dose/cycle = 90 mg/m^2]
May administer a second induction cycle if needed

References

Rai KR, Holland JF, Glidewell OJ, et al, "Treatment of Acute Myelocytic Leukemia: A Study by Cancer and Leukemia Group B," Blood, 1981, 58(6):1203-12.

5 + 2 (Cytarabine-Daunorubicin) (AML Postremission)

Index Terms Cytarabine-Daunorubicin (5 + 2) (AML); Daunorubicin-Cytarabine (5 + 2) (AML)

Use Leukemia, acute myeloid

Regimen

Cytarabine: IV: 100 mg/m^2/day continuous infusion days 1 to 5
[total dose/cycle = 500 mg/m^2]
Daunorubicin: IV: 45 mg/m^2/day IV bolus days 1 and 2
[total dose/cycle = 90 mg/m^2]
Administer 2 courses

References

Wiernik PH, Banks P, Case Jr DC, et al, "Cytarabine Plus Idarubicin or Daunorubicin as Induction and Consolidation Therapy for Previously Untreated Adult Patients With Acute Myeloid Leukemia," Blood, 1992, 79(2):313-9.

5 + 2 (Cytarabine-Idarubicin) (AML Consolidation)

Index Terms Cytarabine-Idarubicin (5 + 2) (AML Consolidation); Idarubicin-Cytarabine (5 + 2) (AML Consolidation)

Use Leukemia, acute myeloid

Regimen

Cytarabine: IV: 100 mg/m^2/day continuous infusion days 1 to 5
[total dose/cycle = 500 mg/m^2]
Idarubicin: IV: 13 mg/m^2/day IV bolus days 1 and 2
[total dose/cycle = 26 mg/m^2]
Administer 2 courses

References

Wiernik PH, Banks P, Case Jr DC, et al, "Cytarabine Plus Idarubicin or Daunorubicin as Induction and Consolidation Therapy for Previously Untreated Adult Patients With Acute Myeloid Leukemia," Blood, 1992, 79(2):313-9.

5 + 2 (Cytarabine-Mitoxantrone) (AML Consolidation)

Index Terms Cytarabine-Mitoxantrone (5 + 2) (AML Consolidation)

Use Leukemia, acute myeloid

Regimen

Cytarabine: IV: 100 mg/m^2/day continuous infusion days 1 to 5
[total dose/cycle = 500 mg/m^2]
Mitoxantrone: IV: 12 mg/m^2/day days 1 and 2
[total dose/cycle = 24 mg/m^2]
Administered every 28 days for a total of 2 cycles

References

Arlin Z, Case DC Jr, Moore J, et al, "Randomized Multicenter Trial of Cytosine Arabinoside With Mitoxantrone or Daunorubicin in Previously Untreated Adult Patients With Acute Nonlymphocytic Leukemia (ANLL). Lederle Cooperative Group," *Leukemia*, 1990, 4(3):177-83.

5 + 2 + 5 (Cytarabine-Daunorubicin-Etoposide) (AML Consolidation)

Index Terms Cytarabine-Daunorubicin-Etoposide (5 + 2 + 5) (AML Consolidation)

Use Leukemia, acute myeloid

Regimen

Cytarabine: IV: 100 mg/m^2/day continuous infusion days 1 to 5
[total dose/cycle = 500 mg/m^2]
Daunorubicin: IV: 50 mg/m^2/day IV bolus days 1 and 2
[total dose/cycle = 100 mg/m^2]
Etoposide: IV: 75 mg/m^2/day over 1 hour days 1 to 5
[total dose/cycle = 375 mg/m^2]
Administer 2 courses

References

Bishop JF, Lowenthal RM, Joshua D, et al, "Etoposide in Acute Nonlymphocytic Leukemia, Australian Leukemia Study Group," *Blood*, 1990, 75(1):27-32.
Bishop JF, Matthews JP, Young GA, et al, "A Randomized Study of High-Dose Cytarabine in Induction in Acute Myeloid Leukemia," *Blood*, 1996, 87(5):1710-7.

7 + 3 (Cytarabine-Daunorubicin) (AML Induction)

Index Terms Cytarabine-Daunorubicin (7 + 3) (AML Induction)

Use Leukemia, acute myeloid

Regimen NOTE: Multiple variations are listed.

Variation 1:
Cytarabine: IV: 100 mg/m^2/day continuous infusion days 1 to 7
[total dose/cycle = 700 mg/m^2]
Daunorubicin: IV: 45 mg/m^2/day IV bolus days 1, 2, and 3
[total dose/cycle = 135 mg/m^2]
May administer a second induction cycle if needed

Variation 2 (≥60 years of age):
Cytarabine: IV: 100 mg/m^2/day continuous infusion days 1 to 7
[total dose/cycle = 700 mg/m^2]
Daunorubicin: IV: 30 mg/m^2/day days 1, 2, and 3
[total dose/cycle = 90 mg/m^2]
May administer a second induction cycle if needed (at a reduced dose of daunorubicin [45 mg/m^2])

Variation 3 (between 17 and 60 years of age):
Cytarabine: IV: 100 mg/m^2/day continuous infusion days 1 to 7
[total dose/cycle = 700 mg/m^2]
Daunorubicin: IV: 90 mg/m^2/day IV bolus days 1, 2, and 3
[total dose/cycle = 270 mg/m^2]
May administer a second induction cycle if needed

Variation 4 (<60 years of age):
Cytarabine: IV: 200 mg/m^2/day continuous infusion days 1 to 7
[total dose/cycle = 1400 mg/m^2]
Daunorubicin: IV: 45 mg/m^2/day IV bolus days 1, 2, and 3
[total dose/cycle = 135 mg/m^2]
May administer a second induction cycle if needed

◀ **References**

Variation 1:

Dillman RO, Davis RB, Green MR, et al, "A Comparative Study of Two Different Doses of Cytarabine for Acute Myeloid Leukemia: A Phase III Trial of Cancer and Leukemia Group B," *Blood*, 1991, 78(10):2520-6.

Rai KR, Holland JF, Glidewell OJ, et al, "Treatment of Acute Myelocytic Leukemia: A Study by Cancer and Leukemia Group B," *Blood*, 1981, 58(6):1203-12.

Yates J, Glidewell O, Wiernik P, et al, "Cytosine Arabinoside With Daunorubicin or Adriamycin® for Therapy of Acute Myelocytic Leukemia: A CALGB Study," *Blood*, 1982, 60(2):454-62.

Variation 2:

Dillman RO, Davis RB, Green MR, et al, "A Comparative Study of Two Different Doses of Cytarabine for Acute Myeloid Leukemia: A Phase III Trial of Cancer and Leukemia Group B," *Blood*, 1991, 78(10):2520-6.

Variation 3:

Fernandez HF, Sun Z, Yao X, et al, "Anthracycline Dose Intensification in Acute Myeloid Leukemia," *N Engl J Med*, 2009, 361(13):1249-59.

Variation 4:

Dillman RO, Davis RB, Green MR, et al, "A Comparative Study of Two Different Doses of Cytarabine for Acute Myeloid Leukemia: A Phase III Trial of Cancer and Leukemia Group B," *Blood*, 1991, 78(10):2520-6.

7 + 3 (Cytarabine-Idarubicin) (AML Induction)

Index Terms Cytarabine-Idarubicin (7 + 3) (AML Induction)

Use Leukemia, acute myeloid

Regimen NOTE: Multiple variations are listed.

Variation 1:

Cytarabine: IV: 100 mg/m^2/day continuous infusion days 1 to 7
  [total dose/cycle = 700 mg/m^2]
Idarubicin: IV: 12 mg/m^2/day slow IV infusion days 1, 2, and 3
  [total dose/cycle = 36 mg/m^2]
May administer a second induction cycle if needed

Variation 2:

Cytarabine: IV: 100 mg/m^2/day continuous infusion days 1 to 7
  [total dose/cycle = 700 mg/m^2]
Idarubicin: IV: 13 mg/m^2/day slow IV infusion days 1, 2, and 3
  [total dose/cycle = 39 mg/m^2]
May administer a second induction cycle if needed

References

Variation 1:

Vogler WR, Velez-Garcia E, Weiner RS, et al, "A Phase III Trial Comparing Idarubicin and Daunorubicin in Combination With Cytarabine in Acute Myelogenous Leukemia: A Southeastern Cancer Study Group Study," *J Clin Oncol*, 1992, 10(7):1103-11.

Variation 2:

Wiernik PH, Banks P, Case Jr DC, et al, "Cytarabine Plus Idarubicin or Daunorubicin as Induction and Consolidation Therapy for Previously Untreated Adult Patients With Acute Myeloid Leukemia," *Blood*, 1992, 79(2):313-9.

7 + 3 (Cytarabine-Mitoxantrone) (AML Induction)

Index Terms Cytarabine-Mitoxantrone (7 + 3) (AML Induction)

Use Leukemia, acute myeloid

Regimen

Induction:

Cytarabine: IV: 100 mg/m^2/day continuous infusion days 1 to 7
  [total dose/cycle = 700 mg/m^2]
Mitoxantrone: IV: 12 mg/m^2/day days 1, 2, and 3
  [total dose/cycle = 36 mg/m^2]

Reinduction if needed:
Cytarabine: IV: 100 mg/m²/day continuous infusion days 1 to 5
[total dose/cycle = 500 mg/m²]
Mitoxantrone: IV: 12 mg/m²/day days 1 and 2
[total dose/cycle = 24 mg/m²]

References

Arlin Z, Case DC Jr, Moore J, et al, "Randomized Multicenter Trial of Cytosine Arabinoside With Mitoxantrone or Daunorubicin in Previously Untreated Adult Patients With Acute Nonlymphocytic Leukemia (ANLL). Lederle Cooperative Group," *Leukemia*, 1990, 4(3):177-83.

◆ **A1 (NEW) (Neuroblastoma)** *see* New A1 (Neuroblastoma) *on page 2043*

7 + 3 + 7 (Cytarabine-Daunorubicin-Etoposide) (AML Induction)

Index Terms Cytarabine-Daunorubicin-Etoposide (7 + 3 + 7) (AML Induction)
Use Leukemia, acute myeloid
Regimen
Cytarabine: IV: 100 mg/m²/day continuous infusion days 1 to 7
[total dose/cycle = 700 mg/m²]
Daunorubicin: IV: 50 mg/m²/day days 1, 2, and 3
[total dose/cycle = 150 mg/m²]
Etoposide: IV: 75 mg/m²/day over 1 hour days 1 to 7
[total dose/cycle = 525 mg/m²]
Up to 3 induction cycles may be given based on individual response

References

Bishop JF, Lowenthal RM, Joshua D, et al, "Etoposide in Acute Nonlymphocytic Leukemia, Australian Leukemia Study Group," *Blood*, 1990, 75(1):27-32.
Bishop JF, Matthews JP, Young GA, et al, "A Randomized Study of High-Dose Cytarabine in Induction in Acute Myeloid Leukemia," *Blood*, 1996, 87(5):1710-7.
Bishop JF, Matthews JP, Young GA, et al, "Intensified Induction Chemotherapy With High Dose Cytarabine and Etoposide for Acute Myeloid Leukemia: A Review and Updated Results of the Australian Leukemia Study Group," *Leuk Lymphoma*, 1998, 28(3-4):315-27.

A3 (Neuroblastoma)

Index Terms Cyclophosphamide, Doxorubicin, Etoposide, Cisplatin (Neuroblastoma); Regimen A3 (Neuroblastoma)
Use Neuroblastoma
Regimen
Cycle 1 (New A1):
Cyclophosphamide: IV: 1200 mg/m² over 6 hours day 1
[total dose/cycle = 1200 mg/m²]
Doxorubicin: IV: 40 mg/m² day 3
[total dose/cycle = 40 mg/m²]
Etoposide: IV: 100 mg/m²/day days 1 to 5
[total dose/cycle = 500 mg/m²]
Cisplatin: IV: 90 mg/m² day 5
[total dose/cycle = 90 mg/m²]
Treatment cycle is 28 days
Cycles 2-5 (A3):
Cyclophosphamide: IV: 1200 mg/m²/day over 6 hours days 1 and 2
[total dose/cycle = 2400 mg/m²]
Doxorubicin: IV: 40 mg/m² day 3
[total dose/cycle = 40 mg/m²]
Etoposide: IV: 100 mg/m²/day days 1 to 5
[total dose/cycle = 500 mg/m²]

Cisplatin: IV: 25 mg/m^2/day continuous infusion days 1 to 5
[total dose/cycle = 125 mg/m^2]
Repeat cycle every 28 days for 5 cycles (total of 6 cycles, cycle 1 administer New A1, cycles 2 to 5 administer A3)

References

Kaneko M, Nishihira H, Mugishima H, et al, "Stratification of Treatment of Stage 4 Neuroblastoma Patients Based on N-myc Amplification Status. Study Group of Japan for Treatment of Advanced Neuroblastoma, Tokyo, Japan," *Med Pediatr Oncol*, 1998, 31(1):1-7.

Kaneko M, Tsuchida Y, Mugishima H, et al, "Intensified Chemotherapy Increases the Survival Rates in Patients With Stage 4 Neuroblastoma With MYCN Amplification," *J Pediatr Hematol Oncol*, 2002, 24(8):613-21.

Abiraterone-Prednisone (Prostate)

Index Terms Prednisone-Abiraterone (Prostate)

Use Prostate cancer

Regimen

Abiraterone acetate: Oral: 1000 mg once daily days 1 to 28
[total dose/cycle = 28,000 mg]
Prednisone: Oral: 5 mg twice a day days 1 to 28
[total dose/cycle = 280 mg]
Repeat cycle every 28 days until disease progression or unacceptable toxicity

References

de Bono JS, Logothetis CJ, Molina A, et al, "Abiraterone and Increased Survival in Metastatic Prostate Cancer," *New Engl J Med*, 2011, 364(21):1995-2005.

Ryan CJ, Smith MR, de Bone JS, et al, "Interim Analysis (IA) Results of COU-AA-302, A Randomized, Phase III Study of Abiraterone Acetate (AA) in Chemotherapy-Naïve Patients (pts) With Metastatic Castration-Resistant Prostate Cancer (mCRPC)," *J Clin Oncol*, 2012, 30 (18):LBA4518 [abstract LBA4518 from 2012 ASCO Annual Meeting].

♦ **Abraxane (Ovarian Regimen)** see Paclitaxel (Protein Bound) (Ovarian Regimen) *on page 2055*

ABVD Early Stage (Hodgkin)

Index Terms Doxorubicin, Bleomycin, Vinblastine, Dacarbazine (Hodgkin)

Use Lymphoma, Hodgkin

Regimen NOTE: Multiple variations are listed.

Variation 1 (newly diagnosed, stage I or II, favorable prognosis with no clinical risk factors):
Doxorubicin: IV: 25 mg/m^2/day days 1 and 15
[total dose/cycle = 50 mg/m^2]
Bleomycin: IV: 10 units/m^2/day days 1 and 15
[total dose/cycle = 20 units/m^2]
Vinblastine: IV: 6 mg/m^2/day days 1 and 15
[total dose/cycle = 12 mg/m^2]
Dacarbazine: IV: 375 mg/m^2/day days 1 and 15
[total dose/cycle = 750 mg/m^2]
Repeat cycle every 28 days for a total of 2 cycles followed by 20 Gy of radiation therapy

Variation 2 (newly diagnosed, stage IA or IIA non-bulky, favorable and unfavorable):
Doxorubicin: IV: 25 mg/m^2/day days 1 and 15
[total dose/cycle = 50 mg/m^2]
Bleomycin: IV: 10 units/m^2/day days 1 and 15
[total dose/cycle = 20 units/m^2]

Vinblastine: IV: 6 mg/m^2/day days 1 and 15
[total dose/cycle = 12 mg/m^2]

Dacarbazine: IV: 375 mg/m^2/day days 1 and 15
[total dose/cycle = 750 mg/m^2]

Repeat cycle every 28 days for a total of 4 to 6 cycles. Patient who had complete remission after 2 cycles received a total of 4 cycles, and if the patient did not have a complete remission after 2 cycles received a total of 6 cycles.

Variation 3 (newly diagnosed, stage I and II with certain risk factors, unfavorable prognosis):

Doxorubicin: IV: 25 mg/m^2/day days 1 and 15
[total dose/cycle = 50 mg/m^2]

Bleomycin: IV: 10 units/m^2/day days 1 and 15
[total dose/cycle = 20 units/m^2]

Vinblastine: IV: 6 mg/m^2/day days 1 and 15
[total dose/cycle = 12 mg/m^2]

Dacarbazine: IV: 375 mg/m^2/day days 1 and 15
[total dose/cycle = 750 mg/m^2]

Repeat cycle every 28 days for a total of 4 cycles followed by 30 Gy of radiation therapy

Variation 4 (newly diagnosed, stage I, II, IIIA, non-bulky):

Doxorubicin: IV: 25 mg/m^2/day days 1 and 15
[total dose/cycle = 50 mg/m^2]

Bleomycin: IV: 10 units/m^2/day days 1 and 15
[total dose/cycle = 20 units/m^2]

Vinblastine: IV: 6 mg/m^2/day days 1 and 15
[total dose/cycle = 12 mg/m^2]

Dacarbazine: IV: 375 mg/m^2/day days 1 and 15
[total dose/cycle = 750 mg/m^2]

Repeat cycle every 28 days for a total of 6 cycles followed by radiation therapy

References

Variation 1:
Engert A, Plütschow A, Eich HT, et al. Reduced treatment intensity in patients with early-stage Hodgkin's lymphoma. *N Engl J Med*. 2010;363(7):640-652.
Variation 2:
Meyer RM, Gospodarowicz MK, Connors JM, et al. ABVD alone versus radiation-based therapy in limited-stage Hodgkin's lymphoma. *N Engl J Med*. 2012;366(5):399-408.
Variation 3:
Eich HT, Diehl V, Görgen H, et al. Intensified chemotherapy and dose-reduced involved-field radiotherapy in patients with early unfavorable Hodgkin's lymphoma: final analysis of the German Hodgkin Study Group HD11 trial. *J Clin Oncol*. 2010;28(27):4199-4206.
Variation 4:
Straus DJ, Portlock CS, Qin J, et al. Results of a prospective randomized clinical trial of doxorubicin, bleomycin, vinblastine, and dacarbazine (ABVD) followed by radiation therapy (RT) versus ABVD alone for stages I, II, and IIIA nonbulky Hodgkin disease. *Blood*. 2004;104 (12):3483-3489.

ABVD (Hodgkin)

Index Terms Doxorubicin-Bleomycin-Vinblastine-Dacarbazine (Hodgkin)
Use Lymphoma, Hodgkin
Regimen

Doxorubicin: IV: 25 mg/m^2/day days 1 and 15
[total dose/cycle = 50 mg/m^2]

Bleomycin: IV: 10 units/m^2/day days 1 and 15
[total dose/cycle = 20 units/m^2]

◄ Vinblastine: IV: 6 mg/m^2/day days 1 and 15
   [total dose/cycle = 12 mg/m^2]
Dacarbazine: IV: 375 mg/m^2/day days 1 and 15
   [total dose/cycle = 750 mg/m^2]
Repeat cycle every 28 days for 6-8 cycles

References

Bonadonna G and Santoro A, "ABVD Chemotherapy in the Treatment of Hodgkin's Disease," *Cancer Treat Rev*, 1982, 9(1):21-35.

Canellos GP, Anderson JR, Propert KJ, et al, "Chemotherapy of Advanced Hodgkin's Disease With MOPP, ABVD, or MOPP Alternating With ABVD," *N Engl J Med*, 1992, 327(21):1478-84.

Viviani S, Zinzani PL, Rambaldi A, et al, "ABVD Versus BEACOPP for Hodgkin's Lymphoma When High-Dose Salvage Is Planned," *N Engl J Med*, 2011, 365(3):203-12.

AC (Breast)

Index Terms Cyclophosphamide-Doxorubicin (Breast); Doxorubicin-Cyclophosphamide (Breast)

Use Breast cancer

Regimen NOTE: Multiple variations are listed.

Variation 1 (adjuvant):
   Doxorubicin: IV: 60 mg/m^2 day 1
      [total dose/cycle = 60 mg/m^2]
   Cyclophosphamide: IV: 600 mg/m^2 day 1
      [total dose/cycle = 600 mg/m^2]
   Repeat cycle every 21 days for 4 cycles
Variation 2 (metastatic):
   Doxorubicin: IV: 60 mg/m^2 day 1
      [total dose/cycle = 60 mg/m^2]
   Cyclophosphamide: IV: 600 mg/m^2 day 1
      [total dose/cycle = 600 mg/m^2]
   Repeat cycle every 21 days for up to 8 cycles

References

Variation 1:

Fisher B, Brown AM, Dimitrov NV, et al, "Two Months of Doxorubicin-Cyclophosphamide With and Without Interval Reinduction Therapy Compared With 6 Months of Cyclophosphamide, Methotrexate, and Fluorouracil in Positive-Node Breast Cancer Patients With Tamoxifen-Nonresponsive Tumors: Results From the National Surgical Adjuvant Breast and Bowel Project B-15," *J Clin Oncol*, 1990, 8(9):1483-96.

Variation 2:

Nabholtz JM, Falkson C, Campos D, et al. Docetaxel and doxorubicin compared with doxorubicin and cyclophosphamide as first-line chemotherapy for metastatic breast cancer: results of a randomized, multicenter, phase III trial. *J Clin Oncol*. 2003;21(6):968-75.

AC (Dose-Dense) followed by Paclitaxel (Dose-Dense) (Breast)

Index Terms Doxorubicin, Cyclophosphamide, Paclitaxel Dose Dense (Breast)

Use Breast cancer

Regimen

Cycles 1-4:
   Doxorubicin: IV: 60 mg/m^2 day 1
      [total dose/cycle = 60 mg/m^2]
   Cyclophosphamide: IV: 600 mg/m^2 day 1
      [total dose/cycle = 600 mg/m^2]

Filgrastim: SubQ: 5 mcg/kg/day days 3 to 10, rounded to either 300 or 480
mcg/day

[total dose/cycle = 40 mcg/kg, 2400-3840 mcg/cycle]

Repeat cycle every 14 days for 4 cycles

followed by

Cycles 5-8:

Paclitaxel: IV: 175 mg/m² day 1

[total dose/cycle = 175 mg/m²]

Filgrastim: SubQ: 5 mcg/kg/day days 3 to 10, rounded to either 300 or 480
mcg/day

[total dose/cycle = 40 mcg/kg, 2400-3840 mcg/cycle]

Repeat cycle every 14 days for 4 cycles

References

Citron ML, Berry DA, Cirrincione C, et al, "Randomized Trial of Dose-Dense Versus Conventionally
Scheduled and Sequential Versus Concurrent Combination Chemotherapy as Postoperative
Adjuvant Treatment of Node-Positive Primary Breast Cancer: First Report of Intergroup Trial
C9741/Cancer Leukemia Group B Trial 9741," *J Clin Oncol*, 2003, 21(8):1431-9.

AC (Dose-Dense) followed by Paclitaxel (Dose-Dense)-Trastuzumab (Breast)

Index Terms Doxorubicin, Cyclophosphamide, Paclitaxel (Dose-Dense), Trastuzumab (Breast)

Use Breast cancer

Regimen

Cycles 1-4 of AC (dose-dense):

Doxorubicin: IV: 60 mg/m² day 1

[total dose/cycle = 60 mg/m²]

Cyclophosphamide: IV: 600 mg/m² day 1

[total dose/cycle = 600 mg/m²]

Pegfilgrastim: SubQ: 6 mg day 2

[total dose/cycle = 6 mg]

Repeat cycle every 14 days for 4 cycles

followed by

Cycle 1 of Paclitaxel (dose-dense)-Trastuzumab:

Paclitaxel: IV: 175 mg/m² day 1

[total dose/cycle 1 = 175 mg/m²]

Pegfilgrastim: SubQ: 6 mg day 2

[total dose/cycle = 6 mg]

Trastuzumab: IV: 4 mg/kg (loading dose) day 1 cycle 1 only

followed by

Trastuzumab: IV: 2 mg/kg day 8

[total dose/cycle 1 = 6 mg/kg]

Treatment cycle is 14 days

followed by

Cycles 2-4 of Paclitaxel (dose-dense)-Trastuzumab:

Paclitaxel: IV: 175 mg/m² day 1

[total dose/cycle 1 = 175 mg/m²]

Pegfilgrastim: SubQ: 6 mg day 2

[total dose/cycle = 6 mg]

Trastuzumab: IV: 2 mg/kg days 1 and 8

[total dose/cycle = 4 mg/kg]

Repeat cycle every 14 days for 3 cycles

followed by

Trastuzumab: IV: 6 mg/kg day 1

[total dose/cycle = 6 mg/kg]

Repeat cycle every 21 days to complete one year of Trastuzumab

References

Dang C, Fornier M, Sugarman S, et al. The safety of dose-dense doxorubicin and cyclophospha-mide followed by paclitaxel with trastuzumab in HER-2/neu overexpressed/amplified breast cancer. *J Clin Oncol*. 2008;26(8):1216-22.

AC (Dose-Dense) followed by Paclitaxel Weekly (Breast)

Index Terms Doxorubicin, Cyclophosphamide, Paclitaxel (Breast)

Use Breast cancer

Regimen

Cycles 1-4 (Citron, 2003):

Doxorubicin: IV: 60 mg/m^2 day 1

[total dose/cycle = 60 mg/m^2]

Cyclophosphamide: IV: 600 mg/m^2 day 1

[total dose/cycle = 600 mg/m^2]

Filgrastim: SubQ: ~5 mcg/kg/day days 3 to 10 (rounded to either 300 or 480 mcg/day)

[total dose/cycle = ~40 mcg/kg, 2400-3840 mcg/cycle]

Repeat cycle every 14 days for 4 cycles

followed by (Sparano, 2008):

Paclitaxel: IV: 80 mg/m^2 over 1 hour day 1

[total dose/cycle = 80 mg/m^2]

Repeat cycle every 7 days for 12 cycles

References

Citron ML, Berry DA, Cirrincione C, et al, "Randomized Trial of Dose-Dense Versus Conventionally Scheduled and Sequential Versus Concurrent Combination Chemotherapy as Postoperative Adjuvant Treatment of Node-Positive Primary Breast Cancer: First Report of Intergroup Trial C9741/Cancer Leukemia Group B Trial 9741," *J Clin Oncol*, 2003, 21(8):1431-9.

Sparano JA, Wang M, Martino S, et al, "Weekly Paclitaxel in the Adjuvant Treatment of Breast Cancer," *N Engl J Med*, 2008, 358(16):1663-71.

AC followed by Docetaxel Every 3 Weeks (Breast)

Index Terms Doxorubicin, Cyclophosphamide, Docetaxel (Breast)

Use Breast cancer

Regimen

Doxorubicin: IV: 60 mg/m^2 over 5-15 minutes day 1

[total dose/cycle = 60 mg/m^2]

Cyclophosphamide: IV: 600 mg/m^2 over 30-60 minutes day 1

[total dose/cycle = 600 mg/m^2]

Repeat cycle every 21 days for 4 cycles

followed by

Docetaxel: IV: 100 mg/m^2 over 1 hour day 1

[total dose/cycle = 100 mg/m^2]

Repeat cycle every 21 days for 4 cycles

References

Sparano JA, Wang M, Martino S, et al, "Weekly Paclitaxel in the Adjuvant Treatment of Breast Cancer," *N Engl J Med*, 2008, 358(16):1663-71.

Swain SM, Jeong JH, Geyer CE, et al, "Longer Therapy, Iatrogenic Amenorrhea, and Survival in Early Breast Cancer, *N Engl J Med*, 2010, 362(22):2053-65.

AC followed by Paclitaxel-Trastuzumab (Breast)

Index Terms Doxorubicin, Cyclophosphamide, Paclitaxel, Trastuzumab (Breast)

Use Breast cancer

Regimen

Cycles 1-4 of AC:

Doxorubicin: IV: 60 mg/m^2 day 1

[total dose/cycle = 60 mg/m^2]

Cyclophosphamide: IV: 600 mg/m^2 day 1

[total dose/cycle = 600 mg/m^2]

Repeat cycle every 21 days for 4 cycles

followed by

Cycle 1 of Paclitaxel-Trastuzumab:

Paclitaxel: IV: 80 mg/m^2 day 1

[total dose/cycle = 80 mg/m^2]

Trastuzumab: IV: 4 mg/kg (loading dose) day 1

[total dose/cycle = 4 mg/kg]

Treatment cycle is 7 days for 1 cycle

followed by

Weekly Paclitaxel-Trastuzumab:

Paclitaxel: IV: 80 mg/m^2 day 1

[total dose/cycle = 80 mg/m^2]

Trastuzumab: IV: 2 mg/kg day 1

[total dose/cycle = 2 mg/kg]

Repeat cycle every 7 days for 11 cycles

followed by

Weekly Trastuzumab:

Trastuzumab: IV: 2 mg/kg day 1

[total dose/cycle = 2 mg/kg]

Repeat cycle every 7 days for 40 cycles (total of 52 weeks of trastuzumab)

References

Romond EH, Perez EA, Bryant J, et al, "Trastuzumab Plus Adjuvant Chemotherapy for Operable HER2-Positive Breast Cancer," *N Engl J Med*, 2005, 353(16):1673-84.

AC followed by Paclitaxel Weekly (Breast)

Index Terms Doxorubicin, Cyclophosphamide, Paclitaxel (Breast)

Use Breast cancer

Regimen

Doxorubicin: IV: 60 mg/m^2 over 5-15 minutes day 1

[total dose/cycle = 60 mg/m^2]

Cyclophosphamide: IV: 600 mg/m^2 over 30-60 minutes day 1

[total dose/cycle = 600 mg/m^2]

Repeat cycle every 21 days for 4 cycles

followed by

Paclitaxel: IV: 80 mg/m^2 over 1 hour day 1

[total dose/cycle = 80 mg/m^2]

Repeat cycle every 7 days for 12 cycles

References
Sparano JA, Wang M, Martino S, et al, "Weekly Paclitaxel in the Adjuvant Treatment of Breast Cancer, *N Engl J Med*, 2008, 358(16):1663-71.

Ado-Trastuzumab Emtansine (Breast)

Index Terms T-DM1 (Breast); Trastuzumab Emtansine (Breast); Trastuzumab-DM1 (Breast); Trastuzumab-MCC-DM1 (Breast)

Use Breast cancer

Regimen

Ado-Trastuzumab Emtansine: IV: 3.6 mg/kg day 1

[total dose/cycle = 3.6 mg/kg]

Repeat cycle every 21 days until disease progression or unacceptable toxicity

References
Hurvitz SA, Dirix L, Kocsis J, et al. Phase II randomized study of trastuzumab emtansine versus trastuzumab plus docetaxel in patients with human epidermal growth factor receptor 2-positive metastatic breast cancer. *J Clin Oncol*. 2013;31(9):1157-1163.

Krop IE, LoRusso P, Miller KD, et al. A phase II study of trastuzumab emtansine in patients with human epidermal growth factor receptor 2-positive metastatic breast cancer who were previously treated with trastuzumab, lapatinib, an anthracycline, a taxane, and capecitabine. *J Clin Oncol*. 2012;30(26):3234-3241.

Verma S, Miles D, Gianni L, et al. Trastuzumab emtansine for HER2-positive advanced breast cancer. *N Engl J Med*. 2012;367(19):1783-1791.

AD (Soft Tissue Sarcoma)

Index Terms Doxorubicin-Dacarbazine (Soft Tissue Sarcoma)

Use Soft tissue sarcoma

Regimen NOTE: Multiple variations are listed.

Variation 1 (metastatic):

Doxorubicin: IV: 15 mg/m^2/day continuous infusion days 1 to 4

[total dose/cycle = 60 mg/m^2]

Dacarbazine: IV: 187.5 mg/m^2/day continuous infusion days 1 to 4

[total dose/cycle = 750 mg/m^2]

Repeat cycle every 21 days; maximum lifetime doxorubicin dose of 450 mg/m^2

Variation 2 (metastatic):

Doxorubicin: IV: 60 mg/m^2 IV bolus day 1

[total dose/cycle = 60 mg/m^2]

Dacarbazine: IV: 750 mg/m^2/day IV bolus day 1

[total dose/cycle = 750 mg/m^2]

Repeat cycle every 21 days; maximum lifetime doxorubicin dose of 450 mg/m^2

Variation 3 (metastatic):

Doxorubicin: IV: 15 mg/m^2/day continuous infusion days 1 to 4

[total dose/cycle = 60 mg/m^2]

Dacarbazine: IV: 250 mg/m^2/day continuous infusion days 1 to 4

[total dose/cycle = 1000 mg/m^2]

Repeat cycle every 21 days

Variation 4 (metastatic):

Doxorubicin: IV: 60 mg/m^2 day 1

[total dose/cycle = 60 mg/m^2]

Dacarbazine: IV: 250 mg/m^2/day days 1 to 5

[total dose/cycle = 1250 mg/m^2]

Repeat cycle every 21 days until disease progression; when maximum lifetime doxorubicin dose received, continue with single agent dacarbazine

References

Variations 1 and 2:

Zalupski M, Metch B, Fletcher WS, et al, "Phase III Comparison of Doxorubicin and Dacarbazine Given by Bolus Versus Infusion in Patients With Soft-Tissue Sarcomas: A Southwest Oncology Group Study," *J Natl Cancer Inst*, 1991, 83(13):926-32.

Variation 3:

Antman K, Crowley J, Balcerzak SP, et al, "An Intergroup Phase III Randomized Study of Doxorubicin and Dacarbazine With or Without Ifosfamide and Mesna in Advanced Soft Tissue and Bone Sarcomas," *J Clin Oncol*, 1993, 11(7):1276-85.

Variation 4:

Borden EC, Amato DA, Rosenbaum C, et al, "Randomized Comparison of Three Adriamycin Regimens for Metastatic Soft Tissue Sarcomas," *J Clin Oncol*, 1987, 5(6):840-50.

Afatinib (NSCLC Regimen)

Use Lung cancer, non-small cell

Regimen

Afatinib: Oral: 40 mg once daily days 1 to 21

[total dose/cycle = 840 mg]

Repeat cycle every 21 days until disease progression or unacceptable toxicity

References

Sequist LV, Yang J C-H, Yamamtoto, et al, "Phase III Study of Afatinib or Cisplatin Plus Pemetrexed in Patients With Metastatic Lung Adenocarcinoma With EGFR Mutations," *J Clin Oncol*, 2013 [epub ahead of print].

AIM (Soft Tissue Sarcoma)

Index Terms Doxorubicin-Ifosfamide (Soft Tissue Sarcoma); Ifosfamide-Doxorubicin (Soft Tissue Sarcoma)

Use Soft tissue sarcoma

Regimen NOTE: Mesna uroprotection should be administered before and 4 and 8 hours after ifosfamide days 1 to 4.

Ifosfamide: IV: 1,500 mg/m^2/day over 2 hours days 1 to 4

[total dose/cycle = 6,000 mg/m^2]

Doxorubicin: IV: 20 mg/m^2/day continuous infusion days 1, 2, and 3

[total dose/cycle = 60 mg/m^2]

Filgrastim: SubQ: 5 mcg/kg/day for 10 days, starting 24 hours after last dose of mesna

[total dose/cycle = 50 mcg/kg]

Repeat cycle every 21 days for a total of 4 cycles for localized disease and 6 cycles for metastatic disease

References

Worden FP, Taylor JM, Biermann JS, et al. Randomized phase II evaluation of 6 g/m^2 of ifosfamide plus doxorubicin and granulocyte colony-stimulating factor (G-CSF) compared with 12 g/m^2 of ifosfamide plus doxorubicin and G-CSF in the treatment of poor-prognosis soft tissue sarcoma. *J Clin Oncol*. 2005;23(1):105-112.

Axitinib (RCC Regimen)

Use Renal cell cancer

Regimen

Axitinib: Oral: Initial: 5 mg twice daily; if tolerated (no adverse reactions higher than grade 2 and blood pressure 150/90 mm Hg or lower without antihypertensive drugs) for 2 consecutive weeks, may escalate to 7 mg twice daily and then if tolerated, may escalate to a maximum dose of 10 mg twice daily

Continue until disease progression or unacceptable toxicity

References

Motzer RJ, Escudier B, Tomczak P, et al. Axitinib versus sorafenib as second-line treatment for advanced renal cell carcinoma: overall survival analysis and updated results from a randomised phase 3 trial. *Lancet Oncol.* 2013;14(6):552-562.

Rini BI, Escudier B, Tomczak P, et al, Comparative effectiveness of axitinib versus sorafenib in advanced renal cell carcinoma (AXIS): a randomised phase 3 trial. *Lancet.* 2011;378 (9807):1931-1939.

Azacitidine (AML Regimen)

Use Leukemia, acute myeloid

Regimen

Azacitidine: SubQ: 75 mg/m^2/day days 1 to 7

[total dose/cycle = 525 mg/m^2]

Repeat cycle every 28 days (for a minimum of 6 cycles [Fenaux, 2010]) as long as tolerated and maintaining response

References

Fenaux P, Mufti GJ, Hellstrom-Lindberg E, et al, "Azacitidine Prolongs Overall Survival Compared With Conventional Care Regimens in Elderly Patients With Low Bone Marrow Blast Count Acute Myeloid Leukemia," *J Clin Oncol*, 2010, 28(4):562-9.

Sudan N, Rossetti JM, Shadduck RK, et al, "Treatment of Acute Myelogenous Leukemia With Outpatient Azacitidine," *Cancer*, 2006, 107(8):1839-43.

Azacitidine (MDS Regimen)

Use Myelodysplastic syndrome

Regimen NOTE: Multiple variations are listed.

Variation 1:

Azacitidine: SubQ: 75 mg/m^2/day days 1 to 7

[total dose/cycle = 525 mg/m^2]

Repeat cycle every 28 days

Variation 2:

Azacitidine: IV: 75 mg/m^2/day days 1 to 7

[total dose/cycle = 525 mg/m^2]

Repeat cycle every 28 days

Variation 3:

Azacitidine: SubQ: 75 mg/m^2/day days 1 to 5 (Mon-Fri), 2 days of rest (Sat, Sun), then 75 mg/m^2/day days 1 and 2 (Mon, Tues)

[total dose/cycle = 525 mg/m^2]

Repeat cycle every 28 days for a total of 6 cycles

Variation 4:

Azacitidine: SubQ: 50 mg/m^2/day days 1 to 5 (Mon-Fri), 2 days of rest (Sat, Sun), then 50 mg/m^2/day days 1 to 5 (Mon-Fri)

[total dose/cycle = 500 mg/m^2]

Repeat cycle every 28 days for a total of 6 cycles

Variation 5:

Azacitidine: SubQ: 75 mg/m^2/day days 1 to 5 (Mon-Fri)

[total dose/cycle = 375 mg/m^2]

Repeat cycle every 28 days for a total of 6 cycles

References

Variation 1:

Fenaux P, Mufti GJ, Hellstrom-Lindberg E, et al, "Efficacy of Azacitidine Compared With That of Conventional Care Regimens in the Treatment of Higher-Risk Myelodysplastic Syndromes: A Randomised, Open-Label, Phase III Study," *Lancet Oncol*, 2009, 10(3):223-32.

Variation 2:

Marcucci G, Silverman L, Eller M, et al, "Bioavailability of Azacitidine Subcutaneous Versus Intravenous in Patients With the Myelodysplastic Syndromes," *J Clin Pharmacol*, 2005, 45 (5):597-602.

Sekeres MA, Maciejewski JP, Donley DW, et al, "A Study Comparing Dosing Regimens and Efficacy of Subcutaneous to Intravenous Azacitidine (ASA) for the Treatment of Myelodysplastic Syndromes (MDS), *Blood*, 2009, 114(22) [abstract 3797 from 2009 ASH Annual Meeting].

Variations 3, 4, and 5:

Lyons RM, Cosgriff TM, Modi SS, et al, "Hematologic Response to Three Alternative Dosing Schedules of Azacitidine in Patients With Myelodysplastic Syndrome," *J Clin Oncol*, 2009, 27 (11):1850-6.

◆ **Baby Brain I** *see* COPE *on page 1926*

◆ **BDR (Waldenstrom Macroglobulinemia)** *see* Bortezomib-Dexamethasone-Rituximab (Waldenstrom Macroglobulinemia) *on page 1848*

BEACOPP-14 (Hodgkin)

Index Terms Bleomycin, Etoposide, Doxorubicin, Cyclophosphamide, Vincristine, Procarbazine, Prednisone (Hodgkin)

Use Lymphoma, Hodgkin

Regimen

Bleomycin: IV: 10 units/m^2 day 8

[total dose/cycle = 10 units/m^2]

Etoposide: IV: 100 mg/m^2/day days 1, 2, and 3

[total dose/cycle = 300 mg/m^2]

Doxorubicin: IV: 25 mg/m^2 day 1

[total dose/cycle = 25 mg/m^2]

Cyclophosphamide: IV: 650 mg/m^2 day 1

[total dose/cycle = 650 mg/m^2]

Vincristine: IV: 1.4 mg/m^2 (maximum dose: 2 mg) day 8

[total dose/cycle = 1.4 mg/m^2; maximum: 2 mg]

Procarbazine: Oral: 100 mg/m^2/day days 1 to 7

[total dose/cycle = 700 mg/m^2]

Prednisone: Oral: 80 mg/m^2/day days 1 to 7
[total dose/cycle = 560 mg/m^2]
Filgrastim: SubQ: 300 mcg/day (patients <75 kg) or 480 mcg/day (patients ≥75 kg) days 8 to13
Repeat cycle every 14 days for a total of 8 cycles

References

Sieber M, Bredenfeld H, Josting A, et al, "14-Day Variant of the Bleomycin, Etoposide, Doxorubicin, Cyclophosphamide, Vincristine, Procarbazine, and Prednisone Regimen in Advanced-Stage Hodgkin's Lymphoma: Results of a Pilot Study of the German Hodgkin's Lymphoma Study Group," *J Clin Oncol*, 2003, 21(9):1734-9.

◆ **BEACOPP Baseline (Hodgkin)** *see* BEACOPP Standard (Hodgkin) on page 1832

BEACOPP Escalated (Hodgkin)

Index Terms Bleomycin, Etoposide, Doxorubicin, Cyclophosphamide, Vincristine, Procarbazine, Prednisone (Hodgkin)

Use Lymphoma, Hodgkin

Regimen

Bleomycin: IV: 10 units/m^2 day 8
[total dose/cycle = 10 units/m^2]
Etoposide: IV: 200 mg/m^2/day days 1, 2, and 3
[total dose/cycle = 600 mg/m^2]
Doxorubicin: IV: 35 mg/m^2 day 1
[total dose/cycle = 35 mg/m^2]
Cyclophosphamide: IV: 1200 mg/m^2 day 1
[total dose/cycle = 1200 mg/m^2]
Vincristine: IV: 1.4 mg/m^2 (maximum dose: 2 mg) day 8
[total dose/cycle = 1.4 mg/m^2: maximum: 2 mg]
Procarbazine: Oral: 100 mg/m^2/day days 1 to 7
[total dose/cycle = 700 mg/m^2]
Prednisone: Oral: 40 mg/m^2/day days 1 to 14
[total dose/cycle = 560 mg/m^2]
Filgrastim: SubQ: 300 or 480 mcg/day (depending on weight of 75 kg) day 8 until leukocyte recovery (3 days at >1000/mm^3)
Repeat cycle every 21 days for a total of 8 cycles

References

Diehl V, Franklin J, Hasenclever D, et al, "BEACOPP, A New Dose-Escalated and Accelerated Regimen, Is at Least as Effective as COPP/ABVD in Patients With Advanced-Stage Hodgkin's Lymphoma: Interim Report From a Trial of the German Hodgkin's Lymphoma Study Group," *J Clin Oncol*, 1998, 16(12):3810-21.

Diehl V, Franklin J, Pfreundschuh M, et al, "Standard and Increased-Dose BEACOPP Chemotherapy Compared With COPP-ABVD for Advanced Hodgkin's disease," *N Engl J Med*, 2003, 348(24):2386-95.

Engert A, Diehl V, Franklin J, et al, "Escalated-Dose BEACOPP in the Treatment of Patients With Advanced-Stage Hodgkin's Lymphoma: 10 Years of Follow-Up of the GHSG HD9 Study," *J Clin Oncol*, 2009, 27(27):4548-54.

BEACOPP Escalated Plus Standard (Hodgkin)

Index Terms Bleomycin, Etoposide, Doxorubicin, Cyclophosphamide, Vincristine, Procarbazine, Prednisone (Hodgkin)

Use Lymphoma, Hodgkin

Regimen NOTE: Multiple variations are listed.

Variation 1: BEACOPP Escalated for 4 cycles **followed by** 2 cycles of BEACOPP Standard

BEACOPP Escalated for 4 cycles:

Bleomycin: IV: 10 units/m^2 day 8
[total dose/cycle = 10 units/m^2]

Etoposide: IV: 200 mg/m^2/day days 1, 2, and 3
[total dose/cycle = 600 mg/m^2]

Doxorubicin: IV: 35 mg/m^2 day 1
[total dose/cycle = 35 mg/m^2]

Cyclophosphamide: IV: 1250 mg/m^2 day 1
[total dose/cycle = 1250 mg/m^2]

Vincristine: IV: 1.4 mg/m^2 (maximum dose: 2 mg) day 8
[total dose/cycle = 1.4 mg/m^2: maximum: 2 mg]

Procarbazine: Oral: 100 mg/m^2/day days 1 to 7
[total dose/cycle = 700 mg/m^2]

Prednisone: Oral: 40 mg/m^2/day days 1 to 14
[total dose/cycle = 560 mg/m^2]

Filgrastim: SubQ: 300 mcg/day day 8 until neutrophil recovery (>500/mm^3)
Repeat cycle every 21 days for a total of 4 cycles

Followed by BEACOPP Standard for 2 cycles:

Bleomycin: IV: 10 units/m^2 day 8
[total dose/cycle = 10 units/m^2]

Etoposide: IV: 100 mg/m^2/day days 1, 2, and 3
[total dose/cycle = 300 mg/m^2]

Doxorubicin: IV: 25 mg/m^2 day 1
[total dose/cycle = 25 mg/m^2]

Cyclophosphamide: IV: 650 mg/m^2 day 1
[total dose/cycle = 650 mg/m^2]

Vincristine: IV: 1.4 mg/m^2 (maximum dose: 2 mg) day 8
[total dose/cycle = 1.4 mg/m^2: maximum: 2 mg]

Procarbazine: Oral: 100 mg/m^2/day days 1 to 7
[total dose/cycle = 700 mg/m^2]

Prednisone: Oral: 40 mg/m^2/day days 1 to 14
[total dose/cycle = 560 mg/m^2]

Filgrastim: SubQ: 300 mcg/day day 8 until neutrophil recovery (>500/mm^3)
Repeat cycle every 21 days for a total of 2 cycles

Variation 2: BEACOPP Escalated for 4 cycles **followed by** 4 cycles of BEACOPP Standard

BEACOPP Escalated for 4 cycles:

Bleomycin: IV: 10 units/m^2 day 8
[total dose/cycle = 10 units/m^2]

Etoposide: IV: 200 mg/m^2/day days 1, 2, and 3
[total dose/cycle = 600 mg/m^2]

Doxorubicin: IV: 35 mg/m^2 day 1
[total dose/cycle = 35 mg/m^2]

Cyclophosphamide: IV: 1250 mg/m^2 day 1
[total dose/cycle = 1250 mg/m^2]

Vincristine: IV: 1.4 mg/m^2 (maximum dose: 2 mg) day 8
[total dose/cycle = 1.4 mg/m^2: maximum: 2 mg]

Procarbazine: Oral: 100 mg/m^2/day days 1 to 7
[total dose/cycle = 700 mg/m^2]

◀

Prednisone: Oral: 40 mg/m²/day days 1 to 14
[total dose/cycle = 560 mg/m²]
Filgrastim: SubQ: 300 mcg/day day 8 until neutrophil count >1000/mm³ for 3
consecutive days)
Repeat cycle every 21 days for a total of 4 cycles
Followed by BEACOPP Standard for 4 cycles:
Bleomycin: IV: 10 units/m² day 8
[total dose/cycle = 10 units/m²]
Etoposide: IV: 100 mg/m²/day days 1, 2, and 3
[total dose/cycle = 300 mg/m²]
Doxorubicin: IV: 25 mg/m² day 1
[total dose/cycle = 25 mg/m²]
Cyclophosphamide: IV: 650 mg/m² day 1
[total dose/cycle = 650 mg/m²]
Vincristine: IV: 1.4 mg/m² (maximum dose: 2 mg) day 8
[total dose/cycle = 1.4 mg/m²: maximum: 2 mg]
Procarbazine: Oral: 100 mg/m²/day days 1 to 7
[total dose/cycle = 700 mg/m²]
Prednisone: Oral: 40 mg/m²/day days 1 to 14
[total dose/cycle = 560 mg/m²]
Filgrastim: SubQ: 300 mcg/day day 8 until neutrophil count >1000/mm³ for 3
consecutive days)
Repeat cycle every 21 days for a total of 4 cycles

References
Variation 1:
Federico M, Luminari S, Iannitto E, et al, "ABVD Compared With BEACOPP Compared With CEC
for the Initial Treatment of Patients With Advanced Hodgkin's Lymphoma: Results From the
HD2000 Gruppo Italiano per lo Studio dei Linfomi Trial," *J Clin Oncol*, 2009, 27(5):805-11.
Variation 2:
Viviani S, Zinzani PL, Rambaldi A, et al, "ABVD Versus BEACOPP for Hodgkin's Lymphoma When
High-Dose Salvage Is Planned," *N Engl J Med*, 2011, 365(3):203-12.

BEACOPP Standard (Hodgkin)

Index Terms BEACOPP Baseline (Hodgkin); Bleomycin, Etoposide, Doxorubicin, Cyclophosphamide, Vincristine, Procarbazine, Prednisone (Hodgkin)
Use Lymphoma, Hodgkin
Regimen
Bleomycin: IV: 10 units/m² day 8
[total dose/cycle = 10 units/m²]
Etoposide: IV: 100 mg/m²/day days 1, 2, and 3
[total dose/cycle = 300 mg/m²]
Doxorubicin: IV: 25 mg/m² day 1
[total dose/cycle = 25 mg/m²]
Cyclophosphamide: IV: 650 mg/m² day 1
[total dose/cycle = 650 mg/m²]
Vincristine: IV: 1.4 mg/m² (maximum dose: 2 mg) day 8
[total dose/cycle = 1.4 mg/m²; maximum: 2 mg]
Procarbazine: Oral: 100 mg/m²/day days 1 to 7
[total dose/cycle = 700 mg/m²]
Prednisone: Oral: 40 mg/m²/day days 1 to 14
[total dose/cycle = 560 mg/m²]
Repeat cycle every 21 days for a total of 8 cycles

References

Diehl V, Franklin J, Hasenclever D, et al, "BEACOPP, a New Dose-Escalated and Accelerated Regimen, Is at Least as Effective as COPP/ABVD in Patients With Advanced-Stage Hodgkin's Lymphoma: Interim Report From a Trial of the German Hodgkin's Lymphoma Study Group," *J Clin Oncol*, 1998, 16(12):3810-21.

Diehl V, Sieber M, Rüffer U, et al, "BEACOPP: An Intensified Chemotherapy Regimen in Advanced Hodgkin's Disease. The German Hodgkin's Lymphoma Study Group," *Ann Oncol*, 1997, 8 (2):143-8.

Bendamustine-Bortezomib-Rituximab (NHL-Follicular)

Index Terms Bortezomib-Bendamustine-Rituximab (NHL-Follicular); Rituximab-Bortezomib-Bendamustine (NHL-Follicular); VBR (NHL-Follicular)

Use Lymphoma, non-Hodgkin (relapsed/refractory follicular NHL)

Regimen NOTE: Multiple variations are listed.

Variation 1:

Bortezomib: IV: 1.3 mg/m^2/day days 1, 4, 8, and 11

[total dose/cycle = 5.2 mg/m^2]

Rituximab: IV: 375 mg/m^2 day 1

[total dose/cycle = 375 mg/m^2]

Bendamustine: IV: 90 mg/m^2/day over 30 to 60 minutes days 1 and 4

[total dose/cycle = 180 mg/m^2]

Repeat cycle every 28 days for 6 cycles

Variation 2:

Cycle 1:

Bortezomib: IV: 1.6 mg/m^2/day days 1, 8, 15, and 22

[total dose/cycle = 6.4 mg/m^2]

Bendamustine: IV: 90 mg/m^2/day over 60 minutes days 1 and 2

[total dose/cycle = 180 mg/m^2]

Rituximab: IV: 375 mg/m^2/day days 1, 8, 15, and 22 cycle 1 only

[total dose/cycle 1 = 1,500 mg/m^2]

Treatment duration for cycle 1 is 35 days

Cycles 2 to 5:

Bortezomib: IV: 1.6 mg/m^2/day days 1, 8, 15, and 22

[total dose/cycle = 6.4 mg/m^2]

Bendamustine: IV: 90 mg/m^2/day over 60 minutes days 1 and 2

[total dose/cycle = 180 mg/m^2]

Rituximab: IV: 375 mg/m^2 day 1

[total dose/cycle = 375 mg/m^2]

Repeat cycle every 35 days for a total of 5 cycles

References

Variation 1:

Friedberg JW, Vose JM, Kelly JL, et al. The combination of bendamustine, bortezomib, and rituximab for patients with relapsed/refractory indolent and mantle cell non-Hodgkin lymphoma. *Blood*. 2011;117(10):2807-2812.

Variation 2:

Fowler N, Kahl BS, Lee P, et al. Bortezomib, bendamustine, and rituximab in patients with relapsed or refractory follicular lymphoma: the phase II VERTICAL study. *J Clin Oncol*. 2011;29 (25):3389-3395.

Bendamustine (CLL Regimen)

Use Leukemia, chronic lymphocytic

Regimen

Bendamustine: IV: 100 mg/m^2/day over 30 minutes days 1 and 2

[total dose/cycle = 200 mg/m^2]

Repeat cycle every 28 days for up to 6 cycles

References

Knauf WU, Lissitchkov T, Aldaoud A, et al. Bendamustine compared with chlorambucil in previously untreated patients with chronic lymphocytic leukaemia: updated results of a randomized phase III trial. *Br J Haematol.* 2012;159(1):67-77.

Knauf WU, Lissichkov T, Aldaoud A, et al. Phase III randomized study of bendamustine compared with chlorambucil in previously untreated patients with chronic lymphocytic leukemia. *J Clin Oncol.* 2009;27(26):4378-4384.

Bendamustine (Hodgkin Regimen)

Use Lymphoma, Hodgkin

Regimen

Benamustine: IV: 120 mg/m^2/day over 30 minutes days 1 and 2
[total dose/cycle = 240 mg/m^2]
Repeat cycle every 28 days (with growth factor support) for up to 6 cycles

References

Moskowitz AJ, Hamlin PA, Perales M-A, et al. Phase II study of bendamustine in relapsed and refractory Hodgkin lymphoma. *J Clin Oncol.* 2013;31(4):456-460.

Bendamustine-Lenalidomide-Dexamethasone (Multiple Myeloma)

Index Terms BLD (Multiple Myeloma); Lenalidomide-Bendamustine-Dexamethasone (Multiple Myeloma)

Use Multiple myeloma

Regimen

Bendamustine: IV: 75 mg/m^2/day days 1 and 2
[total dose/cycle = 150 mg/m^2]
Lenalidomide: Oral: 10 mg once daily days 1 to 21
[total dose/cycle = 210 mg]
Dexamethasone: Oral: 40 mg once daily on days 1, 8, 15, and 22
[total dose/cycle = 160 mg]
Repeat cycle every 28 days for up to a maximum of 8 cycles

References

Lentzsch S, O'Sullivan A, Kennedy RC, et al. Combination of bendamustine, lenalidomide, and dexamethasone (BLD) in patients with relapsed or refractory multiple myeloma is feasible and highly effective: results of phase 1/2 open-label, dose escalation study. *Blood.* 2012;119 (20):4608-4613.

Bendamustine (Multiple Myeloma Regimen)

Use Multiple myeloma

Regimen

Bendamustine: IV: 90-100 mg/m^2/day days 1 and 2
[total dose/cycle = 180-200 mg/m^2]
Repeat cycle every 28 days for at least 2 cycles

References

Knop S, Straka C, Haen M, et al. The efficacy and toxicity of bendamustine in recurrent multiple myeloma after high-dose chemotherapy. *Haematologica.* 2005;90(9):1287-1288.

Bendamustine (NHL-Indolent Regimen)

Use Lymphoma, non-Hodgkin (indolent B-cell refractory)

Regimen

Bendamustine: IV: 120 mg/m^2/day over 60 to 120 minutes days 1 and 2
[total dose/cycle = 240 mg/m^2]
Repeat cycle every 21 days for up to 8 cycles

References

Kahl BS, Bartlett NL, Leonard JP, et al. Bendamustine is effective therapy in patients with rituximab-refractory, indolent B-cell non-Hodgkin lymphoma: results from a Multicenter Study. *Cancer.* 2010;116(1):106-114.

Bendamustine-Rituximab (CLL)

Index Terms B-R (CLL); BR (CLL); Rituximab-Bendamustine (CLL)

Use Leukemia, chronic lymphocytic

Regimen NOTE: Multiple variations are listed.

Variation 1 (relapsed/refractory):

Cycle 1:

Rituximab: IV: 375 mg/m^2 day 0 cycle 1 only
[total dose/cycle 1 = 375 mg/m^2]
Bendamustine: IV: 70 mg/m^2/day days 1 and 2
[total dose/cycle = 140 mg/m^2]

Cycle 2 to 6:

Rituximab: IV: 500 mg/m^2 day 1
[total dose/cycle = 500 mg/m^2]
Bendamustine: IV: 70 mg/m^2/day days 1 and 2
[total dose/cycle = 140 mg/m^2]
Repeat cycle every 28 days for up to 6 cycles

Variation 2 (first-line):

Cycle 1:

Rituximab: IV: 375 mg/m^2 day 0 cycle 1 only
[total dose/cycle 1 = 375 mg/m^2]
Bendamustine: IV: 90 mg/m^2/day days 1 and 2
[total dose/cycle = 180 mg/m^2]

Cycles 2 to 6:

Rituximab: IV: 500 mg/m^2 day 1
[total dose/cycle = 500 mg/m^2]
Bendamustine: IV: 90 mg/m^2/day days 1 and 2
[total dose/cycle = 180 mg/m^2]
Repeat cycle every 28 days for up to 6 cycles

References

Variation 1:

Fischer K, Cramer P, Busch R, et al. Bendamustine combined with rituximab in patients with relapsed and/or refractory chronic lymphocytic leukemia: a multicenter phase II trial of the German Chronic Lymphocytic Leukemia Study Group. *J Clin Oncol.* 2011;29(26):3559-3566.

Variation 2:

Fischer K, Cramer P, Busch R, et al. Bendamustine in combination with rituximab for previously untreated patients with chronic lymphocytic leukemia: a multicenter phase II trial of the German Chronic Lymphocytic Leukemia Study Group. *J Clin Oncol.* 2012;30(26):3209-3216.

Bendamustine-Rituximab (NHL-Follicular)

Index Terms B-R (NHL-Follicular); BR (NHL-Follicular); Rituximab-Bendamustine (NHL-Follicular)

Use Lymphoma, non-Hodgkin (grade 1 and grade 2 follicular NHL)

Regimen NOTE: Multiple variations are listed.

Variation 1 (first-line):

Rituximab: IV: 375 mg/m^2 day 1
[total dose/cycle = 375 mg/m^2]
Bendamustine: IV: 90 mg/m^2/day days 1 and 2
[total dose/cycle = 180 mg/m^2]
Repeat cycle every 28 days for 6 cycles (Rummel, 2013); maximum of 8 cycles (Flinn, 2014)

◀ Variation 2 (refractory):
Pretreatment:
Rituximab: IV: 375 mg/m² 1 week before the start of cycle 1
  [total dose/pretreatment = 375 mg/m²]
Cycles:
Rituximab: IV: 375 mg/m² day 1
  [total dose/cycle = 375 mg/m²]
Bendamustine: IV: 90 mg/m²/day days 2 and 3
  [total dose/cycle = 180 mg/m²]
Repeat cycle every 28 days for up to 4 cycles (Rummel, 2005) or 4 to 6 cycles (Robinson, 2008)
Post-Treatment:
Rituximab: IV: 375 mg/m² 4 weeks after the last cycle
  [total dose/post-treatment = 375 mg/m²]

References

Variation 1:

Flinn IW, van der Jagt R, Kahl BS, et al. Randomized trial of bendamustine-rituximab or R-CHOP/R-CVP in first-line treatment of indolent NHL or MCL: the BRIGHT study. *Blood.* 2014;123 (19):2944-2952.

Rummel MJ, Niederle N, Maschmeyer G, et al. Bendamustine plus rituximab versus CHOP plus rituximab as first-line treatment for patients with indolent and mantle-cell lymphomas: an open-label, multicentre, randomised, phase 3 non-inferiority trial. *Lancet.* 2013;381(9873):1203-1210.

Variation 2:

Robinson KS, Williams ME, van der Jagt RH, et al. Phase II multicenter study of bendamustine plus rituximab in patients with relapsed indolent B-cell and mantle cell non-Hodgkin's lymphoma. *J Clin Oncol,* 2008;26(27):4473-4479.

Rummel MJ, Al-Batran SE, Kim SZ, et al. Bendamustine plus rituximab is effective and has a favorable toxicity profile in the treatment of mantle cell and low-grade non-Hodgkin's lymphoma. *J Clin Oncol.* 2005;23(15):3383-3389.

Bendamustine-Rituximab (NHL-Mantle Cell)

Index Terms B-R (NHL-Mantle Cell); BR (NHL-Mantle Cell); Rituximab-Bendamustine (NHL-Mantle Cell)

Use Lymphoma, non-Hodgkin (Mantle cell)

Regimen NOTE: Multiple variations are listed.
Variation 1 (first-line):
Rituximab: IV: 375 mg/m² day 1
  [total dose/cycle = 375 mg/m²]
Bendamustine: IV: 90 mg/m²/day days 1 and 2
  [total dose/cycle = 180 mg/m²]
Repeat cycle every 28 days for 6 cycles (Rummel, 2013); maximum of 8 cycles (Flinn, 2014)
Variation 2 (refractory):
Pretreatment:
Rituximab: IV: 375 mg/m² 1 week before the start of cycle 1
  [total dose/pretreatment = 375 mg/m²]
Cycles:
Rituximab: IV: 375 mg/m² day 1
  [total dose/cycle = 375 mg/m²]
Bendamustine: IV: 90 mg/m²/day days 2 and 3
  [total dose/cycle = 180 mg/m²]
Repeat cycle every 28 days for up to 4 cycles (Rummel, 2005) or 4 to 6 cycles (Robinson, 2008)

Post-Treatment:
Rituximab: IV: 375 mg/m² 4 weeks after the last cycle
[total dose/post-treatment = 375 mg/m²]

References

Variation 1:

Flinn IW, van der Jagt R, Kahl BS, et al. Randomized trial of bendamustine-rituximab or R-CHOP/R-CVP in first-line treatment of indolent NHL or MCL: the BRIGHT study. *Blood.* 2014;123 (19):2944-2952.

Rummel MJ, Niederle N, Maschmeyer G, et al. Bendamustine plus rituximab versus CHOP plus rituximab as first-line treatment for patients with indolent and mantle-cell lymphomas: an open-label, multicentre, randomised, phase 3 non-inferiority trial. *Lancet.* 2013;381(9873):1203-1210.

Variation 2:

Robinson KS, Williams ME, van der Jagt RH, et al. Phase II multicenter study of bendamustine plus rituximab in patients with relapsed indolent B-cell and mantle cell non-Hodgkin's lymphoma. *J Clin Oncol,* 2008;26(27):4473-4479.

Rummel MJ, Al-Batran SE, Kim SZ, et al. Bendamustine plus rituximab is effective and has a favorable toxicity profile in the treatment of mantle cell and low-grade non-Hodgkin's lymphoma. *J Clin Oncol.* 2005;23(15):3383-3389.

Bendamustine-Rituximab (Waldenstrom Macroglobulinemia)

Index Terms BR (Waldenstrom Macroglobulinemia); Rituximab-Bendamustine (Waldenstrom Macroglobulinemia)

Use Waldenstrom macroglobulinemia

Regimen NOTE: Multiple variations are listed.

Variation 1:
Rituximab: IV: 375 mg/m² day 1 or day 2
[total dose/cycle = 375 mg/m²]
Bendamustine: IV: 90 mg/m²/day days 1 and 2
[total dose/cycle = 180 mg/m²]
Repeat cycle every 28 days for 6 cycles

Variation 2:
Rituximab: IV: 375 mg/m²/day days 1, 7, 35, 63, 91, 120
[total dose = 2250 mg/m²]
Bendamustine: IV: 90 mg/m²/day over 30 minutes days 8 and 9, 36 and 37, 64 and 65, and 92 and 93
[total dose = 720 mg/m²]

References

Variation 1:

Treon SP, Hanzis C, Tripsas C, et al. Bendamustine therapy in patients with relapsed or refractory Waldenström's macroglobulinemia. *Clin Lymphoma Myeloma Leuk.* 2011; 11(1):133-135.

Variation 2:

Rummel MJ, Al-Batran SE, Kim SZ, et al. Bendamustine plus rituximab is effective and has a favorable toxicity profile in the treatment of mantle cell and low-grade non-Hodgkin's lymphoma. *J Clin Oncol.* 2005;23(15):3383-3389.

BEP (Ovarian)

Index Terms Bleomycin-Etoposide-Cisplatin (Ovarian)

Use Ovarian cancer (germ cell tumors)

Regimen

Bleomycin: IV: 30 units once weekly
[total dose/cycle = 90 units]
Etoposide: IV: 100 mg/m²/day days 1 to 5
[total dose/cycle = 500 mg/m²]

Cisplatin: IV: 20 mg/m^2/day days 1 to 5
[total dose/cycle = 100 mg/m^2]
Repeat cycle every 21 days for 3 cycles

References

Williams S, Blessing JA, Liao SY, Ball H, Hanjani P. Adjuvant therapy of ovarian germ cell tumors with cisplatin, etoposide, and bleomycin: a trial of the Gynecologic Oncology Group. *J Clin Oncol.* 1994;12(4):701-706.

BEP (Testicular)

Index Terms Bleomycin-Etoposide-Cisplatin (Testicular)

Use Testicular cancer

Regimen NOTE: Multiple variations are listed.

Variation 1 (good risk):

Bleomycin: IV: 30 units/day days 1, 8, and 15
[total dose/cycle = 90 units]
Etoposide: IV: 100 mg/m^2/day days 1 to 5
[total dose/cycle = 500 mg/m^2]
Cisplatin: IV: 20 mg/m^2/day days 1 to 5
[total dose/cycle = 100 mg/m^2]
Repeat cycle every 21 days for 3 cycles

Variation 2 (intermediate/poor risk):

Bleomycin: IV: 30 units/day days 1, 8, and 15
[total dose/cycle = 90 units]
Etoposide: IV: 100 mg/m^2/day days 1 to 5
[total dose/cycle = 500 mg/m^2]
Cisplatin: IV: 20 mg/m^2/day days 1 to 5
[total dose/cycle = 100 mg/m^2]
Repeat cycle every 21 days for 4 cycles

References

Variation 1:

Einhorn LH, Williams SD, Loehrer PJ, Birch R, Drasga R, Omura G, et al. Evaluation of optimal duration of chemotherapy in favorable-prognosis disseminated germ cell tumors: a Southeastern Cancer Study Group protocol. *J Clin Oncol.* 1989;7(3):387-391.

Garcia-del-Muro X, Maroto P, Gumà J, et al. Chemotherapy as an alternative to radiotherapy in the treatment of stage IIA and IIB testicular seminoma: a Spanish Germ Cell Cancer Group Study. *J Clin Oncol.* 2008;26(33):5416-5421.

Saxman SB, Finch D, Gonin R, Einhorn LH. Long-term follow-up of a phase III study of three versus four cycles of bleomycin, etoposide, and cisplatin in favorable-prognosis germ-cell tumors: the Indian University experience. *J Clin Oncol.* 1998;16(2):702-706.

Variation 2:

Culine S, Kramar A, Théodore C, et al. Randomized trial comparing bleomycin/etoposide/cisplatin with alternating cisplatin/cyclophosphamide/doxorubicin and vinblastine/bleomycin regimens of chemotherapy for patients with intermediate- and poor-risk metastatic nonseminomatous germ cell tumors: Genito-Urinary Group of the French Federation of Cancer Centers Trial T93MP. *J Clin Oncol.* 2008;26(3):421-427.

Nichols CR, Catalano PJ, Crawford ED, Vogelzang NJ, Einhorn LH, Loehrer PJ. Randomized comparison of cisplatin and etoposide and either bleomycin or ifosfamide in treatment of advanced disseminated germ cell tumors: an Eastern Cooperative Oncology Group, Southwest Oncology Group, and Cancer and Leukemia Group B Study. *J Clin Oncol.* 1998;16(4):1287-1293.

Bevacizumab (Angiosarcoma Regimen)

Use Soft Tissue Sarcoma (Angiosarcoma)

Regimen

Bevacizumab: IV: 15 mg/kg day 1
[total dose/cycle = 15 mg/kg]
Repeat cycle every 21 days until disease progression or unacceptable toxicity

References

Agulnik M, Yarber JL, Okuno SH, et al. An open-label, multicenter, phase II study of bevacizumab for the treatment of angiosarcoma and epithelioid hemangioendotheliomas. *Ann Oncol.* 2013;24 (1):257-263.

Bevacizumab-Carboplatin-Gemcitabine (Ovarian)

Index Terms Bevacizumab-Gemcitabine-Carboplatin (Ovarian); Carboplatin-Gemcitabine-Bevacizumab (Ovarian); GC-Bevacizumab (Ovarian)

Use Ovarian cancer

Regimen

Bevacizumab: IV: 15 mg/kg day 1

[total dose/cycle = 15 mg/kg]

Gemcitabine: IV: 1000 mg/m^2/day days 1 and 8

[total dose/cycle = 2000 mg/m^2]

Carboplatin: IV: AUC 4 day 1

[total dose/cycle = AUC = 4]

Repeat cycle every 21 days for 6-10 cycles

followed by

Bevacizumab: IV: 15 mg/kg day 1

[total dose/cycle = 15 mg/kg]

Repeat cycle every 21 days until disease progression or unacceptable toxicity

References

Aghajanian C, Blank SV, Goff BA, et al, "OCEANS: A Randomized, Double-Blind, Placebo-Controlled Phase III Trial of Chemotherapy With or Without Bevacizumab in Patients With Platinum-Sensitive Recurrent Epithelial Ovarian, Primary Peritoneal, or Fallopian Tube Cancer," *J Clin Oncol,* 2012, 30(17):2039-45.

Bevacizumab-Carboplatin-Paclitaxel (NSCLC)

Index Terms Bevacizumab-Paclitaxel-Carboplatin (NSCLC); Carboplatin-Paclitaxel-Bevacizumab (NSCLC)

Use Lung cancer, non-small cell (nonsquamous cell histology)

Regimen

Paclitaxel: IV: 200 mg/m^2 day 1

[total dose/cycle = 200 mg/m^2]

Carboplatin: IV: AUC 6 day 1

[total dose/cycle = AUC = 6]

Bevacizumab: IV: 15 mg/kg day 1

[total dose/cycle = 15 mg/kg]

Repeat cycle every 21 days for 6 cycles

followed by

Bevacizumab: IV: 15 mg/kg day 1

[total dose/cycle = 15 mg/kg]

Repeat cycle every 21 days until disease progression or unacceptable toxicity

References

Sandler A, Gray R, Perry MC, et al, "Paclitaxel-Carboplatin Alone or With Bevacizumab for Nonsmall-Cell Lung Cancer," *N Engl J Med,* 2006, 355(24):2542-50.

Bevacizumab-Carboplatin-Pemetrexed (NSCLC)

Index Terms Carboplatin-Pemetrexed-Bevacizumab (NSCLC); Pemetrexed-Carboplatin-Bevacizumab (NSCLC)

Use Lung cancer, non-small cell

◀ **Regimen**

Pemetrexed: IV: 500 mg/m^2 over 10 minutes day 1
[total dose/cycle = 500 mg/m^2]
Carboplatin: IV: AUC 6 day 1
[total dose/cycle = AUC = 6]
Bevacizumab: IV: 15 mg/kg day 1
[total dose/cycle = 15 mg/kg]
Repeat cycle every 21 days for 6 cycles

followed by

Pemetrexed: IV: 500 mg/m^2 over 10 minutes day 1
[total dose/cycle = 500 mg/m^2]
Bevacizumab: IV: 15 mg/kg day 1
[total dose/cycle = 15 mg/kg]
Repeat cycle every 21 days until disease progression or unacceptable toxicity

References

Patel JD, Hensing TA, Rademaker A, et al, "Phase II Study of Pemetrexed and Carboplatin Plus Bevacizumab With Maintenance Pemetrexed and Bevacizumab as First-Line Therapy for Non-squamous Non-Small-Cell Lung Cancer," *J Clin Oncol*, 2009, 27(20):3284-9.

Bevacizumab (Cervical Regimen)

Use Cervical cancer

Regimen

Bevacizumab: IV: 15 mg/kg day 1
[total dose/cycle = 15 mg/kg]
Repeat cycle every 21 days until disease progression or unacceptable toxicity

References

Monk BJ, Sill MW, Burger RA, Gray HJ, Buekers TE, Roman LD. Phase II trial of bevacizumab in the treatment of persistent or recurrent squamous cell carcinoma of the cervix: a gynecologic oncology group study. *J Clin Oncol*. 2009;27(7):1069-1074.

Bevacizumab-Cisplatin-Gemcitabine (NSCLC)

Index Terms Cisplatin-Gemcitabine-Bevacizumab (NSCLC)

Use Lung cancer, non-small cell

Regimen

Cisplatin: IV: 80 mg/m^2 day 1
[total dose/cycle = 80 mg/m^2]
Gemcitabine: IV: 1250 mg/m^2/day days 1 and 8
[total dose/cycle = 2500 mg/m^2]
Bevacizumab: IV: 7.5 or 15 mg/kg day 1
[total dose/cycle = 7.5 or 15 mg/kg]
Repeat cycle every 21 days for up to 6 cycles

followed by

Bevacizumab: IV: 7.5 or 15 mg/kg day 1
[total dose/cycle = 7.5 or 15 mg/kg]
Repeat cycle every 21 days until disease progression or unacceptable toxicity

References

Reck M, von Pawel J, Zatloukal P, et al, "Overall Survival With Cisplatin-Gemcitabine and Bevacizumab or Placebo as First-Line Therapy for Nonsquamous Non-Small-Cell Lung Cancer: Results From a Randomised Phase III Trial AVAiL," *Ann Oncol*, 2010, 21(9):1804-9.

Reck M, von Pawel J, Zatloukal P, et al, "Phase III Trial of Cisplatin Plus Gemcitabine With Either Placebo or Bevacizumab as First-Line Therapy for Nonsquamous Non-Small-Cell Lung Cancer: AVAiL," *J Clin Oncol*, 2009, 27(8):1227-34.

Bevacizumab-Cisplatin-Paclitaxel (Cervical)

Index Terms Bevacizumab-Paclitaxel-Cisplatin (Cervical); Cisplatin-Paclitaxel-Bevacizumab (Cervical)

Use Cervical cancer

Regimen

Bevacizumab: IV: 15 mg/kg day 1
[total dose/cycle = 15 mg/kg]
Paclitaxel: IV: 135-175 mg/m^2 day 1
[total dose/cycle = 135-175 mg/m^2]
Cisplatin: IV: 50 mg/m^2 day 1
[total dose/cycle = 50 mg/m^2]

Repeat cycle every 21 days until disease progression or unacceptable toxicity

References

Tewari KS, Sill MW, Long HJ 3rd, et al. Improved survival with bevacizumab in advanced cervical cancer. *N Engl J Med.* 2014;370(8):734-743.

◆ **Bevacizumab-Doxil (Ovarian)** *see* Bevacizumab-Doxorubicin (Liposomal) (Ovarian) *on page 1841*

Bevacizumab-Doxorubicin (Liposomal) (Ovarian)

Index Terms Bevacizumab-Doxil (Ovarian); Doxorubicin (Liposomal)-Bevacizumab (Ovarian)

Use Ovarian cancer

Regimen

Bevacizumab: IV: 10 mg/kg days 1 and 15
[total dose/cycle = 20 mg/kg]
Doxorubicin (liposomal): IV: 40 mg/m^2 day 1
[total dose/cycle = 40 mg/m^2]

Repeat cycle every 28 days until disease progression or unacceptable toxicity

References

Pujade-Lauraine E, Hilpert F, Weber B, et al. Bevacizumab combined with chemotherapy for platinum-resistant recurrent ovarian cancer: the AURELIA open-label randomized phase III trial. *J Clin Oncol.* 2014;32(13):1302-1308.

Bevacizumab (Endometrial Regimen)

Use Endometrial cancer

Regimen

Bevacizumab: IV: 15 mg/kg day 1
[total dose/cycle = 15 mg/kg]

Repeat cycle every 21 days until disease progression or unacceptable toxicity

References

Aghajanian C, Sill MW, Darcy KM, et al. Phase II trial of bevacizumab in recurrent or persistent endometrial cancer: a Gynecologic Oncology Group study. *J Clin Oncol.* 2011;29(16):2259-2265.

Bevacizumab-Fluorouracil-Leucovorin (Colorectal)

Index Terms Fluorouracil-Leucovorin-Bevacizumab (Colorectal)

Use Colorectal cancer (metastatic)

Regimen

Bevacizumab: IV: 5 mg/kg/day days 1, 15, 29, and 43
[total dose/cycle = 20 mg/kg]
Leucovorin: IV: 500 mg/m^2/day over 2 hours days 1, 8, 15, 22, 29, and 36
[total dose/cycle = 3,000 mg/m^2]

◀ Fluorouracil: IV bolus: 500 mg/m^2/day days 1, 8, 15, 22, 29, and 36 (administer midway through leucovorin infusion)

[total dose/cycle = 3,000 mg/m^2]

Repeat cycle every 56 days through 96 weeks or until disease progression (bevacizumab monotherapy may continue after confirmed complete response or unacceptable toxicity to fluorouracil/leucovorin)

References

Kabbinavar FF, Schulz J, McCleod M, et al. Addition of bevacizumab to bolus fluorouracil and leucovorin in first-line metastatic colorectal cancer: results of a randomized phase II trial. *J Clin Oncol.* 2005;23(16):3697-3705.

Bevacizumab + FOLFIRI (Colorectal)

Index Terms Bevacizumab, Irinotecan, Leucovorin, Fluorouracil (Colorectal)

Use Colorectal cancer

Regimen

Bevacizumab: IV: 5 mg/kg day 1

[total dose/cycle = 5 mg/kg]

Irinotecan: IV: 180 mg/m^2 over 90 minutes day 1

[total dose/cycle = 180 mg/m^2]

Leucovorin: IV: 400 mg/m^2 over 2 hours day 1

[total dose/cycle = 400 mg/m^2]

Fluorouracil: IV bolus: 400 mg/m^2 day 1

followed by IV: 2400 mg/m^2 continuous infusion (CI) over 46 hours beginning day 1

[total fluorouracil dose/cycle (bolus and CI) = 2800 mg/m^2]

Repeat cycle every 14 days until disease progression or unacceptable toxicity

References

Fuchs CS, Marshall J, Mitchell E, et al, "Randomized, Controlled Trial of Irinotecan Plus Infusional, Bolus, or Oral Fluoropyrimidines in First-Line Treatment of Metastatic Colorectal Cancer: Results From the BICC-C Study," *J Clin Oncol,* 2007, 25(30):4779-86.

Bevacizumab FOLFOX (Colorectal)

Index Terms Bevacizumab-Oxaliplatin-Leucovorin-Fluorouracil (Colorectal); Oxaliplatin-Fluorouracil-Leucovorin-Bevacizumab (Colorectal)

Use Colorectal cancer

Regimen NOTE: Multiple variations are listed below.

Variation 1:

Bevacizumab: IV: 5 mg/kg day 1

[total dose/cycle = 5 mg/kg]

Oxaliplatin: IV: 85 mg/m^2 over 2 hours day 1

[total dose/cycle = 85 mg/m^2]

Leucovorin: IV: 350 mg over 2 hours day 1

[total dose/cycle = 350 mg]

Fluorouracil: IV bolus: 400 mg/m^2 day 1

followed by IV: 2400 mg/m^2 continuous infusion over 46 hours beginning day 1

[total dose/cycle (bolus and continuous infusion) = 2800 mg/m^2]

Repeat cycle every 14 days until disease progression or unacceptable toxicity

Variation 2:

Bevacizumab: IV: 5 mg/kg over 30 to 90 minutes day 1

[total dose/cycle = 5 mg/kg]

Oxaliplatin: IV: 85 mg/m^2 over 2 hours day 1

[total dose/cycle = 85 mg/m^2]

Leucovorin: IV: 200 mg/m^2/day over 2 hours days 1 and 2

[total dose/cycle = 400 mg/m^2]

Fluorouracil: IV bolus: 400 mg/m^2/day days 1 and 2

followed by IV: 600 mg/m^2/day continuous infusion over 22 hours days 1 and 2

[total dose/cycle (bolus and continuous infusion) = 2000 mg/m^2]

Repeat cycle every 14 days; up to a maximum of 24 cycles

Variation 3:

Bevacizumab: IV: 10 mg/kg over 30 to 90 minutes day 1

[total dose/cycle = 10 mg/kg]

Oxaliplatin: IV: 85 mg/m^2 over 2 hours day 1

[total dose/cycle = 85 mg/m^2]

Leucovorin: IV: 200 mg/m^2/day over 2 hours days 1 and 2

[total dose/cycle = 400 mg/m^2]

Fluorouracil: IV bolus: 400 mg/m^2/day days 1 and 2

followed by IV: 600 mg/m^2/day continuous infusion over 22 hours days 1 and 2

[total dose/cycle (bolus and continuous infusion) = 2000 mg/m^2]

Repeat cycle every 14 days

References

Variation 1:

Hochster HS, Hart LL, Ramanathan RK, et al. Safety and efficacy of oxaliplatin and fluoropyrimidine regimens with or without bevacizumab as first-line treatment of metastatic colorectal cancer: results of the TREE Study. *J Clin Oncol*. 2008;26(21):3523-3529.

Variation 2:

Saltz LB, Clarke S, Díaz-Rubio E, et al. Bevacizumab in combination with oxaliplatin-based chemotherapy as first-line therapy in metastatic colorectal cancer: a randomized phase III study. *J Clin Oncol*. 2008;26(12):2013-2019.

Variation 3:

Giantonio BJ, Catalano PJ, Meropol NJ, et al. Bevacizumab in combination with oxaliplatin, fluorouracil, and leucovorin (FOLFOX4) for previously treated metastatic colorectal cancer: results from the Eastern Cooperative Oncology Group Study E3200. *J Clin Oncol*. 2007; 25 (12):1539-1544.

◆ **Bevacizumab-Gemcitabine-Carboplatin (Ovarian)** see Bevacizumab-Carboplatin-Gemcitabine (Ovarian) on page 1839

Bevacizumab (Glioblastoma Regimen)

Use Brain tumors (glioblastoma)

Regimen

Bevacizumab: IV: 10 mg/kg day 1

[total dose/cycle = 10 mg/kg]

Repeat cycle every 14 days until disease progression or unacceptable toxicity

References

Friedman HS, Prados MD, Wen PY, et al. Bevacizumab alone and in combination with irinotecan in recurrent glioblastoma. *J Clin Oncol*. 2009;27(28):4733-4740.

◆ **Bevacizumab-Interferon Alfa 2b (RCC)** see Bevacizumab-Interferon Alfa (RCC) on page 1844

Bevacizumab-Interferon Alfa (RCC)

Index Terms Bevacizumab-Interferon Alfa 2b (RCC); Interferon Alfa 2b-Bevacizumab (RCC); Interferon Alfa-Bevacizumab (RCC)

Use Renal cell cancer

Regimen

Interferon Alfa-2b: SubQ: 9 million units on 3 nonconsecutive days per week
[total dose/cycle = 108 million units]

Bevacizumab: IV: 10 mg/kg days 1 and 15
[total dose/cycle = 20 mg/kg]

Repeat cycle every 28 days until disease progression or unacceptable toxicity

References

Rini BI, Halabi S, Rosenberg JE, et al, "Bevacizumab Plus Interferon Alfa Compared With Interferon Alfa Monotherapy in Patients With Metastatic Renal Cell Carcinoma: CALGB 90206," *J Clin Oncol*, 2008, 26(33):5422-8.

Rini BI, Halabi S, Rosenberg JE, et al, "Phase III Trial of Bevacizumab Plus Interferon Alfa Versus Interferon Alfa Monotherapy in Patients With Metastatic Renal Cell Carcinoma: Final Results of CALGB 90206," *J Clin Oncol*, 2010, 28(13):2137-43.

Bevacizumab-Irinotecan (Glioblastoma)

Index Terms Irinotecan-Bevacizumab (Glioblastoma)

Use Brain tumors

Regimen NOTE: Patients receiving concurrent antiepileptic enzyme-inducing drugs received an increased dose of irinotecan (340 mg/m^2/dose).

Bevacizumab: IV: 10 mg/kg day 1
[total dose/cycle = 10 mg/kg]

Irinotecan: IV: 125 mg/m^2 day 1
[total dose/cycle = 125 mg/m^2]

Repeat cycle every 14 days

References

Vredenburgh JJ, Desjardins A, Herndon JE 2nd, et al, "Bevacizumab Plus Irinotecan in Recurrent Glioblastoma Multiforme," *J Clin Oncol*, 2007, 25(30):4722-9.

♦ **Bevacizumab, Irinotecan, Leucovorin, Fluorouracil (Colorectal)** *see* Bevacizumab + FOLFIRI (Colorectal) *on page 1842*

♦ **Bevacizumab-Oxaliplatin-Leucovorin-Fluorouracil (Colorectal)** *see* Bevacizumab FOLFOX (Colorectal) *on page 1842*

Bevacizumab-Paclitaxel (Breast)

Index Terms Paclitaxel-Bevacizumab (Breast)

Use Breast cancer

Regimen

Paclitaxel: IV: 90 mg/m^2/day days 1, 8, and 15
[total dose/cycle = 270 mg/m^2]

Bevacizumab: IV: 10 mg/kg/day days 1 and 15
[total dose/cycle = 20 mg/kg]

Repeat cycle every 28 days until disease progression or unacceptable toxicity

References

Brufsky AM, Hurvitz S, Perez E, et al, "RIBBON-2 A Randomized, Double-Blind, Placebo-Controlled, Phase III Trial Evaluating the Efficacy and Safety of Bevacizumab in Combination With Chemotherapy for Second-Line Treatment of Human Epidermal Growth Factor 2-Negative Metastatic Breast Cancer," *J Clin Oncol*, 2011, 29(32):4286-93.

Miller K, Wang M, Gralow J, et al, "Paclitaxel Plus Bevacizumab Versus Paclitaxel Alone for Metastatic Breast Cancer," *N Engl J Med*, 2007, 357(26):2666-76.

◆ **Bevacizumab-Paclitaxel-Carboplatin (NSCLC)** *see* Bevacizumab-Carboplatin-Paclitaxel (NSCLC) *on page 1839*

◆ **Bevacizumab-Paclitaxel-Cisplatin (Cervical)** *see* Bevacizumab-Cisplatin-Paclitaxel (Cervical) *on page 1841*

Bevacizumab-Paclitaxel (Ovarian)

Index Terms Paclitaxel-Bevacizumab (Ovarian)

Use Ovarian cancer

Regimen

Bevacizumab: IV: 10 mg/kg days 1 and 15

[total dose/cycle = 20 mg/kg]

Paclitaxel: IV: 80 mg/m^2/day days 1, 8, 15, and 22

[total dose/cycle = 320 mg/m^2]

Repeat cycle every 28 days until disease progression or unacceptable toxicity

References

Pujade-Lauraine E, Hilpert F, Weber B, et al. Bevacizumab combined with chemotherapy for platinum-resistant recurrent ovarian cancer: the AURELIA open-label randomized phase III trial. *J Clin Oncol.* 2014;32(13):1302-1308.

Bevacizumab-Paclitaxel-Topotecan (Cervical)

Index Terms Bevacizumab-Topotecan-Paclitaxel (Cervical); Paclitaxel-Topotecan-Bevacizumab (Cervical)

Use Cervical cancer

Regimen

Bevacizumab: IV: 15 mg/kg day 1

[total dose/cycle = 15 mg/kg]

Topotecan: IV: 0.75 mg/m^2 days 1 to 3

[total dose/cycle = 2.25 mg/m^2]

Paclitaxel: IV: 175 mg/m^2 day 1

[total dose/cycle = 175 mg/m^2]

Repeat cycle every 21 days until disease progression or unacceptable toxicity

References

Tewari KS, Sill MW, Long HJ 3rd, et al. Improved survival with bevacizumab in advanced cervical cancer. *N Engl J Med.* 2014;370(8):734-743.

Bevacizumab (RCC Regimen)

Use Renal cell cancer

Regimen

Bevacizumab: IV: 10 mg/kg day 1

[total dose/cycle = 10 mg/kg]

Repeat cycle every 14 days until disease progression or unacceptable toxicity

References

Yang JC, Haworth L, Sherry RM, et al. "A Randomized Trial of Bevacizumab, an Anti-Vascular Endothelial Growth Factor Antibody, for Metastatic Renal Cancer," *N Engl J Med*, 2003, 349 (5):427-34.

Bevacizumab-Topotecan Daily (Ovarian)

Index Terms Topotecan Daily-Bevacizumab (Ovarian)

Use Ovarian cancer

Regimen
Bevacizumab: IV: 15 mg/kg day 1
[total dose/cycle = 15 mg/kg]
Topotecan: IV: 1.25 mg/m^2/day days 1, 2, 3, 4, and 5
[total dose/cycle = 6.25 mg/m^2]
Repeat cycle every 21 days until disease progression or unacceptable toxicity

References
Pujade-Lauraine E, Hilpert F, Weber B, et al. Bevacizumab combined with chemotherapy for platinum-resistant recurrent ovarian cancer: the AURELIA open-label randomized phase III trial. *J Clin Oncol.* 2014;32(13):1302-1308.

◆ **Bevacizumab-Topotecan-Paclitaxel (Cervical)** *see* Bevacizumab-Paclitaxel-Topotecan (Cervical) *on page 1845*

Bevacizumab-Topotecan Weekly (Ovarian)

Index Terms Topotecan Weekly-Bevacizumab (Ovarian)
Use Ovarian cancer
Regimen
Bevacizumab: IV: 10 mg/kg days 1 and 15
[total dose/cycle = 20 mg/kg]
Topotecan: IV: 4 mg/m^2/day days 1, 8, and 15
[total dose/cycle = 12 mg/m^2]
Repeat cycle every 28 days until disease progression or unacceptable toxicity

References
Pujade-Lauraine E, Hilpert F, Weber B, et al. Bevacizumab combined with chemotherapy for platinum-resistant recurrent ovarian cancer: the AURELIA open-label randomized phase III trial. *J Clin Oncol.* 2014;32(13):1302-1308.

Bevacizumab + XELOX (Colorectal)

Index Terms Bevacizumb-Capecitabine-Oxaliplatin (Colorectal Cancer); Bevacizumb-CapeOx (Colorectal Cancer); Bevacizumb-CAPOX (Colorectal Cancer); Bevacizumb-Oxaliplatin-Capecitabine (Colorectal Cancer)
Use Colorectal cancer
Regimen NOTE: Multiple variations are listed.
Variation 1:
Bevacizumab: IV: 7.5 mg/kg day 1
[total dose/cycle = 7.5 mg/kg]
Oxaliplatin: IV: 130 mg/m^2 day 1
[total dose/cycle = 130 mg/m^2]
Capecitabine: Oral: 850 mg/m^2 twice daily days 1 (beginning with evening dose) to 15 (ending with morning dose)
[total dose/cycle = 23,800 mg/m^2]
Repeat cycle every 21 days
Variation 2:
Bevacizumab: IV: 7.5 mg/kg over 30-90 minutes day 1
[total dose/cycle = 7.5 mg/kg]
Oxaliplatin: IV: 130 mg/m^2 over 2 hours day 1
[total dose/cycle = 130 mg/m^2]
Capecitabine: Oral: 1000 mg/m^2 twice daily days 1 to 14
[total dose/cycle = 28,000 mg/m^2]
Repeat cycle every 21 days

References
Variation 1:

Hochster HS, Hart LL, Ramanathan RK, et al, "Safety and Efficacy of Oxaliplatin and Fluoropyr-imidine Regimens With or Without Bevacizumab as First-Line Treatment of Metastatic Colorectal Cancer: Results of the TREE Study," *J Clin Oncol*, 2008, 26(21):3523-9.

Variation 2:

Saltz LB, Clarke S, Díaz-Rubio E, et al, "Bevacizumab in Combination With Oxaliplatin-Based Chemotherapy as First-Line Therapy in Metastatic Colorectal Cancer: A Randomized Phase III Study," *J Clin Oncol*, 2008, 26(12):2013-9.

◆ **Bevacizumb-Capecitabine-Oxaliplatin (Colorectal Cancer)** *see* Bevacizumab + XELOX (Colorectal) *on page 1846*

◆ **Bevacizumb-CapeOx (Colorectal Cancer)** *see* Bevacizumab + XELOX (Colorectal) *on page 1846*

◆ **Bevacizumb-CAPOX (Colorectal Cancer)** *see* Bevacizumab + XELOX (Colorectal) *on page 1846*

◆ **Bevacizumb-Oxaliplatin-Capecitabine (Colorectal Cancer)** *see* Bevacizumab + XELOX (Colorectal) *on page 1846*

Bexarotene (NHL-CTCL Regimen)

Use Lymphoma, non-Hodgkin (CTCL)

Regimen

Bexarotene: Oral: 300 mg/m^2/day once daily on days 1 to 28 (may increase to 400 mg/m^2/day)

[total dose/cycle = 8,400-11,200 mg/m^2]

Repeat cycle every 28 days until disease progression or unacceptable toxicity

References

Duvic M, Hymes K, Heald P, et al. Bexarotene is effective and safe for treatment of refractory advanced-stage cutaneous T-cell lymphoma: multinational phase II-III trial results. *J Clin Oncol*. 2001;19(9):2456-2471.

◆ **Biweekly Cetlri (Colorectal)** *see* Cetuximab (Biweekly)-Irinotecan (Colorectal) *on page 1879*

◆ **Biweekly Cetuximab (Colorectal Regimen)** *see* Cetuximab Biweekly (Colorectal Regimen) *on page 1879*

◆ **BLD (Multiple Myeloma)** *see* Bendamustine-Lenalidomide-Dexamethasone (Multiple Myeloma) *on page 1834*

◆ **Bleomycin-Etoposide-Cisplatin (Ovarian)** *see* BEP (Ovarian) *on page 1837*

◆ **Bleomycin, Etoposide, Doxorubicin, Cyclophosphamide, Vincristine, Procarbazine, Prednisone (Hodgkin)** *see* BEACOPP-14 (Hodgkin) *on page 1829*

◆ **Bleomycin, Etoposide, Doxorubicin, Cyclophosphamide, Vincristine, Procarbazine, Prednisone (Hodgkin)** *see* BEACOPP Escalated (Hodgkin) *on page 1830*

◆ **Bleomycin, Etoposide, Doxorubicin, Cyclophosphamide, Vincristine, Procarbazine, Prednisone (Hodgkin)** *see* BEACOPP Escalated Plus Standard (Hodgkin) *on page 1830*

◆ **Bleomycin, Etoposide, Doxorubicin, Cyclophosphamide, Vincristine, Procarbazine, Prednisone (Hodgkin)** *see* BEACOPP Standard (Hodgkin) *on page 1832*

◆ **Bleomycin-Etoposide-Cisplatin (Testicular)** *see* BEP (Testicular) *on page 1838*

◆ **Bortezomib-Bendamustine-Rituximab (NHL-Follicular)** *see* Bendamustine-Bortezomib-Rituximab (NHL-Follicular) *on page 1833*

Bortezomib-Dexamethasone (Amyloidosis)

Index Terms Dexamethasone-Bortezomib (Amyloidosis)

Use Systemic light chain amyloidosis

Regimen

Bortezomib: IV: 1.3 mg/m^2/dose days 1, 4, 8, and 11
  [total dose/cycle = 5.2 mg/m^2]
Dexamethasone: Oral: 40 mg/day days 1 to 4
  [total dose/cycle = 160 mg]
Repeat cycle every 21 days

References

Kastritis E, Wechalekar AD, Dimopoulos MA, et al, "Bortezomib With or Without Dexamethasone in Primary Systemic (Light Chain) Amyloidosis," *J Clin Oncol*, 2010, 28(6):1031-7.

Bortezomib-Dexamethasone (Multiple Myeloma)

Index Terms Dexamethasone-Bortezomib (Multiple Myeloma); VD (Multiple Myeloma)

Use Multiple myeloma

Regimen

Cycles 1 and 2:
  Bortezomib: IV: 1.3 mg/m^2/day days 1, 4, 8, and 11
    [total dose/cycle = 5.2 mg/m^2]
  Dexamethasone: Oral: 40 mg/day days 1 to 4 and days 9 to 12
    [total dose/cycle = 320 mg]
  Repeat cycle every 21 days for cycles 1 and 2
Cycles 3 and 4:
  Bortezomib: IV: 1.3 mg/m^2/day days 1, 4, 8, and 11
    [total dose/cycle = 5.2 mg/m^2]
  Dexamethasone: Oral: 40 mg/day days 1 to 4
    [total dose/cycle = 160 mg]
  Repeat cycle every 21 days for cycles 3 and 4

References

Harousseau JL, Attal M, Avet-Loiseau H, et al. Bortezomib plus dexamethasone is superior to vincristine plus doxorubicin plus dexamethasone as induction treatment prior to autologous stem-cell transplantation in newly diagnosed multiple myeloma: results of the IFM 2005-01 phase III trial. *J Clin Oncol*. 2010;28(30):4621-4629.

◆ **Bortezomib-Dexamethasone-Panobinostat (Multiple Myeloma)** *see* Panobinostat-Bortezomib-Dexamethasone (Multiple Myeloma) *on page 2059*

Bortezomib-Dexamethasone-Rituximab (Waldenstrom Macroglobulinemia)

Index Terms BDR (Waldenstrom Macroglobulinemia)

Use Waldenstrom Macroglobulinemia

Regimen

Bortezomib: IV: 1.3 mg/m^2 days 1, 4, 8, and 11
  [total dose/cycle = 5.2 mg/m^2]
Dexamethasone: IV: 40 mg days 1, 4, 8, and 11
  [total dose/cycle = 160 mg]

Rituximab: IV: 375 mg/m^2 day 11
[total dose/cycle = 375 mg/m^2]
Repeat cycle every 21 days for 4 cycles, followed by a 12 week interruption, then repeat cycle every 12 weeks for 4 cycles

References

Treon SP, Ioakimidis L, Soumerai JD, et al, "Primary Treatment of Waldenstrom Macroglobulinemia With Bortezomib, Dexamethasone, and Rituximab: WMCTG Clinical Trial 05-180," *J Clin Oncol*, 2009, 27(23):3830-5.

Bortezomib-Doxorubicin-Dexamethasone (Multiple Myeloma)

Index Terms Dexamethasone-Bortezomib-Doxorubicin (Multiple Myeloma); Doxorubicin-Dexamethasone-Bortezomib (Multiple Myeloma); PAD (Multiple Myeloma)

Use Multiple myeloma (first-line)

Regimen

Induction:
Bortezomib: IV: 1.3 mg/m^2/day days 1, 4, 8, and 11
[total dose/cycle = 5.2 mg/m^2]
Doxorubicin: IV: 9 mg/m^2/day days 1 to 4
[total dose/cycle = 36 mg/m^2]
Dexamethasone: Oral: 40 mg/day days 1 to 4, 9 to 12, and 17 to 20
[total dose/cycle = 480 mg]
Repeat cycle every 28 days for 3 cycles, followed by high-dose melphalan and autologous stem-cell transplantation

Maintenance:
Bortezomib: IV: 1.3 mg/m^2/day day 1 (starting 4 weeks after high-dose melphalan)
[total dose/cycle = 1.3 mg/m^2]
Repeat cycle every 14 days for 2 years

References

Sonneveld P, Schmidt-Wolf IG, van der Holt B, et al. Bortezomib induction and maintenance treatment in patients with newly diagnosed multiple myeloma: results of the randomized phase III HOVON-65/ GMMG-HD4 trial. *J Clin Oncol*. 2012;30(24):2946-2955.

Bortezomib-Doxorubicin (Liposomal)

Index Terms Doxorubicin (Liposomal)-Bortezomib

Use Multiple myeloma

Regimen

Bortezomib: IV: 1.3 mg/m^2/day days 1, 4, 8, and 11
[total dose/cycle = 5.2 mg/m^2]
Doxorubicin (liposomal): IV: 30 mg/m^2 day 4
[total dose/cycle = 30 mg/m^2]
Repeat cycle every 21 days for up to 8 cycles

References

Biehn SE, Moore DT, Voorhees PM, et al, "Extended Follow-Up of Outcome Measures in Multiple Myeloma Patients Treated on a Phase I Study With Bortezomib and Pegylated Liposomal Doxorubicin," *Ann Hematol*, 2007, 86(3):211-6.

Orlowski RZ, Nagler A, Sonneveld P, et al, "Randomized Phase III Study of Pegylated Liposomal Doxorubicin Plus Bortezomib Compared With Bortezomib Alone in Relapsed or Refractory Multiple Myeloma: Combination Therapy Improves Time to Progression," *J Clin Oncol*, 2007, 25(25):3892-901.

Orlowski RZ, Voorhees PM, Garcia RA, et al, "Phase 1 Trial of the Proteasome Inhibitor Bortezomib and Pegylated Liposomal Doxorubicin in Patients With Advanced Hematologic Malignancies," *Blood*, 2005, 105(8):3058-65.

Bortezomib-Doxorubicin (Liposomal)-Dexamethasone

Index Terms Dexamethasone-Bortezomib-Doxorubicin (Liposomal); Doxorubicin (Liposomal)-Dexamethasone-Bortezomib

Use Multiple myeloma

Regimen

Bortezomib: IV: 1.3 mg/m^2/day days 1, 4, 8, and 11
[total dose/cycle = 5.2 mg/m^2]
Doxorubicin (Liposomal): IV: 30 mg/m^2 day 1
[total dose/cycle = 30 mg/m^2]
Dexamethasone: Oral: 40 mg/day days 1 to 4
[total dose/cycle = 160 mg]
Repeat cycle every 28 days for up to 6 cycles

References

Palumbo A, Gay F, Bringhen S, et al, "Bortezomib, Doxorubicin and Dexamethasone in Advanced Multiple Myeloma," *Ann Oncol*, 2008, 19(6):1160-5.

◆ **Bortezomib-Lenalidomide-Dexamethasone (Multiple Myeloma)** *see* Lenalidomide-Bortezomib-Dexamethasone (Multiple Myeloma) *on page 2026*

◆ **Bortezomib-Melphalan-Prednisone (Multiple Myeloma)** *see* Melphalan-Prednisone-Bortezomib (Multiple Myeloma) *on page 2033*

Bortezomib-Melphalan-Prednisone-Thalidomide

Index Terms Melphalan-Prednisone-Bortezomib-Thalidomide; VMPT

Use Multiple myeloma

Regimen

Bortezomib: IV: 1-1.3 mg/m^2/day days 1, 4, 15, and 22
[total dose/cycle = 4-5.2 mg/m^2]
Melphalan: Oral: 6 mg/m^2/day days 1 to 5
[total dose/cycle = 30 mg/m^2]
Prednisone: Oral: 60 mg/m^2/day days 1 to 5
[total dose/cycle = 300 mg/m^2]
Thalidomide: Oral: 50 mg/day days 1 to 35
[total dose/cycle = 1750 mg]
Repeat cycle every 35 days for 6 cycles

References

Palumbo A, Ambrosini MT, Benevolo G, et al, "Bortezomib, Melphalan, Prednisone, and Thalidomide for Relapsed Multiple Myeloma," *Blood*, 2007, 109(7):2767-72.

Bortezomib-Rituximab (Waldenstrom Macroglobulinemia)

Index Terms Rituximab-Bortezomib (Waldenstrom Macroglobulinemia)

Use Waldenstrom Macroglobulinemia

Regimen

Bortezomib: IV: 1.6 mg/m^2/day days 1, 8, and 15 (cycles 1 to 6)
[total dose/cycle = 4.8 mg/m^2]
Rituximab: IV: 375 mg/m^2/day days 1, 8, 15, and 22 (cycles 1 and 4 only)
[total dose/cycle (cycles 1 and 4 only) = 1500 mg/m^2]
Repeat cycle every 28 days for a total of 6 cycles; bortezomib administered for all 6 cycles and rituximab administered cycles 1 and 4 only

References

Ghobrial IM, Hong F, Padmanabhan S, et al, "Phase II Trial of Weekly Bortezomib in Combination With Rituximab in Relapsed or Refractory and Refractory Waldenstrom Macroglobulinemia," *J Clin Oncol*, 2010, 28(8):1422-8.

Bortezomib (Waldenstrom Macroglobulinemia)

Use Waldenstrom Macroglobulinemia

Regimen

Bortezomib: IV: 1.3 mg/m^2/day days 1, 4, 8, and 11
[total dose/cycle = 5.2 mg/m^2]
Repeat cycle every 21 days until disease progression or until 2 cycles after a complete response

References

Chen CI, Kouroukis CT, White D, et al, "Bortezomib is Active in Patients With Untreated or Relapsed Waldenstrom's Macroglobulinemia: A Phase II Study of the National Cancer Institute of Canada Clinical Trials Group," *J Clin Oncol*, 2007, 25(12):1570-5.

Bosutinib (CML Regimen)

Use Leukemia, chronic myelogenous

Regimen

Bosutinib: Oral: 500 mg once daily
[total dose/cycle = 14,000 mg]
Repeat cycle every 28 days until disease progression or unacceptable toxicity

References

Cortes JE, Kim, DW, Kantarjian HM, et al, "Bosutinib Versus Imatinib in Newly Diagnosed Chronic-Phase Chronic Myeloid Leukemia: Results From the BELA Trial," *J Clin Oncol*, 2012, 30 (28):3486-92.

Khoury HJ, Cortes JE, Kantarjian HM, et al, "Bosutinib Is Active in Chronic Phase Chronic Myeloid Leukemia After Imatinib and Dasatinib and/or Nilotinib Therapy Failure," *Blood*, 2012, 199 (5):3403-12.

◆ **Botezomib-Rituximab-Cyclophosphamide-Doxorubicin-Prednisone (NHL-Mantle Cell)** *see* VcR-CAP (NHL-Mantle Cell) *on page* 2106

◆ **B-R (CLL)** *see* Bendamustine-Rituximab (CLL) *on page* 1835

Brentuximab (Hodgkin Regimen)

Use Lymphoma, Hodgkin

Regimen NOTE: Multiple variations are listed.

Variation 1 (relapsed/refractory):
Brentuximab: IV: 1.8 mg/kg (maximum dose: 180 mg) over 30 minutes day 1
[total dose/cycle = 1.8 mg/kg (maximum dose/cycle: 180 mg)]
Repeat cycle every 21 days for up to 16 cycles
Variation 2 (maintenance therapy for unfavorable risk, relapsed or primary refractory who had undergone autologous stem-cell transplantation):
Brentuximab: IV: 1.8 mg/kg (maximum dose: 180 mg) over 30 minutes day 1
(start 30 to 45 days after transplantation)
[total dose/cycle = 1.8 mg/kg (maximum dose/cycle: 180 mg)]
Repeat cycle every 21 days for up to 16 cycles

References

Variation 1:
Younes A, Gopal AK, Smith SE, et al. Results of a pivotal phase II study of brentuximab vedotin for patients with relapsed or refractory Hodgkin's lymphoma. *J Clin Oncol*. 2012;30(18):2183-2189.
Variation 2:
Moskowitz CH, Nademanee A, Masszi T, et al. Brentuximab vedotin as consolidation therapy after autologous stem-cell transplantation in patients with Hodgkin's lymphoma at risk of relapse or progression (AETHERA): a randomised, double-blind, placebo-controlled, phase 3 trial. *Lancet*. 2015;385(9980):1853-1862.

◆ **B-R (NHL-Follicular)** *see* Bendamustine-Rituximab (NHL-Follicular) *on page* 1835

◆ **B-R (NHL-Mantle Cell)** *see* Bendamustine-Rituximab (NHL-Mantle Cell) *on page 1836*

◆ **BR (Waldenstrom Macroglobulinemia)** *see* Bendamustine-Rituximab (Waldenstrom Macroglobulinemia) *on page 1837*

Cabazitaxel-Prednisone (Prostate)

Index Terms Prednisone-Cabazitaxel (Prostate)

Use Prostate cancer

Regimen

Cabazitaxel: IV: 25 mg/m^2 over 1 hour day 1
   [total dose/cycle = 25 mg/m^2]
Prednisone: Oral: 10 mg once daily days 1 to 21
   [total dose/cycle = 210 mg]
Repeat cycle every 21 days

References

De Bono JS, Oudard S, Ozguroglu M, et al, "Prednisone Plus Cabazitaxel or Mitoxantrone for Metastatic Castration-Resistant Prostate Cancer Progressing After Docetaxel Treatment: A Randomised Open-Label Trial," *Lancet*, 2010, 376(9747):1147-54.

CAF IV (Breast)

Index Terms Cyclophosphamide, Doxorubicin, Fluorouracil IV (Breast); FAC IV (Breast)

Use Breast cancer

Regimen NOTE: Multiple variations are listed.

Variation 1:
Fluorouracil: IV: 500 mg/m^2/day days 1 and 8
   [total dose/cycle = 1000 mg/m^2]
Doxorubicin: IV: 50 mg/m^2 over 72 hours days 1-3
   [total dose/cycle = 50 mg/m^2]
Cyclophosphamide: IV: 500 mg/m^2 day 1
   [total dose/cycle = 500 mg/m^2]
Repeat cycle every 21-28 days for up to 6 cycles

Variation 2:
Fluorouracil: IV: 500 mg/m^2/day days 1 and 8
   [total dose/cycle = 1000 mg/m^2]
Doxorubicin: IV: 50 mg/m^2 day 1
   [total dose/cycle = 50 mg/m^2]
Cyclophosphamide: IV: 500 mg/m^2 day 1
   [total dose/cycle = 500 mg/m^2]
Repeat cycle every 21 days for up to 9 cycles

References

Variation 1:
Assikis V, Buzdar A, Yang Y, et al, "A Phase III Trial of Sequential Adjuvant Chemotherapy for Operable Breast Carcinoma: Final Analysis With 10-Year Follow-Up," *Cancer*, 2003, 97 (11):2716-23.
Variation 2:
Hortobagyi GN, Gutterman JU, Blumenschein GR, et al, "Combination Chemoimmunotherapy of Metastatic Breast Cancer With 5-Fluorouracil, Adriamycin, Cyclophosphamide, and BCG," *Cancer*, 1979, 43(4):1225-33.

CAF Oral (Breast)

Index Terms Cyclophosphamide, Doxorubicin, Fluorouracil Oral (Breast); FAC Oral (Breast)

Use Breast cancer

Regimen
Cyclophosphamide: Oral: 100 mg/m²/day days 1 to 14
[total dose/cycle = 1400 mg/m²]
Doxorubicin: IV: 30 mg/m²/day days 1 and 8
[total dose/cycle = 60 mg/m²]
Fluorouracil: IV: 500 mg/m²/day days 1 and 8
[total dose/cycle = 1000 mg/m²]
Repeat cycle every 28 days, until a cumulative doxorubicin dose of 450 mg/m² in the metastatic setting (Bull, 1978), and for a total of 6 cycles in the adjuvant setting (Hutchins, 2005)

References
Bull JM, Tormey DC, Li SH, et al, "A Randomized Comparative Trial of Adriamycin® Versus Methotrexate in Combination Drug Therapy," *Cancer*, 1978, 41(5):1649-57.
Hutchins LF, Green SJ, Ravdin PM, et al, "Randomized, Controlled Trial of Cyclophosphamide, Methotrexate, and Fluorouracil Versus Cyclophosphamide, Doxorubicin, and Fluorouracil With and Without Tamoxifen for High-Risk, Node-Negative Breast Cancer: Treatment Results of Intergroup Protocol INT-0102," *J Clin Oncol*, 2005, 23(33):8313-21.

CALGB 8811 Regimen (ALL)
Index Terms Larson 8811 Regimen (ALL); Larson Regimen 8811 (ALL)
Use Leukemia, acute lymphocytic
Regimen
Induction, patients <60 years of age (4-week cycle):
Cyclophosphamide: IV: 1200 mg/m² day 1
[total dose/cycle = 1200 mg/m²]
Daunorubicin: IV: 45 mg/m²/dose days 1, 2, and 3
[total dose/cycle = 135 mg/m²]
Vincristine: IV: 2 mg/dose days 1, 8, 15, and 22
[total dose/cycle = 8 mg]
Prednisone: Oral: 60 mg/m²/dose days 1 to 21
[total dose/cycle = 1260 mg/m²]
Asparaginase *(E. coli)*: SubQ: 6000 units/m²/dose days 5, 8, 11, 15, 18, and 22
[total dose/cycle = 36,000 units/m²]
Induction, patients ≥60 years of age (4-week cycle):
Cyclophosphamide: IV: 800 mg/m² day 1
[total dose/cycle = 800 mg/m²]
Daunorubicin: IV: 30 mg/m²/dose days 1, 2, and 3
[total dose/cycle = 90 mg/m²]
Vincristine: IV: 2 mg/dose days 1, 8, 15, and 22
[total dose/cycle = 8 mg]
Prednisone: Oral: 60 mg/m²/dose days 1 to 7
[total dose/cycle = 420 mg/m²]
Asparaginase *(E. coli)*: SubQ: 6000 units/m²/dose days 5, 8, 11, 15, 18, and 22
[total dose/cycle = 36,000 units/m²]
Early intensification (4-week cycle; repeat cycle once):
Methotrexate: Intrathecal: 15 mg/dose day 1
[total dose/cycle = 15 mg]
Cyclophosphamide: IV: 1000 mg/m² day 1
[total dose/cycle = 1000 mg/m²]
Mercaptopurine: Oral: 60 mg/m²/dose days 1 to 14
[total dose/cycle = 840 mg/m²]

◄ Cytarabine: SubQ: 75 mg/m²/dose days 1 to 4 and 8 to 11
   [total dose/cycle = 600 mg/m²]
Vincristine: IV: 2 mg/dose days 15 and 22
   [total dose/cycle = 4 mg]
Asparaginase *(E. coli)*: SubQ: 6000 units/m²/dose days 15, 18, 22, and 25
   [total dose/cycle = 24,000 units/m²]
CNS prophylaxis/interim maintenance (12-week duration; with cranial irradiation days 1 to 12):
   Methotrexate: Intrathecal: 15 mg/dose days 1, 8, 15, 22, and 29
      [total dose/cycle = 75 mg]
   Mercaptopurine: Oral: 60 mg/m²/dose days 1 to 70
      [total dose/cycle = 4200 mg/m²]
   Methotrexate: Oral: 20 mg/m²/dose days 36, 43, 50, 57, and 64
      [total dose/cycle = 100 mg/m²]
Late intensification (8-week cycle):
   Doxorubicin: IV: 30 mg/m²/dose days 1, 8, and 15
      [total dose/cycle = 90 mg/m²]
   Vincristine: IV: 2 mg/dose days 1, 8, and 15
      [total dose/cycle = 6 mg]
   Dexamethasone: Oral: 10 mg/m²/dose days 1 to 14
      [total dose/cycle = 140 mg/m²]
   Cyclophosphamide: IV: 1000 mg/m² day 29
      [total dose/cycle = 1000 mg/m²]
   Thioguanine: Oral: 60 mg/m²/dose days 29 to 42
      [total dose/cycle = 840 mg/m²]
   Cytarabine: SubQ: 75 mg/m²/dose days 29 to 32 and 36 to 39
      [total dose/cycle = 600 mg/m²]
Maintenance (continue until 24 months from diagnosis):
   Vincristine: IV: 2 mg/dose day 1 every 4 weeks
      [total dose/4 weeks = 2 mg]
   Prednisone: Oral: 60 mg/m²/dose days 1 to 5 every 4 weeks
      [total dose/4 weeks = 300 mg/m²]
   Methotrexate: Oral: 20 mg/m²/dose days 1, 8, 15, and 22
      [total dose/phase = 80 mg/m²]
   Mercaptopurine: Oral: 60 mg/m²/dose days 1 to 28
      [total dose/phase = 1680 mg/m²]
References
Larson RA, Dodge RK, Burns CP, et al. A five-drug remission induction regimen with intensive consolidation for adults with acute lymphoblastic leukemia: Cancer and Leukemia Group B Study 8811. *Blood.* 1995;85(8):2025-2037.

CALGB 9111 Regimen (ALL)
Index Terms Larson 9111 Regimen (ALL); Larson Regimen 9111 (ALL)
Use Leukemia, acute lymphocytic
Regimen
   Induction, patients <60 years of age (4-week cycle):
   Cyclophosphamide: IV: 1200 mg/m² day 1
      [total dose/cycle = 1200 mg/m²]
   Daunorubicin: IV: 45 mg/m²/dose days 1, 2, and 3
      [total dose/cycle = 135 mg/m²]
   Vincristine: IV: 2 mg/dose days 1, 8, 15, and 22
      [total dose/cycle = 8 mg]
   Prednisone: Oral: 60 mg/m²/dose days 1 to 21
      [total dose/cycle = 1260 mg/m²]

Asparaginase *(E. coli)*: SubQ, IM: 6000 units/m²/dose days 5, 8, 11, 15, 18, and 22
[total dose/cycle = 36,000 units/m²]
Filgrastim: SubQ: 5 mcg/kg/day starting day 4; continue for at least 7 days and until ANC ≥1000/mm³ on two draws, 24 hours apart

Induction, patients ≥60 years of age (4-week cycle):
Cyclophosphamide: IV: 800 mg/m² day 1
[total dose/cycle = 800 mg/m²]
Daunorubicin: IV: 30 mg/m²/dose days 1, 2, and 3
[total dose/cycle = 90 mg/m²]
Vincristine: IV: 2 mg/dose days 1, 8, 15, and 22
[total dose/cycle = 8 mg]
Prednisone: Oral: 60 mg/m²/dose days 1 to 7
[total dose/cycle = 420 mg/m²]
Asparaginase *(E. coli)*: SubQ, IM: 6000 units/m²/dose days 5, 8, 11, 15, 18, and 22
[total dose/cycle = 36,000 units/m²]
Filgrastim: SubQ: 5 mcg/kg/day starting day 4; continue for at least 7 days and until ANC ≥1000/mm³ on two draws, 24 hours apart

Early intensification (4-week cycle; repeat cycle once):
Methotrexate: Intrathecal: 15 mg/dose day 1
[total dose/cycle = 15 mg]
Cyclophosphamide: IV: 1000 mg/m² day 1
[total dose/cycle = 1000 mg/m²]
Mercaptopurine: Oral: 60 mg/m²/dose days 1 to 14
[total dose/cycle = 840 mg/m²]
Cytarabine: SubQ: 75 mg/m²/dose days 1 to 4 and 8 to 11
[total dose/cycle = 600 mg/m²]
Vincristine: IV: 2 mg/dose days 15 and 22
[total dose/cycle = 4 mg]
Asparaginase *(E. coli)*: SubQ, IM: 6000 units/m²/dose days 15, 18, 22, and 25
[total dose/cycle = 24,000 units/m²]
Filgrastim: SubQ: 5 mcg/kg/day starting day 2; continue at least 14 days and until ANC ≥5000/mm³ on two draws, 24 hours apart

CNS prophylaxis/interim maintenance (12-week duration; with cranial irradiation days 1 to 12):
Methotrexate: Intrathecal: 15 mg/dose days 1, 8, 15, 22, and 29
[total dose/cycle = 75 mg]
Mercaptopurine: Oral: 60 mg/m²/dose days 1 to 70
[total dose/cycle = 4200 mg/m²]
Methotrexate: Oral: 20 mg/m²/dose days 36, 43, 50, 57, and 64
[total dose/cycle = 100 mg/m²]

Late intensification (8-week cycle):
Doxorubicin: IV: 30 mg/m²/dose days 1, 8, and 15
[total dose/cycle = 90 mg/m²]
Vincristine: IV: 2 mg/dose days 1, 8, and 15
[total dose/cycle = 6 mg]
Dexamethasone: Oral: 10 mg/m²/dose days 1 to 14
[total dose/cycle = 140 mg/m²]
Cyclophosphamide: IV: 1000 mg/m² day 29
[total dose/cycle = 1000 mg/m²]
Thioguanine: Oral: 60 mg/m²/dose days 29 to 42
[total dose/cycle = 840 mg/m²]

Cytarabine: SubQ: 75 mg/m²/dose days 29 to 32 and 36 to 39
[total dose/cycle = 600 mg/m²]
Maintenance (continue until 24 months from diagnosis):
Vincristine: IV: 2 mg/dose day 1 every 4 weeks
[total dose/4 weeks = 2 mg]
Prednisone: Oral: 60 mg/m²/dose days 1 to 5 every 4 weeks
[total dose/4 weeks = 300 mg/m²]
Mercaptopurine: Oral: 60 mg/m²/dose days 1 to 28
[total dose/phase = 1680 mg/m²]
Methotrexate: Oral: 20 mg/m²/dose days 1, 8, 15, and 22
[total dose/phase = 80 mg/m²]

References

Larson RA, Dodge RK, Linker CA, et al. A randomized controlled trial of filgrastim during remission induction and consolidation chemotherapy for adults with acute lymphoblastic leukemia: CALGB Study 9111. *Blood*. 1998;92(5):1556-1564.

Capecitabine (Breast Regimen)

Use Breast cancer (locally advanced or metastatic breast cancer)

Regimen NOTE: Multiple variations are listed.

Variation 1:
Capecitabine: Oral: 1,000 mg/m² twice daily within 30 minutes of a meal days 1 to 14
[total dose/cycle = 28,000 mg/m²]
Repeat cycle every 21 days

Variation 2:
Capecitabine: Oral: 1,250 mg/m² twice daily within 30 minutes of a meal days 1 to 14
[total dose/cycle = 35,000 mg/m²]
Repeat cycle every 21 days

References

Variation 1:
Bajetta E, Procopio G, Celio L, et al. Safety and efficacy of two different doses of capecitabine in the treatment of advanced breast cancer in older women. *J Clin Oncol*. 2005;23(10):2155-2161.
Rossi D, Alessandroni P, Catalano V, et al. Safety profile and activity of lower capecitabine dose in patients with metastatic breast cancer. *Clinical Breast Cancer*. 2007;7(11):857-860.
Variation 2:
Fumoleau P, Largillier R, Clippe C, et al. Multicentre, phase II study evaluating capecitabine monotherapy in patients with anthracycline- and taxane-pretreated metastatic breast cancer. *Eur J Cancer*. 2004;40(4):536-542.
Kaufman PA, Awada A, Twelves C, et al. Phase III open-label randomized study of eribulin mesylate versus capecitabine in patients with locally advanced or metastatic breast cancer previously treated with an anthracycline and a taxane. *J Clin Oncol*. 2015;33(6):594-601.

◆ **Capecitabine-Cisplatin-Epirubicin (Gastric/Esophageal)** *see* Epirubicin-Cisplatin-Capecitabine (Gastric/Esophageal) *on page 1956*

◆ **Capecitabine-Cisplatin (Esophageal Cancer)** *see* Cisplatin-Capecitabine (Esophageal Cancer) *on page 1889*

◆ **Capecitabine-Cisplatin (Gastric Cancer)** *see* Cisplatin-Capecitabine (Gastric Cancer) *on page 1889*

◆ **Capecitabine-Cisplatin-Trastuzumab (Gastric Cancer)** *see* Trastuzumab-Cisplatin-Capecitabine (Gastric Cancer) *on page 2093*

Capecitabine-Docetaxel (Breast)

Index Terms Docetaxel-Capecitabine (Breast)

Use Breast cancer

Regimen
Capecitabine: Oral: 1250 mg/m^2 twice daily days 1 to 14
[total dose/cycle = 35,000 mg/m^2]
Docetaxel: IV: 75 mg/m^2 over 1 hour day 1
[total dose/cycle = 75 mg/m^2]
Repeat cycle every 21 days until disease progression or unacceptable toxicity

References
O'Shaughnessy J, Miles D, Vukelja S, et al, "Superior Survival With Capecitabine Plus Docetaxel Combination Therapy in Anthracycline-Pretreated Patients With Advanced Breast Cancer: Phase III Trial Results," *J Clin Oncol*, 2002, 20(12):2812-23.

Capecitabine-Docetaxel (Gastric Cancer)

Index Terms Docetaxel-Capecitabine (Gastric Cancer)

Use Gastric cancer

Regimen NOTE: Multiple variations are listed.

Variation 1:
Capecitabine: Oral: 1000 mg/m^2 twice daily days 1 to 14
[total dose/cycle = 28,000 mg/m^2]
Docetaxel: IV: 75 mg/m^2 day 1
[total dose/cycle = 75 mg/m^2]
Repeat cycle every 3 weeks for up to 9 cycles or until disease progression or unacceptable toxicity

Variation 2:
Capecitabine: Oral: 1000 mg/m^2 twice daily days 1 to 14
[total dose/cycle = 28,000 mg/m^2]
Docetaxel: IV: 36 mg/m^2 days 1 and 8
[total dose/cycle = 72 mg/m^2]
Repeat cycle every 3 weeks until disease progression or unacceptable toxicity

Variation 3:
Capecitabine: Oral: 825 mg/m^2 twice daily days 1 to 14
[total dose/cycle = 23,100 mg/m^2]
Docetaxel: IV: 75 mg/m^2 day 1
[total dose/cycle = 75 mg/m^2]
Repeat cycle every 3 weeks until disease progression

Variation 4:
Capecitabine: Oral: 1250 mg/m^2 twice daily days 1 to 14
[total dose/cycle = 35,000 mg/m^2]
Docetaxel: IV: 75 mg/m^2 day 1
[total dose/cycle = 75 mg/m^2]
Repeat cycle every 3 weeks until disease progression for up to a maximum of 6 cycles

References
Variation 1:
Kim JG, Sohn SK, Kim DH, et al, "Phase II Study of Docetaxel and Capecitabine in Patients With Metastatic or Recurrent Gastric Cancer," *Oncology*, 2005, 68(2-3):190-5.
Variation 2:
Chun JH, Kim HK, Lee JS, et al, "Weekly Docetaxel in Combination With Capecitabine in Patients With Metastatic Gastric Cancer," *Am J Clin Oncol*, 2005, 28(2):188-94.
Variation 3:
Giordano KF, Jatoi A, Stella PJ, et al, "Docetaxel and Capecitabine in Patients With Metastatic Adenocarcinoma of the Stomach and Gastroesophageal Junction: A Phase II Study From the North Central Cancer Treatment Group," *Ann Oncol*, 2006, 17(4):652-6.
Variation 4:
Park YH, Ryoo BY, Choi SJ, et al, "A Phase II Study of Capecitabine and Docetaxel Combination Chemotherapy in Patients With Advanced Gastric Cancer," *Br J Cancer*, 2004, 90(7):1329-33.

♦ **Capecitabine-Gemcitabine (Biliary Cancer)** *see* Gemcitabine-Capecitabine (Biliary Cancer) *on page 1990*

Capecitabine-Gemcitabine (Pancreatic)

Index Terms GEM-CAP (Pancreatic); Gemcitabine-Capecitabine (Pancreatic)

Use Pancreatic cancer

Regimen NOTE: Multiple variations are listed.

Variation 1:

Gemcitabine: IV: 1000 mg/m^2/day over 30 minutes days 1 and 8
[total dose/cycle = 2000 mg/m^2]

Capecitabine: Oral: 650 mg/m^2/dose twice daily days 1 to 14
[total dose/cycle = 18,200 mg/m^2]

Repeat cycle every 21 days until disease progression (maximum duration: 24 weeks)

Variation 2:

Gemcitabine: IV: 1000 mg/m^2/day over 30 minutes days 1, 8, and 15
[total dose/cycle = 3000 mg/m^2]

Capecitabine: Oral: 830 mg/m^2/dose twice daily days 1 to 21
[total dose/cycle = 34,860 mg/m^2]

Repeat cycle every 28 days until disease progression or unacceptable toxicity

References

Variation 1:
Herrmann R, Bodoky G, Ruhstaller T, et al, "Gemcitabine Plus Capecitabine Compared With Gemcitabine Alone in Advanced Pancreatic Cancer: A Randomized, Multicenter, Phase III Trial of the Swiss Group for Clinical Cancer Research and the Central European Cooperative Oncology Group," *J Clin Oncol*, 2007, 25(16):2212-7.

Variation 2:
Cunningham D, Chau I, Stocken DD, et al, "Phase III Randomized Comparison of Gemcitabine Versus Gemcitabine Plus Capecitabine in Patients With Advanced Pancreatic Cancer," *J Clin Oncol*, 2009, 27(33):5513-8.

♦ **Capecitabine-Irinotecan (Esophageal Cancer)** *see* Irinotecan-Capecitabine (Esophageal Cancer) *on page 2019*

♦ **Capecitabine-Irinotecan (Gastric Cancer)** *see* Irinotecan-Capecitabine (Gastric Cancer) *on page 2020*

Capecitabine-Ixabepilone (Breast)

Index Terms Ixabepilone-Capecitabine (Breast)

Use Breast cancer

Regimen

Capecitabine: Oral: 1000 mg/m^2 twice daily days 1 to 14
[total dose/cycle = 28,000 mg/m^2]

Ixabepilone: IV: 40 mg/m^2 over 3 hours day 1
[total dose/cycle = 40 mg/m^2]

Repeat cycle every 21 days until disease progression or unacceptable toxicity

References

Sparano JA, Vrdolijak E, Rixe O, et al, "Randomized Phase III Trial of Ixabepilone Plus Capecitabine Versus Capecitabine in Patients With Metastatic Breast Cancer Previously Treated With an Anthracycline and a Taxane," *J Clin Oncol*, 2010, 28(20):3256-63.

Thomas ES, Gomez HL, Li RK, et al, "Ixabepilone Plus Capecitabine for Metastatic Breast Cancer Progressing After Anthracycline and Taxane Treatment," *J Clin Oncol*, 2007, 25(33):5210-7.

Capecitabine + Lapatinib (Breast)

Index Terms Lapatinib-Capecitabine (Breast)

Use Breast cancer
Regimen
Capecitabine: Oral: 1000 mg/m² twice daily days 1 to 14 within 30 minutes
after a meal
[total dose/cycle = 28,000 mg/m²]
Lapatinib: Oral: 1250 mg/day days 1 to 21 one hour before or one hour after
a meal
[total dose/cycle = 26,250 mg]
Repeat cycle every 21 days until disease progression or unacceptable toxicity
References
Bachelot T, Romieu G, Campone M, et al, "Lapatinib Plus Capecitabine in Patients With Previously Untreated Brain Metastases From HER2-Positive Metastatic Breast Cancer (LANDSCAPE): A Single-Group Phase 2 Study," *Lancet Oncol*, 2013, 14(1):64-71.
Cameron D, Casey M, Oliva C, et al, "Lapatinib Plus Capecitabine in Woman With HER-2-Positive Advanced Breast Cancer: Final Survival Analysis of a Phase III Randomized Trial," *Oncologist*, 2010, 15(9):924-34.
Geyer CE, Forster J, Lindquist D, et al, "Lapatinib Plus Capecitabine for HER2-Positive Advanced Breast Cancer," *N Engl J Med*, 2006, 355(26):2733-43.

- **Capecitabine-Oxaliplatin (Biliary Cancer)** *see* CAPOX (Biliary Cancer)
  on page 1860
- **Capecitabine-Oxaliplatin (Colorectal)** *see* XELOX (Colorectal)
  on page 2111
- **Capecitabine-Oxaliplatin-Epirubicin (Gastric/Esophageal)** *see* Epirubicin-Oxaliplatin-Capecitabine (Gastric/Esophageal) *on page 1957*

Capecitabine-Oxaliplatin (Gastric)
Index Terms CAPOX (Gastric); Oxaliplatin-Capecitabine (Gastric); XELOX
(Gastric)
Use Gastric cancer
Regimen
Capecitabine: Oral: 1000 mg/m² twice daily days 1 to 14, taken with water
within 30 minutes after a meal
[total dose/cycle = 28,000 mg/m²]
Oxaliplatin: IV: 130 mg/m² day 1
[total dose/cycle = 130 mg/m²]
Repeat cycle every 21 days for 8 cycles
References
Bang YJ, Kim YW, Yang HK, et al. Adjuvant capecitabine and oxaliplatin for gastric cancer after D2 gastrectomy (CLASSIC): a phase 3 open-label, randomised controlled trial. *Lancet*. 2012;379 (9813):315-321.

- **Capecitabine-Oxaliplatin (Pancreatic)** *see* CAPOX (Pancreatic)
  on page 1861

Capecitabine-Trastuzumab (Breast)
Index Terms Trastuzumab-Capecitabine (Breast)
Use Breast cancer
Regimen NOTE: Multiple variations are listed.
Variation 1:
Cycle 1:
Capecitabine: Oral: 1250 mg/m² twice daily days 1 to 14
[total dose/cycle 1 = 35,000 mg/m²]

◄ Trastuzumab: IV: 4 mg/kg (loading dose) over 90 minutes day 1 cycle 1
followed by IV: 2 mg/kg/day over 30 minute days 8 and 15 cycle 1
[total dose/cycle 1 = 8 mg/kg]
Treatment cycle is 21 days
Subsequent cycles:
Capecitabine: Oral: 1250 mg/m² twice daily days 1 to 14
[total dose/cycle = 35,000 mg/m²]
Trastuzumab: IV: 2 mg/kg/day over 30 minutes days 1, 8, and 15
[total dose/cycle = 6 mg/kg]
Repeat cycle every 21 days until disease progression or unacceptable
toxicity
Variation 2:
Cycle 1:
Capecitabine: Oral: 1250 mg/m² twice daily days 1 to 14
[total dose/cycle·1 = 35,000 mg/m²]
Trastuzumab: IV: 8 mg/kg (loading dose) day 1 cycle 1
[total dose/cycle 1 = 8 mg/kg]
Treatment cycle is 21 days
Subsequent cycles:
Capecitabine: Oral: 1250 mg/m² twice daily days 1 to 14
[total dose/cycle = 35,000 mg/m²]
Trastuzumab: IV: 6 mg/kg day 1
[total dose/cycle = 6 mg/kg]
Repeat cycle every 21 days

References

Variation 1:
Schaller G, Fuchs I, Gonsch T, et al, "Phase II Study of Capecitabine Plus Trastuzumab in Human Epidermal Growth Factor Receptor 2 Overexpressing Metastatic Breast Cancer Pretreated With Anthracyclines or Taxanes," *J Clin Oncol*, 2007, 25(22):3246-50.
Variation 2:
Bartsch R, Wenzel C, Altorjai G, et al, "Capecitabine and Trastuzumab in Heavily Pretreated Metastatic Breast Cancer," *J Clin Oncol*, 2007, 25(25):3853-8.

◆ **CapeOx (Colorectal)** *see* XELOX (Colorectal) *on page* 2111

CAPOX (Biliary Cancer)

Index Terms Capecitabine-Oxaliplatin (Biliary Cancer); Oxaliplatin-Capecitabine (Biliary Cancer)
Use Biliary adenocarcinoma
Regimen
Capecitabine: Oral: 1000 mg/m²/dose twice daily days 1 to 14
[total dose/cycle = 28,000 mg/m²]
Oxaliplatin: IV: 130 mg/m² over 2 hours day 1
[total dose/cycle = 130 mg/m²]
Repeat cycle every 3 weeks
References
Nehls O, Oettle H, Hartmann JT, et al, "Capecitabine Plus Oxaliplatin as First-Line Treatment in Patients With Advanced Biliary System Adenocarcinoma: A Prospective Multicentre Phase II Trial," *Br J Cancer*, 2008, 98(2):309-15.

◆ **CAPOX (Colorectal)** *see* XELOX (Colorectal) *on page* 2111
◆ **CAPOX (Gastric)** *see* Capecitabine-Oxaliplatin (Gastric) *on page* 1859

CAPOX (Pancreatic)

Index Terms Capecitabine-Oxaliplatin (Pancreatic); Oxaliplatin-Capecitabine (Pancreatic); XELOX (Pancreatic)

Use Pancreatic cancer

Regimen NOTE: Multiple variations are listed.

Variation 1 (patients <65 years of age and ECOG PS <2):

Capecitabine: Oral: 1000 mg/m^2 twice daily days 1 to 14
  [total dose/cycle = 28,000 mg/m^2]

Oxaliplatin: IV: 130 mg/m^2 over 2 hours day 1
  [total dose/cycle = 130 mg/m^2]

Repeat cycle every 21 days until disease progression or unacceptable toxicity

Variation 2 (patients >65 years of age, ECOG PS of 2, or significant comorbidities):

Capecitabine: Oral: 750 mg/m^2 twice daily days 1 to 14
  [total dose/cycle = 21,000 mg/m^2]

Oxaliplatin: IV: 110 mg/m^2 over 2 hours day 1
  [total dose/cycle = 110 mg/m^2]

Repeat cycle every 21 days until disease progression or unacceptable toxicity

References

Variations 1 and 2:

Xiong HQ, Varadhachary GR, Blais JC, et al, "Phase 2 Trial of Oxaliplatin Plus Capecitabine (XELOX) as Second-Line Therapy for Patients With Advanced Pancreatic Cancer," *Cancer*, 2008, 113(8):2046-52.

◆ **Carboplatin-Abraxane (NSCLC)** *see* Carboplatin-Paclitaxel (Protein Bound) (NSCLC) *on page 1872*

Carboplatin (Breast Regimen)

Use Breast cancer

Regimen

Carboplatin: IV: AUC 6 day 1
  [total dose/cycle = AUC = 6]

Repeat cycle every 21-28 days

References

Isakoff SJ, Goss PE, Mayer EL, et al, "TBCR009: A Multicenter Phase II Study of Cisplatin or Carboplatin for Metastatic Triple-Negative Breast Cancer and Evaluation of p63/p73 as a Biomarker of Response," *J Clin Oncol*, 2011, 29(15S):1025 [abstract 1025 from 2011 annual ASCO meeting].

Carboplatin-Cetuximab (Head and Neck Cancer)

Index Terms Cetuximab-Carboplatin (Head and Neck Cancer)

Use Head and neck cancer

Regimen

Cycle 1:

Cetuximab: IV: 400 mg/m^2 (loading dose) day 1 (week 1, cycle 1 only)
  [total loading dose = 400 mg/m^2]
    followed by IV: 250 mg/m^2/day days 8 and 15
    [total dose/cycle 1 = 900 mg/m^2]

Carboplatin: IV: AUC 5 day 1
  [total dose/cycle = AUC = 5]

Treatment cycle is 3 weeks

Subsequent cycles:

Cetuximab: IV: 250 mg/m^2/day days 1, 8, and 15

[total dose/cycle = 750 mg/m^2]

Carboplatin: IV: AUC 5 day 1

[total dose/cycle = AUC = 5]

Repeat cycle every 3 weeks until disease progression or unacceptable toxicity for up to a maximum of 8 cycles

References

Chan AT, Hsu MM, Goh BC, et al, "Multicenter, Phase II Study of Cetuximab in Combination With Carboplatin in Patients With Recurrent or Metastatic Nasopharyngeal Carcinoma," *J Clin Oncol*, 2005, 23(15):3568-76.

Carboplatin-Docetaxel (Ovarian)

Index Terms Docetaxel-Carboplatin (Ovarian)

Use Ovarian cancer

Regimen NOTE: Multiple variations are listed.

Variation 1:

Docetaxel: IV: 60 mg/m^2 over 60 minutes day 1

[total dose/cycle = 60 mg/m^2]

Carboplatin: IV: AUC 6 over 30 minutes day 1

[total dose/cycle = AUC = 6]

Repeat cycle every 21 days for 6 cycles

Variation 2:

Docetaxel: IV: 75 mg/m^2 over 60 minutes day 1

[total dose/cycle = 75 mg/m^2]

Carboplatin: IV: AUC 5 over 30-60 minutes day 1

[total dose/cycle = AUC = 5]

Repeat cycle every 21 days for 6 cycles

Variation 3:

Docetaxel: IV: 35 mg/m^2 (maximum dose: 70 mg) over 60 minutes days 1, 8, and 15

[total dose/cycle = 105 mg/m^2, maximum dose/cycle = 210 mg]

Carboplatin: IV: AUC 2 over 30 minutes days 1, 8, and 15

[total dose/cycle = AUC = 6]

Repeat cycle every 28 days until disease progression or unacceptable toxicity or 2 cycles post complete response

References

Variation 1:

Markman M, Kennedy A, Webster K, et al, "Combination Chemotherapy With Carboplatin and Docetaxel in the Treatment of Cancers of the Ovary and Fallopian Tube and Primary Carcinoma of the Peritoneum," *J Clin Oncol*, 2001, 19(7):1901-5.

Variation 2:

Strauss HG, Henze A, Teichmann A, et al, "Phase II Trial of Docetaxel and Carboplatin in Recurrent Platinum-Sensitive Ovarian, Peritoneal, and Tubal Cancer," *Gynecol Oncol*, 2007, 104(3):612-6.

Vasey PA, Jayson GC, Gordon A, et al, "Phase III Randomized Trial of Docetaxel-Carboplatin Versus Paclitaxel-Carboplatin as First-line Chemotherapy for Ovarian Carcinoma," *J Natl Cancer Inst*, 2004, 96(22):1682-91.

Variation 3:

Kushner DM, Connor JP, Sanchez F, et al, "Weekly Docetaxel and Carboplatin for Recurrent Ovarian and Peritoneal Cancer," *Gynecol Oncol*, 2007, 105(2):358-64.

Carboplatin-Docetaxel-Trastuzumab (Breast)

Index Terms TCH (Breast); Trastuzumab-Docetaxel-Carboplatin (Breast)

Use Breast cancer

Regimen

Cycle 1:

Trastuzumab: IV: 4 mg/kg (loading dose) day 1 cycle 1
followed by IV: 2 mg/kg/day days 8 and 15 cycle 1
[total dose/cycle 1 = 8 mg/kg]

Docetaxel: IV: 75 mg/m^2 day 1
[total dose/cycle 1 = 75 mg/m^2]

Carboplatin: IV: AUC 6 day 1
[total dose/cycle 1 = AUC = 6]

Treatment cycle is 21 days

Cycles 2-6:

Trastuzumab: IV: 2 mg/kg/day days 1, 8, and 15
[total dose/cycle = 6 mg/kg]

Docetaxel: IV: 75 mg/m^2 day 1
[total dose/cycle = 75 mg/m^2]

Carboplatin: IV: AUC 6 day 1
[total dose/cycle = AUC = 6]

Repeat cycle every 21 days for a total of 6 cycles

Followed by:

Trastuzumab: IV: 6 mg/kg/day day 1
[total dose/cycle = 6 mg/kg]

Repeat cycle every 21 days for 11 cycles (to complete 1 year of Trastuzumab)

References

Slamon D, Eiermann W, Robert N, et al, "Adjuvant Trastuzumab in HER2-Positive Breast Cancer," *N Engl J Med*, 2011, 365(14):1273-83.

Carboplatin-Docetaxel (Unknown Primary, Adenocarcinoma)

Index Terms Docetaxel-Carboplatin (Unknown Primary, Adenocarcinoma)

Use Unknown primary (adenocarcinoma)

Regimen

Docetaxel: IV: 65 mg/m^2 over 1 hour day 1
[total dose/cycle = 65 mg/m^2]

Carboplatin: IV: AUC 6 over 20 minutes day 1
[total dose/cycle = AUC = 6]

Repeat cycle every 21 days for up to a maximum of 8 cycles

References

Greco FA, Erland JB, Morrissey LH, et al, "Carcinoma of Unknown Primary Site: Phase II Trials With Docetaxel Plus Cisplatin or Carboplatin," *Ann Oncol*, 2000, 11(2):211-5.

Carboplatin-Docetaxel (Unknown Primary, Squamous Cell)

Index Terms Docetaxel-Carboplatin (Unknown Primary, Squamous Cell)

Use Unknown primary (squamous cell)

Regimen

Docetaxel: IV: 75 mg/m^2 over 30 minutes day 1
[total dose/cycle = 75 mg/m^2]

Carboplatin: IV: AUC 5 over 30 minutes day 1
[total dose/cycle = AUC = 5]

Repeat cycle every 21 days for up to a maximum of 8 cycles

References

Pentheroudakis G, Briasoulis E, Kalofonos HP, et al, "Docetaxel and Carboplatin Combination Chemotherapy as Outpatient Palliative Therapy in Carinoma of Unknown Primary: A Multicentre Hellenic Cooperative Oncology Group Phase II Study," *Acta Oncol*, 2008, 47(6):1148-55.

Carboplatin-Doxorubicin (Liposomal) (Ovarian)

Index Terms Doxorubicin (Liposomal)-Carboplatin (Ovarian)

Use Ovarian cancer

Regimen NOTE: Multiple variations are listed.

Variation 1:

Doxorubicin (liposomal): IV: 30 mg/m^2 day 1

[total dose/cycle = 30 mg/m^2]

Carboplatin: IV: AUC 5 day 1

[total dose/cycle = AUC = 5]

Repeat cycle every 28 days until disease progression or unacceptable toxicity

Variation 2:

Doxorubicin (liposomal): IV: 30 mg/m^2 over 60 minutes day 1

[total dose/cycle = 30 mg/m^2]

Carboplatin: IV: AUC 5 over 30 minutes day 1

[total dose/cycle = AUC = 5]

Repeat cycle every 21 days for 6 cycles

References

Variation 1:

Pujade-Lauraine E, Wagner U, Aavall-Lundqvist E, et al, "Pegylated Liposomal Doxorubicin and Carboplatin Compared With Paclitaxel and Carboplatin for Patients With Platinum-Sensitive Ovarian Cancer in Late Relapse," *J Clin Oncol*, 2010, 28(20):3323-9.

Variation 2:

Pignata S, Scambia G, Ferrandina G, et al, "Carboplatin Plus Paclitaxel Versus Carboplatin Plus Pegylated Liposomal Doxorubicin as First-Line Treatment for Patients With Ovarian Cancer: The MITO-2 Randomized Phase III Trial," *J Clin Oncol*, 2011, 29(27):3628-35.

◆ **Carboplatin, Etoposide, Cyclophosphamide, Doxorubicin, Vincristine (Neuroblastoma)** see CE-CAdO (Neuroblastoma) on page 1877

Carboplatin-Etoposide (Ovarian Germ Cell Tumor)

Index Terms Etoposide-Carboplatin (Ovarian Germ Cell Tumor)

Use Ovarian cancer (adjuvant therapy in completely resected stage IB-III dysgerminoma)

Regimen

Etoposide: IV: 120 mg/m^2/day days 1, 2, and 3

[total dose/cycle = 360 mg/m^2]

Carboplatin: IV: 400 mg/m^2 day 1

[total dose/cycle = 400 mg/m^2]

Repeat cycle every 28 days for a total of 3 cycles

References

Williams SD, Kauderer J, Burnett AF, et al. Adjuvant therapy of completely resected dysgerminoma with carboplatin and etoposide: a trial of the Gynecologic Oncology Group. *Gynecol Oncol*. 2004;95(3):496-499.

Carboplatin-Etoposide-Paclitaxel (Unknown Primary, Adenocarcinoma)

Index Terms Paclitaxel-Carboplatin-Etoposide (Unknown Primary)

Use Unknown primary, adenocarcinoma

Regimen

Paclitaxel: IV: 200 mg/m^2 over 1 hour day 1
  [total dose/cycle = 200 mg/m^2]
Carboplatin: IV: AUC 6 over 20-30 minutes day 1
  [total dose/cycle = AUC = 6]
Etoposide: Oral: 50 mg/day days 1, 3, 5, 7, and 9
  and Oral: 100 mg/day days 2, 4, 6, 8, and 10
  [total dose/cycle = 750 mg]
Repeat cycle every 21 days for a total of 4-8 cycles

References

Greco FA, Burris HA 3rd, Erland JB, et al, "Carcinoma of Unknown Primary Site," *Cancer*, 2000, 89 (12):2655-60.

Carboplatin-Etoposide (Retinoblastoma)

Index Terms Etoposide-Carboplatin (Retinoblastoma)
Use Retinoblastoma

Regimen

Etoposide: IV: 100 mg/m^2/day over 1 hour days 1 to 5
  [total dose/cycle = 500 mg/m^2]
Carboplatin: IV: 160 mg/m^2/day over 1 hour days 1 to 5
  [total dose/cycle = 800 mg/m^2]
Repeat cycle in 21 to 28 days for a total of 2 cycles

References

Doz F, Neuenschwander S, Plantaz D, et al, "Etoposide and Carboplatin in Extraocular Retinoblastoma: A Study by the Societe Francaise d'Oncologie Pediatrique," *J Clin Oncol*, 1995, 13 (4):902-9.

Carboplatin-Etoposide (Small Cell Lung Cancer)

Index Terms EC (Small Cell Lung Cancer); Etoposide-Carboplatin (Small Cell Lung Cancer)
Use Lung cancer, small cell
Regimen NOTE: Multiple variations are listed.

Variation 1 (limited stage with thoracic radiotherapy):
  Carboplatin: IV: AUC 6 over 1 hour day 1
    [total dose/cycle = AUC = 6]
  Etoposide: IV: 100 mg/m^2/day over 2 hours days 1, 2, and 3
    [total dose/cycle = 300 mg/m^2]
  Repeat cycle every 21 days for 6 cycles
Variation 2 (extensive):
  Carboplatin: IV: AUC 5 day 1
    [total dose/cycle = AUC = 5]
  Etoposide: IV: 100 mg/m^2/day days 1, 2, and 3
    [total dose/cycle = 300 mg/m^2]
  Repeat cycle every 21 days for 6 cycles
Variation 3 (elderly, limited, and extensive):
  Carboplatin: IV: AUC 5 over 1 hour day 1
    [total dose/cycle = AUC = 5]
  Etoposide: IV: 100 mg/m^2/day over 1 hour days 1, 2, and 3
    [total dose/cycle = 300 mg/m^2]
  Repeat cycle every 28 days for 4 cycles

◀ **References**
Variation 1:

Skarlos DV, Samantas E, Briassoulis E, et al, "Randomized Comparison of Early Versus Late Hyperfractionated Thoracic Irradiation Concurrently With Chemotherapy in Limited Disease Small-Cell Lung Cancer: A Randomized Phase II Study of the Hellenic Cooperative Oncology Group (HeCOG)," *Ann Oncol*, 2001, 12(9):1231-8.

Variation 2:

Socinski MA, Smit EF, Lorigan P, et al, "Phase III Study of Pemetrexed Plus Carboplatin Compared With Etoposide Plus Carboplatin in Chemotherapy-Naïve Patients With Extensive-Stage Small Cell-Cell Lung Cancer," *J Clin Oncol*, 2009, 27(28):4787-92.

Variation 3:

Okamoto H, Watanabe K, Nishiwaki Y, et al, "Phase II Study of Area Under the Plasma-Concentration-Versus-Time Curve-Based Carboplatin Plus Standard-Dose Intravenous Etoposide in Elderly Patients With Small-Cell Lung Cancer," *J Clin Oncol*, 1999, 17(11):3540-5.

Carboplatin-Etoposide-Vincristine (Retinoblastoma)

Index Terms Etoposide-Carboplatin-Vincristine (Retinoblastoma); Vincristine-Carboplatin-Etoposide (Retinoblastoma)

Use Retinoblastoma

Regimen NOTE: Multiple variations are listed.

Variation 1 (<1 year of age):

Carboplatin: IV: 20 mg/kg day 1

[total dose/cycle = 20 mg/kg]

Etoposide Phosphate: IV: 5 mg/kg day 1

[total dose/cycle = 5 mg/kg]

Vincristine: IV: 0.05 mg/kg day 1

[total dose/cycle = 0.05 mg/kg]

Variation 2 (age >1 year):

Carboplatin: IV: 550-600 mg/m^2 day 1

[total dose/cycle = 550-600 mg/m^2]

Etoposide Phosphate: IV: 150 mg/m^2 day 1

[total dose/cycle = 150 mg/m^2]

Vincristine: IV: 1.5-2 mg/m^2 day 1

[total dose/cycle = 1.5-2 mg/m^2]

Variation 3 (≤36 months of age):

Carboplatin: IV: 18.6 mg/kg day 1

[total dose/cycle = 18.6 mg/kg]

Etoposide: IV: 5 mg/kg days 1 and 2

[total dose/cycle = 10 mg/kg]

Vincristine: IV: 0.05 mg/kg day 1 (maximum dose: 2 mg)

[total dose/cycle = 0.05 mg/kg; maximum dose: 2 mg]

Repeat cycle every 28 days for a total of 6 cycles

Variation 4 (>36 months of age):

Carboplatin: IV: 560 mg/m^2 day 1

[total dose/cycle = 560 mg/m^2]

Etoposide: IV: 150 mg/m^2 days 1 and 2

[total dose/cycle = 300 mg/m^2]

Vincristine: IV: 1.5 mg/m^2 day 1 (maximum dose: 2 mg)

[total dose/cycle = 1.5 mg/m^2; maximum dose: 2 mg]

Repeat cycle every 28 days for a total of 6 cycles

References
Variations 1 and 2:

Sussman DA, Escalona-Benz E, Benz MS, et al, "Comparison of Retinoblastoma Reduction for Chemotherapy vs External Beam Radiotherapy," *Arch Ophthalmol*, 2003, 121(7):979-84.

Variations 3 and 4:

Friedman DL, Himelstein B, Shields CL, et al, "Chemoreduction and Local Ophthalmic Therapy for Intraocular Retinoblastoma," *J Clin Oncol*, 2000, 18(1):12-7.

Shields CL, Honavar SG, Meadows AT, et al, "Chemoreduction for Unilateral Retinoblastoma," *Arch Ophthalmol*, 2002, 120(12):1653-8.

◆ **Carboplatin-Fluorouracil-Cetuximab (Head and Neck Cancer)** *see* Cetuximab-Carboplatin-Fluorouracil (Head and Neck Cancer) *on page 1880*

◆ **Carboplatin-Fluorouracil (Head and Neck Cancer)** *see* Fluorouracil-Carboplatin (Head and Neck Cancer) *on page 1977*

◆ **Carboplatin-Gemcitabine-Bevacizumab (Ovarian)** *see* Bevacizumab-Carboplatin-Gemcitabine (Ovarian) *on page 1839*

Carboplatin-Gemcitabine (Bladder)

Index Terms GC (Bladder); Gemcitabine-Carboplatin (Bladder)

Use Bladder cancer

Regimen

Gemcitabine: IV: 1000 mg/m^2/day over 30 minutes days 1 and 8
[total dose/cycle = 2000 mg/m^2]

Carboplatin: IV: AUC 4.5 over 60 minutes day 1
[total dose/cycle = AUC = 4.5]

Repeat cycle every 21 days until disease progression or unacceptable toxicity

References

De Santis M, Bellmunt J, Mead G, et al. Randomized phase II/III trial assessing gemcitabine/carboplatin and methotrexate/carboplatin/vinblastine in patients with advanced urothelial cancer who are unfit for cisplatin-based chemotherapy: EORTC study 30986. *J Clin Oncol*. 2012;30 (2):191-199.

Carboplatin-Gemcitabine (NSCLC)

Index Terms GC (NSCLC); Gemcitabine-Carboplatin (NSCLC)

Use Lung cancer, non-small cell

Regimen NOTE: Multiple variations are listed.

Variation 1:

Gemcitabine: IV: 1000 mg/m^2/day over 30 minutes days 1, 8, and 15
[total dose/cycle = 3000 mg/m^2]

Carboplatin: IV: AUC 5 day 1
[total dose/cycle = AUC = 5]

Repeat cycle every 28 days for up to 4 cycles

Variation 2:

Gemcitabine: IV: 1000 mg/m^2/day days 1 and 8
[total dose/cycle = 2000 mg/m^2]

Carboplatin: IV: AUC 5 day 1
[total dose/cycle = AUC = 5]

Repeat cycle every 21 days for up to 4 cycles

References

Variation 1:

Danson S, Middleton MR, O'Byrne KJ, et al, "Phase III Trial of Gemcitabine and Carboplatin Versus Mitomycin, Ifosfamide, and Cisplatin or Mitomycin, Vinblastine, and Cisplatin in Patients With Advanced Nonsmall Cell Lung Carcinoma," *Cancer*, 2003, 98(3):542-53.

Variation 2:

Grønberg BH, Bremnes RM, Fløtten O, et al, "Phase III Study by the Norwegian Lung Cancer Study Group: Pemetrexed Plus Carboplatin Compared With Gemcitabine Plus Carboplatin as First-Line Chemotherapy in Advanced Non-Small-Cell Lung Cancer," *J Clin Oncol*, 2009, 27 (19):3217-24

Carboplatin-Gemcitabine (Ovarian)

Index Terms Gemcitabine-Carboplatin (Ovarian)

Use Ovarian cancer

Regimen

Gemcitabine: IV: 1000 mg/m²/day days 1 and 8
[total dose/cycle = 2000 mg/m²]
Carboplatin: IV: AUC 4 day 1
[total dose/cycle = AUC = 4]
Repeat cycle every 21 days for 6-10 cycles

References

Pfisterer J, Plante M, Vergote I, et al, "Gemcitabine Plus Carboplatin Compared With Carboplatin in Patients With Platinum-Sensitive Recurrent Ovarian Cancer: An Intergroup Trial of the AGO-OVAR, the NCIC CTG, and the EORTC GCG," *J Clin Oncol*, 2006, 24(29):4699-707.

Carboplatin-Irinotecan (Small Cell Lung Cancer)

Index Terms IC (Small Cell Lung Cancer); IP (Small Cell Lung Cancer); Irinotecan-Carboplatin (Small Cell Lung Cancer)

Use Lung cancer, small cell

Regimen NOTE: Multiple variations are listed.

Variation 1:
Carboplatin: IV: AUC 5 (Calvert formula) day 1
[total dose/cycle = AUC = 5]
Irinotecan: IV: 175 mg/m² day 1
[total dose/cycle = 175 mg/m²]
Repeat cycle every 21 days for a total of 4 cycles

Variation 2:
Carboplatin: IV: AUC 5 (Calvert formula) over 1 hour day 1
[total dose/cycle = AUC = 5]
Irinotecan: IV: 50 mg/m²/day over 30 minutes days 1, 8, and 15
[total dose/cycle = 150 mg/m²]
Repeat cycle every 28 days

References

Variation 1:
Hermes A, Bergman B, Bremnes R, et al, "Irinotecan Plus Carboplatin Versus Oral Etoposide Plus Carboplatin in Extensive Small-Cell Lung Cancer: A Randomized Phase III Trial," *J Clin Oncol*, 2008, 26(26):4261-7.
Variation 2:
Schmittel A, Fischer von Weikersthal L, Sebastian M, et al, "A Randomized Phase II Trial of Irinotecan Plus Carboplatin Versus Etoposide Plus Carboplatin Treatment in Patients With Extended Disease Small-Cell Lung Cancer," *Ann Oncol*, 2006, 17(4):663-7.
Schmittel A, Sebastian M, Fischer von Weikersthal L, et al, "A German Multicenter, Randomized Phase III Trial Comparing Irinotecan-Carboplatin With Etoposide-Carboplatin as First-Line Therapy for Extensive-Disease Small-Cell Lung Cancer," *Ann Oncol*, 2011, 22(8):1798-804.

- ◆ **Carboplatin-nab Paclitaxel (NSCLC)** *see* Carboplatin-Paclitaxel (Protein Bound) (NSCLC) *on page 1872*
- ◆ **Carboplatin-Paclitaxel-Bevacizumab (NSCLC)** *see* Bevacizumab-Carbo-platin-Paclitaxel (NSCLC) *on page 1839*

Carboplatin-Paclitaxel (Cervical Cancer)

Index Terms Paclitaxel-Carboplatin (Cervical Cancer)

Use Cervical cancer

Regimen NOTE: Multiple variations are listed.

Variation 1:

Paclitaxel: IV: 175 mg/m² over 3 hours day 1 (reduce to 155 mg/m² over 3 hours day 1 if prior pelvic irradiation)

[total dose/cycle = 175 (or 155) mg/m²]

Carboplatin: IV: AUC 5 or 6 day 1

[total dose/cycle = AUC = 5 or 6]

Repeat cycle every 28 days for up to a total of 6-9 cycles

Variation 2:

Paclitaxel: IV: 175 mg/m² over 3 hours day 1

[total dose/cycle = 175 mg/m²]

Carboplatin: IV: AUC 5 day 1

[total dose/cycle = AUC = 5]

Repeat cycle every 21 days for 6-9 cycles

References

Variation 1:

Tinker AV, Bhagat K, Swenerton KD, et al, "Carboplatin and Paclitaxel for Advanced and Recurrent Cervical Carcinoma: The British Columbia Cancer Agency Experience," *Gynecol Oncol*, 2005, 98 (1):54-8.

Variation 2:

Pectasides D, Fountzilas G, Papaxoinis G, et al, "Carboplatin and Paclitaxel in Metastatic or Recurrent Cervical Cancer," *Int J Gynecol Cancer*, 2009, 19(4):777-81.

Carboplatin-Paclitaxel (Endometrial)

Index Terms Paclitaxel-Carboplatin (Endometrial); TC (Endometrial)

Use Endometrial cancer

Regimen NOTE: Multiple variations are listed.

Variation 1:

Paclitaxel: IV: 175 mg/m² day 1

[total dose/cycle = 175 mg/m²]

Carboplatin: IV: AUC 6 day 1

[total dose/cycle = AUC = 6]

Repeat cycle every 21 days for a total for 7 cycles

Variation 2:

Paclitaxel: IV: 175 mg/m² over 3 hours day 1

[total dose/cycle = 175 mg/m²]

Carboplatin: IV: AUC 5 over 1 hour day 1

[total dose/cycle = AUC = 5]

Repeat cycle every 21 days for a total of 6 to 9 cycles

Variation 3:

Paclitaxel: IV: 80 mg/m² over 60 minutes days 1, 8, and 15

[total dose/cycle = 240 mg/m²]

Carboplatin: IV: AUC 2 over 30 minutes days 1, 8, and 15

[total dose/cycle = AUC = 6]

Repeat cycle every 28 days until disease progression or unacceptable toxicity

References

Variation 1:

Miller DS, Filiaci G, Fleming G, et al. Randomized phase III noninferiority trial of first line chemotherapy for metastatic or recurrent endometrial carcinoma: A Gynecologic Oncology Group Study. *Gynecol Oncol*. 2012;125(3):771.

Variation 2:

Pectasides D, Xiros N, Papaxoinis G, et al. Carboplatin and paclitaxel in advanced or metastatic endometrial cancer. *Gynecol Oncol*. 2008;109(2):250-254.

Variation 3:
Secord AA, Havrilesky LJ, Carney ME, et al. Weekly low-dose paclitaxel and carboplatin in the treatment of advanced or recurrent cervical and endometrial cancer. *Int J Clin Oncol.* 2007;12 (1):31-36.

◆ **Carboplatin-Paclitaxel (Esophageal Cancer)** *see* Paclitaxel-Carboplatin (Esophageal Cancer) *on page 2050*

Carboplatin-Paclitaxel (NSCLC)

Index Terms Paclitaxel-Carboplatin (NSCLC); PC (NSCLC); TC (NSCLC)

Use Lung cancer, non-small cell

Regimen NOTE: Multiple variations are listed.

Variation 1:
Paclitaxel: IV: 225 mg/m^2 over 3 hours day 1
  [total dose/cycle = 225 mg/m^2]
Carboplatin: IV: AUC 6 day 1
  [total dose/cycle = AUC = 6]
Repeat cycle every 21 days

Variation 2:
Paclitaxel: IV: 200 mg/m^2 over 3 hours day 1
  [total dose/cycle = 200 mg/m^2]
Carboplatin: IV: AUC 6 day 1
  [total dose/cycle = AUC = 6]
Repeat cycle every 21 days

Variation 3:
Paclitaxel: IV: 100 mg/m^2/week over 3 hours for 6 weeks
  [total dose/cycle = 600 mg/m^2]
Carboplatin: IV: AUC 2 weekly over 30 to 60 minutes for 6 weeks
  [total dose/cycle = AUC = 12]
Repeat cycle every 8 weeks

Variation 4:
Paclitaxel: IV: 100 mg/m^2/day days 1, 8, and 15
  [total dose/cycle = 300 mg/m^2]
Carboplatin: IV: AUC 6 day 1
  [total dose/cycle = AUC = 6]
Repeat cycle every 28 days

References

Variation 1:
Belani CP, Ramalingam S, Perry MC, et al. Randomized, phase III study of weekly paclitaxel in combination with carboplatin versus standard every-3-weeks administration of carboplatin and paclitaxel for patients with previously untreated advanced non-small-cell lung cancer. *J Clin Oncol.* 2008;26(3):468-473.

Schiller JH, Harrington D, Belani CP, et al. Comparison of four chemotherapy regimens for advanced non-small-cell lung cancer. *N Engl J Med,* 2002;346(2):92-98.

Variation 2:
Ohe Y, Ohashi Y, Kubota K, et al. Randomized phase III study of cisplatin plus irinotecan versus carboplatin plus paclitaxel, cisplatin plus gemcitabine, and cisplatin plus vinorelbine for advanced non-small-cell lung cancer: Four-Arm Cooperative Study in Japan. *Ann Oncol.* 2007;18 (2):317-323.

Schuette W, Blankenburg T, Guschall W, et al. Multicenter randomized trial for stage IIIB/IV non-small-cell lung cancer using every-3-week versus weekly paclitaxel/carboplatin. *Clin Lung Cancer.* 2006;7(5):338-343.

Variation 3:
Schuette W, Blankenburg T, Guschall W, et al. Multicenter randomized trial for stage IIIB/IV non-small-cell lung cancer using every-3-week versus weekly paclitaxel/carboplatin. *Clin Lung Cancer.* 2006;7(5):338-343.

Variation 4:
Belani CP, Ramalingam S, Perry MC, et al. Randomized, phase III study of weekly paclitaxel in combination with carboplatin versus standard every-3-weeks administration of carboplatin and paclitaxel for patients with previously untreated advanced non-small-cell lung cancer. *J Clin Oncol*. 2008;26(3):468-473.

Carboplatin-Paclitaxel (Ovarian)

Index Terms Paclitaxel-Carboplatin (Ovarian)

Use Ovarian cancer

Regimen NOTE: Multiple variations are listed.

Variation 1:

Paclitaxel: IV: 175 mg/m^2 over 3 hours day 1

[total dose/cycle = 175 mg/m^2]

Carboplatin: IV: AUC 7.5 day 1

[total dose/cycle = AUC = 7.5]

Repeat cycle every 21 days for a total of 6 cycles

Variation 2:

Paclitaxel: IV: 175-185 mg/m^2 over 3 hours day 1

[total dose/cycle = 175-185 mg/m^2]

Carboplatin: IV: AUC 5-6 day 1

[total dose/cycle = AUC = 5-6]

Repeat cycle every 21 days

Variation 3:

Paclitaxel: IV: 175 mg/m^2 over 3 hours day 1

[total dose/cycle = 175 mg/m^2]

Carboplatin: IV: AUC 5 day 1

[total dose/cycle = AUC = 5]

Repeat cycle every 21 days

Variation 4:

Paclitaxel: IV: 175 mg/m^2 over 3 hours day 1

[total dose/cycle = 175 mg/m^2]

Carboplatin: IV: AUC 7.5 over 30 minutes day 1

[total dose/cycle = AUC = 7.5]

Repeat cycle every 21 days for 3-6 cycles

Variation 5:

Paclitaxel: IV: 80 mg/m^2 over 1 hour days 1, 8, and 15

[total dose/cycle = 240 mg/m^2]

Carboplatin: IV: AUC 6 over 1 hour day 1

[total dose/cycle = AUC = 6]

Repeat cycle every 21 days for a total of 6 cycles

References

Variation 1:
Ozols RF, Bundy BN, Greer BE, et al, "Phase III Trial of Carboplatin and Paclitaxel Compared With Cisplatin and Paclitaxel in Patients With Optimally Resected Stage III Ovarian Cancer: A Gynecologic Oncology Group Study," *J Clin Oncol*, 2003, 21(17):3194-200.
Variation 2:
Parmar MK, Ledermann JA, Colombo N, et al, "Paclitaxel Plus Platinum-Based Chemotherapy Versus Conventional Platinum-Based Chemotherapy in Women With Relapsed Ovarian Cancer: The ICON4/AGO-OVAR-2.2 Trial," *Lancet*, 2003, 361(9375):2099-106.
Variation 3:
Neijt JP, Engelholm SA, Tuxen MK, et al, "Exploratory Phase III Study of Paclitaxel and Cisplatin Versus Paclitaxel and Carboplatin in Advanced Ovarian Cancer," *J Clin Oncol*, 2000, 18 (17):3084-92.
Vasey PA, Jayson GC, Gordon A, et al, "Phase III Randomized Trial of Docetaxel-Carboplatin Versus Paclitaxel-Carboplatin as First-Line Chemotherapy for Ovarian Carcinoma," *J Natl Cancer Inst*, 2004, 96(22):1682-91.

Variation 4:
Bell J, Brady MF, Young RC, et al, "Randomized Phase III Trial of Three Versus Six Cycles of Adjuvant Carboplatin and Paclitaxel in Early Stage Epithelial Ovarian Carcinoma: A Gynecologic Oncology Group Study," *Gynecol Oncol*, 2006, 102(3):432-9.
Variation 5:
Katsumata N, Yasuda M, Takahashi F, et al, "Dose-Dense Paclitaxel Once a Week in Combination With Carboplatin Every 3 Weeks for Advanced Ovarian Cancer: A Phase III, Open-Label, Randomised Trial," *Lancet*, 2009, 374(9698):1331-8.

Carboplatin-Paclitaxel (Protein Bound) (NSCLC)

Index Terms Carboplatin-Abraxane (NSCLC); Carboplatin-nab Paclitaxel (NSCLC); nab Paclitaxel-Carboplatin (NSCLC); nab-PC (NSCLC); Paclitaxel (Protein Bound)-Carboplatin (NSCLC)

Use Lung cancer, non-small cell

Regimen

Paclitaxel (Protein Bound): IV: 100 mg/m^2/day over 30 minutes days 1, 8, and 15

[total dose/cycle = 300 mg/m^2]

Carboplatin: IV: AUC 6 day 1

[total dose/cycle = AUC = 6]

Repeat cycle every 21 days for at least 6 cycles or until disease progression or unacceptable toxicity

References

Socinski MA, Bondarenko I, Karaseva NA, et al, "Weekly nab-Paclitaxel in Combination With Carboplatin Versus Solvent-Based Paclitaxel Plus Carboplatin as First-Line Therapy in Patients With Advanced Non-Small-Cell Lung Cancer: Final Results of a Phase III Trial," *J Clin Oncol*, 2012, 30(17):2055-62.

Carboplatin-Paclitaxel (Thymoma/Thymic)

Use Thymoma/thymic carcinoma (advanced previously untreated)

Regimen

Paclitaxel: IV: 225 mg/m^2 over 3 hours day 1

[total dose/cycle = 225 mg/m^2]

Carboplatin: IV: AUC 6 over 30 minutes day 1

[total dose/cycle = AUC = 6]

Repeat cycle every 21 days for up to 6 cycles

References

Lemma GL, Lee JW, Aisner SC, et al. Phase II study of carboplatin and paclitaxel in advanced thymoma and thymic carcinoma. *J Clin Oncol*. 2011;29(15):2060-2065.

Carboplatin-Paclitaxel-Trastuzumab (Breast)

Index Terms Paclitaxel-Carboplatin-Trastuzumab (Breast); TCH (Breast); TPC (Breast); Trastuzumab-Paclitaxel-Carboplatin (Breast)

Use Breast cancer

Regimen

Variation 1:

Cycle 1:

Trastuzumab: IV: 4 mg/kg (loading dose) cycle 1 day 1

followed by IV: 2 mg/kg days 8 and 15

[total dose/cycle 1 = 8 mg/kg]

Paclitaxel: IV: 175 mg/m^2 day 2

[total dose/cycle = 175 mg/m^2]

Carboplatin: IV: AUC 6 day 2

[total dose/cycle = AUC = 6]

Treatment cycle is 21 days

Subsequent cycles:

    Trastuzumab: IV: 2 mg/kg days 1, 8, and 15
      [total dose/cycle = 6 mg/kg]
    Paclitaxel: IV: 175 mg/m^2 day 2
      [total dose/cycle = 175 mg/m^2]
    Carboplatin: IV: AUC 6 day 2
      [total dose/cycle = AUC = 6]
    Repeat cycle every 21 days for a total of at least 6 cycles
    followed by:
    Trastuzumab: IV: 2 mg/kg once weekly until disease progression or unacceptable toxicity

Variation 2:

  Cycle 1:
    Paclitaxel: IV: 80 mg/m^2 over 1 hour days 1, 8, and 15
      [total dose/cycle 1 = 240 mg/m^2]
    Carboplatin: IV: AUC 2 over 15 minutes days 1, 8, and 15
      [total dose/cycle 1 = AUC = 6]
    Trastuzumab: IV: 4 mg/kg (loading dose) over 90 minutes cycle 1 day 1
      followed by IV: 2 mg/kg over 30 minutes days 8, 15, and 22
        [total dose/cycle 1 = 10 mg/kg]
    Treatment cycle is 28 days

  Subsequent cycles:
    Paclitaxel: IV: 80 mg/m^2 over 1 hour days 1, 8, and 15
      [total dose/cycle = 240 mg/m^2]
    Carboplatin: IV: AUC 2 over 15 minutes days 1, 8, and 15
      [total dose/cycle = AUC = 6]
    Trastuzumab: IV: 2 mg/kg over 30 minutes days 1, 8, 15, and 22
      [total dose/cycle = 8 mg/kg]
    Repeat cycle every 28 days for a maximum of 6 cycles
    followed by:
    Trastuzumab: IV: 6 mg/kg every 21 days until disease progression or unacceptable toxicity

References

Variation 1:
Robert N, Leyland-Jones B, Asmar L, et al, "Randomized Phase III Study of Trastuzumab, Paclitaxel, and Carboplatin Compared With Trastuzumab and Paclitaxel in Women With HER-2-Overexpressing Metastatic Breast Cancer," *J Clin Oncol*, 2006, 24(18):2786-92.
Variation 2:
Perez EA, Suman VJ, Rowland KM, et al, "Two Concurrent Phase II Trials of Paclitaxel/Carboplatin/Trastuzumab (Weekly or Every-3-Week Schedule) as First-Line Therapy in Women With HER2-Overexpressing Metastatic Breast Cancer: NCCTG Study 983252," *Clin Breast Cancer*, 2005, 6(5):425-32.

Carboplatin-Paclitaxel (Unknown Primary, Adenocarcinoma)

Index Terms Carbo-Tax (Unknown Primary); Paclitaxel-Carboplatin (Unknown Primary)

Use Unknown primary (adenocarcinoma)

Regimen

  Carboplatin: IV: Target AUC 6 day 1
    [total dose/cycle = AUC = 6]
  followed by
  Paclitaxel: IV: 200 mg/m^2 infused over 3 hours day 1
    [total dose/cycle = 200 mg/m^2]

◄ Filgrastim: SubQ: 300 mcg/day days 5 to 12
[total dose/cycle = 2400 mcg]
Repeat cycle every 21 days for a total of 6 or 8 cycles

References
Briasoulis E, Kalofonos H, Bafaloukos D, et al, "Carboplatin Plus Paclitaxel in Unknown Primary Carcinoma: A Phase II Hellenic Cooperative Oncology Group Study," *J Clin Oncol*, 2000, 18 (17):3101-7.

♦ **Carboplatin-Pemetrexed-Bevacizumab (NSCLC)** *see* Bevacizumab-Carbo-platin-Pemetrexed (NSCLC) *on page 1839*

Carboplatin-Pemetrexed (Mesothelioma)
Index Terms Pemetrexed-Carboplatin (Mesothelioma)
Use Malignant pleural mesothelioma
Regimen
Pemetrexed: IV: 500 mg/m² over 10 minutes day 1
[total dose/cycle = 500 mg/m²]
Carboplatin: IV: AUC 5 over 30 minutes day 1 (start 30 minutes after pemetrexed)
[total dose/cycle = AUC = 5]
Repeat cycle every 21 days

References
Ceresoli GL, Zucali PA, Favaretto AG, et al, "Phase II Study of Pemetrexed Plus Carboplatin in Malignant Pleural Mesothelioma," *J Clin Oncol*, 2006, 24(9):1443-8.
Santoro A, O'Brien ME, Stahel RA, et al, "Pemetrexed Plus Cisplatin or Pemetrexed Plus Carboplatin for Chemonaïve Patients With Malignant Pleural Mesothelioma: Results of the International Expanded Access Program," *J Thorac Oncol*, 2008, 3(7):756-63.

Carboplatin-Pemetrexed (NSCLC)
Index Terms Pemetrexed-Carboplatin (NSCLC)
Use Lung cancer, non-small cell
Regimen
Pemetrexed: IV: 500 mg/m² day 1
[total dose/cycle = 500 mg/m²]
Carboplatin: IV: AUC 5 day 1
[total dose/cycle = AUC = 5]
Repeat cycle every 21 days for a maximum of 4 cycles

References
Gronberg BH, Bremnes RM, Flotten O, et al, "Phase III Study by the Norwegian Lung Cancer Study Group: Pemetrexed Plus Carboplatin Compared With Gemcitabine Plus Carboplatin as First-Line Chemotherapy in Advanced Non-Small-Cell Lung Cancer," *J Clin Oncol*, 2009, 27(19):3217-24.

Carboplatin (Testicular Regimen)
Use Testicular cancer
Regimen NOTE: Multiple variations are listed.
Variation 1:
Carboplatin: IV: AUC 7 day 1
[total dose/cycle = AUC = 7]
This is administered as a one-time infusion
Variation 2:
Carboplatin: IV: AUC 7 day 1
[total dose/cycle = AUC = 7]
Repeat cycle every 21 days for a total of 2 cycles

References

Variation 1:

Oliver RT, Mason MD, Mead GM, et al, "Radiotherapy Versus Single-Dose Carboplatin in Adjuvant Treatment of Stage I Seminoma: A Randomised Trial," *Lancet*, 2005, 366(9482):293-300.

Oliver RT, Mead GM, Rustin G, et al, "Randomized Trial of Carboplatin Versus Radiotherapy for Stage I Seminoma: Mature Results on Relapse and Contralateral Testis Cancer Rates in MRC TE19/EORTC 30982 Study (ISRCTN27163214)," *J Clin Oncol*, 2011, 29(8):957-62.

Variation 2:

Aparicio J, Germa JR, Garcia del Muro X, et al, "Risk-Adapted Management for Patients With Clinical Stage I Seminoma: The Second Spanish Germ Cell Cancer Cooperative Group Study," *J Clin Oncol*, 2005, 23(34):8717-23.

Carboplatin-Vincristine (Retinoblastoma)

Index Terms Vincristine-Carboplatin (Retinoblastoma)

Use Retinoblastoma

Regimen NOTE: Multiple variations are listed.

Variation 1 (GFR >50 mL/minute/m²):

Carboplatin: IV: 560 mg/m² day 1

[total dose/cycle = 560 mg/m²]

Vincristine: IV: 0.05 mg/kg day 1

[total dose/cycle = 0.05 mg/kg]

Repeat for up to a total of 8 cycles

Variation 2 (GFR <50 mL/minute/m²):

Carboplatin: IV: AUC 6.5 day 1

[total dose/cycle = AUC 6.5]

Vincristine: IV: 0.05 mg/kg day 1

[total dose/cycle = 0.05 mg/kg]

Repeat for up to a total of 8 cycles

References

Rodriguez-Galindo C, Wilson MW, Haik BG, et al, "Treatment of Intraocular Retinoblastoma With Vincristine and Carboplatin," *J Clin Oncol*, 2003, 21(10):2019-25.

◆ **Carbo-Tax (Unknown Primary)** *see* Carboplatin-Paclitaxel (Unknown Primary, Adenocarcinoma) *on page 1873*

Carfilzomib, Lenalidomide, Dexamethasone (Multiple Myeloma)

Index Terms CRd (Multiple Myeloma); Lenalidomide, Carfilzomib, Dexamethasone (Multiple Myeloma)

Use Multiple myeloma (relapsed)

Regimen

Cycle 1:

Carfilzomib: IV: 20 mg/m²/day over 10 minutes days 1 and 2 (cycle 1)

followed by: 27 mg/m²/day over 10 minutes days 8, 9, 15, and 16 (cycle 1)

[total dose/cycle = 148 mg/m²]

Lenalidomide: Oral: 25 mg once daily days 1 to 21

[total dose/cycle = 525 mg]

Dexamethasone: Oral: 40 mg once daily on days 1, 8, 15, and 22

[total dose/cycle = 160 mg]

Treatment cycle duration is 28 days

Cycles 2 to 12:

Carfilzomib: IV: 27 mg/m²/day over 10 minutes days 1, 2, 8, 9, 15, and 16

[total dose/cycle = 162 mg/m²]

Lenalidomide: Oral: 25 mg once daily days 1 to 21

[total dose/cycle = 525 mg]

Dexamethasone: Oral: 40 mg once daily on days 1, 8, 15, and 22
  [total dose/cycle = 160 mg]
Treatment cycle duration is 28 days
Cycles 13 to 18:
  Carfilzomib: IV: 27 mg/m²/day over 10 minutes days 1, 2, 15, and 16
    [total dose/cycle = 108 mg/m²]
  Lenalidomide: Oral: 25 mg once daily days 1 to 21
    [total dose/cycle = 525 mg]
  Dexamethasone: Oral: 40 mg once daily on days 1, 8, 15, and 22
    [total dose/cycle = 160 mg]
  Treatment cycle duration is 28 days
Subsequent Cycles:
  Lenalidomide: Oral: 25 mg once daily days 1 to 21
    [total dose/cycle = 525 mg]
  Dexamethasone: Oral: 40 mg once daily on days 1, 8, 15, and 22
    [total dose/cycle = 160 mg]
  Repeat cycle every 28 days until disease progression or unacceptable toxicity

References

Stewart AK, Rajkumar SV, Dimopoulos MA, et al. Carfilzomib, lenalidomide, and dexamethasone for relapsed multiple myeloma. *N Engl J Med.* 2015;372(2):142-152.

Carfilzomib (Multiple Myeloma Regimen)

Use Multiple myeloma

Regimen
Cycle 1:
  Carfilzomib: IV: 20 mg/m²/day over 2-10 minutes days 1, 2, 8, 9, 15, and 16
    [total dose/cycle = 120 mg/m²]
  Treatment cycle is 28 days
Cycles 2-12:
  Carfilzomib: IV: 27 mg/m²/day over 2-10 minutes days 1, 2, 8, 9, 15, and 16
    [total dose/cycle = 162 mg/m²]
  Repeat cycle every 28 days

References

Siegel DS, Martin T, Wang M, et al, "A Phase 2 Study of Single-Agent Carfilzomib (PX-171-003-A01) in Patients With Relapsed and Refractory Multiple Myeloma," *Blood*, 2012, 120:2817-25.
Vij R, Wang M, Kaufman JL, et al, "An Open-Label, Single-Arm, Phase 2 (PX-171-004) Study of Single-Agent Carfilzomib in Bortezomib-Naïve Patients With Relapsed and/or Refractory Multiple Myeloma," *Blood*, 2012, 119:5661-70.

◆ **Carmustine-Etoposide-Cytarabine-Melphalan (Hodgkin)** *see* mini-BEAM (Hodgkin) *on page 2037*

CAV-P/VP (Neuroblastoma)

Index Terms Cyclophosphamide, Doxorubicin, Vincristine, Etoposide, Cisplatin (Neuroblastoma); N6 Protocol (Neuroblastoma)

Use Neuroblastoma

Regimen Note: The interval between courses is not fixed; the next course to begin upon hematologic recovery (ANC ≥500/mm³ and platelets ≥100,000/mm³)
Course 1, 2, 4, and 6 (CAV):
  Cyclophosphamide: IV: 70 mg/kg/day over 6 hours days 1 and 2
    [total dose/cycle = 140 mg/kg]
  Doxorubicin: IV: 25 mg/m²/day continuous infusion days 1, 2, and 3
    [total dose/cycle = 75 mg/m²]

Vincristine: IV: 0.033 mg/kg/day continuous infusion days 1, 2, and 3
  [total dose/cycle = 0.099 mg/kg]
Vincristine: IV: 1.5 mg/m² bolus day 9
  [total dose/cycle = 1.5 mg/m²]
Course 3, 5, and 7 (P/VP):
Etoposide: IV: 200 mg/m²/day over 2 hours days 1, 2, and 3
  [total dose/cycle = 600 mg/m²]
Cisplatin: IV: 50 mg/m²/day over 1 hour days 1 to 4
  [total dose/cycle = 200 mg/m²]

References

Kushner BH, LaQuaglia MP, Bonilla MA, et al, "Highly Effective Induction Therapy for Stage 4 Neuroblastoma in Children Over 1 Year of Age," *J Clin Oncol*, 1994, 12(12):2607-13.

CAV (Small Cell Lung Cancer)

Index Terms Cyclophosphamide, Doxorubicin, Vincristine (Small Cell Lung Cancer)

Use Lung cancer, small cell

Regimen

Cyclophosphamide: IV: 1000 mg/m² day 1
  [total dose/cycle = 1000 mg/m²; maximum: 2000 mg]
Doxorubicin: IV: 45 mg/m² day 1
  [total dose/cycle = 45 mg/m²; maximum: 100 mg]
Vincristine: IV: 2 mg day 1
  [total dose/cycle = 2 mg]
Repeat cycle every 21 days

References

von Pawel J, Schiller JH, Shephard FA, et al, "Topotecan Versus Cyclophosphamide, Doxorubicin, and Vincristine for the Treatment of Recurrent Small-Cell Lung Cancer," *J Clin Oncol*, 1999, 17 (2):658-67.

♦ 2-CDA-Rituximab (NHL-Mantle Cell) *see* Cladribine-Rituximab (NHL-Mantle Cell) *on page 1916*

CDDP/VP-16

Use Brain tumors

Regimen

Cisplatin: IV: 90 mg/m² day 1
  [total dose/cycle = 90 mg/m²]
Etoposide: IV: 150 mg/m²/day days 3 and 4
  [total dose/cycle = 300 mg/m²]
Repeat cycle every 21 days

References

Kovnar EH, Kellie SJ, Horowitz ME, et al, "Preirradiation Cisplatin and Etoposide in the Treatment of High-Risk Medulloblastoma and Other Malignant Embryonal Tumors of the Central Nervous System: A Phase II Study," *J Clin Oncol*, 1990, 8(2):330-6.

CE-CAdO (Neuroblastoma)

Index Terms Carboplatin, Etoposide, Cyclophosphamide, Doxorubicin, Vincristine (Neuroblastoma)

Use Neuroblastoma

◀ **Regimen**
Variation 1:
  Cycles 1 and 2 (CE):
    Carboplatin: IV: 200 mg/m²/day days 1, 2, and 3
      [total dose/cycle = 600 mg/m²]
    Etoposide: IV: 150 mg/m²/day days 1, 2, and 3
      [total dose/cycle = 450 mg/m²]
    Repeat CE cycle once at 21 days, then follow with
  Cycles 3 and 4 (CAdO):
    Cyclophosphamide: IV: 300 mg/m²/day days 1 to 5
      [total dose/cycle = 1500 mg/m²]
    Doxorubicin: IV: 60 mg/m² day 5
      [total dose/cycle = 60 mg/m²]
    Vincristine: IV: 1.5 mg/m² (maximum dose: 2 mg) days 1 and 5
      [total dose/cycle = 3 mg/m² (maximum: 2 mg/dose)]
    Repeat CAdO cycle once at 21 days
Variation 2:
  Cycles 1 and 2 (CE):
    Carboplatin: IV: 6.6 mg/kg/day days 1, 2, and 3
      [total dose/cycle = 19.8 mg/kg]
    Etoposide: IV: 5 mg/kg/day days 1, 2, and 3
      [total dose/cycle = 15 mg/kg]
    Repeat CE cycle once, then follow with
  Cycles 3 and 4 (CAdO):
    Cyclophosphamide: IV: 10 mg/kg/day days 1 to 5
      [total dose/cycle = 50 mg/kg]
    Doxorubicin: IV: 2 mg/kg day 5
      [total dose/cycle = 2 mg/kg]
    Vincristine: IV: 0.05 mg/kg days 1 and 5
      [total dose/cycle = 0.1 mg/kg]
    Repeat CAdO cycle once

References
Variation 1:
Rubie H, Michon J, Plantaz D, et al, "Unresectable Localized Neuroblastoma: Improved Survival After Primary Chemotherapy Including Carboplatin-Etoposide. Neuroblastoma Study Group of the Societe Francaise d'Oncologie Pediatrique (SFOP)," *Br J Cancer*, 1998, 77(12):2310-7.
Variation 2:
Rubie H, Plantaz D, Coze C, et al, "Localised and Unresectable Neuroblastoma in Infants: Excellent Outcome With Primary Chemotherapy. Neuroblastoma Study Group, Société Française d'Oncologie Pédiatrique," *Med Pediatr Oncol*, 2001, 36(1):247-50.

CEPP (NHL-DLBCL)

Index Terms Cyclophosphamide-Etoposide-Procarbazine-Prednisone (NHL-DLBCL)

Use Lymphoma, non-Hodgkin (DLBCL)

Regimen
Cyclophosphamide: IV: 600 to 650 mg/m²/day days 1 and 8
  [total dose/cycle = 1,200 to 1,300 mg/m²]
Etoposide: IV: 70 to 85 mg/m²/day days 1, 2, and 3
  [total dose/cycle = 210 to 255 mg/m²]
Procarbazine: Oral: 60 mg/m²/day days 1 to 10
  [total dose/cycle = 600 mg/m²]
Prednisone: Oral: 60 mg/m²/day days 1 to 10
  [total dose/cycle = 600 mg/m²]
Repeat cycle every 28 days

References

Chao NJ, Rosenberg SA, Horning SJ. CEPP(B): an effective and well-tolerated regimen in poor-risk, aggressive non-Hodgkin's lymphoma. *Blood*. 1990;76(7):1293-1298.

Ceritinib (NSCLC Regimen)

Use Lung cancer, non-small cell (ALK-positive, metastatic)

Regimen

Ceritinib: Oral: 750 mg once daily on empty stomach (at least 2 hours before or 2 hours after a meal)

[total dose/cycle = 21,000 mg]

Repeat cycle every 28 days until disease progression or unacceptable toxicity

References

Shaw AT, Kim DW, Mehra R, et al. Ceritinib in ALK-rearranged non-small-cell lung cancer. *N Engl J Med*. 2014;370(13):1189-1197.

Cetuximab Biweekly (Colorectal Regimen)

Index Terms Biweekly Cetuximab (Colorectal Regimen); Every 2 Weeks Cetuximab (Colorectal Regimen)

Use Colorectal cancer

Regimen

Cetuximab: IV: 500 mg/m² day 1; over 120 minutes for the first infusion, and over 60 minutes for subsequent infusions

[total dose/cycle = 500 mg/m²]

Repeat cycle every 14 days until disease progression or unacceptable toxicity

References

Bouchahda M, Marcarulla T, Liedo G, et al, "Feasibility of Cetuximab Given With a Simplified Schedule of Every 2 Weeks in Advanced Colorectal Cancer: A Multicenter, Retrospective Analysis," *Med Oncol*, 2011, 28(Suppl 1):S253-8.

Tabernero J, Pfeiffer P, and Cervantes A, "Administration of Cetuximab Every 2 Weeks in the Treatment of Metastatic Colorectal Cancer: An Effective, More Convenient, Alternative to Weekly Administration," *Oncologist*, 2008, 13(2):113-9.

Cetuximab (Biweekly)-Irinotecan (Colorectal)

Index Terms Biweekly CetIri (Colorectal); Every 2 Weeks Cetuximab – Irinotecan (Colorectal); Irinotecan-Biweekly Cetuximab (Colorectal)

Use Colorectal cancer

Regimen

Cycle 1:

Cetuximab: IV: 500 mg/m² over 120 minutes day 1 cycle 1

[total dose/cycle 1 = 500 mg/m²]

Irinotecan: IV: 180 mg/m² over 30 minutes day 1 cycle 1

[total dose/cycle 1 = 180 mg/m²]

Treatment cycle is 14 days

Subsequent cycles:

Cetuximab: IV: 500 mg/m² over 60 minutes day 1

[total dose/cycle = 500 mg/m²]

Irinotecan: IV: 180 mg/m² over 30 minutes day 1

[total dose/cycle = 180 mg/m²]

Repeat cycle every 14 days until disease progression or unacceptable toxicity

◀ **References**

Martín-Martorell P, Roselló S, Rodríguez-Braun E, et al, "Biweekly Cetuximab and Irinotecan in Advanced Colorectal Cancer Patients Progressing After at Least One Previous Line of Chemotherapy: Results of a Phase II Single Institution Trial," *Br J Cancer*, 2008, 99(3):455-8.

Pfeiffer P, Nielsen D, Bjerregaard J, et al, "Biweekly Cetuximab and Irinotecan as Third-Line Therapy in Patients With Advanced Colorectal Cancer After Failure to Irinotecan, Oxaliplatin and 5-Fluorouracil," *Ann Oncol*, 2008, 19(6):1141-5.

Cetuximab-Carboplatin-Fluorouracil (Head and Neck Cancer)

Index Terms Carboplatin-Fluorouracil-Cetuximab (Head and Neck Cancer)

Use Head and neck cancer

Regimen

Cycle 1:

Cetuximab: IV: 400 mg/m^2 (loading dose) day 1 (week 1, cycle 1 only)
[total loading dose = 400 mg/m^2]
followed by IV: 250 mg/m^2/day days 8 and 15
[total dose/cycle 1 = 900 mg/m^2]

Carboplatin: IV: AUC 5 day 1
[total dose/cycle = AUC = 5]

Fluorouracil: IV: 1000 mg/m^2/day continuous infusion days 1 to 4
[total dose/cycle = 4000 mg/m^2]

Treatment cycle is 3 weeks

Subsequent cycles:

Cetuximab: IV: 250 mg/m^2/day days 1, 8, and 15
[total dose/cycle = 750 mg/m^2]

Carboplatin: IV: AUC 5 day 1
[total dose/cycle = AUC = 5]

Fluorouracil: IV: 1000 mg/m^2/day continuous infusion days 1 to 4
[total dose/cycle = 4000 mg/m^2]

Repeat cycle every 3 weeks for a total of up to 6 cycles (cetuximab monotherapy may be continued thereafter until disease progression or unacceptable toxicity)

References

Vermorken JB, Mesia R, Rivera F, et al, "Platinum-Based Chemotherapy Plus Cetuximab in Head and Neck Cancer," *N Engl J Med*, 2008, 359(11):1116-27.

♦ **Cetuximab-Carboplatin (Head and Neck Cancer)** *see* Carboplatin-Cetuximab (Head and Neck Cancer) *on page 1861*

Cetuximab-Cisplatin-Fluorouracil (Head and Neck Cancer)

Index Terms Cisplatin-Fluorouracil-Cetuximab (Head and Neck Cancer)

Use Head and neck cancer

Regimen

Cycle 1:

Cetuximab: IV: 400 mg/m^2 (loading dose) day 1 (week 1, cycle 1 only)
[total loading dose = 400 mg/m^2]
followed by IV: 250 mg/m^2/day days 8 and 15
[total dose/cycle 1 = 900 mg/m^2]

Cisplatin: IV: 100 mg/m^2 day 1
[total dose/cycle = 100 mg/m^2]

Fluorouracil: IV: 1000 mg/m^2/day continuous infusion days 1 to 4
[total dose/cycle = 4000 mg/m^2]
Treatment cycle is 3 weeks
Subsequent cycles:
Cetuximab: IV: 250 mg/m^2/day days 1, 8, and 15
[total dose/cycle = 750 mg/m^2]
Cisplatin: IV: 100 mg/m^2 day 1
[total dose/cycle = 100 mg/m^2]
Fluorouracil: IV: 1000 mg/m^2/day continuous infusion days 1 to 4
[total dose/cycle = 4000 mg/m^2]
Repeat cycle every 3 weeks for a total of up to 6 cycles (cetuximab monotherapy may be continued thereafter until disease progression or unacceptable toxicity)

References

Vermorken JB, Mesia R, Rivera F, et al, "Platinum-Based Chemotherapy Plus Cetuximab in Head and Neck Cancer," *N Engl J Med*, 2008, 359(11):1116-27.

◆ **Cetuximab-Cisplatin (Head and Neck Cancer)** *see* Cisplatin-Cetuximab (Head and Neck Cancer) *on page 1889*

Cetuximab-Cisplatin-Vinorelbine (NSCLC)

Index Terms Cisplatin-Vinorelbine-Cetuximab (NSCLC)
Use Lung cancer, non-small cell
Regimen
Cycle 1:
Cetuximab: IV: 400 mg/m^2 (loading dose) over 2 hours day 1 (week 1, cycle 1 only)
[total loading dose = 400 mg/m^2]
followed by IV: 250 mg/m^2/day over 1 hour days 8 and 15
[total dose/cycle 1 = 900 mg/m^2]
Cisplatin: IV: 80 mg/m^2 day 1
[total dose/cycle = 80 mg/m^2]
Vinorelbine: IV: 25 mg/m^2/day days 1 and 8
[total dose/cycle = 50 mg/m^2]
Treatment cycle is 21 days
Cycles 2-6:
Cetuximab: IV: 250 mg/m^2/day over 1 hour days 1, 8, and 15
[total dose/cycle = 750 mg/m^2]
Cisplatin: IV: 80 mg/m^2 day 1
[total dose/cycle = 80 mg/m^2]
Vinorelbine: IV: 25 mg/m^2/day days 1 and 8
[total dose/cycle = 50 mg/m^2]
Repeat cycle every 21 days for a maximum of 6 cycles
followed by
Cetuximab: IV: 250 mg/m^2/day over 1 hour days 1, 8, and 15
[total dose/cycle = 750 mg/m^2]
Repeat cycle every 21 days until disease progression or unacceptable toxicity

References

Pirker R, Pereira JR, Szczesna A, et al, "Cetuximab Plus Chemotherapy in Patients With Advanced Non-Small-Cell Lung Cancer (FLEX): An Open-Label Randomised Phase III Trial," *Lancet*, 2009, 373(9674):1525-31.

Pirker R, Pereira JR, von Pawel J, et al, "EGFR Expression as a Predictor of Survival for First-Line Chemotherapy Plus Cetuximab in Patients With Advanced Non-Small-Cell Lung Cancer: Analysis of Data From the Phase 3 FLEX Study," *Lancet Oncol*, 2012, 13(1):33-42.

Cetuximab (Colorectal Regimen)

Use Colorectal cancer

Regimen

Cycle 1:

Cetuximab: IV: 400 mg/m^2 (loading dose) over 120 minutes day 1 (week 1, cycle 1 only)

followed by IV: 250 mg/m^2/day over 60 minutes days 8, 15, and 22 (cycle 1)

[total dose/cycle 1 = 1150 mg/m^2]

Treatment cycle is 28 days

Subsequent cycles:

Cetuximab: IV: 250 mg/m^2/day over 60 minutes days 1, 8, 15, and 22

[total dose/cycle = 1000 mg/m^2]

Repeat cycle every 28 days until disease progression or unacceptable toxicity

References

Cunningham D, Humblet Y, Siena S, et al, "Cetuximab Monotherapy and Cetuximab Plus Irinotecan in Irinotecan-Refractory Metastatic Colorectal Cancer," *N Engl J Med*, 2004, 351 (4):337-45.

Jonker DJ, O'Callaghan CJ, Karapetis CS, "Cetuximab for the Treatment of Colorectal Cancer," *N Engl J Med*, 2007, 357(20):2040-8.

Karapetis CS, Khambata-Ford S, Jonker DJ, et al, "K-ras Mutations and Benefit From Cetuximab in Advanced Colorectal Cancer," *N Engl J Med*, 2008, 359(17):1757-65.

Cetuximab + FOLFIRI (Colorectal)

Index Terms Cetuximab, Irinotecan, Leucovorin, Fluorouracil (Colorectal)

Use Colorectal cancer

Regimen

Cycle 1:

Cetuximab: IV: 400 mg/m^2 (loading dose) over 120 minutes day 1 (week 1, cycle 1 only)

followed by IV: 250 mg/m^2/day over 60 minutes day 8

[total dose/cycle 1 = 650 mg/m^2]

Irinotecan: IV: 180 mg/m^2 over 30-90 minutes day 1

[total dose/cycle = 180 mg/m^2]

Leucovorin (racemic): IV: 400 mg/m^2 over 120 minutes day 1

[total dose/cycle = 400 mg/m^2]

Fluorouracil: IV bolus: 400 mg/m^2 day 1

followed by IV: 2400 mg/m^2 continuous infusion (CI) over 46 hours beginning day 1

[total fluorouracil dose/cycle (bolus and CI) = 2800 mg/m^2]

Treatment cycle is 14 days

Subsequent cycles:

Cetuximab: IV: 250 mg/m^2/day over 60 minutes days 1 and 8

[total dose/cycle = 500 mg/m^2]

Irinotecan: IV: 180 mg/m^2 over 30-90 minutes day 1

[total dose/cycle = 180 mg/m^2]

Leucovorin (racemic): IV: 400 mg/m^2 over 120 minutes day 1

[total dose/cycle = 400 mg/m^2]

Fluorouracil: IV bolus: 400 mg/m^2 day 1

followed by IV: 2400 mg/m^2 CI over 46 hours beginning day 1

[total fluorouracil dose/cycle (bolus and CI) = 2800 mg/m^2]

Repeat cycle every 14 days until disease progression or unacceptable toxicity

References

Van Custem E, Köhne CH, Hitre E, et al, "Cetuximab and Chemotherapy as Initial Treatment for Metastatic Colorectal Cancer," *N Engl J Med*, 2009, 360(14):1408-17.

Van Custem E, Köhne CH, Láng I, et al, "Cetuximab Plus Irinotecan, Fluorouracil, and Leucovorin as First-Line Treatment for Metastatic Colorectal Cancer: Updated Analysis of Overall Survival According to Tumor KRAS and BRAF Mutation Status," *J Clin Oncol*, 2011, 29(15):2011-9.

Cetuximab-Irinotecan (Colorectal)

Index Terms Irinotecan-Cetuximab

Use Colorectal cancer

Regimen NOTE: Multiple variations are listed.

Variation 1:

Cycle 1:

Cetuximab: IV: 400 mg/m^2 (loading dose) day 1 (week 1, cycle 1 only)
followed by IV: 250 mg/m^2/day days 8, 15, 22, 29, and 36
[total dose/cycle 1 = 1650 mg/m^2]

Irinotecan: IV: 125 mg/m^2/day days 1, 8, 15, and 22
[total dose/cycle = 500 mg/m^2]

Treatment cycle is 42 days (6 weeks)

Subsequent cycles:

Cetuximab: IV: 250 mg/m^2/day days 1, 8, 15, 22, 29, and 36
[total dose/cycle = 1500 mg/m^2]

Irinotecan: IV: 125 mg/m^2/day days 1, 8, 15, and 22
[total dose/cycle = 500 mg/m^2]

Repeat cycle every 42 days (6 weeks) until disease progression or unacceptable toxicity

Variation 2:

Cycle 1:

Cetuximab: IV: 400 mg/m^2 (loading dose) day 1 (week 1, cycle 1 only)
followed by IV: 250 mg/m^2/day days 8 and 15
[total dose/cycle 1 = 900 mg/m^2]

Irinotecan: IV: 350 mg/m^2 day 1
[total dose/cycle = 350 mg/m^2]

Treatment cycle is 21 days

Subsequent cycles:

Cetuximab: IV: 250 mg/m^2/day days 1, 8, and 15
[total dose/cycle = 750 mg/m^2]

Irinotecan: IV: 350 mg/m^2 day 1
[total dose/cycle = 350 mg/m^2]

Repeat cycle every 21 days until disease progression or unacceptable toxicity

References

Variation 1 and 2:

Cunningham D, Humblet Y, Siena S, et al, "Cetuximab Monotherapy and Cetuximab Plus Irinotecan in Irinotecan-Refractory Metastatic Colorectal Cancer," *N Engl J Med*, 2004, 351 (4):337-45.

Variation 2:

Sobrero AF, Maurel J, Fehrenbacher L, et al, "EPIC: Phase III Trial of Cetuximab Plus Irinotecan After Fluoropyrimidine and Oxaliplatin Failure in Patients With Metastatic Colorectal Cancer," *J Clin Oncol*, 2008, 26(14):2311-9.

♦ **Cetuximab, Irinotecan, Leucovorin, Fluorouracil (Colorectal)** *see* Cetuximab + FOLFIRI (Colorectal) *on page 1882*

♦ **Cetuximab-Paclitaxel** *see* Paclitaxel-Cetuximab *on page 2050*

Cetuximab (Squamous Cell Regimen)

Use Squamous cell carcinoma

Regimen

Cycle 1:

Cetuximab: IV: 400 mg/m^2 (loading dose) day 1 cycle 1 only

followed by IV: 250 mg/m^2/day over 60 minutes days 8, 15, 22, 29, and 36 cycle 1

[total dose/cycle 1 = 1650 mg/m^2]

Treatment cycle is 42 days

Subsequent cycles:

Cetuximab: IV: 250 mg/m^2/day over 60 minutes days 1, 8, 15, 22, 29, and 36

[total dose/cycle = 1500 mg/m^2]

Repeat cycle every 42 days

References

Maubec E, Petrow P, Scheer-Senyarich I, et al, "Phase II Study of Cetuximab as First-Line Single-Drug Therapy in Patients With Unresectable Squamous Cell Carcinoma of the Skin," *J Clin Oncol,* 2011, 29(25):3419-26.

◆ **CF (Esophageal Cancer)** *see* Cisplatin-Fluorouracil (Esophageal Cancer) *on page 1897*

◆ **CF (Gastric Cancer)** *see* Cisplatin-Fluorouracil (Gastric Cancer) *on page 1899*

◆ **CF (Head and Neck Cancer)** *see* Cisplatin-Fluorouracil (Head and Neck Cancer) *on page 1900*

◆ **CF (NHL-Mantle Cell)** *see* Fludarabine-Cyclophosphamide (NHL-Mantle Cell) *on page 1973*

Chlorambucil (CLL Regimen)

Use Leukemia, chronic lymphocytic

Regimen NOTE: Multiple variations are listed.

Variation 1:

Chlorambucil: Oral: 0.4 mg/kg day 1 (may increase by 0.1 mg/kg with each treatment course to a maximum dose of 0.8 mg/kg)

[total dose/cycle = 0.4-0.8 mg/kg]

Repeat cycle every 14 days for a maximum of 24 cycles

Variation 2:

Chlorambucil: Oral: 40 mg/m^2 day 1

[total dose/cycle = 40 mg/m^2]

Repeat cycle every 28 days for a maximum of 12 cycles

References

Variation 1:
Eichhorst BF, Busch R, Stilgenbauer S, et al, "First-Line Therapy With Fludarabine Compared With Chlorambucil Does Not Result in a Major Benefit for Elderly Patients With Advanced Chronic Lymphocytic Leukemia," *Blood,* 2009, 114(16):3382-91.
Variation 2:
Rai KR, Peterson BL, Appelbaum FR, et al, "Fludarabine Compared With Chlorambucil as Primary Therapy for Chronic Lymphocytic Leukemia," *N Engl J Med,* 2000, 343(24):1750-7.

Chlorambucil-Obinutuzumab (CLL)

Index Terms Obinutuzumab-Chlorambucil (CLL)

Use Leukemia, chronic lymphocytic

Regimen

Cycle 1:

Obinutuzumab: IV: 100 mg day 1, followed by 900 mg day 2, followed by 1,000 mg days 8 and 15

[total dose/cycle = 3,000 mg]

Chlorambucil: Oral: 0.5 mg/kg/day days 1 and 15

[total dose/cycle = 1 mg/kg]

Treatment cycle duration is 28 days

Cycles 2 to 6:

Obinutuzumab: IV: 1,000 mg day 1

[total dose/cycle = 1,000 mg]

Chlorambucil: Oral: 0.5 mg/kg/day days 1 and 15

[total dose/cycle = 1 mg/kg]

Repeat cycle every 28 days for a total of 6 cycles

References

Gazyva (obinutuzumab) [prescribing information]. South San Francisco, CA: Genentech Inc; December 2014.

Goede V, Fischer K, Busch R, et al. Obinutuzumab plus chlorambucil in patients with CLL and coexisting conditions. *N Engl J Med*. 2014;370(12):1101-1110.

Chlorambucil-Ofatumumab (CLL)

Index Terms O + CHL (CLL); Ofatumumab-Chlorambucil (CLL)

Use Leukemia, chronic lymphocytic

Regimen

Cycle 1:

Chlorambucil: Oral: 10 mg/m^2 days 1 to 7

[total dose/cycle = 70 mg/m^2]

Ofatumumab: IV: 300 mg day 1

followed by:

Ofatumumab: IV: 1000 mg day 8

[total dose/cycle 1 = 1300 mg]

Treatment cycle is 28 days

Cycle 2 to 12:

Chlorambucil: Oral: 10 mg/m^2 days 1 to 7

[total dose/cycle = 70 mg/m^2]

Ofatumumab: IV: 1000 mg day 1

[total dose/cycle = 1000 mg]

Repeat cycle every 28 days for a minimum of 3 cycles and a maximum of 12 cycles

References

Hillmen P, Robak T, Janssens A, et al. Ofatumumab + chlorambucil versus chlorambucil alone in patients with untreated chronic lymphocytic leukemia (CLL): results of the phase III study complement 1 (OMB110911) [published online December 6, 2013]. *Blood*.

Chlorambucil-Prednisone (CLL)

Index Terms Prednisone–Chlorambucil (CLL)

Use Leukemia, chronic lymphocytic

◀ **Regimen**

Chlorambucil: Oral: 30 mg/m^2 day 1

[total dose/cycle = 30 mg/m^2]

Prednisone: Oral: 80 mg/day days 1 to 5

[total dose/cycle = 400 mg]

Repeat cycle every 14 days until disease progression for a maximum duration of 9 months (if no response at 9 months), 15 months (if complete response at 9 months), or 18 months (if partial response at 9 months)

References

Raphael B, Anderson JW, Silber R, et al, "Comparison of Chlorambucil and Prednisone Versus Cyclophosphamide, Vincristine, and Prednisone as Initial Treatment for Chronic Lymphocytic Leukemia: Long-Term Follow-up of an Eastern Cooperative Oncology Group Randomized Clinical Trial," *J Clin Oncol*, 1991, 9(5):770-6.

♦ **Chlorambucil, Vinblastine, Procarbazine, Prednisolone (Hodgkin)** *see* ChlVPP (Hodgkin) *on page 1886*

♦ **Chlorambucil, Vinblastine, Procarbazine, Prednisone (Hodgkin)** *see* ChlVPP (Hodgkin) *on page 1886*

♦ **2-chloro-2'-deoxyadenosine-Rituximab (Waldenstrom Macroglobuline-mia)** *see* Cladribine-Rituximab (Waldenstrom Macroglobulinemia) *on page 1916*

♦ **CHLVPP (Hodgkin)** *see* ChlVPP (Hodgkin) *on page 1886*

ChlVPP (Hodgkin)

Index Terms Chlorambucil, Vinblastine, Procarbazine, Prednisolone (Hodgkin); Chlorambucil, Vinblastine, Procarbazine, Prednisone (Hodgkin); CHLVPP (Hodgkin)

Use Lymphoma, Hodgkin

Regimen NOTE: Multiple variations are listed.

Variation 1:

Chlorambucil: Oral: 6 mg/m^2/day (maximum dose: 10 mg/day) days 1 to 14

[total dose/cycle = 84 mg/m^2; maximum: 140 mg/cycle]

Vinblastine: IV: 6 mg/m^2/day (maximum dose: 10 mg/dose) days 1 and 8

[total dose/cycle = 12 mg/m^2; maximum: 20 mg/cycle]

Procarbazine: Oral: 100 mg/m^2/day (maximum dose: 150 mg/day) days 1 to 14

[total dose/cycle = 1400 mg/m^2; maximum: 2100 mg/cycle]

Prednisone or Prednisolone: Oral: 40 mg/day days 1 to 14

[total dose/cycle = 560 mg]

Repeat cycle every 28 days to complete remission plus 2 cycles; minimum of 6 cycles, maximum of 8 cycles

Variation 2:

Chlorambucil: Oral: 6 mg/m^2/day days 1 to 14

[total dose/cycle = 84 mg/m^2]

Vinblastine: IV: 6 mg/m^2/day days 1 and 8

[total dose/cycle = 12 mg/m^2]

Procarbazine: Oral: 100 mg/m^2/day days 1 to 14

[total dose/cycle = 1400 mg/m^2]

Prednisone: Oral: 40 mg/day days 1 to 14

[total dose/cycle = 560 mg]

Repeat cycle every 28 days for 6 cycles

References

Variation 1:

The International ChIVPP Treatment Group, "ChIVPP Therapy for Hodgkin's Disease: Experience of 960 Patients," *Ann Oncol*, 1995, 6(2):167-72.

Selby P, Patel P, Milan S, et al, "ChIVPP Combination Chemotherapy for Hodgkin's Disease: Long-Term Results," *Br J Cancer*, 1990, 62(2):279-85.

Variation 2:

Vose JM, Bierman PJ, Anderson JR, et al, "CHLVPP Chemotherapy With Involved-Field Irradiation for Hodgkin's Disease: Favorable Results With Acceptable Toxicity," *J Clin Oncol*, 1991, 9 (8):1421-5.

CHOP (NHL)

Use Lymphoma, non-Hodgkin

Regimen NOTE: Multiple variations are listed.

Variation 1:

Cyclophosphamide: IV: 750 mg/m^2 day 1
  [total dose/cycle = 750 mg/m^2]
Doxorubicin: IV: 50 mg/m^2 day 1
  [total dose/cycle = 50 mg/m^2]
Vincristine: IV: 1.4 mg/m^2 (maximum dose: 2 mg) day 1
  [total dose/cycle = 1.4 mg/m^2; maximum: 2 mg]
Prednisone: Oral: 100 mg/day days 1 to 5
  [total dose/cycle = 500 mg]
Repeat cycle every 21 days for 6 to 8 cycles

Variation 2 (dose intensity/dose-dense):

Cyclophosphamide: IV: 1600 mg/m^2 day 1
  [total dose/cycle = 1600 mg/m^2]
Doxorubicin: IV: 65 mg/m^2 day 1
  [total dose/cycle = 65 mg/m^2]
Vincristine: IV: 1.4 mg/m^2 day 1
  [total dose/cycle = 1.4 mg/m^2]
Prednisone: Oral: 100 mg/day days 1 to 5
  [total dose/cycle = 500 mg]
Filgrastim: SubQ: 5 mcg/kg days 2 to 11 or until ANC >10,000/mm^3
Repeat cycle every 14 days for 6 cycles

Variation 3 (dose-dense):

Cyclophosphamide: IV: 750 mg/m^2 day 1
  [total dose/cycle = 750 mg/m^2]
Doxorubicin: IV: 50 mg/m^2 day 1
  [total dose/cycle = 50 mg/m^2]
Vincristine: IV: 2 mg day 1
  [total dose/cycle = 2 mg]
Prednisone: Oral: 100 mg/day days 1 to 5
  [total dose/cycle = 500 mg]
Filgrastim: SubQ: 300 mcg/day (<75 kg patient) or 480 mcg/day (≥75 kg patient) days 4 to 13
Repeat cycle every 14 days for 6 cycles

Variation 4 (localized disease; chemotherapy plus radiotherapy):

Cyclophosphamide: IV: 750 mg/m^2 day 1
  [total dose/cycle = 750 mg/m^2]
Doxorubicin: IV: 50 mg/m^2 day 1
  [total dose/cycle = 50 mg/m^2]
Vincristine: IV: 1.4 mg/m^2 (maximum dose: 2 mg) day 1
  [total dose/cycle = 1.4 mg/m^2; maximum: 2 mg]

◀ Prednisone: Oral: 100 mg/day days 1 to 5
    [total dose/cycle = 500 mg]
Repeat cycle every 21 days for 3 cycles followed by radiation therapy
Variation 5 (HIV-associated NHL):
Cyclophosphamide: IV: 750 mg/m^2 day 1
    [total dose/cycle = 750 mg/m^2]
Doxorubicin: IV: 50 mg/m^2 day 1
    [total dose/cycle = 50 mg/m^2]
Vincristine: IV: 1.4 mg/m^2 (maximum dose: 2 mg) day 1
    [total dose/cycle = 1.4 mg/m^2; maximum: 2 mg]
Prednisone: Oral: 100 mg/day 1 to 5
    [total dose/cycle = 500 mg]
Filgrastim: SubQ: 300 mcg/day (<70 kg patient) or 480 mcg/day (>70 kg patient) days 4 to 13
Repeat cycle every 21 days; minimum of 4 cycles or 2 cycles beyond complete remission

References
Variation 1:
Fisher RI, Gaynor ER, Dahlberg S, et al, "Comparison of a Standard Regimen (CHOP) With Three Intensive Chemotherapy Regimens for Advanced Non-Hodgkin's Lymphoma," *N Engl J Med*, 1993,328(14):1002-6.

McKelvey EM, Gottlieb JA, Wilson HE, et al, "Hydroxyldaunomycin (Adriamycin®) Combination Chemotherapy in Malignant Lymphoma," *Cancer*, 1976, 38(4):1484-93.

van Oers MH, Klasa R, Marcus RE, et al, "Rituximab Maintenance Improves Clinical Outcome of Relapsed/Resistant Follicular Non-Hodgkin's Lymphoma in Patients Both With and Without Rituximab During Induction: Results of a Prospective Randomized Phase 3 Intergroup Trial," *Blood*, 2006, 108(10):3295-301.

Variation 2:
Blayney DW, LeBlanc ML, Grogan T, et al, "Dose-Intense Chemotherapy Every 2 Weeks With Dose-Intense Cyclophosphamide, Doxorubicin, Vincristine, and Prednisone May Improve Survival in Intermediate- and High-Grade Lymphoma: A Phase II Study of the Southwest Oncology Group (SWOG 9349)," *J Clin Oncol*, 2003, 21(13): 2466-73.

Variation 3:
Pfreundschuh M, Trümper L, Kloess M, et al, "Two-Weekly or 3-Weekly CHOP Chemotherapy With or Without Etoposide for the Treatment of Elderly Patients With Aggressive Lymphomas: Results of the NHL-B2 Trial of the DSHNHL," *Blood*, 2004, 104(3):634-41.

Variation 4:
Miller TP, Dahlberg S, Cassady JR, et al, "Chemotherapy Alone Compared With Chemotherapy Plus Radiotherapy for Localized Intermediate- and High-Grade Non-Hodgkin's Lymphoma," *N Engl J Med*, 1998, 339(1):21-6.

Variation 5:
Ratner L, Lee J, Tang S, et al, "Chemotherapy for Human Immunodeficiency Virus-Associated Non-Hodgkin's Lymphoma in Combination With Highly Active Antiretroviral Therapy," *J Clin Oncol*, 2001, 19(8):2171-8.

◆ **CHOP-Rituximab (NHL)** *see* Rituximab-CHOP (NHL) *on page 2077*

◆ **Cisplatin-5FU (Cervical Cancer)** *see* Cisplatin-Fluorouracil (Cervical Cancer) *on page 1897*

Cisplatin (Breast Regimen)
Use Breast cancer
Regimen NOTE: Multiple variations are listed.
Variation 1 (metastatic triple negative):
Cisplatin: IV: 75 mg/m^2 day 1
    [total dose/cycle = 75 mg/m^2]
Repeat cycle every 21-28 days

Variation 2 (neoadjuvant triple-negative):

Cisplatin: IV: 75 mg/m^2 day 1

[total dose/cycle = 75 mg/m^2]

Repeat cycle every 21 days for up to 4 cycles

References

Variation 1:

Isakoff SJ, Goss PE, Mayer EL, et al, "TBCR009: A Multicenter Phase II Study of Cisplatin or Carboplatin for Metastatic Triple-Negative Breast Cancer and Evaluation of p63/p73 as a Biomarker of Response," *J Clin Oncol*, 2011, 29(15S):1025 [abstract 1025 from 2011 annual ASCO meeting].

Variation 2:

Silver DP, Richardson AL, Eklund AC, et al, "Efficacy of Neoadjuvant Cisplatin in Triple-Negative Breast Cancer," *J Clin Oncol*, 2010, 28(7):1145-53.

◆ **Cisplatin-Capecitabine-Epirubicin (Gastric/Esophageal)** *see* Epirubicin-Cisplatin-Capecitabine (Gastric/Esophageal) *on page 1956*

Cisplatin-Capecitabine (Esophageal Cancer)

Index Terms Capecitabine-Cisplatin (Esophageal Cancer)

Use Esophageal cancer

Regimen

Cisplatin: IV: 80 mg/m^2 over 2 hours day 1

[total dose/cycle = 80 mg/m^2]

Capecitabine: Oral: 1000 mg/m^2/dose twice daily, days 1 to 14

[total dose/cycle = 28,000 mg/m^2]

Repeat cycle every 3 weeks until disease progression or unacceptable toxicity

References

Kang YK, Kang WK, Shin DB, et al, "Capecitabine/Cisplatin Versus 5-Fluorouracil/Cisplatin as First-Line Therapy in Patients With Advanced Gastric Cancer: A Randomised Phase III Non-inferiority Trial," *Ann Oncol*, 2009, 20(4):666-73.

Cisplatin-Capecitabine (Gastric Cancer)

Index Terms Capecitabine-Cisplatin (Gastric Cancer)

Use Gastric cancer

Regimen

Cisplatin: IV: 80 mg/m^2 over 2 hours day 1

[total dose/cycle = 80 mg/m^2]

Capecitabine: Oral: 1000 mg/m^2/dose twice daily, days 1 to 14

[total dose/cycle = 28,000 mg/m^2]

Repeat cycle every 3 weeks until disease progression or unacceptable toxicity

References

Kang YK, Kang WK, Shin DB, et al, "Capecitabine/Cisplatin Versus 5-Fluorouracil/Cisplatin as First-Line Therapy in Patients With Advanced Gastric Cancer: A Randomised Phase III Non-inferiority Trial," *Ann Oncol*, 2009, 20(4):666-73.

◆ **Cisplatin-Capecitabine-Trastuzumab (Gastric Cancer)** *see* Trastuzumab-Cisplatin-Capecitabine (Gastric Cancer) *on page 2093*

Cisplatin-Cetuximab (Head and Neck Cancer)

Index Terms Cetuximab-Cisplatin (Head and Neck Cancer)

Use Head and neck cancer

◄ **Regimen** NOTE: Multiple variations are listed.

Variation 1:

Cycle 1:

Cetuximab: IV: 400 mg/m^2 (loading dose) day 1 (week 1, cycle 1 only)

[total loading dose = 400 mg/m^2]

followed by IV: 250 mg/m^2/day days 8, 15, and 22

[total dose/cycle 1 = 1150 mg/m^2]

Cisplatin: IV: 100 mg/m^2 day 1

[total dose/cycle = 100 mg/m^2]

Treatment cycle is 4 weeks

Subsequent cycles:

Cetuximab: IV: 250 mg/m^2/day days 1, 8, 15, and 22

[total dose/cycle = 1000 mg/m^2]

Cisplatin: IV: 100 mg/m^2 day 1

[total dose/cycle = 100 mg/m^2]

Repeat cycle every 4 weeks

Variation 2:

Cycle 1:

Cetuximab: IV: 400 mg/m^2 (loading dose) day 1 (week 1, cycle 1 only)

[total loading dose = 400 mg/m^2]

followed by IV: 250 mg/m^2/day days 8 and 15

[total dose/cycle 1 = 900 mg/m^2]

Cisplatin: IV: 75-100 mg/m^2 day 1

[total dose/cycle = 75-100 mg/m^2]

Treatment cycle is 3 weeks

Subsequent cycles:

Cetuximab: IV: 250 mg/m^2/day days 1, 8, and 15

[total dose/cycle = 750 mg/m^2]

Cisplatin: IV: 75-100 mg/m^2 day 1

[total dose/cycle = 75-100 mg/m^2]

Repeat cycle every 3 weeks

References

Variation 1:

Burtness B, Goldwasser MA, Flood W, et al, "Phase III Randomized Trial of Cisplatin Plus Placebo Compared With Cisplatin Plus Cetuximab in Metastatic/Recurrent Head and Neck Cancer: An Eastern Cooperative Oncology Group Study," *J Clin Oncol*, 2005, 23(34):8646-54.

Variation 2:

Herbst RS, Arquette M, Shin DM, et al, "Phase II Multicenter Study of the Epidermal Growth Factor Receptor Antibody Cetuximab and Cisplatin for Recurrent and Refractory Aquamous Cell Carcinoma of the Head and Neck," *J Clin Oncol*, 2005, 23(24):5578-87.

Cisplatin-Docetaxel-Fluorouracil (Unknown Primary, Squamous Cell)

Index Terms Fluorouracil-Cisplatin-Docetaxel (Unknown Primary); TPF (Unknown Primary)

Use Unknown primary (squamous cell)

Regimen

Docetaxel: IV: 75 mg/m^2 day 1
[total dose/cycle = 75 mg/m^2]
Cisplatin: IV: 75 mg/m^2 day 1
[total dose/cycle = 75 mg/m^2]
Fluorouracil: IV: 750 mg/m^2/day continuous infusion days 1 to 5
[total dose/cycle = 3750 mg/m^2]
Repeat cycle every 21 days for a total of 3 cycles

References

Pointreau Y, Garaud P, Chapet S, et al, "Randomized Trial of Induction Chemotherapy With Cisplatin and 5-Fluorouracil With or Without Docetaxel for Larynx Preservation," *J Natl Cancer Inst*, 2009, 101(7):498-506.

Cisplatin-Docetaxel-Gemcitabine (Bladder)

Index Terms Gemcitabine-Cisplatin-Docetaxel (Bladder)

Use Bladder cancer

Regimen

Docetaxel: IV: 35 mg/m^2/day over 30 minutes days 1 and 8
[total dose/cycle = 70 mg/m^2]
Gemcitabine: IV: 800 mg/m^2/day over 30 minutes days 1 and 8
[total dose/cycle = 1600 mg/m^2]
Cisplatin: IV: 35 mg/m^2/day over 1 hour days 1 and 8
[total dose/cycle = 70 mg/m^2]
Filgrastim: SubQ: 150 mcg/m^2/day days 3 to 6 and days 10 to 15
[total dose/cycle = 1500 mcg/m^2]
Repeat cycle every 21 days for at least 6 cycles, maximum of 8 cycles

References

Pectasides D, Glotsos J, Bountouroglou N, et al, "Weekly Chemotherapy With Docetaxel, Gemcitabine and Cisplatin in Advanced Transitional Cell Urothelial Cancer: A Phase II Trial," *Ann Oncol*, 2002, 13(2):243-50.

Cisplatin-Docetaxel (NSCLC)

Index Terms DC (NSCLC); Docetaxel-Cisplatin (NSCLC)

Use Lung cancer, non-small cell

Regimen

Docetaxel: IV: 75 mg/m^2 day 1
[total dose/cycle = 75 mg/m^2]
Cisplatin: IV: 75 mg/m^2 day 1
[total dose/cycle = 75 mg/m^2]
Repeat cycle every 21 days

References

Fossella F, Pereira JR, von Pawel J, et al. Randomized, multinational, phase III study of docetaxel plus platinum combinations versus vinorelbine plus cisplatin for advanced non-small-cell lung cancer: the TAX 326 study group. *J Clin Oncol*. 2003;21(16):3016-3024.

Schiller JH, Harrington D, Belani CP, et al. Comparison of four chemotherapy regimens for advanced non-small-cell lung cancer. *N Engl J Med*, 2002;346(2):92-98.

Cisplatin-Docetaxel (Unknown Primary, Adenocarcinoma)

Index Terms Docetaxel-Cisplatin (Unknown Primary, Adenocarcinoma)

Use Unknown primary (adenocarcinoma)

◀ **Regimen** NOTE: Multiple variations are listed.

Variation 1:

Docetaxel: IV: 75 mg/m^2 over 1 hour day 1

[total dose/cycle = 75 mg/m^2]

Cisplatin: IV: 75 mg/m^2 over 1 hour day 1

[total dose/cycle = 75 mg/m^2]

Repeat cycle every 21 days for up to a total of 8 cycles

Variation 2:

Docetaxel: IV: 60 mg/m^2 over 1 hour day 1

[total dose/cycle = 60 mg/m^2]

Cisplatin: IV: 80 mg/m^2 over 2 hours day 1

[total dose/cycle = 80 mg/m^2]

Repeat cycle every 21 days

References

Variation 1:

Greco FA, Erland JB, Morrissey LH, et al, "Carcinoma of Unknown Primary Site: Phase II Trials With Docetaxel Plus Cisplatin or Carboplatin," *Ann Oncol*, 2000, 11(2):211-5.

Variation 2:

Mukai H, Katsumata N, Ando M, et al, "Safety and Efficacy of a Combination of Docetaxel and Cisplatin in Patients With Unknown Primary Cancer," *Am J Clin Oncol*, 2010, 33(1):32-5.

Cisplatin-Docetaxel (Unknown Primary, Squamous Cell)

Index Terms Docetaxel-Cisplatin (Unknown Primary, Squamous Cell)

Use Unknown primary (squamous cell)

Regimen

Docetaxel: IV: 60 mg/m^2 over 1 hour day 1

[total dose/cycle = 60 mg/m^2]

Cisplatin: IV: 80 mg/m^2 over 2 hours day 1

[total dose/cycle = 80 mg/m^2]

Repeat cycle every 21 days for up to 6 cycles

References

Mukai H, Katsumata N, Ando M, et al, "Safety and Efficacy of a Combination of Docetaxel and Cisplatin in Patients With Unknown Primary Cancer," *Am J Clin Oncol*, 2010, 33(1):32-5.

Cisplatin-Doxorubicin (Endometrial)

Index Terms AP (Endometrial); DC (Endometrial); Doxorubicin-Cisplatin (Endometrial)

Use Endometrial cancer

Regimen NOTE: Multiple variations are listed.

Variation 1 (≤65 years old with no prior external radiation):

Doxorubicin: IV: 60 mg/m^2 day 1

[total dose/cycle = 60 mg/m^2]

Cisplatin: IV: 50 mg/m^2 day 1

[total dose/cycle = 50 mg/m^2]

Repeat cycle every 21 days; maximum cumulative dose of doxorubicin 500 mg/m^2

Variation 2 (>65 years old and/or prior external radiation):

Doxorubicin: IV: 45 mg/m^2 day 1, may be escalated to 60 mg/m^2 on cycle 2 if no > grade 1 toxicity)

[total dose/cycle = 45 to 60 mg/m^2]

Cisplatin: IV: 50 mg/m² day 1
[total dose/cycle = 50 mg/m²]
Repeat cycle every 21 days; maximum cumulative dose of doxorubicin 500 mg/m²

Variation 3 (≤65 years old with no prior pelvic radiation):
Doxorubicin: IV: 60 mg/m² day 1
[total dose/cycle = 60 mg/m²]
Cisplatin: IV: 50 mg/m² over 1 hour day 1
[total dose/cycle = 50 mg/m²]
Repeat cycle every 21 days up to a maximum of 7 cycles

Variation 4 (>65 years old or prior pelvic radiation):
Doxorubicin: IV: 45 mg/m² day 1
[total dose/cycle = 45 mg/m²]
Cisplatin: IV: 50 mg/m² over 1 hour day 1
[total dose/cycle = 50 mg/m²]
Repeat cycle every 21 days up to a maximum of 7 cycles

References

Variations 1 and 2:
Thigpen JT, Brady MF, Homesley HD, et al. Phase III trial of doxorubicin with or without cisplatin in advanced endometrial carcinoma: a Gynecologic Oncology Group Study. *J Clin Oncol*. 2004;22 (19):3902-3908.

Variations 3 and 4:
Fleming GF, Brunetto VL, Cella D, et al. Phase III trial of doxorubicin plus cisplatin with or without paclitaxel plus filgrastim in advanced endometrial carcinoma: a Gynecologic Oncology Group Study. *J Clin Oncol*. 2004;22(11):2159-2166.

Cisplatin-Doxorubicin-Etoposide-Cyclophosphamide (Neuroblastoma)

Use Neuroblastoma

Regimen
Cisplatin: IV: 60 mg/m² over 6 hours day 0
[total dose/cycle = 60 mg/m²]
Doxorubicin: IV: 30 mg/m² day 2
[total dose/cycle = 30 mg/m²]
Etoposide: IV: 100 mg/m²/day days 2 and 5
[total dose/cycle = 200 mg/m²]
Cyclophosphamide: IV: 1000 mg/m²/day days 3 and 4
[total dose/cycle = 2000 mg/m²]
Repeat cycle every 28 days for a total of 5 cycles

References

Matthay KK, Villablanca JG, Seeger RC, et al, "Treatment of High-Risk Neuroblastoma With Intensive Chemotherapy, Radiotherapy, Autologous Bone Marrow Transplantation, and 13-*cis*-Retinoic Acid. Children's Cancer Group," *N Engl J Med*, 1999, 341(16):1165-73.

Cisplatin-Doxorubicin-Paclitaxel (Endometrial)

Index Terms Paclitaxel-Doxorubicin-Cisplatin (Endometrial); TAP (Endometrial)

Use Endometrial cancer

Regimen
Doxorubicin: IV: 45 mg/m² day 1
[total dose/cycle = 45 mg/m²]
Cisplatin: IV: 50 mg/m² day 1
[total dose/cycle = 50 mg/m²]
Paclitaxel: IV: 160 mg/m² over 3 hours day 2
[total dose/cycle = 160 mg/m²]

Growth Factor:

Filgrastim: SubQ: 5 mcg/kg/day days 3 to 12

or

Pegfilgrastim: SubQ: 6 mg day 3

Repeat cycle every 21 days; maximum of 6 cycles (Homesley, 2009) or a maximum of 7 cycles (Fleming, 2004; Miller, 2012)

References

Fleming GF, Brunetto VL, Cella D, et al. Phase III trial of doxorubicin plus cisplatin with or without paclitaxel plus filgrastim in advanced endometrial carcinoma: a Gynecologic Oncology Group Study. *J Clin Oncol.* 2004;22(11):2159-2166.

Homesley HD, Filiaci V, Gibbons SK, et al. A randomized phase III trial in advanced endometrial carcinoma of surgery and volume directed radiation followed by cisplatin and doxorubicin with or without paclitaxel: A Gynecologic Oncology Group study. *Gynecol Oncol.* 2009;112(3):543-552.

Miller DS, Filiaci G, Fleming G, et al. Randomized phase III noninferiority trial of first line chemotherapy for metastatic or recurrent endometrial carcinoma: A Gynecologic Oncology Group Study. *Gynecol Oncol.* 2012;125(3):771.

Cisplatin-Etoposide (NSCLC)

Index Terms Etoposide-Cisplatin (NSCLC); PE (NSCLC)

Use Lung cancer, non-small cell

Regimen NOTE: Multiple variations are listed.

Variation 1 (adjuvant):

Cisplatin: IV: 80 mg/m^2 day 1

[total dose/cycle = 80 mg/m^2]

Etoposide: IV: 100 mg/m^2/day days 1, 2, and 3

[total dose/cycle = 300 mg/m^2]

Repeat cycle every 21 days for a total of 4 cycles

Variation 2 (adjuvant):

Cisplatin: IV: 100 mg/m^2 day 1

[total dose/cycle = 100 mg/m^2]

Etoposide: IV: 100 mg/m^2/day days 1, 2, and 3

[total dose/cycle = 300 mg/m^2]

Repeat cycle every 28 days for a total of 3 cycles

Variation 3 (adjuvant):

Cisplatin: IV: 100 mg/m^2 day 1

[total dose/cycle = 100 mg/m^2]

Etoposide: IV: 100 mg/m^2/day days 1, 2, and 3

[total dose/cycle = 300 mg/m^2]

Repeat cycle every 28 days for a total of 4 cycles

Variation 4 (adjuvant):

Cisplatin: IV: 120 mg/m^2/day days 1, 29, and 71

[total dose/treatment = 360 mg/m^2]

Etoposide: IV: 100 mg/m^2/day days 1, 2, 3, 29, 30, 31, 71, 72, and 73

[total dose/treatment = 900 mg/m^2]

Variation 5 (concurrent radiation):

Cisplatin: IV: 50 mg/m^2/day days 1 and 8

[total dose/cycle = 100 mg/m^2]

Etoposide: IV: 50 mg/m^2/day days 1 to 5

[total dose/cycle = 250 mg/m^2]

Repeat cycle every 28 days for a total of 2 cycles

References

Variations 1 to 4:

Arriagada R, Bergman B, Dunant A, et al. Cisplatin-based adjuvant chemotherapy in patients with completely resected non-small-cell lung cancer. *N Engl J Med.* 2004;350(4):351-360.

Arriagada R, Dunant A, Pignon JP, et al. Long-term results of the international adjuvant lung cancer trial evaluating adjuvant Cisplatin-based chemotherapy in resected lung cancer. *J Clin Oncol.* 2010;28(1):35-42.

Variation 5:

Albain KS, Crowley JJ, Turrisi AT 3rd, et al. Concurrent cisplatin, etoposide, and chest radiotherapy in pathologic stage IIIB non-small-cell lung cancer: a Southwest Oncology Group phase II study, SWOG 9019. *J Clin Oncol.* 2002;20(16):3454-3460.

Albain KS, Swann RS, Rusch VW, et al. Radiotherapy plus chemotherapy with or without surgical resection for stage III non-small-cell lung cancer: a phase III randomised controlled trial. *Lancet.* 2009;374(9687):379-386.

Cisplatin-Etoposide (Small Cell Lung Cancer)

Index Terms EP (Small Cell Lung Cancer); Etoposide-Cisplatin (Small Cell Lung Cancer); PE (Small Cell Lung Cancer)

Use Lung cancer, small cell

Regimen NOTE: Multiple variations are listed.

Variation 1: (limited stage with concurrent thoracic radiotherapy)
Etoposide: IV: 120 mg/m^2/day days 1, 2, and 3
  [total dose/cycle = 360 mg/m^2]
Cisplatin: IV: 60 mg/m^2 day 1
  [total dose/cycle = 60 mg/m^2]
Repeat cycle every 21 days for 4 cycles

Variation 2: (limited stage with concurrent thoracic radiotherapy)
Etoposide: IV: 100 mg/m^2/day days 1, 2, and 3
  [total dose/cycle = 300 mg/m^2]
Cisplatin: IV: 80 mg/m^2 day 1
  [total dose/cycle = 80 mg/m^2]
Repeat cycle every 28 days for 4 cycles

Variation 3: (extensive stage)
Etoposide: IV: 100 mg/m^2/day days 1, 2, and 3
  [total dose/cycle = 300 mg/m^2]
Cisplatin: IV: 80 mg/m^2 day 1
  [total dose/cycle = 80 mg/m^2]
Repeat cycle every 21 days for 4 cycles

Variation 4: (extensive stage)
Etoposide: IV: 100 mg/m^2 day 1
  [total IV dose/cycle = 100 mg/m^2]
  followed by: Etoposide: Oral: 200 mg/m^2/day days 2, 3, and 4
    [total oral dose/cycle = 600 mg/m^2]
Cisplatin: IV: 75 mg/m^2 day 1
  [total dose/cycle = 75 mg/m^2]
Repeat cycle every 21 days for a maximum of 5 cycles

Variation 5: (extensive stage)
Etoposide: IV: 80 mg/m^2/day days 1, 2, and 3
  [total dose/cycle = 240 mg/m^2]
Cisplatin: IV: 80 mg/m^2 day 1
  [total dose/cycle = 80 mg/m^2]
Repeat cycle every 21 days for maximum of 8 cycles

◀ Variation 6: (extensive stage)
   Etoposide: IV: 100 mg/m^2/day days 1, 2, and 3
     [total dose/cycle = 300 mg/m^2]
   Cisplatin: IV: 25 mg/m^2/day days 1, 2, and 3
     [total dose/cycle = 75 mg/m^2]
   Repeat cycle every 21 to 28 days for 6 cycles
Variation 7: (extensive stage)
   Etoposide: IV: 80 mg/m^2/day days 1 to 5
     [total dose/cycle = 400 mg/m^2]
   Cisplatin: IV: 20 mg/m^2/day days 1 to 5
     [total dose/cycle = 100 mg/m^2]
   Repeat cycle every 21 days for 4 cycles

References

Variation 1:
Turrisi AT, Kyungmann K, Blum R, et al, "Twice-Daily Compared With Once-Daily Thoracic Radiotherapy in Limited Small-Cell Lung Cancer Treated Concurrently With Cisplatin and Etoposide," *N Engl J Med*, 1999, 340(4):265-71.

Variation 2:
Takada M, Fukuoka M, Kawahara M, et al, "Phase III Study of Concurrent Verses Sequential Thoracic Radiotherapy in Combination With Cisplatin and Etoposide for Limited-Stage Small-Cell Lung Cancer: Results of the Japan Clinical Oncology Group Study 9104," *J Clin Oncol*, 2002, 20 (14):3054-60.

Variation 3:
Lara Jr PN, Natale R, Crowley J, et al, "Phase III Trial of Irinotecan/Cisplatin Compared With Etoposide/Cisplatin in Extensive-Stage Small-Cell Lung Cancer: Clinical and Pharmacogenomic Results From SWOG S0124," *J Clin Oncol*, 2009, 27(15):2530-5.

Variation 4:
Sundstrom S, Bremnes RM, Kaasa S, et al, "Cisplatin and Etoposide Regimen Is Superior to Cyclophosphamide, Epirubicin, and Vincristine Regimen in Small-Cell Lung Cancer: Results From a Randomized Phase III Trial With 5 Years' Follow-Up," *J Clin Oncol*, 2002, 20(24):4665-72.

Variation 5:
Ihde DC, Mulshine JL, Kramer BS, et al, "Prospective Randomized Comparison of High-Dose and Standard-Dose Etoposide and Cisplatin Chemotherapy in Patients With Extensive-Stage Small-Cell Lung Cancer," *J Clin Oncol*, 1994, 12(10):2022-34.

Variation 6:
Evans WK, Shepherd FA, Feld R, et al, "VP-16 and Cisplatin as First-Line Therapy for Small-Cell Lung Cancer," *J Clin Oncol*, 1985, 3(11):1471-7.

Variation 7:
Roth BJ, Johnson DH, Einhorn LH, et al, "Randomized Study of Cyclophosphamide, Doxorubicin, and Vincristine Versus Etoposide and Cisplatin Versus Alternation of These Two Regimens in Extensive Small-Cell Lung Cancer: A Phase III Trial of the Southeastern Cancer Study Group," *J Clin Oncol*, 1992, 10(2):281-91.

◆ **Cisplatin-Etoposide (Testicular)** see EP (Testicular) *on page 1961*

Cisplatin-Fluorouracil (Bladder Cancer)

Index Terms Fluorouracil-Cisplatin (Bladder Cancer)

Use Bladder cancer

Regimen In combination with radiation therapy

Note: Begin infusion(s) 2 hours before radiation therapy on days 1, 3, 15, and 17:

Cisplatin: IV: 15 mg/m^2/day over 2 hours days 1, 2, 3, 15, 16, and 17
  [total dose/cycle = 90 mg/m^2]
Fluorouracil: IV: 400 mg/m^2/day over 2 hours days 1, 2, 3, 15, 16, and 17
  [total dose/cycle = 2400 mg/m^2]

References

Housset M, Maulard C, Chretien Y, et al, "Combined Radiation and Chemotherapy for Invasive Transitional-Cell Carcinoma of the Bladder: A Prospective Study," *J Clin Oncol*, 1993, 11 (11):2150-7.

Cisplatin-Fluorouracil (Cervical Cancer)

Index Terms 5FU-Cisplatin (Cervical Cancer); Cisplatin-5FU (Cervical Cancer); Fluorouracil-Cisplatin (Cervical Cancer)

Use Cervical cancer

Regimen NOTE: Multiple variations are listed.

Variation 1 (with concurrent radiation therapy):

Cisplatin: IV: 75 mg/m^2 day 1

[total dose/cycle = 75 mg/m^2]

Fluorouracil: IV: 1000 mg/m^2/day continuous infusion days 1 to 4 (96 hours)

[total dose/cycle = 4000 mg/m^2]

Repeat cycle every 21 days for a total 3 cycles

Variation 2 (with concurrent radiation therapy):

Cisplatin: IV: 50 mg/m^2 day 1 starting 4 hours before radiotherapy

[total dose/cycle = 50 mg/m^2]

Fluorouracil: IV: 1000 mg/m^2/day continuous infusion days 2 to 5 (96 hours)

[total dose/cycle = 4000 mg/m^2]

Repeat cycle every 28 days for a total of 2 cycles

Variation 3 (cycles 1 and 2 are with concurrent radiation therapy):

Cisplatin: IV: 70 mg/m^2 day 1

[total dose/cycle = 70 mg/m^2]

Fluorouracil: IV: 1000 mg/m^2/day continuous infusion days 1 to 4 (96 hours)

[total dose/cycle = 4000 mg/m^2]

Repeat cycle every 21 days for a total of 4 cycles

References

Variation 1:

Morris M, Eifel PJ, Lu J, et al, "Pelvic Radiation With Concurrent Chemotherapy Compared With Pelvic and Para-aortic Radiation for High-Risk Cervical Cancer," *N Engl J Med*, 1999, 340 (15):1137-43.

Variation 2:

Whitney CW, Sause W, Bundy BN, et al, "Randomized Comparison of Fluorouracil Plus Cisplatin Versus Hydroxyurea as an Adjunct to Radiation Therapy in Stage IIB-IVA Carcinoma of the Cervix With Negative Para-aortic Lymph Nodes: A Gynecologic Oncology Group and Southwest Oncology Group Study," *J Clin Oncol*, 1999, 17(5):1339-48.

Variation 3:

Peters WA 3rd, Liu PY, Barrett RJ 2nd, et al, "Concurrent Chemotherapy and Pelvic Radiation Therapy Compared With Pelvic Radiation Therapy Alone as Adjuvant Therapy After Radical Surgery in High-Risk Early-Stage Cancer of the Cervix," *J Clin Oncol*, 2000, 18(8):1606-13.

◆ **Cisplatin-Fluorouracil-Cetuximab (Head and Neck Cancer)** *see* Cetuximab-Cisplatin-Fluorouracil (Head and Neck Cancer) *on page 1880*

◆ **Cisplatin-Fluorouracil-Epirubicin (Gastric/Esophageal)** *see* Epirubicin-Cisplatin-Fluorouracil (Gastric/Esophageal) *on page 1956*

Cisplatin-Fluorouracil (Esophageal Cancer)

Index Terms CF (Esophageal Cancer); Fluorouracil-Cisplatin (Esophageal Cancer)

Use Esophageal cancer

Regimen NOTE: Multiple variations are listed.

Variation 1:

Cisplatin: IV: 100 mg/m^2/dose day 1

[total dose/cycle = 100 mg/m^2]

Fluorouracil: IV: 1000 mg/m^2/day continuous infusion days 1 to 5

[total dose/cycle = 5000 mg/m^2]

Repeat cycle every 28 days until disease progression or unacceptable toxicity.

◀ Variation 2:
  Cycles 1 to 3 (prior to surgery):
    Cisplatin: IV: 100 mg/m^2/dose day 1
    [total dose/cycle = 100 mg/m^2]
    Fluorouracil: IV: 1000 mg/m^2/day continuous infusion days 1 to 5
    [total dose/cycle = 5000 mg/m^2]
    Treatment cycles 1-3 are 28 days each
  Cycles 4 and 5 (postoperative):
    Cisplatin: IV: 75 mg/m^2/dose day 1
    [total dose/cycle = 75 mg/m^2]
    Fluorouracil: IV: 1000 mg/m^2/day continuous infusion days 1 to 5
    [total dose/cycle = 5000 mg/m^2]
    Treatment cycles 4 and 5 are 28 days each
Variation 3 (in combination with radiation therapy):
  Cycle 1:
    Cisplatin: IV: 75 mg/m^2/dose day 1
    [total dose/cycle = 75 mg/m^2]
    Fluorouracil: IV: 1000 mg/m^2/day continuous infusion days 1 to 4
    [total dose/cycle = 4000 mg/m^2]
    Treatment cycle is 28 days
  Cycles 2 to 4:
    Cisplatin: IV: 75 mg/m^2/dose day 1
    [total dose/cycle = 75 mg/m^2]
    Fluorouracil: IV: 1000 mg/m^2/day continuous infusion days 1 to 4
    [total dose/cycle = 4000 mg/m^2]
    Repeat cycle every 21 days for 3 more cycles (total of 4 cycles)
Variation 4 (in combination with radiation therapy):
  Cisplatin: IV: 100 mg/m^2/dose day 1
  [total dose/cycle = 100 mg/m^2]
  Fluorouracil: IV: 1000 mg/m^2/day continuous infusion days 1 to 4
  [total dose/cycle = 4000 mg/m^2]
  Repeat cycle every 28 days for total of 2 cycles
Variation 5 (in combination with radiation therapy):
  Cisplatin: IV: 75 mg/m^2/dose day 1
  [total dose/cycle = 75 mg/m^2]
  Fluorouracil: IV: 1000 mg/m^2/day continuous infusion days 1 to 4
  [total dose/cycle = 4000 mg/m^2]
  Repeat cycle every 28 days for 4 cycles
Variation 6 (in combination with radiation therapy):
  Cycles 1 and 2:
    Cisplatin: IV: 75 mg/m^2/dose day 1
    [total dose/cycle = 75 mg/m^2]
    Fluorouracil: IV: 1000 mg/m^2/day continuous infusion days 1 to 4
    [total dose/cycle = 4000 mg/m^2]
    Treatment cycles 1 and 2 are 28 days each; cycle 2 is followed by a 2-week rest
  Cycles 3 and 4 (begin cycle 3 at week 11):
    Cisplatin: IV: 75 mg/m^2/dose day 1
    [total dose/cycle = 75 mg/m^2]
    Fluorouracil: IV: 1000 mg/m^2/day continuous infusion days 1 to 4
    [total dose/cycle = 4000 mg/m^2]
    Treatment cycles 3 and 4 are 28 days each

Variation 7 (in combination with radiation therapy):
  Cycles 1 to 4:
    Cisplatin: IV: 15 mg/m^2/day days 1 to 5
    [total dose/cycle = 75 mg/m^2]
    Fluorouracil: IV: 800 mg/m^2/day continuous infusion days 1 to 5
    [total dose/cycle = 4000 mg/m^2]
    Repeat cycles 1-4 every 21 days; cycle 4 is followed by a 1-week rest
  Cycles 5 (begin cycle 5 at week 14):
    Cisplatin: IV: 15 mg/m^2/day days 1 to 5
    [total dose/cycle = 75 mg/m^2]
    Fluorouracil: IV: 800 mg/m^2/day continuous infusion days 1 to 5
    [total dose/cycle = 4000 mg/m^2]
Variation 8:
  Cisplatin: IV: 80 mg/m^2/dose day 1
  [total dose/cycle = 80 mg/m^2]
  Fluorouracil: IV: 800 mg/m^2/day continuous infusion days 1 to 5
  [total dose/cycle = 4000 mg/m^2]
  Repeat cycle every 21 days until disease progression or unacceptable toxicity.

References

Variation 1:

Ajani JA, Moiseyenko VM, Tjulandin S, et al, "Quality of Life With Docetaxel Plus Cisplatin and Fluorouracil Compared With Cisplatin and Fluorouracil From a Phase III Trial for Advanced Gastric or Gastroesophageal Adenocarcinoma: The V-325 Study Group," *J Clin Oncol*, 2007, 25 (22):3210-6.

Dank M, Zaluski J, Barone C, et al, "Randomized Phase III Study Comparing Irinotecan Combined With 5-Fluorouracil and Folinic Acid to Cisplatin Combined With 5-Fluorouracil in Chemotherapy Naive Patients With Advanced Adenocarcinoma of the Stomach or Esophagogastric Junction," *Ann Oncol*, 2008, 19(8):1450-7.

Van Cutsem E, Moiseyenko VM, Tjulandin S, et al, "Phase III Study of Docetaxel and Cisplatin Plus Fluorouracil Compared With Cisplatin and Fluorouracil As First-Line Therapy for Advanced Gastric Cancer: A Report of the V325 Study Group," *J Clin Oncol*, 2006, 24(31):4991-7.

Variation 2:

Kelsen DP, Ginsberg R, Pajak TF, et al, "Chemotherapy Followed by Surgery Compared With Surgery Alone for Localized Esophageal Cancer," *N Engl J Med*, 1998, 339(27):1979-84.

Variation 3:

Cooper JS, Guo MD, Herskovic A, et al, "Chemoradiotherapy of Locally Advanced Esophageal Cancer: Long-Term Follow-Up of a Prospective Randomized Trial (RTOG 85-01). Radiation Therapy Oncology Group," *JAMA*, 1999, 281(17):1623-7.

Variation 4:

Tepper J, Krasna MJ, Niedzwiecki D, et al, "Phase III Trial of Trimodality Therapy With Cisplatin, Fluorouracil, Radiotherapy, and Surgery Compared With Surgery Alone for Esophageal Cancer: CALGB 9781," *J Clin Oncol*, 2008, 26(7):1086-92.

Variation 5 and 6:

Minsky BD, Pajak TF, Ginsberg RJ, et al, "INT 0123 (Radiation Therapy Oncology Group 94-05) Phase III Trial of Combined-Modality Therapy for Esophageal Cancer: High-Dose Versus Standard-Dose Radiation Therapy," *J Clin Oncol*, 2002, 20(5):1167-74.

Variation 7:

Bedenne L, Michel P, Bouché O, et al, "Chemoradiation Followed by Surgery Compared With Chemoradiation Alone in Squamous Cancer of the Esophagus: FFCD 9102," *J Clin Oncol*, 2007, 25(10):1160-8.

Variation 8:

Kang YK, Kang WK, Shin DB, et al, "Capecitabine/Cisplatin Versus 5-Fluorouracil/Cisplatin as First-Line Therapy in Patients With Advanced Gastric Cancer: A Randomised Phase III Non-inferiority Trial," *Ann Oncol*, 2009, 20(4):666-73.

Cisplatin-Fluorouracil (Gastric Cancer)

Index Terms CF (Gastric Cancer); Fluorouracil-Cisplatin (Gastric Cancer)
Use Gastric cancer

◄ **Regimen** NOTE: Multiple variations are listed.

Variation 1:

Cisplatin: IV: 100 mg/m² day 1

[total dose/cycle = 100 mg/m²]

Fluorouracil: IV: 1000 mg/m²/day continuous infusion days 1 to 5

[total dose/cycle = 5000 mg/m²]

Repeat cycle every 4 weeks until disease progression or unacceptable toxicity

Variation 2:

Cisplatin: IV: 80 mg/m² over 2 hours day 1

[total dose/cycle = 80 mg/m²]

Fluorouracil: IV: 800 mg/m²/day continuous infusion days 1 to 5

[total dose/cycle = 4000 mg/m²]

Repeat cycle every 21 days until disease progression or unacceptable toxicity

Variation 3:

Fluorouracil: IV: 1000 mg/m²/day continuous infusion days 1 to 5

[total dose/cycle = 5000 mg/m²]

Cisplatin: IV: 100 mg/m² day 2

[total dose/cycle = 100 mg/m²]

Repeat cycle every 4 weeks

References

Variation 1:

Ajani JA, Moiseyenko VM, Tjulandin S, et al, "Clinical Benefit With Docetaxel Plus Fluorouracil and Cisplatin Compared With Cisplatin and Fluorouracil in a Phase III Trial of Advanced Gastric or Gastroesophageal Cancer Adenocarcinoma: The V-325 Study Group," *J Clin Oncol*, 2007, 25 (22):3205-9.

Dank M, Zaluski J, Barone C, et al, "Randomized Phase III Study Comparing Irinotecan Combined With 5-Fluorouracil and Folinic Acid to Cisplatin Combined With 5-Fluorouracil in Chemotherapy Naive Patients With Advanced Adenocarcinoma of the Stomach or Esophagogastric Junction," *Ann Oncol*, 2008, 19(8):1450-7.

Van Cutsem E, Moiseyenko VM, Tjulandin S, "Phase III Study of Docetaxel and Cisplatin Plus Fluorouracil Compared With Cisplatin and Fluorouracil as First-Line Therapy for Advanced Gastric Cancer: A Report of the V325 Study Group," *J Clin Oncol*, 2006, 24(31):4991-7.

Variation 2:

Kang YK, Kang WK, Shin DB, "Capecitabine/Cisplatin Versus 5-Fluorouracil/Cisplatin as First-Line Therapy in Patients With Advanced Gastric Cancer: A Randomised Phase III Noninferiority Trial," *Ann Oncol*, 2009, 20(4):666-73.

Variation 3:

Vanhoefer U, Rougier P, Wilke H, et al, "Final Results of a Randomized Phase III Trial of Sequential High-Dose Methotrexate, Fluorouracil, and Doxorubicin Versus Etoposide, Leucovorin, and Fluorouracil Versus Infusional Fluorouracil and Cisplatin in Advanced Gastric Cancer: A Trial of the European Organization for Research and Treatment of Cancer Gastrointestinal Tract Cancer Cooperative Group," *J Clin Oncol*, 2000, 18(14):2648-57.

Cisplatin-Fluorouracil (Head and Neck Cancer)

Index Terms CF (Head and Neck Cancer); Fluorouracil-Cisplatin (Head and Neck Cancer)

Use Head and neck cancer

Regimen NOTE: Multiple variations are listed.

Variation 1:

Cisplatin: IV: 100 mg/m² day 1

[total dose/cycle = 100 mg/m²]

Fluorouracil: IV: 1000 mg/m²/day continuous infusion days 1 to 4

[total dose/cycle = 4000 mg/m²]

Repeat cycle every 3 weeks

Variation 2:
  Cisplatin: IV: 100 mg/m^2 day 1
    [total dose/cycle = 100 mg/m^2]
  Fluorouracil: IV: 1000 mg/m^2/day continuous infusion days 1 to 4
    [total dose/cycle = 4000 mg/m^2]
  Repeat cycle every 3 or 4 weeks
Variation 3:
  Cisplatin: IV: 100 mg/m^2 day 1
    [total dose/cycle = 100 mg/m^2]
  Fluorouracil: IV: 1000 mg/m^2/day continuous infusion days 1 to 5
    [total dose/cycle = 5000 mg/m^2]
  Repeat cycle every 3 or 4 weeks
Variation 4:
  Cisplatin: IV: 60 mg/m^2 day 1
    [total dose/cycle = 60 mg/m^2]
  Fluorouracil: IV: 800 mg/m^2/day continuous infusion days 1 to 5
    [total dose/cycle = 4000 mg/m^2]
  Repeat cycle every 14 days
Variation 5:
  Cisplatin: IV: 20 mg/m^2/day days 1 to 5
    [total dose/cycle = 100 mg/m^2]
  Fluorouracil: IV: 200 mg/m^2/day days 1 to 5
    [total dose/cycle = 1000 mg/m^2]
  Repeat cycle every 3 weeks
Variation 6:
  Cisplatin: IV: 80 mg/m^2 continuous infusion day 1
    [total dose/cycle = 80 mg/m^2]
  Fluorouracil: IV: 800 mg/m^2/day continuous infusion days 2 to 6
    [total dose/cycle = 4000 mg/m^2]
  Repeat cycle every 3 weeks
Variation 7:
  Cisplatin: IV: 75 mg/m^2 day 1
    [total dose/cycle = 75 mg/m^2]
  Fluorouracil: IV: 1000 mg/m^2/day continuous infusion days 1 to 4
    [total dose/cycle = 4000 mg/m^2]
  Repeat cycle every 4 weeks
Variation 8:
  Cisplatin: IV: 120 mg/m^2 day 1
    [total dose/cycle = 120 mg/m^2]
  Fluorouracil: IV: 1000 mg/m^2/day continuous infusion days 1 to 5
    [total dose/cycle = 5000 mg/m^2]
  Repeat cycle every 3 weeks
Variation 9:
  Cisplatin: IV: 25 mg/m^2/day continuous infusion days 1 to 4
    [total dose/cycle = 100 mg/m^2]
  Fluorouracil: IV: 1000 mg/m^2/day days 1 to 4
    [total dose/cycle = 4000 mg/m^2]
  Repeat cycle every 3 weeks
Variation 10:
  Fluorouracil: IV: 350 mg/m^2/day continuous infusion days 1 to 5
    [total dose/cycle = 1750 mg/m^2]
  Cisplatin: IV: 50 mg/m^2 day 6
    [total dose/cycle = 50 mg/m^2]
  Repeat cycle every 3 weeks

◀ Variation 11:

Cisplatin: IV: 5 mg/m^2/day continuous infusion days 1 to 14

[total dose/cycle = 70 mg/m^2]

Fluorouracil: IV: 200 mg/m^2/day continuous infusion days 1 to 14

[total dose/cycle = 2800 mg/m^2]

With concurrent radiation therapy, cycle does not repeat

Variation 12 (administer during the final 2 weeks of radiation therapy; weeks 6 and 7):

Cisplatin: IV: 10 mg/m^2/day days 1 to 5 beginning week 6

[total dose/week = 50 mg/m^2]

Fluorouracil: IV: 400 mg/m^2/day continuous infusion days 1 to 5 beginning week 6

[total dose/week = 2000 mg/m^2]

Repeat cycle one time in week 7

Variation 13:

Cisplatin: IV: 100 mg/m^2/day day 1 (concurrent with radiation therapy)

[total dose/cycle = 100 mg/m^2]

Repeat cycle every 3 weeks for a total of 3 cycles

Followed by (postradiation chemotherapy; begin 4 weeks after radiotherapy or the last cisplatin dose):

Cisplatin: IV: 80 mg/m^2 day 1

[total dose/cycle = 80 mg/m^2]

Fluorouracil: IV: 1000 mg/m^2/day continuous infusion days 1 to 4

[total dose/cycle = 4000 mg/m^2]

Repeat cycle every 4 weeks for a total of 3 cycles

References

Variation 1:

Forastiere AA, Metch B, Schuller DE, et al, "Randomized Comparison of Cisplatin Plus Fluorouracil and Carboplatin Plus Fluorouracil Versus Methotrexate in Advanced Squamous-Cell Carcinoma of the Head and Neck: A Southwest Oncology Group Study," *J Clin Oncol*, 1992, 10(8):1245-51.

Gibson MK, Li Y, Murphy B, et al, "Randomized Phase III Evaluation of Cisplatin Plus Fluorouracil Versus Cisplatin Plus Paclitaxel in Advanced Head and Neck Cancer (E1395): An Intergroup Trial of the Eastern Cooperative Oncology Group," *J Clin Oncol*, 2005, 23(15):3562-7.

Variation 2:

Kish J, Drelichman A, Jacobs J, et al, "Clinical Trial of Cisplatin and 5-FU Infusion as Initial Treatment for Advanced Squamous Cell Carcinoma of the Head and Neck," *Cancer Treat Rep*, 1982, 66(3):471-4.

Mercier RJ, Neal GD, Mattox DE, et al, "Cisplatin and 5-Fluorouracil Chemotherapy in Advanced or Recurrent Squamous Cell Carcinoma of the Head and Neck," *Cancer*, 1987, 60(11):2609-12.

Variation 3:

Dasmahapatra KS, Citrin P, Hill GJ, et al, "A Prospective Evaluation of 5-Fluorouracil Plus Cisplatin in Advanced Squamous-Cell Cancer of the Head and Neck," *J Clin Oncol*, 1985, 3(11):1486-9.

Rooney M, Kish J, Jacobs J, et al, "Improved Complete Response Rate and Survival in Advanced Head and Neck Cancer After Three-Course Induction Therapy With 120-Hour 5-FU Infusion and Cisplatin," *Cancer*, 1985, 55(5):1123-8.

Variation 4:

Taylor SG 4th, Murthy AK, Showel JL, et al, "Improved Control in Advanced Head and Neck Cancer With Simultaneous Radiation and Cisplatin/5-FU Chemotherapy," *Cancer Treat Rep*, 1985, 69 (9):933-9.

Variation 5:

Merlano M, Tatarek R, Grimaldi A, et al, "Phase I-II Trial With Cisplatin and 5-FU in Recurrent Head and Neck Cancer: An Effective Outpatient Schedule," *Cancer Treat Rep*, 1985, 69(9):961-4.

Variation 6:

Amrein PC and Weitzman SA, "Treatment of Squamous-Cell Carcinoma of the Head and Neck With Cisplatin and 5-Fluorouracil," *J Clin Oncol*, 1985, 3(12):1632-9.

Variation 7:

Adelstein DJ, Li Y, Adams GL, et al, "An Intergroup Phase III Comparison of Standard Radiation and Two Schedules of Concurrent Chemoradiotherapy in Patients With Unresectable Squamous Cell Head and Neck Cancer," *J Clin Oncol*, 2003, 21(1):92-8.

Adelstein DJ, Sharan VM, Earle AS, et al, "Chemoradiotherapy as Initial Management in Patients With Squamous Cell Carcinoma of the Head and Neck," *Cancer Treat Rep*, 1986, 70(6):761-7.

Variation 8:

Paredes J, Hong WK, Felder TB, et al, "Prospective Randomized Trial of High-Dose Cisplatin and Fluorouracil Infusion With or Without Sodium Diethyldithiocarbamate in Recurrent and/or Metastatic Squamous Cell Carcinoma of the Head and Neck," *J Clin Oncol*, 1988, 6(6):955-62.

Variation 9:

Bernal AG, Cruz JJ, Sanchez P, et al, "Four-Day Continuous Infusion of Cisplatin and 5-Fluorouracil in Head and Neck Cancer," *Cancer*, 1989, 63(10):1927-30.

Variation 10:

Denham JW and Abbott RL, "Concurrent Cisplatin, Infusional Fluorouracil, and Conventionally Fractionated Radiation Therapy in Head and Neck Cancer: Dose-Limiting Mucosal Toxicity," *J Clin Oncol*, 1991, 9(3):458-63.

Variation 11:

Arcangeli G, Saracino B, Danesi DT, et al, "Accelerated Hyperfractionated Radiotherapy and Concurrent Protracted Venous Infusion Chemotherapy in Locally-Advanced Head and Neck Cancer," *Am J Clin Oncol*, 2002, 25(5):431-7.

Variation 12:

Garden AS, Harris J, Vokes EE, et al, "Preliminary Results of Radiation Therapy Oncology Group 97-03: A Randomized Phase II Trial of Concurrent Radiation and Chemotherapy for Advanced Squamous Cell Carcinomas of the Head and Neck," *J Clin Oncol*, 2004, 22(14):2856-64.

Variation 13:

Al-Sarraf M, LeBlanc M, Giri PG, et al, "Chemoradiotherapy Versus Radiotherapy in Patients With Advanced Nasopharyngeal Cancer: Phase III Randomized Intergroup Study 0099," *J Clin Oncol*, 1998, 16(4):1310-7.

Cisplatin-Fluorouracil-Paclitaxel (Unknown Primary, Squamous Cell)

Index Terms Cisplatin-Paclitaxel-Fluorouracil (Unknown Primary); PCF (Unknown Primary)

Use Unknown primary (squamous cell)

Regimen

Paclitaxel: IV: 175 mg/m^2 over 3 hours day 1
[total dose/cycle = 175 mg/m^2]

Cisplatin: IV: 100 mg/m^2 day 2
[total dose/cycle = 100 mg/m^2]

Fluorouracil: IV: 500 mg/m^2/day continuous infusion days 2 to 6
[total dose/cycle = 2500 mg/m^2]

Repeat cycle every 21 days for a total of 3 cycles

References

Hitt R, López-Pousa A, Martínez-Trufero J, et al, "Phase III Study Comparing Cisplatin Plus Fluorouracil to Paclitaxel, Cisplatin, and Fluorouracil Induction Chemotherapy Followed by Chemoradiotherapy in Locally Advanced Head and Neck Cancer," *J Clin Oncol*, 2005, 23 (34):8636-45.

◆ **Cisplatin-Fluorouracil-Trastuzumab (Gastric Cancer)** *see* Trastuzumab-Cisplatin-Fluorouracil (Gastric Cancer) *on page 2093*

◆ **Cisplatin-Gemcitabine-Bevacizumab (NSCLC)** *see* Bevacizumab-Cisplatin-Gemcitabine (NSCLC) *on page 1840*

◆ **Cisplatin-Gemcitabine (Biliary Cancer)** *see* Gemcitabine-Cisplatin (Biliary Cancer) *on page 1991*

Cisplatin-Gemcitabine (Bladder)

Index Terms GC (Bladder); Gemcitabine-Cisplatin (Bladder); GP (Bladder)

◀ **Use** Bladder cancer

Regimen NOTE: Multiple variations are listed.

Variation 1 (metastatic):

Gemcitabine: IV: 1000 mg/m^2/day days 1, 8, and 15
[total dose/cycle = 3000 mg/m^2]

Cisplatin: IV: 70 mg/m^2 day 2
[total dose/cycle = 70 mg/m^2]

Repeat cycle every 28 days for a maximum of 6 cycles

Variation 2 (neoadjuvant):

Cisplatin: IV: 70 mg/m^2 day 1
[total dose/cycle = 70 mg/m^2]

Gemcitabine: IV: 1000 mg/m^2/day days 1 and 8
[total dose/cycle = 2000 mg/m^2]

Repeat cycle every 21 days for 4 cycles

Variation 3 (neoadjuvant):

Cisplatin: IV: 35 mg/m^2/day days 1 and 8
[total dose/cycle = 70 mg/m^2]

Gemcitabine: IV: 1000 mg/m^2/day days 1 and 8
[total dose/cycle = 2000 mg/m^2]

Repeat cycle every 21 days for 4 cycles

References

Variation 1:

von der Maase H, Hansen SW, Roberts JT, et al. Gemcitabine and cisplatin versus methotrexate, vinblastine, doxorubicin, and cisplatin in advanced or metastatic bladder cancer: results of a large, randomized, multinational, multicenter, phase III study. *J Clin Oncol.* 2000;18 (17):3068-3077.

Variations 2 and 3:

Dash A, Pettus JA 4th, Herr HW, et al. A role for neoadjuvant gemcitabine plus cisplatin in muscle-invasive urothelial carcinoma of the bladder: a retrospective experience. *Cancer.* 2008;113 (9):2471-2477.

Cisplatin-Gemcitabine (Cervical)

Index Terms Gemcitabine-Cisplatin (Cervical)

Use Cervical cancer

Regimen NOTE: Multiple variations are listed.

Variation 1:

Gemcitabine: IV: 1250 mg/m^2/day over 30 minutes days 1 and 8
[total dose/cycle = 2500 mg/m^2]

Cisplatin: IV: 50 mg/m^2 over 60 minutes day 1
[total dose/cycle = 50 mg/m^2]

Repeat cycle every 21 days for up to a total of 6 cycles

Variation 2:

Gemcitabine: IV: 1000 mg/m^2/day days 1 and 8
[total dose/cycle = 2000 mg/m^2]

Cisplatin: IV: 50 mg/m^2 day 1
[total dose/cycle = 50 mg/m^2]

Repeat cycle every 21 days for up to a total of 6 cycles; responders may continue beyond 6 cycles

Variation 3:

Cisplatin: IV: 30 mg/m^2/day days 1 and 8
[total dose/cycle = 60 mg/m^2]

Gemcitabine: IV: 800 mg/m^2/day days 1 and 8
[total dose/cycle = 1600 mg/m^2]

Repeat cycle every 28 days until disease progression or unacceptable toxicity

References

Variation 1:

Burnett AF, Roman LD, Garcia AA, Muderspach LI, Brader KR, Morrow CP. A phase II study of gemcitabine and cisplatin in patients with advanced, persistent, or recurrent squamous cell carcinoma of the cervix. *Gynecol Oncol.* 2000;76(1):63-66.

Variation 2:

Monk BJ, Sill MW, McMeekin DS, et al. Phase III trial of four cisplatin-containing doublet combinations in stage IVB, recurrent, or persistent cervical carcinoma: a Gynecologic Oncology Group study. *J Clin Oncol.* 2009;27(28):4649-4655.

Variation 3:

Brewer CA, Blessing JA, Nagourney RA, McMeekin DS, Lele S, Zweizig SL. Cisplatin plus gemcitabine in previously treated squamous cell carcinoma of the cervix: a phase II study of the Gynecologic Oncology Group. *Gynecol Oncol.* 2006;100(2):385-388.

Cisplatin-Gemcitabine (Mesothelioma)

Index Terms Gemcitabine-Cisplatin (Mesothelioma)

Use Malignant pleural mesothelioma

Regimen NOTE: Multiple variations are listed.

Variation 1:

Cisplatin: IV: 100 mg/m^2 over 1 hour day 1

[total dose/cycle = 100 mg/m^2]

Gemcitabine: IV: 1000 mg/m^2/day over 30 minutes days 1, 8, and 15

[total dose/cycle = 3000 mg/m^2]

Repeat cycle every 28 days for up to a total of 6 cycles

Variation 2:

Gemcitabine: IV: 1250 mg/m^2/day over 30 minutes days 1 and 8

[total dose/cycle = 2500 mg/m^2]

Cisplatin: IV: 80 mg/m^2 over 3 hours day 1

[total dose/cycle = 80 mg/m^2]

Repeat cycle every 21 days for up to a total of 6 cycles

Variation 3:

Gemcitabine: IV: 1000 mg/m^2/day over 30 minutes days 1, 8, and 15

[total dose/cycle = 3000 mg/m^2]

Cisplatin: IV: 30 mg/m^2/day over 30 minutes days 1, 8, and 15

[total dose/cycle = 90 mg/m^2]

Repeat cycle every 28 days

References

Variation 1:

Nowak AK, Byrne MJ, Williamson R, et al, "A Multicentre Phase II Study of Cisplatin and Gemcitabine for Malignant Mesothelioma," *Br J Cancer,* 2002, 87(5):491-6.

Variation 2:

van Haarst JM, Baas P, Manegold Ch, et al, "Multicentre Phase II Study of Gemcitabine and Cisplatin in Malignant Pleural Mesothelioma," *Br J Cancer,* 2002, 86(3):342-5.

Variation 3:

Kalmadi SR, Rankin C, Kraut MJ, et al, "Gemcitabine and Cisplatin in Unresectable Malignant Mesothelioma of the Pleura: A Phase II Study of the Southwest Oncology Group (SWOG 9810)," *Lung Cancer,* 2008, 60:259-63.

Cisplatin-Gemcitabine (NSCLC)

Index Terms GC (NSCLC); Gemcitabine-Cisplatin (NSCLC)

Use Lung cancer, non-small cell

◄ **Regimen** NOTE: Multiple variations are listed.

Variation 1:

Gemcitabine: IV: 1,000 mg/m²/day over 30 minutes days 1, 8, and 15
[total dose/cycle = 3,000 mg/m²]

Cisplatin: IV: 100 mg/m² day 1
[total dose/cycle = 100 mg/m²]

Repeat cycle every 28 days (for up to 6 cycles Sandler 2000)

Variation 2:

Cisplatin: IV: 100 mg/m² over 60 minutes day 1
[total dose/cycle = 100 mg/m²]

Gemcitabine: IV: 1,250 mg/m²/day over 30 minutes days 1 and 8
[total dose/cycle = 2,500 mg/m²]

Repeat cycle every 21 days for up to 6 cycles

Variation 3:

Gemcitabine: IV: 1,250 mg/m²/day over 30 minutes days 1 and 8
[total dose/cycle = 2,500 mg/m²]

Cisplatin: IV: 80 mg/m² day 1
[total dose/cycle = 80 mg/m²]

Repeat cycle every 21 days for up to 6 cycles

Variation 4:

Gemcitabine: IV: 1,000 mg/m²/day over 30 minutes days 1 and 8
[total dose/cycle = 2,000 mg/m²]

Cisplatin: IV: 80 mg/m² day 1
[total dose/cycle = 80 mg/m²]

Repeat cycle every 21 days until disease progression or unacceptable toxicity

References

Variation 1:

Comella P, Frasci G, Panza N, et al. Randomized trial comparing cisplatin, gemcitabine, and vinorelbine with either cisplatin and gemcitabine or cisplatin and vinorelbine in advanced non-small-cell lung cancer: interim analysis of a phase III trial of the Southern Italy Cooperative Oncology Group. *J Clin Oncol*. 2000;18(7):1451-1457.

Sandler AB, Nemunaitis J, Denham C, et al. Phase III trial of gemcitabine plus cisplatin versus cisplatin alone in patients with locally advanced or metastatic non-small-cell lung cancer. *J Clin Oncol*. 2000;18(1):122-130.

Schiller JH, Harrington D, Belani CP, et al. Comparison of four chemotherapy regimens for advanced non-small-cell lung cancer. *N Engl J Med*. 2002;346(2):92-98.

Variation 2:

Cardenal F, López-Cabrerizo MP, Antón A, et al. Randomized phase III study of gemcitabine-cisplatin versus etoposide-cisplatin in the treatment of locally advanced or metastatic non-small-cell lung cancer. *J Clin Oncol*. 1999;17(1):12-18.

Variation 3:

Smit EF, van Meerbeeck JP, Lianes P, et al. Three-arm randomized study of two cisplatin-based regimens and paclitaxel plus gemcitabine in advanced non-small-cell lung cancer: a phase III trial of the European Organization for Research and Treatment of Cancer Lung Cancer Group–EORTC 08975. *J Clin Oncol*. 2003;21(21):3909-3917.

Variation 4:

Ohe Y, Ohashi Y, Kubota K, et al. Randomized phase III study of cisplatin plus irinotecan versus carboplatin plus paclitaxel, cisplatin plus gemcitabine, and cisplatin plus vinorelbine for advanced non-small-cell lung cancer: Four-Arm Cooperative Study in Japan. *Ann Oncol*. 2007;18(2):317-323.

Cisplatin-Gemcitabine (Pancreatic)

Index Terms GemCis (Pancreatic); Gemcitabine-Cisplatin (Pancreatic)

Use Pancreatic cancer

Regimen NOTE: Multiple variations are listed.
Variation 1:
Cisplatin: IV: 50 mg/m²/day over 1 hour days 1 and 15
[total dose/cycle = 100 mg/m²]
Gemcitabine: IV: 1000 mg/m²/day over 30 minutes days 1 and 15
[total dose/cycle = 2000 mg/m²]
Repeat cycle every 28 days
Variation 2:
Cycle 1:
Cisplatin: IV: 25 mg/m²/day days 1, 8, 15, 29, 36, and 43 (cycle 1 only)
[total dose/cycle 1 = 150 mg/m²]
Gemcitabine: IV: 1000 mg/m²/day over 30 minutes days 1, 8, 15, 22, 29, 36, and 43 (cycle 1 only), 1 hour after cisplatin
[total dose/cycle 1 = 7000 mg/m²]
Treatment cycle is 56 days
Subsequent cycles:
Cisplatin: IV: 25 mg/m²/day days 1, 8, and 15
[total dose/cycle = 75 mg/m²]
Gemcitabine: IV: 1000 mg/m²/day over 30 minutes days 1, 8, and 15, 1 hour after cisplatin
[total dose/cycle = 3000 mg/m²]
Repeat cycle every 28 days until disease progression or unacceptable toxicity

References
Variation 1:
Heinemann V, Quietzsch D, Gieseler F, et al, "Randomized Phase III Trial of Gemcitabine Plus Cisplatin Compared With Gemcitabine Alone in Advanced Pancreatic Cancer," *J Clin Oncol*, 2006, 24(24):3946-52.
Variation 2:
Colucci G, Labianca R, Di Costanzo F, et al, "Randomized Phase III Trial of Gemcitabine Plus Cisplatin Compared With Single-Agent Gemcitabine As First-Line Treatment of Patients With Advanced Pancreatic Cancer: The GIP-1 Study," *J Clin Oncol*, 2010, 28(10):1645-51.

Cisplatin-Gemcitabine (Unknown Primary, Adenocarcinoma)

Index Terms Gemcitabine-Cisplatin (Unknown Primary)
Use Unknown primary (adenocarcinoma)
Regimen
Gemcitabine: IV: 1250 mg/m²/day days 1 and 8
[total dose/cycle = 2500 mg/m²]
Cisplatin: IV: 100 mg/m² day 1
[total dose/cycle = 100 mg/m²]
Repeat cycle every 21 days
References
Culine S, Lortholary A, Voigt JJ, et al, "Cisplatin in Combination With Either Gemcitabine or Irinotecan in Carcinomas of Unknown Primary Site: Results of a Randomized Phase II Study - Trial for the French Study Group on Carcinomas of Unknown Primary (GEFCAPI 01)," *J Clin Oncol*, 2003, 21(18):3479-82.

◆ **Cisplatin-Ifosfamide-Epirubicin (Osteosarcoma)** *see* Ifosfamide-Cisplatin-Epirubicin (Osteosarcoma) *on page 2015*

◆ **Cisplatin-Ifosfamide-Paclitaxel (Penile)** *see* Paclitaxel-Ifosfamide-Cisplatin (Penile) *on page 2052*

◆ **Cisplatin-Ifosfamide-Paclitaxel (Testicular)** *see* TIP (Testicular) *on page 2090*

♦ **Cisplatin-Irinotecan (Esophageal Cancer)** see Irinotecan-Cisplatin (Esophageal Cancer) on page 2021

Cisplatin-Irinotecan (Gastric)

Index Terms Irinotecan-Cisplatin (Gastric)

Use Gastric cancer

Regimen NOTE: Multiple variations are listed.

Variation 1:

Irinotecan: IV: 65 mg/m^2/day over 90 minutes days 1, 8, 15, and 22
[total dose/cycle = 260 mg/m^2]

Cisplatin: IV: 30 mg/m^2/day over 60 minutes days 1, 8, 15, and 22
[total dose/cycle = 120 mg/m^2]

Repeat cycle every 6 weeks until disease progression or unacceptable toxicity

Variation 2:

Irinotecan: IV: 70 mg/m^2/day over 90 minutes days 1 and 15
[total dose/cycle = 140 mg/m^2]

Cisplatin: IV: 70 mg/m^2 over 2 hours day 1
[total dose/cycle = 70 mg/m^2]

Repeat cycle every 28 days for up to 6 cycles

References

Variation 1:
Ajani JA, Baker J, Pisters PW, et al.CPT-11 plus cisplatin in patients with advanced, untreated gastric or gastroesophageal junction carcinoma: results of a phase II study. *Cancer.* 2002;94 (3):641-646.
Variation 2:
Park SH, Choi EY, Bang SM, et al. Salvage chemotherapy with irinotecan and cisplatin in patients with metastatic gastric cancer failing both 5-fluorouracil and taxanes. *Anticancer Drugs.* 2005;16 (6):621-625.

Cisplatin-Irinotecan (NSCLC)

Index Terms Irinotecan-Cisplatin (NSCLC)

Use Lung cancer, non-small cell

Regimen

Cisplatin: IV: 80 mg/m^2 day 1
[total dose/cycle = 80 mg/m^2]

Irinotecan: IV: 60 mg/m^2/dose days 1, 8, and 15
[total dose/cycle = 180 mg/m^2]

Repeat cycle every 28 days for at least 3 more cycles or until disease progression or unacceptable toxicity

References

Ohe Y, Ohashi Y, Kubota K, et al, "Randomized Phase III Study of Cisplatin Plus Irinotecan Versus Carboplatin Plus Paclitaxel, Cisplatin Plus Gemcitabine, and Cisplatin Plus Vinorelbine for Advanced Non-Small-Cell Lung Cancer: Four-Arm Cooperative Study in Japan," *Ann Oncol*, 2007, 18(2):317-23.

Cisplatin-Irinotecan (Small Cell Lung Cancer)

Index Terms IP (Small Cell Lung Cancer); Irinotecan-Cisplatin (Small Cell Lung Cancer)

Use Lung cancer, small cell

Regimen NOTE: Multiple variations are listed.

Variation 1:

Cisplatin: IV: 60 mg/m^2 day 1
[total dose/cycle = 60 mg/m^2]

Irinotecan: IV: 60 mg/m²/day days 1, 8, and 15
[total dose/cycle = 180 mg/m²]
Repeat cycle every 28 days for 4 cycles
Variation 2:
Cisplatin: IV: 30 mg/m²/day days 1 and 8
[total dose/cycle = 60 mg/m²]
Irinotecan: IV: 65 mg/m²/day days 1 and 8
[total dose/cycle = 130 mg/m²]
Repeat cycle every 21 days for at least 4 cycles

References

Variation 1:

Lara PN Jr, Natale R, Crowley J, et al, "Phase III Trial of Irinotecan/Cisplatin Compared With Etoposide/Cisplatin in Extensive-Stage Small-Cell Lung Cancer: Clinical and Pharmacogenomic Results from SWOG S0124," *J Clin Oncol*, 2009, 27(15):2530-5.

Noda K, Nishiwaki Y, Kawahara M, et al, "Irinotecan Plus Cisplatin Compared With Etoposide Plus Cisplatin for Extensive Small-Cell Lung Cancer," *N Engl J Med*, 2002, 346(2):85-91.

Variation 2:

Hanna N, Bunn PA Jr, Langer C, et al, "Randomized Phase III Trial Comparing Irinotecan/Cisplatin With Etoposide/Cisplatin in Patients With Previously Untreated Extensive-Stage Disease Small-Cell Lung Cancer," *J Clin Oncol*, 2006, 24(13):2038-43.

♦ **Cisplatin-Paclitaxel-Bevacizumab (Cervical)** *see* Bevacizumab-Cisplatin-Paclitaxel (Cervical) *on page 1841*

Cisplatin-Paclitaxel (Cervical Cancer)

Index Terms Paclitaxel-Cisplatin (Cervical Cancer)

Use Cervical cancer

Regimen

Paclitaxel: IV: 135 mg/m² continuous infusion over 24 hours day 1
[total dose/cycle = 135 mg/m²]
Cisplatin: IV: 50 mg/m² day 2
[total dose/cycle = 50 mg/m²]
Repeat cycle every 21 days for up to a total of 6 cycles; responders may continue beyond 6 cycles

References

Monk BJ, Sill MW, McMeekin DS, et al, "Phase III Trial of Four Cisplatin-Containing Doublet Combinations in Stage IVB, Recurrent, or Persistent Cervical Carcinoma: A Gynecologic Oncology Group Study," *J Clin Oncol*, 2009, 27(28):4649-55.

Moore DH, Blessing JA, McQuellon RP, et al, "Phase III Study of Cisplatin With or Without Paclitaxel in Stage IVB, Recurrent, or Persistent Squamous Cell Carcinoma of the Cervix: A Gynecologic Oncology Group Study," *J Clin Oncol*, 2004, 22(15):3113-9.

♦ **Cisplatin-Paclitaxel (Esophageal Cancer)** *see* Paclitaxel-Cisplatin (Esophageal Cancer) *on page 2050*

♦ **Cisplatin-Paclitaxel-Fluorouracil (Unknown Primary)** *see* Cisplatin-Fluorouracil-Paclitaxel (Unknown Primary, Squamous Cell) *on page 1903*

Cisplatin-Paclitaxel (Head and Neck Cancer)

Index Terms Paclitaxel-Cisplatin (Head and Neck Cancer)

Use Head and neck cancer

Regimen NOTE: Multiple variations are listed.

Variation 1 (with concurrent radiation therapy):
Paclitaxel: IV: 30 mg/m² day 1
[total dose/week = 30 mg/m²]

Cisplatin: IV: 20 mg/m^2 day 2

[total dose/week = 20 mg/m^2]

Repeat every week for a total of 7 weeks

Variation 2:

Paclitaxel: IV: 175 mg/m^2 dose over 3 hours day 1

[total dose/cycle = 175 mg/m^2]

Cisplatin: IV: 75 mg/m^2/dose day 1

[total dose/cycle = 75 mg/m^2]

Repeat cycle every 3 weeks

References

Variation 1:

Garden AS, Harris J, Vokes EE, et al, "Preliminary Results of Radiation Therapy Oncology Group 97-03: A Randomized Phase II Trial of Concurrent Radiation and Chemotherapy for Advanced Squamous Cell Carcinomas of the Head and Neck," *J Clin Oncol*, 2004, 22(14):2856-64.

Variation 2:

Gibson MK, Li Y, Murphy B, et al, "Randomized Phase III Evaluation of Cisplatin Plus Fluorouracil Versus Cisplatin Plus Paclitaxel in Advanced Head and Neck Cancer (E1395): An Intergroup Trial of the Eastern Cooperative Oncology Group," *J Clin Oncol*, 2005, 23(15):3562-7.

Cisplatin-Paclitaxel Intraperitoneal (Ovarian)

Index Terms Paclitaxel-Cisplatin Intraperitoneal (Ovarian)

Use Ovarian cancer

Regimen Note: I.P. therapies administered in 2 liters warmed saline

Paclitaxel: IV: 135 mg/m^2 continuous infusion over 24 hours day 1

[total IV dose/cycle = 135 mg/m^2]

Cisplatin: I.P.: 100 mg/m^2 day 2

[total I.P. dose/cycle = 100 mg/m^2]

Paclitaxel: I.P.: 60 mg/m^2 day 8

[total I.P. dose/cycle = 60 mg/m^2]

Repeat cycle every 21 days for 6 cycles

References

Armstrong DK, Bundy B, Wenzel L, et al, "Intraperitoneal Cisplatin and Paclitaxel in Ovarian Cancer," *N Engl J Med*, 2006, 354(1):34-43.

Cisplatin-Paclitaxel (NSCLC)

Index Terms Paclitaxel-Cisplatin (NSCLC)

Use Lung cancer, non-small cell

Regimen

Paclitaxel: IV: 135 mg/m^2 continuous infusion over 24 hours day 1

[total dose/cycle = 135 mg/m^2]

Cisplatin: IV: 75 mg/m^2 day 2

[total dose/cycle = 75 mg/m^2]

Repeat cycle every 21 days

References

Schiller JH, Harrington D, Belani CP, et al. Comparison of four chemotherapy regimens for advanced non-small-cell lung cancer. *N Engl J Med*, 2002;346(2):92-98.

Cisplatin-Paclitaxel (Ovarian)

Index Terms Paclitaxel-Cisplatin (Ovarian)

Use Ovarian cancer

Regimen

Paclitaxel: IV: 135 mg/m^2 continuous infusion over 24 hours day 1
[total dose/cycle = 135 mg/m^2]
Cisplatin: IV: 75 mg/m^2 day 2
[total dose/cycle = 75 mg/m^2]
Repeat cycle every 21 days for a total of 6 cycles

References

McGuire WP, Hoskins WJ, Brady MF, et al, "Cyclophosphamide and Cisplatin Compared With Paclitaxel and Cisplatin in Patients With Stage III and Stage IV Ovarian Cancer," *N Engl J Med*, 1996, 334(1):1-6.

Muggia FM, Braly PS, Brady MF, et al, "Phase III Randomized Study of Cisplatin Versus Paclitaxel Versus Cisplatin and Paclitaxel in Patients With Suboptimal Stage III or IV Ovarian Cancer: A Gynecologic Oncology Group Study," *J Clin Oncol*, 2000, 18(1):106-15.

Cisplatin-Pemetrexed (Mesothelioma)

Index Terms Pemetrexed-Cisplatin (Mesothelioma)

Use Malignant pleural mesothelioma

Regimen

Pemetrexed: IV: 500 mg/m^2 over 10 minutes day 1
[total dose/cycle = 500 mg/m^2]
Cisplatin: IV: 75 mg/m^2 over 2 hours day 1 (start 30 minutes after pemetrexed)
[total dose/cycle = 75 mg/m^2]
Repeat cycle every 21 days

References

Santoro A, O'Brien ME, Stahel RA, et al, "Pemetrexed Plus Cisplatin or Pemetrexed Plus Carboplatin for Chemonaïve Patients With Malignant Pleural Mesothelioma: Results of the International Expanded Access Program," *J Thorac Oncol*, 2008, 3(7):756-63.

Vogelzang NJ, Rusthoven JJ, Symanowski J, et al, "Phase III Study of Pemetrexed in Combination With Cisplatin Versus Cisplatin Alone in Patients With Malignant Pleural Mesothelioma," *J Clin Oncol*, 2003, 21(14):2636-44.

Cisplatin-Pemetrexed (NSCLC)

Index Terms Pemetrexed-Cisplatin (NSCLC)

Use Lung cancer, non-small cell

Regimen

Pemetrexed: IV: 500 mg/m^2 day 1
[total dose/cycle = 500 mg/m^2]
Cisplatin: IV: 75 mg/m^2 day 1
[total dose/cycle = 75 mg/m^2]
Repeat cycle every 21 days for up to 6 cycles

References

Scagliotti GV, Parikh P, von Pawel J, et al, "Phase III Study Comparing Cisplatin Plus Gemcitabine With Cisplatin Plus Pemetrexed in Chemotherapy-Naive Patients With Advanced-Stage Non-Small-Cell Lung Cancer," *J Clin Oncol*, 2008, 26(21):3543-51.

Cisplatin-Raltitrexed (Mesothelioma)

Index Terms Raltitrexed-Cisplatin (Mesothelioma)

Use Malignant pleural mesothelioma

Regimen

Raltitrexed: IV: 3 mg/m^2 over 15 minutes day 1
[total dose/cycle = 3 mg/m^2]
Cisplatin: IV: 80 mg/m^2 over 1-2 hours day 1
[total dose/cycle = 80 mg/m^2]
Repeat cycle every 21 days until disease progression or unacceptable toxicity.

References

Bottomley A, Coens C, Efficace F, et al, "Symptoms and Patient-Reported Well-Being: Do They Predict Survival in Malignant Pleural Mesothelioma? A Prognostic Factor Analysis of EORTC-NCIC 08983: Randomized Phase III Study of Cisplatin With or Without Raltitrexed in Patients With Malignant Pleural Mesothelioma," *J Clin Oncol*, 2007, 25(36):5770-6.

van Meerbeeck JP, Gaafar R, Manegold C, et al, "Randomized Phase III Study of Cisplatin With or Without Raltitrexed in Patients With Malignant Pleural Mesothelioma: An Intergroup Study of the European Organisation for Research and Treatment of Cancer Lung Cancer Group and the National Cancer Institute of Canada," *J Clin Oncol*, 2005, 23(23):6881-9.

Cisplatin-Topotecan (Cervical Cancer)

Index Terms Topotecan-Cisplatin (Cervical Cancer)

Use Cervical cancer

Regimen NOTE: Multiple variations are listed.

Variation 1 (Body surface area capped at 2 m² maximum):

Topotecan: IV: 0.75 mg/m²/day days 1, 2, and 3
[total dose/cycle = 2.25 mg/m²]
Cisplatin: IV: 50 mg/m² day 1 only
[total dose/cycle = 50 mg/m²]
Repeat cycle every 21 days for up to a total of 6 cycles; responders may continue beyond 6 cycles

Variation 2:

Topotecan: IV: 0.75 mg/m²/day days 1, 2, and 3
[total dose/cycle = 2.25 mg/m²]
Cisplatin: IV: 50 mg/m² day 1 only
[total dose/cycle = 50 mg/m²]
Repeat cycle every 21 days for up to a total of 6 cycles; responders may continue beyond 6 cycles

References

Variation 1:
Long HJ 3rd, Bundy BN, Grendys EC Jr, et al, "Randomized Phase III Trial of Cisplatin With or Without Topotecan in Carcinoma of the Uterine Cervix: A Gynecologic Oncology Group Study," *J Clin Oncol*, 2005, 23(21):4626-33.
Variation 2:
Monk BJ, Sill MW, McMeekin DS, et al, "Phase III Trial of Four Cisplatin-Containing Doublet Combinations in Stage IVB, Recurrent, or Persistent Cervical Carcinoma: A Gynecologic Oncology Group Study," *J Clin Oncol*, 2009, 27(28):4649-55.

◆ **Cisplatin-Vinblastine-Dacarbazine-Interleukin-Interferon (Melanoma)** see CVD-Interleukin-Interferon (Melanoma) *on page 1926*

Cisplatin-Vinblastine-Dacarbazine (Melanoma)

Index Terms CVD; Dacarbazine-Cisplatin-Vinblastine; Vinblastine-Cisplatin-Dacarbazine

Use Melanoma

Regimen NOTE: Multiple variations are listed.

Variation 1:

Cisplatin: IV: 20 mg/m²/day days 2 to 5
[total dose/cycle = 80 mg/m²]
Vinblastine: IV: 1.6 mg/m²/day days 1 to 5
[total dose/cycle = 8 mg/m²]
Dacarbazine: IV: 800 mg/m² day 1
[total dose/cycle = 800 mg/m²]
Repeat cycle every 21 days

Variation 2:
Cisplatin: IV: 20 mg/m^2/day days 1 to 4
[total dose/cycle = 80 mg/m^2]
Vinblastine: IV: 2 mg/m^2/day days 1 to 4
[total dose/cycle = 8 mg/m^2]
Dacarbazine: IV: 800 mg/m^2 day 1
[total dose/cycle = 800 mg/m^2]
Repeat cycle every 21 days

References

Variation 1:
Legha SS, Ring S, Papadopoulos N, et al, "A Prospective Evaluation of a Triple-Drug Regimen Containing Cisplatin, Vinblastine, and Dacarbazine (CVD) for Metastatic Melanoma," *Cancer*, 1989, 64(10):2024-9.

Variation 2:
Eton O, Legha SS, Bedikian AY, et al, "Sequential Biochemotherapy Versus Chemotherapy for Metastatic Melanoma: Results From a Phase III Randomized Trial," *J Clin Oncol*, 2002, 20 (8):2045-52.

Cisplatin-Vinblastine (NSCLC)

Index Terms Vinblastine-Cisplatin (NSCLC)

Use Lung cancer, non-small cell

Regimen NOTE: Multiple variations are listed.
Variation 1 (concurrent radiation preferred):
Cisplatin: IV: 100 mg/m^2/day days 1 and 29
[total dose/treatment = 200 mg/m^2]
Vinblastine: IV: 5 mg/m^2/week days 1, 8, 15, 22, and 29
[total dose/treatment = 25 mg/m^2]
Variation 2 (sequential radiation):
Cisplatin: IV: 100 mg/m^2/day days 1 and 29
[total dose/treatment = 200 mg/m^2]
Vinblastine: IV: 5 mg/m^2/week days 1, 8, 15, 22, and 29
[total dose/treatment = 25 mg/m^2]
Variation 3 (adjuvant therapy):
Cisplatin: IV: 80 mg/m^2/day days 1, 22, 43, and 64
[total dose/treatment = 320 mg/m^2]
Vinblastine: IV: 4 mg/m^2/day days 1, 8, 15, 22, 29, 43, and 57
[total dose/treatment = 28 mg/m^2]
Variation 4 (adjuvant therapy):
Cisplatin: IV: 100 mg/m^2/day days 1, 29, and 57
[total dose/treatment = 300 mg/m^2]
Vinblastine: IV: 4 mg/m^2/day days 1, 8, 15, 22, 29, 43, and 57
[total dose/treatment = 28 mg/m^2]
Variation 5 (adjuvant therapy):
Cisplatin: IV: 100 mg/m^2/day days 1, 29, 57, and 85
[total dose/treatment = 400 mg/m^2]
Vinblastine: IV: 4 mg/m^2/day days 1, 8, 15, 22, 29, 43, 57, 71, and 85
[total dose/treatment = 36 mg/m^2]

References

Variations 1 and 2:
Curran WJ Jr, Paulus R, Langer CJ, et al. Sequential vs. concurrent chemoradiation for stage III non-small cell lung cancer: randomized phase III trial RTOG 9410. J Natl Cancer Inst. 2011;103 (19):1452-1460.

Variations 3, 4, and 5:
Arriagada R, Bergman B, Dunant A, et al. Cisplatin-based adjuvant chemotherapy in patients with completely resected non-small-cell lung cancer. N Engl J Med. 2004;350(4):351-360.

Cisplatin-Vinorelbine (Adjuvant NSCLC)

Index Terms VC (Adjuvant NSCLC); Vinorelbine-Cisplatin (Adjuvant NSCLC)

Use Lung cancer, non-small cell (adjuvant)

Regimen NOTE: Multiple variations are listed.

Variation 1:

Cisplatin: IV: 50 mg/m^2/day days 1 and 8
  [total dose/cycle = 100 mg/m^2]
Vinorelbine: IV: 25 mg/m^2/day days 1, 8, 15, and 22
  [total dose/cycle = 100 mg/m^2]
Repeat cycle every 28 days for total of 4 cycles

Variation 2:

Vinorelbine: IV: 30 mg/m^2/day days 1, 8, 15, and 22
  [total dose/cycle = 120 mg/m^2]
Cisplatin: IV: 100 mg/m^2 day 1
  [total dose/cycle = 100 mg/m^2]
Repeat cycle every 28 days for total of 4 cycles

Variation 3:

Cisplatin: IV: 80 mg/m^2 day 1
  [total dose/cycle = 80 mg/m^2]
Vinorelbine: IV: 30 mg/m^2/day days 1, 8, and 15
  [total dose/cycle = 90 mg/m^2]
Repeat cycle every 21 days for total of 4 cycles
Note: Vinorelbine treatment is discontinued after day 1 of the final treatment cycle

Variation 4:

Cisplatin: IV: 100 mg/m^2 day 1
  [total dose/cycle = 100 mg/m^2]
Vinorelbine: IV: 30 mg/m^2/day days 1, 8, 15, and 22
  [total dose/cycle = 120 mg/m^2]
Repeat cycle every 28 days for total of 3 or 4 cycles
Note: Vinorelbine treatment is discontinued after day 1 of the final treatment cycle

References

Variation 1:

Butts CA, Ding K, Seymour L, et al. Randomized phase III trial of vinorelbine plus cisplatin compared with observation in completely resected stage IB and II non-small-cell lung cancer: updated survival analysis of JBR-10. *J Clin Oncol.* 2010;28(1):29-34.

Winton T, Livingston R, Johnson D, et al. Vinorelbine plus cisplatin vs. observation in resected non-small-cell lung cancer. *N Engl J Med.* 2005;352(25):2589-2597.

Variation 2:

Douillard JY, Rosell R, De Lena M, et al. Adjuvant vinorelbine plus cisplatin versus observation in patients with completely resected stage IB-IIIA non-small-cell lung cancer (Adjuvant Navelbine International Trialist Association [ANITA]): a randomised controlled trial. *Lancet Oncol.* 2006;7 (9):719-727.

Variations 3 and 4:

Arriagada R, Bergman B, Dunant A, et al. Cisplatin-based adjuvant chemotherapy in patients with completely resected non-small-cell lung cancer. *N Engl J Med.* 2004;350(4):351-360.

Arriagada R, Dunant A, Pignon JP, et al. Long-term results of the international adjuvant lung cancer trial evaluating adjuvant cisplatin-based chemotherapy in resected lung cancer. *J Clin Oncol.* 2010;28(1):35-42.

Cisplatin-Vinorelbine (Cervical Cancer)

Index Terms Vinorelbine-Cisplatin (Cervical Cancer)

Use Cervical cancer

Regimen NOTE: Multiple variations are listed.

Variation 1:

Cisplatin: IV: 50 mg/m² day 1

[total dose/cycle = 50 mg/m²]

Vinorelbine: IV: 30 mg/m²/day days 1 and 8

[total dose/cycle = 60 mg/m²]

Repeat cycle every 21 days for up to a total of 6 cycles; responders may continue beyond 6 cycles

Variation 2:

Cisplatin: IV: 80 mg/m² day 1

[total dose/cycle = 80 mg/m²]

Vinorelbine: IV: 25 mg/m²/day days 1 and 8

[total dose/cycle = 50 mg/m²]

Repeat cycle every 21 days for a total of 3-6 cycles

References

Variation 1:

Monk BJ, Sill MW, McMeekin DS, et al, "Phase III Trial of Four Cisplatin-Containing Doublet Combinations in Stage IVB, Recurrent, or Persistent Cervical Carcinoma: A Gynecologic Oncology Group Study," *J Clin Oncol*, 2009, 27(28):4649-55.

Variation 2:

Gebbia V, Caruso M, Testa A, et al, "Vinorelbine and Cisplatin for the Treatment of Recurrent and/or Metastatic Carcinoma of the Uterine Cervix," *Oncology*, 2002, 63(1):31-7.

Pignata S, Silvestro G, Ferrari E, et al, "Phase II Study of Cisplatin and Vinorelbine as First-Line Chemotherapy in Patients With Carcinoma of the Uterine Cervix," *J Clin Oncol*, 1999, 17 (3):756-60.

◆ **Cisplatin-Vinorelbine-Cetuximab (NSCLC)** see Cetuximab-Cisplatin-Vinorelbine (NSCLC) *on page 1881*

Cisplatin-Vinorelbine (Metastatic NSCLC)

Index Terms VC (Metastatic NSCLC); Vinorelbine-Cisplatin (Metastatic NSCLC)

Use Lung cancer, non-small cell (metastatic)

Regimen NOTE: Multiple variations are listed.

Variation 1:

Cisplatin: IV: 100 mg/m² day 1

[total dose/cycle = 100 mg/m²]

Vinorelbine: IV: 25 mg/m²/day days 1, 8, 15, and 22

[total dose/cycle = 100 mg/m²]

Repeat cycle every 28 days for up to 10 cycles

Variation 2:

Cisplatin: IV: 80 mg/m² day 1

[total dose/cycle = 80 mg/m²]

Vinorelbine: IV: 25 mg/m²/day days 1 and 8

[total dose/cycle = 50 mg/m²]

Repeat cycle every 21 days

References

Variation 1:

Kelly K, Crowley J, Bunn PA Jr, et al. Randomized phase III trial of paclitaxel plus carboplatin versus vinorelbine plus cisplatin in the treatment of patients with advanced non-small-cell lung cancer: a Southwest Oncology Group trial. *J Clin Oncol*. 2001;19(13):3210-3218.

Variation 2:

Ohe Y, Ohashi Y, Kubota K, et al. Randomized phase III study of cisplatin plus irinotecan versus carboplatin plus paclitaxel, cisplatin plus gemcitabine, and cisplatin plus vinorelbine for advanced non-small-cell lung cancer: Four-Arm Cooperative Study in Japan. *Ann Oncol*. 2007;18 (2):317-323.

♦ **Cladribine-Cytarabine-G-CSF** *see* CLAG (AML Induction) *on page 1916*

♦ **Cladribine-Cytarabine-Mitoxantrone-G-CS** *see* CLAG-M (AML Induction) *on page 1917*

Cladribine-Rituximab (NHL-Mantle Cell)

Index Terms 2-CDA-Rituximab (NHL-Mantle Cell); Rituximab-Cladribine (NHL-Mantle Cell)

Use Lymphoma, non-Hodgkin (Mantle cell)

Regimen

Rituximab: IV: 375 mg/m^2 day 1

[total dose/cycle = 375 mg/m^2]

Cladribine: IV: 5 mg/m^2/day over 2 hours days 1 to 5

[total dose/cycle = 25 mg/m^2]

Growth Factor:

Pegfilgrastim: SubQ: 6 mg day 6

or

Filgrastim: SubQ: Days 6 to 15 (no dose specified)

Repeat cycle every 28 days for a total of 2 to 6 cycles

References

Inwards DJ, Fishkin PA, Hillman DW, et al. Long-term results of the treatment of patients with mantle cell lymphoma with cladribine (2-CDA) alone (95-80-53) or 2-CDA and rituximab (N0189) in the North Central Cancer Treatment Group. *Cancer.* 2008;113(1):108-116.

Cladribine-Rituximab (Waldenstrom Macroglobulinemia)

Index Terms 2-chloro-2'-deoxyadenosine-Rituximab (Waldenstrom Macroglobulinemia); Rituximab-Cladribine (Waldenstrom Macroglobulinemia)

Use Waldenstrom macroglobulinemia

Regimen

Rituximab: IV: 375 mg/m^2 day 1

[total dose/cycle = 375 mg/m^2]

Cladribine: SubQ: 0.1 mg/kg/day once daily days 1 to 5

[total dose/cycle = 0.5 mg/kg]

Repeat cycle every 28 days for 4 cycles

References

Laszlo D, Andreola G, Rigacci L, et al. Rituximab and subcutaneous 2-chloro-2'-deoxyadenosine combination treatment for patients with Waldenstrom macroglobulinemia: clinical and biologic results of a phase II multicenter study. *J Clin Oncol.* 2010;28(13):2233-2238.

CLAG (AML Induction)

Index Terms Cladribine-Cytarabine-G-CSF

Use Leukemia, acute myeloid

Regimen

Cladribine: IV: 5 mg/m^2/day over 2 hours days 1 to 5

[total dose/cycle = 25 mg/m^2]

Cytarabine: IV: 2 g/m^2/day over 4 hours days 1 to 5 (begin 2 hours after cladribine)

[total dose/cycle = 10 g/m^2]

Filgrastim: SubQ: 300 mcg daily days 0 to 5 (start 24 hours prior to chemotherapy; for a total of 6 days)

[total dose/cycle = 1800 mcg]

May administer a second induction cycle if needed

References

Robak T, Wrzesień-Kuś A, Lech-Marańda E, et al, "Combination Regimen of Cladribine (2-Chlorodeoxyadenosine), Cytarabine and G-CSF (CLAG) as Induction Therapy for Patients With Relapsed or Refractory Acute Myeloid Leukemia," *Leuk Lymphoma*, 2000, 39(1-2):121-9.

Wrzesień-Kuś A, Robak T, Lech-Marańda E, et al, "A Multicenter, Open, Non-Comparative Phase II Study of the Combination of Cladribine (2-Chlorodeoxyadenosine), Cytarabine, and G-CSF as Induction Therapy in Refractory Acute Myeloid Leukemia – A Report of the Polish Adult Leukemia Group (PALG)," *Eur J Haematol*, 2003;71(3):155–62.

CLAG-M (AML Induction)

Index Terms Cladribine-Cytarabine-Mitoxantrone-G-CS

Use Leukemia, acute myeloid

Regimen

Cladribine: IV: 5 mg/m^2/day over 2 hour days 1 to 5

[total dose/cycle = 25 mg/m^2]

Cytarabine: IV: 2 g/m^2/day over 4 hours days 1 to 5 (begin 2 hours after cladribine)

[total dose/cycle = 10 g/m^2]

Mitoxantrone: IV: 10 mg/m^2/day days 1 to 3

[total dose/cycle = 30 mg/m^2]

Filgrastim: SubQ: 300 mcg daily days 0 to 5 (start 24 hours prior to chemotherapy; for a total of 6 days)

[total dose/cycle = 1800 mcg]

May administer a second induction cycle if needed

References

Wierzbowska A, Robak T, Pluta A, et al, "Cladribine Combined With High Doses of Arabinoside Cytosine, Mitoxantrone, and G-CSF (CLAG-M) is a Highly Effective Salvage Regimen in Patients With Refractory and Relapsed Acute Myeloid Leukemia of the Poor Risk: A Final Report of the Polish Adult Leukemia Group," *Eur J Haematol* 2008; 80(2):115-26.

Clofarabine (ALL Regimen)

Use Leukemia, acute lymphocytic (relapsed/refractory)

Regimen

Induction:

Clofarabine: IV: 40 mg/m^2/day over 1 hour days 1 to 5

[total dose/cycle = 200 mg/m^2]

A second induction cycle may be administered if needed between day 21 to 42 depending on marrow response and recovery, up to a maximum of 2 induction cycles

Consolidation:

Clofarabine: IV: 30 mg/m^2/day over 1 hour days 1 to 5

[total dose/cycle = 150 mg/m^2]

Repeat cycle every 28 days up to a maximum of 6 consolidation cycles

References

Kantarjian H, Gandhi V, Cortes J, et al. Phase 2 clinical and pharmacologic study of clofarabine in patients with refractory or relapsed acute leukemia. *Blood*. 2003;102(7):2379-2386.

Clofarabine-Cytarabine (AML)

Index Terms Cytarabine-Clofarabine (AML); GCLAC (AML)

Use Leukemia, acute myeloid (relapsed/refractory, 18 to 70 years of age) ▶

◀ **Regimen**

Induction:

Filgrastim: SubQ: 5 mcg/kg (round to nearest vial size) once daily beginning day 0 and continuing until the ANC ≥2,000/mm³ for 2 consecutive days

Clofarabine: IV: 25 mg/m²/day over 1 hour days 1 to 5

[total dose/cycle = 125 mg/m²]

Cytarabine: IV: 2,000 mg/m²/day over 2 hours days 1 to 5 (beginning 4 hours after start of clofarabine)

[total dose/cycle = 10,000 mg/m²]

A second induction cycle may be administered after day 21 if needed, up to a maximum of 2 induction cycles

Consolidation:

Filgrastim: SubQ: 5 mcg/kg (round to nearest vial size) once daily beginning day 0 and continuing until the ANC ≥2,000/mm³ for 2 consecutive days

Clofarabine: IV: 20 mg/m²/day over 1 hour days 1 to 5

[total dose/cycle = 100 mg/m²]

Cytarabine: IV: 1,000 mg/m²/day over 2 hours days 1 to 5 (beginning 4 hours after start of clofarabine)

[total dose/cycle = 5,000 mg/m²]

Repeat consolidation every 21 days for 1 or 2 cycles, up to a maximum of 2 consolidation cycles

References

Becker PS, Kantarjian HM, Appelbaum FR, et al. Clofarabine with high dose cytarabine and granulocyte colony-stimulating factor (G-CSF) priming for relapsed and refractory acute myeloid leukaemia. *Br J Haematol.* 2011;155(2):182-189.

CMF Oral (Breast)

Index Terms Cyclophosphamide, Methotrexate, Fluorouracil (Breast)

Use Breast cancer

Regimen NOTE: Multiple variations are listed.

Variation 1 (patients ≤60 years of age):

Methotrexate: IV: 40 mg/m²/day days 1 and 8

[total dose/cycle = 80 mg/m²]

Fluorouracil: IV: 600 mg/m²/day days 1 and 8

[total dose/cycle = 1200 mg/m²]

Cyclophosphamide: Oral: 100 mg/m²/day days 1 to 14

[total dose/cycle = 1400 mg/m²]

Repeat cycle every 28 days for 12 cycles

Variation 1 (patients >60 years of age):

Methotrexate: IV: 30 mg/m²/day days 1 and 8

[total dose/cycle = 60 mg/m²]

Fluorouracil: IV: 400 mg/m²/day days 1 and 8

[total dose/cycle = 800 mg/m²]

Cyclophosphamide: Oral: 100 mg/m²/day days 1 to 14

[total dose/cycle = 1400 mg/m²]

Repeat cycle every 28 days for 12 cycles

Variation 2 (adjuvant treatment):

Methotrexate: IV: 40 mg/m²/day days 1 and 8

[total dose/cycle = 80 mg/m²]

Fluorouracil: IV: 600 mg/m²/day days 1 and 8

[total dose/cycle = 1200 mg/m²]

Cyclophosphamide: Oral: 100 mg/m²/day days 1 to 14

[total dose/cycle = 1400 mg/m²]

Repeat cycle every 28 days for a total of 6 cycles

Variation 3 (metastatic disease):

Methotrexate: IV: 40 mg/m^2/day days 1 and 8
  [total dose/cycle = 80 mg/m^2]

Fluorouracil: IV: 600 mg/m^2/day days 1 and 8
  [total dose/cycle = 1200 mg/m^2]

Cyclophosphamide: Oral: 100 mg/m^2/day days 1 to 14
  [total dose/cycle = 1400 mg/m^2]

Repeat cycle every 28 days until disease progression or unacceptable toxicity

References

Early Breast Cancer Trialists' Collaborative Group (EBCTCG), Peto R, Davies C, et al, "Comparisons Between Different Polychemotherapy Regimens for Early Breast Cancer: Meta-Analysis of Long-Term Outcome Among 100,000 Women in 123 Randomised Trials," Lancet, 2012, 379 (9814):432-44.

Goldhirsch A, Colleoni M, Coates AS, et al, "Adding Adjuvant CMF Chemotherapy to Either Radiotherapy or Tamoxifen: Are All CMFs Alike? The International Breast Cancer Study Group (IBCSG)" Ann Oncol, 1998, 9(5):489-93.

Variation 1:

Bonadonna G, Brusamolino E, Valagussa P, et al, "Combination Chemotherapy as an Adjuvant Treatment in Operable Breast Cancer," N Engl J Med, 1976, 294(8):405-10.

Bonadonna G, Valagussa P, Moliterni A, et al, "Adjuvant Cyclophosphamide, Methotrexate, and Fluorouracil in Node-Positive Breast Cancer: The Results of 20 Years of Follow-Up," N Engl J Med, 1995, 332(14):901-6.

Canellos GP, Pocock SJ, Taylor SG III, et al, "Combination Chemotherapy for Metastatic Breast Carcinoma, Prospective Comparison of Multiple Drug Therapy With L-Phenylalanine Mustard," Cancer, 1976, 38(5):1882-6.

Variation 2:

Hutchins LF, Green SJ, Ravdin PM, et al, "Randomized, Controlled Trial of Cyclophosphamide, Methotrexate, and Fluorouracil Versus Cyclophosphamide, Doxorubicin, and Fluorouracil With and Without Tamoxifen for High-Risk, Node-Negative Breast Cancer: Treatment Results of Intergroup Protocol INT-0102," J Clin Oncol, 2005, 23(33):8313-21.

Variation 3:

Engelsman E, Klijn JC, Rubens RD, et al, "'Classical' CMF Versus a 3-Weekly Intravenous CMF Schedule in Postmenopausal Patients With Advanced Breast Cancer: An EORTC Breast Cancer Co-Operative Group Phase III Trial (10808)," Eur J Cancer, 1991, 27(8):966-70.

C-MOPP/ABV Hybrid (Hodgkin)

Index Terms Cyclophosphamide-Vincristine-Procarbazine-Prednisone-Doxorubicin-Bleomycin-Vinblastine (Hodgkin)

Use Lymphoma, Hodgkin

Regimen

Cyclophosphamide: IV: 650 mg/m^2/day day 1
  [total dose/cycle = 650 mg/m^2]

Vincristine: IV: 1.4 mg/m^2/day (maximum dose: 3 mg) day 1
  [total dose/cycle = 1.4 mg/m^2; maximum dose/cycle: 3 mg]

Procarbazine: Oral: 100 mg/m^2/day days 1 to 7
  [total dose/cycle = 700 mg/m^2]

Prednisone: Oral: 40 mg/m^2/day days 1 to 14
  [total dose/cycle = 560 mg/m^2]

Doxorubicin: IV: 35 mg/m^2/day day 8
  [total dose/cycle = 35 mg/m^2]

Bleomycin: IV: 10 units/m^2/day day 8
  [total dose/cycle = 10 units/m^2]

Vinblastine: IV: 6 mg/m^2/day day 8
  [total dose/cycle = 6 mg/m^2]

Repeat cycles every 28 days for a total of 8 cycles

References

Montoto S, Camós M, López-Guillermo A, et al, "Hybrid Chemotherapy Consisting of Cyclo-phosphamide, Vincristine, Procarbazine, Prednisone, Doxorubicin, Bleomycin, and Vinblastine (C-MOPP/ABV) as First-Line Treatment for Patients With Advanced Hodgkin Disease," *Cancer*, 2000;88(9):2142-8.

CMV (Bladder)

Use Bladder cancer, neoadjuvant

Regimen

Methotrexate: IV: 30 mg/m^2/day days 1 and 8

[total dose/cycle = 60 mg/m^2]

Vinblastine: IV: 4 mg/m^2/day days 1 and 8

[total dose/cycle = 8 mg/m^2]

Cisplatin: IV: 100 mg/m^2 day 2

[total dose/cycle = 100 mg/m^2]

Leucovorin: Oral or IV: 15 mg every 6 hours for 4 doses days 2 and 9, starting 24 hours after day 1 and day 8 methotrexate

[total dose/cycle = 120 mg]

Repeat cycle every 21 days for 3 cycles

References

Neoadjuvant cisplatin, methotrexate, and vinblastine chemotherapy for muscle-invasive bladder cancer: a randomised controlled trial. International collaboration of trialists. *Lancet*. 1999;354 (9178):533-540.

Griffiths G, Hall R, Sylvester R, et al. International phase III trial assessing neoadjuvant cisplatin, methotrexate, and vinblastine chemotherapy for muscle-invasive bladder cancer: long-term results of the BA06 30894 trial. *J Clin Oncol.* 2011;29(16):2171-2177.

CODOX-M/IVAC (NHL-Burkitt)

Index Terms Cyclophosphamide-Doxorubicin-Vincristine-Methotrexate-Cytar-abine-Ifosfamide-Etoposide (NHL-Burkitt)

Use Lymphoma, non-Hodgkin (Burkitt)

Regimen NOTE: Multiple variations are listed.

Variation 1:

CODOX-M (Cycles 1 and 3; cycles begin when ANC >1,000/mm^3)

Cyclophosphamide: IV: 800 mg/m^2 day 1

followed by IV: 200 mg/m^2/day days 2 to 5

[total dose/cycle = 1,600 mg/m^2]

Vincristine: IV: 1.5 mg/m^2/day (no maximum dose) days 1 and 8 (cycle 1) and days 1, 8, and 15 (cycle 3; day 15 in cycle 3 only if no neuropathy)

[total dose/cycle = 3 to 4.5 mg/m^2]

Doxorubicin: IV: 40 mg/m^2 day 1

[total dose/cycle = 40 mg/m^2]

Methotrexate: IV: 1,200 mg/m^2 (loading dose) over 1 hour day 10

followed by IV: 240 mg/m^2/hour for 23 hours day 10

[total dose/cycle = 6,720 mg/m^2]

Leucovorin: IV: 192 mg/m^2 day 11 (begin 36 hours after the start of methotrexate infusion)

followed by IV: 12 mg/m^2 every 6 hours until methotrexate level <5 x 10^{-8} micromolar

Cytarabine: Intrathecal: 70 mg/day (adjust to age-appropriate dose if ≤3 years of age) days 1 and 3

[total dose/cycle = 140 mg]

Methotrexate: Intrathecal: 12 mg (adjust to age-appropriate dose if ≤3 years of age) day 15

[total dose/cycle = 12 mg]

Sargramostim: SubQ: 7.5 mcg/kg/day beginning day 13, continue until ANC >1,000/mm^3

Note: If CNS disease present, administer additional intrathecal treatment in cycle 1: Cytarabine 70 mg (adjust to age-appropriate dose if ≤3 years of age) day 5 and methotrexate 12 mg (adjust to age-appropriate dose if ≤3 years of age) day 17

IVAC (Cycles 2 and 4; cycles begin when ANC >1,000/mm^3)

Ifosfamide: IV: 1,500 mg/m^2/day days 1 to 5

[total dose/cycle = 7,500 mg/m^2]

Mesna: IV: 360 mg/m^2 every 3 hours days 1 to 5

[total dose/cycle = 14,400 mg/m^2]

Etoposide: IV: 60 mg/m^2/day days 1 to 5

[total dose/cycle = 300 mg/m^2]

Cytarabine: IV: 2,000 mg/m^2 every 12 hours, for 4 doses, days 1 and 2

[total dose/cycle = 8,000 mg/m^2]

Methotrexate: Intrathecal: 12 mg day 5

[total dose/cycle = 12 mg]

Sargramostim: SubQ: 7.5 mcg/kg/day beginning day 7, continue until ANC >1000/mm^3

Note: If CNS disease present, administer additional intrathecal treatment in cycle 2: Cytarabine 70 mg/day (adjust to age-appropriate dose if ≤3 years of age) days 7 and 9

Variation 2:

CODOX-M (Cycles 1 and 3; cycles begin when ANC >1,000/mm^3 without growth factor support and an unsupported platelet count >75,000/mm^3)

Cyclophosphamide: IV: 800 mg/m^2 day 1

followed by IV: 200 mg/m^2/day days 2 to 5

[total dose/cycle = 1,600 mg/m^2]

Vincristine: IV: 1.5 mg/m^2/day (maximum dose: 2 mg) days 1 and 8

[total dose/cycle = 3 mg/m^2; maximum: 4 mg/cycle]

Doxorubicin: IV: 40 mg/m^2 day 1

[total dose/cycle = 40 mg/m^2]

Methotrexate: IV: 300 mg/m^2 (100 mg/m^2 if >65 years of age) (loading dose) over 1 hour day 10

followed by IV: 2,700 mg/m^2 (900 mg/m^2 if >65 years of age) over 23 hours day 10

[total dose/cycle = 3,000 mg/m^2 (1,000 mg/m^2 if >65 years of age)]

Leucovorin: IV: 15 mg/m^2 every 3 hours day 11 (begin 36 hours after the start of methotrexate infusion) for 5 doses

followed by IV: 15 mg/m^2 every 6 hours until methotrexate level <5 x 10^{-8} micromolar

Cytarabine: Intrathecal: 70 mg/day days 1 and 3

[total dose/cycle = 140 mg]

Methotrexate: Intrathecal: 12 mg day 15

[total dose/cycle = 12 mg]

Leucovorin: Oral: 15 mg day 16 (24 hours after intrathecal methotrexate)

Filgrastim: SubQ: 5 mcg/kg/day beginning day 13, continue until ANC >1,000/mm^3

Note: If CNS disease present, administer additional intrathecal treatment: Cytarabine 70 mg day 5 and methotrexate 12 mg (with leucovorin rescue) day 17

▶

◄ **IVAC** (Cycles 2 and 4; cycles begin when ANC >1,000/mm^3 without growth
factor support and an unsupported platelet count >75,000/mm^3)

Ifosfamide: IV: 1,500 mg/m^2/day (1,000 mg/m^2/day if >65 years of age) over
1 hour days 1 to 5

[total dose/cycle = 7,500 mg/m^2 (5,000 mg/m^2 if >65 years of age)]

Mesna: IV: 300 mg/m^2/day (200 mg/m^2/day if >65 years of age) over 1 hour
mixed with each ifosfamide dose days 1 to 5

followed by IV: 300 mg/m^2 (200 mg/m^2 if >65 years of age) every 4 hours
for 2 doses/day days 1 to 5

[total dose/cycle = 4,500 mg/m^2 (3,000 mg/m^2 if >65 years of age)]

Etoposide: IV: 60 mg/m^2/day over 1 hour days 1 to 5

[total dose/cycle = 300 mg/m^2]

Cytarabine: IV: 2,000 mg/m^2 (1,000 mg/m^2 if >65 years of age) over 3 hours
every 12 hours, for 4 doses, days 1 and 2

[total dose/cycle = 8,000 mg/m^2 (4,000 mg/m^2 if >65 years of age)]

Methotrexate: Intrathecal: 12 mg day 5

[total dose/cycle = 12 mg]

Leucovorin: Oral: 15 mg day 6 (24 hours after intrathecal methotrexate)

Filgrastim: SubQ: 5 mcg/kg/day beginning day 7, continue until ANC
>1,000/mm^3

Note: If CNS disease present, administer additional intrathecal treatment:
Cytarabine 70 mg/day on days 7 and 9

Variation 3:

CODOX-M (Cycles 1 and 3; cycles begin when ANC >1,000/mm^3 without
growth factor support and an unsupported platelet count >75,000/mm^3)

Cyclophosphamide: IV: 800 mg/m^2 day 1

followed by IV: 200 mg/m^2/day days 2 to 5

[total dose/cycle = 1,600 mg/m^2]

Vincristine: IV: 1.5 mg/m^2/day (maximum dose: 2 mg) days 1 and 8

[total dose/cycle = 3 mg/m^2; maximum: 4 mg/cycle]

Doxorubicin: IV: 40 mg/m^2 day 1

[total dose/cycle = 40 mg/m^2]

Methotrexate: IV: 1,200 mg/m^2 (loading dose) over 1 hour day 10

followed by IV: 240 mg/m^2/hour for 23 hours day 10

[total dose/cycle = 6,720 mg/m^2]

Leucovorin: IV: 192 mg/m^2 day 11 (begin 36 hours after the start of
methotrexate infusion)

followed by IV: 12 mg/m^2 every 6 hours until methotrexate level <5 x 10^{-8}
micromolar

Cytarabine: Intrathecal: 70 mg/day days 1 and 3

[total dose/cycle = 140 mg]

Methotrexate: Intrathecal: 12 mg day 15

[total dose/cycle = 12 mg]

Leucovorin: Oral: 15 mg day 16 (24 hours after intrathecal methotrexate)

Filgrastim: SubQ: 5 mcg/kg/day beginning day 13, continue until ANC
>1,000/mm^3

Note: If CNS disease present, administer additional intrathecal treatment in
cycle 1: Cytarabine 70 mg (15 mg if via Ommaya reservoir) day 5 and
methotrexate 12.5 mg (2 mg if via Ommaya reservoir) day 17

IVAC (Cycles 2 and 4; cycles begin when ANC >1,000/mm³ without growth factor support and an unsupported platelet count >75,000/mm³)

Ifosfamide: IV: 1,500 mg/m²/day over 1 hour days 1 to 5
[total dose/cycle = 7,500 mg/m²]

Mesna: IV: 360 mg/m² mixed with each ifosfamide dose over 1 hour days 1 to 5
followed by IV: 360 mg/m² every 3 hours for 7 doses/day days 1 to 5
[total dose/cycle = 14,400 mg/m²]

Etoposide: IV: 60 mg/m²/day over 1 hour days 1 to 5
[total dose/cycle = 300 mg/m²]

Cytarabine: IV: 2,000 mg/m² over 3 hours every 12 hours, for 4 doses, days 1 and 2
[total dose/cycle = 8,000 mg/m²]

Methotrexate: Intrathecal: 12 mg day 5
[total dose/cycle = 12 mg]

Leucovorin: Oral: 15 mg day 6 (24 hours after intrathecal methotrexate)

Filgrastim: SubQ: 5 mcg/kg/day beginning day 7, continue until ANC >1,000/mm³

Note: If CNS disease present, administer additional intrathecal treatment in cycle 2: Cytarabine 70 mg/day (15 mg if via Ommaya reservoir) days 7 and 9

Variation 4:

CODOX-M (Cycles 1 and 3; cycles begin when ANC >1,000/mm³)

Cyclophosphamide: IV: 800 mg/m²/day days 1 and 2
[total dose/cycle = 1,600 mg/m²]

Vincristine: IV: 1.4 mg/m²/day (maximum dose: 2 mg) days 1 and 10
[total dose/cycle = 2.8 mg/m²; maximum: 4 mg/cycle]

Doxorubicin: IV: 50 mg/m² day 1
[total dose/cycle = 50 mg/m²]

Methotrexate: IV: 3,000 mg/m² day 10
[total dose/cycle = 3,000 mg/m²]

Leucovorin: IV: 200 mg/m² day 11 (24 hours after methotrexate infusion)
followed by Oral, IV: 15 mg/m² every 6 hours until methotrexate level <0.1 micromolar

Cytarabine: Intrathecal: 50 mg/day days 1 and 3
[total dose/cycle = 100 mg]

Hydrocortisone: Intrathecal: 50 mg/day days 1 and 3
[total dose/cycle = 100 mg]

Methotrexate: Intrathecal: 12 mg day 1
[total dose/cycle = 12 mg]

Filgrastim: SubQ: Dose not specified, days 3 to 8 and day 12 until ANC >1,000 mm³

Note: If CNS disease present, administer additional intrathecal treatment in cycle 1: Cytarabine 50 mg day 5 and methotrexate 12 mg day 10

IVAC (Cycles 2 and 4; cycles begin when ANC >1,000/mm³)

Ifosfamide: IV: 1,500 mg/m²/day days 1 to 5
[total dose/cycle = 7,500 mg/m²]

Mesna: IV: 1,500 mg/m²/day (in divided doses) days 1 to 5
[total dose/cycle = 7,500 mg/m²]

Etoposide: IV: 60 mg/m²/day days 1 to 5
[total dose/cycle = 300 mg/m²]

Cytarabine: IV: 2,000 mg/m² every 12 hours, for 4 doses, days 1 and 2
[total dose/cycle = 8,000 mg/m²]

◄ Methotrexate: Intrathecal: 12 mg day 5
   [total dose/cycle = 12 mg]
Hydrocortisone: Intrathecal: 50 mg day 5
   [total dose/cycle = 50 mg]
Filgrastim: SubQ: Dose not specified, daily beginning day 6 until ANC >1,000/mm³
Note: If CNS disease present, administer additional intrathecal treatment in cycle 2: Cytarabine 50 mg/day days 3 and 5

References

Variation 1:

Magrath I, Adde M, Shad A, et al, "Adults and Children With Small Non-Cleaved-Cell Lymphoma Have a Similar Excellent Outcome When Treated With the Same Chemotherapy Regimen," *J Clin Oncol*, 1996, 14(3):925-34.

Variation 2:

Mead GM, Barrans SL, Qian W, et al, "A Prospective Clinicopathologic Study of Dose-Modified CODOX-M/IVAC in Patients With Sporadic Burkitt Lymphoma Defined Using Cytogenetic and Immunophenotypic Criteria (MRC/NCRI LY10 Trial)," *Blood*, 2008, 112(6):2248-60.

Variation 3:

Mead GM, Sydes MR, Walewski J, et al, "An International Evaluation of CODOX-M and CODOX-M Alternating With IVAC in Adult Burkitt's Lymphoma: Results of United Kingdom Lymphoma Group LY06 Study," *Ann Oncol*, 2002, 13(8):1264-74.

Variation 4:

Lacasce A, Howard O, Lib S, et al, "Modified Magrath Regimens for Adults With Burkitt and Burkitt-Like Lymphomas: Preserved Efficacy With Decreased Toxicity," *Leuk Lymphoma*, 2004, 45 (4):761-7.

CODOX-M (NHL-Burkitt)

Index Terms Cyclophosphamide-Doxorubicin-Vincristine-Methotrexate-Cytarabine (NHL-Burkitt)

Use Lymphoma, non-Hodgkin (Burkitt)

Regimen NOTE: Multiple variations are listed.

Variation 1:

Cyclophosphamide: IV: 800 mg/m² day 1
   followed by IV: 200 mg/m²/day days 2 to 5
   [total dose/cycle = 1,600 mg/m²]
Vincristine: IV: 1.5 mg/m²/day (no maximum dose) days 1 and 8
   [total dose/cycle = 3 mg/m²]
Doxorubicin: IV: 40 mg/m² day 1
   [total dose/cycle = 40 mg/m²]
Methotrexate: IV: 1,200 mg/m² (loading dose) over 1 hour day 10
   followed by IV: 240 mg/m²/hour for 23 hours day 10
   [total dose/cycle = 6,720 mg/m²]
Leucovorin: IV: 192 mg/m² day 11 (begin 36 hours after the start of methotrexate infusion)
   followed by IV: 12 mg/m² every 6 hours until methotrexate level <5 x 10⁻⁸ micromolar
Cytarabine: Intrathecal: 70 mg (adjust to age-appropriate dose if ≤3 years of age) day 1
   [total dose/cycle = 70 mg]
Methotrexate: Intrathecal: 12 mg (adjust to age-appropriate dose if ≤3 years of age) day 3
   [total dose/cycle = 12 mg]
Repeat cycle when ANC >1,000/mm³ for a total of 3 cycles

Variation 2:

Cyclophosphamide: IV: 800 mg/m² day 1
followed by IV: 200 mg/m²/day days 2 to 5
  [total dose/cycle = 1,600 mg/m²]

Vincristine: IV: 1.5 mg/m²/day (maximum dose: 2 mg) days 1 and 8
  [total dose/cycle = 3 mg/m²; maximum: 4 mg/cycle]

Doxorubicin: IV: 40 mg/m² day 1
  [total dose/cycle = 40 mg/m²]

Methotrexate: IV: 1,200 mg/m² (loading dose) over 1 hour day 10
followed by IV: 240 mg/m²/hour for 23 hours day 10
  [total dose/cycle = 6,720 mg/m²]

Leucovorin: IV: 192 mg/m² day 11 (begin 36 hours after the start of methotrexate infusion)
followed by IV: 12 mg/m² every 6 hours until methotrexate level <5 x 10⁻⁸ micromolar

Cytarabine: Intrathecal: 70 mg/day days 1 and 3
  [total dose/cycle = 140 mg]

Methotrexate: Intrathecal: 12 mg day 15
  [total dose/cycle = 12 mg]

Leucovorin: Oral: 15 mg day 16 (24 hours after intrathecal methotrexate)

Filgrastim: SubQ: 5 mcg/kg/day beginning day 13, continue until ANC >1,000/mm³

Repeat cycle when ANC >1,000/mm³ without growth factor support and an unsupported platelet count of >75,000/mm³ for a total of 3 cycles

Variation 3:

Cyclophosphamide: IV: 800 mg/m²/day days 1 and 2
  [total dose/cycle = 1,600 mg/m²]

Vincristine: IV: 1.4 mg/m²/day (maximum dose: 2 mg) days 1 and 10
  [total dose/cycle = 2.8 mg/m²; maximum: 4 mg/cycle]

Doxorubicin: IV: 50 mg/m² day 1
  [total dose/cycle = 50 mg/m²]

Methotrexate: IV: 3,000 mg/m² day 10
  [total dose/cycle = 3,000 mg/m²]

Leucovorin: IV: 200 mg/m² day 11 (24 hours after methotrexate infusion)
followed by Oral, IV: 15 mg/m² every 6 hours until methotrexate level <0.1 micromolar

Cytarabine: Intrathecal: 50 mg day 1
  [total dose/cycle = 50 mg]

Hydrocortisone: Intrathecal: 50 mg day 1
  [total dose/cycle = 50 mg]

Methotrexate: Intrathecal: 12 mg day 1
  [total dose/cycle = 12 mg]

Filgrastim: SubQ: Dose not specified; days 3 to 8 and day 12 if ANC <1,000/mm³; administer until ANC >1,000/mm³

Repeat cycle when ANC >1,000/mm³ for a total of 3 cycles

References

Variation 1:

Magrath I, Adde M, Shad A, et al. Adults and children with small non-cleaved-cell lymphoma have a similar excellent outcome when treated with the same chemotherapy regimen. *J Clin Oncol.* 1996;14(3):925-934.

Variation 2:
Mead GM, Sydes MR, Walewski J, et al. An international evaluation of CODOX-M and CODOX-M alternating with IVAC in adult Burkitt's Lymphoma: results of United Kingdom Lymphoma Group LY06 Study. *Ann Oncol.* 2002;13(8):1264-1274.
Variation 3:
Lacasce A, Howard O, Lib S, et al. Modified magrath regimens for adults with burkitt and burkitt-like lymphomas: preserved efficacy with decreased toxicity. *Leuk Lymphoma.* 2004;45(4):761-767.

COPE

Index Terms Baby Brain I
Use Brain tumors
Regimen
Cycle A:
Vincristine: IV: 0.065 mg/kg/day (maximum dose: 1.5 mg) days 1 and 8
  [total dose/cycle = 0.13 mg/kg]
Cyclophosphamide: IV: 65 mg/kg day 1
  [total dose/cycle = 65 mg/kg]
Cycle B:
Cisplatin: IV: 4 mg/kg day 1
  [total dose/cycle = 4 mg/kg]
Etoposide: IV: 6.5 mg/kg/day days 3 and 4
  [total dose/cycle = 13 mg/kg]
Repeat cycle every 28 days in the following sequence: AABAAB

References
Duffner PK, Horowitz ME, Krischer JP, et al "Postoperative Chemotherapy and Delayed Radiation in Children Less Than Three Years of Age With Malignant Brain Tumors," *N Engl J Med*, 1993, 328(24):1725-31.

◆ **CRd (Multiple Myeloma)** *see* Carfilzomib, Lenalidomide, Dexamethasone (Multiple Myeloma) *on page 1875*

Crizotinib (NSCLC Regimen)

Use Lung cancer, non-small cell
Regimen
Crizotinib: Oral: 250 mg twice daily days 1 to 28
  [total dose/cycle = 14,000 mg]
Repeat cycle every 28 days until disease progression or unacceptable toxicity
References
Kwak EL, Bang YJ, Camidge R, et al, "Anaplastic Lymphoma Kinase Inhibition in Non-Small-Cell Lung Cancer," *N Engl J Med*, 2010, 363(18):1693-703.

◆ **CVD** *see* Cisplatin-Vinblastine-Dacarbazine (Melanoma) *on page 1912*

◆ **CVD-IL-2-IFN (Melanoma)** *see* CVD-Interleukin-Interferon (Melanoma) *on page 1926*

CVD-Interleukin-Interferon (Melanoma)

Index Terms Cisplatin-Vinblastine-Dacarbazine-Interleukin-Interferon (Melanoma); CVD-IL-2-IFN (Melanoma)
Use Melanoma
Regimen NOTE: Multiple variations are listed.
Variation 1:
Cisplatin: IV: 20 mg/m^2/day days 1 to 4 and 22 to 25
  [total dose/cycle = 160 mg/m^2]
Vinblastine: IV: 1.5 mg/m^2/day days 1 to 4 and 22 to 25
  [total dose/cycle = 12 mg/m^2]

Dacarbazine: IV: 800 mg/m^2/day days 1 and 22
  [total dose/cycle = 1600 mg/m^2]
Aldesleukin: IV: 9 million units/m^2/day continuous infusion days 5 to 8, 17 to 20, and 26 to 29
  [total dose/cycle = 108 million units/m^2]
Interferon alfa-2b: SubQ: 5 million units/m^2/day days 5 to 9, 17 to 21, and 26 to 30
  [total dose/cycle = 75 million units/m^2]
Repeat every 42 days (maximum of five 21-day cycles for cytokine [interleukin and interferon] component)
Variation 2:
Cisplatin: IV: 20 mg/m^2/day days 1 to 4
  [total dose/cycle = 80 mg/m^2]
Vinblastine: IV: 1.6 mg/m^2/day days 1 to 4
  [total dose/cycle = 6.4 mg/m^2]
Dacarbazine: IV: 800 mg/m^2 day 1
  [total dose/cycle = 800 mg/m^2]
Aldesleukin: IV: 9 million units/m^2/day continuous infusion days 1 to 4
  [total dose/cycle = 36 million units/m^2]
Interferon alfa-2a: SubQ: 5 million units/m^2/day days 1 to 5, 7, 9, 11, and 13
  [total dose/cycle = 45 million units/m^2]
Repeat cycle every 21 days for a total of 6 cycles
Variation 3:
Cisplatin: IV: 20 mg/m^2/day days 1 to 4
  [total dose/cycle = 80 mg/m^2]
Vinblastine: IV: 1.2 mg/m^2/day days 1 to 4
  [total dose/cycle = 4.8 mg/m^2]
Dacarbazine: IV: 800 mg/m^2 day 1
  [total dose/cycle = 800 mg/m^2]
Aldesleukin: IV: 9 million units/m^2/day continuous infusion days 1 to 4
  [total dose/cycle = 36 million units/m^2]
Interferon alfa-2b: SubQ: 5 million units/m^2/day days 1 to 5, 8, 10, and 12
  [total dose/cycle = 40 million units/m^2]
Repeat cycle every 21 days (maximum: 4 cycles)

References

Variation 1:
Eton O, Legha SS, Bedikian AY, et al, "Sequential Biochemotherapy Versus Chemotherapy for Metastatic Melanoma: Results From a Phase III Randomized Trial," *J Clin Oncol*, 2002, 20 (8):2045-52.
Variation 2:
Legha SS, Ring S, Eton O, et al, "Development of a Biochemotherapy Regimen With Concurrent Administration of Cisplatin, Vinblastine, Dacarbazine, Interferon Alfa, and Interleukin-2 for Patients With Metastatic Melanoma," *J Clin Oncol*, 1998, 16(5):1752-9.
Variation 3:
McDermott DF, Mier JW, Lawrence DP, et al, "A Phase II Pilot Trial of Concurrent Biochemotherapy With Cisplatin, Vinblastine, Dacarbazine, Interleukin 2, and Interferon Alpha-2B in Patients With Metastatic Melanoma," *Clin Cancer Res*, 2000, 6(6):2201-8.

◆ **CVP-R (NHL-Follicular)** *see* R-CVP (NHL-Follicular) *on page 2073*

◆ **CyBorD (Multiple Myeloma)** *see* Cyclophosphamide-Bortezomib-Dexamethasone (Multiple Myeloma) *on page 1927*

Cyclophosphamide-Bortezomib-Dexamethasone (Multiple Myeloma)

Index Terms CyBorD (Multiple Myeloma)

◀ **Use** Multiple myeloma

Regimen NOTE: Multiple variations are listed.

Variation 1:

Cycles 1 through 4:

Cyclophosphamide: PO: 300 mg/m^2/day on days 1, 8, 15, and 22
[total dose/cycle = 1200 mg/m^2]

Bortezomib: IV or SubQ: 1.3 mg/m^2/day on days 1, 4, 8, and 11
[total dose/cycle = 5.2 mg/m^2]

Dexamethasone: PO: 40 mg/day on days 1-4, 9-12, and 17-20
[total dose/cycle = 480 mg]

Treatment cycle is 28 days

Variation 2:

Cycles 1 and 2:

Cyclophosphamide: PO: 300 mg/m^2/day on days 1, 8, 15, and 22
[total dose/cycle = 1200 mg/m^2]

Bortezomib: IV or SubQ: 1.5 mg/m^2/day on days 1, 8, 15, and 22
[total dose/cycle = 6 mg/m^2]

Dexamethasone: PO: 40 mg/day on days 1-4, 9-12, and 17-20
[total dose/cycle = 480 mg]

Treatment cycle is 28 days

Cycles 3 and 4:

Cyclophosphamide: PO: 300 mg/m^2/day on days 1, 8, 15, and 22
[total dose/cycle = 1200 mg/m^2]

Bortezomib: IV or SubQ: 1.5 mg/m^2/day on days 1, 8, 15, and 22
[total dose/cycle = 6 mg/m^2]

Dexamethasone: PO: 40 mg/day on days 1, 8, 15, and 22
[total dose/cycle = 160 mg]

Treatment cycle is 28 days

Variation 3:

Cyclophosphamide: PO: 500 mg/m^2/day on days 1, 8, and 15
[total dose/cycle = 1500 mg/m^2]

Bortezomib: IV or SubQ: 1.3 mg/m^2/day on days 1, 4, 8, and 11
[total dose/cycle = 5.2 mg/m^2]

Dexamethasone: PO: 40 mg/day on days 1, 8, and 15
[total dose/cycle = 120 mg]

Repeat cycle every 21 days for up to 8 cycles

Variation 4:

Cyclophosphamide: PO: 500 mg/m^2/day on days 1 and 8
[total dose/cycle = 1000 mg/m^2]

Bortezomib: IV or SubQ: 1.3 mg/m^2/day on days 1, 4, 8, and 11
[total dose/cycle = 5.2 mg/m^2]

Dexamethasone: PO: 40 mg/day on days 1, 8, and 15
[total dose/cycle = 120 mg]

Repeat cycle every 21 days for up to 8 cycles

References

Variations 1 and 2:

Reeder CB, Reece DE, Kukrati V, et al, "Cyclophosphamide, Bortezomib and Dexamethasone Induction for Newly Diagnosed Multiple Myeloma: High Response Rates in a Phase II Clinical Trial," *Leukemia*, 2009, 23(7):1887-41.

Reeder CB, Reece DE, Kukreti V, et al, "Once- Versus Twice-Weekly Bortezomib Induction Therapy With CyBorD in Newly Diagnosed Multiple Myeloma," *Blood*, 2010, 115(16):3416-7.

Variations 3 and 4:
Kumar S, Flinn IW, Richardson PG, et al, "Novel Three- and Four-Drug Combination Regimens of Bortezomib, Dexamethasone, Cyclophosphamide, and Lenalidomide, for Previously Untreated Multiple Myeloma: Results From the Multi-Center, Randomized, Phase 2 EVOLUTION Study," *Blood*, 2010, 116:621 [abstract 621 from ASH 2010 Annual Meeting].

Cyclophosphamide-Epirubicin (Breast)

Index Terms EC (Breast); Epirubicin-Cyclophosphamide (Breast)

Use Breast cancer

Regimen NOTE: Multiple variations are listed.

Variation 1 (metastatic):
Epirubicin: IV: 75 mg/m^2 day 1
[total dose/cycle = 75 mg/m^2]
Cyclophosphamide: IV: 600 mg/m^2 day 1
[total dose/cycle = 600 mg/m^2]
Repeat cycle every 21 days for up to 6 cycles

Variation 2 (adjuvant):
Epirubicin: IV: 100 mg/m^2 day 1
[total dose/cycle = 100 mg/m^2]
Cyclophosphamide: IV: 830 mg/m^2 day 1
[total dose/cycle = 830 mg/m^2]
Repeat cycle every 21 days for up to 8 cycles

References

Variation 1:
Langley RE, Carmichael J, Jones AL, et al, "Phase III Trial of Epirubicin Plus Paclitaxel Compared With Epirubicin Plus Cyclophosphamide As First-Line Therapy for Metastatic Breast Cancer: United Kingdom National Cancer Research Institute Trial AB01," *J Clin Oncol*, 2005, 23 (33):8322-30.

Variation 2:
Piccart MJ, Di Leo A, Beauduin M, et al, "Phase III Trial Comparing Two Dose Levels of Epirubicin Combined With Cyclophosphamide With Cyclophosphamide, Methotrexate, and Fluorouracil in Node-Positive Breast Cancer," *J Clin Oncol*, 2001, 19(12):3103-10.

♦ **Cyclophosphamide-Etoposide-Procarbazine-Prednisone (NHL-DLBCL)**
see CEPP (NHL-DLBCL) *on page* 1878

♦ **Cyclophosphamide-Fludarabine (CLL)** *see* Fludarabine-Cyclophosphamide (CLL) *on page* 1971

♦ **Cyclophosphamide-Fludarabine (NHL-Mantle Cell)** *see* Fludarabine-Cyclophosphamide (NHL-Mantle Cell) *on page* 1973

♦ **Cyclophosphamide, Methotrexate, Fluorouracil (Breast)** *see* CMF Oral
(Breast) *on page* 1918

♦ **Cyclophosphamide-Pentostatin-Rituximab (CLL)** *see* Pentostatin-Cyclophosphamide-Rituximab (CLL) *on page* 2065

Cyclophosphamide-Topotecan (Ewing Sarcoma)

Index Terms TOPO/CYC (Ewing Sarcoma); Topotecan-Cyclophosphamide
(Ewing Sarcoma)

Use Ewing sarcoma

Regimen

Cyclophosphamide: IV: 250 mg/m^2/day over 30 minutes days 1 to 5
[total dose/cycle = 1,250 mg/m^2]
Topotecan: IV: 0.75 mg/m^2/day over 30 minutes days 1 to 5
[total dose/cycle = 3.75 mg/m^2]
Filgrastim: SubQ: 5 mcg/kg daily beginning on day 6 until ANC ≥1,500/mm^3
after time of expected nadir
Repeat cycle every 21 days until disease progression or unacceptable toxicity

References

Hunold A, Weddeling N, Paulussen M, Ranft A, Liebscher C, Jürgens H. Topotecan and cyclophosphamide in patients with refractory or relapsed Ewing tumors. *Pediatr Blood Cancer*.
2006;47(6):795-800.

Saylors RL 3rd, Stine KC, Sullivan J, et al. Cyclophosphamide plus topotecan in children with
recurrent or refractory solid tumors: a Pediatric Oncology Group phase II study. *J Clin Oncol*.
2001;19(15):3463-3469.

Cyclophosphamide-Topotecan (Neuroblastoma)

Index Terms TOPO/CTX (Neuroblastoma); Topotecan-Cyclophosphamide
(Neuroblastoma)

Use Neuroblastoma

Regimen

Cyclophosphamide: IV: 250 mg/m^2/day over 30 minutes days 1 to 5
[total dose/cycle = 1,250 mg/m^2]
Topotecan: IV: 0.75 mg/m^2/day over 30 minutes days 1 to 5
[total dose/cycle = 3.75 mg/m^2]
Filgrastim: SubQ: 5 mcg/kg daily beginning on day 6 until ANC recovery as
defined per study
Repeat cycle every 21 days until disease progression or unacceptable toxicity
(up to 1 year [London 2010])

References

Ashraf K, Shaikh F, Gibson P, Baruchel S, Irwin MS. Treatment with topotecan plus cyclophosphamide in children with first relapse of neuroblastoma. *Pediatr Blood Cancer*. 2013;60
(10):1636-1641.

London WB, Frantz CN, Campbell LA, et al. Phase II randomized comparison of topotecan plus
cyclophosphamide versus topotecan alone in children with recurrent or refractory neuroblastoma:
a Children's Oncology Group study. *J Clin Oncol*. 2010;28(24):3808-3815.

Saylors RL 3rd, Stine KC, Sullivan J, et al. Cyclophosphamide plus topotecan in children with
recurrent or refractory solid tumors: a Pediatric Oncology Group phase II study. *J Clin Oncol*.
2001;19(15):3463-3469.

Cyclophosphamide-Topotecan (Rhabdomyosarcoma)

Index Terms Topotecan-Cyclophosphamide (Rhabdomyosarcoma)

Use Soft tissue sarcoma (rhabdomyosarcoma)

Regimen

Cyclophosphamide: IV: 250 mg/m²/day over 30 minutes days 1 to 5
[total dose/cycle = 1,250 mg/m²]

Topotecan: IV: 0.75 mg/m²/day over 30 minutes days 1 to 5
[total dose/cycle = 3.75 mg/m²]

Filgrastim: SubQ: 5 mcg/kg daily beginning on day 6 until ANC ≥1,500/mm³
after time of expected nadir

Repeat cycle every 21 days until disease progression and unacceptable
toxicity

References

Saylors RL 3rd, Stine KC, Sullivan J, et al. Cyclophosphamide plus topotecan in children with recurrent or refractory solid tumors: a Pediatric Oncology Group phase II study. *J Clin Oncol.* 2001;19(15):3463-3469.

♦ **Cyclophosphamide-Vincristine-Procarbazine-Prednisone-Doxorubicin-Bleomycin-Vinblastine (Hodgkin)** see C-MOPP/ABV Hybrid (Hodgkin) *on page 1919*

♦ **Cytarabine-Clofarabine (AML)** see Clofarabine-Cytarabine (AML) *on page 1917*

♦ **Cytarabine-Daunorubicin (5 + 2) (AML)** see 5 + 2 (Cytarabine-Daunorubicin) (AML Induction) *on page 1816*

♦ **Cytarabine-Daunorubicin (5 + 2) (AML)** see 5 + 2 (Cytarabine-Daunorubicin) (AML Postremission) *on page 1816*

♦ **Cytarabine-Daunorubicin (7 + 3) (AML Induction)** see 7 + 3 (Cytarabine-Daunorubicin) (AML Induction) *on page 1817*

♦ **Cytarabine-Daunorubicin-Etoposide (5 + 2 + 5) (AML Consolidation)** see 5 + 2 + 5 (Cytarabine-Daunorubicin-Etoposide) (AML Consolidation) *on page 1817*

♦ **Cytarabine-Daunorubicin-Etoposide (7 + 3 + 7) (AML Induction)** see 7 + 3 + 7 (Cytarabine-Daunorubicin-Etoposide) (AML Induction) *on page 1819*

♦ **Cytarabine-Etoposide-Mitoxantrone-CSF (AML Induction)** see MEC-G (AML Induction) *on page 2032*

Cytarabine (High Dose)-Daunorubicin (AML Induction)

Index Terms HDAC-Daunorubicin (AML Induction); HIDAC-Daunorubicin (AML Induction)

Use Leukemia, acute myeloid

Regimen

Cytarabine: IV: 2 g/m²/day over 1 hour every 12 hours days 1 to 6 (12 total
doses)
[total dose/cycle = 24 g/m²]

Daunorubicin: IV: 45 mg/m²/day IV bolus days 7 to 9
[total dose/cycle = 135 mg/m²]

References

Weick JK, Kopecky KJ, Appelbaum FR, et al, "A Randomized Investigation of High-Dose Versus Standard-Dose Cytosine Arabinoside With Daunorubicin in Patients With Previously Untreated Acute Myeloid Leukemia: A Southwest Oncology Group Study," *Blood*, 1996, 88(8):2841-51.

Cytarabine (High Dose)-Daunorubicin-Etoposide (AML Induction)

Index Terms HIDAC-3-7 (AML Induction)

Use Leukemia, acute myeloid

Regimen

Daunorubicin: IV: 50 mg/m^2/day days 1, 2, and 3
[total dose/cycle = 150 mg/m^2]

Cytarabine: IV: 3 g/m^2/dose over 3 hours every 12 hours days 1, 3, 5, and 7 (8 total doses)
[total dose/cycle = 24 g/m^2]

Etoposide: IV: 75 mg/m^2/day days 1 to 7
[total dose/cycle = 525 mg/m^2]

Up to 3 induction cycles may be given based on individual response

References

Bishop JF, Matthews JP, Young GA, et al, "A Randomized Study of High-Dose Cytarabine in Induction in Acute Myeloid Leukemia," *Blood*, 1996, 87(5):1710-7.

Cytarabine (High-Dose Single-Agent AML Induction Regimen)

Index Terms HD Cytarabine (Single Agent AML Induction); HIDAC (Single Agent AML Induction)

Use Leukemia, acute myeloid

Regimen NOTE: Multiple variations are listed.

Variation 1 (ages 14 to 50 years):

Cytarabine: IV: 3 g/m^2 over 2 hours every 12 hours days 1 to 6 (total of 12 doses)
[total dose/cycle = 36 g/m^2]

May administer a second induction cycle if needed

Variation 2 (ages >50 years):

Cytarabine: IV: 2 g/m^2 over 2 hours every 12 hours days 1 to 6 (total of 12 doses)
[total dose/cycle = 24 g/m^2]

May administer a second induction cycle if needed

References

Karanes C, Kopecky KJ, Head DR, et al "A Phase III Comparison of High Dose ARA-C (HIDAC) Versus HIDAC Plus Mitoxantrone in the Treatment of First Relapsed or Refractory Acute Myeloid Leukemia - Southwest Oncology Group Study," *Leuk Res*, 1999, 23(9): 787-94.

◆ **Cytarabine-Idarubicin (5 + 2) (AML Consolidation)** see 5 + 2 (Cytarabine-Idarubicin) (AML Consolidation) on page 1816

◆ **Cytarabine-Idarubicin (7 + 3) (AML Induction)** see 7 + 3 (Cytarabine-Idarubicin) (AML Induction) on page 1818

◆ **Cytarabine-Mitoxantrone (5 + 2) (AML Consolidation)** see 5 + 2 (Cytarabine-Mitoxantrone) (AML Consolidation) on page 1816

◆ **Cytarabine-Mitoxantrone (7 + 3) (AML Induction)** see 7 + 3 (Cytarabine-Mitoxantrone) (AML Induction) on page 1818

Cytarabine (Single-Agent AML Consolidation Regimen)

Use Leukemia, acute myeloid

Regimen NOTE: Multiple variations are listed.

Variation 1:

Cytarabine: IV: 3 g/m^2 over 3 hours every 12 hours on days 1, 3, and 5 (total of 6 doses)

[total dose/cycle = 18 g/m^2]

Repeat cycle every 4 to 5 weeks (depending on marrow recovery) for a total of 4 postremission cycles

Variation 2:

Cytarabine: IV: 400 mg/m^2/day continuous infusion on days 1 to 5

[total dose/cycle = 2000 mg/m^2]

Repeat cycle every 4 to 5 weeks (depending on marrow recovery) for a total of 4 postremission cycles

Variation 3:

Cytarabine: IV: 100 mg/m^2/day continuous infusion on days 1 to 5

[total dose/cycle = 500 mg/m^2]

Repeat cycle every 4 to 5 weeks (depending on marrow recovery) for a total of 4 postremission cycles

Variation 4 (≥60 years of age):

Cytarabine: IV: 100 mg/m^2/day continuous infusion on days 1 to 5

[total dose/cycle = 500 mg/m^2]

Repeat cycle every 28 days for a total of 4 consolidation cycles

Variation 5 (≤50 years of age):

Cytarabine: IV: 3 g/m^2 every 12 hours on days 1 to 3 (total of 6 doses)

[total dose/cycle = 18 g/m^2]

Administer a total of 3 consolidation cycles

Variation 6 (>50 years of age)

Cytarabine: IV: 2 g/m^2 every 12 hours on days 1 to 3 (total of 6 doses)

[total dose/cycle = 12 g/m^2]

Administer a total of 3 consolidation cycles

Variation 7 (>65 years of age):

Cytarabine: SubQ: 10 mg/m^2/dose every 12 hours days 1 to 14

[total dose/cycle = 280 mg/m^2]

Repeat cycle every 6 weeks for 18 months

References

Variations 1, 2, and 3:

Mayer RJ, Davis RB, Schiffer CA, et al, "Intensive Postremission Chemotherapy in Adults With Acute Myeloid Leukemia, Cancer and Leukemia Group B," *N Engl J Med*, 1994, 331 (14):896-903.

Variation 4:

Stone RM, Berg DT, George SL, et al, "Postremission Therapy in Older Patients With *de novo* Acute Myeloid Leukemia: A Randomized Trial Comparing Mitoxantrone and Intermediate-Dose Cytarabine With Standard-Dose Cytarabine," *Blood*, 2001, 98(3):548-53.

Variations 5 and 6:

Karanes C, Kopecky KJ, Head DR, et al "A Phase III Comparison of High Dose ARA-C (HIDAC) Versus HIDAC Plus Mitoxantrone in the Treatment of First Relapsed or Refractory Acute Myeloid Leukemia - Southwest Oncology Group Study," *Leuk Res*, 1999, 23(9): 787-94.

Variation 7:

Tilly H, Castaigne S, Bordessoule D, et al, "Low-Dose Cytarabine Versus Intensive Chemotherapy in the Treatment of Acute Nonlymphocytic Leukemia in the Elderly," *J Clin Oncol*, 1990, 8 (2):272-9.

Cytarabine (SubQ Single-Agent AML Induction Regimen)

Use Leukemia, acute myeloid

▶

◀ **Regimen** NOTE: Multiple variations are listed.
Variation 1 (>50 years of age):
Cytarabine: SubQ: 20 mg/m²/day days 1 to 14
  [total dose/cycle = 280 mg/m²]
Repeat cycle every 28 days for at least 4 cycles
Variation 2 (>65 years of age):
Cytarabine: SubQ: 10 mg/m²/day every 12 hours days 1 to 21
  [total dose/cycle = 420 mg/m²]
After 15 days, a second induction course may be administered if needed

References
Variation 1:
Fenaux P, Mufti GJ, Hellstrom-Lindberg E, et al, "Azacitidine Prolongs Overall Survival Compared With Conventional Care Regimens in Elderly Patients With Low Bone Marrow Blast Count Acute Myeloid Leukemia, *J Clin Oncol*, 2010, 28(4):562-9.
Variation 2:
Tilly H, Castaigne S, Bordessoule D, et al, "Low-Dose Cytarabine Versus Intensive Chemotherapy in the Treatment of Acute Nonlymphocytic Leukemia in the Elderly," *J Clin Oncol*, 1990, 8 (2):272-9.

Dabrafenib (Melanoma Regimen)

Use Melanoma
Regimen
Dabrafenib: Oral: 150 mg twice daily days 1 to 28
  [total dose/cycle = 8400 mg]
Repeat cycle every 28 days until disease progression or unacceptable toxicity
References
Hauschild A, Grob JJ, Demidov LV, et al, "Dabrafenib in BRAf-Mutated Metastatic Melanoma: A Multicenter, Open-Label, Phase 3 Randomised Controlled Trial," *Lancet*, 2012, 380 (9839):358-65.

Dabrafenib-Trametinib (Melanoma)

Use Melanoma
Regimen
Dabrafenib: Oral: 150 mg twice daily days 1 to 28
  [total dose/cycle = 8400 mg]
Trametinib: Oral: 2 mg once daily days 1 to 28
  [total dose/cycle = 56 mg]
Repeat cycle every 28 days
References
Flaherty KT, Infante JR, Daud A, et al. Combined BRAF and MEK inhibition in melanoma with BRAF V600 mutations. *N Engl J Med*. 2012;367(18):1694-1703.

◆ **Dacarbazine-Cisplatin-Vinblastine** *see* Cisplatin-Vinblastine-Dacarbazine (Melanoma) *on page 1912*

◆ **Dactinomycin-Vincristine (Wilms' Tumor)** *see* EE-4A (Wilms' Tumor) *on page 1953*

◆ **Dactinomycin-Doxorubicin-Vincristine (Wilms' Tumor)** *see* DD-4A (Wilms' Tumor) *on page 1936*

Dasatinib (ALL Regimen)

Use Leukemia, acute lymphocytic
Regimen
Dasatinib: Oral: 140 mg once daily days 1 to 28
  [total dose/cycle = 3920 mg]
Repeat cycle every 28 days until disease progression or unacceptable toxicity

References

Lilly MB, Ottmann OG, Shah NP, et al, "Dasatinib 140 mg Once Daily Versus 70 mg Twice Daily in Patients With Ph-Positive Acute Lymphoblastic Leukemia Who Failed Imatinib: Results From A Phase 3 Study," *Am J Hematol*, 2010, 85(3):164-70.

Dasatinib (CML Regimen)

Use Leukemia, chronic myelogenous

Regimen NOTE: Multiple variations are listed.

Variation 1 (chronic phase):

Dasatinib: Oral: 100 mg once daily

[total dose/cycle = 2800 mg]

Repeat cycle every 28 days until disease progression or unacceptable toxicity

Variation 2 (accelerated and blast phase resistant or intolerant to imatinib):

Dasatinib: Oral: 140 mg once daily

[total dose/cycle = 3920 mg]

Repeat cycle every 28 days until disease progression or unacceptable toxicity

References

Variation 1:

Kantarjian H, Shah NP, Hochhaus A, et al, "Dasatinib Versus Imatinib in Newly Diagnosed Chronic-Phase Chronic Myeloid Leukemia," *N Engl J Med*, 2010, 362(24):2260-70.

Shah NP, Kantarjian HM, Kim DW, et al, "Intermittent Target Inhibition With Dasatinib 100 mg Once Daily Preserves Efficacy and Improves Tolerability in Imatinib-Resistant and -Intolerant Chronic-Phase Chronic Myeloid Leukemia," *J Clin Oncol*, 2008, 26(19):3204-12.

Variation 2:

Kantarjian H, Cortes J, Kim DW, et al, "Phase 3 Study of Dasatinib 140 mg Once Daily Versus 70 mg Twice Daily in Patients With Chronic Myeloid Leukemia in Accelerated Phase Resistant or Intolerant to Imatinib: 15-Month Median Follow-up," *Blood*, 2009, 113(25):6322-9.

Saglio G, Hochhaus A, Goh YT, et al, "Dasatinib in Imatinib-Resistant or Imatinib-Intolerant Chronic Myeloid Leukemia in Blast Phase After 2 Years of Follow-up in a Phase 3 Study: Efficacy and Tolerability of 140 Milligrams Once Daily and 70 Milligrams Twice Daily," *Cancer*, 2010, 116 (16):3852-61.

Dasatinib (GIST Regimen)

Use Soft Tissue Sarcoma (Gastrointestinal Stromal Tumor [GIST])

Regimen

Dasatinib: Oral: 70 mg twice daily days 1 to 28

[total dose/cycle = 3920 mg]

Repeat cycle every 28 days until disease progression or unacceptable toxicity

References

Montemurro M, Domont J, Blesius A, et al, "Dasatinib First-Line Treatment in Gastrointestinal Stromal Tumors: A Multicenter Phase II Trial of the SAKK (SAKK 56/07)," *J Clin Oncol*, 2012, 30 (15s):10033 [abstract 10033 from 2012 ASCO Annual Meeting].

Trent JC, Wathen J, von Mehren M, et al, "A Phase II Study of Dasatinib for Patients With Imatinib-Resistant Gastrointestinal Stromal Tumor (GIST)," *J Clin Oncol*, 2011, 29(15s):10006 [abstract 10006 from 2011 ASCO Annual Meeting].

- ◆ **DCF (Gastric/Esophageal Cancer)** *see* Docetaxel-Cisplatin-Fluorouracil (Gastric/Esophageal Cancer) *on page 1940*

- ◆ **DC (NSCLC)** *see* Cisplatin-Docetaxel (NSCLC) *on page 1891*

- ◆ **DD4A (Wilms' Tumor)** *see* DD-4A (Wilms' Tumor) *on page 1936*

DD-4A (Wilms' Tumor)

Index Terms Dactinomycin–Doxorubicin–Vincristine (Wilms' Tumor); DD4A (Wilms' Tumor); Regimen DD-4A (Wilms' Tumor)

Use Wilms' tumor

Regimen

Dactinomycin: IV: 45 mcg/kg day 1 of weeks 0, 6, 12, 18, 24, 30, 36, 42, 48, and 54

[total dose = 450 mcg/kg]

Doxorubicin: IV: 45 mg/m² days 1 of weeks 3 and 9

Followed by

Doxorubicin: IV: 30 mg/m² days 1 of weeks 15, 21, 27, 33, 39, 45, and 51

[total dose = 300 mg/m²]

Vincristine: IV: 1.5 mg/m² day 1 of weeks 1 to 10

Followed by

Vincristine: IV: 2 mg/m² day 1 of weeks 12, 15, 18, 21, 24, 27, 30, 33, 36, 39, 42, 45, 48, 51, and 54

[total dose = 45 mg/m²]

Treatment course duration is week 0 through week 54

References

Green DM, Breslow NE, Beckwith JB, et al, "Effect of Duration of Treatment on Treatment Outcome and Cost of Treatment for Wilms' Tumor: A Report From the National Wilms' Tumor Study Group," *J Clin Oncol*, 1998, 16(12):3744-51.

- ◆ **DDM-VAC (Bladder Cancer)** *see* Dose Dense MVAC (Bladder Cancer) *on page 1948*

Decitabine (AML Regimen)

Use Leukemia, acute myeloid

Regimen

Decitabine: IV: 20 mg/m²/day over 1 hour days 1 to 5

[total dose/cycle = 100 mg/m²]

Repeat cycle every 28 days

References

Cashen AF, Schiller GJ, O'Donnell MR, et al, "Multicenter Phase II Study of Decitabine for the First-Line Treatment of Older Patients With Acute Myeloid Leukemia," *J Clin Oncol*, 2010, 28 (4):556-61.

Decitabine (MDS Regimen)

Use Myelodysplastic syndrome

Regimen NOTE: Multiple variations are listed.

Variation 1:

Decitabine: IV: 20 mg/m²/day over 1 hour days 1 to 5

[total dose/cycle = 100 mg/m²]

Repeat cycle every 28 days

Variation 2:

Decitabine: IV: 15 mg/m²/dose over 3 hours every 8 hours days 1 to 3 (total of 45 mg/m²/day)

[total dose/cycle = 135 mg/m²]

Repeat cycle every 6 weeks

References
Variation 1:
Kantarjian H, Oki Y, Garcia-Manero G, et al, "Results of a Randomized Study of 3 Schedules of Low-Dose Decitabine in Higher-Risk Myelodysplastic Syndrome and Chronic Myelomonocytic Leukemia," *Blood*, 2007, 109(1):52-7.
Steensma DP, Baer MR, Slack JL, et al, "Multicenter Study of Decitabine Administered Daily for 5 Days Every 4 Weeks to Adults With Myelodysplastic Syndromes: The Alternative Dosing for Outpatient Treatment (ADOPT) Trial," *J Clin Oncol*, 2009, 27(23):3842-8.
Variation 2:
Kantarjian H, Issa JP, Rosenfeld CS, et al, "Decitabine Improves Patient Outcomes in Myelodysplastic Syndromes," *Cancer*, 2006, 106(8):1794-803.

Degarelix (Prostate Regimen)

Use Prostate cancer

Regimen

Cycle 1:
Degarelix: SubQ: 240 mg (loading dose) day 1 cycle 1
[total dose/cycle = 240 mg]
Treatment cycle is 28 days
Subsequent cycles:
Degarelix: SubQ: 80 mg day 1
[total dose/cycle = 80 mg]
Repeat cycle every 28 days

References
Klotz L, Boccon-Gibod L, Shore ND, et al, "The Efficacy and Safety of Degarelix: A 12-Months, Comparative, Randomized, Open-Label, Parallel-Group Phase III Study in Patients With Prostate Cancer," *BJU Int*, 2008, 102(11):1531-8.

Dexa-BEAM (Hodgkin)

Index Terms Dexamethasone, Carmustine, Etoposide, Cytarabine, Melphalan (Hodgkin)

Use Lymphoma, Hodgkin

Regimen

Dexamethasone: Oral: 8 mg every 8 hours days 1 to 10
[total dose/cycle = 240 mg]
Carmustine: IV: 60 mg/m^2 day 2
[total dose/cycle = 60 mg/m^2]
Etoposide: IV: 75 mg/m^2/day days 4 to 7
[total dose/cycle = 300 mg/m^2]
Cytarabine: IV: 100 mg/m^2/dose every 12 hours days 4 to 7 (total of 8 doses)
[total dose/cycle = 800 mg/m^2]
Melphalan: IV: 20 mg/m^2 day 3
[total dose/cycle = 20 mg/m^2]
Repeat cycle every 28 days; consider stem cell transplantation after 2 cycles in responding patients and a maximum of 4 cycles (total) in nontransplant candidates

References
Pfreundschuh MG, Rueffer U, Lathan B, et al, "Dexa-BEAM in Patients With Hodgkin's Disease Refractory to Multidrug Chemotherapy Regimens: A Trial of the German Hodgkin's Disease Study Group," *J Clin Oncol*, 1994, 12(3):580-6.

◆ **Dexamethasone-Bortezomib (Amyloidosis)** *see* Bortezomib-Dexamethasone (Amyloidosis) *on page 1848*

◆ **Dexamethasone-Bortezomib-Doxorubicin (Liposomal)** *see* Bortezomib-Doxorubicin (Liposomal)-Dexamethasone *on page 1850*

- **Dexamethasone-Bortezomib-Doxorubicin (Multiple Myeloma)** *see* Bortezomib-Doxorubicin-Dexamethasone (Multiple Myeloma) *on page 1849*

- **Dexamethasone-Bortezomib (Multiple Myeloma)** *see* Bortezomib-Dexamethasone (Multiple Myeloma) *on page 1848*

- **Dexamethasone-Bortezomib-Panobinostat (Multiple Myeloma)** *see* Panobinostat-Bortezomib-Dexamethasone (Multiple Myeloma) *on page 2059*

- **Dexamethasone, Carmustine, Etoposide, Cytarabine, Melphalan (Hodgkin)** *see* Dexa-BEAM (Hodgkin) *on page 1937*

- **Dexamethasone-Cisplatin-Cytarabine (Hodgkin)** *see* DHAP (Hodgkin) *on page 1938*

- **Dexamethasone-Cisplatin-Cytarabine (NHL-DLBCL)** *see* DHAP (NHL-DLBCL) *on page 1938*

- **Dexamethasone-Lenalidomide (Multiple Myeloma)** *see* Lenalidomide-Dexamethasone (Multiple Myeloma) *on page 2028*

- **Dexamethasone (Low-Dose)-Lenalidomide (Multiple Myeloma)** *see* Lenalidomide-Dexamethasone (Multiple Myeloma) *on page 2028*

- **Dexamethasone-Thalidomide (MM)** *see* Thalidomide-Dexamethasone (MM) *on page 2088*

DHAP (Hodgkin)

Index Terms Dexamethasone-Cisplatin-Cytarabine (Hodgkin)

Use Lymphoma, Hodgkin

Regimen

Salvage treatment:

Dexamethasone: IV: 40 mg/day days 1 to 4
[total dose/cycle = 160 mg]

Cisplatin: IV: 100 mg/m^2 continuous infusion for 24 hours day 1
[total dose/cycle = 100 mg/m^2]

Cytarabine: IV: 2000 mg/m^2 over 3 hours every 12 hours day 2 (total of 2 doses)
[total dose/cycle = 4000 mg/m^2]

Filgrastim: SubQ: 5 mcg/kg/day beginning 24 hours after last dose of cytarabine, continue until leukocytes ≥2500/mm^3 for 3 days

Administer 2 cycles

References

Josting A, Rudolph C, Reiser M, et al, "Time-Intensified Dexamethasone/Cisplatin/Cytarabine: An Effective Salvage Therapy With Low Toxicity in Patients With Relapsed and Refractory Hodgkin's Disease," *Ann Oncol*, 2002, 13(10):1628-35.

DHAP (NHL-DLBCL)

Index Terms Cisplatin-Cytarabine-Dexamethasone (NHL-DLBCL); Dexamethasone-Cisplatin-Cytarabine (NHL-DLBCL)

Use Lymphoma, non-Hodgkin (DLBCL relapsed/refractory)

Regimen NOTE: Multiple variations are listed.

Variation 1 (patients ≤70 years of age):

Dexamethasone: IV or Oral: 40 mg daily days 1 to 4
[total dose/cycle = 160 mg]

Cisplatin: IV: 100 mg/m^2 continuous infusion over 24 hours day 1
[total dose/cycle = 100 mg/m^2]

Cytarabine: IV: 2,000 mg/m² over 3 hours every 12 hours for 2 doses day 2 (begins at the end of the cisplatin infusion)
  [total dose/cycle = 4,000 mg/m²]
Repeat cycle every 21 to 28 days for 6 to 10 cycles (usually for 4 cycles beyond maximum response)
Variation 2 (patients >70 years of age):
  Dexamethasone: IV or Oral: 40 mg daily days 1 to 4
    [total dose/cycle = 160 mg]
  Cisplatin: IV: 100 mg/m² continuous infusion over 24 hours day 1
    [total dose/cycle = 100 mg/m²]
  Cytarabine: IV: 1,000 mg/m² over 3 hours every 12 hours for 2 doses day 2 (begins at the end of the cisplatin infusion)
    [total dose/cycle = 2,000 mg/m²]
  Repeat cycle every 21 to 28 days for 6 to 10 cycles (usually for 4 cycles beyond maximum response)

References

Variation 1 and 2:
Velasquez WS, Cabanillas F, Salvador P, et al. Effective salvage therapy for lymphoma with cisplatin in combination with high-dose Ara-C and dexamethasone (DHAP). *Blood*. 1988;71 (1):117-122.

◆ **DHAX (NHL Regimen)** *see* Oxaliplatin-Cytarabine-Dexamethasone (NHL Regimen) *on page 2047*

Docetaxel (Bladder Regimen)

Use Bladder cancer
Regimen
Docetaxel: IV: 100 mg/m² over 1 hour day 1
  [total dose/cycle = 100 mg/m²]
Repeat cycle every 21 days until disease progression or unacceptable toxicity
References
McCaffrey JA, Hilton S, Mazumdar M, et al, "Phase II Trial of Docetaxel in Patients With Advanced or Metastatic Transitional-Cell Carcinoma," *J Clin Oncol*, 1997, 15(5):1853-7.

Docetaxel (Breast Regimen)

Use Breast cancer
Regimen NOTE: Multiple variations are listed.
Variation 1:
  Docetaxel: IV: 40 mg/m² over 1 hour days 1, 8, 15, 22, 29, and 36
    [total dose/cycle = 240 mg/m²]
  Repeat every 56 days until disease progression or unacceptable toxicity
Variation 2:
  Docetaxel: IV: 35 mg/m² days 1, 8, and 15
    [total dose/cycle = 105 mg/m²]
  Repeat every 28 days
Variation 3:
  Docetaxel: IV: 60-100 mg/m² over 1 hour day 1
    [total dose/cycle = 60-100 mg/m²]
  Repeat every 21 days until disease progression or unacceptable toxicity
References
Variation 1:
Burstein HJ, Manola J, Younger J, et al, "Docetaxel Administered on a Weekly Basis for Metastatic Breast Cancer," *J Clin Oncol*, 2000, 18(6):1212-9.

Variation 2:
Rivera E, Mejia JA, Arun BK, et al, "Phase 3 Study Comparing the Use of Docetaxel on an Every-3-Week Versus Weekly Schedule in the Treatment of Metastatic Breast Cancer," *Cancer*, 2008, 112 (7):1455-61.
Variation 3:
Harvey V, Mouridsen H, Semiglazov V, et al, "Phase III Trial Comparing Three Doses of Docetaxel For Second-Line Treatment of Advanced Breast Cancer," *J Clin Oncol*, 2006, 24(31):4963-4970.

◆ **Docetaxel-Capecitabine (Breast)** *see* Capecitabine-Docetaxel (Breast) *on page 1856*

◆ **Docetaxel-Capecitabine (Gastric Cancer)** *see* Capecitabine-Docetaxel (Gastric Cancer) *on page 1857*

◆ **Docetaxel-Carboplatin (Ovarian)** *see* Carboplatin-Docetaxel (Ovarian) *on page 1862*

◆ **Docetaxel-Carboplatin (Unknown Primary, Adenocarcinoma)** *see* Carboplatin-Docetaxel (Unknown Primary, Adenocarcinoma) *on page 1863*

◆ **Docetaxel-Carboplatin (Unknown Primary, Squamous Cell)** *see* Carboplatin-Docetaxel (Unknown Primary, Squamous Cell) *on page 1863*

Docetaxel (Cervical Regimen)

Use Cervical cancer

Regimen
Docetaxel: IV: 100 mg/m^2 over 1 hour day 1
[total dose/cycle = 100 mg/m^2]
Repeat cycle every 21 days until disease progression or unacceptable toxicity

References
Garcia AA, Blessing JA, Vaccarell L, et al, "Phase II Clinical Trial of Docetaxel in Refractory Squamous Cell Carcinoma of the Cervix: A Gynecologic Oncology Group Study," *Am J Clin Oncol*, 2007, 30(4):428-31.

Docetaxel-Cisplatin-Fluorouracil (Gastric/Esophageal Cancer)

Index Terms DCF (Gastric/Esophageal Cancer); TCF (Gastric/Esophageal Cancer)

Use Esophageal cancer; Gastric cancer

Regimen NOTE: Multiple variations are listed.
Variation 1:
Docetaxel: IV: 75 mg/m^2 day 1
[total dose/cycle = 75 mg/m^2]
Cisplatin: IV: 75 mg/m^2 day 1
[total dose/cycle = 75 mg/m^2]
Fluorouracil: IV: 750 mg/m^2/day continuous infusion days 1 to 5
[total dose/cycle = 3750 mg/m^2]
Repeat cycle every 21 days until disease progression or unacceptable toxicity
Variation 2:
Docetaxel: IV: 75 mg/m^2 day 1
[total dose/cycle = 75 mg/m^2]
Cisplatin: IV: 75 mg/m^2 over 4 hours day 1
[total dose/cycle = 75 mg/m^2]
Fluorouracil: IV: 300 mg/m^2/day continuous infusion days 1 to 14
[total dose/cycle = 4200 mg/m^2]
Repeat cycle every 21 days until disease progression or unacceptable toxicity for up to a maximum of 8 cycles

References

Variation 1:

Ajani JA, Fodor MB, Tjulandin SA, et al, "Phase II Multi-Institutional Randomized Trial of Docetaxel Plus Cisplatin With or Without Fluorouracil in Patients With Untreated, Advanced Gastric, or Gastroesophageal Adenocarcinoma," *J Clin Oncol*, 2005, 23(24):5660-7.

Ajani JA, Moiseyenko VM, Tjulandin S, et al, "Quality of Life With Docetaxel Plus Cisplatin and Fluorouracil Compared With Cisplatin and Fluorouracil From a Phase III Trial for Advanced Gastric or Gastroesophageal Adenocarcinoma: The V-325 Study Group," *J Clin Oncol*, 2007, 25(22):3210-6.

Van Cutsem E, Moiseyenko VM, Tjulandin S, et al, "Phase III Study of Docetaxel and Cisplatin Plus Fluorouracil Compared With Cisplatin and Fluorouracil as First-Line Therapy for Advanced Gastric Cancer: A Report of the V325 Study Group," *J Clin Oncol*, 2006, 24(31):4991-7.

Variation 2:

Roth AD, Fazio N, Stupp R, et al, "Docetaxel, Cisplatin, and Fluorouracil; Docetaxel and Cisplatin; and Epirubicin, Cisplatin, and Fluorouracil as Systemic Treatment for Advanced Gastric Carcinoma: A Randomized Phase II Trial of the Swiss Group for Clinical Cancer Research," *J Clin Oncol*, 2007, 25(22):3217-23.

Docetaxel-Cisplatin-Fluorouracil (Head and Neck Cancer)

Index Terms TPF

Use Head and neck cancer

Regimen NOTE: Multiple variations are listed.

Variation 1:

Docetaxel: IV: 75 mg/m^2 day 1

[total dose/cycle = 75 mg/m^2]

Cisplatin: IV: 75 mg/m^2 day 1

[total dose/cycle = 75 mg/m^2]

Fluorouracil: IV: 750 mg/m^2/day continuous infusion days 1 to 5

[total dose/cycle = 3750 mg/m^2]

Repeat cycle every 21 days for 4 cycles

Variation 2:

Docetaxel: IV: 75 mg/m^2 day 1

[total dose/cycle = 75 mg/m^2]

Cisplatin: IV: 75-100 mg/m^2 day 1

[total dose/cycle = 75-100 mg/m^2]

Fluorouracil: IV: 1000 mg/m^2/day continuous infusion days 1 to 4

[total dose/cycle = 4000 mg/m^2]

Repeat cycle every 21 days for total of 3 cycles

References

Variation 1:

Schrijvers D, van Herpen C, Kerger J, et al, "Docetaxel, Cisplatin and 5-Fluorouracil in Patients With Locally Advanced Unresectable Head and Neck Cancer: A Phase I-II Feasibility Study," *Ann Oncol*, 2004, 15(4):638-45.

Vermorken JB, Remenar E, van Herpen C, et al, "Cisplatin, Fluorouracil, and Docetaxel in Unresectable Head and Neck Cancer," *N Engl J Med*, 2007, 357(17):1695-1704.

Variation 2:

Posner MR, Glisson B, Frenette G, et al, "Multicenter Phase I-II Trial of Docetaxel, Cisplatin, and Fluorouracil Induction Chemotherapy for Patients With Locally Advanced Squamous Cell Cancer of the Head and Neck," *J Clin Oncol*, 2001, 19(4):1096-104.

Posner MR, Hershock DM, Blajman CR, et al, "Cisplatin and Fluorouracil Alone or With Docetaxel in Head and Neck Cancer," *N Engl J Med*, 2007, 357(17):1705-15.

◆ **Docetaxel-Cisplatin (NSCLC)** *see* Cisplatin-Docetaxel (NSCLC) *on page 1891*

◆ **Docetaxel-Cisplatin (Unknown Primary, Adenocarcinoma)** *see* Cisplatin-Docetaxel (Unknown Primary, Adenocarcinoma) *on page 1891*

Docetaxel Every 3 Weeks-Trastuzumab (Breast)

Index Terms Trastuzumab-Docetaxel Every 3 Weeks (Breast)

Use Breast cancer

Regimen

Cycle 1:

Docetaxel: IV: 100 mg/m² day 1

[total dose/cycle 1 = 100 mg/m²]

Trastuzumab: IV: 4 mg/kg (loading dose) day 1 cycle 1

followed by IV: 2 mg/kg/day days 8 and 15 cycle 1

[total dose/cycle 1 = 8 mg/kg]

Treatment cycle is 21 days

Subsequent cycles:

Docetaxel: IV: 100 mg/m² day 1

[total dose/cycle = 100 mg/m²]

Trastuzumab: IV: 2 mg/kg/day days 1, 8, and 15

[total dose/cycle = 6 mg/kg]

Repeat cycle every 21 days for a total of at least 6 cycles

followed by

Trastuzumab: IV: 2 mg/kg/day days 1, 8, and 15

[total dose/cycle = 6 mg/kg]

Repeat cycle every 21 days until disease progression or unacceptable toxicity

References

Marty M, Cognetti F, Maraninchi D, et al, "Randomized Phase II Trial of the Efficacy and Safety of Trastuzumab Combined With Docetaxel in Patients With Human Epidermal Growth Factor Receptor 2-Positive Metastatic Breast Cancer Administered as First-Line Treatment: The M77001 Study Group," *J Clin Oncol*, 2005, 23(19):4265-74.

Docetaxel-Gemcitabine (Ewing Sarcoma)

Index Terms Gemcitabine-Docetaxel (Ewing Sarcoma)

Use Ewing sarcoma

Regimen

Gemcitabine: IV: 675 mg/m²/day over 90 minutes days 1 and 8

[total dose/cycle = 1,350 mg/m²]

Docetaxel: IV: 100 mg/m² over 60 minutes day 8

[total dose/cycle = 100 mg/m²]

Growth Factor:

Filgrastim: SubQ: 300 mcg once daily days 9 to 15

or

Pegfilgrastim: SubQ: 6 mg administered day 9

Repeat cycle every 21 days

References

Leu KM, Ostruszka LJ, Shewach D, et al. Laboratory and clinical evidence of synergistic cytotoxicity of sequential treatment with gemcitabine followed by docetaxel in the treatment of sarcoma. *J Clin Oncol*. 2004;22(9):1706-1712.

Navid F, Willert JR, McCarville MB, et al. Combination of gemcitabine and docetaxel in the treatment of children and young adults with refractory bone sarcoma. *Cancer*. 2008;113(2):419-425.

Docetaxel-Gemcitabine (NSCLC)

Index Terms GD (NSCLC); Gemcitabine-Docetaxel (NSCLC)

Use Lung cancer, non-small cell

Regimen

Gemcitabine: IV: 1000 mg/m^2 over 30 minutes days 1 and 8
 [total dose/cycle = 2000 mg/m^2]
Docetaxel: IV: 85 mg/m^2 over 60 minutes day 8 (prior to gemcitabine)
 [total dose/cycle = 85 mg/m^2]
Repeat cycle every 21 days for a total of 8 cycles

References

Pujol JL, Breton JL, Gervais R, et al. Gemcitabine-docetaxel versus cisplatin-vinorelbine in advanced or metastatic non-small-cell lung cancer: a phase III study addressing the case for cisplatin. *Ann Oncol.* 2005;16(4):602-610.

Docetaxel-Gemcitabine (Osteosarcoma)

Index Terms Gemcitabine-Docetaxel (Osteosarcoma)

Use Osteosarcoma

Regimen

Gemcitabine: IV: 675 mg/m^2/day over 90 minutes days 1 and 8
 [total dose/cycle = 1,350 mg/m^2]
Docetaxel: IV: 100 mg/m^2 over 60 minutes day 8
 [total dose/cycle = 100 mg/m^2]
Growth Factor:
Filgrastim: SubQ: 300 mcg once daily days 9 to 15
 or
Pegfilgrastim: SubQ: 6 mg administered day 9
Repeat cycle every 21 days

References

Leu KM, Ostruszka LJ, Shewach D, et al. Laboratory and clinical evidence of synergistic cytotoxicity of sequential treatment with gemcitabine followed by docetaxel in the treatment of sarcoma. *J Clin Oncol.* 2004;22(9):1706-1712.

Navid F, Willert JR, McCarville MB, et al. Combination of gemcitabine and docetaxel in the treatment of children and young adults with refractory bone sarcoma. *Cancer.* 2008;113 (2):419-425.

Docetaxel-Gemcitabine (Soft Tissue Sarcoma)

Index Terms Gemcitabine-Docetaxel (Soft Tissue Sarcoma)

Use Soft tissue sarcoma

Regimen NOTE: Multiple variations are listed.

Variation 1:
Gemcitabine: IV: 675 mg/m^2/day over 90 minutes days 1 and 8
 [total dose/cycle = 1350 mg/m^2]
Docetaxel: IV: 100 mg/m^2 over 60 minutes day 8
 [total dose/cycle = 100 mg/m^2]
Growth factor:
Filgrastim: SubQ: 300 mcg once daily days 9 to 15
 or
Pegfilgrastim: SubQ: 6 mg administered day 9
Repeat cycle every 21 days
Variation 2:
Gemcitabine: IV: 900 mg/m^2/day over 90 minutes days 1 and 8
 [total dose/cycle = 1800 mg/m^2]
Docetaxel: IV: 100 mg/m^2 over 60 minutes day 8
 [total dose/cycle = 100 mg/m^2]

◀ **Growth factor:**

Filgrastim: SubQ: 5 mcg/kg once daily, starting day 9 or 10, for 7 to 10 days

or

Pegfilgrastim: SubQ: 6 mg administered day 9 or 10

Repeat cycle every 21 days

References

Variation 1:

Leu KM, Ostruszka LJ, Shewach D, et al. Laboratory and clinical evidence of synergistic cytotoxicity of sequential treatment with gemcitabine followed by docetaxel in the treatment of sarcoma. *J Clin Oncol.* 2004;22(9):1706-1712.

Variation 2:

Maki RG, Wathen JK, Patel SR, et al. Randomized phase II study of gemcitabine and docetaxel compared with gemcitabine alone in patients with metastatic soft tissue sarcomas: results of sarcoma alliance for research through collaboration study 002 [corrected]. *J Clin Oncol.* 2007;25 (19):2755-2763.

Docetaxel-Gemcitabine (Unknown Primary, Adenocarcinoma)

Index Terms Gemcitabine-Docetaxel (Unknown Primary)

Use Unknown primary (adenocarcinoma)

Regimen

Gemcitabine: IV: 1000 mg/m^2/day over 30 minutes days 1 and 8

[total dose/cycle = 2000 mg/m^2]

Docetaxel: IV: 75 mg/m^2 over 1 hour day 8

[total dose/cycle = 75 mg/m^2]

Repeat cycle every 21 days for up to a total of 6 cycles

References

Pouessel D, Culine S, Becht C, et al, "Gemcitabine and Docetaxel as Front-Line Chemotherapy in Patients With Carcinoma of an Unknown Primary Site," *Cancer,* 2004, 100(6):1257-61.

Docetaxel-Gemcitabine (Uterine Leiomyosarcoma)

Index Terms Gemcitabine-Docetaxel (Uterine Leiomyosarcoma)

Use Uterine sarcoma (uterine leiomyosarcoma)

Regimen

Variation 1 (no history of pelvic radiation):

Gemcitabine: IV: 900 mg/m^2/day over 90 minutes days 1 and 8

[total dose/cycle = 1800 mg/m^2]

Docetaxel: IV: 100 mg/m^2 over 60 minutes day 8

[total dose/cycle = 100 mg/m^2]

Growth factor:

Filgrastim: SubQ: 150 mcg/m^2 days 9 to 15

or

Pegfilgrastim: SubQ: 6 mg day 9 or 10

Repeat cycle every 21 days until disease progression or unacceptable toxicity

Variation 2 (prior pelvic radiation):

Gemcitabine: IV: 675 mg/m^2/day over 90 minutes days 1 and 8

[total dose/cycle = 1350 mg/m^2]

Docetaxel: IV: 75 mg/m^2 over 60 minutes day 8

[total dose/cycle = 75 mg/m^2]

Growth factor:

Filgrastim: SubQ: 150 mcg/m^2 days 9 to 15

or

Pegfilgrastim: SubQ: 6 mg day 9 or 10

Repeat cycle every 21 days until disease progression or unacceptable toxicity

References

Variations 1 and 2:

Hensley ML, Blessing JA, Degeest K, Abulafia O, Rose PG, Homesley HD. Fixed-dose rate gemcitabine plus docetaxel as second-line therapy for metastatic uterine leiomyosarcoma: a Gynecologic Oncology Group phase II study. *Gynecol Oncol.* 2008;109(3):323-328.

Hensley ML, Blessing JA, Mannel R, Rose PG. Fixed-dose rate gemcitabine plus docetaxel as first-line therapy for metastatic uterine leiomyosarcoma: a Gynecologic Oncology Group phase II trial. *Gynecol Oncol.* 2008;109(3):329-334.

Docetaxel (NSCLC Regimen)

Use Lung cancer, non-small cell

Regimen NOTE: Multiple variations are listed.

Variation 1:

Docetaxel: IV: 75 mg/m^2 over 1 hour day 1

[total dose/cycle = 75 mg/m^2]

Repeat cycle every 21 days

Variation 2:

Docetaxel: IV: 35 mg/m^2 days 1, 8, and 15

[total dose/cycle = 105 mg/m^2]

Repeat cycle every 28 days for a maximum of 8 cycles

Variation 3:

Docetaxel: IV: 36 mg/m^2/day over 1 hour days 1, 8, 15, 22, 29, and 36

[total dose/cycle = 216 mg/m^2]

Repeat cycle every 56 days for up to 4 cycles

Variation 4 (maintenance therapy):

Docetaxel: IV: 75 mg/m^2 over 1 hour day 1

[total dose/cycle = 75 mg/m^2]

Repeat cycle every 21 days for a maximum of 6 cycles

References

Variation1:

Fossella FV, DeVore R, Kerr RN, et al, "Randomized Phase III Trial of Docetaxel Versus Vinorelbine or Ifosfamide in Patients With Advanced Non-Small-Cell Lung Cancer Previously Treated With Platinum-Containing Chemotherapy Regimens," *J Clin Oncol*, 2000, 18 (12):2354-62.

Variation 2:

Schuette W, Nagel S, Blankenburg T, et al, "Phase III Study of Second-Line Chemotherapy for Advanced Non-Small-Cell Lung Cancer With Weekly Compared With 3-Weekly Docetaxel," *J Clin Oncol*, 2005, 23(33):8389-95.

Variation 3:

Hainsworth JD, Burris HA, Litchy S, et al, "Weekly Docetaxel in the Treatment of Elderly Patients With Advanced Nonsmall Cell Lung Cancer: A Minnie Pearl Cancer Research Network Phase II Trial," *Cancer*, 2000, 89(2):328-33.

Variation 4:

Fidias PM, Dakhill SR, Lyss AP, et al, "Phase III Study of Immediate Compared With Delayed Docetaxel After Front-Line Therapy With Gemcitabine Plus Carboplatin in Advanced Non-Small-Cell Lung Cancer," *J Clin Oncol*, 2009, 27(4):591-8.

Docetaxel (Ovarian Regimen)

Use Ovarian cancer

Regimen

Docetaxel: IV: 100 mg/m^2 over 1 hour day 1
[total dose/cycle = 100 mg/m^2]
Repeat cycle every 21 days

References

Rose PG, Blessing JA, Ball HG, et al, "A Phase II Study of Docetaxel in Paclitaxel-Resistant Ovarian and Peritoneal Carcinoma: A Gynecologic Oncology Group Study," *Gynecol Oncol*, 2003, 88(2):130-5.

Docetaxel-Oxaliplatin-Leucovorin-Fluorouracil (Esophageal Cancer)

Index Terms FLOT (Esophageal Cancer); Oxaliplatin-Docetaxel-Leucovorin-Fluorouracil (Esophageal Cancer)

Use Esophageal cancer

Regimen

Docetaxel: IV: 50 mg/m^2 day 1
[total dose/cycle = 50 mg/m^2]
Oxaliplatin: IV: 85 mg/m^2 day 1
[total dose/cycle = 85 mg/m^2]
Leucovorin: IV: 200 mg/m^2 day 1
[total dose/cycle = 200 mg/m^2]
Fluorouracil: IV: 2600 mg/m^2/day continuous infusion over 24 hours day 1
[total dose/cycle = 2600 mg/m^2]
Repeat cycle every 14 days until disease progression or unacceptable toxicity for up to a total of 8 cycles.

References

Al-Batran SE, Hartmann JT, Hofheinz R, et al, "Biweekly Fluorouracil, Leucovorin, Oxaliplatin, and Docetaxel (FLOT) for Patients With Metastatic Adenocarcinoma of the Stomach or Esophago-gastric Junction: A Phase II Trial of the Arbeitsgemeinschaft Internistische Onkologie," *Ann Oncol*, 2008, 19(11):1882-7.

◆ **Docetaxel-Pertuzumab-Trastuzumab (Metastatic Breast)** *see* Pertuzumab-Trastuzumab-Docetaxel (Metastatic Breast) *on page 2066*

◆ **Docetaxel-Pertuzumab-Trastuzumab (Neoadjuvant Breast)** *see* Pertuzumab-Trastuzumab-Docetaxel (Neoadjuvant Breast) *on page 2067*

Docetaxel-Prednisone (Prostate)

Index Terms Prednisone-Docetaxel (Prostate)

Use Prostate cancer

Regimen

Docetaxel: IV: 75 mg/m^2 over 1 hour day 1
[total dose/cycle = 75 mg/m^2]
Prednisone: Oral: 5 mg twice daily days 1 to 21
[total dose/cycle = 210 mg]
Repeat cycle every 21 days, for a maximum 10 cycles

References

Berthold DR, Pond GR, Soban F, et al, "Docetaxel Plus Prednisone or Mitoxantrone Plus Prednisone for Advanced Prostate Cancer: Updated Survival in the TAX 327 Study," *J Clin Oncol*, 2008, 26(2):242-5.

Tannock IF, de Wit R, Berry WR, et al, "Docetaxel Plus Prednisone or Mitoxantrone Plus Prednisone for Advanced Prostate Cancer," *N Engl J Med*, 2004, 351(15):1502-12.

Docetaxel-Ramucirumab (NSCLC)

Index Terms Ramucirumab-Docetaxel (NSCLC)

Use Lung cancer, non-small cell (second-line, stage IV, disease progression on platinum-based chemotherapy)

Regimen

Ramucirumab: IV: 10 mg/kg over 1 hour day 1
[total dose/cycle = 10 mg/kg]
Docetaxel: IV: 75 mg/m² day 1
[total dose/cycle = 75 mg/m²]
Repeat cycle every 21 days until disease progression or unacceptable toxicity

References

Garon EB, Ciuleanu TE, Arrieta O, et al. Ramucirumab plus docetaxel versus placebo plus docetaxel for second-line treatment of stage IV non-small-cell lung cancer after disease progression on platinum-based therapy (REVEL): a multicentre, double-blind, randomised phase 3 trial. *Lancet*. 2014;384(9944):665-673.

Docetaxel (Small Cell Lung Cancer Regimen)

Use Lung cancer, small cell

Regimen

Docetaxel: IV: 100 mg/m² over 1 hour day 1
[total dose/cycle = 100 mg/m²]
Repeat cycle every 21 days

References

Smyth JF, Smith IE, Sessa C, et al, "Activity of Docetaxel (Taxotere) in Small Cell Lung Cancer," *Eur J Cancer*, 1994, 30A(8):1058-60.

♦ **Docetaxel-Trastuzumab-Fluorouracil-Epirubicin-Cyclophosphamide (Breast)** *see* Docetaxel-Trastuzumab followed by FEC (Breast) *on page 1947*

Docetaxel-Trastuzumab followed by FEC (Breast)

Index Terms Docetaxel-Trastuzumab-Fluorouracil-Epirubicin-Cyclophospha-mide (Breast); Trastuzumab-Docetaxel-FEC (Breast)

Use Breast cancer

Regimen

Cycle 1:

Trastuzumab: IV: 4 mg/kg (loading dose) over 90 minutes day 1 cycle 1
followed by IV: 2 mg/kg/day over 30 minutes days 8 and 15 cycle 1
[total dose/cycle 1 = 8 mg/kg]
Docetaxel: IV: 80-100 mg/m² over 1 hour day 1
[total dose/cycle 1 = 80-100 mg/m²]
Treatment cycle is 21 days

Cycles 2 and 3:

Trastuzumab: IV: 2 mg/kg/day days 1, 8, and 15
[total dose/cycle = 6 mg/kg]
Docetaxel: IV: 80-100 mg/m² over 1 hour day 1
[total dose/cycle = 80-100 mg/m²]
Repeat docetaxel-trastuzumab cycle every 21 days for a total of 3 cycles

Cycles 4, 5, and 6 (FEC):

Fluorouracil: IV: 600 mg/m² day 1
[total dose/cycle = 600 mg/m²]
Epirubicin: IV: 60 mg/m² day 1
[total dose/cycle = 60 mg/m²]
Cyclophosphamide: IV: 600 mg/m² day 1
[total dose/cycle = 600 mg/m²]
Repeat FEC cycle every 21 days for total of 3 cycles

◀ **References**

Joensuu H, Bono P, Kataja V, et al, "Fluorouracil, Epirubicin, and Cyclophosphamide With Either Docetaxel or Vinorelbine, With or Without Trastuzumab, As Adjuvant Treatments of Breast Cancer: Final Results of the FinHer Trial," *J Clin Oncol*, 2009, 27(34):5685-92.

Joensuu H, Kellokumpu-Lehtinen PL, Bono P, et al, "Adjuvant Docetaxel or Vinorelbine With or Without Trastuzumab for Breast Cancer," *N Engl J Med*, 2006, 354(8):809-20.

Docetaxel Weekly-Trastuzumab (Breast)

Index Terms Trastuzumab-Docetaxel Weekly (Breast)

Use Breast cancer

Regimen

Cycle 1:

Docetaxel: IV: 35 mg/m^2/day over 30 minutes days 1, 8, and 15
[total dose/cycle 1 = 105 mg/m^2]

Trastuzumab: IV: 4 mg/kg (loading dose) over 90 minutes day 0 cycle 1
followed by IV: 2 mg/kg/day over 30 minutes days 8, 15, and 22 cycle 1
[total dose/cycle 1 = 10 mg/kg]

Treatment cycle is 28 days

Subsequent cycles:

Docetaxel: IV: 35 mg/m^2/day over 30 minutes days 1, 8, and 15
[total dose/cycle = 105 mg/m^2]

Trastuzumab: IV: 2 mg/kg/day over 30 minutes days 1, 8, 15, and 22
[total dose/cycle = 8 mg/kg]

Repeat cycle every 28 days until disease progression or unacceptable toxicity

References

Esteva FJ, Valero V, Booser D, et al, "Phase II Study of Weekly Docetaxel and Trastuzumab for Patients With HER-2-Overexpressing Metastatic Breast Cancer," *J Clin Oncol*, 2002, 20 (7):1800-8.

◆ **Dose-Adjusted EPOCH (AIDS-Related Lymphoma)** *see* EPOCH Dose-Adjusted (AIDS-Related Lymphoma) *on page 1958*

◆ **Dose-Adjusted EPOCH (NHL)** *see* EPOCH Dose-Adjusted (NHL) *on page 1959*

◆ **Dose-Adjusted Etoposide-Vincristine-Doxorubicin-Cyclophosphamide-Prednisone (NHL)** *see* EPOCH Dose-Adjusted (NHL) *on page 1959*

◆ **Dose Dense M-VAC** *see* Dose Dense MVAC (Bladder Cancer) *on page 1948*

Dose Dense MVAC (Bladder Cancer)

Index Terms DDM-VAC (Bladder Cancer); DDMVAC (Bladder Cancer); Dose Dense M-VAC; HD-MVAC (Bladder Cancer); High-Dose-Intensity M-VAC (Bladder Cancer); MVAC (Bladder Cancer)

Use Bladder cancer

Regimen NOTE: Multiple variations are listed.

Variation 1:

Methotrexate: IV: 30 mg/m^2 day 1
[total dose/cycle = 30 mg/m^2]

Vinblastine: IV: 3 mg/m^2 day 2
[total dose/cycle = 3 mg/m^2]

Doxorubicin: IV: 30 mg/m^2 day 2
[total dose/cycle = 30 mg/m^2]

Cisplatin: IV: 70 mg/m^2 day 2
[total dose/cycle = 70 mg/m^2]

Filgrastim: SubQ: 240 mcg/m^2 days 4 to 10 (discontinue if ANC >30,000/mm^3 or may extend up to a total of 14 days if needed)

Repeat cycle every 14 days until disease progression or unacceptable toxicity

Variation 2:

Methotrexate: IV: 30 mg/m^2 day 1

[total dose/cycle = 30 mg/m^2]

Vinblastine: IV: 3 mg/m^2 day 2

[total dose/cycle = 3 mg/m^2]

Doxorubicin: IV: 30 mg/m^2 day 2

[total dose/cycle = 30 mg/m^2]

Cisplatin: IV: 70 mg/m^2 day 2

[total dose/cycle = 70 mg/m^2]

Filgrastim: SubQ: Days 3 to 7 (dose not specified)

Repeat cycle every 14 days until disease progression or unacceptable toxicity

References

Variation 1:

Sternberg CN, de Mulder PH, Schornagel JH, et al. Randomized phase III trial of high-dose-intensity methotrexate, vinblastine, doxorubicin, and cisplatin (MVAC) chemotherapy and recombinant human granulocyte colony-stimulating factor versus classic MVAC in advanced urothelial tract tumors: European Organization for Research and Treatment of Cancer Protocol no. 30924. *J Clin Oncol.* 2001;19(10):2638-2646.

Variation 2:

Sternberg CN, de Mulder P, Schornagel JH, et al. Seven year update of an EORTC phase III trial of high-dose intensity M-VAC chemotherapy and G-CSF versus classic M-VAC in advanced urothelial tract tumours. *Eur J Cancer.* 2006;42(1):50-54.

Doxorubicin (Breast Regimen)

Use Breast cancer

Regimen NOTE: Multiple variations are listed.

Variation 1:

Doxorubicin: IV: 75 mg/m^2 over 5-15 minutes day 1

[total dose/cycle = 75 mg/m^2]

Repeat cycle every 21 days for up to 7 cycles, cumulative dose 525 mg/m^2

Variation 2:

Doxorubicin: IV: 60 mg/m^2 day 1

[total dose/cycle = 60 mg/m^2]

Repeat cycle every 21 days for up to 8 cycles, cumulative dose 480 mg/m^2

Variation 3:

Doxorubicin: IV: 20 mg/m^2 day 1

[total dose/cycle = 20 mg/m^2]

Repeat cycle every 7 days

References

Variation 1:

Paridaens R, Biganzoli L, Bruning P, et al, "Paclitaxel Versus Doxorubicin as First-Line Single-Agent Chemotherapy For Metastatic Breast Cancer: A European Organization For Research and Treatment of Cancer Randomized Study With Cross-Over," *J Clin Oncol*, 2000, 18(4):724-33.

Variation 2:

Sledge GW, Neuberg D, Bernardo P, et al, "Phase III Trial of Doxorubicin, Paclitaxel, and the Combination of Doxorubicin and Paclitaxel as Front-Line Chemotherapy For Metastatic Breast Cancer: An Intergroup Tiral (E1193)," *J Clin Oncol*, 2003, 21(4):588-92.

Variation 3:

Gundersen S, Kvinnsland S, Klepp O, et al, "Weekly Adriamycin Versus VAC in Advanced Breast Cancer. A Randomized Trial," *Eur J Cancer Clin Oncol*, 1986, 22:1431-4.

Doxorubicin (Liposomal) (Breast Regimen)

Use Breast cancer

Regimen

Doxorubicin (liposomal): IV: 50 mg/m^2 over 1 hour day 1

[total dose/cycle = 50 mg/m^2]

Repeat cycle every 28 days

References

Keller AM, Mennel RG, Georgoulias VA, et al, "Randomized Phase III Trial of Pegylated Liposomal Doxorubicin Versus Vinorelbine or Mitomycin C Plus Vinblastine in Women With Taxane-Refractory Advanced Breast Cancer," *J Clin Onc*, 2004, 22(19):3893-3901

O'Brien MER, Wigler N, Inbar M, et al, "Reduced Cardiotoxicity and Comparable Efficacy in a Phase III Trial of Pegylated Liposomal Doxorubicin HCL (CAELYX™/Doxil®) Versus Conventional Doxorubicin For First-Line Treatment of Metastatic Breast Cancer," *Ann Oncol*, 2004,15 (3):440-9.

Doxorubicin (Liposomal) (Ovarian Regimen)

Use Ovarian cancer

Regimen NOTE: Multiple variations are listed.

Variation 1:

Doxorubicin (liposomal): IV: 50 mg/m^2 over 60 minutes day 1

[total dose/cycle = 50 mg/m^2]

Repeat cycle every 28 days until disease progression or unacceptable toxicity

Variation 2:

Doxorubicin (liposomal): IV: 40 mg/m^2 over 60 minutes day 1

[total dose/cycle = 40 mg/m^2]

Repeat cycle every 28 days until disease progression or unacceptable toxicity

References

Variation 1:

Gordon AN, Tonda M, Sun S, et al, "Long-Term Survival Advantage for Women Treated With Pegylated Liposomal Doxorubicin Compared With Topotecan in a Phase III Randomized Study of Recurrent and Refractory Epithelial Ovarian Cancer," *Gynecol Onc*, 2004, 95(1):1-8.

Mutch DG, Orlando M, Goss T, et al, "Randomized Phase III Trial of Gemcitabine Compared With Pegylated Liposomal Doxorubicin in Patients With Platinum-Resistant Ovarian Cancer," *J Clin Oncol*, 2007, 25(19):2811-8.

Variation 2:

Ferrandina G, Ludovisi M, Lorusso D, et al, "Phase III Trial of Gemcitabine Compared With Pegylated Liposomal Doxorubicin in Progressive or Recurrent Ovarian Cancer," *J Clin Oncol*, 2008, 26(6):890-6.

Rose PG, Maxson JH, Fusco N, et al, "Liposomal Doxorubicin in Ovarian, Peritoneal, and Tubal Carcinoma: A Retrospective Comparative Study of Single-Agent Dosages," *Gynecol Oncol*, 2001, 82(2):323-8.

◆ **Doxorubicin, Bleomycin, Vinblastine, Dacarbazine (Hodgkin)** *see* ABVD Early Stage (Hodgkin) *on page 1820*

◆ **Doxorubicin-Bleomycin-Vinblastine-Dacarbazine (Hodgkin)** *see* ABVD (Hodgkin) *on page 1821*

◆ **Doxorubicin-Cisplatin (Endometrial)** *see* Cisplatin-Doxorubicin (Endometrial) *on page 1892*

◆ **Doxorubicin-Cyclophosphamide (Breast)** *see* AC (Breast) *on page 1822*

◆ **Doxorubicin, Cyclophosphamide, Docetaxel (Breast)** *see* AC followed by Docetaxel Every 3 Weeks (Breast) *on page 1824*

◆ **Doxorubicin, Cyclophosphamide, Docetaxel (Breast)** *see* TAC (Breast) *on page 2086*

Doxorubicin (Liposomal) (Uterine Leiomyosarcoma Regimen)

Use Uterine sarcoma (recurrent/advanced leiomyosarcoma)

Regimen

Doxorubicin (liposomal): IV: 50 mg/m^2 over 60 minutes day 1
[total dose/cycle = 50 mg/m^2]

Repeat cycle every 28 days for 6 cycles (Judson 2001) or disease progression or unacceptable toxicity (Sutton 2005)

References

Judson I, Radford JA, Harris M, et al. Randomised phase II trial of pegylated liposomal doxorubicin (DOXIL/CAELYX) versus doxorubicin in the treatment of advanced or metastatic soft tissue sarcoma: a study by the EORTC Soft Tissue and Bone Sarcoma Group. *Eur J Cancer.* 2001;37 (7):870-877.

Sutton G, Blessing J, Hanjani P, Kramer P; Gynecologic Oncology Group. Phase II evaluation of liposomal doxorubicin (Doxil) in recurrent or advanced leiomyosarcoma of the uterus: a Gynecologic Oncology Group study. *Gynecol Oncol.* 2005;96(3):749-752.

Doxorubicin (Liposomal)-Vincristine-Dexamethasone

Index Terms DVd; DVD

Use Multiple myeloma

◀ **Regimen** NOTE: Multiple variations are listed.

Variation 1:

Doxorubicin, liposomal: IV: 40 mg/m^2 day 1

[total dose/cycle = 40 mg/m^2]

Vincristine: IV: 2 mg day 1

[total dose/cycle = 2 mg]

Dexamethasone: Oral or IV: 40 mg/day days 1 to 4

[total dose/cycle = 160 mg]

Repeat cycle every 4 weeks

Variation 2:

Doxorubicin, liposomal: IV: 40 mg/m^2 day 1

[total dose/cycle = 40 mg/m^2]

Vincristine: IV: 1.4 mg/m^2 (maximum dose: 2 mg) day 1

[total dose/cycle = 1.4 mg/m^2; maximum: 2 mg]

Dexamethasone: Oral: 40 mg/day days 1 to 4

[total dose/cycle = 160 mg]

Repeat cycle every 4 weeks

References

Variation 1:

Hussein MA, Wood L, Hsi E, et al, "A Phase II Trial of Pegylated Liposomal Doxorubicin, Vincristine, and Reduced-Dose Dexamethasone Combination Therapy in Newly Diagnosed Multiple Myeloma Patients," *Cancer*, 2002, 95(10):2160-8.

Variation 2:

Rifkin RM, Gregory SA, Mohrbacher A, et al, "Pegylated Liposomal Doxorubicin, Vincristine, and Dexamethasone Provide Significant Reduction in Toxicity Compared With Doxorubicin, Vincristine, and Dexamethasone in Patients With Newly Diagnosed Multiple Myeloma: A Phase III Multicenter Randomized Trial," *Cancer*, 2006, 106(4):848-58.

DTPACE

Use Multiple myeloma

Regimen

Dexamethasone: Oral: 40 mg/day days 1 to 4

[total dose/cycle = 160 mg]

Thalidomide: Oral: 400 mg/day

[total dose/cycle = 11,200 - 16,800 mg]

Cisplatin: IV: 10 mg/m^2/day continuous infusion days 1 to 4

[total dose/cycle = 40 mg/m^2]

Doxorubicin: IV: 10 mg/m^2/day continuous infusion days 1 to 4

[total dose/cycle = 40 mg/m^2]

Cyclophosphamide: IV: 400 mg/m^2 continuous infusion days 1 to 4

[total dose/cycle = 1600 mg/m^2]

Etoposide: IV: 40 mg/m^2 continuous infusion days 1 to 4

[total dose/cycle = 160 mg/m^2]

Repeat cycle every 4-6 weeks

References

Lee CK, Barlogie B, Munshi N, et al, "DTPACE: An Effective, Novel Combination Chemotherapy With Thalidomide for Previously Treated Patients With Myeloma," *J Clin Oncol*, 2003, 21 (14):2732-9.

◆ **DVd** see Doxorubicin (Liposomal)-Vincristine-Dexamethasone on page 1951

DVP

Use Leukemia, acute lymphocytic

Regimen Induction:

Daunorubicin: IV: 25 mg/m²/day days 1, 8, and 15
[total dose/cycle = 75 mg/m²]

Vincristine: IV: 1.5 mg/m²/day (maximum dose: 2 mg) days 1, 8, 15, and 22
[total dose/cycle = 6 mg/m²]

Prednisone: Oral: 60 mg/m²/day days 1 to 28 then taper over next 14 days
[total dose/cycle = 1680 mg/m² + taper over next 14 days]

Administer single cycle; used in conjunction with intrathecal chemotherapy

References

Belasco JB, Luery N, and Scher C, "Multiagent Chemotherapy in Relapsed Acute Lymphoblastic Leukemia in Children," *Cancer*, 1990, 66(12):2492-7.

◆ **EC (Breast)** *see* Cyclophosphamide-Epirubicin (Breast) *on page 1929*

◆ **ECF (Gastric/Esophageal)** *see* Epirubicin-Cisplatin-Fluorouracil (Gastric/ Esophageal) *on page 1956*

EC (NSCLC)

Use Lung cancer, non-small cell

Regimen

Etoposide: IV: 120 mg/m²/day days 1, 2, and 3
[total dose/cycle = 360 mg/m²]

Carboplatin: IV: AUC 6 day 1
[total dose/cycle = AUC = 6]

Repeat cycle every 21-28 days

References

Birch R, Weaver CH, Hainsworth JD, et al, "A Randomized Study of Etoposide and Carboplatin With or Without Paclitaxel in the Treatment of Small Cell Lung Cancer," *Semin Oncol*, 1997, 24(4 Suppl 12):S12-135, 137.

◆ **EC (Small Cell Lung Cancer)** *see* Carboplatin-Etoposide (Small Cell Lung Cancer) *on page 1865*

◆ **ECX (Gastric/Esophageal)** *see* Epirubicin-Cisplatin-Capecitabine (Gastric/ Esophageal) *on page 1956*

◆ **EE4A (Wilms' Tumor)** *see* EE-4A (Wilms' Tumor) *on page 1953*

EE-4A (Wilms' Tumor)

Index Terms Dactinomycin-Vincristine (Wilms' Tumor); EE4A (Wilms' Tumor); Regimen EE-4A (Wilms' Tumor); Vincristine-Dactinomycin (Wilms' Tumor)

Use Wilms' tumor

Regimen

Dactinomycin: IV: 45 mcg/kg day 1 of weeks 0, 3, 6, 9, 12, 15, and 18
[total dose = 315 mcg/kg]

Vincristine: IV: 1.5 mg/m² day 1 of weeks 1 to 10

Followed by

Vincristine: IV: 2 mg/m² day 1 of weeks 12, 15, and 18
[total dose = 21 mg/m²]

Treatment course duration is week 0 through week 18

References

Green DM, Breslow NE, Beckwith JB, et al, "Effect of Duration of Treatment on Treatment Outcome and Cost of Treatment for Wilms' Tumor: A Report From the National Wilms' Tumor Study Group," *J Clin Oncol*, 1998, 16(12):3744-51.

◆ **EMA (AML)** *see* Mitoxantrone-Etoposide-Cytarabine (AML) *on page 2038*

EMA/CO (Gestational Trophoblastic Tumor)

Index Terms Etoposide-Methotrexate-Dactinomycin-Leucovorin-Cyclophosphamide-Vincristine (Gestational Trophoblastic Tumor)

Use Gestational trophoblastic tumor

Regimen

Dactinomycin: IV: 0.5 mg/day days 1 and 2
   [total dose/cycle = 1 mg]
Etoposide: IV: 100 mg/m^2/day over 30 minutes days 1 and 2
   [total dose/cycle = 200 mg/m^2]
Methotrexate: IV bolus: 100 mg/m^2 day 1

followed by

Methotrexate: IV: 200 mg/m^2 continuous infusion over 12 hours day 1
   [total dose/cycle = 300 mg/m^2]
Leucovorin: Oral, IM: 15 mg every 12 hours for 4 doses (begin 24 hours after
   start of methotrexate) days 2 and 3
   [total dose/cycle = 60 mg]
Vincristine: IV: 1 mg/m^2 day 8
   [total dose/cycle = 1 mg/m^2]
Cyclophosphamide: IV: 600 mg/m^2 day 8
   [total dose/cycle = 600 mg/m^2]
Repeat cycle every 14 days, continue for at least 2 treatment cycles after a
   normal hCG level

References

Escobar PF, Lurain JR, Singh DK, Bozorgi K, Fishman DA. Treatment of high-risk gestational
   trophoblastic neoplasia with etoposide, methotrexate, actinomycin D, cyclophosphamide, and
   vincristine chemotherapy. *Gynecol Oncol.* 2003;91(3):552-557.
Lurain JR, Singh DK, Schink JC. Primary treatment of metastatic high-risk gestational trophoblastic
   neoplasia with EMA-CO chemotherapy. *J Reprod Med.* 2006;51(10):767-772.

EMA/EP (Gestational Trophoblastic Tumor)

Index Terms EP/EMA (Gestational Trophoblastic Tumor); Etoposide-Cisplatin-Methotrexate-Dactinomycin (Gestational Trophoblastic Tumor); Etoposide-Methotrexate-Leucovorin-Dactinomycin-Cisplatin (Gestational Trophoblastic Tumor)

Use Gestational trophoblastic tumor

Regimen

Etoposide: IV: 150 mg/m^2 over 30 minutes day 1
   [total dose/cycle = 150 mg/m^2]
Cisplatin: IV: 25 mg/m^2 over 4 hours each for 3 consecutive doses day 1
   [total dose/cycle = 75 mg/m^2]

Alternate weekly with:

Etoposide: IV: 100 mg/m^2 over 30 minutes day 1
   [total dose/cycle = 100 mg/m^2]
Methotrexate: IV: 300 mg/m^2 over 12 hours day 1
   [total dose/cycle = 300 mg/m^2]
Dactinomycin: IV: 0.5 mg (IV bolus) day 1
   [total dose/cycle = 0.5 mg]
Leucovorin: Oral, IM: 15 mg twice daily for 4 doses days 2 and 3 (begin 24
   hours after the start of methotrexate)
   [total dose/cycle = 60 mg]
Alternate weekly EP and EMA

References

Newlands ES, Bower M, Holden L, et al. Management of resistant gestational trophoblastic tumors. *J Reprod Med.* 1998;43(2):111-118.

Newlands ES, Mulholland PJ, Holden L, Seckl MJ, Rustin GJ. Etoposide and cisplatin/etoposide, methotrexate, and actinomycin D (EMA) chemotherapy for patients with high-risk gestational trophoblastic tumors refractory to EMA/cyclophosphamide and vincristine chemotherapy and patients presenting with metastatic placental site trophoblastic tumors. *J Clin Oncol.* 2000;18(4):854-859.

◆ **EMA-G (AML Induction)** *see* MEC-G (AML Induction) *on page 2032*

EMA (Gestational Trophoblastic Tumor)

Index Terms Etoposide-Methotrexate-Dactinomycin-Leucovorin (Gestational Trophoblastic Tumor); MEA (Gestational Trophoblastic Tumor)

Use Gestational trophoblastic tumor

Regimen

Dactinomycin: IV bolus: 0.5 mg/day days 1 to 5
[total dose/cycle = 2.5 mg]

Etoposide: IV: 100 mg/day over 1 hour days 1 to 5
[total dose/cycle = 500 mg]

Methotrexate: IV bolus: 150 mg day 1
followed by: IV: 300 mg over 4 hours day 1
[total dose/cycle = 450 mg]

Leucovorin: IM: 15 mg every 12 hours for 3 doses beginning on day 2 (24 hours after start of methotrexate)
[total dose/cycle = 45 mg]

Repeat cycle every 14 to 21 days, continue until hCG level decreases to within normal range (<1 mIU/mL)

References

Matsui H, Suzuka K, Iitsuka Y, Seki K, Sekiya S. Combination chemotherapy with methotrexate, etoposide, and actinomycin D for high-risk gestational trophoblastic tumors. *Gynecol Oncol.* 2000;78(1):28-31.

Enzalutamide (Prostate Regimen)

Use Prostate cancer

Regimen

Enzalutamide: Oral: 160 mg once daily days 1 to 28
[total dose/cycle = 4480 mg]

Repeat cycle every 28 days until disease progression or unacceptable toxicity

References

Beer TM, Armstrong AJ, Rathkopf DE, et al. Enzalutamide in metastatic prostate cancer before chemotherapy. *N Engl J Med.* 2014;371(5):424-433.

Scher HI, Fizazi K, Saad F, et al. Increased survival with enzalutamide in prostate cancer after chemotherapy. *N Engl J Med.* 2012;367(13):1187-1197.

◆ **EOF (Gastric/Esophageal)** *see* Epirubicin-Oxaliplatin-Fluorouracil (Gastric/Esophageal) *on page 1958*

◆ **EOX (Gastric/Esophageal)** *see* Epirubicin-Oxaliplatin-Capecitabine (Gastric/Esophageal) *on page 1957*

◆ **EP/EMA (Gestational Trophoblastic Tumor)** *see* EMA/EP (Gestational Trophoblastic Tumor) *on page 1954*

Epirubicin (Breast Regimen)

Use Breast cancer

◀ **Regimen**

Epirubicin: IV: 60-90 mg/m² over 10 minutes day 1

[total dose/cycle = 60-90 mg/m²]

Repeat cycle every 21 days until disease progression, unacceptable toxicity, or to a maximum cumulative dose of 1000 mg/m²

References

Bastholt L, Dalmark M, Gjedde SB, et al, "Dose-Response Relationship of Epirubicin in the Treatment of Postmenopausal Patients With Metastatic Breast Cancer: A Randomized Study of Epirubicin at Four Different Dose Levels Performed by the Danish Breast Cancer Cooperative Group," *J Clin Oncol*, 1996, 14(4):1146-55.

Epirubicin-Cisplatin-Capecitabine (Gastric/Esophageal)

Index Terms Capecitabine-Cisplatin-Epirubicin (Gastric/Esophageal); Cisplatin-Capecitabine-Epirubicin (Gastric/Esophageal); ECX (Gastric/Esophageal)

Use Esophageal cancer; Gastric cancer

Regimen

Epirubicin: IV: 50 mg/m² day 1

[total dose/cycle = 50 mg/m²]

Cisplatin: IV: 60 mg/m² day 1

[total dose/cycle = 60 mg/m²]

Capecitabine: Oral: 625 mg/m² twice daily days 1 to 21; administer within 30 minutes after a meal

[total dose/cycle = 26,250 mg/m²]

Repeat cycle every 21 days for up to 8 cycles

References

Cunningham D, Starling N, Rao S, et al. Capecitabine and oxaliplatin for advanced esophago-gastric cancer. *N Engl J Med*. 2008;358(1):36-46.

Epirubicin-Cisplatin-Fluorouracil (Gastric/Esophageal)

Index Terms Cisplatin-Fluorouracil-Epirubicin (Gastric/Esophageal); ECF (Gastric/Esophageal); Fluorouracil-Cisplatin-Epirubicin (Gastric/Esophageal)

Use Esophageal cancer; Gastric cancer

Regimen NOTE: Multiple variations are listed.

Variation 1:

Epirubicin: IV: 50 mg/m² day 1

[total dose/cycle = 50 mg/m²]

Cisplatin: IV: 60 mg/m² day 1

[total dose/cycle = 60 mg/m²]

Fluorouracil: IV: 200 mg/m²/day continuous infusion days 1 to 21

[total dose/cycle = 4,200 mg/m²]

Repeat cycle every 21 days for up to a maximum of 8 cycles

Variation 2:

Epirubicin: IV: 50 mg/m² day 1

[total dose/cycle = 50 mg/m²]

Cisplatin: IV: 60 mg/m² day 1

[total dose/cycle = 60 mg/m²]

Fluorouracil: IV: 200 mg/m²/day continuous infusion days 1 to 21

[total dose/cycle = 4,200 mg/m²]

Repeat cycle every 21 days for 6 cycles (3 cycles preoperatively and 3 cycles postoperatively)

References

Variation 1:
Cunningham D, Starling N, Rao S, et al. Capecitabine and oxaliplatin for advanced esophago-gastric cancer. *N Engl J Med.* 2008;358(1):36-46.
Variation 2:
Cunningham D, Allum WH, Stenning SP, et al. Perioperative chemotherapy versus surgery alone for resectable gastroesophageal cancer. *N Engl J Med.* 2006;355(1):11-20.

♦ **Epirubicin-Cyclophosphamide (Breast)** *see* Cyclophosphamide-Epirubicin (Breast) *on page* 1929

Epirubicin-Ifosfamide (Soft Tissue Sarcoma)

Index Terms Ifosfamide-Epirubicin (Soft Tissue Sarcoma)

Use Soft tissue sarcoma (adjuvant)

Regimen NOTE: Multiple variations are listed.

Variation 1 (begin no later than 4 weeks after surgery):

Epirubicin: IV: 25 mg/m^2/day days 1, 2, and 3
[total dose/cycle = 75 mg/m^2]

Ifosfamide: IV: 1,200 mg/m^2/day days 1 to 5
[total dose/cycle = 6,000 mg/m^2]

Mesna: IV: 240 mg/m^2 administer before and 4 and 8 hours after ifosfamide (total of 3 doses/day) days 1 to 5
[total dose/cycle = 3,600 mg/m^2]

Repeat cycle every 28 days for a total of 4 cycles

Variation 2:

Epirubicin: IV: 60 mg/m^2/day days 1 and 2
[total dose/cycle = 120 mg/m^2]

Ifosfamide: IV: 1,800 mg/m^2/day over 1 hour days 1 to 5
[total dose/cycle = 9,000 mg/m^2]

Mesna: IV bolus: 360 mg/m^2 administer before and 4 and 8 hours after ifosfamide (total of 3 doses/day) days 1 to 5
[total dose/cycle = 5,400 mg/m^2]

Filgrastim: SubQ: 300 mcg/day days 8 to 15
[total dose/cycle = 2,400 mcg]

Repeat cycle every 21 days for a total of 5 cycles

References

Variation 1:
Petrioli R, Coratti A, Correale P, et al. Adjuvant epirubicin with or without Ifosfamide for adult soft-tissue sarcoma. *Am J Clin Oncol.* 2002;25(5):468-473.
Variation 2:
Frustaci S, Gherlinzoni F, De Paoli A, et al. Adjuvant chemotherapy for adult soft tissue sarcomas of the extremities and girdles: results of the Italian randomized cooperative trial. *J Clin Oncol.* 2001;19(5):1238-1247.

Epirubicin-Oxaliplatin-Capecitabine (Gastric/Esophageal)

Index Terms Capecitabine-Oxaliplatin-Epirubicin (Gastric/Esophageal); EOX (Gastric/Esophageal); Oxaliplatin-Capecitabine-Epirubicin (Gastric/Esophageal)

Use Esophageal cancer; Gastric cancer

Regimen

Epirubicin: IV: 50 mg/m^2 day 1
[total dose/cycle = 50 mg/m^2]

Oxaliplatin: IV: 130 mg/m^2 over 2 hours day 1
[total dose/cycle = 130 mg/m^2]

◄ Capecitabine: Oral: 625 mg/m^2 twice daily days 1 to 21; administer within 30 minutes after a meal

[total dose/cycle = 26,250 mg/m^2]

Repeat cycle every 21 days for up to 8 cycles

References
Cunningham D, Starling N, Rao S, et al. Capecitabine and oxaliplatin for advanced esophago-gastric cancer. *N Engl J Med.* 2008;358(1):36-46.

Epirubicin-Oxaliplatin-Fluorouracil (Gastric/Esophageal)

Index Terms EOF (Gastric/Esophageal); Fluorouracil-Oxaliplatin-Epirubicin (Gastric/Esophageal); Oxaliplatin-Fluorouracil-Epirubicin (Gastric/Esophageal)

Use Esophageal cancer; Gastric cancer

Regimen

Epirubicin: IV: 50 mg/m^2 day 1

[total dose/cycle = 50 mg/m^2]

Oxaliplatin: IV: 130 mg/m^2 over 2 hours day 1

[total dose/cycle = 130 mg/m^2]

Fluorouracil: IV: 200 mg/m^2/day continuous infusion days 1 to 21

[total dose/cycle = 4,200 mg/m^2]

Repeat cycle every 21 days for up to 8 cycles

References
Cunningham D, Starling N, Rao S, et al. Capecitabine and oxaliplatin for advanced esophago-gastric cancer. *N Engl J Med.* 2008;358(1):36-46.

EPOCH Dose-Adjusted (AIDS-Related Lymphoma)

Index Terms Dose-Adjusted EPOCH (AIDS-Related Lymphoma)

Use Lymphoma, AIDS-related

Regimen

Etoposide: IV: 50 mg/m^2/day continuous infusion days 1 to 4

[total dose/cycle = 200 mg/m^2]

Vincristine: IV: 0.4 mg/m^2/day continuous infusion days 1 to 4

[total dose/cycle = 1.6 mg/m^2]

Doxorubicin: IV: 10 mg/m^2/day continuous infusion days 1 to 4

[total dose/cycle = 40 mg/m^2]

Cyclophosphamide: IV: 375 mg/m^2 day 5 for CD4+ cells ≥100/mm^3 **or** 187 mg/m^2 day 5 for CD4+ cells <100/mm^3

[total dose/cycle = 187-375 mg/m^2]

Prednisone: Oral: 60 mg/m^2/day days 1 to 5

[total dose/cycle = 300 mg/m^2]

Filgrastim: SubQ: 5 mcg/kg/day beginning day 6; continue until ANC >5000/mm^3 (past nadir)

Repeat cycle every 21 days for 6 cycles with cyclophosphamide dose adjusted based on previous cycle nadir according to the following schedule:

Nadir ANC >500/mm^3: Increase cyclophosphamide dose by 187 mg/m^2 above previous cycle dose (maximum dose: 750 mg/m^2)

Nadir ANC <500/mm^3 or platelet <25,000/mm^3: Decrease cyclophosphamide dose by 187 mg/m^2 below previous cycle dose

References
Little RF, Pittaluga S, Grant N, et al, "Highly Effective Treatment of Acquired Immunodeficiency Syndrome-Related Lymphoma With Dose-Adjusted EPOCH: Impact of Antiretroviral Therapy Suspension and Tumor Biology," *Blood*, 2003, 101(12):4653-9.

EPOCH Dose-Adjusted (NHL)

Index Terms Dose-Adjusted EPOCH (NHL); Dose-Adjusted Etoposide-Vin-cristine-Doxorubicin-Cyclophosphamide-Prednisone (NHL)

Use Lymphoma, non-Hodgkin

Regimen

Etoposide: IV: 50 mg/m²/day continuous infusion days 1 to 4
[total dose/cycle = 200 mg/m²]

Vincristine: IV: 0.4 mg/m²/day continuous infusion days 1 to 4
[total dose/cycle = 1.6 mg/m²]

Doxorubicin: IV: 10 mg/m²/day continuous infusion days 1 to 4
[total dose/cycle = 40 mg/m²]

Cyclophosphamide: IV: 750 mg/m² day 5
[total dose/cycle = 750 mg/m²]

Prednisone: Oral: 60 mg/m²/day (given once daily or in 2 divided doses) days
1 to 5 or days 1 to 6 (some centers may use 60 mg/m² twice daily days 1 to 5)
[total dose/cycle = 300 to 360 mg/m² or 600 mg/m²]

Filgrastim: SubQ: 5 mcg/kg/day beginning day 6 or 8; continue until ANC
recovery

Repeat cycle every 21 days with etoposide, doxorubicin, and cyclophosphamide dose adjustments (based on CBC 2 times/week) according to the
following schedule:

Nadir ANC ≥500/mm³: 20% to 25% increase (above previous cycle) for
etoposide, doxorubicin, and cyclophosphamide

Nadir ANC <500/mm³ (on 1 or 2 measurements): Same doses as previous
cycle

Nadir ANC <500/mm³ (on ≥3 measurements) or nadir platelet <25,000/mm³
(on 1 measurement): 20% to 25% decrease below previous cycle for
etoposide, doxorubicin, and cyclophosphamide (dosing adjustments below
starting dose levels only apply to cyclophosphamide)

References

Gutierrez M, Chabner BA, Pearson D, et al, "Role of a Doxorubicin-Containing Regimen in
Relapsed and Resistant Lymphomas: An 8-Year Follow-Up Study of EPOCH," *J Clin Oncol*,
2000, 18(21):3633-42.

Wilson WH, Bryant G, Bates S, et al, "EPOCH Chemotherapy: Toxicity and Efficacy in Relapsed
and Refractory Non-Hodgkin's Lymphoma," *J Clin Oncol*, 1993, 11(8):1573-82.

Wilson WH, Grossbard ML, Pittaluga S, et al, "Dose-Adjusted EPOCH Chemotherapy for
Untreated Large B-Cell Lymphomas: A Pharmacodynamic Approach With High Efficacy," *Blood*,
2002, 99(8):2685-93.

EPOCH (Dose-Adjusted)-Rituximab (NHL)

Index Terms EPOCH (Dose-Adjusted)-R (NHL); R-EPOCH Dose Adjusted
(NHL); Rituxan-Etoposide-Prednisone-Vincristine-Cyclophosphamide-Doxoru-
bicin (Dose-Adjusted) (NHL); Rituximab-EPOCH Dose Adjusted (NHL)

Use Lymphoma, non-Hodgkin

Regimen

Rituximab: IV: 375 mg/m² day 1
[total dose/cycle = 375 mg/m²]

Etoposide: IV: 50 mg/m²/day continuous infusion days 1 to 4
[total dose/cycle = 200 mg/m²]

Vincristine: IV: 0.4 mg/m²/day continuous infusion days 1 to 4
[total dose/cycle = 1.6 mg/m²]

Doxorubicin: IV: 10 mg/m²/day continuous infusion days 1 to 4
[total dose/cycle = 40 mg/m²]

Cyclophosphamide: IV: 750 mg/m^2 day 5
[total dose/cycle = 750 mg/m^2]

Prednisone: Oral: 60 mg/m^2/day (given once daily or in 2 divided doses) days 1 to 5 (some centers may use 60 mg/m^2 twice daily days 1 to 5)
[total dose/cycle = 300 mg/m^2 or 600 mg/m^2]

Filgrastim: SubQ: 5 mcg/kg/day beginning day 6; continue until ANC recovery

Repeat cycle every 21 days (for at least 2 cycles beyond best response; minimum of 6 cycles and maximum of 8 cycles) with etoposide, doxorubicin, and cyclophosphamide dose adjustments (based on CBC 2 times/week) according to the following schedule:

Nadir ANC ≥500/mm^3: 20% increase (above previous cycle) for etoposide, doxorubicin, and cyclophosphamide

Nadir ANC <500/mm^3 (on 1 or 2 measurements): Same doses as previous cycle

Nadir ANC <500/mm^3 (on ≥3 measurements): 20% decrease below previous cycle for etoposide, doxorubicin, and cyclophosphamide (dosing adjustments below starting dose levels only apply to cyclophosphamide)

References

García-Suárez J, Bañas H, Arribas I, et al, "Dose-Adjusted EPOCH Plus Rituximab Is an Effective Regimen in Patients With Poor-Prognostic Untreated Diffuse Large B-Cell Lymphoma: Results From a Prospective Observational Study," *Br J Haematol*, 2007, 136(2):276-85.

Wilson WH, Gutierrez M, O'Connor P, et al, "The Role of Rituximab and Chemotherapy in Aggressive B-Cell Lymphoma: A Preliminary Report of Dose-Adjusted EPOCH-R," *Semin Oncol*, 2002, 29(1 Suppl 2):41-7.

◆ **EPOCH (Dose-Adjusted)-R (NHL)** *see* EPOCH (Dose-Adjusted)-Rituximab (NHL) *on page 1959*

EPOCH (NHL)

Use Lymphoma, non-Hodgkin

Regimen NOTE: Multiple variations are listed.

Variation 1:

Etoposide: IV: 50 mg/m^2/day continuous infusion days 1 to 4
[total dose/cycle = 200 mg/m^2]

Vincristine: IV: 0.4 mg/m^2/day continuous infusion days 1 to 4
[total dose/cycle = 1.6 mg/m^2]

Doxorubicin: IV: 10 mg/m^2/day continuous infusion days 1 to 4
[total dose/cycle = 40 mg/m^2]

Cyclophosphamide: IV: 750 mg/m^2 day 5
[total dose/cycle = 750 mg/m^2]

Prednisone: Oral: 60 mg/m^2/day days 1 to 5
[total dose/cycle = 300 mg/m^2]

Repeat cycle (with cyclophosphamide dose adjustments if needed based on ANC) every 21 days (best response seen in a median of 4 cycles)

Variation 2:

Etoposide: IV: 50 mg/m^2/day continuous infusion days 1 to 4
[total dose/cycle = 200 mg/m^2]

Vincristine: IV: 0.4 mg/m^2/day continuous infusion days 1 to 4
[total dose/cycle = 1.6 mg/m^2]

Doxorubicin: IV: 10 mg/m^2/day continuous infusion days 1 to 4
[total dose/cycle = 40 mg/m^2]

Cyclophosphamide: IV: 750 mg/m² day 6
[total dose/cycle = 750 mg/m²]
Prednisone: Oral: 60 mg/m²/day days 1 to 6
[total dose/cycle = 360 mg/m²]
Repeat cycle (with cyclophosphamide dose adjustments if needed based on ANC) every 21 days (best response seen in a median of 4 cycles)

References

Variation 1:
Gutierrez M, Chabner BA, Pearson D, et al, "Role of a Doxorubicin-Containing Regimen in Relapsed and Resistant Lymphomas: An 8-Year Follow-Up Study of EPOCH," *J Clin Oncol*, 2000, 18(21):3633-42.
Variation 2:
Wilson WH, Bryant G, Bates S, et al, "EPOCH Chemotherapy: Toxicity and Efficacy in Relapsed and Refractory Non-Hodgkin's Lymphoma," *J Clin Oncol*, 1993, 11(8):1573-82.

EPOCH-Rituximab (NHL)

Index Terms EPOCH-R (NHL); R-EPOCH (NHL); Rituximab-EPOCH (NHL)
Use Lymphoma, non-Hodgkin
Regimen
Rituximab: IV: 375 mg/m² day 1
[total dose/cycle = 375 mg/m²]
Etoposide: IV: 65 mg/m²/day continuous infusion days 2, 3, and 4
[total dose/cycle = 195 mg/m²]
Vincristine: IV: 0.5 mg/m²/day continuous infusion days 2, 3, and 4
[total dose/cycle = 1.5 mg/m²]
Doxorubicin: IV: 15 mg/m²/day continuous infusion days 2, 3, and 4
[total dose/cycle = 45 mg/m²]
Cyclophosphamide: IV: 750 mg/m² day 5
[total dose/cycle = 750 mg/m²]
Prednisone: Oral: 60 mg/m²/day days 1 to 14
[total dose/cycle = 840 mg/m²]
Repeat cycle every 21 days for 4-6 cycles

References

Jermann M, Jost LM, Taverna Ch, et al, "Rituximab-EPOCH, An Effective Salvage Therapy for Relapsed, Refractory or Transformed B-Cell Lymphomas: Results of a Phase II Study," *Ann Oncol*, 2004, 15(3):511-6.

◆ **EPOCH-R (NHL)** see EPOCH-Rituximab (NHL) *on page 1961*

◆ **EP (Small Cell Lung Cancer)** see Cisplatin-Etoposide (Small Cell Lung Cancer) *on page 1895*

EP (Testicular)

Index Terms Cisplatin-Etoposide (Testicular); Etoposide-Cisplatin (Testicular)
Use Testicular cancer
Regimen
Etoposide: IV: 100 mg/m²/day days 1 to 5
[total dose/cycle = 500 mg/m²]
Cisplatin: IV: 20 mg/m²/day days 1 to 5
[total dose/cycle = 100 mg/m²]
Repeat cycle every 21 days for 4 cycles

References

Culine S, Kerbrat P, Kramar A. et al. Refining the optimal chemotherapy regimen for good-risk metastatic nonseminomatous germ-cell tumors: a randomized trial of the Genito-Urinary Group of the French Federation of Cancer Centers (GETUG T93BP). *Ann Oncol*. 2007;18(5):917-924.
Xiao H, Mazumdar M, Bajorin DF, et al. Long-term follow-up of patients with good-risk germ cell tumors treated with etoposide and cisplatin. *J Clin Oncol*. 1997;15(7):2553-2558.

Eribulin (Breast Regimen)

Use Breast cancer

Regimen

Eribulin: IV: 1.4 mg/m^2/day over 2-5 minutes days 1 and 8

[total dose/week = 2.8 mg/m^2]

Repeat cycle every 21 days until disease progression or unacceptable toxicity

References

Cortes J, O'Shaughnessy J, Loesch D, et al, "Eribulin Monotherapy Versus Treatment of Physician's Choice in Patients With Metastatic Breast Cancer (EMBRACE): A Phase 3 Open-Label Randomised Study," *Lancet*, 2011, 377(9769):914-23.

Erlotinib-Gemcitabine (Pancreatic)

Index Terms Gemcitabine-Erlotinib (Pancreatic)

Use Pancreatic cancer

Regimen

Cycle 1:

Gemcitabine: IV: 1000 mg/m^2/day over 30 minutes days 1, 8, 15, 22, 29, 36, and 43 (cycle 1 only)

[total dose/cycle 1 = 7000 mg/m^2]

Erlotinib: Oral: 100 mg once daily days 1 to 56

[total dose/cycle 1 = 5600 mg]

Treatment cycle is 56 days

Subsequent cycles:

Gemcitabine: IV: 1000 mg/m^2/day over 30 minutes days 1, 8, and 15

[total dose/cycle = 3000 mg/m^2]

Erlotinib: Oral: 100 mg once daily days 1 to 28

[total dose/cycle = 2800 mg]

Repeat cycle every 28 days

References

Moore MJ, Goldstein D, Hamm J, et al, "Erlotinib Plus Gemcitabine Compared With Gemcitabine Alone in Patients With Advanced Pancreatic Cancer: A Phase III Trial of the National Cancer Institute of Canada Clinical Trials Group," *J Clin Oncol*, 2007, 25(15):1960-6.

Erlotinib (NSCLC Regimen)

Use Lung cancer, non-small cell

Regimen NOTE: Multiple variations are listed.

Variation 1 (refractory):

Erlotinib: Oral: 150 mg once daily days 1 to 28

[total dose/cycle = 4200 mg]

Repeat cycle every 28 days

Variation 2 (maintenance):

Erlotinib: Oral: 150 mg once daily days 1 to 28

[total dose/cycle = 4200 mg]

Repeat cycle every 28 days until disease progression or unacceptable toxicity

Variation 3 (first-line):

Erlotinib: Oral: 150 mg once daily days 1 to 28

[total dose/cycle = 4200 mg]

Repeat cycle every 28 days until disease progression or unacceptable toxicity

References

Variation 1:

Ciuleanu T, Stelmakh L, Cicenas S, et al, "Efficacy and Safety of Erlotinib Versus Chemotherapy in Second-Line Treatment of Patients With Advanced, Non-Small-Cell Lung Cancer With Poor Prognosis (TITAN): A Randomised Multicentre, Open-Label, Phase 3 Study," *Lancet Oncol*, 2012, 13(3):300-8.

Sheppherd FA, Pereira JR, Ciuleanu T, et al, "Erlotinib in Previously Treated Non-Small-Cell Lung Cancer," *N Engl J Med*, 2005, 353(2):123-32.

Variation 2:

Cappuzzo F, Ciuleanu T, Stelmakh L, et al, "Erlotinib as Maintenance Treatment in Advanced Non-Small-Cell Lung Cancer: A Multicentre, Randomised, Placebo-Controlled Phase 3 Study," *Lancet Oncol*, 2010, 11(6):521-9.

Variation 3:

Rosell R, Carcereny E, Gervais R, et al, "Erlotinib Versus Standard Chemotherapy as First-Line Treatment for European Patients With Advanced EGFR Mutation-Positive Non-Small-Cell Lung Cancer (EURTAC): A Multicentre, Open-Label, Randomised, Phase 3 Trial," *Lancet Oncol*, 2012, 13(3):239-46.

Zhou C, Wu YL, Chen G, et al, "Erlotinib Versus Chemotherapy as First-Line Treatment for Patients With Advanced EGFR Mutation-Positive Non-Small-Cell Lung Cancer (OPTIMAL, CTONG-0802): A Multicentre, Open-Label, Randomised, Phase 3 Study," *Lancet Oncol*, 2011, 12 (8):735-42.

ESHAP

Use Lymphoma, non-Hodgkin

Regimen NOTE: Multiple variations are listed.

Variation 1:

Etoposide: IV: 40 mg/m^2/day days 1 to 4

[total dose/cycle = 160 mg/m^2]

Methylprednisolone: IV: 250-500 mg/day days 1 to 5

[total dose/cycle = 1250-2500 mg]

Cytarabine: IV: 2000 mg/m^2 day 5

[total dose/cycle = 2000 mg/m^2]

Cisplatin: IV: 25 mg/m^2/day continuous infusion days 1 to 4

[total dose/cycle = 100 mg/m^2]

Repeat cycle every 21-28 days

Variation 2:

Etoposide: IV: 40 mg/m^2/day days 1 to 4

[total dose/cycle = 160 mg/m^2]

Methylprednisolone: IV: 500 mg/day days 1 to 5

[total dose/cycle = 2500 mg]

Cytarabine: IV: 2000 mg/m^2 day 5

[total dose/cycle = 2000 mg/m^2]

Cisplatin: IV: 25 mg/m^2/day continuous infusion days 1 to 4

[total dose/cycle = 100 mg/m^2]

Repeat cycle every 21-28 days

Variation 3:

Etoposide: IV: 60 mg/m^2/day days 1 to 4

[total dose/cycle = 240 mg/m^2]

Methylprednisolone: IV: 500 mg/day days 1 to 4

[total dose/cycle = 2000 mg]

Cytarabine: IV: 2000 mg/m^2 day 5

[total dose/cycle = 2000 mg/m^2]

Cisplatin: IV: 25 mg/m^2/day continuous infusion days 1 to 4

[total dose/cycle = 100 mg/m^2]

Repeat cycle every 21 days

References

Variation 1:

Velasquez WF, McLaughlin P, Tucker S, et al, "ESHAP - An Effective Chemotherapy Regimen in Refractory and Relapsing Lymphoma: A 4-Year Follow-up Study," *J Clin Oncol*, 1994, 12 (6):1169-76.

Variation 2:

Wang WS, Chiou TJ, Liu JH, et al, "ESHAP as Salvage Therapy for Refractory Non-Hodgkin's Lymphoma: Taiwan Experience," *Jpn J Clin Oncol*, 1999, 29(1):33-7.

Variation 3:

Rodriguez MA, Cabanillas FC, Velasquez W, et al, "Results of a Salvage Treatment Program for Relapsing Lymphoma: MINE Consolidated With ESHAP," *J Clin Oncol*, 1995, 13(7):1734-41.

ESHAP (Hodgkin)

Index Terms Etoposide-Methylprednisolone-Cytarabine-Cisplatin (Hodgkin)

Use Lymphoma, Hodgkin

Regimen

Etoposide: IV: 40 mg/m^2/day days 1 to 4
[total dose/cycle = 160 mg/m^2]

Methylprednisolone: IV: 500 mg/day days 1 to 4
[total dose/cycle = 2000 mg]

Cisplatin: IV: 25 mg/m^2/day days 1 to 4
[total dose/cycle = 100 mg/m^2]

Cytarabine: IV: 2000 mg/m^2 day 5
[total dose/cycle = 2000 mg/m^2]

Filgrastim: SubQ: 5 mcg/kg/day days 6 to 18

Repeat cycle every 21 to 28 days for 3 cycles (if transplant candidate) or 6 cycles (nontransplant candidate)

References

Aparicio J, Segura A, Garcerá S, et al, "ESHAP is an Active Regimen for Relapsing Hodgkin's Disease," *Ann Oncol*, 1999, 10(5):593-5.

- **Etoposide-Carboplatin (Ovarian Germ Cell Tumor)** *see* Carboplatin-Etoposide (Ovarian Germ Cell Tumor) *on page 1864*

- **Etoposide-Carboplatin (Retinoblastoma)** *see* Carboplatin-Etoposide (Retinoblastoma) *on page 1865*

- **Etoposide-Carboplatin (Small Cell Lung Cancer)** *see* Carboplatin-Etoposide (Small Cell Lung Cancer) *on page 1865*

- **Etoposide-Carboplatin-Vincristine (Retinoblastoma)** *see* Carboplatin-Etoposide-Vincristine (Retinoblastoma) *on page 1866*

- **Etoposide-Cisplatin-Methotrexate-Dactinomycin (Gestational Trophoblastic Tumor)** *see* EMA/EP (Gestational Trophoblastic Tumor) *on page 1954*

- **Etoposide-Cisplatin (NSCLC)** *see* Cisplatin-Etoposide (NSCLC) *on page 1894*

- **Etoposide-Cisplatin (Small Cell Lung Cancer)** *see* Cisplatin-Etoposide (Small Cell Lung Cancer) *on page 1895*

- **Etoposide-Cisplatin (Testicular)** *see* EP (Testicular) *on page 1961*

- **Etoposide-Ifosfamide-Cisplatin (Testicular)** *see* VIP (Testicular) *on page 2110*

- **Etoposide-Ifosfamide-Mitoxantrone-Dexamethasone (Hodgkin)** *see* VIM-D (Hodgkin) *on page 2107*

- ♦ **Etoposide-Methotrexate-Dactinomycin-Leucovorin-Cyclophosphamide-Vincristine (Gestational Trophoblastic Tumor)** *see* EMA/CO (Gestational Trophoblastic Tumor) *on page 1954*

- ♦ **Etoposide-Methotrexate-Dactinomycin-Leucovorin (Gestational Trophoblastic Tumor)** *see* EMA (Gestational Trophoblastic Tumor) *on page 1955*

- ♦ **Etoposide-Methotrexate-Leucovorin-Dactinomycin-Cisplatin (Gestational Trophoblastic Tumor)** *see* EMA/EP (Gestational Trophoblastic Tumor) *on page 1954*

- ♦ **Etoposide-Methylprednisolone-Cytarabine-Cisplatin (Hodgkin)** *see* ESHAP (Hodgkin) *on page 1964*

Etoposide Oral (Small Cell Lung Cancer Regimen)

Use Lung cancer, small cell

Regimen

Etoposide: Oral: 50 mg/m^2/day in the morning for 21 days
[total oral dose/cycle = 1050 mg/m^2]
Repeat cycle every 21 days

References

Einhorn LH, Pennington K, and McClean J, "Phase II Trial of Daily Oral VP-16 in Refractory Small Cell Lung Cancer: A Hoosier Oncology Group Study," *Semin Oncol*, 1990, 17(1 Suppl 2):32-5.

Johnson DH, Greco FA, Strupp J, et al, "Prolonged Administration of Oral Etoposide in Patients With Relapsed or Refractory Small-Cell Lung Cancer: A Phase II Trial," *J Clin Oncol*, 1990, 8 (10):1613-7.

Etoposide (Ovarian Regimen)

Use Ovarian cancer

Regimen NOTE: Multiple variations are listed.

Variaition 1: (no prior radiation therapy)
Etoposide: Oral: 50 mg/m^2/day days 1 to 21
[total dose/cycle = 1050 mg/m^2]
Repeat cycle every 28 days

Variation 2: (prior radiation therapy)
Etoposide: Oral: 30 mg/m^2/day days 1 to 21
[total dose/cycle = 630 mg/m^2]
Repeat cycle every 28 days

References

Variations 1 and 2:

Rose PG, Blessing JA, Mayer AR, et al, "Prolonged Oral Etoposide as Second-Line Therapy for Platinum-Resistant and Platinum-Sensitive Ovarian Carcinoma: A Gynecologic Oncology Group Study," *J Clin Oncol*, 1998, 16(2):405-10.

Everolimus-Exemestane (Breast)

Index Terms Exemestane-Everolimus (Breast)

Use Breast cancer

Regimen

Everolimus: Oral: 10 mg once daily
Exemestane: Oral: 25 mg once daily
Continue until disease progression or unacceptable toxicity

References

Baselga J, Campone M, Piccart M, et al, "Everolimus in Postmenopausal Hormone-Receptor-Positive Advanced Breast Cancer," *N Engl J Med*, 2012, 366(6):520-9.

Everolimus (RCC Regimen)

Use Renal cell cancer

▶

◄ **Regimen**
Everolimus: Oral: 10 mg once daily
[total dose/cycle = 280 mg]
Repeat cycle every 28 days until disease progression or unacceptable toxicity

References

Motzer RJ, Escudier B, Oudard S, et al, "Efficacy of Everolimus in Advanced Renal Cell Carcinoma: A Double-Blind, Randomised, Placebo-Controlled Phase III Trial," *Lancet*, 2008, 372(9637):449-56.

Motzer RJ, Escudier B, Oudard S, et al, "Phase 3 Trial of Everolimus for Metastatic Renal Cell Carcinoma: Final Results and Analysis of Prognostic Factors," *Cancer*, 2010, 116(18):4256-65.

Everolimus (Waldenstrom Macroglobulinemia)

Use Waldenstrom macroglobulinemia

Regimen
Everolimus: Oral: 10 mg once daily days 1 to 28
[total dose/cycle = 280 mg]
Repeat cycle every 28 days until disease progression or unacceptable toxicity

References

Ghobrial IM, Gertz M, Laplant B, et al. Phase II trial of the oral mammalian target of rapamycin inhibitor everolimus in relapsed or refractory Waldenstrom macroglobulinemia. *J Clin Oncol*. 2010;28(8):1408-1414.

FEC followed by Docetaxel Every 3 Weeks (Breast)

Index Terms Fluorouracil, Epirubicin, Cyclophosphamide, Docetaxel (Breast)

Use Breast cancer

Regimen
Fluorouracil: IV: 500 mg/m² day 1
[total dose/cycle = 500 mg/m²]
Epirubicin: IV: 100 mg/m² day 1
[total dose/cycle = 100 mg/m²]

Cyclophosphamide: IV: 500 mg/m² day 1
[total dose/cycle = 500 mg/m²]
Repeat cycle every 21 days for 3 cycles
followed by
Docetaxel: IV: 100 mg/m² day 1
[total dose/cycle = 100 mg/m²]
Repeat cycle every 21 days for 3 cycles

References

Roche H, Fumoleau P, Spielmann M, et al, "Sequential Adjuvant Epirubicin-Based and Docetaxel Chemotherapy For Node-Positive Breast Cancer Patients: The FNCLCC PACS 01 Trial," *J Clin Oncol*, 2006, 24(36):5664-71.

FEC followed by Paclitaxel Weekly (Breast)

Index Terms FEC-P (Breast); Fluorouracil, Epirubicin, Cyclophosphamide, Paclitaxel (Breast)

Use Breast cancer

Regimen

Fluorouracil: IV: 600 mg/m² day 1
[total dose/cycle = 600 mg/m²]
Epirubicin: IV: 90 mg/m² day 1
[total dose/cycle = 90 mg/m²]
Cyclophosphamide: IV: 600 mg/m² day 1
[total dose/cycle = 600 mg/m²]
Repeat cycle every 21 days for 4 cycles
followed by 3 weeks no treatment, then
Paclitaxel: IV: 100 mg/m² over 1 hour day 1
[total dose/cycle = 100 mg/m²]
Repeat cycle every 7 days for 8 cycles

References

Martín Miguel, Rodríguez-Lescure A, Ruiz A, et al, "Randomized Phase 3 Trial of Fluorouracil, Epirubicin, and Cyclophosphamide Alone or Followed by Paclitaxel for Early Breast Cancer," *J Natl Cancer Inst*, 2008, 100(11):805-814.

FEC IV (Breast)

Index Terms Fluorouracil, Epirubicin, Cyclophosphamide (Breast)

Use Breast cancer

Regimen NOTE: Multiple variations are listed.

Variation 1 (adjuvant):
Fluorouracil: IV: 500 mg/m² day 1
[total dose/cycle = 500 mg/m²]
Cyclophosphamide: IV: 500 mg/m² day 1
[total dose/cycle = 500 mg/m²]
Epirubicin: IV: 100 mg/m² day 1
[total dose/cycle = 100 mg/m²]
Repeat cycle every 21 days for 6 cycles
Variation 2 (metastatic):
Fluorouracil: IV: 500 mg/m² days 1 and 8
[total dose/cycle = 1000 mg/m²]
Cyclophosphamide: IV: 400 mg/m² days 1 and 8
[total dose/cycle = 800 mg/m²]
Epirubicin: IV: 50 mg/m² days 1 and 8
[total dose/cycle = 100 mg/m²]
Repeat cycle every 21-28 days for 6 to 9 cycles

◄ **References**

Variation 1:

Bonneterre J, Roché H, Kerbrat P, et al, "Epirubicin Increases Long-Term Survival in Adjuvant Chemotherapy of Patients With Poor-Prognosis, Node-Positive, Early Breast Cancer: 10-Year Follow-Up Results of the French Adjuvant Study Group 05 Randomized Trial," *J Clin Oncol*, 2005, 23(12):2686-93.

French Adjuvant Study Group. Benefit of a high-dose epirubicin regimen in adjuvant chemotherapy for node-positive breast cancer patients with poor prognostic factors: 5-year follow-up results of French Adjuvant Study Group 05 randomized trial. *J Clin Oncol*. 2001;19(3):602-11.

Variation 2:

Ackland SP, Anton A, Breitbach GP, et al, "Dose-Intensive Epirubicin-Based Chemotherapy is Superior to an Intensive Intravenous Cyclophosphamide, Methotrexate, and Fluorouracil Regimen in Metastatic Breast Cancer: A Randomized Multinational Study," *J Clin Oncol*, 2001, 19 (4):943-53.

FEC Oral (Breast)

Index Terms Fluorouracil, Epirubicin, Cyclophosphamide (Breast)

Use Breast cancer

Regimen NOTE: Multiple variations are listed.

Variation 1 (adjuvant):

Cyclophosphamide: Oral: 75 mg/m^2/day days 1 to 14
  [total dose/cycle = 1050 mg/m^2]

Epirubicin: IV: 60 mg/m^2/day days 1 and 8
  [total dose/cycle = 120 mg/m^2]

Fluorouracil: IV: 500 mg/m^2/day days 1 and 8
  [total dose/cycle = 1000 mg/m^2]

Repeat cycle every 28 days for 6 cycles

Variation 1 (metastatic):

Cyclophosphamide: Oral: 100 mg/m^2/day days 1 to 14
  [total dose/cycle = 1400 mg/m^2]

Epirubicin: IV: 30 mg/m^2/day days 1 and 8
  [total dose/cycle = 60 mg/m^2]

Fluorouracil: IV: 500 mg/m^2/day days 1 and 8
  [total dose/cycle = 1000 mg/m^2]

Repeat cycle every 28 days

References

Variation 1:

Levine MN, Bramwell VH, Pritchard KI, et al, "Randomized Trial of Intensive Cyclophosphamide, Epirubicin, and Fluorouracil Chemotherapy Compared With Cyclophosphamide, Methotrexate, and Fluorouracil in Premenopausal Women With Node-Positive Breast Cancer, National Cancer Institute of Canada Clinical Trials Group," *J Clin Oncol*, 1998, 16(8):2651-8.

Variation 2:

Estaban E, Lacave AJ, Fernández JL. Phase III trial of cyclophosphamide, epirubicin, fluorouracil (CEF) versus cyclophosphamide, mitoxantrone, fluorouracil (CNF) in women with metastatic breast cancer. *Breast Cancer Res Treat*. 1999;58(2):141-50.

◆ **FEC-P (Breast)** *see* FEC followed by Paclitaxel Weekly (Breast) on page 1967

FLAG (AML Induction)

Index Terms Fludarabine-ARAC-GCSF (AML Induction); Fludarabine-Cytarabine-Filgrastim (AML Induction)

Use Leukemia, acute myeloid

Regimen NOTE: Multiple variations are listed.

Variation 1:

Fludarabine: IV: 30 mg/m^2/day over 30 minutes days 1 to 5

[total dose/cycle = 150 mg/m^2]

Cytarabine: IV: 2 g/m^2/day over 4 hours days 1 to 5 (begin 4 hours after fludarabine infusion)

[total dose/cycle = 10 g/m^2]

Filgrastim: SubQ: 300 mcg 12 hours prior to start of fludarabine then 300 mcg/day days 2 through 5

[total dose/cycle = 1500 mcg]

followed by Filgrastim: SubQ: 300 mcg/day beginning one week after the end of treatment and continuing until complete neutrophil recovery

Variation 2:

Fludarabine: IV: 30 mg/m^2/day over 30 minutes days 1 to 5

[total dose/cycle = 150 mg/m^2]

Cytarabine: IV: 2 g/m^2/day over 4 hours days 1 to 5 (begin 3.5 hours after end of fludarabine infusion)

[total dose/cycle = 10 g/m^2]

Filgrastim: SubQ: 5 mcg/kg/day beginning 24 hours prior to start of fludarabine and continuing until ANC >500 mm^3

May repeat cycle one time for partial remission

Variation 3:

Fludarabine: IV: 30 mg/m^2/day over 30 minutes days 1 to 5

[total dose/cycle = 150 mg/m^2]

Cytarabine: IV: 2 g/m^2/day over 2 hours days 1 to 5 (begin 4 hours after the start of fludarabine infusion)

[total dose/cycle = 10 g/m^2]

Filgrastim: SubQ or IV: 300 mcg/day beginning the day prior to start of chemotherapy and continuing during chemotherapy and until ANC >1000 mm^3

May receive a second cycle

Variation 4:

Fludarabine: IV: 25 mg/m^2/day over 30 minutes days 1 to 5

[total dose/cycle = 125 mg/m^2]

Cytarabine: IV: 2 g/m^2/day over 4 hours days 1 to 5 (begin 4 hours after start of fludarabine infusion)

[total dose/cycle = 10 g/m^2]

Filgrastim: SubQ: 5 mcg/kg/day beginning 24 hours prior to start of cytarabine and continuing until ANC >500 mm^3

May repeat cycle in patients with complete remission and partial remission

References

Variation 1:

Clavio M, Carrara P, Miglino M, et al, "High Efficacy of Fludarabine-Containing Therapy (FLAG-FLANG) in Poor Risk Acute Myeloid Leukemia," *Haematologica*, 1996, 81(6):513-20.

Variation 2:

Montillo M, Mirto S, Petti MC, et al, "Fludarabine, Cytarabine, and G-CSF (FLAG) for the Treatment of Poor Risk Acute Myeloid Leukemia," *Am J Hematol*, 1998, 58(2):105-9.

Variation 3:

Virchis A, Koh M, Rankin P, et al, "Fludarabine, Cytosine Arabinoside, Granulocyte-Colony Stimulating Factor With or Without Idarubicin in the Treatment of High Risk Acute Leukaemia or Myelodysplastic Syndromes," *Br J Haematol*, 2004, 124(1):26-32.

Variation 4:

Ossenkoppele GJ, Graveland WJ, Sonneveld P, et al, "The Value of Fludarabine in Addition to ARA-C and G-CSF in the Treatment of Patients With High-Risk Myelodysplastic Syndromes and AML in Elderly Patients," *Blood*, 2004, 103(8):2908-13.

FLAG-IDA (AML Induction)

Use Leukemia, acute myeloid

Regimen NOTE: Multiple variations are listed.

Variation 1:

Fludarabine: IV: 30 mg/m²/day over 30 minutes days 1 to 5
[total dose/cycle = 150 mg/m²]

Cytarabine: IV: 2 g/m²/day over 4 hours days 1 to 5 (begin 4 hours after the start of fludarabine)
[total dose/cycle = 10 g/m²]

Idarubicin: IV: 10 mg/m²/day days 1, 2, and 3
[total dose/cycle = 30 mg/m²]

Filgrastim: SubQ: 5 mcg/kg from day 6 until ANC >500/mm³

Variation 2:

Fludarabine: IV: 30 mg/m²/day over 30 minutes days 1 to 5
[total dose/cycle = 150 mg/m²]

Cytarabine: IV: 2 g/m²/day over 2 hours days 1 to 5 (begin 4 hours after the start of fludarabine infusion)
[total dose/cycle = 10 g/m²]

Idarubicin: IV: 8 mg/m²/day over 30 minutes days 1, 2, and 3
[total dose/cycle = 24 mg/m²]

Filgrastim: SubQ or IV: 300 mcg/day beginning the day prior to start of chemotherapy and continuing during chemotherapy and until ANC >1000/mm³

May receive up to 2 cycles

Variation 3:

Fludarabine: IV: 30 mg/m²/day over 30 minutes days 1 to 4
[total dose/cycle = 120 mg/m²]

Cytarabine: IV: 2 g/m²/day over 4 hours days 1 to 4 (begin 4 hours after fludarabine treatment)
[total dose/cycle = 8 g/m²]

Idarubicin: IV: 10 mg/m²/day days 1, 2, and 3
[total dose/cycle = 30 mg/m²]

Filgrastim: Sub Q: see article for dose and frequency

References

Variation 1:
Pastore D, Specchia G, Carluccio P, et al, "FLAG-IDA in the Treatment of Refractory/Relapsed Acute Myeloid Leukemia: Single-Center Experience," *Ann Hematol*, 2003, 82(4):231-5.
Variation 2:
Virchis A, Koh M, Rankin P, et al, "Fludarabine, Cytosine Arabinoside, Granulocyte-Colony Stimulating Factor With or Without Idarubicin in the Treatment of High Risk Acute Leukaemia or Myelodysplastic Syndromes," *Br J Haematol*, 2004, 124(1):26-32.
Variation 3:
De la Rubia J, Regadera AI, Martin G, et al, "FLAG-IDA Regimen in the Treatment of Patients With High-Risk Myeloid Malignancies," *Leuk Res*, 2002, 26(8):725-30.

◆ **FLO (Gastric/Esophageal)** *see* Fluorouracil-Leucovorin-Oxaliplatin (Gastric/Esophageal) *on page 1982*

◆ **FLOT (Esophageal Cancer)** *see* Docetaxel-Oxaliplatin-Leucovorin-Fluorouracil (Esophageal Cancer) *on page 1946*

FLOX (Colorectal)

Index Terms Oxaliplatin-Leucovorin-Fluorouracil (Colorectal)

Use Colorectal cancer

Regimen

Oxaliplatin: IV: 85 mg/m² over 2 hours days 1, 15, and 29
  [total dose/cycle = 255 mg/m²]
Leucovorin: IV: 500 mg/m²/day over 2 hours weekly for 6 weeks on days 1, 8, 15, 22, 29, and 36
  [total dose/cycle = 3000 mg/m²]
Fluorouracil: IV: 500 mg/m²/day bolus (1 hour after beginning the leucovorin infusion) weekly for 6 weeks on days 1, 8, 15, 22, 29, and 36
  [total dose/cycle = 3000 mg/m²]
Repeat cycle every 8 weeks for a total of 3 cycles

References

Kuebler JP, Wieand HS, O'Connell MJ, et al, "Oxaliplatin Combined With Weekly Bolus Fluorouracil and Leucovorin as Surgical Adjuvant Chemotherapy for Stage II and III Colon Cancer: Results From NSABP C-07," J Clin Oncol, 2007, 25(16):2198-204.

◆ **Fludarabine-ARAC-GCSF (AML Induction)** see FLAG (AML Induction) on page 1968

Fludarabine-Cyclophosphamide (CLL)

Index Terms Cyclophosphamide-Fludarabine (CLL); FC (CLL)
Use Leukemia, chronic lymphocytic
Regimen NOTE: Multiple variations are listed.

Variation 1:
Fludarabine: IV: 25 mg/m²/day days 1, 2, and 3
  [total dose/cycle = 75 mg/m²]
Cyclophosphamide: IV: 250 mg/m²/day days 1, 2, and 3
  [total dose/cycle = 750 mg/m²]
Repeat cycle every 4 weeks for up to 6 cycles

Variation 2:
Fludarabine: IV: 30 mg/m²/day days 1, 2, and 3
  [total dose/cycle = 90 mg/m²]
Cyclophosphamide: IV: 250 mg/m²/day days 1, 2, and 3
  [total dose/cycle = 750 mg/m²]
Repeat cycle every 4 weeks for up to 6 cycles

Variation 3:
Cyclophosphamide: IV: 600 mg/m² day 1
  [total dose/cycle = 600 mg/m²]
Fludarabine: IV: 20 mg/m²/day days 1 to 5
  [total dose/cycle = 100 mg/m²]
Repeat cycle every 4 weeks for up to 6 cycles

Variation 4:
Fludarabine: IV: 30 mg/m²/day days 1, 2, and 3
  [total dose/cycle = 90 mg/m²]
Cyclophosphamide: IV: 300 mg/m²/day days 1, 2, and 3
  [total dose/cycle = 900 mg/m²]
Repeat cycle every 4 weeks for up to 6 cycles

Variation 5:
Fludarabine: IV: 30 mg/m²/day days 1, 2, and 3
  [total dose/cycle = 90 mg/m²]
Cyclophosphamide: IV: 300 mg/m²/day days 1, 2, and 3
  [total dose/cycle = 900 mg/m²]
Repeat cycle every 4-6 weeks for up to 6 cycles

References

Variation 1:

Catovsky D, Richards S, Matutes E, et al, "Assessment of Fludarabine Plus Cyclophosphamide for Patients With Chronic Lymphocytic Leukaemia (The LRF CLL4 Trial): A Randomised Controlled Trial," *Lancet*, 2007, 370(9583):230-9.

O'Brien S, Moore JO, Boyd TE, et al, "Randomized Phase III Trial of Fludarabine Plus Cyclophosphamide With or Without Oblimersen Sodium (Bcl-2 Antisense) in Patients With Relapsed or Refractory Chronic Lymphocytic Leukemia," *J Clin Oncol*, 2007, 25(9):1114-20.

Variation 2:

Eichhorst BF, Busch R, Obwandner T, et al, "Health-Related Quality of Life in Younger Patients With Chronic Lymphocytic Leukemia Treated With Fludarabine Plus Cyclophosphamide or Fludarabine Alone for First-Line Therapy: A Study by the German CLL Study Group," *J Clin Oncol*, 2007, 25(13):1722-31.

Variation 3:

Flinn IW, Neuberg DS, Grever MR, et al, "Phase III Trial of Fludarabine Plus Cyclophosphamide Compared With Fludarabine for Patients With Previously Untreated Chronic Lymphocytic Leukemia: US Intergroup Trial E2997," *J Clin Oncol*, 2007, 25(7):793-8.

Variation 4:

Wierda W, O'Brien S, Faderl S, et al, "A Retrospective Comparison of Three Sequential Groups of Patients With Recurrent/Refractory Chronic Lymphocytic Leukemia Treated With Fludarabine-Based Regimens," *Cancer*, 2006, 106(2):337-45.

Variation 5:

O'Brien SM, Kantarjian HM, Cortes J, et al, "Results of the Fludarabine and Cyclophosphamide Combination Regimen in Chronic Lymphocytic Leukemia," *J Clin Oncol*, 2001, 19(5):1414-20.

Fludarabine-Cyclophosphamide-Mitoxantrone-Rituximab

Index Terms FCMR (NHL); R-FCM (NHL); Rituximab-Fludarabine-Cyclophosphamide-Mitoxantrone

Use Lymphoma, non-Hodgkin

Regimen NOTE: Multiple variations are listed.

Consider pretherapy cytoreduction with cyclophosphamide 200 mg/m^2/day for 3-5 days for patients with high tumor burden and/or lymphocytes >20,000/mm^3

Variation 1:

Rituximab: IV: 375 mg/m^2/dose day 1

[total dose/cycle = 375 mg/m^2]

Fludarabine: IV: 25 mg/m^2/day days 2, 3, and 4

[total dose/cycle = 75 mg/m^2]

Cyclophosphamide: IV: 200 mg/m^2/day days 2, 3, and 4

[total dose/cycle = 600 mg/m^2]

Mitoxantrone: IV: 8 mg/m^2/dose day 2

[total dose/cycle = 8 mg/m^2]

Repeat cycle every 28 days for total of 4 cycles

Variation 2 (with maintenance rituximab):

Rituximab: IV: 375 mg/m^2/dose day 1

[total dose/cycle = 375 mg/m^2]

Fludarabine: IV: 25 mg/m^2/day days 2, 3, and 4

[total dose/cycle = 75 mg/m^2]

Cyclophosphamide: IV: 200 mg/m^2/day days 2, 3, and 4

[total dose/cycle = 600 mg/m^2]

Mitoxantrone: IV: 8 mg/m²/dose day 2
[total dose/cycle = 8 mg/m²]
Repeat cycle every 28 days for total of 4 cycles
followed by:
Maintenance rituximab (begin 3 months after completion of cycle 4):
Rituximab: IV: 375 mg/m²/dose day 1, 8, 15, and 22
[total dose/cycle = 1500 mg/m²]
Repeat maintenance cycle (once) in 6 months

References

Variation 1:

Forstpointner R, Dreyling M, Repp R, et al, "The Addition of Rituximab to a Combination of Fludarabine, Cyclophosphamide, Mitoxantrone (FCM) Significantly Increases the Response Rate and Prolongs Survival as Compared With FCM Alone in Patients With Relapsed and Refractory Follicular and Mantle Cell Lymphomas: Results of a Prospective Randomized Study of the German Low-Grade Lymphoma Study Group," *Blood*, 2004, 104(10):3064-71.

Variation 2:

Forstpointner R, Unterhalt M, Dreyling M, et al, "Maintenance Therapy With Rituximab Leads to a Significant Prolongation of Response Duration After Salvage Therapy With a Combination of Rituximab, Fludarabine, Cyclophosphamide, and Mitoxantrone (R-FCM) in Patients With Recurring and Refractory Follicular and Mantle Cell Lymphomas: Results of a Prospective Randomized Study of the German Low Grade Lymphoma Study Group (GLSG)," *Blood*, 2006, 108 (13):4003-8.

Fludarabine-Cyclophosphamide (NHL-Mantle Cell)

Index Terms CF (NHL-Mantle Cell); Cyclophosphamide-Fludarabine (NHL-Mantle Cell); FC (NHL-Mantle Cell)

Use Lymphoma, non-Hodgkin (Mantle cell)

Regimen NOTE: Multiple variations are listed.
Variation 1:
Fludarabine: IV: 20 mg/m²/day days 1 to 5
[total dose/cycle = 100 mg/m²]
Cyclophosphamide: IV: 800 mg/m²/dose day 1
[total dose/cycle = 800 mg/m²]
Repeat cycle every 3-4 weeks for up to a total of 5 cycles
Variation 2:
Fludarabine: IV: 20 mg/m²/day days 1 to 5
[total dose/cycle = 100 mg/m²]
Cyclophosphamide: IV: 1000 mg/m²/dose day 1
[total dose/cycle = 1000 mg/m²]
Repeat cycle every 3-4 weeks for up to a total of 5 cycles
Variation 3:
Fludarabine: IV: 25 mg/m²/day days 1 to 4
[total dose/cycle = 100 mg/m²]
Cyclophosphamide: IV: 1000 mg/m²/dose day 1
[total dose/cycle = 1000 mg/m²]
Repeat cycle every 3-4 weeks for up to a total of 5 cycles

References

Variations 1-3:

Cohen BJ, Moskowitz C, Straus D, et al, "Cyclophosphamide/Fludarabine (CF) Is Active in the Treatment of Mantle Cell Lymphoma," *Leuk Lymphoma*, 2001, 42(5):1015-22.

Fludarabine-Cyclophosphamide-Rituximab (CLL)

Index Terms FCR (CLL); Rituximab-Fludarabine-Cyclophosphamide (CLL)

Use Leukemia, chronic lymphocytic

▶

◀ **Regimen**

Cycle 1:

Rituximab: IV: 375 mg/m² day 1

[total dose/cycle = 375 mg/m²]

Fludarabine: IV: 25 mg/m²/day days 2, 3, and 4

[total dose/cycle = 75 mg/m²]

Cyclophosphamide: IV: 250 mg/m²/day days 2, 3, and 4

[total dose/cycle = 750 mg/m²]

Treatment cycle is 4 weeks

Cycles 2-6:

Rituximab: IV: 500 mg/m² day 1

[total dose/cycle = 500 mg/m²]

Fludarabine: IV: 25 mg/m²/day days 1, 2, and 3

[total dose/cycle = 75 mg/m²]

Cyclophosphamide: IV: 250 mg/m²/day days 1, 2, and 3

[total dose/cycle = 750 mg/m²]

Repeat cycle every 4 weeks

References

Keating MJ, O'Brien S, Albitar M, et al, "Early Results of a Chemoimmunotherapy Regimen of Fludarabine, Cyclophosphamide, and Rituximab as Initial Therapy for Chronic Lymphocytic Leukemia," *J Clin Oncol*, 2005, 23(18):4079-88.

Wierda W, O'Brien S, Wen S, et al, "Chemoimmunotherapy With Fludarabine, Cyclophosphamide, and Rituximab for Relapsed and Refractory Chronic Lymphocytic Leukemia," *J Clin Oncol*, 2005, 23(18):4070-8.

Fludarabine-Cyclophosphamide-Rituximab (NHL-Follicular)

Index Terms FCR (NHL-Follicular); Rituximab-Fludarabine-Cyclophosphamide (NHL-Follicular)

Use Lymphoma, non-Hodgkin (Follicular lymphoma)

Regimen

Cycle 1:

Rituximab: IV: 375 mg/m² day 15

[total dose/cycle = 375 mg/m²]

Fludarabine: IV: 25 mg/m²/day days 1, 2, and 3

[total dose/cycle = 75 mg/m²]

Cyclophosphamide: IV: 300 mg/m²/day days 1, 2, and 3

[total dose/cycle = 900 mg/m²]

Treatment cycle is 3 weeks

Cycles 2-4:

Rituximab: IV: 375 mg/m² day 1

[total dose/cycle = 375 mg/m²]

Fludarabine: IV: 25 mg/m²/day days 1, 2, and 3

[total dose/cycle = 75 mg/m²]

Cyclophosphamide: IV: 300 mg/m²/day days 1, 2, and 3

[total dose/cycle = 900 mg/m²]

Each treatment cycle is 3 weeks

References

Sacchi S, Pozzi S, Marcheselli R, et al, "Rituximab in Combination With Fludarabine and Cyclophosphamide in the Treatment of Patients With Recurrent Follicular Lymphoma," *Cancer*, 2007, 110(1):121-8.

◆ **Fludarabine-Cytarabine-Filgrastim (AML Induction)** see FLAG (AML Induction) *on page 1968*

Fludarabine-Mitoxantrone-Dexamethasone (NHL)

Index Terms FND (NHL)

Use Lymphoma, non-Hodgkin

Regimen

Fludarabine: IV: 25 mg/m^2/day days 1, 2, and 3

[total dose/cycle = 75 mg/m^2]

Mitoxantrone: IV: 10 mg/m^2/dose day 1

[total dose/cycle = 10 mg/m^2]

Dexamethasone: IV or Oral: 20 mg/day days 1 to 5

[total dose/cycle = 100 mg]

Repeat cycle every 28 days for up to a total of 8 cycles

References

McLaughlin P, Hagemeister FB, Romaguera JE, et al, "Fludarabine, Mitoxantrone, and Dexamethasone: An Effective New Regimen for Indolent Lymphoma," *J Clin Oncol*, 1996, 14(4):1262-8.

Tsimberidou AM, McLaughlin P, Younes A, et al, "Fludarabine, Mitoxantrone, Dexamethasone (FND) Compared With an Alternating Triple Therapy (ATT) Regimen in Patients With Stage IV Indolent Lymphoma," *Blood*, 2002, 100(13):4351-7.

Fludarabine-Mitoxantrone-Dexamethasone-Rituximab

Index Terms FNDR (NHL); Rituximab-Fludarabine-Mitoxantrone-Dexamethasone

Use Lymphoma, non-Hodgkin

Regimen

Cycle 1:

Rituximab: IV: 375 mg/m^2/day days 1 and 8

[total dose/cycle = 750 mg/m^2]

Fludarabine: IV: 25 mg/m^2/day days 1, 2, and 3

[total dose/cycle = 75 mg/m^2]

Mitoxantrone: IV: 10 mg/m^2/dose day 1

[total dose/cycle = 10 mg/m^2]

Dexamethasone: IV or Oral: 20 mg/m^2/day days 1 to 5

[total dose/cycle = 100 mg/m^2]

Treatment cycle is 28 days

Cycles 2-5:

Rituximab: IV: 375 mg/m^2 day 1

[total dose/cycle = 375 mg/m^2]

Fludarabine: IV: 25 mg/m^2/day days 2, 3, and 4

[total dose/cycle = 75 mg/m^2]

Mitoxantrone: IV: 10 mg/m^2/dose day 2

[total dose/cycle = 10 mg/m^2]

Dexamethasone: IV or Oral: 20 mg/m^2/day days 1 to 5

[total dose/cycle = 100 mg/m^2]

Repeat cycle every 28 days

Cycles 6-8:
Fludarabine: IV: 25 mg/m^2/day days 1, 2, and 3
[total dose/cycle = 75 mg/m^2]
Mitoxantrone: IV: 10 mg/m^2/dose day 1
[total dose/cycle = 10 mg/m^2]
Dexamethasone: IV or Oral: 20 mg/m^2/day days 1 to 5
[total dose/cycle = 100 mg/m^2]
Repeat cycle every 28 days
followed by:
Interferon maintenance:
Interferon alfa-2b: SubQ: 3 million units/m^2 days 1 to 14
[total dose/cycle = 42 million units/m^2]
Dexamethasone: Oral: 8 mg/day days 1, 2, and 3
[total dose/cycle = 24 mg]
Repeat cycle every month for 1 year

References
McLaughlin P, Hagemeister FB, Rodriguez MA, et al, "Safety of Fludarabine, Mitoxantrone, and Dexamethasone Combined With Rituximab in the Treatment of Stage IV Indolent Lymphoma," *Semin Oncol*, 2000, 27(6 Suppl 12):37-41.

Fludarabine-Rituximab (CLL)

Index Terms Rituximab-Fludarabine (CLL)
Use Leukemia, chronic lymphocytic
Regimen
Cycle 1:
Rituximab: IV: 375 mg/m^2/day days 1 and 4 (or 50 mg/m^2 day 1, followed by 325 mg/m^2 day 3, and then 375 mg/m^2 day 5)
[total dose/cycle = 750 mg/m^2]
Fludarabine: IV: 25 mg/m^2/day over 20 to 30 minutes days 1 to 5
[total dose/cycle = 125 mg/m^2]
Treatment cycle is 28 days
Cycle 2 to 6:
Rituximab: IV: 375 mg/m^2 day 1
[total dose/cycle = 375 mg/m^2]
Fludarabine: IV: 25 mg/m^2/day over 20 to 30 minutes days 1 to 5
[total dose/cycle = 125 mg/m^2]
Repeat cycle every 28 days for a total of 6 cycles

References
Byrd JC, Peterson BL, Morrison VA, et al. Randomized phase 2 study of fludarabine with concurrent vs sequential treatment with rituximab in symptomatic, untreated patients with B-cell chronic lymphocytic leukemia: results from cancer and leukemia group B 9712 (CALGB 9712). *Blood*. 2003;101(1):6-14.

Woyach JA, Ruppert AS, Heerema NA, et al. Chemoimmunotherapy with fludarabine and rituximab produces extended overall survival and progression-free survival in chronic lymphocytic leukemia: long-term follow-up of CALGB study 9712. *J Clin Oncol*. 2011;29(10):1349-1355.

Fludarabine-Rituximab (NHL-Follicular)

Index Terms Rituximab-Fludarabine (NHL-Follicular)
Use Lymphoma, non-Hodgkin (Follicular lymphoma)
Regimen
Week 1:
Rituximab: IV: 375 mg/m^2/dose for 2 doses 4 days apart
[total dose/week = 750 mg/m^2]

Week 2:
  Fludarabine: IV: 25 mg/m^2/day days 1 to 5
    [total dose/week = 125 mg/m^2]
Week 5:
  Rituximab: IV: 375 mg/m^2/dose day 5
    [total dose/week = 375 mg/m^2]
Week 6:
  Fludarabine: IV: 25 mg/m^2/day days 1 to 5
    [total dose/week = 125 mg/m^2]
Week 10:
  Fludarabine: IV: 25 mg/m^2/day days 1 to 5
    [total dose/week = 125 mg/m^2]
Week 13:
  Rituximab: IV: 375 mg/m^2/dose day 5
    [total dose/week = 375 mg/m^2]
Week 14:
  Fludarabine: IV: 25 mg/m^2/day days 1 to 5
    [total dose/week = 125 mg/m^2]
Week 18:
  Fludarabine: IV: 25 mg/m^2/day days 1 to 5
    [total dose/week = 125 mg/m^2]
Week 21:
  Rituximab: IV: 375 mg/m^2/dose day 5
    [total dose/week = 375 mg/m^2]
Week 22:
  Fludarabine: IV: 25 mg/m^2/day days 1 to 5
    [total dose/week = 125 mg/m^2]
Week 26:
  Rituximab: IV: 375 mg/m^2/dose for 2 doses 4 days apart
    [total dose/week = 750 mg/m^2]

References

Czuczman MS, Koryzna A, Mohr A, et al, "Rituximab in Combination With Fludarabine Chemotherapy in Low-Grade or Follicular Lymphoma," *J Clin Oncol*, 2005, 23(4):694-704.

Fluorouracil-Carboplatin (Head and Neck Cancer)

Index Terms Carboplatin-Fluorouracil (Head and Neck Cancer)

Use Head and neck cancer

Regimen NOTE: Multiple variations are listed.
  Variation 1:
  Fluorouracil: IV: 600 mg/m^2/day continuous infusion days 1 to 4
    [total dose/cycle = 2400 mg/m^2]
  Carboplatin: IV: 70 mg/m^2/day days 1 to 4
    [total dose/cycle = 280 mg/m^2]
  Repeat cycle every 3 weeks for 3 cycles
  Variation 2:
  Fluorouracil: IV: 1000 mg/m^2/day continuous infusion days 1 to 4
    [total dose/cycle = 4000 mg/m^2]
  Carboplatin: IV: 300 mg/m^2/dose day 1 (may escalate to 360 mg/m^2/dose in future cycles for grade 0 or 1 hematologic toxicity)
    [total dose/cycle = 300-360 mg/m^2]
  Repeat cycle every 28 weeks

◀ Variation 3:

Carboplatin: IV: 400 mg/m² day 1

[total dose/cycle = 400 mg/m²]

Fluorouracil: IV: 1000 mg/m²/day continuous infusion days 1 to 4

[total dose/cycle = 4000 mg/m²]

Repeat cycle every 28 days for a total of 2 or 3 cycles

References

Variation 1:

Denis F, Garaud P, Bardet E, et al, "Final Results of the 94-01 French Head and Neck Oncology and Radiotherapy Group Randomized Trial Comparing Radiotherapy Alone With Concomitant Radiochemotherapy in Advanced-Stage Oropharynx Carcinoma," *J Clin Oncol*, 2004, 22 (1):69-76.

Variation 2:

Forastiere AA, Metch B, Schuller DE, et al, "Randomized Comparison of Cisplatin Plus Fluorouracil and Carboplatin Plus Fluorouracil Versus Methotrexate in Advanced Squamous-Cell Carcinoma of the Head and Neck: A Southwest Oncology Group Study," *J Clin Oncol*, 1992, 10(8):1245-51.

Gregoire V, Beauduin M, Humblet Y, et al, "A Phase I-II Trial of Induction Chemotherapy With Carboplatin and Fluorouracil in Locally Advanced Head and Neck Squamous Cell Carcinoma: A Report From the UCL-Oncology Group, Belgium," *J Clin Oncol*, 1991, 9(8):1385-92.

Fluorouracil-Hydroxyurea (Head and Neck Cancer)

Index Terms Hydroxyurea-Fluorouracil (Head and Neck Cancer)

Use Head and neck cancer

Regimen NOTE: Administered with concurrent radiation therapy
  Fluorouracil: IV: 800 mg/m^2/day continuous infusion days 1 to 5
    [total dose/cycle = 4000 mg/m^2]
  Hydroxyurea: Oral: 1000 mg/dose every 12 hours for 11 doses beginning day 1
    [total dose/cycle = 11,000 mg]
  Repeat cycle every other week for a total therapy duration of 13 weeks
References
Garden AS, Harris J, Vokes EE, et al, "Preliminary Results of Radiation Therapy Oncology Group 97-03: A Randomized Phase II Trial of Concurrent Radiation and Chemotherapy for Advanced Squamous Cell Carcinomas of the Head and Neck," *J Clin Oncol*, 2004, 22(14):2856-64.

Fluorouracil-Leucovorin

Index Terms F-CL; FU-LV; FU/Leucovorin
Use Colorectal cancer
Regimen NOTE: Multiple variations are listed.
  Variation 1 (Mayo Regimen):
  Fluorouracil: IV: 370-425 mg/m^2/day days 1 to 5
    [total dose/cycle = 1850-2125 mg/m^2]
  Leucovorin: IV: 20 mg/m^2/day days 1 to 5
    [total dose/cycle = 100 mg/m^2]
  Repeat cycle at 4 weeks, 8 weeks, and every 5 weeks thereafter
  Variation 2:
  Fluorouracil: IV: 400 mg/m^2/day days 1 to 5
    [total dose/cycle = 2000 mg/m^2]
  Leucovorin: IV: 20 mg/m^2/day days 1 to 5
    [total dose/cycle = 100 mg/m^2]
  Repeat cycle every 28 days
  Variation 3:
  Fluorouracil: IV: 500 mg/m^2 day 1
    [total dose/cycle = 500 mg/m^2]
  Leucovorin: IV: 20 mg/m^2 (2-hour infusion) day 1
    [total dose/cycle = 20 mg/m^2]
  Repeat cycle weekly
  Variation 4:
  Fluorouracil: IV: 600 mg/m^2 weekly for 6 weeks
    [total dose/cycle = 3600 mg/m^2]
  Leucovorin: IV: 500 mg/m^2 (3-hour infusion) weekly for 6 weeks
    [total dose/cycle = 3000 mg/m^2]
  Repeat cycle every 8 weeks
  Variation 5:
  Fluorouracil: IV: 600 mg/m^2 weekly for 6 weeks
    [total dose/cycle = 3600 mg/m^2]
  Leucovorin: IV: 500 mg/m^2 (2-hour infusion) weekly for 6 weeks
    [total dose/cycle = 3000 mg/m^2]
  Repeat cycle every 8 weeks
  Variation 6:
  Fluorouracil: IV: 600 mg/m^2 weekly
    [total dose/cycle = 600 mg/m^2]
  Leucovorin: IV: 500 mg/m^2 (2-hour infusion) weekly
    [total dose/cycle = 500 mg/m^2]
  Repeat cycle weekly

◄ Variation 7:
  Fluorouracil: IV: 2600 mg/m^2 continuous infusion over 24 hours day 1
    [total dose/cycle = 2600 mg/m^2]
  Leucovorin: IV: 500 mg/m^2 continuous infusion over 24 hours day 1
    [total dose/cycle = 500 mg/m^2]
  Repeat cycle weekly
Variation 8:
  Fluorouracil: IV: 2600 mg/m^2 continuous infusion over 24 hours day 1
    [total dose/cycle = 2600 mg/m^2]
  Leucovorin: IV: 300 mg/m^2 (maximum dose: 500 mg) continuous infusion
    over 24 hours day 1
    [total dose/cycle = 300 mg/m^2; maximum: 500 mg]
  Repeat cycle weekly
Variation 9:
  Fluorouracil: IV: 2600 mg/m^2 continuous infusion over 24 hours once weekly
    for 6 weeks
    [total dose/cycle = 15,600 mg/m^2]
  Leucovorin: IV: 500 mg/m^2 over 2 hours once weekly for 6 weeks
    [total dose/cycle = 3000 mg/m^2]
  Repeat cycle every 8 weeks
Variation 10:
  Fluorouracil: IV: 2300 mg/m^2 continuous infusion over 24 hours day 1
    [total dose/cycle = 2300 mg/m^2]
  Leucovorin: IV: 50 mg/m^2 continuous infusion over 24 hours day 1
    [total dose/cycle = 50 mg/m^2]
  Repeat cycle weekly
Variation 11:
  Fluorouracil: IV: 200 mg/m^2/day continuous infusion days 1 to 14
    [total dose/cycle = 2800 mg/m^2]
  Leucovorin: IV: 5 mg/m^2/day continuous infusion days 1 to 14
    [total dose/cycle = 70 mg/m^2]
  Repeat cycle every 28 days
Variation 12:
  Cycle 1:
    Fluorouracil: IV: 200 mg/m^2/day continuous infusion for 4 weeks
      [total dose/cycle = 5600 mg/m^2]
    Leucovorin: IV: 20 mg/m^2/day days 1, 8, 15, 22
      [total dose/cycle = 80 mg/m^2]
    Treatment cycle is 6 weeks
  Subsequent cycles (starting week 7):
    Fluorouracil: IV: 200 mg/m^2 continuous infusion days 1 to 21
      [total dose/cycle = 4200 mg/m^2]
    Leucovorin: IV: 20 mg/m^2/day days 1, 8, and 15
      [total dose/cycle = 60 mg/m^2]
    Repeat cycle every 4 weeks

References

Variation 1:
Poon MA, O'Connell MJ, Moertel CG, et al, "Biochemical Modulation of Fluorouracil: Evidence of Significant Improvement of Survival and Quality of Life in Patients With Advanced Colorectal Carcinoma," *J Clin Oncol*, 1989, 7(10):1407-18.
Variation 2:
Borner MM, Castiglione M, Bacchi M, et al "The Impact of Adding Low-Dose Leucovorin to Monthly 5-Fluorouracil in Advanced Colorectal Carcinoma: Results of a Phase III Trial. Swiss Group for Clinical Cancer Research (SAKK)," *Ann Oncol*, 1998, 9(5):535-41.

Variation 3:
Jager E, Heike M, Bernhard H, et al, "Weekly High-Dose Leucovorin Versus Low-Dose Leucovorin Combined With Fluorouracil in Advanced Colorectal Cancer: Results of a Randomized Multicenter Trial. Study Group for Palliative Treatment of Metastatic Colorectal Cancer Study Protocol 1," *J Clin Oncol*, 1996, 14(8):2274-9.

Variation 4:
Leichman CG, Fleming TR, Muggia FM, et al, "Phase II Study of Fluorouracil and Its Modulation in Advanced Colorectal Cancer: A Southwest Oncology Group Study," *J Clin Oncol*, 1995, 13 (6):1303-11.

Variation 5:
Buroker TR, O'Connell MJ, Wieand HS, et al, "Randomized Comparison of Two Schedules of Fluorouracil and Leucovorin in the Treatment of Advanced Colorectal Cancer," *J Clin Oncol*, 1994, 12(1):14-20.

Variation 6:
Nobile MT, Rosso R, Sertoli MR, et al, "Randomised Comparison of Weekly Bolus 5-Fluorouracil With or Without Leucovorin in Metastatic Colorectal Carcinoma," *Eur J Cancer*, 1992, 28A (11):1823-7.

Variation 7:
Ardalan B, Chua L, Tian EM, et al, "A Phase II Study of Weekly 24-Hour Infusion With High-Dose Fluorouracil With Leucovorin in Colorectal Carcinoma," *J Clin Oncol*, 1991, 9(4):625-30.

Variation 8:
Yeh KH, Cheng AL, Lin MT, et al, "A Phase II Study of Weekly 24-Hour Infusion of High-Dose 5-Fluorouracil and Leucovorin (HDFL) in the Treatment of Recurrent or Metastatic Colorectal Cancers," *Anticancer Res*, 1997, 17(5B):3867-72.

Variation 9:
Kohne CH, Schoffski P, Wilke H, et al, "Effective Biomodulation by Leucovorin of High-Dose Infusion Fluorouracil Given as a Weekly 24-Hour Infusion: Results of a Randomized Trial in Patients With Advanced Colorectal Cancer," *J Clin Oncol*, 1998, 16(2):418-26.

Variation 10:
Haas NB, Schilder RJ, Nash S, et al, "A Phase II Trial of Weekly Infusional 5-Fluorouracil in Combination With Low-Dose Leucovorin in Patients With Advanced Colorectal Cancer," *Invest New Drugs*, 1995, 13(3):229-33.

Variation 11:
Falcone A, Allegrini G, Lencioni M, et al, "Protracted Continuous Infusion of 5-Fluorouracil and Low-Dose Leucovorin in Patients With Metastatic Colorectal Cancer Resistant to 5-Fluorouracil Bolus-Based Chemotherapy: A Phase II Study," *Cancer Chemother Pharmacol*, 1999, 44 (2):159-63.

Variation 12:
Leichman CG, Leichman L, Spears CP, et al, "Prolonged Continuous Infusion of Fluorouracil With Weekly Bolus Leucovorin: A Phase II Study in Patients With Disseminated Colorectal Cancer," *J Natl Cancer Inst*, 1993, 85(1):41-4.

◆ **Fluorouracil-Leucovorin-Bevacizumab (Colorectal)** *see* Bevacizumab-Fluorouracil-Leucovorin (Colorectal) *on page 1841*

◆ **Fluorouracil-Leucovorin-Irinotecan (Esophageal Cancer)** *see* Irinotecan-Fluorouracil-Leucovorin (Esophageal Cancer) *on page 2022*

◆ **Fluorouracil-Leucovorin-Irinotecan (Gastric Cancer)** *see* Irinotecan-Leucovorin-Fluorouracil (Gastric Cancer) *on page 2023*

Fluorouracil-Leucovorin-Irinotecan (Saltz Regimen) (Colorectal)

Index Terms 5FU-LV-CPT-11 (Saltz Regimen) (Colorectal); Irinotecan-Fluorouracil-Leucovorin (Saltz Regimen) (Colorectal); Saltz Regimen (Colorectal)

Use Colorectal cancer

Regimen

Irinotecan: IV: 125 mg/m^2/day over 90 minutes days 1, 8, 15, and 22
[total dose/cycle = 500 mg/m^2]

Leucovorin: IV bolus: 20 mg/m^2/day days 1, 8, 15, and 22
[total dose/cycle = 80 mg/m^2]

◄ Fluorouracil: IV bolus: 500 mg/m^2/day days 1, 8, 15, and 22
  [total dose/cycle = 2000 mg/m^2]
Repeat cycle every 42 days until disease progression or unacceptable toxicity
References
Saltz LB, Cox JV, Blanke C, et al. Irinotecan plus fluorouracil and leucovorin for metastatic colorectal cancer. Irinotecan study group. *N Engl J Med.* 2000;343(13):905-914.

◆ **Fluorouracil, Leucovorin, Oxaliplatin (Colorectal)** *see* FOLFOX4 (Colorectal) *on page 1985*

◆ **Fluorouracil-Leucovorin-Oxaliplatin (Colorectal)** *see* FOLFOX6 and mFOLFOX6 (Colorectal) *on page 1986*

Fluorouracil-Leucovorin-Oxaliplatin (Gastric/Esophageal)

Index Terms FLO (Gastric/Esophageal); FOLFOX (Gastric/Esophageal); Oxaliplatin-Leucovorin-Fluorouracil (Gastric/Esophageal)

Use Esophageal cancer; Gastric cancer

Regimen NOTE: Multiple variations are listed.
  Variation 1:
    Oxaliplatin: IV: 85 mg/m^2 over 2 hours day 1
    [total dose/cycle = 85 mg/m^2]
    Leucovorin: IV: 200 mg/m^2 over 2 hours day 1
    [total dose/cycle = 200 mg/m^2]
    Fluorouracil: IV: 2,600 mg/m^2 continuous infusion over 24 hours day 1
    [total dose/cycle = 2,600 mg/m^2]
    Repeat cycle every 14 days until disease progression or unacceptable toxicity
  Variation 2:
    Oxaliplatin: IV: 85 mg/m^2 over 2 hours day 1
    [total dose/cycle = 85 mg/m^2]
    Leucovorin: IV: 200 mg/m^2 over 2 hours day 1
    [total dose/cycle = 200 mg/m^2]
    Fluorouracil: IV bolus: 400 mg/m^2 over 10 minutes day 1
    followed by IV: 1,600 mg/m^2 continuous infusion over 48 hours beginning day 1
    [total dose/cycle = 2,000 mg/m^2]
    Repeat cycle every 14 days for a total of 6 cycles; cycles 1 to 3 were administered with radiation therapy and cycles 4 to 6 were administered after completion of radiation therapy

References
Variation 1:
Al-Batran SE, Hartmann JT, Probst S, et al. Phase III trial in metastatic gastroesophageal adenocarcinoma with fluorouracil, leucovorin plus either oxaliplatin or cisplatin: a study of the arbeitsgemeinschaft internistische onkologie. *J Clin Oncol.* 2008;26(9):1435-1442.
Variation 2:
Conroy T, Galais MP, Raoul JL, et al. Definitive chemoradiotherapy with FOLFOX versus fluorouracil and cisplatin in patients with oesophageal cancer (PRODIGE5/ACCORD17): final results of a randomised, phase 2/3 trial. *Lancet Oncol.* 2014;15(3):305-314.

◆ **Fluorouracil, Leucovorin, Oxaliplatin (Pancreatic)** *see* FOLFOX (Pancreatic) *on page 1988*

Fluorouracil-Leucovorin (Pancreatic)

Index Terms 5FU-Folinic Acid (Pancreatic); 5FU-Leucovorin (Pancreatic); 5FU-LV (Pancreatic)

Use 5FU-Folinic Acid (Pancreatic)

Regimen

Leucovorin: IV: 20 mg/m^2/day bolus days 1 to 5
[total dose/cycle = 100 mg/m^2]
Fluorouracil: IV: 425 mg/m^2/day bolus days 1 to 5
[total dose/cycle = 2125 mg/m^2]
Repeat cycle every 28 days for 6 cycles

References

Neoptolemos JP, Stocken DD, Bassi C, et al, "Adjuvant Chemotherapy With Fluorouracil Plus Folinic Acid Vs Gemcitabine Following Pancreatic Cancer Resection: A Randomized Controlled Trial," *JAMA*, 2010, 304(10):1073-81.

Neoptolemos JP, Stocken DD, Friess H, et al, "A Randomized Trial of Chemoradiotherapy and Chemotherapy After Resection of Pancreatic Cancer," *N Engl J Med*, 2004, 350(12):1200-10.

Neoptolemos JP, Stocken DD, Smith CT, et al, "Adjuvant 5-Fluorouracil and Folinic Acid Vs Observation for Pancreatic Cancer: Composite Data From the ESPAC-1 and -3 (v1) Trials," *Br J Cancer*, 2009, 100(2):246-50.

Fluorouracil-Mitomycin (Anal Cancer)

Index Terms Mitomycin–Fluorouracil (Anal Cancer)

Use Anal cancer

Regimen NOTE: Multiple variations are listed.

Variation 1 (in combination with radiotherapy):
Fluorouracil: IV: 1000 mg/m^2/day continuous infusion days 1 to 4 and days 29 to 32
[total dose/cycle = 8000 mg/m^2]
Mitomycin: IV: 10 mg/m^2/day (maximum dose: 20 mg) days 1 and 29
[total dose/cycle = 20 mg/m^2; maximum: 40 mg]
Variation 2 (in combination with radiotherapy):
Fluorouracil: IV: 1000 mg/m^2/day continuous infusion days 1 to 4
[total dose/cycle = 4000 mg/m^2]
Mitomycin: IV: 10 mg/m^2/dose (maximum dose: 20 mg) day 1
[total dose/cycle = 10 mg/m^2; maximum: 20 mg]
Repeat cycle in 28 days (total of 2 cycles)

References

Variation 1:
Ajani JA, Winter KA, Gunderson LL, et al, "Fluorouracil, Mitomycin, and Radiotherapy vs Fluorouracil, Cisplatin, and Radiotherapy for Carcinoma of the Anal Canal: A Randomized Controlled Trial," *JAMA*, 2008, 299(16):1914-21.

Variation 2:
Flam M, John M, Pajak TF, et al, "Role of Mitomycin in Combination With Fluorouracil and Radiotherapy, and of Salvage Chemoradiation in the Definitive Nonsurgical Treatment of Epidermoid Carcinoma of the Anal Canal: Results of a Phase III Randomized Intergroup Study," *J Clin Oncol*, 1996, 14(9):2527-39.

◆ **Fluorouracil-Oxaliplatin-Epirubicin (Gastric/Esophageal)** *see* Epirubicin-Oxaliplatin-Fluorouracil (Gastric/Esophageal) *on page 1958*

◆ **Fluorouracil-Paclitaxel (Esophageal Cancer)** *see* Paclitaxel-Fluorouracil (Esophageal Cancer) *on page 2052*

◆ **FND (NHL)** *see* Fludarabine-Mitoxantrone-Dexamethasone (NHL) *on page 1975*

◆ **FNDR (NHL)** *see* Fludarabine-Mitoxantrone-Dexamethasone-Rituximab *on page 1975*

FOLFIRI (Colorectal)

Use Colorectal cancer

Regimen
Irinotecan: IV: 180 mg/m² over 90 minutes day 1
  [total dose/cycle = 180 mg/m²]
Leucovorin: IV: 400 mg/m² over 2 hours day 1
  [total dose/cycle = 400 mg/m²]
Fluorouracil: IV bolus: 400 mg/m² day 1
  followed by IV: 2400 mg/m² continuous infusion over 46 hours beginning day 1
  [total fluorouracil dose/cycle (bolus and continuous infusion) = 2800 mg/m²]
Repeat cycle every 14 days until disease progression or unacceptable toxicity

References
Fuchs CS, Marshall J, Mitchell E, et al. Randomized, controlled trial of irinotecan plus infusional, bolus, or oral fluoropyrimidines in first-line treatment of metastatic colorectal cancer: results from the BICC-C study. *J Clin Oncol.* 2007;25(30):4779-4786.

FOLFIRINOX (Pancreatic)

Index Terms Irinotecan-Oxaliplatin-Fluorouracil-Leucovorin (Pancreatic); Oxaliplatin-Irinotecan-Fluorouracil-Leucovorin (Pancreatic)

Use Pancreatic cancer

Regimen
Oxaliplatin: IV: 85 mg/m² over 2 hours day 1
  [total dose/cycle = 85 mg/m²]
Leucovorin: IV: 400 mg/m² over 2 hours day 1
  [total dose/cycle = 400 mg/m²]
Irinotecan: IV: 180 mg/m² over 90 minutes day 1
  [total dose/cycle = 180 mg/m²]
Fluorouracil: IV bolus: 400 mg/m² day 1
  followed by IV: 2400 mg/m² continuous infusion (CI) over 46 hours beginning day 1
  [total fluorouracil dose/cycle (bolus and CI) = 2800 mg/m²]
Note: Bolus and CI fluorouracil are both given on day 1
Repeat cycle every 14 days until disease progression or unacceptable toxicity, 12 cycles recommended

References
Conroy T, Desseigne F, Ychou M, et al, "FOLFIRINOX Versus Gemcitabine for Metastatic Pancreatic Cancer," *N Engl J Med*, 2011, 364(19):1817-25.

Conroy T, Paillot B, François E, et al, "Irinotecan Plus Oxaliplatin and Leucovorin-Modulated Fluorouracil in Advanced Pancreatic Cancer–A Groupe Tumeurs Digestives of the Federation Nationale des Centres de Lutte Contre le Cancer Study," *J Clin Oncol*, 2005, 23(6):1228-36.

◆ **FOLFOX 6 (Pancreatic)** *see* FOLFOX (Pancreatic) *on page* 1988

FOLFOX1 (Colorectal)

Index Terms Oxaliplatin-Leucovorin-Fluorouracil (Colorectal)

Use Colorectal cancer

Regimen
Oxaliplatin: IV: 130 mg/m² over 2 hours day 1 (every other cycle)
  [total dose/cycle = 130 mg/m²]
Leucovorin: IV: 500 mg/m²/day over 2 hours days 1 and 2
  [total dose/cycle = 1000 mg/m²]
Fluorouracil: IV: 1500-2000 mg/m²/day continuous infusion over 22 hours days 1 and 2
  [total dose/cycle = 3000-4000 mg/m²]
Repeat cycle every 14 days until disease progression or unacceptable toxicity

References

de Gramont A, Tournigand C, Louvet C, et al, "Oxaliplatin, Folinic Acid, and 5-Fluorouracil (FOLFOX) in Pretreated Patients With Metastatic Advanced Cancer, The GERCOD," *Rev Med Interne*, 1997, 18(10):769-75.

FOLFOX2 (Colorectal)

Index Terms Oxaliplatin-Leucovorin-Fluorouracil (Colorectal)

Use Colorectal cancer

Regimen

Oxaliplatin: IV: 100 mg/m^2 over 2 hours day 1

[total dose/cycle = 100 mg/m^2]

Leucovorin: IV: 500 mg/m^2/day over 2 hours days 1 and 2

[total dose/cycle = 1000 mg/m^2]

Fluorouracil: IV: 1500-2000 mg/m^2/day continuous infusion over 22 hours days 1 and 2

[total dose/cycle = 3000-4000 mg/m^2]

Repeat cycle every 14 days until disease progression or unacceptable toxicity

References

de Gramont A, Tournigand C, Louvet C, et al, "Oxaliplatin, Folinic Acid and 5-Fluorouracil (Folfox) in Pretreated Patients With Metastatic Advanced Cancer. The GERCOD," *Rev Med Interne*, 1997, 18(10):769-75.

de Gramont A, Vignoud J, Tournigand C, et al, "Oxaliplatin With High-Dose Leucovorin and 5-Fluorouracil 48-Hour Continuous Infusion in Pretreated Metastatic Colorectal Cancer," *Eur J Cancer*, 1997, 33(2):214-9.

FOLFOX3 (Colorectal)

Index Terms Oxaliplatin-Leucovorin-Fluorouracil (Colorectal)

Use Colorectal cancer

Regimen

Oxaliplatin: IV: 85 mg/m^2 over 2 hours day 1

[total dose/cycle = 85 mg/m^2]

Leucovorin: IV: 500 mg/m^2/day over 2 hours days 1 and 2

[total dose/cycle = 1000 mg/m^2]

Fluorouracil: IV: 1500-2000 mg/m^2/day continuous infusion over 22 hours days 1 and 2

[total dose/cycle = 3000-4000 mg/m^2]

Repeat cycle every 14 days until disease progression or unacceptable toxicity

References

de Gramont A, Tournigand C, Louvet C, et al, "Oxaliplatin, Folinic Acid, and 5-Fluorouracil (FOLFOX) in Pretreated Patients With Metastatic Advanced Cancer, The GERCOD," *Rev Med Interne*, 1997, 18(10):769-75.

FOLFOX4 (Colorectal)

Index Terms Fluorouracil, Leucovorin, Oxaliplatin (Colorectal); Oxaliplatin, Leucovorin, Fluorouracil (Colorectal)

Use Colorectal cancer

Regimen NOTE: Multiple variations are listed.

Variation 1:

Oxaliplatin: IV: 85 mg/m^2 over 2 hours day 1

[total dose/cycle = 85 mg/m^2]

Leucovorin: IV: 200 mg/m^2/day over 2 hours days 1 and 2

[total dose/cycle = 400 mg/m^2]

◄ Fluorouracil: IV bolus: 400 mg/m^2/day days 1 and 2

    followed by IV: 600 mg/m^2/day continuous infusion (CI) over 22 hours days 1 and 2

    [total dose/cycle (bolus and CI) = 2000 mg/m^2]

Repeat cycle every 14 days for a total of 12 cycles in the adjuvant setting; and until disease progression or unacceptable toxicity in the metastatic setting.

Variation 2:

Oxaliplatin: IV: 85 mg/m^2 over 2 hours day 1

    [total dose/cycle = 85 mg/m^2]

Leucovorin (L-isomer): IV: 100 mg/m^2/day over 2 hours days 1 and 2

    [total dose/cycle = 200 mg/m^2]

Fluorouracil: IV bolus: 400 mg/m^2/day days 1 and 2

    followed by IV: 600 mg/m^2/day continuous infusion (CI) over 22 hours days 1 and 2

    [total dose/cycle (bolus and CI) = 2000 mg/m^2]

Repeat cycle every 14 days

References

Variation 1:

Andre T, Boni C, Mounedji-Boudiaf L, et al, "Oxaliplatin, Fluorouracil, and Leucovorin as Adjuvant Treatment for Colon Cancer," *N Engl J Med*, 2004, 350(23):2343-51.

Andre T, Boni C, Navarro M, et al, "Improved Overall Survival With Oxaliplatin, Fluorouracil, and Leucovorin as Adjuvant Treatment in Stage II or III Colon Cancer in the MOSAIC Trial," *J Clin Oncol*, 2009, 27(19):3109-16.

de Gramont A, Figer A, Seymour M, et al, "Leucovorin and Fluorouracil With or Without Oxaliplatin as First-Line Treatment in Advanced Colorectal Cancer," *J Clin Oncol*, 2000, 18(16):2938-47.

Variation 2:

Colucci G, Gebbia V, Paoletti G, et al, "Phase III Randomized Trial of FOLFIRI Versus FOLFOX4 in the Treatment of Advanced Colorectal Cancer: A Multicenter Study Gruppo Oncologico Dell'Italia Meridionale," *J Clin Oncol*, 2005, 23(22):4866-75.

FOLFOX6 and mFOLFOX6 (Colorectal)

Index Terms Fluorouracil-Leucovorin-Oxaliplatin (Colorectal); mFOLFOX6 and FOLFOX6 (Colorectal); Modified Fluorouracil-Leucovorin-Oxaliplatin (Colorectal); Modified FOLFOX6 (Colorectal); Oxaliplatin-Leucovorin-Fluorouracil (Colorectal)

Use Colorectal cancer

Regimen NOTE: Multiple variations are listed.

Variation 1:

Cycles 1 and 2:

Oxaliplatin: IV: 100 mg/m^2 over 2 hours day 1

    [total dose/cycle = 100 mg/m^2]

Leucovorin: IV: 400 mg/m^2 over 2 hours day 1

    [total dose/cycle = 400 mg/m^2]

Fluorouracil: IV bolus: 400 mg/m^2 day 1

    followed by IV: 2400 mg/m^2 continuous infusion (CI) over 46 hours beginning day 1

    [total fluorouracil dose/cycle (bolus and CI) = 2800 mg/m^2]

Repeat cycle every 14 days for 2 cycles

Subsequent Cycles:

Oxaliplatin: IV: 100 mg/m^2 over 2 hours day 1

    [total dose/cycle = 100 mg/m^2]

Leucovorin: IV: 400 mg/m^2 over 2 hours day 1

    [total dose/cycle = 400 mg/m^2]

Fluorouracil: IV bolus: 400 mg/m^2 day 1

followed by IV: 3000 mg/m^2 continuous infusion (CI) over 46 hours beginning day 1

[total fluorouracil dose/cycle (bolus and CI) = 3400 mg/m^2]

Repeat cycle every 14 days until disease progression or unacceptable toxicity

Variation 2:

Oxaliplatin: IV: 85 mg/m^2 over 2 hours day 1

[total dose/cycle = 85 mg/m^2]

Leucovorin: IV: 350 mg over 2 hours day 1

[total dose/cycle = 350 mg]

Fluorouracil: IV bolus: 400 mg/m^2 day 1

followed by IV: 2400 mg/m^2 continuous infusion (CI) over 46 hours beginning day 1

[total fluorouracil dose/cycle (bolus and CI) = 2800 mg/m^2]

Repeat cycle every 14 days until disease progression or unacceptable toxicity

References

Variation 1:

Maindrault-Goebel F, Louvet C, Andre T, et al, "Oxaliplatin Added to the Simplified Bimonthly Leucovorin and 5-Fluorouracil Regimen as Second-Line Therapy for Metastatic Colorectal Cancer (FOLFOX6), GERCOR," *Eur J Cancer*, 1999, 35(9):1338-42.

Tournigand C, André T, Achille E, et al, "FOLFIRI Followed by FOLFOX6 or the Reverse Sequence in Advanced Colorectal Cancer: A Randomized GERCOR Study," *J Clin Oncol*, 2004, 22 (2):229-37.

Variation 2:

Cheeseman SL, Joel SP, Chester JD, et al, "A 'Modified de Gramont' Regimen of Fluorouracil, Alone and With Oxaliplatin, for Advanced Colorectal Cancer," *Br J Cancer*, 2002, 87(4): 393-9.

Hochster HS, Hart LL, Ramanathan RK, et al, "Safety and Efficacy of Oxaliplatin and Fluoropyrimidine Regimens With or Without Bevacizumab as First-Line Treatment of Metastatic Colorectal Cancer: Results of the TREE Study," *J Clin Oncol*, 2008, 26(21):3523-9.

FOLFOX7 (Colorectal)

Use Colorectal cancer

Regimen

Oxaliplatin: IV: 130 mg/m^2 over 2 hours day 1

[total dose/cycle = 130 mg/m^2]

Leucovorin: IV: 400 mg/m^2 over 2 hours day 1

[total dose/cycle = 400 mg/m^2]

Fluorouracil: IV bolus: 400 mg/m^2 day 1

followed by IV: 2400 mg/m^2 continuous infusion (CI) over 46 hours beginning on day 1

total fluorouracil dose/cycle (bolus and CI) = 2800 mg/m^2

Repeat cycle every 14 days for a total of 8 cycles; evaluate every 2 months; may resume if disease progression

References

Maindrault-Goebel F, de Gramont A, Louvet C, et al, "High-Dose Intensity Oxaliplatin Added to the Simplified Bimonthly Leucovorin and 5-Fluorouracil Regimen as Second-Line Therapy for Metastatic Colorectal Cancer (FOLFOX 7)," *Eur J Cancer*, 2001, 37(8):1000-5.

◆ **FOLFOX (Gastric/Esophageal)** *see* Fluorouracil-Leucovorin-Oxaliplatin (Gastric/Esophageal) *on page 1982*

FOLFOXIRI (Colorectal)

Index Terms Irinotecan, Oxaliplatin, Leucovorin, Fluorouracil (Colorectal)

Use Colorectal cancer

▶

◀ **Regimen**
Irinotecan: IV: 165 mg/m² over 1 hour day 1
[total dose/cycle = 165 mg/m²]
Oxaliplatin: IV: 85 mg/m² over 2 hours day 1
[total dose/cycle = 85 mg/m²]
Leucovorin: IV: 200 mg/m² over 2 hours day 1
[total dose/cycle = 200 mg/m²]
Fluorouracil: IV: 3200 mg/m² continuous infusion over 48 hours beginning day 1
[total dose/cycle = 3200 mg/m²]
Repeat cycle every 14 days for a maximum of 12 cycles

References
Falcone A, Ricci S, Brunetti I, et al, "Phase III Trial of Infusional Fluorouracil, Leucovorin, Oxaliplatin, and Irinotecan (FOLFOXIRI) Compared With Infusional Fluorouracil, Leucovorin, and Irinotecan (FOLFIRI) as First-Line Treatment for Metastatic Colorectal Cancer: The Gruppo Oncologico Nord Ovest," *J Clin Oncol*, 2007, 25(13):1670-6.

FOLFOX (Pancreatic)

Index Terms Fluorouracil, Leucovorin, Oxaliplatin (Pancreatic); FOLFOX 6 (Pancreatic); Oxaliplatin, Fluorouracil, Leucovorin (Pancreatic)
Use Pancreatic cancer
Regimen
Oxaliplatin: IV: 100 mg/m² day 1
[total dose/cycle = 100 mg/m²]
Leucovorin: IV: 400 mg/m² day 1
[total dose/cycle = 400 mg/m²]
Fluorouracil: IV bolus: 400 mg/m² day 1
followed by IV: 3000 mg/m² continuous infusion (CI) over 46 hours beginning day 1
[total fluorouracil dose/cycle (bolus and CI) = 3400 mg/m²]
Repeat cycle every 14 days until disease progression or unacceptable toxicity

References
Ghosn M, Farhat, Kattan J, et al, "FOLFOX-6 Combination as the First-Line Treatment of Locally Advanced and/or Metastatic Pancreatic Cancer," *Am J Clin Oncol*, 2007, 30(1):15-20.

- ◆ **GCD (Hodgkin)** *see* Gemcitabine-Dexamethasone-Carboplatin (Hodgkin) *on page 1991*

- ◆ **GCLAC (AML)** *see* Clofarabine-Cytarabine (AML) *on page 1917*

- ◆ **GC (NSCLC)** *see* Carboplatin-Gemcitabine (NSCLC) *on page 1867*

- ◆ **GC (NSCLC)** *see* Cisplatin-Gemcitabine (NSCLC) *on page 1905*

- ◆ **GDC (Hodgkin)** *see* Gemcitabine-Dexamethasone-Carboplatin (Hodgkin) *on page 1991*

- ◆ **GD (NSCLC)** *see* Docetaxel-Gemcitabine (NSCLC) *on page 1943*

GDP (Hodgkin)

Index Terms Gemcitabine-Dexamethasone-Cisplatin (Hodgkin)

Use Lymphoma, Hodgkin

Regimen

Gemcitabine: IV: 1000 mg/m^2 over 30 minutes days 1 and 8
[total dose/cycle = 2000 mg/m^2]

Dexamethasone: Oral: 40 mg/day (divided doses) days 1 to 4
[total dose/cycle = 160 mg]

Cisplatin: IV: 75 mg/m^2 over 1 hour day 1, administer after gemcitabine
[total dose/cycle = 75 mg/m^2]

Repeat cycle every 21 days; consider stem cell transplantation after 2 cycles in responding patients; and a maximum of 6 cycles in nontransplant candidates

References

Baetz T, Belch A, Couban S, et al, "Gemcitabine, Dexamethasone and Cisplatin is an Active and Non-Toxic Chemotherapy Regimen in Relapsed or Refractory Hodgkin's Disease: A Phase II Study by the National Cancer Institute of Canada Clinical Trials," *Ann Oncol*, 2003, 14 (12):1762-7.

- ◆ **GDP (NHL-DLBCL)** *see* Gemcitabine-Dexamethasone-Cisplatin (NHL-DLBCL) *on page 1992*

Gefitinib (NSCLC Regimen)

Use Lung cancer, non-small cell (first-line in patients with metastatic disease and EGFR exon 19 deletions or exon 21 [L858R] substitution mutations)

Regimen

Gefitinib: Oral: 250 mg once daily (administer with or without food)
[total dose/cycle = 7,000 mg]

Repeat cycle every 28 days until disease progression or unacceptable toxicity

References

Fukuoka M, Wu YL, Thongprasert S, et al. Biomarker analyses and final overall survival results from a phase III, randomized, open-label, first-line study of gefitinib versus carboplatin/paclitaxel in clinically selected patients with advanced non-small-cell lung cancer in Asia (IPASS). *J Clin Oncol*. 2011;29(21):2866-2874.

- ◆ **GEM-CAP (Pancreatic)** *see* Capecitabine-Gemcitabine (Pancreatic) *on page 1858*

- ◆ **GemCis (Pancreatic)** *see* Cisplatin-Gemcitabine (Pancreatic) *on page 1906*

- ◆ **Gemcitabine-Abraxane (Pancreatic)** *see* Gemcitabine-Paclitaxel (Protein Bound) (Pancreatic) *on page 1996*

Gemcitabine (Breast Regimen)

Use Breast cancer

◄ **Regimen** NOTE: Multiple variations are listed.

Variation 1:

Gemcitabine: IV: 1000 mg/m² over 30 minutes days 1, 8, and 15

[total dose/cycle = 3000 mg/m²]

Repeat cycle every 28 days

Variation 2:

Gemcitabine: IV: 800 mg/m² over 30 minutes days 1, 8, and 15

[total dose/cycle = 2400 mg/m²]

Repeat cycle every 28 days

Variation 3:

Gemcitabine: IV: 1200 mg/m² over 30 minutes days 1, 8, and 15

[total dose/cycle = 3600 mg/m²]

Repeat cycle every 28 days

References

Variation 1:

Possinger K, Kaufmann M, Coleman R, at al, "Phase II Study of Gemcitabine As First-Line Chemotherapy in Patients With Advanced or Metastatic Breast Cancer," *Anticancer Drugs*, 1999; 10(2):152-62.

Variation 2:

Carmichael J, Possinger K, Phillip P, et al, "Advanced Breast Cancer: A Phase II Trial With Gemcitabine," *J Clin Oncol*, 1995, 13(11):2731-6.

Variation 3:

Blackstein M, Vogel CL, Ambinder R, et al, "Gemcitabine As First-Line Therapy in Patients With Metastatic Breast Cancer: A Phase II Trial," *Oncology*, 2002, 62(1):2-8.

Gemcitabine-Capecitabine (Biliary Cancer)

Index Terms Capecitabine-Gemcitabine (Biliary Cancer)

Use Biliary adenocarcinoma

Regimen

Gemcitabine: IV: 1000 mg/m²/day over 30 minutes days 1 and 8

[total dose/cycle = 2000 mg/m²]

Capecitabine: Oral: 650 mg/m² twice daily days 1 to 14

[total dose/cycle = 18,200 mg/m²]

Repeat cycle every 21 days until disease progression or unacceptable toxicity

References

Knox JJ, Hedley D, Oza A, et al, "Combining Gemcitabine and Capecitabine in Patients With Advanced Biliary Cancer: A Phase II Trial," *J Clin Oncol*, 2005, 23(10):2332-8.

◆ **Gemcitabine-Capecitabine (Pancreatic)** *see* Capecitabine-Gemcitabine (Pancreatic) *on page 1858*

◆ **Gemcitabine-Carboplatin (Bladder)** *see* Carboplatin-Gemcitabine (Bladder) *on page 1867*

◆ **Gemcitabine-Carboplatin (NSCLC)** *see* Carboplatin-Gemcitabine (NSCLC) *on page 1867*

◆ **Gemcitabine-Carboplatin (Ovarian)** *see* Carboplatin-Gemcitabine (Ovarian) *on page 1868*

Gemcitabine (Cervical Regimen)

Use Cervical cancer

Regimen

Gemcitabine: IV: 800 mg/m²/day over 30 minutes days 1, 8, and 15

[total dose/cycle = 2400 mg/m²]

Repeat cycle every 28 days until disease progression or unacceptable toxicity

References

Schilder RJ, Blessing JA, Cohn D. Evaluation of gemcitabine in previously treated patients with non-squamous cell carcinoma of the cervix: a phase II study of the Gynecologic Oncology Group. *Gynecol Oncol*. 2005;96(1):103-107.

Gemcitabine-Cisplatin (Biliary Cancer)

Index Terms Cisplatin-Gemcitabine (Biliary Cancer)

Use Biliary adenocarcinoma

Regimen NOTE: Multiple variations are listed.

Variation 1:

Gemcitabine: IV: 1250 mg/m^2/dose days 1 and 8

[total dose/cycle = 2500 mg/m^2]

Cisplatin: IV: 75 mg/m^2/dose day 1

[total dose/cycle = 75 mg/m^2]

Repeat cycle every 3 weeks

Variation 2:

Gemcitabine: IV: 1000 mg/m^2/dose days 1 and 8

[total dose/cycle = 2000 mg/m^2]

Cisplatin: IV: 70 mg/m^2/dose day 1

[total dose/cycle = 70 mg/m^2]

Repeat cycle every 3 weeks (maximum: 6 cycles)

References

Variation 1:
Thongprasert S, Napapan S, Charoentum C, et al, "Phase II Study of Gemcitabine and Cisplatin as First-Line Chemotherapy in Inoperable Biliary Tract Carcinoma," *Ann Oncol*, 2005, 16(2):279-81.
Variation 2:
Doval DC, Sekhon JS, Gupta SK, et al, "A Phase II Study of Gemcitabine and Cisplatin in Chemotherapy-Naive, Unresectable Gall Bladder Cancer," *Br J Cancer*, 2004, 90(8):1516-20.

- ◆ **Gemcitabine-Cisplatin (Bladder)** *see* Cisplatin-Gemcitabine (Bladder) *on page 1903*

- ◆ **Gemcitabine-Cisplatin (Cervical)** *see* Cisplatin-Gemcitabine (Cervical) *on page 1904*

- ◆ **Gemcitabine-Cisplatin-Dexamethasone (NHL-DLBCL)** *see* Gemcitabine-Dexamethasone-Cisplatin (NHL-DLBCL) *on page 1992*

- ◆ **Gemcitabine-Cisplatin-Dexamethasone-Rituximab (NHL-DLBCL)** *see* Rituximab-Gemcitabine-Dexamethasone-Cisplatin (NHL-DLBCL) *on page 2081*

- ◆ **Gemcitabine-Cisplatin-Docetaxel (Bladder)** *see* Cisplatin-Docetaxel-Gemcitabine (Bladder) *on page 1891*

- ◆ **Gemcitabine-Cisplatin (Mesothelioma)** *see* Cisplatin-Gemcitabine (Mesothelioma) *on page 1905*

- ◆ **Gemcitabine-Cisplatin (NSCLC)** *see* Cisplatin-Gemcitabine (NSCLC) *on page 1905*

- ◆ **Gemcitabine-Cisplatin (Pancreatic)** *see* Cisplatin-Gemcitabine (Pancreatic) *on page 1906*

- ◆ **Gemcitabine-Cisplatin (Unknown Primary)** *see* Cisplatin-Gemcitabine (Unknown Primary, Adenocarcinoma) *on page 1907*

Gemcitabine-Dexamethasone-Carboplatin (Hodgkin)

Index Terms GCD (Hodgkin); GDC (Hodgkin); Gemcitabine-Dexamethasone-Carboplatin (Hodgkin)

Use Lymphoma, Hodgkin (relapsed refractory)

◀ **Regimen**

Gemcitabine: IV: 1,000 mg/m^2/day over 30 minutes days 1 and 8
  [total dose/cycle = 2,000 mg/m^2]
Dexamethasone: Oral: 40 mg/day days 1 to 4
  [total dose/cycle = 160 mg]
Carboplatin: IV: AUC 5 over 30 minutes day 1
  [total dose/cycle = AUC = 5]
Repeat cycle every 21 days for up to 4 cycles

References

Gopal AK, Press OW, Shustov AR, et al. Efficacy and safety of gemcitabine, carboplatin, dexamethasone, and rituximab in patients with relapsed/refractory lymphoma: a prospective multi-center phase II study by the Puget Sound Oncology Consortium. *Leuk Lymphoma.* 2010;51 (8):1523-1529.

◆ **Gemcitabine-Dexamethasone-Carboplatin (Hodgkin)** *see* Gemcitabine-Dexamethasone-Carboplatin (Hodgkin) *on page 1991*

◆ **Gemcitabine-Dexamethasone-Carboplatin-Rituximab (NHL-DLBCL)** *see* Rituximab-Gemcitabine-Dexamethasone-Carboplatin (NHL-DLBCL) *on page 2081*

◆ **Gemcitabine-Dexamethasone-Cisplatin (Hodgkin)** *see* GDP (Hodgkin) *on page 1989*

Gemcitabine-Dexamethasone-Cisplatin (NHL-DLBCL)

Index Terms GDP (NHL-DLBCL); Gemcitabine-Cisplatin-Dexamethasone (NHL-DLBCL)

Use Lymphoma, non-Hodgkin (DLBCL recurrent/refractory)

Regimen

Gemcitabine: IV: 1,000 mg/m^2 over 30 minutes days 1 and 8
  [total dose/cycle = 2,000 mg/m^2]
Dexamethasone: IV or Oral: 40 mg/day in divided doses days 1 to 4
  [total dose/cycle = 160 mg]
Cisplatin: IV: 75 mg/m^2 over 1 hour day 1
  [total dose/cycle = 75 mg/m^2]
Repeat cycle every 21 days for 2 to 6 cycles; eligible patients proceeding to transplant received 2 cycles and nontransplant eligible patients received up to 6 cycles

References

Crump M, Baetz T, Couban S, et al. Gemcitabine, dexamethasone, and cisplatin in patients with recurrent or refractory aggressive histology B-cell non-Hodgkin lymphoma: a Phase II study by the National Cancer Institute of Canada Clinical Trials Group (NCIC-CTG). *Cancer.* 2004;101 (8):1835-1842.

◆ **Gemcitabine-Dexamethasone-Cisplatin-Rituximab (NHL-DLBCL)** *see* Rituximab-Gemcitabine-Dexamethasone-Cisplatin (NHL-DLBCL) *on page 2081*

◆ **Gemcitabine-Docetaxel-Capecitabine (Pancreatic)** *see* GTX (Pancreatic) *on page 2001*

◆ **Gemcitabine-Docetaxel (Ewing Sarcoma)** *see* Docetaxel-Gemcitabine (Ewing Sarcoma) *on page 1942*

◆ **Gemcitabine-Docetaxel (NSCLC)** *see* Docetaxel-Gemcitabine (NSCLC) *on page 1943*

◆ **Gemcitabine-Docetaxel (Osteosarcoma)** *see* Docetaxel-Gemcitabine (Osteosarcoma) *on page 1943*

♦ **Gemcitabine-Docetaxel (Soft Tissue Sarcoma)** *see* Docetaxel-Gemcitabine (Soft Tissue Sarcoma) *on page 1943*

♦ **Gemcitabine-Docetaxel (Unknown Primary)** *see* Docetaxel-Gemcitabine (Unknown Primary, Adenocarcinoma) *on page 1944*

♦ **Gemcitabine-Docetaxel (Uterine Leiomyosarcoma)** *see* Docetaxel-Gemcitabine (Uterine Leiomyosarcoma) *on page 1944*

♦ **Gemcitabine-Erlotinib (Pancreatic)** *see* Erlotinib-Gemcitabine (Pancreatic) *on page 1962*

Gemcitabine Fixed Dose Rate (Pancreatic Regimen)
Use Pancreatic cancer
Regimen
Gemcitabine: IV: 1500 mg/m^2/day over 150 minutes (10 mg/m^2/minute) days 1, 8, and 15
[total dose/cycle = 4500 mg/m^2]
Repeat cycle every 28 days until disease progression or unacceptable toxicity
References
Poplin E, Feng Y, Berlin J, et al, "Phase III, Randomized Study of Gemcitabine and Oxaliplatin Versus Gemcitabine (Fixed-Dose Rate Infusion) Compared With Gemcitabine (30-Minute Infusion) in Patients With Pancreatic Carcinoma E6201: A Trial of the Eastern Cooperative Oncology Group," *J Clin Oncol*, 2009, 27(23):3778-85.
Tempero M, Plunkett W, Ruiz van Haperen VW, et al, "Randomized Phase II Comparison of Dose-Intense Gemcitabine: Thirty-Minute Infusion and Fixed Dose Rate Infusion in Patients With Pancreatic Adenocarcinoma," *J Clin Oncol*, 2003, 21(18):3402-8.

Gemcitabine (Head and Neck Regimen)
Use Head and neck cancer (nasopharyngeal)
Regimen
Gemcitabine: IV: 1000 mg/m^2/day over 30 minutes days 1, 8, and 15
[total dose/cycle = 3000 mg/m^2]
Repeat cycles every 28 days until disease progression or unacceptable toxicity
References
Zhang L, Zhang Y, Huang PY, Xu F, Peng PJ, Guan ZZ. Phase II clinical study of gemcitabine in the treatment of patients with advanced nasopharyngeal carcinoma after the failure of platinum-based chemotherapy. *Cancer Chemother Pharmacol*. 2008;61(1):33-38.

Gemcitabine (Hodgkin Regimen)
Use Lymphoma, Hodgkin
Regimen NOTE: Multiple variations are listed.
Variation 1:
Gemcitabine: IV: 1250 mg/m^2/day over 30 minutes days 1, 8, and 15
[total dose/cycle = 3750 mg/m^2]
Repeat cycles every 28 days
Variation 2:
Gemcitabine: IV: 1200 mg/m^2/day over 30 minutes days 1, 8, and 15
[total dose/cycle = 3600 mg/m^2]
Repeat cycles every 28 days for a total of 6 cycles
Variation 3:
Cycle 1:
Gemcitabine: IV: 1000 mg/m^2/day over 30 minutes weekly for 7 weeks, followed by one week rest
[total dose/cycle = 7000 mg/m^2]
Treatment cycle is 8 weeks

◀ Subsequent Cycles:

Gemcitabine: IV: 1000 mg/m^2/day over 30 minutes days 1, 8, and 15
[total dose/cycle = 3000 mg/m^2]

Repeat cycle every 28 days until disease progression or drug intolerance

References

Variation 1:

Santoro A, Bredenfeld H, Devizzi L, et al, "Gemcitabine in the Treatment of Refractory Hodgkin's Disease: Results of a Multicenter Phase II Study," *J Clin Oncol*, 2000, 18(13):2615-9.

Variation 2:

Zinzani PL, Bendandi M, Stefoni V, et al, "Value of Gemcitabine Treatment in Heavily Pretreated Hodgkin's Disease Patients," *Haematologica*, 2000, 85(9):926-9.

Variation 3:

Savage DG, Rule SA, Tighe M, et al, "Gemcitabine for Relapsed or Resistant Lymphoma," *Ann of Oncol*, 2000, 11(5):595-7.

Gemcitabine (Mesothelioma Regimen)

Use Malignant pleural mesothelioma

Regimen

Gemcitabine: IV: 1250 mg/m^2/day over 30 minutes days 1, 8, and 15
[total dose/cycle = 3750 mg/m^2]

Repeat cycle every 28 days for up to a total of 10 cycles

References

van Meerbeeck JP, Baas P, Debruyne C, et al, "A Phase II Study of Gemcitabine in Patients With Malignant Pleural Mesothelioma," *Cancer*, 1999, 85(12):2577-82.

♦ **Gemcitabine-nab Paclitaxel (Pancreatic)** *see* Gemcitabine-Paclitaxel (Protein Bound) (Pancreatic) *on page 1996*

Gemcitabine (Ovarian Regimen)

Use Ovarian cancer

Regimen NOTE: Multiple variations are listed.

Variation 1:

Gemcitabine: IV: 1000 mg/m^2/dose over 30-60 minutes days 1 and 8
[total dose/cycle = 2000 mg/m^2]

Repeat cycle every 21 days until disease progression or unacceptable toxicity

Variation 2:

Gemcitabine: IV: 1000 mg/m^2/dose over 30 minutes days 1, 8, and 15
[total dose/cycle = 3000 mg/m^2]

Repeat cycle every 28 days until disease progression or unacceptable toxicity

References

Variation 1:

Mutch DG, Orlando M, Goss T, et al, "Randomized Phase III Trial of Gemcitabine Compared With Pegylated Liposomal Doxorubicin in Patients With Platinum-Resistant Ovarian Cancer," *J Clin Oncol*, 2007, 25(19):2811-8.

Variation 2:

Ferrandina G, Ludovisi M, Lorusso D, et al, "Phase III Trial of Gemcitabine Compared With Pegylated Liposomal Doxorubicin in Progressive or Recurrent Ovarian Cancer," *J Clin Oncol*, 2008, 26(6):890-6.

Gemcitabine-Oxaliplatin-Paclitaxel (Testicular)

Index Terms GOP (Testicular); Oxaliplatin-Gemcitabine-Paclitaxel (Testicular); Paclitaxel-Gemcitabine-Oxaliplatin (Testicular)

Use Testicular cancer

Regimen

Gemcitabine: IV: 800 mg/m^2/day over 30 minutes days 1 and 8
   [total dose/cycle = 1600 mg/m^2]
Paclitaxel: IV: 80 mg/m^2/day over 1 hour days 1 and 8
   [total dose/cycle = 160 mg/m^2]
Oxaliplatin: IV: 130 mg/m^2 over 2 hours day 1
   [total dose/cycle = 130 mg/m^2]
Repeat cycle every 21 days for 2 cycles beyond best response, maximum of 8 cycles

References

Bokemeyer C, Oechsle K, Honecker F, et al, "Combination Chemotherapy With Gemcitabine, Oxaliplatin, and Paclitaxel in Patients With Cisplatin-Refractory or Multiply Relapsed Germ-Cell Tumors: A Study of the German Testicular Cancer Study Group," *Ann Oncol*, 2008, 19(3):448-53.

♦ **Gemcitabine-Oxaliplatin-Rituximab (NHL-DLBCL)** *see* GEMOX-R (NHL-DLBCL) *on page* 2000

♦ **Gemcitabine-Oxaliplatin-Rituximab (NHL-Mantle Cell)** *see* GEMOX-R (NHL-Mantle Cell) *on page* 2000

♦ **Gemcitabine-Oxaliplatin (Testicular)** *see* GEMOX (Testicular) *on page* 2000

Gemcitabine-Paclitaxel (Bladder)

Index Terms Paclitaxel-Gemcitabine (Bladder)

Use Bladder cancer

Regimen NOTE: Multiple variations are listed.

Variation 1:
   Paclitaxel: IV: 200 mg/m^2 over 1 hour day 1
      [total dose/cycle = 200 mg/m^2]
   Gemcitabine: IV: 1000 mg/m^2/day over 30 minutes days 1, 8, and 15
      [total dose/cycle = 3000 mg/m^2]
   Repeat cycle every 21 days for 6 cycles

Variation 2:
   Gemcitabine: IV: 2500 to 3000 mg/m^2 day 1
      [total dose/cycle = 2500 to 3000 mg/m^2]
   Paclitaxel: IV: 150 mg/m^2 day 1
      [total dose/cycle = 150 mg/m^2]
   Repeat cycle every 14 days

Variation 3:
   Paclitaxel: IV: 150 mg/m^2 over 3 hours day 1
      [total dose/cycle = 150 mg/m^2]
   Gemcitabine: IV: 2500 mg/m^2 over 30 minutes day 1
      [total dose/cycle = 2500 mg/m^2]
   Repeat cycle every 14 days up to a maximum of 12 cycles

References

Variation 1:
Meluch AA, Greco FA, Burris HA 3rd, et al. Paclitaxel and gemcitabine chemotherapy for advanced transitional-cell carcinoma of the urothelial tract: a phase II trial of the Minnie pearl cancer research network. *J Clin Oncol*. 2001;19(12):3018-3024.
Variation 2:
Sternberg CN, Calabrò F, Pizzocaro G, Marini L, Schnetzer S, Sella A. Chemotherapy with an every-2-week regimen of gemcitabine and paclitaxel in patients with transitional cell carcinoma who have received prior cisplatin-based therapy. *Cancer*. 2001;92(12):2993-2998.
Variation 3:
Calabrò F, Lorusso V, Rosati G, et al. Gemcitabine and paclitaxel every 2 weeks in patients with previously untreated urothelial carcinoma. *Cancer*. 2009;115(12):2652-2659.

Gemcitabine-Paclitaxel (Breast)

Index Terms GT (Breast); Paclitaxel-Gemcitabine (Breast)

Use Breast cancer

Regimen

Paclitaxel: IV: 175 mg/m^2 over 3 hours day 1
[total dose/cycle = 175 mg/m^2]
Gemcitabine: IV: 1250 mg/m^2 over 30 minutes days 1 and 8
[total dose/cycle = 2500 mg/m^2]
Repeat cycle every 21 days until disease progression or unacceptable toxicity

References

Albain KS, Nag SM, Calderillo-Ruiz G, et al, "Gemcitabine Plus Paclitaxel Versus Paclitaxel Monotherapy in Patients With Metastatic Breast Cancer and Prior Anthracycline Treatment," *J Clin Oncol*, 2008, 26(24):3950-7.

◆ **Gemcitabine-Paclitaxel (nanoparticle albumin bound) (Pancreatic)** *see* Gemcitabine-Paclitaxel (Protein Bound) (Pancreatic) *on page 1996*

Gemcitabine-Paclitaxel (Protein Bound) (Pancreatic)

Index Terms Gemcitabine-Abraxane (Pancreatic); Gemcitabine-nab Paclitaxel (Pancreatic); Gemcitabine-Paclitaxel (nanoparticle albumin bound) (Pancreatic); Paclitaxel (Protein Bound)-Gemcitabine (Pancreatic)

Use Pancreatic cancer

Regimen NOTE: Multiple variations are listed.

Variation 1:

Cycle 1:

Paclitaxel (protein bound): IV: 125 mg/m^2/day days 1, 8, 15, 29, 36, and 43
[total dose/cycle = 750 mg/m^2]
Gemcitabine: IV: 1000 mg/m^2/day days 1, 8, 15, 29, 36, and 43
[total dose/cycle = 6000 mg/m^2]
Cycle 1 duration is 8 weeks

Subsequent cycles:

Paclitaxel (protein bound): IV: 125 mg/m^2/day days 1, 8, and 15
[total dose/cycle = 375 mg/m^2]
Gemcitabine: IV: 1000 mg/m^2/day days 1, 8, and 15
[total dose/cycle = 3000 mg/m^2]
Repeat cycle every 28 days until disease progression or unacceptable toxicity

Variation 2:

Gemcitabine: IV: 1000 mg/m^2/day days 1, 8, and 15
[total dose/cycle = 3000 mg/m^2]
Paclitaxel (protein bound): IV: 125 mg/m^2/day days 1, 8, and 15
[total dose/cycle = 375 mg/m^2]
Repeat cycle every 28 days until disease progression or unacceptable toxicity

References

Variation 1:
Von Hoff DD, Ervin T, Arena FP, et al. Increased Survival in Pancreatic Cancer with nab-Paclitaxel plus Gemcitabine. *N Engl J Med*. 2013 [epub ahead of print].
Variation 2:
Von Hoff DD, Ramanathan RK, Borad MJ, et al, "Gemcitabine Plus Nab-Paclitaxel Is an Active Regimen in Patients With Advanced Pancreatic Cancer: A Phase I/II Trial," *J Clin Oncol*, 2011, 29 (34):4548-54.

Gemcitabine-Paclitaxel (Testicular)

Index Terms Paclitaxel-Gemcitabine (Testicular)

Use Testicular cancer

Regimen

Paclitaxel: IV: 100 mg/m^2/day over 1 hour days 1, 8, and 15
[total dose/cycle = 300 mg/m^2]

Gemcitabine: IV: 1000 mg/m^2/day over 30 minutes days 1, 8, and 15
[total dose/cycle = 3000 mg/m^2]

Repeat cycle every 28 days for a maximum of 6 cycles

References

Einhorn LH, Brames MJ, Juliar B, et al, "Phase II Study of Paclitaxel Plus Gemcitabine Salvage Chemotherapy for Germ Cell Tumors After Progression Following High-Dose Chemotherapy With Tandem Transplant," *J Clin Oncol*, 2007, 25(5):513-6.

Mulherin BP, Brames MJ, Einhorn LH, at el, "Long-Term Survival With Paclitaxel and Gemcitabine for Germ Cell Tumors After Progression Following High-Dose Chemotherapy With Tandem Transplants," *J Clin Oncol*, 2011, 29:4562 [abstract 4562 from 2011 ASCO Annual Meeting].

Gemcitabine (Small Cell Lung Cancer Regimen)

Use Lung cancer, small cell

Regimen NOTE: Multiple variations are listed.

Variation 1:

Gemcitabine: IV: 1000 mg/m^2/day over 30 minutes days 1, 8, and 15
[total dose/cycle = 3000 mg/m^2]

Repeat cycle every 28 days

Variation 2:

Gemcitabine: IV: 1250 mg/m^2/day over 30 minutes days 1 and 8
[total dose/cycle = 2500 mg/m^2]

Repeat cycle every 21 days

References

Variation1:

Masters GA, Declerck L, Blanke C, et al, "Phase II Trial of Gemcitabine in Refractory or Relapsed Small-Cell Lung Cancer: Eastern Cooperative Oncology Group Trial 1597," *J Clin Oncol*, 2003, 21(8):1550-5.

van der Lee I, Smit EF, van Putten JWG, et al, "Single-Agent Gemcitabine in Patients With Resistant Small-Cell Lung Cancer," *Ann Oncol*, 2001, 12(4):557-61.

Variation 2:

Hoang T, Kim K, Jaslowski A, et al, "Phase II Study of Second-Line Gemcitabine in Sensitive or Refractory Small Cell Lung Cancer," *Lung Cancer*, 2003, 42(1):97-102.

Gemcitabine Standard Infusion (Pancreatic Regimen)

Use Pancreatic cancer

Regimen NOTE: Multiple variations are listed.

Variation 1: (advanced)

Cycle 1:

Gemcitabine: IV: 1000 mg/m^2/day over 30 minutes days 1, 8, 15, 22, 29, 36, and 43 (cycle 1 only)
[total dose/cycle 1 = 7000 mg/m^2]

Treatment cycle is 56 days

Subsequent cycles:

Gemcitabine: IV: 1000 mg/m^2/day over 30 minutes days 1, 8, and 15
[total dose/cycle = 3000 mg/m^2]

Repeat cycle every 28 days until disease progression or unacceptable toxicity

Variation 2: (adjuvant)

Gemcitabine: IV: 1000 mg/m^2/day over 30 minutes days 1, 8, and 15
[total dose/cycle = 3000 mg/m^2]

Repeat cycle every 28 days until for 6 cycles

◀ **References**

Variation 1:

Burris HA 3rd, Moore MJ, Andersen J, et al, "Improvements in Survival and Clinical Benefit With Gemcitabine as First-Line Therapy for Patients With Advanced Pancreas Cancer: A Randomized Trial," *J Clin Oncol*, 1997, 15(6):2403-13.

Variation 2:

Neoptolemos JP, Stocken DD, Bassi C, et al, "Adjuvant Chemotherapy With Fluorouracil Plus Folinic Acid Vs Gemcitabine Following Pancreatic Cancer Resection: A Randomized Controlled Trial," *JAMA*, 2010, 304(10):1073-81.

Oettle H, Post S, Neuhaus P, et al, "Adjuvant Chemotherapy With Gemcitabine Vs Observation in Patients Undergoing Curative-Intent Resection of Pancreatic Cancer: A Randomized Controlled Trial," *JAMA*, 2007, 297(3):267-77.

Gemcitabine (Uterine Leiomyosarcoma Regimen)

Use Uterine sarcoma (uterine leiomyosarcoma)

Regimen

Gemcitabine: IV: 1000 mg/m^2/day over 30 minutes days 1, 8, and 15

[total dose/cycle = 3000 mg/m^2]

Repeat cycle every 28 days

References

Look KY, Sandler A, Blessing JA, Lucci JA 3rd, Rose PG. Phase II trial of gemcitabine as second-line chemotherapy of uterine leiomyosarcoma: a Gynecologic Oncology Group (GOG) Study. *Gynecol Oncol*. 2004;92(2):644-647.

◆ **Gemcitabine-Vinorelbine-Doxorubicin (Liposomal) (Hodgkin)** *see* GVD (Hodgkin) *on page 2002*

Gemcitabine-Vinorelbine (Head and Neck)

Index Terms GV (Head and Neck); Vinorelbine-Gemcitabine (Head and Neck)

Use Head and neck cancer (nasopharyngeal)

Regimen

Vinorelbine: IV: 25 mg/m^2/day days 1 and 8

[total dose/cycle = 50 mg/m^2]

Gemcitabine: IV: 1000 mg/m^2/day over 30 minutes days 1 and 8

[total dose/cycle = 2000 mg/m^2]

Repeat cycle every 21 days for 6 cycles

References

Chen C, Wang FH, Wang ZQ, et al. Salvage gemcitabine-vinorelbine chemotherapy in patients with metastatic nasopharyngeal carcinoma pretreated with platinum-based chemotherapy. *Oral Oncol*. 2012;48(11):1146-1151.

Gemcitabine-Vinorelbine (NSCLC)

Index Terms GemVin (NSCLC); GV (NSCLC); Vinorelbine-Gemcitabine (NSCLC)

Use Lung cancer, non-small cell

Regimen NOTE: Multiple variations are listed.

Variation 1:

Gemcitabine: IV: 1000 mg/m^2/day days 1, 8, and 15

[total dose/cycle = 3000 mg/m^2]

Vinorelbine: IV: 25 mg/m^2/day days 1, 8, and 15

[total dose/cycle = 75 mg/m^2]

Repeat cycle every 28 days for up to 6 cycles

Variation 2:

Vinorelbine: IV: 25 mg/m^2/day over 10 minutes days 1, 8, and 15
 [total dose/cycle = 75 mg/m^2]

Gemcitabine: IV: 900 mg/m^2/day over 30 minutes days 1, 8, and 15
 [total dose/cycle = 2700 mg/m^2]

Repeat cycle every 28 days for a recommended 6 cycles, further treatment could be administered until disease progression or unacceptable toxicity

Variation 3:

Gemcitabine: IV: 1000 mg/m^2/day over 30 minutes days 1 and 8
 [total dose/cycle = 2000 mg/m^2]

Vinorelbine: IV: 25 mg/m^2/day over 15 minutes days 1 and 8, one hour after completion of gemcitabine
 [total dose/cycle = 50 mg/m^2]

Repeat cycle every 21 days for up to 6 cycles

References

Variation 1:

Greco FA, Spigel DR, Kuzur ME, et al. Paclitaxel/carboplatin/gemcitabine versus gemcitabine/vinorelbine in advanced non-small-cell lung cancer: a phase II/III study of the Minnie Pearl Cancer Research Network. *Clin Lung Cancer.* 2007;8(8):483-487.

Variation 2:

Herbst RS, Khuri FR, Lu C, et al. The novel and effective nonplatinum, nontaxane combination of gemcitabine and vinorelbine in advanced nonsmall cell lung carcinoma: potential for decreased toxicity and combination with biological therapy. *Cancer.* 2002;95(2):340-353.

Variation 3:

Gridelli C, Gallo C, Shepherd FA, et al. Gemcitabine plus vinorelbine compared with cisplatin plus vinorelbine or cisplatin plus gemcitabine for advanced non-small-cell lung cancer: a phase III trial of the Italian GEMVIN Investigators and the National Cancer Institute of Canada Clinical Trials Group. *J Clin Oncol.* 2003;21(16):3025-3034.

Laack E, Dickgreber N, Müller T, et al. Randomized phase III study of gemcitabine and vinorelbine versus gemcitabine, vinorelbine, and cisplatin in the treatment of advanced non-small-cell lung cancer: from the German and Swiss Lung Cancer Study Group. *J Clin Oncol.* 2004;22(12):2348-2356.

Gemcitabine-Vinorelbine (Soft Tissue Sarcoma)

Index Terms Vinorelbine-Gemcitabine (Soft Tissue Sarcoma)

Use Soft tissue sarcoma

Regimen

Vinorelbine: IV: 25 mg/m^2/day over 10 minutes days 1 and 8
 [total dose/cycle = 50 mg/m^2]

Gemcitabine: IV: 800 mg/m^2/day over 90 minutes days 1 and 8
 [total dose/cycle = 1600 mg/m^2]

Repeat cycle every 21 days until disease progression or unacceptable toxicity

References

Dileo P, Morgan JA, Zahrieh D, et al. Gemcitabine and vinorelbine combination chemotherapy for patients with advanced soft tissue sarcomas: results of a phase II trial. *Cancer.* 2007;109(9):1863-1869.

GEMOX (Biliary Cancer)

Use Biliary adenocarcinoma

Regimen

Gemcitabine: IV: 1000 mg/m^2 day 1
 [total dose/cycle = 1000 mg/m^2]

Oxaliplatin: IV: 100 mg/m^2 day 2
 [total dose/cycle = 100 mg/m^2]

Repeat cycle every 2 weeks

◄ **References**

Andre T, Tournigand C, Rosmorduc O, et al, "Gemcitabine Combined With Oxaliplatin (GEMOX) in Advanced Biliary Tract Adenocarcinoma: A GERCOR Study," *Ann Oncol*, 2004, 15(9):1339-43.

GEMOX-R (NHL-DLBCL)

Index Terms Gemcitabine-Oxaliplatin-Rituximab (NHL-DLBCL); Oxaliplatin-Gemcitabine-Rituximab (NHL-DLBCL); Rituximab-Gemcitabine-Oxaliplatin (NHL-DLBCL)

Use Lymphoma, non-Hodgkin (DLBCL)

Regimen

Rituximab: IV: 375 mg/m^2 day 1
[total dose/cycle = 375 mg/m^2]
Gemcitabine: IV: 1000 mg/m^2 day 1
[total dose/cycle = 1000 mg/m^2]
Oxaliplatin: IV: 100 mg/m^2 day 1
[total dose/cycle = 100 mg/m^2]
Repeat cycle every 21 days for a total of 6 to 8 cycles

References

López A, Gutiérrez A, Palacios A, et al, "GEMOX-R Regimen is a Highly Effective Salvage Regimen in Patients With Refractory/Relapsing Diffuse Large-Cell Lymphoma: A Phase II Study," *Eur J Haematol*, 2008, 80(2):127-32.

GEMOX-R (NHL-Mantle Cell)

Index Terms Gemcitabine-Oxaliplatin-Rituximab (NHL-Mantle Cell); Oxaliplatin-Gemcitabine-Rituximab (NHL-Mantle Cell); Rituximab-Gemcitabine-Oxaliplatin (NHL-Mantle Cell)

Use Lymphoma, non-Hodgkin (Mantle cell)

Regimen

Rituximab: IV: 375 mg/m^2 day 1
[total dose/cycle = 375 mg/m^2]
Gemcitabine: IV: 1000 mg/m^2 day 1
[total dose/cycle = 1000 mg/m^2]
Oxaliplatin: IV: 100 mg/m^2 day 1
[total dose/cycle = 100 mg/m^2]
Repeat cycle every 21 days for a maximum of 8 cycles

References

Rodríguez J, Gutierrez A, Palacios A, et al, "Rituximab, Gemcitabine and Oxaliplatin: An Effective Regimen in Patients With Refractory and Relapsing Mantle Cell Lymphoma," *Leuk Lymphoma*, 2007, 48(11):2172-8.

GEMOX (Testicular)

Index Terms Gemcitabine-Oxaliplatin (Testicular); Oxaliplatin-Gemcitabine (Testicular)

Use Testicular cancer

Regimen NOTE: Multiple variations are listed.

Variation 1:

Gemcitabine: IV: 1000 mg/m^2/day over 30 minutes days 1 and 8
[total dose/cycle = 2000 mg/m^2]
Oxaliplatin: IV: 130 mg/m^2 over 2 hours day 1
[total dose/cycle = 130 mg/m^2]
Repeat cycle every 21 days for a total of at least 2 cycles (maximum: 6 cycles)

Variation 2:
 Gemcitabine: IV: 1250 mg/m^2/day over 30 minutes days 1 and 8
  [total dose/cycle = 2500 mg/m^2]
 Oxaliplatin: IV: 130 mg/m^2 over 2 hours day 1
  [total dose/cycle = 130 mg/m^2]
 Repeat cycle every 21 days for a maximum of 6 cycles

References
Variation 1:
Kollmannsberger C, Beyer J, Liersch R, et al, "Combination Chemotherapy With Gemcitabine Plus Oxaliplatin in Patients With Intensively Pretreated or Refractory Germ Cell Cancer: A Study of the German Testicular Cancer Study Group," *J Clin Oncol*, 2004, 22(1):108-14.

Pectasides D, Pectasides M, Farmakis D, et al, "Gemcitabine and Oxaliplatin (GEMOX) in Patients With Cisplatin-Refractory Germ Cell Tumors: A Phase II Study," *Ann Oncol*, 2004, 15(3):493-7.

Variation 2:
De Giorgi U, Rosti G, Aieta M, et al, "Phase II Study of Oxaliplatin and Gemcitabine Salvage Chemotherapy in Patients With Cisplatin-Refractory Nonseminomatous Germ Cell Tumor," *Eur Urol*, 2006, 50(5):1032-8.

◆ **GemVin (NSCLC)** *see* Gemcitabine-Vinorelbine (NSCLC) *on page 1998*

◆ **GOP (Testicular)** *see* Gemcitabine-Oxaliplatin-Paclitaxel (Testicular) *on page 1994*

◆ **GP (Bladder)** *see* Cisplatin-Gemcitabine (Bladder) *on page 1903*

◆ **GT (Breast)** *see* Gemcitabine-Paclitaxel (Breast) *on page 1996*

GTX (Pancreatic)

Index Terms Gemcitabine-Docetaxel-Capecitabine (Pancreatic)
Use Pancreatic cancer
Regimen NOTE: Multiple variations are listed.
 Variation 1:
 Gemcitabine: IV: 750 mg/m^2/day over 75 minutes days 4 and 11
  [total dose/cycle = 1500 mg/m^2]
 Docetaxel: IV: 30 mg/m^2/day over 60 minutes days 4 and 11
  [total dose/cycle = 60 mg/m^2]
 Capecitabine: Oral: 750 mg/m^2/dose twice daily days 1 to 14
  [total dose/cycle = 21,000 mg/m^2]
 Repeat cycle every 21 days
 Variation 2:
 Gemcitabine: IV: 600 mg/m^2/day over 60 minutes days 4 and 11
  [total dose/cycle = 1200 mg/m^2]
 Docetaxel: IV: 30 mg/m^2/day over 60 minutes days 4 and 11
  [total dose/cycle = 60 mg/m^2]
 Capecitabine: Oral: 500 mg/m^2/dose twice daily days 1 to 14
  [total dose/cycle = 14,000 mg/m^2]
 Repeat cycle every 21 days until disease progression or unacceptable toxicities

References
Variation 1:
Fine RL, Fogelman DR, Schreibman SM, et al, "The Gemcitabine, Docetaxel,and Capecitabine (GTX) Regimen for Metastatic Pancreatic Cancer: A Retrospective Analysis," *Cancer Chemother Pharmacol*, 2008, 61(1):167-75.

Variation 2:
Dakik HK, Moskovic DJ, Carlson PJ, et al. The use of GTX as second-line and later chemotherapy for metastatic pancreatic cancer: a retrospective analysis. *Cancer Chemother Pharmacol*. 2012;69(2):425-30.

GVD (Hodgkin)

Index Terms Gemcitabine-Vinorelbine-Doxorubicin (Liposomal) (Hodgkin)
Use Lymphoma, Hodgkin
Regimen NOTE: Multiple variations are listed.

Variation 1 (for transplant-naive patients):

Vinorelbine: IV: 20 mg/m^2/day over 6-10 minutes days 1 and 8
[total dose/cycle = 40 mg/m^2]
Gemcitabine: IV: 1000 mg/m^2/day over 30 minutes days 1 and 8
[total dose/cycle = 2000 mg/m^2]
Doxorubicin liposomal: IV: 15 mg/m^2/day over 30-60 minutes days 1 and 8
[total dose/cycle = 30 mg/m^2]
Repeat cycle every 21 days for a total of 2 to 6 cycles

Variation 2 (for patients with prior transplant):

Vinorelbine: IV: 15 mg/m^2/day over 6-10 minutes days 1 and 8
[total dose/cycle = 30 mg/m^2]
Gemcitabine: IV: 800 mg/m^2/day over 30 minutes days 1 and 8
[total dose/cycle = 1600 mg/m^2]
Doxorubicin liposomal: IV: 10 mg/m^2/day over 30-60 minutes days 1 and 8
[total dose/cycle = 20 mg/m^2]
Repeat cycle every 21 days for a total of 2 to 6 cycles

References

Variations 1 and 2:
Bartlett NL, Niedzwiecki D, Johnson JL, et al, "Gemcitabine, Vinorelbine, and Pegylated Liposomal Doxorubicin (GVD), A Salvage Regimen in Relapsed Hodgkin's Lymphoma: CALGB 59804," *Ann Oncol*, 2007, 18(6):1071-9.

◆ **GV (Head and Neck)** see Gemcitabine-Vinorelbine (Head and Neck) on page 1998

◆ **GV (NSCLC)** see Gemcitabine-Vinorelbine (NSCLC) on page 1998

◆ **HDAC-Daunorubicin (AML Induction)** see Cytarabine (High Dose)-Daunorubicin (AML Induction) on page 1931

◆ **HD Cytarabine (Single Agent AML Induction)** see Cytarabine (High-Dose Single-Agent AML Induction Regimen) on page 1932

HDMTX

Use Osteosarcoma
Regimen

Methotrexate: IV: 12 g/m^2/week for 2-12 weeks
[total dose/cycle = 24-144 g/m^2]
Leucovorin calcium rescue: Oral, IV: 15 mg/m^2 every 6 hours (beginning 30 hours after the beginning of the 4-hour methotrexate infusion) for 10 doses; **serum methotrexate levels must be monitored**
[total dose/cycle = 150 mg/m^2]

References

Camitta BM and Holcenberg JS, "Safety of Delayed Leucovorin 'Rescue' Following High-Dose Methotrexate in Children," *Med Pediatr Oncol*, 1978, 5(1):55-9.

◆ **HD-MVAC (Bladder Cancer)** see Dose Dense MVAC (Bladder Cancer) on page 1948

◆ **HIDAC-3-7 (AML Induction)** see Cytarabine (High Dose)-Daunorubicin-Etoposide (AML Induction) on page 1932

◆ **HIDAC-Daunorubicin (AML Induction)** see Cytarabine (High Dose)-Daunorubicin (AML Induction) on page 1931

- ◆ **HIDAC (Single Agent AML Induction)** *see* Cytarabine (High-Dose Single-Agent AML Induction Regimen) *on page 1932*

- ◆ **High-Dose-Intensity M-VAC (Bladder Cancer)** *see* Dose Dense MVAC (Bladder Cancer) *on page 1948*

High Dose Methotrexate (CNS Lymphoma)

Use Primary CNS lymphoma

Regimen NOTE: Start leucovorin 24 hours after methotrexate infusion and until methotrexate level <0.1 µM

Induction:

Methotrexate: IV: 8000 mg/m^2 over 4 hours day 1

[total dose/cycle = 8000 mg/m^2]

Repeat cycle every 14 days until complete response or a maximum of 8 cycles

Consolidation (for patients in complete response after induction):

Methotrexate: IV: 8000 mg/m^2 over 4 hours day 1

[total dose/cycle = 8000 mg/m^2]

Repeat cycle every 14 days for 2 cycles

Maintenance:

Methotrexate: IV: 8000 mg/m^2 over 4 hours day 1

[total dose/cycle = 8000 mg/m^2]

Repeat cycle every 28 days for 11 cycles

References

Batchelor T, Carson K, O'Neill A, et al. Treatment of primary CNS lymphoma with methotrexate and deferred radiotherapy: a report of NABTT 96-07. *J Clin Oncol*. 2003;21(6):1044-1049.

Histrelin (Prostate Regimen)

Use Prostate cancer

Regimen

Histrelin: SubQ: 50 mg implant surgically, insert every 12 months

Remove old implant prior to insertion of replacement implant.

References

Shore N, Cookson MS, and Gittelman MC. Long-term efficacy and tolerability of once-yearly histrelin acetate subcutaneous implant in patients with advanced prostate cancer. *BJU Int*. 2012;109(2):226-232.

Hydroxyurea (AML Regimen)

Use Leukemia, acute myeloid

Regimen

Hydroxyurea: Oral: 25 mg/kg/dose 4 times/day for a maximum of 30 days

[total maximum dose/cycle = 3000 mg/kg]

Administer treatment until achievement of bone marrow aplasia, for a maximum of 30 days

References

Petti MC, Tafuri A, Latagliata R, et al, "High-Dose Hydroxyurea in the Treatment of Poor-Risk Myeloid Leukemias," *Ann Hematol*, 2003, 82(8):476-80.

- ◆ **Hydroxyurea-Fluorouracil (Head and Neck Cancer)** *see* Fluorouracil-Hydroxyurea (Head and Neck Cancer) *on page 1978*

Hyper-CVAD Alternating With High-Dose Methotrexate-Cytarabine + Rituximab + CNS Prophylaxis (NHL-Burkitt)

Index Terms Rituximab, Cyclophosphamide, Vincristine, Doxorubicin, Dexamethasone, Methotrexate, Cytarabine (NHL-Burkitt); Rituximab-Hyper-CVAD Alternating With High-Dose Methotrexate-Cytarabine (NHL-Burkitt)

Use Lymphoma, non-Hodgkin (Burkitt)

Regimen

Cycle A (Cycles 1, 3, 5, and 7):

Rituximab: IV: 375 mg/m^2/day over 2 to 6 hours days 1 and 11 cycles 1 and 3 only

[total dose/cycle = 750 mg/m^2]

Cyclophosphamide: IV: 300 mg/m^2 every 12 hours, for 6 doses, days 1, 2, and 3

[total dose/cycle = 1800 mg/m^2]

Mesna: IV: 600 mg/m^2 continuous infusion days 1, 2, and 3

[total dose/cycle = 1800 mg/m^2]

Vincristine: IV: 2 mg/day days 4 and 11

[total dose/cycle = 4 mg]

Doxorubicin: IV: 50 mg/m^2 continuous infusion over 24 hours day 4

[total dose/cycle = 50 mg/m^2]

Dexamethasone: Oral, IV: 40 mg/day days 1 to 4 and 11 to 14

[total dose/cycle = 320 mg]

CNS Prophylaxis

Methotrexate: Intrathecal: 12 mg (6 mg by Ommaya reservoir) day 2

Cytarabine: Intrathecal: 100 mg day 7

CNS prophylaxis to be given with each course (total of 16 Intrathecal treatments)

Filgrastim: SubQ: 10 mcg/kg daily, starting 24 hours after completion of chemotherapy and continuing until WBC ≥3000/mm^3

Cycle B (Cycles 2, 4, 6, and 8):

Rituximab: IV: 375 mg/m^2/day over 2 to 6 hours days 2 and 8 on cycles 2 and 4 only

[total dose/cycle = 750 mg/m^2]

Methotrexate: IV: 1000 mg/m^2 continuous infusion over 24 hours day 1

[total dose/cycle = 1000 mg/m^2]

Leucovorin: IV: 50 mg (start 12 hours after the end of the methotrexate infusion)

followed by IV: 15 mg every 6 hours, for 8 doses or until methotrexate level ≤0.1 mmol/L

[total dose/cycle = 170 mg]

Cytarabine: IV: 3000 mg/m^2 every 12 hours, for 4 doses, day 2 and 3

[total dose/cycle = 12,000 mg/m^2]

CNS Prophylaxis

Methotrexate: Intrathecal: 12 mg (6 mg by Ommaya reservoir) day 2

Cytarabine: Intrathecal: 100 mg day 7

CNS prophylaxis to be given with each course (total of 16 Intrathecal treatments)

Filgrastim: SubQ: 10 mcg/kg daily, starting 24 hours after completion of chemotherapy and continuing until WBC ≥3000/mm^3

Repeat every 14 to 21 days (depending on count recovery) in the following sequence: ABABABAB

References

Thomas DA, Faderl S, O'Brien S, et al. Chemoimmunotherapy with hyper-CVAD plus rituximab for the treatment of adult Burkitt and Burkitt-type lymphoma or acute lymphoblastic leukemia. *Cancer.* 2006;106(7):1569-1580.

Thomas DA, Kantarjian HM, Cortes J, et al. Long-Term Outcome after Hyper-CVAD and Rituximab Chemoimmunotherapy for Burkitt (BL) or Burkitt-Like (BLL) Leukemia/Lymphoma and Mature B-Cell Acute Lymphocytic Leukemia (ALL). *Blood.* 2008;112:1929 [abstract 1929 from 2008 ASH Annual Meeting].

Hyper-CVAD + Imatinib

Use Leukemia, acute lymphocytic

Regimen

Cycle A (Cycles 1, 3, 5, and 7):

Imatinib: Oral: 400 mg/day days 1 to 14
[total dose/cycle = 5600 mg]

Cyclophosphamide: IV: 300 mg/m^2 every 12 hours, for 6 doses, days 1, 2, and 3
[total dose/cycle = 1800 mg/m^2]

Mesna: IV 600 mg/m^2/day continuous infusion days 1, 2, and 3
[total dose/cycle = 1800 mg/m^2]

Vincristine: IV: 2 mg/day days 4 and 11
[total dose/cycle = 4 mg]

Doxorubicin: IV: 50 mg/m^2/day continuous infusion day 4
[total dose/cycle = 50 mg/m^2]

Dexamethasone: Oral, IV: 40 mg/day days 1 to 4 and 11 to 14
[total dose/cycle = 320 mg]

Cycle B (Cycles 2, 4, 6, and 8):

Imatinib: Oral: 400 mg/day days 1 to 14
[total dose/cycle = 5600 mg]

Methotrexate: IV: 1 g/m^2/day continuous infusion day 1
[total dose/cycle = 1 g/m^2]

Leucovorin: IV: 50 mg then 15 mg every 6 hours, for 8 doses (start 12 hours after the end of the methotrexate infusion)
[total dose/cycle = 170 mg]

Cytarabine: IV: 3 g/m^2 every 12 hours for 4 doses, days 2 and 3
[total dose/cycle = 12 g/m^2]

Repeat every 6 weeks in the following sequence: ABABABAB

CNS Prophylaxis

Methotrexate: Intrathecal: 12 mg/day day 2
[total dose/cycle = 12 mg/day]

or 6 mg into Ommaya day 2
[total dose/cycle = 6 mg/day]

Cytarabine: Intrathecal: 100 mg/day day 7 or 8
[total dose/cycle = 100 mg/day]

Repeat cycle every 3 weeks for 3 or 4 cycles

Maintenance (POMP)

Imatinib: Oral: 600 mg/day
[total dose/cycle = 18,000 mg]

Vincristine: IV: 2 mg/day day 1
[total dose/cycle = 2 mg]

Prednisone: Oral: 200 mg/day days 1 to 5
[total dose/cycle = 1000 mg/m^2]

Repeat cycle every month (except months 6 and 13) for 13 months

◄ **Intensification**

Imatinib: Oral: 400 mg/day days 1 to 14

[total dose/cycle = 5600 mg]

Cyclophosphamide: IV: 300 mg/m^2 every 12 hours, for 6 doses, days 1, 2, and 3

[total dose/cycle = 1800 mg/m^2]

Mesna: IV: 600 mg/m^2/day continuous infusion days 1, 2, and 3

[total dose/cycle = 1800 mg/m^2]

Vincristine: IV: 2 mg/day days 4 and 11

[total dose/cycle = 4 mg]

Doxorubicin: 50 mg/m^2/day continuous infusion day 4

[total dose/cycle = 50 mg/m^2]

Dexamethasone: IV or Oral: 40 mg/day days 1 to 4 and 11 to 14

[total dose/cycle = 320 mg]

Cycle is given in months 6 and 13 during maintenance

References

Thomas DA, Faderl S, Cortes J, et al, "Treatment of Philadelphia Chromosome-Positive Acute Lymphocytic Leukemia With Hyper-CVAD and Imatinib Mesylate," *Blood*, 2004, 103 (12):4396-407.

Hyper-CVAD (Leukemia, Acute Lymphocytic)

Use Leukemia, acute lymphocytic

Regimen NOTE: Multiple variations are listed.

Variation 1:

Cycle A (Cycles 1, 3, 5, and 7):

Cyclophosphamide: IV: 300 mg/m^2 every 12 hours, for 6 doses, days 1, 2, and 3

[total dose/cycle = 1800 mg/m^2]

Mesna: IV: 1200 mg/m^2/day continuous infusion days 1, 2, and 3

[total dose/cycle = 3600 mg/m^2]

Vincristine: IV: 2 mg/day days 4 and 11

[total dose/cycle = 4 mg]

Doxorubicin: IV: 50 mg/m^2 day 4

[total dose/cycle = 50 mg/m^2]

Dexamethasone: (route not specified): 40 mg/day days 1 to 4 and 11 to 14

[total dose/cycle = 320 mg]

Cycle B (Cycles 2, 4, 6, and 8):

Methotrexate: IV: 1 g/m^2 continuous infusion day 1

[total dose/cycle = 1g/m^2]

Leucovorin: (route not specified): 15 mg every 6 hours, for 8 doses (start 12 hours after end of methotrexate infusion)

[total dose/cycle = 120 mg]

Cytarabine: IV: 3 g/m^2 every 12 hours, for 4 doses, days 2 and 3

[total dose/cycle = 12 g/m^2]

Methylprednisolone: IV: 50 mg twice daily, for 6 doses, days 1, 2, and 3

[total dose/cycle = 300 mg/m^2]

Repeat every 6 weeks in the following sequence: ABABABAB

CNS Prophylaxis

Methotrexate: Intrathecal: 12 mg/day day 2

[total dose/cycle = 12 mg]

or 6 mg/day into Ommaya day 2

[total dose/cycle = 6 mg]

Cytarabine: Intrathecal: 100 mg day 8
  [total dose/cycle = 100 mg]
Repeat cycle every 3 weeks
Maintenance (POMP)
  Mercaptopurine: Oral: 50 mg 3 times/day
    [total dose/cycle = 4200-4650 mg]
  Vincristine: IV: 2 mg day 1
    [total dose/cycle = 2 mg]
  Methotrexate: Oral: 20 mg/m^2/day days 1, 8, 15, and 22
    [total dose/cycle = 80 mg/m^2]
  Prednisone: Oral: 200 mg/day days 1 to 5
    [total dose/cycle = 1000 mg/m^2]
  or
  Mercaptopurine: IV: 1 g/m^2/day days 1 to 5
    [total dose/cycle = 5 g/m^2]
  Vincristine: IV: 2 mg day 1
    [total dose/cycle = 2 mg]
  Methotrexate: IV: 10 mg/m^2/day days 1 to 5
    [total dose/cycle = 50 mg/m^2]
  Prednisone: Oral: 200 mg/day days 1 to 5
    [total dose/cycle = 1000 mg/m^2]
  Repeat cycles every month for 2 years
Variation 2:
  Cycle A (Cycles 1, 3, 5, and 7):
  Cyclophosphamide: IV: 300 mg/m^2 every 12 hours, for 6 doses, days 1, 2, and 3
    [total dose/cycle = 1800 mg/m^2]
  Mesna: IV: 600 mg/m^2/day continuous infusion days 1, 2, and 3
    [total dose/cycle = 1800 mg/m^2]
  Vincristine: IV: 2 mg/day days 4 and 11
    [total dose/cycle = 4 mg]
  Doxorubicin: IV: 50 mg/m^2 day 4
    [total dose/cycle = 50 mg/m^2]
  Dexamethasone: Oral, IV: 40 mg/day days 1 to 4 and 11 to 14
    [total dose/cycle = 320 mg]
  Cycle B (Cycles 2, 4, 6, and 8):
  Methotrexate: IV: 1 g/m^2 continuous infusion day 1
    [total dose/cycle = 1 g/m^2]
  Leucovorin: IV: 50 mg (start 12 hours after end of methotrexate infusion)
    followed by IV: 15 mg every 6 hours, for 8 doses
    [total dose/cycle = 170 mg]
  Cytarabine: IV: 3 g/m^2 every 12 hours, for 4 doses, days 2 and 3
    [total dose/cycle = 12 g/m^2]
  Repeat every 6 weeks in the following sequence: ABABABAB
CNS Prophylaxis
  Methotrexate: Intrathecal: 12 mg day 2
    [total dose/cycle = 12 mg]
  or 6 mg into Ommaya day 2
    [total dose/cycle = 6 mg]
  Cytarabine: Intrathecal: 100 mg day 7
    [total dose/cycle = 100 mg]
  Repeat cycle every 3 weeks

2007

◀ Variation 3:

Cycle A (Cycles 1, 3, 5, and 7):

Cyclophosphamide: IV: 300 mg/m^2 every 12 hours, for 6 doses, days 1, 2, and 3
[total dose/cycle = 1800 mg/m^2]

Mesna: IV: 600 mg/m^2/day continuous infusion days 1, 2, and 3
[total dose/cycle = 1800 mg/m^2]

Vincristine: IV: 2 mg/day days 4 and 11
[total dose/cycle = 4 mg]

Doxorubicin: IV: 50 mg/m^2 continuous infusion day 4
[total dose/cycle = 50 mg/m^2]

Dexamethasone: Oral, IV: 40 mg/day days 1 to 4 and 11 to 14
[total dose/cycle = 320 mg]

Cycle B (Cycles 2, 4, 6, and 8):

Methotrexate: IV: 200 mg/m^2 day 1
followed by IV: 800 mg/m^2 continuous infusion day 1
[total dose/cycle = 1 g/m^2]

Leucovorin: IV: 50 mg (start 12 hours after end of methotrexate infusion)
followed by IV: 15 mg every 6 hours, for 8 doses
[total dose/cycle = 170 mg/m^2]

Cytarabine: IV: 3 g/m^2 every 12 hours, for 4 doses, days 2 and 3
[total dose/cycle = 12 g/m^2]

Repeat every 6 weeks in the following sequence: ABABABAB

CNS Prophylaxis

Methotrexate: Intrathecal: 12 mg day 2
[total dose/cycle = 12 mg]

or 6 mg into Ommaya day 2
[total dose/cycle = 6 mg]

Cytarabine: Intrathecal: 100 mg day 7 **or** 8
[total dose/cycle = 100 mg]

Repeat cycles every 3 weeks for 6 or 8 cycles

Maintenance (POMP)

Mercaptopurine: Oral: 50 mg 3 times/day
[total dose/cycle = 4200-4650 mg]

Vincristine: IV: 2 mg day 1
[total dose/cycle = 2 mg]

Methotrexate: Oral, I V: 20 mg/m^2/ day days 1, 8, 15, and 22
[total dose/cycle = 80 mg/m^2]

Prednisone: Oral: 200 mg/day days 1 to 5
[total dose/cycle = 1000 mg/m^2]

or

Mercaptopurine: IV: 1 g/m^2/day days 1 to 5
[total dose/cycle = 5 g/m^2]

Vincristine: IV: 2 mg day 1
[total dose/cycle = 2 mg]

Methotrexate: IV: 10 mg/m^2/day days 1 to 5
[total dose/cycle = 50 mg/m^2]

Prednisone: Oral: 200 mg/day days 1 to 5
[total dose/cycle = 1000 mg]

Repeat cycles every month (except months 7 and 11 or 9 and 12) for 2 years

Intensification

Etoposide: IV: 100 mg/m^2/day days 1 to 5
　[total dose/cycle = 500 mg/m^2]
Pegaspargase: IV: 2500 units/m^2 day 1
　[total dose/cycle = 2500 units/m^2]
Given during months 9 and 12 of maintenance
or
Methotrexate: IV: 100 mg/m^2/day days 1, 8, 15, and 22
　[total dose/cycle = 400 mg/m^2]
Asparaginase: IV: 20,000 units/day days 2, 9, 16, and 23
　[total dose/cycle = 80,000 units]
Given during months 7 and 11 of maintenance

Variation 4:

Cycle A (Cycles 1, 3, 5, and 7):

Cyclophosphamide: IV: 300 mg/m^2 every 12 hours, for 6 doses, days 1, 2, and 3
　[total dose/cycle = 1800 mg/m^2]
Mesna: IV: 600 mg/m^2/day continuous infusion days 1, 2, and 3
　[total dose/cycle = 1800 mg/m^2]
Vincristine: IV: 2 mg/day days 4 and 11
　[total dose/cycle = 4 mg]
Doxorubicin: IV: 50 mg/m^2 day 4
　[total dose/cycle = 50 mg/m^2]
Dexamethasone: (route not specified): 40 mg/day days 1 to 4 and 11 to 14
　[total dose/cycle = 320 mg]

Cycle B (Cycles 2, 4, 6, and 8):

Methotrexate: IV: 200 mg/m^2 day 1
　followed by IV: 800 mg/m^2 continuous infusion day 1
　　[total dose/cycle = 1 g/m^2]
Leucovorin: (route not specified): 15 mg every 6 hours, for 8 doses (start 24 hours after end of methotrexate infusion)
　[total dose/cycle = 120 mg]
Cytarabine: IV: 3 g/m^2 every 12 hours, for 4 doses, days 2 and 3
　[total dose/cycle = 12 g/m^2]
Repeat every 6 weeks in the following sequence: ABABABAB

CNS Prophylaxis

Methotrexate: Intrathecal: 12 mg day 2
　[total dose/cycle = 12 mg]
Cytarabine: Intrathecal: 100 mg day 8
　[total dose/cycle = 100 mg]
Repeat cycle every 3 weeks for 4 or 8 cycles

Maintenance (POMP)

Mercaptopurine: Oral: 50 mg 3 times/day
　[total dose/cycle = 4200-4650 mg]
Vincristine: IV: 2 mg day 1
　[total dose/cycle = 2 mg]
Methotrexate: Oral: 20 mg/m^2/day days 1, 8, 15, and 22
　[total dose/cycle = 80 mg/m^2]
Prednisone: Oral: 200 mg/day days 1 to 5
　[total dose/cycle = 1000 mg/m^2]
or
Mercaptopurine: IV: 1 g/m^2/day days 1 to 5
　[total dose/cycle = 5 g/m^2]

◀

Vincristine: IV: 2 mg day 1
  [total dose/cycle = 2 mg]
Methotrexate: IV: 10 mg/m^2/day days 1 to 5
  [total dose/cycle = 50 mg/m^2]
Prednisone: Oral: 200 mg/day days 1 to 5
  [total dose/cycle = 1000 mg/m^2]
or
Interferon alfa: SubQ: 5 million units/m^2 daily
  [total dose/cycle = 140-155 million units/m^2]
Cytarabine: SubQ: 10 mg daily
  [total dose/cycle = 280-310 mg]
Repeat cycles every month for 2 years
Variation 5:
 Cycle A (Cycles 1, 4, 6, and 8):
  Cyclophosphamide: IV: 300 mg/m^2 every 12 hours, for 6 doses, days 1, 2, and 3
   [total dose/cycle = 1800 mg/m^2]
  Mesna: IV: 600 mg/m^2/day continuous infusion days 1, 2, and 3
   [total dose/cycle = 1800 mg/m^2]
  Vincristine: IV: 2 mg/day days 4 and 11
   [total dose/cycle = 4 mg]
  Doxorubicin: IV: 50 mg/m^2 continuous infusion day 4
   [total dose/cycle = 50 mg/m^2]
  Dexamethasone: Oral, IV: 40 mg/day days 1 to 4 and 11 to 14
   [total dose/cycle = 320 mg]
 Cycle B (Cycles 3, 5, 7, and 9):
  Methotrexate: IV: 200 mg/m^2 day 1
   followed by IV: 800 mg/m^2 continuous infusion day 1
    [total dose/cycle = 1 g/m^2]
  Leucovorin: IV: 50 mg (start 12 hours after end of methotrexate infusion)
   followed by IV: 15 mg every 6 hours, for 8 doses
    [total dose/cycle = 170 mg]
  Cytarabine: IV: 3 g/m^2 every 12 hours, for 4 doses, days 2 and 3
   [total dose/cycle = 12 g/m^2]
 Cycle C: Liposomal Daunorubicin/Cytarabine (Cycle 2):
  Daunorubicin, liposomal: IV: 150 mg/m^2/day days 1 and 2
   [total dose/cycle = 300 mg/m^2]
  Cytarabine: IV: 1.5 g/m^2/day continuous infusion days 1 and 2
   [total dose/cycle = 3 g/m^2]
  Prednisone: Oral: 200 mg/day days 1 to 5
   [total dose/cycle = 1000 mg]
  Administer in the following sequence: ACBABABA (Cycle C does not repeat)
 CNS Prophylaxis
  Methotrexate: Intrathecal: 12 mg day 2
   [total dose/cycle = 12 mg]
  or 6 mg into Ommaya day 2
   [total dose/cycle = 6 mg]
  Cytarabine: Intrathecal: 100 mg day 7 **or** 8
   [total dose/cycle = 100 mg]
  Repeat cycle every 3 weeks for 6 or 8 cycles

Maintenance (POMP)
Mercaptopurine: IV: 1 g/m^2/day days 1 to 5
  [total dose/cycle = 5 g/m^2]
Vincristine: IV: 2 mg day 1
  [total dose/cycle = 2 mg]
Methotrexate: IV: 10 mg/m^2/day days 1 to 5
  [total dose/cycle = 50 mg/m^2]
Prednisone: Oral: 200 mg/day days 1 to 5
  [total dose/cycle = 1000 mg]
Repeat cycles monthly, except months 6, 7, 18, and 19 for 3 years

Intensification
Methotrexate: IV: 100 mg/m^2/day days 1, 8, 15, and 22
  [total dose/cycle = 400 mg/m^2]
Asparaginase: IV: 20,000 units/day days 2, 9, 16, and 23
  [total dose/cycle = 80,000 units]
Given during months 6 and 18 of maintenance
Cyclophosphamide: IV: 300 mg/m^2 every 12 hours, for 6 doses, days 1, 2, and 3
  [total dose/cycle = 1800 mg/m^2]
Mesna: IV: 600 mg/m^2/day continuous infusion days 1, 2, and 3
  [total dose/cycle = 1800 mg/m^2]
Vincristine: IV: 2 mg/day days 4 and 11
  [total dose/cycle = 4 mg]
Doxorubicin: IV: 50 mg/m^2/day continuous infusion day 4
  [total dose/cycle = 50 mg/m^2]
Dexamethasone: Oral, IV: 40 mg/day days 1 to 4 and 11 to 14
  [total dose/cycle = 320 mg]
Given during months 7 and 19 of maintenance

References

Variation 1:
Kantarjian H, Thomas D, O'Brien S, et al, "Long-Term Follow-Up Results of Hyperfractionated Cyclophosphamide, Vincristine, Doxorubicin, and Dexamethasone (Hyper-CVAD), A Dose-Intensive Regimen, in Adult Acute Lymphocytic Leukemia," *Cancer*, 2004, 101(12):2788-2801.
Variation 2:
Thomas DA, Cortes J, O'Brien S, et al, "Hyper-CVAD Program in Burkitt's-Type Adult Acute Lymphoblastic Leukemia," *J Clin Oncol*, 1999, 17(8):2461-70.
Variation 3:
Thomas DA, O'Brien S, Cortes J, et al, "Outcome With the Hyper-CVAD Regimens in Lymphoblastic Lymphoma," *Blood*, 2004, 104(6):1624-30.
Variation 4:
Kantarjian HM, O'Brien S, Smith TL, et al, "Results of Treatment With Hyper-CVAD, A Dose-Intensive Regimen, in Adult Acute Lymphocytic Leukemia," *J Clin Oncol*, 2000, 18(3): 547-61.
Variation 5:
Thomas DA, O'Brien S, Cortes J, et al, "Outcome With the Hyper-CVAD Regimens in Lymphoblastic Lymphoma," *Blood*, 2004, 104(6):1624-30.

Hyper-CVAD (Lymphoma, non-Hodgkin)

Use Lymphoma, non-Hodgkin

Regimen

Cycle A (Cycles 1, 3, 5, and 7):
Cyclophosphamide: IV: 300 mg/m^2 every 12 hours, for 6 doses, days 1, 2, and 3
  [total dose/cycle = 1800 mg/m^2]
Vincristine: IV: 2 mg/day days 4 and 11
  [total dose/cycle = 4 mg]

◄ Doxorubicin: IV: 25 mg/m^2/day continuous infusion days 4 and 5
[total dose/cycle = 50 mg/m^2]
Dexamethasone: Oral, IV: 40 mg/day days 1 to 4 and 11 to 14
[total dose/cycle = 320 mg]:
Cycle B (Cycles 2, 4, 6, and 8):
Methotrexate: IV: 200 mg/m^2 day 1
followed by IV: 800 mg/m^2 continuous infusion day 1
[total dose/cycle = 1 g/m^2]
Leucovorin: Oral: 50 mg
followed by Oral: 15 mg every 6 hours, for 8 doses (start 24 hours after end of methotrexate infusion)
[total dose/cycle = 170 mg]
Cytarabine: IV: 3 g/m^2 every 12 hours, for 4 doses, days 2 and 3
[total dose/cycle = 12 g/m^2]
Repeat every 6 weeks in the following sequence: ABABABAB

References

Khouri IF, Romaguera J, Kantarjian H, et al, "Hyper-CVAD and High-Dose Methotrexate/Cytarabine Followed by Stem-Cell Transplantation: An Active Regimen for Aggressive Mantle-Cell Lymphoma," *J Clin Oncol*, 1998, 16(12):3803-9.

Hyper-CVAD (Multiple Myeloma)

Use Multiple myeloma

Regimen

Cyclophosphamide: IV: 300 mg/m^2 every 12 hours, for 6 doses, days 1, 2, and 3
[total dose/cycle = 1800 mg/m^2]
Mesna: IV: 600 mg/m^2/day continuous infusion days 1, 2, and 3
[total dose/cycle = 1800 mg/m^2]
Doxorubicin: IV: 25 mg/m^2/day continuous infusion days 4 and 5
[total dose/cycle = 50 mg/m^2]
Vincristine: IV: 1 mg/day continuous infusion days 4 and 5
followed by IV: 2 mg day 11
[total dose/cycle = 4 mg]
Dexamethasone: Oral, IV: 20 mg/m^2/day days 1 to 5 and 11 to 14
[total dose/cycle = 180 mg/m^2]
Repeat cycle once if ≥50% reduction in myeloma protein

Maintenance

Cyclophosphamide: Oral: 125 mg/m^2 every 12 hours, for 10 doses, days 1 to 5
[total dose/cycle = 1250 mg/m^2]
Dexamethasone: Oral: 20 mg/m^2/day days 1 to 5
[total dose/cycle = 100 mg/m^2]
Repeat maintenance cycle every 5 weeks

References

Dimopoulos MA, Weber D, Kantarjian H, et al, "HyperCVAD for VAD-Resistant Multiple Myeloma," *Am J Hematol*, 1996, 52(2):77-81.

Ibrutinib (CLL Regimen)

Use Leukemia, chronic lymphocytic

Regimen

Ibrutinib: Oral: 420 mg once daily days 1 to 28
[total dose/cycle = 11,760 mg]
Repeat cycle every 28 days until disease progression or unacceptable toxicity

References

Byrd JC, Brown JR, O'Brien S, et al. Ibrutinib versus ofatumumab in previously treated chronic lymphoid leukemia. *N Engl J Med.* 2014;371(3):213-223.

Ibrutinib (NHL-Mantle Cell Regimen)
Use Lymphoma, non-Hodgkin (Mantle cell)
Regimen
Ibrutinib: Oral: 560 mg once daily days 1 to 28
  [total dose/cycle = 15,680 mg]
Repeat cycle every 28 days until disease progression or unacceptable toxicity
References

Wang ML, Rule S, Martin P, et al. Targeting BTK with ibrutinib in relapsed or refractory mantle-cell lymphoma. *N Engl J Med.* 2013;369(6):507-516.

Ibrutinib (Waldenstrom Macroglobulinemia Regimen)
Use Waldenstrom macroglobulinemia
Regimen
Ibrutinib: Oral: 420 mg once daily days 1 to 28
  [total dose/cycle = 11,760 mg]
Repeat cycle every 28 days until disease progression or unacceptable toxicity
References

Treon SP, Tripsas CK, Meid K, et al. Ibrutinib in previously treated Waldenström's macroglobulinemia. *N Engl J Med.* 2015;372(15):1430-1440.

♦ **ICE (Ewing Sarcoma)** see Ifosfamide-Carboplatin-Etoposide (Ewing Sarcoma) on page 2014

ICE (Hodgkin)
Index Terms Ifosfamide-Carboplatin-Etoposide (Hodgkin)
Use Lymphoma, Hodgkin
Regimen
Etoposide: IV: 100 mg/m^2/day days 1 to 3
  [total dose/cycle = 300 mg/m^2]
Carboplatin: IV: AUC 5 day 2 (maximum dose: 800 mg)
  [total dose/cycle = AUC 5, maximum dose/cycle: 800 mg]
Ifosfamide: IV: 5 g/m^2/day continuous infusion for 24 hours day 2
  [total dose/cycle = 5 g/m^2]
Mesna: IV: 5 g/m^2/day continuous infusion for 24 hours day 2
  [total dose/cycle = 5 g/m^2]
Filgrastim: 5 mcg/kg/day days 5 to 12 (except during PBPC mobilization)
Repeat cycle every 14 days for 2 cycles
References

Moskowitz CH, Nimer SD, Zelenetz AD, et al, "A 2-Step Comprehensive High-Dose Chemoradiotherapy Second-Line Program for Relapsed and Refractory Hodgkin Disease: Analysis by Intent to Treat and Development of a Prognostic Model," *Blood*, 2001, 97(3):616-23.

ICE (Lymphoma, non-Hodgkin)
Use Lymphoma, non-Hodgkin
Regimen
Etoposide: IV: 100 mg/m^2/day days 1, 2, and 3
  [total dose/cycle = 300 mg/m^2]
Carboplatin: IV: AUC 5 (maximum dose: 800 mg) day 2
  [total dose/cycle = AUC = 5]
Ifosfamide: IV: 5000 mg/m^2 continuous infusion day 2
  [total dose/cycle = 5000 mg/m^2]

Mesna: IV: 5000 mg/m² continuous infusion day 2
[total dose/cycle = 5000 mg/m²]
Filgrastim: SubQ: 5 mcg/kg/day days 5-12 (cycles 1 and 2 only)
[total dose/cycle = 40 mcg/kg]
followed by SubQ: 10 mcg/kg/day day 5 through completion of leukaphoresis (cycle 3 only)
Repeat cycle every 2 weeks for 3 cycles

References

Moskowitz CH, Bertino JR, Glassman JR, et al, "Ifosfamide, Carboplatin, and Etoposide: A Highly Effective Cytoreduction and Peripheral-Blood Progenitor-Cell Mobilization Regimen for Transplant-Eligible Patients With Non-Hodgkin's Lymphoma," *J Clin Oncol*, 1999, 17(12):3776-85.

♦ **ICE (Osteosarcoma)** *see* Ifosfamide-Carboplatin-Etoposide (Osteosarcoma) *on page 2015*

♦ **IC (Small Cell Lung Cancer)** *see* Carboplatin-Irinotecan (Small Cell Lung Cancer) *on page 1868*

♦ **Idarubicin-ATRA (APL)** *see* Tretinoin-Idarubicin (APL) *on page 2099*

♦ **Idarubicin-Cytarabine (5 + 2) (AML Consolidation)** *see* 5 + 2 (Cytarabine-Idarubicin) (AML Consolidation) *on page 1816*

♦ **Idarubicin-Tretinoin (APL)** *see* Tretinoin-Idarubicin (APL) *on page 2099*

Idelalisib (NHL-Follicular Regimen)

Use Lymphoma, non-Hodgkin (follicular)
Regimen
Idelalisib: Oral: 150 mg twice daily days 1 to 28, taken with or without food
[total dose/cycle = 8400 mg]
Repeat cycle every 28 days until disease progression or unacceptable toxicity

References

Gopal AK, Kahl BS, de Vos S, et al. PI3Kδ inhibition by idelalisib in patients with relapsed indolent lymphoma. *N Engl J Med*. 2014;370(11):1008-1018.

Idelalisib-Rituximab (CLL)

Index Terms Rituximab-Idelalisib (CLL)
Use Leukemia, chronic lymphocytic
Regimen
Idelalisib: Oral: 150 mg twice daily starting day 1, continue until disease progression or unacceptable toxicity
Rituximab: IV: 375 mg/m² day 1
followed by: IV: 500 mg/m² every 2 weeks for 4 doses
followed by: IV: 500 mg/m² every 4 weeks for 3 doses
Total of 8 Rituximab infusions.

References

Furman RR, Sharman JP, Coutre SE, et al. Idelalisib and rituximab in relapsed chronic lymphocytic leukemia. *New Engl J Med*. 2014;370(11):997-1007.

Ifosfamide-Carboplatin-Etoposide (Ewing Sarcoma)

Index Terms ICE (Ewing Sarcoma)
Use Ewing sarcoma (recurrent, refractory)
Regimen NOTE: Mesna uroprotection should be administered.
Ifosfamide: IV: 1,800 mg/m²/day days 1 to 5
[total dose/cycle = 9,000 mg/m²]
Carboplatin: IV: 400 mg/m²/day days 1 and 2
[total dose/cycle = 800 mg/m²]

Etoposide: IV: 100 mg/m^2/day days 1 to 5
  [total dose/cycle = 500 mg/m^2]
Filgrastim: SubQ: 5 to 10 mcg/kg/day days 6 to 18 if ANC ≥1,000/mm^3 or until
  post nadir ANC ≥1,000/mm^3
  [total dose/cycle = up to 65 to 130 mcg/kg]
Repeat cycle every 21 days for up to 12 cycles

References

Van Winkle P, Angiolillo A, Krailo M, et al. Ifosfamide, carboplatin, and etoposide (ICE) reinduction chemotherapy in a large cohort of children and adolescents with recurrent/refractory sarcoma: the Children's Cancer Group (CCG) experience. *Pediatr Blood Cancer.* 2005;44(4):338-347.

◆ **Ifosfamide-Carboplatin-Etoposide (Hodgkin)** *see* ICE (Hodgkin)
  on page 2013

Ifosfamide-Carboplatin-Etoposide (Osteosarcoma)

Index Terms ICE (Osteosarcoma)

Use Osteosarcoma (recurrent, refractory)

Regimen NOTE: Mesna uroprotection should be administered.
Ifosfamide: IV: 1,800 mg/m^2/day days 1 to 5
  [total dose/cycle = 9,000 mg/m^2]
Carboplatin: IV: 400 mg/m^2/day days 1 and 2
  [total dose/cycle = 800 mg/m^2]
Etoposide: IV: 100 mg/m^2/day days 1 to 5
  [total dose/cycle = 500 mg/m^2]
Filgrastim: SubQ: 5 to 10 mcg/kg/day days 6 to 18 if ANC ≥1,000/mm^3 or until
  post nadir ANC ≥1,000/mm^3
  [total dose/cycle = up to 65 to 130 mcg/kg]
Repeat cycle every 21 days for up to 12 cycles

References

Van Winkle P, Angiolillo A, Krailo M, et al. Ifosfamide, carboplatin, and etoposide (ICE) reinduction chemotherapy in a large cohort of children and adolescents with recurrent/refractory sarcoma: the Children's Cancer Group (CCG) experience. *Pediatr Blood Cancer.* 2005;44(4):338-347.

Ifosfamide-Cisplatin-Epirubicin (Osteosarcoma)

Index Terms Cisplatin-Ifosfamide-Epirubicin (Osteosarcoma)

Use Bone sarcoma (osteosarcoma, pre and postoperative)

Regimen
Cycles 1 to 3 (prior to surgery):
Epirubicin: IV: 90 mg/m^2 over 15 minutes day 1
  [total dose/cycle = 90 mg/m^2]
Cisplatin: IV: 100 mg/m^2 over 2 hours day 1
  [total dose/cycle = 100 mg/m^2]
Ifosfamide: IV: 2,000 mg/m^2/day over 4 hours days 2, 3, and 4
  [total dose/cycle = 6,000 mg/m^2]
Mesna: IV: 2,000 mg/m^2/day over 4 hours days 2, 3, and 4
  [total dose/cycle = 6,000 mg/m^2]
Repeat cycle every 21 days for 3 cycles
Cycles 4 to 6 (after surgery):
Epirubicin: IV: 90 mg/m^2 over 15 minutes day 1
  [total dose/cycle = 90 mg/m^2]
Cisplatin: IV: 100 mg/m^2 over 2 hours day 1
  [total dose/cycle = 100 mg/m^2]
Ifosfamide: IV: 2,000 mg/m^2/day over 4 hours days 2, 3, and 4
  [total dose/cycle = 6,000 mg/m^2]

Mesna: IV: 2,000 mg/m^2/day over 4 hours days 2, 3, and 4
[total dose/cycle = 6,000 mg/m^2]
Repeat cycle every 28 days for 3 cycles

References

Basaran M, Bavbek ES, Saglam S, et al. A phase II study of cisplatin, ifosfamide and epirubicin combination chemotherapy in adults with nonmetastatic and extremity osteosarcomas. *Oncology*. 2007;72(3-4):255-260.

♦ **Ifosfamide-Doxorubicin (Soft Tissue Sarcoma)** *see* AIM (Soft Tissue Sarcoma) *on page 1827*

♦ **Ifosfamide-Epirubicin (Soft Tissue Sarcoma)** *see* Epirubicin-Ifosfamide (Soft Tissue Sarcoma) *on page 1957*

Ifosfamide-Etoposide (Ewing Sarcoma)

Use Bone sarcoma (Ewing sarcoma)
Regimen NOTE: Mesna uroprotection should be administered.
Etoposide: IV: 100 mg/m^2/day over 1 hour days 1 to 5
[total dose/cycle = 500 mg/m^2]
Ifosfamide: IV: 1,800 mg/m^2/day days 1 to 5
[total dose/cycle = 9,000 mg/m^2]
Repeat cycle every 21 days for a total of 12 cycles

References

Miser JS, Kinsella TJ, Triche TJ, et al. Ifosfamide with mesna uroprotection and etoposide: an effective regimen in the treatment of recurrent sarcomas and other tumors of children and young adults. *J Clin Oncol*. 1987;5(8):1191-1198.

♦ **Ifosfamide, Gemcitabine, Vinorelbine, Prednisolone (Hodgkin)** *see* IGEV (Hodgkin) *on page 2016*

IGEV (Hodgkin)

Index Terms Ifosfamide, Gemcitabine, Vinorelbine, Prednisolone (Hodgkin)
Use Lymphoma, Hodgkin
Regimen
Ifosfamide: IV: 2000 mg/m^2/day over 2 hours days 1 to 4
[total dose/cycle = 8000 mg/m^2]
Mesna: IV: 2600 mg/m^2/day days 1 to 4
[total dose/cycle = 10,400 mg/m^2]
Gemcitabine: IV: 800 mg/m^2 days 1 and 4
[total dose/cycle = 1600 mg/m^2]
Vinorelbine: IV: 20 mg/m^2 day 1
[total dose/cycle = 20 mg/m^2]
Prednisolone: IV: 100 mg days 1 to 4
[total dose/cycle = 400 mg/m^2]
Filgrastim: Days 7 to 12 of each course or up to apheresis in the course of mobilization
Repeat cycle every 21 days for a total of 4 cycles

References

Santoro A, Magagnoli M, Spina M, et al, "Ifosfamide, Gemcitabine, and Vinorelbine: A New Induction Regimen for Refractory and Relapsed Hodgkin's Lymphoma," *Haematologica*, 2007, 92(1):35-41.

♦ **IL-2-Interferon Alfa 2 (RCC)** *see* Interleukin 2-Interferon Alfa-2 (RCC) *on page 2018*

Imatinib (CML Regimen)

Use Leukemia, chronic myelogenous

Regimen NOTE: Multiple variations are listed.

Variation 1 (chronic phase):

Imatinib: Oral: 400 mg once daily

[total dose/cycle = 11,200 mg]

Repeat cycle every 28 days until disease progression or unacceptable toxicity

Variation 2 (accelerated phase and blast crisis):

Imatinib: Oral: 600 mg once daily

[total dose/cycle = 16,800 mg]

Repeat cycle every 28 days until disease progression or unacceptable toxicity

Variation 3 (chronic phase high dose):

Imatinib: Oral: 400 mg twice daily

[total dose/cycle = 22,400 mg]

Repeat cycle every 28 days until disease progression or unacceptable toxicity

References

Variation 1:

Deininger M, O'Brien SG, Guilhot F, et al, "International Randomized Study of Interferon Vs STI571 (IRIS) 8-Year Follow Up: Sustained Survival and Low Risk for Progression or Events in Patients With Newly Diagnosed Chronic Myeloid Leukemia in Chronic Phase (CML-CP) Treated With Imatinib," *Blood*, 2009, 114:abstract 1126.

Druker BJ, Guilhot F, O'Brien SG, et al, "Five-Year Follow-Up of Patients Receiving Imatinib for Chronic Myeloid Leukemia," *N Engl J Med*, 2006, 355(23):2408-17.

O'Brien SG, Guilhot F, Larson RA, et al, "Imatinib Compared With Interferon and Low-Dose Cytarabine for Newly Diagnosed Chronic-Phase Chronic Myeloid Leukemia," *N Engl J Med*, 2003, 348(11):994-1004.

Variation 2:

Sawyers CL, Hochhaus A, Feldman E, et al, "Imatinib Induces Hematologic and Cytogenetic Responses in Patients With Chronic Myelogenous Leukemia in Myeloid Blast Crisis: Results of a Phase II Study," *Blood*, 2002, 99(10):3530-9.

Talpaz M, Silver RT, Druker BJ, et al, "Imatinib Induces Durable Hematologic and Cytogenetic Responses in Patients With Accelerated Phase Chronic Myeloid Leukemia: Results of a Phase 2 Study," *Blood*, 2002, 99(6):1928-37.

Variation 3:

Cortes JE, Baccarani M, Guilhot F, et al, "Phase III, Randomized, Open-Label Study of Daily Imatinib Mesylate 400 mg Versus 800 mg in Patients With Newly Diagnosed, Previously Untreated Chronic Myeloid Leukemia in Chronic Phase Using Molecular End Points: Tyrosine Kinase Inhibitor Optimization and Selectivity Study," *J Clin Oncol*, 2010, 28(3):424-30.

Imatinib (GIST Regimen)

Use Soft Tissue Sarcoma (Gastrointestinal Stromal Tumor [GIST])

Regimen NOTE: Multiple variations are listed.

Variation 1 (metastatic):

Imatinib: Oral: 400 mg once daily days 1 to 28

[total dose/cycle = 11,200 mg]

Repeat cycle every 28 days until disease progression or unacceptable toxicity

Variation 2 (adjuvant):

Imatinib: Oral: 400 mg once daily days 1 to 28

[total dose/cycle = 11,200 mg]

Repeat cycle every 28 days for 3 years

References
Variation 1:

Blanke CD, Rankin C, Demetri GD, et al. Phase III randomized, intergroup trial assessing imatinib mesylate at two dose levels in patients with unresectable or metastatic gastrointestinal stromal tumors expressing the kit receptor tyrosine kinase: S0033. *J Clin Oncol.* 2008;26(4):626-32.

Variation 2:

Joensuu H, Eriksson M, Sundby Hall K, et al, "One vs Three Years of Adjuvant Imatinib for Operable Gastrointestinal Stromal Tumor: A Randomized Trial," *JAMA*, 2012, 307(12):1265-72.

♦ **Interferon Alfa 2b-Bevacizumab (RCC)** *see* Bevacizumab-Interferon Alfa (RCC) *on page 1844*

♦ **Interferon Alfa 2-Interleukin (RCC)** *see* Interleukin 2-Interferon Alfa-2 (RCC) *on page 2018*

♦ **Interferon Alfa-Bevacizumab (RCC)** *see* Bevacizumab-Interferon Alfa (RCC) *on page 1844*

Interleukin 2-Interferon Alfa-2 (RCC)

Index Terms Aldesleukin-Interferon Alfa-2 (RCC); IL-2-Interferon Alfa 2 (RCC); Interferon Alfa 2-Interleukin (RCC)

Use Renal cell cancer

Regimen

Induction (2 cycles):

Aldesleukin: IV: 18 million units/m^2/day continuous infusion days 1 to 5 and days 12 to 16

[total dose/cycle = 180 million units/m^2]

Repeat aldesleukin induction cycle one time (total of 2 cycles) after a 3-week rest between cycles

Interferon Alfa-2: SubQ: 6 million units/dose 3 times weekly continuously (no rest break) during induction cycles

[total dose/week = 18 million units/week]

Maintenance (begin after a 3-week aldesleukin rest):

Aldesleukin: IV: 18 million units/m^2/day continuous infusion days 1 to 5

[total dose/cycle = 90 million units/m^2]

Repeat aldesleukin maintenance cycle 3 times (total of 4 maintenance cycles) after 3-week rest between cycles

Interferon Alfa-2: SubQ: 6 million units/dose 3 times weekly continuously (no rest break) during maintenance cycles

[total dose/week = 18 million units/week]

References
Negrier S, Escudier B, Lasset C, et al, "Recombinant Human Interleukin-2, Recombinant Human Interferon Alfa-2a, or Both in Metastatic Renal-Cell Carcinoma. Groupe Français d'Immunothérapie," *N Engl J Med*, 1998, 338(18):1272-8.

IPA

Use Hepatoblastoma

Regimen

Ifosfamide: IV: 500 mg/m^2 day 1

[total dose/cycle = 500 mg/m^2]

followed by IV: 1000 mg/m^2/day continuous infusion days 1 to 3

[total dose/cycle = 3000 mg/m^2]

Cisplatin: IV: 20 mg/m^2/day days 4 to 8

[total dose/cycle = 100 mg/m^2]

Doxorubicin: IV: 30 mg/m^2/day continuous infusion days 9 and 10

[total dose/cycle = 60 mg/m^2]

Repeat cycle every 21 days

References

von Schweinitz D, Byrd DJ, Hecker H, et al, "Efficiency and Toxicity of Ifosfamide, Cisplatin, and Doxorubicin in the Treatment of Childhood Hepatoblastoma. Study Committee of the Cooperative Paediatric Liver Tumour Study HB89 of the German Society for Paediatric Oncology and Haematology," *Eur J Cancer*, 1997, 33(8):1243-9.

Ipilimumab (Melanoma Regimen)

Use Melanoma

Regimen

Ipilimumab: IV: 3 mg/kg day 1

[total dose/cycle = 3 mg/kg]

Repeat cycle every 21 days for 4 cycles

References

Hodi FS, O'Day SJ, McDermott DF, et al, "Improved Survival With Ipilimumab in Patients With Metastatic Melanoma," *N Engl J Med*, 2010, 363(8):711-23.

Ipilimumab-Nivolumab (Melanoma)

Index Terms Nivolumab-Ipilimumab (Melanoma)

Use Melanoma (unresectable, metastatic, first-line)

Regimen

Cycles 1 to 4:

Nivolumab: IV: 1 mg/kg day 1

[total dose/cycle = 1 mg/kg]

Ipilimumab: IV: 3 mg/kg day 1

[total dose/cycle = 3 mg/kg]

Repeat cycle every 21 days for 4 cycles

Subsequent Cycles:

Nivolumab: IV: 3 mg/kg day 1

[total dose/cycle = 3 mg/kg]

Repeat cycle every 14 days until disease progression or unacceptable toxicity; treatment beyond progression was allowed in patients tolerating drug and experiencing clinical benefit

References

Larkin J, Hodi FS, Wolchok JD. Combined nivolumab and ipilimumab or monotherapy in untreated melanoma. *N Engl J Med.* 2015;373(13):1270-1271.

◆ **IP (Small Cell Lung Cancer)** *see* Carboplatin-Irinotecan (Small Cell Lung Cancer) *on page 1868*

◆ **IP (Small Cell Lung Cancer)** *see* Cisplatin-Irinotecan (Small Cell Lung Cancer) *on page 1908*

◆ **Irinotecan-Bevacizumab (Glioblastoma)** *see* Bevacizumab-Irinotecan (Glioblastoma) *on page 1844*

◆ **Irinotecan-Biweekly Cetuximab (Colorectal)** *see* Cetuximab (Biweekly)-Irinotecan (Colorectal) *on page 1879*

Irinotecan-Capecitabine (Esophageal Cancer)

Index Terms Capecitabine-Irinotecan (Esophageal Cancer)

Use Esophageal cancer

◀ **Regimen** NOTE: Multiple variations are listed.

Variation 1:

Irinotecan: IV: 250 mg/m^2/dose day 1

[total dose/cycle = 250 mg/m^2]

Capecitabine: Oral: 1000 mg/m^2/dose twice daily days 1 to 14

[total dose/cycle = 28000 mg/m^2]

Repeat cycle every 21 days until disease progression or unacceptable toxicity

Variation 2:

Irinotecan: IV: 250 mg/m^2/dose day 1

[total dose/cycle = 250 mg/m^2]

Capecitabine: Oral: 1000 mg/m^2/dose twice daily days 1 to 14

[total dose/cycle = 28000 mg/m^2]

Repeat cycle every 21 days for up to 24 weeks

References

Variation 1:

Moehler M, Kanzler S, Geissler M, et al, "A Randomized Multicenter Phase II Study Comparing Capecitabine With Irinotecan or Cisplatin in Metastatic Adenocarcinoma of the Stomach or Esophagogastric Junction," *Ann Oncol*, 2010, 21(1):71-7.

Variation 2:

Leary A, Assersohn L, Cunningham D, et al, "A Phase II Trial Evaluating Capecitabine and Irinotecan as Second Line Treatment in Patients With Oesophago-Gastric Cancer Who Have Progressed on, or Within 3 Months of Platinum-Based Chemotherapy," *Cancer Chemother Pharmacol*, 2009, 64(3):455-62.

Irinotecan-Capecitabine (Gastric Cancer)

Index Terms Capecitabine-Irinotecan (Gastric Cancer)

Use Gastric cancer

Regimen NOTE: Multiple variations are listed.

Variation 1:

Irinotecan: IV: 250 mg/m^2/dose day 1

[total dose/cycle = 250 mg/m^2]

Capecitabine: Oral: 1000 mg/m^2/dose twice daily days 1 to 14

[total dose/cycle = 28000 mg/m^2]

Repeat cycle every 21 days until disease progression or unacceptable toxicity

Variation 2:

Irinotecan: IV: 250 mg/m^2/dose day 1

[total dose/cycle = 250 mg/m^2]

Capecitabine: Oral: 1000 mg/m^2/dose twice daily days 1 to 14

[total dose/cycle = 28000 mg/m^2]

Repeat cycle every 21 days for up to 24 weeks

References

Variation 1:

Moehler M, Kanzler S, Geissler M, et al, "A Randomized Multicenter Phase II Study Comparing Capecitabine With Irinotecan or Cisplatin in Metastatic Adenocarcinoma of the Stomach or Esophagogastric Junction," *Ann Oncol*, 2010, 21(1):71-7.

Variation 2:

Leary A, Assersohn L, Cunningham D, et al, "A Phase II Trial Evaluating Capecitabine and Irinotecan as Second Line Treatment in Patients With Oesophago-Gastric Cancer Who Have Progressed on, or Within 3 Months of Platinum-Based Chemotherapy," *Cancer Chemother Pharmacol*, 2009, 64(3):455-62.

◆ **Irinotecan-Carboplatin (Small Cell Lung Cancer)** see Carboplatin-Irinotecan (Small Cell Lung Cancer) on page 1868

Irinotecan (Cervical Regimen)

Use Cervical cancer

Regimen

Irinotecan: IV: 125 mg/m^2/day over 90 minutes days 1, 8, 15, and 22; followed by a 2 week rest

[total dose/cycle = 500 mg/m^2]

Repeat cycle every 42 days until disease progression or unacceptable toxicity

References

Verschraegen CF, Levy T, Kudelka AP, et al. Phase II study of irinotecan in prior chemotherapy-treated squamous cell carcinoma of the cervix. *J Clin Oncol.* 1997;15(2):625-631.

♦ **Irinotecan-Cetuximab** *see* Cetuximab-Irinotecan (Colorectal) *on page 1883*

Irinotecan-Cisplatin (Esophageal Cancer)

Index Terms Cisplatin-Irinotecan (Esophageal Cancer)

Use Esophageal cancer

Regimen NOTE: Multiple variations are listed.

Variation 1:

Cisplatin: IV: 30 mg/m^2/dose days 1, 8, 15, and 22

[total dose/cycle = 120 mg/m^2]

Irinotecan: IV: 65 mg/m^2/dose days 1, 8, 15, and 22

[total dose/cycle = 260 mg/m^2]

Repeat cycle every 6 weeks until disease progression.

Variation 2 (with concurrent radiation therapy):

Cisplatin: IV: 30 mg/m^2/dose on day 1 and 8

[total dose/cycle = 60 mg/m^2]

Irinotecan: IV: 65 mg/m^2/dose day 1 and 8

[total dose/cycle = 130 mg/m^2]

Treatment cycle is 21 days; cycle is not repeated.

Variation 3:

Cisplatin: IV: 30 mg/m^2/dose on days 1, 8, 22, and 29

[total dose/cycle = 120 mg/m^2]

Irinotecan: IV: 50 mg/m^2/dose on days 1, 8, 22, and 29

[total dose/cycle = 200 mg/m^2]

Administered (with concurrent radiation therapy) over one 5-week treatment cycle.

Followed by: Postoperative therapy:

Cisplatin: IV: 30 mg/m^2/dose on days 1 and 8

[total dose/cycle = 60 mg/m^2]

Irinotecan: IV: 65 mg/m^2/dose on days 1 and 8

[total dose/cycle = 130 mg/m^2]

Repeat postop cycle every 21 days for a total of 3 cycles.

Variation 4:

Cisplatin: IV: 30 mg/m^2/dose on day 1 and 8

[total dose/cycle = 60 mg/m^2]

Irinotecan: IV: 65 mg/m^2/dose day 1 and 8

[total dose/cycle = 130 mg/m^2]

Repeat cycle every 21 days.

References

Variation 1

Ilson DH, Saltz L, Enzinger P, et al, "Phase II Trial of Weekly Irinotecan Plus Cisplatin in Advanced Esophageal Cancer," *J Clin Oncol*, 1999, 17(10):3270-5.

Variation 2:
Sharma R, Yang GY, Nava HR, et al, "A Single Institution Experience With Neoadjuvant Chemo-radiation (CRT) With Irinotecan (I) and Cisplatin (C) in Locally Advanced Esophageal Carcinoma (LAEC)," *J Clin Oncol*, 2009, 27(15S):e15619 [abstract e15619 from 2009 annual ASCO meeting].

Variation 3:
Kleinberg L, Powell ME, Forastiere AA, et al, "Survival Outcome of E1201: An Eastern Cooperative Oncology Group (ECOG) Randomized Phase II Trial of Neoadjuvant Preoperative Paclitaxel/Cisplatin/Radiotherapy (RT) or Irinotecan/Cisplatin/RT in Endoscopy With Ultrasound (EUS) Staged Esophageal Adenocarcinoma," *J Clin Oncol*, 2008, 26(15S):4532 [abstract 4532 from 2008 annual ASCO meeting].

Variation 4:
Ilson DH, "Phase II Trial of Weekly Irinotecan/Cisplatin in Advanced Esophageal Cancer," *Oncology (Williston Park)*, 2004, 18(14 Supp14):22-5.

◆ **Irinotecan-Cisplatin (Gastric)** *see* Cisplatin-Irinotecan (Gastric) *on page 1908*

◆ **Irinotecan-Cisplatin (NSCLC)** *see* Cisplatin-Irinotecan (NSCLC) *on page 1908*

◆ **Irinotecan-Cisplatin (Small Cell Lung Cancer)** *see* Cisplatin-Irinotecan (Small Cell Lung Cancer) *on page 1908*

Irinotecan (Colorectal Regimen)

Use Colorectal cancer

Regimen NOTE: Multiple variations are listed.

Variation 1:
Irinotecan: IV: 125 mg/m^2/week over 90 minutes weekly for 4 weeks on days 1, 8, 15, and 22
[total dose/cycle = 500 mg/m^2]
Repeat cycle every 6 weeks until disease progression or unacceptable toxicity

Variation 2:
Irinotecan: IV: 350 mg/m^2 over 90 minutes day 1
[total dose/cycle = 350 mg/m^2]
Repeat cycle every 21 days until disease progression or unacceptable toxicity

Variation 3 (patients ≥70 years, ECOG PS 2, previous pelvic irradiation):
Irinotecan: IV: 300 mg/m^2 over 90 minutes day 1
[total dose/cycle = 300 mg/m^2]
Repeat cycle every 21 days until disease progression or unacceptable toxicity

References

Variation 1, 2, 3:
Fuchs CS, Moore MR, Harker G, et al, "Phase III Comparison of Two Irinotecan Dosing Regimens in Second-Line Therapy of Metastatic Colorectal Cancer," *J Clin Oncol*, 2003, 21(5):807-14.

Irinotecan-Fluorouracil-Leucovorin (Esophageal Cancer)

Index Terms Fluorouracil-Leucovorin-Irinotecan (Esophageal Cancer); Irinotecan-Leucovorin-Fluorouracil (Esophageal cancer)

Use Esophageal cancer

Regimen NOTE: Multiple variations are listed.

Variation 1:
Irinotecan: IV: 80 mg/m^2/dose days 1, 8, 15, 22, 29, and 36
[total dose/week = 480 mg/m^2]

Fluorouracil: IV: 2000 mg/m^2/dose continuous infusion over 24 hours days 1, 8, 15, 22, 29, and 36

[total dose/cycle = 12,000 mg/m^2]

Leucovorin: IV: 500 mg/m^2/dose continuous infusion over 24 hours days 1, 8, 15, 22, 29, and 36

[total dose/week = 3000 mg/m^2]

Repeat cycle every 8 weeks until disease progression or unacceptable toxicity.

Variation 2:

Irinotecan: IV: 80 mg/m^2/dose day 1

[total dose/cycle = 80 mg/m^2]

Leucovorin: IV: 500 mg/m^2/dose over 2 hours day 1

[total dose/cycle = 500 mg/m^2]

Fluorouracil: IV: 2000 mg/m^2/dose continuous infusion over 22 hours day 1 (begin immediately after leucovorin)

[total dose/cycle = 2000 mg/m^2]

Repeat every week for 6 weeks followed by a 1-week rest, continue until disease progression or unacceptable toxicity.

References

Variation 1:

Wolff K, Wein A, Reulbach U, et al, "Weekly High-Dose 5-Fluorouracil as a 24-h Infusion and Sodium Folinic Acid (AIO Regimen) Plus Irinotecan in Patients With Locally Advanced Non-resectable and Metastatic Adenocarcinoma or Squamous Cell Carcinoma of the Oesophagus: A Phase II Trial," *Anticancer Drugs*, 2009, 20(3):165-73.

Variation 2:

Dank M, Zaluski J, Barone C, et al, "Randomized Phase III Study Comparing Irinotecan Combined With 5-Fluorouracil and Folinic Acid to Cisplatin Combined With 5-Fluorouracil in Chemotherapy Naive Patients With Advanced Adenocarcinoma of the Stomach or Esophagogastric Junction," *Ann Oncol*, 2008, 19(8):1450-7.

◆ **Irinotecan-Fluorouracil-Leucovorin (Saltz Regimen) (Colorectal)** *see* Fluorouracil-Leucovorin-Irinotecan (Saltz Regimen) (Colorectal) *on page 1981*

◆ **Irinotecan-Leucovorin-Fluorouracil (Esophageal cancer)** *see* Irinotecan-Fluorouracil-Leucovorin (Esophageal Cancer) *on page 2022*

Irinotecan-Leucovorin-Fluorouracil (Gastric Cancer)

Index Terms Fluorouracil-Leucovorin-Irinotecan (Gastric Cancer)

Use Gastric cancer

Regimen NOTE: Multiple variations are listed.

Variation 1:

Irinotecan: IV: 80 mg/m^2/dose day 1

[total dose/week = 80 mg/m^2]

Leucovorin: IV: 500 mg/m^2/dose over 2 hours day 1

[total dose/week = 500 mg/m^2]

Fluorouracil: IV: 2000 mg/m^2/dose continuous infusion over 22 hours day 1

[total dose/week = 2000 mg/m^2]

Repeat cycle weekly for 6 weeks followed by a 1-week rest; repeat until disease progression or unacceptable toxicity

Variation 2:

Irinotecan: IV: 180 mg/m^2/dose day 1

[total dose/cycle = 180 mg/m^2]

Leucovorin: IV: 200 mg/m^2/dose over 2 hours days 1 and 2

[total dose/cycle = 400 mg/m^2]

◀   Fluorouracil: IV bolus: 400 mg/m² days 1 and 2
    followed by IV: 600 mg/m²/dose continuous infusion over 22 hours days 1
    and 2
    [total dose/cycle = 2000 mg/m²]
  Repeat cycle every 14 days for at least 4 cycles or until disease progression
  or unacceptable toxicity

References
Variation 1:
Dank M, Zaluski J, Barone C, et al, "Randomized Phase III Study Comparing Irinotecan Combined With 5-Fluorouracil and Folinic Acid to Cisplatin Combined With 5-Fluorouracil in Chemotherapy Naive Patients With Advanced Adenocarcinoma of the Stomach or Esophagogastric Junction," *Ann Oncol*, 2008, 19(8):1450-7.
Variation 2:
Bouché O, Raoul JL, Bonnetain F, et al, "Randomized Multicenter Phase II Trial of a Biweekly Regimen of Fluorouracil and Leucovorin (LV5FU2), LV5FU2 Plus Cisplatin, or LV5FU2 Plus Irinotecan in Patients With Previously Untreated Metastatic Gastric Cancer: A Federation Francophone de Cancerologie Digestive Group Study–FFCD 9803," *J Clin Oncol*, 2004, 22 (21):4319-28.

♦ **Irinotecan-Oxaliplatin-Fluorouracil-Leucovorin (Pancreatic)** *see* FOLFIR-INOX (Pancreatic) *on page* 1984

♦ **Irinotecan, Oxaliplatin, Leucovorin, Fluorouracil (Colorectal)** *see* FOL-FOXIRI (Colorectal) *on page* 1987

Irinotecan (Small Cell Lung Cancer Regimen)
Use Lung cancer, small cell
Regimen
Irinotecan: IV: 100 mg/m²/day over 90 minutes days 1, 8, 15, and 22
  [total dose/cycle = 400 mg/m²]
Repeat cycle every 28 days

References
Masuda N, Fukuoka M, Kusunoki Y, et al, "CPT-11: A New Derivative of Camptothecin for the Treatment of Refractory or Relapsed Small-Cell Lung Cancer," *J Clin Oncol*, 1992, 10(8):1225-9.

Irinotecan-Temozolomide (Ewing Sarcoma)
Index Terms Temozolomide-Irinotecan (Ewing Sarcoma)
Use Ewing sarcoma
Regimen
Irinotecan: IV: 20 mg/m²/dose days 1 to 5 and days 8 to 12
  [total dose/cycle = 200 mg/m²]
Temozolomide: Oral: 100 mg/m²/dose days 1 to 5
  [total dose/cycle = 500 mg/m²]
Repeat cycle every 21 days

References
Casey DA, Wexler LH, Merchant MS, et al, "Irinotecan and Temozolomide for Ewing Sarcoma: The Memorial Sloan-Kettering Experience," *Pediatr Blood Cancer*, 2009, 53(6):1029-34.

Ixabepilone (Breast Regimen)
Use Breast cancer
Regimen
Ixabepilone: IV: 40 mg/m² over 3 hours day 1
  [total dose/cycle = 40 mg/m²]
Repeat cycle every 21 days until disease progression or unacceptable toxicity,
for up to a maximum of 18 cycles

References

Pérez EA, Lerzo G, Pivot X, et al, "Efficacy and Safety of Ixabepilone (BMS-247550), in a Phase II Study of Patients With Advanced Breast Cancer Resistant to an Anthracycline, a Taxane and Capecitabine," *J Clin Oncol*, 2007, 25(23):3407-14.

♦ **Ixabepilone-Capecitabine (Breast)** *see* Capecitabine-Ixabepilone (Breast) *on page 1858*

Ixabepilone (Endometrial Regimen)

Use Endometrial cancer (advanced, recurrent)

Regimen

Ixabepilone: IV: 40 mg/m^2 over 3 hours day 1

[total dose/cycle = 40 mg/m^2]

Repeat cycle every 21 days until disease progression or unacceptable toxicity

References

Dizon DS, Blessing JA, McMeekin DS, Sharma SK, Disilvestro P, Alvarez RD. Phase II trial of ixabepilone as second-line treatment in advanced endometrial cancer: gynecologic oncology group trial 129-P. *J Clin Oncol*. 2009;27(19):3104-3108.

♦ **Lapatinib-Capecitabine (Breast)** *see* Capecitabine + Lapatinib (Breast) *on page 1858*

Lapatinib-Letrozole (Breast)

Index Terms Letrozole-Lapatinib (Breast)

Use Breast cancer

Regimen

Lapatinib: Oral: 1500 mg once daily days 1 to 28

[total dose/cycle = 42,000 mg]

Letrozole: Oral: 2.5 mg once daily days 1 to 28

[total dose/cycle = 70 mg]

Repeat cycle every 28 days until disease progression or unacceptable toxicity

References

Johnston S, Pippen J Jr, Pivot X, et al, "Lapatinib Combined With Letrozole Versus Letrozole and Placebo as First-Line Therapy for Postmenopausal Hormone Receptor-Positive Metastatic Breast Cancer," *J Clin Oncol*, 2009, 27(33):5538-46.

Lapatinib-Trastuzumab (Breast)

Index Terms Trastuzumab-Lapatinib (Breast)

Use Breast cancer

Regimen

Cycle 1:

Trastuzumab: IV: 4 mg/kg (loading dose) day 1 cycle 1 only

[total dose/cycle 1 = 4 mg/kg]

Lapatinib: Oral: 1000 mg/day days 1 to 7, take on an empty stomach 1 hour before or 1 hour after a meal

[total dose/cycle = 7000 mg]

Treatment cycle is 7 days

Subsequent cycles:

Trastuzumab: IV: 2 mg/kg day 1

[total dose/cycle = 2 mg/kg]

Lapatinib: Oral: 1000 mg/day days 1 to 7, take on an empty stomach 1 hour before or 1 hour after a meal

[total dose/cycle = 7000 mg]

Repeat cycle every 7 days

◀

References

Blackwell KL, Burstein HJ, Stomiolo AM, et al. Overall survival benefit with lapatinib in combination with trastuzumab for patients with human epidermal growth factor receptor 2-positive metastatic breast cancer: final results from the EGF104900 Study. *J Clin Oncol*. 2012;30(21):2585-2592.

Blackwell KL, Burstein HJ, Stomiolo AM, et al. Randomized study of lapatinib alone or in combination with trastuzumab in women with ErbB2-positive, trastuzumab-refractory metastatic breast cancer. *J Clin Oncol*. 2010;28(7):1124-1130.

◆ **Larson 8811 Regimen (ALL)** *see* CALGB 8811 Regimen (ALL) on page *1853*

◆ **Larson 9111 Regimen (ALL)** *see* CALGB 9111 Regimen (ALL) *on page 1854*

◆ **Larson Regimen 8811 (ALL)** *see* CALGB 8811 Regimen (ALL) on page *1853*

◆ **Larson Regimen 9111 (ALL)** *see* CALGB 9111 Regimen (ALL) *on page 1854*

◆ **Lenalidomide-Bendamustine-Dexamethasone (Multiple Myeloma)** *see* Bendamustine-Lenalidomide-Dexamethasone (Multiple Myeloma) *on page 1834*

Lenalidomide-Bortezomib-Dexamethasone (Multiple Myeloma)

Index Terms Bortezomib-Lenalidomide-Dexamethasone (Multiple Myeloma); RVD (Multiple Myeloma); VDR (Multiple Myeloma); VRd (Multiple Myeloma)

Use Multiple myeloma (first-line, transplant eligible or relapsed/refractory)

Regimen NOTE: Multiple variations are listed.

Variation 1 (first-line, transplant eligible):

Induction cycles 1 to 4:

Lenalidomide: Oral: 25 mg daily days 1 to 14
[total dose/cycle = 350 mg]

Bortezomib: IV: 1.3 mg/m^2/day days 1, 4, 8, and 11
[total dose/cycle = 5.2 mg/m^2]

Dexamethasone: Oral: 20 mg daily days 1, 2, 4, 5, 8, 9, 11, and 12
[total dose/cycle = 160 mg]

Repeat cycle every 21 days for 4 cycles; patients with at least a partial response could proceed to autologous stem cell transplantation (after at least 4 cycles) or continue 4 more cycles of induction

Induction cycles 5 to 8:

Lenalidomide: Oral: 25 mg daily days 1 to 14
[total dose/cycle = 350 mg]

Bortezomib: IV: 1.3 mg/m^2/day days 1, 4, 8, and 11
[total dose/cycle = 5.2 mg/m^2]

Dexamethasone: Oral: 10 mg daily days 1, 2, 4, 5, 8, 9, 11, and 12
[total dose/cycle = 80 mg]

Repeat cycle every 21 days for 4 cycles (total of 8 induction cycles); patients with at least a partial response could proceed to autologous stem cell transplantation or proceed to maintenance therapy

Maintenance:

Lenalidomide: Oral: 25 mg daily days 1 to 14 (or dose tolerated at end of cycle 8 induction)
[total dose/cycle = 350 mg]

Bortezomib: IV: 1.3 mg/m^2/day days 1 and 8 (or dose tolerated at end of cycle 8 induction)
[total dose/cycle = 2.6 mg/m^2]

    Dexamethasone: Oral: 10 mg daily days 1, 2, 8, and 9
    [total dose/cycle = 40 mg]
    Repeat cycle every 21 days
Variation 2 (first-line, transplant eligible):
Induction:
    Lenalidomide: Oral: 25 mg daily days 1 to 14
    [total dose/cycle = 350 mg]
    Bortezomib: IV: 1.3 mg/m^2/day days 1, 4, 8, and 11
    [total dose/cycle = 5.2 mg/m^2]
    Dexamethasone: Oral: 40 mg daily days 1, 8, and 15
    [total dose/cycle = 120 mg]
    Repeat cycle every 21 days for up to 8 cycles then proceed to maintenance
    therapy. Alternatively, patients could undergo autologous stem cell trans-
    plantation any time after 4 cycles.
Maintenance:
    Bortezomib: IV: 1.3 mg/m^2/day days 1, 8, 15, and 22
    [total dose/cycle = 5.2 mg/m^2]
    Repeat cycle every 42 days for a total of 4 cycles
Variation 3 (first-line, transplant eligible):
Induction:
    Lenalidomide: Oral: 25 mg daily days 1 to 14
    [total dose/cycle = 350 mg]
    Bortezomib: IV: 1.3 mg/m^2/day days 1, 8, and 15
    [total dose/cycle = 3.9 mg/m^2]
    Dexamethasone: Oral: 40 mg daily days 1, 8, 15, and 22
    [total dose/cycle = 160 mg]
    or
    Dexamethasone: Oral: 20 mg daily days 1, 2, 8, 9, 15, and 16
    [total dose/cycle = 120 mg]
    Repeat cycle every 21 days
Variation 4 (relapsed or relapsed/refractory):
Induction cycles 1 to 4:
    Lenalidomide: Oral: 15 mg daily days 1 to 14
    [total dose/cycle = 210 mg]
    Bortezomib: IV: 1 mg/m^2/day days 1, 4, 8, and 11
    [total dose/cycle = 4 mg/m^2]
    Dexamethasone: Oral: 20 mg daily days 1, 2, 4, 5, 8, 9, 11, and 12
    [total dose/cycle = 160 mg]
    Repeat cycle every 21 days for 4 cycles
Induction cycles 5 to 8:
    Lenalidomide: Oral: 15 mg daily days 1 to 14
    [total dose/cycle = 210 mg]
    Bortezomib: IV: 1 mg/m^2/day days 1, 4, 8, and 11
    [total dose/cycle = 4 mg/m^2]
    Dexamethasone: Oral: 10 mg daily days 1, 2, 4, 5, 8, 9, 11, and 12
    [total dose/cycle = 80 mg]
    Repeat cycle every 21 days for 4 cycles (total of 8 induction cycles); patients
    with response or stable disease could proceed to maintenance therapy

Maintenance:

Lenalidomide: Oral: 15 mg daily days 1 to 14 (or dose tolerated at end of cycle 8 induction)

[total dose/cycle = 210 mg]

Bortezomib: IV: 1 mg/m^2/day days 1 and 8 (or dose tolerated at end of cycle 8 induction)

[total dose/cycle = 2 mg/m^2]

Dexamethasone: Oral: 10 mg daily days 1, 2, 8, and 9

[total dose/cycle = 40 mg]

Repeat cycle every 21 days until disease progression or unacceptable toxicity (may selectively discontinue any component while continuing the balance of maintenance therapy)

References

Variation 1:

Richardson PG, Weller E, Lonial S, et al, "Lenalidomide, Bortezomib, and Dexamethasone Combination Therapy in Patients With Newly Diagnosed Multiple Myeloma," *Blood*, 2010, 116 (5):679-86.

Variation 2:

Kumar S, Flinn I, Richardson PG, et al. Randomized, multicenter, phase 2 study (EVOLUTION) of combinations of bortezomib, dexamethasone, cyclophosphamide, and lenalidomide in previously untreated multiple myeloma. *Blood*. 2012;119(19):4375-4382.

Variation 3:

Rajkumar SV. Multiple myeloma: 2011 update on diagnosis, risk-stratification, and management. *Am J Hematol*. 2011;86(1):57-65.

Variation 4:

Richardson PG, Xie W, Jagannath S, et al. A phase 2 trial of lenalidomide, bortezomib, and dexamethasone in patients with relapsed and relapsed/refractory myeloma. *Blood*. 2014;123 (10):1461-1469.

◆ **Lenalidomide, Carfilzomib, Dexamethasone (Multiple Myeloma)** *see* Carfilzomib, Lenalidomide, Dexamethasone (Multiple Myeloma) *on page 1875*

Lenalidomide-Dexamethasone (Multiple Myeloma)

Index Terms Dexamethasone (Low-Dose)-Lenalidomide (Multiple Myeloma); Dexamethasone-Lenalidomide (Multiple Myeloma); Rd (Multiple Myeloma)

Use Multiple myeloma

Regimen NOTE: Multiple variations are listed.

Variation 1 (low dose dexamethasone):

Lenalidomide: Oral: 25 mg/day days 1 to 21

[total dose/cycle = 525 mg]

Dexamethasone: Oral: 40 mg/day days 1, 8, 15, and 22

[total dose/cycle = 160 mg]

Repeat cycle every 28 days

Variation 2:

Cycles 1 to 4:

Lenalidomide: Oral: 25 mg/day days 1 to 21

[total dose/cycle = 525 mg]

Dexamethasone: Oral: 40 mg/day days 1 to 4, 9 to 12, and 17 to 20 (cycles 1 to 4)

[total dose/cycle = 480 mg]

Repeat cycle every 28 days for 4 cycles

Subsequent cycles:
Lenalidomide: Oral: 25 mg/day days 1 to 21
[total dose/cycle = 525 mg]
Dexamethasone: Oral: 40 mg/day days 1 to 4
[total dose/cycle = 160 mg]
Repeat cycle every 28 days until disease progression or unacceptable toxicity

References

Variation 1:

Rajkumar SV, Jacobus S, Callander NS, et al. Lenalidomide plus high-dose dexamethasone versus lenalidomide plus low-dose dexamethasone as initial therapy for newly diagnosed multiple myeloma: an open-label randomised controlled trial. *Lancet Oncol.* 2010;11(1):29-37.

Variation 2:

Dimopoulos MA, Chen C, Spencer A, et al. Long-term follow-up on overall survival from the MM-009 and MM-010 phase III trials of lenalidomide plus dexamethasone in patients with relapsed or refractory multiple myeloma. *Leukemia.* 2009;23(11):2147-2152.

Dimopoulos M, Spencer A, Attal M, et al. Lenalidomide plus dexamethasone for relapsed or refractory multiple myeloma. *N Engl J Med.* 2007;357(21):2123-2132.

Weber DM, Chen C, Niesvizky R, et al. Lenalidomide plus dexamethasone for relapsed multiple myeloma in North America. *N Engl J Med.* 2007;357(21):2133-2142.

Lenalidomide (NHL-DLBCL Regimen)

Use Lymphoma, non-Hodgkin (DLBCL recurrent/refractory)
Regimen
Lenalidomide: Oral: 25 mg once daily on days 1 to 21
[total dose/cycle = 525 mg]
Repeat cycle every 28 days for up to one year of treatment
References

Wiernik PH, Lossos IS, Tuscano JM, et al. Lenalidomide monotherapy in relapsed or refractory aggressive non-Hodgkin's lymphoma. *J Clin Oncol.* 2008;26(30):4952-4957.

Lenalidomide (NHL-Mantle Cell Regimen)

Use Lymphoma, non-Hodgkin (Mantle cell)
Regimen
Lenalidomide: Oral: 25 mg once daily on days 1 to 21
[total dose/cycle = 525 mg]
Repeat cycle every 28 days until disease progression or unacceptable toxicity
References

Goy A, Sinha R, Williams ME, et al. Single-Agent Lenalidomide in Patients With Mantle-Cell Lymphoma Who Relapsed or Progressed After or Were Refractory to Bortezomib: Phase II MCL-001 (EMERGE) Study. *J Clin Oncol.* 2013;31(29):3688-95.

Lenalidomide-Rituximab (CLL)

Index Terms Rituximab-Lenalidomide (CLL)
Use Leukemia, chronic lymphocytic (relapsed/refractory)
Regimen
Cycle 1:
Rituximab: IV: 375 mg/m^2/day days 1, 8, 15, and 22
[total dose/cycle = 1,500 mg/m^2]
Lenalidomide: Oral: 10 mg daily starting on day 9 of cycle 1
[total dose/cycle = 200 mg]
Treatment duration of cycle 1 is 28 days
Cycle 2:
Lenalidomide: Oral: 10 mg daily days 1 to 28
[total dose/cycle = 280 mg]
Treatment duration of cycle 2 is 28 days

Cycles 3 to 12:
Rituximab: IV: 375 mg/m^2 day 1
[total dose/cycle = 375 mg/m^2]
Lenalidomide: Oral: 10 mg daily days 1 to 28
[total dose/cycle = 280 mg]
Repeat cycle every 28 days for a total of 12 cycles; if patients experienced ongoing partial or complete response lenalidomide could be continued beyond 12 cycles

References
Badoux XC, Keating MJ, Wen S, et al. Phase II study of lenalidomide and rituximab as salvage therapy for patients with relapsed or refractory chronic lymphocytic leukemia. *J Clin Oncol.* 2013;31(5):584-591.

Lenvatinib (Thyroid Regimen)

Use Thyroid cancer (radioiodine-refractory differentiated thyroid cancer)
Regimen
Lenvatinib: Oral: 24 mg once daily days 1 to 28, with or without food
[total dose/cycle = 672 mg]
Repeat cycle every 28 days until disease progression or unacceptable toxicity
References
Schlumberger M, Tahara M, Wirth LJ, et al. Lenvatinib versus placebo in radioiodine-refractory thyroid cancer. *N Engl J Med.* 2015;372(7):621-630.

♦ **Letrozole-Lapatinib (Breast)** *see* Lapatinib-Letrozole (Breast) *on page* 2025

♦ **Letrozole-Palbociclib (Breast)** *see* Palbociclib-Letrozole (Breast) *on page* 2058

Linker Protocol (ALL)

Use Leukemia, acute lymphocytic
Regimen
Remission induction:
Daunorubicin: IV: 50 mg/m^2/day days 1, 2, and 3
[total dose/cycle = 150 mg/m^2]
Vincristine: IV: 2 mg/day days 1, 8, 15, and 22
[total dose/cycle = 8 mg]
Prednisone: Oral: 60 mg/m^2/day days 1 to 28
[total dose/cycle = 1680 mg/m^2]
Asparaginase: IM: 6000 units/m^2/day days 17 to 28
[total dose/cycle = 72,000 units/m^2]
If residual leukemia in bone marrow on day 14:
Daunorubicin: IV: 50 mg/m^2 day 15
[total dose/cycle = 50 mg/m^2]
If residual leukemia in bone marrow on day 28:
Daunorubicin: IV: 50 mg/m^2/day days 29 and 30
[total dose/cycle = 100 mg/m^2]
Vincristine: IV: 2 mg/day days 29 and 36
[total dose/cycle = 4 mg]
Prednisone: Oral: 60 mg/m^2/day days 29 to 42
[total dose/cycle = 840 mg/m^2]
Asparaginase: IM: 6000 units/m^2/day days 29 to 35
[total dose/cycle = 42,000 units/m^2]

Consolidation therapy:
Treatment A (cycles 1, 3, 5, and 7):
Daunorubicin: IV: 50 mg/m^2/day days 1 and 2
[total dose/cycle = 100 mg/m^2]
Vincristine: IV: 2 mg/day days 1 and 8
[total dose/cycle = 4 mg]
Prednisone: Oral: 60 mg/m^2/day days 1 to 14
[total dose/cycle = 840 mg/m^2]
Asparaginase: IM: 12,000 units/m^2/day days 2, 4, 7, 9, 11, and 14
[total dose/cycle = 72,000 units/m^2]
Treatment B (cycles 2, 4, 6, and 8):
Teniposide: IV: 165 mg/m^2/day days 1, 4, 8, and 11
[total dose/cycle = 660 mg/m^2]
Cytarabine: IV: 300 mg/m^2/day days 1, 4, 8, and 11
[total dose/cycle = 1200 mg/m^2]
Treatment C (cycle 9):
Methotrexate: IV: 690 mg/m^2 continuous infusion over 42 hours day 1
[total dose/cycle = 690 mg/m^2]
Leucovorin: IV: 15 mg/m^2 every 6 hours for 12 doses (start at end of methotrexate infusion)
[total dose/cycle = 180 mg/m^2]
Administer remission induction regimen for one cycle only. Repeat consolidation cycle every 28 days.

References
Linker CA, Levitt LJ, O'Donnell M, et al, "Treatment of Adult Acute Lymphoblastic Leukemia With Intensive Cyclical Chemotherapy: A Follow-up Report," *Blood*, 1991 78(11):2814-22.

MAC (Gestational Trophoblastic Tumor)

Index Terms Methotrexate-Leucovorin-Cyclophosphamide-Dactinomycin (Gestational Trophoblastic Tumor)
Use Gestational trophoblastic tumor
Regimen
Methotrexate: IM: 1 mg/kg/day days 1, 3, 5, and 7
[total dose/cycle = 4 mg/kg]
Leucovorin: IM: 0.1 mg/kg/day (begin 24 hours after each methotrexate injection) days 2, 4, 6, and 8
[total dose/cycle = 0.4 mg/kg]
Dactinomycin: IV: 12 mcg/kg/day days 1 to 5
[total dose/cycle = 60 mcg/kg]
Cyclophosphamide: IV: 3 mg/kg/day days 1 to 5
[total dose/cycle = 15 mg/kg]
Repeat cycle every 21 days, continue until 3 consecutive normal hCG levels and then 1 more cycle

References
Berkowitz RS, Goldstein DP, Bernstein MR. Modified triple chemotherapy in the management of high-risk metastatic gestational trophoblastic tumors. *Gynecol Oncol*. 1984;19(2):173-181.

MAID (Soft Tissue Sarcoma)

Index Terms Doxorubicin-Dacarbazine-Ifosfamide-Mesna (Soft Tissue Sarcoma); Mesna-Doxorubicin-Ifosfamide-Dacarbazine (Soft Tissue Sarcoma)
Use Soft tissue sarcoma (metastatic, unresectable)

◀ **Regimen** NOTE: Multiple variations are listed. Mesna uroprotection should be administered.

Variation 1 (no prior radiation):

Doxorubicin: IV: 20 mg/m^2/day continuous infusion days 1, 2, and 3
[total dose/cycle = 60 mg/m^2]

Ifosfamide: IV: 2,500 mg/m^2/day infusion days 1, 2, and 3
[total dose/cycle = 7,500 mg/m^2]

Dacarbazine: IV: 300 mg/m^2/day continuous infusion days 1, 2, and 3
[total dose/cycle = 900 mg/m^2]

Repeat cycle every 21 days (delay 1 week if WBC <3,000/mm^3 or platelets <100,000/mm^3)

Variation 2 (if prior pelvic irradiation):

Doxorubicin: IV: 20 mg/m^2/day continuous infusion days 1, 2, and 3
[total dose/cycle = 60 mg/m^2]

Ifosfamide: IV: 1,500 mg/m^2/day infusion days 1, 2, and 3
[total dose/cycle = 4,500 mg/m^2]

Dacarbazine: IV: 300 mg/m^2/day continuous infusion days 1, 2, and 3
[total dose/cycle = 900 mg/m^2]

Repeat cycle every 21 days (delay 1 week if WBC <3,000/mm^3 or platelets <100,000/mm^3)

Variation 3:

Doxorubicin: IV: 15 mg/m^2/day continuous infusion days 1 to 4
[total dose/cycle = 60 mg/m^2]

Ifosfamide: IV: 2,000 mg/m^2/day continuous infusion days 1, 2, and 3
[total dose/cycle = 6,000 mg/m^2]

Dacarbazine: IV: 250 mg/m^2/day continuous infusion days 1 to 4
[total dose/cycle = 1,000 mg/m^2]

Repeat cycle every 21 days (or when WBC ≥3,000/mm^3 and platelets ≥100,000/mm^3)

References

Variations 1 and 2:

Elias A, Ryan L, Sulkes A, et al. Response to mesna, doxorubicin, ifosfamide, and dacarbazine in 108 patients with metastatic or unresectable sarcoma and no prior chemotherapy. *J Clin Oncol.* 1989;7(9):1208-1216.

Variation 3:

Antman K, Crowley J, Balcerzak SP, et al. An intergroup phase III randomized study of doxorubicin and dacarbazine with or without ifosfamide and mesna in advanced soft tissue and bone sarcomas. *J Clin Oncol.* 1993;11(7):1276-1285.

◆ **MEA (Gestational Trophoblastic Tumor)** *see* EMA (Gestational Trophoblastic Tumor) *on page 1955*

◆ **MEC (AML)** *see* Mitoxantrone-Etoposide-Cytarabine (AML) *on page 2038*

MEC-G (AML Induction)

Index Terms Cytarabine-Etoposide-Mitoxantrone-CSF (AML Induction); EMA-G (AML Induction)

Use Leukemia, acute myeloid

Regimen

Variation 1:

Mitoxantrone: IV: 12 mg/m^2/day days 1, 2, and 3
[total dose/cycle = 36 mg/m^2]

Cytarabine: IV: 500 mg/m^2/day continuous infusion days 1, 2, and 3 and days 8, 9, and 10
[total dose/cycle = 3000 mg/m^2]

Etoposide: IV: 200 mg/m^2/day continuous infusion days 8, 9, and 10
  [total dose/cycle = 600 mg/m^2]
Sargramostim: IV: 5 mcg/kg/day over 6 hours days 4 to 8
Variation 2:
Mitoxantrone: IV: 12 mg/m^2/day IV bolus days 1, 2, and 3
  [total dose/cycle = 36 mg/m^2]
Cytarabine: IV: 500 mg/m^2/day continuous infusion days 1, 2, and 3 and days 8, 9, and 10
  [total dose/cycle = 3000 mg/m^2]
Etoposide: IV: 200 mg/m^2/day continuous infusion days 8, 9, and 10
  [total dose/cycle = 600 mg/m^2]
Filgrastim: SubQ: 5 mcg/kg/day starting on day 4 til ANC >500/mm^3 for 2 consecutive days
Administer one cycle only

References

Variation 1:
Archimbaud E, Fenaux P, Reiffers J, et al, "Granulocyte-Macrophage Colony-Stimulating Factor in Association to Timed-Sequential Chemotherapy With Mitoxantrone, Etoposide, and Cytarabine for Refractory Acute Myelogenous Leukemia," *Leukemia*, 1993, 7(3):372-7.
Variation 2:
He XY, Elson P, Pohlman B, et al, "Timed Sequential Chemotherapy With Concomitant Granulocyte Colony-Stimulating Factor for High-Risk Acute Myelogenous Leukemia: A Single Arm Clinical Trial," *BMC Cancer*, 2002, 2:12.
He XY, Pohlman B, Lichtin A, et al, "Timed-Sequential Chemotherapy With Concomitant Granulocyte Colony-Stimulating Factor for Newly Diagnosed De Novo Acute Myelogenous Leukemia," *Leukemia*, 2003, 17(6):1078-84.

◆ **Mechlorethamine, Doxorubicin, Vinblastine, Vincristine, Bleomycin, Etoposide, Prednisone (Hodgkin)** see Stanford V (Hodgkin) on page 2085

◆ **Mechlorethamine, Vincristine, Procarbazine, Prednisone, Doxorubicin, Bleomycin, Vinblastine, Dacarbazine (Hodgkin)** see MOPP/ABVD (Hodgkin) on page 2039

◆ **Mechlorethamine, Vincristine, Procarbazine, Prednisone, Doxorubicin, Bleomycin, Vinblastine (Hodgkin)** see MOPP/ABV Hybrid (Hodgkin) on page 2040

◆ **Mechlorethamine, Vincristine, Procarbazine, Prednisone (Hodgkin)** see MOPP (Hodgkin) on page 2041

Melphalan-Prednisone-Bortezomib (Multiple Myeloma)

Index Terms Bortezomib-Melphalan-Prednisone (Multiple Myeloma); VMP (Multiple Myeloma)

Use Multiple myeloma

Regimen NOTE: Multiple variations are listed.
Variation 1:
Bortezomib: IV: 1.3 mg/m^2/day days 1, 4, 8, 11, 22, 25, 29, and 32
  [total dose/cycle = 10.4 mg/m^2]
Melphalan: Oral: 9 mg/m^2/day days 1 to 4
  [total dose/cycle = 36 mg/m^2]
Prednisone: Oral: 60 mg/m^2/day days 1 to 4
  [total dose/cycle = 240 mg/m^2]
Repeat cycle every 42 days for 4 cycles
followed by
Bortezomib: IV: 1.3 mg/m^2/day days 1, 8, 22, and 29
  [total dose/cycle = 5.2 mg/m^2]

◀ Melphalan: Oral: 9 mg/m^2/day days 1 to 4
 [total dose/cycle = 36 mg/m^2]
Prednisone: Oral: 60 mg/m^2/day days 1 to 4
 [total dose/cycle = 240 mg/m^2]
Repeat cycle every 42 days for 5 cycles
Variation 2:
 Bortezomib: IV: 1-1.3 mg/m^2/day days 1, 4, 8, 11, 22, 25, 29, and 32
 [total dose/cycle = 8-10.4 mg/m^2]
 Melphalan: Oral: 9 mg/m^2/day days 1 to 4
 [total dose/cycle = 36 mg/m^2]
 Prednisone: Oral: 60 mg/m^2/day days 1 to 4
 [total dose/cycle = 240 mg/m^2]
 Repeat cycle every 42 days for 4 cycles
 followed by
 Bortezomib: IV: 1-1.3 mg/m^2/day days 1, 8, 15, and 22
 [total dose/cycle = 4-5.2 mg/m^2]
 Melphalan: Oral: 9 mg/m^2/day days 1 to 4
 [total dose/cycle = 36 mg/m^2]
 Prednisone: Oral: 60 mg/m^2/day days 1 to 4
 [total dose/cycle = 240 mg/m^2]
 Repeat cycle every 35 days for 5 cycles

References

Variation 1:

Dimopoulos MA, Richardson PG, Schlag R, et al, "VMP (Bortezomib, Melphalan, and Prednisone) Is Active and Well Tolerated in Newly Diagnosed Patients With Multiple Myeloma With Moderately Impaired Renal Function, and Results in Reversal of Renal Impairment: Cohort Analysis of the Phase III VISTA Study," *J Clin Oncol*, 2009, 27(36):6086-93.

San Miguel JF, Schlag R, Khuageva NK, et al, "Bortezomib Plus Melphalan and Prednisone for Initial Treatment of Multiple Myeloma," *N Engl J Med*, 2008, 359(9):906-17.

Variation 2:

Mateos MV, Hernández JM, Hernández MT, et al, "Bortezomib Plus Melphalan and Prednisone in Elderly Untreated Patients With Multiple Myeloma: Results of a Multicenter Phase 1/2 Study," *Blood*, 2006, 108(7):2165-72.

Mateos MV, Hernández JM, Hernández MT, et al, "Bortezomib Plus Melphalan and Prednisone in Elderly Untreated Patients With Multiple Myeloma: Updated Time-to-Events Results and Prognostic Factors for Time to Progression," *Haematologica*, 2008, 93(4):560-5.

◆ **Melphalan-Prednisone-Bortezomib-Thalidomide** *see* Bortezomib-Melphalan-Prednisone-Thalidomide *on page 1850*

Melphalan-Prednisone (Multiple Myeloma)

Index Terms MP (Multiple Myeloma)
Use Multiple myeloma
Regimen NOTE: Multiple variations are listed.
 Variation 1:
 Melphalan: Oral: 0.25 mg/kg/dose days 1 to 4
 [total dose/cycle = 1 mg/kg]
 Prednisone: Oral: 2 mg/kg/dose days 1 to 4
 [total dose/cycle = 8 mg/kg]
 Repeat cycle every 6 weeks for a total of 12 cycles
 Variation 2:
 Melphalan: Oral: 4 mg/m^2/dose days 1 to 7
 [total dose/cycle = 28 mg/m^2]
 Prednisone: Oral: 40 mg/m^2/dose days 1 to 7
 [total dose/cycle = 280 mg/m^2]
 Repeat cycle every 4 weeks for a total of 6 cycles

Variation 3:

Melphalan: Oral: 9 mg/m^2/dose days 1 to 4
[total dose/cycle = 36 mg/m^2]

Prednisone: Oral: 60 mg/m^2/dose days 1 to 4
[total dose/cycle = 240 mg/m^2]

Repeat cycle every 6 weeks for a total of 9 cycles

Variation 4:

Melphalan: Oral: 6 mg/m^2/dose days 1 to 7
[total dose/cycle = 42 mg/m^2]

Prednisone: Oral: 60 mg/m^2/dose days 1 to 7
[total dose/cycle = 420 mg/m^2]

Repeat cycle every 4 weeks for a total of 6 cycles

Followed by (in responders):

Interferon alfa: SubQ: 3 million units/dose 3 times/week until relapse

Dexamethasone: Oral: 40 mg/dose days 1 to 4 every 2 months until relapse

References

Variation 1:

Facon T, Mary JY, Hulin C, et al, "Melphalan and Prednisone Plus Thalidomide Versus Melphalan and Prednisone Alone or Reduced-Intensity Autologous Stem Cell Transplantation in Elderly Patients With Multiple Myeloma (IFM 99-06): A Randomised Trial," *Lancet*, 2007, 370 (9594):1209-18.

Facon T, Mary JY, Pégourie B, et al, "Dexamethasone-Based Regimens Versus Melphalan-Prednisone for Elderly Multiple Myeloma Patients Ineligible for High-Dose Therapy," *Blood*, 2006, 107(4):1292-8.

Variation 2:

Palumbo A, Bringhen S, Caravita T, et al, "Oral Melphalan and Prednisone Chemotherapy Plus Thalidomide Compared With Melphalan and Prednisone Alone in Elderly Patients With Multiple Myeloma: Randomised Controlled Trial," *Lancet*, 2006, 367(9513):825-31.

Palumbo A, Bringhen S, Liberati AM, et al, "Oral Melphalan, Prednisone, and Thalidomide in Elderly Patients With Multiple Myeloma: Updated Results of a Randomized Controlled Trial," *Blood*, 2008, 112(8):3107-14.

Variation 3:

San Miguel JF, Schlag R, Khuageva NK, et al, "Bortezomib Plus Melphalan and Prednisone for Initial Treatment of Multiple Myeloma," *N Engl J Med*, 2008, 359(9):906-17.

Variation 4:

Palumbo A, Bringhen S, Petrucci MT, et al, "Intermediate-Dose Melphalan Improves Survival of Myeloma Patients Aged 50 to 70: Results of a Randomized Controlled Trial," *Blood*, 2004, 104 (10):3052-7.

Melphalan-Prednisone-Thalidomide (Multiple Myeloma)

Index Terms MPT (Multiple Myeloma)

Use Multiple myeloma

Regimen NOTE: Multiple variations are listed.

Variation 1:

Melphalan: Oral: 4 mg/m^2/day days 1 to 7
[total dose/cycle = 28 mg/m^2]

Prednisone: Oral: 40 mg/m^2/day days 1 to 7
[total dose/cycle = 280 mg/m^2]

Thalidomide: Oral: 100 mg/day days 1 to 28
[total dose/cycle = 2800 mg]

Repeat cycle every 28 days for 6 cycles

followed by

Thalidomide: Oral: 100 mg daily (as maintenance)

Variation 2:
Melphalan: Oral: 0.25 mg/kg/dose days 1 to 4
[total dose/cycle = 1 mg/kg]
Prednisone: Oral: 2 mg/kg/day days 1 to 4
[total dose/cycle = 8 mg/kg]
Thalidomide: Oral: 100-400 mg/day days 1 to 42
[total dose/cycle = 4200-16,800 mg]
Repeat cycle every 6 weeks for a total of 12 cycles (discontinue thalidomide on day 4 of the last cycle)

References

Variation 1:

Palumbo A, Bertola A, Musto P, et al, "Oral Melphalan, Prednisone, and Thalidomide for Newly Diagnosed Patients With Myeloma," *Cancer* , 2005, 104(7):1428-33.

Palumbo A, Bringhen S, Caravita T, et al, "Oral Melphalan and Prednisone Chemotherapy Plus Thalidomide Compared With Melphalan and Prednisone Alone in Elderly Patients With Multiple Myeloma: Randomised Controlled Trial," *Lancet*, 2006, 367(9513):825-31.

Palumbo A, Bringhen S, Liberati AM, et al, "Oral Melphalan, Prednisone, and Thalidomide in Elderly Patients With Multiple Myeloma: Updated Results of a Randomized Controlled Trial," *Blood*, 2008, 112(8):3107-14.

Variation 2:

Facon T, Mary JY, Hulin C, et al, "Melphalan and Prednisone Plus Thalidomide Versus Melphalan and Prednisone Alone or Reduced-Intensity Autologous Stem Cell Transplantation in Elderly Patients With Multiple Myeloma (IFM 99-06): A Randomised Trial," *Lancet*, 2007, 370 (9594):1209-18.

◆ **Mesna-Doxorubicin-Ifosfamide-Dacarbazine (Soft Tissue Sarcoma)** *see* MAID (Soft Tissue Sarcoma) *on page 2031*

◆ **Mesna-Ifosfamide-Mitoxantrone-Etoposide and Etoposide-Methylprednisolone-Cytarabine-Cisplatin (Hodgkin)** *see* MINE-ESHAP (Hodgkin) *on page 2036*

◆ **Methotrexate-Leucovorin-Cyclophosphamide-Dactinomycin (Gestational Trophoblastic Tumor)** *see* MAC (Gestational Trophoblastic Tumor) *on page 2031*

◆ **Methotrexate-Vinblastine-Doxorubicin-Cisplatin (Bladder)** *see* MVAC (Bladder) *on page 2042*

Methotrexate-Vinblastine (Soft Tissue Sarcoma)

Index Terms Vinblastine-Methotrexate (Soft Tissue Sarcoma)

Use Soft tissue sarcoma (desmoid tumor, aggressive fibromatosis)

Regimen

Methotrexate: IV: 30 mg/m² day 1 (dose usually rounded to 50 mg)
[total dose/cycle = 30 mg/m²]
Vinblastine: IV: 6 mg/m² day 1 (dose usually rounded to 10 mg)
[total dose/cycle = 6 mg/m²]
Repeat cycle every 7 to 10 days for 1 year (52 treatments)

References

Azzarelli A, Gronchi A, Bertulli R, et al. Low-dose chemotherapy with methotrexate and vinblastine for patients with advanced aggressive fibromatosis. *Cancer.* 2001;92(5):1259-1264.

◆ **mFOLFOX6 and FOLFOX6 (Colorectal)** *see* FOLFOX6 and mFOLFOX6 (Colorectal) *on page 1986*

MINE-ESHAP (Hodgkin)

Index Terms Mesna-Ifosfamide-Mitoxantrone-Etoposide and Etoposide-Methylprednisolone-Cytarabine-Cisplatin (Hodgkin)

Use Lymphoma, Hodgkin

Regimen
Refractory disease (alternate MINE regimen with ESHAP regimen for a total of 2 MINE cycles and 2 ESHAP cycles):

MINE Regimen:
Mesna: IV: 2250 mg/m^2/day days 1, 2, and 3
  [total dose/cycle = 6750 mg/m^2]
Ifosfamide: IV: 1500 mg/m^2/day days 1, 2, and 3
  [total dose/cycle = 4500 mg/m^2]
Mitoxantrone: IV: 10 mg/m^2 day 1
  [total dose/cycle = 10 mg/m^2]
Etoposide: IV: 80 mg/m^2/day days 1, 2, and 3
  [total dose/cycle = 240 mg/m^2]
Treatment cycle is 28 days

ESHAP Regimen:
Etoposide: IV: 40 mg/m^2/day days 1 to 4
  [total dose/cycle = 160 mg/m^2]
Methylprednisolone: IV: 250 mg/day days 1 to 4
  [total dose/cycle = 1000 mg]
Cisplatin: IV: 25 mg/m^2/day continuous infusion over 21 hours days 1 to 4
  [total dose/cycle = 100 mg/m^2]
Cytarabine: IV: 2000 mg/m^2 day 5
  [total dose/cycle = 2000 mg/m^2]
Treatment cycle is 28 days

References
Fernandez de Larrea C, Martinez C, Gaya A, et al, "Salvage Chemotherapy With Alternating MINE-ESHAP Regimen in Relapsed or Refractory Hodgkin's Lymphoma Followed By Autologous Stem-Cell Transplantation," *Ann Oncol*, 2010, 21(6):1211-6.

mini-BEAM (Hodgkin)
Index Terms Carmustine-Etoposide-Cytarabine-Melphalan (Hodgkin)
Use Lymphoma, Hodgkin
Regimen
Carmustine: IV: 60 mg/m^2 over 30 minutes day 1
  [total dose/cycle = 60 mg/m^2]
Etoposide: IV: 75 mg/m^2/day over 30 minutes days 2 to 5
  [total dose/cycle = 300 mg/m^2]
Cytarabine: IV: 100 mg/m^2 every 12 hours days 2 to 5 (total of 8 doses)
  [total dose/cycle = 800 mg/m^2]
Melphalan: IV: 30 mg/m^2 over 15 minutes day 6
  [total dose/cycle = 30 mg/m^2]
Repeat cycle every 4 to 6 weeks

References
Colwill R, Crump M, Couture F, et al, "Mini-BEAM as Salvage Therapy for Relapsed or Refractory Hodgkin's Disease Before Intensive Therapy and Autologous Bone Marrow Transplantation," *J Clin Oncol*, 1995, 13(2):396-402.

Martín A, Fernández-Jiménez MC, Caballero MD, et al. "Long-Term Follow-Up in Patients Treated With Mini-BEAM as Salvage Therapy for Relapsed or Refractory Hodgkin's Disease," *Br J Haematol*, 2001, 113(1):161-71.

◆ **Mitomycin–Fluorouracil (Anal Cancer)** *see* Fluorouracil-Mitomycin (Anal Cancer) *on page 1983*

Mitoxantrone-Etoposide (AML Induction)
Index Terms MV (AML Induction)
Use Leukemia, acute myeloid

Regimen

Mitoxantrone: IV: 10 mg/m^2/day over ≤15 minutes days 1 to 5
  [total dose/cycle = 50 mg/m^2]
Etoposide: IV: 100 mg/m^2/day over 30 minutes days 1 to 5
  [total dose/cycle = 500 mg/m^2]
May administer a second induction cycle if needed

References

Ho AD, Lipp T, Ehninger G, et al, "Combination of Mitoxantrone and Etoposide in Refractory Acute Myelogenous Leukemia an Active and Well-Tolerated Regimen," *J Clin Oncol*, 1988, 6(2):213-17.

Mitoxantrone-Etoposide-Cytarabine (AML)

Index Terms EMA (AML); MEC (AML)
Use Leukemia, acute myeloid (relapsed, refractory)
Regimen NOTE: Multiple variations are listed.

Variation 1 (induction):

Etoposide: IV: 80 mg/m^2/day over 1 hour days 1 to 6
  [total dose/cycle = 480 mg/m^2]
Cytarabine: IV: 1,000 mg/m^2/day over 6 hours days 1 to 6
  [total dose/cycle = 6,000 mg/m^2]
Mitoxantrone: IV: 6 mg/m^2/day days 1 to 6 (3 hours after the end of the cytarabine infusion)
  [total dose/cycle = 36 mg/m^2]
Patients in complete remission proceeded to consolidation therapy

Variation 2:

Etoposide: IV: 100 mg/m^2/day over 2 hours days 1 to 5
  [total dose/cycle = 500 mg/m^2]
Cytarabine: IV: 1,000 mg/m^2/day days 1 to 5
  [total dose/cycle = 5,000 mg/m^2]
Mitoxantrone: IV: 8 mg/m^2/day days 1 to 5
  [total dose/cycle = 40 mg/m^2]

References

Variation 1:
Amadori S, Arcese W, Isacchi G, et al. Mitoxantrone, etoposide, and intermediate-dose cytarabine: an effective and tolerable regimen for the treatment of refractory acute myeloid leukemia. *J Clin Oncol*. 1991;9(7):1210-1214.
Variation 2:
Döhner H, Weisdorf DJ, Bloomfield CD. Acute myeloid leukemia. *N Engl J Med*. 2015;373 (12):1136-1152.
Kohrt HE, Patel S, Ho M, et al. Second-line mitoxantrone, etoposide, and cytarabine for acute myeloid leukemia: a single-center experience. *Am J Hematol*. 2010;85(11):877-881.

Mitoxantrone-Prednisone (Prostate)

Index Terms MP (Prostate); Prednisone-Mitoxantrone (Prostate)
Use Prostate cancer
Regimen NOTE: Multiple variations are listed.

Variation 1:

Mitoxantrone: IV: 12 mg/m^2 day 1
  [total dose/cycle = 12 mg/m^2]
Prednisone: Oral: 5 mg twice daily
  [total dose/cycle = 210 mg]
Repeat cycle every 21 days, for up to a cumulative mitoxantrone dose of 140 mg/m^2 (Tannock, 1996); or for a total of 6 cycles (Berry, 2002); or for up to a total of 10 cycles (Tannock, 2004)

Variation 2:
  Cycle 1:
    Mitoxantrone: IV: 12 mg/m^2 day 1
      [total dose/cycle = 12 mg/m^2]
    Prednisone: Oral: 5 mg twice daily
      [total dose/cycle = 210 mg]
    Treatment cycle is 21 days
  Cycles 2-8:
    Mitoxantrone: IV: 12-14 mg/m^2 day 1 (increase to 14 mg/m^2 if granulocyte
      nadir is >1000/mm^3 and platelet nadir >50,000/mm^3)
      [total dose/cycle = 12-14 mg/m^2]
    Prednisone: Oral: 5 mg twice daily
      [total dose/cycle = 210 mg]
    Repeat cycle every 21 days for a maximum of 8 cycles

References

Variation 1:
Berry W, Dakhil S, Modiano M, et al, "Phase III Study of Mitoxantrone Plus Low Dose Prednisone Versus Low Dose Prednisone Alone in Patients With Asymptomatic Hormone Refractory Prostate Cancer," *J Urol*, 2002, 168(6):2439-43.
Tannock IF, de Wit R, Berry WR, et al, "Docetaxel Plus Prednisone or Mitoxantrone Plus Prednisone for Advanced Prostate Cancer," *N Engl J Med*, 2004, 351(15):1502-12.
Tannock IF, Osoba D, Stockler MR, et al, "Chemotherapy With Mitoxantrone Plus Prednisone or Prednisone Alone For Symptomatic Hormone-Resistant Prostate Cancer: A Canadian Randomized Trial With Palliative End Points," *J Clin Oncol*, 1996, 14(6):1756-64.
Variation 2:
Moore MJ, Osoba D, Murphy K, et al, "Use of Palliative Endpoints to Evaluate the Effects of Mitoxantrone and Low-Dose Prednisone in Patients With Hormonally Resistant Prostate Cancer," *J Clin Oncol*, 1994, 12(4):689-94.

♦ **Modified Fluorouracil-Leucovorin-Oxaliplatin (Colorectal)** *see* FOLFOX6 and mFOLFOX6 (Colorectal) *on page 1986*

♦ **Modified FOLFOX6 (Colorectal)** *see* FOLFOX6 and mFOLFOX6 (Colorectal) *on page 1986*

MOPP/ABVD (Hodgkin)

Index Terms Mechlorethamine, Vincristine, Procarbazine, Prednisone, Doxorubicin, Bleomycin, Vinblastine, Dacarbazine (Hodgkin)

Use Lymphoma, Hodgkin

Regimen NOTE: Multiple variations are listed.
  Variation 1:
    Mechlorethamine: IV: 6 mg/m^2/day days 1 and 8
      [total dose/cycle = 12 mg/m^2]
    Vincristine: IV: 1.4 mg/m^2/day days 1 and 8
      [total dose/cycle = 2.8 mg/m^2]
    Procarbazine: Oral: 100 mg/m^2/day days 1 to 14
      [total dose/cycle = 1400 mg/m^2]
    Prednisone: Oral: 40 mg/m^2/day days 1 to 14 (during cycles 1, 4, 7, and
      10 **only**)
      [total dose/cycle = 560 mg/m^2]
    Doxorubicin: IV: 25 mg/m^2/day days 29 and 43
      [total dose/cycle = 50 mg/m^2]
    Bleomycin: IV: 10 units/m^2/day days 29 and 43
      [total dose/cycle = 20 units/m^2]
    Vinblastine: IV: 6 mg/m^2/day days 29 and 43
      [total dose/cycle = 12 mg/m^2]

◄ Dacarbazine: IV: 375 mg/m^2/day days 29 and 43
  [total dose/cycle = 750 mg/m^2]
  Repeat cycle every 56 days for a total of 6 cycles.
Variation 2:
  Mechlorethamine: IV: 6 mg/m^2/day days 1 and 8
  [total dose/cycle = 12 mg/m^2]
  Vincristine: IV: 1.4 mg/m^2/day (maximum dose: 2 mg) days 1 and 8
  [total dose/cycle = 2.8 mg/m^2; maximum dose/cycle: 4 mg]
  Procarbazine: Oral: 100 mg/m^2/day days 1 to 14
  [total dose/cycle = 1400 mg/m^2]
  Prednisone: Oral: 40 mg/m^2/day days 1 to 14 (during cycles 1 and 7 **only**)
  [total dose/cycle = 560 mg/m^2]
  Doxorubicin: IV: 25 mg/m^2/day days 29 and 43
  [total dose/cycle = 50 mg/m^2]
  Bleomycin: IV: 10 units/m^2/day days 29 and 43
  [total dose/cycle = 20 units/m^2]
  Vinblastine: IV: 6 mg/m^2/day days 29 and 43
  [total dose/cycle = 12 mg/m^2]
  Dacarbazine: IV: 375 mg/m^2/day days 29 and 43
  [total dose/cycle = 750 mg/m^2]
  Repeat cycle every 56 days for a total of 6 cycles.

References

Variation 1:
Bonadonna G, Valagussa P, and Santoro A, "Alternating Noncross-Resistant Combination Chemotherapy or MOPP in State IV Hodgkin's Disease. A Report of 8-Year Results," *Ann Int Med*, 1986, 104(6):739-46.
Variation 2:
Canellos, GP, Anderson JR, Propert KJ, et al, "Chemotherapy of Advanced Hodgkin's Disease With MOPP, ABVD, or MOPP Alternating With ABVD," *N Engl J Med*, 1992, 327(21):1478-84.

MOPP/ABV Hybrid (Hodgkin)

Index Terms Mechlorethamine, Vincristine, Procarbazine, Prednisone, Doxorubicin, Bleomycin, Vinblastine (Hodgkin)

Use Lymphoma, Hodgkin

Regimen
  Mechlorethamine: IV: 6 mg/m^2 day 1
  [total dose/cycle = 6 mg/m^2]
  Vincristine: IV: 1.4 mg/m^2 (maximum dose: 2 mg) day 1
  [total dose/cycle = 1.4 mg/m^2; maximum: 2 mg/cycle]
  Procarbazine: Oral: 100 mg/m^2/day days 1 to 7
  [total dose/cycle = 700 mg/m^2]
  Prednisone: Oral: 40 mg/m^2/day days 1 to 14
  [total dose/cycle = 560 mg/m^2]
  Doxorubicin: IV: 35 mg/m^2 day 8
  [total dose/cycle = 35 mg/m^2]
  Bleomycin: IV: 10 units/m^2 day 8
  [total dose/cycle = 10 units/m^2]
  Vinblastine: IV: 6 mg/m^2 day 8
  [total dose/cycle = 6 mg/m^2]
  Repeat cycle every 28 days for a maximum of 8 cycles

References

Conners JM, Klimo P, Adams G, et al, "Treatment of Advanced Hodgkin's Disease With Chemotherapy – Comparison of MOPP/ABV Hybrid Regimen With Alternating Courses of MOPP and ABVD: A Report From the National Cancer Institute of Canada Clinical Trials," *J Clin Oncol*, 1997, 15(4):1638-45.

Klimo P and Connors JM, "MOPP/ABV Hybrid Program: Combination Chemotherapy Based on Early Introduction of Seven Effective Drugs for Advanced Hodgkin's Disease," *J Clin Oncol*, 1985, 3(9):1174-82.

MOPP (Hodgkin)

Index Terms Mechlorethamine, Vincristine, Procarbazine, Prednisone (Hodgkin)

Use Lymphoma, Hodgkin

Regimen NOTE: Multiple variations are listed.

Variation 1:

Mechlorethamine: IV: 6 mg/m^2/day days 1 and 8
  [total dose/cycle = 12 mg/m^2]

Vincristine: IV: 1.4 mg/m^2/day days 1 and 8
  [total dose/cycle = 2.8 mg/m^2]

Procarbazine: Oral: 100 mg/m^2/day days 1 to 14
  [total dose/cycle = 1400 mg/m^2]

Prednisone: Oral: 40 mg/m^2/day days 1 to 14 (cycles 1 and 4)
  [total dose/cycle = 560 mg/m^2]

Repeat cycle every 28 days for 6 cycles

Variation 2:

Mechlorethamine: IV: 6 mg/m^2/day days 1 and 8
  [total dose/cycle = 12 mg/m^2]

Vincristine: IV: 1.4 mg/m^2/day (maximum dose: 2 mg) days 1 and 8
  [total dose/cycle = 2.8 mg/m^2; maximum dose/cycle: 4 mg]

Procarbazine: Oral: 100 mg/m^2/day days 1 to 14
  [total dose/cycle = 1400 mg/m^2]

Prednisone: Oral: 40 mg/m^2/day days 1 to 14 (cycles 1 and 4)
  [total dose/cycle = 560 mg/m^2]

Repeat cycle every 28 days for 6-8 cycles

References

Variation 1:
Devita VT Jr, Serpick AA, and Carbone PP, "Combination Chemotherapy in the Treatment of Advanced Hodgkin's Disease," *Ann Intern Med*, 1970, 73(6):881-95.
Variation 2:
Canellos GP, Anderson JR, Propert KJ, et al, "Chemotherapy of Advanced Hodgkin's Disease With MOPP, ABVD, or MOPP Alternating With ABVD," *N Engl J Med*, 1992, 327(21):1478-84.

◆ **MP (Multiple Myeloma)** see Melphalan-Prednisone (Multiple Myeloma) on page 2034

◆ **MP (Prostate)** see Mitoxantrone-Prednisone (Prostate) on page 2038

◆ **MPT (Multiple Myeloma)** see Melphalan-Prednisone-Thalidomide (Multiple Myeloma) on page 2035

MTX/6-MP/VP (Maintenance)

Use Leukemia, acute lymphocytic

Regimen

Methotrexate: Oral: 20 mg/m^2 weekly
  [total dose/cycle = 80 mg/m^2]

Mercaptopurine: Oral: 75 mg/m^2/day
  [total dose/cycle = 2250 mg/m^2]

Vincristine: IV: 1.5 mg/m^2 day 1
  [total dose/cycle = 1.5 mg/m^2]

Prednisone: Oral: 40 mg/m^2/day days 1 to 5
  [total dose/cycle = 200 mg/m^2]

Repeat monthly for 2-3 years

References

Bleyer WA, Sather HN, Nickerson HJ, et al, "Monthly Pulses of Vincristine and Prednisone Prevent Bone Marrow and Testicular Relapse in Low-Risk Childhood Acute Lymphoblastic Leukemia: A Report of the CCG-161 Study by the Childrens Cancer Study Group," *J Clin Oncol*, 1991, 9 (6):1012-21.

MVAC (Bladder)

Index Terms M-VAC (Bladder); Methotrexate-Vinblastine-Doxorubicin-Cisplatin (Bladder)

Use Bladder cancer

Regimen NOTE: Multiple variations are listed.

Variation 1 (neoadjuvant):

Methotrexate: IV: 30 mg/m^2/day days 1, 15, and 22
[total dose/cycle = 90 mg/m^2]

Vinblastine: IV: 3 mg/m^2/day days 2, 15, and 22
[total dose/cycle = 9 mg/m^2]

Doxorubicin: IV: 30 mg/m^2 day 2
[total dose/cycle = 30 mg/m^2]

Cisplatin: IV: 70 mg/m^2 day 2
[total dose/cycle = 70 mg/m^2]

Repeat cycle every 28 days for a total of 3 cycles

Variation 2 (metastatic):

Methotrexate: IV: 30 mg/m^2/day days 1, 15, and 22
[total dose/cycle = 90 mg/m^2]

Vinblastine: IV: 3 mg/m^2/day days 2, 15, and 22
[total dose/cycle = 9 mg/m^2]

Doxorubicin: IV: 30 mg/m^2 day 2
[total dose/cycle = 30 mg/m^2]

Cisplatin: IV: 70 mg/m^2 day 2
[total dose/cycle = 70 mg/m^2]

Repeat cycle every 28 days; for up to a total of 6 cycles (von der Maase 2000) or until disease progression or unacceptable toxicity (Sternberg 2001)

Variation 3 (metastatic):

Methotrexate: IV: 30 mg/m^2/day days 1, 15, and 22
[total dose/cycle = 90 mg/m^2]

Vinblastine: IV: 3 mg/m^2/day days 1, 15, and 22
[total dose/cycle = 9 mg/m^2]

Doxorubicin: IV: 30 mg/m^2 day 1
[total dose/cycle = 30 mg/m^2]

Cisplatin: IV: 70 mg/m^2 day 1
[total dose/cycle = 70 mg/m^2]

Filgrastim was administered on days 7, 8, 9, 25, and 26

Repeat cycle every 28 days for a total of 6 cycles

References

Variation 1:

Grossman HB, Natale RB, Tangen CM, et al. Neoadjuvant chemotherapy plus cystectomy compared with cystectomy alone for locally advanced bladder cancer. *N Engl J Med.* 2003;349 (9):859-866.

Variation 2:

Sternberg CN, de Mulder PH, Schornagel JH, et al. Randomized phase III trial of high-dose-intensity methotrexate, vinblastine, doxorubicin, and cisplatin (MVAC) chemotherapy and recombinant human granulocyte colony-stimulating factor versus classic MVAC in advanced urothelial tract tumors: European Organization for Research and Treatment of Cancer Protocol no. 30924. *J Clin Oncol.* 2001;19(10):2638-2646.

Sternberg CN, de Mulder P, Schornagel JH, et al. Seven year update of an EORTC phase III trial of high-dose intensity M-VAC chemotherapy and G-CSF versus classic M-VAC in advanced urothelial tract tumours. *Eur J Cancer.* 2006;42(1):50-54.

von der Maase H, Hansen SW, Roberts JT, et al. Gemcitabine and cisplatin versus methotrexate, vinblastine, doxorubicin, and cisplatin in advanced or metastatic bladder cancer: results of a large, randomized, multinational, multicenter, phase III study. *J Clin Oncol.* 2000;17 (17):3068-3077.

Variation 3:

Bamias A, Aravantinos G, Deliveliotis C, et al. Docetaxel and cisplatin with granulocyte colony-stimulating factor (G-CSF) versus MVAC with G-CSF in advanced urothelial carcinoma: a multicenter, randomized, phase III study from the Hellenic Cooperative Oncology Group. *J Clin Oncol.* 2004;22(2):220-228.

◆ **M-VAC (Bladder)** *see* MVAC (Bladder) *on page 2042*

◆ **MVAC (Bladder Cancer)** *see* Dose Dense MVAC (Bladder Cancer) *on page 1948*

◆ **MV (AML Induction)** *see* Mitoxantrone-Etoposide (AML Induction) *on page 2037*

◆ **N6 Protocol (Neuroblastoma)** *see* CAV-P/VP (Neuroblastoma) *on page 1876*

◆ **nab Paclitaxel (NSCLC Regimen)** *see* Paclitaxel (Protein Bound) (NSCLC Regimen) *on page 2055*

◆ *nab* **Paclitaxel (Ovarian Regimen)** *see* Paclitaxel (Protein Bound) (Ovarian Regimen) *on page 2055*

◆ **nab Paclitaxel–Carboplatin (NSCLC)** *see* Carboplatin-Paclitaxel (Protein Bound) (NSCLC) *on page 1872*

◆ **nab-PC (NSCLC)** *see* Carboplatin-Paclitaxel (Protein Bound) (NSCLC) *on page 1872*

◆ **NEW A1 (Neuroblastoma)** *see* New A1 (Neuroblastoma) *on page 2043*

New A1 (Neuroblastoma)

Index Terms A1 (NEW) (Neuroblastoma); Cyclophosphamide, Doxorubicin, Etoposide, Cisplatin (Neuroblastoma); NEW A1 (Neuroblastoma); Regimen new A1 (Neuroblastoma)

Use Neuroblastoma

Regimen

Cyclophosphamide: IV: 1200 mg/m^2 over 6 hours day 1
  [total dose/cycle = 1200 mg/m^2]
Doxorubicin: IV: 40 mg/m^2 day 3
  [total dose/cycle = 40 mg/m^2]
Etoposide: IV: 100 mg/m^2/day days 1 to 5
  [total dose/cycle = 500 mg/m^2]
Cisplatin: IV: 90 mg/m^2 day 5
  [total dose/cycle = 90 mg/m^2]
Repeat cycle every 28 days for up to a total of 6 cycles

References

Kaneko M, Nishihira H, Mugishima H, et al, "Stratification of Treatment of Stage 4 Neuroblastoma Patients Based on N-myc Amplification Status. Study Group of Japan for Treatment of Advanced Neuroblastoma, Tokyo, Japan," *Med Pediatr Oncol.* 1998, 31(1):1-7.

Kaneko M, Tsuchida Y, Mugishima H, et al, "Intensified Chemotherapy Increases the Survival Rates in Patients With Stage 4 Neuroblastoma With MYCN Amplification," *J Pediatr Hematol Oncol.* 2002, 24(8):613-21.

Nilotinib (CML Regimen)

Use Leukemia, chronic myelogenous

◀ **Regimen** NOTE: Multiple variations are listed.

Variation 1 (newly diagnosed chronic phase):

Nilotinib: Oral: 300 mg twice daily

[total dose/cycle = 16,800 mg]

Repeat cycle every 28 days until disease progression or unacceptable toxicity

Variation 2 (chronic or accelerated phase resistant or intolerant to imatinib):

Nilotinib: Oral: 400 mg twice daily

[total dose/cycle = 22,400 mg]

Repeat cycle every 28 days until disease progression or unacceptable toxicity

References

Variation 1:

Larson RA, Kim D, Rosti G, et al, "Comparison of Nilotinib and Imatinib in Patients (Pts) With Newly Diagnosed Chronic Myeloid Leukemia in Chronic Phase (CML-CP): ENESTnd 24-Month Follow-Up," *J Clin Oncol*, 2011, 29(Suppl 15):6511 [abstract].

Saglio G, Kim DW, Issaragrisil S, et al, "Nilotinib Versus Imatinib for Newly Diagnosed Chronic Myeloid Leukemia," *N Engl J Med*, 2010, 362(24):2251-9.

Variation 2:

Kantarjian HM, Giles F, Gattermann N, et al, "Nilotinib (Formerly AMN107), a Highly Selective BCR-ABL Tyrosine Kinase Inhibitor, Is Effective in Patients With Philadelphia Chromosome-Positive Chronic Myelogenous Leukemia in Chronic Phase Following Imatinib Resistance and Intolerance," *Blood*, 2007, 110(10):3540-6.

Kantarjian HM, Giles FJ, Bhalla KN, et al, "Nilotinib Is Effective in Patients With Chronic Myeloid Leukemia in Chronic Phase After Imatinib Resistance or Intolerance: 24-Month Follow-up Results," *Blood*, 2011, 117(4):1141-5.

le Coutre P, Ottmann OG, Giles F, et al, "Nilotinib (Formerly AMN107), a Highly Selective BCR-ABL Tyrosine Kinase Inhibitor, Is Active in Patients With Imatinib-Resistant or -Intolerant Accelerated-Phase Chronic Myelogenous Leukemia," *Blood*, 2008, 111(4):1834-9.

Nilotinib (GIST Regimen)

Use Soft Tissue Sarcoma (Gastrointestinal Stromal Tumor [GIST])

Regimen

Nilotinib: Oral: 400 mg twice daily days 1 to 28

[total dose/cycle = 22,400 mg]

Repeat cycle every 28 days

References

Montemurro M, Schöffski P, Reichardt P, et al, "Nilotinib in the Treatment of Advanced Gastrointestinal Stromal Tumours Resistant to Both Imatinib and Sunitinib," *Eur J Cancer*, 2009, 45(13):2293-7.

Reichardt P, Blay JY, Gelderblom H, et al, "Phase III Study of Nilotinib Versus Best Supportive Care With or Without a TKI in Patients With Gastrointestinal Stromal Tumors Resistant to or Intolerant of Imatinib and Sunitinib," *Ann Oncol*, 2012, 23(7):1680-7.

♦ **Nivolumab-Ipilimumab (Melanoma)** see Ipilimumab-Nivolumab (Melanoma) on page 2019

Nivolumab (Melanoma Regimen)

Use Melanoma

Regimen NOTE: Multiple variations are listed.

Variation 1 [second or later-line therapy; unresectable stage IIIC or IV meta-static, ipilimumab and/or BRAF inhibitor (if BRAF^{V600} mutation-positive) refractory]:

Nivolumab: IV: 3 mg/kg day 1

[total dose/cycle = 3 mg/kg]

Repeat cycle every 14 days until disease progression or unacceptable toxicity; treatment beyond progression was allowed in patients tolerating drug and experiencing clinical benefit

Variation 2 (first-line therapy; unresectable stage III or IV, without BRAF mutation):

Nivolumab: IV: 3 mg/kg day 1

[total dose/cycle = 3 mg/kg]

Repeat cycle every 14 days until disease progression or unacceptable toxicity; treatment beyond progression was allowed in patients tolerating drug and experiencing clinical benefit

References

Variation 1:

Weber JS, D'Angelo SP, Minor D, et al. Nivolumab versus chemotherapy in patients with advanced melanoma who progressed after anti-CTLA-4 treatment (CheckMate 037): a randomised, controlled, open-label, phase 3 trial. *Lancet Oncol.* 2015;16(4):375-384.

Variation 2:

Robert C, Long GV, Brady B, et al. Nivolumab in previously untreated melanoma without BRAF mutation. *N Engl J Med.* 2015;372(4):320-330.

Nivolumab (NSCLC Regimen)

Use Lung cancer, non-small cell

Regimen NOTE: Multiple variations are listed.

Variation 1 (advanced, squamous cell):

Nivolumab: IV: 3 mg/kg day 1

[total dose/cycle = 3 mg/kg]

Repeat cycle every 14 days until disease progression or unacceptable toxicity

Variation 2 (advanced, non-squamous cell):

Nivolumab: IV: 3 mg/kg day 1

[total dose/cycle = 3 mg/kg]

Repeat cycle every 14 days until disease progression or unacceptable toxicity

References

Variation 1:

Brahmer J, Reckamp KL, Baas P, et al. Nivolumab versus docetaxel in advanced squamous-cell non-small-cell lung cancer. *N Engl J Med.* 2015;373(2):123-135.

Variation 2:

Paz-Ares L, Horn L, Borghaei H, et al. Phase III, randomized trial (CheckMate 057) of nivolumab (NIVO) versus docetaxel (DOC) in advanced non-squamous cell (non-SQ) non-small cell lung cancer [abstract]. *J Clin Oncol.* 2015;33(18s); abstr LBA109.

◆ **Obinutuzumab-Chlorambucil (CLL)** see Chlorambucil-Obinutuzumab (CLL) on page 1884

◆ **O + CHL (CLL)** see Chlorambucil-Ofatumumab (CLL) on page 1885

OFAR (CLL)

Index Terms Oxaliplatin-Fludarabine-Cytarabine-Rituximab (CLL)

Use Leukemia, chronic lymphocytic

◀ **Regimen**

Cycle 1:

Oxaliplatin: IV: 25 mg/m^2/dose day 1 to 4
   [total dose/cycle = 100 mg/m^2]
Fludarabine: IV: 30 mg/m^2/dose days 2 and 3
   [total dose/cycle = 60 mg/m^2]
Cytarabine: IV: 1000 mg/m^2/dose over 2 hours days 2 and 3
   [total dose/cycle = 2000 mg/m^2]
Rituximab: IV: 375 mg/m^2 day 3
   [total dose/cycle = 375 mg/m^2]
Treatment cycle is 4 weeks

Cycles 2-6:

Oxaliplatin: IV: 25 mg/m^2/dose day 1 to 4
   [total dose/cycle = 100 mg/m^2]
Fludarabine: IV: 30 mg/m^2/dose days 2 and 3
   [total dose/cycle = 60 mg/m^2]
Cytarabine: IV: 1000 mg/m^2/dose over 2 hours days 2 and 3
   [total dose/cycle = 2000 mg/m^2]
Rituximab: IV: 375 mg/m^2 day 1
   [total dose/cycle = 375 mg/m^2]
Repeat cycle every 4 weeks (maximum: 6 cycles)

References

Tsimberidou AM, Wierda WG, Plunkett W, et al, "Phase I-II Study of Oxaliplatin, Fludarabine, Cytarabine, and Rituximab Combination Therapy in Patients With Richter's Syndrome or Fludarabine-Refractory Chronic Lymphocytic Leukemia," *J Clin Oncol*, 2008, 26(2):196-203.

♦ **Ofatumumab-Chlorambucil (CLL)** *see* Chlorambucil-Ofatumumab (CLL)
on page 1885

Ofatumumab (CLL Regimen)

Use Leukemia, chronic lymphocytic

Regimen

Dose 1 (week 1):
   Ofatumumab: IV: 300 mg day 1
Doses 2 to 8 (beginning day 8):
   Ofatumumab: IV: 2000 mg once weekly
   Repeat weekly for 7 weeks (followed by 4 weeks off treatment)
Doses 9 to 12 (beginning week 13):
   Ofatumumab: IV: 2000 mg day 1 of each month for 4 months
   [total dose/treatment course = 22,300 mg]

References

Wierda WG, Kipps TJ, Mayer J, et al. Ofatumumab as single-agent CD20 immunotherapy in fludarabine-refractory chronic lymphocytic leukemia. *J Clin Oncol*. 2010;28(10):1749-1755.

Omacetaxine (CML Regimen)

Use Leukemia, chronic myelogenous

Regimen

Induction Phase:
   Omacetaxine: SubQ: 1.25 mg/m^2 twice daily days 1 to 14
   [total dose/cycle = 35 mg/m^2]
   Repeat cycle every 28 days until achievement of hematologic response, up to
   a maximum of 6 cycles

Maintenance Phase:
Omacetaxine: SubQ: 1.25 mg/m² twice daily days 1 to 7
[total dose/cycle = 17.5 mg/m²]
Repeat cycle every 28 days

References

Cortes J, Digumarti R, Parikh PM, et al, "Phase 2 Study of Subcutaneous Omacetaxine Mepesuccinate for Chronic-Phase Chronic Myeloid Leukemia Patients Resistant to or Intolerant of Tyrosine Kinase Inhibitors," *Am J Hem*, 2013, 88(5):350-4.

Cortes J, Lipton JH, Rea D, et al, "Phase 2 Study of Subcutaneous Omacetaxine Mepesuccinate After TKI Failure in Patients With Chronic-Phase CML With T315I Mutation," *Blood*, 2012, 120 (13):2573-80.

◆ **Oxaliplatin-Capecitabine (Biliary Cancer)** *see* CAPOX (Biliary Cancer) *on page 1860*

◆ **Oxaliplatin-Capecitabine (Colorectal)** *see* XELOX (Colorectal) *on page 2111*

◆ **Oxaliplatin-Capecitabine-Epirubicin (Gastric/Esophageal)** *see* Epirubicin-Oxaliplatin-Capecitabine (Gastric/Esophageal) *on page 1957*

◆ **Oxaliplatin-Capecitabine (Gastric)** *see* Capecitabine-Oxaliplatin (Gastric) *on page 1859*

◆ **Oxaliplatin-Capecitabine (Pancreatic)** *see* CAPOX (Pancreatic) *on page 1861*

Oxaliplatin-Cytarabine-Dexamethasone (NHL Regimen)

Index Terms DHAX (NHL Regimen)
Use Lymphoma, non-Hodgkin
Regimen
Dexamethasone: IV or Oral: 40 mg/day days 1 to 4
[total dose/cycle = 160 mg]
Oxaliplatin: IV: 130 mg/m² over 2 hours day 1
[total dose/cycle = 130 mg/m²]
Cytarabine: IV: 2000 mg/m² over 3 hours every 12 hours for 2 doses day 2
[total dose/cycle = 4000 mg/m²]
Repeat cycle every 3 weeks
References

Chau I, Webb A, Cunningham D, et al, "An Oxaliplatin-Based Chemotherapy in Patients With Relapsed or Refractory Intermediate and High-Grade Non-Hodgkin's Lymphoma," *Br J Haematol*, 2001, 115(4):786-92.

◆ **Oxaliplatin-Docetaxel-Leucovorin-Fluorouracil (Esophageal Cancer)** *see* Docetaxel-Oxaliplatin-Leucovorin-Fluorouracil (Esophageal Cancer) *on page 1946*

◆ **Oxaliplatin-Fludarabine-Cytarabine-Rituximab (CLL)** *see* OFAR (CLL) *on page 2045*

◆ **Oxaliplatin-Fluorouracil-Epirubicin (Gastric/Esophageal)** *see* Epirubicin-Oxaliplatin-Fluorouracil (Gastric/Esophageal) *on page 1958*

◆ **Oxaliplatin-Fluorouracil-Leucovorin-Bevacizumab (Colorectal)** *see* Bevacizumab FOLFOX (Colorectal) *on page 1842*

◆ **Oxaliplatin, Fluorouracil, Leucovorin (Pancreatic)** *see* FOLFOX (Pancreatic) *on page 1988*

◆ **Oxaliplatin-Gemcitabine-Paclitaxel (Testicular)** *see* Gemcitabine-Oxaliplatin-Paclitaxel (Testicular) *on page 1994*

PA-CI

Use Hepatoblastoma

Regimen NOTE: Multiple variations are listed.
Variation 1:
Cisplatin: IV: 90 mg/m^2 day 1
[total dose/cycle = 90 mg/m^2]
Doxorubicin: IV: 20 mg/m^2/day continuous infusion days 2 to 5
[total dose/cycle = 80 mg/m^2]
Repeat cycle every 21 days
Variation 2:
Cisplatin: IV: 20 mg/m^2/day days 1 to 4
[total dose/cycle = 80 mg/m^2]
Doxorubicin: IV: 100 mg/m^2 continuous infusion day 1
[total dose/cycle = 100 mg/m^2]
Repeat cycle every 21-28 days

References

Variation 1:
Ortega JA, Douglass EC, Feusner JH, et al, "Randomized Comparison of Cisplatin/Vincristine/Fluorouracil and Cisplatin/Continuous Infusion Doxorubicin for Treatment of Pediatric Hepatoblastoma: A Report From the Children's Cancer Group and the Pediatric Oncology Group," *J Clin Oncol*, 2000, 18(14):2665-75.
Variation 2:
Ortega JA, Krailo MD, Haas JE, et al, "Effective Treatment of Unresectable or Metastatic Hepatoblastoma With Cisplatin and Continuous Infusion Doxorubicin Chemotherapy: A Report From the Childrens Cancer Study Group," *J Clin Oncol*, 1991, 9(12):2167-76.

Paclitaxel (Angiosarcoma Regimen)

Use Soft tissue sarcoma (advanced, unresectable angiosarcoma)

Regimen NOTE: Multiple variations are listed.
Variation 1:
  Paclitaxel: IV: 80 mg/m²/day over 60 minutes days 1, 8, and 15
    [total dose/cycle = 240 mg/m²]
  Repeat cycle every 28 days for 6 cycles
Variation 2:
  Paclitaxel: IV: 75 to 100 mg/m²/day days 1, 8, 15, 22
    [total dose/cycle = 300 to 400 mg/m²]
  Repeat cycle every 28 days
Variation 3:
  Paclitaxel: IV: 135 to 175 mg/m² over 3 hours day 1
    [total dose/cycle = 135 to 175 mg/m²]
  Repeat cycle every 21 days

References

Variation 1:
Penel N, Bui BN, Bay JO, et al. Phase II trial of weekly paclitaxel for unresectable angiosarcoma:
  the ANGIOTAX Study. *J Clin Oncol.* 2008;26(32):5269-5274.
Variations 2 and 3:
Schlemmer M, Reichardt P, Verweij J. et al. Paclitaxel in patients with advanced angiosarcomas of
  soft tissue: a retrospective study of the EORTC soft tissue and bone sarcoma group. *Eur J
  Cancer.* 2008;44(16):2433-2436.

◆ **Paclitaxel-Bevacizumab (Breast)** *see* Bevacizumab-Paclitaxel (Breast)
on page 1844

◆ **Paclitaxel-Bevacizumab (Ovarian)** *see* Bevacizumab-Paclitaxel (Ovarian)
on page 1845

Paclitaxel (Breast Regimen)

Use Breast cancer

Regimen NOTE: Multiple variations are listed.
Variation 1 (weekly [preferred]):
  Paclitaxel IV: 80 mg/m² over 1 hour day 1
    [total dose/cycle = 80 mg/m²]
  Repeat cycle every 7 days until disease progression or unacceptable toxicity
Variation 2 (every 3 weeks):
  Paclitaxel IV: 175 mg/m² over 3 hours day 1
    [total dose/cycle = 175 mg/m²]
  Repeat cycle every 21 days

References

Variation 1:
Mauri D, Kamposioras K, Tsali L, et al, "Overall Survival Benefit For Weekly Vs. Three-Weekly
  Taxanes Regimens in Advanced Breast Cancer: A Meta-Analysis," *Cancer Treat Rev,* 2010; 36
  (1):69-74.
Perez EA, Vogel CL, Irwin DH, et al, "Multicenter Phase II Trial of Weekly Paclitaxel in Women With
  Metastatic Breast Cancer," *J Clin Oncol,* 2001:19(22):4216-23.
Seidman AD, Berry D, Cirrincione C, et al, "Randomized Phase III Trial of Weekly Compared With
  Every-3-Weeks Paclitaxel for Metastatic Breast Cancer, With Trastuzumab for all HER-2 Over-
  expressors and Random Assignment to Trastuzumab or Not in HER-2 Nonoverexpressors: Final
  Results of Cancer and Leukemia Group B Protocol 9840," *J Clin Oncol,* 2008, 26(10):1642-9.
Variation 2:
Winer EP, Berry DA, Woolf S, et al, "Failure of Higher-Dose Paclitaxel to Improve Outcome in
  Patients With Metastatic Breast Cancer: Cancer and Leukemia Group B Tiral 9342," *J Clin Oncol,*
  2004, 22(11):2061-8.

◆ **Paclitaxel-Carboplatin (Cervical Cancer)** *see* Carboplatin-Paclitaxel (Cervical Cancer) *on page 1868*

♦ **Paclitaxel-Carboplatin (Endometrial)** *see* Carboplatin-Paclitaxel (Endometrial) *on page 1869*

Paclitaxel-Carboplatin (Esophageal Cancer)

Index Terms Carboplatin-Paclitaxel (Esophageal Cancer)

Use Esophageal cancer

Regimen

Paclitaxel: IV: 50 mg/m^2/dose over 1 hour days 1, 8, 15, 22, and 29
[total dose/cycle = 250 mg/m^2]
Carboplatin: IV: AUC = 2 days 1, 8, 15, 22, and 29
[total dose/cycle = AUC = 10]
Administer with concurrent radiation therapy; cycle does not repeat.

References

van Meerten E, Muller K, Tilanus HW, et al ""Neoadjuvant Concurrent Chemoradiation With Weekly Paclitaxel and Carboplatin for Patients With Oesophageal Cancer: A Phase II Study," *Br J Cancer*, 2006, 94(10):1389-94.

♦ **Paclitaxel-Carboplatin-Etoposide (Unknown Primary)** *see* Carboplatin-Etoposide-Paclitaxel (Unknown Primary, Adenocarcinoma) *on page 1864*

♦ **Paclitaxel-Carboplatin (Ovarian)** *see* Carboplatin-Paclitaxel (Ovarian) *on page 1871*

♦ **Paclitaxel-Carboplatin-Trastuzumab (Breast)** *see* Carboplatin-Paclitaxel-Trastuzumab (Breast) *on page 1872*

♦ **Paclitaxel-Carboplatin (Unknown Primary)** *see* Carboplatin-Paclitaxel (Unknown Primary, Adenocarcinoma) *on page 1873*

Paclitaxel-Cetuximab

Index Terms Cetuximab-Paclitaxel

Use Head and neck cancer

Regimen

Week 1:
Paclitaxel: IV: 80 mg/m^2 day 1
[total dose/week 1 = 80 mg/m^2]
Cetuximab: IV: 400 mg/m^2 (loading dose) day 1 (week 1 only)
[total loading dose (week 1) = 400 mg/m^2]
Subsequent weeks:
Paclitaxel: IV: 80 mg/m^2 day 1
[total dose/week = 80 mg/m^2]
Cetuximab: IV: 250 mg/m^2 day 1
[total dose/week = 250 mg/m^2]

References

Hitt R, Irigoyen H, Nunez J, et al, "Phase II Study of Combination Cetuximab and Weekly Paclitaxel in Patients With Metastatic/Recurrent Squamous Cell Carcinoma of Head and Neck (SCCHN): Spanish Head and Neck Cancer Group (TTCC)," *J Clin Oncol*, 2007, 25(18S) [abstract 6012 from 2007 ASCO Annual Meeting].

♦ **Paclitaxel-Cisplatin (Cervical Cancer)** *see* Cisplatin-Paclitaxel (Cervical Cancer) *on page 1909*

Paclitaxel-Cisplatin (Esophageal Cancer)

Index Terms Cisplatin-Paclitaxel (Esophageal Cancer)

Use Esophageal cancer

Regimen NOTE: Multiple variations are listed.

Variation 1:

Paclitaxel: IV: 50 mg/m^2/dose over 1 hour days 1, 8, 15, 22, and 29
[total dose/cycle = 250 mg/m^2]

Cisplatin: IV: 30 mg/m^2/dose days 1, 8, 15, 22, and 29
[total dose/cycle = 150 mg/m^2]

Administered (with concurrent radiation therapy) over one 5-week treatment cycle.

Followed by: Postoperative therapy:

Paclitaxel: IV: 175 mg/m^2/dose day 1
[total dose/cycle = 175 mg/m^2]

Cisplatin: IV: 75 mg/m^2/dose day 1
[total dose/cycle = 75 mg/m^2]

Repeat postop cycle every 21 days for a total of 3 cycles.

Variation 2:

Paclitaxel: IV: 60 mg/m^2/dose over 3 hours days 1, 8, 15, and 22
[total dose/cycle = 240 mg/m^2]

Cisplatin: IV: 75 mg/m^2/dose over 2 hours day 1
[total dose/cycle = 75 mg/m^2]

Filgrastim: SubQ: 5 mcg/kg/day starting day 23; continue until ANC >10,000/mm^3

Administer with concurrent radiation therapy; cycle does not repeat.

Variation 3:

Paclitaxel: IV: 90 mg/m^2/dose over 3 hours day 1
[total dose/cycle = 90 mg/m^2]

Cisplatin: IV: 50 mg/m^2/dose over 1 hour day 1
[total dose/cycle = 50 mg/m^2]

Repeat cycle every 14 days until disease progression or unacceptable toxicity.

References

Variation 1:

Kleinberg L, Powell ME, Forastiere AA, et al, "Survival Outcome of E1201: An Eastern Cooperative Oncology Group (ECOG) Randomized Phase II Trial of Neoadjuvant Preoperative Paclitaxel/Cisplatin/Radiotherapy (RT) or Irinotecan/Cisplatin/RT in Endoscopy With Ultrasound (EUS) Staged Esophageal Adenocarcinoma," *J Clin Oncol*, 2008, 26(15S):4532 [abstract 4532 from 2008 annual ASCO meeting].

Variation 2:

Urba SG, Orringer MB, Ianettonni M, et al, "Concurrent Cisplatin, Paclitaxel, and Radiotherapy as Preoperative Treatment for Patients With Locoregional Esophageal Carcinoma," *Cancer*, 2003, 98(10):2177-83.

Variation 3:

Petrasch S, Welt A, Reinacher A, et al, "Chemotherapy With Cisplatin and Paclitaxel in Patients With Locally Advanced, Recurrent or Metastatic Oesophageal Cancer," *Br J Cancer*, 1998, 78(4):511-4.

Paclitaxel-Cisplatin-Fluorouracil (Esophageal Cancer)

Index Terms Paclitaxel-Fluorouracil-Cisplatin (Esophageal Cancer); TCF (Esophageal Cancer)

Use Esophageal cancer

Regimen

Paclitaxel: IV: 175 mg/m^2 over 3 hours day 1
[total dose/cycle = 175 mg/m^2]

Cisplatin: IV: 20 mg/m^2/day days 1 to 5 for cycles 1, 2, and 3
[total dose/cycle = 100 mg/m^2]
then 15 mg/m^2/day days 1 to 5
[total dose/cycle = 75 mg/m^2]

◄ Fluorouracil: IV: 750 mg/m^2/day continuous infusion days 1 to 5
[total dose/cycle = 3750 mg/m^2]

Repeat cycle every 28 days

References

Ilson DH, Ajani J, Bhalla K, et al, "Phase II Trial of Paclitaxel, Fluorouracil, and Cisplatin in Patients With Advanced Carcinoma of the Esophagus," *J Clin Oncol*, 1998, 16(5):1826-34.

◆ **Paclitaxel-Cisplatin-Gemcitabine (Bladder)** *see* PCG (Bladder) *on page 2060*

◆ **Paclitaxel-Cisplatin (Head and Neck Cancer)** *see* Cisplatin-Paclitaxel (Head and Neck Cancer) *on page 1909*

◆ **Paclitaxel-Cisplatin Intraperitoneal (Ovarian)** *see* Cisplatin-Paclitaxel Intraperitoneal (Ovarian) *on page 1910*

◆ **Paclitaxel-Cisplatin (NSCLC)** *see* Cisplatin-Paclitaxel (NSCLC) *on page 1910*

◆ **Paclitaxel-Cisplatin (Ovarian)** *see* Cisplatin-Paclitaxel (Ovarian) *on page 1910*

◆ **Paclitaxel-Doxorubicin-Cisplatin (Endometrial)** *see* Cisplatin-Doxorubicin-Paclitaxel (Endometrial) *on page 1893*

◆ **Paclitaxel-Fluorouracil-Cisplatin (Esophageal Cancer)** *see* Paclitaxel-Cisplatin-Fluorouracil (Esophageal Cancer) *on page 2051*

Paclitaxel-Fluorouracil (Esophageal Cancer)

Index Terms Fluorouracil-Paclitaxel (Esophageal Cancer)

Use Esophageal cancer

Regimen

Paclitaxel: IV: 45 mg/m^2/dose over 3 hours day 1
[total dose/cycle = 45 mg/m^2]

Fluorouracil: IV: 300 mg/m^2/day continuous infusion days 1 to 5
[total dose/cycle = 1500 mg/m^2]

Repeat cycle weekly for 5 weeks; administer concurrent with radiation therapy; cycle does not repeat.

References

Schnirer II, Komaki R, Yao JC, et al, "Pilot Study of Concurrent 5-Fluorouracil/Paclitaxel Plus Radiotherapy in Patients With Carcinoma of the Esophagus and Gastroesophageal Junction," *Am J Clin Oncol*, 2001, 24(1):91-5.

◆ **Paclitaxel-Gemcitabine (Bladder)** *see* Gemcitabine-Paclitaxel (Bladder) *on page 1995*

◆ **Paclitaxel-Gemcitabine (Breast)** *see* Gemcitabine-Paclitaxel (Breast) *on page 1996*

◆ **Paclitaxel-Gemcitabine-Oxaliplatin (Testicular)** *see* Gemcitabine-Oxaliplatin-Paclitaxel (Testicular) *on page 1994*

◆ **Paclitaxel-Gemcitabine (Testicular)** *see* Gemcitabine-Paclitaxel (Testicular) *on page 1996*

Paclitaxel-Ifosfamide-Cisplatin (Penile)

Index Terms Cisplatin-Ifosfamide-Paclitaxel (Penile)

Use Penile cancer (squamous cell, neoadjuvant)

Regimen
Paclitaxel: IV: 175 mg/m^2 over 3 hours day 1
  [total dose/cycle = 175 mg/m^2]
Ifosfamide: IV: 1,200 mg/m^2/day over 2 hours days 1, 2, and 3
  [total dose/cycle = 3,600 mg/m^2]
Cisplatin: IV: 25 mg/m^2/day over 2 hours days 1, 2, and 3
  [total dose/cycle = 75 mg/m^2]
Mesna: IV: 400 mg/m^2 prior to each ifosfamide dose and 200 mg/m^2 at 4 and 8 hours after each ifosfamide dose, days 1, 2, and 3
  [total dose/cycle = 2,400 mg/m^2]
Repeat cycle every 21 to 28 days for 4 cycles. **Note:** The cycle was repeated on day 22 if the patient's absolute neutrophil count was at least 1,400/mm^3 and platelet count was at least 100,000/mm^3).

References
Pagliaro LC, Williams DL, Daliani D, et al. Neoadjuvant paclitaxel, ifosfamide, and cisplatin chemotherapy for metastatic penile cancer: a phase II study. *J Clin Oncol.* 2010;28 (24):3851-3857.

- ◆ **Paclitaxel-Ifosfamide-Cisplatin (Testicular)** *see* TIP (Testicular) *on page 2090*
- ◆ **Paclitaxel (nanoparticle albumin bound) (Ovarian Regimen)** *see* Paclitaxel (Protein Bound) (Ovarian Regimen) *on page 2055*

Paclitaxel (Ovarian Regimen)
Use Ovarian cancer
Regimen NOTE: Multiple variations are listed.
Variation 1:
  Paclitaxel: IV: 80 mg/m^2/day days 1, 8, and 15
    [total dose/cycle = 240 mg/m^2]
  Repeat cycle every 28 days for 6-9 cycles or until disease progression or unacceptable toxicity
Variation 2:
  Paclitaxel: IV: 80 mg/m^2/day over 1 hour days 1, 8, 15, and 21
    [total dose/cycle = 320 mg/m^2]
  Repeat cycle every 28 days for 3 cycles
  Followed by:
  Paclitaxel: IV: 80 mg/m^2/day days 1, 8, and 15
    [total dose/cycle = 240 mg/m^2]
  Repeat cycle every 28 days until disease progression or unacceptable toxicity
Variation 3:
  Paclitaxel: IV: 175 mg/m^2 over 3 hours day 1
    [total dose/cycle = 175 mg/m^2]
  Repeat cycle every 21 days for 6-10 cycles
Variation 4 (heavily pretreated or poor performance status patients):
  Paclitaxel: IV: 135 mg/m^2 over 3 hours day 1
    [total dose/cycle = 135 mg/m^2]
  Repeat cycle every 21 days for 6-10 cycles

References
Variation 1:
Lortholary A, Largiller R, Weber B, et al, "Weekly Paclitaxel as a Single Agent or in Combination With Carboplatin or Weekly Topotecan in Patients With Resistant Ovarian Cancer: The CARTAXHY Randomized Phase II Trial From Groupe d'Investigateurs Nationaux pour l'Etude des Cancers Ovarianens (GINECO)," *Ann Oncol*, 2012, 23(2):346-52.

Variation 2:
Markman M, Blessing J, Rubin SC, et al, "Phase II Trial of Weekly Paclitaxel (80mg/m²) in Platinum and Paclitaxel-Resistant Ovarian and Primary Peritoneal Cancers: A Gynecologic Group Study," *Gynecol Oncol*, 2006, 101(3):436-40.
Variation 3 and 4:
Bruzzone M, Catsafados E, Miglietta L, et al, "Salvage Chemotherapy With Paclitaxel in Platinum-Resistant Advanced Ovarian Cancer Patients," *Oncology*, 1996, 53(5):349-53.

Paclitaxel-Pertuzumab-Trastuzumab (Breast)

Index Terms Pertuzumab-Trastuzumab-Paclitaxel (Breast); Trastuzumab-Pertuzumab-Paclitaxel (Breast)

Use Breast cancer

Regimen

Cycle 1:
Trastuzumab: IV: 8 mg/kg (loading dose) day 1 cycle 1
[total dose/cycle 1 = 8 mg/kg]
Paclitaxel: IV: 80 mg/m² days 1, 8, and 15
[total dose/cycle 1 = 240 mg/m²]
Pertuzumab: IV: 840 mg (loading dose) day 1 cycle 1
[total dose/cycle 1 = 840 mg]
Treatment cycle is 21 days
Subsequent cycles:
Trastuzumab: IV: 6 mg/kg day 1
[total dose/cycle = 6 mg/kg]
Paclitaxel: IV: 80 mg/m² days 1, 8, and 15
[total dose/cycle = 240 mg/m²]
Pertuzumab: IV: 420 mg day 1
[total dose/cycle = 420 mg]
Repeat cycle every 21 days

References

Datko FM, D'Andrea G, Dickler MN, et al, "Phase II Study of Pertuzumab, Trastuzumab, and Weekly Paclitaxel in Patients With HER2-Overexpressing Metastatic Breast Cancer (MBC)," *J Clin Oncol*, 2012, 30(27s)134:[abstract 134 from 2012 ASCO Annual Meeting]

Paclitaxel (Protein Bound) (Breast Regimen)

Use Breast cancer

Regimen NOTE: Multiple variations are listed.

Variation 1:
Paclitaxel (Protein Bound): IV: 260 mg/m² over 30 minutes day 1
[total dose/cycle = 260 mg/m²]
Repeat cycle every 21 days
Variation 2:
Paclitaxel (Protein Bound): IV: 150 mg/m² over 30 minutes days 1, 8, and 15
[total dose/cycle = 450 mg/m²]
Repeat cycle every 28 days
Variation 3:
Paclitaxel (Protein Bound): IV: 100 mg/m² over 30 minutes days 1, 8, and 15
[total dose/cycle = 300 mg/m²]
Repeat cycle every 28 days

References

Variation 1:
Gradishar WJ, Tjulandin S, Davidson N, et al, "Phase III Trial of Nanoparticale Albumin-Bound Paclitaxel Compared With Polyethylated Castor Oil-Based Paclitaxel in Woman With Breast Cancer, *J Clin Oncol*, 2005, 23(31):7794-7803.

Variation 2 and 3:

Gradishar WJ, Krasnojon D, Cheporov S, et al, "Significantly Longer Progression-Free Survival With *nab*-Paclitaxel Compared With Docetaxel as First-Line Therapy for Metastatic Breast Cancer," *J Clin Oncol*, 2009, 27(22):3611-3619.

◆ **Paclitaxel (Protein Bound)-Carboplatin (NSCLC)** *see* Carboplatin-Paclitaxel (Protein Bound) (NSCLC) *on page 1872*

◆ **Paclitaxel (Protein Bound)-Gemcitabine (Pancreatic)** *see* Gemcitabine-Paclitaxel (Protein Bound) (Pancreatic) *on page 1996*

Paclitaxel (Protein Bound) (NSCLC Regimen)

Index Terms nab Paclitaxel (NSCLC Regimen)

Use Lung cancer, non-small cell

Regimen NOTE: Multiple variations are listed.

Variation 1:

Paclitaxel (Protein Bound): IV: 260 mg/m^2 over 30 minutes day 1
[total dose/cycle = 260 mg/m^2]

Repeat cycle every 21 days until disease progression or unacceptable toxicity

Variation 2:

Paclitaxel (Protein Bound): IV: 125 mg/m^2/day over 30 minutes days 1, 8, and 15
[total dose/cycle = 375 mg/m^2]

Repeat cycle every 28 days until disease progression or unacceptable toxicity

References

Variation 1:

Green MR, Manikhas GM, Orlov S, et al, "Abraxane®, a Novel Cremophor®-Free, Albumin-Bound Particle Form of Paclitaxel for the Treatment of Advanced Non-Small-Cell Lung Cancer," *Ann Oncol*, 2006, 17(8):1263-8.

Variation 2:

Rizvi NA, Riely GJ, Azzoli CG, et al, "Phase I/II Trial of Weekly Intravenous 130-nm Albumin-Bound Paclitaxel As Initial Chemotherapy in Patients With Stage IV Non-Small-Cell Lung Cancer," *J Clin Oncol*, 2008, 26(4):639-43.

Paclitaxel (Protein Bound) (Ovarian Regimen)

Index Terms *nab* Paclitaxel (Ovarian Regimen); Abraxane (Ovarian Regimen); Paclitaxel (nanoparticle albumin bound) (Ovarian Regimen)

Use Ovarian cancer

Regimen NOTE: Multiple variations are listed.

Variation 1:

Paclitaxel (Protein Bound): IV: 260 mg/m^2 over 30 minutes day 1
[total dose/cycle = 260 mg/m^2]

Repeat cycle every 21 days for 6 cycles, or up to a maximum of 8 cycles

Variation 2:

Paclitaxel (Protein Bound): IV: 100 mg/m^2 over 30 minutes days 1, 8 and 15
[total dose/cycle = 300 mg/m^2]

Repeat cycle every 28 days until disease progression or unacceptable toxicity

References

Variation 1:

Teneriello MG, Tseng PC, Crozier M, et al, "Phase II Evaluation of Nanoparticle Albumin-Bound Paclitaxel in Platinum-Sensitive Patients With Recurrent Ovarian, Peritoneal, or Fallopian Tube Cancer," *J Clin Oncol*, 2009, 27(9):1426-31.

Variation 2:
Coleman RL, Brady WE, McMeekin DS, et al, "A Phase II Evaluation of Nanoparticle Albumin-Bound (Nab) Paclitaxel in the Treatment of Recurrent or Persistent Platinum-Resistant Ovarian, Fallopian Tube, or Primary Peritoneal Cancer: A Gynecologic Oncology Group Study," *Gynecol Oncol*, 2011, 122 (1): 111-115.

Paclitaxel-Ramucirumab (Gastric)

Index Terms Ramucirumab-Paclitaxel (Gastric)

Use Gastric cancer

Regimen

Ramucirumab: IV: 8 mg/kg days 1 and 15
[total dose/cycle = 16 mg/kg]
Paclitaxel: IV: 80 mg/m² days 1, 8, and 15
[total dose/cycle = 240 mg/m²]

Repeat cycle every 28 days until disease progression or unacceptable toxicity

References

Wilke H, Muro K, Van Cutsem E, et al. Ramucirumab plus paclitaxel versus placebo plus paclitaxel in patients with previously treated advanced gastric or gastro-oesophageal junction adenocarcinoma (RAINBOW): a double-blind, randomised phase 3 trial. *Lancet Oncol*. 2014;15 (11):1224-1235.

Paclitaxel (Small Cell Lung Cancer Regimen)

Use Lung cancer, small cell

Regimen NOTE: Multiple variations are listed.

Variation 1:
Paclitaxel: IV: 175 mg/m² over 3 hours day 1
[total dose/cycle = 175 mg/m²]
Repeat cycle every 21 days

Variation 2:
Paclitaxel: IV: 80 mg/m²/day over 1 hour days 1, 8, 15, 22, 29, and 36
[total dose/cycle = 480 mg/m²]
Repeat cycle every 56 days

References

Variation 1:
Smit EF, Fokkema E, Biesma B, et al, "A Phase II Study of Paclitaxel in Heavily Pretreated Patients With Small-Cell Lung Cancer," *Br J Cancer*, 1998, 77(2):347-51.

Variation 2:
Yamamoto N, Tsurutani J, Yoshimura N, et al, "Phase II Study of Weekly Paclitaxel for Relapsed and Refractory Small Cell Lung Cancer," *Anticancer Res*, 2006, 26(1B):777-82.

♦ **Paclitaxel-Topotecan-Bevacizumab (Cervical)** *see* Bevacizumab-Paclitaxel-Topotecan (Cervical) *on page 1845*

Paclitaxel-Trastuzumab (Breast)

Index Terms Trastuzumab-Paclitaxel (Breast)

Use Breast cancer

Regimen NOTE: Multiple variations are listed.

Variation 1 (weekly [preferred]):
Cycle 1:
Trastuzumab: IV: 4 mg/kg (loading dose) over 90 minutes day 0 cycle 1 only
[total dose/cycle 1 = 4 mg/kg]
Paclitaxel: IV: 90 mg/m² over 1 hour day 1
[total dose/cycle 1 = 90 mg/m²]
Treatment cycle 1 is 7 days

Subsequent cycles:
Paclitaxel: IV: 90 mg/m^2 over 1 hour day 1
[total dose/cycle = 90 mg/m^2]
Trastuzumab: IV: 2 mg/kg over 30 minutes day 1
[total dose/cycle = 2 mg/kg]
Repeat cycle every 7 days until disease progression or unacceptable toxicity

Variation 2 (weekly [preferred]):
Cycle 1:
Trastuzumab: IV: 4 mg/kg (loading dose) over 90 minutes day 1 cycle 1 only
[total dose/cycle 1 = 4 mg/kg]
Paclitaxel: IV: 80 mg/m^2 over 1 hour day 1
[total dose/cycle 1 = 80 mg/m^2]
Treatment cycle 1 is 7 days
Subsequent cycles:
Trastuzumab: IV: 2 mg/kg over 30 minutes day 1
[total dose/cycle = 2 mg/kg]
Paclitaxel: IV: 80 mg/m^2 over 1 hour day 1
[total dose/cycle = 80 mg/m^2]
Repeat cycle every 7 days

Variation 3 (every 3 weeks):
Cycle 1:
Trastuzumab: IV: 4 mg/kg (loading dose) over 90 minutes day 1 cycle 1 only
followed by:
Trastuzumab: IV: 2 mg/kg/day over 30 minutes days 8, 15
[total dose/cycle 1 = 8 mg/kg]
Paclitaxel: IV: 175 mg/m^2 over 3 hours day 1
[total dose/cycle 1 = 175 mg/m^2]
Treatment cycle 1 is 21 days
Subsequent cycles:
Trastuzumab: IV: 2 mg/kg/day over 30 minutes days 1, 8, 15
[total dose/cycle = 6 mg/kg]
Paclitaxel: IV: 175 mg/m^2 over 3 hours day 1
[total dose/cycle = 175 mg/m^2]
Repeat cycle every 21 days

References

Variation 1:
Seidman AD, Fornier MN, Esteva FJ, et al, "Weekly Trastuzumab and Paclitaxel Therapy for Metastatic Breast Cancer With Analysis of Efficacy by HER2 Immunophenotype and Gene Amplification," *J Clin Oncol*, 2001, 19(10):2587-95.

Variation 2 and 3:
Seidman AD, Berry D, Cirrincione C, et al, "Randomized Phase III Trial of Weekly Compared With Every-3-Weeks Paclitaxel for Metastatic Breast Cancer, With Trastuzumab for all HER-2 Overexpressors and Random Assignment to Trastuzumab or Not in HER-2 Nonoverexpressors: Final Results of Cancer and Leukemia Group B Protocol 9840," *J Clin Oncol*, 2008, 26(10):1642-9.

◆ **Paclitaxel-Carboplatin (NSCLC)** *see* Carboplatin-Paclitaxel (NSCLC) *on page 1870*

◆ **PAD (Multiple Myeloma)** *see* Bortezomib-Doxorubicin-Dexamethasone (Multiple Myeloma) *on page 1849*

Palbociclib-Fulvestrant (Breast)

Index Terms Fulvestrant-Palbociclib (Breast)

Use Breast cancer, advanced second-line endocrine-based therapy (ER-Positive, HER2-Negative, relapsed or progressed during prior endocrine therapy)

◀ **Regimen** NOTE: In the study, premenopausal and perimenopausal patients also received goserelin (starting at least 4 weeks prior to randomization and then every 28 days) for the duration of therapy.

Cycle 1:

Palbociclib: Oral: 125 mg once daily (with food) for 21 days, followed by 7 days off treatment

[total dose/cycle = 2,625 mg]

Fulvestrant: IM: 500 mg days 1 and 15

[total dose/cycle = 1,000 mg]

Treatment cycle is 28 days

Subsequent Cycles:

Palbociclib: Oral: 125 mg once daily (with food) for 21 days, followed by 7 days off treatment

[total dose/cycle = 2,625 mg]

Fulvestrant: IM: 500 mg day 1

[total dose/cycle = 500 mg]

Repeat cycle every 28 days until disease progression or unacceptable toxicity

References

Turner NC, Ro J, André F, et al. Palbociclib in Hormone-Receptor-Positive Advanced Breast Cancer. *N Engl J Med.* 2015;373(3):209-219.

Palbociclib-Letrozole (Breast)

Index Terms Letrozole-Palbociclib (Breast)

Use Breast cancer, advanced (ER-Positive, HER2-Negative)

Regimen

Palbociclib: Oral: 125 mg once daily (with food) for 21 days, followed by 7 days off treatment

[total dose/cycle = 2,625 mg]

Letrozole: Oral: 2.5 mg once daily days 1 to 28

[total dose/cycle = 70 mg]

Repeat cycle every 28 days until disease progression or unacceptable toxicity

References

Finn RS, Crown JP, Lang I, et al. The cyclin-dependent kinase 4/6 inhibitor palbociclib in combination with letrozole versus letrozole alone as first-line treatment of oestrogen receptor-positive, HER2-negative, advanced breast cancer (PALOMA-1/TRIO-18): a randomised phase 2 study. *Lancet Oncol.* 2015;16(1):25-35.

Panitumumab (Colorectal Regimen)

Use Colorectal cancer

Regimen

Panitumumab: IV: 6 mg/kg over 60 minutes day 1

[total dose/cycle = 6 mg/kg]

Repeat cycle every 14 days until disease progression or unacceptable toxicity

References

Amado RG, Wolf M, Peeters M, et al, "Wild-Type *KRAS* Is Required for Panitumumab Efficacy in Patients With Metastatic Colorectal Cancer," *J Clin Oncol,* 2008, 26(10):1626-34.

Van Cutsem E, Peeters M, Siena S, et al, "Open-Label Phase III Trial of Panitumumab Plus Best Supportive Care Compared With Best Supportive Care Alone in Patients With Chemotherapy-Refractory Metastatic Colorectal Cancer," *J Clin Oncol,* 2007, 25(13):1658-64.

Panitumumab + FOLFIRI (Colorectal)

Use Colorectal cancer

Regimen

Panitumumab: IV: 6 mg/kg over 30-60 minutes day 1
  [total dose/cycle = 6 mg/kg]
Irinotecan: IV: 180 mg/m^2 day 1
  [total dose/cycle = 180 mg/m^2]
Leucovorin (racemic): IV: 400 mg/m^2 day 1
  [total dose/cycle = 400 mg/m^2]
Fluorouracil: IV bolus: 400 mg/m^2 day 1
  followed by IV: 2400 mg/m^2 continuous infusion (CI) over 46 hours beginning day 1
  [total fluorouracil dose/cycle (bolus and CI) = 2800 mg/m^2]
Repeat cycle every 14 days until disease progression or unacceptable toxicity

References

Peeters M, Price TJ, Cervantes A, et al, "Randomized Phase III Study of Panitumumab With Fluorouracil, Leucovorin, and Irinotecan (FOLFIRI) Compared With FOLFIRI Alone as Second-Line Treatment in Patients With Metastatic Colorectal Cancer," *J Clin Oncol*, 2010, 28 (31):4706-13.

Panitumumab + FOLFOX4 (Colorectal)

Use Colorectal cancer

Regimen

Panitumumab: IV: 6 mg/kg over 30-60 minutes day 1
  [total dose/cycle = 6 mg/kg]
Oxaliplatin: IV: 85 mg/m^2 day 1
  [total dose/cycle = 85 mg/m^2]
Leucovorin: IV: 200 mg/m^2/day days 1 and 2
  [total dose/cycle = 400 mg/m^2]
Fluorouracil: IV bolus: 400 mg/m^2/day days 1 and 2
  followed by IV: 600 mg/m^2 continuous infusion (CI) over 22 hours days 1 and 2
  [total fluorouracil dose/cycle (bolus and CI) = 2000 mg/m^2]
Note: Bolus fluorouracil and continuous infusion fluorouracil are both given on each day
Repeat cycle every 14 days until disease progression or unacceptable toxicity

References

Douillard JY, Siena S, Cassidy J, et al, "Randomized, Phase III Trial of Panitumumab With Infusional Fluorouracil, Leucovorin, and Oxaliplatin (FOLFOX4) Versus FOLFOX4 Alone as First-Line Treatment in Patients With Previously Untreated Metastatic Colorectal Cancer: The PRIME Study," *J Clin Oncol*, 2010, 28(31):4697-705.

Panobinostat-Bortezomib-Dexamethasone (Multiple Myeloma)

Index Terms Bortezomib-Dexamethasone-Panobinostat (Multiple Myeloma); Dexamethasone-Bortezomib-Panobinostat (Multiple Myeloma)
Use Multiple myeloma (relapsed/refractory)

Regimen

Phase I: Cycles 1 to 8:
  Panobinostat: Oral: 20 mg days 1, 3, 5, 8, 10, and 12
    [total dose/cycle = 120 mg]
  Bortezomib: IV: 1.3 mg/m^2/day days 1, 4, 8, and 11
    [total dose/cycle = 5.2 mg/m^2]

Dexamethasone: Oral: 20 mg daily days 1, 2, 4, 5, 8, 9, 11, and 12
  [total dose/cycle = 160 mg]
Repeat cycle every 21 days for 8 cycles; if patient derives clinical benefit then proceed to phase II
Phase II: Cycles 9 to 12:
Panobinostat: Oral: 20 mg days 1, 3, 5, 8, 10, 12, 22, 24, 26, 29, 31, and 33
  [total dose/cycle = 240 mg]
Bortezomib: IV: 1.3 mg/m^2/day days 1, 8, 22, and 29
  [total dose/cycle = 5.2 mg/m^2]
Dexamethasone: Oral: 20 mg daily days 1, 2, 8, 9, 22, 23, 29, and 30
  [total dose/cycle = 160 mg]
Repeat cycle every 42 days for 4 cycles

References
San-Miguel JF, Hungria VT, Yoon SS, et al. Panobinostat plus bortezomib and dexamethasone versus placebo plus bortezomib and dexamethasone in patients with relapsed or relapsed and refractory multiple myeloma: a multicentre, randomised, double-blind phase 3 trial. *Lancet Oncol.* 2014;15(11):1195-1206.

Pazopanib (RCC Regimen)
Use Renal cell cancer
Regimen
Pazopanib: Oral: 800 mg once daily
  [total dose/cycle = 22,400 mg]
Repeat cycle every 28 days until disease progression or unacceptable toxicity
References
Sternberg CN, Davis ID, Mardiak J, et al, "Pazopanib in Locally Advanced or Metastatic Renal Cell Carcinoma: Results of a Randomized Phase III Trial," *J Clin Oncol*, 2010, 28(6): 1061-8.

Pazopanib (Soft Tissue Sarcoma Regimen)
Use Soft tissue sarcoma (advanced, refractory)
Regimen
Pazopanib: Oral: 800 mg once daily
  [total dose/cycle = 22,400 mg]
Repeat cycle every 28 days until disease progression or unacceptable toxicity
References
van der Graaf WT, Blay JY, Chawla SP, et al. Pazopanib for metastatic soft-tissue sarcoma (PALETTE): a randomised, double-blind, placebo-controlled phase 3 trial. *Lancet.* 2012;379 (9829):1879-1886.

Pazopanib (Thyroid Regimen)
Use Thyroid cancer
Regimen
Pazopanib: Oral: 800 mg once daily
  [total dose/cycle = 22,400 mg]
Repeat cycle every 28 days until disease progression or unacceptable toxicity
References
Bible KC, Suman VJ, Molina JR, et al. Efficacy of pazopanib in progressive, radioiodine-refractory, metastatic differentiated thyroid cancers: results of a phase 2 consortium study. *Lancet Oncol*, 2010;11(10): 962-972.

◆ **PCF (Unknown Primary)** see Cisplatin-Fluorouracil-Paclitaxel (Unknown Primary, Squamous Cell) on page 1903

PCG (Bladder)
Index Terms Paclitaxel-Cisplatin-Gemcitabine (Bladder)

Use Bladder cancer (locally advanced, metastatic)
Regimen
Paclitaxel: IV: 80 mg/m^2/day days 1 and 8
[total dose/cycle = 160 mg/m^2]
Cisplatin: IV: 70 mg/m^2 day 1
[total dose/cycle = 70 mg/m^2]
Gemcitabine: IV: 1,000 mg/m^2/day days 1 and 8
[total dose/cycle = 2,000 mg/m^2]
Repeat cycle every 21 days until disease progression, unacceptable toxicity, or a maximum of up to 6 cycles

References
Bellmunt J, von der Maase H, Mead GM, et al. Randomized phase III study comparing paclitaxel/cisplatin/gemcitabine (PCG) and gemcitabine/cisplatin (GC) in patients with locally advanced (LA) or metastatic (M) urothelial cancer without prior systemic therapy; EORTC30987/Intergroup Study. *J Clin Oncol.* 2007;25(suppl 18):LBA5030.

Bellmunt J, von der Maase H, Mead GM, et al. Randomized phase III study comparing paclitaxel/cisplatin/gemcitabine and gemcitabine/cisplatin in patients with locally advanced or metastatic urothelial cancer without prior systemic therapy: EORTC Intergroup Study 30987. *J Clin Oncol.* 2012;30(10):1107-1113.

◆ **PC (NSCLC)** *see* Carboplatin-Paclitaxel (NSCLC) *on page 1870*
◆ **PCR (CLL)** *see* Pentostatin-Cyclophosphamide-Rituximab (CLL) *on page 2065*

PCV (Brain Tumor Regimen)

Index Terms Procarbazine-CCNU-Vincristine; Procarbazine-Lomustine-Vincristine
Use Brain tumors
Regimen NOTE: Multiple variations are listed.
Variation 1:
Lomustine: Oral: 110 mg/m^2 day 1
[total dose/cycle = 110 mg/m^2]
Procarbazine: Oral: 60 mg/m^2/day days 8 to 21
[total dose/cycle = 840 mg/m^2]
Vincristine: IV: 1.4 mg/m^2/day (maximum dose: 2 mg) days 8 and 29
[total dose/cycle = 2.8 mg/m^2; maximum: 4 mg]
Repeat cycle every 6 weeks for a total of 6 cycles
Variation 2:
Lomustine: Oral: 110 mg/m^2 day 1
[total dose/cycle = 110 mg/m^2]
Procarbazine: Oral: 60 mg/m^2/day days 8 to 21
[total dose/cycle = 840 mg/m^2]
Vincristine: IV: 1.4 mg/m^2/day (maximum dose: 2 mg) days 8 and 29
[total dose/cycle = 2.8 mg/m^2; maximum: 4 mg]
Repeat cycle every 6 weeks for a total of 7 cycles
Variation 3:
Procarbazine: Oral: 75 mg/m^2/day days 8 to 21
[total dose/cycle = 1050 mg/m^2]
Lomustine: Oral: 130 mg/m^2 day 1
[total dose/cycle = 130 mg/m^2]
Vincristine: IV: 1.4 mg/m^2/day (no maximum) days 8 and 29
[total dose/cycle = 2.8 mg/m^2; no maximum]
Repeat cycle every 6 weeks for a total of 6 cycles

◀ Variation 4:

Procarbazine: Oral: 75 mg/m^2/day days 8 to 21
[total dose/cycle = 1050 mg/m^2]

Lomustine: Oral: 130 mg/m^2 day 1
[total dose/cycle = 130 mg/m^2]

Vincristine: IV: 1.4 mg/m^2/day (no maximum) days 8 and 29
[total dose/cycle = 2.8 mg/m^2; no maximum]

Repeat cycle every 6 weeks for up to a total of 4 cycles

Variation 5:

Lomustine: Oral: 110 mg/m^2 day 1
[total dose/cycle = 110 mg/m^2]

Procarbazine: Oral: 60 mg/m^2/day days 8 to 21
[total dose/cycle = 840 mg/m^2]

Vincristine: IV: 1.4 mg/m^2/day days 8 and 29
[total dose/cycle = 2.8 mg/m^2]

Repeat cycle every 6-8 weeks for 1 year

References

Variation 1:

van den Bent MJ, Carpentier AF, Brandes AA, et al, "Adjuvant Procarbazine, Lomustine, and Vincristine Improves Progression-Free Survival But Not Overall Survival in Newly Diagnosed Anaplastic Oligodendrogliomas and Oligoastrocytomas: A Randomized European Organisation for Research and Treatment of Cancer Phase III Trial," *J Clin Oncol*, 2006, 24(18):2715-22.

Variation 2:

Levin VA, Uhm JH, Jaeckle KA, et al, "Phase III Randomized Study of Postradiotherapy Chemotherapy With Alpha-Difluoromethylornithine-Procarbazine, N-(2-Chloroethyl)-N'-Cyclohexyl-N-Nitrosurea, Vincristine (DFMO-PCV) Versus PCV for Glioblastoma Multiforme," *Clin Cancer Res*, 2000, 6(10):3878-84.

Variation 3:

Cairncross G, Macdonald D, Ludwin S, et al, "Chemotherapy for Anaplastic Oligodendroglioma. National Cancer Institute of Canada Clinical Trials Group," *J Clin Oncol*, 1994, 12(10):2013-21.

Variation 4:

Intergroup Radiation Therapy Oncology Group Trial 9402, Cairncross G, Berkey B, et al, "Phase III Trial of Chemotherapy Plus Radiotherapy Compared With Radiotherapy Alone for Pure and Mixed Anaplastic Oligodendroglioma: Intergroup Radiation Therapy Oncology Group Trial 9402," *J Clin Oncol*, 2006, 24(18):2707-14.

Variation 5:

Levin VA, Silver P, Hannigan J, et al, "Superiority of Post-Radiotherapy Adjuvant Chemotherapy With CCNU, Procarbazine, and Vincristine (PCV) Over BCNU for Anaplastic Gliomas: NCOG 6G61 Final Report," *Int J Radiat Oncol Biol Phys*, 1990, 18(2):321-4.

Pemetrexed (Bladder Cancer Regimen)

Use Bladder cancer

Regimen

Pemetrexed: IV: 500 mg/m^2 infused over 10 minutes day 1
[total dose/cycle = 500 mg/m^2]

Repeat cycle every 21 days

References

Sweeney CJ, Roth BJ, Kabbinavar FF, et al, "Phase II Study of Pemetrexed for Second-Line Treatment of Transitional Cell Cancer of the Urothelium," *J Clin Oncol*, 2006, 24(21):3451-7.

♦ **Pemetrexed-Carboplatin-Bevacizumab (NSCLC)** *see* Bevacizumab-Carboplatin-Pemetrexed (NSCLC) *on page 1839*

♦ **Pemetrexed-Carboplatin (Mesothelioma)** *see* Carboplatin-Pemetrexed (Mesothelioma) *on page 1874*

♦ **Pemetrexed-Carboplatin (NSCLC)** *see* Carboplatin-Pemetrexed (NSCLC) *on page 1874*

Pemetrexed (Cervical Regimen)

Use Cervical cancer

Regimen NOTE: Multiple variations are listed.

Variation 1:

Pemetrexed: IV: 500 mg/m^2 over 10 minutes day 1

[total dose/cycle = 500 mg/m^2]

Repeat cycle every 21 days until disease progression or unacceptable toxicity

Variation 2 (no prior radiation):

Pemetrexed: IV: 900 mg/m^2 over 10 minutes day 1

[total dose/cycle = 900 mg/m^2]

Repeat cycle every 21 days until disease progression or unacceptable toxicity

Variation 3 (prior radiation):

Pemetrexed: IV: 700 mg/m^2 over 10 minutes day 1

[total dose/cycle = 700 mg/m^2]

Repeat cycle every 21 days until disease progression or unacceptable toxicity

References

Variation 1:

Lorusso D, Ferrandina G, Pignata S, et al, "Evaluation of Pemetrexed (Alimta, LY231514) as Second-Line Chemotherapy in Persistent or Recurrent Carcinoma of the Cervix: The CERVIX 1 Study of the MITO (Multicentre Italian Trials in Ovarian Cancer and Gynecologic Malignancies) Group," *Ann Oncol*, 2010, 21(1):61-6.

Variation 2 and 3:

Miller DS, Blessing JA, Bodurka DC, et al, "Evaluation of Pemetrexed (Alimta, LY231514) as Second Line Chemotherapy in Persistent or Recurrent Carcinoma of the Cervix: A Phase II Study of the Gynecologic Oncology Group," *Gynecol Oncol*, 2008, 110(1):65-70.

♦ **Pemetrexed-Cisplatin (Mesothelioma)** *see* Cisplatin-Pemetrexed (Mesothelioma) *on page 1911*

♦ **Pemetrexed-Cisplatin (NSCLC)** *see* Cisplatin-Pemetrexed (NSCLC) *on page 1911*

Pemetrexed (Mesothelioma Regimen)

Use Malignant pleural mesothelioma

Regimen

Pemetrexed: IV: 500 mg/m^2 over 10 minutes day 1

[total dose/cycle = 500 mg/m^2]

Repeat cycle every 21 days

References

Jassem J, Ramlau R, Santoro A, et al, "Phase III Trial of Pemetrexed Plus Best Supportive Care Compared With Best Supportive Care in Previously Treated Patients With Advanced Malignant Pleural Mesothelioma," *J Clin Oncol*, 2008, 26(10):1698-1704.

Taylor P, Castagneto B, Dark G, et al, "Single-Agent Pemetrexed for Chemonaïve and Pretreated Patients With Malignant Pleural Mesothelioma: Results of an International Expanded Access Program," *J Thorac Oncol*, 2008, 3(7):764-71.

Pemetrexed (NSCLC Regimen)

Use Lung cancer, non-small cell

◄ **Regimen** NOTE: Multiple variations are listed.

Variation 1 (second-line):

Pemetrexed: IV: 500 mg/m^2 over 10 minutes day 1

[total dose/cycle = 500 mg/m^2]

Repeat cycle every 21 days until disease progression or unacceptable toxicity

Variation 2 (maintenance therapy):

Pemetrexed: IV: 500 mg/m^2 day 1

[total dose/cycle = 500 mg/m^2]

Repeat cycle every 21 days until disease progression or unacceptable toxicity

References

Variation 1:

Hanna N, Shephard FA, Fossella FV, et al, "Randomized Phase III Trial of Pemetrexed Versus Docetaxel in Patients With Non-Small-Cell Lung Cancer Previously Treated With Chemotherapy," *J Clin Oncol*, 2004, 22(9):1589-97.

Variation 2:

Ciuleanu T, Brodowicz T, Zielinski C, et al, "Maintenance Pemetrexed Plus Best Supportive Care Versus Palcebo Plus Best Supportive Care For Non-Small-Cell Lung Cancer: A Randomised, Double-Blind, Phase 3 Study," *Lancet*, 2009, 374(9699):1432-40.

Pemetrexed (Ovarian Regimen)

Use Ovarian cancer

Regimen NOTE: Multiple variations are listed.

Variation 1:

Pemetrexed: IV: 500 mg/m^2 day 1

[total dose/cycle = 500 mg/m^2]

Repeat cycle every 21 days

Variation 2 (no prior radiation):

Pemetrexed: IV: 900 mg/m^2 over 10 minutes day 1

[total dose/cycle = 900 mg/m^2]

Repeat cycle every 21 days until disease progression or unacceptable toxicity

Variation 3 (prior radiation):

Pemetrexed: IV: 700 mg/m^2 over 10 minutes day 1

[total dose/cycle = 700 mg/m^2]

Repeat cycle every 21 days until disease progression or unacceptable toxicity

References

Variation 1:

Vergote I, Calvert H, Kania M, et al, "A Randomised, Double-Blind, Phase II Study of Two Doses of Pemetrexed in the Treatment of Platinum-Resistant, Epithelial Ovarian or Primary Peritoneal Cancer," *Eur J Cancer*, 2009, 45(8):1415-23.

Variation 2 and 3:

Miller DS, Blessing JA, Krasner CN, et al, "Phase II Evaluation of Pemetrexed in the Treatment of Recurrent or Persistent Platinum-Resistant Ovarian or Primary Peritoneal Carcinoma: A Study of the Gynecologic Oncology Group," *J Clin Oncol*, 2009, 27(16):2686-91.

Pemetrexed (Thymoma/Thymic Regimen)

Use Thymoma/thymic carcinoma (recurrent)

Regimen

Pemetrexed: IV: 500 mg/m^2 day 1

[total dose/cycle = 500 mg/m^2]

Repeat cycle every 21 days for up to 6 cycles

References

Loehrer PJ, Yiannoutsos CT, Dropcho S, et al. A phase II trial of pemetrexed in patients with recurrent thymoma or thymic carcinoma. *J Clin Oncol*. 2006;24(suppl):7079 [abstract 7079 from 2006 ASCO Annual Meeting].

◆ **PE (NSCLC)** *see* Cisplatin-Etoposide (NSCLC) *on page 1894*

Pentostatin-Cyclophosphamide-Rituximab (CLL)

Index Terms Cyclophosphamide-Pentostatin-Rituximab (CLL); PCR (CLL)

Use Leukemia, chronic lymphocytic

Regimen NOTE: Multiple variations are listed.

Variation 1 (refractory):

Cycle 1:

Cyclophosphamide: IV: 600 mg/m^2 day 1
  [total dose/cycle = 600 mg/m^2]
Pentostatin: IV: 4 mg/m^2 day 1
  [total dose/cycle = 4 mg/m^2]
Filgrastim: SubQ: 300 mcg (patients ≤70 kg) or 480 mcg (patients >70 kg)
  daily beginning 2 days after each treatment and continued until ANC
  >5,000/mm^3 or >1,500/mm^3 for 2 days
Treatment cycle duration is 21 days

Cycles 2 to 6:

Cyclophosphamide: IV: 600 mg/m^2 day 1
  [total dose/cycle = 600 mg/m^2]
Pentostatin: IV: 4 mg/m^2 day 1
  [total dose/cycle = 4 mg/m^2]
Rituximab: IV: 375 mg/m^2 day 1
  [total dose/cycle = 375 mg/m^2]
Filgrastim: SubQ: 300 mcg (patients ≤70 kg) or 480 mcg (patients >70 kg)
  daily beginning 2 days after each treatment and continued until ANC
  >5,000/mm^3 or >1,500/mm^3 for 2 days
Repeat cycle every 21 days for total of 3 cycles, if at a least partial
  response, continue for a total of 6 cycles

Variation 2 (first-line):

Cycle 1:

Cyclophosphamide: IV: 600 mg/m^2 day 1
  [total dose/cycle = 600 mg/m^2]
Pentostatin: IV: 2 mg/m^2 day 1
  [total dose/cycle = 2 mg/m^2]
Rituximab: IV: 100 mg/m^2 day 1 cycle 1 only
  followed by IV: 375 mg/m^2/day days 3 and 5 cycle 1 only
    [total dose/cycle 1 = 850 mg/m^2]
Filgrastim: SubQ: Daily (dose not specified) beginning day 3 and continued
  for 10 consecutive days or until ANC >1,000/mm^3 for 2 consecutive days
Treatment cycle duration is 21 days

Cycles 2 to 6:

Cyclophosphamide: IV: 600 mg/m^2 day 1
  [total dose/cycle = 600 mg/m^2]
Pentostatin: IV: 2 mg/m^2 day 1
  [total dose/cycle = 2 mg/m^2]
Rituximab: IV: 375 mg/m^2 day 1
  [total dose/cycle = 375 mg/m^2]

◀   Filgrastim: SubQ: Daily (dose not specified) beginning day 3 and continued for 10 consecutive days or until ANC >1,000/mm^3 for 2 consecutive days

    Repeat cycle every 21 days for a total of 6 cycles

References

Variation 1:

Lamanna N, Kalaycio M, Maslak P, et al. Pentostatin, cyclophosphamide, and rituximab is an active, well-tolerated regimen for patients with previously treated chronic lymphocytic leukemia. *J Clin Oncol.* 2006;24(10):1575-1581.

Variation 2:

Kay NE, Geyer SM, Call TG, et al. Combination chemoimmunotherapy with pentostatin, cyclophosphamide, and rituximab shows significant clinical activity with low accompanying toxicity in previously untreated B chronic lymphocytic leukemia. *Blood.* 2007;109(2):405-411.

Shanafelt TD, Lin T, Geyer SM, et al. Pentostatin, cyclophosphamide, and rituximab regimen in older patients with chronic lymphocytic leukemia. *Cancer.* 2007;109(11):2291-2298.

PEP-C (NHL)

Index Terms Prednisone, Etoposide, Procarbazine, Cyclophosphamide (NHL)

Use Lymphoma, non-Hodgkin

Regimen

Prednisone: Oral: 20 mg once daily after breakfast (morning dose)

Cyclophosphamide: Oral: 50 mg once daily after lunch (afternoon dose)

Etoposide: Oral: 50 mg once daily after dinner (evening dose)

Procarbazine: Oral: 50 mg once daily at bedtime (night dose)

Length of cycle and frequency depends on phase of treatment and blood counts

References

Coleman M, Martin P, Ruan J, et al, "Prednisone, Etoposide, Probarbazine, And Cyclophosphamide (PEP-C) Oral Combination Chemotherapy Regimen For Recurring/Refractory Lymphoma: Low-Dose Metronomic, Multidrug Therapy," *Cancer*, 2008, 112(10):2228-32.

Pertuzumab-Trastuzumab-Docetaxel (Metastatic Breast)

Index Terms Docetaxel-Pertuzumab-Trastuzumab (Metastatic Breast); Trastuzumab-Pertuzumab-Docetaxel (Metastatic Breast)

Use Breast cancer, metastatic (HER2-positive, first-line treatment)

Regimen

Cycle 1:

Pertuzumab: IV: 840 mg (loading dose) day 1 cycle 1

[total dose/cycle 1 = 840 mg]

Trastuzumab: IV: 8 mg/kg (loading dose) day 2 cycle 1

[total dose/cycle 1 = 8 mg/kg]

Docetaxel: IV: 75 mg/m^2 day 2 (administer after trastuzumab on day 2)

[total dose/cycle 1 = 75 mg/m^2]

Treatment cycle duration is 21 days

Subsequent cycles:

Pertuzumab: IV: 420 mg day 1

[total dose/cycle = 420 mg]

Trastuzumab: IV: 6 mg/kg day 1

[total dose/cycle = 6 mg/kg]

Docetaxel: IV: 75 mg/m² day 1 (may escalate to 100 mg/m² if tolerated; administer after trastuzumab and pertuzumab)
[total dose/cycle = 75 to 100 mg/m²]

Repeat cycle every 21 days until disease progression or unacceptable toxicity (minimum of 6 cycles of docetaxel). In the case of discontinuation of chemotherapy owing to toxic effects, antibody therapy may be continued until disease progression.

References

Baselga J, Cortés J, Kim SB, et al. Pertuzumab plus trastuzumab plus docetaxel for metastatic breast cancer. N Engl J Med. 2012;366(2):109-119.

Swain SM, Baselga J, Kim SB, et al. Pertuzumab, trastuzumab, and docetaxel in HER2-positive metastatic breast cancer. N Engl J Med. 2015;372(8):724-734.

Pertuzumab-Trastuzumab-Docetaxel (Neoadjuvant Breast)

Index Terms Docetaxel-Pertuzumab-Trastuzumab (Neoadjuvant Breast); Trastuzumab-Pertuzumab-Docetaxel (Neoadjuvant Breast)

Use Breast cancer, neoadjuvant

Regimen

Cycle 1:

Trastuzumab: IV: 8 mg/kg (loading dose) day 1 cycle 1
[total dose/cycle 1 = 8 mg/kg]

Pertuzumab: IV: 840 mg (loading dose) day 1 cycle 1
[total dose/cycle 1 = 840 mg]

Docetaxel: IV: 75 mg/m² day 1 (administer after trastuzumab and pertuzumab)
[total dose/cycle 1 = 75 mg/m²]

Treatment cycle is 21 days

Cycles 2-4:

Trastuzumab: IV: 6 mg/kg day 1
[total dose/cycle = 6 mg/kg]

Pertuzumab: IV: 420 mg day 1
[total dose/cycle = 420 mg]

Docetaxel: IV: 75 mg/m² day 1 (may escalate to 100 mg/m² if tolerated; administer after trastuzumab and pertuzumab)
[total dose/cycle = 75-100 mg/m²]

Repeat cycle every 21 days for a total of 4 cycles

References

Gianni L, Pienkowski T, Im YH, et al. Efficacy and safety of neoadjuvant pertuzumab and trastuzumab in women with locally advanced, inflammatory, or early HER2-positive breast cancer (NeoSphere): a randomised multicentre, open-label, phase 2 trial. Lancet Oncol. 2012;13 (1):25-32.

◆ **Pertuzumab-Trastuzumab-Paclitaxel (Breast)** see Paclitaxel-Pertuzumab-Trastuzumab (Breast) *on page 2054*

◆ **PE (Small Cell Lung Cancer)** see Cisplatin-Etoposide (Small Cell Lung Cancer) *on page 1895*

POC

Use Brain tumors

Regimen

Prednisone: Oral: 40 mg/m²/day days 1 to 14
[total dose/cycle = 560 mg/m²]

◄ Vincristine: IV: 1.5 mg/m^2/day (maximum dose: 2 mg) days 1, 8, and 15
[total dose/cycle = 4.5 mg/m^2]
Lomustine: Oral: 100 mg/m^2 day 1
[total dose/cycle = 100 mg/m^2]
Repeat cycle every 6 weeks

References

Finlay JL, Boyett JM, Yates AJ, et al, "Randomized Phase III Trial in Childhood High-Grade Astrocytoma Comparing Vincristine, Lomustine, and Prednisone With the Eight-Drugs-In-1-Day Regimen. Childrens Cancer Group," *J Clin Oncol*, 1995, 13(1):112-23.

Pomalidomide-Dexamethasone (Multiple Myeloma)

Index Terms POM-LoDEX (Multiple Myeloma); Pomalidomide-Low-Dose Dexamethasone (Multiple Myeloma)

Use Multiple myeloma

Regimen
Pomalidomide: Oral: 4 mg once daily days 1 to 21
[total dose/cycle = 84 mg]
Dexamethasone: Oral: 40 mg once daily on days 1, 8, 15, and 22
[total dose/cycle = 160 mg]
Repeat cycle every 28 days until disease progression or unacceptable toxicity

References

Richardson PG, Siegel DS, Vij R, et al. Pomalidomide alone or in combination with low-dose dexamethasone in relapsed and refractory multiple myeloma: a randomized phase 2 study. *Blood*. 2014;123(12):1826-1832.

San Miguel J, Weisel K, Moreau P, et al. Pomalidomide plus low-dose dexamethasone versus high-dose dexamethasone alone for patients with relapsed and refractory multiple myeloma (MM-003): a randomised, open-label, phase 3 trial. *Lancet Oncol*. 2013;14(11):1055-1066.

◆ **Pomalidomide-Low-Dose Dexamethasone (Multiple Myeloma)** *see* Pomalidomide-Dexamethasone (Multiple Myeloma) *on page* 2068

◆ **POM-LoDEX (Multiple Myeloma)** *see* Pomalidomide-Dexamethasone (Multiple Myeloma) *on page* 2068

POMP

Use Leukemia, acute lymphocytic

Regimen Maintenance:
Mercaptopurine: Oral: 50 mg 3 times/day
[total dose/cycle = 4200-4600 mg]
Methotrexate: Oral: 20 mg/m^2 once weekly
[total dose/cycle = 80 mg/m^2]
Vincristine: IV: 2 mg day 1
[total dose/cycle = 2 mg]
Prednisone: Oral: 200 mg/day days 1 to 5
[total dose/cycle = 1000 mg]
Repeat cycle monthly for 2 years

References

Kantarjian HM, O'Brien S, Smith TL, et al, "Results of Treatment With Hyper-CVAD, a Dose-Intensive Regimen, in Adult Acute Lymphocytic Leukemia," *J Clin Oncol*, 2000, 18(3):547-61.

Ponatinib (ALL Regimen)

Use Leukemia, acute lymphocytic

Regimen
Ponatinib: Oral: 45 mg once daily days 1 to 28
[total dose/cycle = 1260 mg]
Repeat cycle every 28 days until disease progression or unacceptable toxicity

References

Cortes JE, Kim DW, Pinilla-Ibarz J, et al. A phase 2 trial of ponatinib in Philadelphia chromosome-positive leukemias. *N Engl J Med.* 2013;369(19):1783-1796.

Ponatinib (CML Regimen)

Use Leukemia, chronic myelogenous
Regimen
Ponatinib: Oral: 45 mg once daily days 1 to 28
[total dose/cycle = 1260 mg]
Repeat cycle every 28 days until disease progression or unacceptable toxicity
References

Cortes JE, Kim DW, Pinilla-Ibarz J, et al. A phase 2 trial of ponatinib in Philadelphia chromosome-positive leukemias. *N Engl J Med.* 2013;369(19):1783-1796.

PVA (POG 8602)

Index Terms AlinC 14
Use Leukemia, acute lymphocytic
Regimen
Induction:
Prednisone: Oral: 40 mg/m^2/day (maximum dose: 60 mg) given in 3 divided doses days 0 to 28
[total dose/cycle = 1160 mg/m^2]
Vincristine: IV: 1.5 mg/m^2/day (maximum dose: 2 mg) days 0, 7, 14, and 21
[total dose/cycle = 6 mg/m^2; maximum: 8 mg]
Asparaginase: IM: 6000 units/m^2 3 times per week for 2 weeks
[total dose/cycle = 36,000 units/m^2]
Intrathecal therapy (triple): Days 0 and 22
Leucovorin: Route and dose not specified: Single dose 24 hours after every intrathecal treatment days 1 and 23
Administer one cycle only

◄ **CNS consolidation:**
Mercaptopurine: Oral: 75 mg/m^2/day days 29 to 43
[total dose/cycle = 1125 mg/m^2]
Intrathecal therapy (triple): Days 29 and 36
Leucovorin: Route and dose not specified: Single dose 24 hours after every
intrathecal treatment days 30 and 37
Administer one cycle only
Intensification:
Regimen A:
Methotrexate: IV: 1000 mg/m^2 continuous infusion over 24 hours day 1
[total dose/cycle = 1000 mg/m^2]
Cytarabine: IV: 1000 mg/m^2 continuous infusion over 24 hours day 1 (start 12
hours after start of methotrexate)
[total dose/cycle = 1000 mg/m^2]
Leucovorin: IM, IV, or Oral: 30 mg/m^2 at 24 and 36 hours after the start of
methotrexate
[total dose/cycle = 60 mg/m^2]
followed by IM, IV, or Oral: 3 mg/m^2 at 48, 60, and 72 hours after the start
of methotrexate
[total dose/cycle = 9 mg/m^2]
Repeat cycle every 3 weeks for 6 cycles (administered weeks 7, 10, 13, 16,
19, and 22)
Intrathecal therapy (triple): Weeks 9, 12, 15, and 18
Leucovorin: Route and dose not specified: Single dose 24 hours after every
intrathecal treatment weeks 9, 12, 15, and 18
or
Regimen B:
Methotrexate: IV: 1000 mg/m^2 continuous infusion over 24 hours day 1
[total dose/cycle = 1000 mg/m^2]
Cytarabine: IV: 1000 mg/m^2 continuous infusion over 24 hours day 1 (start 12
hours after methotrexate)
[total dose/cycle = 1000 mg/m^2]
Leucovorin: IM, IV, or Oral: 30 mg/m^2 at 24 and 36 hours after the start of
methotrexate
[total dose/cycle = 60 mg/m^2]
followed by IM, IV, or Oral: 3 mg/m^2 at 48, 60, and 72 hours after the start
of methotrexate
[total dose/cycle = 9 mg/m^2]
Repeat cycle every 12 weeks for 6 cycles (administer weeks 7, 19, 31, 43, 55,
and 67)
Intrathecal therapy (triple): Weeks 9, 12, 15, and 18
Leucovorin: Route and dose not specified: Single dose 24 hours after every
intrathecal treatment weeks 9, 12, 15, and 18
Maintenance:
Regimen A:
Methotrexate: IM: 20 mg/m^2 weekly, weeks 25 to 156
[total dose/cycle = 2640 mg/m^2]
Mercaptopurine: Oral: 75 mg/m^2 daily, weeks 25 to 156
[total dose/cycle = 69,300 mg/m^2]
Intrathecal therapy (triple): Every 8 weeks, weeks 26 through 105
Leucovorin: Route and dose not specified: Single dose 24 hours after every
intrathecal treatment weeks 26 through 105

Prednisone: Oral: 40 mg/m^2/day (maximum dose: 60 mg) days 1 to 7 (given in 3 divided doses), weeks 8, 17, 25, 41, 57, 73, 89, and 105
[total dose/cycle = 2240 mg/m^2; maximum: 3360 mg]

Vincristine: IV: 1.5 mg/m^2/day (maximum dose: 2 mg) day 1, weeks 8, 9, 17, 18, 25, 26, 41, 42, 57, 58, 73, 74, 89, 90, 105, and 106
[total dose/cycle = 24 mg/m^2; maximum: 32 mg]

or

Regimen B:

Methotrexate: IM: 20 mg/m^2 weekly, weeks 22-28, 34-40, 46-52, and 58-64
[total dose/cycle = 560 mg/m^2]

Mercaptopurine: Oral: 75 mg/m^2 daily for 7 weeks, weeks 22-28, 34-40, 46-52, and 58-64
[total dose/cycle = 14700 mg/m^2]

followed by

Methotrexate: IM: 20 mg/m^2 weekly, weeks 70 to 156
[total dose/cycle = 1720 mg/m^2]

Mercaptopurine: Oral: 75 mg/m^2 daily, weeks 70 to 156
[total dose/cycle = 45,150 mg/m^2]

Intrathecal therapy (triple): Every 8 weeks, weeks 26 through 105

Leucovorin: Route and dose not specified: Single dose 24 hours after every intrathecal treatment weeks 26 through 105

Prednisone: Oral: 40 mg/m^2/day (maximum dose: 60 mg) days 1 to 7 (given in 3 divided doses), weeks 8, 17, 25, 41, 57, 73, 89, and 105
[total dose/cycle = 2240 mg/m^2]

Vincristine: IV: 1.5 mg/m^2/day (maximum dose: 2 mg) day 1, weeks 8, 9, 17, 18, 25, 26, 41, 42, 57, 58, 73, 74, 89, 90, 105, and 106
[total dose/cycle = 24 mg/m^2; maximum dose: 32 mg]

References

Land VJ, Shuster JJ, Crist WM, et al, "Comparison of Two Schedules of Intermediate-Dose Methotrexate and Cytarabine Consolidation Therapy for Childhood B-Precursor Cell Acute Lymphoblastic Leukemia: A Pediatric Oncology Group Study," *J Clin Oncol*, 1994, 12(9):1939-45.

PVDA

Use Leukemia, acute lymphocytic

Regimen Induction:

Prednisone: Oral: 60 mg/m^2/day days 1 to 28
[total dose/cycle = 1680 mg/m^2]

Vincristine: IV: 1.5 mg/m^2/day days 1, 8, 15, and 22
[total dose/cycle = 6 mg/m^2]

Daunorubicin: IV: 25 mg/m^2/day days 1, 8, 15, and 22
[total dose/cycle = 100 mg/m^2]

Asparaginase: IM, SubQ, or IV: 5000 units/m^2/day days 1 to 14
[total dose/cycle = 70,000 units/m^2]

Administer one cycle only; used in conjunction with intrathecal chemotherapy

References

Hoelzer D, Thiel E, Loffler H, et al, "Intensified Therapy in Acute Lymphoblastic and Acute Undifferentiated Leukemia in Adults," *Blood*, 1984, 64(1):38-47.

♦ **Raltitrexed-Cisplatin (Mesothelioma)** *see* Cisplatin-Raltitrexed (Mesothelioma) *on page 1911*

♦ **Ramucirumab-Docetaxel (NSCLC)** *see* Docetaxel-Ramucirumab (NSCLC) *on page 1946*

Ramucirumab-FOLFIRI (Colorectal)

Index Terms Ramucirumab-Irinotecan-Leucovorin-Fluorouracil (Colorectal Cancer)

Use Colorectal cancer (relapsed, refractory)

Regimen

Ramucirumab: IV: 8 mg/kg over 60 minutes day 1
  [total dose/cycle = 8 mg/kg]
Irinotecan: IV: 180 mg/m^2 over 90 minutes day 1
  [total dose/cycle = 180 mg/m^2]
Leucovorin: IV: 400 mg/m^2 over 2 hours day 1
  [total dose/cycle = 400 mg/m^2]
Fluorouracil: IV bolus: 400 mg/m^2 day 1
  followed by IV: 2,400 mg/m^2 continuous infusion over 48 hours beginning day 1
  [total fluorouracil dose/cycle (bolus and continuous infusion) = 2,800 mg/m^2]
Repeat cycle every 14 days until disease progression or unacceptable toxicity

References

Tabernero J, Yoshino T, Cohn AL, et al. Ramucirumab versus placebo in combination with second-line FOLFIRI in patients with metastatic colorectal carcinoma that progressed during or after first-line therapy with bevacizumab, oxaliplatin, and a fluoropyrimidine (RAISE): a randomised, double-blind, multicentre, phase 3 study. *Lancet Oncol.* 2015;16(5):499-508.

Ramucirumab (Gastric Regimen)

Use Gastric cancer

Regimen

Ramucirumab: IV: 8 mg/kg day 1
  [total dose/cycle = 8 mg/kg]
Repeat cycle every 14 days

References

Fuchs CS, Tomasek J, Yong CJ, et al. Ramucirumab monotherapy for previously treated advanced gastric or gastro-oesophageal junction adenocarcinoma (REGARD): an international, randomised, multicentre, placebo-controlled, phase 3 trial. *Lancet.* 2014;383(9911):31-39.

◆ **Ramucirumab-Irinotecan-Leucovorin-Fluorouracil (Colorectal Cancer)** *see* Ramucirumab-FOLFIRI (Colorectal) *on page* 2072

◆ **Ramucirumab-Paclitaxel (Gastric)** *see* Paclitaxel-Ramucirumab (Gastric) *on page* 2056

◆ **R-CHOP (NHL)** *see* Rituximab-CHOP (NHL) *on page* 2077

R-CHOP (Waldenstrom Macroglobulinemia)

Index Terms Rituximab-Cyclophosphamide-Doxorubicin-Vincristine-Prednisone (Waldenstrom Macroglobulinemia)

Use Waldenstrom Macroglobulinemia

Regimen

Rituximab: IV: 375 mg/m^2 day 1
  [total dose/cycle = 375 mg/m^2]
Cyclophosphamide: IV: 750 mg/m^2 day 1
  [total dose/cycle = 750 mg/m^2]
Doxorubicin: IV: 50 mg/m^2 day 1
  [total dose/cycle = 50 mg/m^2]
Vincristine: IV: 1.4 mg/m^2 (maximum dose: 2 mg) day 1
  [total dose/cycle = 1.4 mg/m^2; maximum: 2 mg]

Prednisone: Oral: 100 mg/day days 1 to 5
  [total dose/cycle = 500 mg]
Repeat cycle every 21 days for 6 cycles

References

Ioakimidis L, Patterson CJ, Hunter ZR, et al. Comparative outcomes following CP-R, CVP-R, and CHOP-R in Waldenström's macroglobulinemia. *Clin Lymphoma Myeloma.* 2009;9(1):62-6.

R-CVP (NHL-Follicular)

Index Terms CVP-R (NHL-Follicular); RCVP (NHL-Follicular); Rituximab-CVP (NHL-Follicular); Rituximab-Cyclophosphamide-Vincristine-Prednisone (NHL-Follicular)

Use Lymphoma, non-Hodgkin (first-line therapy for advanced follicular lymphoma)

Regimen

Rituximab: IV: 375 mg/m^2 day 1
  [total dose/cycle = 375 mg/m^2]
Cyclophosphamide: IV: 750 mg/m^2 day 1
  [total dose/cycle = 750 mg/m^2]
Vincristine: IV: 1.4 mg/m^2 (maximum dose: 2 mg) day 1
  [total dose/cycle = 1.4 mg/m^2 (maximum: 2 mg/cycle)]
Prednisone: Oral: 40 mg/m^2/day days 1 to 5
  [total dose/cycle = 200 mg/m^2]
Repeat cycle every 21 days for up to 8 cycles

References

Federico M, Luminari S, Dondi A, et al. R-CVP versus R-CHOP versus R-FM for the initial treatment of patients with advanced-stage follicular lymphoma: results of the FOLL05 trial conducted by the Fondazione Italiana Linfomi. *J Clin Oncol.* 2013;31(12):1506-1513.

Marcus R, Imrie K, Belch A, et al. CVP chemotherapy plus rituximab compared with CVP as first-line treatment for advanced follicular lymphoma. *Blood.* 2005;105(4):1417-1423.

◆ **RCVP (NHL-Follicular)** *see* R-CVP (NHL-Follicular) *on page 2073*

R-DHAP (NHL-DLBCL)

Index Terms Cisplatin-Cytarabine-Dexamethasone-Rituximab (NHL-DLBCL); Rituximab-Dexamethasone-Cisplatin-Cytarabine (NHL-DLBCL)

Use Lymphoma, non-Hodgkin (DLBCL relapsed/refractory transplant eligible)

Regimen

Rituximab: IV: 375 mg/m^2 day 1
  [total dose/cycle = 375 mg/m^2]
Dexamethasone: Oral: 40 mg daily days 1 to 4
  [total dose/cycle = 160 mg]
Cisplatin: IV: 100 mg/m^2 continuous infusion over 24 hours day 1
  [total dose/cycle = 100 mg/m^2]
Cytarabine: IV: 2,000 mg/m^2 over 3 hours every 12 hours for 2 doses day 2 (begins at the end of the cisplatin infusion)
  [total dose/cycle = 4,000 mg/m^2]
Repeat cycle every 21 days for 2 cycles followed by autologous stem-cell transplant; patients without complete or partial response were allowed 1 additional cycle

References

Crump M, Kuruvilla J, Couban S, et al. Randomized comparison of gemcitabine, dexamethasone, and cisplatin versus dexamethasone, cytarabine, and cisplatin chemotherapy before autologous stem-cell transplantation for relapsed and refractory aggressive lymphomas: NCIC-CTG LY.12. *J Clin Oncol.* 2014;32(31):3490-3496.

- ◆ **Rd (Multiple Myeloma)** *see* Lenalidomide-Dexamethasone (Multiple Myeloma) *on page 2028*

- ◆ **Regimen DD-4A (Wilms' Tumor)** *see* DD-4A (Wilms' Tumor) *on page 1936*

- ◆ **Regimen A3 (Neuroblastoma)** *see* A3 (Neuroblastoma) *on page 1819*

- ◆ **Regimen EE-4A (Wilms' Tumor)** *see* EE-4A (Wilms' Tumor) *on page 1953*

Regimen I (Wilms' Tumor)

Index Terms Vincristine, Doxorubicin, Cyclophosphamide, Mesna, Etoposide
Use Wilms' tumor
Regimen NOTE: Multiple variations are listed.

Variation 1 (patients ≤30 kg):

Vincristine: IV: 0.05 mg/kg (maximum dose: 2 mg) IV push day 1 of weeks 1, 2, 4 to 8, 10 and 11
Followed by
Vincristine 0.067 mg/kg (maximum dose: 2 mg) IV push day 1 of weeks 12, 13, 18, and 24
[total dose = 0.718 mg/kg; maximum: 26 mg]
Doxorubicin: IV: 1.5 mg/kg IV push day 1 of weeks 0, 6, 12, 18, and 24
[total dose = 7.5 mg/kg]
Cyclophosphamide: IV: 14.7 mg/kg/day days 1 to 5 of weeks 3, 9, 15, and 21
[total dose = 294 mg/kg]
Mesna: IV: 3 mg/kg/dose 4 doses/day (after cyclophosphamide) days 1 to 5 of weeks 3, 9, 15, and 21
[total dose = 240 mg/kg]
Cyclophosphamide: IV: 14.7 mg/kg/day days 1 to 3 of weeks 6, 12, 18, and 24
[total dose = 176.4 mg/kg]
Mesna: IV: 3 mg/kg/dose 4 doses/day (after cyclophosphamide) days 1 to 3 of weeks 6, 12, 18, and 24
[total dose = 144 mg/kg]
Etoposide: IV: 3.3 mg/kg/day days 1 to 5 of weeks 3, 9, 15, and 21
[total dose = 66 mg/kg]
Filgrastim: SubQ: 5 mcg/kg/day beginning 24 hours after last dose of chemotherapy and continued until ANC ≥10,000/mm^3 or for a minimum of 1 week
Treatment course duration is week 0 through week 24

Variation 2 (patients >30 kg):

Vincristine: IV: 1.5 mg/m^2 (maximum dose: 2 mg) IV push day 1 of weeks 1, 2, 4 to 8, 10 and 11
Followed by
Vincristine 2 mg/m^2 (maximum dose: 2 mg) IV push days 1 of weeks 12, 13, 18, and 24
[total dose = 21.5 mg/m^2; maximum: 26 mg]
Doxorubicin: IV: 45 mg/m^2 IV push day 1 of weeks 0, 6, 12, 18, and 24
[total dose = 225 mg/m^2]
Cyclophosphamide: IV: 440 mg/m^2/day days 1 to 5 of weeks 3, 9, 15, and 21
[total dose = 8800 mg/m^2]
Mesna: IV: 90 mg/m^2/dose 4 doses/day (after cyclophosphamide) days 1 to 5 of weeks 3, 9, 15, and 21
[total dose = 7200 mg/m^2]
Cyclophosphamide: IV: 440 mg/m^2/day days 1 to 3 of weeks 6, 12, 18, and 24
[total dose = 5280 mg/m^2]

Mesna: IV: 90 mg/m^2/dose 4 doses/day (after cyclophosphamide) days 1 to 3 of weeks 6, 12, 18, and 24
[total dose = 4320 mg/m^2]

Etoposide: IV: 100 mg/m^2/day days 1 to 5 of weeks 3, 9, 15, and 21
[total dose = 2000 mg/m^2]

Filgrastim: SubQ: 5 mcg/kg/day beginning 24 hours after last dose of chemotherapy and continued until ANC ≥10,000/mm^3 or for a minimum of 1 week

Treatment course duration is week 0 through week 24

References

Variations 1 and 2:

Green DM, Cotton CA, Malogolowkin M, et al, "Treatment of Wilms Tumor Relapsing After Initial Treatment With Vincristine and Actinomycin D: A Report From the National Wilms Tumor Study Group," *Pediatr Blood Cancer*, 2007, 48(5):493-9.

◆ **Regimen new A1 (Neuroblastoma)** *see* New A1 (Neuroblastoma) *on page 2043*

Regorafenib (Colorectal Regimen)

Use Colorectal cancer

Regimen

Regorafenib: Oral: 160 mg once daily for 21 days
[total dose/cycle = 3360 mg]

Repeat cycle every 28 days, continue until disease progression or unacceptable toxicity

References

Grothey A, Van Cutsem E, Sobrero A, et al, "Regorafenib Monotherapy for Previously Treated Metastatic Colorectal Cancer (CORRECT): An International, Multicenter, Randomized, Placebo-Controlled, Phase 3 Trial," *Lancet*, 2013, 381(9863):303-12.

Regorafenib (GIST Regimen)

Use Soft Tissue Sarcoma (Gastrointestinal Stromal Tumor [GIST])

Regimen

Regorafenib: Oral: 160 mg once daily days 1 to 21
[total dose/cycle = 3360 mg]

Repeat cycle every 28 days, continue until disease progression or unacceptable toxicity

References

Demetri GD, Reichardt P, Kang YK, et al, "Efficacy and Safety of Regorafenib for Advanced Gastrointestinal Stromal Tumours After Failure of Imatinib and Sunitinib (GRID): An International, Multicenter, Randomized, Placebo-Controlled, Phase 3 Trial," *Lancet*, 2013, 381(9863):295-302.

◆ **R-EPOCH Dose Adjusted (NHL)** *see* EPOCH (Dose-Adjusted)-Rituximab (NHL) *on page 1959*

◆ **R-EPOCH (NHL)** *see* EPOCH-Rituximab (NHL) *on page 1961*

◆ **R-FCM (NHL)** *see* Fludarabine-Cyclophosphamide-Mitoxantrone-Rituximab *on page 1972*

◆ **R-GCD (NHL-DLBCL)** *see* Rituximab-Gemcitabine-Dexamethasone-Carboplatin (NHL-DLBCL) *on page 2081*

◆ **R-GDC (NHL-DLBCL)** *see* Rituximab-Gemcitabine-Dexamethasone-Carboplatin (NHL-DLBCL) *on page 2081*

◆ **R-GDP (NHL-DLBCL)** *see* Rituximab-Gemcitabine-Dexamethasone-Cisplatin (NHL-DLBCL) *on page 2081*

R-ICE (NHL-DLBCL)

Index Terms R-ICE (NHL-DLBCL); RICE (NHL-DLBCL); Rituximab-ICE (NHL-DLBCL); Rituximab-Ifosfamide-Carboplatin-Etoposide (NHL-DLBCL)

Use Lymphoma, non-Hodgkin (before autologous stem cell transplantation for relapsed or primary refractory DLBCL)

Regimen

Forty-eight hours prior to cycle 1:

Rituximab: IV: 375 mg/m^2 48 hours prior to initiation of cycle 1
[total dose/cycle = 375 mg/m^2]

Cycles 1 and 2:

Rituximab: IV: 375 mg/m^2 day 1
[total dose/cycle = 375 mg/m^2]

Etoposide: IV: 100 mg/m^2/day days 3, 4, and 5
[total dose/cycle = 300 mg/m^2]

Carboplatin: IV: AUC = 5 (maximum dose: 800 mg) day 4
[total dose/cycle = AUC = 5 (maximum dose/cycle: 800 mg)]

Ifosfamide: IV: 5,000 mg/m^2 continuous infusion over 24 hours beginning on day 4
[total dose/cycle = 5,000 mg/m^2]

Mesna: IV: 5,000 mg/m^2 continuous infusion over 24 hours beginning on day 4
[total dose/cycle = 5,000 mg/m^2]

Filgrastim: SubQ: 5 mcg/kg/day days 7 to 14
[total dose/cycle = 40 mcg/kg]

Repeat cycle every 14 days for 2 cycles

Cycle 3:

Rituximab: IV: 375 mg/m^2 day 1
[total dose/cycle = 375 mg/m^2]

Etoposide: IV: 100 mg/m^2/day days 3, 4, and 5
[total dose/cycle = 300 mg/m^2]

Carboplatin: IV: AUC = 5 (maximum dose: 800 mg) day 4
[total dose/cycle = AUC = 5 (maximum dose/cycle: 800 mg)]

Ifosfamide: IV: 5,000 mg/m^2 continuous infusion over 24 hours beginning on day 4
[total dose/cycle = 5,000 mg/m^2]

Mesna: IV: 5,000 mg/m^2 continuous infusion over 24 hours beginning on day 4
[total dose/cycle = 5,000 mg/m^2]

Filgrastim: SubQ: 10 mcg/kg/day days 7 until end of leukapheresis

Treatment cycle is 14 days

References

Kewalramani T, Zelenetz AD, Nimer SD, et al. Rituximab and ICE as second-line therapy before autologous stem cell transplantation for relapsed or primary refractory diffuse large B-cell lymphoma. *Blood.* 2004;103(10):3684-3688.

- ◆ **Rituximab-Bendamustine (NHL-Mantle Cell)** *see* Bendamustine-Rituximab (NHL-Mantle Cell) *on page 1836*
- ◆ **Rituximab-Bendamustine (Waldenstrom Macroglobulinemia)** *see* Bendamustine-Rituximab (Waldenstrom Macroglobulinemia) *on page 1837*
- ◆ **Rituximab-Bortezomib-Bendamustine (NHL-Follicular)** *see* Bendamustine-Bortezomib-Rituximab (NHL-Follicular) *on page 1833*
- ◆ **Rituximab-Bortezomib-Cyclophosphamide-Doxorubicin-Prednisone (NHL-Mantle Cell)** *see* VcR-CAP (NHL-Mantle Cell) *on page 2106*
- ◆ **Rituximab-Bortezomib (Waldenstrom Macroglobulinemia)** *see* Bortezomib-Rituximab (Waldenstrom Macroglobulinemia) *on page 1850*

Rituximab-CHOP (NHL)

Index Terms CHOP-Rituximab (NHL); R-CHOP (NHL); RCHOP (NHL)

Use Lymphoma, non-Hodgkin

Regimen NOTE: Multiple variations are listed.

Variation 1 (diffuse large B-cell lymphoma):
Rituximab: IV: 375 mg/m² day 1
[total dose/cycle = 375 mg/m²]
Cyclophosphamide: IV: 750 mg/m² day 1
[total dose/cycle = 750 mg/m²]
Doxorubicin: IV: 50 mg/m² day 1
[total dose/cycle = 50 mg/m²]
Vincristine: IV: 1.4 mg/m² (maximum dose: 2 mg) day 1
[total dose/cycle = 1.4 mg/m²; maximum: 2 mg]
Prednisone: Oral: 40 mg/m²/day days 1 to 5
[total dose/cycle = 200 mg/m²]
Repeat cycle every 21 days for a total of 8 cycles

Variation 2 (low-grade or follicular lymphoma):
Rituximab: IV: 375 mg/m² administer 7 and 2 days prior to the start of cycle 1 of CHOP, 2 days prior to the start of cycles 3 and 5 of CHOP, and after the 6th cycle of CHOP on days 134 and 141 (total of 6 doses of rituximab)
CHOP:
Cyclophosphamide: IV: 750 mg/m² day 1
[total dose/cycle = 750 mg/m²]
Doxorubicin: IV: 50 mg/m² day 1
[total dose/cycle = 50 mg/m²]
Vincristine: IV: 1.4 mg/m² (maximum dose: 2 mg) day 1
[total dose/cycle = 1.4 mg/m²; maximum: 2 mg]
Prednisone: Oral: 100 mg/m²/day days 1 to 5
[total dose/cycle = 500 mg/m²]
Repeat each CHOP cycle every 21 days for a total of 6 CHOP cycles

Variation 3 (dose-dense R-CHOP in aggressive CD20-expressing B-cell lymphomas):
Pre-treatment (to improve performance status and diminish adverse effects to cycle 1):
Vincristine: IV: 1 mg 1 week before cycle 1
Prednisone: Oral: 100 mg/day for 7 days 1 week before cycle 1
Rituximab: IV: 375 mg/m² day 1
[total dose/cycle = 375 mg/m²]
Cyclophosphamide: IV: 750 mg/m² day 1
[total dose/cycle = 750 mg/m²]

Doxorubicin: IV: 50 mg/m^2 day 1
  [total dose/cycle = 50 mg/m^2]
Vincristine: IV: 2 mg day 1
  [total dose/cycle = 2 mg]
Prednisone: Oral: 100 mg/day days 1 to 5
  [total dose/cycle = 500 mg]
Filgrastim (dose and route not specified): Daily beginning day 4 until
  leukocyte recovery
Repeat cycle every 14 days for a total of 6 cycles
Variation 4 (diffuse large B-cell lymphoma):
 Rituximab: IV: 375 mg/m^2 days -7, 1, 22, and 43
  [total dose/cycle = 1400 mg/m^2]
 Cyclophosphamide: IV: 750 mg/m^2 days 3, 24, and 45
  [total dose/cycle = 2250 mg/m^2]
 Doxorubicin: IV: 50 mg/m^2 days 3, 24, and 45
  [total dose/cycle = 150 mg/m^2]
 Vincristine: IV: 1.4 mg/m^2 (maximum dose: 2 mg) days 3, 24, and 45
  [total dose/cycle = 4.2 mg/m^2; maximum: 6 mg/cycle]
 Prednisone: Oral: 100 mg/day for 5 days starting on days 3, 24, and 45
  [total dose/cycle = 1500 mg]
 Cycle does not repeat; followed by radiation therapy beginning on day 66
Variation 5 (diffuse large B-cell lymphoma):
 Rituximab: IV: 375 mg/m^2 administer 7 and 3 days prior to the start of cycle 1
  of CHOP, 2 days prior to the start of cycles 3 and 5 of CHOP, and 2 days
  before cycle 7 (if administered)
 CHOP:
 Cyclophosphamide: IV: 750 mg/m^2 day 1
  [total dose/cycle = 750 mg/m^2]
 Doxorubicin: IV: 50 mg/m^2 day 1
  [total dose/cycle = 50 mg/m^2]
 Vincristine: IV: 1.4 mg/m^2 (maximum dose: 2 mg) day 1
  [total dose/cycle = 1.4 mg/m^2; maximum: 2 mg]
 Prednisone: Oral: 100 mg/m^2/day days 1 to 5
  [total dose/cycle = 500 mg/m^2]
 Repeat each CHOP cycle every 21 days for a total of 6 CHOP cycles
Variation 6 (mantle cell lymphoma):
 Rituximab: IV: 375 mg/m^2 day 0 (administer the day before CHOP)
  [total dose/cycle = 375 mg/m^2]
 Cyclophosphamide: IV: 750 mg/m^2 day 1
  [total dose/cycle = 750 mg/m^2]
 Doxorubicin: IV: 50 mg/m^2 day 1
  [total dose/cycle = 50 mg/m^2]
 Vincristine: IV: 1.4 mg/m^2 (maximum dose: 2 mg) day 1
  [total dose/cycle = 1.4 mg/m^2; maximum: 2 mg]
 Prednisone: Oral: 100 mg/m^2/day days 1 to 5
  [total dose/cycle = 500 mg/m^2]
 Repeat cycle every 21 days for a total of 6 cycles
Variation 7 (follicular lymphoma):
 Rituximab: IV: 375 mg/m^2 day 0 (administer the day before CHOP)
  [total dose/cycle = 375 mg/m^2]
 Cyclophosphamide: IV: 750 mg/m^2 day 1
  [total dose/cycle = 750 mg/m^2]
 Doxorubicin: IV: 50 mg/m^2 day 1
  [total dose/cycle = 50 mg/m^2]

Vincristine: IV: 1.4 mg/m^2 (maximum dose: 2 mg) day 1
  [total dose/cycle = 1.4 mg/m^2; maximum: 2 mg]
Prednisone: Oral: 100 mg/m^2/day days 1 to 5
  [total dose/cycle = 500 mg/m^2]
Repeat cycle every 21 days for a total of 6-8 cycles
Variation 8 (follicular lymphoma):
Rituximab: IV: 375 mg/m^2 day 1
  [total dose/cycle = 375 mg/m^2]
Cyclophosphamide: IV: 750 mg/m^2 day 1
  [total dose/cycle = 750 mg/m^2]
Doxorubicin: IV: 50 mg/m^2 day 1
  [total dose/cycle = 50 mg/m^2]
Vincristine: IV: 1.4 mg/m^2 (maximum dose: 2 mg) day 1
  [total dose/cycle = 1.4 mg/m^2; maximum: 2 mg]
Prednisone: Oral: 100 mg/day days 1 to 5
  [total dose/cycle = 500 mg]
Repeat cycle every 21 days for a total of 6 cycles
followed by (maintenance rituximab):
Rituximab: IV: 375 mg/m^2 day 1
  [total dose/cycle = 375 mg/m^2]
Repeat every 3 months until relapse or for a maximum of 2 years

References

Variation 1:

Coiffier B, Lepage E, Briere J, et al, "CHOP Chemotherapy Plus Rituximab Compared With CHOP Alone in Elderly Patients With Diffuse Large-B-Cell Lymphoma," *N Engl J Med*, 2002, 346 (4):235-42.

Coiffier B, Thieblemont C, Van Den Neste E, et al, "Long-Term Outcome of Patients in the LNH-98.5 Trial, the First Randomized Study Comparing Rituximab-CHOP to Standard CHOP Chemotherapy in DLBCL Patients: A Study by the Groupe d'Etudes des Lymphomes de l'Adulte," *Blood*, 2010, 116(12):2040-5.

Feugier P, Van Hoof A, Sebban C, et al, "Long-Term Results of the R-CHOP Study in the Treatment of Elderly Patients With Diffuse Large B Cell Lymphoma: A Study by the Groupe d'Etude des Lymphomes de l'Adulte," *J Clin Oncol*, 2005, 23(18):4117-26.

Variation 2:

Czuczman MS, Grillo-López AJ, White CA, et al, "Treatment of Patients With Low-Grade B-Cell Lymphoma With the Combination of Chimeric Anti-CD20 Monoclonal Antibody and CHOP Chemotherapy," *J Clin Oncol*, 1999, 17(1):268-76.

Czuczman MS, Weaver R, Alkuzweny B, et al, "Prolonged Clinical and Molecular Remission in Patients With Low-Grade or Follicular Non-Hodgkin's Lymphoma Treated With Rituximab Plus CHOP Chemotherapy: 9-Year Follow-Up," *J Clin Oncol*, 2004, 22(23):4711-6.

Variation 3:

Pfreundschuh M, Schubert J, Ziepert M, et al, "Six Versus Eight Cycles of Bi-Weekly CHOP-14 With or Without Rituximab in Elderly Patients With Aggressive CD20+ B-cell Lymphomas: A Randomised Controlled Trial (RICOVER-60)," *Lancet Oncol*, 2008, 9(2):105-16.

Variation 4:

Persky DO, Unger JM, Spier CM, et al, "Phase II Study of Rituximab Plus Three Cycles of CHOP and Involved-Field Radiotherapy for Patients With Limited-Stage Aggressive B-Cell Lymphoma: Southwest Oncology Group Study 0014," *J Clin Oncol*, 2008, 26(14):2258-63.

Variation 5:

Habermann TM, Weller EA, Morrison VA, et al, "Rituximab-CHOP Versus CHOP Alone or With Maintenance Rituximab in Older Patients With Diffuse Large B-cell Lymphoma," *J Clin Oncol*, 2006, 24(19):3121-7.

Variation 6:

Lenz G, Dreyling M, Hoster E, et al, "Immunochemotherapy With Rituximab and Cyclophosphamide, Doxorubicin, Vincristine, and Prednisone Significantly Improves Response and Time to Treatment Failure, but Not Long-Term Outcome in Patients With Previously Untreated Mantle Cell Lymphoma: Results of a Prospective Randomized Trial of the German Low Grade Lymphoma Study Group (GLSG)," *J Clin Oncol*, 2005, 23(9):1984-92

Variation 7:

Hiddemann W, Kneba M, Dreyling M, et al, "Frontline Therapy With Rituximab Added to the Combination of Cyclophosphamide, Doxorubicin, Vincristine, and Prednisone (CHOP) Significantly Improves the Outcome for Patients With Advanced-Stage Follicular Lymphoma Compared With Therapy With CHOP Alone: Results of a Prospective Randomized Study of the German Low-Grade Lymphoma Study Group," *Blood*, 2005, 106(12):3725-32.

Variation 8:

van Oers MH, Klasa R, Marcus RE, et al, "Rituximab Maintenance Improves Clinical Outcome of Relapsed/Resistant Follicular Non-Hodgkin Lymphoma in Patients Both With and Without Rituximab During Induction: Results of a Prospective Randomized Phase 3 Intergroup Trial," *Blood*, 2006, 108(10):3295-301.

van Oers MH, Van Glabbeke M, Giurgea L, et al, "Rituximab Maintenance Treatment of Relapsed/Resistant Follicular Non-Hodgkin's Lymphoma: Long-Term Outcome of the EORTC 20981 Phase III Randomized Intergroup Study," *J Clin Oncol*, 2010, 28(17):2853-8.

♦ **Rituximab-Cladribine (NHL-Mantle Cell)** *see* Cladribine-Rituximab (NHL-Mantle Cell) *on page 1916*

♦ **Rituximab-Cladribine (Waldenstrom Macroglobulinemia)** *see* Cladribine-Rituximab (Waldenstrom Macroglobulinemia) *on page 1916*

♦ **Rituximab-CVP (NHL-Follicular)** *see* R-CVP (NHL-Follicular) *on page 2073*

♦ **Rituximab-Cyclophosphamide-Doxorubicin-Vincristine-Prednisone (Waldenstrom Macroglobulinemia)** *see* R-CHOP (Waldenstrom Macroglobulinemia) *on page 2072*

♦ **Rituximab, Cyclophosphamide, Vincristine, Doxorubicin, Dexamethasone, Methotrexate, Cytarabine (NHL-Burkitt)** *see* Hyper-CVAD Alternating With High-Dose Methotrexate-Cytarabine + Rituximab + CNS Prophylaxis (NHL-Burkitt) *on page 2004*

♦ **Rituximab-Cyclophosphamide-Vincristine-Doxorubicin-Methotrexate-Cytarabine (NHL-Mantle Cell)** *see* Rituximab-Hyper-CVAD (NHL-Mantle Cell) *on page 2082*

♦ **Rituximab-Cyclophosphamide-Vincristine-Prednisone (NHL-Follicular)** *see* R-CVP (NHL-Follicular) *on page 2073*

♦ **Rituximab-Dexamethasone-Cisplatin-Cytarabine (NHL-DLBCL)** *see* R-DHAP (NHL-DLBCL) *on page 2073*

♦ **Rituximab-EPOCH Dose Adjusted (NHL)** *see* EPOCH (Dose-Adjusted)-Rituximab (NHL) *on page 1959*

♦ **Rituximab-EPOCH (NHL)** *see* EPOCH-Rituximab (NHL) *on page 1961*

♦ **Rituximab-Fludarabine (CLL)** *see* Fludarabine-Rituximab (CLL) *on page 1976*

♦ **Rituximab-Fludarabine-Cyclophosphamide (CLL)** *see* Fludarabine-Cyclophosphamide-Rituximab (CLL) *on page 1973*

♦ **Rituximab-Fludarabine-Cyclophosphamide-Mitoxantrone** *see* Fludarabine-Cyclophosphamide-Mitoxantrone-Rituximab *on page 1972*

♦ **Rituximab-Fludarabine-Cyclophosphamide (NHL-Follicular)** *see* Fludarabine-Cyclophosphamide-Rituximab (NHL-Follicular) *on page 1974*

♦ **Rituximab-Fludarabine-Mitoxantrone-Dexamethasone** *see* Fludarabine-Mitoxantrone-Dexamethasone-Rituximab *on page 1975*

♦ **Rituximab-Fludarabine (NHL-Follicular)** *see* Fludarabine-Rituximab (NHL-Follicular) *on page 1976*

Rituximab-Gemcitabine-Dexamethasone-Carboplatin (NHL-DLBCL)

Index Terms Gemcitabine-Dexamethasone-Carboplatin-Rituximab (NHL-DLBCL); R-GCD (NHL-DLBCL); R-GDC (NHL-DLBCL)

Use Lymphoma, non-Hodgkin (DLBCL relapsed refractory)

Regimen

Gemcitabine: IV: 1,000 mg/m^2/day over 30 minutes days 1 and 8
  [total dose/cycle = 2,000 mg/m^2]

Dexamethasone: Oral: 40 mg/day days 1 to 4
  [total dose/cycle = 160 mg]

Carboplatin: IV: AUC 5 over 30 minutes day 1
  [total dose/cycle = AUC = 5]

Rituximab: IV: 375 mg/m^2 day 8
  [total dose/cycle = 375 mg/m^2]

Repeat cycle every 21 days for up to 4 cycles

References

Gopal AK, Press OW, Shustov AR, et al. Efficacy and safety of gemcitabine, carboplatin, dexamethasone, and rituximab in patients with relapsed/refractory lymphoma: a prospective multi-center phase II study by the Puget Sound Oncology Consortium. *Leuk Lymphoma.* 2010;51 (8):1523-1529.

Rituximab-Gemcitabine-Dexamethasone-Cisplatin (NHL-DLBCL)

Index Terms Gemcitabine-Cisplatin-Dexamethasone-Rituximab (NHL-DLBCL); Gemcitabine-Dexamethasone-Cisplatin-Rituximab (NHL-DLBCL); R-GDP (NHL-DLBCL)

Use Lymphoma, non-Hodgkin (DLBCL recurrent/refractory, transplant eligible patients)

Regimen

Rituximab: IV: 375 mg/m^2 day 1
  [total dose/cycle = 375 mg/m^2]

Gemcitabine: IV: 1,000 mg/m^2/day over 30 minutes days 1 and 8
  [total dose/cycle = 2,000 mg/m^2]

Dexamethasone: Oral: 40 mg/day days 1 to 4
  [total dose/cycle = 160 mg]

Cisplatin: IV: 75 mg/m^2 day 1
  [total dose/cycle = 75 mg/m^2]

Repeat cycle every 21 days for 2 cycles followed by autologous stem-cell transplant; patients without complete or partial response were allowed 1 additional cycle

References

Crump M, Kuruvilla J, Couban S, et al. Randomized comparison of gemcitabine, dexamethasone, and cisplatin versus dexamethasone, cytarabine, and cisplatin chemotherapy before autologous stem-cell transplantation for relapsed and refractory aggressive lymphomas: NCIC-CTG LY.12. *J Clin Oncol.* 2014;32(31):3490-3496.

♦ **Rituximab-Gemcitabine-Oxaliplatin (NHL-DLBCL)** *see* GEMOX-R (NHL-DLBCL) *on page* 2000

♦ **Rituximab-Gemcitabine-Oxaliplatin (NHL-Mantle Cell)** *see* GEMOX-R (NHL-Mantle Cell) *on page* 2000

♦ **Rituximab-Hyper-CVAD Alternating With High-Dose Methotrexate-Cytar-abine (NHL-Burkitt)** *see* Hyper-CVAD Alternating With High-Dose Metho-trexate-Cytarabine + Rituximab + CNS Prophylaxis (NHL-Burkitt) *on page 2004*

Rituximab-Hyper-CVAD (NHL-Mantle Cell)

Index Terms Rituximab-Cyclophosphamide-Vincristine-Doxorubicin-Metho-trexate-Cytarabine (NHL-Mantle Cell)

Use Lymphoma, non-Hodgkin (Mantle cell)

Regimen

Cycle A (Cycles 1, 3, 5 [and 7, if needed]):

Rituximab: IV: 375 mg/m^2 day 1

[total dose/cycle = 375 mg/m^2]

Cyclophosphamide: IV: 300 mg/m^2 over 3 hours every 12 hours for 6 doses days 2, 3, and 4

[total dose/cycle = 1,800 mg/m^2]

Mesna: IV: 600 mg/m^2/day continuous infusion over 24 hours days 2, 3, and 4, beginning 1 hour prior to start of cyclophosphamide and finishing 12 hours after last dose of cyclophosphamide

[total dose/cycle = 1,800 mg/m^2]

Vincristine: IV: 1.4 mg/m^2/day (maximum dose: 2 mg) days 5 (12 hours after last dose of cyclophosphamide) and 12

[total dose/cycle = 2.8 mg/m^2; maximum: 4 mg]

Doxorubicin: IV: 16.7 mg/m^2/day continuous infusion over 24 hours days 5, 6, and 7 (12 hours after last dose of cyclophosphamide)

[total dose/cycle = 50.1 mg/m^2]

Dexamethasone: Oral, IV: 40 mg/day days 2 to 5 and days 12 to 15

[total dose/cycle = 320 mg]

Filgrastim: SubQ: 5 mcg/kg daily starting 24 to 36 hours after completion of doxorubicin infusion and continuing for 10 days

Treatment cycle is 21 days

Cycle B (Cycles 2, 4, 6 [and 8, if needed]):

Rituximab: IV: 375 mg/m^2 day 1

[total dose/cycle = 375 mg/m^2]

Methotrexate: IV: 200 mg/m^2 over 2 hours day 2 (50% dose reduction for patients with serum creatinine >1.5 mg/dL)

followed by IV: 800 mg/m^2 continuous infusion over 22 hours day 2

[total dose/cycle = 1,000 mg/m^2]

Leucovorin: Oral: 50 mg (start 12 hours after the end of the methotrexate infusion)

followed by Oral: 15 mg every 6 hours for 8 doses

[total dose/cycle = 170 mg]

Cytarabine: IV: 3,000 mg/m^2 over 2 hours every 12 hours for 4 doses days 3 and 4 (or 1,000 mg/m^2 in patients >60 years old and in patients with serum creatinine >1.5 mg/dL)

[total dose/cycle = 12,000 mg/m^2]

Filgrastim: SubQ: 5 mcg/kg daily starting 24 to 36 hours after completion of cytarabine infusion and continuing for 10 days

Treatment cycle is 21 days

Alternate cycles A and B every 21 days in the following sequence: ABABA-BAB. Patients who achieved a complete remission after 2 cycles (AB) received a total of 6 cycles (ABABAB). Patients who achieved a partial response after 2 cycles and a complete remission after 6 cycles received a total of 8 cycles.

References

Romaguera JE, Fayad L, Rodriguez MA, et al. High rate of durable remissions after treatment of newly diagnosed aggressive mantle-cell lymphoma with rituximab plus hyper-CVAD alternating with rituximab plus high-dose methotrexate and cytarabine. *J Clin Oncol.* 2005;23 (28):7013-7023.

- ◆ **Rituximab-ICE (NHL-DLBCL)** *see* R-ICE (NHL-DLBCL) *on page 2076*
- ◆ **Rituximab-Idelalisib (CLL)** *see* Idelalisib-Rituximab (CLL) *on page 2014*
- ◆ **Rituximab-Ifosfamide-Carboplatin-Etoposide (NHL-DLBCL)** *see* R-ICE (NHL-DLBCL) *on page 2076*
- ◆ **Rituximab-Lenalidomide (CLL)** *see* Lenalidomide-Rituximab (CLL) *on page 2029*
- ◆ **Rituximab-Temozolomide (CNS Lymphoma)** *see* Temozolomide-Rituximab (CNS Lymphoma) *on page 2087*
- ◆ **RVD (Multiple Myeloma)** *see* Lenalidomide-Bortezomib-Dexamethasone (Multiple Myeloma) *on page 2026*
- ◆ **Saltz Regimen (Colorectal)** *see* Fluorouracil-Leucovorin-Irinotecan (Saltz Regimen) (Colorectal) *on page 1981*

Sonidegib (Basal Cell Regimen)

Use Basal cell carcinoma (locally advanced, metastatic)

Regimen

Sonidegib: Oral: 200 mg once daily (1 hour before or 2 hours after a meal) [total dose/cycle = 5,600 mg]

Repeat cycle every 28 days until disease progression or unacceptable toxicity

References

Migden MR, Guminski A, Gutzmer R, et al. Treatment with two different doses of sonidegib in patients with locally advanced or metastatic basal cell carcinoma (BOLT): a multicentre, randomised, double-blind phase 2 trial. *Lancet Oncol.* 2015;16(6):716-728.

Sorafenib (Angiosarcoma Regimen)

Use Soft Tissue Sarcoma (Angiosarcoma)

Regimen

Sorafenib: Oral: 400 mg twice daily days 1 to 28 [total dose/cycle = 22,400 mg]

Repeat cycle every 28 days

References

Maki RG, D'Adamo DR, Keohan ML, et al. Phase II study of sorafenib in patients with metastatic or recurrent sarcomas. *J Clin Oncol.* 2009;27(19):3133-3140.

Sorafenib (GIST Regimen)

Use Soft Tissue Sarcoma (Gastrointestinal Stromal Tumor [GIST])

◀ **Regimen**

Sorafenib: Oral: 400 mg twice daily days 1 to 28

[total dose/cycle = 22,400 mg]

Repeat cycle every 28 days

References

Campbell NP, Wroblewski K, Maki RG, et al. Final results of a University of Chicago phase II consortium trial of sorafenib (SOR) in patients (pts) with imatinib (IM)- and sunitinib (SU)-resistant (RES) gastrointestinal stromal tumors (GIST). *J Clin Oncol*. 2011;29(4s):4 [abstract 4 from the 2011 Gastrointestinal Cancers Symposium].

Montemurro M, Gelderblom H, Bitz U, et al. Sorafenib as third- or fourth-line treatment of advanced gastrointestinal stromal tumour and pretreatment including both imatinib and sunitinib, and nilotinib: a retrospective analysis. *Eur J Cancer*. 2013;49(5):1027-1031.

Sorafenib (Hepatocellular Regimen)

Use Hepatocellular cancer

Regimen

Sorafenib: Oral: 400 mg twice daily days 1 to 28

[total dose/cycle = 22,400 mg]

Repeat cycle every 28 days until disease progression or unacceptable toxicity

References

Llovet JM, Ricci S, Mazzaferro V, et al. Sorafenib in advanced hepatocellular carcinoma. *N Engl J Med*. 2008;359(4):378-390.

Sorafenib (RCC Regimen)

Use Renal cell cancer

Regimen NOTE: Multiple variations are listed.

Variation 1 (refractory):

Sorafenib: Oral: 400 mg twice daily

Continue until disease progression or unacceptable toxicity.

Variation 2 (first-line):

Sorafenib: Oral: 400 mg twice daily; if disease progression, may escalate to 600 mg twice daily

Continue until disease progression or unacceptable toxicity.

References

Variation 1:

Escudier B, Eisen T, Stadler WM, et al, "Sorafenib for Treatment of Renal Cell Carcinoma: Final Efficacy and Safety Results of the Phase III Treatment Approaches in Renal Cancer Global Evaluation Trial," *J Clin Oncol*, 2009, 27(20):3312-8.

Escudier B, Eisen T, Stadler WM, et al, "Sorafenib in Advanced Clear-Cell Renal-Cell Carcinoma," *N Engl J Med*, 2007, 356(2):125-34.

Variation 2:

Escudier B, Szczylik C, Hutson TE, et al, "Randomized Phase II Trial of First-Line Treatment With Sorafenib Versus Interferon Alfa-2a in Patients With Metastatic Renal Cell Carcinoma," *J Clin Oncol*, 2009, 27(8):1280-9.

Sorafenib (Thyroid Regimen)

Use Thyroid cancer

Regimen

Sorafenib: Oral: 400 mg twice daily days 1 to 28, take on an empty stomach 1 hour before or 2 hours after a meal

[total dose/cycle = 22,400 mg]

Repeat cycle every 28 days until disease progression or unacceptable toxicity

References

Brose MS, Nutting CM, Jarzab B, et al. Sorafenib in radioactive iodine-refractory, locally advanced or metastatic differentiated thyroid cancer: a randomised, double-blind, phase 3 trial. *Lancet*. 2014;384(9940):319-328.

Stanford V (Hodgkin)

Index Terms Mechlorethamine, Doxorubicin, Vinblastine, Vincristine, Bleomycin, Etoposide, Prednisone (Hodgkin)

Use Lymphoma, Hodgkin

Regimen NOTE: Multiple variations are listed.

Variation 1 (advanced or locally extensive disease with bulky mediastinal adenopathy):

Mechlorethamine: IV: 6 mg/m^2 day 1 on weeks 1, 5, and 9
  [total dose/cycle = 18 mg/m^2]

Doxorubicin: IV: 25 mg/m^2 day 1 on weeks 1, 3, 5, 7, 9, and 11
  [total dose/cycle = 150 mg/m^2]

Vinblastine: IV: 6 mg/m^2 day 1 on weeks 1, 3, 5, 7, 9, and 11
  [total dose/cycle = 36 mg/m^2]

Vincristine: IV: 1.4 mg/m^2 (maximum dose: 2 mg) day 1 on weeks 2, 4, 6, 8, 10, and 12
  [total dose/cycle = 8.4 mg/m^2; maximum: 12 mg]

Bleomycin: IV: 5 units/m^2 day 1 on weeks 2, 4, 6, 8, 10, and 12
  [total dose/cycle = 30 units/m^2]

Etoposide: IV: 60 mg/m^2/day days 1 and 2 on weeks 3, 7, and 11
  [total dose/cycle = 360 mg/m^2]

Prednisone: Oral: 40 mg/m^2 every other day for 10 weeks
  [total dose prior to taper = 1,400 mg/m^2]
    followed by tapering of prednisone dose during weeks 11 and 12

Treatment cycle is 12 weeks, followed by radiation 2 to 3 weeks after completion of chemotherapy

Variation 2 (stage I to IIA nonbulky):

Mechlorethamine: IV: 6 mg/m^2 day 1 on weeks 1 and 5
  [total dose/cycle = 12 mg/m^2]

Doxorubicin: IV: 25 mg/m^2 day 1 on weeks 1, 3, 5, and 7
  [total dose/cycle = 100 mg/m^2]

Vinblastine: IV: 6 mg/m^2 day 1 on weeks 1, 3, 5, and 7
  [total dose/cycle = 24 mg/m^2]

Vincristine: IV: 1.4 mg/m^2 (maximum dose: 2 mg) day 1 on weeks 2, 4, 6, and 8
  [total dose/cycle = 5.6 mg/m^2; maximum: 8 mg]

Bleomycin: IV: 5 units/m^2 day 1 on weeks 2, 4, 6, and 8
  [total dose/cycle = 20 units/m^2]

Etoposide: IV: 60 mg/m^2/day days 1 and 2 on weeks 3 and 7
  [total dose/cycle = 240 mg/m^2]

Prednisone: Oral: 40 mg/m^2 every other day for 6 weeks
  [total dose prior to taper = 840 mg/m^2]
    followed by tapering of prednisone 10 mg/day during weeks 7 and 8

Treatment cycle is 8 weeks, followed by radiation 1 to 3 weeks after completion of chemotherapy

References

Variation 1:

Gordon LI, Hong F, Fisher RI, et al. Randomized phase III trial of ABVD versus Stanford V with or without radiation therapy in locally extensive and advanced-stage Hodgkin lymphoma: an intergroup study coordinated by the Eastern Cooperative Oncology Group (E2496). *J Clin Oncol.* 2013;31(6):684-691.

Horning SJ, Hoppe RT, Breslin S, et al. Stanford V and radiotherapy for locally extensive and advanced Hodgkin's disease: mature results of a prospective clinical trial. *J Clin Oncol.* 2002;20 (3):630-637.

Variation 2:

Advani RH, Hoppe RT, Baer D, et al. Efficacy of abbreviated Stanford V chemotherapy and involved-field radiotherapy in early-stage Hodgkin lymphoma: mature results of the G4 trial. *Ann Oncol.* 2013;24(4):1044-1048.

Sunitinib (GIST Regimen)

Use Soft Tissue Sarcoma (Gastrointestinal Stromal Tumor [GIST])

Regimen NOTE: Multiple variations are listed.

Variation 1:

Sunitinib: Oral: 50 mg once daily for 4 weeks, followed by 2 weeks rest

[total dose/cycle = 1400 mg]

Repeat cycle every 6 weeks

Variation 2:

Sunitinib: Oral: 37.5 mg once daily days 1 to 28

[total dose/cycle = 1050 mg]

Repeat cycle every 28 days

References

Variation 1:

Demetri GD, van Oosterom AT, Garrett CR, et al, "Efficacy and Safety of Sunitinib in Patients With Advanced Gastrointestinal Stromal Tumour After Failure of Imatinib: A Randomised Controlled Trial," *Lancet*, 2006, 9544(368):1329-38.

Variation 2:

George S, Blay JY, Casali PG, et al, "Clinical Evaluation of Continuous Daily Dosing of Sunitinib Malate in Patients With Advanced Gastrointestinal Stromal Tumour After Imatinib Failure," *Eur J Cancer*, 2009, 45(11):1959-68.

Sunitinib (RCC Regimen)

Use Renal cell cancer

Regimen

Sunitinib: Oral: 50 mg once daily for 4 weeks, followed by 2 weeks of rest

[total dose/cycle = 1400 mg]

Repeat cycle every 6 weeks until disease progression or unacceptable toxicity

References

Motzer RJ, Hutson TE, Tomczak P, et al, "Overall Survival and Updated Results for Sunitinib Compared With Interferon Alfa in Patients With Metastatic Renal Cell Carcinoma," *J Clin Oncol*, 2009, 27(22):3584-90.

Motzer RJ, Hutson TE, Tomczak P, et al, "Sunitinib Versus Interferon Alfa in Metastatic Renal-Cell Carcinoma," *N Engl J Med*, 2007, 356(2):115-24.

Sunitinib (Soft Tissue Sarcoma Regimen)

Use Soft tissue sarcoma (Non-gastrointestinal stromal tumor sarcomas)

Regimen

Sunitinib: Oral: 37.5 mg once daily days 1 to 28

[total dose/cycle = 1050 mg]

Repeat cycle every 28 days until disease progression or unacceptable toxicity

References

George S, Merriam P, Maki RG, et al. Multicenter phase II trial of sunitinib in the treatment of nongastrointestinal stromal tumor sarcomas. *J Clin Oncol.* 2009;27(19):3154-3160.

TAC (Breast)

Index Terms Docetaxel, Doxorubicin, Cyclophosphamide (Breast); Doxorubicin, Cyclophosphamide, Docetaxel (Breast)

Use Breast cancer

Regimen

Doxorubicin: IV: 50 mg/m² over 15 minutes day 1
  [total dose/cycle = 50 mg/m²]
Cyclophosphamide: IV: 500 mg/m² day 1
  [total dose/cycle = 500 mg/m²]
Docetaxel: IV: 75 mg/m² over 1 hour day 1, administered 1 hour after cyclophosphamide
  [total dose/cycle = 75 mg/m²]
Repeat cycle every 21 days for 6 cycles

References

Mackey JR, Martin M, Pienkowski T, et al, "Adjuvant Docetaxel, Doxorubicin, and Cyclophosphamide in Node-Positive Breast Cancer: 10-Year Follow Up of the Phase III Randomised BCIRG 001 Trial," *Lancet Oncol*, 2013, 14(1):72-80.

Martin M, Pienkowski T, Mackey J, et al, "Adjuvant Docetaxel for Node-Positive Breast Cancer," *N Engl J Med*, 2005, 352(22):2302-13.

◆ **TAP (Endometrial)** *see* Cisplatin-Doxorubicin-Paclitaxel (Endometrial)
  on page 1893

TC (Breast)

Index Terms Cyclophosphamide-Docetaxel (Breast); Docetaxel-Cyclophosphamide (Breast)
Use Breast cancer

Regimen

Docetaxel: IV: 75 mg/m² day 1
  [total dose/cycle = 75 mg/m²]
Cyclophosphamide: IV: 600 mg/m² day 1
  [total dose/cycle = 600 mg/m²]
Repeat cycle every 21 days for 4 cycles

References

Jones SE, Savin MA, Holmes FA, et al, "Phase III Trial Comparing Doxorubicin Plus Cyclophosphamide With Docetaxel Plus Cyclophosphamide as Adjuvant Therapy for Operable Breast Cancer," *J Clin Oncol*, 2006, 24(34):5381-7.

Jones S, Holmes FA, O'Shaughnessy JO, et al, "Docetaxel With Cyclophosphamide Is Associated With an Overall Survival Benefit Compared With Doxorubicin and Cyclophophosphamide: 7-Year Follow-Up of US Oncology Research Trial 9735," *J Clin Oncol*, 2009, 27(8):1177-83.

◆ **TC (Endometrial)** *see* Carboplatin-Paclitaxel (Endometrial) *on page 1869*

◆ **TCF (Esophageal Cancer)** *see* Paclitaxel-Cisplatin-Fluorouracil (Esophageal Cancer) *on page 2051*

◆ **TCF (Gastric/Esophageal Cancer)** *see* Docetaxel-Cisplatin-Fluorouracil (Gastric/Esophageal Cancer) *on page 1940*

◆ **TCH (Breast)** *see* Carboplatin-Docetaxel-Trastuzumab (Breast) *on page 1862*

◆ **TCH (Breast)** *see* Carboplatin-Paclitaxel-Trastuzumab (Breast) *on page 1872*

◆ **TC (NSCLC)** *see* Carboplatin-Paclitaxel (NSCLC) *on page 1870*

◆ **T-DM1 (Breast)** *see* Ado-Trastuzumab Emtansine (Breast) *on page 1826*

◆ **Temozolomide-Irinotecan (Ewing Sarcoma)** *see* Irinotecan-Temozolomide (Ewing Sarcoma) *on page 2024*

Temozolomide-Rituximab (CNS Lymphoma)

Index Terms Rituximab-Temozolomide (CNS Lymphoma)
Use Primary CNS lymphoma

▶

◄ **Regimen** NOTE: Multiple variations are listed.

Variation 1:

Induction therapy (cycles 1 to 4):

Rituximab: IV: 375 mg/m^2 day 1

[total dose/cycle = 375 mg/m^2]

Temozolomide: Oral: 150 mg/m^2/day days 1 to 5

[total dose/cycle = 750 mg/m^2]

Repeat cycle every 28 days for a total of 4 cycles

followed by

Maintenance therapy:

Temozolomide: Oral: 150 mg/m^2/day days 1 to 5

[total dose/cycle = 750 mg/m^2]

Repeat cycle every 28 days for a total of 8 cycles

Variation 2:

Induction therapy (cycles 1 and 2):

Rituximab: IV: 750 mg/m^2 days 1, 8, 15, and 22

[total dose/cycle = 3000 mg/m^2]

Temozolomide: Oral: 150 mg/m^2/day days 1 to 7 and days 15 to 21

[total dose/cycle = 2100 mg/m^2]

Administer cycle every 28 days for a total of 1 or 2 cycles

followed by

Maintenance therapy:

Temozolomide: Oral: 150 mg/m^2/day days 1 to 5

[total dose/cycle = 750 mg/m^2]

Repeat cycle every 28 days

References

Variation 1:
Wong ET, Tishler R, Barron L, Wu JK. Immunochemotherapy with rituximab and temozolomide for central nervous system lymphomas. *Cancer.* 2004;101(1):139-145.
Variation 2:
Enting RH, Demopoulos A, DeAngelis LM, Abrey LE. Salvage therapy for primary CNS lymphoma with a combination of rituximab and temozolomide. *Neurology.* 2004;63(5):901-903.

Temsirolimus (RCC Regimen)

Use Renal cell cancer

Regimen

Temsirolimus: IV: 25 mg over 30 minutes day 1

[total dose/cycle = 25 mg]

Repeat cycle every week until disease progression or unacceptable toxicity

References

Hudes G, Carducci M, Tomczak P, et al, "Temsirolimus, Interferon Alfa, or Both for Advanced Renal-Cell Carcinoma," *N Engl J Med*, 2007, 356(22):2271-81.

Thalidomide-Dexamethasone (MM)

Index Terms Dexamethasone-Thalidomide (MM)

Use Multiple myeloma

Regimen NOTE: Multiple variations are listed.

Variation 1 (refractory):

Thalidomide: Oral: 100 mg/day days 1 to 28

[total dose/cycle = 2800 mg]

Dexamethasone: Oral: 40 mg/day days 1 to 4

[total dose/cycle = 160 mg]

Repeat cycle every 28 days

Variation 2 (refractory):
  Thalidomide: Oral: 200 mg/day days 1 to 14 (cycle 1)
    followed by Oral: 400 mg/day days 15 to 28 (cycle 1)
    [total dose/cycle = 8400 mg]
  Thalidomide: Oral: 400 mg/day days 1 to 28 (subsequent cycles)
    [total dose/cycle = 11,200 mg]
  Dexamethasone: Oral: 20 mg/m^2/day days 1 to 4, 9 to 12, and 17 to 20
  (cycle 1)
    [total dose/cycle = 240 mg/m^2]
    followed by Oral: 20 mg/m^2/day days 1 to 4 (subsequent cycles)
      [total dose/cycle = 80 mg/m^2]
  Repeat cycle every 28 days
Variation 3 (newly diagnosed):
  Thalidomide: Oral: 200 mg/day days 1 to 28
    [total dose/cycle = 5600 mg]
  Dexamethasone: Oral: 40 mg/day days 1 to 4, 9 to 12, and 17 to 20
    [total dose/cycle = 480 mg]
  Repeat cycle every 28 days
Variation 4 (newly diagnosed):
  Thalidomide: Oral: 50 mg/day days 1 to 14
    followed by Oral: 100 mg/day days 15 to 28 (cycle 1)
    [total dose/cycle 1 = 2100 mg]
      followed by Oral: 200 mg/day days 1 to 28 (starting with cycle 2 and
      subsequent cycles)
        [total dose/cycle = 5600 mg]
  Dexamethasone: Oral: 40 mg/day days 1 to 4, 9 to 12, and 17 to 20 (cycles 1
  to 4)
    [total dose/cycle 1 to 4 = 480 mg]
      followed by Oral: 40 mg/day days 1 to 4 (starting with cycle 5 and
      subsequent cycles)
        [total dose/cycle = 160 mg]
  Repeat cycle every 28 days until disease progression or unacceptable
  toxicity
Variation 5 (newly diagnosed):
  Thalidomide: Oral: 100 mg/day days 1 to 14
    followed by Oral: 200 mg/day days 15 to 28 (cycle 1)
    [total dose/cycle = 4200 mg]
      followed by Oral: 200 mg/day days 1 to 28 (starting with cycle 2 and
      subsequent cycles)
        [total dose/cycle = 5600 mg]
  Dexamethasone: Oral: 40 mg/day days 1 to 4, 9 to 12, and 17 to 20 (odd
  cycles)
    [total dose/cycle = 480 mg]
  Dexamethasone: Oral: 40 mg/day days 1 to 4 (even cycles)
    [total dose/cycle = 160 mg]
  Repeat cycle every 28 days for a total of 4 cycles
Variation 6 (newly diagnosed induction):
  Thalidomide: Oral: 50 mg/day; may escalate by 50 mg per week to a
  maximum dose of 400 mg/day
    [total dose/cycle = up to 14,000 mg]
  Dexamethasone: Oral: 40 mg/day days 1 to 4, 9 to 12, and 17 to 20
    [total dose/cycle = 480 mg]
  Repeat cycle every 35 days for a total of 3 cycles

◀ **References**

Variation 1:
Palumbo A, Giaccone L, Bertola A, et al, "Low-Dose Thalidomide Plus Dexamethasone Is an Effective Salvage Therapy for Advanced Myeloma," *Haematologica*, 2001, 86(4):399-403.
Variation 2:
Dimopoulos MA, Zervas K, Kouvatseas G, et al, "Thalidomide and Dexamethasone Combination for Refractory Multiple Myeloma," *Ann Oncol*, 2001, 12(7):991-5.
Variation 3:
Rajkumar SV, Blood E, Vesole D, et al, "Phase III Clinical Trial of Thalidomide Plus Dexamethasone Compared With Dexamethasone Alone in Newly Diagnosed Multiple Myeloma: A Clinical Trial Coordinated by the Eastern Cooperative Oncology Group," *J Clin Oncol*, 2006, 24(3):431-6.
Variation 4:
Rajkumar SV, Rosiñol L, Hussein M, et al, "Multicenter, Randomized, Double-Blind, Placebo-Controlled Study of Thalidomide Plus Dexamethasone Compared With Dexamethasone as Initial Therapy for Newly Diagnosed Multiple Myeloma," *J Clin Oncol*, 2008, 26(13):2171-7.
Variation 5:
Cavo M, Zamagni E, Tosi P, et al, "Superiority of Thalidomide and Dexamethasone Over Vincristine-Doxorubicin-Dexamethasone (VAD) as Primary Therapy in Preparation for Autologous Transplantation for Multiple Myeloma," *Blood*, 2005, 106(1):35-9.
Variation 6:
Hussein MA, Bolejack V, Zonder JA, et al, "Phase II Study of Thalidomide Plus Dexamethasone Induction Followed by Tandem Melphalan-Based Autotransplantation and Thalidomide-Plus-Prednisone Maintenance for Untreated Multiple Myeloma: A Southwest Oncology Group Trial (S0204)," *J Clin Oncol*, 2009, 27(21):3510-7.

TIP (Testicular)

Index Terms Cisplatin-Ifosfamide-Paclitaxel (Testicular); Paclitaxel-Ifosfamide-Cisplatin (Testicular)

Use Testicular cancer

Regimen

Paclitaxel: IV: 250 mg/m^2 continuous infusion day 1
[total dose/cycle = 250 mg/m^2]
Ifosfamide: IV: 1500 mg/m^2/day over 60 minutes days 2 to 5
[total dose/cycle = 6000 mg/m^2]
Cisplatin: IV: 25 mg/m^2/day over 30 minutes days 2 to 5
[total dose/cycle = 100 mg/m^2]
Mesna: IV: 500 mg/m^2 prior to ifosfamide and every 4 hours for 2 doses, days 2 to 5
[total dose/cycle = 6000 mg/m^2]
Filgrastim SubQ: 5 mcg/kg daily days 7 to 18 (discontinue if WBC >10,000/mm^3 for 2 days)
Repeat cycle every 21 days for 4 cycles

References

Kondagunta GV, Bacik J, Donadio A. et al. Combination of paclitaxel, ifosfamide, and cisplatin is an effective second-line therapy for patients with relapsed testicular germ cell tumors. *J Clin Oncol.* 2005;23(27):6549-6555.

- ◆ **TOPO/CTX (Neuroblastoma)** *see* Cyclophosphamide-Topotecan (Neuroblastoma) *on page 1930*

- ◆ **TOPO/CYC (Ewing Sarcoma)** *see* Cyclophosphamide-Topotecan (Ewing Sarcoma) *on page 1930*

- ◆ **Topotecan-Cisplatin (Cervical Cancer)** *see* Cisplatin-Topotecan (Cervical Cancer) *on page 1912*

- ◆ **Topotecan-Cyclophosphamide (Ewing Sarcoma)** *see* Cyclophosphamide-Topotecan (Ewing Sarcoma) *on page 1930*

- ◆ **Topotecan-Cyclophosphamide (Neuroblastoma)** *see* Cyclophosphamide-Topotecan (Neuroblastoma) *on page 1930*

- ◆ **Topotecan-Cyclophosphamide (Rhabdomyosarcoma)** *see* Cyclophosphamide-Topotecan (Rhabdomyosarcoma) *on page 1931*
- ◆ **Topotecan Daily-Bevacizumab (Ovarian)** *see* Bevacizumab-Topotecan Daily (Ovarian) *on page 1845*

Topotecan Intravenous (Small Cell Lung Cancer Regimen)

Use Lung cancer, small cell

Regimen

Topotecan: IV: 1.5 mg/m^2/day over 30 minutes days 1 to 5
[total dose/cycle = 7.5 mg/m^2]
Repeat cycle every 21 days

References

Eckardt JR, von Pawel J, Pujol JL, et al, "Phase III Study of Oral Compared With Intravenous Topotecan as Second-Line Therapy in Small-Cell Lung Cancer," *J Clin Oncol*, 2007, 25 (15):2086-92.

van Pawel J, Gatzemeier U, Pujol JL, et al, "Phase II Comparator Study of Oral Versus Intravenous Topotecan in Patients With Chemosensitive Small-Cell Lung Cancer," *J Clin Oncol*, 2001, 19 (6):1743-9.

von Pawel J, Schiller JH, Shephard FA, et al, "Topotecan Versus Cyclophosphamide, Doxorubicin, and Vincristine for the Treatment of Recurrent Small-Cell Lung Cancer," *J Clin Oncol*, 1999, 17 (2):658-67.

Topotecan Oral (Small Cell Lung Cancer Regimen)

Use Lung cancer, small cell

Regimen

Topotecan: Oral: 2.3 mg/m^2/day days 1 to 5
[total dose/cycle = 11.5 mg/m^2]
Repeat cycle every 21 days

References

Eckardt JR, von Pawel J, Pujol JL, et al, "Phase III Study of Oral Compared With Intravenous Topotecan as Second-Line Therapy in Small-Cell Lung Cancer," *J Clin Oncol*, 2007, 25 (15):2086-92.

O'Brien ME, Ciuleanu TE, Tsekov H, et al, "Phase III Trial Comparing Supportive Care Alone With Supportive Care With Oral Topotecan in Patients With Relapsed Small-Cell Lung Cancer," *J Clin Oncol*, 2006, 24(34):5441-7.

Topotecan (Ovarian Cancer Regimen)

Use Ovarian cancer

Regimen NOTE: Multiple variations are listed.

Variation 1:

Topotecan: IV: 1.25 mg/m^2/day over 30 minutes days 1, 2, 3, 4, and 5
[total dose/cycle = 6.25 mg/m^2]
Repeat cycle every 21 days until disease progression or unacceptable toxicity; maximum of 12 months

Variation 2:

Topotecan: IV: 1.5 mg/m^2/day over 30 minutes days 1, 2, 3, 4, and 5
[total dose/cycle = 7.5 mg/m^2]
Repeat cycle every 21 days

References

Variation 1:

Herzog TJ, Sill MW, Walker JL, et al. A phase II study of two topotecan regimens evaluated in recurrent platinum-sensitive ovarian, fallopian tube or primary peritoneal cancer: a Gynecologic Oncology Group Study (GOG 146Q). *Gynecol Oncol*. 2011;120(3):454-458.

Sehouli J, Stengel D, Harter P, et al. Topotecan weekly versus conventional 5-day schedule in patients with platinum-resistant ovarian cancer: a randomized multicenter phase II trial of the North-Eastern German Society of Gynecological Oncology Ovarian Cancer Study Group. *J Clin Oncol.* 2011;29(2):242-248.
Variation 2:
Gordon AN, Fleagle JT, Guthrie D, Parkin DE, Gore ME, Lacave AJ. Recurrent epithelial ovarian carcinoma: a randomized phase III study of pegylated liposomal doxorubicin versus topotecan. *J Clin Oncol.* 2001;19(14):3312-3322.

Gordon AN, Tonda M, Sun S, Rackoff W; Doxil Study 30-49 Investigators. Long-term survival advantage for women treated with pegylated liposomal doxorubicin compared with topotecan in a phase 3 randomized study of recurrent and refractory epithelial ovarian cancer. *Gynecol Oncol.* 2004;95(1):1-8.

◆ **Topotecan Weekly-Bevacizumab (Ovarian)** *see* Bevacizumab-Topotecan Weekly (Ovarian) *on page 1846*

Topotecan Weekly (Ovarian Cancer Regimen)

Use Ovarian cancer

Regimen

Topotecan: IV: 4 mg/m^2/day over 30 minutes days 1, 8, and 15
[total dose/cycle = 12 mg/m^2]
Repeat cycle every 28 days until disease progression or unacceptable toxicity; maximum of 12 months

References

Herzog TJ, Sill MW, Walker JL, et al. A phase II study of two topotecan regimens evaluated in recurrent platinum-sensitive ovarian, fallopian tube or primary peritoneal cancer: a Gynecologic Oncology Group Study (GOG 146Q). *Gynecol Oncol.* 2011;120(3):454-458.

Sehouli J, Stengel D, Harter P, et al. Topotecan weekly versus conventional 5-day schedule in patients with platinum-resistant ovarian cancer: a randomized multicenter phase II trial of the North-Eastern German Society of Gynecological Oncology Ovarian Cancer Study Group. *J Clin Oncol.* 2011;29(2):242-248.

◆ **TPC (Breast)** *see* Carboplatin-Paclitaxel-Trastuzumab (Breast) *on page 1872*

◆ **TPF** *see* Docetaxel-Cisplatin-Fluorouracil (Head and Neck Cancer) *on page 1941*

◆ **TPF (Unknown Primary)** *see* Cisplatin-Docetaxel-Fluorouracil (Unknown Primary, Squamous Cell) *on page 1890*

Trabectedin-Doxorubicin (Liposomal) (Ovarian Cancer)

Index Terms Doxorubicin Liposomal-Trabectedin (Ovarian Cancer)

Use Ovarian cancer

Regimen

Doxorubicin (liposomal): IV: 30 mg/m^2 over 90 minutes day 1
[total dose/cycle = 30 mg/m^2]
Trabectedin: IV: 1.1 mg/m^2 over 3 hours (via central line) day 1
[total dose/cycle = 1.1 mg/m^2]
Repeat cycle every 3 weeks until disease progression or for 2 cycles beyond confirmed complete response.

References

Monk BJ, Herzog TJ, Kaye SB, et al, "Trabectedin Plus Pegylated Liposomal Doxorubicin in Recurrent Ovarian Cancer," *J Clin Oncol*, 2010, 28(19):3107-14.

Trametinib (Melanoma Regimen)

Use Melanoma

Regimen

Trametinib: Oral: 2 mg once daily days 1 to 28

[total dose/cycle = 56 mg]

Repeat cycle every 28 days until disease progression or unacceptable toxicity

References

Flaherty KT, Robert C, Hersey P, et al. Improved survival with MEK inhibition in BRAF-mutated melanoma. *N Engl J Med.* 2012;367(2):107-114.

◆ **Trastuzumab-MCC-DM1 (Breast)** *see* Ado-Trastuzumab Emtansine (Breast) *on page 1826*

◆ **Trastuzumab-Capecitabine (Breast)** *see* Capecitabine-Trastuzumab (Breast) *on page 1859*

Trastuzumab-Cisplatin-Capecitabine (Gastric Cancer)

Index Terms Capecitabine-Cisplatin-Trastuzumab (Gastric Cancer); Cisplatin-Capecitabine-Trastuzumab (Gastric Cancer)

Use Gastric cancer

Regimen

Cycle 1:

Capecitabine: Oral: 1000 mg/m^2/dose twice daily days 1 to 14

[total dose/cycle = 28,000 mg/m^2]

Cisplatin: IV: 80 mg/m^2/dose day 1

[total dose/cycle = 80 mg/m^2]

Trastuzumab: IV: 8 mg/kg/dose (loading dose) day 1

[total dose/cycle 1 = 8 mg/kg]

Treatment cycle is 21 days

Cycles 2-6:

Capecitabine: Oral: 1000 mg/m^2/dose twice daily days 1 to 14

[total dose/cycle = 28,000 mg/m^2]

Cisplatin: IV: 80 mg/m^2/dose day 1

[total dose/cycle = 80 mg/m^2]

Trastuzumab: IV: 6 mg/kg/dose day 1

[total dose/cycle = 6 mg/kg]

Treatment cycle is 21 days

Subsequent cycles:

Trastuzumab: IV: 6 mg/kg/dose day 1

[total dose/cycle = 6 mg/kg]

Repeat cycle every 3 weeks until disease progression or unacceptable toxicity

References

Bang YJ, Van Cutsem E, Feyereislova A, et al, "Trastuzumab in Combination With Chemotherapy Versus Chemotherapy Alone for Treatment of HER2-Positive Advanced Gastric or Gastro-Oesophageal Junction Cancer (ToGA): A Phase 3, Open-Label, Randomised Controlled Trial," *Lancet*, 2010, 376(9742):687-97.

Trastuzumab-Cisplatin-Fluorouracil (Gastric Cancer)

Index Terms Cisplatin-Fluorouracil-Trastuzumab (Gastric Cancer); Fluorouracil-Cisplatin-Trastuzumab (Gastric Cancer)

Use Gastric cancer

◄ **Regimen**
Cycle 1:
   Fluorouracil: IV: 800 mg/m²/day continuous infusion days 1 to 5
      [total dose/cycle = 4000 mg/m²]
   Cisplatin: IV: 80 mg/m²/dose day 1
      [total dose/cycle = 80 mg/m²]
   Trastuzumab: IV: 8 mg/kg/dose (loading dose) day 1
      [total dose/cycle 1 = 8 mg/kg]
   Treatment cycle is 21 days
Cycles 2-6:
   Fluorouracil: IV: 800 mg/m²/day continuous infusion days 1 to 5
      [total dose/cycle = 4000 mg/m²]
   Cisplatin: IV: 80 mg/m²/dose day 1
      [total dose/cycle = 80 mg/m²]
   Trastuzumab: IV: 6 mg/kg/dose day 1
      [total dose/cycle = 6 mg/kg]
   Treatment cycle is 21 days
Subsequent cycles:
   Trastuzumab: IV: 6 mg/kg/dose day 1
      [total dose/cycle = 6 mg/kg]
   Repeat cycle every 3 weeks until disease progression or unacceptable
   toxicity

References
Bang YJ, Van Cutsem E, Feyereislova A, et al, "Trastuzumab in Combination With Chemotherapy Versus Chemotherapy Alone for Treatment of HER2-Positive Advanced Gastric or Gastro-Oesophageal Junction Cancer (ToGA): A Phase 3, Open-Label, Randomised Controlled Trial," *Lancet*, 2010, 376(9742):687-97.

◆ **Trastuzumab-Pertuzumab-Paclitaxel (Breast)** *see* Paclitaxel-Pertuzumab-Trastuzumab (Breast) *on page 2054*

Trastuzumab-Vinorelbine (Breast)

Index Terms Vinorelbine-Trastuzumab (Breast)

Use Breast cancer

Regimen NOTE: Multiple variations are listed.

Variation 1:

Cycle 1:

Trastuzumab: IV: 4 mg/kg (loading dose) over 90 minutes day 1 cycle 1
[total dose/cycle 1 = 4 mg/kg]

Vinorelbine: IV: 25 mg/m^2 over 6-10 minutes day 1
[total dose/cycle 1 = 25 mg/m^2]

Treatment cycle is 7 days

Subsequent cycles:

Trastuzumab: IV: 2 mg/kg over 30 minutes day 1
[total dose/cycle = 2 mg/kg]

Vinorelbine: IV: 25 mg/m^2 over 6-10 minutes day 1
[total dose/cycle = 25 mg/m^2]

Repeat cycle every 7 days until disease progression or unacceptable toxicity

Variation 2:

Cycle 1:

Trastuzumab: IV: 8 mg/kg (loading dose) over 90 minutes day 1 cycle 1
[total dose/cycle 1 = 8 mg/kg]

Vinorelbine: IV: 30-35 mg/m^2/day days 1 and 8
[total dose/cycle 1 = 60-70 mg/m^2]

Treatment cycle is 21 days

Subsequent cycles:

Trastuzumab: IV: 6 mg/kg over 30 minutes day 1
[total dose/cycle = 6 mg/kg]

Vinorelbine: IV: 30-35 mg/m^2/day days 1 and 8
[total dose/cycle = 60-70 mg/m^2]

Repeat cycle every 21 days until disease progression or unacceptable toxicity

References

Variation 1:

Burstein HJ, Keshaviah A, Baron AD, et al, "Trastuzumab Plus Vinorelbine or Taxane Chemotherapy for HER2-Overexpressing Metastatic Breast Cancer: The Trastuzumab and Vinorelbine or Taxane Study," *Cancer*, 2007, 110(5):965-72.

Burstein HJ, Kuter I, Campos SM, et al, "Clinical Activity of Trastuzumab and Vinorelbine in Women With HER2-Overexpressing Metastatic Breast Cancer," *J Clin Oncol*, 2001, 19(10):2722-30.

Variation 2:

Andersson M, Lidbrink E, Bjerre K, et al, "Phase III Randomized Study Comparing Docetaxel Plus Trastuzumab With Vinorelbine Plus Trastuzumab as First-Line Therapy of Metastatic or Locally Advanced Human Epidermal Growth Factor Receptor 2-Positive Breast Cancer: The HERNATA Study," *J Clin Oncol*, 2011, 29(3):264-71.

Tretinoin-Arsenic Trioxide (APL)

Index Terms Arsenic Trioxide-ATRA (APL); ATRA-Arsenic Trixoide (APL)

Use Leukemia, acute promyelocytic

◀ **Regimen**

Induction (continue until <5% blasts in marrow and no abnormal promyelo-cytes):

Tretinoin: Oral: 45 mg/m^2/day (in 2 divided doses) day 1 up to day 85

[total induction dose = up to 3825 mg/m^2]

Arsenic Trioxide: IV: 0.15 mg/kg/day over 1 hour beginning day 10 up to day 85

[total induction dose = up to 11.25 mg/kg]

Postremission therapy (beginning with complete remission):

Tretinoin: Oral: 45 mg/m^2/day weeks 1, 2, 5, 6, 9, 10, 13, 14, 17, 18, 21, 22, 25, 26

[total postremission dose = 4410 mg/m^2]

Arsenic Trioxide: IV: 0.15 mg/kg/day Monday through Friday weeks 1 to 4, 9 to 12, 17 to 20, and 25 to 28

[total postremission dose = 12 mg/kg]

References

Estey E, Garcia-Manero G, Ferrajoli A, et al, "Use of All-*Trans* Retinoic Acid Plus Arsenic Trioxide as an Alternative to Chemotherapy in Untreated Acute Promyelocytic Leukemia," *Blood*, 2006, 107(9):3469-73.

Ravandi F, Estey E, Jones D, et al, "Effective Treatment of Acute Promyelocytic Leukemia With All-*Trans*-Retinoic Acid, Arsenic Trioxide, and Gemtuzumab Ozogamicin," *J Clin Oncol*, 2009, 27 (4):504-10.

Tretinoin-Daunorubicin (APL)

Index Terms ATRA-Daunorubicin (APL); Daunorubicin-ATRA (APL); Daunor-ubicin-Tretinoin (APL)

Use Leukemia, acute promyelocytic

Regimen

Induction:

Tretinoin: Oral: 45 mg/m^2/day (in 2 divided doses) day 1 until hematologic complete remission

Daunorubicin: IV: 60 mg/m^2/day days 1, 2, and 3

[total dose/cycle = 180 mg/m^2]

Consolidation:

Course 1:

Daunorubicin: IV: 60 mg/m^2/day days 1, 2, and 3

[total dose/cycle = 180 mg/m^2]

Course 2:

Daunorubicin: IV: 45 mg/m^2/day days 1, 2, and 3

[total dose/cycle = 135 mg/m^2]

Maintenance:

Mercaptopurine: Oral: 90 mg/m^2 daily

[total dose/cycle = 8100 mg/m^2 (90 days)]

Methotrexate: Oral: 15 mg/m^2 weekly

[total dose/cycle = 180 mg/m^2]

Tretinoin: Oral: 45 mg/m^2/day (in 2 divided doses) days 1 to 15

[total dose/cycle = 675 mg/m^2]

Repeat cycle every 3 months for 2 years

References

Adès L, Chevret S, Raffoux E, et al, "Is Cytarabine Useful in the Treatment of Acute Promyelocytic Leukemia? Results of a Randomized Trial From the European Acute Promyelocytic Leukemia Group," *J Clin Oncol*, 2006, 24(36):5703-10.

Tretinoin-Daunorubicin-Cytarabine Induction, Consolidation, Maintenance (APL)

Index Terms Arsenic Trioxide-ATRA-Daunorubicin-Cytarabine (APL); ATRA-Daunorubicin-AraC (APL); ATRA-Daunorubicin-Cytarabine (APL); ATRA-Daunorubicin-Cytarabine-Arsensic Trioxide (APL)

Use Leukemia, acute promyelocytic

Regimen NOTE: Multiple variations are listed.

Variation 1:

Induction:

Tretinoin: Oral: 45 mg/m^2/day (in 2 divided doses) day 1 until complete remission or day 90

Daunorubicin: IV: 50 mg/m^2/day days 3, 4, 5, and 6

[total dose/cycle = 200 mg/m^2]

Cytarabine: IV: 200 mg/m^2/day continuous infusion for 7 days beginning on day 3

[total dose/cycle = 1,400 mg/m^2]

Consolidation (begin within 2 to 4 weeks of hematologic remission):

Cycles 1 and 2:

Arsenic Trioxide: IV: 0.15 mg/kg/day over 1 hour days 1 to 5 for 5 weeks followed by 2 weeks off

[total dose/cycle = 3.75 mg/kg]

Repeat cycle in 49 days (7 weeks) for a total of 2 cycles

Cycles 3 and 4:

Tretinoin: Oral: 45 mg/m^2/day (in 2 divided doses) days 1 to 7

[total dose/cycle = 315 mg/m^2]

Daunorubicin: IV: 50 mg/m^2/day days 1, 2, and 3

[total dose/cycle = 150 mg/m^2]

Repeat for a total of 2 cycles

Maintenance (if patient remains in complete remission, begin 2 to 4 weeks after recovery from consolidation):

Mercaptopurine: Oral: 60 mg/m^2 daily for 1 year

[total dose/maintenance = 21,900 mg/m^2]

Methotrexate: Oral: 20 mg/m^2 weekly for 1 year

[total dose/maintenance = 1,040 mg/m^2]

Tretinoin: Oral: 45 mg/m^2/day (in 2 divided doses) days 1 to 7, every other week for 1 year

[total dose/maintenance = 8,190 mg/m^2]

or maintenance with:

Tretinoin: Oral: 45 mg/m^2/day (in 2 divided doses) days 1 to 7, every other week for 1 year

[total dose/maintenance = 8,190 mg/m^2]

Variation 2 (patients ≤60 years of age and WBC <10,000/mm^3):

Induction:

Tretinoin: Oral: 45 mg/m^2/day (in 2 divided doses) day 1 until hematologic complete remission

Daunorubicin: IV: 60 mg/m^2/day days 3, 4, and 5

[total dose/cycle = 180 mg/m^2]

Cytarabine: IV: 200 mg/m^2/day continuous infusion for 7 days beginning on day 3

[total dose/cycle = 1,400 mg/m^2]

◄

Consolidation:
Course 1:
Daunorubicin: IV: 60 mg/m^2/day days 1, 2, and 3
[total dose/cycle = 180 mg/m^2]
Cytarabine: IV: 200 mg/m^2/day days 1 to 7
[total dose/cycle = 1,400 mg/m^2]
Course 2:
Daunorubicin: IV: 45 mg/m^2/day days 1, 2, and 3
[total dose/cycle = 135 mg/m^2]
Cytarabine: IV: 1,000 mg/m^2 every 12 hours for 8 doses days 1 to 4
[total dose/cycle = 8,000 mg/m^2]
Maintenance:
Mercaptopurine: Oral: 50 or 90 mg/m^2 daily
[total dose/12 week maintenance cycle = 4,200 or 7,560 mg/m^2 (84 days)]
Methotrexate: Oral: 15 mg/m^2 weekly
[total dose/12 week maintenance cycle = 180 mg/m^2]
Tretinoin: Oral: 45 mg/m^2/day (in 2 divided doses) days 1 to 15
[total dose/12 week maintenance cycle = 675 mg/m^2]
Repeat cycle every 12 weeks for 2 years
Variation 3 (patients ≤60 years of age and WBC ≥10,000/mm^3):
Induction:
Tretinoin: Oral: 45 mg/m^2/day (in 2 divided doses) day 1 until hematologic complete remission
Daunorubicin: IV: 60 mg/m^2/day days 3, 4, and 5
[total dose/cycle = 180 mg/m^2]
Cytarabine: IV: 200 mg/m^2/day continuous infusion for 7 days beginning on day 3
[total dose/cycle = 1,400 mg/m^2]
Consolidation:
Course 1:
Daunorubicin: IV: 60 mg/m^2/day days 1, 2, and 3
[total dose/cycle = 180 mg/m^2]
Cytarabine: IV: 200 mg/m^2/day days 1 to 7
[total dose/cycle = 1,400 mg/m^2]
Course 2:
Daunorubicin: IV: 45 mg/m^2/day days 1, 2, and 3
[total dose/cycle = 135 mg/m^2]
Cytarabine: IV: 2,000 mg/m^2 every 12 hours for 10 doses days 1 to 5 (Ades 2006; patients <50 years; Ades 2008) or 1,500 mg/m^2 every 12 hours for 10 doses days 1 to 5 (patients 50 to 60 years; Ades 2008)
[total dose/cycle = 15,000 mg/m^2 to 20,000 mg/m^2]
Intrathecal prophylaxis: Five intrathecal injections: First dose in between induction and consolidation and 2 doses during each consolidation phase:
Methotrexate (preservative free): Intrathecal: 15 mg
Cytarabine (preservative free): Intrathecal: 50 mg
Corticosteroids (preservative free): Intrathecal: Dose unspecified
Maintenance:
Mercaptopurine: Oral: 50 or 90 mg/m^2 daily
[total dose/12 week maintenance cycle = 4,200 or 7,560 mg/m^2 (84 days)]
Methotrexate: Oral: 15 mg/m^2 weekly
[total dose/12 week maintenance cycle = 180 mg/m^2]
Tretinoin: Oral: 45 mg/m^2/day (in 2 divided doses) days 1 to 15
[total dose/12 week maintenance cycle = 675 mg/m^2]
Repeat cycle every 12 weeks for 2 years

Variation 4 (patients >60 years of age and WBC >10,000/mm^3):
Induction:
Tretinoin: Oral: 45 mg/m^2/day (in 2 divided doses) day 1 until hematologic complete remission
Daunorubicin: IV: 60 mg/m^2/day days 3, 4, and 5
[total dose/cycle = 180 mg/m^2]
Cytarabine: IV: 200 mg/m^2/day continuous infusion for 7 days beginning on day 3
[total dose/cycle = 1,400 mg/m^2]
Consolidation:
Course 1:
Daunorubicin: IV: 60 mg/m^2/day days 1, 2, and 3
[total dose/cycle = 180 mg/m^2]
Cytarabine: IV: 200 mg/m^2/day days 1 to 7
[total dose/cycle = 1,400 mg/m^2]
Course 2:
Daunorubicin: IV: 45 mg/m^2/day days 1, 2, and 3
[total dose/cycle = 135 mg/m^2]
Cytarabine: IV: 1,000 mg/m^2 every 12 hours for 8 doses days 1 to 4
[total dose/cycle = 8,000 mg/m^2]
Intrathecal prophylaxis: Five intrathecal injections: First dose in between induction and consolidation and 2 doses during each consolidation phase:
Methotrexate (preservative free): Intrathecal: 15 mg
Cytarabine (preservative free): Intrathecal: 50 mg
Corticosteroids (preservative free): Intrathecal: Dose unspecified
Maintenance:
Mercaptopurine: Oral: 50 or 90 mg/m^2 daily
[total dose/12 week maintenance cycle = 4,200 or 7,560 mg/m^2 (84 days)]
Methotrexate: Oral: 15 mg/m^2 weekly
[total dose/12 week maintenance cycle = 180 mg/m^2]
Tretinoin: Oral: 45 mg/m^2/day (in 2 divided doses) days 1 to 15
[total dose/12 week maintenance cycle = 675 mg/m^2]
Repeat cycle every 12 weeks for 2 years

References

Variation 1:
Powell BL, Moser B, Stock W, et al. Arsenic trioxide improves event-free and overall survival for adults with acute promyelocytic leukemia: North American Leukemia Intergroup Study C9710. *Blood.* 2010;116(19):3751-3757.

Variations 2, 3, and 4:
Adès L, Chevret S, Raffoux E, et al, "Is Cytarabine Useful in the Treatment of Acute Promyelocytic Leukemia? Results of a Randomized Trial From the European Acute Promyelocytic Leukemia Group," *J Clin Oncol,* 2006, 24(36):5703-10.
Adès L, Sanz MA, Chevret S, et al. Treatment of newly diagnosed acute promyelocytic leukemia (APL): a comparison of French-Belgian-Swiss and PETHEMA results. *Blood.* 2008;111 (3):1078-1084.

Tretinoin-Idarubicin (APL)

Index Terms ATRA-Idarubicin (APL); Idarubicin-ATRA (APL); Idarubicin-Tretinoin (APL)

Use Leukemia, acute promyelocytic

◀ **Regimen** NOTE: Multiple variations are listed.
Variation 1:
Induction:
Tretinoin: Oral: 45 mg/m^2/day (in 2 divided doses) day 1 up to 90 days
[total dose/cycle = up to 4050 mg/m^2]
≤20 years: Oral: 25 mg/m^2/day (in 2 divided doses) day 1 up to 90 days
[total dose/cycle = up to 2250 mg/m^2]
Idarubicin: IV: 12 mg/m^2/day days 2, 4, 6, and 8 (omit day 8 for patients >70
years of age)
[total dose/cycle = 36-48 mg/m^2]
Consolidation (administer courses sequentially at 1-month intervals for 3
months):
Course 1:
Idarubicin: IV: 5 mg/m^2/day days 1 to 4
[total dose/cycle = 20 mg/m^2]
or
Idarubicin: IV: 7 mg/m^2/day days 1 to 4
[total dose/cycle = 28 mg/m^2]
Tretinoin: Oral: 45 mg/m^2/day (in 2 divided doses) days 1 to 15
[total dose/cycle = 675 mg/m^2]
Course 2:
Mitoxantrone: IV: 10 mg/m^2/day days 1 to 5
[total dose/cycle = 50 mg/m^2]
or
Mitoxantrone: IV: 10 mg/m^2/day days 1 to 5
[total dose/cycle = 50 mg/m^2]
Tretinoin: Oral: 45 mg/m^2/day (in 2 divided doses) days 1 to 15
[total dose/cycle = 675 mg/m^2]
Course 3:
Idarubicin: IV: 12 mg/m^2 day 1
[total dose/cycle = 12 mg/m^2]
or
Idarubicin: IV: 12 mg/m^2/day days 1 and 2
[total dose/cycle = 24 mg/m^2]
Tretinoin: Oral: 45 mg/m^2/day (in 2 divided doses) days 1 to 15
[total dose/cycle = 675 mg/m^2]
Maintenance:
Mercaptopurine: Oral: 50 mg/m^2 daily
[total dose/cycle = 4500 mg/m^2 (90 days)]
Methotrexate: IM: 15 mg/m^2 weekly
[total dose/cycle = 180 mg/m^2]
Tretinoin: Oral: 45 mg/m^2/day (in 2 divided doses) days 1 to 15
[total dose/cycle = 675 mg/m^2]
Repeat cycle every 3 months for 2 years
Variation 2:
Induction:
Tretinoin: Oral: 45 mg/m^2/day (in 2 divided doses) day 1 up to 90 days
[total dose/cycle = up to 4050 mg/m^2]
<15 years: Oral: 25 mg/m^2/day (in 2 divided doses) day 1 up to 90 days
[total dose/cycle = up to 2250 mg/m^2]
Idarubicin: IV: 12 mg/m^2/day days 2, 4, 6, and 8
[total dose/cycle = 48 mg/m^2]

Consolidation (administer courses sequentially at 1-month intervals for 3 months):
Course 1:
 Idarubicin: IV: 5 mg/m^2/day days 1 to 4
  [total dose/cycle = 20 mg/m^2]
Course 2:
 Mitoxantrone: IV: 10 mg/m^2/day days 1 to 5
  [total dose/cycle = 50 mg/m^2]
Course 3:
 Idarubicin: IV: 12 mg/m^2 day 1
  [total dose/cycle = 12 mg/m^2]
Maintenance:
 Mercaptopurine: Oral: 90 mg/m^2 daily
  [total dose/cycle = 8100 mg/m^2 (90 days)]
 Methotrexate: IM: 15 mg/m^2 weekly
  [total dose/cycle = 180 mg/m^2]
 Tretinoin: Oral: 45 mg/m^2/day (in 2 divided doses) days 1 to 15
  [total dose/cycle = 675 mg/m^2]
 Repeat cycle every 3 months for 2 years
Variation 3 (patients ≥60 years of age):
Induction:
 Tretinoin: Oral: 45 mg/m^2/day (in 2 divided doses) day 1 up to 90 days
  [total dose/cycle = up to 4050 mg/m^2]
 Idarubicin: IV: 12 mg/m^2/day days 2, 4, 6, and 8 (omit day 8 for patients ≥70 years of age)
  [total dose/cycle = 36-48 mg/m^2]
Consolidation (administer courses sequentially at 1-month intervals for 3 months):
Course 1:
 Idarubicin: IV: 5 mg/m^2/day days 1 to 4
  [total dose/cycle = 20 mg/m^2]
 Tretinoin: Oral: 45 mg/m^2/day (in 2 divided doses) days 1 to 15 (if intermediate or high risk)
  [total dose/cycle = 675 mg/m^2]
Course 2:
 Mitoxantrone: IV: 10 mg/m^2/day days 1 to 5
  [total dose/cycle = 50 mg/m^2]
 Tretinoin: Oral: 45 mg/m^2/day (in 2 divided doses) days 1 to 15 (if intermediate or high risk)
  [total dose/cycle = 675 mg/m^2]
Course 3:
 Idarubicin: IV: 12 mg/m^2 day 1
  [total dose/cycle = 12 mg/m^2]
 Tretinoin: Oral: 45 mg/m^2/day (in 2 divided doses) days 1 to 15 (if intermediate or high risk)
  [total dose/cycle = 675 mg/m^2]
Maintenance:
 Mercaptopurine: Oral: 50 mg/m^2 daily
  [total dose/cycle = 4500 mg/m^2 (90 days)]
 Methotrexate: IM: 15 mg/m^2 weekly
  [total dose/cycle = 180 mg/m^2]
 Tretinoin: Oral: 45 mg/m^2/day (in 2 divided doses) days 1 to 15
  [total dose/cycle = 675 mg/m^2]
 Repeat cycle every 3 months for 2 years

References
Variation 1:

Sanz MA, Martin G, Gonzalez M, et al, "Risk-Adapted Treatment of Acute Promyelocytic Leukemia With All-*Trans*-Retinoic Acid and Anthracycline Monochemotherapy: A Multicenter Study by the PETHEMA Group," *Blood*, 2004, 103(4):1237-43.

Variation 2:

Sanz MA, Martin G, Rayon C, et al, "A Modified AIDA Protocol With Anthracycline-Based Consolidation Results in High Antileukemic Efficacy and Reduced Toxicity in Newly Diagnosed PML/RARalpha-Positive Acute Promyelocytic Leukemia," *Blood*, 1999, 94(9):3015-21.

Variation 3:

Sanz MA, Vellenga E, Rayón C, et al, "All-*Trans* Retinoic Acid and Anthracycline Monochemo-therapy for the Treatment of Elderly Patients With Acute Promyelocytic Leukemia," *Blood*, 2004, 104(12):3490-3.

VAC Alternating With IE (Ewing Sarcoma)

Use Ewing sarcoma

Regimen

Cycle A (Odd numbered cycles):

Cyclophosphamide: IV: 1200 mg/m^2 day 1 (followed by mesna; dose not specified)

[total dose/cycle = 1200 mg/m^2]

Vincristine: IV: 2 mg/m^2 (maximum dose: 2 mg) day 1

[total dose/cycle = 2 mg/m^2; maximum: 2 mg]

Doxorubicin: IV: 75 mg/m^2 day 1, for 5 cycles (maximum cumulative dose: 375 mg/m^2)

[total dose/cycle = 75 mg/m^2; maximum cumulative dose: 375 mg/m^2]

Dactinomycin: IV: 1.25 mg/m^2 day 1, begin cycle 11 (after reaching maximum cumulative doxorubicin dose)

[total dose/cycle = 1.25 mg/m^2]

Cycle B (Even numbered cycles):

Ifosfamide: IV: 1800 mg/m^2/day days 1 to 5 (given with mesna)

[total dose/cycle = 9000 mg/m^2]

Etoposide: IV: 100 mg/m^2/day days 1 to 5

[total dose/cycle = 500 mg/m^2]

Alternate Cycles A and B, administering a cycle every 3 weeks (alternating in the following sequence: ABABAB) for 17 cycles

References
Grier HE, Krailo MD, Tarbell NJ, et al, "Addition of Ifosfamide and Etoposide to Standard Chemotherapy for Ewing's Sarcoma and Primitive Neuroectodermal Tumor of Bone," *N Engl J Med*, 2003, 348(8):694-701.

VAC (Ovarian)

Index Terms Vincristine, Dactinomycin, Cyclophosphamide (Ovarian)

Use Ovarian cancer (germ cell tumor)

Regimen

Vincristine: IV: 1.5 mg/m^2/day (maximum dose: 2 mg) days 1, 8, 15, and 22 for 2-3 cycles

[total dose/cycle = 6 mg/m^2 (maximum: 8 mg)] for 2-3 cycles

Dactinomycin: IV: 300 mcg/m^2/day days 1 to 5

[total dose/cycle = 1500 mcg/m^2]

Cyclophosphamide: IV: 150 mg/m^2/day days 1 to 5

[total dose/cycle = 750 mg/m^2]

Repeat cycle every 28 days for at least 10 cycles; vincristine is only administered for 2-3 cycles

References
Slayton RE, Park RC, Silverberg SG, et al, "Vincristine, Dactinomycin, and Cyclophosphamide in the Treatment of Malignant Germ Cell Tumors of the Ovary. A Gynecologic Oncology Group Study (A Final Report)," *Cancer*, 1985, 56(2):243-8.

VAC Pulse
Use Soft tissue sarcoma (rhabdomyosarcoma)
Regimen
Vincristine: IV: 2 mg/m^2/dose (maximum dose: 2 mg/dose) every 7 days, for 12 weeks

Dactinomycin: IV: 0.015 mg/kg/day (maximum dose: 0.5 mg/day) days 1 to 5, every 3 months for 5 courses

Cyclophosphamide: Oral, IV: 10 mg/kg/day for 7 days, repeat every 6 weeks
References
Wilbur JR, Sutow WW, Sullivan MP, et al, "Chemotherapy of Sarcomas," *Cancer*, 1975, 36 (2):765-9.

VAC (Rhabdomyosarcoma)
Use Soft tissue sarcoma (rhabdomyosarcoma)
Regimen
Induction (weeks 1 to 17):
Vincristine: IV push: 1.5 mg/m^2 (maximum dose: 2 mg) day 1 of weeks 1 to 13, then one dose at week 17

Dactinomycin: IV push: 0.015 mg/kg/day (maximum dose: 0.5 mg) days 1 to 5 of weeks 1, 4, 7, and 17

Cyclophosphamide: IV: 2.2 g/m^2 day 1 of weeks 1, 4, 7, 10, 13, and 17
Continuation (weeks 21 to 44):
Vincristine: IV push: 1.5 mg/m^2 (maximum dose: 2 mg) day 1 of weeks 21 to 26, 30 to 35, and 39 to 44

Dactinomycin: IV push: 0.015 mg/kg/day (maximum dose: 0.5 mg) days 1 to 5 of weeks 21, 24, 30, 33, 39, and 42

Cyclophosphamide: IV: 2.2 g/m^2 day 1 of weeks 21, 24, 30, 33, 39, and 42
References
Baker KS, Anderson JR, Link MP, et al, "Benefit of Intensified Therapy for Patients With Local or Regional Embryonal Rhabdomyosarcoma: Results From the Intergroup Rhabdomyosarcoma Study IV," *J Clin Oncol*, 2000, 18(12):2427-34.

VAD
Use Multiple myeloma
Regimen
Vincristine: IV: 0.4 mg/day continuous infusion days 1 to 4
[total dose/cycle = 1.6 mg]
Doxorubicin: IV: 9 mg/m^2/day continuous infusion days 1 to 4
[total dose/cycle = 36 mg/m^2]
Dexamethasone: Oral: 40 mg/day days 1 to 4, 9 to 12, and 17 to 20
[total dose/cycle = 480 mg]
Repeat cycle every 28-35 days
References
Barlogie B, Smith L, and Alexanian R, "Effective Treatment of Advanced Multiple Myeloma Refractory to Alkylating Agents," *N Engl J Med*, 1984, 310(21):1353-6.

VAD/CVAD
Use Leukemia, acute lymphocytic

◄ **Regimen** Induction cycle:
Vincristine: IV: 0.4 mg/day continuous infusion days 1 to 4 and 24 to 27
[total dose/cycle = 3.2 mg]
Doxorubicin: IV: 12 mg/m^2/day continuous infusion days 1 to 4 and 24 to 27
[total dose/cycle = 96 mg/m^2]
Dexamethasone: Oral: 40 mg/day days 1 to 4, 9 to 12, 17 to 20, 24 to 27, 32 to
35, and 40 to 43
[total dose/cycle = 960 mg]
Cyclophosphamide: IV: 1 g/m^2 day 24
[total dose/cycle = 1 g/m^2]
Administer one cycle only

References
Kantarjian H, Walters RS, Keating MJ, et al, "Results of the Vincristine, Doxorubicin, and Dexamethasone Regimen in Adults With Standard and High-Risk Acute Lymphocytic Leukemia," *J Clin Oncol*, 1990, 8(6):994-1004.

VAD (Wilms' Tumor)

Index Terms Vincristine, Dactinomycin, Doxorubicin (Wilms' Tumor)
Use Wilms' tumor
Regimen NOTE: Multiple variations are listed.
Variation 1 (Stage III favorable disease; children ≥1 year):
Vincristine: IV: 1.5 mg/m^2 weekly for 10 to 11 weeks
Followed by:
Vincristine: IV: 1.5 mg/m^2 every 3 weeks
Dactinomycin: IV: 1.5 mg/m^2 every 6 weeks
Doxorubicin: IV: 40 mg/m^2 every 6 weeks
NOTE: Alternate dactinomycin and doxorubicin; administer dactinomycin at 3
weeks and doxorubicin in 3 weeks
Treatment continued for 1 year
Variation 2 (Stage III favorable disease; children <1 year):
Vincristine: IV: 0.75 mg/m^2 weekly for 10 to 11 weeks
Followed by:
Vincristine: IV: 0.75 mg/m^2 every 3 weeks
Dactinomycin: IV: 0.75 mg/m^2 every 6 weeks
Doxorubicin: IV: 20 mg/m^2 every 6 weeks
NOTE: Alternate dactinomycin and doxorubicin; administer dactinomycin at 3
weeks and doxorubicin in 3 weeks
Treatment continued for 1 year

References
Variations 1 and 2:
Pritchard J, Imeson J, Barnes J, et al, "Results of the United Kingdom Children's Cancer Study Group First Wilms' Tumor Study," *J Clin Oncol*, 1995, 13(1):124-33.

VAMP (Hodgkin)

Index Terms Vinblastine, Doxorubicin, Methotrexate, Prednisone (Hodgkin)
Use Lymphoma, Hodgkin
Regimen NOTE: Patients <21 years old
Vinblastine: IV: 6 mg/m^2/day days 1 and 15
[total dose/cycle = 12 mg/m^2]
Doxorubicin: IV: 25 mg/m^2/day days 1 and 15
[total dose/cycle = 50 mg/m^2]
Methotrexate: IV: 20 mg/m^2/day days 1 and 15
[total dose/cycle = 40 mg/m^2]

Prednisone: Oral: 40 mg/m²/day days 1 to 14 (omit after mediastinal radiation)
[total dose/cycle = 560 mg/m²]
Repeat cycle every 28 days for a total of 4 cycles

References

Donaldson SS, Link MP, Weinstein HJ, et al, "Final Results of a Prospective Clinical Trial With VAMP and Low-Dose Involved Radiation for Children With Low-Risk Hodgkin's Disease," *J Clin Oncol*, 2007, 25(3):332-7.

Vandetanib (Thyroid Regimen)

Use Thyroid cancer

Regimen

Vandetanib: Oral: 300 mg once daily days 1 to 28
[total dose/cycle = 8400 mg]
Repeat cycle every 28 days until disease progression or unacceptable toxicity

References

Wells SA Jr, Gosnell JE, Gagel RF, et al, "Vandetanib for the Treatment of Patients With Locally Advanced or Metastatic Hereditary Medullary Thyroid Cancer," *J Clin Oncol*, 2010, 28(5):767-72.

VBMCP (Multiple Myeloma)

Use Multiple myeloma

Regimen NOTE: Multiple variations are listed.

Variation 1:
Vincristine: IV: 1.2 mg/m² day 1
[total dose/cycle = 1.2 mg/m²]
Carmustine: IV: 20 mg/m² day 1
[total dose/cycle = 20 mg/m²]
Melphalan: Oral: 8 mg/m²/day days 1 to 4
[total dose/cycle = 32 mg/m²]
Cyclophosphamide: IV: 400 mg/m² day 1
[total dose/cycle = 400 mg/m²]
Prednisone: Oral: 40 mg/m²/day days 1 to 7
[total dose/cycle = 280 mg/m²]
Repeat cycle every 35 days for up to 2 years or until disease progression

Variation 2:
Vincristine: IV: 1.2 mg/m² (maximum dose: 2 mg) day 1
[total dose/cycle = 1.2 mg/m²; maximum: 2 mg]
Carmustine: IV: 20 mg/m² day 1
[total dose/cycle = 20 mg/m²]
Melphalan: Oral: 8 mg/m²/day days 1 to 4
[total dose/cycle = 32 mg/m²]
Cyclophosphamide: IV: 400 mg/m² day 1
[total dose/cycle = 400 mg/m²]
Prednisone: Oral: 40 mg/m²/day days 1 to 7 (all cycles)
[total dose/cycle = 280 mg/m²]
followed by Oral: 20 mg/m²/day days 8 to 14 (first 3 cycles only)
[total dose/cycle = 140 mg/m²]
Repeat cycle every 35 days

References

Variation 1:
Kyle RA, Leong T, Li S, et al, "Complete Response in Multiple Myeloma: Clinical Trial E9486, an Eastern Cooperative Oncology Group Study Not Involving Stem Cell Transplantation," *Cancer*, 2006, 106(9):1958-66.

◀ Variation 2:
Oken MM, Harrington DP, Abramson N, et al, "Comparison of Melphalan and Prednisone With Vincristine, Carmustine, Melphalan, Cyclophosphamide, and Prednisone in the Treatment of Multiple Myeloma: Results of Eastern Cooperative Oncology Group Study E2479," *Cancer*, 1997, 79(8):1561-7.

♦ **VBR (NHL-Follicular)** *see* Bendamustine-Bortezomib-Rituximab (NHL-Follicular) *on page 1833*

♦ **VC (Adjuvant NSCLC)** *see* Cisplatin-Vinorelbine (Adjuvant NSCLC) *on page 1914*

♦ **VC (Metastatic NSCLC)** *see* Cisplatin-Vinorelbine (Metastatic NSCLC) *on page 1915*

VcR-CAP (NHL-Mantle Cell)

Index Terms Botezomib-Rituximab-Cyclophosphamide-Doxorubicin-Prednisone (NHL-Mantle Cell); Rituximab-Bortezomib-Cyclophosphamide-Doxorubicin-Prednisone (NHL-Mantle Cell); VR-CAP (NHL-Mantle Cell)

Use Lymphoma, non-Hodgkin (first-line, transplant ineligible, stage 2 to 4 mantle cell)

Regimen

Bortezomib: IV: 1.3 mg/m^2/day days 1, 4, 8, and 11
  [total dose/cycle = 5.2 mg/m^2]
Rituximab: IV: 375 mg/m^2 day 1
  [total dose/cycle = 375 mg/m^2]
Cyclophosphamide: IV: 750 mg/m^2 day 1
  [total dose/cycle = 750 mg/m^2]
Doxorubicin: IV: 50 mg/m^2 day 1
  [total dose/cycle = 50 mg/m^2]
Prednisone: Oral: 100 mg/m^2/day days 1 to 5
  [total dose/cycle = 500 mg/m^2]

Repeat cycle every 21 days for 6 to 8 cycles. If response first documented at cycle 6, treatment could continue for an additional 2 more cycles.

References

Robak T, Huang H, Jin J, et al. Bortezomib-based therapy for newly diagnosed mantle-cell lymphoma. *N Engl J Med*. 2015;372(10):944-953.

♦ **VD (Multiple Myeloma)** *see* Bortezomib-Dexamethasone (Multiple Myeloma) *on page 1848*

♦ **VDR (Multiple Myeloma)** *see* Lenalidomide-Bortezomib-Dexamethasone (Multiple Myeloma) *on page 2026*

VelP (Testicular)

Index Terms Vinblastine-Ifosfamide-Cisplatin (Testicular); VIP (Vinblastine) (Testicular)

Use Testicular cancer

Regimen

Vinblastine: IV: 0.11 mg/kg/day days 1 and 2
  [total dose/cycle = 0.22 mg/kg]
Ifosfamide: IV: 1200 mg/m^2/day days 1 to 5
  [total dose/cycle = 6000 mg/m^2]
Cisplatin: IV: 20 mg/m^2/day days 1 to 5
  [total dose/cycle = 100 mg/m^2]

Mesna: IV: 400 mg/m^2 prior to ifosfamide day 1
followed by IV: 1200 mg/m^2/day continuous infusion days 1 to 5
[total dose/cycle = 6400 mg/m^2]
Repeat cycle every 21 days for 4 cycles

References

Loehrer PJ Sr, Gonin R, Nichols CR, Weathers T, Einhorn LH. Vinblastine plus ifosfamide plus cisplatin as initial salvage therapy in recurrent germ cell tumor. *J Clin Oncol*. 1998;16 (7):2500-2504.

Loehrer PJ Sr, Lauer R, Roth BJ, Williams SD, Kalasinski LA, Einhorn LH. Salvage therapy in recurrent germ cell cancer: ifosfamide and cisplatin plus either vinblastine or etoposide. *Ann Intern Med*. 1988;109(7):540-546.

Correction: incomplete dosage information in article on germ cell cancer. *Ann Intern Med*. 1988;109 (10):846.

Vemurafenib (Melanoma Regimen)

Use Melanoma

Regimen

Vemurafenib: Oral: 960 mg twice daily
Continue until disease progression or unacceptable toxicity

References

Chapman PB, Hauschild A, Robert C, et al, "Improved Survival With Vemurafenib in Melanoma With BRAF V600E Mutation," *N Engl J Med*, 2011, 364(26):2507-16.

Sosman JA, Kim KB, Schuchter L, et al, "Survival in BRAF V600-Mutant Advanced Melanoma Treated With Vemurafenib," *N Engl J Med*, 2012, 366(8):707-14.

VIM-D (Hodgkin)

Index Terms Etoposide-Ifosfamide-Mitoxantrone-Dexamethasone (Hodgkin)

Use Lymphoma, Hodgkin

Regimen

Etoposide: IV: 100 mg/m^2 over 30 minutes day 1
[total dose/cycle = 100 mg/m^2]
Ifosfamide: IV: 4 g/m^2 continuous infusion over 24 hours day 1
[total dose/cycle = 4 g/m^2]
Mesna: IV: 1 g/m^2 IV bolus day 1
followed by: Mesna: IV: 6 g/m^2 continuous infusion over 36 hours
[total dose/cycle = 7 g/m^2]
Mitoxantrone: IV: 10 mg/m^2 IV bolus day 1
[total dose/cycle = 10 mg/m^2]
Dexamethasone: Oral: 40 mg/day days 1 to 5
[total dose/cycle = 200 mg]
Repeat cycle every 28 days; treat 3 cycles post remission

References

Phillips JK, Spearing RL, Davies JM, et al, "VIM-D Salvage Chemotherapy in Hodgkin's Disease," *Cancer Chemother Pharmacol*, 1990, 27(2):161-3.

◆ **Vinblastine-Cisplatin-Dacarbazine** *see* Cisplatin-Vinblastine-Dacarbazine (Melanoma) *on page 1912*

◆ **Vinblastine-Cisplatin (NSCLC)** *see* Cisplatin-Vinblastine (NSCLC) *on page 1913*

◆ **Vinblastine, Doxorubicin, Methotrexate, Prednisone (Hodgkin)** *see* VAMP (Hodgkin) *on page 2104*

Vinblastine (Hodgkin Regimen)

Use Lymphoma, Hodgkin

◄ **Regimen**

Vinblastine: IV: 4-6 mg/m^2/day IV bolus day 1

[total dose/cycle = 4-6 mg/m^2]

Repeat cycle every 1 to 2 weeks until disease progression

References

Little R, Wittes RE, Longo DL, et al, "Vinblastine for Recurrent Hodgkin's Disease Following Autologous Bone Marrow Transplant," *J Clin Oncol*, 1998, 16(2):584-8.

◆ **Vinblastine-Ifosfamide-Cisplatin (Testicular)** *see* VeIP (Testicular) *on page 2106*

◆ **Vinblastine-Methotrexate (Soft Tissue Sarcoma)** *see* Methotrexate-Vinblastine (Soft Tissue Sarcoma) *on page 2036*

◆ **Vincristine-Carboplatin-Etoposide (Retinoblastoma)** *see* Carboplatin-Etoposide-Vincristine (Retinoblastoma) *on page 1866*

◆ **Vincristine-Carboplatin (Retinoblastoma)** *see* Carboplatin-Vincristine (Retinoblastoma) *on page 1875*

◆ **Vincristine, Dactinomycin, Cyclophosphamide (Ovarian)** *see* VAC (Ovarian) *on page 2102*

◆ **Vincristine, Dactinomycin, Doxorubicin (Wilms' Tumor)** *see* VAD (Wilms' Tumor) *on page 2104*

◆ **Vincristine-Dactinomycin (Wilms' Tumor)** *see* EE-4A (Wilms' Tumor) *on page 1953*

◆ **Vincristine, Doxorubicin, Cyclophosphamide, Mesna, Etoposide** *see* Regimen I (Wilms' Tumor) *on page 2074*

Vinorelbine (Cervical Regimen)

Use Cervical cancer

Regimen

Vinorelbine: IV: 30 mg/m^2/day days 1 and 8

[total dose/cycle = 60 mg/m^2]

Repeat cycle every 21 days

References

Muggia FM, Blessing JA, Method M, et al, "Evaluation of Vinorelbine in Persistent or Recurrent Squamous Cell Carcinoma of the Cervix: A Gynecologic Oncology Group Study," *Gynecol Oncol*, 2004, 92(2):639-43.

Muggia FM, Blessing JA, Waggoner S, et al, "Evaluation of Vinorelbine in Persistent or Recurrent Nonsquamous Carcinoma of the Cervix: A Gynecologic Oncology Group Study," *Gynecol Oncol*, 2005, 96(1):108-11.

◆ **Vinorelbine-Cisplatin (Adjuvant NSCLC)** *see* Cisplatin-Vinorelbine (Adjuvant NSCLC) *on page 1914*

◆ **Vinorelbine-Cisplatin (Cervical Cancer)** *see* Cisplatin-Vinorelbine (Cervical Cancer) *on page 1914*

◆ **Vinorelbine-Cisplatin (Metastatic NSCLC)** *see* Cisplatin-Vinorelbine (Metastatic NSCLC) *on page 1915*

◆ **Vinorelbine-Gemcitabine (Head and Neck)** *see* Gemcitabine-Vinorelbine (Head and Neck) *on page 1998*

◆ **Vinorelbine-Gemcitabine (NSCLC)** *see* Gemcitabine-Vinorelbine (NSCLC) *on page 1998*

◆ **Vinorelbine-Gemcitabine (Soft Tissue Sarcoma)** *see* Gemcitabine-Vinorelbine (Soft Tissue Sarcoma) *on page 1999*

Vinorelbine (Hodgkin Regimen)

Use Lymphoma, Hodgkin

Regimen

Vinorelbine: IV: 30 mg/m^2/day day 1

[total dose/cycle = 30 mg/m^2]

Repeat cycle every 7 days, maximum of 24 doses

References

Devizzi L, Santoro A, Bonfante V, et al, "Vinorelbine: An Active Drug for the Management of Patients With Heavily Pretreated Hodgkin's Disease," *Ann Oncol*, 1994, 5(9):817-20.

Vinorelbine (Mesothelioma Regimen)

Use Malignant pleural mesothelioma

Regimen

Vinorelbine: IV: 30 mg/m^2 (maximum dose: 60 mg) weekly for 6 weeks

[total dose/cycle = 180 mg/m^2; maximum 360 mg]

Repeat cycle every 42 days

References

Stebbing J, Powles T, McPherson K, et al. The efficacy and safety of weekly vinorelbine in relapsed malignant pleural mesothelioma. *Lung Cancer*. 2009;63(1):94-97.

Vinorelbine (NSCLC Regimen)

Use Lung cancer, non-small cell

Regimen NOTE: Multiple variations are listed.

Variation 1 (elderly ≥70 years old):

Vinorelbine: IV: 30 mg/m^2/day days 1 and 8

[total dose/cycle = 60 mg/m^2]

Repeat cycle every 21 days for up to 6 cycles

Variation 2 (elderly ≥70 years old):

Vinorelbine: IV: 25 mg/m^2/day days 1 and 8

[total dose/cycle = 50 mg/m^2]

Repeat cycle every 21 days for 4 cycles

Variation 3:

Vinorelbine: IV: 30 mg/m^2/day days 1, 8, and 15

[total dose/cycle = 90 mg/m^2]

Repeat cycle every 21 days

References

Variation 1:

Effects of vinorelbine on quality of life and survival of elderly patients with advanced non-small-cell lung cancer. The Elderly Lung Cancer Vinorelbine Italian Study Group. *J Natl Cancer Inst*. 1999;91(1):66-72.

Variation 2:

Kudoh S, Takeda K, Nakagawa K, et al. Phase III study of docetaxel compared with vinorelbine in elderly patients with advanced non-small-cell lung cancer: results of the West Japan Thoracic Oncology Group Trial (WJTOG 9904). *J Clin Oncol*. 2006;24(22):3657-3663.

Variation 3:

Fossella FV, DeVore R, Kerr RN, et al. Randomized phase III trial of docetaxel versus vinorelbine or ifosfamide in patients with advanced non-small-cell lung cancer previously treated with platinum-containing chemotherapy regimens. The TAX 320 Non-Small Cell Lung Cancer Study Group. *J Clin Oncol*. 2000;18(12):2354-2362.

Vinorelbine (Ovarian Regimen)

Use Ovarian cancer

Regimen NOTE: Multiple variations listed.
Variation 1:
Vinorelbine: IV: 30 mg/m^2/day days 1 and 8
[total dose/cycle = 60 mg/m^2]
Repeat cycle every 21 days until disease progression or unacceptable toxicity
Variation 2:
Vinorelbine: IV: 25 mg/m^2/day days 1, 8, and 15
[total dose/cycle = 75 mg/m^2]
Repeat cycle every 21 days until disease progression or unacceptable toxicity

References
Variation 1:
Rothenberg ML, Liu PY, Wilczynski S, et al, "Phase II Trial of Vinorelbine for Relapsed Ovarian Cancer: A Southwest Oncology Group Study," *Gynecol Oncol*, 2004, 95(3):506-12.
Variation 2:
Bajetta E, Di Leo A, Biganzoli L, et al, "Phase II Study of Vinorelbine in Patients With Pretreated Advanced Ovarian Cancer: Activity in Platinum-Resistant Disease," *J Clin Oncol*, 1996, 14 (9):2546-51.

Vinorelbine (Small Cell Lung Cancer Regimen)

Use Lung cancer, small cell

Regimen NOTE: Multiple variations are listed:
Variation 1:
Vinorelbine: IV: 30 mg/m^2 day 1
[total dose/cycle = 30 mg/m^2]
Repeat cycle every 7 days until disease progression or unacceptable toxicity
Variation 2:
Vinorelbine: IV: 25 mg/m^2 day 1
[total dose/cycle = 25 mg/m^2]
Repeat cycle every 7 days until disease progression, no response after 4 cycles, or unacceptable toxicity

References
Variation 1:
Jassem J, Karnicka-Mlodkowska H, van Pottelsberghe C, et al, "Phase II Study of Vinorelbine (Navelbine) in Previously Treated Small Cell Lung Cancer Patients. EORTC Lung Cancer Cooperative Group," *Eur J Cancer*, 1993, 29(12):1720-2.
Variation 2:
Furuse K, Kubota K, Kawahara M, et al, "Phase II Study of Vinorelbine in Heavily Previously Treated Small Cell Lung Cancer. Japan Lung Cancer Vinorelbine Study Group," *Oncology*, 1996, 53(2):169-172.

◆ **Vinorelbine-Trastuzumab (Breast)** see Trastuzumab-Vinorelbine (Breast) on page 2095

◆ **VIP (Etoposide) (Testicular)** see VIP (Testicular) on page 2110

VIP (Testicular)

Index Terms Etoposide-Ifosfamide-Cisplatin (Testicular); VIP (Etoposide) (Testicular)

Use Testicular cancer

Regimen
Etoposide: IV: 75 mg/m^2/day days 1 to 5
[total dose/cycle = 375 mg/m^2]
Ifosfamide: IV: 1200 mg/m^2/day days 1 to 5
[total dose/cycle = 6000 mg/m^2]

Cisplatin: IV: 20 mg/m^2/day days 1 to 5
[total dose/cycle = 100 mg/m^2]
Mesna: IV: 120 mg/m^2 prior to ifosfamide day 1
followed by IV: 1200 mg/m^2/day continuous infusion days 1 to 5
[total dose/cycle = 6120 mg/m^2]
Filgrastim: SubQ: 5 mcg/kg daily days 7 to 16
Repeat cycle every 21 days for 4 cycles

References

Nichols CR, Catalano PJ, Crawford ED, Vogelzang NJ, Einhorn LH, Loehrer PJ. Randomized comparison of cisplatin and etoposide and either bleomycin or ifosfamide in treatment of advanced disseminated germ cell tumors: an Eastern Cooperative Oncology Group, Southwest Oncology Group, and Cancer and Leukemia Group B Study. *J Clin Oncol.* 1998;16(4):1287-1293.

◆ **VIP (Vinblastine) (Testicular)** *see* VeIP (Testicular) *on page 2106*

Vismodegib (Basal Cell Regimen)

Use Basal cell carcinoma

Regimen

Vismodegib: Oral: 150 mg once daily
[total dose/cycle = 4200 mg]
Repeat cycle every 28 days until disease progression or unacceptable toxicity

References

Sekulic A, Migden MR, Oro AE, et al, "Efficacy and Safety of Vismodegib in Advanced Basal-Cell Carcinoma," *N Engl J Med*, 2012, 366(23):2171-9.

◆ **VMP (Multiple Myeloma)** *see* Melphalan-Prednisone-Bortezomib (Multiple Myeloma) *on page 2033*

◆ **VMPT** *see* Bortezomib-Melphalan-Prednisone-Thalidomide *on page 1850*

Vorinostat (NHL-CTCL Regimen)

Use Lymphoma, non-Hodgkin (CTCL)

Regimen

Vorinostat: Oral: 400 mg once daily on days 1 to 28
[total dose/cycle = 11,200 mg]
Repeat cycle every 28 days until disease progression or unacceptable toxicity

References

Duvic M, Olsen EA, Breneman D, et al. Evaluation of the long-term tolerability and clinical benefit of vorinostat in patients with advanced cutaneous T-cell lymphoma. *Clin Lymphoma Myeloma*. 2009;9(6):412-416.

Duvic M, Talpur R, Ni X, et al. Phase 2 trial of oral vorinostat (suberoylanilide hydroxamic acid, SAHA) for refractory cutaneous T-cell lymphoma (CTCL). *Blood*. 2007;109(1):31-39.

Olsen EA, Kim YH, Kuzel TM, et al. Phase IIb multicenter trial of vorinostat in patients with persistent, progressive, or treatment refractory cutaneous T-cell lymphoma. *J Clin Oncol*. 2007;25(21):3109-3115.

◆ **VR-CAP (NHL-Mantle Cell)** *see* VcR-CAP (NHL-Mantle Cell) *on page 2106*

◆ **VRd (Multiple Myeloma)** *see* Lenalidomide-Bortezomib-Dexamethasone (Multiple Myeloma) *on page 2026*

XELOX (Colorectal)

Index Terms Capecitabine-Oxaliplatin (Colorectal); CapeOx (Colorectal); CAPOX (Colorectal); Oxaliplatin-Capecitabine (Colorectal)
Use Colorectal cancer

◀ **Regimen** NOTE: Multiple variations are listed.

Variation 1 (adjuvant):

Oxaliplatin: IV: 130 mg/m² over 2 hours day 1

[total dose/cycle = 130 mg/m²]

Capecitabine: Oral: 1000 mg/m² twice daily days 1 to 14

[total dose/cycle = 28,000 mg/m²]

Repeat cycle every 21 days for 8 cycles

Variation 2 (metastatic):

Oxaliplatin: IV: 130 mg/m² over 2 hours day 1

[total dose/cycle = 130 mg/m²]

Capecitabine: Oral: 1000 mg/m² twice daily days 1 (beginning with evening dose) to 15 (ending with morning dose)

[total dose/cycle = 28,000 mg/m²]

Repeat cycle every 21 days

Variation 3 (metastatic):

Oxaliplatin: IV: 130 mg/m² day 1

[total dose/cycle = 130 mg/m²]

Capecitabine: Oral: 850 mg/m² twice daily days 1 (beginning with evening dose) to 15 (ending with morning dose)

[total dose/cycle = 23,800 mg/m²]

Repeat cycle every 21 days

References

Variation 1:

Haller DG, Tabernero J, Maroun J, et al, "Capecitabine Plus Oxaliplatin Compared With Fluorouracil and Folinic Acid as Adjuvant Therapy for Stage III Colon Cancer," *J Clin Oncol*, 2011, 29 (11):1465-71.

Variation 2:

Cassidy J, Clarke S, Díaz-Rubio E, et al, "Randomized Phase III Study of Capecitabine Plus Oxaliplatin Compared With Fluorouracil/Folinic Acid Plus Oxaliplatin as First-Line Therapy for Metastatic Colorectal Cancer," *J Clin Oncol*, 2008, 26(12):2006-12.

Cassidy J, Tabernero J, Twelves C, et al, "XELOX (Capecitabine Plus Oxaliplatin): Active First-Line Therapy for Patients With Metastatic Colorectal Cancer," *J Clin Oncol*, 2004, 22(11):2084-91.

Variation 3:

Hochster HS, Hart LL, Ramanathan RK, et al, "Safety and Efficacy of Oxaliplatin and Fluoropyrimidine Regimens With or Without Bevacizumab as First-Line Treatment of Metastatic Colorectal Cancer: Results of the TREE Study," *J Clin Oncol*, 2008, 26(21):3523-9.

◆ **XELOX (Gastric)** *see* Capecitabine-Oxaliplatin (Gastric) *on page 1859*

◆ **XELOX (Pancreatic)** *see* CAPOX (Pancreatic) *on page 1861*

Ziv-Aflibercept + FOLFIRI (Colorectal)

Index Terms Ziv-Aflibercept, Irinotecan, Leucovorin, Fluorouracil (Colorectal)

Use Colorectal cancer

Regimen

Ziv-Aflibercept: IV: 4 mg/kg over 1 hour day 1

[total dose/cycle = 4 mg/kg]

Irinotecan: IV: 180 mg/m² over 90 minutes day 1

[total dose/cycle = 180 mg/m²]

Leucovorin: IV: 400 mg/m² over 2 hours day 1

[total dose/cycle = 400 mg/m²]

Fluorouracil: IV bolus: 400 mg/m^2 day 1
  followed by IV: 2400 mg/m^2 continuous infusion (CI) over 46 hours beginning day 1
    [total fluorouracil dose/cycle (bolus and CI) = 2800 mg/m^2]
Repeat cycle every 14 days until disease progression or unacceptable toxicity

References

Van Cutsem E, Tabernero J, Lakomy R, et al, "Addition of Aflibercept to Fluorouracil, Leucovorin, and Irinotecan Improves Survival in a Phase III Randomized Trial in Patients With Metastatic Colorectal Cancer Previously Treated With an Oxaliplatin-Based Regimen," *J Clin Oncol*, 2012 [epub ahead of print].

◆ **Ziv-Aflibercept, Irinotecan, Leucovorin, Fluorouracil (Colorectal)** *see* Ziv-Aflibercept + FOLFIRI (Colorectal) *on page 2112*

SPECIAL TOPICS

CHEMOTHERAPY-INDUCED PERIPHERAL NEUROPATHY

INTRODUCTION

Chemotherapy-induced peripheral neuropathy (CIPN) is a common dose-related cumulative toxicity associated with many chemotherapeutic agents. CIPN occurs in close to 40% of patients receiving cancer therapy, although the actual incidence rate and severity varies depending on the chemotherapy regimen and dosing, duration of exposure, concomitant use of other neurotoxic drugs, and assessment methodology (Hershman 2014; Piccolo 2014). CIPN may adversely affect patient quality of life (QOL) and toxicity may necessitate chemotherapy dose reduction or therapy cessation, possibly compromising cancer outcomes. In many instances, CIPN may be partially or wholly reversible after therapy discontinuation; however, if it is not identified early and managed appropriately, permanent toxicity may occur. It is crucial that health care providers alert patients of the signs and symptoms of this condition in order to promptly identify its development and treat accordingly.

Chemotherapy agents frequently associated with CIPN include the platinum agents, taxanes, vinca alkaloids, bortezomib (route-specific), thalidomide, ixabepilone, and dinutuximab. Neuropathy symptoms in patients receiving chemotherapy are primarily sensory in nature and may include numbness, tingling/burning, paresthesias, hyperalgesia, and loss of tendon reflexes. The distribution of symptoms is mostly symmetric and distal and the condition spreads to the extremities in a "stocking and glove" pattern as it worsens (Hershman 2014; Piccolo 2014). Motor nerve function generally remains intact in patients with CIPN.

In addition to CIPN, taxanes and oxaliplatin may cause an acute neuropathy syndrome that is clinically separate from CIPN. Oxaliplatin-induced acute neuropathy occurs in the hours to days following administration; manifestations include throat discomfort, muscle cramps, discomfort swallowing cold liquids, and sensitivity to touching cold items or being exposed to cool temperatures. Patients receiving paclitaxel, particularly those administered higher individual doses, may develop an acute pain syndrome consisting of arthralgia/myalgia symptoms. This acute syndrome typically develops 1 to 3 days after administration and mostly resolves within a week.

While prevention and treatment of CIPN are often managed similarly to other neuropathic conditions such as diabetic peripheral neuropathy or postherpetic neuralgia, high-quality data with consistent evidence that supports such therapy is limited in the cancer patient population. Further research needs to be conducted to provide guidance on the management of this serious and potentially debilitating toxicity.

PREVENTION

Many agents have been investigated for the prevention of CIPN, but minimal efficacy and lack of consistent evidence supporting these options limits their use. A recently published guideline by the American Society of Clinical Oncology (ASCO) does not support the use of acetyl-L-carnitine (ALC), amifostine, amitriptyline, calcium/magnesium infusions (for oxaliplatin-induced neuropathy), diethyldithio-carbamate (DDTC), glutathione, nimodipine, Org 2766, all-*trans*-retinoic acid, rhuLIF, or vitamin E for CIPN prevention (Hershman 2014). No recommendations can be made on the use of N-acetylcysteine, carbamazepine, glutamate, goshajinkigan, omega-3 fatty acids, or oxcarbazepine for CIPN prevention at this time (Hershman 2014). The following discussion is a brief summary of the data for CIPN prevention of select agents.

Venlafaxine

Venlafaxine, a serotonin and norepinephrine reuptake inhibitor (SNRI), was studied in a randomized, double-blind, placebo-controlled phase 3 trial in 48 patients with oxaliplatin-induced acute neurotoxicity (EFFOX trial). Eligible patients included those who experienced acute neuropathy after oxaliplatin therapy; patients with preexisting neuropathy or diabetes were excluded. Patients were randomized to receive venlafaxine 50 mg orally 1 hour prior to oxaliplatin on day 1 and extended release venlafaxine 37.5 mg orally twice daily on days 2 through 11 or placebo; oxaliplatin was administered every 14 days. The primary end point was the percentage of patients with complete relief of acute neuropathy; secondary endpoints included percentage of patients with ≥50% pain relief, mean Neuropathic Pain Symptom Inventory (NPSI) and numeric rating scale (NRS) score variations during treatment, and percentage of patients with grade 0 and grade 3 neuropathy at 3 months (Durand 2012).

Venlafaxine-treated patients were significantly more likely than placebo-treated patients to achieve complete symptom relief (31.3% vs 5.3%, respectively; p=0.03). At 3 months after conclusion of oxaliplatin treatment, 38.5% of venlafaxine-treated patients reported no neuropathy compared with 5.6% of patients in the placebo group (p=0.06). In addition, significantly fewer patients with grade 3 neuropathy were observed in the venlafaxine group (0% vs 33.3%; p=0.03) at 3 months after treatment (Durand 2012).

While these data suggest that venlafaxine may be beneficial in the prevention of oxaliplatin-associated CIPN, its routine use in clinical practice is not currently recommended until additional data becomes available (Hershman 2014).

Calcium/Magnesium Infusions

Many clinical trials have been performed to evaluate the use of calcium and magnesium infusions for the prevention of oxaliplatin-associated neuropathy. Calcium and magnesium infusions are thought to prevent neuropathy by increasing the extracellular concentrations of these electrolytes, thereby decreasing the hyperexcitability of oxaliplatin-subjected neurons (Piccolo 2014). Its use is controversial; while some data support the efficacy of calcium and magnesium infusions for this indication, questions regarding its effect on tumor control remain.

The CONcePT trial (Combined Oxaliplatin Neurotoxicity Prevention Trial) evaluated whether patients receiving FOLFOX/bevacizumab for the treatment of metastatic colorectal cancer allowed patients to remain on therapy longer with intermittent oxaliplatin administration compared to a conventional oxaliplatin schedule (Hochster 2014). Patients were also randomized to calcium/magnesium infusion (administered at a dose of 1 g each, given pre- and post-oxaliplatin) or placebo for neurotoxicity prophylaxis. Randomization was conducted in a 2x2 factorial design (intermittent vs conventional oxaliplatin; calcium/magnesium vs placebo). The study was terminated early due to a decreased tumor response rate in patients receiving calcium and magnesium; however, retrospective review of computed tomography scans collected during the study did not demonstrate an inferior response in patients receiving calcium and magnesium (Hochster 2014).

Subsequent to the CONcePT trial, several other prospective clinical trials studying calcium/magnesium for prevention of oxaliplatin-associated neuropathy were closed. Grothey and colleagues studied 102 patients with colon cancer receiving adjuvant therapy with FOLFOX; patients were randomly assigned to receive calcium/magnesium infusions pre- and post-oxaliplatin or placebo (Grothey 2011). Calcium and magnesium significantly decreased the incidence of chronic, cumulative, ≥ grade 2 sensory neuropathy (p=0.018). Acute muscle spasms attributed to oxaliplatin were also reduced (p=0.01), but calcium/magnesium infusions did not appear to decrease cold sensitivity toxicities (Grothey 2011). Additionally, a large, randomized trial in 353 patients receiving FOLFOX as adjuvant therapy for colon cancer failed to show statistically significant differences in neuropathy scores in patients who received calcium and magnesium pre- and post-oxaliplatin compared to placebo (Loprinzi 2014).

Until further data is available to confirm that administering calcium and magnesium does not decrease tumor response rates, the use of this strategy to prevent oxaliplatin-induced peripheral neuropathy is not recommended (Hershman 2014).

Amifostine

The chemoprotective effects of amifostine are thought to be due to its binding of toxic chemotherapy metabolites, thus preventing damage to normal tissue. To investigate its chemoprotective benefits, 242 patients with stage III or IV ovarian cancer were randomized to receive amifostine 910 mg/m^2 or placebo prior to cyclophosphamide and cisplatin administration (Kemp 1996). After six cycles of therapy, severity of cisplatin-associated peripheral neuropathy was significantly decreased in the amifostine arm as compared to placebo (p=0.029). Amifostine was also studied in ovarian cancer patients receiving carboplatin and paclitaxel (Lorusso 2003). Similar to the previous trial, patients were randomly assigned to receive amifostine at 910 mg/m^2 prior to chemotherapy. The incidence of grade 3 or 4 neurotoxicity was significantly reduced in the amifostine arm as compared to placebo (3.7% vs 7.2%, respectively; p=0.02); however, other studies utilizing amifostine have not demonstrated significant efficacy for prevention of CIPN (Hilpert 2005; Openshaw 2004). Given the adverse effect profile of amifostine (including cardiovascular, dermatologic, and gastrointestinal toxicities), as well as conflicting and limited efficacy data, this agent is not recommended for CIPN prevention (Hershman 2014).

Vitamin E

Vitamin E has been studied in CIPN prevention for its antioxidant and free radical scavenging properties. A phase 3, randomized, double-blind, placebo-controlled study was performed in 189 patients receiving neurotoxic chemotherapy (taxanes, platinum agents, or a combination of agents) (Kottschade 2011). Patients were randomized to receive vitamin E 400 mg twice daily or placebo; the primary study objective was the incidence of ≥ grade 2 sensory neuropathy. The results did not show a statistically significant difference between the groups; the incidence of ≥ grade 2 sensory neuropathy was 34% in the vitamin E arm vs 29% in the placebo group (p=0.43). In addition, no significant differences were seen in time to neuropathy onset or chemotherapy dose reductions due to neuropathy (Kottschade 2011).

Other small studies have shown a positive benefit of using vitamin E for CIPN prevention, but limited patient numbers and methodological concerns reduce their applicability (Pace 2003; Pace 2010). Further research is needed to recommend vitamin E for CIPN prevention.

TREATMENT

Treatment options for CIPN include therapy interruption or discontinuation, chemotherapy dose reduction, alteration of the route of administration (bortezomib) or use of an adjuvant medication to provide symptomatic pain relief. Reducing, interrupting, or discontinuing chemotherapy is not an ideal management option (particularly in the curative setting), as patient outcomes could be adversely affected by decreasing chemotherapy dose intensity. Identifying viable CIPN treatment options is crucial in order to optimize cancer-related care. While data for management of other neuropathic conditions is plentiful, data for treatment of CIPN remains limited. Currently, the ASCO guidelines recommend duloxetine for CIPN treatment; tricyclic antidepressants (eg, nortriptyline or desipramine), gabapentin or pregabalin, or a topical gel containing baclofen, amitriptyline, and ketamine may be offered to select patients if the risk/benefit ratio is acceptable (Hershman 2014). The following discussion provides a brief summary of the data for CIPN treatment of select agents.

Duloxetine

Duloxetine was evaluated in a randomized, double-blind, placebo-controlled, crossover trial of patients with a diagnosis of ≥ grade 1 sensory neuropathy and a pain score of ≥4 on a Brief Pain Inventory-Short Form scale of 1 to 10 after receiving therapy with paclitaxel, another taxane, cisplatin, or oxaliplatin (Smith 2013). Patients received either placebo for 5 weeks or duloxetine 30 mg daily for the first week, followed by duloxetine 60 mg daily for 4 additional weeks; the crossover study design also included a 2-week washout between treatment periods. After 5 weeks of therapy, patients receiving duloxetine reported a mean decrease in pain score of 1.06 (95% CI, 0.72 to 1.40) vs 0.34 (95% CI, 0.01 to 0.66) in patients receiving placebo (p=0.003) (Smith 2013). Analysis of secondary outcomes showed that duloxetine-treated patients experienced a greater decrease in pain interfering with daily activities and an increased quality of life as compared to patients who received placebo.

A subgroup analysis of the interaction between treatment group and chemotherapy class suggests that duloxetine may be of most benefit in patients receiving oxaliplatin therapy compared to those who received taxanes, although the results were not statistically significant (p=0.13). Overall, duloxetine was well tolerated, with fatigue, nausea, and insomnia being the most commonly reported adverse events (Smith 2013).

Gabapentin

Gabapentin is commonly used to treat diabetic neuropathy and postherpetic pain, and due to its largely favorable side effect profile, it has been used frequently for CIPN management despite limited trial data for this indication. Rao et al conducted a multicenter, double-blind, randomized, crossover trial in 115 patients with symptomatic CIPN to evaluate the effect of gabapentin on CIPN pain (Rao 2007). Eligible patients were those with an average daily reported pain score of ≥4 on a scale of 1 to 10 or those with a score of ≥1 on the Eastern Cooperative Oncology Group Neuropathy scale (ENS). Patients were stratified according to the class of neurotoxic chemotherapy regimen received and then randomized to either gabapentin (target dose of 2,700 mg daily) or placebo. After taking the maximum tolerated dose for 3 weeks, gabapentin was weaned off and patients crossed over to the opposite arm. The primary efficacy measure was the self-reported average daily pain score, measured by the numeric rating scale and the

◀ ENS. While gabapentin was well-tolerated, no statistically significantly change in the pain score was observed as compared to placebo (Rao 2007).

Despite a lack of data demonstrating a benefit of using gabapentin for CIPN treatment, the current ASCO guidelines suggest that it may still be a reasonable option to offer patients suffering from this condition. Given its acceptable side effect profile, its efficacy in treating other types of neuropathic pain, and limited options for CIPN management, gabapentin (or the mechanistically similar pregabalin) may provide benefit to select patients (Hershman 2014).

Tricyclic Antidepressants

Tricyclic antidepressants such as amitriptyline and nortriptyline have shown efficacy in the management of other neuropathic conditions. While amitriptyline has been studied in small trials for CIPN, efficacy was not seen due to insufficient statistical power (Kautio 2008; Kautio 2009). Nortriptyline was studied in a randomized, double-blind, placebo-controlled, crossover trial to evaluate its efficacy in treating cisplatin-induced neuropathy (Hammack 2002). Eligible patients had evidence of sensory peripheral neuropathy due to cisplatin on exam and had painful paresthesiae for at least 1 month. Fifty-one patients were randomly assigned to receive either nortriptyline (starting dose of 25 mg daily, titrated at weekly intervals to a target dose of 100 mg daily) or placebo for 4 weeks, after which they were crossed over to the opposite arm. No significant differences between nortriptyline and placebo was observed with respect to paresthesiae (mean scores of 49 and 55, respectively, on a 100-point visual analog scale; p=0.78), nor was quality of life improved with nortriptyline use (Hammack 2002).

Given the lack of efficacy data and significant adverse event profile, tricyclic antidepressants are not considered first-line therapy for treatment of CIPN (Piccolo 2014). However, the ASCO guidelines state that they may still be considered in select patients if the possible benefit outweighs the toxicity risk (Hershman 2014).

REFERENCES

Durand JP, Deplanque G, Montheil V, et al. Efficacy of venlafaxine for the prevention and relief of oxaliplatin-induced acute neurotoxicity: results of EFFOX, a randomized, double-blind, placebo-controlled phase III trial. *Ann Oncol.* 2012;23(1):200-205.

Grothey A, Nikcevich DA, Sloan JA, et al. Intravenous calcium and magnesium for oxaliplatin-induced sensory neurotoxicity in adjuvant colon cancer: NCCTG N04C7. *J Clin Oncol.* 2011;29 (4):421-427.

Hammack JE, Michalak JC, Loprinzi CL, et al. Phase III evaluation of nortriptyline for alleviation of symptoms of cis-platinum-induced peripheral neuropathy. *Pain.* 2002;98(1-2):195-203.

Hershman DL, Lacchetti C, Dworkin RH, et al. Prevention and management of chemotherapy-induced peripheral neuropathy in survivors of adult cancers: American Society of Clinical Oncology clinical practice guideline. *J Clin Oncol.* 2014;32(18):1941-1967.

Hilpert F, Stähle A, Tomé O, et al. Neuroprotection with amifostine in the first-line treatment of advanced ovarian cancer with carboplatin/paclitaxel-based chemotherapy – a double-blind, placebo-controlled, randomized phase II study from the Arbeitsgemeinschaft Gynäkologische Onkologoie (AGO) Ovarian Cancer Study Group. *Support Care Cancer.* 2005;13(10):797-805.

Hochster HS, Grothey A, Hart L, et al. Improved time to treatment failure with an intermittent oxaliplatin strategy: results of CONcePT. *Ann Oncol.* 2014;25(6):1172-1178.

Kautio AL, Haanpää M, Leminen A, Kalso E, Kautiainen H, Saarto T. Amitriptyline in the prevention of chemotherapy-induced neuropathic symptoms. *Anticancer Res.* 2009;29(7):2601-2606.

Kautio AL, Haanpää M, Saarto T, Kalso E. Amitriptyline in the treatment of chemotherapy-induced neuropathic symptoms. *J Pain Symptom Manage.* 2008;35(1):31-39.

Kemp G, Rose P, Lurain J, et al. Amifostine pretreatment for protection against cyclophosphamide-induced and cisplatin-induced toxicities: results of a randomized control trial in patients with advanced ovarian cancer. *J Clin Oncol.* 1996;14(7):2101-2112.

Kottschade LA, Sloan JA, Mazurczak MA, et al. The use of vitamin E for the prevention of chemotherapy-induced peripheral neuropathy: results of a randomized phase III clinical trial. *Support Care Cancer*. 2011;19(11):1769-1777.

Loprinzi CL, Qin R, Dakhil SR, et al. Phase III randomized, placebo-controlled, double-blind study of intravenous calcium and magnesium to prevent oxaliplatin-induced sensory neurotoxicity (N08CB/Alliance). *J Clin Oncol*. 2014;32(10):997-1005.

Lorusso D, Ferrandina G, Greggi S, et al. Phase III multicenter randomized trial of amifostine as cytoprotectant in first-line chemotherapy in ovarian cancer patients. *Ann Oncol*. 2003;14(7):1086-1093.

Openshaw H, Beamon K, Synold TW, et al. Neurophysiological study of peripheral neuropathy after high-dose Paclitaxel: lack of neuroprotective effect of amifostine. *Clin Cancer Res*. 2004;10(2):461-467.

Pace A, Giannarelli D, Galiè E, et al. Vitamin E neuroprotection for cisplatin neuropathy: a randomized, placebo-controlled trial. *Neurology*. 2010;74(9):762-766.

Pace A, Savarese A, Picardo M, et al. Neuroprotective effect of vitamin E supplementation in patients treated with cisplatin chemotherapy. *J Clin Oncol*. 2003;21(5):927-931.

Piccolo J, Kolesar JM. Prevention and treatment of chemotherapy-induced peripheral neuropathy. *Am J Health Syst Pharm*. 2014;71(1):19-25.

Rao RD, Michalak JC, Sloan JA, et al. Efficacy of gabapentin in the management of chemotherapy-induced peripheral neuropathy: a phase 3 randomized, double-blind, placebo-controlled, cross-over trial (N00C3). *Cancer*. 2007;110(9):2110-2118.

Smith EM, Pang H, Cirrincione C, et al. Effect of duloxetine on pain, function, and quality of life among patients with chemotherapy-induced painful peripheral neuropathy: a randomized clinical trial. *JAMA*. 2013;309(13):1359-1367.

COMMON TOXICITY CRITERIA

Selected Common Toxicity Criteria[1]

Toxicity	Grade 0	Grade 1	Grade 2	Grade 3	Grade 4
Hematologic					
Leukocytes (WBC)	WNL	3,000/mm^3 to <LLN	2,000 to <3,000/mm^3	1,000 to <2,000/mm^3	<1,000/mm^3
Neutrophils (ANC)	WNL	1,500/mm^3 to <LLN	1,000 to <1,500/mm^3	500 to <1,000/mm^3	<500/mm^3
Lymphocytes	WNL	800/mm^3 to <LLN	500 to <800/mm^3	200 to <500/mm^3	<200/mm^3
Anemia (Hgb)	WNL	10 g/dL to <LLN	8 to <10 g/dL	v3: 6.5 to <8 g/dL v4: <8 g/dL	v3: <6.5 g/dL v4: Life-threatening
Platelets	WNL	75,000/mm^3 to <LLN	50,000 to <75,000/mm^3	25,000 to <50,000/mm^3	<25,000/mm^3
Hemorrhage	None	Mild, no intervention indicated	Intervention indicated (symptomatic or medical)	Transfusion (and/or other intervention) indicated	Life-threatening; major intervention indicated
Cardiovascular					
Acute coronary syndrome	None		Symptomatic; progressive angina; normal cardiac enzymes; hemodynamically stable	Symptomatic, unstable angina and/or acute MI; abnormal cardiac enzymes; hemodynamically stable	Symptomatic, unstable angina and/or acute MI; abnormal cardiac enzymes; hemodynamically unstable
Atrial fibrillation	None	Asymptomatic; intervention not indicated	Medical intervention indicated (nonurgent)	Symptomatic; incomplete medical control or controlled with device or ablation	Life-threatening; urgent intervention required
Chest pain (cardiac)	None	Mild pain	Moderate pain; limits instrumental ADL	Pain at rest; limits self-care ADL	
Heart failure	None	Asymptomatic with laboratory (eg, B-Natriuretic Peptide [BNP]) or cardiac imaging abnormalities	Symptoms with mild to moderate activity or exertion	Symptoms (severe) at rest or with minimal activity/exertion; intervention indicated	Life-threatening; urgent intervention indicated

Selected Common Toxicity Criteria[1] *continued*

Toxicity	Grade 0	Grade 1	Grade 2	Grade 3	Grade 4
Hypotension	None	v3: Changes v4: Asymptomatic; no treatment required	v3: Brief (<24 hours) treatment (eg, fluid replacement or other therapy) required v4: Nonurgent medical intervention indicated	v3: Sustained (>24 hours) treatment required; resolves without persisting physiologic consequences v4: Medical intervention indicated	v3: Shock v4: Life-threatening; urgent intervention indicated
Hypertension	None	v3: Increase of DBP >20 mm Hg or to >150/100; treatment not required v4: Prehypertension (SBP 120 to 139 mm Hg or DBP 80 to 89 mm Hg)	v3: Recurrent or persistent grade 1 level; may require monotherapy treatment v4: Stage 1 (SBP 140 to 159 mm Hg or DBP 90 to 99 mm Hg); medical intervention indicated; recurrent or persistent (≥24 hours); symptomatic increase of >20 mm Hg (DBP) or to >140/90; monotherapy indicated	v3: More intensive treatment or >1 drug required v4: Stage 2 (SBP ≥16 mm Hg or DBP ≥100 mm Hg); medical intervention indicated; >1 drug or more intensive therapy indicated	v3: Life-threatening (eg, hypertensive crisis) v4: Life-threatening (eg, malignant hypertension, hypertensive crisis); urgent intervention indicated
Left ventricular systolic dysfunction	None	v3: Asymptomatic; resting ejection fraction (EF) >50% to <60%; shortening fraction (SF) >24% to <30%	v3: Asymptomatic; resting EF >40% to <50%; SF >15% to <24%	v3: Symptomatic heart failure (HF) responsive to intervention; EF >20% to <50%, SF <15% v4: Symptomatic due to decreased ejection fraction; responsive to intervention	v3: Refractory or poorly controlled HF; EF <20%; intervention indicated v4: Refractory or poorly controlled HF due to decreased ejection fraction; intervention indicated

Selected Common Toxicity Criteria[1] *continued*

Toxicity	Grade 0	Grade 1	Grade 2	Grade 3	Grade 4
Myocardial infarction (MI)	None	v3: Asymptomatic arterial narrowing without ischemia	v3: Asymptomatic; testing suggestive of ischemia; stable angina v4: Asymptomatic; cardiac enzymes minimally abnormal; no evidence of ischemic ECG changes	v3: Symptomatic; testing consistent with ischemia; unstable angina; intervention indicated v4: Severely symptomatic; abnormal cardiac enzymes; hemodynamically stable; ECG changes consistent with infarction	v3: Acute MI v4: Life-threatening; hemodynamically unstable
Pericardial effusion	None	v3: Asymptomatic effusion	v4: Small- to moderate-sized asymptomatic effusion	Physiologic consequences	Life-threatening consequences; urgent intervention indicated
Pericarditis	None	Asymptomatic, ECG or physical findings consistent with diagnosis	Symptomatic (eg, chest pain)	Physiologic consequences (eg, pericardial constriction)	Life-threatening; urgent intervention indicated
QTc prolongation	WNL	v3: QTc >450 to 470 msec v4: QTc >450 to 480 msec	v3: QTc >470 to 500 msec; ≥60 msec increase from baseline v4: QTc 481 to 500 msec	v3: QTc >500 msec v4: QTc ≥501 msec (on 2 separate ECGs)	v3: QTc >500 msec with life-threatening signs or symptoms (eg, arrhythmia, CHF, hypotension, shock, syncope); Torsades de pointes v4: QTc ≥501 msec or >60 msec change from baseline and Torsades de pointes or polymorphic ventricular tachycardia or signs/ symptoms of serious arrhythmia

Selected Common Toxicity Criteria[1] *continued*

Toxicity	Grade 0	Grade 1	Grade 2	Grade 3	Grade 4
Sinus bradycardia	None	Asymptomatic; intervention not indicated	v3: Medical intervention indicated (nonurgent) v4: Symptomatic; medical intervention indicated	v3: Symptomatic; incomplete medical control or controlled with device v4: Severe, medically significant; medical intervention indicated	v3: Life-threatening v4: Life-threatening; urgent intervention indicated
Sinus tachycardia	None	Asymptomatic; intervention not indicated	Symptomatic; medical intervention indicated (nonurgent)	v3: Symptomatic; incomplete medical control or controlled with device v4: Urgent medical intervention indicated	v3: Life-threatening
Supraventricular tachycardia	None	Asymptomatic; intervention not indicated	Symptomatic; medical intervention indicated (nonurgent)	v3: Symptomatic; incomplete medical control or controlled with device v4: Medical intervention indicated	v3: Life-threatening v4: Life-threatening; urgent intervention indicated
Syncope	Absent			v3: Present v4: Fainting; orthostatic collapse	Life-threatening consequences
Thrombosis/embolism	None	v4: Superficial	v3: DVT or cardiac thrombosis; intervention not indicated v4: Venous thrombosis (uncomplicated DVT); medical intervention indicated	v3: DVT or cardiac thrombosis; intervention indicated v4: Thrombosis (eg, uncomplicated pulmonary embolism, nonembolic cardiac mural thrombus); medical intervention indicated	v3: Pulmonary embolism/life threatening thrombus v4: Life-threatening (eg, pulmonary embolism, cerebrovascular event, arterial insufficiency); hemodynamic or neurologic instability; urgent intervention indicated

Selected Common Toxicity Criteria[1] *continued*

Toxicity	Grade 0	Grade 1	Grade 2	Grade 3	Grade 4
			Dermatologic		
Rash (acne/acneiform)	None	v3: Intervention not indicated v4: Papules and/or pustules covering <10% of BSA	v3: Intervention indicated v4: Papules and/or pustules covering 10% to 30% of BSA; limits ADL	v3: Pain, disfigurement, ulceration, desquamation v4: Papules and/or pustules covering >30% of BSA; limits self-care ADL; local superinfection requiring oral antibiotics	v4: Papules or pustules associated with extensive superinfection with IV antibiotics indicated; life-threatening consequences
Rash	None	v3: Macular or papular eruption v4: Macules or papules covering <10% of BSA	v3: Macular or papular eruption or erythema w/ pruritus affecting <50% of BSA v4: Macules or papules covering 10% to 30% of BSA; limits ADL	v3: Severe erythema/ desquamation/macular, papular, or vesicular eruption covering ≥50% of BSA v4: Macules or papules covering >30% of BSA; limits self-care ADL	v3: Generalized exfoliative, ulcerative, or bullous dermatitis
Rash (erythema multiforme)	None	v4: Lesions covering <10% of BSA	v3: Scattered eruption v4: Lesions covering 10% to 30% of BSA, associated with skin tenderness	v3: Severe eruption; IV fluids, tube feeding, or TPN indicated v4: Lesions covering >30% of BSA, associated with oral or genital erosions	v3: Life-threatening eruption; disabling v4: Lesions covering >30% of BSA, associated with fluid or electrolyte abnormality; ICU or burn unit indicated

Selected Common Toxicity Criteria[1] continued

Toxicity	Grade 0	Grade 1	Grade 2	Grade 3	Grade 4
Hand-foot syndrome	None	Minimal skin changes or dermatitis without pain	v3: Skin changes or pain not interfering with ADL v4: Skin changes with pain; limits ADL	v3: Ulcerative dermatitis or skin changes with pain; interferes with ADL v4: Severe skin changes (peeling, blisters, bleeding, edema, hyperkeratosis) with pain; limits self-care ADL	
Alopecia	None	v3: Thinning or patchy v4: Hair loss <50% (of normal)	v3: Complete v4: Hair loss ≥50% (of normal)		
Gastrointestinal					
Nausea	None	Loss of appetite/able to eat	v3: Oral intake decreased, no significant weight loss, dehydration, or malnutrition; IV fluids indicated <24 hours v4: Oral intake decreased, no significant weight loss, dehydration, or malnutrition	v3: Inadequate oral caloric or fluid intake/IV fluids required ≥24 hours v4: Inadequate oral caloric or fluid intake; tube feeding, TPN, or hospitalization indicated	Life-threatening consequences
Vomiting	None	v3: 1 episode per 24 hours v4: 1 to 2 episodes per 24 hours	v3: 2 to 5 episodes per 24 hours; IV fluids indicated <24 hours v4: 3 to 5 episodes per 24 hours	v3: ≥6 episodes per 24 hours, IV fluids, or TPN required ≥24 hours v4: ≥6 episodes per 24 hours, IV fluids, tube feeding, or TPN required	Life-threatening consequences

Selected Common Toxicity Criteria[1] *continued*

Toxicity	Grade 0	Grade 1	Grade 2	Grade 3	Grade 4
Diarrhea	None	<4 stools/day increase over baseline	v3: 4 to 6 stools/day increase over baseline; IV fluids indicated <24 hours; does not limit ADL v4: 4 to 6 stools/day increase over baseline	v3: ≥7 stools/day increase over baseline; IV fluids required ≥24 hours; hospitalization; interferes with ADL v4: ≥7 stools/day increase over baseline; incontinence; hospitalization; limits self-care ADL	v3: Life-threatening consequences v4: Life-threatening consequences; urgent intervention indicated
Mucositis/stomatitis	None	v3: Mucosal erythema v4: Asymptomatic or mild	v3: Patchy ulcerations v4: Moderate pain; does not interfere with oral intake; modified diet needed	v3: Confluent ulceration, bleeding with minor trauma v4: Severe pain, interferes with oral intake	v3: Tissue necrosis/ bleeding; life-threatening v4: Life-threatening; urgent intervention indicated
GI bleeding	None	Mild; intervention not indicated	Symptomatic; mild intervention indicated	Transfusion required; intervention indicated	Life-threatening consequences; urgent intervention indicated
Amylase elevation	None	>ULN to 1.5 x ULN	>1.5 to 2 x ULN	>2 to 5 x ULN	>5 x ULN
Lipase elevation	None	>ULN to 1.5 x ULN	>1.5 to 2 x ULN	>2 to 5 x ULN	>5 x ULN
Ascites	None	Asymptomatic	Symptomatic; intervention indicated	Symptomatic; invasive intervention indicated	v3: Life-threatening consequences v4: Life-threatening consequences; urgent operative intervention indicated

Selected Common Toxicity Criteria[1] *continued*

Toxicity	Grade 0	Grade 1	Grade 2	Grade 3	Grade 4
			Hepatic		
Alkaline phosphatase elevation	WNL	>ULN to 2.5 x ULN	>2.5 to 5 x ULN	>5 to 20 x ULN	>20 x ULN
AST elevation	WNL	v3: >ULN to 2.5 x ULN v4: >ULN to 3 x ULN	v3: >2.5 to 5 x ULN v4: >3 to 5 x ULN	>5 to 20 x ULN	>20 x ULN
ALT elevation	WNL	v3: >ULN to 2.5 x ULN v4: >ULN to 3 x ULN	v3: >2.5 to 5 x ULN v4: >3 to 5 x ULN	>5 to 20 x ULN	>20 x ULN
Hyperbilirubinemia	WNL	>ULN to 1.5 x ULN	>1.5 to 3 x ULN	>3 to 10 x ULN	>10 x ULN
			Metabolic		
Hypoalbuminemia	WNL	3 g/dL to <LLN	2 to <3 g/dL	<2 g/dL	v4: Life-threatening; urgent intervention indicated
Hypercholesteremia	None	>ULN to 300 mg/dL	>300 to 400 mg/dL	>400 to 500 mg/dL	>500 mg/dL
Hyperglycemia	WNL	>ULN to 160 mg/dL	>160 to 250 mg/dL	>250 to 500 mg/dL	>500 mg/dL
Hypertriglyceridemia	None	v3: >ULN to 2.5 x ULN v4: 150 to 300 mg/dL	v3: >2.5 to 5 x ULN v4: >300 to 500 mg/dL	v3: >5 to 10 x ULN v4: >500 to 1000 mg/dL	v3: >10 x ULN v4: >1000 mg/dL; life-threatening
Hyperuricemia	WNL	>ULN to 10 mg/dL (without physiologic consequences)	>ULN to 10 mg/dL (without physiologic consequences)	>ULN to 10 mg/dL (with physiologic consequences)	>10 mg/dL.; life-threatening
Hypoglycemia	WNL	55 mg/dL to <LLN	40 to <55 mg/dL	30 to <40 mg/dL	<30 mg/dL

Selected Common Toxicity Criteria[1] *continued*

Toxicity	Grade 0	Grade 1	Grade 2	Grade 3	Grade 4
Hypocalcemia	WNL	Corrected calcium: 8 mg/dL to <LLN	Corrected calcium: 7 to <8 mg/dL	v3: Corrected calcium: 6 to <7 mg/dL v4: Corrected calcium: 6 to <7 mg/dL; hospitalization indicated	v3: Corrected calcium: <6 mg/dL v4: Corrected calcium: <6 mg/dL; life-threatening
Hypokalemia	WNL	3 mmol/L to <LLN	v3: 3 mmol/L to <LLN v4: 3 mmol/L to <LNN; symptomatic; intervention indicated	v3: 2.5 to <3 mmol/L v4: 2.5 to <3 mmol/L; hospitalization indicated	v3: <2.5 mmol/L v4: <2.5 mmol/L; life-threatening
Hypomagnesemia	WNL	1.2 mg/dL to <LLN	0.9 to <1.2 mg/dL	0.7 to <0.9 mg/dL	v3: <0.7 mg/dL v4: <0.7 mg/dL; life-threatening
Hypophosphatemia	WNL	2.5 mg/dL to <LLN	2 to <2.5 mg/dL	1 to <2 mg/dL	v3: <1 mg/dL v4: <1 mg/dL; life-threatening
Ocular					
Cataract		Asymptomatic; detected on exam only	Symptomatic with moderate decrease in visual acuity (20/40 or better); decreased visual function (correctable with glasses)	Symptomatic with marked decrease in visual acuity (worse than 20/40 but better than 20/200); operative intervention (cataract surgery) indicated	v4: Blindness (20/200 or worse) in affected eye

Selected Common Toxicity Criteria[1] continued

Toxicity	Grade 0	Grade 1	Grade 2	Grade 3	Grade 4
Conjunctivitis		Mild symptoms or asymptomatic; intervention not indicated	v3: Symptomatic; topical intervention (eg, antibiotics or other topical intervention) indicated; interferes with function but not ADL v4: Symptomatic; topical intervention (eg, antibiotics) indicated; limits instrumental ADL	v3: Symptomatic; interferes with ADL; operative intervention indicated v4: Limits self-care ADL	
Corneal ulceration			v3: Symptomatic; interferes with function but not ADL v4: Symptomatic; intervention indicated (eg, topical agents); limits instrumental ADL	v3: Symptomatic; interferes with ADL; operative intervention indicated v4: Limits self-care ADL; declining vision (worse than 20/40 but better than 20/200)	Perforation or blindness (worse than 20/200) in the affected eye
Eye dryness		v3: Mild; intervention not indicated v4: Asymptomatic; clinical or diagnostic observations only; mild symptoms relieved by lubricants	v3: Symptomatic; interferes with function but not ADL; medical intervention indicated v4: Symptomatic; multiple agents indicated; limits instrumental ADL	v3: Symptomatic or decrease in visual acuity; interferes with ADL; operative intervention indicated v4: Decrease in visual acuity (worse than 20/40); limits self-care ADL	
Eye pain		Mild pain	Moderate pain; limits instrumental ADL	Severe pain; limits self-care ADL	

Selected Common Toxicity Criteria[1] *continued*

Toxicity	Grade 0	Grade 1	Grade 2	Grade 3	Grade 4
Glaucoma		Elevated intraocular pressure (EIOP); intervention indicated (single topical agent); no visual field deficit	EIOP causing early visual field deficits; intervention indicated (multiple topical/oral agents); limits instrumental ADL	EIOP causing marked visual field deficits (eg, involving both superior and inferior visual fields); operative intervention indicated; limits self-care ADL	v3: Blindness (20/200 or worse); enucleation indicated v4: Blindness (20/200 or worse) in affected eye
Keratitis			v3: Symptomatic and interferes with function but does not interfere with ADL v4: Symptomatic; medical intervention indicated (eg, topical agents); limits instrumental ADL	v3: Symptomatic; interferes with ADL; operative intervention indicated v4: Decline in vision (worse than 20/40 but better than 20/200); limits self-care ADL	Perforation or blindness (20/200 or worse) in affected eye
Photophobia		Symptomatic; does not limit ADL	v3: Symptomatic and interferes with function but does not interfere with ADL v4: Symptomatic; limits instrumental ADL	v3: Symptomatic; limits ADL v4: Limits self-care ADL	
Retinal detachment		Asymptomatic	Exudative and visual acuity 20/40 or better	Rhegmatogenous or exudative detachment; operative intervention indicated; decline in vision (worse than 20/40 but better than 20/200)	Blindness (20/200 or worse) in affected eye
Retinopathy		Asymptomatic; clinical or diagnostic observations only	Symptomatic with moderate decrease in visual acuity (20/40 or better); limits instrumental ADL	Symptomatic with marked decrease in visual acuity (worse than 20/40 but better than 20/200); disabling; limits self-care ADL	Blindness (20/200 or worse) in affected eye

Selected Common Toxicity Criteria[1] *continued*

Toxicity	Grade 0	Grade 1	Grade 2	Grade 3	Grade 4
Uveitis		Asymptomatic; clinical or diagnostic observations only	Anterior uveitis; medical intervention indicated	Posterior or pan-uveitis	Blindness (20/200 or worse) in affected eye
Watering eyes		Intervention not indicated	v4: Intervention indicated	v4: Operative intervention indicated	
Renal/Genitourinary					
Hematuria	None	v3: Minimal or microscopic; intervention not indicated v4: Asymptomatic; intervention not indicated	v3: Gross bleeding; intervention or irrigation required v4: Symptomatic; catheter or irrigation indicated; limits ADL	v3: Transfusion or intervention indicated v4: Gross hematuria, transfusion, IV medications, or hospitalization indicated; limits self-care ADL	Life-threatening consequences; urgent intervention indicated
Serum creatinine elevation	WNL	v3: >ULN to 1.5 x ULN v4: Increase of >0.3 mg/dL; 1.5 to 2 x baseline	v3: >1.5 to 3 x ULN v4: >2 to 3 x baseline	v3: >3 to 6 x ULN v4: >3 x baseline or >4 mg/dL; hospitalization indicated	v3: >6 x ULN v4: Life-threatening; dialysis indicated
Respiratory					
Dyspnea	None	v3: Dyspnea on exertion (can walk 1 flight of stairs without stopping) v4: Dyspnea with moderate exertion	v3: Dyspnea on exertion (cannot walk 1 flight of stairs or 1 city block without stopping) v4: Dyspnea with minimal exertion; limits ADL	v3: Dyspnea with ADL v4: Dyspnea at rest; limits self-care ADL	v3: Dyspnea at rest; intubation/ventilator support indicated v4: Life-threatening; urgent intervention indicated
Epistaxis	None	Mild; no intervention indicated	Symptomatic; intervention indicated	Transfusion required; intervention indicated	Life-threatening consequences; urgent intervention indicated

Selected Common Toxicity Criteria[1] continued

Toxicity	Grade 0	Grade 1	Grade 2	Grade 3	Grade 4
Pleural effusion	None	Asymptomatic	v3: Symptomatic; intervention required (diuretics or up to 2 thoracenteses)	v3: Symptomatic, oxygen, thoracentesis, tube drainage, or pleurodesis required	Life-threatening; intubation or urgent intervention required
			v4: Symptomatic; intervention required (thoracentesis or tube drainage)	v4: Severe symptoms; intervention indicated	
Pneumonitis/ pulmonary infiltrates	None	Asymptomatic; radiographic findings only	Symptomatic but does not interfere with ADL	Symptomatic; interferes with ADL; oxygen indicated	Life-threatening; ventilator support indicated
CNS/Neurologic					
Fatigue/weakness	None	v3: Mild fatigue over baseline	v3: Moderate; some difficulty with ADL	v3: Severe; interferes with ADL	Disabling
		v4: Fatigue relieved by rest	v4: Fatigue not relieved by rest; limits ADL	v4: Fatigue not relieved by rest; limits self-care ADL	
Neuropathy, motor	Normal	Asymptomatic; weakness on exam	Symptomatic weakness; mild difficulty with function	Weakness; interferes with ADL	Life-threatening/ disabling
Neuropathy, sensory	Normal	Asymptomatic; paresthesia/deep tendon reflex loss	v3: Paresthesia/sensory loss; interferes with function but not ADL	v3: Sensory loss/ paresthesia; interferes w/ ADL	v3: Disabling
			v4: Moderate symptoms; limits ADL	v4: Severe symptoms; limits self-care ADL	v4: Life-threatening/ disabling

Selected Common Toxicity Criteria[1] *continued*

Toxicity	Grade 0	Grade 1	Grade 2	Grade 3	Grade 4
			Miscellaneous		
Allergic reaction	None	Transient flushing or rash, drug fever <38°C	v3: Rash, flushing, urticaria, dyspnea, drug fever ≥38°C v4: Intervention or interruption of infusion indicated	v3: Symptomatic bronchospasm; parenteral medications indicated v4: Prolonged recurrence of symptoms after initial improvement	Life-threatening; urgent intervention indicated
Anaphylaxis	None			Symptomatic bronchospasm; parenteral treatment required; allergy-related edema, angioedema, hypotension	Life-threatening; urgent intervention indicated
Infusion-related reaction	None	Mild, transient; infusion interruption or intervention not indicated	Interruption indicated; responds promptly to symptomatic treatment; prophylactic medications indicated ≤24 hours	Prolonged reaction (not initially responding to symptomatic treatment); symptoms recur following initial improvement; hospitalization indicated	Life-threatening; urgent intervention indicated

Selected Common Toxicity Criteria[1] *continued*

Toxicity	Grade 0	Grade 1	Grade 2	Grade 3	Grade 4
Fever	None	38°C to 39°C (100.4°F to 102.2°F)	>39°C to 40°C (102.3°F to 104°F)	>40°C (104°F) for ≤24 h	>40°C (104°F) for >24 h
Neutropenic fever	None			v3: ANC <1,000/mm³ with temperature ≥38.3°C (101.3°F) v4: ANC <1,000/mm³ with single temperature >38.3°C (101.3°F) or sustained temperature ≥38°C (100.4°F) for >1 hour	Life-threatening; urgent intervention indicated

DBP = diastolic blood pressure, SBP = systolic blood pressure, BSA = body surface area, ADL = activities of daily living, WNL = within normal limits, LLN = lower limits of normal, ULN = upper limits of normal

[1] The National Cancer Institute (NCI) Cancer Therapy Evaluation Program (CTEP) has developed version 4.0 of the Common Terminology Criteria for Adverse Events (CTCAE). While version 4 is transitioning into practice, protocols and/or dosage reduction recommendations may be based on version 3. When version 4 differs from version 3, the differences are noted.

Adapted from the NCI Common Terminology Criteria for Adverse Events (CTCAE) versions 3.0 and 4.0. http://ctep.cancer.gov/protocolDevelopment/electronic_applications/ctc.htm#ctc_40_conversion. Accessed May 2013.

FERTILITY AND CANCER THERAPY

Antineoplastic therapy (chemotherapy, radiation, surgery) or cancer itself can affect fertility and/or sexual function in both men and women. Temporary or permanent sequelae that impact pregnancy outcomes, neonatal development, pubertal development, and gonadal function are possible in cancer survivors. Factors influencing fertility and reproduction in cancer survivors include the type and intensity of therapy, duration of therapy, age, and gender.

Table 1. Primary Antineoplastic Agents Associated With Sterility

Women	Men
Busulfan	Busulfan
Chlorambucil	Chlorambucil
Cyclophosphamide	Cyclophosphamide
Mechlorethamine	Mechlorethamine
Melphalan	Nitrosoureas
Procarbazine	Procarbazine
Other alkylating agents	Other alkylating agents
	Cisplatin
DOXOrubicin	DOXOrubicin
Everolimus	Everolimus
	Enzalutamide

Recommendations from the American Society for Clinical Oncology (ASCO) for preservation of fertility in cancer patients are presented in Table 2 (Loren 2013).

Table 2. ASCO Clinical Practice Guidelines for Preservation of Fertility in Cancer Patients

Intervention
• Discuss infertility risk and fertility preservation options with cancer patients anticipating treatment(s) which may affect fertility
Key Recommendations
• If infertility is a potential risk of therapy, discuss fertility preservation with all patients of reproductive age (for children or adolescents, discuss with parents/guardians)
• Refer patients who express an interest in fertility preservation to reproductive specialists (also refer patients who are unsure)
• Address fertility preservation as early as possible, prior to treatment initiation
• Document fertility preservation discussions in the medical record

Table 2. ASCO Clinical Practice Guidelines for Preservation of Fertility in Cancer Patients *(continued)*

• Answer basic questions about whether fertility preservation may impact successful cancer treatment
• Refer patients to psychosocial providers if they experience distress regarding potential infertility
• Encourage patient participation in registries and clinical studies
Adult Females
• Describe both embryo and oocyte cryopreservation as established fertility preservation methods
• If pelvic radiation therapy is part of cancer treatment, discuss the option of ovarian transposition (oophoropexy)
• Inform patients of conservative gynecologic surgery and radiation therapy alternatives
• Inform patients that evidence is insufficient regarding the effectiveness of ovarian suppression (gonadotropin-releasing hormone analogs) as fertility preservation, and these agents should not be relied on for fertility preservation
• Inform patients that other methods (eg, ovarian tissue cryopreservation [which does not require sexual maturity] for future transplantation) are still experimental
Adult Males
• Describe sperm cryopreservation (sperm banking) as the only established fertility preservation method
• Do not recommend hormonal therapy in men, as it is not successful for fertility preservation
• Inform patients that other methods (eg, testicular tissue cryopreservation [which does not require sexual maturity] for future re-implantation or grafting of human testicular tissue) are experimental
• Advise men of the potential for a higher risk of genetically damaged sperm if collected after the start of chemotherapy
Children
• Use established fertility preservation methods (semen cryopreservation and oocyte cryopreservation) for post-pubertal minor children, with patient agreement (if appropriate) and parent/guardian consent
• Present information on additional methods that are available for children, although still investigational
• When available, refer for experimental protocols

FEMALES

Antineoplastic drugs can stop the development of follicles (vesicles within ovarian that contain oocytes) or damage oocytes (female egg cells). Prepubertal gonads may be more resistant than postpubertal gonads, possibly due to a larger number of follicles as compared to ovaries in older patients. Gonadal destruction causes clinical findings associated with estrogen deficiency such as amenorrhea, endometrial hypoplasia, vaginal atrophy and dryness, and hot flashes. Follicle stimulating hormone (FSH) levels become elevated and estrogen levels decrease with impaired ovarian function. The onset and duration of symptoms is both dose-related and age-related. Younger patients are able to tolerate higher doses of chemotherapy before symptoms develop and have a higher likelihood of the return of menses when therapy is stopped.

The effect of radiation on fertility depends on the age of the patient, the number of remaining oocytes at the time of radiation, and the exposure dose and field. Childhood cancer survivors who have received a hypothalamic/pituitary radiation dose of 30 gray (Gy) (RR = 0.61) or more or an ovarian uterine radiation dose exceeding 5 Gy (RR = 0.56) are less likely to ever become pregnant than their female siblings.

In vitro fertilization with embryo cryopreservation is an option for circumventing the gonadotoxic effect of antineoplastic therapy. Ovarian stimulation for oocyte collection generally involves estrogenic therapy and may be risky in women with hormonally-responsive cancers. In addition, this method can only be used when the consequent delay in chemotherapy administration is not deleterious to the expected outcome of anticancer therapy. Some women may choose to make use of a gestational surrogate to carry their child through pregnancy. Investigational procedures for fertility preservation may be considered when in vitro fertilization is not advisable for medical reasons or impractical for women without a partner to provide sperm. Pertinent investigational techniques include oocyte cryopreservation, ovarian follicle cryopreservation, ovarian tissue cryopreservation, and in vitro follicle maturation. It should be noted that potential risks to the patient and prospective offspring from investigational fertility preservation are still being identified and delineated. Inadvertent reimplantation of cancer cells is possible with autotransplantation of cryopreserved ovarian tissue. Genetic and in vivo analysis of frozen ovarian tissue from patients with acute lymphoblastic leukemia and chronic myeloid leukemia have demonstrated the presence of viable malignant cells in the cryopreserved specimens.

Gonadotropin releasing hormone (GnRH) agonists are under investigation as a tool to preserve female fertility throughout chemotherapy administration. GnRH agonists cause medical castration which may provide a gonadoprotective effect by decreasing the number of follicles entering the differentiation phase, the stage most sensitive to chemotherapy. In addition, decreased serum estrogen concentrations reduce ovarian perfusion, thereby reducing ovarian exposure to systemic chemotherapy. Additional proposed mechanisms of GnRh agonist gonadoprotection during chemotherapy administration include a direct effect of the GnRH on the ovary, indirect antiapoptotic effects, and protection of germ line cells. Women older than 36 years of age may not have an adequate follicular reserve to benefit from gonadoprotection from GnRh therapy during chemotherapy administration. One comparative trial evaluated return of spontaneous menstruation and ovulation in 80 women with breast cancer undergoing treatment with chemotherapy with or without goserelin. All women were younger than 40 years of age and received treatment with FAC (fluorouracil-doxorubicin-cyclophosphamide). Following completion of treatment, menses returned within 3 to 8 months for 90% of women in the cohort treated with chemotherapy and goserelin and 33% of women receiving chemotherapy alone. Ovulation returned for 69% of women in the goserelin cohort and 26% the control patients. This trial suggests a positive effect of GnRH agonist therapy for protection of female fertility during chemotherapy; however, continued research is required to substantiate these findings in a broader patient population and with longer follow-up. At present, most clinical evidence supporting use of a GnRh agonist to protect female fertility during chemotherapy is based on noncomparative phase II trials, case series, and case reports.

◀ MALES

Antineoplastic drugs and radiation destroy epithelial germ cells in a dose-dependent fashion. This damage results in increased FSH levels, decreased testosterone levels, oligospermia, or azoospermia. Spermatogenesis is more susceptible than testosterone production; and postpubertal testes are more susceptible to damage than prepubertal testes. Azoospermia may or may not be reversible. When it does recover, return of spermatogenesis may take up to 49 months.

Effects of radiation therapy on the testes are dependent on the dose, stage of germ cell development, and pubertal stage of the patient. Spermatogonia (precursor cell for spermatocyte) are the most sensitive to radiation damage, followed in decreasing sensitivity by spermatocytes (produce spermatid by meiosis) and spermatids (precursor for spermatozoa that fertilize ovum). Prepubertal boys may have oligo- or azoospermia once they reach sexual maturation. They may also have delayed sexual maturation due to destruction of Leydig cells and thus decreased testosterone production. Prolonged azoospermia generally occurs following a cumulative radiation dose of 2.5 Gy to the testis.

Surgery can affect male sexuality and fertility. Surgery for testicular cancer includes orchiectomy (surgical castration) and retroperitoneal lymph node resection which can result in decreased semen volume, erectile dysfunction, and low sexual desire. Prostate cancer surgery can also produce erectile dysfunction and changes in semen volume or ejaculatory problems.

Impaired spermatogenesis is present at the time of diagnosis for 60% to 70% men with testicular cancer. Elevated serum levels of beta-human chorionic gonadotropin (beta-hCG), which is a finding in many cases of testicular cancer, is associated with inferior spermatogenesis relative to cases with normal beta-hCG levels.

In men, cryopreservation of sperm is a viable alternative and should be offered. The clinical pregnancy success rate of cryopreserved sperm is 36% by intrauterine insemination and 50% with in vitro fertilization and intracytoplasmic sperm injection. During in vitro fertilization sperm fertilize ovum in a liquid medium. Intracytoplasmic sperm injection is a more advanced process that injects one sperm into one oocyte for fertilization.

OUTCOMES OF PREGNANCY

Improved survival for cancer patients introduces the concern of long term treatment- and disease-related sequelae, including pregnancy outcome. The Childhood Cancer Survivor Study is a collaborative effort involving 25 health care institutions in the United States and Canada to facilitate research pertaining to the long term health outcomes of childhood cancer survivors. Over 14,000 subjects surviving 5 years or more following the diagnosis of childhood cancer are participating in this project.

Analysis of data from the Childhood Cancer Survivor Study demonstrated that offspring of female cancer survivors were more likely to be born preterm (OR, 1.9; P<0.001) than offspring from their female siblings. Moreover, previous treatment with a cumulative radiation dose exceeding 0.5 Gy to the uterus was associated with preterm birth (OR, 3.5; P=0.003), low birth weight (<2.5 g) (OR, 6.8; P=0.001), and small for gestational age (OR, 4; P=0.003). Data from the Childhood Cancer Survivor Study was also evaluated to assess pregnancy outcome for the female partners of male cancer survivors. Pregnant partners of male cancer survivors were less likely to yield a live born infant (RR, 0.77) than the control group (P=0.007). This was particularly evident when anticancer treatment included radiation with the treatment field affecting the testicles with or without shielding. The offspring of male cancer survivors treated with nonalkylating chemotherapy were more likely to have low birth weight than offspring from the survivor's male siblings (RR, 3.03; P=0.025). Otherwise, there was no difference in birth weight between offspring of the male cancer survivors in comparison to the control group. The male:female ratio of offspring fathered by male cancer survivors was 1:1.03; whereas, the male:female ratio of offspring from the survivor's male siblings was 1.24:1.0 (P=0.016).

A British survey of 10,483 childhood cancer survivors examined pregnancy outcome and reported that women treated with radiation to the abdomen or brain produced markedly fewer offspring than expected. Women treated with abdominal radiation were threefold and twofold more likely to have preterm or low birth weight babies. In addition, the risk of miscarriage was slightly increased in this group.

The impact of malignant disease and antineoplastic treatment on pregnancy outcome is not fully defined. However, patients with cancer should be informed of the known risks and potential options for fertility and reproduction.

SELECTED READINGS

Badawy A, Elnashar A, El-Ashry M, Shahat M Gonadotropin-releasing hormone agonists for prevention of chemotherapy-induced ovarian damage: prospective randomized study. *Fertil Steril.* 2009;91(3):694-697.

Blumenfeld Z. How to preserve fertility in young women exposed to chemotherapy? The role of GnRH agonist cotreatment in addition to cryopreservation of embrya, oocytes, or ovaries. *Oncologist.* 2007;12(9):1044-1054.

de Bruin D, de Jong IJ, Arts EG, et al. Semen quality in men with disseminated testicular cancer: relation with human chorionic gonadotropin beta-subunit and pituitary gonadal hormones. *Fertil Steril.* 2009;91(6):2481-2486.

Dolmans MM, Marinescu C, Saussoy P, Van Langendonckt A, Amorim C, Donnez J. Reimplantation of cryopreserved ovarian tissue from patients with acute lymphoblastic leukemia is potentially unsafe. *Blood.* 2010;116(16):2908-2914.

Green DM, Kawashima T, Stovall M, et al. Fertility of female survivors of childhood cancer: a report from the childhood cancer survivor study. *J Clin Oncol.* 2009;27(16):2677-2685.

Green DM, Whitton JA, Stovall M, et al. Pregnancy outcome of partners of male survivors of childhood cancer: a report from the childhood cancer survivor study. *J Clin Oncol.* 2003;21 (4):716-721.

Krychman ML, King T. Pregnancy after breast cancer: a case study resolving the reproductive challenge with a gestational surrogate. *Breast J.* 2006;12(4):363-365.

Lee SJ, Schover LR, Partridge AH, et al. American Society of Clinical Oncology recommendations on fertility preservation in cancer patients. *J Clin Oncol.* 2006;24(18):2917-2931.

Loren AW, Mangu PB, Beck LN, et al. Fertility preservation for patients with cancer: American Society of Clinical Oncology clinical practice guideline update. *J Clin Oncol.* 2013;31 (19):2500-2510. Available at http://jco.ascopubs.org/cgi/doi/10.1200/JCO.2013.49.2678. Accessed September 29, 2014.

Neal MS, Nagel K, Duckworth J, et al. Effectiveness of sperm banking in adolescents and young adults with cancer: a regional experience. *Cancer.* 2007;110(5):1125-1129.

Pentheroudakis G, Pavlidis N, Castiglione M. Cancer, fertility and pregnancy: ESMO clinical recommendations for diagnosis, treatment and follow-up. *Ann Oncol.* 2009;20(Suppl 4):178-181.

Reulen RC, Zeegers MP, Wallace WH, et al. Pregnancy outcomes among adult survivors of childhood cancer in the British childhood cancer survivor study. *Cancer Epidemiol Biomarkers Prev.* 2009;18(8):2239-2247.

Robison LL, Mertens AC, Boice JD, et al. Study design and cohort characteristics of the childhood cancer survivor study: a multi-institutional collaborative project. *Med Pediatr Oncol.* 2002;38 (4):229-239.

Signorello LB, Cohen SS, Bosetti C, et al. Female survivors of childhood cancer: preterm birth and low birth weight among their children. *J Natl Cancer Inst.* 2006;98(20):1453-1461.

MANAGEMENT OF CHEMOTHERAPY-INDUCED NAUSEA AND VOMITING IN ADULTS

> **Nausea:** The feeling or sensation of an imminent desire to vomit.
>
> **Vomiting:** The forceful upward expulsion of gastric contents.
>
> **Retching:** Rhythmic, labored, spasmodic respiratory movements involving the diaphragm, chest wall, and abdominal muscles.

Nausea and vomiting are common side effects of many antineoplastic agents. Studies, both prior to the advent of serotonin antagonists and after their introduction, have been conducted asking chemotherapy patients to rank the five most distressing symptoms in order from most to least severe. Nausea and vomiting remained among the top three most distressing symptoms, despite the use of serotonin antagonists for prevention or management of acute chemotherapy-induced nausea and vomiting. Uncontrolled nausea and vomiting can have a significant impact on a patient's overall attitude, quality of life, compliance, and response to treatment. Uncontrolled nausea and vomiting can result in dehydration, electrolyte imbalances, weight loss, and malnutrition. Prolonged vomiting and retching can cause esophageal and/or gastric ruptures (Mallory-Weiss tears, Boerhaave syndrome) and bleeding. Even in the absence of actual emesis, patients may experience varying degrees of nausea, often accompanied by anorexia.

Table 1. Other Causes of Nausea or Vomiting

Abdominal Emergencies
  Appendicitis
  Cholecystitis
  GI obstruction
  Peritonitis
Acute Systemic Infections
  Bacterial
  Parasitic
  Viral
Cardiovascular Disorders
  Congestive heart failure
  Hypotension
  Myocardial infarction
  Syncope
Neurologic
  Increased intracranial pressure
  Mènière's disease
  Otitis interna
  Severe or chronic pain
  Anticipatory nausea and vomiting
  Vestibular dysfunction
Drugs
  Anesthetics
  Antibiotics
  Antineoplastics
  Aspirin
  Cardiac glycosides
  Ethanol

Levodopa
Nonsteroidal anti-inflammatory agents
Opioids
Quinidine
Steroids
Theophylline
Endocrine Disorders
  Adrenal insufficiency
  Diabetes mellitus
Gastrointestinal Disorders
  Dyspepsia
  Gastric outlet obstruction
  Gastroparesis
  Heartburn
  Partial or complete bowel obstruction
  Constipation
  Hepatic metastases
Metabolic
  Hypercalcemia
  Hyperglycemia
  Hyponatremia
  Uremia
Pregnancy
Psychogenic Stimuli
Therapy-Related
  Postsurgical
  Radiation Therapy

Patterns of Drug-Induced Nausea / Vomiting

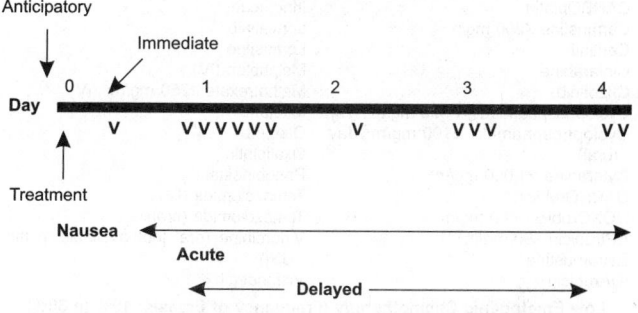

Table 2 describes the emetogenic potential of many of the antineoplastic agents. This table has been developed based on various guidelines and publications including: American Society of Clinical Oncology (ASCO), Multinational Association of Supportive Care in Cancer (MASCC), and National Comprehensive Cancer Network (NCCN). Several factors affect the emetic potential of these agents. For some drugs, such as cyclophosphamide or methotrexate, the dose administered has a significant effect on the drug's emetogenicity. Higher doses of these agents are much more emetogenic than low doses. The method of administration can also affect the incidence of nausea. Cytarabine, when given as a continuous infusion, is generally moderately emetogenic; however, higher cytarabine doses with short infusion times can produce a much higher incidence and severity of nausea and vomiting. Patient-related risk factors for nausea and vomiting include: Age (<50 years), female gender, prior experiences with chemotherapy, psychosocial factors (anxiety, depression), history of morning sickness with pregnancies, and history of motion sickness.

Table 2. Emetogenic Potential of Antineoplastic Agents

Highly Emetogenic Chemotherapy (Frequency of Emesis: >90%)

AC (either DOXOrubicin or EPIrubicin in combination with cyclophosphamide)	Dacarbazine
	DACTINomycin
Altretamine	DOXOrubicin ≥60 mg/m²
Carmustine >250 mg/m²	EPIrubicin >90 mg/m²
CISplatin	Mechlorethamine
Cyclophosphamide ≥1,500 mg/m²	Procarbazine (oral)
	Streptozocin

Moderately Emetogenic Chemotherapy (Frequency of Emesis: 30% to 90%)

Aldesleukin >12 to 15 million units/m²	Amifostine >300 mg/m²
Alemtuzumab	Arsenic trioxide

MANAGEMENT OF CHEMOTHERAPY-INDUCED NAUSEA AND VOMITING IN ADULTS

AzaCITIDine
Bendamustine
Busulfan (IV) or ≥4 mg/day (oral)
CARBOplatin
Carmustine ≤250 mg/m²
Ceritinib
Clofarabine
Crizotinib
Cyclophosphamide <1,500 mg/m² (IV)
Cyclophosphamide ≥100 mg/m²/day (oral)
Cytarabine >1,000 mg/m²
DAUNOrubicin
DOXOrubicin <60 mg/m²
EPIrubicin ≤90 mg/m²
Estramustine
IDArubicin
Ifosfamide
Imatinib
Interferon alfa ≥10 million units/m²
Irinotecan
Lenvatinib
Lomustine
Melphalan (IV)
Methotrexate ≥250 mg/m² (IV)
Mitotane
Olaparib
Oxaliplatin
Panobinostat
Temozolomide (IV)
Temozolomide (oral)
Vinorelbine (oral [not available in the US])
Vismodegib

Low Emetogenic Chemotherapy (Frequency of Emesis: 10% to 30%)

Ado-trastuzumab emtansine
Aldesleukin ≤12 million units/m²
Amifostine ≤300 mg
Belinostat
Bexarotene (oral)
Blinatumomab
Bortezomib
Brentuximab vedotin
Cabazitaxel
Capecitabine
Carfilzomib
Cytarabine ≤1,000 mg/m²
DAUNOrubicin (liposomal)
DOCEtaxel
DOXOrubicin (liposomal)
EriBULin
Etoposide (IV)
Etoposide (oral)
Everolimus
Floxuridine
Fludarabine (oral)
Fluorouracil
Gemcitabine
Ibrutinib
Idelalisib
Interferon alfa >5 million to <10 million units/m²
Ixabepilone
Lapatinib
Lenalidomide
Methotrexate >50 to <250 mg/m² (IV)
MitoMYcin
MitoXANtrone
Nilotinib
Omacetaxine
PACLitaxel
PACLitaxel protein bound
Palbociclib
Panitumumab
PEMEtrexed
Pentostatin
PRALAtrexate
RomiDEPsin
SUNItinib
Tegafur and Uracil
Temsirolimus
Teniposide
Thalidomide
Thiotepa
Topotecan
Trastuzumab
Tretinoin
Vandetanib
Vorinostat
Ziv-aflibercept

Minimal Emetogenic Chemotherapy (Frequency of Emesis: <10%)

Afatinib
Asparaginase
Axitinib
Bevacizumab
Bleomycin
Bosutinib
Busulfan <4 mg/day
Cabozantinib
Cetuximab
Chlorambucil

Cladribine
Cyclophosphamide <100 mg/m²/day (oral)
Cytarabine <100 mg/m²
Dabrafenib
Dasatinib
Decitabine
Denileukin diftitox
Dexrazoxane
Erlotinib
Fludarabine (IV)
Gefitinib
Gemtuzumab ozogamicin
Hydroxyurea
Interferon alfa <5 million units/m²
Ipilimumab
Melphalan (oral)
Mercaptopurine
Methotrexate ≤50 mg/m² (IV)
Methotrexate (oral)
Nelarabine
Nivolumab
Obinutuzumab

Ofatumumab
PAZOPanib
Pegaspargase
Peginterferons
Pembrolizumab
Pertuzumab
Pomalidomide
PONATinib
Ramucirumab
Regorafenib
RiTUXimab
Ruxolitinib
Siltuximab
SORAfenib
Thioguanine (oral)
Trametinib
Valrubicin
Vemurafenib
VinBLAStine
VinCRIStine
VinCRIStine (liposomal)
Vinorelbine (IV)

Types of Chemotherapy-Associated Nausea and Vomiting

Nausea and vomiting caused by cytotoxic therapy generally falls into one of five categories: Acute, delayed, anticipatory, breakthrough, or refractory.

Acute nausea or vomiting is seen within the first 18 to 24 hours of drug administration, with the peak incidence seen at 4 to 6 hours. Acute nausea and vomiting tends to be responsive to drug therapy. Guidelines support the use of a neurokinin-1 receptor antagonist, serotonin antagonist, and dexamethasone combination for the prevention of acute nausea and vomiting in a patient receiving a highly emetogenic regimen. Patients receiving regimens classified as moderately emetogenic are recommended to be given a serotonin antagonist and dexamethasone. For multi-day chemotherapy regimens, antiemetics should be administered for each day of chemotherapy and for 2 days after (Basch 2011).

Delayed nausea or vomiting usually begins after the first 18 to 24 hours of drug administration but may occur up to 7 days after chemotherapy, with the peak incidence in 2 to 3 days. The classic causative agent for delayed nausea and vomiting is cisplatin; however the phenomenon has also been described with cyclophosphamide, doxorubicin, carboplatin, and ifosfamide administration. The exact cause of this side effect is not clear; however, it is believed to have a separate mechanism from acute nausea or vomiting. Gastritis, tissue destruction, electrolyte fluctuations, or effects on the central or peripheral nervous system have all been postulated as possible mechanisms for delayed nausea and vomiting.

Delayed nausea and vomiting is not as responsive to drug therapy when
compared to acute nausea and vomiting. The MASCC guidelines recommend
the use of dexamethasone and aprepitant (or fosaprepitant) for the prevention of
delayed emesis associated with high emetic risk chemotherapy (MASCC 2013;
Roila 2010).

While not drug-induced *per se*, anticipatory nausea and vomiting is also a
relatively common complication of antineoplastic therapy. Anticipatory nausea
and vomiting occurs due to inadequate control of nausea and vomiting in the past.
Sights, smells, or sounds can also trigger anticipatory nausea and vomiting. This
type of nausea and vomiting occurs before the administration of chemotherapy
and has a variable response to drug therapy. The most active antiemetic regimen
appropriate for the chemotherapy treatment is recommended; these antiemetics
should be administered with the initial chemotherapy, as opposed to retrospective
assessment of response with a less active antiemetic regimen (Basch 2011).

Breakthrough nausea and vomiting is defined as nausea and/or vomiting despite
adequate prophylaxis therapy and requires rescue therapy. Refractory nausea
and vomiting on the other hand occurs during subsequent cycles of chemotherapy when antiemetic prophylaxis or rescue therapy (or both) has failed in
earlier cycles.

Before changing a patient's antiemetic regimen, it is important to determine when
the patient experienced the nausea and vomiting. Basing the decision on the
timing of the episode(s) will help guide the change(s) in the regimen. If the patient
experienced nausea and vomiting within the first 24 hours, it would be appropriate
to change the patient's prophylactic acute regimen. If the patient had no episodes
until day 2, it would be more appropriate to change the delayed regimen for the
patient.

A number of possible alternatives exist when changing a patient's acute regimen,
including switching to another serotonin antagonist, adding a neurokinin receptor
antagonist (eg, aprepitant, fosaprepitant) to the previous serotonin antagonist/
steroid regimen, switching to a nonserotonin modulating antiemetic, or adding an
benzodiazepine prophylactically. When changing the delayed regimen, there are
numerous possibilities including: Adding a neurokinin receptor antagonist, dopamine antagonists, benzodiazepines, or cannabinoids, depending on the specific
patient situation. Olanzapine is a thienobenzodiazepine antipsychotic that blocks
multiple receptors associated with nausea or vomiting, including dopamine,
histamine, muscarinic, and serotonin receptors. A few small trials have reported
olanzapine effective (in combination with a steroid and serotonin antagonist) for
prevention of delayed nausea and vomiting.

Table 3. Classification of Antiemetic Agents

Antihistamines	DiphenhydrAMINE, hydrOXYzine, promethazine
Anticholinergics	Scopolamine
Benzodiazepines	Diazepam, LORazepam
Butyrophenones	Droperidol, haloperidol
Cannabinoids	Dronabinol, nabilone
Corticosteroids	Dexamethasone, methylPREDNISolone
Neurokinin antagonists	Aprepitant, fosaprepitant, netupitant[1]
Phenothiazines	ChlorproMAZINE, perphenazine, prochlorperazine, thiethylperazine, triflupromazine[2], (promethazine)
Serotonin antagonists	Dolasetron, granisetron, ondansetron, palonosetron, tropisetron[2]
Substituted benzamides	Metoclopramide, trimethobenzamide
Thienobenzodiazepines	OLANZapine

[1]Netupitant and palonosetron (oral) available as a fixed combination oral agent

[2]Not commercially available in the United States

Table 4. Site of Action of Antiemetic Agents

Emetic center	Antihistamines, anticholinergics, serotonin antagonists, thienobenzodiazepines(?)
Chemoreceptor trigger zone (CTZ)	Benzamides, butyrophenones, phenothiazines, thienobenzodiazepines(?)
Cerebral cortex	Antihistamines, benzodiazepines, cannabinoids, (corticosteroids), neurokinin antagonists(?), thienobenzodiazepines(?)
Peripheral	Metoclopramide, neurokinin antagonists, serotonin antagonists, thienobenzodiazepines(?)
Unknown	Corticosteroids

Table 5. Typical Serotonin Antagonist Doses

Drug	Oral	IV	Transdermal
Dolasetron	100 mg	(contraindicated)	
Granisetron	1 or 2 mg	0.01 mg/kg or 1 mg (maximum: 1 mg)	3.1 mg per 24 h
Ondansetron	16 to 24 mg or 8 mg twice daily	8 mg or 0.15 mg/kg (maximum: 16 mg)	
Palonosetron	0.5 mg*	0.25 mg	

*Netupitant and palonosetron (oral) available as a fixed combination oral agent

Receptors for a large number of different neurotransmitters, including dopamine, serotonin, substance P, endocannabinoids, acetylcholine, histamine, opioids, and benzodiazepines, are involved in the vomiting reflex. Blockade of one or more of these receptors is the basic mechanism of action of most antiemetic agents.

Anticholinergics. Alkaloids (eg, atropine and scopolamine) exhibit some antiemetic activity, primarily postoperative nausea and vomiting, and motion sickness. The apparent mechanism of action is blockage of central muscarinic receptors. Toxicities, such as sedation, restlessness, blurred vision, and dry mouth, limit the systemic use of these agents. Transdermal application of scopolamine is most useful in patients whose nausea is positional or due to motion. Scopolamine is also helpful as an adjunct in chemotherapy-induced delayed nausea or in treating prolonged mild nausea.

Antihistamines. The antihistamines block H_1 receptors both centrally and in the middle ear. A number of drugs in this class are effective against motion sickness and labyrinth disorders, but only diphenhydramine, hydroxyzine, and promethazine seem to have any activity against chemotherapy-induced nausea or vomiting. The major toxicities seen with these drugs are drowsiness, sedation, and dry mouth. These agents are most commonly used to enhance the efficacy of combination antiemetic regimens, although hydroxyzine or promethazine are occasionally used to treat mild to moderate nausea in patients who cannot tolerate, or are refractory to, other antiemetics. Diphenhydramine can be used in combination with dopamine antagonists to prevent extrapyramidal reactions seen with these agents at high doses.

Benzodiazepines. The exact antiemetic mechanism or location of action of the benzodiazepines is unclear. An inhibitory effect on the vomiting center, anxiolytic activity, and general CNS depression have all been postulated. Possible sites of action include the limbic system, vomiting center, cerebrum, and brain stem. The most common side effects include sedation, drowsiness, disinhibition, motor incoordination, and amnesia. In this setting, the anterograde amnesia induced by the benzodiazepine is usually considered a desired therapeutic effect rather than an adverse reaction. Benzodiazepines are commonly used as adjuncts to conventional antiemetics in the prophylaxis and treatment of chemotherapy-induced acute, breakthrough, and refractory nausea and vomiting. The benzodiazepines are also highly effective in the prevention of anticipatory nausea and vomiting. As single agents, the benzodiazepines have only mild antiemetic activity. Lorazepam is the most commonly used benzodiazepine for chemotherapy induced nausea and vomiting, but midazolam and diazepam have also been used.

Butyrophenones. A group of dopamine antagonists that can be effective in treating chemotherapy-induced nausea and vomiting are the butyrophenones. Both haloperidol and droperidol have been reported to have antiemetic activity against highly, moderately, and mild emetogenic chemotherapy, although their use may be reserved for management of breakthrough nausea and vomiting. Droperidol has been associated with cardiovascular toxicities, particularly QT prolongation and torsade de points. These toxicities, some fatal, occurred in patients receiving recommended doses or lower and also in patients with no known risk factors, which has ultimately limited the use of this agent. However, one trial comparing ondansetron and droperidol found no difference in the incidence or severity of QTc interval changes between the two drugs. As with most other antiemetics, the optimum response to the butyrophenones is seen in multidrug regimens. Like other dopamine blockers, extrapyramidal reactions, restlessness, sedation, and hypotension are relatively common side effects.

Cannabinoids. Proper evaluation of the antiemetic activity of cannabinoid derivatives has been hindered by social and political stigmas associated with marijuana use. Tetrahydrocannabinol, levonantradol, and nabilone are all reported to be effective in treating chemotherapy-induced nausea and vomiting. The specific site and mechanism of activity is unclear. Inhibition of endorphins in the emetic center, suppression of prostaglandin synthesis, and inhibition of medullary activity through an unspecified cortical action have all been postulated. Cannabinoids can inhibit buildup of cyclic adenosine monophosphate and cannabinoid receptors have been identified in the hippocampus, hypothalamus, and cortex. Cannabinoids used by the oral route seem to be most effective against mild to moderately emetogenic chemotherapy. Blurred vision, hypotension, and tachycardia, and a number of CNS complications, including euphoria, dysphoria, hallucinations, and sedation can be seen with cannabinoid therapy. Cannabinoids offer an alternative in patients unable to tolerate, or who are refractory to, other antiemetic agents.

Corticosteroids. The mechanism of antiemetic activity for the steroids is unknown, although alterations of cell permeability and inhibition of prostaglandin activity have been postulated. In spite of this uncertainty, corticosteroids, particularly dexamethasone, are frequent components of combination antiemetic regimens for high to moderately emetogenic chemotherapy. Studies have demonstrated a synergistic activity with metoclopramide and serotonin antagonists resulting in a 20% increase in effectiveness. For delayed nausea and vomiting, monotherapy dexamethasone appears to be more effective than serotonin antagonists for delayed nausea and vomiting. Side effects from single or short term dosing of dexamethasone are infrequent, but may include euphoria, anxiety, insomnia, increased appetite, and hyperglycemia. For patients in whom a corticosteroid is not clearly contraindicated, these agents are an important component of antiemetic therapy.

Neurokinin-1 (NK$_1$) Receptor Antagonists. Neurokinin, or substance P, antagonists are the latest class of antiemetics. Substance P is a tachykinin (neurokinin) located in neurons of the central and peripheral nervous system. It is associated with a variety of functions, including emesis, depression, inflammatory pain and inflammatory/immune responses in asthma, and other diseases. Substance P's activity is mediated by the NK$_1$ receptor, a G-protein receptor coupled to the inositol phosphate signal pathway. Blocking this receptor is a mechanism to treat conditions mediated at least in part by substance P. Several neurokinin receptor antagonists, including aprepitant (MK-869, L-754030), its prodrug L-758298, ezlopitant (CJ-11974), fosaprepitant, rolapitant (SCH-619734), vofopitant (GR-205171), and CP-122721 have been studied. Aprepitant, fosaprepitant, and rolapitant are approved for marketing; netupitant is approved as a combination product with palonosetron (oral fixed combination containing netupitant 300 mg and palonosetron 0.5 mg).

NK$_1$ antagonists are effective in preventing cisplatin-induced nausea and vomiting, when used in conjunction with a serotonin antagonist and steroid. Addition of a neurokinin antagonist to a serotonin antagonist and steroid combination increases control of acute nausea by 10% to 15%, and control of delayed nausea by 20% to 30%. Most studies indicate the neurokinin receptors are less effective than serotonin antagonists, particularly for prevention of acute nausea within the first 8 to 12 hours. However, the neurokinin antagonists appear to be more effective than serotonin antagonists in preventing delayed nausea (days 2 to 5). Aprepitant has a very complex metabolism. Aprepitant is a substrate of 3A4 and when administered for 3 days is an inhibitor of 3A4, and an inducer of 3A4 and 2C9 if administered for more than 14 days. Caution should be used when administering with oral contraceptives, warfarin, dexamethasone, midazolam, and 3A4 inhibitors and inducers. Side effects, although similar to placebo, may include asthenia/fatigue, dizziness, hiccups, gastritis/heartburn, diarrhea, and mild and transient increase in LFTs. Rolapitant is a moderate inhibitor of CYP2D6; due to the long half-life, the inhibitory effect may persist for at least 7 days (concurrent use of rolapitant with thioridazine is contraindicated due to a significant increase in plasma concentrations of thioridizine). Current guidelines recommend aprepitant, fosaprepitant, or rolapitant as initial therapy for highly emetogenic regimens (including high dose cisplatin) or moderately emetogenic regimens that contain both doxorubicin and cyclophosphamide.

Phenothiazines. Phenothiazines were the first class of drugs accepted as antiemetic therapy for antineoplastic chemotherapy. Blockade of dopamine (D_2) receptors in the area postrema (chemoreceptor trigger zone and vomiting center) appears to be their primary mechanism of action. A number of different drugs, including chlorpromazine, perphenazine, prochlorperazine, promethazine, and thiethylperazine (no longer marketed in the United States), have antiemetic activity. Common toxicities such as extrapyramidal reactions, restlessness, sedation, and hypotension limit the use of these drugs. Phenothiazines are most effective against mild to moderate nausea or vomiting, but have little impact on emesis from highly emetogenic agents such as dacarbazine or cisplatin. Higher doses of these agents may have increased activity, but the increased incidence and severity of side effects prohibits their use. Since the serotonin antagonists became available, use of the phenothiazines generally has been limited to prevention of nausea from mildly emetogenic chemotherapy, treatment of breakthrough nausea or vomiting in patients refractory to a serotonin blocker, or in association with dexamethasone to treat delayed nausea.

Serotonin (5-HT$_3$) Antagonists. A major advance in antiemetic therapy was the introduction of the serotonin (5-HT$_3$) antagonists. These agents have been shown to block serotonin in two ways: Peripheral antagonism by blocking release from enterochromaffin cells in the GI tract and central antagonism of receptors in the medulla. The high efficacy rate of these agents in preventing acute nausea and vomiting for highly and moderately emetogenic agents, coupled with their low incidence of side effects, has made them the standard of care in these settings.

Studies comparing serotonin antagonist plus dexamethasone with dexamethasone monotherapy or serotonin antagonist monotherapy have demonstrated that the combination regimen is significantly better than either agent alone. The addition of corticosteroids is synergistic and results in an increase in response of approximately 20%. Conversely, serotonin antagonists are not as efficacious as corticosteroids for delayed nausea and vomiting.

A transdermal patch formulation of the serotonin antagonist granisetron is available. The patch contains 34.3 mg of granisetron and releases 3.1 mg/day. The patch was approved based on a noninferiority study compared to oral granisetron in the setting of highly and moderately emetogenic chemotherapy. The patch is recommended to be applied 24 to 48 hours prior to chemotherapy.

The currently available serotonin antagonists have relatively flat dose/response curves. Dose response studies have demonstrated that granisetron's efficacy seems to reach a plateau at 0.01 mg/kg. There appears to be no difference in efficacy between granisetron doses of 0.01 mg/kg and 0.04 mg/kg. A few small studies suggest higher doses of granisetron (3 mg IV or 0.04 to 0.24 mg/kg) may be effective in treating breakthrough nausea; however, none of these reports found the improvement to be statistically significant. A similar limitation exists for dolasetron, ondansetron, and palonosetron. Data are also lacking on the value of using a different serotonin antagonist to treat nausea or vomiting resulting from the failure of the initial serotonin antagonist regimen.

Toxicities with these agents, including headache, constipation or diarrhea, and elevated transaminases, have been minimal. QTc prolongation and/or ECG abnormalities have been observed with dolasetron, granisetron, ondansetron, and palonosetron. Due to the risk for torsade de points, the use of the IV formulation of dolesetron is contraindicated in the prevention of chemotherapy-induced nausea and vomiting and the maximum recommended single IV ondansetron dose is 16 mg.

Substituted Benzamides. Metoclopramide is the most commonly used antiemetic drug in this category. Prior to introduction of the serotonin antagonists, high-dose (1 to 3 mg/kg) metoclopramide was the preferred drug for prevention of nausea or vomiting from highly emetogenic chemotherapy. Metoclopramide's ability to block central and peripheral dopamine receptors was believed to be the mechanism of its antiemetic activity. Recognition that high doses also blocked peripheral serotonin receptors in the intestines led to the identification of the role serotonin inhibition has in preventing nausea or vomiting, and, ultimately, to development of the serotonin antagonists. Like the phenothiazines, use of metoclopramide is complicated by extrapyramidal reactions, restlessness, sedation, and hypotension. Diarrhea is also a significant side effect, especially with the high doses used for antiemetic therapy. Also like the phenothiazines, the current use of metoclopramide is generally limited, although may be for prevention of nausea from mild to moderately emetogenic chemotherapy, prophylaxis of delayed nausea or vomiting, or treatment of breakthrough nausea and vomiting.

Olanzapine is a thienobenzodiazepine antipsychotic that blocks multiple receptors associated with nausea or vomiting, including dopamine, histamine, muscarinic, and serotonin receptors. A few small trials have reported olanzapine effective (in combination with a steroid and $5-HT_3$-antagonist) for prevention of delayed nausea and vomiting.

◀ # REPRESENTATIVE ANTIEMETIC REGIMENS

HIGHLY EMETOGENIC CHEMOTHERAPY

Neurokinin 1 antagonist-containing regimen:

Aprepitant 125 mg orally day 1, followed by aprepitant 80 mg orally days 2 and 3 **or** fosaprepitant 150 mg IV on day 1 only **or** rolapitant 180 mg orally ~1 to 2 hours prior to chemotherapy on day 1 only **plus**

Dexamethasone 12 mg orally or IV day 1, followed by 8 mg orally once daily days 2 to 4 (with aprepitant) or dexamethasone 12 mg orally or IV day 1, followed by 8 mg orally day 2, followed by 8 mg orally twice daily days 3 and 4 (with fosaprepitant 150 mg) **or** dexamethasone 20 mg orally or IV day 1, followed by 8 mg orally or IV twice daily days 2 to 4 (if no aprepitant, fosaprepitant, or with rolapitant) **plus**

Serotonin antagonist as follows:

- Dolasetron 100 mg orally day 1 **or**

- Granisetron 2 mg daily or 1 mg twice daily orally or 0.01 mg/kg (maximum: 1 mg) IV day 1 or 34.3 mg transdermal patch (3.1 mg/24 hours; maximum duration: 7 days) applied 24 to 48 hours prior to first chemotherapy dose **or**

- Ondansetron 16 to 24 mg orally or 8 to 16 mg IV or 0.15 mg/kg (maximum dose: 16 mg) IV day 1 **or**

- Palonosetron 0.25 mg IV day 1

NK$_1$ fixed combination: Netupitant 300 mg/palonosetron 0.5 mg orally 1 hour prior to chemotherapy on day 1 plus dexamethasone 12 mg orally 30 minutes prior to chemotherapy day 1, followed by dexamethasone 8 mg orally days 2 to 4

± LORazepam 0.5 to 2 mg orally, IV, or sublingual every 6 hours days 1 to 4, if needed

± H$_2$-blocker or proton pump inhibitor (PPI)

or

OLANZapine-containing regimen:

OLANZapine 10 mg orally days 1 to 4 **plus** palonosetron 0.25 mg IV day 1 **plus** dexamethasone 20 mg IV day 1

± LORazepam 0.5 to 2 mg orally, IV, or sublingual every 6 hours days 1 to 4, if needed

± H$_2$-blocker or proton pump inhibitor (PPI)

MODERATELY EMETOGENIC CHEMOTHERAPY

Palonosetron 0.25 mg IV day 1 (may substitute granisetron or ondansetron if palonosetron not available), **plus** dexamethasone days 1 to 3, ± aprepitant **or**:

Day 1:

Aprepitant 125 mg orally **or** fosaprepitant 150 mg IV (in selected patients) **or** rolapitant 180 mg orally ~1 to 2 hours prior to chemotherapy **plus**

Dexamethasone 8 to 12 mg orally or IV **or** dexamethasone 20 mg orally or IV (with rolapitant) **plus**

Serotonin antagonist as follows:

* Dolasetron 100 mg orally **or**

* Granisetron 2 mg daily or 1 mg twice daily orally or 0.01 mg/kg (maximum: 1 mg) IV or 34.3 mg transdermal patch (3.1 mg/24 hours; maximum duration: 7 days) applied 24 to 48 hours prior to first chemotherapy dose **or**

* Ondansetron 16 to 24 mg orally or 8 to 16 mg IV or 0.15 mg/kg IV (maximum dose: 16 mg IV) **or**

* Palonosetron 0.25 mg IV

± LORazepam 0.5 to 2 mg orally, IV, or sublingual every 6 hours, if needed

± H_2 blocker or PPI

Day 2 (and beyond):

Aprepitant 80 mg orally days 2 and 3 (if oral aprepitant included day 1) **or**

± Dexamethasone 8 mg daily orally or IV for 2 days or 8 mg daily or 4 mg twice daily for 2 to 3 days **or**

Serotonin antagonist as follows:

* Dolasetron 100 mg daily orally **or**

* Granisetron 1 to 2 mg daily or 1 mg twice daily orally or 0.01 mg/kg (maximum: 1 mg) IV **or**

* Ondansetron 8 mg twice daily or 16 mg daily orally or 8 to 16 mg IV or 0.15 mg/kg (maximum dose: 16 mg) IV

± LORazepam 0.5 to 2 mg orally, IV, or sublingual every 6 hours, if needed

± H_2 blocker or PPI

or

OLANZapine-containing regimen:

Day 1:

OLANZapine 10 mg orally **plus** dexamethasone 20 mg IV **plus** palonosetron 0.25 mg IV

± LORazepam 0.5 to 2 mg orally, IV, or sublingual every 6 hours, if needed

± H_2 blocker or PPI

◀ **Day 2 (and beyond):**

OLANZapine 10 mg orally days 2 and 3 (if given day 1)

± LORazepam 0.5 to 2 mg orally, IV, or sublingual every 6 hours, if needed

± H_2 blocker or PPI

LOW EMETOGENIC CHEMOTHERAPY

Dexamethasone 12 mg orally or IV daily or 4 to 8 mg orally or IV daily prior to chemotherapy **or**

Prochlorperazine 10 mg orally or IV prior to chemotherapy and then every 6 hours if needed (maximum: 40 mg/day) **or**

Serotonin antagonists (oral): Dolasetron 100 mg daily or granisetron 2 mg daily or 1 mg twice daily or ondansetron 8 to 16 mg daily

± LORazepam 0.5 to 2 mg orally, IV, or sublingual every 6 hours if needed

± H_2 blocker or PPI

MINIMAL EMETOGENIC CHEMOTHERAPY

No routine prophylaxis is necessary.

ORAL CHEMOTHERAPY

High to moderate emetogenic risk:

Serotonin antagonists (oral): Dolasetron 100 mg daily or granisetron 2 mg daily or 1 mg twice daily or ondansetron 16 to 24 mg daily

± LORazepam 0.5 to 2 mg orally or sublingual every 6 hours, if needed

± H_2 blocker or PPI

Low to minimal emetogenic risk:

Prochlorperazine 10 mg orally prior to chemotherapy and then every 6 hours (maximum: 40 mg/day) as needed **or**

Serotonin antagonists (oral): Dolasetron 100 mg daily (if needed) or granisetron 1 to 2 mg daily (if needed) or 1 mg twice daily (if needed) or ondansetron 8 to 16 mg daily (if needed)

± LORazepam 0.5 to 2 mg orally every 6 hours, if needed

± H_2 blocker or PPI

BREAKTHROUGH TREATMENT OPTIONS

Prochlorperazine 25 mg rectally every 12 hours or 10 mg orally or IV every 6 hours **or**

Promethazine 12.5 to 25 mg orally or IV every 4 to 6 hours **or**

Haloperidol 0.5 to 1 mg orally every 6 hours as needed **or**

LORazepam 0.5 to 2 mg orally every 6 hours **or**

Dolasetron 100 mg orally **or**

Granisetron 1 to 2 mg daily or 1 mg twice daily orally or 0.01 mg/kg (maximum: 1 mg) IV or 34.3 mg transdermal patch (3.1 mg/24 hours; maximum duration: 7 days) **or**

Ondansetron 16 mg daily orally or IV **or**

Dronabinol 5 mg 3 to 4 times daily **or** 5 to 10 mg orally every 6 to 8 hours **or** 2.5 to 10 mg 3 or 4 times daily **or** (manufacturer labeling) 5 mg/m² to 15 mg/m² orally 1 to 3 hours prior to chemotherapy, then every 2 to 4 hours after chemotherapy (for a total of 4 to 6 doses per day) **or**

Nabilone 1 to 2 mg orally twice a day **or**

Dexamethasone 12 mg orally or IV daily **or**

OLANZapine 10 mg daily for 3 days **or**

Scopolamine transdermal one patch every 72 hours **or**

Metoclopramide:

 Low dose: 10 to 20 mg orally or IV every 6 hours

 High dose: 1 to 2 mg/kg/dose IV before chemotherapy and repeat 2 hours after chemotherapy (for nausea and vomiting refractory or intolerant to antiemetics with a higher therapeutic index) or 0.5 mg/kg orally every 6 hours on days 2 to 4

General Principles for Managing Nausea and Vomiting

Key to prevention is aggressively prescribing the most effective antiemetic regimen during initial therapy.

A. **Prevention**

 a. **Antiemetics are most effective when given prophylactically.**

 b. Depending on the antiemetic agent(s) and route(s) of administration, pretreatment may range from 1 hour to 5 minutes prior to administration of the antineoplastic agent(s).

 c. **Emetogenic potential is additive and may be different on different days of the regimen.**

 d. **Provide patient with delayed nausea regimen for 2 to 3 days and PRN antiemetics while at home.**

 e. In most cases, **combination antiemetics are required for optimum control of nausea.** Two or more agents, from *different pharmacologic categories*, may be required to achieve optimal results.

f. **Avoid duplication of agents from the same pharmacologic category.**

g. **Doses and intervals of the antiemetic regimen need to be individualized for each patient.** "PRN" regimens should not be used for highly and moderately emetogenic chemotherapy. A fixed schedule of drug administration is preferable.

h. **If a patient has had no nausea for 24 hours** while on their scheduled antiemetic regimen, **it is usually possible to switch to a "PRN" regimen.** The patient should be advised to resume the fixed schedule *at the FIRST sign of recurrent nausea*, and continue it until they have had at least 24 hours without nausea.

i. **Titrate antiemetic dose to patient tolerance.**

j. **Anticipatory nausea and vomiting can often be minimized if the patient receives effective prophylaxis against nausea from the first cycle of therapy.**

k. **If anticipatory nausea does develop, an anxiolytic agent is usually the drug of choice.**

l. **"If it's not broken – DON'T fix it!"** Regardless of your own preferences, if the patient's current antiemetic regimen is working, don't change it.

B. **Antiemetics**

a. **The serotonin antagonists have a "ceiling" dose,** above which there is little or no added antiemetic effect.

b. **Serotonin antagonists are most effective within the first 24 hours.** Most studies of multiple day dosing show a sharp decline in the efficacy of the serotonin antagonists after the second or third day.

c. **Neurokinin antagonists are not very effective as single agents**, and should only be used in combination with a serotonin antagonist and steroid.

d. **Serotonin and neurokinin blockers are most effective in scheduled prophylactic regimens;** rather than in "PRN" regimens to chase existing vomiting.

e. **Serotonin and neurokinin antagonists have limited efficacy in stopping nausea or vomiting once it has begun.** A dopamine blocker may be more effective.

f. **Other antiemetics, such as cannabinoids, antihistamines, or anticholinergics, have limited use as initial therapy.** They are best used in combination with more effective agents (steroids, dopamine, or serotonin blockers); or, as second- or third-line therapy.

SELECTED READINGS

Aapro M. 5-HT$_3$-receptor antagonists in the management of nausea and vomiting in cancer and cancer treatment. *Oncology.* 2005;69(2):97-109.

Basch E, Prestrud AA, Hesketh PJ, et al. Antiemetics: American Society of Clinical Oncology clinical practice guideline update. *J Clin Oncol.* 2011;29(31):4189-4198.

Dupuis LL, Boodhan S, Sung L, et al. Guideline for the classification of the acute emetogenic potential of antineoplastic medication in pediatric cancer patients. *Pediatr Blood Cancer.* 2011;57(2):191-198.

Feyer PC, Maranzano E, Molassiotis A, et al. Radiotherapy-induced nausea and vomiting (RINV): MASCC/ESMO guideline for antiemetics in radiotherapy: update 2009. *Support Care Cancer.* 2011;19(Suppl 1):S5-S14.

Geling O, Eichler HG. Should 5-hydroxytryptamine-3 receptor antagonists be administered beyond 24 hours after chemotherapy to prevent delayed emesis? Systematic re-evaluation of clinical evidence and drug cost implications. *J Clin Oncol.* 2005;23(6):1289-1294.

Gralla RJ, Bosnjak SM, Hontsa A, et al. A phase III study evaluating the safety and efficacy of NEPA, a fixed-dose combination of netupitant and palonosetron, for prevention of chemotherapy-induced nausea and vomiting over repeated cycles of chemotherapy. *Ann Oncol.* 2014;25(7):1333-1339.

Graves T. Emesis as a complication of cancer chemotherapy: pathophysiology, importance, and treatment. *Pharmacotherapy.* 1992;12(4):337-345.

Grunberg SM, Hesketh PJ. Control of chemotherapy-induced emesis. *N Engl J Med.* 1993;329(24):1790-1796.

Grunberg SM, Warr D, Gralla RJ, et al. Evaluation of new antiemetic agents and definition of antineoplastic agent emetogenicity – state of the art. *Support Care Cancer.* 2011;19(Suppl 1):S43-S47.

Hesketh PJ. Chemotherapy-induced nausea and vomiting. *N Engl J Med.* 2008;358(23):2482-2494.

Hesketh PJ, Kris MG, Grunberg SM, et al. Proposal for classifying the acute emetogenicity of cancer chemotherapy. *J Clin Oncol.* 1997;15(1):103-109.

Hesketh PJ, Van Belle S, Aapro M, et al. Differential involvement of neurotransmitters through the time course of cisplatin-induced emesis as revealed by therapy with specific receptor antagonists. *Eur J Cancer.* 2003;39(8):1074-1080.

Holdsworth MT. Ethical issues regarding study designs used in serotonin-antagonist drug development. *Ann Pharmacother.* 1996;30(10):1182-1184.

Horiot JC. Antiemetic therapy in cancer: an update. *Expert Opin Pharmacother.* 2005;6(10):1713-1723.

Jordan K, Schmoll HJ, Aapro MS. Comparative activity of antiemetic drugs. *Crit Rev Oncol Hematol.* 2007;61(2):162-175.

Kris MG, Hesketh PJ, Somerfield MR, et al. American Society of Clinical Oncology guideline for antiemetics in oncology: update 2006. *J Clin Oncol.* 2006;24(18):2932-2947.

Lohr L. Chemotherapy-induced nausea and vomiting. *Cancer J.* 2008;14(2):85-93.

Multinational Association of Supportive Care in Cancer. MASCC/ESMO antiemetic guideline 2013. http://www.mascc.org/assets/documents/mascc_guidelines_english_2013.pdf. Accessed October 2013.

National Comprehensive Cancer Network (NCCN). NCCN clinical practice guidelines in oncology: antiemesis. v.1.2015. http://www.nccn.org/professionals/physician_gls/PDF/antiemesis.pdf

Navari RM, Gray SE, Kerr AC. Olanzapine versus aprepitant for the prevention of chemotherapy-induced nausea and vomiting: a randomized phase III trial. *J Support Oncol.* 2011;9(5):188-195.

Navari RM. Prevention of emesis from multiple-day and high-dose chemotherapy regimens. *J Natl Compr Canc Netw.* 2007;5(1):51-59.

Oo TH, Hesketh PJ. Drug insight: new antiemetics in the management of chemotherapy-induced nausea and vomiting. *Nat Clin Pract Oncol.* 2005;2(4):196-201.

Rapoport BL, Chasen MR, Gridelli C, et al. Safety and efficacy of rolapitant for prevention of chemotherapy-induced nausea and vomiting after administration of cisplatin-based highly emetogenic chemotherapy in patients with cancer: two randomised, active-controlled, double-blind, phase 3 trials. *Lancet Oncol.* 2015;16(9):1079-1089.

Roila F, Herrstedt J, Aapro M, et al. Guideline update for MASCC and ESMO in the prevention of chemotherapy- and radiotherapy-induced nausea and vomiting: results of the Perugia Consensus Conference. *Ann Oncol.* 2010;21(Suppl 5):v232-v243.

Roscoe JA, Heckler CE, Morrow GR, et al. Prevention of delayed nausea: a University of Rochester Cancer Center Community Clinical Oncology Program study of patients receiving chemotherapy. *J Clin Oncol.* 2012;30(27):3389-3395.

Schwartzberg LS, Modiano MR, Rapoport BL, et al. Safety and efficacy of rolapitant for prevention of chemotherapy-induced nausea and vomiting after administration of moderately emetogenic chemotherapy or anthracycline and cyclophosphamide regimens in patients with cancer: a randomised, active-controlled, double-blind, phase 3 trial. *Lancet Oncol.* 2015;16(9):1071-1078.

Trigg ME, Higa GM. Chemotherapy-induced nausea and vomiting: antiemetic trials that impacted clinical practice. *J Oncol Pharm Pract.* 2010;16(4):233-244.

MANAGEMENT OF DRUG EXTRAVASATIONS

A potential complication of drug therapy is extravasation. A variety of symptoms, including erythema, ulceration, pain, tissue sloughing, and necrosis, are possible. A variety of drugs have been reported to cause tissue damage if extravasated.

DEFINITIONS

- **Extravasation:** Unintentional or inadvertent leakage (or instillation) of fluid out of a blood vessel into surrounding tissue

- **Irritant:** An agent that causes aching, tightness, and phlebitis with or without inflammation, but does not typically cause tissue necrosis. Irritants can cause necrosis if the extravasation is severe or left untreated.

- **Vesicant:** An agent that has the potential to cause blistering, severe tissue injury, or tissue necrosis when extravasated

- **Flare:** Local, nonpainful, possibly allergic reaction often accompanied by reddening along the vein

PREVENTING EXTRAVASATIONS

Although it is not possible to prevent all extravasations, a few precautions can minimize the risk to the patient. The vein used should be a large, intact vessel with good blood flow. Veins in the forearm (ie, basilic, cephalic, and median antebrachial) are usually good options for peripheral infusions. To minimize the risk of dislodging the catheter, avoid using veins in the hands, dorsum of the foot, and any joint space (eg, antecubital). It is important to remember to not administer chemotherapy distal to a recent venipuncture.

A frequently recommended precaution against drug extravasation is the use of a central venous catheter. Use of a central line has several advantages, including high patient satisfaction, reliable venous access, high flow rates, and rapid dilution of the drug. Many institutions encourage or require use of a vascular access device for administration of vesicant agents. Despite their benefit, central lines are not an absolute solution. Vascular access devices are subject to a number of complications. Misplacement/migration of the catheter or improper placement of the needle in accessing injection ports, and cuts, punctures, infections, or rupture of the catheter itself have all been reported.

Education of both the patient and practitioner is imperative. Educate the patient to immediately report any signs of pain, itching, tingling, burning, redness, swelling, or discomfort, all of which could be early signs of extravasation. Symptoms of extravasation which may appear later include blistering, ulceration, and necrosis. Ensure the health care team is informed of the risks and management strategies for both prevention and treatment of extravasations. Absence of blood return, resistance upon administration, or interruption of the IV flow should raise suspicion of potential extravasation.

INITIAL EXTRAVASATION MANAGEMENT

1. **Stop the infusion:** At the first suspicion of extravasation, the drug infusion and IV fluids should be stopped.

2. **Do NOT remove the catheter/needle:** The IV tubing should be disconnected, but the catheter/needle should be left in place to facilitate aspiration of fluid from the extravasation site and, if appropriate, administration of an antidote.

3. **Aspirate fluid:** To the extent possible, the extravasated drug solution should gently be removed from the subcutaneous tissues. It is important to avoid any friction or pressure to the area.

4. **Do NOT flush the line:** Flooding the infiltration site with saline or dextrose in an attempt to dilute the drug solution is not recommended.

5. **Remove the catheter/needle:** If an antidote is not going to be administered into the extravasation site, the catheter/needle should be removed. If an antidote is to be injected into the area, it should be injected through the catheter to ensure delivery of the antidote to the extravasation site. When this has been accomplished, the catheter should then be removed.

6. **Elevate:** The affected extremity should be elevated.

7. **Compresses:** If indicated, apply dry compress to area of extravasation (either cold or warm, depending on vesicant extravasated).

8. **Monitor and document:** Mark the extravasation site (using a surgical felt pen, gently draw an outline on the skin of the extravasation area) and photograph if possible. Monitor and document the event and follow-up activities according to institutional policy.

Table 1: Vesicant Agents and Extravasation Management

Extravasated Medication	Preferred Antidote	Antidote Administration	Supportive Management	Comments
Amino Acids (4.25%)/ parenteral nutrition	Hyaluronidase	Hyaluronidase: Intradermal or SubQ: Inject a total of 1 mL (15 units/mL) as five separate 0.2 mL injections (using a 25-gauge needle) into area of extravasation at the leading edge in a clockwise manner (MacCara 1983; Zenk 1981)	Apply dry cold compresses (Hurst 2004)	
Aminophylline	Hyaluronidase	Hyaluronidase: Intradermal or SubQ: Inject a total of 1 mL (15 units/mL) as five separate 0.2 mL injections (using a 25-gauge needle) into area of extravasation at the leading edge in a clockwise manner (MacCara 1983; Zenk 1981)	Apply dry cold compresses (Hurst 2004)	
Amsacrine	No known antidote	No known antidote	Apply dry warm compresses (Schulmeister 2011)	Not commercially available in the US
Bendamustine	Sodium Thiosulfate	May be managed in the same manner as mechlorethamine extravasation (Schulmeister 2011); Sodium thiosulfate 1/6 M solution: Inject subcutaneously into extravasation area using 2 mL for each mg of mechlorethamine suspected to have extravasated (Pérez Fidalgo 2012; Polovich 2009)	Apply dry cold compresses for 20 minutes 4 times/day for 1 to 2 days (Pérez Fidalgo 2012)	Irritant with vesicant-like properties (reports of both irritant and vesicant reactions)
Calcium Chloride (≥10%)	Hyaluronidase	Hyaluronidase: Intradermal or SubQ: Inject a total of 1 mL (15 units/mL) as five separate 0.2 mL injections (using a 25-gauge needle) into area of extravasation at the leading edge in a clockwise manner (MacCara 1983; Zenk 1981)	Apply dry cold compresses (Hurst 2004)	
Calcium Gluconate	Hyaluronidase	Hyaluronidase: Intradermal or SubQ: Inject a total of 1 mL (15 units/mL) as five separate 0.2 mL injections (using a 25-gauge needle) into area of extravasation at the leading edge in a clockwise manner (MacCara 1983; Zenk 1981)	Apply dry cold compresses (Hurst 2004)	

Table 1: Vesicant Agents and Extravasation Management *continued*

Extravasated Medication	Preferred Antidote	Antidote Administration	Supportive Management	Comments
CISplatin (>0.4 mg/mL)	Sodium Thiosulfate	Sodium thiosulfate 1/6 M solution: Inject 2 mL into existing IV line for each 100 mg of cisplatin extravasated; then consider also injecting 1 mL as 0.1 mL subcutaneous injections (clockwise) around the area of extravasation; may repeat subcutaneous injections several times over the next 3 to 4 hours (Ener 2004) Dimethyl sulfoxide (DMSO) may also be considered an option. Apply topically to a region covering twice the affected area every 8 hours for 7 days; begin within 10 minutes of extravasation; do not cover with a dressing (Pérez Fidalgo 2012).	Information conflicts regarding use of warm or cold compresses	
Contrast Media	Hyaluronidase	Hyaluronidase: Intradermal or SubQ: Inject a total of 1 mL (15 units/mL) as five separate 0.2 mL injections (using a 25-gauge needle) into area of extravasation at the leading edge in a clockwise manner (MacCara 1983; Zenk 1981) The injection of a total of 5 mL (150 units/mL) as five separate 1 mL injections around the extravasation site has been also used successfully (Rowlett 2012)	Apply dry cold compresses (Hurst 2004)	
DACTINomycin	No known antidote	No known antidote	Apply dry cold compress for 20 minutes 4 times/ day for 1 to 2 days (Pérez Fidalgo 2012)	
Dantrolene	No known antidote	No known antidote	No recommendation	

Table 1: Vesicant Agents and Extravasation Management *continued*

Extravasated Medication	Preferred Antidote	Antidote Administration	Supportive Management	Comments
DAUNOrubicin (Conventional)	Dexrazoxane or topical Dimethyl Sulfoxide (DMSO)	Adults: Dexrazoxane 1,000 mg/m² (maximum dose: 2,000 mg) IV (administer in a large vein remote from site of extravasation) over 1 to 2 hours days 1 and 2, then 500 mg/m² (maximum dose: 1,000 mg) IV over 1 to 2 hours day 3; begin within 6 hours after extravasation (Mouridsen 2007; Pérez Fidalgo 2012). **Note:** Reduce dexrazoxane dose by 50% in patients with moderate to severe renal impairment (CrCl <40 mL/min). Pediatrics and Adults: DMSO: Apply topically to a region covering twice the affected area every 8 hours for 7 days; begin within 10 minutes of extravasation; do not cover with a dressing (Pérez Fidalgo 2012)	Apply dry cold compress for 20 minutes 4 times/day for 1 to 2 days (Pérez Fidalgo 2012). Withhold cooling for 15 minutes before and after dexrazoxane.	If using dexrazoxane, do not use DMSO. Administer dexrazoxane through a large vein remote from area of the extravasation.
Dextrose (≥10%)	Hyaluronidase	Hyaluronidase: **Dextrose 10%:** Intradermal or SubQ: Inject a total of 1 mL (15 units/mL) as five separate 0.2 mL injections (using a 25-gauge needle) into area of extravasation at the leading edge in a clockwise manner (MacCara 1983; Zenk 1981). **Dextrose 50%:** Injection of a total of 1 mL (150 units/mL) as five separate 0.2 mL injections administered along the leading edge of erythema has been used successfully (Wiegand 2010)	Apply dry cold compresses (Hurst 2004)	
Diazepam	No known antidote	No known antidote	Apply dry cold compresses (Hurst 2004)	
Digoxin	No known antidote	No known antidote	No recommendation	
DOCEtaxel	No known antidote	No known antidote	Information conflicts regarding use of warm or cold compresses	Irritant with vesicant-like properties (reports of both irritant and vesicant reactions)

Table 1: Vesicant Agents and Extravasation Management *continued*

Extravasated Medication	Preferred Antidote	Antidote Administration	Supportive Management	Comments
DOPamine	Phentolamine	Phentolamine: Dilute 5 to 10 mg in 10 to 15 mL NS and administer into extravasation site as soon as possible after extravasation (Peberdy 2010) *Alternatives to phentolamine (due to shortage):* Nitroglycerin topical 2% ointment (based on limited case reports in neonates/infants): Apply 4 mm/kg as a thin ribbon to the affected areas; may repeat after 8 hours if needed (Wong 1992) **or** apply a 1-inch strip on the affected site (Denkler 1989) Terbutaline (based on limited case reports): Infiltrate extravasation area using a solution of terbutaline 1 mg diluted to 10 mL in NS (large extravasation site; administration volume varied from 3 to 10 mL) **or** 1 mg diluted in 1 mL 0.9% NS (small/distal extravasation site; administration volume varied from 0.5 to 1 mL) (Stier 1999)	Apply dry warm compresses (Hurst 2004)	
DOXOrubicin (Conventional)	Dexrazoxane or topical DMSO	Adults: Dexrazoxane 1,000 mg/m² (maximum dose: 2,000 mg) IV (administer in a large vein remote from site of extravasation) over 1 to 2 hours days 1 and 2, then 500 mg/m² (maximum dose: 1,000 mg) IV over 1 to 2 hours day 3; begin within 6 hours after extravasation (Mouridsen 2007; Pérez Fidalgo 2012). **Note:** Reduce dexrazoxane dose by 50% in patients with moderate to severe renal impairment (CrCl <40 mL/min). Pediatrics and Adults: DMSO: Apply topically to a region covering twice the affected area every 8 hours for 7 days; begin within 10 minutes of extravasation; do not cover with a dressing (Pérez Fidalgo 2012)	Apply dry cold compress for 20 minutes 4 times/ day for 1 to 2 days (Pérez Fidalgo 2012). Withhold cooling for 15 minutes before and after dexrazoxane.	If using dexrazoxane, do not use DMSO. Administer dexrazoxane through a large vein remote from area of the extravasation.

Table 1: Vesicant Agents and Extravasation Management *continued*

Extravasated Medication	Preferred Antidote	Antidote Administration	Supportive Management	Comments
EPINEPHrine	Phentolamine	Phentolamine: Dilute 5 to 10 mg in 10 to 15 mL NS and administer into extravasation site as soon as possible after extravasation (Peberdy 2010) *Alternatives to phentolamine (due to shortage):* Nitroglycerin topical 2% ointment (based on limited case reports in neonates/infants): Apply 4 mm/kg as a thin ribbon to the affected areas; may repeat after 8 hours if needed (Wong 1992) **or** apply a 1-inch strip on the affected site (Denkler 1989) Terbutaline (based on limited case reports): Infiltrate extravasation area using a solution of terbutaline 1 mg diluted to 10 mL in NS (large extravasation site; administration volume varied from 3 to 10 mL) **or** 1 mg diluted in 1 mL NS (small/distal extravasation site; administration volume varied from 0.5 to 1 mL) (Stier 1999)	Apply dry warm compresses (Hurst 2004)	
EPIrubicin	Dexrazoxane or topical DMSO	Adults: Dexrazoxane 1,000 mg/m² (maximum dose: 2,000 mg) IV (administer in a large vein remote from site of extravasation) over 1 to 2 hours days 1 and 2, then 500 mg/m² (maximum dose: 1,000 mg) IV over 1 to 2 hours day 3; begin within 6 hours after extravasation (Mouridsen 2007; Pérez Fidalgo 2012). **Note:** Reduce dexrazoxane dose by 50% in patients with moderate to severe renal impairment (CrCl <40 mL/min). Pediatrics and Adults: DMSO: Apply topically to a region covering twice the affected area every 8 hours for 7 days; begin within 10 minutes of extravasation; do not cover with a dressing (Pérez Fidalgo 2012)	Apply dry cold compress for 20 minutes 4 times/ day for 1 to 2 days (Pérez Fidalgo 2012). Withhold cooling for 15 minutes before and after dexrazoxane.	If using dexrazoxane, do not use DMSO. Administer dexrazoxane through a large vein remote from area of the extravasation.
Esmolol	No known antidote	No known antidote	No recommendation	

Table 1: Vesicant Agents and Extravasation Management *continued*

Extravasated Medication	Preferred Antidote	Antidote Administration	Supportive Management	Comments
HydrOXYzine	No known antidote	No known antidote	No recommendation	**Note:** Labeled route of administration for parenteral hydroxyzine is by IM injection only; IV administration is contraindicated.
IDArubicin	Dexrazoxane or topical DMSO	Adults: Dexrazoxane 1,000 mg/m^2 (maximum dose: 2,000 mg) IV (administer in a large vein remote from site of extravasation) over 1 to 2 hours days 1 and 2, then 500 mg/m^2 (maximum dose: 1,000 mg) IV over 1 to 2 hours day 3; begin within 6 hours after extravasation (Mouridsen 2007; Pérez Fidalgo 2012). **Note:** Reduce dexrazoxane dose by 50% in patients with moderate to severe renal impairment (CrCl <40 mL/min). Pediatrics and Adults: DMSO: Apply topically to a region covering twice the affected area every 8 hours for 7 days; begin within 10 minutes of extravasation; do not cover with a dressing (Pérez Fidalgo 2012)	Apply dry cold compress for 20 minutes 4 times/day for 1 to 2 days. (Pérez Fidalgo 2012). Withhold cooling for 15 minutes before and after dexrazoxane.	If using dexrazoxane, do not use DMSO. Administer dexrazoxane through a large vein remote from area of the extravasation.
Mannitol (>5%)	Hyaluronidase	Hyaluronidase: SubQ: Administer multiple 0.5 to 1 mL injections of a 15 units/mL solution around the periphery of the extravasation (Kumar 2003)	No recommendation	
Mechlorethamine	Sodium Thiosulfate	Sodium thiosulfate $^1/_6$ M solution: Inject subcutaneously into extravasation area using 2 mL for each mg of mechlorethamine suspected to have extravasated (Pérez Fidalgo 2012; Polovich 2009)	Apply ice for 6 to 12 hours after sodium thiosulfate administration (Mustargen prescribing information 2012; Polovich 2009) **or** may apply dry cold compresses for 20 minutes 4 times/day for 1 to 2 days (Pérez Fidalgo 2012)	

Table 1: Vesicant Agents and Extravasation Management *continued*

Extravasated Medication	Preferred Antidote	Antidote Administration	Supportive Management	Comments
Methylene Blue	Nitroglycerin topical 2% ointment	Nitroglycerin topical 2% ointment (based on mechanism of extravasation injury **[has not been clinically evaluated]**): Apply a 1-inch strip on the site of ischemia; may redose every 8 hours as necessary (Reynolds 2014)	Apply dry, warm compresses (based on mechanism of extravasation injury **[has not been clinically evaluated]**) proximal to the infection site (Reynolds 2014)	
MitoMYcin	Topical DMSO	DMSO: Apply topically to a region covering twice the affected area every 8 hours for 7 days; begin within 10 minutes of extravasation; do not cover with a dressing (Pérez Fidalgo 2012)	Apply dry cold compress for 20 minutes 4 times/ day for 1 to 2 days (Pérez Fidalgo 2012)	
MitoXANtrone	Dexrazoxane or topical DMSO	Adults: Dexrazoxane 1,000 mg/m² (maximum dose: 2,000 mg) IV (administer in a large vein remote from site of extravasation) over 1 to 2 hours days 1 and 2, then 500 mg/m² (maximum dose: 1,000 mg) IV over 1 to 2 hours day 3; begin within 6 hours after extravasation (Mouridsen 2007; Pérez Fidalgo 2012). **Note:** Reduce dexrazoxane dose by 50% in patients with moderate to severe renal impairment (CrCl <40 mL/min). Pediatrics and Adults: DMSO: Apply topically to a region covering twice the affected area every 8 hours for 7 days; begin within 10 minutes of extravasation; do not cover with a dressing (Pérez Fidalgo 2012)	Apply dry cold compress for 20 minutes 4 times/ day for 1 to 2 days (Pérez Fidalgo 2012)	Irritant with vesicant-like properties (reports of both irritant and vesicant reactions). Administer dexrazoxane through a large vein remote from area of the extravasation.
Nafcillin	Hyaluronidase	Hyaluronidase: Intradermal or SubQ: Inject a total of 1 mL (15 units/mL) as five separate 0.2 mL injections (using a 25-gauge needle) into area of extravasation at the leading edge in a clockwise manner (MacCara 1983; Zenk 1981)	Apply dry cold compresses (Hurst 2004)	

Table 1: Vesicant Agents and Extravasation Management *continued*

Extravasated Medication	Preferred Antidote	Antidote Administration	Supportive Management	Comments
Norepinephrine	Phentolamine	Phentolamine: Dilute 5 to 10 mg in 10 to 15 mL NS and administer into extravasation site as soon as possible after extravasation (Peberdy 2010) **or** dilute 5 to 10 mg in 10 mL NS and administer into extravasation area (within 12 hours of extravasation) (Phentolamine product information 1999) *Alternatives to phentolamine (due to shortage):* Nitroglycerin topical 2% ointment (based on limited case reports in neonates/infants): Apply 4 mm/kg as a thin ribbon to the affected areas; may repeat after 8 hours if needed (Wong 1992) **or** apply a 1-inch strip on the affected site (Denkler 1989) Terbutaline (based on limited case reports): Infiltrate extravasation area using a solution of terbutaline 1 mg diluted to 10 mL in NS (large extravasation site; administration volume varied from 3 to 10 mL) **or** 1 mg diluted in 1 mL NS (small/distal extravasation site; administration volume varied from 0.5 to 1 mL) (Stier 1999)	Apply dry warm compresses (Hurst 2004)	
Oxaliplatin	No known antidote	No known antidote	Information conflicts regarding use of warm or cold compresses Cold compresses could potentially precipitate or exacerbate peripheral neuropathy (de Lemos 2005)	Irritant with vesicant-like properties (reports of both irritant and vesicant reactions)
PACLitaxel	Hyaluronidase	Hyaluronidase: *If needle/cannula still in place:* Administer 1 to 6 mL (150 units/mL) into existing IV line; usual dose is 1 mL for each 1 mL of extravasated drug; if needle/cannula has been removed, inject subcutaneously in a clockwise manner around area of extravasation; may repeat several times over the next 3 to 4 hours (Ener 2004)	Information conflicts regarding use of warm or cold compresses	Irritant with vesicant-like properties (reports of both irritant and vesicant reactions)

Table 1: Vesicant Agents and Extravasation Management *continued*

Extravasated Medication	Preferred Antidote	Antidote Administration	Supportive Management	Comments
Pentamidine	No known antidote	No known antidote	Dry warm compresses (Reynolds 2014)	Irritant with vesicant-like properties (reports of both irritant and vesicant reactions)
Phenylephrine	Phentolamine	Phentolamine: Dilute 5 to 10 mg in 10 to 15 mL NS and administer into extravasation site as soon as possible after extravasation (Peberdy 2010) *Alternatives to phentolamine (due to shortage):* Nitroglycerin topical 2% ointment (based on limited case reports in neonates/infants): Apply 4 mm/kg as a thin ribbon to the affected areas; may repeat after 8 hours if needed (Wong 1992) **or** apply a 1-inch strip on the affected site (Denkler 1989) Terbutaline (based on limited case reports): Infiltrate extravasation area using a solution of terbutaline 1 mg diluted to 10 mL in NS (large extravasation site; administration volume varied from 3 to 10 mL) **or** 1 mg diluted in 1 mL NS (small/distal extravasation site; administration volume varied from 0.5 to 1 mL). (Stier 1999)	Apply dry warm compresses (Hurst 2004)	
Phenytoin	No antidote **or** Hyaluronidase	*Conflicting information:* Do not use antidotes (pediatrics) (Montgomery 1999) Hyaluronidase: SubQ: Inject four separate 0.2 mL injections of 15 units/mL (using a 25-gauge needle) into area of extravasation (Sokol 1998)	No recommendation	
Potassium Acetate (>0.1 mEq/mL)	Hyaluronidase	Hyaluronidase: Intradermal or SubQ: Inject a total of 1 mL (15 units/mL) as five separate 0.2 mL injections (using a 25-gauge needle) into area of extravasation at the leading edge in a clockwise manner (MacCara 1983; Zenk 1981)	Apply dry cold compresses (Hurst 2004)	Reports of both irritant and vesicant reactions

2169

Table 1: Vesicant Agents and Extravasation Management *continued*

Extravasated Medication	Preferred Antidote	Antidote Administration	Supportive Management	Comments
Potassium Chloride (>0.1 mEq/mL)	Hyaluronidase	Hyaluronidase: Intradermal or SubQ: Inject a total of 1 mL (15 units/mL) as five separate 0.2 mL injections (using a 25-gauge needle) into area of extravasation at the leading edge in a clockwise manner (MacCara 1983; Zenk 1981)	Apply dry cold compresses (Hurst 2004)	Reports of both irritant and vesicant reactions
Potassium Phosphate (may depend on concentration)	Hyaluronidase	Hyaluronidase: Intradermal or SubQ: Inject a total of 1 mL (15 units/mL) as five separate 0.2 mL injections (using a 25-gauge needle) into area of extravasation at the leading edge in a clockwise manner (MacCara 1983; Zenk 1981)	Apply dry cold compresses (Hurst 2004)	May be an irritant
Promethazine	No known antidote	No known antidote	Apply dry cold compresses (Hurst 2004)	**Note:** Preferred route of administration for promethazine is by deep intramuscular (IM) injection. If IV route is used, discontinue infusion immediately with onset of burning/pain; evaluate for inadvertent arterial injection or extravasation.
Sodium Bicarbonate (≥8.4%)	Hyaluronidase	Hyaluronidase: SubQ: Inject four to five separate 0.2 mL injections of 15 units/mL around area of extravasation (Hurst 2004)	Apply dry cold compresses (Hurst 2004)	
Sodium Chloride (>1%)	No known antidote	No known antidote	Apply dry warm compresses (Hastings-Tolsma 1993)	
Streptozocin	No known antidote	No known antidote	No recommendation	Irritant with vesicant-like properties (reports of both irritant and vesicant reactions)
Trabectedin	No known antidote	No known antidote	No recommendation	

Table 1: Vesicant Agents and Extravasation Management *continued*

Extravasated Medication	Preferred Antidote	Antidote Administration	Supportive Management	Comments
Tromethamine	No known antidote	No known antidote	No recommendation	
Vasopressin	Phentolamine	Phentolamine: Dilute 5 to 10 mg in 10 to 15 mL NS and administer into extravasation site as soon as possible after extravasation (Peberdy 2010) *Alternatives to phentolamine (due to shortage):* Nitroglycerin topical 2% ointment (based on limited case reports in neonates/infants): Apply 4 mm/kg as a thin ribbon to the affected areas; may repeat after 8 hours if needed (Wong 1992) **or** apply a 1-inch strip on the affected site (Denkler 1989) Terbutaline (based on limited case reports): Infiltrate extravasation area using a solution of terbutaline 1 mg diluted to 10 mL in NS (large extravasation site; administration volume varied from 3 to 10 mL), **or** 1 mg diluted in 1 mL NS (small/distal extravasation site; administration volume varied from 0.5 to 1 mL) (Stier 1999)	No recommendation	

Table 1: Vesicant Agents and Extravasation Management *continued*

Extravasated Medication	Preferred Antidote	Antidote Administration	Supportive Management	Comments
VinBLAStine	Hyaluronidase	Hyaluronidase: *If needle/cannula still in place:* Administer 1 to 6 mL (150 units/mL) into existing IV line; usual dose is 1 mL for each 1 mL of extravasated drug (Pérez Fidalgo 2012; Schulmeister 2011) *If needle/cannula was removed:* Inject 1 to 6 mL (150 units/mL) subcutaneously in a clockwise manner using 1 mL for each 1 mL of drug extravasated (Schulmeister 2011) or administer 1 mL (150 units/mL) as five separate 0.2 mL injections (using a 25-gauge needle) into the extravasation site (Polovich 2009)	Apply dry warm compress for 20 minutes 4 times/day for 1 to 2 days (Pérez Fidalgo 2012)	
VinCRIStine	Hyaluronidase	Hyaluronidase: *If needle/cannula still in place:* Administer 1 to 6 mL (150 units/mL) into existing IV line; usual dose is 1 mL for each 1 mL of extravasated drug (Pérez Fidalgo 2012; Schulmeister 2011) *If needle/cannula was removed:* Inject 1 to 6 mL (150 units/mL) subcutaneously in a clockwise manner using 1 mL for each 1 mL of drug extravasated (Schulmeister 2011) **or** administer 1 mL (150 units/mL) as five separate 0.2 mL injections (using a 25-gauge needle) into the extravasation site (Polovich 2009)	Apply dry warm compress for 20 minutes 4 times/day for 1 to 2 days (Pérez Fidalgo 2012)	

Table 1: Vesicant Agents and Extravasation Management *continued*

Extravasated Medication	Preferred Antidote	Antidote Administration	Supportive Management	Comments
Vindesine	Hyaluronidase	Hyaluronidase: *If needle/cannula still in place:* Administer 1 to 6 mL (150 units/mL) into existing IV line; usual dose is 1 mL for each 1 mL of extravasated drug (Pérez Fidalgo 2012; Schulmeister 2011) *If needle/cannula was removed:* Inject 1 to 6 mL (150 units/mL) subcutaneously in a clockwise manner using 1 mL for each 1 mL of drug extravasated (Schulmeister 2011) **or** administer 1 mL (150 units/mL) as five separate 0.2 mL injections (using a 25-gauge needle) into the extravasation site (Polovich 2009)	Apply dry warm compress for 20 minutes 4 times/day for 1 to 2 days (Pérez Fidalgo 2012)	Not commercially available in the US
Vinorelbine	Hyaluronidase	Hyaluronidase: *If needle/cannula still in place:* Administer 1 to 6 mL (150 units/mL) into existing IV line; usual dose is 1 mL for each 1 mL of extravasated drug (Pérez Fidalgo 2012; Schulmeister 2011) *If needle/cannula was removed:* Inject 1 to 6 mL (150 units/mL) subcutaneously in a clockwise manner using 1 mL for each 1 mL of drug extravasated (Schulmeister 2011) **or** administer 1 mL (150 units/mL) as five separate 0.2 mL injections (using a 25-gauge needle) into the extravasation site (Polovich 2009)	Apply dry warm compress for 20 minutes 4 times/day for 1 to 2 days (Pérez Fidalgo 2012)	

◀ **SUPPORTIVE MANAGEMENT**

Compresses: Two issues for which there is less consensus are the application of warm or cold compresses and the use of various antidotes for extravasation management. A variety of recommendations exists for each of these concerns; however, there is no consensus concerning the proper approach.

Cold: Intermittent cooling of the area of extravasation results in vasoconstriction, potentially restricting the spread of the drug and decreasing the pain and inflammation in the area. Application of dry cold compresses for 20 minutes 4 times/day for 1 to 2 days is usually recommended as immediate treatment for most drug extravasations, including anthracycline, antibiotic (eg, mitomycin or dactinomycin), or alkylating agent extravasation (Pérez Fidalgo 2012). Cold dry compresses may also be utilized in the management of nonvesicant extravasations.

Warm: Application of dry warm compresses results in a localized vasodilation and increased blood flow. Increased circulation is believed to facilitate removal of the drug from the area of extravasation. Application of dry warm compresses for 20 minutes 4 times/day for 1 to 2 days is generally recommended for extravasation of vinca alkaloid, taxane, and platinum derivatives (Pérez Fidalgo 2012). Avoid moist heat. Most data are from animal studies with relatively few human case reports. Animal models indicate application of heat exacerbates the damage from anthracycline extravasations.

For some agents, such as oxaliplatin and taxanes, there are conflicting recommendations. Some reports recommend application of cold; others recommend warm.

For most vasopressors (dopamine, ephedrine, norepinephrine, and phenylephrine), dry, warm compresses may be applied (Hurst 2004). Cool compresses should be avoided with vasopressor extravasation as cooling may exacerbate vasoconstrictive effects (Reynolds 2014).

Table 2: Antineoplastic Agents Associated With Irritation or Occasional Extravasation Reactions

Arsenic Trioxide	Gemcitabine
Bendamustine[1]	Ibritumomab
Bleomycin	Ifosfamide
Bortezomib	Irinotecan
Busulfan	Ixabepilone
CARBOplatin	Melphalan
Carmustine	MitoXANtrone[1]
CISplatin (≤0.4 mg/mL)	Oxaliplatin[1]
Cladribine	PACLitaxel[1]
Cyclophosphamide	PACLitaxel (Protein Bound)
Dacarbazine	Pentamidine[1]
DAUNOrubicin Citrate (Liposomal)	Streptozocin[1]
DOCEtaxel[1]	Teniposide
DOXOrubicin (Liposomal)	Thiopental[1]
Etoposide	Thiotepa
Etoposide Phosphate	Topotecan
Fluorouracil	

[1] Irritant with vesicant-like properties (there have been reports of both irritant and vesicant reactions)

The nurse administering the vesicant agent should monitor the patient and IV site frequently. Prior to drug administration, verify the patency of the IV line. The line should be flushed with 5 to 10 mL of a saline or dextrose solution (depending on compatibility) and the drug(s) infused through the side of a free-flowing IV line over 2 to 5 minutes. If an extravasation occurs, it is important to monitor the site closely at 24 hours, 1 week, 2 weeks, and as necessary for any signs and symptoms of extravasation.

EXTRAVASATION-SPECIFIC ANTIDOTES

Dexrazoxane: Dexrazoxane, a derivative of EDTA, is an intracellular chelating agent initially approved as a cardioprotective agent in patients receiving anthracycline therapy. It is believed that the cardioprotective effect of dexrazoxane is a result of chelating iron following intracellular hydrolysis. Dexrazoxane is not an effective chelator itself but is hydrolyzed intracellularly to an open-ring chelator form, which complexes with iron, other heavy metals, and doxorubicin complexes to inhibit the generation of free radicals. In the management of anthracycline-induced extravasation, dexrazoxane may act by reversibly inhibiting topoisomerase II, protecting tissue from anthracycline cytotoxicity, thereby decreasing tissue damage.

Dexrazoxane is administered as 3 IV infusions over 1 to 2 hours through a different venous access location: 1,000 mg/m^2 within 6 hours, 1,000 mg/m^2 after 24 hours, and 500 mg/m^2 after 48 hours of the actual extravasation up to a maximum total dose of 2,000 mg on days 1 and 2 and 1,000 mg on day 3, respectively (Mouridsen 2007). Localized cooling was permitted (except within 15 minutes before and after dexrazoxane infusion). Prior to administering dexrazoxane, discontinue DMSO as studies suggest the single agent is more effective than when used in combination with DMSO. **Note:** Reduce dexrazoxane dose by 50% in patients with moderate to severe renal impairment (CrCl <40 mL/minute).

Dimethyl sulfoxide (DMSO): Case reports and small studies have suggested that DMSO is an effective treatment for certain chemotherapy extravasations (anthracyclines, mitomycin, and mitoxantrone). DMSO has free-radical scavenger properties, which increases removal of vesicant drugs from tissues to minimize tissue damage in extravasation management (Pérez Fidalgo 2012). Common dosing is to apply topically by gently painting DMSO 50% solution onto an area twice the size of the extravasation with a saturated gauze pad or cotton swab every 8 hours for 7 days (Pérez Fidalgo 2012). Allow the site to dry. Do not cover with a dressing, as severe blistering may result. During application, DMSO may cause local erythema. Clinical reports of DMSO use are difficult to interpret due to variations in DMSO concentration (50% to 99%); the product is only commercially available in the United States at a concentration of 50% (vol/vol) solution in water.

Hyaluronidase: Hyaluronidase is an enzyme that destroys hyaluronic acid, an essential component of connective tissue. This results in increased permeability of the tissue, facilitating diffusion and absorption of fluids. It is postulated that increasing the diffusion of extravasated fluids results in more rapid absorption, thereby limiting tissue damage. In individual case reports, hyaluronidase has been reported effective in preventing tissue damage from a wide variety of agents, including vinca alkaloids, epipodophyllotoxins, and taxanes. The ESMO/EONS guidelines suggest that 150 to 900 units may be administered subcutaneously around the area of chemotherapy extravasation (Pérez Fidalgo 2012). Administration as 5 separate 0.2 mL (15 units/mL) SubQ or intradermal injections into the extravasation site has been reported (MacCara 1983). A 24-gauge or smaller needle should be used. It is recommended to use a new syringe for each injection site. If needle/cannula still in place, administration of a 1 to 6 mL hyaluronidase (150 units/mL) has been reported in the management of plant alkaloid extravasation (Pérez Fidalgo 2012; Schulmeister 2011) and paclitaxel extravasation (Ener 2004). Refer to Table 1 for vesicant-specific management.

Phentolamine: Phentolamine minimizes tissue injury due to extravasation of norepinephrine and other sympathomimetic vasoconstrictors. Inject 5 to 10 mg diluted in 10 to 15 mL normal saline and inject/infiltrate into the extravasation area; begin as soon as possible after extravasation but within 12 hours.

Topical nitroglycerin or terbutaline (alternatives to phentolamine): Terbutaline and topical nitroglycerin have been used (case reports) as alternatives to phentolamine in the event of phentolamine supply shortages. Topical nitroglycerin (2% ointment) is reported to reverse the vasoconstriction at the extravasation site caused by infiltration of sympathomimetic vasoconstrictors; case reports for use in neonates/infants suggest resolution of ischemia (Denkler 1989; Wong 1992).

Sodium thiosulfate: Sodium thiosulfate ($^1/_6$ molar) has been recommended for treatment of mechlorethamine, concentrated cisplatin, and bendamustine extravasations. Sodium thiosulfate provides a substrate for alkylation by mechlorethamine, preventing the alkylation and subsequent destruction in subcutaneous tissue.

Preparation of a $^1/_6$ molar solution of sodium thiosulfate:

- Dilute 4 mL of a sodium thiosulfate 10% solution into a syringe with 6 mL of sterile water for injection, resulting in 10 mL of $^1/_6$ molar solution

  or

- Dilute 1.6 mL of a sodium thiosulfate 25% solution with 8.4 mL of sterile water for injection, resulting in 10 mL of $^1/_6$ molar solution

Inject the $^1/_6$ molar sodium thiosulfate solution either into the existing needle/cannula or subcutaneously around the edge of the extravasation site using a tuberculin syringe, using a new syringe for each injection site. The dose of sodium thiosulfate and route of administration depend on the amount of drug extravasated. Refer to Table 1 for vesicant-specific dosing.

REFERENCES

Albanell J, Baselga J. Systemic therapy emergencies. *Semin Oncol.* 2000;27(3):347-361.

Bellin MF, Jakobsen JA, Tomassin I, et al. Contrast medium extravasation injury: guidelines for prevention and management. *Eur Radiol.* 2002;12(11):2807-2812.

Bertelli G. Prevention and management of extravasation of cytotoxic drugs. *Drug Saf.* 1995;12 (4):245-255.

Boyle DM, Engelking C. Vesicant extravasation: myths and realities. *Oncol Nurs Forum.* 1995;22 (1):57-67.

de Lemos ML. Role of dimethylsulfoxide for mangement of chemotherapy extravasation. *J Oncol Pharm Practice*. 2004;10(4):197-200.

de Lemos ML, Walisser S. Management of extravasation of oxaliplatin. *J Oncol Pharm Pract*. 2005;11(4):159-162.

Denkler KA, Cohen BE. Reversal of dopamine extravasation injury with topical nitroglycerin ointment. *Plast Reconstr Surg*. 1989;84(5):811-813.

Doellman D, Hadaway L, Bowe-Geddes LA, et al. Infiltration and extravasation: update on prevention and management. *J Infus Nurs*. 2009;32(4):203-211.

Dorr RT. Antidotes to vesicant chemotherapy extravasations. *Blood Rev*. 1990;4(1):41-60.

Dorr RT, Soble M, Alberts DS. Efficacy of sodium thiosulfate as a local antidote to mechlorethamine skin toxicity in the mouse. *Cancer Chemother Pharmacol*. 1988;22(4):299-302.

Dumbarton TC, Gorman SK, Minor S, Loubani O, White F, Green R. Local cutaneous necrosis secondary to a prolonged peripheral infusion of methylene blue in vasodilatory shock. *Ann Pharmacother*. 2012;46(3):e6.

Ener RA, Meglathery SB, Styler M. Extravasation of systemic hemato-oncological therapies. *Ann Oncol*. 2004;15(6):858-862.

Hadaway L. Infiltration and extravasation. *Am J Nurs*. 2007;107(8):64-72.

Hastings-Tolsma MT, Yucha CB, Tompkins J, Robson L, Szeverenyi N. Effect of warm and cold applications on the resolution of IV infiltrations. *Res Nurs Health*. 1993;16(3):171-178.

Hurst S, McMillan M. Innovative solutions in critical care units: extravasation guidelines. *Dimens Crit Care Nurs*. 2004;23(3):125-128.

Kumar MM, Sprung J. The use of hyaluronidase to treat mannitol extravasation. *Anesth Analg*. 2003;97(4):1199-1200.

Kurul S, Saip P, Aydin T. Totally implantable venous-access ports: local problems and extravasation injury. *Lancet Oncol*. 2002;3(11):684-692.

Larson DL. Alterations in wound healing secondary to infusion injury. *Clin Plast Surg*. 1990;17(3):509-517.

Larson DL. Treatment of tissue extravasation by antitumor agents. *Cancer*. 1982;49(9):1796-1799.

Larson DL. What is the appropriate management of tissue extravasation by antitumor agents? *Plast Reconstr Surg*. 1985;75(3):397-405.

MacCara ME. Extravasation: a hazard of intravenous therapy. *Drug Intell Clin Pharm*. 1983;17(10):713-717.

Montgomery LA, Hanrahan K, Kottman K, Otto A, Barrett T, Hermiston B. Guideline for IV infiltrations in pediatric patients. *Pediatr Nurs*. 1999;25(2):167-169, 173-180.

Mouridsen HT, Langer SW, Buter J, et al. Treatment of anthracycline extravasation with savene (dexrazoxane): results from two prospective clinical multicentre studies. *Ann Oncol*. 2007;18(3):546-550.

Mustargen product information, Lundbeck, 2012

Peberdy MA, Callaway CW, Neumar RW, et al. Part 9: post-cardiac arrest care: 2010 American Heart Association guidelines for cardiopulmonary resuscitation and emergency cardiovascular care. *Circulation*. 2010;122(18 Suppl 3):S768-S786.

Pérez Fidalgo JA, García Fabregat L, Cervantes A, et al. Management of chemotherapy extravasation: ESMO-EONS clinical practice guidelines. *Ann Oncol*. 2012;23(Suppl 7):vii167-173.

Perry MC. Extravasation. *The Chemotherapy Source Book*. 4th ed. Philadelphia, PA; 2008.

Phentolamine [prescribing information]. Eatontown, NJ: West-Ward Pharmaceuticals; September 2015.

Polovich M, Whitford JN, Olsen M. *Chemotherapy and Biotherapy Guidelines and Recommendations for Practice*. 3rd ed. Pittsburgh, PA: Oncology Nursing Society; 2009.

Reynolds PM, Maclaren R, Mueller SW, Fish DN, Kiser TH. Management of extravasation injuries: a focused evaluation of noncytotoxic medications. *Pharmacotherapy*. 2014;34(6):617-632.

Rowlett J. Extravasation of contrast media managed with recombinant human hyaluronidase. *Am J Emerg Med*. 2012;30(9):2102.

Schrijvers DL. Extravasation: a dreaded complication of chemotherapy. *Ann Oncol*. 2003;14(Suppl 3):iii26-iii30.

Schulmeister L, Camp-Sorrell D. Chemotherapy extravasation from implanted ports. *Oncol Nurs Forum*. 2000;27(3):531-538.

Schulmeister L. Extravasation management: clinical update. *Semin Oncol Nurs*. 2011;27(1):82-90.

Schulmeister L. Preventing and managing vesicant chemotherapy extravasations. *J Support Oncol*. 2010;8(5):212-215.

Sokol DK, Dahlmann A, Dunn DW. Hyaluronidase treatment for intravenous phenytoin extravasation. *J Child Neurol*. 1998;13(5):246-247.

Stanford BL, Hardwicke F. A review of clinical experience with paclitaxel extravasations. *Support Care Cancer*. 2003;11(5):270-277.

Stier PA, Bogner MP, Webster K, Leikin JB, Burda A. Use of subcutaneous terbutaline to reverse peripheral ischemia. *Am J Emerg Med*. 1999;17(1):91-94.

Wang CL, Cohan RH, Ellis JH, Adusumilli S, Dunnick NR. Frequency, management, and outcome of extravasation of nonionic iodinated contrast medium in 69,657 intravenous injections. *Radiology*. 2007;243(1):80-87.

Wiegand R, Brown J. Hyaluronidase for the management of dextrose extravasation. *Am J Emerg Med*. 2010;28(2):257.

Wong AF, McCulloch LM, Sola A. Treatment of peripheral tissue ischemia with topical nitroglycerin ointment in neonates. *J Pediatr*. 1992;121(6):980-983.

Zenk KE. Management of intravenous extravasations. *Infusion*. 1981;5(4):77-79.

MANAGEMENT OF EGFR INHIBITOR TOXICITIES: DERMATOLOGIC, OCULAR, AND GASTROINTESTINAL

BACKGROUND

Epidermal growth factor receptor inhibitor (EGFRI) therapy is used in the treatment of advanced and metastatic malignant diseases arising from epithelial tissue, such as non-small cell lung cancer, colorectal cancer, squamous cell cancer of the head and neck, pancreatic cancer, and breast cancer. The epidermal growth factor receptor (EGFR) is found on the surface of most human cells. The EGFR is a transmembrane protein belonging to the ErbB-2 (avian erythroblastosis oncogene B-like) family of membrane-bound receptor protein tyrosine kinases (EGFR/ErbB1, Her2/ErbB2, Her3/ErbB3, and Her4/ErbB4). Receptor activation is preceded by ligand binding to the extracellular domain of EGFR which facilitates dimerization of the EGFR-ligand and another EGFR or ErbB family monomer. Following dimerization, the internal tyrosine kinase domain becomes activated which generates molecular second messaging within the cell (Berlanga-Acosta 2009; Ciardiello 2008). Receptor activation yields intracellular signaling that promotes cell proliferation and inhibits apoptosis. Cellular motility is also modulated by EGFR functionality. EGFR is overexpressed and activated in many cancers that arise from epithelial tissue, making it an attractive target for anticancer therapy.

Common adverse effects from pharmacologic inhibition of EGFR generally represent perturbation of this molecule's role in the homeostasis of epithelial tissue, including skin, mucosa, hair, nails, and various other epithelial surfaces (Agero 2006; Berlanga-Acosta 2009). Effective management of adverse effects with EGFRI therapy is important to maintain optimal dose intensity of anticancer therapy and improve patient quality of life (Baas 2012). Most adverse effects attributed to EGFRI administration are mild to moderate in severity; however, the chronic nature of these side effects can become unbearable to the patient.

Commercially available EGFRI therapy includes small molecules that inhibit the EGFR intracellular protein tyrosine kinase domain (afatinib, erlotinib, gefitinib, lapatinib, vandetanib) and monoclonal antibodies (cetuximab, panitumumab) that bind and block the external ligand binding domain.

DERMATOLOGIC TOXICITIES

Rash

Rash is the most common dermatologic adverse effect reported with EGFRI therapy. Patients may experience physical and psychosocial discomfort with EGFRI rash due to its distribution in cosmetically sensitive anatomic locations (Lacouture 2011). Dermatologic descriptions of EGFRI rash include monomorphous erythematous maculopapules, acneiform, acneiform-follicular, acne-like, sterile form of suppurative folliculitis, inflammatory follicular papules and pustules, and rosacea-like reaction (Agero 2006). The rash appearance often resembles acne vulgaris; however, it is important to recognize that the pathophysiology and etiology of EGFRI rash is not the same as acne vulgaris (Agero 2006; Pérez-Soler 2005). Rash description based on anatomic location and using the phenotypic terms pustular papular rash, pustular eruption, or follicular and intrafollicular pustular eruption is recommended by experts in the field (Pérez-Soler 2005). Dry skin generally accompanies rash with EGFRI therapy (Agero 2006; Lacouture 2011). Rash severity is graded using the National Cancer Institute Common Toxicity Criteria for Adverse Events. Most cases of rash are mild to moderate in severity and cause some pain, burning, and itching (Agero 2006; Lacouture 2011). The face (specifically nose, cheeks, nasolabial folds, chin, and forehead) and areas of the upper torso are the most commonly affected locations; additional anatomic sites affected by EGFRI rash include the scalp, abdomen, buttocks, arms, and legs (Agero 2006). Rash onset is generally 7 to 21 days following initiation of therapy with maximal rash severity generally noted by weeks 3 to 5. Rash from EGFRI therapy is considered reversible; resolution generally occurs within 4 weeks following discontinuation of the causative agent (Agero 2006). Hyperpigmentation and erythema may persist for months to years in some cases (Lacouture 2011). Rash recurrence may occur with medication rechallenge. In some cases, rash resolves or waxes and wanes with continued EGFRI administration. The occurrence and severity of follicular rash is proposed as a surrogate marker for response to EGFRI therapy; findings from pharmacokinetic studies suggest that rash may be an indicator of pharmacologic activity that correlates with EGFR occupancy and blockage (Agero 2006).

Skin toxicity occurs more commonly with EGFRI monoclonal antibody administration than with the small molecule TKIs (Baas 2012; Lacouture 2011). Severe skin toxicity occurs more frequently with addition of radiotherapy (Niyazi 2011). EGFRI rash is a dose-related adverse effect, for both incidence and severity (Balagula 2011). Age may be a factor for risk of dermatologic toxicity with EGFRI therapy. Age over 70 years is a reported risk factor for skin toxicity with erlotinib therapy in patients with non-small cell lung cancer. Age under 70 years is a reported risk factor for skin toxicity with cetuximab therapy in patients with colorectal cancer (Lacouture 2011). Risk of rash with erlotinib therapy is greater in nonsmokers, which probably corresponds to increased bioavailability in this group (Balagula 2011; Lacouture 2011). Skin phototype may modulate the severity of EGFRI rash. One retrospective analysis reported the greatest rate of serious rash with erlotinib therapy occurred in fair-skinned patients with a lower rate in medium-skinned patients and the lowest rate noted in dark-skinned patients. This study also reported similar rate of rash development throughout all four seasons with a trend towards more frequent grade 3 to 4 rashes during the winter months (Luu 2011). One study identified an increased density of *Demodex folliculorum* (DF) in skin biopsies taken from patients treated with EGFRI therapy. DF is a transparent mite that colonizes human hair follicles; increased concentrations of DF are implicated in the pathogenesis of various dermatologic diseases, including papulopustular rosacea and related conditions, pityriasis folliculorum, and blepharitis (Gerber 2011). Dermatologic toxicity with EGFRI therapy may affect the scalp and yield hair loss. Hair loss is considered a transient effect; resolution is generally expected following discontinuation of therapy. In cases of severe scalp inflammation, known as scarring alopecia, hair may not grow back. Management of scalp toxicity follows the same recommendations as general rash management (Lacouture 2011). EGFRI therapy may yield changes in hair texture, such as making it curlier, finer, or brittle.

Secondary infections at affected anatomic sites were noted in 38% of 221 patients receiving treatment for EGFRI skin toxicity. The most frequently isolated organisms were *Staphylococcus aureus* (60% of infectious diagnoses) and methicillin-resistant *Staphylococcus aureus* (14% of infectious diagnoses); less frequent infectious diagnoses included dermatophytes, *Herpes simplex*, and

Herpes zoster (Eilers 2010). Another study isolated *Staphylococcus aureus* in 55% of cultures taken from papulopustular eruptions in patients treated with erlotinib (17 patients) or cetuximab (12 patients) (Amitay-Laish 2010). Additional serious complications attributed to dermatologic toxicity with EGFRI therapy include exfoliative dermatitis, bullous dermatitis, and rash covering >50% of the patient's body surface area (Agero 2006).

Pre-emptive therapy beginning with EGFRI initiation is recommended due to the predictable occurrence of rash in most patients (Lacouture 2011). The usual constituents of preventive therapy are orally administered minocycline 100 mg once daily or doxycycline 100 mg twice daily in combination with twice daily application of a topical moisturizing agent (alcohol-free, thick emollient cream), hydrocortisone 1% cream, and sunscreen (para-aminobenzoic acid-free, sun protection factor ≥15, UVA and UVB protective) (Balagula 2011; Lacouture 2011). The recommended duration of preventive therapy is 6 to 8 weeks. Administration of oral doxycycline 100 mg twice daily in combination with the aforementioned topical therapy reduced the rate of grade 2 or greater skin toxicity by 50% during weeks 1 to 6 of panitumumab therapy relative to observation and reactive treatment. Quality of life scores were better in the group receiving pre-emptive skin care (Lacouture 2011). Administration of minocycline 100 mg daily during weeks 1 to 8 of cetuximab therapy reduced moderate to severe facial rash and significantly reduced moderate to severe itching (p=0.05) relative to placebo (Scope 2007). Doxycycline is preferred for patients with impaired renal function. Minocycline is considered to be less photosensitizing than other tetracyclines (Lacouture 2011). Tetracycline is not recommended for EGFRI rash prevention; a placebo-controlled trial conducted by the North Central Cancer Treatment Group demonstrated overall efficacy for this intervention to be similar to placebo (Jatoi 2008). Topical administration of tazarotene 0.05% cream did not improve skin tolerance to panitumumab therapy in a placebo-controlled trial. Moreover, one-third of patients treated with tazarotene discontinued therapy due to local irritation (Scope 2007). The topical calcineurin inhibitor pimecrolimus did not improve the severity of facial rash or patient perception of symptomatology when tested as a preventive measure with cetuximab therapy (Scope 2009). Lifestyle modifications to support skin health during EGFRI therapy include avoiding the sun, bathing with tepid water, and avoiding prolonged showering in hot water (Balagula 2011).

Treatment of EGFRI rash is based primarily on anecdotal information. The MASCC Skin Study Group recommendations include application of a moderate-to high-potency topical corticosteroid and clindamycin 1% to affected areas (Lacouture 2011). The MASCC Skin Study Group guidelines also discuss the use of systemic isotretinoin. One small noncomparative study evaluated the use of oral clindamycin (450 mg daily days 1 to 10, 300 mg daily days 11 to 20) in combination with oral isotretinoin (20 mg daily on days 11 to 20) for treatment of grade 2 to 3 rash with erlotinib therapy. Rash resolution within 14 days of beginning the intervention was reported for 6 of 7 patients (Bidoli 2010). The use of oral tretinoin (20 to 30 mg daily for 20 days; 30 to 40 mg daily) for management of EGFRI skin toxicity is also described in case reports (Gutzmer 2005; Vezzoli 2008). Systemically administered retinoids must be used cautiously because they are associated with dermatologic toxicities (mucocutaneous xerosis, desquamation, paronychia, photosensitization) and liver dysfunction (Balagula 2011). Routine use of systemic corticosteroids is discouraged due to the toxicity associated with repeated administration. Additional ancillary treatments, such as antimicrobials, should be utilized as warranted by the patient's clinical history and symptomatology.

Pruritus

Pruritus occurring with EGFRI therapy often accompanies other dermatologic adverse effects. Effective management of the underlying dermatologic pathology is an essential aspect of managing pruritus in these patients. Recommendations from the MASCC Skin Study Group (Lacouture 2011) include application of topical products, such as moderate- to high-potency corticosteroids, menthol 0.5%, pramoxine 1%, or doxepin creams. Topical lidocaine and topical antihistamine creams are not recommended due to the systemic absorption that occurs with these products. Systemic antihistamines can be used as warranted for symptom control; nonsedating products are preferable for patient safety. Additional agents to consider when systemic antihistamines do not provide adequate relief from pruritus include gabapentin, pregabalin, or oral doxepin. A correspondence describes two cases of refractory erlotinib-associated pruritus that were managed with oral aprepitant therapy (Vincenzi 2010). However, the use of aprepitant for EGFRI pruritus is not recommended by the MASCC Skin Study Group due to the risks of drug-drug interactions and lack of safety data for continuous administration. Patients should be instructed to treat their skin gently and wear comfortable, loose-fitting clothing.

Miscellaneous Dermatologic Adverse Effects

Other dermatologic adverse effects attributed to EGFRI administration include brittle hair, facial hirsutism, onycholysis or onychodystrophy, paronychia (nail fold inflammation), skin fissures, and tympanic membrane rupture (Garden 2012; Lee 2008). Such side effects are managed as appropriate for the severity, symptomatology, and patient's clinical condition.

Ocular Adverse Effects

Ocular adverse effects attributed to EGFRI therapy are reported. The most common ocular symptoms in 45 patients presenting to an ophthalmology clinic were foreign body sensation (38%), dryness (32%), itchiness (28%), rash (22%), redness (14%), eyelash changes (12%), blurry vision (7%), tearing (6%), burning (3%), and photophobia (3%) (Borkar 2013). Many reports of ocular adverse effects were associated with cetuximab or erlotinib therapy (Borkar 2013; Cohen 2011). These are presumably an extension of the pharmacologic effect of EGFRI because EGFR is normally expressed in basal epithelial cells of the cornea and conjunctiva. EGFRI therapy can weaken the cornea, which is evidenced by corneal thinning, ulceration, melting, perforation, punctate keratitis (pinpoint distribution of epithelial damage), blepharitis, dysfunctional tear syndrome (symptoms from tear film with abnormal composition) (Borkar 2013; Saint-Jean 2012). Lower lid ectropion (outward lid orientation due to tissue weakening) is reported with erlotinib therapy (Saint-Jean 2012). Infectious keratitis with *Staphylococcus epidermidis* is attributed to a nonhealing corneal ulcer arising during chronic erlotinib administration (Johnson 2009). Corneal damage with EGFRI therapy can also be due to direct abrasion secondary to irregular eyelash growth, resulting from trichomegaly (elongation of the eyelashes) and misdirected eyelash growth (Saif 2010; Saint-Jean 2012). The median onset to trichomegaly is 12 weeks after starting therapy; however, onset may occur as early as 3 weeks to as long as 8 months after therapy initiation. Trichomegaly and other eyelash abnormalities are transient effects that resolve with discontinuation of EGFRI administration (Cohen 2011). Hypertrichosis can also affect the eyebrows; however, medical sequelae to this side effect have not been reported (Cohen 2011). Symptoms warranting prompt referral to an ophthalmologist include sustained ocular pain or loss of vision; severe eye redness or light sensitivity; lack of response within 1 week of beginning therapy for blepharitis, meibomitis, or dysfunctional tear syndrome; and misdirected eyelash growth. In addition, ophthalmologic management is indicated to rule out infection and monitor intraocular pressure when corticosteroid eye drops are utilized. Approaches to the management of EGFRI ocular toxicity are presented in the table below (Borkar 2013).

Management of EGFRI-Associated Ocular Adverse Effects (Borkar 2013)

Adverse Effect	Recommendation
Dry eyes	Mild symptoms: Supplemental ophthalmic artificial tears solution
	Moderate to severe or persistent symptoms: Refer to ophthalmologist for evaluation of tear film or concomitant contributing conditions, and for ocular anti-inflammatory medications
Blepharitis (eyelid margin inflammation); meibomitis (eyelid margin sebaceous gland inflammation)	Gentle lid scrubs and warm compress (5-minute application duration) twice daily
	Hyperemia or crust formation: Ocular neomycin-polymyxin B-dexamethasone ointment applied at bedtime for 2 weeks
	Severe or persistent hyperemia or crust formation: Oral doxycycline 50 mg twice daily for 2 weeks, followed by 50 mg once daily for 4 weeks
Trichomegaly	Refer patient to ophthalmologist for trimming and removal of excessively curled, misdirected, or irritating eyelashes
Eyelid skin rash/ hyperemia	Acute reactions: Fluorometholone 0.1% ointment applied to affected eyelid skin and margin 1 to 3 times daily for 1 week (maximum duration of 2 weeks). Ophthalmologic evaluation of intraocular pressure recommended within 4 weeks of treatment initiation.
	Chronic reactions: Tacrolimus 0.03% ointment or pimecrolimus 1% cream applied to external eyelid skin twice daily. Tacrolimus 0.1% may be used for insufficient response to lower concentration. Topical calcineurin products should be applied to the skin only; they are not formulated for administration to the eyelid margin. Maximum duration of therapy is 6 months.

Gastrointestinal Toxicities

Gastrointestinal adverse effects may arise with EGFRI therapy. Diarrhea frequently occurs and may be dose-limiting, either due to secondary complications such as dehydration or to patient intolerance. Other common side effects include stomatitis, mucositis, xerostomia, pharyngitis, dysphagia, and taste alteration (Watters 2011).

Diarrhea may alter gastrointestinal integrity and affect the pharmacokinetics of oral medications, nutritional agents, and fluids. The onset of diarrhea with EGFRI administration is generally within 1 week of beginning therapy and the severity is usually mild to moderate. The duration of diarrhea may be 1 to 2 weeks or this adverse effect may persist for the duration of therapy (Loriot 2008). Diarrhea is a common dose-limiting side effect for erlotinib, gefitinib, and lapatinib (Cherny 2008; Loriot 2008). In general, diarrhea occurs more frequently with orally administered therapy than with monoclonal antibody administration (Loriot 2008). Coadministration of capecitabine, fluorouracil, or irinotecan can increase the risk and severity of diarrhea (Cherny 2008). Diarrhea associated with EGFRI therapy is presumably secretory in nature (Loriot 2008).

◀ Loperamide is recommended as initial therapy for treatment-related diarrhea; EGFRI dose reduction may also be instituted, if appropriate (Loriot 2008). The usual dose of loperamide is 4 mg to initiate therapy, followed by 2 mg every 2 to 4 hours or following each unformed stool. Loperamide is the preferred medication for use in management of diarrhea because it is minimally absorbed from the gastrointestinal tract; however, other opioids, such as tincture of opium, codeine, and morphine, can also be used (Cherny 2008). Octreotide is useful for the management of severe or refractory diarrhea occurring with cytotoxic chemotherapy; however, the utility of this product has not been tested in the management of diarrhea from molecularly targeted anticancer therapy (Loriot 2008). Medications (eg, laxatives, antacids, stool softeners, antimicrobials) and dietary habits (eg, high fiber content, lactose-containing) that may be contributing to diarrhea should be modified whenever possible (Loriot 2008). Oral or parenteral hydration and rehydration with electrolyte repletion are essential for prevention of medical consequences of diarrhea, including dehydration and major organ dysfunction (Benson 2004; Cherny 2008). Medical conditions, such as infection or partial bowel obstruction, that may promote diarrhea should be identified and managed.

Stomatitis associated with EGFRI therapy is characterized by erythema and pain without extensive ulceration to nonkeratinized tissue. Oral ulceration becomes more prominent when EGFRI therapy is used in combination with radiotherapy or cytotoxic therapy (Watters 2011). Refer to Mucositis and Stomatitis on page 2186 for additional information about the management of stomatitis.

REFERENCES

Agero AL, Dusza SW, Benvenuto-Andrade C, Busam KJ, Myskowski P, Halpern AC. Dermatologic side effects associated with the epidermal growth factor receptor inhibitors. *J Am Acad Dermatol*. 2006;55(4):657-670.

Amitay-Laish I, David M, Stemmer SM. Staphylococcus coagulase-positive skin inflammation associated with epidermal growth factor receptor-targeted therapy: an early and a late phase of papulopustular eruptions. *Oncologist*. 2010;15(9):1002-1008.

Baas JM, Krens LL, Guchelaar HJ, et al. Recommendations on management of EGFR inhibitor-induced skin toxicity: a systematic review. *Cancer Treat Rev*. 2012;38(5):505-514.

Balagula Y, Garbe C, Myskowski PL, et al. Clinical presentation and management of dermatological toxicities of epidermal growth factor receptor inhibitors. *Int J Dermatol*. 2011;50(2):129-146.

Benson AB 3rd, Ajani JA, Catalano RB, et al. Recommended guidelines for the treatment of cancer treatment-induced diarrhea. *J Clin Oncol*. 2004;22(14):2918-2926.

Bidoli P, Cortinovis DL, Colombo I, et al. Isotretinoin plus clindamycin seem highly effective against severe erlotinib-induced skin rash in advanced non-small cell lung cancer. *J Thorac Oncol*. 2010;5(10):1662-1663.

Borkar DS, Lacouture ME, Basti S. Spectrum of ocular toxicities from epidermal growth factor receptor inhibitors and their intermediate-term follow-up: a five-year review. *Support Care Cancer*. 2013;21(4):1167-1174.

Cherny NI. Evaluation and management of treatment-related diarrhea in patients with advanced cancer: a review. *J Pain Symptom Manage*. 2008;36(4):413-423.

Ciardiello F, Tortora G. EGFR antagonists in cancer treatment. *N Engl J Med*. 2008;358(11):1160-1174.

Cohen PR, Escudier SM, Kurzrock R. Cetuximab-associated elongation of the eyelashes: case report and review of eyelash trichomegaly secondary to epidermal growth factor receptor inhibitors. *Am J Clin Dermatol*. 2011;12(1):63-67.

Eilers RE Jr, Gandhi M, Patel JD, et al. Dermatologic infections in cancer patients treated with epidermal growth factor receptor inhibitor therapy. *J Natl Cancer Inst*. 2010;102(1):47-53.

Garden BC, Wu S, Lacouture ME. The risk of nail changes with epidermal growth factor receptor inhibitors: a systematic review of the literature and meta-analysis. *J Am Acad Dermatol*. 2012;67(3):400-408.

Gerber PA, Kukova G, Buhren BA, Homey B. Density of *Demodex folliculorum* in patients receiving epidermal growth factor receptor inhibitors. *Dermatology*. 2011;222(2):144-147.

Gutzmer R, Werfel T, Mao R, Kapp A, Elsner J. Successful treatment with oral isotretinoin of acneiform skin lesions associated with cetuximab therapy. *Br J Dermatol*. 2005;153(4):849-851.

Jatoi A, Rowland K, Sloan JA, et al. Tetracycline to prevent epidermal growth factor receptor inhibitor-induced skin rashes: results of a placebo-controlled trial from the North Central Cancer Treatment Group (N03CB). *Cancer.* 2008;113(4):847-853.

Johnson KS, Levin F, Chu DS. Persistent corneal epithelial defect associated with erlotinib treatment. *Cornea.* 2009;28(6):706-707.

Lacouture ME, Anadkat MJ, Bensadoun RJ, et al. Clinical practice guidelines for the prevention and treatment of EGFR inhibitor-associated dermatologic toxicities. *Support Care Cancer.* 2011;19(8):1079-1095.

Lee SM, Buchler T, Joseph T, Lai C. Bilateral eardrum perforation after long-term treatment with erlotinib. *J Clin Oncol.* 2008;26(15):2582-2584.

Loriot Y, Perlemuter G, Malka D, et al. Drug insight: gastrointestinal and hepatic adverse effects of molecular-targeted agents in cancer therapy. *Nat Clin Pract Oncol.* 2008;5(5):268-278.

Luu M, Boone SL, Patel J, et al. Higher severity grade of erlotinib-induced rash is associated with lower skin phototype. *Clin Exp Dermatol.* 2011;36(7):733-738.

Niyazi M, Maihoefer C, Krause M, Rödel C, Budach W, Belka C. Radiotherapy and "new" drugs-new side effects? *Radiat Oncol.* 2011;6:177.

Pastore S, Lulli D, Girolomoni G. Epidermal growth factor receptor signalling in keratinocyte biology: implications for skin toxicity of tyrosine kinase inhibitors. *Arch Toxicol.* 2014;88 (6):1189-1203.

Pérez-Soler R, Delord JP, Halpern A, et al. HER1/EGFR inhibitor-associated rash: future directions for management and investigation outcomes from the HER1/EGFR inhibitor rash management forum. *Oncologist.* 2005;10(5):345-356.

Saif MW, Gnanaraj J. Erlotinib-induced trichomegaly in a male patient with pancreatic cancer. *Cutan Ocul Toxicol.* 2010;29(1):62-66.

Saint-Jean A, Sainz de la Maza M, Morral M, et al. Ocular adverse events of systemic inhibitors of the epidermal growth factor receptor: report of 5 cases. *Ophthalmology.* 2012;119(9):1798-1802.

Scope A, Agero AL, Dusza SW, et al. Randomized double-blind trial of prophylactic oral minocycline and topical tazarotene for cetuximab-associated acne-like eruption. *J Clin Oncol.* 2007;25(34):5390-5396.

Scope A, Lieb JA, Dusza SW, et al. A prospective randomized trial of topical pimecrolimus for cetuximab-associated acnelike eruption. *J Am Acad Dermatol.* 2009;61(4):614-620.

Vezzoli P, Marzano AV, Onida F, et al. Cetuximab-induced acneiform eruption and the response to isotretinoin. *Acta Derm Venereol.* 2008;88(1):84-86.

Vincenzi B, Tonini G, Santini D. Aprepitant for erlotinib-induced pruritus. *N Engl J Med.* 2010;363 (4):397-398.

Voigt M, Braig F, Göthel M, et al. Functional dissection of the epidermal growth factor receptor epitopes targeted by panitumumab and cetuximab. *Neoplasia.* 2009;14(11):1023-1031.

Watters AL, Epstein JB, Agulnik M. Oral complications of targeted cancer therapies: a narrative literature review. *Oral Oncol.* 2011;47(6):441-448.

MUCOSITIS AND STOMATITIS

Mucositis and stomatitis (also known as mucosal barrier injury) are general terms for the erythema, edema, desquamation, and ulceration of the gastrointestinal tract caused by many antineoplastic drugs and external beam radiation therapy (radiotherapy). Stomatitis refers to the finding of mucositis in the mouth or oropharynx. Gastrointestinal complications of mucositis include pain, xerostomia, bloating, diarrhea, malabsorption, and dysmotility. Airway compromise can develop from severe tissue damage and inflammation. Mucositis is defined as severe (grade 3 to 4) when the pain and anatomic damage prevent adequate oral hydration and oral nutrition, or airway compromise is evident (Table 1). Severe mucositis increases the risk of infectious complications. Moreover, some opportunistic infections, such as herpesvirus, cause and exacerbate mucositis. In addition, severe and prolonged mucositis contributes to anticancer treatment dosage reductions and delays, and increases the cost of therapy.

Table 1. National Cancer Institute (NCI) Common Toxicity Criteria Grading for Mucositis

Grade 0	Grade 1	Grade 2	Grade 3	Grade 4
No signs or symptoms	v3: Mucosal erythema v4: Asymptomatic or mild symptoms; intervention not indicated	v3: Patchy ulcerations v4: Moderate pain; not interfering with oral intake; modified diet indicated	v3: Confluent ulceration, bleeding with minor trauma v4: Severe pain; interfering with oral intake	v3: Tissue necrosis/ bleeding; life-threatening v4: Life-threatening consequences; urgent intervention indicated

The severity of chemotherapy-associated mucositis is related to drug selection, increased dose amount, combination versus single agent chemotherapy, administration rate (eg, extended infusion of cell cycle-specific chemotherapy drugs), route of administration, concurrent radiotherapy, and female gender. Genetic polymorphisms and comorbidities (eg, malnutrition) may also contribute to the risk for mucositis. The frequency of severe mucositis for patients undergoing standard dose therapy and high dose therapy is 5% to 40% and 60% to 100%, respectively. Major organ impairment that prolongs the clearance of anticancer treatments can increase the likelihood and severity of mucositis. Patients with Down syndrome or carriers of the methylenetetrahydrofolate reductase *677 TT* genotype have an increased risk of severe mucositis following methotrexate administration. The severity of mucositis secondary to radiotherapy is related to the anatomic site of radiation exposure, radiation dose, and dosage fractionation. Grade 3 to 4 mucositis occurs in more than 50% of patients undergoing radiotherapy to the head and neck, abdomen, or pelvis. Table 2 lists various anticancer treatments associated with severe mucositis. The duration and severity of regimen-related mucositis can be increased by concurrent infections from opportunistic bacterial or viral pathogens affecting the gastrointestinal tract. Moreover, graft-versus-host disease can worsen regimen-related mucositis following allogeneic hematopoietic stem cell transplantation.

Table 2. Standard Dose Regimens Associated With Grade 3 to 4 Mucositis

Occurring in ≥30% of Patients	Occurring in ≥10% of Patients
Anthracycline + DOCEtaxel + fluorouracil	Anthracycline + cyclophosphamide
Taxane + radiotherapy	Anthracycline + taxane
DOCEtaxel + fluorouracil	Anthracycline + cyclophosphamide + DOCEtaxel
PACLitaxel + fluorouracil + radiotherapy	Anthracycline + cyclophosphamide + PACLitaxel
Taxane + platinum + radiotherapy	
Taxane + platinum + fluorouracil	Anthracycline + DOCEtaxel + platinum
Oxaliplatin + radiotherapy	Capecitabine + DOCEtaxel
Platinum + taxane + radiotherapy	DOCEtaxel
Fluorouracil CIV[1] + platinum + radiotherapy	Platinum + radiotherapy
Fluorouracil + leucovorin + taxane	Platinum + gemcitabine + taxane
Irinotecan	Platinum + taxane + irinotecan
Irinotecan + fluorouracil + radiotherapy	Platinum + methotrexate + leucovorin
Irinotecan + fluorouracil + leucovorin	Fluorouracil CIV[1]
Irinotecan + fluorouracil + leucovorin + platinum	Fluorouracil CIV[1] + radiotherapy
	Fluorouracil CIV[1] + platinum
	Fluorouracil + leucovorin
	Fluorouracil + leucovorin + mitoMYcin
	Irinotecan + taxane
	PRALAtrexate

[1]CIV, continuous intravenous infusion; adapted from Sonis ST, Elting LS, Keefe D, et al. Perspectives on cancer therapy-induced mucosal injury: pathogenesis, measurement, epidemiology, and consequences for patients. *Cancer.* 2004;100(9 Suppl):1995-2025.

MUCOSITIS PREVENTION AND TREATMENT

Evidence-based clinical practice guidelines for management of regimen-related mucositis have been published by the Mucositis Study Group of the Multinational Association of Supportive Care in Cancer and International Society of Oral Oncology (MASCC/ISOO). Recommendations and suggestions from the Mucositis Study Group for and against specific interventions in the management of oral mucositis are presented in Table 3 and Table 4, respectively (Lalla 2014). Recommendations and suggestions for and against specific interventions in the management of gastrointestinal mucositis are presented in Table 7 and Table 8, respectively (Lalla 2014).

Table 3. MASCC/ISOO Oral Mucositis Recommended Interventions

Recommendations supported by level I and II evidence
1. Oral cryotherapy (30 minutes) for prevention of oral mucositis in patients receiving bolus fluorouracil chemotherapy
2. Palifermin to prevent oral mucositis for patients receiving high-dose chemotherapy and total body irradiation, followed by autologous hematopoietic stem cell transplantation (HSCT) for a hematological malignancy
3. Low-level laser therapy to prevent oral mucositis for patients receiving high-dose chemotherapy, (with or without total body irradiation) for HSCT
4. Patient-controlled analgesia using morphine for management of pain due to oral mucositis in patients undergoing HSCT
5. Benzydamine mouthwash to prevent oral mucositis for patients with head and neck cancer receiving moderate-dose radiation therapy (up to 50 Gy) without concomitant chemotherapy (benzydamine is available in Canada; not approved in the US)

(continued) ▶

Table 3. MASCC/ISOO Oral Mucositis Recommended Interventions *(continued)*

Suggestions supported by level III and IV evidence
1. Oral care procedures for prevention of oral mucositis in all age groups and across all cancer treatment settings
2. Oral cryotherapy to prevent oral mucositis for patients receiving high-dose melphalan, with or without total body irradiation, prior to HSCT
3. Low-level laser therapy to prevent oral mucositis for patients undergoing radiotherapy, without concomitant chemotherapy, for head and neck cancer
4. Transdermal fentanyl may be effective to treat pain due to oral mucositis in patients receiving conventional or high-dose chemotherapy, with or without total body irradiation * The patient's opioid tolerance and expected duration of moderate to severe pain must be considered prior to use of transdermal fentanyl.
5. Morphine 2% mouthwash may be effective to treat pain due to oral mucositis in patients receiving chemoradiation for head and neck cancer.
6. Doxepin 0.5% mouthwash may be effective to treat pain due to oral mucositis.
7. Systemic zinc supplements administered orally may be used to prevent oral mucositis in oral cancer patients receiving radiation therapy or chemoradiation.

Good oral hygiene is an essential constituent of routine supportive care for stomatitis and mucositis. Regular, gentle brushing with a soft toothbrush or cotton swab several times a day is helpful in removing dental plaque. Rinsing the mouth with water rinses or a saline/bicarbonate solution helps remove debris and increases the pH, slowing the growth of oral flora. Use of mouthwashes containing alcohol may be painful or may dry the oral mucosa; phenol may promote mucosal ulceration.

Guidelines from the European Society of Medical Oncology (ESMO) on management of oral and gastrointestinal mucosal injury (Peterson 2015) also recommend eliminating sources of oral mucosal trauma (eg, sharp edges or ill-fitting dentures), avoiding hot foods and drinks, and avoiding hard, sharp/crusty, or spicy foods. The ESMO guidelines also recommend regular dental examinations, daily oral mucosa inspections, adequate hydration, and lip balm. Smoking and alcohol should be avoided.

Palifermin is a recombinant human keratinocyte growth factor that works in a receptor-mediated manner to reduce the duration and severity of mucositis by promoting epithelial cell proliferation, differentiation, and migration. Palifermin is indicated to decrease the incidence and duration of severe oral mucositis in patients with hematologic malignancies receiving myelotoxic therapy requiring hematopoietic stem cell support. The 2008 American Society of Clinical Oncology (ASCO) guidelines for the use of chemotherapy and radiotherapy protectants recommend palifermin to decrease the incidence of severe mucositis in patients undergoing autologous stem-cell transplantation with a total body irradiation (TBI) conditioning regimen. Additionally, palifermin may be considered in patients undergoing myeloablative allogeneic stem-cell transplantation with a TBI conditioning regimen. (Goldberg 2013; Hensley 2009). Data are insufficient however, for autologous and allogeneic transplant, to recommend palifermin when the conditioning regimen is chemotherapy only (Hensley 2009). The manufacturer instructs against use of palifermin in patients receiving melphalan 200 mg/m^2 as a conditioning regimen prior to autologous hematopoietic stem cell transplantation due to a lack of efficacy demonstrated in a placebo-controlled trial. The labeled dose for palifermin is 60 mcg/kg/day IV for 3 doses prior to myelotoxic therapy, with the third dose given at least 24 hours before the chemotherapy and then 60 mcg/kg/day for 3 doses after myelotoxic therapy beginning on the same day as hematopoietic stem cell infusion.

Weekly administration of palifermin for reduction of mucositis secondary to chemoradiotherapy for head and neck cancer was tested in two randomized, double-blind, placebo-controlled clinical trials (Henke 2011; Le 2011). In both studies, palifermin administration reduced the incidence, time to onset, and duration of severe mucositis. However, in both studies, patient reported mouth soreness scores and interruptions in therapy were similar for palifermin- and placebo-treated cohorts. Overall survival and disease response were similar for the palifermin- and placebo-treated patients. An exploratory phase II trial testing weekly palifermin versus placebo to reduce dysphagia with chemoradiotherapy for stage III non-small cell lung cancer suggests decreased regimen-related toxicity and improved dose intensity with palifermin administration (Schuette 2012). Single-dose palifermin prior to doxorubicin-based chemotherapy for the treatment of soft tissue sarcoma reduced patient-reported symptoms of oral mucositis (Vandhan-Raj 2010).

Administration of palifermin concurrently with chemotherapy can cause increased severity of mucositis because epithelial cells are stimulated to proliferate when exposed to the systemic cytotoxic therapy. Precautions from the manufacturer include the lack of safety and efficacy data in patients with solid tumors. The effect of palifermin on tumor growth in patients has not been established; however, palifermin promotes in vitro and in vivo epithelial tumor growth in experimental models.

Amifostine has been studied for reduction of chemotherapy-associated mucositis; however, the findings are equivocal. Due to insufficient data, the ASCO guidelines for the use of chemotherapy and radiotherapy protectants do not recommend amifostine to reduce the incidence of radiation therapy-induced mucositis associated with head and neck cancer or to prevent esophagitis due to concurrent chemoradiotherapy in patients with non-small cell lung cancer. Amifostine use to prevent xerostomia in patients with head and neck cancer receiving concurrent platinum-based chemotherapy is not supported; however, the guidelines suggest that the use of amifostine may be considered to reduce the incidence of xerostomia in patients with head and neck cancer undergoing radiation therapy alone (Hensley 2009).

Regular gum chewing by pediatric patients to promote salivation as a means for preventing chemotherapy-induced mucositis did not reduce the rate of severe stomatitis following administration of intensive treatment regimens. However, the frequency of grades 1 to 4 stomatitis was significantly reduced with gum chewing five times daily with lower intensity chemotherapy regimens. In the multivariate analysis, the risk of oral mucositis was related only to the type of chemotherapy regimen used. There is lack of sufficient evidence to support routine use of celecoxib, vitamin E, or allopurinol rinse for prevention of mucositis.

Cryotherapy reduces oral mucositis associated with intravenous bolus administration of fluorouracil, methotrexate, and high-dose melphalan. Cryotherapy requires that the patient hold ice in their mouth for 30 to 60 minutes before and following chemotherapy administration. Cryotherapy purportedly reduces local oromucosal blood flow and consequently reduces chemotherapy exposure to the affected area. Patient tolerance limits the duration of cryotherapy treatments and reduces the utility of cryotherapy for chemotherapy with prolonged systemic clearance or drugs administered by protracted continuous infusion.

◀ **MUCOSITIS OR STOMATITIS DUE TO TARGETED AGENTS**

Oral care for patients taking targeted agents should align with basic oral care for mucositis due to standard chemotherapy. Due to the risk for infections, saline mouth rinses are recommended for these patients (Peterson 2015).

Table 4. Interventions NOT Recommended by MASCC/ISOO for Oral Mucositis

Lack of efficacy supported by level I and II evidence
1. PTA (polymyxin, tobramycin, amphotericin B) and BCoG (bacitracin, clotrimazole, gentamicin) antimicrobial lozenges and PTA paste are not recommended in patients receiving radiation therapy for head and neck cancer.
2. Iseganan antimicrobial mouthwash is not recommended in patients receiving high-dose chemotherapy (with or without total body irradiation) for HSCT or in patients receiving radiation therapy or concomitant chemoradiation for head and neck cancer.
3. Sucralfate mouthwash is not recommended for prevention of oral mucositis in patients receiving chemotherapy for cancer or in patients receiving radiation therapy or chemoradiotherapy for head and neck cancer.
4. Sucralfate mouthwash is not recommended for treatment of oral mucositis in patients receiving chemotherapy for cancer or in patients receiving radiation therapy for head and neck cancer.
5. Intravenous glutamine is not recommended for prevention of oral mucositis in patients receiving high-dose chemotherapy (with or without total body irradiation) for HSCT.
Lack of efficacy supported by level III and IV evidence
1. Chlorhexidine mouthwash is not recommended for prevention of oral mucositis in patients receiving radiation therapy for head and neck cancer.
2. Sargramostim (GM-CSF) mouthwash is not recommended for prevention of oral mucositis in patients receiving high-dose chemotherapy for autologous or allogeneic HSCT.
3. Misoprostol mouthwash is not recommended for prevention of oral mucositis in patients receiving radiation therapy for head and neck cancer.
4. Systemic pentoxifylline, administered orally, is not recommended for prevention of oral mucositis in patients undergoing bone marrow transplantation.
5. Systemic pilocarpine, administered orally, is not recommended for prevention of oral mucositis in patients receiving radiation therapy for head and neck cancer or in patients receiving high-dose chemotherapy (with or without total body irradiation) for HSCT.

Therapy of stomatitis consists primarily of symptomatic support.

Pain control is a crucial part of stomatitis therapy. In addition to making the patient more comfortable, adequate pain control allows the patient to communicate and eat normally, thereby improving quality of life and reducing nutritional complications. Opioid analgesia is frequently required for management of moderate to severe pain from mucositis. Gabapentin may be useful as an adjunct to opioid therapy when additional analgesia is warranted (Bar 2010). Topical application of local anesthetics is the most common approach to management of mild to moderate pain from stomatitis. Local application of cold sometimes provides adequate relief. Diphenhydramine has been used, but may cause drying of local tissues and sedation. Most products also contain significant amounts of alcohol which can exacerbate symptomatology. Local anesthetics (eg, benzocaine, lidocaine, tetracaine) are more potent than diphenhydramine, and are not associated with significant drying of local tissues. However, the numbing effect of these agents can impair swallowing. In addition, most of these products are unpalatable, and some are relatively expensive. The following table lists some of the commonly used agents.

Table 5. Various Mouth Care Products

Product	Concentration(s)	Dosage
Anesthetics		
Benzocaine	5% to 20%	1 to 5 mL; swish and expectorate q4 to 6h
DiphenhydrAMINE	12.5 mg per 5 mL	5 mL; swish and expectorate (or swallow) q4 to 6h
Lidocaine	1%	5 mL; swish and expectorate (or swallow) q2 to 3h
Antimicrobials		
Amphotericin B	100 mg/mL	1 mL qid; swish in mouth as long as possible; swallow or expectorate
Clotrimazole	10 mg	1 troche tid (prophylaxis) One 5 times/day for 14 days (treatment)
Nystatin	100,000 units/mL	5 mL; swish and expectorate (or swallow) q4 to 6h
	100,000 units (vaginal tablet)	1 q4 to 6h (dissolve in mouth)
Mouth Rinses		
Sodium bicarbonate (8.4 g per 50 mEq per 0.9% NaCl [1,000 mL] mixture)	0.5 mEq per 10 mL	5 to 15 mL q3 to 4h
Sodium chloride	0.9%	5 to 15 mL q3 to 4h

Many institutions and prescribers use locally compounded anesthetic formulations for treatment of stomatitis pain. Although the exact formulae may vary tremendously, the general rubric includes a local anesthetic to which one or more of the following are added: A second anesthetic, aluminum hydroxide/magnesium hydroxide suspension, diphenhydramine, hydrocortisone, kaolin/pectin suspension, sucralfate suspension, nystatin, tetracycline, and/or water. Controlled trials comparing various formulations with each other, or with the various individual ingredients are not available. However, these products often form the mainstay of symptomatic treatment for stomatitis. Examples of recipes for a few such formulations are found in Table 6.

A number of groups have studied sucralfate as a therapy for various oral ulcerative conditions with equivocal results. Although the results published to date do not demonstrate a real advantage to sucralfate therapy, some patients may experience subjective benefit from its use. Sucralfate is commercially available as a tablet (1 g) or suspension (1 g/10 mL). When placed into water, the tablet readily absorbs the fluid and forms a gelatinous suspension.

Table 6. Examples of Extemporaneously Compounded Oral Stomatitis Products

Anesthetics

Diphenhydramine syrup 5 mL + lidocaine 2% 5 to 10 mL + aluminum/magnesium hydroxide suspension 5 to 15 mL (Maalox/Mylanta) (may also be referred to as "BMX"). **Note:** Avoid diphenhydramine products containing alcohol.

Lidocaine 2% 45 mL + diphenhydramine elixir 30 mL + sodium bicarbonate 8.4 g + 0.9% sodium chloride qs 1,000 mL

Intubation: Nondepolarizing neuromuscular blockade should be used for the patient with severe mucositis requiring intubation to support the airway. One case report describes succinylcholine-induced hyperkalemia in a patient with severe mucositis following treatment chemotherapy.

Xerostomia

Xerostomia often accompanies stomatitis, particularly in patients who have received radiation to the neck and lower jaw. The condition can result in severe pain, dysphagia, malnutrition, and secondary infections. Subcutaneous or intravenous push administration of amifostine 200 mg/m^2 15 to 30 minutes prior to radiotherapy of the head and neck reduces acute and chronic xerostomia. The dose of amifostine for reduction of radiation-associated xerostomia and mucositis can be standardized to 500 mg in 0.9% sodium chloride 2.5 mL. Benzydamine oral rinse (not available in the United States), which has local anesthetic and anti-inflammatory properties, may be used for the prevention of radiation-induced mucositis in head and neck cancer patients. Artificial saliva substitutes can provide symptomatic relief from dry mouth and throat discomfort following chemotherapy and radiotherapy. Saliva substitutes, which generally contain a mixture of electrolytes, sugar(s), and carboxymethylcellulose, are available without a prescription.

Infections

In spite of good oral hygiene, some patients develop oral infections. This is particularly common in the patient with additional sources of immunosuppression, such as severe neutropenia, treatment with exogenous immunosuppressants, or disease-related immune impairment. One organism most commonly seen in such infections is *Candida albicans*. Topical treatment with nystatin or clotrimazole is usually sufficient to control these infections. Such treatments are usually well tolerated and produce minimal systemic effects. Nystatin 400,000 to 600,000 units (4 to 6 mL) four times a day, swished in the mouth for at least 2 minutes, then swallowed is recommended. Alternatively, nystatin vaginal tablets can be used orally. Clotrimazole 10 mg five times a day is another effective treatment for these infections. Troches are placed under the tongue or in a buccal cavity and allowed to dissolve. In some patients, clotrimazole used three times a day is an effective prophylaxis against oral *Candida* infections. Patients with significant xerostomia may have trouble dissolving the nystatin or clotrimazole tablets, and may require an artificial saliva product to moisten the mouth. Oral or intravenous administration of fluconazole 100 to 200 mg daily may be necessary for treatment of microbiologically documented or presumed oromucosal candidiasis in the patient with moderate to severe mucositis extending proximally beyond the mouth or the patient with additional sources of immune suppression. Fluconazole should be continued for at least 2 weeks, and until microbiologic and clinical evidence of infectious disease have resolved and the patient's immune recovery is considered adequate. Alternative systemic antifungal agents that can be considered for treatment of oromucosal and esophageal candidiasis include anidulafungin, caspofungin, itraconazole, micafungin, posaconazole, voriconazole, and amphotericin B products.

Herpes simplex virus is another common pathogen causing oral and other gastrointestinal infections in the patient with moderate to severe mucositis. The risk for oral Herpes simplex infection is greatest in patients with an additional source of immune compromise. Systemic treatment with acyclovir, famciclovir, or valacyclovir is required for oromucosal or gastrointestinal Herpes simplex infection. Alternative systemic antiviral agents for treatment of resistant Herpes simplex infections include ganciclovir, valganciclovir, and foscarnet.

Gastrointestinal Mucositis

Symptoms of gastrointestinal mucositis include pain, nausea, vomiting, and diarrhea. The following are recommendations/suggestions for and against specific interventions in the management of gastrointestinal mucositis (Lalla 2014).

Table 7. MASCC/ISOO Gastrointestinal Mucositis (Not Including the Oral Cavity) Recommended Interventions

Recommendations supported by level I and II evidence
1. Intravenous amifostine (≥ 340 mg/m^2) is recommended to prevent proctitis in patients receiving radiation treatment
2. Subcutaneous octreotide (≥ 100 mcg twice daily) is recommended to treat chemotherapy-induced diarrhea associated with HSCT (if loperamide is ineffective)
Suggestions supported by level III and IV evidence
1. Intravenous amifostine may be used to prevent esophagitis due to concomitant chemotherapy and radiation therapy in patients with non-small cell lung cancer
2. Sucralfate enemas may be used to treat chronic radiation-induced proctitis in patients with rectal bleeding
3. Systemic sulfasalazine (500 mg orally twice daily) may be used to prevent radiation-induced enteropathy in patients receiving radiation therapy to the pelvis
4. Probiotics containing *Lactobacillus* species may be used to prevent diarrhea in patients receiving chemotherapy and/or radiation therapy for a pelvic malignancy
5. Hyperbaric oxygen may be used to treat radiation-induced proctitis in patients receiving radiation therapy for solid tumors

Table 8. Interventions NOT Recommended by MASCC/ISOO for Gastrointestinal Mucositis

Lack of efficacy supported by level I and II evidence
1. Systemic oral sucralfate is not recommended to treat gastrointestinal mucositis in patients receiving radiation therapy for a solid tumor
2. Oral aspirin (ASA), mesalazine, and olsalazine are not recommended to prevent acute radiation-induced diarrhea in patients receiving radiation therapy for a pelvic malignancy
3. Misoprostol suppositories are not recommended to prevent acute radiation-induced proctitis in patients receiving radiation therapy for prostate cancer

◀ REFERENCES AND SELECTED READINGS

Aisa Y, Mori T, Kudo M, et al. Oral cryotherapy for the prevention of high-dose melphalan-induced stomatitis in allogeneic hematopoietic stem cell transplant recipients. *Support Care Cancer.* 2005;13(4):266-269.

Al-Khafaji AH, Dewhirst WE, Cornell CJ Jr, Quill TJ. Succinylcholine-induced hyperkalemia in a patient with mucositis secondary to chemotherapy. *Crit Care Med.* 2001;29(6):1274-1276.

Alterio D, Jereczek-Fossa BA, Zuccotti GF, et al. Tetracaine oral gel in patients treated with radiotherapy for head-and-neck cancer: final results of a phase II study. *Int J Radiat Oncol Biol Phys.* 2006;64(2):392-395.

Bar Ad V, Weinstein G, Dutta PR, Chalian A, Both S, Quon H. Gabapentin for the treatment of pain related to radiation-induced mucositis in patients with head and neck tumors treated with intensity-modulated radiation therapy. *Head Neck.* 2010;32(2):173-177.

Chan A, Ignoffo RJ. Survey of topical oral solutions for the treatment of chemo-induced oral mucositis. *J Oncol Pharm Pract.* 2005;11(4):139-143.

El-Housseiny AA, Saleh SM, El-Masry AA, Allam AA. The effectiveness of vitamin "E" in the treatment of oral mucositis in children receiving chemotherapy. *J Clin Pediatr Dent.* 2007;31 (3):167-170.

Gandemer V, Le Deley MC, Dollfus C, et al. Multicenter randomized trial of chewing gum for preventing oral mucositis in children receiving chemotherapy. *J Pediatr Hematol Oncol.* 2007;29 (2):86-94.

Garre ML, Relling MV, Kalwinsky D, et al. Pharmacokinetics and toxicity of methotrexate in children with down syndrome and acute lymphocytic leukemia. *J Pediatr.* 1987;111(4):606-612.

Goldberg JD, Zheng J, Castro-Malaspina H, et al. Palifermin is efficacious in recipients of TBI-based but not chemotherapy-based allogeneic hematopoietic stem cell transplants. *Bone Marrow Transplant.* 2013;48(1):99-104.

Gori E, Arpinati M, Bonifazi F, et al. Cryotherapy in the prevention of oral mucositis in patients receiving low-dose methotrexate following myeloablative allogeneic stem cell transplantation: a prospective randomized study of the Gruppo Italiano Trapianto Di Midollo Osseo Nurses group. *Bone Marrow Transplant.* 2007;39(6):347-352.

Henke M, Alfonsi M, Foa P, et al. Palifermin decreases severe oral mucositis of patients undergoing postoperative radiochemotherapy for head and neck cancer: a randomized, placebo-controlled trial. *J Clin Oncol.* 2011;29(20):2815-2820.

Hensley ML, Hagerty KL, Kewalramani T, et al. American Society of Clinical Oncology 2008 clinical practice guideline update: use of chemotherapy and radiotherapy protectants. *J Clin Oncol.* 2009;27(1):127-145.

Javle MM, Cao S, Durrani FA, et al. Celecoxib and mucosal protection: translation from an animal model to a phase I clinical trial of celecoxib, irinotecan, and 5-fluorouracil. *Clin Cancer Res.* 2007;13(3):965-971.

Kepivance (palifermin) [prescribing information]. Stockholm, Sweden: Swedish Orphan Biovitrum; May 2013.

Lalla RV, Bowen J, Barasch A, et al. MASCC/ISOO clinical practice guidelines for the management of mucositis secondary to cancer therapy. *Cancer.* 2014;120(10):1453-1461.

Le QT, Kim HE, Schneider CJ, et al. Palifermin reduces severe mucositis in definitive chemo-radiotherapy of locally advanced head and neck cancer: a randomized, placebo-controlled study. *J Clin Oncol.* 2011;29(20):2808-2814.

Lilleby K, Garcia P, Gooley T, et al. A prospective, randomized study of cryotherapy during administration of high-dose melphalan to decrease the severity and duration of oral mucositis in patients with multiple myeloma undergoing autologous peripheral blood stem cell trans-plantation. *Bone Marrow Transplant.* 2006;37(11):1031-1035.

Mori T, Yamazaki R, Aisa Y, et al. Brief oral cryotherapy for the prevention of high-dose melphalan-induced stomatitis in allogeneic hematopoietic stem cell transplant recipients. *Support Care Cancer.* 2006;14(4):392-395.

National Cancer Institute common terminology criteria for adverse events (CTCAE) version 3. Available at http://ctep.cancer.gov/protocolDevelopment/electronic_applications/docs/ctcaev3. pdf. Accessed October 13, 2014.

National Cancer Institute common terminology criteria for adverse events (CTCAE) version 4.03. Available at http://evs.nci.nih.gov/ftp1/CTCAE/CTCAE_4.03_2010-06-14_QuickReferen-ce_8.5x11.pdf. Accessed September 29, 2014.

Peterson DE, Boers-Doets CB, Bensadoun RJ, Herrstedt J; ESMO Guidelines Committee. Management of oral and gastrointestinal mucosal injury: ESMO Clinical Practice Guidelines for diagnosis, treatment, and follow-up. *Ann Oncol.* 2015;26(Suppl 5):v139-v151.

Potting CM, Uitterhoeve R, Op Reimer WS, Van Achterberg T. The effectiveness of commonly used mouthwashes for the prevention of chemotherapy-induced oral mucositis: a systematic review. *Eur J Cancer Care (Engl).* 2006;15(5):431-439.

Quintiliani R, Owens NJ, Quercia RA, Klimek JJ, Nightingale CH. Treatment and prevention of oropharyngeal candidiasis. *Am J Med*. 1984;77(4D):44-48.

Schuette W, Krzakowski MJ, Massuti B, et al. Randomized phase II study of palifermin for reducing dysphagia in patients receiving concurrent chemoradiotherapy for locally advanced unresectable non-small cell lung cancer. *J Thorac Oncol*. 2012;7(1):157-164.

Sonis ST, Elting LS, Keefe D, et al. Perspectives on cancer therapy-induced mucosal injury: pathogenesis, measurement, epidemiology, and consequences for patients. *Cancer*. 2004;100(9 Suppl):1995-2025.

Stokman MA, Wachters FM, Koopmans P, et al. Outcome of local application of amifostine (WR-1065) on epirubicin-induced oral mucositis. A phase II study. *Anticancer Res*. 2004;24 (5B):3263-3267.

Sung L, Tomlinson GA, Greenberg ML, et al. Serial controlled N-of-1 trials of topical vitamin E as prophylaxis for chemotherapy-induced oral mucositis in paediatric patients. *Eur J Cancer*. 2007;43(8):1269-1275.

Ulrich CM, Yasui Y, Storb R, et al. Pharmacogenetics of methotrexate: toxicity among marrow transplantation patients varies with the methylenetetrahydrofolate reductase C677T polymorphism. *Blood*. 2001;98(1):231-234.

Vadhan-Raj S, Trent J, Patel S, et al. Single-dose palifermin prevents severe oral mucositis during multicyle chemotherapy in patients with cancer: a randomized trial. *Ann Intern Med*. 2010;153 (6):358-367.

Vokurka S, Bystricka E, Koza V, et al. Higher incidence of chemotherapy induced oral mucositis in females: a supplement of multivariate analysis to a randomized multicentre study. *Support Care Cancer*. 2006;14(9):974-976.

Yokomizo H, Yoshimatsu K, Hashimoto M, et al. Prophylactic efficacy of allopurinol ice ball for leucovorin/5-fluorouracil therapy-induced stomatitis. *Anticancer Res*. 2004;24(2C):1131-1134.

PREVENTION AND MANAGEMENT OF INFECTIONS

Certain oncology patients are at increased risk of morbidity and mortality from infectious complications secondary to disease- or treatment-related loss of immunity (see table). Impaired immunity is generally associated with malignancies that arise from hematologic cells and lymphoid tissues. The most common iatrogenic reasons for impaired immunity are repeated courses of chemotherapy, biotherapy, or radiation which are toxic to normal cells of the immune system, the loss of an innate barrier (such as mucositis), and central venous access device placement. Patients undergoing allogeneic hematopoietic stem cell (blood or marrow) transplantation are at great risk for infectious complications because they generally have a hematologic malignancy, receive intensive chemotherapy prior to the bone marrow transplant, and require chronic immunosuppression to prevent graft-versus-host disease.

Table 1. Disease-Related Risks for Infections

Cancer	Corresponding Normal Cell	Infectious Risk
Hodgkin lymphoma	Reed Sternberg cell (B lymphocyte origin)	Encapsulated bacteria; *Pneumocystis jirovecii*; herpes simplex virus and varicella zoster virus; extensive chemotherapy/radiation
Non-Hodgkin lymphoma	B cells (90% of cases) T cells (10% of cases)	*Pneumocystis jirovecii*; herpes simplex virus and varicella zoster virus; extensive chemotherapy/biotherapy/radiation/corticosteroid therapy
Acute lymphoblastic leukemia	B cells (90% of cases) T cells (10% of cases)	Extensive chemotherapy/radiation/corticosteroid therapy
Acute myeloid leukemia	Myeloid blood cell(s)	Extensive chemotherapy/radiation
Chronic lymphocytic leukemia	B cells (90% of cases) T cells (10% of cases)	Atypical infections secondary to chronic immune impairment with protracted indolent course of disease; chemotherapy/biotherapy

Neutropenia increases the risk of developing infection. The likelihood of morbidity or mortality from infection escalates as the severity, rate of decline, and duration of neutropenia increase. The underlying cause of neutropenia is often anticancer treatment; however, it can also be secondary to the patient's malignant disease. It is important to distinguish the neutrophil count from the white blood cell count. The white blood cell count represents the sum of different types of white blood cells, including neutrophils, monocytes, lymphocytes, basophils, and mast cells. Patients with leukemias can present with a normal or markedly elevated white blood cell count, and at the same time, be profoundly neutropenic because the vast majority of their circulating blood cells are blasts (malignant hematologic cells). An absolute neutrophil count (ANC) <500 cells/mm^3 blood increases the risk of infectious complications. In fact, patients are considered "high-risk" neutropenics when the ANC is ≤100 cells/mm^3 blood for ≥7 days. Additional clinical criteria for identification of patients at high risk for infection-related morbidity include unstable vital signs, pneumonia, new onset abdominal pain, and neurologic changes. The ANC is calculated as follows:

ANC = WBC x [(% segmented neutrophils + % band neutrophils) / 100]

Most anticancer treatments reduce immunity by causing neutropenia and mucositis. However, some drugs also impair the adaptive arm of immunity, which includes cell-mediated immunity and antibody production. Examples include monoclonal antibodies (eg, alemtuzumab, rituximab), denileukin diftitox, bortezomib, the cytotoxic purine nucleotides (eg, clofarabine, fludarabine, nelarabine), and corticosteroids (eg, dexamethasone, methylprednisolone, prednisone). Anti-CD20 antibodies (eg, rituximab, ofatumumab, obinutuzumab) increase the risk of hepatitis B virus (HBV) reactivation and disease. Severe and lethal cases of fulminant hepatitis and hepatic failure are attributed to HBV reactivation and disease during and following anti-CD20 antibody therapy. HBV reactivation occurring up to 12 months following discontinuation of anti-CD20 antibody therapy has been reported. The American Society of Clinical Oncology (ASCO) provisional clinical opinion update on hepatitis B virus screening (Hwang 2015) recommends screening patients for HBV prior to initiation of anti-CD20 antibody therapy to identify patients with chronic or clinically resolved HBV infection. Serologic tests to detect HBV virus include Hepatitis B surface antigen (HBsAg) and hepatitis B core antibody (anti-HBc) measurements; either a total anti-HBc (with both IgG and IgM) or anti-HBc IgG test should be used to screen for chronic or unresolved HBV infection (do not use anti-HBc IgM as it may only confirm acute HBV infection). In addition, clinical and laboratory signs of hepatitis or HBV should be monitored during and for several months after treatment with anti-CD20 antibodies. The ASCO provisional clinical opinion recommends initiation of prophylactic antiviral treatment for patients with chronic HBV infection (HBsAg-positive/anti-HBc-positive) without delaying anticancer therapy. Selection of antiviral therapy should be based on products with low rates of viral resistance. Antiviral therapy should be continued for ~6- to 12-months following completion of anti-CD20 antibody therapy. Providers should monitor patients with a clinically resolved HBV infection (HBsAg-negative/anti-HBc-positive) by serial analysis of serum alanine aminotransferase or HBV DNA approximately every 3 months with prompt initiation of antiviral therapy as warranted by laboratory findings. In addition, patients with risk factors for HBV infection (eg, residence in a geographic location with ≥2% HBV prevalence, household or sexual contact with HBV-infected patients, high-risk behaviors [eg, intravenous drug use], HIV infection) should also be screened and monitored for HBV infection or reactivation prior to beginning anti-CD20 antibody administration.

The most frequent source of opportunistic pathogens is the patient or close human contacts. Common causes of gram-positive bacterial infections include *Staphylococcus aureus*, *Staphylococcus epidermidis*, *Streptococcus pneumoniae*, *Streptococcus pyogenes*, *Streptococcus viridans*, *Enterococcus faecalis*, *Enterococcus faecium*, and *Corynebacterium* spp. Common causes of gram-negative bacterial infections include *Escherichia coli*, *Klebsiella pneumoniae*, and *Pseudomonas* spp. *Candida albicans* generally colonizes mucous membranes of the gastrointestinal and urogenital tract. Environmental sources of opportunistic pathogens include the surface of fresh fruits and vegetables (bacteria), dried foliage, tobacco, marijuana leaves (*Aspergillus* spp); recent construction or renovation (*Aspergillus* spp); and tap water (*Legionella* spp). Rarely, viruses can be transmitted by blood products (packed red blood cells, platelets, stem cells) or plasma-derived products (intravenous immune globulin).

Thorough and frequent handwashing and sanitation reduce the risk of transmitting opportunistic pathogens to neutropenic patients. In addition, limiting the number of visitations and personal contacts also reduces opportunity for transmission of opportunistic pathogens. Additional preventive measures which are generally implemented to reduce the risk of infection in patients at greatest risk (eg, allogeneic bone marrow transplant patients) include hospital room-specific supplies and instrumentation, HEPA filtration of patient rooms or nursing units, total room clean following discharge, low microbial diets, and diligent mouth care. HEPA filtration involves circulation of room air through a filter 8 to 12 times/hour to remove small airborne particles. Low microbial diets prohibit ingestion of fresh fruits and vegetables, or undercooked meat. Diligent mouth care requires swishing and expectoration of mouthwash 4 to 6 times daily. Mouthwashes may be 0.9% NaCl or dilute bicarbonate solution (sodium bicarbonate 50 mEq/L in sterile water); frequent use is important in order to remove oral debris and thereby prohibit microbial growth. Nonpharmacologic methods for reducing risk of opportunistic infection should be risk-based and guided by institutional policy due to the limited availability of clinical literature stringently supporting the efficacy of some interventions.

Selective gut decontamination with sulfamethoxazole-trimethoprim or a fluoroquinolone is used to reduce gram-negative colonization in patients undergoing intensive chemotherapy. Selective gut decontamination allows continued colonization of the lower gastrointestinal tract with anaerobic bacteria, which lessens the possibility of fungal overgrowth. Judicious use of antibacterial prophylaxis (antibacterial and antifungal) for patients with severe neutropenia expected to last more than 7 days is recommended by ASCO clinical practice guidelines for outpatient management of fever and neutropenia in adults (Flowers 2013). Antibacterial prophylaxis may be considered for certain patients with hematologic malignancies. Cautious (vs routine) use of antibacterial prophylaxis is recommended due to the associated risk of *Clostridium difficile* diarrhea and emergence of resistance organisms. High-risk patients undergoing treatment with intensive chemotherapy, such as allogeneic hematopoietic stem cell transplant recipients, or patients with acute myeloid leukemia receiving induction chemotherapy, may also receive prophylactic acyclovir (or an equivalent antiviral) and antifungal prophylaxis. An oral triazole antifungal agent is generally used for antifungal prophylaxis; agent selection is based on the risk for invasive fungal disease and oromucosal candidiasis. Allogeneic bone marrow transplant recipients at risk for cytomegalovirus infection may receive prophylactic ganciclovir following engraftment. Sulfamethoxazole-trimethoprim is administered chronically to prevent *Pneumocystis jirovecii* pneumonia in some patients undergoing repeated chemotherapy treatments or alemtuzumab therapy for lymphoid malignancies. Alternative agents used for pneumocystis prophylaxis in patients allergic to sulfanilamide-type antibacterials include pentamidine, dapsone, and atovaquone.

Guidelines from the Infectious Diseases Society of America (IDSA) for vaccination of the immunocompromised host (Rubin 2014) endorse that the responsibility for ensuring appropriate immunization of patients with cancer is shared by the specialists providing oncology care and the primary care provider. Annual administration of inactivated influenza vaccine (IIV) is recommended for all patients ≥6 months with malignant disease, except for patients receiving anti-B-cell antibodies, such as rituximab, ofatumumab, or obinutuzumab, or intensive chemotherapy, such as induction or consolidation chemotherapy for acute leukemia. Administration of a single dose of 13-valent pneumococcal conjugate vaccine (PCV13) is recommended for newly diagnosed adult cancer patients. In addition, a single dose of pneumococcal polysaccharide vaccine-23 (PPSV23) should be given at least 8 weeks following administration of the PCV13 vaccination (in patients ≥2 years). For patients who have previously received PPSV23, a single dose of PCV13 may be administered one year or longer after PPSV23 administration. Immunosuppression caused by anticancer therapy may reduce the efficacy of immunization. Vaccinations administered during chemotherapy should not be considered protective without testing for protective antibody level(s). Live viral vaccines should not be administered to patients receiving chemotherapy. In addition to reduced immunization efficacy, there is a potential risk for opportunistic infection secondary to administration of live virus vaccines to profoundly immunocompromised patients. According to the IDSA guidelines, patients should be vaccinated 3 months after completion of chemotherapy and at least 6 months following administration of anti-B-cell antibodies with inactivated and live vaccines for varicella, measles, mumps, and rubella according to the schedule recommended routinely for immunocompetent patients by the Centers for Disease Control (available at http://www.cdc.gov/vaccines/schedules/).

The management of microbiologically identified infections in cancer patients is directed by the nature and degree of immune compromise and the identified or suspected pathogen(s). Cancer patients without disease-related or treatment-related immune suppression are managed as appropriate for the type and severity of infection. A comprehensive discussion on all potential infections in cancer patients is outside of the scope of this chapter.

Fever is frequently the only sign of infection in the neutropenic patient. Febrile neutropenic patients are empirically managed for presumed infection. Fever is defined as single oral temperature exceeding 38.3°C (101°F), or oral temperature 38°C (100.4°F) for at least 60 minutes. Evaluation of the febrile neutropenic patient should determine whether the individual is at high risk or low risk (table 2) for infection-related morbidity and mortality. The evaluation should include medical history and physical examination, chest radiograph, blood cultures drawn from the central venous line (all ports), blood cultures drawn by peripheral venipuncture, specimens of urine and diarrheal stool, plus additional specimens as indicated by history and physical examination. Blood cultures must be drawn prior to initiation of antimicrobials to increase the likelihood of acquiring a positive culture; although, blood cultures generally remain negative due to the small inoculum of microbes needed to cause infection in the neutropenic host and due to the early initiation of broad spectrum antibacterials. Empiric treatment with broad spectrum, bactericidal antibiotics should be initiated as soon as possible after blood cultures have been collected. Clinical practice guidelines recommend the administration of antimicrobial therapy within one hour of fever documentation. Choice of therapy greatly depends on the clinical status of the patient (ie, high vs low risk), as well as the presumed origin of infection based on clinical presentation. Hospitalization with the administration of intravenous antimicrobials is warranted for most patients with febrile neutropenia. Oral therapy (eg, amoxicillin/clavulanate plus a fluoroquinolone) can be considered for patients at low risk for medical complications from febrile neutropenia. ASCO guidelines caution that any and all clinical conditions and comorbidities must be considered in addition to those listed in the MASCC Scoring System when considering whether a patient is at high risk or low risk for morbidity and mortality from febrile neutropenia (Flowers 2013). Intravenous antimicrobials should be infused through alternating central venous line ports.

Table 2. MASCC Scoring System to Identify Patients at Low Risk of Medical Complications From Febrile Neutropenia

Characteristic	Weight
Burden of febrile neutropenia	
No or mild symptoms	5
Moderate symptoms	3
Severe symptoms or moribund	0
No hypotension (SBP >90 mmHg)	5
No chronic obstructive pulmonary disease	4
Solid tumor or hematologic malignancy with no previous fungal infection	4
No dehydration requiring parenteral fluids	3
Outpatient status	3
Age <60 years	2

Score of ≥21 = low risk for medical complications from febrile neutropenia

Monotherapy (eg, cefepime, meropenem, piperacillin/tazobactam) or dual therapy (aminoglycoside or ciprofloxacin plus an antipseudomonal penicillin) should be initiated for treatment of high-risk febrile neutropenia. Dual therapy is generally reserved for patients with hemodynamic instability or evidence of a gram-negative bacterial infection. The antipseudomonal beta lactam can be replaced with aztreonam for severely penicillin-allergic patients; an antimicrobial with activity against gram-positive organisms must be added to aztreonam to provide broad spectrum antibacterial activity. The choice of monotherapy vs dual therapy is determined by the patient's history and physical examination. The effect of antimicrobial therapy should be assessed in 72 hours or as indicated by the patient's clinical status.

Vancomycin is not recommended as a routine component of initial empiric therapy in the neutropenic patient due to concerns of emerging resistant organisms. Vancomycin should only be considered for patients considered high-risk for serious gram-positive infections. Criteria for use of vancomycin in the febrile neutropenia patient are listed in the table below. Vancomycin should be used in combination with a bactericidal agent that has activity against gram-negative organisms, including *Pseudomonas* spp (eg, cefepime, a carbapenem, or piper-acillin/tazobactam). To minimize the development of resistant organisms, treatment with vancomycin should be discontinued in 2 to 3 days if resistant gram-positive organisms have not been identified. If history or cultures suggest vancomycin-resistant organisms (eg, enterococci), treatment options include daptomycin or linezolid. Monitor serum creatine kinase (CPK) levels at baseline and at least once weekly for patients receiving daptomycin treatment. Myelosuppression is a reported side effect of linezolid. Use of this product in patients undergoing treatment with chemotherapy is reported in the medical literature; however, linezolid should be used with caution in any patients with additional risk factors for leukopenia, thrombocytopenia, or anemia.

Criteria for Use of Vancomycin in Febrile Neutropenia

- Clinically apparent, serious, catheter-related infection
- Positive blood cultures for gram positive bacteria prior to final identification and susceptibility testing
- Colonization with penicillin/cephalosporin-resistant pneumococci or methicillin resistant *Staphylococcus aureus*
- Clinically unstable (eg, hypotension, shock) without an identified pathogen
- Soft tissue infection; health care-associated pneumonia

The low-risk febrile neutropenic patient who defervesces within 72 hours following appropriate antibiotic therapy and is free of signs and symptoms of infection, may be converted to oral antimicrobials (second generation cephalosporin or fluoroquinolone). Criteria for considering a patient high risk and continuing intravenous antimicrobials include signs and symptoms of sepsis at presentation, additional signs of infection such as pneumonia or endocarditis, moderate to severe mucositis, dermal or mucosal loss of integrity, impending invasive procedure(s), or impending immunosuppressive therapy. If the patient remains febrile despite 72 hours of broad spectrum antibiotic coverage, the selection of antimicrobials can be changed or additional agents can be started. Vancomycin can be discontinued in patients who are clinically stable with no positive gram-positive cultures. Additional antimicrobials should be added to patients who appear acutely ill from infection or are at high risk for infectious complications. The choice of antibiotic, which is dependent on current antimicrobial therapy in addition to the patient's history and physical examination, may include vancomycin, second gram-negative agent, antifungal with activity against invasive mold infections (voriconazole, isavuconazonium, caspofungin, an amphotericin product), or antianaerobic agent (metronidazole). Atypical pathogens, including *Legionella pneumoniae*, invasive molds (*Aspergillus* spp, *Fusarium* spp, mucormycoses), and viruses (cytomegalovirus [CMV], adenovirus, herpes simplex), should be considered in the chronically immunosuppressed patient. An echinocandin antifungal agent (anidulofungin, caspofungin, micafungin) or fluconazole are used for the treatment of mucocutaneous candidiasis in the neutropenic patient. Treatment with an antifungal should be started for patients with persistent fevers, despite 5 to 7 days of appropriate empiric antibiotic therapy, as prolonged and persistent neutropenia is a risk factor for invasive aspergillosis. Initial antifungal therapy for presumed or microbiologically documented aspergillosis is a triazole antifungal with antiaspergillus activity (isavuconazonium, posaconazole, voriconazole), an amphotericin product, or an echinocandin. Itraconazole has activity against *Aspergillus* spp; however, characteristics of the formulation(s) make it a less attractive option to use than posaconazole or voriconazole. Isavuconazonium is approved for the treatment of invasive aspergillosis and mucormycosis. Appropriate empiric treatment for suspected viral infection would include acyclovir, but valacyclovir or famciclovir are reasonable alternatives. Treatment with ganciclovir, valganciclovir, or foscarnet is recommended if there is concern for CMV. Ganciclovir plus intravenous immune globulin are administered for CMV pneumonitis. Cidofovir or ribavirin are options for treatment of adenovirus infections (Tomblyn 2009). Positive cultures and antibiotic sensitivity reports may streamline therapy in the stable patient. However, the high-risk patient may continue receiving broad spectrum antibacterials because the finding of a specific pathogen does not exclude the possibility of additional infecting organisms in the neutropenic patient.

◄ Central venous line removal is done judiciously due to the ongoing need for intravenous fluids, drugs, and blood products in the neutropenic and thrombocytopenic patient, and the risk of infection or bleeding with insertion of a new central venous line. Empiric antimicrobials should be continued until the patient is afebrile and clinically stable. Empiric antimicrobials can be discontinued after 7 days in the low-risk neutropenic patient. One may consider discontinuation of empiric antimicrobials in the high-risk neutropenic patient following 5 to 7 days without fever. Although, antimicrobials should be continued until the ANC is at least 500 cells/mm^3 and severe mucositis, or signs and symptoms of sepsis have resolved. Four to 5 days following resolution of neutropenia, discontinuation of antimicrobials may be considered in the low-risk, neutropenic, clinically stable patient with persistent fevers. With close observation and follow-up, antimicrobials may be discontinued after 2 weeks of therapy in the clinically stable patient with persistent fever and persistent neutropenia.

Myeloid growth factors, which reduce the duration of neutropenia, are helpful in reducing hospital admission for neutropenic fevers in patients with a history of febrile neutropenia or prolonged neutropenia following outpatient chemotherapy. The ASCO guidelines for the use of WBC growth factors (Smith 2015) recommend primary prophylaxis with myeloid growth factors after administration of chemotherapy with a ≥20% risk of febrile neutropenia and, if appropriate, in patients receiving dose-dense chemotherapy. Secondary prophylaxis is recommended by the ASCO WBC guidelines for patients who experience a neutropenic complication from a prior chemotherapy cycle (where primary WBC growth factors were not employed) and when a dose reduction or treatment delay may affect overall survival or treatment outcome.

Patients with chronic lymphocytic leukemia do not produce antibodies effectively and may require periodic administration of intravenous immune globulin to maintain normal serum immunoglobulin levels. Impaired production of endogenous immunoglobulins also occurs with administration of monoclonal antibodies directed against the CD20 ligand (ofatumumab, obinutuzumab, rituximab) and following allogeneic hematopoietic stem cell transplantation.

SELECTED READINGS

Centers for Disease Control and Prevention (CDC). Immunization schedules. Available at http://www.cdc.gov/vaccines/schedules/. Last accessed August 3, 2015.

Flowers CR, Seidenfeld J, Bow EJ, et al. Antimicrobial prophylaxis and outpatient management of fever and neutropenia in adults treated for malignancy: American Society of Clinical Oncology clinical practice guideline. *J Clin Oncol.* 2013;31(6):794-810.

Freifeld AG, Bow EJ, Sepkowitz KA, et al. Clinical practice guideline for the use of antimicrobial agents in neutropenic patients with cancer: 2010 update by the Infectious Diseases Society of America. *Clin Infect Dis.* 2011;52(4):427-431.

Hwang JP, Somerfield MR, Alston-Johnson DE, et al. Hepatitis B virus screening for patients with cancer before therapy: American Society of Clinical Oncology provisional clinical opinion update. *J Clin Oncol.* 2015;33(19):2212-2220.

Rubin LG, Levin MJ, Ljungman P, et al. 2013 IDSA clinical practice guideline for vaccination of the immunocompromised host. *Clin Infect Dis.* 2014;58(3):309-318.

Smith TJ, Bohlke K, Lyman GH, et al. Recommendations for the use of WBC growth factors: American Society of Clinical Oncology clinical practice guideline update [published online July 13, 2015]. *J Clin Oncol.*

Tomblyn M, Chiller T, Einsele H, et al. Guidelines for preventing infectious complications among hematopoietic cell transplantation recipients: a global perspective. *Biol Blood Marrow Transplant.* 2009;15(10):1143-1238.

PREVENTION OF CHEMOTHERAPY-INDUCED NAUSEA AND VOMITING IN CHILDREN

Note: Unless otherwise specified, emetogenic potential listed is for single agent treatment. For multi-agent regimens, if not otherwise specified, emetogenic potential should be based on the component with the higher emetic potential.

Highly Emetogenic Chemotherapy (Frequency of Emesis: >90%)

Altretamine
CARBOplatin
Carmustine >250 mg/m^2
CISplatin
Cyclophosphamide ≥1,000 mg/m^2
Cytarabine 3,000 mg/m^2
Dacarbazine
DACTINomycin
Mechlorethamine
Methotrexate ≥12 g/m^2
Procarbazine (oral)
Streptozocin

Thiotepa ≥300 mg/m^2
Multi-agent regimens:
    Cyclophosphamide + Anthracycline
    (doxorubicin or epirubicin)
    Cyclophosphamide + Etoposide
    Cytarabine 150 to 200 mg/m^2 +
    Daunorubicin
    Cytarabine 300 mg/m^2 + Etoposide
    Cytarabine 300 mg/m^2 + Teniposide
    Doxorubicin + Ifosfamide
    Doxorubicin + Methotrexate 5 g/m^2
    Etoposide + Ifosfamide

Moderately Emetogenic Chemotherapy (Frequency of Emesis: 30% to 90%)

Aldesleukin >12 to 15 million units/m^2
Amifostine >300 mg/m^2
Arsenic trioxide
AzaCITIDine
Bendamustine
Busulfan (IV)
Carmustine ≤250 mg/m^2
Clofarabine
Cyclophosphamide <1,000 mg/m^2 (IV)
Cyclophosphamide (oral)
Cytarabine >200 mg/m^2 to
   <3,000 mg/m^2
DAUNOrubicin
DOXOrubicin
EPIrubicin

Etoposide (oral)
IDArubicin
Ifosfamide
Imatinib
Intrathecal treatment (methotrexate
   and/or cytarabine ± hydrocortisone)
Irinotecan
Lomustine
Melphalan >50 mg/m^2
Methotrexate ≥250 **mg**/m^2 to <12 **g**/m^2
Mitotane
Oxaliplatin ≥75 mg/m^2
Temozolomide (IV)
Temozolomide (oral)

Low Emetogenic Chemotherapy (Frequency of Emesis: 10% to <30%)

Aldesleukin ≤12 million units/m^2
Amifostine ≤300 mg/m^2
Bexarotene (oral)
Busulfan (oral)
Capecitabine
Cytarabine ≤200 mg/m^2
DOCEtaxel
DOXOrubicin (liposomal)
Etoposide (IV)
Everolimus
Fludarabine (oral)
Fluorouracil

Gemcitabine
Ixabepilone
Methotrexate >50 to <250 mg/m^2
MitoMYcin
MitoXANtrone
Nilotinib
PACLitaxel
PACLitaxel (protein bound)
PEMEtrexed
Teniposide
Thiotepa <300 mg/m^2
Topotecan
Tretinoin
Vorinostat

◀ **Minimal Emetogenic Chemotherapy (Frequency of Emesis: <10%)**

Alemtuzumab
Asparaginase
Bevacizumab
Bleomycin
Bortezomib
Cetuximab
Chlorambucil
Cladribine
Dasatinib
Decitabine
Denileukin diftitox
Dexrazoxane
Erlotinib
Fludarabine (IV)
Gefitinib
Gemtuzumab ozogamicin
Hydroxyurea
Interferon alfa
Lapatinib
Lenalidomide

Melphalan (oral, low dose)
Mercaptopurine (oral)
Methotrexate ≤50 mg/m^2
Methotrexate (oral)
Nelarabine
Panitumumab
Pegaspargase
Peginterferon alfa
Pentostatin
RiTUXimab
SORAfenib
SUNITtinib
Temsirolimus
Thalidomide
Thioguanine (oral)
Trastuzumab
Valrubicin
VinBLAStine
VinCRIStine
Vinorelbine (IV)

Prevention of Acute Nausea and Vomiting

Acute nausea and vomiting includes vomiting, retching, or nausea which occurs within 24 hours of administration of chemotherapeutic agents. Guidelines for prevention of acute nausea and vomiting from the Pediatric Oncology Group of Ontario (POGO) recommend the following for pediatric patients ages 1 month to 18 years (Dupuis 2013):

For prevention of acute nausea and vomiting due to chemotherapy with **highly** emetogenic risk:
Children ≥12 years and Adolescents receiving chemotherapy agents that do **not** potentially interact with aprepitant: Ondansetron or granisetron plus dexamethasone plus aprepitant
Children ≥12 years and Adolescents receiving chemotherapy agents that **potentially** interact with aprepitant: Ondansetron or granisetron plus dexamethasone
Infants and Children <12 years: Ondansetron or granisetron plus dexamethasone
Pediatric patients receiving highly emetogenic chemotherapeutic agents who cannot receive corticosteroids (due to contraindications): Ondansetron or granisetron plus chlorpromazine or nabilone

For prevention of acute nausea and vomiting due to chemotherapy with **moderately** emetogenic risk:
Infants, Children, and Adolescents: Ondansetron or granisetron plus dexamethasone
Pediatric patients receiving moderately emetogenic chemotherapeutic agents who cannot receive corticosteroids (due to contraindications): Ondansetron or granisetron plus chlorpromazine or metoclopramide or nabilone

For prevention of acute nausea and vomiting due to chemotherapy with **low** emetogenic risk:
Infants, Children, and Adolescents: Ondansetron or granisetron

For prevention of acute nausea and vomiting due to chemotherapy with **minimal** emetogenic risk: No routine prophylaxis

Pediatric Antiemetic Dosing Based on Emetogenic Potential

Name	Chemotherapy Emetogenic Potential	Route/Dose
Serotonin Antagonists		
Granisetron	High	IV: 40 mcg/kg/dose as a single daily dose
	Moderate or low	IV: 40 mcg/kg/dose as a single daily dose
		Oral: 40 mcg/kg/dose every 12 hours
Ondansetron	High	IV, Oral: 0.15 mg/kg/dose (5 mg/m^2/dose); prior to chemotherapy and then every 8 hours (maximum recommended IV dose: 16 mg)
	Moderate	IV, Oral: 0.15 mg/kg/dose (5 mg/m^2/dose); prior to chemotherapy and then every 12 hours (maximum: 8 mg/dose)
	Low	IV, Oral: 0.3 mg/kg/dose (10 mg/m^2/dose); prior to chemotherapy (maximum IV dose: 16 mg)
Substance P/Neurokinin 1 Receptor Antagonist		
Aprepitant	High or moderate*	Children's <12 years and ≥30 kg*, Children ≥12 years, and Adolescents: Oral: 125 mg on day 1, followed by 80 mg once daily on days 2 and 3
Corticosteroid		
Dexamethasone	High	IV, Oral: 6 mg/m^2/dose every 6 hours. **Note:** If administering with aprepitant, reduce dexamethasone dose by 50%
	Moderate	IV, Oral: ≤0.6 m^2: 2 mg every 12 hours; >0.6 m^2 4 mg every 12 hours. **Note:** If administering with aprepitant, reduce dexamethasone dose by 50%
Phenothiazine		
ChlorproMAZINE	High or moderate	IV: 0.5 mg/kg/dose every 6 hours
Dopamine Receptor Antagonist		
Metoclopramide	Moderate	IV, Oral: 1 mg/kg/dose IV prior to chemotherapy, then 0.0375 mg/kg/dose orally every 6 hours (administer concomitantly with diphenhydramine or benztropine)
Cannabinoid		
Nabilone	High or moderate	Oral: <18 kg: 0.5 mg twice daily; 18 to 30 kg: 1 mg twice daily; >30 kg: 1 mg 3 times daily. Maximum daily dose: 0.06 mg/kg/**day**

*Aprepitant for moderate emetogenic potential and for children <12 years and ≥30 kg is from the prescribing information.

◀ **Prevention and Treatment of Anticipatory Nausea and Vomiting**

The risk for anticipatory nausea and vomiting will be minimized if acute and delayed nausea and vomiting associated with chemotherapy are optimally managed. If anticipatory nausea and vomiting develop, interventions including hypnosis and/or systematic desensitization (eg, deep muscle relaxation with imagery) may be offered to help manage symptoms (Dupuis 2014; Roila 2010). Guidelines for prevention and treatment of anticipatory nausea and vomiting from POGO recommend the following for pediatric patients ages 1 month to 18 years (Dupuis 2014): Lorazepam 0.04 to 0.08 mg/kg/dose (maximum dose: 2 mg) administered orally once at bedtime the evening prior to chemotherapy and once prior to chemotherapy the next day may be used to prevent or treat anticipatory nausea and vomiting.

REFERENCES

Basch E, Prestrud AA, Hesketh PJ, et al. Antiemetics: American Society of Clinical Oncology clinical practice guideline update. *J Clin Oncol.* 2011;29(31):4189-4198.

Dupuis LL, Boodhan S, Holdsworth M, et al. Guideline for the prevention of acute nausea and vomiting due to antineoplastic medication in pediatric cancer patients. *Pediatr Blood Cancer.* 2013;60(7):1073-1082.

Dupuis LL, Boodhan S, Sung L, et al. Guideline for the classification of the acute emetogenic potential of antineoplastic medication in pediatric cancer patients. *Pediatr Blood Cancer.* 2011;57 (2):191-198.

Dupuis LL, Robinson PD, Boodhan S, et al. Guideline for the prevention and treatment of anticipatory nausea and vomiting due to chemotherapy in pediatric cancer patients. *Pediatr Blood Cancer.* 2014;61(8):1506-1512.

Emend (aprepitant) [prescribing information]. Whitehouse Station, NJ: Merck & Co; August 2015.

Multinational Association of Supportive Care in Cancer. MASCC/ESMO antiemetic guideline 2013. http://www.mascc.org/assets/documents/mascc_guidelines_english_2013.pdf. Accessed October 2013.

National Comprehensive Cancer Network (NCCN). Clinical practice guidelines in oncology: antiemesis. v.2.2014. http://www.nccn.org/professionals/physician_gls/PDF/antiemesis.pdf

Roila F, Herrstedt J, Aapro M, et al. Guideline update for MASCC and ESMO in the prevention of chemotherapy- and radiotherapy-induced nausea and vomiting: results of the Perugia consensus conference. *Ann Oncol.* 2010;21(Suppl 5):v232-v243.

TUMOR LYSIS SYNDROME

INTRODUCTION

Tumor lysis syndrome (TLS) is a potentially life-threatening disorder that is characterized as an acute metabolic disturbance resulting from the rapid destruction of tumor cells. Cellular destruction releases intracellular constituents (nucleic acids, anions, cations, peptides) that overwhelm the body's normal mechanisms for their utilization, excretion, and elimination. Signs and symptoms of TLS often develop within 72 hours of beginning cytotoxic chemotherapy in patients with newly diagnosed acute leukemias (acute lymphoblastic leukemia [ALL] and acute myeloid leukemia [AML]) or lymphoproliferative malignancies (Burkitt's and non-Burkitt's lymphomas). Moreover, TLS can occur spontaneously in malignant diseases with vigorous cell turnover. Although most commonly reported in patients with hematologic and lymphoid malignancies, TLS has also been reported with solid tumors such as breast cancer, colon cancer, melanoma, ovarian cancer, prostate cancer, small cell lung cancer, and testicular cancer. Acute TLS attributed to administration of a corticosteroid, imatinib, rituximab, sorafenib, and zoledronic acid in patients with treatment-sensitive tumors have been reported in the medical literature. Additional treatment and diagnostic procedures attributed with causing tumor lysis syndrome include total body irradiation, splenic irradiation, staging laparotomy, laparoscopic splenectomy preceded by splenic artery embolization, and radiofrequency interstitial thermal ablation of metastatic hepatic lesions. Metabolic abnormalities associated with acute TLS include hyperphosphatemia, hyperkalemia, hyperuricemia, azotemia, hypocalcemia, and metabolic acidosis. Cardiac arrhythmias, seizures, and major organ failure can occur in severe cases of TLS. Hyperkalemia, hyperuricemia, and hypocalcemia can produce cardiac arrhythmias, tetany, and sudden death. Acute renal failure can occur due to precipitation of uric acid and calcium phosphate in the renal tubules.

PREDISPOSING FACTORS

1. Leukemia with high white blood cell count (>25,000/mm^3) or rapidly increasing peripheral blast count

2. Solid tumors with bulky disease (>10 cm), high tumor cell proliferation rate, wide metastatic dispersal, and/or bone marrow involvement

3. Acute myeloid leukemia with history of chronic myelomonocytic leukemia

4. Marked sensitivity of the tumor to a particular treatment modality

5. Renal impairment, including preexisting volume depletion

6. Elevated pretreatment lactic dehydrogenase (LDH) serum concentrations (>2 times ULN)

7. Elevated pretreatment uric acid (>7.5 mg/dL), potassium, and/or phosphate serum concentrations independent of renal impairment

CLINICAL FEATURES AND TREATMENT

Classification and Risk Stratification

TLS can be described as either laboratory (LTLS) or clinical (CTLS) type. LTLS is the presence of 2 or more abnormal lab values or a 25% change in lab values within 3 days before or 7 days after chemotherapy. Laboratory values to monitor include uric acid, potassium, phosphorus, and calcium. CTLS is defined as LTLS with at least one clinical manifestation such as renal insufficiency, seizures, cardiac arrhythmias, or sudden death.

Certain patients have greater risk for developing LTLS and/or CTLS and should be treated more aggressively to prevent its occurrence. Risk stratification guides what type of prophylaxis and management therapies should be used for which patients. Patients classified as high risk should have aggressive prophylactic treatment with hydration and rasburicase while being monitored closely in an ICU or similarly monitored setting. Intermediate risk patients should receive prophylactic treatment with hydration and allopurinol; if hyperuricemia does develop in these patients, consider rasburicase. Initial management of pediatric patients at intermediate risk may include rasburicase. Patients at low risk for developing TLS require no prophylactic therapy but should be monitored closely and treated as necessary.

Risk Stratification

Type of Cancer	High Risk	Intermediate Risk	Low Risk
Non-Hodgkin lymphoma (NHL)	Burkitt's, Burkitt's-ALL (B-ALL), lymphoblastic lymphoma	Diffuse large B-cell lymphoma (DLBCL)	Indolent NHL
Acute lymphoblastic leukemia (ALL)	WBC ≥100,000 cells/mm^3	WBC 50,000 to 100,000 cells/mm^3	WBC ≤50,000 cells/mm^3
Acute myeloid leukemia (AML)	WBC ≥50,000 cells/mm^3; monoblastic; rapidly increasing peripheral blast count	WBC 10,000 to 50,000 cells/mm^3	WBC ≤10,000 cells/mm^3
Chronic lymphocytic leukemia (CLL)		WBC 10,000 to 100,000 cells/mm^3; treatment with fludarabine	WBC ≤10,000 cells/mm^3
Other hematologic malignancies (chronic myeloid leukemia [CML], multiple myeloma) and solid tumors		Rapid proliferation with expected rapid response to therapy	Remainder of patients

LDH ≥2 x ULN, renal impairment, or elevated uric acid, potassium, or phosphate serum concentrations increases risk level (Sarno 2013)

Monitoring

High risk patients should have laboratory and clinical parameters (serum uric acid, phosphate, calcium, creatinine, LDH, and fluid input and output) monitored 4 to 6 hours after initiating chemotherapy. For all patients treated with rasburicase, monitor serum uric acid 4 hours after administration, then every 6 to 8 hours thereafter until resolution of TLS occurs. Frequent assessment of serum chemistries and fluid balance is necessary to avert pathophysiologic adverse events and guide the duration of rasburicase therapy. Electrolyte and fluid abnormalities must be addressed at the time that they are identified. However, rasburicase is administered no more frequently than once daily to achieve uric acid control for a duration of 5 to 7 doses (has also been administered as a single dose schedule with repeat doses, if needed, based on serum uric acid level).

Intermediate risk patients should be monitored throughout and for at least 24 hours after completion of chemotherapy. If rasburicase is not used, laboratory parameters should be monitored 8 hours after initiation of chemotherapy and regularly thereafter according to the patient's clinical condition and institutional practice.

Low risk patients should be monitored as determined by the institution and patient factors. If TLS has not occurred within 2 days, development is very unlikely.

General Principles

Prevention and early management of TLS are aimed at decreasing the risk of morbidity and mortality from cardiac arrhythmias, seizures, and organ failure. In patients with high or intermediate risk, vigorous hydration is the cornerstone of the initial management for acute or potential TLS. Patients should be hydrated with 2 to 3 $L/m^2/day$ (200 mL/kg/day if $\leq$10 kg) intravenous fluid (Children: $D_5W1/4NS$; Adults: Not specified) to maintain urine output of 80 to 100 $mL/m^2/hour$ (4 to 6 mL/kg/hour if $\leq$10 kg), with diuretic use if necessary (avoid or minimize diuretic use in patients with hypovolemia or obstructive uropathy). Due to the tendency for calcium phosphate nephrocalcinosis and the potential for metabolic alkalosis, urinary alkalinization with sodium bicarbonate is no longer universally recommended for the treatment and prevention of TLS (Coiffier 2008).

Allopurinol should be administered to intermediate risk patients to decrease endogenous uric acid production and reduce associated urinary obstruction; dose reductions may be required for renal dysfunction (Coiffier 2008). In adult or pediatric patients, give 150 to 300 $mg/m^2/day$ (or 10 mg/kg/day in pediatric patients) divided every 8 hours (maximum: 800 mg/day) orally or 200 to 400 $mg/m^2/day$ IV (in 1 to 3 divided doses; maximum: 600 mg/day). The time to maximum effect of allopurinol is 27 hours. While allopurinol decreases uric acid production, it is ineffective in reducing markedly elevated uric acid concentrations which may allow renotubular crystal formation and obstruction despite its administration. In addition, allopurinol impedes the clearance of purine analogues such as mercaptopurine and azathioprine.

Rasburicase is administered to rapidly reduce uric acid concentrations; significant reduction in plasma uric acid concentrations is measurable four hours following drug administration. Rasburicase, which is a recombinant form of urate oxidase produced in *Saccharomyces cerevisiae*, catalyzes the degradation of uric acid to allantoin, which is more soluble and readily excreted by the kidneys. Rasburicase is reserved for patients at high risk for TLS (or considered in intermediate risk pediatric patients), patients with elevated uric acid concentrations, or patients with signs of moderate to severe renal impairment or other major organ dysfunction. The major risks associated with administration of rasburicase include anaphylaxis, hypersensitivity reactions, methemoglobinemia, and hemolysis. Rasburicase is contraindicated in patients with glucose-6-phosphate dehydrogenase deficiency due to an increased risk of hemolysis. An additional concern with rasburicase administration is the development of neutralizing antibodies. This phenomenon was observed in 64% of 28 normal, healthy volunteers studied; the effect of neutralizing antibodies on the efficacy of this product with repeated usage is unknown. Rasburicase appears to be less immunogenic in patients with hematologic or lymphoid malignancies receiving chemotherapy. One study reported detection of neutralizing antibodies in 2% of 184 patients with hematologic or lymphoid malignancies treated with rasburicase before and throughout chemotherapy (Cortes 2010).

Rasburicase is approved for use in pediatric and adult patients, with the labeled dose of 0.2 mg/kg/dose daily for up to five days. Due to the costs and risks of therapy plus the immediate and measurable effects of rasburicase, some centers administer a single dose which is repeated daily as warranted by plasma uric acid concentrations. The following doses (based on risk for TLS) and duration of treatment based on plasma uric acid concentrations have been recommended for children: 0.2 mg/kg once daily (duration based on plasma uric acid concentrations) for high risk patients, 0.15 mg/kg once daily (duration based on plasma uric acid concentrations) for intermediate risk, and 0.05 to 0.1 mg/kg once daily (duration based on clinical judgment) if used for low-risk patients (Coiffier 2008). Weight- and risk-based dosing as detailed above has been reported in adults. Fixed-dose rasburicase, ranging from 3 to 7.5 mg as a single dose (Hutcherson 2006; McDonnell 2006; Reeves 2008; Trifilio 2006) with doses (1.5 to 6 mg) repeated if needed (based on serum uric acid concentrations) has also been reported in adults. The optimal timing of rasburicase administration (with respect to chemotherapy administration) is not specified in the manufacter's labeling. In some studies, chemotherapy was administered 4 to 24 hours after the first rasburicase dose (Cortes 2010; Kikuchi 2009; Vadhan-Raj 2012); however, rasburicase generally may be administered irrespective of chemotherapy timing.

Upon rasburicase administration, serum uric acid levels generally decrease within 4 hours. In order to allow for appropriate therapeutic effect and to accurately assess the need for a repeat dose, repeat uric acid levels should be drawn no earlier than 4 hours post-rasburicase dose. Rasburicase will degrade uric acid in vitro when the blood sample is stored at room temperature. Consequently, to prevent artifactually depressed uric acid concentrations, plasma samples must be collected in prechilled tubes, then immediately placed in an ice water bath until centrifuged at 4°C. Plasma must be analyzed within four hours of collection.

Clinical features and treatment for specific metabolic disorders are discussed in the following sections.

Hyperuricemia

Cytolysis during TLS releases purine and pyrimidine nucleotides into the bloodstream and extracellular tissues. Oxidation of the purines hypoxanthine and xanthine yields uric acid, which can precipitate in the renal tubules and cause oliguric renal failure. A high concentration of uric acid and an acidic urine pH promote uric acid crystallization and renotubular precipitation. Maintenance of urine flow is utilized to reduce purine precipitation and preserve renal function. Allopurinol blocks the endogenous production of uric acid by inhibiting the enzyme xanthine oxidase, which oxidizes hypoxanthine and xanthine to uric acid. Allopurinol is used prophylactically during the early management of TLS in intermediate risk patients. Rasburicase decreases existing uric acid concentrations by conversion of this molecule to the inactive and soluble metabolite allantoin, which is readily excreted by the kidneys. Rasburicase should be used prophylactically in high risk patients or in patients with preexisting hyperuricemia or acute renal impairment.

Hyperkalemia

Potassium is primarily an intracellular ion that is released during massive cellular breakdown. Increasing concentrations of serum potassium can be dangerous, leading to cardiac arrhythmias or sudden death, especially in the presence of hypocalcemia (see following discussion). Standard treatments to remove potassium from the blood stream and extracellular fluids should be initiated as warranted by the patient's serum potassium concentration and electrocardiographic abnormalities. Other sources of potassium intake (including nutritional sources, medications, and intravenous solutions) should be eliminated in patients at risk for or with TLS. Pharmaceutical measures routinely used to manage hyperkalemia in patients with TLS include volume expansion with forced diuresis, administration of insulin with glucose, and the cation exchange product sodium polystyrene sulfonate. Sodium bicarbonate can be administered IV push to induce influx of potassium into cells. Textbook algorithms for management of hyperkalemia include instructions for administration of calcium as a cardioprotective measure; however, this is **not** a standard intervention in the setting of TLS. Calcium gluconate administration must be done judiciously in the patient with TLS as it can precipitate as calcium phosphate in highly perfused tissues. Monitor patient ECG and cardiac rhythm closely for arrhythmias.

Hyperphosphatemia

The release of intracellular inorganic phosphate following massive cellular breakdown sets into motion several important clinical features. Serum phosphate concentrations will quickly exceed the threshold for normal renal excretion, with phosphate excretion becoming limited by the glomerular filtration rate. Any azotemia that develops during therapy will hinder phosphate excretion. Treatment includes the use of phosphate binders such as aluminum hydroxide, sevelamer, calcium carbonate (avoid use in patients with hypercalcemia and limit use to pediatric patients), or lanthanum carbonate (avoid use in pediatric patients). In severe cases of hyperphosphatemia, hemodialysis or hemofiltration may be necessary.

Hypocalcemia

High phosphate concentrations will also cause reciprocal hypocalcemia. Although generally asymptomatic, hypocalcemia may cause neuromuscular irritation, tetany, and cardiac dysrhythmias. Symptomatic patients may receive calcium gluconate intravenously (slowly, with ECG monitoring) to increase serum calcium concentrations. Unfortunately, despite hypocalcemia, the solubility product of calcium and phosphate may be exceeded in acute TLS due to high concentrations of phosphate, resulting in tissue calcification and organ failure. For this reason, calcium gluconate should be administered cautiously and only if necessary.

Hemodialysis/Hemofiltration

Due to the unpredictability of TLS, renal replacement therapy may be needed and can be lifesaving. Hemodialysis or hemofiltration may be used to control and maintain fluid volume and/or to remove uric acid, phosphate, and potassium from serum. Intermittent hemodialysis, continuous arteriovenous hemodialysis, or continuous veno-venous hemodiafiltration should be considered as warranted by the severity of serum chemistry abnormalities, major organ dysfunction, and the patient's response to pharmaceutical treatments.

Leukoreduction/Plasmapheresis

Leukoreduction, which utilizes plasmapheresis and hydroxyurea to rapidly decrease the peripheral white blood cell count, is performed in some cases of acute myeloid leukemia. The primary goal of leukoreduction is to reduce the risk of complications from serum hyperviscosity syndrome consequent to a very high white blood cell count. However, leukoreduction can indirectly reduce the risk of TLS as removal of circulating blasts diminishes the primary source of cells undergoing lysis in patients with acute myeloid leukemia. Plasmapheresis is used infrequently and very cautiously in patients with acute promyelocytic leukemia due to the inherent disease-related risks of coagulopathy, hemorrhage, and hypotension in this population. Plasmapheresis is rarely used for leukoreduction in patients with lymphocytic or lymphoblastic leukemias as these patients are at lower risk for hyperviscosity syndrome despite a high white blood cell count. This is because lymphocytes do not have the same 'sticky' quality as myeloid cells. Hydroxyurea can be used without plasmapheresis to achieve leukoreduction.

REFERENCES

Abu-Alfa AK, Younes A. Tumor lysis syndrome and acute kidney injury: evaluation, prevention, and management. *Am J Kidney Dis.* 2010;55(5 Suppl 3):S1-S13.

Al-Kali A, Farooq S, Tfayli A. Tumor lysis syndrome after starting treatment with gleevec in a patient with chronic myelogenous leukemia. *J Clin Pharm Ther.* 2009;34(5):607-610.

Arnold TM, Reuter JP, Delman BS, Shanholtz CB. Use of single-dose rasburicase in an obese female. *Ann Pharmacother.* 2004;38(9):1428-1431.

Barry BD, Kell MR, Redmond HP. Tumor lysis syndrome following endoscopic radiofrequency interstitial thermal ablation of colorectal liver metastases. *Surg Endosc.* 2002;16(7):1109.

Cairo MS, Bishop M. Tumour lysis syndrome: new therapeutic strategies and classification. *Br J Haematol.* 2004;127(1):3-11.

Cairo MS, Coiffier B, Reiter A, Younes A; TLS Expert Panel. Recommendations for the evaluation of risk and prophylaxis of tumour lysis syndrome (TLS) in adults and children with malignant diseases: an expert TLS panel consensus. *Br J Haematol.* 2010;149(4):578-586.

Chen SW, Hwang WS, Tsao CJ, Liu HS, Huang GC. Hydroxyurea and splenic irradiation-induced tumour lysis syndrome: a case report and review of the literature. *J Clin Pharm Ther.* 2005;30(6):623-625.

Coiffier B, Altman A, Pui CH, Younes A, Cairo MS. Guidelines for the management of pediatric and adult tumor lysis syndrome: an evidence-based review. *J Clin Oncol.* 2008;26(16):2767-2778.

Coiffier B, Mounier N, Bologna S, et al. Efficacy and safety of rasburicase (recombinant urate oxidase) for the prevention and treatment of hyperuricemia during induction chemotherapy of aggressive non-hodgkin's lymphoma: results of the GRAAL1 (Groupe d'Etude Des Lymphomes De l'Adulte trial on rasburicase activity in adult lymphoma) study. *J Clin Oncol.* 2003;21(23):4402-4406.

Cortes J, Moore JO, Maziarz RT, et al. Control of plasma uria acid in adults at risk for tumor lysis syndrome: efficacy and safety of rasburicase alone and rasburicase followed by allopurinol compared with allopurinol alone – results of a multicenter phase III study. *J Clin Oncol.* 2010;28(27):4207-4213.

Duzova A, Cetin M, Gümrük F, Yetgin S. Acute tumour lysis syndrome following a single-dose corticosteroid in children with acute lymphoblastic leukaemia. *Eur J Haematol.* 2001;66(6):404-407.

Gemici C. Tumour lysis syndrome in solid tumours. *Clin Oncol (R Coll Radiol).* 2006;18(10):773-780.

Habib GS, Saliba WR. Tumor lysis syndrome after hydrocortisone treatment in metastatic melanoma: a case report and review of the literature. *Am J Med Sci.* 2002;323(3):155-157.

Huang WS, Yang CH. Sorafenib induced tumor lysis syndrome in an advanced hepatocellular carcinoma patient. *World J Gastroenterol.* 2009;15(35):4464-4466.

Hutcherson DA, Gammon DC, Bhatt MS, Faneuf M. Reduced-dose rasburicase in the treatment of adults with hyperuricemia associated with malignancy. *Pharmacotherapy.* 2006;26(2):242-247.

Jabr FI. Acute tumor lysis syndrome induced by rituximab in diffuse large B-cell lymphoma. *Int J Hematol.* 2005;82(4):312-314.

Kikuchi A, Kigasawa H, Tsurusawa M, et al. A study of rasburicase for the management of hyperuricemia in pediatric patients with newly diagnosed hematologic malignancies at high risk for tumor lysis syndrome. *Int J Hematol.* 2009;90(4):492-500.

Kurt M, Onal IK, Elkiran T, Altun B, Altundag K, Gullu I. Acute tumor lysis syndrome triggered by zoledronic acid in patient with metastatic lung adenocarcinoma. *Med Oncol*. 2005;22(2):203-206.

Lee AC, Li CH, So KT, Chan R. Treatment of impending tumor lysis with single-dose rasburicase. *Ann Pharmacother*. 2003;37(11):1614-1617.

Lee MH, Cheng KI, Jang RC, Hsu JH, Dai ZK, Wu JR. Tumour lysis syndrome developing during an operation. *Anaesthesia*. 2007;62(1):85-87.

Leibowitz AB, Adamsky C, Gabrilove J, Labow DM. Intraoperative acute tumor lysis syndrome during laparoscopic splenectomy preceded by splenic artery embolization. *Surg Laparosc Endosc Percutan Tech*. 2007;17(3):210-211.

Lerza R, Botta M, Barsotti B, et al. Dexamethazone-induced acute tumor lysis syndrome in a T-cell malignant lymphoma. *Leuk Lymphoma*. 2002;43(5):1129-1132.

Linck D, Basara N, Tran V, et al. Peracute onset of severe tumor lysis syndrome immediately after 4 Gy fractionated TBI as part of reduced intensity preparative regimen in a patient with T-ALL with high tumor burden. *Bone Marrow Transplant*. 2003;31(10):935-937.

Liu CY, Sims-McCallum RP, Schiffer CA. A single dose of rasburicase is sufficient for the treatment of hyperuricemia in patients receiving chemotherapy. *Leuk Res*. 2005;29(4):463-465.

Mato AR, Riccio BE, Qin L, et al. A predictive model for the detection of tumor lysis syndrome during AML induction therapy. *Leuk Lymphoma*. 2006;47(5):877-883.

McBride A, Westervelt P. Recognizing and managing the expanded risk of tumor lysis syndrome in hematologic and solid malignancies. *J Hematol Oncol*. 2012;5:75.

McDonnell AM, Lenz KL, Frei-Lahr DA, Hayslip J, Hall PD. Single-dose rasburicase 6 mg in the management of tumor lysis syndrome in adults. *Pharmacotherapy*. 2006;26(6):806-812.

National Comprehensive Cancer Network (NCCN). Practice guidelines in oncology: acute myeloid leukemia, version 1.2011. http://www.nccn.org/professionals/physician_gls/PDF/aml.pdf

Oztop I, Demirkan B, Yaren A, et al. Rapid tumor lysis syndrome in a patient with metastatic colon cancer as a complication of treatment with 5-fluorouracil/leucoverin and irinotecan. *Tumori*. 2004;90(5):514-516.

Reeves DJ, Bestul DJ. Evaluation of a single fixed dose of rasburicase 7.5 mg for the treatment of hyperuricemia in adults with cancer. *Pharmacother*. 2008;28(6):685-690.

Riccio B, Mato A, Olson EM, Berns JS, Luger S. Spontaneous tumor lysis syndrome in acute myeloid leukemia: two cases and a review of the literature. *Cancer Biol Ther*. 2006;5 (12):1614-1617.

Rostom AY, El-Hussainy G, Kandil A, Allam A. Tumor lysis syndrome following hemi-body irradiation for metastatic breast cancer. *Ann Oncol*. 2000;11(10):1349-1351.

Sarno J. Prevention and management of tumor lysis syndrome in adults with malignancy. *J Adv Pract Oncol*. 2013;4(2):101-106.

Sorscher SM. Tumor lysis syndrome following docetaxel therapy for extensive metastatic prostate cancer. *Cancer Chemother Pharmacol*. 2004;54(2):191-192.

Theodorou D, Lagoudianakis E, Pattas M, et al. Pretreatment tumor lysis syndrome associated with bulky retroperitoneal tumors. Recognition is the mainstay of therapy. *Tumori*. 2006;92 (6):540-541.

Trifilio S, Gordon L, Singhal S, et al. Reduced-dose rasburicase (recombinant xanthine oxidase) in adult cancer patients with hyperuricemia. *Bone Marrow Transplant*. 2006;37(11):997-1001.

Vadhan-Raj S, Fayad LE, Fanale MA, et al. A randomized trial of a single-dose rasburicase versus five-daily doses in patients at risk for tumor lysis syndrome. *Ann Oncol*. 2012;23(6):1640-1645.

Wagner J, Arora S. Oncologic metabolic emergencies. *Emerg Med Clin North Am*. 2014;32 (3):509-525.

Yahata T, Nishikawa N, Aoki Y, Tanaka K. Tumor lysis syndrome associated with weekly paclitaxel treatment in a case with ovarian cancer. *Gynecol Oncol*. 2006;103(2):752-754.

Zigrossi P, Brustia M, Bobbio F, Campanini M. Flare and tumor lysis syndrome with atypical features after letrozole therapy in advanced breast cancer. A case report. *Ann Ital Med Int*. 2001;16(2):112-117.

CHEMOTHERAPY AND CANCER TREATMENT DURING PREGNANCY

Cancer is the second leading cause of death in women between the ages of 20 to 39 years and it complicates up to 1 in 1,000 pregnancies. The most common malignancies occurring during pregnancy are the same as those diagnosed in comparative nonpregnant females: Breast cancer, cervical cancer, lymphoma, and melanoma. Medical management of the pregnant patient with cancer must consider both maternal and fetal outcomes. Disease prognosis, natural history, and symptomatology are important considerations with respect to maternal outcome because these determine the urgency of treatment initiation. In addition, hematologic and major organ toxicity from anticancer treatment increases the risk of maternal complications from pregnancy and delivery. Anticancer therapy can be delayed until after delivery when this is not deleterious to the patient's prognosis or does not unacceptably exacerbate cancer-related morbidity (Pereg 2008). Unfortunately, in some cases, the risks of anticancer treatments to fetal or maternal health are considered unacceptable; in such cases, therapeutic abortion is generally recommended (Pereg 2008).

One retrospective analysis of data from an international registry evaluated pregnancy outcome in 215 women from Belgium (68%), Netherlands (26%), and Czech Republic (6%) diagnosed with cancer while pregnant (Van Calsteren 2010). The leading diagnosis was breast cancer, affecting 46% of the women, followed by hematologic malignancy (18%), dermatologic cancer (10%), and cervical cancer (9%). The mean maternal age at cancer diagnosis was 33 years ± 5 years. The diagnosis of cancer was made in the first, second, and third trimesters in 24%, 43%, and 33% of cases, respectively. Fifty-eight women (27%) were able to delay treatment until after delivery. For 122 patients (57%), anticancer treatment (single agent or combination therapy) was initiated at mean gestational age 20 weeks ± 9 weeks. Spontaneous miscarriage occurred prior to initiation of anticancer therapy in five women (2%) at mean gestational age of 11 weeks ± 5 weeks. Pregnancy was terminated at mean gestational age of 11 weeks ± 7 weeks for 30 cases (14%). Treatment included chemotherapy, non-cytotoxic anticancer therapy, and/or radiation therapy for 73 women (60% of treated patients). Surgery was the only treatment for 49 women (40% of treated patients). A gestational complication occurred in 27 (15%) of the 180 pregnancies that progressed to delivery. The rate of preterm labor was increased for women treated with chemotherapy or radiation therapy relative to the general population (p=0.012). The incidence of preterm premature rupture of membranes was similar to that of the general population (p=0.668). Delivery occurred at gestational age of <32 weeks, 32 to 37 weeks, and at term for 8%, 46%, and 46% of children, respectively. More babies exposed *in utero* to anticancer treatment were small for their gestational age (p=0.012) in comparison to infants not exposed to anticancer treatment *in utero*. Low birth weight was noted in 24% of babies born following *in utero* exposure to chemotherapy or radiation treatment. The frequency of major and minor congenital physical abnormalities for babies born to treated and untreated mothers were similar to that expected of the general population. Two infants born following 2 weeks of maternal chemotherapy treatment for acute leukemia required white blood cell colony stimulating factor support for neutropenia. Neonatal intensive care unit admission was required by 75 babies for prematurity.

Gestational age is an important consideration with respect to fetal outcome. Gestation refers to the period of time that the fetus is developing in the uterus, which is normally a period of about 38 weeks. Pertinent phases of fetal development include implantation, organogenesis, and growth. Implantation, which begins with conception and lasts for about 2 weeks, often ends in spontaneous abortion subsequent to toxic drug or radiation exposure. Organogenesis begins shortly after implantation and continues throughout the first trimester. During this period, toxic drug or radiation exposure can yield organ dysgenesis (malformation) and fetal death. The fetal liver can metabolize medications as early as gestational weeks 7 to 8; however, the degree to which this contributes to drug detoxification is unknown. The fetal growth phase occurs from the second trimester to term. Toxic exposures during this period of fetal development can lead to growth retardation with low birth weight and complications, including abnormal brain development with learning disabilities (Pereg 2008).

There is a great degree of interpatient variability for systemic exposure to most pharmaceutical anticancer treatments (Baker 2002). Physiologic changes that occur normally in pregnancy can enhance pharmacokinetic variability by influencing the systemic exposure to anticancer treatments. Pregnancy increases plasma volume and alters plasma protein expression. In addition, systemic medication elimination is increased due to enhanced mixed function oxidase activity and increased glomerular filtration rate. The intestinal absorption of medications is reduced in pregnant patients due to delayed gastric emptying and reduced gut motility. Enterohepatic circulation is increased with pregnancy, which increases the absorption of certain medications.

Limited data is available describing the effects of pregnancy on the pharmacokinetics of chemotherapy. One study evaluated the pharmacokinetics of doxorubicin (14 patients), epirubicin (10 patients), docetaxel (3 patients), and paclitaxel (5 patients) in pregnant women with median gestational age of 23 to 33 weeks (van Hasselt 2014). The pharmacokinetic parameters were compared to those analyzed in nonpregnant women receiving the same chemotherapy drugs: Doxorubicin (59 patients), epirubicin (57 patients), docetaxel (32 patients), and paclitaxel (105 patients). The AUC in pregnant women was reduced relative to the AUC in nonpregnant women by ~5%, ~8%, ~15%, and ~27% for doxorubicin, epirubicin, docetaxel, and paclitaxel, respectively. In addition, for paclitaxel the time above 0.1 micromolar (85.39 ng/mL) was analyzed; for pregnant patients, the time for paclitaxel >0.1 micromolar was reduced ~11% in comparison to the nonpregnant cohort.

Systemic anticancer treatments are generally mutagenic, teratogenic, or fetotoxic in preclinical models. The true risk of chemotherapy administration during pregnancy is not well-delineated because relevant clinical information is based primarily on case series and anecdotal reports. Controlled clinical trials evaluating the risks of chemotherapy administration throughout pregnancy are not always feasible because of the relatively infrequent and sporadic occurrence of cancer diagnosis during pregnancy and the ethical concerns related to chemotherapy administration during certain gestational periods. The overall risk of major fetal malformations attributed to chemotherapy administration during the first trimester of pregnancy is 10% to 20% (Pereg 2008). Successful pregnancy despite systemic anticancer therapy during pregnancy is reported; however, it is imperative to recognize that due to the lack of stringently evaluated scientific data, these cases **do not verify** the safety of systemic anticancer therapy during pregnancy. In fact, one report describes *in utero* exposure of fraternal twins to cyclophosphamide and prednisone throughout the first 33 weeks of gestation with

▶

divergent outcomes for the male and female offspring. The male twin was affected with multiple congenital anomalies affecting the right arm, esophagus, inferior vena cava, and renal collecting system (Zemlickis 1993). In addition, the male twin was diagnosed with papillary thyroid cancer at 11 years of age and neuroblastoma at 14 years of age. In contrast, the female twin was born without congenital anomalies and demonstrated normal growth and development until her last follow-up at 22 years of age. The greatest risk for spontaneous abortion occurs with systemic anticancer therapy or radiation administered during the first 2 to 3 weeks of pregnancy (Azim 2010). The greatest risk of congenital abnormalities occurs with anticancer treatment during organogenesis and the first trimester of pregnancy. Following organogenesis, the central nervous system, eyes, hematopoietic system, and genitalia remain sensitive to the toxic effects of systemic anticancer therapy and radiation exposure (Pereg 2008). Anticancer treatments given after the first trimester should be scheduled in such a manner as to reduce the risk of complications at the time of delivery.

The most common abnormality attributed to *in utero* exposure to anticancer therapy is low birth weight for gestational age (Briggs 2011). *In utero* exposure to cytotoxic chemotherapy during the second and third trimesters can yield growth retardation and premature delivery. Numerous congenital anomalies affecting bone and cartilage, major organs, gastrointestinal tract, vascular system, and limbs have been identified after *in utero* exposure to anticancer therapy during the first trimester. Congenital anomalies have occurred following first trimester exposure to cyclophosphamide, cytarabine, doxorubicin, fluorouracil, imatinib, methotrexate, procarbazine, tamoxifen, thalidomide, thioguanine, and vincristine (Briggs 2011; Paskulin 2005; Vaux 2003). Medication-specific congenital abnormalities are implicated with *in utero* exposure to methotrexate, imatinib, and tretinoin (Briggs 2011; Pye 2008). Methotrexate is an abortifacient, fetotoxic, and teratogenic compound. The fetal aminopterin/methotrexate syndrome is characterized by fetal growth deficiency, severe lack of ossification of the calvarium (portion of the skull), prominent eyes due to defective supraorbital ridge formation, small low-set ears, micrognathia (undersized jaw), and limb abnormalities (Del Campo 1999). Mispositioned heart, anomalous ribs, and digit malformations are also reported following *in utero* methotrexate exposure (Briggs 2011). Mental retardation, motor impediment, and postnatal growth delay can occur from prenatal exposure to methotrexate. Tretinoin is a retinoid, so it carries the class risk of retinoic acid embryopathy characterized by growth delays, skull and facial malformations, central nervous system abnormalities, and cardiac anomalies (Briggs 2011). Microphthalmos (small eye diameter), polyhydramnios (increased amniotic fluid volume), and oligohydramnios (reduced amniotic fluid volume) are reported after *in utero* exposure to cisplatin (Mir 2008). Doxorubicin and daunorubicin concentrations have been detected in amniotic fluid, placental tissue, and fetal tissues (Germann 2004). Albeit for many anticancer treatments, including the aforementioned products, congenital anomalies do not conform to a medication-specific array of abnormalities (Briggs 2011).

Molecularly targeted therapy and endocrine therapy also present a risk to the mother and fetus. Pregnancy and fetal outcome in 125 women treated with imatinib included normal delivery (50%), elective pregnancy termination (28%), spontaneous abortion (14%), live birth with congenital anomaly (6%), and stillbirth with fetal abnormalities (1%) (Pye 2008). Six of eight live births with congenital anomalies and the single case of stillbirth occurred following *in utero* exposure to imatinib during the first trimester of pregnancy. Birth defects demonstrated by more than one child were exomphalos (umbilical protrusion), right renal dysgenesis, and scoliosis or vertebral anomalies. Oligohydramnios has been reported with *in utero* exposure to erlotinib, lapatinib, and trastuzumab (Robinson 2007). Craniofacial abnormalities are attributed to *in utero* exposure to tamoxifen and retinoids, such as tretinoin (Berger 2008). Thalidomide is a known teratogen. Absent or short limbs, bone defects, external ear abnormalities, eye defects, and congenital heart defects are attributed to *in utero* exposure to thalidomide exposure (Briggs 2011). Due to similar pharmacology and preclinical teratogenicity, lenalidomide is presumed to carry the same risks.

One retrospective series describes fetal outcome following maternal treatment with chemotherapy for breast cancer during (one patient) and after the first trimester (27 patients) (Ring 2005). Chemotherapy regimens used were cyclophosphamide/methotrexate/fluorouracil (CMF), doxorubicin/cyclophosphamide (AC), and epirubicin/cyclophosphamide (EC) for 43%, 39%, and 18% of cases, respectively. The median gestational age at birth was 37 weeks (range: 30 to 40 weeks); no fetal anomalies were identified for the 28 births, none of the infants had a birth weight lower than the 10th percentile for their gestational age, and five newborns required neonatal intensive care unit support. Another case report describes congenital anomalies in a child born at 38 weeks gestational age following *in utero* exposure (during the first 16 weeks of pregnancy) to cyclophosphamide/doxorubicin/fluorouracil (CAF) for treatment of maternal breast cancer; the abnormalities included high-arched palate, small head circumference, a flat nasal bridge, bilateral syndactyly (skin webbing between fingers), and finger nail dystrophy (Paskulin 2005). This child had a low birth weight and retarded postnatal development. The use of trastuzumab during pregnancy is associated with reports with oligohydroamnios (Pant 2008; Sekar 2007).

Chemotherapy administration during the second and third trimester of pregnancy can cause treatment-related toxicity to the fetus due to drug distribution through the placental barrier (Briggs 2011). Transient renal impairment with resolution on postpartum day 8 was noted following *in utero* exposure to cisplatin (Mir 2008). Cases of cardiotoxicity are reported following second and third trimester *in utero* exposure to anthracyclines (Germann 2004). Fetal myelosuppression can occur secondary to maternal chemotherapy treatments during the second and third trimesters. Hematologic abnormalities are reported in some babies born to women receiving rituximab for the treatment of non-Hodgkin lymphoma and management of nonmalignant disorders (Chakravarty 2011). Neonatal lymphopenia, B cell lymphopenia or depletion, leukopenia, thrombocytopenia, and anemia have been reported in babies born following *in utero* exposure to rituximab. In addition, perinatal infectious complications, including cytomegalovirus infection (vertical transmission), bronchiolitis, acute chorioamnionitis (diagnosed in placental pathology), and fever (presumably from viral infection), have been reported following *in utero* exposure to rituximab. Detectable levels of cisplatin have been measured in neonatal blood (Mir 2008).

The threshold dose of radiation for inducing congenital abnormalities during fetal organogenesis is 0.1 to 0.2 Gy; a decrease in intelligence quotient can result from fetal central nervous system exposure to radiation 0.1 Gy during gestational weeks 8 to 25 and there is a 40% risk of severe mental retardation if the fetus is exposed to radiation 1 Gy during gestation weeks 8 to 25 (Pereg 2008). Fetal exposure to radiation therapy increases the risk of developing malignant disease during the first ten years of life. Therapeutic radiation should be delayed until the postpartum period whenever possible. Radiation to the flank area for the treatment of pediatric unilateral Wilms tumor can yield pathophysiologic changes affecting pregnancies that occur decades following treatment. These cancer survivors are more likely to have hypertension complicating pregnancy, fetal malposition, and premature labor and their babies are more likely to be born prematurely and have a low birth weight for their gestational age (Green 2010).

Guideline Recommendations

The European Society for Medical Oncology (ESMO) has published guidelines for diagnosis, treatment, and follow-up of cancer during pregnancy (Peccatori 2013). The ESMO guidelines recommend referral to a facility with expertise in cancer during pregnancy and a multidisciplinary team (obstetrician, neonatologist, oncology team) is encouraged. No chemotherapy treatment should be administered in the first trimester; may begin in the second trimester; there should be a 3-week time period between the last chemotherapy dose and anticipated delivery, although because spontaneous delivery may occur any time after 34 weeks of gestation, chemotherapy should not be administered beyond week 33 of gestation. These pregnancies should be considered high-risk and regular fetal monitoring during gestation should be considered; placental histologic examination is also recommended. Standard protocols for dose calculations should be followed, although pharmacokinetics may be altered in pregnancy. The Society of Obstetricians and Gynaecologists of Canada (SOGC) has also published guidelines, which recognize that exposure to chemotherapy after the first trimester has not been associated with increased risk of malformation, although there is a risk of stillbirth, intrauterine growth restriction, and fetal toxicities; a 2- to 3-week time frame should be permitted between the last dose of chemotherapy and expected delivery to allow for bone marrow recovery. As neonates have limited ability to metabolize and excrete drugs due to renal and/or hepatic immaturity, allowing a 2- to 3-week time frame between chemotherapy administration and delivery may reduce possible toxicity in the infant. In addition, a multidisciplinary team is recommended (Koren 2013).

REFERENCES

Amant F, Loibl S, Neven P, Van Calsteren K. Breast cancer in pregnancy. *Lancet.* 2012;379 (9815):570-579.

Azim HA Jr, Peccatori FA, Pavlidis N. Treatment of the pregnant mother with cancer: a systematic review on the use of cytotoxic, endocrine, targeted agents and immunotherapy during pregnancy. Part I: solid tumors. *Cancer Treat Rev.* 2010;36(2):101-109.

Baker SD, Verweij J, Rowinsky EK, et al. Role of body surface area in dosing of investigational anticancer agents in adults, 1991-2001. *J Natl Cancer Inst.* 2002;94(24):1883-1888.

Berger JC, Clericuzio CL. Pierre Robin sequence associated with first trimester fetal tamoxifen exposure. *Am J Med Genet A.* 2008;146A(16):2141-2144.

Briggs GG, Freeman RK, Yaffe SJ. Drugs in pregnancy and lactation. 9th ed. Philadelphia, PA: Lipincott Williams & Wilkins; 2011.

Chakravarty EF, Murray ER, Kelman A, Farmer P. Pregnancy outcomes after maternal exposure to rituximab. *Blood.* 2011;117(5):1499-1506.

Del Campo M, Kosaki K, Bennett FC, Jones KL. Developmental delay in fetal aminopterin/ methotrexate syndrome. *Teratology.* 1999;60(1):10-12.

Germann N, Goffinet F, Goldwasser F. Anthracyclines during pregnancy: embryo-fetal outcome in 160 patients. *Ann Oncol.* 2004;15(1):146-150.

Green DM, Lange JM, Peabody EM, et al. Pregnancy outcome after treatment for wilms tumor: a report from the national wilms tumor long-term follow-up study. *J Clin Oncol.* 2010;28 (17):2824-2830.

Koren G, Carey N, Gagnon R, et al. Cancer chemotherapy and pregnancy. *J Obstet Gynaecol Can.* 2013;35(3):263-280.

Mir O, Berveiller P, Ropert S, Goffinet F, Goldwasser F. Use of platinum derivatives during pregnancy. *Cancer.* 2008;113(11):3069-3074.

Pant S, Landon MB, Blumenfeld M, Farrar W, Shapiro CL. Treatment of breast cancer with trastuzumab during pregnancy. *J Clin Oncol.* 2008;26(9):1567-1569.

Paskulin GA, Gazzola Zen PR, de Camargo Pinto LL, Rosa R, Graziadio C. Combined chemotherapy and teratogenicity. *Birth Defects Res A Clin Mol Teratol.* 2005;73(9):634-637.

Peccatori FA, Azim HA Jr, Orecchia R, et al. Cancer, pregnancy and fertility: ESMO Clinical Practice Guidelines for diagnosis, treatment and follow-up. *Ann Oncol.* 2013;24(Suppl 6): vi160-170.

Pereg D, Koren G, Lishner M. Cancer in pregnancy: gaps, challenges and solutions. *Cancer Treat Rev.* 2008;34(4):302-312.

Pye SM, Cortes J, Ault P, et al. The effects of imatinib on pregnancy outcome. *Blood.* 2008;111 (12):5505-5508.

Reynoso EE, Shepherd FA, Messner HA, Farquharson HA, Garvey MB, Baker MA.. Acute leukemia during pregnancy: the Toronto Leukemia Study Group experience with long-term follow-up of children exposed *in utero* to chemotherapeutic agents. *J Clin Oncol.* 1987;5 (7):1098-1106.

Ring AE, Smith IE, Jones A, Shannon C, Galani E, Ellis PA. Chemotherapy for breast cancer during pregnancy: an 18-year experience from five London teaching hospitals. *J Clin Oncol.* 2005;23(18):4192-4197.

Robinson AA, Watson WJ, Leslie KK. Targeted treatment using monoclonal antibodies and tyrosine-kinase inhibitors in pregnancy. *Lancet Oncol.* 2007;8(8):738-743.

Sekar R, Stone PR. Trastuzumab use for metastatic breast cancer in pregnancy. *Obstet Gynecol.* 2007;110(2 Pt 2):507-510.

Van Calsteren K, Heyns L, De Smet F, et al. Cancer during pregnancy: an analysis of 215 patients emphasizing the obstetrical and the neonatal outcomes. *J Clin Oncol.* 2010;28(4):683-689.

van Hasselt JG, van Calsteren K, Heyns L, et al. Optimizing anticancer drug treatment in pregnant cancer patients: pharmacokinetic analysis of gestation-induced changes for doxorubicin, epirubicin, docetaxel and paclitaxel. *Ann Oncol.* 2014;25(10):2059-2065.

Vaux KK, Kahole NC, Jones KL. Cyclophosphamide, methotrexate, and cytarabine embryopathy: is apoptosis the common pathway? *Birth Defects Res A Clin Mol Teratol.* 2003;67(6):403-408.

Zemlickis D, Lishner M, Erlich R, Koren G. Teratogenicity and carcinogenicity in a twin exposed *in utero* to cyclophosphamide. *Teratog Carcinog Mutagen.* 1993;13(3):139-143.

CHEMOTHERAPY AND OBESITY

Obesity increases the risk for development of certain cancers and is often associated with poorer outcomes. The World Health Organization defines obesity in terms of body mass index (BMI): Underweight, <18.5 kg/m^2; normal weight, 18.5 to 24.9 kg/m^2; overweight, 25 to 29.9 kg/m^2; moderately obese, 30 to 34.9 kg/m^2; severely obese, 35 to 39.9 kg/m^2; morbidly obese, >40 kg/m^2. For the purpose of this text, the term obese refers to any BMI ≥30 kg/m^2, unless specified otherwise.

The American Society of Clinical Oncology (ASCO) has established an initiative intended to reduce the deleterious effect of obesity on cancer risk, management, and outcome (Ligibel 2014). The fundamentals of this initiative are: 1) increase education and awareness of the evidence pertaining to obesity and cancer; 2) offer oncology providers tools and resources to address obesity with their patients; 3) support robust research program(s) to improve the scientific, clinical, and epidemiologic knowledgebase related to obesity and cancer; and 4) advocate for policy and systems changes that improve societal management of obesity. ASCO encourages oncology provider-directed management of obesity because the diagnosis of cancer often produces very teachable moments that motivate patients and significant others to make lifestyle changes. Moreover, the oncology team maintains a close relationship with cancer patients and their significant others throughout the duration of active cancer treatment and survivorship. The ASCO position statement recommends routine calculation of patient BMI and use of this parameter as a tool to begin dialogue about obesity and weight management at any time from cancer diagnosis through long-term follow-up.

The relationship between body size and the pharmacokinetics of chemotherapy is variable and not fully delineated. Chemotherapy has a narrow therapeutic index and is generally administered at a dosage one level below the amount associated with unacceptable toxicity. Presumably, the safety and efficacy of treatment correlate with systemic drug exposure. Much of the data defining systemic exposure to chemotherapy and other medications is based on pharmacokinetic studies performed in nonobese patients. Obesity can alter chemotherapy pharmacokinetics due to increased vasculature within excess adipose tissue and blood flow redistribution with respect to major organs, such as the liver, kidneys, and heart (Hall 2013). With respect to medication absorption, obesity can prolong the systemic absorption of subcutaneously administered medications (Jain 2011). Volume of distribution is often altered in obesity due to increased vascular space (Jain 2011). Additionally, obese patients may have increased or decreased alpha-1-acid glycoprotein concentrations, which can impact the distribution of basic drugs; however, there is inconsistent data in the primary literature regarding this matter (Jain 2011). The findings of altered alpha-1-acid glycoprotein levels in obesity are also confounded by comorbidities commonly affecting this population that increase the expression of this plasma protein (Jain 2011). Hepatic fatty infiltration can yield liver damage in morbidly obese patients; thus, obesity may affect enzymatic drug metabolism (Jain 2011). The activity of CYP2E1, which metabolizes fatty acids, ketones, and ethanol, increases proportionally with obesity; the effect of obesity on other CYP isoforms is confounded by inconsistent data in the primary literature (Jain 2011). Lean body mass correlates well with drug clearance for many medications (Jain 2011); however, several chemotherapy drugs demonstrate increased or decreased drug clearance, depending on the drug and the patient's body size (Sparreboom 2007). According to one study, glomerular filtration rate (GFR) determined by inulin clearance is increased in obese patients, although the difference abates when normalized for lean body mass (Janmahasatian 2008).

Obesity confounds optimal dosing of chemotherapy. Most chemotherapy doses are calculated using body surface area (BSA). The calculated value of this parameter increases disproportionately less than weight with increasing obesity. For example, in a patient whose actual body weight (ABW) is double that of their ideal body weight (IBW), the BSA increases ~1.4-fold instead of 2-fold. Utilization of body size for calculation of chemotherapy dose(s) is historically based on adaptation of preclinical dose amounts (administered to animal models) for use in humans. Methods for adjusting body weight in obese patients aim to estimate body size relative to lean body weight or augmented extravascular space and can be used as tools for chemotherapy dose calculation. Body size may be replaced by more precise tools for chemotherapy dose calculation in obesity as knowledge in this discipline progresses.

The American Society of Clinical Oncology (ASCO) Clinical Practice Guidelines provide evidence-based recommendations for dosing chemotherapy to treat cancer in obese patients (Griggs 2012). The ASCO Clinical Practice Guidelines are based on clinical evidence that the use of actual body weight for chemotherapy dose calculation does not increase acute or chronic regimen-related toxicity. Interestingly, when chemotherapy doses are calculated using actual body weight, the subsequent myelosuppression is similar or reduced in obese patients relative to their nonobese counterparts. In addition, the ASCO guidelines inherently support the premise that the use of actual body weight to calculate chemotherapy doses for obese patients improves the efficacy of treatment. The ASCO guidelines are based on clinical evidence from administration of regimens using standard chemotherapy dosages; novel targeted agents, biologic agents (immunotherapies and monoclonal antibodies), and treatment of leukemias were excluded from the guideline. The American Society for Blood and Marrow Transplantation (ASBMT) position statement provides recommendations for dose calculation of high-dose chemotherapy and agents used in conditioning regimens, which are presented later in this chapter.

Key Points of the ASCO Clinical Practice Guidelines for Dosing Chemotherapy in Obesity

- Calculate chemotherapy doses using actual body weight; this is especially important for curative therapy.

- Manage regimen-related toxicities in obese patients in the same manner as for nonobese patients.

- If chemotherapy dose reduction is utilized in response to toxicity, resumption of full actual body weight-based dosing should be considered as possible by the patient's clinical status and major organ function. There is no evidence to support greater dose reductions for obese patients compared to nonobese patients.

- Use of fixed-dose cytotoxic chemotherapy is rarely justified, except for a few agents. Stated exceptions:

    - Carboplatin dose calculated using Calvert formula and maximum creatinine clearance of 150 mL/minute

    - Vincristine dose cap for neurotoxicity

    - Bleomycin set dose (due to pulmonary toxicity)

Well-intentioned empiric adjustment of chemotherapy dosage in obese patients carries the risk of lessening therapeutic efficacy without improving safety. Ultimately, the decision of whether to empirically adjust chemotherapy dosages for obesity must take into consideration the same factors that are considered for the nonobese cancer patient: the goal of treatment (curative vs palliative), the patient's ability to tolerate treatment, and the nature of regimen-related toxicity (transient vs potentially debilitating).

A meta-analysis examining outcomes in obese versus nonobese adult cancer patients receiving chemotherapy dosed using actual body weight determined that obese patients experienced similar or lower rates of toxic effects compared with normal weight patients, without a difference in survival outcomes. The relative rates of toxic effects in obese patients for grades 3/4 hematologic toxicity, grades 3/4 nonhematologic toxicity, and any grade 3/4 adverse event were OR 0.73 (95% CI 0.55 to 0.98), OR 0.98 (95% CI 0.76 to 1.26), and OR 0.75 (95% CI 0.65 to 0.87), respectively. This analysis included data from 12 studies representing 9,314 pooled patients. Overall, 13 different types of cancer were represented, although the majority of subjects had colorectal cancer (55%) or breast cancer (29%). Treatment regimens included 21 different chemotherapy agents, which represented the major chemotherapy classes (Hourdequin 2013).

Administration of adjuvant chemotherapy for breast cancer using actual body weight in the dose calculations for obese women is reported. Substituting actual body weight in body surface area-based chemotherapy dose calculations did not yield greater toxicity in 408 obese patients (BMI ≥ 27.3 kg/m^2) receiving FAC (fluorouracil-doxorubicin-cyclophoshamide) as adjuvant therapy for breast cancer relative to their 818 nonobese counterparts in the clinical trial CALBG 8541 (Rosner 1996); severe hematologic and nonhematologic adverse events were similar with the first treatment cycle and throughout the entire course of therapy for all patients. In addition, one retrospective analysis evaluated toxicity in 662 women with breast cancer receiving adjuvant FEC (fluorouracil-epirubicin-cyclo-phosphamide). The population consisted of underweight (1%), normal weight (44%), overweight (37%), obese (16%), and morbidly obese (2%) patients (Jenkins 2007). The relative dose intensity (RDI) for FEC was >92.6% for all patients. In this report, patients with BMI >25 kg/m^2 were less likely to experience cycle delays due to prolonged myelosuppression (p <0.001), particularly toward the end of the treatment course.

In clinical trial NSABP B-14, the rate of breast cancer recurrence and mortality were similar for 3,385 women receiving adjuvant therapy with tamoxifen for breast cancer; ~50% of the women enrolled in this study were overweight or obese (Dignam 2003). Breast cancer recurrence was not significantly increased for obese women [HR 0.98, 95% CI 0.8 to 1.18] and breast cancer mortality was not significantly increased for obese women (HR 1.20, 95% CI 0.97 to 1.49); however, the obese women in this study did fare worse with respect to develop-ment of contralateral breast cancer (HR 1.58, 95% CI 1.1 to 2.25), risk of other primary cancers (HR 1.62, 95% CI 1.16 to 2.24), all cause mortality (HR 1.31, 95% CI 1.12 to 1.54), and risk of mortality unrelated to breast cancer (HR 1.49, 95% CI 1.15 to 1.92) (Dignam 2003).

Obesity may influence the pharmacodynamics of aromatase inhibitor therapy. The augmented amount of peripheral adipose tissue in obese patients increases aromatase activity for peripheral estradiol production. The clinical significance of this effect is not fully established. A disparity of breast cancer recurrence rate relative to BMI was identified in the ATAC (Arimidex, Tamoxifen Alone or in

Combination) trial, which prospectively compared anastrozole 1 mg daily (n=3,125) vs tamoxifen 20 mg daily (n=3,116) vs the combination of these products (n=3,125) as adjuvant therapy for postmenopausal breast cancer in a prospective, randomized, and double-blind manner (Baum 2002); the combination arm failed to demonstrate benefit compared to tamoxifen and was terminated after the first analysis (Baum 2003). A secondary analysis of outcome relative to body size reported that disease recurrence occurred more often in women with BMI >35 kg/m^2 vs women with BMI <23 kg/m^2 (adjusted hazard ratio [HR 1.39, 95% CI 1.06 to 1.82; P$_{heterogeneity}$=0.03) (Sestak 2010). The analysis reported similar efficacy for tamoxifen across all BMI values when compared to the lowest weight quintile (P$_{heterogeneity}$=0.54); however, the efficacy of anastrozole was superior for women with BMI <28 kg/m^2 than for women with BMI >30 kg/m^2 (P$_{heterogeneity}$=0.01) (Sestak 2010). A retrospective analysis of results from the Austrian Breast and Colorectal Cancer Study Group (ABCSG)-12 trial reported divergent outcome data for obese vs nonobese women (Pfeiler 2011). The ABCSG-12 trial compared anastrozole 1 mg daily vs tamoxifen 20 mg daily as adjuvant therapy for premenopausal women with breast cancer receiving ovarian ablation (goserelin 3.6 mg monthly) with or without zoledronic acid 4 mg monthly. For patients receiving anastrozole, women with BMI >25 kg/m^2 had an increased risk of disease recurrence (HR 1.6, 95% CI 1.06 to 2.41; p=0.02) or death (HR 2.14, 95% CI 1.17 to 3.92; p=0.01) compared to their nonobese counterparts. Overweight or obese patients treated with anastrozole had an increased risk of disease recurrence (HR 1.49, 95% CI 0.93 to 2.38; p=0.08) or death (HR 3.03, 95% CI 1.35 to 6.82; p=0.004) compared to all women treated with tamoxifen (Pfeiler 2011). One small study compared estradiol suppression in 44 postmenopausal women who received therapy with anastrozole 1 mg daily and letrozole 2.5 mg daily for 3-month intervals in a treatment crossover manner. Both treatments reduced endogenous estradiol concentrations, although mean estradiol levels were greater for five women with BMI >35 kg/m^2 in comparison to their leaner counterparts. Estradiol suppression was more pronounced with letrozole treatment for all body sizes (Folkerd 2012).

Empiric dosage reduction of chemotherapy used for the adjuvant treatment of breast cancer is reported. One analysis of socioeconomic status and BMI in 764 women found that RDI of ordered treatment versus standard therapy was <0.85 for 10%, 14%, 18%, and 27% of normal or underweight, overweight, obese, and morbidly obese patients, respectively (Griggs 2007). A retrospective analysis of 9,672 breast cancer patients receiving adjuvant therapy with AC (doxorubicin-cyclophosphamide) demonstrated reduced RDI for obese patients; empiric first cycle dose reductions to <0.9-times the standard dose were done for 9%, 11%, 20%, and 37% of healthy weight, overweight, obese, and very obese women, respectively. Reduced RDI is also suggested based on fewer admissions for febrile neutropenia in the very obese patients (Griggs 2005).

A retrospective analysis of 333 women treated with chemotherapy for advanced epithelial ovarian cancer examined the relationship between BMI, RDI, overall survival, and progression free survival (PFS). RDI was defined as the administered dose intensity relative to the dose intensity calculated using ABW for all administrations. In this analysis, 303 patients were treated with carboplatin (target AUC 5 to 6) and paclitaxel (175 mg/m^2) and 30 were treated with single agent carboplatin (target AUC 5 to 6). The study population included 27% overweight (BMI 25 to 29.9 kg/m^2) and 21% obese (BMI ≥30 kg/m^2) women. Overall chemotherapy RDI as well as carboplatin RDI was <0.85 more often in obese patients relative to their nonobese counterparts (p=0.02 and p<0.001, respectively). The RDI comparison for paclitaxel was not statistically different (p=0.76). Progression free survival was poorer for patients receiving carboplatin RDI <0.85 (PFS 11 months vs 15 months, HR 1.29, p=0.04). Otherwise, there was not a statistical difference in patient outcomes (OS and PFS) relative to BMI (Ae-Yeung 2014).

The pharmacokinetics of carboplatin, cisplatin, docetaxel, doxorubicin, irinotecan, paclitaxel, topotecan, and troxcitabine in obese patients (n=162) relative to nonobese patients (n=1,044) were analyzed with respect to BSA calculations. The body size descriptors actual body weight, body mass index, ideal body weight, adjusted ideal body weight, lean body mass, and predicted normal weight were used (Sparreboom 2007). This study identified significantly increased absolute clearance for cisplatin (p=0.007), paclitaxel (p=0.023), and troxcitabine (p=0.016) for obese patients by a factor of 13%, 20%, and 19%, respectively; however, statistical significance was not sustained when drug clearance for the aforementioned products was normalized to body surface area using actual body weight for the calculation. The relative systemic exposure was increased 1.25-fold for doxorubicin and 1.33-fold for docetaxel in obese patients. Interestingly, doxorubicin clearance in obese patients relative to nonobese patients was 0.69 for women and 1.11 for men. Another study reported a positive correlation between BSA and docetaxel clearance in 69 males patients (p=0.039) that was not statistically significant in 83 female subjects (p=0.27) (Rudek 2004). The study by Sparreboom et al (2007) did not identify an advantage to using parameters other than actual body weight for irinotecan, carboplatin, or topotecan dosage calculation. In addition, the findings of this study suggest the risk of notable underdosing with use of parameters other than actual body weight for calculation of cisplatin, paclitaxel, and troxcitabine doses.

Anthracycline pharmacokinetics in obesity have been examined in small clinical studies, in addition to the previously mentioned gender difference findings reported by Sparreboom et al (2007). Reduced doxorubicin clearance with increased area under the plasma concentration-time curve (AUC) and mean half-life were demonstrated in 7 obese (>130% IBW) patients compared to 14 nonobese patients receiving doxorubicin 50 to 70 mg/m^2 in combination with other chemotherapy drugs. A noteworthy finding in this study was that the clearance and half-life of the active metabolite doxorubicinol were similar for obese and nonobese patients. Furthermore, doxorubicin and doxorubicinol volume of distribution were similar for all patients in this study (Rodvold 1988). Another study reported reduced doxorubicin AUC and increased volume of distribution in 7 overweight (BMI >25 kg/m^2) breast cancer patients relative to 3 normal weight counterparts. Caveats to pharmacokinetic studies evaluating doxorubicin pharmacokinetics in obesity include small sample size(s) and inadequate analysis of concurrent medications that can influence anthracycline pharmacokinetics, such as cyclophosphamide (Rudek 2004). The maximum plasma concentration of epirubicin did not correlate with weight in 60 women with breast cancer who received a 2-hour infusion of single agent epirubicin 60 mg/m^2; the average body weight in this population was 68 kg, which represented mean 127% IBW (Eksborg 1992). Administration of a set dose of epirubicin 150 mg by continuous intravenous infusion over 120 hours to 20 chemotherapy-naïve women did not demonstrate a relationship between body size and systemic blood concentrations (Gurney 1998).

Clinical studies and reports indicate that body size impacts the accuracy of pharmacokinetically based carboplatin dose calculations. The Calvert method of dosing carboplatin calculates a patient's dose according to a target AUC and the patient's GFR. In clinical practice, the patient's GFR is generally estimated by the calculated creatinine clearance. Carboplatin with dosage calculation using the Calvert method to achieve an AUC of 7.5 (in combination with paclitaxel) was administered to 358 women enrolled in the GOG 158 clinical trial (Wright 2008). The women in this cohort were normal weight (50%), overweight (32%), and obese (18%). To estimate GFR, GOG 158 utilized the Jelliffe formula [creatinine clearance = {98 - [0.8 x (age - 20)]} / creatinine} x 0.9], which, notably, does not include a factor for body size. Consequently, for a given GFR calculation, overweight and obese patients received a lower surface area-based carboplatin dose than the normal weight patients. Patient tolerance in this trial suggested that the obese women received a less intensive systemic exposure than their normal weight counterparts. The proportional decrease in platelet count was less for obese (25% reduction) than normal weight (61% reduction) patients (p=0.01). Treatment-related reduction in hemoglobin (p=0.006) and hematocrit (p=0.002) were also less for the obese patients. Chemotherapy dose reductions due to adverse events were less in obese (21%) than normal weight (34%) patients (p=0.004). The obese women were also less likely to experience moderate to severe thrombocytopenia, leukopenia, and neutropenia during the entire treatment course than the normal weight subjects. Treatment schedule delays and dose reductions were more common in the normal weight women.

The Cockcroft-Gault formula is another GFR estimation tool used in the Calvert method for carboplatin dose calculation. The Cockcroft-Gault formula utilizes weight, age, gender, and serum creatinine as variable factors for calculation of creatinine clearance. The utility of various body weight descriptors for use in the Cockcroft-Gault equation was tested with pharmacokinetic data from 240 patients and 380 carboplatin administrations (Ekhart 2009). For normal body weight and underweight individuals, lean body weight provided the best fit dose calculation for target AUC; for obese and very obese patients (with normal renal function), adjusted ideal body weight provided the best fit dose calculation for target AUC. Interestingly, the study demonstrated that the best fit for all patients was the use of actual body weight with a maximum creatinine clearance value of 140 mL/minute (Ekhart 2009). This finding is aligned with the Food and Drug Administration recommendation to cap the creatinine clearance value at 125 mL/minute when used for pharmacokinetically-derived carboplatin doses. A case illustrating the inaccuracy of using actual body weight for calculation of creatinine clearance with the Cockcroft-Gault formula for AUC-based carboplatin dosing is presented in the arena of high-dose chemotherapy (De Jonge 2002). The measured carboplatin AUC was 1.7-fold greater than the targeted AUC for a 167 cm, 130 kg patient (BSA 2.34 m^2 and BMI 47 kg/m^2) receiving CTC (cyclophosphamide-thiotepa-carboplatin) prior to autologous hematopoietic stem cell transplantation. This patient's actual body weight was used for the calculation of creatinine clearance using the Cockcroft-Gault equation. Another study evaluating patient gender, weight, creatinine, and age as variables predicting carboplatin clearance demonstrated that the mean value between actual and ideal body weight was the most accurate weight variable for use in overweight and obese patients; this study analyzed carboplatin pharmacokinetics in 25 subjects who were 1.2- to 1.7-times their ideal body weight (Bénézet 1997). The good correlation of carboplatin AUC and total body clearance supports a role for use of population-based clearance parameters as a tool for AUC-based dose calculations, such as the Calvert method (Ekhart 2009).

A position statement by the ASBMT Practice Guidelines Committee (Bubalo 2014) provides recommendations for dose calculation of high-dose chemotherapy used prior to hematopoietic stem cell transplantation. The ASBMT position statement cautions that its recommendations are not based on Level 1 and Level 2 clinical evidence. Limitations to reports evaluated by the committee included retrospective data collection, case series, insufficient reporting of pertinent patient data (height, weight, and BMI), and variable use of pharmaco-kinetic-based targeting of chemotherapy drugs.

Recommendations From the ASBMT Position Statement for Dosing High-Dose Chemotherapy and Conditioning Regimen Agents in Obesity

Product(s)	Recommendations
Alemtuzumab	Set dose (flat dose) according to regimen
Antithymocte globulin (equine), Antithymocte globulin (rabbit)	Weight-based (mg/kg) using actual body weight (ABW)
Busulfan >12 mg/kg; oral administration	Surface area-based (BSA) using ABW to calculate BSA
	For adults: Weight-based (mg/kg) using ABW25 for obese and nonobese patients
	For pediatrics: Weight-based (mg/kg) using ABW
	Pharmacokinetically targeted dosage as appropriate for disease state
Busulfan ≤12 mg/kg; oral administration	BSA using ABW to calculate BSA
	For adults: Weight-based (mg/kg) using ABW25 for obese and nonobese patients*
	For pediatrics: Weight-based (mg/kg) using ABW
Carboplatin, clofarabine, cytarabine, fludarabine, melphalan, pentostain	BSA using ABW to calculate BSA
Carmustine	For patients ≤120% ideal body weight (IBW), utilize BSA with ABW to calculate BSA.
	For patients >120% IBW, utilize BSA with ABW25 to calculate BSA.
Cyclophosphamide*	For weight-based (mg/kg) cyclophosphamide total dose 200 mg/kg, use the lesser of IBW or ABW.
	For weight-based (mg/kg) cyclophosphamide total dose 120 mg/kg, use either IBW or ABW for patients ≤120% IBW (preferred method for adults of all body sizes); use ABW25 for patients >120% IBW (preferred for pediatric patients).
Etoposide	BSA using ABW to calculate BSA
	Weight-based (mg/kg) using ABW25
Thiotepa	For patients ≤120% IBW, utilize BSA with ABW to calculate BSA.
	For patients >120% IBW, utilize BSA using with ABW40 to calculate BSA.

*The ASBMT position statement does not include a specific recommendation for surface area-based dosing of cyclophosphamide.

ABW25: Adjusted wt (kg) = ideal body weight (kg) + 0.25 [actual wt (kg) - ideal body weight (kg)]

ABW40: Adjusted wt (kg) = ideal body weight (kg) + 0.4 [actual wt (kg) - ideal body weight (kg)]

REFERENCES

Au-Yeung G, Webb PM, DeFazio A, Fereday S, Bressel M, Mileshkin L. Impact of obesity on chemotherapy dosing for women with advanced stage serous ovarian cancer in the Australian Ovarian Cancer Study (AOCS). *Gynecol Oncol.* 2014;133(1):16-22.

Baum M, Buzdar A, Cuzick J, et al. Anastrozole alone or in combination with tamoxifen versus tamoxifen alone for adjuvant treatment of postmenopausal women with early-stage breast cancer: results of the ATAC (arimidex, tamoxifen alone or in combination) trial efficacy and safety update analyses. *Cancer.* 2003;98(9):1802-1810.

Baum M, Budzar AU, Cuzick J, et al. Anastrozole alone or in combination with tamoxifen versus tamoxifen alone for adjuvant treatment of postmenopausal women with early breast cancer: first results of the ATAC randomised trial. *Lancet.* 2002;359(9324):2131-2139.

Bénézet S, Guimbaud R, Chatelut E, Chevreau C, Bugat R, Canal P. How to predict carboplatin clearance from standard morphological and biological characteristics in obese patients. *Ann Oncol.* 1997;8(6):607-609.

Bubalo J, Carpenter PA, Majhail N, et al. Conditioning chemotherapy dose adjustment in obese patients: a review and position statement by the American Society for Blood and Marrow Transplantation practice guideline committee. *Biol Blood Marrow Transplant.* 2014;20 (5):600-616.

Centers for Disease Control and Prevention (CDC). About BMI for adults. http://www.cdc.gov/healthyweight/assessing/bmi/adult_bmi/index.html. Accessed April 5, 2014.

De Jonge ME, Mathôt RA, Van Dam SM, Beijnen JH, Rodenhuis S. Extremely high exposures in an obese patient receiving high-dose cyclophosphamide, thiotepa and carboplatin. *Cancer Chemother Pharmacol.* 2002;50(3):251-255.

Dignam JJ, Wieand K, Johnson KA, Fisher B, Xu L, Mamounas EP. Obesity, tamoxifen use, and outcomes in women with estrogen receptor-positive early-stage breast cancer. *J Natl Cancer Inst.* 2003;95(19):1467-1476.

Efstathiou JA, Bae K, Shipley WU, et al. Obesity and mortality in men with locally advanced prostate cancer: analysis of RTOG 85-31. *Cancer.* 2007;110(12):2691-2699.

Ekhart C, Rodenhuis S, Schellens JH, Beijnen JH, Huitema AD. Carboplatin dosing in overweight and obese patients with normal renal function, does weight matter? *Cancer Chemother Pharmacol.* 2009;64(1):115-122.

Eksborg S, Hardell L, Bengtsson NO, Sjödin M, Elfsson B. Epirubicin as a single agent therapy for the treatment of breast cancer – a pharmacokinetic and clinical study. *Med Oncol Tumor Pharmacother.* 1992;9(2):75-80.

Ewertz M, Jensen MB, Gunnarsdóttir KÁ, et al. Effect of obesity on prognosis after early-stage breast cancer. *J Clin Oncol.* 2011;29(1):25-31.

Folkerd EJ, Dixon JM, Renshaw L, A'Hern RP, Dowsett M. Suppression of plasma estrogen levels by letrozole and anastrozole is related to body mass index in patients with breast cancer. *J Clin Oncol.* 2012;30(24):2977-2980.

Geyer SM, Morton LM, Habermann TM, et al. Smoking, alcohol use, obesity, and overall survival from non-Hodgkin lymphoma: a population-based study. *Cancer.* 2010;116(12):2993-3000.

Gong Z, Agalliu I, Lin DW, Stanford JL, Kristal AR. Obesity is associated with increased risks of prostate cancer metastasis and death after initial cancer diagnosis in middle-aged men. *Cancer.* 2007;109(6):1192-1202.

Griggs JJ, Culakova E, Sorbero ME, et al. Effect of patient socioeconomic status and body mass index on the quality of breast cancer adjuvant chemotherapy. *J Clin Oncol.* 2007;25(3):277-284.

Griggs JJ, Mangu PB, Anderson H, et al. Appropriate chemotherapy dosing for obese adult patients with cancer: American Society of Clinical Oncology clinical practice guideline. *J Clin Oncol.* 2012;30(13):1553-1561.

Griggs JJ, Sorbero ME, Lyman GH. Undertreatment of obese women receiving breast cancer chemotherapy. *Arch Intern Med.* 2005;165(11):1267-1273.

Gurney H. Dose calculation of anticancer drugs: a review of the current practice and introduction of an alternative. *J Clin Oncol.* 1996;14(9):2590-2611.

Gurney HP, Ackland S, Gebski V, Farrell G. Factors affecting epirubicin pharmacokinetics and toxicity: evidence against using body-surface area for dose calculation. *J Clin Oncol.* 1998;16 (7):2299-2304.

Hall RG 2nd, Jean GW, Sigler M, Shah S. Dosing considerations for obese patients receiving cancer chemotherapeutic agents. *Ann Pharmacother.* 2013;47(12):1666-1674.

Hourdequin KC, Schpero WL, McKenna DR, Piazik BL, Larson RJ. Toxic effect of chemotherapy dosing using actual body weight in obese versus normal-weight patients: a systematic review and meta-analysis. *Ann Oncol.* 2013;24(12):2952-2962.

Jain R, Chung SM, Jain L, et al. Implications of obesity for drug therapy: limitations and challenges. *Clin Pharmacol Ther.* 2011;90(1):77-89.

Janmahasatian S, Duffull SB, Chagnac A, Kirkpatrick CM, Green B. Lean body mass normalizes the effect of obesity on renal function. *Br J Clin Pharmacol.* 2008;65(6):964-965.

Jenkins P, Elyan S, Freeman S. Obesity is not associated with increased myelosuppression in patients receiving chemotherapy for breast cancer. *Eur J Cancer.* 2007;43(3):544-548.

Key TJ, Appleby PN, Reeves GK, et al. Body mass index, serum sex hormones, and breast cancer risk in postmenopausal women. *J Natl Cancer Inst.* 2003;95(16):1218-1226.

Ligibel JA, Alfano CM2, Courneya KS, et al. American Society of Clinical Oncology position statement on obesity and cancer. *J Clin Oncol.* 2014;32(31):3568-3574.

Litton JK, Gonzalez-Angulo AM, Warneke CL, et al. Relationship between obesity and pathologic response to neoadjuvant chemotherapy among women with operable breast cancer. *J Clin Oncol.* 2008;26(25):4072-4077.

McWilliams RR, Matsumoto ME, Burch PA, et al. Obesity adversely affects survival in pancreatic cancer patients. *Cancer.* 2010;116(21):5054-5062.

Park SM, Lim MK, Shin SA, Yun YH. Impact of prediagnosis smoking, alcohol, obesity, and insulin resistance on survival in male cancer patients: National Health Insurance Corporation study. *J Clin Oncol.* 2006;24(31):5017-5024.

Pavelka JC, Brown RS, Karlan BY, et al. Effect of obesity on survival in epithelial ovarian cancer. *Cancer.* 2006;107(7):1520-1524.

Pfeiler G, Königsberg R, Fesl C, et al. Impact of body mass index on the efficacy of endocrine therapy in premenopausal patients with breast cancer: an analysis of the prospective ABCSG-12 trial. *J Clin Oncol.* 2011;29(19):2653-2659.

Rodvold KA, Rushing DA, Tewksbury DA. Doxorubicin clearance in the obese. *J Clin Oncol.* 1988;6(8):1321-1327.

Rosner GL, Hargis JB, Hollis DR, et al. Relationship between toxicity and obesity in women receiving adjuvant chemotherapy for breast cancer: results from cancer and leukemia group B study 8541. *J Clin Oncol.* 1996;14(11):3000-3008.

Rudek MA, Sparreboom A, Garrett-Mayer ES, et al. Factors affecting pharmacokinetic variability following doxorubicin and docetaxel-based therapy. *Eur J Cancer.* 2004;40(8):1170-1178.

Sestak I, Distler W, Forbes JF, Dowsett M, Howell A, Cuzick J. Effect of body mass index on recurrences in tamoxifen and anastrozole treated women: an exploratory analysis from the ATAC trial. *J Clin Oncol.* 2010;28(21):3411-3415.

Sparreboom A, Wolff AC, Mathijssen RH, et al. Evaluation of alternate size descriptors for dose calculation of anticancer drugs in the obese. *J Clin Oncol.* 2007;25(30):4707-4713.

Wright JD, Tian C, Mutch DG, et al. Carboplatin dosing in obese women with ovarian cancer: a gynecologic oncology group study. *Gynecol Oncol.* 2008;109(3):353-358.

CHRONIC PAIN MANAGEMENT (CANCER)

DEFINITION AND INCIDENCE

Pain is defined by the International Society for the Study of Pain as "an unpleasant sensory and emotional experience associated with actual or potential tissue damage, or described in terms of such damage". The reported incidence of pain in cancer patients varies with the method used to determine the presence of pain, and the type and stage of cancer. It is estimated that 51% of patients with various stages of cancer experience pain, and patients with advanced disease are more likely to have severe pain. Pain in cancer patients may be due to the disease itself (eg, metastatic bone disease, visceral involvement); it may be secondary to some treatments (eg, painful neuropathy from vincristine or paclitaxel, or postoperative pain); it may result from complications associated with cancer (eg, postherpetic neuralgia); or it may have been present prior to the diagnosis of cancer and be unrelated to cancer (eg, arthritis). Most often, treatment guidelines and discussions focus on the management of chronic pain associated with progressive disease.

PAIN MEASUREMENT

The severity of pain is generally measured using a visual analogue scale (VAS), a numeric rating scale (NRS), or a verbal rating scale (VRS). A similar scale that uses facial expressions representing pain severity instead of numerals can be used for pediatric or cognitively impaired patients (faces pain scale [FPS]). The aforementioned pain scales are all considered to be valid and reliable measures of pain severity and changes in pain severity.

The VAS uses a 100 millimeter line to represent the range of pain severity from no pain to worst imaginable pain. Patients are instructed to mark a spot on the line that best correlates with their perceived pain severity. The NRS uses a numeric scale of 0 (no pain) to 10 (worst imaginable pain) for patients to select which number best represents their perceived pain severity. Numerical ratings of 1 to -3, 4 to -6, and 7 to -10 are generally considered mild, moderate, and severe, respectively. The VRS offers 5 phrases representing pain severity ratings as a measurement tool. The FPS consists of 6 facial expressions representing pain severity from no pain to very high pain.

◀ **Visual Analogue Scale (VAS)**

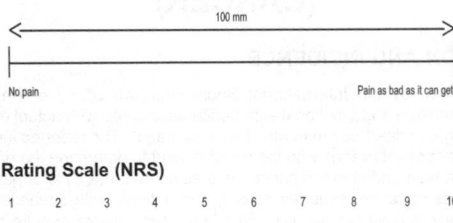

No pain   Pain as bad as it can get

Numeric Rating Scale (NRS)

1   2   3   4   5   6   7   8   9   10

No pain   Pain as bad as it can get

Verbal Rating Scale (VRS)

[ ] No pain
[ ] Mild pain
[ ] Moderate pain
[ ] Intense pain
[ ] Maximum pain

NONOPIOID ANALGESICS

The World Health Organization recommends a stepwise approach to the management of cancer pain (see figure).

WHO Three-Step Analgesic Ladder

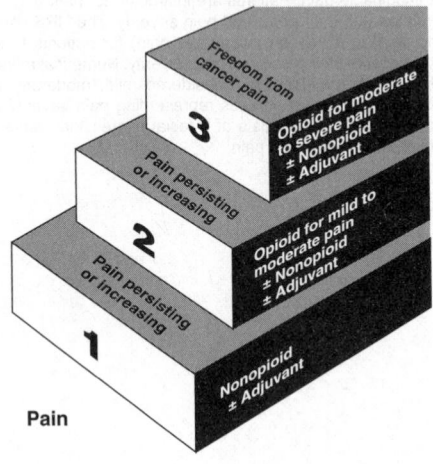

This approach recommends that the choice of therapy match the severity of pain (ie, strong opioids for moderate to severe pain). Nonopioids for (mild) cancer pain include acetaminophen, nonsteroidal anti-inflammatory drugs (NSAIDs), and aspirin. All of these have a ceiling above which increasing the dose will not enhance pain relief and will increase the likelihood of side effects. Although nonopioid analgesics are traditionally WHO step 1 products, they do have a role in the management of moderate to severe cancer pain. One blinded, placebo-controlled study reports that acetaminophen added to a strong opioid regimen in cancer patients improves pain control and well being.

Acetaminophen is commonly used for the management of mild to moderate pain. Use (including amounts contained in combination products) should be limited to a maximum daily dose of acetaminophen 4,000 mg per 24 hours (acute use) or 3,000 mg per 24 hours (chronic use) to reduce the risk of hepatotoxicity. Concerns regarding the use of NSAIDs in chronic cancer pain include the reversible inhibition of platelet aggregation, and the potential for gastropathy and nephrotoxicity. Aspirin is frequently avoided because of the potential for gastropathy and inhibition of platelet aggregation. Platelets exposed to aspirin become acetylated and permanently impaired. Celecoxib and nonacetylated salicylates, such as choline salicylate and magnesium salicylate, do not inhibit platelet aggregation.

OPIOID ANALGESICS

Opioid analgesic therapy should be initiated when adequate doses of nonopioid analgesics provide inadequate pain control or they are poorly tolerated.

Opioid analgesics for severe, persistent pain should be given "around-the-clock", not on an "as needed" or "PRN" basis. It is easier to prevent pain from recurring than to treat it once it has recurred. Titration of opioids to pain relief is easiest and safest using short-acting drugs (average duration of pain relief of 4 hours) or a continuous parenteral infusion. Once adequate pain relief is achieved, the 24-hour opioid dose can be given as a long-acting preparation (eg, sustained release morphine or oxycodone, transdermal fentanyl). In fact, opioid requirements can be increased in a similar manner for patients with worsening chronic pain daily. Short-acting medication for breakthrough pain, which is a transient worsening of otherwise stable pain in a patient taking an opioid, should always be available. Doses for breakthrough pain (ie, rescue doses) are commonly 5% to 15% of the 24-hour opioid dose, and may be administered every 1 to 2 hours as needed.

The oral route of administration for opioid analgesics is preferred whenever possible. All opioids undergo a high first-pass effect, which must be considered when converting from one route of administration to another. The parenteral to oral ratios for effectiveness of the different opioids vary from 1:2 to 1:6. The parenteral to oral dose ratio for morphine is 1:3 and 1:6 for the treatment of chronic pain and acute pain, respectively. Opioid equianalgesic doses are listed in the table that follows. Dose titration of opioid analgesics is based on pain control and patient tolerance; there is no maximum dosage for administration of opioid analgesics. Tolerance develops to most of the medication-related adverse effects, except constipation and myoclonus.

Table 1. Opioid Analgesics

Drug	Route of Administration	Approximate Equianalgesic Dose (mg)	Approximate Duration[1] (h)
Codeine	IM, IV	100 to 130	4 to 6
	Oral	200	
FentaNYL[2]	IV	0.1	0.5 to 2
HYDROcodone	Oral	30 to 45	4 to 6
HYDROmorphone	IM, IV, SubQ	1.5	2 to 5
	Oral, rectal	7.5	
Meperidine	IM, IV, SubQ	75	2 to 4
	Oral	300	
Methadone	IM, IV, SubQ	Variable	6 to 12
	Oral	See Guidelines for Conversion to Oral Methadone in Adults	
Morphine	IM, IV, SubQ	10	3 to 4[3]
	Oral, rectal	30	
OxyCODONE	Oral	20	4 to 6[3]
Oxymorphone	Oral	10	3 to 6[3]

Guidelines for Conversion to Oral Methadone in Adults[4]	
Oral Morphine Dose or Equivalent (mg/day)	Oral Morphine:Oral Methadone (Conversion Ratio)
<90	4:1
90 to 300	8:1
>300	12:1

[1]Parenteral or immediate-release products

[2]Transdermal fentanyl conversion presented in separate table that follows

[3]Duration for sustained release dosage forms is 8 to 12 hours (MS Contin, Oramorph SR), 24 hours (Kadian), 12 hours (OxyCONTIN), unknown (Opana ER)

[4]Conversion of higher doses may be guided by the following (consult a pain or palliative care specialist if unfamiliar with methadone prescribing): As the total daily chronic dose of morphine increases, the equianalgesic dose ratio (morphine:methadone) changes (American Pain Society 2008). Total daily dose should be divided by 3; delivered every 8 hours. Methadone is significantly more potent with repetitive dosing (due to its active metabolite). Begin methadone at lower doses and gradually titrate. Applicability to pediatric patients is unknown.

Meperidine is not recommended for chronic use. This is because of the potential for accumulation of a neurotoxic metabolite, normeperidine (see following information). Meperidine administration is best reserved for incident pain (ie, before a painful manipulation or procedure).

Tolerance is characterized by the requirement for a higher dose of opioid in order to produce the same effect previously seen with a lower dose. Tolerance develops to many side effects of opioids: respiratory depression, sedation, nausea, and vomiting. Tolerance does not usually develop to constipation or myoclonus. When a given dose of opioid is not effective, for whatever reason, and if side effects are tolerable, the dose can be increased. Physical dependence occurs with regular use of opioids, but is only of clinical importance if the opioid is abruptly discontinued or an opioid antagonist (eg, naloxone) is administered, in which cases a withdrawal syndrome can be seen. Opioids should be tapered in patients whose pain improves. Signs and symptoms of withdrawal can be reduced by maintaining at least 25% of the previous day's opioid dose. The opioid can be discontinued when the total daily dose is the equivalent of 10 to 15 mg of intramuscular morphine. Psychological dependence is defined as a "pattern of compulsive drug use characterized by a continued craving for an opioid and the need to use the opioid for effects other than pain relief." Unlike tolerance and physical dependence, psychological dependence is a characteristic of the patient, and is a function of environmental, social, economic, and personality factors. Psychological dependence or addiction, can develop in patients requiring management of chronic pain; however, this is **not** a valid reason to undertreat pain.

The most troublesome side effect associated with chronic opioid use is constipation, and, as noted above, tolerance to constipation does not occur. Regular use of stimulant laxatives is often required.

Tolerance does develop to opioid-induced respiratory depression, allowing safe dose escalation. In the event of an acute overdose, or in the case of respiratory depression not responding to supportive measures, naloxone can be used. Naloxone administration is reserved for serious situations because it precipitates withdrawal symptoms and the prompt return of pain in patients physically dependent on opioids. Other side effects of naloxone administration include nausea, vomiting, sedation, sweating, itching, dry mouth, and tremulousness. Initiate naloxone therapy with low doses (0.1 to 0.2 mg) repeated and increased as warranted by respiratory rate and patient comfort. Naltrexone is only available as an oral formulation, which limits its utility for acute reversal of opioid toxicity. Tolerance develops to nausea and vomiting, and these effects are more likely to occur when opioid therapy is initiated. Phenothiazines can be used to treat nausea and vomiting. Dimenhydrinate or meclizine can also be used to treat this side effect. Tolerance usually develops to sedation. For those patients in whom persistent or profound sedation limits opioid dose escalation and therefore pain relief, the use of stimulants (eg, dextroamphetamine, methylphenidate) should be considered. Sweating and itching are thought to be due to histamine release. Morphine and meperidine are notable for causing histamine release. Switching to another opioid should be considered for patients with intolerable sweating or itching. Seizures associated with opioids are generally attributed to accumulation of neurotoxic metabolites or large overdoses that presumably cause hypoxia. Normeperidine, a metabolite of meperidine that can accumulate with frequent repeated doses or in patients with renal insufficiency, is the most well known of these neurotoxic metabolites. Distinct from seizures, myoclonic jerks may be seen with the use of high doses of opioids. Occasional reports indicate that they may also be seen with relatively lower doses. Benzodiazepines have been suggested to control this side effect as tolerance does not typically develop to this adverse event.

Opioid-induced hyperalgesia (OIH) should be suspected when analgesic efficacy is inexplicably lost or when generalized or worsening pain develops during aggressive opioid titration. OIH is a rare consequence of opioid therapy in cancer patients, and most often seen with aggressive morphine titration. The underlying mechanism is thought to be related to inhibition of glycinergic activity at the level of the spinal cord by phenanthrene-type opioids that promotes a strychnine-like excitatory effect. Additional biochemical mechanisms implicated in OIH include upregulation of intracellular phosphokinase C which activates the NMDA receptor

◀ system, and intraspinal dynorphin-mediated substance P and glutamate release. In the scenario of OIH, continued dose escalation aggravates pain which then improves with dose reduction. Management of OIH includes dose reduction or interruption of treatment with the offending agent. Replacing a phenanthrene derivative to a piperidine-type opioid, such as fentanyl or methadone, is recommended. The addition of low-dose methadone to chronically administered phenanthrene derivative opioid analgesia has been suggested as a strategy to mitigate OIH.

As previously noted, the oral route of administration for opioids is generally preferred. When oral administration is not possible, several other routes are available (see Table 1). Morphine and hydromorphone are also available in rectal suppositories. The recommended rectal dose is the same as the oral dose. Continuous subcutaneous or intravenous infusions administered with an infusion control device are useful when oral administration is impossible. Continuous parenteral infusion of opioids provides more consistent pain relief and patient tolerance compared to intermittent injections which result in peaks and valleys of pain relief or side effects. Continuous infusions also allow for quick titration of opioid in patients with uncontrolled pain. Patient-controlled analgesia provides a continuous infusion of opioid with a capacity for patient-administered bolus injections for breakthrough pain. This is not unlike the concept of regularly scheduled sustained release oral opioid with immediate release tablets for breakthrough, as previously discussed. Assessment of the use of breakthrough doses, whether oral or parenteral, provides a basis for adjusting the dose/rate of the underlying opioid. Transdermal fentanyl is another alternative, long-acting, analgesic for patients unable to take oral opioids. Transdermal fentanyl should be avoided when initiating chronic analgesia in opioid-naïve patients to reduce the risk of profound respiratory depression. As is the case with sustained release oral opioids, it is preferable to titrate to pain relief using short-acting drugs, and then switch to transdermal fentanyl. The manufacturer recommends equianalgesic conversion to the fentanyl patch as presented in Table 2. This schema represents a conservative conversion from an oral or parenteral opioid to the fentanyl transdermal system, so the tabulated information should **not** be used to convert from fentanyl transdermal to an oral or parenteral opioid analgesic.

Table 2. Dosing Guidelines for Conversion to FentaNYL Transdermal Systems

Current Analgesic	Daily Dosage (mg/day)			
Morphine (oral)	60 to 134	135 to 224	225 to 314	315 to 404
Morphine (parenteral)	10 to 22	23 to 37	38 to 52	53 to 67
HYDROmorphone (oral)	8 to 17	17.1 to 28	28.1 to 39	39.1 to 51
HYDROmorphone (parenteral)	1.5 to 3.4	3.5 to 5.6	5.7 to 7.9	8 to 10
OxyCODONE (oral)	30 to 67	67.5 to 112	112.5 to 157	157.5 to 202
Meperidine (parenteral)	75 to 165	166 to 278	279 to 390	391 to 503
FentaNYL transdermal recommended dose[1]	25 mcg/h	50 mcg/h	75 mcg/h	100 mcg/h

[1]Recommendations are based on US product labeling and differ from Canadian transdermal product labeling; see current Canadian product label.

One method for switching transdermal fentanyl and oral methadone is described by using the transdermal fentanyl:oral methadone conversion factor of 1:20 (daily dose:daily dose) to change patients (n=31) with inadequate pain control from one product to another (Mercandante 2005). Oral methadone was administered in divided doses every eight hours. Fentanyl patches were removed when the first dose of methadone was administered. Conversely, for patients transitioning to transdermal fentanyl, the patch was applied with administration of the last methadone dose. This method was used successfully in 24 of 31 patients (78%) with improved pain control reported within 24 hours of product conversion and acceptable patient tolerance. Inadequate symptom control (6 patients) and adverse effects (1 patient) were the reasons for unsuccessful switching in seven patients. Using this conversion ratio, treatment with transdermal fentanyl 200 mcg/hour is switched to oral methadone 96 mg daily administered in divided doses as 30 mg every eight hours.

A similar method has been described which calculates the appropriate methadone dose using two steps (Benitez-Rosario 2004). First, the patient's daily transdermal fentanyl dose is converted to the equivalent oral morphine dose using a ratio of fentanyl:oral morphine of 1:100. The resultant value is converted to the equivalent daily dose of oral methadone using the ratio of oral morphine: oral methadone ratio of 5:1 or 10:1. The calculated methadone dose is divided for administration every 8 to 12 hours beginning 8 to 24 hours following removal of the transdermal fentanyl system. Using this method, a patient with adequate pain control from transdermal fentanyl 100 mcg/hour would be receiving a daily dose of fentanyl 2.4 mg every 24 hours, which converts to oral morphine 240 mg per 24-hour, which converts to oral methadone 24 to 48 mg per 24 hours. So, 8 to 24 hours after removing the fentanyl patch, a dosage of oral methadone 15 mg administered every 8 or 12 hours can be started.

Intraspinal administration of opioids should be reserved for patients in whom systemic administration of opioids results in unacceptable or unmanageable toxicity. Epidural morphine is 5 to 10 times more potent than parenteral morphine, and intrathecal morphine is 10 times more potent than epidural morphine. Bupivacaine, clonidine, and ketamine have been added to epidural morphine infusions to enhance effectiveness.

Partial opioid agonists (eg, buprenorphine) or agonist-antagonists (eg, pentazocine, butorphanol, dezocine, nalbuphine) are generally not recommended for use in chronic cancer pain management. They have a ceiling for analgesic effectiveness, above which side effects are much more likely to increase, and they may precipitate withdrawal in patients receiving opioid agonists (eg, morphine). Naloxone may not be effective in reversing respiratory depression caused by buprenorphine.

Tramadol is a synthetic opioid that inhibits the neuronal reuptake of norepinephrine and serotonin. This product is indicated for the management of moderate pain and it has been tested in the management of mild to moderate cancer pain. Its use is limited by the risk of seizures which have occurred in patients taking the usual and recommended dosage. One comparative study reported that the rate of vomiting, dizziness, anorexia, and weakness was greater with tramadol than codeine or hydrocodone when used for cancer pain (Rodriguez, 2007). Abrupt discontinuation of tramadol can precipitate withdrawal symptoms, such as tremors, sweating, diarrhea, upper respiratory symptoms, and rarely, hallucinations. The dosage of tramadol must be adjusted for impaired renal function.

◀ # ADJUVANT ANALGESICS

Adjuvant analgesics are frequently used in addition to, rather than instead of, opioid analgesics. Adjuvants are often drugs that have primary indications other than pain, but may provide pain relief in certain situations. NSAIDs are commonly used for pain due to bone metastases (see individual NSAID monographs). Gabapentin and pregabalin are commonly used as adjunctive therapy for neuropathic pain. Additional drugs that have been used for this purpose include tricyclic antidepressants (eg, amitriptyline, nortriptyline), anticonvulsants (eg, carbamazepine), corticosteroids, and antiarrhythmics (eg, topical lidocaine). Methadone and ketamine are thought to improve neuropathic pain through blockade of the N-methyl-D-aspartate (NMDA) receptor. Neuropathic pain, often characterized by sharp, shooting, lancinating sensations, may result from nerve compression, infiltration, or destruction by tumor or from other associated conditions (eg, postherpetic neuralgia). Pain relief is usually not complete and, as is the case with NSAIDs in bone pain, these drugs are generally used in addition to opioids. Baclofen has also been used as an adjuvant analgesic for various types of neuropathic pain. Strontium-89 is a radiopharmaceutical that is reported to decrease the need for analgesics in patients with osteoblastic bone metastases. Prostate cancer is the most frequent malignancy associated with painful osteoblastic lesions. The bisphosphonates pamidronate and zoledronic acid are used to decrease pain and adverse skeletal events in patients with multiple myeloma and breast cancer. Capsaicin is a topically applied adjuvant analgesic that depletes substance P, a "painful" neurotransmitter. Capsaicin is recommended for use in postherpetic neuralgia and other painful neuropathies.

REFERENCES

Axelrod DJ, Reville B. Using methadone to treat opioid-induced hyperalgesia and refractory pain. *J Opioid Manag.* 2007;3(2):113-114.

Benítez-Rosario MA, Feria M, Salinas-Martín A, Martínez-Castillo LP, Martín-Ortega JJ. Opioid switching from transdermal fentanyl to oral methadone in patients with cancer pain. *Cancer.* 2004;101(12):2866-2873.

Benrath J, Scharbert G, Gustorff B, Adams HA, Kress HG. Long-term intrathecal S(+)-ketamine in a patient with cancer-related neuropathic pain. *Br J Anaesth.* 2005;95(2):247-249.

Berenson JR, Lichtenstein A, Porter L, et al. Efficacy of pamidronate in reducing skeletal events in patients with advanced multiple myeloma. Myeloma aredia study group. *N Engl J Med.* 1996;334 (8):488-493.

Cordell GA, Araujo OE. Capsaicin: identification, nomenclature, and pharmacotherapy. *Ann Pharmacother.* 1993;27(3):330-336.

Davis MP, Shaiova LA, Angst MS. When opioids cause pain. *J Clin Oncol.* 2007;25(28):4497-4498.

Elsner F, Radbruch L, Loick G, Gaertner J, Sabatowski R. Intravenous versus subcutaneous morphine titration in patients with persisting exacerbation of cancer pain. *J Palliat Med.* 2005;8 (4):743-750.

Ferreira-Valente MA, Pais-Ribeiro JL, Jensen MP. Validity of four pain intensity rating scales. *Pain.* 2011;152(10):2399-2404.

Fromm GH. Baclofen as an adjuvant analgesic. *J Pain Symptom Manage.* 1994;9(8):500-509.

Højsted J, Sjøgren P. Addiction to opioids in chronic pain patients: a literature review. *Eur J Pain.* 2007;11(5):490-518.

Holdsworth MT, Adams VR, Chavez CM, Vaughan LJ, Duncan MH. Continuous midazolam infusion for the management of morphine-induced myoclonus. *Ann Pharmacother.* 1995;29 (1):25-29.

Jackson KC 2nd. Pharmacotherapy for neuropathic pain. *Pain Pract.* 2006;6(1):27-33.

Jacox A, Carr DB, Payne R, et al. Management of cancer pain. *Clinical Practice Guideline No. 9, AHCPR Publication No. 94-0592.* Rockville, MD: Agency for Health Care Policy and Research, US Department of Health and Human Services, Public Health Service; 1994.

Laizure SC. Considerations in morphine therapy. *Am J Hosp Pharm.* 1994;51(16):2042-2043.

Levy MH, Chwistek M, Mehta RS. Management of chronic pain in cancer survivors. *Cancer J.* 2008;14(6):401-409.

Levy MH. Pharmacologic treatment of cancer pain. *N Engl J Med.* 1996;335(15):1124-1132.

Lossignol DA, Obiols-Portis M, Body JJ. Successful use of ketamine for intractable cancer pain. *Support Care Cancer*. 2005;13(3):188-193.

Mercadante SL, Berchovich M, Casuccio A, Fulfaro F, Mangione S. A prospective randomized study of corticosteroids as adjuvant drugs to opioids in advanced cancer patients. *Am J Hosp Palliat Care*. 2007;24(1):13-19.

Mercadante S, Ferrera P, Villari P, Casuccio A.. Rapid switching between transdermal fentanyl and methadone in cancer patients. *J Clin Oncol*. 2005;23(22):5229-5234.

Potter JM, Reid DB, Shaw RJ, Hackett P, Hickman PE. Myoclonus associated with treatment with high doses of morphine: the role of supplemental drugs. *BMJ*. 1989;299(6692):150-153.

Principles of analgesic use in the treatment of acute pain and cancer pain. 6th ed. Glenview, IL: American Cancer Pain Society; 2008.

Robinson RG, Preston DF, Baxter KG, Dusing RW, Spicer JA. Clinical experience with strontium-89 in prostatic and breast cancer patients. *Semin Oncol*. 1993;20(3 Suppl 2):44-48.

Rodriguez RF, Bravo LE, Castro F, et al. Incidence of weak opioids adverse events in the management of cancer pain: a double-blind comparative trial. *J Palliat Med*. 2007;10(1):56-60.

Rodriguez RF, Castillo JM, Del Pilar Castillo M, et al. Codeine/acetaminophen and hydrocodone/acetaminophen combination tablets for the management of chronic cancer pain in adults: a 23-day, prospective, double-blind, randomized, parallel-group study. *Clin Ther*. 2007;29(4):581-587.

Salpeter SR, Buckley JS, Bruera E. The use of very-low-dose methadone for palliative pain control and the prevention of opioid hyperalgesia. *J Palliat Med*. 2013;16(6):616-622.

Stearns L, Boortz-Marx R, Du Pen S, et al. Intrathecal drug delivery for the management of cancer pain: a multidisciplinary consensus of best clinical practices. *J Support Oncol*. 2005;3 (6):399-408.

Stockler M, Vardy J, Pillai A, Warr D. Acetaminophen (paracetamol) improves pain and well-being in people with advanced cancer already receiving a strong opioid regimen: a randomized, double-blind, placebo-controlled cross-over trial. *J Clin Oncol*. 2004;22(16):3389-3394.

Svendsen KB, Andersen S, Arnason S, et al. Breakthrough pain in malignant and non-malignant diseases: a review of prevalence, characteristics and mechanisms. *Eur J Pain*. 2005;9 (2):195-206.

Szeto HH, Inturrisi CE, Houde R, Saal S, Cheigh J, Reidenberg MM. Accumulation of normeperidine, an active metabolite of meperidine in patients with renal failure of cancer. *Ann Intern Med*. 1977;86(6):738-741.

Tsavaris N, Kopterides P, Kosmas C, et al. Analgesic activity of high-dose intravenous calcitonin in cancer patients with bone metastases. *Oncol Rep*. 2006;16(4):871-875.

Vranken JH, van der Vegt MH, Kal JE, Kruis MR. Treatment of neuropathic cancer pain with continuous intrathecal administration of S +-ketamine. *Acta Anaesthesiol Scand*. 2004;48 (2):249-252.

Wallace E, Ridley J, Bryson J, Mak E, Zimmermann C. Addition of methadone to another opioid in the management of moderate to severe cancer pain: a case series. *J Palliat Med*. 2013;16 (3):305-309.

Wellington K, Goa KL. Zoledronic acid: a review of its use in the management of bone metastases and hypercalcaemia of malignancy. *Drugs*. 2003;63(4):417-437.

Yucel A, Ozyalcin S, Koknel Talu G, et al. The effect of venlafaxine on ongoing and experimentally induced pain in neuropathic pain patients: a double blind, placebo controlled study. *Eur J Pain*. 2005;9(4):407-416.

HOSPICE (END OF LIFE) CARE

Hospice care is provided to maintain comfort and control symptoms in the dying patient. Most patients receiving hospice care have a life expectancy of less than a few months. The pharmaceutical component of hospice care is one aspect pertaining to the quality of dying and death. The quality of dying and death entails the physical experience, psychological experience, social and cultural comprehension, spiritual or existential understanding, life closure and death preparation, and the circumstances of death. For cancer patients the type and stage of malignant disease and their health care experience impact the quality of dying and death.

Important communications between the patient and loved one or the patient and health care professional is best conducted early during hospice care rather than later. Many people are unable to effectively communicate within hours to days before death occurs. The percentage of patients who are awake, drowsy, or comatose one week prior to death is 56%, 44%, and zero, respectively. In comparison, 24 hours before death 26% of patients are awake, 62% of patients are drowsy, and 12% are comatose. And within 6 hours of death 8% of patients are awake, 42% of patients are drowsy, and 50% are comatose.

It is difficult to predict the expected time of impending death. Some patients become progressively less responsive until they die; whereas, other experience symptomatology portending death. Noisy respirations (also known as death rattle) occur when patients are obtunded or too weak to expectorate secretions. The noise is generated by secretions that accumulate in the hypopharynx and bronchial tree and oscillate with the movement of air during inspiration and exhalation. Noisy respirations generally develop within 2 to 3 days of death. Respiration with involuntary mandibular movement, cyanosis of the extremities, and loss of radial pulse occur approximately eight hours, five hours, and three hours, respectively, prior to death. Interestingly, the time from respiration with mandibular movement or cyanosis to death is markedly prolonged in patients with primary lung cancer or metastatic malignant disease affecting the lungs. Additional adverse events associated with dying include agitation or restlessness, delirium, dyspnea, incontinence of urine or stool, irregular breathing including gasping or 20- to 30-second interruptions in respiration, nausea, and swelling of the extremities.

It is important to provide safe and appropriate therapy relative to the expected outcome of therapy. Medications utilized in hospice care are often for off-label uses and are administered outside of the usual dosage range. In addition, many medications used for symptom control are prone to diversion for recreational use. In order to effectively deliver pharmacologic medication therapy for hospice care, it is important for institutions to develop policies and procedures governing the management and use of drugs for end of life care.

Noisy respirations are generally managed by placement of the patient in a semiprone position, reduction of parenteral hydration, explanation of the situation to family members and visitors, gentle nasopharyngeal or tracheal suctioning, and administration of anticholinergic medications. Transdermal scopolamine and parenteral glycopyrrolate are used in the management of noisy respirations. The commercially available patch delivers scopolamine 1 mg over 72 hours. A single patch may be sufficient for reduction of noisy respirations; however, additional patches can be applied without exceeding the daily dose of subcutaneous scopolamine administered to European hospice patients. Administration of scopolamine 1.2 mg per 24 hours by continuous subcutaneous infusion for reduction of noisy respirations is reported in the medical literature. Application of four patches is expected to deliver scopolamine 1.3 mg per 24 hours. Parenteral scopolamine is not licensed for use in the United States. Glycopyrrolate 0.2 mg can be administered by subcutaneous or intravenous bolus. Administration of glycopyrrolate 0.6 mg per 24 hours by continuous subcutaneous infusion for management of noisy respirations is reported in the medical literature. Administration of parenteral medications can be difficult for patients who are dying at home or outside of a hospital. In such circumstances, ipratropium bromide 0.03% nasal solution may provide an alternative to glycopyrrolate. Sublingual administration of ipratropium bromide 0.03% nasal solution two sprays 1 to 3 times daily is reportedly effective for reduction of drug induced sialorrhea. One drawback to sublingual administration may be erratic absorption for patients with excess secretions in the oral cavity. Atropine 1% ophthalmic drops are a suboptimal selection because each drop of solution delivers 0.5 mg of atropine, which is a pharmacologic dose that can modulate heart rate.

Opioid therapy is the cornerstone of treatment for pain and dyspnea in hospice care. Opioid requirements tend to increase in the dying patient. The proportion of dying patients requiring opioids expands from 42% one week before death to 78% during the final 48 hours of life. In addition, the daily opioid dose increases 2- to 3-fold during the same time frame. Increased opioid requirements are thought to be due to progression of the patient's underlying pathophysiologic problems instead of the development of tolerance. (Refer to Chronic Pain Management (Cancer) on page 2229 and Palliative Care Medicine (Cancer) on page 2252.)

Pharmacologic sedation is often required for end of life delirium restlessness and agitation. Normally the goal of sedation is to manage symptoms without appreciably reducing the patient's level of consciousness. End of life sedation has not been shown to shorten survival. Sedation during hospice care can include proportional palliative sedation (PPS) or, less commonly, palliative sedation to achieve unconsciousness (PSU). The goal of PPS is to provide an adequate amount of sedation for symptom control and maintain consciousness, as much as possible. Gradual titration of a benzodiazepine is commonly used for PPS. Two of the most commonly studied benzodiazepines for end of life sedation are midazolam and lorazepam. Additional drugs that have been utilized for end of life sedation are propofol and phenobarbital. Respiratory depression caused by phenobarbital should be considered when this product is administered. Limited information describes use of chlorpromazine and haloperidol for end of life restlessness and agitation. Chlorpromazine is suboptimal because it lowers the seizure threshold. Haloperidol should be reserved for use in patients with concurrent delirium. The potential for QTc interval prolongation with haloperidol should be considered with use of this product. The goal of PSU is to induce unconsciousness. This is reserved for refractory cases with unbearable symptoms. PSU is generally accomplished by rapid titration of a benzodiazepine to the state of unconsciousness, with continuation of adequate doses to maintain unconsciousness.

Medication administration can be problematic in the hospice setting. Oral administration, which is the preferred route whenever possible, can be ineffective and dangerous for the obtunded, delirious, or actively dying patient. Intravenous medication administration is often problematic for patients who choose to die outside of the hospital. Moreover, venous access can become difficult in all care environments with reduced peripheral blood circulation in the dying patient. Intramuscular administration is too painful for repeated use. Subcutaneous administration of medications is feasible if it can be accomplished without causing undue discomfort for the patient. Repeated subcutaneous bolus of medications can cause discomfort for some patients. Certain opioids, such as morphine, hydromorphone, and fentanyl, can be administered by continuous subcutaneous infusion. The utility of continuous subcutaneous infusion of medications is generally limited by the rate of fluid volume administration required for drug delivery. Rectal administration of medications can be used in the hospice setting. The Macy Catheter is a device that facilitates discreet and hygienic rectal administration. This device consists of two lumens, one for medication administration and the other for inflation of a retention balloon. The retention balloon can be deflated for device removal or left in place for device expulsion by defecation. Transdermal administration is an option for selected medications, such as scopolamine and fentanyl.

SELECTED READINGS

Back IN, Jenkins K, Blower A, Beckhelling J. A study comparing hyoscine hydrobromide and glycopyrrolate in the treatment of death rattle. *Palliat Med.* 2001;15(4):329-336.

Hales S, Zimmermann C, Rodin G. The quality of dying and death. *Arch Intern Med.* 2008;168 (9):912-918.

Hugel H, Ellershaw J, Gambles M. Respiratory tract secretions in the dying patient: a comparison between glycopyrronium and hyoscine hydrobromide. *J Palliat Med.* 2006;9(2):279-284.

Kåss RM, Ellershaw J. Respiratory tract secretions in the dying patient: a retrospective study. *J Pain Symptom Manage.* 2003;26(4):897-902.

Kehl KA. Treatment of terminal restlessness: a review of the evidence. *J Pain Palliat Care Pharmacother.* 2004;18(1):5-30.

Kintzel PE, Chase SL, Thomas W, Vancamp DM, Clements EA. Anticholinergic medications for managing noisy respirations in adult hospice patients. *Am J Health Syst Pharm.* 2009;66 (5):458-464.

Maltoni M, Scarpi E, Rosati M, et al. Palliative sedation in end-of-life care and survival: a systematic review. *J Clin Oncol.* 2012;30(12):1378-1383.

Morita T, Ichiki T, Tsunoda J, Inoue S, Chihara S. A prospective study on the dying process in terminally ill cancer patients. *Am J Hosp Palliat Care.* 1998;15(4):217-222.

Pantilat SZ, Isaac M. End-of-life care for the hospitalized patient. *Med Clin North Am.* 2008;92 (2):349-370.

Quill TE, Lo B, Brock DW, Meisel A. Last-resort options for palliative sedation. *Ann Intern Med.* 2009;151(6):421-424.

HYPERCALCEMIA OF MALIGNANCY

INTRODUCTION

Hypercalcemia of malignancy (HCM) affects 20% to 30% of patients with advanced cancer. It is the most frequently occurring life-threatening metabolic disorder in this patient population. The highest incidence is seen in patients with lung, breast, and renal cell cancers. In addition to these solid tumors, HCM is also commonly observed in patients with the hematologic malignancies multiple myeloma and human T-cell lymphotropic virus type I (HTLV-1)-associated T-cell lymphoma. Even with appropriate treatment, 30-day mortality rates following the HCM diagnosis approach 50% (Stewart 2005). Poor prognostic indicators include corrected serum calcium exceeding 11.3 mg/dL (hazard ratio [HR]: 2.21), serum albumin <3.6 g/dL (HR: 2.41), squamous cell carcinoma (HR: 2.64), and metastatic disease affecting the bone (HR: 1.44) or liver (HR: 2.22) (Penel 2008).

PATHOPHYSIOLOGY

The primary cause of HCM is increased bone resorption secondary to osteoclast activation which is mediated by proteins and cytokines released by tumor cells or their microenvironment. HCM can be classified into 4 types (local humoral, osteolytic, calcitriol secreting lymphomas, and ectopic hyperparathyroidism). Parathyroid-hormone-related protein (PTHrP)-mediated hypercalcemia (or humoral HCM) is the most common cause in solid tumors without bone metastasis. PTHrP released by the tumor initially stimulates osteoblasts to secrete receptor activator of nuclear factor-kappa ligand (RANKL). RANKL activates osteoclasts, resulting in increased bone resorption. PTHrP also promotes calcium renal tubular reabsorption. In patients with bone metastasis, local osteoclastic bone resorption is increased in the areas surrounding the tumor within the marrow space. Some lymphomas produce calcitriol ($1,25[OH]_2D3$), leading to hypercalcemia due to increased osteoclastic bone resorption and enhanced intestinal absorption of calcium. Lastly, a very rare cause of HCM is ectopic secretion of parathyroid hormone (PTH).

SYMPTOMS AND DIAGNOSIS

One early sign of hypercalcemia is polyuria, which develops as the body tries to eliminate excess ionized calcium from the serum. Polyuria causes intravascular volume depletion and dehydration, which signals the body to retain sodium. The ensuing renotubular reabsorption of sodium promotes concurrent reabsorption of calcium which fuels the hypercalcemia. Acute renal impairment may occur due to intravascular volume depletion and calcium-phosphate precipitation in the renal tubules. Neurologic adverse effects are generally the most serious sequelae of hypercalcemia. Confusion is common and patients can progress to somnolence and coma. Malaise and muscle weakness occur. Gastrointestinal adverse effects include anorexia, constipation, ileus, nausea, and vomiting. Cardiac effects include bradycardia and other dysrhythmias. Symptom severity is related to the degree of hypercalcemia and the rate at which the serum calcium increased.

Diagnosis of HCM is confirmed with laboratory measurement of serum calcium levels. As total calcium levels are associated with patients' albumin stores, it is important to calculate the serum ionized calcium level using the equation [corrected Ca++ (mg/dL) = measured serum Ca++ (mg/dL) + 0.8 x (4 - measured serum albumin in g/dL)]. However, this equation may not always accurately reflect true ionized calcium levels; in such cases, directly measuring serum ionized calcium is prudent. PTH and PTHrP may be measured in the occasional cases in which the cause of hypercalcemia is not clear. Likewise, $1,25(OH)_2D3$ levels may be assessed if sarcoidosis or other granulomatous conditions, or the $1,25(OH)_2D3$ lymphoma syndrome, is in the differential diagnosis.

Body System	Symptoms
General	Dehydration, weight loss, pruritis, polydipsia
Neuromuscular	Fatigue, lethargy, muscle weakness, hyporeflexia, confusion, psychosis, seizure, obtundation, coma
Gastrointestinal	Anorexia, nausea, vomiting, constipation, ileus
Renal	Polyuria, renal insufficiency
Cardiac	Bradycardia, prolonged PR, shortened QT, wide T wave, arrhythmias

MANAGEMENT

The first treatment priority of HCM is reversal of dehydration to reduce the serum calcium concentration and preserve renal function. Once normovolemia is restored, furosemide is often added; however, the primary role of a loop diuretic in this situation is to prevent volume overload. First-line therapies to reduce bone resorption include bisphosphonates and calcitonin. Second-line therapies include corticosteroids for multiple myeloma and lymphoid malignancies. Hemodialysis may be necessary in severe cases of hypercalcemia. Treatment of the underlying malignancy is also an option for reducing HCM for some patients. However, the metabolic benefits of effective anticancer treatment may not be clinically evident for a period of weeks to months. Unfortunately, many patients with HCM have cancer that has progressed despite the standard anticancer therapies.

Treatment is based on symptomatology and the serum calcium level. The criteria for initiation of treatment are generally hypercalcemia with signs of toxicity (polyuria, mental status changes, renal dysfunction, cardiac dysrhythmias) attributed to hypercalcemia. A total calcium level exceeding 13 mg/dL is cited as criteria for initiation of therapy; although, it is unusual for HCM to present without related symptomatology.

0.9% Sodium Chloride

The intravenous fluid used for rehydration is 0.9% sodium chloride because it effectively improves intravascular volume and promotes renal excretion of calcium. The rate of administration of sodium chloride depends on the degree of dehydration, the severity of hypercalcemia, and the cardiopulmonary status of the patient. Ideally, patients should receive 0.9% sodium chloride at a rate of 2 to 3 L/m^2 per 24 hours; however, this often must be attenuated relative to what the patient's cardiopulmonary status can accommodate. Hydration rates as high as 5 L/m^2 per 24 hours have been used in severe cases. Following rehydration, proximal tubular reabsorption of sodium, and therefore calcium, will decrease. Further, other treatments for hypercalcemia require prior volume replacement in order to minimize toxicities. Sodium chloride can lower serum calcium by approximately 2 mg/dL. Saline hydration has an immediate but transient effect. Even if normocalcemia is achieved, serum calcium will increase again unless additional treatments aimed at reducing bone resorption or treating the underlying malignancy are administered.

Furosemide

The major use of furosemide in the management of cancer-associated hyper-calcemia is to prevent and manage fluid overload in order to facilitate the administration of sodium chloride for volume replacement. A usual starting dose of furosemide is 10 to 20 mg by intravenous push every 6 to 12 hours around the clock or as needed to maintain an acceptable rate of urine output. Loop diuretics are not effective agents for enhancing renal excretion of calcium. Loop diuretics should be used with caution to avoid intravascular volume depletion with exacerbation of hypercalcemia and renal impairment.

Bisphosphonates

Bisphosphonates bind to hydroxyapatite in bone and inhibit osteoclastic bone resorption. Pamidronate and zoledronic acid are the most commonly used bisphosphonates for management of HCM. Intravenous ibandronate is also a treatment option for this condition. The dose of intravenous ibandronate used for HCM in clinical trials is 2 mg or 4 mg. In a randomized, double-blind comparison with 275 of 287 subjects evaluable for efficacy zoledronic acid was superior to pamidronate for normalization of serum calcium by day 4 (50% vs 33% of patients) and day 10 (88% vs 70% of patients) of therapy. The median duration of normocalcemia was 32 days for zoledronic acid 4 mg and 18 days for pamidronate 90 mg. However, the frequency of renal impairment was greater in the zoledronic acid treatment arm.

Bisphosphonates should be used with caution in patients with severe renal impairment because these products are eliminated by the kidneys and can cause nephrotoxicity. Pamidronate has not been studied in patients with serum creatinine exceeding 3 mg/dL or creatinine clearance <30 mL/minute. Renal dosage adjustment of zoledronic acid administered for the treatment of HCM is not warranted when the serum creatinine is <4.5 mg/dL. The manufacturer of intravenous ibandronate recommends against use of this product for serum creatinine exceeding 2.3 mg/dL or creatinine clearance <30 mL/min.

Common side effects of bisphosphonates are mild and include fever and infusion site reactions, such as phlebitis. Avascular osteonecrosis of the jaw (ONJ) is an infrequent but serious adverse effect of bisphosphonate therapy. ONJ can be an extremely painful condition. Most reported cases of ONJ involve cancer patients receiving intravenous bisphosphonate therapy while undergoing dental procedures. Risk factors for ONJ during bisphosphonate therapy include cancer, chemotherapy, radiotherapy, corticosteroids, poor oral hygiene, preexisting dental disease or infection, anemia, and coagulopathy. Patients should maintain good oral hygiene and have a dental examination with preventive dentistry prior to treatment with bisphosphonates. Another adverse effect identified in women receiving bisphosphonate therapy for postmenopausal osteoporosis is severe musculoskeletal pain that develops within days, weeks or months of beginning treatment. This condition may become debilitating and necessitate discontinuation of bisphosphonate therapy.

Denosumab

Denosumab, a monoclonal antibody which binds to RANKL and inhibits osteoclast formation, function, and survival, is approved for hypercalcemia of malignancy that is refractory to bisphosphonate therapy. Denosumab is effective in reducing the serum calcium in nearly 2/3 of bisphosphonate-refractory (corrected serum calcium remaining ≥11.5 mg/dL 7 to 30 days after IV bisphosphonate treatment) patients; the median time to response was 9 days, the median duration of response was 104 days, and the median duration of complete response was 34 days (Hu 2014). Hypocalcemia has been reported with denosumab use; monitor serum calcium levels accordingly.

Calcitonin

Calcitonin works in a receptor-mediated manner to inhibit bone resorption and enhance urinary excretion of calcium. It is the fastest acting of the agents used to treat hypercalcemia and may be given safely before rehydration is complete. The usual starting dose of calcitonin is 4 units/kg by subcutaneous injection every 12 hours. Side effects are mild and infrequent and include nausea, abdominal cramps, and flushing. Calcitonin lowers serum calcium by ~2 mg/dL. Resistance to the pharmacologic effects of calcitonin generally develops with a few days of therapy. In fact, this can become apparent clinically as rebound hypercalcemia.

Corticosteroids

Corticosteroid administration is added to therapy when the underlying malignancy is a steroid-responsive disease, such as multiple myeloma, and lymphoma.

Other

Bortezomib has a dual anticancer and bone stabilizing effect. This medication, which is used in the treatment of multiple myeloma and mantle cell lymphoma, stimulates osteoblast differentiation, and inhibits osteoclast formation and bone resorption independently of its anticancer effect.

Drug	Usual Dose	Onset of Effect (h)	Duration of Effect
Bisphosphonates (IV)			
Pamidronate	60 or 90 mg	24 to 48	Median: 10 days (1 to 30)
Zoledronic acid	4 mg	24 to 48	Median: 10 days (1 to 30)
Calcitonin (SubQ)	4 units/kg q12h	4	Median: 2 day (1 to 6)
Denosumab (SubQ)	120 mg every 4 weeks; during the first month, give an additional 120 mg on days 8 and 15	Median: 9 days; time to complete response: 23 days	Median: 104 days; duration of complete response: 34 days
0.9% sodium chloride (IV)	2 to 3 L/m^2 per 24 h	12 to 48	Transient

Treatments are listed in alphabetical order. See text for guidance on priority and order of use.

REFERENCES

Hu MI, Glezerman IG, Leboulleux S, et al. Denosumab for treatment of hypercalcemia of malignancy. *J Clin Endocrinol Metab*. 2014;99(9):3144-3152.

LeGrand SB, Leskuski D, Zama I. Narrative review: furosemide for hypercalcemia: an unproven yet common practice. *Ann Intern Med*. 2008;149(4):259-263.

Lumachi F, Brunello A, Roma A, Basso U. Cancer-induced hypercalcemia. *Anticancer Res*. 2009;29(5):1551-1555.

Major P, Lortholary A, Hon J, et al. Zoledronic acid is superior to pamidronate in the treatment of hypercalcemia of malignancy: a pooled analysis of two randomized, controlled clinical trials. *J Clin Oncol*. 2001;19(2):558-567.

Nussbaum SR, Younger J, Vandepol CJ, et al. Single-dose intravenous therapy with pamidronate for the treatment of hypercalcemia of malignancy: comparison of 30-, 60-, and 90-mg dosages. *Am J Med*. 1993;95(3):297-304.

Penel N, Dewas S, Doutrelant P, Clisant S, Yazdanpanah Y, Adenis A. Cancer-associated hypercalcemia treated with intravenous diphosphonates: a survival and prognostic factor analysis. *Support Care Cancer.* 2008;16(4):387-392.

Perlia CP, Gubisch NJ, Wolter J, Edelberg D, Dederick MM, Taylor SG 3rd. Mithramycin treatment of hypercalcemia.*Cancer.* 1970;25:389-394.

Shemerdiak WP, Kukreja SC, Lad TE, York PA, Henderson WJ. Evaluation of routine ionized calcium determination in cancer patients. *Clin Chem.* 1981;27:1621-1622.

Stewart AF. Clinical practice. Hypercalcemia associated with cancer. *N Engl J Med.* 2005;352 (4):373-379.

MALIGNANT PLEURAL EFFUSIONS

Malignant pleural effusion is an accumulation of fluid in the pleural space separating the lung and chest wall. It may be attributed to primary tumor growth, direct extension of tumor from an adjacent anatomic structure, or metastatic dissemination to the affected area. By definition, malignant pleural effusion must contain cancer cells. Breast, lung, and lymphoid malignancies account for two-thirds of malignant pleural effusions, but they are also found with gastric cancer, ovarian carcinomas, and mesothelioma. Case reports describe malignant pleural effusions with juvenile granulose cell tumor, pulmonary leiomyosarcoma, pleural liposarcoma, malignant melanoma, primitive neuroendocrine tumor, renal medullary carcinoma, and salivary gland cancer. A malignant pleural effusion may be the presenting sign of cancer, but most often it is a complication of a previously diagnosed malignancy. The median duration of survival following the diagnosis of malignant pleural effusion is 4 months; however, prolonged survival is possible in some cases. Predictors of less favorable outcome include high-risk tumors, poor performance status, lower pleural fluid glucose levels, leukocytosis, hypoxemia, and hypoalbuminemia.

PATHOPHYSIOLOGY

The pleura is a thin membrane that covers the lungs and chest wall. It is composed of the visceral pleura (covering the surface of the lungs) and the parietal pleura (covering the thoracic cavity). The interface between the two surfaces is the pleural space. Normally, pleural fluid production is <100 mL/day. Movement of fluid within the pleural space is governed by hydrostatic and oncotic pressures that follow Starling's law of transcapillary exchange. Hydrostatic pressure in the parietal capillaries is higher, causing a net movement into the pleural space. Reabsorption of the fluid occurs primarily through lymphatics on the parietal surface and less prominently via lymphatics on the visceral surface. Changes in pleural fluid production, reabsorption, or both produce a pleural effusion.

Malignancies can cause a fluid imbalance within the pleural space in several ways. Malignant cells in the pleural space can cause an inflammatory response that increases both capillary permeability and the net filtration of fluid, proteins, and cells into the pleural space. In addition, malignant obstruction of lymphatic channels and changes in pleural fluid protein content can impair reabsorption and drainage of fluid from the pleural space. The resulting fluid accumulation is exudative and is characterized by an increased concentration of protein and cells, decreased glucose levels compared to the serum, and an absence of eosinophils.

CLINICAL SYMPTOMS AND DIAGNOSIS

The most common symptom is dyspnea, often in conjunction with cough, chest pain, tachypnea, and reduced exercise tolerance. Symptoms are often related not to the amount of pleural fluid present, but to the rate of fluid accumulation. Patients with pleural effusions may be asymptomatic. A diagnosis often begins with a chest x-ray, which will demonstrate fluid accumulation on the poster-oanterior (PA) and lateral decubitus film. Physical findings include dullness to percussion, decreased breath sounds, decreased diaphragmatic excursion, and possible contralateral tracheal deviation. In asymptomatic patients, malignant pleural effusion is generally diagnosed incidentally from radiographic imaging performed for other reasons.

TREATMENT PRINCIPLES

The goal of treatment is to effectively provide symptomatic relief with the least amount of risk and discomfort to the patient. Mainstays of therapy include fluid drainage (thoracentesis) with prevention of fluid reaccumulation by way of pleurodesis or an implanted pleural catheter. Successful palliation of dyspnea is possible with either pleurodesis or chronic drainage. Not all patients benefit from treatment. Some patients with effusions are asymptomatic and may not require treatment until symptoms develop. Individuals with a life expectancy of <1 month might only require oxygen, opioids, and possibly thoracentesis.

SYSTEMIC AND RADIATION THERAPY

Malignant pleural effusions arising from treatment-sensitive cancers are managed with systemic or radiation therapy intended to reduce the effusion by treating the underlying malignant cause. Improvement of malignant pleural effusions with systemic or radiation therapy is most likely to occur when the underlying cause is lymphoma, small cell lung cancer, germ cell tumor, breast cancer, ovarian cancer, prostate cancer, or thyroid cancer. Systemic therapy may be administered in addition to local therapy (effusion drainage) and pleurodesis (local instillation of treatment).

LOCAL THERAPY

Thoracentesis is the process of removing fluid from the pleural space using a specialized catheter and syringe under local anesthetic. This procedure can be done at the bedside and is utilized frequently for symptomatic patients. Thoracentesis is ineffective for long-term control of the malignant pleural effusion. Recurrence is frequent and repeated procedures carry a risk of increased complications, such as pneumothorax; ultrasound-guided thoracentesis can be performed to reduce this risk.

Tube thoracostomy (chest tube) is effective in controlling a malignant pleural effusion for a short period of time. Its 30-day success rate is ~70%. However, it is ineffective in the long-term control of effusions. Tubal thoracostomy is most useful in draining the fluid from the pleural space prior to instilling a sclerosing agent.

Indwelling pleural catheters with small bore tubing can be placed subcutaneously to provide long-term drainage of malignant pleural effusions. Patients can be educated to drain the catheters on a routine basis or as needed for symptom relief. The most common complication is pain or other symptoms due to intrapleural loculations, which occur in approximately 8% of cases. Additional complications reported in <5% of cases include unsuccessful insertion, asymptomatic loculations, cellulitis, empyema, and pneumothorax. Pleuroperitoneal shunts represent another tool that can be used for management of malignant pleural effusion.

PLEURODESIS

Pleurodesis, or sclerosis, should be considered in patients who experience symptomatic relief from thoracentesis with complete lung re-expansion and who have a life expectancy of at least weeks to months. The primary goals of pleurodesis are prevention of effusion reaccumulation and reduced hospitalizations for thoracentesis. Sclerosing agents act by promoting an inflammatory response in the pleura that causes fibrin adhesions of the visceral and parietal pleura. This results in fixed obliteration of the pleural space, which is prohibitive to recurrent effusion accumulation. Sclerosing agents are administered via a ▶

thoracostomy tube following demonstration of adequate effusate drainage (<200 mL/day).

The efficacy of pleurodesis is categorized as complete success, partial success, or failure. Criteria for complete success are long-term symptom relief and absence of fluid reaccumulation. Criteria for partial success are improved symptomatology with <50% of fluid reaccumulation without additional thoracentesis. Any less of a response is categorized as pleurodesis failure.

Successful use of a sclerosing agent depends on its uniform distribution in the pleural space and the dose of selected drug. The presence of loculations within the pleural space can interfere with distribution of the sclerosing agent. Immediate and complete lung expansion is desirable for pleurodesis. However, the clinical outcome for patients experiencing partial lung expansion is similar with respect to quality of life, procedure-related complications, extent of effusion drainage, hospital stay duration, and overall survival. Effective lung expansion and durable prevention of effusion reaccumulation may be related to tumor type. Patients with lung cancer and mesothelioma tend to have a less favorable response to pleurodesis in comparison to patients with breast or other cancers. Another factor that influences the efficacy of pleurodesis is the extent of tumor involving the pleural space. Preclinical data suggests that inhibition of vascular endothelial growth factor is deleterious to successful pleurodesis due to impeded adhesion formation (Teixeira 2011).

SCLEROSING AGENTS

Sterile talc is one of the oldest and most effective sclerosing agents for treatment of malignant pleural effusions. Successful talc pleurodesis is achieved in 70% to 96% of patients. Meta-analysis infers that talc is a more effective sclerosing agent than bleomycin or tetracycline and tetracycline analogues. Pharmaceutical grade sterile asbestos-free talc is commercially available for use as a sclerosing agent. Talc powder is prepared as a sterile suspension for bedside administration through a chest tube. The usual dose of talc suspension is 5 g in 100 mL of 0.9% sodium chloride. Powdered talc is also available in a pressurized spray canister for administration under video-assisted thoracic surgery (VATS, thoracoscopy) or open thoracotomy. Aerosolized talc is available in single-use 4 g canisters; the usual dose is 4 to 8 g. Pain and fever are the most common acute side effects of pleurodesis. Rare serious adverse effects of talc pleurodesis include adult respiratory distress syndrome (ARDS), pneumonia, empyema, hemoptysis, bronchopleural fistula, tachycardia, hypotension, and infection. Cases of ARDS have usually occurred in patients receiving instillations of talc suspension at doses of 10 g.

The TIME2 study compared symptom control with talc pleurodesis vs an indwelling pleural catheter in 106 cases of previously untreated malignant pleural effusion. A 100 mm visual analogue scale (VAS) was used to measure dyspnea; a score of 0 mm indicated no dyspnea and a score of 100 mm indicated maximal dyspnea. Dyspnea was similarly improved in both groups for the initial 6 weeks of therapy (p=0.96). Assessment at 6 months identified a mean VAS score difference of 14 mm favoring symptom palliation in the group with implanted pleural catheters. This finding was statistically significant (p=0.01); however, it did not translate into a difference in quality of life between the two groups (p=0.14). More patients treated with talc pleurodesis (22%) required additional pleural procedures for symptom control compared to those with implanted pleural catheters (6%) (p=0.03). In addition, pleurodesis required hospitalization for a median 4 days (interquartile range: 2 to 6 days); whereas, catheter implantation was generally an entirely outpatient procedure (initial hospitalization for median 0 days [interquartile range: 0 to 1 days]). Treatment-related adverse events were more common in patients with implanted pleural catheters (40%) than in patients treated with pleurodesis (13%) (p=0.002) (Davies 2012).

Bleomycin 1 mg/kg (1 unit/kg) in 100 mL of 0.9% sodium chloride is an effective agent for controlling malignant pleural effusions. The range of intrapleural bleomycin doses reported in the literature is 24 to 240 mg. However, due to a lack of increased efficacy at doses >60 mg, some authors have recommended limiting the dose to 60 mg or 1 mg/kg body weight. Bleomycin has not demonstrated an efficacy advantage over talc and the acquisition cost of bleomycin is substantially greater than that of talc (Haddad 2004). Common toxicities associated with intrapleural bleomycin include pain, fever, and gastrointestinal adverse effects (nausea, vomiting, diarrhea). Serious adverse effects are more common in patients with elderly age or reduced renal function.

Parenteral tetracycline was one of the most widely used sclerosing agents prior to its removal from the market in the mid-1990s. Doxycycline 500 mg injection mixed in 50 to 100 mL of 0.9% sodium chloride effectively treats pleural effusions in 50% to 75% of patients; however, repeated instillations are generally required to achieve results similar to tetracycline. Intrapleural minocycline following VATS for spontaneous pneumothorax reduced prolonged postoperative air leaks, chest drainage, and hospital days for 313 patients relative to 51 consecutive historical controls (Chen 2004). The author reported administration of minocycline 300 to 400 mg injection in 20 mL of 0.9% sodium chloride through a chest tube. Due to a lack of stability information, this dose of minocycline should be prepared immediately before use. Chest pain was a common complaint after pleurodesis with minocycline.

Additional products that have been used as sclerosing agents for pleurodesis are povidone iodine, silver nitrate, distilled water, quinacrine, *Corynebacterium parvum*, interferon-alpha, and interferon-beta.

OTHER

Intrapleural administration of cytotoxic chemotherapy is reported. Its use is based on the premise that cytotoxic chemotherapy can exert anticancer and proinflammatory actions. In addition, intrapleural administration of chemotherapy may yield a regional advantage with intrapleural drug levels greatly exceeding drug levels in the plasma (Heffner 2008; Lombardi 2010). The reader is cautioned that the safety and efficacy of intrapleural administration of cytotoxic chemotherapy is not extensively tested.

A phase II study tested intrapleural administration of paclitaxel 120 mg/m^2 for the treatment of malignant pleural effusion in 18 patients with ovarian cancer (11 patients) or breast cancer (7 patients). Paclitaxel was infused after thoracentesis. The catheter used for paclitaxel administration was clamped for a period of 24 hours, after which it remained in place until drainage was <200 mL over 24 hours. Objective response (complete plus partial success rate) at 1 month and 2 months following treatment was reported in 78% and 89% of patients, respectively. Common side effects included chest pain, fever, and dyspnea. Pleural fluid paclitaxel concentrations were approximately 10,000-fold greater than those measured in the plasma. The half-life of intrapleural paclitaxel was approximately 68 hours (Lombardi 2012). A phase I study with pharmacokinetic analysis of intrapleural docetaxel 50 to 125 mg/m^2 reported a 1,000-fold difference in concurrent drug concentrations measured in the pleural fluid relative to those in the plasma. This relative AUC from 0 to 36 hours for docetaxel in pleural fluid was 2,000 to 7,000 times greater than the corresponding plasma AUC (Jones 2010).

GENERAL PLEURODESIS PROCEDURE

Effusate is drained via a chest tube until the fluid production is <200 mL/day. The patient is premedicated with systemic analgesia (usually a parenteral opioid), sedation, and intrapleural administration of a topical anesthetic (typically lidocaine 1%). The sclerosing agent is instilled through the chest tube and the tube is clamped for 1 to 2 hours; the tube is then unclamped to drain the pleural fluid. The chest tube can be removed when drainage is <100 to 150 mL per 24 hours (Dresler 2005; Kvale 2007). Some procedures include frequent repositioning of the patient during the time that the chest tube is clamped to facilitate uniform distribution of the sclerosing agent, although the efficacy of repositioning is untested and its use is controversial.

COMPLICATIONS

Management of malignant pleural effusions is associated with several complications. Pain from insertion of the chest tube or instillation of the sclerosing agent should be pretreated with parenteral opioids. Traction pneumothorax results from repeated attempts to re-expand the lung. Cough is caused by lung re-expansion and is self-limiting. Fluid loculation is associated with drainage and pleurodesis. Lysis of adhesions may be necessary prior to pleurodesis. Empyema (purulent fluid) formation from contamination or bronchopulmonary communication should be treated with appropriate antibiotics.

REFERENCES

Antonangelo L, Rosa AG, Corá AP, Acencio MM, Moreira LC, Suso FV. Uncommon pleural effusion: pleuropulmonary metastasis from primitive neuroectodermal tumor. *J Bras Pneumol.* 2009;35(6):606-609.

Bielsa S, Hernández P, Rodriguez-Panadero F, Taberner T, Salud A, Porcel JM. Tumor type influences the effectiveness of pleurodesis in malignant effusions. *Lung.* 2011;189(2):151-155.

Chen JS, Hsu HH, Kuo SW, et al. Effects of additional minocycline pleurodesis after thoracoscopic procedures for primary spontaneous pneumothorax. *Chest.* 2004;125(1):50-55.

Dagli AF, Pehlivan S, Ozercan AR. Pleural liposarcoma mimicking carcinoma in pleural effusion cytology: a case report. *Acta Cytol.* 2010;54(4):601-604.

Davies HE, Mishra EK, Kahan BC, et al. Effect of an indwelling pleural catheter vs chest tube and talc pleurodesis for relieving dyspnea in patients with malignant pleural effusion: the TIME2 randomized controlled trial. *JAMA.* 2012;307(22):2383-2389.

Dresler CM, Olak J, Herndon JE 2nd, et al. Phase III intergroup study of talc poudrage vs talc slurry sclerosis for malignant pleural effusion. *Chest.* 2005;127(3):909-915.

Ellis CL, Burroughs F, Michael CW, Li QK. Cytology of metastatic renal medullary carcinoma in pleural effusion: a study of two cases. *Diagn Cytopathol.* 2009;37(11):843-848.

Haddad FJ, Younes RN, Gross JL, Deheinzelin D. Pleurodesis in patients with malignant pleural effusions: talc slurry or bleomycin? Results of a prospective randomized trial. *World J Surg.* 2004;28(8):749-753.

Heffner JE, Klein JS. Recent advances in the diagnosis and management of malignant pleural effusions. *Mayo Clin Proc.* 2008;83(2):235-250.

Hirata T, Yonemori K, Hirakawa A, et al. Efficacy of pleurodesis for malignant pleural effusions in breast cancer patients. *Eur Respir J.* 2011;38(6):1425-1430.

Jones DR, Taylor MD, Petroni GR, et al. Phase I trial of intrapleural docetaxel administered through an implantable catheter in subjects with a malignant pleural effusion. *J Thorac Oncol.* 2010;5 (1):75-81.

Kaifi JT, Toth JW, Gusani NJ, et al. Multidisciplinary management of malignant pleural effusion. *J Surg Oncol.* 2012;105(7):731-738.

Kaur H, Bagga R, Saha SC, et al. Juvenile granulosa cell tumor of the ovary presenting with pleural effusion and ascites. *Int J Clin Oncol.* 2009;14(1):78-81.

Kriegel I, Daniel C, Falcou MC, et al. Use of a subcutaneous implantable pleural port in the management of recurrent malignant pleurisy: five-year experience based on 168 subcutaneous implantable pleural ports. *J Palliat Med.* 2011;14(7):829-834.

Kubo A, Koh Y, Kawaguchi T, et al. Malignant pleural effusion from lung adenocarcinoma treated by gefitinib. *Intern Med.* 2011;50(7):745-748.

Kvale PA, Selecky PA, Prakash UB; American College of Chest Physicians. Palliative care in lung cancer: ACCP evidence-based clinical practice guidelines (2nd edition). *Chest.* 2007;132(3 Suppl):368S-403S.

Lombardi G, Nicoletto MO, Gusella M, et al. Intrapleural paclitaxel for malignant pleural effusion from ovarian and breast cancer: a phase II study with pharmacokinetic analysis. *Cancer Chemother Pharmacol.* 2012;69(3):781-787.

Lombardi G, Zustovich F, Nicoletto MO, Donach M, Artioli G, Pastorelli D. Diagnosis and treatment of malignant pleural effusion: a systematic literature review and new approaches. *Am J Clin Oncol.* 2010;33(4):420-423.

Mitra S, Kundu S, Pattari SK, Ghosal AG. Metastatic pleural effusion: a rare presentation of salivary gland adenoid cystic carcinoma. *Indian J Chest Dis Allied Sci.* 2011;53(2):107-110.

Ozyurtkan MO, Balci AE, Cakmak M. Predictors of mortality within three months in the patients with malignant pleural effusion. *Eur J Intern Med.* 2010;21(1):30-34.

Passamonte PM, Luger AM. Primary pulmonary leiomyosarcoma with digital clubbing and pleural effusion. Case report. *Mo Med.* 1984;81(10):667-668.

Pilling JE, Dusmet ME, Ladas G, Goldstraw P. Prognostic factors for survival after surgical palliation of malignant pleural effusion. *J Thorac Oncol.* 2010;5(10):1544-1550.

Rodriguez-Panadero F, Montes-Worboys A. Mechanisms of pleurodesis. *Respiration.* 2012;83(2):91-98.

Shameem M, Akhtar J, Baneen U, et al. Malignant melanoma presenting as an isolated pleural effusion. *Monaldi Arch Chest Dis.* 2011;75(2):138-140.

Shaw P, Agarwal R. Pleurodesis for malignant pleural effusions. *Cochrane Database Syst Rev.* 2004;(1):CD002916.

Suzuki K, Servais EL, Rizk NP, et al. Palliation and pleurodesis in malignant pleural effusion: the role for tunneled pleural catheters. *J Thorac Oncol.* 2011;6(4):762-767.

Teixeira LR, Vargas FS, Acencio MM, et al. Blockage of vascular endothelial growth factor (VEGF) reduces experimental pleurodesis. *Lung Cancer.* 2011;74(3):392-395.

Terra RM, Junqueira JJ, Teixeira LR, Vargas FS, Pégo-Fernandes PM, Jatene FB. Is full postpleurodesis lung expansion a determinant of a successful outcome after talc pleurodesis? *Chest.* 2009;136(2):361-368.

PALLIATIVE CARE MEDICINE (CANCER)

SCOPE OF PALLIATIVE CARE MEDICINE

The primary objective of palliative care is to improve quality of life through prevention of and relief from suffering (Herman 2013). Palliative care addresses symptoms arising from serious, life-threatening diseases and intractable symptoms caused by benign conditions that depreciate quality of life. Palliative care is often used in the management of patients with life expectancies extending months, years, or decades; however, it can also be an essential part of end-of-life (hospice) care. The scope of palliative care embraces improving quality of life for patients and their significant others. In addition to traditional disease-based medical treatments, comprehensive provision of palliative care strives to optimize functional capabilities, facilitate decision-making, and extend opportunities for personal growth. Elements of effective palliative care include an appropriate philosophy of care plus a well-organized infrastructure to address physical, psychological, social, cultural, and spiritual aspects of health.

The American Society of Clinical Oncology (ASCO) published a provisional clinical opinion stating that palliative care should be offered in addition to standard anticancer therapy at the time of initial diagnosis of metastatic non-small cell lung cancer (NSCLC) (Smith 2012). In several randomized controlled trials, demonstration of improved patient and caregiver outcomes with the addition of palliative care to standard therapy provided the impetus for this ASCO statement. Advantages conferred with palliative care in the management of metastatic NSCLC include improvement in symptom control, mood, patient satisfaction, and reduced caregiver burden (Pirl 2012; Smith 2012). In addition, appropriate utilization of hospice services and reduced futile intensive terminal care were substantiated with early initiation of palliative care. Longer median survival, despite less aggressive end-of-life care, was reported for 77 patients with metastatic NSCLC randomized to receive palliative care (in addition to standard anticancer therapy) at the time of initial diagnosis vs a cohort of 74 patients randomized to receive standard anticancer therapy alone (p=0.02) (Temel 2010). Palliative care achieves these benefits without causing harm to the patient or caregiver, and without increasing the overall cost of care (Smith 2012). In fact, a prospective, observational study that examined 969 patient cases in five hospitals determined that direct health care costs are reduced with earlier palliative care consultation for hospitalized patients with advanced cancers. The cost of hospitalization was reduced 14% and 24% when the consultation was placed within six days and two days, respectively, of hospital admission in comparison to patients not receiving palliative care consultations (May 2015). Despite these positive findings, the ASCO provisional clinical opinion acknowledges that stringently performed palliative care research is in its infancy. To facilitate the integration of palliative care into standard oncology practice, ASCO recommends the following investigative priorities: Optimal timing and venue (inpatient, outpatient/community) for palliative care, reimbursement models, interventions providing greatest benefit, benefit in diseases other than lung cancer, and impact of palliative care across the continuum of care (especially during the delivery of anticancer therapy).

Palliative care is provided most effectively by an interdisciplinary team specializing in this area of medicine. One central aspect of palliative care is symptom control for intractable situations following an adequate trial of the therapeutic standard of care. Subsequently, medications may be prescribed for off-label indications at doses outside of the norm and for administration by atypical routes. Due to this unique practice approach, clinical and regulatory challenges related to the delivery of pharmaceutical products for palliative care directly impact the pharmacy department. Moreover, since palliative care medicine is an evolving field, medical literature supporting the safety and efficacy of certain interventions may be scant. Some medications used for symptom management are controlled substances or medications prone to diversion, so the pharmacy department and all members of the palliative care team must adhere to stringent methods of drug accountability. To address these challenges, pharmacy departments should formalize policies and procedures that support the legitimate and uniform delivery of palliative pharmaceutical care.

SYMPTOM MANAGEMENT

Pain

The management of pain, including both opioid and nonopioid analgesic therapy, should be optimized as per standard clinical practice; for more information, refer to Chronic Pain Management (Cancer) on page 2229. Nonopioid analgesic therapy for cancer-related pain may include both pharmaceutical and nonpharmaceutical interventions. Nonsteroidal anti-inflammatory drugs (NSAIDs), bisphosphonates, and radiotherapy should be used as appropriate for bone pain. External beam radiation may be helpful for tumor size reduction with pain relief in some cases. NSAIDs or corticosteroids should be used as warranted for inflammatory pain. Gabapentin, pregabalin, and antidepressants may improve neuropathic pain.

In cases of intractable pain, high doses of opioid analgesia may be required for adequate pain management. The oral route of administration is preferred whenever possible. Opioid administration by continuous subcutaneous or intravenous infusion (with or without patient-controlled PRN boluses) is also an option; however, subcutaneous infusion of methadone should be avoided due to local irritation. Some patients may require intraspinal opioid administration to achieve and tolerate adequate pain control.

Methadone can be administered by continuous intravenous infusion and patient-controlled analgesia; however, this intervention is often reserved for select patients as a bridge to intraspinal therapy because methadone prolongs the QTc interval and exhibits discordance between its pharmacokinetics and pharmacodynamics. The risk of torsade de pointes is increased when the QTc interval exceeds 500 milliseconds. Consensus guidelines (Shaiova 2008) pertaining to intravenous administration of methadone recommend assessment of the QTc interval at baseline, 24 hours, and 4 days after initiation of methadone, as well as assessment following any significant dose increase or at the discretion of the practitioner. More frequent monitoring of the QTc interval should be considered for patients with a QTc interval exceeding 450 milliseconds. Patients should be advised of the risk of dysrhythmias with methadone so that they may make an informed decision about their therapy. Since the half-life of methadone exceeds the duration of analgesia, the consensus guidelines state that the initial rate titration must be performed at least 12 hours after initiation of the infusion to allow evolution of side effects prior to increasing systemic drug concentrations.

Subsequent rate titrations should be executed once daily. The consensus guidelines also recommend liberal use of PRN boluses before and between rate titration of methadone by continuous intravenous infusion. Due to incomplete cross-tolerance between methadone and high-dose morphine, a 25% to 50% reduction in the calculated methadone dose at infusion initiation is recommended for patients requiring >50 mg/hour of morphine. In addition, the consensus guidelines recommend the following conversion factors (Shaiova 2008):

| Opioid | Basal Rate (mg/h) | Methadone | |
		Basal Rate (mg/h)	PRN Bolus Available Every 15 Minutes
Morphine	10	1	1
HYDROmorphone	1.5	0.3	0.3
FentaNYL	0.25	1.25	1.25

Intravenous lidocaine is used for severe intractable neuropathic pain. The efficacy of lidocaine is greater in the treatment of peripheral sensory neuropathy vs symptoms caused by a central pain syndrome. Small studies report administration of intravenous lidocaine 1 to 5 mg/kg over a period of 30 minutes to 6 hours. Alternatively, some centers use a set dose of 100 to 150 mg infused intravenously over a period of 30 to 60 minutes. Analgesia superior to placebo is reported in crossover design trials. The reported time to maximum analgesia is 1 to 6 hours, with the reported duration of analgesia ranging from hours to days to weeks. Common adverse effects include lightheadedness, vertical nystagmus, feeling drunk, and sedation. Administration of intravenous lidocaine 1 to 5 mg/kg over a period of 30 minutes to 6 hours without demonstration of cardiac or central nervous system toxicity is reported; the lack of serious side effects is probably explained by the rapid metabolism of systemic lidocaine. Caution should be exercised when using intravenous lidocaine in patients who are elderly, debilitated, or have poor hepatic function. Instead of intravenous lidocaine infusion, one case series of three patients with neuropathic cancer pain describes chronic administration of lidocaine 100 to 160 mg/hour by continuous subcutaneous infusion (Brose 1991). With administration by continuous infusion via any route, periodic assessment of serum lidocaine levels should be considered.

Ketamine is used as an adjunct to opioid therapy for intractable cancer pain and neuropathic pain. Ketamine can be administered orally, intravenously, and subcutaneously. Ketamine can also be administered intramuscularly; however, this route is rarely used for repeated administration. The recommended dose of oral ketamine is 20 to 60 mg 3 to 4 times daily plus PRN administration of ketamine 20 mg every 3 hours. When ketamine is being discontinued, tapering the dose at a rate of 25% per 24 hours may reduce the likelihood of dysphoria. Ketamine is commercially available as a parenteral formulation and the oral dose can be mixed in cola immediately prior to ingestion. To reduce the risk of drug diversion or inadvertent ingestion by a family member, some institutions have the nurse squirt the dose of ketamine from an oral syringe into the patient's mouth with cola or another beverage to follow. Intravenous ketamine is generally given as a continuous infusion starting at 1 to 2 mg/hour; administration as an intravenous bolus of 0.1 to 0.4 mg/kg is also reported in the literature. Ketamine may cause hallucinations, drowsiness, and confusion. At anesthetic doses (1 to 4.5 mg/kg via intravenous bolus), ketamine causes hypertension and tachycardia. Common adverse effects described with infusional ketamine for palliative care include nausea (63%), vomiting (47%), and central nervous system effects (93%)

(psychomimetic effects, hallucinations, dizziness, feeling of inebriation). Cystitis attributed to ketamine administration is primarily reported with repeated oral administration. A case of markedly elevated blood pressure is also described following repeated oral administration of ketamine (Van Hecke 2014). Cases of hepatotoxicity, which are common with ketamine-based substance abuse, are reported with ketamine administered by continuous intravenous infusion to manage chronic regional pain syndrome.

Dyspnea

The sensation of dyspnea is a complex disorder that is influenced by many pathophysiologic changes within and outside of the cardiopulmonary system. Opioid (usually morphine) administration is the cornerstone of medication therapy for reducing the sensation of chronic dyspnea in advanced cancer patients. Opioid medications should always be used cautiously; however, medical literature supports the safety and efficacy of opioid administration for the management of chronic dyspnea in this patient population. Morphine (or an equivalent opioid) can be administered to cancer patients with mild to severe dyspnea for symptom control without having a deleterious effect on SaO_2, $PaCO_2$, or heart rate. These findings are consistent when evaluated relative to whether the patient was opioid-naïve or hypoxic (SaO_2 <90%) at baseline. For opioid-naïve patients, morphine doses in the range of 1 to 3 mg by intravenous push or 5 to 10 mg orally PRN every 4 hours may be sufficient to improve dyspnea; opioid-tolerant patients will need higher doses to relieve dyspnea. There is no advantage to morphine administration by nebulization vs use of the subcutaneous, intravenous, or oral routes.

The identification and management of comorbid conditions also contributes to the relief of dyspnea symptoms. Treatment of anxiety using lorazepam or another suitable product may improve the sensation of dyspnea. The addition of furosemide to therapy should be considered when heart failure may be a contributing factor. For patients with chronic obstructive pulmonary disease, long acting beta-agonists improve dyspnea. The use of oxygen therapy in all patients with dyspnea is controversial due to conflicting information about its efficacy in the medical literature; patients with chronic obstructive pulmonary disease are most likely to benefit from oxygen therapy.

Cough/Hiccups

Initial symptomatic treatment of persistent cough due to chronic disease affecting the lungs includes guaifenesin, dextromethorphan, and benzonatate. For intractable cough despite usual therapies, nebulized lidocaine may provide relief. Symptomatic relief from nebulized lidocaine occurs rapidly for responding patients. Common adverse effects of this therapy include oropharyngeal numbness and an unpleasant taste. It is also important to note that nebulized lidocaine causes a transient loss of gag reflex. Nebulized lidocaine for intractable cough is often administered as follows:

Nebulized Lidocaine for Intractable Cough Administration

Lidocaine 4% preservative-free 2.5 mL

Administer by nebulization every 4 hours as needed.

Note: Patient should have nothing by mouth for 30 minutes before and 2 hours after each dose.

Intractable hiccups, which are generally defined as hiccups lasting more than 1 month, impair the quality and activities of daily life. Hiccups are caused by repeated, involuntary, spasmodic contractions of the diaphragm, followed by a sudden closure of the glottis, which blocks incoming air to produce the characteristic sounds. Hiccups can present secondary to gastric extension and diaphragmatic irritation. Drugs credited with causing intractable hiccups include aprepitant, dexamethasone, doxycycline, etoposide, megestrol acetate, and perphenazine. When hiccups are thought to be medication-related, interruption of therapy should be tried. Nonpharmacologic methods for hiccup cessation should be attempted prior to drug therapy. Examples of nonpharmacologic therapy include holding one's breath, breathing inside of a paper (nonplastic) grocery bag, gasping with sudden fright, the Valsalva maneuver, hyperventilation, slowly drinking water, and drinking water from the "wrong side" of a glass.

Medications used to manage intractable hiccups include chlorpromazine, metoclopramide, baclofen, and gabapentin. Chlorpromazine may be administered orally or intravenously at a dosage of 25 to 50 mg 3 to 4 times daily as needed or around the clock. Chlorpromazine may also be administered intramuscularly; however, this route is seldom utilized for repeated administration. Metoclopramide, baclofen, and gabapentin are administered on a scheduled basis around the clock (instead of PRN) for this indication. Metoclopramide 10 mg is generally administered 4 times daily (orally or intravenously) for control of hiccups. The dosage of baclofen for intractable hiccups is 5 to 10 mg by mouth 3 to 4 times daily. Gabapentin administered 300 to 400 mg 3 times daily by mouth for control of hiccups is reported in the medical literature, but gabapentin has a wide margin of safety and doses up to 3,600 mg/day are well-tolerated in patients with adequate renal function. Combination therapy using drugs with different pharmacologic mechanisms of action and nonoverlapping toxicity may be tried for patients not responding to single-agent therapy.

Hiccups that continue despite an adequate trial of chlorpromazine, metoclopramide, and baclofen may respond to nebulized lidocaine. The dosage, time to effect, and safety of nebulized lidocaine is described in the preceding section pertaining to management of intractable cough.

Fatigue

Cancer-related fatigue (CRF) is a persistent sensation of physical, emotional, or cognitive tiredness or exhaustion attributed to oncologic disease or its treatment that exceeds the usual severity for associated actions and hinders normal activities. The foundation for management of CRF is routine screening with evaluation of related symptomatology and contributing factors, such as pain, anemia, sleep disorders, emotional distress, nutritional deficits, decreased functional status, and medical comorbidities. Nonpharmacologic interventions supersede medication use for management of CRF; examples of applicable nonpharmacologic treatment options include physical therapy, massage therapy, psychosocial interventions, nutrition counseling, and cognitive behavioral therapy. Ancillary pharmacologic treatments may be added for management of CRF once the aforementioned therapies have been optimized. Stimulant medications used to manage fatigue in cancer patients are modafinil, methylphenidate, and dexmethylphenidate. The use of corticosteroids, progestational steroids, antidepressants, and vitamins for the management of CRF has also been reported (Campos 2011).

A multicenter, randomized, double-blind, placebo-controlled trial evaluated modafinil 200 mg daily (n=315) vs placebo (n=316) for the treatment of cancer-related fatigue. Patient condition was evaluated using the following scales: Brief Fatigue Inventory (BFI), Epworth Sleepiness Scale, and Center for Epidemiological Study-Depression Profile of Mood States-Depression/Dejection. Patients with severe baseline fatigue benefited from modafinil (p=0.017); however, patients with mild or moderate baseline fatigue did not experience significant improvement in their fatigue scores with modafinil. Modafinil did not positively impact depression scores (p>0.05). The frequency and severity of adverse effects were similar between the two treatment groups (Jean-Pierre 2010). Another randomized, double-blind study compared modafinil (n=104) vs placebo (n=104) in patients with NSCLC, a baseline WHO performance status of 0 to 2, and moderate to severe fatigue reported using a numeric rating scale (Spathis 2014). Modafinil 100 mg daily was administered for 14 days and was then escalated to 200 mg daily for an additional 14 days. The primary study endpoint was change in Functional Assessment of Chronic Illness Therapy-Fatigue (FACIT-Fatigue) subscale score from baseline (day 0) to treatment day 28. Secondary efficacy endpoints included patient-reported measures of depression, daytime sleepiness, and quality of life (QOL). The study results supported a significant placebo effect in that the FACIT-Fatigue scores improved similarly for both treatment groups: Modafinil 5.29 (95% CI, 2.57 to 8.02) vs placebo 5.09 (95% CI, 2.54 to 7.65). There was no difference between the treatment groups for secondary outcome measures and side effects were similar between the treatment groups. In addition to these findings, a randomized, double-blind study demonstrated modafinil 200 mg daily (n=56) did not improve M.D. Anderson Symptom Inventory scores in comparison to placebo (n=28) for patients undergoing treatment with docetaxel for advanced breast cancer or prostate cancer (Hovey 2014).

A meta-analysis conducted using five randomized clinical trials (with a total of 498 enrolled patients) concluded that existing studies provide limited evidence for the use of methylphenidate for management of CRF (Gong 2014). The meta-analysis determined that a large placebo effect was demonstrated. Adverse effects with methylphenidate were similar to placebo control across the five studies, although the rate of vertigo, anxiety, anorexia, and nausea was greater in the active treatment arms. One randomized, double-blind study using a cross-over design compared sequential administration of methylphenidate then placebo vs placebo then methylphenidate in a total of 38 patients who served as their own controls (Escalante 2014). The study used an active treatment dosage of methylphenidate 18 mg sustained release once daily. No difference in improvement of fatigue (ascertained using the BFI) was observed between the two groups from baseline to end of treatment (4 weeks duration). Interestingly, during the active treatment phases, patients missed significantly less time from work due to illness relative to the placebo treatment phases.

A randomized, double-blind study compared dexmethylphenidate 5 mg twice daily (n=75) to placebo (n=77) for the management of chemotherapy-related fatigue and cognitive impairment in breast cancer (78% of patients), ovarian cancer (13% of patients), or other cancer (9% of patients) (Lower 2009). Patients receiving dexmethylphenidate demonstrated improved fatigue scores according to the FACIT-Fatigue subscale (p=0.02) and Clinical Global Impression-Severity Scores (p=0.02). Cognitive function was not significantly improved in either cohort during the 8-week follow-up period. Adverse effects attributed to medication therapy occurred more commonly in patients treated with dexmethylphenidate (63% vs 28%) and discontinuation of medication therapy due to regimen-related adverse effects occurred more frequently in the active treatment group (11% vs 1.3%). Headache was a common side effect in both treatment groups, nausea and xerostomia occurred more commonly in the dexmethylphenidate cohort, and diarrhea and insomnia occurred more commonly in the placebo cohort.

Several studies have assessed treatment with corticosteroids for management of CRF. The efficacy of a 14-day course of oral dexamethasone 4 mg twice daily (n=43) vs placebo (n=41) was evaluated in a randomized, double-blind study that enrolled patients with advanced cancer and at least 3 CRF-related symptoms (Yennurajalingam 2013). The improvement in FACIT-Fatigue subscale score from baseline to day 15 was significantly greater for the dexamethasone group (9 ± 10.3) than the placebo group (3.1 ± 9.59) (p=0.008). In addition, the dexamethasone group demonstrated superior improvement in FACIT-Fatigue total quality of life scores (p=0.03) and mean Edmonton Symptom Assessment Scale (ESAS) physical distress scores at day 15 (p=0.013). The dexamethasone and placebo groups demonstrated similar ESAS overall symptom distress (p=0.22) and psychological distress scores (p=0.76) at day 15. The rate of adverse effects was similar between the dexamethasone and placebo groups in this study. In another randomized, double-blind study, the effect of a 7-day course of oral methylprednisolone 16 mg twice daily (n=25) vs placebo (n=22) for CRF was examined as a secondary outcome; the primary outcome measure was the efficacy of methylprednisolone for cancer-related chronic pain (Paulsen 2014). The methylprednisolone group demonstrated significantly improved scores for fatigue (p=0.003) and appetite loss (p=0.003) from baseline to treatment day 7 using the European Organization for Research and Treatment of Cancer-Quality of Life Questionnaire C30. In addition, patient satisfaction with treatment assessed using a scale of 1 to -10 was significantly better in the methylprednisolone group (mean 5.4, 95% CI 4.05 to 6.7) compared to the placebo group (mean 2, 95% CI 0.74 to 3.29) (p=0.001). Results regarding pain intensity and opioid consumption were similar between the two groups. The aforementioned studies report a positive effect of short-term corticosteroid administration for symptoms of CRF; however, when considering use of a corticosteroid for symptom management, it is essential to consider the potential adverse effects associated with corticosteroids that can contribute to fatigue (such as muscle loss and glucose intolerance) and other types of morbidity.

Effective anticancer therapy may provide the optimal treatment for CRF. This was demonstrated in a phase III clinical trial evaluating the efficacy of abiraterone plus prednisone (n=797) vs placebo plus prednisone (n=398) for the treatment of metastatic castration-resistant prostate cancer with progression after docetaxel therapy (Sternberg 2013). Low-dose oral prednisone (5 mg twice daily) was administered concurrently with abiraterone to prevent adrenocorticoid insufficiency secondary to the adrenolytic effects of abiraterone. In patients reporting clinically significant fatigue at baseline, a benefit in intensity of CRF was observed in the group receiving abiraterone plus prednisone (p=0.0001). Additional outcome measures improved in the abiraterone plus prednisone group included interference of fatigue on activities (p=0.0075) and time to improvement of fatigue (p=0.0155). Notably, this phase III trial demonstrated a prolonged duration of survival in patients treated with abiraterone plus prednisone vs the placebo plus prednisone arm.

Anemia is a common condition affecting cancer patients that may cause fatigue. Patients with anemia should be evaluated for underlying contributing factors, such as iron deficiency, vitamin B_{12} or folate deficiency, hemolysis, blood loss, renal dysfunction, and treatment with myelosuppressive therapy. Initial management of anemia focuses on treatment of these relevant contributing factors; patients with anemia that persists despite correction of treatable causes may benefit from blood transfusions or erythropoietin-stimulating agents (ESAs). Blood transfusions are advantageous to ESAs when rapid improvement in hemoglobin is warranted, but risks specific to blood transfusions for anemia must be considered, including blood-borne infection(s) and immune-mediated adverse effects. The use of ESAs can reduce the need for blood transfusions; however, ESA use in cancer patients confers an increased risk of thromboembolic disorders and shortened survival. ESA therapy is guided by a Food and Drug Administration-mandated Risk-Evaluation-Mitigation-Strategy (REMS) program that was implemented to support informed decision-making by health care professionals and patients with regard to medication-related risks. The ESA APPRISE Oncology Program is a piece of the REMS program intended to reduce the risk of decreased survival or worse tumor outcomes in cancer patients. The ESAs epoetin and darbepoetin are considered to be therapeutically equivalent for the management of anemia in cancer patients and benefit from ESAs is greatest for cases in which the baseline hemoglobin is ≤10 g/dL. ESAs should be administered at the lowest possible dose to achieve a hemoglobin value greater than 10 g/dL. An adequate trial of ESA use is considered to be 6 to 8 weeks; patients without an adequate response to ESAs administered according to the product labeling should not continue to receive treatment with these agents beyond a period of 6 to 8 weeks. Guidelines for the use of ESAs in cancer patients are jointly published by the American Society of Clinical Oncology and the American Socieity of Hematology (Rizo 2010). In line with the preceding recommendations, the ASCO ASH guidelines support the use of ESAs for cancer patients undergoing treatment with myelosuppressive therapy who have baseline hemoglobin <10 g/dL. The guidelines also support the use of ESAs for patients with low-risk myelodysplastic syndromes who are not undergoing treatment with chemotherapy.

REFERENCES

Attal N, Rouaud J, Brasseur L, Chauvin M, Bouhassira D. Systemic lidocaine in pain due to peripheral nerve injury and predictors of response. *Neurology.* 2004;62(2):218-225.

Brose WG, Cousins MJ. Subcutaneous lidocaine for treatment of neuropathic cancer pain. *Pain.* 1991;45(2):145-148.

Campos MP, Hassan BJ, Riechelmann R, Del Giglio A. Cancer-related fatigue: a practical review. *Ann Oncol.* 2011;22(6):1273-1279.

Clemens KE, Quednau I, Klaschik E. Use of oxygen and opioids in the palliation of dyspnoea in hypoxic and nonhypoxic palliative care patients: a prospective study. *Support Care Cancer.* 2009;17(4):367-377.

Clinical Practice Guidelines for Quality Palliative Care. 2nd ed. Pittsburgh, PA: National Consensus Project for Quality Palliative Care; 2009. http://www.nationalconsensusproject.org/guideline.pdf

Dy SM, Lorenz KA, Naeim A, Sanati H, Walling A, Asch SM. Evidence-based recommendations for cancer fatigue, anorexia, depression, and dyspnea. *J Clin Oncol.* 2008;26(23):3886-3895.

Enarson MC, Hays H, Woodroffe MA. Clinical experience with oral ketamine. *J Pain Symptom Manage.* 1999;17(5):384-386.

Escalante CP, Meyers C, Reuben JM, et al. A randomized, double-blind, 2-period, placebo-controlled crossover trial of a sustained-release methylphenidate in the treatment of fatigue in cancer patients. *Cancer J.* 2014;20(1):8-14.

Gong S, Sheng P2, Jin H, et al. Effect of methylphenidate in patients with cancer-related fatigue: a systematic review and meta-analysis. *PLoS One.* 2014;9(1):e84391.

Herman C. National Consensus Project Updates Palliative Care Guidelines. *Aging Today Online.* September 26, 2013. Available at http://asaging.org/blog/national-consensus-project-updates-palliative-care-guidelines

Hovey E, de Souza P, Marx G, et al. Phase III, randomized, double-blind, placebo-controlled study of modafinil for fatigue in patients treated with docetaxel-based chemotherapy. *Support Care Cancer.* 2014;22(5):1233-1242.

Jean-Pierre P, Morrow GR, Roscoe JA, et al. A phase 3 randomized, placebo-controlled, double-blind, clinical trial of the effect of modafinil on cancer-related fatigue among 631 patients receiving chemotherapy: a University of Rochester Cancer Center community clinical oncology program research base study. *Cancer.* 2010;116(14):3513-3520.

Kannan TR, Saxena A, Bhatnagar S, Barry A. Oral ketamine as an adjuvant to oral morphine for neuropathic pain in cancer patients. *J Pain Symptom Manage.* 2002;23(1):60-65.

Kerr CW, Drake J, Milch RA, et al. Effects of methylphenidate on fatigue and depression: a randomized, double-blind, placebo-controlled trial. *J Pain Symptom Manage.* 2012;43(1):68-77.

Lower EE, Fleishman S, Cooper A, et al. Efficacy of dexmethylphenidate for the treatment of fatigue after cancer chemotherapy: a randomized clinical trial. *J Pain Symptom Manage.* 2009;38 (5):650-662.

May P, Garrido MM, Cassel JB, et al. Prospective cohort study of hospital palliative care teams for inpatients with advanced cancer: earlier consultation is associated with larger cost-saving effect. *J Clin Oncol.* 2015;33(25):2745-2752.

Midgren B, Hansson L, Karlsson JA, Simonsson BG, Persson CG. Capsaicin-induced cough in humans. *Am Rev Respir Dis.* 1992;146(2):347-351.

Neeno TA, Rosenow EC 3rd. Intractable hiccups. Consider nebulized lidocaine. *Chest.* 1996;110 (4):1129-1130.

Paulsen O, Klepstad P, Rosland JH, et al. Efficacy of methylprednisolone on pain, fatigue, and appetite loss in patients with advanced cancer using opioids: a randomized, placebo-controlled, double-blind trial. *J Clin Oncol.* 2014;32(29):3221-3228.

Pirl WF, Greer JA, Traeger L, et al. Depression and survival in metastatic non-small-cell lung cancer: effects of early palliative care. *J Clin Oncol.* 2012;30(12):1310-1315.

Qaseem A, Snow V, Shekelle P, et al. Evidence-based interventions to improve the palliative care of pain, dyspnea, and depression at the end of life: a clinical practice guideline from the American College of Physicians. *Ann Intern Med.* 2008;148(2):141-146.

Rizzo JD, Brouwers M, Hurley P, et al. American Society of Clinical Oncology/American Society of Hematology clinical practice guideline update on the use of epoetin and darbepoetin in adult patients with cancer. *J Clin Oncol.* 2010;28(33):4996-5010.

Shaiova L, Berger A, Blinderman CD, et al. Consensus guideline on parenteral methadone use in pain and palliative care. *Palliat Support Care.* 2008;6(2):165-176.

Smith TJ, Temin S, Alesi ER, et al. American Society of Clinical Oncology provisional clinical opinion: the integration of palliative care into standard oncology care. *J Clin Oncol.* 2012;30 (8):880-887.

Spathis A, Fife K, Blackhall F, et al. Modafinil for the treatment of fatigue in lung cancer: results of a placebo-controlled, double-blind, randomized trial. *J Clin Oncol.* 2014;32(18):1882-1888.

Sternberg CN, Molina A, North S, et al. Effect of abiraterone acetate on fatigue in patients with metastatic castration-resistant prostate cancer after docetaxel chemotherapy. *Ann Oncol.* 2013;24(4):1017-1025.

Temel JS, Greer JA, Muzikansky A, et al. Early palliative care for patients with metastatic non-small-cell lung cancer. *N Engl J Med.* 2010;363(8):733-742.

Tremont-Lukats IW, Hutson PR, Backonja MM. A randomized, double-masked, placebo-controlled pilot trial of extended IV lidocaine infusion for relief of ongoing neuropathic pain. *Clin J Pain.* 2006;22(3):266-271.

van Hecke O, Guthrie B. Oral ketamine analgesia in chronic pain and problematic rise in blood pressure. *BMJ Case Rep.* 2014;2014.

Yennurajalingam S, Frisbee-Hume S, Palmer JL, et al. Reduction of cancer-related fatigue with dexamethasone: a double-blind, randomized, placebo-controlled trial in patients with advanced cancer. *J Clin Oncol.* 2013;31(25):3076-3082.

PRINCIPLES OF ANTICANCER THERAPY

Treatment options for cancer include systemic therapy, radiation therapy, and surgical procedures. The wide array of treatment options is warranted by the great complexity of treating cancer. The diagnosis of cancer actually encompasses a multitude of malignant diseases with differing symptomatology and prognosis relative to the tumor's site of origin, natural history, and biologic characteristics. In addition, the intent of therapy can be curative, palliative, or supportive, or it may be investigational. Curative therapy is expected to eradicate cancer from the body, whereas palliative therapy is intended to reduce the body's tumor burden to improve disease-related adverse events. A greater degree of transient and supportable treatment-related toxicity is considered acceptable with curative therapy than with palliative therapy. Best supportive care, which is provided when curative therapy and palliative therapy are not established for a particular cancer, manages disease-related symptomatology without impacting the progression of malignant disease. Investigational therapy adds to the body of knowledge directing the standard of care for cancer patients.

Selection of specific anticancer treatment options is based on disease-related and patient-specific factors. Resource availability is also a consideration. Primary disease-related factors that determine selection of anticancer therapy are the cancer type, stage, and biologic characteristics. The type of cancer (breast cancer, lymphoma, sarcoma) is defined by the cell of origin and is determined by pathologic analysis of tissue or hematology specimens. The stage of disease refers to the body's tumor burden and how advanced the disease process has become. Early stage cancer tends to be localized in the area of initial growth, whereas advanced cancer has often spread to distant sites within the body. Biologic characteristics of cancer can vary, even within a particular tumor type. As an example, breast cancer specimens are tested to determine the amount of estrogen receptor, progesterone receptor, and HER-2 expression. These characteristics vary between patients and influence the selection of treatment options.

The patient's ability to withstand anticancer treatments is an important consideration. Comorbidities that impair major organ function increase the likelihood of serious treatment-related adverse events because the body is more sensitive to drug toxicity and may be less able to effectively eliminate systemic therapies. Life expectancy guides selection of anticancer therapy. As an example, androgen deprivation therapy for localized prostate cancer is generally deferred for patients with a life expectancy of less than 10 years because the chronic cardiovascular and endocrine side effects of therapy outweigh its benefits. Patient and family wishes also factor into treatment-related decisions for cancer patients.

Resource availability that affects selection of anticancer therapy includes reimbursement and accessible level of care. The product acquisition cost of anticancer therapy spans a sizable range from economical to very expensive. Optimal treatment of malignant disease is provided by trained oncologists and an interdisciplinary team. Some treatments, such as hematopoietic stem cell transplantation and major surgeries, are performed only at regional treatment centers.

Systemic therapy is used for the treatment of localized and metastatic sites of disease. The most extensively used type of systemic therapy is cytotoxic chemotherapy. Cytotoxic chemotherapy has a narrow therapeutic index and the overall ▶

efficacy of therapy is often based on a balance of tumor sensitivity and patient tolerance. In order to optimize anticancer treatment, cytotoxic chemotherapy is generally administered as combination therapy. Combination of specific chemotherapy drugs (see Table 1) is based on principles intended to provide the greatest anticancer effect with acceptable regimen-related toxicity. Proven efficacy against the tumor type being treated is essential to justify inclusion of a particular agent in combination therapy. Combination of chemotherapy drugs with different pharmacologic mechanisms of action yields increased sites of pharmacologic damage to the cancer. In addition, an increased number of pharmacologic mechanisms of action provides stronger overall anticancer efficacy when the malignant cells comprising a patient's tumor vary with respect to drug target sensitivity. Administration of chemotherapy drugs susceptible to different mechanisms of anticancer drug resistance improves treatment efficacy because a specific mechanism of cellular resistance will only impede a proportion of the regimen's overall anticancer activity. Selection of anticancer drugs with non-overlapping serious nonhematologic toxicities for use in combination therapy is important in order to maintain acceptable toxicity with respect to anticipated outcome and to allow administration of the maximum dose for each drug in the regimen. The anticancer activity of most chemotherapy drugs correlates with the dose amount administered, so use of the maximum tolerated dose of each drug within a regimen is generally warranted for optimal efficacy. The maximum tolerated dose of chemotherapy drugs is often lower when administered in combination vs single agent therapy. In addition, combination chemotherapy must be scheduled such that cycles are repeated with the shortest possible time interval between administrations. The time interval should be adequate to allow recovery of nonmalignant tissues, such as gastrointestinal mucosa and bone marrow, and otherwise as short as possible to impede malignant cellular repair and tumor progression.

Table 1: Principles of Combination Chemotherapy

- Proven efficacy against the tumor type being treated
- Different pharmacologic mechanisms of action
- Different spectrum of drug resistance
- Nonoverlapping serious nonhematologic toxicities
- Maximum tolerated dose
- Shortest possible interval between cyclic administrations

Additional models used for evaluating and optimizing the delivery of efficacious anticancer therapy include dose intensity, alternating or sequential noncross-resistant chemotherapy, and dose density. Dose intensity is mathematically defined by the equation $mg/m^2/week$ of chemotherapy. Increased dose intensity was initially investigated for its correlation with disease response and relapse-free survival in the treatment of localized and metastatic breast cancer and has since been examined in other tumor types. Initial findings supported a correlation of increased dose intensity with improved disease response and relapse-free survival in breast cancer patients. Several aspects of the initial work evaluating dose intensity have been criticized, including its retrospective evaluation of protocol-directed vs actual drug administration and failure to consider the impact of different administration routes. However, dose intensity provides a useful tool for assessing the efficacy and safety of chemotherapy administration. Relative dose intensity is used to evaluate the efficacy and safety of varying the dose amount or interval between administrations of a particular chemotherapy regimen (see Table 2). In addition, the relative dose intensity of planned vs actual drug administration provides a measure of patient tolerance relative to treatment efficacy. Alternating or sequential noncross-resistant chemotherapy delivers alternating or sequentially repeated cycles of chemotherapy with known activity against a particular tumor type at the full doses tested to demonstrate anticancer efficacy. This approach utilizes the efficacy advantage of combination chemotherapy without the need to reduce chemotherapy doses for patient tolerance. An example of sequential chemotherapy is AC → T which administers four cycles of cyclophosphamide 600 mg/m^2/dose and doxorubicin 60 mg/m^2/dose every 21 days, followed by four cycles of paclitaxel 175 mg/m^2/dose administered every 21 days for the treatment of breast cancer. Dose density refers to the practice of shortening the interval between chemotherapy administration to reduce the time allowed for malignant cellular repair and tumor progression. Patient tolerance is maintained throughout administration of dose-dense chemotherapy by the use of white blood cell colony-stimulating factors. An example of dose-dense chemotherapy is AC → T with chemotherapy cycles shortened to 14-day intervals and white blood cell colony-stimulating factor support.

Table 2: Relative Dose Intensity of AC Regimen Administered at 21-Day or 28-Day Intervals

Dose intensity of AC with 21-day administration schedule:
  Cyclophosphamide 600 mg/m^2/dose every 21 days x 4 cycles = 200 mg/m^2/week
  Doxorubicin 60 mg/m^2/dose every 21 days x 4 cycles = 20 mg/m^2/week

Dose intensity of AC with 28-day administration schedule:
  Cyclophosphamide 600 mg/m^2/dose every 28 days x 4 cycles = 150 mg/m^2/week
  Doxorubicin 60 mg/m^2/dose every 28 days x 4 cycles = 15 mg/m^2/week

Relative dose intensity of cyclophosphamide: 200 mg/m^2/week *divided by* 150 mg/m^2/week = 1.33
Relative dose intensity of doxorubicin: 20 mg/m^2/week *divided by* 15 mg/m^2/week = 1.33

Endocrine therapy is effective in cancers that utilize a hormone-dependent pathway for growth and survival. The greatest utility of endocrine therapy is in the treatment of breast cancer and prostate cancer. A major advantage to endocrine therapy is patient tolerance of these products relative to the side effect profile of cytotoxic chemotherapy. Antiestrogenic therapy is part of curative therapy for most cases of estrogen-receptor positive localized breast cancer and it is utilized as primary therapy for many estrogen-receptor positive advanced and metastatic cases of breast cancer. Medical castration using LHRH agonist, LHRH antagonist, and androgen-receptor blocking therapy is the initial systemic therapy for prostate cancer that is advancing or metastatic. Most side effects from endocrine therapy are transient and manageable, consisting of hot flashes, fatigue, fluid retention, vaginal discharge, and mood changes. However, for some patients, the immediate side effects can be dose-limiting and other sequelae can occur with chronic administration. A troublesome and sometimes dose-limiting side effect of aromatase inhibitor therapy is arthralgias. Chronic administration of aromatase inhibitors is associated with loss of bone mineral density. Chronic administration of tamoxifen is associated with endometrial cancer, thromboembolic disorders, and cataract formation. Chronic androgen deprivation is associated with the development of metabolic syndrome and increased cardiovascular morbidity.

◀ Targeted anticancer therapy is designed to inactivate or disrupt a molecular process or biochemical pathway that is unique to malignant cell growth and viability. The efficacy of molecularly targeted anticancer agents is related to their ability to interfere with an essential malignant process. The utility of targeted therapy may be limited by redundancies occurring in some cellular processes that circumvent the damage done by these agents. Small molecule tyrosine kinase inhibitors and multikinase inhibitors represent the largest number of targeted products that are commercially available (see Table 3). Additional molecules and pathways targeted by commercially available anticancer therapy include angiogenesis, histone deacetylase, and proteasome activity (see Table 3). Many types of biologic therapy have a targeted mechanism of action (see Table 4). Targeted therapy is less toxic than cytotoxic chemotherapy because it does not predictably exert the classic severe dose-related effects of bone marrow suppression, mucositis, and emesis. However, side effects associated with targeted therapy that are mild-to-moderate in severity can be dose-limiting due to the negative impact on quality of life with the chronic nature of drug administration. Examples include diarrhea and skin problems from tyrosine kinase inhibitor therapy. In addition, targeted therapy with antiVEGF activity can cause or exacerbate adverse effects deleterious to cardiovascular, endocrine, and renal function, which can limit the use of these products.

Table 3: Molecularly Targeted Anticancer Therapy: Small Molecular Entities

Drug	Molecular Target-Mechanism
Abiraterone	CYP17 inhibitor
Afatinib	Epidermal growth factor receptor (EGFR) tyrosine kinase inhibitor (TKI), HER-2 TKI
Axitinib	Vascular endothelial growth factor (VEGF) TKI
Belinostat	Histone deactylase inhibitor
Bortezomib	Proteosome inhibitor
Bosutinib	BCR-ABL TKI
Cabozatinib	Multityrosine kinase inhibitor (MTKI)
Carfilzomib	Proteosome inhibitor
Ceritinib	ALK TKI
Crizotinib	ALK TKI
Dabrafenib	BRAF TKI
Dasatinib	BCR-ABL TKI
Erlotinib	EGFR TKI
Everolimus	m-TOR inhibitor
Ibrutinib	Bruton's TKI
Idelalisib	PI3K TKI
Imatinib	BCR-ABL TKI
Lapatinib	EGFR TKI, HER-2 TKI
Lenalidomide	Multiple mechanisms

Table 3: Molecularly Targeted Anticancer Therapy: Small Molecular Entities *(continued)*

Drug	Molecular Target-Mechanism
Lenvatinib	MTKI
Nilotinib	BCR-ABL TKI
Olaparib	Poly (ADP-ribose) polymerase (PARP) inhibitor
Palbociclib	Cyclin-dependent kinase (CDK) inhibitor
Panobinostat	Histone deactylase inhibitor
Pazopanib	MTKI
Pomalidomide	Multiple mechanisms
Ponatinib	Pan-BCR-ABL TKI
Regorafinib	MTKI
Romidepsin	Histone deactylase inhibitor
Sonidegib	Hedgehog pathway inhibitor
Sorafenib	MTKI
Sunitinib	MTKI
Temsirolimus	m-TOR inhibitor
Thalidomide	Multiple mechanisms
Trametinib	MEK TKI
Tretinoin	Nuclear retinoic acid receptor isotypes alpha, beta, gamma
Vandetanib	MTKI
Vemurafenib	BRAF TKI
Vismodegib	Hedgehog pathway inhibitor
Vorinostat	Histone deactylase inhibitor

Table 4: Molecularly Targeted Anticancer Therapy: Biologic Products

Drug	Product Type	Molecular Target-Mechanism
Ado-trastuzumab	Conjugated monoclonal antibody	HER-2 ligand, tubulin
Aldesleukin	Recombinant cytokine	Interleukin-2 receptor agonist
Alemtuzumab	Monoclonal antibody	CD52 ligand
Bevacizumab	Monoclonal antibody	VEGF inhibitor
Blinatumomab	Bispecific T-cell engager	CD 19 ligand and CD 3 ligand
Brentuximab vedotin	Conjugated monoclonal antibody	CD30, tubulin
Cetuximab	Monoclonal antibody	EGFR inhibitor
Denileukin diftitox	Fusion protein	CD25 ligand
Dinutuximab	Monoclonal antibody	Disialoganglioside GD2
Ipilimumab	Monoclonal antibody	CTLA-4 ligand

Table 4: Molecularly Targeted Anticancer Therapy: Biologic Products *(continued)*

Drug	Product Type	Molecular Target-Mechanism
Nivolumab	Monocloncal antibody	Programmed cell death-1 (PD-1) receptor
Obinutuzumab	Monoclonal antibody	CD20 ligand
Ofatumumab	Monoclonal antibody	CD20 ligand
Panitumumab	Monoclonal antibody	EGFR inhibitor
Pembrolizumab	Monoclonal antibody	PD-1 receptor
Pertuzumab	Monoclonal antibody	HER-2 ligand
Ramucirumab	Monoclonal antibody	VEGF-2R inhibitor
Rituximab	Monoclonal antibody	CD20 ligand
Siltuximab	Monoclonal antibody	Interleukin-6
Trastuzumab	Monoclonal antibody	HER-2 ligand
Ziv-aflibercept	Recombinant fusion protein	VEGF ligand

REFERENCES

Citron ML, Berry DA, Cirrincione C, et al. Randomized trial of dose-dense versus conventionally scheduled and sequential versus concurrent combination chemotherapy as postoperative adjuvant treatment of node-positive primary breast cancer: first report of intergroup trial C9741/cancer and leukemia group B trial 9741. *J Clin Oncol.* 2003;21(8):1431-1439.

DeVita VT Jr, Young RC, Canellos GP. Combination versus single agent chemotherapy: a review of the basis for selection of drug treatment of cancer. *Cancer.* 1975;35(1):98-110.

Felson DT, Cummings SR. Aromatase inhibitors and the syndrome of arthralgias with estrogen deprivation. *Arthritis Rheum.* 2005;52(9):2594-2598.

Hryniuk W, Bush H. The importance of dose intensity in chemotherapy of metastatic breast cancer. *J Clin Oncol.* 1984;2(11):1281-1288.

Hryniuk W, Levine MN. Analysis of dose intensity for adjuvant chemotherapy trials in stage II breast cancer. *J Clin Oncol.* 1986;4(8):1162-1170.

Kintzel PE, Chase SL, Schultz LM, O'Rourke TJ. Increased risk of metabolic syndrome, diabetes mellitus, and cardiovascular disease in men receiving androgen deprivation therapy for prostate cancer. *Pharmacotherapy.* 2008.28(12):1511-1522.

Marill J, Idres N, Capron CC, Nguyen E, Chabot GG. Retinoic acid metabolism and mechanism of action: a review. *Curr Drug Metab.* 2003;4(1):1-10.

VENOUS THROMBOEMBOLISM IN THE CANCER PATIENT

INTRODUCTION

Venous thromboembolism (VTE) is a common and life-threatening complication in cancer patients. Overall, ~500,000 new cases of VTE are diagnosed annually, 1 in 5 of which are diagnosed in cancer patients. Patients with active cancer have at least a 6- to 7-fold increased risk of VTE. Development of VTE is a major cause of mortality in this population; it may increase the likelihood of death by up to 47-fold in certain patients (Khorana 2007). Diagnosis of VTE or superficial venous thrombosis in a young or middle-aged person without an identifiable cause raises suspicion for underlying malignancy. VTE is generally diagnosed in cancer patients within the first few months of malignant disease and may be related to a number of intrinsic (eg, tumor aggressiveness) or extrinsic (eg, surgery, radiation) factors. Pathophysiologic causes for VTE in cancer patients include hypercoagulability, vessel wall damage, and vessel stasis from direct compression by tumors. Given the significant morbidity and mortality caused by VTE, it is important for the clinician to recognize patients at risk for VTE and to offer appropriate prophylactic and treatment strategies. In addition, clinicians should provide patients with proper education regarding signs and symptoms of VTE.

VTE RISK ASSESSMENT

VTE risk should be assessed in all cancer patients at the time of chemotherapy initiation and periodically thereafter. VTE risk factors in this patient population can be separated into three categories: patient-related (ie, intrinsic and extrinsic factors), cancer-related, and treatment-related. Patient-related factors include an active cancer diagnosis, previous VTE, hypercoagulable state (eg, factor V Leiden, lupus anticoagulant, anticardiolipin antibodies), >70 years of age, obesity (BMI $\geq$30 kg/m^2), hospitalization, and bed rest/immobility (for at least 3 days). Increased comorbid burden defined by coexisting conditions, such as pulmonary disease, kidney disease, and infections, is also associated with a greater risk of VTE.

The type of cancer also influences VTE risk. A diagnosis of metastatic cancer arising from the pancreas, stomach, bladder, uterus, kidney, and lung confers a greater risk for VTE, as do diagnoses of acute leukemia, multiple myeloma, and non-Hodgkin lymphoma. Lower risk for VTE is associated with breast cancer, prostate cancer, and head and neck cancers. In addition, histologic subtype also plays a role in VTE prevalence, with adenocarcinomas having a higher risk compared to squamous cell cancers. Advanced stage of disease, poor patient performance status, and the finding of leukocytosis or thrombocytosis (platelet count >350,000/microliter) at presentation all may put patients at risk for thrombosis. Lastly, VTE risk factors specific to multiple myeloma include M-spike >1.6 g/dL, progressive disease, and hyperviscosity syndrome.

Treatment-related and iatrogenic factors, such as surgery, the presence of a central venous access device (CVAD), and chemotherapy and/or radiotherapy administration, place cancer patients in jeopardy of developing VTE. The reported incidence of ultrasound-detected upper extremity deep venous thrombosis (DVT) is variable (2% to 67%) (Rooden 2005) and the incidence of pulmonary embolism (PE) on autopsy reports was up to 50% (Verso 2003) in cancer patients with

CVADs. The 3 main classes of cancer drugs which may lead to VTE include cytotoxic chemotherapy, hormonal therapy with estrogenic properties, and anti-angiogenic medications. Administration of cytotoxic chemotherapy is associated with a 2- to 6-fold increased risk of VTE. Selective estrogen receptor modulator (tamoxifen) administration is associated with 2- to 5-fold increased risk of VTE among women with breast cancer (Kahn 2012). The findings of one meta-analysis indicate that the incidence of VTE (all grades) is ~11% with bevacizumab (in combination with chemotherapy or immunotherapy) administration (Hurwitz 2011). The immune modulating products lenalidomide and thalidomide are thrombogenic, especially when administered in combination with a corticosteroid or cytotoxic chemotherapy. Treatment of multiple myeloma and lymphoid malignancies often involves chronic or episodic corticosteroid administration, which further increases the risk of VTE. Ancillary therapies used to prevent and manage disease and treatment-related adverse events can also increase the likelihood of VTE. Two such examples are erythropoietin-stimulating agents (ESA) administered for anemia and corticosteroids, which may be administered for antiemesis, as well as other indications.

VTE PROPHYLAXIS

Due to the high risk of VTE in hospitalized patients with cancer, prophylactic anticoagulation using a low molecular weight heparin (LMWH), fondaparinux, or unfractionated heparin should be administered to all hospitalized patients with active cancer and acute medical illness or reduced mobility (in the absence of bleeding or other contraindications) according to standard guidelines. Prophylaxis with LMWH or unfractionated heparin is also recommended in patients with cancer prior to undergoing major surgery and continuing for at least 7 to 10 days postoperatively (unless contraindicated). In patients for whom anticoagulation is absolutely or relatively contraindicated (eg, recent central nervous system bleeding, major active bleeding, recent lumbar puncture, low platelet count), intermittent pneumatic venous compression devices (IPCs) may be considered for VTE prophylaxis. There is not enough evidence to support or oppose routine thromboprophylaxis in patients hospitalized for short chemotherapy courses, minor procedures, or for hematopoietic stem cell transplantation.

Criteria for VTE prophylaxis in the outpatient cancer setting are not clearly delineated. Routine pharmacologic thromboprophylaxis is not recommended for most ambulatory cancer patients; however, some surgical and medical oncology patients are at high risk for VTE and may benefit from extended outpatient prophylaxis. For surgical oncology patients (particularly high-risk patients undergoing abdominal or pelvic surgery), continued administration of VTE prophylaxis after hospital discharge for a period of up to 4 weeks following major surgery may be recommended. Multiple myeloma patients receiving thrombotic anticancer therapy (lenalidomide or thalidomide in combination with dexamethasone >480 mg monthly or doxorubicin or multiagent chemotherapy) also may require outpatient VTE prophylaxis. LMWHs, unfractionated heparin, and warfarin are the primary agents used for VTE prophylaxis in cancer patients. Aspirin can be considered for VTE prophylaxis in patients with multiple myeloma at relatively low-risk for VTE (no more than one VTE risk factor). Risk stratification criteria based on tumor site, prechemotherapy platelet count, prechemotherapy leukocyte count, anemia and ESA administration, and body size have been proposed (Dutia, 2012). Overall, primary pharmacologic prophylaxis for VTE in ambulatory cancer patients remains controversial because it increases the risk of bleeding with indeterminate efficacy for prevention of VTE.

VTE TREATMENT

Initial treatment of VTE in cancer patients is similar to that of noncancer patients, with unfractionated heparin, LMWHs, and warfarin (vitamin K antagonist [VKA]) providing the cornerstone of anticoagulant therapy. Initial assessment and management of VTE in cancer patients is conducted according to clinical practice guidelines and institutional policy. The minimum duration of anticoagulant therapy is 3 months for DVT and PE; anticoagulation for a 6-month duration is recommended for proximal DVT, PE, and recurrent VTE in patients with advanced or metastatic cancer. The use of LMWH is preferred over a VKA for the first 6 months of treatment in cancer patients who develop DVT of the leg or PE. If long-term therapy with LMWH is not feasible, the use of VKAs is an acceptable alternative. For patients with active cancer or continuing VTE risk factors, anticoagulation should be continued indefinitely. For treatment of a catheter-related DVT, the recommended duration of treatment is at least 3 months and for as long as the catheter remains in place.

Special situations related to cancer and its treatments may complicate delivery of safe and effective therapeutic anticoagulation. Low platelet counts due to hematologic malignancies or cytotoxic treatments may be present in cancer patients requiring anticoagulation. Unfortunately, limited options exist for patients with an active clotting process, despite a low platelet count, so management of therapeutic anticoagulation in the setting of thrombocytopenia must be handled judiciously on a case-by-case basis. Inferior vena cava (IVC) filter placement is one method for reducing the risk of PE in patients with DVT who have contraindications to anticoagulant therapy. Drawbacks to IVC filter placement include lack of systemic anticoagulant effect and increased risk of recurrent DVT. Cancer patients requiring anticoagulation may also need intrathecal administration of chemotherapy. Anticoagulation must be interrupted for spinal injection and intrathecal medication administration. The American Society of Regional Anesthesia and Pain Medicine (ASRA) recommends withholding LMWH for at least 24 hours and unfractionated heparin for at least 1 hour before spinal injection for the delivery of analgesia. Warfarin should be held for 4 to 5 days prior to spinal injection.

ANTICOAGULANT SELECTION

Anticoagulant selection may be influenced by cancer and its treatments. The anticoagulant activity of warfarin is readily affected by diet, drug interactions, liver function, and certain physiologic stressors. Food intake in the cancer patient can vary relative to disease- and treatment-related factors that alter taste sensation, reduce appetite, and cause adverse gastrointestinal events. Numerous therapeutic and ancillary medications used in the management of cancer interact with the anticoagulant intensity of warfarin. Due to the extensive and expanding list of medications that interact with warfarin, the reader should refer to specific drug monographs for detailed information about particular medications. Hepatic function in the cancer patient can be impaired due to primary or metastatic tumor growth in the liver. In addition, any physiologic stressor, such as infection, can alter the anticoagulant effect of warfarin in this patient population.

LMWHs are not prone to altered anticoagulant intensity by the myriad of dietary, drug, and physiologic factors affecting warfarin therapy. However, all commercially available LMWHs are excreted renally and may require dosage adjustments in patients with renal dysfunction; anti-Xa monitoring may facilitate appropriate administration in this clinical scenario. Unfractionated heparin should be considered as an alternative to LMWH for use in patients with severely impaired renal function.

The use of novel oral anticoagulants (eg, dabigatran, rivaroxaban, apixaban) is not currently recommended for either prevention or treatment of VTE in cancer patients (Lyman 2015). While some oral anticoagulants are approved for selected VTE prevention/treatment indications, trials using these agents included few patients with malignancies. There is growing data that support the efficacy of these agents in cancer patients (Vedovati 2015); however, it is important to note that most trials in cancer patients have used UFH or warfarin as a comparator and trials comparing oral agents to LMWH are lacking. Unpredictable absorption, potential for increased adverse events, alterations in metabolism, and potential drug interactions are among concerns with the use of novel oral anticoagulants in patients with malignancies (Lyman 2013). Further data from randomized controlled trials including patients with malignancies are needed to confirm the safety and efficacy of these agents in cancer patients.

Anticoagulant Comparison Table

Name	Use	DVT and PE Dose	Adjust Dose for Renal Impairment?
Low Molecular Weight Heparins			
Dalteparin	Prophylaxis	SubQ: 2,500 to 5,000 units once daily	Yes
	Treatment	SubQ: Month 1: 200 units/kg once daily (maximum dose: 18,000 units) Months 2 to 6: 150 units/kg once daily (maximum dose: 18,000 units)	
Enoxaparin	Prophylaxis	SubQ: 30 mg q12h or 40 mg once daily	Yes
	Treatment	SubQ: 1 mg/kg q12h	
Heparin			
Heparin	Prophylaxis	SubQ: 5,000 units q8 to 12h	No
	Treatment	IV: 80 units/kg (bolus), then 18 units/kg/h	
Selective Anti-Xa Inhibitor			
Fondaparinux	Prophylaxis	SubQ: ≥50 kg: 2.5 mg once daily (prophylactic use is contraindicated in patients <50 kg)	Yes
	Treatment	SubQ: <50 kg: 5 mg once daily 50 to 100 kg: 7.5 mg once daily >100 kg: 10 mg once daily	
Vitamin K Antagonists			
Warfarin	Prophylaxis	Oral: Variable	No
	Treatment	Oral: Variable; adjust dose to maintain INR 2 to 3	

REFERENCES

Battinelli EM, Murphy DL, Connors JM. Venous thromboembolism overview. *Hematol Oncol Clin North Am.* 2012;26(2):345-367.

Dutia M, White RH, Wun T. Risk assessment models for cancer-associated venous thromboembolism. *Cancer.* 2012;118(14):3468-3476.

Horlocker TT, Wedel DJ, Rowlingson JC, et al. Regional anesthesia in the patient receiving antithrombotic or thrombolytic therapy: American Society of Regional Anesthesia and Pain Medicine evidence-based guidelines (third edition). *Reg Anesth Pain Med.* 2010;35(1):64-101.

Hurwitz HI, Saltz LB, Van Cutsem E, et al. Venous thromboembolic events with chemotherapy plus bevacizumab: a pooled analysis of patients in randomized phase II and III studies. *J Clin Oncol.* 2011;29(13):1757-1764.

Kahn SR, Lim W, Dunn AS, et al. Prevention of VTE in nonsurgical patients: antithrombotic therapy and prevention of thrombosis, 9th ed: American College of Chest Physicians evidence-based clinical practice guidelines. *Chest*. 2012;141(2 Suppl):e195S-e226S.

Kearon C, Akl EA, Comerota AJ, et al. Antithrombotic therapy for VTE disease: antithrombotic therapy and prevention of thrombosis, 9th ed: American College of Chest Physicians evidence-based clinical practice guidelines. *Chest*. 2012;141(2 Suppl):e419S-e494S.

Khorana AA, Francis CW, Culakova E, Kuderer NM, Lyman GH. Thromboembolism is a leading cause of death in cancer patients receiving outpatient chemotherapy. *J Thromb Haemost*. 2007;5 (3):632-634.

Lyman GH, Bohlke K, Khorana AA, et al. Venous thromboembolism prophylaxis and treatment in patients with cancer: american society of clinical oncology clinical practice guideline update 2014. *J Clin Oncol*. 2015;33(6):654-656.

Lyman GH, Khorana AA, Kuderer NM, et al. Venous thromboembolism prophylaxis and treatment in patients with cancer: American Society of Clinical Oncology clinical practice guideline update. *J Clin Oncol*. 2013;31(17):2189-2204.

Palumbo A, Cavo M, Bringhen S, et al. Aspirin, warfarin, or enoxaparin thromboprophylaxis in patients with multiple myeloma treated with thalidomide: a phase III, open-label, randomized trial. *J Clin Oncol*. 2011;29(8):986-993.

Rooden CJ, Tesselaar ME, Osanto S, Rosendaal FR, Huisman MV. Deep vein thrombosis associated with central venous catheters – a review. *J Thromb Haemost*. 2005;3(11):2409-2419.

Sørensen HT, Sværke C, Farkas DK, et al. Superficial and deep venous thrombosis, pulmonary embolism and subsequent risk of cancer. *Eur J Cancer*. 2012;48(4):586-593.

Vedovati MC, Germini F, Agnelli G, Becattini C. Direct oral anticoagulants in patients with VTE and cancer: a systematic review and meta-analysis. *Chest*. 2015;147(2):475-483.

Verso M, Agnelli G. Venous thromboembolism associated with long-term use of central venous catheters in cancer patients. *J Clin Oncol*. 2003;21(19):3665-3675.

HEMATOPOIETIC STEM CELL TRANSPLANTATION

INTRODUCTION

Hematopoietic stem cell transplantation (HSCT) involves the infusion of hematopoietic stem and progenitor cells into a patient in order to treat malignant disease and nonmalignant hematologic, lymphopoietic, congenital, and other disorders. Hematopoietic stem cells are immature cells that mature and differentiate into the various functional myeloid (eg, neutrophils, monocytes, macrophages, megakaryocytes, erythrocytes) and lymphoid cells (eg, T lymphocytes, B lymphocytes, natural killer cells) of the hematopoietic system. Hematopoietic stem cells are transplanted in order to replace diseased hematopoietic cells, reduce the duration of pancytopenia following administration of high dose chemotherapy, or to generate antitumor immunity in cancer patients. Allogeneic stem cell transplants require donation of stem cells from a healthy donor; whereas, autologous transplantation uses stem cells previously collected from the patient undergoing treatment. Allogeneic stem cell transplants are further classified as related transplants (donor and recipient are siblings or first-degree relatives), unrelated transplants (donor and recipient are not related by pedigree), or syngeneic transplants (donor and recipient are identical twins). Immunologic likeness of the donor and recipient is determined by comparison of the genotype of donor and recipient class I and class II major histocompatibility (MHC) antigens. MHC Class I antigens (HLA-A, HLA-B, HLA-C) are present on all nucleated cells in the body and provide a means for the immune system to differentiate self vs nonself. MHC Class II proteins (HLA-D) are present on antigen presenting cells, such as macrophages, dendritic cells, B lymphocytes, and activated endothelial cells, and are critical in initiation and maintenance of long-lasting immunity and tolerance.

Stem cell transplants are classified according to the intensity of the pretransplant preparative regimen. Myeloablative chemotherapy regimens administer the highest possible dose of chemotherapy, with the doses limited by regimen-related nonhematologic toxicity. The goal of the myeloablative regimen is to achieve the maximum anticancer effect and complete immunosuppression through the effects of the high dose cytotoxic agents. The goal of the nonmyeloablative preparative or reduced intensity conditioning (RIC) regimen is to inhibit the recipient immune system adequately to allow engraftment of the donated hematopoietic cells. Complete donor engraftment following nonmyeloablative transplantation typically occurs after a period of mixed chimerism (coexistence of donor and recipient hematologic cells) and is associated with antitumor effect mediated by donor immune cells.

Terms that are synonymous with hematopoietic stem cell transplantation include bone marrow transplantation, peripheral blood cell transplantation, and peripheral blood cell rescue. The following table lists clinical uses for allogeneic and autologous myeloablative hematopoietic stem cell transplantation.

Condition	Allogeneic	Autologous
Acute lymphocytic leukemia (ALL)	+	+
Acute myelogenous leukemia (AML)	+	+
Myelodysplastic syndrome	+	-
Chronic lymphocytic leukemia (CLL)	+	-
Chronic myelogenous leukemia (CML)	+	-
Non-Hodgkin's lymphoma (NHL)	+	+
Hodgkin's lymphoma	+	+
Multiple myeloma (MM)	+	+
Severe aplastic anemia (SAA)	+	-
Sickle cell disease (SCD)	+	-
Congenital immunodeficiency syndromes	+	-
Adult autoimmune disorders (eg, scleroderma, multiple sclerosis, rheumatoid arthritis)	-	+
Germ cell/testicular cancer	-	+
Neuroblastoma	-	+
Congenital hematopoietic disorders	+	-
Inborn errors of metabolism	+	-
Paroxysmal nocturnal hemoglobinuria	+	-
Thalassemia major	+	-
Wiskott-Aldrich syndrome	+	-

SOURCES, COLLECTION, AND PROCESSING OF HEMATOPOIETIC PROGENITOR CELLS

Hematopoietic progenitor cells used for transplantation are generally gathered from the peripheral blood. The hematopoietic stem and progenitor cells are removed via leukapheresis, which is routinely done in an ambulatory setting. Cells collected for autologous transplantation are processed and cryopreserved for future use. Cells collected for allogeneic transplantation are processed and infused immediately (within 24 hours). Leukapheresis involves the processing of ~10 L of peripheral blood over a 2- to 6-hour period. The usual goal is a product containing at least 2×10^6/kg and ideally 5×10^6/kg of recipient weight of CD34$^+$ cells, which closely correlate with the content of stem and progenitor cells collected. This may be accomplished by 1 or several leukaphereses. Donors may require calcium supplementation during leukapheresis due to the citrate anticoagulant used during the procedure. Common medical risks to the allogeneic donor of peripheral hematopoietic stem cells include adverse effects from treatment with a colony-stimulating factor (bone pain) and adverse events associated with leukapheresis (acute hypocalcemia, catheter-related discomfort). Although no long-term toxicity has been reported in donors treated with colony-stimulating factors, rare serious toxicity such as splenic rupture can occur and the donor must be screened carefully prior to donation.

The peripheral blood concentration of hematopoietic stem cells and progenitor cells must be increased to facilitate successful collection. This process is known as peripheral progenitor cell mobilization. After administration of chemotherapy, colony-stimulating factors, or a combination of the two agents, the numbers of circulating early and late progenitor cells expands. A colony-stimulating factor, such as filgrastim or sargramostim, is used for this purpose in the healthy allogeneic donor. For the autologous donor, a colony-stimulating factor is administered alone or prescribed following chemotherapy. Mobilization of hematopoietic progenitor cells can be more difficult in patients with hematologic malignancies or a history of extensive treatment with chemotherapy and radiation. Plerixafor can be used in combination with filgrastim to enhance hematopoietic stem cell mobilization in heavily pretreated autologous donors. The following table provides the dosage and schedule for some of the more commonly used mobilization regimens. Selection of the chemotherapy for mobilization in the autologous donor is primarily based on the type of cancer being treated.

Mobilization Agent	Dosage and Duration
Filgrastim (G-CSF)	10 mcg/kg/day SubQ for 5 to 7 days or until target WBC; dose escalation to 16 to 32 mcg/kg/day has been used to improve inadequate mobilization
Sargramostim (GM-CSF)	250 mg/m^2/day SubQ for 5 to 7 days or until target WBC
Etoposide (VP-16)	2 g/m^2 IV over 2 hours, followed in 24 hours by G-CSF or GM-CSF until target WBC
Cyclophosphamide	4 g/m^2 (range of 1.5 to 7 g/m^2) IV over 2 hours followed at 24 hours by G-CSF 5 to 10 mcg/kg/day until target WBC; higher doses are also used (7 g/m^2)
Cytarabine plus etoposide	2 g/m^2 IV q12h x 8 doses + 40 mg/kg VP-16 over 4 days then G-CSF 10 mcg/kg/day from day 14 until cells collected
Plerixafor (in combination with filgrastim)	0.24 mg/kg SubQ once daily for up to 4 consecutive days beginning ~11 hours prior to apheresis; maximum dose: 40 mg/day

Historically, the bone marrow was the primary source of hematopoietic stem cells for transplantation and it still represents an equivalent, if not better, stem cell source in the setting of allogeneic transplantation. The bone marrow contains populations of hematopoietic cells ranging from the pluripotent stem cell, early progenitor cells, and later, more differentiated progenitor cells that all exist within and are supported by the bone marrow stroma (matrix composed of connective tissue, reticuloendothelial cells, adipose cells). Compared to blood, the concentration of T lymphocytes is significantly lower in the marrow. Bone marrow can be harvested by removing an adequate volume of marrow (~10 mL/kg) from the posterior iliac crests of the donor or patient. This is generally done in an operating room and requires general or local anesthesia. Common medical risks to the donor of bone marrow include the risks of undergoing anesthesia, and transient moderate pain in the area of cell harvesting. Severe anemia can also develop. The frequency of life-threatening complications, which have included thromboembolic disorders, aspiration pneumonia, and cardiac dysrhythmias, is ≤0.3%. Hematopoietic engraftment (normalization of the peripheral white blood cell count) occurs earlier following peripheral stem cell transplantation than following bone marrow transplantation. However, chronic graft-versus-host disease (GVHD) risk is lower with the bone marrow source.

Umbilical cord blood (UCB) is another source of hematopoietic progenitor cells. The product, which is harvested from the placenta and umbilical cord immediately after birth, can be processed and transplanted or frozen for future use. The product obtained from UCB contains a high proportion of pluripotent stem cells and natural killer cells, and a low proportion of mature lymphocytes. The time to engraftment is generally longer following UCB transplantation than following peripheral blood or bone marrow hematopoietic stem cell transplantation. Moreover, UCB transplantation is generally reserved for children and small adults because the number of stem cells that can be collected from cord blood may be inadequate to support timely engraftment for larger patients. The risk for severe GVHD is lower with UCB even when HLA matching is not perfect. The process of harvesting UCB does not present a medical risk to the donor, because the actual collection of cells is done after the placenta is extruded as part of the birthing process. One investigational strategy for expanding the pool of UCB is to transplant UCB from two donors instead of a single donor. Preliminary data (in children and adolescents) demonstrates similar survival rates between cohorts receiving 2-unit vs 1-unit UCB transplantation with increased grade III to IV GVHD and longer time to platelet recovery with infusion of the 2-unit product (Wagner 2014).

The hematopoietic progenitor cells may be treated prior to transplantation to eradicate tumor cell contamination in the product following autologous donation or reduce the number of T lymphocytes that may promote graft-versus-host disease in an allogeneic recipient. The term purging refers to the removal of tumor cells by various techniques such as binding to specific monoclonal antibodies or incubation with cytotoxic drugs, such as 4-hydroperoxycyclophosphamide, that spare the immature stem cells. *Ex vivo* T lymphocyte reduction, also known as T cell depletion, is generally achieved using monoclonal antibodies directed against surface proteins expressed on T lymphocytes. Engraftment is generally delayed following transplantation of hematopoietic progenitor cells that have undergone *ex vivo* purging or T cell depletion.

AUTOLOGOUS MYELOABLATIVE TRANSPLANTATION

Chemotherapy and dosage selection for autologous myeloablative HSCT is based on three important principles:

1. Certain drugs such as alkylating agents and etoposide exhibit steep dose-response curves when used to treat susceptible malignancies. Therefore, when the dose-limiting adverse effect of these drugs is myelosuppression, high doses can be administered with hematopoietic stem cell rescue to achieve high response rates.

2. High doses of chemotherapy with nonoverlapping nonhematologic major organ toxicity can be combined without compromising dose.

3. Cryopreserved bone marrow and/or blood progenitor cells can rescue the patient from the myeloablative effects of the high-dose chemotherapy.

Administration of filgrastim or sargramostim following reinfusion of the autologous hematopoietic progenitor cells significantly shortens the duration of neutropenia associated with myeloablative chemotherapy (refer to Filgrastim or Sargramostim monographs for dosing, etc). The hematopoietic recovery period following HSCT is generally 1 to 2 weeks, which is shorter than that for bone marrow or UCB transplants which require 2 to 4 weeks. The monocytes and neutrophils engraft first followed by the platelets about a week later. The most common complications associated with autologous HSCT are febrile neutropenia, serum electrolyte abnormalities, infection, bleeding, gastrointestinal toxicities (mucositis, nausea, vomiting, and diarrhea), and less commonly, other organ toxicities that are related to the specific chemotherapy administered. Palifermin is approved for use to decrease the incidence and duration of severe oral mucositis in patients with hematologic malignancies undergoing HSCT. The following table lists commonly used chemotherapy agents with their dose-limiting toxicities in SCT.

Chemotherapy	Standard Dose[1]	Maximum SCT Dose as Single Agent[2]	Maximum SCT Dose in Combination[2]	Dose-Limiting Toxicity
Busulfan (oral)	4 mg/d	16 mg/kg	16 mg/kg	GI, liver (SOS), CNS (seizure), pulmonary
Busulfan (IV)		12 mg/kg	12 mg/kg	GI, liver (SOS), CNS (seizure), pulmonary
CARBOplatin	400 mg/m²	2,000 mg/m²	1,800 mg/m²	Liver, renal
Carmustine	200 mg/m²	800 mg/m²	600 mg/m²	Liver, pulmonary
CISplatin	50 to 100 mg/m²	180 to 200 mg/m²	165 to 200 (in BEP) mg/m²	Renal, neuropathy
Cyclophosphamide	600 to 1,875 mg/m²	200 mg/kg or 7.5 g/m²	200 mg/kg or 7.5 g/m²	Cardiac, hemorrhagic cystitis, liver (SOS)
Etoposide	100 mg/m²/dose x 1 to 5 days	2,400 mg/m²	2,400 mg/m²	GI, hypotension
Melphalan	40 mg/m²	220 mg/m²	140 to 180 mg/m²	GI
MitoXANtrone	12 mg/m²/d x 3	90 mg/m²	60 to 80 mg/m²	GI, cardiac

[1]Usual dose for therapy that does not include HSCT

[2]Maximum dose is divided for administration over 2 or more days

ALLOGENEIC MYELOABLATIVE TRANSPLANTATION

The principle behind allogeneic myeloablative hematopoietic stem cell transplantation is that hematological disease can be cured by complete marrow ablation with profound immunosuppression so that the donor cells can engraft and successfully replace the patient's diseased hematopoietic system. Post-transplant immunosuppressive therapy is essential for successful engraftment of donor cells and prevention of GVHD. Preparative regimens for allogeneic transplantation are based on the need for both marrow ablation and immunosuppression. Commonly used regimens are listed below.

Acronym	Chemotherapy Drugs (Total Dose)	Dosages and Scheduling
BuCy	Busulfan (12 to 16 mg/kg); dose determined using patient-specific pharmacokinetics	0.875 to 1 mg/kg/dose PO q6h x 16 doses; or 1 mg/kg/dose PO q6h x 12 doses; or 0.8 mg/kg IV q6h x 16 doses
	Cyclophosphamide (120 mg/kg)	60 mg/kg/dose IV q24h x 2 doses
FTBI/Cy or CyTBI	Fractionated total body irradiation	1,200 to 1,500 cGy divided bid over 3 to 5 days
	Cyclophosphamide (120 to 200 mg/kg)	50 mg/kg/dose IV q24h x 4 doses or 60 mg/kg/dose IV q24h x 2 doses
TBI-VP16-Cy	Fractionated total body irradiation	1,200 to 1,400 cGy divided bid over 3 to 5 days
	Etoposide (30 mg/kg)	30 mg/kg/dose IV x 1 dose
	Cyclophosphamide (120 mg/kg)	60 mg/kg/dose IV q24h x 2 doses
Bu/Mel	Busulfan (16 mg/kg); dose determined using patient-specific pharmacokinetics	1 mg/kg/dose PO q6h x 16 doses
	Melphalan (135 to 140 mg/m^2)	45 mg/m^2/dose IV q24h x 3, or 140 mg/m^2 once
FTBI/Mel	Fractionated total body irradiation	1,200 to 1,500 cGy divided bid over 3 to 5 days
	Melphalan (135 to 140 mg/m^2)	45 mg/m^2/dose IV q24h x 2, 70 mg/m^2/dose IV q24h x 2, or 140 mg/m^2 once
CyATG	Cyclophosphamide (200 mg/kg)	50 mg/kg/dose IV q24h x 4
	Lymphocyte immune globulin (90 to 160 mg/kg)	30 to 40 mg/kg/dose IV q24 to 48h x 3 to 4 doses

The systemic exposure to busulfan correlates with safety and efficacy of therapy. Busulfan area under the plasma concentration versus time curve (AUC) exceeding 1,500 micromole/minutes per dose (24,000 micromole/minutes per total course of therapy) is associated with an increased risk of regimen-related toxicity, including sinusoidal obstruction syndrome (SOS) and seizures. Busulfan AUC lower than 900 micromole/minutes per dose (14,400 micromole/minutes per total course of therapy) correlates with graft failure and disease recurrence (Ciurea 2009). Use of patient-specific pharmacokinetics to determine the optimal dose of oral busulfan is warranted due to the extreme interpatient variability of oral absorption and pharmacokinetic parameters. Pharmacokinetics can also be used to optimize the delivery of intravenous busulfan therapy (Ciurea 2009).

Lymphocyte immune globulin or antithymocyte globulin is included in the preparative regimen for patients with severe aplastic anemia. Lymphocyte immune globulin or antithymocyte globulin is often added to the preparative regimen for allogeneic transplants when the donor and recipient are immunologically mismatched or unrelated, and for umbilical cord blood transplants. This added immunosuppression improves engraftment and may decrease acute GVHD.

Hematopoietic growth factors (filgrastim or sargramostim) are usually administered after infusion of allogeneic donor blood cells. The doses range from 5 to 10 mcg/kg/day and administration is begun either on day 0 or +1 or may be delayed up to 6 days post-cell infusion. The colony stimulating factors are discontinued when the absolute neutrophil count reaches a designated target, which is often in the range of 5,000 to 10,000/mm^3.

Allogeneic HSCT recipients are at risk for all of the common complications associated with administration of high-dose chemotherapy, including febrile neutropenia, serum electrolyte abnormalities, infection, bleeding, gastrointestinal toxicities (mucositis, nausea, vomiting, and diarrhea), and less commonly, other organ toxicities that are related to the specific chemotherapy administered. The risk of posttransplant complications is greater in allogeneic transplant recipients due to the chronic immunosuppression required to prevent GVHD.

NONMYELOABLATIVE TRANSPLANTS

Nonmyeloablative or RIC HSCT is achieved by administration of immunosuppressive conditioning regimens that are less directly cytotoxic to bone marrow and nonhematopoietic tissue(s). Nonmyeloablative transplantation utilizes the graft-versus-leukemia effect as part of the overall treatment. The safety impetus for use of RIC is to allow allogeneic HSCT in patients unable to tolerate the myeloablative preparative regimens, such as elderly patients, or patients with an extensive history of chemotherapy treatment, impaired major organ function, or comorbid conditions. Clinical trials and case series describe use of nonmyeloablative hematopoietic stem cell transplantation for the following diseases: Congenital immunodeficiency syndromes, acute myelogenous leukemia, myelodysplastic syndrome, acute lymphocytic leukemia, multiple myeloma, non-Hodgkin's lymphoma, Hodgkin's disease, sickle cell disease, renal cell carcinoma, and various advanced solid tumors. Most of the published studies and case series report use of this procedure in patients with relapsed or refractory disease, elderly patients, or those unable to tolerate myeloablative preparative regimens.

The premise supporting nonmyeloablative transplantation is that nonmyeloablative, but sufficiently immunosuppressive conditioning regimens, yield a state of mixed chimerism in the recipient, which gradually converts to full donor chimerism. The chimeric engraftment supports a graft-versus-malignancy effect. Complete donor engraftment, also known as 100% donor chimerism, occurs when all of the detectable hematopoietic cells are of donor origin. Complete donor chimerism occurring within 30 to 90 days following transplantation is generally associated with disease response. Because antitumor effects of nonmyeloablative allogeneic transplants appear somewhat late (2 to 3 months after the procedure), patients with active or poorly controlled malignancies do not appear to be optimal candidates for this type of transplantation.

Examples of reduced-intensity preparative regimens are listed in the following table.

Acronym	Chemotherapy Drugs (Total Dose)	Dosages and Scheduling
Flu/ATG	Lymphocyte immune globulin 40 mg/kg (Atgam)	10 mg/kg/day IV on 4 consecutive days
	Antithymoglobulin 10 mg/kg (Thymoglobulin)	2.5 mg/kg/day IV on 4 consecutive days
	Fludarabine 125 mg/m^2	25 mg/m^2/day IV on 5 consecutive days
FC-ATG	Fludarabine 125 mg/m^2	25 mg/m^2/day IV on days -6 to -2
	Cyclophosphamide 120 mg/kg	60 mg/kg/day IV on days -3 and -2
	Lymphocyte immune globulin 60 mg/kg (Atgam)	20 mg/kg/day IV on 3 consecutive days
TBI/Flu	Total body irradiation 4 Gy	2 Gy/day on days -8 and -7
	Fludarabine 125 mg/m^2	25 mg/m^2/day IV on days -6 to -2
Flu/Mel/ATG	Fludarabine 125 mg/m^2	25 mg/m^2/day IV on days -6 to -2
	Melphalan 140 to 180 mg/m^2	70 to 90 mg/m^2/day IV on days -3 and -2
	Lymphocyte immune globulin 120 mg/kg (Atgam)	30 mg/kg/day IV on days -4 to -1
Bu/Flu/ATG	Busulfan 8 mg/kg	1 mg/kg/dose PO q6h X8 doses on days -6 and -5
	Fludarabine 125 mg/m^2	25 mg/m^2/day IV on days -6 to -2
	Antithymocyte globulin (Fresnius) 10 mg/kg	2.5 mg/kg/day IV on 4 consecutive days
Cy/Flu/TBI	Cyclophosphamide 50 mg/kg	50 mg/kg IV on day -6
	Fludarabine 200 mg/m^2	40 mg/m^2/day IV on days -6 to -2
	TBI 200 cGy	TBI 200 cGy on day -1

Most complications following nonmyeloablative hematopoietic stem cell transplantation are related to GVHD and the immunosuppression required for treatment of GVHD. Infectious complications from cytomegalovirus, herpes virus, candidiasis, aspergillosis, and other opportunistic microbes are common. Treatment of moderate to severe GVHD is similar to the approach taken for that of GVHD following myeloablative allogeneic hematopoietic stem cell transplantation (see Posttransplant Complications).

Less regimen-related toxicity occurs with RIC, so it is considered as an alternative therapeutic modality for patients unable to tolerate the adverse effects inherent to myeloablative therapy. However, patients undergoing nonmyeloablative transplantation must have adequate organ function and physiologic reserve for chronic administration of immunosuppressive therapy and management of opportunistic infections that may arise.

DONOR LYMPHOCYTE INFUSION

Donor lymphocyte infusion (DLI) is a technique that involves transfusion of lymphocytes from the original HSCT donor in order to treat relapsed or refractory hematologic cancers following allogeneic HSCT. The donor lymphocytes are contained within a white blood cell product obtained by apheresis (leukapheresis) from the donor. The anticancer effect of DLI is secondary to a graft-versus-tumor effect triggered when the donor lymphocytes recognize antigens on the malignant cells as nonself. A surrogate marker for graft-versus-leukemia is clinical evidence of GVHD. The efficacy of DLI is related to the type of cancer being treated, the dose of infused lymphocytes, and the demonstration of a graft-versus-host response. Durable responses to DLI are reported with chronic myeloid leukemia; lesser responses are reported with lymphomas, multiple myeloma, and acute myeloid leukemia.

POSTTRANSPLANT COMPLICATIONS

Graft-Versus-Host Disease

GVHD is an immune-mediated reaction initiated by donor T-cell recognition of recipient tissues as nonself. GVHD which occurs before 100 days post-transplant is classified as acute GVHD, and after 100 days, it is classified as chronic GVHD. Acute GVHD primarily affects the skin, gastrointestinal tract, and liver. It is graded based on extent of organ involvement from grade I (mild) to grade IV (life-threatening). Chronic GVHD affects the skin, gastrointestinal tract, liver, and other organs and tissues, including the lungs, lacrimal glands, and connective tissue. Chronic GVHD is generally graded as limited or extensive disease. Mortality ranges from 10% to 30%. There is a strong positive correlation between development of acute or chronic GVHD and decreased risk of malignancy recurrence due to associated graft vs malignancy effect.

Given the high morbidity and mortality associated with severe GVHD, post-transplant care is directed to prevent this complication. A combination of 2 to 3 immunosuppressants is used to prevent GVHD. The selection of prophylactic immunosuppressants used is based on the degree of risk for GVHD and the risk of malignant relapse. In general, as the depth and duration of immunosuppression increase, so does the risk of malignant relapse, and infectious disease. Commonly used prophylactic immunosuppressants include cyclosporine or tacrolimus plus methotrexate, with addition of a methylprednisolone for patients at high risk for GVHD.

GVHD Prophylactic Agents	Usual Dose and Schedule
CycloSPORINE	2.5 to 4 mg/kg/day IV continuous infusion or divided q12h over 2 to 6 hours. Adjust dose according to toxicity and blood concentrations. Convert to oral dose when appropriate.
Tacrolimus	0.02 to 0.03 mg/kg/day IV continuous infusion. Adjust dose according to toxicity and blood concentrations. Transition (using appropriate conversion) to oral dose when appropriate.
Methotrexate	15 mg/m^2/dose on day +1, 10 mg/m^2/dose on days +3, +6, and +11; give IV push.
MethylPREDNISolone	Variable; 0.5 to 1 mg/kg/day divided q6 to 12h then taper. May start day +1 up to +7; increase dose for acute GVHD reactions.
Mycophenolate mofetil	1 g/dose IV or PO q12h; or 15 mg/kg/dose IV or PO q12h
Sirolimus	12 mg PO on day -3, then 4 mg PO daily

Initial treatment of GVHD includes addition of a corticosteroid or a dosage increase of ongoing corticosteroid treatment. Other agents used for the treatment of steroid-refractory acute GVHD include lymphocyte immune globulin or antithymocyte globulin, interleukin-2 receptor antagonists (basiliximab), tumor necrosis factor antagonists (etanercept, infliximab), sirolimus, and pentostatin. Thalidomide, pentostatin, PUVA (8-methoxypsoralen plus UV-A radiation), and rituximab also have been utilized in the setting of steroid-refractory GVHD.

Infection

Allogeneic stem cell transplantation is associated with a wide range of infectious complications that occur during identifiable time periods after the transplant. The early period of neutropenia is most commonly associated with bacterial infections, fungal infections (*Candida* species), and herpes simplex virus (HSV) reactivation. *Pneumocystis jirovecii pneumoniae* (PCP) risk increases with duration of immunosuppressive therapy. Other life-threatening opportunistic infections typically occurring 2 to 3 months post-transplant include aspergillosis and CMV (disseminated or pneumonitis). Other serious atypical viral and fungal infections can also be seen at this later time. Infections with rhinovirus and coronavirus are common during the first 100 days following allogeneic HSCT and tend to present as symptoms of rhinorrhea, congestion, postnasal drip, sputum production, and cough. Lower respiratory tract infections attributed to rhinovirus or coronavirus occur in ~2% of infected patients.

Prophylaxis for certain infections is routine while others are treated when they are diagnosed. Trimethoprim-sulfamethoxazole or a fluoroquinolone is given during the preparative regimen for selective gut decontamination. Trimethoprim-sulfamethoxazole is also administered after hematopoietic recovery on a 2 to 3 times weekly schedule as PCP prophylaxis. The major concern with trimethoprim-sulfamethoxazole is the myelosuppressive effect. Alternative antimicrobials for patients allergic to sulfonamide antimicrobials include inhaled pentamidine or oral dapsone. Fungal prophylaxis is routinely given as well. This generally consists of fluconazole, voriconazole, or an amphotericin B product. Inhalational amphotericin B can also be used to decrease risk of pulmonary aspergillosis. Acyclovir is routinely used to prevent HSV reinfection. The role of acyclovir for prevention of CMV infection is controversial. Some centers routinely prescribe acyclovir immediately following the transplant for prevention of CMV or HSV infection. After cellular recovery, the patient may be switched to ganciclovir or valganciclovir therapy. The hematologic toxicity of ganciclovir and valganciclovir precludes its routine use at an earlier point in the transplant; however, CMV therapy is started preemptively before engraftment with the finding of CMV DNA by polymerase chain reaction in the peripheral white blood cells. The role of antibacterial prophylaxis or continued gut decontamination varies with transplant centers but is often used in some form. Prophylactic antimicrobials are generally administered throughout the duration of exogenous immunosuppression following allogeneic hematopoietic stem cell transplantation. The American Society of Clinical Oncology (ASCO) provisional clinical opinion update on hepatitis B virus (HBV) screening recommends screening patients for HBV prior to HSCT or initiation of anti-CD20 antibody therapy to identify patients with chronic or clinically resolved HBV infection. Serologic tests to detect HBV virus include hepatitis B surface antigen (HBsAg) and hepatitis B core antibody (anti-HBc) measurements; either a total anti-HBc (with both IgG and IgM) or anti-HBc IgG test should be used to screen for chronic or unresolved HBV infection (do not use anti-HBc IgM as it may only confirm acute HBV infection). In addition, clinical and laboratory signs of hepatitis or HBV should be monitored until patients are considered immunocompetent following HSCT. The ASCO provisional clinical opinion recommends initiation of prophylactic antiviral treatment for patients with chronic HBV infection (HBsAg-positive/anti-HBc-positive) without delaying anticancer therapy. Selection of antiviral therapy should be based on products with low rates of viral resistance.

Antiviral therapy should be continued for 6 to 12 months following completion of cancer therapy. Providers should monitor patients with a clinically resolved HBV infection (HBsAg-negative/anti-HBc-positive) by serial analysis of serum alanine aminotransferase or HBV DNA approximately every 3 months with prompt initiation of antiviral therapy as warranted by laboratory findings. In addition, patients with risk factors for HBV infection (eg, residence in a geographic location with ≥2% HBV prevalence, household or sexual contact with HBV-infected patients, high-risk behaviors [eg, intravenous drug use], HIV infection) should also be screened and monitored for HBV infection or reactivation prior to beginning immunosuppressive therapy.

Sinusoidal Obstruction Syndrome

Hepatic sinusoidal obstruction syndrome (SOS), formerly known as hepatic veno-occlusive disease (VOD), can occur as a result of the pretransplant conditioning regimen. Risk factors for hepatic SOS include preexisting liver disease, malignant involvement of the liver, serum ferritin level exceeding 1,000 ng/mL, malnutrition, prior extensive chemotherapy treatment, and previous treatment with busulfan, imatinib, or gemtuzumab ozogamicin. SOS, which usually presents within the first 3 weeks after transplant, results from obstruction of blood flow in the small hepatic veins. Signs and symptoms include right upper quadrant pain or tenderness, hepatomegaly, weight gain, ascites, hyperbilirubinemia, and thrombocytopenia. Treatment options include supportive care and the investigational agent defibrotide, which has antithrombotic, thrombolytic, and anti-ischemic properties. Low-dose heparin, ursodiol, and defibrotide have also been used for SOS prophylaxis.

FUTURE DIRECTIONS

Improved methods for prevention of GVHD following allogeneic HSCT will benefit posttransplant quality of life and promote prolonged survival. Preliminary clinical trials demonstrate efficacy for prevention of severe acute and chronic GVHD with postranplant administration of high-dose cyclophosphamide as the only GVHD prophylaxis or with a short course of sirolimus following HLA-matched allogeneic HSCT with a myeloablative conditioning regimen (Kanakry 2014; Solomon 2014). Clinical trials are evaluating the immunomodulatory and anti-inflammatory effects of atorvastatin as a modulator of GVHD (Choi 2014). The proteasome inhibitor bortezomib demonstrated clinical efficacy for reduction of GVHD; however, the outcome may not be improved with this agent due to toxicity (Choi 2014). Histone deacetylase inhibitors, such as vorinostat, are being tested for immunoregulatory and anti-inflammatory effects that may reduce the severity of GVHD (Choi 2014).

REFERENCES

Anasetti C, Logan BR, Lee SJ, et al. Peripheral-blood stem cells versus bone marrow from unrelated donors. N Engl J Med. 2012;367(16):1487-1496.

Bacigalupo A. Second EBMT workshop on reduced intensity allogeneic hemopoietic stem cell transplants (RI-HSCT). Bone Marrow Transplant. 2002;29:191-195.

Ballen KK, Gluckman E, Broxmeyer HE. Umbilical cord blood transplantation: the first 25 years and beyond. Blood. 2013;122(4):491-498.

Carreras E. How I manage sinusoidal obstruction syndrome after haematopoietic cell transplantation. Br J Haematol. 2015;168(4):481-491.

Chang YJ, Huang XJ. Donor lymphocyte infusions for relapse after allogeneic transplantation: when, if and for whom? Blood Rev. 2013;27(1):55-62.

Choi SW, Reddy P. Current and emerging strategies for the prevention of graft-versus-host disease. Nat Rev Clin Oncol. 2014;11(9):536-547.

Ciurea SO, Andersson BS. Busulfan in hematopoietic stem cell transplantation. Biol Blood Marrow Transplant. 2009;15(5):523-536.

Copelan EA. Hematopoietic stem-cell transplantation. N Engl J Med. 2006;354(17):1813-1826.

Cutler C, Logan B, Nakamura R, et al. Tacrolimus/sirolimus vs tacrolimus/methotrexate as GVHD prophylaxis after matched, related donor allogeneic HCT. *Blood.* 2014;124(8):1372-1377.

Deol A, Lum LG. Role of donor lymphocyte infusions in relapsed hematological malignancies after stem cell transplantation revisited. *Cancer Treat Rev.* 2010;36(7):528-538.

Ho VT, Soiffer RJ. The history and future of t-cell depletion as graft-versus-host disease prophylaxis for allogeneic hematopoietic stem cell transplantation. *Blood.* 2001;98:3192-3204.

Hwang JP, Somerfield MR, Alston-Johnson DE, et al. Hepatitis B virus screening for patients with cancer before therapy: American Society of Clinical Oncology provisional clinical opinion update. *J Clin Oncol.* 2015;33(19):2212-2220.

Kanakry CG, Tsai HL, Bolaños-Meade J, et al. Single-agent GVHD prophylaxis with posttransplantation cyclophosphamide after myeloablative, HLA-matched BMT for AML, ALL, and MDS. *Blood.* 2014;124(25):3817-3827.

Klingebiel T, Schlegel PG. GVHD: overview on pathophysiology, incidence, clinical and biological features. *Bone Marrow Transplant.* 1998;21(Suppl 2):S45-S49.

Maradei SC, Maiolino A, de Azevedo AM, Colares M, Bouzas LF, Nucci M. Serum ferritin as risk factor for sinusoidal obstruction syndrome of the liver in patients undergoing hematopoietic stem cell transplantation. *Blood.* 2009;114(6):1270-1275.

Martin PJ, Rizzo JD, Wingard JR, et al. First- and second-line systemic treatment of acute graft-versus-host disease: recommendations of the American Society of Blood and Marrow Transplantation. *Biol Blood Marrow Transplant.* 2012;18(8):1150-1163.

McClune BL, Weisdorf DJ, Pedersen TL, et al. Effect of age on outcome of reduced-intensity hematopoietic cell transplantation for older patients with acute myeloid leukemia in first complete remission or with myelodysplastic syndrome. *J Clin Oncol.* 2010;28(11):1878-1887.

Milano F, Campbell AP, Guthrie KA, et al. Human rhinovirus and coronavirus detection among allogeneic hematopoietic stem cell transplantation recipients. *Blood.* 2010;115(10):2088-2094.

Mogul MJ. Unrelated cord blood transplantation vs matched unrelated donor bone marrow transplantation: the risks and benefits of each choice. *Bone Marrow Transplant.* 2000;25(Suppl 2):S58-S60.

Ringdén O, Labopin M, Ehninger G, et al. Reduced intensity conditioning compared with myeloablative conditioning using unrelated donor transplants in patients with acute myeloid leukemia. *J Clin Oncol.* 2009;27(27):4570-4577.

Rowe JM, Ciobanu N, Ascensao J, et al. Recommended guidelines for the management of autologous and allogeneic bone marrow transplantation. A report from the Eastern Cooperative Oncology Group (ECOG). *Ann Intern Med.* 1994;120:143-158.

Ruutu T, Gratwohl A, de Witte T, et al. Prophylaxis and treatment of GVHD: EBMT-ELN working group recommendations for a standardized practice. *Bone Marrow Transplant.* 2014;49 (2):168-173.

Solomon SR, Sanacore M, Zhang X, et al. Calcineurin inhibitor – free graft-versus-host disease prophylaxis with post-transplantation cyclophosphamide and brief-course sirolimus following reduced-intensity peripheral blood stem cell transplantation. *Biol Blood Marrow Transplant.* 2014;20(11):1828-1834.

Storb R, Gyurkocza B, Storer BE, et al. Allogeneic hematopoietic cell transplantation following minimal intensity conditioning: predicting acute graft-versus-host disease and graft-versus-tumor effects. *Biol Blood Marrow Transplant.* 2013;19(5):792-798.

Vogelsang GB, Arai S. Mycophenolate mofetil for the prevention and treatment of graft-versus-host disease following stem cell transplantation: preliminary findings. *Bone Marrow Transplant.* 2001;27:1255-1262.

Wagner JE Jr, Eapen M, Carter S, et al. One-unit versus two-unit cord-blood transplantation for hematologic cancers. *N Engl J Med.* 2014;371(18):1685-1694.

DRUG DEVELOPMENT PROCESS

Drug development describes the process required to bring a drug from its original identity to becoming a commercially available product for use in human beings. The drug development process involves scientific, clinical, and regulatory activities. Bringing a new molecular entity or new active substance through the drug development process takes years of time and hundreds of millions to billions of dollars.

SCIENTIFIC CONTRIBUTION

The major scientific contribution is drug discovery and drug design. Candidates for drug development arise from biotechnologic or chemical synthesis and natural product extraction. Selection of drug candidates is often based on their ability in vitro to bind a molecular target or exert a biologic effect. This is an inefficient low-yield process despite the use of automated high throughput screening methods that can test thousands of drug candidates daily. A challenge of drug discovery is the myriad of factors that can abrogate the utility or efficacy of drug candidates as they proceed through preclinical and clinical testing.

Preclinical testing is done in several species of animals to evaluate toxicity, pharmacodynamics, and pharmacokinetics. Acute toxicity, chronic toxicity, feto-toxicity, teratogenicity, and carcinogenicity are tested in animals to identify common sites of toxicity and potentially use-limiting harm, such as neurologic adverse effects or carcinogenicity. Drug pharmacodynamics and pharmacokinetics are evaluated in animals to extrapolate a first in human (FIH) dose when the drug advances to clinical trials.

Additional scientific contributions to drug development include chemical characterization and pharmaceutical development of drug candidates.

REGULATORY PROCESS

In the United States, clinical trials administering drugs to human beings are regulated by the Food and Drug Administration (FDA). Regulation is directed and implemented through an application process required for various levels of clinical drug development. The Investigational New Drug (IND) application is required prior to testing a drug in human subjects or distributing it across state lines. The IND (Form 1571) contains preclinical data, proposed clinical protocol, investigator's brochure (if available), and manufacturing information. An Exploratory IND allows administration of subtherapeutic doses to a small number of subjects to assess whether the preclinically tested drug-target interaction occurs in humans. An Emergency IND allows distribution of an investigational drug on a patient-specific basis for management of a serious condition. Investigational drugs must have demonstrated a certain degree of efficacy and safety for an Emergency IND application to be granted. The New Drug Application (NDA) is reviewed by the FDA to determine whether drug testing is sufficient for product approval and consumer use. The NDA is a comprehensive document containing data supporting all of the chemical, pharmacologic, pharmaceutical, preclinical, therapeutic, safety, and pharmacokinetic information and claims required for product approval. Approval of generic equivalents can be achieved with an Abbreviated New Drug Application (ANDA). Generic drugs are reviewed using the ANDA because the efficacy and safety of these products was previously established by the original brand (innovator drug). Approval of a generic drug is based on scientific data demonstrating that the generic product is bioequivalent to the innovator product. Biologic products, such as monoclonal antibodies and vaccines, are approved for commercial use using a Biologic License Application (BLA). Biological products that are "biosimilar" to or "interchangeable" with an FDA-licensed biological product can be approved under an abbreviated licensure pathway. The biosimilar must meet rigorous standards for safety and efficacy and the manufacturer must demonstrate that the new product is "highly similar" to the reference product. The reference product is an already approved biologic product that was licensed for commercial use by way of a BLA.

The conduct of clinical trials is approved, monitored, and reviewed by an institutional review board (IRB), also known as human subjects committee, independent ethics committee, ethical review board, etc. The IRB is responsible for overseeing the conduct of biomedical and behavioral research involving human subjects. The IRB ensures that biomedical and behavioral research is ethical, informed consent is sufficient, and appropriate safeguards are established. The FDA Department of Health and Human Services Office for Human Research Protection empowers IRBs to approve, require modifications, or disapprove research conducted under their domain. Most IRBs are based at academic institutions or health care systems. However, independent commercial for profit IRBs exist that adhere to the same federal regulations as local committees. Research misconduct identified by IRB oversight or an FDA inspection can result in regulatory action, such as a warning letter, an injection prohibiting a researcher or institution from conducting research, or even criminal charges. One caveat to regulatory oversight of clinical trials is that research misconduct addressed by the FDA is rarely mentioned in publications reporting the results of these trials (Seife 2015).

CLINICAL TRIALS

Clinical trials include Phase 0, Phase I, Phase II, and Phase III analysis of a drug in humans. Phase 0 studies evaluate clinical drug-target interaction(s). Phase I testing is done to assess drug safety and pharmacokinetics. Phase 0 and Phase I clinical trials are FIH drug studies that are unlikely to provide any therapeutic benefit to the participating subjects. Phase II clinical trials test the efficacy of a drug in the management of a specific disease or pathophysiologic process. The purpose of Phase III clinical trials is to compare the investigational treatment to the standard of care. Phase IV testing (postmarketing surveillance) generally involves pharmacovigilance or additional pharmacokinetic or drug interaction characterization in FDA-approved medications. Phase IV testing is often done independently by academic investigators or it may be a requirement imposed by the FDA.

Oncology Agents

Phase 0 clinical trials are an attempt to reduce the consumption of valuable time and resources that occur when promising preclinical candidates fail in Phase II clinical trials. Specifically, small doses of drug are administered to 15 or fewer subjects for a short period of time to evaluate whether the therapeutic drug-target interaction occurs in human beings. Drugs tested in Phase 0 clinical trials must have a wide margin of safety and a validated method for testing drug-target interaction(s).

Phase I clinical trials for anticancer treatments are used to identify safety. For cytotoxic products, phase I studies determine the maximum tolerated dose (MTD). The FIH dose of cytotoxic chemotherapy is generally a small fraction (1/10th) of the preclinical dose that produced lethality in 10% of the most sensitive animal model. The dose is increased in a stepwise fashion until the dose-limiting toxicity (DLT) is reached in >33% of a patient cohort. The dose at which <33% of patients have DLT is utilized in Phase II studies. Dose calculation based on body surface area or weight is used as a tool to extrapolate clinical doses from those administered to animals in preclinical testing. Unlike Phase I clinical trials for nononcology medications conducted in healthy human subjects, only patients with advanced cancer refractory to treatment and with normal organ function, are utilized for Phase I oncology studies. The MTD is rarely determined for biologic and targeted anticancer treatments, such as monoclonal antibodies and tyrosine kinase inhibitors. For these products, the dose designated for Phase II testing is generally based on receptor saturation or another surrogate marker of efficacy instead of MTD. Phase I methodology should be used when anticancer treatments with an established dose for single agent therapy or administered as combination therapy.

Phase II trials evaluate drug safety and efficacy in a group of patients with a disease the drug is intended to treat. Data is collected on adverse effects and response to the therapy. Phase II clinical trials may report efficacy based on tumor response (tumor shrinkage), which is a much less stringent measure of efficacy than survival. An increasing proportion of phase II studies in oncology are precision cancer medicine trials (Roper 2015). Precision cancer medicine trials prospectively test the efficacy of targeted therapy in patients with tumors demonstrating the targetable genetic trait. Generally, these studies are conducted in a multicenter, open-label manner and enroll patients with breast cancer, colorectal cancer, and skin cancer.

Phase III studies involve a larger number of patients with a particular tumor. Patients are randomized to the new treatment or the current standard of care. A placebo arm is used for Phase III analysis of novel treatments for which there is no comparable standard of care; use of placebo can be controversial when studying treatments for life-threatening diseases. Primary endpoints for Phase III clinical trials evaluating anticancer treatments generally include disease response, duration of disease-free survival, duration of overall survival, and safety. As was the case with gemcitabine in pancreatic cancer, a clinical benefit response may be an endpoint that is measured.

COST(S)

Investigational new drugs are generally provided free of charge to the patient. However, there are cases when the manufacturer can seek FDA authorization to charge for use of an investigational new drug to recover costs necessary to continue drug development.

SELECTED READINGS

Daugherty CK, Ratain MJ, Emanuel EJ, Farrell AT, Schilsky RL. Ethical, scientific, and regulatory perspectives regarding the use of placebos in cancer clinical trials. *J Clin Oncol.* 2008;26 (8):1371-1378.

The drug development process. Available at http://www.fda.gov/forpatients/approvals/drugs/default.htm. Accessed September 2015.

Egorin MJ. Horseshoes, hand grenades, and body-surface area-based dosing: aiming for a target. *J Clin Oncol.* 2003;21(2):182-183.

Fojo T, Grady C. How much is life worth: cetuximab, non-small cell lung cancer, and the $440 billion question. *J Natl Cancer Inst.* 2009;101(15):1044-1048.

Hamberg P, Verweij J. Phase I drug combination trial design: walking the tightrope. *J Clin Oncol.* 2009;27(27):4441-32009.

Health and Human Services, Office for Human Research Protections (OHRP). Available at http://www.hhs.gov/ohrp

Le Tourneau C, Stathis A, Vidal L, Moore MJ, Siu LL. Choice of starting dose for molecularly targeted agents evaluated in first-in-human phase I cancer clinical trials. *J Clin Oncol*. 2010;28 (8):1401-1407.

Roper N, Stensland KD, Hendricks R, Galsky MD. The landscape of precision cancer medicine clinical trials in the United States. *Cancer Treat Rev*. 2015;41(5):385-390.

Rowan K. Oncology's first phase 0 trial. *J Natl Cancer Inst*. 2009;101(14):978-979.

Seife C. Research misconduct identified by the US Food and Drug Administration: out of sight, out of mind, out of the peer-reviewed literature. *JAMA Intern Med*. 2015;175(4):567-577.

Tosi D, Laghzali Y, Vinches M, et al. Clinical development strategies and outcomes in first-in-human trials of monoclonal antibodies. *J Clin Oncol*. 2015;33(19):2158-2165.

INVESTIGATIONAL DRUG SERVICE

An Investigational Drug Service (IDS) should be used for management of investigational medications administered under the direction of clinical trials. The IDS is an organized pharmacy-based service that controls the procurement, inventory, preparation, and dispensing of investigational drugs. Investigational drugs are administered only to patients who have, in an informed manner, signed a consent form to participate in the particular study using these investigational drugs. A patient formally enrolled to participate in a clinical study is known as a "subject". Investigational drugs used in this manner are frequently new drugs undergoing First in Human, Phase I, Phase II, or Phase III evaluation prior to Food and Drug Administration (FDA) approval for a medical purpose. In addition, investigational drugs can be commercially available drugs used under the direction of a protocol for an off-label indication or as a supportive measure for a new drug. An IDS should be under the direction of an appropriately trained pharmacist with additional professional and supportive staff as warranted by the workload. The IDS should operate under the direction of institutional and departmental policies and procedures delineating appropriate investigational drug management. Computer software programs should be utilized to support investigational drug management.

A study protocol is the document describing the scientific background providing the basis for doing the study, specific study objectives and endpoints, treatments and tests done as part of the study, study drug information, statistical methodology, means for assurance of patient confidentiality, and the subject consent form. Some studies provide an Investigator's Drug Brochure, which presents very detailed and comprehensive study drug information. Each study is assigned a unique identifier (eg, SWOG S0927) that generally includes an abbreviation for the research consortium (Southwest Oncology Group), a truncation of the year of study development (2009), and its position within a series of studies (27). Study protocols and Investigator's Drug Brochures are confidential, and frequently proprietary documents. Prior to study activation at an institution, the planned research must be approved by the institutional investigational review board. All departments needed to provide personnel or resources for study implementation should review the protocol prior to study implementation to ensure that study activities can reasonably be supported with available resources. The IDS pharmacist should scrutinize each study protocol prior to study activation to determine the impact of study implementation on pharmacy department personnel and resources.

IDS pharmacists play an integral role in study protocol development, implementation, and management. Pharmacists should write and/or review protocol sections pertaining to medication use, such as the medication information section, supportive care guidelines, and any medication-related information utilized in the informed consent process (Goldspiel 2014). In addition, pharmacists should participate in scientific review and/or IRB committee meetings. Investigational drug medication counseling, adherence assessment, and adverse reaction and protocol deviation monitoring are also responsibilities that should be performed by a pharmacist.

Meticulous investigational drug inventory management is an IDS activity that is essential for maintaining the integrity of clinical trial results. Investigational drug inventory must be stored at the appropriate conditions and separate from commercial drug inventory. An ongoing drug-specific inventory must be maintained for all investigational drugs housed within a pharmacy. Some studies will require lot number-specific, or subject-specific inventory for study drugs. Minimal inventory documentation should include study identification number, study drug dosage form and lot number, study drug expiration date or date of preparation, transaction date, transaction type (receipt, dispensing, return, waste), and current number of dosage forms available. Although it may be kept separately from individual study drug inventories, the pharmacy must maintain an ongoing refrigerator, freezer, and ambient temperature log for study drug storage facilities. Product shelf life might not be established prior to use of some investigational agents in clinical trials. The IDS should formalize a process for tracking the expiration dating of investigational drugs. All inventory records should be kept in a secure, yet accessible, location by the pharmacy, even after study closure. In addition, study drug should be shipped directly to the Pharmacy Department rather than the Principal Investigator's office. This will ensure that the Pharmacy Department has shipping receipts and shipment invoices to verify receipt of the packaged contents. This will also support the documentation of continuous drug management within the instructed storage and handling conditions.

Only designated study personnel can order investigational treatments for use under the direction of a clinical trial. A list of authorized prescribers for each study should be easily accessible by IDS and pharmacy staff. Protocol-specific medication order templates should be used for prescribing investigational drugs. The IDS should delineate a method for confirming that a patient has formally consented to participate in a research study before beginning preparation of the first dose of an investigational drug and as warranted afterwards.

Pharmacy support of blinded studies can involve additional responsibilities and challenges. Pharmacy-related activities may include randomization (treatment assignment) of subjects when the Principal Investigator and other study personnel are blinded to the study treatment. Randomization for treatment assignment can be done for some studies by simply following a list of treatment assignments sequentially for consecutive subjects. However, randomization for large multi-center studies may require contacting a central randomization center with provision of patient-specific information. When pharmacy activities include randomization, it is important for the IDS to ensure that a workable plan is in place prior to study activation. Moreover, labeling of blinded study drug doses can be challenging since the traditional role of pharmacy labeling is to provide a completely clear description of the dosage form. In contrast, to maintain a study blind, the specific contents of a study dosage form must be omitted from the pharmacy label. The IDS must develop a plan such that study drug doses are labeled in the manner directed by the study, are consistent with institutional policies and procedures, and are in accordance with state and federal regulations.

Study drug preparation should be described in the protocol or Investigator's Drug Brochure. Institutional methods of handling precautions should be adhered to as appropriate for the hazardous potential of each investigational product. Many investigational drugs will not yet have been evaluated for addition to the National Institute for Occupational Safety and Health (NIOSH) list of antineoplastic and other hazardous drugs in health care settings. Subsequently, it is important for the IDS to have a standard process for assessing the hazardous potential of investigational drugs. Unfortunately, extensive admixture stability and compatibility information is not available for many injectable study drugs. Subsequently, these may have to be prepared on a dose-by-dose basis. Departmental inservices to acquaint professional and technical personnel with each new study are helpful tools for increasing staff familiarity with new studies and study drug preparation. Pharmacy department personnel should have 24-hour access to information about study drug preparation. Ideally, this is in the form of an easy-to-read and readily accessible fast facts sheet. Study protocols and Investigator's Drug Brochures should also be available to Pharmacy Department personnel around the clock for questions that arise outside of standard business hours.

Study drug doses prepared for administration within a hospital or clinic should be dispensed directly to the study or institutional nurse for delivery to the patient's bedside for administration or placed directly into the subject's secured medication bin on the nursing unit. Generally, study drug doses should not be intermixed with standard medication doses transported via the routine intrainstitutional delivery system. Although the risk of inadvertent misplacement of a study drug dose may be low, the consequences can have ethical and legal implications. As an example, a study drug dose inadvertently transported to the wrong nursing unit may be mistakenly administered to a patient with a name similar to that of the actual study subject. Consequently, the study drug dose could potentially be administered to a person who did not consent to receive an investigational drug. The IDS should ensure that interdisciplinary staff caring for patients receiving an investigational drug have access to pertinent educational material regarding the study and investigational medication.

The IDS plays a crucial role in episodic or situational audits performed by study sponsors and regulatory bodies to check the integrity of investigational drug management. The IDS also assists local study personnel with formal study closeout to ensure that all investigational drug inventory is returned or destroyed as instructed by the study sponsor and that all investigational drug records are complete.

Investigational drugs are generally supplied free-of-charge by the study sponsor for use according to a predefined protocol. However, there are limited circumstances whereby a study sponsor can charge for use of an investigational drug. In select predetermined situations, the FDA will allow a manufacturer to charge for direct drug costs when it would be otherwise impossible for drug development to proceed. In addition, a drug manufacturer can charge for costs related to expanded access (compassionate use) of investigational products. The IDS determines fair charges for Pharmacy Department personnel time and resources utilized in the support of study activities. As a rule, routine pharmacy charges to the patient's bill cannot be generated for investigational new drugs, or study drugs provided free-of-charge by the study sponsor. The IDS must charge the study funds. This is generally achieved at the institutional level by generating charges to the local Principal Investigator or Clinical Trials Office.

REFERENCES

Additional information about handling investigational drugs is available from the National Cancer Institute Pharmaceutical Management Branch. http://ctep.cancer.gov/branches/pmb/default.htm. Accessed October 9, 2015.

Information from the FDA regarding access to investigational drugs is available at http://www.fda.gov/downloads/AboutFDA/Transparency/Basics/UCM202331.pdf. Accessed October 9, 2015.

HOPA investigational drug service best practice standards. Goldspiel BR, ed. Chicago, IL: Hematology/Oncology Pharmacy Association; 2014. Available at http://www.hoparx.org/uploads/files/2014/HOPA14_IDS_Guidelines_Final.pdf. Accessed October 9, 2015.

SAFE HANDLING OF HAZARDOUS DRUGS

Early concerns regarding the identification and exposure risk of hazardous drugs in health care setting were primarily focused on antineoplastic medications, but now have expanded to numerous other agents (eg, antivirals, hormones, bio-engineered medications). The criteria for a hazardous drug include one or more of the following characteristics:

*   Carcinogenic

*   Teratogenic (or other developmental toxicity)

*   Causing reproductive toxicity

*   Organotoxic at low doses

*   Genotoxic

*   New agents with structural or toxicity profiles similar to existing hazardous agents

Agencies have developed definitions, created lists, and generated guidelines to minimize risk of exposure to products considered hazardous. The Environmental Protection Agency (EPA), National Institute for Occupational Safety and Health (NIOSH), and American Society of Health-System Pharmacists (ASHP) have created definitions of hazardous agents (table 1) which may be useful. Based on their definitions, these agencies developed lists of agents which are identified as hazardous drugs or should be handled as hazardous (table 2).

Table 1. Criteria for Defining Hazardous Agents

EPA	NIOSH	ASHP
Meets one of the following criteria: Ignitability: Create fire (under certain conditions) or are spontaneously combustible and have a flash point <60°C (140°F) Corrosivity: Acids or bases (pH ≤2 or ≥12.5) capable of corroding metal containers Reactivity: Unstable under "normal" conditions; may cause explosions, toxic fumes, gases, or vapors if heated, compressed, or mixed with water Toxicity: Harmful or fatal if ingested or absorbed; may leach from the waste and pollute ground water when disposed of on land **OR**	Carcinogenic Teratogenic or other developmental toxicity Reproductive toxicity Organotoxic at low doses Genotoxic New drugs with structural and toxicity profiles similar to existing hazardous agents	Genotoxic Carcinogenic Teratogenic or impairs fertility Causes serious organ or other toxicity at low doses
Appears on one of the following lists: F: Wastes (nonspecific) from common or industrial manufacturing processes from nonspecific sources K: Specific (source) wastes from specific industries (eg, petroleum or pesticides) P (acutely toxic) or U (toxic): Wastes (unused form) from certain discarded commercial chemical products		

When considering the effects of agents on reproductive and developmental toxicity and carcinogenicity, NIOSH evaluated the dose at which adverse effects occurred. If observed at, near, or below the maximum recommended dose for humans, it was considered relevant; if occurred at doses well above the maximum human dose, then NIOSH did not consider it in the hazardous drug evaluation.

NIOSH updated its list of antineoplastic and hazardous drugs in 2014. Medications with special handling precautions in the product labeling and medications with hazardous characteristics or with structural/toxicity profiles similar to agents on the NIOSH list are also listed in Table 2. In order to account for hazardous nonantineoplastic medications, as well as varying dosage forms, the 2014 update categorized hazardous drugs into three groups to account for the diversity of potential exposures:

- NIOSH Group 1: Antineoplastic drugs (may also pose a reproductive risk)

- NIOSH Group 2: Nonantineoplastic drugs that meet at least one of the NIOSH criteria (may also pose a reproductive risk)

- NIOSH Group 3: Nonantineoplastic drugs with adverse reproductive effects; pose a reproductive risk to men and/or women who are actively attempting conception and to women who are pregnant or breast-feeding

Medications listed in group 3 may not pose as serious a risk to personnel not at risk for reproductive toxicity due to age or infertility, although they should still be handled as hazardous. It is important to note that for medications in groups 1 and 2, in addition to meeting the NIOSH hazardous drug criteria, some may also pose a reproductive risk in susceptible populations. According to the NIOSH document, definitions for hazardous drugs may not accurately reflect toxicity criteria associated with newer or recently developed biologic or targeted agents. While biologic and targeted agents may pose a risk to patients, a risk to health care workers may not be present.

Table 2. Drugs Listed as or Considered Hazardous

	NIOSH List[1]			EPA List[2,3]	Product Labeling[4]	Structure or Toxicity Profile Similar to Existing Hazardous Agents	Radiopharmaceutical	Not on NIOSH List, but Meets NIOSH Criteria[5]
	Group 1	Group 2	Group 3					
Abacavir		X						
Abiraterone	X							
Acitretin			X					
Ado-Trastuzumab Emtansine					X			X
Afatinib	X					X		
Alefacept		X						
Alitretinoin			X		X			
Altretamine	X				X			
Ambrisentan					X			
Amsacrine	X							
Anastrozole	X							
Apomorphine		X						
Arsenic Trioxide	X			P-listed	X	X		X
Axitinib	X				X			
AzaCITIDine		X			X			
AzaTHIOprine					X			
BCG Vaccine	X				X	X		
Belinostat					X			
Bendamustine	X							
Bexarotene	X							X
Bicalutamide	X							
Bleomycin	X				X			
Bortezomib	X				X			

Table 2. Drugs Listed as or Considered Hazardous *continued*

	NIOSH List[1]			EPA List[2,3]	Product Labeling[4]	Structure or Toxicity Profile Similar to Existing Hazardous Agents	Radio-pharmaceutical	Not on NIOSH List, but Meets NIOSH Criteria[5]
	Group 1	Group 2	Group 3					
Bosentan			X					
Bosutinib					X	X		X
Brentuximab Vedotin	X				X			
Buserelin						X		X
Busulfan	X				X			
Cabazitaxel	X				X			
Cabergoline			X		X			
Cabozantinib						X		X
Capecitabine	X				X			
CarBAMazepine		X						
Carbon 14 Urea							X	
CARBOplatin	X				X			
Carfilzomib					X	X		X
Carmustine	X				X			
Ceritinib						X		X
Cetrorelix			X					
Chlorambucil	X			U-listed	X			
Chloramphenicol		X						
Choline C 11							X	
Choriogonadotropin Alfa			X		X			
Chromic Phosphate P 32					X		X	
Cidofovir		X			X			
CISplatin	X				X			

Table 2. Drugs Listed as or Considered Hazardous *continued*

	NIOSH List[1]			EPA List[2,3]	Product Labeling[4]	Structure or Toxicity Profile Similar to Existing Hazardous Agents	Radio-pharmaceutical	Not on NIOSH List, but Meets NIOSH Criteria[5]
	Group 1	Group 2	Group 3					
Cladribine	X				X			
Clofarabine	X				X			
ClomiPHENE						X		X
ClonazePAM			X					
Cobimetinib						X		X
Colchicine			X					
Crizotinib	X							
Cyclophosphamide	X			U-listed	X			
CycloSPORINE		X				X		X
Cyproterone						X		
Cytarabine	X				X			
Cytarabine (Liposomal)	X				X			
Dabrafenib						X		X
Dacarbazine	X				X			
DACTINomycin	X				X			
Dasatinib	X				X			
DAUNOrubicin	X			U-listed	X			
DAUNOrubicin (Liposomal)	X			U-listed	X			
Decitabine	X				X			
Deferiprone		X						
Degarelix	X				X			
Desogestrel		X						
Dexrazoxane		X						

Table 2. Drugs Listed as or Considered Hazardous *continued*

	NIOSH List[1]			EPA List[2,3]	Product Labeling[4]	Structure or Toxicity Profile Similar to Existing Hazardous Agents	Radio-pharmaceutical	Not on NIOSH List, but Meets NIOSH Criteria[5]
	Group 1	Group 2	Group 3					
Dichlorodifluoromethane				U-listed				
Diethylstilbestrol		X		U-listed				
Dinoprostone			X					
Divalproex		X						
DOCEtaxel	X				X			
DOXOrubicin	X				X			
DOXOrubicin (Liposomal)	X				X			
Dronedarone			X		X			
Dutasteride			X		X			
Dydrogesterone		X						
Efavirenz						X		X
Entecavir		X						
Enzalutamide						X		X
EPINEPHrine (does not include epinephrine salts)				P-listed				
EPIrubicin	X				X			
Ergonovine/Methylergonovine			X					
Eribulin	X							
Erlotinib	X							
Eslicarbazepine						X		X
Estradiol		X						
Estramustine	X			X				

2297

Table 2. Drugs Listed as or Considered Hazardous *continued*

	NIOSH List[1]			EPA List[2,3]	Product Labeling[4]	Structure or Toxicity Profile Similar to Existing Hazardous Agents	Radio-pharmaceutical	Not on NIOSH List, but Meets NIOSH Criteria[5]
	Group 1	Group 2	Group 3					
Estrogen-Progestin Combinations		X						
Estrogens (Conjugated)		X						
Estrogens (Esterified)		X						
Estropipate		X						
Etoposide	X				X			
Etoposide Phosphate	X				X			
Everolimus	X				X			
Exemestane	X							
Finasteride			X		X			
Fingolimod		X						
Florbetaben F18					X		X	
Florbetapir F18					X		X	
Floxuridine	X				X			
Fluconazole			X					
Fludarabine	X				X			
Fludeoxyglucose F 18					X		X	
Fluorouracil	X				X			
Fluoxymesterone		X						
Flutamide	X							
Flutemetamol F18					X		X	
Formaldehyde				U-listed				
Fosphenytoin		X						
Fulvestrant	X							

Table 2. Drugs Listed as or Considered Hazardous *continued*

	NIOSH List[1]			EPA List[2,3]	Product Labeling[4]	Structure or Toxicity Profile Similar to Existing Hazardous Agents	Radio-pharmaceutical	Not on NIOSH List, but Meets NIOSH Criteria[5]
	Group 1	Group 2	Group 3					
Gallium Citrate Ga-67							X	
Ganciclovir		X			X			
Ganirelix			X		X			
Gefitinib						X		X
Gemcitabine	X				X			
Gemtuzumab Ozogamicin	X				X			
Gonadotropin, Chorionic			X					
Goserelin	X							
Hexachlorophene				U-listed				
Histrelin						X		X
Hydroxyurea	X				X			X
Ibritumomab					X		X	
Ibrutinib					X	X		X
Icatibant			X					
IDArubicin	X				X			
Idelalisib								X
Ifosfamide	X				X			
Imatinib	X				X			
Indium 111 Capromab Pendetide					X		X	
Indium 111 Oxyquinoline					X		X	
Indium In-111 Pentetreotide					X		X	
Iobenguane I 123					X		X	
Iodinated I 131 Albumin					X		X	

Table 2. Drugs Listed as or Considered Hazardous *continued*

	NIOSH List[1]			EPA List[2,3]	Product Labeling[4]	Structure or Toxicity Profile Similar to Existing Hazardous Agents	Radio-pharmaceutical	Not on NIOSH List, but Meets NIOSH Criteria[5]
	Group 1	Group 2	Group 3					
Iodine I-125 Human Serum Albumin							X	
Iodine I-125 Iothalamate					X		X	
Ioflupane I 123					X		X	
Irinotecan	X				X			
Irinotecan (Liposomal)	X				X			
Isotretinoin						X		X
Ixabepilone	X				X			
Lapatinib						X		X
Leflunomide		X						
Lenalidomide		X			X			
Lenvatinib						X		X
Letrozole	X							
Leuprolide	X							
Lindane				U-listed				
Liraglutide		X						
Lomustine	X				X			
Macitentan						X		
Mechlorethamine	X				X			
MedroxyPROGESTERone		X						
Megestrol	X							
Melphalan	X			U-listed	X			
Menotropins			X					
Mercaptopurine	X				X			

Table 2. Drugs Listed as or Considered Hazardous *continued*

	NIOSH List[1]			EPA List[2,3]	Product Labeling[4]	Structure or Toxicity Profile Similar to Existing Hazardous Agents	Radio-pharmaceutical	Not on NIOSH List, but Meets NIOSH Criteria[5]
	Group 1	Group 2	Group 3					
Mercury				U-listed				
Methimazole						X		X
Methotrexate	X				X			
MethylTESTOSTERone			X					
Mifepristone			X					
Misoprostol			X					
MitoMYcin	X			U-listed	X			
Mitotane	X				X			
MitoXANtrone	X				X			
Mycophenolate		X			X			
Nafarelin			X					
Nelarabine	X				X			
Nevirapine		X						
Nicotine				P-listed				
Nilotinib	X							
Nilutamide						X		X
Nintedanib						X		X
Nitrogen 13 Ammonia							X	
Nitroglycerin (doses in "finished form" are excluded)				P-listed	X			
Olaparib								X
Omacetaxine	X				X			
Osimertinib						X		X
Ospemifene						X		X

2301

Table 2. Drugs Listed as or Considered Hazardous *continued*

	NIOSH List[1]			EPA List[2,3]	Product Labeling[4]	Structure or Toxicity Profile Similar to Existing Hazardous Agents	Radio-pharmaceutical	Not on NIOSH List, but Meets NIOSH Criteria[5]
	Group 1	Group 2	Group 3					
Oxaliplatin	X				X			
OXcarbazepine		X						
Oxytocin			X					
PACLitaxel	X				X			
PACLitaxel (Protein Bound)	X				X			
Palbociclib								X
Palifermin		X						
Paliperidone						X		X
Pamidronate						X		X
Panobinostat				U-listed	X	X		X
Paraldehyde				U-listed				
PARoxetine			X					
PAZOPanib	X							
PEMEtrexed	X				X			
Pentetate Calcium Trisodium			X					
Pentetate Indium Disodium In 111					X		X	
Pentostatin	X				X			
Pertuzumab						X		X
Phenacetin				U-listed				
Phenol				U-listed				
Phenoxybenzamine		X						
Physostigmine				P-listed				
Phenytoin		X						

Table 2. Drugs Listed as or Considered Hazardous *continued*

	NIOSH List[1]			EPA List[2,3]	Product Labeling[4]	Structure or Toxicity Profile Similar to Existing Hazardous Agents	Radio-pharmaceutical	Not on NIOSH List, but Meets NIOSH Criteria[5]
	Group 1	Group 2	Group 3					
Pimecrolimus						X		X
Pipobroman		X						
Plerixafor			X					
Pomalidomide					X	X		X
PONATinib						X		X
Porfimer					X			X
PRALAtrexate	X				X			
Procarbazine	X				X			
Progesterone		X			X			
Progestins		X						
Propylthiouracil		X						
Radium Ra 223 Dichloride							X	
Raloxifene		X			X			
Raltitrexed					X	X		
Rasagiline		X						
Regorafenib						X		X
Reserpine				U-listed				
Resorcinol				U-listed				
Ribavirin			X					
Riociguat								X
RisperiDONE		X						
RomiDEPsin	X				X			
Rubidium-82 Chloride					X		X	

2303

Table 2. Drugs Listed as or Considered Hazardous *continued*

	NIOSH List[1]			EPA List[2,3]	Product Labeling[4]	Structure or Toxicity Profile Similar to Existing Hazardous Agents	Radio-pharmaceutical	Not on NIOSH List, but Meets NIOSH Criteria[5]
	Group 1	Group 2	Group 3					
Ruxolitinib						X		X
Saccharin				U-listed				
Samarium Sm 153 Lexidronam					X		X	
Selenium Sulfide				U-listed				
Sirolimus		X						
Sodium Fluoride F18					X		X	
Sodium Iodide I123					X		X	
Sodium Iodide I131					X		X	
Sonidegib						X		X
SORAfenib	X							
Spironolactone		X						
Streptozocin	X			U-listed	X			
Strontium-89					X		X	
Sunitinib	X							
Tacrolimus		X						
Talimogene Laherparepvec					X			X
Tamoxifen	X							
Technetium Tc 99m Albumin Aggregated					X		X	
Technetium Tc 99m Bicisate					X		X	
Technetium Tc 99m Disofenin					X		X	
Technetium Tc 99m Exametazime					X		X	

Table 2. Drugs Listed as or Considered Hazardous *continued*

	NIOSH List[1]			EPA List[2,3]	Product Labeling[4]	Structure or Toxicity Profile Similar to Existing Hazardous Agents	Radio-pharmaceutical	Not on NIOSH List, but Meets NIOSH Criteria[5]
	Group 1	Group 2	Group 3					
Technetium Tc 99m Gluceptate					X		X	
Technetium Tc 99m–Labeled Red Blood Cells					X		X	
Technetium Tc 99m Mebrofenin					X		X	
Technetium Tc 99m Medronate					X		X	
Technetium Tc 99m Mertiatide					X		X	
Technetium Tc 99m Oxidronate					X		X	
Technetium Tc 99m Pentetate					X		X	
Technetium Tc 99m Pyrophosphate					X		X	
Technetium Tc 99m Sestamibi					X		X	
Technetium Tc 99m Succimer					X		X	
Technetium Tc 99m Sulfur Colloid					X		X	
Technetium Tc 99m Tetrofosmin					X		X	
Technetium Tc 99m Tilmanocept					X		X	
Tegafur and Uracil					X	X		X
Tegafur, Gimeracil, and Oteracil					X	X		X

Table 2. Drugs Listed as or Considered Hazardous *continued*

	NIOSH List[1]			EPA List[2,3]	Product Labeling[4]	Structure or Toxicity Profile Similar to Existing Hazardous Agents	Radio-pharmaceutical	Not on NIOSH List, but Meets NIOSH Criteria[5]
	Group 1	Group 2	Group 3					
Televancin			X					
Temozolomide	X				X			
Temsirolimus	X				X			
Teniposide	X				X			
Teriflunamide						X		X
Testosterone			X					
Thalidomide		X			X			
Thallous Chloride TI 201					X		X	
Thioguanine	X				X			
Thiotepa	X				X			
Tibolone		X						X
Tofacitinib						X		
Topiramate			X					
Topotecan	X				X			
Toremifene	X							
Tositumomab					X		X	X
Trabectedin					X			X
Trametinib						X		X
Trastuzumab			X					
Tretinoin			X					
Trichloromonofluoromethane				U-listed				
Trifluridine and Tipiracil					X	X		X
Triptorelin	X							

Table 2. Drugs Listed as or Considered Hazardous *continued*

	NIOSH List[1]			EPA List[2,3]	Product Labeling[4]	Structure or Toxicity Profile Similar to Existing Hazardous Agents	Radio-pharmaceutical	Not on NIOSH List, but Meets NIOSH Criteria[5]
	Group 1	Group 2	Group 3					
Ulipristal			X					
Uracil Mustard		X		U-listed				
ValGANciclovir		X			X			
Valproic Acid			X					
Valrubicin	X				X			
Vandetanib	X				X			
Vemurafenib	X							
Vigabatrin			X					
VinBLAStine	X				X			
VinCRIStine	X				X			
VinCRIStine (Liposomal)					X			
Vindesine					X	X		
Vinorelbine	X				X			X
Vismodegib								X
Voriconazole			X					
Vorinostat	X				X			

Table 2. Drugs Listed as or Considered Hazardous *continued*

	NIOSH List[1]			EPA List[2,3]	Product Labeling[4]	Structure or Toxicity Profile Similar to Existing Hazardous Agents	Radio-pharmaceutical	Not on NIOSH List, but Meets NIOSH Criteria[5]
	Group 1	Group 2	Group 3					
Warfarin			X	<0.3%: U-listed; >0.3%: P-listed				
Xenon Xe 133 Gas					X		X	
Zidovudine		X						
Ziprasidone			X					
Zoledronic Acid			X					
Zonisamide			X					

[1] US Department of Health and Human Services; Centers for Disease Control and Prevention; National Institute for Occupational Safety and Health. NIOSH list of antineoplastic and other hazardous drugs in the healthcare settings, 2014. Available at http://www.cdc.gov/niosh/docs/2014-138/pdfs/2014-138.pdf. Updated September 2014. Accessed September 15, 2014.

[2] Healthcare Environmental Resource Center (HERC). Pharmaceutical wastes in healthcare facilities. Available at http://www.hercenter.org/hazmat/pharma.cfm#listed. Accessed September 15, 2010.

[3] Healthcare Environmental Resource Center (HERC). Hazardous waste determination. http://www.hercenter.org/hazmat/hazdeterm.cfm. Accessed September 15, 2010.

[4] Product labeling (prescribing information) indicates precautions for safe handling and disposal should be followed.

[5] Meets one or more of the NIOSH characteristics for defining hazardous agents: Carcinogenicity, Teratogenicity (or other developmental toxicity), Reproductive toxicity, Organ toxicity (at low doses), Genotoxicity, and/or New drugs with structural and toxicity profiles similar to existing hazardous agents (http://www.cdc.gov/niosh/docs/2014-138/pdfs/2014-138.pdf)

NIOSH has developed guidance on personal protective equipment when working with various dosage forms of hazardous drugs within the health care setting. These recommendations are listed in Table 3.

Table 3. Personal Protection for Handling Hazardous Drugs

Formulation	Activity	Gloving	Protective Gown	Eye Protection	Respiratory Protection	Ventilation Controls
Intact tablet or capsule	Administration from a unit dose package	Single	No	No	No	N/A
Tablets or capsules	Cutting, crushing, or manipulating	Double	Yes	No	Yes (if not done in a controlled device)	Yes
	Administration	Double	Yes	No	Yes (if powder is generated)	N/A
Oral liquid	Compounding	Double	Yes	Yes (if not done in a controlled device)	Yes (if not done in a controlled device)	Yes
	Administration	Double	Yes	No	No	N/A
Topical product	Compounding	Double	Yes	Yes	Yes (if not done in a controlled device)	Yes
	Administration	Double	Yes	Yes (if liquid could splash)	Yes (if potential inhalation)	N/A
Ampule	Opening	Double	Yes	Yes (if not done in a controlled device)	Yes (if not done in a controlled device)	Yes (BSC or CACI)
SubQ or IM injection	Preparation for administration	Double	Yes	Yes (if not done in a controlled device)	Yes (if not done in a controlled device)	Yes (BSC or CACI)
	Administration	Double	Yes	Yes (if liquid could splash)	Yes (if potential inhalation)	N/A
IV solutions	Compounding	Double	Yes	Yes (if not done in a controlled device)	Yes (if not done in a controlled device)	Yes (BSC or CACI; CSTD recommended)
	Administration	Double	Yes	Yes (if liquid could splash)	Yes (if potential inhalation)	N/A (CSTD recommended)

Table 3. Personal Protection for Handling Hazardous Drugs *continued*

Formulation	Activity	Gloving	Protective Gown	Eye Protection	Respiratory Protection	Ventilation Controls
Irrigation solutions	Compounding	Double	Yes	Yes (if not done in a controlled device)	Yes (if not done in a controlled device)	Yes (BSC or CACI; CSTD recommended)
	Administration	Double	Yes	Yes	Yes	N/A
Inhalation powder or solution	Inhalation	Double	Yes	Yes	Yes	Yes (if applicable)

BSC = biologic safety cabinet (class II), CACI = compounding aseptic containment isolator, CSTD = closed system transfer device

US Department of Health and Human Services; Centers for Disease Control and Prevention; National Institute for Occupational Safety and Health. NIOSH list of antineoplastic and other hazardous drugs in the healthcare settings, 2014. Available at http://www.cdc.gov/niosh/docs/2014-138/pdfs/2014-138.pdf. Updated September 2014. Accessed September 15, 2014.

Hazardous drugs must be stored, transported, prepared, administered, and disposed of under conditions that protect the health care worker from either acute or chronic/low level exposure. Institutional policies or guidelines to minimize occupational exposure to hazardous drugs should include a focus on the following areas:

- Development and maintenance of a facility-specific hazardous drugs list

    - Working definition/criteria of a hazardous drug

    - Volumes, formulations, and frequency of hazardous drugs handled: Injection, oral (liquid, solid), topical

    - Oral dosage forms and administration (uncoated tablets or alteration of forms by crushing or preparation of oral solutions may result in exposure; coated tablets or capsules administered intact may pose a lower exposure risk)

Each institution or facility must create its own policy or guideline, including a facility-specific list of drugs deemed hazardous. According to the Joint Commission standards, organizations should minimize risks associated with handling hazardous medications. Orientation and routine training related to safe handling of hazardous drugs is recommended. Until proven otherwise, most institutions consider investigational drugs to be hazardous and to be handled accordingly, particularly if the mechanism of action suggests a potential for concern. Hazardous drug procedures must include all possible routes of administration.

Additional information regarding development and implementation of an institutional policy/guideline, areas at risk, personnel at risk, risk management, spill management, personnel training, surveillance, and medicine disposal may be found at:

ASHP Guidelines on Handling Hazardous Drugs:
http://www.ashp.org/DocLibrary/BestPractices/PrepGdlHazDrugs.aspx

Environmental Protection Agency Recommendations:
http://hercenter.org/hazmat/hazdeterm.cfm
http://hercenter.org/hazmat/pharma.cfm

Food and Drug Administration Safe Medicine Disposal Options:
http://www.fda.gov/Drugs/NewsEvents/ucm464197.htm

NIOSH List of Antineoplastic and Other Hazardous Drugs in Health Care Settings:
http://www.cdc.gov/niosh/docs/2014-138/pdfs/2014-138.pdf

US Nuclear Regulatory Commission (radiopharmaceuticals, such as ibritumomab or tositumomab):
http://www.nrc.gov/materials/miau/med-use.html

- Identification of personnel and locations in the facility at risk for occupational exposure to hazardous drugs

    - Pharmacy

        - Receiving storage and inventory

        - Dose preparation and dispensing

        - Drug waste disposal

- Nursing Unit
  - Drug administration
  - Drug waste disposal
  - Patient waste disposal

- Other areas
  - Laboratory
  - Operating/procedure rooms
  - Veterinary department
  - Facility shipping/receiving
  - Environmental/laundry services
  - Maintenance services

While the greatest risk of occupational exposure to hazardous drugs occurs during preparation and administration of these agents, it is important to recognize that a risk of exposure can occur throughout the facility from the moment of delivery through the disposal of product and contaminated human waste. Drug preparation and administration may occur in nontraditional areas of the institution including the operating room and in veterinary facilities. Procedures should address the importance of proper labeling and packaging and separation of hazardous vs nonhazardous inventories throughout the facility. Drug containers should be examined upon their arrival at the pharmacy. Containers that show signs of damage should be handled carefully and may require quarantine and decontamination before being placed in stock. Give consideration to routinely quarantining and decontaminating all hazardous drug containers as part of the inspection process before placing in stock.

- Mechanisms/routes of occupational exposure
  - Inhalation of dust or aerosolized droplets (most common)
  - Absorption through skin (most common)
  - Ingestion from contaminated food/drink
  - Accidental injection during preparation/administration/disposal

- Potential adverse effects of hazardous exposure
  - Skin disorders
  - Reproductive effects (eg, spontaneous abortion, stillbirth, congenital malformation)
  - Leukemia and other cancers

- Risk management
  - Use and maintenance of equipment designed to minimize exposure during handling
    - Buffer/Ante transition area
    - Biological safety cabinets, isolators
    - Closed system drug-transfer devices
    - Personal protective equipment
    - Deactivation, decontamination, and cleaning procedures

Barrier protection through the use of ventilation controls and personal protective equipment is the current standard to minimize exposure when handling hazardous drugs. NIOSH and ASHP recommend the use of Class II biological safety cabinets (type B2 preferred), but other options include the totally enclosed Class III biological safety cabinets, appropriate isolators, and robotic systems. Self-contained or closed system devices have been recommended to minimize workplace contamination by preventing escape of drug or vapor out of the device. Devices available include PhaSeal, ONGARD, TEVADAPTOR, Equashield, and CLAVE systems; other systems may also be commercially available. Gloves, gowns, respiratory protection, hair and shoe covers, and eye protection represent the core of personal protective equipment. Guidelines for choice of gowns and gloving, and the circumstances to employ this protection are published by ASHP, NIOSH, and in USP 797.

Procedures for safe handling should be followed with oral dosage forms of antineoplastics (Goodin 2011). Appropriate personal protective equipment should be worn, automatic counting machines should not be utilized, compounding should be performed in a biologic safety cabinet, separate equipment (eg, counting trays) should be used, disposable equipment should be used if possible, cytotoxic waste should be disposed of, and non-disposable equipment used for preparation should be appropriately decontaminated.

  - Hazardous drug spill management
    - Size and location
    - Spill kit use
    - Worker contamination

Procedures for handling spills throughout a facility are well described by ASHP and NIOSH. Institutional procedures should focus on location and size of the spill, how to handle a spill when a spill kit is not available, and how to respond to a worker contamination (emergent treatment, follow-up care).

  - Personnel training in the handling of hazardous drugs
    - Prior to handling hazardous drugs
    - Periodic and ongoing testing

Personnel throughout a facility must have training in the handling of hazardous drugs that are relevant to their job description. Pharmacy personnel who compound and dispense hazardous drugs must be fully trained in the storing, preparation, dispensing, and disposal of these agents. Such training should include didactic, as well as demonstrating hands-on technique, and such validation should be repeated on a regular schedule. Special training may be necessary for hazardous drugs administered by routes outside of traditional administration routes and when administered in settings outside of traditional settings (eg, at home).

- Environmental and medical surveillance

  - Components of a comprehensive medical surveillance program

  - Reproductive and health questionnaires (at time of hire and periodically)

  - Drug handling history (to estimate current and prior exposure)

  - Baseline clinical evaluation plan (including related medical history, physical exam, lab work)

  - Follow-up plan (for those with health changes suggestive of toxicity or acute exposure)

  - Potential use of environmental sampling techniques

  - Use of common marker hazardous drugs for assay purposes

The goal of medical surveillance is to minimize adverse effects on the health of workers exposed to hazardous drugs. NIOSH recommends that medical surveillance be employed by the facility, and may include the basic observation of employee symptom complaints or monitoring for changes in health status as part of routine checkups. Some programs follow the employee more closely and procedures may include periodic lab studies (eg, blood cell counts), physical exam, detailed medical history and occupational exposure history, and/or biologic studies. Environmental sampling to look for surface contamination in hazardous drug preparation and administration areas may be considered, particularly in institutions with high volumes. Certain hazardous drugs serve as markers which allow for assay for measurable contamination, and can alert the facility for proper follow-up.

- Work practices regarding reproductive risks to health care workers

  - Alternative duty options

Since hazardous drugs are associated with reproductive risks, policies and guidelines should address health care workers whom are pregnant, attempting to conceive or father a child, and whom are breast-feeding. Workers of reproductive capability should acknowledge in writing that they understand the risk of handling hazardous drugs and be given the opportunity for reassignment or alternate work duty.

REFERENCES

American Society of Hospital Pharmacists. ASHP guidelines on handling hazardous drugs. 2006;63(12):1172-1193.

Baker ES, Connor TH. Monitoring occupational exposure to cancer chemotherapy drugs. *Am J Health Syst Pharm.* 1996;53(22):2713-2723.

Bos RP, Sessink PJ. Biomonitoring of occupational exposures to cytostatic anticancer drugs. *Rev Environ Health.* 1997;12(1):43-58.

Connor TH, Anderson RW, Sessink PJ, Broadfield L, Power LA. Surface contamination with antineoplastic agents in six cancer treatment centers in Canada and the United States. *Am J Health Syst Pharm.* 1999;56(14):1427-1432.

Connor TH, DeBord DG, Pretty JR, et al. Evaluation of antineoplastic drug exposure of health care workers at three university-based US cancer centers. *J Occup Environ Med.* 2010;52 (10):1019-1027.

Connor TH, McDiarmid MA. Preventing occupational exposures to antineoplastic drugs in health care settings. *CA Cancer J Clin.* 2006;56(6):354-365.

Connor TH. Permeability of nitrile rubber, latex, polyurethane, and neoprene gloves to 18 antineoplastic drugs. *Am J Health Syst Pharm.* 1999;56(23):2450-2453.

Connor TH, Sessink PJ, Harrison BR, et al. Surface contamination of chemotherapy drug vials and evaluation of new vial-cleaning techniques: results of three studies. *Am J Health Syst Pharm.* 2005;62(5):475-484.

Goodin S, Griffith N, Chen B, et al. Safe handling of oral chemotherapeutic agents in clinical practice: recommendations from an international pharmacy panel. *J Oncol Pract.* 2011;7(1):7-12.

Healthcare Environmental Resource Center (HERC). Hazardous waste determination. http://www.-hercenter.org/hazmat/hazdeterm.cfm. Accessed September 15, 2010.

Healthcare Environmental Resource Center (HERC). Pharmaceutical wastes in healthcare facilities. http://www.hercenter.org/hazmat/pharma.cfm#listed. Accessed September 15, 2010.

Lawson CC, Rocheleau CM, Whelan EA, et al. Occupational exposures among nurses and risk of spontaneous abortion. *Am J Obstet Gynecol.* 2012;206(4):327.

McDiarmid MA, Oliver MS, Roth TS, Rogers B, Escalante C. Chromosome 5 and 7 abnormalities in oncology personnel handling anticancer drugs. *J Occup Environ Med.* 2010;52(10):1028-1034.

National Institute for Occupational Safety and Health (NIOSH). Medical surveillance for healthcare workers exposed to hazardous drugs. 2012. http://www.cdc.gov/niosh/docs/wp-solutions/2013-103/. Accessed January 22, 2013.

National Institute for Occupational Safety and Health (NIOSH). Preventing occupational exposure to antineoplastic and other hazardous drugs in health care settings. http://www.cdc.gov/niosh/docs/2004-165/2004-165d.html#o. Accessed October 1, 2007.

Polovich M. *Safe Handling of Hazardous Drugs.* 2nd ed. Pittsburgh, PA: Oncology Nursing Society; 2011.

Sessink PJ, Bos RP. Drugs hazardous to healthcare workers. Evaluation of methods for monitoring occupational exposure to cytostatic drugs. *Drug Saf.* 1999;20(4):347-359.

Sessink PJ, Anzion RB, Van den Broek PH, Bos RP. Detection of contamination with antineoplastic agents in a hospital pharmacy department. *Pharm Weekbl Sci.* 1992;14(1):16-22.

Sessink PJ, Boer KA, Scheefhals AP, Anzion RB, Bos RP. Occupational exposure to antineoplastic agents at several departments in a hospital. Environmental contamination and excretion of cyclophosphamide and ifosamide in urine of exposed workers. *Int Arch Occup Environ Health.* 1992;64(2):105-112.

Sorsa M, Anderson D. Monitoring of occupational exposure to cytostatic anticancer agents. *Mutat Res.* 1996;355(1-2):253-261.

US Department of Health and Human Services; Centers for Disease Control and Prevention; National Institute for Occupational Safety and Health. NIOSH list of antineoplastic and other hazardous drugs in healthcare settings, 2014. Available at http://www.cdc.gov/niosh/docs/2014-138/pdfs/2014-138.pdf. Updated September 2014. Accessed September 18, 2014.

APPENDIX TABLE OF CONTENTS

MILLIEQUIVALENT AND MILLIMOLE CALCULATIONS AND CONVERSIONS

DEFINITIONS AND CALCULATIONS

Definitions

mole	=	gram molecular weight of a substance (aka molar weight)
millimole (mM)	=	milligram molecular weight of a substance (a millimole is 1/1,000 of a mole)
equivalent weight	=	gram weight of a substance which will combine with or replace 1 gram (1 mole) of hydrogen; an equivalent weight can be determined by dividing the molar weight of a substance by its ionic valence
milliequivalent (mEq)	=	milligram weight of a substance which will combine with or replace 1 milligram (1 millimole) of hydrogen (a milliequivalent is 1/1,000 of an equivalent)

Calculations

moles	=	$\dfrac{\text{weight of a substance (grams)}}{\text{molecular weight of that substance (grams)}}$
millimoles	=	$\dfrac{\text{weight of a substance (grams) x 1,000}}{\text{molecular weight of that substance (grams)}}$
equivalents	=	moles x valence of ion
milliequivalents	=	millimoles x valence of ion
moles	=	$\dfrac{\text{equivalents}}{\text{valence of ion}}$
millimoles	=	$\dfrac{\text{milliequivalents}}{\text{valence of ion}}$
millimoles	=	moles x 1,000
milliequivalents	=	equivalents x 1,000

Note: Use of equivalents and milliequivalents is valid only for those substances which have fixed ionic valences (eg, sodium, potassium, calcium, chlorine, magnesium, bromine, etc). For substances with variable ionic valences (eg, phosphorous), a reliable equivalent value cannot be determined. In these instances, one should calculate millimoles (which are fixed and reliable) rather than milliequivalents.

MILLIEQUIVALENT CONVERSIONS

To convert mg/100 mL to mEq/L the following formula may be used:

$$\frac{(mg\ per\ 100\ mL) \times 10 \times valence}{atomic\ weight} = mEq/L$$

To convert mEq/L to mg/100 mL the following formula may be used:

$$\frac{(mEq/L) \times atomic\ weight}{10 \times valence} = mg\ per\ 100\ mL$$

To convert mEq/L to volume of percent of a gas the following formula may be used:

$$\frac{(mEq/L) \times 22.4}{10} = volume\ percent$$

Valences and Atomic Weights of Selected Ions

Substance	Electrolyte	Valence	Molecular Wt
Calcium	Ca^{++}	2	40
Chloride	Cl^-	1	35.5
Magnesium	Mg^{++}	2	24
Phosphate	HPO_4^{--} (80%)	1.8	96[1]
pH = 7.4	$H_2PO_4^-$ (20%)	1.8	96[1]
Potassium	K^+	1	39
Sodium	Na^+	1	23
Sulfate	SO_4^{--}	2	96[1]

[1]The molecular weight of phosphorus only is 31 and sulfur only is 32.

Approximate Milliequivalents — Weights of Selected Ions

Salt	mEq/g Salt	mg Salt/mEq
Calcium carbonate [$CaCO_3$]	20	50
Calcium chloride [$CaCl_2 \cdot 2H_2O$]	14	74
Calcium gluceptate [$Ca(C_7H_{13}O_8)_2$]	4	245
Calcium gluconate [$Ca(C_6H_{11}O_7)_2 \cdot H_2O$]	5	224
Calcium lactate [$Ca(C_3H_5O_3)_2 \cdot 5H_2O$]	7	154
Magnesium gluconate [$Mg(C_6H_{11}O_7)_2 \cdot H_2O$]	5	216
Magnesium oxide [MgO]	50	20
Magnesium sulfate [$MgSO_4$]	17	60
Magnesium sulfate [$MgSO_4 \cdot 7H_2O$]	8	123
Potassium acetate [$K(C_2H_3O_2)$]	10	98
Potassium chloride [KCl]	13	75

Approximate Milliequivalents — Weights of Selected Ions (continued)

Salt	mEq/g Salt	mg Salt/mEq
Potassium citrate [$K_3(C_6H_5O_7) \cdot H_2O$]	9	108
Potassium iodide [KI]	6	166
Sodium acetate [$Na(C_2H_3O_2)$]	12	82
Sodium acetate [$Na(C_2H_3O_2) \cdot 3H_2O$]	7	136
Sodium bicarbonate [$NaHCO_3$]	12	84
Sodium chloride [NaCl]	17	58
Sodium citrate [$Na_3(C_6H_5O_7) \cdot 2H_2O$]	10	98
Sodium iodine [NaI]	7	150
Sodium lactate [$Na(C_3H_5O_3)$]	9	112
Zinc sulfate [$ZnSO_4 \cdot 7H_2O$]	7	144

ACID-BASE ASSESSMENT

Henderson-Hasselbalch Equation

$pH = 6.1 + \log ([HCO_3^-] / (0.03) [PaCO_2])$

Normal arterial blood pH: 7.4 (normal range: 7.35 to 7.45)

Where:

$[HCO_3^-]$ = Serum bicarbonate concentration

$PaCO_2$ = Arterial carbon dioxide partial pressure

Alveolar Gas Equation

P_iO_2 $= F_iO_2 \times$ (total atmospheric pressure – vapor pressure of H_2O at 37°C)

$= F_iO_2 \times (760 \text{ mm Hg} - 47 \text{ mm Hg})$

PAO_2 $= P_iO_2 - (PaCO_2 / R)$

Alveolar-arterial oxygen (A-a) gradient = $PAO_2 - PaO_2$

or

A-a gradient = $[(F_iO_2 \times 713) - (PaCO_2/0.8)] - PaO_2$

A-a gradient normal ranges:

Children   15 to 20 mm Hg

Adults   20 to 25 mm Hg

where:

P_iO_2 = Oxygen partial pressure of inspired gas (mm Hg) (150 mm Hg in room air at sea level)

F_iO_2 = Fractional pressure of oxygen in inspired gas (0.21 in room air)

PAO_2 = Alveolar oxygen partial pressure

PaO_2 = Arterial oxygen partial pressure

$PaCO_2$ = Arterial carbon dioxide partial pressure

R = Respiratory exchange quotient (typically 0.8, increases with high carbohydrate diet, decreases with high fat diet)

Acid-Base Disorders

Acute metabolic acidosis:
$PaCO_2$ expected = 1.5 ($[HCO_3^-]$) + 8 ± 2 **or**
Expected decrease in $PaCO_2$ = 1.3 (1-1.5) x decrease in $[HCO_3^-]$

Acute metabolic alkalosis:
Expected increase in $PaCO_2$ = 0.6 (0.5-1) x increase in $[HCO_3^-]$

Acute respiratory acidosis (<6 h duration):
For every $PaCO_2$ increase of 10 mm Hg, $[HCO_3^-]$ increases by 1 mEq/L

Chronic respiratory acidosis (>6 h duration):
  For every $PaCO_2$ increase of 10 mm Hg, $[HCO_3^-]$ increases by 4 mEq/L

Acute respiratory alkalosis (<6 h duration):
  For every $PaCO_2$ decrease of 10 mm Hg, $[HCO_3^-]$ decreases by 2 mEq/L

Chronic respiratory alkalosis (>6 h duration):
  For every $PaCO_2$ decrease of 10 mm Hg, $[HCO_3^-]$ increases by 5 mEq/L

SELECTED CLINICAL EQUATIONS

CORRECTED SODIUM

Corrected Na^+ = measured Na^+ + [1.5 x (glucose − 150 divided by 100)]

Note: Do not correct for glucose <150.

WATER DEFICIT

Water deficit = 0.6 x body weight [1 − (140 divided by Na^+)]

Note: Body weight is estimated weight in kg when fully hydrated; **Na^+** is serum or plasma sodium. Use corrected Na^+ if necessary. Consult medical references for recommendations for replacement of deficit.

TOTAL SERUM CALCIUM CORRECTED FOR ALBUMIN LEVEL

[(Normal albumin − patient's albumin) x 0.8] + patient's measured total calcium

OSMOLALITY

Definition: The summed concentrations of all osmotically active solute particles.

Predicted serum osmolality =

$$mOsm/L = (2 \times serum\ Na^{++}) + \frac{serum\ glucose}{18} + \frac{BUN}{2.8}$$

The normal range of serum osmolality is 285 to 295 mOsm/L.

Calculated Osm

Note: Osm is a term used to reconcile osmolality and osmolarity

Osmol gap = measured Osm − calculated Osm

0 to +10: Normal
>10: Abnormal
<0: Probable lab or calculation error

Drugs Causing Osmolar Gap
(by freezing-point depression, gap is >10 mOsm)
Ethanol
Ethylene glycol
Glycerol
Iodine (questionable)
Isopropanol (acetone)
Mannitol
Methanol
Sorbitol

BICARBONATE DEFICIT

HCO_3^- deficit = (0.4 x wt in kg) x (HCO_3^- desired − HCO_3^- measured)

Note: In clinical practice, the calculated quantity may differ markedly from the actual amount of bicarbonate needed or that which may be safely administered.

ANION GAP

Definition: The difference in concentration between unmeasured cation and anion equivalents in serum.

Anion gap = $Na^+ - (Cl^- + HCO_3^-)$
(The normal anion gap is 10 to 14 mEq/L)

Differential Diagnosis of Increased Anion Gap Acidosis

Organic anions
  Lactate (sepsis, hypovolemia, seizures, large tumor burden)
  Pyruvate
  Uremia
  Ketoacidosis (β-hydroxybutyrate and acetoacetate)
  Amino acids and their metabolites
  Other organic acids

Inorganic anions
  Hyperphosphatemia
  Sulfates
  Nitrates

Differential Diagnosis of Decreased Anion Gap

Organic cations
  Hypergammaglobulinemia

Inorganic cations
  Hyperkalemia
  Hypercalcemia
  Hypermagnesemia

Medications and toxins
  Lithium

Hypoalbuminemia

RETICULOCYTE INDEX

(% retic divided by 2) x (patient's Hct divided by normal Hct) **or**
(% retic divided by 2) x (patient's Hgb divided by normal Hgb)

Normal index: 1
Good marrow response: 2 to 6

CORRECTED QT INTERVAL EQUATIONS

Bazett (B) Formula:

  QTcB: $QTc = QT/(R - R \text{ interval}^{0.5})$

  or

  QTcB: QTc = QT/Square root of (R - R interval)

Frederica (F) Formula:

  QTcF: $QTc = QT/(R - R \text{ interval}^{0.33})$

BODY SURFACE AREA

Body Surface Area (BSA) – Adults and Pediatric

$$BSA\ (m^2) = \frac{kg^{0.425} \times cm^{0.725} \times 71.84}{10,000}$$

or

$$log\ BSA\ (m^2) = \frac{(log\ kg \times 0.425) + (log\ cm \times 0.725) + 1.8564}{10,000}$$

DuBois D, DuBois EF. A formula to estimate the approximate surface area if height and weight be known. *Arch Intern Med.* 1916;17:863-871.

$$BSA\ (m^2) = \sqrt{\frac{ht\ (in) \times wt\ (lb)}{3131}} \quad or \quad BSA\ (m^2) = \sqrt{\frac{ht\ (cm) \times wt\ (kg)}{3600}}$$

Lam TK, Leung DT. More on simplified calculation of body-surface area. *N Engl J Med.* 1988;318 (17):1130 (letter).
Mosteller RD. Simplified calculation of body surface area. *N Engl J Med.* 1987;317:1098 (letter).

Ideal Body Weight

Men: 50 kg + 2.3 kg/inch >5 ft
Women: 45 kg + 2.3 kg/in >5 ft

Devine BJ. Gentamicin therapy. *Drug Intelligence and Clinical Pharmacy.* 1974;8:650-655.

or

Men: 51.65 kg + 1.85 kg/in >5 ft
Women: 48.67 kg + 1.7 kg/in >5 ft

Robinson JD, Lupkiewicz SM, Palenik L, Lopez LM, Ariet M. Determination of ideal body weight for drug dosage calculations. *Am J Hosp Pharm.* 1983;40(6):1016-1019.

Adjusted Body Weight

Adjusted wt (kg) = ideal body weight (kg) + 0.25 [actual wt (kg) - ideal body weight (kg)]

Adjusted wt (kg) = ideal body weight (kg) + 0.4 [actual wt (kg) – ideal body weight (kg)]

Bubalo J, Carpenter PA, Majhail N, et al. Conditioning chemotherapy dose adjustment in obese patients: a review and position statement by the American Society for Blood and Marrow Transplantation practice guideline committee. *Biol Blood Marrow Transplant.* 2014;20 (5):600-616.

Area Under the Curve (AUC) for Carboplatin Dosing

Carboplatin (mg) = desired AUC x (25 + GFR)

GFR = creatinine clearance (measured or estimated)

Calvert AH, Newell DR, Gumbrell LA, et al. Carboplatin dosage: prospective evaluation of a simple formula based on renal function. *J Clin Oncol.* 1989;7(11):1748-1756.

RENAL FUNCTION ESTIMATION IN ADULT PATIENTS

Evaluation of a patient's renal function often includes the use of equations to estimate glomerular filtration rate (GFR) (eg, estimated GFR [eGFR] creatinine clearance [CrCl]) using an endogenous filtration marker (eg, serum creatinine) and other patient variables. For example, the Cockcroft-Gault equation estimates renal function by calculating CrCl and is typically used to steer medication dosing. Equations which calculate eGFR are primarily used to categorize chronic kidney disease (CKD) staging and monitor progression. The rate of creatinine clearance does not always accurately represent GFR; creatinine may be cleared by other renal mechanisms in addition to glomerular filtration and serum creatinine concentrations may be affected by nonrenal factors (eg, age, gender, race, body habitus, illness, diet). In addition, these equations were developed based on studies in limited populations and may either over- or underestimate the renal function of a specific patient.

Nevertheless, most clinicians estimate renal function using CrCl as an indicator of actual renal function for the purpose of adjusting medication doses. For medications that require dose adjustment for renal impairment, utilization of eGFR (ie, Modification of Diet in Renal Disease [MDRD]) may overestimate renal function by up to 40% which may result in supratherapeutic medication doses (Hermsen 2009). These equations should only be used in the clinical context of patient-specific factors noted during the physical exam/work-up. The 2012 National Kidney Foundation (NKF)-Kidney Disease Improving Global Outcomes (KDIGO) CKD guidelines state that drug dosing should be based on an e-GFR which is **not** adjusted for body surface area (BSA) (ie, reported in units of mL/minute per 1.73 m^2) since the effect of eGFR adjusted for BSA compared to eGFR without adjustments for BSA has not been extensively studied. **Decisions regarding drug therapy and doses must be based on clinical judgment.**

RENAL FUNCTION ESTIMATION EQUATIONS

Commonly used equations to estimate renal function utilizing the endogenous filtration marker serum creatinine include the Cockcroft-Gault, Jelliffe, four-variable Modification of Diet in Renal Disease (MDRD), six-variable MDRD (aka, MDRD extended), and Chronic Kidney Disease Epidemiology Collaboration (CKD-EPI). All of these equations, except for the CKD-EPI, were originally developed using a serum creatinine assay measured by the alkaline picrate-based (Jaffe) method. Many substances, including proteins, can interfere with the accuracy of this assay and overestimate serum creatinine concentration. The NKF and The National Kidney Disease Education Program (NDKEP) advocated for a universal creatinine assay, in order to ensure an accurate estimate of renal function in patients. As a result, a more specific enzymatic assay with an isotope dilution mass spectrometry (IDMS)-traceable international standard was developed. Compared to the older methods, IDMS-traceable assays may report lower serum creatinine values and may, therefore, overestimate renal function when used in the original equations not re-expressed for use with a standardized serum creatinine assay (eg, Cockcroft-Gault, Jelliffe, original MDRD). Updated four-variable MDRD and six-variable MDRD equations based on serum creatinine measured by the IDMS-traceable method has been proposed for adults (Levey 2006); the Cockcroft-Gault and Jelliffe equations have not been re-expressed and may overestimate renal function when used with a serum creatinine measured by the IDMS-traceable method. However, at this point, all laboratories should be using creatinine methods calibrated to be IDMS traceable.

The CKD-EPI creatinine equation, published in 2009, uses the same four variables as the four-variable MDRD (serum creatinine, age, sex, and race), but allows for more precision when estimating higher GFR values (eg, eGFR >60 mL/minute per 1.73 m^2) as compared to the MDRD equation. The NKDEP has not made a recommendation on the general implementation of the CKD-EPI equation but does suggest that laboratories which report numeric values for eGFR >60 mL/minute per 1.73 m^2 should consider the use of CKD-EPI. The NKD-KDIGO 2012 CKD guidelines recommend that clinicians use a creatinine-derived equation for the evaluation and management of CKD and specifically recommend that clinical laboratories use the 2009 CKD-EPI equation when reporting eGFR in adults.

The following factors may contribute to an inaccurate estimation of renal function (Stevens 2006):

- Increased creatinine generation (may underestimate renal function):
    - Black patients
    - Muscular body habitus
    - Ingestion of cooked meats
- Decreased creatinine generation (may overestimate renal function):
    - Increased age
    - Female patients
    - Hispanic patients
    - Asian patients
    - Amputees
    - Malnutrition, inflammation, or deconditioning (eg, cancer, severe cardiovascular disease, hospitalized patients)
    - Neuromuscular disease
    - Vegetarian diet
- Rapidly changing serum creatinine (either up or down): In patients with rapidly rising serum creatinines (ie, increasing by >0.5 to 0.7 mg/dL/day), it is best to assume that the patient's renal function is severely impaired

Use extreme caution when estimating renal function in the following patient populations:

- Low body weight (actual body weight < ideal body weight)
- Liver transplant
- Elderly patients (>90 years of age)
- Dehydration
- Recent kidney transplantation (serum creatinine values may decrease rapidly and can lead to renal function underestimation; conversely, delayed graft function may be present)

◄ **Note:** In most situations, the use of the patient's ideal body weight (IBW) is recommended for estimating renal function, except when the patient's actual body weight (ABW) is less than ideal. Use of actual body weight (ABW) in obese patients (and possibly patients with ascites) may significantly overestimate renal function. Some clinicians prefer to use an adjusted body weight in such cases [eg, IBW + 0.4 (ABW - IBW)]; the adjustment factor may vary based on practitioner and/or institutional preference.

IDMS-traceable methods

Method 1: MDRD equation[1]:

$$eGFR = 175 \times (Creatinine)^{-1.154} \times (Age)^{-0.203} \times (Gender) \times (Race)$$

where:
  eGFR = estimated GFR; calculated in mL/minute per 1.73 m^2
  Creatinine is input in mg/dL
  Age is input in years
  Gender: Females: Gender = 0.742; Males: Gender = 1
  Race: Black: Race = 1.212; White or other: Race = 1

Method 2: MDRD Extended equation:

$$eGFR = 161.5 \times (Creatinine)^{-0.999} \times (Age)^{-0.176} \times (SUN)^{-0.170} \times (Albumin)^{0.318} \times (Gender) \times (Race)$$

where:
  eGFR = estimated GFR; calculated in mL/minute per 1.73 m^2
  Creatinine is input in mg/dL
  Age is input in years
  SUN = Serum Urea Nitrogen; input in mg/dL
  Albumin = Serum Albumin; input in g/dL
  Gender: Females: Gender = 0.762; Males: Gender = 1
  Race: Black: Race = 1.18; White or other: Race = 1

Method 3: CKD-EPI equation[2]:

$$eGFR = 141 \times (Creatinine/k)^{Exp} \times (0.993)^{Age} \times (Gender) \times (Race)$$

where:
  eGFR = estimated GFR; calculated in mL/minute per 1.73 m^2
  (Creatinine/k):
    Creatinine is input in mg/dL
    k: Females: k = 0.7; Males: k = 0.9
    Exp:
      When (Creatinine/k) is ≤1: Females: Exp = -0.329; Males: Exp = -0.411
      When (Creatinine/k) is >1: Exp = -1.209
  Age is input in years
  Gender: Females: Gender = 1.018; Males: Gender = 1
  Race: Black: Race = 1.159; White or other: Race = 1

Alkaline picrate-based (Jaffe) methods

Note: These equations have not been updated for use with serum creatinine methods traceable to IDMS. Use with IDMS-traceable serum creatinine methods may overestimate renal function; use with caution.

Method 1: MDRD equation:

$$eGFR = 186 \times (Creatinine)^{-1.154} \times (Age)^{-0.203} \times (Gender) \times (Race)$$

where:
eGFR = estimated GFR; calculated in mL/minute per 1.73 m^2
Creatinine is input in mg/dL
Age is input in years
Gender: Females: Gender = 0.742; Males: Gender = 1
Race: Black: Race = 1.212; White or other: Race = 1

Method 2: MDRD Extended equation:

$$eGFR = 170 \times (Creatinine)^{-0.999} \times (Age)^{-0.176} \times (SUN)^{-0.170} \times (Albumin)^{0.318} \times (Gender) \times (Race)$$

where:
eGFR = estimated GFR; calculated in mL/minute per 1.73 m^2
Creatinine is input in mg/dL
Age is input in years
SUN = Serum Urea Nitrogen; input in mg/dL
Albumin = Serum Albumin; input in g/dL
Gender: Females: Gender = 0.762; Males: Gender = 1
Race: Black: Race = 1.18; White or other: Race = 1

Method 3: Cockroft-Gault equation[3]

Males: CrCl = [(140 - Age) X Weight] / (72 X Creatinine)
Females: CrCl = {[(140 - Age) X Weight] / (72 X Creatinine)} X 0.85
where:
CrCl = creatinine clearance; calculated in mL/minute
Age is input in years
Weight is input in kg
Creatinine is input in mg/dL

Method 4: Jelliffe equation

Males: CrCl = {98 - [0.8 X (Age - 20)]} / (Creatinine)
Females: CrCl = Use above equation, then multiply result by 0.9
where:
CrCl = creatinine clearance; calculated in mL/minute per 1.73 m^2
Age is input in years
Creatinine is input in mg/dL

FOOTNOTES
[1] Preferred equation for CKD staging National Kidney Disease Education Program
[2] Recommended equation for the reporting of eGFR by the NKD-KDIGO guidelines
[3] Equation typically used for adjusting medication doses

REFERENCES

Cockcroft DW, Gault MH. Prediction of creatinine clearance from serum creatinine. *Nephron.* 1976;16(1):31-41.

Dowling TC, Matzke GR, Murphy JE, Burckart GJ. Evaluation of renal drug dosing: prescribing information and clinical pharmacist approaches. *Pharmacotherapy.* 2010;30(8):776-786.

Hermsen ED, Maiefski M, Florescu MC, Qiu F, Rupp ME. Comparison of the modification of diet in renal disease and Cockcroft-Gault equations for dosing antimicrobials. *Pharmacotherapy.* 2009;29(6):649-655.

Jelliffe RW. Letter: creatinine clearance: bedside estimate. *Ann Intern Med.* 1973;79(4):604-605.

Kidney disease: improving global outcomes (KDIGO) CKD work group. KDIGO 2012 clinical practice guidelines for the evaluation and management of chronic kidney disease. *Kidney Inter.* 2013;3:1-150. http://www.kdigo.org/clinical_practice_guidelines/pdf/CKD/KDIGO_2012_CKD_GL.pdf

Levey AS, Bosch JP, Lewis JB, Greene T, Rogers N, Roth D. A more accurate method to estimate glomerular filtration rate from serum creatinine: a new prediction equation. Modification of diet in renal disease study group. *Ann Intern Med.* 1999;16;130(6):461-470.

Levey AS, Coresh J, Greene T, et al. Using standardized serum creatinine values in the modification of diet in renal disease study equation for estimating glomerular filtration rate. *Ann Intern Med.* 2006;145(4):247-254.

Levey AS, Stevens LA, Schmid CH, et al. A new equation to estimate glomerular filtration rate. *Ann Intern Med.* 2009;150(9):604-612.

National Kidney Disease Education Program. GFR calculators. http://www.nkdep.nih.gov/professionals/gfr_calculators. Accessed April 24, 2013.

Stevens LA, Coresh J, Greene T, Levey AS. Assessing kidney function – measured and estimated glomerular filtration rate. *N Engl J Med.* 2006;354(23):2473-2483.

RENAL FUNCTION ESTIMATION IN PEDIATRIC PATIENTS

Evaluation of a patient's renal function often includes the use of equations to estimate glomerular filtration rate (GFR) (eg, estimated GFR [eGFR] creatinine clearance [CrCl]) using an endogenous filtration marker (eg, serum creatinine) and other patient variables. For example, the Schwartz equation estimates renal function by calculating eGFR and is typically used to steer medication dosing or categorize chronic kidney disease (CKD) staging and monitor progression. The rate of creatinine clearance does not always accurately represent GFR; creatinine may be cleared by other renal mechanisms in addition to glomerular filtration and serum creatinine concentrations may be affected by nonrenal factors (eg, age, gender, race, body habitus, illness, diet). In addition, these equations were developed based on studies in limited populations and may either over- or underestimate the renal function of a specific patient.

Nevertheless, most clinicians use an eGFR or CrCl as an indicator of renal function in pediatric patients for the purposes of adjusting medication doses. These equations should be used in the clinical context of patient-specific factors noted during the physical exam/work-up. **Decisions regarding drug therapy and doses must be made on clinical judgment.**

RENAL FUNCTION ESTIMATION EQUATIONS

Commonly used equations to estimate renal function utilizing the endogenous filtration marker serum creatinine include the Schwartz and Traub-Johnson equations. Both equations were originally developed using a serum creatinine assay measured by the alkaline picrate-based (Jaffe) method. Many substances, including proteins, can interfere with the accuracy of this assay and overestimate serum creatinine concentration. The National Kidney Foundation and The National Kidney Disease Education Program advocated for a universal creatinine assay, in order to ensure an accurate estimate of GFR in patients. As a result, a more specific enzymatic assay with an isotope dilution mass spectrometry (IDMS)-traceable international standard was developed. Compared to the older methods, IDMS-traceable assays may report lower serum creatinine values and may, therefore, overestimate renal function when used in the original equations. An updated Schwartz equation (eg, Bedside Schwartz) based on serum creatinine measured by the IDMS-traceable method has been proposed for pediatrics (Schwartz 2009); the Traub-Johnson equation has not been re-expressed. The original Schwartz and Traub-Johnson equations may overestimate renal function when used with a serum creatinine measured by the IDMS-traceable method. However, at this point, all laboratories should be using creatinine methods calibrated to be IDMS traceable.

The following factors may contribute to an inaccurate estimation of renal function (Stevens 2006):

- Increased creatinine generation (may underestimate renal function):

    - Black patients

    - Muscular body habitus

    - Ingestion of cooked meats

- Decreased creatinine generation (may overestimate renal function):

    - Increased age

    - Female patients

    - Asian patients

    - Amputees

    - Malnutrition, inflammation, or deconditioning (eg, cancer, severe cardiovascular disease, hospitalized patients)

    - Neuromuscular disease

    - Vegetarian diet

- Rapidly changing serum creatinine (either up or down):

    - In patients with rapidly rising serum creatinines (ie, increasing by >0.5 to 0.7 mg/dL/day), it is best to assume that the patient's renal function is severely impaired

Use extreme caution when estimating renal function in the following patient populations:

- Low body weight (actual body weight < ideal body weight)

- Liver transplant

- Prematurity (especially very low birth weight)

- Dehydration

- Recent kidney transplantation (serum creatinine values may decrease rapidly and can lead to renal function underestimation; conversely, delayed graft function may be present)

IDMS-traceable method: Bedside Schwartz[1]

Note: This equation is for use in ages 1 to 16 years.

eGFR = (0.413 X Height) / Creatinine

where:

eGFR = estimated GFR; calculated in mL/minute per 1.73 m^2

Height (length) is input in cm

Creatinine = Sr_{Cr} input in mg/dL

Alkaline picrate-based (Jaffe) methods

Note: These equations have not been updated for use with serum creatinine methods traceable to IDMS. Use with IDMS-traceable serum creatinine methods may overestimate renal function; use with caution.

Method 1: Schwartz equation

> **Note:** This equation may not provide an accurate estimation of creatinine clearance for infants <6 months of age or for patients with severe starvation or muscle wasting.

eGFR = (k X Height) / Creatinine

where:

eGFR = estimated GFR; calculated in mL/minute per 1.73 m^2

Height (length) is input in cm

k = constant of proportionality that is age-specific

<1 year preterm: 0.33

<1 year full-term: 0.45

1 to 12 years: 0.55

>12 years female: 0.55

>12 years male: 0.7

Creatinine is input in mg/dL

Method 2: Traub-Johnson equation

> **Note:** This equation is for use in ages 1 to 18 years.

CrCl = (0.48 X Height) / Creatinine

where:

CrCl = estimated creatinine clearance; calculated in mL/minute per 1.73 m^2

Height (length) is input in cm

Creatinine = Sr$_{Cr}$ input in mg/dL

FOOTNOTES

[1] National Kidney Disease Education Program preferred equation

REFERENCES

Dowling TC, Matzke GR, Murphy JE, Burckart GJ. Evaluation of renal drug dosing: prescribing information and clinical pharmacist approaches. *Pharmacotherapy.* 2010;30(8):776-786.

Myers GL, Miller WG, Coresh J, et al. Recommendations for improving serum creatinine measurement: a report from the laboratory working group of the National Kidney Disease Education Program. *Clin Chem.* 2006;52(1):5-18.

National Kidney Disease Education Program. GFR calculators. http://www.nkdep.nih.gov/professionals/gfr_calculators. Accessed April 24, 2013.

Pottel H, Mottaghy FM, Zaman Z, Martens F. On the relationship between glomerular filtration rate and serum creatinine in children. *Pediatr Nephrol.* 2010;25(5):927-934.

Schwartz GJ, Brion LP, Spitzer A. The use of plasma creatinine concentration for estimating glomerular filtration rate in infants, children, and adolescents. *Pediatr Clin North Am.* 1987;34 (3):571-590.

Schwartz GJ, Haycock GB, Edelmann CM Jr, Spitzer A. A simple estimate of glomerular filtration rate in children derived from body length and plasma creatinine. *Pediatrics.* 1976;58(2):259-263.

Schwartz GJ, Muñoz A, Schneider MF, et al. New equations to estimate GFR in children with CKD. *J Am Soc Nephrol.* 2009;20(3):629-637.

Staples A, LeBlond R, Watkins S, Wong C, Brandt J. Validation of the revised Schwartz estimating equation in a predominantly non-CKD population. *Pediatr Nephrol.* 2010;25(11):2321-2326.

Stevens LA, Coresh J, Greene T, Levey AS. Assessing kidney function – measured and estimated glomerular filtration rate. *N Engl J Med.* 2006;354(23):2473-2483.

Traub SL, Johnson CE. Comparison of methods of estimating creatinine clearance in children. *Am J Hosp Pharm.* 1980;37(2):195-201.

CORTICOSTEROIDS SYSTEMIC EQUIVALENCIES

Glucocorticoid	Approximate Equivalent Dose (mg)	Routes of Administration	Relative Anti-inflammatory Potency	Relative Mineralocorticoid Potency	Protein Binding (%)	Half-life Plasma (min)
Short-Acting						
Cortisone	25	PO, IM	0.8	0.8	90	30
Hydrocortisone	20	IM, IV	1	1	90	90
Intermediate-Acting						
MethylPREDNISolone[1]	4	PO, IM, IV	5	0	—	180
PrednisoLONE	5	PO, IM, IV, intra-articular, intradermal, soft tissue injection	4	0.8	90 to 95	200
PredniSONE	5	PO	4	0.8	<50	120 to 180
Triamcinolone[1]	4	IM, intra-articular, intradermal, intrasynovial, soft tissue injection	5	0	—	300
Long-Acting						
Betamethasone	0.75	PO, IM, intra-articular, intradermal, intrasynovial, soft tissue injection	25	0	64	100 to 300
Dexamethasone	0.75	PO, IM, IV, intra-articular, intradermal, soft tissue injection	25 to 30	0	—	100 to 300
Mineralocorticoids						
Fludrocortisone	—	PO	10	125	42	200

[1] May contain propylene glycol as an excipient in injectable forms

Asare K. Diagnosis and treatment of adrenal insufficiency in the critically ill patient. *Pharmacotherapy.* 2007;27(11):1512-1528.

Frey BM, Frey FJ. Clinical pharmacokinetics of prednisone and prednisolone. *Clin Pharmacokinet.* 1990;19(2):126-146.

IMMUNE GLOBULIN PRODUCT COMPARISON

Brand Name	Concentration	pH	Initial Rate IV	Initial Rate SubQ[1]	Max Rate IV[2]	Max Rate SubQ[1]	IgA Content (mcg/mL)	Osmolarity/ Osmolality (mOsmol/kg)	Comments
Bivigam	10%	4 to 4.6	0.3 mL/kg/h	–	3.6 mL/kg/h	–	≤200	Not available	Contains polysorbate 80
Carimune NF[3]	3%	6.4 to 6.8	1 mL/kg/h	–	6 mL/kg/h	–	Trace[4]	192 to 498[5]	Contains sucrose
	12%		0.24 mL/kg/h		1.5 mL/kg/h			768 to 1,074[5]	
Flebogamma DIF	5%	5 to 6	0.6 mL/kg/h	–	6 mL/kg/h	–	<50	240 to 370	
	10%		0.6 mL/kg/h		4.8 mL/kg/h		<100		
GamaSTAN S/D	15% to 18%	6.4 to 7.2	–	–	–	–	Not available	Not available	For IM use
Gammagard S/D	5%	6.4 to 7.2	0.5 mL/kg/h	–	4 mL/kg/h	–	≤1[6]	636	Contains polysorbate 80
	10%		0.5 mL/kg/h		8 mL/kg/h		≤2[6]	1,250	
Gammagard Liquid	10%	4.6 to 5.1	0.5 mL/kg/h	<40 kg: 15 mL/h/site with a maximum of 8 sites; ≥40 kg: 20 mL/h/site with a maximum of 8 sites	5 mL/kg/h; 5.4 mL/kg/h (MMN only)	<40 kg: 20 mL/h/site with a maximum of 8 sites; maximum total rate: 160 mL/h; ≥40 kg: 30 mL/h/site with a maximum of 8 sites; maximum total rate: 240 mL/h	37	240 to 300	
Gammaked	10%	4 to 4.5	0.6 mL/kg/h; 1.2 mL/kg/h (CIDP only)	20 mL/h/site with a maximum of 8 sites	4.8 mL/kg/h	Not determined	46	258	
Gammaplex	5%	4.8 to 5	0.6 mL/kg/h	–	4.8 mL/kg/h	–	<10	420 to 500	Contains polysorbate 80
Gamunex-C	10%	4 to 4.5	0.6 mL/kg/h; 1.2 mL/kg/h (CIDP only)	20 mL/h/site with a maximum of 8 sites	4.8 mL/kg/h	Not determined	46	258	
Hizentra	20%	4.6 to 5.2	–	15 mL/h/site with a maximum of 4 sites	–	Up to 25 mL/h/site with a maximum of 4 sites; maximum total rate: 50 mL/h	≤50	380	Contains L-proline and polysorbate 80

Brand Name	Concentration	pH	Initial Rate		Max Rate		IgA Content (mcg/mL)	Osmolarity/ Osmolality (mOsmol/kg)	Comments
			IV	SubQ[1]	IV[2]	SubQ[1]			
HyQvia	10%	4.6 to 5.1	–	*First 2 infusions:* <40 kg: 5 mL/h for 5 to 15 min; 10 mL/h for 5 to 15 min; 20 mL/h for 5 to 15 min; 40 mL/h for 5 to 15 min; then 80 mL/h for remainder of infusion ≥40 kg: 10 mL/h for 5 to 15 min; 30 mL/h for 5 to 15 min; 60 mL/h for 5 to 15 min; 120 mL/h for 5 to 15 min; then 240 mL/h for remainder of infusion *Next 2 or 3 infusions:* <40 kg: 10 mL/h for 5 to 15 min; 20 mL/h for 5 to 15 min; 40 mL/h for 5 to 15 min; 80 mL/h for 5 to 15 min; then 160 mL/h for remainder of infusion ≥40 kg: 10 mL/h for 5 to 15 min; 30 mL/h for 5 to 15 min; 120 mL/h for 5 to 15 min; 240 mL/h for 5 to 15 min; then 300 mL/h for remainder of infusion	–	<40 kg: 160 mL/h ≥40 kg: 300 mL/h	37	240 to 300	Supplied with hyaluronidase (human recombinant)
Octagam	5%	5.1 to 6	0.6 mL/kg/h	–	4 mL/kg/h	–	≤200	310 to 380	Contains maltose

Brand Name	Concentration	pH	Initial Rate		Max Rate		IgA Content (mcg/mL)	Osmolarity/ Osmolality (mOsmol/kg)	Comments
			IV	SubQ[1]	IV[2]	SubQ[1]			
Octagam	10%	4.5 to 5	0.6 mL/kg/h	–	7.2 mL/kg/h	–	106	310 to 380	Sucrose-free
Privigen	10%	4.6 to 5	0.3 mL/kg/h	–	2.4 mL/kg/h (ITP) 4.8 mL/kg/h	–	≤25	240 to 440	Contains L-proline

CIDP = chronic inflammatory demyelinating polyneuropathy, ITP = immune (idiopathic) thrombocytopenic purpura, MMN = multifocal motor neuropathy

[1]Subcutaneous administration **only** for the treatment of primary humoral immunodeficiency (PI)

[2]Lower infusion rates should be used in patients at risk for renal dysfunction or thrombotic complications; see specific product information for details.

[3]Other concentrations may be prepared; see product information for additional details.

[4]Per product information; other sources list IgA content as 1,000 to 2,000 mcg/mL for 6% solution (Siegel J. Immune globulins: therapeutic, pharmaceutical, cost, and administration considerations. *Pharm Pract News*. 2013).

[5]Osmolarity depends on concentration and diluent used; see product information for details.

[6]Data presented is based on the maximum concentration that can be prepared. The 5% solution with IgA content <2.2 mcg/mL has been discontinued. The lower IgA product (ie, IgA <1 mcg/mL for the 5% prepared solution) is available by special request; contact manufacturer or see specific product information for details.

ORAL ANTICOAGULANT COMPARISON CHART

Medication	Mechanism of Action	Metabolism	Monitoring Parameters	Pharmacotherapy Pearls	Reversal Strategies[1]	Preoperative/ Preprocedure Management (General Guide)
Warfarin	Inhibits formation of vitamin K-dependent clotting factors II, VII, IX, X, and proteins C and S	CYP2C9 CYP1A2 CYP3A4 CYP2C19	PT/INR (individualized; depends on INR stability)	CYP1A2, 3A4, 2C9, and 2C19 drug interactions and vitamin K-containing food interactions Full therapeutic effect usually seen within 5 to 7 days Half-life is ~40 hours	Vitamin K (route and dose will depend on clinical situation and INR) For major bleeding (at any INR): Consider PCC with vitamin K ± FFP	Hold at least 5 days before surgery; depending on urgency of surgery/procedure, may administer low-dose IV or oral vitamin K Minor dental and minor dermatological procedures or cataract surgery: Continue warfarin (with hemostatic agent [dental] or local hemostasis [dermatological]); may also discontinue use 2 to 3 days prior to dental procedures. Patients with prior stroke undergoing dental procedures should routinely continue warfarin.
Dabigatran (Pradaxa)	Directly inhibits thrombin	Hepatic glucuronidation P-gp substrate	Routine lab monitoring not required; aPTT, ECT (if available), TT (most sensitive) may be used to detect presence of dabigatran Renal function	Compliance issues (BID dosing) Specific conversions to/from warfarin, parenteral anticoagulants Renal dosing adjustment required; per ACCP, contraindicated with CrCl ≤30 mL/minute Use with caution in patients ≥80 years of age Dose reduction or avoidance required if used with dronedarone, ketoconazole, P-gp inhibitors P-gp drug interactions Half-life is 12 to 17 hours; considerably prolonged with severe renal impairment	No specific antidote; for major bleeding, may consider activated PCC (ie, FEIBA NF), recombinant factor VIIa[2], or concentrates of factors II, IX, or X[3] Dabigatran is ~60% dialyzable Activated charcoal may be used if ingestion occurred <2 hours prior to presentation	CrCl ≥50 mL/minute: Hold 1 to 2 days before surgery CrCl <50 mL/minute: Hold 3 to 5 days before surgery May consider holding for >5 days in patients undergoing major surgery, spinal puncture, or insertion of a spinal or epidural catheter or port

Medication	Mechanism of Action	Metabolism	Monitoring Parameters	Pharmacotherapy Pearls	Reversal Strategies[1]	Preoperative/ Preprocedure Management (General Guide)
Edoxaban (Savaysa)	Directly inhibits factor Xa	CYP3A4 (minor) Hydrolysis (minimal) P-gp substrate	Routine lab monitoring not required	Specific conversions to/from warfarin, parenteral anticoagulants DVT/PE: Dose reduction necessary for patients <60 kg, concomitant P-gp inhibitor, or if CrCl 15 to 50 mL/min. Not recommended if CrCl <15 mL/min NVAF: **Do not use if CrCl >95 mL/min.** Dose reduction necessary if CrCl 15 to 50 mL/min. Not recommended if CrCl <15 mL/min	No specific antidote Edoxaban is **not** dialyzable	Discontinue at least 24 hours prior to elective surgery or invasive procedures
Rivaroxaban (Xarelto)	Directly inhibits factor Xa	CYP3A4 CYP3A5 CYP2J2 P-gp substrate	Routine lab monitoring not required; may use PT to detect presence of rivaroxaban Renal and hepatic function	Administer doses ≥15 mg/day with food Dosing frequency depends on indication Specific conversions to/from warfarin, parenteral anticoagulants Renal dosing adjustment required Avoid in moderate or severe hepatic impairment CYP3A4 and P-gp drug interactions Half-life is 5 to 9 hours; slightly prolonged with renal impairment	No specific antidote; for major bleeding, may consider PCC, activated PCC (ie, FEIBA NF), or recombinant factor VIIa[3] Rivaroxaban is **not** dialyzable	Hold at least 24 hours before surgery; longer duration of treatment cessation may be necessary based on individual patient situation and physician clinical judgment
Apixaban (Eliquis)	Directly inhibits factor Xa	CYP3A4 P-gp substrate	Routine lab monitoring not required; PT, INR, and aPTT may be used to detect presence of apixaban	Compliance issues (BID dosing) Specific conversions to/from warfarin, parenteral anticoagulants Renal dosing adjustment required (NVAF); the AHA/ASA recommends to avoid use with CrCl <25 mL/minute Not recommended in patients with severe liver impairment CYP3A4 and P-gp drug interactions Half-life is ~8 to 15 hours; slightly prolonged with renal impairment	No specific antidote; for major bleeding, may consider PCC, activated PCC (ie, FEIBA NF), or recombinant factor VIIa Apixaban is **not** dialyzable Activated charcoal may be used if ingestion occurred within 2 to 6 hours of presentation	Hold at least 24 to 48 hours, depending on risk or location of bleeding, before elective surgery or invasive procedures.

Footnotes for Oral Anticoagulant Comparison Chart

Abbreviations: ACCP = American College of Chest Physicians, AHA/ASA = American Heart Association/American Stroke Association, aPTT = activated partial thromboplastin time, BID = twice daily, DVT = deep venous thrombosis, ECT = ecarin clotting time, FFP = fresh frozen plasma, INR = international normalized ratio, NVAF = nonvalvular atrial fibrillation, PCC = prothrombin complex concentrate, PE = pulmonary embolism, P-gp = P-glycoprotein, PT = prothrombin time, TT = thrombin time

Note: Recommendations listed reflect only the US labeling or US clinical practice guidelines.

[1] Management of anticoagulant-associated bleeding requires careful consideration of the indication for anticoagulant therapy and bleeding extent (eg, epistaxis vs intracranial hemorrhage); minor bleeding may only require local hemostasis.

[2] The use of rFVIIa in healthy subjects treated with another direct thrombin inhibitor, melagatran (not FDA-approved), did not reverse the anticoagulant effects of melagatran.

[3] The evidence in support of these reversal strategies is limited; an exception to this may be the use of a 4-factor PCC for rivaroxaban reversal. The only available 4-factor PCC currently in the US is Kcentra. Other 4-factor PCCs **not** available in the US include Beriplex P/N, Cofact, and Octaplex. Beriplin VH and Profilnine SD **do not** contain adequate levels of factor VII and are considered 3-factor PCCs.

Armstrong MJ, Gronseth G, Anderson DC, et al. Summary of evidence-based guideline: periprocedural management of antithrombotic medications in patients with ischemic cerebrovascular disease: report of the Guideline Development Subcommittee of the American Academy of Neurology. *Neurology.* 2013;80 (22):2065-2069.

Furie KL, Goldstein LB, Albers GW, et al. Oral antithrombotic agents for the prevention of stroke in nonvalvular atrial fibrillation: a science advisory for health care professionals from the American Heart Association/American Stroke Association. *Stroke.* 2012;43(12):3442-3453.

Guyatt GH, Akl EA, Crowther M, et al. Executive summary: antithrombotic therapy and prevention of thrombosis, 9th ed: American College of Chest Physicians evidence-based clinical practice guidelines. *Chest.* 2012;141(2 Suppl):7S-47S.

Kaatz S, Kouides PA, Garcia DA, et al. Guidance on the emergent reversal of oral thrombin and factor Xa inhibitors. *Am J Hematol.* 2012;87(Suppl 1):S141-S145.

Levi M, Eerenberg E, Kamphuisen PW. Bleeding risk and reversal strategies for old and new anticoagulants and antiplatelet agents. *J Thromb Haemost.* 2011;9(9):1705-1712.

Poulsen BK, Grove EL, Husted SE. New oral anticoagulants: a review of the literature with particular emphasis on patients with impaired renal function. *Drugs.* 2012;72(13):1739-1753.

Wolzt M, Levi M, Sarich TC, et al. Effect of recombinant factor VIIa on melagatran-induced inhibition of thrombin generation and platelet activation in healthy volunteers. *Thromb Haemost.* 2004;91(6):1090-1096.

ORAL ANTIPLATELET COMPARISON CHART

Medication	Mechanism of Action	Reversible Platelet Inhibition	Prodrug	Metabolism	Pharmacotherapy Pearls	Reversal Strategies[1]	Preoperative/Preprocedure Management (General Guide)
Aspirin	Inhibits cyclooxygenase-1 and 2	No	No	CYP2C9	Chronic NSAID use can compromise antiplatelet effects Monitor for GI ulceration	No specific antidote Consider platelet transfusion ± DDAVP Normal platelet function returns within 7 to 10 days after discontinuation	Hold 7 to 10 days before surgery May be continued through surgery for CABG or noncardiac surgery in patients with moderate to high cardiac risk Minor dental or dermatological procedures or cataract surgery: Continue through procedure. AAN recommends continuation when undergoing any dental procedure for patients taking aspirin for ischemic stroke prevention.
Cilostazol (Pletal)	Inhibits platelet phosphodiesterase III	Yes	No	CYP3A4 CYP2C19 CYP1A2 CYP2D6	Administer before or 2 hours after meals Contraindicated in patients with heart failure of any severity CYP3A4 and 2C19 drug interactions	No specific antidote Normal platelet function returns within 4 days after discontinuation	Hold 2 to 3 days before surgery
Clopidogrel (Plavix)	Inhibits P2Y$_{12}$ component of ADP receptors	No	Yes	CYP2C19 CYP3A4	CYP2C19 inhibitors may reduce concentrations of active metabolite CYP2C19 polymorphisms may affect clopidogrel efficacy	No specific antidote Consider platelet transfusion ± DDAVP Normal platelet function returns within 7 to 10 days after discontinuation	Hold 5 to 10 days before surgery[2]

Medication	Mechanism of Action	Reversible Platelet Inhibition	Prodrug	Metabolism	Pharmacotherapy Pearls	Reversal Strategies[1]	Preoperative/Preprocedure Management (General Guide)
Prasugrel (Effient)	Inhibits $P2Y_{12}$ component of ADP receptors	No	Yes	CYP3A4 CYP2B6	Reduce maintenance dose to 5 mg in patients <60 kg Contraindicated in patients with history of stroke, TIA Not recommended in patients ≥75 years of age	No specific antidote Consider platelet transfusion ± DDAVP Normal platelet function returns within 5 to 9 days after discontinuation	Hold 5 to 7 days before surgery[2]
Ticagrelor (Brilinta)	Inhibits $P2Y_{12}$ component of ADP receptors	Yes	No	CYP3A4 CYP3A5	Used in combination with aspirin; daily maintenance aspirin dose should not exceed 81 mg CYP3A4 drug interactions BID dosing Monitor closely for dyspnea, bradyarrhythmia (including ventricular pauses)	No specific antidote Consider aminocaproic acid, tranexamic acid, recombinant factor VIIa Normal platelet function returns within 3 to 5 days after discontinuation	Hold at least 5 days before surgery[2]

Medication	Mechanism of Action	Reversible Platelet Inhibition	Prodrug	Metabolism	Pharmacotherapy Pearls	Reversal Strategies[1]	Preoperative/Preprocedure Management (General Guide)
Ticlopidine	Inhibits $P2Y_{12}$ component of ADP receptors	No	Yes	CYP3A4	Black Box warning on hematologic toxicities (aplastic anemia, TTP) Frequent CBC monitoring required BID dosing	No specific antidote Consider platelet transfusion ± DDAVP Normal platelet function returns within 5 to 10 days after discontinuation	Hold 10 to 14 days before surgery
Vorapaxar	Inhibits PAR-1	Yes[3]	No	CYP3A4 CYP2J2	Use in combination with aspirin and/ or clopidogrel Contraindicated in patients with history of stroke, TIA, or ICH Extremely long effective half-life of 3 to 5 days	No specific antidote Significant inhibition of platelet aggregation remains 4 weeks after discontinuation	No recommendation can be made

[1] Management of antiplatelet-associated bleeding requires careful consideration of the indication for antiplatelet therapy and bleeding extent (eg, epistaxis vs intracranial hemorrhage); minor bleeding may only require local hemostasis.

[2] When urgent CABG is necessary, the ACCF/AHA CABG guidelines recommend discontinuation for at least 24 hours prior to surgery (Hillis 2011).

[3] Due to the very long half-life, vorapaxar is effectively irreversible.

Armstrong MJ, Gronseth G, Anderson DC, et al. Summary of evidence-based guideline: periprocedural management of antithrombotic medications in patients with ischemic cerebrovascular disease: report of the Guideline Development Subcommittee of the American Academy of Neurology. *Neurology*. 2013;80 (22):2065-2069.

Hillis LD, Smith PK, Anderson JL, et al. 2011 ACCF/AHA guideline for coronary artery bypass graft surgery: executive summary: a report of the American College of Cardiology Foundation/American Heart Association task force on practice guidelines. *Circulation*. 2011;124(23):2610-2642.

Levi M, Eerenberg E, Kamphuisen PW. Bleeding risk and reversal strategies for old and new anticoagulants and antiplatelet agents. *J Thromb Haemost*. 2011;9(9):1705-1712.

Patrono C, Andreotti F, Arnesen H, et al. Antiplatelet agents for the treatment and prevention of atherothrombosis. *Eur Heart J*. 2011;32(23):2922-2932.

REFERENCE VALUES FOR ADULTS

CHEMISTRY

Test	Values	Remarks
Serum/Plasma		
Acetone	Negative	
Albumin	3.2 to 5 g/dL	
Alcohol, ethyl	Negative	
Aldolase	1.2 to 7.6 IU/L	
Ammonia	20 to 70 mcg/dL	Specimen to be placed on ice as soon as collected.
Amylase	30 to 110 units/L	
Bilirubin, direct	0 to 0.3 mg/dL	
Bilirubin, total	0.1 to 1.2 mg/dL	
Calcium	8.6 to 10.3 mg/dL	
Calcium, ionized	2.24 to 2.46 mEq/L	
Chloride	95 to 108 mEq/L	
Cholesterol, total	≤200 mg/dL	Fasted blood required – normal value affected by dietary habits. This reference range is for a general adult population.
HDL cholesterol	40 to 60 mg/dL	Fasted blood required – normal value affected by dietary habits
LDL cholesterol	<160 mg/dL	If triglyceride is >400 mg/dL, LDL cannot be calculated accurately (Friedewald equation). Target LDL-C depends on patient's risk factors.
CO_2	23 to 30 mEq/L	
Creatine kinase (CK) isoenzymes		
CK-BB	0%	
CK-MB (cardiac)	0% to 3.9%	
CK-MM (muscle)	96% to 100%	

CK-MB levels must be both ≥4% and 10 IU/L to meet diagnostic criteria for CK-MB positive result consistent with myocardial injury.

Test	Values	Remarks
Creatine phosphokinase (CPK)	8 to 150 IU/L	
Creatinine	0.5 to 1.4 mg/dL	
Ferritin	13 to 300 ng/mL	
Folate	3.6 to 20 ng/dL	

CHEMISTRY *(continued)*

Test	Values	Remarks
GGT (gamma-glutamyltranspeptidase)		
male	11 to 63 IU/L	
female	8 to 35 IU/L	
GLDH	To be determined	
Glucose (preprandial)	<115 mg/dL	Goals different for diabetics
Glucose, fasting	60 to 110 mg/dL	Goals different for diabetics
Glucose, nonfasting (2-h postprandial)	<120 mg/dL	Goals different for diabetics
Hemoglobin A_{1c}	<8	
Hemoglobin, plasma free	<2.5 mg per 100 mL	
Hemoglobin, total glycosolated (HbA_1)	4% to 8%	
Iron	65 to 150 mcg/dL	
Iron binding capacity, total (TIBC)	250 to 420 mcg/dL	
Lactic acid	0.7 to 2.1 mEq/L	Specimen to be kept on ice and sent to lab as soon as possible
Lactate dehydrogenase (LDH)	56 to 194 IU/L	
Lactate dehydrogenase (LDH) isoenzymes		
LD_1	20% to 34%	
LD_2	29% to 41%	
LD_3	15% to 25%	
LD_4	1% to 12%	
LD_5	1% to 15%	

Flipped LD_1/LD_2 ratios (>1 may be consistent with myocardial injury) particularly when considered in combination with a recent CK-MB positive result.

Lipase	23 to 208 units/L	
Magnesium	1.6 to 2.5 mg/dL	Increased by slight hemolysis
Osmolality	289 to 308 mOsm/kg	
Phosphatase, alkaline		
Adults 25 to 60 y	33 to 131 IU/L	
Adults ≥61 y	51 to 153 IU/L	
Infancy-adolescence	Values range up to 3 to 5 times higher than adults	
Phosphate, inorganic	2.8 to 4.2 mg/dL	
Potassium	3.5 to 5.2 mEq/L	Increased by slight hemolysis
Prealbumin	>15 mg/dL	
Protein, total	6.5 to 7.9 g/dL	

CHEMISTRY *(continued)*

Test	Values	Remarks
AST	<35 IU/L (20 to 48)	
ALT (10 to 35)	<35 IU/L	
Sodium	134 to 149 mEq/L	
Thyroid stimulating hormone (TSH)		
Adults ≤20 y	0.7 to 6.4 milliunits/L	
21 to 54 y	0.4 to 4.2 milliunits/L	
55 to 87 y	0.5 to 8.9 milliunits/L	
Transferrin	>200 mg/dL	
Triglycerides	45 to 155 mg/dL	Fasted blood required
Troponin I	<1.5 ng/mL	
Urea nitrogen (BUN)	7 to 20 mg/dL	
Uric acid		
Male	2 to 8 mg/dL	
Female	2 to 7.5 mg/dL	
Cerebrospinal Fluid		
Glucose	50 to 70 mg/dL	
Protein	15 to 45 mg/dL	CSF obtained by lumbar puncture

Note: Bloody specimen gives erroneously high value due to contamination with blood proteins

Urine
(24-hour specimen is required for all these tests unless specified)

Amylase	32 to 641 units/L	The value is in units/L and **not** calculated for total volume.
Amylase, fluid (random samples)		Interpretation of value left for physician, depends on the nature of fluid
Calcium	Depends upon dietary intake	
Creatine		
Male	150 mg per 24 h	Higher value on children and during pregnancy
Female	250 mg per 24 h	
Creatinine	1,000 to 2,000 mg per 24 h	
Creatinine clearance (endogenous)		
Male	85 to 125 mL/min	A blood sample must accompany urine specimen.
Female	75 to 115 mL/min	
Glucose	1 g per 24 h	
5-hydroxyindoleacetic acid	2 to 8 mg per 24 h	

CHEMISTRY (continued)

Test	Values	Remarks
Iron	0.15 mg per 24 h	Acid washed container required
Magnesium	146 to 209 mg per 24 h	
Osmolality	500 to 800 mOsm/kg	With normal fluid intake
Oxalate	10 to 40 mg per 24 h	
Phosphate	400 to 1,300 mg per 24 h	
Potassium	25 to 120 mEq per 24 h	Varies with diet; the interpretation of urine electrolytes and osmolality should be left for the physician
Sodium	40 to 220 mEq per 24 h	
Porphobilinogen, qualitative	Negative	
Porphyrins, qualitative	Negative	
Proteins	0.05 to 0.1 g per 24 h	
Salicylate	Negative	
Urea clearance	60 to 95 mL/min	A blood sample must accompany specimen.
Urea N	10 to 40 g per 24 h	Dependent on protein intake
Uric acid	250 to 750 mg per 24 h	Dependent on diet and therapy
Urobilinogen	0.5 to 3.5 mg per 24 h	For qualitative determination on random urine, send sample to urinalysis section in Hematology Lab.
Xylose absorption test		
Children	16% to 33% of ingested xylose	

Feces

Fat, 3-day collection	<5 g/d	Value depends on fat intake of 100 g/d for 3 days preceding and during collection

Gastric Acidity

Acidity, total, 12 h	10 to 60 mEq/L	Titrated at pH 7

Blood Gases

	Arterial	Capillary	Venous
pH	7.35 to 7.45	7.35 to 7.45	7.32 to 7.42
pCO_2 (mm Hg)	35 to 45	35 to 45	38 to 52
pO_2 (mm Hg)	70 to 100	60 to 80	24 to 48
HCO_3 (mEq/L)	19 to 25	19 to 25	19 to 25
TCO_2 (mEq/L)	19 to 29	19 to 29	23 to 33
O_2 saturation (%)	90 to 95	90 to 95	40 to 70
Base excess (mEq/L)	-5 to +5	-5 to +5	-5 to +5

HEMATOLOGY

Complete Blood Cell Count

Age	Hgb (g/dL)	Hct (%)	RBC (mill/mm³)	RDW
0 to 3 d	15 to 20	45 to 61	4 to 5.9	<18
1 to 2 wk	12.5 to 18.5	39 to 57	3.6 to 5.5	<17
1 to 6 mo	10 to 13	29 to 42	3.1 to 4.3	<16.5
7 mo to 2 y	10.5 to 13	33 to 38	3.7 to 4.9	<16
2 to 5 y	11.5 to 13	34 to 39	3.9 to 5	<15
5 to 8 y	11.5 to 14.5	35 to 42	4 to 4.9	<15
13 to 18 y	12 to 15.2	36 to 47	4.5 to 5.1	<14.5
Adult male	13.5 to 16.5	41 to 50	4.5 to 5.5	<14.5
Adult female	12 to 15	36 to 44	4 to 4.9	<14.5

Age	MCV (fL)	MCH (pg)	MCHC (%)	Plts (x 10³/mm³)
0 to 3 d	95 to 115	31 to 37	29 to 37	250 to 450
1 to 2 wk	86 to 110	28 to 36	28 to 38	250 to 450
1 to 6 mo	74 to 96	25 to 35	30 to 36	300 to 700
7 mo to 2 y	70 to 84	23 to 30	31 to 37	250 to 600
2 to 5 y	75 to 87	24 to 30	31 to 37	250 to 550
5 to 8 y	77 to 95	25 to 33	31 to 37	250 to 550
13 to 18 y	78 to 96	25 to 35	31 to 37	150 to 450
Adult male	80 to 100	26 to 34	31 to 37	150 to 450
Adult female	80 to 100	26 to 34	31 to 37	150 to 450

WBC and Differential

Age	WBC (x 10³/mm³)	Segs	Bands	Lymphs	Monos
0 to 3 d	9 to 35	32 to 62	<18	19 to 29	5 to 7
1 to 2 wk	5 to 20	14 to 34	<14	36 to 45	6 to 10
1 to 6 mo	6 to 17.5	13 to 33	<12	41 to 71	4 to 7
7 mo to 2 y	6 to 17	15 to 35	<11	45 to 76	3 to 6
2 to 5 y	5.5 to 15.5	23 to 45	<11	35 to 65	3 to 6
5 to 8 y	5 to 14.5	32 to 54	<11	28 to 48	3 to 6
13 to 18 y	4.5 to 13	34 to 64	<11	25 to 45	3 to 6
Adults	4.5 to 11	35 to 66	<11	24 to 44	3 to 6

Age	Eosinophils	Basophils	Atypical Lymphs	No. of NRBCs
0 to 3 d	0 to 2	0 to 1	0 to 8	0 to 2
1 to 2 wk	0 to 2	0 to 1	0 to 8	0
1 to 6 mo	0 to 3	0 to 1	0 to 8	0
7 mo to 2 y	0 to 3	0 to 1	0 to 8	0
2 to 5 y	0 to 3	0 to 1	0 to 8	0
5 to 8 y	0 to 3	0 to 1	0 to 8	0
13 to 18 y	0 to 3	0 to 1	0 to 8	0
Adults	0 to 3	0 to 1	0 to 8	0

Bands = band neutrophils, lymphs = lymphocytes, monos = monocytes, segs = segmented neutrophils

Erythrocyte Sedimentation Rates and Reticulocyte Counts

Sedimentation rate, Westergren	Children	0 to 20 mm/h
	Adult male	0 to 15 mm/h
	Adult female	0 to 20 mm/h
Sedimentation rate, Wintrobe	Children	0 to 13 mm/h
	Adult male	0 to 10 mm/h
	Adult female	0 to 15 mm/h
Reticulocyte count	Newborns	2% to 6%
	1 to 6 mo	0% to 2.8%
	Adults	0.5% to 1.5%

PHARMACOLOGIC CATEGORY INDEX

Other Lexicomp Offerings

Drug Information Handbook

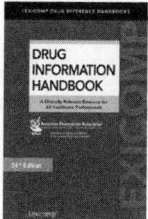

An easy-to-use reference for pharmacists, physicians and other healthcare professionals requiring fast access to relevant drug information, this handbook presents over 1500 drug monographs, each with up to 40 fields of information. A valuable appendix includes hundreds of charts and reviews of special topics such as guidelines for treatment and therapy recommendations. A pharmacologic category index is also provided.

Geriatric Dosage Handbook

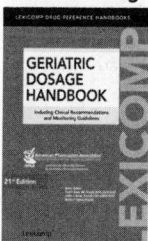

Designed for healthcare professionals managing geriatric patients. Includes: Detailed adult and geriatric dosing; special geriatric considerations; up to 40 key fields of information in each monograph, including medication safety issues; extensive information on drug interactions, as well as dosing for patients with renal/hepatic impairment.

Pediatric & Neonatal Dosage Handbook

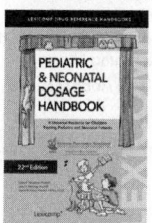

This book is designed for healthcare professionals requiring quick access to relevant pediatric drug information. Each monograph contains multiple fields of content, including usual dosage by age group, indication and route of administration. Drug interactions, adverse reactions, extemporaneous preparations, pharmacodynamics/pharmacokinetics data and medication safety issues are covered.

Drug Information Handbook for Nursing

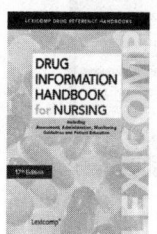

Designed for registered professional nurses and upper-division nursing students requiring dosing, administration, monitoring and patient education information.
Includes: Over 4800 generic and brand name drugs, cross-referenced by page number; drug names and specific nursing fields highlighted in RED for easy reference; Nursing Actions field includes Physical Assessment and Patient Education guidelines.

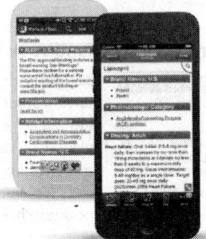